D0883346

SURGERY OF THE ANUS, RECTUM AND COLON

SECOND EDITION

DEDICATION

This book is dedicated to our long suffering wives Margaret and Linda and our children.

VOLUME ONE

SURGERY OF THE ANUS, RECTUM AND COLON

MICHAEL R B KEIGHLEY MS, FRCS
Barling Professor of Surgery, and
Head of Department of Surgery
University of Birmingham
Queen Elizabeth Hospital · Birmingham · England

NORMAN S WILLIAMS MS, FRCS
Professor of Surgery and Director of the Academic Department of Surgery
St Bartholomew's and The Royal London School of Medicine and Dentistry
Queen Mary and Westfield College
The Royal London Hospital · London · England

SECOND EDITION

W. B. Saunders
London · Edinburgh · New York · Philadelphia · Sydney · Toronto

WB SAUNDERS
A Division of Harcourt Brace and Company Limited

ISBN 0–7020–2335–3

First edition 1993
Reprinted 1997

British Library Cataloguing in Publication Data
A catalogue record for this book is available from the British Library

Library of Congress Cataloging in Publication Data
A catalog record for this book is available from the Library of Congress

Medical knowledge is constantly changing. As new information becomes available, changes in treatment, procedures, equipment and the use of drugs become necessary. The authors and Publishers have, as far as it is possible, taken care to ensure that the information given in the text is accurate and up to date. However, readers are strongly advised to confirm that the information, especially with regard to drug usage, complies with latest legislation and standards of practice.

The Publishers and authors have made every effort to trace the copyright holders for borrowed material. If they have inadvertently overlooked any, they will be pleased to rectify the matter at the first opportunity.

Typeset by Phoenix Photosetting, Chatham, Kent
Printed and bound in China

The
Publisher's
policy is to use
paper manufactured
from sustainable forests

CONTENTS

Volume Two

INFLAMMATORY BOWEL DISEASE

ULCERATIVE COLITIS

CROHN'S DISEASE

LAPAROSCOPY FOR IBD

EMERGENCIES

INFECTIONS

SPECIALIST CONSIDERATIONS

PAEDIATRIC COLORECTAL SURGERY

CONTRIBUTORS

J.P. Blandy CBE, MA, DM, Mch, FACS, FRCSI(Hon)
Emeritus Professor of Urology
St Bartholomew's and The Royal London School of Medicine and Dentistry
London
United Kingdom

(with C.G. Fowler)
Urological Considerations in Colorectal Surgery

C.M. Doig CHM, FRCSE, FRCS
Senior Lecturer in Paediatric Surgery
Booth Hall Children's Hospital
Manchester
United Kingdom

Other Paediatric Disorders

S. Dorudi BSc, PhD, FRCS
Consultant Colorectal Surgeon and Senior Lecturer in Surgery
St Bartholomew's and The Royal London School of Medicine and Dentistry
Queen Mary and Westfield College
Royal London & St Bartholomew's Hospitals
London
United Kingdom

Molecular Biology of Colorectal Cancer

M.J.G. Farthing MD, FRCP
Professor of Gastroenterology and Honorary Consultant Physician
St Bartholomew's and The Royal London School of Medicine and Dentistry
Queen Mary and Westfield College
Department of Gastroenterology
St Bartholomew's Hospital
London
United Kingdom

Tropical Colorectal Surgery

C.G. Fowler MS, FRCP, FRCS(Urol), FEBU
Consultant Urological Surgeon and Senior Lecturer in Urology
St Bartholomew's and The Royal London School of Medicine and Dentistry
Queen Mary and Westfield College
Royal London Hospital
London, United Kingdom

(with J.P. Blandy)
Urological Considerations in Colorectal Surgery

S. Glandiuk MD, FACS
Associate Professor
Department of Surgery
University of Louisville School of Medicine
Louisville, USA

Injuries to the Colon and Rectum

L. Gottesman MD, FACS, FASCRS
Director, Division of Colon and Rectal Surgery
St Luke's-Roosevelt Hospital Center
New York
Assistant Professor of Clinical Surgery
Columbia University, College of Physicians and Surgeons
New York, USA

(with J.D. Wishner)
Sexually Transmitted Disease in Colorectal Surgery

P. Hutton PhD, FRCA
Professor of Anaesthesia
Department of Anaesthesia and Intensive Care
University of Birmingham
Queen Elizabeth Hospital
Birmingham
United Kingdom

(with A.D. Wilkey)
Anaesthesia for Colorectal Surgery

G.J. Jarvis MA, FRCS, FRCOG
Consultant Obstetrician and Gynaecologist
St James University Hospital
Leeds, United Kingdom

(with A.M. Lower and J.H. Shepherd)
Gynaecological Conditions Relevant to the Colorectal Surgeon

M.L. Kennedy BSc
Research Fellow
Department of Colorectal Surgery
St George Hospital
Sydney, Australia

(with D.Z. Lubowski)
Anatomy & Physiology Investigations

H. Moreira Jr. MD
Research Fellow
Department of Colorectal Surgery
Cleveland Clinic Florida, USA

(with S.D. Wexner)
Role of Laparoscopy for Inflammatory Bowel Disease

A.M. Lower BMedSc, Bmbs, MRCOG
Consultant Gynaecologist and Minimal Access Surgeon
St Bartholomew's Hospital
London, United Kingdom

(with G.J. Jarvis and J.H. Shepherd)
Gynaecological Conditions Relevant to the Colorectal Surgeon

D.Z. Lubowski FRACS
Consultant Surgeon and Director Anorectal Physiology Unit
Department of Colorectal Surgery
St George Private Hospital
Sydney, Australia

(with M.L. Kennedy)
Anatomy & Physiology Investigations

J.H. Shepherd FRCS, FRCOG
Consultant Gynaecological Surgeon and Oncologist
St Bartholomew's Hospital
Royal Marsden Hospital
London, United Kingdom

(with G.J. Jarvis and A.M. Lower)
Gynaecological Conditions Relevant to the Colorectal Surgeon

M.D. Stringer MS, FRCS, FRCS (Paed.)
Consultant Paediatric Surgeon
Leeds Teaching Hospitals NHS Trust
Leeds
Honorary Senior Lecturer, Leeds University
Leeds, United Kingdom

Anorectal Malformations
Hirschprung's Disease

S.D. Wexner MD, FACS, FASCRS, FACG
Chief of Staff Cleveland Clinic Florida
Chairman, Division of Research and Education
Chairman and Residency Program Director, Department of Colorectal Surgery
Professor of Surgery, The Cleveland Clinic Foundation Sciences Center of the Ohio State University
USA

Laparoscopic Construction of Stomas
Laparoscopy for Colorectal Cancer
Laparoscopic techniques in Colonic Diverticular Disease
Role of Laparoscopy for Inflammatory Bowel Disease (with H. Moreira Jr.)

A.D. Wilkey FRCA
Consultant Anaesthetist
Department of Anaesthesia and Intensive Care
University of Birmingham
Queen Elizabeth Hospital
Birmingham
United Kingdom

(with P. Hutton)
Anaesthesia for Colorectal Surgery

J.D. Wishner MD, FACS, FASCRS
Associate Program Director
Colon and Rectal Surgery Training Program
St. Luke's Roosevelt Hospital Center
New York
Assistant Clinical Professor of Surgery
Columbia University, College of Physicians and Surgeons
New York, USA

(with L. Gottesman)
Sexually Transmitted Disease in Colorectal Surgery

FOREWORD

And so the second edition of the highly successful *"Surgery of the Anus, Rectum, and Colon"* has arrived. There is a nebulous aspect to the optimal timing of a second ... or new edition of any text book. Publishers tend to be aggressively proactive and persuasive in getting the authors "up" for another go at it. Authors rightly point out that their physical and emotional energy reserves need a bit more time to be recharged before tackling the next edition. We, the readers, are the beneficiaries of this acquiescence of our authors, Michael Keighley and Norman Williams, in marshaling their energies and talent, and producing an excellent reprise of their first joint contribution.

As we are fast approaching the end of the century and a new millennium, the burgeoning knowledge base required of the colorectal surgical specialist – or indeed the general surgeon with an interest in major abdominal or rectal surgery – is intimidating. Text books typically lag several years behind the "cutting edge" literature. E-mail "chat rooms" and, list servers are appearing in multiple disciplines, and could challenge the relevance of textbooks generally. And so, frequency of publications of new editions will be a key feature for those prominent, authoritative and successful text books, in keeping us surgeons aware of the spectrum of the specialty of colon and rectal surgery, as well as putting into perspective the new information acquired in the time from previous editions. It is this perspective "thing" that really can be best provided by a text book. And one cannot think of a better time to produce the second edition . . . as this century comes to an end.

This edition has been improved in many ways. Much of this has been listed in the Preface but several areas bear emphasis. The inclusion of specialized chapters from international experts on topics such as sexually transmitted diseases, laparoscopic bowel surgery and anorectal physiology adds value and authority to the second edition. Over a third of the book has been rewritten entirely with particularly useful additions to the colonic neoplasia section, molecular biology and heredity aspects of colorectal cancer, and newer technologies for the treatment of functional anorectal and colonic disorders.

But the book still looks and "feels" like the first edition – maintaining the successful formula of clear and explicit description of the problem; an objective review of the published work on the subject; a description of the authors experience and scholarly ventures into this area and finally, the author's overview, summarizing, collating and weighing the data. This might well be called the Goligher method, a formula that has been tried and tested over many editions of John Goligher's textbook, and which brought the reader to acquire each new edition with anticipation and delight.

Michael Keighley and Norman Williams are to be congratulated on the authorship of this excellent second edition of *Surgery of the Anus, Rectum and Colon*. I recommend it to all serious students or practitioners of the treatment of diseases of the large intestine.

Victor W. Fazio
Rupert B. Turnbull Jr., Chairman
Department of Colorectal Surgery
The Cleveland Clinic Foundation
Cleveland, Ohio

PREFACE TO SECOND EDITION

Spurred on by the apparent success of the 1st Edition, which has been reprinted twice and translated into Spanish and Italian, we were persuaded by our publishers to produce a 2nd Edition.

Despite supportive reviews for the 1st Edition, we were aware of some deficiencies. Neither of us felt able to write on colorectal trauma with authority and we are grateful for Dr Susan Galandiuk's contribution to this subject. We also felt the need to expand the gynaecological section, not only colorectal and gynaecological malignancy but also in functional and inflammatory disease. We are, therefore, grateful to Messrs John Shepherd, Adrian Lower and Gerry Jarvis for their contributions to this area. Mr Jeremy Lawson and Mr Neil Freeman have now retired and the paediatric section has been rewritten by Mr Mark Stringer and Caroline Doig. We were aware that the 1st Edition did not include a separate section on disordered physiology, although physiological aspects of disease were incorporated throughout the text where appropriate. We are grateful, therefore, to Dr David Lubowski for putting together an overview of the role of anorectal physiology in our introductory chapter. Dr Steven Wexner graciously gave up his contribution on sexually transmitted diseases which is now taken over by Dr Lester Gottesman who has an extensive practice in this subject which allows him to write on the subject with great authority. On the other hand, Dr Wexner has expanded his critique of laparoscopic procedures in inflammatory disease, stoma construction and colorectal malignancy as we are now beyond the learning curve and into regular practice in benign disease in some institutes. We are grateful for the support of Dr Tony Wilkey with Professor Peter Hutton in providing a chapter on anaesthesia. Likewise, we are grateful for Professor Michael Farthing's overview on tropical diseases. Mr Sina Dorudi has provided a chapter on the rapidly developing field of molecular biology in colorectal malignancy. Mr Chris Fowler has taken over the urological chapter from Professor John Blandy who has retired. The rest of the text has been produced by the two of us. As before we have exchanged manuscripts and constructively criticized each other's contributions.

At least a third of the book has been rewritten for this 2nd Edition. Areas of major change include:

- The medical management of anal fissure
- The physiological impact of anal fistula surgery
- New treatments for bowel incontinence
- Multidisciplinary management of constipation with particular reference to outlet obstruction, rectocele and techniques for improving impaired rectal evacuation
- The aetiopathology of inflammatory bowel disease and its medical treatment, particularly the role of newer agents
- Restorative proctocolectomy with particular reference to pouch salvage procedures
- The biology and natural history of cancer
- Hereditary colon cancer
- The polyposis syndromes
- The role of adjuvant therapy in colorectal cancer
- The surgical management of recurrent rectal cancer and hepatic metastases
- The management of anal cancer and anal intraepithelial neoplasia (AIN)
- The role of laparoscopy in colorectal disease

As in the 1st Edition, we have continued to adopt the Socratic principle of reviewing all the available evidence and giving our balanced views on what we consider the most appropriate method of management based on our own clinical experience. This approach is one of the features that so endeared readers to John Goligher's book, which carries the same title. Sadly, Professor J C Goligher died during preparation of the 2nd Edition. Before his death he wrote to us expressing great enthusiasm for the 1st Edition and gratitude that his original style was being incorporated in this book. Needless to say, Professor Goligher's inspiration has continued to be a beacon in the preparation of this new edition.

Our professional responsibilities do not diminish with the years, particularly those of an administrative nature. Clinical practice must still go on, often in an increasingly demanding and judgmental society. Yet without our respective practices, we could not have contemplated a revision to our work. We are also extremely grateful for the continued support of our long suffering wives who have allowed us to withdraw from some of our family responsibilities in order to make this 2nd Edition possible.

PREFACE TO FIRST EDITION

We have been conscious of the need to produce an up-to-date reference work on the ever-expanding and now internationally recognized specialty of coloproctology. We believe that the concept of a book primarily based on the experience of two individuals has certain advantages over an edited text contributed to by numerous experts to cover particular fields of the subject.

We have based our management policies on experience gained when we were both in Leeds, and subsequently in Birmingham and London. The ties with Leeds, particularly with Professor John Goligher, his teaching and his clinical material, have been an inspiration to both of us. We are privileged to be able to continue his tradition and to retain the title of the book which bore his name for five editions.

The entire book, apart from 11 specialized chapters (anaesthesia, sexually transmitted disease, urology, gynaecology, tropical disease, laparoscopic colectomy and five paediatric chapters) have been written by one of us, and then read and amended by the other. We have attempted to approach controversial issues in a Socratic manner, but we hope we have made it clear where our preferences lie. Occasionally, where a difference of opinion remains between us, we have made it obvious and leave readers to make up their own mind.

Work began several years ago, but the entire text has been rewritten during preparation in order to bring it completely up-to-date. There is some repetition, since we see this work as providing a reference to the management of specific diseases rather than a book which is likely to be read in its entirely. We have deliberately chosen to provide a book which is heavily illustrated so that there can be no confusion over the techniques of operative management. We have also tried to provide a comprehensive bibliography throughout so that the reader can draw from the experience of others in understanding the disease and its optimum therapy.

Apart from extensive writing from our own libraries, much has also been compiled during travel, sabbatical appointments and at overseas conferences. This has provided us with an international perspective of the clinical management of coloproctological disorders. Nevertheless, it has been necessary to include experts to address specific subjects about which we cannot write from personal experience. Such contributions include: Anaesthesia – Professor Peter Hutton; Paediatrics – Mr Jeremy Lawson and Mr Neil Freeman; Gynaecological aspects of coloproctology – Mr Charlic Chan; Urological aspects of coloproctology – Professor John Blandy; Tropical and infectious diseases – Professor Michael Farthing, including sub-sections on Bilharzia by Professor Mageed Barsoum, and Chagas' disease by Professor Angelita Habr-Gama; and Sexually transmitted disease – Dr Hiliary Andrews, Professor Andrew Sim and Dr Steven Wexner. Since the USA experience in laparoscopic colectomy was more advanced than our own we asked Dr Steven Wexner to cover the subject. We are also grateful to the following for their critique in relation to specific surgical procedures: Dr Stanley Goldberg – haemorrhoidectomy; Dr Bob Beart – restorative proctocolectomy; Mr Mark Coldman – tuberculosis; Dr Marvin Corman – graciloplasty; Mr David Cant – colorectal trauma; and Dr Michael Veidenheimer – diverticular disease.

Throughout the text we have attempted both to review the available data from the world literature, which has been tabulated where possible, as well as to draw on personal experience from our own clinical practice particularly in the operative treatment of colorectal disorders. One of us (MRBK) has a personal practice which has been entirely based in Birmingham since 1976. The other (NSW) has been on the staff at Leeds before moving to The Royal London Hospital in 1986. We hope you enjoy reading this book as much as we have in gathering the information for you.

M.R.B. Keighley
N.S. Williams

ACKNOWLEDGEMENTS

The second edition has been no less of a commitment than the first. We are extremely fortunate to have been able to engage the talents of Gillian Lee for this 2nd edition. The clarity of and sensitivity of her artwork was much appreciated in the 1st edition and we are glad of her continued expertise in this respect. We are also grateful to the Publishing team of WB Saunders at Harcourt Brace and Company Limited, London on its advice and technical support. We thank Dr S Scott Sanders who has kindly supplied some more histopathology illustrations; other colleagues who contributed illustrations have been appropriately acknowledged at the end of legends.

In addition to all those junior and senior colleagues who contributed advice and assistance in the first and second editions, we should like to acknowledge in particular the support in the second edition of John Abercrombie, Janet Ansell, Alex Buttafuoco, Mark Chapman, Andrew Connelly, Dominic Corry, Sina Dorudi, James Eccersley, Rodney Hallan, Hiro Hasegawa, Frances Hughes, Charlie Knowles, Stephan Korsgen, Peter Lunniss, James Mander, Andrew Maw, Gunju Ogunbiyi, Shaun Purkiss, Simon Radley, Rita Ratani, Mark Scott, Hugo Taylor, Heng Tee Tan, Jonathan Tilsed, Steve Warren and Taka Yamamoto.

We are indebted to the following companies for their generous support towards the artwork in this second edition:

American Medical Systems
B-K Medical
Ethicon Endo-Surgical
Genzyme Therapeutics
Hollister Limited
Medtronic

We very much appreciate the support of our secretaries – Janet Mutch and Andrea Hickey in London and Lynne Hopwood, Jayne Hamill, Julia Reeves and Yvette Young in Birmingham. Finally we know that the task would never have been accomplished without the patience of our long suffering wives.

1

ANATOMY AND PHYSIOLOGY INVESTIGATIONS

PART ONE: SURGICAL ANATOMY

The anatomy of the colon, rectum and anus will not be described in detail here: specific anatomy is described in relation to diseases of the colon and rectum and can be found throughout this book. The purpose of this chapter is to give an overall description of the anatomy of the region and to highlight particular aspects of surgical importance.

GENERAL POSITION AND RELATIONS OF THE COLON

The large bowel is easily recognized and distinguished from the small intestine by its larger diameter and the presence of appendices epiploicae and taeniae coli. The three taeniae consist of condensations of longitudinal smooth muscle fibres commencing at the base of the appendix and continuing throughout the colon; in the upper rectum these three bands disappear as they fuse to the continuous longitudinal muscle of the rectum (Figure 1.1).

The caecum is the widest part of the large bowel and lies in the right iliac fossa just above the lateral half of the inguinal ligament on the iliacus muscle; it is variable in position since, unlike the ascending colon, it is usually completely intraperitoneal. It is therefore at risk of becoming involved by volvulus. The appendix lies at the lower pole of the caecum and the ileum joins the medial and posterior aspect of the viscus. The ileum, 5–10 cm proximal to the ileocaecal valve, often adheres to the posterior abdominal wall by an anterior peritoneal attachment. This must be freed in order to mobilize the ileocaecal region.

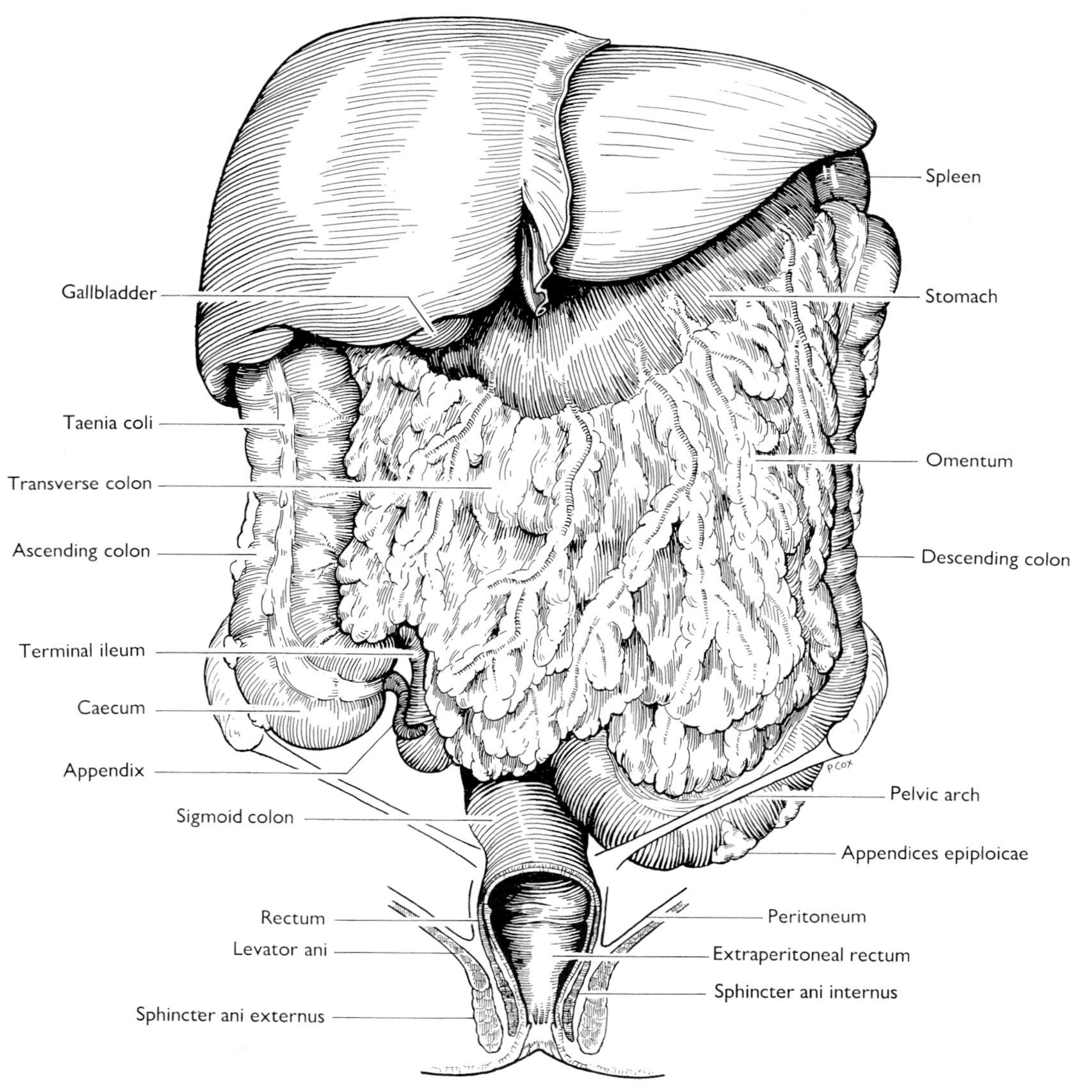

Figure 1.1 General topography of the large bowel and rectum. The relations of the large bowel to the omentum, stomach, liver, gall bladder and pelvis are demonstrated.

The ascending colon is fixed by adherent anterior peritoneum throughout its length. At the hepatic flexure numerous veins lie immediately underneath the peritoneum and these may have to be diathermized when dividing the peritoneum during mobilization of the hepatic flexure. These veins enlarge considerably in portal hypertension. The lower part of the ascending colon lies on the iliopsoas muscle with the genital branch of the genitofemoral nerve. The upper part of the right colon lies on the quadratus lumborum muscle and the origin of the transversus abdominis (Figure 1.2).

The hepatic flexure lies over the lower pole of the right kidney, medial to which are the second and third parts of the duodenum. The second or third part of the duodenum may be damaged during mobilization of the hepatic flexure, particularly when resecting colonic Crohn's disease with an associated abscess.

The transverse colon is variable in length and its middle part may reach into the pelvis. Proximally, the first 5–10 cm is retroperitoneal but the rest of the transverse colon has a complete peritoneal covering. The greater omentum, arising from the greater curvature of the stomach, lies over the transverse colon. The inferior peritoneal coat of the omentum is adherent to the anterior surface of the transverse colon and the transverse mesocolon containing the middle colic vessels and lymphatics. These peritoneal layers can be divided so that the transverse colon and mesocolon can be freed from the omentum (Figure 1.3).

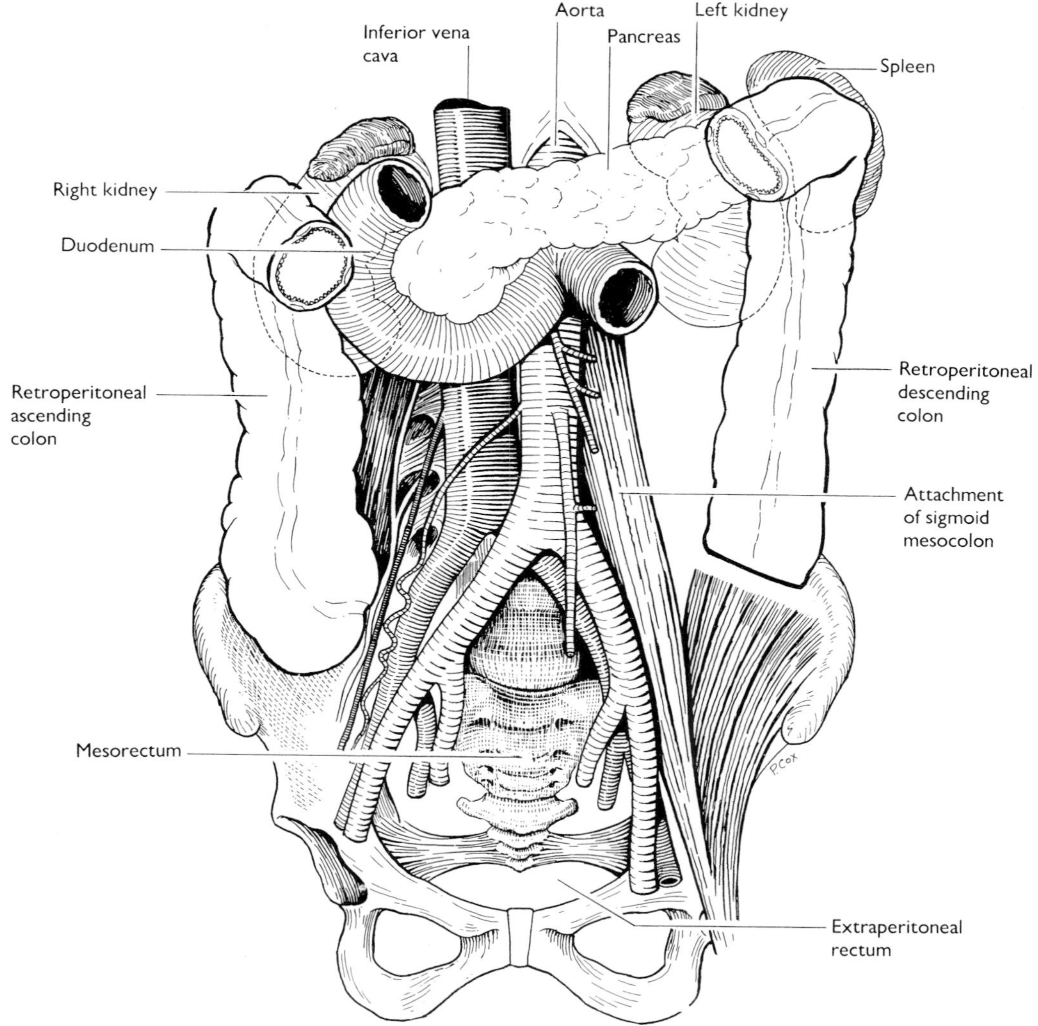

Figure 1.2 The posterior relations of the colon and rectum are demonstrated, particularly (1) the relations of the right colon to the right kidney, the duodenum and the iliopsoas muscle, (2) the descending colon to the spleen, the tail of the pancreas, the left kidney, the transversus abdominis and iliacus, and (3) the mesorectum to the bifurcation of the aorta, the left iliac vein and the sacrum.

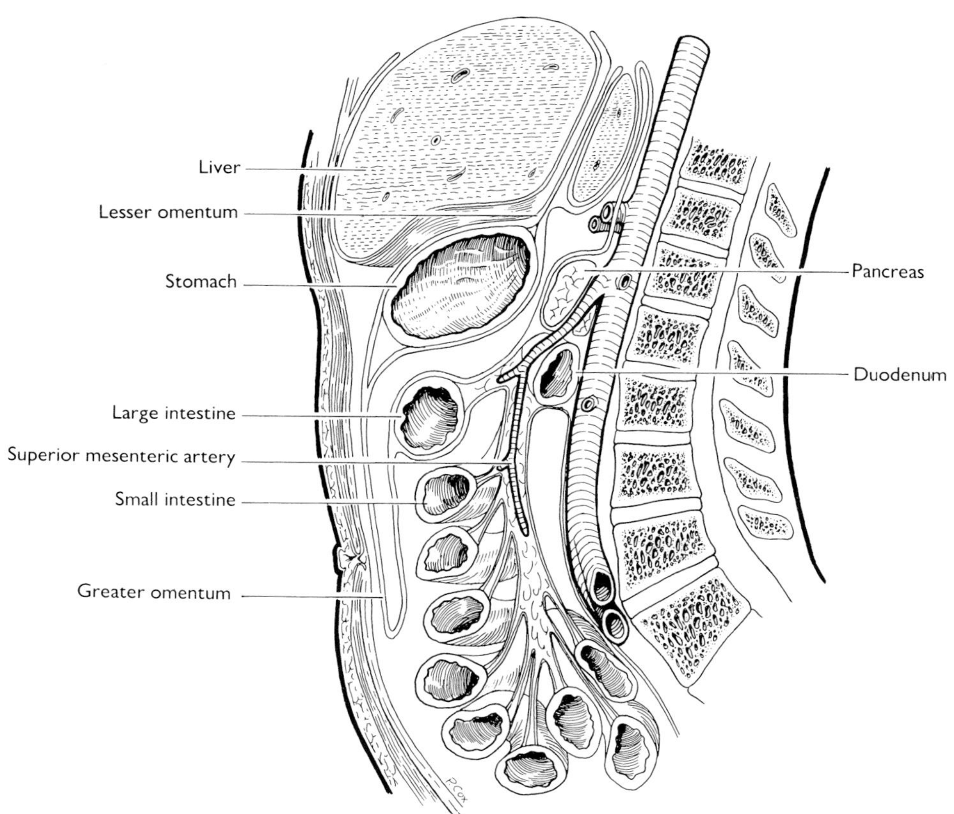

Figure 1.3 Sagittal section of the abdomen to demonstrate the blood supply to the transverse colon and small bowel, the greater omentum, the greater sac and the lesser sac.

The splenic flexure is usually situated at a higher level than the hepatic flexure and it lies more laterally, making it less accessible. The splenic flexure lies over the lower pole of the left kidney and may touch the lower border of the spleen, which usually lies just above and lateral to it. The spleen may become damaged either by the tip of a retractor during mobilization of the splenic flexure or by excessive traction on the gastrosplenic ligament. The splenic flexure lies retroperitoneally and there is a condensation of loose connective tissue arising laterally which connects the colon to the under-surface of the diaphragm: this is termed the phrenicocolic ligament. The blood supply to the splenic flexure lies medially to it and is not normally in danger during mobilization and division of the peritoneum.

The descending colon is firmly adherent to the posterior abdominal wall, being entirely retroperitoneal. It lies on the transverse abdominis, quadratus lumborum and, lower down, on the iliopsoas muscle.

The sigmoid colon is intraperitoneal and very variable in length; it is the narrowest part of the large bowel. The sigmoid commences just below the pelvic brim and terminates at the upper rectum, just below the sacral promontory. The sigmoid mesocolon is V-shaped, running upwards and medially over the psoas muscle, the genital vessels and the ureter to the aortic bifurcation. It then runs downwards over the sacrum to the upper rectum. The sigmoid colon is subject to volvulus.

THE RECTUM AND ITS RELATIONS

The rectum commences where the taenia coli fuse to form a continuous longitudinal muscle coat. The upper third of the rectum is surrounded by peritoneum, apart from a small segment posteriorly through which the mesorectum provides its blood supply from the superior haemorrhoidal vessels

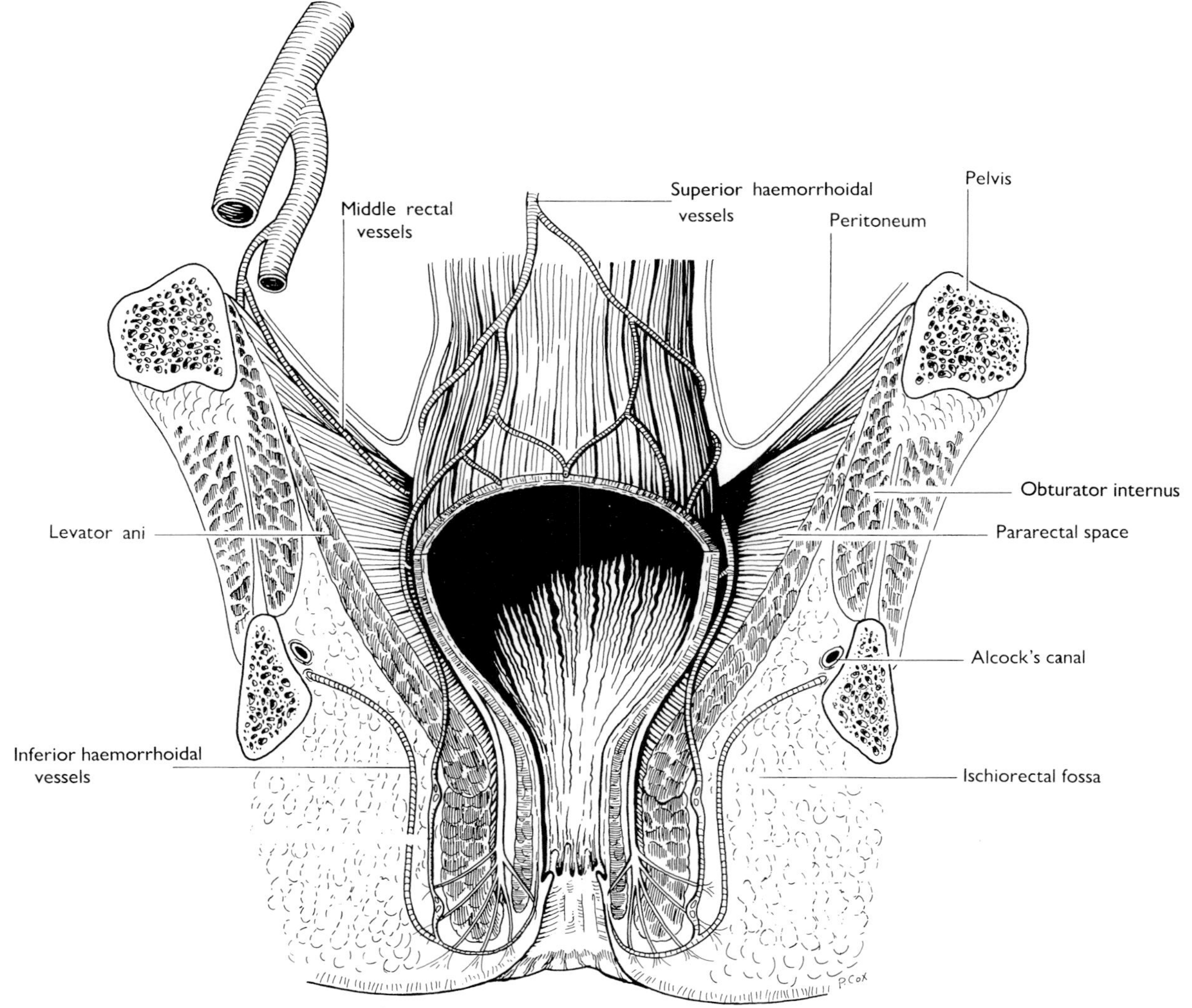

Figure 1.4 Coronal section of the anorectum to demonstrate (1) the relations of the rectum to the levator ani, and (2) the arterial supply to the rectum from the superior haemorrhoidal vessels and the inferior haemorrhoidal vessels.

(Figure 1.4). The middle third of the rectum is essentially retroperitoneal and is only covered anteriorly by peritoneum. At this point the mesorectum becomes wider and the posterior rectum is entirely devoid of peritoneum. At the base of the rectovesical or rectouterine pouch the rectum becomes completely infraperitoneal. On account of the obliquity of the levator ani, the rectum is intimately related laterally to the pararectal space, but below and laterally to the pelvic diaphragm and to the apex of the ischiorectal fossa. The pararectal space is formed by the peritoneum above, the obturator internus and the side walls of the pelvis laterally, by the rectum medially and by the levator ani below. The ischiorectal fossa is roofed by the sloping levator ani above the anorectum, with the external and internal sphincters forming the medial boundary. Laterally lies the ischium with Alcock's canal which transmits the pudendal nerve and the inferior haemorrhoidal vessels. The space is deficient below.

The rectum follows the curve of the sacral hollow in its lower two-thirds but at the level of the levator ani, where it enters the anal canal, it turns abruptly backwards and downwards (Figure 1.5). This anorectal angle, which is maintained by the puborectalis sling, has in the past been regarded as an important mechanism in maintaining continence.

The posterior relations of the rectum are the sacrum, the coccyx, the puborectalis muscles and the middle sacral vessels. The sacral plexus and the autonomic nerve fibres in the pelvis, together with

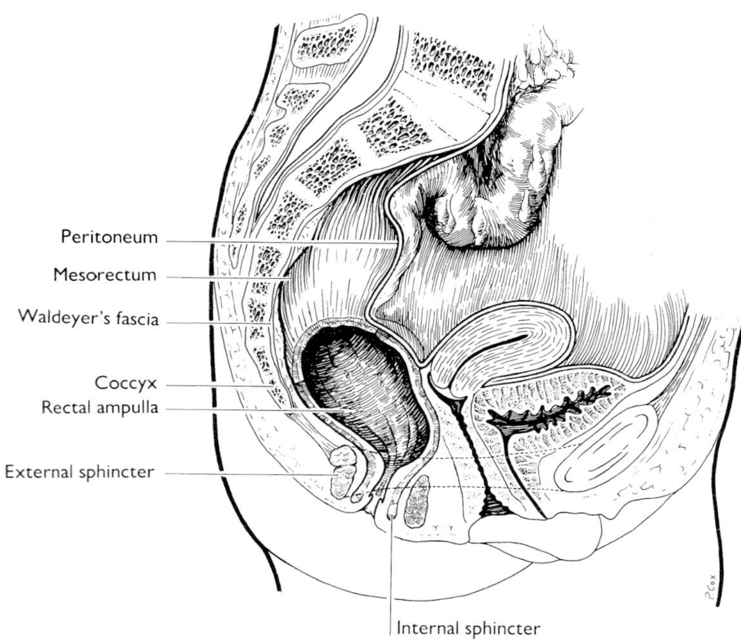

Figure 1.5 Sagittal section of the female pelvis to demonstrate the relations of the rectum anteriorly to the pouch of Douglas, the uterus, the vagina and the bladder and posteriorly to the tip of the coccyx.

the pelvic lymphatics, lie behind the upper rectum. Lateral relations include the uterine appendages above the peritoneal reflection; below the peritoneal reflection lie the ureters, the iliac vessels and the lateral ligaments with the middle rectal artery within them; lower still lie the pubococcygeus, ischiococcygeus and iliococcygeus (components of the levator ani). The anterior relations differ according to sex (Figures 1.5 and 1.6). In males the extraperitoneal rectum is related from below upwards to the prostate, seminal vesicles, vas and bladder. In the female the infraperitoneal rectum lies immediately behind the posterior vaginal wall. Above the peritoneal reflection the rectum is related to the upper vagina, with the uterus above. Loops of small bowel, the ovaries, the fallopian tubes and the sigmoid colon frequently intervene anteriorly above the pouch of Douglas.

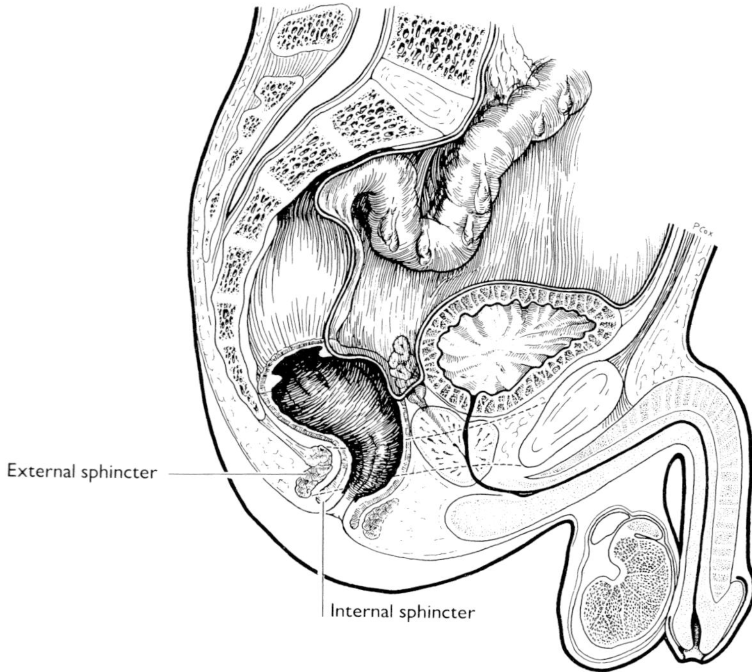

Figure 1.6 Sagittal section of the male pelvis to demonstrate the relations of the rectum anteriorly to the seminal vesicles, prostate and bladder and posteriorly to the tip of the coccyx and sacrum.

The endopelvic fasciae form important relations with the rectum. These fascial components consist of condensations of fibrous tissue below the peritoneal reflection attached to the parietal pelvic fascia. There is a condensation of tissue around the middle rectal artery forming the lateral ligaments. Posteriorly there is a thickened area of parietal pelvic fascia over the sacrum and coccyx (Waldeyer's fascia); this must be divided during perineal and abdominal mobilization of the rectum. If this is not done correctly, the fascia may be stripped from the sacrum, resulting in damage to the presacral veins lying between the sacrum and the fascia, and to the nervi irrigentes, causing impotence in men. Anteriorly the visceral pelvic fascia is expanded from the peritoneal reflection to the urogenital triangle, where it is known as Denonvilliers' fascia. In the male it intervenes between the rectum and the prostate. In the female it is less prominent and divides the rectum from the vagina.

THE ANAL CANAL

The anal canal is 3–4 cm long; it commences at the anorectal angle and ends at the anal verge. Normally the anus is closed. Posteriorly the anal canal is related to the coccyx, the puborectalis and the sphincters. Laterally lies the ischiorectal fossa with the inferior haemorrhoidal vessels and pudendal nerve in Alcock's canal (see Figure 1.4). Anteriorly the anal canal is related to the bulb of the urethra and the urogenital triangle in the male, and to the perineal body and vagina in the female (see Figure 1.5) (Goligher et al, 1955; Hughes, 1957; Nivatvongs et al, 1981).

The anal canal is lined by columnar (mucosal) epithelium above the anal valves, and squamous epithelium (skin) below (Figures 1.7 and 1.8). The dentate or pectinate lines are synonymous and represent the site of the anal valves, which mark the mucocutaneous junction. These valves are remnants of the proctodeal membrane separating the post-allantoic hind-gut from the proctodeum. Above each anal valve is a pit, known as an anal crypt or sinus, formed by the orifices of the anal glands. These glands lie in the intersphincteric plane and help to lubricate the anal canal. The mucosa above the dentate line is thrown into a number of longitudinal columns, beneath which lies the internal haemorrhoidal plexus. The epithelium is loose above but becomes adherent to the internal sphincter at the anal valves via the mucosal suspensory ligament of Parks. For a distance of 0.5–2 cm above the anal valves the mucosa is cuboidal (not columnar): this is known as the anal transition zone (Duthie and Bennett, 1963). This area is richly innervated with sensory nerve endings (Duthie and Gairns, 1960). Below the anal valves the epithelium is squamous but devoid of hair, sebaceous and sweat glands. Only at the anal verge does the epithelium and subcutaneous tissue resemble those of normal skin.

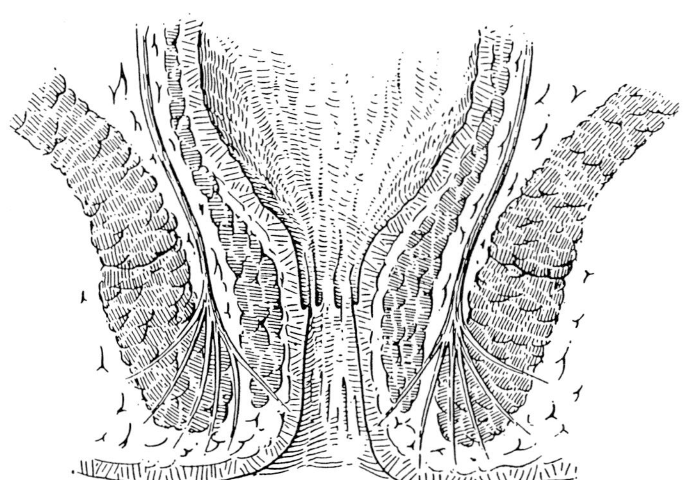

Figure 1.7 A coronal section of the anorectum to demonstrate the distribution of the internal anal sphincter as a continuation of the circular muscle of the rectum, the levator ani and the external anal sphincter. The conjoint longitudinal ligaments are demonstrated in the intersphincteric plane.

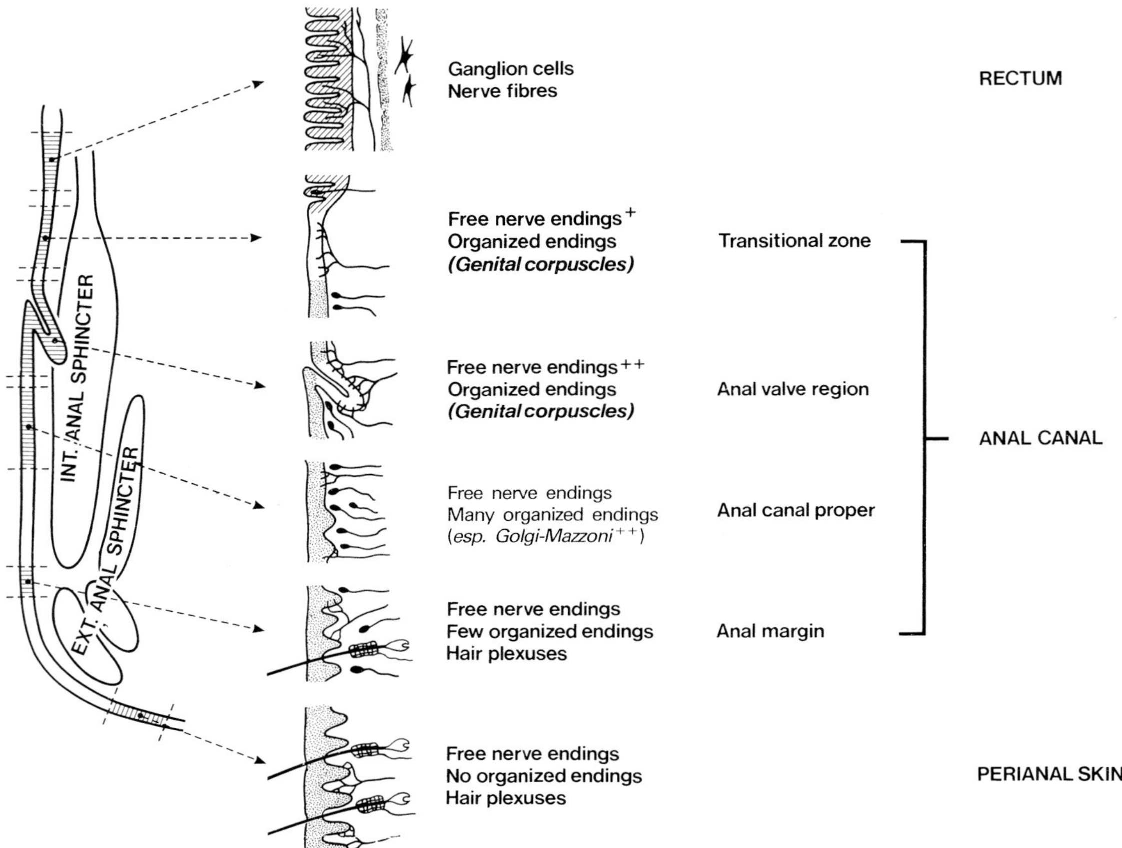

Figure 1.8 A diagrammatic representation of the innervation of the anal canal and perianal skin. The nerve endings characteristic of the transitional zone and the anal valve region are shown.

THE SPHINCTERS

The internal anal sphincter is merely a thickening of the circular fibres surrounding the gut. It is visceral in origin and consists of smooth muscle innervated by the pelvic autonomic plexus. The internal sphincter is 0.2–0.3 cm thick and surrounds the entire anal canal, extending at least 1 cm below it. The lower margin is quite distinct.

The external sphincter is somatic in origin and consists of skeletal muscle arranged circumferentially around the anal canal. Posteriorly the upper fibres of the external sphincter merge imperceptibly with the inner fibres of the puborectalis. Fibres of the external sphincter surround the anal canal, some of which are inserted into the pubis anteriorly and with the puborectalis. There are some fibres which are attached to the coccyx (Shafik, 1975; Handley, 1978). Although in fixed specimens the external sphincter may appear to descend lower in the anal canal than the internal sphincter, at the operation of internal sphincterotomy or anorectal myectomy the internal sphincter is usually found to be the lower of the two. Conventional anatomical texts describe three components to the external anal sphincter: surgically, these are indistinguishable (Ayoub, 1979).

In the lower anal canal there is a longitudinal band (known by some as the longitudinal conjoined ligament) which fans out to form a number of septa: these extend radially through the lower fibres of the external sphincter to the perianal skin. The longitudinal bands consist of longitudinal smooth muscle fibres and elastic tissue which are inferior extensions of the longitudinal fibres of the rectum.

THE LEVATOR ANI

The levator ani forms the pelvic diaphragm, separating the pelvis from the perineum. It consists of a funnel arising from the sides of the pelvis through which the urethra, vagina and anorectum pass to enter the perineum. The levator ani is quite thin and the pelvic surface is covered by endopelvic fascia, lymphatics and fat. The inner fibres consist of the puborectalis which arises from the symphysis pubis. These fibres surround the vagina (or prostate) and the anorectum, just above the sphincters, to be inserted into the opposite side of the symphysis pubis, creating a sling which is deficient anteriorly (Figure 1.9). Fibres of the pubococcygeus arise from the pubic ramus and the fascia over the obturator internus and are inserted into the coccyx. The iliococcygeus also arises from the arcus

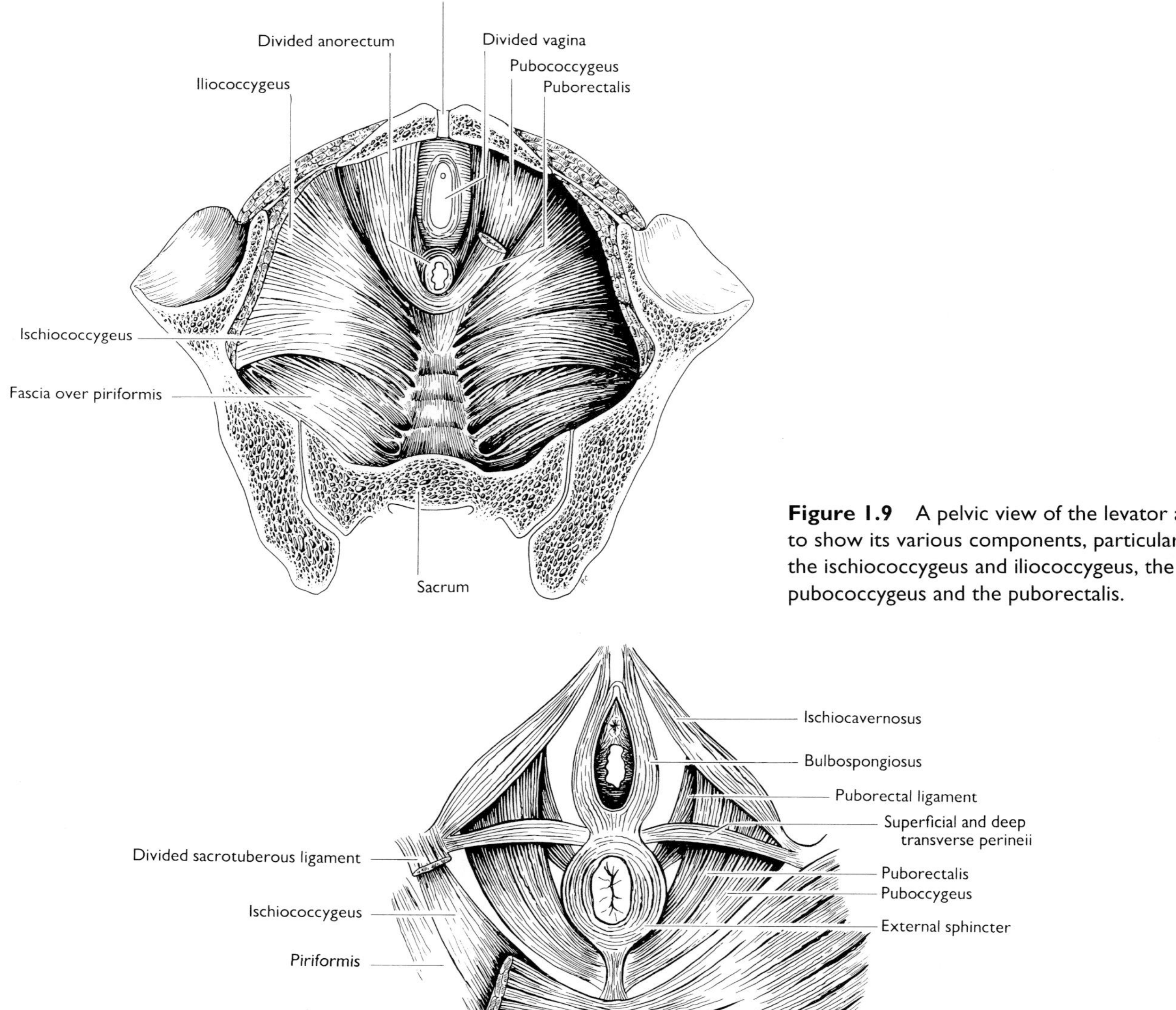

Figure 1.9 A pelvic view of the levator ani to show its various components, particularly the ischiococcygeus and iliococcygeus, the pubococcygeus and the puborectalis.

Figure 1.10 The levator ani viewed from the perineum. The relationship of the ischiococcygeus to the gluteus maximus is shown, together with the puborectalis and pubococcygeus. The puborectal fibres of the pubococcygeus, the bulbospongiosus, the transverse perineii and the ischiocavernosus are demonstrated.

tendineus and is inserted into the coccyx and the anococcygeal raphe. The ischiococcygeus arises from the tip of the ischial spine and is inserted into the coccyx and the lower part of the sacrum. The perineal surface of the ischiococcygeus is covered by the sacrotuberous ligament and the gluteus maximus (Figure 1.10). Anteriorly, the pubococcygeus forms two separate raphes which are inserted into the prostate, bladder or anterior rectum and are known as the puboprostatic, pubovesical and puborectal ligaments respectively. A similar, though less pronounced condensation of striated muscle is seen running from the pubis to the anterior aspect of the rectum in the female. These muscle fibres are always encountered during anterior dissection of the anorectum at proctectomy.

ARTERIAL SUPPLY

The colon and rectum are supplied from the territory of the superior and inferior mesenteric arteries (Figure 1.11). The pattern of vascular supply is variable and for a detailed description of these variations readers are encouraged to consult the excellent articles on the subject by Griffiths (1956), Goligher (1951), Vandamme et al (1982), Ayoub (1978) and Michels et al (1965).

The superior mesenteric artery arises from the front of the aorta just below the coeliac axis. It

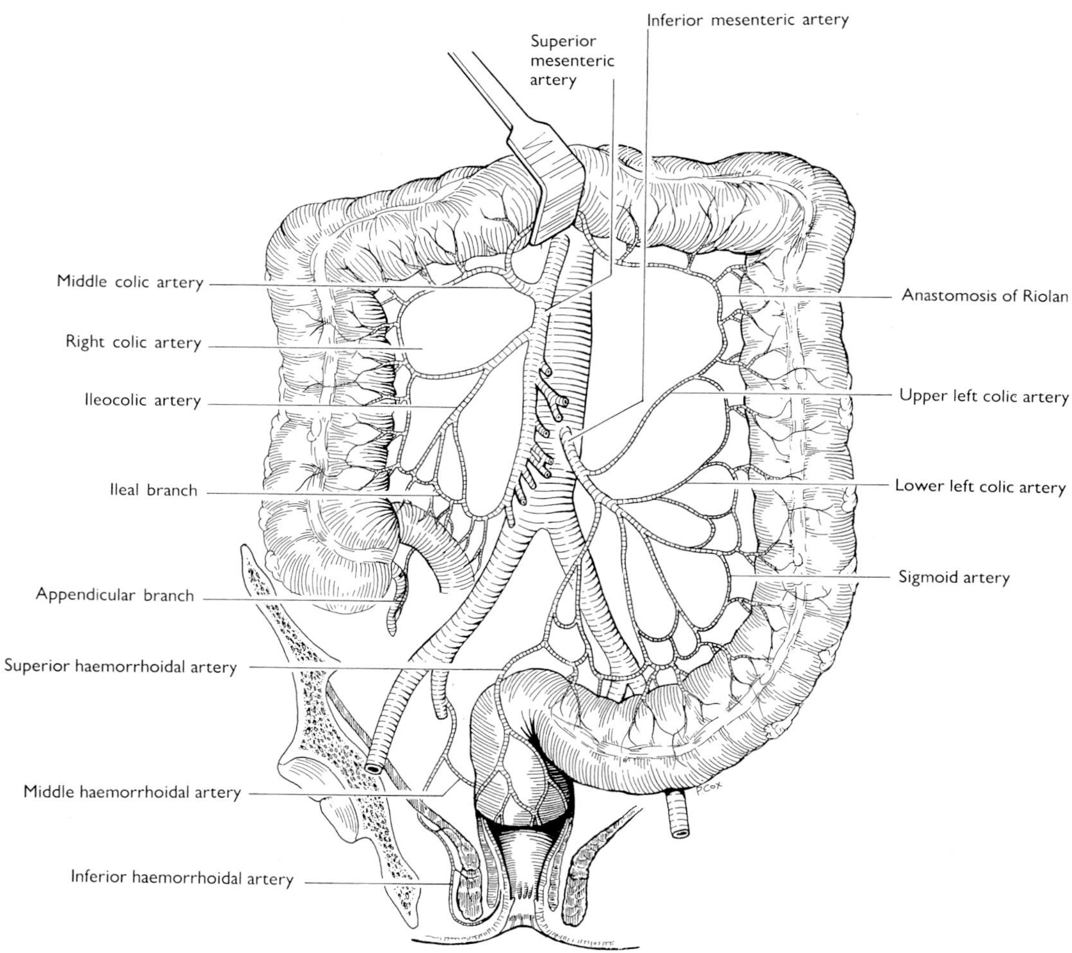

Figure 1.11 The arterial supply to the colon and rectum. The normal distribution of supply to the ileum, right colon and right side of transverse colon from the middle colic artery and ileocolic arteries is shown. The distribution of the arterial supply from the inferior mesenteric artery to the left side of the transverse colon, the descending colon, the sigmoid and the upper rectum is also demonstrated.

emerges under the pancreas, with the superior mesenteric vein on its right, where it lies in association with lymphatics and sympathetic nerve fibres. The main artery is very short since it divides, soon after its origin, into the middle colic artery and its parent trunk. The middle colic artery subdivides to produce two or three large arcades in the mesocolon. The parent trunk then subdivides into the right colic artery and the ileocolic artery, the terminal portion of the parent vessel lying in the free edge of the small bowel mesentery. The arrangement of the terminal branches to the caecum and ileum have now assumed great importance for the construction of ileal pouches (Figure 1.12). The ileocolic artery forms a pericolic arcade with the right colic artery about 2 cm medial to the ascending aorta. The terminal portion of the ileocolic artery divides into an anterior and a posterior caecal branch, an appendicular branch running in the free border of the mesoappendix and an ileal branch which forms arcades with the ileal branches of the superior mesenteric artery. Provided the arcades in the small bowel mesentery are patent and they are of sufficient calibre it is possible to divide the main superior mesenteric arterial pedicle distal to a satisfactory ileal arcade, as well as the ileocolic artery, without jeopardizing the blood supply to the terminal ileum.

The inferior mesenteric artery arises from the aorta on the under-surface of the third part of the duodenum. In atherosclerotic patients it is frequently occluded by thrombus. The exact anatomical arrangement of the origin of the inferior mesenteric artery is variable. There is often a branch running upwards to the splenic flexure (upper left colic) as well as one running transversely (lower left colic). There are three or four sigmoid arcades from which further arcades are formed before end arteries supply the sigmoid colon and upper rectum. The terminal portion of the inferior mesenteric artery continues down over the pelvic brim in the mesocolon as the superior haemorrhoidal artery and divides into right and left branches before subdividing into terminal anterior and posterior end arteries supplying the rectum.

The middle haemorrhoidal artery arises from the anterior division of the internal iliac artery or from the vesical branch of this vessel. The middle haemorrhoidal artery traverses the infraperitoneal pelvis in the lateral ligaments and supplies the middle

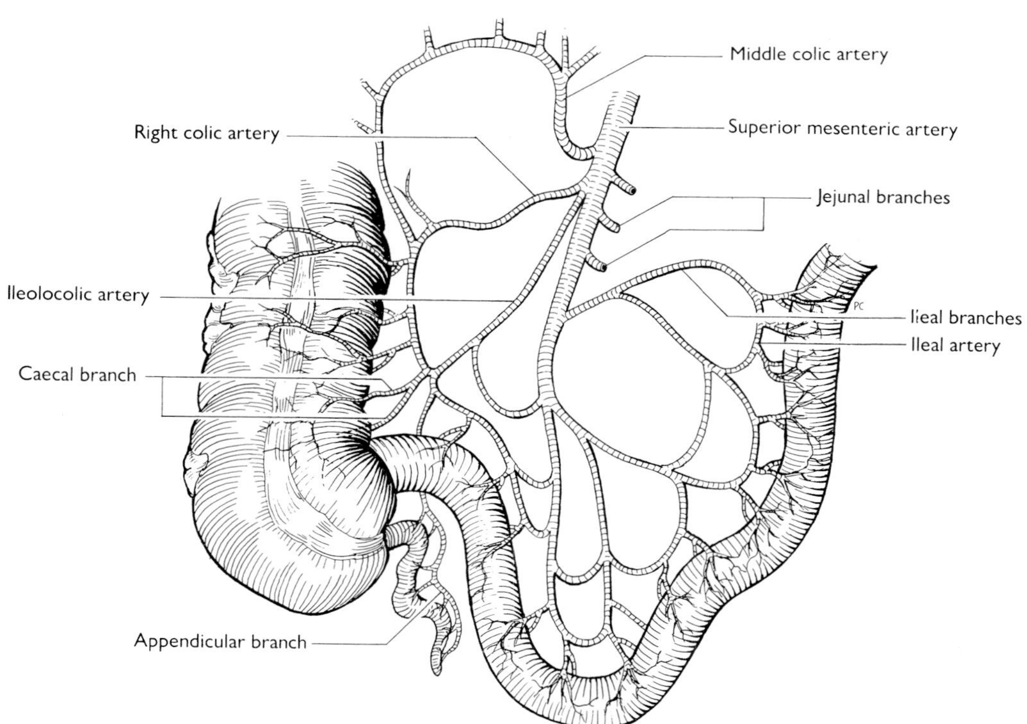

Figure 1.12 Detailed anatomy of the arterial supply to the terminal ileum and right colon is shown. In particular, the normal divisions of the ileocolic artery and arcade with the middle colic artery are demonstrated.

third of the rectum. The inferior haemorrhoidal artery is also a branch of the anterior division of the internal iliac artery. It is invested by endopelvic fascia as it passes out of the pelvis, below the piriformis, through the greater sciatic foramen. It pursues a short course in the buttock and re-enters the pelvis, after passing over the sacrospinous ligament, to enter Alcock's canal in the lateral wall of the ischiorectal fossa. The vessel crosses the ischiorectal fossa where it may cause considerable bleeding if encountered during abdominoperineal excision of the rectum. The vessel supplies the levator ani and sphincters as well as the lower rectum and anal canal. The three haemorrhoidal vessels form a comprehensive anastomosis in the submucosa of the anal canal and lower rectum.

The colon is supplied by a marginal artery known as the marginal artery of Riolan (Drummond, 1913). The proximity of this vessel to the colon is variable but it provides an important communication between the superior and inferior mesenteric arteries. The vessel is usually present and provides the arterial supply to the entire left colon. When the origin of the inferior mesenteric artery is occluded by atheroma or following aortic surgery, the marginal artery is the only means of maintaining a blood supply to the descending colon and sigmoid. If this vessel is present, radical high ligation of the inferior mesenteric artery can be performed without jeopardizing the viability of the left colon (Morgan and Griffiths, 1959). The marginal artery provides terminal end arteries which supply the colon. These are either short vasa recta supplying the adjacent colonic wall and mucosa or long vasa recta which supply the appendices epiploicae and the antimesenteric border of the colon (Figure 1.13).

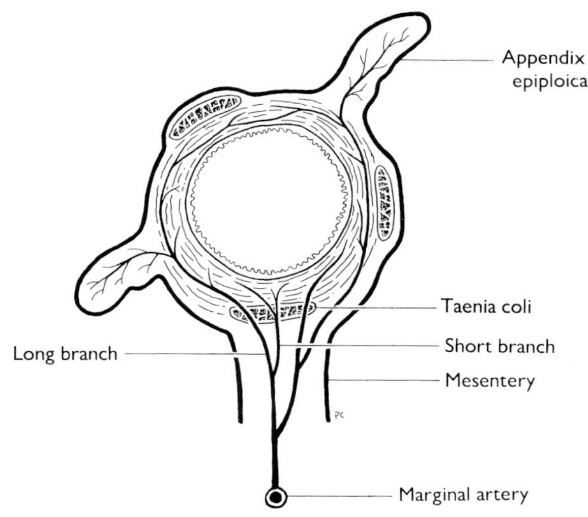

Figure 1.13 The terminal arterial supply to the colon and its relation to the taenia coli and appendices epiploicae is demonstrated.

VENOUS DRAINAGE

Essentially the venous drainage mirrors the arterial supply with three major exceptions (Figure 1.14). First, there is a much freer venous communication between the middle haemorrhoidal veins and the veins around the base of the vagina (or prostate) and the bladder. In fact the contribution of the middle rectal veins to rectal venous drainage is small. The second difference is that there is a very free communication between the superior and inferior haemorrhoidal veins in the submucosal plexus of the anorectum. Blood from the inferior haemorrhoidal veins enters the systemic circulation through the internal iliac vein, whereas the superior haemorrhoidal veins drain into the portal system. It is said that these veins enlarge in portal hypertension, but the incidence of haemorrhoids is not always increased in patients with this condition (Keighley et al, 1973). Finally, drainage of the superior mesenteric vein and the inferior mesenteric vein is through the portal distribution, hence the inferior mesenteric vein drains into the splenic vein and, in so doing, runs far higher and more laterally than the inferior mesenteric artery. In high vascular ligation for large bowel cancer the vein must be ligated separately, and preferably traced to its confluence with the splenic vein.

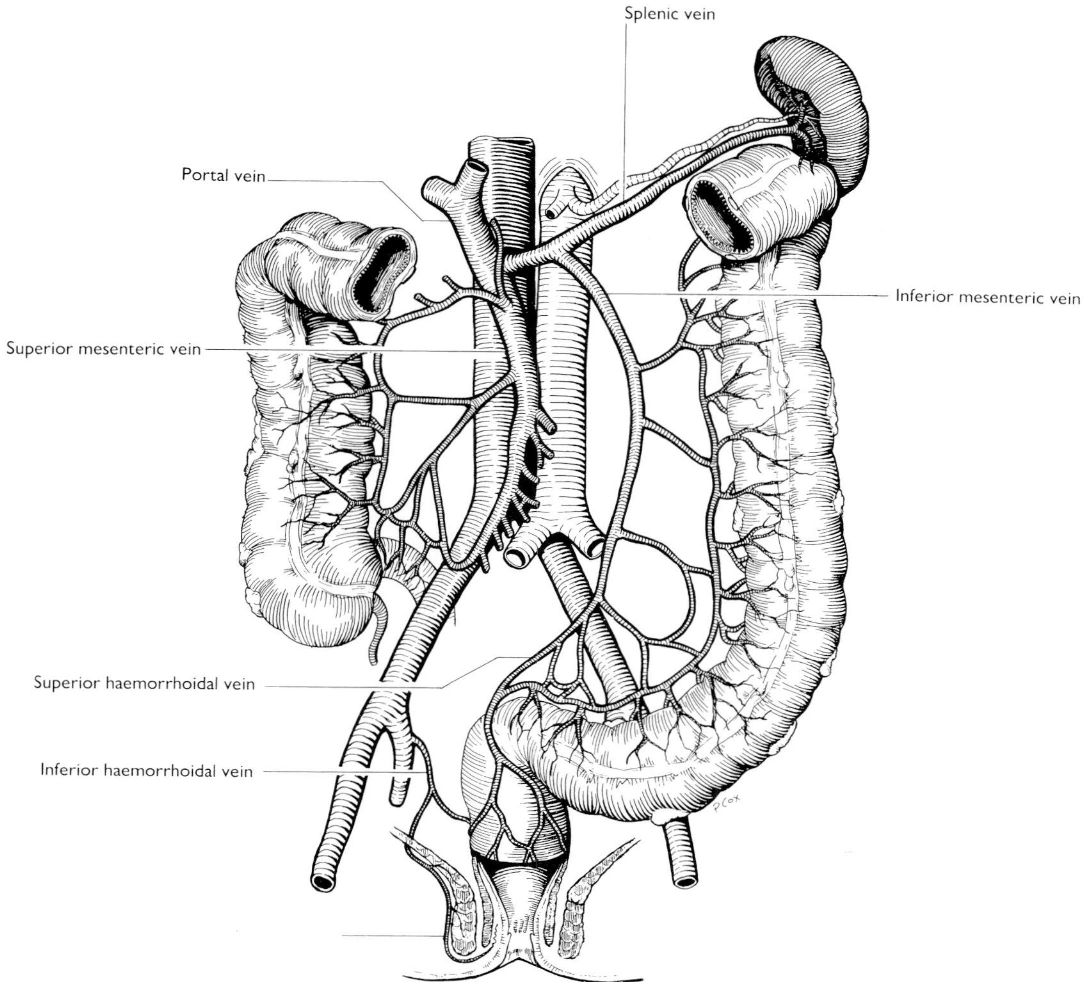

Figure 1.14 The venous drainage of the large bowel and rectum is illustrated, in particular the drainage of the left colon via the inferior mesenteric vein to the splenic vein is shown.

LYMPHATIC DRAINAGE

The lymphatic drainage of the large bowel follows its vascular supply (Figure 1.15). There are four tiers of lymphatics draining the colon and rectum: the lymphatic channels from the submucosal and subserosal plexus first pass through the lymph nodes lying adjacent to the colon, known as epicolic nodes; the next filter is through nodes found adjacent to the marginal artery or its terminal branches, known as paracolic nodes; the intermediate nodes are found along the main branches of the superior mesenteric artery and the inferior mesenteric artery; finally, the principal nodes surround the origin of these vessels on the front of the aorta. Lymphatic channels may bypass one or two of these tiers of nodes but lymphatic involvement by malignancy outside the distribution of the colonic lymphatics is rare, hence involvement of splenic hilar nodes or gastroepiploic nodes is unusual in malignant disease. Lymphatic drainage of the anorectum also mirrors its blood supply. The upper anal canal and rectum drains cephalad through lymphatic channels that coalesce around the rectum where they are interrupted by perirectal nodes; proximal drainage is along the inferior mesenteric artery to the preaortic nodes. The lower anal canal below the dentate line drains caudally to a perianal plexus of lymphatics and hence to the inguinal nodes.

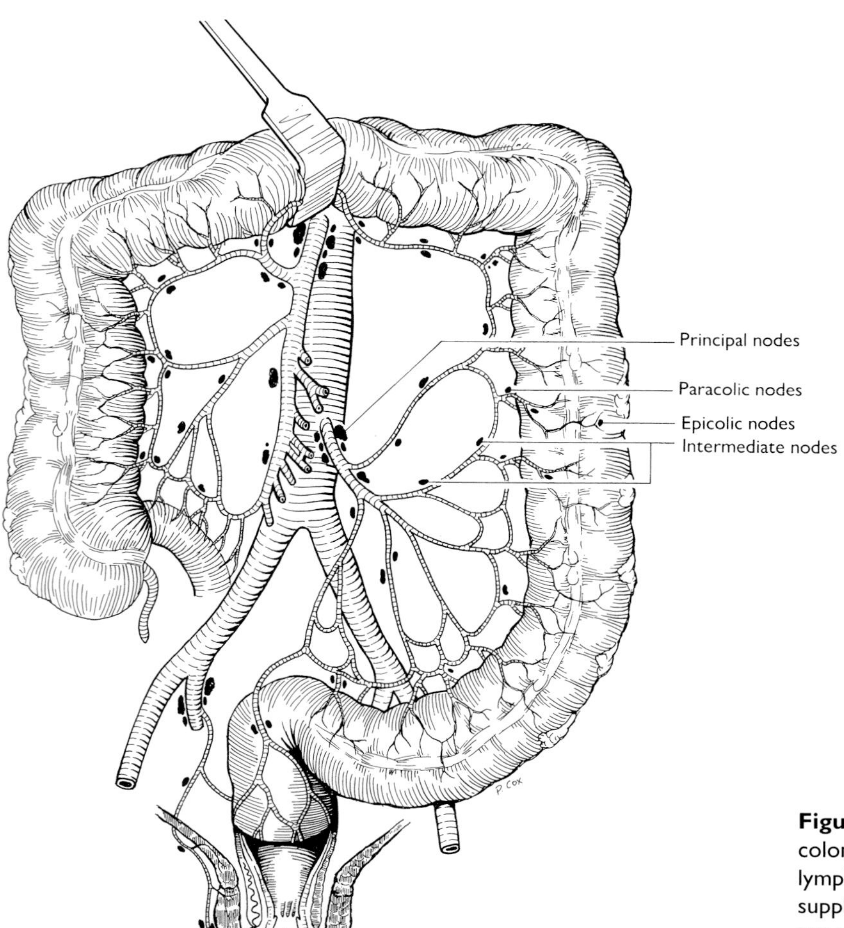

Figure 1.15 The lymphatic drainage of the colon and rectum is illustrated, showing that the lymph nodes are distributed around the arterial supply to the large intestine. Four tiers of nodes are recognized: paracolic, epicolic, intermediate and principal lymph nodes.

NERVE SUPPLY

Sympathetics

The sympathetic supply to the right side of the colon is derived from connector cells in the lower six thoracic segments of the spinal cord, from which preganglionic white fibres pass out to the paravertebral sympathetic chain. This chain lies behind the inferior vena cava on the right and to the side of the aorta on the left (Figure 1.16). The outflow for the left colon takes its origin from the first three lumbar segments of the cord. Fibres leave the ganglionated sympathetic trunks to form a plexus around the superior and inferior mesenteric arteries. It is only in the perivascular ganglia that synapses form, from which nerves follow the arteries to supply the gut.

Sympathetic innervation to the pelvic viscera differs, however, since it is not derived from the inferior mesenteric plexus. Preganglionic fibres from the sympathetic trunk converge over the sacral promontory at the bifurcation of the aorta to form the hypogastric plexus. Fibres leave the hypogastric plexus together with the pelvic parasympathetics to form the presacral nerves. The presacral nerves are easily visible during rectal dissection: they lie behind and below the pelvic peritoneum running from below the aortic bifurcation laterally to the side wall of the pelvis. They therefore lie behind the mesorectum and the superior haemorrhoidal veins. The presacral nerves are closely associated with the middle haemorrhoidal arteries at their origin from the internal iliac artery. Fibres from the hypogastric plexus travel with the arteries to supply the urethra, prostate, seminal vesicles, penis, vagina and base of the bladder as well as the rectum and anal canal.

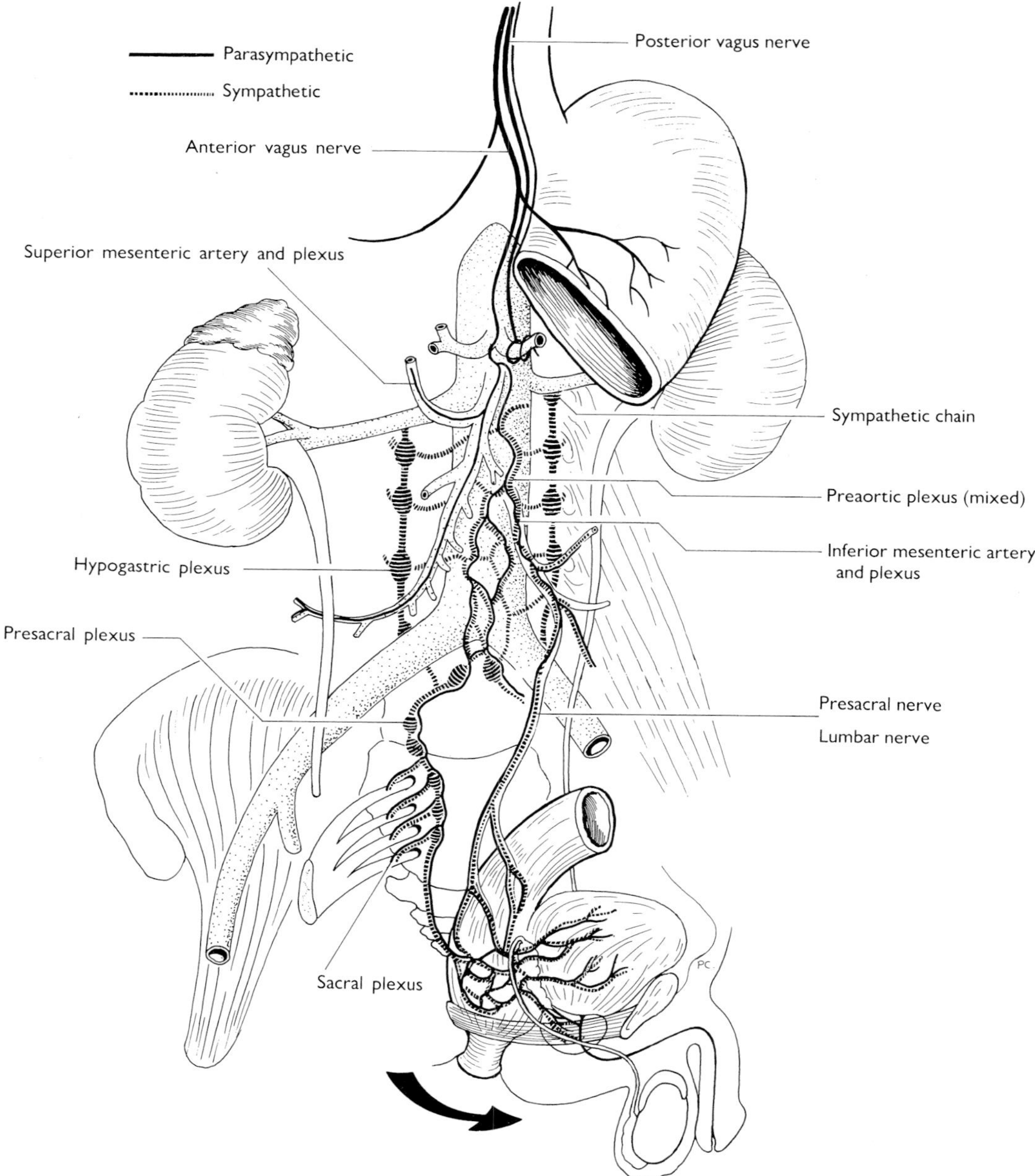

Figure 1.16 The autonomic supply to the colon and rectum is diagrammatically illustrated in an oblique plane. The contribution of the vagus nerve and the nervi erigentes to the parasympathetic supply to the pelvis is demonstrated. The sympathetic chain is shown together with the perivascular plexus to provide the autonomic innervation to the large bowel and rectum.

Parasympathetics

The parasympathetic nerve supply to the right colon is probably from the posterior vagus, the fibres of which join the superior mesenteric plexus. The parasympathetic supply to the left colon, rectum and anal canal, as well as the pelvic viscera, is from the second, third and fourth sacral nerve roots as they emerge on the piriformis from the sacral foramina. The parasympathetic fibres continue laterally as the nervi erigentes to join the presacral nerves which, with the sympathetics, supply the genital organs, bladder and anorectum. A few fibres join the hypogastric plexus and run over the aortic birfurcation to accompany the inferior mesenteric plexus supplying the sigmoid and descending colon.

The nervi erigentes lie behind Waldeyer's fascia before they join the presacral nerves and may be damaged by stripping the fascia off the sacrum. Damage to the presacral nerves may also occur during clearance of the internal iliac artery for malignant disease or lateral division of the lateral ligaments. Some fibres may also be damaged in front of the aortic bifurcation (see Chapter 11).

Somatic nerve supply to the pelvic floor and external sphincters

The levator ani has a dual nerve supply (Figure 1.17). It receives direct innervation from the perineal branch of the third and fourth sacral nerves as they pass from the pelvis to the perineum through the pelvic floor between the ischiococcygeus and iliococcygeus. The perineal branch of S4 supplies the puborectalis and has afferent nerve fibres supplying the anal canal and perianal skin. The external anal sphincter by contrast, as well as the peripheral part of the levator ani, is supplied by the pudendal nerve. This also has afferent fibres in the anal canal and perianal skin. The pudendal nerve is formed from the anterior divisions of S2–S4. The nerve passes out of the pelvis between the piriformis and the ischiococcygeus. It has a short course in the buttocks and re-enters the pelvis over the sacrospinous ligament, together with the nerve to obturator internus and the internal pudendal artery, through the lesser sciatic foramen. At this juncture it enters Alcock's canal in the lateral aspect of the ischiorectal fossa. The pudendal nerve runs forwards on the under-surface of the levator ani and gives origin to the inferior haemorrhoidal nerve, the main pudendal nerve dividing into the perineal nerve and the dorsal nerve of the penis. The inferior haemorrhoidal nerve runs forwards under the puborectalis and then enters the external anal sphincter which it supplies in association with the perianal skin. The perianal branch of the pudendal nerve may supply some fibres of the levator ani as well as the vagina, the base of the bladder, ischiocavernosus and bulbospongiosus.

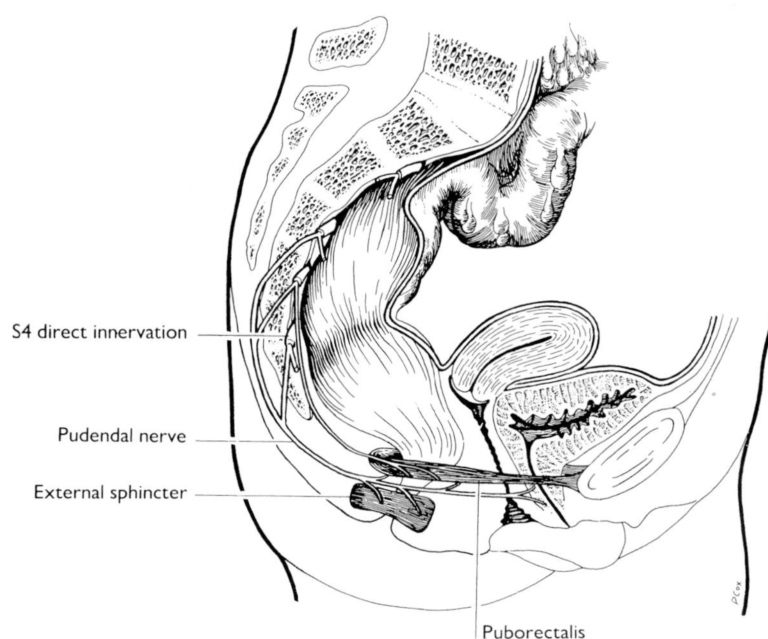

Figure 1.17 Sagittal section of the pelvis to show the innervation of the sphincters and puborectalis from the pudendal nerve and from a direct branch from S4.

PART TWO: TESTS OF ANORECTAL PHYSIOLOGY

Normal anorectal function is dependent upon an intact anatomy and is a complex physiological process, unique in that somatic and visceral function are intimately linked. The mechanisms of continence and defecation, although apparently separate functional entities, are interdependent and neither process can be completely normal without the other. Continence and defecation both involve colonic and anorectal function, and the term 'anorectal physiology' has become a misnomer, since any discussion on anorectal function must now include the colon in order to have clinical relevance.

A variety of tests have evolved to study anorectal and colonic function. Some have proved to be useful in everyday clinical practice, while other tests have played a role in adding to the large body of research that has contributed to our understanding of disease processes. This section describes the available physiological tests, and places each test in a clinical context. It is important to select carefully those tests which will provide useful clinical information for an individual patient, since each patient has a tolerance level for anorectal tests above which he or she will become less compliant, and exceeding this level with unhelpful tests will be counterproductive.

ANORECTAL MANOMETRY

Technique

The high-pressure zone around the anal canal is the most important component of the continence mechanism. There are a variety of methods for recording anal pressure. Pressure may be measured simultaneously or sequentially at different levels in the anal canal. Traditionally this is done at about 1-cm intervals. Simultaneous recording is somewhat simpler and quicker since the resting pressure must only equilibrate once rather than separately at each level. Several recording devices are available: perfusion catheters, microballoons, sleeve catheters, or strain gauge transducers. The maximum diameter of the recording device should be no greater than 5 mm since large-diameter catheters artificially raise anal pressure (Duthie and Watts, 1965; Gutierrez et al, 1975; Gibbons et al, 1986). Computerized acquisition of data is now the standard method, being more convenient for analysis as well as storage of recordings. Chart recorders may still be used, but those setting up a new service or replacing equipment would be advised to use a computerized system.

Perfusion systems

The perfusion catheter comprises a series of low-compliance tubes that are perfused with water at a constant rate, varying from 0.4 to 0.6 mL/min. Most commercially produced catheters have six to eight channels, although only four pressure channels are generally required for clinical studies. Each channel terminates at a side-hole, the first being 2 cm proximal to the tip for recording rectal pressure. Three centimetres proximal to this is the first of three side-holes placed 1 cm apart for recording anal pressure. One channel opens at the tip and is used to inflate a rectal balloon.

The catheter is placed so that the distal recording side-hole is in the lower anal canal. Basal resting pressure is allowed to stabilize for 1–3 min. The subject then maximally contracts the sphincter for 3–5 seconds three times at 10-second intervals. The resting pressure is again allowed to stabilize, and the subject is asked to cough forcefully three times at 10-second intervals (Figure 1.18). In this way internal and external sphincter strength are assessed. The length of the high-pressure zone is measured by initially examining the pressure in the most cranial of the three anal channels. If this side-hole lies within the high-pressure zone then the catheter is inserted further in 1-cm intervals until the upper limit of the high-pressure zone is reached; the length of the high-pressure zone is calculated as the sum of this length and the initial 3 cm in the distal anal canal. If a recording system containing more than three anal channels is used then this manoeuvre is not necessary. The high-pressure zone length is a mean of 2.5 cm in men and 2.0 cm in women (Sun and Read, 1989) and can reach 5 cm in men (Nivatvongs et al, 1981).

A perfusion catheter can also be used with a pull-through technique. In this case, pressure is recorded sequentially at different levels. This is usually done to assess radial variation in pressure. Resting and squeeze pressures in the upper anal canal are lower anteriorly than posteriorly due to the anterior deficiency of the puborectalis muscle (Collins et al, 1969; Taylor et al, 1984) (Figure 1.19). Radial pressure

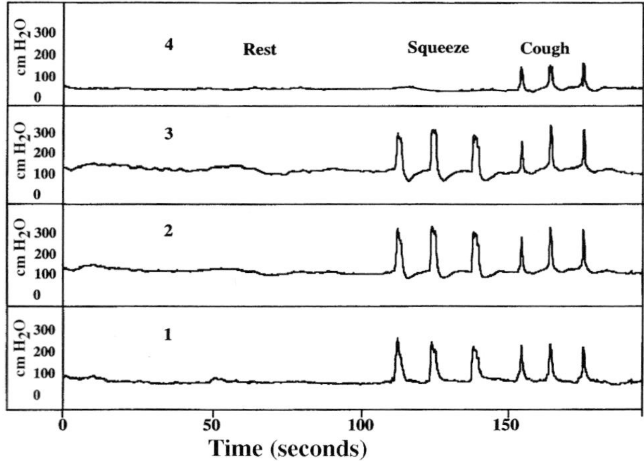

Figure 1.18 Anorectal manometry using a perfusion system. Channel 1 is recording just within the anal verge, and channels 2 and 3 progressively more proximally in the anal canal. Channel 4 is rectal pressure. Pressures at rest, during muscle contraction and then during coughing are shown. Rectal pressure increases during coughing but not with voluntary contraction.

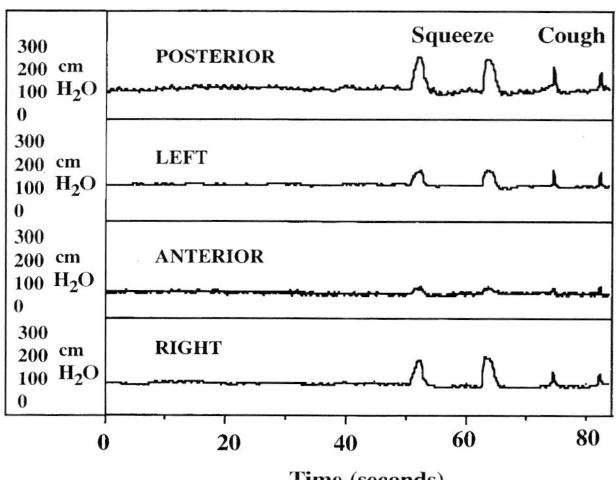

Figure 1.19 Radial variation in anal pressure in the upper anal canal. Recording with a perfusion catheter containing four side-holes arranged radially at one level. Squeeze and cough pressures are lowest anteriorly due to the anterior absence of the puborectalis muscle. Resting pressure is also lower anteriorly in this recording.

is recorded with a catheter which has four side-holes at the same level, using either a station pull-through technique or a continuous pull-through. With a station technique the catheter is inserted with the side-holes positioned in the rectum, then withdrawn into the high-pressure zone in the upper anal canal. Basal pressure is allowed to stabilize and then the subject is asked to maximally contract the sphincter for 3–5 seconds three times at 10-second intervals. The catheter is then withdrawn at 1-cm intervals and the procedure is repeated at each interval. Using a continuous pull-through the catheter is withdrawn through the anal canal at a constant rate, to produce a continuous pressure profile (Coller, 1987; Keck et al, 1995). This pressure profile allows clear visualization of the length of the high-pressure zone. Movement during the pull-through technique may stimulate reflex contraction of the external sphincter and artificially raise resting pressure, and therefore the catheter should be withdrawn by a motorized device to ensure a constant rate (Coller, 1987).

Balloon systems

Early balloon systems used large-diameter balloons. Balloons over 1 cm in diameter artificially raise anal pressure, and therefore only a microballoon 4 mm in diameter should be used. The balloon is attached to a fine non-distensible tube and thence to a pressure transducer. Water-filled balloons are usually used but an air-filled system produces comparable pressures (Miller et al, 1989; Orrom et al, 1990). A station pull-through technique is used as described above. Information about radial pressure variation is not obtained since the microballoon records only the maximal pressure at each site.

Sleeve catheters

A sleeve catheter consists of a fine silastic membrane fixed over a catheter to enclose a chamber through which water is perfused (Dent, 1976). The sleeve spans the entire anal canal length and therefore records the maximal anal pressure, wherever that may occur. Anal sleeve catheters were adapted from those used for recording lower oesophageal pressure where they are useful because of the vertical movement of the abdominal diaphragm. Similarly, they have a place for recordings of anal pressure during defecation with the patient seated on a commode, where there may be considerable downward movement of the anus. Sleeve catheters have generally been restricted to research studies.

Strain gauge catheters

Modern strain gauge transducers evolved from those using a cantilever and semiconductor set in a resistance bridge (Wankling et al, 1968). Commercially available strain gauge transducers now contain resistors placed on a metal diaphragm within a vacuum. Pressure on the diaphragm changes resistance in the system which is converted to a pressure measurement (Roberts and Williams, 1992). Recording catheters may have a single transducer or multiple transducers, used respectively with a station pull-through technique or simultaneous recording technique. Either a static recording system or an ambulatory system with real-time recording may be used (see Ambulatory manometry and electromyography).

Vector manometry

Using a perfusion catheter recording radial pressures, a three-dimensional computer-generated image of anal sphincter tone may be obtained. The catheter has eight side-holes and either a station pull-through (Perry et al, 1990) or continuous pull-through (Yang and Wexner, 1994) is used (Figure 1.20a,b). Vector manometry may help to determine whether sphincter weakness is due to a sphincter defect or neurogenic weakness with an intact sphincter ring (Figure 1.20c). Perry et al (1990) calculated a vector symmetry index (range 0–1.0), all normal sphincters being symmetrical with index greater than 0.6, and all cases of sphincter injury having an index less than 0.6. Theoretically, this has the potential to help select patients for sphincter repair, although Yang and Wexner (1994) found that only 13% of sphincter defects on vector manometry correlated with electromyography and 11% with endoanal ultrasound.

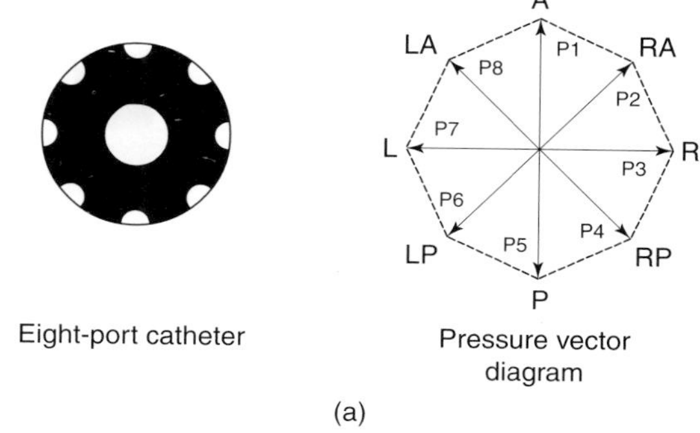

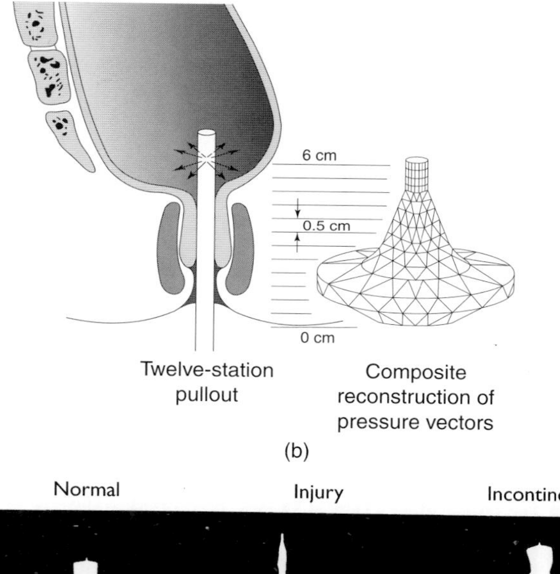

Normal Injury Incontinent

(c)

Figure 1.20 Vector manometry. (a) Perfusion catheter for vector manometry. Eight side-holes are arranged radially. (b) Pressure data collected at each level are used to construct a three-dimensional image of the sphincter. (c) Images during voluntary squeeze. Left: normal symmetrical sphincter; centre: sphincter defect producing asymmetrical image; right: neurogenic weakness producing a global symmetrical weakness. Reproduced with permission from Excerpta Medica Inc. (Perry et al, 1990).

Normal recordings

Resting anal pressure

Resting anal pressure is largely due to the internal sphincter (Figure 1.18). The muscle is in a state of continuous intrinsic contraction (Frenckner and von Euler, 1975; Gutierrez et al, 1975; Lestar et al, 1989), which has phasic variation known as slow waves. These are more commonly observed when resting pressure is high and occur at a rate of 6–20 per minute with amplitude 10–25 cmH_2O (Kerremans, 1969; Hancock and Smith, 1975). Additionally, ultra-slow waves are high-pressure waves with a frequency of 1–3 per minute found in 5% of normal subjects (Hancock, 1976, 1977a) but in almost 50% when maximum resting pressure is greater than 100 cmH_2O (Figure 1.21) (Haynes and Read, 1982). They are frequently present in conditions caused by internal sphincter spasm, including haemorrhoids (Hancock, 1976; Deutsch et al, 1987; Sun et al, 1990a) and anal fissure (Hancock, 1977b; Gibbons and Read, 1986; McNamara et al, 1990). There is no consensus as to which part of the ultra-slow wave should be regarded as the maximal resting pressure and it is best to document peak and trough pressures as well as mean pressure. There is wide variation in resting and squeeze pressure, depending on the recording system and methodology, and there are also variations in repeatability studies

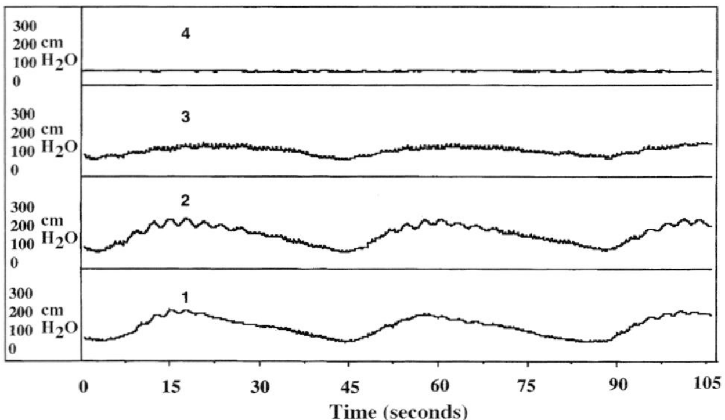

Figure 1.21 Anal manometry showing ultra-slow waves at 1 per 45 seconds. Channels 1, 2, 3 in lower, mid and upper anal canal respectively. Channel 4 is rectal pressure. Slow waves are superimposed on the ultra-slow waves, seen best in channel 2.

(Ryhammer et al, 1997a). Resting pressure is lower in women than in men (Loening-Baucke and Anuras, 1985; Sun and Read, 1989) and decreases with age (Read et al, 1979; Matheson and Keighley, 1981; Ryhammer et al, 1997b). Generally a pressure of 50–100 cmH_2O is considered normal (Table 1.1).

Spontaneous relaxation of the internal sphincter has been shown to occur at a mean of 7 times per hour (Miller et al, 1988a,b; Kumar et al, 1989, 1990; Orkin et al, 1991) providing support for the original hypothesis of Duthie and Bennet (1963) that a 'sampling reflex' allows the upper anal canal mucosa to discriminate gas from stool. Spontaneous relaxations occur more frequently than normal in patients with faecal incontinence (Miller et al, 1988b; Sun et al, 1990b). It is caused by a rise in rectal pressure due to rectal distension or contraction (Denny-Brown and Robertson, 1935; Naudy et al, 1984), mediated via an intramural neural pathway (Gowers, 1877; Lubowski et al, 1987) and known as the rectoanal inhibitory reflex.

The reflex is tested in the laboratory by balloon distension of the rectum while simultaneously recording anal pressure. A fully deflated party balloon, attached to the tip of a perfusion catheter or to a separate catheter if a microballoon system is used, is inserted into the rectum. Resting anal pressure is allowed to stabilize, and the rectal balloon is then inflated with 20-mL increments of air. A fall in resting anal pressure of 20%, followed by return to the resting level constitutes a positive reflex (Figure 1.22). Care must be taken to ensure that the record-

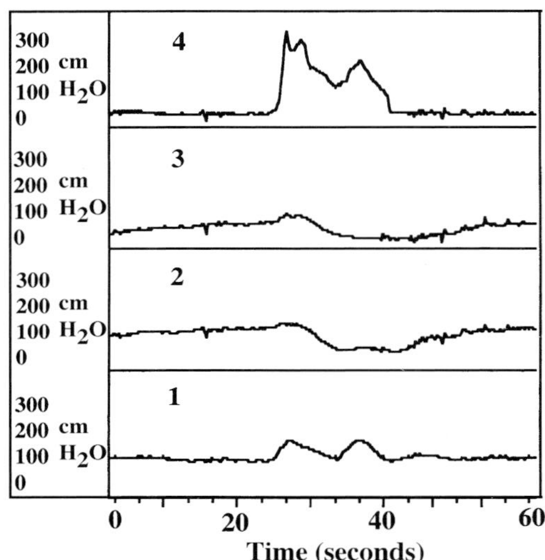

Figure 1.22 Rectoanal reflex. With distension of the rectal balloon there is a rise in rectal pressure (channel 4). Pressure falls in the upper- and mid-anal canal (channels 3 and 2) due to internal sphincter relaxation, and then returns toward the basal level. Pressure in the lowest part of the anal canal rises (channel 1) due to reflex contraction of the subcutaneous external sphincter.

Table 1.1 Normal mean anal pressures.

	Sun and Read (1989) (cmH_2O)	*Loening-Baucke and Anuras (1985)* (mmHg)	*Williams et al (1995)* (mmHg)
Resting pressure			
Mean		60 (13)	
Mean male	91 (5)	63 (12)	62 (5)
Mean female	61 (6)	50 (13)	64 (5)
Squeeze pressure			
Mean		204 (54)	
Mean male	257 (20)	238 (38)	189 (10)
Mean female	107 (13)	159 (45)	142 (7)
Method	Perfusion	Strain gauge	Perfusion

Values in parentheses are standard deviations.

ing catheter is not displaced upwards into the rectum. This would cause a fall in pressure without return to the baseline and may be incorrectly interpreted as a positive reflex. The reflex is absent in Hirschsprung's disease (Lawson and Nixon, 1967). A false negative reflex may be obtained when the basal pressure is low, or if an insufficient distension volume is used in a patient with megarectum. The reflex is absent after rectal excision with ileoanal or coloanal anastomosis but recovers after several months in some patients (Lane and Parks, 1977; Nicholls et al, 1988) due to regeneration of nerves across the anastomosis (Brookes et al, 1996).

Voluntary contraction pressure

The external sphincter is in a state of tonic partial contraction, even during sleep (Floyd and Walls, 1953; Taverner and Smiddy, 1959; Ruskin and Davis, 1969) and contributes about 15% of the resting pressure (Frenckner and von Euler, 1975; Lestar et al, 1989). This involuntary external sphincter tone is controlled by the spinal Onuf nucleus. The external sphincter produces the voluntary contraction pressure (Keighley et al, 1989) and is measured as the increase above the resting pressure (see Figure 1.18). Like the resting pressure, it is lower in women and reduces with age (Loening-Baucke and Anuras, 1985). The external sphincter undergoes reflex contraction in response to a rise in abdominal pressure, and this is tested as the cough pressure. In some cases the voluntary contraction pressure may be artificially low if the patient is unable to contract the external sphincter in the laboratory setting. In such cases a more accurate measure of external sphincter strength is obtained with the cough pressure (Meagher et al, 1993) (Figure 1.23), which should be routinely tested during anal manometry. Movement of the pelvic floor may be measured

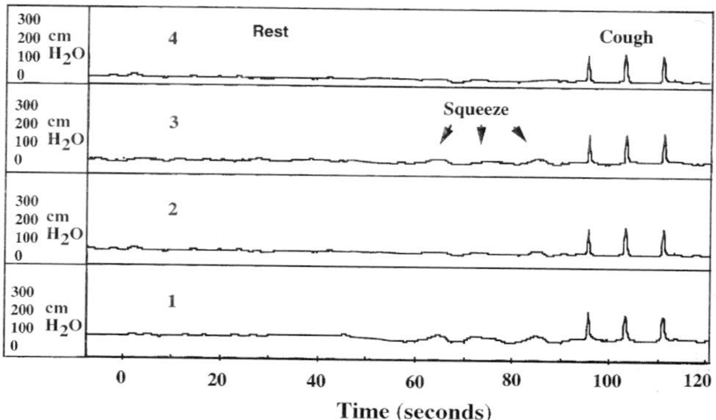

Figure 1.23 Anorectal manometry showing very weak squeeze pressure due to poor patient compliance. External sphincter weakness is excluded by the presence of normal cough pressure. Channels 1, 2, 3: anal canal; channel 4: rectum.

MEASUREMENT OF PERINEAL DESCENT

radiologically or with the perineometer (Henry et al, 1982; Oettle et al, 1985) (see Figure 20.28). Using the perineometer, the anal verge is taken as a convenient reference point although it of course does not represent the position of the pelvic floor. The perineometer is placed with the two lateral beams firmly pressed on the ischial tuberosities, and the central cylinder is positioned on the anal verge to measure the perineal position at rest. The subject is then asked to strain down firmly and perineal descent is recorded. The perineum lies at a mean of 2.5 cm above the level of the ischial tuberosities in normal subjects, and descends up to 2.0 cm on maximal straining down (Henry et al, 1982; Ambrose and Keighley, 1986; Beevors et al, 1991). Perineal descent of more than 3 cm is abnormal (Oettle et al, 1985; Bartolo et al, 1986; Jones et al, 1987a).

Manometry provides a measure of sphincter func-

ELECTROPHYSIOLOGY

tion and will help determine whether sphincter weakness or dysfunction is likely to be the cause of symptoms. Other tests such as electromyography or ultrasound are needed to determine the underlying pathology. A variety of such tests are now available and are used routinely in clinical anorectal physiology laboratories. Electrophysiological studies are a non-invasive way of determining whether spinal or pelvic nerve damage is present, usually in a patient with faecal or urinary incontinence. This nerve damage, and the resulting neurogenic muscle changes are known to occur from histological studies of the anal sphincter (Parks et al, 1977; Beersiek et al, 1979). The levator ani derives its nerve supply from

ANATOMICAL CONSIDERATIONS

branches of the third and fourth sacral nerves, the perineal branch of S4, and also from the pudendal nerves. The external anal sphincter is innervated only by the pudendal nerves (Percy et al, 1981), deriving fibres from the S2–S4 ventral rami. The pudendal nerves leave the pelvis through the greater sciatic foramen and pass below the ischial spines to enter the perineum. The nerves are fixed at the ischial spines but distal to this are free to move as the position of the muscular pelvic floor changes. Excessive descent of the pelvic floor causes stretch-induced damage to the pudendal nerves (Kiff and Swash, 1984a). Normal somatic nerves can withstand stretching up to 12% of their length, and above this amount nerve damage results (Sunderland, 1978). Abnormal perineal descent may result in stretching the pudendal nerves up to 20% of their length (Beersiek et al, 1979) with consequent nerve damage.

MOTOR NERVE CONDUCTION STUDIES

Pudendal nerve motor latency

Stretch-induced damage to the pudendal nerve may be measured using motor conduction studies. Electrical stimulation of the portion of the pudendal nerve distal to the ischial spine is achieved using the technique described by Kiff and Swash (1984a). Initially, a custom-built fingerstall was used (Kiff and Swash, 1984a,b) but subsequently a disposable electrode (Dantec 13L40, Skovlunde, Denmark) was considered necessary to guarantee sterility. The electrode contains an adhesive backing and is mounted on the gloved index finger with anode immediately proximal to the finger-tip (Rogers et al, 1988a) (Figure 1.24).

Technique and stimulation parameters

With the patient in the left lateral position, the finger is inserted into the rectum and the tip of the finger is placed in the region of the left ischial spine. Square wave stimuli of duration 0.1 ms are delivered at one-second intervals using a constant current stimulator, and the amplitude is progressively increased to 20 mA. The finger-tip is repositioned until it lies over the pudendal nerve, at which time a reproducible tracing with shortest possible pudendal latency is obtained. When the anode at the finger-tip is distant from the nerve, the latency is artificially prolonged by passage of the current through the soft tissues to reach the nerve. The ischial spine cannot be accurately palpated in many subjects and the correct position of the finger is determined by a reproducible tracing with minimum latency. The latency is defined as the time from stimulus to the point of take-off when the impulse reaches the recording electrode at the external sphincter. The polarity of the contraction is mirror-imaged on the left and right sides because of the orientation of the electrodes (Figure 1.25). Filter settings on the electro-

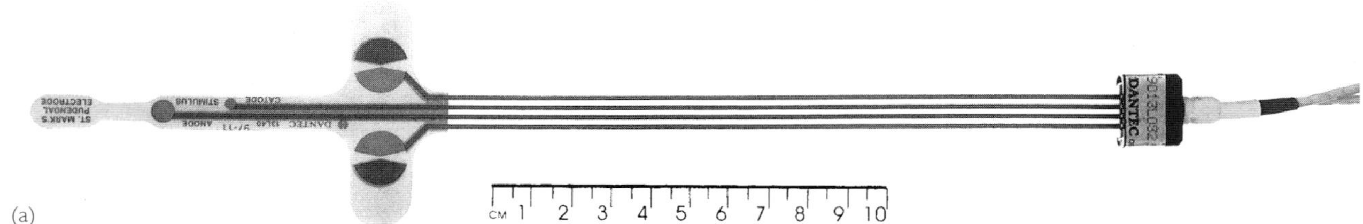

(a)

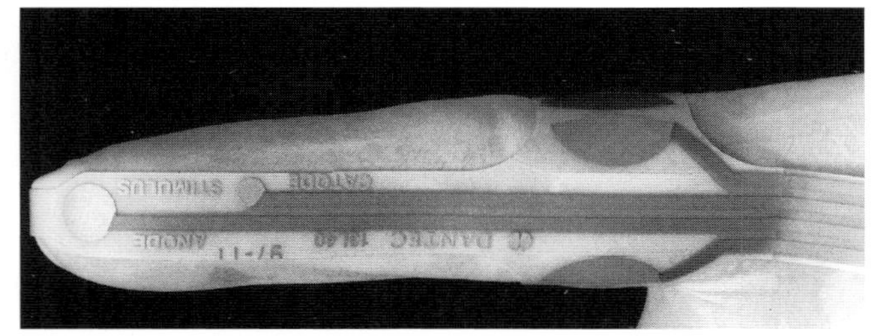
(b)

Figure 1.24 (a) Disposable pudendal electrode and connector (Dantec, Denmark). (b) The electrode is mounted on the right index finger with the anode at the finger-tip, and the recording electrodes at the base of the finger.

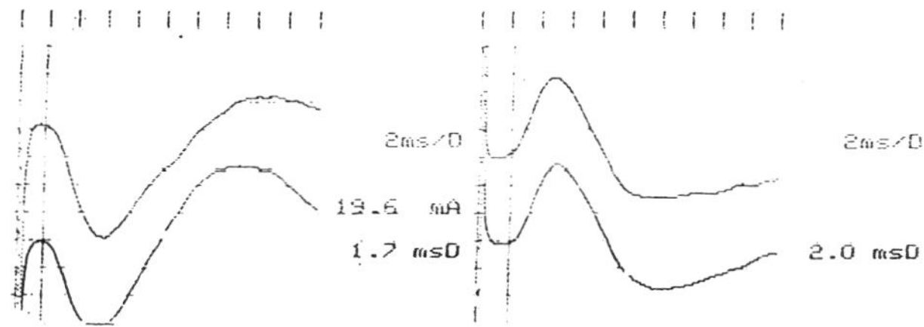

Figure 1.25 Pudendal nerve motor latency. The two cursors (vertical lines) on each trace mark the point of the stimulus and the onset of arrival of the electrical impulse in the external sphincter. The left and right pudendal latencies are shown respectively as the left (1.7 ms) and right (2.0 ms) traces. The traces are mirror-imaged because of the reversed position of the recording electrodes when testing on each side. Note that the trace is reproducible on each side.

myography machine are set at low frequency 20 Hz, high frequency 5 kHz, and sweep speed 2 ms/division.

Normal recordings

Initially, the average of the left and right pudendal latencies was calculated (Kiff and Swash, 1984a,b). However, nerve damage is often asymmetrical and the latencies should be documented separately (Lubowski et al, 1988a; Sangwan et al, 1996a). Normal pudendal latencies are shown in Table 1.2. In normal subjects, latencies are slightly higher in men than women (Jameson et al, 1994), and increase with age (Laurberg and Swash, 1989; Ryhammer et al, 1997b). Sex differences were not observed in patients with chronic constipation (Vaccaro et al, 1994). There is a significant relationship between the amount of perineal descent and pudendal latency (Jones et al, 1987a; Laurberg et al, 1988; Jameson et al, 1994; Roig et al, 1995; Ho and Goh, 1995) although one large study did not confirm these findings (Jorge et al, 1993). It is thought that either an acute severe stretch injury during vaginal delivery (Snooks et al, 1984a, 1986, 1990; Sultan et al, 1994a), or a repetitive injury due to chronic straining at stool (Kiff et al, 1984; Snooks et al, 1985a) results in nerve damage. This is supported by evidence of acute prolongation of pudendal latency during straining in patients with abnormal perineal descent (Lubowski et al, 1988b; Engel and Kamm, 1994). Prolonged pudendal latencies are found in several disorders associated with difficult vaginal delivery or chronic straining at stool, including faecal incontinence (Kiff and Swash, 1984b; Snooks et al, 1985b; Jones et al, 1987a; Lubowski et al, 1988c; Rogers et al, 1988b; Vernava et al, 1993; Tjandra et al, 1994; Roig et al, 1995), combined urinary and faecal incontinence (Swash et al, 1985; Snooks et al, 1984b, 1985c), severe constipation (Snooks et al, 1985a; Vaccaro et al, 1995), haemorrhoids (Bruck et al, 1988), uterine prolapse (Beevors et al, 1991; Benson and McClellan, 1993; Spence-Jones et al, 1994) and solitary rectal ulcer syndrome (Snooks et al, 1985d; Speakman et al, 1991a). Prolonged pudendal latencies differentiated minor soiling from major incontinence (Kafka et al, 1997).

Table 1.2 Normal mean pudendal latencies.

Reference	*Pudendal motor latency* (ms)
Kiff and Swash (1984a)	2.1 (0.2)
Snooks et al (1986)	1.9 (0.2)
Rogers et al (1988c)	1.95 (1.7–2.25)
Beevors et al (1991)	Right 1.9 (0.2) Left 2.0 (0.2)

Values in parentheses are standard deviation or range.

Perineal nerve motor latency

The perineal branch of the pudendal nerve passes forward to innervate the periurethral striated sphincter (see Figure 20.7). This nerve may also undergo a stretch-induced injury, and the perineal latency is increased in patients with urinary stress incontinence (Snooks et al, 1984b, 1985e; Smith et al, 1989) as well as faecal incontinence.

The perineal nerve latency is measured by intrarectal stimulation as for pudendal motor latency, and the muscle contraction is recorded in the periurethral muscle rather than external sphincter using a ring electrode (Dantec 21L10, Skovlunde, Denmark) mounted immediately proximal to the balloon on a Foley catheter (Figure 1.26). The balloon is inflated in the bladder and the catheter is drawn down so that the electrode lies within the urethral muscle. Mean perineal latency

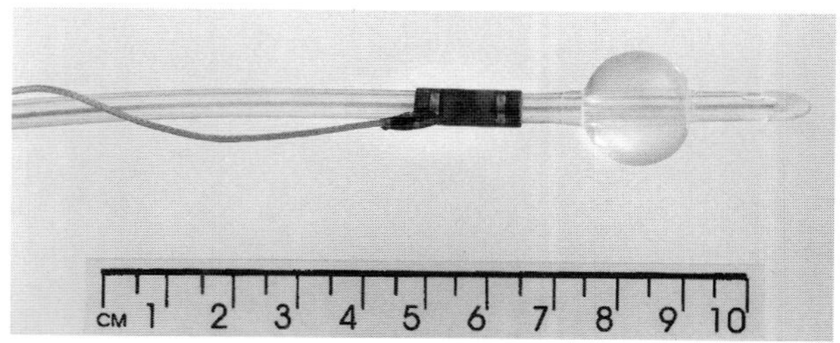

Figure 1.26 Ring electrode for measuring perineal latency (Dantec, Denmark). The same electrode is used for measuring anal and rectal mucosal electrosensitivity.

in normal subjects is 2.4 ms (SD 0.2) (Snooks et al, 1984b).

Spinal motor latency

In neurogenic faecal incontinence the site of nerve injury is the distal portion of the pudendal nerves in most cases. In a small proportion of patients a proximal lesion in the pelvis or spinal column is the cause of neurogenic weakness. A proximal lesion should be considered in patients who have pelvic floor weakness and normal pudendal latencies and mucosal electrosensitivity, particularly when single-fibre electromyography in the external sphincter is abnormal or when there are no predisposing factors to distal pudendal nerve injury. Proximal nerve injuries may be considered as supranuclear (upper motor neurone) or infranuclear (lower motor neurone) depending on their relation to the Onuf nucleus (Lubowski et al, 1988d). Infranuclear injuries are more common and are due to: (1) lesions of the cauda equina such as trauma, disc prolapse, tumours; or (2) lesions of the pelvis such as presacral tumours or cysts.

Spinal motor latency is carried out by transcutaneous stimulation of the cauda equina at the L1 and L4 vertebral levels (Snooks et al, 1985f; Swash and Snooks, 1986). Recording of the impulse may be made at the external sphincter, puborectalis or periurethral sphincter. Recording at the external sphincter is the most simple, using the recording electrodes of the disposable pudendal nerve device. Disorders affecting the spinal nerve pathways will prolong the spinal latency.

The test is carried out using a high-voltage low-impedance stimulator (Digitimer, Hertfordshire, UK) (Figure 1.27a). With the patient in the left lateral position and a ground electrode on the thigh, the skin is shaved over the lower back at the L1 and L4 levels in the midline and marks are placed at these two points. An impulse of 1500 V, 0.5 ms duration, and decaying with a time constant of 50 μs is delivered using a transcutaneous electrode containing two small saline-soaked pads (Figure 1.27b). The cathode is placed at the L1 level with the anode cranially. The procedure is then repeated with the cathode electrode moved to the L4 level. The patient is not aware of an electrical impulse because of the rapid decay, and experiences only a slight jolt on the back and a lower limb muscle twitch. Filter settings are the same as for pudendal latencies.

A spinal latency ratio (SLR) is calculated as follows:

$$\text{SLR} = \frac{\text{Latency (ms) from L1}}{\text{Latency (ms) from L4}}$$

For lesions in the pelvis, the latency from the L1 and L4 levels will be increased and SLR will be normal (Figure 1.28). Lesions affecting the cauda equina will only prolong the L1 latency and SLR will be increased. If there is also delay in the distal part of the pudendal nerves then both L1 and L4 latency

(a)

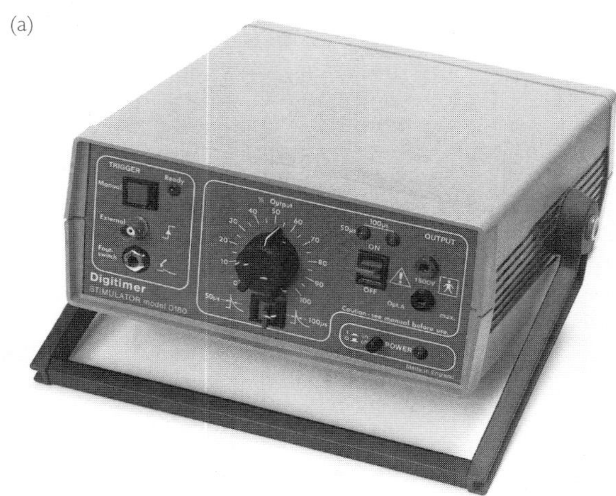

(b)

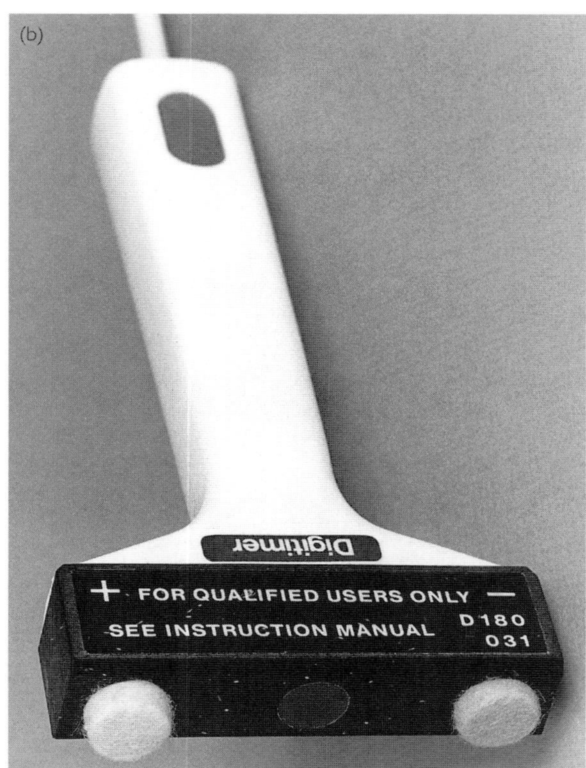

Figure 1.27 Spinal stimulator. (a) High-voltage stimulator. The stimulating impulse from the machine is triggered by interfacing with the EMG machine, which in turn records the muscle contraction. (b) Electrode with two pads for stimulation over the lumbar spine.

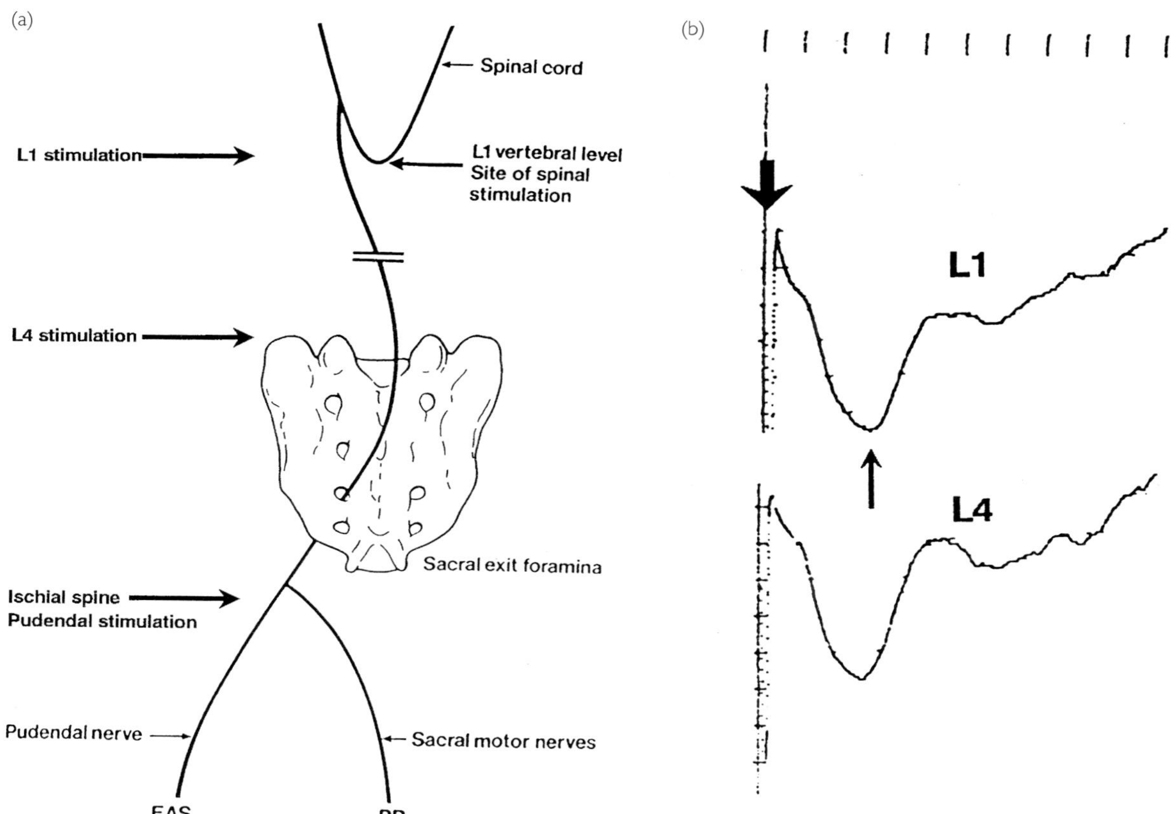

Figure 1.28 Spinal motor latency. (a) Spinal stimulation at the L1 and L4 levels to show the position of the spinal cord and cauda equina relative to the stimulating points. (b) Spinal latency recording. The latency from L1 is the upper trace, and from L4 the lower trace. The onset of the stimulus is the cursor at the broad arrow, and arrival of the impulse at the external sphincter is at the narrow arrow. Note the L4 latency is shorter than L1 latency.

will be increased but SLR will be normal. Mean normal spinal latencies to the external anal sphincter are:

L1 latency 5.5 ms (SD 0.4)
L4 latency 4.4 ms (SD 0.4)
SLR 1.33 (SD 0.1).

ELECTROMYOGRAPHY

Electromyography (EMG) was applied to the clinical study of skeletal muscle after the introduction of the concentric needle electrode (Adrian and Bronk, 1929). The electrode records action potentials in depolarizing muscle motor units. The motor unit comprises the axon, its branches, and the group of muscle fibres innervated by these branches. There are two types of muscle fibres, type 1 which are slow twitch fatigue-resistant, and type 2 which are fast twitch. Peripheral skeletal muscles have a predominance of type 2 fibres, while 78% of the fibres in the external sphincter are type 1 (Swash, 1992). All the fibres in a motor unit are of the same type (Stalberg and Ekstedt, 1973; Stalberg et al, 1976). The electrical activity recorded from a contracting motor unit is called the motor unit action potential (MUP).

Concentric needle electromyography

Concentric needle EMG is used to record overall muscle activity, or to test for denervation. Recording of overall muscle activity is used for mapping of sphincter defects and for assessment of pelvic floor dysfunction. The needle electrode consists of a central platinum wire insulated within a stainless steel cannula. The recording surface at the tip of the wire is 0.5×0.15 mm.

Motor unit potential duration

The motor unit potential duration (MUPD) is measured to assess denervation and reinnervation of the muscle. The normal motor unit action potential is biphasic and 5–7.5 ms in duration (Petersen and Franksson, 1955). MUPD increases with age (Bartolo et al, 1983a) and when there is muscle denervation such as in neurogenic incontinence (Bartolo et al, 1983b).

The needle electrode is inserted into the external sphincter once on each side and ten different motor potentials are recorded. The mean MUPD is calculated. Filter settings are low frequency 20 Hz, high frequency 5 kHz. A rapid sweep speed (2 ms/div) is used to separate recordings of individual motor unit potentials.

Sphincter mapping

Mapping of sphincter defects correlates well with clinical and histological findings (Sultan et al, 1994b). After a careful digital examination of the sphincter, the needle is first inserted into healthy muscle at the edge of the apparent defect. Successive passes are then made into the defect, and finally into healthy muscle on the opposite side (Figure 1.29). Local anaesthetic should not be used. Filter settings are 20 Hz, 5 kHz. Sweep speed is slow, 100 ms/div, to compress the potentials and give an overall pattern. The test can be painful although this is less so if there is an associated sensory pudendal neuropathy. In many centres endoanal ultrasound has replaced sphincter mapping.

Assessment of pelvic floor dysfunction

The external sphincter and puborectalis are in a state of continuous partial contraction, which is usually inhibited during defecation straining (Porter, 1961) in normal subjects. Muscle contraction during straining down has been observed in a variety of clinical conditions and symptoms have been attributed to paradoxical muscle activity (Lane, 1974; Rutter, 1974; Rutter and Riddell, 1975; Kuijpers and Bleijenberg, 1985; Snooks et al, 1985d). This test is now considered to be unphysiological and muscle contraction is likely to be a laboratory artefact in some subjects (Jones et al, 1987b; Duthie et al, 1991; Duthie and Bartolo, 1992; Lubowski et al, 1992).

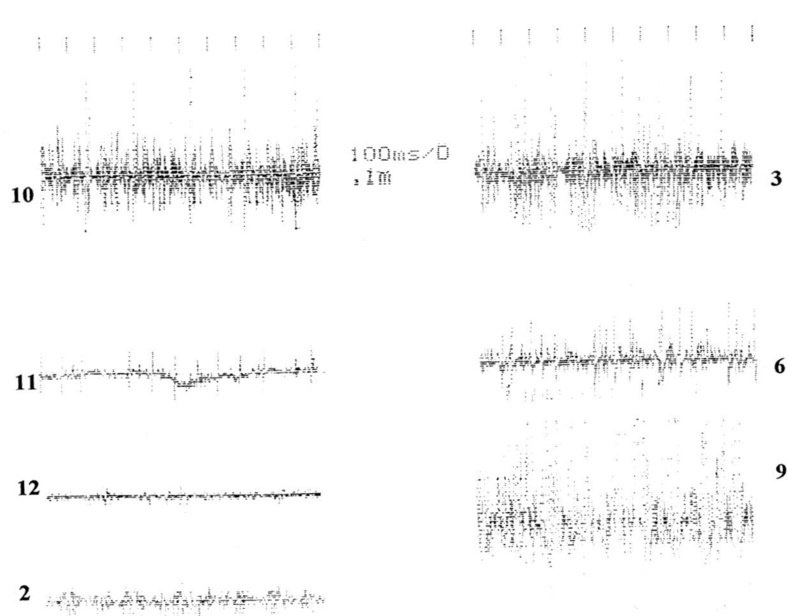

Figure 1.29 Concentric needle EMG sphincter mapping. There is marked reduction in electrical activity between 11 o'clock and 2 o'clock, indicating an anterior defect in the external sphincter. Elsewhere there is normal muscle activity.

Single-fibre electromyography

When a stretch-induced nerve injury occurs, action potentials pass down the fastest conducting remaining nerve fibres. Therefore significant nerve damage may occur before motor latencies become prolonged. Examination of the innervated muscle provides evidence of nerve damage at an earlier stage (Strijers et al, 1989). Single-fibre EMG is the most accurate method of testing for denervation and reinnervation of skeletal muscle, by recording action potentials from individual muscle fibres (Stalberg and Ekstedt, 1973; Lubowski et al, 1988d; Swash, 1992; Sangwan et al, 1996b).

Denervation of skeletal muscle is accompanied by reinnervation from neighbouring axons. Histological and histometric studies show the normal random distribution of type 1 and type 2 fibres replaced by type 1 and type 2 grouping (Parks et al, 1977; Beersiek et al, 1979). These changes can be measured accurately with single-fibre EMG. The single-fibre EMG electrode consists of a platinum wire 25 µm in diameter, insulated in a stainless steel cannula, and terminating end-on at the side of the cannula 5 mm proximal to the tip. Hence the recording surface is 25 µm in diameter (Figure 1.30a).

The changes of denervation and reinnervation can be quantified by calculating the fibre density, which is a measure of the number of muscle fibres in a motor unit within the area of uptake of the single-fibre electrode (Trontelj and Stalberg, 1995; Stalberg and Thiele, 1975) (Figure 1.30b). The mean fibre density is the average number of fibres recorded at 20 sites in the muscle. With reinnervation, the number of muscle fibres within this area increases and the number of recorded spikes in the action potentials increases correspondingly (Figure 1.30c). Normal fibre density in the external anal sphincter is 1.5 (SD 0.16) (Neill and Swash, 1980); fibre density greater than 2.0 indicates denervation and reinnervation.

Method of recording

Interference from distant muscle fibres is eliminated by using appropriate filter settings, allowing recording of individual action potentials. The trigger on the EMG machine is set to record only potentials with amplitude greater than 100 µV. Electrical energy from single action potentials lies between 100 Hz and 10 kHz with peak 1.01 kHz (Gath and Stalberg, 1975). Filters are therefore set at low frequency 500 Hz, high frequency 2 kHz, sweep speed 2 ms/div.

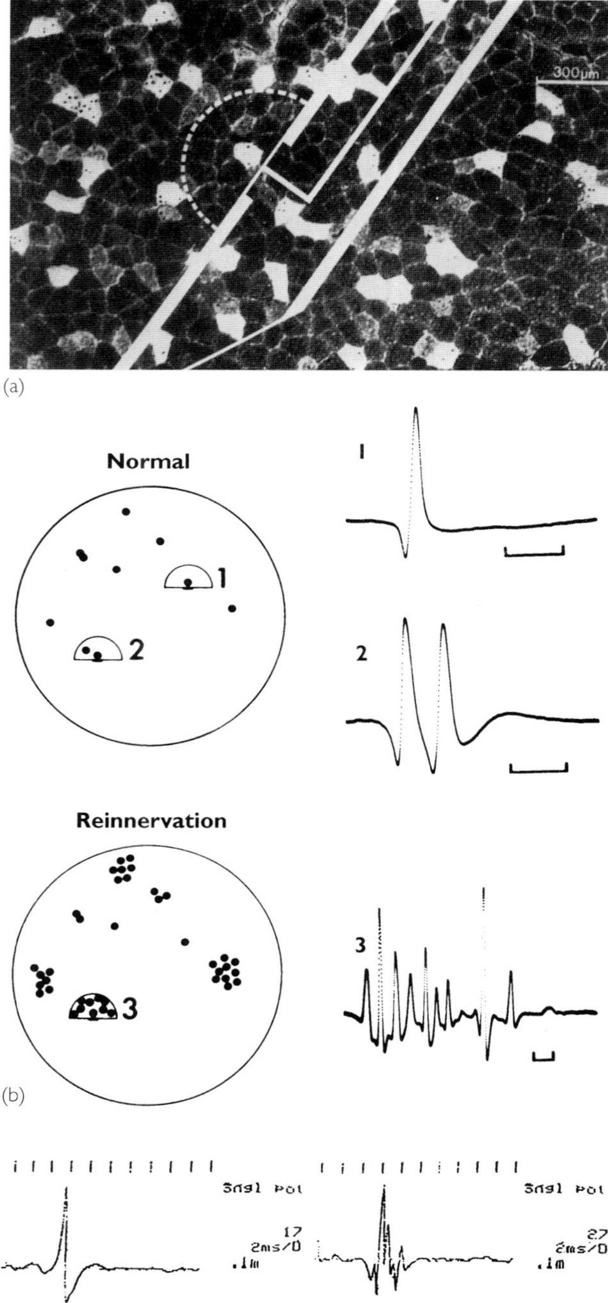

Figure 1.30 Single-fibre EMG. (a) Single-fibre electrode shown superimposed on normal muscle to demonstrate the recording surface of the wire electrode on the side of cannula. The field of electrical uptake involves only a small number of muscle fibres. From Stalberg and Trontelj (1979). (b) Recording of muscle fibres in a normal muscle (above) and a denervated muscle (below). The denervated and reinnervated muscle has fibre grouping, resulting in a larger number of muscle fibres in the motor unit, and hence the polyphasic action potentials shown diagramatically. (c) Single-fibre EMG recording from a reinnervated muscle showing a normal action potential (left) and a polyphasic action potential (right).

Clinical application

Single-fibre EMG is a reproducible test (Rogers et al, 1989). Fibre density increases with age (Laurberg and Swash, 1989). It is increased in a variety of conditions associated with stretch-induced pudendal neuropathy, including faecal incontinence (Neill and Swash, 1980; Neill et al, 1981; Lubowski et al, 1988c; Fink et al, 1992), rectal prolapse (Neill et al, 1981), urinary stress incontinence (Snooks et al, 1984b; Smith et al, 1989), haemorrhoids (Bruck et al, 1988), solitary rectal ulcer syndrome (Snooks et al, 1985d) and uterine prolapse (Beevors et al, 1991). Single-fibre EMG is more invasive than motor and sensory testing of pudendal function. Therefore although it is more accurate, it is often used selectively in those patients in whom there is clinical evidence of neurogenic muscle weakness but pudendal latency and mucosal electrosensitivity are normal.

Internal sphincter electromyography

Internal sphincter activity can be recorded with an intra-anal surface electrode (Lubowski et al, 1988c) or with a fine wire electrode. For surface recording a ring electrode similar to that used for measuring perineal nerve latency is suitable (Dantec 21L11, Dantec, Denmark). The electrode is mounted on a Foley catheter and the balloon is left deflated. Wire electrodes (Basmajian and Stecko, 1963) have been used for static (Sorensen et al, 1994) and ambulatory recordings (Farouk et al, 1992) (see Ambulatory manometry and electromyography).

Electrical activity of the adjacent external sphincter must be filtered in order to isolate and display internal sphincter activity. Special filter settings are needed: low frequency 0.05 Hz, high frequency 2 kHz and sweep speed 500 ms/div. Internal sphincter electrical activity is recorded as slow waves of frequency 20–30 per minute although occasionally up to 40 per minute (Wankling et al, 1968; Lubowski et al, 1988c). Others have recorded slow waves with a higher frequency of 34–55 (mean 47) per minute (Sorensen et al, 1994) but this was carried out using a rectified EMG signal so that some negative waves would have registered above the baseline. Additionally, a low pass filter of 0.5 kHz was used and all electrical activity of the external sphincter may not have been filtered out.

EMG activity corresponds with manometric slow wave activity. In neurogenic faecal incontinence there is loss of internal anal sphincter (IAS) EMG activity, and this is accompanied by a fall in resting anal pressure (Lubowski et al, 1988c).

AMBULATORY MANOMETRY AND ELECTROMYOGRAPHY

Static measurements of anorectal function carried out in the left lateral position are somewhat unphysiological and do not provide complete information. Anal pressure varies with posture (Johnson et al, 1990), and anal pressure alone is not always an accurate predictor of incontinence. Studying patients with incontinence or obstructed defecation using ambulatory techniques provides additional information.

Equipment and technique

Manometry

The development of small portable data recording systems which are able to collect and digitally compress data, have allowed this technique to be applicable in clinical practice (Gaeltec, Isle of Skye, UK) (Figure 1.31). Recordings from multichannel manometry catheters for 24 hours is possible. Currently available pressure systems use strain gauge transducers. These are easy to use but probes with multiple transducers are very expensive and ambulatory perfusion systems are under development. The probe should contain three transducers, one at the tip for recording rectal pressure, and two for anal pressure. Current technology determines that the minimum distance between the transducers in a flexible probe is 2 cm (Figure 1.31). It may not be possible to use both recording sites if the anal canal is short. If a single anal transducer is used then this must be positioned in the mid anal canal since upward or downward displacement out of the high-pressure zone may occur.

The probe is inserted and secured with adhesive tape at the anal verge and along the natal cleft. Recordings of rest, squeeze and cough pressures are taken in real time to confirm that the catheter is correctly positioned. The data recording box is subsequently carried in a portable case with a shoulder strap for ambulatory recording. An event marker is used and a diary is kept to record sitting, running, passage of flatus, episodes of incontinence, urge to defecate and defecation. At the end of recording, the data are downloaded for computer analysis.

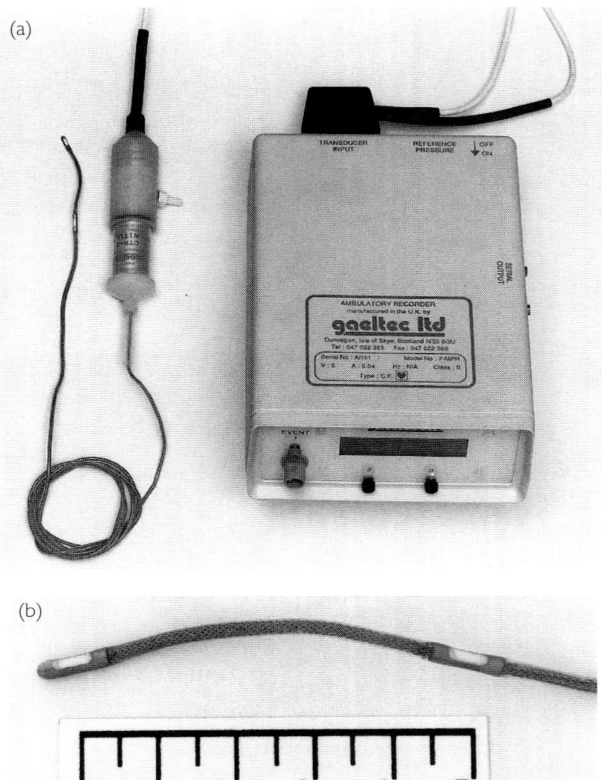

Figure 1.31 Ambulatory recording system for manometry and electromyography. (a) Portable data recording box. (b) Manometric strain-gauge recording catheter showing two sensors.

Electromyography

Ambulatory EMG recordings may be made in the external sphincter, puborectalis and the internal sphincter. The technique is carried out using bipolar fine wire electrodes. Two electrodes each 0.1 mm in diameter are passed through a 23-G needle and the protruding 3 mm are hooked back. The needle is inserted into the muscle and then withdrawn, leaving the hooked electrodes in position. The electrodes are connected to the data recording box. If recordings from one muscle are taken then filter settings are the same as described previously for static internal sphincter EMG. Simultaneous recordings from all three muscles have been made, in which case a low-frequency channel <10 Hz and two high-frequency channels 10 Hz–1 kHz are used (Farouk et al, 1993).

Clinical results

Internal sphincter slow pressure waves occur intermittently in normal subjects but are present for 35% of the time in patients with haemorrhoids (Waldron et al, 1989). In patients undergoing ileoanal pouch surgery, preoperative EMG slow wave activity was normal with a mean of 30 cycles per minute, and frequency reduced postoperatively by 70% to 13 per minute (Farouk et al, 1994a). This was accompanied by a 50% reduction in resting anal pressure. Conversely, restoration of internal sphincter pressure after abdominal rectopexy for prolapse is associated with a significant increase in internal sphincter EMG slow wave frequency (Farouk et al, 1992).

Spontaneous relaxations of the internal sphincter were first demonstrated by Miller et al (1988a) and these are accompanied by inhibition of internal sphincter EMG (Farouk et al 1994b). These episodes may play an important role in the continence mechanism and ambulatory recordings have been a powerful tool to study this. Abnormalities of sphincter relaxation have been shown using EMG and manometry in patients with neurogenic faecal incontinence (Miller et al, 1988b; Farouk et al, 1993) and prolonged episodes of relaxation have been found in patients with pruritis ani (Farouk et al, 1994b).

In many instances, patients with faecal incontinence may be found to have anal pressures which fall within normal defined limits. Using static recordings, the cause for incontinence may be obscure in these cases. High-amplitude proximal pressure waves may be associated with a feeling of urgency (Roberts and Williams, 1992), and have been observed in patients with incontinence after restorative proctocolectomy (Miller et al, 1990; Farouk et al, 1994a). High-pressure waves have been observed in incontinent subjects after rectal excision with coloanal anastomosis, and after coloperineal anastomosis and stimulated graciloplasty (Figure 1.32).

Laboratory investigation of patients with obstructed defecation demonstrates apparent para-

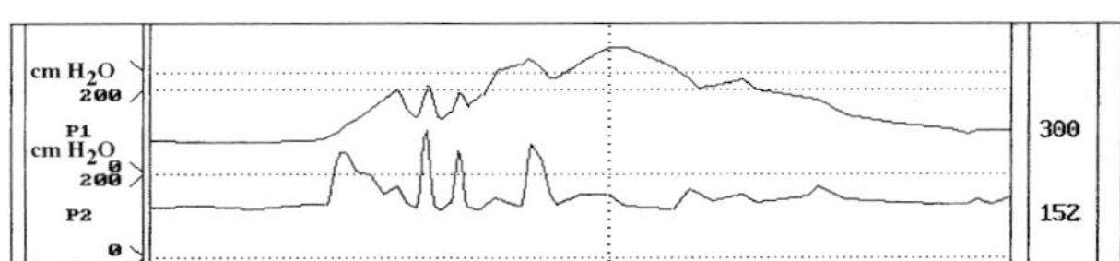

Figure 1.32 Ambulatory anorectal manometry showing a 30-second segment of a recording in a patient after low anterior resection. Top trace is neorectal pressure; bottom trace is mid-anal canal pressure. A high-amplitude pressure wave reaches the neorectum, producing a sensation of urgency and several voluntary contractions of the external sphincter. The cursor shows neorectal pressure exceeding anal pressure, and this was accompanied by soiling.

doxical contraction of the external sphincter and puborectalis on straining down (anismus) (Kuijpers and Bleijenberg, 1985; Preston and Lennard-Jones, 1985). This is also observed in some subjects when the test is carried out with the patient in the seated position (Womack et al, 1985). Other studies have questioned whether this may be an artefact due to the unphysiological nature of the laboratory tests (Jones et al, 1987a; Roberts et al, 1991; Duthie and Bartolo, 1992), and using ambulatory manometry and EMG it was shown that 8 of 11 patients with anismus diagnosed in the laboratory had normal pelvic floor relaxation when tested at home under physiological conditions (Duthie et al, 1991).

ANAL AND RECTAL SENSATION

Anal sensation

The anal mucosa is richly innervated with free and organized nerve endings and is sensitive to touch, pain, temperature and movement (Duthie and Gairns, 1960). Pain sensation extends 0.5–1.5 cm above the level of the dentate line, an important consideration during the treatment of haemorrhoids. Sensory fibres travel via the pudendal nerves to the S2–S4 nerve roots.

Anal sensation is assessed by testing temperature sensation or mucosal electrosensitivity. Temperature sensation is measured using a probe containing three channels for perfusion of water, each at a different temperature (Miller et al, 1987). The temperature is rapidly increased or decreased and this change is detected by the anal mucosa. The equipment is complex and is not commercially available.

In 1986 Roe et al described the technique of testing sensitivity to electrical stimulation. A tiny current is applied to the anal mucosa and the sensory threshold can be quantitatively measured. The test is very simple to perform and complements tests of pudendal motor nerve conduction. Mucosal electrosensitivity is carried out using a constant current stimulator, which delivers a current that is not varied by the surrounding tissue resistance. A ring electrode as described for perineal nerve motor latency (Dantec, Skovlunde, Denmark) is placed on a Foley catheter with the balloon deflated. The stimulator machine is set to deliver a current of duration 0.1 ms at a rate of 5 cycles per second, and the amplitude is increased from zero in 0.1 mA increments using a rheostat. The length of the anal canal should be measured manometrically prior to the procedure, in order to place the electrosensitivity electrode in the upper, mid and lower anal canal. Three recordings are taken at each level and the mean electrosensitivity calculated. The test is reproducible (Rogers et al, 1989; Ryhammer et al, 1997a) and provides an accurate measure of anal sensation. Normal median values and range (Roe et al, 1986) are:

Lower anal canal (mA)	4.8 (3.0–7.0)
Mid anal canal (mA)	4.2 (2.0–6.0)
Upper anal canal (mA)	5.7 (3.3–7.3)

Anal sensation is an important part of the continence mechanism and is reduced in patients with neurogenic incontinence (Roe et al, 1986; Rogers et al, 1988c). However, when the anal transitional zone has been removed after restorative proctocolectomy, loss of sensation is not always accompanied by impaired continence (Keighley et al, 1987), and other factors such as an alteration in the sampling reflex may contribute to the incontinence.

Rectal sensation

Rectal sensation plays an important role in the continence mechanism, and a sensation of rectal filling is also an integral part of normal defecation. The rectum is sensitive to distension but lacks pain receptors (Duthie and Gairns, 1960). There is debate about the site of receptors for rectal sensation. Distension of the rectum produces a sensation of pelvic filling, whereas distension of the lower sigmoid causes an abdominal visceral sensation (Goligher and Hughes, 1951). This suggests that the stretch receptors may be in the pelvic floor rather than the rectal wall. Indeed stretch receptors (Winckler, 1958; Walls, 1959) and muscle spindles (Swash, 1992) are found in the pelvic floor muscles, and a similar ‘rectal’ sensation is found after rectal excision and balloon distension of the colon anastomosed to the anus (Lane and Parks, 1977; Nicholls et al, 1988). Similarly, mucosal electrosensitivity testing of the colon anastomosed to the anus produces a sensation similar to when testing with the rectum intact (Meagher et al, 1996). Rectal sensation is tested by balloon distension of the rectum or with mucosal electrosensitivity.

Balloon distension

A balloon attached to a fine catheter is inserted into the rectum, with the lower edge of the balloon, once

Table 1.3 Rectal sensation showing balloon distension volumes in normal subjects.

Reference	*Mean age (years)*	*Balloon distension volume (ml)*			*Method*
		RST	*Urge to defecate*	*MTV*	
Loening-Baucke and Anuras (1985)	29	17 (8)	173 (64)		Bolus air
	72	17 (9)	151 (61)		Bolus air
Sun et al (1990c)	22	12 (1)	75 (10)	110 (10)	Bolus air
		20 (5)	128 (10)	178 (20)	Continuous air 20 ml/min
		20 (6)	130 (12)	176 (20)	Continuous water 20 ml/min
		43 (10)	167 (7)	230 (21)	Continuous air 100 ml/min
		40 (10)	175 (10)	216 (20)	Continuous water 100 ml/min

Values in parentheses are standard deviations.

inflated, lying on the pelvic floor. Three endpoints are taken: rectal sensitivity threshold (RST) being the volume first felt; volume producing the urge to defecate; and the volume causing intolerable pain, called the maximum tolerable volume (MTV). There are several methods used to inflate the balloon. Air and water produce similar thresholds of sensation (Sun et al, 1990c), and air is more commonly used. Inflation with 10 mL-increments of air is easiest. The threshold of sensation is lower when small incremental volumes are used or with slow inflation. It is also lower with bolus inflation compared with continuous inflation using a pump (Sun et al, 1990c). Normal values for RST, urge to defecate and MTV are shown in Table 1.3.

Rectal mucosal electrosensitivity

This test was described by Kamm and Lennard-Jones (1990). Equipment is the same as for anal mucosal electrosensitivity. A ring electrode mounted on a Foley catheter is inserted 6 cm above the anorectal junction. Stimulation parameters are 10 cycles per second, stimulus 500 μs, increasing from zero in 0.5-mA increments until a tingling or tapping sensation is felt.

RECTAL BALLOON EXPULSION

The ability to evacuate the rectum may be tested by rectal balloon expulsion. With the patient in the left lateral position a deflated party balloon attached to a catheter is inserted into the rectum and inflated with 50 mL warm water. The subject is instructed to expel the balloon, and if this cannot be done then it is inflated further up to the volume producing the urge to defecate.

Patients with anismus have been found to be unable to expel a rectal balloon (Preston and Lennard-Jones, 1985; Barnes and Lennard-Jones, 1985; Fleshman et al, 1992) and this has been used as a measure of rectal outlet obstruction caused by failure of relaxation of the pelvic floor muscles. Although initial studies showed normal subjects able to expel a balloon and patients with anismus unable to do so, more recent work has questioned the validity of the test since normal subjects and patients with incontinence in addition to patients with obstructed defecation were unable to expel a balloon (Schouten et al, 1997). The test has been carried out with the patient seated, in an attempt to make it more physiological. However, balloon expulsion is an unphysiological test and should be interpreted with caution.

MEASUREMENT OF COLONIC FUNCTION

Constipation is a common clinical problem and objective measurement of function is essential. Additionally, symptoms apparently referable to the anorectal region may have their origin higher in the colon in some patients, and anorectal function cannot always be taken in isolation.

Colonic transit studies

Earliest studies of transit employed barium (Alvarez and Freedlander, 1924; Manousos et al, 1967; Ritchie et al, 1971) but these do not give a quantitative measure, and barium may alter colonic transit time. Current techniques use radio-opaque markers or radioisotopes.

Radio-opaque markers

A simple test to measure colonic transit was described by Hinton et al (1969). All laxatives are ceased for at least 48 hours and 20 markers are swallowed. A single radiograph is taken on day 5 and in normal subjects at least 14 (80%) have been passed (Figure 1.33). The test is a measure of whole gut transit time but since colonic transit time forms a large component of this, it is a useful simple method of assessing colonic transit time.

Further information is obtained by assessing segmental colonic transit. This can be done by taking daily X-rays after ingestion of 20 markers. The colon is divided into three segments on the abdominal X-ray: right colon, left colon, and pelvis (sigmoid/rectum) (Martelli et al, 1978; Arhan et al, 1981). Segmental transit time as well as total transit time are calculated. Radiation exposure is minimized by ingesting 20 markers of different shapes daily on three consecutive days and taking a single radiograph on day 4 (Metcalf et al, 1987). Mean total colonic transit time in hours is: males 30.7 (SD 3.0), females 38.3 (SD 2.9).

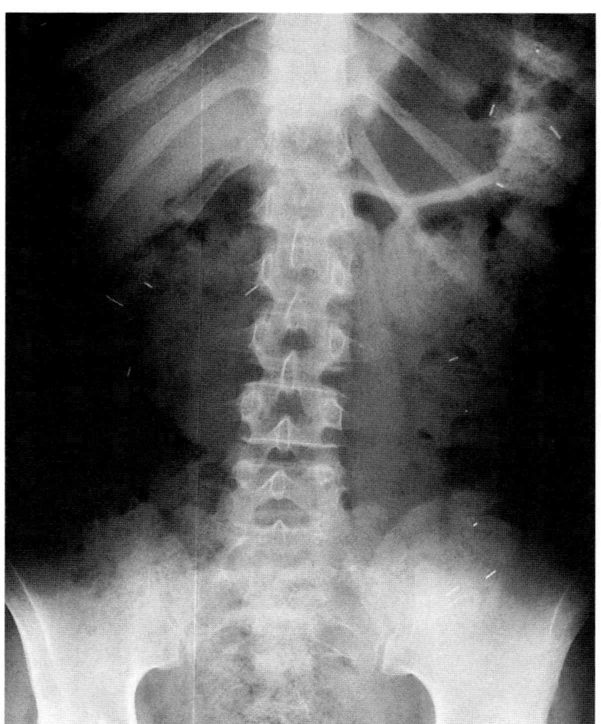

Figure 1.33 Radio-opaque marker study, showing retention of markers on day 5 in a patient with constipation.

Colonic scintigraphy

Radioisotope techniques are used in some centres as an alternative to markers. They are more complex and more expensive but provide clear quantitative information about segmental transit, and are particularly useful if colectomy for constipation is being considered. Early techniques involved delivering isotope to the caecum either via a nasocaecal tube or a colonoscopically placed tube (Krevsky et al, 1986; Spiller et al, 1986; Kamm et al, 1988). Based on the observation in an animal model, that when iodine-131 bound to cellulose was ingested to assess small bowel transit the colon was also visualized, this technique was adapted for use in humans (McLean

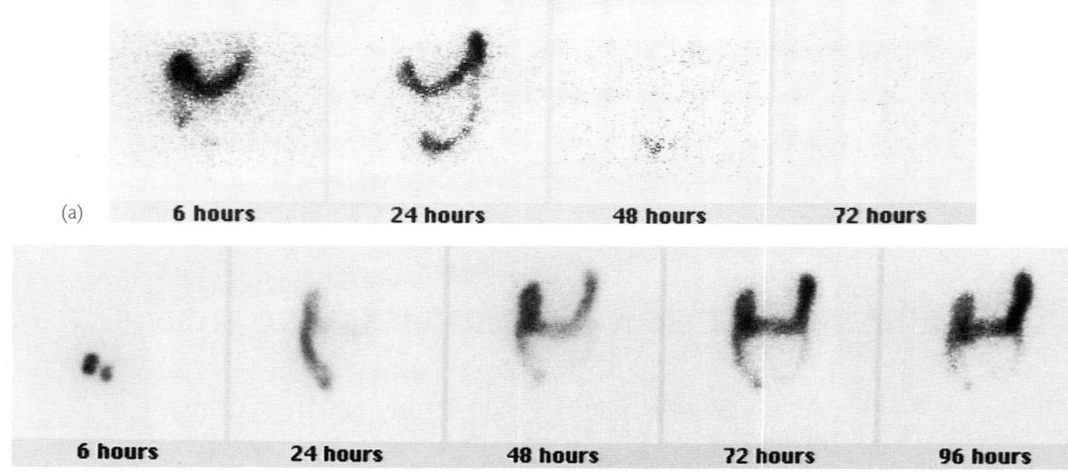

Figure 1.34 Radioisotope colon transit study. (a) Normal subject. At 6 hours after ingestion isotope has reached the right colon. There is normal passage of isotope through the colon over 48 hours. (b) Subject with severe constipation. There is prolonged retention of isotope in the colon to 96 hours.

et al, 1990; Stivland et al, 1991; Kamm et al, 1992). To simplify the test and avoid the step of binding iodine to cellulose, indium-111-DTPA can be used (Smart et al, 1991).

The isotope is given orally and the abdomen is scanned with a wide-field-of-view gamma camera 6, 24, 48, 72 and 96 hours after ingestion (Figure 1.34). The colon is divided in right, left and sigmoid/rectal segments for analysis. Segmental transit is expressed in one of two ways: the percentage of isotope retained in each segment and total percentage retained; or as the midpoint of the isotope column (mean activity position) (Smart et al, 1991; van der Sijp et al, 1993). Segmental and total percentage retention in normal subjects is shown in Table 1.4. Total percentage retention is significantly increased in patients with severe idiopathic constipation (Smart et al, 1991) (Figure 1.35). The total percentage retained is a simple measure for clinical use and can be plotted for comparison with normal data (Figure 1.36).

Table 1.4 Mean segmental and total percentage retention of isotope in the colon in normal subjects.

	Right colon	*Left colon*	*Rectosigmoid*	*Total colon*
24 hours	16 (7)	26 (17)	15 (9)	48 (28)
48 hours	3 (3)	5 (5)	6 (7)	11 (11)
72 hours	0.8 (1)	1 (2)	0.5 (0.5)	2 (4)
96 hours	0.2 (0.6)	0.1 (0.3)	0	0.3 (0.9)

Values in parentheses are standard deviations.
From Smart et al (1991).

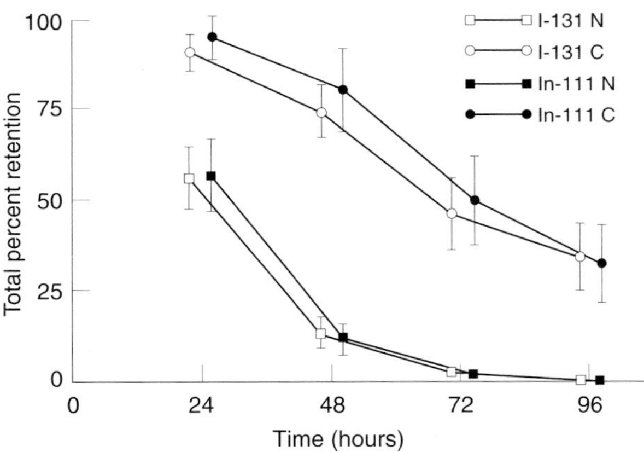

Figure 1.35 Percentage retention of isotope in the colon in normal subjects (N) and patients with severe idiopathic constipation (C). Both indium-111 (In-111) and iodine-131 (I-131) were given for comparison. There was no significant difference between the two tracers. There was a significant difference between the normal and constipated groups in the percentage isotope retained at each time interval. Reproduced with permission from the Society of Nuclear Medicine (Smart et al, 1991).

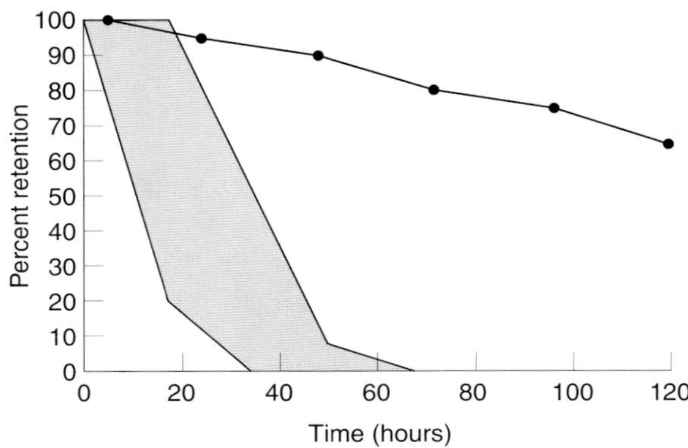

Figure 1.36 Total percentage isotope retained in a patient with severe constipation. Normal values (McLean et al, 1992) are shown within the shaded area. Retention of isotope is increased, indicating slow colonic transit.

Defecation scintigraphy

Recently, colon transit scintigraphy has been adapted to assess the rectum and colon during defecation. The impetus for this arose out of the hypotheses that in some patients with obstructed defecation there may be an underlying diffuse colonic abnormality. Oral indium-111-DTPA (4 MBq) is given as for standard colon scintigraphy, and then on the following day, when the subject develops a normal call to stool, the colon and rectum are screened immediately before, during and after defecation. Software is modified to allow rapid accumulation of data during defecation (Lubowski et al, 1995). Examination in cine mode showed partial evacuation of the left colon during defecation in 13 of 14 subjects (Figure 1.37). The mean percentage isotope evacuation from the rectum during defecation was 67% (range 30–97%), from the left colon 32% (range 4–86%), and right colon 20% (range 0–76%). Hence normal defecation was shown to include partial evacuation of the left colon in the majority of subjects, and even the right colon in some. This test is readily applied to the study of patients with defecatory disorders.

Colonic manometry

Colonic function is integrated with anorectal function. There is evidence from ambulatory anorectal manometry that vigorous colonic propulsion may cause faecal incontinence (see page 29), so that an apparently 'anorectal' condition may have its origin more proximally. Similarly, defecation is not only a process of rectal evacuation but involves propulsive

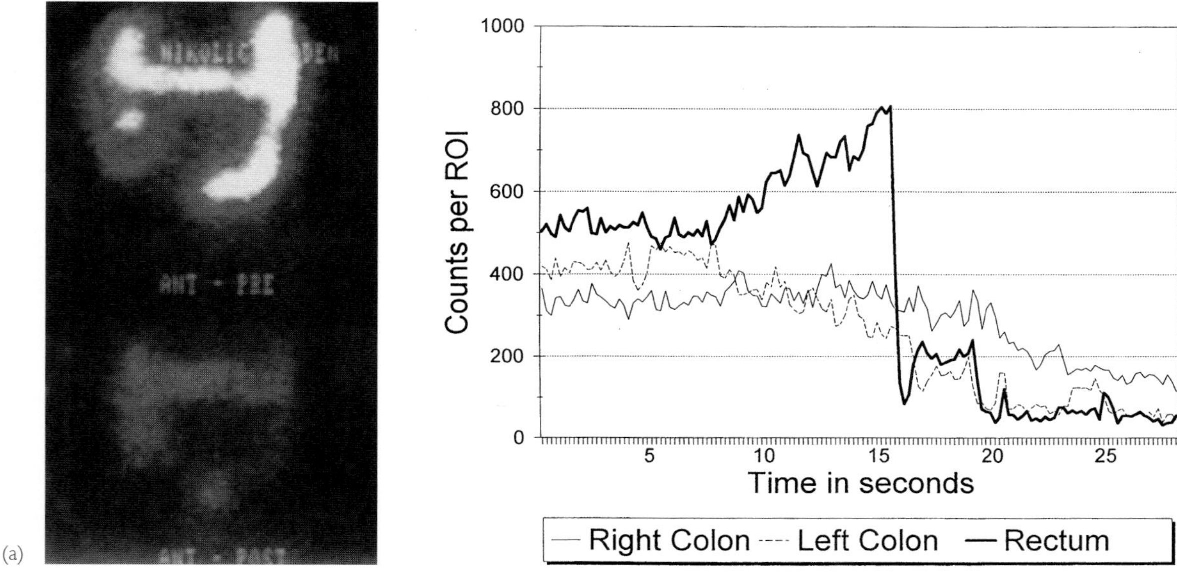

Figure 1.37 Colonic scintigraphy to study defecation under physiological conditions. (a) Images before (above) and after (below) defecation, showing emptying of the left and right colonic segments in this subject. (b) Dynamic segmental isotope counts in the right, left and rectosigmoid segments taken during defecation in the same subject. Initial emptying of the left colon is accompanied by filling of the rectum. Rectal emptying then occurs, together with continued emptying of the left colon, and emptying of the right colon. Reproduced with permission from Lubowski et al (1995).

activity in the colon. Difficulty with access to the colon has produced an obvious barrier to the study of propagated pressure waves in the colon. Additionally, long-term studies are needed because of the infrequent nature of manometric events in the colon.

Colonic manometry has been studied by placing a catheter colonoscopically into the prepared colon (Narducci et al, 1987; Bassotti et al, 1988; Furukawa et al, 1994). Low-amplitude non-propagating contractions, often occurring in bursts, are observed particularly on awakening and after eating (Narducci et al, 1987). High-amplitude propagating waves with a frequency of 4 per 24 hours and an amplitude of 100–200 mmHg are also found. Retrograde placement of a catheter into the prepared colon is an unphysiological test. Solid-state transducer systems have been inserted in an antegrade fashion (Soffer et al, 1989) but little information was obtained because of the long distances (up to 45 cm) between recording sites. We have developed a 16-channel catheter with side-holes 7.5 cm apart, passed transnasally to the rectum for recording from the unprepared colon (Dinning et al, 1997a). The catheter is 5 m long, with a total outside diameter of 3.5 mm (Figure 1.38). The catheter channels are connected to pressure transducers and signals are amplified and digitized (10 Hz) by preamplifiers (Accqknowledge 111 software, Biopac Systems Inc., Santa Barbara, CA, USA). The catheter tip is positioned in the duodenum under fluoroscopy and a balloon on the tip is inflated to a diameter of 2 cm. The catheter is fed manually through the nose and checked fluoroscopically to prevent curling in the stomach. Recording is begun when the catheter tip reaches the rectum. Using this technique antegrade propagating waves with mean

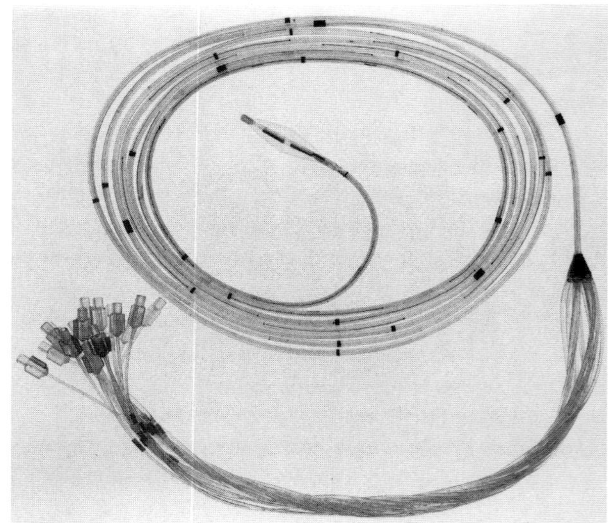

Figure 1.38 Sixteen-channel perfusion catheter for manometry of the unprepared colon.

frequency 1.53 per hour (SD 0.13) were found, originating most commonly in the caecum. Retrograde propagating waves were observed much less commonly. Non-propagating activity was also found, particularly after meals.

Of more interest, the motor events surrounding normal defecation were recorded under physiological conditions (Dinning et al, 1996, 1997b). In 10 of 13 subjects in the hour preceding 'defecation', a series of up to three propagating waves arose in the proximal colon, with the site of origin of each wave arising progressively more distally. In the 15 minutes prior to

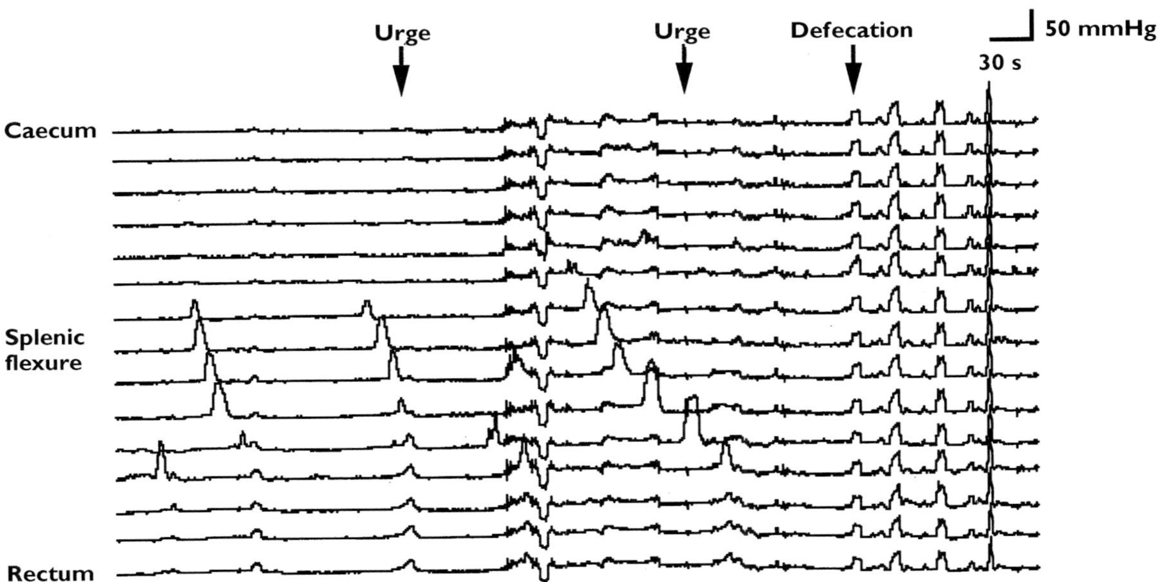

Figure 1.39 Manometric recording from the unprepared colon during defecation in a normal subject. Pressure channels are from the caecum (top trace) to the rectum. Three propagated waves are seen; the second and third are associated with an urge to defecate. There is a straining effort between the two urges, seen as a small rise in pressure in all channels. Defecation follows the second urge, with four straining efforts seen as a rise in each channel with each strain. Reproduced with permission from Bampton et al (1998).

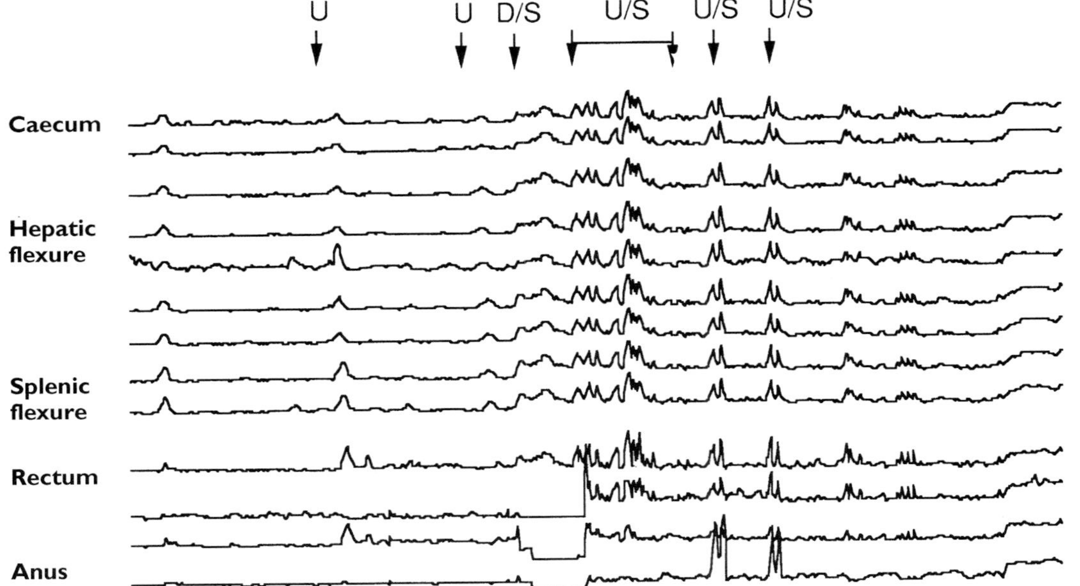

Figure 1.40 Manometric recording during attempted defecation in a patient with symptoms of obstructed defecation. There are no normal propagated pressure waves. Several straining efforts are seen in association with the urge to defecate. A small amount of stool was passed (D) at one straining effort. Anal pressure is shown in the lowest two traces. With one straining effort there is a fall in anal pressure, and with the subsequent strain there is a rise in pressure. Reproduced with permission from Bampton et al (1998).

defecation, up to three propagating sequences were again seen but the reverse pattern was present, with each successive propagating wave having its point of origin at a more proximal site. These propagating waves were associated with the urge to defecate at the end of the wave, namely when the wave had propagated to its most distal point (Figure 1.39). There was a marked reduction, or even absence of propagating sequences both in the distal and proximal colon in patients with obstructed defecation including those with anismus, suggesting a more diffuse colonic abnormality rather than an anorectal abnormality alone (Figure 1.40). Measurement of total anorectal and colonic function under physiological conditions is likely to give new insights into a variety of conditions.

DYNAMIC IMAGING OF THE RECTUM

Several methods are available to image the rectum. Scintigraphic methods provide a quantitative measure of rectal evacuation but do not demonstrate the anatomy of the anorectum, and defecography using barium has therefore been more widely used.

Defecography

Dynamic imaging of the rectum has been used for over 30 years (Burhenne, 1964; Broden and Snellman, 1968). More recently a large literature has grown around the syndrome of obstructed defecation and a variety of anatomical abnormalities and disorders of function have been identified. It should however be recognized that defecography does not assess defecation under physiological conditions since it ignores the normal sensory responses as well as the colonic motor events during defecation.

Technique

The barium mixture used varies widely. Theoretically, it would be best to use a mixture which approximates the volume and consistency of stool, but these parameters are variable in normal subjects. A solid artificial stool might alter the process of evacuation (Bannister et al, 1987) and a standard mixture has not been established (Finlay, 1988). Mahieu et al (1984) described barium diluted 1.5 to 4 in water and mixed with potato starch to form a thick paste, injected using a special plunger instrument. A softer mixture which is readily instilled using a syringe and Foley catheter has been more popular. One hundred millilitres will outline the rectum and lower sigmoid, but the volume has also not been standardized and 50–300 mL are reported (Finlay, 1988).

The mixture is instilled while the patient lies in the lateral position. The line of the anal canal can be defined using a metal chain, or more simply by injecting the mixture while withdrawing the catheter from the anus. Lateral radiographs are obtained with the subject sitting on a water-filled balloon ring or plastic commode to eliminate an air interface. X-rays are obtained at rest, while coughing, during a Valsalva manoeuvre, and during evacuation of the barium. Images are stored on video or static film. The examination room should be darkened and the number of observers limited as much as possible.

Normal evacuation (Figure 1.41)

During normal rectal emptying the following changes are observed: (1) As straining begins, abdominal pressure produces a slight concavity of the anterior rectal wall. (2) The pelvic floor descends. (3) The anorectal angle widens. (4) The anal canal begins to open, shortens, and becomes funnel shaped. (5) Rectal evacuation begins and emptying is completed. (6) A slight degree of rectal wall intussusception may occur.

Despite the widespread use of defecography in clinical practice, there are very few studies in normal controls, particularly in young women because of the radiation exposure. From the available studies there is wide variation in normal values (Mahieu et al, 1984; Skomorowska et al, 1987; Shorvon et al, 1989; Goei et al, 1989), and certain changes which were initially considered abnormal, particularly intussusception, are seen in asymptomatic subjects and are now considered normal.

Anorectal angle

The anorectal angle is measured at rest, during contraction of the pelvic floor muscles, and during rectal evacuation. The angle measures about 90 degrees at rest, is more acute (range 60–80 degrees) during contraction, and more obtuse (mean 130 degrees, range 120–145 degrees) during evacuation (Finlay, 1988). The angle is measured using either the line of the posterior wall, or the central axis of the rectum. There is subjectivity in this measurement, with inter- and intraobserver variance (Penninckx et al, 1990; Jorgensen et al, 1993). A computerized method of determining the central axis has been suggested (Keighley et al, 1989), but has not been widely used (see Figure 20.34a,b). In an individual subject the exact measurement is not as important as the change which occurs from the rest to straining positions.

Position of the pelvic floor

This is represented by the position of the anorectal junction, and is measured against a reference point, either the pubococcygeal line (see Figure 20.34a,b) or the plane of the ischial tuberosities (Figure 1.42). The latter is simpler to use. The pelvic floor lies about 2 cm above the plane of the tuberosities at

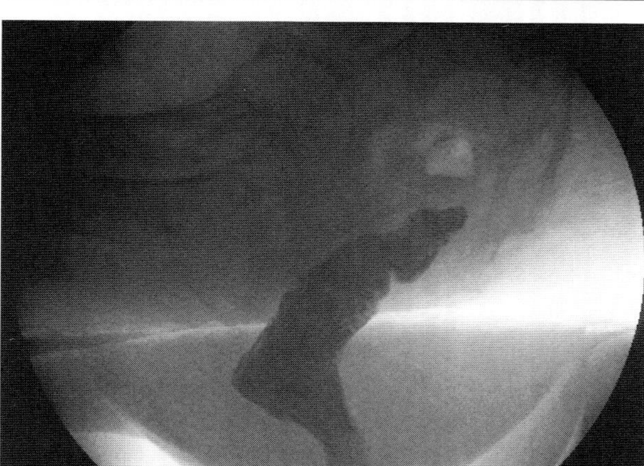

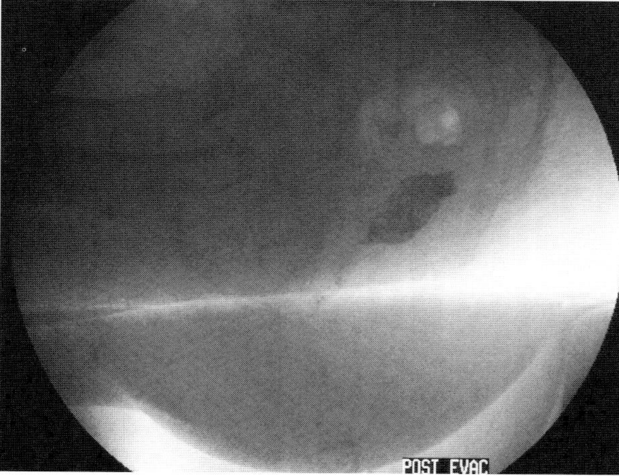

Figure 1.41 Defecography. Normal evacuation of barium. Slight concavity of the anterior rectal wall is seen on straining down; the anal canal opens and funnels; evacuation is complete.

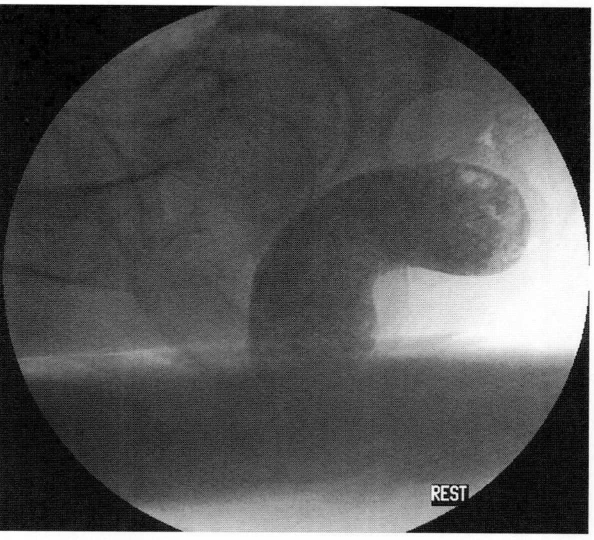

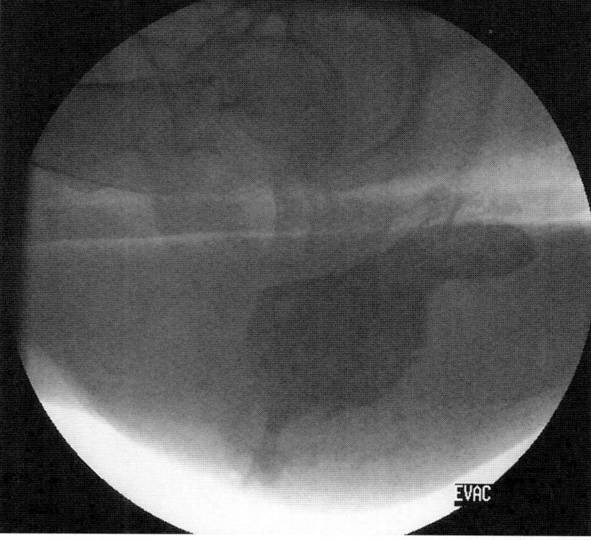

Figure 1.42 Proctogram showing descent of the perineum from the resting to the straining position. Descent is measured in relation to the line of the ischial tuberosities which are usually clearly visualized.

rest, and may be up to 2 cm below this level during straining (Bartram et al, 1988; Shorvon et al, 1989). It should not descend more than 3 cm. Pelvic floor descent is found in the elderly (Pinho et al, 1990), and in patients with obstructed defecation and chronic straining at stool (Bartolo et al, 1988) and faecal incontinence (Pinho et al, 1991).

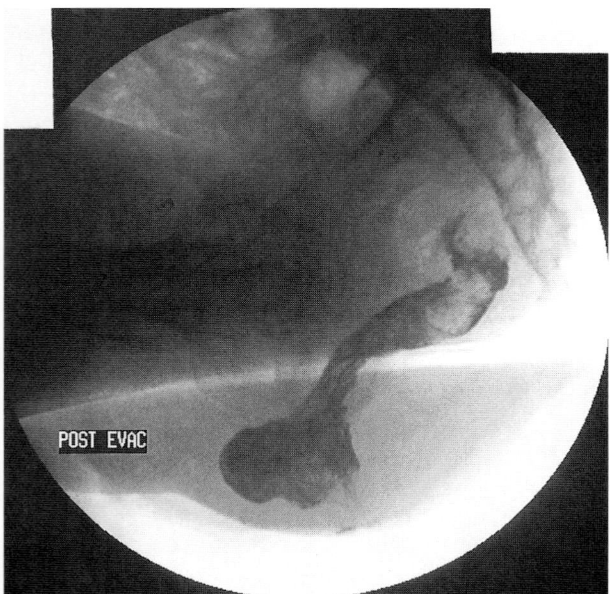

Figure 1.43 Proctogram showing anterior rectocele which fails to empty after evacuation.

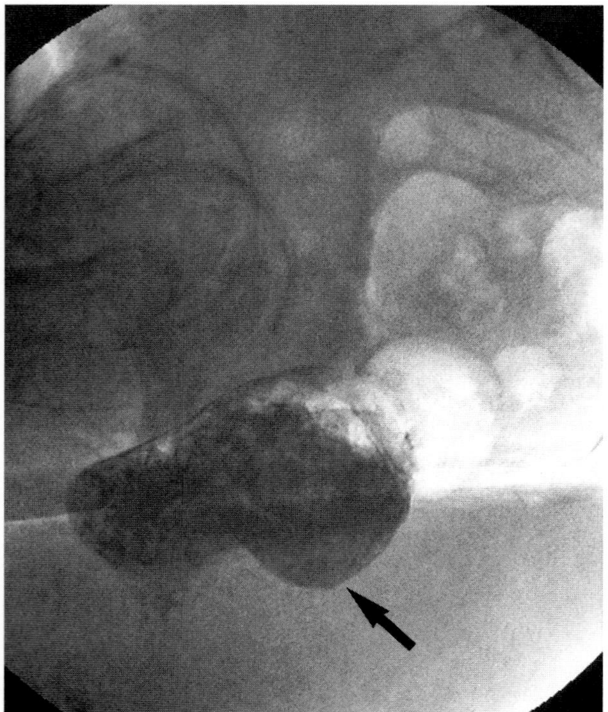

Figure 1.44 Posterior rectocele (arrow), formed by weakness of the levators.

Rectocele

Small rectoceles are a normal finding in asymptomatic women (Finlay, 1988). The size is measured anteriorly from a line drawn upwards from the anterior wall of the anal canal. Precisely what size rectocele will cause symptoms is not defined but a bulge greater than 2–3 cm is considered abnormal. Of more importance is failure of the rectocele to empty (Figure 1.43). Posterior wall rectoceles are much less common and are caused by a weakness in the supporting pelvic floor muscles (Figure 1.44) (Halligan and Bartram, 1996).

Intussusception

Prolapse of the rectal wall occurs within the rectum (rectorectal), within the anal canal (rectoanal), or there may be external rectal prolapse (Figure 1.45). Minor infoldings of the rectal wall are seen in up to 45% of asymptomatic subjects (Shorvon et al, 1989) and are considered normal. There is debate about the clinical importance of intussusception, particularly in relation to symptoms of obstructed defecation (van Tets and Kuijpers, 1995). There is a clear association in patients with the solitary rectal ulcer syndrome (Womack et al, 1987a,b; Nicholls and Simson, 1986) and surgery to correct internal intussusception in this condition is effective in some patients (van Tets and Kuijpers, 1995; Nicholls and Simson, 1986), but not for internal intussusception without solitary rectal ulcer syndrome (van Tets and Kuijpers, 1995; Orrom et al, 1991).

Incontinence

Neurogenic incontinence is associated with perineal descent and a widened anorectal angle at rest (Pinho et al, 1991). There may be leakage of barium during coughing or a Valsalva manoeuvre, which is a useful simple test to help determine whether sphincter weakness is the cause of the incontinence (Figure 1.46).

Dynamic synchronous defecography

In an attempt to correlate rectal evacuation with muscle activity, Womack et al (1985) developed a technique of synchronous defecography, electromyography and manometry. During defecography, external sphincter and puborectalis EMG is recorded using fine wire electrodes and rectal pressures are recorded; the EMG and pressure traces are integrated with the video defecography.

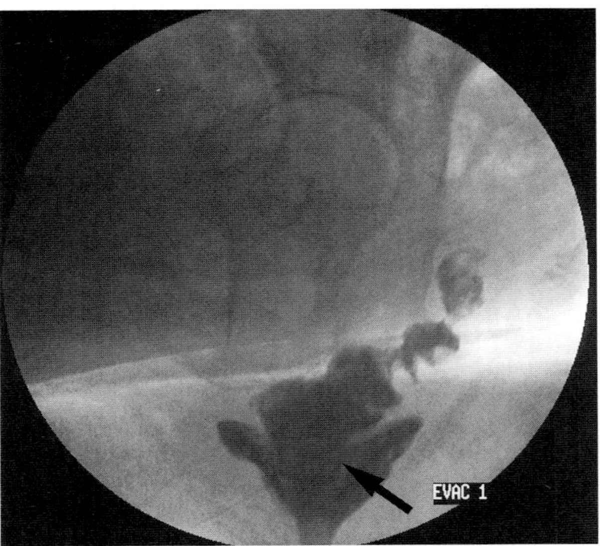

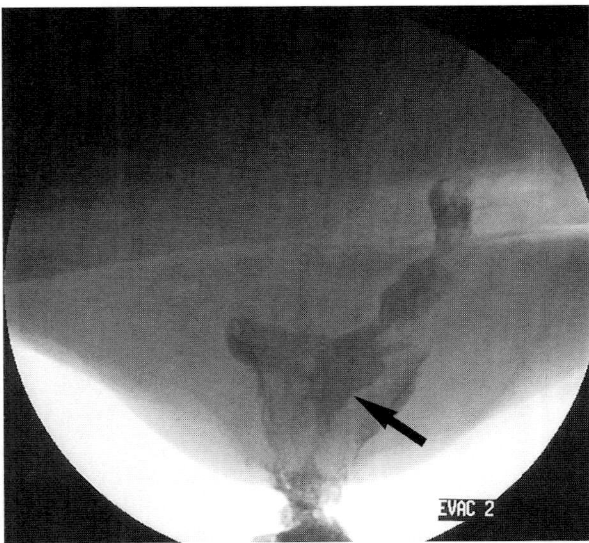

Figure 1.45 Intussusception of the rectum. The typical double shadow formed by circumferential intussusception is seen (arrow).

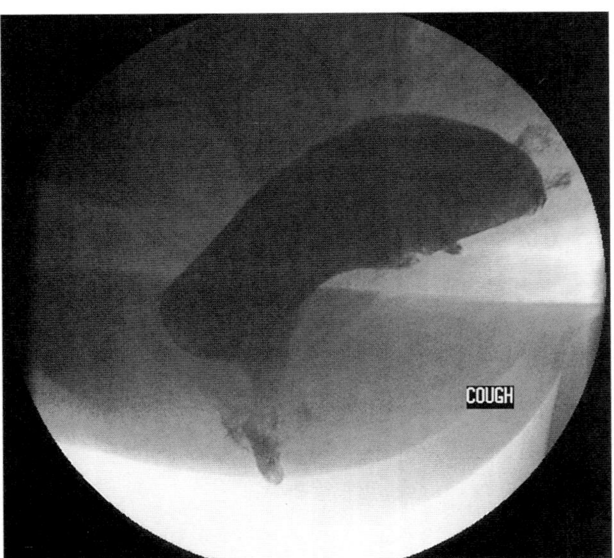

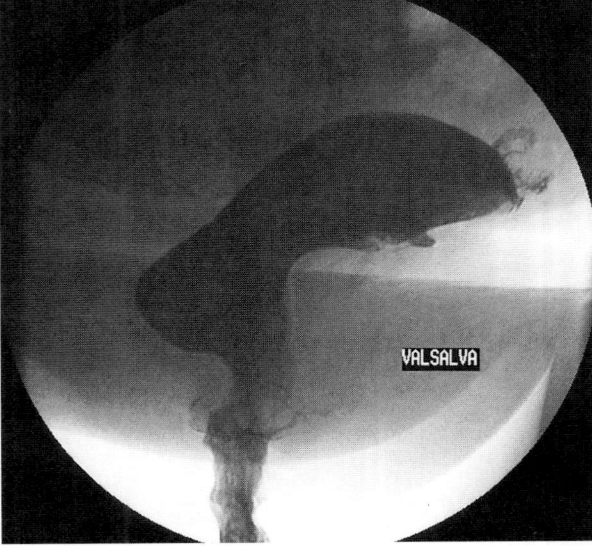

Figure 1.46 Proctogram showing incontinence during a cough and Valsalva manoeuvre due to anal sphincter weakness.

The technique is more complex than individual tests, but assesses pressure and EMG in the more physiological seated position. This test has shown high rectal voiding pressure in association with intussusception as the cause of ulceration in the solitary rectal ulcer syndrome (Womack et al, 1987a).

Scintigraphic defecography

With conventional defecography it can be difficult to quantitatively assess the degree of emptying since barium coating of the rectal wall gives the impression of incomplete evacuation. By using a radioisotope, accurate quantitative assessment of rectal emptying is possible. Indium-111-DTPA (2 Mbq) mixed in 100 mL potato mash or oatmeal porridge is instilled into the rectum, and then passed with the patient seated comfortably on a commode. Isotope counts are then taken over the rectum before and after evacuation and the percentage retained is calculated.

Differing results of evacuation in normal subjects are reported, apparently depending upon the technique used. Isotope instilled to the volume producing a sensation of fullness resulted in 90% (SD 3%) evacuation (Heppell et al, 1987), but if instilled to the maximum tolerated volume only 60% (SD 6%) was evacuated (O'Connell et al, 1986).

ENDOANAL ULTRASOUND

The anal sphincters may be visualized very clearly using an endoanal probe. Two systems are available: a rotating 7 MHz or 10 MHz probe housed within a water-filled plastic cone (Bruel and Kjaer, Gentofte, Denmark) (Figure 1.47), or a static linear 7 MHz probe. The linear probe may be used with an inexpensive small portable ultrasound machine (Aloka SSD-500, Tokyo, Japan) (Figure 1.48). Since the static probe is non-rotating, the recording surface is allowed to interface directly with the anal mucosa and a surrounding cone is therefore unnecessary. The rotating probe provides a 360 degree horizontal cross-sectional image at each level, and is inserted into the rectum, and then withdrawn from the top of the anal canal to the anal verge. The linear probe produces a longitudinal image of the entire sphincter length and recordings are taken at several points in each quadrant.

Normal recordings

Rotating probe

The surrounding cone forms two central echoes. The internal sphincter is a well-defined hypoechoic layer. Beyond this is the thick echogenic external sphincter ring (Figure 1.49). The internal sphincter ring is absent in the lowest part of the anal canal. In the upper anal canal the puborectalis is seen above the upper limit of the external sphincter.

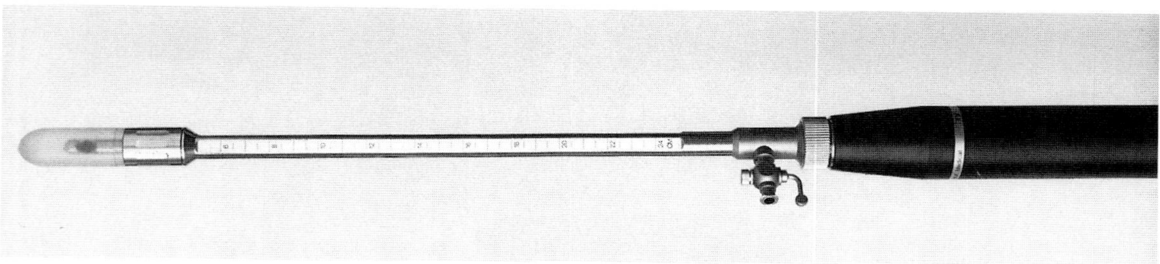

Figure 1.47 Rotating 10 MHz probe and surrounding cone for endoanal ultrasound (Bruel and Kjaer, Denmark).

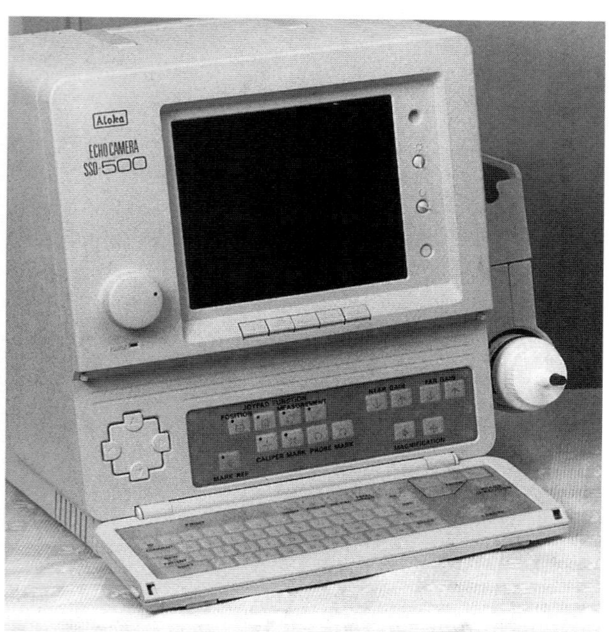

(a)

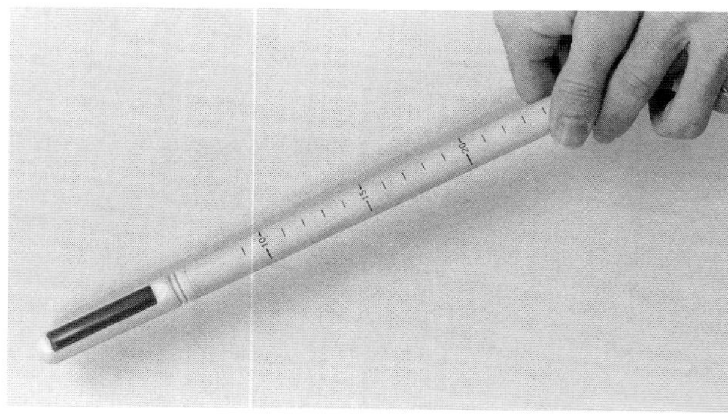

(b)

Figure 1.48 Portable ultrasound machine (a) and 7 MHz linear probe (b) (Aloka, Japan).

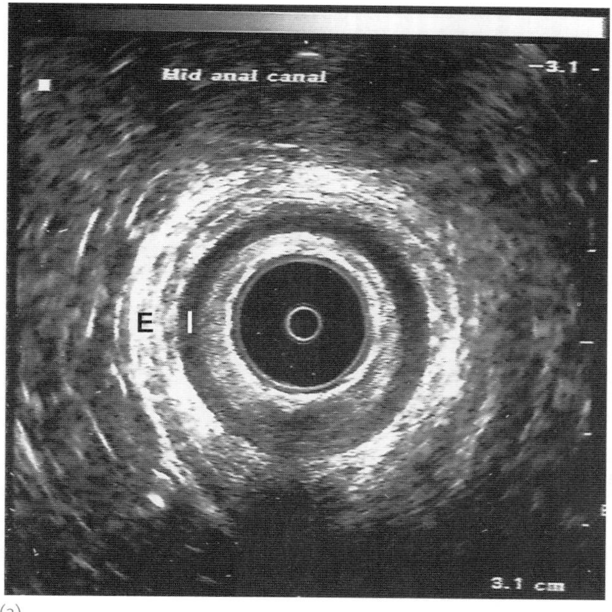

(a)

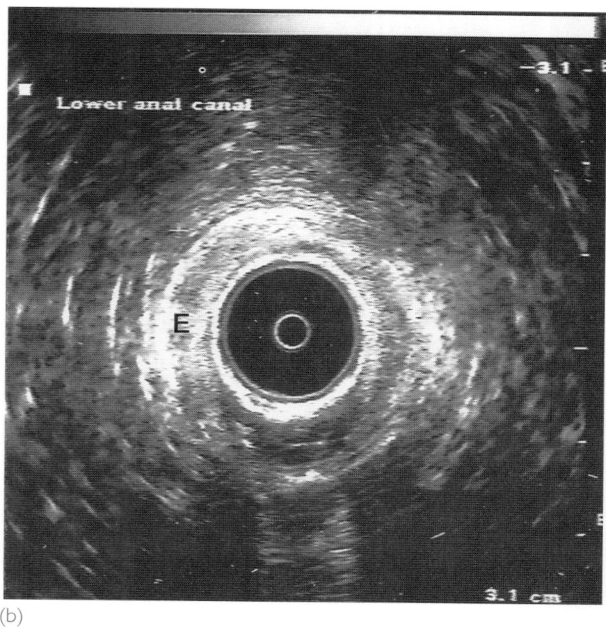

(b)

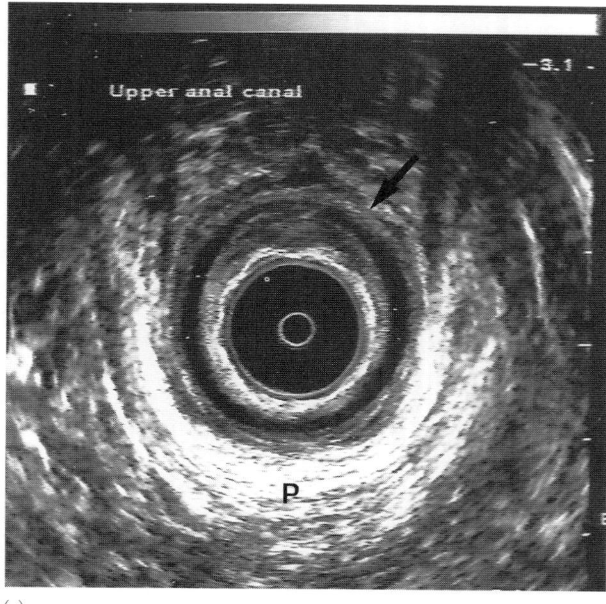

(c)

Figure 1.49 Normal ultrasound, rotating probe. (a) Mid-anal canal. Internal sphincter (I), external sphincter (E). (b) Lowest level of anal canal. Internal sphincter is absent at this level. Subcutaneous external sphincter seen (E). (c) Upper-anal canal. The puborectalis (P) is deficient anteriorly (arrow). (Courtesy of Dr Peter Stewart, Sydney.)

Linear probe

The internal and external sphincter layers have a similar appearance to the rotating probe (Figure 1.50). The subcutaneous part of the external sphincter is seen to extend beyond the lower limit of the internal sphincter. Anteriorly the striated muscle layer is shorter than posteriorly or laterally because of the absence of the puborectalis ring.

Abnormal findings

The normal internal sphincter thickness increases with age from 1 mm under 20 years to 2–3 mm in the elderly (Burnett and Bartram, 1991). The sphincter is stretched and becomes thinner with a large-diameter probe (Papachrysostomou et al, 1992). Therefore a 3-mm internal sphincter in a young patient is abnormal. A thickened internal sphincter may be due to rectal intussusception in the solitary rectal ulcer syndrome (Halligan et al, 1995). It is thin in patients undergoing restorative proctocolectomy (Silvis et al, 1995), and is also sometimes thin in patients with neurogenic incontinence, in keeping with the known muscle atrophy in that condition (Swash et al, 1988).

A defect is found in the internal sphincter following fistulotomy (Figure 1.51), lateral sphincterotomy (Figure 1.52), and in some cases after vaginal delivery in association with external sphincter injury (Figure 1.53) (Sultan et al, 1993a,b). Disruption in one or more places may occur after anal dilatation (Speakman et al, 1991b).

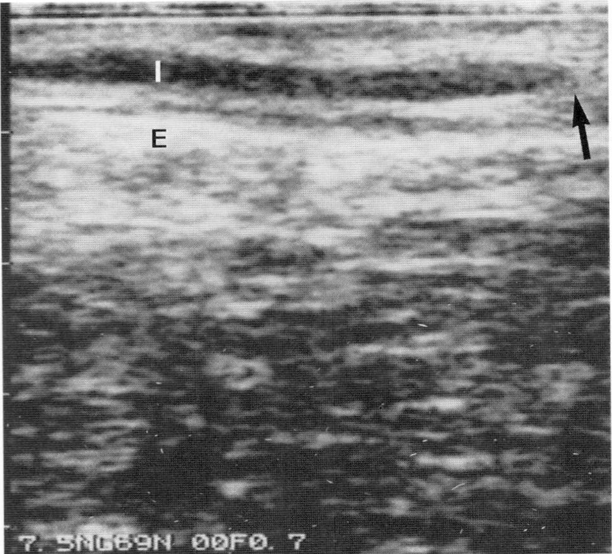

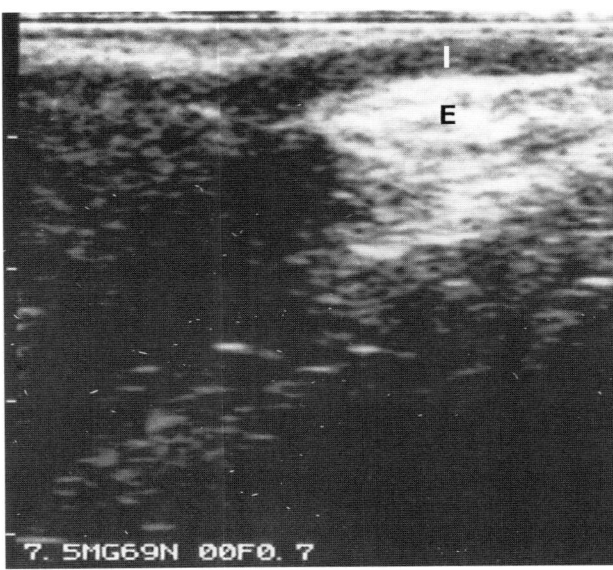

Figure 1.50 Normal ultrasound, linear probe. Longitudinal image with anal verge to the right of the screen. (a) Posterior image. Internal sphincter (I), external sphincter (E). The subcutaneous external sphincter (arrow) extends beyond the lower limit of internal sphincter. (b) Anterior image. The external sphincter length is much shorter than laterally or posteriorly due to the absence of the puborectalis. Internal sphincter (I), external sphincter (E).

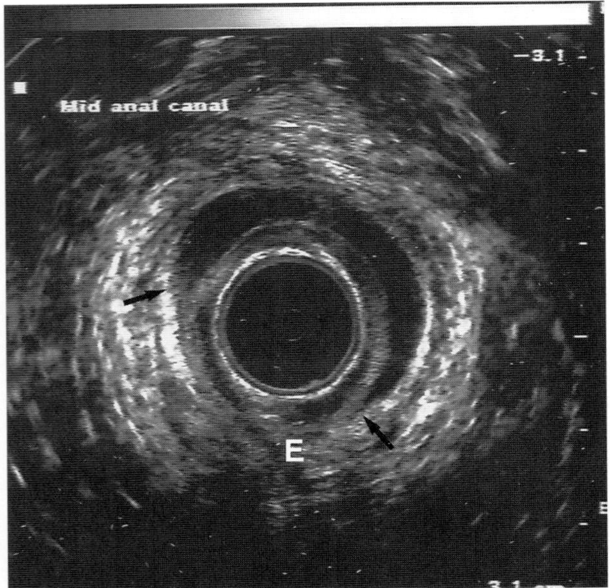

Figure 1.51 Rotating probe. Sphincter defect following fistulotomy. Mid-anal canal. Internal sphincter defect (between arrows). There is also some deficiency in the external sphincter at this level (E).

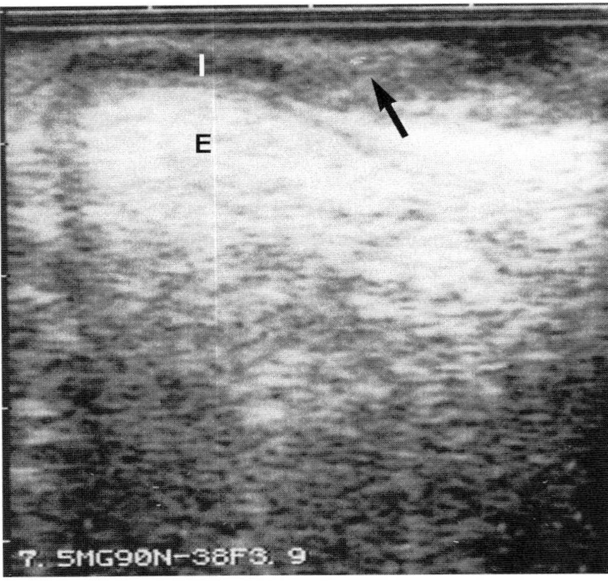

Figure 1.52 Linear probe. Loss of the lower half of internal sphinter following lateral sphincterotomy (arrow). Internal sphincter (I), external sphincter (E).

Endoanal ultrasound detects external sphincter defects as accurately as EMG (Tjandra et al, 1993; Sultan et al, 1994b) and surgery (Deen et al, 1993), and has become the procedure of choice for sphincter mapping since it causes much less discomfort than EMG. However, it should not be forgotten that a high percentage of multiparous women have a sphincter defect on ultrasound (Sultan et al, 1993a) and therefore until further data are available to predict which patients will benefit from sphincter repair, ultrasound should not be regarded as a discriminatory test and can only be used in conjunction with clinical assessment to select patients for surgery.

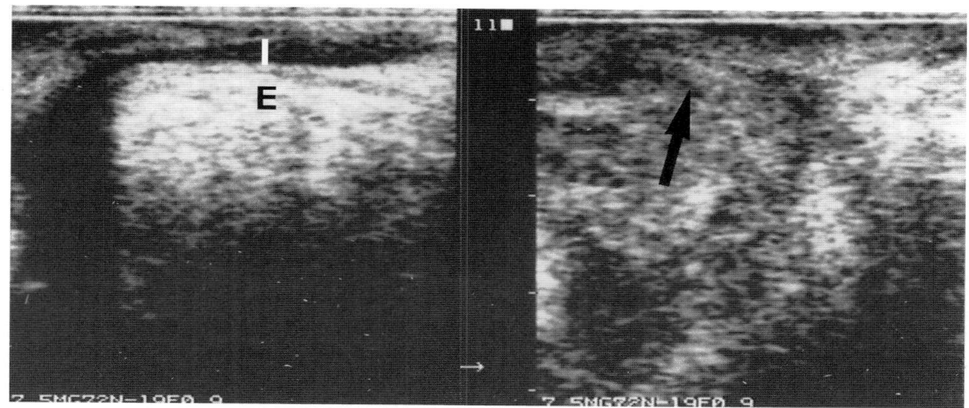

Figure 1.53 Linear probe. Normal internal sphincter (I) and external sphincter (E) at 5 o'clock (left); anterior sphincter defect (arrow) involving internal and external sphincters at 11 o'clock (right).

REFERENCES

Adrian ED & Bronk DV (1929) Discharge of impulses in motor nerve fibres. *J Physiol* **67**: 119–151.

Alvarez WC & Freedlander BL (1924) The rate of progress of food residues through the bowel. *JAMA* **83**: 576–580.

Ambrose S & Keighley MRB (1986) Outpatient measurement of perineal descent. *Ann R Coll Surg Engl* **67**: 306–308.

Arhan P, Devroede G, Jehannin B et al (1981) Segmental colonic transit time. *Dis Colon Rectum* **24**: 625–629.

Ayoub SF (1978) Arterial supply to the human rectum. *Acta Anat* **100**: 317–327.

Ayoub SF (1979) Anatomy of the external sphincter in man. *Acta Anat* **105**: 25–36.

Bampton PA, Dinning PG, Kennedy ML, Lubowski DZ & Cook IJ (1998) The manometric correlates of spontaneous defecation in patients with obstructed defecation. Evidence of a pancolonic disorder. *Gastroenterology* **114**: A716.

Bannister JJ, Davison P, Timms JM, Gibbons C & Read NW (1987) Effect of stool size and consistency on defecation. *Gut* **28**: 1246–1250.

Barnes PRH & Lennard-Jones JE (1985) Balloon expulsion from the rectum in constipation of different types. *Gut* **26**: 1049–1052.

Bartolo DCC, Jarrett JA & Read NW (1983a) The use of conventional electromyography to assess external sphincter neuropathy in man. *J Neurol Neurosurg Psychiatry* **46**: 1115–1118.

Bartolo DCC, Jarratt JA, Read MG, Donnelly TC & Read NW (1983b) The role of partial denervation of the puborectalis in idiopathic faecal incontinence. *Br J Surg* **70**: 664–667.

Bartolo DCC, Roe AM & Mortensen NJMcC (1986) The relationship between perineal descent and denervation of the puborectalis in incontinent patients. *Int J Colorectal Dis* **1**: 91–95.

Bartolo DCC, Roe AM, Virjee J, Mortensen NJ & Locke-Edmunds JC (1988) An analysis of rectal morphology in obstructive defaecation. *Int J Colorectal Dis* **3**: 17–22.

Bartram CI, Turnbull GK & Lennard-Jones JE (1988) Evacuation proctography: an investigation of rectal expulsion in 20 subjects without defecatory disturbance. *Gastrointest Radiol* **13**: 72–80.

Basmajian JV & Stecko G (1963) New bipolar electrode for electromyography. *J Appl Physiol* **17**: 849.

Bassotti G, Gaburri M, Imbimbo BP et al (1988) Colonic mass movements in idiopathic chronic constipation. *Gut* **29**: 1173–1179.

Beersiek F, Parks AG & Swash M (1979) Pathogenesis of ano-rectal incontinence. A histometric study of the anal sphincter musculature. *J Neurol Sci* **42**: 111–127.

Beevors MA, Lubowski DZ, King DW & Carlton MA (1991) Pudendal nerve damage in women with symptomatic utero-vaginal prolapse. *Int J Colorectal Dis* **6**: 24–28.

Benson JT & McClellan E (1993) The effect of vaginal dissection on the pudendal nerve. *Obstet Gynecol* **82**: 387–389.

Broden B & Snellman B (1968) Procidentia of the rectum studied with cineradiography: A contribution to the discussion of causative mechanism. *Dis Colon Rectum* **11**: 330–347.

Brookes SJH, Lam TCF, Lubowski DZ, Costa M & King DW (1996) Regeneration of nerves across a colonic anastomosis in the guinea-pig. *J Gastroenterol Hepatol* **11**: 325–334.

Bruck CE, Lubowski DZ & King DW (1988) Do patients with haemorrhoids have pelvic floor denervation? *Int J Colorectal Dis* **3**: 210–214.

Burhenne HJ (1964) Intestinal evacuation study: A new roentgenologic technique. *Radiol Clin* **33**: 79–84.

Burnett SJ & Bartram CI (1991) Endosonographic variations in the normal internal anal sphincter. *Int J Colorectal Dis* **6**: 2–4.

Coller JA (1987) Clinical application of anorectal manometry. *Gastroenterol Clin North Am* **16**: 17–33.

Collins CD, Brown BH, Whittaker GE & Duthie HL (1969) New method of measuring forces in the anal canal. *Gut* **10**: 160–163

Deen KI, Kumar D, Williams JG, Olliff J & Keighley MR (1993) Anal sphincter defects. Correlation between endoanal ultrasound and surgery. *Ann Surg* **218**: 201–205.

Denny-Brown D & Robertson EG (1935) An investigation of the nervous control of defaecation. Brain **58**: 256–310.

Dent J (1976) A new technique for continuous sphincter pressure measurement. *Gastroenterology* **71**: 263–267

Deutsch AA, Moshkovitz M, Nudelman I, Dinari G & Reiss R (1987) Anal pressure measurements in the study of hemorrhoid etiology and their relation to treatment. *Dis Colon Rectum* **30**: 855–857.

Dinning PG, Kennedy ML, Lubowski DZ, deCarle DJ & Cook IJ (1996) Manometric findings in the unprepared proximal colon in patients with severe obstructed defaecation. *Gastroenterology* **110**: 657.

Dinning PG, Bampton PA, Kennedy ML et al (1997a) Prolonged, closely spaced, multipoint perfusion manometry of the entire unprepared human colon. *J Gastroenterol Hepatol* **12**: A105.

Dinning PG, Kennedy ML, Lubowski DZ, deCarle DJ & Cook IJ (1997b) Nasocolonic manometry recordings of the unprepared proximal colon from patients with severe obstructed defecation. *J Gastroenterol Hepatol* **11**: A111.

Drummond H (1913) The arterial supply of the rectum and pelvic colon. *Br J Surg* **1**: 677–685.

Duthie GS & Bartolo DCC (1992) Anismus: The cause of constipation? Results of investigation and treatment. *World J Surg* **16**: 831–835.

Duthie HL & Bennett RC (1963) The relations of sensation in the anal canal to the functional anal sphincter: a possible factor in anal continence. *Gut* **4**: 179–182.

Duthie HL & Gairns FW (1960) Sensory nerve endings and sensation in the anal region of man. *Br J Surg* **47**: 585–595.

Duthie HL & Watts JM (1965) Contribution of the external anal sphincter to the pressure zone in the anal canal. *Gut* **6**: 64–68.

Duthie HL, Bartolo DCC & Miller R (1991) Estimation of the incidence of anismus by laboratory tests. *Br J Surg* **78**: 747.

Engel AF & Kamm MA (1994) The acute effect of straining on pelvic floor neurological function. *Int J Colorectal Dis* **9**: 8–12.

Farouk R, Duthie GS, Bartolo DC & MacGregor AB (1992) Restoration of continence following rectopexy for rectal prolapse and recovery of the internal anal sphincter electromyogram. *Br J Surg* **79**: 439–440.

Farouk R, Duthie GS, Pryde A, McGregor AB & Bartolo DCC (1993) Internal anal sphincter dysfunction in neurogenic faecal incontinence. *Br J Surg* **80**: 259–261.

Farouk R, Duthie GS & Bartolo DCC (1994a) Recovery of the internal anal sphincter and continence after restorative proctocolectomy. *Br J Surg* **81**: 1065–1068.

Farouk R, Duthie GS, Pryde A & Bartolo DCC (1994b) Abnormal transient internal sphincter relaxation in idiopathic pruritis ani: physiological evidence from ambulatory monitoring. *Br J Surg* **81**: 603–606.

Fink RL, Roberts LJ & Scott M (1992) The role of manometry, electromyography and radiology in the assessment of faecal incontinence. *Aust N Z J Surg* **62**: 951–958.

Finlay IG (moderator) (1988) Symposium: Proctography. *Int J Colorectal Dis* **3**: 67–89.

Fleshman JW, Dreznick Z, Cohen E, Fry RP & Kodner IJ (1992) Balloon expulsion test facilitates diagnosis of pelvic floor outlet obstruction due to nonrelaxing puborectalis muscle. *Dis Colon Rectum* **35**: 1019–1025.

Floyd WF & Walls EW (1953) Electromyography of the sphincter ani externum in man. *J Physiol* **122**: 599–609.

Frenckner B & von Euler C (1975) Influence of pudendal block on the function of the anal sphincters. *Gut* **16**: 482–489.

Furukawa Y, Cook IJ, Panagopoulos V, McEvoy RD, Sharp DJ & Simula M (1994) Relationship between sleep patterns and human colonic motor patterns. *Gastroenterology* **107**: 1372–1381.

Gath I & Stalberg E (1975) Frequency and time domain characteristics of single muscle fibre action potential. *Electroencephalogr Clin NeuroPhysiol* **39**: 371–376.

Gibbons CP & Read NW (1986) Anal hypertonia in fissures: cause or effect? *Br J Surg* **73**: 443–445.

Gibbons CP, Bannister JJ, Trowbridge GA & Read NW (1986) An analysis of anal sphincter pressure and anal compliance in normal subjects. *Int J Colorectal Dis* **1**: 231–237.

Goei R, van Engelshoven J, Schouten H, Baeten C & Stassen C (1989) Anorectal function: defecographic measurement in asymptomatic subjects. *Radiology* **173**: 137–141.

Goligher JC (1951) The functional results after sphincter saving resections of the rectum. *Ann R Coll Surg Engl* **8**: 421–439.

Goligher J & Hughes F (1951) Sensibility of the rectum and colon: its role in the mechanism of anal continence. *Lancet* **i**: 543–548.

Goligher JC, Leacock AG & Brossy JJ (1955) The surgical anatomy of the anal canal. *Br J Surg* **43**: 51–61.

Gowers WR (1877) The autonomic action of the sphincter ani. *Proc R Soc Med* **26**: 77–84.

Griffiths JD (1956) Surgical anatomy of the blood supply of the distal colon. *Ann R Coll Surg Engl* **19**: 241–256.

Gutierrez JG, Oliai A & Chey WY (1975) Manometric profile of the internal anal sphincter in man. *Gastroenterology* **68**: 907.

Halligan S & Bartram CI (1996) Is barium trapping in rectoceles significant? *Dis Colon Rectum* **38**: 764–768.

Halligan S, Sultan A, Rottenberg G & Bartram CI (1995) Endosonography of the anal sphincters in solitary rectal ulcer syndrome. *Int J Colorectal Dis* **10**: 79–82.

Hancock BD (1976) Measurement of anal pressure and motility. *Gut* **17**: 645–651.

Hancock BD (1977a) Internal sphincter and the nature of haemorrhoids. *Gut* **18**: 651–655.

Hancock BD (1977b) The internal anal sphincter and anal fissure. *Br J Surg* **64**: 92–95.

Hancock BD & Smith K (1975) The internal sphincter and Lord's procedure for haemorrhoids. *Br J Surg* **62**: 833–866.

Handley PH (1978) Rubber band seton in the management of abscess-anal fistula. *Ann Surg* **187**: 435–437.

Haynes WG & Read NW (1982) Anorectal activity in man during rectal infusion of saline: a dynamic assessment of the anal continence mechanism. *J Physiol* **330**: 45–56.

Henry MM, Parks AG & Swash M (1982) The pelvic floor musculature in the descending perineum syndrome. *Br J Surg* **69**: 470–472.

Heppell J, Bellivaeu P, Taillefer R, Dube S & Derbekyan V (1987) Quantitative assessment of pelvic ileal reservoir emptying with a semisolid radionuclide enema. *Dis Colon Rectum* **30**: 81–85

Hinton JM, Lennard-Jones JE & Young AC (1969) A new method for studying gut transit times using radio-opaque markers. *Gut* **10**: 842–847.

Ho YH & Goh HS (1995) The neurophysiological significance of perineal descent. *Int J Colorectal Dis* **10**: 107–111.

Hughes ESR (1957) Surgical anatomy of the anal canal. *Aust NZ J Surg* **26**: 48–55.

Jameson JS, Chia YW, Kamm MA, Speakman CT, Chye YH & Henry MM (1994) Effect of age, sex and parity on anorectal function. *Br J Surg* **81**: 1689–1692.

Johnson GP, Pemberton JH, Ness J, Samson N, Zinsmeister AR (1990) Transducer manometry and the effect of body position on anal canal pressures. *Dis Colon Rectum* **33**: 469–475.

Jones PN, Lubowski DZ, Swash M & Henry MM (1987a) Relation between perineal descent and pudendal nerve damage in idiopathic faecal incontinence. *Int J Colorectal Dis* **2**: 93–95.

Jones PN, Lubowski DZ, Swash M & Henry MM (1987b) Is paradoxical contraction of puborectalis muscle of functional importance? *Dis Colon Rectum* **30**: 667–670.

Jorge JM, Wexner SD, Ehrempreis ED, Nogueras JJ & Jagelman DG (1993) Does perineal descent correlate with pudendal neuropathy? *Dis Colon Rectum* **36**: 475–483.

Jorgensen J, Stein P, King DW & Lubowski DZ (1993) The anorectal angle is not a reliable parameter on defaecating proctography. *Aust N Z J Surg* **63**: 105–108.

Kafka NJ, Coller JA, Barrett RC, Murray JJ, Roberts PL, Rusin LC & Schoetz DJ Jr (1997) Pudendal neuropathy is the only parameter differentiating leakage from solid stool incontinence. *Dis Colon Rectum* **40**: 1220–1227.

Kamm MA & Lennard-Jones JE (1990) Rectal mucosal electrosensitivity testing – evidence for a rectal sensory neuropathy in idiopathic constipation. *Dis Colon Rectum* **33**: 419–423.

Kamm MA, Lennard-Jones JE, Thompson DG, Sobnack R, Garvie NW & Granowska M (1988) Dynamic scanning defines a colonic defect in severe idiopathic constipation. *Gut* **29**: 1085–1092.

Kamm MA, van der Sijp JRM & Lennard-Jones JE (1992) Observations of the characteristics of stimulated defaecation in severe idiopathic constipation. *Int J Colorectal Dis* **7**: 197–201.

Keck JO, Staniunas RJ, Coller JA, Barrett RC & Oster ME (1995) Computer-generated profiles of the anal canal in patients with anal fissure. *Dis Colon Rectum* **38**: 72–79.

Keighley MRB, Ionesue MI & Wooler GH (1973) Late results of elective and emergency portocaval anastomosis: with particular reference to the type of stoma used. *Am J Surg* **126**: 601–606.

Keighley MRB, Winslet MC, Yoshioka K & Lightwood R (1987) Discrimination is not impaired by excision of the anal transitional zone after restorative proctocolectomy. *Br J Surg* **74**: 1118–1121.

Keighley MRB, Henry MM, Bartolo DCC & Mortensen NJMcC (1989) Anorectal physiology measurement: report of a working party. *Br J Surg* **76**: 356–357.

Kerremans R (1969) *Morphological and Physiological Aspects of Anal Continence and Defaecation*. Brussels: Editions Arscia.

Kiff ES & Swash M (1984a) Slowed conduction in the pudendal nerves in idiopathic (neurogenic) faecal incontinence. *Br J Surg* **71**: 614–616.

Kiff ES & Swash M (1984b) Normal proximal and delayed distal conduction in the pudendal nerves of patients with idiopathic (neurogenic) faecal incontinence. *J Neurol Neurosurg Psychiatry* **47**: 820–823.

Kiff ES, Barnes P & Swash M (1984) Evidence of pudendal neuropathy in patients with perineal descent and chronic straining at stool. *Gut* **25**: 1279–1282.

Krevsky B, Malmud LS, D'Ercole F, Maurer AH & Fisher RS (1986) Colonic transit scintigraphy: a physiologic approach to the quantitative measurement of colonic transit in humans. *Gastroenterology* **91**: 1102–1112.

Kuijpers HC & Bleijenberg G (1985) The spastic pelvic floor syndrome. *Dis Colon Rectum* **28**: 669–672.

Kumar D, Williams NS, Waldron D & Wingate DL (1989) Prolonged manometric recording of anorectal motor activity in ambulant human subjects: evidence of periodic activity. *Gut* **30**: 1007–1011.

Kumar D, Waldron D & Williams NS (1990) Prolonged anorectal manometry and external sphincter electromyography in ambulant human subjects. *Dig Dis Sci* **35**: 641–648.

Lane RHS (1974) Clinical application of anorectal physiology. *Proc R Soc Med* **68**: 28–30.

Lane RHS & Parks AG (1977) Function of the anal sphincters following coloanal anastomosis. *Br J Surg* **64**: 596–599.

Laurberg S & Swash M (1989) Effects of ageing on the anorectal sphincters and their innervation. *Dis Colon Rectum* **32**: 734–742.

Laurberg S, Swash M, Snooks SJ & Henry MM (1988) Neurologic cause of idiopathic incontinence. *Arch Neurol* **45**: 1250–1253.

Lawson JON & Nixon HH (1967) Anal canal pressure in the diagnosis of Hirschsprung's disease. *J Pediatr Surg* **2**: 544–552.

Lestar B, Penninckx F & Kerremans R (1989) The composition of anal basal pressure: An in vivo and in vitro study in man. *Int J Colorectal Dis* **4**: 118–122.

Loening-Baucke V & Anuras S (1985) Effects of age and sex on anorectal manometry. *Am J Gastroenterol* **80**: 50–53.

Lubowski DZ, Nicholls RJ, Swash M & Jordan MJ (1987) Neural control of internal anal sphincter function. *Br J Surg* **74**: 668–670.

Lubowski DZ, Jones PN, Swash M & Henry MM (1988a) Asymmetrical pudendal nerve damage in pelvic floor disorders. *Int J Colorectal Dis* **3**: 158–160.

Lubowski DZ, Swash M, Nicholls RJ & Henry MM (1988b) Increase in pudendal nerve terminal motor latency with defaecation straining. *Br J Surg* **75**: 1095–1097.

Lubowski DZ, Nicholls RJ, Burleigh DE & Swash M (1988c) Internal anal sphincter in neurogenic fecal incontinence. *Gastroenterology* **95**: 997–1002.

Lubowski DZ, Swash M & Henry MM (1988d) Neural mechanisms in disorders of defaecation, pp. 201–203. In Grundy D & Read NW (eds) *Clinical Gastroenterology. Gastrointestinal Neurophysiology*. London: Baillière Tindall, WB Saunders.

Lubowski DZ, King DW & Finlay IG (1992) Electromyography of the pubococcygeus muscle in patients with obstructed defaecation. *Int J Colorectal Dis* **7**: 184–187.

Lubowski DZ, Meagher AP, Smart RC & Butler SP (1995) Scintigraphic assessment of colonic function during defaecation. *Int J Colorectal Dis* **10**: 91–93.

McLean RG, Smart RC, Gaston-Parry D et al (1990) Colon transit scintigraphy in health and constipation using I-131-cellulose. *J Nucl Med* **31**: 985–989.

McLean RG, Smart RC, Lubowski DZ, King DW, Barbagello S & Talley NA (1992) Oral colon transit scintigraphy using indium-III DTPA: variability in healthy subjects. *Int J Colorectal Dis* **7**: 173–176.

McNamara MJ, Percy JP & Fielding IR (1990) A manometric study of anal fissure treated by subcutaneous lateral internal sphincterotomy. *Ann Surg* **211**: 235–238.

Mahieu P, Pringot J & Bodart P (1984) I. Description of a new procedure and results in normal patients. *Gastrointestinal Radiol* **9**: 247–251.

Manousos ON, Truelove SC & Lumsden K (1967) Transit times of food in patients with diverticulosis or irritable colon syndrome and normal subjects. *BMJ* **3**: 760–762.

Martelli H, Devroede G, Arhan P, Duguay C, Dornic C & Faverdin C (1978) Some parameters of large bowel motility in normal man. *Gastroenterology* **75**: 612–618.

Matheson DM & Keighley MRB (1981) Manometric evaluation of rectal prolapse and faecal incontinence. *Gut* **22**: 126–129.

Meagher AP, Lubowski DZ & King DW (1993) The cough response of the anal sphincter. *Int J Colorectal Dis* **8**: 217.

Meagher AP, Kennedy ML & Lubowski DZ (1996) Rectal mucosal electrosensitivity – what is being tested? *Int J Colorectal Dis* **11**: 29–33.

Metcalf AM, Phillips SF, Zinsmeister AR, MacCarty RL, Beart RW & Wolff BG (1987) Simplified assessment of segmental colonic transit. *Gastroenterology* **92**: 40–47.

Michels NA, Siddarth P, Kornblith PL & Park WW (1965) The variant blood supply to the descending colon, rectosigmoid dissections: a review of medical literature. *Dis Colon Rectum* **8**: 251–278.

Miller R, Bartolo DCC, Cervero F & Mortensen NJMcC (1987) Anorectal temperature sensation: a comparison of normal and incontinent patients. *Br J Surg* **74**: 511–515.

Miller R, Lewis GT, Bartolo DCC, Cervero F & Mortensen NJMcC (1988a) Sensory discrimination and dynamic activity in the anorectum: evidence using a new ambulatory technique. *Br J Surg* **75**: 1003–1007.

Miller R, Bartolo DCC, Cervero F & Mortensen NJMcC (1988b) Anorectal sampling: a comparison of normal and incontinent patients. *Br J Surg* **75**: 44–47.

Miller R, Bartolo DCC, James D & Mortensen NJMcC (1989) Air-filled microballoon manometry for use in anorectal physiology. *Br J Surg* **76**: 72–75.

Miller R, Orrom WJ, Duthie G, Bartolo DCC & Mortensen NJMcC (1990) Ambulatory anorectal physiology in patients following restorative proctocolectomy for ulcerative colitis: comparison with normal controls. *Br J Surg* **77**: 895–897.

Morgan CN & Griffiths JD (1959) High ligation of the inferior mesenteric artery during operations for carcinoma of the distal colon and rectum. *Surg Gynecol Obstet* **108**: 641–650.

Narducci F, Bassotti G, Gaburri M & Morelli A (1987) Twenty four hour manometric recording of colonic motor activity in healthy man. *Gut* **28**: 17–25.

Naudy B, Planche D, Monges B & Salducci J (1984) Relaxations of the internal anal sphincter elicited by rectal and extra-rectal distensions in man. In Roman C (ed.) *Gastrointestinal Motility*, pp 451–458. London: MTP Press.

Neill ME & Swash M (1980) Increased motor unit fibre density in the external sphincter muscle in anorectal incontinence: a single fibre EMG study. *J Neurol Neurosurg Psychiatry* **43**: 343–347.

Neill ME, Parks AG & Swash M (1981) Physiological studies of the pelvic floor in idiopathic faecal incontinence and rectal prolapse. *Br J Surg* **68**: 531–536.

Nicholls RJ & Simson JNL (1986) Anteroposterior rectopexy in the treatment of solitary rectal ulcer syndrome without overt rectal prolapse. *Br J Surg* **73**: 222–224.

Nicholls RJ, Lubowski DZ & Donaldson DR (1988) Comparison of colonic reservoir and straight coloanal reconstruction following rectal excision. *Br J Surg* **75**: 318–320.

Nivatvongs S, Stern HS & Fryd DS (1981) The length of the anal canal. *Dis Colon Rectum* **24**: 600–601.

O'Connell PR, Kelly KA & Brown ML (1986) Scintigraphic assessment of neorectal motor function. *J Nucl Med* **27**: 460–464.

Oettle GJ, Roe AM, Bartolo DCC & Mortensen NJMcC (1985) What is the best way of measuring perineal descent? A comparison of radiographic and clinical methods. *Br J Surg* **72**: 999–1001.

Orkin BA, Hanson RB, Kelly KA, Phillips SF & Dent J (1991) Human anal motility while fasting, after feeding and during sleep. *Gastroenterology* **100**: 1016–1023.

Orrom WJ, Wong WD, Rothenberger DA & Jensen LL (1990) Evaluation of an air-filled microballoon and mini-transducer in the clinical practice of anorectal manometry. *Dis Colon Rectum* **33**: 594–597.

Orrom WJ, Bartolo DCC, Miller R, Mortensen NJMcC & Roe AM (1991) Rectopexy is an effective treatment for obstructed defaecation. *Dis Colon Rectum* **34**: 41–46.

Papachrysostomou M, Pye SD, Wild SR & Smith AN (1992) Anal endosonography: which endprobe? *Br J Radiol* **65**: 715–717.

Parks AG, Swash M & Urich H (1977) Sphincter denervation in ano-rectal incontinence and rectal prolapse. *Gut* **18**: 656–665.

Penninckx F, Debruyne C, Lestar B & Kerremans R (1990) Observer variation in the radiological measurement of the anorectal angle. *Int J Colorectal Dis* **5**: 94–97.

Percy JP, Neill ME, Swash M & Parks AG (1981) Electrophysiological study of motor nerve supply of pelvic floor. *Lancet* **i**: 16–17 (see also *Lancet* 1981 **i**: 999–1000)

Perry RE, Blatchford GJ, Christensen MA, Thorson AG & Attwood SEA (1990) Manometric diagnosis of anal sphincter injuries. *Am J Surg* **159**: 112–117.

Petersen I & Franksson EE (1955) Electromyographic study of the striated muscles of the male urethra. *Br J Urol* **27**: 148–153.

Pinho M, Yoshioka K, Ortiz J, Oya M & Keighley MRB (1990) The effect of age on pelvic floor dynamics. *Int J Colorectal Dis* **5**: 207–208.

Pinho M, Yoshioka K & Keighley MRB (1991) Are pelvic floor movements abnormal in disordered defaecation? *Dis Colon Rectum* **34**: 1117–1119.

Porter NH (1961) Physiological study of the pelvic floor in rectal prolapse. *Ann R Soc Med* **286**: 379–404.

Preston DM & Lennard-Jones JE (1985) Anismus in chronic constipation. *Dig Dis Sci* **30**: 413–418.

Read NW, Harford WV, Schmulen AC, Read MG, Santa Ana C & Fordtran JS (1979) A clinical study of patients with fecal incontinence and diarrhea. *Gastroenterology* **76**: 747–756.

Ritchie JA, Truelove SC, Ardan GM & Tuckey MS (1971) Propulsion and retropulsion of normal colonic contents. *Dig Dis* **16**: 697–704.

Roberts JP, Thorpe AC & Williams NS (1991) The assessment of defective rectal evacuation by dynamic integrated proctography. *Br J Surg* **78**: 747.

Roberts JP & Williams NS (1992) The role and technique of ambulatory manometry. *Baillière's Clin Gastroenterol* **6**: 163–178.

Roe AM, Bartolo DCC & Mortensen NJMcC (1986) New method for assessment of anal sensation in various anorectal disorders. *Br J Surg* **73**: 310–312.

Rogers J, Henry MM & Misiewicz JJ (1988a) Disposable pudendal nerve stimulator: evaluation of the standard instrument and the new device. *Gut* **29**: 1131–1133.

Rogers J, Levy DM, Henry MM & Misiewicz JJ (1988b) Pelvic floor neuropathy: a comparative study of diabetes mellitus and idiopathic faecal incontinence. *Gut* **29**: 756–761.

Rogers J, Henry MM & Misiewicz JJ (1988c) Combined sensory and motor deficit in primary neuropathic faecal incontinence. *Gut* **29**: 5–9.

Rogers J, Laurberg S, Misiewicz JJ, Henry MM & Swash M (1989) Anorectal physiology validated: a repeatability study of the motor and sensory tests of anorectal function. *Br J Surg* **76**: 607–609.

Roig JV, Villoslada C, Lledo S, Solana A, Buch E, Alos R & Hinojosa J (1995) Prevalence of pudendal neuropathy in faecal incontinence. Results of a prospective study. *Dis Colon Rectum* **38**: 952–958.

Ruskin AP & Davis JE (1969) Anal sphincter electromyography. *Electroencephalogr Clin NeuroPhysiol* **27**: 713.

Rutter KR (1974) Electromyographic changes in certain pelvic floor abnormalities. *Proc R Soc Med* **67**: 53–56.

Rutter KR & Riddell RH (1975) The solitary ulcer syndrome of the rectum. *Clin Gastroenterology* **4**: 503–530.

Ryhammer AM, Laurberg S & Hermann AP (1997a) Test-retest repeatability of anorectal physiology tests in healthy volunteers. *Dis Colon Rectum* **40**: 287–292.

Ryhammer AM, Laurberg S & Sorensen FH (1997b) Effects of age on anal function in normal women. *Int J Colorectal Dis* **12**: 225–229.

Sangwan YP, Coller JA, Barrett RC et al (1996a) Unilateral pudendal neuropathy. Impact on outcome of anal sphincter repair. *Dis Colon Rectum* **39**: 686–689.

Sangwan YP, Coller JA, Barrett RC, Murray JJ, Roberts PL & Schoetz DJ (1996b) Prospective comparative study of abnormal distal rectoanal excitatory reflex, pudendal nerve terminal motor latency, and single fiber density as markers of pudendal neuropathy. *Dis Colon Rectum* **39**: 794–798.

Schouten WR, Briel JW, Auwerda JJ et al (1997) Anismus: fact or fiction? *Dis Colon Rectum* **40**: 1033–1041.

Shafik A (1975) A new concept of the anatomy of the anal sphincter mechanism of the physiology of defaecation. The external anal sphincter: a triple-loop system. *Invest Urol* **12**: 412–419.

Shorvon PJ, McHugh S, Diament NE, Somers S & Stevenson GW (1989) Defecography in normal volunteers: normal results and implications. *Gut* **30**: 1737–1749.

Silvis R, van Eekelen JW, Delemarre JB & Gooszen HG (1995) Endosonography of the anal sphincter after ileal pouch–anal anastomosis. Relation with anal manometry and fecal incontinence. *Dis Colon Rectum* **38**: 383–388.

Skomorowska E, Henrichsen S, Christiansen J & Hegedus V (1987) Videodefaecography combined with measurement of the anorectal angle and perineal descent. *Acta Radiol* **28**: 559–562.

Smart RC, McLean RG, Gaston-Parry D et al (1991) Comparison of oral iodine-131-cellulose and Indium-111 DTPA as tracers for colon transit scintigraphy: analysis by colon activity profiles. *J Nucl Med* **32**: 1668–1674.

Smith ARB, Hosker GL & Warrell DW (1989) The role of partial denervation of the pelvic floor in the aetiology of genitourinary prolapse and stress incontinence of urine. A neurophysiological study. *Br J Obstet Gynaecol* **96**: 24–28.

Snooks SJ, Setchell M, Swash M & Henry MM (1984a) Injury to the innervation of the pelvic floor musculature in childbirth. *Lancet* **ii**: 546–550.

Snooks SJ, Barnes RPH & Swash M (1984b) Damage to the innervation of the voluntary anal and periurethral sphincter musculature in incontinence: an electrophysiological study. *J Neurol Neurosurg Psychiatry* **47**: 1269–1273.

Snooks SJ, Barnes PRH, Swash M & Henry MM (1985a) Damage to the innervation of the pelvic floor musculature in chronic constipation. *Gastroenterology* **89**: 977–981.

Snooks SJ, Henry MM & Swash M (1985b) Faecal incontinence due to urethral anal sphincter division in childbirth is associated with damage to the innervation of the pelvic floor musculature: a double pathology. *Br J Obstet Gynaecol* **92**: 824–828.

Snooks SJ, Henry MM & Swash M (1985c) Abnormalities in central and peripheral nerve conduction in anorectal incontinence. *J R Soc Med* **78**: 294–300.

Snooks SJ, Nicholls RJ, Henry MM & Swash M (1985d) Electrophysiological and manometric assessment of the pelvic floor in the solitary rectal ulcer syndrome. *Br J Surg* **72**: 131–133.

Snooks SJ, Badenoch D, Tiptaft R & Swash M (1985e) Perineal nerve damage in genuine stress urinary incontinence: an electrophysiological study. *Br J Urol* **57**: 422–426.

Snooks SJ, Henry MM & Swash M (1985f) Anorectal incontinence and rectal prolapse: differential assessment of the innervation to puborectalis and external anal sphincter muscles. *Gut* **26**: 470–476.

Snooks SJ, Swash M, Henry MM & Setchell M (1986) Risk factors in childbirth causing damage to the pelvic floor innervation: a precursor of stress incontinence. *Int J Colorectal Dis* **1**: 20–24.

Snooks SJ, Swash M, Mathers SE & Henry MM (1990) Effect of vaginal delivery on the pelvic floor: a 5 year follow-up. *Br J Surg* **77**: 1358–1360.

Soffer EE, Saalabrini P & Wingate DL (1989) Prolonged ambulant monitoring of human colonic motility. *Am J Physiol* **257**: G601–G606.

Sorensen M, Nielsen MB, Pedersen JF & Christiansen J (1994) Electromyography of the internal anal sphincter performed under endosonographic guidance. Description of a new method. *Dis Colon Rectum* **37**: 138–143.

Speakman CTM, Madden MV, Nicholls RJ & Kamm MA (1991a) Lateral ligament division during rectopexy causes constipation but prevents recurrence: results of a prospective randomized study. *Br J Surg* **78**: 1431–1433.

Speakman CT, Burnett SJ, Kamm MA & Bartram CI (1991b) Sphincter injury after anal dilatation demonstrated by anal endosonography. *Br J Surg* **78**: 1429–1430.

Spence-Jones C, Kamm MA, Henry MM & Hudson CN (1994) Bowel dysfunction: a pathogenic factor in uterovaginal prolapse and urinary stress incontinence. *Br J Obstet Gynaecol* **101**: 147–152.

Spiller RC, Brown ML & Phillips SF (1986) Decreased fluid intolerance accelerated transit and abnormal motility of the human colon induced by oleic acid. *Gastroenterology* **91**: 100–107.

Stalberg E & Ekstedt J (1973) Single fibre EMG and microphysiology of the motor unit in normal and diseased human muscle. In Desmedt JE (ed.) *New Developments in Electromyography and Clinical NeuroPhysiology, Vol. 1*, pp 113–129. Basel: Karger.

Stalberg E & Thiele B (1975) Motor unit fibre density in the extensor digitorum communis muscle. *J Neurol Neurosurg Psychiatry* **38**: 874–880.

Stalberg E & Trontelj J (1979) *Single Fibre Electromyography*. Surrey: Mirvalle Press.

Stalberg E, Schwartz B, Thiele B & Schiller HH (1976) The normal motor unit in man. A single fibre EMG multielectrode investigation. *J Neurol Sci* **27**: 291–301.

Stivland T, Camilleri M, Vassallo M et al (1991) Scintigraphic measurement of regional gut transit in idiopathic constipation. *Gastroenterology* **101**: 107–115.

Strijers RL, Felt-Bersma RJ, Visser SL & Meuwissen SG (1989) Anal sphincter EMG in anorectal disorders. *Electromyogr Clin NeuroPhysiol* **29**: 405–408.

Sultan AH, Kamm MA, Hudson CN, Thomas JM & Bartram CI (1993a) Anal-sphincter disruption during vaginal delivery. *N Engl J Med* **329**: 1905–1911.

Sultan AH, Kamm MA, Bartram CI & Hudson CN (1993b) Anal sphincter trauma during instrumental delivery. *Int J Gynaecol Obstet* **43**: 263–270.

Sultan AH, Kamm MA & Hudson CN (1994a) Pudendal nerve damage during labour: prospective study before and after childbirth. *Br J Obstet Gynaecol* **101**: 22–28.

Sultan AH, Kamm MA, Talbot IC, Nicholls RJ & Bartram CI (1994b) Anal sphincter endosonography for identifying external sphincter defects confirmed histologically. *Br J Surg* **81**: 463–465.

Sun WM & Read NW (1989) Anorectal function in normal subjects: the effect of gender. *Int J Colorectal Dis* **4**: 188–196.

Sun WM, Read NW & Shorthouse AJ (1990a) The hypertensive anal cushion as a cause of the high anal pressures in patients with haemorrhoids. *Br J Surg* **77**: 458–462.

Sun WM, Read NW, Miner PB, Kerrigan DD & Donnelly TC (1990b) The role of transient internal sphincter relaxation in faecal incontinence. *Int J Colorectal Dis* **5**: 31–36.

Sun WM, Read NW, Prior A, Daly JA, Cheah SK & Grundy D (1990c) Sensory and motor responses to rectal distension vary according to rate and pattern of balloon inflation. *Gastroenterology* **99**: 1008–1015.

Sunderland S (1978) *Nerves and Nerve Injuries*, 2nd edn, pp 82–86. Edinburgh: Churchill Livingstone.

Swash M (1992) Histopathology of pelvic floor muscles in pelvic floor disorders. In Henry MM & Swash M (eds) *Coloproctology and the Pelvic Floor*, 2nd edn, pp 173–183. Oxford: Butterworth-Heinemann.

Swash M & Snooks SJ (1986) Slowed motor conduction in lumbosacral nerve roots in cauda equina lesions: a new diagnostic technique. *J Neurol Neurosurg Psychiatry* **49**: 808–816.

Swash M, Snooks SJ & Henry MM (1985) Unifying concept of pelvic floor disorders and incontinence. *J R Soc Med* **78**: 906–911.

Swash M, Gray A, Lubowski DZ & Nicholls RJ (1988) Ultrastructural changes in internal sphincter in neurogenic faecal incontinence. *Gut* **29**: 1692–1698.

Taverner D & Smiddy FG (1959) An electromyographic study of the normal function of the external anal sphincter and pelvic diaphragm. *Dis Colon Rectum* **2**: 153–160.

Taylor BM, Beart RW & Phillips SF (1984) Longitudinal and radial variations of pressure in the human anal sphincter. *Gastroenterology* **86**: 693–697.

Tjandra JJ, Milson JW, Schroeder T & Fazio VW (1993) Endoluminal ultrasound is preferable to electromyography in mapping anal sphincter defects. *Dis Colon Rectum* **36**: 689–692.

Tjandra JJ, Sharma ER, McKirdy HC, Lowndes RH & Mansel RE (1994) Anorectal physiological testing in defecatory disorders: a prospective study. *Aust N Z J Surg* **64**: 322–326.

Trontelj JV & Stalberg E (1995) Single fiber electromyography in studies of neuromuscular function. *Adv Exp Med Biol* **384**: 109–119.

Vaccaro CA, Cheong DM, Wexner SD, Salanga VD, Phillips RC & Hansen MR (1994) Role of pudendal nerve terminal motor latency assessment in constipated patients. *Dis Colon Rectum* **37**: 1250–1254.

Vaccaro CA, Wexner SD, Teoh TA, Choi SK, Cheong DM & Salanga VD (1995) Pudendal neuropathy is not related to physiologic pelvic outlet obstruction. *Dis Colon Rectum* **38**: 630–634.

Vandamme JP, Bonte J & van der Schueren G (1982) Re-evaluation of the colic irrigation from the inferior mesenteric artery. *Acta Anat* **112**: 18–30.

van der Sijp JR, Kamm MA, Nightingale JM et al (1993) Radioisotope determination of regional colonic transit in severe constipation: comparison with radio opaque markers. *Gut* **34**: 402–408.

van Tets WF & Kuijpers JHC (1995) Internal rectal intussusception – fact or fancy? *Dis Colon Rectum* **38**: 1080–1083.

Vernava AM, Longo WE & Daniel GL (1993) Pudendal neuropathy and the importance of EMG evaluation of faecal incontinence. *Dis Colon Rectum* **36**: 23–27.

Waldron DJ, Kumar D, Hallan RI & Williams NS (1989) Prolonged ambulant assessment of anorectal function in patients with prolapsing haemorrhoids. *Dis Colon Rectum* **32**: 968–974.

Walls EW (1959) Recent observations on the anatomy of the anal canal. *Proc R Soc Med* **52**: 85–87.

Wankling WJ, Brown BH, Collins CD & Duthie HL (1968) Basal electrical activity in the anal canal in man. *Gut* **9**: 457–460.

Williams N, Barlow J, Hobson A, Scott N & Irving M (1995) Manometric asymmetry in the anal canal in controls and patients with fecal incontinence. *Dis Colon Rectum* **38**: 1275–1280.

Winckler G (1958) Remarques sur la morphologie et l'innervation du muscle releveur de l'anus. *Arch d'Anatom d'Histol d'Embryol* **41**: 77–95.

Womack NR, Williams NS, Holmfield JHM, Morrison JFB & Simpkins KC (1985) New method for the dynamic assessment of anorectal function in constipation. *Br J Surg* **72**: 994–998.

Womack NR, Williams NS, Holmfield JHM & Morrison JF (1987a) Pressure and prolapse – the cause of solitary rectal ulcer syndrome. *Gut* **28**: 1228–1233.

Womack NR, Williams NS, Holmfield JHM, Mist JH & Morrison JF (1987b) Anorectal function in the solitary rectal ulcer syndrome. *Dis Colon Rectum* **30**: 319–323.

Yang YK & Wexner SD (1994) Anal pressure vectography is of no apparent benefit for sphincter evaluation. *Int J Colorectal Dis* **9**: 92–95.

2

RUNNING A COLORECTAL SURGERY SERVICE

The principal aims of providing a colorectal surgery service are to make a diagnosis, to counsel the patient with all available information and support, to treat the disorder and to liaise with primary care physicians regarding surveillance, education and follow-up. The manner in which this is achieved has a profound effect on a person's attitude to their disorder, on their ability to cope with illness and on their quality of life. The delivery of this process involves the dissemination of information and education (Goligher, 1996).

PRINCIPLES

Collaborative approach

In the past, surgery and medicine existed in separate camps and there were structural, political and economic barriers separating the medical personnel who would be needed to provide a colorectal surgery service. Now, however, we are witnessing the provision of system-based medical services involving the integration of surgeons, physicians, radiologists, histopathologists, nurses and counsellors. In gastroenterology, for example, there are subunits of paediatric gastroenterology, hepatopancreatico-biliary disease, gastro-oesophageal disease and colorectal surgery.

Both in Birmingham and at the Royal London we are fortunate in having a group of committed physicians, surgeons, radiologists and histopathologists, nurses, nutritionalists and counsellors who have created colorectal surgery units, working closely with basic sciences and oncology. Some aspects of our work are undertaken in a common geographical location but our units are evolving and, as yet, are not in purpose-built facilities. There are separate ward, theatre, outpatient and endoscopy components. Nevertheless, we recognize the enormous savings that could be made if these activities had been planned together.

Having said this, it is not the 'bricks and mortar' but the people that work together to create the right environment that make a colorectal surgery unit. Industry, compassion, sensitivity, enthusiasm, teamwork and enquiring minds are some of the attributes needed to make this venture succeed. Most clinicians trained in colorectal surgery are endoscopists, physiologists and diagnosticians; some are surgeons with an emphasis on therapy, while others are trained as physicians who play a greater role in endoscopy. Within colorectal surgery we now see focused, multidisciplinary teams providing specialist oncology care, services for inflammatory bowel disease, counselling for functional bowel disease and screening in patients at risk of familial colorectal cancer. These teams also include nurse specialists (Moshakis et al, 1996), physiotherapists, dietitians (Wright and Scott, 1997), stoma care nurses, audit clerks, those involved with nutritional therapy, radiologists, specialist histopathologists and counsellors (Wiig et al, 1996), anaesthetists and pain control experts (Kamm, 1997).

The doctor–patient relationship

There are few other fields of practice where communication between the doctor and the patient is more important. Many patients are terrified that their symptoms are due to cancer growing in the anorectum which will necessitate the construction of a stoma (Bass et al, 1997). The thought of cancer is bad enough, but the concept of treatment involving a stoma that uncontrollably discharges wind and waste, that smells and can be seen, is completely shattering to self-esteem. Patients will probably be aware of the impact of colorectal disease and its treatment on sexual behaviour and function which may be devastating (Rapkin et al, 1990; Wood et al, 1990; Brook, 1991). Many also have gynaecological or urological symptoms (Farquhar et al, 1990; Steege and Stout, 1991).

Before seeing the colorectal surgeon, a patient may not only have been suffering from pain, diarrhoea or bleeding but may have had episodes of incontinence. Clearly it is unkind to treat a patient even with a minor colorectal disorder in the same manner as, for instance, a patient with a hernia or gallstones. Patients referred with colorectal symptoms, however minor, must be adequately assessed so that they may be reassured that they do not have a malignancy. If malignancy is identified, an honest appraisal of the clinical outcome and its natural history should be provided in collaboration with oncology counsellors. Most patients will require information and dietary advice. It may be necessary to trace members of a family; most patients will need some form of endoscopy involving a bowel preparation, some will be offered outpatient or day-case surgery. A dedicated psychologist is essential to assess and advise on treatment, especially in functional bowel disease but also in those with malignancy and inflammatory disease. For all these reasons, the method, attitude taken and extent of the communication between the doctor and the patient is crucial to the success or failure of treating the whole person (Ward et al, 1979; Svedlund et al, 1983; Whorwell et al, 1987; Peters et al, 1991).

Dissemination of information

Patients should understand why they may have developed their disease, what we know about the condition, the available therapeutic options and the consequences of treatment. Booklets and videos should be available on all the common colorectal disorders and their treatment, particularly on subjects such as haemorrhoids, fissure, fistula, pilonidal sinus, warts, the irritable bowel syndrome, colostomy, ileostomy, Crohn's disease, ulcerative

colitis, Kock and pelvic pouches, bowel cancer and hereditary bowel cancer. In certain circumstances videos are useful in reinforcing the information provided, particularly as books are often not read or fully understood. Today the public can gain up-to-the-minute information through the Internet. This practice should be encouraged and its impact on outcome is being assessed in our oncology patients, particularly to evaluate the impact of education packages on coping and psychological morbidity.

Teaching

Teaching of undergraduates and particularly of postgraduate medical staff can be conducted in a stimulating and informative way in the right environment. An undergraduate can assess a symptom complex, he or she can then be taken through the most cost-effective process of diagnosis using radiological and endoscopic techniques, and assessment of the histopathology, before deciding on the optimum therapy and follow-up, all in the one clinical environment. Colorectal surgeons have a responsibility to educate students from other disciplines, particularly nurses, nutritionalists, physiotherapists and stoma care nurses. Postgraduate education can take place at various levels: regular ward management rounds with case presentations, audit, surgical skills workshops, logbook-based activity, and joint weekly meetings with histopathologists, radiologists and physiologists in oncology inflammatory and function bowel disease.

In Birmingham we run courses for trainees and established clinicians. There is Continued Medical Education (CME) approval for accreditation and credentialling purposes for the licensing bodies to monitor professional standards. We also have regular multidisciplinary case presentations followed by journal clubs to keep us abreast with the latest developments and technology (Ziemer, 1983; Bartlett, 1986; Karam et al, 1986; Kreps et al, 1987).

Assessment

A great deal of treatment can be delivered on an outpatient or day-case basis. However, because not all patients are suitable for this, either because of coexisting pathology, unsatisfactory home circumstances or incompatible personality, a thorough assessment of the patient and the patient's environment is needed. Special forms have been devised to determine suitability for day-case management (Table 2.1). The patients are then screened by the day-case nursing team and if necessary are reviewed by the anaesthetist to ensure that they are suitable for this form of treatment.

Information systems

Information retrieval is necessary both for financial and auditing purposes. Appropriate software will provide a fail-safe follow-up procedure (Kjeldsen et al, 1997) and will generate information for hospital staff, the patient, the general practitioner and medical colleagues. Computer programs will provide admission dates, identify operating theatre facilities, screen for day-case suitability, code for cost and generate files for research. For these reasons, data sheets must be completed and updated regularly. Interlinked terminals should be available in outpatients departments, the stoma care suite, endoscopy, the operating theatre and the ward for updating and extracting patient information.

Much of the information required for computer purposes can be derived from a patient questionnaire, completed by the patient, a research fellow, a junior doctor or a member of the nursing staff. This provides a checklist for the surgeon, logs data for audit and ensures that severity of illness indices, ethnic variables and coding are accurate for financial purposes.

Colorectal surgery and the law

Increasingly we live in a world dominated by litigation. The principal areas of potential negligence in colorectal surgery seem to be: (a) inadequate counselling leading to unacceptable informed consent, (b) delayed diagnosis of colonic perforation or malignancy leading to complications or reduced life expectancy, (c) iatrogenic bowel perforation at colonoscopy, laparoscopy or laparotomy, (d) failure of diagnosis by clinical acumen, endoscopy or radiology, (e) iatrogenic incontinence following inappropriate colorectal excision or sphincter damage during anal surgery, and (f) inadequate training or experience of certain procedures such as laparoscopy, pouch surgery or low rectal excision. We are frequently involved, though not directly liable for postobstetric incontinence or fistulas, and for bowel damage leading to sepsis, fistulas and sometimes death caused by our colleagues in urology or gynaecology.

Table 2.1 Questionnaire used to assess suitability for day surgery (to be completed by the DSU Staff).

Physiological assessment		
1. Have you had an operation before? Specify:	☐ YES	☐ NO
2. Have you had any problems with anaesthetics? Specify:	☐ YES	☐ NO
3. Have any of your relatives had any problems with anaesthetics? Specify:	☐ YES	☐ NO
4. Have you any allergies? Specify:	☐ YES	☐ NO
5. Have you had any serious illness in the past? Specify:	☐ YES	☐ NO
6. Do you have blackouts or faint easily?	☐ YES	☐ NO
7. Have you ever had a convulsion or fit?	☐ YES	☐ NO
8. Do you have high blood pressure?	☐ YES	☐ NO
9. Do you get chest pain, indigestion or heartburn?	☐ YES	☐ NO
10. Do you get breathless easily?	☐ YES	☐ NO
11. Do you have asthma or bronchitis?	☐ YES	☐ NO
12. Do you have anaemia or other blood disorders?	☐ YES	☐ NO
13. Do you know your sickle status (if relevant) Specify:	☐ YES	☐ NO
14. Have you been jaundiced?	☐ YES	☐ NO
15. Do you have diabetes?	☐ YES	☐ NO
16. Are you taking any medicines? Specify:	☐ YES	☐ NO
17. Are you taking the contraceptive pill or hormone replacement therapy?	☐ YES	☐ NO
18. Do you smoke?	☐ YES	☐ NO
19. Do you drink alcohol? Regularly ☐ Rarely ☐ Never ☐		
Observations		
BP: Pulse: Weight (kg) Urinalysis		
If the patient is found to be unsuitable, please state the reason and refer back to the referring doctor.		

Few physicians would ascribe to defensive medicine, but all of us should be aware of potential pitfalls which can be minimized or avoided. Most would not wish to delegate complex surgery to trainees unless they can be properly supervised. Availability and appropriate supervision of emergency procedures is mandatory. Proper accreditation and continued monitoring of performance is necessary, hence a personal audit of workload and outcome has become essential to deflect criticism and claims of incompetence. Attendance at regular meetings for CME accreditation is now essential in all areas of clinical practice.

Thorough counselling and explanation of procedures must now become a part of preoperative assessment, and information on likely outcome and risks must be explained. Booklets, videos and handouts can be useful. Many practitioners regularly send patients copies of the correspondence to their referring clinician. In this correspondence an estimate of risk and likely outcome is stated. Patients requiring more information must be offered further consultations before embarking on surgical operations. The consent form should signify that the patient understands what is proposed in the statement that he or she is asked to sign.

AUDIT

Audit is essential in monitoring standards and providing information for planning future structures, resource management and education (Holm et al, 1997; Kjeldsen et al, 1997; Singh et al, 1997). It also facilitates greater links with primary care. Audit may be undertaken globally or at a local level. Total activity audits are generally fairly superficial but essential for resource management and service allocation. More detailed local audit may be undertaken short term to examine specific events or therapies; for instance an audit may be taken on the efficacy of glyceryl trinitrate in anal fissure or on the outcome of seton fistulotomy. Some specific local audits will necessitate financial information, for instance to examine the cost effectiveness of surgical treatments for bowel incontinence or to assess the cost benefits of stapling low coloanal anastomosis. Other local audits may be deliberately short term so as to provide education to other groups. This has been the case in a city-wide audit of the provision and delivery of colorectal cancer services being directed mainly to health-care planning, collaboration with primary care and reappraisal of emergency services (Phillips et al, 1984; Allum et al, 1994).

There may be more robust local audits to cover areas of particular interest, for instance outcome after pouch operations or recurrence rates in Crohn's disease. These specialist audits provide much more information than the resource management package and are important for postgraduate education.

National audits organized through training bodies regularly examine specific areas of practice. These are currently voluntary and do not necessarily capture total practice since the information is derived from enthusiasts and specialists. Subjects recently scrutinized have included operations for rectal prolapse, treatments of anal fissure and restorative proctocolectomy. They are short term but provide a snapshot of current practice.

Most local and national trials require a robust database which provides extremely useful information for audit purposes (Fielding et al, 1978; Umpleby et al, 1984; McArdle and Hole, 1991; Gordon et al, 1993; Ubhi and Kent, 1995).

DIAGNOSIS

History

A comprehensive history, paying particular attention to the patient's own description of symptoms, is essential. A brief obstetric, gynaecological and urinary tract history should be taken. Details of the key proctological symptoms: pain, bleeding, altered bowel habit, incontinence, swelling, discharge and irritation should be obtained. A family history is essential. Thorough documentation of previous gynaecological, urological, abdominal and anal operations must be recorded. A list of risk factors for anaesthesia and contraindications for day-case surgery should be checked: hypertension, diabetes, angina, chronic renal disease, valvular heart disease, previous coronary thrombosis and cerebrovascular accident, epilepsy and others. Coexisting medical therapy, especially anticoagulants, diabetic therapy, anticonvulsants, antihypertensives and immunosuppressants should be recorded. Social circumstances should also be assessed.

Some symptoms must be explored in some depth. Abdominal pain is an important symptom and the clinician will need to know its site, whether it is meal related, what relieving factors there are, whether the pain is constant or colicky, and whether there is relief from posture, defecation or medication. Duration of symptoms must be recorded but severity is difficult to quantify. Anal and perineal pain may be related to defecation, posture or sexual activity, and may radiate.

Details of bowel habit are best ascertained by encouraging the patient to provide the history spontaneously. Normal periodicity and factors influencing frequency are noted. Details of consistency, characteristics of the stool and defecatory difficulty must be sought. A history of straining, self-digitation, rectal sensation, urgency, assisted defecation by perineal or vaginal pressure may provide valuable information about the pathophysiological problem.

Bleeding is always worrying to the patient. The relationship between bleeding, defecation, straining, scratching, prolapse, constipation and diarrhoea is noted, as is the colour of the blood loss and its presence in relation to the stool. Whether blood is on the surface or mixed with the faeces provides a pointer to the pathology. Other important symptomatic clues can be gained by ascertaining whether blood is on the paper only, drips into the pan on straining or is lost as clots. The relationship of blood loss to pain or altered bowel habit needs to be sought.

Table 2.2 Score of incontinence (Cleveland Clinic) (0–20).

Type of incontinence	*Frequency*				
	Never	*Rarely*[a]	*Sometimes*[b]	*Usually*[c]	*Always*[d]
Solid	0	1	2	3	4
Liquid	0	1	2	3	4
Gas	0	1	2	3	4
Requires pad	0	1	2	3	4
Lifestyle	0	1	2	3	4

From Oliveira et al (1996).
[a] Less than once a month.
[b] More than once a month; less than once a week.
[c] More than once a week; less than every day.
[d] Every day.

Information on incontinence must be asked as it is rarely volunteered. A distinction must be made between the patient being truly unaware of passing stool and urgency. Similarly, it is essential to distinguish soiling from true incontinence. Frequency of incontinence and the relationship between it and stool consistency and lifestyle helps to define the severity of the problem. An incontinence grade that is widely used is outlined in Table 2.2. The relationship of symptoms due to obstetric, gynaecological and urinary tract symptoms and their treatment must be included.

Other specific proctological symptoms which will need to be explored include discharge, soiling, irritation and prolapse.

The interview may involve relatives and friends; some questions are extremely personal and should only be discussed on a one-to-one basis. Above all, this conversation must be undertaken in a place where there is privacy, available counselling and a relaxed environment.

Examination

General considerations

The way in which the history, and particularly the examination, is conducted often sets a seal on the entire future communication process. The patient must be made to feel at ease. The room should be clean but not too clinical, well ventilated and warm with adequate lighting, provided preferably by a fibreoptic cord light. The couch should have height and backrest adjustment, and there should be a stool on which the doctor can sit on during the examination. A handbasin for the patient and doctor is necessary. There should be separate examination and treatment trollies. The patient should be left alone to undress and, if possible, given a light bathrobe to wear. He or she must be covered when lying on the couch.

The first part of the examination should help to reassure the patient while general clinical information is obtained. The clinician should make the patient feel at ease while checking for anaemia, cyanosis, clubbing, jaundice and lymphadenopathy and inspecting and palpating the abdomen.

Position

Views differ about the best position for the anorectal assessment. It could be argued that more information can be obtained in the knee–elbow position; however, most patients find this position undignified and will not readily allow the examination to be repeated. By contrast, the left lateral position enables most conditions to be diagnosed with all except the patient's perineum covered.

The patient lies on the left side on the examining table or bed with buttocks protruding over the edge, hips flexed, knees slightly extended, and right shoulder rotated anteriorly. The examiner may sit or stand depending on the height of the table or bed. Although this position is the easiest for the patient, it is not as convenient for the examiner as the prone position. There is no evidence to suggest that position influences the ability to pass a sigmoidoscope to its full length.

Inspection

Inspection is critical and may reveal scars, a fistula, a fissure, tags, a patulous anus, vaginal and rectal prolapse, or dermatological problems (including pruritic changes). The position of the perineum at rest is noted, as is the movement of the perineum in relationship to the ischial tuberosities during pelvic floor contraction and straining. During straining a rectocele, haemorrhoids and anal polyps, intra-anal warts or a rectal prolapse may become visible. Parting of the buttocks may reveal an anal fissure. If the clinician suspects a rectal prolapse it may be necessary to examine the patient during straining on a toilet.

Rectal examination

If a satisfactory and reasonably comfortable examination is to be achieved, thereby obtaining the maximum information, it is essential to inform the patient continually of what is to be expected and what is happening. Rectal examination may be a frustratingly unsuccessful experience if proper explanation is not provided, particularly in view of the patient's understandable reluctance to submit to such an unpleasant intrusion. Having applied a water-soluble lubricant to the gloved index finger, the pulp of the finger should be placed gently over the anal orifice and pressure exerted until the sphincter relaxes, allowing the finger to enter the anal canal and rectum. The anal canal and rectum and their surrounding structures should then be examined in an organized manner. This examination should usually be combined with a vaginal examination in women.

First, the resting tone of the anal sphincters is assessed, then the presence of scars, induration, local pain and discharge. The patient is then asked to contract the sphincters and pelvic floor maximally to gauge their activity, degree of movement and position in relation to the rectal ampulla and vagina. The rectovaginal septum must be carefully palpated from both sides. Deeper palpation is needed to feel for the prostate and most rectal tumours. The clinician should then sweep the examining finger from anterior to posterior, consciously thinking of a possible lesion that might be present. The conscious thought process is emphasized because too often this phase of the examination is simply performed as a routine. In the case of a tumour, its position, size and characteristics, especially whether it is polypoidal, sessile or ulcerated, together with its depth of bowel wall involvement, mobility, fixity and relationship to local anatomy, must be recorded, preferably on a chart. Finally, as the finger is withdrawn, the presence of additional anal pathology is noted (e.g. hypertrophied papilla, thrombosed haemorrhoid, stenosis, scarring, etc.).

Proctosigmoidoscopy

The present authors almost always pass a rigid sigmoidoscope at the completion of the digital examination in the unprepared patient provided there is no painful anal lesion. If the colorectal surgery practice comprises potentially at-risk patients with human immunodeficiency virus (HIV) infection, disposable instruments are advisable. The limit of the 25-cm instrument can usually be reached in 40% of examinations and in over half of these the presence of stool does not prevent adequate inspection of the anorectum. The sigmoidoscope is one of our most valuable diagnostic tools and the rigid sigmoidoscope is the best instrument available for evaluation of the rectum. The purpose of the examination is to identify polyps, benign strictures, vascular abnormalities, malignancy and colitis. Any visible lesion or abnormality should be biopsied, any palpable lesion should be scraped for cytopathology and biopsied and in patients with diarrhoea the stool should be cultured.

Equipment

There are numerous rigid sigmoidoscopes available: reusable and disposable; with proximal or with distal lighting; with and without fibreoptics (Figure 2.1). If only a few examinations a day are

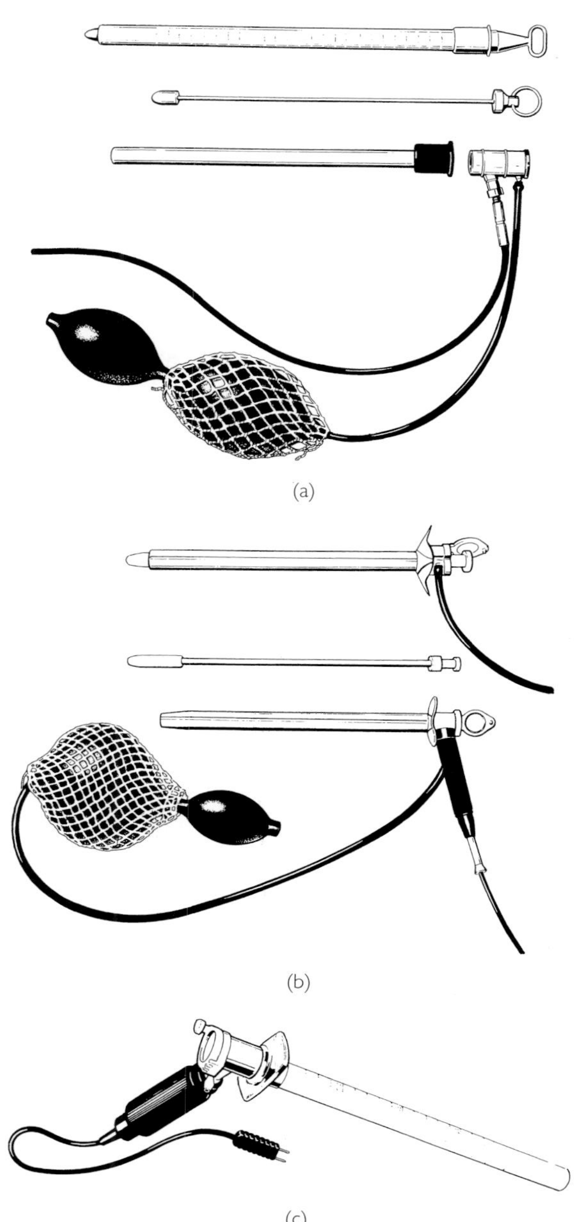

Figure 2.1 (a) A Lloyd–Davies rigid sigmoidoscope with obturator and eyepiece. (b) A Welsh Allen rigid sigmoidoscope with bellows, eyepiece, obturator and light source. (c) A disposable transparent Perspex rigid sigmoidoscope.

performed, the reusable instrument may be most appropriate. If many examinations are undertaken every day, unless one can afford the luxury of having a number of instruments and can justify the labour and expense of cleansing them, the disposable instrument is usually preferred. When using plastic disposable instruments be generous with the lubricant gel – they do not glide like cold steel.

Instruments are available in a number of diameters ranging from 1.1 to 2.7 cm; the 1.9-cm instrument is an excellent compromise. The large-bore instrument is less useful for screening because of greater patient discomfort but may be invaluable for removing large polyps. The narrow sigmoidoscope is a good screening tool and is particularly useful if an anal stricture precludes the use of the larger diameter instrument or if the patient has had a previous anal anastomosis. In addition to the tube itself, the instrumentation includes a light source, a proximal magnifying lens, and an attachment for the insufflation of air. Suction facilities should be available for banding piles and removal of liquid stool.

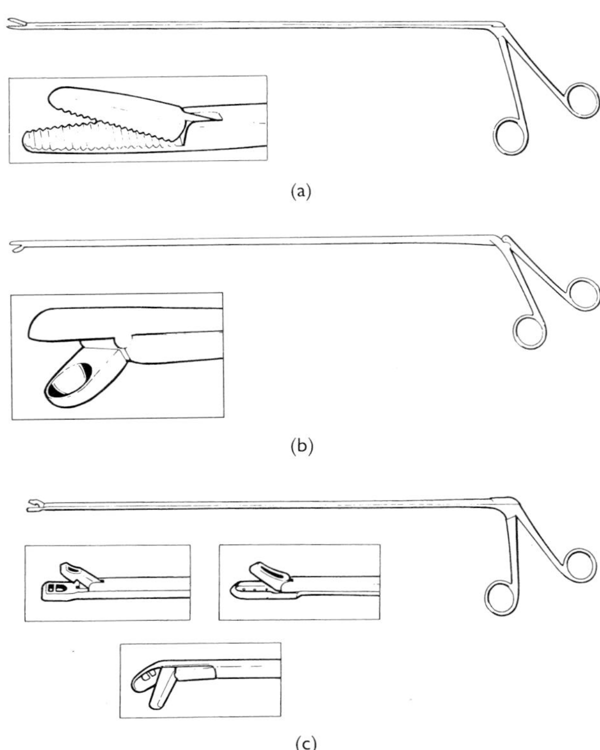

Figure 2.2 (a) Long alligator forceps used for swabbing out the bowel during sigmoidoscopy. (b) Lloyd–Davies biopsy forceps. (c) Cutting biopsy forceps (Mueller design).

Method

Bowel preparation is not normally necessary, although a digital rectal examination should always precede instrumentation. The well-lubricated, warmed sigmoidoscope is inserted and passed to the maximum height under vision as quickly as possible without causing discomfort. Air insufflation may be of value in demonstrating the lumen and is of even greater benefit in visualizing the mucosa, but it should be kept to a minimum because it tends to cause pain. Most information is obtained as the sigmoidoscope is withdrawn, when the entire circumference of the bowel wall can be inspected.

Biopsy

Various biopsy forceps are available (Siegel et al, 1983; Yang et al, 1990). Some instruments are electrified for biopsy and coagulation. The authors prefer the Lloyd–Davies biopsy forceps which has very strong blades (Figure 2.2). The lesion is grasped with the forceps which is then rotated to prevent bleeding when shearing the mucosa. Cytology smears may be prepared from potentially malignant lesions to gain an immediate diagnosis. Random biopsies for inflammatory bowel disease should always be performed on the posterior rectal wall and from the valve of Houston where possible. Biopsies should be orientated on a card with the mucosa uppermost before placement in fixative.

Proctoscopy, vaginal speculum examination and outpatient therapy

Proctoscopy

Proctoscopy allows thorough inspection of the anal canal at rest and during straining to exclude an internal opening of a fistula, a discharging intersphincteric abscess, haemorrhoids, condylomata acuminata and a chronic fissure.

There are a number of proctoscopes, most of which have fittings for a fibreoptic light source. The authors generally use a proctoscope with a separate proximal oblique tunnel for a fibreoptic light source connector. The instrument is 7 cm long with a diameter of 22 mm. A bivalve speculum is sometimes preferred to the tubular proctoscope of the Goligher or Eisenhammer design. Proctoscopes with a seg-

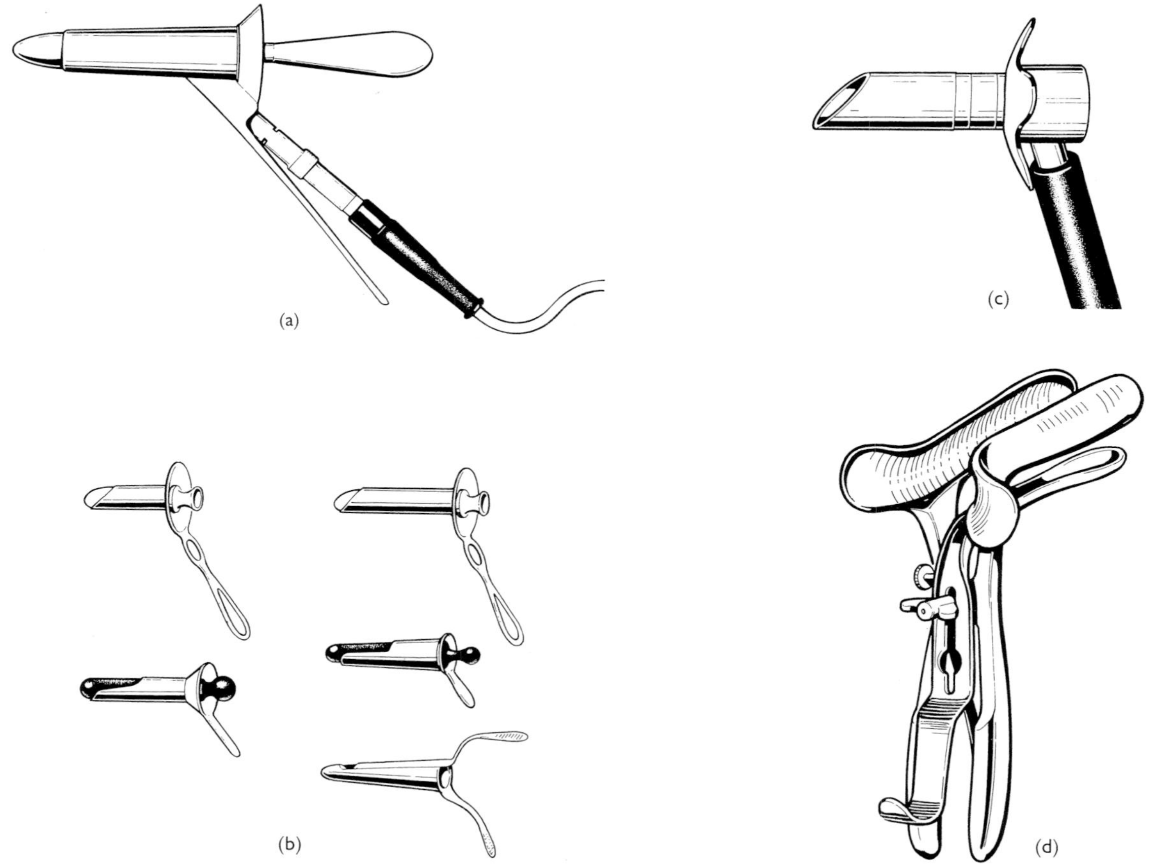

Figure 2.3 (a) Rigid proctoscope with light source of the St Mark's variety. (b) Proctoscopes widely used in clinical practice. (c) Welsh Allen fibreoptic proctoscope with an oblique tip. (d) Bivalve anal speculum with attachable third blade for intra-anal surgery.

ment removed from one side of the instrument to allow a side view of the anal canal are available (Figure 2.3a). These instruments have been used in the past for cryotherapy but are rarely used in diagnosis. When rotating the anoscope around the circumference of the anal cavity it is helpful to reinsert the obturator. The site of any pathology should be recorded.

Vaginal speculum examination

A speculum examination of the vagina is often carried out to exclude a fistula, to assess uterine descent, to evaluate a cystocele or rectocele and to swab a chronic discharge to exclude specific causes of vaginitis.

Outpatient therapy

After a complete clinical assessment, certain disorders can be treated at the same time as the initial consultation, provided the patient has been informed and is agreeable. Thus rapid outpatient therapy is eminently feasible at the first consultation. Outpatient or office procedures include: polypectomy, photocoagulation, cryotherapy, injection or rubber-band ligation of haemorrhoids, application of podophyllin for condylomata, and curettage of a pilonidal sinus.

Different organizations have their own specific facilities. Thus in countries offering office diagnosis and therapy there is often a well-equipped minor operating theatre adjacent to the office with specialized nursing personnel who are able to provide a wider range of outpatient therapy. In other countries the culture is geared to day-case surgical procedures usually not undertaken at the time of the first consultation but booked on a minor or day-case list. With the provision of a minor operating theatre equipped for colorectal surgery, the range of outpatient therapeutic options increases considerably. Under these circumstances, internal anal sphincterotomy either as an open or closed technique may be practised under local or regional anaesthesia. Likewise, an office facility enables the clinician to drain anorectal sepsis under local or regional anaesthesia; furthermore, low-lying anorectal fistulas may be laid open or encircled with a seton as an outpatient procedure. Certainly skin tags can be excised and minor operations such as the Bascomb operation for pilonidal sinus are eminently feasible.

PHYSIOLOGY

There are certain conditions, notably faecal incontinence, previous anorectal fistula surgery, prolapse, constipation, rectovaginal fistula, solitary ulcer and megarectum, in which physiological assessment is necessary for assessment and diagnosis. In other disorders selective physiological testing is needed to determine optimum therapy, particularly sphincter preservation in colitis, cancer or Crohn's disease, or the avoidance of sphincter damage in the treatment of fissure, fistula and haemorrhoids.

Physiological assessment is performed in a separate room, hence the patient needs to stay in the bathrobe and be transferred to the physiology laboratory. However, if sufficient information can be derived from measurement of sphincter pressures alone, it may be possible to use a mobile unit for this purpose so that transfer of the patient is unnecessary.

Details of anorectal physiological investigation are described in Chapter 1. The organizational aspects and available information are included here to describe the running of a colorectal surgery service. Our physiological systems were initially driven by research staff who were engaged in measurement in functional disease. Many different, often homemade systems were developed and used for research purposes only. Over the years, many tests have become essential for clinical assessment, hence equipment has become more standardized and physiology personnel undertake many of the routine investigations. The physiologists often have a nursing background and see their role in measurement, counselling, research and psychological support. There are organizations and courses for these individuals who have now established a recognized professional role with links to stoma therapy, psychology, medical physics and clinical colorectal surgery.

Manometry

Most systems are modular and fully computerized so that they can be used for ambulatory measurement, biofeedback and static diagnostic purposes. The essential manometric assessments include resting and squeeze anal canal pressures, rectomanometry with station pull-through techniques using circumferential perfusion channels, combined anal and rectal manometry during pelvic floor contraction and defecation and motility measurements in the colon (or ileum in the case of pouch patients) to evaluate evacuation disorders (Loening-Baucke and Anuras, 1984; Matheson and Keighley, 1981; McHugh and Diamant, 1987).

Electromyography

Surface electromyography may be used for biofeedback. Pudendal nerve conduction studies are used widely in incontinent and constipated patients and may help to predict outcome. Fine wire needle electrodes may be used to measure internal anal sphincter EMG activity, external anal sphincter and puborectalis activity in incontinence and in patients with evacuatory disorders. Fibre density is still used by some to quantify the extent of sphincter and pelvic floor neuropathy (Kiff and Swash, 1984; Swash et al, 1985; Snooks et al, 1986; Birnbaum et al, 1996).

Sensory parameters

Anorectal anaesthesia is a feature of pudendal neuropathy that has a major impact on function and which may help to predict outcome.

Rectal sensibility can be evaluated by balloon distension or by electrosensitivity. Likewise anal sensation to an electrical or temperature stimulus may identify anaesthesia involving the anal transition zone (Rao et al, 1997).

Evacuatory assessment

Most evacuatory measurements are now performed with isotopic techniques in nuclear medicine or by evacuatory proctography in the X-ray suite. It is possible to integrate EMG measurements and manometry as part of videoproctography, a technique that is particularly useful in assessing rectal evacuatory disorders, but there is a potentially high radiation dose in these studies which are often needed in young women. Simple physical assessment by evacuation of cellulose paste from the rectum may be performed in the physiology laboratory. Administration of markers for transit studies are also arranged through the physiology nurse (Ryhammer et al, 1996).

Anorectal imaging

It is largely a matter of logistics where anal and rectal ultrasound is performed. The authors believe that these investigations in selected cases should be performed by medical staff. Anal ultrasound allows imaging of the internal and external sphincter to detect injury, fistulas or abscess. Rectal ultrasound is available for imaging rectal filling defects particularly polyps and tumours (Waizer et al, 1991; Sultan et al, 1993).

ENDOSCOPY

Most endoscopies are planned to be performed at a separate session but there are certain situations where an urgent assessment is needed, particularly where rigid sigmoidoscopy has been unsatisfactory. Under these circumstances a disposable phosphate enema is given at the end of the examination; the patient uses the lavatory 10–20 minutes later and the bowel is then usually sufficiently well prepared to allow a flexible sigmoidoscopy to be performed without sedation in the endoscopy suite. This policy has proved invaluable in distinguishing ulcerative colitis from Crohn's disease, has helped in the quick assessment of pouchitis so that treatment can be started and, most importantly, has provided a means of biopsying a tumour that could not be adequately seen on rigid sigmoidoscopy.

All other endoscopies are performed on fully prepared patients who have been booked in for total colonoscopy or small bowel endoscopy under sedation. These patients therefore require transport after recovery from the examination.

Flexible sigmoidoscopy

Flexible fibreoptic sigmoidoscopy has developed as an offshoot of colonoscopy in order to simplify the former procedure and yet permit more bowel to be examined than is possible with a rigid instrument (Figure 2.4). The examination requires skill and patience. The lateral Sims' position is preferred for patient comfort and the examination takes 2–5 minutes (Atkins et al, 1993; British Society of Gastroenterology, 1994; Vipond and Moshakis, 1996).

Complications such as haemorrhage or perforation occur more frequently with the flexible instrument than with the rigid (see Chapter 61), thus care is required whenever the procedure is undertaken in the presence of bowel disease, especially active inflammatory disease. Minimal air should be used under these circumstances and no attempt should be made to force the instrument into the sigmoid colon. The limited bowel preparation combined with a closed system provides a potential hazard from explosion. Biopsies should be carried out only with 'cold' forceps but brush cytology may provide additional information in suspicious lesions that are difficult to biopsy. Flexible sigmoidoscopy may prove to be a useful relatively cost-effective screening tool in the asymptomatic population and is the subject of rigorous scrutiny at this time. Flexible sigmoidoscopy is not the procedure of choice for evaluating the colon in symptomatic patients or in those known to have polyps or a family history of colon cancer.

The examination requires only a limited bowel preparation. We use a single disposable phosphate

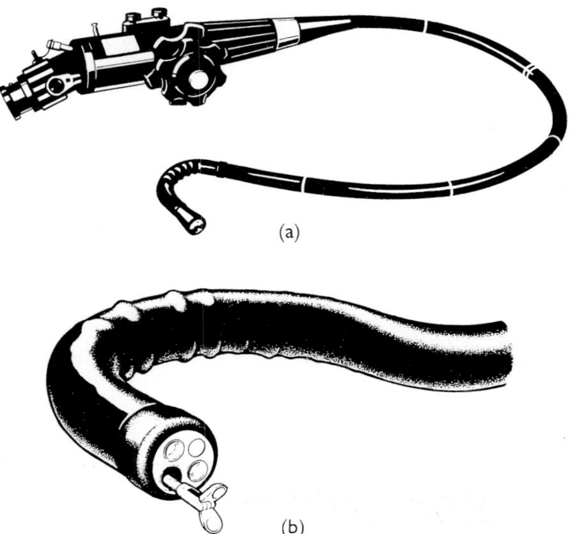

Figure 2.4 (a) Flexible fibreoptic sigmoidoscope (ACMI pattern). (b) Close-up of the bending section of a flexible sigmoidoscope with biopsy forceps.

enema. A well-lubricated finger is passed into the rectum, the instrument is then inserted and passed under direct vision. The tip of the instrument is deflected by rotation of the larger dial in each direction. The small dial deflects the tip from side to side. If passage is impeded, the instrument is withdrawn slightly, the lumen is searched out by dial manipulation and rotation, and the instrument is advanced again. Negotiation of the sigmoid colon is the most difficult part of the procedure. Counterclockwise rotation of the instrument produces the so-called 'alpha loop'. Clockwise rotation results in relative straightening of the sigmoid colon and the opportunity to advance the instrument into the descending colon. Another means of proceeding up the descending colon when the sigmoid loop has already been traversed is to withdraw the instrument while rotating clockwise.

After the instrument has been passed to its full length, or as far as is possible, it is carefully and slowly withdrawn. It is important to remember that flexible sigmoidoscopy and colonoscopy are poor tools for evaluation of rectal pathology.

Colonoscopy

As with barium enema examination, the importance of an adequately cleansed colon cannot be overemphasized. We have previously used two sachets of sodium picosulphate but recent evidence suggests that sodium sulphate is superior. Sedation is advised whenever total colonoscopy is contemplated. The insufflation of air and traction on the bowel from the instrument may cause considerable discomfort and anxiety. A combination of pethidine and medazolam is used for analgesia and sedation.

Most instruments now use video imaging which greatly facilitates training. It also enables patients to observe their colon if they wish, and lawyers may also access tapes to ensure that the examination of the colon is complete. Video recordings are useful in assessing polyp density in polyposis syndromes and as a means of comparing the appearances of the colon before and after therapy for inflammatory bowel disease.

There is an unresolved debate concerning the staffing of endoscopy facilities. The increasing emphasis on screening programmes, surveillance of polyps and individuals at risk of cancer with a much greater use of endoscopy over contrast radiology has highlighted a manpower problem in some countries. Nurse endoscopists are at the moment less expensive than medical staff. However, the potential legal implications of missed pathology even by fully trained and accredited nurse endoscopists is hotly debated. A robust risk analysis will be needed before agreed policies on staffing of colonoscopy services is resolved (British Society of Gastroenterology, 1994; Moshakis et al, 1996).

The examination can be performed by one or two persons. The left lateral decubitus position is recommended by most endoscopists. The well-lubricated end of the colonoscope (Figure 2.5) is pressed gently but firmly against the anal orifice and the scope passes into the rectum. A little air is now introduced and viewing starts. It is better to continue the advancement of the instrument under vision. The important principle is to keep the lumen constantly in view by a certain amount of inflation combined with angulation and rotation of the instrument. If a so-called 'red-out' develops and a clear view of the lumen and mucosa is lost, it can always be regained by withdrawing the scope slightly. By the judicious use of these manoeuvres the rectosigmoid flexure can usually be negotiated and the scope passed along the sigmoid loop into the descending colon and round the splenic flexure to the transverse and right colon and caecum.

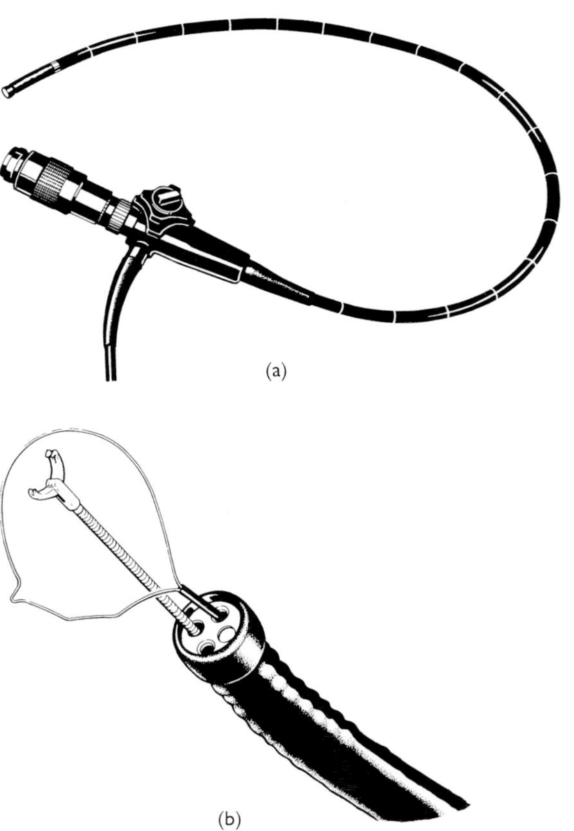

Figure 2.5 (a) Olympus colonoscope. (b) Distal extremity of the Olympus two-channel colonoscope with biopsy forceps and snare projecting from the channels.

One of the most difficult areas in colonoscopy is the sigmoid loop, and particularly the angle which it makes with the descending colon. There are two ways of dealing with this difficulty. One is to try to fix the distal end of the scope by strong angulation of it in the upper end of the sigmoid and then under X-ray control to withdraw the shaft of the instrument so as to straighten and shorten the sigmoid loop. If the tip of the instrument is then unhooked, it can often be advanced. The other plan for dealing with an initially impassable sigmoido-descending angle is to employ what is known as the 'alpha manoeuvre'. The scope is withdrawn to approximately 25 cm from the anus and the distal end is angulated to the patient's left. Then, while the instrument is strongly rotated approximately 180° in an anticlockwise direction, to turn the tip to the patient's right, it is again advanced. If the manoeuvre is successful the scope makes a loop to the patient's right and proceeds from below up the descending colon. Once the tip of the instrument has reached the upper descending colon or beyond the splenic flexure, the alpha loop in the sigmoid can be undone by a combination of slight withdrawal and clockwise rotation.

Another way in which the sigmoid may give rise to difficulty during colonoscopy is by its forming a very large loop which 'uses up' a certain amount of the length of the colonoscope and gives rise to considerable discomfort to the patient. The loop can be undone by fixing the distal end of the instrument in the descending colon by forcibly flexing it and then withdrawing the shaft of the scope. When the sigmoid has thus been straightened out, it may be possible, by undoing the terminal loop, to advance the instrument along the descending and transverse colon and from there round to the caecum (Figures 2.6–2.10).

The really detailed and comprehensive survey of the lining of the bowel is reserved until after the colonoscopist has reached what is considered to be the limit of the examination, which should be the caecum. Then, during the phase of slow withdrawal, every effort is made by bending and rotating the scope to view the mucosa of all parts of the circumference of the bowel throughout the length examined. Fluoroscopy is quite useful but is not mandatory.

There are many articles that describe in detail the techniques for passage of the colonoscope (Macrae et al, 1983; Greenstein and Sachar, 1989; Kavin et al, 1992) and the reader is referred to specific texts on this subject (Hunt and Way, 1981). The role of therapeutic colonoscopy is discussed in the section on colorectal polyps (Chapter 28).

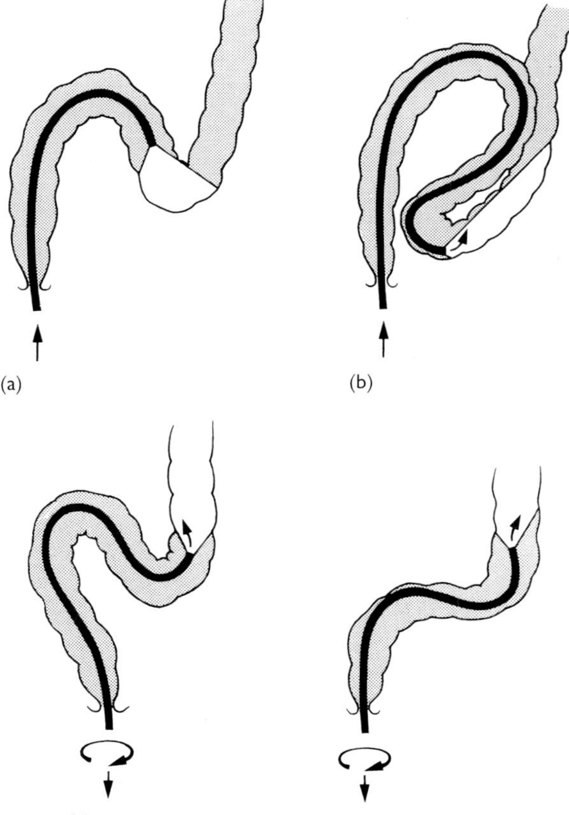

Figure 2.6 The configuration of the colonoscope which may occur at the junction of the descending colon with the sigmoid colon. Advancement is achieved by wriggling and jiggling into the lower descending colon followed by withdrawal with clockwise torque. Straightening of the instrument allows advancement into the descending colon.

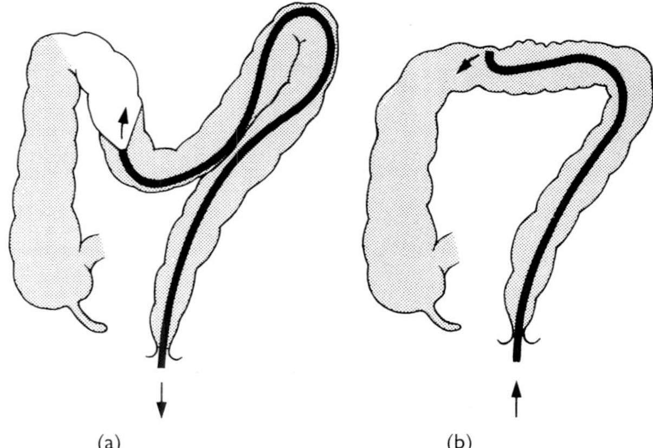

Figure 2.7 Looping in the mid transverse colon. When the tip has not reached the hepatic flexure this may be resolved by hooking the tip against the bowel wall and withdrawing. On straightening of the tip a paradoxical advance towards the hepatic flexure is achieved.

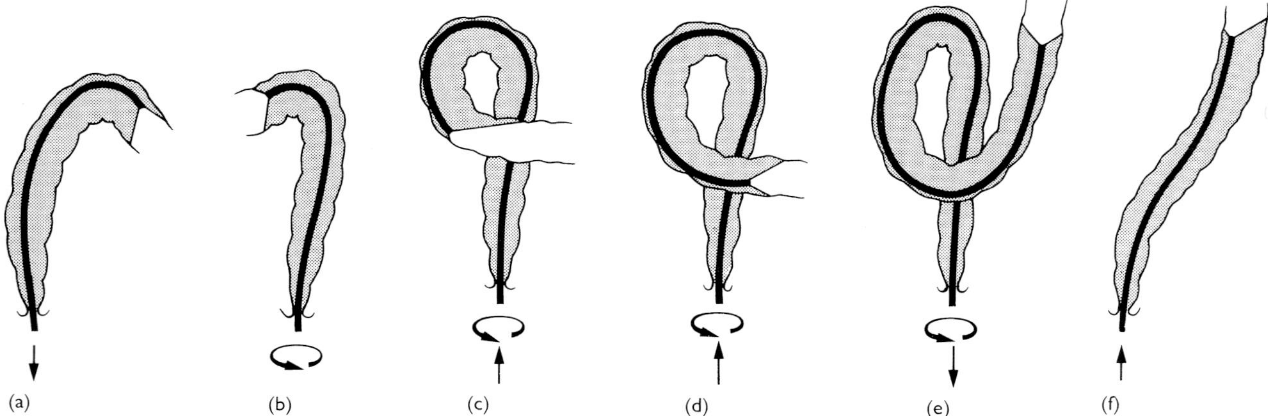

Figure 2.8 The alpha loop may be created by withdrawal of the instrument tip to the apex of the sigmoid colon. Initial anticlockwise rotation through 180° is followed by advance of the instrument with torque. Once the colonoscope tip is inserted well into the descending colon the instrument is straightened by clockwise rotation and simultaneous withdrawal before further advancement.

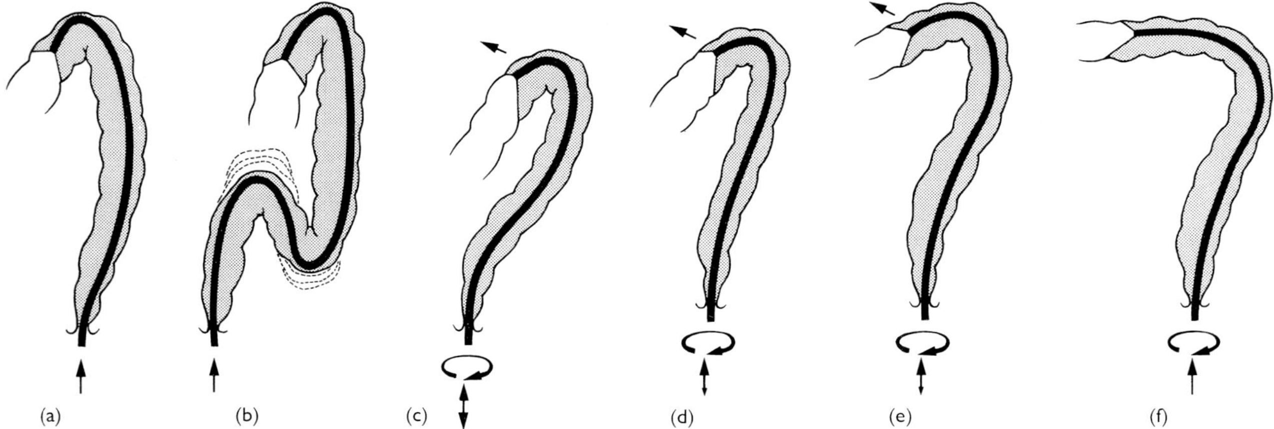

Figure 2.9 Negotiation of the splenic flexure. Insertion of the colonoscope with the tip at the splenic flexure may stretch both the flexure and the sigmoid colon. In order to negotiate the flexure the instrument is withdrawn with clockwise torque and reintroduction of the instrument. Further advance is achieved by bringing the acutely angled flexure downward with each withdrawal and reducing flexion on the tip with each reinsertion. Clockwise torque is maintained with each advance to prevent recurrence of loops in the sigmoid.

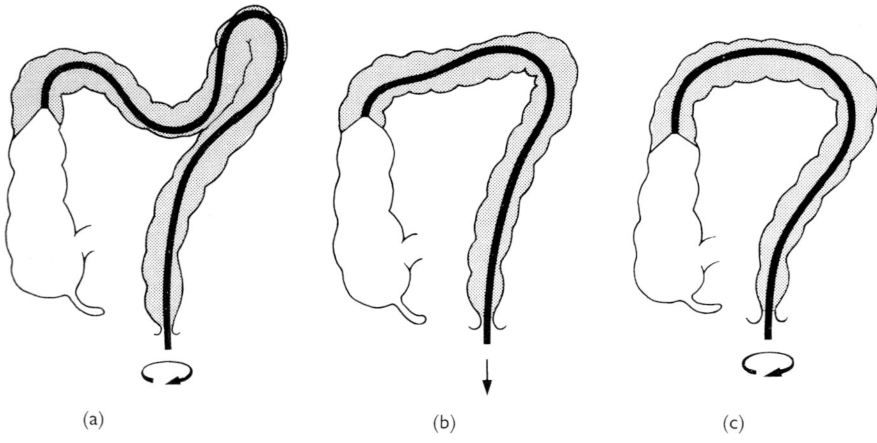

Figure 2.10 At the hepatic flexure careful steering to avoid the prominent folds will usually allow the ascending colon to be seen. Withdrawal to reduce the transverse loop produces a paradoxical advance.

Endoscopic ultrasound

Endoscopic ultrasound may be helpful in scrutinizing filling defects, staging malignancies and assessing strictures (Ramirez et al, 1994; Novell et al, 1997). The rotating probe will provide images which define the extent of bowel wall and extraluminal involvement and may provide information on the pericolonic lymph nodes (Hunerbein and Schlag, 1997).

Laparoscopy

Diagnostic laparoscopy may be invaluable in staging some tumours, identifying serosal and peritoneal deposits from gynaecological malignancy and for the diagnosis of endometriosis involving the bowel. Details of laparoscopy are provided in Chapter 6.

RADIOLOGY

Details of radiological diagnosis and management are provided in each section; this merely provides an overview of need for colorectal surgery services.

Contrast radiology

Barium enema examination is still widely used as the primary diagnostic facility in bowel disease. It has the advantage of imaging the whole of the large bowel whereas colonoscopy achieves satisfactory examination of the caecum in less than 70%. Barium enema provides hard copy evidence of pathology which can be digitized for storage and transmission to other centres. Both barium enema and colonoscopy depend on rigorous bowel preparation. Barium enema provides information on panmural pathology and is thus particularly useful in distingushing ulcerative colitis from Crohn's colitis, evaluating complicated diverticular disease and assessing the extent of malignancy. Colonoscopy, on the other hand, allows biopsy and polypectomy and does not involve ionizing radiation (Simpkins and Young, 1971; Nolan and Gourtsoyiannis, 1980; Joffe, 1981; Hooyman et al, 1987).

Small bowel enema or barium follow-through is immensely useful for diagnosing and assessing small bowel Crohn's disease, but after the first resection, barium enema is usually preferred (Herlinger, 1978; Maglinte et al, 1987; Jabra et al, 1991).

Contrast radiology is helpful in assessing enterocutaneous fistulas by fistulography or gut radiology. Likewise perineal sinograms will define the extent and ramifications of a persistent perineal sinus. Pouchography provides invaluable information in pouch dysfunction or pouch-related fistulas, but the peranal catheter should be removed before imaging the pouch anal anastomosis. Cystograms and tubograms are sometimes used when there is urinary involvement from disease or following colorectal surgery. Retrograde ileograms are the best way of identifying recurrent Crohn's disease and pathology in the ileum after ileostomy. Kock pouchography is useful to assess the integrity of the nipple valve and pouch-related complications.

Ultrasonography

Abdominal ultrasound is the most cost-effective method of detecting hepatic metastases in asymptomatic patients after potentially curative bowel resection. The examination is cheap, non-invasive and repeatable. Hence its value in detecting postoperative sepsis, pelvic cysts, gynaecological pathology, liver disease, as well as facilitating biopsy of a tumour or drainage of an inflammatory mass. Vaginal ultrasound is helpful in excluding gynaecological pathology. Surface hepatic ultrasonography may provide better definition and anatomical location of hepatic deposits.

Endoscopic and rectal ultrasonography is extremely accurate in terms of staging the bowel involvement in malignancy but is less sensitive for identifying perirectal or pericolonic lymph node metastases. Rectal ultrasonography is operator dependent in terms of accuracy. It is more useful for smaller lesions rather than circumferential involvement and cannot be used for obstructing lesions (Dubbins, 1984; Kimi et al, 1990; Khaw et al, 1991).

Computerized tomography

CT is still the best method of staging colorectal cancer, providing information on the primary tumour as well as any hepatic metastases. It is probably still the best investigation for detecting locoregional and distant recurrence, although differentiation between inflammatory reaction or postoperative fibrosis and tumour recurrence is still unresolved. Lymphatic involvement is judged on size and architecture but is not necessarily specific for tumour deposits. Increasingly, CT scanning is used for assessing inflammatory bowel disease and recurrent Crohn's in particular (Ambrosetti et al, 1997).

Cross-sectional imaging with contrast provides evidence of panmural involvement which can be very helpful in distinguishing Crohn's disease from ulcerative colitis. CT can demonstrate fistulating disease and localize paraenteric abscess, thus facilitating preoperative percutaneous drainage. CT remains the most useful imaging technique for diagnosis and localization of postoperative sepsis (Frager et al, 1983; Goldberg et al, 1983; Halvorsen et al, 1984).

Magnetic resonance imaging

MRI has a specific role in colorectal surgery. It is the imaging investigation of choice in defining septic conditions in the pelvis, pelvic floor and peritoneum, particularly in distinguishing them from neurological abnormalities such as meningocele. Thus MRI has a unique role in imaging complex anorectal fistulas. It may provide better imaging of desmoids or of recurrent malignancy than CT. MRI provides exclusive anatomic detail of the pelvic floor and perineum. Functional studies are being developed to delineate the anatomy of the pelvis and perineum in functional bowel disease. Intrarectal MRI coils are being developed for staging rectal carcinoma as well as providing functional imaging (Koelber et al, 1989; Frager et al, 1983; de Souza et al, 1996; Hadfield et al, 1997).

Angiography

The role of angiography for staging tumours has been largely taken over by improved CT, but angiography is still the best method for preoperative localization of arteriovenous malformations involving the large bowel (Van der Vliet et al, 1985; Browder et al, 1986; Pennoyer et al, 1996; Ng et al, 1997).

Videoproctography

Pelvic floor studies with conventional radiology involve quite high radiation exposure as high penetration of the perineum is necessary. Furthermore, most patients are young women. Contrast can be introduced into the vagina, bladder, small bowel and the peritoneum if necessary to provide greater anatomical information in the investigation of defecatory disorders, especially enterocele, sigmoidocele, intussusception and associated gynaecological prolapse (Bartolo et al, 1985). Videoproctography may be combined with simultaneous sphincter EMG and manometry in patients with evacuatory disorders.

NUCLEAR MEDICINE

Dynamic isotope measurements of the colon give more precise information on disordered transit than marker studies. Likewise isotopic rectal or pouch emptying provides objective measurement of the speed of evacuation and residual volume (Krevsky et al, 1986; Pemberton et al, 1991).

Isotopic imaging of bone and the liver may be useful in staging or defining advanced malignancy. Labelling of autologous blood products may help to localize the source of bleeding from the gut.

Leucocyte scans with indium or technetium can be helpful in assessing disease activity in Crohn's disease and in distingushing bowel disease from abscess.

Positron emission tomography is still being evaluated in colorectal surgery. It may have a role in staging malignancy but is more likely to be useful in distinguishing recurrence from postoperative fibrosis.

ONCOLOGY

Colorectal surgery may be a standalone subject, but there are great advantages to patients if they are in close proximity to chemotherapy services and radiotherapy, particularly as these disciplines are usually supported by palliative care, chemotherapy personnel, first-class imaging, basic science laboratories and national databanks. Quality assurance, appraisal and rigorous audit of diagnostic facilities also enhances high standards and a multidisciplinary approach to clinical services for patients with colorectal cancer (Davies et al, 1984; Jarvinen et al, 1988; Lopez and Monafo, 1993).

HISTOPATHOLOGY AND CYTOPATHOLOGY

Most outpatient histopathology is obtained from biopsies which are fixed, embedded, sectioned and stained in the laboratories. There is a small call for cryostat sections, particularly in tumours of uncertain origin, but unlike the Mayo Clinic, at Birmingham frozen section is rarely used in theatre. If an urgent oncological diagnosis is required, scrape cytology is employed, using either a serrated fingered glove or a wooden spatula for palpable lesions. Alternatively, multiple biopsies are obtained, one of which is transected for smear or imprint cytology; the glass slide is then fixed in alcohol and stained by the Papanicolaou technique and instantly reported while the remainder is examined by conventional histopathology. Likewise, fine needle aspiration cytology is used for subcutaneous, hepatic and perineal lesions (Bemvenuti et al, 1974; Mortensen et al, 1984; Ehya and O'Hara, 1990; Farouk et al, 1996, 1997).

Histology and cytopathology reporting should be confined to personnel who are committed to oncology protocols for accurate staging and who have a special interest in inflammatory bowel disease (Winawer et al, 1978; Danesh et al, 1985; Jeevanandam et al, 1987; Lessells et al, 1994).

MULTIDISCIPLINARY TEAM APPROACH

One of the most exciting outcomes of a cancer services appraisal process in the UK has been the development of a rapid access team approach for the early diagnosis of colorectal disease. One of the essential components of designated cancer units and central referral cancer centres has been a multidisciplinary approach to patient care which is closely scrutinized by external quality assurance. We have established a six-person team of surgeons supported by four gastroenterologists (to deliver endoscopy), two dedicated histopathologists, two radiologists, two oncologists (one majoring in radiotherapy, the other in chemotherapy), three colorectal nurses, two cancer counsellors, two nutritionists and a psychologist, with audit and secretarial support. The colorectal cancer team provides rapid access consultation (within a week). Visible malignancy is biopsied and staged by CT in the week; probable malignancy is endoscoped or X-rayed for diagnosis. Lesions requiring more detailed evaluation are examined under anaesthesia and biopsied on a dedicated day-case list. There are diagnostic sessions linked with the clinic manned by the team.

Each week, all the pathology and radiology results from patients seen in the previous clinic are reviewed by the team. This alerts staff to particular patients returning for review who may need additional investigation or counselling. The preclinic meeting is attended by trainees and nurses. Each week there is a journal club so that the recent literature can be reviewed.

The majority of patients with colorectal symptoms do not have malignant disease. Many have minor anal conditions which can be treated in the clinic or in the day unit. The majority of patients with these conditions are treated and discharged.

All follow-up is undertaken in parallel clinics. Thus known malignancy, once initially treated by surgery with or without chemotherapy or radiotherapy, is followed up in specific oncology clinics. The follow-up process depends on whether the patient has been entered in a national trial or not. Trials have their own protocol. Potentially curable non-trial patients are seen at 12 months to make sure there is no synchronous lesion if a colonoscopy was not accomplished successfully before surgery, and to check using ultrasound or CT that there is no asymptomatic hepatic metastases. This is then repeated at 24 months and, if clear, the patient is discharged to the primary care physician with specific follow-up advice depending on the site and nature of the tumour. There are multidisciplinary parallel clinics for patients with established inflammatory bowel disease and a separate clinic for patients with functional bowel disease (incontinence, prolapse and constipation) that might be amenable to surgical treatment.

SCREENING

Asymptomatic screening is undertaken within the context of a national multicentre trial of once only flexible sigmoidoscopy (aged 55–65). A national screening policy for colorectal cancer has not yet been agreed.

Screening of high-risk patients with a family history of colorectal cancer is undertaken through special family cancer screening clinics. Screening of patients at risk of colorectal cancer with longstanding colitis is undertaken through our inflammatory bowel disease clinic by regular colonoscopy (Hardcastle et al, 1989; Lieberman, 1990; Jatzko et al, 1992; Atkins et al, 1993).

FACILITIES

Ideally there should be a single, self-contained unit comprising an outpatient facility, counselling rooms, follow-up and screening areas, adjacent to an endoscopy suite, radiology, oncology and anorectal physiology rooms. There should be purpose-built recovery and waiting areas, a dedicated day-case unit and theatre offices, a single theatre suite and the ward. The entire network should be linked by telephone and computers. The colorectal surgery unit should incorporate changing areas, toilets and teaching and seminar rooms. The plan should provide offices for physicians, surgeons, nursing staff, stoma care nurses, dietitians and, if possible, dedicated radiologists, histopathologists and a psychologist.

Outpatient area

There should be sufficient waiting room space and plenty of examination cubicles. Separate rooms are needed to lay up trolleys, a sluice, a pathology laboratory, a linen room, a sterilizing room, counselling rooms, rooms for stomatherapy and follow-up, with a booking clerk who enters and extracts information from the computer. There should be a good seminar room which is fully equipped for teaching. Booklets should be available, preferably in a reading room with video and information technology facilities. There must be plenty of good changing and lavatory facilities.

Diagnostic and therapeutic trolleys must contain a light source, anal and vaginal specula, a sigmoidoscope with biopsy forceps, local anaesthetic agents and syringes, a cataract blade, dressings, rubber-band ligators, photocoagulation and injection sclerosants. There must be microscope slides, cytology fixative, bottles of formaldehyde, culture swabs, stool culture bottles, haematology and biochemistry tubes, as well as lubricant jelly, skin preparation and gloves.

Endoscopy

There must be a large waiting area, two or three endoscopy suites, good changing, washing and lavatory facilities, a sterilization area, a room for bowel preparation, a sluice, linen cupboards, a patient trolley store and a recovery area. Video teaching bays should be a part of the facility since explanatory video programmes are useful for those patients who have never had an endoscopy before. Reporting facilities and computer linkage are now features of most modern endoscopy suites.

Ward

The ward area should be bright, light and attractively decorated. Ideally this zone should include the data manager's office, the admissions unit and the secretarial and academic offices with a library, a small lecture theatre and several seminar rooms. There should be office space for stoma care nurses, the nursing staff and other paramedical staff. There should be a room in which the staff can relax. Hard copies of patients' notes should also be easily available and storage facilities for appliances, stationery, linen and toilet requisites should be supplied. The patients will need a waiting area and a reading room. There should be an area for preadmission registration and clerking. There should be a small kitchen and easy access to a coffee shop.

It is wise to incorporate some flexibility over the use of beds. Substantial financial savings can be made if some beds are staffed only from Monday to Friday. This provides a useful buffer for emergency admissions and allows operations to be performed on patients who would not be suitable candidates for day-case surgery. Many intra-anal procedures, complex anal fistulas, stoma resitings, perineal proctectomies and even pelvic floor repairs can be performed from 5-day units.

The main ward area will need a central nursing station, plenty of lavatories, showers, baths, bidets and washing facilities. Most beds will be in single or four-bedded cubicles. Most units need a small high-dependency unit in case there are patients who require intensive care monitoring or high-dependency nursing care. There is also an argument for placing all patients needing parenteral nutrition in a specific area. There should be close access to an intensive care unit to accommodate those patients needing ventilation or cardiovascular support. We prefer to admit all emergencies to a triage unit for resuscitation, investigation and observation; many can be discharged the following day while those needing operation or admission are transferred to the colorectal unit.

Operating theatres

There should be separate day theatre, emergency theatre and elective theatre suites. In Birmingham we are extremely fortunate in having a dedicated colorectal theatre adjacent to the ward with specialized instruments, stapling devices, leg poles, Allan stirrups, trays and a purpose-built operating table. Furthermore, the staff are trained specifically in the disciplines of colorectal procedures. There is a computer terminal in the office. Separate anaesthetic and recovery bays, stores and offices are incorporated into the theatre suite.

Day-case unit

There should be a dedicated day-case unit, which must include its own operating theatre, anaesthetic room and recovery area and have space for prepacked instrument trays, patient changing facilities with lockers, and a kitchen with an adjacent sitting room. This allows patients to have a meal and a drink once they have recovered and are ready to return home. There should be public telephones. There is considerable teaching potential in a day-case unit. A system must be incorporated into a day-case unit to provide primary care physicians and nurses with information about the procedures.

Patients should only be booked into the day unit after they have been carefully screened by the medical and nursing staff to ensure that they are fit for day-case surgery and that their home facilities are adequate for recovery purposes. A drug history is crucial, since diabetics, those on anticoagulants, patients receiving antihypertensives and cardiotropic agents may not be suitable. Patients with unstable epilepsy or those suffering from asthma will need to be carefully screened. Thus there must be a preadmission assessment unit as well as the day ward. Details of the day-case assessment are shown in Table 2.1. The following procedures can be performed as day-case procedures on selected patients: ileostomy refashioning, haemorrhoidectomy, sphincterotomy, laying open of low anal fistula and pilonidal sinus, excision of skin tags and warts, drainage of abscess and examination under anaesthesia.

Emergency admission

A third of colorectal cancers still present as emergencies with obstructive symptoms, pain, advanced disease or perforation. The outlook in such patients is poor and the facilities for rapid resuscitation, early imaging and rapid surgical treatment is often suboptimal (Irvin and Greaney, 1977; Phillips et al, 1985; Chester and Britton, 1989; Serpell et al, 1989; Rumkel et al, 1991; Anderson et al, 1992). Likewise the majority of patients with diverticular disease present with sepsis or obstruction. At least a third of all inflammatory bowel disease present to the front door with acute symptoms. A small number of patients with lower gastroinstestinal bleeding will require urgent admission and investigation. Civil violence when it affects the large bowel will also need to be managed through the emergency admission unit. Thus it is essential that a colorectal unit should be in easy access of the emergency facilities with a dedicated intensive care unit and an emergency operating theatre suite.

STOMA CARE

Stoma care is a recognized component of colorectal surgery. Despite this, the need for appropriately trained nursing personnel to supervise the management of stomas in hospital and the rehabilitation of patients into the community is still threatened by funding constraints (IAET Standards Committee, 1983; Cheung, 1995; Londono-Schimmer et al, 1994). The role of the stoma care nurse includes fistula management, counselling patients with incontinence and colitics being considered for pouch surgery, as well as care of patients with colorectal cancer irrespective of their stoma requirements.

History

Stoma care really began in the late 1950s when Norma Gill at the Cleveland Clinic envisioned a proper service to support patients who were having to adjust to life with a permanent colostomy or ileostomy. She realized that there was a need not only for the provision of a counselling and advisory service, but for a proper training programme to teach the essential skills of stoma management (Devlin, 1982). Later, Barbara Saunders and Josephine Plant established training programmes in the UK (Plant and Devlin, 1968).

Function

The function of an enterostomal therapy service is to advise patients about the management of any intestinal stoma. In practical terms this involves preoperative counselling of patients, marking a stoma site, interviewing relatives and arranging for someone with a stoma to visit the patient. In the immediate postoperative period, the stoma care nurse will be involved in teaching the patient to look after their stoma, whilst providing advice on the management of any complications and the choice of appliance. When patients are confident in changing and emptying their appliance and are ready to be discharged from hospital, they will need to know where they can seek advice if there are difficulties in the future. They will also require advice on diet, medication and skin care.

Patients with any additional disability, such as a paralysed patient with spina bifida, may need the support of the stoma care nurse in their home, particularly if there are social and housing problems. The stoma care nurse may need to liaise with the social services, employment agencies and pharmacies as well as the primary care physician and district nursing services. Stoma care nurses will need to establish close links with all intestinal surgeons, medical gastroenterologists, appliance manufacturers and voluntary stoma organizations.

Stoma care nurses have now expanded their role beyond the management of the stoma patient to the care of patients with an intestinal fistula, colorectal cancer, inflammatory bowel disease and incontinence. They are invaluable to help with counselling patients before pouch construction, resections for malignancy and operations for incontinence.

An experienced stoma care nurse will need to fulfil the role of a psychologist in the assessment of factors which will influence the attitude of a patient to a stoma, such as age, personality, intelligence and marital status. Psychological adjustment will depend on sexual attitudes, emotional stability and psychosomatic illness as well as on whether the stoma is permanent or temporary. The reaction of the patient will also be influenced by the underlying disorder, particularly malignant disease. Potential physical disorders causing management problems include arthritis, neurological disease, poor eyesight, scars and obesity (Bierman, 1966; Druss et al, 1969; Prudden, 1971; Rowbotham, 1971; Breckman, 1977; Briggs et al, 1977; Burnham et al, 1977).

Physical needs

A stoma care service will need a consultation suite, either in an outpatient department or adjacent to a surgical ward. This facility must be easily accessible to patients within the hospital and to patients attending from the community. There must be good access by public transport and parking facilities nearby for ambulances and private vehicles. Physical links within the hospital to the gastrointestinal unit, as well as to patients attending other outpatient clinics, is essential. A stoma care nurse may have to provide advice for children with anorectal agenesis and Hirschsprung's disease.

There should be an examination suite and a teaching room for seminars where local courses can be conducted. There must be a room for private discussion and counselling with facilities for preparing beverages. There must be space for patients who are waiting and space for storage. The entire area should be well ventilated with regular waste disposal and with hot and cold water. The area should have adequate lighting, particularly for removal of sutures and examination of perineal wounds. A lavatory and sluice is clearly essential. It is desirable to be able to modify the area so that patients may be taught colostomy irrigation techniques, management of a reservoir ileostomy, and wound management.

The consultation room should have a wide variety of literature. There are useful booklets produced by the patient support associations, and the pharmaceutical industry on life with a stoma. Written advice is also available regarding sexual adjustment, stoma management during pregnancy and advice for the elderly. It may be helpful to display wallcharts in the teaching area.

Records

It is essential to have some simple yet reliable way of keeping essential independent records on stoma patients. It is quite unsatisfactory to request hospital notes every time a patient with a stoma problem seeks advice. The record system devised by Devlin (1983) is particularly useful in this regard. We use a card system since this is easily transferred to the computer on which information for all our stoma patients is stored. The computer database records name, address and telephone number of the patient, the name and address of the primary care physician and the names of the hospital consultants who have been involved in management. A record is kept of the hospital registration number, the diagnosis and the date and type of surgical procedure performed. The record identifies the type of stoma (ileostomy, colostomy, ileal conduit and whether it is a loop or end stoma) and its site. The type of appliance used is recorded, with the prescription given to the patient on discharge since the dispensing of supplies is undertaken by our stoma care nurse and not the pharmacy staff. Any problems encountered with the stoma are identified with a note of their management. We also record any psychological and sexual problems associated with the stoma as well as the attitude of the patient to the appliance. Physical disabilities and problems associated with the perineal wound are also noted. The database will be needed for counselling purposes so that potential ostomates can be put in touch with appropriate patients who have a stoma.

Personnel

A senior stoma care nurse should be a person with experience in teaching, administration and close liaison between senior medical and nursing staff, both in the outpatient, ward and theatre environment of the hospital and in the community. The person concerned should have experience of looking after patients with inflammatory bowel disease and malignancy of the colon and rectum, as well as having served on a surgical unit. Some experience and training in physiology, sociology, psychology and therapeutics, counselling, dermatology, oncology and nutrition is desirable. There is potential for research. A successful stoma care nurse needs to have basic knowledge and training in a variety of areas.

It is important that the person in charge of a stoma care service, apart from commanding respect and being a good communicator, should also be a teacher. There will be a need to educate ward staff, theatre personnel and district nurses about stoma care and to run courses. Hence, knowledge of anatomy as well as physiology and surgery will be required.

It is usually necessary to have other members of staff in the team. The number depends upon the size of the hospital and its community. Indeed, it is probably never desirable to have one person working in isolation unless the person concerned does so in close liaison with other groups. Often part-time staff help with outpatient clinics and they may be supplemented by personnel from industry.

If the organization is responsible for running courses, trainees may provide some help with the care of patients but they cannot and should not be relied upon to provide the clinic services. Trainees must be properly supervised; therefore, rather than needing less staff, a training unit will need more personnel in order to provide the level of supervision and teaching needed to fulfil the daily functions of a unit. Teaching of stoma care to medical and nursing staff and attending surgical and gastroenterological courses may be required. There may even be a place for teaching in the primary care environment.

Some secretarial help will also be required, both to organize course curricula and to furnish reports and letters.

Although not core members of a service, patients with a stoma and employees of stoma appliance manufacturers often comprise important members of the team.

Emergency cover

Provision of a 24-hour service is an ideal that few stoma care services can offer. Arrangements must therefore be made to provide for patients who present with stoma complications out of hours. One way to overcome these problems is to have a cohort of nursing staff on the gastroenterology, surgery and urology units who have been trained in counselling and the siting of a stoma. These individuals should have access to the database of patients with a stoma who would be prepared to visit patients facing an emergency operation.

Ethical considerations and open access clinics

Apart from the follow-up of their own patients, most stoma care nurses provide an open access clinic for anybody in the community with a stoma. One in four of all ostomates have had their operations performed elsewhere, having since moved for various reasons to a different area. These patients may experience stoma complications or need advice. For this reason, attendance at stoma clinics is often by open access; this explains the need for a separate system for clinical information on patients, as already described.

Voluntary organizations

There are a number of voluntary organizations throughout the world that are extremely supportive to patients with a stoma. The principal organizations in the UK are the I.A.: Ileostomy and Internal Pouch Support Group and the Colostomy Welfare Group. There is also a Urinary Diversion Group (Urostomy Association). The reasons for the existence of three separate organizations are largely historical. For instance, many patients having a colostomy have malignant disease where long-term prognosis is poor. For these patients annual meetings are inappropriate since the fall-off of supporters only reinforces to the others the natural history of their disease. By contrast, the I.A. caters for young patients with inflammatory bowel disease who may have metabolic problems and psychological readjustments which they may find helpful to discuss with others. Regular meetings are therefore supportive and appropriate for patients with an ileostomy or a pouch.

In North America, the stoma associations have amalgamated to become the United Ostomy Association. This organization caters for all patients and is closely affiliated to the International Ostomy Association, an international organization aimed at supporting national societies in disseminating information and stoma development.

The voluntary organizations are invaluable agencies for encouraging early rehabilitation after operation. Much of the information produced by the United Ostomy Association and its sister organizations in the UK is of the highest standard and extremely practical, having been prepared by people who have first-hand experience of life with a stoma (Bartlett et al, 1994). These organizations also provide useful consumer audit on new appliances. They may also identify individuals who might be recruited as 'visitors'. These individuals are carefully selected and trained to visit patients before operation. All are patients who are chosen because they take a positive attitude towards their stoma and usually provide valuable support to patients who are about to face the prospect of a stoma.

The voluntary organizations provide guidance to ostomates who are seeking employment or retraining. They also provide advice on legal and insurance matters which seem to be unfair to the ostomate.

REFERENCES

Allum WH, Slaney G, McConkey CC & Powell J (1994) Cancer of the colon and rectum in the West Midlands. *Br J Surg* **81**: 1060–1063.

Ambrosetti P, Grossholz M, Becker C, Terrier F & Morel Ph (1997) Computed tomography in acute left colonic diverticulitis. *Br J Surg* **84**: 532–534.

Anderson JH, Hole D & McArdle CS (1992) Elective versus emergency surgery for patients with colorectal cancer. *Br J Surg* **79**: 706–709.

Atkins WS, Cuzick J, Northover JMA & Whynes DK (1993) Prevention of colorectal cancer by once only sigmoidoscopy. *Lancet* **341**: 736.

Bartlett EE (1986) How can patient education contribute to improved health care under prospective pricing? *Health Policy* **6**: 283–294.

Bartlett EE, Katam JA, Kreps GL, IAET & Ziemer MM (1994) National Guidelines for Enterostomal Patient Education. *Dis Colon Rectum* **37**: 559–563.

Bartolo DCC, Roe AM, Virjee J & Mortensen NJMcC (1985) Evacuation proctography in obstructed defaecation and rectal intussusception. *Br J Surg* S111–116.

Bass EM, Del Pino A, Tan A, Pearl RK, Orsay CP & Abcarian H (1997) Does preoperative stoma marking and education by the enterostomal therapist affect outcome? *Dis Colon Rectum* **40**: 440–442.

Bemvenuti GA, Prolla JC, Kirsner JB & Reilly RW (1974) Direct vision brushing cytology in the diagnosis of colo-rectal malignancy. *Acta Cytol* **18**: 477–481.

Bierman HJ (1966) Statistical survey of problems in patients with colostomy or ileostomy. *Am J Surg* **112**: 647–650.

Birnbaum EH, Stamm L, Rafferty JF, Fry RD, Kodner IJ & Fleshman JW (1996) Pudendal nerve terminal motor latency influences surgical outcome in treatment of rectal prolapse. *Dis Colon Rectum* **39**: 1215–1221.

Breckman BE (1977) Care of the stoma patient. *Nurs Mirror* (Suppl) 13 October: 1–10.

Briggs MK, Plant J & Devlin HB (1977) Labelling the stigmatised: the career of the colostomist. *Ann R Coll Surg Engl* **59**: 248–250.

British Society of Gastroenterology (1994) *The Nurse Endoscopist. Report of the BSG Working Party*. London: BSG.

Brook A (1991) Bowel distress and emotional conflict. *J R Soc Med* **84**: 39–42.

Browder W, Cerise EJ & Litwin MS (1986) Impact of emergency angiography in massive lower gastrointestinal bleeding. *Ann Surg* **204**: 530–536.

Burnham WR, Lennard-Jones JE & Brooke BN (1977) Sexual problems among married ileostomists. *Gut* **18**: 673–677.

Chester J & Britton D (1989) Elective and emergency surgery for colorectal cancer in a district general hospital: impact of surgical training on patient survival. *Ann R Coll Surg Engl* **71**: 370–374.

Cheung MT (1995) Complications of an abdominal stoma: an analysis of 322 stomas. *Aust NZ J Surg* **65**: 808–811.

Danesh BJ, Burke M, Newman J, Aylott A, Whitfield P & Cotton PB (1985) Comparison of weight, depth and diagnostic adequacy of specimens obtained with 16 different biopsy forceps designed for upper gastrointestinal endoscopy. *Gut* **26**: 227–231.

Davies NC, Evans EB, Cohen JR & Thiele DE (1984) Staging of colorectal cancer. The Australian clinico-pathological staging (ACPS) system compared with Dukes' system. *Dis Colon Rectum* **27**: 707–713.

de Souza NM, Hall AS, Puni R, Gilderdale DJ, Young IR & Kmiot WA (1996) High resolution magnetic resonance imaging of the anal sphincter using a dedicated endoanal coil: comparison of magnetic resonance imaging with surgical findings. *Dis Colon Rectum* **39**: 926–934.

Devlin HB (1982) Stomatherapy review, part 2. *Coloproctology* **4**: 250.

Devlin HB (1983) The stoma clinic. In Allan RN, Keighley MRB, Alexander-Williams J & Hawkins C (eds) *Inflammatory Bowel Diseases*, pp 262–267. London: Churchill Livingstone.

Druss RG, O'Connor JF & Stern LO (1969) Psychological response to colectomy: II. Adjustment of a permanent colostomy. *Arch Gen Psychiatr* **20**: 419–427.

Dubbins PA (1984) Ultrasound demonstration of bowel wall thickness in inflammatory bowel disease. *Clin Radiol* **35**: 227.

Ehya H & O'Hara (1990) Brush cytology in the diagnosis of colonic neoplasms. Cancer **66**: 1563–1567.

Farouk R, Edwards J, MacDonald AW et al (1996) Brush cytology for rectal cancer. *Br J Surg* **83**: 1456–1458.

Farouk R, Dodds J, MacDonald AW et al (1997) Feasibility study for use of brush cytology as a complementary method for diagnosis of rectal cancer. *Dis Colon Rectum* **40**: 609–613.

Farquhar CM, Hoghton GBS & Beard RW (1990) Pelvic pain – pelvic congestion or the irritable bowel syndrome? *Eur J Obstet Gynecol Reprod Biol* **37**: 71–75.

Fielding LP, Stewart-Brown S & Dudley HAF (1978) Surgeon-related variables and clinical trial. *Lancet* **ii**: 778–779.

Frager DH, Goldman M & Beneventano TC (1983) Computed tomography in Crohn's disease. *J Comput Assist Tomogr* **7**: 819–824.

Goldberg HT, Gore RM, Margulis AR et al (1983) Computed tomography in the evaluation of Crohn's disease. *Am J Roentgenol* **140**: 277–282.

Goligher JC (1996) Colorectal surgery as a specialty. *J R Soc Med* **89**: 601–602.

Greenstein AJ & Sachar DB (1989) Surveillance of Crohn's disease for carcinoma. In Seitz HK, Simanowski VA & Wright NA (eds) *Colorectal Cancer, from Pathogenesis to Prevention*. New York: Springer-Verlag.

Gordon NL, Dawson AA, Bennett B, Innes G, Eremin O & Jones PF (1993) Outcome in colorectal adenocarcinoma: two seven year studies of a population. *BMJ* **307**: 707–710.

Hadfield MB, Nicholson AA, MacDonald AWM et al (1997) Preoperative staging of rectal carcinoma by magnetic resonance imaging with a pelvic phased-array coil. *Br J Surg* **84**: 529–531.

Halvorson RA, Korobkin M, Foster WL, Silverman PM & Thompson WM (1994) The variable CT appearance of hepatic abscess. *Am J Roentgenol* **142**: 941–946.

Hardcastle JD, Thomas WM, Chamberlain J et al (1989) Randomised controlled trial of faecal occult blood screening for colorectal cancer. Results for first 107 349 subjects. *Lancet* **i**: 1160–1164.

Holm T, Johansson H, Cedermark B, Ekelund G & Rutovist LE (1997) Influence of hospital and surgeon-related factors on outcome after treatment of rectal cancer with or without preoperative radiotherapy. *Br J Surg* **84**: 657–663.

Herlinger H (1978) A modified technique for the double contrast small bowel enema. *Gastrointest Radiol* **3**: 201–207.

Hooyman JR, MacCarty RL, Carpenter HA, Schroeder KW & Carlson HC (1987) Radiographic appearance of mucosal dysplasia associated with ulcerative colitis. *Am J Roentgenol* **149**: 47–51.

Hunerbein M & Schlag PM (1997) Three-dimensional endosonography for staging of rectal cancer. *Ann Surg* **225**: 432–438.

Hunt RH & Way ED (eds) (1981) *Colonoscopy*. London: Chapman & Hall.

IAET Standards Committee (1983) Outcome standards for the ostomy client. *J Enterostomal Ther* **10**: 128–131.

Irvin TT & Greaney MG (1977) The treatment of colonic cancer presenting with intestinal obstruction. *Br J Surg* **64**: 741–744.

Jabra O, Fishman EK & Taylor GA (1991) Crohn's disease in the paediatric patient: CT evaluation. *Radiology* **179**: 495–498.

Jarvinen HJ, Ovaska J & Mecklin JP (1988) Improvements in the treatment and prognosis of colorectal carcinoma. *Br J Surg* **75**: 25–27.

Jatzko G, Lisborg P & Wette V (1992) Improving survival rates for patients with colorectal cancer. *Br J Surg* **79**: 588–591.

Jeevanandam V, Treat MR & Forde KA (1987) A comparison of direct brush cytology and biopsy in the diagnosis of colorectal cancer. *Gastrointest Endosc* **33**: 370–371.

Joffe N (1981) Diffuse mucosal granularity in double contrast studies of Crohn's disease of the colon. *Clin Radiol* **32**: 85–90.

Kamm MA (1997) Chronic pelvic pain in women-gastroenterological, gynaecological or psychological? *Int J Colorect Dis* **12**: 57–62.

Karam JA, Sundre SM & Smith GA (1986) Cost/benefit analysis of patient education. *Hosp Health Serv Adm* **31**: 82–90.

Kavin H, Sinicrope F & Esker AH (1992) Management of perforation of the colon at colonoscopy. *J Gastroenterol* **8**: 161–167.

Khaw KT, Yeoman LJ, Saverymutu SH et al (1991) Ultrasonic patterns in inflammatory bowel disease. *Clin Radiol* **43**: 171.

Kiff ES & Swash M (1984) Slowed conduction in the pudendal nerves in idiopathic (neurogenic) faecal incontinence. *Br J Surg* **71**: 614–616.

Kimi MB, Wang KY, Huggett RC et al (1990) Diagnosis of inflammatory bowel disease with ultrasound: an in-vitro study. *Invest Radiol* **25**: 1085.

Kjeldsen BJ, Kronborg O, Fenger C & Jorgensen OD (1997) A prospective randomized study of follow-up after radical surgery for colorectal cancer. *Br J Surg* **84**: 666–669.

Koelber G, Schmiedl G, Majer MC et al (1989) Diagnosis of fistulae and sinus tracts in patients with Crohn's disease: value of MR imaging. *Am J Roentgenol* **152**: 999–1003.

Kreps GL, Ruben BD, Baker MW & Rosenthal SR (1987) Survey of public health knowledge about digestive health and diseases: implications for health education. *Public Health Rep* **102**: 270–277.

Krevsky B, Malmud LS, D'Ercole F, Maurer AH & Fisher RS (1986) Colonic transit scintigraphy: a physiologic approach to the quantitative measurement of colonic transit in humans. *Gastroenterology* **91**: 1102–1112.

Lessells AM, Beck JS, Burnett RA et al (1994) Observer variability in the histopathological reporting of abnormal rectal biopsy specimens. *J Clin Pathol* **47**: 48–52.

Lieberman DA (1990) Colon cancer screening: the dilemma of positive screening tests. *Arch Int Med* **150**: 740–744.

Loening-Baucke V & Anuras S (1984) Anorectal manometryin healthy elderly subjects. *J Am Geriatr Soc* **32**: 636–639.

Londono-Schimmer EE, Leong AP & Phillips RK (1994) Life table analysis of stomal complications following colostomy. *Dis Colon Rectum* **37**: 916–920.

Lopez MJ & Monafo WW (1993) Role of extended resection in initial treatment of locally advanced colorectal carcinoma. *Surgery* **113**: 365–372.

McArdle CS & Hole D (1991) Impact of variability among surgeons on post operative morbidity and mortality and ultimate survival. *BMJ* **302**: 1501–1505.

McHugh SM & Diamant NE (1987) Effect of age, gender and parity on anal canal pressures: contribution of impaired anal sphincter function to fecal incontinence. *Dig Dis Sci* **32**: 726–736.

Macrae FA, Tan KG & Williams CB (1983) Towards safer colonoscopy: a report on the complications of 5000 diagnostic or therapeutic colonoscopies. *Gut* **24**: 376–383.

Maglinte DDJ, Lappas JC, Delvin FM, Rex D & Chermish SM (1987) Small bowel radiography: how, when and why? *Radiology* **163**: 297–305.

Matheson DM & Keighley MRB (1981) Manometric evaluation of rectal prolapse and faecal incontinence. *Gut* **22**: 126–129.

Mortensen NJ, Eltringham WK, Mountford RA & Lever JV (1984) Direct vision brush cytology with colonoscopy: an aid to the accurate diagnosis of colonic strictures. *Br J Surg* **71**: 930–932.

Moshakis V, Ruban R & Wood G (1996) Role of the nurse endoscopist in colorectal practice. *Br J Surg* **83**: 1399.

Ng DA, Opelka FG, Beck DE et al (1997) Predictive value of technetium Tc 99m-labeled red blood cell scintigraphy for positive angiogram in massive lower gastrointestinal hemorrhage. *Dis Colon Rectum* **40**: 471–477.

Nolan DJ & Gourtsoyiannis NC (1980) Crohn's disease of the small intestine: a review of the radiological appearances in 100 consecutive patients examined by a barium infusion technique. *Clin Radiol* **31**: 597–603.

Novell F, Pascual S, Viella P & Trias M (1997) Endorectal ultrasonography in the follow-up of rectal cancer. Is it a better way to detect early local recurrence? *Int J Colorectal Dis* **12**: 78–81.

Oliveira L, Pfeifer J & Wexner SD (1996) Physiological and clinical outcome of anterior sphincteroplasty. *Br J Surg* **83**: 502–505.

Pemberton JH, Rath DM & Iistrup DM (1991) Evaluation and surgical treatment of severe chronic constipation. *Ann Surg* **214**: 403–413.

Pennoyer WP, Vignati PV & Cohen JL (1996) Management of angiogram positive lower gastrointestinal hemorrhage: long term follow-up of non-operative treatments. *Int J Colorectal Dis* **11**: 279–282.

Peters AA, van Dorst E, Jellis B, van Zuuren E, Hermans J & Trimbos JB (1991) A randomised clinical trial to compare two different approaches in women with chronic pelvic pain. *Obstet Gynecol* **77**: 740–744.

Phillips RKS, Hittinger R, Blesovsky L, Fry JS & Fielding LP (1984) Local recurrence following 'curative' surgery for large bowel cancer: II The rectum and sigmoid. *Br J Surg* **71**: 17–20.

Phillips RSK, Hittinger R, Fry JS & Fielding LP (1985) Malignant large bowel obstruction. *Br J Surg* **72**: 296–302.

Plant JA & Devlin HB (1968) Ileostomy and its management. *Nurs Times* **24**: 711–714.

Prudden JF (1971) Psychological problems following ileostomy and colostomy. *Cancer* **28**: 236–238.

Ramirez JM, Mortensen NJMcC, Takeuchi N & Smilgin Humphreys MM (1994) Endoluminal ultrasonography in the follow-up of patients with rectal cancer. *Br J Surg* **81**: 692–694.

Rao GN, Drew PJ, Monson JRT & Duthie GS (1997) Physiology of rectal sensations: a mathematic approach. *Dis Colon Rectum* **40**: 298–306.

Rapkin AJ, Kames LD, Darke LL, Stampler FM & Naliboff BD (1990) History of physical and sexual abuse in women with chronic pelvic pain. *Obset Gynecol* **76**: 92–96.

Rowbotham JL (1971) Colostomy problems: dietary and colostomy management. *Cancer* **28**: 222–225.

Rumkel NS, Schlag P, Schwarz V & Herfarth C (1991) Outcome after emergency surgery for cancer of the large intestine. *Br J Surg* **78**: 183–188.

Ryhammer AM, Laurberg S & Hermann AP (1996) Long-term effect of vaginal deliveries on anorectal function in normal peri-menopausal women. *Dis Colon Rectum* **39**: 852–859.

Serpell JW, McDermott FT, Katrivessis H & Hughes ESR (1989) Obstructing carcinomas of the colon. *Br J Surg* **76**: 965–969.

Siegel M, Barkin JS, Rogers AI, Thomsen S & Clerk R (1983) Gastric biopsy: a comparison of biopsy forceps. *Gastrointest Endosc* **29**: 35–36.

Simpkins KC & Young AC (1971) The differential diagnosis of large bowel strictures. *Clin Radiol* **22**: 449–457.

Singh KK, Barry MK, Ralston P et al (1997) Audit of colorectal cancer surgery by non-specialist surgeons. *Br J Surg* **84**: 343–347.

Snooks SJ, Swash M, Henry MM & Setchell M (1986) Risk factors in childbirth causing damage to the pelvic floor innervation. *Int J Colorectal Dis* **1**: 20–24.

Steege JF & Stout AL (1991) Resolution of chronic pelvic pain after laparoscopic lysis of adhesions. *Am J Obstet Gynecol* **165**: 278–281.

Sultan AH, Kamm MA, Hudson CN, Thomas JM & Bartram CI (1993) Anal sphincter disruption during vaginal delivery. *N Engl J Med* **329**: 1905–1911.

Svedlund J, Sjodin I, Ottoson JD et al (1983) Controlled study of psychotherapy in irritable bowel syndrome. *Lancet* **ii**: 589–591.

Swash M, Snooks SJ & Henry MM (1985) Unifying concept of pelvic floor disorders and incontinence. *J R Soc Med* **78**: 906–911.

Ubhi SS & Kent SJS (1995) Which surgeons in a district general hospital should treat patients with carcinoma of the rectum? *J R Coll Surg Edinb* **40**: 52–54.

Umpleby HC, Bristol JB, Rainey JB & Williamson RCN (1984) Survival of 727 patients with single carcinomas of the large bowel. *Dis Colon Rectum* **27**: 803–810.

van der Vliet AH, Kalff V, Sacharias N & Kelly MJ (1985) The role of contrast angiography in gastrointestinal bleeding with the advent of technetium labelled red blood cell scans. *Australas Radiol* **29**: 29–33.

Vipond M & Moshakis V (1996) Four-year evaluation of a direct-access fibreoptic sigmoidoscopy service. *Ann R Coll Surg Engl* **78**: 23–26.

Waizer A, Powsner E, Russo I et al (1991) Prospective comparative study of magnetic resonance imaging versus transrectal ultrasound for preoperative staging and follow-up rectal cancer. Preliminary report. *Dis Colon Rectum* **34**: 1068–1072.

Ward NG, Bloom VL & Friedel RO (1979) The effectiveness of tricyclic antidepressants in the treatment of coexisting pain and depression. *Pain* **7**: 331–341.

Whorwell PJ, Prior A & Colgan SM (1987) Hypnotherapy in severe irritable bowel syndrome. *Gut* **28**: 423–425.

Wiig JN, Berner A, Tveit KM & Giercksky EK (1996) Evaluation of digitally guided fine needle aspiration cytology versus fine needle core biopsy for the diagnosis of recurrent rectal cancer. *Int J Colorect Dis* **11**: 272–275.

Winawer SJ, Leidner SD, Hajdu SI & Sherlock P (1978) Colonoscopic biopsy and cytology in the diagnosis of colon cancer. *Cancer* **42**: 2849–2853.

Wood DP, Wiesner MG & Reiter RC (1990) Psychogenic chronic pelvic pain: diagnosis and management. *Clin Obstet Gynecol* **33**: 179–195.

Wright N & Scott BB (1997) Dietary treatment of active Crohn's disease. *BMJ* **314**: 454–455.

Yang R, Vuitch F, Wright K & McCarthy J (1990) Adequacy of disposable biopsy forceps for gastrointestinal endoscopy: a direct comparison with reusable forceps. *Gastrointest Endosc* **36**: 379–381.

Ziemer MM (1983) Effects of information on postsurgical patient coping. *Nurs Res* **32**: 282–287.

3 MECHANICAL BOWEL PREPARATION

It is necessary to clear the colon and rectum of faecal material for the diagnosis and treatment of many large bowel disorders, but requirements often differ. Radiologists prefer a dry mucosa to allow adequate mucosal coating by barium, whereas the colonoscopist is able to aspirate clear fluid and a dry mucosa is therefore not a necessity. If endoscopic or surgical therapy is planned, other factors besides the elimination of faecal material must be considered: these include fluid and electrolyte homeostasis or the risk of explosion if electrocautery is to be used.

Obstructing lesions have a profound influence on the requirements of mechanical preparation. Although the majority of patients requiring barium enema examination or colonoscopy do not have obstructing lesions, surgical patients often do. There are certain situations in which vigorous mechanical bowel preparation should be avoided because of the risk of perforation or the exacerbation of dormant sepsis. In some patients bowel preparation usually will not succeed, for instance in gross megarectum with a faecaloma. It is argued by some that bowel preparation is not necessary in patients having a proctocolectomy where the entire large bowel is being removed without an anastomosis. Finally, there are a few patients in whom preoperative preparation may be impossible, as in patients with complete obstruction or active bleeding in whom intraoperative techniques may have to be used.

Some authors have challenged the need and even the desirability of bowel preparation for colorectal resection. Hughes (1972), for instance, claimed that risks of sepsis and anastomotic breakdown were no greater in the unprepared bowel than after bowel preparation. His view that solid stool was less dangerous than liquid bowel contents after bowel preparation held little support however until recently, when conventional bowel preparation was again challenged by Irving and Scrimgeour (1987), who concluded that it was not necessary. Two recent randomized trials comparing outcomes with and without bowel preparation came to the same conclusion. Santos et al (1994) in a study from Brazil used a phenothallin laxative or nothing in patients with a high incidence of Chagas' disease and malignancy. They showed that complications were more common in the bowel preparation group (Table 3.1). In Ireland, Burke et al (1994) reported on a trial of Picolax against no preparation and showed no difference in outcome even in patients undergoing anterior resection (Table 3.2). They concluded that bowel preparation does not influence outcome.

Despite this, most colorectal surgeons use bowel preparation and in the majority of patients there is minimal contamination from liquid stool (Lee et al, 1996). The majority of colorectal surgeons still believe that contamination results in an increased risk of sepsis, that there are fewer defunctioning stomas after successful bowel preparation for low rectal anastomosis and that bowel management is easier postoperatively (Wolters et al, 1994; Oliveira et al, 1997).

Table 3.1 Impact of any bowel preparation on outcome of colorectal surgery.

	Mechanical bowel preparation (laxatives) (*n* = 72)	*No mechanical bowel preparation* (*n* = 77)
Total number of patients with complications	21 (29%)	11 (14%)
Total number with anastomotic dehiscence	7 (10%)	4 (5%)
Surgical management	4	1
Conservative management	3	3
Total number with wound sepsis	17 (24%)	9 (12%)

From Santos et al (1994).

Table 3.2 Impact of bowel preparation on outcome of colorectal surgery.

	Bowel preparation (*n* = 82)	*No bowel preparation* (*n* = 87)
Deaths	2	0
Complications		
Cardiorespiratory	8	9
Wound sepsis	4	3
Anastomotic dehiscence	3	4

From Burke et al (1994).

AIMS

Indications

Bowel preparation is always used for barium enema examinations, over 3 million of which are performed per annum in the USA (National Center for Health Statistics, 1973). Preparation of the large bowel is necessary for colonoscopy and the number of examinations for diagnostic or therapeutic purposes is increasing annually (Hunt and Way, 1981). Distal preparation of the rectosigmoid region is necessary for flexible sigmoidoscopy, and some clinicians feel that an enema, with or without a rectal washout, is desirable for rigid sigmoidoscopy.

In the surgical treatment of large bowel malignancy it is desirable to utilize preoperative measures which will reduce morbidity; good quality bowel preparation is one of these (American Cancer Society, 1973; Miller, 1975a; Turnbull, 1975). Vigorous mechanical preparation is not always indicated or desirable in acute inflammatory bowel disease, but bowel preparation is used by most surgeons in patients with chronic disease requiring elective restorative resection (Barker et al, 1971; Allan et al, 1983; Allan and Keighley, 1988).

Some patients require forms of bowel preparation such as enemata for the management of incontinence or chronic constipation (Dresen and Kratzer, 1959; Woo et al, 1976; Smith and Currie, 1978).

Bowel preparation in diagnosis

A clean colon is crucial to the accuracy of diagnosis in large bowel disorders (Miller, 1976). Eyler (1973) believes that 75% of the tumours missed during barium enema examination are due to excessive faecal residue. In view of the slow growth of many of these tumours (Welin et al, 1963; Ekelund et al, 1974; Morson, 1974), any malignant tumour identified in the large bowel within 3 years of a 'normal' barium enema must be regarded as a missed lesion (Figiel et al, 1965). A good barium enema examination should be able to detect 98% of the polyps identified by colonoscopy (Williams et al, 1974) but this can only be achieved by meticulous bowel preparation (Welin, 1958, 1967; Lee et al, 1981; Keighley, 1982). The medicolegal consequences of a missed malignant lesion are well known and, as up to 20% of lesions may not be seen on double contrast radiology, the number of colonoscopy examinations has risen considerably, and with it a more critical appraisal of bowel preparation (Saunders and MacEwen, 1971; Williams et al, 1974; Ernstoff et al, 1983; Kohler et al, 1990; Adams et al, 1994; Cohen et al, 1994; Berry and DiPalma, 1994; Golub et al, 1995).

Bowel preparation prior to therapy

Bowel preparation is practised by most surgeons performing elective operations in the belief that sepsis and anastomotic breakdown may be minimized by operating on an empty colon (Nichols and Condon, 1971). However, as discussed above, this concept has been challenged in recent years (Irving and Scrimgeour, 1987) and the evidence that leak rates and infection are reduced by successful bowel preparation is contradictory. Before assuming that mechanical bowel preparation is desirable, the impact of bowel preparation on infections, anastomotic dehiscence and safety must be assessed critically.

Reducing the risk of sepsis

Although it is assumed that a clean colon is associated with a significant reduction in sepsis, the evidence that this is true among patients having mechanical preparation alone, without antibiotic cover, is lacking (Burton, 1973). If an efficient method of bowel preparation is used with antibiotic cover, the quality of bowel preparation is an independent variable in reducing sepsis (Morris et al, 1983). There are some forms of mechanical bowel preparation, such as the oligosaccharide mannitol, that may increase the risk of sepsis (Hares et al, 1981a). Nevertheless there is now substantial evidence that efficient mechanical bowel preparation will protect against the risk of sepsis if it is combined with some form of systemic antibiotic cover (Chung et al, 1979; Gottrup et al, 1985; Panton et al, 1985; Raahave et al, 1986). In this regard, oral whole bowel irrigation or nasogastric irrigation is not necessarily superior to traditional forms of preparation in minimizing sepsis (Christensen and Kronberg, 1981; Fleites et al, 1985).

Reducing the risk of anastomotic breakdown

There is also evidence that the quality of mechanical bowel preparation is closely related to anastomotic dehiscence (Goligher et al, 1970; Rosenberg et al, 1971). Irvin and Goligher (1973), in their retrospective review of 204 hand-sutured large bowel anastomoses, showed that the most powerful determinant of anastomotic leakage was the quality of mechanical bowel preparation. There were nine leaks from 116 anastomoses when mechanical preparation was of good quality (8%), compared with 19 leaks from 59 anastomoses when faecal residue was present at the operation (32%). Morris et al (1983) reported anastomotic leaks or perianastomotic abscess in 1 of 76 patients who had a good bowel preparation compared with 6 of 13 in those in whom there was gross faecal residue in the colon. Similar observations have been made by others (Schrock et al, 1973; Walls, 1980; Christensen and Kronberg, 1981). Animal studies indicate that the bursting pressure at a colonic anastomosis is reduced if there is increased faecal residue (Smith et al, 1983; O'Dwyer et al, 1989), possibly due to increased collagenase activity (Hawley et al, 1970; Ryan, 1970).

Safety

It is obviously important that mechanical bowel preparation is safe and does not cause unnecessary discomfort or anxiety to the patient. Serious changes in body composition and acid–base balance, which are potentially dangerous to elderly patients and those with cardiac, renal or hepatic disease, are now recognized as occurring with certain forms of preparations. These will be discussed later. Vigorous mechanical bowel preparation may occasionally be complicated by perforation and bacteraemia, hence the use of bowel preparation should be avoided in acute colitis and possibly in patients with a localized pericolic abscess (Galloway et al, 1982).

AVAILABLE METHODS

Development of bowel preparation

The need for some method of bowel preparation became recognized soon after the introduction of colonic resection rather than colostomy for the management of large bowel disease (Reybar, 1844; Wilkie, 1938). In the past, clinicians relied upon a period of starvation (allowing liquids only for 4–5 days), purgation (usually with magnesium salts), enemata and rectal washouts (Rogers, 1971; Miller, 1975b).

During the 1970s and 1980s new techniques were introduced, largely to improve patient compliance and reduce the length of preoperative hospital stay, or even to allow preparation at home before elective surgery (Huddy et al, 1990; Lee et al, 1996). These developments have included elemental diets, whole bowel irrigation and methods which dispense with enemas and rectal washouts altogether. Lee and others (1996) compared preparation at home with conventional preparation in hospital using polyethylene glycol electrolyte solution or sodium phosphate. They reported comparable quality of preparation and reduced hospital stay in the home preparation group but emphasized the importance of increased preoperative fluid requirements after preparation.

Traditional methods

Traditional bowel preparation, which involves starvation, purgation, enemata and washouts, is time consuming, exhausting to the patient and demanding on nursing time, requiring supervision for 5–7 days before operation (Duthie et al, 1990; Santos et al, 1994).

Food intake is discontinued for a variable period. Patients are encouraged to drink plenty, both to avoid dehydration and to overcome the feeling of hunger (Binder, 1977; Fingl and Freston, 1979). To avoid faecal residue, only clear fluids should be consumed since low-residue diets result in the production of some faeces (Winitz et al, 1966; Cooney et al, 1974; Johnson, 1974). Milk products should not be allowed and oral iron therapy must be discontinued (Teague and Manning, 1977). This form of preparation is clearly unsuitable for diabetics.

A variety of purgatives have been employed. They may be used once, in a large dose, or repeatedly. Magnesium salts have been used extensively in the past. These reduce sodium and water absorption and produce some secretion into the lumen of the small bowel, hence a large-volume hyperosmolar fluid load is presented to the caecum. Consequently, although magnesium salts produce excellent clearance of the right colon, they cause considerable abdominal colic (Forth et al, 1972; Jauch et al, 1975). The dose of magnesium sulphate varies from 5 to 15 g; in some institutions 10 mg is given 2-hourly on the day before operation. Magnesium citrate causes less colic and is usually effective using only two 13 g doses. Sodium sulphate has a similar action to magnesium citrate and inhibits sodium reabsorption (Tsang et al, 1992).

Senna compounds are activated by colonic bacteria and have no laxative effect until they reach the large bowel, hence their clearance of the right colon is inferior to that achieved with magnesium salts (Hardcastle and Wilkins, 1970). Senna also causes vigorous mass contractions in the colon which result in some discomfort (Laurence, 1973). Sodium picosulphate (10 mg), which is often given with magnesium citrate (Picolax), is another purgative whose action depends on bacterial activation. The anthraquinones such as bisacodyl or oxyphenisatin may be given orally and are also activated by colonic bacteria. They may be given rectally as a stimulant enema.

Castor oil may be used as a stool softener (Levy et al, 1976; Beck et al, 1985) in a dose of 45 mL on the evening before operation, with saline enemata and a fluid diet (Margulis, 1967; Barnes, 1968; Irwin et al, 1974). Alternatives to castor oil include dioctyl sodium sulphosuccinate (100 mg 8-hourly for 3–4 days prior to the enemata) and washouts.

Most traditional preparations conclude with enemata and a washout. Saline enemata are said to cause less electrolyte disturbance than tapwater or soap enemata (Turrell and Landau, 1959; Tyson and Spaulding, 1959; Mikal, 1965). Phosphate or bisacodyl enemata stimulate mass contraction of the rectosigmoid. Corman (1984) considers that the tapwater enema is the most important part of bowel preparation and should be continued until the returns are completely clear. The most aggressive form of distal clearance is by the Henderson or Suda irrigating machines or using pulsed irrigation evacuation (Kokoszka et al, 1994). Like most forms of distal preparation, the quality is largely determined by the commitment of the nurse. Both De Lacey et al (1982) and Lee and Ferrando (1984) came to the conclusion that these forms of rectal washout had no influence on quality of preparation for barium enema. Furthermore, rectal washout produced a wet colon which resulted in poor mucosal coating by barium.

Elemental diets

Elemental diets maintain nitrogen balance and reduce faecal residue (Gurry and Ellis-Pegler, 1976); however, they must be used for at least 5–7 days and some method of distal preparation is essential to clear residue from the large bowel. If elemental diets are used without enemata or washouts the quality of preparation is very poor (Matheson et al, 1978; Keighley, 1982). Most patients find elemental diets unpalatable when taken by mouth and although delivery can be achieved via a fine bore nasogastric tube, most patients do not like tubes passed before operation.

The vogue of using elemental diets for mechanical bowel preparation seems to be over (Winitz et al, 1965, 1970; Atterbery et al, 1972; Crowther et al, 1973; Glotzer et al, 1973; Bounnos and Devroede, 1974). In our view the only possible role for elemental diets is in a malnourished patient with a stenosing tumour or an inflammatory mass in whom vigorous bowel preparation may precipitate obstruction or sepsis.

Nasogastric whole bowel irrigation

Irrigation of the bowel with an electrolyte solution was first proposed for the treatment of cholera (Hewitt et al, 1973) and for the investigation of bidirectional ionic flux in the colon (Love et al, 1968). The technique was subsequently modified as a method of bowel preparation. The procedure involves passing a fine nasogastric tube. An intravenous dose of metoclopramide may be given to minimize nausea and vomiting and to accelerate gastric emptying (Crapp et al, 1975). Advancement of the tube through the pylorus into the duodenum does not alleviate abdominal distension and nausea (Christensen and Kronberg, 1981).

The irrigation solution does not have to be sterile: Walls (1980) recommended adding 90 g of salt to 10 L of tapwater. The solution should be warmed to room temperature and infused at a constant rate using a roller pump. After about 30 minutes the patient usually wants to defecate and should then be seated on a commode. Preparation should be in a separate room with some form of call device connected to the nursing station. The preparation should not be terminated until completely clear fluid has been passed for at least half an hour. It is usually necessary to infuse 10–12 L of fluid and the procedure takes between 4 and 6 hours. If nothing is passed after one hour, if the patient's abdomen becomes distended or if there is repeated vomiting, the infusion should be stopped. Sometimes the usual response is merely delayed but in some patients the procedure must be abandoned for fear of causing obstruction.

Not surprisingly, patients do not like this form of bowel preparation. They often express fear and complain of fatigue and embarrassment. Despite the use of metoclopramide, nausea and vomiting are frequent side-effects. Above all, patients hate the passage of a nasogastric tube (Downing et al, 1979). Nevertheless whole bowel irrigation still provides high quality of bowel preparation. A recent study, however, failed to demonstrate superior results over polyethylene glycol electrolyte solution or sodium phosphate with bisacodyl (Wolters et al, 1994).

An advantage of the technique is that enemata, washouts and dietary restriction are unnecessary and the preparation can be completed on the day before operation.

Electrolyte solution

Originally, isotonic saline was used for irrigation (Hewitt et al, 1973), but it consistently caused fluid and sodium retention and was contraindicated in elderly patients with renal, cardiac or hepatic failure unless used with frusemide (Crapp et al, 1975). The infusion also caused a loss of potassium and the use of a diuretic further increased the risk of hypokalaemia. Hence Gilmore et al (1981) recommended a solution containing less sodium (125 mmol/L) but including potassium and bicarbonate. Ringer's lactate was therefore recommended by those still enthusiastic about the technique (Wolters et al, 1994), but water retention of between 1 and 8 L is a serious complication in patients with cardiac or renal disease and should not be used.

Electrolyte solution and osmotic agents

Combining an osmotic agent with saline irrigation reduced the volume required to achieve an empty colon (Donovan et al, 1980). Furthermore, the fluid and sodium retention which accompanied saline lavage alone was eliminated when an osmotic agent was used before the saline irrigation (Minervini et al, 1980). A balanced electrolyte solution with polyethylene glycol as an osmotic agent was developed and achieved an excellent quality of mechanical preparation with only 4–5 L of fluid, so that the procedure could be completed in 2–3 hours without disturbance of fluid or electrolyte balance (Ambrose et al, 1983).

Nasogastric whole bowel irrigation using an osmotic agent and a balanced electrolyte solution is still an excellent method of preparing the colon (Kohler et al, 1990). It is certainly better than traditional bowel preparation (Christensen and Kronberg, 1981) but the method is disliked by most patients. Furthermore, the technique is contraindicated in acute colitis, in megarectum with gross constipation and in obstructing tumours of the large bowel. An alternative approach which reduces the duration of preparation is to use Picolax before whole gut irrigation (Grace, 1988).

Oral whole bowel irrigation

Electrolyte solution

The principal objection to whole bowel irrigation has been the use of a nasogastric tube. For this reason, Levy et al (1976) proposed the use of an electrolyte solution by mouth but patients found it extremely nauseating and four of 37 patients could not complete the preparation. Not surprisingly, patients also complained of abdominal fullness, but found oral irrigation less of an ordeal than traditional preparation.

Osmotic agents

Newstead and Morgan (1979) introduced the concept of drinking an osmotic agent. They chose the oligosaccharide mannitol since it was not absorbed or digested during rapid transit through the small bowel, thereby achieving an osmotic catharsis (Hindle and Code, 1962; Nasrullah and Iber, 1969; Kreel, 1975; Nagy, 1981). Mannitol, although rather sweet, was in fact well tolerated if served chilled with peppermint flavouring or with fruit juice. However, it soon became apparent that mannitol was associated with dehydration and sodium loss (Gilmore et al, 1981). There were also reports of occasional fatal explosion with mannitol bowel preparation, probably due to methane production as a result of its fermentation by *Escherichia coli* (Bigarde et al, 1979; Keighley et al, 1981; Taylor et al, 1981; Zanoni et al, 1982). Mannitol was therefore discontinued.

Electrolyte solution and osmotic agents

Gilmore et al (1981) suggested that if osmotic agents were combined with an electrolyte solution there should be no fluid and electrolyte disturbance. A formulation which used sodium sulphate rather than sodium chloride was therefore developed (Davis et al, 1980). Sulphate inhibits sodium reabsorption, thereby minimizing the risk of sodium and water retention. The mannitol was replaced by polyethylene glycol, an inert, non-absorbable, non-fermentable compound which acted as the osmotic agent. The formulation also included sodium bicarbonate to prevent acidosis and some sodium supplements to minimize potassium loss (Table 3.3). The formulation may be prepared in any pharmacy but it is now marketed in many different preparations, such as sulphate free, Nulytely, Calyte, CP100, many of which are flavoured for improved palatability (Diab and Marshall, 1996; Berry and DiPalma, 1994).

Table 3.3 Formulation and preparation of the polyethylene glycol electrolyte solution.

Sodium chloride BP	17.7 g
Potassium chloride BP	9.0 g
Sodium sulphate BP	154.8 g
Sodium bicarbonate BP	20.1 g
BPC PEG 4000	600.0 g
BPC peppermint emulsion	36.0 mL
BPC saccharin sodium solution	24.0 mL
Made up to 12 L with sterile water	
(Total osmolarity 259–275 mosmol/L)	

Polyethylene glycol electrolyte solutions are safe and generally achieve a high quality of preparation (Kolts et al, 1993; Lazzaroni et al, 1993; Chia et al, 1995). However, 4 L of fluid must be taken which some patients find difficult to tolerate (Goldman and Reichelderfer, 1982; Thomas et al, 1982; Girard et al, 1984). There is no need to administer metoclopramide (Rhodes et al, 1978) but bisacodyl reduces the fluid intake from 4 to 2 L, which is easier for elderly patients to cope with, without compromising the quality of preparation (Adams et al, 1994). The risk of explosion is only related to the amount of faecal residue in the colon and there is no disturbance in electrolyte balance or acidosis (Ambrose et al, 1983). The preparation is more efficient than conventional preparation for colonoscopy (Rhodes et al, 1977; Thomas et al, 1982; Ernstoff et al, 1983; DiPalma et al, 1984; Beck et al, 1985) but all forms of gut lavage seem to be disappointing when used for barium enema examination (Skucas et al, 1976; Backran et al, 1977; King et al, 1979; Ernstoff et al, 1983). Completion of a 4-L preparation is only achieved in 50–65% of patients and causes considerable nausea and distress to many patients (Vanner et al, 1990; Marshall et al, 1993; Adams et al, 1994; Chia et al, 1995; Golub et al, 1995).

We found that oral irrigation with electrolyte and polyethylene glycol is preferred by most patients to conventional preparation and nasogastric whole bowel irrigation (Ambrose et al, 1983). However, in our experience, compliance is much higher with Picolax or sodium phosphate (Takada et al, 1989; Yoshioka et al, 1998).

Although oral bowel irrigation seemed to be the logical approach to bowel preparation for both diagnostic and therapeutic procedures, the technique has not been as popular in the UK as in North

America. The reasons for this are various. Radiologists find that whole gut irrigation leaves the colon too wet for optimum mucosal coating (Skucas et al, 1976; Backran et al, 1977; Lee et al, 1981; Ernstoff et al, 1983). Outpatient compliance to the polyethylene glycol electrolyte solution is variable. Many elderly patients will not drink a sufficient volume to ensure that the faecal effluent is completely clear. Hence the technique may be unsuitable except for patients who are properly supervised in hospital. Finally, the technique may precipitate large bowel obstruction, whereas it is sometimes still possible to achieve preparation of the bowel in patients with stenotic lesions using purgatives alone.

Purgation alone

Sodium picosulphate and magnesium citrate (Picolax)

A variety of purgatives have been used to prepare the bowel. In a series of studies we showed that sodium picosulphate with magnesium citrate (Picolax) gives better results than either sennosides or mannitol because the right colon is cleared better (Lee and Ferrando, 1984). Picolax is substantially more effective than conventional preparation with enemas and washouts (Roe et al, 1984). It also appears that rectal washout is not necessary (Dodds et al, 1977) (Table 3.4). However, clear fluids for 24 hours seems essential to achieve an adequate bowel preparation.

Until recently our practice has been to use Picolax exclusively, using two sachets given 4 hours apart, 24 hours before operation, endoscopy or double contrast barium enema, followed by clear fluids thereafter. Compliance is good, colic is troublesome but is usually transient and generally a high-quality preparation is achieved. In a physiological assessment of Picolax we found that dehydration was common unless patients were given an i.v. infusion or encouraged to take extra fluids (Takada et al, 1993). Tsang et al (1992) found that Picolax was superior to a balanced oral electrolyte solution (CP100) but inferior to sodium sulphate, which is marginally less expensive. The importance of intravenous replacement with Picolax administration was stressed by Barker and others (1992) who showed that when Picolax was used alone there was a substantial reduction in intravascular volume.

Table 3.4 Dodds' method of barium enema assessment.

Score	*Description*
Excellent	No retained faecal matter
Good	Minimal faecal material, few line particles, 1–2 mm in diameter
Fair	Moderate faecal debris, particles 5 mm or less, not sufficient to invalidate examination
Poor	Considerable faecal material, particles less than 1 cm, sufficient to compromise examination
Unacceptable	Abundant faecal material, particles 1 cm or more

From Dodds et al (1977).

Sodium phosphate

Sodium phosphate is marketed as Fleet phospho-soda. Its advantage is that a much smaller volume is required compared with the polyethylene glycol electrolyte solutions: 45 mL of the highly osmolic cathartic is mixed with 90 mL of water and taken twice (Chia et al, 1995). The only drawback to sodium phosphate is the small risk of hyperphosphataemia and hypocalcaemia. Hyperphosphataemia is dose related and more common in patients with renal failure (Afridi et al, 1995). Patients may encounter a modest reduction in serum potassium and increased serum sodium with sodium phosphate preparation (Lieberman et al, 1996) and it is therefore contraindicated in congestive cardiac failure, ascites and renal failure (Aradhye & Brensilver, 1991).

With the exception of a small colonoscopy study from California (Marshall et al, 1993), five other colonoscopy studies found that sodium phosphate was cheaper, better tolerated, more likely to be completed and more effective than polyethylene glycol electrolyte lavage for bowel preparation (Vanner et al, 1990; Kolts et al, 1993; Cohen et al, 1994; Chia et al, 1995; Golub et al, 1995). Transient minor elevation of serum phosphate was recorded by some who examined body composition, but there were no recorded side-effects and calcium levels were uninfluenced by the preparation. Sodium phosphate is thus gaining popularity for colonoscopy in the USA because of its competitive price, ease of administration and greater patient compliance. A recent surgical trial to compare sodium phosphate with polyethylene glycol based oral lavage also reported greater compliance, less pain, fatigue and bloating with comparable efficacy but both preparations resulted in a significant decrease in serum calcium (Oliveira et al, 1997).

We have just completed a colonoscopy trial and a surgery trial to compare sodium phosphate with sodium picosulphate magnesium citrate (Picolax), the most widely used preparation in the UK (Tables 3.5 and 3.6). Both studies indicate that the quality of

Table 3.5 Randomized trial of sodium phosphate versus sodium picosulphate for colonoscopy.

	Sodium phosphate (n = 51)		*Sodium picosulphate (n = 55)*
Faecal residue score			
Right colon	1.1 +/– 1.0	*	1.5 +/– 1.0
Transverse colon	0.8 +/– 0.9		1.0 +/– 1.0
Left colon	0.3 +/– 0.6	*	0.7 +/– 0.9
Rectum	0.3 +/– 0.6		0.5 +/– 0.8
Total	2.0 +/– 2.2	*	3.1 +/– 2.9

* $P < 0.05$.

Table 3.6 Randomized trial of sodium phosphate versus sodium picosulphate for colorectal surgery.

	Sodium sulphate (n = 76)	*Sodium picosulphate (n = 77)*
Linear analogue score		
Abdominal pain	1.2 +/– 1.8	2.0 +/– 2.1
Nausea	1.7 +/– 2.8	1.1 +/– 2.1
Vomiting	0.5 +/– 1.8	0.2 +/– 0.7
Fear	1.3 +/– 2.1	0.9 +/– 2.0
Fatigue	1.9 +/– 2.5	2.0 +/– 2.6
Surgical assessment of bowel preparation		
Excellent	18	16
Good	43	38
Poor	5	11
Awful	0	2
Not assessed	1	4
Faecal residue (g/cm)	0.18 +/– 0.28	0.45 +/– 0.69*

* $P < 0.05$.

bowel preparation with sodium phosphate was superior to that with Picolax; there was a transient rise of serum phosphate with sodium phosphate but no change in calcium levels with either group. We believe, therefore, that phospho-soda should be evaluated by others, and if it is consistently superior it should replace Picolax (Yoshioka et al, in prep.).

Distal preparation

Enemata are useful if sigmoidoscopy is impossible because of gross faecal residue in patients attending outpatient clinics. Devlin et al (1979) compared dioctyl sodium sulphosuccinate (1% w/v) with sodium acid phosphate (10%) and with soap enemata (5% w/v). All three preparations were equally successful for rigid sigmoidoscopy. Although the dioctyl and phosphate enemata were more expensive compared with soap enemata, the added cost of the proprietary preparations was justified in terms of reduced nursing time. We usually find that an outpatient flexible sigmoidoscopy is desirable in a patient with a suspected carcinoma in the sigmoid which cannot be visualized or biopsied with the rigid instrument. In this situation we have shown that a disposable phosphate enema is superior to the small volume Microlax (Silverman and Keighley, 1985).

On-table preparation

Antegrade irrigation

Peroperative preparation has been accepted as a method of ensuring that the colon is empty prior to primary anastomosis. This procedure may be used either during an emergency operation for bleeding, localized perforation or obstruction, or when preoperative bowel preparation is unsatisfactory (Muir, 1968; Dudley et al, 1980).

Indications

The concept of intraoperative irrigation for large bowel obstruction stems from the knowledge that staged procedures are attended by a high mortality (Hughes, 1966; Fielding and Wells, 1974; Irvin and Greaney, 1977; Stewart et al, 1984; Phillips et al, 1985). The aim is therefore to resect diseased bowel and perform a primary anastomosis after removing all faecal residue from the proximal colon.

Patients with localized sepsis from a walled-off perforation of the colon constitute a group in whom on-table lavage might also be advised, since conventional bowel preparation may result in a free perforation. If the proximal colon can be rendered empty, a safe primary anastomosis can be performed (Mealy et al, 1988).

In patients with severe repeated colonic haemorrhage on-table lavage should facilitate total gut endoscopy and bleeding lesions may be more easily identified.

Technique

A no. 14 Foley catheter is inserted through a purse-string suture placed in the caecum, either through the base of the appendix, if it is still present, or where the taenia coli converge. The Foley catheter is attached to an infusion set and a 3-L bag of Hartmann's solution (Munro et al, 1987). Some authors use tapwater but there is a risk of excessive water absorption if an isotonic solution is not used (Jones and Siwek, 1986; Pollock et al, 1987).

The splenic flexure, left colon and sigmoid are mobilized, taking great care not to injure the distended and obstructed bowel or to damage the vascular arcade. The bowel is isolated below the site of obstruction with a tape or curved aortic clamp, and an on-table rectal washout is performed until the rectum is completely clean (see below). The obstructed or locally perforated bowel is resected. If the lesion is a carcinoma, the inferior mesenteric artery is ligated flush with the aorta and the vein divided at its junction with the splenic vein. The vascular arcade supplying the colon from the middle colic artery is carefully preserved. The bowel is divided above and below the tumour between clamps (Figure 3.1). The descending colon can then be delivered out of the wound and two further clamps are placed across it. A purse-string is placed around the anterior aspect of the colon to secure a length of anaesthetic scavenger tubing. A strong Nylon tape should also be passed under the colon at this point to secure the position of the tube within the colon. A transverse incision corresponding to about half of the circumference of the bowel is then made between the clamps. Anaesthetic scavenger tubing is connected to a transparent plastic bag or a purpose-built unit (Koruth et al, 1985) and is then inserted into the proximal colon through the purse-string and secured by a second Nylon tape (Figure 3.2). Irrigation through the Foley catheter can now commence. It may be necessary to break up any solid faecal matter in the descending colon in order to allow it to pass through the tubing into the collecting bag and to vent the tubing with a wide bore needle if a negative pressure develops in the closed irrigation system.

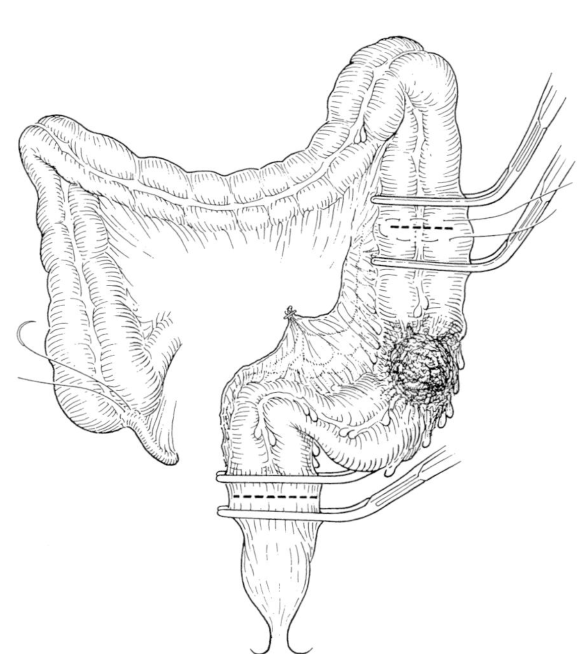

Figure 3.1 On-table colonic lavage. A purse-string suture has been placed around the base of the appendix for the insertion of a Foley catheter after appendicectomy. Bowel clamps have been placed above and below the obstructing lesion and an enterotomy has been placed between bowel clamps proximal to the obstruction for the insertion of anaesthetic scavenger tubing.

The irrigation should continue until clear effluent emerges. In acute obstruction this may require 7–15 L of fluid and the procedure may take up to one hour. The irrigation fluid should be at room temperature. Jones and Siwek (1986) use a mercuric perchloride rectal irrigation at the completion of the proximal colonic lavage. Pollock et al (1987) use 10% povidone-iodine through the proximal colon as a 'last wash' (Banich and Mendak, 1989). When the irrigation is complete and the colon is no longer contracting vigorously the tumour-bearing segment with its scavenger tubing is resected. A stapled or sutured anastomosis should be possible with an empty rectum and proximal colon. The duration of colonic on-table lavage for patients with acute bleeding or when preoperative preparation has been unsatisfactory is much shorter; usually only 2–4 L of fluid is necessary and the procedure takes less than 20 minutes.

There are several reported series of patients who have had antegrade on-table colonic irrigation; most of these studies are not confined to patients with acute obstruction but include those in whom preoperative bowel preparation was inadequate. The mortality in patients having primary resection and anastomosis under emergency surgical conditions with on-table lavage ranges from 3 to 17% (Radcliffe and Dudley, 1983: 3%; Koruth et al, 1985: 13%; Thomson and Carter, 1986: 4%; Weaver and Khawaja, 1986: 3%; Pollock et al, 1987: 17%). In a few patients the procedure had to be abandoned because solid faeces would not drain through the tubing. Some authors advise decompressing the anastomosis (tube ileostomy or tube caecostomy, depending on the site of enterotomy) by inflating the balloon after securing the serosa of the bowel to the parietal peritoneum and the catheter to the abdominal wall. However, since tube decompression has been complicated by sepsis and fatal peritonitis we do not recommend it. If proximal decompression is considered necessary we would advise raising a proximal loop ileostomy.

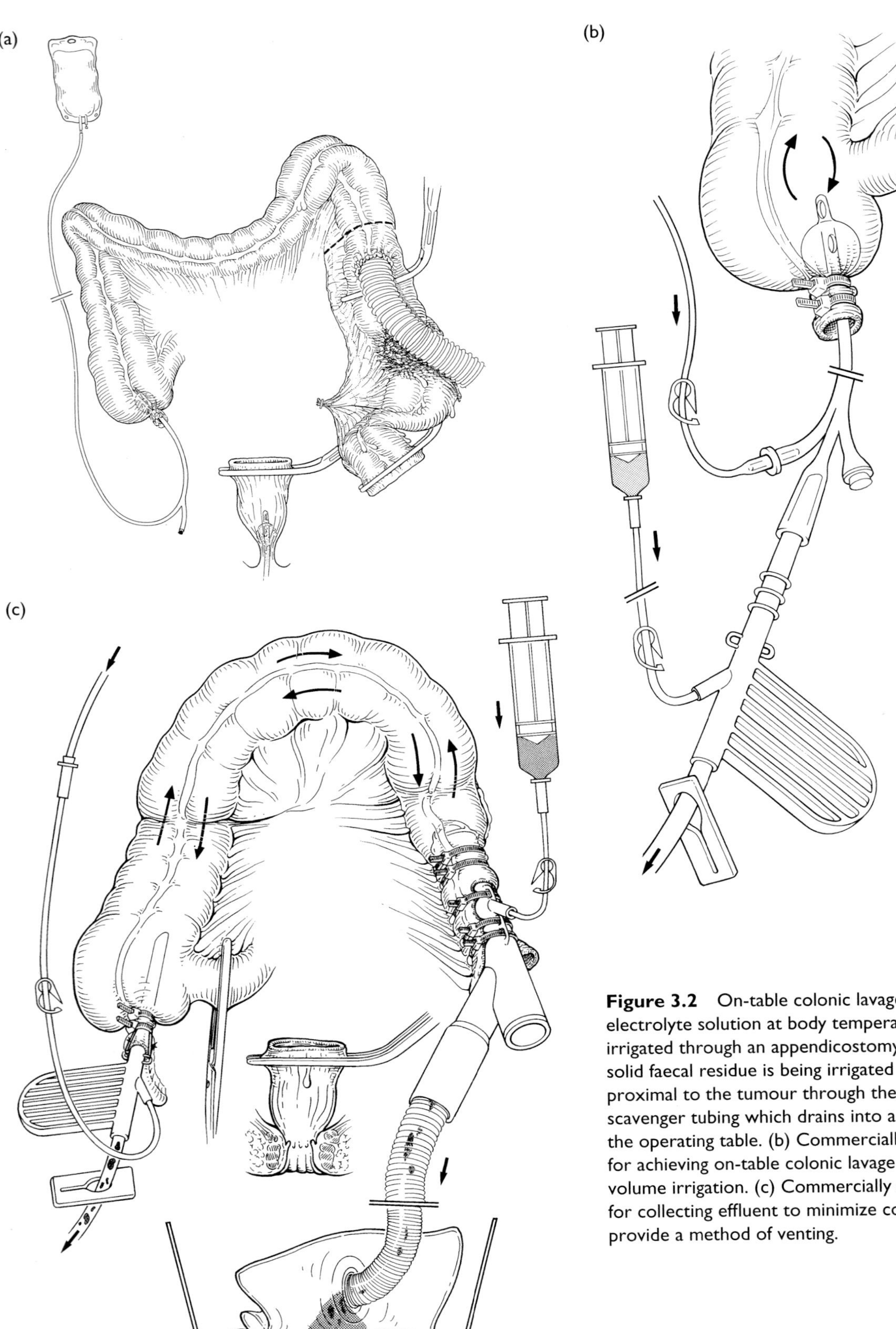

Figure 3.2 On-table colonic lavage in progress. (a) An electrolyte solution at body temperature is being irrigated through an appendicostomy purse-string and solid faecal residue is being irrigated from the colon proximal to the tumour through the anaesthetic scavenger tubing which drains into a plastic bag below the operating table. (b) Commercially available device for achieving on-table colonic lavage to achieve rapid volume irrigation. (c) Commercially available technique for collecting effluent to minimize contamination and to provide a method of venting.

Rectal washout

On-table rectal washout should always be a therapeutic option when operating on the left colon or rectum. Accordingly, all patients should be placed in the Lloyd–Davies position and a large 30 Foley catheter inserted into the rectal ampulla.

Indications

It is not appropriate in this section to discuss the relative merits of cytocidal washout as a means of preventing implantation of malignant cells into the site of a colorectal anastomosis. Nevertheless, if the reader believes that this is important, all patients having a pelvic anastomosis for neoplasia should have a rectal washout during the procedure.

If a stapled rectal anastomosis is used, rectal washout is always advised to ensure that the rectal ampulla is free from any faecal material. Passage of a stapling instrument through an inadequately prepared rectal ampulla increases the risk of pelvic contamination.

Technique

The rectum is cross-clamped after full mobilization and, in the case of rectal cancer, the clamp should be applied just below the tumour. The washout is performed using a large no. 30 Foley catheter or, if very low, a 50 mL syringe and should continue until the effluent is completely clear of any faecal residue (Figure 3.3). We have found that although povidone-iodine achieved a significant reduction in the aerobic counts within the rectal ampulla, 0.3% hypochlorite solution eliminated both aerobes and anaerobes from the rectal stump (Scammell et al, 1985). There is no evidence that rectal washout reduces the anastomotic leak rates after low anterior resection (Cade, 1981; Tagart, 1981).

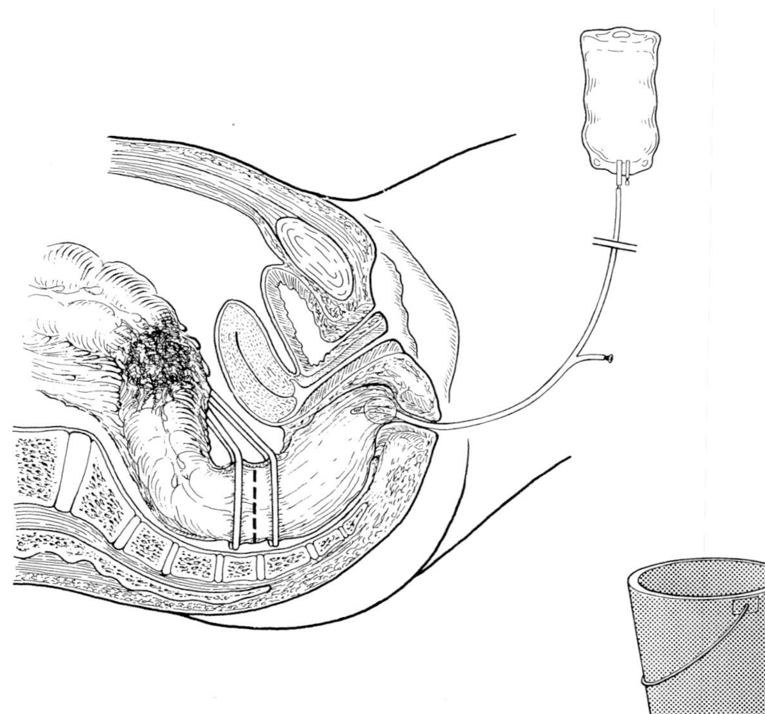

Figure 3.3 On-table rectal washout. The patient is in the Lloyd–Davies position. Bowel clamps have been placed below the obstructing lesion. A Foley catheter has been inserted into the rectal stump. The rectal stump is being irrigated with an antiseptic solution.

QUALITY OF BOWEL PREPARATION

Evaluation

Most assessments of the quality of mechanical bowel preparation are based upon subjective evaluation by the operating surgeon and are likely to be unreliable. Christensen and Kronberg (1981) recorded whether or not the small and large bowel were collapsed. Others have scored the contents of the small bowel and large bowel (fluid, air or soft faeces) (Chung et al, 1979). Most authors refer to the quality of mechanical preparation as poor, fair, good or excellent (Beck et al, 1985).

Preoperative sigmoidoscopic assessment merely provides some non-quantifiable information about the quality of preparation below the pathology in the large bowel. The amount of faecal residue above a tumour can be assessed by washing out the luminal contents from a known length of the resected specimen. However, this takes no account of the surgeon milking faecal residue into the segment of bowel which is to be resected. The amount of faecal residue in the colon can obviously be measured more accurately if on-table irrigation is used routinely during colorectal resections.

Evaluation by barium enema examination may be used to compare bowel preparations for diagnostic radiology and has been described by Dodds et al (1977). The colon is divided into four segments (ascending, transverse, descending and sigmoid) and classified according to five criteria (Table 3.4).

Quality of bowel preparation can be scored during colonoscopy and this is more precise than barium enema since the volume of liquid inside the lumen of the colon can be aspirated for measurement. The colon is divided into segments and scored according to the area of mucosa visualized (>75% = 0; 50–75% = 1; 25–50% = 2; <25% = 3) and the material within the lumen of the colon (0 = nothing; 1 = lavage fluid only; 2 = liquid; 3 = solid).

One method that we have used to assess bowel preparation relies on giving the patient 75 radio-opaque markers 5 days before bowel preparation (Ambrose and Keighley, 1986). The number of markers present in the colon and on the morning of operation after bowel preparation is recorded from plain X-rays. We found that the percentage reduction of markers did not correlate either with the surgeon's assessment of the quality of bowel preparation (Figure 3.4) or with the amount of residue within the resected colon (Figure 3.5). We concluded that a radio-opaque marker assessment of bowel preparation was unreliable.

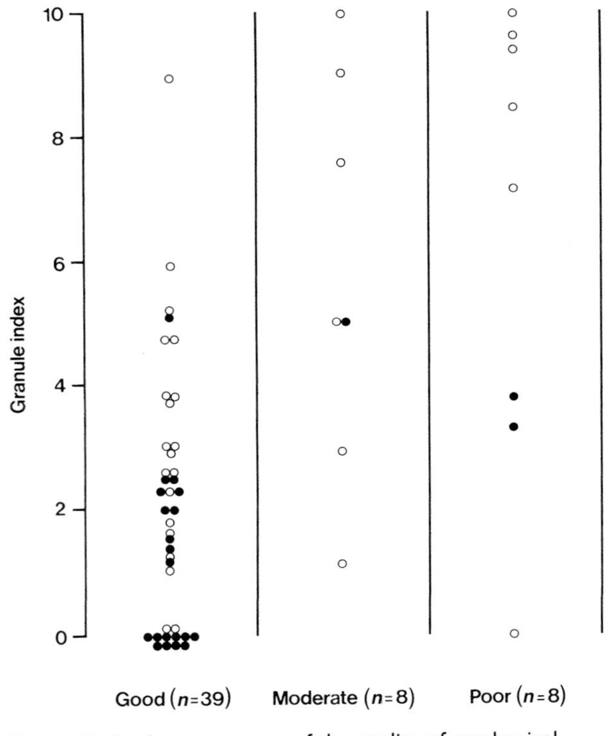

Granule index

Good (n=39) Moderate (n=8) Poor (n=8)

Figure 3.4 An assessment of the quality of mechanical bowel preparation using radio-opaque markers. The granule index is a measure of the number of markers present in the proximal colon in patients with obstructive and non-obstructive disease. Results have been correlated with the quality of mechanical bowel preparation as assessed by the surgeon at the time of the operation. It can be seen that there is a reasonable correlation between granule index and subjective assessment of bowel preparation. ○, Potentially obstructed; ●, not obstructed.

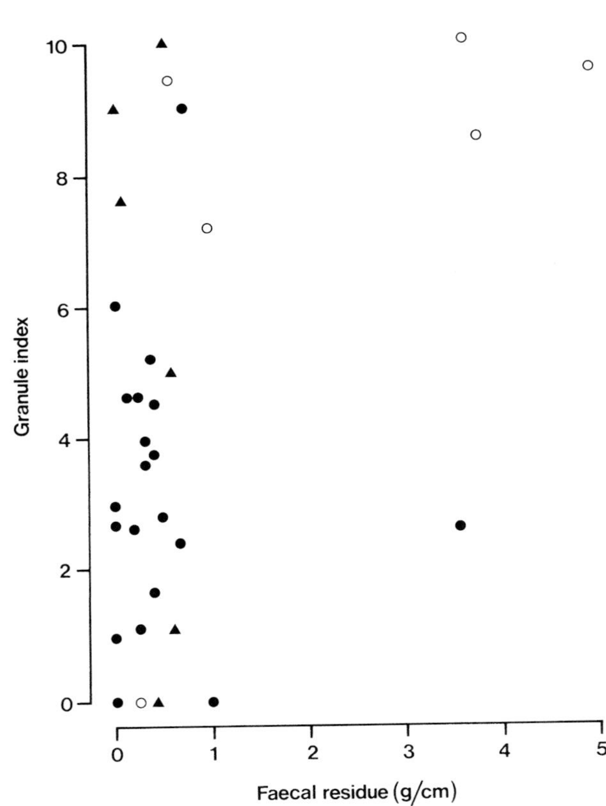

Figure 3.5 A correlation between faecal residue, as assessed by weighing the amount of faecal material per centimetre of colon proximal to the obstructing lesion, and a radio-opaque marker index of proximal faecal residue. Preparation: ●, good; ▲, moderate; ○, poor.

Comparisons of methods of bowel preparation

Barium enema

X-Prep was shown to be superior to mannitol (Lee et al, 1981) for barium enema preparation. We, and others, have found that sodium picosulphate and magnesium citrate (Picolax) is superior to X-Prep or mannitol in preparing the bowel for barium enema (Cargill and Hately, 1978; Lee et al, 1981) (Tables 3.7 and 3.8). Restriction of oral intake to clear fluids only was shown to be essential for successful bowel preparation. Rectal washout was associated with no significant benefit over Picolax and starvation alone (Lee and Ferrando, 1984). Mannitol produces excessive amounts of gas and a wet mucosal surface and is not advised for barium enema examination (Palmer and Khan, 1979).

Most studies indicate that nasogastric and oral whole bowel irrigation is unsatisfactory for barium enema examination because the colon is too wet, resulting in poor mucosal coating (Levy et al, 1976; Backran et al, 1977; Ernstoff et al, 1983). Hence, most radiologists prefer senna and castor oil (Slanger, 1979) or Picolax (Lee et al, 1981) for bowel preparation.

Colonoscopic preparations

Polyethylene glycol electrolyte oral lavage was reported to be superior to conventional purgation with enemas (Ernstoff et al, 1983). In addition, traditional mechanical preparation appears to influence the histology of the colon and is associated with flattening of the surface epithelial cells, goblet cell depletion and increased oedema in the lamina propria (Gaginella and Phillips, 1976; Saunders et al, 1977). Likewise, enemata are known to cause sloughing of the surface epithelium (Meisel et al, 1977). By contrast, Golytely was associated with minimal changes on light microscopy (Pockros and Foroozan, 1985). Recent trial data however suggest that sodium phosphate is superior to oral polyethylene glycol electrolyte lavage (Adams et al, 1994; Cohen et al, 1994; Chia et al, 1995; Golub et al, 1995). However, two publications suggest that sodium phosphate can produce aphthous ulcers and that they are more common than in patients prepared with polyethylene glycol electrolyte solutions (Hixson, 1995; Zwas et al, 1996). Nevertheless, these lesions have not been observed by others either at endoscopy or from resection specimens (Kolts et al, 1993; Cohen et al, 1994; Oliveira et al, 1997). Furthermore, oral whole bowel irrigation is often poorly tolerated and cannot be completed in a high proportion of patients (Burbridge et al, 1978; King et al, 1979; Thomas et al, 1982; Ernstoff et al, 1983; Adler et al, 1984; DiPalma et al, 1984; Kohler et al, 1990; Cohen et al, 1994; Chia et al, 1995; Oliveira et al, 1997).

Surgical evaluation

Objective evaluation of the efficacy of bowel preparation is unsatisfactory (Ambrose and Keighley,

Table 3.7 Radiological study of X-Prep and Picolax with or without starvation and rectal washout: evaluation of bowel cleanliness.

	Laxative alone		*Laxative + starvation*		*Laxative + colonic lavage*		*Laxative + starvation + colonic lavage*	
Evaluation	*X-Prep*	*Picolax*	*X-Prep*	*Picolax*	*X-Prep*	*Picolax*	*X-Prep*	*Picolax*
Excellent	0	0	0	3	0	0	1	1
Good	22	22	35	46	24	33	38	59
Fair	25	25	30	20	28	21	24	13
Poor	24	15	11	8	13	17	15	5
Unacceptable	9	18	4	3	15	9	2	2

Table 3.8 Assessment of bowel preparation for each anatomical site in the colon for all four groups of patients receiving either X-Prep or Picolax.

	Right colon		*Transverse colon*		*Left colon*		*Sigmoid and rectum*	
Evaluation	*X-Prep*	*Picolax*	*X-Prep*	*Picolax*	*X-Prep*	*Picolax*	*X-Prep*	*Picolax*
Excellent	0	0	0	1	0	1	1	2
Good	3	17	22	44	48	51	46	48
Fair	24	19	40	15	23	19	20	26
Poor	32	23	13	13	7	6	11	3
Unacceptable	21	21	5	7	2	3	3	1

Table 3.9 Operative assessment of faecal residue.

	Magnesium sulphate + enemas + fluids only (n = 56)	*Elemental diet only (n = 48)*	*Nasogastric whole bowel irrigation only (n = 46)*	*Oral whole bowel irrigation only (n = 58)*	*Picolax + fluids only (n = 63)*
No residue	13 (23)	0	28 (61)	24 (41)	35 (55)
Small amount of residue	24 (43)	8 (17)	10 (22)	24 (41)	18 (28)
Gross residue	19 (34)	40 (83)	8 (17)	10 (17)	10 (16)

Values in parentheses are percentages.

1986). Using a variety of parameters, Picolax or whole bowel irrigation through a nasogastric tube seems to give the best results (Table 3.9). Poor results occur in patients with potentially obstructing lesions.

Failure of bowel irrigation seems to be due either to intolerance of the preparation or a luminal diameter of less than 1.2 cm (Arabi et al, 1978). The best surgical results seem to occur among patients who have a short nasogastric electrolyte irrigation after 1 L of an osmotic agent (Minervini et al, 1980) or after Picolax (Grace, 1988). Oral polyethylene glycol electrolyte lavage is effective provided the high fluid load can be tolerated and may be improved by prior bisacodyl administration (Chung et al, 1979; Ambrose et al, 1983; Beck et al, 1985; Fleites et al, 1985; Panton et al, 1985; Adams et al, 1994) (Table 3.10). Picolax, however, is well tolerated, cheap and at least as effective as oral or nasogastric irrigation but fluid replacement preoperatively is advised (Takada et al, 1989; Barker et al, 1992).

Recent data, however, suggest that sodium phosphate is superior to oral lavage with polyethylene glycol and electrolytes and is also superior to Picolax (Oliveira et al, 1997; Yoshioka et al, in prep.) (Table 3.11). We found that the proportion of patients with a completely empty colon was related to luminal diameter, being 28% when the diameter was less than 1.2 cm compared with 77% when the diameter was greater than 1.8 cm (Table 3.12).

Since on-table irrigation can be used if bowel preparation is less than ideal, we are certainly prepared to accept that 10% of patients may have a suboptimal preparation and may require peroperative lavage as well. Until the results of our sodium phosphate trial was known it had been our practice to give patients Picolax to take at home 24–36 hours before operation and to administer i.v. fluids to correct fluid and electrolyte losses before surgical treatment. We may now switch to sodium phosphate if the cost benefits are confirmed by others.

Table 3.10 Comparison between Golytely and traditional preparation.

Evaluation	*Golytely*	*Magnesium + enemas + liquid diet + X-Prep*
Poor	0	0
Fair	0	9
Good	11	7
Excellent	18	9

From Beck et al (1985).

Table 3.11 Randomized comparison of PEG against sodium phosphate.

	Sodium phosphate (n = 100)	*PEG/electrolyte (n = 100)*
Acceptable or excellent/good	87	76
Unacceptable or fair/poor	13	24

From Oliveira et al (1997).

Table 3.12 Effect of obstruction of bowel preparation: results of whole bowel irrigation or oral mannitol according to diameter of the obstructing tumour.

	Diameter of tumour		
Result	*>1.8 cm (n = 35)*	*1.2–1.8 cm (n = 17)*	*<1.2 cm (n = 18)*
No residue	27 (77)	7 (41)	5 (28)
Small amount of residue	6 (17)	9 (53)	7 (39)
Gross residue	2 (6)	1 (6)	6 (33)

Values in parentheses are percentages.

DISTURBANCES IN BODY COMPOSITION

Reference has already been made to the fluid and electrolyte imbalance which may occur in patients receiving certain preparations. These disturbances will now be discussed in greater detail.

Traditional preparation

The changes in body composition with conventional preparation are variable. Levy et al (1976) showed that the use of castor oil was associated with a mean weight loss of 1.4 kg. Unless patients are encouraged to drink large volumes of clear fluid there is usually some dehydration, with sodium loss, and this is further exacerbated by the pre-anaesthetic period of starvation (Takada et al, 1989). In some units intravenous fluids are deliberately commenced on the afternoon prior to operation.

Elemental diet

As far as we are aware there are no serious metabolic disturbances among patients taking an elemental diet, provided that diarrhoea does not persist (Glotzer et al, 1973).

Nasogastric irrigation

Irrigating of 10–12 L of isotonic saline through the gastrointestinal tract results in profound changes in body composition. We recorded a total fluid gain of 2.7 L, as well as retention of 500 mmol of sodium. There is an overall loss of 50–70 mmol of potassium which is not prevented by adding KCl to the saline irrigation fluid (Crapp et al, 1975). There is also a risk of acidosis with saline lavage (Chung et al, 1979). Gilmore et al (1981) reported a mean weight gain of 0.75 kg, a rise in plasma volume and a rise in blood pressure after saline lavage (Figure 3.6). These changes are due to the very large fluid load presented to the colon (Love et al, 1973), where sodium and water are absorbed in exchange for potassium (Dillard et al, 1965; Phillips and Giller, 1973).

The combination of osmotic agents such as mannitol or polyethylene glycol or the use of a balanced electrolyte solution such as Ringer's lactate or Hartmann's solution has almost eliminated any metabolic and electrolyte disturbance but water retention may still occur and the method should not be used in patients with cardiac or renal disease (Donovan et al, 1980; Thomas et al, 1982; Ambrose et al, 1983; Wolters et al, 1994).

Oral irrigation and osmotic agents

Severe dehydration occurs with 20% mannitol and most patients require the addition of intravenous fluids to achieve an adequate urine output (Hares et al, 1981b). Even with a 10% mannitol solution there is sodium and potassium loss and some dehydration (Minervini et al, 1980), resulting in increased haematocrit and a fall in plasma volume, loss of weight and hypotension (Figure 3.6) (Gilmore et al, 1981). For these reasons most clinicians who still use mannitol usually accept that a larger volume of a 5% solution is desirable (Nasrullah and Iber, 1969).

Formulations, such as Golytely, that combine an osmotic agent such as mannitol or polyethylene glycol with an electrolyte solution cause no dehydration and minimal change in sodium balance (Ambrose et al, 1983; Ernstoff et al, 1983; Beck et al, 1985; Fleites et al, 1985). Sodium phosphate is an osmotic agent: 45 mL is mixed with 90 mL of water and administered twice. This causes dehydration unless oral fluids are given, hence patients are instructed to drink 480 mL of fluid during the

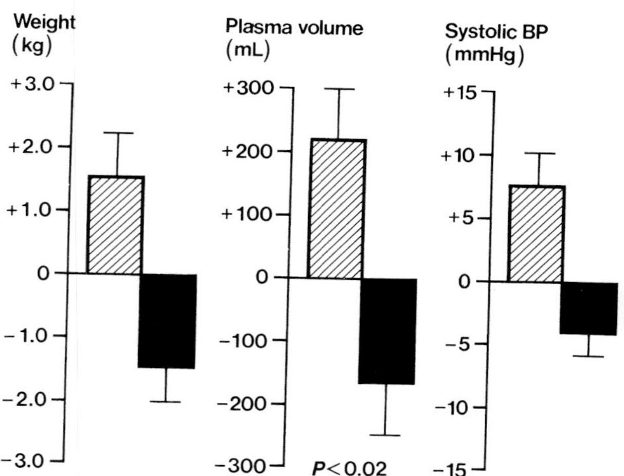

Figure 3.6 Changes in body weight, plasma volume and systolic blood pressure following bowel preparation with nasogastric saline whole bowel irrigation compared with oral mannitol. ▨, Saline; ■, mannitol.

preparation. Provided these instructions are followed fluid homeostasis is achieved and dehydration is rare. In this dose sodium phosphate administration is associated with asymptomatic and transient hyperphosphataemia (Cohen et al, 1994) and there is a risk of hypokalaemia and hypocalcaemia; however we did not encounter any such changes in surgical patients (Yoshioka et al, in prep.). Nevertheless, sodium phosphate preparation is probably contraindicated in patients with cardiac or renal disease (Oliveira et al, 1997).

Laxatives

Sodium picosulphate with magnesium citrate (Picolax) will dehydrate. Administration of Picolax is associated with a profound fall in intravascular volume (Barker et al, 1992); hence, oral fluid replacement must be encouraged and we commence an intravenous infusion overnight before operation the following day. If preparation is given at home, patients should be admitted 4 hours before operation to receive a litre of saline preoperatively.

EFFECT ON FAECAL FLORA

Most forms of mechanical bowel preparation alone have little if any influence on the faecal flora (Nichols and Condon, 1971; Arabi et al, 1978; Santos et al, 1994), although whole bowel irrigation may be associated with a 10 000-fold reduction in *E. coli* and *Bacteroides fragilis* (Bornside and Cohn, 1969; Hewitt et al, 1973; Bond et al, 1976), which is almost certainly a dilutional effect. Elemental diets result in a 10 000-fold reduction in the counts of aerobic bacteria. By contrast, mannitol is associated with a 100 000-fold increase in the counts of *E. coli* (Keighley et al, 1979) and an increased risk of sepsis due to *E. coli* (Hares et al, 1981a). Golytely has no influence on faecal flora (Ambrose et al, 1983). However, colonic lavage may result in bacteraemia from translocation of *E. coli* across the bowel wall (Horgan et al, 1994). Consequently, antibiotic cover is always advised during on-table lavage.

In vitro studies from the Royal London Hospital have shown that some laxatives have an influence on the growth of obligate anaerobes. Thus polyethylene glycol and Picolax had no influence on counts of *B. fragilis* whereas senna inhibited *B. fragilis*. As senna is poorly absorbed and as *Bacteroides* spp. are the principal polysaccharide-fermenting bacteria, long-term ingestion of senna by patients with constipation might lower butyrate levels and could increase the risk of adenoma formation (Chapman et al, 1995). The impact of senna on reducing faecal flora in bowel preparation is speculative.

Bowel preparation also has some impact on the mucosa-associated bacterial population. Thus, Bleday et al (1993) from the Deaconess Hospital found higher counts of aerobes and anaerobes on the mucosa of the proximal bowel than on the rectum after oral polyethylene glycol electrolyte lavage.

RISKS OF EXPLOSION

Faeces produce combustible gas, principally hydrogen and methane, in the lumen of the colon. These gases are not explosive unless they are in high concentration and present with air or oxygen. The critical potentially explosive concentrations for hydrogen are 4–74% and for methane are 5–15%. These gases are produced by colonic bacteria (Bond et al, 1976) and may cause explosion, which can be fatal if a diathermy current is used during colonoscopy or open surgical procedures (Carter, 1952; Aspinall, 1964; Ragins et al, 1971; Bigarde et al, 1979; Shinagawa et al, 1985; de Wilt et al, 1996).

The problem of explosion is not a new one and has been described in association with rigid sigmoidoscopy for over four decades (Lambling and Truffert, 1944; Lieberman, 1944; Moutier, 1946; Kirk, 1949; Zimmerman, 1959), as well as with flexible colonoscopy (Bond and Levitt, 1975).

The risk of explosive gas being present during operation or colonoscopy appears to be related to the quality of mechanical bowel preparation, the use of compounds such as mannitol which can be fermented by faecal bacteria (La Brooy et al, 1981; Taylor et al, 1981; Ambrose et al, 1983) and the resident flora in the bowel (Takada et al, 1993). Poor preparation increases the risk of combustible gas (Ambrose et al, 1983; Takada et al, 1993). Oral antimicrobials such as neomycin and metronidazole eliminate the risk, provided that there is a reduction in faecal flora (Nichols et al, 1972; Keighley et al, 1981). Similarly Golytely is safe as it is not fermented by intestinal bacteria and appears to have no influence on the faecal flora (Beck et al, 1985; Fleites et al, 1985). However no form of preparation, even Picolax, is immune from risk of explosion if the quality of preparation is poor (Takada et al, 1993).

The risk of explosion at colonoscopic polypectomy can be avoided by insufflation with carbon dioxide (Arnous, 1945; Levy, 1954; Woodward, 1961; Rogers, 1974; Bond et al, 1976).

PATIENT ACCEPTABILITY

We, and others, have analysed the views expressed by patients about a variety of mechanical bowel preparations prior to surgical operation (Table 3.13 and Figure 3.7). No preparation is pleasant but Picolax and fluid intake only over 24–36 hours seem to be associated with the lowest incidence of troublesome side-effects (Lee and Ferrando, 1984; Tsang et al, 1992). Traditional bowel preparation is poorly tolerated (Beck et al, 1985). Golytely is more acceptable but patients do not like drinking large volumes of fluid (Ernstoff et al, 1983). Recent evidence suggests that oral sodium phosphate is well tolerated and comparable to Picolax. It also has advantages over oral polyethylene glycol electrolyte lavage (Oliveira et al, 1997; Yoshioka et al, in prep.).

The main discomfort associated with whole bowel irrigation relates to the nasogastric tube and the indignity of sitting on a lavatory for 3–4 hours (Chung et al, 1979; Downing et al, 1979; Gottrup et al, 1985; Panton et al, 1985; Kohler et al, 1990).

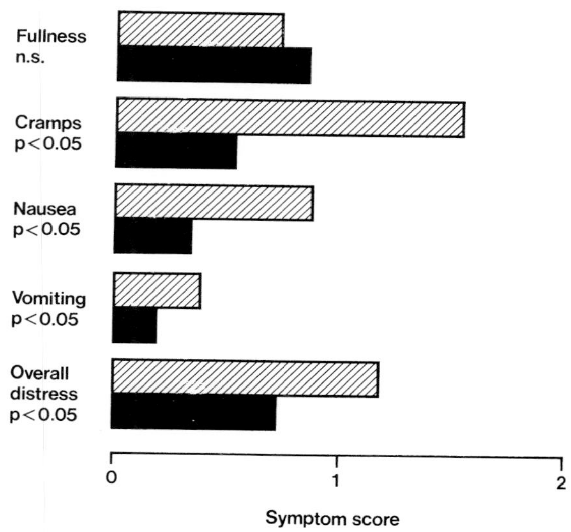

Figure 3.7 Symptoms when conventional mechanical bowel preparation (group 1) was compared with oral Golytely (group 2). n.s., Not significant. Group 1, ▨; group 2, ■.

Table 3.13 Patient acceptability of bowel preparation.

Reaction	*Traditional preparation* (*n* = 56)	*Elemental diet* (*n* = 48)	*Nasogastric irrigation* (*n* = 46)	*Oral bowel irrigation* (*n* = 58)	*Picolax and starvation* (*n* = 62)
Abdominal pain	40 (71)	4 (8)	13 (28)	7 (12)	21 (34)
Anal pain	7 (12)	3 (6)	12 (26)	8 (14)	3 (5)
Nausea	13 (23)	20 (42)	29 (63)	16 (28)	14 (22)
Vomiting	10 (18)	16 (33)	24 (52)	14 (24)	11 (18)
Fear	20 (36)	3 (6)	30 (65)	13 (22)	10 (16)
Embarrassment	22 (39)	2 (4)	36 (78)	12 (21)	11 (18)
Extreme fatigue	28 (50)	3 (6)	34 (74)	18 (31)	7 (11)

Values in parentheses are percentages.

CURRENT PRACTICE

Barium enema

It is not the practice of our radiologists to use oral whole bowel irrigation for barium enema examination as compliance amongst outpatients is poor and the mucosa too wet to achieve optimum coating with contrast. They now advise two sachets of Picolax 36–48 hours prior to examination, without enemas or washouts insisting that only clear fluids be allowed after the first dose of Picolax (Lee et al, 1981; Lee and Ferrando, 1984). If patients are diabetic, they are admitted to hospital for a 5% dextrose insulin infusion and the regimen described above, but blood glucose levels are monitored.

Flexible sigmoidoscopy and colonoscopy

We accept that there are a group of patients who attend outpatient clinics with an unprepared bowel and in whom rigid sigmoidoscopy is unsatisfactory but in whom the clinician suspects a lesion of the sigmoid colon. Using a disposable phosphate enema, we have found that an adequate view of the rectum and lower sigmoid can be obtained in 70% of patients during the initial outpatient visit.

We have now come to the conclusion that all patients who require a planned flexible sigmoidoscopic examination should be prepared in exactly the same manner as for colonoscopy with total dietary restriction for 36 hours and two sachets of magnesium citrate with sodium picosulphate (Picolax). Although sodium phosphate seems to give a marginally better preparation it is more expensive and much more difficult to dispatch by post. Thus, Picolax is likely to remain our standard outpatient preparation for colonoscopy.

Surgical resection

Non-obstructed

In patients with non-obstructed colorectal disease we use two sachets of Picolax and starvation for 36 hours preoperatively. We do not use enemata or rectal washouts. If the preparation is poor, on-table lavage is used prior to primary anastomosis. If others confirm a cost benefit with sodium phosphate as a result of better clearance of stool, lower incidence of complications and reduced hospital stay, we will switch to phospho-soda preparation.

Partially obstructed

If the patient has a large bowel carcinoma and if conventional bowel preparation for barium enema or endoscopy has resulted in adequate preparation, we use our standard Picolax preoperative preparation.

If a patient with a colorectal carcinoma has a history of partial obstruction it may not be possible to prepare the colon by conventional means. Sometimes, small daily doses of Picolax may be successful especially if elemental diets have been used for a few days before. If, on the other hand, there is no result after a single sachet of Picolax, or if the patient becomes distended or vomits, the preoperative preparation must be abandoned.

Completely obstructed

If preoperative preparation fails or if a patient is admitted with abdominal pain and a contrast enema confirms an obstructing lesion, peroperative colonic lavage is used if a resection with primary anastomosis is to be performed (see Chapter 60).

Inflammatory bowel disease

Vigorous mechanical bowel preparation may be undesirable in some patients with inflammatory bowel disease. The risks of perforation and intra-abdominal sepsis are almost entirely confined to patients with acute colitis or those with a localized perforation and a coexisting abscess. In almost all other groups routine preoperative preparation is desirable to reduce the risk of faecal contamination (McDonagh et al, 1989). There are, however, two exceptions: we do not use any form of mechanical bowel preparation in patients requiring operation for acute fulminating colitis or in elective cases if no anastomosis is being performed, as in proctocolectomy.

Diabetes

Diabetic patients are admitted for bowel preparation. Insulin or oral agents are discontinued; patients requiring insulin are given an insulin/dextrose infusion and regular bowel preparation with blood sugar monitoring.

Colonic bleeding

Acute bleeding from the large bowel may sometimes require emergency laparotomy without the source of bleeding being identified preoperatively. With the patient in the Lloyd–Davies position and using the technique of on-table antegrade colonic lavage and an anal speculum, the bowel can be completely cleared of blood so that an on-table panendoscopy can be performed to identify the bleeding source.

REFERENCES

Adams WJ, Meagher AP, Lubowski DZ & King DW (1994) Bisacodyl reduces the volume of polyethylene glycol solution required for bowel preparation. *Dis Colon Rectum* **37**: 229–234.

Adler M, Quenon M, Even-Adin D et al (1984) Whole gut lavage for colonoscopy: a comparison between two solutions. *Gastrointest Endosc* **30**: 65.

Afridi SA, Barthel JS, King PD, Pineda JJ & Marshall JB (1995) Prospective randomized trial comparing a new sodium phosphate-bisacodyl regimen with conventional PED-ES lavage for outpatient colonoscopy preparation. *Gastrointest Endosc* **41**: 485–489.

Allan RN & Keighley MRB (1988) Operative approaches to the distal rectum. In Decosse JJ & Todd IP (eds) *Clinical Surgery International, Vol. 15, Anorectal Surgery*, pp 213–238. London: Churchill Livingstone.

Allan RN, Keighley MRB, Alexander-Williams J & Hawkins C (eds) (1983) *Inflammatory Bowel Diseases*. London: Churchill Livingstone.

Ambrose NS & Keighley MRB (1986) An aid to the assessment of bowel preparation prior to colon resection. *Ann R Coll Surg Engl* **68**: 34–36.

Ambrose NS, Hohnson M, Burdon DW & Keighley MRB (1983) A physiological appraisal of polyethylene glycol and a balanced electrolyte solution as bowel preparation. *Br J Surg* **70**: 428–430.

American Cancer Society (1973) 74 facts and figures. 21 October.

Arabi Y, Dimock F, Burdon DW, Alexander-Williams J & Keighley MRB (1978) Influence of bowel preparation and antimicrobials on colonic microflora. *Br J Surg* **65**: 555–559.

Aradhye S & Brensilver JM (1991) Sodium phosphate-induced hypernatraemia in an elderly patient: a complex pathophysiologic state. *Am J Kidney Dis* **18**: 1018–1019.

Arnous J (1945) Annscope permettant les electro-coagulation intra-rectales sous une atmosphere de gaz inerte. *Arch Mal Appa Dig Nutr* **34**: 277–279.

Aspinall DL (1964) Unusual explosion during electrosurgery. *BMJ* **2**: 1178.

Atterbery HR, Sutter VL & Finegold SM (1972) Effect of a partially chemically defined diet on normal faecal flora. *Am J Clin Nutr* **25**: 1391–1398.

Backran A, Bradley JA, Bresnihan E et al (1977) Whole gut irrigation. An adequate preparation for double contrast barium enema examination. *Gastroenterology* **73**: 28–30.

Banich FE & Mendak SJ Jr (1989) Intraoperative colonic irrigation with povidone iodine: an effective method of wound sepsis prevention. *Dis Colon Rectum* **32**: 219–222.

Barker K, Graham NG, Mason MC et al (1971) The relative significance of preoperative oral antibiotics, mechanical bowel preparation and preoperative peritoneal contamination in the avoidance of sepsis, after radical surgery for UC and Crohn's disease of the large bowel. *Br J Surg* **58**: 270–273.

Barker P, Hanning C & Trotter T (1992). A study of the effect of Picolax on body weight, cardiovascular variables and haemoglobin concentration. *Ann R Coll Surg Engl* **74**: 318–319.

Barnes MR (1968) How to get a clean colon – with less effort. *Radiology* **91**: 948–953.

Beck DE, Hartford FJ & DiPalma JA (1985) Comparison of cleansing methods in preparation for colonic surgery. *Dis Colon Rectum* **28**: 491–495.

Berry MA & DiPalma JA (1994) Review article: orthograde gut lavage for colonoscopy. *Aliment Pharmacol Ther* **8**: 391–395.

Bigarde MA, Gaucher P & Lassalle C (1979) Fatal colonic explosion during colonoscopic polypectomy. *Gastroenterology* **77**: 1307–1310.

Binder HJ (1977) Pharmacology of laxatives. *Ann Rev Pharmacol Toxicol* **17**: 355–367.

Bleday R, Braidt J, Ruoff K, Shellito PC & Ackroyd FW (1993) Quantitative cultures of the mucosal-associated bacteria in the mechanically prepared colon and rectum. *Dis Colon Rectum* **36**: 844–849.

Bond JH & Levitt MD (1975) Factors affecting the concentration of combustible gases in the colon during colonoscopy. *Gastroenterology* **68**: 1445–1448.

Bond JH, Levy M & Levy MD (1976) Explosion of hydrogen gas in the colon during proctosigmoidoscopy. *Gastrointest Endosc* **23**: 41–42.

Bornside GH & Cohn I Jr (1969) Intestinal antisepsis: stability of fecal flora during mechanical cleansing. *Gastroenterology* **57**: 569–573.

Bounnos G & Devroede GJ (1974) Effects of an elemental diet on human faecal flora. *Gastroenterology* **66**: 210–214.

Burbridge EJ, Bourke E & Tarder G (1978) Effect of preparation for colonoscopy on fluid and electrolyte balance. *Gastrointest Endosc* **24**: 286–287.

Burke P, Mealy K, Gillen P, Joyce W, Traynor O & Hyland J (1994) Requirement for bowel preparation in colorectal surgery. *Br J Surg* **81**: 907–910.

Burton RC (1973) Postoperative wound infections in colonic and rectal surgery. *Br J Surg* **60**: 363–365.

Cade D (1981) Complications of anterior resection of the rectum using the EEA stapling device. *Br J Surg* **68**: 339–340.

Cargill A & Hately W (1978) Preparation of the colon prior to radiology: a comparison of the effectiveness of castor oil, dulcodos and X-Prep liquid. *Br J Radiol* **51**: 910–912.

Carter HG (1952) Explosion in the colon during electrodesiccation of polyps. *Am J Surg* **84**: 514–517.

Chapman MAS, Abercrombie J, Livermore DM & Williams NS (1995). Antibacterial activity of bowel-cleansing agents: implications of antibacteroides activity of senna. *Br J Surg* **82**: 1053.

Chia YW, Cheng LC, Goh PMY et al (1995) Role of oral sodium phosphate and its effectiveness in large bowel preparation for out-patient colonoscopy. *J R Coll Surg Edinb* **40**: 374–376.

Christensen PB & Kronberg O (1981) Whole gut irrigation versus enema in elective colorectal surgery: a prospective randomised study. *Dis Colon Rectum* **24**: 592–595.

Chung RS, Gurll NJ & Bergland EM (1979) A controlled clinical trial of whole gut lavage as a method of bowel preparation for colonic operations. *Am J Surg* **137**: 75–81.

Cohen SM, Wexner SD, Binderow SR et al (1994) Prospective, randomized, endoscopic-blinded trial comparing precolonoscopy bowel cleansing methods. *Dis Colon Rectum* **37**: 689–696.

Cooney DR, Wassner JD, Grosfeld JL et al (1974) Are elemental diets useful in bowel preparation? *Arch Surg* **109**: 206–210.

Corman ML (1984) *Colon and Rectal Surgery*. Philadelphia: Lippincott.

Crapp AR, Powis SJA, Tillotson P, Cooke WT & Alexander-Williams J (1975) Preparation of the bowel by whole gut irrigation. *Lancet* **ii**: 1239–1240.

Crowther JS, Droser BS, Goddard P et al (1973) The effect of a chemically defined diet on the faecal flora and faecal steroid concentration. *Gut* **14**: 790–793.

Davis GR, Santa Ana CA, Molawski SG & Frodstran JS (1980) Development of a lavage solution associated with minimal water and electrolyte absorption or secretion. *Gastroenterology* **78**: 991–995.

De Lacey G, Beason M, Wilkins R, Spencer J & Cramer B (1982) Routine colonic lavage is unnecessary for double contrast barium enema in outpatients. *BMJ* **284**: 1021–1022.

Devlin HB, Sharm SD, MacRae CA & Walton EW (1979) Enema: an old remedy – brought up to date. *Coloproctology* **1**: 43–45.

DeWilt JHW, Rinks IHMB & Brouwer KJ (1996) Gas explosion during colonic surgery. *J R Coll Surg Edinb* **41**: 419–422.

Diab FH & Marshall JB (1996) The palatability of five colonic lavage solutions. *Aliment Pharmacol Ther* **10**: 815–819.

Dillard RL, Eastman H & Fordtran JS (1965) Volume-flow relationship during the transport of fluid through the human small intestine. *Gastroenterology* **49**: 55–56.

DiPalma JA, Brady CE, Steward DL et al (1984) Comparison of colon cleansing methods in preparation for colonoscopy. *Gastroenterology* **86**: 856–860.

Dodds WJ, Scanlon GT, Shaw T, Steward E, Yorker JE & Metter GE (1977) An evaluation of the colon cleansing regimens. *Am J Roentgenol* **128**: 57–59.

Donovan IA, Arabi Y, Keighley MRB & Alexander-Williams J (1980) Modification of the physiological disturbances produced by whole gut irrigation by preliminary mannitol administration. *Br J Surg* **67**: 138–139.

Downing R, Dorricott NJ, Keighley MRB, Oates GD & Alexander-Williams J (1979) Whole gut irrigation: a survey of patient opinion. *Br J Surg* **88**: 201–202.

Dresen KA & Kratzer GL (1959) Fecal impaction in modern practice. *JAMA* **170**: 644–647.

Dudley HAF, Radcliffe AG & McGeehan D (1980) Intraoperative irrigation of the colon to permit primary anastomosis. *Br J Surg* **67**: 80–81.

Duthie GS, Foster ME, Price-Thomas JM & Leaper DJ (1990) Bowel preparation or not for elective colorectal surgery. *J R Coll Surg Edinb* **35**: 169–171.

Ekelund G, Lindstrom C & Rosengren JE (1974) Appearance and growth of early carcinomas of the colon-rectum. *Acta Radiol* **15**: 670–679.

Ernstoff JJ, Howard De Grasia A, Marshall JB et al (1983) A randomised blinded clinical trial of a rapid colonic lavage solution (Golytely) compared with standard preparation for colonoscopy and barium enema. *Gastroenterology* **84**: 1412–1516.

Eyler W (1973) In *Detection of Colon Lesions, First Standardisation Conference, 1969*, p 108. Chicago: American College of Radiology.

Fielding LP & Wells BW (1974) Survival after primary and after staged resection of the colon. *Br J Surg* **61**: 16–18.

Figiel LS, Figiel SJ & Wietersen FK (1965) Roentgenologic observations of growth rates of colonic polyps and carcinomas. *Acta Radiol* **3**: 417–429.

Fingl E & Freston JW (1979) Anti-diarrhoeal agents and laxatives: changing concepts. *Clin Gastroenterol* **8**: 161–185.

Fleites RA, Marshall JB, Eckhauser ML, Mansour EG, Imbembo AL & McCullough AJ (1985) The efficacy of polyethylene glycol-electrolyte lavage solution versus traditional mechanical bowel preparation for elective colonic surgery: a randomised, prospective blinded clinical trial. *Surgery* **98**: 708–717.

Forth WK, Nell G, Rummel W & Andres H (1972) The hydragogue and laxative effect of the sulphuric acid ester and the free diphenol of 4,4-dihydroxydiphenyl (pyridyl-2)-methane. *Naunyn Schmiedebergs Arch Pharmacol* **274**: 46–53.

Gaginella TS & Phillips SF (1976) Riconoleic acid (castor oil) alters intestinal surface structure: a scanning electron microscopic study. *Mayo Clin Proc* **51**: 6–12.

Galloway D, Burns HJG, Moffat LEF et al (1982) Faecal peritonitis after laxative preparation for barium enema. *BMJ* **284**: 472.

Gilmore IT, Ellis WR, Barrett GS, Pendower JEH & Parkins RA (1981) A comparison of two methods of whole gut lavage for colonoscopy. *Br J Surg* **68**: 388–389.

Girard CM, Rugh KS, DiPalma JA, Brody CE III & Pierson WP (1984) Comparison of Golytely lavage with standard diet/cathartic preparation for double contrast barium enema. *Am J Roentgenol* **142**: 1147–1149.

Glotzer DJ, Boyle PL & Silen WS (1973) Preoperative preparation of the colon with an elemental diet. *Surgery* **74**: 703–707.

Goldman J & Reichelderfer M (1982) Evaluation of rapid colonoscopy preparation using a net gut lavage solution. *Gastrointest Endosc* **28**: 9–11.

Goligher JC, Graham NC & De Dombal FT (1970) Anastomotic dehiscence after anterior resection of rectum and sigmoid. *Br J Surg* **57**: 109–118.

Golub RW, Kerner BA, Wise WE et al (1995). Colonoscopic bowel preparations – Which one? A blinded, prospective randomized trial. *Dis Colon Rectum* **38**: 594–599.

Gottrup F, Diederich P, Sorensen K, Nielson SV, Ornsholt J & Brandborg O (1985) Prophylaxis with whole gut irrigation and antimicrobials in colorectal surgery. *Am J Surg* **149**: 317–322.

Grace RH (1988) The role of Picolax before whole gut irrigation in the preparation of the colon for large bowel surgery. *Ann R Coll Surg Engl* **70**: 322–323.

Gurry JF & Ellis-Pegler RB (1976) An elemental diet as preoperative preparation of the colon. *Br J Surg* **63**: 969–972.

Hardcastle TD & Wilkins JL (1970) The action of sennosides and related compounds on the human colon and rectum. *Gut* **11**: 1038–1042.

Hares MM, Green F, Ylungs D et al (1981a) Failure of antimicrobial prophylaxis with cefoxitin or metronidazole and gentamicin: is mannitol to blame? *J Hosp Infect* **2**: 127–133.

Hares MM, Nevah E, Minervini E et al (1981b) An attempt to reduce the side effects of mannitol bowel preparation by intravenous infusion. *Dis Colon Rectum* **24**: 289–291.

Hawley PJ, Hunt TK & Dunphy JE (1970) Aetiology of colonic anastomotic leaks. *Proc R Soc Med* **63** (Suppl): 28–30.

Hewitt J, Reeve J, Rigby J & Cox AG (1973) Whole gut irrigation in preparation for large bowel surgery. *Lancet* **ii**: 337–340.

Hindle W & Code CF (1962) Some differences between duodenal and ileal sorption. *Am J Physiol* **203**: 215–220.

Hixson LJ (1995) Colorectal ulcers associated with sodium phosphate catharsis. *Gastrointest Endosc* **42**: 101–102.

Horgan AF, Stuart RC, O'Shaughnessy EM, Cryan B & Kirwan WO (1994) Bacterial translocation during peroperative colonic lavage of the obstructed rat colon. *Br J Surg* **81**: 1796–1798.

Huddy SPJ, Rayter Z, Webber PP & Southam JA (1990) Preparation of the bowel before elective surgery using a polyethylene glycol solution at home and in hospital compared with conventional preparation using magnesium sulphate. *J Coll Surg Edinb* **35**: 16–20.

Hughes ESR (1966) Mortality of acute bowel obstruction. *Br J Surg* **53**: 593–594.

Hughes ESR (1972) A sepsis in large-bowel surgery. *Ann R Coll Surg Engl* **51**: 347–356.

Hunt RH & Way ED (eds) (1981) *Colonoscopy*. London: Chapman & Hall.

Irvin TT & Goligher JC (1973) Aetiology of disruption of intestinal anastomoses. *Br J Surg* **60**: 461–464.

Irvin TT & Greaney MG (1977) The treatment of colonic cancer presenting with intestinal obstruction. *Br J Surg* **64**: 741–744.

Irving AD & Scrimgeour D (1987) Mechanical bowel

preparation for colonic resection and anastomosis. *Br J Surg* **74**: 580–581.

Irwin GAL, Sheilds JE & Wolff W (1974) Clearer roentgenographic visualisation of the colon. *Gastroenterology* **67**: 47–50.

Jauch R, Hawkwitz R, Beschke K & Pelzer H (1975) Bis-(*p*-hydroxyphenyl)-pyridyl-2-methane: the common laxative principle of bisacodyl and sodium sulphate. *Arzneimittelforschung* **25**: 1796–1800.

Johnson WC (1974) Oral elemental diet: a new bowel preparation. *Arch Surg* **108**: 32–34.

Jones PF & Siwek RJP (1986) *A Colour Atlas of Colorectal Surgery*. London: Wolfe Medical.

Keighley MRB (1982) A clinical and physiological evaluation of bowel preparation for elective colorectal surgery. *World J Surg* **6**: 464–470.

Keighley MRB, Arabi Y, Alexander-Williams J, Youngs D & Burdon DW (1979) Comparison between systemic and oral antimicrobial prophylaxis in colorectal surgery. *Lancet* **i**: 894–897.

Keighley MRB, Taylor EW, Hares MM et al (1981) Influence of oral mannitol bowel preparation on colonic microflora and the risk of explosion during endoscopic diathermy. *Br J Surg* **68**: 554–556.

King DM, Downes MO & Heddle RM (1979) An alternative method of bowel preparation for barium enemas. *Br J Radiol* **52**: 388–389.

Kirk E (1949) The quantity and composition of human colonic flatus. *Gastroenterology* **12**: 782–794.

Kohler L, Vestweber KH, Menningen R, Sommer H & Troidl H (1990) Whole gut irrigation and Prepacol laxative preparation for colonoscopy: a comparison. *Br J Surg* **77**: 527–529.

Kolts BE, Lyles WE, Achem SR, Burton L, Geller AJ & MacMath T (1993). A comparison of the effectiveness and patient tolerance of oral sodium phosphate, castor oil and standard electrolyte lavage for colonoscopy or sigmoidoscopy preparation. *Am J Gastroenterol* **88**: 1218–1223.

Kokoszka J, Nelson R, Falconio M & Abcarian H (1994) Treatment of fecal impaction with pulsed irrigation enhanced evacuation. *Dis Colon Rectum* **37**: 161–164.

Koruth NM, Hunter DC, Krukowski ZH & Matheson NA (1985) Immediate resection in emergency large bowel surgery: a 7 year audit. *Br J Surg* **72**: 708–711.

Kreel L (1975) Pharmaco-radiology in barium examinations with special reference to glucagon. *Br J Radiol* **48**: 691–703.

La Brooy SJ, Averginos A, Fendick CL & Williams CB (1981) Potentially explosive colonic concentrations of hydrogen after bowel preparation with mannitol. *Lancet* **i**: 634–636.

Lambling A & Truffert L (1944) L'explosion des gaz intestinaux au cours de l'electro-coagulation intrarectale. Un cas de rupture sigmoidienne mortelle. *Arch Mal Appar Digestif Nutr* **33**: 148–152.

Laurence DR (1973) *Clinical Pharmacology*, pp 21.9–21.14. Edinburgh: Churchill Livingstone.

Lazzaroni M, Petrillo M, Desideri S & Bianchi Porro G (1993) Efficacy and tolerability of polyethylene glycos-electrolyte lavage solution with and without simethicone in the preparation of patients with inflammatory bowel disease for colonoscopy. *Aliment Pharmacol Ther* **7**: 655–659.

Lee EC, Roberts PL, Taranto R, Schoetz DJ, Murray JJ & Coller JA (1996) Inpatient vs. outpatient bowel preparation for elective colorectal surgery. *Dis Colon Rectum* **39**: 369–373.

Lee JR & Ferrando JR (1984) Variables in the preparation of the large intestine for double contrast barium enema examination. *Gut* **25**: 69–72.

Lee JR, Hares MM & Keighley MRB (1981) A randomised trial to investigate X-Prep, oral mannitol and colonic washout for double contrast barium enema. *Clin Radiol* **32**: 591–594.

Levy AG, Benson JW, Hewlett EL, Herdt JR, Doppman JL & Gordon RS (1976) Saline lavage: a rapid, effective and acceptable method for cleansing the gastrointestinal tract. *Gastroenterology* **70**: 157–161.

Levy EI (1954) Explosions during lower bowel electrosurgery: a method of prevention. *Am J Surg* **88**: 754–758.

Lieberman DA, Ghormley J & Flora K (1996) Effect of oral sodium phosphate colon preparation on serum electrolytes in patients with normal serum creatinine. *Gastrointest Endosc* **43**: 467–469.

Lieberman W (1944) Inflammable physiologic gases in the rectum and colon. *Rev Gastroenterol Mex* **11**: 259–261.

Love AHG, Mitchell NG & Phillips RA (1968) Water and sodium absorption in the human intestine. *J Physiol* **195**: 133–140.

Love AHG, Rohde JE, Abrams ME et al (1973) The measurement of bidirectional sodium fluxes across the intestinal wall in man using whole gut perfusion. *Clin Sci* **44**: 267–278.

McDonagh AJG, Singh P, Pilbrow WJ & Youngs GR (1989) Safety of Picolax (sodium picosulphate-magnesium citrate) in inflammatory bowel disease. *BMJ* **299**: 776–777.

Margulis AR (1967) Some new approaches to the examination of the gastrointestinal tract. *Am J Roentgenol Radium Ther Nucl Med* **101**: 265–286.

Marshall JB, Barthel JS & King PD (1993). Short report: prospective, randomized trial comparing a single dose sodium phosphate regimen with PEG-electrolyte lavage for colonoscopy preparation. *Aliment Pharmacol Ther* **7**: 679–682.

Matheson DM, Arabi Y, Baxter-Smith D, Alexander-Williams J & Keighley MRB (1978) Randomised multicentre trial of oral bowel preparation and antimicrobials in elective colorectal operation. *Br J Surg* **65**: 597–600.

Mealy K, Salman A & Arthur G (1988) Definitive one-stage emergency large bowel surgery. *Br J Surg* **75**: 1216–1219.

Meisel JL, Bergman D, Graney D, Saunders DR & Rubin CE (1977) Human rectal mucosa: proctoscopic and morphological changes caused by laxatives. *Gastroenterology* **72**: 1274–1279.

Mikal S (1965) Metabolic effects of preoperative intestinal preparation. *Am J Proctol* **16**: 437–442.

Miller RE (1975a) Examination of the colon. *Curr Probl Radiol* **5**: 1–40.

Miller RE (1975b) The cleansing enema. *Radiology* **117**: 483–485.

Miller RE (1976) The clean colon. *Gastroenterology* **70**: 289–290.

Minervini S, Alexander-Williams J, Donovan I, Bentley S & Keighley MRB (1980) Comparison of three methods of whole bowel irrigation. *Am J Surg* **140**: 399–402.

Morris DL, Hares MM, Voogt RJ, Burden DW & Keighley MRB (1983) Metronidazole need not be combined with an aminoglycoside when used for prophylaxis in elective colorectal surgery. *J Hosp Infect* **4**: 65–69.

Morson B (1974) The polyp-cancer sequence in the large bowel. *Proc Soc Med* **67**: 451–457.

Moutier F (1946) Un nouveau cas d'explosion intra-rectale au cours d'une electro-coagulation. *Arch Med Appar Digest Par* **35**: 240–242.

Muir EG (1968) Safety in colonic resection. *J R Soc Med* **61**: 401–408.

Munro A, Steele RJC & Logie JRC (1987) Technique for intra-operative colonic irrigation. *Br J Surg* **75**: 1039–1040.

Nagy GS (1981) Preparing the patient. In Hunt RH & Way JR (eds) *Colonoscopy*, pp 36–44. London: Chapman & Hall.

Nasrullah SM & Iber FL (1969) Mannitol absorption and metabolism in man. *Am J Med Sci* **258**: 80–88.

National Center for Health Statistics (1973) *Volume of X-ray visits, United States, April–September 1970*. Rockville, MD: National Center for Health Statistics, Office of Information Public Health Service.

Newstead G & Morgan BP (1979) Bowel preparation with mannitol. *Med J Aust* **2**: 591–593.

Nichols RL & Condon RE (1971) Antibiotic preparation of the colon: failure of commonly used regimens. *Surg Clin North Am* **51**: 223–227.

Nichols RL, Condon RE, Gorbach SL & Nyhus LM (1972) Efficacy of pre-operative antimicrobial preparation of the bowel. *Ann Surg* **176**: 217–232.

Oliveira L, Wexner SD, Daniel N et al (1997) Mechanical bowel preparation for elective colorectal surgery. *Dis Colon Rectum* **40**: 585–591.

O'Dwyer PJ, Conway E, McDermott EWM & O'Higgins NJ (1989) Effect of mechanical bowel preparation on anastomotic integrity following low anterior resection in dogs. *Br J Surg* **76**: 756–758.

Palmer KR & Khan AN (1979) Oral mannitol: a simple and effective bowel preparation for barium enema. *BMJ* **2**: 1038.

Panton ONM, Atkinson KG, Crichton EP, Schulzer M, Beaujoy A & Gormann E (1985) Mechanical preparation of the large bowel for elective surgery. Comparison of whole gut lavage with the conventional enema and purgative technique. *Am J Surg* **149**: 615–619.

Phillips RKS, Hittinger R, Fry JS & Fielding LP (1985) Malignant large bowel obstruction. *Br J Surg* **72**: 296–302.

Phillips SF & Giller J (1973) The contribution of the colon to electrolyte and water conservation in man. *J Lab Clin Med* **81**: 733–746.

Pockros PJ & Foroozan P (1985) Golytely lavage versus a standard colonoscopy preparation. Effect on normal colonic mucosal histology. *Gastroenterology* **88**: 545–548.

Pollock AV, Playforth MJ & Evans M (1987) Peroperative lavage of the obstructed left colon to allow safe primary anastomosis. *Dis Colon Rectum* **30**: 270–274.

Raahave D, Bulow S, Jakobsen BH, Knudsen J & Nilsson T (1986) Whole bowel irrigation: a bacteriologic assessment. *Infect Surg* **5**: 12–23.

Radcliffe AG & Dudley HAF (1983) Intraoperative antegrade irrigation of the large intestine. *Surg Gynecol Obstet* **156**: 721–723.

Ragins HR, Shinya H & Wolff WI (1971) The explosive potential of colonic gas during colonoscopic electrosurgical polypectomy. *Surg Gynecol Obstet* **138**: 554–556.

Reybar JF (1844) *Bull Acad Med (Paris)* **9**: 1031.

Rhodes JB, Zvargulis JE & Williams CH (1977) Oral electrolyte overload to clean the colon for colonoscopy. *Gastrointest Endosc* **24**: 24–26.

Rhodes JB, Engstrom J & Stone KF (1978) Metoclopramide reduces the distress associated with colon cleansing by an oral electrolyte overload. *Gastrointest Endosc* **24**: 162–163.

Roe AM, Jamison MH & MacLennan I (1984). Colonoscopy preparation with Picolax. *J R Coll Surg Edinb* **29**: 103–104.

Rogers BGH (1974) The safety of carbon dioxide insufflation during colonoscopic electrosurgical polypectomy. *Gastrointest Endosc* **20**: 115–117.

Rogers CW (1971) Radiology's stepchild – the colon. *JAMA* **216**: 1855–1856.

Rosenberg IL, Graham NG, De Dombal FT & Goligher JC (1971) Preparation of the intestine in patients undergoing major large bowel surgery, mainly for neoplasms of the colon and rectum. *Br J Surg* **58**: 266–269.

Ryan P (1970) The effect of surrounding infection upon the leaking of colonic wounds: experimental studies and clinical experiences. *Dis Colon Rectum* **13**: 124–126.

Santos JCM, Batista J, Sirimarco MT, Guimaraes AS & Levy CE (1994). Prospective randomized trial of mechanical bowel preparation in patients undergoing elective colorectal surgery. *Br J Surg* **81**: 1673–1676.

Saunders CG & MacEwan DW (1971) Delay in diagnosis of colonic cancer – a continuing challenge. *Radiology* **101**: 207–208.

Saunders DR, Sillery J, Rachmilewitz D, Rubin CE & Tygot GN (1977) Effects of bisacodyl on the structure and function of rodent and human intestine. *Gastroenterology* **72**: 849–856.

Scammell BE, Phillips RP, Brown R, Burdon DW & Keighley MRB (1985) Influence of rectal washout on bacterial counts in the rectal stump. *Br J Surg* **72**: 548–550.

Schrock TR, Daveney CW & Dunphy JE (1973) Factors contributing to leakage of colonic anastomoses. *Ann Surg* **177**: 513–518.

Shinagawa N, Mizuno H, Shibata Y et al (1985) Gas explosion during diathermy colotomy. *Br J Surg* **72**: 306.

Silverman SH & Keighley MRB (1985) Rapid bowel preparation for outpatient flexible sigmoidoscopy. *Gut* **26**: A1156.

Skucas J, Cutliff W & Fischer HW (1976) Whole gut irrigation as a means of cleaning the colon. *Radiology* **121**: 303–305.

Slanger A (1979) Comparative study of a radiographic examination of the colon. *Dis Colon Rectum* **22**: 356–359.

Smith AG & Currie AEJ (1978) Whole gut irrigation: a new treatment for constipation. *BMJ* **3**: 296–297.

Smith SRG, Connolly JC & Gilmore OJA (1983) The effect of faecal loading on colonic anastomosis healing. *Br J Surg* **70**: 49–50.

Stewart J, Finan PJ, Courtney DF & Brennan TG (1984) Does a water soluble contrast enema assist in the management of acute large bowel obstruction: a prospective study of 117 cases. *Br J Surg* **71**: 799–801.

Tagart REB (1981) Colorectal anastomosis: factors influencing success. *J R Soc Med* **74**: 111–118.

Takada H, Ambrose NS, Galbraith K, Alexander-Williams J & Keighley MRB (1989) Quantitative appraisal of Picolax (sodium picosulfate/magnesium citrate) in the preparation of the large bowel for elective surgery. *Dis Colon Rectum* **33**: 679–683.

Takada H, Hioki K, Ambrose NS, Alexander-Williams J & Keighley MRB (1993) Potentially explosive colonic gas is not eliminated by successful mechanical bowel preparation. *Dig Surg* **10**: 20–23.

Taylor EW, Bentley S, Youngs D & Keighley MRB (1981) Bowel preparation and the safety of colonoscopic polypectomy. *Gastroenterology* **81**: 1–4.

Teague RH & Manning AP (1977) Preparation of the large bowel for endoscopy. *J Int Med Res* **5**: 374–377.

Thomas G, Brozinsky S & Isenberg JI (1982) Patient acceptance and effectiveness of a balanced lavage solution (Golytely) versus the standard preparation for colonoscopy. *Gastroenterology* **82**: 435–437.

Thomson WHF & Carter SStC (1986) On-table lavage to achieve safe restorative rectal and emergency left colonic resection. *Br J Surg* **73**: 61–63.

Tsang GMK, Bacelar T & Keighley MRB (1992) Sodium sulphate is cheaper and at least as good as 'Picolax' as an oral whole bowel irrigation solution (CP100) for bowel preparation. *Dig Surg* **9**: 209–211.

Turnbull RB Jr (1975) The no-touch isolation technique of resection. *JAMA* **231**: 1181–1182.

Turrell R & Landau SJ (1959) Antibiotics in the preoperative preparation of the colon. *J Int Coll Surg* **31**: 215–224.

Tyson RR & Spaulding EH (1959) Should antibiotics be used in large bowel preparation? *Surg Gynecol Obstet* **108**: 623–626.

Vanner SJ, MacDonald PH, Paterson WG, Prentice RSA, DaCosta LR & Beck IT (1990) A randomized prospective trial comparing oral sodium phosphate with standard polyethylene glycol-based lavage solution (Golytely) in the preparation of patients for colonoscopy. *Am J Gastroenterol* **85**: 422–427.

Walls ADF (1980) Colon preparation. *J R Coll Surg Edinb* **25**: 26–31.

Weaver PC & Khawaja HT (1986) Intra-operative colonic irrigation. *Br J Surg* **73**: 83–84.

Welin S (1958) Modern trends in diagnostic roentgenology of the colon. *Br J Radiol* **31**: 453–464.

Welin S (1967) Results of the Malmo technique of colon examination. *JAMA* **199**: 369–371.

Welin S, Youker J & Spratt JS (1963) The rates and patterns of growth of 375 tumours of the large intestine and rectum observed serially by double contrast enema study (Malmo technique). *Am J Roentgenol Radium Ther Nucl Med* **90**: 673–687.

Wilkie D (1938) *Edinburgh Postgraduate Lectures in Medicine.* Edinburgh: Oliver & Boyd.

Williams CB, Hunt RH, Loose H et al (1974) Colonoscopy in the management of colon polyps. *Br J Surg* **61**: 673–682.

Winitz M, Graff J, Gallagher N et al (1965) Evaluation of chemical diets as nutrition for man-in-space. *Nature* **205**: 741–743.

Winitz M, Adams RF, Seedman DA et al (1966) Regulation of intestinal flora patterns with chemical diets. *Fed Proc* **25**: 343.

Winitz M, Adams RF, Seedman DA et al (1970) Studies in metabolic nutrition employing chemically defined diets: II. Effect on gut microflora populations. *Am J Clin Nutr* **23**: 546–559.

Wolters U, Keller HW, Sorgatz S, Raab A & Pichlmaier H (1994) Prospective randomized study of preoperative bowel cleansing for patients undergoing colorectal surgery. *Br J Surg* **81**: 598–600.

Woo P, Hatfield A, Green JR & Hamilton SM (1976) Whole gut perfusion for therapeutic purgation. *BMJ* **1**: 433–434.

Woodward NW (1961) Prevention of explosion while fulgurating polyps of the colon. *Dis Colon Rectum* **4**: 32.

Yoshioka K, Connolly AB, Ogunbiyi OA, Hasegawa H, Morton DG & Keighley MRB (1998) Randomized trials of oral sodium phosphate compared with sodium picosulphate in colonoscopy and colorectal surgery. *Ann R Coll Surg Engl* (in preparation).

Zanoni CE, Gergamini C, Bertoncini M, Bertoncini L & Garbini A (1982) Whole gut lavage for surgery: a case of intra-operative colonic explosion after administration of mannitol. *Dis Colon Rectum* **25**: 580–581.

Zimmerman K (1959) Detonation of intestinal gas by an electrosurgical unit. *South Med J* **52**: 605–608.

Zwas FR, Cirillo NW, El-Serag HB & Eisen RN (1996) Colonic mucosal abnormalities associated with oral sodium phosphate solution. *Gastrointest Endosc* **42**: 463–466.

4 NUTRITIONAL CARE

In the past 25 years great advances have been made in the nutritional care of the surgical patient. The introduction of parenteral nutrition in particular has revolutionized the treatment of those patients who cannot rely on their gastrointestinal tract for adequate nutrition. Patients with colorectal disease who require surgery may fall into this category. Nutritional support may be needed preoperatively or postoperatively, especially if a complication intervenes, and in certain circumstances nutrition alone may prevent surgical intervention. Nutrition can be supplied by the parenteral, enteral and oral routes. If nutritional support is needed in colorectal patients the parenteral route is often required. Further details are provided in the chapters devoted to intestinal fistulas (Chapter 65) and Crohn's disease (Chapters 50–58).

PARENTERAL NUTRITION

Preoperative indications

There is considerable debate as to the indications, and indeed the necessity, for intravenous feeding of patients before elective surgery. Most surgeons would, however, agree with Studley (1936) that those patients who have lost more than 20% of their bodyweight are at particular risk of sepsis and anastomotic dehiscence and would benefit from a period of feeding. The difficulty arises in patients who have lost less than this amount of weight.

Numerous indices in addition to bodyweight have been studied as markers for nutritional depletion, perhaps the most common being the plasma proteins. Low plasma concentrations of albumin (Hickman et al, 1980; Brown et al, 1982; Klidjian et al, 1982), transferrin (Kamminski et al, 1977) and prealbumin (Pettigrew and Hill, 1986), and combinations of these (Harvey et al, 1981; Simms et al, 1982; Rainey-MacDonald et al, 1983), have been shown to identify groups of high-risk patients in whom postoperative complications are likely to occur. Similarly, anthropometric measurements such as arm circumference, triceps skin-fold thickness and body mass index have been used to identify such high-risk patients (Studley, 1936; Klidjian et al, 1980). Muscle function may also be measured by voluntary hand grip and electrical stimulation, both of which have been shown to be useful prognostic indicators (Sutton and Karran, 1985). Various immunological tests, such as low absolute lymphocyte counts and decreased response to recall antigens and delayed hypersensitivity, have also been used to assess nutritional state (Dowd and Heatley, 1984). Despite these numerous studies there is considerable scepticism as to the accuracy of these indices. Although they may indicate those patients who may have a poor outcome from surgery, it is possible that they reflect other problems apart from the nutritional state.

A study by Pettigrew and Hill (1986) is of particular importance in this context. These authors looked prospectively at a number of the predictors of surgical outcome discussed above. They compared these predictors with a global assessment of risk made by the operating surgeon and with the results of a more complex clinical assessment rating derived from a detailed history and examination of the patient. Plasma proteins were reasonably accurate in identifying the high-risk groups but the authors concluded that a careful examination of the patient before surgery was by far the most important predictor of outcome. The preoperative plasma protein concentrations were most often decreased as a result of preoperative sepsis rather than nutritional deprivation.

It would appear that the surgeon should not interpret these so-called 'nutritional markers' in isolation. The chances are they are altered for reasons other than the nutritional state.

In the light of present knowledge it seems sensible to recommend preoperative feeding only in the patient who is obviously grossly malnourished. We take weight loss of 20% or more as being a strong indication for nutritional support. If other nutritional markers, in particular plasma proteins, indicate a poor prognosis, it seems wise to correct other factors such as sepsis which might be responsible for these abnormalities before proceeding to surgery.

It is perhaps worth mentioning that there are very few controlled trials which have demonstrated any clinical benefit from routine preoperative intravenous nutrition for patients undergoing elective colorectal surgery.

Postoperative indications

The indications for feeding patients intravenously in the postoperative period can broadly be classified into three categories:

1. The gut cannot cope because there has been a complication following major surgery; for instance, intra-abdominal abscess complicating proctocolectomy.
2. The gastrointestinal tract is too short. In the context of colorectal surgery, this is usually because an external fistula has developed from the small intestine.
3. The gastrointestinal tract is blocked, either because of mechanical obstruction or paralytic ileus.

Nutritional requirements

As with nutritional indicators, there is debate concerning the nutritional requirements of surgical patients. Rhoads et al (1981) in Philadelphia were among the first to use parenteral nutrition in surgical patients, and they laid the foundation for its widespread use by surgeons around the world. Dudrick et al (1970) noted weight gain, positive nitrogen balance and clinical improvement with intakes of 2000–4000 kcal and nitrogen intakes equivalent to 125–170 g of protein, amounts which are well above levels currently recommended for normal adult subjects. For this reason this form of parenteral nutrition was referred to as intravenous hyperalimentation (IVH). In recent years the consensus of opinion is that for most general surgical patients such high requirements are unnecessary and indeed may be harmful. The vogue is to match intake fairly closely to requirements (Skenkin and Wretlind, 1978), a technique now referred to as total parenteral nutrition (TPN). Patients with colorectal problems who may require nutritional support can be subdivided into three categories, as recommended by Hill and Church (1984), each with separate requirements. (Note that 'stress' in these patients is defined as major sepsis or a major operation.)

1. *Nutritional depletion without stress.* This results simply from an overall deficit in intake or utilization of food. Weight loss may be as much as 40%, with skeletal muscle, adipose tissue, skin and liver accounting for much of this. Wasting of depot fat and skeletal muscle is generalized and plasma albumin is normal. The patient is not hypercatabolic (Wilmore, 1977). A common cause in colorectal surgery is the patient with widespread carcinoma.
2. *Nutritional depletion with stress.* Patients may vary from those with relatively little wasting of subcutaneous fat to those with virtually non-existent fat stores. Muscle wasting and low plasma albumin are constant findings. Patients who are already wasted and in addition suffer postoperative complications almost always suffer from sepsis (Hill, 1981). A normally nourished patient may develop this syndrome as well if a major complication develops after surgery and nutritional therapy is inadequate (Hill and Church, 1984).
3. *Normal nutritional state with added stress.* In this syndrome the patient has normal quantities of fat and muscle but there is a rapid fall in plasma albumin. The patient is hypermetabolic. This

state is seen when a major postoperative septic complication occurs in a previously well-nourished patient.

The category to which the patient belongs will dictate the energy and protein requirements. Table 4.1 indicates the approximate amounts of energy and nitrogen required per 24 hours in the various groups.

The table is based on recommendations made by Hill and Church (1984) and for further details as to the rationale for these amounts the reader is strongly urged to read their excellent review.

Most of the energy requirements will be met by using glucose. The main disadvantage of glucose is its hyperosmolarity but this is outweighed by lack of serious metabolic side-effects. The alternative carbohydrate energy substrates are fructose, maltose and the polyols sorbitol, xylitol and glycerol. The use of these agents in clinical practice has effectively been ruled out because of their serious side-effects, which include metabolic acidosis, hyperuricaemia, hypophosphataemia, renal damage and a decrease in adenine nucleotides in the liver (Skenkin and Wretlind, 1978). The optimum utilization of glucose occurs when it is administered at a rate of 7 mg/kg bodyweight per minute (equivalent to 40 kcal/kg per day). Above this level undesirable effects occur and it is recommended that if more energy is required it should be given as fat (Hill and Church, 1984).

Indeed, there are many nutritional experts (Elwyn et al, 1980; MacFie et al, 1981) who recommend that some of the energy requirements should routinely be given as fat. The advantages of fat as an energy source are the lack of osmotic activity, a high energy value (9 kcal/g) and the supply of essential fatty acids. The only barrier to the routine use of fat until recently was its adverse side-effects and, in particular, its effect on the reticuloendothelial system, the coagulation mechanism and pulmonary function. However, the introduction of soyabean oil–egg yolk emulsions has virtually eliminated these problems. The only problem with the administration of fat is that it makes the whole process more complicated and time consuming for the nursing staff. For this reason it is recommended that fat administration is limited to three groups of colorectal patients (Hill and Church, 1984):

1. Patients having intravenous nutrition for periods of more than one week who therefore require a source of essential fatty acids.
2. Patients who need their energy intake topped up. Since it is believed that when amounts of glucose above 40 kcal/kg per 24 hours are administered they are poorly utilized, fat is given if further energy is required.
3. Patients being weaned from ventilatory assistance. Some patients receiving high glucose loads cannot easily be weaned from ventilation because of carbon dioxide retention. The giving of fat can reduce the respiratory quotient to less than unity and by so doing spontaneous ventilation can be more easily achieved (Askanazi et al, 1981).

Table 4.1 Guidelines for intravenous administration of energy and nitrogen in different categories of surgical patients.

Nutritional and metabolic category	*Energy (kcal/kg/day)*	*Nitrogen (mg/kg/day)*
Normally nourished: preoperative	40	260
Normally nourished: postoperative	40	300
Depleted: no stress	40	300
Depleted and stressed	45	350
Normally nourished and stressed	50	400

Stress = major sepsis or major operation.
Adapted from Hill and Church (1984).

Protein requirements are nowadays supplied universally as synthetic crystalline amino acids. There are several commercially available solutions and there seems to be little difference between them. The most important considerations in the composition of an amino acid solution include the quantities of essential and non-essential amino acids, the ratio of essential amino acids (EAA) to total nitrogen, the balance of the mixture, its toxicity (glycine content) and its biological value (Hegsted, 1978). The proportion of EAA is important for optimum nutrition and is generally expressed as grams per gram of total nitrogen (Skenkin and Wretlind, 1978). Nutritionally depleted individuals require approximately three times the EAA requirements of normal subjects. Anderson et al (1974) state that normal subjects need 81 mg/kg EAA, whereas the nutritionally depleted patient needs 219 mg/kg. Amino acids for intravenous nutrition need to have an EAA content similar to that of proteins with a high biological value, approximately 40%. Commercial preparations of crystalline amino acid solutions contain a range of EAA proportions from 27 to 47%.

It has been shown (Rudman et al, 1975) that sodium, potassium and phosphate are all essential for nitrogen retention from infused amino acids. To be fully effective intravenous nutrition must therefore be balanced with respect to electrolytes, vitamins and trace metals, as well as nitrogen and calories. The importance of some trace elements has only recently been realized. Thus, lack of selenium over the long term can result in muscle damage (Watson et al, 1985). Similarly, the importance of certain vitamins needs emphasizing. Until recently biotin was not added to TPN mixtures until a biotin deficiency syndrome was recognized. This manifested itself by loss of hair, rash and changes in facial fat distribution (Mock et al, 1985).

Methods of administration

The practice of parenteral nutrition requires the skills of medical, nursing and pharmacy staff and dieticians. This is best organized, in our view, by having a nutritional support team which includes a member from each department which it serves. After consultation with the surgeon in charge of the patient the team remains responsible for the administration and day-to-day nutritional requirements. Nehme (1980) compared the results in patients managed during parenteral nutrition by a nutritional support team with those managed by a variety of physicians. Mechanical problems of catheter insertion, sepsis and metabolic fluid and electrolyte complications were all more common in the latter group.

TPN can be administered either by the peripheral or more commonly the central route. Early attempts to use peripheral veins were thwarted by their inability to accept hypertonic solutions. However, with the development of isotonic fat solutions, energy requirements can be met more easily utilizing the peripheral route. By combining amino acids and fat with a small quantity of isotonic glucose, the nutritional needs of the average patient can be provided. However, there are problems. Peripheral lines are more cumbersome for the patient, and despite meticulous care and the use of heparin or hydrocortisone, phlebitis and occlusion still occur, even with the use of fine bore silicone rubber or polyurethane catheters (Madan et al, 1992; Kohlhardt and Smith, 1989; Kohlhardt et al, 1994; Everitt et al, 1993; Everitt and McMahon, 1997). In colorectal surgery, we use this form of administration for a few days postoperatively when we wish to prevent early bowel actions which might contaminate a perineal wound, e.g. after sphincter repair for incontinence. Occasionally, the peripheral route is required when a central line is contraindicated or is impossible to insert.

Insertion of a central venous catheter for feeding can be achieved in one of two ways, either by percutaneous puncture (Powell Tuck, 1978a) or under direct vision by cut down (Oosterlee and Dudley, 1980). The aim is to position the catheter under X-ray control in the superior vena cava; the vein used to introduce the catheter is either the internal jugular or subclavian. It is debatable which is superior but we prefer the subclavian. Cut down to the veins is preferred by some to prevent damage to adjacent structures but the percutaneous method utilizing a subcutaneous tunnel appears quite satisfactory if due care is employed (Figure 4.1) (Powell Tuck, 1978a; Nehme, 1980).

Complications which may occur include pneumothorax, venous thrombosis, arterial injury, nerve damage and haemothorax, but the most important of all is catheter sepsis which has been recognized since the early days of parenteral feeding. *Staphylococcus epidermidis* is the most common pathogen isolated and it may gain access to the bloodstream down the subcutaneous tract of the catheter (Garden and Sim, 1983; Keohane et al, 1983) or through the connector hub (Sitges-Serra and Linares, 1984). Provided catheter care is conducted under strict aseptic conditions the catheter sepsis rate should be less than 5% (McIntyre et al, 1984; Irving et al, 1985; Pettigrew et al, 1985). If catheter sepsis is suspected it is quite safe to change the catheter over a guidewire unless the catheter has been proven to be infected (Pettigrew et al, 1985).

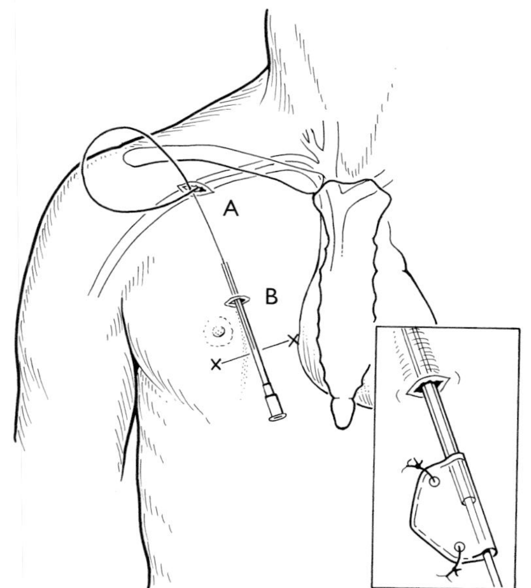

Figure 4.1 Subclavian catheterization with a skin tunnel AB. The sedated patient is placed in a head-down position. The procedure is carried out in a clean room using strict aseptic technique. Insert: the plastic clip which grips the emerging catheter at B and sleeve is anchored with sutures.

Quantitative cultures of the withdrawn catheter tips should be made before a new catheter is introduced over a guidewire. In most cases it is inappropriate to treat catheter-related sepsis with antibiotics since septicaemia often recurs as a consequence of bacteria remaining adherent to the tip of the catheter. Removal of the catheter is almost always necessary and eradicates the septicaemia (Sitges-Serra et al, 1984). However, if feeding must continue and other sites of venous access are not available, long-term treatment with vancomycin may be successful.

Studies investigating the development of venous thrombosis in relation to TPN have concluded that the main cause is the material from which the catheter is made. Polyvinylchloride is most frequently associated with thrombosis, whereas silicone rubber seems to be the safest material in this respect (Laidlow et al, 1983). There is also a higher risk of thrombosis of major veins when attempts are made to replace catheters, in particular when a guidewire is used.

Pneumothorax is always a risk of catheter insertion but in an experienced unit the incidence should be no greater than 2%. Between 1979 and 1982 the Oxford parenteral nutrition team administered a total of 190 courses of parenteral nutrition to 179 patients, and the incidence of pneumothorax was 1.5% (Oxford Parenteral Nutrition Team, 1983).

Metabolic complications

In addition to the trace element deficiencies which have already been mentioned, hypophosphataemia may be common, particularly amongst patients who have been seriously ill before parenteral nutrition is commenced. Thus Thompson and Hodges (1984) noted that 12% of their patients were found to have hypophosphataemia prior to TPN, and 42% developed the problem during therapy. Sixty per cent of the 42% of patients developed hypophosphataemia within 3 days of commencing TPN. Provided the patients are monitored carefully and replacement is undertaken promptly this deficiency should be eradicated. It should be pointed out that no related morbidity or mortality has been demonstrated in relation to hypophosphataemia.

Modern TPN regimens do not contain the amino acid taurine, deficiency of which causes retinal dysfunction. Reduced taurine levels have been found in patients on long-term TPN (Geggel et al, 1984). Another non-essential nutrient, carnitine C1, appears to be needed during the metabolic response to injury. It is required for fatty acid oxidation in skeletal and cardiac muscles. Hyperbilirubinaemia, generalized skeletal weakness and reactive hypoglycaemia may result from its deficiency (Worthley et al, 1983). Recognition of this problem may be complicated by the failure of plasma carnitine to reflect tissue carnitine status. Red cell carnitine levels should be measured in addition to the plasma carnitine (Meguid and Borum, 1984).

Apart from deficiency of nutrients, nutrient excess may lead to problems, the most frequent of which is hyperglycaemia, and patients on TPN should always be on a sliding scale of insulin. A less common problem is hyperoxaluria, which appears to be related to the excessive availability of ascorbic acid in TPN regimens. Other factors include pyridoxine deficiency and excesses of other precursors such as glycine, hydroxyproline or xylitol. Renal impairment may result from hyperoxaluria (Swartz et al, 1984).

The infusion of fat in amounts greater than 4 g/kg per day may lead to a bleeding diathesis characterized by fever, hyperlipidaemia, hepatic dysfunction, diarrhoea and spontaneous haemorrhage (Heyman et al, 1981).

Administration of high doses of glucose to patients with borderline respiratory function may increase carbon dioxide production, which may in turn compromise their respiratory function (Elwyn, 1980).

Cholestasis is a common complication during parenteral nutrition. It seems to result from impaired biliary motor function, which in turn leads to sludge formation and the development of gallstones. Both calculous and acalculous cholecystitis may occur (Pitt et al, 1983). It has been suggested that patients on long-term TPN, even if asymptomatic, should undergo elective cholecystectomy (Roslyn et al, 1984). This seems to be somewhat unnecessary although with laparoscopic cholecystectomy it may be more acceptable. Perhaps regular treatment with cholecystokinin or ursodeoxycholic acid may be a compromise.

Home parenteral nutrition

Occasionally patients with a colorectal disease require long-term intravenous nutrition. This treatment is most likely to be required for a young patient who has widespread small bowel Crohn's disease and who has undergone a massive small bowel resection. In these circumstances, in order to sustain life and allow the patient to be rehabilitated, he or she may be fed at home. The decision to follow this treatment regimen is a difficult one, both from the practical and the ethical point of view. Provided the patient is reasonably intelligent and physically able to master the technique of changing the dressing, connecting the catheter and adjusting the pump, and provided the prognosis is reasonable, we believe that appropriate patients should be offered home parenteral nutrition. The cost is high but it is not in our opinion the responsibility of the surgeon to base his decision on financial considerations. The situation is akin to patients being managed on long-term renal dialysis except that the option of small bowel transplantation is not yet sufficiently developed for this to be a realistic clinical option for these patients (Mitchell et al, 1984).

A prodigious experience of home parenteral nutrition has been reported by Dudrick and his colleagues (1984) in the USA. One hundred and thirty-three patients were treated at home for a total of more than 100 catheter-years. Catheter sepsis rates were acceptable, being 1 in every 3 catheter-years. This review indicated that home parenteral nutrition was likely to become a widespread and safe procedure for a minority of patients who required protracted or indefinite TPN and who could be relied upon to manage their own therapies. This prophesy has indeed been borne out. Most large colorectal centres have several patients managed in this way. Solutions are prepared in pharmacy and given intermittently, usually overnight, so the patient is free of the infusion apparatus during the day. A vest with a small pump may be used to enable continuous infusion of nutrients throughout the day if required (Dudrick et al, 1979).

There have been several studies assessing quality of life of patients on home parenteral nutrition (Detsky et al, 1986; Richards and Irving, 1997). The consensus seems to be that the health status profile of young patients on home parenteral nutrition is good compared with the normal population. The poorest scores occur in older patients and those dependent on narcotic drugs. The cost of treating a patient with intestinal failure in this way has been carefully calculated. In the UK the cost per quality adjusted life year (QALY) for an average person was approximately £68 975, but the value for patients over 55 years of age was about £126 865 compared with approximately £58 233 for those under 44 years (Richards and Irving, 1996). Treating a patient in hospital rather than at home increased the estimated cost per QALY to approximately £190 000. Thus, home parenteral nutrition is about 65% more cost effective than the same care provided in hospital.

The possibility of small bowel transplantation (Thompson et al, 1995) for patients with intestinal failure maintained on TPN has certainly increased optimism for such patients, and their medical attendants. However, there are still major problems which have delayed widespread adoption of the operation. At present young, well-adjusted patients on home parenteral nutrition are being advised to continue on this course until outcomes of small bowel transplantation improve (Richards and Irving, 1997). However, it is interesting to note that in a study by Carlson et al (1998) it was the young patients (with the best quality of life scores) who were most keen on a small bowel transplantation, indicating an unwillingness to accept long-term home parenteral nutrition.

ENTERAL NUTRITION

Enteral nutrition is defined as the administration of nutrients to the gastrointestinal tract (Silk, 1985) and is to be preferred to the parenteral route of administration whenever possible. In certain units approximately 75% of patients with medical and surgical disorders are fed via the enteral route (Silk, 1983). Most colorectal surgeons, however, use this route relatively infrequently, either because the patient's condition does not allow such therapy or because they wish to ensure that the patient receives all the nutrition prescribed. In view of the simplicity of administration it should perhaps be used more often than at present.

Clearly patients with concomitant small bowel disease or patients with enteric fistulas are unsuitable for enteral feeding. Patients with colorectal disease who need supplementary feeding preoperatively and in certain cases postoperatively may be ideal candidates for such therapy if time allows. This is particularly so in view of the recently demonstrated effect that enteral nutrition has been shown to have on preventing bacterial translocation in the gut. Absence or inadequate enteral nutrition results in a failure of gut barrier function. Translocation occurs which is associated with activation of macrophages both in mesenteric lymph nodes and the liver with subsequent release of interleukins 1 and 6 and tumour necrosis factor (Alexander et al, 1990). Such changes may have a profound effect on the incidence of sepsis and cancer immunology.

There are three principal methods of administering enteral nutrition: by nasogastric or nasoenteric tube, tube enterostomy or fine needle catheter jejunostomy. The nasogastric tubes are of fine bore and have weighted ends to allow them to be positioned at the appropriate site. As these tubes may permit aspiration their position needs to be checked by X-ray before feeding commences. Feeding tubes can become blocked when the consistency of the nutrient is too thick but they can be irrigated with water to overcome the obstruction. Regurgitation may still occur with fine bore tubes, particularly at night, and patients should be advised to sleep in a semirecumbent position. With regard to the nasogastric or nasoenteric routes of enteral feeding, most authorities recommend the former route whenever possible (Silk, 1985). The advocates of nasogastric feeding point out that the pylorus acts as a brake. Direct delivery of a hypertonic enteral diet into the duodenum or jejunum is therefore likely to increase the incidence of gastrointestinal side-effects, including diarrhoea.

Tube enterostomy can be used in the stomach or jejunum. Traditionally, large tubes were used and they were inserted at operation when enteral feeding was to be prolonged for more than 4–6 weeks. Nowadays fine tubes are available and they can be inserted by percutaneous endoscopic techniques or in the case of jejunostomies also by a fine needle technique. A jejunostomy is used when there is a risk of aspiration; otherwise, a gastrostomy is used. For endoscopic placement of the tube a 'pull method' is used (Ponsky and Gauderer, 1989). The endoscope is passed and the stomach is fully inflated, the room lights are dimmed, allowing transillumination of the stomach. An intravenous cannula is then passed percutaneously into the transilluminated stomach to lie within a snare loop which is tightened around the cannula, when the needle is removed and replaced with a thread of Nylon about 150 cm in length. The endoscope, snare and Nylon are then pulled up through the oesophagus and out of the patient's mouth. The Nylon is then attached to the pointed end of a specially constructed gastrostomy tube, which is drawn through into the stomach and out through its wall and through the abdominal wall (Figure 4.2). A balloon on the 'stomach side' of the tube is inflated and delivered through the abdominal wall to abut against the stomach wall and the tube is anchored to the abdominal wall.

Those patients requiring jejunostomy have another tube which passes into the stomach via the gastrostomy tube and out of the pylorus to lie in the upper jejunum. Alternatively, a jejunostomy can be constructed with a fine needle technique (Figure 4.3). This is a technique which has been used mainly during the postoperative period. The catheter is placed at the time of operation by inserting a needle tunnelled submucosally along a 10-cm length of jejunum and the bowel segment is secured to the anterior abdominal wall (Yeung et al, 1979). There are, however, dangers; in particular, the catheters may leak into the abdominal cavity. Despite this risk, for those surgeons who do not have access to safe parenteral nutrition, the technique, if used properly, can be a valuable aid in selected patients.

It is customary to administer 3 L of a nutrient solution via the tube, be it nasogastric or jejunal. Although gravity can be used for instillation, a pump is generally used to ensure a more constant infusion. Continuous infusion is required because nursing care is easier and there is less diarrhoea and

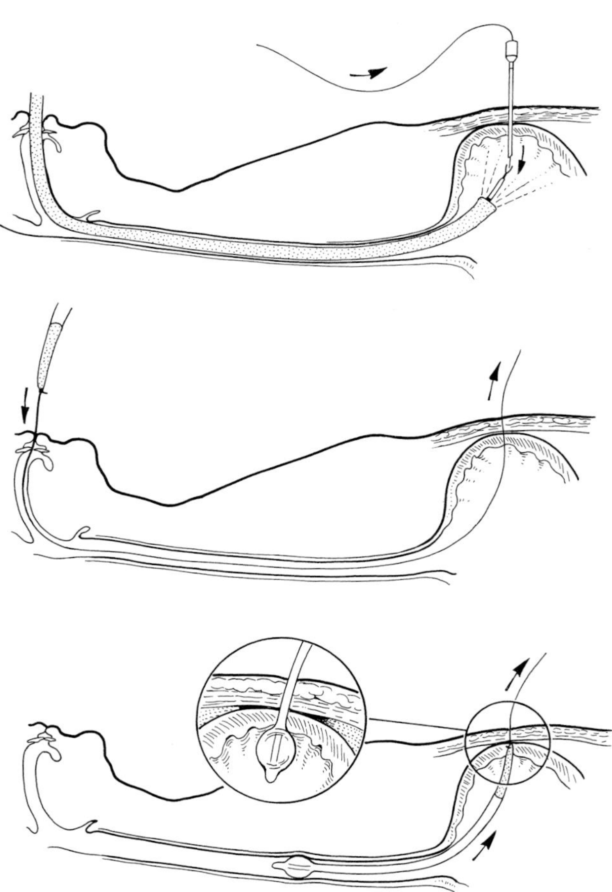

Figure 4.2 The 'pull' technique for endoscopic gastrostomy. The gastrostomy tube is pulled in a retrograde fashion down the oesophagus into the stomach and out through the abdominal wall using the Nylon thread.

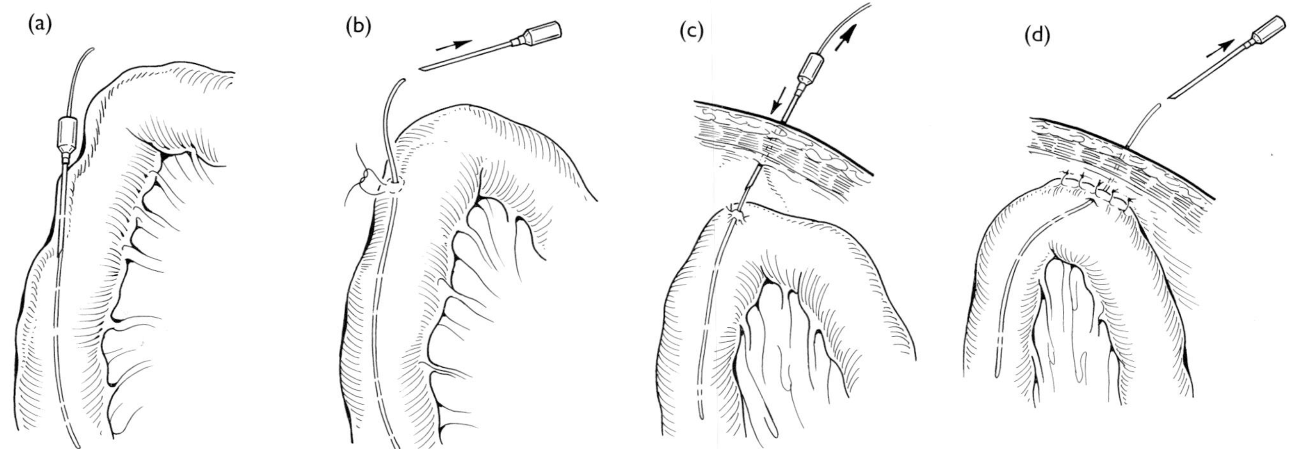

Figure 4.3 Fine needle jejunostomy. (a) A large-bore needle is inserted obliquely through the wall of the jejunum into its lumen. A catheter with a stylet is then passed through the needle into the jejunum (b). The needle is taken out and the catheter is fixed in place with a surrounding anchor stitch after removal of the stylet. (c) The end of the catheter is brought out through another large-bore needle inserted through the abdominal wall. (d) The jejunum is secured to the anterior abdominal wall.

fewer problems with nausea and vomiting. Enteral feeding should be commenced gradually, usually with quarter strength solutions progressing to a full nutrient load over the next 2 days if the patient's tolerance allows. The patient must be monitored carefully, ensuring that fluid overload or electrolyte imbalance do not occur. Diarrhoea is a common problem and is one cogent reason why many colorectal surgeons do not use enteral feeding regimens extensively. Diarrhoea can be controlled to some extent by slowing the rate of infusion or reducing the osmotic load. There are many types of liquid feeding regimens available. It is perhaps best to have a regimen made up by the hospital pharmacy to fulfil the individual patient's needs. The ideal complete formula should have about 1000 kcal/L with a nitrogen:energy ratio (g:kg) of approximately 1:840 (Pettigrew and Hill, 1984).

ORAL NUTRITION

Although the oral route is the cheapest, most efficient and preferred route for the ingestion and assimilation of nutrients, it is not always possible for patients with colorectal disease to utilize this route. Furthermore, it is rarely possible to replenish a major nutritional deficit prior to operation by the oral route, since time is too short and the patient cannot usually take sufficient by mouth. Postoperative complications also rarely allow the oral route to be used since it is usually a prerequisite for their treatment that the gut needs to be rested. In addition, the patient is usually too sick to ingest the required calories. The oral route may, however, be of use in certain situations for patients with colorectal disease or those who undergo elective operations for it.

An elemental diet may be used as an alternative technique of bowel preparation and the same diet may be used to induce a 'medical colostomy' when the distal gut needs to be rested for a period of time in the postoperative course. Elemental diets have also been used in patients with the short bowel syndrome, inflammatory bowel disease, faecal fistula, chronic intestinal obstruction, diverticulitis and various diarrhoeas.

Elemental diets were developed in the 1960s for astronauts in order to eliminate problems of storage, ingestion and waste disposal. They are composed of amino acids or small peptides as the nitrogen source with up to 30% of the energy as fat. Elemental diets have no lactose or digestive residues and have added trace metals and vitamins. They can maintain nitrogen and energy balance in normal subjects for up to 6 months (Pettigrew and Hill, 1984). A variety of products are available, including Vivonex, Flexical, Aminoid (essential amino acids) and Hapeticoid (branched-chain enriched amino acids).

The clinical application of elemental diets has been based on the premise that they are more easily absorbed, do not stimulate gastrointestinal secretions and have a low residue. While oral residue is reduced, we are not convinced that improved absorption or reduced secretion is achieved by these dietary regimens. A number of side-effects have been reported, including gastric retention, fluid balance problems, hyperglycaemia and deficiencies of vitamins or fatty acids. While most can be corrected by careful attention to the composition of the diet or by slowing delivery to the gut, we have found that diarrhoea can remain a persistent problem. Diarrhoea may well defeat the object of elemental diet if the aim is to rest the distal bowel and create a medical colostomy. Although the problem of diarrhoea occurs more frequently with hyperosmotic feeds, dilution does not necessarily remedy the situation. Diarrhoea does not seem to affect all patients and there is considerable individual variability in response. However, in our view it occurs with sufficient frequency such that we cannot recommend the widespread use of elemental diets, although for selected patients with certain problems, particularly extensive Crohn's disease, these diets may have an important therapeutic role.

DIETARY FIBRE AND THE LARGE INTESTINE

While the relationship between dietary fibre, diverticular disease, colorectal cancer, haemorrhoids and other coloproctological disorders is discussed in the appropriate chapters, it is convenient to discuss the principles of dietary fibre in this section. Fibre was thought to be a component of food which was inert and of no nutritional value. However, enthusiasts had for centuries propounded the virtues of wholemeal foods which were rich in fibre for better health, for treatment of many diseases and particularly for the relief of constipation. In 1941, Surgeon Captain Cleave RN was one of the first to define in scientific terms a specific role for dietary fibre in the treatment of constipation (Cleave, 1983).

Major scientific interest in dietary fibre really started in the 1960s when a number of independent reports suggested that dietary fibre altered the incidence of diseases. Most of the evidence was epidemiological, based mainly on diet and disease patterns in tropical countries where many other factors may have contributed. Many papers were published by various authors (Cleave and Campbell, 1966; Burkitt, 1969; Trowell et al, 1974) to popularize the 'fibre hypothesis', which proposed that a diet low in fibre and high in refined carbohydrates may be responsible for many of the Western diseases that have increased during the past 100 years. Despite circumstantial evidence, 'hard data' are lacking, most studies being poorly controlled or even anecdotal. A further problem is that 'dietary fibre' is a generic name for all plant polysaccharides and lignin that are resistant to hydrolysis by the digestive enzymes of humans. They have widely diverse chemical structures and physical properties. They vary from one source to another and even from batch to batch. Their properties are influenced by methods of purification, particle size, the presence of impurities and formulation. Consequently much of the literature on the short-term effects of dietary fibre is confusing, sometimes conflicting and not always reproducible. Long-term controlled trials are very difficult to perform. As yet the only evidence of the role of dietary fibre in the aetiology of colorectal disease is epidemiological, therefore a causal relationship remains speculative (Taylor, 1985).

Despite these criticisms most authors agree that an increase in dietary fibre can only be beneficial for patients. Dietary fibre can normalize bowel function, particularly in constipation (Cummings, 1984), and can relieve the symptoms of diverticular disease. The long-term effects on the wide range of diseases implicated in the fibre hypothesis are still unknown. The types and balance of fibres eaten may also be important. Long-term epidemiological evidence is influenced by many factors, including extrinsic and dietary factors, unrelated to fibre intake. It would appear, however, that a diet containing more fibre certainly confers short-term benefits and may also have long-term advantages, although these remain unproven (Jones, 1984; Taylor, 1984).

The mode of action of fibre is to increase faecal bulk, shorten transit time through the gut and hence reduce intraluminal colonic pressure and reduce the pressure required to effect defecation. The bulking effect of fibre appears to be due to a combination of its water-holding properties and its ability to be degraded by colonic bacteria (Stephen and Cummings, 1980).

A major problem in the therapeutic use of dietary fibre is its palatability and consequently patient compliance. Formulation and presentation appears to be almost as important as the type and dose of fibre used. Older people in particular find it difficult to change their dietary habit. An increase in dietary fibre may not be tolerated. It may cause abdominal symptoms because microbial fermentation of the available carbohydrate releases gas which causes distension and flatulence, and because osmotically active residues may cause loose bulky stools or even watery diarrhoea. Such symptoms may limit the use of fibre but patients should be advised that they do improve with time (O'Donnell and Fleming, 1984). A detailed account on the impact of fibre on colonic function is provided in the chapter devoted to diverticular disease (Chapter 37).

REFERENCES

Alexander JW, Boyce ST, Babcock GF et al (1990) The process of microbial translocation. *Ann Surg* **212**: 496–512.

Anderson GH, Patel DG & Jeejeebhoy KN (1974) Design and evaluation by nitrogen balance and blood aminograms of an amino acid mixture for total parenteral nutrition of adults with gastrointestinal disease. *J Clin Invest* **53**: 904–912.

Askanazi J, Norderstom J, Rosenbaum SH et al (1981) Nutrition for the patient with respiratory failure: glucose vs fat. *Anesthesiology* **54**: 373–377.

Brown R, Bancewicz J, Hamid J et al (1982) Failure of delayed hypersensitivity skin testing to predict postoperative sepsis and mortality. *BMJ* **284**: 851–853.

Burkitt DP (1969) Related disease – related cause? *Lancet* **ii**: 1229–1231.

Carlson GL, Maguire G, Williams N et al (1998) Quality of life on home parenteral nutrition and attitudes towards intestinal transplantation. A single centre study of 37 patients. *Clin Nutr* (in press).

Cleave TL (1983) Obituary. *BMJ* **287**: 1145.

Cleave TL & Campbell GD (1966) *Diabetes, Coronary Thrombosis and the Saccharine Disease*. London: Wright.

Cummings JH (1984) Constipation, dietary fibre and the control of large bowel function. *Postgrad Med J* **60**: 811–819.

Dowd PS & Heatley RV (1984) The influence of under-nutrition on immunity. *Clin Sci* **66**: 241–248.

Detsky A, McLaughlin JR, Abrams HB et al (1986) Quality of life of patients on long term total parenteral nutrition at home. *J Gen Intern Med* **1**: 26–33.

Dudrick SJ, Long JM, Steiger E & Rhoads JE (1970) Intravenous hyperalimentation. *Med Clin North Am* **54**: 577–589.

Dudrick SJ, Englert DM, Van Buren CT et al (1979) New concepts of ambulatory home hyperalimentation. *J Parenter Enteral Nutr* **3**: 72–76.

Dudrick SJ, O'Donnell JJ & Englert DM (1984) One hundred years of ambulatory home total parenteral nutrition. *Ann Surg* **199**: 770–781.

Elwyn DH (1980) Nutritional requirements of adult surgical patients. *Crit Care Med* **8**: 9–20.

Elwyn DH, Kinney JM, Gump FE et al (1980) Some metabolic effects of fat infusions in depleted patients. *Metabolism* **29**: 125–132.

Everitt NJ & McMahon MJ (1997) Influence of fine bore catheter length on infusion thrombophlebitis in peripheral intravenous nutrition: a randomised controlled trial. *Ann R Coll Surg Engl* **79**: 221–224.

Everitt NJ, Madan M, Alexander D & McMahon MJ (1993) Fine bore silicone rubber and polyurethane catheters for the delivery of complete intravenous nutrition via a peripheral vein. *Clin Nutr* **12**: 261–265.

Garden OJ & Sim AJW (1983) A comparison of tunnelled and non-tunnelled subclavian vein catheters: a prospective study of complications during parenteral feeding. *Clin Nutr* **2**: 49–52.

Geggel HS, Ament ME, Heckenliveley JR, Martin DA & Kopple JD (1984) Nutritional requirements for taurine in patients receiving long term parenteral nutrition. *N Engl J Med* **312**: 142–145.

Harvey KB, Moldawer LL, Bistrian BS & Blackburn GL (1981) Biological measures for the formulation of a hospital prognostic index. *Am J Clin Nutr* **34**: 2013–2022.

Hegsted DM (1978) Assessment of nitrogen requirements. *Am J Clin Nutr* **31**: 1669–1677.

Heyman MB, Storch S & Ament ME (1981) The fat overload syndrome. Report of a case and literature review. *Am J Dis Child* **135**: 628–630.

Hickman DM, Miller RA, Rombeau JL, Twomey PL & Frey CF (1980) Serum albumin and body weight as predictors of postoperative course in colorectal cancer. *J Parenter Enteral Nutr* **4**: 315–316.

Hill GL (1981) Surgically created nutritional problems. *Surg Clin North Am* **61**: 721–728.

Hill GL & Church J (1984) Energy and protein requirements of general surgical patients requiring intravenous nutrition. *Br J Surg* **7**: 1–9.

Irving M, White R & Tresarden J (1985) Three years experience with an intestinal failure unit. *Ann R Coll Surg Engl* **67**: 2–5.

Jones FA (1984) Refined food and dietary fibre, two sides of the same coin. *Saudi Med J* **5**: 119–122.

Kamminski MV, Fitzgerald MJ, Murphy RJ et al (1977) Correlation of mortality with serum transferrin and energy. *J Parenter Enteral Nutr* **1**: 27.

Keohane P, Jones BJM, Attrill H et al (1983) Effect of catheter tunnelling and a nutrition nurse on catheter sepsis during parenteral nutrition. *Lancet* **ii**: 1388–1389.

Klidjian AM, Foster KJ, Kammerling RM, Cooper A & Karran SJ (1980) Relation of anthropometric and dynamometric variables to serious postoperative complications. *Br Med J* **281**: 899–901.

Klidjian AM, Archer TJ, Foster KJ & Karran SJ (1982) Detection of dangerous malnutrition. *J Parenter Enteral Nutr* **6**: 119–121.

Kohlhardt SR & Smith RC (1989) Fine bore silicone catheters for peripheral intravenous nutrition in adults. *BMJ* **299**: 1380–1381.

Kohlhardt SR, Smith RC & Wright CR (1994) Peripheral versus central intravenous nutrition: comparison of two delivery systems. *Br J Surg* **81**: 66–70.

Laidlow JM, McIntyre PB, Wood SR, Bartram CI & Lennard Jones JE (1983) A radiological study after parenteral nutrition through silicone rubber catheters: fibrin sleeves without thrombosis. *Clin Nutr* **1**: 305–311.

MacFie J, Smith RC & Hill GL (1981) Glucose or fat as a non protein energy source? A controlled clinical trial in gastroenterological patients requiring intravenous nutrition. *Gastroenterology* **80**: 103–107.

McIntyre PB, Ritchie JK, Hawley PR, Bartrum C & Lennard-Jones JE (1984) Management of enterocutaneous fistulas: a review of 132 cases. *Br J Surg* **71**: 293–296.

Madan M, Alexander DJ, McMahon MJ (1992) Influence of catheter type on occurrence of thrombophlebitis during peripheral intravenous nutrition. *Lancet* **339**: 101–103.

Meguid MM & Borum P (1984) Carnitine deficiency with hyperbilirubinaemia, generalised skeletal muscle weakness and reactive hypoglycaemia in a patient on long term TPN. *J Parenter Enteral Nutr* **8**: 51.

Mitchell A, Watkins RM & Collins J (1984) Surgical treatment of the short bowel syndrome. *Br J Surg* **71**: 329–332.

Mock DM, Baswell DI, Baker H, Holman RT & Sweetman L (1985) Biotin deficiency complicating parenteral alimentation: diagnosis, metabolic repercussions and treatment. *J Pediatr* **106**: 762–769.

Nehme AE (1980) Nutritional support of the hospitalized patient. The team concept. *JAMA* **243**: 1906–1908.

O'Donnell AU & Fleming SE (1984) Influence of frequent and long-term consumption of legume seeds on excretion of intestinal gases. *Am J Clin Nutr* **40**: 48–57.

Oosterlee J & Dudley HAF (1980) Central catheter placement by puncture of exposed subclavian vein. *Lancet* **i**: 19–20.

Oxford Parenteral Nutrition Team (1983) Total parenteral nutrition: value of a standard feeding regimen. *BMJ* **286**: 1323–1327.

Pettigrew RA & Hill GL (1984) Therapeutic nutrition. In Bouchier IAD, Allan RN, Hodgson HJF & Keighley MRB (eds) *Textbook of Gastroenterology*, pp 1227–1249. London: Baillière Tindall.

Pettigrew RA & Hill GL (1986) Indicators of surgical risk and clinical judgement. *Br J Surg* **73**: 27–51.

Pettigrew RA, Lang JDR, Haydock DA et al (1985) Catheter related sepsis in patients on intravenous nutrition: a prospective study of quantitative catheter cultures and guideline changes for suspected sepsis. *Br J Surg* **72**: 52–55.

Pitt HA, King WIII, Mann LL et al (1983) Increased risk of cholelithiasis with prolonged total parenteral nutrition. *Am J Surg* **145**: 106–112.

Ponsky JL, Gauderer MWL (1989) Percutaneous endoscopic gastrostomy indications, limitations and results. *World J Surg* **13**: 165–170.

Powell Tuck J (1978a) Skin tunnel for central venous catheter: non-operative technique. *BMJ* **1**: 625.

Powell Tuck J (1978b) Team approach to long term intravenous feeding in patients with gastrointestinal disorders. *Lancet* **ii**: 825–828.

Rainey-MacDonald CG, Holliday RL, Wells G & Donner AP (1983) Validity of a two variable nutritional index for use in selecting candidates for nutritional support. *J Parenter Enteral Nutr* **7**: 15–20.

Rhoads JE, Vars HM & Dudrick SJ (1981) The development of intravenous hyperalimentation. *Surg Clin North Am* **61**: 429–435.

Richards DM & Irving MH (1996) Cost-utility analysis of home parenteral nutrition. *Br J Surg* **83**: 1226–1229.

Richards DM & Irving MH (1997) Assessing the quality of life of patients with intestinal failure on home parenteral nutrition. *Gut* **40**: 218–222.

Roslyn JJ, Pitt HA, Mann L, Fonkalsrud EW & Denbesten L (1984) Parenteral nutrition induced gall bladder disease: a reason for early cholecystectomy. *Am J Surg* **148**: 58–63.

Rudman D, Millikan WJ, Richardson TJ et al (1975) Elemental balances during intravenous hyperalimentation of underweight adult subjects. *J Clin Invest* **55**: 94–104.

Silk DBA (1983) Nutritional support. In Silk DBA (ed.) *Hospital Practice*, pp 102. Oxford: Blackwell Scientific.

Silk DBA (1985) Enteral nutrition. *Curr Opin Gastroenterol* **1**: 295–301.

Simms JM, Smith JAR & Woods HF (1982) A modified prognostic index based upon nutritional measurements. *Clin Nutr* **1**: 71–79.

Sitges-Serra A & Linares J (1984) Tunnels do not protect against venous-catheter-related sepsis. *Lancet* **i**: 459 (letter).

Sitges-Serra A, Puig P, Linares J et al (1984) Hub colonisation as the initial step in an outbreak of catheter related sepsis due to a coagulase negative staphylococci during parenteral nutrition. *J Parenter Enteral Nutr* **8**: 688–692.

Skenkin A & Wrettind A (1978) Parenteral nutrition. *World Rev Nutr Diet* **28**: 1–111.

Stephen AM & Cummings JH (1980) Mechanism of action of dietary fibre in the human colon. *Nature* **284**: 283–284.

Studley HO (1936) Percentage of weight loss: basic indicator of surgical risk in patients with chronic peptic ulcer. *JAMA* **106**: 458–460.

Sutton G & Karran SJ (1985) The diagnosis of malnutrition: nutritional parameters. *Curr Opin Gastroenterol* **1**: 281–287.

Swartz RD, Wesley JR, Somermeyer MG & Lau K (1984) Hyperoxoluria and renal insufficiency due to ascorbic acid administration during total parenteral nutrition. *Ann Intern Med* **100**: 530.

Taylor RH (1984) Bran yesterday . . . bran tomorrow? *BMJ* **289**: 69–70.

Taylor RH (1985) Dietary fibre, *Gastroenterology* and nutrition. *Curr Opin Gastroenterol* **1**: 330–335.

Thompson JS & Hodges RE (1984) Preventing hypophosphataemia during total parenteral nutrition. *J Parenter Enteral Nutr* **8**: 137–139.

Thompson JS, Langnas AN, Pinch LW et al (1995) Surgical approach to the short bowel syndrome. Experience in a population of 160 patients. *Ann Surg* **222**: 600–607.

Trowell H, Pointer N & Burkitt D (1974) Aspects of the epidemiology of diverticular disease and ischemic heart disease. *Am J Dig Dis* **19**: 864–873.

Watson RD, Cannon RA, Kurland GS, Cox KL & Frates RC (1985) Selenium responsive myosites during prolonged home total parenteral nutrition in cystic fibrosis. *J Parenter Enteral Nutr* **9**: 58–60.

Wilmore DW (1977) *The Metabolic Management of the Critically Ill.* New York: Plenum Publishing.

Worthley LI, Fishlock RC & Snoswell AM (1983) Carnitine deficiency with hyperbilirubinemia, generalized skeletal muscle weakness and reactive hypoglycemia in a patient on long term total parenteral nutrition: treatment with intravenous L. carnitine. *J Parenter Enteral Nutr* **7**: 176–180.

Yeung CK, Young GA, Hackett AF & Hill GL (1979) Fine needle jejunostomy: an assessment of a new method of nutritional support after major gastrointestinal surgery. *Br J Surg* **66**: 727–732.

5

SEPSIS AND THE USE OF ANTIBIOTIC COVER IN COLORECTAL SURGERY

Sepsis still remains the most common cause of hospital death in colorectal surgery (Stephen and Loewenthal, 1978; Keighley and Burdon, 1979; Fry et al, 1980b; Windsor et al, 1995; Varty et al, 1994) from multiorgan failure, septicaemia, peritonitis, abscess and synergistic gangrene. Apart from the associated mortality and morbidity, infections are expensive (Hughes et al, 1982; de la Hunt et al, 1986; Davey et al, 1992). This chapter aims to review the factors responsible for sepsis and its prevention; therapy for patients with established sepsis is discussed in Chapter 66.

THE PROBLEM

Wound infections

Abdominal wounds

Infection in abdominal wounds may be superficial or deep seated (Lawrence, 1994). Deep wound infection may be complicated by wound dehiscence. Classification of abdominal wound sepsis has been the subject of considerable debate (National Research Council, 1964; Gibson, 1974; Cruse, 1975; Williams et al, 1976; Sanderson, 1983). We recognize three groups: (1) erythema of the wound without any detectable pus; (2) pus in part of the incision; and (3) sepsis deep to the linea alba, rectus sheath or external oblique.

Perineal wounds

Perineal wound infection after proctocolectomy or abdominoperineal excision is common and may be associated with a presacral cavity. Synergistic gangrene is an occasional complication of perineal wound sepsis, particularly in diabetic patients (DeGennaro et al, 1978; Goodson and Hunt, 1979; Kirk et al, 1988).

Incidence

Abdominal wounds

The incidence of abdominal wound sepsis in colorectal surgery without antibiotic cover is usually reported to be greater than 35% (Table 5.1), being highest after abdominoperineal excision of the rectum. High wound infection rates are common following ileostomy or colostomy closure (Belliveau, 1995; Hackam and Rotstein, 1995). Left-sided restorative resection carries a higher infection rate than right hemicolectomy and sepsis is more frequent after emergency operations (Table 5.2). Careful follow-up is needed to document sepsis rates since most now occur after patients' early discharge from hospital (Keeling and Morgan, 1995). There has been a real reduction in sepsis rates after colorectal surgery, due to some extent to the use of prophylactic antibiotics but also to increasing specialization in surgery and surgical audit (Hancock, 1990; Leaper, 1994; Avery et al, 1995). Wound sepsis rates should be now less than 10% (Krukowski et al, 1984; Krukowski and Matheson, 1988; Coco et al, 1993; Kwok et al, 1993) (Table 5.3), but higher rates continue to be reported (Karran et al, 1993; Keeling and Morgan, 1995).

Perineal wounds

The incidence of infection in the perineal wound was reported to be 47% by Hojer and Wetterfors (1978) when antibiotic cover was not used. It still remains high despite prophylaxis.

Table 5.1 Sepsis rates (%) in patients receiving no antibiotic cover.

Reference	*No.*	*Wound*	*Abscess*	*Septicaemia*	*Peritonitis*	*Anastomotic dehiscence*
Burton (1973)	105	61	8	35	NS	3
Keighley et al (1976)	29	38	10	10	NS	NS
Everett et al (1969)	16	62	0	6	8	8
Kippax and Thomas (1966)	143	46	NS	NS	NS	NS
Nash and Hugh (1967)	34	41	NS	NS	NS	NS
Barker et al (1979)	50	38	4	4	NS	NS
Goldring et al (1975)	25	44	16	8	0	16
Washington et al (1974)	63	43	8	6	8	8
Clarke et al (1977)	60	35	17	10	0	17
Gurry and Ellis-Pegler (1976)	51	47	NS	NS	NS	14
Matheson et al (1978)	59	42	5	12	0	12

NS, not stated.

Table 5.2 Incidence of sepsis (%) in colorectal surgery (no antibiotic cover).

	Cancer		*Inflammatory bowel disease*	
	Elective	*Emergency*	*Elective*	*Emergency*
Wound sepsis (abdominal)	40	60	37	42
Wound sepsis (perineal)	79	–	69	–
Abscess	5	13	12	22
Septicaemia	10	12	7	8

Dashes, no data.

Table 5.3 Ten-year audit of sepsis in abdominal surgery.

	Elective		*Emergency*	
	No.	*%*	*No.*	*%*
Ileocolic anastomosis	67	3	47	11
Colocolic/rectal anastomosis	185	2	27	7
Hartmann/total colectomy	13	0	51	8
Abdominal-perineal excision/ panproctocolectomy (PPC)	31	6	2	50
Loop colostomy	4	0	5	20
Total	328	3	148	9

From Krukowski and Matheson (1988).

Organisms

Sepsis in colorectal surgery is due to mixed cultures of enterobacteriaceae and obligate anaerobes (Table 5.4). The importance of transport medium and rapid delivery to a laboratory for anaerobic culture must still be emphasized (Van Houte and Gibbons, 1966; Leigh, 1974; Eykyn et al, 1979; Taylor et al, 1979; Pollock et al, 1986; Nichols and Smith, 1994; Krepel et al, 1995).

Table 5.4 Bacterial isolates in colorectal surgery (no antibiotic cover).

	Frequency of isolates from postoperative infections
Aerobes	
Staphylococcus aureus	7
Staphylococcus albus	15
Streptococcus faecalis	6
Haemolytic streptococci	6
Streptococcus viridans	7
Nonhaemolytic streptococci	7
Escherichia coli	46
Proteus spp.	10
Klebsiella aerogenes	8
Pseudomonas aeruginosa	9
Anaerobes	
Peptostreptococcus spp.	7
Peptococcus spp.	5
Clostridium spp.	13
Bacteroides fragilis	56

Specialized wound sepsis

Synergistic gangrene

Synergistic necrotizing fasciitis is a rapidly spreading infection caused by a combination of obligate anaerobes, fusobacteria, clostridia and peptostreptococci (Smith et al, 1996). Infections are associated with gas production, odour and rapid proliferation in the subcutaneous tissues or within subfascial planes. Characteristically, these synergistic infections occur in the perineum and spread rapidly into the scrotum, abdominal wall, the thigh and buttocks (Badrinath et al, 1994). Malnourished, obese, diabetic and immunocompromised patients are particularly susceptible. There is a wide spectrum of non-clostridial infective gangrene, associated with eponyms such as Meleney's synergistic gangrene and Fournier's gangrene (Keighley and Burdon, 1979). Treatment is by wide surgical debridement and systemic antimicrobial agents. Frequent, repeated desloughing procedures, topical antiseptics and eventual skin grafting are commonly required. Hyperbaric oxygen may play a role in therapy (Brown et al, 1994).

Gas gangrene

Gas gangrene is a clinical syndrome associated with *Clostridium perfringens* which carries a high mortality unless treated early (Parker, 1969). Most infections are endogenous, but other species of *Clostridium*, such as *Cl. sporogenes* and *Cl. paraputrificum*, may be responsible. Gas gangrene requires the presence of devitalized or anaerobic tissue. Exotoxins are released into the tissues causing necrosis and increased capillary permeability with the accumulation of fluid and impaired venous return. Clostridia invade and multiply in necrotic tissue. End-stage infections are characterized by septicaemia, shock, haemolysis and renal failure. The cardinal features are rapidly spreading cellulitis with crepitus associated with oliguria, hypotension and acidosis. Fever is not always present (Nichols and Smith, 1975). Gas gangrene is more common in diabetics. Sometimes other gas-forming organisms such as coliforms, fusobacteria, bifidobacteria, peptostreptococci and *Bacteroides* may be responsible (Rodeheaver et al, 1974).

The mortality is high in elderly diabetic patients with chronic renal disease and malignancy. Septicaemia, disseminated intravascular coagulation, respiratory or renal failure and thromboembolism are associated with a poor prognosis (Altemeier et al, 1967; Howe, 1969).

Treatment is by wide debridement, high-dose penicillin or, preferably, metronidazole; hyperbaric oxygen is also advised.

Sepsis in the immunocompromised host

Some patients with colorectal diseases are on drugs such as steroids, azathioprine or chemotherapy for cancer or have diseases such as Crohn's or AIDS which render them susceptible to microorganisms that are harmless to healthy individuals. Furthermore, antimicrobial agents are less effective in the absence of normal defence mechanisms. The common presentations include septicaemia, endocarditis, septic arthritis, encephalitis and respiratory, biliary or urinary infection (Hong and Davis, 1996).

The most important bacterial infections are from staphylococci, aerobic Gram-negative bacteria and *Mycobacterium tuberculosis*. Viral infections include herpes zoster, cytomegalovirus and heptatis B.

Protozoal infections, particularly *Pneumocystis carinii*, and fungal overgrowth by candida are common.

Opportunistic infections frequently occur in neutropenic patients (Iberti et al, 1986). These infections are poorly localized and pus is often not present. Where possible they are best managed by high-dose antimicrobial therapy (Tartter, 1988; Jensen et al, 1990). Perianal sepsis in neutropenic patients is discussed in Chapter 15.

Septicaemia

Presentation

Septicaemia or bacteraemia usually presents with fever, leucocytosis and signs of localized sepsis but may result in profound cardiovascular disturbance, causing hypotension, hypovolaemia, oliguria, impaired tissue perfusion and acidosis, which may be complicated by disseminated intravascular coagulation and multiple system organ failure (Bullard and Dunn, 1996). Septicaemia still carries a high mortality, particularly when associated with these complications (Gelb and Seligman, 1970; Bodner et al, 1972; Wilson et al, 1972; Leigh, 1974, 1975; MacKenzie and Litton, 1974; Lawrence et al, 1977; Eykyn, 1982).

Incidence

Routine blood cultures indicate that bacteraemia may complicate sigmoidoscopy (Le Frock et al, 1973), barium enema examination (Le Frock et al, 1975) and polypectomy (Lal and Levitan, 1972; Burton, 1973; Anonymous, 1975). Sykes et al (1983) reported a 47% rate of bacteraemia after peranal diathermy of rectal tumours and found that *Bacteroides fragilis* was the most common isolate. Burton (1973) recorded a 35% incidence following colorectal operations. The incidence of bacteraemia rises with age (Figure 5.1) (Eykyn, 1982).

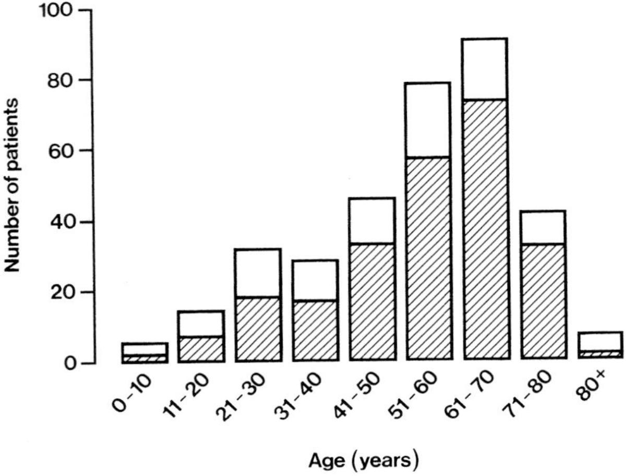

Figure 5.1 Frequency of episodes of septicaemia related to the age of the patients. ▨ Male; □ female. From Eykyn, 1982.

Organisms

Bacteroides fragilis appears to be the dominant organism from blood cultures after large bowel surgery (Eykyn, 1982). McHenry et al (1971) also reported that *Escherichia coli*, *Klebsiella* spp. and *Pseudomonas aeruginosa* are frequent isolates (Bullard and Dunn, 1996). Fungal septicaemia is an important isolate in immunocompromised patients (Solomkin, 1996).

There has been an increased awareness of streptococcal septicaemia in patients with colorectal disease, possibly due to the increasing use of cephalosporins. *Streptococcus bovis* seems to be associated with colorectal cancer and may cause endocarditis (Klein et al, 1977; Steinberg and Naggar, 1977; Noble et al, 1978; Hossenbux et al, 1983; Silver, 1984). *S. milleri* has also been recognized as an occasional isolate from blood cultures in patients with colorectal disease (Bateman et al, 1975; Nagler and Poticha, 1979; Tresadern et al, 1983).

Bacteroides septicaemia is associated with a high mortality (Gillespie and Guy, 1956; Gunn, 1956; Okubadejo et al, 1973; Leigh, 1974; MacKenzie and Litton, 1974).

Intra-abdominal abscess

Intra-abdominal abscess or pelvic abscess is commonly associated with anastomotic failure, advanced inflammatory or neoplastic disease, and presents with fever, leucocytosis and severe systemic illness (CS Higgens et al, 1980; Jensen et al, 1990; Nathens and Rotstein, 1996). Most collections are associated with a mixed growth of aerobic organisms, such as *E. coli*, *Klebsiella* spp., *Proteus* spp., *Ps. aeruginosa* and, occasionally, *S. milleri*. However, the obligate anaerobes, particularly *B. fragilis*, peptostreptococci and *Cl. perfringens* are almost universal after intestinal surgery (Bartlett, 1981). Mortality of intra-abdominal abscess depends on the site of the abscess, the age of the patient, the nature of the underlying disease (Fry et al, 1980a), the extent of malnutrition and anergy (Christou et al, 1985; Pollock, 1988). Localization with ultrasound or CT and percutaneous drainage have been associated with a reduced mortality. Treatment strategies for abdominal sepsis complicating colorectal disease are discussed in Chapter 66.

AVAILABLE ANTIMICROBIAL AGENTS

Penicillins

Most penicillins are highly active against streptococci, oral anaerobes and clostridia. They have a fairly short half-life when administered systemically and anaphylaxis, urticaria and hypersensitivity reactions are recognized complications. Many variations of penicillin have been prepared; they differ in their spectrum and their susceptibility to penicillinases, which destroy the β-lactam ring and thereby abolish its antibacterial activity. Penicillinases are produced by some staphylococci, coliforms, *Proteus* spp. and *Bacteroides* spp.

The instability of ampicillin to β-lactamases has rendered it ineffective unless used for treatment of severe streptococcal sepsis. Although penicillin was considered to be the treatment of choice for clostridial infections, particularly gas gangrene, there is now some evidence that metronidazole is more effective, particularly if there might be a mixed infection causing synergistic gangrene.

The ureidopenicillins have a much wider spectrum of activity and are more stable to β-lactamases (Paradisi and Corti, 1992). However, like all penicillins they may be inactivated by staphylococci and some obligate anaerobes (Niinikoski et al, 1993). These compounds are also active against all pathogenic streptococci, but activity against staphylococci is poor. Piperacillin is active, however, and used widely now in Gram-negative sepsis (Barie et al, 1994; Vestweber and Grundel, 1994), but *in vivo* activity against the anaerobic bacteria is modest, and in clinical practice both mezlocillin and piperacillin should be used in combination with a nitroimidazole (Ambrose et al, 1983; Eklund et al, 1993; Taylor and Lindsay, 1994). Azlocillin is a penicillin which is now reserved for treatment of gentamicin-resistant pseudomonal infections.

The use of sulbactam with ampicillin or clavulanic acid with ampicillin (Augmentin) provides a rational approach to therapy against bowel organisms (Brown, 1984; de la Hunt and Karran, 1986).

Cephalosporins

With the exception of cefoxitin, which is a cephamycin, the cephalosporins are semisynthetic derivatives of cephalosporin. The cephalosporin nucleus has a β-lactam ring like the penicillins and is therefore susceptible to degradation by β-lactamases (Solomkins et al, 1984).

Most cephalosporins are inactive when given by mouth and have a half-life of less than 2 hours when given intravenously. They are generally free from serious side-effects, although some third-generation cephalosporins such as latamoxef and cefotetan are associated with disturbance of clotting, particularly prolongation of prothrombin times and abnormal values of factors II, VII, VIII, IX and XII (Baxter et al, 1985; Bowcock et al, 1986). Although these effects may be reversed by vitamin K, serious bleeding may occur with latamoxef (Morris et al, 1984), particularly amongst patients with inflammatory bowel disease (Smith and Lipsky, 1983; Weitekamp and Aber, 1983; Fabricus et al, 1984).

Most of the third-generation cephalosporins have a profound inhibitory effect on intestinal microflora (Heimdahl et al, 1982; Ambrose et al, 1985), which may be accompanied by the emergence of *Cl. difficile*. Pseudomembranous colitis is now more frequently recorded after cephalosporin administration than after clindamycin therapy (Hares et al, 1981; Morris et al, 1984; Marts et al, 1994; Settle and Wilcox, 1996).

Most cephalosporins are less susceptible than the penicillins to β-lactamases but protection, even among the β-lactam group of agents, is not absolute.

The first-generation cephalosporins (e.g. cephaloridine, cephazolin and cephalexin) are not effective against Gram-negative anaerobic organisms.

The second-generation cephalosporins (e.g. cefuroxime, cephamandole and ceftriaxone) are bactericidal against the Gram-negative aerobic intestinal organisms, but are not effective against *Pseudomonas* spp. or the anaerobes (Ambrose et al, 1983). Ceftriaxone has an extremely long half-life (Shepherd et al, 1986) and when used in combination with metronidazole is very effective in colorectal surgery (Morris, 1993; Matikainen and Hiltunen, 1993).

The third-generation cephalosporins (e.g. cefoxitin, latamoxef, cefotetan, cefotaxime and ceftizoxime) are active against 70–80% of strains of anaerobes and most Gram-negative aerobes but their activity against aerobic Gram-positive organisms is poor (Stone, 1983).

The cephalosporins have been used extensively and provide effective prophylaxis in colorectal surgery, particularly when combined with agents effective against gut anaerobes (Polk and Lopez-Mayor, 1969; Stone et al, 1976; Kaiser et al, 1983; Condon et al, 1979; Hares et al, 1981; Morris et al, 1984; de la Hunt and Karran, 1986; Tudor et al,

Table 5.5 Sepsis from *B. fragilis*.

Reference	*Agent*	*No. of serious infections/no. of patients treated*
Hall et al (1989)	Augmentin alone	13/183
	Metronidazole + gentamicin	4/176
Hares et al (1981)	Cefoxitin alone	5/35
	Metronidazole + gentamicin	0/33
Morris et al (1984)	Latamoxef alone	4/53
	Latamoxef + metronidazole	1/54
Tudor et al (1988)	Cefotetan	6/76
	Metronidazole + gentamicin	1/74

1988; Jones, 1992). We remain convinced that even the third-generation cephalosporins must be used with metronidazole in colorectal surgery (Hakansson et al, 1993) (Table 5.5).

Aminoglycosides

The principal aminoglycosides are streptomycin, kanamycin, gentamicin, neomycin, tobramycin and amikacin. The aminoglycosides are excreted by the kidney and delayed excretion in patients with poor renal function may result in toxic serum levels. All aminoglycosides show variable degrees of ototoxicity and may interfere with reversal of non-depolarizing muscle relaxants (Wylie and Churchill-Davidson, 1966).

Aminoglycosides are potentially nephrotoxic, particularly when used in combination with cephalosporins. They have a short half-life and a second dose of the drug should be given if an operation takes longer than 2 hours. Most aminoglycosides have good antistaphylococcal activity and are effective against most strains of *E. coli*, *Klebsiella* spp., *Proteus* spp. and *Ps. aeruginosa* (Eykyn, 1982). The preoperative use of oral aminoglycosides such as neomycin has been associated with the emergence of resistant organisms (Hartley and Richmond, 1975; Keighley et al, 1976; Valtonen et al, 1977; Handelsman et al, 1993). Nevertheless, high-dose aminoglycosides in combination with metronidazole are associated with low rates of sepsis (Waterworth, 1972; Drasar et al, 1976; Burdon et al, 1985) although the use of gentamicin with metronidazole for prophylaxis has been largely discontinued because of the risks of renal failure, ototoxicity and bacterial resistance. Amikacin is used for gentamicin-resistant *E. coli* and *Pseudomonas* infections.

Nitroimidazoles

The nitroimidazoles include metronidazole and tinidazole. They are unique as they are only active against obligate anaerobes. Unlike other agents used for the treatment of anaerobic infections, resistance to metronidazole is almost unheard of (Finegold, 1985; Joiner and Bartlett, 1985; Ueno, 1985; Willis, 1985). The nitroimidazoles have no activity against aerobic pathogens and must therefore be used in combination with an aminoglycoside or a cephalosporin (Bartlett et al, 1978a; Willis and Jones, 1979; Stone, 1983; Carr et al, 1984; Morris et al, 1984; Cunliffe et al, 1985; Roland et al, 1985, 1986). The nitroimidazoles have a long track record of safety (Roe, 1985) and neurotoxicity is only experienced when they are used for prolonged periods at high dose, as for instance in perianal Crohn's disease.

Alternative agents with activity against the obligate anaerobes include clindamycin, rifampicin and erythromycin (Kislak, 1972; Leigh, 1975) but none are as effective as metronidazole (Gorbach, 1975; Britz and Wilkinson, 1984). As metronidazole is not destroyed by β-lactamases it is the drug of choice for *B. fragilis*, *Cl. perfringens* and *Cl. tetani*. Metronidazole has a long half-life and can be relied upon to provide adequate serum levels but poor levels in fat, even when administered by suppository in critically ill patients (Hobbis et al, 1988; Badia et al, 1995).

Other agents

Co-trimoxazole

Co-trimoxazole is a mixture of trimethoprim and sulphamethoxazole. Resistance is relatively uncommon but there are side-effects such as rashes and neutropenia from the sulphonamides. It has been used for prophylaxis with low rates of sepsis in colorectal surgery (AF Higgens et al, 1980).

Quinolones

The quinolones (e.g. ciprofloxacin, perfloxacin, ofloxacin and norfloxacin) are active against most Gram-negative infections and have some activity against the obligate anaerobes (Reeves et al, 1984; Silverman et al, 1986). These agents have a profound inhibitory effect on the intestinal microflora, yet emergence of *Cl. difficile* diarrhoea is rare. Tissue penetration is very high (Silverman et al, 1986). In combination with metronidazole, ciprofloxacin may be used for treatment and prophylaxis in colorectal surgery (Yoshioka et al, 1991). Alternatively, oral ciprofloxacin may be used to reduce faecal flora (selective decontamination) in combination with systemic antimicrobials for prophylaxis in large bowel surgery (Taylor and Lindsay, 1994; McArdle et al, 1995).

Clindamycin

Clindamycin is active against many Gram-positive aerobic bacteria and most anaerobes. Resistance of bacteroides to clindamycin is becoming more common (Phillips et al, 1981; Ueno, 1985). Clindamycin is often complicated by antibiotic-associated diarrhoea and pseudomembranous colitis (Mogg et al, 1979; Keighley, 1980).

Chloramphenicol

Chloramphenicol is cheap and resistance is uncommon; it would be used much more widely were it not for occasional bone marrow depression which may be irreversible and fatal (Brumfitt and Hamilton-Miller, 1980). Chloramphenicol has excellent activity against Gram-negative aerobic bacteria and a high proportion of anaerobic organisms are also sensitive to this agent.

Tetracycline

Tetracycline has been used extensively for prophylaxis in Scandinavia (Goransson et al, 1984; Norwegian Study Group, 1985; Bergman and Solhaug, 1987) and by a few enthusiasts of tetracycline peritoneal lavage (Krukowski and Matheson, 1988). Since the introduction of tetracycline in 1948, resistance has increased against streptococci, staphylococci, haemophilus, coliform bacilli, clostridia and bacteroides species (Steigbigel et al, 1968). Despite these observations, it has been claimed that high doses of tetracycline used topically in the peritoneal cavity is effective against faecal organisms (Stewart and Matheson, 1978; Krukowski and Matheson, 1983). However, topical tetracycline may cause renal failure (Sandle and Mandell, 1980) and be responsible for adhesions (Phillips and Dudley, 1984).

Monobactams

The monobactams include agents such as aztreonam. They have a narrow spectrum of activity against Gram-negative aerobic organisms.

Imipenems

This group of antibiotics have a broad spectrum of activity, being effective against most aerobic and anaerobic intestinal pathogens. They are relatively stable to β-lactamases and are effective as prophylactic and therapeutic agents in colorectal surgery (Karran et al, 1993) but they are expensive and are usually reserved for treating serious infections (Fry, 1996).

FACTORS RESPONSIBLE FOR SEPSIS

Patient factors

Renal disease

Chronic renal failure is associated with an increased incidence of sepsis, often from opportunistic infections in immunosuppressed patients (Barnes, 1979). Infection may be associated with arteriovenous shunts or peritoneal dialysis catheters. The principal organisms are staphylococcal and Gram-negative, particularly *Ps. aeruginosa* (Kuruvila and Bevan, 1971; Ralston et al, 1971; Dobkin et al, 1978). There is also an increased risk of viral and fungal infections in patients with chronic renal failure on dialysis programmes and in immunosuppressed patients after transplantation.

Malignancy

Patients with advanced malignancy have an increased susceptibility to infection (Hell et al, 1995). Late presentation is often associated with complications such as abscess, local perforation and obstruction (DeGennaro et al, 1978). In advanced malignancy, host defence mechanisms are also impaired, although anergy is not necessarily increased (Pietsch et al, 1977; Brown et al, 1982).

Age

Older patients have a higher risk of infection (Davidson et al, 1971; Cruse and Foord, 1973; Claesson and Holmlund, 1988) (Figure 5.2).

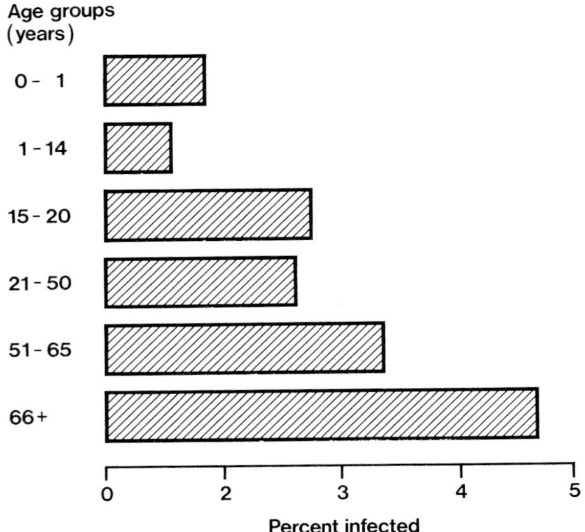

Figure 5.2 Impact of age on overall infection rates in gastrointestinal surgical practice.

Colorectal operations in children carry low rates of infection (Swenson et al, 1975).

Nutrition

Malnourished patients are more susceptible to sepsis but they are often septic themselves (Figure 5.3). It has been suggested by some that preoperative nutritional support might be justified in an attempt to reduce the risk of infection (Williams et al, 1976; Mullen et al, 1980), but this is only justified if any sepsis is controlled at the same time (Holter et al,

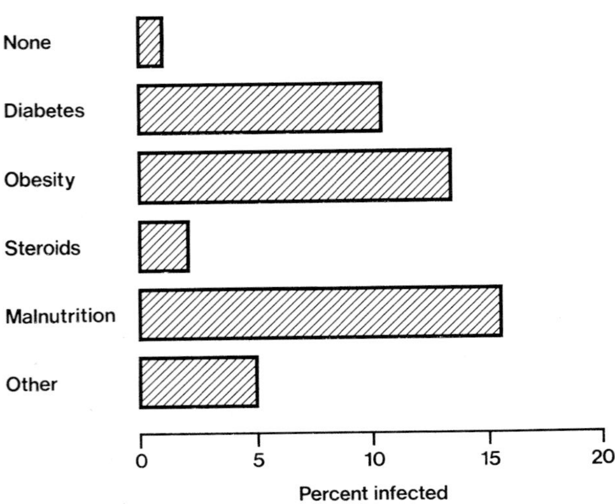

Figure 5.3 Influence of diabetes, obesity, steroids, malnutrition and other high-risk factors on infection rates in gastrointestinal surgical practice.

Table 5.6 Sepsis after resection for Crohn's disease related to percentage ideal bodyweight.

		Sepsis			
% Ideal body weight	*No. of patients*	*Minor* (%)	*Major* (%)	*None* (%)	*Hospital stay* (days)
Less than 80%	38	10	16	74	21
80–90%	38	8	13	79	20
More than 90%	51	12	14	74	17

From Higgens et al (1984).

1976; Goodgame, 1980). In Crohn's disease percentage ideal weight does not correlate with sepsis (Table 5.6) (Higgens et al, 1984). Obesity is associated with higher sepsis rates (Burton, 1973; DeGennaro et al, 1978; Stone, 1983).

Diabetes

Diabetes mellitus is a risk factor, particularly amongst patients requiring emergency operations or rectal excision (DeGennaro et al, 1978; Goodson and Hunt, 1979). Diabetics have defective phagocytic function and an increased risk of bacterial and fungal infections (Bybee and Rogers, 1964).

Reticuloendothelial and neutrophil function

Impairment of phagocytosis is evident in severe sepsis (Saba and Cho, 1979; Fry et al, 1980a,b; Saba and Joffe, 1980; Richards et al, 1983). Other determinants of sepsis include low serum antithrombin III, prealbumin and transferrin (Rubli et al, 1983). Numerical deficiency of neutrophils as well as impaired motility and defective leucocyte function increases susceptibility to infection (Holmes et al, 1966; Clark and Kimball, 1971; Alexander, 1974). Acquired defects in neutrophil function occur with trauma, sepsis, malignancy, anaemia and diabetes mellitus.

Anergy

MacLean et al (1975) showed that anergy was associated with a significantly higher incidence of sepsis and mortality (De Cree et al, 1974; Meakins et al, 1977, 1978; Kune, 1978; Johnson et al, 1979; Christou et al, 1985) (Table 5.7). Pietsch et al (1977) found that anergic patients tended to be older, had advanced malignancy and were more frequently malnourished. Sequential testing may be valuable in predicting infection risk. Anergy may be reversible by parenteral nutrition, relief of obstruction or drainage of infection. Levamisole in anergic

Table 5.7 Immunosuppression, sepsis and mortality.

	No. of patients	*Sepsis (%)*	*Death (%)*
Reactive	1373	8	4
Relative anergy	306	21	15
Anergy	523	33	31

From Christou et al (1985).

patients increased sepsis but not mortality (Meakins et al, 1979). Despite these observations Brown et al (1982) found that anergy was not associated with an increased risk of sepsis, but was a marker of nutritional disturbance. Innate immunological deficiency such as hypogammaglobulinaemia may be associated with recurrent episodes of infection and is an indication for immunoglobulin prophylaxis during operation.

Preoperative function scores may be helpful in identifying groups in whom there is a high risk of sepsis (Playforth et al, 1987; Ponting et al, 1987).

Trauma and emergency operations

Emergency colonic surgery (Cruse and Foord, 1973) is universally associated with a much higher rate of infection than elective surgery (DeGennaro et al, 1978; Hughes et al, 1982; Krukowski et al, 1984), particularly in elderly obstructed septic patients.

Drugs

Antimicrobials

Antimicrobial agents themselves may be responsible for an increased susceptibility to infection, particularly with prolonged use or when taken orally or applied topically since bacterial resistance is encouraged (Selden et al, 1971). Antimicrobials increase the risk of fungal sepsis, and high levels of some antibiotics may inhibit phagocytosis.

Steroids and immunosuppression

There is controversy regarding the potential risk of infection among patients receiving steroid therapy (Ehrlich et al, 1973; Fauci, 1975; Fuenfer et al, 1975; Knudsen et al, 1976; Allsop and Lee, 1978; Ziv et al, 1996). Both long-term and short-term steroid therapy cause a depression in the inflammatory response and interference with the phagocytic activity (David et al, 1970; Fauci et al, 1976). Azathioprine may increase the risk of sepsis if therapy is associated with leucopenia or thrombocytopenia.

Blood transfusion

Blood transfusion has been associated with increased sepsis rates (Tartter, 1988; Jensen et al, 1990). This was independent of age, blood loss, type of operation, admission haematocrit, tumour characteristics, duration of operation, but more common in patients requiring emergency operation.

Cancer chemotherapy

All forms of chemotherapy are capable of suppressing erythropoiesis and leucocyte, lymphocyte and macrophage function.

Radiotherapy

Theoretically, radiotherapy should increase the susceptibility to infection: marrow function is depressed and treatment causes mucosal ulceration and decreased host defence mechanisms. There may be impaired leucocyte function and reticuloendothelial activity, with depressed wound healing and malnutrition from enteric damage. In practice, preoperative short-term low-dose megavoltage radiotherapy does not appear to increase the risk of sepsis in colonic surgery (Localio et al, 1983; Påhlman and Glimelius, 1990), whereas larger doses of adjuvant radiotherapy have been attended by higher rates of sepsis and impaired wound healing (Sparso et al, 1984; Thomas et al, 1986).

Surgical factors

Contamination

The risk of sepsis is related to the degree of intestinal contamination (Davidson et al, 1971; Burton, 1973; Cruse and Foord, 1973; Allsop and Lee, 1978; Pollock, 1979; Scammell et al, 1985). The prediction of postoperative sepsis can be made from wound or peritoneal cultures taken at the end of operation (Evans and Pollock, 1973; Kelly and Warren, 1978; Fry et al, 1985; Pollock et al, 1986). Two studies report reduced postoperative infection rates with prolonged antibiotic cover in patients, with more than 10^5 colony forming units per mL in peritoneal fluid (Claesson et al, 1986; Tornqvist et al, 1987).

Duration of operation

Rates of infection may be greater after long operations (Davidson et al, 1971; DeGennaro et al, 1978). Long operations can be associated with inadequate serum concentrations if single-dose prophylaxis is used with agents with a short half-life (Burdon et al, 1985). Higher glove puncture rates are also associated with longer operations (Wastell, 1992; Hartley et al, 1996). Long operations may result in hypothermia, carrying potentially a greater risk of wound sepsis (Kurz et al, 1996).

Wound protection

Many workers advocate the use of plastic wound protectors (Maxwell et al, 1969; Jackson et al, 1971; Krukowski and Matheson, 1983) to reduce the counts of bacteria recovered from the wound at the end of the operation (Cole and Bernard, 1967; Raahave, 1974). However, there is no evidence that they reduce the risk of sepsis (Bernard and Cole, 1964; Psaila et al, 1977; Nystrom et al, 1984; Gamble and Hopton, 1985).

Shaving

The increased risk of sepsis from shaving is usually related to exogenous organisms. Clippers are preferable to razors and depilatory creams have an advantage over both (Powis et al, 1976; Seropian and Reynolds, 1981).

Drains

Open drains increase rather than minimize sepsis in elective colonic surgery (Davidson et al, 1971; Gilmore and Martin, 1974; Irvin et al, 1975; DeGennaro et al, 1978; Krukowski and Matheson, 1983; Simchen et al, 1984; Abussaud and Megden, 1986; Bibby et al, 1986; Claesson and Holmlund, 1988). In one of the few randomized trials of drains in colorectal surgery, Higson and Kettlewell (1978) found that drains increased the risk of sepsis. Most clinicians now only use drains for patients with established intra-abdominal abscess. In elective operation, closed suction drainage reduces the risk of haematoma and probably, therefore, the incidence of pelvic abscess. This subject is discussed more fully in Chapter 6.

Blood loss

Operative blood loss correlates closely with the incidence of sepsis (DeGennaro et al, 1978). Units claiming a low rate of sepsis in large bowel surgery generally report a low rate of transfusion (Fikri and McAdams, 1975; Hughes et al, 1982; Rietz et al, 1984).

Audit

There is growing evidence that morbidity can be substantially reduced by audit (Leaper, 1994). The process of accountability and regular review improves surgical discipline (Cruse and Foord, 1973; Dudley and Fielding, 1980; Krukowski and Matheson, 1983; Grundmann et al, 1984).

The wound

Incisions using diathermy gave marginally lower rates of sepsis in contaminated wounds than scalpal incisions (Johnson and Serpell, 1990). In elective, uncontaminated operations the abdominal wall and skin are usually sutured. If there is sepsis or gross contamination the skin and subcutaneous fat may be left open, particularly in obese patients or diabetics (Pollock et al, 1979; Forrester, 1980). Delayed primary closure may not be a particularly useful alternative to leaving wounds open (Grosfield, 1968). Open wound management certainly has a role in severely contaminated perineal wounds (Delalande et al, 1994). Elastomer foam is still useful in some open wounds (Hunt et al, 1975; Wood et al, 1977; Goodson and Hunt, 1979; Young and Wheeler, 1982; Marks et al, 1983; Stone, 1983; Gingold et al, 1984) but hydro-colloid dressings (Granuflex) are increasingly replacing silicone foam (Lawrence, 1994). In severe intra-abdominal sepsis or where closure of the abdominal wall is difficult, temporary closure with Marlex or Teflon mesh may have a role (Mathes and Stone, 1975; Boyd, 1977). The use of a zipper in severe abdominal sepsis also has its advocates (Singh and Chhina, 1993).

PROPHYLAXIS OR THERAPY

The term 'prophylaxis' should be confined to colorectal surgery undertaken in the absence of established sepsis (Wittmann and Schein, 1996). Hence, antibiotic cover for disease complicated by pericolic abscess, a fistula or active perianal disease cannot be classified as prophylaxis and the term 'therapy' should be used.

PROPHYLAXIS

Principles

Bowel preparation

As discussed in Chapter 3, the quality of mechanical bowel preparation is an important determinant of the risk of sepsis in colorectal surgery (Matheson et al, 1978; Barker et al, 1979; Eykyn et al, 1979; Pollock, 1979, 1981b; Hughes et al, 1982; Morris et al, 1983; Olivera et al, 1997) (Tables 5.8 and 5.9), but most preparations have little influence on the faecal microflora (Nichols et al, 1972; Arabi et al, 1978; Bleday et al, 1993). Recent studies, however, have questioned whether mechanical preparation for left-sided disease really reduces the risk of sepsis and anastomotic breakdown (Memon et al, 1997). Irvin and Goligher (1973) also showed that anastomotic dehiscence was increased with poor mechanical bowel preparation. If mechanical bowel preparation is suboptimal on-table colonic lavage may be used (Devine and Devine, 1948; Muir, 1968; Dudley and Fielding, 1980; Krukowski et al, 1984).

Hypochlorite rectal washout is advised for low stapled anastomosis since this has been found to virtually eliminate *B. fragilis* and *E. coli* from the rectal stump and to be more effective than povidone-iodine (Figure 5.4) (Scammell et al, 1985).

Table 5.8 Influence of mechanical bowel preparation on sepsis in colorectal surgery.

	n	*Wound sepsis*	*Abscess*	*Anastomotic dehiscence*
Empty colon at operation	76	14 (18)	0	1 (1)
Inadequate bowel preparation	13	7 (54)	2 (15)	6 (46)

Values in parentheses are percentages.
From Morris et al (1983).

Table 5.9 Influence of mechanical bowel preparation on wound sepsis.

	Right-sided resection		*Left-sided resection*	
	n	*Wound sepsis (%)*	*n*	*Wound sepsis (%)*
Satisfactory preparation	13	0	25	8
Poor preparation	48	31	83	33
No preparation possible (emergency operation)	67	37	16	44

From Pollock (1981b).

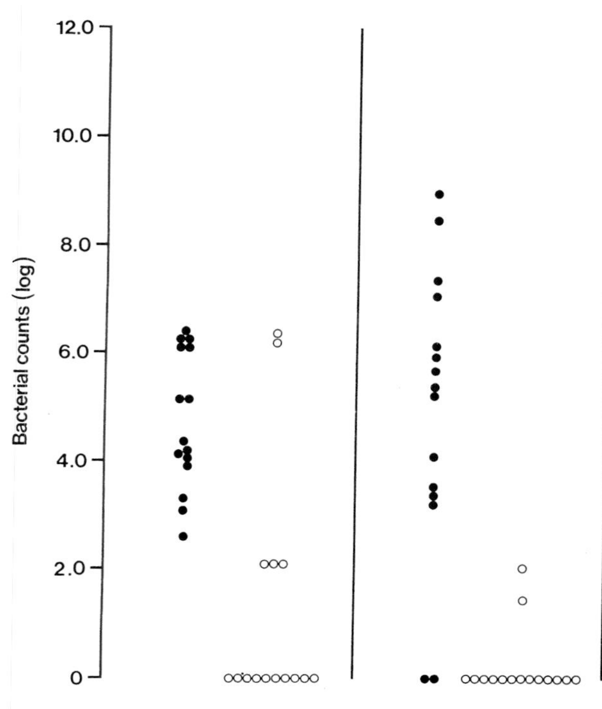

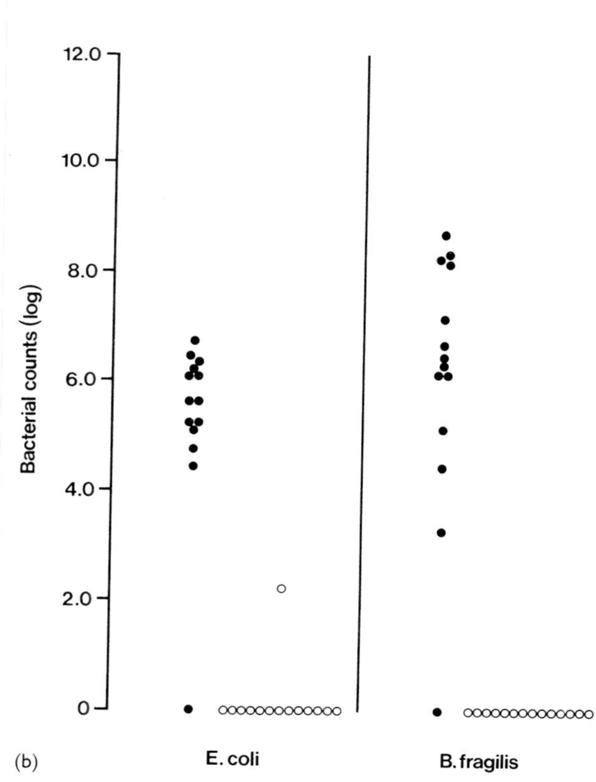

Figure 5.4 Impact of rectal washout with (a) povidone-iodine and (b) a 0.3% hypochlorite solution on counts of *E. coli* and *B. fragilis*. ● Before washout; ○ after washout.

Theatre discipline

Quite apart from surgical technique, operating theatre discipline is believed by many to reduce the risk of contamination, and consequently the incidence of sepsis (Hughes, 1972; Krukowski et al, 1984). Simple matters such as ensuring that division of the bowel is the last event in a colonic resection and the use of occluding tapes and staples reduces the duration and the extent of contamination (Keighley et al, 1996). Ensuring that an adequate sucker is available when the bowel is divided and the use of large gauze swabs soaked in an antiseptic solution helps to minimize contamination (Rietz et al, 1984).

Other simple measures include protecting the end of the bowel prior to construction of a stoma with a Cope's or Potts' clamp or by staples to reduce contamination of the wound and the stoma trephine. The stoma should not be constructed until the abdominal incision has been closed and covered.

Gentleness in handling tissues, adequate perfusion of the gut and avoidance of local ischaemia are important surgical principles (Fawcett et al, 1996). Avoidance of tension at an anastomosis or a stoma and preserving an adequate blood supply to the colon are crucial. Meticulous haemostasis and avoidance of contamination have already been mentioned. Other surgical expedients such as avoiding an anastomosis if there is gross contamination or established infection cannot be overstressed (Fikri and McAdams, 1975; Hughes et al, 1982; Krukowski and Matheson, 1983; Ahrendt et al, 1994, 1996). Using these principles, Krukowski et al (1984) reported an infection rate of only 1.8% in elective colorectal surgery and a rate of 6.7% in emergency procedures. Synchronous surgical procedures increase the risk of sepsis (Simchen et al, 1984).

Clinical trials: quality

Chodak and Plaut (1977) reviewed the quality of clinical trials and were critical of many published studies. Essential elements of trials include: a satisfactory method of randomization, independent assessment, consent, matched pathology in the comparator groups, adequate numbers, few exclusions, stratification for risk factors, appropriate choice and dose of trial drugs, and sufficient information on microbial isolates (Evans and Pollock, 1984, 1985).

Methods

Antiseptics

The availability of antibiotics has questioned the need for antiseptics in intestinal surgery (Gilmore, 1977). Most colorectal surgeons accept the need for antiseptic skin preparation and as protection against bowel contamination during resection (Ambrose et al, 1983; McDonald et al, 1984). Skin preparation should be performed with two applications of an alcohol-based preparation which should be given adequate time to dry between applications (Lilly and Lowbury, 1971; Lowbury and Lilly, 1973; Lowbury et al, 1974). Hexachlorophane may cause hypersensitivity reactions (Cruse and Foord, 1973). Chlorhexidine or iodine solutions in an alcohol base are usually preferred.

Intraperitoneal antiseptics

Antiseptics can damage small blood vessels, collagen synthesis and rapidly dividing cells (Brennan et al, 1986). Kuijpers (1985) questioned the wisdom of using povidone-iodine in patients with peritonitis, since they can cause serious peritoneal damage. On the other hand, povidone-iodine may be useful if there has been inadvertent faecal contamination (Browne and Stoller, 1970; Gilmore et al, 1978b; Ahrenholz and Simmons, 1979; Flint et al, 1979; Sindelar and Mason, 1979). Most authorities believe that antiseptic lavage is unsafe if there is established inflammation, as in faecal or purulent peritonitis (Lagarde et al, 1978; McAvinchey et al, 1983). Neither continuous saline nor antiseptic lavage influenced postoperative sepsis in colorectal surgery (Hallerback and Andersson, 1986; Leiboff and Soroff, 1987; Baker et al, 1994).

Intraluminal antiseptics

Intraluminal antiseptics may be used for rectal washouts as they reduce the counts of luminal bacteria (Jones et al, 1976; Scammell et al, 1985).

Intraincisional antiseptics

Antiseptics have been applied to the wound at the end of the operation in order to minimize the consequences of inadvertent contamination (Gilmore and Sanderson, 1975; Gilmore, 1977; Gilmore et al, 1978a; Stokes et al, 1977; Sindelar and Mason, 1979; Galle and Homersley, 1980; de Jong et al, 1982) but this practice is now rarely used.

Topical antibiotics

Topical antibiotics have been explored but administration is rarely advised in colorectal procedures (Nash and Hugh, 1967; Anderson et al, 1972; Evans and Pollock, 1973; Stone and Hester, 1973; Evans et al, 1974; Holder, 1976; Lord et al, 1977; Greenhall et al, 1979; Brumfitt and Hamilton-Miller, 1980; Pitt et al, 1980; Pollock, 1981a). In intestinal surgery, topical cephradine was inferior to systemic antibiotic administration (Finch et al, 1979). The combination of broad-spectrum systemic antibiotic cover and topical agents conferred no benefit over intravenous administration alone in colorectal surgery (Moesgaard et al, 1988; Raahave et al, 1989).

Intraincisional antibiotics

Antibiotics may be administered by injection into the subcutaneous tissues and the rectus muscle immediately prior to laparotomy (Armstrong et al, 1982; Taylor et al, 1982; Chalkiadakis et al, 1995). This method of antibiotic delivery is associated with more sustained serum levels than if the same agent is given intravenously. Clinical trials indicate that this method of antibiotic cover may be comparable to systemic antibiotic cover in prevention of wound sepsis in large bowel surgery (Pollock et al, 1989).

Antibiotic peritoneal lavage

Antibiotic peritoneal lavage is controversial in colorectal practice both for prophylaxis and treatment of intra-abdominal sepsis (Krukowski and Matheson, 1983; Krukowski et al, 1984). Lavage with saline alone may be dangerous since microorganisms may be disseminated by peritoneal lavage (Minervini et al, 1980; Ambrose et al, 1982a). Antibiotic lavage may be dangerous in faecal or purulent peritonitis since absorption is much more rapid and toxic serum levels have been reported (Ericsson et al, 1978). Renal failure and adhesive obstruction may occur if tetracycline lavage is used in acute peritonitis (Sandle and Mandell, 1980; Phillips and Dudley, 1984).

Washington et al (1974) reported a significantly reduced rate of residual abdominal sepsis with erythromycin lavage compared with saline alone in diffuse bacterial peritonitis. Stephen and Loewenthal (1979) claimed that peritoneal lavage with gentamicin, cephalothin and lincomycin improved survival and reduced the risk of residual abscess. Others maintain that lavage with a broad-spectrum antibiotic is effective (Rambo, 1972; Moukhtar and Romney, 1980; Jennings et al, 1982). Tetracycline lavage is reported by some to reduce sepsis in peritonitis from appendicitis and in colorectal surgery because of the very high peritoneal concentrations of tetracycline achieved in this way. However, these studies were not randomized (Steigbigel et al, 1968; Stewart and Matheson, 1978; Krukowski et al, 1984). In a randomized trial of tetracycline lavage in contaminated colorectal surgery, wound infection rates were reduced but there was no influence on intra-abdominal sepsis despite a sustained reduction in the counts of aerobic and anaerobic organisms in the peritoneal cavity (Silverman et al, 1986). As most antibiotics administered systemically achieve high concentrations in peritoneal fluid the intravenous route is generally preferred for antibiotic administration in the treatment of established intra-abdominal sepsis (Schiessel et al, 1984). Furthermore, Sauven et al (1986) reported that short-term antibiotic cover was superior to tetracycline lavage.

Oral antimicrobial agents

Antimicrobial prophylaxis in elective colorectal surgery used to be exclusively by oral agents, such as neomycin or the sulphonamides, which are poorly absorbed and are thought to be capable of reducing the faecal flora but none were clinically effective because they had no influence on the gut anaerobes (Poth and Knotts, 1942; Everett et al, 1969; Washington et al, 1974; Varquish et al, 1978; Taylor et al, 1979).

Neomycin with metronidazole, however, caused a profound fall in the counts of aerobic and anaerobic flora in the colon (Arabi et al, 1978), with a significant reduction in postoperative sepsis (Matheson et al, 1978). Neomycin and erythromycin base also reduced the counts of streptococci, coliforms and *Bacteroides* spp. and clinical studies indicated that these agents were capable of achieving a significant reduction in the rates of infection in elective colorectal surgery (Nichols et al, 1971, 1972; Clarke et al, 1977; Bartlett et al, 1978a).

Stenosing tumours of the large bowel did not adversely effect the reduction in faecal microflora achieved by oral antimicrobial agents (Figure 5.5; Table 5.10).

A significant reduction in faecal flora and postoperative sepsis was observed using kanamycin and metronidazole (Goldring et al, 1975; Keighley et al, 1979). However, metronidazole alone had no influence on the faecal flora unless there was severe diarrhoea (Lewis et al, 1977; Arabi et al, 1978).

The results of trials to test the efficacy of oral antimicrobials for prophylaxis in colorectal surgery are summarized in Table 5.11.

Table 5.10 Influence of mechanical preparation and antimicrobials on colonic flora.

	Staphylococci	*Streptococci*	*Coliforms*	*Bacteroides*	*Peptostreptococci*	*Clostridia*
Nichols et al (1972)						
Controls	1.6	7.1	7.5	9.6	9.2	3.8
Mechanical preparation	1.8	5.5	4.3	9.0	8.5	2.9
Kanamycin	1.0	3.4	3.1	9.4	7.6	2.0
Neomycin	1.0	1.9	1.2	3.2	2.6	1.7
Neomycin + phthalylsulphathiazole	1.0	1.0	1.7	3.3	4.4	2.3
Neomycin + erythromycin	1.0	1.0	1.4	1.7	1.0	1.7
Arabi et al (1978)						
Control	0.4	6.1	7.5	7.2	3.2	3.8
Mechanical preparation	0.5	3.1	7.1	8.4	1.0	2.1
Vivonex 5 days	0.5	2.2	5.7	6.9	0.3	1.6
Whole bowel irrigation	0.5	5.2	7.5	8.2	1.6	3.1
Neomycin + metronidazole	0.8	2.8	2.4	0.5	0.5	0.5
Bartlett et al (1978b)						
Control	5.1	5.5	6.9	8.5	7.6	7.4
Neomycin + erythromycin	4.7	5.6	4.4	4.3	4.6	4.6

Values shown are log counts.

Table 5.11 Influence of oral antimicrobials on sepsis rates in elective colorectal resection.

Agent (duration)	*No. of patients*	*Sepsis in treatment group (%)*	*Sepsis controls (%)*	*Reference*
Colistin + phthalylsulphathiazole (5 days)	100	32	38	Barker et al (1979)
Neomycin + erythromycin (1 day)	116	9	43	Clarke et al (1977)
Neomycin (3 days)	29	62	56	Everett et al (1969)
Kanamycin + metronidazole (3 days)	50	8	44	Goldring et al (1975)
Neomycin + metronidazole (3 days)	110	17	42	Matheson et al (1978)
Neomycin + bacitracin (5 days)	35	21	65	Sellwood et al (1969)
Neomycin (2 days)		41		
Neomycin + tetracycline (2 days)	196	5	43	Washington et al (1974)
Phthalylsulphathiazole (3 days)		38		
Neomycin + bacitracin + nystatin (3 days)	36	35	None	Sellwood et al (1969)
Phthalylsulphathiazole		49		
Metronidazole + phthalylsulphathiazole	120	13	None	Taylor et al (1979)
Erythromycin + neomycin (1 day)		25		
Metronidazole + neomycin (1 day)	79	5	None	Brass et al (1978)
Neomycin (2 days)		12.5		
Neomycin + phthalylsulphathiazole (2 days)		10		
Neomycin + erythromycin (2 days)	91	10	None	Varquish et al (1978)
Kanamycin (2 days)		41		
Kanamycin + erythromycin (2 days)	77	38	None	Wapnick et al (1979)

Although the combination of neomycin with erythromycin still has a considerable impact in North America we are uncertain that this is the best form of antibiotic prophylaxis and most clinicians still using the method add systemic antibiotics to the regimen (Handelsman et al, 1993). Recent evidence suggests that if antibiotics are to be used to reduce gut flora, ciprofloxacin may be more effective because it is rapidly absorbed (Taylor and Lindsay, 1994; McArdle et al, 1995).

In a prospective multicentre randomized controlled study involving 11 centres, Clarke et al (1977) reported that oral neomycin and erythromycin reduced sepsis from 43% to 9% but 407 patients were excluded, leaving only 116 for eventual analysis. Brass et al (1978) found that the combination of neomycin and erythromycin was inferior to neomycin with metronidazole. Varquish et al (1978) showed that neomycin and erythromycin was no better than neomycin alone.

When Weaver et al (1986) compared oral erythromycin–neomycin against systemic antibiotic cover the study had to be discontinued after entry of only 60 patients because of a 48% sepsis rate with

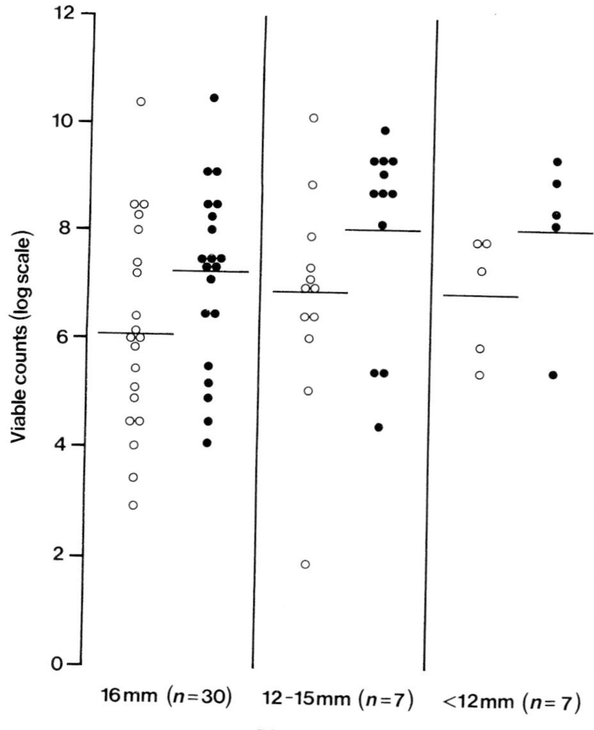

Figure 5.5 Impact of luminal diameter on counts of *E. coli* and *B. fragilis* in the large bowel. ○ *E. coli* (NS); ● *B. fragilis* (NS).

the oral regimen. Serious disadvantages of oral agents are the promotion of antibiotic resistance (Hartley and Richmond, 1975; Keighley and Burdon, 1979; Lacey, 1980), the risk of superinfection from yeasts or staphylococci and the risk of antibiotic-associated colitis (Keighley et al, 1979). For these reasons, systemic antibiotic prophylaxis is advised in colorectal surgery.

Systemic antimicrobials: justification for systemic antimicrobial prophylaxis

It would be impossible to review the results of all the clinical trials on systemic antibiotic prophylaxis in colorectal surgery, we therefore intend merely to highlight the important principles. The early studies compared antibiotic prophylaxis with no antibiotic cover at all and, almost without exception, these indicated that some form of prophylaxis is better than no cover at all (Table 5.12) (Stokes et al, 1974; Griffiths et al, 1976; Keighley and Crapp, 1976; Keighley et al, 1976; Downing et al, 1977; Willis et al, 1977; Hojer and Wetterfors, 1978; Eykyn et al, 1979).

Principles of systemic antibiotic prophylaxis

Timing of antibiotic administration

Antibiotics are only effective when given immediately prior to the inoculation of bacteria into wounds (Burke, 1961). These principles were confirmed clinically by Stone and his colleagues (1976), who showed that if antibiotic administration was delayed for 1–4 hours after operation, the rate of sepsis was the same as if no antibiotic cover had been given at all. Systemic antibiotics should be administered immediately before the start of an operation, either in the anaesthetic room or in the theatre (Bates et al, 1989).

Route of administration: oral or systemic?

A few studies have compared oral against systemic antimicrobial prophylaxis (Table 5.13). In three, oral administration was inferior to systemic antibiotic cover (Keighley et al, 1979; Weaver et al, 1986; Lau et al, 1988), whereas two studies showed no difference (Aeberhard et al, 1979; Beggs et al, 1982). The combination of oral and systemic antibiotic cover was shown to be superior to intravenous administration alone in three studies (Kaiser et al, 1983; Playforth et al, 1988; Taylor and Lindsay, 1994), equivalent in one study (Lau et al, 1988) and inferior in another (Coppa and Eng, 1988). In view of the dangers of resistance, superinfection and *Cl. difficile* colitis we would recommend using systemic antibiotic administration alone in elective colorectal surgery and firmly believe that it is the only logical route of administration in emergency large bowel surgery.

Table 5.12 Results of randomized controlled trials of systemic antibiotic prophylaxis.

Reference	*No. of patients*	*Agent*	*Antibiotic % sepsis*	*No antibiotic % sepsis*
Downing et al (1977)	60	Lincomycin: 3 doses	16	38
Keighley et al (1976)	62	Lincomycin: 5 days	12	33
Griffiths et al (1976)	60	Lincomycin + tobramycin: 1 dose	5	34
Willis et al (1977)	46	Metronidazole + gentamicin: 7 days	15	63
Hojer and Wetterfors (1978)	116	Doxycycline: 5 days	12	45
Eykyn et al (1979)	83	Metronidazole: 3 doses	13	51

Table 5.13 Results of randomized trials on optimum routes of antibiotic administration.

Reference	No. of patients	% sepsis Oral	i.v.	Oral + i.v.
Beggs et al (1982)	97	13	9	–
Aeberhard et al (1979)	72	10	9	–
Keighley et al (1979)	93	36	6	–
Kaiser et al (1983)	119	–	12	3
Weaver et al (1986)	60	48	9	–
Lau et al (1988)*	194	27	12	12
Coppa and Eng (1988)	350	–	5	11
Playforth et al (1988)	119	–	28	15
Taylor and Lindsay (1994)	327	–	23	11
McArdle et al (1995)	169	–	22	9

*Cancer only.

Influence on faecal flora

In view of the dangers of disturbing the normal faecal flora, it is appropriate to consider the influence of intravenous antibiotic administration on colonic microflora. Intravenous doxycycline and many of the third-generation cephalosporins suppress faecal microflora with the emergence of *Cl. difficile* (Ambrose et al, 1985), whereas tinidazole, metronidazole and most of the penicillins have little, if any, influence (Heimdahl and Nord, 1979; Heimdahl et al, 1982; Kager et al, 1985).

Dose of antimicrobial

The antibiotics chosen for prophylaxis should provide adequate serum concentrations throughout the duration of the operation. Some cephalosporins, penicillins and aminoglycosides have extremely short half-lives. Therefore, for complex colorectal procedures involving excessive blood loss or prolonged operation, repeated intraoperative antibiotic administration may be indicated (Burdon et al, 1985).

Optimum duration of antibiotic cover

With the exception of a study with four major variables and small numbers (McArdle et al, 1995) most now indicate that, provided antibiotics with an adequate half-life are used for prophylaxis, single-dose cover is as effective as prolonged antibiotic cover for 24 hours or even several days (AF Higgens et al, 1980; Giercksky et al, 1982; Goransson et al, 1984; Juul et al, 1987; Rowe-Jones et al, 1990) (Table 5.14). However, this policy can only be justified if there has been minimal endogenous bacterial contamination (Claesson et al, 1986) and under these circumstances single-dose antibiotic cover is effective in elective colorectal surgery (Dipiro et al, 1986; Jensen et al, 1990; Wittmann and Schein, 1996). Agents such as ceftriaxone, with a long serum half-life, have been particularly effective in large bowel surgery (Shepherd et al, 1986; Weaver et al, 1986; Morris, 1993; Matikainen and Hiltunen, 1993).

Choice of antimicrobials: role of a specific anaerobicidal agent

Several studies have compared the use of a nitroimidazole alone or in combination with a broad-spectrum antibiotic (Morris et al, 1984; Cunliffe et al, 1985; Norwegian Study Group, 1985; Roland et al, 1986; Bergman and Solhaug, 1987). The overall trend is in favour of combined antibiotic cover (Table 5.15). Other studies have compared single-agent, broad-spectrum antibiotic cover against a combination of two antibiotics, one of which has specific anaerobicidal activity. So far, single-agent, broad-spectrum antibiotic cover does not seem to be sufficiently reliable to be advised in colorectal surgery (Hares et al, 1981; de la Hunt and Karran, 1986; McCulloch et al, 1986; Tudor et al, 1988; Walker et al, 1988; Kingston et al, 1989; Hall et al, 1989; Taylor and Lindsay, 1994). Furthermore, detailed microbiological evaluation of anaerobic

Table 5.14 Single-dose or multiple-dose antibiotic cover in colorectal surgery.

Reference	No. of patients	Agent	Incidence of wound sepsis (%) Single dose	Multiple doses
AF Higgens et al (1980)	59	Metronidazole + co-trimoxazole	8	9
Giercksky et al (1982)	234	Tinidazole + doxycycline	4	11
Goransson et al (1984)	102	Doxycycline	10	10
Juul et al (1987)	294	Metronidazole + ampicillin	7	7
Shepherd et al (1986)	124	Metronidazole + ceftriaxone: 1 dose	9	
		Metronidazole + gentamicin: 3 doses		22
Hakansson et al (1993)	600	Cefotaxime + metronidazole	7	16 (3 days)
McArdle et al (1995)	169	Metronidazole + gentamicin or metronidazole + ciprofloxacin	19 (24 hours)	11 (3 days)

Table 5.15 Spectrum of antimicrobial agents: is the addition of an anaerobicide necessary?

		Incidence of wound sepsis (%)			
Reference	*No. of patients*	*Anaerobicide alone*	*With a broad-spectrum agent*	*Broad-spectrum agent alone*	*With anaerobicide*
Morris et al (1984)	100	Metronidazole (27)	+ Gentamicin (23)	–	–
Cunliffe et al (1985)	90	Metronidazole (25)	+ Cefuroxime (15)	–	–
Norwegian Study Group (1985)	47	Tinidazole (10)	+ Doxycycline (3)		
Roland et al (1986)	358	Metronidazole (13)	+ Doxycycline (or ampicillin) (3)	–	–
Morris et al (1984)	109	–	–	Latamoxef (21)	+ Metronidazole (23)
Bergman and Solhaug (1987)	261			Doxycycline (16)	+ Metronidazole (3)
Morris et al (1993)	260	–	–	Ceftriaxone (6)	Gentamicin + metronidazole (17)

infections, particularly from *B. fragilis*, provides convincing evidence of the need to use a nitroimidazole with a broad-spectrum antibiotic. What is also clear is that a specific anaerobicide alone is inadequate for prophylaxis (Cunliffe et al, 1985; Roland et al, 1986; Khubchandani et al, 1989).

Clinical trials also seem to imply that single agents, particularly cephalosporins or penicillins in combination with a β-lactamase inhibitor, are less effective than their use in combination with metronidazole because they are not sufficiently active *in vivo* against faecal anaerobes (Condon et al, 1979; Hoffmann et al, 1981; Kager et al, 1981; Ivarsson et al, 1982; Kaiser et al, 1983; Peck et al, 1984; Baker et al, 1985; Drumm and Donovan, 1985; de la Hunt and Karran, 1986; Hall et al, 1989; Hakansson et al, 1993). We still believe, therefore, that prophylaxis in colorectal surgery should include metronidazole in combination with an agent providing broad-spectrum cover against the aerobic Enterobacteriaceae.

Policy for contaminated operations

Two studies have now demonstrated that if the degree of bacterial colonization in the peritoneum exceeds 10^5 colony-forming units per mL, prolonged exposure to antimicrobials is justified on the grounds of reduced postoperative morbidity (Claesson et al, 1986; Tornqvist et al, 1987). On the other hand, newer agents capable of high tissue penetration may perform almost as well when given for shorter periods (Tudor et al, 1988; Hall et al, 1989; Yoshioka et al, 1991).

INFLAMMATORY BOWEL DISEASE

There are only a few trials of antimicrobial prophylaxis in inflammatory bowel disease (Hares et al, 1982). Generally, rates of sepsis are lower than those for patients with malignancy. This may reflect a younger population. On the other hand, patients with inflammatory bowel disease often have coexisting infection (intra-abdominal sepsis or intestinal fistula), hence there is a higher risk of contamination. However, the impact of the obligate anaerobes may be less in patients with inflammatory bowel disease, provided the ileum is not partially obstructed (Ambrose et al, 1982b; Ambrose, 1984).

Incidence of sepsis

Ulcerative colitis

The incidence of sepsis in ulcerative colitis is largely determined by presentation. Emergency colectomy for toxic megacolon or perforation carries a high morbidity and mortality from sepsis (Watts et al, 1966; Jalan et al, 1970).

Elective proctocolectomy for ulcerative colitis has a low rate of abdominal wound infection (Ritchie, 1972; Goligher, 1984) but perineal sepsis may be high, especially if the rectum has been inadvertently

Table 5.16 Influence of contamination on sepsis rates in patients with inflammatory bowel disease.

	Contaminated		*Non-contaminated*	
	No.	*Sepsis (%)*	*No.*	*Sepsis (%)*
Abdominal wound	39	46	123	10
Perineal wound	27	81	36	36
Postoperative abscess	39	41	123	6

From Allsop and Lee (1978).

damaged during excision (Allsop and Lee, 1978) (Table 5.16). Sepsis rates appear to be much lower after colectomy and ileorectal anastomosis, and restorative proctocolectomy (Jones et al, 1977; Dozois, 1986; Nicholls, 1987; Keighley et al, 1989; Cohen et al, 1992) (see Chapters 47 and 49).

Diverticular disease

In the UK, most operations on diverticular disease are for its complications, hence a high proportion of patients require emergency procedures. Even staged resections for abscess and peritonitis are attended by high rates of infection, both at the time of the emergency procedure and when restoring intestinal continuity (Madden and Tan, 1961; Wara et al, 1981; Eisenstat et al, 1983; Weston-Underwood and Marks, 1984; Tudor et al, 1986a,b) (see Chapter 37).

Crohn's disease

High rates of infection are reported following emergency operations for Crohn's disease (Farmer et al, 1976). Elective operations performed for complications such as fistula and abscess, or on patients with active disease are associated with a high risk of infection (Table 5.17) (CS Higgens et al, 1980) but steroid therapy did not increase the risk of sepsis. A high rate of sepsis occurs in Crohn's surgery especially after proctocolectomy (De Dombal et al, 1971; Ritchie and Lockhart-Mummery, 1973; Higgens and Allan, 1980; CS Higgens et al, 1980; Ambrose et al, 1984a; Scammell et al, 1986) (Table 5.18).

Table 5.17 Factors associated with sepsis in resection for Crohn's disease.

	Factor present (%)	*Factor absent (%)*
Increased incidence		
Fistula present (*n* = 20)	50	22
Abscess present (*n* = 15)	67	21
Seromucoids > 400 mg/dL (*n* = 20)	55	21
Albumin < 3.0 g/dL (*n* = 17)	65	20
No increased incidence		
Fever present (*n* = 21)	24	28
WBC >10 000/cm (*n* = 34)	32	25
Age > 50 years (*n* = 26)	31	26
Steroid cover (*n* = 49)	28	26

From CS Higgens et al (1980).

Table 5.18 Incidence of sepsis in resections for Crohn's disease.

Operation	*Incidence (%)*
Small bowel resection and ileocaecal resection	28
Ileostomy revision	21
Colectomy and ileorectal anastomosis	7
Proctocolectomy	44

From CS Higgens et al (1980).

Flora

The intestinal flora in ulcerative colitis and diverticular disease does not differ from that of the normal colon, provided that the patient is not receiving sulphasalazine (Drasar et al, 1969; Gorbach and Tabaqchali, 1969; Gorbach, 1971; Jacomina et al, 1975; Keighley et al, 1978). In patients with Crohn's disease the counts of *E. coli* and *B. fragilis* in the terminal ileum are significantly higher than in normal subjects (Figure 5.6). Surprisingly, these changes are not related to disease activity, luminal diameter, previous excision of the ileocaecal valve, macroscopic colitis or enteroenteric fistula (Keighley et al, 1978; Ambrose et al, 1984b). In quiescent Crohn's colitis, counts of *E. coli* in the large bowel are significantly higher than in normal subjects. However, in acute colitis counts of faecal organisms are significantly lower than those with quiescent disease (Ambrose et al, 1982a).

Factors related to the incidence of postoperative sepsis

Contamination

The Oxford experience highlights the importance of contamination in the pathogenesis of postoperative sepsis (Allsop and Lee, 1978) (see Table 5.16). These observations are in agreement with our own, where significantly higher rates of sepsis were observed in patients with intra-abdominal abscess,

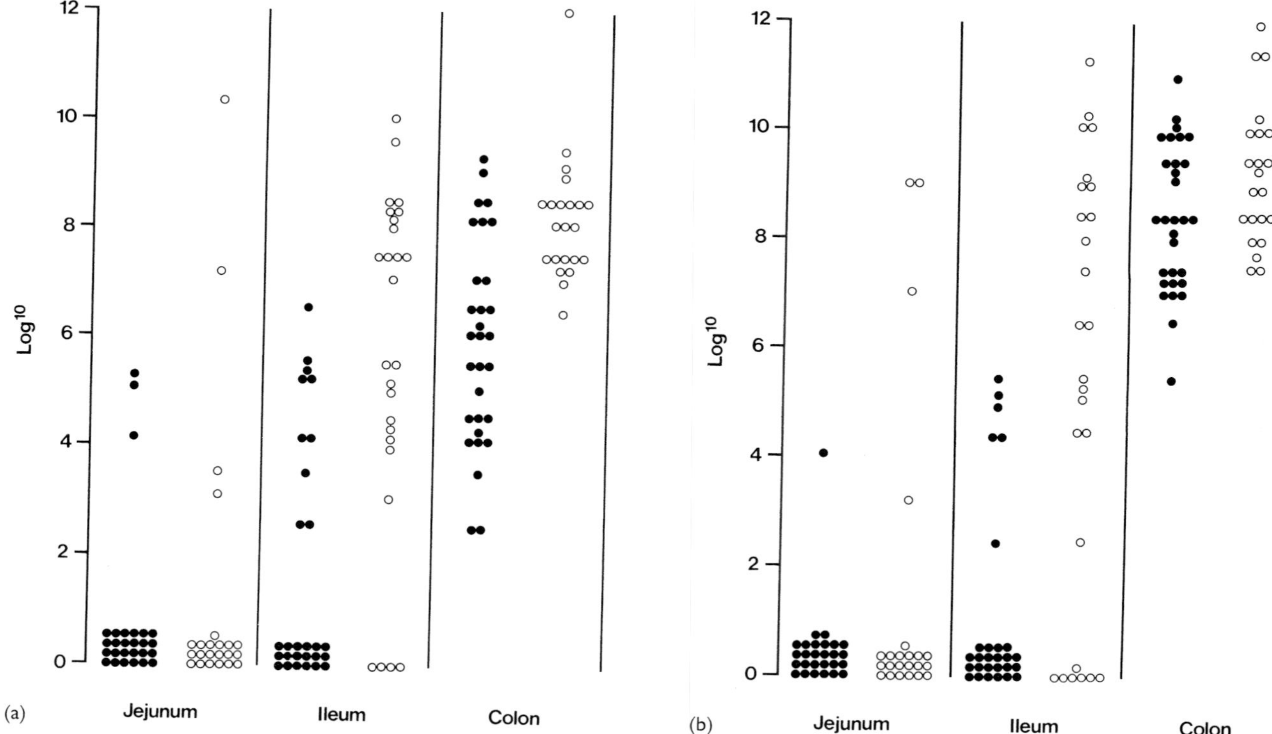

Figure 5.6 Impact of Crohn's disease on counts of (a) *E. coli* and (b) *B. fragilis* in the jejunum, ileum and colon compared with controls. ● Control; ○ Crohn's disease.

enterocutaneous fistula and active bowel disease (see Table 5.17). Furthermore, pathogenic bacteria were present significantly more frequently on the serosa of the bowel or in the regional lymph nodes in non-contaminated Crohn's disease than in controls (Ambrose et al, 1984b) (Table 5.19) and may explain the increased infection rate in elective Crohn's resection (Barker et al, 1979; Keighley, 1982).

Table 5.19 Occurrence (%) of pathogenic bacteria outside the lumen of the bowel and in the lymph nodes.

	Crohn's disease (n = 46)	*Control (n = 43)*
Serosa	27	15
Lymph nodes	33	5

From Ambrose et al (1984b).

Steroids

There is no evidence that steroids increase the risk of sepsis (Seneca and Peer, 1966) in Crohn's disease (Fauci, 1975; Allsop and Lee, 1978; Hares et al, 1982; Higgens et al, 1981).

Weight loss

Weight loss has been regarded as a high-risk factor in patients with inflammatory bowel disease, but gross hypoproteinaemia may be a manifestation of intra-abdominal sepsis (Bistrian et al, 1974; Keighley, 1982). Evidence that preoperative nutrition reduces the morbidity from sepsis is conflicting (Holter et al, 1976; Williams et al, 1976; Goodgame, 1980; Mullen et al, 1980). The risk of sepsis was not increased in patients weighing less than 80% of their ideal bodyweight (Higgens et al, 1984). Anthropometric parameters improved more following operation in those patients who were badly malnourished than in patients of normal body stature (Figure 5.7).

Duration of antibiotic cover

There have been few trials of antimicrobial prophylaxis in inflammatory bowel disease. Prophylactic antibiotics appeared to have little influence on postoperative sepsis (Allsop and Lee, 1978; Barker et al, 1979; CS Higgens et al, 1980). Hares et al (1982) found that only prolonged antibiotic cover reduced sepsis rates in Crohn's surgery (Table 5.20). It appears that prolonged exposure to antimicrobials is necessary in inflammatory bowel disease because of the high risk of contamination and established sepsis at the time of resection (Ambrose et al, 1984a).

Table 5.20 Duration of antibiotic cover in Crohn's disease.

	Metronidazole + gentamicin		
	No antibiotic (*n* = 27)	*24-hour cover* (*n* = 30)	*5-day cover* (*n* = 30)
Wound sepsis	37%	23%	13%
Perineal sepsis	4/6	1/8	3/6
Abscess	11%	10%	3%
Septicaemia	7%	10%	0%

From Hares et al (1982).

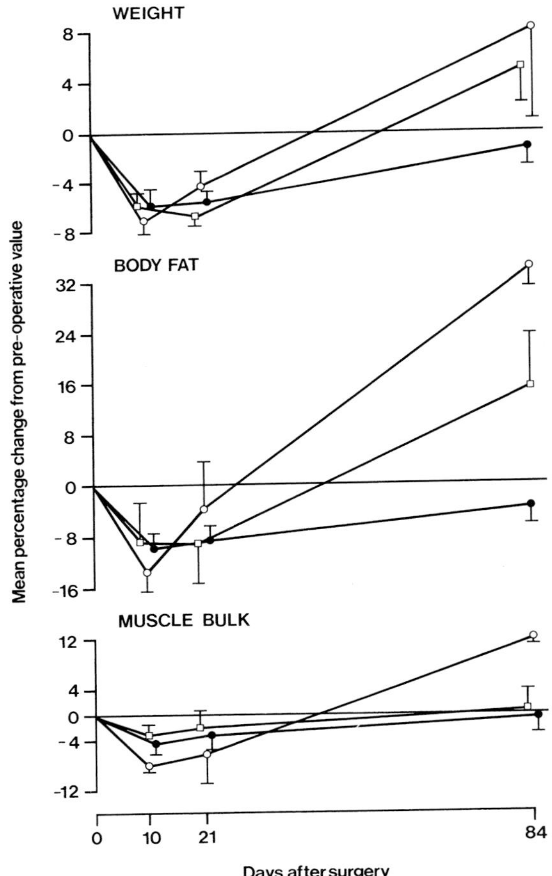

Figure 5.7 Mean percentage change of weight, body fat and muscle bulk compared with percentage ideal body weight (IBW). Percent IBW group: ○—○ <90; □—□ 80–90; ●—● >90.

AUTHORS' RECOMMENDATION

Sepsis rates in elective colorectal surgery should be less than 10%. This can be achieved by meticulous mechanical bowel preparation, operating theatre discipline, avoidance of anastomosis in the presence of sepsis and short-term antibiotic cover using metronidazole and cephalosporin. Prolonged antibiotic cover would be recommended in Crohn's disease and whenever there is gross contamination or established sepsis.

REFERENCES

Abussaud MJ & Megdem MM (1986) A study of some factors associated with wound infection. *J Hosp Infect* **8**: 300–304.

Aeberhard P, Berger J & Casey P (1979) A comparison of oral bowel preparation and intravenous chemotherapy given at the time of operation. *R Soc Med Int Cong Symp Ser* **18**: 173–177.

Ahrendt GM, Gardner K & Barbul A (1994) Loss of colonic structural collagen impairs healing during intra-abdominal sepsis. *Arch Surg* **129**: 1179–1183.

Ahrendt GM, Tantry US & Barbul A (1996) Intra-abdominal sepsis impairs colonic reparative collagen synthesis. *Am J Surg* **171**: 102–108.

Ahrenholz DH & Simmons RL (1979) Povidone-iodine in peritonitis: I. Adverse effects of local instillation in experimental *E. coli* peritonitis. *J Surg Res* **26**: 458–463.

Alexander JW (1974) Emerging concepts in control of clinical infection. *Surgery* **74**: 934–946.

Allsop JR & Lee ECG (1978) Factors which influenced post-operative complications in patients with UC or Crohn's disease of the colon on corticosteroids. *Gut* **19**: 729–734.

Altemeier WA, Todd JC & Ince WW (1967) Gram-negative septicaemia: a growing threat. *Ann Surg* **166**: 530–542.

Ambrose NS (1984) Antimicrobials, intestinal flora and

colorectal disease. Intestinal microflora: physiology of bowel preparation and sepsis in colorectal surgery. MS thesis, University of London.

Ambrose NS, Donovan IA, Derges S, Minervini S & Harding LK (1982a) The efficacy of peritoneal lavage at elective abdominal operations. *Br J Surg* **69**: 143–144.

Ambrose NS, Youngs D, Burdon DW & Keighley MRB (1982b) Changes in intestinal microflora in Crohn's disease. *Br J Surg* **69**: 681.

Ambrose NS, Burdon DW & Keighley MRB (1983) A prospective randomized trial to compare mezlocillin and metronidazole with cefuroxime and metronidazole as prophylaxis in elective colorectal operations. *J Hosp Infect* **4**: 375–382.

Ambrose NS, Alexander-Williams J & Keighley MRB (1984a) Audit of sepsis in operations for IBD. *Dis Colon Rectum* **27**: 602–604.

Ambrose NS, Johnson M, Burdon DW & Keighley MRB (1984b) Incidence of pathogenic bacteria from mesenteric lymph nodes and ileal serosa during Crohn's disease surgery. *Br J Surg* **71**: 623–625.

Ambrose NS, Johnson M, Burdon DW & Keighley MRB (1985) The influence of single dose intravenous antibiotics on faecal flora and emergence of *Clostridium difficile*. *J Antimicrob Chemother* **15**: 319–326.

Anderson B, Bendtsen A, Holbraad L et al (1972) Wound infections after appendicectomy. I. A controlled trial on the prophylactic efficacy of topical ampicillin in non-perforated appendicitis. II. A controlled trial on the prophylactic efficacy of delayed primary suture and topical ampicillin in perforated appendicitis. *Acta Chir Scand* **138**: 531–536.

Anonymous (1975) Bacteraemia from the bowel. *BMJ* **2**: 396–397.

Arabi Y, Dimock F, Burdon DW, Alexander-Williams J & Keighley MRB (1978) Influence of bowel preparation and antimicrobials on colonic microflora. *Br J Surg* **65**: 555–559.

Armstrong CP, Taylor TV & Reeves DS (1982) Pre-incisional intraparietal injection of cefamandole; a new approach to wound infection prophylaxis. *Br J Surg* **69**: 459–460.

Avery CME, Jamieson N & Calne RY (1995) Effective administration of heparin and antibiotic prophylaxis. *Br J Surg* **82**: 1136–1137.

Badia JM, De la Torre R, Farre M et al (1995) Inadequate levels of metronidazole in subcutaneous fat after standard prophylaxis. *Br J Surg* **82**: 479–482.

Badrinath K, Jairam N & Ravi HR (1994) Spreading extraperitoneal cellulitis following perirectal sepsis. *Br J Surg* **81**: 297–298.

Baker DM, Jones JA, Nguyen-Van-Tam JS et al (1994) Taurolidine peritoneal lavage as prophylaxis against infection after elective colorectal surgery. *Br J Surg* **81**: 1054–1056.

Baker RJ, Donahue PE, Finegold S et al (1985) A prospective double-blind comparison of piperacillin, cephalothin and cefoxitin in the prevention of post-operative infections in patients undergoing intra-abdominal operations. *Surg Gynecol Obstet* **161**: 409–415.

Barie PS, Bennion RS & Cheadle WG (1994) Results of the North American trial of piperacillin/tazobactam compared with clindamycin and gentamicin in the treatment of severe intra-abdominal infections. *Eur J Surg* Suppl 573: 61–66.

Barker K, Graham NG, Mason MC, De Dombal FT & Goligher JC (1979) The relative significance of pre-operative oral antibiotics, mechanical bowel preparation and pre-operative peritoneal contamination in the avoidance of sepsis after radical surgery for UC and Crohn's disease of the large bowel. *Br J Surg* **58**: 270–274.

Barnes AD (1979) Dialysis and transplantation. In Keighley MRB & Burdon DW (eds) *Antimicrobial Prophylaxis in Surgery*, pp 197–212. Tunbridge Wells: Pitman Medical.

Bartlett JG (1981) The pathophysiology of intra-abdominal sepsis. In Watt JMcK, McDonald P, O'Brien P, Marshall V & Finlay-Jones D (eds) *Infections in Surgery*, pp 47–58. Edinburgh: Churchill Livingstone.

Bartlett JG, Onderdont AB, Louie T et al (1978a) A review: lessons from an animal model of intra-abdominal sepsis. *Arch Surg* **113**: 853–857.

Bartlett JG, Condon RE, Gorbach SL, Clarke JS, Nichols RL & Ochi S (1978b) Veterans administration co-operative study on bowel preparation for elective colorectal operations: impact of oral antibiotic regimen on colonic flora, wound irrigation cultures and bacteriology of septic complications. *Ann Surg* **188**: 249–254.

Bateman NT, Eykyn SJ & Phillips I (1975) Pyrogenic liver abscess caused by *Streptococcus milleri*. *Lancet* **i**: 657–659.

Bates T, Siller G, Crathern BC et al (1989) Timing of prophylactic antibiotics in abdominal surgery: trial of a pre-operative versus an intra-operative first dose. *Br J Surg* **76**: 52–56.

Baxter JG, Marble DA, Whitfield LR, Wels PB, Walczak P & Scheatag JJ (1985) Clinical risk factors for prolonged PT.PTT in abdominal sepsis patients treated with moxalactam or tobramycin plus clindamycin. *Ann Surg* **201**: 96–102.

Beggs FD, Jobanputra RS & Holmes JT (1982) A comparison of intravenous and oral metronidazole as prophylactic in colorectal surgery. *Br J Surg* **69**: 226–227.

Belliveau P (1995) Defining wound infection in stoma closure. *Can J Surg* **39**: 108–109.

Bergman L & Solhaug JH (1987) Single-dose chemoprophylaxis in elective colorectal surgery. A comparison between doxycycline plus metronidazole and doxycycline. *Ann Surg* **205**: 77–82.

Bernard H & Cole W (1964) The prophylaxis of surgical infection: the effect of prophylactic antimicrobial drugs on incidence of infection following potentially contaminated wounds. *Surgery* **56**: 151–157.

Bibby BA, Collins BJ & Ayliffe GA (1986) A mathematical model for assessing risk of postoperative wound infection. *J Hosp Infect* **8**: 31–39.

Bistrian BR, Blackburn GL, Holwell H & Heddle RJ (1974) Protein status of general surgical patients. *JAMA* **230**: 858–860.

Bleday R, Braidt J, Ruoff K, Shellito PC & Ackroyd FW (1993) Quantitative cultures of the mucosal-associated bacteria in the mechanically prepared colon and rectum. *Dis Colon Rectum* **36**: 844–849.

Bodner SJ, Koenig MG, Treanor LL & Goodman JS (1972) Antibiotic susceptibility testing of *Bacteroides*. *Antimicrob Agents Chemother* **2**: 57–60.

Bowcock S, Mackie IJ, Ho D, Moulsdale M, Billings P & Machin SJ (1986) Effects of various doses of latamoxef (moxalactam) on haemostasis. *J Hosp Infect* **8**: 193–199.

Boyd WC (1977) Use of merlex mesh in acute loss of the abdominal wall due to infection. *Surg Gynecol Obstet* **144**: 251–252.

Brass C, Richards GK, Ruedy J, Prentis J & Hinchey EJ (1978) The effect of metronidazole on the incidence of post-operative wound infection in elective colon surgery. *Am J Surg* **135**: 91–96.

Brennan SS, Foster ME & Leaper DJ (1986) Antiseptic toxicity in wounds healing by secondary intention. *J Hosp Infect* **8**: 263–267.

Britz ML & Wilkinson RG (1984) Metronidazole resistance in *Bacteroides fragilis*. *J Antimicrob Chemother* **13**: 393–403.

Brown EM (1984) The in vitro susceptibility of *Bacteroides fragilis* group to amoxycillin-clavulanic acid. *J Antimicrob Chemother* **14**: 367–372.

Brown R, Bancewicz J, Hamid J, Patel NJ et al (1982) Failure of delayed hypersensitivity skin testing to predict post-operative sepsis and mortality. *BMJ* **284**: 851–853.

Brown DR, Davis NL, Lepawsky M, Cunningham J & Kortbeek J (1994) A multicenter review of the treatment of major truncal necrozing infections with and without hyperbaric oxygen therapy. *Am J Surg* **167**: 485–489.

Browne MK & Stoller JL (1970) Intraperitoneal noxythiolin in faecal peritonitis. *Br J Surg* **57**: 525–529.

Brumfitt W & Hamilton-Miller JMT (1980) Dangers of chemoprophylaxis. In Karran S (ed.) *Controversies in Surgical Sepsis*, pp 76–86. Dorset: Praeger.

Bullard KM & Dunn DL (1996) Diagnosis and treatment of bacteremia and intravascular catheter infections. *Am J Surg* **172** (Suppl 6A): 13S–19S.

Burdon DW, Youngs DJ, Silverman SH & Keighley MRB (1985) Serum pharmacokinetics of prophylactic antibiotics during colorectal surgery. *Proceedings of the 14th International Congress of Chemotherapy*, pp 2431–2432, Kyoto.

Burke J (1961) Effective period of preventive antibiotic action in experimental excisions and dermal lesions. *Surgery* **50**: 161–168.

Burton RC (1973) Post operative wound infection in colonic rectal surgery. *Br J Surg* **60**: 363–365.

Bybee JD & Rogers DE (1964) The phagocytic activity of polymorphonuclear leukocytes obtained from patients with diabetes mellitus. *J Lab Clin Med* **64**: 1–13.

Carr ND, Hobbis J & Cade D (1984) A double-blind dose ranging study of intravenous metronidazole in the prevention of sepsis after elective colorectal surgery. *J R Coll Surg Edinb* **29**: 139–142.

Chalkiadakis GE, Gonnianakis C, Tsatsakis A, Tsakalof A & Michalodimitrakis M (1995) Preincisional single-dose Ceftriaxone for the prophylaxis of surgical wound infection. *Am J Surg* **170**: 353–355.

Chodak GW & Plaut ME (1977) Use of systemic antibiotics for prophylaxis in surgery. A critical review. *Arch Surg* **112**: 326–334.

Christou NV, Boisvert G, Broadhead M & Meakins JL (1985) The techniques of measurement of the delayed hypersensitivity skin test response for the assessment of bacterial host resistance. *World J Surg* **9**: 798–806.

Claesson BEB & Holmlund DEW (1988) Predictors of intraoperative bacterial contamination and postoperative infection in elective colorectal surgery. *J Hosp Infect* **11**: 127–135.

Claesson BEB, Filipsson S, Holmlund DEW, Matzsch TW & Wahlby L (1986) Selective cefuroxime prophylaxis following colorectal surgery based on intra-operative dipslide culture. *Br J Surg* **73**: 953–957.

Clark RA & Kimball HR (1971) Defective granulocyte chemotaxis in the Chediak–Higashi syndrome. *J Clin Invest* **50**: 2645–2652.

Clarke JS, Condon RE, Bartlett JG et al (1977) Preoperative oral antibiotics reduce septic complications of colon operations: results of prospective, randomized, double-blind clinical study. *Ann Surg* **186**: 251–259.

Coco C, Roncolini G, Perrotti P et al (1993) Antimicrobial prophylaxis with ceftriaxone in colorectal surgery. *Coloproctology* **1**: 59–62.

Cohen Z, McLeod RS, Stephen W, Stern HS, O'Connor B & Reznick R (1992) Continuing evolution of the pelvic pouch procedure. *Ann Surg* **216**: 506–512.

Cole WR & Bernard HR (1967) Wound isolation in the prevention of post operative wound infection. *Surg Gynecol Obstet* **125**: 257–260.

Condon RE, Bartlett JG, Nichols RL et al (1979) Preoperative prophylactic cephalothin fails to control septic complications of colorectal operations: results of controlled clinical trial. *Am J Surg* **137**: 68–74.

Coppa GF & Eng K (1988) Factors involved in antibiotic selection in elective colon and rectal surgery. *Surgery* **104**: 853–858.

Cruse PJE (1975) Incidence of wound infection on surgical services. *Surg Clin North Am* **55**: 1269–1276.

Cruse PJE & Foord R (1973) A five year prospective study of 23 649 surgical wounds. *Arch Surg* **107**: 206–210.

Cunliffe WJ, Carr N & Schofield PF (1985) Prophylactic metronidazole with and without cefuroxime in elective colorectal surgery. *J R Coll Surg Edinb* **30**: 123–125.

Davey P, Malek M & Thomas P (1992) Measuring the cost-effectiveness of antibiotic prophylaxis in surgery. *Am J Surg* **164**(4A) (Suppl): 395–435.

David DS, Grieco MH & Cushman P (1970) Adrenal glucocorticoids after 20 years. A review of their clinically relevant consequences. *J Chron Dis* **22**: 637–711.

Davidson AIG, Clark C & Smith G (1971) Postoperative wound infection: a computer analysis. *Br J Surg* **58**: 333–337.

De Cree J, Verhaegen H, De Cock W et al (1974) Impaired neutrophil phagocytosis. *Lancet* **ii**: 294–295.

De Dombal FT, Burton I & Goligher JC (1971) The early and late results of surgical treatment for Crohn's disease. *Br J Surg* **58**: 807–811.

DeGennaro VA, Corman ML, Coller JA, Pribek MC & Veidenheimer MC (1978) Wound infections after colectomy. *Dis Colon Rectum* **21**: 567–572.

de Jong TE, Vierhout RJ & van Vroonhovea TJ (1982) Povidone-iodine irrigation of the subcutaneous tissue to prevent surgical wound infections. *Surg Gynecol Obstet* **155**: 221.

de la Hunt MN & Karran SJ (1986) Sylbactam/ampicillin compared with cefoxitin for chemoprophylaxis in elective colorectal surgery. *Dis Colon Rectum* **29**: 157–159.

de la Hunt MN, Chan AYC & Karran SJ (1986) Postoperative complications: how much do they cost? *Ann R Coll Surg Engl* **68**: 199–202.

Delalande JP, Hay JM, Fingerhut A, Kohlmann G & Paquet JC (for the French Association of Surgical Research) (1994) Perineal wound management after abdominoperineal rectal excision for carcinoma with unsatisfactory hemostasis or gross septic contamination: primary closure vs. packing. A multicenter, controlled trial. *Dis Colon Rectum* **37**: 890–896.

Devine HB & Devine J (1948) *Surgery of the Colon and Rectum*. Bristol: Wright.

Dipiro JT, Cheung RPF, Bowden TA Jr & Mansberger JA (1986) Single dose systemic antibiotic prophylaxis of surgical wound infections. *Am J Surg* **152**: 552–559.

Dobkin JF, Miller MH & Steigbigel NH (1978) Septicaemia in patients on chronic haemodialysis. *Ann Intern Med* **88**: 28–33.

Downing R, McLeish AR, Buralon DW, Alexander-Williams J & Keighley MRB (1977) Duration of systemic prophylactic antibiotic cover against anaerobic sepsis of intestinal surgery. *Dis Colon Rectum* **20**: 401–404.

Dozois R (1986) Ileoanal anastomosis for colitis with special reference to a straight anastomosis with a J-shaped pouch. *Proceedings of the World Congress of Gastroenterology*, San Paulo.

Drasar BS, Shiner M & McLeod GM (1969) Studies on the intestinal flora. The bacterial flora of the gastrointestinal tract in healthy achlorhydric persons. *Gastroenterology* **56**: 71–79.

Drasar FA, Farrell W, Maskell J & Williams JD (1976) Tobramycin, amikacin, sissomicin and gentamicin resistant Gram-negative rods. *BMJ* **2**: 1284–1287.

Drumm J & Donovan IA (1985) Metronidazole and Augmentin in the prevention of sepsis after appendicectomy. *Br J Surg* **72**: 571–573.

Dudley HAF & Fielding LP (1980) Management of patients undergoing colorectal surgery with particular reference to sepsis. In Karran S (ed.) *Controversies in Surgical Sepsis*, pp 303–370. Dorset: Praeger.

Ehrlich HP, Tarver H & Hunt TK (1973) Effects of vitamin A and glucocorticoids upon inflammation and collagen synthesis. *Ann Surg* **177**: 222–227.

Eklund AE, Nord CE & Swedish Study Group (1993) A randomized multicenter trial of piperacillin/tazobactam versus imipenem/cilastatin in the treatment of severe intra-abdominal infections. *J Antimicrob Chemother* **31** (Suppl A): 79–85.

Eisenstat TE, Rubin RJ & Salvati EP (1983) Surgical management of diverticulitis: the role of the Hartmann procedure. *Dis Colon Rectum* **26**: 429–432.

Ericsson CD, Duke JH Jr & Pickering LK (1978) Clinical pharmacology of intravenous and intraperitoneal aminoglycoside antibiotics in the prevention of wound infections. *Ann Surg* **188**: 66–70.

Evans C & Pollock AV (1973) The reduction of surgical wound infection by prophylactic parenteral cephaloridiae. *Br J Surg* **60**: 434–437.

Evans C, Pollock AV & Rosenberg IL (1974) The reduction of surgical wound infection by topical cephaloridine: a controlled clinical trial. *Br J Surg* **61**: 133–135.

Evans M & Pollock AV (1984) Trials on trial: a review of trials of antibiotic prophylaxis. *Arch Surg* **119**: 109–113.

Evans M & Pollock AV (1985) A score system for evaluating random control clinical trials of prophylaxis of abdominal surgical wound infection. *Br J Surg* **72**: 256–260.

Everett MT, Brogan TD & Nettleton J (1969) The place of antibiotics in colonic surgery: a clinical study. *Br J Surg* **56**: 679–684.

Eykyn SJ (1982) The microbiology of postoperative bacteremia. *World J Surg* **6**: 268–272.

Eykyn SJ, Jackson BT, Lockhart-Mummery HE & Phillips I (1979) Prophylactic peroperative intravenous metronidazole in elective colorectal surgery. *Lancet* **ii**: 761–764.

Fabricus PJ, Morris DL, Ozuner G, Scammell B, Allan RN & Keighley MRB (1984) Postoperative bleeding and latamoxef prophylaxis in surgery for colorectal and IBD. *Gut* **25A**: 553–554.

Farmer RG, Hawk WA & Turnbull RB Jr (1976) Indications for surgery in Crohn's disease: analysis of 500 cases. *Gastroenterology* **71**: 245–252.

Fauci AS (1975) Mechanisms of corticosteroid action on lymphocyte subpopulations. *Immunology* **28**: 669–680.

Fauci AS, Dale DC & Balow JE (1976) Glucocorticoid therapy: mechanisms of action and clinical considerations. *Ann Intern Med* **84**: 304–315.

Fawcett A, Shembekar M, Church JS, Vashisht R, Springall RG & Nott DM (1996) Smoking, hypertension and colonic anastomotic healing; a combined clinical and histopathological study. *Gut* **38**: 714–718.

Fikri E & McAdams AJ (1975) Wound infection in colonic surgery. *Ann Surg* **182**: 724–726.

Finch DRA, Taylor L & Morris PJ (1979) Wound sepsis following gastrointestinal surgery: a comparison of topical and two dose systemic cephradine. *Br J Surg* **66**: 580–582.

Finegold SM (1985) Comparison of agents available for treating anaerobic infections. *Southeast Asian J Surg* **8** (Suppl 1): 113–120.

Flint LM Jr, Beasley DJ, Richardson JD & Polk HC (1979) Topical povidone-iodine reduces mortality from bacterial peritonitis. *J Surg Res* **26**: 280–284.

Forrester JC (1980) Sutures and sepsis. In Karran S (ed.) *Controversies in Surgical Sepsis*, pp 43–52. Dorset: Praeger.

Fry DE (1996) The importance of antibiotic pharmacokinetics in critical illness. *Am J Surg* **172** (Suppl 6A): 20S–25S.

Fry DE, Garrison RN, Heitsch RC et al (1980a) Determinants of death in patients with intra-abdominal abscess. *Surgery* **88**: 517–523.

Fry DE, Pearlstein L, Folton RL & Polk HC Jr (1980b) Multiple system organ failure: the role of uncontrolled infection. *Arch Surg* **115**: 16–140.

Fry DE, Garrison RN, Trachtenberg L & Polk HC Jr (1985) Bacterial inoculum and the activity of antimicrobial agents. *Surg Gynecol Obstet* **160**: 105–108.

Fuenfer MM, Olsen GE & Polk HC Jr (1975) Effect of various corticosteroids upon phagocytic bactericidal activity of neutrophils. *Surgery* **78**: 27–33.

Galle PC & Homersley HD (1980) Ineffectiveness of povidone-iodine irrigation of abdominal incisions. *Obstet Gynecol* **55**: 744–747.

Gamble SS & Hopton DS (1985) Plastic ring wound drapes in elective colorectal surgery. *J R Coll Surg Edinb* **29**: 232–233.

Garrod LP (1975) Chemoprophylaxis. *BMJ* **2**: 561–564.

Gelb AF & Seligman SJ (1970) Bacteroidaceae bacteremia. Effect of age and focus of infection upon clinical course. *JAMA* **212**: 1038–1041.

Gibson GL (1974) *Infection in Hospital: A Code of Practice*. London: Churchill Livingstone.

Giercksky KE, Danielson S, Garberg O et al (1982) A single dose tinidozole and doxycycline prophylaxis in elective surgery of colon and rectum. *Ann Surg* **195**: 227–231.

Gillespie WA & Guy J (1956) *Bacteroides* in intra-abdominal sepsis. *Lancet* **i**: 1039–1042.

Gilmore OJA (1977) A reappraisal of the use of antiseptics in surgical practice. *Ann R Coll Surg Engl* **59**: 93–102.

Gilmore OJA & Martin TDM (1974) The aetiology and prevention of wound infection after appendicectomy. *Br J Surg* **61**: 281–287.

Gilmore OJA & Sanderson PJ (1975) Prophylactic interparenteral povidone-iodine in abdominal surgery. *Br J Surg* **62**: 792–799.

Gilmore OJA, Reid C, Honang ET & Shaw EJ (1978a) Prophylactic intraperitoneal povidone-iodine in alimentary tract surgery. *Am J Surg* **135**: 156–159.

Gilmore OJA, Reid C, Honang ET & Shaw EJ (1978b) Intraperitoneal povidone-iodine in peritonitis. *J Surg Res* **25**: 471–476.

Gingold BS, Berardis J & Knight P (1984) Reducing the risk of wound infection in operations upon the colon. *Surg Gynecol Obstet* **158**: 9–12.

Goldring J, Scott A, McNaught W & Gillespie G (1975) Prophylactic oral antimicrobial agents in elective colonic surgery. *Lancet* **ii**: 997–1000.

Goligher JC (1984) In *Surgery of the Anus, Rectum and Colon*, 5th edn, pp 914–916. Eastbourne: Baillière Tindall.

Goodgame JT (1980) A critical assessment of the indication for total parenteral nutrition. *Surg Gynecol Obstet* **151**: 433–441.

Goodson WH III & Hunt TK (1979) Wound healing and the diabetic patient. *Surg Gynecol Obstet* **149**: 600–608.

Goransson G, Nilsson-Ehle I, Olsson SA et al (1984) Single versus multiple dose doxycycline prophylaxis in elective colorectal surgery. *Acta Chir Scand* **150**: 245–249.

Gorbach SL (1971) Intestinal microflora. *Gastroenterology* **60**: 1110–1129.

Gorbach SL (1975) Management of anerobic infections:

intra-abdominal sepsis (UCLA Conference). *Ann Intern Med* **83**: 377–379.

Gorbach SL & Tabaqchali S (1969) Bacteria, bile and the small bowl. *Gut* **10**: 963–972.

Greenhall MJ, Froom K, Evans M & Pollock AY (1979) The influence of intra-incisional clindamycin on the incidence of wound sepsis after abdominal operations. *J Antimicrob Chemother* **5**: 511–516.

Griffiths DA, Simpson RA, Shorey BA & Speller DCE (1976) Single dose preoperative antibiotic prophylaxis in gastrointestinal surgery. *Lancet* **ii**: 325–328.

Grosfield JL (1968) Prevention of wound infection in perforated appendicitis. Experience with delayed primary wound closure. *Ann Surg* **168**: 891–893.

Grundmann R, Rimer P & Pichlmaier H (1984) Benefits of regular documentation of wound infection and complication rates after gastric and colon resection. *Dis Surg* **1**: 50–54.

Gunn AA (1956) *Bacteroides* septicaemia. *J R Coll Surg Edinb* **2**: 41–46.

Gurry JF & Ellis-Pegler RB (1976) An elemental diet as preoperative preparation of the colon. *Br J Surg* **63**: 969–972.

Hackam DJ & Rotstein OD (1995) Stoma closure and wound infection: an evaluation of risk factors. *Can J Surg* **38**: 144–148.

Hakansson T, Raahave D, Hansen OH & Pedersen T (1993) Effectiveness of single dose prophylaxis with cefotaxime and metronidazole compared with three doses of cefotaxime alone in elective colorectal surgery. *Eur J Surg* **159**: 177–180.

Hall C, Curran F, Burdon DW & Keighley MRB (1989) A randomized trial to compare (Augmentin) amoxycillin/clavulanate with metronidazole and gentamicin in prophylaxis in elective colorectal surgery. *J Antimicrob Chemother* **24**: 1195–1202.

Hallerback B & Andersson C (1986) A prospective randomized study of continuous peritoneal lavage postoperatively in the treatment of purulent peritonitis. *Surg Gynecol Obstet* **163**: 433–436.

Hancock BD (1990) Audit of major colorectal and biliary surgery to reduce rates of wound infection. *BMJ* **301**: 911–912.

Handelsman JC, Zeiler S, Coleman J, Dooley W & Walrath JM (1993) Experience with ambulatory preoperative bowel preparation at the Johns Hopkins Hospital. *Arch Surg* **128**: 441–444.

Hares MM, Green F, Youngs D, Bentley S, Burdon DW & Keighley MRB (1981) Failure of antimicrobial prophylaxis with cefoxitin or metronidazole and gentamicin in colorectal surgery: is mannitol to blame? *J Hosp Infect* **2**: 127–133.

Hares MM, Bentley S, Burdon DW, Allan RN & Keighley MRB (1982) Clinical trials of the efficacy and duration of antibacterial cover for elective resection in IBD. *Br J Surg* **69**: 215–217.

Hartley CL & Richmond MH (1975) Antibiotic resistance and survival of *E. coli* in the alimentary tract. *BMJ* **4**: 71–74.

Hartley JE, Ahmed S, Milkins R, Naylor G, Monson JRT & Lee PWR (1996) Randomized trial of blunt-tipped versus cutting needles to reduce glove puncture during mass closure of the abdomen. *Br J Surg* **83**: 1156–1157.

Heimdahl A & Nord CE (1979) Effect of phenoxymethyl-penicillin and clindamycin on the oral, throat and faecal microflora of man. *Scand J Infect Dis* **11**: 233–242.

Heimdahl A, Kager L, Malmborg AS & Nord CE (1982) Impact of different betalactam antibiotics on the normal human flora: a colonisation of the oral cavity, throat and colon. *Infection* **10**: 120–124.

Hell K, Gastinger I, Lippert H & Winter M (1995) Antibiotic administration in operations on 1927 patients with colorectal carcinoma. *Coloproctology* **17**: 18–26.

Higgens AF, Lewis A, Moore P & Hole M (1980) Single and multiple dose cotrimoxazole and metronidazole in colorectal surgery. *Br J Surg* **67**: 90–92.

Higgens CS & Allan RN (1980) Crohn's disease of the distal ileum. *Gut* **21**: 933–940.

Higgens CS, Allan RN, Keighley MRB, Arabi Y & Alexander-Williams J (1980) Sepsis following operation for inflammatory intestinal disease. *Dis Colon Rectum* **23**: 102–105.

Higgens CS, Keighley MRB & Allan RN (1981) Impact of pre-operative weight loss on post-operative morbidity. *J R Soc Med* **74**: 511–573.

Higgens CS, Keighley MRB & Allan RN (1984) Impact of preoperative weight loss and body composition changes on postoperative outcome in surgery for IBD. *Gut* **25**: 732–736.

Higson RH & Kettlewell MGW (1978) Parietal wound drainage in abdominal surgery. *Br J Surg* **65**: 326–329.

Hobbis JH, Carr ND & Schofield PF (1988) Are we using the correct dose of metronidazole in colorectal surgery? *J R Soc Med* **81**: 95–97.

Hoffmann CEJ, McDonald PJ & Watts JM (1981) Use of preoperative cefoxitin to prevent infection after colonic and rectal surgery. *Ann Surg* **193**: 353–356.

Hojer H & Wetterfors J (1978) Systemic prophylaxis with doxycycline in surgery of the colon and rectum. *Ann Surg* **187**: 362–368.

Holder IA (1976) Gentamycin resistant *Pseudomonas aeruginosa* in a burns unit. *Antimicrob Chemother* **2**: 309–311.

Holmes B, Quie PG, Windhorst DB & Good RA (1966) Fatal granulomatous disease of childhood. *Lancet* **i**: 1225–1228.

Holter AR, Rosen HM & Fischer JE (1976) The effects of hyperalimentation on major surgery in patients with malignant diseases: a prospective study. *Acta Chir Scand Suppl* **466**: 86–87.

Hong J & Davis JM (1996) Nosocomial infections and nosocomial pneumonia. *Am J Surg* **172** (Suppl 6A): 33S–37S.

Hossenbux K, Dale BAS, Walls ADF & Lawrene JR (1983) *Streptococcus bovis* endocarditis and colonic carcinoma: a neglected association. *BMJ* **3**: 21.

Howe CW (1969) Experimental wound sepsis from transient *Escherichia coli* bacteremia. *Surgery* **66**: 570–574.

Hughes ESR (1972) Asepsis in large bowel surgery. *Ann R Coll Surg Engl* **51**: 347–354.

Hughes ESR, Hardy KJ, Cuthbertson AM et al (1970) Chemoprophylaxis in large bowel surgery. I. Effect of intravenous administration of penicillin on incidence of postoperative infection. *Med J Aust* **1**: 305–311.

Hughes ESR, McDermott FT, Polglase AL et al (1982) Sepsis and asepsis in large bowel cancer surgery. *World J Surg* **6**: 160–165.

Hunt TK, Connolly WB, Aronson SB & Goldstine P (1975) Anaerobic metabolism and wound healing: a hypothesis for initiation and cessation of collagen synthesis in wounds. *Am J Surg* **130**: 328–332.

Iberti TJ, Rand JH, Benjamin E et al (1986) Thrombocytopenia following peritonitis in surgical patients. *Ann Surg* **204**: 341–345.

Irvin TT & Goligher JC (1973) Aetiology of disruption of intestinal anastomoses. *Br J Surg* **60**: 461–464.

Irvin TT, Goligher JC & Johnston D (1975) A controlled trial of three different methods of perineal wound management following excision of the rectum. *Br J Surg* **62**: 287–291.

Ivarsson L, Darle N, Kewenter JG et al (1982) Short-term systemic prophylaxis with cefoxitin and doxycycline in colorectal surgery. *Am J Surg* **144**: 257–261.

Jackson DW, Pollock AV & Tindal DS (1971) The value of a plastic adhesive drape in the prevention of wound infection. A controlled trial. *Br J Surg* **58**: 340–342.

Jacomina AA, Van der Wiel-Korstanje & Winkler KC (1975) The faecal flora of UC. *J Med Microbiol* **8**: 491–501.

Jalan KM, Prescott RJ, Smith AM et al (1970) The influence of corticosteroids on the results of surgical treatment for UC. *N Engl J Med* **282**: 588–594.

Jennings WC, Wood CD & Guernsey JM (1982) Continuous postoperative lavage in the treatment of peritoneal sepsis. *Dis Colon Rectum* **25**: 641–643.

Jensen LS, Anderson A, Fristrup SC et al (1990) Comparison of one dose versus three doses of prophylactic antibiotics, and the influence of blood transfusion, on infectious complications in acute and elective colorectal surgery. *Br J Surg* **77**: 513–518.

Johnson CD & Serpell JW (1990) Wound infection after abdominal incision with scalpel or diathermy. *Br J Surg* **77**: 626–627.

Johnson WC, Ulrich F, Meguid MM et al (1979) Role of delayed hypersensitivity in predicting postoperative morbidity and mortality. *Am J Surg* **137**: 536–542.

Joiner KA & Bartlett JG (1985) Evaluation of antimicrobial agents in animal models of infections involving *Bacteroides fragilis*. *Southeast Asian J Surg* **8** (Suppl 1): 96–102.

Jones FE, De Cosse JJ & Condon RE (1976) Evaluation of 'instant' preparation of the colon with povidone iodine. *Ann Surg* **184**: 74–79.

Jones PF, Munro A & Ewen WB (1977) Colectomy and ileorectal anastomosis for colitis: report on a personal series with a critical review. *Br J Surg* **64**: 615–621.

Jones RN (1992) Antibiotic prophylaxis for surgical infections: summation. *Am J Surg* **164**: 485–495.

Juul P, Klaaborg KE & Kronborg O (1987) Single or multiple doses of metronidazole and ampicillin in elective colorectal surgery. A randomized trial. *Dis Colon Rectum* **30**: 526–528.

Kager L, Ljungdahl I, Malmborg AS et al (1981) Antibiotic prophylaxis with cefoxitin in colorectal surgery. *Ann Surg* **193**: 277–282.

Kager L, Brismar B, Malmborg AS & Nord CE (1985) Effect of imipenem prophylaxis on colon microflora in patients undergoing colorectal surgery. *Proceedings of the 14th International Congress of Chemotherapy*, Kyoto.

Kaiser AB, Herrington JL, Jacobs JK, Mulherin JL Jr, Roach AC & Sawyers JL (1983) Cefoxitin versus erythromycin, neomycin and cefazolin in colorectal operations. *Ann Surg* **198**: 525–530.

Karran SJ, Sutton G, Gartell P, Karran SE, Finnis D & Blenkinsop J (1993) Imipenem prophylaxis in elective colorectal surgery. *Br J Surg* **80**: 1196–1198.

Keeling NJ & Morgan MWE (1995) Inpatient and post-discharge wound infections in general surgery. *Ann R Coll Surg Engl* **77**: 245–247.

Keighley MRB (1980) Antibiotic associated pseudomembranous colitis: pathogenesis and management. *Drugs* **20**: 49–56.

Keighley MRB (1982) Prevention and treatment of infection in colorectal surgery. *World J Surg* **6**: 312–320.

Keighley MRB & Burdon DW (eds) (1979) *Antimicrobial Prophylaxis in Surgery*. Tunbridge Wells: Pitman Medical.

Keighley MRB & Crapp AR (1976) Short-term prophylaxis with tobramycin and lincomycin in bowel surgery. *Scott Med J* **21**: 70–72.

Keighley MRB, Crapp AR, Burdon DW et al (1976) Prophylaxis against anaerobic sepsis in bowel surgery. *Br J Surg* **63**: 538–542.

Keighley MRB, Arabi Y, Dikock F, Burdon DW, Allan RN & Alexander-Williams J (1978) Influence of IBD on intestinal microflora. *Gut* **19**: 1099–1104.

Keighley MRB, Alexander-Williams J, Arabi Y & Youngs D (1979) Comparison between systemic and oral antimicrobial prophylaxis in colorectal surgery. *Lancet* **i**: 894–897.

Keighley MRB, Winslet MC, Flinn R & Kmiot W (1989) Multivariate analysis of factors influencing the results of restorative proctocolectomy. *Br J Surg* **76**: 740–744.

Keighley MRB, Pemberton JH, Fazio VW & Parc R (1996) *Atlas of Colorectal Surgery*. Churchill Livingstone: New York, Edinburgh, London.

Kelly MJ & Warren RE (1978) The value of an operative wound swab sent in transport medium in the prediction of later clinical wound infection: a controlled clinical and bacteriological evaluation. *Br J Surg* **65**: 81–88.

Khubchandani IT, Karamchandani MC, Sheets JA, Stasik JJ, Rosen L & Reither RD (1989) Metronidazole vs erythromycin, neomycin and cefazolin in prophylaxis for colonic surgery. *Dis Colon Rectum* **32**: 17–20.

Kingston RD, Kiff RS, Duthie JS, Walsh S, Spicer A & Jeacock J (1989) Comparison of two prophylactic single-dose intravenous antibiotic regimes in the treatment of patients undergoing elective colorectal surgery in a district general hospital. *J R Coll Surg Edinb* **34**: 208–211.

Kippax PW & Thomas ET (1966) Surgical wound sepsis in a general hospital. *Lancet* **ii**: 1297–1300.

Kirk CR, Dorgan JC & Hart CA (1988) Gas gangrene: a cautionary tale. *BMJ* **296**: 1236–1237.

Kislak JW (1972) The susceptibility of *Bacteroides fragilis* to 24 antibiotics. *J Infect Dis* **125**: 295–304.

Klein RS, Rose A, Recco MD et al (1977) Association of *Streptococcus bovis* with carcinoma of the colon. *N Engl J Med* **297**: 800–802.

Knudsen L, Christiansen L & Jarnum S (1976) Early complications in patients previously treated with corticosteroids. *Scand J Gastroenterol* **11** (Suppl 27): 123–128.

Krepel CJ, Gohr CM, Edmiston CE & Condon RE (1995) Surgical sepsis: constancy of antibiotic susceptibility of causative organisms. *Surgery* **117**: 505–509.

Krukowski ZH & Matheson MA (1983) The management of peritoneal and parietal contamination in abdominal surgery. *Br J Surg* **70**: 440–441.

Krukowski ZH & Matheson MA (1988) Ten-year computerized audit of infection after abdominal surgery. *Br J Surg* **75**: 857–861.

Krukowski ZH, Stewart MPM, Alsayer HM & Matheson NA (1984) Infection after abdominal surgery: 5 years prospective study. *BMJ* **288**: 278–280.

Kuijpers HC (1985) Is prophylactic abdominal irrigation with polyvinyl pyrrolidone iodine (PVPI) safe? *Dis Colon Rectum* **28**: 481–483.

Kune GA (1978) Life threatening surgical infection: its development and prediction. *Ann R Coll Surg Engl* **60**: 92–98.

Kuruvila KC & Bevan EG (1971) Arteriovenous shunts and fistulas for haemodialysis. *Surg Clin North Am* **51**: 1219–1234.

Kurz A, Sessler DI & Lenhardt R (1996) Perioperative normothermia to reduce the incidence of surgical-wound infections and shorten hospitalization. *N Engl J Med* **334**: 1209–1215.

Kwok SPY, Lau WY, Leung KL, Ku KW, Ho WS & Li AKC (1993) Amoxycillin and clavulanic acid versus cefotaxime and metronidazole as antibiotic prophylaxis in elective colorectal resectional surgery. *Chemotherapy* **39**: 135–139.

Lacey RW (1980) Deployment of antibiotics to prevent resistance. In Karran S (ed.) *Controversies in Surgical Sepsis*, pp 95–105. Dorset: Praeger.

Lagarde MC, Bolton JS & Cohn I (1978) Intraperitoneal povidone-iodine in experimental peritonitis. *Ann Surg* **187**: 613–619.

Lal D & Levitan R (1972) Bacteremia following proctoscopic biopsy of a rectal polyp. *Arch Intern Med* **130**: 127–128.

Lau WY, Chu KW, Poon GP & Ho KK (1988) Prophylactic antibiotics in elective colorectal surgery. *Br J Surg* **75**: 782–785.

Lawrence JC (1994) Dressings and wound infection. *Am J Surg* **167** (Suppl): 21S–24S.

Lawrence PF, Tietjen GW, Gingrich S & Thomas TC (1977) *Bacteroides* bacteremia. *Ann Surg* **186**: 559–561.

Leaper DJ (1994) Prophylactic and therapeutic role of antibiotics in wound care. *Am J Surg* **167** (Suppl): 15–20.

Le Frock J, Ellis CA, Turchik JB & Weinstein L (1973) Transient bacteremia associated with sigmoidoscopy. *N Engl J Med* **289**: 457–469.

Le Frock J, Ellis CA, Klainer AS & Weinstein L (1975) Transient bacteremia association with barium enema. *Arch Intern Med* **135**: 835–837.

Leiboff AR & Soroff HS (1987) The treatment of generalized peritonitis by closed postoperative peritoneal lavage. A critical review of the literature. *Arch Surg* **122**: 1005–1010.

Leigh DA (1974) Clinical importance of infections due to *Bacteroides fragilis* and role of antibiotic therapy. *BMJ* **3**: 225–228.

Leigh DA (1975) Wound infections due to *Bacteroides fragilis* following intestinal surgery. *Br J Surg* **62**: 375–378.

Lewis RP, Wideman P, Sutter VL & Finegold SM (1977) The effect of metronidazole on human faecal flora. *Proceedings of the International Metronidazole Conference*, pp 307–309, Montreal, 1976.

Lilly EJ & Lowbury EJL (1971) Disinfection of the skin: Assessment of some new preparations. *BMJ* **3**: 674–680.

Localio SA, Nealon W, Newell J & Valensi Q (1983) Adjuvant postoperative radiation therapy for Dukes C adenocarcinoma of the rectum. *Ann Surg* **198**: 18–24.

Lord JW Jr, Rossi G & Daliana M (1977) Intraoperative antibiotic wound lavage: an attempt to eliminate postoperative infection in arterial and general surgical procedures. *Ann Surg* **185**: 634–641.

Lowbury EJL & Lilly HA (1973) Use of 4% chlorhexidine detergent (Hibiscrub) and other methods of skin disinfection. *BMJ* **1**: 510–515.

Lowbury EJL, Lilly HA, Ayliffe GAJ et al (1974) Preoperative disinfection of surgeons' hands: use of alcoholic solutions and effects of gloves on skin flora. *BMJ* **4**: 369–372.

McArdle CS, Morran CG, Pettit L, Gemmell CG, Sleigh JD & Tillotson GS (1995). Value of oral antibiotic prophylaxis in colorectal surgery. *Br J Surg;* **82**: 1046–1048.

McAvinchey DJ, McCollum PT, McElearney NG, Mundinger G & Lynch G (1983) Antiseptics in the treatment of bacterial peritonitis in rats. *Br J Surg* **70**: 158–160.

McCulloch PG, Blamey SL, Finlay IG et al (1986) A prospective comparison of gentamicin and metronidazole and moxalactam in the prevention of septic complications associated with elective operations of the colon and rectum. *Surg Gynecol Obstet* **162**: 521–524.

McDonald PJ, Watts JMcK & Finlay-Jones JJ (1984) The antimicrobial management of gut derived sepsis complicating surgery and cancer chemotherapy. In Goodwin CS (ed.) *Microbes and Infections of the Gut*, pp 307–326. Oxford: Blackwell Scientific.

McHenry MC, Turnbull RB Jr, Weakley FL & Hawk WA (1971) Septicaemia in surgical patients with intestinal disease. *Dis Colon Rectum* **14**: 195–199.

MacKenzie I & Litton A (1974) *Bacteroides* bacteraemia in surgical patients. *Br J Surg* **61**: 287–290.

MacLean LD, Meakins JL, Taguchi K et al (1975) Host resistance in sepsis and trauma. *Ann Surg* **182**: 207–217.

Madden JL & Tan PY (1961) Primary resection and anastomosis in the treatment of perforated lesions of the colon, with abscess or diffusing peritonitis. *Surg Gynecol Obstet* **113**: 646–650.

Marks J, Hughes LE, Harding KG, Campbell H & Ribeiro CD (1983) Prediction of healing time as an aid to the management of open granulating wounds. *World J Surg* **7**: 641–645.

Marts BC, Longo WE, Vernava AM, Kennedy DJ, Daniel GL & Jones I (1994) Patterns and prognosis of *Clostridium difficile* colitis. *Dis Colon Rectum* **37**: 837–845.

Mathes SJ & Stone HH (1975) Acute traumatic losses of abdominal wall substance. *J Trauma* **15**: 386.

Matheson DM, Arabi Y, Baxter-Smith D, Alexander-Williams J & Keighley MRB (1978) Randomised multicentre trial of oral bowel preparation and antimicrobials for elective colorectal operations. *Br J Surg* **65**: 597–600.

Matikainen M & Hiltunen KM (1993) Parenteral single dose ceftriaxone with tinidatsole versus aminoglycoside with tinidatsole in colorectal surgery: a prospective single-blind randomized multicentre study. *Int J Colorectal Dis* **8**: 148–150.

Maxwell JG, Ford CR, Peterson DE & Richards RC (1969) Abdominal wound infections and plastic drape protectors. *Am J Surg* **118**: 844–848.

Meakins JL, Pietsch JB, Buberik O et al (1977) Delayed hypersensitivity: indicator of acquired failure of host defences in sepsis and trauma. *Ann Surg* **186**: 241–250.

Meakins JL, McLean APH, Kelly R et al (1978) Delayed hypersensitivity and neutrophil chemotaxis: effect of trauma. *J Trauma* **18**: 240–247.

Meakins JL, Christou NV, Shizgal HM & McLean LD (1979) Therapeutic approaches to energy in surgical patients. *Ann Surg* **190**: 286–296.

Memon MA, Devine J, Freeney J & From SG (1997) Is mechanical bowel preparation really necessary for elective left-sided colon and rectal surgery. *Int J Colorectal Dis* **12**: 298–302.

Minervini S, Bentley S, Youngs D, Alexander-Williams J, Burdon DW & Keighley MRB (1980) Prophylactic saline peritoneal lavage in elective colorectal operations. *Dis Colon Rectum* **23**: 392–394.

Moesgaard F, Lykkegaard & Nielsen M (1988) Failure of topically applied antibiotics, added to systemic prophylaxis, to reduce perineal wound infection in abdominoperineal excision of the rectum. *Acta Chir Scand* **154**: 589–592.

Mogg GAG, Keighley MRB, Burdon JW et al (1979) Antibiotic associated colitis: a review of 66 cases. *Br J Surg* **66**: 738–742.

Morris DL, Hares MM, Voogt RJ, Burdon DW & Keighley MRB (1983) Metronidazole need not be combined with an aminoglycoside when used for prophylaxis in elective colorectal surgery. *J Hosp Infect* **4**: 65–69.

Morris DL, Fabricius PJ, Ambrose NS, Scammell B, Burdon DW & Keighley MRB (1984) A high incidence of bleeding is observed in a trial to determine whether addition of metronidazole is needed with latamoxef for prophylaxis in colorectal surgery. *J Hosp Infect* **5**: 398–408.

Morris WT (1993) Ceftriaxone is more effective than gentamicin/metronidazole prophylaxis in reducing wound and urinary tract infections after bowel operations. Results of a controlled, randomized, blind clinical trial. *Dis Colon Rectum* **36**: 826–833.

Moukhtar M & Romney S (1980) Continuous intraperitoneal antibiotic lavage in the management of purulent sepsis of the pelvis. *Surg Gynec Obstet* **150**: 548–550.

Muir EG (1968) Safety in colonic resection. *Proc R Soc Med* **61**: 401–408.

Mullen JL, Buzby GP, Matthews DC, Smales BF & Rosato EF (1980) Reduction of operative morbidity and mortality by combined preoperative and postoperative nutritional support. *Ann Surg* **192**: 604–613.

Nagler SM & Poticha SM (1979) Intra-abdominal abscess in regional enteritis. *Am J Surg* **137**: 350–354.

Nash AG & Hugh TB (1967) Topical ampicillin and wound infection in colon surgery. *BMJ* **1**: 471–472.

Nathens AB & Rotstein OD (1996) Antimicrobial therapy for intraabdominal infection. *Am J Surg* **172**(Suppl 6A): 1S–6S.

National Research Council (1964) Postoperative wound infections, the influence of ultraviolet irradiation of the operating room and various other factors. *Ann Surg* **160** (Suppl): 1–192.

Nicholls RJ (1987) Restorative proctocolectomy with various types of reservoir. *World J Surg* **11**: 751–762.

Nichols RL & Smith JW (1994) Anaerobes from a surgical perspective. *Clin Infect Dis* **18**: S280–S286.

Nichols RL & Smith JW (1975) Gas in the wound: what does it mean? *Surg Clin North Am* **55**: 1289–1296.

Nichols RL, Gorbach SL & Condon RE (1971) Alteration of intestinal microflora following preoperative mechanical preparation of the colon. *Dis Colon Rectum* **4**: 123–127.

Nichols RL, Condon RE, Gorbach SL & Hughes LM (1972) Efficacy of preoperative antimicrobial preparation of the bowel. *Ann Surg* **176**: 227–232.

Niinikoski J, Havia T, Alhava E et al (1993) Piperacillin/tazobactam versus imipenem/cilastatin in the treatment of intra-abdominal infections. *Surg Gynecol Obstet* **176**: 255–261.

Noble CJ, Ohley AMC, Falk RH & Richardson PJ (1978) *Streptococcus bovis* endocarditis and colonic cancer. *Lancet* **i**: 766.

Norwegian Study Group for Colorectal Surgery (1985) Should antimicrobial prophylaxis in colorectal surgery include agents effective against both anaerobic and aerobic microorganisms? A double-blind, multicentre study. *Surgery* **97**: 402–407.

Nystrom PO, Broome A, Hojer H & Ling L (1984) A controlled trial of a plastic wound ring drape to prevent contamination and infection in colorectal surgery. *Dis Colon Rectum* **27**: 451–453.

Okubadejo OA, Green PJ & Payne DJH (1973) *Bacteroides* infection among hospital patients. *BMJ* **2**: 212–214.

Oliviera L, Wexner SD, Daniel N et al (1997) Mechanical bowel preparation for elective colorectal surgery. *Dis Colon Rectum* **40**: 585–591.

Påhlman L & Glimelius B (1990) Pre- or postoperative radiotherapy in rectal and rectosigmoid carcinoma. *Ann Surg* **211**: 187–195.

Paradisi F & Corti G (1992) Which prophylactic regimen for which surgical procedure? *Am J Surg* **164** (Suppl): 2–5.

Parker MT (1969) Post-operative clostridial infections in Britain. *BMJ* **3**: 671–676.

Peck JJ, Fuchs PC & Gustafson ME (1984) Antimicrobial prophylaxis in elective colon surgery. *Am J Surg* **147**: 633–637.

Phillips I, Warren C, Taylor E, Timewell R & Eykeyn S (1981) The antimicrobial susceptibility of anaerobic bacteria in a London teaching hospital. *J Antimicrob Chemother* **8** (Suppl D): 17–26.

Phillips RKS & Dudley HA (1984) The effect of tetracycline lavage and trauma on visceral and parietal peritoneal ultrastructure and adhesion formation. *Br J Surg* **71**: 537–539.

Pietsch JB, Meakins JL & McLean LD (1977) The delayed hypersensitivity response: application in clinical surgery. *Surgery* **82**: 349–355.

Pitt HA, Postier RG, MacGowen WAL et al (1980) Prophylactic antibiotics in vascular surgery. *Ann Surg* **192**: 356–364.

Playforth MJ, Smith GMR, Evans M & Pollock AV (1987) Pre-operative assessment of fitness score. *Br J Surg* **74**: 890–892.

Playforth MJ, Smith GMR, Evans M & Pollock AV (1988) Antimicrobial bowel preparation: oral, parenteral or both? *Dis Colon Rectum* **31**: 90–93.

Polk HC & Lopez-Mayor J (1969) Post-operative wound infections: a prospective study of determinant factors and prevention. *Surgery* **66**: 97–103.

Pollock AV (1979) Surgical wound sepsis. *Lancet* **i**: 1283–1286.

Pollock AV (1981a) Antibiotic prophylaxis in general surgery. A comparison of single-dose intravenous and single-dose intraincisional cephaloridine. *Aktuel Probl Chir Orthop* **19**: 71–76.

Pollock AV (1981b) Laparotomy. *J R Soc Med* **74**: 480–484.

Pollock AV (1988) Immunological implications of surgery. *Surg Immun* **1**: 3–12.

Pollock AV, Greenhall MJ & Evans M (1979) Single layer mass closure of major laparotomies by continuous suturing. *J R Soc Med* **72**: 889–893.

Pollock AV, Evans M & Parida S (1986) The prediction of abdominal surgical wound infection: the value of an enrichment broth for initial culture of operative parietal swabs. *J Hosp Infect* **8**: 242–247.

Pollock AV, Evans M & Smith GMR (1989) Preincisional intraparietal Augmentin in abdominal operations. *Ann R Coll Surg* **71**: 97–100.

Ponting GA, Sim AJW & Dudley HAF (1987) Comparison of local and systemic effects of sepsis in predicting survival. *Br J Surg* **74**: 750–752.

Poth EJ & Knotts TL (1942) Clinical use of succinylsulfathiazole. *Arch Surg* **44**: 208–222.

Powis SJA, Waterworth TA & Arkell DG (1976) Preoperative skin preparation: clinical evaluation of depilatory cream. *BMJ* **2**: 1166–1168.

Psaila JV, Wheeler MH & Crosby DL (1977) The role of plastic wound drapes in the prevention of wound infection following abdominal surgery. *Br J Surg* **64**: 729–732.

Raahave D (1974) Aseptic barriers of plastic to prevent bacterial contamination of operation wounds. *Acta Chir Scand* **140**: 603–610.

Raahave D, Hesselfeldt P, Pedersen T, Zachariassen A, Kann D & Hasen OH (1989) No effect of topical ampicillin prophylaxis in elective operations of the colon or rectum. *Surg Gynecol Obstet* **168**: 112–114.

Ralston AT, Harlow GR, Jones DM & Davis P (1971) Infections of Scribner and Bescia arteriovenous shunts. *BMJ* **3**: 408–409.

Rambo WM (1972) Irrigation of the peritoneal cavity with cephalothin. *Am J Surg* **123**: 192–195.

Reeves DS, Bywater MJ, Holt HA & White LO (1984) In vitro studies with ciprofloxacin, a new 4-quinolone compound. *J Antimicrob Chemother* **13**: 333–346.

Richards WO, Scovill WA & Shin B (1983) Opsonic fibronectin deficiency in patients with intra-abdominal infection. *Surgery* **94**: 210–217.

Rietz KA, Altman B & Lahnborg G (1984) A simple regimen for control of postoperative sepsis in colorectal surgery. *Dis Colon Rectum* **27**: 519–522.

Ritchie JK (1972) UC-treatment by ileostomy and excisional surgery. Fifteen years' experience at St Mark's Hospital. *Br J Surg* **59**: 345–350.

Ritchie JK & Lockhart-Mummery HE (1973) Non-restorative surgery in the treatment of Crohn's disease of the large bowel. *Gut* **14**: 263–266.

Rodeheaver G, Pettry D, Turnbull V, Edgerton M & Edlich R (1974) Identification of wound infection: potentiating factors in soil. *Am J Surg* **128**: 8–14.

Roe F (1985) Toxicological aspects of metronidazole. *Southeast Asian J Surg* **8** (Suppl 1): 87–94.

Roland M, Bergen T, Bjerkeset T et al (1985) Prophylactic regimens in colorectal surgery: comparisons between metronidazole used alone or with ampicillin for one or three days. *World J Surg* **9**: 626–632.

Roland M, Wiig JN, Odegard O et al (1986) Prophylactic regimens in colorectal surgery: an open, randomized, consecutive trial on metronidazole used alone or in combination with ampicillin or doxycycline. *World J Surg* **10**: 1003–1008.

Rowe-Jones DC, Peel ALG, Kingston JFL, Shaw C, Teasdale C & Cole DS (1990) Single dose cefotaxime plus metronidazole versus three dose cefuroxime plus metronidazole as prophylaxis against wound infection in colorectal surgery: multicentre prospective randomized study. *BMJ* **300**: 18–22.

Rubli E, Bussard S, Frei E, Langsgaard-Hansen P & Pappova E (1983) Plasma fibronectin and associated variables in surgical intensive care patients. *Ann Surg* **197**: 310–317.

Saba TM & Cho E (1979) Reticuloendothelial systemic response to operative trauma as influenced by cryoprecipitate or cold-insoluble globulin therapy. *J Reticuloendothel Soc* **26**: 171–186.

Saba TM & Joffe E (1980) Plasma fibronectin (opsonic glycoprotein): its synthesis by vascular endothelial cells and role in cardiopulmonary integrity after trauma as related to reticuloendothelial function. *Am J Med* **68**: 577–594.

Sanderson PJ (1983) *Antibiotics for Surgical Infections.* Hertfordshire: Research Studies Press.

Sandle MA & Mandell GL (1980) Antimicrobial agents: tetracycline and chloramphenicol. In Gilman AG, Goodman LS & Gilman A (eds) *The Pharmacological Basis of Therapeutics*, 6th edn, pp 1181–1199. New York: Macmillan.

Sauven P, Playforth MJ, Smith GMR, Evans M & Pollock AV (1986) Single-dose antibiotic prophylaxis of abdominal surgical wound infection: a trial of preoperative latamoxef against preoperative tetracycline lavage. *J R Soc Med* **79**: 137–141.

Scammell BE, Phillips RP, Brown R, Burdon DW & Keighley MRB (1985) Influence of rectal washout on bacterial counts in the rectal stump. *Br J Surg* **72**: 548–550.

Scammell B, Allan RN & Keighley MRB (1986) Reoperation rates following resection and anastomosis compared with resection and ileostomy for Crohn's disease. *Dig Dis Sci* **31** (Suppl): 10S.

Schiessel R, Huk I, Starlinger M et al (1984) Postoperative infections in colonic surgery after enteral bacitracin-neomycin-clindamycin or parenteral mezlocillin-oxacillin prophylaxis. *J Hosp Infect* **5**: 289–297.

Selden R, Lee S, Wang WLL et al (1971) Nosocomial *Klebsiella* infections: intestinal colonisation as a reservoir. *Ann Intern Med* **74**: 657–664.

Sellwood RA, Bon JI, Waterworth PM & Wellbourne RB (1969) A second clinical trial to compare two methods of preoperative preparations of the large bowel. *Br J Surg* **56**: 610–612.

Seneca H & Peer P (1966) Effect of antibacterials, antibiotics, enzymes and steroids on phagocytosis. *J Am Geriatr Soc* **14**: 187–193.

Seropian R & Reynolds BM (1981) Wound infections after preoperative depilatory versus razor preparation. *Am J Surg* **121**: 251–254.

Settle CD & Wilcox MH (1996) Review article: antibiotic-induced *Clostridium difficile* infection. *Aliment Pharmacol Ther* **10**: 835–841.

Shepherd A, Roberts A, Ambrose NS, Youngs D, Burdon DW & Keighley MRB (1986) Ceftriaxone (a long acting cephalosporin) with metronidazole as single dose prophylaxis in colorectal surgery. *Colo-proctology* **8**: 90–94.

Silver SC (1984) *Streptococcus bovis* endocarditis and its association with colonic carcinoma. *Dis Colon Rectum* **27**: 613–614.

Silverman SH, Ambrose NS, Youngs DJ, Shepherd AFI, Roberts AP & Keighley MRB (1986) The effect of peritoneal lavage with tetracycline solution in postoperative infection. *Dis Colon Rectum* **29**: 165–169.

Simchen E, Shapiro M, Sacks TG, Michel J, Durst A & Eyal Z (1984) Determinants of wound infection after colon surgery. *Ann Surg* **199**: 260–265.

Sindelar WF & Mason GR (1979) Intraperitoneal irrigation with povidone-iodine solution for the prevention of intra-abdominal abscesses in the bacterially contaminated abdomen. *Surg Gynecol Obstet* **148**: 409–411.

Singh K & Chhina RS (1993) Role of zipper in the management of abdominal sepsis. *Indian J Gastroenterol* **12**: 1–4.

Smith AJ, Daniels T & Bohnen JMA (1996) Soft tissue infections and the diabetic foot. *Am J Surg* **172** (Suppl 6A): 7S–12S.

Smith CR & Lipsky JJ (1983) Hypothrombinaemia and platelet dysfunction caused by cephalosporin and exalactam antibiotics. *J Antimicrob Chemother* **11**: 496–497.

Solomkins JS (1996) Timing of treatment for nonneutropenic patients colonized with *Candida. Am J Surg* **172** (Suppl 6A): 44S–48S.

Solomkins JS, Meakins JL, Allo MD, Dellinger EP & Simmons RL (1984) Antibiotic trials in intra-abdominal infections. A critical evaluation of study design and outcome reporting. *Ann Surg* **200**: 29–39.

Sparso BH, Van der Masse H, Kristensen D et al (1984) Complications following postoperative combined radiation and chemotherapy in adenocarcinoma of the rectum and rectosigmoid. *Cancer* **54**: 2363–2366.

Steigbigel NH, Reed CW & Finland M (1968) Susceptibility of common pathogenic bacteria to seven tetracycline antibiotics in vitro. *Am J Med Sci* **255**: 179–195.

Steinberg D & Naggar CZ (1977) *Streptococcus bovis* endocarditis with carcinoma of colon. *N Engl J Med* **297**: 1354–1355.

Stephen M & Loewenthal J (1978) Generalised infective peritonitis. *Surg Gynecol Obstet* **147**: 231–234.

Stephen M & Loewenthal J (1979) Continuing peritoneal lavage in high-risk peritonitis. *Surgery* **85**: 603–606.

Stewart DJ & Matheson NA (1978) Peritoneal lavage in appendicular peritonitis. *Br J Surg* **65**: 54–56.

Stokes EJ, Waterworth PM, Franks V et al (1974) Short term routine antibiotic prophylaxis in surgery. *Br J Surg* **61**: 739–742.

Stokes EJ, Peters JL, Howard E, Milne SE & Witherow RO (1977) Comparison of antibiotic and antiseptic prophylaxis of wound infection in acute abdominal surgery. *World J Surg* **1**: 777–782.

Stone HH (1983) Antibiotics in colon surgery. *Surg Clin North Am* **63**: 3–9.

Stone HH & Hester TR Jr (1973) Incisional and peritoneal infection after emergency celiotomy. *Ann Surg* **177**: 669–678.

Stone HH, Hooper CA, Kolb LB et al (1976) Antibiotic prophylaxis in gastric, biliary and colonic surgery. *Ann Surg* **184**: 443–452.

Swenson O, Sherman JO, Fisher JH & Cohen E (1975) The treatment and postoperative complications of congenital megacolon. A 25 year follow up. *Ann Surg* **182**: 266–273.

Sykes PA, Jones DM & Ostick G (1983) Bacteraemia during anorectal surgery. *J R Coll Surg Edinb* **28**: 178–181.

Tartter PI (1988) Blood transfusion and infection complications following colorectal cancer surgery. *Br J Surg* 75: 789–792.

Taylor EW & Lindsay G (1994) Selective decontamination of the colon before elective colorectal surgery. *World J Surg* **18**: 926–932.

Taylor SA, Candery HM & Smith J (1979) The use of metronidazole in the preparation of the bowel for surgery. *Br J Surg* **66**: 191–192.

Taylor TV, Walker WS, Mason RC, Richmond J & Lee D (1982) Preoperative intraparietal (intra-incisional) cefoxitin in abdominal surgery. *Br J Surg* **69**: 461–462.

Thomas PRM, Lindblad AS, Stablein DM et al (1986) Toxicity associated with adjuvant postoperative therapy for adenocarcinoma of the rectum. *Cancer* **57**: 1130–1134.

Tornqvist A, Forsgren A, Leandoer L & Ursing J (1987) Identification and antibiotic prophylaxis of high-risk patients in elective colorectal surgery. *World J Surg* **11**: 115–119.

Tresadern JC, Farrand RJ & Irving MH (1983) *Streptococcus milleri* and surgical sepsis. *Ann R Coll Surg Engl* **65**: 77–79.

Tudor RG, Oates GD & Keighley MRB (1986a) Outcome after the Hartmann procedure for complicated diverticular disease. *Gut* **27**: 626.

Tudor RG, Oates GD & Keighley MRB (1986b) Outcome following the Hartmann procedure for complicated diverticular disease. *Dig Dis Sci* **31** (Suppl): 503s.

Tudor RG, Haynes I, Youngs DJ, Burdon DW & Keighley MRB (1988) Comparison of short-term antibiotic cover with a third-generation cephalosporin against conventional five-day therapy using metronidazole with an aminoglycoside in emergency and complicated colorectal surgery. *Dis Colon Rectum* **31**: 28–32.

Ueno K (1985) Anaerobic infections in Japan: progress in culture and identification. *Southeast Asian J Surg* **8** (Suppl 1): 35–37.

Valtonen MV, Suomalainen RJ, Ylikohri RH et al (1977) Selection of multiresistant coliforms by long term treatment of hypercholesterolaemia with neomycin. *BMJ* **1**: 683–684.

Van Houte J & Gibbons RJ (1966) Studies of the cultivable flora of normal human faeces. *Antonie van Leeuwenhoek* **32**: 212–222.

Varquish T, Crawford LC, Stallings RA, Wasilaustas BL & Myers RT (1978) A randomised prospective evaluation of orally administered antibiotics in operations on the colon. *Surg Gynecol Obstet* **146**: 193–198.

Varty PP, Linehan IP & Boulos PB (1994) Intra-abdominal sepsis and survival after surgery for colorectal cancer. *Br J Surg* **81**: 915–918.

Vestweber KH & Grundel E (1994) Efficacy and safety of piperacillin/tazobactam in intra-abdominal infections. *Eur J Surg* Suppl 573: 57–60.

Walker AJ, Taylor EW, Lindsay G, Dewar EP and the West of Scotland Surgical Infection Study Group (1988) Sepsis in colorectal surgery. *J Hosp Infect* **11**: 340–348.

Wapnick S, Guinto R, Reizis I & Lee Veen HH (1979) Reduction of postoperative infection in elective colon surgery with preoperative administration of kanamycin and erythromycin. *Surgery* **85**: 317–320.

Wara P, Sorensen K, Berg V & Amdrup E (1981) The outcome of staged management of complicated diverticular disease of the sigmoid colon. *Acta Chir Scand* **147**: 209–214.

Washington JA, Dearing WH, Judd ES & Elveback LR (1974) Effect of preoperation antibiotic regimen on development of infection after intestinal surgery. *Ann Surg* **180**: 567–572.

Wastell C (1992) Glove punctures and wet gowns: no room for complacency. *Ann R Coll Surg Engl* **74**: 305.

Waterworth PM (1972) The in vitro activity of tobramycin compared with that of other aminoglycosides. *J Clin Pathol* **25**: 979–983.

Watts JMcK, De Dombal FT & Goligher JC (1966) Long term complications and prognosis following major surgery for UC. *Br J Surg* **53**: 1014–1019.

Weaver M, Burdon DW, Youngs DJ & Keighley MRB (1986) Oral neomycin and erythromycin compared with single dose systemic metronidazole and ceftriaxone prophylaxis in elective colorectal surgery. *Am J Surg* **151**: 437–442.

Weitekamp MR & Aber RC (1983) Prolonged bleeding times and bleeding diathesis associated with moxalactam administration. *JAMA* **249**: 69–71.

Weston-Underwood J & Marks CG (1984) The septic complications of sigmoid diverticular disease. *Br J Surg* **71**: 209–211.

Williams RHP, Heatley RV, Lewis MH & Hughes LE (1976) A randomised controlled trial of preoperative intravenous nutrition in patients with stomach cancer. *Br J Surg* **63**: 667.

Willis AT (1985) Antimicrobial prophylaxis of anaerobic infections: an overview. *Southeast Asian J Surg* **8** (Suppl 1): 157–164.

Willis AT & Jones PH (1979) The prophylactic role of metronidazole in colorectal surgery. In *Proceedings of the Second International Symposium on Metronidazole*, pp 137–148, 25–27 April, Geneva.

Willis AT, Ferguson IR, Jones PH et al (1977) Metronidazole in prevention and treatment of *Bacteroides* infections in elective colonic surgery. *BMJ* **1**: 607–610.

Wilson WR, Martin WJ, Wilkowske CJ & Washington JA (1972) Anaerobic bacteraemia. *Mayo Clin Proc* **47**: 649–656.

Windsor ACJ, Klava A, Somers SS, Guillou PJ & Reynolds JV (1995) Manipulation of local and systemic host defence in the prevention of perioperative sepsis. *Br J Surg* **82**: 1460–1467.

Wittmann DH & Schein M (1996) Let us shorten antibiotic prophylaxis and therapy in surgery. *Am J Surg* **172** (Suppl 6A): 26S–32S.

Wood RAB, Williams PHP & Hughes LE (1977) Foam elastomer dressing in the management of open granulating wounds: experience with 250 patients. *Br J Surg* **64**: 554–557.

Wylie WD & Churchill-Davidson HC (1966) In *A Practice of Anaesthesia*, 2nd edn, p 728. London: Lloyd-Luke.

Yoshioka K, Youngs DJ & Keighley MRB (1991) A randomised prospective controlled study of ciprofloxacin with metronidazole versus amoxicillin/clavulanic acid with metronidazole in the treatment of intraabdominal infection. *Infection* **19**: 25–29.

Young HL & Wheeler MH (1982) Report of a prospective trial: dextranomer beads (Debrisan) and silicone foam elastomer (silastic) dressings in surgical wounds. *Br J Surg* **69**: 33–34.

Ziv Y, Church JM, Fazio VW, King TM & Lavery IC (1996) Effect of systemic steroids on ileal pouch-anal anastomosis in patients with ulcerative colitis. *Dis Colon Rectum* **39**: 504–508.

6

SURGICAL PRINCIPLES

The majority of colorectal operations are performed by open operation. However, in recent years, the laparoscopic approach has been introduced. Initially, there was great enthusiasm for this approach, as the feasibility of performing many colorectal procedures laparoscopically was demonstrated. The benefits of such minimally invasive procedures were thought to include less postoperative pain, quicker return to normal function and shorter hospital stay, with consequent economic benefits. However, this initial enthusiasm has been tempered by realism. Most colorectal surgeons accept that although the laparoscope may have certain benefits, with present technology major colorectal procedures are difficult, and in certain situations may be dangerous. Whereas research progresses to make this approach easier, at present the laparoscopic revolution within colorectal surgery has not yet taken place. For this reason, we concentrate primarily on the open approach in this chapter.

Nevertheless, it is important for the colorectal surgeon to be aware of how the laparoscope may be used in the speciality. We have therefore included the principles relating to laparoscopic surgery at the end of this chapter. Elsewhere in the book, the reader will find how certain procedures can be performed laparoscopically and, where applicable, how they compare with the conventional open approach.

INCISIONS

The three principles that the surgeon should bear in mind when making the incision for the surgical treatment of a colorectal problem are:

1. Accessibility
2. Extensibility
3. Security (Maingot, 1969).

Opinions differ as to how the various types of incision achieve these aims and naturally there is a degree of individual preference. Vertical incisions are used most frequently for both elective and emergency work and these are usually either midline or paramedian (Figure 6.1). Although muscle-splitting vertical incisions have enjoyed a vogue in the past,

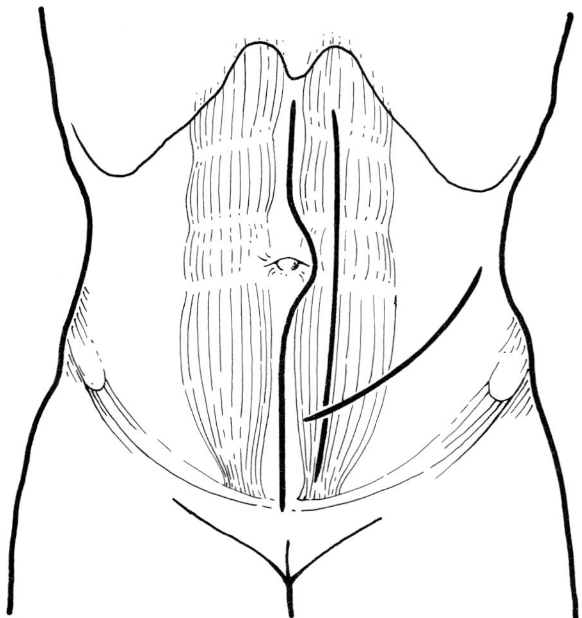

Figure 6.1 Abdominal incisions: midline, paramedian and oblique for access to the abdomen in colorectal surgery.

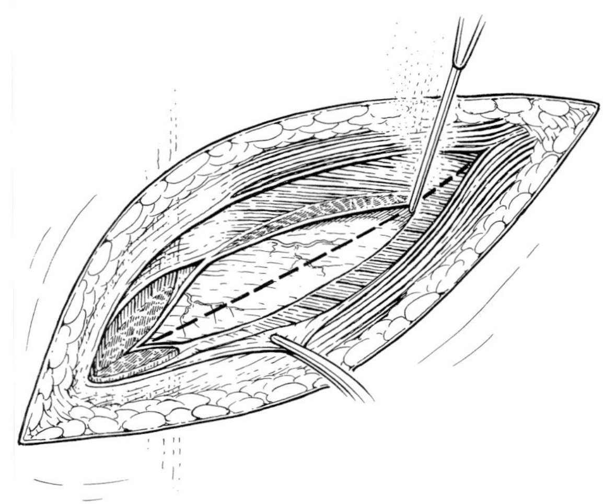

Figure 6.2 Anatomy of oblique muscle cutting incision. The external oblique aponeurosis has been divided in the line of its fibres. The internal oblique and transverse muscles have been cut across their fibres, exposing the peritoneum. The rectus has been partially divided at the medial end of the wound.

they are no longer popular. Similarly, pararectal incisions through the linea semilunaris are virtually never used today. Such incisions sever the motor nerves supplying the rectus muscle as they run transversely into its lateral edge. As a result the rectus muscle, and in certain cases even adjacent portions of the external and internal oblique muscles, become partially or completely paralysed and then waste, leaving a hernia. In certain circumstances transverse or oblique incisions may be the surgeon's preference (Figure 6.2).

For resection of the right or left colon, Lockart-Mummery (1934) and Turner (1955) recommended a long oblique muscle-cutting incision from the tip of the 12th rib to below the umbilicus. This gave excellent exposure to the splenic and hepatic flexures but was not ideal for access to the main vessels, particularly at their origin from the aorta. Transverse incisions have been strongly recommended by some surgeons (Goldberg et al, 1980; Bloch, 1981) who claim that they provide good access to the abdominal cavity as well as superior strength after closure and result in less postoperative pulmonary problems for the patient. While these points may be true, controlled trials indicate that there is no significant difference in wound dehiscence and respiratory complications between midline and transverse incisions (Greenall et al, 1980a,b). In Birmingham the midline incision was compared with the transverse incision for rectopexy. Although the cosmetic results of transverse incision were superior to a midline approach, there was more postoperative pain and haematoma with a transverse incision. Transverse incisions are also not ideal if a stoma may be needed in the future.

The choice between the two most commonly used vertical incisions, paramedian (Figure 6.3) and midline, is very much a personal one but in recent years the midline seems to be proving more popular. The apparent advantages of the paramedian over the midline incision are that it gives slightly better access to one or other side of the abdomen and that having the rectus muscle intervening between the anterior and posterior rectus sheaths makes it a stronger incision. There may be some truth in the first point but since the conventional paramedian technique places the incision 2–3 cm from the midline the advantage is relatively small, particularly with the use of the modern muscle relaxants. With regard to strength there are no controlled data which have shown that the conventional paramedian incision results in a stronger wound than that placed in the midline. However, controlled studies using a very lateral paramedian incision, i.e. at least 5 cm from the midline, have shown a significant reduction in incisional hernias compared to midline and conventional paramedian incisions (Guillou et al, 1980; Donaldson et al, 1982). The lateral paramedian incision is unlikely to be generally adopted,

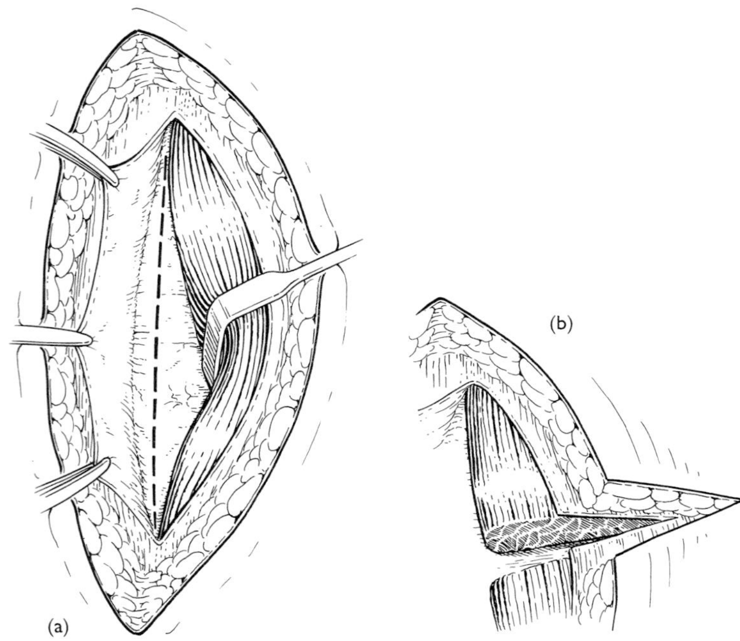

Figure 6.3 (a) Anatomy of the paramedian incision. (b) Occasionally transverse section of the rectus muscle is required to give adequate access to a difficult splenic or hepatic flexure. The same can be done with a midline incision.

however, since the dissection of the anterior rectus sheath off the muscle is tedious and increases the risk of haemorrhage and wound infection. In addition it limits exposure to the opposite side of the abdominal cavity if this is subsequently required.

For the above reasons we prefer a long midline vertical incision for virtually all colorectal procedures. In addition to the points discussed above, the midline incision has the merits of speed, less trauma and ease of extension in either the vertical or transverse directions. Furthermore, potential stoma sites are never compromised by this approach. Although the supraumbilical portion of a midline incision is said to be weaker than with other techniques, this has not been borne out in practice. The security of an incision depends more on the method and materials of closure rather than its site (Dudley, 1977).

The exact length and site of the midline incision will depend on the portion of the colon and rectum which are to be dealt with. For procedures involving the rectum and sigmoid the incision commences approximately 5 cm above the umbilicus, passes downwards, skirting it, and continues down to the pubic symphysis. For lesions elsewhere the extension downwards as far as the pubis is not usually necessary but extension upwards is invariably required.

Short transverse and oblique incisions are still sometimes required for the construction of defunctioning loop stomas.

WOUND CLOSURE

The abdominal wound may be closed in one of two ways: either by single layer mass closure or by layered closure. Mass closure involves the insertion of wide sutures through the entire musculoaponeurotic layers of the abdominal wall, including the peritoneum but not the subcutaneous fat or skin. Layered closure involves the insertion of two rows of sutures in the musculoaponeurotic layers, one in the posterior rectus sheath, including the anterior parietal peritoneum, and the other in the anterior sheath.

Mass closure may employ interrupted or continuous sutures but whichever is chosen it is usual to use a non-absorbable material. For many years stainless steel wire was the material of choice (Jones et al, 1941; Spencer et al, 1963). However, wire is not easy to work with and the knots can produce a pricking sensation for the patient. For these reasons most surgeons today use monofilament Prolene or Nylon. One problem associated with the use of these materials is the tendency for wound sinuses to develop around the knots. Although this complication may be reduced if the knots are buried beneath the peritoneum, sinus formation may remain a problem and hence there has been a vogue more recently to use either Dexon or PDS (polydioxane). These materials last for several weeks but are eventually absorbed. Leaper et al (1976) compared mass suture with Dexon or wire and found that there was no significant difference in the dehiscence or incisional hernia rates between the two types of material. Similarly, in a controlled trial using the continuous technique of mass suture, Pollock and Evans (1977) found no difference in wound breakdown rates between stainless steel wire, monofilament Nylon and Dexon. Although the incisional hernia rate was relatively high, at approximately 9%, it was similar for all three materials.

As a consequence of sinus formation with Prolene wound closure, we adopted a policy of mass closure with Dexon. However, there was a high rate of incisional hernia as well as keloid formation, especially if subcuticular Dexon was used as well. For these reasons we have returned to using Prolene or Nylon for abdominal wall closure.

Layered closure implies the insertion of two layers of sutures into the musculoaponeurotic layers of the abdominal wall. In vertical incisions the first or deepest layer is into the posterior rectus sheath together with the anterior parietal peritoneum. The second layer is through the anterior rectus sheath. Both layers are usually closed with a continuous suture, although some surgeons use interrupted sutures for the anterior layer. Although in the past chromic catgut was employed for both layers, this material results in unacceptable dehiscence and incisional hernia rates (Goligher et al, 1975). It is now usual to close at least the anterior rectus sheath with a continuous non-absorbable material such as Prolene or monofilament Nylon. Some surgeons in fact prefer to use these materials for both layers (Jenkins, 1976). Others have tended to use the stronger but nevertheless absorbable materials of Dexon, Vicryl (Irvin et al, 1976) or PDS. Although Dexon (polyglycolic acid) and Vicryl (polyglactin) have been demonstrated by Irvin et al (1976) to be no different to Prolene as far as healing is concerned, the incidence of wound infection and subsequent stitch sinus is much less with the absorbable materials. It is unnecessary to close the anterior parietal peritoneum when a layered technique is used, provided the anterior and posterior sheaths are closed with a non-absorbable material (Ellis and Heddle, 1977).

Which type of closure to use is a matter of personal choice and although layered closure seems theoretically more secure than mass suture there are no data to support this contention. Thus Irvin and his colleagues (1977), in a randomized controlled trial of the two techniques in 200 patients, using non-absorbable material, found an overall dehiscence rate of 1% and an incisional hernia rate of 4.7% but there was no significant difference in these complications between the two techniques of closure. It would also appear from experimental work that mass sutures are less likely to cut out of the tissue than layered sutures (Leaper et al, 1977). There are no data either to indicate whether continuous mass suture is as secure as interrupted mass suture. In spite of this, the vogue is to close midline incisions with a continuous mass suture of a non-absorbable material, either Prolene or monofilament nylon. This in fact is our own practice and we use two double loops of 1/0 Nylon or Prolene. Each is inserted at the extremity of the wound and anchored by placing the needle through the loop. The mass closure continues from each end of the wound until the centre is reached, whereupon the two sutures are tied and the knot buried below the peritoneum.

If a paramedian incision has been used, most surgeons still close this by the layered technique using continuous non-absorbable material, if not for both layers at least for the anterior sheath. The use of interrupted through and through non-absorbable tension sutures is advocated by some to add security to abdominal wall closure. There is no evidence, however, of any benefit from such sutures; indeed there is a danger of damage to loops of small bowel which may become adherent to the wound. Furthermore, as the tissues of the abdominal wall swell, the sutures may cut out and cause dehiscence. For these reasons we do not use reinforcing deep tension sutures; indeed the use of this closure technique has almost disappeared.

Closure of the wound in septic cases

In patients with severe septic complications such as faecal peritonitis there is a high risk of intra-abdominal abscess and wound infection. In patients in whom re-laparotomy is the policy or where re-operation is likely some surgeons have recommended the insertion of a patch of polypropylene mesh into the abdominal wall with a 'zipper' (Stone et al, 1981; Voyles et al, 1981). This is claimed to allow re-laparotomy to be undertaken with relative ease and also permits 'give' in the abdominal wall without the risk of necrosis from sutures cutting out of the abdominal wall (Dudley, 1984). The technique described by Dudley (1984) is as follows. At the end of the procedure and after peritoneal toilet has been completed the anaesthetist provides complete relaxation. The gap that then exists is measured and an oblong piece of polypropylene mesh is cut to approximately one and a half times the size of the wound. The mesh is then sutured 1.5–2 cm under the peritoneal edge with interrupted 1/0 polypropylene sutures. Suction drains are laid across the mesh to scavenge exudate for the first 48 hours. Gauze dressings are then applied and changed as necessary. In most circumstances a fibrinous membrane forms, granulation tissue replaces this and the wound heals by second intention. Alternatively, the wound may be skin grafted, though a delayed flap closure is preferable. We have used this technique on a number of occasions and have found it to be of considerable benefit.

Where the patient is fat and there has been moderate or severe contamination by intestinal contents and when the risk of wound sepsis is considerable, it is a good policy to leave the skin and subcutaneous tissues unsutured. The wound is then packed and may be filled with elastomer foam. Some surgeons recommend delayed primary suture after 7–8 days, while others find that granulation proceeds rapidly and that secondary closure is unnecessary. Although we have sometimes used delayed primary suture, we would not advocate the technique as a routine in all large bowel cases, as was recommended by Turnbull (1966).

WOUND BREAKDOWN

Surgical technique and the materials used to close the abdominal wall are perhaps the most important factors influencing healing of the abdominal wall. However, other factors cannot be ignored. Persistent postoperative abdominal distension due to ileus, mechanical obstruction or ascites increases the risk of abdominal dehiscence. Similarly, other causes of persistent raised intra-abdominal pressure, such as a chronic respiratory disease, repeated hiccups or vomiting, may produce a similar result. Wound infection is a particularly important reason for abdominal wound breakdown, especially if associated with an enterocutaneous fistula or gross malnutrition. In addition to these local factors, systemic factors such as anaemia, jaundice, advanced age, malignant disease, steroid treatment, deficient nutrition, particularly hypoalbuminaemia and low vitamin C intake, all retard healing of abdominal wall incisions. Patients with colorectal disease have a high incidence of these risk factors and are therefore more prone to dehiscence than other groups.

The management of a burst abdomen following a colorectal procedure is the same as that following wound dehiscence after any other major abdominal procedure. This involves reopening the entire incision and resuture with the interrupted mass closure technique. The skin is often left open.

TO DRAIN OR NOT TO DRAIN?

The use of drains is a much discussed and a largely unresolved subject. The aim of leaving a drain within the peritoneal cavity is to ensure that potentially infected fluid or blood is evacuated. A secondary aim is the evacuation of infected or faecal material if there is breakdown of an anastomosis or suture line so that the result is a fistula rather than peritonitis. The potential dangers are that open drains may allow entry of bacteria, resulting in intra-abdominal infection rather than its prevention. There is the added fear that a drain may encourage an inflammatory reaction or erode through various structures, such as arteries or an intestinal anastomosis, resulting in such complications as secondary haemorrhage and anastomotic dehiscence. Scientific evaluation of the benefit of drains in clinical practice is complicated by the many variables that may influence complications, such as open or closed drainage systems, the type of material used to manufacture the drain and the methods of extracting fluid within drains, for example high or low negative pressure suction, syphonage or static systems.

Much of the available information about the value of intraperitoneal drains in clinical practice emanates from studies that investigated their efficacy following cholecystectomy and appendicectomy. Furthermore, most of the studies relating to open drains are retrospective in nature; however, several points emerge. If drainage is to be used, the critical period appears to be during the first 48 hours after the operation. Drainage for longer is associated with a greater incidence of postoperative complications such as chest and wound infections (Gordon et al, 1976; Man et al, 1977; Stone et al, 1978; Fraser et al, 1982; Mittelman and Doberneck, 1982). Other complications, such as herniation (Gordon et al, 1976), fistulas (Hanna, 1970), loss of the drain (Kambouris et al, 1973) and knotting of the drain and bowel injury (Benjamin, 1980; Woodforde Scott, 1981), have all been described. Hence exposure of the patient to these risks by prolonged drainage is unwarranted. Large volumes of intra-abdominal fluid are retrieved only in the first 24–48 hours and experimental evidence suggests that drains cease to function satisfactorily after that period (Santos et al, 1962; Hanna, 1970; Agrama et al, 1976). Even though as much as 2 L of fluid may drain in the first 8 hours after cholecystectomy, fluid collections are rare and are usually rapidly absorbed (Elboim et al, 1983; Truedson, 1983). Two prospective studies in patients undergoing simple cholecystectomy have shown no significant benefit from drainage after this operation (Ragoonan et al, 1983; Playforth et al, 1985). Similarly in the higher risk group of patients with perforated appendicitis, Greenall et al (1978), in a carefully conducted, prospective, randomized trial, showed no significant difference in intra-abdominal sepsis between those patients who had intra-abdominal drainage with a rubber drain and those who had no drain. David et al (1982) and Haller et al (1973) came to similar conclusions in their trials on children with ruptured appendicitis. In controlled studies following splenectomy, however, the incidence of septic problems was significantly greater in the drained group (Cohn, 1965; Cerise et al, 1970).

Studies on the use of drains in colonic surgery are sparse and there are few adequate controlled trials in the literature. In a retrospective analysis of 454 colonic resections conducted by Berliner et al (1967), 390 patients had intraperitoneal anastomoses, 67 with open drainage; 64 patients had an anterior resection, 29 of whom had an extraperitoneal drain inserted. The authors found a significantly higher overall complication rate among patients with drains compared with those without drains (25% no drains; 45% intraperitoneal drains; 38% extraperitoneal drains). Three of the 29 (10%) who were drained extraperitoneally developed an anastomotic leak, compared with five of 67 (7%) who were drained intraperitoneally. These figures compare with nine leaks in the 358 patients (2.5%) who were not drained.

There are perhaps only two prospective controlled trials of drainage after colonic resection. Johnson et al (1989) randomized 106 patients to a test group (n = 49), who received a corrugated Silastic drain placed next to the colonic anastomosis, or a control group (n = 57) who had no drain. There was no significant difference in outcome between the two groups (Table 6.1). Baillet et al (1995) performed a multicentre trial which randomized 813 patients having both emergency and elective procedures for the whole gamut of colorectal diseases. The method was sump drainage in the pelvis and a dependent tube or corrugated drain in the abdomen. Once again, there was no significant difference between the two groups with regard to mortality or morbidity, and the authors concluded that prophylactic drainage was useless.

Irvin and Goligher (1973) drained all but 12 of their 215 patients who underwent large bowel resection using open tube drains. Two (16.7%) of the undrained anastomoses developed clinical leaks compared with an overall clinical leak rate of 13.8%. Schrock et al (1973), on the other hand, only inserted a drain in exceptional circumstances and their overall leakage rate was 4.5% in 1763 cases. Interestingly, Koruth et al (1985) found a similar low incidence of leaks (2.2%) when drains were not used in 15 emergency left colonic anastomoses.

The inference from some of these clinical studies is that intraperitoneal drainage may in fact be harmful after colorectal procedures, particularly when placed adjacent to an anastomosis. This suspicion is supported by experimental studies. Manz et al (1970) and Crowson and Wilson (1973) found that rubber drains in dogs predisposed to colonic anastomotic breakdown. Smith (1986) has confirmed

Table 6.1 Complications of colonic anastomosis in a prospective controlled trial of drain versus no drain.

	Drain	*No drain*
No. of patients	49	57
Wound infection	10	10
Anastomotic leak	6	6
Intra-abdominal sepsis (apart from leakage)	0	1
Other	3	5
Death	2	1

From Johnson et al (1989).

these findings in rats and has shown that, in addition to latex rubber, drains of polyvinylchloride (PVC), Teflon and Silastic also may lead to anastomotic problems, although the risk is not as great as with rubber.

Despite the above findings, many surgeons have not been persuaded to stop using drains. Smith (1986) in the UK investigated the practice of over 80 surgeons in the North East Thames region: 30% of surgeons reported that they did not use drains following right hemicolectomy but 47% routinely used them. In left hemicolectomy approximately two-thirds of surgeons favoured drainage, and after low anterior resection only 15% did not use them.

Our policy over the last decade has reflected a change in philosophy: we no longer believe that drains prevent complications of anastomotic breakdown, indeed they may precipitate them. We believe drains principally reduce the risk of infected haematoma which can be responsible for anastomotic dehiscence. Our policy therefore has been to reserve the use of drains for removal of pelvic or intraperitoneal blood before it can clot, thereby reducing the risk of infected haematoma. If drainage is required we select a suction drain made of Silastic or PVC and leave it in place for no longer than 48 hours if possible, provided the drainage volume is not excessive.

PRINCIPLES OF LARGE BOWEL ANASTOMOSIS

The principles of large bowel anastomosis do not differ from those applied to an anastomosis constructed elsewhere in the gastrointestinal tract. The surgeon needs good access and exposure to the two ends of bowel, the blood supply must be adequate, the technique must be meticulous and there must be no tension on the anastomosis. Ideally the patient should be well nourished and there should have been no faecal contamination. These principles should be adhered to whenever possible because the morbidity attending anastomotic breakdown in the colon can be considerable. Thus in a multicentre study of 1466 patients who underwent large bowel anastomosis, Fielding et al (1980) found there was a hospital mortality of 22% in 191 patients with an anastomotic leak compared with 7.1% of 1275 patients without a leak. The morbidity was also higher, as might be expected, in the group that leaked, which resulted in a more prolonged inpatient stay: 45.7 days compared with 25.4 days.

Access and exposure

The surgeon must ensure that access to both ends of the bowel is adequate. This will be achieved by appropriately sited and sufficiently long incisions, adequate mobilization of the bowel, correct positioning of assistants and retractors and appropriate illumination. Also, there must be adequate muscle relaxation. Adequate mobilization may be impossible in certain circumstances when the low rectum is involved. If access is limited, it may be possible to improve matters by extending the incision or converting it into another type, but if this approach fails, the question as to whether an anastomosis is appropriate or whether an alternative technique should be adopted will need to be asked.

Blood supply

A good blood supply is essential for satisfactory healing of an anastomosis. Until recently it was thought that provided the bowel ends were pink and there was no blanching or cyanosis and there was no sign of dark venous bleeding, the surgeon could be satisfied that the blood supply was adequate for anastomotic healing. However, evidence in both animals and humans suggests that clinical observations concerning the blood supply to bowel may be misleading (Sheridan et al, 1987). Tissue oxygen measurements have shown that the colon might look viable at operation even when the blood supply is insufficient to allow anastomotic healing. It remains to be seen whether anastomotic breakdown can be reduced by routine measurement of tissue oxygen and by laser Doppler velocimetry.

In order to achieve optimum vascularization there are some important operative precautions to be followed. Although mobilization must be adequate so that there is no tension on the anastomosis and its blood supply, it is essential that critical vessels are not divided in order to achieve adequate mobilization since this will result in ischaemia of the bowel ends. Sutures used for the anastomosis must not be placed too deeply or too tightly so as to avoid strangulation of tissue. In this respect the interrupted extramucosal suture has certain theoretical advantages. Any bleeding from the cut ends of bowel should not be controlled by excessive diathermy as tissue necrosis may result. It is preferable to ligate any bleeding point individually. For open anastomoses it is usual to place bowel clamps proximal to the bowel ends in order to avoid faecal contamination. Such clamps must always be of the non-crushing variety; they should be lightly applied and should not include the mesentery since this may compromise the blood supply.

Manual sutured anastomosis

The principles of anastomotic technique were established over 150 years ago when early surgeons considered that it was essential to obtain serosal apposition and that mucosal eversion was dangerous as it resulted in leakage (Travers, 1812; Lembert, 1826; Leonardo, 1943). In the early days these principles were achieved by using a two-layer technique, as recommended by Czerny (1880). The first layer was an inner through and through suture which was either continuous or interrupted and the second layer was an outer seromuscular or Lembert stitch. The latter was usually interrupted and produced inversion and opposed the serosa. Halsted (1887) showed that the submucosa was the strongest layer of the intestinal wall and that a single-layer anastomosis could be used provided the suture included a good bite of the submucosa. Gambee (1951) also believed this principle and supported the single-layer technique. Although both Halsted and Gambee felt that too much inversion should be avoided, they both believed that eversion was dangerous and that end-to-end apposition of bowel ends was necessary.

The view that eversion should be avoided was challenged in the mid-1960s by several authors who demonstrated that eversion techniques were quite safe (Getzen et al, 1966; Ravitch, 1967; Healey et al, 1967; Hamilton, 1967; Loeb, 1967; Ravitch et al, 1967a,b; Buyers and Meier, 1968). However, numerous other clinical and experimental studies which followed demonstrated the reverse (Canalis and Ravitch, 1968; Hargreaves and Keddie, 1968; Mellish et al, 1968; Singleton et al, 1968; Gill et al, 1969; McAdam et al, 1969; Orr, 1969; Rusca et al, 1969; Trueblood et al, 1969; Goligher et al, 1970b). The currently accepted view is that eversion should be avoided at all costs and that inversion techniques should be employed for large bowel anastomosis.

Controversy exists, however, on the need for a one- or two-layer anastomosis and the optimum type of suture material. These issues are particularly relevant now that staples have become so popular. Theoretically, the two-layer technique might be expected to produce more ischaemia and tissue necrosis and more narrowing of the intestinal lumen than the one-layer technique. In practice, there are no consistent data which demonstrate the benefit of the one-layer anastomosis over a two-layer anastomosis. Most of the experimental and clinical studies that have compared the single- or two-layer intraperitoneal colonic anastomoses demonstrate no significant difference between the methods (McAdam et al, 1969; Irvin and Edwards, 1973; Irvin and Goligher, 1973). Controversy still exists, however, concerning low colorectal anastomoses. Everett (1975), in a series of anterior resections, compared a one-layer inverting suture of interrupted 4/0 Supramid with knots tied on the mucosa with a two-layer inverting suture of inner continuous catgut and outer interrupted 4/0 Supramid. Although there was no significant difference in leak rates between the techniques for intraperitoneal anastomosis, the single-layer technique resulted in significantly less dehiscence than the two-layer technique for low anastomoses on the extraperitoneal rectum. On the other hand, Goligher et al (1977) in a similar study found a significantly greater dehiscence rate with the one-layered technique.

It has always seemed to us that a one-layer anastomosis is far easier to perform within the pelvis where access may be restricted. At the Royal London the policy has been to perform a two-layer anastomosis whenever it is reasonable to do so, reserving a one-layer technique for low colorectal anastomoses. In Birmingham, on the other hand, a two-layer anastomosis for colorectal surgery has virtually been abandoned. For low anastomoses a one-layer manual anastomosis is deemed to be easier to perform than a two-layer technique. However, in both centres we, like most surgeons, opt to use the circular stapling instrument for virtually all colorectal anastomoses.

Suture material

The basic types of suture material are absorbable and non-absorbable. In general terms it is usual to perform a two-layer anastomosis using an inner layer of absorbable material and an outer layer of non-absorbable material. A single-layer technique normally utilizes a non-absorbable suture. Chromic catgut on a round-bodied needle is the most popular absorbable suture but some surgeons prefer polyglycolic acid (Dexon) or polyglactin (Vicryl) as these are reputed to last longer. Indeed there is some evidence from controlled studies that polyglycolic acid is superior to catgut as the inner layer of a conventional two-layer colonic or colorectal anastomosis in preventing anastomotic breakdown (Deveney and Way, 1976; Clark et al, 1978). Despite these obvious advantages, many surgeons still use chromic catgut as their absorbable suture of choice since they prefer its handling qualities. If polyglactin is used, many lubricate the material with liquid paraffin to prevent it from cutting through the bowel wall.

Various non-absorbable sutures are available and these include silk, linen, polypropylene and synthetic polyesters. There has been a vogue when performing a single-layer anastomosis to use interrupted sutures of non-absorbable material, even 5/0 stainless steel wire (Kratzer and Onsanit, 1974; Trimpi et al, 1976). Wire, however, has never been universally adopted since it is technically difficult to work with and has never been put to the test in a formal clinical trial. One advantage of monofilament non-absorbable sutures, such as Nylon or polypropylene or even wire, is that they cause much less tissue reaction than braided material, particularly when this is absorbable. This difference does not seem to be as obvious in the intestine as it is on peritoneal surfaces or in muscle. Since braided material is easier to handle, most surgeons prefer it (Fontaine and Dudley, 1978).

The size or gauge of the suture material is usually 00 or 000 for adult intestinal anastomosis and the needle is of the round-bodied type.

Techniques

A colocolic, colorectal or enterocolic anastomosis may be made end-to-end, end-to-side or side-to-side. Although techniques exist to perform closed anastomoses, most surgeons prefer an open technique. There are numerous variations in technique but a brief description of the more common methods follows.

End-to-end anastomosis

Two-layer technique (Figure 6.4)

The divided ends of the bowel are occluded by crushing clamps and light occlusion clamps are applied across the bowel approximately 5–10 cm from the crushing clamps, taking care not to occlude the mesentery. The anastomosis is commenced by inserting the posterior outer layer of sutures. This usually consists of a layer of interrupted sutures such as Vicryl or PDS. After these sutures have been inserted and tied, the sutures at the mesenteric and antimesenteric borders of the anastomosis are left long and grasped in the jaws of a small arterial clamp. The remainder are cut. For ease of insertion it is our practice to ensure that each suture is waxed. The crushing clamps are then removed by cutting the bowel below them with a knife and thus the bowel lumen is opened. The two open ends of bowel are then irrigated with a dilute antibiotic solution; at the Royal London we use a cefuroxime solution, in Birmingham an antiseptic such as proflavine is used.

After achieving haemostasis of the bowel ends the inner layer of catgut or Vicryl is next inserted as a continuous, full-thickness suture. This suture commences at the antimesenteric border and is inserted so that, when tied, the knot lies on the serosal surface. An artery forceps is then placed on the short end of the suture. The needle is passed back into the lumen of the gut and the posterior layer of the anastomosis constructed by insertion of an over-and-over continuous all-coats suture. The mesenteric corner of the anastomosis is then invaginated using a Connell (loop on mucosa) stitch, and the latter is continued on the anterior wall of the anastomosis. Alternatively a simple over-and-over suture may be used, preferably using a double-ended suture with two needles commencing at the centre of the back row. When the antimesenteric aspect of the anastomosis is reached, the corner is invaginated using the Connell stitch and the suture is tied to its other end. The anterior outer layer of the anastomosis is then performed in an identical fashion to the posterior outer layer.

Some surgeons prefer initially to insert the inner layer, using a continuous suture. When this layer is complete they insert the anterior outer layer and, by rotating the anastomosis, insert the posterior outer layer. Whereas this is usually easily achieved for small bowel anastomosis, it is less applicable to large bowel anastomosis. It is often difficult, particularly in rectal resections, to rotate the anastomosis and we would not recommend this approach.

A modified two-layer technique may be used for low colorectal anastomoses. In these cases, where access is usually limited, it is easier to insert the outer posterior seromuscular sutures as horizontal mattress sutures instead of the more conventional vertical sutures. They are easier to place and have the added advantage that, being placed at right-angles to the longitudinal muscle fibres, they are less likely to cut out than vertical sutures. None of the sutures is tied until all have been placed. Once tied, secure inversion of the suture line is achieved. Although it may be feasible to use the two-layer technique for low colorectal anastomoses, we prefer to use a one-layer technique or the circular stapling device.

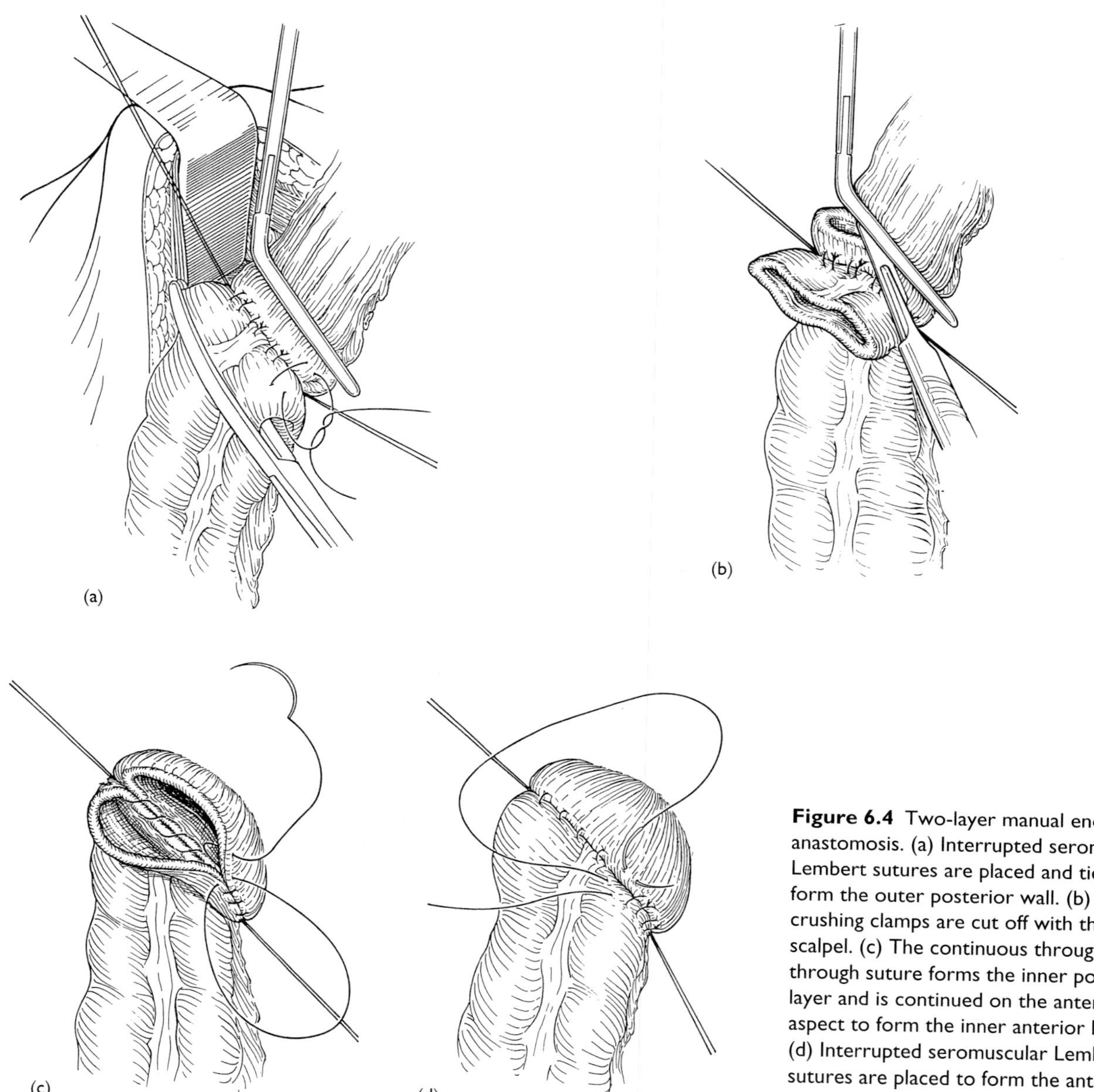

Figure 6.4 Two-layer manual end-to-end anastomosis. (a) Interrupted seromuscular Lembert sutures are placed and tied to form the outer posterior wall. (b) The crushing clamps are cut off with the scalpel. (c) The continuous through-and-through suture forms the inner posterior layer and is continued on the anterior aspect to form the inner anterior layer. (d) Interrupted seromuscular Lembert sutures are placed to form the anterior outer layer.

Single-layer full-thickness technique (Figure 6.5)

Although at the Royal London we prefer to use the single-layer technique only for the low colorectal anastomoses, many surgeons as in the Birmingham Unit prefer to use it routinely for all large bowel anastomoses. The usual technique is to employ interrupted non-absorbable sutures such as linen or silk but many surgeons now prefer Vicryl or PDS. The anastomosis begins with the insertion of the posterior layer of sutures. These are through-and-through sutures which incorporate all layers of the bowel wall and they are usually inserted as simple vertical sutures or as vertical mattress sutures. Each is left long and clipped, and tied only when all have been inserted. The space between each suture should be relatively small, otherwise there is a tendency for eversion to occur when the sutures are tied. The anterior layer of the anastomosis may be constructed either using interrupted through-and-through sutures, inserted from within out so that when they are tied the knot lies on the mucosa, or as vertical mattress Connell sutures. It is usual to insert these sutures in a lateral to medial direction alternately. A small gap in the suture line

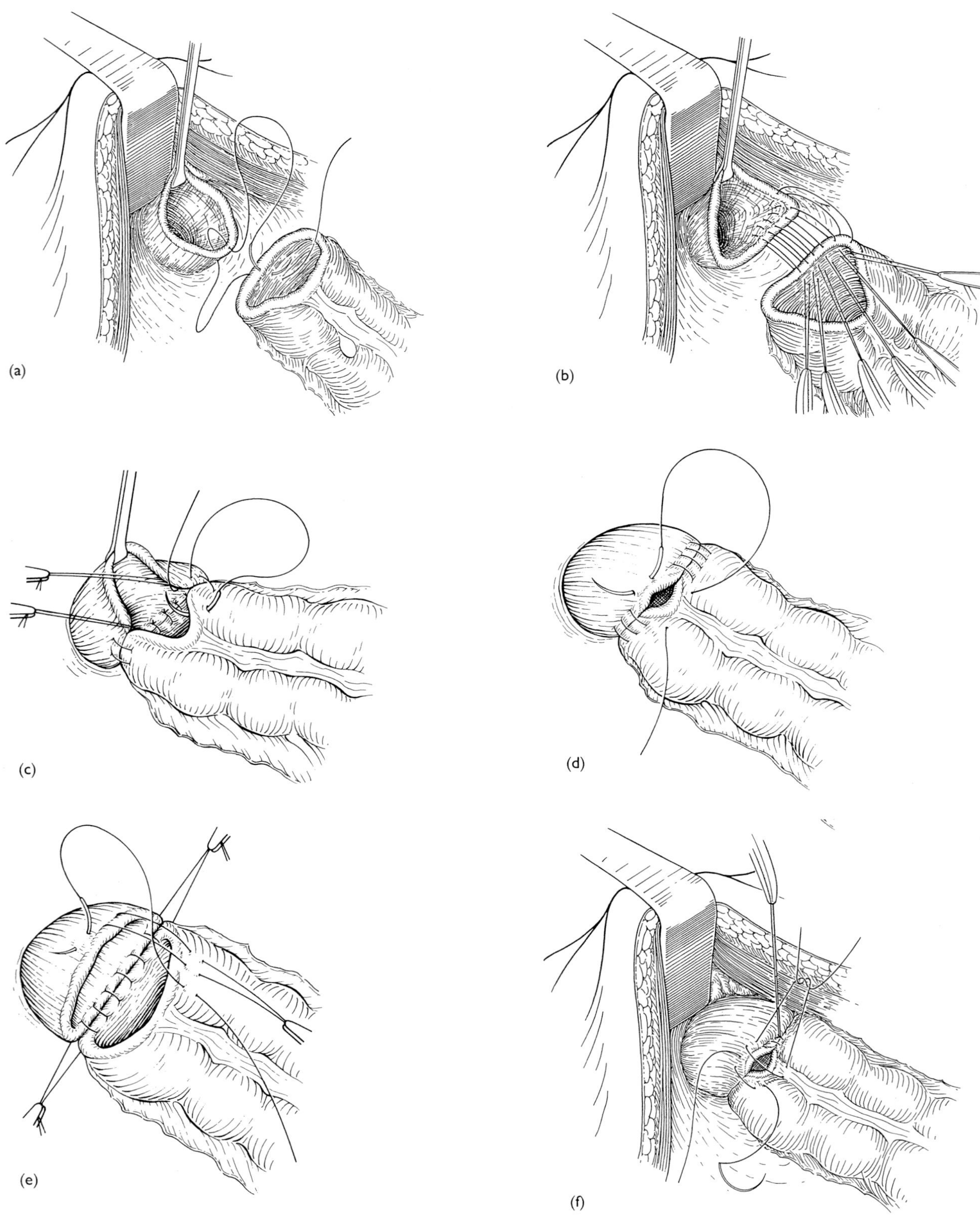

Figure 6.5 One-layer manual end-to-end anastomosis. (a,b) Interrupted mattress through-and-through sutures are inserted to form the posterior layer. (c) Interrupted through-and-through sutures are inserted from within out to form the anterior layer. (d) Central seromuscular suture placed to complete anterior layer. (e) Alternative method of constructing anterior layer using interrupted seromuscular Lembert sutures. (f) Another method of constructing anterior layer using interrupted Connell (loop on mucosa) sutures. This has the advantage of inverting the mucosa with the knot on the outside of the bowel.

finally remains in the centre of the anterior layer and this is closed with a submucosal suture inserted parallel to the edge of the suture line. Alternatively, the anterior layer may be closed with a series of submucosal Lembert type sutures, as used for the outer layer of a two-layer anastomosis. Finally, after all sutures have been inserted and tied the anastomosis is gently rotated and any defects within it are closed by extra sutures.

Single-layer extramucosal anastomosis
In order to avoid strangulating submucosal end arteries a vertical interrupted anastomosis technique which excludes the mucosa is being used increasingly for intestinal anastomosis (Figure 6.5c). This provides excellent inversion. Provided the sutures are not pulled too tightly, the same technique may be used as a continuous suture using PDS which runs easily.

No matter whether the end-to-end anastomosis is performed as a one-layer or two-layer technique, it is normal practice, if feasible, to close the defect in the mesentery. This is usually done after right hemicolectomy or transverse colectomy but is not possible for left-sided anastomoses. When closing the mesenteric defect care is required not to damage the blood supply to the bowel ends.

Disparity between the lumen size of the two bowel ends may be overcome by various manoeuvres. The end of bowel with the smaller lumen can be sectioned more obliquely than the end of bowel with the larger lumen, or it may be enlarged by a longitudinal cut of 1–2 cm along its antimesenteric border (Figure 6.6).

Disparity can also be overcome by fashioning the anastomosis in such a way as to space the sutures wider on the larger lumen and closer together on the smaller bowel end. Another method to overcome disparity between bowel lumens is to abandon an end-to-end anastomosis and perform an end-to-side anastomosis.

End-to-side anastomosis

Many surgeons prefer to perform an end-to-side anastomosis following right hemicolectomy. The same anastomosis may also be useful for ileorectal or ileosigmoid anastomoses. When constructing an end-to-side ileotransverse anastomosis following right hemicolectomy it is normal practice to close the end of the transverse colon and construct the anastomosis between the end of ileum and side of colon. Closure of the end of colon may be performed manually or by stapling. Most surgeons who prefer a manual technique use a two-layer inverting procedure (Figure 6.7). There are a variety of ways of performing this closure and our preference is as follows. The end of the bowel is held in a crushing clamp and a chromic catgut or lubricated Vicryl suture on a straight needle is inserted through all layers of bowel at the antimesenteric end and then tied. The suture is then continued to the mesenteric end of the bowel as a continuous horizontal mattress suture inserted through all layers of bowel beneath the crushing clamp. It is then tied and the crushing clamp is removed. The suture is returned to the antimesenteric end of the bowel as a continuous over-and-over suture and tied at the end. Finally, the outer layer is inserted as interrupted seromuscular Lembert sutures using either Vicryl or non-absorbable braided material. This technique ensures that the closed bowel end is securely invaginated into the colonic lumen. After the end of colon has been closed in the manner described, a longitudinal colotomy is created along one of the taenia by cutting diathermy 2–3 cm from the closed end of

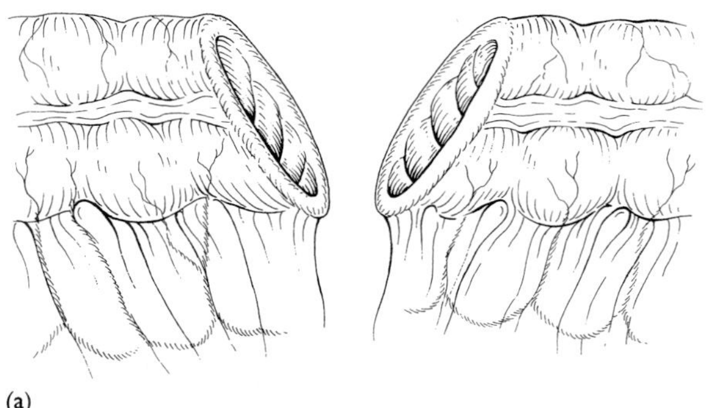
(a)

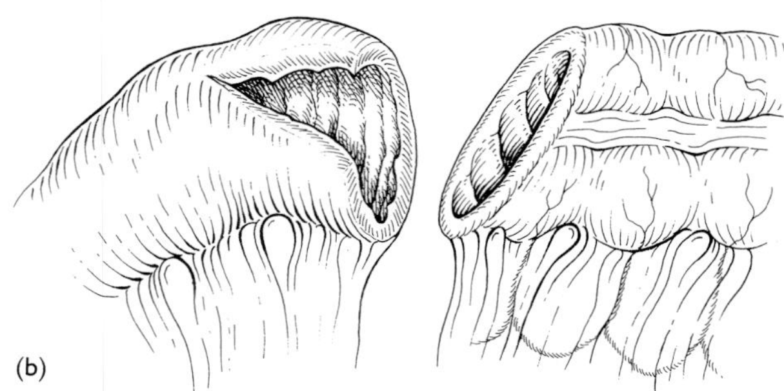
(b)

Figure 6.6 Techniques to overcome disparity between two ends of colon. (a) Colon is divided obliquely. (b) Enlargement of one lumen by division along the antimesenteric border for 2–2.5 cm.

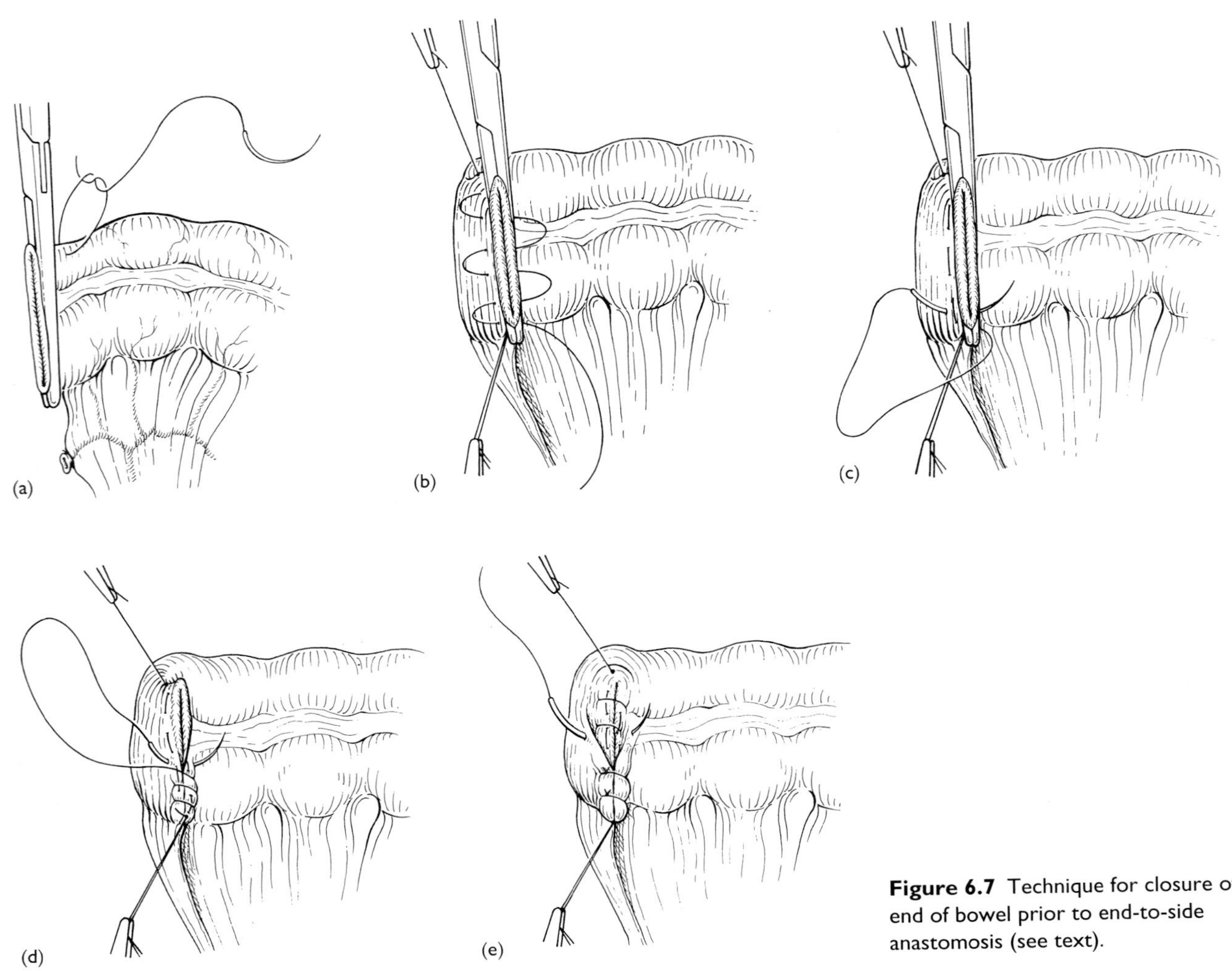

Figure 6.7 Technique for closure of end of bowel prior to end-to-side anastomosis (see text).

colon and its length is matched approximately with the diameter of the ileum. The end of ileum is anastomosed to the colon by a standard two- or one-layer technique, depending on the preference of the surgeon (Figure 6.8).

Side-to-side anastomosis (Figure 6.9)

Some surgeons prefer this type of anastomosis, in particular for ileocolic or ileorectal anastomoses. It has the theoretical advantage that it uses only completely peritonealized surfaces of bowel for the anastomosis. It does, however, use more bowel than the more conventional end-to-end anastomosis. It has been said that the blind ends are subsequently liable to undergo dilatation, which may give rise to discomfort and, on occasion, perforation (Goligher, 1984). Although perforation can occur in the blind ends of bowel, there is no scientific evidence that complications from side-to-side anastomoses are significantly more common than after either end-to-side or end-to-end anastomoses.

Stapling techniques

An alternative to manual techniques of suturing is the use of stapling instruments. The introduction of these instruments has allowed colonic closure and anastomosis to be performed more quickly than the manual alternative. Whether such techniques are safer than the more conventional methods, as suggested by some authors, is open to debate. The instruments were primarily developed in Russia during the 1950s but were not introduced into North America and Western Europe until the 1970s (Steichen, 1968, 1971; Ravitch and Steichen, 1972; Ravitch, 1974; Fain et al, 1975). The design was

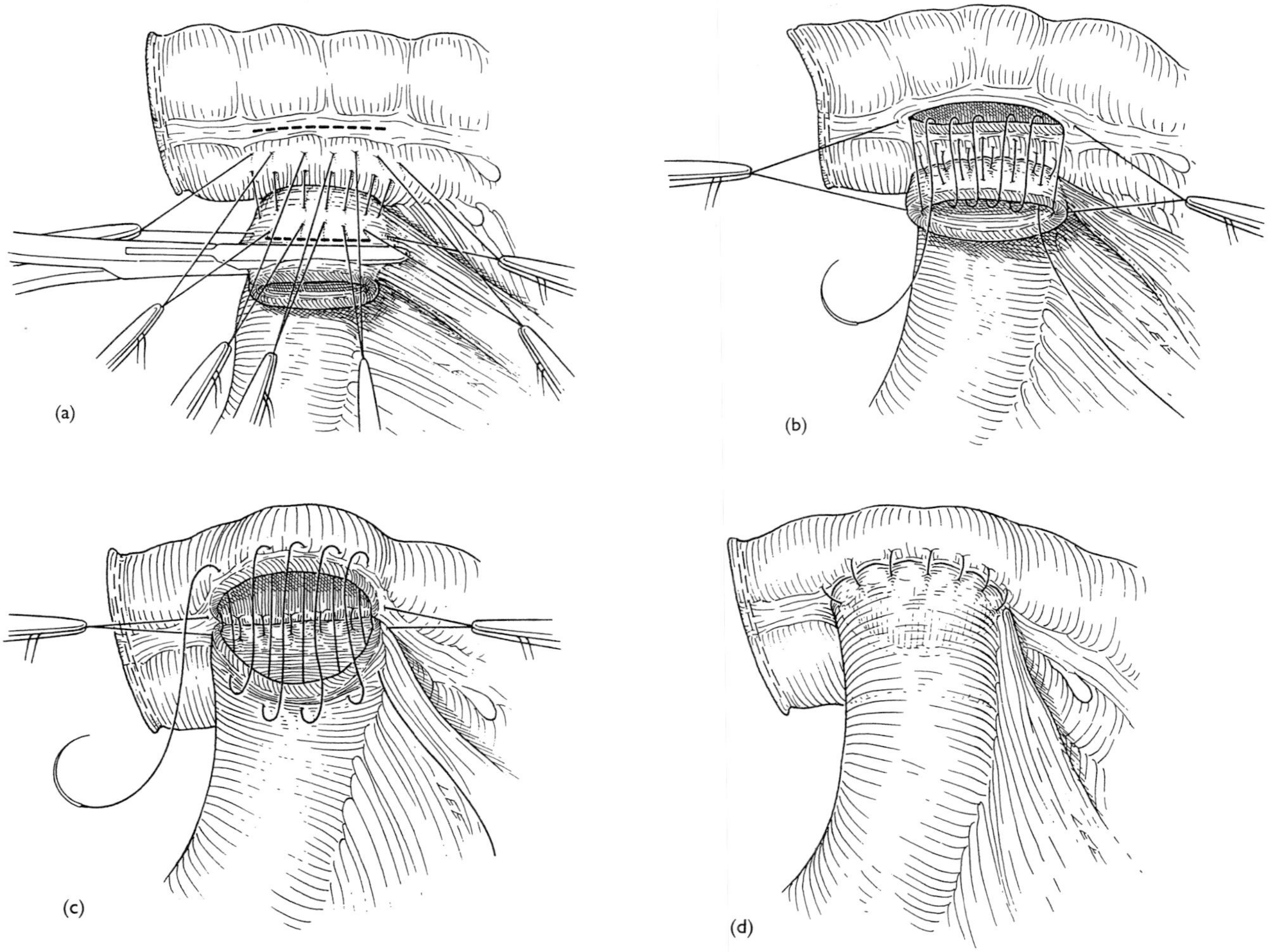

Figure 6.8 Construction of end-to-side ileocolic anastomosis in two layers.

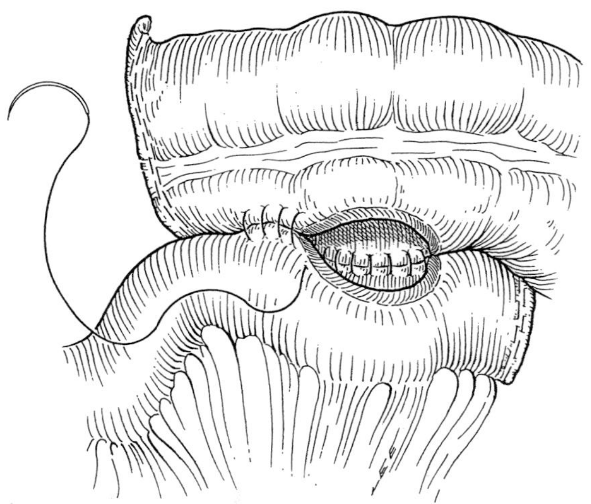

Figure 6.9 Construction of side-to-side ileocolic anastomosis.

based on the original gastrointestinal stapling device invented at the beginning of this century in Hungary by Hurll, who was a surgeon, and Fischer, who was an instrument maker (Robiscek, 1980). At present there are various companies that manufacture these instruments, the main ones being the United States Surgical Corporation (USSC), Ethicon Ltd and 3M. When the instruments were first introduced, only the cartridges which housed the staples were disposable; the rest of the instrument had to be resterilized prior to use. Nowadays, all manufacturers make entirely disposable instruments.

There are three types of stapling instrument with applications in colorectal surgery: linear staplers (TA or TL), linear cutters (GIA, TLC or ILA) and circular stapling instruments (EEA or its modifications and ILS).

Linear staplers

The TA instrument (USSC) or linear stapler, TL model (Ethicon Ltd) is designed to close and seal the end of a viscus (Figure 6.10). It does so by first apposing the two walls of the viscus within the jaws of the clamp without crushing them. When apposition is complete the instrument is 'fired', driving a double row of fine, stainless steel staples through the tissues held in the clamp. Before the staples are inserted they have a '⊔' configuration, but after firing of the instrument the perpendicular prongs are compressed so that the staple represents a capital B lying on its side 'ꓭ'. This allows the edges of the tissue to be firmly apposed and held together but at the same time prevents occlusion of the small blood vessels (Smith et al, 1981). Hence, although stapling does not produce ischaemia of the two edges of the viscus, it is not as haemostatic as a continuous manual suture. If haemostasis is a problem, the suture line can always be under-run or the bleeding vessels in the cut edge may be lightly diathermied.

There are three sizes of TA or TL instrument available, which differ in the length of the jaws. These are the TA or TL 30, TA or TL 55 and TA or TL 90, although the 90 is rarely used in colorectal surgery. Two sizes of staples are normally supplied with the USSC instruments: 3.5 mm and 4.8 mm. The larger 4.8-mm staples should be used for all colorectal work. With the Ethicon (TL) instruments the height of the staples before they become bent over during firing can be adjusted according to the thickness of the tissues.

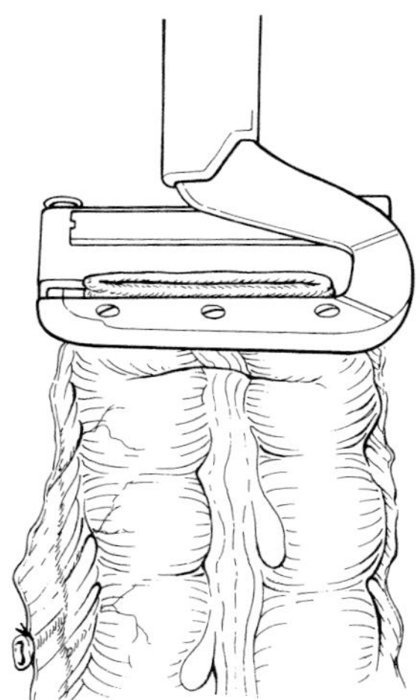

Figure 6.10 Transverse stapling instrument being used to close the end of the colon.

There are certain practical considerations that must be observed by the surgeon when using the TA or TL instrument. The TA and TL instruments should not be fired until the retaining pins are well in place. The TL instrument has a mobile ratchet device that is closed until the tissue is firmly compressed and the narrow green band on the inner frame is completely within the confines of the wider black band on the outer frame. The instrument handle must be squeezed as far as it will go and a 'stapling crunch' must be felt by the surgeon.

The linear stapler instrument can be used for colorectal work in a variety of ways. Where an end-to-side anastomosis is constructed the TA or TL instrument can be used to close off the end of the colon. Similarly, the distal end of the bowel can be stapled transversely, either to close the upper rectum as part of the Hartmann's procedure or the low rectum or anus is transected prior to a low colorectal or coloanal anastomosis, with the circular stapling device. Occasionally an end-to-end colocolic anastomosis can be constructed with the TA or TL instrument in the following way (Figure 6.11). The posterior walls of the open colon are approximated with Allis or Babcock forceps and two traction sutures to align the mesenteric and antimesenteric borders are inserted. Traction on these allows the posterior wall of the anastomosis to be drawn into the jaws of the TA or TL 55. The pin is then placed, the jaws closed and the instrument fired. The excess tissue above the jaws of the instrument is excised with the knife prior to release of the jaws. A traction suture is placed in the centre of the two walls of bowel which will form the anterior wall of the anastomosis. Traction on this suture creates a triangle based on the posterior wall. The two sides of this triangle are then stapled in turn with the TA or TL 55. Excess tissue is once again excised. The anastomosis is checked for deficiencies which, if located, are repaired with interrupted manual sutures.

Linear staple cutter

The GIA, TLC or ILA are linear staple cutters. These instruments place four rows of staples across a viscus or viscera and divide it or them between the two double rows. There are various sizes: the GIA range, which may be made of steel or disposable plastic, are 50, 70 or 90 mm long, while the TLC range are 50, 75 or 100 mm in length. They can be used simply to divide the intestine neatly and cleanly without spillage. Combined with the TA or TL instrument they may also be used for constructing an anastomosis with a wide lumen or constructing an ileal or colonic pouch.

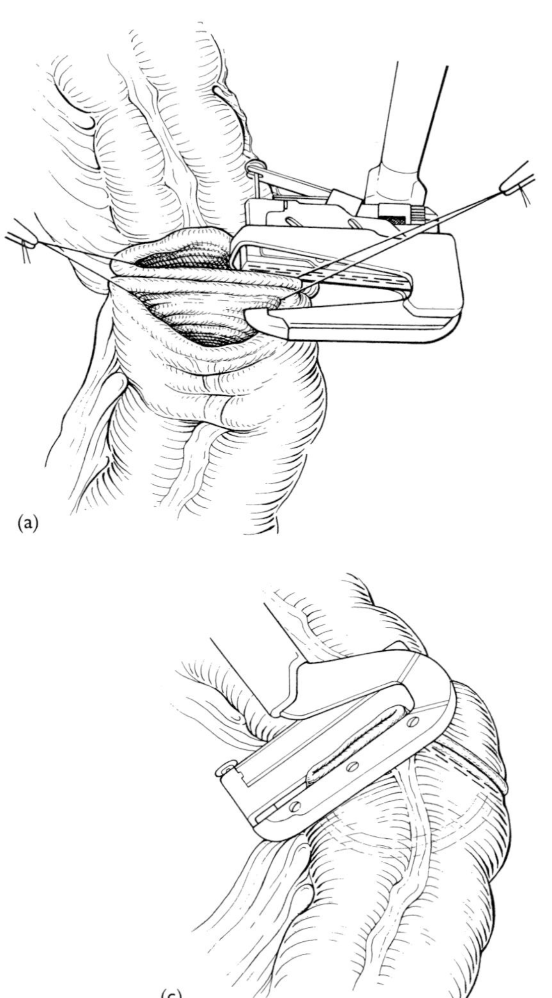

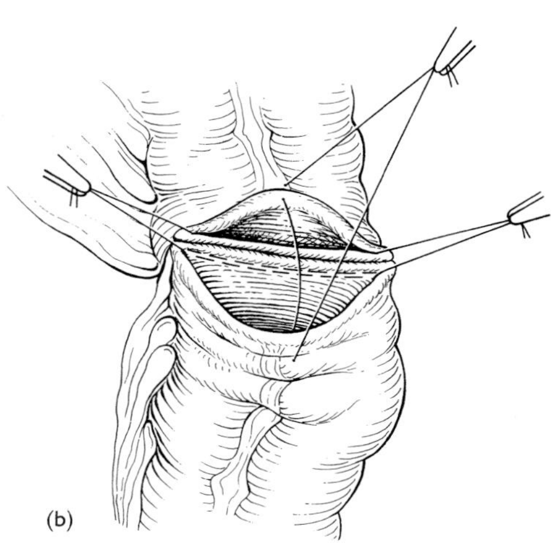

Figure 6.11 End-to-end colocolic anastomosis constructed using the transverse stapling instrument.

The ability of the GIA, TLC or ILA instrument to divide bowel makes it useful for resection of intestine (Figure 6.12).

An opening is first made in the mesocolon or mesentery at the point at which the proximal bowel is to be divided immediately adjacent to the intestine so that one of the jaws of the GIA, TLC or ILA instrument can be placed under the loop. The smaller, lower jaw of the instrument is then slid at right-angles under the intestine at the point of transection and the larger jaw is placed on the upper surface so that the bowel is in the middle of the anvil. The instrument is then closed, the lock lever engaging with a click. Care is taken to ensure that no mesentery or omentum is caught within the jaws of the instrument, otherwise troublesome bleeding may ensue. The push-bar knife assembly is then advanced, dividing the intestine while the two divided ends are simultaneously stapled. The

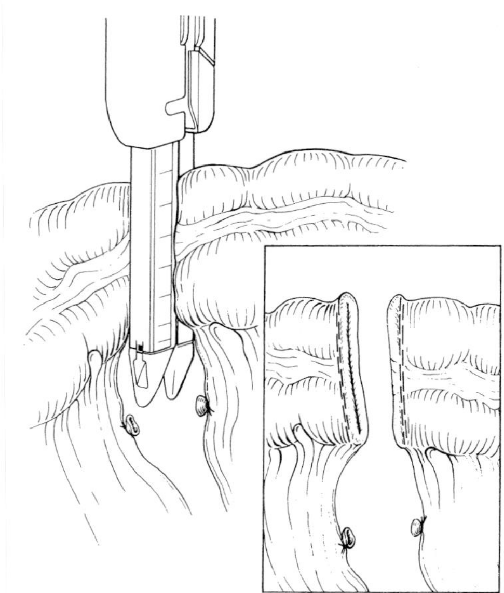

Figure 6.12 Transection and simultaneous stapling of colon using the GIA instrument makes it useful for resection.

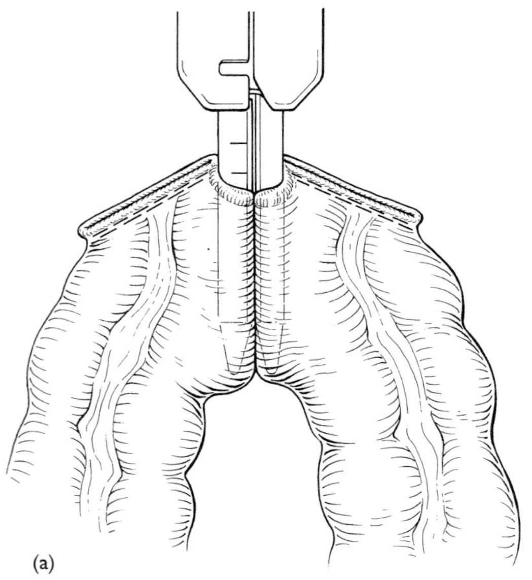

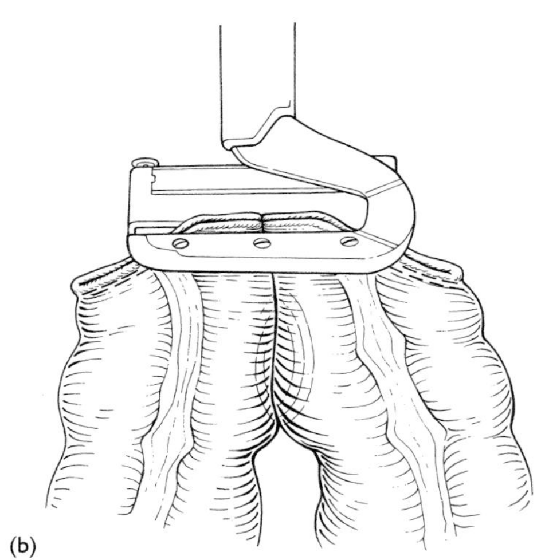

Figure 6.13 (a) Colocolic anastomosis using the GIA instrument (see text). (b) The anterior wall of the newly constructed colocolic anastomosis is closed using the transverse stapling instrument.

procedure is repeated at a point distal to the lesion and after division and ligation of the mesentery the involved segment can be removed. This technique reduces the risk of contamination.

The GIA, TLC or ILA instrument can then be used to make the anastomosis in the following way (Figure 6.13a,b). The antimesenteric corners of the two loops of bowel to be anastomosed are excised. It is often helpful to stabilize the two loops with a 3/0 suture placed in the antimesenteric border. The forks of the instrument are inserted into the two loops of bowel and the antimesenteric borders are carefully approximated. The instrument is then closed and the knife assembly advanced, thereby achieving a long side-to-side anastomosis. This should be checked for bleeding, which, if present, is controlled by under-running with a continuous suture. The anastomosis is completed by closing the two open corners with the TA or TL 55 instrument. The open edges are grasped with sutures and are drawn into the jaws of the stapler. The previous stapled line is overlapped and the instrument fired; protruding tissue is then excised.

A slight modification of the technique involves totally dividing the mesentery in the line of the proposed resection and placing the edges of the bowel to form the side-to-side anastomosis adjacent to one another with stay sutures. Non-crushing clamps are applied to the two bowel ends to be resected, beyond which two small antimesenteric enterotomies are made to facilitate the insertion of the GIA 70 or TLC 75. Once the side-to-side anastomosis is completed, the enterotomy and resection specimen are stapled across transversely with a TA 90 or TL 90.

The GIA, TLC or ILA instrument can also be used for an anterior resection. In these circumstances a modified side-to-side anastomosis may be achieved. It can only be used in this way when a reasonable length of anorectum remains. If this technique is to be used the proximal colon should be divided so that its distal end is stapled transversely with the TA or TL instrument. A stab wound is made in the antimesenteric border of the proximal colon approximately 5 cm proximal to the closed end. The colon is placed into the sacral hollow posterior to the anorectal remnant. The GIA or TLC instrument is then inserted into the two bowel lumens and closed and fired. As a result of this manoeuvre there is now a colorectal cavity. The anterior portion of the anastomosis is completed with an inverted line of continuous or interrupted sutures.

End-to-end circular staplers

End-to-end colocolic or colorectal anastomoses may be achieved by using the third major type of stapling device, the circular stapling 'gun'. This particular instrument has revolutionized the place of sphincter-preserving operations for the treatment of low rectal cancer and ulcerative colitis. It is particularly useful in performing a low colorectal, ileoanal or coloanal anastomosis that cannot be performed, under normal circumstances, by a manual technique. It differs from the instruments so far described in that it produces a circumferential inverted anastomosis.

The basic design of the instrument is shown in Figure 6.14. It consists of the anvil, proximal to which is the shoulder or cartridge segment which contains the staples. In the early versions of the instrument, both the anvil and cartridge segments were mounted on a central shaft and could not be separated. At the other end of the central shaft was a rotating wheel or knob. Anticlockwise rotation caused the anvil and cartridge segment to approximate. Purse-string sutures were placed around the cut edge of each bowel lumen (Figure 6.15). The instrument was inserted through one lumen of the bowel, either via the anus or through an enterotomy. The instrument was opened and the purse-string placed around the open bowel was tied on to the shaft. The cut end of the other segment of bowel, with a second purse-string around the bowel end, was eased over the anvil and the purse-string

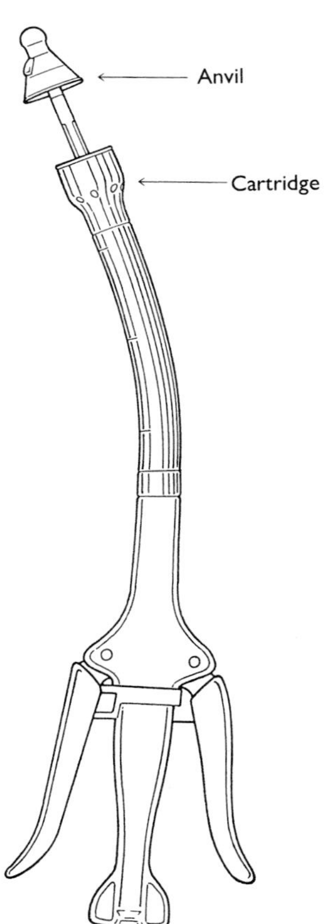

Figure 6.14 Early version of disposable CEEA circular stapling instrument.

was securely tied. The rotating wheel or wing-nut was then turned in a clockwise direction so that the anvil and the cartridge were apposed and separated only by the two purse-strings. When the safety catch was released and the handle of the instrument was compressed, a circular knife protruded from the centre of the cartridge and cut through the two bowel ends, thus producing 'doughnuts' of tissue contained within the purse-string sutures. Simultaneously, a circular row of staples on the outer circumference of the circular knife was advanced with the prongs upwards. These were inserted across the two bowel ends and, as they impacted on the base of the anvil, they were forced into a 'B' configuration. In this manner an inverting circular anastomosis was produced.

The first circular stapling device to be used in the West came from Russia and was known as the SPTU Russian gun (Fain et al, 1975). The problems with this instrument were that it needed very careful maintenance, the staples had to be loaded by hand and only one row of staples was inserted. The American Auto Suture Company (ASC) next produced their disposable factory-packed cartridge gun which consisted of a metal frame and a disposable plastic cartridge with preloaded staples. The EEA stapling instrument was introduced in 1979, and became so successful that the Russian instrument was soon discarded by most surgeons. During 1982 and 1983 Ethicon introduced their ILS range of straight, totally disposable circular cartridge stapling devices. ASC did the same a little later on, producing instruments with curved or straight shafts.

In 1987, USSC produced a modified EEA instrument known as the Premium CEEA and subsequently a Premium plus CEEA (Figure 6.16). This instrument has a detachable anvil and central shaft, which ensures that the anvil can be inserted accurately into the proximal colonic lumen and makes tying of the purse-string suture more reliable, thereby avoiding the cumbersome task of threading bowel over an anvil in awkward situations, as in the bottom of the pelvis. The anvil can then be inserted into the shaft and the anastomosis can proceed in the manner described for the older version EEA. Another advantage is the detachable pin which can be engaged into the cartridge section to facilitate end-to-side or double stapling end-to-end techniques.

The latest modification involves a tilting anvil which flips from horizontal to vertical on disengaging it from the cartridge holder (Figure 6.17). This advance greatly facilitates withdrawal through the rectum and anus. Ethicon also now produce a similarly designed circular stapling instrument with a

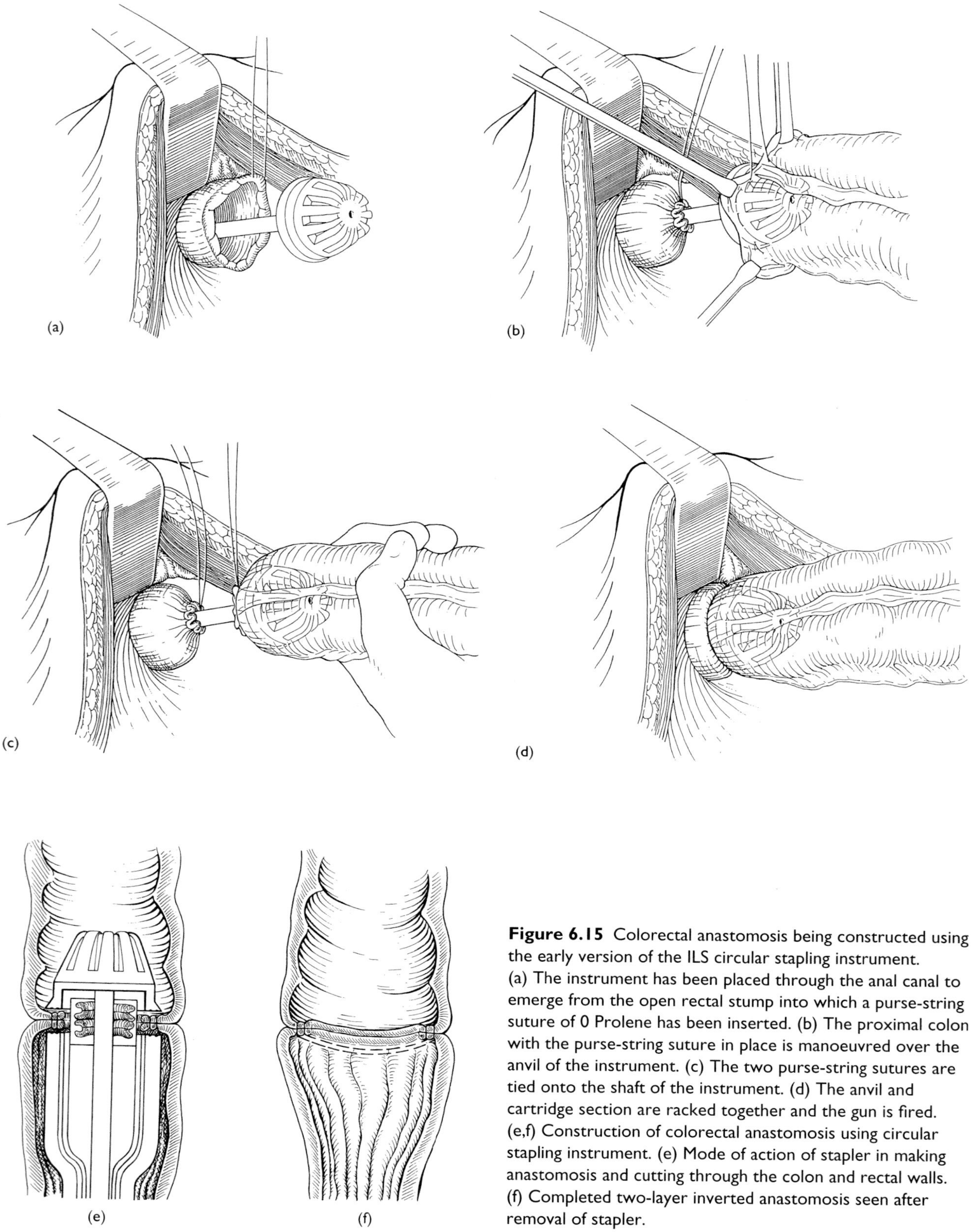

(a)

(b)

(c)

(d)

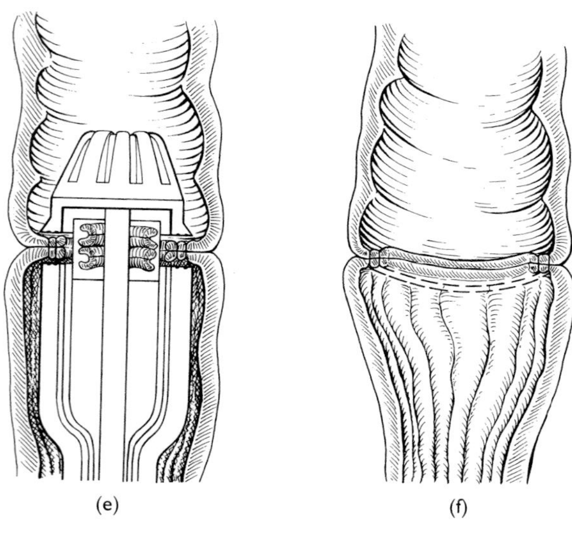

Figure 6.15 Colorectal anastomosis being constructed using the early version of the ILS circular stapling instrument. (a) The instrument has been placed through the anal canal to emerge from the open rectal stump into which a purse-string suture of 0 Prolene has been inserted. (b) The proximal colon with the purse-string suture in place is manoeuvred over the anvil of the instrument. (c) The two purse-string sutures are tied onto the shaft of the instrument. (d) The anvil and cartridge section are racked together and the gun is fired. (e,f) Construction of colorectal anastomosis using circular stapling instrument. (e) Mode of action of stapler in making anastomosis and cutting through the colon and rectal walls. (f) Completed two-layer inverted anastomosis seen after removal of stapler.

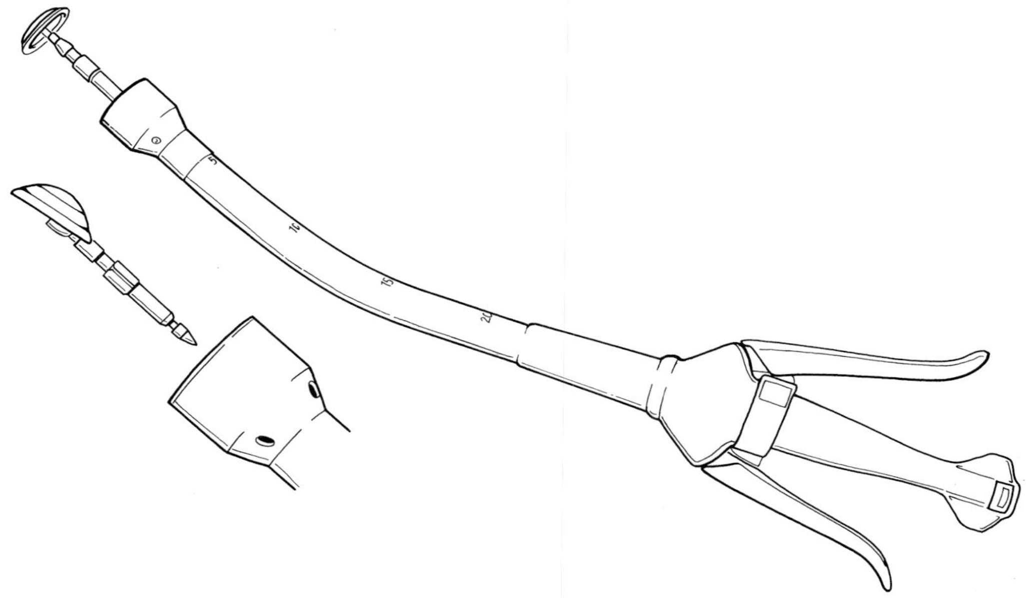

Figure 6.16 Modern circular stapling instruments: Premium Plus CEEA instrument with the tilt top for easy removal (Auto Suture).

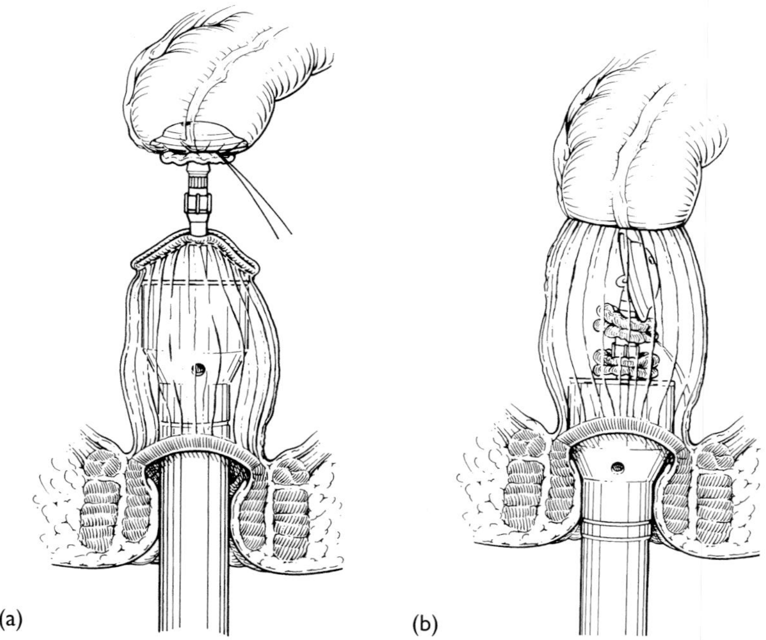

Figure 6.17a–b Double-stapled circular end-to-end anastomosis.

detachable anvil known as the Proximate ILS instrument (Figure 6.18).

It should be noted that the circular stapling instrument can be used in conjunction with the other instruments previously mentioned. Thus a popular method for low colorectal anastomosis is to close the low anorectal stump transversely with a TA or TL instrument. Using the Premium Plus CEEA instrument, a spiked shaft can be placed in the centre of the cartridge segment of the instrument, which can be advanced and retracted by turning the rotating wheel. The cartridge segment is inserted to the transected anorectum and the spike advanced so that it pierces the centre of the staple line (Figure 6.17a). The spike is then removed, revealing the hollow shaft. The detached anvil of the instrument is then inserted into the lumen of the proximal colon and the purse-string tied. The shaft connected to the

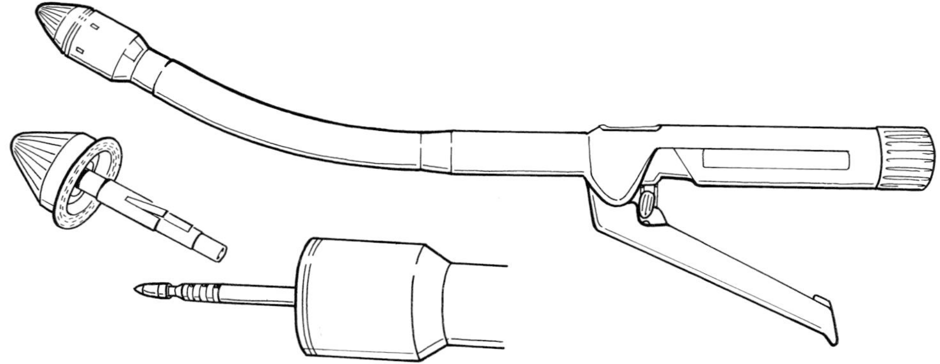

Figure 6.18 Modern circular stapling instruments: Proximate ILS instrument (Ethicon).

anvil is then inserted into the hollow shaft of the cartridge segment so that it clicks home. The gun is racked together and fired (Figure 6.19).

This technique seems to be a safer method of effecting a low anastomosis than the conventional gun technique. As noted previously, Ethicon produced a similar detachable ILS and a stainless steel central pin. The anvil incorporates a hollow shaft that slides over the central pin.The circular stapling cartridges come in three sizes: 25 mm, 29 mm and either 31 mm (USSC) or 33 mm (Ethicon). Only the two larger sizes are widely used in coloproctological practice: the 29-mm cartridge for ileoanal and coloanal anastomosis and the 31-mm or 33-mm instrument for colorectal anastomosis.

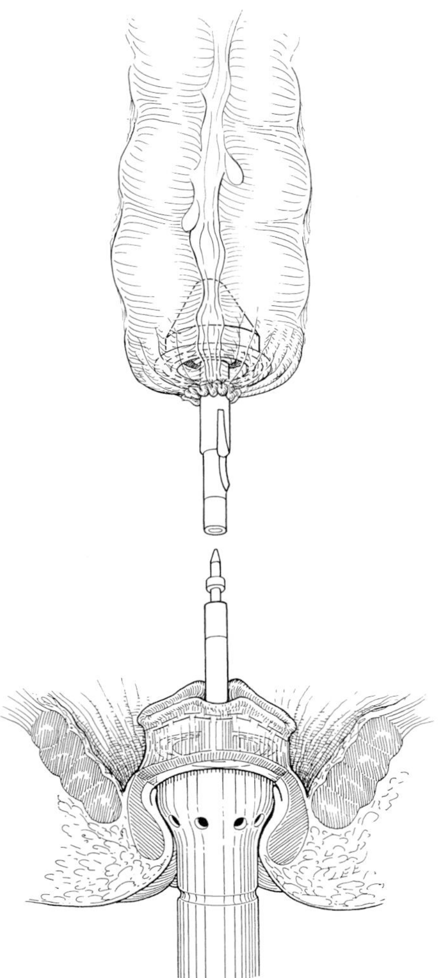

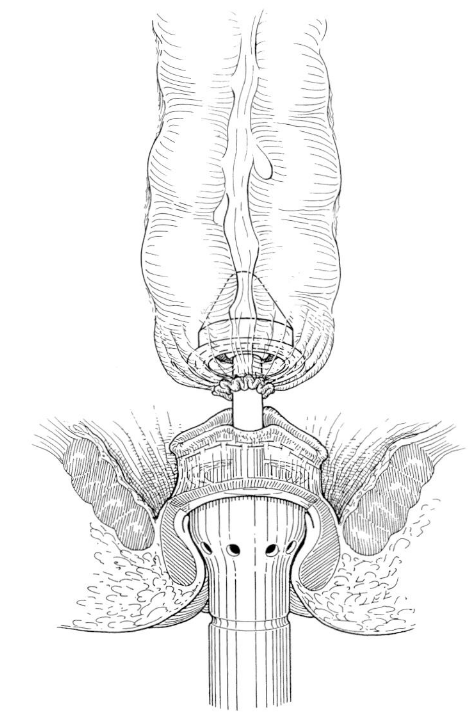

Figure 6.19 Colorectal anastomosis using the Proximate ILS instrument (see text).

The circular stapling instruments have enabled safe colorectal anastomoses to be made at much lower levels in the pelvis than can be performed by hand (Moran, 1996). There are therefore real cost benefits of circular stapling instruments, despite the capital outlay, if the sphincter can be preserved and stomas avoided. The disposable circular stapling instruments are expensive. This poses an important question for the use of stapling instruments in situations where it is just as easy to perform a manual anastomosis. Some justification can be made with respect to operating theatre time since in most situations use of the instruments does save 30–40 minutes of operating time, during which other patients could be operated upon. There are no data to show that stapled anastomoses are safer than conventional techniques (Brennan et al, 1982; Didolkar et al, 1986), although several controlled trials show they are as safe (Everett et al, 1986; West of Scotland and Highland Anastomosis Study Group, 1991; Fingerhut et al, 1994). Nevertheless, it does seem that stapled anastomoses are more prone to stricture formation than manual anastomosis (Fingerhut et al, 1994). All in all it would seem that unless a conventional hand-sewn anastomosis is not feasible, or if there is a very valid reason for shortening the operative time, a stapled procedure should be the second option. The only exception to this policy is that if by using a stapling device a protecting stoma is not needed, then the avoidance of a second hospital admission more than justifies the capital outlay of the stapling instrument.

Other anastomotic techniques

Biofragmentable ring (Valtrac)

This technique is based on the Murphy button (Murphy, 1892) concept, whereby a compression device approximates the two ends of bowel and after several days becomes free in the lumen to be passed per rectum at a later date, leaving the ends of bowel joined together. The advantage of the biofragmentable ring or Valtrac system is that it does not produce necrosis, but fragments during the third week following implantation.

First introduced by Hardy et al in 1985, the ring consists of two segments containing polyglycolic acid (Dexon) and 12% barium sulphate. By producing an anastomosis without sutures, it eliminates any potential problems there might be with the latter. For instance, some regard any foreign material left in an anastomosis, particularly staples, as a potential source for implantation of cancer cells (Phillips and Cooke, 1986). Although there are experimental data to support this, in our opinion the suggestion is scientifically flawed, and, because of the extremely low incidence of suture line recurrence in patients, is unlikely to be important. The Valtrac procedure is said to be more rapid than conventional suturing; however, as presently designed, it is quite limiting with respect to a low rectal anastomosis, especially when compared with the circular stapling device. On the other hand, several prospective controlled trials have demonstrated its safety compared with conventional techniques (Corman et al, 1989; Bubrick et al, 1991; Pahlman et al, 1997). Although this technique may have potential benefits, it has not gained universal popularity; we include it here for the sake of completeness.

Technique (Figure 6.20a–e)

The bowel is mobilized in the usual way. Purse-string sutures of monofilament material are placed in both ends of the bowel to be anastomosed. If a colorectal anastomosis is to be constructed, the device is placed in the proximal end of the colon first because it is easier to pull the rectum onto the ring rather than push the proximal bowel down. If the anastomosis is to be performed well out of the pelvis, it does not matter whether the proximal or distal end is secured first. Triangulation of the lumen using Allis or Babcock clamps helps to slide the proximal end of the bowel over the ring. The purse-string is then tied. The ring is then inserted into the distal bowel and the second purse-string is tied. The ring is snapped shut with an audible and tactile click, and an inverted serosa-to-serosa anastomosis is formed (Corman, 1993).

Other compression devices

Rosati et al (1988) introduced a mechanical device for creating a circular anastomosis through compression. The apparatus consists of three moulded polypropylene rings that are carried by a gun which introduces them into the bowel. Rebuffat et al (1990) used the technique in 56 patients for a variety of colorectal conditions. There was one operative death and an anastomotic dehiscence. Jansen et al (1981) used a similar device consisting of two magnetic rings embedded in polyester. This progressively compressed and necrosed the intervening bowel as the magnetic force gradually increased and healing took place. There are no long-term reports on this method, and neither this nor the Rosati device are widely used.

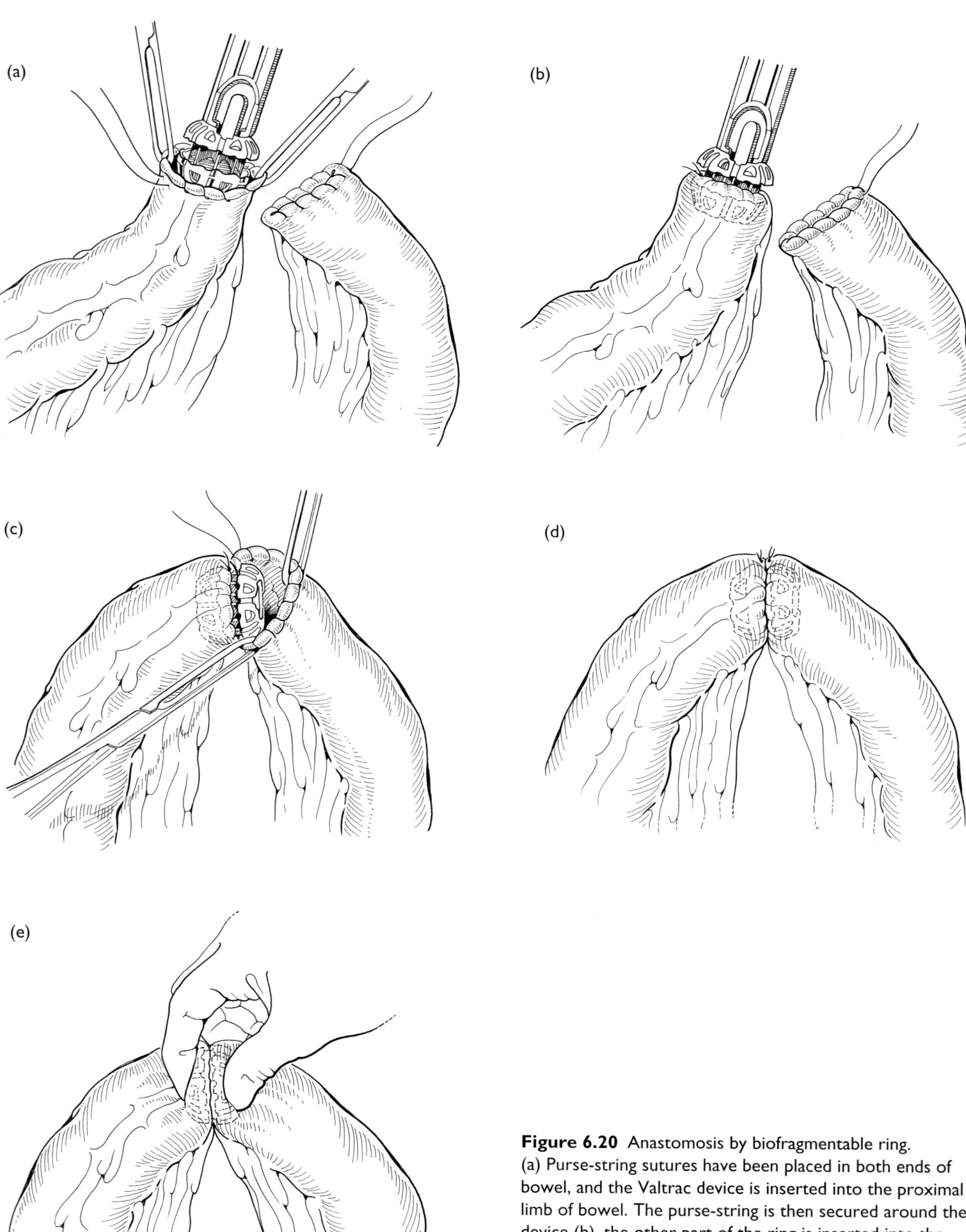

Figure 6.20 Anastomosis by biofragmentable ring. (a) Purse-string sutures have been placed in both ends of bowel, and the Valtrac device is inserted into the proximal limb of bowel. The purse-string is then secured around the device (b), the other part of the ring is inserted into the distal bowel (c) and the purse-string tied (d). (e) The ring is then closed using the thumb and index finger.

Factors affecting anastomotic healing

Anastomotic dehiscence is an important source of morbidity after construction of a large bowel anastomosis. Such a complication can only be prevented if the causes are understood. Many factors may be implicated, including poor surgical technique, lack of judgement and various local and systemic complications. It would appear from the data of Fielding et al (1980) that surgeon-related variables are some of the most important factors.

Local factors

Sepsis

Local sepsis has been shown experimentally to cause a reduction in collagen synthesis and increased lysis of collagen at a colonic anastomosis (Irvin, 1976; Hunt et al, 1980). It is not surprising, therefore, that dehiscence rates tend to be higher if a large bowel anastomosis is performed in the presence of local sepsis. The risk of anastomotic breakdown is increased if a primary anastomosis is performed after colonic resection for perforated diverticulitis, a perforated carcinoma or in some cases of colonic trauma. Faecal contamination is also a potential cause of sepsis and may therefore be responsible for dehiscence.

Bowel preparation

It has been generally accepted that faecal loading has an adverse effect on the healing of colonic anastomoses. Thus retrospective studies (Goligher et al, 1970a; Irvin and Goligher, 1973) have reported an increased anastomotic leakage rate associated with gross faecal contamination. However, a much larger review of 1703 patients by Schrock et al (1973) was unable to demonstrate a relationship between anastomotic disruption and either the method or adequacy of mechanical preparation. Similarly, in two prospective studies (Barker et al, 1971; Rosenberg et al, 1971), the leak rate was not increased when bowel preparation was poor.

The results of experimental studies are equally confusing, although the data are scanty. Thus preoperative evacuation of the bowel may improve survival of devascularized bowel and is equally effective in this respect as preoperative antibiotics (Cohn and Rives, 1955; Cohn et al, 1957). Faecal soiling of the peritoneum increased the leak rate of colonic anastomoses performed in rabbits (Hawley et al, 1970a,b) but similar experiments in dogs produced no significant difference. Despite the conflicting reports concerning the relationship between bowel preparation and anastomotic dehiscence, it seems common sense to ensure that the bowel is empty at the time of anastomosis. Even if faecal loading proves not to be so important in the aetiology of anastomotic breakdown there is little doubt that it is safer to leak from an empty bowel than one that is full of faeces. In addition, the incidence of wound infection is considerably lower when the bowel is adequately prepared preoperatively.

A more extreme method of preventing faecal contamination of an anastomosis during the postoperative period is the construction of a defunctioning stoma. There is no evidence, however, that proximal faecal diversion prevents anastomotic dehiscence. On the contrary, experimental evidence in rats (Blomquist et al, 1985; Uden et al, 1987) demonstrates that a defunctioning stoma results in a 50% reduction of collagen metabolism in left-sided colonic anastomoses, with a concomitant reduction in anastomotic strength. On the other hand it can be argued that if an anastomic dehiscence does take place and a defunctioning stoma has been constructed, the septic complications resulting from it are considerably reduced.

Drains

The effect of drainage of the peritoneal cavity on the healing of large bowel anastomoses has already been considered.

Role of the peritoneum and omentum

The properties of the peritoneum and omentum seem to be important in the healing of large intestinal anastomoses. Exclusion of experimental anastomoses from the peritoneal cavity by wrapping bowel in a variety of materials such as gelatin or oxidized cellulose (Laufman and Method, 1948), polyurethane (Trowbridge and Howes, 1967), Silastic gauze (Canalis and Ravitch, 1968), polyethylene (Rusca et al, 1969) or latex (Hawley, 1970) results in a greater incidence of dehiscence than control anastomoses that are not excluded from the peritoneal cavity. The results of these experiments have been explained on the basis that under normal circumstances bacteria liberated during the construction of an anastomosis are usually satisfactorily eliminated by the peritoneal macrophages and local defence mechanisms. Exclusion of the anastomosis by one of the above methods inhibits these defence mechanisms, resulting in sepsis and an increased risk of anastomotic disruption. It appears that infection adjacent to an anastomosis results in an increase of collagenase activity (Hawley et al, 1970a,b), resulting in anastomotic breakdown. This explanation, however, appears to be too simplistic; in other experiments (Ryan, 1970), when the areas around anastomoses which had been exteriorized from the peritoneal cavity were deliberately infected, dehiscence was a rare event. Clearly, in these experiments the defence mechanism of the peritoneal cavity played no part in the prevention of anastomotic breakdown. These divergent results cast doubt, therefore, on the role of the peritoneal cavity in the healing of anastomoses.

Similar reservations must be expressed concerning the value of the omentum. It is the common belief of many surgeons that wrapping an anastomosis with omentum prevents breakdown. However, several groups have demonstrated in experimental animals that such a manoeuvre is of no benefit (Carter et al, 1972; McLachlin and Denton, 1973), provided the blood supply to the anastomosis is satisfactory. Conversely, McLachlin et al (1976) demonstrated that dehiscence can be prevented by this technique if the anastomosis is first rendered ischaemic. It would appear, therefore, that the omentum improves the blood supply and assists the healing process. Thus, although it may not act as a bacteriological barrier it may still be worth wrapping an anastomosis with omentum, particularly if the surgeon is concerned about the blood supply. Certainly many surgeons throughout the world routinely use this technique (Turner-Warwick et al, 1967; Localio and Eng, 1975; Goldsmith, 1977) for a variety of anastomoses, but the technique is rarely used for large bowel anastomoses. Our own practice at The Royal London Hospital was to use the manoeuvre whenever we were concerned about the integrity of an anastomosis, particularly in elderly patients and those with severe atherosclerosis. However, we have stopped this practice following the results of the first controlled trial which examined this question. Celicout et al (1995) on behalf of the French Association of Surgical Research randomized 705 patients in 19 centres to omental protection (n = 341) or not (n = 364) after colorectal anastomosis. Thirty-five patients (4.9%) had postoperative anastomotic leakage, 16 (4.7%) in the omental protection group and 19 (5.2%) in the control arm. There was also no significant difference in mortality.

Effect of drugs used during anaesthesia

Anaesthetists frequently use neostigmine to reverse the effects of curare-type muscle relaxants at the end of colorectal operations. This is combined with atropine administration, which blocks the muscarinic effects of neostigmine on smooth muscle. Bell and Lewis (1968), working at the Gordon Hospital in London, suggested that there was a risk that the atropine would not entirely block the action of neostigmine and the subsequent active contraction of the intestine after completion of the anastomosis might result in its disruption. They showed that the anastomotic dehiscence rate in a series of patients undergoing colectomy and ileorectal anastomoses and anaesthetized in this way was 36%, which was considerably higher than the leak rate recorded with other anaesthetic techniques. They also claimed that they had visualized the terminal ileum undergoing vigorous peristalsis after curare administration in many of their patients.

The results of a study carried out by Wilkins et al (1970) are therefore of particular interest in this context. These workers recorded intraluminal pressure in the ileum, colon and rectum in conscious and anaesthetized patients and found that neostigmine and atropine when given together or separately (the atropine given before) in doses used during anaesthesia caused significant increase in bowel motility. This response also occurred in a high proportion of patients who were not anaesthetized with halothane. The maximum activity seemed to occur in the ileum. Halothane anaesthesia, however, abolished this abnormal response. Current evidence therefore does suggest that neostigmine should be avoided when a colonic anastomosis is performed, particularly when anaesthesia has not been induced with halothane. This subject is discussed further in Chapter 7.

Systemic factors

The exact role of systemic factors in the aetiology of anastomotic dehiscence has not been clearly defined but it would seem that local factors and surgeon-related variables are far more important. The systemic factors that do seem to play a role are malnutrition, advanced malignancy and excessive blood loss.

Nutritional state

Severe malnutrition in experimental animals results in reduced collagen synthesis at colonic anastomoses (Irvin and Hunt, 1974a,b) and consequently a reduction in tensile strength (Mukerjee et al, 1969; Daly et al, 1970). Furthermore, there is circumstantial evidence from a variety of uncontrolled studies in humans that provision of energy and amino acids, usually in the form of parenteral nutrition, can reverse this process and prevent anastomotic dehiscence. Suffice it to say that there are precious few prospective data confirming this clinical impression, although there are abundant biochemical data which suggest that it should be the case (Sagar et al, 1979; Yeung et al, 1979).

Blood loss

Blood loss during a large bowel operation may affect the healing of an anastomosis in a number of ways. If haemorrhage is excessive, the resulting hypovolaemia leads to reduced colonic flow with subsequent tissue necrosis. In dogs a 10% reduction in blood volume leads to a 28% fall in colonic blood flow. Such a reduction, if uncorrected for any length of time, must lead to tissue hypoxia, which may be sufficient to interfere with adequate colonic healing (Gilmour et al, 1980; Sheridan et al, 1987).

If a tumour is locally advanced its removal will inevitably lead to local tissue damage and blood loss. Such trauma will naturally predispose to peritoneal infection, which in turn may cause dehiscence. A third factor must also be considered. Blood loss inevitably leads to transfusion, which in turn has been shown to decrease the patient's immunocompetence (Burrows and Tartter, 1982; Moffat and Sunderland, 1985; Blumberg et al, 1985). Such an effect may also influence the ability of the anastomosis to heal satisfactorily.

Surgeon-related variables

Until recently there was little information on the relationship of the individual surgeon to the outcome of the anastomosis. In a most revealing study, Fielding et al (1980), as part of the St Mary's large bowel study, found that the dehiscence rates amongst 84 surgeons in 23 hospitals who had performed 1466 large bowel anastomoses ranged from 0.5 to 30%. Similar variability was found by McArdle and Hole (1991), who collected data independently on the complications and outcome in 645 consecutive colorectal cancer patients operated upon by 13 individual surgeons. The anastomotic leakage rates varied between 0% and 25% and postoperative mortality varied between 8% and 30%. These data cannot all be explained by population differences, although presumably a greater proportion of some surgeons' practice involves emergency work, where the risks of anastomotic breakdown are greater. Nevertheless, it seems hard to escape from the conclusion that some surgeons perform colorectal anastomoses badly. Presumably the causes for poor performance relate to individual surgical technique and lack of judgement.

Prevention of adhesions

Adhesions cause a significant morbidity following all abdominal procedures, and colorectal operations are no exception. Our understanding of the pathogenesis of adhesions has improved in recent years (Thompson and Whawell, 1995). Injury to a mesothelial surface leads to an inflammatory response with exudation into the tissues and body cavity. Fibrin is deposited and results in fibrinous adhesions between adjacent surfaces which may then be organized into permanent fibrous adhesions, a process that starts about 4–5 days after injury (Thompson, 1995). Normal mesothelial surfaces possess fibrinolytic activity, but this is lost in inflammation because of cytokine-initiated production and rapid release of plasminogen activator inhibitors (Vipond et al, 1990).

Theoretically, it is possible to interrupt this sequence of events, although attempts to do so up to now have been difficult to carry out and even more difficult to assess. However, the introduction of starch-free glues is now accepted in clinical practice, and barrier methods that rely on physical separation of surfaces with liquid gels or membranes are becoming more prevalent (Wiseman, 1994). Thus, several recent randomized trials of barrier membranes have shown striking reductions in adhesions after laparotomy (Sekiba et al, 1992; di Zerega, 1994; Becker et al, 1995), as assessed by second-look laparotomy or laparoscopy. These agents are either absorbable, examples being regenerated oxidized cellulose (Interceed and hyaluronic acid (HAL-F, Genzyme)) or permanent polytetrafluoroethylene (GoreTex Surgical Membranes). They produce minimal inflammatory response, and prevent the early fibrinous adherence of adjacent surfaces by producing a slow-release lubricant or providing a non-stick surface (Becker et al, 1996). It is likely that these agents will be used far more frequently in the future in colorectal surgery (see Chapter 49). Indications and contraindications relative to laparo-

PRINCIPLES AND TECHNIQUES OF LAPAROSCOPIC SURGERY

scopic surgery of the colon, rectum and anus are discussed in the appropriate sections elsewhere within this textbook. However, it is important to realize that there are major differences between laparoscopic colorectal surgery and other laparoscopic procedures. These critical differences include the following:

1. Laparoscopic colorectal surgery necessitates work in more than one anatomic region because of the position of the colon, thereby requiring relocation of instruments, monitors and personnel.
2. Removal of a small organ or suturing a defect without organ removal enables the entire procedure to be performed through 5–10-mm ports. In contrast, most colorectal procedures require specimen retrieval through large-calibre ports or a small incision.
3. Unlike other procedures, where specimen retrieval brings the procedure to its conclusion, with most colorectal procedures creation of a tension-free, well-vascularized, circumferentially intact anastomosis is required.
4. In contrast to other laparoscopic procedures in which no or few vessels are divided, in most of the colorectal procedures a large number of large mesenteric vessels must be divided in a safe, inexpensive, timely fashion.
5. The loss of tactile sensation is critical in colorectal procedures. Therefore additional procedures such as intraoperative colonoscopy or preoperative colonic tattooing for marking of the lesion are mandatory.
6. Unlike most other laparoscopic procedures, colorectal procedures necessitate the use of advanced instrumentation such as laparoscopic stapling devices, which dramatically increase the cost of these procedures. Like all mechanical devices, these instruments can misfire, adding further time and morbidity to the procedure. Verification of the integrity of all vascular and enteric staple lines is crucial to limit the occurrence of such problems.
7. Finally, perhaps the most serious way in which colorectal procedures differ from others is in the management of cancer. None of the other laparoscopic procedures is performed for the cure of cancer and therefore issues such as local or distant recurrences, long-term survival, and the recently alarming phenomenon of tumour implantation at port sites are relevant to these procedures.

Nevertheless, many principles and tenets of preoperative, intraoperative and postoperative management are uniform regardless of the indication or procedure. To avoid repetition, areas which are germane to multiple diagnoses or operations are discussed within this chapter. These certain similarities include informed consent, adjunct preoperative studies, patient preparation, patient positioning, port placement, operative technique, available instrumentation and postoperative management.

Patient-informed consent

Whether being given prior to an abdominal operation by laparotomy or laparoscopy, consent for an anorectal endoscopic procedure should include the same basic details. Specifically, the various risks, benefits, alternatives and possible complications should be discussed with the patient and preferably also family members. In the United States, it is customary to also use a lengthy signed informed consent as well as documenting this conversation in the patient's medical record. While it is unreasonable for anyone to expect an in-depth discussion of all of the various rare complications (such as parotitis or diabetes insipidus), it is important for the patient to be made aware of the 'standard', more frequently seen problems such as intraoperative haemorrhage, organ injury and cardiopulmonary complications, as well as the more common postoperative complications such as sepsis, anastomotic leak, deep venous thrombosis, myocardial infarction, pulmonary embolism and haemorrhage. In addition, the specific management alternatives for these problems should be mentioned, such as opening an infected wound, percutaneously draining a pelvic abscess or creating a stoma for an anastomotic leak. It is certainly appropriate to mention that, although rare, death can ensue either during or after any operation.

Clearly, this type of informed consent, while traditionally 'American', has become more commonplace elsewhere in the world due to a variety of external forces including increased permeation of lawyers in other societies, increased patient awareness of the possibility of malpractice litigation, and increased exposure of non-American patients to American patients on television and in other media forms.

Several fundamental differences exist relative to the laparoscopic surgical consent form. First, the surgeon who has little experience in laparoscopic colorectal surgery should freely admit this fact to the patient rather than trying to convince the patient of pre-existing expertise. Once again, in the event of any complication, such lack of honesty will virtually ensure major problems. Secondly, if the procedure is being performed for attempted cure of carcinoma, it should be done only within a prospective, randomized trial. In this instance, the patient will need to be given a separate informed consent approved by the local institutional review board or ethics committee. The patient must be made aware of the fact that the 'standard of care' for cure of colorectal carcinoma is currently laparotomy. The patient should certainly be informed of the potential benefits of laparoscopy, as discussed in many places within this textbook. However, they should also be aware of the fact that the curative nature of the procedure has not yet been proven in scientifically valid, prospective, randomized trials.

Thirdly, the patient should be made aware of the fact that conversion to laparotomy may be necessary. The patient should never be promised a laparoscopy to the exclusion of the possibility of a laparotomy becoming necessary either to avert or to solve intraoperative complications. Fourthly, the patient needs to know that additional adjunct procedures may be necessary to facilitate the laparoscopic approach. Although laparoscopic surgery may be beneficial, the patient may opt for laparotomy to avoid additional radiologic or intraoperative measures. It is crucial to employ specific definitions to enable other surgeons to understand what type of procedure is being performed. It is rather clear during a laparoscopic cholecystectomy or herniorrhaphy if the procedure is converted as a non-trocar standard incision was made. However, given the fact that a large specimen needs to be removed during laparoscopic colorectal surgery, the terms used are often more vague and confusing. Some surgeons have suggested definitions other than those proposed here in Table 6.2 (Phillips, 1994). Senagore et al (1995) and Fleshman et al (1996) have included in their definition of 'successful laparoscopic' procedures, those performed through 15–25-cm-long incisions.

Adjunct studies

Whether the procedure is being performed by laparotomy or laparoscopy, if the diagnosis is an inflammatory disorder such as terminal ileal Crohn's disease or sigmoid diverticulitis, preoperative CT scanning is helpful to exclude an abscess. In addition, if a phlegmon is present in the iliac fossa, intraoperative ureteric catheters may be desirable whether the procedure is being performed by laparotomy or laparoscopy. Placement of ureteric catheters may delay the commencement of the colorectal portion of the procedure by 20–30 minutes, but may save more than that amount of time during the operation if the ureteric catheter is readily appreciated, despite intense inflammation. In a recent study, Parameswaran et al (1997) sought to evaluate the results of elective intraoperative ureteric catheterization in patients who underwent

Table 6.2 Differences between resectional laparoscopic colorectal surgery and other laparoscopic procedures.

Considerations	*Variable*	*Colon*	*Other procedures: cholecystectomy herniorrhaphy fundoplication*
Anatomy	Quadrants	Multiple	Single
Vascular	Vascularity	Multiple	Single
	Vascular ligation	Complex	Rapid
Procedures	Resection	At least two sites	One
	Anastomosis	Usually required	Never required
Result	Specimen	Large: Requires enlargement of port site extirpation	Small: (cholecystectomy, appendectomy) can be retrieved through 10-mm port or None: (herniorrhaphy, fundoplication)

either re-operative pelvic surgery or had prior pelvic sepsis or radiation. The retrospective review of 189 patients who underwent intraoperative catheterization during a 4-year period showed that catheterization was deemed necessary for various diagnoses including diverticular disease, Crohn's disease and mucosal ulcerative colitis, rectal cancer, pelvic radiation, ischaemia, endometriosis and recurrent rectal prolapse. Of the 189 procedures 16.4% (31) were laparoscopic or laparoscopic-assisted procedures, while the remainder were done by laparotomy. Results showed that the ureters in all patients were intraoperatively identified and that there were no intraoperative ureteric complications attributable either to the catheters or to the colorectal procedure. There was only a 1% post-operative morbidity and there was only an additional cost of $450.00 to the procedure. It was therefore concluded that elective ureteric catheterization is rapid, inexpensive and safe in patients who are potentially at increased risk of ureteric injury.

Because of the lack of tactile sensation during laparoscopic colorectal procedures, a variety of early studies reported the wrong section of colon having been excised because of the inability to palpate and therefore verify the location of the pathology (Monson et al, 1992; Larach et al, 1993). Perhaps even more disconcerting are the cases in which following surgery to remove the segment known to contain what was preoperatively and intraoperatively thought to have been the only neoplastic lesion, several patients presented with bowel obstruction soon after the index operation. In each instance, a preoperatively and intraoperatively unrecognized, synchronous, proximal tumour was the cause of the obstruction (McDermott et al, 1994; Fingerhut, 1996). Although such problems occur during laparotomy, they certainly intuitively seem more likely to occur in the setting in which manual palpation is impossible. These problems seem to occur early in one's experience.

It seems clear that although a certain amount of information can be gleaned by the experience of the laparoscopist using 'clamp palpation', other more accurate means of lesion identification are desirable. These measures include the standard availability of intraoperative colonoscopy. In this instance, informed consent should be given by the patient, the consent form should include the possibility of intraoperative colonoscopy, and the equipment should be readily available in the operating room. For this reason, all patients are placed in the modified lithotomy position, in case colonoscopy is necessary.

Another alternative is the routine performance of an air contrast barium enema prior to surgery. The patient needs to be informed that this additional measure would not generally be undertaken if the procedure were to be performed by laparotomy. A third alternative includes preoperative marking of the area around the lesion with either India ink, indocyanine green, or methylene blue. The first agent is probably superior in terms of longevity and lack of diffusion throughout the mesentery. However, great care must be taken to inject all four sites at 90° intervals as it is impossible to tell during colonoscopy which of the areas represents the mesenteric margin. Thus, regardless of which method is employed, some additional thought must be given to ensure that the lesion will be appropriately identified and resected at the time of surgery.

Preoperative patient preparation

A variety of issues need to be considered prior to surgery. Once again, some of these concerns parallel those outlined elsewhere in this chapter for patients scheduled to undergo laparotomy. For example, if a stoma may be necessary, because of a diagnosis such as diverticulitis, Crohn's disease, mucosal ulcerative colitis or an obstructing neoplasm, then the patient should be preoperatively counselled and marked. No differences exist between either the counselling procedure or the localization for the stoma, as noted elsewhere. Bowel preparation for laparoscopy includes a mechanical cathartic preparation as well as both oral and parenteral antibiotic administration.

In the late 1980s, a survey of the American Society of Colon and Rectal Surgeons revealed that 100% of members employed some form of mechanical bowel preparation (Solla and Rothenberger, 1990). Unfortunately, this survey was undertaken at a time when polyethylene glycol preparation was most commonly used. Since then, two prospective, randomized trials have been carried out comparing polyethylene glycol to the supposedly better-tasting sulphate-free (but also 4 L) polyethylene glycol and in turn comparing both of these solutions to two 45 mL doses of sodium phosphate (Cohen et al, 1994; Oliveira et al, 1997).

The first study included 450 consecutive patients scheduled to undergo colonoscopy. Before and after bowel preparation, all patients were weighed and serum electrolytes as well as phosphate, magnesium, calcium and osmolarity were measured. In addition, a detailed patient questionnaire was used to assess side-effects and patient satisfaction. Endoscopists blinded to the type and quantity of preparation used scored the type of residual stool and the percentage of bowel wall visualized for each segment of colon and for the overall examination. Nurses recorded all procedure times as well as the quality of irrigation and aspiration route utilized. Four hundred and twenty-two age- and gender-matched patients completed all phases of the trial. Overall, endoscopists scored sodium phosphate as 'excellent' or 'good' in 90% versus 70% and 73% after the polyethylene glycol or sulphate-free polyethylene glycol lavage, respectively ($P<0.01$). Moreover, particulate or solid stool was found in all segments of the colon, more frequently after both of the two large-volume preparations than after the small-volume sodium phosphate ($P<0.05$). Eighty-three per cent of the patients who received the sodium phosphate preparation stated that they would take the same preparation again versus only 19% and 33% for polyethylene glycol and the sulphate-free polyethylene glycol lavage, respectively ($P<0.01$). The conclusion of the study was that the small-volume oral sodium phosphate solution was not associated with any clinically significant problems, caused no increase in the incidence of side-effects, was vastly preferred by patients, and was more effective in colonic cleansing in this endoscopist-blinded trial (Cohen et al, 1994).

As a result of that trial, a second group of 200 consecutive patients scheduled to undergo colorectal resection by either laparotomy or laparoscopy were prospectively randomized between the 4 L of polyethylene glycol and the two 45-ml volumes of sodium phosphate preparation (Oliveira et al, 1997). The findings of the trial were virtually identical to those of the earlier one. There was no increased septic sequelae with the smaller volume preparation, that preparation was vastly preferred by patients, and surgeons detected no difference in the cleansing ability. Based upon the overwhelming superiority of the sodium phosphate preparation in both of these prospective, randomized, blinded trials, it has become our routine preparation of choice prior to both laparotomy and laparoscopy.

Specifically, all patients are instructed to consume liquids only, commencing at 1.00 p.m. on the day prior to surgery. The polyethylene glycol preparation is taken as 45 mL followed by a 230-mL glass of water at 4.00 p.m., repeating this regimen at 10.00 p.m. the day before the procedure. In addition to this mechanical bowel preparation, a modified Condon–Nicholls preparation is used, wherein patients receive 1 g each of metronidazole and neomycin, by mouth, at 1.00 p.m., 2.00 p.m. and 10.00 p.m., the day before surgery. On arrival in the operating room, patients receive 2 g of cefotaxime and 1 g of metronidazole. The cefotaxime is repeated every 8 hours for 24 hours; the metronidazole is repeated as 500 mg every 8 hours, also for 24 hours.

Other standard measures which are useful in laparoscopy include placement of a nasogastric tube and urinary bladder catheter after induction of anaesthesia. The nasogastric tube is generally removed at the conclusion of the procedure, although the bladder catheter is left in for a variable period of time, contingent upon the dissection performed. These details are discussed below.

Any intra-abdominal or intrapelvic surgery is associated with the risk of deep venous thrombosis. Since laparoscopic procedures entail elevation of the legs in Lloyd Davies position for long periods of time, consideration of antiembolic manoeuvres is important. At the very least, sequential compression stockings should be used in all patients. Furthermore, many surgeons advocate routine use of 5000 units of subcutaneous heparin every 12 hours, commencing on arrival in the operating room and continuing until the patient is either fully ambulatory or even discharged from hospital. The newer low molecular weight single-dose heparin is discussed elsewhere in this textbook. Regardless of the regimen employed, care should be taken to limit the possibility of a venous thrombosis. It is the author's preference to employ both sequential compression stockings and subcutaneous heparin in all patients (SAGES, 1998).

Patient positioning

As previously mentioned, it is desirable to have transanal access to facilitate intraoperative colonoscopy. Furthermore, the position between the legs may be a useful one for either the assistant or camera-holder, particularly when dissecting the splenic flexure. Accordingly, all patients are placed in the modified lithotomy position in Allen stirrups (Allen Medical Corp., Bedford Heights, OH, USA) with no more than 15° flexion in each knee and hip (Figure 6.21). Any additional flexion may impede the axis of motion of the instruments in the iliac fossa ports. Our preference is to utilize the Allen rather than the traditional Lloyd Davies stirrups; the former obviates the potential for direct compression of the peroneal nerve, as the boot-like configuration does not exert any pressure upon the fibular head.

It is important for the operating room table to have the capacity to tilt into the steep Trendelenburg and anti-Trendelenburg positions as

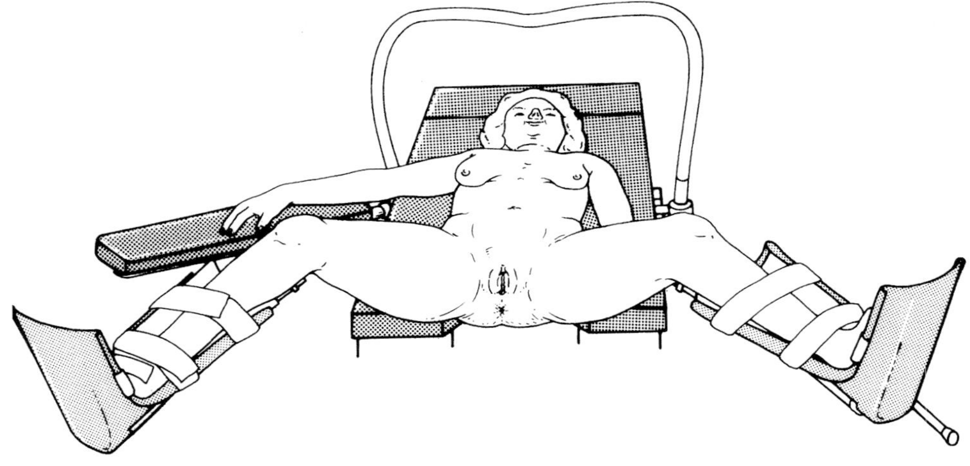

Figure 6.21 The Lloyd Davies position modified to include the use of Allen stirrups.

well as steep left- and right-side-down positions, respectively. These manoeuvres provide the means for laparoscopic bowel retraction, and table position and gravity are the best means by which loops of bowel can be removed from the operative field. Clearly, the patient must be secured to the table in some manner to prevent injury during these positions. In addition, in order to maximize access, both the arms should be tucked into the sides but obviously well padded to prevent injury to the ulnar nerve or other areas. The previously mentioned nasogastric tube will decompress the stomach and should prevent injury during Veress needle and/or trocar insertion (Figure 6.22). Similarly, the indwelling urinary bladder catheter should help to prevent injury to that structure. Also, as previously outlined, if an iliac fossa phlegmon is either clinically suspected or discovered by preoperative CT, then ureteric stents may be placed after induction of general endotracheal anaesthetic, but prior to commencement of the laparoscopic phase of the procedure.

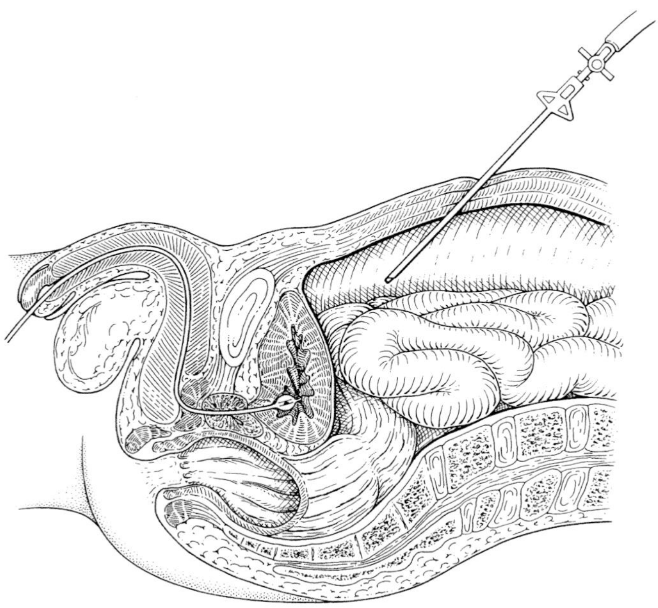

Figure 6.22 Use of a Veress needle technique to establish a pneumoperitoneum. A bladder catheter helps decompress the urinary bladder and prevent injury to it.

Instruments

'Standard' laparoscopy instrumentation such as a 0 degree camera, light source and insufflator are important. A minimum of two monitors is important for laparoscopic colorectal surgery. The size of the operating field and the need to reposition personnel frequently during the operation, as well as the number of people often required to perform this operation, necessitates multiple monitors. It is our preference to utilize all 10–12-mm ports so that three to four ports are used for most resections and two to three ports for stoma creation.

Various companies sell both disposable and reusable 10-mm diameter instruments. In general, either electrocautery scissors or, preferably, a harmonic (ultrasonic) scalpel (Ethicon Endosurgery Inc., Cincinnatti, OH, USA) along with two 'atraumatic' Babcock-type clamps, a modified Allis anvil grasping clamp, clips for ligation, a 10-mm-diameter non-crushing bowel clamp, and pretied sutures are important.

Other surgeons have advocated the neodymium YAG contact laser instead of monopolar electrosurgery in laparoscopic intestinal surgery (Bohm et al, 1994). Previous publications have detailed a wide array of ports, trocars, stapling devices, retractors, suturing devices and even camera holders commercially available (Simmang and Rosenthal, 1994).

Other frequently used adjuncts, as described below, include both 35-mm and 60-mm endoscopic linear cutters. The former size is generally used for vascular ligation and division and the latter for transection of the rectosigmoid junction. The dedicated laparoscopic operating theatre should include a colonoscope readily available at all times.

Port placement and technique

The vast majority of laparoscopic resections can be successfully performed through 10–12-mm ports. The only difference between the right- and left-sided procedures is that because of the need for intracorporeal vascular division of the inferior mesenteric, left colic or sigmoidal arteries and veins, an infraumbilical camera port is favoured for left-sided resections. Conversely, such a camera port position for right-sided resections would greatly limit visibility as that site would place the camera almost directly over the ileocaecal valve. Therefore, for right-sided resections, a supraumbilical camera port is chosen. Mirror-image port configurations are then used for the right and left side; for right-sided resections a left iliac fossa and left paraumbilical port are used. In obese patients or patients with tremendous redundancy, a left upper quadrant port can be used for flexure mobilization or retraction. The mirror-image configuration is utilized for sigmoid resections. For right-sided resections the surgeon stands to the patient's left and vice versa.

For all of these procedures, most of the dissection is accomplished with a 10-mm (relatively) atraumatic Babcock-type grasping forceps and a 10-mm-diameter ultrasonic scalpel; occasionally, a 10-mm-diameter electrocautery scissors is utilized. Using these tools, the right or left side of the colon is dissected commencing in the respective iliac fossa and proceeding in a cephalad direction around the flexure. To dissect the colon with the exception of the flexures, significant Trendelenburg and contralateral table tilt is essential. To dissect the flexures, reverse Trendelenburg position with maintenance of contralateral table tilt is exceedingly useful. Once again, in markedly obese patients, patients with significant adhesions, or patients with tremendous colonic redundancy, the optional third contralateral upper quadrant 10–12-mm port may be useful. A 10-mm grasping instrument through that port can facilitate this component of the dissection.

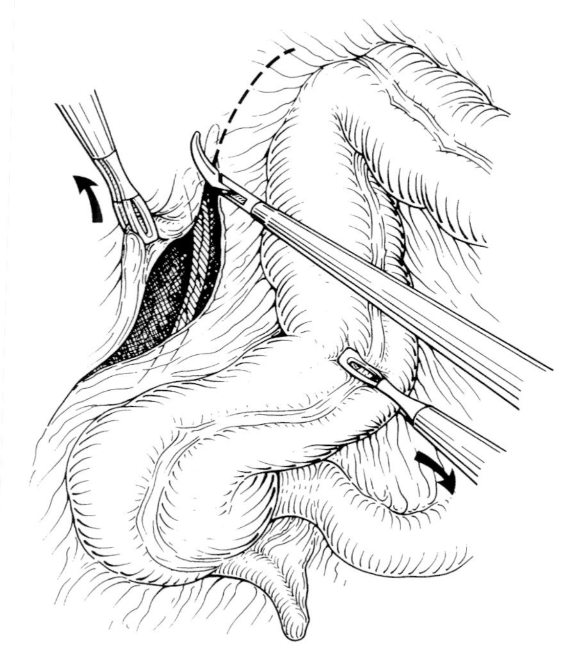

Figure 6.23 Babcock-type clamps used in the dissection of the hepatic flexure. The right ureter should be identified.

Full mobilization of the right colon is acknowledged when the right ureter and the duodenum have been utilized and reflected posteriorly and the dissection has proceeded to the level of the middle colic vessels (Figures 6.23 and 6.24). Similarly, the left-sided dissection is completed when the left ureter has been reflected posteriorly, common splenic flexures have been mobilized, and the gastrocolic omentum has been divided to the level of the middle colic vessels (Figure 6.25).

The transverse colon poses unique problems, especially if the mesentery is fat or if the gastrocolic omentum is fused to the ventral aspect of the transverse mesocolon. In this latter instance, it may be advantageous to retain the omentum *in situ* by mobilizing the colon along the avascular embryological attachment to the omentum. The preference of the author is to perform an *en bloc* omentectomy with the ultrasonic scalpel commencing at the respective flexure and proceeding in a contralateral direction remaining sufficiently caudal of the gastroepiploic vessels to prevent injury to those structures.

The rectum is best accessed by ventral traction. If the uterus and round ligaments interfere with the dissection, a suture on a Keith needle can be passed transabdominally to intracorporeally encircle the round ligament and then be delivered back through the abdominal wall to retract the uterus against the abdominal wall. Although some surgeons have described the use of the uterus sonde for this procedure, the author feels more comfortable with the suture method. The rectal mobilization can occasionally be facilitated by a transanally placed proctoscope or colonoscope. Once again, like the uterine fixation sutures, this method saves the use of a port. The ultrasonic scalpel is well suited to total mesorectal excision.

After full mobilization of the right colon, the right colic vessels can be either intracorporeally or extracorporeally divided. Our preference after full right colonic mobilization is to extend the supraumbilical port site from the initially placed 10-mm vertical incision to a 3–5-cm vertical supraumbilical incision through which the specimen can be delivered. Patients with caecal polyps can usually have this manoeuvre accomplished through the smaller incision while patients with phlegmonous ileal Crohn's disease generally require the larger incision. If appropriate mobilization has been undertaken, the superior mesenteric vessels can be seen and a high ligation performed for a malignant disease or a more distal blood supply preserving ligation for patients with inflammatory bowel disease. In the patients with inflammatory bowel disease, complete intracorporeal inspection of the entire

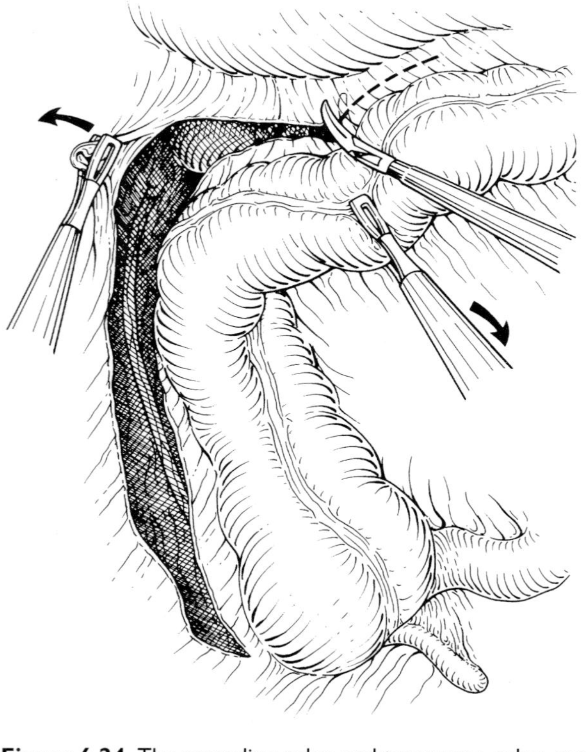

Figure 6.24 The ascending colon and transverse colon can be retracted inferiorly and medially so that the omentum is separated from the colon relatively easily.

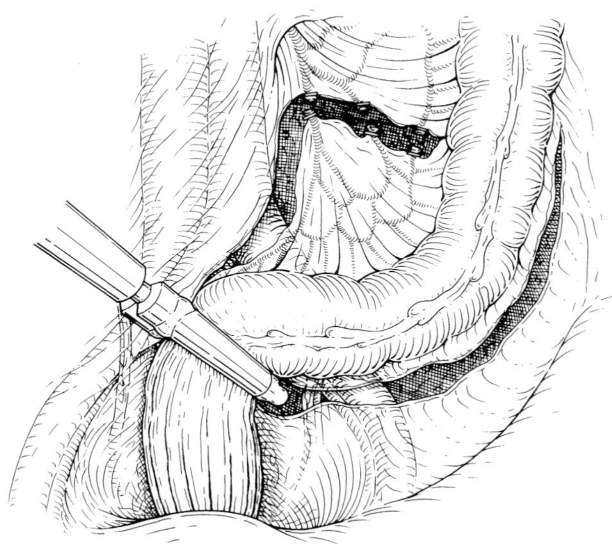

Figure 6.25 The proximal rectum is divided using one (or more) applications of the 60-mm linear stapler.

length of the small bowel from the duodeno-jejunal flexure to the ileocaecal valve will have been performed at the commencement of the procedure. Full inspection should not be performed extracorporeally as delivery of the small bowel through this small incision may result in trauma to the bowel or its mesentery, venous congestion, or significant postoperative ileus due to the amount of handling and force necessary to inspect all of the bowel through this small site.

Although intracorporeal vascular division, bowel transection and anastomosis are technically feasible, it is our belief that such a manoeuvre presents a triumph of technique over common sense. Since after appropriate mobilization the ligation can be rapidly, safely and inexpensively performed, as can the bowel transection anastomosis, there is no reason to prolong the procedure and increase the expense merely to facilitate a laparoscopic intracorporeal right-sided procedure. This is confirmed when one considers that even if the intracorporeal procedure is completed as performed, the incision must still be made in order to ultimately deliver the specimen.

One additional technical pointer is important: the mesentery should be divided first and the mesenteric defect partially closed prior to transection of the bowel and performance of an anastomosis. This precaution is necessary as anecdotal reports have noted malrotation of the bowel because of malalignment. If the bowel is transected prior to mesenteric division, it is easy to understand how the limbs can become twisted through such a small opening.

The inferior mesenteric vessels cannot be delivered through the skin as can right colic vessels. The inferior mesenteric artery at its junction with the aorta must be intracorporeally transected either individually with clips or with the endoscopic linear vascular stapler/cutter. Similar treatment of the inferior mesenteric vein at the duodeno-jejunal flexure and tail of the pancreatic junction is necessary. After left-sided intracorporeal vascular division, the laparoscope affords excellent visualization of the sympathetic nerves. Either the harmonic scalpel or the 10-mm-diameter electrocautery scissors can be used to continue the dissection in a distal direction beyond the sacral promontory distally to the rectum, laterally along the pelvic side-walls, and into the levator hiatus. Similarly, the vagina can be ventrally retracted by transvaginal digitation, facilitating ultrasonic dissection of the anterior wall from the posterior vaginal wall. In this manner, the laparoscopic dissection can proceed to the same level as dissection during laparotomy. The only limiting feature is that although the dissection can proceed as distally, the currently available laparoscopic stapler cannot be placed as low as the 30-mm stapler during a laparotomy.

After full left-sided rectal or rectosigmoid mobilization, the procedures are directed by the surgical indication. Cases to include an anastomosis are accomplished by inserting a 33-mm port (Ethicon Endosurgery Inc., Cincinnati, OH, USA) in the left upper quadrant or left paraumbilical region. Prior to delivery of the specimen through the site, intracorporeal verification of sufficient length to achieve an anastomosis is undertaken. Also prior to delivery of the specimen, the rectosigmoid junction or desired level of the rectum is identified and transected with a 60-mm stapler introduced through the right iliac fossa port. Obviously, the 10–12-mm port will have been exchanged for an 18-mm port to facilitate introduction of a 60-mm stapler.

The extracorporeal phase of the left-sided procedure consists only of division of the marginal vessels, division of the bowel, introduction of the anvil, and returning the bowel and anvil into the peritoneum. However, if a stoma is to be created, the procedure concludes after bowel transection by construction of the colostomy. If anastomosis is necessary, either the 33-mm port can be maintained in place, or the fascia at that site can be closed after reinsufflation to a pressure of 15 mmHg. This specially designed anvil-grasping clamp is utilized to place the anvil under direct vision onto the trocar of the stapler (Figure 6.26). The stapler closure procedure should be observed through the right iliac fossa camera port to ensure exclusion of extraneous structures and to ensure proper orientation of the descending colon and its mesentery. After the anastomosis is complete, the pelvis is filled with water, and an atraumatic (non-crushing) bowel clamp is placed across the descending colon; an endoscopic evaluation of the anastomosis with air insufflation is undertaken to verify the anastomotic level, its haemostasis and its integrity.

If an abdominoperineal resection is to be performed, the perineal phase proceeds in the standard manner, after which the colostomy is constructed. In cases of Hartmann's reversal, the procedure is undertaken according to the guidelines given in Chapter 9 for anastomotic creation. The only technical caveat is that in initial stoma mobilization the author performs as much enterolysis as possible through the stoma site prior to returning the stoma with the *in situ* stapler anvil into the peritoneal cavity.

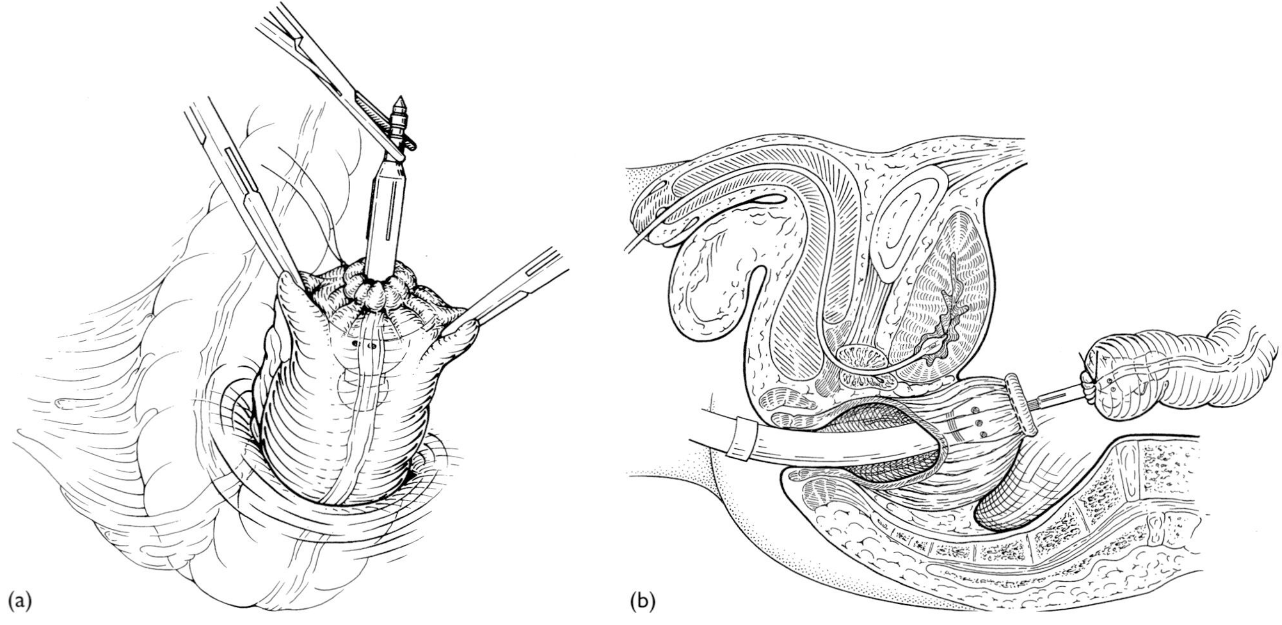

Figure 6.26 (a) After the bowel is resected, the anvil of a circular stapler is secured in the proximal bowel. (b) The bowel and anvil are returned to the abdominal cavity, the circular stapler is introduced per anus, and a double-stapled anastomosis is performed.

Postoperative management

A recent meta-analysis of over 4000 patients evaluated in trials meant to assess the need or lack of need for nasogastric tube suction after elective colorectal surgery clearly demonstrated that these tubes were not necessary in approximately 90% of patients (Reiver and Wexner, in press). It has been this author's practice for the last 10 years to remove nasogastric tubes even after laparotomy. Prior to the advent of laparoscopy, other measures were undertaken to expedite bowel recovery and hospital discharge (Cheape et al, 1991). In one prospective, surgeon-blinded randomized trial the two groups of patients either received or did not receive metaclopromide intravenously administered every 8 hours from the completion of surgery until a solid food diet was able to be tolerated. Assessment of the 100 consecutive patients who underwent elective abdominal colorectal procedures in this group failed to reveal any differences in the length of time between the two groups relative to the intake of either oral fluid or solid food. Accordingly, metaclopromide did not allow for expedited bowel recovery.

Many enthusiasts of laparoscopy have claimed more expeditious gut function than after laparotomy (Bohm et al, 1995). However, although electromyographic and other laboratory parameters may reveal a more rapid bowel recovery after laparoscopy than after laparotomy, the majority of clinical studies that have revealed marked improvements in speed of discharge in the laparoscopic group have been imbalanced. Specifically, most of these investigators have kept their patients 'nil per os' following laparotomy while allowing their laparoscopic patients to eat food commencing either on the day of surgery or the day after. Similarly, the same laparoscopic enthusiasts often allow their patients in the laparoscopy groups to be discharged home prior to having a bowel movement, whereas patients in the laparotomy group are kept in hospital until after bowel movement.

We performed two prospective, randomized trials to assess the possibility of early postoperative feeding (claimed as a unique benefit of laparoscopic surgery) after laparotomy and colorectal resection (Binderow et al, 1994; Reissman et al, 1995). The first trial included 64 consecutive patients who underwent laparotomy with either a colonic or ileal resection. In all cases, the nasogastric tube was removed immediately after the operation. The two groups of 32 patients each were well matched for age by both mean and range of age, diagnosis and procedure type. In the 'traditional' group, patients were kept 'nil per os' until they passed flatus. At that point, a clear fluid diet was administered until the patient had a bowel movement, after which a regular diet was permitted. Patients were kept in hospital until they were tolerating a regular diet, moving their bowels, and had no abdominal distension, nausea or vomiting. Patients in the early oral intake group were permitted a regular diet on the first postoperative morning. A nasogastric tube was reinserted in patients in either group if they had more than a single, self-limiting episode of more than 100 mL of vomiting within 24 hours. The rate of nasogastric tube reinsertion for distension with persistent vomiting was 18.7% in the traditional group and 12.5% in the early oral feeding group. There was no difference relative to the duration of postoperative ileus. Patients in the early oral feeding group who did not require a nasogastric tube were discharged sooner than were other patients.

A second trial, also prospectively randomized, included 161 consecutive patients again well matched between the two groups for a mean age and age range, diagnosis and procedure. The only difference in the second trial was that the early oral feeding group was permitted clear fluids rather than a solid food diet immediately after surgery and had their diet advanced, as it was also in the traditional feeding group. As in the first study, in both groups of patients, hospital discharge was not permitted until the patient had had at least one bowel movement, tolerated at least three solid meals and had no nausea, vomiting or abdominal distension. Nasogastric tube reinsertion was necessary in 11% of patients in the early feeding group and 10% in the traditional feeding group. The length of hospital stay was reduced from 6.8 to 6.2 days and the overall complication rate was the same in the two groups at 7.5% and 6.1% respectively.

These two trials reached the same conclusion. Specifically, early oral feeding need not be denied to patients after either laparoscopy or colorectal resection by laparotomy. Thus, our standard practice is to remove the nasogastric tube in the operating room, to allow a clear fluid diet to commence on the morning after surgery, to advance to a regular diet as requested by the patient, and to discharge home when the patient is having bowel movements, tolerating a solid food diet and not experiencing nausea, vomiting or abdominal distension.

As mentioned earlier, antibiotics are continued after surgery for 24 hours in the empiric prophylactic manner or longer if clinically indicated as a therapeutic measure. The pneumatic sequential compression stockings and subcutaneous heparin are maintained until the patient is discharged from hospital. If the patient experiences more than two episodes of 100 mL emesis within 24 hours, a nasogastric tube is inserted. As outlined above, this manoeuvre is necessary in approximately 10% of patients.

If a low pelvic dissection has been performed, the indwelling catheter remains for approximately 4–5 days. If no pelvic dissection has been performed, the bladder catheter is generally removed the morning after surgery, regardless of whether the patient has had a laparoscopy or laparotomy.

One of the reasons for performing laparoscopic colorectal surgery is to reduce the risk of adhesion formation. Indeed, in a prospectively randomized porcine model, we have confirmed that laparoscopic anterior resection was associated with only minimal, insignificant adhesions, none of which were at the port sites. These findings were clearly different from the 100% rate of severe adhesions noted at all of the laparotomy incisions (Reissman et al, 1996).

Avoidance of complications

Two reasons for conversion exist. If conversion is undertaken to avoid anticipated complications, the patient's outcome will be no worse than if a laparotomy had been performed rather than laparoscopy. If, however, conversion is undertaken as an emergency because of an enterotomy or massive haemorrhage, then clearly an increased postoperative morbidity will result.

A variety of surgeons have described the learning curve as ranging anywhere from 30 to 70 cases (Wishner et al, 1995). This number of cases refers to the *per surgeon* experience rather than group experience. Like most knowledge in the world, technical expertise in laparoscopy is not transmissible in a group mode. Since Wheeler (1993) has noted that the average American general surgeon performs seven colorectal operations per year, it would take 10 years to pass the learning curve of laparoscopic colorectal surgery, even if all 100% of the surgeon's practice was performed laparoscopically (Wexner et al, 1997). Realistically, even enthusiastic laparoscopic colorectal surgeons perform only 15–30% of their practice by laparoscopy. It is not known whether the case number of 70 for the learning curve would still apply if more than a decade was required to reach this goal. Accordingly, laparoscopic colorectal surgery need not be performed by every surgeon and it may, in fact, be in the patient's best interest if such surgery is delegated to a specific member of each group or a specific individual within a geographic region. However, the learning curve may change with time as current trainees and recent graduates have become expert in a variety of laparoscopic procedures including 'advanced' laparoscopic procedures such as splenectomy, Nissen fundoplication and herniorrhaphy (See et al, 1993).

Not surprisingly, because of the high morbidity associated with laparoscopic surgery (Ramos, 1994; Larach et al, 1997), especially early in the learning curve (Larach et al, 1993), a variety of credentialling programmes have been suggested (Dent, 1991; Jakimowicz, 1994; European Association for Endoscopic Surgery Guidelines, 1994; Schwaitzberg et al, 1996; Ooi, 1996; SAGES, 1997). It is imperative that preceptorship and observation follow animal experimentation as it is inappropriate to proceed directly from the animal lab to the patient.

REFERENCES

Agrama H, Blackwood J, Brown C, Machiedo G & Ruch B (1976) Functional longevity of intraperitoneal drains. *Am J Surg* **132**: 418–421.

Baillet P, Merad F & N'Gbama R (1995) Is drainage after colonic resection anastomosis useful? A multicentre controlled trial on 800 patients. *Br J Surg* **82** (Suppl 1): 24 (Abstract).

Barker K, Graham NG, Mason MC, de Dombal FJ & Goligher JC (1971) The relative significance of pre-operative oral antibiotics, mechanical bowel preparation and per-operative peritoneal contamination in the avoidance of sepsis after radical surgery for ulcerative colitis and Crohn's disease of the large bowel. *Br J Surg* **58**: 270–273.

Becker JM, Dayton MT, Fazio VW et al (1995) Sodium hyaluronate-based bioresorbable membrane (HAL-F) in the prevention of post-operative abdominal adhesions: a prospective randomised double-blinded multicenter study. American College of Surgeons Clinical Congress, New Orleans, October 1995.

Becker JM, Dayton MT, Fazio VW et al (1996) Prevention of postoperative abdominal adhesions by a sodium hyaluronate-based bioresorbable membrane: a prospective, randomized, double-blind multicenter study. *J Am Coll Surg* **183**: 297–306.

Bell CMA & Lewis CB (1968) Effect of neostigmine on integrity of ileo-rectal anastomoses. *BMJ* **3**: 587.

Benjamin PJ (1980) Faeculent peritonitis: a complication of vacuum drainage. *Br J Surg* **67**: 453–454.

Berliner SD, Burson LC & Lear PE (1967) Intraperitoneal drains in surgery of the colon. Clinical evaluation of 454 cases. *Am J Surg* **113**: 646–647.

Binderow SR, Cohen SM, Wexner SD & Nogueras JJ (1994) Must early oral feeding be limited to laparoscopy? *Dis Colon Rectum* **37**: 584–589.

Bloch G (1981) Personal communication quoted in Goligher JC *Surgery of the Anus, Rectum and Colon*, 4th edn, p 485. London: Baillière Tindall.

Blomquist P, Jiborn H & Zederfeldt B (1985) Effect of diverting colostomy on collagen metabolism in the colonic wall. *Am J Surg* **149**: 330–333.

Blumberg N, Agarwal M & Chuang C (1985) Relation between recurrence of cancer of the colon and blood transfusion. *BMJ* **290**: 1037–1038.

Bohm B, Milsom JW, Kitago K, Brand M & Fazio VW (1994) Monopolar electrosurgery and Nd:YAG contact laser™ in laparoscopic intestinal surgery. *Surg Endosc* **8**: 677–681.

Bohm M, Milsom J & Fazio VW (1995) Postoperative intestinal motility following conventional and laparoscopic intestinal surgery. *Arch Surg* **130**: 415–419.

Brennan SJ, Pilkford IR, Evans M & Pollock AV (1982) Staples or sutures for colonic anastomosis: a controlled clinicial trial. *Br J Surg* **69**: 722–724.

Bubrick MP, Corman ML, Cahill CJ et al (1991) Prospective randomized trial of the biofragmentable anastomosis ring. *Am J Surg* **161**: 136–140.

Burrows L & Tartter PI (1982) Effect of blood transfusion on colonic malignant recurrence rate (letter). *Lancet* **ii**: 662.

Buyers RA & Meier LA (1968) Everting suture of the bowel: experimental and clinical experience in duodenal closure and colorectal anastomosis. *Surgery* **63**: 475.

Canalis F & Ravitch MM (1968) Study of healing of inverting and everting anastomoses. *Surg Gynecol Obstet* **126**: 109.

Carter DC, Jenkins DHR & Whitfield HN (1972) Omental reinforcement of intestinal anastomoses. *Br J Surg* **59**: 10.

Celicout AB, Hay JM, Fingerhut A & Flamant Y (1995) Omental protection of anastomosis after colonic or rectal resection. *Br J Surg* **82** (Suppl): 25 (Abstract).

Cerise EJ, Pierce WA & Diamond DL (1970) Abdominal drains: their role as a source of infection following splenectomy. *Ann Surg* **171**: 764–769.

Cheape JD, Wexner SD, James K & Jagelman DG (1991) Does metaclopramide reduce the length of ileus after colorectal surgery. A prospective randomized trial. *Dis Colon Rectum* **34**: 437–441.

Clark CG, Wyllie JH, Haggie SJ & Renton P (1978) Comparison in colonic anastomosis. *World J Surg* **1**: 501.

Cohen SM, Wexner SD, Binderow SR et al (1994) Prospective randomized endoscopic blinded trial comparing precolonoscopy bowel cleansing methods. *Dis Colon Rectum* **37**: 689–696.

Cohn I (1965) Intestinal antisepsis. *Dis Colon Rectum* **8**: 18.

Cohn I, Langford D & Rives JD (1957) Antibiotic support of colon anastomoses. *Surg Gynecol Obstet* **104**: 1–7.

Cohn R & Rives JD (1955) Antibiotic protection of colon anastomoses. *Ann Surg* **141**: 707–717.

Corman ML (1993) *Colon and Rectal Surgery*, 3rd edn, pp 540–541. Philadelphia: JB Lippincott.

Corman ML, Prager ED, Hardy TG Jr et al (1989) Comparison of the Valtrac biofragmentable anastomosis ring with conventional suture and stapled anastomosis in colon surgery. Results of a prospective randomized clinical trial. *Dis Colon Rectum* **32**: 183–186.

Crowson WN & Wilson CS (1973) An experimental study of the effect of drains on colonic anastomoses. *Am Surg* **39**: 567–601.

Czerny V (1880) Zur Darmresektion. *Berl Klin Wochenschr* **17**: 637.

Daly JM, Vars HM & Dindrick SJ (1970) Correlation of protein depletion with colonic anastomotic strength in rats. *Surg Forum* **21**: 77–78.

David IB, Buck JR & Filler RM (1982) Rational use of antibiotics for perforated appendicitis in childhood. *J Paediatr Surg* **17**: 494–499.

Dent TL (1991) Training, credentialling, and granting of clinical privileges for laparoscopic general surgery. *Am J Surg* **161**: 399–403.

Deveney KE & Way LW (1976) Effect of different absorbable sutures on healing of gastrointestinal anastomoses. *Am J Surg* **133**: 86.

Di Zerega GS (1994) Contemporary adhesion prevention. *Fertil Steril* **61**: 219–235.

Didolkar M, Reed WP & Elias GE (1986) A prospective randomised study of sutured versus stapled bowel anastomosis in patients with cancer. *Cancer* **57**: 456–460.

Donaldson DR, Hall TJ, Zoltowski JA et al (1982) Does the type of suture material contribute to the strength of the lateral paramedian incision? *Br J Surg* **69**: 163.

Dudley HAF (1977) *Operative Surgery: Abdomen*, 3rd edn. London: Butterworth.

Dudley HAF (1984) Alimentary tract and abdominal wall. 1. Principles. In Dudley HAF, Pories W & Carter DC (eds) *Robb and Smith's Operative Surgery*, 4th edn, pp 45–46. London: Butterworth.

Elboim CM, Goldman L, Hann L, Palestract AM & Silver W (1983) The significance of post cholecystectomy subhepatic fluid collections. *Ann Surg* **198**: 137–141.

Ellis H & Heddle R (1977) Does the peritoneum need to be closed at laparotomy? *Br J Surg* **64**: 733–736.

European Association for Endoscopic Surgery Guidelines (1994) Training and assessment of competence. *Surg Endosc* **8**: 721–722.

Everett WG (1975) A comparison of one layer and two layer technique for colorectal anastomosis. *Br J Surg* **56**: 135–140.

Everett WG, Friend PJ & Forty J (1986) Comparison of stapling and hand suture for left sided large bowel anastomosis. *Br J Surg* **73**: 345–348.

Fain SN, Patin CS & Morganstern L (1975) Use of mechanical suturing apparatus in low colorectal anastomosis. *Arch Surg* **110**: 1079.

Fielding LP, Stewart Brown S, Blesowsky L & Kearney G (1980) Anastomotic integrity after operations for large bowel cancer: a multicentre study. *BMJ* **282**: 411–414.

Fingerhut A (1996) Laparoscopic assisted colonic resection: the French experience. In: Jager R & Wexner SD (eds) *Laparoscopic Colorectal Surgery*, pp. 253–257. Churchill-Livingstone: New York.

Fingerhut A, Elhadad A, Hay JM et al (1994) Intraperitoneal colorectal anstomosis: hand-sewn versus circular staples. A controlled clinical trial. *Surgery* **78**: 337–341.

Fleshman JW, Fry RD, Birnbaum EH & Kodner IJ (1996) Laparoscopic assisted and minilaparotomy: approaches to colorectal diseases are similar in early outcome. *Dis Colon Rectum* **39**: 15–22.

Fontaine CJ & Dudley HAF (1978) Assessment of suture materials for intestinal use by an extramucosal implant technique and a quantitative histological evaluation. *Br J Surg* **65**: 288–290.

Fraser I, Everson NW & Nash JR (1982) A randomised prospective trial of two drainage methods after cholecystectomy. *Ann R Coll Surg Engl* **64**: 183–185.

Gambee LP (1951) Single layer open intestinal anastomosis applicable to small as well as large intestine. *West J Surg Obstet Gynecol* **59**: 1.

Getzen LC, Roe RD & Holloway CI (1966) Comparative study of intestinal anastomotic healing in inverted and everted closures. *Surg Gynecol Obstet* **123**: 1219.

Gill W, Fraser J, Carter DC & Hill R (1969) Colonic anastomosis. A clinical and experimental study. *Surg Gynecol Obstet* **128**: 1297.

Gilmour DG, Aitkenhead AR, Hothersall AP & Ledingham IMcA (1980) The effect of hypovolaemia on colonic blood flow in the dog. *Br J Surg* **67**: 82.

Goldberg SM, Gordon PH & Nivatvongs S (1980) *Essentials of Anorectal Surgery*. Philadelphia: JB Lippincott.

Goldsmith HS (1977) Protection of low rectal anastomosis with intact omentum. *Surg Gynecol Obstet* **144**: 584.

Goligher JC (1984) *Surgery of the Anus, Rectum and Colon*, 5th edn. London: Baillière Tindall.

Goligher JC, Graham NG & De Dombal FT (1970a) Anastomotic dehiscence after anterior resection of rectum and sigmoid. *Br J Surg* **57**: 109–118.

Goligher JC, Morris C, McAdam WAF, De Dombal FT & Johnson D (1970b) A controlled clinical trial of inverting versus everting intestinal suture in clinical large bowel surgery. *Br J Surg* **57**: 817.

Goligher JC, Irvin TT, Johnson D et al (1975) A controlled clinical trial of three methods of closure of laparatomy wounds. *Br J Surg* **62**: 823.

Goligher JC, Lee PWG, Simpkins KC & Lintott DJ (1977) A controlled comparison of one and two layer techniques of suture for high and low colorectal anastomoses. *Br J Surg* **64**: 823–826.

Gordon AB, Bates T & Fiddian RV (1976) A controlled trial of drainage after cholecystectomy. *Br J Surg* **63**: 278–282.

Greenall MJ, Evans M & Pollock AV (1978) Should you drain a perforated appendix? *Br J Surg* **65**: 880–882.

Greenall MJ, Evans M & Pollock AV (1980a) Midline or transverse laparotomy? A random controlled clinical trial. Part 1: Influence on healing. *Br J Surg* **67**: 188–190.

Greenall MJ, Evans M & Pollock AV (1980b) Midline or transverse laparotomy. A random controlled trial. Part 2: Influence on post-operative pulmonary complications. *Br J Surg* **67**: 191–194.

Guillou PJ, Hall TJ, Donaldson DR et al (1980) Vertical abdominal incisions: a choice. *Br J Surg* **67**: 395.

Haller JA, Shaker IJ, Donahoo JS, Schaufer L & White JJ (1973) Peritoneal drainage in ruptured appendicitis in children. *Ann Surg* **177**: 595–600.

Halsted WS (1887) Circular suture of the intestine: an experimental study. *J Med Sci* **94**: 436.

Hamilton JE (1967) Reappraisal of open intestinal anastomoses. *Ann Surg* **165**: 917.

Hanna EA (1970) Efficiency of peritoneal drainage. *Surg Gynecol Obstet* **131**: 983–985.

Hardy TG Jr, Pace WG, Maney JW et al (1985) A biofragmentable ring for sutureless bowel anastomosis. *Dis Colon Rectum* **28**: 484–488.

Hargreaves AW & Keddie NC (1968) Colonic anastomosis: a clinical and experimental study. *Br J Surg* **55**: 774.

Hawley PR (1970) Infection – the cause of anastomotic breakdown; an experimental study. *Proc R Soc Med* **63**: 752.

Hawley PR, Page Faulk W, Hunt TK & Dunphy JE (1970a) Collagenase activity in the gastrointestinal tract. *Br J Surg* **57**: 896–900.

Hawley PR, Hunt TK & Dunphy JE (1970b) Aetiology of colonic anastomotic leaks. *Proc R Soc Med* **63**: 28–30.

Healey JE Jr, McBride CM & Gallagher HS (1967) Bowel anastomosis by inverting and everting techniques. *J Surg Res* **7**: 299.

Hunt TK, Hawley PR, Hale J, Goodson W & Thakral KK (1980) Colonic repair; the collagenous equilibrium. In Hunt TK (ed.) *Wound Healing and Wound Infection: Theory and Surgical Practice*, p 153. New York: Appleton-Century-Crofts.

Irvin TT (1976) Collagen metabolism in infected colonic anastomoses. *Surg Gynecol Obstet* **143**: 220–224.

Irvin TT & Edwards JP (1973) Comparison of single layer inverting and everting anastomoses in the rabbit colon. *Br J Surg* **60**: 453–457.

Irvin TT & Goligher JC (1973) Aetiology of disruption of intestinal anastomoses. *Br J Surg* **60**: 461–464.

Irvin TT & Hunt TK (1974a) Pathogenesis and prevention of disruption of colonic anastomoses in traumatized rats. *Br J Surg* **67**: 437–439.

Irvin TT & Hunt TK (1974b) Reappraisal of the healing process of anastomoses of the colon. *Surg Gynecol Obstet* **138**: 741–746.

Irvin TT, Koffman CG & Duthie HL (1976) Layer closure of laparotomy wounds with absorbable and non-absorbable suture materials. *Br J Surg* **63**(10): 793–796.

Irvin TT, Stoddard CJ, Greaney MG & Duthie HL (1977) Abdominal wound healing: prospective clinical study. *BMJ* **2**: 351.

Jakimowicz JJ (1994) The European Association for Endoscopic Surgery Recommendations for Training in Laparoscopic Surgery. *Ann Chir Gynaecol* **83**: 137–141.

Jansen A, Brummelkamp WH, Davies GA et al (1981) Clinical applications of magnetic rings in colorectal anastomosis. *Surg Gynaecol Obstet* **153**: 537–540.

Jenkins TPN (1976) The burst abdominal wound: a mechanical approach. *Br J Surg* **63**: 873.

Johnson CD, Lamont PM, Orr N & Lennox M (1989) Is a drain necessary after colonic anastomosis. *J R Soc Med* **82**: 661–664.

Jones TE, Newell ET & Brubaker RE (1941) The use of alloy steel wire in the closure of abdominal wounds. *Surg Gynecol Obstet* **71**: 1056.

Kambouris AA, Carpenter WS & Accaben RD (1973) Cholecystectomy without drainage. *Surg Gynecol Obstet* **137**: 613–617.

Koruth NM, Krukowski ZH, Youngson GG et al (1985) Intraoperative colonic irrigation in the management of left-sided large bowel emergencies. *Br J Surg* **72**: 708–711.

Kratzer GL & Onsanit T (1974) Single layer steel wire anastomosis of the intestine. *Surg Gynecol Obstet* **139**: 93.

Larach SW, Salomon MC, Williamson PR & Goldstein E (1993) Laparoscopic assisted colectomy: experience during the learning curve. *Coloproctology* **1**: 38–41.

Larach SW, Patankar SK, Ferrara A, Williamson PR, Perozo S & Lord AS (1997) Complications of laparoscopic colorectal surgery. Analysis and comparison of early versus later experience. *Dis Colon Rectum* **40**: 592–596.

Laufman H & Method H (1948) Effects of absorbable foreign substance on bowel anastomosis. *Surg Gynecol Obstet* **86**: 669.

Leaper DJ, Rosenberg IL, Evans M et al (1976) The influence of suture materials on abdominal wound healing assessed by controlled clinical trials. *Eur Surg Res* **8** (Suppl 1): 75.

Leaper DJ, Pollock AV & Evans M (1977) Abdominal wound closure, a trial of nylon polyglycolic acid and steel sutures. *Br J Surg* **64**: 603–606.

Lembert A (1826) Memoire sur l'enterophie avec la description d'un procede nouveau pour practiquer cette operation chirurgicale. *Rep Gen Anat Physiol Path* **2**: 100.

Leonardo RA (1943) *History of Surgery*, p 281. New York: Froden.

Localio SA & Eng K (1975) Malignant tumours of the rectum. *Curr Prob Surg* **12**: 1.

Lockart-Mummery JP (1934) *Disease of the Rectum and Colon*, 2nd edn. London: Baillière.

Loeb MJ (1967) Comparative strength of inverted, everted and end on intestinal anastomoses. *Surg Gynecol Obstet* **125**: 301.

McAdam AJ, Meikle G & Medina R (1969) An experimental comparison of inversion and eversion colonic anastomoses. *Dis Colon Rectum* **12**: 1.

McArdle CS & Hole D (1991) Impact of variability among surgeons on post-operative morbidity and mortality and ultimate survival. *BMJ* **302**: 1501–1505.

McDermott JP, Devereaux DA & Caushaj PF (1994) Pitfall of laparoscopic colectomy. An unrecognized synchronous tumor. *Dis Colon Rectum* **37**: 602–603.

McLachlin AD & Denton DW (1973) Omental protection of intestinal anastomoses. *Am J Surg* **125**: 134.

McLachlin AD, Olsson LS & Pitt DF (1976) Anterior anastomosis of the rectosigmoid colon; an experimental study. *Surgery* **3**: 306–311.

Maingot R (1969) *Abdominal Operations*, 5th edn. New York: Appleton-Century-Crofts.

Man B, Kraus L & Motovic A (1977) Cholecystectomy without drainage, nasogastric suction and intravenous fluids. *Am J Surg* **133**: 312–314.

Manz CW, La Tendress C & Sako Y (1970) The detrimental effects of drains on colonic anastomosis: an experimental study. *Dis Colon Rectum* **13**: 17–25.

Mellish RW, Ty TC & Keller DJ (1968) A study of intestinal healing. *J Pediatr Surg* **3**: 286.

Mittelman JS & Doberneck RC (1982) Drains and antibiotics perioperatively for elective cholecystectomy. *Surg Gynecol Obstet* **155**: 653–654.

Moffat LEF & Sunderland GT (1985) Relation between recurrence of cancer and blood transfusion. *BMJ* **291**: 971.

Monson JR, Darzi A, Carey PD et al (1992) Prospective evaluation of laparoscopic assisted colectomy in an unsuspected group of patients. *Lancet* **340**: 831–833.

Moran BJ (1996) Stapling instruments for intestinal anastomosis in colorectal surgery. *Br J Surg* **83**: 902–909.

Mukerjee P, Mepham JA, Wapnick S et al (1969) The effect of protein deprivation on alimentary healing. *J Surg Res* **9**: 283–288.

Murphy JB (1892) Cholecysto-intestinal, gastrointestinal and entero-intestinal anastomoses and approximation without sutures. *Med Rec NY* **42**: 665–669.

Oliveira L, Wexner SD, Daniel N, DeMarta D, Weiss EG, Nogueras JJ & Bernstein M (1997) Mechanical bowel preparation for elective colorectal surgery. A prospective, randomized, surgeon-blinded trial comparing sodium phosphate and polyethylene glycol based oral lavage solutions. *Dis Colon Rectum* **40**: 585–591.

Ooi LLPJ (1996) Training in laparoscopic surgery: have we got it right yet? *Ann Acad Med Singapore* **25**: 732–736.

Orr NWM (1969) A single layer intestinal anastomosis. *Br J Surg* **56**: 77.

Pahlman L, Ejerblad S, Graf W et al (1997) Randomised trial of a biofragmentable bowel anastomosis ring in high-risk colonic resection. *Br J Surg* **84**: 1291–1294.

Parameswaran S, Gilliland R, Iroatulam A et al (1997) Role of elective ureteric catheterization in colorectal surgery (abstract). *Dis Colon Rectum* **40**: A48.

Phillips EH (1994) Laparoscopic colon surgery: who, what, where and when? *Semin Colon Rectal Surg* **5**: 218–223.

Phillips RKS & Cooke HT (1986) Effect of steel wire sutures on the incidence of chemically induced rodent colonic tumours. *Br J Surg* **73**: 671–674.

Playforth MJ, Sauven P, Evans M & Pollock AV (1985) Suction drainage of the gall bladder bed does not prevent complications after cholecystectomy: random control clinical trial. *Br J Surg* **72**: 269–271.

Pollock AV & Evans M (1977) Abdominal wound closure: a trial of nylon polyglycolic acid and steel sutures. *Br J Surg* **64**: 603.

Ragoonan C, Crosby DL, Morgan WP & Rees BI (1983) Peritoneal drainage following cholecystectomy: a controlled trial. *Ann R Coll Surg Engl* **65**: 403.

Ramos R (1994) Complications in laparoscopic colon surgery: prevention and management. *Semin Colon Rectal Surg* **5**: 239–243.

Ravitch MM (1967) In discussion of paper by Bronwell AW,

Rutledge R & Dalton ML: Single layer open gastrointestinal anastomosis. *Ann Surg* **165**: 925–932.

Ravitch MM (1974) Sewing with staples. *Clin Med* **81**: 17.

Ravitch MM & Steichen FM (1972) Techniques of staple suturing in the gastrointestinal tract. *Ann Surg* **175**: 815.

Ravitch MM, Canalis F, Weinschelbaum A & McCormack J (1967a) Studies of intestinal healing. III. Observations on everting intestinal anastomosis. *Ann Surg* **166**: 670–680.

Ravitch MM, Rivarola A & Vangrov J (1967b) Studies of intestinal healing. I. Preliminary study of mechanism of healing of the inverting intestinal anastomosis. *Johns Hopkins Med J* **121**: 343.

Rebuffat C, Rosati R, Montorsi M et al (1990). Clinical application of a new compression anastomotic device for colorectal surgery. *Am J Surg* **159**: 330–335.

Reissman P, Teoh T-A, Cohen SM, Weiss EG, Nogueras JJ & Wexner SD (1995) Is early oral feeding safe after elective colorectal surgery? *Ann Surg* **222**: 73–77.

Reissman P, Teoh T-A, Skinner K, Burns J & Wexner SD (1996) Adhesion formation after laparoscopic anterior resection in a porcine model. *Surg Laparosc Endosc* **6**: 136–139.

Reiver D & Wexner SD (1999) Postoperative oral feeding after gastrointestinal surgery. *Nutrition* (in press).

Robiscek F (1980) The birth of the surgical stapler. *Surg Gynecol Obstet* **150**: 579.

Rosati R, Rebuffat C & Pezzuoli G (1988) A new mechanical device for circular compression anastomosis. *Ann Surg* **207**: 245–249.

Rosenberg IL, Graham NG, DeDombal FT & Goligher JC (1971) Preparation of the intestine in patients undergoing major large bowel surgery, mainly for neoplasm of the colon and rectum. *Br J Surg* **58**: 266–268.

Rusca JA, Bornside GH & Cohn I (1969) Everting versus inverting gastrointestinal anastomoses: bacterial leakage and anastomotic disruption. *Ann Surg* **169**: 343.

Ryan P (1970) The effect of surrounding infection upon the healing of colonic wounds: experimental studies and clincial experiences. *Dis Colon Rectum* **13**: 124.

Sagar S, Harland P & Shields R (1979) Early postoperative feeding with elemental diet. *BMJ* **1**: 293–294.

SAGES Committee on Credentialling (1997) Granting of privileges for laparoscopic and/or thoracoscopic general surgery. Policy Statement.

SAGES Position Statement. Global statement on deep venous thrombosis prophylaxis during laparoscopic surgery. August 1998.

Santos OA, Hastings FW & Mazuji MK (1962) Effectiveness of silicone as an abdominal drain. *Arch Surg* **84**: 643–645.

Schrock TR, Deveney CW & Dunphy JE (1973) Factors contributing to leakage of colonic anastomoses. *Ann Surg* **177**: 513–518.

Schwaitzberg SD, Connolly RJ, Sant GR, Reindollar R & Cleveland RJ (1996) Planning, development, and execution of an international training program in laparoscopic surgery. *Surg Laparosc Endosc* **6**: 10–15.

See WA, Cooper CS & Fisher RJ (1993) Predictors of laparoscopic complications after formal training in laparoscopic surgery. *JAMA* **270**: 2689–2692.

Sekiba K and the Obstetric and Gynaecology Adhesions Prevention Committee (1992) Use of Interceed (TC7) absorbable adhesion barrier to reduce post-operative adhesion reformation in infertility and endometriosis surgery. *Obstet Gynaecol* **79**: 518–522.

Senagore AJ, Luchtefeld MA & MacKeigan JM (1995) What is the learning curve for laparoscopic colectomy? *Am Surg* **6**: 681–685.

Sheridan WG, Lownes RH & Young HL (1987) Tissue oxygen measurement as a predictor of colonic anastomotic healing. *Dis Colon Rectum* **30**: 867–871.

Simmang CL & Rosenthal D (1994) Tools for laparoscopic colectomy. *Semin Colon Rectal Surg* **5**: 228–238.

Singleton AO Jr, White D & Montalbo P (1968) A comparative study of intestinal anastomoses. *Arch Surg* **96**: 563.

Smith CR, Cockelet GR, Adams JT et al (1981) Vascularity of gastrointestinal staple lines demonstrated with silicone rubber injects. *Am J Surg* **142**: 563.

Smith SRG (1986) The effect of surgical drainage materials on the healing of colonic anastomoses. MS thesis, University of London.

Solla JA & Rothenberger DA (1990) Preoperative bowel preparation: a survey of colon and rectal surgeons. *Dis Colon Rectum* **33**: 154–159.

Spencer FC, Sharp EH & Jude JR (1963) Experiences with wire closure or abdominal incisions in 293 selected patients. *Surg Gynecol Obstet* **117**: 235.

Steichen FM (1968) The use of staples in anatomical side to side and functional end to end entero-anastomosis. *Surgery* **64**: 948.

Steichen FM (1971) Clinical experience with auto suture instruments. *Surgery* **69**: 609.

Stone HH, Fabin TC, Turkleson ML & Jurkiewicz MJ (1981) Management of acute full thickness losses of the abdominal wall. *Ann Surg* **193**: 612–616.

Stone HH, Hooper CA & Millikan WJ (1978) Abdominal drainage following appendicectomy and cholecystectomy. *Ann Surg* **187**: 606–612.

Thompson JN (1995) Preventing adhesions. *Lancet* **346**: 1382.

Thompson JN & Whawell SA (1995) Pathogenesis and prevention of adhesion formation. *Br J Surg* **82**: 3–5.

Travers B (1812) *An Enquiry into the Process of Nature in Repairing Injuries of the Intestine*, p 12. London: Longman, Rees, Orme, Brown & Green.

Trimpi HD, Khubchandani T, Sheets JA & Stasik JJ (1976) Advances in intestinal anastomosis: experimental study with an analysis of 984 patients. *Dis Colon Rectum* **20**: 107.

Trowbridge PR & Howes EL (1967) Reinforcement of colon anastomosis using polyurethane foam treated with neomycin: an experimental study. *Am J Surg* **113**: 236.

Trueblood HW, Nelson TS, Kohatsu S & Oberhelman HA (1969) Wound healing in the colon: comparison of inverted and everted closure. *Surgery* **65**: 919.

Truedson H (1983) Cholecystectomy with and without intraperitoneal drains. *Acta Chir Scand* **149**: 393–399.

Turnbull R Jr (1966) Personal communication cited in Goligher JC: *Surgery of the Anus, Rectum and Colon*, 4th edn, p 539. London: Baillière Tindall.

Turner C (1955) Operations for intestinal obstruction. In *Modern Operative Surgery*, 4th edn, p 1017. London: Cassell.

Turner-Warwick RT, Wynne EJC & Handley-Ashken M (1967) The use of the omental pedicle graft in the repair and reconstruction of the urinary tract. *Br J Surg* **54**: 55.

Uden P, Blomquist P, Jiborn H & Zederfeldt B (1987) Influence of proximal colostomy on the healing of a left colon anastomosis: an experimental study in the rat. *Br J Surg* **75(4)**: 325–329.

Vipond MN, Whawell SA, Thompson JN & Dudley HAE (1990) Peritoneal fibrinolytic activity and intra-abdominal adhesions. *Lancet* **335**: 1120–1122.

Voyles CR, Richardson JD, Bland KI, Tobin GR, Flint IM & Polk HC (1981) Emergency abdominal wall reconstruction with polypropylene mesh. Short benefits versus long term complications. *Ann Surg* **194**: 219–223.

West of Scotland and Highland Anastomosis Study Group (1991) Suturing or stapling in gastrointestinal surgery: a prospective randomised study. *Br J Surg* **78**: 337–341.

Wexner SD, Latulippe JF, Nogueras JJ & Weiss EG (1997) The effect of colorectal board certification and volume on the costs of large bowel surgery (abstract). *Int J Colorectal Dis* **12**: 183.

Wheeler HB (1993) Myth and reality in general surgery. *Am Coll Surg Bull* **78**: 21–27, 42.

Wilkins JL, Hardcastle JD, Mann CV & Kaufmann L (1970) Effects of neostigmine and atropine on motor activity of ileum, colon and rectum of anaesthetised subjects. *BMJ* **1**: 793.

Wiseman D (1994) Polymers for the prevention of surgical adhesions. In Domb AJ (ed.) *Polymeric Site Specific Pharmacotherapy*, pp 369–421. Chichester: John Wiley.

Wishner JD, Baker JW Jr, Hoffman GC et al (1995) Laparoscopic-assisted colectomy. The learning curve. *Surg Endosc* **9**: 1179–1183.

Woodforde Scott J (1981) Suction drainage complication. *Br J Surg* **68**: 825–826.

Yeung CK, Young GA, Hackett AF & Hill GL (1979) Fine needle catheter jejunostomy: an assessment of a new method of nutritional support after major gastrointestinal surgery. *Br J Surg* **66**: 727–732.

7

ANAESTHESIA FOR COLORECTAL SURGERY

PREOPERATIVE ASSESSMENT

Anaesthesia has improved dramatically over the past 20 years and it is now difficult to find patients who are 'unfit for anaesthesia'. There are, however, many patients who are ill-suited for the stress of the intended procedure and some in whom the recovery from anaesthesia will predictably be slow or stormy. There are others who have intercurrent disease which puts them at special risk in the perioperative period. No matter how sophisticated the colonic surgery, if the large bowel has a dubious life support system the outcome is always in question. Careful preoperative assessment of all patients is therefore crucial to overall operative success.

Whatever operation is to be carried out, hypoxia is obviously to be avoided, although it has a propensity to occur in the postoperative period. Initially, in patients who have been anaesthetized with nitrous oxide there is an unimportant, transient decrease in the $Pa\text{O}_2$ of up to 10 mmHg (1.3 kPa) which lasts for 10 minutes when they resume breathing air. It can be prevented by giving 100% oxygen for 2 minutes at the end of the operation.

The major effects of anaesthesia on pulmonary gas exchange in the postoperative period depend upon the site of surgery. In the operative and immediate postoperative period the functional residual capacity (FRC) is reduced with alveolar gas trapping and there is an increased right-to-left shunt. The cause is unknown but it can produce a fall in $Pa\text{O}_2$ of up to 30 mmHg (4.0 kPa) when breathing air compared with the preoperative level. It is easily corrected by giving 30–40% oxygen through a facemask. After the first hour or two most patients reverse these changes and effectively return to their normal preoperative state. However, when patients with previously healthy lungs undergo abdominal surgery this reduction in oxygenation continues for at least 48 hours and may extend for up to 5 days. This effect is worst with upper abdominal, thoracic and paramedian incisions and least with lower abdominal incisions. Factors known to exacerbate these effects are wound pain (prevents deep breathing, can reduce vital capacity by up to 50% and reduces expiratory force), abdominal distension (splints the diaphragm), the supine position (when the relationship of FRC to closing volume is least favourable) and overtransfusion (tendency to pulmonary oedema).

All the above changes are intensified in patients with poor preoperative lung function, cigarette smokers, the obese and the aged. They are also the groups most at risk from infection and segmental collapse secondary to sputum retention.

It is inappropriate to discuss detailed preoperative assessment here and general references are given at the end of the chapter. It is, however, sensible to list some of the common problems that affect the management of anaesthesia and recovery, many of which not infrequently slip through the net.

Cardiovascular disease

Ischaemic heart disease

Ischaemic heart disease is common, often occult, and there may well be no signs or symptoms present. Any maintenance therapy should be continued peroperatively. Postoperative hypoxia can precipitate cardiac ischaemia and compromise pump function. Cardiac pain may be masked by postoperative analgesia and the episode can present as an acute confusional state. Diagnosis is clinical and by ECG and isoenzyme changes. Because of the relatively high incidence of incidental abnormalities, all patients over 60 years old should have a recent preoperative ECG available for comparison.

Hypertension

Hypertensive patients (both treated and untreated) are at risk during the perioperative period. When hypertension is detected, approximately 10% will have an associated condition such as renal disease, endocrine disease, coarctation or pregnancy. They are often symptom free. The problems specific to hypertensive patients are the following:

- There is a greater fall in blood pressure after a normal dose of induction agent than in a normotensive patient.
- There is an exaggerated response to laryngoscopy and surgical stimulation, resulting in hypertension, tachycardias, dysrhythmias and myocardial ischaemia.
- High left ventricular pressures and tachycardias can produce subendocardial ischaemia. This highlights the importance of continuous ECG and arterial pressure monitoring during induction.
- Interactions may be anticipated between calcium channel blockers and inhalational agents and patients receiving ACE inhibitors may suffer from increased hypotension at induction. However, most of these interactions are relatively mild and antihypertensive agents should be continued up to and including the day of surgery.
- The most common spontaneous dysrhythmia is the conversion from sinus to junctional rhythm, often associated with abrupt hypotension. This may occur more easily in the presence of hypercapnia and volatile agents.
- Atropine may cause a tachycardia leading to ischaemia. It may be preferable to use glycopyrrolate when reversing neuromuscular blockade.
- The recovery period is very important to the hypertensive patient because the blood pressure can suddenly reach dangerously high levels. Such postoperative hypertension is more common in patients who have a previous history of severe hypertension, regardless of whether the arterial pressure was under control prior to anaesthesia. Thus, the blood pressure needs to be monitored closely as the patient becomes more aware and pain is experienced. If appropriate, analgesic agents should be given before embarking on vasoactive drugs.

Do not forget to prescribe postoperative maintenance therapy. Since the oral route is usually inappropriate following colonic surgery this implies a change to a parenteral or alternative preparation.

What is to be done if the blood pressure is found to be elevated preoperatively? Reasonable recommendations would appear to be as follows:

- Repeated measurements should be undertaken.
- All non-urgent cases with diastolic blood pressures persistently over 110 mmHg should be referred for investigation and treatment.
- All non-urgent cases with a diastolic pressure up to 110 mmHg are probably acceptable, provided that there is nothing abnormal in the history (especially episodic states suggestive of phaeochromocytoma) and careful clinical examination reveals no evidence of end organ damage (especially no signs of left ventricular failure) or pregnancy.

In addition, the following should be normal:

- ECG (no evidence of left ventricular hypertrophy, conduction abnormalities or dysrhythmias)
- Chest X-ray (no evidence of ventricular dilatation)
- Full blood count (no evidence of polycythaemia)
- Urea and electrolytes (no evidence of renal/endocrine involvement). Mild hypokalaemia is unlikely to be associated with intraoperative

dysrhythmias but levels below 3 mmol/L should probably be treated.
- Serum glucose (not diabetic).

If any of these findings are positive then the patient should be referred for investigations and treatment. This may include echocardiography, which is a cheap and non-invasive procedure that allows assessment of left ventricular size, movement and ejection fraction – a reduction of which may be associated with increased perioperative morbidity.

With urgent cases, no choice is available to the anaesthetist. The only indications for a rapid reduction of blood pressure (over a period of a few hours) are encephalopathy, acute left ventricular failure (LVF) and very severe pre-eclampsia or eclampsia. Otherwise, the dangers of rapid reduction of blood pressure (blindness and cerebral episodes) are not outweighed by the benefits.

Pulmonary disease

Chronic obstructive airways disease (COAD)

The importance of pulmonary disease is that it results in a reduced ability to provide oxygen to healing tissues. Usually, the history of breathlessness and recurrent infection and clinical examination give a good indication of the patient's pulmonary function. The patients themselves are almost always aware of the dangers which they face following major surgery.

Although in many cases the likely outcome is easy to predict, to our knowledge, there is no study employing large numbers of patients which relates the results of preoperative lung function tests to postoperative complications and eventual outcome (apart from those assessing the feasibility of pneumonectomy). Some general deductions can, however, be made. If the tidal volume (V_T) is close to the vital capacity (VC), then there is little 'ventilatory reserve' and the adequacy of postoperative ventilation easily deteriorates with opioids and residual neuromuscular block (including that provided by a thoracic epidural). Irrespective of the cause, perhaps the most important feature of low values of the forced expiratory volume in 1 second (FEV_1) and the peak expiratory flow rate (PEFR) is an indication that the patient cannot expel air rapidly. Although these tests are not a direct measure of the 'power' of a cough, they are closely related to the ability to expel sputum. An FEV_1 of less than 2 litres or an FEV_1:VC ratio of less than 50% are sometimes quoted as values which define serious disease. The lower the value recorded, the more important it is to optimize the patient's state preoperatively, to monitor closely in the postoperative period, and to subject the patient to vigorous and frequent physiotherapy.

When lung function tests reveal abnormal results it is obviously important to combine them with blood gas estimation. It is only this that demonstrates the effect which the ventilatory defect has on the efficacy of gas exchange.

The patterns of blood gas derangement fall into three main subdivisions: hyperventilation, alveolar hypoventilation and a shunt or gas transfer defect. Often the latter two categories are mixed.

In *hyperventilation* the Pao_2 is normal or elevated and the $Paco_2$ is reduced. These changes are almost invariably due to anxious overventilation on the part of the patient and merely indicate healthy lungs. It is usually of no clinical importance. Exceptions are the hyperventilation of cerebral origin and the low $Paco_2$ which compensates for a metabolic acidosis.

Alveolar hypoventilation can result from COAD, impaired mechanical ventilation (acute airways obstruction, stiff lungs, flail chest, pneumothorax), muscular weakness (myopathy, neuropathy) or central depression from drugs. In essence there is insufficient alveolar ventilation to both oxygenate the blood and to wash out the carbon dioxide so that the $Paco_2$ is elevated and the Pao_2 is reduced. It is important to recognize the presence of alveolar hypoventilation because the Pao_2 (but not the $Paco_2$) can be greatly improved by increasing the concentration of inspired oxygen (Fio_2). If the failure of alveolar ventilation is secondary to chronic abnormal neuromuscular function the patient often shows little clinical distress, but if it is secondary to a mechanical problem vigorous efforts to increase the tidal and minute volumes will be made.

Shunt or gas transfer defects describe those situations in which there is no airways obstruction and the lungs are expanded normally but there is an imperfect interface between pulmonary blood and alveolar air. This can arise from both generalized parenchymal conditions (sarcoidosis, fibrosing alveolitis, shock lung) and localized problems (pulmonary embolus, lobar collapse, lobar pneumonia). This collection of circumstances results in a situation where the $Paco_2$ is normal (because hyperventilation can wash out carbon dioxide adequately from the normal lung tissue) but, because of the necessary mixing of blood with varying oxygen tensions in the pulmonary veins and because of the shape of the oxygen dissociation curve, the Pao_2 is reduced. In the presence of a 50% shunt cardiac output, there is very little to be gained from increasing the FIO_2 to very high levels. This merely increases the risk of pulmonary oxygen toxicity without improving the PaO_2.

All patients with significant pulmonary dysfunction need to be cared for postoperatively in an appropriate setting. This care needs to include regular observations to detect and treat hypoxia and meticulous attention to fluid balance and analgesia. Pulse oximetry can be invaluable.

Asthma

Asthma is difficult to define accurately but an adequate description is 'a clinical syndrome of multifactorial origin, the predominant features of which are dyspnoea and wheeze of fluctuating severity and in which reversibility of airflow obstruction can be demonstrated by objective measures'. The two main clinical groups are extrinsic (childhood, allergic, atopic) asthma and intrinsic (late onset, non-atopic) asthma, although the margin between them is blurred.

The most sensitive indices of bronchial tone are the PEFR and FEV_1. Ideally, the patient should be at their best for surgery but this is not always possible in emergencies. It is important to allow patients to continue their normal medication up to the time of operation and to bring their inhaler to theatre with them. In severe asthmatics prophylactic antibiotic therapy is indicated. All patients need a chest X-ray, both as a baseline and to show the presence of bullae and hyperinflation.

Despite its prevalence in the community, there are very few articles dealing with anaesthesia for asthmatics. The three most common problems are: bronchospasm on intubation or during gas induction, the risk of a pneumothorax when on intermittent positive pressure ventilation (IPPV), and bronchospasm secondary to thiopentone or other histamine-releasing drugs such as curare, suxamethonium, morphine, etc.

Adequate premedication is important if the patient is nervous, because an attack can be precipitated by fear.

An asthmatic attack in the postoperative period should be treated in the normal way. Maintenance therapy may need to be changed from the inhalation to the parenteral route in the immediate postoperative period.

Diabetes

Approximately one-quarter of all diabetic patients undergoing surgery are undiagnosed on admission to hospital. Almost all of these fall into the 'adult onset' type who have a small but insufficient insulin production. It is therefore necessary to have a high index of suspicion that diabetes may be present in any patient, especially if obese and over 60 years old. The stress of surgery may precipitate frank diabetes in a previously undiagnosed patient.

Diabetes has widespread physiological effects relevant to preoperative assessment, the most important of which are listed systemically below.

- *Cardiovascular effects*. Evidence of angina, myocardial infarction, intermittent claudication, gangrene and postural hypotension (systolic fall of >30 mmHg on standing) should be sought.
- *Neurological complications*. Neurological involvement may be evident as numbness, pain, paraesthesia, leg ulcers, strokes, transient ischaemic attacks, impotence or gustatory sweating. Postural hypotension is a late sign of autonomic neuropathy; loss of heart rate variability during deep breathing is the most reliable early sign.
- *Renal complications*. Symptoms may include polyuria (glycosuria or renal failure), frequency, dysuria, pruritus, or the secondary symptoms of anaemia and/or hypertension.
- *Skin*. Staphyloccal infections are common and there is an increased risk of sepsis, especially over the pressure areas.

The perioperative management of diabetes is well described in other texts listed under Further Reading at the end of the chapter and will not be considered further here.

Bowel preparation

Bowel preparation agents (e.g. Picolax) may lead to marked dehydration and subsequent hypotension and oliguria intraoperatively. Patients should be encouraged to drink adequate amounts orally or receive intravenous fluids preoperatively.

Selection for day-case surgery

Many minor surgical procedures may be considered to be appropriate for admission as day cases. The surgical procedures should usually last no longer than an hour although no absolute time limit is necessary. Patients should be assessed for their suitability on both medical and social criteria and this requires preoperative screening and consistent protocols in each unit. They should be in good general health, any chronic disease (e.g. asthma, diabetes, epilepsy) should be well controlled. Grossly obese patients should be excluded. Patients need to be accompanied home, have an adult carer for at least 24 hours, have access to a telephone and be able to return easily to the hospital if problems occur.

INTRAOPERATIVE TECHNIQUES

For the well-prepared elective bowel resection the requirements are abdominal muscle relaxation and lack of response to surgical stimulae, preferably with contracted intestines. This state of anaesthesia can be achieved by general or local techniques, or by a combination of both. In the UK the majority of colonic resections are done under general anaesthesia using nitrous oxide, opioids and relaxants. This gives a smooth intraoperative course but can produce problems during reversal and postoperatively (see below). Increasingly, anaesthetists are combining light general anaesthesia (to achieve unconsciousness) with some form of regional blockade (to achieve analgesia) which can be carried into the postoperative period for pain relief. Patients with a dense regional blockade who are awake during surgery are rarely seen in the UK, although it is not uncommon in some other European countries such as Sweden. In certain instances (e.g. intestinal obstruction) the condition dictates specific techniques (e.g. rapid sequence induction with cricoid pressure in order to prevent aspiration pneumonitis).

Although often regarded as less physiologically insulting, surgery on the anal region produces severe pain, reflex bodily movements, an increase in ventilatory activity and laryngeal spasm. To overcome the pain requires effective analgesia; prevention of muscle movement requires deep anaesthesia or a relaxant; and avoidance of laryngeal spasm requires deep anaesthesia, a relaxant or a tracheal tube. Light anaesthesia with a spontaneously breathing patient usually spells trouble. All the problems can be overcome with a local or regional block but this relaxes the anal sphincters, which some surgeons dislike.

Local anaesthetic techniques

Local anaesthetic techniques have an undeserved reputation for safety (particularly in the compromised patient) which tends to obscure their dangers. All local anaesthetics can produce direct toxicity and adverse side-effects. It is important that those who employ them can recognize and treat these complications. In order that this can be so, local anaesthetics should only be used in environments where full resuscitation facilities and the staff who know how to use them are available. Local techniques are usually combined with a light general anaesthetic. A surgical procedure in a fully conscious patient should not be pushed on to unwilling or nervous patients and all members of the operating theatre staff need to know and to be constantly reminded that the patient is awake.

For colorectal surgery there are only a limited number of ways in which local blocks can be used and none of them interrupt the vagus nerve. This can be a nuisance since traction on the mesentery and viscera often results in unwanted bradycardia and, in the awake patient, can produce intense nausea.

Infiltration

This is suitable only for operations on the anal canal, where it can be very successful. From a point 2.5 cm posterior to the anus (with the index finger of the left hand in the rectum), 25 mL of 1.5% lignocaine-adrenaline solution is injected. Only one site of injection is necessary and the anus and anal canal are ensheathed by a cylinder of solution.

Caudal block

This is a form of epidural blockade achieved through the sacral hiatus. It is usually performed as a one-shot procedure and requires proper sterile precautions to be taken. The sacral canal, in addition to housing the nerves to be blocked, also contains the dural sac (usually attached to the 2nd sacral vertebrae), and a venous plexus. It is therefore quite possible to inject large quantities of local anaesthetic solution both intravascularly and into the subarachnoid space: both of these events can be disastrous if not detected and treated promptly.

When local anaesthetic solution is injected into the sacral canal it ascends upwards in the extradural space for a distance proportional to the volume of the solution, the force of injection, the amount of leakage through the eight sacral foramina, and the consistency of the connective tissue in the sacral space. While the first two are controllable, the last two are not and unexpected results can occur. Lignocaine 1–2% and bupivacaine 0.25–0.5% both work well. In an average man, 30 mL will block to L2–L4 (whole of perineal area) and 20 mL will suffice for haemorrhoids or anal fissure. If surgeons do not like a relaxed anal sphincter for surgery the block can be instituted after surgery but before awakening, for postoperative pain relief. Urinary retention is an easily missed complication of the block which, in the elderly, can present as confusion.

Epidural block

This is blockage of the nerve roots outside the dura. Within the relevant peripheral nerve distribution it gives relaxation of muscles, analgesia and a degree of hypotension dependent upon the extent of sympathetic blockade. Unless the block goes to an unpredictably high level it allows spontaneous respiration with the diaphragm, although the intercostals may be compromised. Like other forms of regional blockade it suppresses afferent impulses secondary to painful stimuli and the hormonal and autonomic responses to surgery. In the UK it is usually used in combination with light general anaesthesia. Often catheters are introduced into the epidural space so that the block can be continued into the postoperative period. One of the advantages of epidural blockade is that it allows a 'band' of analgesia to be established without paralysis of the lower limbs.

Once the epidural space has been identified the extent of the block is influenced by the volume and concentration of solution injected, the age of the patient (the aged need less), the location of the catheter (thoracic segments need less than lumbar segments for each dermatome), the length of the vertebral column, and the presence of large abdominal tumours. The exact extent of block secondary to a given volume of local anaesthetic is unpredictable to a high degree of accuracy.

Epidural blockade has several complications which can occur during 'top-ups' on the postoperative ward as well as at the time of insertion. Those most likely to cause problems are the following:

- Inadequate block, unilateral block or missed segments.
- Hypotension and cardiovascular depression from sympathetic blockade. This requires oxygen, intravenous solutions, pressor drugs and, if there is a bradycardia, atropine.
- Toxicity due to absorption of the injected drug (either local anaesthetic or opioid).
- Unexpected respiratory depression.
- Unexpected total spinal anaesthesia, sometimes from migration of the catheter into the subarachnoid space. This is life threatening and requires immediate action. A typical dose of epidural local anaesthetic (10 mL) is approximately five times the volume of drug required to produce the same level of block when injected into the subarachnoid space.
- Nausea, vomiting and shivering.
- Unexpectedly prolonged analgesia.

Because of the potential complications of epidural analgesia, all patients receiving it postoperatively should be nursed in a suitable environment with ready access to anaesthetic support. Epidural opioid analgesia is considered below (Epidural techniques).

All catheters should be inspected after removal and recorded as being intact. Although extradural abscesses are rare, because they may be metastatic many anaesthetists are reluctant to establish or continue with epidural analgesia in the presence of systemic sepsis.

Other absolute contraindications to regional blockade are local sepsis, patient refusal and the presence of a coagulopathy or therapeutic anticoagulation because of the risk of epidural haematoma formation and subsequent neurological damage. There is controversy concerning the use of these techniques in patients receiving prophylactic low-dose heparin or aspirin. There is no firm evidence that this will increase the risk of epidural haematoma and a balanced judgement as to the risks and benefits of the technique needs to be taken in each patient. If possible, regional anaesthesia should be undertaken before the first dose of unfractionated heparin is given or delayed until 6 hours after the previous dose (Bullingham and Strunin, 1995). A 12-hour interval has been recommended following low molecular weight heparin. Similarly, some would consider that aspirin therapy should ideally be stopped for 7–10 days before instituting a regional block or before a bleeding time is performed.

Other relative contraindications include neurological disease and some forms of cardiac disease (e.g. aortic stenosis).

Subarachnoid (spinal) block

Subarachnoid block entails performing a lumbar puncture and injecting local anaesthetic directly into the cerebrospinal fluid (CSF). Although the use of very fine catheters has been reported, spinal block is essentially a single shot technique. As with epidural block, in the UK it is usually combined with general anaesthesia or sedation.

In contrast to epidural block, when local anaesthetics are injected into the subarachnoid space they effectively produce a pharmacological transection of the cauda equina and spinal cord at the upper level of the solution. There is no sparing of any fibres or tracts, and if the abdomen is to be anaesthetized then the lower limbs are automatically paralysed. The highest dermatome reached depends upon the volume and concentration of solution, the force and rate of injection, the position of the patient, the interspace chosen and the specific gravity of the solution.

The most common intraoperative complication is a fall in blood pressure from sympathetic blockade, which, if necessary, is treated with fluid and vasoconstrictors. As long as the block is acting, retention of urine remains a possibility and the immobility of the patient may lead to ischaemia over pressure areas. If the block does not start to regress at the expected time the anaesthetist should be contacted at once.

The most common postoperative complication is headache. The classical spinal headache is a low pressure headache that is worse in the upright posture and relieved by lying down, and may be associated with meningism and photophobia. It is seen most commonly in young adults (females more than males), and is closely related to the size and type of needle used. The larger the needle, the greater the incidence of headache. The majority of spinal headaches can be managed by the following simple measures:

- Bed rest
- Good hydration via i.v. or oral fluids
- Simple analgesics
- Nursing in a darkened room if photophobia is a problem.

If the headache does not settle within a day or so consideration should be given to performing an epidural blood patch.

The introduction of pencil point needle tips and finer gauge needles have significantly lowered the risk of postdural puncture headaches and hence spinal techniques may be satisfactory for day patients. The use of spinal opioids is described below (Spinal techniques).

Anastomosis and anaesthesia

Morbidity and mortality from gastrointestinal complications can result indirectly from the effects of anaesthesia on cardiovascular and respiratory function, or directly from the effects of drugs and anaesthetic manoeuvres on the bowel. The effect of anaesthesia on the bowel is a very unresearched area with a considerable amount of anecdotal and apocryphal opinion overshadowing fact. Anaesthesia can affect both gastrointestinal activity and intestinal blood flow.

Drugs and gastrointestinal activity

There are many drugs administered intraoperatively which can potentially affect intestinal activity.

The anticholinesterase neostigmine increases motor activity in the ileum very considerably but increased colonic or rectal activity occurs in only 20% of patients anaesthetized with nitrous oxide (Wilkins et al, 1970). Neostigmine has long had a reputation for disrupting anastomoses (Bell and Lewis, 1968) but the increased activity of the colon following neostigmine can be inhibited by using large doses of atropine or by using halothane during the course of anaesthesia (Wilkins et al, 1970). It has also been suggested that neostigmine increases intraluminal pressure, thus increasing the risk of suture line dehiscence, and that the reduction in colonic blood flow it induces (up to 50%) puts the anastomotic area at risk (Whittaker, 1968). To the authors' knowledge, there are no large, well-controlled series which assess the detailed effect of neostigmine or the anticholinesterases atropine or glycopyrollate on the human colon in clinical practice.

Halothane depresses intestinal and colonic contractions and antagonizes the effect of morphine and neostigmine on the bowel (Marshall et al, 1961). Diazepam depresses gastrointestinal motility (Birnbaum et al, 1970), and metoclopramide, although it generates contractions, may prolong ileus because the contractions are uncoordinated and non-propulsive (Jepsen et al, 1986).

Morphine increases the tone of the small and large intestine but decreases motility. The effects can be antagonized experimentally with naloxone. It has been suggested that in patients with diverticular disease morphine should be avoided because of the risk of colonic spasm and diverticular perforation (Painter and Truelove, 1964a). It has also been suggested that because of its spasmolytic effects pethidine may be the analgesic of choice following intestinal anastomosis; on the other hand it may contribute to postoperative ileus in view of its atropine-like action (Painter and Truelove, 1964b; Ekbom et al, 1980).

Spinal and epidural anaesthesia increase motility

in the colon because blockade of the sympathetic nerves allows the parasympathetic to act unopposed. Disruption of a colonic anastomosis in the early postoperative period has been attributed to the increased contractility associated with extradural blockade (Bigler et al, 1985).

Colonic blood flow

Whittaker and colleagues (Whittaker, 1968; Whittaker et al, 1970) concluded that the blood flow to the bowel was the most important factor in the healing of an anastomosis and that a 10% reduction in blood volume from haemorrhage markedly increased the risk of anastomotic breakdown. Schrock et al (1973) found a high anastomotic leakage rate when the blood pressure fell below 50 mmHg. Blood viscosity is cited as being an important factor in wound healing and there is a theoretical optimal haematocrit at which the balance between oxygen carriage and viscosity maximizes the oxygen delivery to the tissues: this is about 11 g/dL, which corresponds to a haematocrit of 35% (Gruber, 1970).

Colonic perfusion is regulated extrinsically by the sympathetic and parasympathetic systems: intrinsically, arteriolar and precapillary tone are modulated by cellular metabolites, and arteriolar smooth muscle contractility responds to stretch, providing some myogenic autoregulation. There are thus many ways in which anaesthesia and its effects can affect colonic blood flow.

Halothane decreases vascular resistance and increases mesenteric blood flow. Enflurane produces little change but isoflurane, surprisingly, was found to increase splanchnic vascular resistance (Tverskoy et al, 1985). Isoflurane can however suppress the reflex vasoconstriction in the renal and intestinal blood vessels in response to surgical stimulation, and to this end its effects were beneficial (Ostman et al, 1986). All these effects of volatile agents are dose dependent and motility returns to normal as the drug is eliminated. Thus, volatile agents are unlikely to alter the postoperative course by effects on gut motility, although they may modify the effects of other drugs given during the operation. Nitrous oxide diffuses into gas-containing viscera more rapidly than nitrogen diffuses out, with resultant distension of the bowel. This distension may hamper abdominal wall closure, predispose to ileus and interfere with colonic blood flow (Lewis, 1975); there are no hard data to quantify these theoretical problems in patients.

If it is necessary to administer vasoactive agents there is considerable potential for altering colonic blood flow. Direct or indirect action on the splanchnic and lumbar colonic nerves decreases blood flow by vasoconstriction. Adrenaline and noradrenaline increase colonic vascular resistance and decrease blood flow and oxygen uptake; isoprenaline increases colonic perfusion but appears to have no effect on oxygen uptake. Vagal stimulation has little effect on colonic blood flow, but activity in the parasympathetic pelvic nerves causes intense hyperaemia.

Spinal and epidural anaesthesia vasodilate the body caudal to the height of the block. Blood flow to the bowel reflects the balance between the degree of vasodilatation and the reduction in systemic arterial perfusion pressure. In dog models a 22% increase in colonic blood flow has been recorded with the onset of epidural block (Aitkenhead et al, 1980). In humans, although retrospective studies have suggested a reduction in anastomotic breakdown with the use of spinal block, this has not been confirmed by prospective studies (Worsley et al, 1988). Although spinal block may well improve colonic blood flow, any improvement may be negated by haemorrhage or the use of vasoconstrictors.

In summary, there are therefore no definite conclusions to be drawn which can at present recommend any one particular intraoperative anaesthetic technique as being superior to another, given that patients are well oxygenated and hydrated.

Perioperative blood transfusion

Adequate perioperative fluid replacement is necessary to maintain vital organ function. Blood transfusion may be associated with many unwanted sequelae including infection and allergic reactions. Subsequent immunosuppression is well described, probably due to donor leucocytes carrying foreign antigens and this may be associated with increased tumour recurrence rate after colorectal surgery (Wheatley and Veitch, 1997). To reduce this risk, leucocyte-depleted blood has been used, as have a variety of methods to reduce the requirement for homologous blood transfusion. There has also been a move, over the past few years, towards accepting a lower perioperative haemoglobin level in otherwise fit patients. This may even improve tissue perfusion, providing that the circulating fluid volume is maintained.

Anaesthesia for minimally invasive surgery

Laparoscopic techniques for abdominal surgery offer a number of advantages, including reduced postoperative pain, low postoperative pulmonary dysfunction and a quicker recovery. However, the effects of a pneumoperitoneum, changes in position and prolonged surgery may have significant adverse effects, especially in patients with pre-existing cardiorespiratory disease.

A steep Trendelenburg position will cause a cephalad movement of the diaphragm leading to a reduced functional residual capacity, reduced lung volume and pulmonary compliance and possibly a deterioration in ventilation/perfusion matching. The pneumoperitoneum will exacerbate these changes. If carbon dioxide is used as the insufflating gas, this will be absorbed systemically, leading to a progressive rise in carbon dioxide excretion which usually plateaus after 20 minutes. This is an important period for careful monitoring since intravascular carbon dioxide can be fatal. A significant gas embolus is characterized by a sudden fall in expired carbon dioxide and cardiovascular collapse. Monitoring with capnography is essentially mandatory as is good communication between anaesthetist and surgeon.

The Trendelenburg position produces an increased venous return and central venous pressure which may produce deleterious effects in those with coronary artery disease or ventricular dysfunction. Intra-abdominal insufflation is associated with a marked reduction in cardiac output due to a diminution of venous return and increased systemic vascular resistance. Splenic and mesenteric blood flow may also be deleteriously affected.

In addition, the anaesthetist may have to deal with the other consequences of surgical complications such as pneumothorax and vascular trauma (Brichant, 1995).

POSTOPERATIVE CARE

All patients recovering from general or regional anaesthesia should be admitted to a properly staffed and equipped recovery room until they are in a satisfactory condition to return to the general ward. There should be adequate provision of high-dependency beds for patients undergoing major surgery or for those with significant intercurrent disease, thereby allowing appropriate analgesia and physiological support postoperatively. The use of high-dependency beds allows proper intensive therapy facilities to be used only for those patients requiring a higher level of respiratory or cardiovascular support.

POSTOPERATIVE PAIN RELIEF

A number of reports have highlighted the unsatisfactory management of postoperative pain (Royal College of Surgeons of England and College of Anaesthetists, 1990). There has been a great deal of recent interest in this area and many hospitals have set up an acute pain service to improve treatment, education and research.

There is a tremendous variability in individual requirements for postoperative analgesia (Figure 7.1). This is related to the site of surgery, pharmacokinetic and pharmacodynamic variability, the psychological make-up of the patient and the expectations of the ward staff. It is commonly stated that thoracic surgery is the most painful, followed by upper abdominal surgery, then lower abdominal surgery, with body surface and limb surgery the least painful.

Although there are as yet few 'hard data' to confirm that effective postoperative pain relief assists the rate of recovery from surgery, there are nevertheless good reasons to improve our management. These include the following:

- Pain should be relieved for humanitarian reasons.
- Pain relief can aid rapid mobilization, thus reducing the complications of bed rest (deep vein thromboses and pressure sores).
- There is no doubt that a painful abdomen reflexly impairs the bellows function of the lungs. This can result in hypoxia and the development of chest infections. Good pain relief also facilitates effective physiotherapy.
- Pain produces hypertension and tachycardia and inhibits sleep. This can produce tiredness, irritability and myocardial ischaemia in susceptible persons.
- There is also good evidence that effective pain relief reduces the detrimental components of the metabolic stress response to surgery.

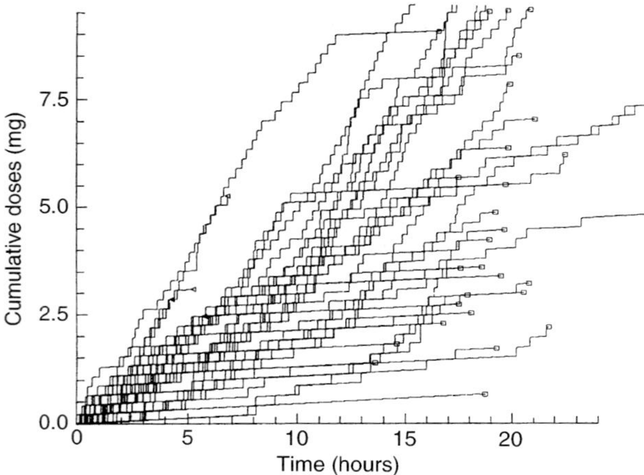

Figure 7.1 Cumulative dose plots of 40 patients treated with alfentanil for postoperative patient-controlled analgesia, demonstrating the variability in opiate requirement. From Lehmann (1985), with permission.

Regular recording of pain postoperatively allows proper assessment and audit of the problem and may, in itself, improve the administration of analgesia (Gould et al, 1992). Recording may take the form of a visual analogue scale or a simple scoring system. A typical example of this is shown in Figure 7.2. It is preferable that the pain scores are recorded on the same sheet as a sedation score and other routine postoperative observations including respiratory rate, pulse and blood pressure.

Pre-emptive analgesia

Tissue injury that occurs during surgery produces both a peripheral and a central sensitization to pain so that subsequent, previously innocuous, stimuli will be perceived to be painful, noxious stimuli will be more painful and the area of sensitivity will be widened. Peripheral sensitization involves the local release of chemical mediators. Central sensitization is related to an increase in the sensitivity of the pain transmitting dorsal horn neurones.

Experimental evidence suggests that administration of analgesics prior to the tissue injury will reduce these changes. However, clinical studies have not confirmed that current analgesic regimens commenced before surgery have a marked impact on subsequent analgesic consumption or pain scores (Dahl and Kehlet, 1993).

There are several ways in which postoperative pain can be managed, as described briefly below.

Non-steroidal anti-inflammatory drugs

These agents are useful for relieving the pain of minor surgery and may also be used after major surgery for their morphine sparing effect. The relative efficacy of these drugs is unclear but only a few are available for parenteral administration. Side-effects may include renal dysfunction, bronchospasm and peptic ulceration. Recent clinical guidelines on their use have been published by the Royal College of Anaesthetists (Royal College of Anaesthetists, 1998).

Intramuscular opioids

The administration of an opioid drug on a p.r.n. i.m. basis is still the most common method of prescribed postoperative analgesia in the UK. Almost all surveys have found it to be ineffective in the control of pain, although often patients have not complained since they expected little else. It is felt by many medical and nursing staff to be 'safe' since the patient has to be awake enough to request a further dose. An algorithm has been produced which allows nursing staff to administer more frequent doses of intramuscular opiates depending on pain and sedation scores and this may improve the efficacy of the method (Figure 7.2).

Intravenous opioid infusions

These are best established with an intraoperative loading dose and then continued into the postoperative period. Properly managed they can be very effective and have the advantage of being able to be titrated to individual need by the nursing staff. The major danger is the risk of serious respiratory depression occurring and respiratory monitoring is mandatory. It is the view of many anaesthetists that this form of analgesia should not be used outside an intensive therapy unit, high-dependency unit or other specialized environment.

Patient-controlled analgesia (PCA)

The basis of PCA is that patients are able to control how much analgesia they receive, within the limits set by the prescribing doctor. In order to set a PCA regimen it is necessary to decide upon several factors, e.g. type of drug, size of bolus dose, lockout interval, background infusion rate (if any) and total dose permissible within a given time interval. PCA may be used to administer drugs intravenously, intramuscularly, subcutaneously or extradurally, but to date almost all the work has been done with intravenous opioids. Several studies have shown

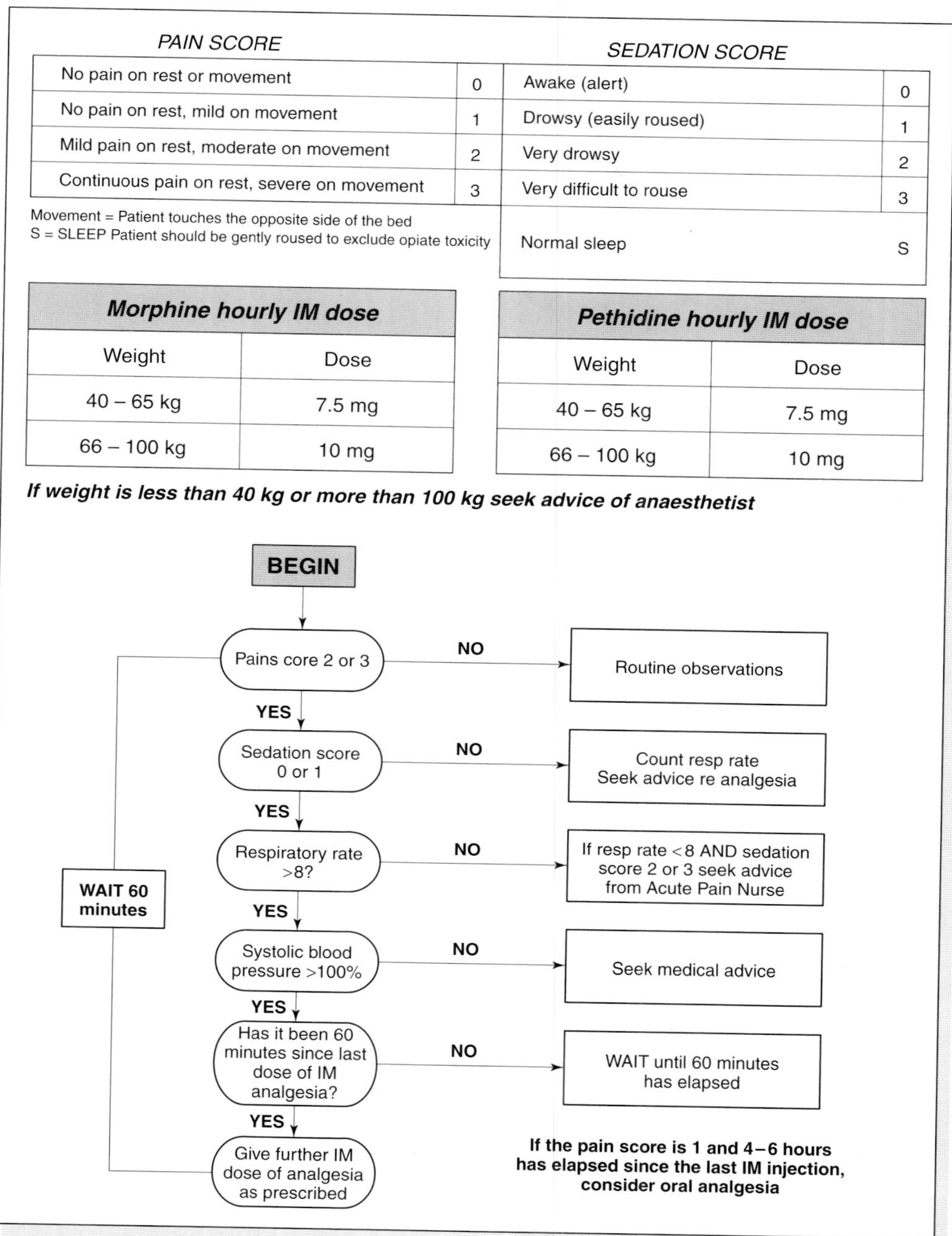

PAIN SCORE	
No pain on rest or movement	0
No pain on rest, mild on movement	1
Mild pain on rest, moderate on movement	2
Continuous pain on rest, severe on movement	3

Movement = Patient touches the opposite side of the bed
S = SLEEP Patient should be gently roused to exclude opiate toxicity

SEDATION SCORE	
Awake (alert)	0
Drowsy (easily roused)	1
Very drowsy	2
Very difficult to rouse	3
Normal sleep	S

Morphine hourly IM dose	
Weight	Dose
40 – 65 kg	7.5 mg
66 – 100 kg	10 mg

Pethidine hourly IM dose	
Weight	Dose
40 – 65 kg	7.5 mg
66 – 100 kg	10 mg

If weight is less than 40 kg or more than 100 kg seek advice of anaesthetist

Figure 7.2 Guidelines for intramuscular analgesia. Every patient receiving opioid analgesia must have an intravenous cannula *in situ*.

that the use of PCA is associated with a lower total dose of drug and superior patient satisfaction. The true reason for this is not yet clear, however, and may in some way be related to the sense of control which the patient has over his or her own therapy.

Caudal blocks

These have been described above and, using bupivacaine on a single shot basis, provide several hours of effective analgesia for all operations on the anus and perineum.

Spinal techniques

Only spinal opioids are relevant to postoperative pain control since local anaesthetics are short acting and spinal blocks cannot be topped up. Spinal opioid receptors exist, probably in the substantia gelatinosa, and their action is thought to be presynaptic, reducing the release of substance P from the first-order pain neurones. In some centres spinal opioids (e.g. 1 or 2 mg morphine in 10 mL saline injected into the cerebrospinal fluid) are used frequently on an empirical basis but there is still a paucity of literature on the subject. One dose typically lasts for 24 hours and the major danger is respiratory depression, which may not occur maximally for several hours. Some of the complications of spinal anaesthesia have been given above (Subarachnoid (spinal) block). Following the administration of spinal opioids careful monitoring of respiration is essential; the side-effects of spinal opioids are similar to those of epidural opioids.

Epidural techniques

Epidural techniques are technically more difficult to perform than spinal techniques and the thoracic epidural space is more difficult to identify than the lumbar space. Furthermore, there is more chance of accidental neurological damage being produced by the needle in the thoracic space because the spinal cord has not divided to form the cauda equina. The advantage of thoracic blockade is that it can provide analgesia for upper abdominal incisions whilst sparing the lumbar and sacral roots.

Although some epidural blocks are done as a 'single shot', in the majority of cases a plastic catheter is introduced into the epidural space. This allows greater control over the duration and extent of analgesia, repeated dosing and the possibility of infusions. Local anaesthetics, opioids, or a combination of both can be used postoperatively. Aficionados of the technique are increasingly moving to combination therapy given by infusion and there are now several reports of successful epidural PCA.

The administration of epidural opioids is now widespread. Experimental human studies are difficult but animal models have shown that following the epidural injection of morphine the concentration in lumbar CSF can peak at 2 hours. This cannot be assumed for other opioids since they have different fat solubilities. There is a considerable concentration gradient of the drug in the CSF and its distribution can be affected by activities such as coughing. Systemic absorption also takes place and contributes to the analgesic effect.

Following administration, epidural opioids start to act in 20–40 minutes and can last from 4 to 36 hours. The effective dose range is wide but is typically 2–5 mg of morphine or diamorphine made up in 10 mL of saline. Some of the complications of epidural blockade have already been given. Complications specific to the use of opioids are respiratory depression (which may be severe and delayed), itching (particularly on the face), urinary retention and nausea. All patients receiving postoperative epidural analgesia need to be monitored in an appropriate setting with particular attention being paid to respiration. In some patients postoperative epidural analgesia is superb. When it is only partially effective great care must be exercised in superimposing intramuscular or intravenous opioids because of synergy producing unpredictable and profound respiratory depression. It is likely that with the development of high-dependency units and postoperative care wards the use of postoperative epidural analgesia will increase.

POSTOPERATIVE NAUSEA AND VOMITING

Many patients consider nausea and vomiting to be the most unpleasant aspect of their postoperative course and may, for example, desist from using a patient-controlled analgesia pump to avoid this complication. There may also be more serious effects including wound dehiscence, bleeding, dehydration, electrolyte imbalance and economic sequelae from increased recovery room stay and unanticipated admission after day surgery (Reynolds and Blogg, 1999). The reported incidence of postoperative nausea and vomiting (PONV) is very variable but is increased in obesity, females, those with a past history of PONV and the administration of opiates. The type of surgery is also important: abdominal and laparoscopic surgery are associated with a higher incidence. Anaesthetic technique and agents have relatively little effect although propofol may be associated with a lower incidence. Avoidance of opiate analgesia should be considered for those at risk from PONV.

A variety of drugs are available for prophylaxis and treatment. These act at different receptor sites and a combination of agents may occasionally be considered appropriate. The phenothiazines (e.g. prochlorperazine) are an effective treatment but have side-effects that include sedation, hypotension and extrapyramidal reactions. Butyrophenones (e.g. droperidol) have a similar mode of action, are effective when given prophylactically but have similar side-effects to the phenothiazines. Metoclopramide also acts via dopamine receptors and has prokinetic effects which may be undesirable after bowel surgery. Although widely used, the evidence for its efficacy is relatively weak. Dystonic reactions are common and cardiovascular side-effects may occur after intravenous injection. Antihistamines (e.g. cyclizine) are effective. Side-effects include sedation and dry mouth. Anticholinergic drugs such as hyoscine have some value but commonly give rise to dry mouth, sedation and visual disturbance. A hyoscine patch has been used to reduce these effects.

Much recent interest has centred on 5-hydroxytryptamine antagonists such as ondansetron. This was introduced to reduce the nausea and vomiting of chemotherapy but has also proved to be useful in the prophylaxis and treatment of PONV, although its efficacy compared to other antiemetic agents has yet to be proved. It has a long period of action and a good side-effect profile but its expense prevents its use as a routine first-line agent.

REFERENCES

Aitkenhead AR, Gilmour DG, Hothershall AP & Ledingham IMcA (1980) Effects of sub-arachnoid spinal nerve block and arterial Pco_2 on colon blood flow in the dog. *Br J Anaesth* **52**: 1071–1077.

Bell CMA & Lewis CB (1968) Effect of neostigmine on integrity of ileorectal anastomosis. *BMJ* **3**: 587–588.

Bigler D, Hjortso N-C & Kehlet H (1985) Disruption of colonic anastomosis during continuous epidural analgesia. An early post-operative complication. *Anaesthesia* **40**: 278–280.

Birnbaum D, Ben-Menachem J & Schwartz A (1970) The influence of oral diazepam on gastrointestinal motility. *Am J Proctol* **21**: 263–267.

Brichant JF (1995) Anaesthesia for minimally invasive abdominal surgery. In Adams AP & Cashman JP (eds) *Recent Advances in Anaesthesia and Analgesia 19*, pp 33–53. Edinburgh: Churchill Livingstone.

Bullingham A & Strunin L (1995) Prevention of postoperative venous thromboembolism. *Br J Anaesth* **75**: 622–630.

Dahl JB & Kehlet H (1993) The value of pre-emptive analgesia in the treatment of postoperative pain. *Br J Anaesth* **70**: 434–439.

Ekbom G, Schulte WJ, Condon RE, Woods JH & Cowles V (1980) Effects of narcotic analgesics on bowel motility in subhuman primates. *J Surg Res* **28**: 293–296.

Gould TH, Crosby DL, Harmer M et al (1992) Policy for controlling pain after surgery: effect of sequential changes in management. *BMJ* **305**: 1187–1193.

Gruber UF (1970) Recent developments in the investigation and treatment of hypovolaemic shock. *Br J Hosp Med* **4**: 631–638.

Jepsen S, Klaerke A, Nielsen PH & Simonsen O (1986) Negative effect of metoclopramide in post-operative adynamic ileus. A prospective, randomised, double blind study. *Br J Surg* **73**: 290–291.

Lehmann KA (1985) The pharmacokinetics of opioid analgesics – discussion. In Harmer M, Rosen M & Vickers MD (eds) *Patient Controlled Analgesia*, p 27. Oxford: Blackwell.

Lewis GBH (1975) Intestinal distension during nitrous oxide anaesthesia. *Can Anaesth Soc J* **22**: 200–201.

Marshall FN, Pittinger CB & Long JP (1961) Effects of halothane on gastrointestinal motility. *Anesthesiology* **22**: 363–366.

Ostman M, Biber B, Martner J & Reiz S (1986) Influence of isoflurane on renal and intestinal vascular responses to stress. *Br J Anaesth* **58**: 630–638.

Painter NS & Truelove SC (1964a) The intraluminal pressure patterns in diverticulosis of the colon. Part II: The effect of morphine. *Gut* **5**: 201–213.

Painter NS & Truelove SC (1964b) The intraluminal pressure patterns in diverticulosis of the colon. Part IV: The effect of pethidine and probanthine. *Gut* **5**: 369–373.

Reynolds DJM & Blogg CE (1995) Prevention and treatment of postoperative nausea and vomiting. *Prescribers J* **35**: 111–116.

Royal College of Anaesthetists (1998) *Guidelines for the Use of NSAIDs in the Post-operative Period*. London: Royal College of Anaesthetists.

Royal College of Surgeons of England, the College of Anaesthetists (1990) *Report of the Working Party on Pain after Surgery*. Commission on the Provision of Surgical Services. London: Royal College of Surgeons.

Schrock TR, Devene CW & Dunphy JE (1973) Factors contributing to colonic anastomosis. *Ann Surg* **177**: 513–517.

Tverskoy CB, Gelman S, Fowler KC & Bradley EL (1985) Intestinal circulation and anaesthesia. *Anesthesiology* **62**: 462–469.

Wheatley T & Veitch PS (1997) Effects of blood transfusion on postoperative immunocompetence. *Br J Anaesth* **78**: 490–492.

Whittaker BL (1968) Observations on the blood flow in the inferior mesenteric arterial system and the healing of colonic anastomoses. *Ann R Coll Surg Engl* **43**: 89–110.

Whittaker BL, Dixon RD & Greatorex G (1970) Anastomosis failure in relation to blood transfusion and blood flow. *Proc R Soc Med* **63**: 751–752.

Wilkins JL, Hardcastle JD, Mann CV & Kaufman L (1970) Effects of neostigmine and atropine on the motor activity of ileum, colon, and rectum of anaesthetised subjects. *BMJ* **1**: 793–794.

Worsley MH, Wishart HY, Peebles Brown DA & Aitkenhead AR (1988) High spinal nerve block for large bowel anastomosis. A prospective study. *Br J Anaesth* **60**: 836–840.

FURTHER READING

Aitkenhead AR (1988) Anaesthesia and the gastro-intestinal system. *Eur J Anaesthesiol* **5**: 73–112.

Healy TEJ & Cohen PJ (1995) *Wylie and Churchill Davidson's A Practice of Anaesthesia*, 6th edn, Chapters 34, 36 and 76. London: Edward Arnold.

Kaufman L (1983) Anaesthesia for large bowel surgery: a review. *J R Soc Med* **76**: 693–696.

Prys-Roberts C & Brown BR (1996) *International Practice of Anaesthesia*, Chapters 41, 64, 140. Oxford: Butterworth-Heinemann.

8

ILEOSTOMY

Ileostomy is a necessary outcome of certain colorectal operations. The ileostomy may be permanent or temporary. It may be a loop stoma or an end ileostomy. Complications and social morbidity are high in ileostomy patients (Pearl et al, 1985). Specific ileostomy complications include retraction, prolapse, hernia, fistula, ulceration, stenosis, bleeding and profuse ileostomy diarrhoea causing serious fluid and electrolyte loss. The rate of complications depends on length of follow-up and may be as high as 59–76% after 20 years (Leong et al, 1994). These complications are found to be more common after loop ileostomy than end ileostomy (Pearl et al, 1985). Complications of loop ileostomy closure are less frequent than those following loop colostomy closure; however, intestinal obstruction, abscess and fistula occur in 10–15% after closing a covering ileostomy after restorative proctocolectomy and pouch anal anastomosis (Hosie et al, 1992; Wexner et al, 1993).

HISTORY

The history of ileostomy is quite short. Ileostomy became a practical method of surgical therapy only when appliances became available which provided a hermetic seal to fluid and gas. Modern appliances emerged following the report by Strauss and Strauss on the Koernig bag (Strauss and Strauss, 1944). Koernig, a chemistry student who had an ileostomy for ulcerative colitis, designed a bag made of rubber and fixed the appliance to the skin with a latex preparation so that the effluent no longer came into contact with the skin. However, at this time the ileum was either sutured flush with the skin or was left protruding from the abdominal wall on its mesentery. The earliest ileostomies were placed either in the incision or through the abdominal wall well lateral to the rectus muscle. Indeed the fate of patients requiring ablative operations for ulcerative colitis early in this century was so dismal that death from untreated disease or an ill-advised ileorectal anastomosis was regarded by some patients as preferable to an ileostomy.

John Young Brown of St Louis first introduced ileostomy into the management of ulcerative colitis in 1913 (Brown, 1913). He suggested that an ileostomy might be used as a temporary measure to allow the inflammatory process in the colon to abate.

Ileostomy was a controversial operation in the 1920s and 1930s and many clinicians preferred appendicostomy as a temporary stoma for colitis. Total proctocolectomy and end ileostomy was popularized as the optimum operation for ulcerative colitis by Gavin Miller, and many still regard this as the best surgical therapy for severe proctocolitis (Miller et al, 1949; Lee & Truelove, 1980). Nevertheless, in the 1940s the place of total ablative surgery for fulminating colitis was questioned and the more cautious approach of subtotal colectomy with ileostomy and mucous fistula became widely accepted as the best surgical option for patients with fulminating colitis who had not responded to aggressive medical therapy (Brooke, 1983). Even so, the early ileostomies were difficult to manage as they were either flush with the skin or, even if they protruded from the skin, they were not everted and there was a high incidence of stenosis. Ileal fluid frequently leaked causing damage to the skin and to the end of the ileum. Scarring of the tissues around the stoma resulted in ileal stenosis and obstruction which caused severe ileostomy dysfunction. Dragstedt et al (1941) tried to resolve this by placing skin grafts over the ileostomy. Warren and McKittrick (1951) were the first to recognize that the symptoms of intestinal colic, dehydration and intermittent profuse ileostomy output were the result of sepsis and obstruction because the ileum and skin were not protected. In order to resolve this problem, Crile and Turnbull (1954) proposed that mucosal grafts should be placed on the scarified serosa of the ileum as a means of protecting it against enzymatic digestion from the bowel. In this manner the skin adjacent to the ileum could also be protected by karaya gum. However, it was Brooke in 1952 (Brooke, 1952) who resolved the problem by designing the eversion ileostomy. This ingenious technique of turning the end of the ileum back over itself provided an immediate solution to problems of ileostomy stenosis and excoriated peristomal skin.

INCIDENCE

Permanent ileostomy

It was estimated by Hawley and Ritchie (1979) that about 10 000 patients with an ileostomy were alive in England and Wales and that at the time of survey 400–500 new ileostomies were being constructed every year. If temporary ileostomies are also taken into consideration it is likely that these numbers have increased significantly in recent years (Office of Population Censuses and Surveys, 1970). Reasons for the increase include the rising incidence of inflammatory bowel disease in northern Europe (Devlin et al, 1980; Langman and Burnham, 1983), surgery for ulcerative colitis has become more attractive now that there are acceptable alternatives to a permanent stoma (Cohen et al, 1985; Dozois et al, 1986) and the increased use of loop ileostomy as an alternative to loop colostomy for the protection of an anastomosis or as primary therapy for inflammatory bowel disease (Fasth et al, 1980; Raimes et al, 1984). Over 5000 ileostomates are registered in Great Britain and Ireland with the Ileostomy Association but it is likely that rather less than half of all patients with a permanent stoma join this organization (Whates and Irving, 1984).

The number of patients with an ileostomy in the USA is not known, but it has been estimated that approximately 4000 ileostomies were created in 1968 (Grogan and Smith, 1973). It is likely, therefore, that the total number of patients with a permanent ileostomy in the USA exceeds 100 000.

Age and sex

Most ileostomies constructed for ulcerative colitis are undertaken in patients in their second or third decade. In Crohn's disease the age spectrum is wider, with a bimodal distribution having an early peak in the second decade and a small peak in the fifth decade. The male to female ratio of ileostomies is approximately 1:1.4 (Devlin, 1982).

INDICATIONS

End ileostomy

End ileostomy is often constructed as a permanent stoma for patients with ulcerative colitis, Crohn's disease, familial adenomatous polyposis or multiple large bowel cancer (Figure 8.1). It is usually the outcome of proctocolectomy (Goligher, 1983a). However, end ileostomy may be used following subtotal colectomy if an ileorectal anastomosis is undesirable. Under these circumstances, the rectal stump may have been oversewn or raised as a mucous fistula. This arrangement should not be regarded as permanent, since the rectal stump may continue to be the source of serious ill-health from inflammatory disease and there is a persistent, though small risk of malignancy (Hughes and Russell, 1967). A decision should be taken in such cases, usually within a year of subtotal colectomy, on whether (1) to proceed with an ileorectal anastomosis on the understanding that close surveillance is mandatory, (2) to advise a restorative proctocolectomy with ileoanal anastomosis, or (3) to remove the rectum leaving the ileostomy as a permanent stoma.

An end ileostomy may be used as a temporary stoma and is preferred by some over a loop ileostomy to protect a colorectal or ileorectal anastomosis or an ileoanal pouch (Fonkaldsrud, 1980; Delaney and Mulholland, 1983; Metcalf et al, 1986a). An end ileostomy is also constructed as part of the operation of split ileostomy so as to ensure complete diversion of the faecal stream. This procedure has been used for patients with Crohn's colitis or severe perianal Crohn's disease (Lee, 1975; Harper et al, 1983), to protect an anastomosis or a pouch, or as an emergency measure for patients who have sustained injury or operative damage to the small or large intestine (Pearl et al, 1985).

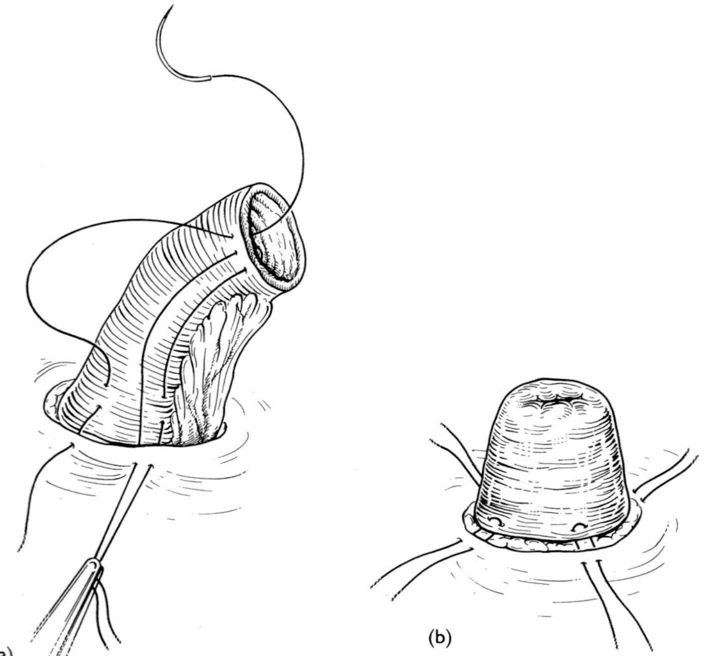

Figure 8.1 Construction of an end ileostomy. In (a) the terminal ileum has been delivered through a circular trephine in the abdominal wall, and in (b) is being everted prior to completion by mucocutaneous sutures.

Loop ileostomy

Loop ileostomy was introduced by Turnbull (1961, 1971, 1975) as a means of providing a more satisfactory stoma for patients with a short or fat ileal mesentery and in the obese patient where the blood supply of a permanent end stoma might become compromised. The distal end of the ileum was oversewn and a loop of proximal ileum raised to the surface and everted over a rod (Figure 8.2a–c). However, the use of a rod is not always necessary (Unti et al, 1991). This stoma proved very effective when the terminal ileum could not be delivered through the abdominal wall without the risk of ischaemia and necrosis of the stoma. The technique is still widely used for this reason (Fazio et al, 1975; Fazio, 1983).

It was soon realized by Alexander-Williams (1974) and others (Devlin, 1982; Rombeau et al, 1978; Todd, 1978; Fasth and Hulten, 1984) that a loop ileostomy could be used not only as a permanent stoma but also as a means of decompressing the distal ileum and colon (Figure 8.3a–c). It has become popular as a means of protecting Kock pouches, ileoanal pouches, and an ileorectal anastomosis if the rectum is diseased and where there is a risk of leak from a suture line (Aylett, 1966; Parks and Nicholls, 1978; Telender and Perrault, 1980; Hulten and Fasth, 1981; Ambrose et al, 1984; Fasth and Hulten, 1984; Alexander-Williams and Haynes, 1985). The scope of the loop ileostomy has been extended to include the management of anal and abdominal fistula as a definitive therapy for megacolon (Raimes et al, 1984) and for protecting reconstructive anorectal procedures. Many now use a loop ileostomy in preference to split ileostomy as a

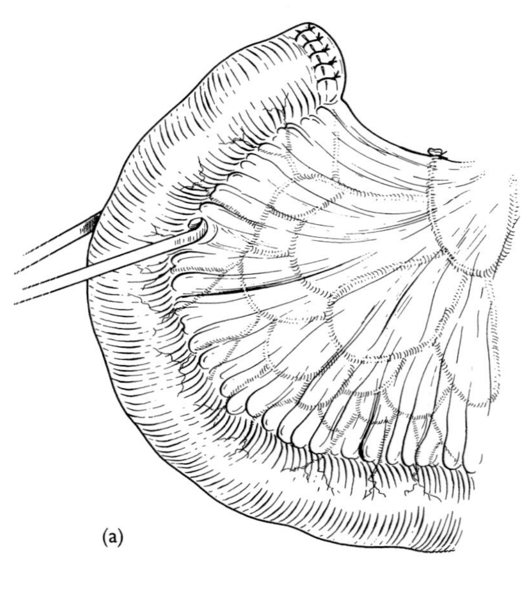

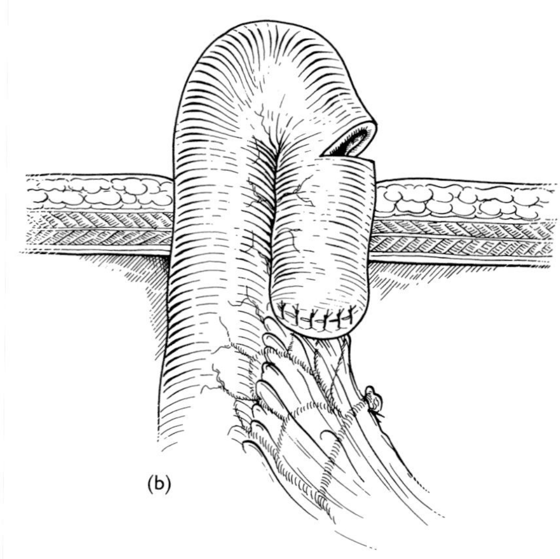

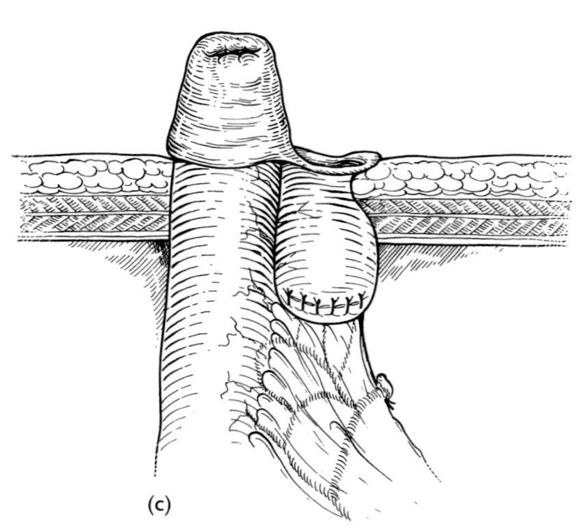

Figure 8.2a–c Construction of a loop ileostomy from a closed end of ileum. This can be a useful technique if the mesentery is short and the abdominal wall is thick, when a conventional end ileostomy is difficult. (a) A tape is placed around the mesenteric surface of the ileum approximately 5 cm from the closed end of the bowel. An adequate blood supply has already been established. (b) A small enterotomy is made 2–3 cm from the end of the bowel after the apex has been delivered through a trephine in the abdominal wall. (c) The proximal end of the loop is everted and sutured to the skin.

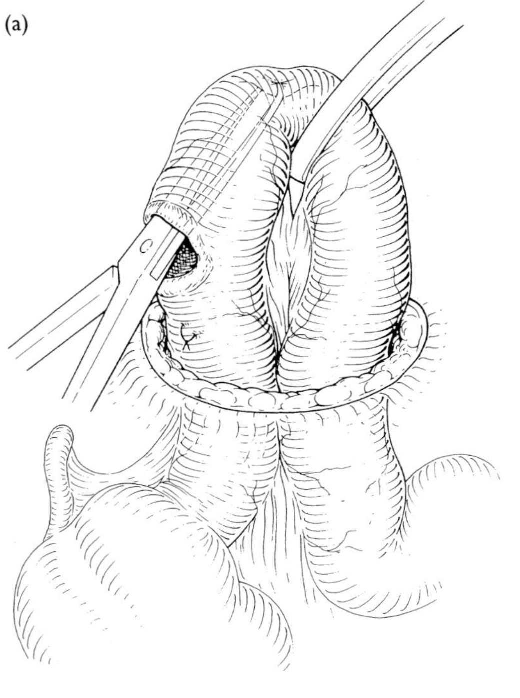

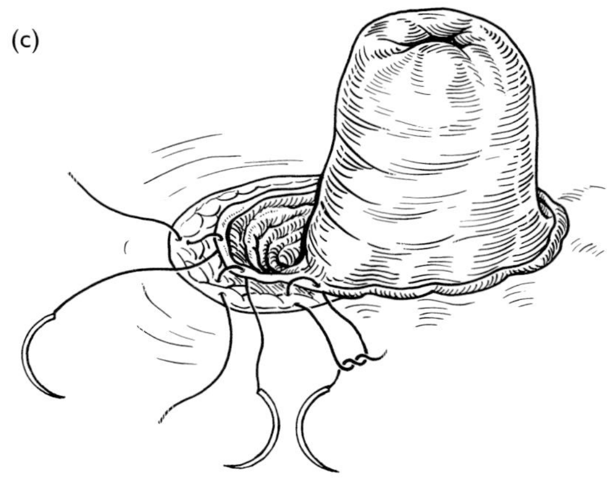

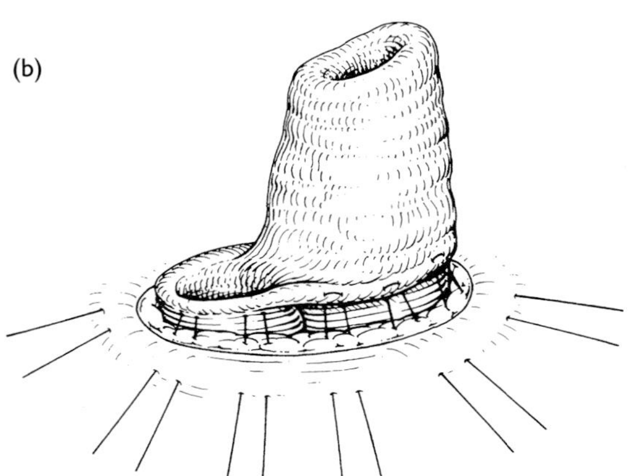

Figure 8.3a–c (a) A loop ileostomy is constructed by delivering a loop of terminal ileum through the abdominal wall trephine. The distal end of the bowel is marked with a suture. A small antemesenteric enterotomy is made in the distal limb and, using a pair of Alice tissue forceps, the antemesenteric portion of the apex of the loop is grasped so that the proximal limb can be everted. (b) Once the loop ileostomy has been everted, there is a distal flush limb and an everted proximal limb. Mucocutaneous apposition can be undertaken without the use of a rod, using full-thickness bites of the bowel and taking the non-absorbable sutures well away from the skin edge as this facilitates their removal. (c) Mucocutaneous apposition can be achieved by a subcuticular mucosal technique with PDS which avoids the need for removing sutures in the future.

means of defunctioning the colon, particularly in Crohn's disease (McIlrath, 1971; Zelas and Jagelman, 1980; Harper et al, 1982). Loop ileostomy may be an alternative to a loop colostomy as a method of decompressing the large bowel or protecting a colorectal anastomosis provided the colon is empty (Fasth et al, 1980; Williams et al, 1986). Even in large bowel obstruction, decompression is possible by passing a catheter down the distal limb through the ileocaecal valve to facilitate washing out the proximal colon (Fasth and Hulten, 1984). Some authors have suggested that tube ileostomy may have advantages over loop ileostomy (Jhittay and Obeid, 1986; Yaque, 1986), but that is uncertain.

Loop ileostomy may cause less skin excoriation than loop transverse colostomy (Rowbotham, 1981); it is certainly less bulky and there is a lower incidence of peristomal sepsis and parastomal hernia (Wright, 1979; Fazio, 1984). Perhaps the most compelling attraction of loop ileostomy over loop colostomy is the lower incidence of complications following closure of the stoma (Knox et al, 1971; Mirelman et al, 1978; Larkin and Fazio, 1980; Garber et al, 1982; Williams et al, 1986).

CONSTRUCTION

Siting the stoma

Counselling

Two detailed audits have examined the lack of counselling among patients having an ileostomy. The first reports the outcome in 51 patients who had a proctocolectomy in Oxford (Kennedy et al, 1982a). None of the patients considered that they had been given sufficient information concerning their stoma. Nearly two-thirds of the patients (63%) expressed the view that they had not been told what life with an ileostomy would really be like; 57% explained that they had never seen a patient with an ileostomy to discuss with them the potential problems of everyday life with a stoma; 39% stated that none of their relatives had been interviewed; and 16% of patients had apparently never changed their appliance before being discharged from hospital. The only gratifying aspect of this survey seems to be that the stoma site itself was generally satisfactory and the incidence of revision and management problems due to poor siting was low. The authors thus advise a checklist (Table 8.1) which they now attach to patients' notes to ensure that these aspects of stoma management are not omitted.

The second report is from Birmingham, where Phillips et al (1985) found that only 83% of ileostomy patients were adequately counselled preoperatively. Patients receiving inadequate counselling were mainly those having an emergency colectomy. Some of these patients were so ill that detailed explanation of the finer management problems encountered by ileostomists was considered to be unwarranted and misplaced. Few would now disagree with the sentiment that all patients having an ileostomy should be seen by a stomatherapist or a nursing sister trained in stoma management before going to theatre *even if this is an emergency operation* and, if possible, should see a patient who has an ileostomy. Acceptance of colorectal surgery as a speciality in most of Europe and North America has ensured that for most patients, inadequate counselling before ileostomy construction is now largely a thing of the past.

Marking a site

The optimum stoma site will vary between individuals because it must be visible and accessible to the patient. These aims will be compromised if the patient has poor eyesight, severe arthritis or is grossly obese (Meguid et al, 1997). Sites must be modified according to scars, skin creases, obesity and patchy skin disorders (Figure 8.4a,b). In obese patients, management of the stoma may only be possible by the use of a mirror. The skin around the stoma site should be flat. The stoma should probably traverse the rectus muscle, although this dogma has been challenged (Leong et al, 1994). If it does not, there may be a higher risk of prolapse, hernia

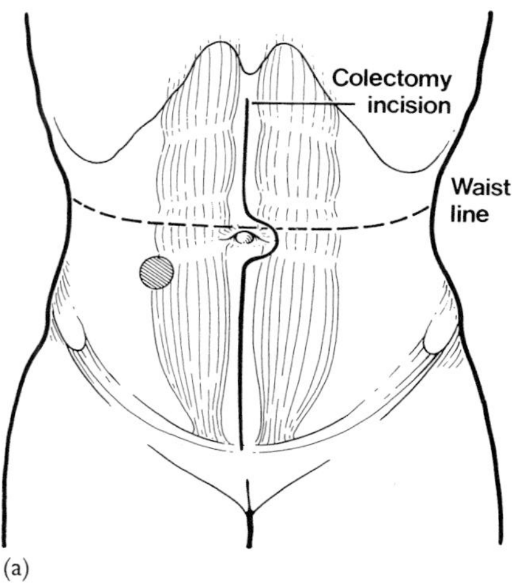

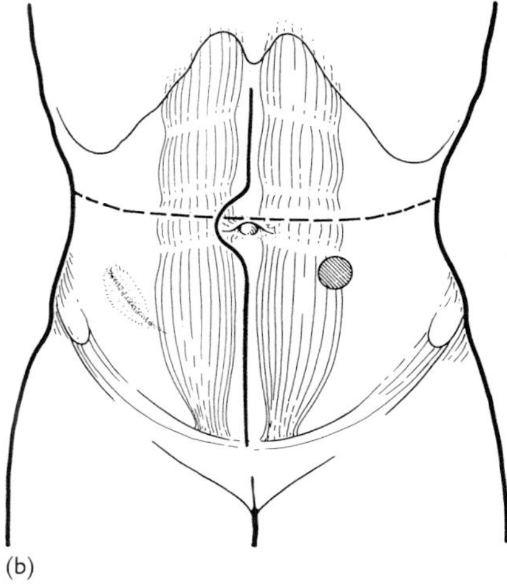

Figure 8.4a–b The usual site for an ileostomy is through a trephine placed over the right rectus muscle approximately half way between the umbilicus and the anterior superior iliac spine, lying just below the midline and well away from the symphysis pubis and costal margin. It should also be as far away as possible from any previous abdominal wall incision. (b) If a patient has already had a gridiron incision it may be preferable to place an ileostomy through a trephine in the left rectus muscle at an equivalent site on the opposite side.

Table 8.1 Checklist for stoma counselling.

Whenever an elective proctocolectomy is planned the following should be carried out well in advance of the operation. When the proctocolectomy is an urgent or emergency procedure, as much explanation as is feasible should be given.

		Please tick
Explanation by physician and surgeon (preferably together)	: the patient	( )
	: the spouse or parents	( )
Explanation by stoma care nurse/ward sister to reinforce the above	: the patient	( )
	: the spouse or parents	( )
Interview arranged between the patient and a suitable ileostomist		( )

The explanation should cover the following points:

	Doctor	Stoma care nurse
1. Reasons for operation	( )	( )
2. The operation and early postoperative period (i.v. infusion, nasogastric tube, urinary catheter, how long in bed, how long before eating, how long in hospital and how long off work)	( )	( )
3. Nature, appearance and function of the stoma and ileostomy effluent (including odour)	( )	( )
4. General discussion about appliance (types, availability, disposal and frequency of changing)	( )	( )
NB Do not forget to mark suitable site on abdomen for stoma		
5. Effect of ileostomy on:		
work	( )	( )
diet and fluid intake	( )	( )
social activities	( )	( )
clothing	( )	( )
sports and hobbies	( )	( )
swimming	( )	( )
sex	( )	( )
bathing or showering	( )	( )
6. Tell the patient about Ileostomy Association	( )	( )

Postoperative care in hospital

	Doctor	Stoma care nurse
1. Repeat preoperative explanations to patient and to spouse or patient	( )	( )
2. Select appliance with the patient from a limited choice of the best makes		( )
3. Show patient and family how to change and empty the appliance		( )
4. Teach the patient how to care for the stoma and the appliance until confident to manage alone		( )
5. Give details of how to obtain appliances and equipment and give adequate supplies to take home		( )
6. Ask patient and family if there are any questions		( )
7. Inform GP and district nurse of discharge and arrange outpatient appointment for surgical and stoma care	( )	( )
8. Attendance at surgical and stoma care clinics. The staff of these clinics must have time to listen to the problems of the patient and family. Go through checklist again, in particular in relation to work, social activities, sports, sex and stoma/appliance problems	( )	( )

From Kennedy et al (1982a).

and retraction, but more fundamentally the appliance often will not adhere properly to the skin.

The proposed stoma site should be well away from the umbilicus, groin, waist and iliac crest. The site should be tested preoperatively, first by applying an empty bag to it and then, if it is apparently satisfactory, retesting with the patient fully clothed. Whether clothing is worn around the waist or hips will have a profound influence on stoma siting (Figure 8.5a,b). The stoma appliance should also be tested while the patient is seated (Figure 8.6a,b) (Devlin, 1984).

Once the ideal site has been identified, it should be marked. Although marking is usually performed with an indelible felt-tipped pen, there is much to recommend the technique of intradermal subcutaneous and intermuscular injection of methylene blue, as described by Turnbull and Weekley (1967), so that each layer of the abdominal wall is identified with dye to ensure construction of a straight trephine. It is the preference of one of the authors (MRBK) to construct a trephine for a permanent stoma before opening the abdomen so as to ensure a straight course from the peritoneal cavity to the abdominal wall.

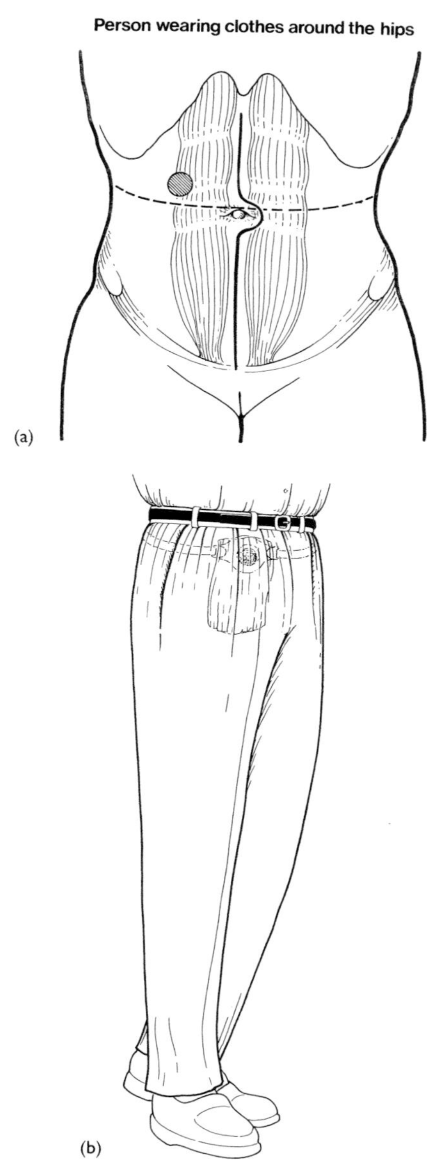

Figure 8.5a–b (a) The position of an ileostomy should be rechecked when the patient is wearing clothing. For some individuals who wear tight-fitting clothing around the waistline it is preferable to place the stoma at a higher level. In such instances the stoma may be placed through the right rectus muscle above the umbilicus but at a distance from the costal margin. (b) It is essential that a potential ileostomy site is tested, before construction of a stoma, when the patient is wearing an appliance with normal clothing.

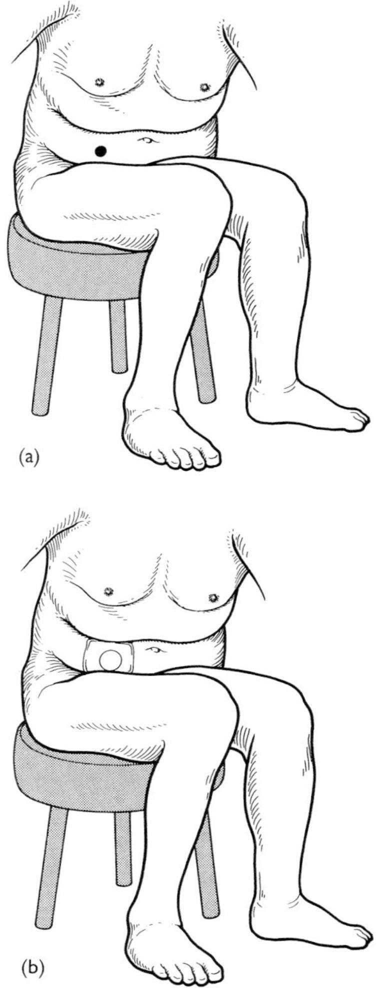

Figure 8.6a–b (a) The selection of an optimum stoma site should also be performed while the patient is seated. (b) Folds of subcutaneous fat on the abdominal wall may make an adequate seal impossible if it lies within a skin crease.

Open surgical techniques

Principles

The bowel must traverse the abdominal wall and protrude beyond the skin so that it can be everted without tension. The mesentery should not be stretched for fear of rendering the stoma ischaemic. The trephine in the abdominal wall should be straight and admit the thumb for an end ileostomy and two fingers for a loop ileostomy. It is therefore advisable to excise a cylinder of subcutaneous fat as well as skin (Figure 8.7a,b) which is cut over a disc or simply after lifting the skin with a pair of tissue forceps (Clifton, 1983).

After the anterior rectus sheath has been divided, the rectus muscle may be divided over cholecystectomy forceps with diathermy if the patient is very muscular (Figure 8.7c,d). Alternatively, and preferably, the rectus muscle is split longitudinally (Figure 8.7e). The posterior rectus sheath is then divided (Figure 8.7f). The small bowel mesentery should be transilluminated so that an appropriate arcade can be preserved to supply the terminal ileum (Figure 8.7g). In view of the metabolic sequelae of small bowel resection, the ileum should be divided as close to the ileocaecal valve as possible. Immediate mucocutaneous suture should then be performed. In Birmingham, Prolene sutures are often used and removed 5–7 days later. However, with an aggressive policy of early hospital discharge, subcuticular to serosal PDS sutures are now frequently used (Figure 8.3c). At the Royal London, interrupted catgut or Vicryl sutures on a taper-cut needle are used. In order to stabilize the stoma, the serosa on the emerging ileum is incorporated into

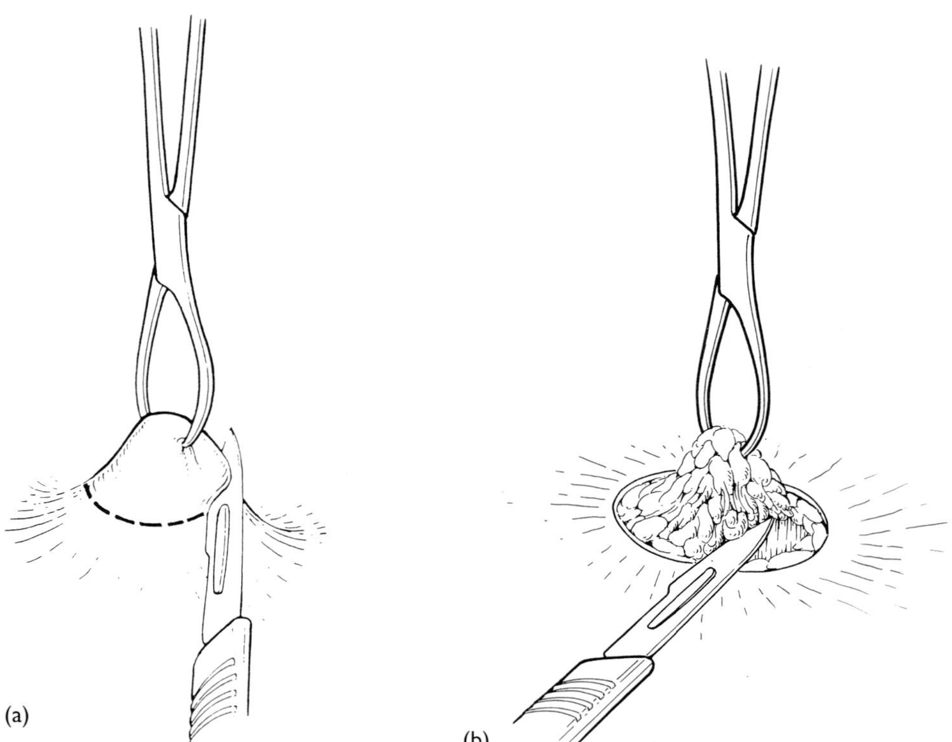

Figure 8.7a–i Construction of an end ileostomy. (a) A trephine is made by excising a disc of skin and subcutaneous tissue. The skin is elevated from the rest of the abdominal wall with a Littlewoods tissue forceps and a disc of skin is excised. (b) Subcutaneous fat is then excised down to the level of the rectus sheath. (c) A cruciate incision is made in the anterior rectus sheath; a curved vascular or bowel clamp is then introduced under the rectus muscle to facilitate its division. (d) The rectus muscle is partially divided with diathermy over the vascular or bowel clamp, taking care to control haemostasis and secure the inferior epigastric vessels if they are encountered (alternatively the muscle may be split: not shown). (e) Rather than dividing the rectus muscle, the muscle fibres may be split longitudinally which allows the fibres to lie in close proximity to the bowel, thereby reducing the risk of parastomal hernia. (f) The peritoneal cavity is opened with cutting diathermy. (g) The serosa of the ileum is loosely tacked to the rectus muscle once the end of the ileum has been delivered through the abdominal wall for a sufficient length. (h)–(i) The ileostomy is everted using an Alice forceps and interrupted sutures are placed between the skin and full thickness of the end of the bowel at a sufficient distance from the skin edge to facilitate the removal of non-absorbable sutures.

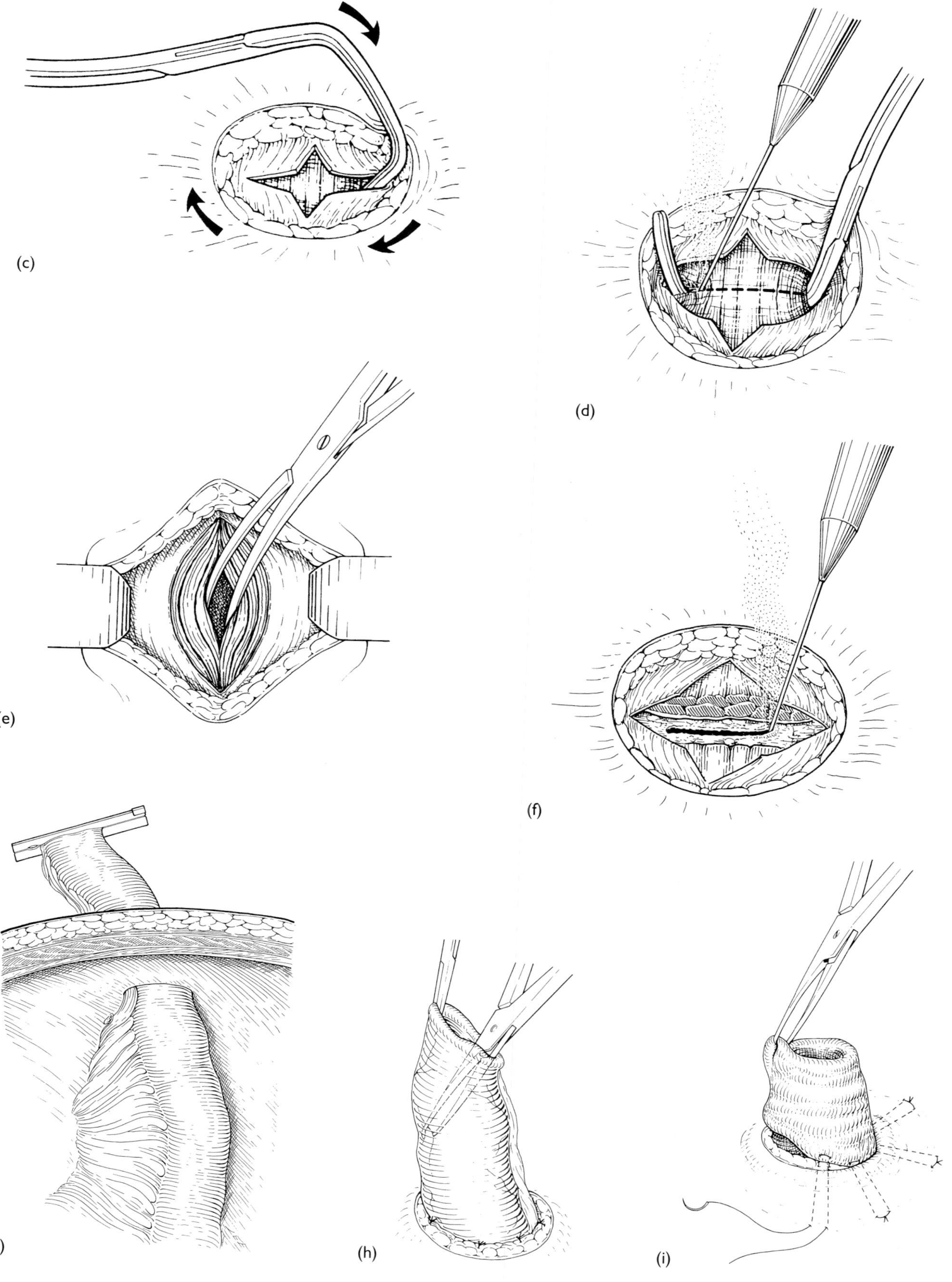
(c)
(d)
(e)
(f)
(g)
(h)
(i)

the suture technique as well as the free edge of the bowel and skin to achieve mucocutaneous apposition (Figures 8.7i and 8.3c). The ileostomy is everted to produce a 2–3 cm stoma. If there is any tension on the terminal ileum despite these manoeuvres, the surgeon should have no hesitation in constructing a loop ileostomy proximal to the divided ileum or simply as a loop ileostomy alone.

End ileostomy

A midline laparotomy incision should be used whenever possible since this leaves both iliac fossae undisturbed if a revision procedure or resiting of the stoma is ever needed in the future. The trephine is constructed by excising a circle of skin and a disc of subcutaneous fat, dividing the rectus sheath, and either splitting or dividing a part of the rectus muscle before opening the peritoneum. The trephine should be constructed as a straight cylinder (Figure 8.7a–h). In ulcerative colitis, the terminal ileum can usually be divided 2 cm from the ileocaecal valve, but in Crohn's disease a segment of ileum will usually require excision. The marginal vessels should be preserved. The space between the distal ileal arcade and the ileocaecal vessels is opened and the marginal artery is ligated opposite the proposed site of ileal transection. In this way a 5–10 cm length of ileum with a good blood supply can be delivered to the abdominal wall to allow a 2–3 cm eversion ileostomy to be made.

The ileum is divided between Nylon tapes (Figure 8.8a) so that the end can be safely delivered through the trephine in the abdominal wall. Stapling techniques minimize the risks of contamination and are often used prior to ileostomy construction (Figure 8.8b).

A decision must be taken regarding the lateral gutter: this can be left widely opened or securely closed. Many surgeons do not attempt to close the space between the free edge of the ileal mesentery and the lateral parietal peritoneum (Figure 8.9a). This potential space may be obliterated if the ileum is delivered through the extraperitoneal route (Figure 8.9b) (Goligher, 1958). Extraperitoneal ileostomy may be associated with a higher incidence of mechanical difficulties than the use of the more direct route but the risk of prolapse and hernia may be less (Whittaker and Goligher, 1976). If the lateral gutter is closed in the conventional way, it is wise to place the lateral purse-string between the stoma and the free edge of the ileal mesentery before withdrawing the ileum through the abdominal wall. An alternative technique is to suture the cut edge of the ileal mesentery to the ligamentum teres and to the anterior abdominal wall. If this method is used, care must be taken not to include the ileal mesentery in the suture during closure of the abdominal wall.

The laparotomy incision should be closed before removing the Potts clamp over the ileum, to minimize intestinal contamination of the wound. It is not

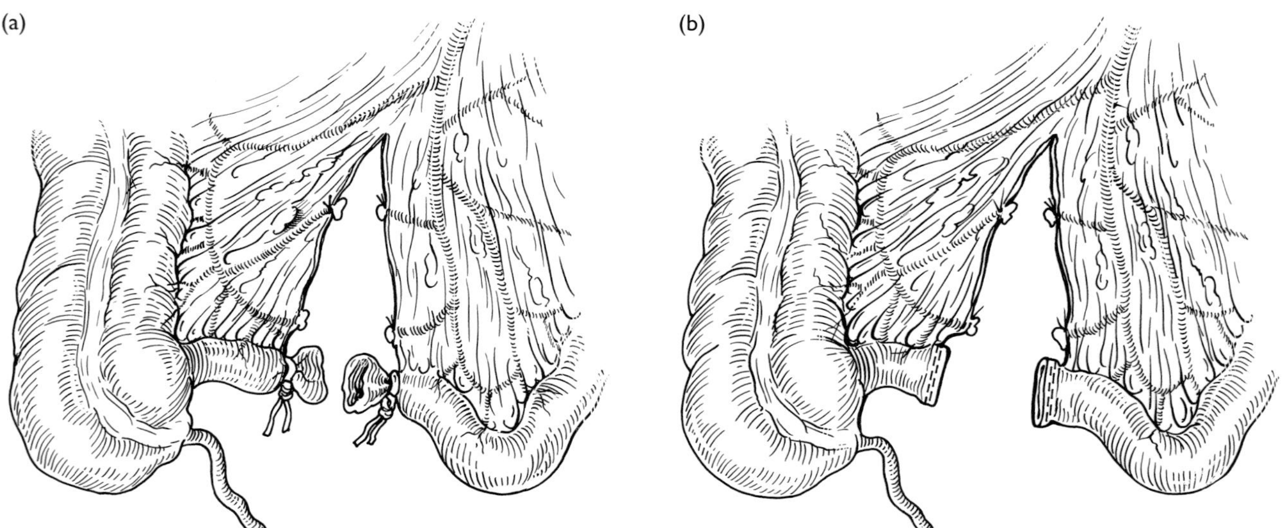

Figure 8.8a–b (a) The bowel ends may be occluded by means of Nylon tapes. (b) An alternative and preferred method of occluding the bowel ends is to use a linear staple cutter which reduces contamination when the distal ileum is divided for ileostomy construction.

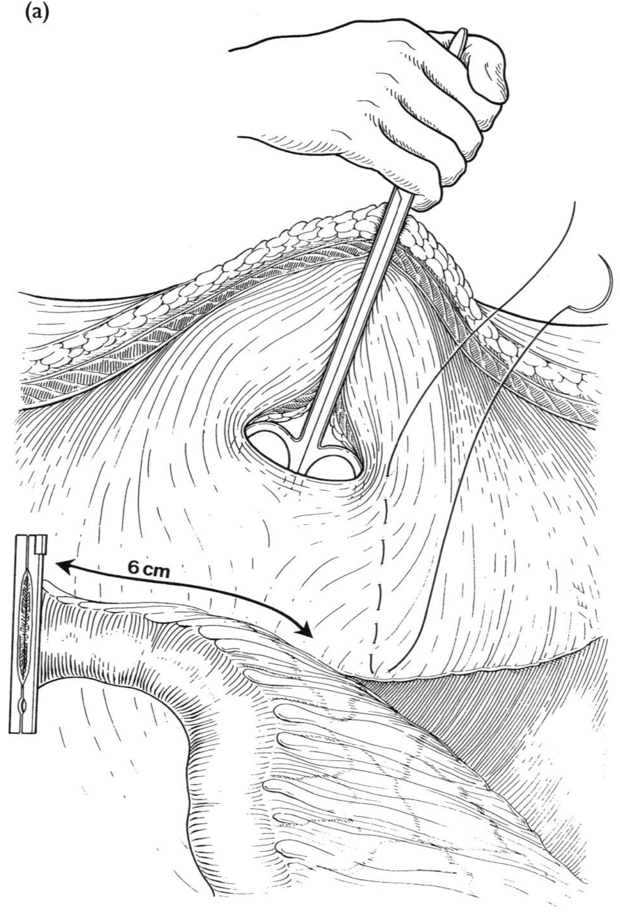

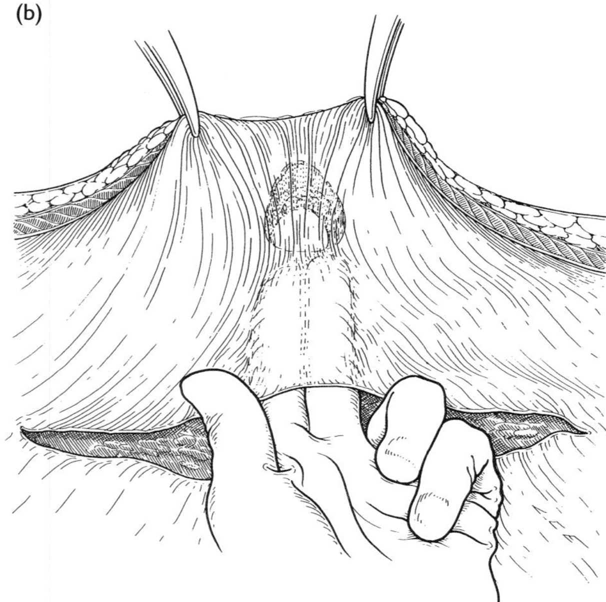

Figure 8.9a–b (a) Closure of the lateral gutter. The lateral gutter should be closed before the ileum is delivered through the abdominal wall trephine. By placement of a long pair of scissors through the trephine in the abdominal wall, lateral retraction is achieved. A purse-string suture is placed from the edge of the trephine to the cut edge of the peritoneum and then to the mesenteric surface of the ileum approximately 6–7 cm from its divided end. Further closure of the lateral gutter is achieved by approximating the cut edge of the lateral parietal peritoneum to the cut edge of the small bowel mesentery (not shown). (b) Closure of the lateral gutter using a retroperitoneal tunnel. The lateral cut edge of the parietal peritoneum is raised and a tunnel is developed between it and the abdominal wall trephine to accommodate the ileum.

usual to suture the serosa of the ileum to the rectus sheath: only the stomal sutures are used to prevent retraction. Interrupted Prolene mucocutaneous sutures or PDS subcuticular to serosal sutures are placed through the skin, the emerging bowel, the cut edge of the ileum and (in the case of Prolene) back through the skin (Figure 8.7h,i). Fixing the bag to the skin around the stoma completes the procedure.

Loop ileostomy

A few technical points are worth emphasizing (see Figure 8.3a–c). The trephine must admit two fingers. The distal loop of the ileum must be marked for identification before it is delivered through the abdominal wall trephine (Raimes et al, 1984). The loop is delivered through the abdominal wall by placing a tape under the mesenteric margin between the ileum and the marginal arcade. The use of a rod under the loop of ileum, described by Turnbull and Weekley (1966), to prevent retraction is rarely advised in the early postoperative period (Shirley et al, 1984). A rod may be responsible for ileal damage or skin excoriation; it is painful to remove and the stoma usually remains adequately everted without its use (Utley and Macbeth, 1984), particularly if a small enterotomy is made for eversion on the antimesenteric border of the ileum. Anderson et al (1994) have advised suture fixation of the ileum to the abdominal wall to prevent stomal volvulus, but the present author does not subscribe to this. The distal limb of the loop should be sutured to the skin preferably before securing the proximal everted stoma. These sutures are clipped until they have all been accurately placed and are tied loosely (Unti et al, 1991). Either Prolene sutures may be used at a distance from the stoma (Figure 8.7i), or subcuticular to serosal sutures with PDS may be used (Figure 8.3c). The type of suture material does not appear to effect long-term outcome (Bagi et al, 1992).

Orientation of a loop ileostomy so that the proximal limb is dependent has attracted some debate (Fasth and Hulten, 1984; Shirley et al, 1984; Utley and Macbeth, 1984). The position of the proximal limb is unlikely to influence its ability to defunction the distal bowel, but some have found that orientation influences the incidence of small bowel obstruction after pouch construction (see Chapter 49). Spillover, if it is going to occur, is most likely when the patient is supine, when the configuration of the stoma is unimportant. When Winslet et al (1991b) assessed the defunctioning capacity of a loop ileostomy, orientation had no influence on its ability to defunction the distal bowel, and ileal contents could be recovered only distal to the stoma if the proximal limb had retracted.

An advantage of the loop ileostomy over a split ileostomy is that it can be raised, refashioned and closed without a laparotomy. However, it may not always be advisable to perform loop ileostomy without laparotomy if there has been previous abdominal surgery, or where the rest of the bowel must be carefully examined, for instance following abdominal trauma. If a loop ileostomy is being raised to defunction Crohn's colitis, laparotomy can sometimes be avoided. Some might argue that laparoscopic stoma construction should be used (Hershman and Kiff, 1997). Alternatively, trephine ileostomy can be achieved especially in thin patients, provided the terminal ileum can be orientated and identified (Figure 8.10). A small trephine is made through the rectus and the peritoneal cavity opened. A Langenbeck retractor is inserted and the terminal ileum and caecum identified by the fold of Treves and the appendix. Once the distal end of the ileum is verified, the loop ileostomy is formed as already described.

Sometimes there may be difficulty orientating a loop ileostomy in patients with pelvic sepsis requiring urgent diversion, as for instance in a patient with a pouch anal anastomosis. The distal limb of the loop can easily be confirmed with air insufflation through a large Foley catheter passed per anum into the distal bowel (Figure 8.11).

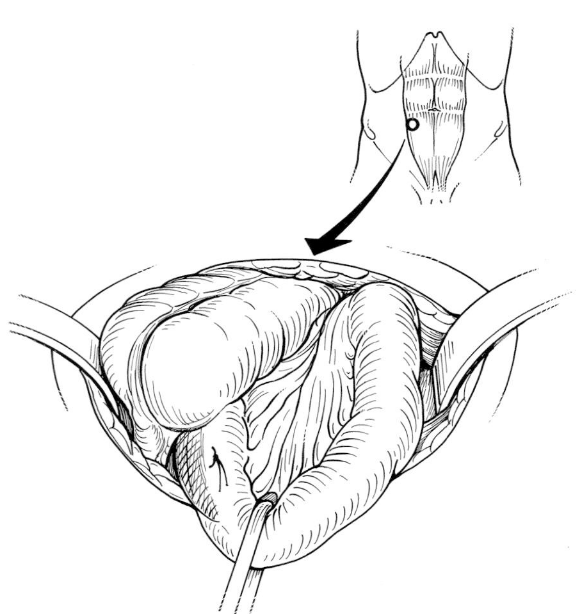

Figure 8.10 Trephine loop ileostomy construction in a patient who has never had a resection. The site having been marked, the trephine is made in the abdominal wall by excising a disc of skin and splitting the rectus muscle. The peritoneal cavity is opened and the ileocaecal junction is identified by the fold of Treves. The distal end of the ileum is marked and the loop is delivered with a sling under the bowel through a mesenteric window.

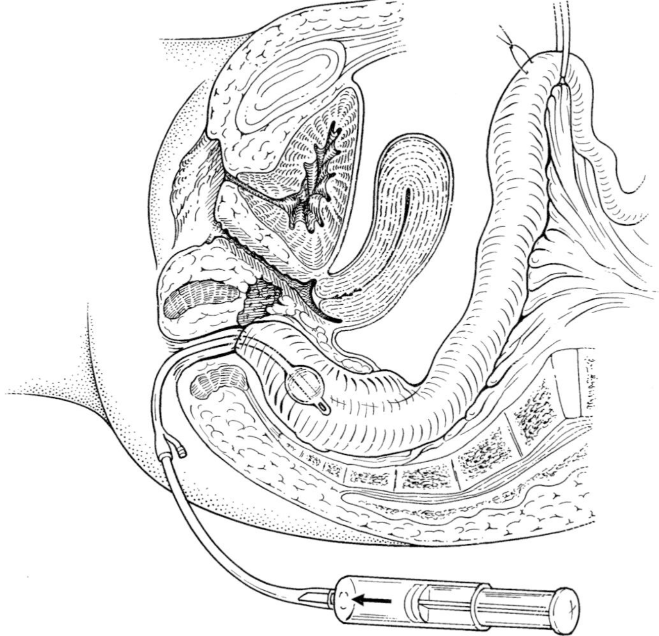

Figure 8.11 Orientating a loop ileostomy in a patient requiring urgent diversion for pelvic sepsis complicating anastomotic breakdown, as in leakage from an ileal pouch. The laparotomy is often difficult owing to dense adhesions, and orientation of a loop of ileum above the dehiscence is facilitated by air insufflation through a catheter placed per anum and distended with air. The distal limb of ileum is marked with a suture.

Split ileostomy

This is not a stoma commonly recommended since the patient has to manage an end ileostomy and a mucous fistula, which is often placed at the end of the wound (Lee, 1975; Harper et al, 1983). Although a split ileostomy completely defunctions the distal bowel, sometimes it is technically difficult to separate the two ends of the bowel and the procedure requires a laparotomy to restore intestinal continuity.

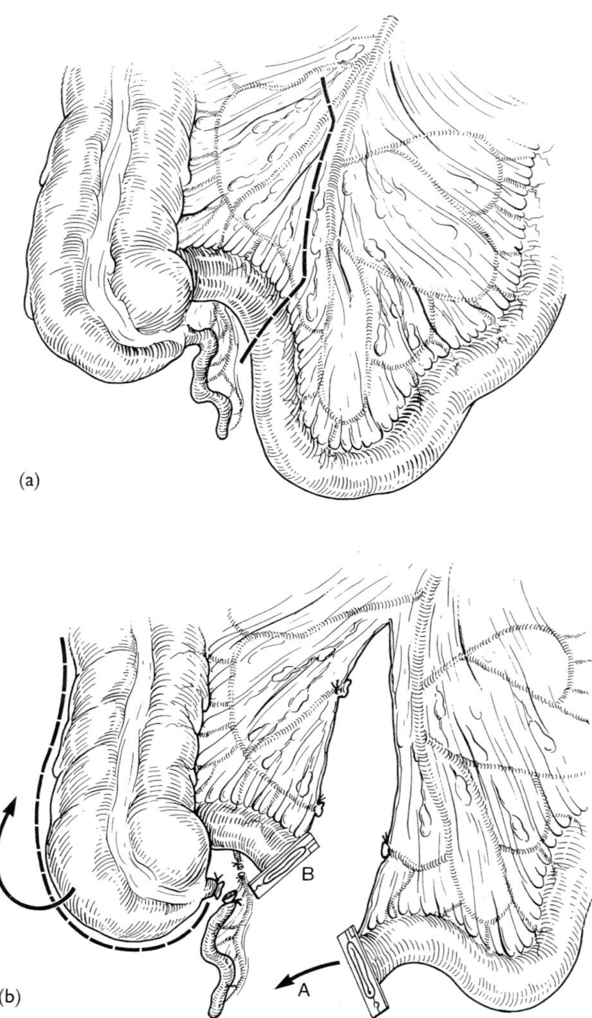

Figure 8.12a–b Split ileostomy. (a) The mesentery of the terminal ileum is divided, ensuring that there are adequate collateral vessels to supply the right colon and caecum from the middle colic artery. (b) The ileum is divided approximately 5 cm proximal to the ileocaecal valve. It is usual to remove the appendix. The proximal end of the ileum is delivered to the abdominal wall as an eversion ileostomy in the right iliac fossa.

If the site of ileal division lies close to the ileocaecal valve, the right colon must be mobilized (Figure 8.12a). The mesentery must be quite extensively divided, leaving the ileum supplied by ileal arcades and the mucous fistula from the middle colic artery (Figure 8.12b). Transillumination of the mesentery may be helpful but can be difficult if there is extensive mesenteric lymphadenopathy and mesenteric thickening. The proximal end of the ileum is delivered through a trephine in the right rectus muscle and the mucous fistula is either raised through the abdominal incision or, preferably, through a separate trephine in the ipsilateral or contralateral muscle (Figure 8.13).

Alternative stoma

Stapling techniques

A loop ileostomy is considered by some as unsatisfactory for defunctioning purposes (Prasad et al, 1984). The ileal loop can be completely divided with a linear staple cutter. The proximal end of bowel is everted and a small enterotomy placed over the summit of the distal limb for decompression or irrigation (Figure 8.14a–c).

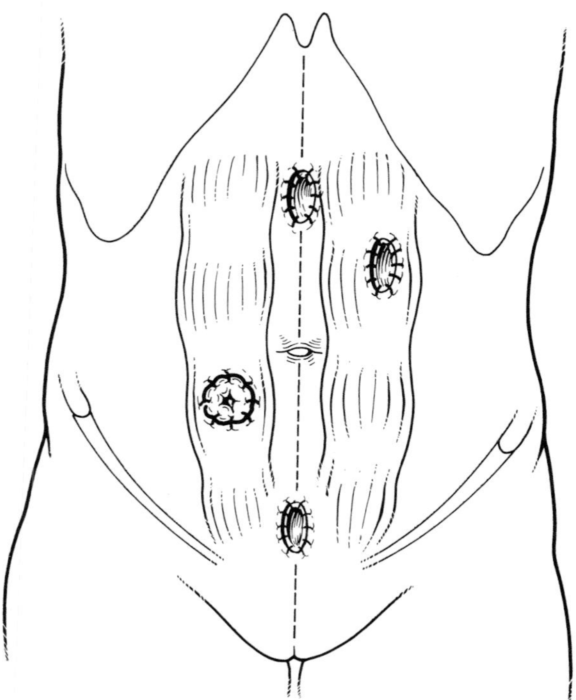

Figure 8.13 The distal end of the ileum, which acts as a mucous fistula, may either be delivered to the lower end of a midline laparotomy or to the upper end of a midline laparotomy or through a separate trephine in the left rectus muscle.

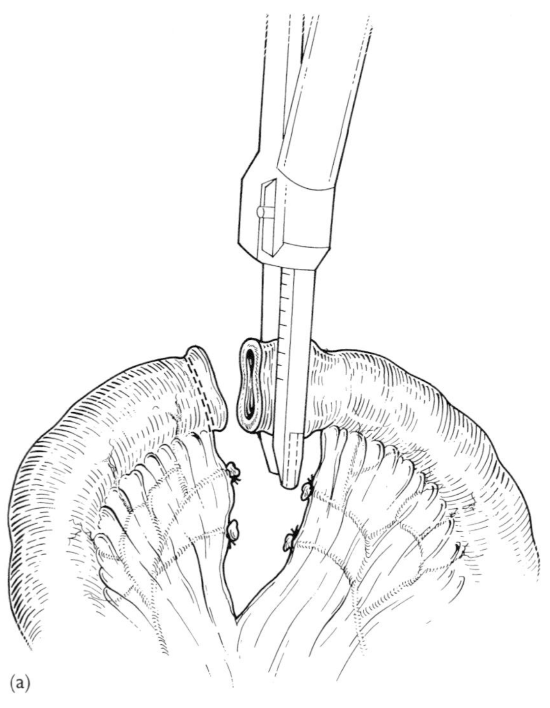

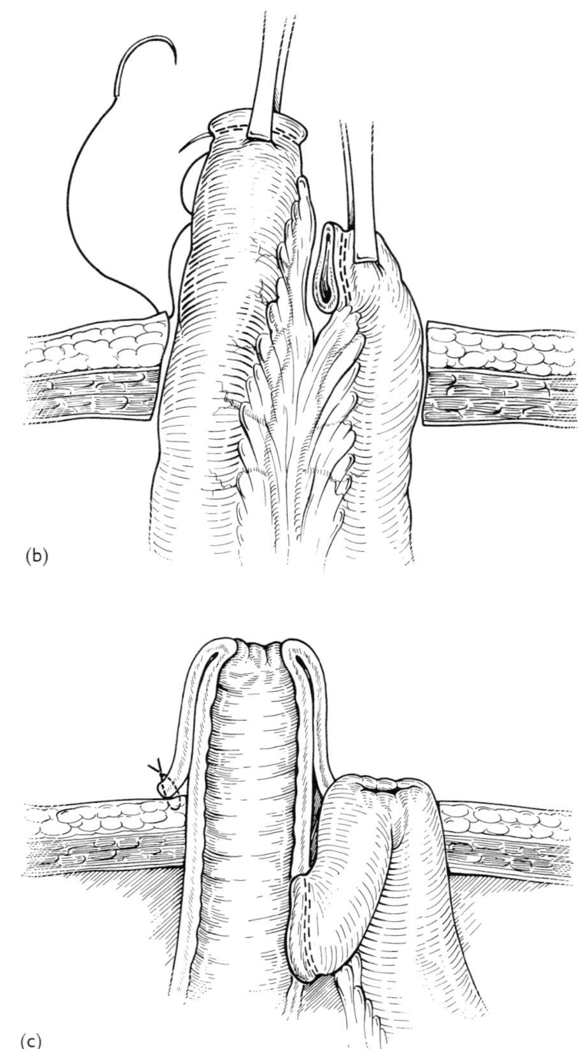

Figure 8.14a–c Divided loop ileostomy. An alternative to split ileostomy is a technique which completely divides the bowel but only utilizes a single trephine in the abdominal wall, making subsequent stoma management easier. (a) The mesentery of the terminal ileum is divided. The ileum is transected using a linear staple cutter. (b) The distal divided loop of ileum is allowed to remain in the peritoneal cavity while the proximal limb is delivered through the abdominal wall trephine and everted. (c) The apex of a loop distal to the distal closure line is opened as a mucous fistula.

Ileostomy construction has been described by others using the circular stapling device. A purse-string is placed around the skin defect and around the ileum (Chung, 1986). Eversion is achieved using tissue forceps and staples (Figure 8.15a–c). No complications were reported in 26 stomas constructed in this way.

Side-to-side temporary end ileostomy

Delaney and Mulholland (1983) describe a method of completely defunctioning the bowel which does not require a laparotomy for closure. The bowel is completely divided. The proximal end is everted as a conventional end ileostomy and after closure of the distal end the serosa of the distal limb is sutured to the side of the emerging bowel (Figure 8.16a,b). Closure of the stoma does not require a laparotomy. The stoma is mobilized, and either an end-to-end anastomosis is performed after straightening out the ileostomy bud (Figure 8.16c,d), or the ileostomy bud is excised and a side-to-side anastomosis is constructed using sutures or the linear staple cutter after closing the end of the proximal bowel (Figure 8.16e,f). This stoma completely defunctions the bowel and has been used to protect a distal intestinal anastomosis.

Appliances used in current practice are illustrated in Figure 8.16g.

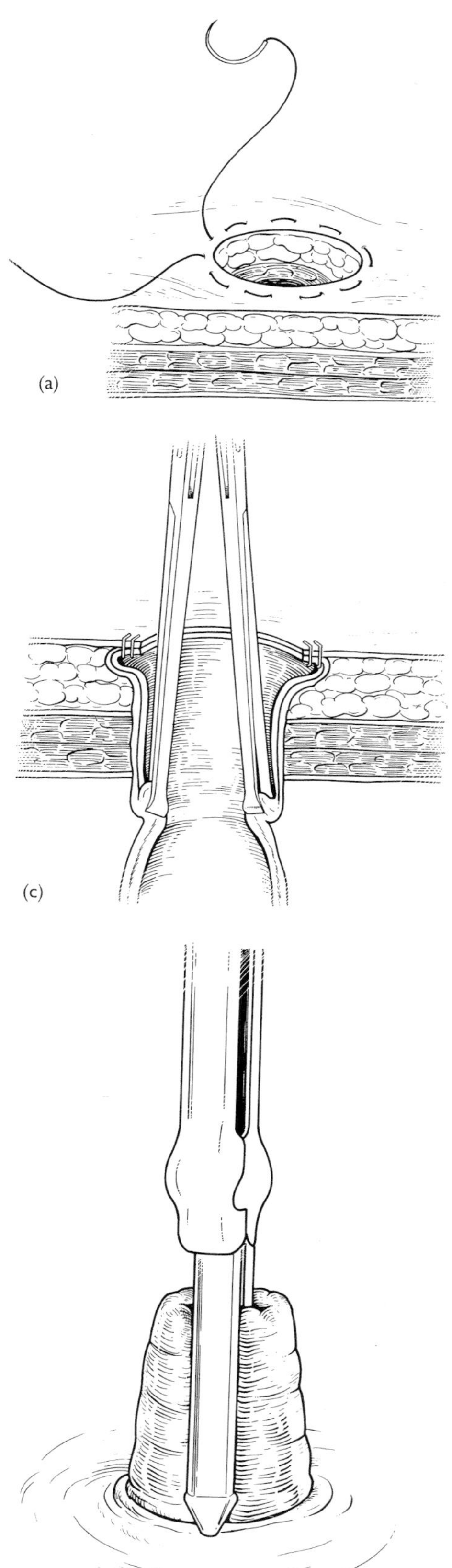

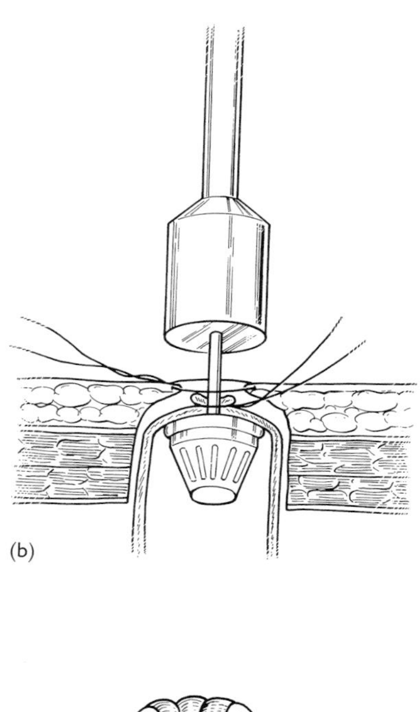

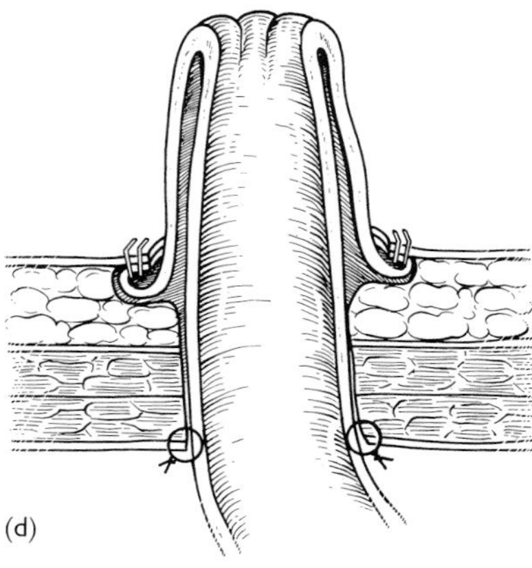

Figure 8.15a–e Totally stapled end ileostomy. (a) A trephine is made in the abdominal wall and a purse-string is placed around the skin edge using a whip stitch. A further purse-string is placed around the end of the ileum. (b) Stapled mucocutaneous apposition is then achieved using a circular stapling device between the end of the ileum and the skin of the abdominal wall. (c) The bowel proximal to the stapled mucocutaneous closure is grasped with Allis tissue forceps and everted. (d) The everted stoma is stabilized by (e) placing three or four rows of staples between the two limbs of the ileostomy using a linear stapler (without cutter).

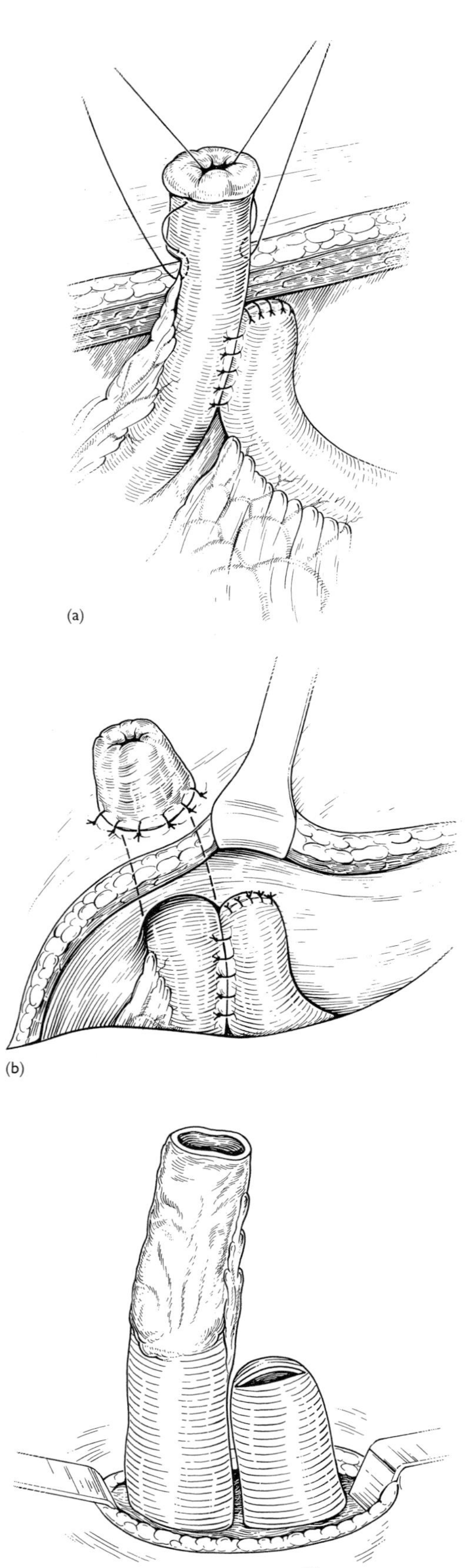
(a)
(b)
(c)

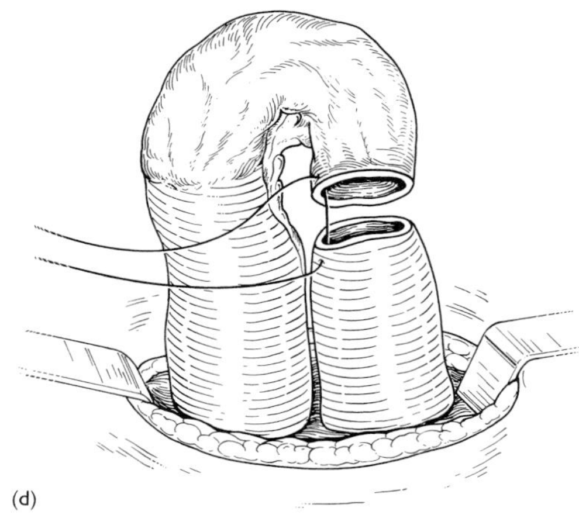
(d)

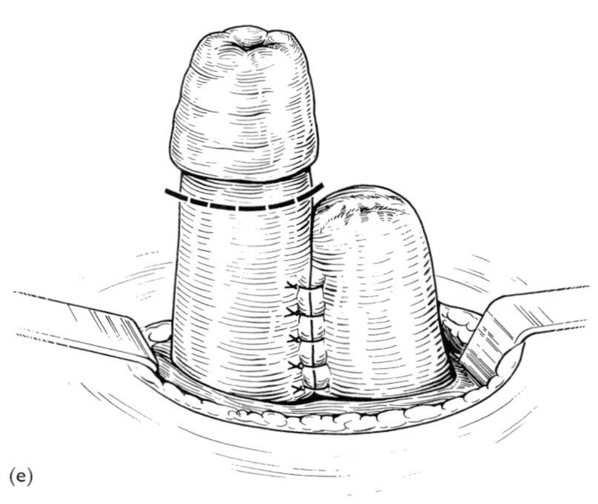
(e)

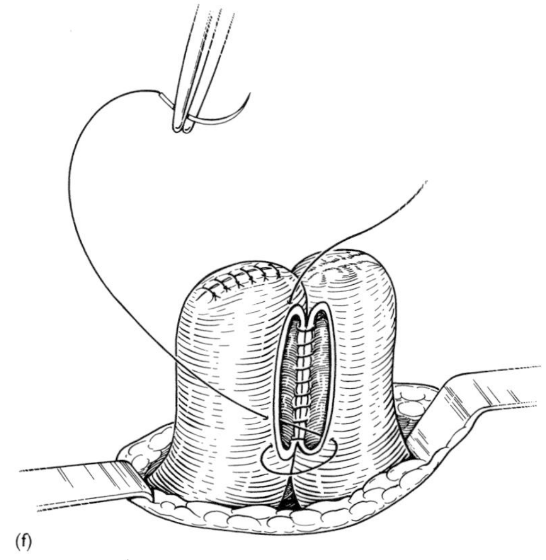
(f)

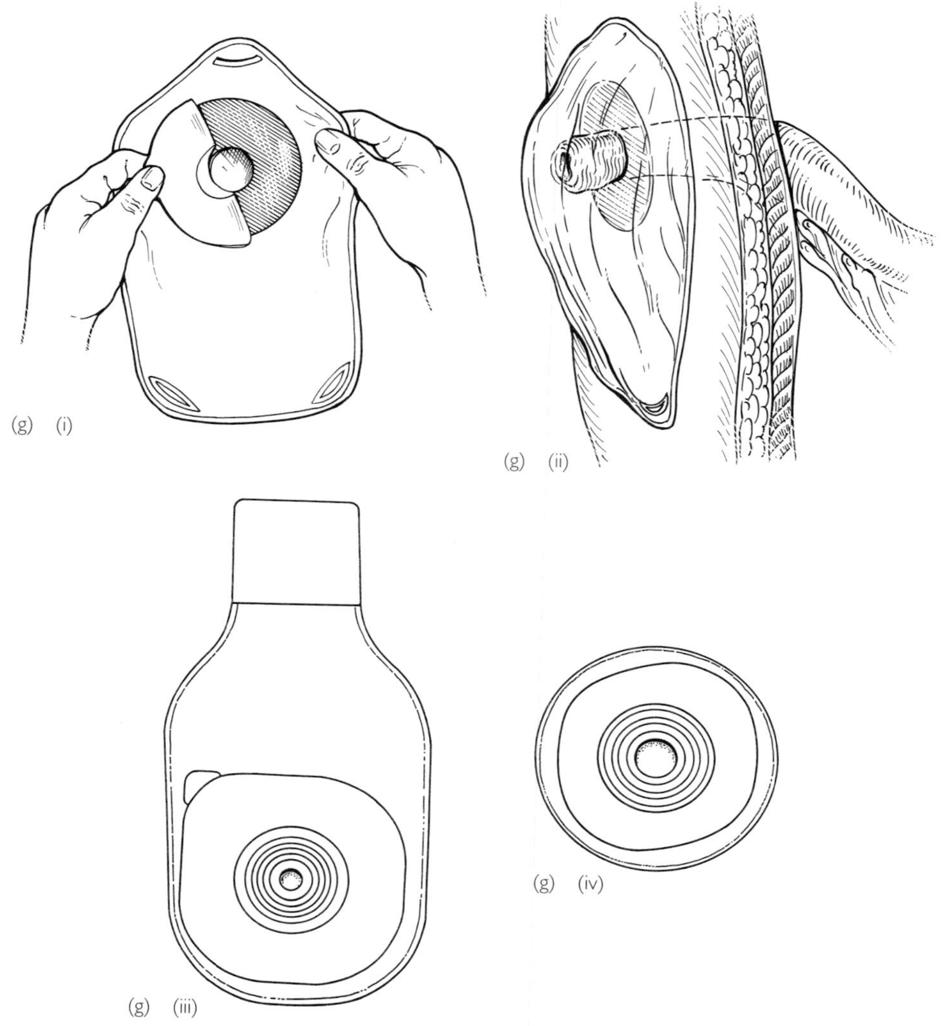

Figure 8.16a–g Construction and closure of divided loop ileostomy. (a) The two ends of ileum have been divided and the distal end oversewn. (b) The proximal end is delivered through an abdominal wall trephine and everted. This achieves proximal defunction without the fear of spillover into the distal bowel. (c) Closure is achieved by dissecting the everted stoma from the abdominal wall, straightening the end of the ileum, opening the closed distal ileum, and (d) performing an end-to-end anastomosis. (e) Construction and closure of divided loop ileostomy. Alternatively the stoma may be closed, after it has been fully mobilized from the abdominal wall, by excising the everted ileostomy bud and closing the end of the proximal ileum. (f) Intestinal continuity is then restored by a side-to-side ileoileal anastomosis and the abdominal wall is closed. (g) An assortment of ileostomy bags: (i) and (ii) show one-piece devices using lightweight material and peel-off adherent seals; (iii) and (iv) show a convex incorporated disc to control a flush ileostomy.

Laparoscopic method

The theoretical advantages of laparoscopic stoma construction include reduced length of ileus and hospital stay, reduced surgical trauma from limiting the number and size of incisions, and consequently a potential reduction in long-term bowel obstruction secondary to adhesions caused by fewer incisions. Although none of these advantages have been proven in prospective, randomized, scientifically valid trials, the data presented here will highlight some of the convincing evidence relative to these features.

Whereas laparoscopic colectomy may be accomplished through ports, ultimately, a large area must be dissected which may require a considerable time. Furthermore, an incision may be necessary to remove the large specimen. Therefore, the advantages of laparoscopy versus laparotomy may be less obvious than in a situation like stoma construction. In this instance, instead of a standard laparotomy incision being followed by stoma construction, a 'trephine' celiotomy is the result. Opponents of laparoscopy will cite the trephine stoma as the preferred approach, thereby avoiding an incision. However, laparoscopy allows complete intracorporeal visualization and such potentially necessary manoeuvres as enterolysis and bowel mobilization. These other steps are not possible through the trephine opening. Furthermore, inspection of potential synchronous sites of Crohn's disease, easily achieved by laparoscopy, are impossible through a trephine opening. Assessing the status of disease in patients with malignancy is also only possible through laparoscopy or laparotomy and not through the trephine stoma. Lastly, it is much easier to ensure appropriate orientation relative to the proximal and distal loop when the procedure is done by laparoscopy instead of a trephine stoma. Clearly, however, the major difference between no incision at all and limiting the surgical insult to port placement and stoma hole construction is vastly different from creation of a standard laparotomy incision merely to construct a stoma.

The potential indications for laparoscopic ileostomy construction are identical to those already described earlier in this chapter. Specifically they are: patients with severe Crohn's disease who are not candidates for, or are not ready to accept, a total proctocolectomy; patients with obstructing distal carcinomas who are not candidates for resection; patients with faecal incontinence as either definitive treatment or as part of a staged treatment such as the artificial bowel sphincter or the dynamic myoplasty/stimulated graciloplasty; and patients for other reasons already described in this chapter.

The only absolute contraindication is diffuse faecal peritonitis. Relative contraindications include a recent low pelvic anastomosis when it may be desirable to perform a laparotomy for a complete mobilization and possibly take-down, redo, or resection of the anastomosis with construction of an end colostomy rather than loop ileostomy. This latter procedure may be easier, especially for the inexperienced laparoscopist, when done by laparotomy. Diffuse carcinomatosis with bowel obstruction is another relative contraindication, especially early in the surgeon's learning curve. Similarly, the patient in whom multiple prior laparotomies, particularly for sepsis, have been undertaken, or the patient with known enterocutaneous fistulas in whom the stoma is being constructed, are best having these procedures performed by laparotomy for reasons of safety in order to limit intraoperative injury.

Patient preparation for laparoscopic ileostomy construction is exactly the same as for laparotomy. No particular oral cathartic preparation is utilized, although patients are given both oral and parenteral antibiotics. These topics are further discussed in Chapter 6. Informed consent includes alerting the patient that laparoscopy may not be possible, and if it is not possible, a standard laparotomy will be undertaken in order to facilitate completion of the operation. All patients must therefore have consented to an eventual laparotomy.

Patient positioning is discussed in Chapter 6. However, particularly germane to stoma construction is the fact that the patient should be in the modified, low, Lloyd Davies lithotomy position (Figure 8.17). As for all laparoscopic procedures, both arms should be carefully tucked at the patient's side to allow maximal movement of the surgeon, assistant and camera-holder around the patient. Allen stirrups are superior to Lloyd Davies stirrups as they function in a 'boot-like' configuration, letting pressure rest upon the dorsum of the foot, heel and calf – thus avoiding pressure on the peroneal nerve. The patients are placed in thigh-high antiembolic stockings and sequential compression device stockings prior to placement in the stirrups. No more than 15 degrees of hip and knee flexion, respectively, should be utilized as more acute angulation may hamper the access of movement of the laparoscopic instruments. If a bladder catheter and a nasogastric tube are placed during the procedure, they can be removed at the time of extubation.

The important facet of port placement for laparoscopic stoma construction is that, if a standard periumbilical position is utilized, the instruments placed through that port will be too close to the instruments placed through the stoma site port and will not allow adequate ergonometric or visual advantage during the dissection. Accordingly, Figure 8.18 shows a suggested port placement schema.

Specifically, the first port is placed in the upper midline, approximately midway between the xiphoid and umbilicus. Remembering that the falciform ligament is located in this vicinity, it is helpful to make the skin incision at the midline, but then aim the Veress needle or Hasson cannula slightly lateral to either side of the falciform ligament to facilitate placement. All patients will, of course, have been preoperatively marked for stoma position as already indicated earlier in this chapter. If cosmetic advantage is a major goal of the surgery, then the initial supraumbilical port can be placed

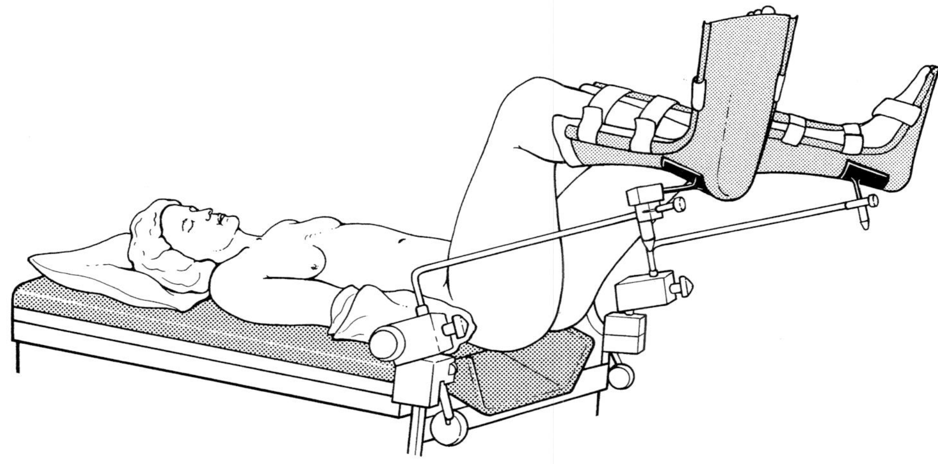

Figure 8.17 Patient positioning for laparoscopy.

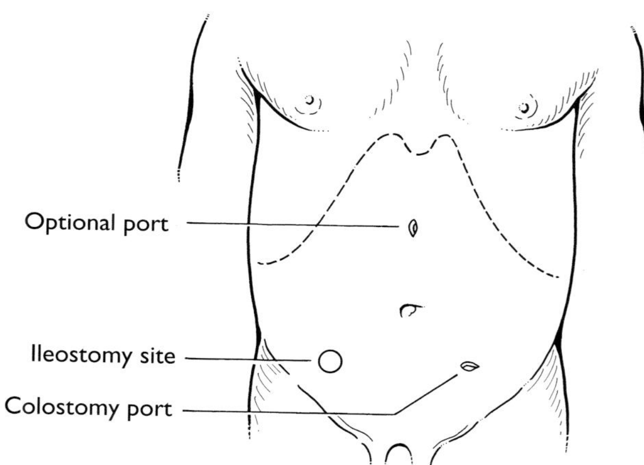

Figure 8.18 Port site placement for laparoscopy.

through a horizontal rather than vertical 1 cm incision. In cases of construction of a loop ileostomy in patients in whom the indication is not Crohn's disease, the second port can be placed through a 10 mm horizontally placed stab wound. Avoidance of the epigastric vessels can be facilitated by both skin transillumination and internal visualization of the peritoneum. In patients with Crohn's disease a potential future stoma site may be best substituted by another midline site.

After port placement, the patient can be placed in steep Trendelenburg and left side down position. A 10 mm Babcock clamp can be placed through the ileostomy site and the terminal ileum and ileocaecal valve can be identified using the standard landmarks of the ligaments of Treitz, the appendix, and the caecum. The loop can be traced back to a point approximately 10–15 cm proximal to the ileocaecal valve which can be selected for the stoma (Figure 8.19). Choosing a site too close to the ileocaecal valve will add considerable difficulty to subsequent ileostomy closure. Conversely, selection of a proximal loop of bowel may result in ileostomy flux, dehydration, and the need for intravenous hydration.

If no adhesions are present and mobility is adequate then the port sleeve is withdrawn over the Babcock forceps. Insufflation is maintained and while the camera operator visualizes the posterior sheath and peritoneum, the surgeon excises two crescents of skin above and below the Babcock forceps which continues to gently grasp the bowel loop. The bowel loop is maintained in its anatomic orientation position. Right-angled retractors are then used to score the fat, anterior rectal sheath and rectus muscle along the axis of its fibres. Ultimately, the Babcock forceps is angled to allow electrocautery to score the posterior sheath and peritoneum along the insulated sheath (Figure 8.20a). Once again, the camera operator continues to visualize the peritoneal cavity to ensure no injury occurs to other structures and to ensure maintenance of proper orientation of the loop.

The scoring of the posterior sheath and peritoneum is facilitated with right-angled retractors introduced through the lower part of the incision. Next, the Babcock clamp is angled in a cephalad manner, again allowing the right-angled retractor to be introduced through the cephalad component of the wound. The manoeuvre of scoring the posterior sheath and peritoneum under direct camera and external visualization is repeated (Figure 8.20b). At this point, the stoma should allow passage of two of the surgeon's fingers. The loop is then withdrawn, maintaining anatomic orientation as proven both intracorporeally by the camera operator and extracorporeally by the surgeon. Several additional means of verifying appropriate bowel loop orientation include delivering the efferent limb into the incision until the ligament of Treitz is delivered or until the camera operator sees the caecum beginning to lift up. Alternatively, a narrow instrument such as an artery forceps can be introduced along the presumed afferent limb, verifying orientation of that position. At this point, the abdomen is desufflated, a rod is placed under the stoma, and standard maturation can occur after the supraumbilical port site is closed.

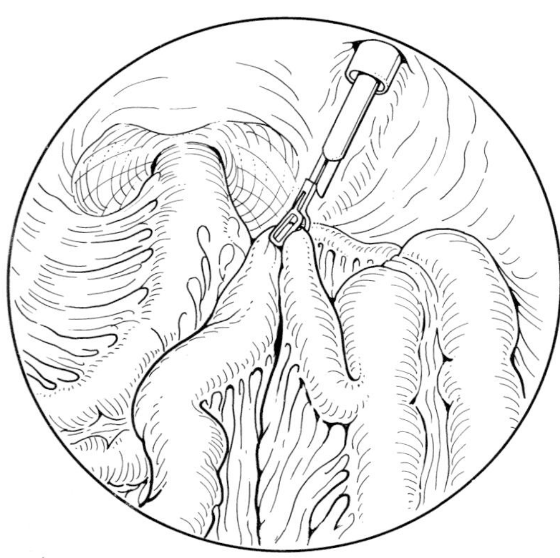

Figure 8.19 Stoma construction by laparoscopy.

Using these techniques, an end stoma can be constructed. Specifically, instead of placing a rod under the mesenteric margin for loop stoma construction, the bowel can be divided with a linear staple cutting device. The efferent limb can be buried in the subcutaneous layers and the stoma matured as an end Brooke ileostomy. Alternatively an Abcarian-type, antimesenteric, efferent limb, blowhole, mucous fistula stoma can be constructed (Unti et al, 1991).

If the indication for stoma construction is perianal Crohn's disease in a patient who is not a candidate for, or does not wish to undergo, a total proctocolectomy, then it is desirable to inspect the entire length of the small bowel to exclude synchronous lesions such as more proximal strictures. Specifically, two left-sided ports are placed, one in the left periumbilical region and one in the left iliac fossa. Through these 10–12 mm ports, each placed through 1 cm horizontal stab wounds lateral to the epigastric

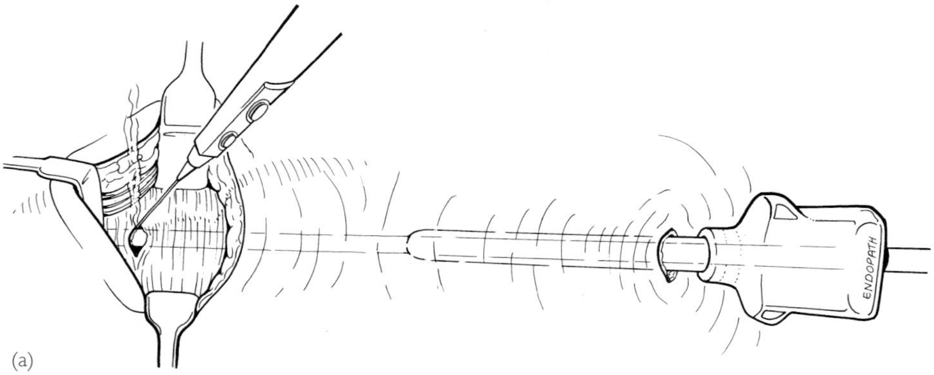

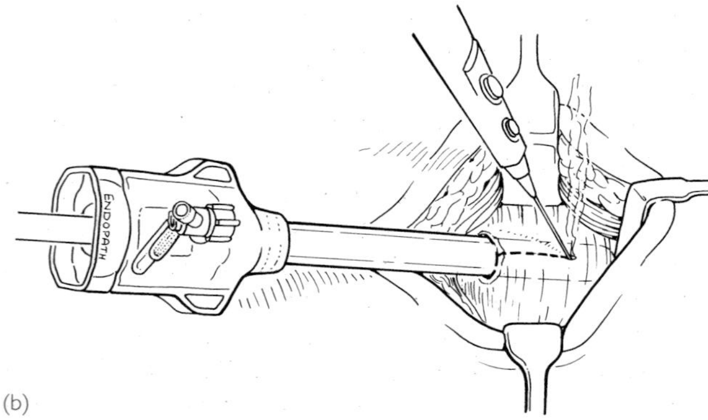

Figure 8.20a–b Laparoscopy: scoring the posterior sheath and peritoneum along the insulated shaft of the Babcock forceps in (a) the inferior aspect and (b) the superior aspect.

vessels, the entire small bowel can be inspected. Any synchronous strictures can be marked and delivered through the stoma site for strictureplasty prior to construction of the stoma itself. Such an approach is also useful in patients in whom, after placement of the right iliac fossa stoma port, adhesions are noted necessitating enterolysis in order to deliver the loop or end stoma into position. Specifically, patients who have undergone prior surgery in whom the terminal ileum loop is fixed to the pelvis secondary to adhesions can benefit from these additional two ports in order to facilitate enterolysis. Other scenarios in which two left-sided ports are useful include leaked anastomoses in which mobilization and irrigation are necessary. Once again, in general it is probably not optimal to operate upon such patients laparoscopically.

Postoperative management

All patients are allowed a clear, liquid diet ad lib commencing the morning after surgery. As tolerated and requested by the patient, the diet is advanced to include solids. Intermediate steps such as 'full fluid' or 'mechanical soft' diets are not employed. Dietary consultation is obtained to assist the patients with their choices.

The determining step in hospital discharge after laparoscopic ileostomy construction is generally not a dietary advancement or stoma function, but rather the patient's comfort level with management of their newly created stoma. For this reason, all patients will have met with the enterostomal care nurse preoperatively at the time of stoma marking. At that time, they will have been provided with literature, videos, and the chance to speak with patients who have stomas. After surgery, intensive consultation and support by the enterostomal care nurse is important. Once the patient is comfortable with stoma management, they are discharged home. Information is provided with regard to stoma support groups, and the health services agency arranges for home visits by the enterostomal care nurse.

Results

The technique of laparoscopic loop ileostomy was described by Khoo et al (1993) and subsequently modified by Teoh et al (1994). The difference in technique between the two series was that Khoo and colleagues stated that 'the fascia was stretched to two fingers breadth to allow easy passage of loop of ileum'. Teoh and colleagues noted that stretching the fascia with a Babcock clamp in place was difficult and insufficient. One patient developed a postoperative fascial outlet obstruction which necessitated prolonged initial hospital stay as well as readmission. The patient was managed without surgery, but required stoma catheterization for evacuation as if she had a continent (Kock) ileostomy. After one month, presumably when the oedema resolved, the catheterization was discontinued. Teoh and coworkers therefore advised that the stoma opening should not have been created by stretching the fascia around an 18 mm port or by two fingers, but rather by incising the fascia under direct vision to ensure an adequate stoma opening. It was agreed that laparoscopic loop ileostomy for temporary faecal diversion was a very worthwhile procedure and a good use of laparoscopy (Fleshman, 1992; Beck, 1994; Roe et al, 1994).

Oliveira et al (1997) described the experience from Cleveland Clinic Florida between March 1993 and January 1996. During that period, 32 patients underwent elective laparoscopic faecal diversion (a loop ileostomy in 25 cases). Indications for faecal diversion are listed in Table 8.2. Conversion was required in five patients (16%) owing to the presence of adhesions in three, enterotomy in one and/or colotomy in one. All of these five patients had undergone previous abdominal surgery and were operated on early in the experience. Major postoperative complications incurred in two patients (6%) and in both cases consisted of stoma outlet obstruction after construction of a loop ileostomy. One of the two patients had undergone prior surgery, in whom reoperation revealed rotation of the terminal ileum at the stoma site. The other patient had a narrow fascial opening which was successfully managed with self-intubation of the stoma as already described. The mean operative time was 76 minutes (range 30–210), the mean length of hospital stay was 6.2 days (range 2–13), and stoma function started after a mean of 3.1 days (range 1–6). The authors concluded that laparoscopic creation of intestinal stomas was safe, feasible and effective. The admonitions were to ensure adequate fascial opening and correct limb orientation.

Ludwig et al (1996) described a two-cannula technique by which 24 stomas, including 16 loop ileostomies, were constructed. Indications for diversion are listed in Table 8.2. Median operative time was 60 minutes (range 20–120) and the median blood loss was 50 mL (range 0–150). There were no intraoperative complications; one patient had the procedure converted to laparotomy because of dense adhesions. The median for the passage of both flatus and stool was 1 day (range 1–3) for ileostomy patients. The median time to discharge

Table 8.2 Indications for laparoscopic stomas

Indication	*Oliveira et al (1997)*	*Ludwig et al (1996)*
Faecal incontinence	11	4
Perianal sepsis or Crohn's disease	6	7
Unresectable rectal carcinoma	4	4
Rectal or pouch–vaginal fistula	4	7
Colonic inertia	2	0
Anal stenosis	1	0
Kaposi's sarcoma	1	0
Tuberculous fistula	1	0
Radiation proctitis	1	0
Complicated pelvic sepsis	0	1

was 6 days (range 2–28) and, as noted earlier, was often delayed by the stoma teaching process. One major complication, a pulmonary embolus, occurred 8 days after the operation in a patient with an obstructing, widely metastatic colon carcinoma; that patient later died of pulmonary failure. All the stomas functioned well with no revisions required during the short follow-up period (Beck, 1994; Luchtefeld and MacKeigan, 1997). In the light of the results presented above, laparoscopic stoma formation can generally be effected very quickly and with surprisingly low postoperative morbidity (Tables 8.3 and 8.4). The outcome certainly compared favourably with that described earlier in this chapter and in the colostomy chapter of this book (Chapter 9).

Iroatulam et al (1998) compared all patients who underwent faecal diversion without any other abdominal procedures. Neither prior laparotomy, inflammatory bowel disease, nor recurrent or metastatic carcinoma were considered absolute contraindications. Parameters evaluated included age, indications for stoma, prior abdominal surgery, operative time, time until stoma function, and the length of postoperative hospital stay. Between March 1993 and October 1996, 41 stomas were constructed by laparoscopy and 11 by laparotomy. There were no significant differences between the two groups relative to mean age of the patient (46 years (18–80) for laparoscopy compared with 58 years (36–81) for laparotomy) or a history of previous abdominal surgery (9 (22%) laparoscopy versus 3 (27%) laparotomy). The stomas began to function more quickly in the laparoscopic group (2.3 days (1–4) versus 4.5 days (3–8); $P<0.05$). Similarly, length of postoperative hospital stay in the laparoscopic group was shorter (5.3 days (2–12) versus 7.6 days (5–19); $P<0.05$). An interesting and unexpected finding was that at a mean follow-up of 22 months (range 2–43) in both groups, none of the patients in the laparoscopic versus two patients in the laparotomy group had stomal prolapse.

Table 8.3 Laparoscopic stomas: outcomes.

Author	*Number*	*Operative morbidity* (%)	*Procedure length* (min)	*Postoperative morbidity* (%)	*Mean length of Hospital stay* (days)
Lange et al (1991)	1	0	100	0	12
Romero et al (1992)	1	0	NS	0	5
Roe et al (1994)	4	0	NS	0	10
Oliveira et al (1997)	32	6	76 (30–210)	6	6.2 (1–13)
Ludwig et al (1996)	24	0	60 (20–120)	4	6 (2–28)

Table 8.4 Laparoscopic stoma: types.

Author	*Number*	*Loop ileostomy*	*Loop colostomy*	*End colostomy*
Lange et al (1991)	1	0	1	0
Romero et al (1992)	1	0	0	1
Khoo et al (1993)	1	1	0	0
Roe et al (1994)	4	1	3	0
Jess and Christiansen (1994)	1	1	0	0
Lyerly and Mautt (1994)	4	1	2	1
Fuhrman and Ota (1994)	0	2	8	0
Oliveira et al (1997)	32	25	4	3
Ludwig et al (1996)	24	16	2	6

Another interesting finding was that the mean duration of surgery in patients who had had prior abdominal surgery was 98 minutes (range 85–210) in the laparoscopy group and 95 minutes (range 65–113) in the laparotomy group. In patients who had *not* had prior abdominal surgery, the mean and range times were respectively 78 (35–125) and 63 (50–80) minutes. Thus, regardless of whether a prior laparotomy had been performed, the laparoscopic approach did not take significantly longer and resulted in a lower incidence of postoperative stomal prolapse. Although it is easy to understand why, especially after ascent of the learning curve, it takes no longer to perform a stoma by laparoscopy than by laparotomy, it is difficult to understand why the incidence of stomal prolapse would be less. Possible reasons include less bowel mobilization by the laparoscopic approach, a different means of stoma creation utilizing the Babcock clamp and trocar technique as earlier described, or merely the shorter length of follow-up in this group than in historical groups of patients who have undergone laparotomy. Nonetheless, considering the large denominator of patients in this group, 0% versus 20% represents an important difference.

THE QUEST FOR CONTINENCE

The advances of the past two decades have allowed many patients to avoid wearing a permanent ileostomy appliance by construction of a reservoir ileostomy, or even to dispense with a stoma by sphincter-preserving operations. Even for those with an intact sphincter, age, coexisting disease and the risk of potential complications cause some patients to choose a conventional proctocolectomy, even after careful counselling (Rothernberger et al, 1983; Fonkalsrud, 1984; Nicholls and Pezim, 1984; Metcalf et al, 1985; Metcalf et al, 1986a). On the other hand, conventional ileostomy is not perfect: leakage occurs in almost half of all ileostomy patients, despite modern appliances (Carlson and Bergan, 1995). Sexual and psychological problems are common (Roy et al, 1970; Bone and Sorensen, 1974; Burnham et al, 1977; Carlstedt et al, 1987; Abcarian and Pearl, 1988; Morowitz and Kirsner, 1981) and there are potentially serious metabolic sequelae from conventional ileostomy, as well as the complications of the stoma itself (Leenen and Kuypers, 1989; Hellman and Lago, 1990; Carlsen et al, 1991).

Kock ileostomy

In experienced hands, the Kock pouch may still provide the best chance of obtaining control over liquid and gaseous discharge from the small bowel (Mullen et al, 1995). However, the revision rate for valve slippage ranges from 7% to 25% and serious complications such as obstruction, sepsis and fistula may jeopardize pouch function in 5–15% (Kock et al, 1981; Beahrs, 1975; Goldman and Rombeau, 1978; Dozois et al, 1980; Goligher, 1983b; Mullen et al, 1995; Ecker et al, 1996). Furthermore, although the quality of life and sexual harmony are greatly improved in young patients who have been converted from a conventional to a reservoir ileostomy (Nilsson et al, 1981; Gerber et al, 1984; McLeod and Fazio, 1984), there is sometimes a high price to pay from slippage of the nipple valve, metabolic sequelae and inflammatory change in the reservoir (Nilsson et al, 1979; Kelly et al, 1980; Bonelo et al, 1981; Beahrs et al, 1981).

Gerber et al (1984) reported on the outcome of conversion from a conventional to a continent ileostomy in 80 patients: sport opportunities were improved in almost all patients; social activities which had previously been restricted were now possible in 96%; and improved sexual harmony was reported in 76%. Although almost all patients stated that they spent less time in managing a continent ileostomy compared with a conventional one, and clothing restrictions were less, many patients find that irrigation of the Medina catheter – to clear the reservoir of particulate matter – distasteful and unacceptable. Nevertheless there are economic advantages for patients who have a Kock pouch, with considerable financial savings in not having to purchase new appliances.

Restorative proctocolectomy

Most patients with a normal anal sphincter and rectal sensation and normal rectal evacuation without Crohn's disease will generally prefer a restorative proctocolectomy to a permanent ileostomy. There are exceptions, particularly the elderly, those who would prefer a stoma to the prospect of 7–10 bowel movements, and those who want one operation with a more certain outcome. These issues are discussed fully in Chapter 49.

Balloon occlusion without a reservoir

Most studies on ileostomy occlusive devices have only been carried out in animals. Chandler et al (1985) achieved increased capacitance by repeated occlusion, but ischaemic necrosis was observed in some animals. Sanada et al (1982) showed that increased ileal volume was only possible following occlusion of a pouch and that catheter obstruction of the normal ileum rarely increased ileal volume. Obstruction of the ileum by balloon occlusion is probably feasible only in patients with a reservoir (Orangio et al, 1984).

Magnetic device

Following the introduction of a magnetic occlusive device for colostomy, application of the same principle for ileostomy was investigated in animals (Sandei et al, 1979). Salmon et al (1980) subsequently reported on its use in two patients with a reservoir ileostomy who had an unsatisfactory nipple valve. Both patients achieved continence. In view of the outcome of the magnetic device for colostomy, it seems unlikely that this approach will be pursued further.

MANAGEMENT OF AN ILEOSTOMY

Immediate postoperative care: routine management

The appliance

The surgeon should be responsible for the fitting of the appliance around an ileostomy at the end of the operation. The appliance should be transparent so that the stoma can be visualized (see Figure 8.16g). A good seal around the stoma is critical since confidence can be destroyed if leakage occurs early during convalescence. If possible, the base of the appliance should be left undisturbed for 4–6 days to allow intestinal contents to drain during the early postoperative period.

Fluids

Prolonged restriction of fluids is unnecessary in most patients who have had an end or loop ileostomy, provided that ileus is not prolonged. The stoma will usually emit gas and then some fluid on the second or third postoperative day. As soon as this event has occurred, the patient may be allowed increased oral fluids and then a light diet, provided the ileostomy continues to function. No special precautions are necessary when replacing fluids and electrolytes in the immediate postoperative period, provided that there are no serious complications and that the patient was not suffering from gross electrolyte disturbance preoperatively. If there is severe ileostomy diarrhoea, this should be replaced by the same volume of normal saline and 40 mmol/L of potassium, in addition to normal fluid and electrolyte requirements.

Steroids

Many patients having an ileostomy have recently been on or are receiving steroids. The usual regimen in such patients is to provide reducing doses of hydrocortisone while they need intravenous fluid replacement. Soon after commencing food, steroids can be given by mouth and discontinued over the next 7–10 days.

Blood

Haemoglobin and haematocrit should be measured before discontinuing the intravenous infusion after surgery since some patients may have been bleeding slowly from the pelvis or perineum and a few may need transfusion.

Management of the stoma

The patient should be encouraged to take a positive interest in the stoma as soon as possible after the operation. Once the stoma begins to act, the patient should learn to empty the bag. The appliance will usually have to be replaced once or twice during the first week. On each occasion the patient should be involved in the removal and replacement of the appliance. After a week all non-absorbable peristomal sutures can be removed. This is another opportunity for the patient to see how the width of the stoma is assessed, to cut out the hole in the appliance to the correct size and to apply the bag with the peel-off backing to the peristomal skin. The patient should be fully mobile by the second or third postoperative day and should be encouraged to change the bag under supervision at this stage so as to facilitate early discharge, particularly in fit young patients with functional or inflammatory bowel disease.

Stoma counselling and follow-up

The patient, and sometimes in the case of children or the elderly an immediate close relative, should be taught stoma management. This is particularly important for patients in the extremes of life, or for those with a mental or physical disability. Advice should be given concerning diet and disposal of and ordering appliances (Irving and Hulme, 1992).

The type of appliance will vary according to many different factors such as the dexterity and intellect of the patient, the volume of the 24-hour ileostomy output, skin creases, scars and body wall. It is fair to say that very few patients now appear for follow-up with their time-honoured black rubber devices with tubes of cream, Karya paste and micropore tape for the plastic base-plate. Even elastic belts are largely a thing of the past. Modern appliances are lightweight one- or two-piece bags with peel-off single-release Perspex covers to the adherent skin discs which really do stick! Different hydrocolloid adhesives are used by the various manufacturers so that Karya, belts and paste are no longer used. Some manufacturers use oval or round discs of adhesive that need to be cut to size, while common sizes are manufactured for specific stoma diameters. One-piece bags have different capacities depending on the volume output of the ileostomy. Women tend to prefer shorter bags. Two-piece appliances often incorporate a floating flange so that the patient can insert his or her fingers under the flange to apply pressure when fitting the base. Attachment of the bag to the flange is usually with a press-on locking device.

If the ileostomy is flush, convex bases are incorporated into one- and two-piece systems which help to evert the stoma (see Figure 8.16g). The days of metal flanges are almost over. The one-piece convex bags are built to a range of sizes and the base provides constant pressure which minimizes the risk of dislodgement. By contrast, the two-piece convex appliances are easier to fit and more versatile but require considerable manual dexterity, intelligence and a belt may be needed.

Two flushable bags are available but they are not biodegradable and therefore must be an environmental hazard, even using the flushable two-piece device where the base is discarded in the dustbin. These flushable appliances consist of an inner paper-like bag containing the waste which can be flushed away and an outer plastic coat which is tossed into the bin. Disposal of all other devices is rather crude and involves emptying the contents down the lavatory and placing the rest in a plastic bag for the dustbin.

Patients should be provided with a list of their own stoma requirements and an explanation of where they can be obtained. Adequate supplies of equipment should be provided for the patient before leaving hospital. The general practitioner should be notified of the operation and type of appliance used. Contact should be made with the district nursing service before the patient is sent home. Information should be available about the activities of the Ileostomy Association or any other stoma support groups. The stoma care nurse will want to talk to the patient and the spouse about the effect of the ileostomy on occupation, social function, clothing, sporting interests and sexual activities. Details of self-referral stomal clinics should be given so that the patient knows how to seek help if needed. The importance of seeking medical advice early if the stoma ceases to function or if the patient develops severe abdominal pain should be reinforced. The consequences of dehydration and acute adrenal insufficiency if a patient develops severe ileostomy diarrhoea must also be explained (Turnbull, 1961).

The principal manufacturers of ileostomy appliances are: Convatec (formerly Squibb Surgicare), Coloplast, Dansac, Hollister, Simcare and Salts.

Special considerations

Prolonged ileus or mechanical obstruction

After operation some patients may experience prolonged ileus with abdominal distension and vomiting. Sometimes the stoma may become oedematous. This event is nearly always associated with profound dehydration, hyponatraemia, hypokalaemia, poor urine output and rising serum creatinine. Causes of the ileus include: retroperitoneal and intraperitoneal bleeding, sepsis, small bowel ischaemia, electrolyte disturbance, traumatic perforation, regional anaesthesia or coexisting medication. Ileus may be difficult to distinguish from mechanical obstruction due to:

- adhesions
- entrapment of bowel through the lateral gutter, in the perineum or through the pelvic peritoneal closure line

- a volvulus around the stoma or where the bowel has become adherent to the abdominal wall closure
- an abscess
- a walled-off perforation.

Immediate management of ileus or obstruction is by nasogastric decompression and replacement of large volumes of intravenous fluid using physiological saline and added potassium. Steroids should be recommenced in full dose if the patient has received steroid therapy within a month of operation. The fluid and electrolyte requirements should be titrated against urine output, central venous pressure and the results of measured electrolyte losses. A catheter can be placed into the stoma to ensure there is no stomal occlusion. In grossly malnourished patients who are septic it may be necessary to replace calories and electrolyte requirements through a subclavian catheter.

It may be quite difficult to know how best to proceed if after 7–10 days there is no return of ileostomy output. If after 10 days of intensive conservative management there is no improvement, serious consideration should be given to repeat laparotomy, provided there is no evidence of an intraperitoneal abscess which might be drained percutaneously. If there is any clinical suspicion of infarction, immediate laparotomy is advised. One of the greatest tragedies for an ileostomate is to lose a substantial length of small bowel from infarction. When laparotomy is performed in these patients, there is usually a mechanical problem which has supervened, such as adherence of small bowel to an abscess or obstruction from an internal hernia. These reoperations are extremely difficult and must be undertaken by the most experienced member of the surgical team, preferably during daylight hours, having set aside sufficient time to display the anatomy of the small bowel. Internal tube stents as advocated by Jones et al (1977) are rarely required. If there is any suspicion of damage to the distal small bowel, a loop proximal jejunostomy can be raised and a gastrostomy inserted. The wound is closed with interrupted mass closure sutures, to include the rectus sheath and muscle, and the skin is left open if there has been gross faecal contamination. With this policy, deep tension sutures are rarely necessary; they can create problems when applying stoma bags.

Retraction

Early retraction of an ileostomy is troublesome since there is a much greater risk of leakage and skin excoriation. Furthermore, retraction of a loop ileostomy usually results in inadequate function. Most stoma care nurses can protect the skin, hence urgent revision is rarely needed. If a retracted stoma can be resolved, for instance using the convex appliances already referred to, there may be no need for surgical correction. Alternatively, if a loop ileostomy used to protect an anastomosis retracts, then serious consideration should be given to closing the loop ileostomy at an earlier date since retraction under these circumstances no longer achieves faecal diversion. Using a small dose of diazepam or Hypnovel and an opiate analgesic, it is often possible to re-evert the stoma after applying tissue forceps to the ileum just below the skin level (Figure 8.21a,b). If this can be achieved, but the stoma does not remain everted, one or two catgut sutures placed between both walls of the ileostomy may retain the stoma in its correct position (Figure 8.21c,d), alternatively the everted bud may be stapled (Figure 8.21e,f). If the stoma re-everts after applying pressure around the ileostomy, a convex flange now incorporated into a two piece appliance can be applied to encourage it to remain in the everted position. If, despite these measures, the stoma retracts again, the situation should be managed conservatively until it is safe to consider a refashioning procedure. Early attempts at refashioning usually result in damage to the small bowel unless stapling refashioning is used (Speakman et al, 1991).

Ischaemia

A great deal of concern is usually expressed when an ileostomy appears purple, or even black, when viewed through a transparent ileostomy appliance within 48 hours of the operation. Provided the patient's general condition is satisfactory it is usually prudent to adopt a conservative policy. It is rarely necessary to reoperate for an infarcted ileostomy. The appearances are usually due to venous congestion and oedema from a relatively narrow abdominal wall or a tight appliance. Adequate postoperative analgesia should be provided and the appliance checked to ensure that it is not obstructing the stoma. In nearly all cases the stoma will resume its normal colour within 48 hours. At worst, there may be some stenosis of the stoma at a later stage, but the need for immediate intervention and resection is rare. Postoperative discolouration appears to have no effect on long-term function (Carlsen and Bergan, 1995).

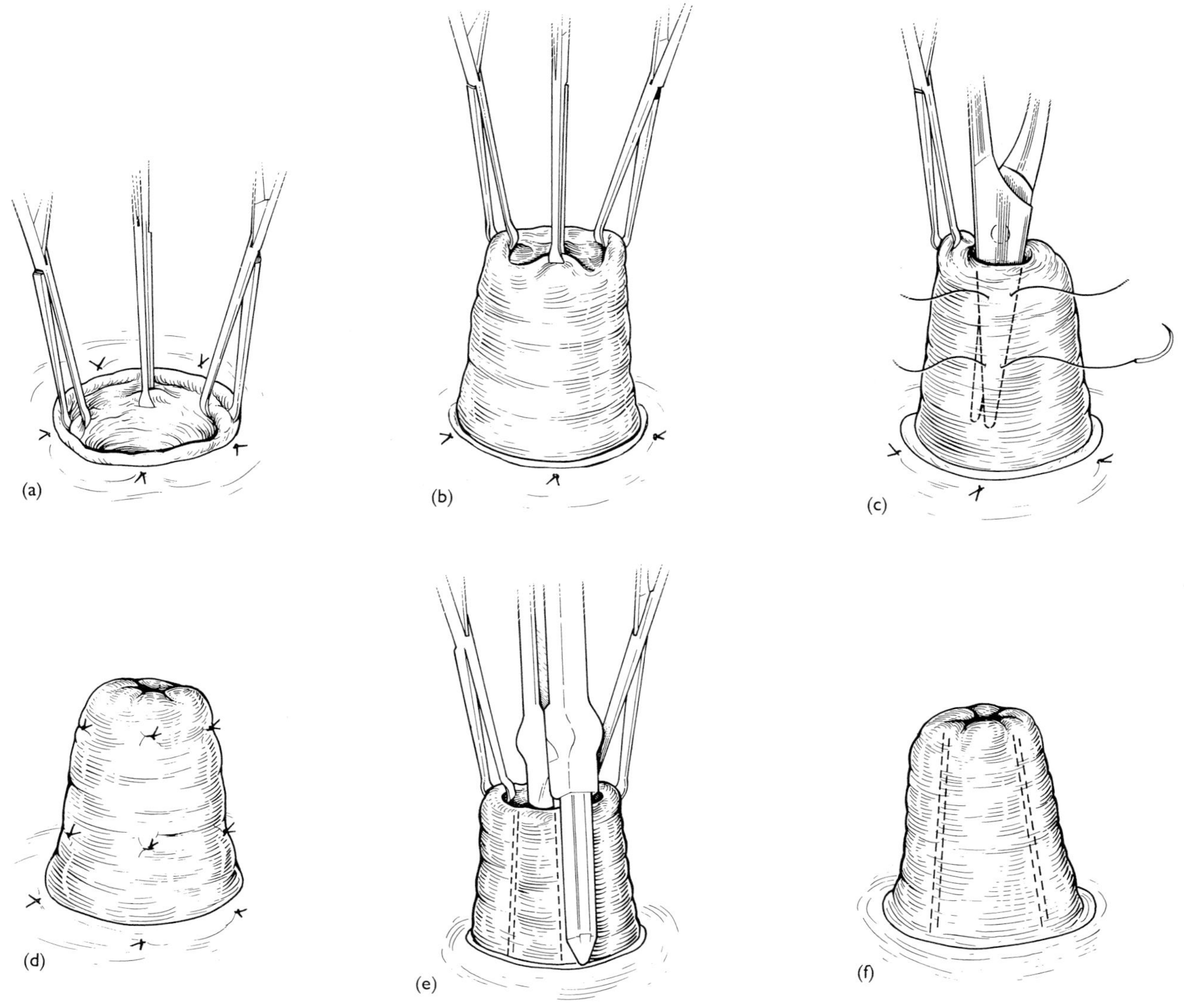

Figure 8.21a–f Revision of a retracted stoma. (a) The retracted stoma is re-everted by grasping the bowel wall deep to the abdominal trephine. (b) Once a sufficient length of everted ileum has been delivered, the stoma may be stabilized by (c) placement of a series of full thickness sutures between the two limbs of the ileostomy over (d) a flat surface acting as an anvil. (e)–(f) Alternatively the stoma may be stabilized by placement of three or four rows of linear staples between the two components of the ileostomy using a linear stapler (without cutter).

Dysfunction

Ileostomy dysfunction was a term coined by Warren and McKittrick (1951) to describe a syndrome of abdominal pain, high-volume ileostomy output and vomiting, irregular ileostomy action occurring about a week after operation. This syndrome is caused by a functional obstruction at the ileostomy spout and occurred almost exclusively in patients who did not have an eversion ileostomy. For this reason the syndrome is now rare. Relief of symptoms can be achieved rapidly by passing a soft Foley catheter through the stoma to relieve the obstruction and subsequent refashioning of the stoma with an everted stoma.

Appliances

The skin must be protected from the digestive action of intestinal enzymes in patients with an ileostomy. A seal must be achieved around the stoma which will be protective, non-allergenic and adherent so that the collecting device will not become dislodged. Small bowel contents must be collected in bags which can accommodate discharge of 200–300 mL of liquid over a few minutes without the appliance becoming dislodged. The two sealants widely used in the past for stoma appliances were karaya and Stomahesive, but these have now been entirely superseded by artificial hydrocolloids.

Karaya

Karaya gum is a partially acetylated polysaccharide characterized by a high affinity for water absorption, having a low pH. It is the dried product of the *Sterculia urens* tree found in India (Goldstein and Alter, 1973). At concentrations of 20–50% in water, karaya exhibits strong adhesive properties. Blending with a mild alkali improves adhesiveness of the gum. Stomal sealants combine the gum with gelatin to form a solid base which can be moulded into a ring. Karaya rings and plates can remain in place on the skin for 8–12 hours before disintegrating. The material can be bonded with plastic. Skin reactions to karaya may occur but are rare. Karaya powder can be applied directly to excoriated skin around the stoma or fistula.

Stomahesive

Stomahesive is a commercially developed product and consists of gelatin, sodium carboxymethylcellulose, pectin and polyisobutylene. It is resistant to heat, perspiration and small bowel enzyme activity (Evans et al, 1976). No hypersensivity to this product has so far been reported. Beernaerts et al (1977) report that Stomahesive can remain around the stoma for periods of 1–15 days. Marks et al (1978) compared Stomahesive with karaya gum and found no difference in skin response over a weeks' application. However, when the adhesive was left in contact with the skin for more than 15 days Stomahesive was found to be much less irritant. Karaya tends to break up and requires replacement more frequently than Stomahesive (Devlin and Plant, 1975). Comfeel, a commercially developed absorbent cellulose derivative used for stoma appliances and akin to Stomahesive, is very elastic and easily moulded; it provides non-elastic skin adhesion and can be helpful in physically very active patients and in patients suffering from skin allergy.

Commercially produced hydrocolloids

Strong adherent hydrocolloids are now manufactured which are largely non-allergenic. They are extremely efficient adhesives that conform to skin contours, their adherence to skin is strong and there are few if any long-term skin complications despite constant application.

Rubber devices

Modern ileostomy appliances are made of lightweight plastics and the bags are constructed with soft pliable material which do not sweat and which no longer needs to be encased with cotton surrounding covers. The old black rubber devices are heavy and bulky, but they have obvious economic advantages over the current disposable appliances; however, they have now virtually disappeared from use even in third world countries.

Single-piece or two-piece?

All appliances consist of a flange with an aperture for the stoma and a bag or pouch. As discussed the flange and pouch may be constructed as a one- or two-piece device (Figure 8.22a,b).

Two-piece devices have the advantage that once the flange is applied and fixed to the skin it can be left in place for up to a week or more. As removal of the flange involves traumatizing the skin, two-piece appliances were generally more gentle to the skin, but with modern sealants this argument no longer usually applies. In a two-piece device a snaplock is used to achieve a hermetic seal between the flange and the bag which must be pushed together with some force to achieve a proper seal. This manoeuvre may be painful in the early postoperative period and impossible for some patients with arthritis and failing sight.

Hill and Pickford (1979) reported the outcome of the then new two-piece device in 11 patients after operation. The Stomahesive base adhered well to the skin (Kyle and Hughes, 1970). The flange did not need to be disturbed for a mean of 5 days; dislodgement of the appliance occurred on ten occasions during 204 patient-days and ten of 11 patients chose to continue using the device. There was no allergy to the Stomahesive, and/or the plastic, which had a low transmission to gas, and was odour-proof.

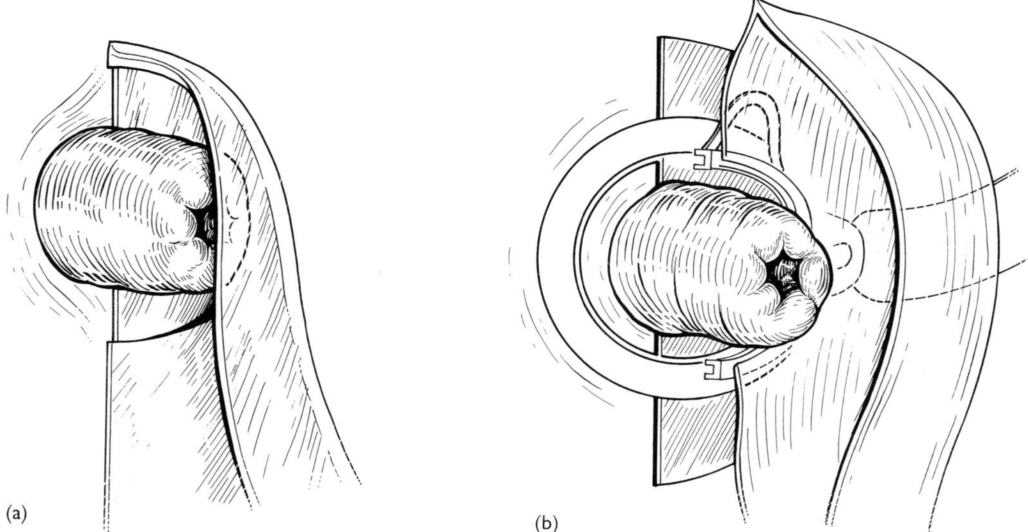

Figure 8.22a–b (a) A one-piece ileostomy bag with an adhesive seal incorporated in the drainage device. (b) A two-piece ileostomy appliance. A flange is incorporated into a Stomahesive base around the ileostomy and a clip-on attachment facilitates attachment of the bag to the Stomahesive base.

One disadvantage of the two-piece device is that it is more bulky under clothing and tends to protrude more than a single-piece appliance. For some patients a single-piece appliance is more attractive, particularly now that reliable sealants have been developed in combination with drainable systems.

Drainable bags

For many ileostomy patients a single-piece drainable system is preferred. This may have to be emptied 3–10 times a day, depending on: the size of the bag, the volume of ileostomy output and thus the proximity of the ileostomy to the ileocaecal junction, the presence of residual bowel disease, the anxiety of the patient, previous operations such as gastrectomy or cholecystectomy-associated metabolic disorders, and the amount of small bowel resected. Drainable bags may be occluded by wire-incorporated plastic seal strips, polypropylene clips, or in the old days by a rubber-band to the rubber drainage spout.

Choice and supply

The choice of appliance is a personal one. There is so much choice that the stoma care nurse will need to advise the patient which appliance will best suit his or her needs. This is particularly important today as there are considerable commercial pressures to attract patients to a particular product. The size of the bag will depend on the ileostomy output and clothing considerations. The flange must achieve a secure fit, the appliance should protect against odour and the device must be strong yet comfortable.

The patient must be given a checklist for reordering purposes with the manufacturer's name, the size of the appliance and the product number.

The cost of appliances varies considerably. Hospital stocks are governed by patient requirements, designs most preferred by the stoma care nurse, and cost. The selection of hospital stocks are usually comprehensive and free as most manufacturers are keen to introduce new ileostomy patients to their own products. Under the British health service, all patients are entitled to free appliances. In most other countries, patients may claim against cost; in the USA patients cannot always obtain insurance against stoma therapy appliances and these costs must therefore be borne by the patient. McLeod et al (1985) calculated that the cost of supplies averaged US$400 per patient per year. These costs were met by the patient in 32% of cases, entirely by the insurance company in only 4%, partly by the insurance company in 41%, by Medicaid or Medicare in 16%, and by other sources in 7%.

Disposal

Disposal of appliances is still a problem. Only two flushable bags are currently available in the UK, and as yet none of the devices is biodegradable. Some authorities provide dirty-dressing collections. The contents of the ileostomy bags are flushed down the lavatory but plastic bags should either be burned (not recommended) or discarded wrapped in a plastic bag for the refuse bins which are taken to land refuse tips.

Changing appliances

Appliances are usually changed in a toilet or bathroom, preferably where there is a small hand-basin. A small cupboard in the bathroom should be used to store appliance materials. A large sponge bag is also desirable for storing spare appliances and materials when travelling.

The flange is gently lifted off the skin around the ileostomy. Carbon tetrachloride or ether is rarely used today unless patients still use the older rubber devices, in which case these agents help to remove grease from the peristomal skin. Karaya, Stomahesive and modern hydrocolloids peel easily from the skin, which can then be washed with water and carefully dried before applying a new flange.

The patient will already know the size of the flange and bag. Most bags are now supplied cut to a particular size and shape and only rarely does the patient have to cut his or her flange. With the single-release paper backing to the adhesive flange, confident application of the device around the ileostomy is rarely a problem. Tape is not necessary and belts are rarely used. For the two-piece appliance, gentle pressure on the floating flange secures a good skin seal. The bag is then clipped on to the flange with the press-on locking device.

Problems

Skin problems

Skin excoriation from leakage remains the most common complication of an ileostomy (Phillips et al, 1985), particularly in a badly sited stoma, if the ileostomy has retracted and if the length of residual small bowel is short. Effluent dermatitis is characterized by peristomal excoriation which delineates any skin furrows and scars near the ileostomy. Faecal dermatitis will cause marked erythema and desquamation and may encourage secondary skin sepsis. Treatment involves careful cleaning of the skin, which is washed with water and dried with a towel or a hair dryer. Any furrows in the skin may be filled with Stomahesive paste, but in practice this is rarely necessary. If the skin or granulation tissue surrounding the stoma is grossly distorted, a Stomahesive base can be constructed to act as a face-plate. During this procedure the ileostomy can be occluded with a catheter balloon while the paste or base is applied (Devlin, 1982). If the ileostomy contents are very liquid it is advisable to prescribe antidiarrhoeal preparations. In some cases local corticosteroid preparations with or without antibiotics or with antifungal agents may be beneficial, these preparations should be used sparingly and only when a diagnosis of infection or fungal infestation has been confirmed.

Other forms of dermatitis include fungal infections and pre-existing skin disorders. Fungal dermatitis can be identified from culture swabs and a history of recent antibiotic administration. The skin disorders which most frequently complicate stoma management include psoriasis and exfoliative dermatitis, both of which may complicate the underlying inflammatory bowel disease. Some skin problems appear to be due to Crohn's disease affecting peristomal skin, or to patient interference.

Gas

Gas is derived from swallowed air or from bacterial fermentation of various dietary products. Pneumogenic foods include eggs, beans, onions, cabbage and sprouts. Agents which may reduce odour by preventing bacterial overgrowth include chlorophyll tablets and bismuth subgallate.

Gaseous odours are less troublesome for patients with an ileostomy than with a colostomy. Nevertheless, audible flatus discharging into an ileostomy bag is a source of great embarrassment. Passage of large amounts of gas may dislodge the appliance from the skin. Flatus patches consisting of activated carbon or charcoal are now available and widely used. Insertion of aspirin tablets into the bag is said to reduce bacterial fermentation, and various commercial products have been developed specifically for the same purpose; their efficacy is unknown.

Diet

There are few dietary studies in ileostomates; most have been based on questionnaires with low response rates (Kramer et al, 1962; Thomson et al, 1970). Gazzard et al (1978) found that although 70% of patients accepted that they could eat any food, in practice over half excluded certain items from their diet, particularly vegetables such as cabbage, cauliflower and beans because they caused excessive flatus, and 68% avoided fish or eggs because of the odour (Table 8.5).

Table 8.5 Influence of various dietary products on ileostomy function ($n = 50$).

	Flatus	*Odour*	*Liquid*
Green vegetables	16	3	9
Onion	6	6	2
Fruit	1	0	6
Eggs	3	13	1
Fish	0	17	3
Cheese	1	7	2
Spices	2	3	1

From Gazzard et al (1978).

Women seem to be more fussy about diet than men. More patients adhere to a highly restrictive diet before proctocolectomy than with the ileostomy afterwards (McLeod and Fazio, 1984). Unfortunately the cheapest vegetable foods cause most stomal upset. Beer but not concentrated alcohol causes diarrhoea. Ileostomies are most active about an hour after the main meal of the day. Obstruction may be precipitated by eating raw fruit, vegetables and nuts. These foods should be thoroughly chewed and eaten in small amounts (Turnbull, 1961).

Drugs

Some drugs are inadequately absorbed in patients with an ileostomy, particularly when they have a short bowel. Enteric-coated tablets should not, therefore, be prescribed in ileostomy patients. Oral medication should also be discouraged in the ileostomy patient unless absolutely necessary. In some patients, particularly those with Crohn's disease, replacement therapy with oral iron, folate and other vitamins may be desirable. Fortunately, most haematinics are adequately absorbed. Antibiotics should be avoided because of the risk of bacterial and fungal overgrowth. Diuretics should be prescribed sparingly in ileostomy patients for fear of dehydration.

In patients who have had an ileal resection, codeine phosphate with added salt may reduce ileostomy output by minimizing water, sodium and potassium losses (Hill et al, 1975a). For patients with the short gut syndrome, water restriction and a balanced glucose electrolyte solution may be needed to maintain fluid and electrolyte homeostasis (Newton et al, 1985). A sipped electrolyte solution is the optimum mode of sodium replacement in these patients (Nightingale et al, 1992).

Antidiarrhoeal agents should be available for ileostomy patients in case they develop ileostomy diarrhoea. Opium and its derivatives act by reducing small bowel transit time, thus preventing water and electrolyte reabsorption. Codeine phosphate in a dose of 30 mg 6-hourly can usually control diarrhoea in 24 hours (Newton, 1978).

Loperamide (2–4 mg three times a day) is usually less effective than codeine but it may be combined with an opiate to enhance its effect (Tytgat et al, 1976). Diphenoxylate with atropine often causes colic and should be used sparingly.

Other drugs which reduce ileostomy output include the tricyclic antidepressants and the phenothiazine derivatives; anticholinergic agents such as disopyramide and quinidine also reduce intestinal motility.

Bulking agents such as methylcellulose, ispaghula or Metamucil are hydrophobic and attract water into the gut. They may therefore cause dehydration. Since the ileostomy patient is chronically sodium- and water-depleted, these compounds should theoretically be sparingly used. However, in practice they seem to be therapeutically beneficial and rarely cause electrolyte disturbances (Kennedy et al, 1982a).

Contraception and pregnancy

Sexual function in ileostomy patients is considered in detail in Chapter 11. The contraceptive options available will need to be discussed with the patient. Although there is a higher incidence of infertility due to tubal occlusion in women who have had a proctocolectomy, this is not sufficiently common for couples to avoid normal contraceptive methods. Male ileostomates with apparent propulsive ejaculatory failure are not necessarily sterile. Furthermore, the incidence of autonomic nerve damage in males is now very low (Kennedy et al, 1982a).

The ideal approach for female ileostomy patients is for their partner to agree either to vasectomy or to use a condom. Contraceptive pills, particularly low-dose agents, are inadequately absorbed; hence ovulation will not be suppressed and the pill is ineffective (Hudson and Lennard-Jones, 1978). There is an increased risk of thromboembolism and failure of menstruation after discontinuing the pill. Barrier methods in the female are compromised by altered pelvic anatomy, since the uterus often becomes retroverted and occlusive methods are therefore insecure. Intrauterine contraceptive devices are difficult to insert if the uterus is retroflexed, and long-term use of the intrauterine device exacerbates chronic pelvic sepsis. Finally, female sterilization may be difficult and potentially dangerous following proctocolectomy. For these reasons the male partner should accept the responsibility for contraception.

Pregnancy usually proceeds normally in women with an ileostomy (Roy et al, 1970; Bone and Sorensen, 1974; Burnham et al, 1977). There may be complications from renal calculi, dehydration or electrolyte deficiency but these are uncommon. Anaemia will need to be monitored carefully and absorption of iron supplements may pose a problem. Most patients with Crohn's disease will require folate and vitamin B_{12} supplements as well as iron. The stoma is usually displaced upwards and laterally by the enlarging gravid uterus, so maintaining an effective seal around the ileostomy may be troublesome. There is an increased incidence of ileostomy prolapse and retraction during pregnancy and a mirror may have to be used to facilitate changing the appliance (Hudson, 1972). Perhaps the most worrying complication is that of intestinal obstruction. It is important that close liaison be established between the obstetrician, gastroenterologist and surgeon since cessation of ileostomy function is an event that requires careful and urgent attention. Most women will be able to have a normal vaginal delivery, but forceps or ventouse assisted delivery may be required. A generous episiotomy is usually required because of previous perineal scarring. Caesarian section may be difficult and best avoided unless absolutely necessary. Problems of perineal wound healing are rarely exacerbated by delivery and this should not be a contraindication to vaginal delivery.

QUALITY OF LIFE WITH AN ILEOSTOMY

Most patients with an ileostomy have a normal life expectancy and enjoy good health (Daly, 1968; Ritchie, 1971). Nevertheless, there are problems in terms of physical well-being, emotional stability and time lost from normal activities (Huibregste et al, 1977; Turnberg et al, 1978; Kennedy et al, 1982a, b; McLeod et al, 1985; Pemberton, 1988; Irvine et al, 1994; Moody and Maybury, 1996) (Table 8.6).

Psychological adjustment

Women seem to suffer less psychological disturbance than men following proctocolectomy. In a study of 51 patients, men became introverted, defensive and had high 'lie scores', as evidenced by a high incidence of 'fake good' in which they seemed unwilling to admit to maladjustment (Kennedy et al, 1982a). Biermann et al (1966) identified an increased incidence of emotional problems among patients with an ileostomy. McLeod et al (1985) found that 22% of their patients felt less attractive, and many overtly resented their stoma. Resentment was greatest among those who had received inadequate stoma counselling before operation, a deficiency which was identified in 52% of patients. Psychological adjustment closely correlated with the function of the ileostomy. In a later study, McLeod et al (1986) recorded that 73% of patients were glad to have had the operation and had accepted their stoma, 22% stated that they were pleased to have had the disease removed but did not like their stoma, and 3% generally regretted having an operation at all.

Table 8.6 Result of ileostomy (permanent) for inflammatory bowel disease.

	Before ileostomy (%)	*After ileostomy* (%)
Physical well-being		
Excellent/good	18	79
Fair	15	18
Poor	67	3
Emotional well-being		
Excellent/good	34	76
Fair	31	15
Poor	33	7
Time lost from normal activities		
Less than 1 week	15	39
1 week–3 months	41	24
More than 3 months	36	24

From McLeod et al (1986).

Sexual sequelae

Although male sexual function may be impaired after rectal excision, from damage to the autonomic supply of the bladder, seminal vesicles, prostate and penis (Watts et al, 1966; Burnham et al, 1977; Gruner et al, 1977), currently accepted methods of rectal excision for inflammatory bowel disease have resulted in an extremely low incidence of impotence or retrograde ejaculation (Lee and Dowling, 1972; Lytle and Parks, 1977; Lee and Truelove, 1980; Kennedy et al, 1982a; Leicester et al, 1984). Nevertheless, there are sexual problems in men which are mainly of an emotional and psychological nature. Although in the study from Oxford (Kennedy et al, 1982a) there was no case of impotence, emotional problems prevented normal intercourse in up to 60% of male patients after proctocolectomy. This observation is most important because it has always been assumed in the past that the psychological problems in the male were the result of autonomic damage. These emotional difficulties do not appear to be present after ileorectal anastomosis for ulcerative colitis, so one must conclude that it is the presence of the stoma itself and not the rectal surgery which is to blame (Jones et al, 1977).

In women the situation is much more complex and less well understood: commonly, sexual dysfunction is never recognized. Detailed information on sexual performance in women after proctocolectomy is poorly documented; however, it seems that between 2% and 22% complain of dysparunia and impaired libido (Watts et al, 1966; Daly, 1968; Burnham et al, 1977). Following proctocolectomy the uterus may become retroverted, there may be vaginal stenosis, or even a vaginoperineal fistula. In some patients the introitus becomes rigid and there may be chronic perineal discomfort following rectal excision (Johnson, 1969; Devlin and Plant, 1979). It is hardly surprising, therefore, that dysparunia and chronic pelvic sepsis are common (Fasth et al, 1978; Johnson, 1979). In the Oxford survey dysparunia was reported in three of 14 women and three women said that they felt less feminine. Hence, anatomical reasons for impaired sexual function are more common in women than men, but emotional factors seem important in both sexes.

Patients with an ileostomy fear that they will not be attractive to the opposite sex. This is probably most true in patients who have newly acquired a stoma and appears to be a greater problem among women than men. Fewer females than males marry after proctocolectomy (Gruner et al, 1977).

Social activities

Patients have a less restricted social life with an ileostomy than when they were ill with colitis before the proctocolectomy (Table 8.7), particularly with respect to diet, sport, hobbies and travel. However, patients with an ileostomy have a more restricted social life than age- and sex-matched normal healthy individuals. In both the Oxford and Cleveland Clinic series, more patients – particularly women – were restricted in the types of clothing they can wear. There was no correlation between the ability to enjoy normal social activities and age, sex, length of symptoms, aetiology of disease and time since operation.

Table 8.7 Severe limitations in life-style.

	Before ileostomy (%)	*After ileostomy* (%)
Diet	30	12
Sports	27	10
Hobbies	19	8
Travel	24	8
Clothing	10	9

From McLeod et al (1985).

Physical problems

Minor problems related to the stoma itself were recorded in over a half of the ileostomy patients reviewed at the Cleveland Clinic but only 9% developed major complications (McLeod et al, 1985). Minor problems included skin irritation (49%), odour and noise (42%) and a feeling that the appliance was visible (17%). A similar experience was recorded by Morowitz and Kirsner (1981) and by Biermann et al (1966). Most patients spend at least an hour a day on the management of their stoma.

Work prospects

The work prospects among ileostomates were analysed from a questionnaire to patients registered with the Ileostomy Association (Whates and Irving, 1984). Although 86% of patients had been employed before their proctocolectomy, approximately a third had had to give up their job preoperatively through illness. After ileostomy, 77% returned to full employment. The shortfall was almost entirely due to patients who were approaching retirement age at the time of their operation and who had decided not to return to work afterwards. The majority of those who returned to work did so with their original employer. A few (6%) began work for the first time after operation. In most cases successful career advancement was possible. Less than 3% were positively discriminated against by their employer because of the stoma.

These data support earlier studies suggesting that job prospects were not impaired by having an ileostomy (Daly and Brooke, 1967; Lennenberg and Rowbotham, 1970; Roy et al, 1970; Watts et al, 1966). The only exception was an Australian survey in

Table 8.8 Aftermath of ileostomy: work status (n = 273).

	Before ileostomy (%)	*After ileostomy* (%)
Full-time job/student	58	49
Housewife	16	13
Part-time employment	8	11
Retired/unemployed	7	10
Disabled due to illness	10	10

From McLeod et al (1986).

Table 8.9 Morbidity (%) of ileostomy in the elderly.

	Less than 60 years	*60 years or more*
Reoperation		
Revision	12	6
Intestinal obstruction	8	3
Skin excoriation	40	37
Problems with stoma management	6	18
Frequency of emptying (per 24 hours)	7.4 ± 0.2	6.6 ± 0.3
Appliance change (no. per week)	2.7–1.0	2.2–0.3
Occupation changed	6	9
Restriction in household jobs	12	18
Restriction in social activity	20	24
Restriction in sexual activity	28	24
Restriction in travel	25	33
Restriction in diet	28	34
Satisfied with stoma	89	97

From Stryker et al (1985).

which only two-thirds of patients returned to their original job (Wilson, 1964). The position in the USA today also seems to be less encouraging than in the UK. McLeod et al (1986) found that a third of patients were prevented from pursuing their career of first choice. Fifteen per cent lost their job and 23% felt that they were discriminated against as far as normal promotion in their employment was concerned (Table 8.8). Wyke et al (1988) found that employment prospects were not hindered in ileostomy patients but that almost a year elapsed before patients were capable of returning to full employment after proctocolectomy. A recent questionnaire indicates that many ileostomy patients are discriminated against by insurance companies offering life cover even though life tables indicate a low mortality in these patients with inflammatory bowel disease (Moody and Mayberry, 1996).

Young and elderly patients

It is remarkable how well children adapt to an ileostomy. They seem to manage the stoma themselves without difficulty. It is only when they reach adolescence that they discover the social consequences of having an ileostomy (Jones et al, 1977).

Data on the quality of life among elderly patients with an ileostomy are scanty (Law et al, 1961; Beahrs, 1971; Ritchie, 1971). As these patients have a high incidence of arthritis, poor eyesight and general ill-health, it is important to know how well elderly patients fare after proctocolectomy. Elderly patients find a stoma less easy to accept than younger patients (Abrams et al, 1975) and there seems to be a higher incidence of dermatitis, but none of the elderly patients from the Lahey Clinic required special nursing care. Stryker et al (1985) reviewed all the patients who were alive after proctocolectomy; 67 (10%) were over 60 years of age. Comparisons with the younger age group (Table 8.9) revealed a lower rate of complications needing revision in the elderly. The only feature which distinguished the older population was that 18%, compared with 6%, had technical difficulties with the management of their stoma. Despite this, restriction in lifestyle was no greater in the older patients (Dlin and Perlman, 1971). These data indicate that elderly patients need more stoma care supervision than the young but that the quality of life is not inferior (Ellor and Rizzo, 1978; Ellor and Ellor, 1982).

METABOLIC SEQUELAE

Haematological sequelae

Many early studies suggested that haemoglobin (Daly, 1968), serum B_{12} and folate levels were normal in patients with an ileostomy (Jagenburg et al, 1971; Miettinen and Peltokallio, 1971; Lenz, 1976). The Oxford group, however, showed that haemoglobin levels, when corrected for dehydration, were low in patients with an ileostomy, irrespective of the underlying disease. Low values for mean corpuscular volume (MCV) and mean corpuscular haemoglobin (MCH) were also found, suggesting a mild iron deficiency anaemia in colitics with an ileostomy (Table 8.10). Despite these findings, serum iron and iron binding capacity were normal. However, there was increased retention of orally administered iron and low ferritin levels, indicative of a mild iron deficiency anaemia. It is suggested,

Table 8.10 Abnormal haematological and biochemical parameters in ileostomy patients.

	Ileostomy (UC)	*Controls*	*Ileostomy (Crohn's)*
Corrected haemoglobin (g/dl)	13.4 ± 1.4*	14.1 ± 13.1	12.1 ± 1.3*
Mean corpuscular volume (fl)	86.1 ± 4.4*	89.6 ± 3.8	89.1 ± 6.2
Mean corpuscular haemoglobin (pg)	29.5 ± 2.0*	30.7 ± 1.5	30.1 ± 2.6
Erythrocyte sedimentation rate (mm/h)	7.5 ± 6.5	6.3 ± 5.1	19.3 ± 14.5*
Serum ferritin (mg/l)	41.3 ± 33.7*	78.6 ± 68.4	–
Iron retention (%)	26.5 ± 17.6*	12.9 ± 7.5	25.5 ± 21.1*
Total protein (g/l)	74.8 ± 4.8*	70.1 ± 4.3	71.5 ± 4.0
Albumin (g/l)	44.2 ± 2.9*	42.7 ± 2.2	41.3 ± 3.0
Alkaline phosphatase (I.U.)	211.7 ± 64.1*	181.9 ± 40.1	232.0 ± 55.2*

UC, ulcerative colitis.
Normal: Haemoglobin, iron, iron binding capacity, mean corpuscular haemaglobin concentration (MCHC), iron loss, sodium, potassium, chloride, bicarbonate, urea, creatinine, calcium, phosphate, bilirubin, aspartate transaminase.
From Kennedy et al (1982b).
* Differ significantly from controls.

therefore, that ileostomy patients should be given prophylactic iron from time to time to correct this abnormality (Kennedy et al, 1982b). Serum folate and red cell folate levels were normal. Although serum B_{12} levels were normal, reduced absorption of B_{12} was demonstrated in ileostomates with Crohn's disease (Figure 8.23). By contrast, absorption was increased in patients with ulcerative colitis who had an ileostomy.

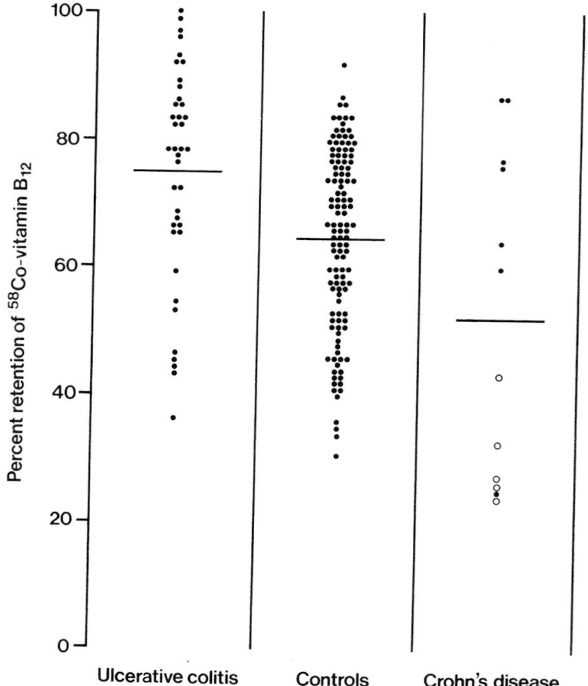

Figure 8.23 Percentage retention of [^{58}Co] vitamin B_{12} in patients with an ileostomy for ulcerative colitis, in control subjects and in patients with an ileostomy for Crohn's disease. The open circles represent patients in whom a segment of ileum has already been resected for Crohn's disease (17–67 cm ileum resected).

Fluid and electrolyte deficiency

The Oxford patients had significantly higher values for serum proteins, albumin and alkaline phosphatase than controls. All other results were normal. It was concluded that the increased serum protein values reflected a state of mild dehydration (Kennedy et al, 1982a). It has been known for some time that healthy patients with an ileostomy are in a state of chronic sodium and water depletion (Crawford and Brooke, 1957; Smiddy et al, 1960; Nuguid et al, 1961; Gallagher et al, 1962; Kramer et al, 1962; Kanaghinis et al, 1963; Clarke et al, 1967; Hill et al, 1975a). The homeostatic response to this deficiency is to actively retain sodium by the kidney (Singer et al, 1973) and the gastrointestinal tract, a phenomenon which one might expect to be mediated by aldosterone. Despite this, earlier studies of aldosterone levels in ileostomy patients revealed normal values (Isaacs et al, 1976; Turnberg et al, 1978). However, Kennedy et al (1983) confirmed that resting levels of both aldosterone and renin were significantly raised in ileostomy patients compared with controls. Although the bowel also tries to conserve sodium, it appears that this mechanism is not due to an increase in antidiuretic hormone (ADH) secretion (Le Veen et al, 1962). The reason for chronic salt and water depletion in ileostomy patients is apparent when the composition of ileostomy effluent is analysed. The normal losses through a healthy ileostomy are in the range 600–640 mL/day and the total loss of sodium is 70–80 mmol/day. Normal subjects excrete only 150 mL of water a day and the sodium content of faeces is less than 5 mmol/day (Wrong, 1970). Hence, ileostomy patients lose in excess of 500 mL of fluid and 70 mmol of sodium. As a result, the kidney conserves sodium at the expense of potassium,

Table 8.11 Abnormal biochemical values in ileostomy patients (ulcerative colitis only).

	Ileostomy	*Control*
pH	5.29 ± 1.04*	5.95 ± 1.05
Sodium (mmol/day)	113 ± 65*	142 ± 59
Potassium (mmol/day)	79 ± 25*	58 ± 20
Sodium:potassium	1.5 –0.8*	2.5 –0.8

Normal: 24 h volume urea, creatinine, creatinine clearance, calcium, phosphate.
From Kennedy et al (1983).
* Differ significantly from controls.

which is lost in excess, resulting in a low urinary sodium/potassium ratio (Table 8.11). There is a further loss of potassium from the ileostomy in exchange for sodium and water (Ladas et al, 1986).

The Leeds group compared ileostomy losses in patients having a minimal small bowel resection with patients who had lost between 30 cm and 120 cm in small bowel (Table 8.12). The volume and total losses of sodium and potassium were much greater after small bowel resection (Hill et al, 1975b) and were proportional to the extent of resection. The mechanism of the increased fluid loss following small bowel resection is due to a loss of absorptive surface area (Hill et al, 1975a), bile salt malabsorption and loss of the ileal brake mechanism. The result is a secretory diarrhoea from high bile salt concentrations in the ileum, which is influenced by long-chain triglycerides (Ladas et al, 1986). Not only is there excessive loss of water and salt after small bowel resection (Hill et al, 1974) but there is excessive loss of fat as well (Neal et al, 1984). Further studies revealed that ileostomy output was not only a function of the available small bowel but was also related to body composition (Hill et al, 1979). Hence, ileostomy output correlated with bodyweight (Figure 8.24), height, free fat mass and total body nitrogen.

Studies on body composition in ileostomy patients have revealed low values for total body nitrogen and potassium, even in patients who have had less than 10 cm of ileum resected. Surprisingly, total body water was normal compared with predicted values (Cooper et al, 1986a). By contrast, after resection (50–120 cm) of the terminal ileum, bodyweight, total

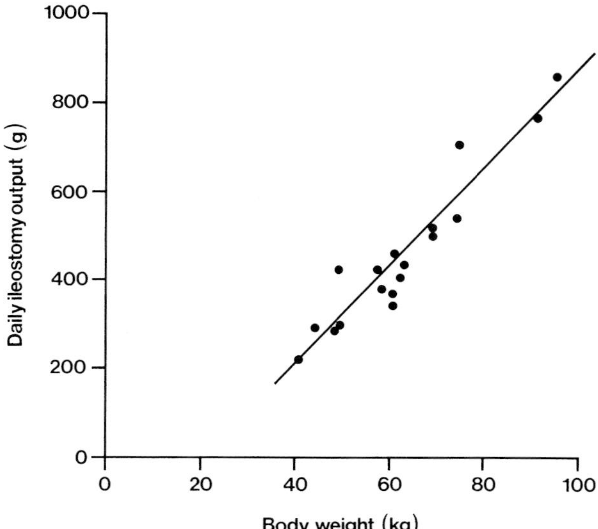

Figure 8.24 Correlation between daily ileostomy output and bodyweight.

body fat, total body nitrogen and total body potassium were depleted but total body water remained normal. These data cast some doubt on the concept that ileostomy patients are in a state of chronic dehydration. There seems to be little doubt that patients with an ileostomy are also nutritionally depleted (Zeiderman et al, 1985) and that fat malabsorption occurs even after minimal small bowel resection (Jeffries et al, 1969; Cooper et al, 1982), presumably due to impaired bile salt absorption and a reduction in the bile salt pool (Heuman et al, 1982). Depletion of total body sodium and total body potassium is no greater after moderate small bowel resection than in those patients whose terminal ileum has been preserved. Moreover, patients having massive small bowel resection compensate by consuming more calories. Codeine, Lomotil and electrolyte supplements minimize the fluid and electrolyte losses in ileostomy patients. Isogel has the opposite effect (Newton, 1978). Steroids also reduce the volume and electrolyte content of ileostomy effluent (Goligher and Lintott, 1975; Feretis et al, 1984).

Table 8.12 Ileostomy chemistry according to extent of small bowel resection.

	Less than 9 cm resected (*n* = 6)	*30–120 cm ileal resected* (*n* = 6)
Ileostomy volume (mL/24 hours)	401 ± 92	1202 ± 284
Sodium loss (mmol/day)	43 ± 12	143 ± 53
Potassium loss (mmol/day)	4.0 ± 0.9	12.7 ± 9.0
Percentage water content (%)	89.0 ± 2.5	93.0 ± 1.8
Sodium:potassium	10.8 ± 2.4	15.6 ± 7.7

From Hill et al (1975b).

Ileostomy patients with the short gut syndrome

There are some patients who lose such enormous quantities of fluid and electrolyte from the ileostomy that they can remain in health only by repeated intravenous infusion of fluid and electrolytes. These patients have either had an extensive small bowel resection, pancreatic insufficiency, chronic obstruction, sepsis or recurrent Crohn's disease (Hill, 1976). In some patients the problem is exacerbated by increased small bowel transit (Fallingborg et al, 1990). It has been proposed that the use of oral glucose–electrolyte solutions might avoid the need for intermittent saline transfusions (Griffen et al, 1980, 1982; Ward et al, 1981; Gore et al, 1992; Nightingale et al, 1992). Studies in seven such patients revealed that four could exist without parenteral support with a regimen containing 60 mmol/L of NaCl, 30 mmol/L of $NaHCO_3$ and 110 mmol/L of glucose (Newton et al, 1985). Potassium was not added to the regimen because losses were small and potassium made the solutions unpalatable (Newton et al, 1985). Losses were reduced by substituting maltose for glucose (72.5 mmol/L NaCl, 52.5 mmol/L $NaHCO_3$, 55 mmol/L maltose). Patients needing parenteral support were easily identified by an oral glucose–electrolyte challenge when over 50% of the volume was passed from the stoma within 3 hours of administration. Some patients, particularly those with Crohn's disease, may become calcium or magnesium deficient owing to excessive losses and poor absorption. Similarly there may be trace element deficiencies such as zinc and others (Allan, 1997).

The administration of a somatostatin analogue may be the only effective therapy in some ileostomy patients with the short gut syndrome. This has a prolonged half-life, 10–12 times greater than its parent compound (Williams et al, 1984). Somatostatin promotes salt and water reabsorption in the small bowel by reducing motility and transit time (Efendic and Mattsson, 1978; Johansson et al, 1978; Dharmasthaphorn et al, 1980; Ruskone et al, 1982). It also inhibits the release of several gut hormones which may cause diarrhoea (Bloom, 1978; Gerich and Patton, 1978; Wood et al, 1983; Kraenzlin et al, 1984; Maton et al, 1985). Somatostatin inhibits exocrine pancreatic secretion, impairs gallbladder emptying and reduces acid secretion (Kayasseh et al, 1978; Meyers et al, 1979). As a result there is impaired fat absorption, which may be further compromised by bacterial overgrowth in the small bowel as a consequence of delayed transit (Gray and Shiner, 1967; Draser et al, 1969; Vantrappen et al, 1977; Spiller et al, 1984). Cooper et al (1986b) undertook a crossover study of somatostatin infusion compared with placebo in five patients. The volume of ileostomy output, water excretion and sodium loss from the ileostomy were significantly reduced (Table 8.13). Fat excretion was increased and transit times prolonged. Unfortunately, when somatostatin was retested under more physiological conditions over 3 days, many of these differences failed to achieve statistical significance. Furthermore, only two of five patients achieved control of their ileostomy diarrhoea in the long term. Hence, somatostatin may be therapeutically effective in some patients with profuse ileostomy diarrhoea but it is expensive and long-term control may not be achieved.

Table 8.13 Absolute values (medians) of ileostomy loss in a crossover study of somatostatin in profuse ileostomy diarrhoea.

	Somatostatin analogue	*Placebo*
Ileostomy output (g)	505	948
Water excretion (mL)	490	885
Potassium loss (mmol)	10	11
Sodium loss (mmol)	74	108
Fat excretion (g)	25	13
Transit time (min)	266	157

From Cooper et al (1986b).

Urolithiasis

There is a reported increased incidence of urinary stones in ileostomy patients but this is extremely variable, ranging from 0.7% to 12.0% (Table 8.14) (Daren et al, 1962; Maratka and Nedbal, 1964; Bennett and Jepson, 1966; Gelzayd et al, 1968; Alexander, 1970; Ritchie, 1971; Bennett and Hughes, 1972; Goligher, 1984). These data are compared with the prevalence figure of 3.8% for urinary stones in subjects living in the UK (Scott et al, 1977). Earlier studies in Birmingham suggested a very low incidence of urolithiasis (Alexander, 1970), but a more recent evaluation (Dew et al, 1979) disclosed a 2.7% incidence. An initial review from Leeds suggested a low incidence of 1.3% (Goligher, 1984), whereas Bambach et al (1981) later reported an 8.9% incidence of stones. Hence, duration of follow-up is an important variable. The incidence of stones in the study by Bambach and co-workers was only 6.7%, if there had been no loss of small bowel, compared with 14.8% where 20–300 cm of terminal ileum had been resected. Serum calcium, vitamin D (Kennedy

Table 8.14 Incidence of urolithiasis in patients with an ileostomy.

Author	*Country*	*Number*	*Disease*	*Incidence (%)*
Daren et al (1962)	USA	163	Both	7.4
Maratka and Nedbal (1964)	Czechoslovakia	74	UC	12.0
Gelzayd et al (1968)	USA	79	Both	18.0
Bennett and Hughes (1972)	Australia	333	UC	8.4
Bennett and Jepson (1966)	Australia	72	UC	8.3
Alexander (1970)	UK	300	UC	0.7
Goligher (1984)	UK	150	UC	1.3
Ritchie (1971)	UK	311	Both	4.3
Kennedy et al (1982a)	UK	39	UC	10.3
Bambach et al (1981)	UK	305	Both	8.9

UC, ulcerative colitis.

et al, 1982a) and urinary calcium levels are usually normal in ileostomy patients with stones. However, high uric acid levels have been reported (Daren et al, 1962; Clarke and McKenzie, 1969) and this presumably is the cause for the high incidence of uric acid stones in these patients (Bennett and Jepson, 1966; Bennett and Hughes, 1972; Kennedy et al, 1982c). All patients with an ileostomy should probably have their uric acid levels monitored and, if raised, a prophylactic course of allopurinol therapy might be justified.

Although radiolucent stones may be more common, a high proportion of renal stones in ileostomy patients contain calcium and are radio-opaque (Grossman and Nugent, 1967; Ritchie, 1971). It has been suggested that hyperuricaemia results in calcium-containing stones (Gutman and Yu, 1968; Smith et al, 1969). Uric acid crystals may act as a nucleus for the precipitation of calcium salts; alternatively, hyperuricaemia may lower the saturation index to initiate calcium oxalate crystal formation (Coe, 1978; Prien and Prien, 1968). The mechanism of stone formation in ileostomates is protean. One important factor is the lower urinary output of these patients, particularly in tropical climates, and it is necessary to stress to these patients the importance of a high fluid intake. A persistently acid urine favours the precipitation of uric acid (Gelzayd et al, 1968). Certain solutes, such as sodium, potassium, magnesium and urea, also help to maintain calcium and urate in solution. The mean 24-hour urinary sodium and magnesium levels are low in ileostomates, so another mechanism may operate to increase the risk of urolithiasis (Modlin, 1967).

In Crohn's disease, proctocolectomy may protect patients from stone formation. After small bowel resection, oxalate is poorly absorbed and there is a high oxalate load in the colon. In the colon, malabsorbed fatty acids combine with calcium oxalate, leaving free oxalate available for absorption (Hoffman et al, 1970; Dowling et al, 1971; Chadwick et al, 1973). Resection of the colon overcomes this mechanism and hyperoxaluria is prevented in patients with an ileostomy. In Crohn's disease other factors exist which may favour stone formation, such as low urine output, low urinary pH and low levels of sodium and magnesium in the urine (Kennedy et al, 1982c).

Gallstones

Controversy persists as to whether there is an increased incidence of gallstones in patients with ulcerative colitis who have an ileostomy when less than 10 cm of small bowel has been resected. Hill et al (1975c) compared the incidence of gallstones in ileostomy patients with data from an autopsy survey. Only in patients with an ileal resection of more than 10 cm was there an increased incidence of gallstones (Table 8.15). This observation is as expected, since ileal resection results in loss of bile salts and a reduction in the size of the bile acid pool, which adversely affects cholesterol solubility (Heaton and Read, 1969; Cohen et al, 1971; Dowling et al, 1972). As expected, ileostomy patients with Crohn's disease have a 5–7 fold increased incidence of gallstones, the risk being related to the extent of small bowel resection and the extent of ileal disease. It is known that patients with Crohn's disease have an increased saturation index for cholesterol owing to the decreased molar percentage of bile acids in bile. This bile acid deficiency is secondary to ileal malabsorption of bile acids and a reduction in the bile acid pool (Hill et al, 1975c). Ursodeoxycholic acid is potentially useful in these patients since it desaturates cholesterol in bile without provoking diarrhoea (Chadwick and Camilleri, 1983).

Table 8.15 Incidence of gallstones in patients with an ileostomy.

Amount of ileum resection	*Number*	*Incidence* Observed (%)	Expected (%)	*Observed:Expected*
More than 10 cm				
Ulcerative colitis	18	33	10	3.2:1
Crohns disease	22	32	5	6.8:1
Less than 10 cm				
Ulcerative colitis	54	15	9	1.6:1
Crohn's disease	11	45	9	4.9:1

From Hill et al (1975c).

Thus many patients with an ileostomy have an increased incidence of gallstones (Jones et al, 1976), particularly those with Crohn's disease (Baker et al, 1974). Kurchin et al (1984) reported a 23% incidence identified from ultrasound examination of the gallbladder. They even suggested that there might be a place for prophylactic cholecystectomy, but that is not a view that many would wish to endorse; not only would morbidity increase but cholecystectomy alone can precipitate metabolic problems of its own.

COMPLICATIONS OF ILEOSTOMY

Overall incidence

There are remarkably few data on the overall incidence of complications after ileostomy. Pearl et al (1985) reported that ileostomy was attended by a much higher morbidity than colostomy, with a complication rate exceeding 40%. The highest morbidity was in patients requiring emergency operation where the stoma was unplanned. In these emergency situations the stoma was often badly sited and the operations were performed by relatively inexperienced surgeons. An even higher morbidity (70%) may occur in patients requiring emergency ileostomy. In some of these patients the bowel was obstructed and the blood supply consequently compromised. In others there was longstanding malnutrition or established sepsis.

Data from Birmingham (Phillips et al, 1985) indicate an overall complication rate of 57% following ileostomy in 1975 patients reviewed prospectively over 3 years (Table 8.16). However, only 18% of these patients required ileostomy revision. To some extent this is a reflection of the stoma management service, since many of the ileostomy problems could be resolved by conservative means. The most common problems were excoriation, leakage around the stoma, ileostomy flux, retraction and parastomal hernia (Table 8.17).

Generally complications are more common in patients with Crohn's disease compared with those with ulcerative colitis (75% and 44% respectively) (Watts et al, 1966; Carlstedt et al, 1987). This is principally due to recurrent disease causing stenosis (31% versus 4%: Carlsen and Bergan, 1995) and fistula. Despite this the St Mark's data report a 20-year complication rate of 76% in ulcerative colitis (Table 8.18) compared with 59% for Crohn's disease (Leong et al, 1994). Other complications such as prolapse and recession are also more common in Crohn's disease. Complications are unrelated to the method of construction, extent of ileal resection, weight gain or previous ileitis. An actuarial analysis of the long-term complication rates is provided in Table 8.19.

In ulcerative colitis, ileostomy complications are more common after restorative proctocolectomy than proctocolectomy. This is largely due to the use of a loop ileostomy and complications of closure; nevertheless, dehydration, retraction, obstruction and skin sepsis are also common in these patients (Feinberg et al, 1987; Winslet et al, 1991a).

Lubbers and Devlin (1984) reported that 33 of 102 patients who developed complications required some form of surgical correction. Carlsen and Bergan (1995) reported a 12% re-operation rate for primary ileostomy construction and a further 7% for reconstruction with a laparotomy compared with 8% for a local revision. Re-operations were needed more frequently after emergency rather than elective operation (13% versus 9%). Closing the lateral gutter or fixation of the ileum to the rectus fascia had no influence on re-operation rates. The incidence of complications are listed in Table 8.20.

Table 8.16 Ileostomy complications (Birmingham).

	Number
Surviving patients	175
Total number with complications	99 (57)
Total number requiring reoperation	32 (18)
Skin excoriation	49 (28)
Ileostomy flux	31 (18)
Sepsis around stoma	18 (10)
Leakage	17 (10)
Retraction	16 (9)
Hernia	8 (5)
Bleeding	7 (4)
Prolapse	6 (3)
Stenosis	3 (2)

Values in parentheses are percentages.
From Phillips et al (1985).

Table 8.17 Incidence of ileostomy complications in 115 patients.

Complication	*Number*
Skin irritation	30 (26)
Retraction	22 (19)
Sliding	13
Fixed	9
Flux	4
Hernia	3
Abscess	2
Stitch sinus	2
Prolapse	3

Values in parentheses are percentages.
From Watts et al (1966).

Table 8.18 Complications of ileostomy and revisional surgery in ulcerative colitis and Crohn's disease (cumulative probabilities).

	Number	*Ulcerative colitis (%)*	*Number*	*Crohn's disease (%)*
Overall complications	27	76	27	59
Revisional surgery	15	28	9	16
Multiple revisions	6	8	5	9

Leong et al, 1994.

Table 8.19 Life-table analysis of stoma complications.

Complications	*Number*	*Crude (%)*	*Cumulative probability (%)*
Necrosis	1	1	1
Stenosis	6	4	5
Prolapse	12	8	11
Retraction	19	13	17
Obstruction	27	18	23
Fistula or Suppuration	11	7	12
Hernia	16	11	16
Skin problem	44	29	34
Any one complication	85	57	68

Leong et al, 1994.

Table 8.20 Complications after end ileostomy (n = 358).

Stenosis	10.3%
Peristomal fistulas	9.4%
Dermatitis	8.0%
Retraction	2.7%
Prolapse	1.8%
Parastomal hernia	1.8%

Carlsen & Bergan (1995).

Revisional operation rates in the St Mark's series were surprisingly higher in ulcerative colitis than in Crohn's disease: 28% versus 16% (Leong et al, 1994). Complications may occur any time after ileostomy construction and follow-up of these patients is therefore advised (Devlin 1986). The need for follow-up is recognized in Crohn's disease, but some clinicians believe that after proctocolectomy for ulcerative colitis follow-up is unnecessary. Not only may these patients develop stomal complications or metabolic sequelae, but some will eventually prove to have Crohn's disease. Many problems such as stenosis, bleeding, fistula and leakage in patients with Crohn's disease are due to recurrence, hence over half of all stomal revisions in Crohn's disease require resection (Roy et al, 1970). In ulcerative colitis, the majority of stoma revisions are necessary because the ileostomy has been badly sited (Taylor et al, 1978).

Revision rates range from 4% to 43% (Warren and McKittrick, 1951; Bargen, 1956; Brooke, 1956; Ritchie, 1971; Steinberg et al, 1975). Ritchie (1971) found that revision rates were lower among more experienced surgical units. Data from institutions having extensive surgical experience in inflammatory bowel disease report reoperation rates which are usually less than 15% (Gruner et al, 1976; Corman et al, 1976; Lee and Truelove, 1980).

Management of ileostomy complications

Options

Although a well-trained stomatherapist can resolve many stoma complications, approximately one-third will require surgical reconstruction (Corman et al, 1976; Goldblatt et al, 1977) (Table 8.21).

Ileostomy reconstruction may be difficult and experience is needed in deciding which approach is most appropriate. The stoma may occasionally be refashioned locally, with or without its mobilization from the abdominal wall, with sutures or staples. The ileostomy, however, usually requires some form of reconstruction of the abdominal wall and fixation of the ileum to it. For technical reasons it is sometimes advisable to perform a laparotomy to facilitate safe stomal mobilization and a more thorough fixation procedure; alternatively, a laparotomy may be needed to achieve reconstruction of the abdominal wall if it is deficient. The ileostomy may need to be resited if it is in a bad position or if there is a parastomal hernia, or an unstable stoma. A resiting procedure usually requires a laparotomy but some describe transperitoneal resiting without laparotomy (Taylor et al, 1978). In a number of patients, stomal complications will be due to recurrent Crohn's disease, where the disease will have to be resected. The new stoma can be brought through either the old site or a new trephine in the abdominal wall. If there is a deficiency in the abdominal wall adjacent to the stoma resulting in prolapse, retraction or hernia, this may be managed locally by reinforcing the abdominal wall, by suture or a mesh implant, or the stoma may be resited and the defect closed.

Weaver et al (1988) reviewed ileostomy revisions in 48 patients (Table 8.22). The principal indications were obstruction (15), retraction (10), hernia (8), prolapse (8) and fistula (4). Obstruction, retraction and fistula were common in Crohn's disease; local revision without laparotomy was used frequently and was even feasible for a parastomal hernia. A laparotomy was usually necessary for obstruction and parastomal fistula and was required in most patients with Crohn's disease (Table 8.23). It was found that the same site could usually be used again unless the stoma was badly sited outside the rectus.

Carlstedt et al (1987) found that 81% of ileostomy revisions could be performed as a local procedure, the exceptions were, almost exclusively, among patients with Crohn's disease. Goldblatt et al (1977) reported that resiting procedures were used in only 13 of 85 revisions (15%) but some form of resection proved necessary in 36% (see Table 8.21).

Assessment of stoma complications

Evaluation of the most appropriate refashioning procedure involves careful assessment with the

Table 8.21 Procedures needed for ileostomy complications.

Complication (n)	*Local refashioning*	*Local refashioning + laparotomy*	*Resiting + laparotomy*	*Part of abdominal operation*
Stenosis (20)	11	4	1	4
Fistula (12)	3	4	3	2
Prolapse (10)	2	1	3	4
Retraction (10)	5	3	0	2
Recurrent disease (8)	0	2	1	5
Small bowel obstruction (8)	0	0	0	8
Poor siting (6)	4	0	2	0
Stomal bleeding (3)	1	0	0	2
Dermatitis (2)	0	0	1	1
Necrosis (2)	0	0	0	2
Stomal pain (2)	1	0	0	1
Hernia (1)	0	0	1	0
Abscess (1)	0	0	1	0

From Goldblatt et al (1977).

Table 8.22 Ileostomy revision: Birmingham.

Complication (n)	*Local refashioning*	*Local refashioning and laparotomy*	*Resiting and laparotomy*
Obstruction (15)	5	6	4
Retraction (10)	8	2	0
Prolapse (8)	8	0	0
Hernia (8)	6	1	1
Fistula (4)	0	3	1
Abscess (1)	0	1	0
Ulceration (1)	1	0	0
Bad siting (1)	0	0	1

From Weaver et al (1988).

Table 8.23 Ileostomy revision: Birmingham. Late complications requiring further revision.

	Ulcerative colitis			*Crohn's disease*		
	No.	*Subsequent revision*	*%*	*No.*	*Subsequent revision*	*%*
Local revision	17	2	12	11	5	45
Laparotomy, same stoma site	7	3 }	30	7	1 }	9
Laparotomy, relocation of stoma	3	0 }		4	0 }	
Total	27	5	19	22	6	27

From Weaver et al (1988).

stoma care nurse. Factors which will have to be considered include the siting of the stoma, evidence of recurrent disease, the potential dangers of another laparotomy and the presence of any abdominal wall deficiency. The proposed new site should be well away from the groin, scars, the umbilicus, the anterior superior iliac spine, and skin creases.

If the ileostomy is deformed from stenosis, ulceration or polyps, the possibility of Crohn's disease must be considered. In these circumstances it may be prudent to arrange radiology of the small bowel. Often the diagnosis of Crohn's disease can best be made by a retrograde ileogram or even endoscopy through the stoma, but this may be impossible if there are strictures or deformity. If there is a fistula or chronic abscess adjacent to the stoma, CT or fistulography may provide useful information.

Principles of refashioning

Antibiotic cover should be used because of the risk of contamination, the abdomen may need to be opened, and a resection might be necessary

The abdomen should be prepared and draped so that a laparotomy may be performed or access to the opposite side of the abdomen is available if necessary. The best possible alternative site should have been selected and marked preoperatively. In view of the importance of preserving access to the opposite side of the abdomen, midline incisions should always be used. If the patient already has a paramedian or muscle cutting incision, the surgeon should probably explore the abdomen through the previous scar.

Whenever a stoma site is closed, non-absorbable sutures are used to coapt the defect in the rectus sheath and muscle. Occasionally the skin can be kept open to minimize sepsis if there is gross contamination, but normally the skin is closed by excising the lateral edges of the skin defect to produce a transverse scar. Although implantation of mesh has been used successfully to repair a parastomal defect (Leslie, 1984), foreign materials around a stoma should be avoided whenever possible because of the fear of chronic sepsis.

Surgical procedures for ileostomy refashioning

Local refashioning procedures

Without stoma mobilization

If an ileostomy has retracted in the early postoperative period, it may be possible to re-evert the spout and suture the stoma in the everted position by passing a row of sutures through the inner and outer components of the ileostomy (see Figure 8.21a–d). However, this technique is rarely successful in the long term. An alternative, to stabilize a retracted end or loop ileostomy, is to apply three rows of staples to the everted stoma bud (Winslet et al, 1990) (see Figure 8.21e,f). The end result is not particularly aesthetically pleasing, but the staples become less obvious with time and cause little concern to the patient. The procedure can be performed using intravenous midazolam or diazepam, though many patients prefer a light general anaesthetic.

The ileostomy is gently everted by traction on three pairs of Allis forceps placed around the circumference of the bowel wall. Three rows of staples are then placed longitudinally across both mucosal surfaces, using the linear stapler without a cutter (see Figure 8.21e,f) (be sure that the cartridge does not include a blade). Care must be taken during this procedure to avoid stapling the mesentery. This technique has been used quite extensively in Birmingham. It is not always successful but is worth considering where retraction occurs, often early after stoma construction, and where laparotomy or ileal stoma mobilization is contraindicated. The great advantage of this operation is that it can be performed under a local anaesthetic as day case surgery. Some units have not been impressed with the outcome of this procedure (Speakman et al, 1991). However, satisfactory defunction of the distal bowel has been demonstrated using this technique (Winslet et al, 1991b). Early results implied that the technique was successful in 25 of 38 patients; however, the overall impression of the long-term results is that only about a third of patients require no further procedure.

Complete stoma mobilization

This technique is most appropriate for the retracted stoma which cannot be everted. The approach is not usually recommend for repair of a parastomal hernia if there is a suitable alternative stoma site or if the stoma is not through the rectus muscle. If no other site is available, local repair and refashioning can be attempted. Local refashioning may be used for ileostomy prolapse. In certain circumstances resection may be feasible through the ileostomy trephine, but it is surely much easier and safer to do this via a laparotomy.

A general anaesthetic with full muscle relaxation is required. Using a small blade the mucocutaneous junction is opened and the stoma mobilized at skin level throughout its circumference (Figure 8.25a). A pair of Allis forceps or stay sutures are placed on the bowel. Keeping close to the ileum and using a fine pair of McIndoes scissors or a small scalpel blade, the serosa of the ileum is gently dissected away from the subcutaneous fat to the anterior rectus sheath. The rectus sheath adjacent to the ileum is freed around the bowel, taking care not to damage the mesentery (Figure 8.25b). Often the ileum is found to be concertinaed between layers of the abdominal wall and will need to be straightened to avoid damage during the operation. By retraction inside the rectus muscle it is possible to open the peritoneal cavity around the entire circumference of the stoma until it is completely free. The skin and subcutaneous fat which are adherent to the free edge of the ileum are then excised (Figure 8.25b). The unstable stoma must now be fixed to the rectus sheath by placing a series of interrupted absorbable sutures from the rectus sheath to the serosa of the ileum. These sutures should not be tied until they have all been placed around the circumference of the defect. Once tied, the stoma is everted in the usual way (Figure 8.25c). If the spout is too long the end of the ileum is resected and the mucocutaneous junction is sutured either with non-absorbable sutures to include the serosa of the emerging bowel (Figure 8.25d) and tied away from the bowel, or with absorbable sutures from the serosa of the bowel to the subcuticular skin edge.

Ileal mobilization may be difficult if there has been previous peristomal sepsis or if the lateral space has been closed with non-absorbable sutures. It is unwise to attempt mobilization of an ileostomy stoma within 6–8 weeks of the original operation unless there are overriding clinical considerations, since the risk of damage to the bowel is considerable.

If there is a prolapse, the redundant bowel will need to be excised, usually using diathermy. It is possible to free quite long segments of ileum in this way (Figure 8.26). The bowel is then fixed and everted as described. The optimum length of ileostomy spout is 2–3 cm, so it is acceptable to leave no more than 6 cm of ileum protruding above the skin level prior to eversion. During local resection of redundant terminal ileum it is important to dissect out the mesentery carefully and divide the mesenteric arcade at the site of bowel transection.

If there is a parastomal defect causing an unstable stoma or a hernia, care must be exercised in mobilizing the ileostomy from loops of bowel adherent to it and to the abdominal wall (Figure 8.27a). The loops of bowel should be gently dissected free from the stoma and the abdominal wall, after which they can be replaced into the peritoneal cavity. It is normally advisable to resite the stoma, but if there is no suitable alternative site the defect can be closed with a series of interrupted Prolene sutures (Figure 8.27b). Care must be taken not to damage the

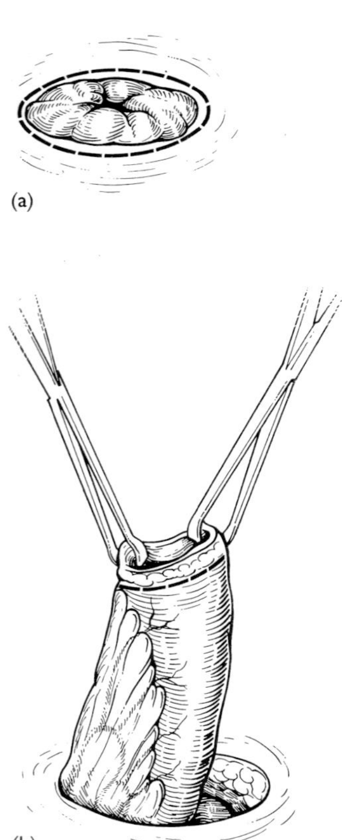

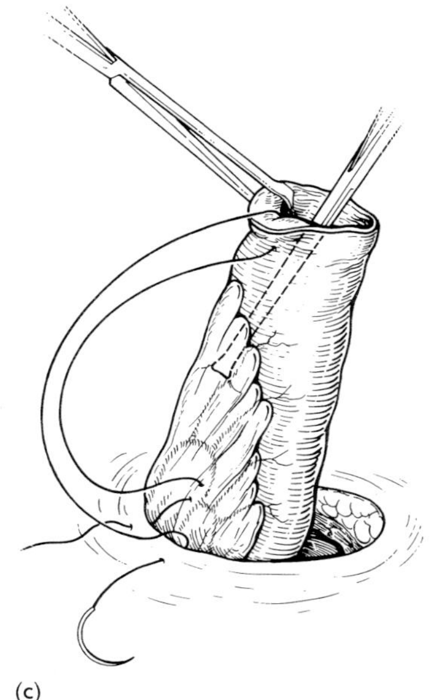

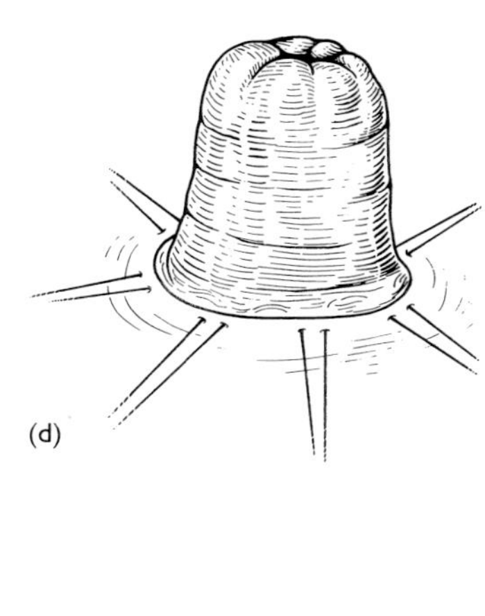

Figure 8.25a–d Surgical correction of retracted ileostomy. (a) A circumstomal incision is made. (b) The stoma is completely mobilized. (c) The ileostomy bud is re-everted and (d) sutured to the skin. In some patients it may not be feasible to evert the stoma and stabilize it as described in Figure 8.21a–f. Under these circumstances the ileostomy must be extensively mobilized from the abdominal wall and within the peritoneal cavity so that 8 cm of ileum can be delivered beyond the skin of the abdominal wall (see Figure 8.26). If there is excess length of ileum after mobilization the end of the ileum is then excised, the ileum is re-everted and sutured to the skin in the usual way.

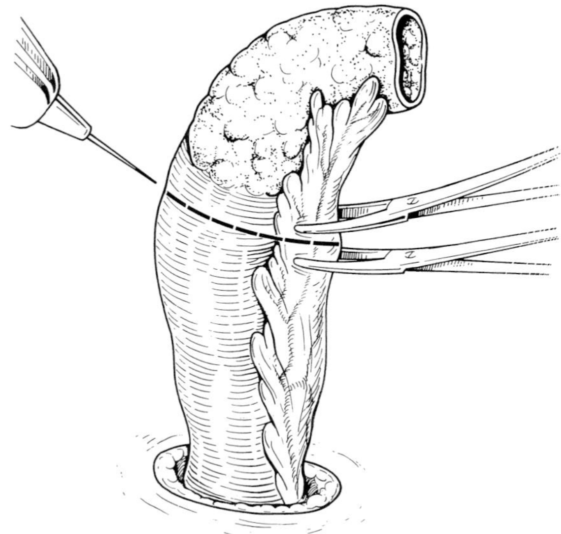

Figure 8.26 Local excision of stoma for prolapse, stenosis or recurrent disease. The ileostomy is taken down and thoroughly mobilized from the abdominal wall so that 10–12 cm of ileum can be delivered through the abdominal wall trephine. The mesentery of the terminal ileum is divided at a point opposite the proposed transection of the ileum, the diseased terminal ileum is excised and the ileostomy is refashioned in the usual way.

mesentery or create an obstruction at the level of the abdominal wall by making the closure too tight. The repair usually results in some discrepancy in size between the edge of the ileum and the skin margin (Figure 8.27c), but the stoma generally often sits in a favourable position and the open peristomal margins rapidly granulate under the protection of a Stomahesive wafer.

Sometimes it is necessary to enlarge the incision to afford better exposure if a local refashioning procedure is preferred. A small longitudinal incision is made above or below the stoma (Figure 8.28a,b). The ileostomy is mobilized and if a parastomal hernia is present this is repaired by suture (Figure 8.28c) or by mesh (Figure 8.28d). Sometimes it is possible to perform a local repair without using an extending incision beside the trephine. A scar adjacent to the stoma may make stoma management difficult, so if the skin disc around the stoma provides inadequate exposure, it is preferable to undertake a laparotomy in order to achieve better access rather than distort a satisfactory stoma site by a peristomal incision (Fig 8.28e). Repair of the abdominal wall defect can then be performed either externally or through the laparotomy. Mesh should be

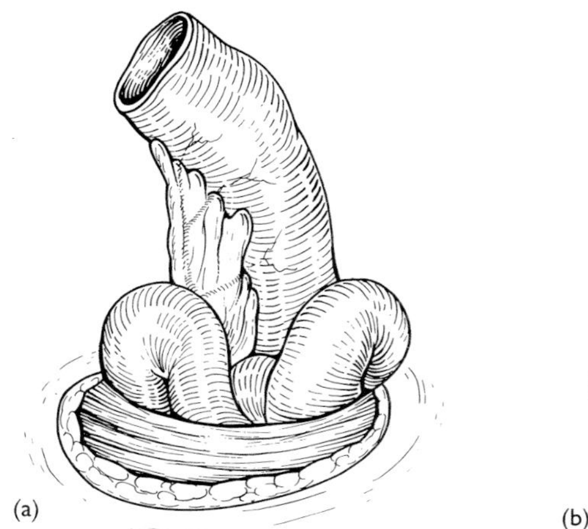

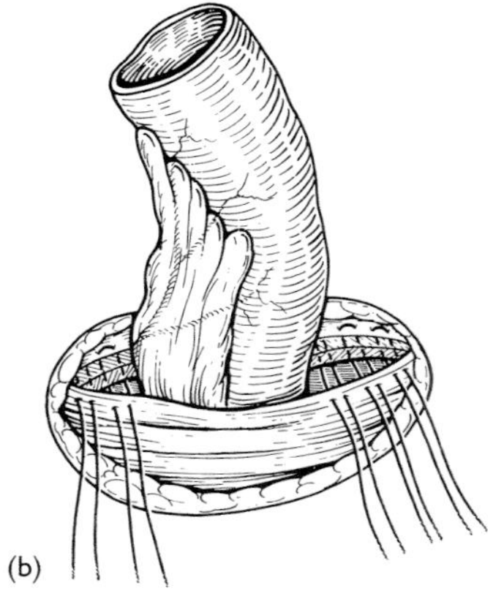

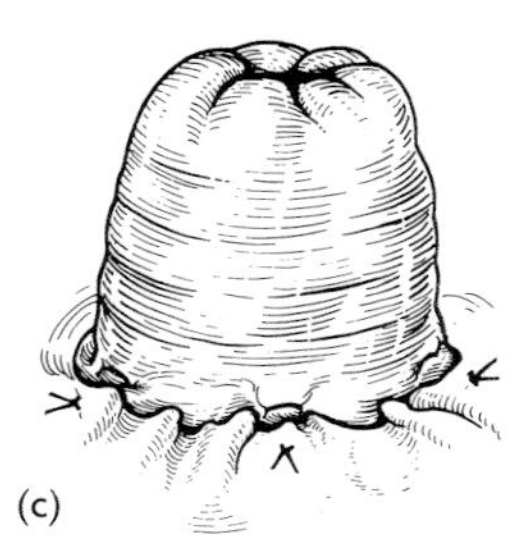

Figure 8.27a–c Local repair of a paraileostomy hernia. (a) The ileostomy is mobilized from the abdominal wall in the usual way. The peritoneal pouch of the parastomal hernia is identified and opened, and the contents of the peritoneal sac are returned to the general peritoneal cavity. (b) The defect in the abdominal wall is identified and repaired using interrupted Prolene sutures on either side of the ileostomy to reconstruct the abdominal wall. (c) The ileostomy is everted and sutured to skin in the usual way.

avoided whenever possible because of the risk of sepsis.

Local stoma refashioning and laparotomy

Laparotomy often facilitates more complete fixation of the ileum to the abdominal wall (Figure 8.29a) if the stoma is unstable (Figure 8.29b), since sutures may be placed from within and without to anchor the ileum to the abdominal wall (Figure 8.29c,d). Laparotomy also allows a more satisfactory closure of the abdominal wall defect around a stoma and the stoma may also be resited if necessary (Figure 8.30a,b). Laparotomy also makes resection much safer and allows full inspection of the blood supply of the ileum (Figure 8.31). Resection may be necessary to remove a segment of recurrent Crohn's disease, excise a fistula, remove damaged small bowel or resect a stricture.

Laparotomy is performed in the usual manner and the contents of the peritoneal cavity are thoroughly inspected. The mesentery of the terminal ileum is identified and any adhesions divided. Adhesions between the peritoneum and the stoma are divided and a plane gently developed between the ileum and the rectus muscle around the full circumference of the bowel. Provided there is no peristomal sepsis, it is usually quite easy to dissect the subcutaneous fat from around the ileum so that through the circumstomal incision, stabilized by pressure against the index finger of the surgeon's left hand, complete separation of the ileum from the abdominal wall is achieved. A thimble may assist this manoeuvre.

Once a sufficient length of ileum has been freed from the abdominal wall for adequate eversion, the serosa of the ileum is then anchored to the peritoneum and the posterior aspect of the rectus using a series of interrupted absorbable sutures. It is not usually necessary to attempt closure of the lateral space during refashioning procedures: it is left wide open. In this way the risk of internal herniation and small bowel obstruction is minimized. The serosa is then sutured to the anterior rectus sheath, as illustrated in Figure 8.29c, and the everted stoma is sutured in the usual way after closure of the abdomen.

Resiting of the ileostomy

Resiting of the ileostomy is arguably the optimum management for a parastomal hernia, a prolapsed stoma, ileostomy, stenosis or a fistula associated with parastomal sepsis, and whenever the original stoma site is badly located (Figure 8.28f). Ileostomies located outside the rectus sheath are inadequately supported, so there is a high incidence of hernia, prolapse or retraction. In addition, appliances are difficult to manage because they tend to lift off during movement. If a badly sited stoma (Figure 8.32) gives rise to leakage and skin excoriation it should be repositioned through the rectus muscle on the opposite side of the abdomen.

Resiting without laparotomy is not advised if

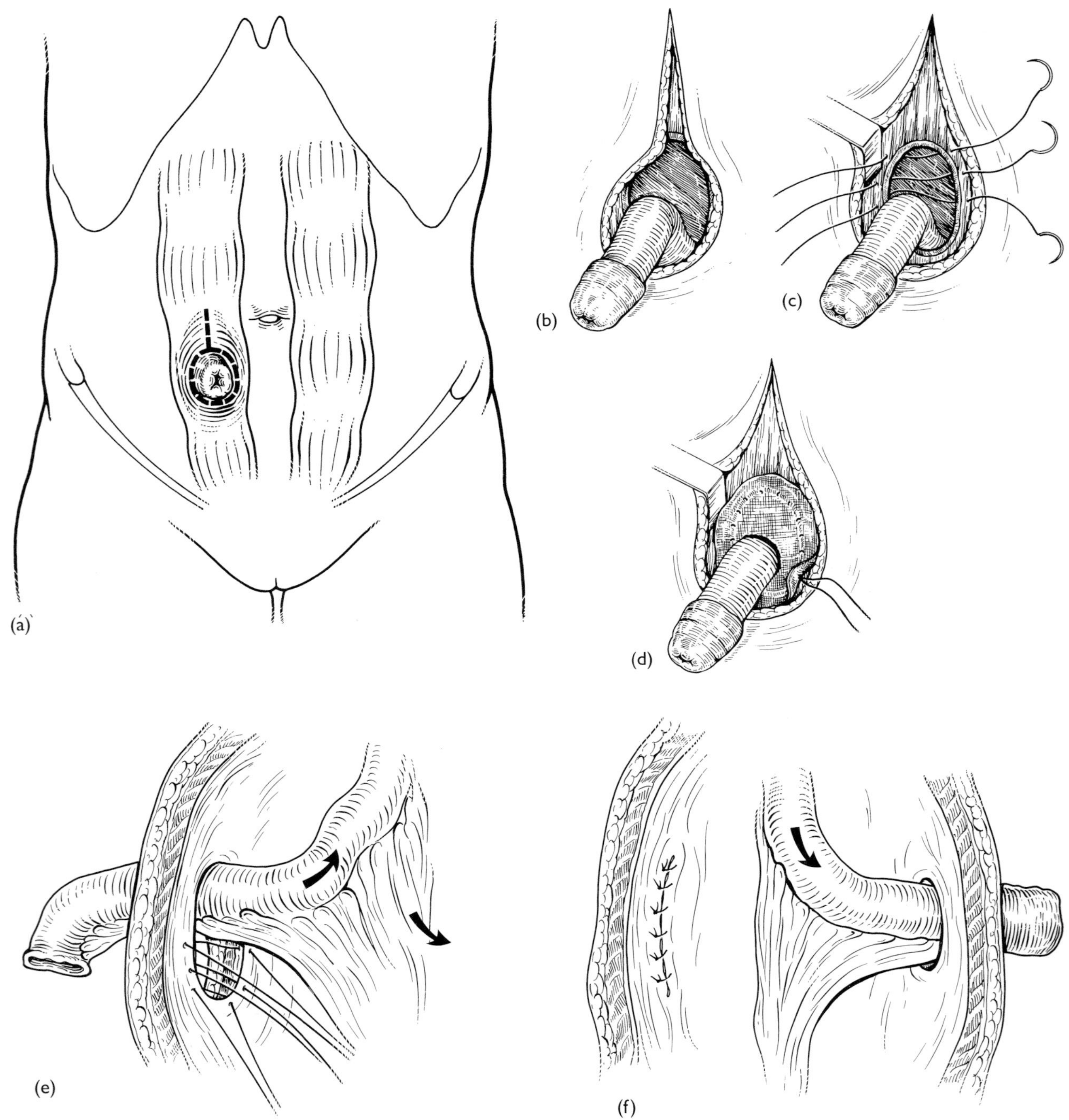

Figure 8.28a–f Enlarging the stoma site to facilitate local repair of a paraileostomy hernia. (a) In some cases access is compromised unless the skin of the abdominal wall is divided beyond the circumstomal incision using a longitudinal extension. (b) The defect in the abdominal wall is defined, and (c) the defect is closed either with a series of interrupted Prolene sutures or (d) by the insertion of a non-absorbable mesh around the defect in the abdominal wall. The skin extension is closed and the ileostomy sutured back to the skin in the usual way. (e) In order to avoid an unsatisfactory local stoma refashioning, the ileostomy has been thoroughly mobilized by a circumstomal incision, and the defect in the rectus muscle is repaired with a series of interrupted Prolene sutures, taking care not to narrow the opening too much, thereby obstructing the bowel or compromising its blood supply. (f) A new trephine is made on the opposite side of the abdomen and the ileostomy is delivered through it.

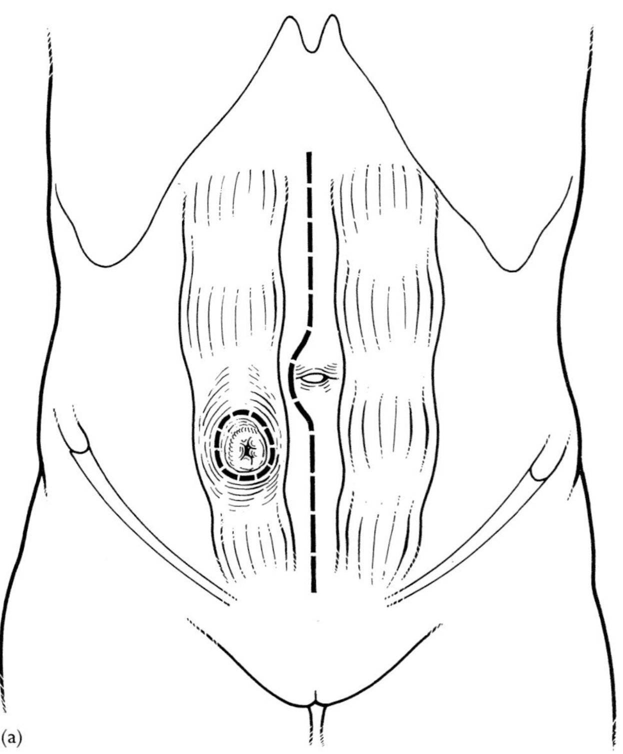

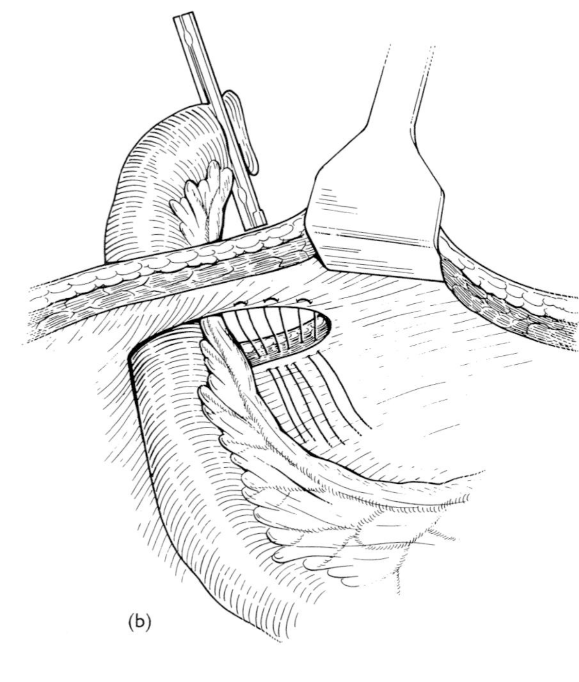

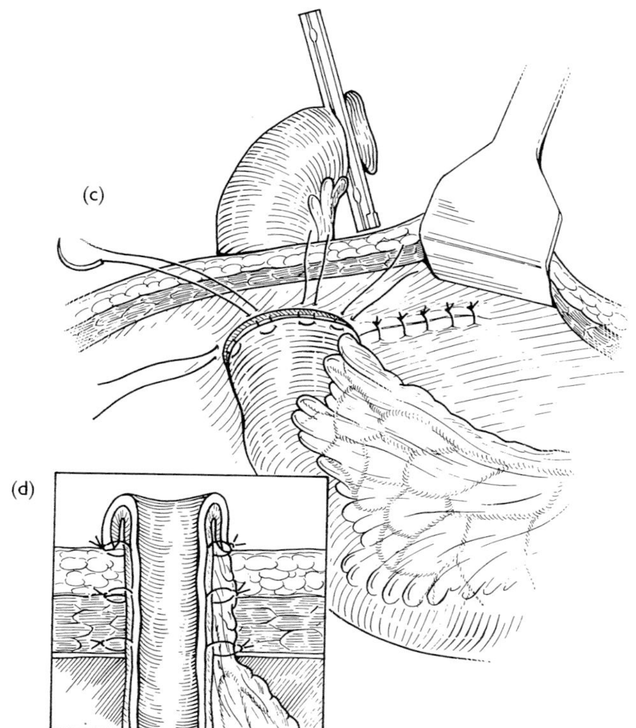

Figure 8.29a–d Laparotomy and repair of parastomal hernia. (a) In some cases a more secure repair may be achieved by a small laparotomy combined with a circumstomal incision and full stomal mobilization. (b) The defect in the abdominal wall is closed both from outside and within the peritoneal cavity. (c) Stabilizing sutures are also placed between the serosa of the ileum and abdominal wall, both at the level of the peritoneum and the rectus sheath, and (d) the ileostomy is completed by mucocutaneous sutures.

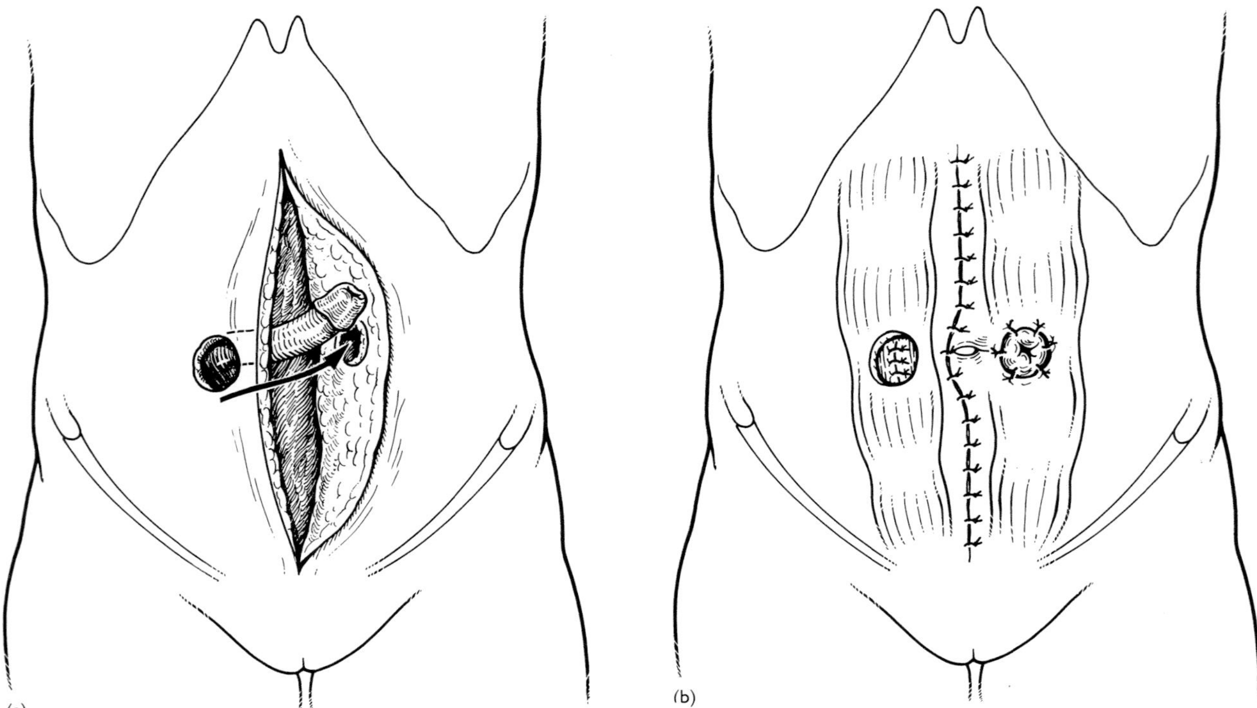

Figure 8.30a–b Relaparotomy and resiting of ileostomy for parastomal hernia. (a) The ileostomy is mobilized through a circumstomal incision and a laparotomy is performed so that the ileum can be delivered through a new trephine on the opposite side of the abdominal wall. (b) The ileostomy is everted and sutured to the skin in the usual way and the laparotomy wound is closed.

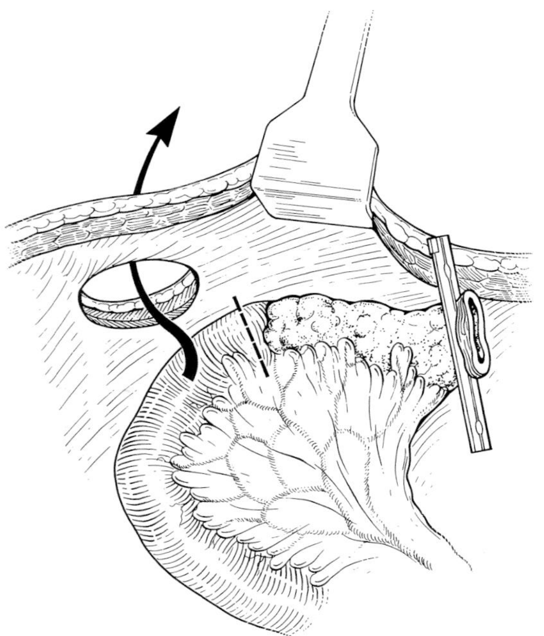

Figure 8.31 Ileal resection for recurrent disease. A laparotomy has been performed, the ileostomy is being mobilized from the abdominal wall, the diseased segment is resected and a new end ileostomy is fashioned through the previous trephine.

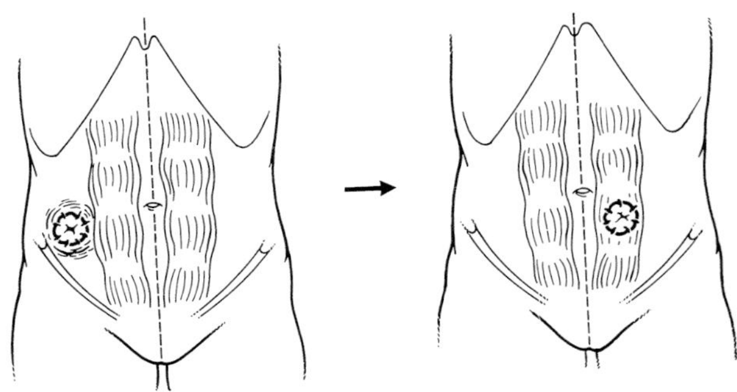

Figure 8.32 Resiting of ileostomy. If an ileostomy is placed outside the rectus muscle and is associated with a prolapse or hernia or causes difficulty with stoma appliances, it should be resited, either with or without a laparotomy, through a trephine on the opposite side of the abdominal wall.

there are dense adhesions, because of the risk of damaging the bowel. In thin subjects with a peritoneal cavity devoid of adhesions the technique may have advantage over using a laparotomy, but under these circumstances laparotomy is usually straightforward and safer anyway.

When a laparotomy is used to resite the stoma, the abdomen is opened through the previous abdominal incision and, after exploration of the peritoneal cavity, the ileostomy site is mobilized from the abdominal wall from within (Figure 8.33a). Since a high proportion of these patients will have a deficiency in the abdominal wall at the stoma site, great care must be exercised to avoid damage to adherent loops of small bowel in a hernia. The ileum is mobilized within the rectus muscle and freed from the peristomal skin, as previously described. A Potts clamp is placed over the end of the ileum to prevent further contamination, or it may be closed with a linear stapler. If the ileum has been damaged or is diseased it should be resected after the ileostomy has been withdrawn from the abdominal wall (Figure 8.33b). A swab soaked in local anaesthetic, placed through the old ileostomy trephine, both protects the wound from contamination and secures some haemostasis by tamponade. If there is a parastomal hernia, the edges of the defect are defined and the defect closed, taking deep bites to include the rectus sheath (Figure 8.28c). If on the other hand there is no defect in the abdominal wall, the stoma site can be closed by placing 3–4 interrupted Prolene or PDS sutures through the rectus sheath and muscle. These sutures are tied only when all have been accurately placed.

A new trephine is then made in the previously selected site, excising a disc of skin and a cylinder of fat; the rectus sheath is opened using a cruciate incision. A segment of rectus muscle is divided or the rectus muscle is split along the line of its fibres. After haemostasis has been secured, the ileum is delivered through the trephine and the abdomen is closed (Figure 8.33c). No attempt is made to close the lateral space. The skin over the previous trephine may be left open and packed with ribbon gauze soaked in proflavine in liquid paraffin if contaminated (Figure 8.33d) or closed by excising the lateral skin edges to provide a cosmetically acceptable transverse scar (Figure 8.33e,f). The ileostomy is tacked to the rectus sheath (if this is felt to be necessary), everted and sutured to the skin as already described. The present author used to leave the skin and subcutaneous tissues of the laparotomy wound open if there had been any contamination during the operation, but with appropriate antibiotic cover and in healthy patients many of these wounds are now closed.

Postoperative management

Patients who have had a local refashioning procedure without laparotomy need only stay in hospital for 48 hours, provided there is no damage to the small bowel. By this stage the ileostomy is usually acting and the patient is able to take a normal diet. Arrangements are then made for the patient to attend the stoma clinic for the removal of the stomal sutures. Many local stoma refashioning procedures are suitable for day case surgery.

Naturally, if there is any concern about viability or trauma to the bowel the patient should be detained in hospital for a longer period of observation. As soon as the stoma has acted and the patient is able to eat and drink there is no need to detain the patient, provided that it is understood that the patient must contact the hospital in the event of a complication.

For patients who have had a laparotomy, hospital stay will depend on clinical progress and their desire to return home. As there is no anastomosis patients can be allowed home as soon as the stoma has acted and they are able to tolerate fluids and a light diet. The wound is managed by the patient, another member of the family or the district nursing service.

Postoperative complications

Apart from ileus and the complications of any abdominal procedure, the most frequent surgical morbidity is sepsis.

Peristomal sepsis is common; drainage can usually be achieved merely by removing a peristomal suture so that pus can discharge into the ileostomy appliance. Occasionally this is inadequate if there is a large cavity, in which case it may be necessary to insert a drain through the peristomal incision. This may be placed either adjacent to the stoma, to allow pus to drain into the appliance, or well beyond the margin of the ileostomy flange (Figure 8.34a,b). If the peristomal sepsis is very severe, drainage may necessitate building a protective barrier of Stomahesive around the ileostomy to separate it from the drainage site. If the stoma is found to be floating free in a collection of pus, as may occasionally happen in fat, elderly, diabetic patients on steroids, it may be necessary to intubate the stoma until healthy granulation tissue has formed around it (Figure 8.34c). Occasionally it may be necessary to divert the faecal stream by raising a proximal loop jejunostomy or by bringing the stoma out through a separate site.

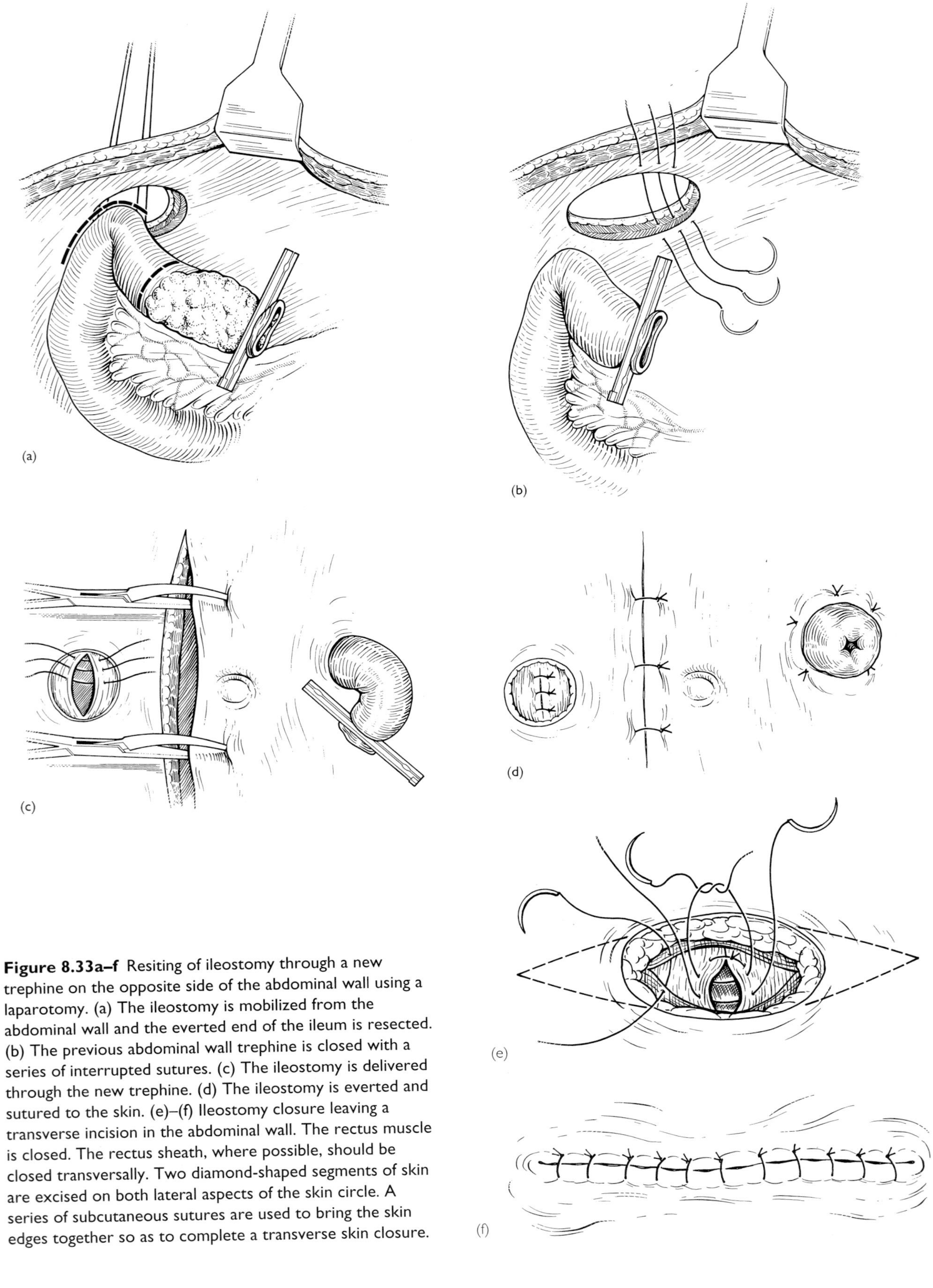

(a)

(b)

(c)

(d)

(e)

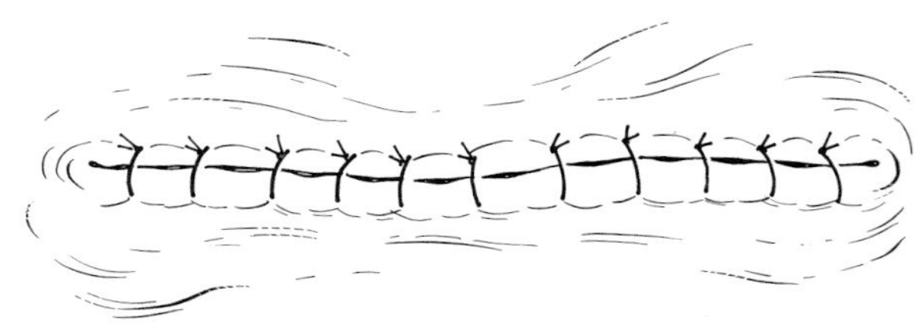

(f)

Figure 8.33a–f Resiting of ileostomy through a new trephine on the opposite side of the abdominal wall using a laparotomy. (a) The ileostomy is mobilized from the abdominal wall and the everted end of the ileum is resected. (b) The previous abdominal wall trephine is closed with a series of interrupted sutures. (c) The ileostomy is delivered through the new trephine. (d) The ileostomy is everted and sutured to the skin. (e)–(f) Ileostomy closure leaving a transverse incision in the abdominal wall. The rectus muscle is closed. The rectus sheath, where possible, should be closed transversally. Two diamond-shaped segments of skin are excised on both lateral aspects of the skin circle. A series of subcutaneous sutures are used to bring the skin edges together so as to complete a transverse skin closure.

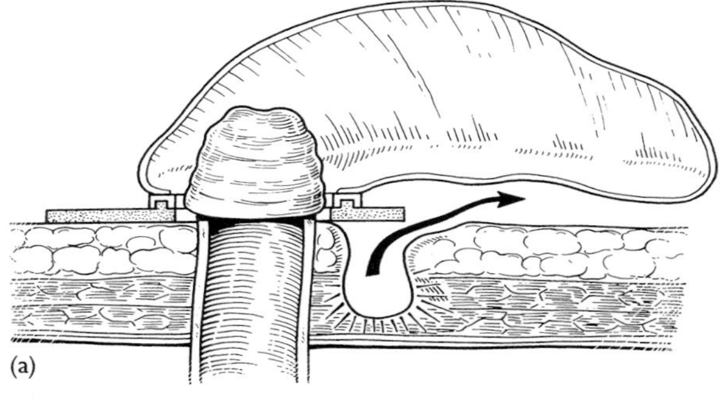

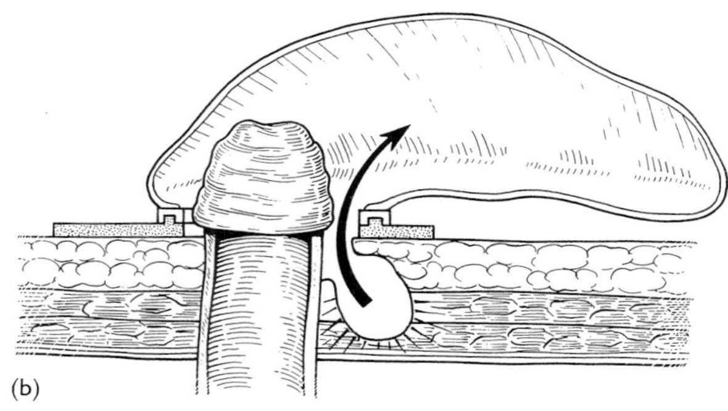

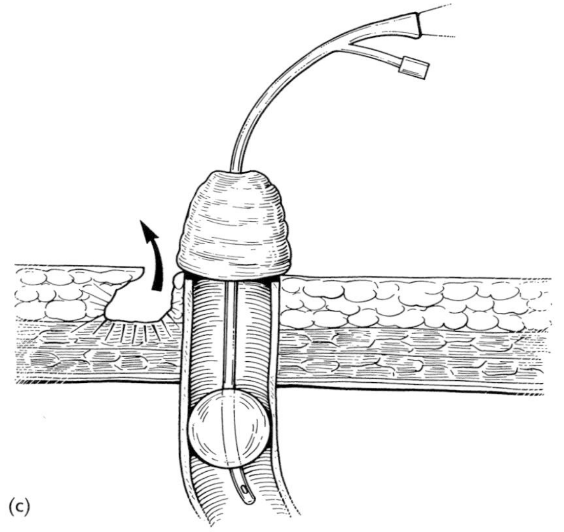

Figure 8.34a–c Management of a paraileostomy abdominal wall abscess. (a) If the abscess is allowed to drain beneath the flange it usually becomes dislodged and is unsatisfactory. (b) The abscess can be drained adjacent to the ileostomy, in which case its contents can be contained within the ileostomy bag. (c) If it proves difficult to achieve drainage with a bag during the early management of a paraileostomy abscess, small bowel contents may be allowed to drain through a Foley catheter placed in the ileostomy while inflating the balloon beyond the abdominal wall.

Results

There are few reports on the outcome of revision procedures. Goligher (1984) refers to a series of 106 cases in whom 16 developed peristomal cellulitis, of whom five also had serious peristomal sepsis. In 13 patients early results were unsatisfactory, and 12 of the remaining 90 cases developed a prolapse or recession at a later stage. Hence approximately a quarter were unsatisfactory and required further attention.

Dew et al (1979), when reviewing 70 of the Birmingham series with ulcerative colitis who required stomal revision, found that 48 eventually needed further surgery. Weaver et al (1988) prospectively studied 49 patients in Birmingham who had a stoma revision between 1976 and 1984. He found that five of 27 patients with ulcerative colitis (19%) and six of 22 patients (27%) with Crohn's disease needed repeat revisions (Table 8.23). The repeat revision rate was 45% for patients with Crohn's disease having a local resection without laparotomy, compared with 12% of colitics having a local procedure. By contrast, repeat revisions were needed in 30% of colitics having a laparotomy, compared with only 9% of those with Crohn's disease. It seems clear, therefore, that it is unwise to attempt local refashioning procedures in Crohn's disease, whereas this approach is often the method of choice in ulcerative colitis. Another finding was that 50% of patients requiring stomal refashioning procedures in Crohn's disease were found to have recurrent disease. Complications of repeat revision procedures included sepsis in two, retraction of the stoma in six, hernia in one, stenosis in two and fistula in one. Sepsis, fistula and stenosis all occurred in patients with Crohn's disease.

MANAGEMENT OF SPECIFIC COMPLICATIONS

Retraction

A retracted stoma is often responsible for leakage and peristomal excoriation (Goldblatt et al, 1977). Retraction may be managed by the local stapling procedure illustrated in Figure 8.21e, but more commonly it is corrected by a local refashioning procedure, with fixation of the serosa of the ileum to the rectus sheath (see Figure 8.29d). If retraction is associated with a peristomal hernia, or is due to insufficient buttressing from the abdominal wall because the stoma is sited lateral to the rectus muscle, the best option is to resite the stoma (see Figure 8.32c).

The Birmingham results for refashioning a retracted ileostomy are frankly unsatisfactory: 50% were found to have retracted again after revisional operations. Retraction is probably the most common reason for revision and is also associated with the worst results (Whates and Irving, 1984). The surgeons at the Lahey Clinic advise resiting the stoma for retraction, and that seems sensible. On the other hand, Todd (1983) felt that resiting was not the answer. He believed that scarification of the serosa of the ileum and meticulous fixation of the serosa to the rectus sheath and the everted limb with tight skin closure are the key to success. In order to achieve a tight closure of the skin, since the skin trephine is almost always widened both from the retraction of the stoma and following its mobilization for refashioning, he advised excising three triangles of skin around the stoma. The edges of each skin wedge are sutured preferably by subcuticular stitch before completing the mucocutaneous closure (Figure 8.35).

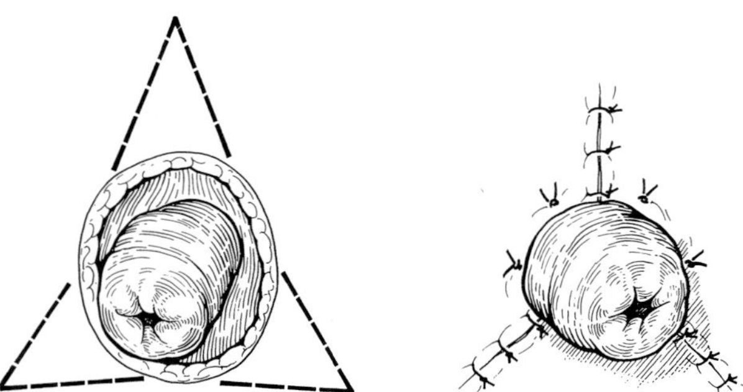

Figure 8.35 Reconstruction of the stoma if the skin disc is much wider than the diameter of the ileum. Under these circumstances three triangles can be excised from the edge of the skin disc and sutured together in the Mercedes manoeuvre.

Prolapse

Ileostomy prolapse, while uncommon, is usually associated with inadequate fixation between the ileostomy and the abdominal wall; it may be associated with a peristomal hernia. Goldblatt et al (1977) classified prolapse as fixed or sliding. This is a useful distinction since the fixed prolapse can be expected to resolve by amputation alone, whereas the sliding variety may have to be resited. The fixed type of prolapse is probably an error of original construction, in that the stoma was made too long.

The sliding prolapse is capricious; one minute it may be flush, and the next it protrudes so much that the appliance becomes dislodged. By contrast, the fixed prolapse is ungainly, causing embarrassment (especially to women) because of its size and the fact that it is impossible to conceal under clothing. Either form of prolapse may be associated with trauma and bleeding.

Amputation of a fixed prolapse is comparable to rectosigmoidectomy for rectal prolapse. The junction between the skin and the mucosa is carefully divided without mobilizing the emerging ileum. The everted limb is straightened. An appropriate length of ileum is excised, usually leaving 5–6 cm projecting above the skin, which is then everted and sutured to the skin (see Figure 8.26).

For sliding prolapse, careful local revision with fixation of the serosa to the rectus and or stapling of the everted ileostomy bud is possible (see Figure 8.29d). Preferably, the stoma should be resited if a suitable alternative position can be found (see Figure 8.30a,b). Todd (1983) considers that mesenteric fixation is crucial to the success of treating a stomal prolapse, in the belief that the condition is due to complete disruption of the mesenteric attachment to the abdominal wall. He therefore believes that the mesentery must be fixed again or that the bowel should be pulled taut so that the mesentery can stretch no more and then the redundant bowel excised. All of the prolapsed ileostomies requiring revision at Birmingham have been managed by local refashioning; none has recurred and the only complication was minor stenosis in one patient.

Turnbull and Weekley (1967) used split skin grafts to correct ileostomy prolapse. Sohn et al (1983) describe a repair using bidirectional myotomy and a meshed split thickness skin graft on the amputated but non-everted ileum. Four patients were reported to have had a successful operation, but the procedure seems to be unnecessarily complex.

Hernia

Parastomal hernias are usually the result of a badly sited stoma (particularly those placed outside the rectus muscle), obesity, a wide abdominal trephine, or chronic obstructive airways disase (Turnbull and Weekley, 1967; Hulten et al, 1976; Todd, 1978) (see Figure 8.32). The importance of a transrectal trephine has been challenged by Leong et al (1994), on the basis that parastomal hernias were just as common when placed through the rectus muscle. In the past, parastomal hernias were associated with ileostomies which had been brought out through the wound (Leslie, 1984), and were often associated with prolapse. Parastomal hernias are more common in patients who are obese or who have had a hernia repair elsewhere. Parastomal hernias may be classified as being interstitial, subcutaneous or intrastomal (Figure 8.36). Stomal hernias may cause dislodgment of ileostomy appliances. Moreover, the small bowel may be damaged during ileostomy closure or refashioning because of adherent loops in the hernia sac. Strangulation and infarction of small bowel within the sac is rare but obstruction is a common indication for surgical correction.

Paraileostomy hernia is an unusual complication (Ritchie, 1971; Goligher, 1984), and was encountered in 16% of Birmingham patients requiring revision. Local repair is usually considered unsatisfactory (Goldblatt et al, 1977); however, five of six local repairs performed were successful (Weaver et al, 1988). Local repair may be performed by resuture of the musculoaponeurotic defect (Todd, 1982) or by placement of a mesh support around the stoma to repair the defect (Rosin and Bonardi, 1977; Abdu, 1982; Leslie, 1984) (see Figure 8.28d). Nonabsorbable mesh (polypropylene or Teflon) carries with it the risk of chronic sepsis, but absorbable (Vicryl) mesh might overcome these disadvantages. If local repair is the best option, because there is no available alternative site, interrupted Prolene sutures can be used to close the defect, usually through a laparotomy (see Figure 8.29a–d).

Resiting is the optimum method of management, by taking down the ileostomy, repairing the defect and constructing a new trephine on the opposite side of the abdomen – the reason being that the cause of the hernia is usually a badly sited stoma (Brooke, 1952; Cuthbertson and Collins, 1977).

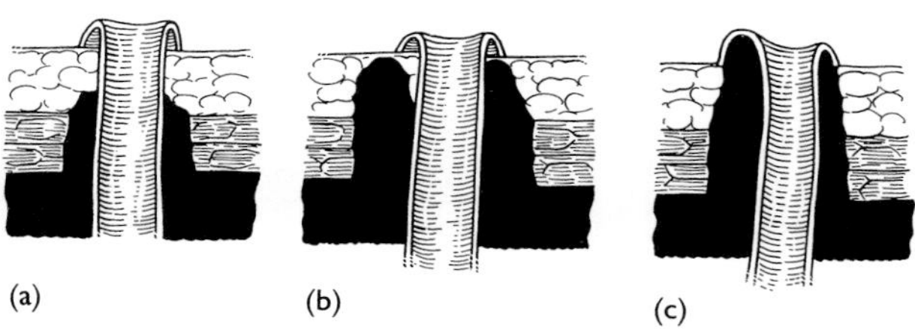

Figure 8.36a–c Types of paraileostomy hernia. These may be (a) through the abdominal wall only, (b) involving the abdominal wall and the subcutaneous tissues, or (c) involving the abdominal wall, subcutaneous tissues and the everted ileum.

Fistula

Paraileostomy fistula occurred in 14% of patients in the Lahey Clinic series (Goldblatt et al, 1977) and in 10% of Birmingham patients. Not all of these patients had recurrent Crohn's disease. Fistulas in ulcerative colitis or familial adenomatous polyposis are nearly always due to a non-absorbable suture which has caused chronic sepsis and has eroded through the ileum. Alternatively, the fistula may be due to trauma to the ileostomy, often as a result of erosion by the flange (Figure 8.37). These non-Crohn's fistulas are either superficial or traverse the anterior rectus sheath. The track is straight, the stoma itself is healthy and the fistula is single. By contrast, fistulas complicating recurrent Crohn's disease are often multiple, associated with recurrent sepsis, the stoma is deformed or stenotic, and there are episodes of intermittent obstruction and flux.

Fistulas usually require surgical correction because of the difficulties encountered with stoma management. Even if the orifice lies adjacent to the stoma, intestinal discharge dislodges the flange and

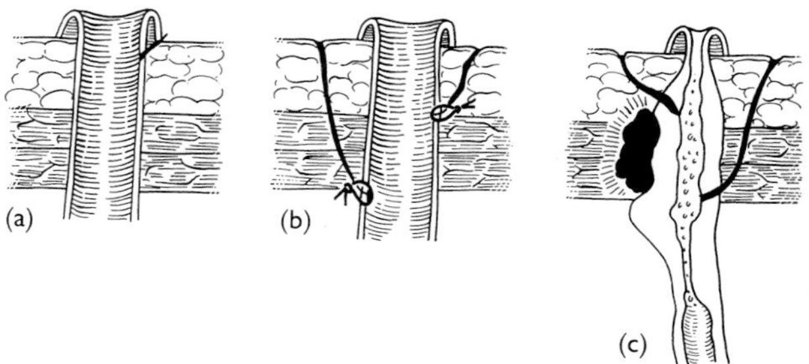

Figure 8.37a–c Paraileostomy fistulas. Paraileostomy fistulas may be (a) superficial. (b) They may involve the rectus sheath particularly if a non-absorbable suture has been used to secure the serosa of the ileum to the peritoneum.
(c) Alternatively, they may be due to disease of the ileum, particularly Crohn's disease where abscess and fistulas are common.

usually lifts the seal within a few hours of application. If, on the other hand, the orifice of the fistula is underneath the flange or outside it, skin excoriation rapidly ensues because intestinal loss either dislodges the appliance immediately or discharges on to the skin beside it.

Re-operation involves mobilizing the stoma from the abdominal wall, a procedure which may be extremely difficult if there is chronic peristomal sepsis and non-absorbable sutures surrounded by an abscess. Since it may be difficult to exclude Crohn's disease, a laparotomy is advisable, both to ensure that the ileum is not damaged when taken down and because resection is usually needed (see Figure 8.31). If the original stoma site is satisfactory and has not been excessively stretched or distorted by disease or operation, the new stoma may be fashioned at the same site. On the other hand there is usually chronic sepsis, a wide deficiency of the abdominal wall at the stoma site or the original stoma site is badly placed. Under these circumstances the new stoma should be resited. All cases of fistula at Birminham have required laparotomy but only 25% required resiting. A more conservative approach for simple non-Crohn's fistula has been described by Greatorex (1988), involving cleaning out the sepsis with a pipe-cleaner soaked in phenol; resolution was reported in two of three cases.

Ulceration, sinus and stricture

Ulceration, polypoidal granulomas and sinuses usually indicate recurrent Crohn's disease. However, ulcers may be traumatic from a badly fitting appliance or from self-induced injury (Wilkinson and Humphreys, 1978). Sinuses may develop around non-absorbable sutures. Strictures usually indicate recurrent Crohn's disease. Before the eversion ileostomy became standard practice, stenosis was a common complication in patients who did not have a matured stoma. Occasionally, stenosis occurs because the opening in the abdominal wall has been made too small following overzealous local repair of a parastomal hernia, or due to ischaemia.

Stomal stenosis usually requires laparotomy and resection, with reconstruction of the ileostomy through the original stoma site (see Figure 8.31). Malt et al (1984) have described four-quadrant subcutaneous fasciotomy around the stoma for stricture in the abdominal wall, but the risk of damage to the ileum must be high and the approach cannot be recommended.

Bleeding

Bleeding may be from ulceration, trauma, polyps, recurrent Crohn's disease or peristomal varices. Traumatic bleeding is nearly always associated with a long stoma, patient interference or too tight an ileostomy appliance. Polyps may appear on the ileostomy of patients with familial adenomatous polyposis and in inflammatory bowel disease. Bleeding is usually minimal in recurrent Crohn's disease. Bleeding from varices around the ileostomy in patients with inflammatory bowel disease and sclerosing cholangitis with cirrhosis is usually profuse, recurrent, unheralded and extremely frightening to the patient (Lewis et al, 1990).

Variceal bleeding from the ileostomy of patients with portal hypertension is a manifestation of progressive underlying liver disease and is discussed fully in Chapter 43. The complication is fortunately uncommon (Eade et al, 1969; Adson and Fulton, 1977; Dew et al, 1979; Cooper et al, 1981). An extensive shunt between the ileal veins and veins of the abdominal wall develops. This caput medusa protects against the formation of gastro-oesophageal varices (Resnick et al, 1968; Hamlyn et al, 1974). Although bleeding is usually profuse, a diffuse ooze sometimes complicates trauma to the stoma (Peck and Boyden, 1985).

Initial treatment of bleeding parastomal varices in patients with portal hypertension is by compression around the stoma, but the patient should be transferred to hospital as soon as possible. Injection sclerotherapy may be used (Mosquera et al, 1988) but this rarely provides long-term control and initial management is often unsatisfactory because tamponade is usually ineffective. The simplest procedure is to detach the mucocutaneous junction, thereby disconnecting the portosystemic collaterals. The mucosal edge is oversewn to control bleeding and the divided mucocutaneous margin is then resutured as in the technique for ileostomy construction (Figure 8.38a,b; see also Figure 43.4a–c) (Beck et al, 1988).

Unfortunately, although local peristomal portosystemic disconnection usually controls bleeding in the short term, recurrent haemorrhage is common (Cameron and Fone, 1970; Graeber et al, 1976; Ackerman et al, 1980). Beck et al (1988), however, reported satisfactory control in seven of nine patients followed up for a mean of 2.5 years. Since local control is often unsatisfactory, and as there may be considerable blood loss causing deterioration of liver function, a number of centres have advised portosystemic decompression by splenorenal or portocaval shunts (Adson and Fulton, 1977;

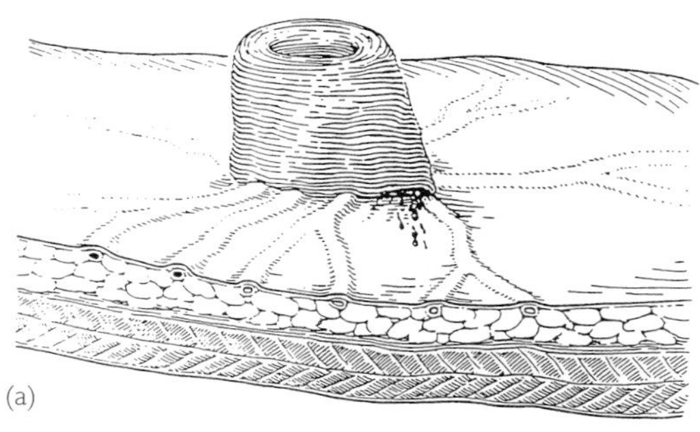

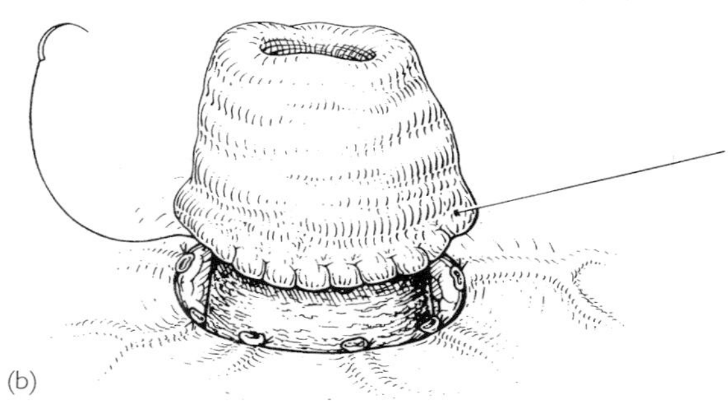

Figure 8.38a–b (a) Under-running of paraileostomy varices. Varices adjacent to the mucocutaneous suture of an ileostomy may be the source of massive haemorrhage and can usually be managed by under-running the vessel after disconnecting the mucocutaneous junction (not shown). (b) New interrupted mucocutaneous sutures applied to the mobilized stoma. The free edge of the ileum is oversewn.

Ackerman et al, 1980; Ricci et al, 1980; Larusso et al, 1984) or even a liver transplantation if bleeding recurs. Colectomy does not protect against encephalopathy, and 20–30% of patients develop neuropsychiatric complications following shunt surgery. Local disconnection may therefore be the safest form of management (Peck and Boyden, 1985) and was successful in three of five patients at Birmingham.

Ileostomy flux

Flux is used to describe profuse ileostomy diarrhoea. This is a common and important complication since patients may rapidly become very dehydrated, hyponatraemic and hypokalaemic and may develop an Addisonian crisis if they have been receiving steroids. At least two patients in our experience have died from steroid depletion complicating ileostomy flux during the past four decades. Patients who have been on steroids in the previous year should be told that they may need further steroid therapy if they develop severe ileostomy flux.

Ileostomy flux is characterized by a watery fluid discharge that requires the pouch to be emptied repeatedly. Flux may be precipitated by local or systemic sepsis. Other causes include gastroenteritis, bacterial overgrowth, obstruction or recurrent Crohn's disease (Hill et al, 1975b). Before eversion ileostomy, flux was a frequent complication of ileostomy stenosis. In many patients the cause of flux is never found.

Apart from profuse ileostomy discharge, the patient often feels weak, light-headed, thirsty and becomes oliguric. The metabolic features of ileostomy flux are the same as those of the short bowel syndrome. Any patient who passes more than 1000 mL of fluid ileostomy contents in 24 hours is in danger of becoming rapidly salt- and water-depleted. Large volume losses from the ileostomy predispose to leakage from the bag unless the patient is extremely vigilant and manages to keep the pouch empty.

Any patient who loses more than 1.5 L of fluid rapidly from their ileostomy should be told to come into hospital immediately. On average, 18 patients a year with this complication are admitted to our unit at Birmingham. After a brief clinical examination to ensure that there are no signs of gastroenteritis, viral infection, intra-abdominal sepsis or intestinal obstruction, an intravenous infusion is commenced, replacing ileostomy losses with normal saline and added potassium. A patient who has received steroids within the previous year is given 100 mg hydrocortisone 6-hourly for 24 hours. A sample of ileostomy fluid is despatched to the microbiology laboratory to ensure that there are no enteric pathogens.

Although intravenous fluid replacement rapidly restores fluid and electrolyte homeostasis, this often aggravates the losses of sodium and water from the stoma so the infusion should not be discontinued too early. The volume of ileostomy effluent usually falls to less than 1200 mL within 48–72 hours and during this time the intravenous infusion should be the only source of fluid and electrolytes, since drinking fluids or even taking salt by mouth merely exacerbates the fluid and electrolyte losses (Kramer, 1966; Newton et al, 1985). Steroids further reduce the fluid and sodium losses (Feretis et al, 1984; Goligher and Lintott, 1975).

Once the fluid losses abate, oral fluids may be slowly administered, but it is wiser to use a glucose–electrolyte solution rather than water (Gore et al, 1992; Nightingale et al, 1995). Sweetened drinks with added oral salt should be encouraged when the patient is discharged. The main uses of glucose–electrolyte solutions are for the patient who cannot be admitted to hospital when travelling, or for those patients with the short bowel syndrome who are habitually on the brink of dehydration.

Drugs such as codeine and Lomotil will reduce ileostomy output and conserve sodium (Newton, 1978; Tytgat and Huibregtse, 1975). These drugs may be used after withdrawing intravenous fluids or be taken as a reserve if the ileostomy suddenly becomes overactive. Somatostatin analogues may have a place in patients with recurrent flux.

Operations for repeated or persistent ileostomy diarrhoea have been advocated by some. The problem is that most of these patients have only a limited amount of small bowel, hence reoperations which might prejudice the limited small bowel available if complications supervene are hazardous. Most would resist re-operating on these patients unless certain long-term benefits would accrue. Reversal of a 10–12 cm segment of terminal ileum has been used for ileostomy diarrhoea (Ellis and Coll, 1968; Javett and Brooke, 1971; Cohen et al, 1975; Matolo and Wolfman, 1976). The length of the reversed segment is critical: if it is too long there is a risk of small bowel obstruction, whereas too short a segment does not adequately reduce small intestinal transit time (Sako and Blackman, 1962; Shepard, 1966). The reversed segment is excised on its vascular pedicle, rotated and re-anastomosed 30 cm proximal to the ileostomy. Matolo and Wolfman (1976) reported prolongation of intestinal transit from 12 to 150 minutes by this procedure. An alternative idea has been to implant a smooth muscle collar around the terminal ileum to act as a brake (Schiller et al, 1967), but there are no long-term results of this procedure (Stacchini et al, 1982).

The idea of constructing a reservoir ileostomy in these patients is not one that should be lightly entertained. The short bowel syndrome is more commonly caused by attempts to make a Kock pouch than resolved by its construction. Any form of reoperation for profuse ileostomy diarrhoea is not advisable unless there is a stricture causing incomplete obstruction that is amenable to strictureplasty. Most procedures potentially jeopardize small bowel and are often unsuccessful.

Replacement of fluid and electrolytes can be achieved by peritoneal dialysis (August and Sugarbaker, 1985). H_2-receptor antagonists should be considered in patients with the short bowel syndrome if there is marked hyperchlorhydria. Oral antibiotics might also be advisable if there is evidence of bacterial overgrowth. Pancreatic enzyme replacement may be indicated if there is exocrine deficiency, and cholestyramine if there is gross bile salt malabsorption.

COMPLICATIONS OF LOOP ILEOSTOMY CLOSURE

Incidence

One of the potential advantages of loop ileostomy over loop colostomy is that complications following closure are less common than after closure of a colostomy (Williams et al, 1986). Furthermore, a loop ileostomy is often easier to manage than a loop colostomy. Khoury et al (1986) reported 34% and 52% complication rates respectively following closure of ileostomy and colostomy. Fasth et al (1980) reported that only one of 21 patients developed complications after closure of a loop ileostomy, compared with six of 21 after loop colostomy closure.

The complication rate of loop ileostomy closure is shown in Table 8.24. A much higher complication rate is recorded following closure of a loop ileostomy for defunction of a pelvic ileal pouch, since there may be persistent pelvic sepsis, stricture, or a fistula from the pouch or the ileoanal anastomosis (Babcock et al, 1980; Metcalf et al, 1985). Moreover, there appears to be a high incidence of small bowel obstruction after ileostomy closure for pelvic pouch. Metcalf et al (1986a) reviewed their experience of loop ileostomy closure compared with a Brooke ileostomy to decompress an ileoanal pouch (Table 8.25). Complications of the stoma itself and closure were fewer using the Brooke ileostomy, and they argue that a loop ileostomy might not be the most appropriate stoma for decompression. On the other hand, although the morbidity of closing a loop ileostomy is greater for patients with an ileoanal pouch than it is when used to protect an ileorectal anastomosis, their view that an end ileostomy is necessarily superior to a loop ileostomy for these patients cannot be supported. Decompression may be achieved by techniques other than loop ileostomy, and tube ileostomy has been proposed by passing a Foley catheter through the ileocaecal valve using a caecostomy. The procedure achieves good decompression when the balloon is inflated but the complication rate is not known (Jhittay and Obeid, 1986).

Table 8.24 Complications of closure of loop ileostomy.

	No.	*Incidence*	*Fistula/leak*	*Sepsis*
Fasth et al (1980)	21	1*	0	1
Raimes et al (1984)	22	3*	2	1
Shirley et al (1984)	15	2*	1	1
Fasth and Hulten (1984)	89	6*	0	5
Williams et al (1986)	23	0*	0	0
Metcalf et al (1986a,b)	122	31*	9	2
Feinberg et al (1987)†	117	16*	4	4

*Many due to obstruction.
†A high proportion for restorative proctocolectomy.

Table 8.25 Comparison of complication rate using two methods of faecal diversion for ileoanal pouch anastomosis.

	Loop ileostomy (*n* = 157)	*Brooke ileostomy* (*n* = 23)
Complications of stoma		
Retraction	25	2
Prolapse	2	0
Fistula	1	0
Abscess	1	1
Obstruction	10	0
Skin excoriation	84	6
Leakage	12	1
High volume output	6	0
Incomplete diversion	9	0
	Loop ileostomy (*n* = 122)	*Brooke ileostomy* (*n* = 27)
Complications of closure		
Obstruction	18	1
Laparotomy needed	2	0
Peritonitis	9	1
Wound infection	2	0
Intestinal bleeding	2	0

From Metcalf et al (1986a,b).

Assessment

Patients requiring ileostomy closure should be assessed appropriately beforehand. Clinical examination, particularly rectal examination, should be used to exclude stenosis which must be treated prior to closure. Sigmoidoscopy should exclude stricture, fistula or severe residual disease, all of which may contraindicate ileostomy. Patency of the bowel to the loop stoma can usually be verified by air insufflation. If there is still any doubt about the integrity of an anastomosis, the pouch, or a stenosis beyond the reach of the sigmoidoscope, a contrast study should be performed, either per anum or through the distal limb of the ileostomy, to ensure that there is no anatomical obstruction, fistula, abscess or contained leak (Figure 8.39). If there is any fear that the patient might be incontinent after closure, anal manometry can be helpful.

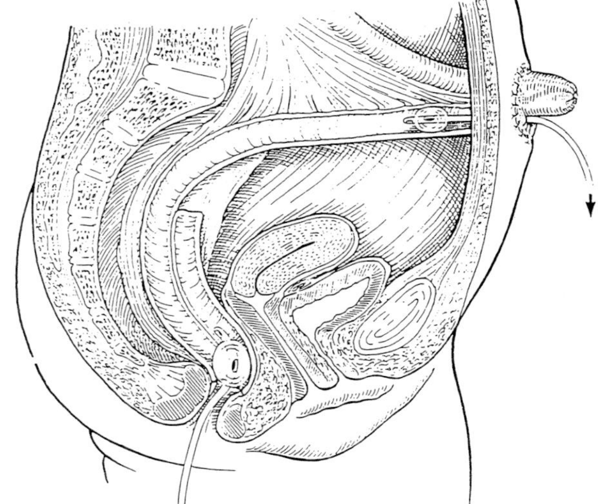

Figure 8.39 Management of a contained leak after ileoanal anastomosis. Catheterization of the pouch, local drainage and proximal loop ileostomy.

Method of closure

It is usually unwise to attempt closure of a loop ileostomy within 6 weeks of construction. A longer period of decompression would be advisable if there has been any postoperative peristomal sepsis, peritonitis or pelvic sepsis. Reliable intravenous access should be established during the operation because of the need to restrict oral fluids postoperatively. Unlike ileostomy revision, closure involves an intra-abdominal anastomosis and there may be a functional or anatomical obstruction at or below the closure. Hence, fluids may need to be restricted for up to a week after closure. Single-dose antibiotic cover is used and the patient is given a general anaesthetic with complete muscle relaxation.

It should not normally be necessary to perform a laparotomy to close a loop ileostomy safely unless there has been technical difficulty during mobilization, a loop of bowel becomes damaged and requires resection, or there is a distal obstruction that needs to be dealt with. Even if one of these problems does arise, adequate access can usually be accomplished by enlarging the peristomal incision laterally which, unlike stoma revision, is always permissable in order to close the stoma safely (see Figures 8.28a and 8.33e). Wexner et al (1993) regard loop ileostomy closure as much safer than loop colostomy closure. Closure was possible through the stomal incision in 64 of 67 patients and a laparotomy was needed in only three. They used a stapling technique for closure in 49 patients and suture closure in 18. The operation time was 56 minutes and hospital stay 5 days. Two patients developed leakage following closure, causing an enterocutaneous fistula which closed spontaneously in 5 and 7 days.

Ileostomy closure may be by suture or staples. In a non-randomized study, Bain et al (1996) found that operating time was less using staples but morbidity was equivalent. Conversely, Hull et al (1996) at the Cleveland Clinic abandoned a randomized trial because morbidity was substantially less with stapled closure, particularly from small bowel obstruction. At Birmingham a randomized trial to compare suture with stapled ileostomy closure has been completed. The final results indicate shorter operating time and fewer complications – particularly bowel obstruction – with stapled closure (Hasegawa et al, 1999). Despite the capital outlay of the stapler, the overall costs were no greater with stapled compared with sutured closure (Table 8.26).

A circumstomal incision is made between the ileostomy and the skin, keeping as close to the bowel as possible (Figure 8.40a). The serosa of the two limbs of the ileostomy are freed from the subcutaneous fat, the rectus sheath and, finally, the peritoneum (Figure 8.40b). Traction is applied to the ileostomy throughout the procedure. The ileum must be completely freed so that the peritoneal cavity can be opened around the entire circumference of the bowel. This ensures that the ileum can be easily replaced into the peritoneal cavity after closure. The everted ileostomy bud is turned back by scissor and gauze dissection. Any residual skin or untidy edges adherent to the ileum are excised and bleeding is controlled by diathermy.

Table 8.26 Randomized trial of loop ileostomy closure.

	Sutured (n = 68)	*Stapled* (n = 69)
Duration of operation (min)	46.2 ± 24.2	37.8 ± 10.5
Complications	18	9
Wound sepsis	3	3
Ileus >7 days	2	2
Intestinal obstruction	10	2
Clinical leak	3	0
Abscess	2	0

From Hasegawa et al, 1999.

The opening on the antimesenteric border of the ileum is closed, using a series of single-layer inverting interrupting sutures or a continuous extramucosal suture (Figure 8.40c). At Birmingham a continuous single-layer extramucosal PDS suture is preferred. The abdominal wall is closed using Prolene to the rectus muscle and rectus sheath, preferably transversally. The lateral skin edges are excised so that the skin wound can be closed transversally. Loop ileostomy closure is now usually performed with a linear staple cutter to achieve a side-to-side enteroenterostomy (Figure 8.41a), then excising the opening with a linear stapler (Figure 8.41b) (Kusunoki et al, 1996).

The ileum is gently eased back into the peritoneal cavity through the trephine in the rectus muscle. The rectus sheath is then closed using interrupted sutures (Figure 8.41c) and the skin defect is either left open and packed with proflavine in liquid paraffin or preferably closed excising the lateral skin edges leaving a transverse incision (see Figure 8.33e,f). If the ileostomy bud becomes traumatized when the everted stoma is turned back, or if there is any iatrogenic injury to the ileal loop, it may be wiser to resect the segment and construct either an end-to-end sutured anastomosis (Figure 8.42a) or a stapled functional end-to-end anastomosis with one of the linear staple cutters (Figure 8.42b,c).

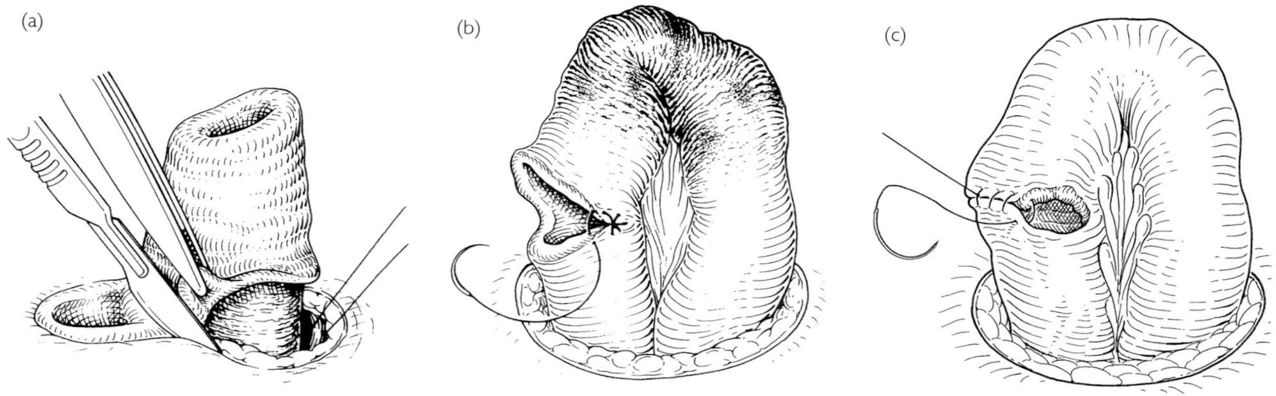

Figure 8.40a–c Mobilization of a loop ileostomy prior to closure. (a) A circumstomal incision is made, and the ileum is gently mobilized from the subcutaneous fat in the rectus sheath so as to open the peritoneal cavity all the way round the loop of bowel. (b) The everted segment of the ileum is reverted and the defect in the antemesenteric portion of the bowel is closed using continuous extramucosal sutures. (c) The skin is best closed transversely, excising the lateral defects of the trephine circle.

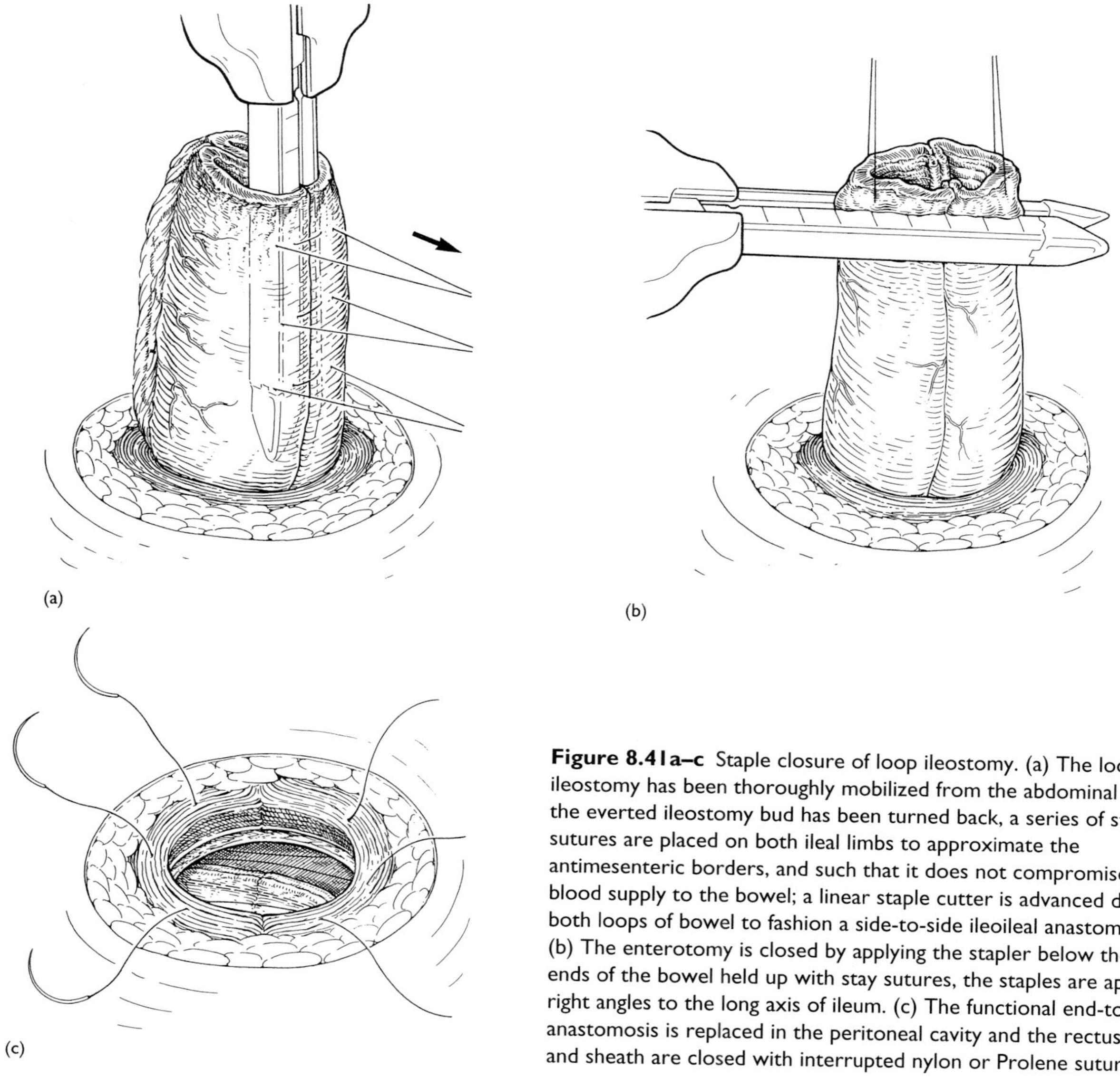

Figure 8.41a–c Staple closure of loop ileostomy. (a) The loop ileostomy has been thoroughly mobilized from the abdominal wall, the everted ileostomy bud has been turned back, a series of stay sutures are placed on both ileal limbs to approximate the antimesenteric borders, and such that it does not compromise the blood supply to the bowel; a linear staple cutter is advanced down both loops of bowel to fashion a side-to-side ileoileal anastomosis. (b) The enterotomy is closed by applying the stapler below the open ends of the bowel held up with stay sutures, the staples are applied at right angles to the long axis of ileum. (c) The functional end-to-end anastomosis is replaced in the peritoneal cavity and the rectus muscle and sheath are closed with interrupted nylon or Prolene sutures.

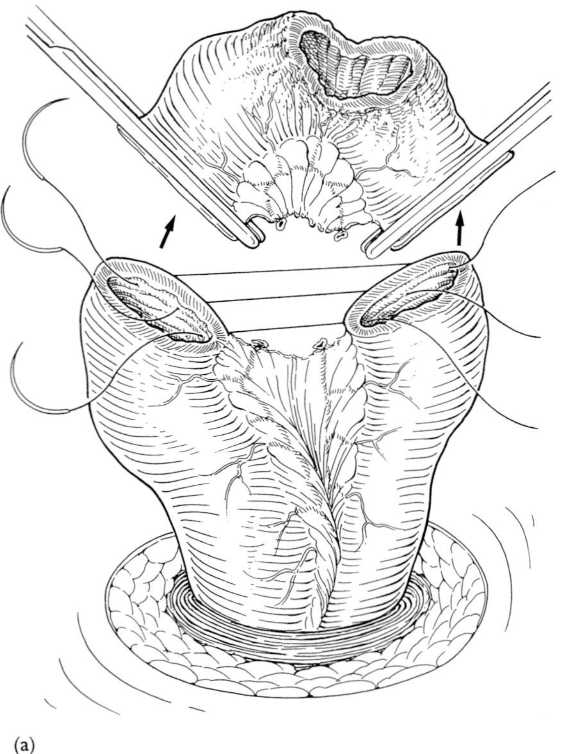

(a)

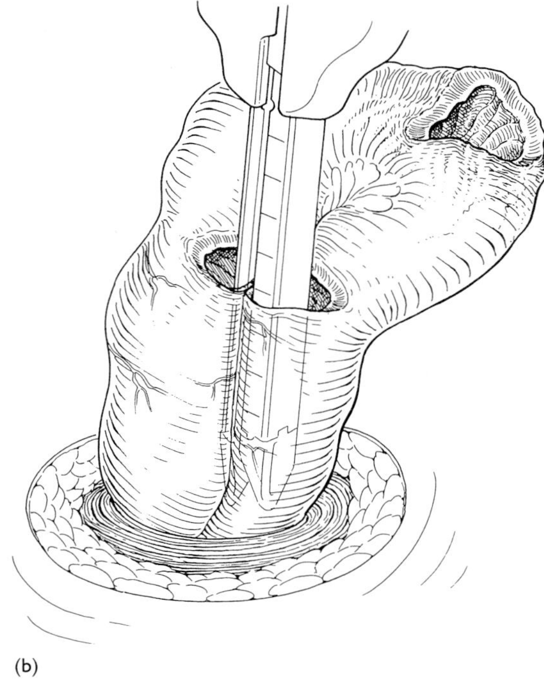

(b)

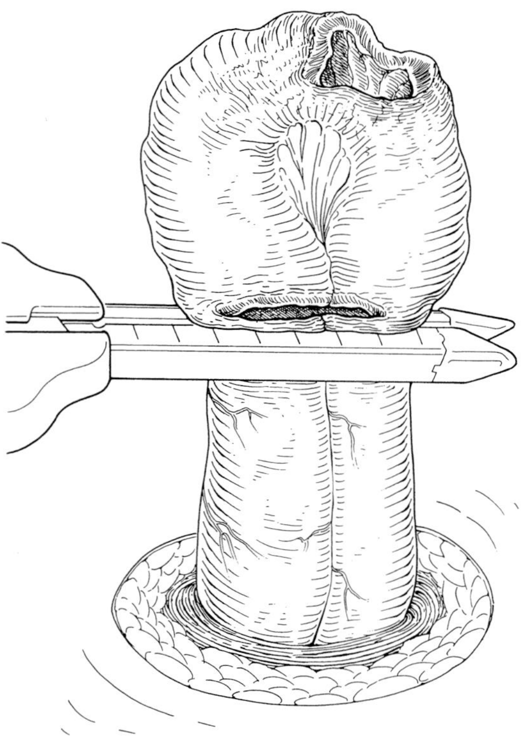

(c)

Figure 8.42a–c Closure of loop ileostomy by resection. (a) The loop has been thoroughly mobilized from the abdominal wall through a circumstomal incision. The loop has been damaged due to fibrosis around the bowel and abdominal wall. Under these circumstances it is often safer to resect the traumatized segment between bowel clamps after dividing the small bowel mesentery; a single layer end-to-end anastomosis is then fashioned. (b) Alternatively, a stapled anastomosis may be constructed by passing a linear staple cutter down the two adjacent loops of bowel through an enterotomy in each of the ileal segments. (c) The damaged segment and the two enterotomies are then resected by a second firing of the stapler at right-angles to the long axis of the bowel as shown; the bowel is then replaced in the peritoneal cavity and the defect in the abdominal wall is closed.

Postoperative management

Oral fluids are restricted until flatus has passed and the risk of obstruction or leakage seems to be over. Usually the intravenous infusion is maintained for 4–7 days while slowly increasing the amount of oral fluid. Most patients will be able to leave hospital 7–10 days after closure.

Antidiarrhoeals may precipitate obstruction and increase the risk of leakage from the suture line. These agents should therefore be avoided in the first 2 weeks after closure, despite severe diarrhoea and perianal excoriation. If antidiarrhoeals have to be prescribed, ispaghula or methylcellulose are preferred in the early postoperative period.

Postoperative complications

Wound sepsis is rare if stoma wounds are left open. If infection occurs in a sutured wound the stitches should be removed and the wound opened. Dehiscence from the closure site is usually heralded by abdominal pain and fever, and signs of peritonitis, abscess, ileus, or a fistula through the wound obstruction. The dehiscence usually resolves spontaneously, unless there is an abscess, a type-2 fistula or peritonitis. In the first instance, conservative treatment with intravenous fluids and antibiotics is advised. In a high proportion of patients no further treatment is necessary. Any abscess should be drained. If a fistula does develop, it usually closes spontaneously if there is no obstruction and provided there is no cavity between the hole in the ileum and the skin. Management should involve withholding oral fluids, total parenteral nutrition, drainage of any abscess and appropriate stoma therapy to contain the fistula.

Intestinal obstruction is a common complication following ileostomy closure, particularly after decompression for a pelvic pouch, and should be treated conservatively by intravenous fluids and nasogastric decompression. If there is no resolution with medical therapy there may be a distal mechanical obstruction. Under these circumstances, laparotomy should then be performed early because of the risks of infarction (see Chapter 49).

Other complications of ileostomy closure include hernia at the abdominal wall trephine, fistula from the original operation site, and chronic sepsis around a non-absorbable suture.

REFERENCES

Abcarian H & Pearl RK (1988) Stomas. *Surg Clin North Am* **68**: 1295–1304.

Abdu RA (1982) Repair of paracolostomy hernias with Marlex mesh. *Dis Colon Rectum* **25**: 529–531.

Abrams AV, Corman ML & Verdenheimer MC (1975) Ileostomy in the elderly. *Dis Colon Rectum* **18**: 115–117.

Ackerman NB, Graeber GM & Fey J (1980) Enterstomal varices secondary to portal hypertension. *Arch Surg* **115**: 1154–1155.

Adson MA & Fulton RE (1977) The ileal stoma and portal hypertension. *Arch Surg* **112**: 501–504.

Alexander FG (1970) Personal communication, cited in Ritchie (1971) *Gut* **12**: 536–540.

Alexander-Williams J (1974) Loop ileostomy and colostomy for faecal diversion. *Ann R Coll Surg Engl* **54**: 141–148.

Alexander-Williams J & Haynes IG (1985) Conservative operations for Crohn's disease of the small bowel. *World J Surg* **9**: 945–951.

Allan RN (1997) Crohn's disease of the small intestine in diffuse jejunal ileitis. In Allan RN, Rhodes JM, Hanauer SB, Keighley MRB, Alexander-Williams J & Fazio VW (eds) *Inflammatory Bowel Diseases*, 3rd edn, p 597. London: Churchill Livingstone.

Ambrose NS, Keighley MRB, Alexander-Williams J & Allan RN (1984) Clinical impact of colectomy and ileorectal anastomosis in the management of Crohn's disease. *Gut* **25**: 223–227.

Anderson DN, Driver CP, Park KGM, Davidson AI & Keenan RA (1994) Loop ileostomy fixation: a simple technique to minimize the risk of stoma volvulus. *Int J Colorect Dis* **9**: 138–140.

August DA & Sugarbaker PH (1985) Tenkhoff catheter administration of intraperitoneal fluid and electrolytes for long-term management of intractable ileostomy diarrhoea: a case report. *Surgery* **97**: 237–239.

Aylett SO (1966) 300 cases of diffuse UC treated by total colectomy and ileorectal anastomosis. *BMJ* **1**: 1001–1005.

Babcock G, Bivins BA & Sachatello CR (1980) Technical complications of ileostomy. *South Med J* **73**: 329–331.

Bagi P, Jendresen M & Kirkegaard P (1992) Early local stoma complications in relation to the applied suture material: comparison between monofilament and multifilament sutures. *Dis Colon Rectum* **35**: 739–742.

Bain IM, Patel R, Keighley MRB (1996) Comparison of sutured and stapled closure of loop ileostomy after restorative proctocolectomy. *Ann R Coll Surg Engl* **78**: 555–556.

Baker A, Kaplan MM, Norton A & Paterson J (1974) Gallstone in IBD. *Dig Dis Sci* **19**: 109–112.

Bambach CP, Robertson WG, Peacock M & Hill GL (1981) Effect of intestinal surgery on the risk of urinary stone formation. *Gut* **22**: 257–263.

Bargen JA (1956) Editorial. Should the indication for surgery in UC be broadened? *Gastroenterology* **30**: 316–317.

Beahrs OH (1971) The acceptability of ileostomies. *Dis Colon Rectum* **14**: 460–463.

Beahrs OH (1975) Use of ileal reservoir following proctocolectomy. *Surg Gynecol Obstet* **185**: 179–184.

Beahrs OH, Bess MA, Beart RW & Pemberton JH (1981) Indwelling ileostomy valve device. *Am J Surg* **141**: 111–115.

Beck DE (1994) Creation and take down of intestinal stomas by laparoscopy. *Semin Colon Rectal Surg* **5**: 244–250.

Beck DE, Fazio VW & Grundfest-Broniatowski S (1988) Surgical management of bleeding stomal varices. *Dis Colon Rectum* **31**: 343–346.

Beernaerts J, Bouffioux C, Chantrie M et al (1977) The management of abdominal wall stomata skin particularly peritoneal wound healing and support for collecting bag. *Acta Chir Belg* **76**: 533–537.

Bennett RC & Hughes ESR (1972) Urinary calculi and UC. *BMJ* **2**: 494–496.

Bennett RC & Jepson RP (1966) Uric acid stone formation following ileostomy. *Aust NZ J Surg* **36**: 153–158.

Biermann HJ, Tocker AM & Tocker LR (1966) Statistical survey of problems in patients with colostomy or ileostomy. *Am J Surg* **112**: 647–649.

Bloom SR (1978) Somatostatin and the gut. *Gastroenterology* **75**: 145-147.

Bone J & Sorensen FH (1974) Life with a conventional ileostomy. *Dis Colon Rectum* **17**: 194–199.

Bonelo JC, Thow GG & Manson RR (1981) Mucosal entertitis: a complication of the continent ileostomy. *Dis Colon Rectum* **24**: 37–41.

Brooke BN (1952) The management of an ileostomy including its complications. *Lancet* **ii**: 102–104.

Brooke BN (1956) Outcome of surgery for UC. *Lancet* **ii**: 532–536.

Brooke BN (1983) Indications for emergency and elective surgery. In Allan RN, Keighley MRB, Alexander-Williams J & Hawkins C (eds) *Inflammatory Bowel Diseases*, pp 240–246. London: Churchill Livingstone.

Brown JY (1913) The value of complete physiological rest of the large bowel in the treatment of certain ulcerative and obstructive lesions of this organ. *Surg Gynecol Obstet* **16**: 610–613.

Burnham WR, Lennard-Jones JE & Brooke BN (1977) Sexual problems among married ileostomists. Survey conducted by the Ileostomy Association of Great Britain and Ireland. *Gut* **18**: 673–677.

Cameron AD & Fone DJ (1970) Portal hypertension and bleeding ileal varices after colectomy and ileostomy for chronic UC. *Gut* **11**: 755–759.

Carlsen E & Bergan A (1995) Technical aspects and complications of end ileostomies. *World J Surg* **19**: 632–636.

Carlsen E, Flatmark A & Bergan A (1991) The epidemiology of ileostomies. *Scand J Gastroenterol* **26** (Suppl 183): 70.

Carlstedt A, Fasth S, Hulten L, Nordgren S & Palselius I (1987) Long term ileostomy complications in patients with ulcerative colitis and Crohn's disease. *Int J Colorect Dis* **1**: 22–25.

Chadwick VS & Camilleri M (1983) Pathophysiology of small intestine function and the effect of Crohn's disease. In Allan RN, Keighley MRB, Alexander-Williams J & Hawkins C (eds) *Inflammatory Bowel Disease*, pp 29-42. London: Churchill Livingstone.

Chadwick VS, Modha K & Dowling RH (1973) Mechanism of hyperoxaluria in patients with ileal dysfunction. *N Engl J Med* **289**: 172–176.

Chandler JG, Adams RB, Friedman CJ, Marcella KL & Guerrant RL (1985) Assessment of an implantable ileostomy sphincter. *Surgery* **98**: 72–80.

Chung RS (1986) End colectomy and Brooks' ileostomy constructed by surgical stapler. *Surg Gynecol Obstet* **162**: 63–64.

Clarke AM & McKenzie RG (1969) Ileostomy and the risk of urinary acid stones. *Lancet* **ii**: 395–397.

Clarke AM, Chirnside A, Hill GL & Pope G (1967) Chronic dehydration and sodium depletion with established ileostomies. *Lancet* **ii**: 740–743.

Clifton M (1983) A simple stoma wafer cutter. *Ann R Coll Surg Engl* **65**: 172.

Coe FL (1978) Hyperuricosuric calcium oxalate nephrolithiasis. *Kidney Int* **13**: 418–426.

Cohen S, Kaplan M, Gottlieb C & Patterson J (1971) Liver disease and gall-stones in regional enteritis. *Gastroenterology* **60**: 237–245.

Cohen SE, Matolo NM, Michas CA & Wolfman EF Jr (1975) Antiperistaltic ileal segment in the prevention of ileostomy diarrhoea. *Arch Surg* **110**: 829–832.

Cohen Z, McLeod RS, Stern H, Grant D & Nordgren S (1985) The pelvic pouch and ileoanal anastomosis procedure: surgical technique and initial results. *Ann Surg* **150**: 601–604.

Cooper G, Abel BJ, Hutchinson AG & MacKay C (1982) What length of terminal ileum is required for bile salt absorption? *Gut* **23**: A892–893.

Cooper JC, Laughland A, Gunning EJ, Burkinshaw L & Williams NS (1986a) Body composition in ileostomy patients with and without ileal resection. *Gut* **27**: 680–685.

Cooper JC, Williams NS, King RFGL & Barker MCJ (1986b) Effects of a long-acting somatostatin analogue in patients with severe ileostomy diarrhoea. *Br J Surg* **73**: 128–131.

Cooper MJ, Muckie CR, Dhorajivala J et al (1981) Haemorrhage from ileal varices after total proctocolectomy. *Am J Surg* **141**: 178–179.

Corman ML, Verdenheimer MC & Coller JA (1976) Ileostomy complications: prevention and treatment. *Contemp Surg* **8**: 36–39.

Crawford N & Brooke BN (1957) Ileostomy chemistry. *Lancet* **i**: 864–867.

Crile G Jr & Turnbull RB Jr (1954) The mechanism and prevention of ileostomy dysfunction. *Ann Surg* **140**: 459–465.

Cuthbertson AM & Collins JP (1977) Strangulated para-ileostomy hernia. *Aust NZ J Surg* **47**: 86–87.

Daly DW (1968) The outcome of surgery for UC. *Ann R Coll Surg Engl* **42**: 38–57.

Daly DW & Brooke BN (1967) Ileostomy and excision of the large intestine for UC. *Lancet* **ii**: 62–64.

Daren JJ, Parish JG, Lewitt MF & Khilnani M (1962) Nephrolithiasis as a complication of UC and regional enteritis. *Ann Intern Med* **56**: 843–853.

Delaney JP & Mulholland MW (1983) The temporary intestinal stoma. *Am J Surg* **146**: 668–670.

Devlin HB (1982) Stoma therapy review: II. *Coloproctology* **4**: 250–259.

Devlin HB (1984) Stomas and stoma care. In Bouchier IA, Allan RN, Hodgson H & Keighley MRB (eds) *Textbook of Gastroenterology*, pp 1009–1021. London: Baillière Tindall.

Devlin HB (1986) Invited commentary: quality of life with ileostomy. *World J Surg* **10**: 479–480.

Devlin HB & Plant JA (1975) Disposal of disposable colostomy appliances. *BMJ* **4**: 705.

Devlin HB & Plant JA (1979) Sexual function in aspects of stoma care. *Br J Sex Med* **6**: 33–37.

Devlin HB, Datta D & Dellipiani AW (1980) The incidence and prevalence of IBD in North Tees Health District. *World J Surg* **4**: 183–193.

Dew MJ, Thompson J & Allan RN (1979) The spectrum of hepatic dysfunction in IBD. *Q J Med* **48**: 113–135.

Dharmasthaphorn K, Binder HJ & Dobbins JW (1980) Somatostatin stimulates sodium and chloride adsorption in the rabbit ileum. *Gastroenterology* **78**: 1559–1565.

Dlin BM & Perlman A (1971) Emotional response to ileostomy and colostomy in patients over the age of 50. *Geriatrics* **26**: 113–118.

Dowling RH, Rose GA & Suter DL (1971) Hyperoxaluria and renal calculi in ileal disease. *Lancet* **i**: 1103–1106.

Dowling RH, Bell GD & White J (1972) Lithogenic bile in patients with ileal dysfunction. *Gut* **13**: 415–420.

Dozois RR, Goldberg SM, Rotherberger DA et al (1986) Symposium: restorative proctocolectomy with ileal reservoir. *Colorect Dis* **1**: 2–19.

Dozois RR, Kelly KA, Beart RW Jr & Beahrs OH (1980) Improved results with continent ileostomy. *Am Surg* **192**: 319–324.

Dragstedt LR, Dack GL & Kirsner JB (1941) Chronic UC. *Ann Surg* **114**: 653–662.

Draser BSM, Shiner M & McLeod GM (1969) Studies on the intestinal flora. The bacterial flora of the gastrointestinal tract in healthy and achlorhydric persons. *Gastroenterology* **66**: 71–79.

Eade MH, Williams JA & Cooke WT (1969) Bleeding from the ileostomy caput medusae. *Lancet* **ii**: 1160–1168.

Ecker KW, Hildebrandt U, Haberer M & Feifel G (1996) Biomechanical stabilization of the nipple valve in continent ileostomy. *Br J Surg* **83**: 1582–1585.

Efendic S & Mattsson O (1978) Effect of somatostatin on intestinal motility. *Acta Radiol Diagn* **19**: 348–352.

Ellis H & Coll I (1968) Antiperistaltic segment for profuse diarrhoea. *BMJ* **1**: 556–557.

Ellor JW & Ellor JR (1982) Concerns of the ET in the care of the elderly osteomate: a survey. *J Enterostom Ther* **9**: 14–19.

Ellor JW & Rizzo M. (1978) Aging is *not* a disease: caring for the elderly ostomate. *J Enterostom Ther* **4**: 4–7.

Evans G, Wood RAB & Hughes LE (1976) Comparative trial of two enterostomy sealants. *BMJ* **1**: 1510–1511.

Fallingborg J, Christensen LA, Imgeman-Nielsen M et al (1990) Gastrointestinal pH and transit times in healthy subjects with ileostomy. *Aliment Pharmacol Therap* **4**: 247–253.

Fasth S & Hulten L (1984) Loop ileostomy: a superior diverting stoma in colorectal surgery. *World J Surg* **8**: 401–407.

Fasth S, Filipsson S, Hellberg R, Hulten L, Lindhagen J & Norgren S (1978) Sexual dysfunction following proctocolectomy. *Ann Chir Gynaecol* **67**: 8–12.

Fasth S, Hulten L & Palselius I (1980) Loop ileostomy: an attractive alternative to a temporary transverse colostomy. *Acta Chir Scand* **146**: 203–207.

Fazio VW (1983) Loop ileostomy and loop-end ileostomy. In Dudley H, Pories W & Carter D (eds) *Rob & Smiths Operative Surgery*, 4th edn, pp 54–64. London: Butterworth.

Fazio VW (1984) Invited commentary: loop ileostomy. *World J Surg* **8**: 405–407.

Fazio V, Turnbull RB & Goldsmith MG (1975) Ileorectal anastomosis: a safe surgical technique. *Dis Colon Rectum* **18**: 107–114.

Feinberg SM, McLeod RS & Cohen Z (1987) Complications of loop ileostomy. *Am J Surg* **153**: 102–106.

Feretis CB, Vyssoulis GP, Pararas BM et al (1984) The influence of corticosteroids on ileostomy discharge of patients operated for UC. *Am Surg* **50**: 433–436.

Fleshman JW (1992) Loop ileostomy. *Surg Rounds* **15**: 129–140.

Fonkalsrud EW (1980) Total colectomy and endorectal ileal pull-through with internal ileal reservoir for UC. *Surg Gynecol Obstet* **150**: 1–8.

Fonkalsrud EW (1984) Endorectal ileoanal anastomosis with isoperistaltic ileal reservoir after colectomy and mucosal proctectomy. *Ann Surg* **199**: 151–157.

Fuhrman GM & Ota DM (1994) Laparoscopic intestinal stomas. *Dis Colon Rectum* **37**: 444–449.

Gallagher ND, Harrison DD & Skyring AP (1962) Fluid and electrolyte disturbances in patients with long established ileostomies. *Gut* **3**: 219–223.

Garber HI, Morris DM, Eisenlat TE, Coker DD & Annous MO (1982) Factors influencing the morbidity of colostomy closure. *Dis Colon Rectum* **25**: 464–470.

Gazzard BG, Saunders B & Dawson AM (1978) Diets and stoma function. *Br J Surg* **65**: 642–644.

Gelzayd EA, Brener RI & Kirsner JB (1968) Nephrolithiasis in IBD. *Am J Dig Dis* **13**: 1027–1034.

Gerber A, Apt MK & Craig PH (1984) The improved quality of life with the Kock continent ileostomy. *J Clin Gastroenterol* **6**: 513–517.

Gerich JE & Patton GS (1978) Somatostatin: physiology and clinical applications. *Med Clin North Am* **62**: 375–392.

Goldblatt MC, Corman ML, Haggitt RC, Coller JA & Veidenheimer MC (1977) Ileostomy complications regarding revision: Lahey Clinic experience 1964–1973. *Dis Colon Rectum* **20**: 209–214.

Goldman SL & Rombeau JL (1978) The continent ileostomy: a collective review. *Dis Colon Rectum* **21**: 594–599.

Goldstein AM & Alter EN (1973) Gum karaya. In Whisler RL & Bemiller JN (eds) *Industrial Gums, Polysaccharides and their Derivatives*. New York: Academic Press.

Goligher JC (1958) Extraperitoneal colostomy or ileostomy. *Br J Surg* **46**: 97–103.

Goligher JC (1983a) Proctocolectomy and ileostomy for UC. In Allan RN, Keighley MRB, Alexander-Williams J & Hawkins C (eds) *Inflammatory Bowel Diseases*, pp 247–255. London: Churchill Livingstone.

Goligher JC (1983b) Procedures concerning continence in the surgical management of UC. *Surg Clin North Am* **63**: 49–60.

Goligher JC (1984) *Surgery of the Anus, Rectum and Colon*, 5th edn, p. 912. London: Baillière Tindall.

Goligher JC & Lintott DJ (1975) Experience with 26 reservoir ileostomies. *Br J Surg* **68**: 893–900.

Gore SM, Fontaine O & Pierce NF (1992) Impact of rice based oral rehydration solution on stool output and duration of diarrhoea: meta-analysis of 13 clinical trials. *BMJ* **304**: 287–291.

Graeber GM, Ratner MH & Ackerman MB (1976) Massive haemorrhage from ileostomy and colostomy stomas due to mucocutaneous varices in patients with coexisting cirrhosis. *Surgery* **79**: 107–110.

Gray JDA & Shiner M (1967) Influence of gastric pH on gastric and jejunal flora. *Gut* **8**: 574–581.

Greatorex RA (1988) Simple method of closing a paraileostomy fistula. *Br J Surg* **75**: 543.

Griffen GE, Hodgson HJ & Chadwick VS (1980) Metabolic sequelae of ileostomy. *Clin Sci* **53**: 3–10.

Griffen GE, Fagan EF, Hodgson HJ & Chadwick VS (1982) Enteral therapy in the management of massive gut resection complicated by chronic fluid and electrolyte depletion. *Dig Dis Sci* **27**: 902–908.

Grogan JE & Smith MC (1973) The economic cost of UC: a national estimate for 1968. *Inquiry* **10**: 61–68.

Grossman MC & Nugent FW (1967) Urolithiasis as a complication of chronic diarrhoeal disease. *Am J Dig Dis* **12**: 491–498.

Gruner OPN, Nass R, Flatmark A, Fretnein B & Gjone E (1976) Ileostomy in UC: results in 149 patients. *Scand J Gastroenterol* **11**: 777–784.

Gruner OPN, Nass R, Fretheim B & Gjone E (1977) Marital status and sexual adjustment after colectomy. Results in 178 patients operated on for UC. *Scand J Gastroenterol* **12**: 193–197.

Gutman AB & Yu T (1968) Uric acid nephrolithiasis. *Am J Med* **45**: 756–779.

Hamlyn AN, Lanzer MR, Morris JS et al (1974) Portal hypertension with varices in unusual sites. *Lancet* **ii**: 1531–1534.

Harper PH, Kettlewell MGW & Lee ECG (1982) The effect of split ileostomy on perianal Crohn's disease. *Br J Surg* **69**: 608–610.

Harper PH, Truelove SC, Lee EGC, Kettlewell MGW & Jewell DP (1983) Split-ileostomy and ileo-colostomy for Crohn's disease of the colon and UC. *Gut* **24**: 106–113.

Hasegawa H, Radley S, Morton DG & Keighley MRB (1999) Randomised trial of stapled vs sutured closure of loop ileostomy (final results) Accepted for presentation, Tripartite Meeting of American Society of Colorectal Surgeons, Washington, USA. 1–6 May, 1999.

Hawley PR & Ritchie JK (1979) Complications of ileostomy and colostomy following excisional surgery. *Clin Gastroenterol* **8**: 403–414.

Heaton KW & Read AE (1969) Gallstones in patients with disorders of the terminal ileum and disturbed bile salt metabolism. *BMJ* **3**: 494–496.

Hellman J & Lago CP (1990) Dermatologic complications in colostomy and ileostomy patients. *Int J Dermatol* **29**: 129.

Hershman MF, Kiff RS (1997) The role of laparoscopy. In Allan RN, Rhodes JM, Hanauer SB, Keighley MRB, Alexander-Williams J & Fazio VW (eds) *Inflammatory Bowel Diseases*, 2nd edn, pp 717–726. London: Churchill Livingstone.

Heuman R, Sjodahl R, Tobiasson C & Tagesson C (1982) Postprandial serum bile acids in resected and non-resected patients with Crohn's disease. *Scand J Gastroenterol* **17**: 137–140.

Hill GL (1976) *Ileostomy: Surgery, Physiology and Management*. New York: Grune & Stratton.

Hill GL & Pickford IR (1979) A new appliance for collecting ileostomy and jejunostomy fluid in the postoperative period. *Br J Surg* **66**: 203–206.

Hill GL, Mair WSJ & Goligher JC (1974) Impairment of ileostomy adaptation in patients after ileal resection. *Gut* **15**: 982–987.

Hill GL, Mair WS & Goligher JC (1975a) Cause and management of high volume output salt-depleting ileostomy. *Br J Surg* **62**: 720–726.

Hill GL, Goligher JC, Smith AH & Mair WSJ (1975b) Long-term changes in total body water, total exchangeable sodium and total body potassium before and after ileostomy. *Br J Surg* **62**: 524–527.

Hill GL, Mair WSJ & Goligher JC (1975c) Gallstones after ileostomy and ileal resection. *Gut* **16**: 932–936.

Hill GL, Millward SF, King RFG & Smith RC (1979) Normal ileostomy output: close relation to body size. *BMJ* **4**: 831–832.

Hoffman AF, Thomas PJ, Smith LH et al (1970) Pathogenesis of secondary hyperoxaluria in patients with ileal resection and diarrhoea. *Gastroenterology* **58**: 960.

Hosie KB, Grobler SP & Keighley MRB (1992) Temporary loop ileostomy following restorative proctocolectomy. *Br J Surg* **79**: 33–34.

Hudson CN (1972) Ileostomy in pregnancy. *Proc R Soc Med* **65**: 281–283.

Hudson CN & Lennard-Jones JE (1978) Sexual relationships and childbirth. In Todd IP (ed.) *Intestinal Stomas*. London: Heinemann.

Hughes ESR & Russell IS (1967) Ileorectal anastomosis for UC. *Dis Colon Rectum* **10**: 35–39.

Huibregtse K, Hock F, Sanders GTB & Tytgat GNJ (1977) Bile acid metabolism in ileostomy patients. *Eur J Clin Invest* **7**: 137–140.

Hull TL, Kobe I & Fazio VW (1996) Comparison of handsewn with stapled loop ileostomy closures. *Dis Colon Rectum* **39**: 1086–1089.

Hulten L & Fasth S (1981) Loop ileostomy for protection of the newly constructed ileostomy reservoir. *Br J Surg* **68**: 11–13.

Hulten L, Kewenter J & Kock NG (1976) Komplikationen der Ileostomie und Colostomie und ihre Behandlung. *Chirurg* **47**: 16–21.

Iroatulam AJ, Potenti F, Oliveira L & Wexner SD (1998) Laparoscopic versus conventional open stoma creation. *Int J Colorectal Dis* (submitted).

Irvine EJ, Feagan B, Rochon J, Archambault A, Fedorak RN, Groll A, Kinnear D, Saibil F & McDonald JWD (1994) Quality of life: a valid and reliable measure of therapeutic efficacy in the treatment of inflammatory bowel disease. *Gastroenterology* 106: 287–296.

Irving MH, Hulme O (1992) Intestinal stomas. *BMJ* **304**: 1679–1781.

Isaacs PET, Horth CE & Turnberg LA (1976) The electrical potential difference across human ileostomy mucosa. *Gastroenterology* **70**: 52–58.

Jagenburg R, Dotevall G, Kewenter J, Kock NG & Philipson B (1971) Absorption studies in patients with intra-abdominal ileostomy reservoirs and in patients with conventional ileostomies. *Gut* **12**: 437–441.

Javett SE & Brooke BN (1971) Reversed ileal segment for ileostomy diarrhoea. *Lancet* **i**: 291.

Jeffries GH, Weser E & Slensenger MH (1969) Malabsorption. *Gastroenterology* **56**: 777–797.

Jess P & Christiansen J (1994) Laparoscopic loop ileostomy for fecal diversion. *Dis Colon Rectum* **37**: 721–722.

Jhittay PS & Obeid ML (1986) Ileostomy in situ. *Surg Gynecol Obstet* **162**: 587–588.

Johansson C, Efendic S, Wisen O, Uvnas-Wallensten K & Luft R (1978) Effects of short-time somatostatin infusion on the gastric and intestinal propulsions in humans. *Scand J Gastroenterol* **13**: 481–483.

Johnson GW (1969) A modification in the perineal dissection in excision of the rectum in females. *Br J Surg* **56**: 530–532.

Johnson GW (1979) The results of vaginoplasty in excision of the rectum. *Br J Surg* **66**: 628–629.

Jones MR, Evans GKT & Rhodes J (1976) The prevalence of gallbladder disease in patients with ileostomy. *Clin Radiol* **27**: 561–562.

Jones PF, Munro A & Ewan SWB (1977) Colectomy and ileorectal anastomosis for colitis: report on a personal series, with a critical review. *Br J Surg* **64**: 615–623.

Kanaghinis T, Lubran M & Cogbill NF (1963) The composition of ileostomy fluid. *Gut* **4**: 322–338.

Kayasseh L, Gyr K, Stalder GA, Rittman WW & Girard J (1978) Effect of somatostatin on exocrine pancreatic secretion stimulated by pancreozymin secretion or by a test meal in the dog. *J Surg Res* **9**: 176–184.

Kelly DG, Branon ME, Phillips SF & Kelly KA (1980) Diarrhoea after continent ileostomy. *Gut* **21**: 711–716.

Kennedy HJ, Lee EGS, Claridge G & Truelove SC (1982a) The health of subjects living with a permanent ileostomy. *Q J Med* **203**: 341–357.

Kennedy HJ, Callender ST, Truelove SC & Warner GT (1982b) Haematological aspects of life with an ileostomy. *Br J Haematol* **52**: 445–454.

Kennedy HJ, Fletcher EWL & Truelove SC (1982c) Urinary stones in subjects with a permanent ileostomy. *Br J Surg* **69**: 661–664.

Kennedy HJ, Al-Dujaili EAS, Edwards CRW & Truelove SC (1983) Water and electrolyte balance in subjects with a permanent ileostomy. *Gut* **24**: 702–705.

Khoo REH, Montrey J & Cohen MM (1993) Laparoscopic loop ileostomy for temporary fecal diversion. *Dis Colon Rectum* **36**: 966–968.

Khoury GA et al (1986) Colostomy or ileostomy after colorectal anastomosis? A randomized trial. *Ann R Coll Surg Engl* **68**: 5–7.

Knox AJS, Birkett FOH & Collins CD (1971) Closure of colostomy. *Br J Surg* **58**: 669–672.

Kock NG, Myrvold HE, Nilsson LO & Philipson BM (1981) Continent ileostomy. *Acta Chir Scand* **147**: 67–72.

Kraenzlin ME, Chng JLC, Wood SM & Bloom SR (1984) Remission of symptoms and shrinkage of metastasis with long term treatment with somatostatin analogue. *Gut* **25**: A576.

Kramer P (1966) The effect of varying sodium loads on the ileal excreta of human ileostomized subjects. *J Clin Invest* **45**: 1710–1718.

Kramer P, Kearney MM & Ingelfinger FJ (1962) The effect of specific foods and water loading on the ileal excreta of ileostomized human subjects. *Gastroenterology* **42**: 535–546.

Kurchin A, Ray JE, Bluth EI et al (1984) Cholelithiasis in ileostomy patients. *Dis Colon Rectum* **27**: 585–588.

Kusunoki M, Yanagi H, Shoji Y & Yamamura T (1996) Modification of the stapled functional end-to-end anastomosis for ileostomy closure. *Jpn J Surg* **26**: 1033–1035.

Kyle EM & Hughes ESR (1970) Peristomal skin protection with 'Orahesive'. *Med J Aust* **2**: 186–187.

Ladas, SD, Isaacs PET, Murphy GM & Sladen GE (1986) Fasting and postprandial ileal function in adapted ileostomates and normal subjects. *Gut* **27**: 906–912.

Lange V, Meyer G, Schardey HM & Schildberg FW (1991) Laparoscopic creation of loop colostomy. *J Laparoendosc Surg* **5**: 307–312.

Langman MJS & Burnham WR (1983) Epidemiology of IBD. In Allan RN, Keighley MRB, Alexander-Williams J & Hawkins C (eds) *Inflammatory Bowel Disease*, pp 17–23. London: Churchill Livingstone.

Larkin K & Fazio VW (1980) Closure of loop ileostomy. VIIIth Biennial Congress of the International Society of Colon and Rectal Surgeons 10 September, Melbourne.

Larusso MF, Wiesner RH, Ludwig J et al (1984) Primary sclerosing cholangitis. *N Engl J Med* **310**: 899–903.

Law DH, Sernberg H & Slesinger MH (1961) UC with onset after the age of fifty. *Gastroenterology* **41**: 457–464.

Lee E (1975) Split ileostomy in the treatment of Crohn's disease of the colon. *Ann R Coll Surg Engl* **56**: 94–102.

Lee ECG & Dowling BL (1972) Perimuscular excision of the rectum for Crohn's disease and UC. *Br J Surg* **59**: 29–32.

Lee ECG & Truelove SC (1980) Proctocolectomy for UC. *World J Surg* **4**: 195–201.

Leenn LP & Kuypers JH (1989) Some factors influencing the outcome of stoma surgery. *Dis Colon Rectum* **32**: 500–504.

Leicester RJ, Ritchie JK, Wadsworth J, Thomson JPS & Hawley PR (1984) Sexual function and perineal wound healing after intersphincteric excision of the rectum for IBD. *Dis Colon Rectum* **27**: 244–248.

Lennenberg E & Rowbotham J (1970) *The Ileostomy Patient*. Springfield, IL: CC Thomas.

Lenz K (1976) Bile acid metabolism and vitamin B_{12} absorption in UC. *Scand J Gastroenterol* **11**: 769–775.

Leong APK, London-Schimmer E, Phillips RKS (1994) Life table analysis of stoma complications following ileostomy. *Br J Surg* **81**: 727–729.

Leslie D (1984) The parastomal hernia. *Surg Clin North Am* **64**: 407–415.

Le Veen HH, Lyons A & Becker E (1962) Physiological adaption to ileostomy. *Am J Surg* **103**: 35–43.

Lewis P, Warren BF & Bartolo DCC (1990) Massive gastrointestinal haemorrhage due to ileal varices. *Br J Surg* **77**: 1277–1278.

Lubbers EJC & Devlin HB (1984) The complications of a permanent ileostomy. Poster. 8th World Congress of the Colleginan Internationale Chirurgiae Digestivae 11–14 September, Amsterdam.

Ludwig KA, Milsom JW, Garcia-Ruiz A & Fazio VW (1996) Laparoscopic fecal diversion. *Dis Colon Rectum* **39**: 285–288.

Luchtefeld MA & MacKeigan JM (1997) Laparoscopic assisted colostomy. In Jager R & Wexner SD (eds) *Laparoscopic Colorectal Surgery*, pp 228–233. New York: Churchill Livingstone.

Lyerly HK & Mautt JR (1994) Laparoscopic ileostomy and colostomy. *Ann Surg* **219**: 317–322.

Lytle JA & Parks AG (1977) Intersphincteric excision of rectum. *Br J Surg* **64**: 413–416.

Malt RA, Bartlett MK & Wheelock FC (1984) Subcutaneous fasciotomy for relief of stricture of the ileostomy. *Surg Gynecol Obstet* **159**: 175–176.

Maratka Z & Nedbal J (1964) Urolithiasis as a complication of the surgical treatment of UC. *Gut* **5**: 214–217.

Marks R, Evans E & Clarke TK (1978) The effects on normal skin of adhesives from stoma appliances. *Curr Med Res Opin* **5**: 720–725.

Matolo NM & Wolfman EF Jr (1976) Reversed ileal segment for treatment of ileostomy dysfunction. *Arch Surg* **11**: 891–892.

Maton PN, O'Dorisio TM, Howe BA et al (1985) Effect of a long acting somatostatin analogue (SMS 201-995) in a patient with pancreatic cholera. *N Engl J Med* **312**: 17–21.

McIlrath DC (1971) Diverting ileostomy or colostomy in the management of Crohn's disease of the colon. *Arch Surg* **103**: 308–310.

McLeod RS & Fazio VW (1984) Quality of life with the continent ileostomy. *World J Surg* **8**: 90–95.

McLeod RS, Lavery IC, Leatherman JR et al (1985) Patient evaluation. *Dis Colon Rectum* **28**: 152–154.

McLeod RS, Lavery IC, Leatherman JR et al (1986) Factors affecting quality of life with a conventional ileostomy. *World J Surg* **10**: 474–480.

Meguid MM, McIvor A & Xenos L (1997) Creation of a neoabdominal wall to facilitate emergency placement of a terminal ileostomy in a morbidly obese patient. *Am J Surg* **173**: 298–300.

Metcalf AM, Dozois RR, Kelly KA, Beart RW & Wolff BC (1985) Ileal 'J' pouch–anal anastomosis; clinical outcome. *Ann Surg* **202**: 735–739.

Metcalf AM, Dozois RR, Beart RW Jr, Kelly KA & Wolff BG (1986a) Temporary ileostomy for ileal pouch–anal anastomosis: function and complications. *Dis Colon Rectum* **29**: 300–303.

Metcalf AM, Dozois RR, Kelly KA & Wolff BG (1986b) Ileal pouch–anal anastomosis without temporary diverting ileostomy. *Dis Colon Rectum* **29**: 33–35.

Meyers WC, Hanks JB & Jones RS (1979) Inhibition of basal and meal stimulated choleresis by somatostatin. *Surgery* **86**: 301–306.

Miettinen TA & Peltokallio P (1971) Bile salt, fat, water and vitamin B_{12} excretion after ileostomy. *Scand J Gastroenterol* **6**: 543–552.

Miller GG, Gardner CMcG & Ripstein CB (1949) Primary resection of the colon in UC. *Can Med Assoc J* **60**: 584–585.

Mirelman D, Corman ML, Veidenheimer MC et al (1978) Colostomies: indications and contraindications. Lahey Clinic experience 1963–1974. *Dis Colon Rectum* **21**: 172–176.

Modlin M (1967) The aetiology of renal stones: a new concept arising from studies of a stone free population. *Ann R Coll Surg Engl* **40**: 155–178.

Moody GA & Mayberry JF (1996) Life insurance and inflammatory bowel disease: is there discrimination against patients? *Int J Colorect Dis* **11**: 276–278.

Morowitz DA & Kirsner JB (1981) Ileostomy in UC: a questionnaire study of 1803 patients. *Am J Surg* **141**: 370–375.

Mosquera DA, Walker SJ & McFarland JB (1988) Bleeding stomal varices treated by sclerotherapy. *J R Coll Surg Edinb* **33**: 337.

Mullen P, Behrens D, Chalmers T, Berkey C, Paris M, Wynn M, Fabito D, Gaskin R, Hughes T, Schiller D, Veninga F, Vilar P & Pollack J (1995) Barnett continent intestinal reservoir. *Dis Colon Rectum* **38**: 573–582.

Neal DE, Williams NS, Barker M and King RFGL (1984) The effect of resection of the distal ileum on gastric emptying and small bowel transit and absorption after proctocolectomy. *Br J Surg* **71**: 666–670.

Newton CR (1978) Effect of codeine phosphate, Lomotil and Isogel on ileostomy function. *Gut* **19**: 377–383.

Newton CR, Gonvers JJ, McIntyre PB, Preseton DM & Lennard-Jones JE (1985) Effects of different drinks on fluid and electrolyte losses from a jejunostomy. *J R Soc Med* **78**: 27–34.

Nicholls RJ & Pezim ME (1984) Restorative proctocolectomy with ileal reservoir: a comparison between the three loop and two loop reservoir. *Dis Colon Rectum* **27**: 565 (abstract).

Nightingale JMD, Lennard-Jones JE, Walker ER & Farthing MJG (1992) Oral salt supplements to compensate for jejunostomy losses: comparison of sodium chloride capsules, glucose electrolyte solution, and glucose polymer electrolyte solution. *Gut* **33**: 759–761

Nilsson LO, Andersson H, Hulten L et al (1979) Absorption studies in patients six to ten years after construction of ileostomy reservoirs. *Gut* **20**: 499–503.

Nilsson LO, Kock NG, Klyberg F, Myrvold H & Palsilius I (1981) Sexual adjustment in ileostomy patients before and after conversion to a continent ileostomy. *Dis Colon Rectum* **24**: 287–290.

Nilsson LO, Andersson H, Bosalus P & Myrvold HE (1982) Total body water and total potassium in patients with continent ileostomies. *Gut* **23**: 589–593.

Nuguid TP, Bacon HE & Boulwell J (1961) An investigation of the volume of output and chemical content of ileal discharges following total colectomy and ileostomy. *Surg Gynecol Obstet* **113**: 733–742.

Office of Population Censuses and Surveys (1970) *Report on Hospital Inpatient Enquiry for the Year 1967. 1: Tables*. London: HMSO.

Oliveira L, Reissman P, Nogueras JJ & Wexner SD (1997) Laparoscopic creation of stomas. *Surg Endosc* **11**: 19–23.

Orangio GR, Bronsther B, Abrams M & Wise L (1984) A new type of continent ileostomy. *Dis Colon Rectum* **27**: 238–243.

Parks AG & Nicholls J (1978) Proctocolectomy without ileostomy for UC. *BMJ* **1**: 85–88.

Pearl RK, Prasad ML, Orsay CP, Abcarian H, Tao AB & Melzl MT (1985) Early complications from intestinal stomas. *Arch Surg* **120**: 1145–1147.

Peck JJ & Boyden AM (1985) Exigent ileostomy hemorrhage: a complication of proctocolectomy in patients with chronic UC and primary sclerosing cholangitis. *Am J Surg* **150**: 153–158.

Pemberton JH (1988) Management of conventional ileostomies. *World J Surg* **12**: 203–210.

Phillips R, Pringle W, Evans C & Keighley MRB (1985) Analysis of a hospital-based stomatherapy service. *Ann R Coll Surg Engl* **67**: 37–40.

Prasad ML, Pearl RK, Orsay CP & Abcarian H (1984) Rodless ileostomy: a modified loop ileostomy. *Dis Colon Rectum* **27**: 270–271.

Prien EL & Prien EL Jr (1968) Composition and structure of urinary stones. *Am J Med* **45**: 654–672.

Raimes SA, Mathew VV & Devlin HB (1984) Temporary loop ileostomy. *J R Soc Med* **77**: 738–741.

Resnick RH, Ishihara A, Chalmers TC et al (1968) A controlled trial of colon bypass in chronic hepatic encephalopathy. *Gastroenterology* **54**: 1057–1069.

Ricci RL, Lee KR & Greenberger NJ (1980) Chronic gastrointestinal bleeding from ileal varices after total proctocolectomy for UC: correction of mesocaval shunt. *Gastroenterology* **78**: 1053–1058.

Ritchie KJ (1971) Ileostomy and excisional surgery of chronic inflammatory disease of the colon: a survey of one hospital region. II: The health of ileostomists. *Gut* **12**: 536–540.

Roe AM, Barlow AP, Durdey P, Eltringham WK & Espiner HJ (1994) Indications for laparoscopic formation of intestinal stomas. *Surg Laparosc Endosc* **4**: 345–347.

Rombeau JL, Wilk PJ, Turnbull RB Jr & Fazio VW (1978) Total fecal diversion by the temporary skin-level loop transverse colostomy. *Dis Colon Rectum* **21**: 223–226.

Romero CA, James KM, Cooperstone LM, Mishrick AS & Ger R (1992) Laparoscopic sigmoid colostomy for perianal Crohn's disease. *Surg Laparosc Endosc* **2**: 148–151.

Rosin JD & Bonardi RA (1977) Paracolostomy hernia repair with Marlex mesh. *Dis Colon Rectum* **20**: 299–302.

Rothernberger DA, Vermeulen FD, Christenson CE et al (1983) Restorative proctocolectomy with ileal reservoir and ileoanal anastomosis. *Am J Surg* **145**: 82–87.

Rowbotham JL (1981) Stomal care. *N Engl J Med* **279**: 90–92.

Roy PH, Sauer WG, Beahrs OH & Farrow GM (1970) Experiences with ileostomies. Evaluation of long term rehabilitation in 497 patients. *Am J Surg* **119**: 77–86.

Ruskone A, Rene E, Chayvialle JA et al (1982) Effect of somatostatin on diarrhoea and on small intestine water and electrolyte transport in a patient with pancreatic cholera. *Dig Dis Sci* **27**: 459–466.

Sako K & Blackman DE (1962) The use of a reversed jejunal segment after massive resection of the small bowel. *Am J Surg* **103**: 202–205.

Salmon R, Block P & Loygue J (1980) Magnetic closure of a reservoir ileostomy. *Dis Colon Rectum* **23**: 242–243.

Sanada Y, Foutalsand EW & Kojima Y (1982) Intermittent ileostomy occlusion for fecal storage using balloon catheter. *Surgery* **91**: 459–466.

Sandei F, Terranova O, Rebuffat C, Settembrine PG, Fiore D & Bortolozzi F (1979) Continent ileostomy: a new technique in the dog. *Dis Colon Rectum* **22**: 87–92.

Schiller WR, Didio LJA & Anderson MC (1967) Production of artificial sphincters. Ablation of the longitudinal layer of the intestine. *Arch Surg* **95**: 436–442.

Scott R, Freeland R, Mowat W et al (1977) The prevalence of calcified urinary tract stone disease in a random population: Cumbernauld Health Survey. *Br J Urol* **49**: 589–595.

Shepard D (1966) Antiperistaltic bowel segment in the treatment of the short bowel syndrome. *Ann Surg* **163**: 850–855.

Shirley F, Kodner IJ & Fry RD (1984) Loop ileostomy: technique and indications. *Dis Colon Rectum* **27**: 382–386.

Singer AM, Bennett RC, Carter NG & Hughes ESR (1973) Blood and urinary changes in patients with ileostomies and ileorectal anastomosis. *BMJ* **3**: 141–143.

Smiddy FH, Gregory SD, Smith IB & Goligher JC (1960) Faecal loss of fluid, electrolytes and nitrogen in colitis before and after ileostomy. *Lancet* **i**: 14–19.

Smith MJV, Hunt LD, King JS et al (1969) Uricaemia and urolithiasis. *J Urol* **101**: 637–642.

Sohn N, Schulman N, Weinstein MA & Robbins RD (1983) Ileostomy prolapse repair utilizing bidirectional myotomy and a meshed split-thickness skin graft. *Am J Surg* **145**: 807–808.

Speakman CTM, Parker MC & Northover JMA (1991) Outcome

of stapled revision of retracted ileostomy. *Br J Surg* **78**: 935–936.

Spiller RC, Trotman IF, Higgins BE et al (1984) The ileal brake: inhibition of jejunal motility after ileal fat perfusion in man. *Gut* **25**: 365–374.

Stacchini A, Didio LJA, Primo MLS et al (1982) Artificial sphincters as surgical treatment for experimental massive resection of small intestine. *Am J Surg* **143**: 721–726.

Steinberg DM, Allan RN, Brooke BN, Cooke WT & Alexander-Williams J (1975) Sequelae of colectomy and ileostomy: comparison between Crohn's colitis and UC. *Gastroenterology* **68**: 33–39.

Strauss AA & Strauss SF (1944) Surgical treatment of UC. *Surg Clin North Am* **24**: 211–224.

Stryker SJ, Pemberton JH & Zinsmeister AR (1985) Long term results of ileostomy in older patients. *Dis Colon Rectum* **28**: 844–846.

Taylor RL, Rombeau JL & Turnbull RB (1978) Transperitoneal relocation of the ileal stoma without formal laparotomy. *Surg Gynecol Obstet* **146**: 953–958.

Telender RL & Perrault J (1980) Total colectomy with rectal mucosectomy and ileoanal anastomosis for chronic UC in children and young adults. *Mayo Clin Proc* **55**: 420–425.

Teoh T-A, Reissman P, Cohen SM, Weiss EG & Wexner SD (1994) Laparoscopic loop ileostomy (letter). *Dis Colon Rectum* **37**: 514.

Thomson TJ, Runce J & Khan A (1970) The effect of diet on ileostomy functions. *Gut* **11**: 482–485.

Todd IP (1978) *Intestinal Stomas*. London: Heinemann.

Todd IP (1982) Mechanical complications of ileostomy. *Clin Gastroenterol* **11**: 268–273.

Todd IP (1983) The resolution of stoma problems. In Allan RN, Keighley MRB, Alexander-Williams J & Hawkins C (eds) *Inflammatory Bowel Disease*, pp 256–261. London: Churchill Livingstone.

Turnberg LA, Morris AI, Hawker PC, Herman KJ, Shields RA & Horth CE (1978) Intracellular electrolyte depletion in patients with ileostomies. *Gut* **19**: 563–568.

Turnbull RB Jr (1961) Instructions to ileostomy patient: use and care of the ileostomy appliance. *Cleve Clin Q* **28**: 213–228.

Turnbull RB (1971) Surgical treatment of toxic megacolon: ileostomy and colostomy to prepare patients for colectomy. *Am J Surg* **122**: 325–331.

Turnbull RB (1975) The surgical approach to the treatment of IBD: a personal view of techniques and prognosis. In Kirsner JB & Shorter RG (eds) *Inflammatory Bowel Disease*. Philadelphia: Lea & Febiger.

Turnbull RB & Weekley FL (1966) Ileostomy techniques and indications for surgery. *Rev Surg Year Book* 310–314.

Turnbull RB & Weekley FL (1967) *An Atlas of Intestinal Stomas*, p. 97. St Louis: CV Mosby.

Tytgat GN & Huibregtse K (1975) Loperamide and ileostomy output: placebo controlled double-blind crossover study. *BMJ* **2**: 667.

Tytgat GN, Huibregtse K & Mevwissen SGM (1976) Loperamide in chronic diarrhoea and after ileostomy. *Arch Surg Neer Pandicum* **28**: 13–20.

Unti JA, Abcarian H, Pearl RK et al (1991) Rodless end-loop stomas. *Dis Colon Rectum* **34**: 999–1004.

Utley RJ & Macbeth WAAG (1984) The split ileostomy. *J R Coll Surg Edinb* **29**: 93–95.

Vantrappen G, Janseens J, Hellemans J & Ghoos Y (1977) The interdigestive motor complex of normal subjects and patients with bacterial overgrowth of the small intestine. *J Clin Invest* **59**: 1158–1166.

Ward K, Murray B, Feighery C, Neale G & Weir DG (1981) Salt losing ileostomy diarrhoea: long term treatment with a glucose electrolyte solution. *Gut* **22**: A864 (T8).

Warren R & McKittrick LS (1951) Ileostomy for UC: technique, complications and management. *Surg Gynecol Obstet* **93**: 555–567.

Watts JMcK, De Dombal FT & Goligher JC (1966) Long term complications and prognosis following major surgery for UC. *Br J Surg* **53**: 1014–1023.

Weaver RM, Alexander-Williams J & Keighley MRB (1988) Indications and outcome of reoperations for ileostomy complications in inflammatory bowel disease. *Int J Colorectal Dis* **3**: 38–42.

Wexner SD, Taranow DA, Johansen OB, Itzkowitz F, Daniel N, Nogueras JJ, Jagelman DG (1993) Loop ileostomy is a safe option for fecal diversion. *Dis Colon Rectum* **36**: 349–354.

Whates PD & Irving M (1984) Return to work following ileostomy. *Br J Surg* **71**: 619–622.

Whittaker M & Goligher JC (1976) A comparison of the results of extraperitoneal and intraperitoneal techniques for construction of terminal iliac colostomies. *Dis Colon Rectum* **19**: 342–344.

Wilkinson AJ & Humphreys (1978) Seatbelt injury to ileostomy. *BMJ* **3**: 1249.

Williams JG, Etherington R, Hayward MWJ & Hughes LE (1990) Paraileostomy hernia: a clinical and radiological study. *Br J Surg* **77**: 1355–1357.

Williams NS, Cooper JC, Axon ATR, King RFGJ & Barker M (1984) Use of a long-acting somatostatin analogue in controlling life threatening ileostomy diarrhoea. *BMJ* **4**: 1027–1028.

Williams NS, Masmyth DG, Jones D & Smith AH (1986) Defunctioning stomas: a prospective controlled trial comparing loop ileostomy with loop transverse colostomy. *Br J Surg* **73**: 566–570.

Wilson E (1964) The rehabilitation of patients with an ileostomy established for UC. *Med J Aust* **1**: 842–844.

Winslet M (1986) Loop ileostomy for Crohn's colitis. Proceedings of the World Congress of Gastroenterology, September, San Paulo.

Winslet MC, Alexander-Williams J & Keighley MRB (1990) Ileostomy revision with a GIA stapler under intravenous sedation. *Br J Surg* **77**: 647.

Winslet MC, Kmiot W & Keighley MRB (1991a) The complications of a loop ileostomy after ileal pouch anal anastomosis. *Dis Colon Rectum* **34**: 1–18.

Winslet MC et al (1991b) Assessment of the defunctioning efficiency of the loop ileostomy. *Dis Colon Rectum* **34**: 699–703.

Wood SM, Kraenzlin ME & Bloom SR (1983) New somatostatin analogue for home treatment of endocrine tumours. *Gut* **24**: A984–985.

Wright HK (1979) Improving transverse colostomy function. *Am J Surg* **137**: 475–477.

Wrong OM (1970) Disorders of the gastrointestinal tract. In Thompson RHS & Wootton IDP (eds) *Biochemical Disorders in Human Disease*, pp 661–688. London: Churchill Livingstone.

Wyke RJ, Edwards FC and Allan RN (1988) Employment problems and prospects for patients with inflammatory bowel disease. *Gut* **29**: 1229–1235.

Yaque S (1986) A new technique for temporary transparietocecal ileal diversion in the prevention of anastomotic leakage in colonic operations. *Surg Gynecol Obstet* **162**: 381–382.

Zeiderman MR, Cooper JC, Williams NS & McMahon MJ (1985) Nutritional status of apparently healthy ileostomy patients. *Br J Surg* **72**: 409.

Zelas P & Jagelman DG (1980) Loop ileostomy in the management of Crohn's colitis in the debilitated patient. *Ann Surg* **191**: 164–168.

9

COLOSTOMY

A colostomy may be permanent or temporary. A permanent colostomy may be constructed for patients with low rectal cancer, anorectal inflammatory bowel disease, persistent incontinence despite attempted surgical correction, neurological disorders or anorectal agenesis. The risk of restoring intestinal continuity may be so high, or the functional results considered to be so poor in some patients, that a stoma initially planned to be temporary may have to become permanent.

Many colostomies are temporary: to protect a distal anastomosis, to bypass severe anorectal sepsis, to manage colorectal trauma, or to decompress large bowel obstruction. Temporary colostomies are usually loop stomas or an end colostomy if a Hartmann resection is performed for emergency resection (Devlin, 1990; Mealy et al, 1996).

Two or three decades ago it was estimated that there were approximately 100 000 patients with a colostomy in the UK (Jones, 1956; Office of Population Censuses and Surveys, 1970; Griffiths et al, 1976). In 1966 over 7600 patients were diagnosed as having a rectal carcinoma; of whom over two-thirds underwent abdominoperineal excision of the rectum (Doran and Hardcastle, 1981). Similarly in the United States, colorectal cancer annually affects 46.5 males per 100 000 inhabitants and 332 females per 100 000, of whom approximately half have rectosigmoid cancer where over half were being treated by constructing a permanent colostomy. The present position is now quite the reverse, although the disease incidence is unchanged (Parkin et al, 1992); fewer than 10% of patients with rectal cancer referred to specialist units have a permanent stoma (Heald and Leicester, 1981; Beart and Wolff, 1982; Blamey and Lee, 1982; Lazorthes and Chiotassal, 1986; Finan, 1987; Dixon et al, 1991; Lewis et al, 1992; Karanjia et al, 1992; Pelissier et al, 1992). In the USA, abdominoperineal excision is performed in approximately 50 000 patients each year (Mazier et al, 1976). Furthermore on both sides of the Atlantic the number of permanent stomas for diverticular disease has fallen considerably in the last 30 years (Khan et al, 1994; Khoury et al, 1996)

Colostomy carries with it a high social and psychological morbidity (White and Hunt, 1997). Physical complications from leakage, odour and noise are common (Sprangers et al, 1995). Revisional procedures may be needed for parastomal hernia, prolapse, obstruction, stricture, fistula retraction or chronic sepsis (Londono-Schimmer et al, 1994). Restoration of bowel continuity after Hartmann resection is attended by the risk of anastomotic leakage, sepsis, fistula and imperfect continence. Even closure of a loop colostomy may be complicated by sepsis, fistula and incisional hernia.

HISTORY

The first record of a colostomy was in 1710 by Littre for an obstructing colonic carcinoma managed by an iliac fossa stoma (Bryant, 1882). Cheselden (1784) later recorded a spontaneous colostomy due to a strangulated umbilical hernia which sloughed, leaving the colon protruding through the umbilicus; this patient survived. Later, colostomy was introduced for relief of intestinal obstruction in children with rectal agenesis, but not all were successful (Duret, 1789; Allan, 1797). Management of battle injuries involving the colon by exteriorization was sometimes associated with long-term survival (Heister, 1743). Some exteriorized loops closed spontaneously (Le Dran, 1781; Larrey, 1823). Extraperitoneal colostomy was devised by Amussat (1839) to reduce the high mortality from peritonitis which occurred following intraperitoneal colostomy. However, retroperitoneal flank colostomy was difficult to manage and stricture was common. In 1884, Maydl revived the practice of intraperitoneal loop colostomy using a goose quill to support the stoma (Devlin and Plant, 1969). Allingham (1887) sutured the seromuscular layer of the colon to the abdominal wall to prevent retraction before opening the antimesenteric surface of the bowel. Surprisingly, immediate colocutaneous suture was not commonly practised until 1950 (Patey, 1951). Although extraperitoneal end colostomy was popularized again by Sames (1958) and Goligher (1958), and may reduce the risk of stomal hernia (Martin and Foster, 1996), intraperitoneal colostomy is now usually regarded as the optimum form of end colostomy (Londono-Schimmer et al, 1994).

INDICATIONS

End colostomy

Permanent colostomy

The principal indication for abdominoperineal excision and an end colostomy is for the treatment of a rectal cancer which is either too low or too bulky to be suitable for restorative resection. Advanced low rectal neoplasms, particularly those that are fixed and which have been treated initially by radiotherapy, may require treatment by abdominoperineal excision (Miller and Allbritten, 1976; Fitzgibbons et al, 1977; Nicholls et al, 1979; Williams, 1984). In some patients with rectal carcinoma the functional results of anterior resection are judged to be so poor that restorative resection is not advised (see Chapter 32). In a few well-selected patients, total anorectal reconstruction with or without a colonic conduit may avoid a permanent stoma for favourable low rectal cancer (Abercrombie and Williams, 1995; Hughes and Williams, 1995; Cavina, 1996; Mander et al, 1996).

Severe anorectal Crohn's disease may be treated by rectal excision (Williams et al, 1979); but there is a risk of recurrence in the proximal colon and a rather wet flush colostomy (see Chapter 57). Some patients with high defects from anorectal agenesis may decide to have a permanent end colostomy (see Chapter 72). Severe perirectal sepsis from trauma or previous surgery may sometimes be managed by total anorectal excision and end colostomy (see Chapter 61). Similarly, some patients with faecal incontinence may be best served by a permanent colostomy (see Chapter 21).

Temporary colostomy

Complicated diverticular disease is probably the principal indication for Hartmann resection and end colostomy, but the operation may be used in obstructing and advanced rectosigmoid carcinoma. (see Chapters 37 and 60). The Hartmann procedure is probably the operation of choice for faecal peritonitis complicating diverticular disease, but fewer than a third of patients actually have their stoma closed (Anderson et al, 1979; Varnell and Pemberton, 1981; Pittman and Smith, 1985; Roe et al, 1991; Mealy et al, 1996). Moreover, even after colorectal anastomosis the functional results are often poor owing to a contracted rectum and poor sphincter function (Tudor et al, 1986). Temporary end colostomy may be appropriate for some penetrating colonic injuries, as a staged approach in imperforate anus, infant Hirschsprung's disease and some forms of inflammatory bowel disease. The distal bowel is oversewn or stapled and an end stoma constructed

Loop colostomy

A loop colostomy may be placed in the right or left side of the transverse colon or in the apex of the sigmoid loop. Loop colostomies may be used to palliate an inoperable tumour, to relieve adult or neonatal obstruction, or as a means of treating complicated diverticular disease, or to protect an anastomosis. However, loop colostomies, particularly loop transverse colostomies, are difficult to manage because of their bulk and are associated with a high incidence of hernia, retraction and prolapse. Their contents are only semiformed, leakage from the appliance may be troublesome, and many patients complain of odour. A loop colostomy does not always completely divert the faecal stream (Fontes et al, 1988; Merrett and Gartell, 1993) and may not be the optimum stoma to protect a colorectal anastomosis if the bowel is empty and the marginal artery is critical for the blood supply of the distal colon (Keighley and Matheson, 1980; Williams et al, 1986). For these reasons, and because alternative surgical options are available such as loop ileostomy, caecostomy, Hartmann resection and on-table lavage with primary anastomosis, transverse colostomy is regarded by some as being an outmoded operation (Rosin, 1987). Some surgeons now prefer a double-barrel end colostomy rather than a loop stoma (Gervin et al, 1987). Thus, if the inferior mesenteric artery has been ligated flush with the aorta, the blood supply of the bowel proximal to the anastomosis is dependent upon the marginal artery supplied by the middle colic artery and this may be compromised by a left-sided transverse or sigmoid colostomy (Keighley and Matheson, 1980).

CONSTRUCTION

Site

The importance of locating the optimum site for a colostomy cannot be overstressed. The site will depend upon the anatomical position and type of stoma, previous incisions, scars, the patient's build and the patient's clotting habits (Figure 9.1a–d). An end left iliac fossa colostomy and a sigmoid loop colostomy are usually placed at the same site: through the left rectus muscle and generally below the umbilicus. A loop stoma will need to be wider. The trephine should be well away from the umbilicus, the iliac spine, previous incisions and the symphysis pubis; it should avoid folds of skin and should be visible to the patient. The final position must be checked preoperatively on the patient while wearing a bag over the proposed site, with their clothing on, and while sitting, standing and walking about (Figure 9.1e; see also Figure 8.5a,b and 8.6a,b). Stoma sites for a transverse colostomy may need to be rather higher but must be well away from the costal margin and the umbilicus. We often advise marking both sides for an ileostomy site as well as a potential colostomy site in case a loop ileostomy proves to be more appropriate. A caecostomy will usually be sited as for an ileostomy.

Aitken et al (1986) undertook a 12-month audit on the quality of stoma counselling in 108 patients requiring a colostomy: only 48% of all patients were seen by a stoma care nurse before operation. Although elective preoperative counselling was achieved in 86%, only 15% were seen before emergency operations requiring a stoma, so many of the stomas constructed as an emergency were considered unsatisfactory. Today in most specialized units all patients will have been counselled and marked by a qualified enterostomal therapist even before emergency operations.

Open surgical techniques

End colostomy

Intraperitoneal

The left colon with its vascular supply should be mobilized adequately before the colon is delivered through the abdominal wall (Figure 9.1f). A disc of skin and subcutaneous fat is excised over the

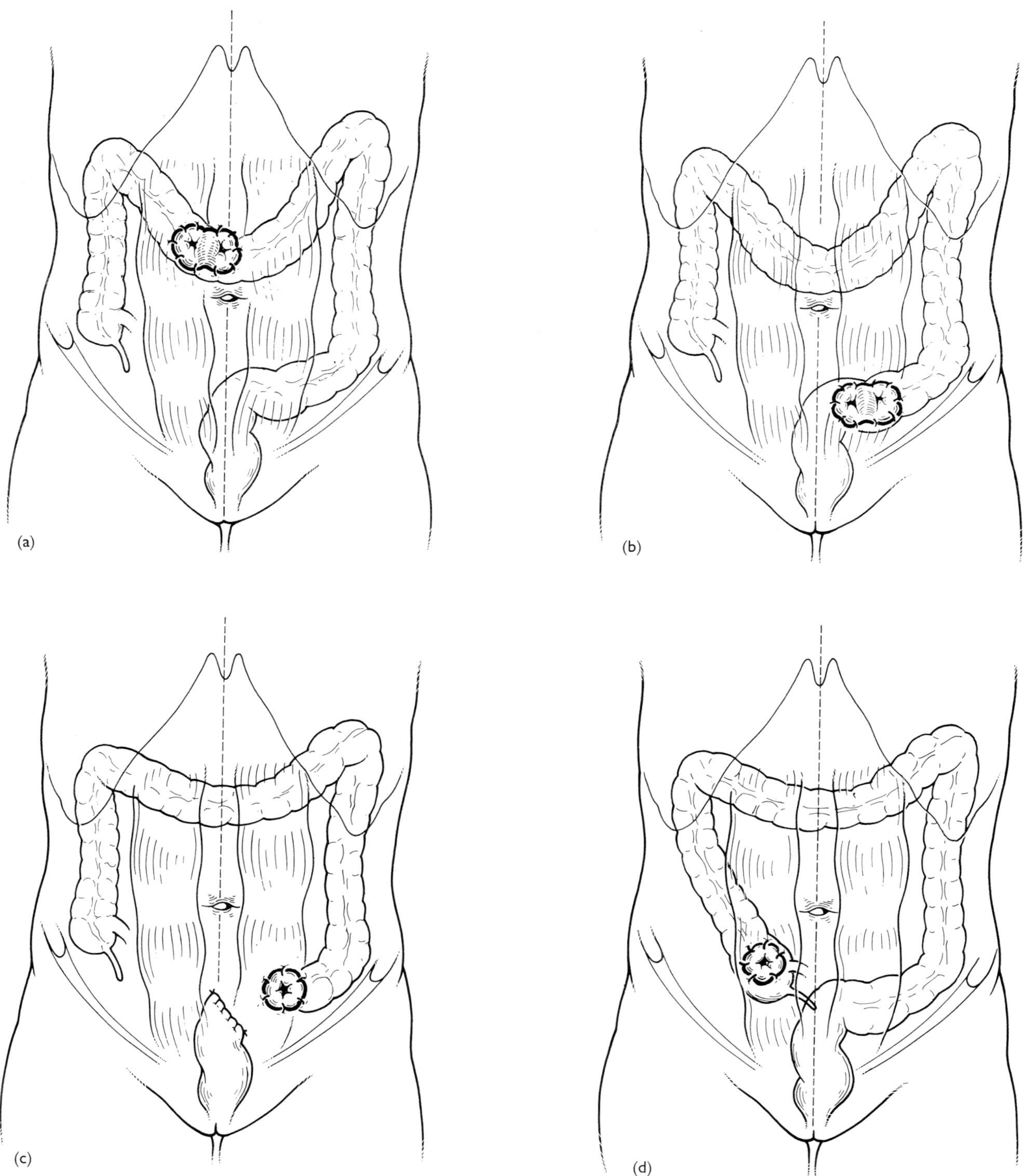

Figure 9.1a–d Siting of a colostomy. (a) Usual siting of a transverse colostomy. A loop transverse colostomy is usually raised through the rectus muscle just to the right of the midline well above the umbilicus through the rectus muscle. (b) Siting of a loop sigmoid colostomy. A loop sigmoid colostomy is usually delivered through a trephine in the left rectus muscle, preferably well above the inguinal ligament. (c) Usual siting of an end left iliac fossa colostomy. An end colostomy is usually delivered through the left rectus muscle away from the inguinal ligament and approximately midway between the umbilicus and the anterior superior iliac spine. This stoma is used particularly following sigmoid resection and the Hartmann procedure. (d) Caecostomy. A caecostomy is usually raised using a trephine through the right rectus muscle (we rarely use it).

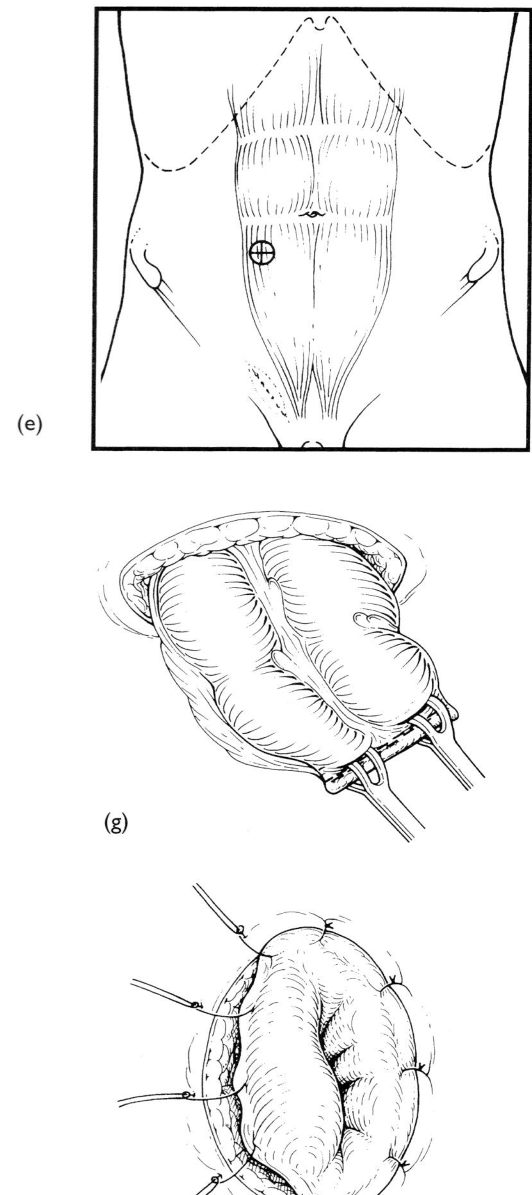

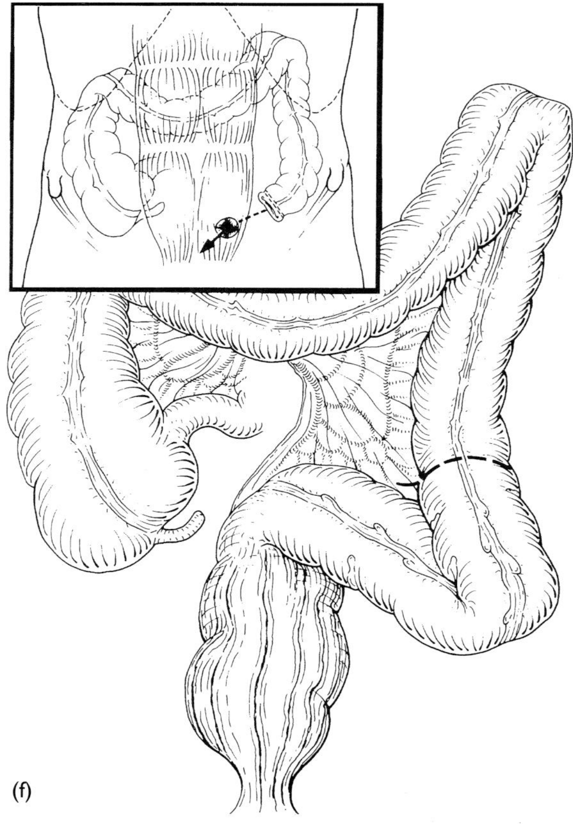

Figure 9.1e–h (e) The ideal colostomy site should be through the rectus muscle but as far away from the umbilicus and the anterior superior iliac spine as possible. The best position should be identified with the patient seated as well as standing and lying. (f) An end colostomy should be delivered through the trephine in the abdominal wall. Stapled closure of the end of the colostomy minimizes contamination. (g) The end of the colon is gently levered out through the abdominal wall using Babcock forceps. (h) Completion of the colostomy is achieved by direct mucocutaneous suture between the wall of the colon and the subcutaneous fat and skin.

selected site (Figure 9.2a,b). This is usually achieved by lifting the centre of the circle of skin away from the abdominal wall; a metal disc may allow a more standardized circle to be removed. Adjustable circular skin cutters have also been advocated for this purpose (Resnick, 1986) but the disc should not be too wide (Martin and Foster, 1996). A cruciate incision is made over the anterior rectus sheath, the rectus muscle is divided or preferably split in the line of the muscle fibres, haemostasis is achieved and the peritoneum is opened (Figure 9.2f).

If the colon is to be brought out as an intraperitoneal stoma directly through the abdominal wall, the lateral gutter is left open in Birmingham (Figure 9.3a) but routinely closed at the Royal London Hospital (Figure 9.3b) by a purse-string then by closure of the residual lateral and infracolic peritoneal defect with a running suture when the bowel has been taken through the abdominal wall.

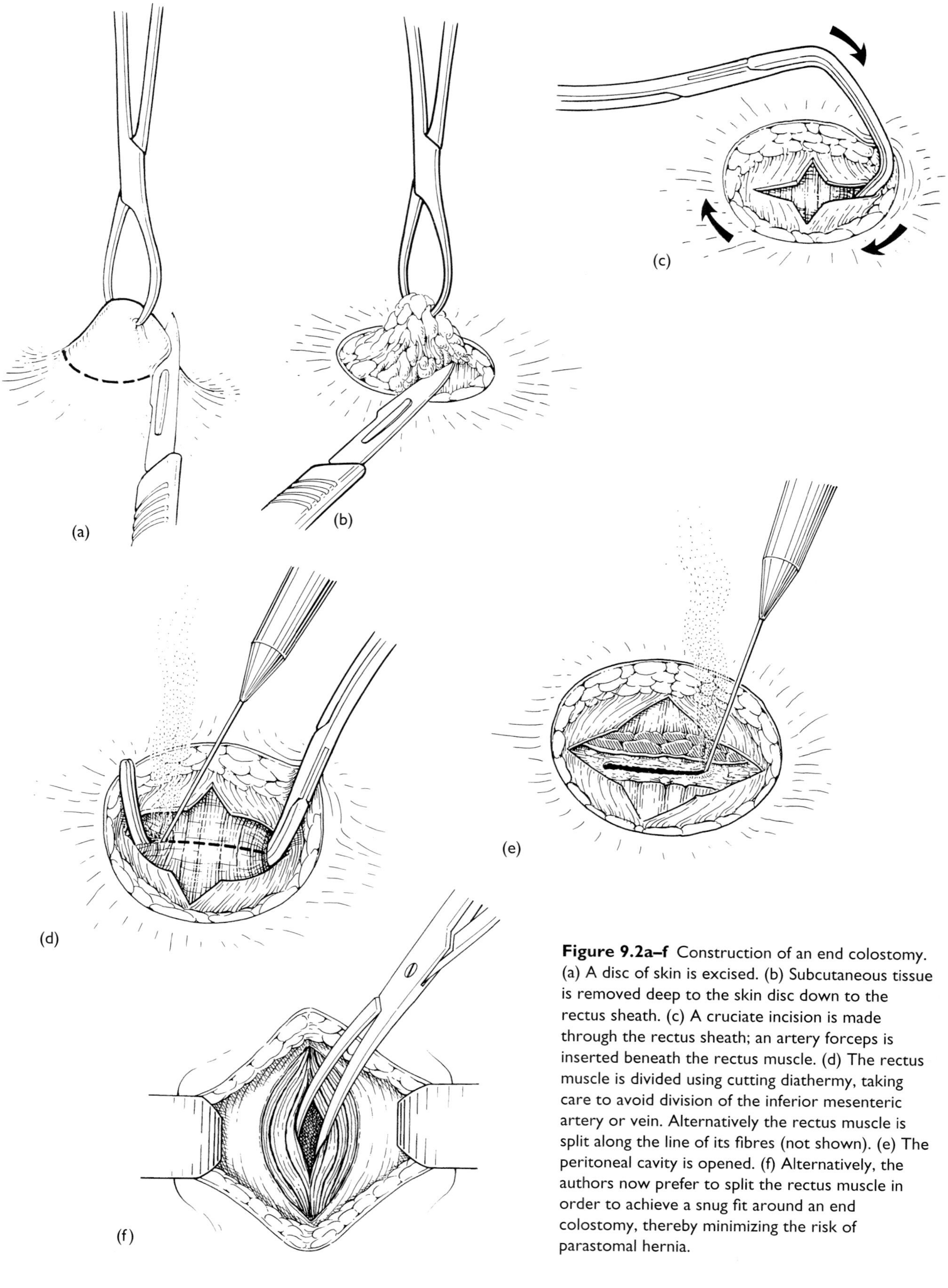

(a)

(b)

(c)

(d)

(e)

(f)

Figure 9.2a–f Construction of an end colostomy. (a) A disc of skin is excised. (b) Subcutaneous tissue is removed deep to the skin disc down to the rectus sheath. (c) A cruciate incision is made through the rectus sheath; an artery forceps is inserted beneath the rectus muscle. (d) The rectus muscle is divided using cutting diathermy, taking care to avoid division of the inferior mesenteric artery or vein. Alternatively the rectus muscle is split along the line of its fibres (not shown). (e) The peritoneal cavity is opened. (f) Alternatively, the authors now prefer to split the rectus muscle in order to achieve a snug fit around an end colostomy, thereby minimizing the risk of parastomal hernia.

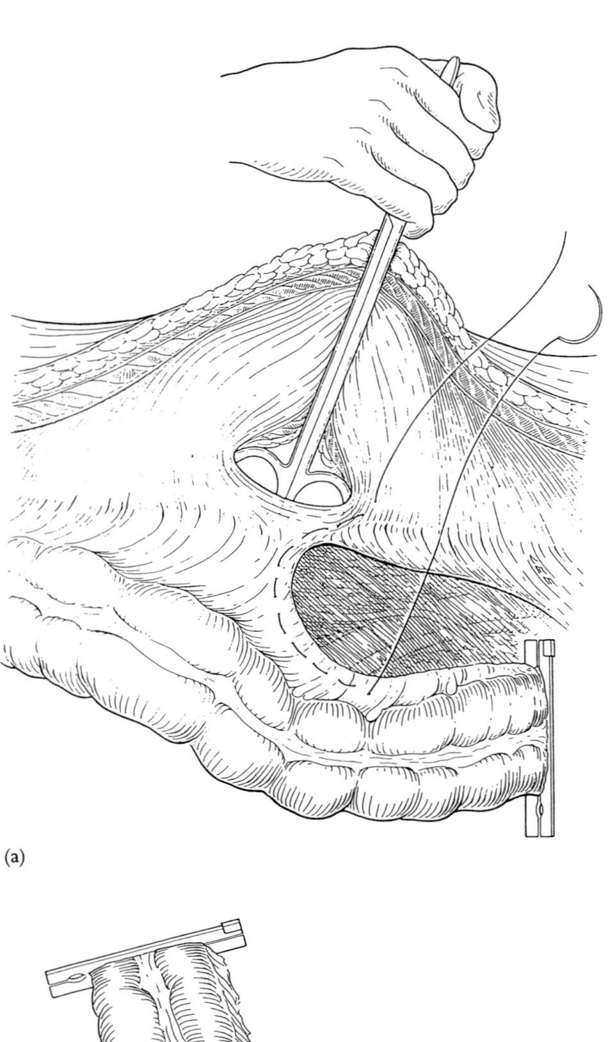

(a)

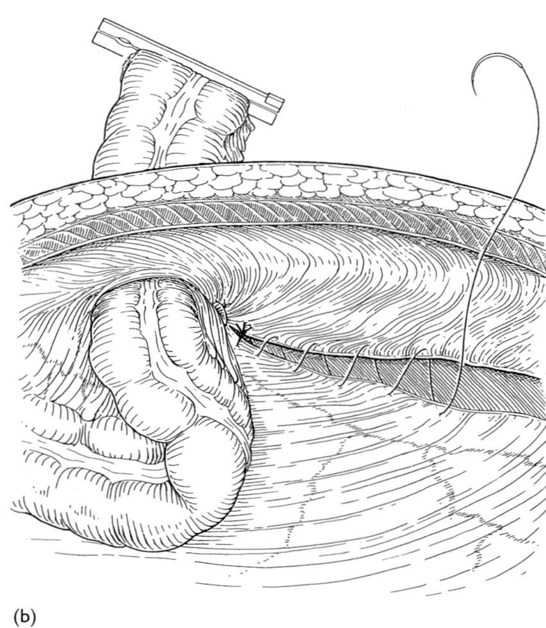

(b)

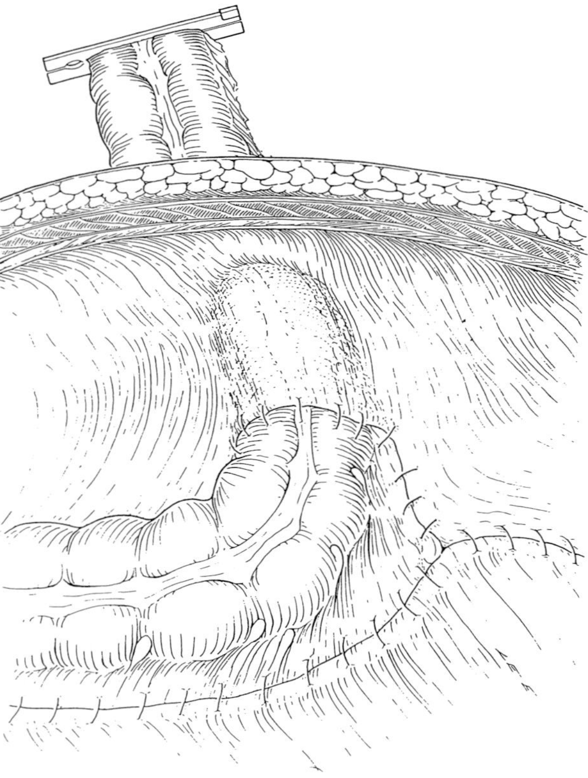

(c)

Figure 9.3a–c Closure of the lateral gutter after end colostomy construction. (a) A purse-string suture is placed from the inner aspect of the abdominal wall trephine to the cut edge of the mesentery of the colon. (b) The end of the colon is delivered through the abdominal wall trephine and the purse-string suture is tied. Closure of the lateral gutter is then completed by approximating the cut edge of the lateral peritoneum to the cut edge of the mesentery. (c) A series of sutures between the serosa of the colon and the abdominal wall completes the lateral wall closure when a retroperitoneal colostomy is fashioned.

1995). Nevertheless in suitably selected cases it is quick and effective though we would accept that the incidence of parastomal hernia may be higher than with conventional stoma construction. Anderson et al (1992) reviewed the results of trephine stomas in 24 patients, this procedure proved impossible in three. The procedure was shorter in terms of operating time than laparotomy and stoma construction, patients were in hospital for fewer days and there was less postoperative pain. Complications were not increased, but two patients developed a colostomy prolapse and one a parastomal hernia. Likewise, Stephenson et al (1997) from Pennsylvania reviewed the outcome in 36 patients who had attempted stoma construction through the trephine in the abdominal wall. Four were unsuccessful and required a laparotomy, the failures tended to be obese and had all had previous

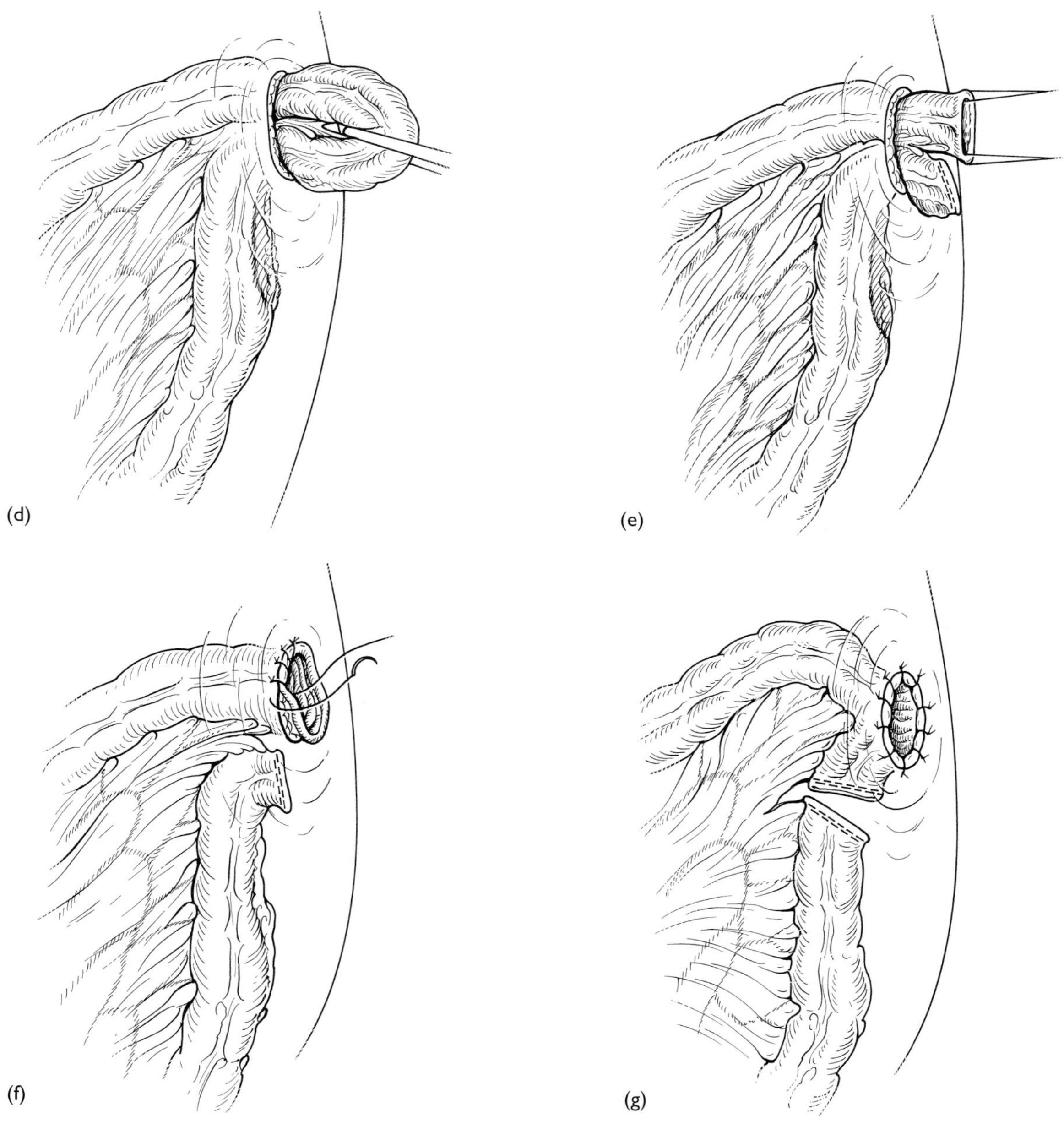

Figure 9.5d–g (d) A tape is placed under the sigmoid colon so that it can be delivered through the trephine and the sigmoid arcade divided. (e) Once the distal end is verified by air insufflation this can be closed by staples. (f) The distal end is dropped back and the proximal end is sutured to the skin, achieving direct mucocutaneous maturation. (g) An alternative technique is to divide the distal and proximal bowel with staples. If there is insufficient length to bring out the end of the colon, a loop above it might be under less tension. A colotomy is therefore made and direct mucocutaneous apposition achieved.

abdominal surgery, whereas only 37% of the successful trephine stomas had had previous abdominal surgery. These authors all concluded that the technique is useful but that cases should be carefully selected.

The patient is placed in the Allan stirrups so that the colon can be insufflated with a sigmoidoscope to identify the distal loop of bowel (Figure 9.5b). A trephine is made, as described, in the abdominal wall. The sigmoid colon is identified and its lateral peritoneal attachments divided so as to deliver a loop through the abdominal wall (Figure 9.5c). The sigmoid arcade is divided between clips. The distal bowel end (having been identified by insufflation with air (Fig 9.5d)) is transected with a double row of staples dividing the colon above the staples between stay sutures (Figure 9.5e). The distal colon is dropped back into the peritoneal cavity and direct mucocutaneous sutures applied between the bowel wall and subcuticular skin edge (Figure 9.5f) (Rose et al, 1985). Occasionally, if the mesentery is short, the distal end of the proximal colon may also be closed by dividing the colon with a linear staple cutter to deliver the side of the bowel above the closed end as a loop end colostomy (Bumin and Yerdel, 1996) (Figure 9.5g).

Loop colostomy

For a loop colostomy, the abdominal wall trephine must be wide enough to admit two fingers. A loop colostomy may be fashioned for large bowel obstruction without performing a laparotomy, as previously described (see Chapter 60), provided the segment of bowel can be correctly identified (Senapati and Phillips, 1991) and there is no fear of colonic perforation or ischaemia. We do not practise constructing a colostomy through a transverse incision, as commonly described, but prefer to excise a disc of skin and subcutaneous fat, as in an end colostomy (see Figure 9.2). Once the appropriate loop of colon has been identified, a small window is opened in the mesentery adjacent to the bowel, without damage to the vascular arcade (Figure 9.6a), and a nylon tape is placed under the colon to facilitate its delivery through the abdominal wall (Figure 9.6b). In the case of a transverse loop colostomy, a window must be opened between the omentum and the colon through the transverse mesocolon and gastrocolic ligament (Figure 9.6c). For the sigmoid colon a small opening is made near the bowel in the sigmoid mesentery (Figure 9.6d). Once the bowel has been opened, immediate muco-

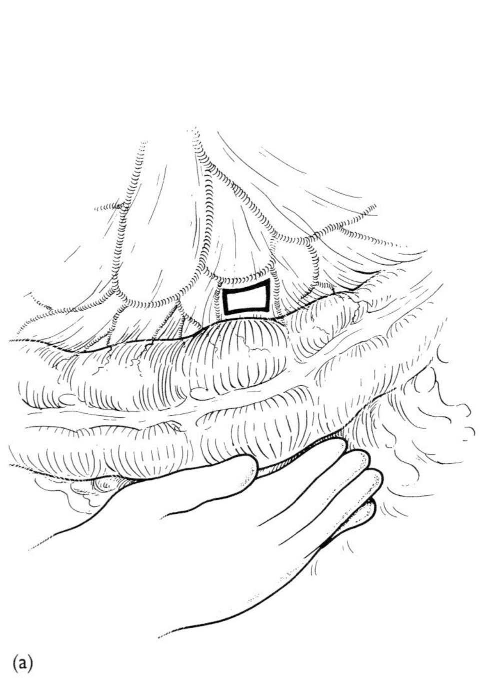

(a)

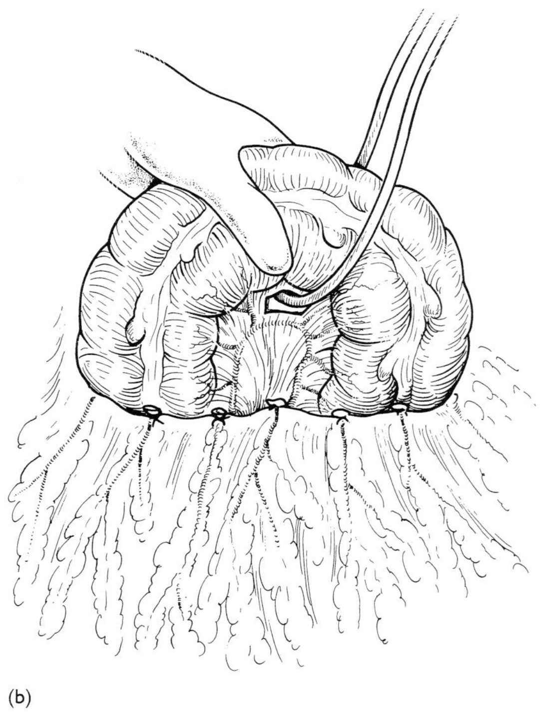

(b)

Figure 9.6a–b Construction of a loop colostomy. (a) The optimum site for loop colostomy is selected. The mesentery is divided between two vascular arcades. (b) A soft rubber tube is placed underneath the colon through the mesenteric window.

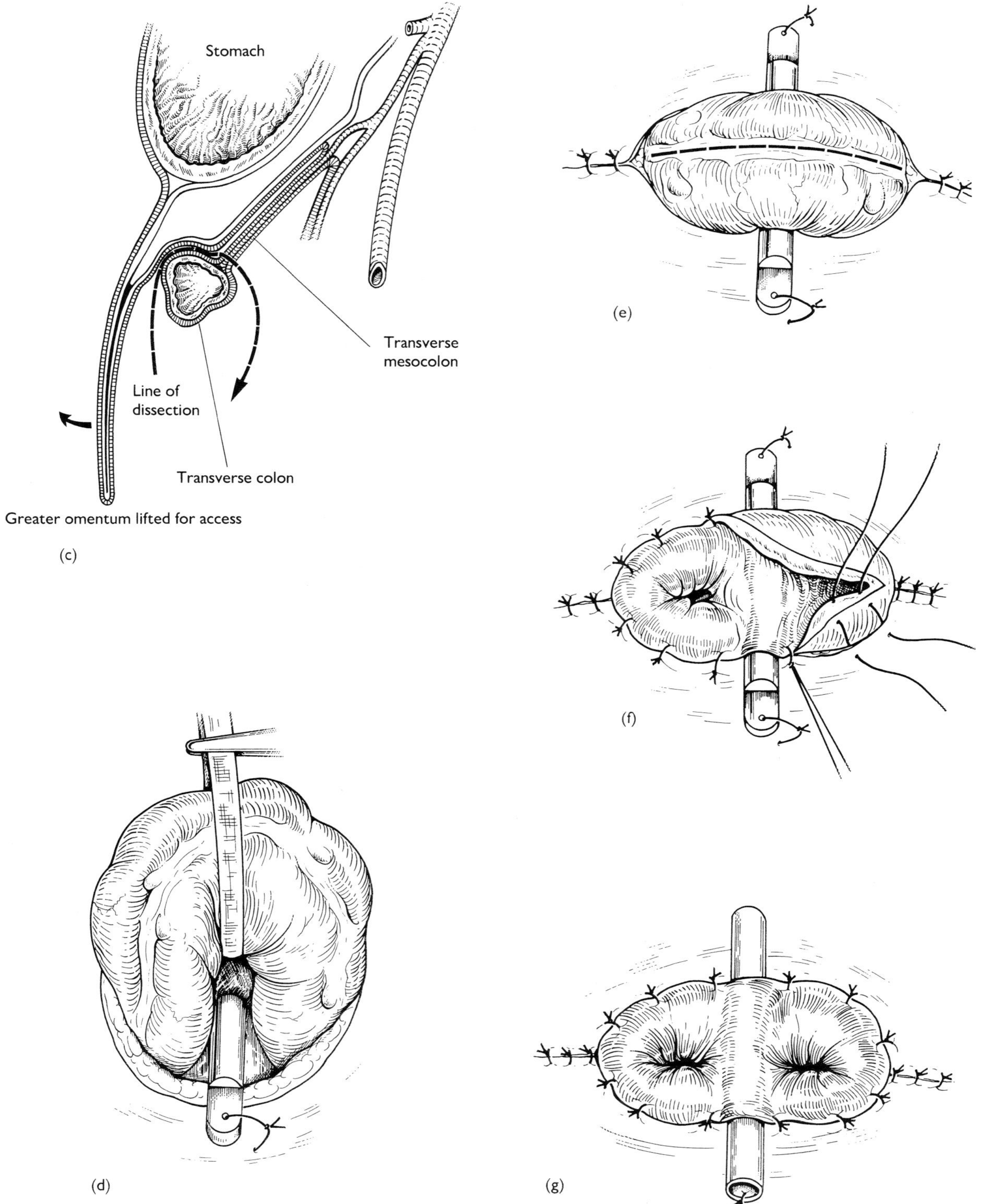

Figure 9.6c–g (c) The omentum is either partially divided or is dissected off the transverse colon to facilitate delivery of the colon through the abdominal wall. (d) A trephine is made in the abdominal wall and the colonic loop is delivered to the surface by traction on the rubber tubing; a rod is then inserted through the window and sutured to the skin to prevent retraction. (e) The colon is opened along the taenia. (f) Mucocutaneous apposition is achieved by a series of sutures. (g) Completed transverse colostomy.

cutaneous suture is performed using absorbable sutures between the skin and bowel wall. (Figure 9.6e–g). A rod may be placed under the colostomy if it is under tension and may retract (Aitken et al, 1986).

Delayed colotomy

Few surgeons today delay colotomy when constructing a loop colostomy, but the technique was frequently used in large bowel obstruction, when immediate mucocutaneous suture increased the risk of sepsis (Lafreniere and Ketcham, 1985). If delayed colotomy is used it is advisable to support the stoma with a rod to prevent retraction (Durst and Freund, 1980). If the stoma is not opened for 3–4 days it is usually impossible to perform a direct mucocutaneous suture. A colotomy is made over a taenia so that the bowel contents can discharge immediately into a bag (Figure 9.7).

Some authorities have advocated the unopened colostomy to protect a distal anastomosis (Vaxman et al, 1993), but Dixon and Thompson (1996) reported problems with obstruction, rod erosion and failure to protect anastomotic breakdown. The GIA stapler can be used to open the colon to prevent bleeding (Figure 9.8a,b) (Chapman et al, 1984).

Immediate mucocutaneous maturation

Immediate mucocutaneous suture allows an appliance to be fitted around the stoma straight away. This is the preferred technique for construction of an end colostomy and is frequently used for loop colostomy. The technique can be used in acute large bowel obstruction but complete apposition cannot be achieved if there is a rod beneath the loop protruding over the skin edges (Figure 9.6g). There are some advocates of mucocutaneous apposition with skin staples (Antrum and Rice, 1988) (Figure 9.9a,b); however, we usually suture the bowel wall to the skin with 3/0 or 4/0 Prolene (Figure 9.10). Although Prolene must be removed, it causes little if any tissue reaction. PDS may have advantages in young patients who dislike sutures being removed, and they also allow apposition of the bowel wall to the subcuticular skin edge; but they remain *in situ* for so long that most patients complain of irritation and discomfort, necessitating removal anyway.

Chung (1985) describes the use of the circular stapling device for mucocutaneous apposition. A similar technique has been described for treatment of skin level colostomy stenosis (Figure 9.11a–d) (Ramia et al, 1996).

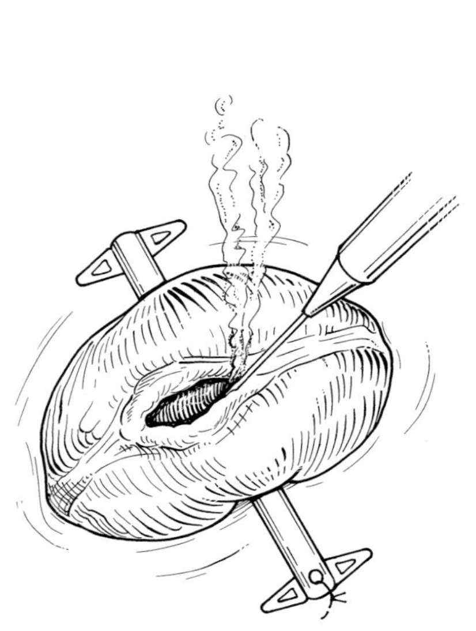

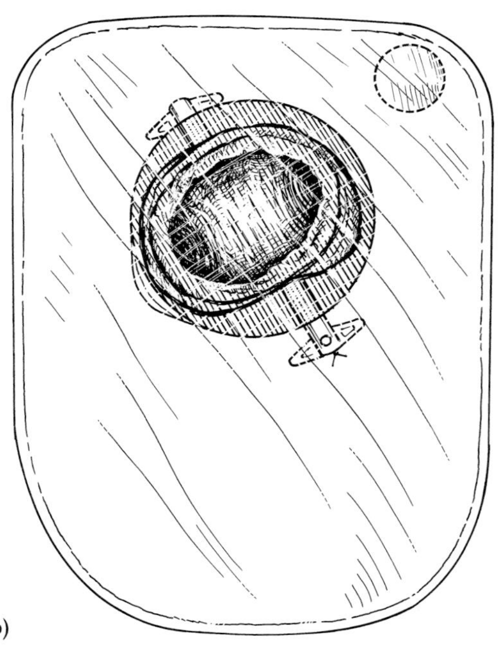

Figure 9.7a–b (a) When an emergency loop transverse colostomy is constructed, it is wise to place a rod underneath the loop to prevent retraction. The colon is opened along the taenia with diathermy. (b) No attempt is made to suture the mucosa to the skin, and a large colostomy appliance is attached to seal the skin around it.

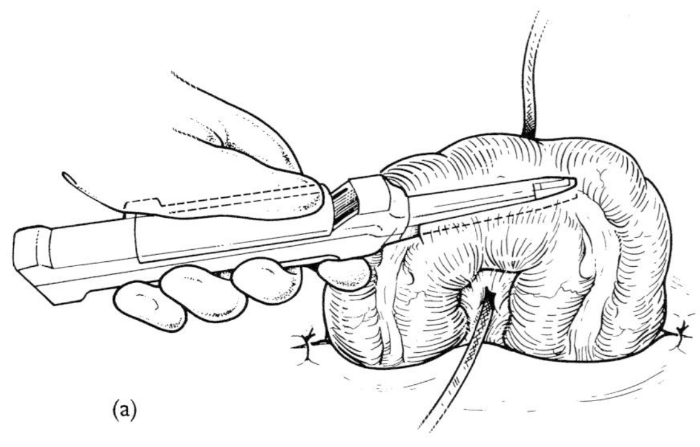
(a)

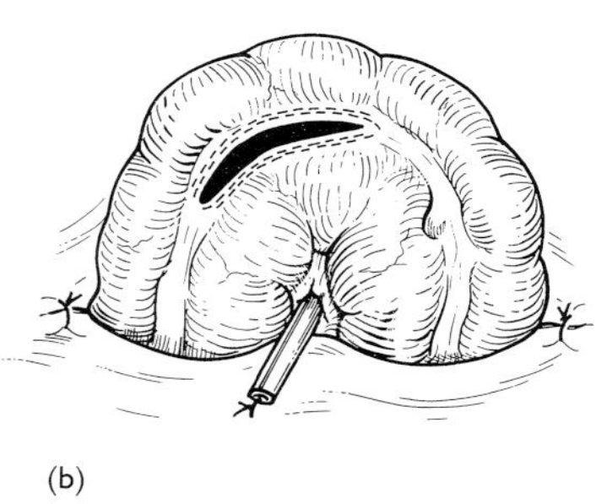
(b)

Figure 9.8a–b Opening of a loop colostomy with the linear staple cutter. A relatively haemostatic form of colotomy can be achieved using a linear staple cutter through a small enterotomy. (a) Insertion of the stapler. (b) Completion of the colotomy.

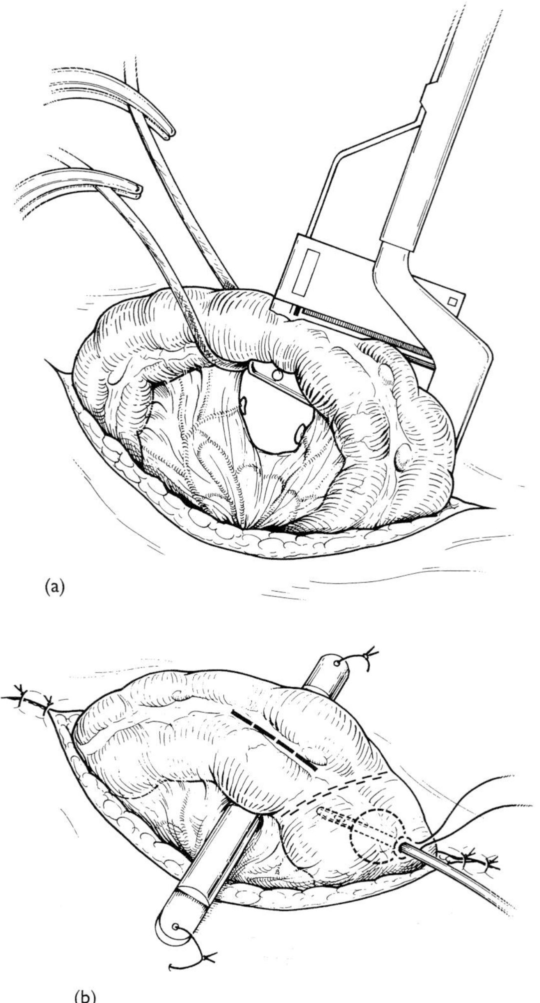
(a)

(b)

Figure 9.9a–b Transection loop colostomy with linear stapler. (a) A loop of colon is delivered to the surface through an abdominal incision. A linear stapler is applied through a mesenteric window to close the distal limb of the colon. (b) A small colotomy is made proximal to the linear staple closure for decompression and distal decompression is achieved using a small Foley catheter inserted through a distal colotomy.

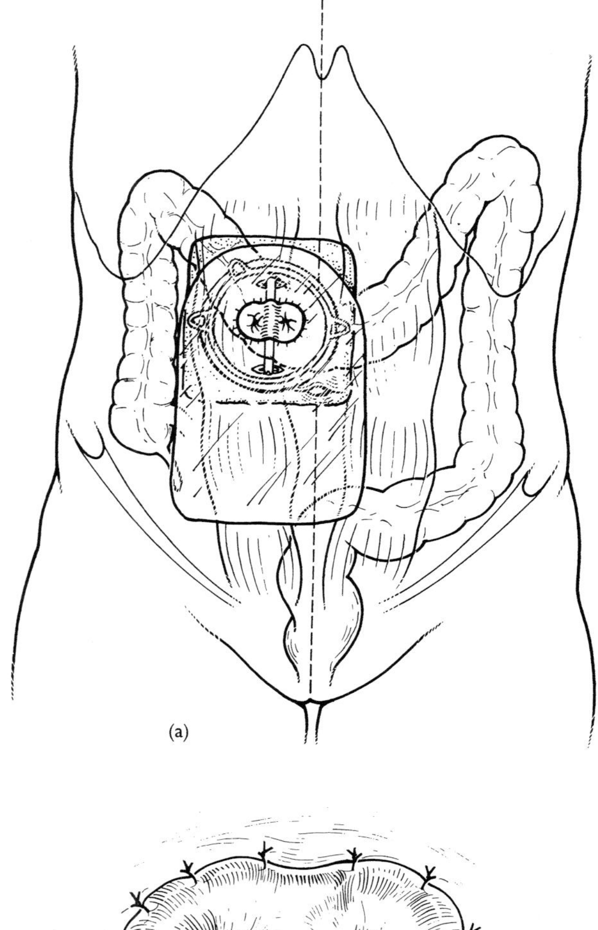
(a)

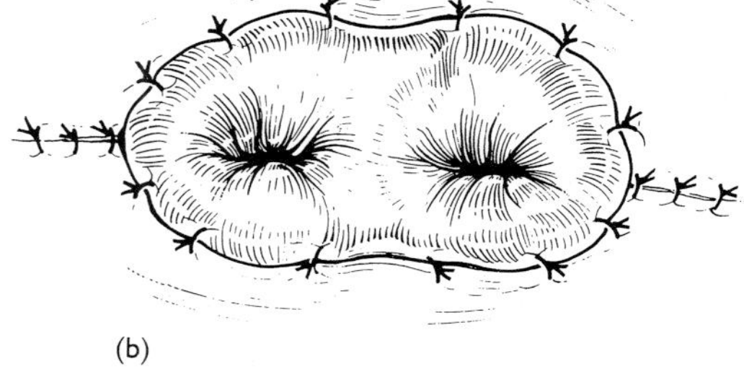
(b)

Figure 9.10a–b Direct mucocutaneous suture of a loop colostomy with and without a rod. (a) Demonstrates immediate mucocutaneous suture over a rod. (b) Shows direct mucocutaneous suture without the use of a rod.

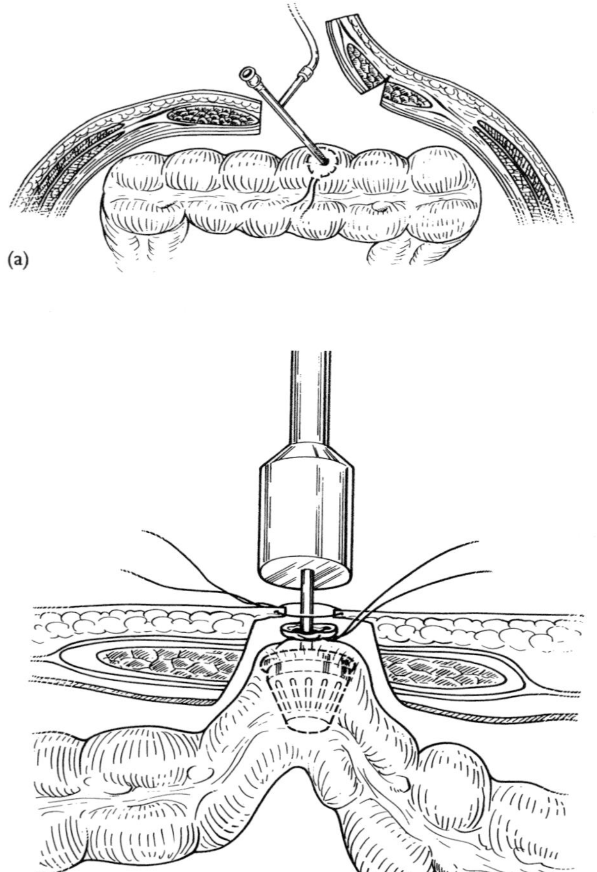

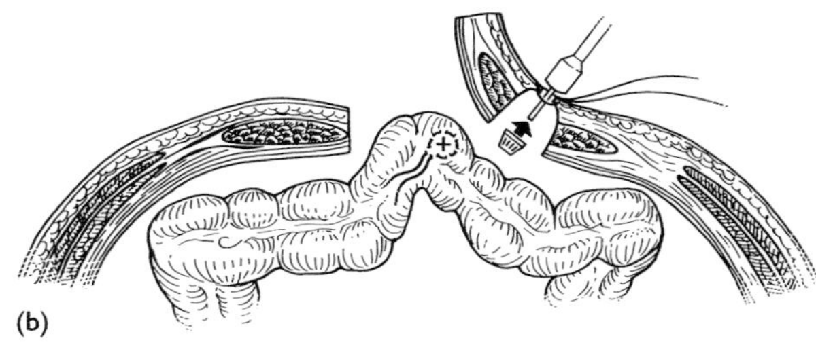

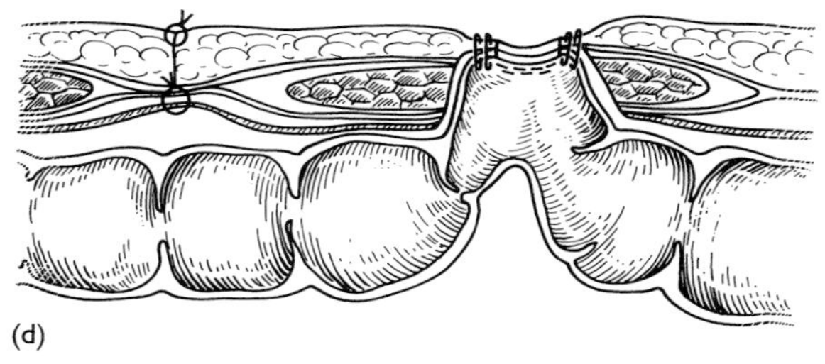

Figure 9.11a–d Stapled mucocutaneous apposition for loop colostomy. (a) A trochar is inserted into the transverse colon through a laparotomy to achieve immediate decompression. A trephine is made in the abdominal wall and a purse-string suture is placed around the skin edges of the stoma site. (b) A circular stapler is then inserted through the abdominal wall and the anvil through the purse-string in the transverse colon. (c) The circular stapling device is closed. (d) Stapled mucocutaneous apposition is achieved.

Defunctioned loop colostomy

A bulky loop colostomy is often difficult to manage. Avoidance of such a stoma can be achieved by closing the distal limb of a divided loop colostomy below the abdominal wall; the proximal colon is sutured to the skin (Figure 9.12) (Delaney and Mulholland, 1983). A conical trephine also achieves a much smaller stoma but may be complicated by recession (Eng and Localio, 1981; Sigurdson et al, 1986).

Rod or bridge beneath the stoma?

Although we frequently avoid using a rod beneath a loop colostomy, we recognize that in some patients – particularly those with large bowel obstruction in whom adequate defunctioning is essential – some form of support behind the loop is desirable.

A glass rod underneath the colon makes stoma management difficult (Wangensteen, 1947) and this practice is rarely used now (Gabriel and Lloyd-Davies, 1935; Hurwitz, 1971). An alternative is to pass a short length of polyethylene tubing under the colon and suture it to the skin (Lee, 1968), but this may be too pliable and allows some retraction (see Figure 9.6b); we prefer a thin Teflon rod if support is desirable (Alexander-Williams, 1974) (see Figure 9.6f). Browning and Parks (1983) use a deep tension suture through a length of polyvinyl tubing to support the colostomy. Schofield et al (1980) use a rubber sling and rotate the stoma so that the proximal limb is dependent, on the basis that the distal bowel is defunctioned more effectively – a theory that we have been unable to substantiate.

The use of a rod or tubing placed at a distance from the skin edges through a subcutaneous tunnel has been used as a means of preventing retraction of the stoma while leaving the skin edges free for mucocutaneous apposition (Rickett, 1969; Vogel

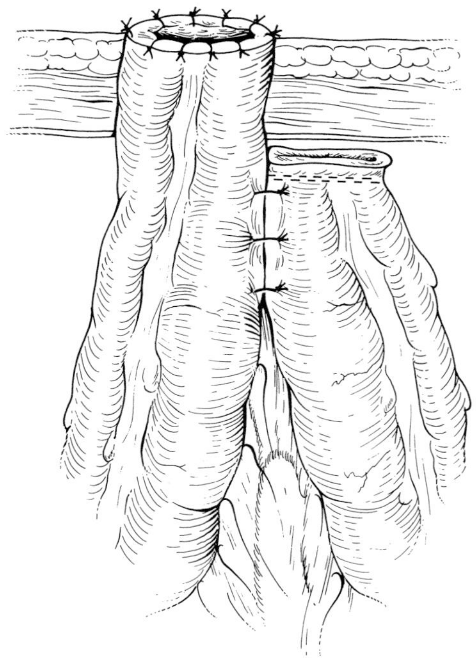

Figure 9.12 End colostomy with closure of the distal loop. An alternative to loop clostomy is to divide the colon, stapling the distal limb with a linear staple device and opening the proximal limb, which is sutured to the skin edges of an abdominal wall trephine.

and Maher, 1986; Fitzgibbons et al, 1987); unfortunately, the subcutaneous tunnel may be associated with sepsis (Abeyatunge, 1972; Galofre and Ponseti, 1983). A subcutaneous bridge has been manufactured from bovine fibrin (Capperauld et al, 1977; Jenkinson et al, 1984), which is completely absorbed in 21 days, leaving a small plaque of fibrous tissue (Simkin, 1980). This method of support is particularly advantageous in obese patients with a short mesocolon.

Some plastic rods supplied by appliance manufacturers (Figure 9.13a–c) are bulky (Greene, 1971; Aries, 1973; Corman and Veidenheimer, 1974; Poticha, 1974). Large rods present difficulties with the fitting of bags, and some of the polymers that are used are too hard with the potential risk of bowel erosion causing bleeding or perforation (Hansen et al, 1974).

Many surgeons are of the opinion that a rod is usually unnecessary when constructing an elective loop colostomy with immediate mucocutaneous suture. Others argue that support is necessary, both to prevent retraction and to achieve complete defunctioning of the distal bowel. There are alternative methods of support. A fascial bridge similar to that used in colonic trauma may be an alternative (Kirkpatrick and Rajpal, 1975; Rombeau and Turnbull, 1978). Baker (1975) and later Jarpa (1986) described the use of a skin bridge.

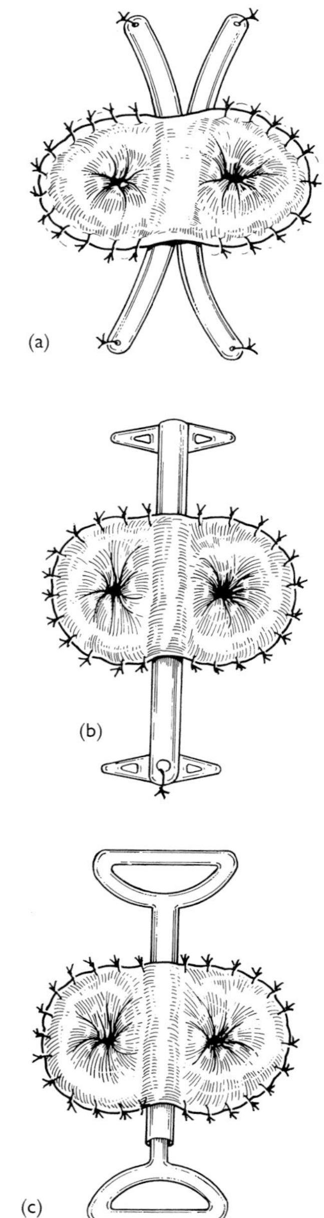

Figure 9.13a–c Commercially available rods for loop colostomy.

Double-barrel colostomy

The double-barrel colostomy is a legacy of the days when malignant tumours were exteriorized and

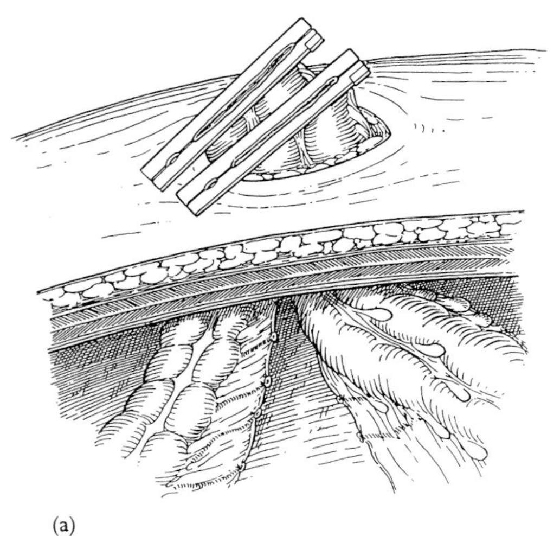
(a)

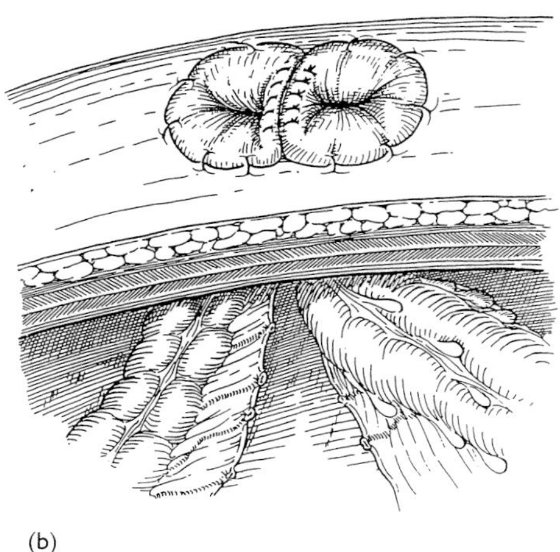
(b)

Figure 9.14a–b Double-barrel colostomy. (a) Two limbs of the colon have been delivered to the abdominal wall through a large stoma site. (b) The two stomata are sutured to the skin and to each other.

later resected. Today the only real advantages of this procedure are that the stoma is less bulky than a loop colostomy (Figure 9.14a,b) and can be easily closed, not with an enterome but after mobilization from the abdominal wall using a linear staple cutter to divide the spur and a linear staple cutter to divide the open bowel ends (Figure 9.15a–d) (Miskowiak, 1983). The double-barrel stoma may be useful in patients presenting with bowel ischaemia from volvulus and in trauma.

Alternatives to a colostomy

Tube colostomy

The theoretical advantage of tube colostomy is that it may provide temporary decompression without the need for a closure procedure (Rickett 1978). Caecostomy is the widest application of this principle. It has been suggested that the technique might be applicable in patients with an empty colon where the device is merely used to vent a distal anastomosis. Shafik (1982) compared results in 180 patients with obstructing carcinoma with those having conventional loop colostomy and showed that the outcome was comparable. He admits that tube decompression is not feasible in the left colon because solid stool blocks the catheter. Sykes (1979) used a similar technique in the right side of the transverse colon to defunction a distal anastomosis. This procedure was not advised for the management of large bowel obstruction.

Caecostomy and appendicostomy

Caecostomy is still a controversial procedure for decompressing a distal anastomosis, for acute large bowel obstruction or for fixation in caecal volvulus (Hunt, 1960; Clarke and Hubay, 1972; Benacci and Wolff, 1995). Caecostomy for large bowel obstruction carried a mortality of 50% between 1938 and 1943 and a 44% mortality in the years 1947–55 (Goligher and Smiddy, 1957). A high mortality was reported by Maynard and Turell (1955) and by Wangensteen (1942) but this reflects the debility of the patients studied. Later evidence reports mortality figures that ranged from 55 to 11% (Polk et al, 1964; King et al, 1966; Jackson and Baird, 1967; Clarke and Hubey, 1972). Mortality figures are generally higher in large bowel obstruction (Gerber and Thompson, 1965). The results of caecostomy in diverticular disease have been disappointing: often the caecostomy does not close spontaneously and peridiverticular sepsis persists (Jackson and Baird, 1967). Even when the obstructing lesion had been resected, 24% of patients had a faecal fistula (Clarke and Hubey, 1972) and sepsis was reported in 16%. Surgical closure of a persistent caecostomy fistula was necessary in 3–10% of patients having caecostomy for decompression (Edmiston and Birnbaum, 1955; King et al, 1966; Jackson and Baird, 1967; Clarke and Hubey, 1972).

Caecostomy has been largely discontinued in acute large bowel obstruction (Fallis, 1946; Becker, 1953; Gerber and Thompson, 1965), but is still

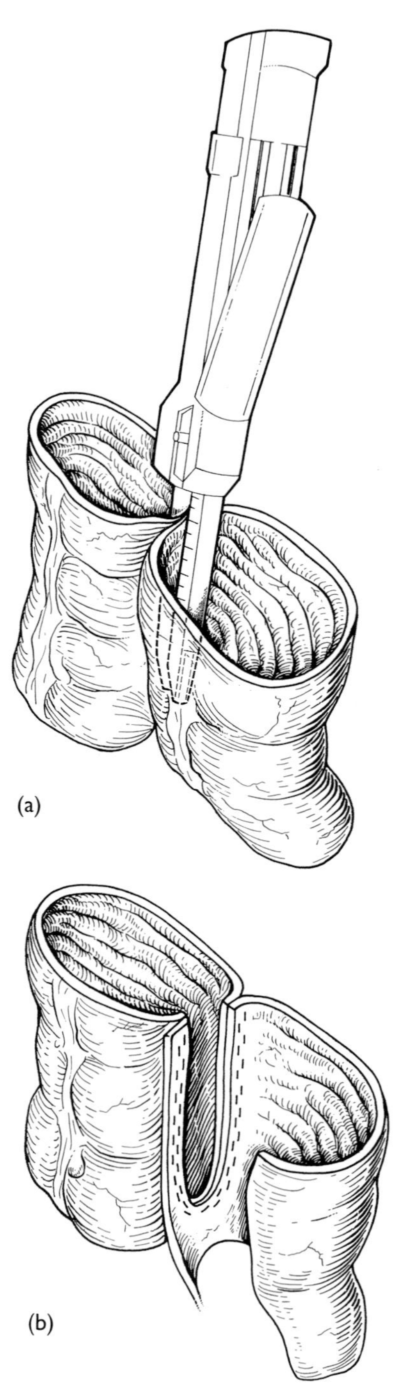

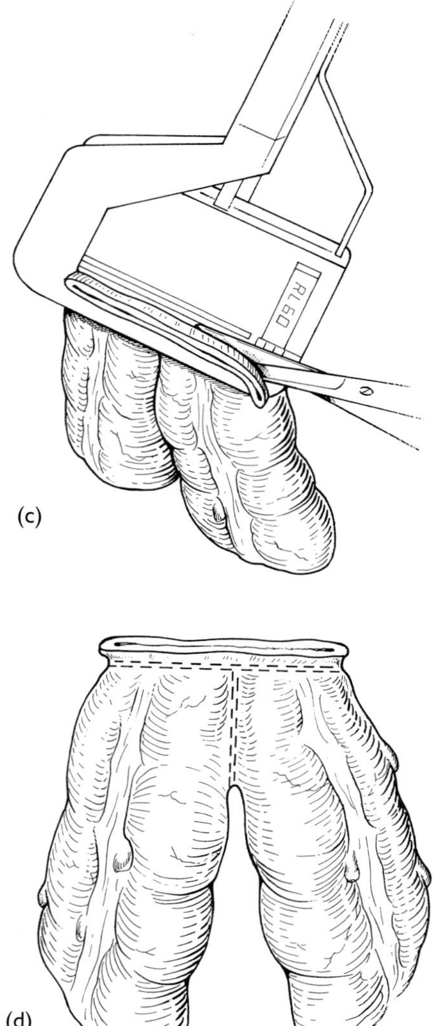

Figure 9.15a–d (a) Closure of a double-barrel colostomy can be achieved after mobilization of the two limbs of the colon from the abdominal wall, using the linear staple cutter to achieve a side-to-side anastomosis. (b) The completed side-to-side anastomosis. (c) A method of closing the two open limbs of colon using a linear stapler. (d) The completed colostomy closure.

practised to decompress bowel anastomoses (Graham, 1948; Stainback and Christiansen, 1962; Hughes, 1963; Jackson and Baird, 1967; Wolff and Wolff, 1980), particularly in children having pull-through procedures for imperforate anus and Hirschsprung's disease (Guttman, 1985). Goldstein and colleagues (1986) are still strong advocates of caecostomy for postoperative decompression, but emphasize the importance of extraperitonealization of the caecum and the use of a large de Pezzer catheter. Benacci and Wolff (1995) reviewed the results of caecostomy in 67 patients at the Mayo Clinic; the indications were pseudo-obstruction (26), obstruction (11), caecal perforation (10), caecal volvulus (9), anastomotic diversion (8), and three others. Pericatheter leak occurred in 15%, wound sepsis in 12%, ventral hernia in 12%, catheter occlusion in 7%, skin excoriation in 4%, premature catheter dislodgement in 4%, and there were two caecocutaneous fistulas that closed spontaneously. None of the patients required re-operation or formal closure. They concluded that tube caecostomy is still a useful procedure for refractory pseudo-obstruction, caecal volvulus and caecal perforation, and in some patients with distal colonic obstruction.

The technique is performed either percutaneously through a small muscle-cutting approach, as in appendicostomy (Stainback and Christiansen, 1962), or during laparotomy (Hughes, 1963). The right iliac fossa is explored with care in patients with large bowel obstruction, for fear of causing caecal rupture. If there is faecal or purulent peritonitis the surgical strategy should be modified and the abdomen explored. If feasible, the seromuscular wall of the caecum should be sutured to the peritoneum (Maynard and Turell, 1955), but this may be unwise if the caecum is on the point of perforation. The use of suction on a trocar and cannula is probably the safest method of initial decompression (Figure 9.16a). Sometimes it is possible to place a purse-string suture around the trocar only after its insertion. After decompression a non-crushing clamp is placed across the caecotomy and a de Pezzer or Foley catheter (with the tip excised) is introduced into the caecum (Figure 9.16b). Two purse-string sutures should be used to close the caecal wall snugly around the tube. If not already performed, the serosa of the caecum is sutured to the peritoneum, the balloon of the Foley catheter is inflated, the wound is closed and the catheter is sutured to the skin and attached to a drainage tube. In certain cases decompression can be achieved through the stump of the appendix rather than the wall of the caecum.

The advantage of caecostomy is that it can be performed under local anaesthesia, and spontaneous closure usually occurs after the catheter has been removed. The disadvantage of the procedure is that decompression is often incomplete and the tube may have to be irrigated to prevent bolus obstruction. We do not believe that caecostomy has an important place in the management of large bowel obstruction or colonic decompression.

Loop ileostomy

We have already stated our preference for loop ileostomy over loop colostomy to protect a distal anastomosis if the bowel has been adequately prepared. There is less risk of compromising the blood supply to the colon. The stoma fits within an appliance much more easily than a loop colostomy, a rod is not required, closure is attended by a lower morbidity (Fasth et al, 1980) (Table 9.1), and decompression is usually complete (Winslet et al, 1991). Williams et al (1986) compared loop ileostomy and loop colostomy in a randomized trial (Table 9.2). Loop ileostomy was associated with less odour,

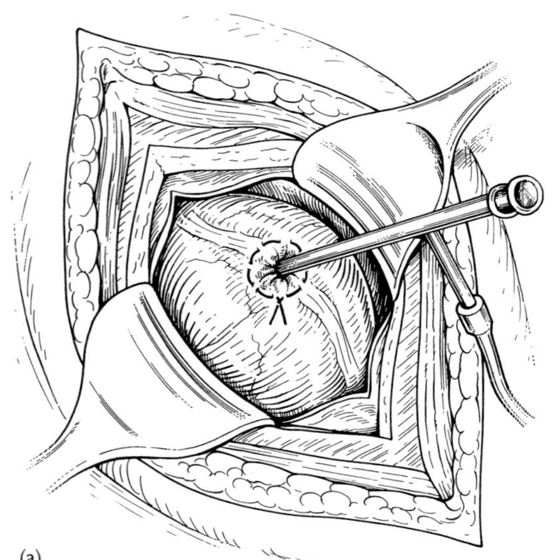

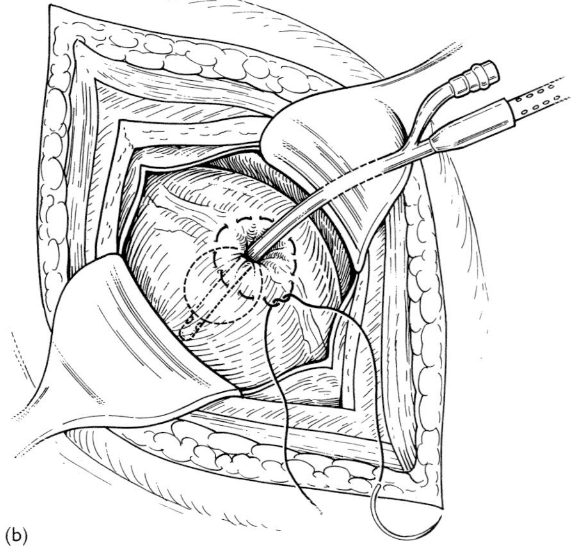

Figure 9.16a–b Caecostomy. (a) An oblique incision has been made in the abdominal wall; the caecum has been identified. A purse-string suture has been placed around a taenia and a trochar has been inserted for decompression. (b) Demonstrates a Foley catheter that has been passed through the purse-string with the balloon inflated for decompression.

Table 9.1 Comparison of complications arising from loop ileostomy and loop colostomy – I*.

	Ileostomy (*n* = 21)	*Colostomy* (*n* = 21)
Postoperative complications		
Wound sepsis	0	1
Stoma problems	4	5
Postclosure complications		
Wound sepsis	1	4
Faecal fistula	0	1

* From Fasth et al (1980).

Table 9.2 Comparison of complications arising from loop ileostomy and loop colostomy – II*.

	Ileostomy (*n* = 23)	*Colostomy* (*n* = 24)
Postoperative complications		
Wound sepsis	3	8
Intestinal obstruction	2	2
Prolapse	0	2
Leakage around appliance	5	5
Skin excoriation	3	7
Late complications		
Bleeding	2	6
Prolapse	1	4
Skin excoriation	7	9
Leakage	3	6
Odour	1	10
Complications of closure		
Infection	0	6
Obstruction	1	0
Hospital stay	9 days	10 days

* From Williams et al (1986).

required fewer appliance changes and only 18% reported stoma management difficulties, compared with 58% of patients who had a loop colostomy. The loop colostomy was more bulky and effluent more difficult to contain, with a higher rate of skin excoriation and more frequent leakage from the appliance than with ileostomy.

Laparoscopic method

The theoretical advantages, indications, contraindications and informed consent relative to colostomy are identical to those precepts already described in ileostomy. One fundamental difference with a colostomy is that, whereas a loop ileostomy is preferred for ease of subsequent closure, an end colostomy is much easier for the patient to manage and has a much lower complication rate related to colostomy hernia and stomal prolapse. Patients with an end colostomy can therefore manage pouching and appliance management much easier than can patients with a loop colostomy.

A few differences exist between the colostomy and ileostomy in terms of patient preparation and informed consent. First, depending on the indications for colostomy construction, colonoscopy may be desirable. Thus, the patient should give consent for possible intraoperative colonoscopy, and the instrumentation should be immediately available. Second, colonoscopic verification of the appropriate orientation of the afferent and efferent limbs of bowel may be a useful adjunctive manoeuvre, again emphasizing the importance of both informed consent and instrument availability.

Another difference between colostomy and ileostomy is that, whereas in the latter group no cathartic preparation is given, for the former group the standard sodium phosphate preparation is utilized as described in Chapter 6. In addition, the modified Nicholls–Condon oral antibiotic preparation including metronidazole and neomycin is administered along with perioperative cefotaxime and metronidazole.

Patient positioning, equipment/instrumentation and port positioning are mostly the same as for ileostomy (see Chapter 8). The fundamental difference is that, in order to facilitate limb orientation, it may be desirable to mark appendices epiploicae intracorporeally with endoscopic clips. It is the author's practice to mark the proximal direction with one clip and the distal direction with two clips to help ensure appropriate bowel orientation after delivery of the loop through the stoma site. As with ileostomy construction, the only other instruments necessary are one or two 10-mm diameter Babcock clamps and the zero-degree camera. If enterolysis is necessary, as has been described for ileostomy and in Chapter 6 in 'patient preparation', our preferred method is no longer the diathermy/electrocautery but instead the 10-mm diameter harmonic scalpel (Ethicon Endosurgery Inc., Cincinnati, OH). With regard to port placement, mirror-image concepts apply to colostomy as those tenets described in Chapter 8 for ileostomy. Specifically, if enterolysis is required or if the sigmoid loop is not redundant and it is necessary to mobilize the left colon in order to deliver the left or sigmoid colon out of the preoperatively marked left iliac fossa stoma site, then mobilization of the line of Toldt with a 10-mm diameter harmonic scalpel may be necessary. Such mobilization is best effected by placing two ports on the patient's right side – one on the right iliac fossa and one on the right periumbilical region, both lateral to the epigastric vessels through 1 cm stab wounds placed under direct vision. Once again, optimal mobilization of the left colon and visualization of the sigmoid loop is best achieved using steep Trendelenburg and a right-side tilted down position.

There are several ways by which an end colostomy can be constructed laparoscopically. If there is limited mobility of the sigmoid colon and a Hartmann's type procedure is desired, then the inferior mesenteric vessels can be divided as they would be for an anterior resection (see Chapter 37). The left ureter is identified and reflected posteriorly on the dissection field. The inferior mesenteric artery is identified and isolated at the aorta. The vessel is then divided with one of the commercially available laparoscopic endoscopic linear cutting staplers which applies two or three rows of vascular type staples. Other manoeuvres for vascular control include absorbable polydioxane clips (Ethicon GmbH, Hamburg, Germany), vascular clips, or endoscopic pre-tied loops. The mesentery is then scored with the harmonic scalpel and the marginal arcade can then be divided by any of the means already listed for inferior mesenteric artery control. Lastly, the rectosigmoid junction is isolated and the right iliac fossa port is exchanged using the Seldinger technique for an 18 mm port (Ethicon Endosurgery Inc., Cincinnati, OH). A 60 mm laparoscopic cutting and stapling device (ELC60, Ethicon Endosurgery Inc) is placed through the 18 mm port and used to transect the rectosigmoid junction (Figure 9.17). The proximal loop of colon is gently grasped at the staple line. The left iliac fossa port is withdrawn and the crescents of skin are excised above and below the shaft of the 10-mm diameter Babcock instrument. The laparoscopic Babcock forceps is then inferiorly angled. Utilizing right-angled retractors, the underlying fat, anterior rectal sheath, rectus fibres along their axis, and posterior sheath of the peritoneum are incised in a cephalad to caudad direction. The manoeuvre is then repeated, again utilizing the insulated shaft of the Babcock clamps and intracorporeal visualization by the camera operator to prevent injury to surrounding structures during widening of the stoma site. Failure to appropriately widen the site could lead to postoperative obstruction. After the stoma site is constructed to allow two of the surgeon's fingers to fit easily, the proximal colon segment is then delivered through the site (Figure 9.18). After irrigation and verification of meticulous haemostasis, the abdomen is desufflated, ports are withdrawn and all port sites are closed. Ultimately, the colostomy is matured in the standard fashion (Figure 9.19), as previously described in this chapter.

An alternative means of stoma construction is more akin to that described for ileostomy. When more redundancy exists, the entire loop of colon can be delivered through the site. Construction of the stoma itself is no different from that already described, utilizing the insulated component of the laparoscopic Babcock forceps to protect underlying structures. After the loop is delivered, it can be divided extracorporeally with a standard stapling device. The distal end can then be reduced under

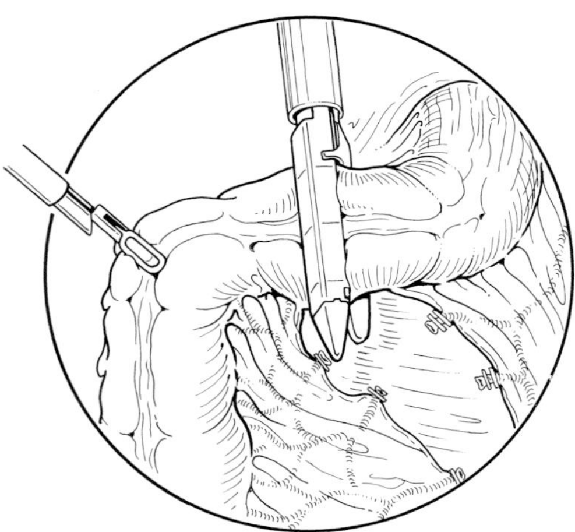

Figure 9.17 A 60 mm laparoscopic cutting and stapling device is placed through the right iliac fossa 18 mm port and used to transect the rectosigmoid junction.

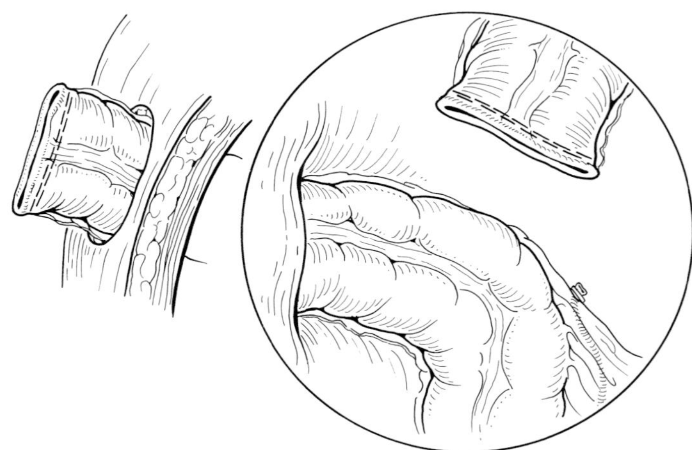

Figure 9.18 The proximal colon segment is delivered through the stoma site.

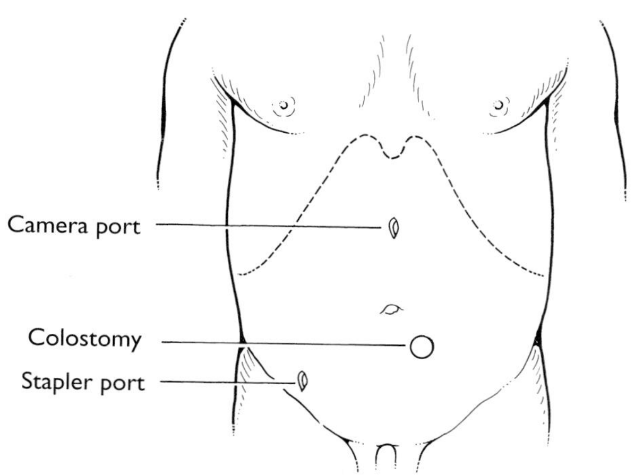

Figure 9.19 The site of the ports and the matured colostomy.

the skin or matured as an Abcarian-type stoma (Unti et al, 1991). The proximal limb is matured as a standard colostomy.

Depending on the surgical indication, on the patient's internal anatomy with regard to sigmoid loop redundancy, and on the presence of underlying adhesions, a colostomy may be performed through as few as two ports (one for the camera and one for the Babcock forceps) or through as many as four ports if enterolysis and/or intracorporeal bowel resection are necessary or desired.

Verification of orientation of the limbs is easily achieved by either passing a colonoscope prior to transsection, by insufflating air per anum, or by simple camera visualization. An adjunctive manoeuvre is, as described for loop ileostomy, the placement of an artery forceps along the serosa of the afferent limb in order to verify intracorporeally the absence of inappropriate limb rotation.

Postoperative management

The postoperative management is identical to that for ileostomy (see Chapter 8). Once again, fundamentally important tenets include extensive preoperative consultation with a stoma care nurse, keeping the patient in hospital until they are comfortable with managing the stoma, and arranging for home stoma care visits and membership of an ostomy support group.

CONTINENT COLOSTOMY

The quest for continence in patients with an end colostomy has been explored for over at least two decades. No device has yet proved satisfactory. Reservoir colostomy is inferior to reservoir ileostomy (Kock et al, 1985) and has largely been abandoned. Implantable devices suffer the risks of sepsis and the quality of continence is disappointing (Goligher et al, 1977; Kewenter, 1978). The smooth muscle collar popularized by Schmidt (1982) relies on colostomy irrigation and there is real doubt as to whether the collar adds anything to the continence achieved. The quality of continence with hydraulic pressure prostheses and most colostomy plugs is disappointing (Wulff, 1953; Ruf et al, 1977; Schwemmle et al, 1982). Recent developments offer no apparent improvement particularly for controlling flatus (Burcharth et al, 1986; Soliani et al, 1992; Codina Cazador et al, 1993). As a result there have been new initiatives to explore total anorectal reconstruction with coloperineal anastomosis surrounded by the electrically stimulated gracilis neosphincter after abdominoperineal excision of the rectum (Mander et al, 1996; Cavina, 1996). A brief account of the development of continent devices is provided here, but details of their construction and surgical management will be omitted since the best method of controlling colostomy activity is still by colostomy irrigation (Williams and Johnston, 1980; Shu-wen Jao et al, 1985).

Reservoir colostomy

Reservoir colostomy was conceived in 1974. The principle of the pouch was to use an intussusception valve of proximal large bowel in a loop of sigmoid colon. Although the device gave good results in dogs (Kock et al, 1974), the results in five patients were absolute failures. Continence was not achieved owing to slippage of the nipple valve, the incidence of sepsis was high, and the irrigation took a long time; hence the method was abandoned (Kock et al, 1985).

In view of the consistency of stool in the left colon it was suggested that the caecum might be used as a reservoir and that anastomosis of an intussuscepted segment of ileum might provide a better valve (Figure 9.20a–d). Results in 30 patients were reported: at the time of review 63% still had a continent pouch; in the remainder the pouch had been removed because of poor function or sepsis. Most patients irrigated twice a day and spent 20–45 minutes daily emptying the

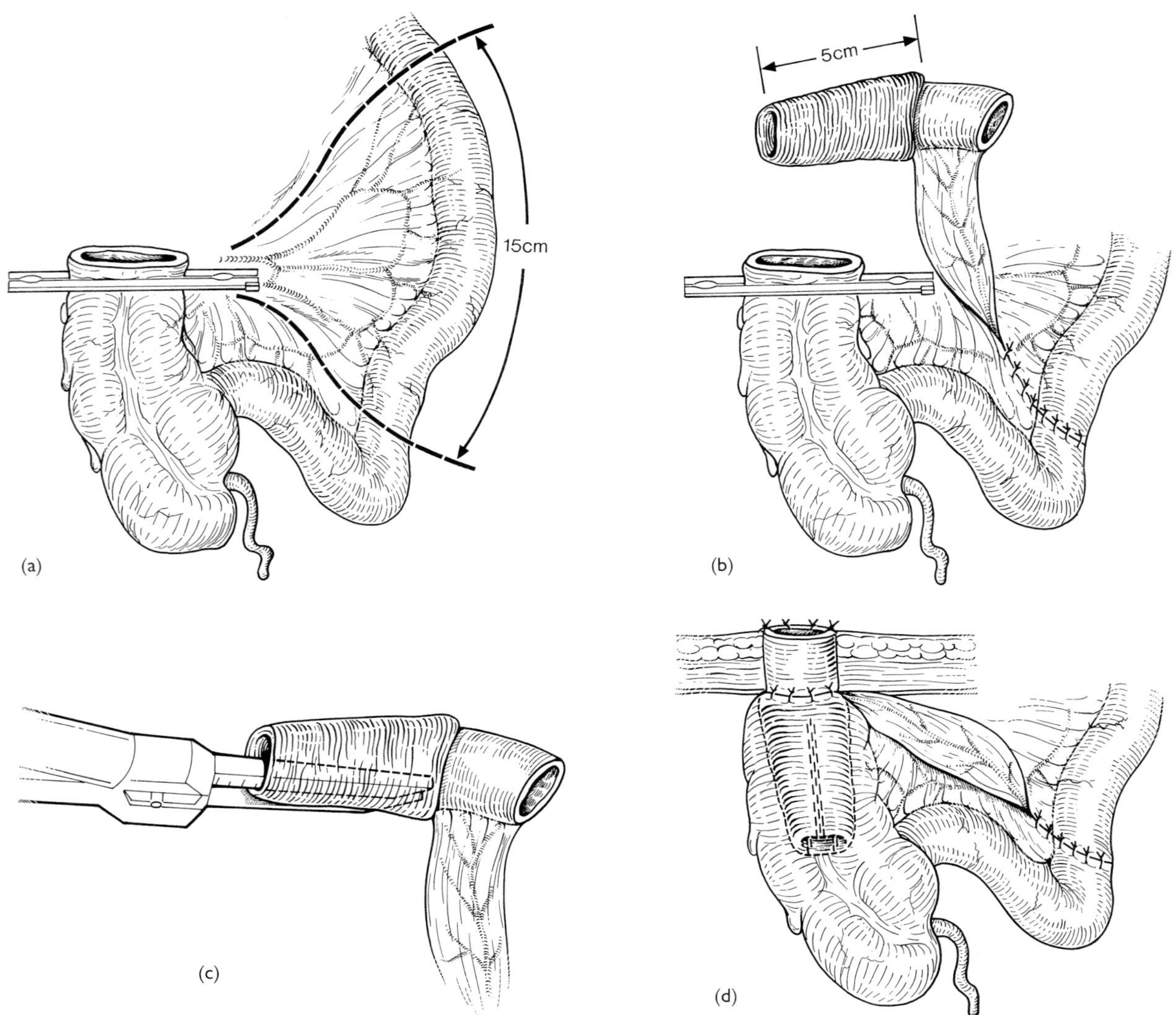

Figure 9.20a–d Reservoir colostomy. (a) A 15 cm limb of terminal ileum is mobilized on a vascular pedicle and the ends of limb are divided. (b) The isolated segment of ileum is fashioned into a nipple valve after ileoileal anastomosis. (c) The nipple valve is stabilized using the linear stapler without cutter. (d) The isolated ileal pedicle is sutured into the end of the colon and to the abdominal wall to achieve a nipple valve into the colon which acts as a reservoir. (This procedure has largely been abandoned.)

pouch. When the results of continent ileostomy and colostomy were compared, complication rates were 8% and 23% respectively and revision rates were 8% and 67% respectively (Kock et al, 1985). The authors concluded that continent ileostomy was superior to colostomy and that reservoir ileostomy should be offered to patients who wished to avoid wearing a bag.

Smooth muscle collar

Schmidt (1982) described placing a smooth muscle collar around the end of the colon. The smooth muscle was obtained from the descending colon during excision of the rectum. The mucosa was dissected from the smooth muscle, the muscle was then stretched and sutured around the distal segment of colon (Figure 9.21a–d). The theory behind the procedure was that the smooth muscle acted as a free smooth muscle graft and functioned as a sphincter. The free graft was said to develop a secondary blood supply from the colon, and electron-microscopy studies suggested that the muscle architecture was maintained (Schmidt et al, 1979; Schmidt, 1981; Zoltan, 1982). Although 509 patients underwent the procedure, critical results have never been presented. Schwemmle et al (1982)

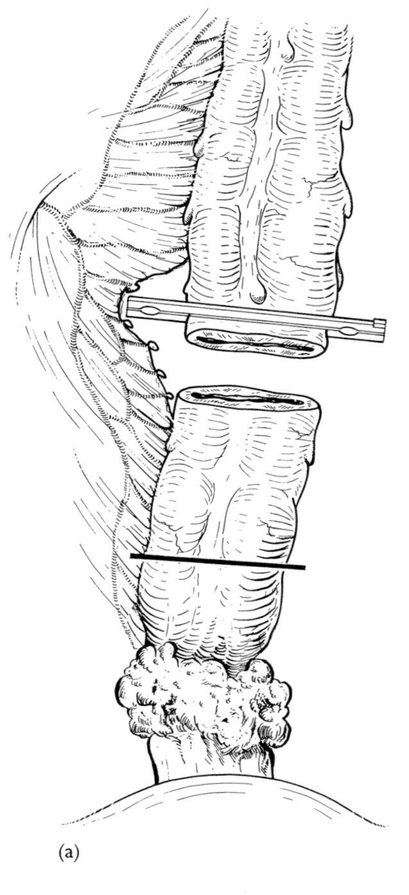

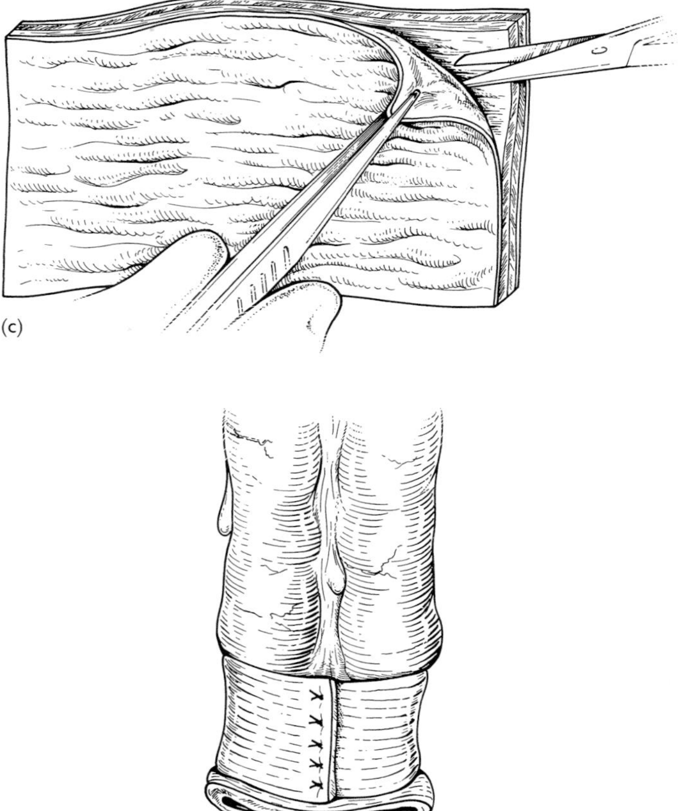

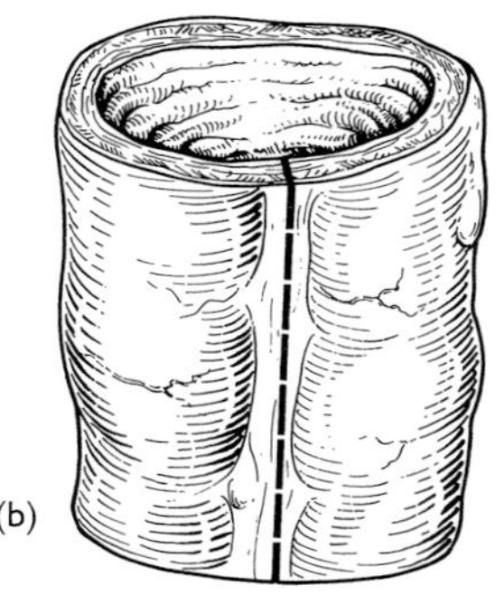

Figure 9.21a–d Smooth muscle collar in an attempt to achieve continence of an end colostomy. (a) A segment of colon has been resected proximal to the site of obstruction. (b) The segment of isolated colon is opened longitudinally along the taenia coli. (c) The mucosa of the colonic segment is removed. (d) The smooth muscle collar is sutured to the end of the colon which is fashioned in the usual way as an end colostomy. (This procedure is rarely used.)

imply that continence is achieved only in patients using colostomy irrigation. We consider this procedure to be obsolete.

Magnetic colostomy device

The magnetic colostomy was developed in Erlangen. The device consists of a ring and a cap containing a central spigot (Figure 9.22). The ring is implanted into the anterior abdominal wall, either at the time of abdominoperineal excision or as a secondary procedure.

The quality of continence with this device was reviewed by Schwemmle et al (1982) but duration of follow-up was short (Table 9.3). Alexander-Williams and eight other surgeons (1977) reported the collective UK experience in 61 patients. There were six deaths, only one of which was related to sepsis. The device had to be removed in 12 patients because of necrosis and sepsis. Twenty-two patients soon stopped using the device because of incontinence, disinterest or dislodgement of the cap. Only 21 patients used the cap regularly, of whom 15 were continent. Most patients used a conventional bag at night. The colostomy is often bulky and the magnet

Table 9.3 Comparison of results achieved with the magnetic colostomy device.

Authors	*n*	*Incontinent*	*Partly incontinent*	*Continent*
Alexander-Williams et al (1977)	43	22	6	15
Goligher et al (1977)	13	5	4	4
Messinetti et al (1977)	12	0	3	9
Skeie (1977)	10	0	0	10
Franchini et al (1978)	7	0	0	7
Kewenter (1978)	16	3	3	10
Kuld-Hansen (1978)	25	6	2	17
Saubier (1978)	7	1	2	4
Stock et al (1978)	27	3	6	18
Hager and Schellerer (1979)	99	35	0	64
Khubchandani et al (1981)	14	7	0	7
Schwemmle et al (1982)	68	23	7	38

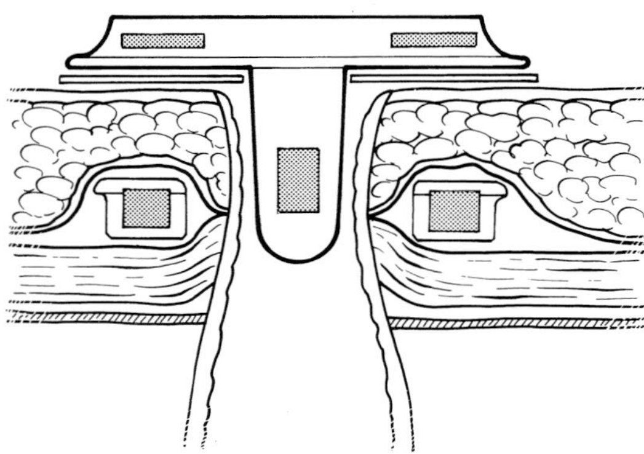

Figure 9.22 A magnetic colostomy device.

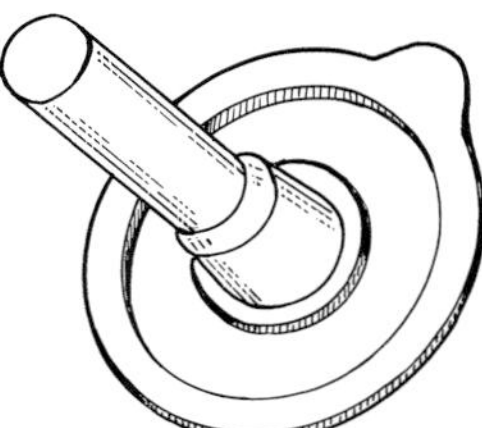

Figure 9.23 A colostomy plug.

may be a nuisance. Late follow-up indicates that most patients have abandoned use of the magnetic cap because of its unreliability. We consider this technique to be obsolete.

Colostomy plug

Although a variety of other appliances to occlude a colostomy stoma have been tried, none has been completely reliable and most have been abandoned (Heiblum and Cordoba, 1978; Prager, 1984). A more recent development has been a two-piece occlusive device. The faceplate consists of a circular clip on a flange. To this is attached a plug. The plug expands inside the stoma so as to occlude it and prevent both solid and liquid contents escaping; gas is absorbed via a filter which is incorporated into the plug. Flatus control has been reported as complete in 90% of patients (Burcharth et al, 1986; Cerdan et al, 1991). Later reviews seem less enthusiastic, however. Soliani et al (1992) compared the one-piece plug with a two-piece device (Figure 9.23). There were technical difficulties in inserting the plug with the two-piece system. Furthermore, all patients were expected to irrigate, and inserting the cone of the irrigator was difficult in many cases. Thus compliance was poor with the two-piece system, frequency of daily irrigations remained unchanged, but in both groups control of flatus was achieved in all except one patient. A similar study from Spain reported that 26 of 37 patients preferred the one-piece plug over a conventional colostomy bag (Codina Cazador et al, 1993).

Total anorectal reconstruction

Total anorectal reconstruction is the ultimate development of a continent perineal colostomy and is described fully in Chapter 32.

The Schmidt smooth muscle collar was first applied to the coloperineal anastomosis (Torres and Gonzalez, 1988), and in a series of 24 patients all of whom were taught to irrigate the colon, a degree of continence was achieved (Elias et al, 1993). A similar experience from Moscow (Fedorov et al, 1989) claimed that the smooth muscle collar resulted in a 38% increase in intraluminal pressure. Skeletal muscle transpositions around the perineal colostomy have also been explored. Chittenden (1930) used gluteus maximus, Fedorov and Shelygin (1989) tried adductor longus, but only the gracilis transposition has really stood the test of time (Simonsen et al, 1976; Cavina et al, 1987; Williams et al, 1990b; Mercati et al, 1991). The non-stimulated muscle wrap was unreliable. Long-term neural stimulation with an implantable device transformed type-2 fast twitch to type-1 slow twitch muscle which achieved sphincteric function during stimulation associated with an improved level of continence. Nevertheless, patients needed to wear pads for soiling and suffered episodes of incontinence. Despite this, none of these patients was willing to return to a conventional colostomy (Mander et al, 1996). However, all of these patients have impaired neorectal sensation (Abercrombie et al, 1996) and all need to empty the colon using either colonic irrigation or a colonic conduit (Hughes and Williams, 1995). Time will tell whether this quest for continence is acceptable and affordable. However, the role of colonic or colostomy irrigation must not be ignored in these patients. Chiotasso et al (1992) reported satisfaction in all their long-term follow-ups using daily irrigation alone without a neosphincter through a perineal colostomy.

MANAGEMENT OF THE COLOSTOMY

Early postoperative care

Early postoperative management is greatly improved if patients have been counselled preoperatively (White and Hunt, 1997). This may be difficult in patients needing emergency operation. For this reason all staff dealing with colorectal patients should have attended a stoma care course so that they are in a better position before the operation to explain to patients the consequences of life with a stoma. Sadly, Phillips et al (1985) found that only 45% of patients having a colostomy had been properly counselled beforehand. Postoperative physical complications should be minimized where possible and dealt with sympathetically since a bad operative experience is associated with a greater risk of psychological problems associated with the stoma (Thomas et al, 1987a,b; Oberst and Scott, 1988).

An appliance should be attached to the skin surrounding the edges of the stoma as soon as it has been sutured in theatre. A good seal is important for morale in the early days after operation. It is preferable to use a transparent bag for observing the stoma in the immediate postoperative period.

Loop colostomy

Loop colostomies are much more difficult to manage than end stomas. The problems are bulk, adjacent skin sutures and the rod. Bulk can be reduced by excision of a wide circular disc of skin and fat with immediate mucocutaneous suture and avoidance of a rod. Use of a transverse skin incision for a loop colostomy may involve lateral skin sutures, which can make fitting of an appliance difficult in the early postoperative period. (see Figure 9.10a,b). A rod should be used only if necessary and preferably should be short (Browning and Parks, 1983). Rods are particularly difficult to manage if they are sutured to the skin.

For most loop colostomies the flange will need to be 75–100 mm diameter. The aperture must be cut to fit snugly around the bowel and under the rod. Most appliances for immediate management of a loop colostomy are one- or two-piece drainable bags often with a plastic winged rod which is either sutured to the skin with a rotatable T-piece to prevent dislodgement or with a clip to facilitate easy removal (see Figure 9.13). Various colostomy appliances are available (Figure 9.7b), Karaya is hardly ever used and each manufacturer has its own formulation of hydrocolloids similar to Stomahesive. The flanges all consist of self-adhesive, protected by single-release paper. There are size-specific oval and round flanges, or patients may have to cut a disc to size from a template. The appliance may be one- or two-piece and the bags may be one-piece or drainable. For transverse loop colostomy, clip-on bags are often used initially as they can be drained in the early postoperative period and replaced by a one-piece device when the effluent becomes solid (Hill and Pickford, 1979). The principal manufacturers are Convatec (formerly Squibb Surgicare), Coloplast, Dansac, Hollister, Simcare and Salts-Welland. Illustrations of some current appliances appear in Figure 8.16.

End colostomy

A much smaller flange can be used for an end colostomy; the aperture should be cut to fit the diameter of the colon at the completion of the operation and a bag with a drainage clip should be used.

Although the two-piece System 2 bags are very convenient, removal and reapplication may be painful early after operation. The floating flange allows improved application which may be less painful than a press-on two-piece locking device (see Figure 8.16). The bags will need to be of different size depending on the site of the colostomy and the likely volume and consistency of the effluent. Bags may have to be vented to remove gas and liquid faeces once ileus has resolved. Subsequently, discardable (usually small one-piece) bags will be used as the faecal discharge becomes solid.

Patient involvement

We believe that it is important to encourage active patient participation as soon as the person is mobile after operation. Patients should first learn to change the bag and drain its contents through the clip. Later they should be taught to shower and bath with their appliance. Finally, practical sessions should be arranged so that patients can learn to cut the flanges, clean the skin, use barrier pastes where appropriate, apply belts and fit covers when needed.

Appliances

Modern appliances have greatly improved the quality of life for colostomy patients. For patients with a left-sided colostomy, bags may be avoided altogether if irrigation is successful, but this form of management is not acceptable in all patients. In Britain, irrigation is often unpopular because of the time factor and is only attractive to those interested in body image and lifestyle. The situation is quite different in Europe and North America where irrigation is the norm and anything else unacceptable. Controlled natural evacuation by dietary restriction and drug therapy may allow a small number of patients who have undergone abdominoperineal excision to dispense with appliances altogether (Grier et al, 1964; Shu-wen Jao et al, 1985); most, however, need to wear an appliance at all times. After abdominoperineal excision, 46% of patients have more than two bowel actions per day; indeed, in 19% the stoma acts more than five times per day and 15% report that they suffer from continuous diarrhoea (Devlin et al, 1971). With a transverse colostomy, frequency of defecation is much greater and episodes of diarrhoea and leakage from the appliance are more common.

Absorption of gas can be achieved with activated charcoal filters, which are usually fitted to colostomy caps and to drainable and non-drainable bags. The basis of all modern appliances is a reliable non-irritant seal which will protect the skin and allow adhesion so that gas and liquid cannot escape. Sealants include Karaya (Plant, 1971; Sparberg, 1974), now replaced by Stomahesive or similar hydrocolloids.

Colostomy bags should be lightweight, easily disposable and odour-proof through the use of impermeable plastic and filters. It is largely up to patients to decide whether they prefer a drainable or a non-drainable bag and a one-piece or two-piece appliance. Their choice will depend upon the consistency of the stool, the size and appearance of the stoma, the control of gas and ease of management. Most appliances have a cover to the plastic made of artificial fibres in order to prevent the plastic sticking to the skin. Control of gas is most important for the colostomy patient: passage of flatus is embarrassing and distension of bags by gas may dislodge the appliance, quite apart from the patient being aware of a visible swelling underneath clothing. There should be an adequate supply of a full range of appliances. Most stoma care nurses who are not funded by a particular appliance manufacturer have a wide selection of free appliances from the rival companies. Each patient should have a checklist of their requirements so that these can be obtained from the pharmacist, or more usually direct from the manufacturers. Some colostomy bags are capable of disposal down the lavatory, there is an inner bag containing stool and an outer plastic surround which can be thrown away as for any plastic bag. At the moment there are no biodegradable appliances. Disposal of conventional bags remains unsatisfactory. The contents are emptied into the lavatory while the appliance is placed in a Jiffy bag and discarded in a dustbin as with disposable nappies. This waste is disposed of in land dumps.

Problems

Skin problems and odour

Skin protection is usually critical only to patients with a loop transverse colostomy. Between 200 and 2000 mL of intestinal gas is passed per day, the amount varying enormously with diet, activity, altitude and eating habits. Most flatus is swallowed air; some is produced by bacterial fermentation of organisms resident in the bowel; the remainder is from dietary intake (Sykes et al, 1976; Arabi et al, 1978; Keighley and Burdon, 1979).

Colostomy patients find that odour is a much greater problem than do ileostomy patients (Levine et al, 1970). Emission of gas, particularly during social functions, is one of the greatest fears to the incontinent ostomate. The problem may be minimized by avoiding aerated drinks and by the use of filters. Filters are now incorporated into most drainable and almost all non-drainable stoma appliances. Diet will modify the amount of gas produced in the colon. Malodorous compounds include amines, indole, methane and hydrogen sulphide. Excessive flatus will be produced by non-absorbed carbohydrates such as stachyose and raffinose in beans and non-digestible oligosaccharides in onions and green vegetables. Eggs produce hydrogen sulphide and methane. Many of these food products are therefore avoided by the more fastidious patient (Bingham et al, 1977; Gazzard et al, 1978).

Oral preparations which may be used to control flatus include chlorophyll tablets, charcoal biscuits and bismuth subgallate. Bismuth subgallate may inhibit growth of the colonic flora by altering intestinal motility but it can sometimes cause constipation (Sparberg, 1974). An alternative is to place compounds such as aspirin in the stoma bag. Commercial preparations are now available for this purpose and include sodium-phenylphenate tetrahydrate (0.3%) with parachlorometaxylenol (0.2%), oxychlorosene or benzalkonium chloride. Filters made of activated carbon or charcoal are effective provided they do not become damp, which renders them useless.

Diet

Dietary advice for colostomy patients is often lacking or imprecise (Thomson et al, 1970; Devlin et al, 1971). Devlin found that no dietary restriction was practised in 47% of patients after rectal excision, whereas 14% avoided at least six foods. A restricted diet was more common among elderly manual workers (Devlin et al, 1971). Foods which are often avoided include onions, salads, beer and eggs. Very little data are available on the effect of different diets on stoma function (Kramer et al, 1962; Gazzard et al, 1978). The influence of certain foods on frequency of flatus, odour and liquid stool is shown in Table 9.4.

Drugs

Very few patients with a colostomy are given advice on the use of antidiarrhoeal preparations (Turnbull, 1961; Devlin and Plant, 1975). Methylcellulose may be used to thicken the effluent in patients with a transverse colostomy. Kaolin, alone or with morphine, should be held in reserve for treatment during an episode of diarrhoea, but small doses of codeine or loperamide are now used regularly by some (Devlin, 1973).

Spontaneous action

Control of a colostomy is rarely achieved by diet, medication or lifestyle. Over 80% of patients therefore need to wear a bag unless they practise colostomy irrigation.

Colostomy irrigation

Although colostomy irrigation has been popular in North America for the last three decades, it has never gained the same wide acceptance in the UK (Turnbull, 1961; Williams and Johnston, 1980). One factor may have been early reports of perforation, when cruder apparatus than currently available was used for irrigation (Seargeant, 1966; Spiro and Hertz, 1966; Isa and Quan, 1975; Griffiths et al, 1976; Mazier et al, 1976). However, the principal reason for the difference is in attitude, expectation and a person's direct involvement with their bowel. There appears to be a real cultural difference between

Table 9.4 Diets and stoma function: patients (%) producing excess flatus, odour or liquid stomal contents.

	Ileostomy			*Colostomy*		
Foodstuff	*Flatus*	*Odour*	*Liquid*	*Flatus*	*Odour*	*Liquid*
Green vegetables	32	6	18	46	28	26
Onions	12	12	4	26	10	4
Fruit	2	0	12	10	0	42
Eggs	6	23	2	4	4	2
Fish	0	34	6	2	6	4
Cheese	2	14	4	2	2	0
Spices	2	6	2	4	2	8

From Gazzard et al (1978).

countries even within Europe and among patients with different educational, ethnic and intellectual background. Irrigation is not a suitable method for all patients since it requires a level of dexterity, intelligence, toilet facilities and stoma design which may not be available to all patients (Venturini et al, 1990). Recent popularity has been helped by the design of a safe, cone-shaped delivery device and equipment which is easy to handle (Dini et al, 1991).

The apparatus needed for colostomy irrigation is illustrated in Figure 9.24. This consists of a one-piece reservoir and delivery tube with a control device and a cone-shaped end, a drainage system and a belt. The drainage system consists of a flange which adheres to the skin around the stoma, a long dependent drainage conduit which will hang between the legs to discharge its contents into a lavatory pan, and a sealable open upper end for access to the stoma. The reservoir is filled with a variable volume of tepid tapwater and suspended above the patient so that the bottom of the reservoir is at shoulder height. The delivery tube is primed with water. The volume of fluid used will depend on the tolerance of the patient and the frequency of irrigation. The flange of the sleeve is attached around the stoma and the patient sits on the lavatory with the conduit in the lavatory pan. After lubricating the cone, the upper end of the conduit is opened, the cone is applied firmly to the stomal orifice and the control device regulating the flow of the irrigation fluid is opened. The flow should not be too fast otherwise troublesome intestinal colic will occur. The water should be at room temperature. Some patients find that they cannot tolerate more than 500 mL but the quality of washout tends to be inferior with small volumes (Meyhoff et al, 1990). Where possible, 1.5 L should be introduced but 500 mL is preferred by some patients. Once the irrigation is complete, the cone is removed, the upper end of the conduit is sealed and the colon is allowed to empty its contents. Irrigation is performed at approximately the same time each day. Most patients irrigate on alternate days, some manage a regime which is only once every three days. Patients with colostomy prolapse or hernia rarely find that irrigation is possible.

Williams and Johnston (1980) assessed irrigation in 30 patients with an end colostomy who had been using the spontaneous action approach prior to irrigation. After training, eight patients (27%) abandoned the technique because they found it to be too much trouble. In the remaining 22 patients the time spent in irrigation was almost as long as the time taken for the management of a conventional colostomy (Table 9.5). The frequency of bowel movements was reduced by irrigation from 13 to 6 per week. Following irrigation, 16 patients (73%) found that dietary restriction and antidiarrhoeal agents were no longer needed and none complained of difficulty with the stoma at work. Lack of control of flatus was reported in 90% of patients during irrigation. Nevertheless, 81% felt that the use of irrigation was more conducive to participating in social functions that had previously been avoided. Four patients started swimming for the first time. Half of the patients irrigated daily, while a third found that alternate daily irrigation was adequate. The most interesting aspect of this report was that only 15 of

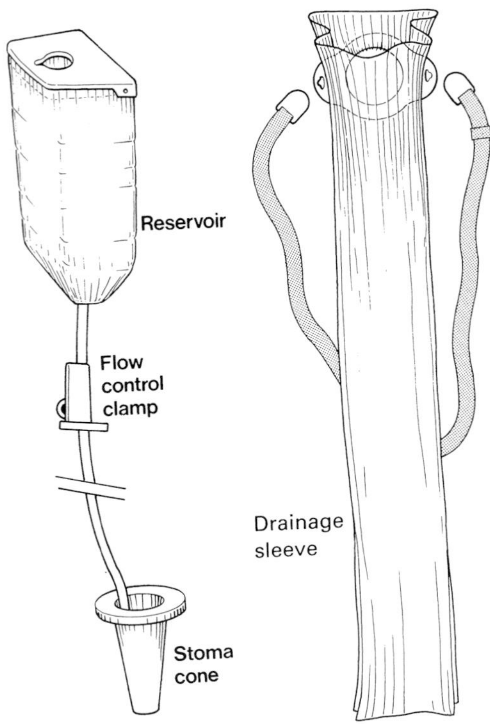

Figure 9.24 The principle of colostomy irrigation.

Table 9.5 Controlled trial of colostomy irrigation compared with spontaneous action.

	Spontaneous action (*n* = 22)	*Irrigation* (*n* = 22)
Time taken (min)	45 ± 9	53 ± 9
Frequency (per week)	13 ± 2	6 ± 1
Dietary restriction	16 (73%)	6 (27%)
Drugs needed	18 (81%)	6 (27%)
Problems at work	8/14 (57%)	0/14 (0%)

From Williams and Johnston (1980).

Table 9.6 Comparison between irrigation and natural evacuation of left-sided end colostomy.

Complication	*Natural evacuation* (*n* = 130)	*Colostomy irrigation** (*n* = 210)
Leakage of stool (use of bag)	130 (100)	54 (26)
Leakage of gas	65 (50)	42 (20)
Irrigation of skin	24 (18)	0
Psychological problems	25 (19)	17 (8)

* One perforation.
Values in parentheses are percentages.
From Terranova et al (1979).

22 patients regularly persisted with the technique, although some of the remainder still used it for special occasions.

Terranova et al (1979) reported that 74% of patients were continent using irrigation, only 20% complained of leakage of gas and 71% irrigated on alternate days only. In 72% irrigation time was less than an hour (Table 9.6). Contraindications to irrigation included age, previous radiotherapy, poor housing, loop colostomy, invisible stomas, prolapse, stenosis, kinking of the colon in or beneath the abdominal wall, hernia, disease in the proximal colon, lack of motivation, poor intelligence, psychotic personality and general disability.

Doran and Hardcastle (1981) undertook a crossover trial to investigate whether a laxative enema (dioctyl sodium sulphosuccinate) might provide superior results to tapwater washout. Both methods reduced the frequency of colostomy action, from 17 to 6 actions per week with water and to 10 actions per week with the enema. Time spent with irrigation was less than the time spent in managing a conventional stoma. Increased flatus and leakage of the enema fluid made this technique inferior to simple tapwater irrigation. Kjaegaard et al (1984) found that the addition of bisacodyl (doses used 1.25, 2.5 and 5.0 mg) or a prostaglandin E2 analogue did not influence the duration of irrigation; furthermore, high-dose bisacodyl caused pain and diarrhoea.

Shu-wen Jao et al (1985) found that irrigation was acceptable in 82% of patients attending the Mayo Clinic, but 74% complained of minor leaks and 26% needed to wear a bag. Women and young patients with a previous history of constipation achieved better results than other patients. In this survey of over 500 patients only one perforation was reported in a patient who did not use a cone device. None suffered from water toxicity, although concern has been voiced that irrigation with water may be contraindicated in patients with cardiac disease because of the risk of precipitating fluid overload.

The great advantage of irrigation is that bulky appliances are not needed, the stoma is simply covered by a cap. Furthermore the practice is cost-effective and enhances body image and self-esteem. Despite positive counselling by our stoma care nurses, the majority of the British public find irrigation time-consuming and unnecessary. In other countries, particularly North America, Scandanavia and Latin European states, the practice is widespread and strongly supported.

Biofeedback

It has been suggested that biofeedback might improve continence among patients with a colostomy. Reboa et al (1985) found that biofeedback achieved objective improvement in the pressure (from 15 to 47 mmH_2O) within the intra-abdominal course of the colostomy. Furthermore, they found that balloon inflation decreased threshold sensation from 62 to 24 mL of air. It is claimed that the colon is capable of generating reflex abdominal wall contraction in response to distension (Reboa et al, 1980) and the principle of biofeedback is therefore applicable, even in the absence of a sphincter (Ceruli et al, 1979; Wald, 1981; McLeod, 1983).

AFTERMATH OF COLOSTOMY

The difficulties encountered by patients with a colostomy were largely dismissed and ignored by the medical and nursing professions until the beginning of the 1970s. Devlin et al (1971) highlighted the enormous physical, psychological and social isolation which some patients face after abdominoperineal excision of the rectum. Conscious of the need for self-help, colostomy patients in North America and the UK established groups to identify problems that patients might encounter after operation (Goligher, 1958). In the UK the British Colostomy Association was founded; it sought to rehabilitate patients with a colostomy.

Three decades ago only 64% of patients lived in housing conditions adequate to facilitate management of their stoma. At that time there was no recognition for preferential housing reallocation on health grounds (Devlin and Plant, 1969). Although housing may have improved, there is still a real problem with respect to disposal of waste and bags. Many patients discard their bags, wrapped in Jiffy bags, in the dustbin. Some appliances have an inner disposable component which can be flushed through the domestic lavatory while the plastic surround is placed into regular waste bins. In the past some appliances were flushed through toilets. Not only did this create problems for the sewage authorities, but it was also held to be partly responsible for pollution to the coastline (Devlin and Plant, 1975). Some patients try to burn their waste but the bags are not inflammable, the plastics smell unpleasant and the solid plastic components are non-degradable. Some local authorities provide a dirty dressing collection service but many patients prefer not to use it. Furthermore, privatization of waste disposal and water has increased the logistical problems of disposal for colostomy patients. Skeet (1970) found that disposal was inadequate for 45% of patients, 25% used the dustbin and 48% pushed articles other than stool down the lavatory.

Apart from often self-imposed dietary restrictions, a certain ritualism seems to have developed among colostomy patients, particularly in the elderly, which increases their social and physical isolation. There is a reluctance to indulge in social activities and evidence of isolationism have been recorded in 51% of colostomy patients compared with 10% of a similar age- and sex-matched normal population (Townsend, 1957; Plant, 1971). Isolationism was even more pronounced in elderly patients in the poor-income bracket and was a feature in both men and women, particularly after rectal excision.

The sexual implications of colostomy, particularly after rectal excision, are discussed elsewhere (see Chapter 11). Although it is acknowledged that sexual interest and performance is often depressed before operation, particularly in inflammatory disease, there is a change in body image which influences affect and sexual behaviour. These patients often consider themselves to be outcasts in society (Briggs et al, 1977). Approximately 25% of patients have severe depressive illnesses, resulting occasionally in suicide (Orbach et al, 1957; Orbach and Tallent, 1965; Druss et al, 1969; George et al, 1975). The incidence of major psychological disturbance was assessed as being 23% following abdominoperineal excision compared with 2% after restorative anterior resection. Physical complications often coexist and include phantom rectal and bladder symptoms. White and Hunt (1997) found that 18–26% of stoma patients experienced psychological problems during the first three months after operation, and that this prevalence persisted for at least the first year (Thomas et al, 1984; Wade 1990). The most common were adjustment disorders with anxiety, depressed mood, clinical depression, panic attacks, social phobia and agoraphobia. Long-term studies indicate that early adjustment disorders often persist and are of the same magnitude as those observed after mastectomy (Maguire, 1978). The prevalence of psychological morbidity does not appear to have changed despite advances in stoma care management. These psychological symptoms often compromise patient recovery after operation and may have an impact on social activity and occupation. Recognition and treatment of these psychological problems after hospital discharge is often poor and may be hindered by poor consultation facilities, fear by patients of expressing symptoms that may be trivialized or used as barriers to return to the workplace.

Factors which appear to have no association with this psychological morbidity are: age, marital status, gender, type of stoma, preoperative diagnosis and severity of illness before operation (Thomas et al, 1987a,b; Wade, 1989a; Klopp, 1990; Marsh, 1994). By contrast, previous psychiatric illness, inadequate preoperative preparation and physical postoperative complications have a major impact on psychological illness after colostomy construction (Wade, 1989b). Thus, stoma patients must be screened before operation to exclude major psychological instability. They must be thoroughly counselled, and if postoperative complications develop they must be managed sympathetically.

Although 56% of men who held jobs before rectal excision were able to return to work, 89% of them had to change to a less demanding form of employment that usually resulted in a loss of income. Furthermore, the time off work was almost twice as long after rectal excision (31 weeks) compared with restorative resection (18 weeks) (Devlin et al, 1971).

The dilemma might not seem to be as great for patients with diverticular disease having a loop colostomy or a Hartmann procedure, but we found that only 56% of patients having a Hartmann operation had their stoma closed. Some died in hospital, others were too ill for closure and a few refused any further operations (Phillips et al, 1985). This experience has been confirmed both by retrospective and prospective observations (Shepherd and Keighley, 1986; Tudor et al, 1986). It might be thought that the prospect of restoring intestinal continuity in loop colostomy patients was greater, but our experience suggests otherwise. Of 104 patients with a temporary loop colostomy, 17 died in hospital, ten died before colostomy closure or resection as a complication of a second operation, seven were too ill for resection, and seven refused further operation, leaving only 63 (60%) who actually had their loop stoma closed. Wara et al (1981) reported that intestinal continuity was restored in 84% of patients having a temporary stoma for malignant disease, in 65% of patients with a stoma for diverticular disease, and in as few as 9% of patients after radiotherapy. Factors associated with a failure to restore intestinal continuity included age, general debility and associated illness.

The most alarming finding of one survey was that only 47% of patients with a colostomy were visited at home by a district nurse to ensure there were no stomal problems and only 36% of patients were seen by their general practitioner after hospital discharge. Many patients felt that general practitioners lacked knowledge about their stoma and considered that the responsibility for their welfare lay with the hospital. Few, if any, provided advice on diet or antidiarrhoeal agents, and 41% of patients had seen neither a nurse nor a doctor after discharge from hospital. Until recently surveillance of the colon after abdominoperineal excision was rare. Patients may attend follow-up for detection of local and distant recurrence, for which little can often be done to improve survival. On the other hand, metachronous cancer or polyps may be present in 2–19% and go undetected and untreated (Zilli et al, 1987).

A recent metanalysis compared the outcome of rectal cancer patients having a stoma with those who could be treated by a sphincter-preserving procedure (Sprangers et al, 1995). Where possible, quality of life was assessed by the patients themselves in relation to physical, psychological, social and sexual function. Both groups suffered from frequent irregular bowel movements and diarrhoea. Stoma patients had a much higher incidence of poor flatus control (50%) and urinary symptoms (20–30%) than the sphincter-preserved group (15–37% and 0–14% respectively). Stoma patients had a much higher level of generalized forms of distress (10–54%) and negative body image (60%) than the non-stoma patients (3–43% and 5%) respectively.

Feelings of unpleasant odour were more prevalent in colostomy patients (37% versus 19%). Concerns about appearance were reported in 20% of stoma patients compared with 9% in the non-stoma group. Generally, colostomy patients have more restrictions in terms of social function, employment, friendships and partners than those without a colostomy. Sexual function in men was consistently more impaired in patients with a colostomy, and women with a colostomy had more dyspareunia and greater interference with intercourse than those having a sphincter-preserving operation (Table 9.7).

Table 9.7 Morbidity of colostomy in rectal cancer.

	Colostomy (%)	*Sphincter-preserving operation* (%)
Problems with flatus (Macdonald and Anderson, 1995)	49	37
Feeling of unpleasant odour (Frigell et al, 1990)	37	19
Concern for appearance (MacDonald and Anderson, 1984)	20	9
Return to work (Cardoen et al, 1984)	20	79
Visiting friends less (Wirsching et al, 1975)	27	17
Less participation in activities (MacDonald and Anderson, 1984)	63	49

From Sprangers et al (1995).

COMPLICATIONS OF COLOSTOMY

Complications of colostomy can for convenience be divided into early and late. Complications are particularly common in children. Wara et al (1981) found that prolapse and colostomy hernia occurred much more commonly in children and that 50% of infants, compared with 26% of adults, developed stomal complications (Table 9.8). The incidence of complications in these two groups will therefore be reviewed separately.

Children

Mollitt et al (1980) reviewed the incidence of colostomy complications in 146 children with Hirschsprung's disease or imperforate anus. The majority were transverse colostomies (82%) and the rest were placed in the sigmoid colon. The complications are listed in Table 9.9. Sepsis, which occurred in 18% of children, was the principal cause

Table 9.8 Complications following construction of a transverse colostomy.

Complication	*Adults* (*n* = 235)	*Infants* (*n* = 22)
Parastomal infection	34 (14)	4 (18)
Stomal necrosis	5 (2)	1 (5)
Stomal prolapse	13 (6)	5 (23)
Stomal retraction	12 (5)	3 (14)
Parastomal hernia	7 (3)	3 (14)
Total with complications	62 (26)	11 (50)

Values in parentheses are percentages.
From Wara et al (1981).

of early complications. Late stomal complications were recorded in 48%, with skin excoriation being the most common. Prolapse occurred in 12% and stenosis in 6%. The revision rate was 16%, being principally related to appliance problems and prolapse. The incidence of complications was similar to the findings reported by MacMahon et al (1963) but rather higher than those reported by Brenner and Swenson (1967). Factors which seemed to be related to an increased risk of complications were the use of transverse as compared with sigmoid colon, and the policy of using loop as compared with divided stomas. Age and underlying diagnosis were not found to be important factors.

Prolapse is the complication which is considerably more prevalent in children than adults. Colostomy prolapse did not occur in the first year of life, but 11 of 19 children (58%) aged between 1 and 13 years developed a prolapse (Chandler and Evans, 1978). By contrast, only 58 of 448 patients (13%) over 13 years of age developed colostomy prolapse. Prolapse was more common in loop colostomy, particularly those in the right side of the transverse colon (Birnbaum and Ferrier, 1952; Cain and Kiesewetter, 1965; Green, 1966; Burns, 1970; Pelok and Nigro, 1973; Saha et al, 1973).

Table 9.9 Colostomy complications in 146 children.

Complication	*Number*
Early	
Postoperative sepsis	14 (2†)
Small bowel herniation	4 (3*) (1†)
Wound infection	2
Intestinal obstruction	1
Pulmonary embolus	1 (1†)
Late	
Skin excoriation	29
Prolapse	17 (5*)
Stenosis	9 (2*)
Colocutaneous fistula	5 (1*)
Retraction	5 (2*)
Wound hernia	2
Bleeding	1
Suture sinus	1
Persistent sepsis	1 (1*)

* Number needing revision; a further ten needed revision for bad siting.
† Deaths.
From Mollitt et al (1980).

Adults

We reviewed the outcome in 276 patients who had had a colostomy (Phillips et al, 1985). The majority of patients had a carcinoma of the large bowel (72%); in 141 (51%) the stoma was temporary and in 48 cases (34%) had been performed as an emergency procedure for obstruction, perforation or sepsis. Of the patients who survived hospital admission, 60 (25%) developed complications (Table 9.10). The most common complications were skin excoriation (12%), leakage (7%) and stomal sepsis (8%). Only 25 of the 60 patients with complications needed surgical refashioning procedures. Porter et al (1989) report very similar observations, with skin excoriation (13%), stomal sepsis (9%), hernia (11%) and stenosis (9%) as the most common complications.

Pearl et al (1985) found that the incidence of stomal complications was more common with loop colostomy than end colostomy, and this is now a fairly universal observation (Porter et al, 1989). Complications were more common following emergency surgery and operations performed by inexperienced personnel. Stothert et al (1982) reviewed the morbidity of stomas constructed as emergency procedures for obstruction, sepsis or trauma. The overall morbidity was over 50%; nine patients died (18%) and four deaths were directly due to the stoma (Table 9.11). Porter et al (1989) reported complications in 44% of patients with a colostomy; hernia was the most common, followed by stricture, sepsis, small bowel obstruction and prolapse, in that order. In addition, 15% suffered from skin excoriation. They found that the incidence of complications was unrelated to site, urgency of operation or underlying disease; 13% required surgical correction. The very high incidence of complications in this report may have been influenced by the large number of stomas (over half) which were brought out through the abdominal incision. Londono-Schimmer et al (1994) at St Marks reviewed the crude and actuarial complication rates of end sigmoid colostomy. They found that the complication rate increased with duration of follow-up, with a figure exceeding 50% ten years after construction (Figure 9.25). Paracolostomy hernia was the single

Table 9.10 Incidence of colostomy complications.

Complication	*Phillips et al (1985)* (*n* (surviving) = 243)	*Porter et al (1989)* (*n* = 126)	*Londono-Schimmer et al (1994)* (*n* = 203)
Skin excoriation	30 (12)	17 (13)	24 (12)
Leakage	18 (7)	0	NS
Stomal sepsis	20 (8)	11 (9)	NS
Hernia	11 (5)	14 (11)	43 (21)
Prolapse	5 (2)	4 (3)	11 (5)
Retraction	5 (2)	0	3 (1.5)
Stenosis	3 (1)	11 (9)	10 (5)
Infarction	3 (1)	0	NS
Bleeding	2 (1)	0	NS
Small bowel obstruction	0	9 (7)	11 (5)
Fistula	0	1 (1)	2 (1)
Total number with complications	60 (25)	NS	NS
Total number requiring stomal refashioning	25 (10)	NS	NS

Values in parentheses are percentages. NS = not stated.

Table 9.11 Morbidity of emergency stomas.

Complication	*Ileostomy* (*n* = 10)	*Transverse colostomy* (*n* = 23)	*Sigmoid colostomy* (*n* = 18)
Intra-abdominal abscess	2	4	1
Peristomal abscess	0	3	0
Necrotizing fasciitis	1	1	0
Obstruction	1	0	0
Necrosis of stoma	2 (1*)	2 (2*)	0
Fascial dehiscence	1	1	0
Peristomal hernia	0	2 (1*)	0
Prolapse	0	1	0
Ulceration of skin	5	2	1
Pressure necrosis of skin	0	1	0

* Deaths associated with stomal complications.
From Stothert et al (1982).

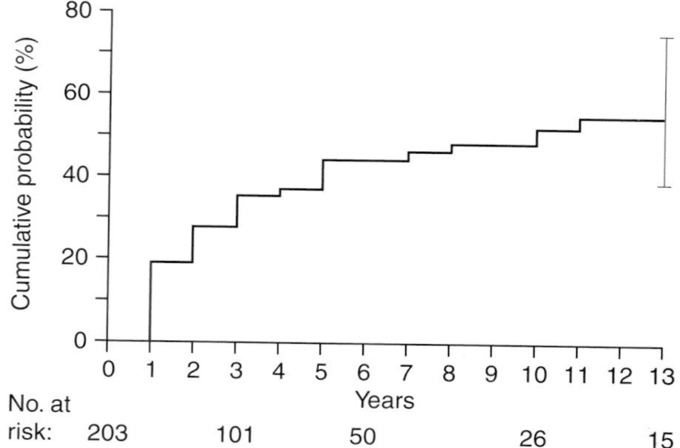

Figure 9.25 The cumulative probability of complication. Error bars represent 95% confidence limits. Complications continue to occur over time at a slower rate (Londono-Schimmer et al, 1994).

most common complication (37% at 10 years). Siting the stoma through the rectus did not reduce the risk of hernia, but the extraperitoneal course had a significantly lower risk of herniation. Hernias were more common in the elderly. Skin complications occurred in 17% at 10 years. Prolapse occurred in 12% at 13 years and was not reduced by mesenteric fixation. At 10 years, 7% had developed skin level stenosis (Table 9.10).

Early complications

Sepsis is a potentially serious early complication. It may be associated with impaired blood supply, either because a loop has been exteriorized under tension or because the vascular arcades supplying the end of the colon have been damaged or divided. Under these circumstances the stoma is liable to retract or slough and may cause faecal contamination within the abdominal wall or the peritoneal cavity, resulting in secondary peritonitis or intra-abdominal abscess. In an obese and immunologically compromised patient with malignant disease, abdominal wall contamination may result in synergistic gangrene which is potentially fatal (see Chapter 5). Secondary peritonitis is equally dangerous, and both events require early laparotomy, resection of non-viable bowel and construction of a stoma sometimes at a new site. Furthermore it may be necessary to perform a radical debridement of the abdominal wall, which may need to be left open (Abrams et al, 1979; Pearl et al, 1985). In view of the danger of infarction it is advisable not to excise appendices epiploicae. Complications such as prolapse and small bowel evisceration may occur through the abdominal trephine. Mirelman et al (1978) reported a 4% incidence of intra-abdominal abscess, and retraction in 3% of their patients; evisceration was less common but carried a high mortality. Minor sepsis is common but relatively unimportant, frequently being caused by contamination and breakdown of the mucocutaneous sutures. Occasionally sepsis is associated with local trauma from a rod which may compromise the blood supply to the colon. If the rod erodes the bowel, the consequences can be serious with intra-abdominal sepsis.

Late complications

Late complications include prolapse, hernia, stenosis and skin excoriation. Skin excoriation is associated with liquid stomal effluent and a badly fitting appliance, which is most common with a loop transverse colostomy. Wright (1979) compared the output of loop compared with end transverse colostomy 9–12 months after construction. The mean 24-hour weight of the stool output from a loop colostomy was 880 g, compared with 560 g from an end stoma, and was independent of the length of colon. Patients with skin excoriation should be managed in the same manner as those with an ileostomy, by cutting a Stomahesive wafer close to the circumference of the stoma and filling in any skin depressions if leakage occurs beneath the flange.

Stenosis

Colostomy stenosis occurs almost exclusively in end colostomies and may be the result of peristomal sepsis, retraction or, more commonly, ischaemia (Green, 1966; Mollitt et al, 1980). Dilatation rarely achieves satisfactory long-term resolution and a stenotic stoma will generally require refashioning, usually with a laparotomy in order to mobilize a sufficient length of viable colon.

Parastomal hernia

Aetiology

Colostomy parastomal hernia is usually caused by peristomal infection, poor abdominal wall support, as in the obese, steroid medication or a wide abdominal defect. A large trephine is frequently needed to raise a loop colostomy, particularly in patients with large bowel obstruction. Poor siting of the stoma outside the rectus sheath has long been considered to be a common cause of herniation and/or prolapse (Thorlakson, 1965; Green, 1966; Saha et al, 1973). Prian et al (1975) report that seven of nine cases of parastomal hernia were sited outside the rectus muscle. Some data now challenge the dogma that stomas must be constructed through the rectus in order to prevent paracolostomy hernia. Sjodahl et al (1988) reported hernia in 3% of rectus-sited stomas compared with 22% in laterally placed colostomies. By contrast, Williams et al (1990a) found no difference, with rates of 37% and 33% respectively. Likewise, Ortiz et al (1994) also reported rates of 52% in the pararectal postition compared with 46% in transrectal colostomies. Nevertheless, surgeons still prefer to locate a stoma through the rectus muscle (Birnbaum and Ferrier, 1952; Turnbull and Weekley, 1967; Hulten et al, 1976; Rosin and Bonardi, 1977; Martin and Foster, 1996). Colostomy hernia may also be associated with increased intra-abdominal pressure, as in prostatic hypertrophy, chronic bronchitis, constipation and ascites (Ray et al, 1960).

Classification and incidence

Leslie (1984) classified colostomy parastomal hernia as being interstitial, subcutaneous, intrastomal or associated with a prolapse. The reported incidence ranges from 42%, in children with temporary stomas, to 1% (Burns, 1970; Saha et al, 1973; Boman-Sandelin and Fenyo, 1985; Pearl et al, 1985). Paracolostomy hernia is usually more common in the first few months after loop colostomy construction than an end colostomy. On the other hand, end stomas usually remain for much longer and some authors therefore report a higher incidence of herniation in the long term with an end colostomy (Saha et al, 1973; Londono-Schimmer et al, 1994).

Complications

Complications of paracolostomy hernia are usually mechanical. Colostomy appliances dislodge; irrigation may be difficult or impossible. Obstructive symptoms are common owing to entrapment of small bowel or omentum within the hernia, but strangulation is rare (Cuthbertson and Collins, 1977; Daniell, 1981).

Treatment

In a temporary stoma, treatment of the hernia merely involves closing the defect when the colostomy is closed or when intestinal continuity is restored. With a permanent colostomy, surgical treatment is indicated if there are appliance problems or recurrent abdominal pain from obstruction (Brooke, 1952; Prian et al, 1975; Devlin, 1983). Resiting of the stoma is usually advisable because

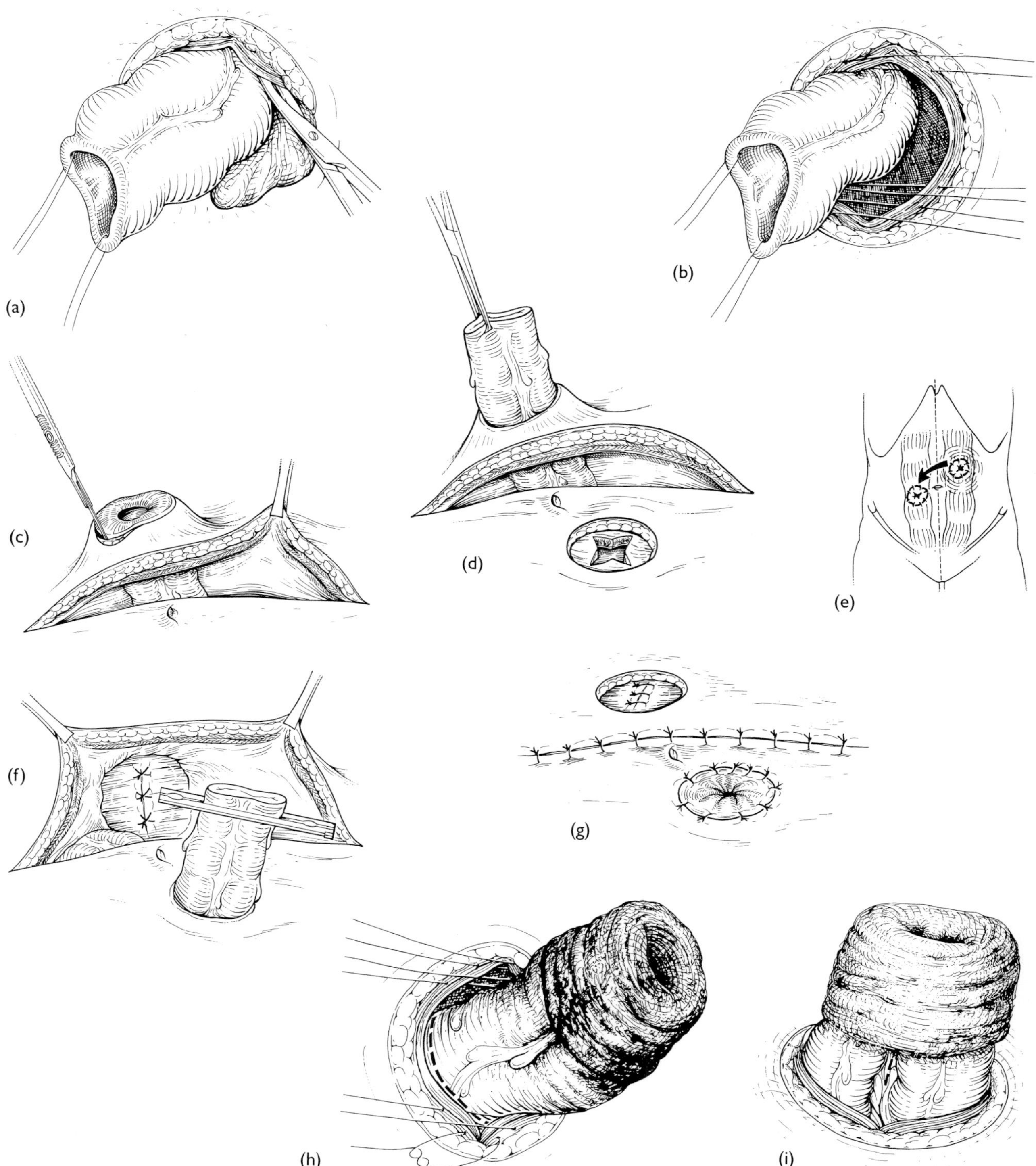

Figure 9.26a–i Local repair of a parastomal hernia: (a) The colostomy is mobilized from the abdominal wall and the peritoneal sac is identified and excised. (b) The defect in the rectus muscle is then defined and repaired with interrupted Prolene sutures prior to new mucocutaneous stoma maturation. Resiting a colostomy for parastomal hernia: (c) A laparotomy has been performed. The colon is being mobilized from the skin and abdominal wall using a circumstomal incision. (d) A new trephine is constructed in the opposite side of the abdominal wall and the colon is completely mobilized from the abdominal wall. (e) The new position. (f) The colostomy hernia site is closed and the colon delivered through the new abdominal wall trephine. (g) The completed procedure. Treatment of colostomy prolapse: (h) One method of treating an end colostomy prolapse. A segment of the distal colon may have to be excised. (i) If a loop transverse colostomy prolapses it may be wiser to close the loop.

local repair is often unsuccessful and there is a risk of local sepsis. The stoma is often incorrectly sited in the first place and needs to be repositioned through the rectus muscle. Repair is not always successful, even if the stoma has been correctly resited, in the obese, if there has been sepsis, in those with chronic obstructive airways disease, and in patients on steroids or with a collagen disorder. Late recurrence of malignancy usually with ascites may present as a parastomal hernia in patients who have had their original operation for malignant disease.

Local repair without resiting the stoma may be occasionally successful and is advocated by some (Botet et al, 1996; Ruiter and Bijnen, 1992). This approach may be the only option in patients who have had multiple operations, or in whom a previous stoma site on the other side of the abdomen has already been used (Todd, 1982; Leslie, 1984). The stoma is completely mobilized, the hernia excised and the defect in the abdominal wall repaired, leaving the sutures long so that the bowel can be brought out through the repaired trephine (Figure 9.26a,b). It is most important that the repair sutures do not occlude the colostomy when it is redelivered through the repaired defect. If suture of the defect is not possible, Abdu (1982) advises the use of a disc of polypropylene mesh. This technique may be successful in some patients (Rosin and Bonardi, 1977; Bayer et al, 1986; Ruiter and Bihnen, 1992), but it may be complicated by persistent sepsis, necessitating removal of the mesh (Prian et al, 1975).

If the stoma can be resited, which is the optimum approach, the previous abdominal incision is reopened under antibiotic cover and the stoma brought out through a new trephine in the opposite rectus muscle. The original stoma is mobilized (Figure 9.26c) through a circumstomal incision; the peritoneal cavity is entered soon after dividing the skin and care must be taken not to damage loops of small bowel within the hernia sac. Once the colon has been mobilized from the abdominal wall (Figure 9.26d), the end of the bowel is occluded, either by a non-crushing clamp or a row of staples, to prevent faecal soiling. The defect in the abdominal wall is then defined and a series of interrupted Prolene or PDS mattress sutures are used to repair the defect, but the skin is left open. It is usually easier to repair the defect from within the abdomen. The colon is then mobilized and delivered through a new trephine (Figure 9.26e,f). In Birmingham the lateral space is usually left open, but at the Royal London it is invariably closed. The abdomen is then closed and the stoma is sutured to the skin (Figure 9.26g). Fluids are usually commenced on the day after operation and food is allowed once the colostomy has acted.

Prolapse

Aetiology

Prolapse is thought to develop in patients with obstruction because of a discrepancy between the eventual size of the colon and the defect in the abdominal wall (Saha et al, 1973). Surprisingly, prolapse and hernia rarely coexist (Burns, 1970). Sutures placed between the rectus sheath and the serosa of the bowel do not appear to prevent prolapse (Pelok and Nigro, 1973).

Incidence

The incidence of prolapse varies from 4% to 13% in adults and may be as high as 58% in children (Chandler and Evans, 1978; Mirelman et al, 1978; Boman-Sandelin and Fenyo, 1985). It is more common in right-sided loop colostomy. The incidence is unrelated to age or sex or to the underlying diagnosis.

Features

Prolapse is usually intermittent and will reduce spontaneously. In loop colostomy, both limbs may prolapse; if so the proximal limb is usually more prominent than the distal one. Prolapse of a transverse colostomy may be complicated by bleeding. Most patients find that a prolapse is unaesthetic, causes colicky pain and is associated with difficulties in stoma management.

Treatment

Manual reduction may be necessary in patients who present with acute prolapse. This may be difficult if the prolapse has become oedematous and occasionally requires amputation or surgical reduction. Conservative treatment consists of reduction and maintaining the prolapse in a reduced state.

Colmer and Fox (1981) described a cone-shaped device which they attached to a colostomy appliance and which was invaginated into the stoma over the colostomy bag. This approach is acceptable only in elderly high-risk patients in whom surgical treatment is contraindicated.

Button colopexy has also been advocated for elderly patients with a prolapsing loop colostomy. The intussuscepting bowel is fixed to the abdominal wall with through-and-through sutures but long-term control by colopexy is poor (Chandler and Evans, 1978; Zinkin and Rosin, 1981).

The prolapse may be treated by amputation in the same way as in rectal prolapse (Figure 9.26h), but recurrence is high because there is a persistent defect in the abdominal wall and a freely mobile colon within it. An alternative approach is to perform a Delorme procedure on the prolapse (Abulafi et al, 1989).

In our opinion a colostomy prolapse should be managed by the same surgical approach as in colostomy hernia, by resiting the stoma through a small transrectus trephine on the opposite side of the abdomen (Figure 9.26c–g). If the prolapse involves a temporary stoma, early closure or restoration of intestinal continuity, if at all possible, would be advocated (Figure 9.26i).

COMPLICATIONS OF COLOSTOMY CLOSURE

Incidence

Sepsis

Closure of a colostomy is not a procedure devoid of problems. The incidence of sepsis ranges from 2% to 37% with a mean incidence of 10%. The frequency of this complication is the same in adults as in children (Tables 9.12 and 9.13).

Fistula

Leakage of intestinal contents from the colostomy closure site is a less common but more serious complication. The incidence of faecal fistula varies from 0% to 23% (Samhouri and Grodsinsky, 1979; Table 9.13), depending on whether this is a loop colostomy closure or closure following a Hartmann operation. The faecal fistula will close spontaneously in over half of patients after loop colostomy closure, provided there is no distal obstruction, since the colostomy closure site lies near the surface of the abdomen and a complex fistula with a chronic abscess cavity is unusual (Finch, 1976; Wheeler and Barker, 1977; Henry and Everett, 1979; Boman-Sandelin and Fenyo, 1985). The fistulas which do not spontaneously resolve are usually complicated, or the distal colon is obstructed (Yajko et al, 1976; Mirelman et al, 1978; Anderson et al, 1979; Salley et al, 1983; Parks and Hastings, 1985). The outcome may be fatal in some patients, particularly in the elderly who develop secondary faecal peritonitis after closure of a Hartmann procedure.

Table 9.12 Complications of colostomy closure in 109 children.

Complication	*Number*
Wound infection	11
Small bowel obstruction	2
Infarction	1
Volvulus	1
Leakage	0
Abscess	0
Incisional hernia	0

From Mollitt et al (1980).

Death

Mortality ranges from nil to 5% and may be incidental due to coexisting cardiorespiratory disease,

Table 9.13 Immediate complications of colostomy closure.

Authors	*n*	*Deaths (%)*	*Leaks (%)*	*Wound sepsis (%)*
Knox et al (1971)	179	2.2	23.0	10.0
Thompson and Hawley (1972)	139	0	2.9	14.4
Thibodeau (1974)	81	1.2	12.0	12.0
Adeyemo et al (1975)	43	0	4.6	4.6
Beck and Conklin (1975)	77	0	2.6	7.6
Yakimets (1975)	71	2.8	2.8	37.0
Barnett et al (1976)	110	4.5	7.3	36.4
Finch (1976)	213	0.5	8.9	21.1
Tomlinson et al (1976)	26	0	7.6	22.0
Yajko et al (1976)	100	1.0	4.0	10.0
Jarret et al (1977)	82	1.5	11.0	17.0
Wheeler and Barker (1977)	74	2.7	17.6	23.0
Garnjobst et al (1978)	125	0	0	1.6
Mirelman et al (1978)	118	4.2	14.4	21.2
Mitchell et al (1978)	89	2.2	5.6	17.9
Smit and Walt (1978)	167	0	3.6	17.5
Anderson et al (1979)	69	0	4.3	14.5
Dolan et al (1979)	118	0	0.8	10.0
Henry and Everett (1979)	74	1.3	5.4	13.5
Samhouri and Grodsinsky (1979)	304	0.3	2.3	9.5
Todd et al (1979)	206	0.9	5.3	11.7
Cabasares and Schoffstall (1980)	100	1.0	2.0	9.0
Rosen and Friedman (1980)	153	1.4	5.2	7.0
Varnell and Pemberton (1981)	69	0	7.2	27.5
Freund et al (1982)	114	0	8.3	29.7
Gerber et al (1982)	80	0	4.0	14.0
Lewis and Weedon (1982)	60	1.0	6.7	10.0
Oluwole et al (1982)	86	1.1	3.5	7.0
Perry et al (1983)	104	0	4.8	29.8
Salley et al (1983)	166	0	1.2	2.4
Boman-Sandelin and Fenyo (1985)	98	0	8.1	10.2
Foster et al (1985)	113	0.9	16.5	33.9
Parks and Hastings (1985)	83	0	10.0	33.0
Pittman and Smith (1985)	126	0	8.7	14.2
Irvin (1987)	98	0	0.	3.0
Demetriades et al (1988)	110	0	2.7	11.8
Livingstone et al (1989)	121	0	3.3	6.6

but half the deaths are related to closure of the stoma, usually from overwhelming sepsis or persistent fistula.

Other early complications

These include obstruction of the colon at the closure site from oedema or mechanical factors, which may be responsible for a persistent fistula (Anderson et al, 1979; Todd et al, 1979). Small bowel obstruction may develop, necessitating surgical treatment if conservative measures of decompression and intravenous fluid therapy fail (Foster et al, 1985). Dehiscence of the abdominal incision around the colostomy may result in evisceration of omentum or small bowel (Mitchell et al, 1978).

Late complications

Late complications include hernia at the closure site in 1–16%, chronic sepsis, usually associated with a non-absorbable suture, and episodes of intestinal obstruction (Table 9.14). Late obstructive episodes are reported in 1–7%, and 2–10% of patients develop a stitch sinus (Adeyemo et al, 1975; Samhouri and Grodsinski, 1979; Varnell and Pemberton, 1981; Perry et al, 1983; Porter et al, 1989).

Children

The complication rate for closure of colostomy in children is similar to adults except for the incidence of sepsis, which is lower. Fistula, obstruction and hernia are less common in children and are unrelated to the method of closure (MacMahon et al, 1963; Brenner and Swenson, 1967).

Table 9.14 Late complications of colostomy closure.

	n	*Hernia* (%)	*Obstruction* (%)	*Stitch sinus* (%)
Adeyemo et al (1975)	43	2	2	*
Finch (1976)	213	11	1	2
Yajko et al (1976)	100	1	7	*
Mirelman et al (1978)	118	16	2	3
Samhouri and Grodsinsky (1979)	304	1	1	*
Todd et al (1979)	206	5	*	*
Varnell and Pemberton (1981)	69	3	1	3
Perry et al (1983)	104	11	*	*
Salley et al (1983)	166	1	2	*
Foster et al (1985)	113	9	1	*
Parks and Hastings (1985)	83	4	6	8
Porter et al (1989)	43	13	4	10

* Not stated.

End colostomy

Morbidity after staged resection and the Hartmann procedure are described in Chapters 32 and 37. It is sometimes assumed, and there are some supporting data, that anastomosis of a closed rectal stump to an end colostomy or staged resection with colostomy closure carries a higher morbidity and mortality than simple closure of the loop stoma in the large bowel (Foster et al, 1985; Parks and Hastings, 1985; Pittman and Smith, 1985). This has certainly not been found to be the case in relation to sepsis. However, Wara et al (1981) showed that sepsis rates did not differ between loop colostomy closure and intra-abdominal anastomosis. Beck and Conklin (1975) came to a similar conclusion in colonic trauma.

Factors influencing complications after colostomy closure

Age, sex and underlying disease

Age, sex or the underlying diagnosis do not seem to influence the rate of complications after colostomy closure (Finch, 1976; Wheeler and Barker, 1977; Demetriades et al, 1988). Complications in patients with carcinoma (22%), diverticular disease (30%) or a traumatic injury (27%) were almost the same (Anderson et al, 1979). Some have reported that complications are less common after traumatic injury requiring colostomy (Varnell and Pemberton, 1981; Pittman and Smith, 1985) but this has not been a universal finding (Williams et al, 1987). Complications after colostomy closure were more common if the original stoma had been raised as an emergency, particularly if the stoma was an end stoma placed in the left colon (Anderson et al, 1979). Closure of loop transverse colostomy gave rise to more complications than closure of a sigmoid loop (Todd et al, 1979). Indeed, some reports record that the incidence of complications after closing a loop colostomy (35%) was higher than intraperitoneal colorectal anastomosis after a Hartmann procedure (26%) (Pittman and Smith, 1985). Although some claim that resection of a loop stoma causes fewer complications than simple closure (Barron and Fallis, 1958), the evidence suggests otherwise – either that there is no difference (Beck and Conklin, 1975; Todd et al, 1979), or that resection of a loop stoma is positively dangerous (Mirelman et al, 1978; Salley et al, 1983). The decison to resect or simply to close a loop colostomy will depend on individual factors, such as whether the stoma was raised for trauma, whether there is evidence of obstruction, the presence of chronic sepsis, the blood supply to the colon and the ease of the dissection. All things being equal, simple closure is a wiser strategy than resection unless there are local factors that might suggest otherwise (Aston and Everett, 1984).

Intraperitoneal closure and use of drains

Extraperitoneal closure has been advocated in the past in the belief that complications are less frequent and less dangerous. All recent reports, however, indicate that intraperitoneal closure is safer (Adeyemo et al, 1975; Finch, 1976). Some advise drainage adjacent to the site of colostomy closure to minimize the consequences of suture line leakage; however, drains appear to have no influence on morbidity (Mirelman et al, 1978; Samhouri and Grodsinski, 1979; Livingstone et al, 1989).

Bowel preparation and distal colonic disease

Patients should be assessed by endoscopy or contrast radiology before closure of a loop stoma so as to ensure that there is no evidence of distal obstruction or persistent colorectal disease (Devlin, 1973; Yajko et al, 1976). The distal colon should be cleared of faecal residue or inspissated mucus before closure (Henry and Everett, 1979). This can usually be achieved adequately by distal colostomy washouts in a loop stoma or rectal washouts if the distal bowel has been oversewn. The proximal bowel should be prepared in the usual way; the vogue for elemental diets before colostomy closure is no longer justified on grounds of expense and inadequate bowel preparation (Tomlinson et al, 1976).

Experience of the surgeon

The experience of the surgeon is a most important factor in determining the incidence of suture line breakdown after colostomy closure. Closure of a stoma is often relegated to the end of an operating list, is delegated to a junior member of the staff, the theatre staff and surgical team are tired and the procedure is not accorded the priority that it deserves. Henry and Everett (1979) concluded that the experience of the surgeon was the most important determinant of anastomotic breakdown.

Closure technique

Suture technique was considered to be less important than surgical experience. However, in a later study the same group reported a 14% complication rate after single-layer closure compared with 37% after two-layer closure. We prefer continuous single-layer extramucosal sutures unless the stapled closure is used with the lineal staple cutter to construct a side-to-side anastomosis completed by stapling the two open bowel ends (Figure 9.15a–d).

Timing of closure

The timing of the colostomy closure is controversial. Early closure of a loop colostomy is considered by many to be dangerous (Thomson and Hawley, 1972; Finch, 1976; Wheeler and Barker, 1977; Henry and Everett, 1979; Wheeler, 1982; Foster et al, 1985; Parks and Hastings, 1985). Mirelman and others (1978) reported a 51% complication rate when stomas were closed within 3 months, compared with a 34% complication rate if more than 3 months had elapsed following construction. On the other hand, data from a prospective survey (Aston and Everett, 1984) implied that the timing of closure had no influence on morbidity (Table 9.15). Other surgeons also advocate early closure when indicated, on the basis that morbidity is not increased (Finch, 1976; Anderson et al, 1979; Todd et al, 1979; Lewis and Weedon, 1982; Salley et al, 1983; Pittman and Smith, 1985). We take the view that if a stoma needs to be closed early it is probably safe to do so, provided there is no distal obstruction and an experienced surgeon performs the operation.

Blood supply

An important factor affecting suture line breakdown relates to the adequacy of the blood supply to the colon (Billings et al, 1986). It has been suggested that early closure might be dangerous because the blood supply to the suture line is often compromised by oedema and distal obstruction. Forrester et al (1981) showed that the mean blood flow 7 days

Table 9.15 Influence of timing on complications of closing transverse loop colostomy.

Complication	*Early closure: 2 weeks (n = 38)*	*Late closure: 8–12 weeks (n = 62)*
Death	0	2 (3)
Faecal fistula	4 (11)	6 (10)
Wound sepsis	1 (3)	4 (6)
Total complications	6 (16)	12 (19)
Hospital stay	10.3 days	10.8 days

Values in parentheses are percentages.
From Aston and Everett (1984).

after construction of a loop colostomy was only 6.9 mL/min, but had improved to 31.1 mL/min by 28 days (Figure 9.27). In two of eight patients, flow even at 28 days was less than 15 mL/min. Forty patients were then studied to correlate the intra-operative blood flow with suture line dehiscence. Five of eight patients with a blood flow of less than 15 mL/min developed a leak. The suture line remained intact in all of the patients with higher flow rates (Figure 9.28).

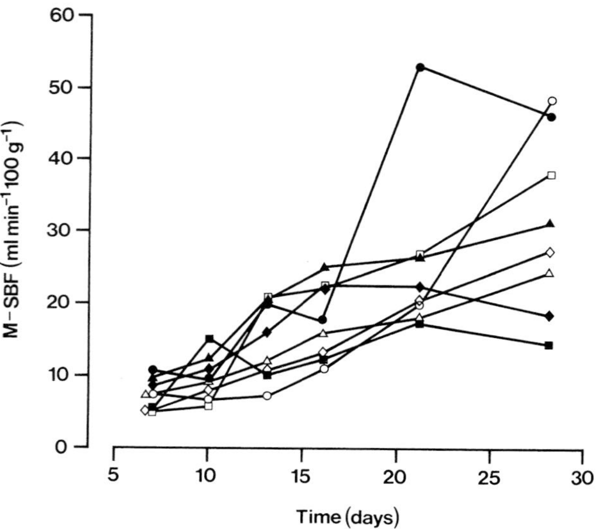

Figure 9.27 Colostomy blood flow changes with time after colostomy construction.

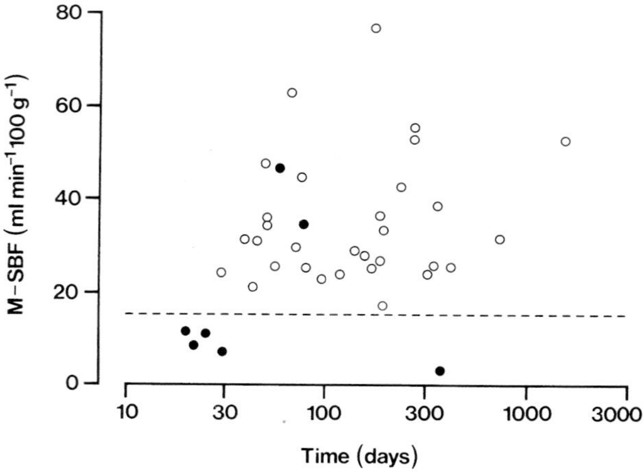

Figure 9.28 Colostomy fistula in relation to blood flow. • Successful closure; o fistula formation following closure.

These findings imply that blood flow is important in the pathogenesis of breakdown after colostomy closure, particularly if there is constriction from a tight trephine in the abdominal wall, an oedematous bowel or early closure in some patients. Foster and Leaper (1985) studied blood flow using laser Doppler velocimetry. Flow was proportional to the bursting pressure and associated with impaired collagen synthesis (Billings et al, 1986). Flow also increased with time after colostomy construction, from 19 units at 1 week to 44 units 8 weeks later (Billings and Leaper, 1987).

Wound sepsis

Antimicrobial prophylaxis has a relatively minor role in preventing colostomy sepsis (Varnell and Pemberton, 1981; Perry et al, 1983): the method of wound closure is probably more important. Todd et al (1979) reported sepsis rates of 27% after wound closure, compared with 5% when the wound was left open. These findings are supported by many others (Mitchell et al, 1978; Perry et al, 1983; Pittman and Smith, 1985). Wound infection rates are generally higher after delayed primary closure than they are after immediate closure (Thal and Yeary, 1980; Berne et al, 1985). Pittman and Smith (1985) found that the rate of sepsis was only 3% in open wounds, 19% in sutured wounds, but 21% after delayed primary closure.

Methods of colostomy closure

General principles

Meticulous mechanical preparation of the proximal and distal colon should minimize the risks of colostomy closure; this is particularly relevant if a contrast enema through the anus or the distal limb of a loop stoma has been performed preoperatively. There should be no evidence of obstruction distal to the stoma or residual disease on sigmoidoscopy or contrast radiology. Residual diverticular disease should be resected before attempting to close a proximal stoma or restore intestinal continuity after a Hartmann operation.

We advise intraperitoneal closure of a loop colostomy, provided there are no local contraindications, and prefer simple closure rather than resection. We also prefer a continuous single-layer extramucosal suture technique. Single-dose, intravenous antibiotic cover is given to all patients. Drains are not used. The skin over the closure site may be left open to granulate if there is contamination or excessive subcutaneous fat, but many wounds are closed primarily. Details of restoring intestinal continuity after Hartmann resection can be found in Chapter 37.

Suture closure of a loop colostomy

Preparation

Sodium picosulphate is given by mouth to clear the proximal bowel. A distal colostomy irrigation is used after a rectal washout to clear the distal bowel. All patients aged over 45 years receive subcutaneous heparin. Single-dose antibiotic prophylaxis is given in the anaesthetic room. A general anaesthetic is used with a muscle relaxant. Bladder catheterization and nasogastric intubation are unnecessary, but reliable intravenous access is important since fluids will have to be restricted after operation.

Operative technique

The mucocutaneous junction is incised around the circumference of the stoma with a small blade. The colon is dissected from the subcutaneous fat and the rectus sheath around its circumference (Figure 9.29a–c). The rectus muscle is then dissected free from the stoma so that it is completely mobile and can be replaced in the peritoneal cavity with ease. The edges of the colostomy are excised with diathermy (Figure 9.29d). A series of Connell or extramucosal sutures are placed transversely to close the antimesenteric defect, but they are not tied until they have all been correctly positioned (Figure 9.29e–g). Alternatively a continuous extramucosal closure technique may be used (Figure 9.29h).

The anastomosis, if it lies in the sigmoid, can be tested by insufflating air through the rectum. The colon is then replaced into the peritoneal cavity and the defect in the rectus muscle is closed by interrupted Prolene or PDS sutures to oppose the rectus sheath. These sutures are also left long until they have been placed correctly and then tied. The skin may be left open and packed with a proflavine swab or it may be closed.

Postoperative management

An intravenous infusion is maintained usually for 3–5 days until flatus and stool have been passed. The patient is then allowed free fluids, and diet 48 hours later. We are deliberately cautious after closing a loop stoma and maintain patients on intravenous fluids; laxatives and enemas are forbidden. If a fistula should develop, it will generally close spontaneously and all that is necessary is to place an appliance around it. If the fistula persists for more than a week we arrange a fistulogram to exclude an abscess cavity between the bowel and the skin or a distal obstruction which may require more urgent surgical attention. Parenteral nutrition is rarely needed for management of colostomy fistula, and fine-bore feeding with a liquid diet is generally advised.

Alternatives

Resection

Although resection is not necessarily superior to simple closure (Barron and Fallis, 1958; Adeyemo et al, 1975; Beck and Conkin, 1975), there are occasions when simple closure is suboptimal. Resection of the colostomy is indicated if the loop of colon is damaged during mobilization from the abdominal wall, if there is evidence of stenosis or an abscess or ischaemia, or if there is a fistula adjacent to the colostomy (Devlin, 1973).

If resection of the loop colostomy is indicated, it is important to completely mobilize the bowel so that an anastomosis can be undertaken without tension on the suture line. If there is any difficulty in mobilizing the bowel, the abdomen should be explored through a laparotomy incision, the bowel ends completely freed and the stoma resected so that the ends can be safely anastomosed.

Resection and anastomosis through the trephine is usually performed using a continuous or interrupted single-layer inverting anastomosis, as illustrated in Figure 9.30a–e. The mesentery is then closed and the abdominal wall sutured as already described.

Stapling

Reference has already been made to stapling techniques used for closure of a loop colostomy (see Figures 9.14a,b and 9.15a,b) (Miskowiak, 1983). The principle is to perform a side-to-side anastomosis using a linear staple cutter through the colotomy followed by closure of the mucocutaneous junction with a transverse stapler. Alternatively the mobilized mucocutaneous bowel ends can simply be closed with a lineal stapler (Figure 9.30f) and the abdominal wall defect repaired with sutures (Figure 9.30g).

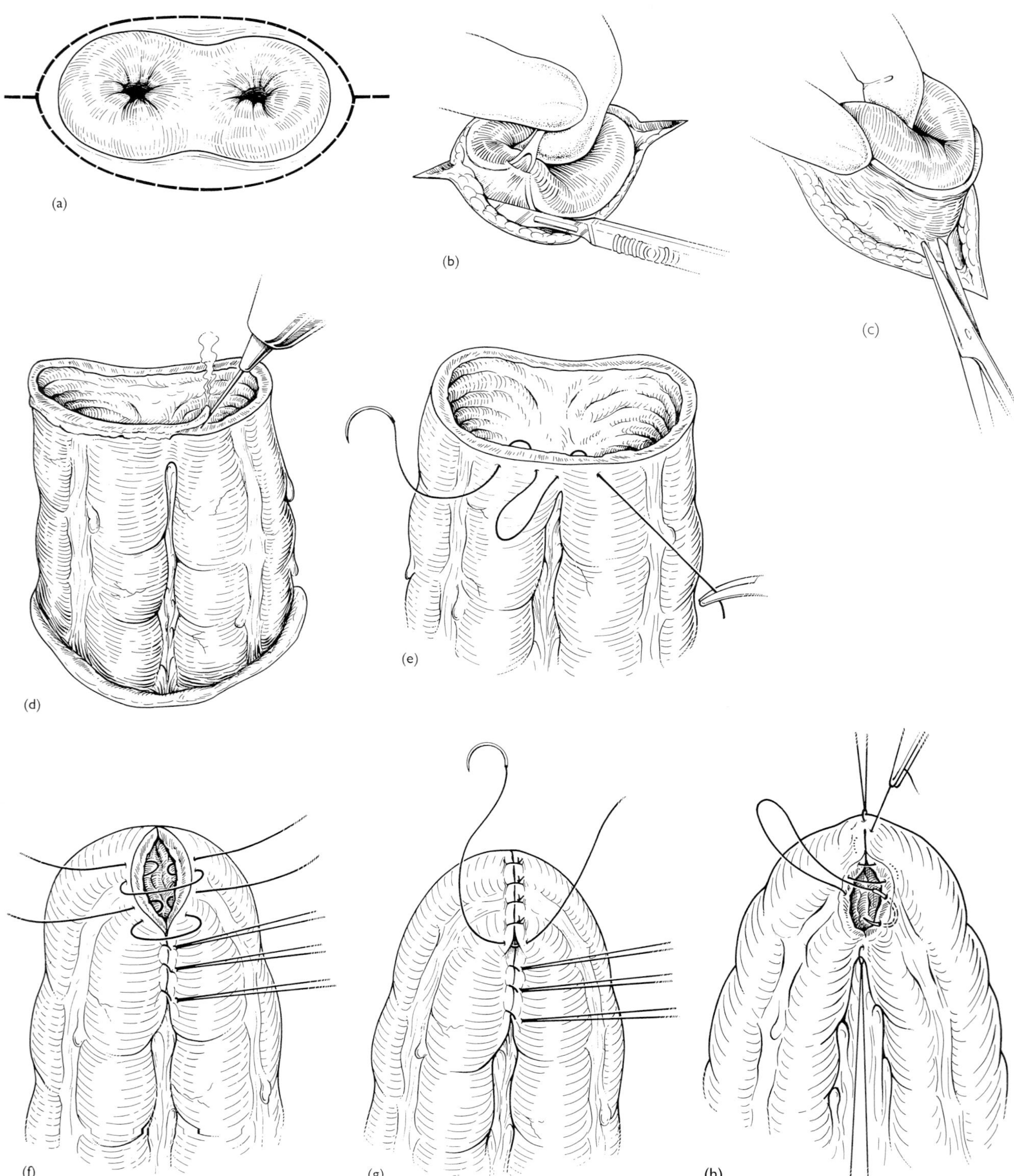

Figure 9.29a–h Closure of a loop colostomy. (a) A circumstomal incision is made. (b) The colon is mobilized from the skin. (c) The colon is then mobilized from the subcutaneous fat and the abdominal wall. (d) The edges of the colostomy are excised. (e) The colostomy is closed transversely using an inverting suture technique. (f) Partial closure. (g) Completed closure of the colostomy. (h) An alternative method of closing the loop colostomy is by continuous extramucosal PDS suture.

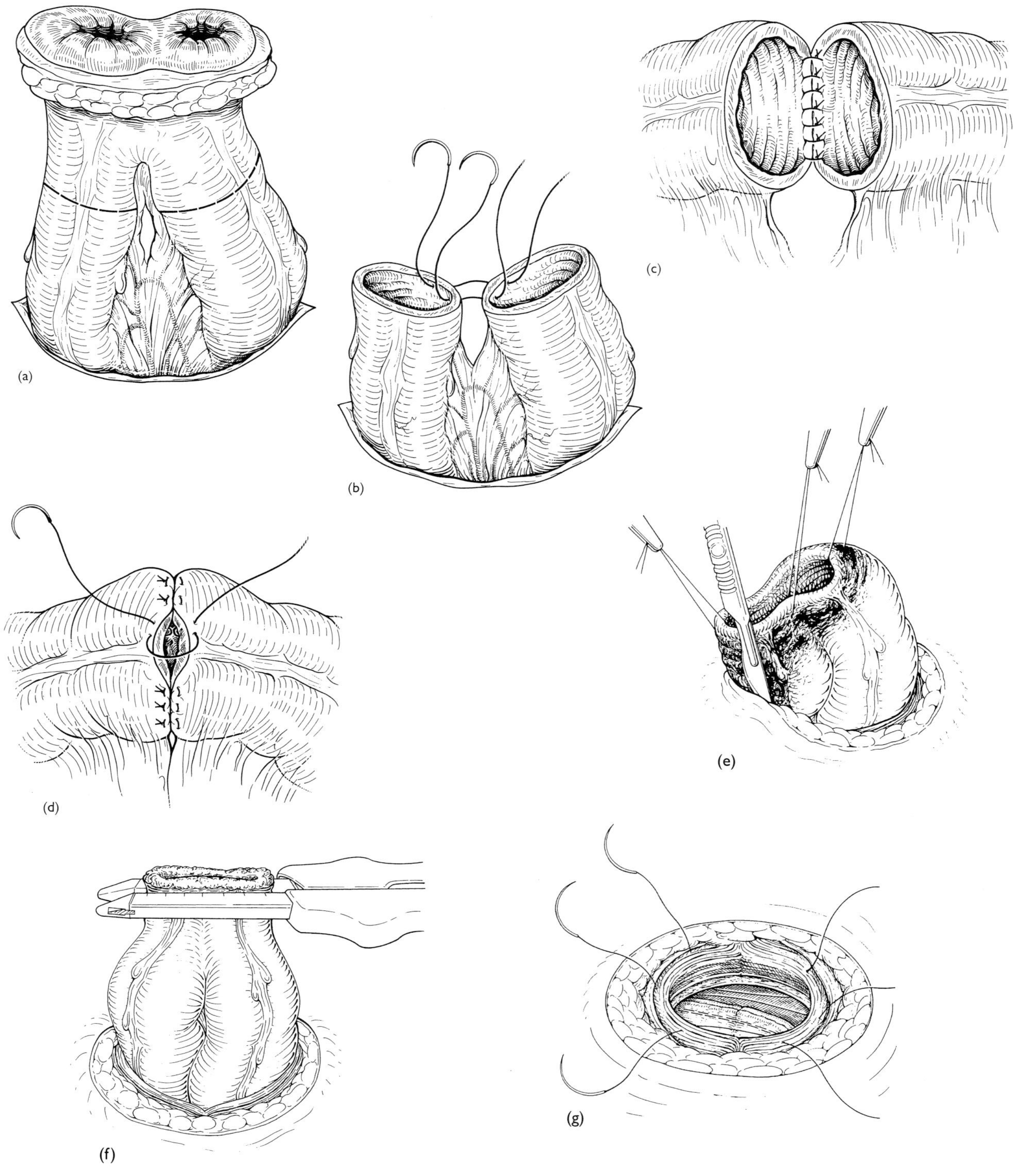

Figure 9.30a–g Resection and anastomosis for closure of loop colostomy: (a) The loop colostomy has been mobilized from the abdominal wall. The two limbs of colon are excised. (b) An end-to-end colocolonic anastomosis is fashioned. (c) Completion of the posterior wall. (d) Completion of the anterior wall. Stapled closure of a loop colostomy: (e) Mobilization of the colostomy. (f) The loop transverse colostomy is closed by a single firing of the linear staple cutter. (g) Closure of the abdominal wall.

REFERENCES

Abdu RA (1982) Repair of paracolostomy hernias with marlex mesh. *Dis Colon Rectum* **25**: 529–531.

Abercrombie JF, Rogers J & Williams NS (1996) Total anorectal reconstruction results in complete anorectal sensory loss. *Br J Surg* **83**: 57–59.

Abercrombie JE & Williams NS (1995) Total anorectal reconstruction. *Br J Surg* **82**: 438–442.

Abeyatunge LR (1972) A modified technique of colostomy. *Br J Surg* **59**: 99–100.

Abrams BL, Alskafi FH & Waterman HG (1979) Colostomy: a new look at morbidity and mortality. *Am J Surg* **45**: 462–464.

Abulafi AM, Sherman IW & Fiddian RV (1989) Delorme operation for collapsed colostomy. *Br J Surg* **76**: 1321–1322.

Adeyemo A, Gaillard WE Jr, Subhi D Ali, Calhoun T & Kurtz LH (1975) Colostomy: intraperitoneal or extraperitoneal closure? *Am J Surg* **130**: 273–274.

Aitken RJ, Stevens PJ d'E, Preez N du & Elliot MS (1986) Raising a colostomy: results of a prospective surgical audit. *Int J Colorect Dis* **1**: 244–247.

Alexander-Williams J (1974) Loop ileostomy and colostomy for faecal diversion. *Ann R Coll Surg Engl* **54**: 141–148.

Alexander-Williams J, Amery AH, Devlin HB et al (1977) Magnetic continent colostomy device. *BMJ* **2**: 1269–1270.

Allan R (1797) Rapport sur les observations et réflexion de Dumas, relatives aux imperforations de l'anus. *Recueil Périodique de la Société de Médicine de Paris* **3**: 123 (reprinted in Amussat (1839), pp. 100–102).

Allingham HW Jr (1887) Inguinal colotomy: its advantages over lumbar operation with special reference to a method of preventing faeces passing below an artificial anus. *BMJ* **2**: 874–878.

Amussat JZ (1839) Mémoire sur la Possibilité d'Etablir un Anus Artificiel dans la Region Lombaire sans Penetrer dans le Peritoine. Paris: Baillière.

Anderson E, Carey LC & Cooperman M (1979) Colostomy closure: a simple procedure? *Dis Colon Rectum* **22**: 466–468.

Anderson ID, Hill J, Vohra R, Schofield PF, Kiff ES (1992) An improved means of faecal diversion: the trephine stoma. *Br J Surg* **79**: 1080–1081.

Antrum RM & Rice JJ (1988) Use of skin staples for fashioning colotomies. *Br J Surg* **75**: 736.

Arabi Y, Dimock F & Burdon DW (1978) Influence of bowel preparation and antimicrobials on colonic microflora. *Br J Surg* **65**: 555–559.

Aries LJ (1973) Colostomy and ileostomy retainer. *Int Surg* **58**: 490.

Aston C & Everett WG (1984) Comparison of early and late closure of transverse loop colostomies. *Ann R Coll Surg Engl* **66**: 331–333.

Baker FS (1975) The rodless loop colostomy. *Dis Colon Rectum* **18**: 528.

Barnett JE, Endrey-Walder P & Rheils MJ (1976) Closure of colostomy. *Aust NZ J Surg* **46**: 131–133.

Barron J & Fallis LS (1958) Colostomy closure by the intraperitoneal method. *Dis Colon Rectum* **1**: 466–470.

Bayer I, Kyzer S & Chaimoff CL (1986) A new approach to primary strengthening of colostomy with Marlex mesh to prevent paracolostomy hernia. *Surg Gynecol Obstet* **163**: 579–580.

Beart RW Jr & Wolff BG (1982) The use of staplers for anterior anastomoses. *World J Surg* **6**: 525–530.

Beck PH & Conklin HB (1975) Closure of colostomy. *Ann Surg* **181**: 795–798.

Becker WF (1953) Acute obstruction of the colon: an analysis of 205 cases. *Surg Gynecol Obstet* **96**: 677–682.

Benacci JC & Wolff BG (1995) Cecostomy: therapeutic indications and results. *Dis Colon Rectum* **38**: 530–534.

Berne TV, Griffith CN, Hill J & Lo Guidice P (1985) Colostomy wound closure. *Arch Surg* **120**: 957–959.

Billings PJ, Foster ME & Leaper DJ (1986) A clinical and experimental study of colostomy blood flow and healing after closure. *Int J Colorect Dis* **1**: 108–112.

Billings PJ & Leaper DJ (1987) Laser doppler velocimetry and the measurement of colostomy blood flow. *Dis Colon Rectum* **30**: 376–380.

Bingham S, McNeill NI & Cummings JH (1977) Diet for the ileostomist. *J Hum Nutr* **31**: 365–366.

Birnbaum W & Ferrier P (1952) Complications of abdominal colostomy. *Am J Surg* **83**: 64–67.

Blamey SL & Lee PWR (1982) A comparison of circular stapling devices in colorectal anastomosis. *Br J Surg* **69**: 19–22.

Boman-Sandelin K & Fenyo G (1985) Construction and closure of the transverse loop colostomy. *Dis Colon Rectum* **28**: 772–774.

Botet X, Boldo E & Llaurado JM (1996) Colonic parastoma hernia repair by translocation without formal laparotomy. *Br J Surg* **83**: 981.

Brenner RW & Swenson O (1967) Colostomy in infants and children. *Surg Gynecol Obstet* **124**: 1239–1244.

Briggs MK, Plant JA & Devlin HB (1977) Labelling the stigmatised: the career of the colostomist. *Ann R Coll Surg Engl* **59**: 247–250.

Brooke BM (1952) The management of an ileostomy including its complications. *Lancet* **ii**: 102–104.

Browning GCP & Parks AG (1983) A method and the results of loop colostomy. *Dis Colon Rectum* **26**: 223–226.

Bryant TA (1882) Case of excision of a stricture of the descending colon through an incision made for a left lumbar colotomy: with remarks. *Proc R Med Chir Soc* **9**: 149–153.

Bumin C, Yerdel MA (1996) Loop end colostomy: a new technique. *Br J Surg* **83**: 810–811.

Burcharth F, Kylberg F, Ballan A & Rasmussen SN (1986) The colostomy plug: a new disposable device for a continent colostomy. *Lancet* **ii**: 1062–1063.

Burns FJ (1970) Complications of colostomy. *Dis Colon Rectum* **13**: 448–450.

Cabasares HV & Schoffstall RO (1980) Low complication rate of colostomy closures. *South Med J* **73**: 1572–1575.

Cain WS & Kiesewetter WB (1965) Infant colostomy: its role and complications. *Arch Surg* **91**: 314–320.

Capperauld A, Lawrie P & French DA (1977) Properties of bovine fibrin absorbable implants. *Surg Gynecol Obstet* **144**: 3–7.

Cardoen G, Daelen van den L & Boeckx G (1984) Argumentatie: houding en resultaten in de behandeling van het rectumcarcinoma. *Acta Chir Belg* **82**: 41–50.

Caruso D, Kassir AA, Robles RA et al (1996) Use of trephine stoma in sigmoid volvulus. *Dis Colon Rectum* **39**: 1222–1226.

Cavina E (1996) Outcome of restorative perineal graciloplasty with simultaneous excision of the anus and rectum for cancer: a ten-year experience with 81 patients. *Dis Colon Rectum* **39**: 182–190.

Cavina E, Seccia M, Evangelista G et al (1987) Construction of a continent perineal colostomy by using electrostimulated gracilis muscles after abdominoperineal resection: personal technique and experience with 32 cases. *Ital J Surg Sci* **17**: 305–314.

Cerdan FJ, Dez M, Campo J et al (1991) Continent colostomy by means of a new one-piece disposable device: preliminary report. *Dis Colon Rectum* **34**: 886–890.

Ceruli MA, Mikoomanesh P & Schuster MM (1979) Progress in biofeedback conditioning for fecal incontinence. *Gastroenterology* **76**: 742–746.

Chandler JG & Evans BP (1978) Colostomy prolapse. *Surgery* **84**: 577–582.

Chapman TP, Davis DR & Woods SD (1984) Bedside loop colostomy. *Surg Gynecol Obstet* **159**: 161.

Cheselden W (1784) Colostomy for strangulated umbilical hernia. In *Anatomy*. London.

Chiotasso P, Schmitt L, Juricic M & Lazorthes F (1992) Acceptation des stomies perineales. Gastroenterol Clin Biol **16**: 200 (abstract).

Chittenden AS (1930) Reconstruction of an anal sphincter by muscle strips from the glutei. *Ann Surg* **92**: 152–154.

Chung RS (1985) Loop ileostomy with the intraluminal stapler (ILS). *Dis Colon Rectum* **28**: 464–465.

Clarke DD & Hubay CA (1972) Tube caecostomy: an evaluation of 161 cases. *Ann Surg* **175**: 55–61.

Codina Cazador A, Pinol M, Marti Rague J, Montane J, Nogueras FM, Sunal J (1993) Multicentre study of a continent colostomy plug. *Br J Surg* **80**: 930–932.

Colmer ML & Fox MJ (1981) A device for the control of colostomy prolapse. *Surg Gynecol Obstet* **152**: 827–828.

Corman ML & Veidenheimer MC (1974) An appliance for management of the diverting loop colostomy. *Arch Surg* **108**: 742–743.

Cuthbertson AM & Collins JP (1977) Strangulated para-ileostomy hernia. *Aust NZ J Surg* **47**: 86–87.

Daniell SJ (1981) Strangulated small bowel hernia within a prolapsed colostomy stoma. *J R Soc Med* **74**: 687–688.

Delaney JP & Mulholland MW (1983) The temporary intestinal stoma? *Am J Surg* **146**: 668–670.

Demetriades D, Pezikis A, Melissas J, Parekh D & Pickles G (1988) Factors influencing the morbidity of colostomy closure. *Am J Surg* **155**: 594–596.

Devlin HB (1973) Colostomy. Indications, management and complications. *Ann R Coll Surg Engl* **52**: 392–407.

Devlin HB (1983) Peristomal hernia. In Dudley H (ed.) *Operative Surgery*, 4th edn, vol. 1, p. 441. London: Butterworth.

Devlin HB (1990) Colostomy: past and present. *Ann R Coll Surg Engl* **72**: 175–176.

Devlin HB & Plant JA (1969) Colostomy and its management. *Nurs Times* **65**: 231–234.

Devlin HB & Plant JA (1975) Disposal of disposable colostomy appliances. *BMJ* **4**: 705.

Devlin HB, Plant JA & Griffen M (1971) Aftermath of surgery for anorectal cancer. *BMJ* **3**: 413–418.

Dini D, Venturini M, Forno G et al (1991) Irrigation for colostomized cancer patients: a rational approach. *Int J Colorect Dis* **6**: 9–11.

Dixon AR, Maxwell WA & Holmes JT (1991) Carcinoma of the rectum: a 10-year experience. *Br J Surg* **78**: 196–198.

Dixon AR, Thomson WHF (1996) Failure of the unopened colostomy to protect high risk rectal anastomoses. *Br J Surg* **83**: 45.

Dolan PA, Caldwell FT, Thompson CH & Westbrook KC (1979) Problems of colostomy closure. *Am J Surg* **137**: 188–191.

Doran J & Hardcastle JD (1981) A controlled trial of colostomy management by natural evacuation, irrigation and foam enema. *Br J Surg* **68**: 731–733.

Druss RG, O'Connor JF & Stern LO (1969) Psychological response to colectomy: adjustment to a permanent colostomy. *Arch Gen Psychiatry* **20**: 419–427.

Duret C (1789) Observations sur un enfant né sans anus, et auguel il a été fait une onverture pour y suppléer. *Recueil Périodique de la Société de Médecine de Paris* **4**: 45–50.

Durst AL & Freund H (1980) Protecting the high-risk rectal anastomosis. *Arch Surg* **115**: 214–215.

Edmiston JM & Birnbaum W (1955) Complications from resection of colon: an evaluation of complementary cecostomy. *Am J Surg* **90**: 12–17.

Elias D, Lasser P, Leroux A et al (1993) Colostomies perineales pseudo-continente aprés amputation rectal pour cancer. *Gastroenterol Clin Biol* **17**: 181–186.

Eng K & Localio A (1981) Simplified complementary transverse colostomy for low colorectal anastomosis. *Surg Gynecol Obstet* **153**: 735.

Fallis LS (1946) Transverse colostomy. *Surgery* **20**: 249–256.

Fasth S, Hulten L & Palselius I (1980) Loop ileostomy: an attractive alternative to a temporary transverse colostomy. *Acta Chir Scand* **146**: 203–207.

Federov VD, Odaryuk TS, Shelygin YS et al (1989) Method of creation of a smooth muscle cuff at the site of the perineal colostomy after extirpation of the rectum. *Dis Colon Rectum* **32**: 562–566.

Federov VD & Shelygin YA (1989) Treatment of patients with rectal cancer. *Dis Colon Rectum* **32**: 138–145.

Finan PJ (1987) Stoma avoidance in rectal cancer. *Br J Hosp Med* **38**: 294–298.

Finch DRA (1976) The results of colostomy closure. *Br J Surg* **63**: 397–399.

Fitzgibbons RJ Jr, Harkrider WW & Cohn I Jr (1977) Review of abdominoperineal resection for cancer. *Am J Surg* **134**: 624–629.

Fitzgibbons RJ, Schmitz GD & Bailey RT (1987) A simple technique for constructing a loop enterostomy which allows immediate placement of an ostomy appliance. *Surg Gynecol Obstet* **164**: 79–81.

Fontes B, Fontes W, Utiyama EM & Birotini D (1988) Efficacy of loop colostomy for complete fecal diversion. *Dis Colon Rectum* **31**: 298–302.

Forrester DW, Spence VA & Walker WF (1981) Colonic mucosal–submucosal blood flow and the incidence of faecal fistula formation following colostomy closure. *Br J Surg* **68**: 541–544.

Foster ME & Leaper DJ (1985) A clinical and experimental study of complications after colostomy closure. *Br J Surg* **72**: 398.

Foster ME, Leaper DJ & Williamson RCN (1985) Changing patterns in colostomy closure: the Bristol experience 1975–82. *Br J Surg* **72**: 142–145.

Franchini A, Cola B, Giardano R, Farella S & Urbani G (1978) Continent colostomies: Italian experience with magnetic ring: I. World Congress of Coloproctology, Madrid.

Freund HR, Daniel J & Muggia-Salam M (1982) Factors affecting the morbidity of colostomy closure: a retrospective study. *Dis Colon Rectum* **25**: 712–715.

Frigell A, Ottander M, Stenbeck H et al (1990) Quality of life of patients treated with abdominoperineal resection or anterior resection for rectal carcinoma. *Ann Chir Gynaecol* **79**: 26–30.

Gabriel WB & Lloyd-Davies OV (1935) Colostomy. *Br J Surg* **22**: 520–528.

Galofre M & Ponseti JM (1983) A simplified method of transverse loop colostomy. *Surg Gynecol Obstet* **156**: 798–799.

Garnjobst W, Leaverton GH & Sullivan ES (1978) Safety of colostomy closure. *Am J Surg* **136**: 85–89.

Gazzard BG, Saunders B & Dawson AM (1978) Diets of stoma function. *Br J Surg* **65**: 642–644.

George WD, Bordley A, Davis FN et al (1975) Problems of a permanent colostomy. *Gut* **16**: 409–410.

Gerber A & Thompson RJ Jr (1965) Use of a tube cecostomy to lower the mortality in acute large intestinal obstruction due to carcinoma. *Am J Surg* **110**: 893–896.

Gerber HI, Morris DM, Eisenstat TE, Coke DD & Annons MO (1982) Factors influencing the morbidity of colostomy closure. *Dis Colon Rectum* **25**: 464–470.

Gervin AS, Hoffman MJ & Fischer RP (1987) Modified Paul–Mikulicz ileocolostomy. *Am J Surg* **154**: 648–650.

Goldstein SD, Salvati EP, Rubin RJ & Eisenstat TE (1986) Tube cecostomy with cecal extraperitonealization in the management of obstructing left-sided carcinoma of the large intestine. *Surg Gynecol Obstet* **162**: 379–380.

Goligher JC (1958) Extraperitoneal colostomy or ileostomy. *Br J Surg* **46**: 97–103.

Goligher JC & Smiddy FG (1957) The treatment of acute obstruction or perforation with carcinoma of the colon and rectum. *Br J Surg* **45**: 270–274.

Goligher JC, Lee PWR, McMahon MJ & Pollard M (1977) The Erlanger magnetic colostomy control device: technique of use and results in 22 patients. *Br J Surg* **64**: 501–507.

Graham AS (1948) Current trends in surgery of the distal colon and rectum for cancer. *Ann Surg* **127**: 1022–1034.

Green EW (1966) Colostomies and their complications. *Surg Gynecol Obstet* **122**: 1230–1232.

Greene HG (1971) Loop colostomy: bar versus rod. *Dis Colon Rectum* **14**: 308–309.

Grier WRN, Postel AH, Jyarse A & Localio SA (1964) An evaluation of colonic stone management. *Surg Gynecol Obstet* **118**: 1234–1242.

Griffiths DA, Philpotts E, Espiner HS & Eltringham WK (1976) The continent colostomy. *Gut* **17**: 385–402.

Guttman FM (1985) Proximal decompression by tube appendicostomy with pull through procedures in pediatric operations. *Surg Gynecol Obstet* **160**: 169–170.

Hager T & Schellerer W (1979) Der erlanger Magnetverschluss. Ein Uberblick uber 2½ Jahre implantations zeit. *Therapiewoche* **29**: 727–732.

Hansen JB, Hoier-Madsen K & Lindenberg J (1974) Loop transverse colostomy. *Acta Chir Scand* **140**: 658–659.

Heald RJ & Leicester RJ (1981) The low stapled anastomosis. *Br J Surg* **68**: 333–337.

Heiblum M & Cordoba A (1978) An artificial sphincter: preliminary report. *Dis Colon Rectum* **21**: 562–566.

Heister L (1743) A General System of Surgery in Three Parts (book 1, chap. V, p. 63; part II, sect. V, p. 53) (Translated into English from the Latin – Inys, Dabrs, Clark, Manby, Whiston, London.) (Original German edition 1718.)

Henry MM & Everett WG (1979) Loop colostomy closure. *Br J Surg* **66**: 275–277.

Hill GL & Pickford IR (1979) A new appliance for collecting ileostomy and jejunostomy in the postoperative period. *Br J Surg* **66**: 203–206.

Hughes ESR (1963) Cecostomy: a part of an efficient method of decompressing the colon obstructed by cancer. *Dis Colon Rectum* **6**: 454–459.

Hughes SF & Williams NS (1995) Continent colonic conduit for the treatment of faecal incontinence associated with disordered evacuation. *Br J Surg* **82**: 1318–1320.

Hulten L, Kewentier J & Kock NG (1976) Komplikatinen der und colostomie und Ihre Behandlung. *Chirurg* **47**: 20–26.

Hunt GJ (1960) Surface cecostomy versus right colon colostomy as the procedure of choice in decompressing the acute obstructed colon due to extensive cancer. *J Med Assoc State Ala* **29**: 244–248.

Hurwitz A (1971) Transverse colostomy. *Am J Surg* **122**: 834.

Irvin TT (1987) Recent results of colostomy closure: a prospective study of 98 operations. *J R Coll Surg Edinb* **32**: 352–354.

Isa S & Quan SHQ (1975) Colostomy perforation. *Dis Colon Rectum* **21**: 92–93.

Jackson PP & Baird RM (1967) Cecostomy: an analysis of 102 cases. *Am J Surg* **114**: 297–301.

Jarpa S (1986) Transverse or sigmoid loop colostomy. *Surg Gynecol Obstet* **163**: 372–373.

Jarret LN, Balfour TW & Bourke JB (1977) Mortality and morbidity in transverse loop colostomy closure. *J R Coll Surg Edinb* **22**: 208–213.

Jenkinson LR, Houghton PWJ, Steele KV, Donaldson LA & Crumplin MKH (1984) The Brethinin Bridge: an advance in stoma care. *Ann R Coll Surg Engl* **66**: 420–422.

Jones EC (1956) Colostomy. *Med Press* **235**: 55.

Karanjia ND, Schache DJ & Heald RJ (1992) Function of the distal rectum after low anterior resection for carcinoma. *Br J Surg* **79**: 114–116.

Keighley MRB & Burdon DW (eds) (1979) *Antimicrobial Prophylaxis in Surgery*. London: Pitman Medical.

Keighley MRB & Matheson D (1980) Functional results of rectal excision and endo-anal anastomosis. *Br J Surg* **67**: 757–761.

Kewenter J (1978) Continent colostomy with the aid of a magnetic closing system: a preliminary report. *Dis Colon Rectum* **21**: 46–51.

Khan AL, Ah-See AK, Crofts TJ, Heys SD, Eremin O (1994) Reversal of Hartmann's Colostomy. *J R Coll Surg Edinb* **39**: 239–242.

Khoury DA, Beck DE, Opelka FG, Hicks TC, Timmcke AE, Gathright JB (1996) Colostomy closure: Ochsner Clinic experience. *Dis Colon Rectum* **39**: 605–609.

Khubchandani IT, Trimpi HD, Sheets JA, Stasik JJ Jr & Belcavage CA (1981) The magnetic stoma device: a continent colostomy. *Dis Colon Rectum* **24**: 344–350.

King RD, Kaiser GC, Lempke RE & Shumacker HB Jr (1966) An evaluation of catheter cecostomy. *Surg Gynecol Obstet* **123**: 779–786.

Kirkpatrick JR & Rajpal SG (1975) The injured colon: therapeutic considerations. *Am J Surg* **129**: 187–191.

Kjaergaard J, Christensen U, Stadil F & Anderson B (1984) Colostomy irrigation with prostaglandin E_2 and bisacodyl: a double-blind crossover study. *Br J Surg* **71**: 556–557.

Klop AL (1990) Body image and self-concept among individuals with stomas. *J Enterostomal Ther* **17**: 98–105.

Knox AJS, Birkett FDH & Collins CD (1971) Closure of colostomy. *Br J Surg* **58**: 669–672.

Kock NG, Geroulanos S, Hahnloser P, Schauwecker H & Sauberli H (1974) Continent colostomy: an experimental study in dogs. *Dis Colon Rectum* **17**: 727–734.

Kock NG, Myrvold HE, Philipson BM, Svaninger G & Ojerskog B (1985) Continent cecostomy. *Dis Colon Rectum* **28**: 705–708.

Kramer P, Kearney MM & Ingelfinger FJ (1962) The effects of specific foods and water loading on the ideal excreta of ileostomised human subjects. *Gastroenterology* **42**: 535–546.

Kuld-Hansen L (1978) Continent colostomy by means of a magnetic stoma seal – experiences of 2½ years: I. World Congress of Coloproctology, Madrid.

Lafreniere R & Ketcham AS (1985) The Penrose drain: a safe, atraumatic colostomy bridge. *Am J Surg* **149**: 288–291.

Larrey DJ (1823) *Some Observations on Wounds of the Intestines. Surgical Essays*. (Translated from the French by J Reveve.) Baltimore: Maxwell.

Lazorthes F & Chiotassal P (1986) Stapled colorectal anastomoses: preoperative integrity of the anastomosis and risk of postoperative leakage. *Int J Colorectal Dis* **1**: 96–98.

Le Dran HF (1781) *The Operations in Surgery* 5th edn, pp. 59–60 (translated by Mr Gataker). London: Dodsley & Law. (Original French edition 1742.)

Lee YN (1968) A simple technique for fixing loop colostomy. *Am J Surg* **116**: 138–139.

Leslie D (1984) The parastomal hernia. *Surg Clin North Am* **64**: 407–415.

Levine SM, Gelford M, Hersh T, Wyshak G, Spiro H & Flock MH (1970) Intestinal bacterial flora after total and partial colon resection. *Am J Dig Dis* **15**: 523–528.

Lewis A & Weedon D (1982) Early closure of transverse loop colostomies. *Ann R Coll Surg Engl* **64**: 57–58.

Lewis WG, Holdsworth PJ, Stephenson BM, Finan PJ, Johnston D (1992) Role of the rectum in the physiological and clinical results of coloanal and colorectal anastomosis after anterior resection for rectal carcinoma. *Br J Surg* **79**: 1082–1086.

Livingstone DH, Miller FB & Richardson JD (1989) Are the risks after colostomy closure exaggerated? *Am J Surg* **158**: 17–20.

Loder PB, Thomson JPS (1995) Trephine colostomy: a warning. *Ann R Coll Surg Engl* **77**: 462.

Londono-Schimmer EE, Leong APK, Phillips RKS (1994) Life table analysis of stoma complications following colostomy. *Dis Colon Rectum* **37**: 916–920.

Ludwig KA, Milsom JW, Garcia-Ruiz A & Fazio VW (1996) Laparascopic techniques for fecal diversion. *Dis Colon Rectum* **39**: 285–288.

McLeod JH (1983) Biofeedback in the management of partial anal incontinence. *Dis Colon Rectum* **26**: 244–246.

MacDonald LD & Anderson HR (1984) Stigma in patients with rectal cancer: a community study. *J Epidemiol Commun Health* **38**: 284–290.

MacDonald LD & Anderson HR (1985) The health of rectal cancer patients in the community. *Eur J Surg Oncol* **11**: 235–241.

MacMahon RA, Cohen SJ & Eckstein HB (1963) Colostomies in infancy and childhood. *Arch Dis Child* **38**: 114–117.

Maguire GP et al (1978) Psychiatric problems in the first year after mastectomy. *BMJ* **1**: 963–965.

Mander BJ, Abercrombie JF, George BD & Williams NS (1996) The electrically stimulated gracilis neosphincter incorporated as part of total anorectal reconstruction after abdominoperineal excision of the rectum. *Ann Surg* **224**: 702–711.

Marsh N (1994) Psychological adaptation to stoma surgery: the relationship of body image to depression. Doctor of Clinical Psychology thesis, University of Birmingham.

Martin L & Foster G (1996) Parastomal hernia. *Ann R Coll Surg Engl* **78**: 81–84.

Maynard A de L & Turell R (1955) Acute left colon obstruction with special reference to cecostomy versus transverostomy. *Surg Gynecol Obstet* **100**: 667–674.

Mazier WP, Dignon RD, Capehart RJ & Smith BG (1976) Effective colostomy irrigation. *Surg Gynecol Obstet* **142**: 905–909.

Mealy K, O'Broine, Donohue J, Tanner A & Keane V (1996) Reversible colostomy: what is the outcome? *Dis Colon Rectum* **39**: 1227–1231.

Mercati U, Trancanelli V, Castagnoli GP, Mariotti A & Ciaccarini R (1991) Use of the gracilis muscle for sphincteric construction after abdominoperineal resection: technique and preliminary results. *Dis Colon Rectum* **34**: 1085–1089.

Merrett ND & Gartell PC (1993) A totally diverting loop colostomy. *Ann R Coll Surg Engl* **75**: 272–274.

Messinetti S, Battisti G & Latorre F (1977) Magnetic prosthesis in patients with a permanent colostomy: Rendic. *Gastroenterology* **9**: 211–216.

Meyhoff HH, Andersen B & Nielson SL (1990) Colostomy irrigation: a clinical and scintigraphic comparison between three different irrigation volumes. *Br J Surg* **77**: 1185–1186.

Miller DR & Allbritten FF Jr (1976) Carcinoma of the colon and rectum. *Arch Surg* **111**: 692–696.

Mirelman D, Corman ML, Veidenheimer MC & Coller JA (1978) Colostomies: indications and contraindications: Lahey Clinic experience 1963–74. *Dis Colon Rectum* **21**: 172–176.

Miskowiak J (1983) Closure of colostomy using GIA stapler. *Dis Colon Rectum* **26**: 550–551.

Mitchell WH, Kovalcik PJ & Cross GH (1978) Complications of colostomy closure. *Dis Colon Rectum* **21**: 180–182.

Mollitt DL, Malangoni MA, Ballantine VN et al (1980) Colostomy complications in children. *Arch Surg* **115**: 455–458.

Nicholls RJ, Ritchie JK, Wadsworth J & Parks AG (1979) Total excision or restorative resection for carcinoma of the middle third of rectum. *Br J Surg* **66**: 625–627.

Oberst MT & Scott DW (1988) Post-discharge distress in surgically treated cancer patients and their spouses. *Res Nurs Health* **11**: 223–233.

Office of Population Censuses and Surveys (1970) *Report on Hospital Inpatient Enquiry for the 1967. I: Tables.* London: HMSO.

Oluwole SF, Freeman HP & Davis K (1982) Morbidity of colostomy closure. *Dis Colon Rectum* **25**: 422–426.

Orbach CE & Tallent N (1965) Modification of perceived body and of body concepts following the construction of a colostomy. *Arch Gen Psychiatr* **12**: 126–135.

Orbach CE, Bard M & Sutherland AM (1957) Fears and defensive adaptations to the loss of anal sphincter control. *Psychoanal Rev* **44**: 121–175.

Ortiz H, Sara MJ, Armendariz P, di Miguel M, Marti J & Chocarro C (1994) Does the frequency of paracolostomy hernias depend on the position of the colostomy in the abdominal wall? *Int J Colorect Dis* **9**: 65–67.

Parkin DM, Muir CS, Whelan SL et al (1992) *Cancer Incidence in Five Continents*, Vol. VI. Lyon: IARC Scientific Publications.

Parks SE & Hastings PR (1985) Complications of colostomy closure. *Am J Surg* **149**: 672–675.

Patey DH (1951) Primary epithelial apposition in colostomy. *Proc R Soc Med* **44**: 423–424.

Pearl RK, Prasad LM, Orsay CP, Abcarian H, Tan AB & Melzil MJ (1985) Early local complications from intestinal stomas. *Arch Surg* **120**: 1145–1147.

Pelissier EP, Blum B, Bachour A et al (1992) Functional results of coloanal anastomosis with reservoir. *Dis Colon Rectum* **35**: 843–846.

Pelok LR & Nigro ND (1973) Colostomy in the trauma patient: experience in 55 cases. *Dis Colon Rectum* **16**: 290–295.

Perry GJ, Payne JE, Chapuis PH, Bokey EL & Pleils MJ (1983) Complications in colostomy closure. *J R Coll Surg Edinb* **28**: 174–177.

Phillips R, Pringle W, Evans MA & Keighley MRB (1985) Analysis of a hospital based stoma therapy service. *Ann R Coll Surg Engl* **67**: 37–40.

Pittman DM & Smith LE (1985) Complications of colostomy closure. *Dis Colon Rectum* **28**: 836–843.

Plant JA (1971) Dissertation, University of London.

Polk HC Jr, Spratt JS Jr, Bernett D, Copher GH & Butcher HR Jr (1964) Surgical mortality and survival from colonic cancer. *Arch Surg* **89**: 16–23.

Porter JA, Salvati EP, Rubin RJ & Eisenstat TE (1989) Complications of colostomies. *Dis Colon Rectum* **32**: 299–303.

Poticha SM (1974) A new technique for loop colostomy with use of a plastic bridge. *Am J Surg* **127**: 620–621.

Prager E (1984) The continent colostomy. *Dis Colon Rectum* **27**: 235–237.

Prian GW, Sawyer RB & Sawyer KC (1975) Repair of peristomal colostomy hernias. *Am J Surg* **133**: 694–696.

Ramia JM, Ibarra A & Alcalde J (1996) Resection of an end-colostomy stricture with a circular stapling device. *Br J Surg* **83**: 1581.

Ray JE, Hine MO & Haley PH (1960) Postoperative problems of ileostomy and colostomy. *JAMA* **174**: 2118–2123.

Reboa G, Ginsto F, Terrizzi A, Secco GB & Berti Riboli E (1980) Concetti orginali sulla motilita intestinale: premesse fisiopatalogiche, diagnostiche e terapeutiche. *Ann Gastroenterol Hepatol* **16**: 363–370.

Reboa G, Frascio M, Zanella R, Pitto G & Riboli EG (1985) Biofeedback training to obtain continence in permanent colostomy. *Dis Colon Rectum* **28**: 419–421.

Resnick S (1986) New method of bowel stoma formation. *Am J Surg* **152**: 545–548.

Rickett JWS (1969) Subcutaneous colostomy rod. *BMJ* **3**: 466.

Rickett JWS (1978) Obturating balloon colostomy (Torbay colostomy): preliminary communication. *J R Soc Med* **71**: 31–32.

Roe AM, Prabhu S, Ali A, Brown C & Brodribb AJM (1991) Reversal of Hartmann's procedure: timing and operative technique. *Br J Surg* **78**: 1167–1170.

Rombeau JL & Turnbull RB (1978) Hidden loop colostomy. *Dis Colon Rectum* **21**: 177–179.

Rose D, Keniges F & Frazier TG (1985) A simplified technique for a totally diverting transverse loop colostomy and distal irrigation. *Surg Gynecol Obstet* **161**: 593.

Rosen L & Friedman IH (1980) Morbidity and mortality following intraperitoneal closure of transverse loop colostomy. *Dis Colon Rectum* **23**: 508–512.

Rosin JD & Bonardi RA (1977) Paracolostomy hernia repair with Marlex mesh: a new technique. *Dis Colon Rectum* **20**: 299–302.

Rosin RD (1987) An obituary to the transverse colostomy. *J R Soc Med* **80**: 728–729.

Ruf W, Hottenrott C & Doertenbach J (1977) Ein prennatischer anus-praeterverschl. *Langenbecks Arch Chir* (Suppl) 189.

Ruiter P de, Bijnen AB (1992) Successful local report of paracolostomy hernia with a newly developed prosthetic device. *Int J Colorect Dis* **7**: 132–134.

Saha SP, Rao H & Stephenson SE Jr (1973) Complications of colostomy. *Dis Colon Rectum* **16**: 515–516.

Salley RK, Butcher RM & Rodning CB (1983) Colostomy closure: morbidity reduction employing a semi-standardised protocol. *Dis Colon Rectum* **26**: 319–322.

Sames CP (1958) Extraperitoneal colostomy. *Lancet* **i**: 567–568.

Samhouri F & Grodsinsky C (1979) The morbidity and mortality of colostomy closure. *Dis Colon Rectum* **22**: 312–314.

Saubier EC (1978) Fermeture magnetique des colostomies: a propros de 12 observations. *Lyon Chir* **74**: 393–397.

Schmidt E (1981) Sphincter kontinenz – plasfik: indikation – technik und Ergebnisse. *Dtsch Med Wochenschr* **1**: 12–14.

Schmidt E (1982) The continent colostomy. *World J Surg* **6**: 805–809.

Schmidt E, Bruch HP, Genlich N, Rothhammer A & Rowen W (1979) Kontinente colostomie durch freie transplantation autologer Diekdarmmuskalatic. *Chirurg* **50**: 96–100.

Schofield PF, Cade D & Lambert M (1980) Dependent proximal loop colostomy: does it defunction the distal colon? *Br J Surg* **67**: 201–202.

Schwemmle K, Kuaze H-H & Padberg W (1982) Management of the colostomy. *World J Surg* **6**: 554–559.

Seargeant PW (1966) Colostomy management by the irrigation technique: review of 165 cases. *BMJ* **2**: 25–26.

Senapati A & Phillips RKS (1991) The trephine colostomy: a permanent left iliac fossa end colostomy without recourse to laparotomy. *Ann R Coll Surg Engl* **73**: 305–306.

Shafik A (1982) 'Tube' and 'marsupialisation' colostomy: a simplified technique for colostomy. *Am J Proctol Gastroenterol Colon Rect Surg* **36**: 14–30.

Shepherd AA & Keighley MRB (1986) Audit on complicated diverticular disease. *Ann R Coll Surg Engl* **68**: 8–10.

Shu-wen Jao, Beart RWJF, Wendorf LJ & Ustrup DM (1985) Irrigation management of sigmoid colostomy. *Arch Surg* **120**: 916–917.

Sigurdson E, Myers E & Stern H (1986) A modification of the transverse loop colostomy. *Dis Colon Rectum* **29**: 65–66.

Simkin EP (1980) Human tissue response to ox-fibrin (Biethium) with special reference to use as absorbable colostomy rods. *Br J Surg* **67**: 376.

Simonsen OS, Stolf NAG, Aun F, Raia A & Habr-Gama A (1976) A rectal sphincter reconstruction in perineal colostomies after abdominoperineal resection for cancer. *Br J Surg* **63**: 389–391.

Sjodahl R, Anderberg B & Boin T (1988) Parastomal hernia in relation to site of the abdominal stoma. *Br J Surg* **75**: 339–341.

Skeet M (1970) Home from Hospital. Dan Mason Nursing Research Committee.

Skeie E (1977) Kontinent kolostomi ved hjaelp at magnetlukning. (Continent colostomy with the aid of magnetic stoma seal.) *Ugeskr Laeger* **139**: 2884.

Smit R & Walt AJ (1978) The morbidity and cost of the temporary colostomy. *Dis Colon Rectum* **21**: 558–561.

Soliani P, Carbognani P, Piccolo P, Sabbagh R & Cudazzo E (1992) Colostomy plug devices: a possible new approach to the problem of incontinence. *Dis Colon Rectum* **35**: 969–974.

Sparberg M (1974) Bismuth subgallate as an effective means to control ileostomy odour: a double-blind study. *Gastroenterology* **66**: 476.

Spiro RH & Hertz RE (1966) Colostomy perforation. *Surgery* **60**: 590–597.

Sprangers MAG, Taal BG, Aaronson NK & te Velde A (1995) Quality of life in colorectal cancer: stoma vs nonstoma patients. *Dis Colon Rectum* **38**: 360–369.

Stainback WC & Christiansen KH (1962) The value of Foley catheter cecostomy in conjunction with resection of the left colon and rectosigmoid. *Surg Clin North Am* **42**: 1475–1479.

Stephenson BM, Myers C & Phillips RKS (1995) Minimally raised end colostomy. *Int J Colorect Dis* **10**: 232–233.

Stephenson ER, Ilahi O & Koltun WA (1997) Stoma creation through the stoma site: a rapid, safe technique. *Dis Colon Rectum* **40**: 112–115.

Stock W, Fiedel U & Muller J (1978) Kolostomie versorgung dureh den Erlanger magnetveschluss. *Dtsch Med Wochenschr* **103**: 327–328.

Stothert JC Jr, Brubacher L & Simonowitz DA (1982) Complications of emergency stoma formation. *Arch Surg* **117**: 307–309.

Sykes FR (1979) Transcutaneous defunctioning colostomy. *Br J Surg* **66**: 505–506.

Sykes PA, Boulter KH & Schofield PF (1976) The microflora of the obstructed bowel. *Br J Surg* **63**: 721–725.

Terranova O, Sandei F, Rebuffat C, Maroutii R & Bortolozzi E (1979) Irrigation vs natural evacuation of left colostomy. *Dis Colon Rectum* **22**: 32–34.

Thal ER & Yeary EC (1980) Morbidity of colostomy closure following colon trauma. *J Trauma* **20**: 287–291.

Thibodeau OA (1974) Colostomy closure: a simple procedure? *J Maine Med Assoc* **65**: 208–210.

Thomas C, Madden F, Jehu D (1984) Psychosocial morbidity in the first three months following stoma surgery. *J Psychosom Res* **28**: 251–257.

Thomas C, Madden F & Jehu D (1987a) Psychological effects of stomas. I: Psychosocial morbidity one year after surgery. *J Psychosom Res* **31**: 311–316.

Thomas C, Madden F, Jehu D (1987b) Psychological effects of stomas. II: Factors influencing outcome. *J Psychosom Res* **31**: 317–323.

Thomson JPS & Hawley PR (1972) Results of closure of loop transverse colostomies. *BMJ* **3**: 459–462.

Thomson TJ, Runce J & Khan A (1970) The effect on ileostomy functions. *Gut* **11**: 482–485.

Thorlakson RH (1965) Technique of repair of herniations associated with colonic stomas. *Surg Gynecol Obstet* **120**: 347–350.

Todd GJ, Kutcher LM & Markowitz AM (1979) Factors influencing the complications of colostomy closure. *Am J Surg* **137**: 749–751.

Todd IP (1982) Mechanical complications of ileostomy. *Clin Gastroenterol* **11**: 268–273.

Tomlinson RJ, Newman BM & Schofield PF (1976) Is colostomy closure a hazardous procedure? A comparison of elemental diet and routine bowel preparation. *Br J Surg* **63**: 799–800.

Torres RA & Gonzalez MA (1988) Perineal continent colostomy: report of a case. *Dis Colon Rectum* **31**: 957–960.

Townsend P (1957) *The Family Life of Old People: An Enquiry in East London*, ch. 13. London: Routledge & Kegan Paul.

Tudor RG, Oates GD & Keighley MRB (1986) Outcome after the Hartmann procedure for complicated diverticular disease. *Gut* **27**: 626.

Turnbull RB (1961) Instructions to the colostomy patient: management of the colostomy. *Cleve Clin Q* **28**: 132–140.

Turnbull RB & Weekley FL (1967) *An Atlas of Instestinal Stomas*, p. 97. St Louis: CV Mosby.

Unti JA, Abcarian H, Pearl RK et al (1991) Rodless end-loop stomas: seven-year experience. *Dis Colon Rectum* **34**: 999–1004.

Varnell J & Pemberton LM (1981) Risk factors in colostomy closure. *Surgery* **89**: 683–868.

Vaxman F, Ionescu C, Volkmar P, Pambou O & Grenier JF (1993) The unopened colostomy: a procedure to protect colonic anastomosis. *Int J Colorectal Dis* **8**: 48–50.

Venturini M, Bertelli G, Forno G et al (1990) Colostomy irrigation in the elderly: effective recovery regardless of age. *Dis Colon Rectum* **33**: 1031–1033.

Vogel SL & Maher JW (1986) An improved method for construction of loop colostomy. *Surg Gynecol Obstet* **162**: 377–378.

Wade BE (1989a) *A Stoma is for Life*. London: Scutari Press.

Wade BE (1989b) Ostomates: the case for a thorough patient assessment. *Senior Nurse* **9**: 12–14.

Wade BE (1990) Colostomy patients: psychological adjustment at 10 weeks and 1 year after surgery in districts which employed stoma-care nurses and districts which did not. *J Adv Nurs* **15**: 1297–1304.

Wald A (1981) Biofeedback therapy for fecal incontinence. *Ann Intern Med* **89**: 683–686.

Wangensteen OH (1942) *Intestinal Obstruction*, 2nd edn. Springfield, IL: CC Thomas.

Wangensteen OH (1947) Complete fecal diversion achieved by a simple loop colostomy. *Surg Gynecol Obstet* **84**: 409–414.

Wara P, Sorensen K & Berg V (1981) Proximal fecal diversion: review of ten years' experience. *Dis Colon Rectum* **24**: 114–119.

Wheeler MH (1982) Early closure of transverse loop colostomies. *Ann R Coll Surg Engl* **64**: 203–204.

Wheeler MH & Barker J (1977) Closure of colostomy: a safe procedure? *Dis Colon Rectum* **20**: 29–32.

White CA & Hunt JC (1997) Psychological factors in postoperative adjustment to stoma surgery. *Ann R Coll Surg Engl* **79**: 3–7.

Williams JG, Etherington R, Hayward MWJ & Hughes LE (1990a) Paraileostomy hernia: a clinical and radiological study. *Br J Surg* **77**: 1355–1357.

Williams NS (1984) The rationale for preservation of the anal sphincter in patients with low rectal cancer. *Br J Surg* **71**: 575–581.

Williams NS & Johnston D (1980) Prospective controlled trial comparing colostomy irrigation with 'spontaneous-action' method. *BMJ* **3**: 107–109.

Williams NS, Macfie J & Celestin LR (1979) Anorectal Crohn's disease. *Br J Surg* **66**: 743–748.

Williams NS, Masmyth DG, Jones D & Smith AH (1986) De-functioning stomas: a prospective controlled trial comparing ileostomy with loop transverse colostomy. *Br J Surg* **73**: 566–570.

Williams NS, Hallan RI, Koeze TH & Watkins ES (1990b) Restoration of gastrointestinal continuity and continence after abdomino-perineal excision of the rectum using an electrically stimulated neoanal sphincter. *Dis Colon Rectum* **33**: 561–565.

Williams RA, Csepanyi E, Hiatt J & Wilson SE (1987) Analysis of the morbidity, mortality and cost of colostomy closure in traumatic compared with non-traumatic colorectal diseases. *Dis Colon Rectum* **30**: 164–167.

Winslet MC, Drolc Z, Allan A & Keighley MRB (1991) Assessment of the defunctioning efficiency of the loop ileostomy. *Dis Colon Rectum* **34**: 699–703.

Wirsching M, Druner HU & Herrmann F (1975) Results of psychosocial adjustment to long term colostomy. *Psychother Psychosom* **26**: 245–256.

Wolff LH & Wolff LH Jr (1980) A re-evaluation of tube cecostomy. *Surg Gynecol Obstet* **151**: 257–259.

Wright HK (1979) Improving transverse colostomy function. *Am J Surg* **137**: 475–477.

Wulff HB (1953) Erfahrungen mit einem ventilkolosto-weversehlub. *Chirurg* **24**: 484–485.

Yajko RD, Morton LW, Bleomendal L & Eiseman B (1976) Morbidity of colostomy closure. *Am J Surg* **132**: 304–306.

Yakimets WW (1975) Complications of closure of loop colostomy. *Can J Surg* **18**: 366–370.

Zilli L, Pietroinski M & Bertario L (1987) Colonoscopy in ostomy patients: results at the first postoperative examination. *Dis Colon Rectum* **30**: 687–691.

Zinkin LD & Rosin JD (1981) Button colopexy for colostomy prolapse. *Surg Gynecol Obstet* **152**: 89–90.

Zoltan J (1982) *Die Anwendung des Spalthautlappens in de Chirurgie*. Jena: Fischer.

10

PERSISTENT PERINEAL SINUS

Primary perineal wound healing is the process of complete healing of a wound that has been closed by suture at the time of rectal excision. Impaired primary healing may result from a wound haematoma or sepsis. *Secondary* healing is complete healing of the perineum when the wound has been deliberately left open to granulate. This process is usually complete by 12–14 weeks but may be delayed in irradiated tissues, if there has been sepsis or advanced malignancy, or where the cavity is large. *Delayed* wound healing is defined here as a wound that has not healed in 4–6 months but which eventually heals. The term *persistent sinus* is confined to patients whose perineal wound remains unhealed at one year.

HEALING OF PERINEAL WOUNDS

Primary healing

If the pelvic floor and sphincters have been retained after rectal excision, they may be sutured together in the midline prior to closure of the skin and subcutaneous tissue. Closure is usually over suction drains in an attempt to obliterate any dead space. If the wound heals by first intention this is usually rapid, and skin sutures can be removed after 7–10 days. Primary healing is delayed if the wound becomes infected or if a haematoma develops. A common sequence of delayed healing is the development of a deep cavity which does not drain adequately owing to a partially healed skin wound. If aware of this complication, the clinician may deliberately convert the attempted primary closure into an open wound by removal of all superficial and deep sutures so that it can heal by secondary intention. In this way a persistent cavity may be eliminated as a cause of delayed perineal wound healing.

Secondary healing

Surgeons who have audited perineal wound healing accept that morbidity is substantially reduced by leaving wounds open in patients with known risk factors associated with low healing rates. These risk factors include established perianal sepsis, high fistulas, anorectal abscess or extensive perianal cellulitis, diabetes mellitus, locally advanced neoplastic disease or previous radiotherapy. The pelvic peritoneum may be sutured, but this is not always possible or prudent. Usually the perineum is packed with an antiseptic solution soaked in large gauze packs which are removed approximately a week later. The cavity is then either repacked, left open or filled with elastomer foam. The aim of secondary healing is to allow the cavity to granulate from its deeper aspect to the surface. The speed of healing is dependent upon the size of the cavity, the presence of pathogenic bacteria, and the host defence mechanisms, particularly radiotherapy, previous malnutrition and advanced malignancy. Most open wounds have completely healed 3 months after operation.

Delayed healing

A perineal wound which persists after 4–6 months causes considerable morbidity. Patients not only complain of a persistent discharge, but there may be dyspareunia, pain, urinary symptoms and psychiatric sequelae. Delayed healing may be due to residual neoplasia, persistent sepsis, a poorly draining cavity or coexisting disease at the time of rectal excision, particularly rectovaginal fistula, a high fistula-in-ano or perineal sepsis (Scammell and Keighley, 1986).

Persistent sinus

A sinus which persists 12 months after proctectomy may be due to a retained foreign body such as barium (after a previous perineal sinogram), nonabsorbable sutures, retained rectal mucosa, persistent granuloma in the perineal sinus track in Crohn's disease, unsuspected hidradenitis suppurativa, radiation damage, recurrent malignancy or an enteroperineal fistula. Perineal wounds that persist 12 months after rectal excision rarely heal with conservative therapy but some can be successfully managed by re-operation (Lees and Everett, 1991).

Vaginoperineal fistula

Vaginoperineal fistula is a form of persistent perineal sinus which is seen particularly in women after rectal excision for Crohn's disease. It usually consists of a low communication between a perineal sinus and the vagina or vulva, often with a higher sinus extending to the mid sacrum (Figure 10.1).

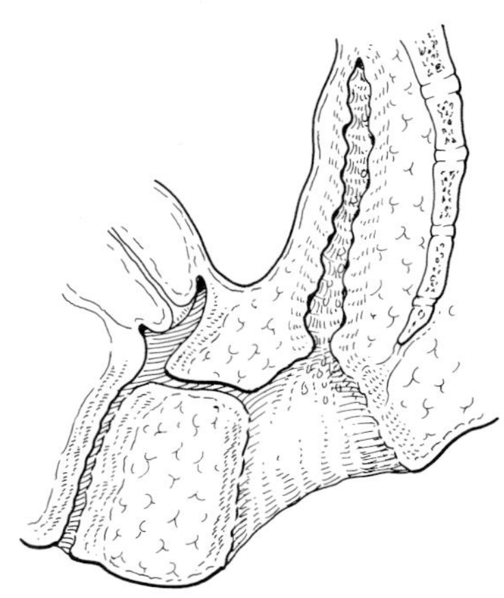

Figure 10.1 Vaginoperineal fistula is a form of persistent perineal sinus occurring in women after proctocolectomy.

PRIMARY PERINEAL WOUND HEALING

After abdominoperineal excision for malignancy

The incidence of primary healing of the perineal wound following abdominoperineal excision is listed in Table 10.1 and ranges from 37% to 92% (Crile and Robert, 1950; Schofield, 1970; Hulten et al, 1971; Kronberg et al, 1974; Irvin and Goligher, 1975; Marks et al, 1976; Saha and Robinson, 1976; Terranova et al, 1979; Alpsan et al, 1980; Aubrey et al, 1984; Lieberman and Feldman, 1984). This variation reflects widely differing patient selection. For instance, our own figure of 41% primary healing is for all patients, but in 12% the perineal wound was deliberately left open because of the risk of sepsis. By contrast, the series reported by Altemeier et al (1974), giving a 92% primary healing rate, is confined to patients having primary closure who were carefully selected because risk factors were absent. For instance in this series, primary suture was not attempted if the rectum had been damaged at the time of operation, if the tumour was extensive, or when preoperative radiotherapy had been used.

After rectal excision for inflammatory bowel disease

Primary healing is achieved less frequently after rectal excision for inflammatory bowel disease than for malignancy. Manjoney et al (1983) showed that, although the incidence of sepsis, haematoma and wound dehiscence was similar, healing 6 weeks after operation was achieved in 64% of patients who had undergone a resection for malignancy, compared with only 39% having proctectomy for inflammatory bowel disease (Table 10.2). We found that primary healing was very infrequent in inflammatory bowel disease (Baudot et al, 1980) compared with rectal excision for malignancy (Table 10.3).

Ulcerative colitis

At the Lahey Clinic, 89% of 90 patients with ulcerative colitis eventually achieved perineal wound healing, but only two wounds healed by first intention (Corman et al, 1978). Our own experience is not much better: only 27 of 33 wounds in ulcerative colitis were closed and the primary healing rate was only 8% (Baudot et al, 1980); but most eventually healed without further intervention. At the Cleveland Clinic, only 34% of 326 patients were reported as having achieved perineal wound healing 1 month after rectal excision for ulcerative colitis (Oakley et al, 1985). Irvin and Goligher (1975) reported primary healing in 45% of patients with

Table 10.1 Incidence of primary perineal wound healing after abdominoperineal excision of the rectum for cancer with primary closure over suction drains.

Authors	*Incidence* (%)
Crile and Robert (1950)	78
Schofield (1970)	77
Hulten et al (1971)	75
Altemeier et al (1974)	92
Broader et al (1974)	69
Kronberg et al (1974)	37
Irvin and Goligher (1975)	45
Marks et al (1976)	56
Saha and Robinson (1976)	88
Terranova et al (1979)	63
Alpsan et al (1980)	65
Baudot et al (1980)	41
Aubrey et al (1984)	56
Lieberman and Feldman (1984)	85

Table 10.2 Comparison of the incidence (%) of perineal wound complications in malignancy and inflammatory bowel disease.

	Cancer (*n* = 58)	*Inflammatory bowel disease* (*n* = 28)
Infection	16	18
Haematoma	3	4
Dehiscence	3	4
Healed at 6 weeks	64	39
Healed at 3 months	84	71
Healed at 1 year	100	86

From Manjoney et al (1983).

Table 10.3 Comparative rates of healing of perineal wounds in Birmingham.

	Ulcerative carcinoma (*n* = 35)	*Crohn's colitis* (*n* = 33)	*Malignant disease* (*n* = 35)
Primary closure of the wound	31	27	31
Primary healing (%)	41	8	18
Healed at 3 months (%)	72	45	45
Healed at 6 months (%)	86	68	64
Persistent sinus (over 6 months) (%)	14	32	36

From Baudot et al (1980).

ulcerative colitis. The best results are those reported by Tompkins and Warshaw (1985), who found that 48 of 50 perineal wounds (96%) healed after primary closure over suction drains (Table 10.4). The incidence of primary healing is higher (54%) after intersphincteric excision (Leicester et al, 1984).

Table 10.4 Primary healing in inflammatory bowel disease.

Authors	*Primary healing* (%)
Ulcerative colitis	
Irvin and Goligher (1975)	45
Leicester et al (1984)	54
Oakley et al (1985)	34
Tompkins and Warshaw (1985)	96
Crohn's disease	
Irvin and Goligher (1975)	36
Leicester et al (1984)	37
Scammell and Keighley (1986)	34

Crohn's disease

Primary healing of the perineal wound may be achieved in Crohn's disease in appropriately selected patients, but persistent perineal sinus is much more common. The Leeds group (Irvin and Goligher, 1975) achieved primary healing in 36% of patients with Crohn's disease. In Birmingham the data were almost identical; among 116 patients having rectal excision for Crohn's disease, only 34% of patients achieved primary healing (Scammell and Keighley, 1986). Primary healing after intersphincteric excision in Crohn's disease was reported in 37% of patients at St Mark's Hospital (Leicester et al, 1984); however, intersphincteric excision is feasible only in those patients without extensive rectal fibrosis, sepsis and fistulas.

FACTORS INFLUENCING THE SUCCESS OF PRIMARY PERINEAL WOUND HEALING

Faecal contamination

Avoidance of faecal contamination is crucial to the success of primary wound healing, so every effort should be made to prevent breaching the anorectum during proctectomy. Meticulous care should be taken in sealing the anus by a reliable purse-string suture as well as in the dissection of the anterior rectal wall from the vagina in women (Figures 10.2 and 10.3). The risk of contamination can be minimized, particularly if mechanical bowel preparation is less than perfect, by stapling the mid-rectum after milking away any faecal material within it (Figure 10.4).

Rectal damage commonly occurs when the abdominal and perineal operators fail to work in harmony. Traction by one with counter-traction by the other and attempted resection by both can lead to damage. We used to believe that the abdominal surgeon should be responsible for the posterior dissection so that the perineal surgeon can concentrate on the anterior plane, while lateral clearance can be accomplished by both under direct vision. However, one of us (MRBK) is firmly of the view that there is far less risk of rectal damage if the entire rectal dissection is performed from above as in restorative proctocolectomy and very low anterior resection. The same surgeon then removes the anal stump from below while the assistant constructs the stoma. In this way the incidence of iatrogenic anorectal perforation has virtually disappeared. Excision of the posterior aspect of the vagina in selected cases may reduce the risk of

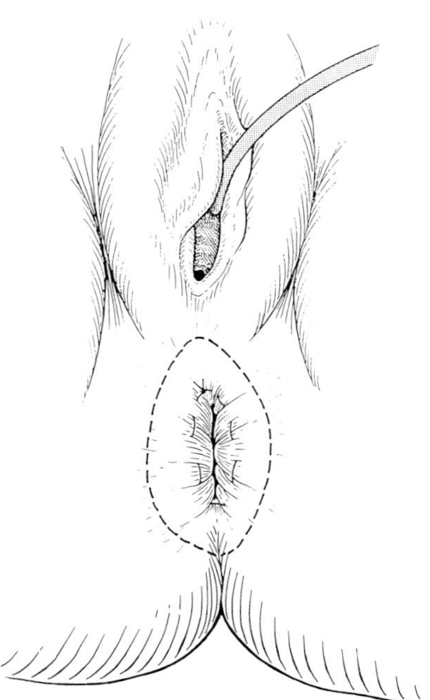

Figure 10.2 A purse-string has been placed around the anal canal to prevent contamination during rectal excision.

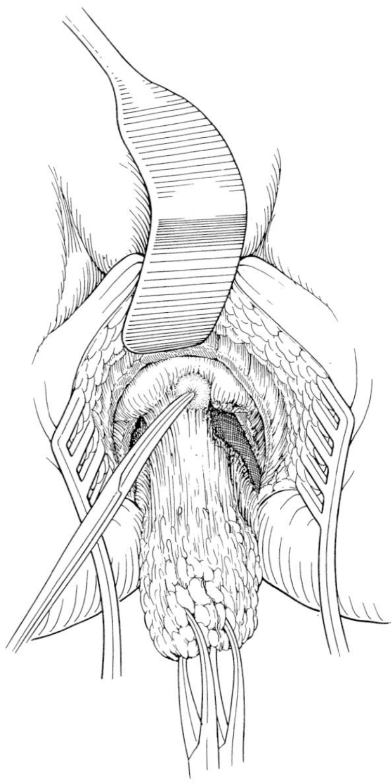

Figure 10.3 Anterior rectal dissection in a female patient during perineal proctectomy. The anus has been completely dissected from the perineum; the anterior rectal dissection involves opening the rectovaginal septum and dividing the medial fibres of the puborectalis.

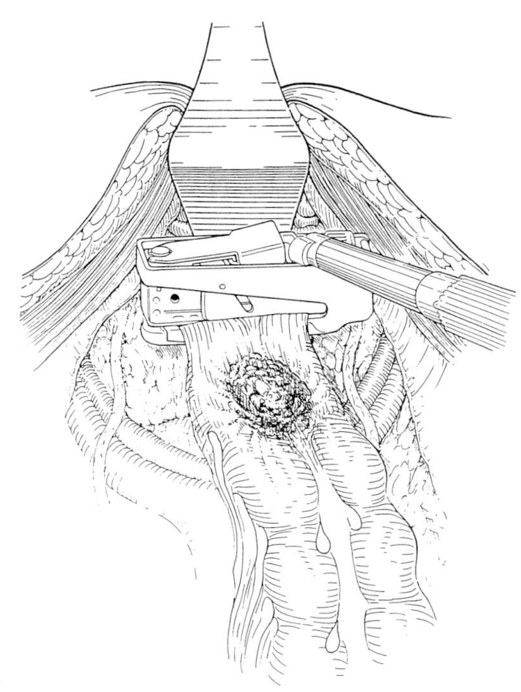

Figure 10.4 Staple transection of the lower third of the rectum to minimize contamination during abdominoperineal excision. A stapling technique across the upper anal canal can be used as an alternative to proctectomy.

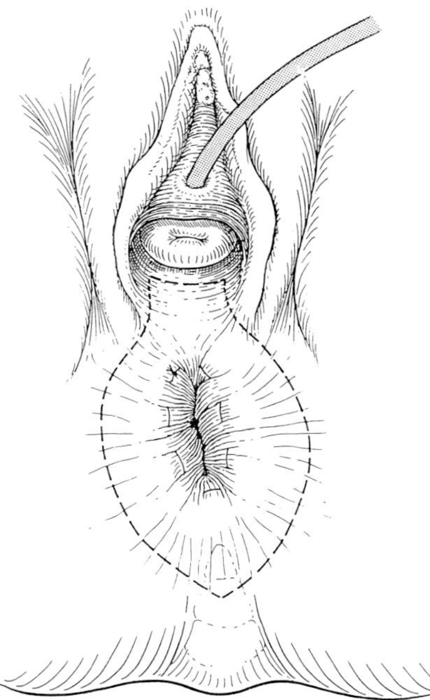

Figure 10.5 Excision of the posterior vaginal wall in continuity with the rectum for malignant disease involving the rectovaginal septum.

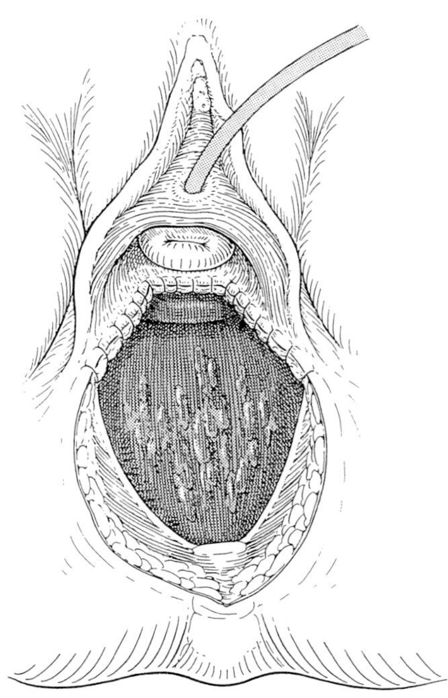

Figure 10.6 Completion of an *en bloc* excision of the rectum and the posterior vaginal wall.

faecal contamination, but we do not think that vaginal excision should ever be practised in young, sexually active women with inflammatory bowel disease. In our view, vaginal excision should be performed only for oncological reasons in women with anterior rectal neoplasms (Figures 10.5 and 10.6). Using vaginal excision, Johnston (1979) reported primary healing in 43 of 45 patients, none of whom developed a persistent perineal sinus.

Haemostasis

Haematoma is often a precursor to sepsis. Meticulous haemostasis is essential while ensuring that the patient is not hypotensive at the time of perineal closure.

Suction drainage

Efficient suction drainage is crucial to the success of primary perineal wound closure. Suction drains are needed to eliminate dead space and to prevent haematoma to ensure immediate evacuation of blood suction; it should be applied before wound closure.

Walton and Mallik (1975) used two Winsbury white catheters, one placed on suction and the other on free drainage, and reported primary healing rates of 94% after excision for malignancy and 75% after excision for inflammatory bowel disease. Lieberman and Feldman (1984) achieved an 85% primary healing rate using a system of closed irrigation suction drainage after primary wound closure (Figure 10.6). The practice of closed suction minimizes the risk of exogenous bacterial contamination.

Aubrey and others (1984) achieved only a 56% primary healing rate in 43 patients after abdominoperineal excision for carcinoma using irrigation suction, but 89% had healed by 6 weeks. Elliot and Todd (1985), using a continuous closed irrigation suction device, reported primary healing in 76% of 34 patients with inflammatory bowel disease. We have found serious design faults with some systems: the air filters may become waterlogged and, if so, suction will not be maintained; irrigation suction cannot be continued while transferring patients from the operating theatre to the ward; and early mobilization is restricted.

We do not advise placing drains through the perineal wound and prefer the transabdominal route. Saha and Robinson (1976) reported a primary wound healing rate of only 34% compared with 85% when drainage was through the abdomen. Tompkins and Warshaw (1985) report the highest primary wound healing rate, which they attribute to closing all defects in the pelvic floor over closed suction drains after rectal excision. The pelvic peritoneum is left open and the omentum and the small bowel obliterates the dead space (Figure 10.7). If there has been any contamination, the pelvic floor is closed but the skin is left open. In a personal series of 57 rectal excisions, using intersphincteric dissection whenever feasible, they report only two infections with a 96% primary healing rate in 50 wounds among patients with inflammatory bowel disease. Of the seven wounds in which the skin was left open, all had healed by 2 months and none developed a perineal sinus.

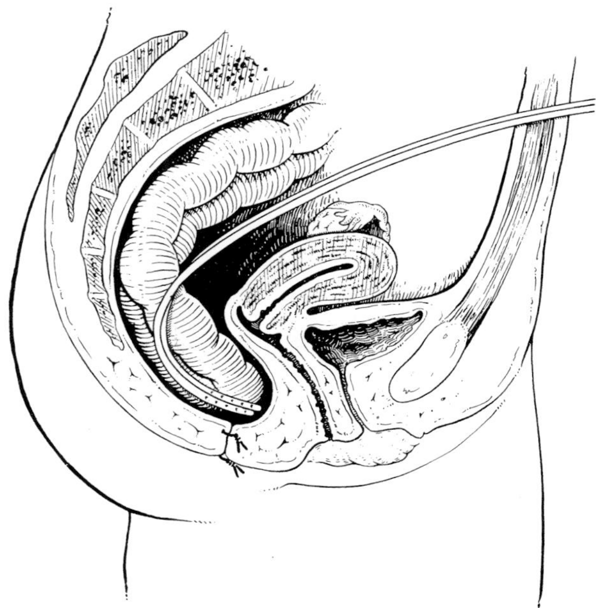

Figure 10.7 Closed pelvic suction drainage or pelvic irrigation. Two suction catheters have been placed above the pelvic floor closure site after rectal excision, to prevent a pelvic abscess.

THE CASE FOR PRIMARY CLOSURE OF PERINEAL WOUNDS AND LEAVING THE PELVIC PERITONEUM OPEN

There is overwhelming evidence to support the superiority of primary perineal wound closure over suction drainage compared with leaving wounds open, provided there is no pre-existing sepsis and there has been no faecal contamination during rectal excision. Unfortunately, almost all the comparisons are based upon retrospective data. It is hardly surprising, therefore, that Oakley et al (1985) reported healing 1 month after operation in 48% of wounds that were sutured, compared with only 11% in wounds left open, but faecal contamination was the reason for open wounds. Similarly, Terranova et al (1979) reported 91% healing at 3 months in 91% of patients after primary closure, compared with only 59% in wounds which were left open because of contamination. Alpsan et al (1980) record healing rates at 6 months of 98% and 54% for closed and open wounds respectively; they also suggested that results were better when the pelvic peritoneum was left unsutured so that the small bowel and omentum could fill the cavity below the sacral promontory (Ruckley et al, 1970).

The only reliable data regarding the optimum method of perineal and peritoneal closure emanate from the one clinical trial designed to answer these questions (Irvin and Goligher, 1975). Although the numbers studied were small, at 6 months twice as many patients (37%) had an unhealed perineal wound when the perineal defect was left open, compared with those whose wounds had been closed primarily (19%). Suture of the pelvic peritoneum conferred no advantage over leaving it open (Table 10.5); indeed, small bowel obstruction was more common after pelvic peritoneal closure. We therefore recommend primary closure of all perineal wounds over suction drains, provided that there is no faecal contamination. Despite modern antibiotics, attempted closure is still not justified in the face of gross contamination because of the risk of pelvic abscess and prolonged hospital stay.

Table 10.5 Results of a trial to compare three methods of perineal closure.

		Primary closure	
	Open wound (n = 24)	*Pelvic peritoneal closure* (n = 31)	*Pelvic peritoneum not sutured* (n = 42)
Cancer	11 (46)	14 (45)	19 (45)
Crohn's disease	8 (33)	3 (10)	8 (19)
Ulcerative colitis	5 (21)	14 (45)	15 (36)
Primary healing	0	14 (45)	18 (43)
Perineal wound unhealed at 6 months	9 (37)	6 (19)	8 (19)
Hospital stay (days)	27.6 ± 2.2	27.4 ± 1.9	27.7 ± 1.51
Postoperative intestinal obstruction	6 (25)	6 (19)	12 (29)
Secondary operation on perineum	5 (21)	8 (26)	8 (19)

Values in parentheses are percentages.
From Irvin and Goligher (1975).

SECONDARY PERINEAL WOUND HEALING

Conditions under which open wound management would be advised

Factors shown to be associated with breakdown of sutured perineal wounds where open wound management is advised include: faecal contamination, pre-existing perineal sepsis, age, high complex anorectal fistulas, previous radiotherapy, advanced malignancy, and inadequate haemostasis (Jalan et al, 1969; Marks et al, 1976; Warshaw et al, 1977; Keighley and Burdon, 1979; Oakley et al, 1985). Irving and Lyall (1984) showed that emergency proctectomy was associated with a higher breakdown rate than after elective operation. Steroids do not adversely influence the rate of primary healing (Tolstedt et al, 1961; Marks et al, 1976; Irving and Lyall, 1984; Leicester et al, 1984; Scammell and Keighley, 1986).

Table 10.6 Primary perineal wound healing and tumour description in 63 male patients after abdominoperineal excision.

	Primary healing	*Delayed healing*
Site of tumour		
Lower third (%)	63	60
Ampullary tumours (%)	29	24
Upper third (%)	8	16
Number of quadrants involved	2.86	2.86
Size (cm)	4.83	5.07
Dukes' classification*	2.26	2.71
Extent of spread†	1.46	1.89

* A = 1; B = 2; C1 = 3; C2 = 4.
† Scored as: n = 0; slight = 1; moderate = 2; extensive = 3.
From Marks et al (1976).

Marks et al (1976) showed that delayed healing was associated with more advanced tumours (Dukes' classification), the size of the tumour, extrarectal spread and site of the tumour (Table 10.6). There is no consensus on the relationship between the Dukes' classification and perineal healing (Manjoney et al, 1983; Saha, 1983; Aubrey et al, 1984). Faecal contamination is probably the most important indication for leaving the perineal wound open. Saha (1983) reported that all wounds healed by first intention when there was no contamination, but that 26% broke down in contaminated wounds. Irvin and Goligher (1975) also reported that operative contamination was the most important factor in failing to achieve primary healing and was more important than the use of steroids or the underlying pathology.

It may be advisable to leave the perineal wound open if rectal excision is being performed after a previous colectomy and ileostomy. Two reports showed that staged proctectomy was associated with a far lower perineal healing rate than primary proctocolectomy (Bartholdson and Hulten, 1975; Oakley et al, 1975). There is a greater risk of unsuccessful primary healing if the operation takes a long time, according to Leicester et al (1984); these authors also report that the outcome is not influenced by age, sex, steroids, underlying pathology or perineal irrigation.

Management of the open wound

The risk of sepsis and wound breakdown is very high if contaminated wounds are sutured. We therefore advise that in such wounds the pelvis and perineum should be left open so that pus can drain adequately and not pocket. This policy eliminates the risk of synergistic gangrene and local sepsis in the perineum. The problem with this approach is that there is a large cavity which can be difficult to manage and necessitates a prolonged hospital stay. Wood et al (1977) suggested that these large granulating cavities could be filled by an elastomer foam dressing, although the mean healing was 5.5 months (7–92 weeks). Macfie and McMahon (1980), in a prospective trial, compared gauze packing with elastomer foam and found no difference in the time to complete healing (9.9 and 8.6 weeks respectively). However, the use of foam reduced the number of visits by the district nurse, and the analgesic requirement in patients with the foam was lower.

We strongly recommend using elastomer foam in open perineal wounds and find it the optimum method of management in this circumstance. There has been a vogue in the past for attempting delayed primary closure but we have found that this option is rarely feasible. The edges of the cavity are so stiff and non-compliant that it is usually impossible to bring the edges of the pelvic floor together.

DELAYED PERINEAL WOUND HEALING

Some wounds which have still not healed by 4–6 months after proctectomy may still eventually close. However, in our experience, most wounds which remain unhealed at a year usually persist. A similar finding was reported by the Lahey Clinic (Corman et al, 1978) (Table 10.7).

Incidence

The incidence of unhealed perineal wounds at 6 months is very variable and is much higher in

Table 10.7 Healing rates following proctectomy for inflammatory bowel disease.

	Ulcerative colitis (*n* = 90)	*Crohn's disease* (*n* = 61)
Primary healing	2 (2)	0
Healed by 6 months	39 (43)	17 (28)
Healed by 12 months	53 (59)	23 (38)
Healed by 18 months	68 (76)	32 (52)
Healed with reoperation	12 (13)	8 (13)
Total healed	80 (89)	40 (66)

Values in parentheses are percentages.
From Corman et al (1978).

patients with inflammatory bowel disease than in those who have undergone excision for malignancy (Watts et al, 1966; Oates and Alexander-Williams, 1970; Broader et al, 1974; Schwab and Kelly, 1974) (Table 10.8).

Table 10.8 Incidence (%) of perineal wounds unhealed at 6 months.

	Cancer	*Ulcerative colitis*	*Crohn's disease*
Watts et al (1966)	—	25	—
Strahan et al (1967)	—	58	—
Jalan et al (1969)	—	55	—
Hulten et al (1971)	—	0	—
Broader et al (1974)	0	—	—
Irvin and Goligher (1975)	9	30	36
Corman et al (1978)	—	57	72
Eftaiha and Abcarian (1978)	4	—	—
Alpsan et al (1980)	16	—	—
Baudot et al (1980)	14	32	36
Lubbers (1982)	—	6	40
Oakley et al (1985)	—	23	—
Scammell and Keighley (1986)	—	—	22

Factors

Factors found to be associated with delayed perineal wound healing included underlying pathology and faecal contamination (Baudot et al, 1980). Among patients with Crohn's disease (Scammell and Keighley, 1986), faecal contamination, pre-existing perineal infection and complex recto-vaginal or anorectal fistulas were associated with delayed healing (Table 10.9). In patients with ulcerative colitis (Oakley et al, 1985), delayed healing was associated with age over 30 years, staged proctectomy, severe proctitis and perineal disease (Table 10.10). Others generally agree with these findings (Altemeier et al, 1974; Anderson and Turnbull, 1976; Corman et al, 1978; Hurwitz et al, 1980; Maruyama et al, 1980; Lubbers, 1982).

Management

The results of local procedures such as curettage, excision and attempted secondary closure are usually very disappointing in patients with delayed perineal wound healing (Corman et al, 1978). Our advice, therefore, is to encourage local hygiene and a full return to normal activities with a sense of optimism, since over half of these wounds will heal by doing nothing (Scammell and Keighley, 1986).

Table 10.9 Factors associated with delayed healing (more than 12 weeks) in Crohn's disease.

Factor	*Delay (%)*	*Factor*	*Delay (%)*
Severe rectal disease	41	Quiescent disease	25
Rectal stricture	40	None	36
Severe perianal disease	37	Absent/mild perianal disease	37
High fistula in ano or rectovaginal fistula*	66	None	28
Faecal contamination*	100	None	31
Perineal wound sepsis*	81	None	19
Antibiotic cover	44	None	31

* Significant differences.
From Scammell and Keighley (1986).

Table 10.10 Factors influencing perineal wound healing at 6 months in ulcerative colitis.

Factor	*Unhealed (%)*	*Factor*	*Unhealed (%)*
Open wound*	43	Primary closure	11
Male	24	Female	21
Age <30 years*	36	Age >30 years	21
Symptoms <3 years	32	Symptoms >3 years	21
Steroids	21	No steroids	25
Two-stage proctectomy*	30	One-stage proctectomy	16
Severe residual proctitis*	34	Minimal proctitis	18
Perineal disease*	44	No perineal disease	24

* Significant differences.
From Oakley et al (1985).

PERSISTENT PERINEAL SINUS

Aetiology

A perineal sinus usually persists because there is a rigid cavity which is narrow at the pelvic floor, preventing adequate drainage (Watts et al, 1966; Silen and Glotzer, 1974; Shaw and Futrell, 1978; Cohen and Ryan, 1979) (Figure 10.8).

This rigid cavity is formed above by pelvic peritoneum, in which lie the omentum and the small bowel. Laterally and posteriorly lie the ischium, coccyx and sacrum and the remains of the levator ani. The urogenital structures lie anteriorly: in the female the vagina, cervix and uterus, and in the male the seminal vesicles, prostate and bladder. Some sinuses can be long, tracking behind the pelvic peritoneum in front of the sacrum, but they usually stop if they are blind tracks at the level of S3. Occasionally, a perineal sinus may persist because there is a communication with the small intestine, the vagina, the urethra or the bladder. Enteroperineal fistulas may be extremely small and difficult to demonstrate radiographically.

Other causes of persistent sinus include recurrent malignancy, tuberculosis, retained rectal mucosa, a foreign body, hidradenitis suppurativa, granulomas or a pilonidal sinus. In Birmingham we found a cause for persistent sinus in six of eight patients after operation for ulcerative colitis, and in 12 of 13 of those with Crohn's disease (Table 10.11).

Table 10.11 Causes of persistent perineal sinus in unhealed wounds: 1973–1986.

Cause	*Ulcerative colitis (n = 8)*	*Crohn's disease (n = 13)*
Sutures (non-absorbed)	1	0
Malignancy	1	1
Urethral fistula	0	1
Vesical fistula	0	1
Enteric fistula	0	2
Retained rectal mucosa	0	2
Granuloma	0	2
Vaginal fistula	1	1
Hidradenitis suppurativa	1	1
Pilonidal sinus	2	1

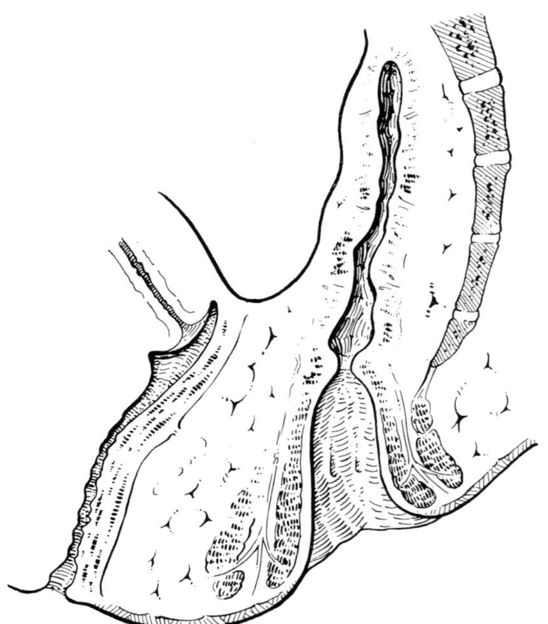

Figure 10.8 Typical anatomy of a perineal sinus. There is a persistent discharging sinus at the site of the previous anal sphincters, with a narrowed component, usually at the level of the pelvic floor, above which there is a presacral cavity of variable dimensions.

A persistent perineal sinus occasionally presents a long time after the original operation. Lubbers (1982) reported that in some of his patients the perineum had remained healed for many years and then intermittently discharged, with long periods of healing between episodes of drainage. Late discharge after initial complete perineal wound healing was reported in eight patients by Smith et al (1978). We believe that late discharge after previous long-term healing is highly suggestive of Crohn's disease or recurrent malignancy. The majority of persistent perineal sinuses occur in patients with inflammatory bowel disease, not malignancy (Hurwitz, 1980; Se-min Baek et al, 1981; Kasper, 1984).

Incidence

After abdominoperineal excision for malignancy

The incidence of unhealed perineal wounds 6 months after abdominoperineal excision for malignancy ranges from nil to 16% (Broader et al, 1974; Irvin and Goligher, 1975; Eftaiha and Abcarian, 1978; Alpsan et al, 1980; Baudot et al, 1980); however, most of these wounds were healed at 12 months (Marks et al, 1976; Eftaiha and Abcarian, 1978; Lubbers, 1982; Manjoney et al, 1983; Lieberman and Feldman, 1984). If a sinus persists, recurrent malignancy should be excluded by CT or

MRI imaging, biopsy or fine needle aspiration cytology.

After proctocolectomy for ulcerative colitis

Unhealed perineal wounds are recorded 6 months after proctocolectomy in 0–58% of patients (Watts et al, 1966; Strahan et al, 1967; Jalan et al, 1969; Hulten et al, 1971; Irvin and Goligher, 1975; Corman et al, 1978; Baudot et al, 1980; Lubbers, 1982; Oakley et al, 1985). Unlike malignancy, not all perineal wounds are healed at 1 year. In fact, Oakley et al (1985) reported that 18% of their 326 patients had an unhealed perineal wound 1 year after operation; furthermore 35 of these 59 patients underwent a secondary surgical procedure in order to try to achieve healing.

Corman et al (1978) reported a very similar experience: 50% of wounds being healed at a year, 76% by 18 months, and only 13% requiring re-operations in an attempt to achieve healing.

After rectal excision for Crohn's disease

The incidence of unhealed perineal wounds in Crohn's disease ranges from 22% to 72% (Irvin and Goligher, 1975; Corman et al, 1978; Baudot et al, 1980; Lubbers, 1982; Scammell and Keighley, 1986). As in ulcerative colitis, there is a slow decline in the incidence with time. At 1 year, only 21 of our patients (18%) had perineal wounds which remained unhealed and, of these, 11 eventually resolved, leaving only 9% with a persistent sinus. Corman reports healing rates at 12 and 18 months of 38% and 52% respectively, but in their experience only 66% eventually achieved healing.

Crohn's disease is associated with a much higher incidence of persistent sinus than ulcerative colitis, and these persistent sinuses are much more difficult to resolve by re-operations (Jalan et al, 1969; Silen and Glotzer, 1974; Warshaw et al, 1977; Corman et al, 1978; Ferrari and DenBesten, 1980). One reason for the higher incidence in Crohn's disease is the presence of anorectal sepsis at proctectomy. Lesions particularly associated with persistent sinus are rectal stricture, high fistula-in-ano, rectovaginal fistula and perirectal abscess (Ritchie and Lockhart-Mummery, 1973; Kasper, 1984).

Clinical features

A persistent perineal sinus causes an intermittent purulent discharge, often associated with perineal discomfort. Pain may be prominent if the cavity is full of mucopus and is relieved by spontaneous discharge. There may be vaginal symptoms if there is a communication with the vagina, resulting in menstrual loss and a chronic vaginal discharge between menstruation. Frequently there are urinary symptoms. The skin around the sinus becomes excoriated and the perineum becomes moist. Secondary infection from yeasts or low-grade pathogens is common. Most patients wear perineal pads which require repeated changing. Underclothes become soiled and personal hygiene is compromised. Some patients irrigate the cavity with an antiseptic solution through a fine catheter to control the accumulation of pus in the cavity. A persistent sinus may cause dyspareunia, and reduced libido if there is chronic sepsis. Some patients develop chronic perineal pain.

Radiological appearances

Perineal sinograms may be used to evaluate the length and extent of the sinus (Figure 10.9a,b). There is usually a rather narrow opening on the skin, leading to a wide granuating cavity below the pelvic floor measuring about 5 cm in length and having a capacity of about 10 mL. The sinus is often strictured at the level of the pelvic floor, beyond which a cavity usually extends to about 12 cm from the perineal skin and lies immediately in front of the sacrum. Perineal sinuses rarely extend above the sacral promontory. There may be a communication with the vagina but, if so, it is usually low.

Fistulous communication with the small bowel may be difficult to demonstrate unless contrast can be injected under pressure. Unfortunately, this procedure is not only painful but is frequently complicated by an episode of bacteraemia. Contrast examination of the small bowel by retrograde ileogram or a barium follow-through may occasionally demonstrate a small enteroperineal fistula. Fistulas to the bladder and the urethra are more frequently demonstrated by perineal sinogram than by intravenous urogram or by cystourethroscopy.

Histology

Most perineal sinus tracks are lined by granulation tissue. It is important, however, to biopsy the sinus in an attempt to exclude malignancy, tuberculosis, active Crohn's disease, or giant cell granulomas that may be due to a foreign body.

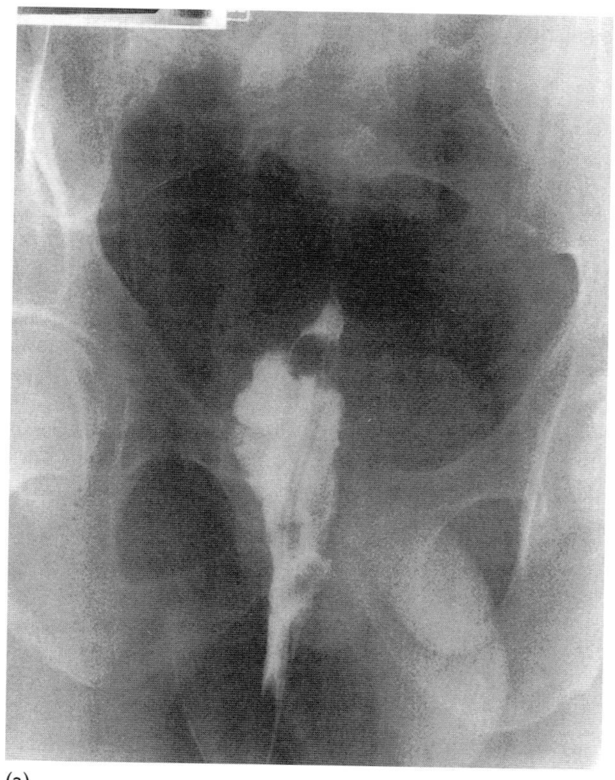
(a)

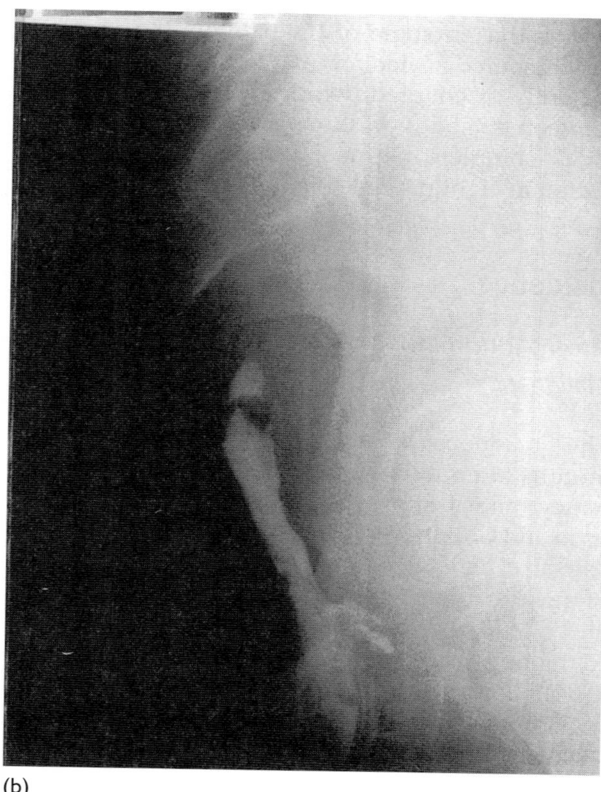
(b)

Figure 10.9 Perineal sinogram. (a) Anteroposterior radiograph demonstrating a large cavity extending to the level of the midsacrum. (b) Lateral radiograph showing an extensive presacral cavity.

Differential diagnosis

Tuberculosis, malignancy, Crohn's disease, pilonidal sinus, hidradenitis and the presence of a foreign body must be considered in the differential diagnosis. There are other disorders which might be responsible for pain, such as sarcoid, herpes zoster, prostatitis, neuroma of a branch of the perineal or pudendal nerve, urinary tract infection or trauma.

PREVENTION OF PERINEAL WOUNDS

In view of the morbidity associated with an unhealed wound, particularly in Crohn's disease, there may be some merit in avoiding distal proctectomy altogether. The rectal stump may be closed by staples in the anal canal at the pelvic floor or in the lower third of the rectum, leaving the levator ani, sphincters and anal canal and a variable length of rectum intact (Figure 10.10a–c). The morbidity of the operation is thought to be generally less than that of a proctocolectomy, particularly if the latter is complicated by a perineal sinus. The retained anorectum is claimed to give rise to very few symptoms, but if it does continue to cause problems it can be excised as a perineal procedure at a later stage.

We recently analysed the results of conservative proctectomy with retention of the anal canal and sphincters. Somewhat to our surprise we found at that time the procedure was associated with a high morbidity, especially in Crohn's disease, because pelvic abscess frequently occurred and drainage was poor because of the retained innervated anal sphincters (Winslet et al, 1990). The St Mark's group came to the same conclusion (Talbot et al, 1989). Since this small series was published we have found that in some people the results were satisfactory; we have therefore adopted a selective approach but warn patients that, while a conservative proctectomy will protect from the problems of a perineal wound, pelvic sepsis and discharge from the anal stump may occur – and if it does, a perineal proctectomy will be

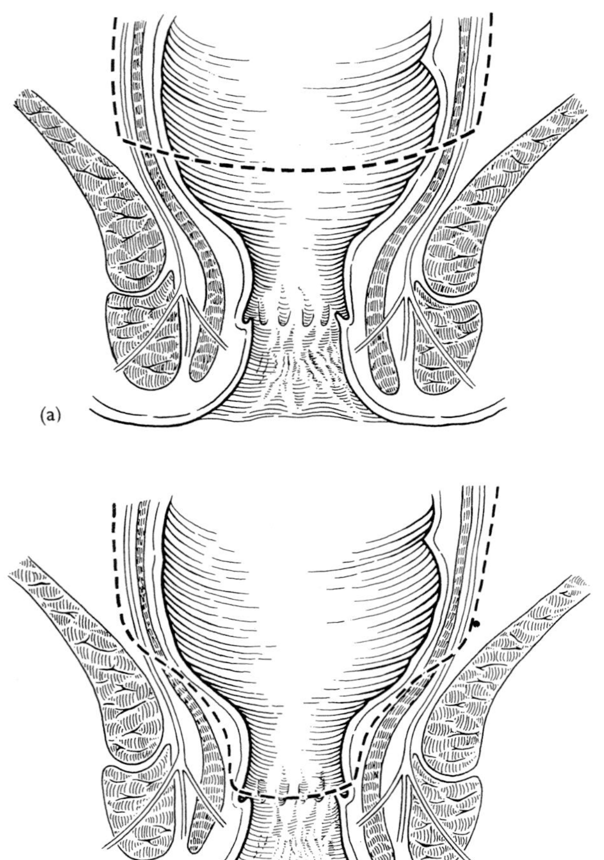

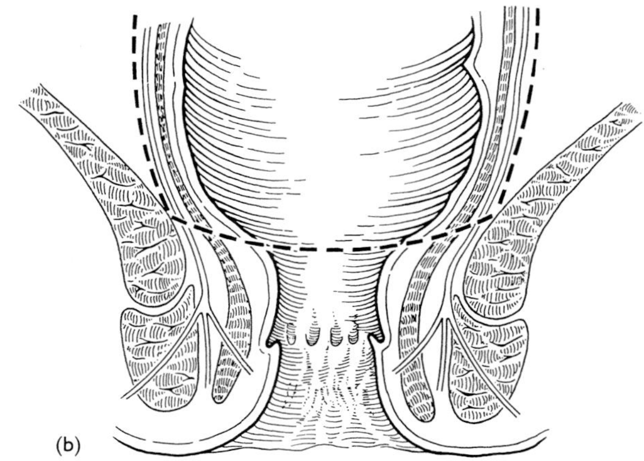

Figure 10.10a–c Conservative proctectomy with or without mucosectomy. (a) The rectum is oversewn just above the levator ani leaving the anal canal and the lower 2 cm of rectum intact. (b) A more radical form of conservative proctectomy, in which the rectum is transected within the levator ani at the top of the anal column. (c) Conservative proctectomy with anal mucosectomy. Here the rectum is removed at the level of the levator ani and the mucosa of the anorectum is also removed in continuity down to the dentate line.

necessary. In ulcerative colitis, conservative proctocolectomy gives much better results and we prefer, where possible, to preserve the sphincters and the anal canal so that there is no perineal wound.

We and others have also been attracted to doing even less than conservative proctocolectomy, particularly in Crohn's patients with complex anorectal sepsis, fistulas and stricture. Some of these patients, usually adolescents or patients who have not yet come to terms with a proctocolectomy, have been offered a proximal loop ileostomy, leaving the colon and the rectum intact (Winslet et al, 1987). We prefer a loop ileostomy to the split ileostomy advocated by the Oxford group (Harper et al, 1983) (see Chapter 58). A loop ileostomy has been shown to defunction the bowel efficiently (Williams et al, 1986; Winslet et al, 1991), the procedure can be performed without a laparotomy, or if desired laparoscopically, a laparotomy is not required for the ileostomy closure, and a stapling technique can be used under sedation without a general anaesthetic if the stoma retracts. Construction of a loop ileostomy in Crohn's disease has been associated with an immediate 76% remission rate and a sustained remission in 70%, as evidenced by a fall in erythrocyte sedimentation rate (ESR), a rise in serum albumin and a fall in acute-phase proteins. Patients gained weight and their general health improved, but after a variable follow-up some patients developed symptoms from defunctioned proctitis or disease relapse (see Chapter 57). Restoration of intestinal continuity was achieved in only 14%. Over a third (39%) of the patients have now undergone proctectomy, but there are still a group of patients (47%) with a loop ileostomy with bad rectal disease who remain in remission and who do not wish to consider ablative surgery. This is particularly true of patients with rectal strictures and those with complex anorectal fistulas in whom rectal excision might result in pelvic nerve damage and a persistent perineal sinus (Keighley and Allan, 1988; Linares et al, 1988). A recent analysis of faecal diversion alone for Crohn's disease has indicated that 23% required no further operation and a further 23% achieved a remission for more than 2 years.

TREATMENT OF PERSISTENT PERINEAL SINUS

Overview of outcome in the author's experience

When we took a snapshot of persistent perineal sinus we found that the only cases which occurred in rectal cancer were associated with recurrent malignancy. Furthermore, failure of perineal healing 18 months after rectal excision for inflammatory bowel disease invariably indicated unrecognized or overt Crohn's disease. We found that the outcome of surgery for persistent sinus in Crohn's disease was a very dismal story: 21 patients had had 56 operations (mean of 2.5 per patient), but only 4 patients (19%) were cured of their perineal sinus by operation. Gracilis transposition achieved healing in 2 of 3 cases and rectus abdominis myocutaneous flap in only 2 of 4 cases. We have had some recent spectacular results with omentoplasty.

Conservative management

Spontaneous healing can occur in about half of all patients who still have an unhealed wound 12 months after rectal excision if the diagnosis is ulcerative colitis (Corman et al, 1978; Lubbers, 1982; Scammell and Keighley, 1986). Indeed, provided the underlying diagnosis is malignancy or ulcerative colitis, almost all persistently discharging wounds will have healed in 18–24 months. Even in Crohn's disease, some perineal sinuses can heal spontaneously up to a year after proctocolectomy. Since the results of secondary procedures are so disappointing and morbidity is considerable, every encouragement should be given to persist with simple non-invasive therapy for at least 2–3 years.

We believe that it is usually worthwhile to examine the sinus under anaesthesia, define its exact position and to dilate any strictures present so that an irrigation catheter can be passed to the apex of the cavity. In this way pus can be sampled for culture, and appropriate antibiotics prescribed if systemic sepsis develops. If the patient can be instructed to pass a catheter daily to the apex of the cavity so that it can be thoroughly irrigated by antiseptic solution, there is at least a chance of reducing the amount of purulent discharge; furthermore, the risk of restricturing is minimized.

A short course of metronidazole is said to be helpful in reducing the volume of discharge in patients with Crohn's disease and a chronically infected perineal sinus (Bernstein et al, 1980), but we have been disappointed with oral metronidazole therapy for this condition. Even a small dose of steroids might be worth considering, particularly if biopsies from the sinus show that there are non-caseating giant cell granulomas. Some claim that azathioprine or 6-mercaptopurine may achieve healing and may reduce sepsis in patients with granulomas in the sinus tract (Korelitz and Present, 1985; Markowitz et al, 1990).

Curettage

In our experience, results of treatment by curettage are poor; if healing does occur it often takes a long time. Nevertheless, Lubbers (1982) reported healing in 3 of 9 patients who underwent curettage, and Oakley et al (1985) achieved healing in 8 of 16 patients similarly treated. Corman and others (1978), who were more persistent than some, stated that all patients with ulcerative colitis and 10 of 11 patients with Crohn's disease achieved healing but that curettage had to be repeated on three or four occasions in each patient.

Excision and primary closure

Wide excision (Figures 10.11 and 10.12) and primary closure, even when performed over closed suction drains (Figure 10.13), is usually unsuccessful because the defect cannot be closed and the dead space becomes infected (Campos et al, 1992). All of the fibrous track must be removed and this may be technically very difficult in high presacral cavities. It is sometimes necessary to excise the coccyx and the lower two sacral bodies to ensure wide excision of all fibrous tissue. If the defect cannot be closed by suture over suction drains, it may be filled with a muscle (Figure 10.14) or a myocutaneous flap (Leahy and Peel, 1984), or it may be marsupialized (Silen and Glotzer, 1974).

Excision and primary closure achieved healing in all five patients reported by Lubbers (1982), and in two of three patients in the Cleveland Clinic series (Oakley et al, 1985). Ferrari and DenBesten (1980) report healing in six of seven patients, but in our group of Crohn's patients, excision and primary suture was successful in only three of 17 patients (Scammell and Keighley, 1986).

Excision and primary suture may be used for vaginoperineal fistula, particularly as it is sometimes the case that the perineal component is not particularly high. The entire perineal sinus should be excised and the defect in the vagina closed or

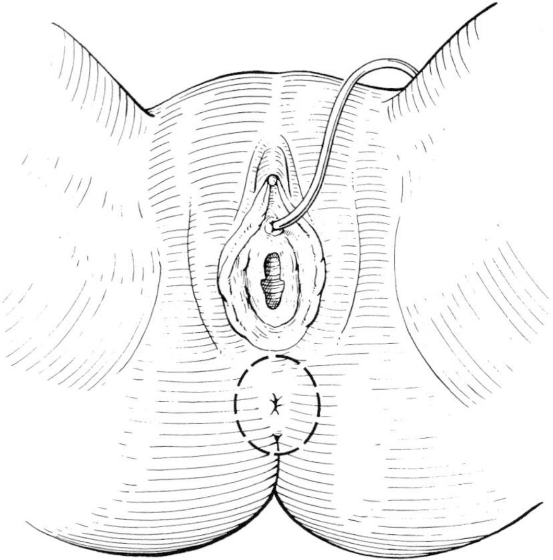

Figure 10.11 Incision used for excision of a persistent perineal sinus. A wide disc of skin is excised outside the sphincters in order to achieve adequate exposure and satisfactory drainage.

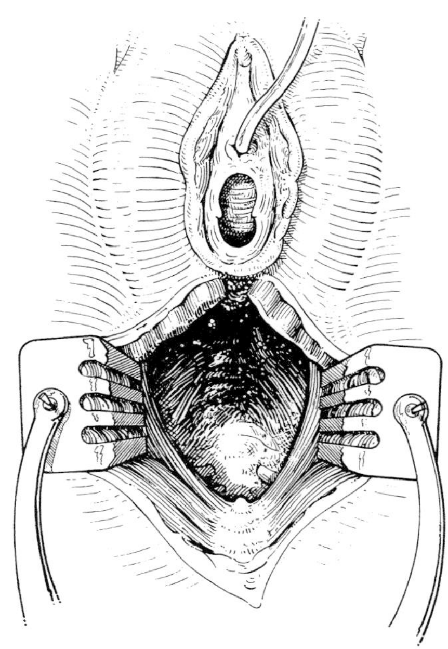

Figure 10.12 Completion of an excised perineal sinus. There is a large cavity above the levators which cannot usually be obliterated by sutures.

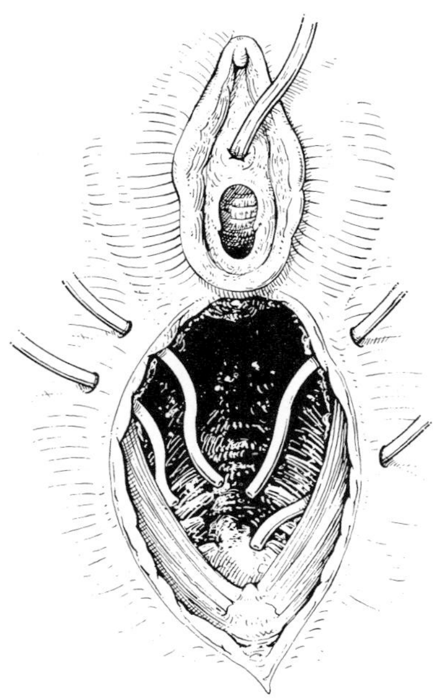

Figure 10.13 An attempt may be made to close the dead space over closed suction drains, but this is only applicable to small cavities.

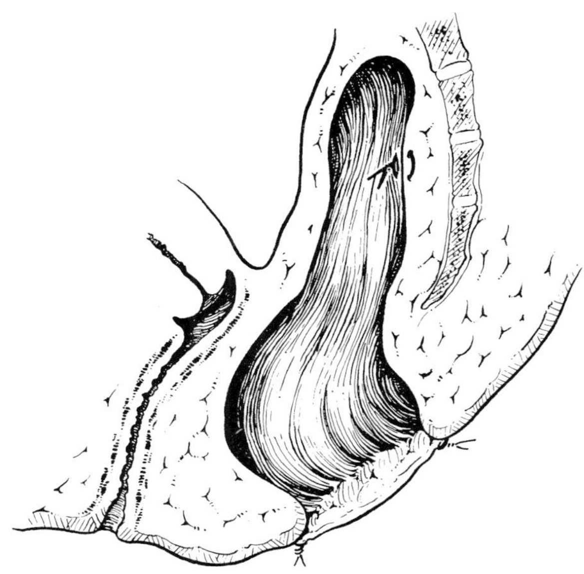

Figure 10.14 In many instances the cavity which remains after excision of a persistent perineal sinus must be filled in order to prevent the collection of serous exudate or blood, which may become infected. In this instance the cavity is filled with a pedicle muscle graft.

preferably excised and reconstructed as a vaginal advancement flap (Figure 10.15a,b). A wide vaginal flap is cut and only undermined enough to bring the upper edge down to the lower limit of the excision without being under tension.

Fibrin adhesive

A dual-component fibrin seal is available to provide a fibrin plug through which fibroblastic activity and collagen synthesis can proceed, allowing fibrous

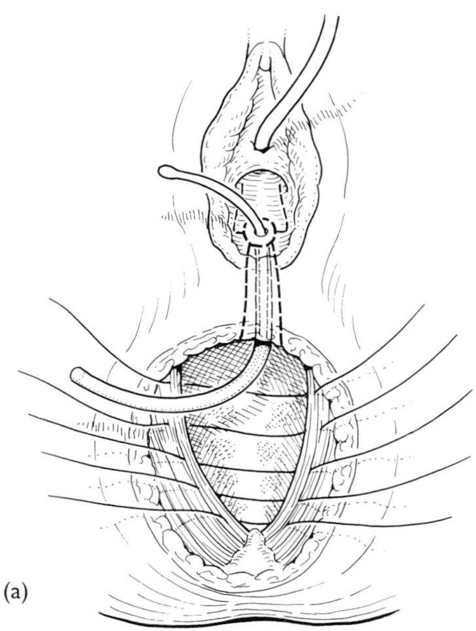

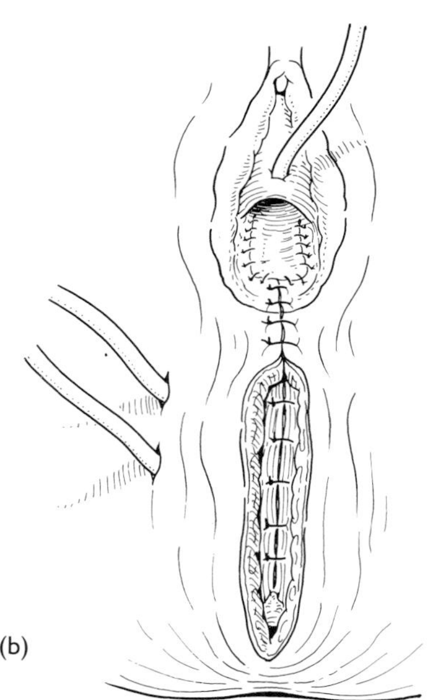

Figure 10.15a–b (a) Repair of a vaginoperineal fistula involves raising a vaginal flap, excising the sinus, repairing the levator where possible, and closing the vaginal orifice with a vaginal flap. (b) The skin is closed over suction drains.

tissue to develop and obliterate a cavity which is resistant to healing by granulation tissue. One component of the sealant consists of concentrated fibrinogen, factor XIII and plasma proteins. The second component, which acts as a hardener, is a solution of thrombin and calcium chloride. When the two components are mixed, coagulation is initiated and within 15–60 minutes a rigid fibrin clot develops. Aprotinin is added to the system in order to prevent early fibrinolytic degradation (Bruhn et al, 1980; Stanek et al, 1980; Turowiski et al, 1980). Kirkegaard and Madsen (1983) treated ten patients with a persistent perineal sinus using the product Tisseel (Immuno Ltd). In most patients the sinus was pretreated by irrigation with aprotinin or tranexamic acid and antibiotic solution. (The two components are applied using a double syringe so that they can be mixed and applied simultaneously. The sinus should be gently dilated beforehand since the solution must reach the apex of the sinus. The syringe is slowly withdrawn during injection so that the sinus is completely filled. The patient should remain in the knee–elbow position until the clot has developed.)

Kirkegaard and Madsen (1983) reported that in two patients this form of therapy was unsuccessful: one had a large cavity, the other had a fistula into the vagina. In the remaining eight patients, the sinus healed immediately in six and after a second application in two. Unfortunately the follow-up of these patients was very short. In Birmingham we used this method of treatment in 13 patients. In two, the application was complicated by an entero-perineal fistula. Nine patients achieved spectacular early healing but in four of them the sinus recurred after 3 months, leaving only five which healed completely. In six patients (46%) treatment was unsuccessful (Ambrose and Alexander-Williams, 1988). We no longer use this form of treatment

Skin grafting

Skin grafting has been used in an attempt to achieve healing after excision of a perineal sinus (Seckel et al, 1985). Anderson and Turnbull (1976) used a combination of wide local saucerization, skin grafting and treatment with adrenocorticotrophic hormone (ACTH) over 2–3 months; however, in their series of 48 patients complete healing was achieved in only seven. In our view, this approach is feasible only in patients with a very superficial sinus with a small cavity. Most perineal sinuses are long and deep, hence some method of filling the dead space is needed (Oakley et al, 1985). Skin grafting may be required if the skin of a myocutaneous flap becomes ischaemic while the muscle remains viable. Sometimes full-thickness cover can be achieved for wide skin defects using V–Y flaps (Marti et al, 1994) (Figure 10.16a–c).

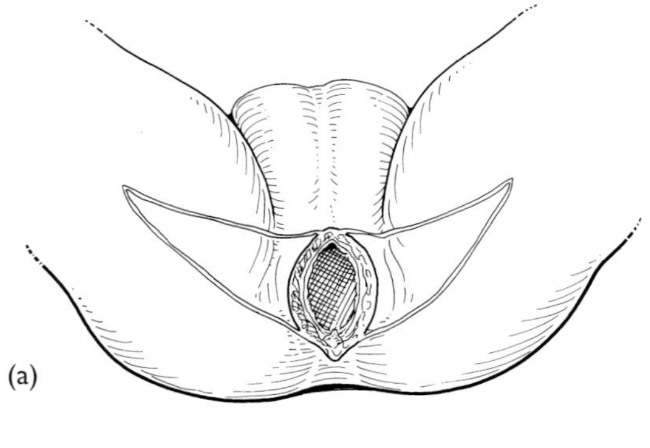

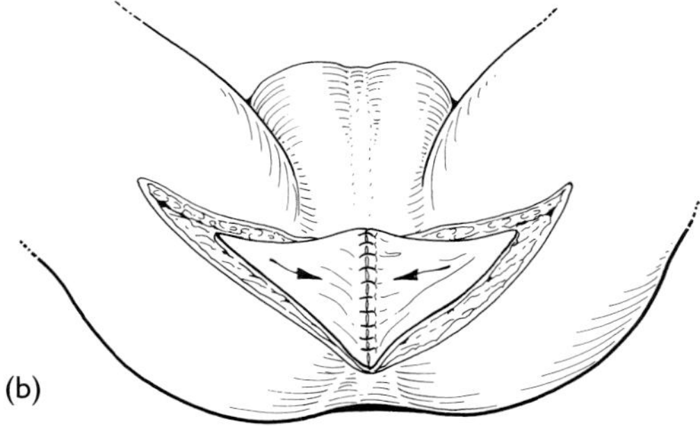

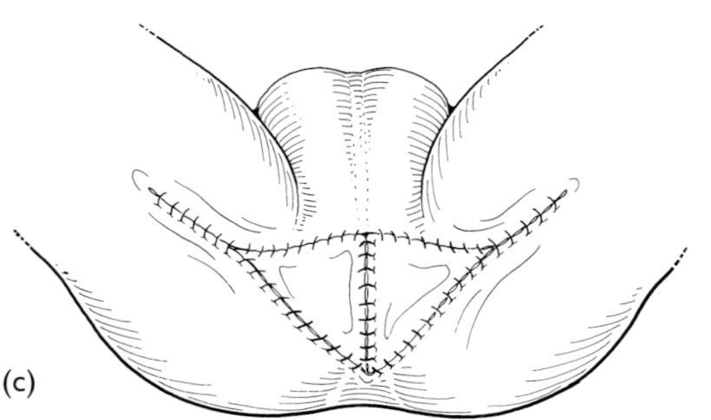

Figure 10.16a–c V–Y flaps may be used to achieve primary skin healing after excision of a persistent perineal sinus. (a) Two large triangular flaps are marked, extending to the inner aspects of the thighs. (b) The skin, subcutaneous fat and deep fascia are incised. The flaps are mobilized 4–6 cm medially on each side. (c) Closure.

Muscle and myocutaneous flaps

A variety of muscle transposition procedures have been advocated for the treatment of a persistent perineal sinus. The procedure may be performed synchronously with wide excision of the sinus as already described, usually removing the coccyx and lower sacrum, or a few days after excision when healthy granulation tissue lines the cavity. The gracilis muscle with or without adjacent skin, or the rectus abdominis, are the ones most widely used for myocutaneous flaps.

Gracilis transposition

The gracilis muscle is frequently used as a pedicle graft for filling the cavity created after excising a long perineal sinus (Baek et al, 1981; Labanter, 1980). Usually, however, the muscle alone is used, without overlying skin, since the blood supply to the latter is precarious and it may easily be sheared. Furthermore, the donor site may be difficult to close (Mathes and Mahai, 1982). Nevertheless Solomon et al (1996) reported successful gracilis myocutaneous flap reconstruction for five patients with a persistent sinus for recurrent perineal malignancy.

The operation must be performed in the Lloyd-Davies position. An island of skin can be raised from the thigh immediately superficial to the gracilis muscle (Figure 10.17). In practice it is sometimes difficult to secure the skin island to the muscle when the gracilis is divided distally, rotated and delivered through the subcutaneous tunnel to the perineal

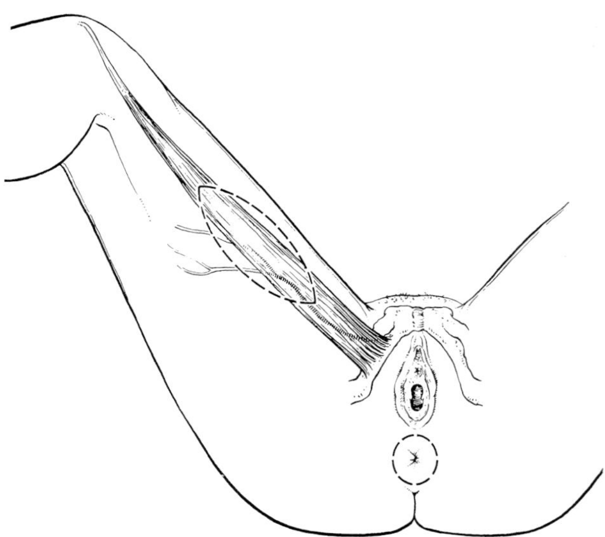

Figure 10.17 A gracilis myocutaneous flap may be used to fill the defect and to achieve primary closure of the skin defect.

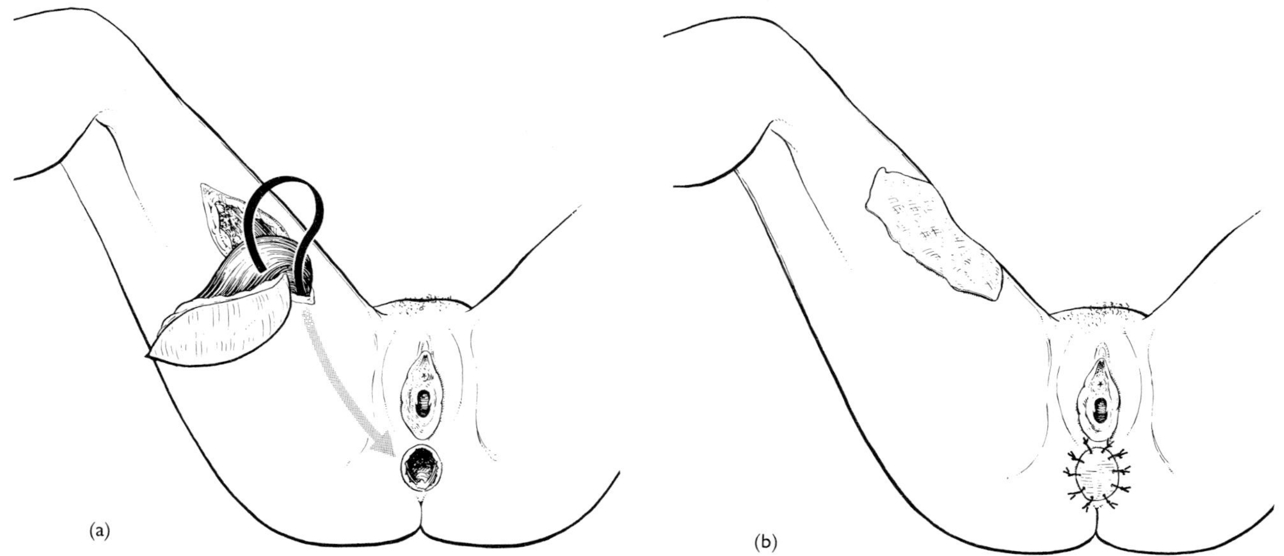

Figure 10.18a–b Rerouting of the gracilis as a myocutaneous flap. (a) The gracilis muscle has been mobilized distal to its neurovascular pedicle and an ellipse of overlying skin has been raised with the underlying muscle. The distal end of the gracilis is divided and the myocutaneous flap is delivered to the perineum through a subcutaneous tunnel. (b) Completion of the myocutaneous flap by skin sutures and closure of the skin defect in the thigh by a skin graft.

sinus (Bartholdson and Hulten, 1975; Se-min Baek et al, 1981) (Figure 10.18a,b). The technique has been successfully applied to radiation fistulas and used as a method of covering other urogenital defects (Inglemann-Sundberg, 1960; Graham, 1965; Orticochea, 1972; McGraw et al, 1976).

Cohen and Ryan (1979) reported complete healing in three patients, but a later report (Ryan, 1984) paints a less enthusiastic picture, with primary healing being achieved in only 3 of 15 patients and delayed healing being reported in nine patients. In none of Ryan's series was it possible to use adjacent skin. By contrast, Ward et al (1982) reported a completely successful outcome in two patients with Crohn's disease and a vaginoperineal fistula treated by myocutaneous flap. We have used the gracilis muscle alone to fill the dead space in the perineum after excising a perineal sinus and have found it to be a useful method of dealing with post-irradiation perineal sinuses. However, patients should be warned about the long and potentially painful thigh incision with the risk of some sensory loss. To avoid the relatively avascular gracilis tendon being used, we try to take only the proximal muscular part of the gracilis through a short incision, dividing the tendon well proximal to the knee. Damage to the saphenous nerve or its branches should be avoided.

Gluteal flaps

The inferior gluteal artery and posterior cutaneous nerve of the thigh supply the inferior portion of gluteus maximus and the skin of the posterior thigh (Figure 10.19a,b). Excision of the lower aspect of the gluteus maximus results in no functional deficit; the donor site can be closed primarily and the muscle is sufficiently bulky to fill the cavity (Shaw and Futrell, 1978; Hurwitz et al, 1980; Achauer et al, 1983).

Hurwitz and Zwiebel (1985) reported results in five patients using two flaps, one of which was de-epithelialized to fill the apex of the cavity; the second was laid superficially to close the skin defect. Primary healing was recorded in four patients. The operation is best performed in the prone jack-knife position (Maruyama et al, 1980). We have no experience of using the gluteus for filling a perineal defect.

Rectus abdominis flaps

The rectus abdominis flap and an ellipse of skin overlying the upper fibres of the muscle based on the inferior epigastric artery provide an excellent method of closing a large perineal defect (Figure 10.20a–d). The rectus abdominis myocutaneous flap may be used at the time of abdominoperineal excision for a large neoplasm, when extensive perineal excision is needed in Crohn's disease, or when the combined approach is used to excise a large perineal sinus in Crohn's disease or after radiotherapy (Shukla and Hughes, 1984; Erdmann and Waterhouse, 1995). However, this is a much more extensive procedure than a perineal approach alone.

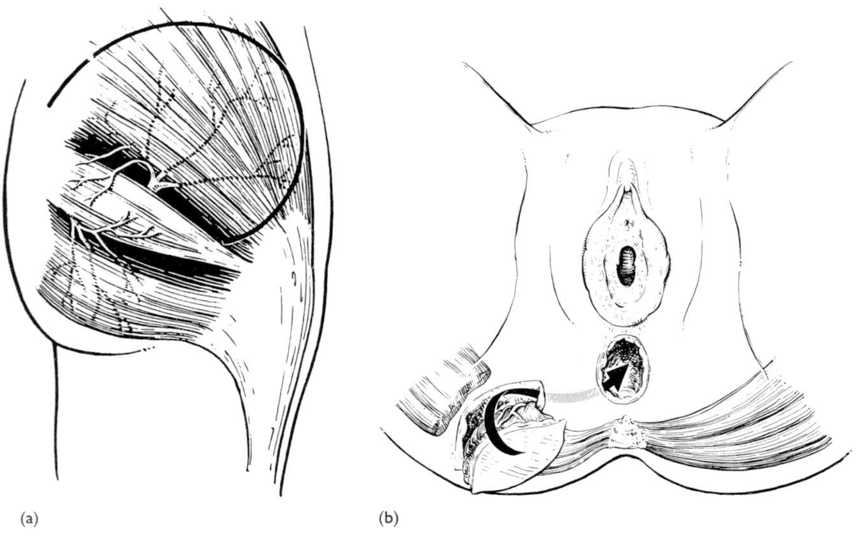

Figure 10.19a–b Gluteal myocutaneous flap. (a) The blood supply and innervation of the gluteus is shown together with the skin incision used for a gluteal flap. (b) The myocutaneous gluteus flap is being delivered to the perineum using a subcutaneous tunnel prior to direct primary skin closure.
(The operation is much easier in the prone jack-knife position: not shown.)

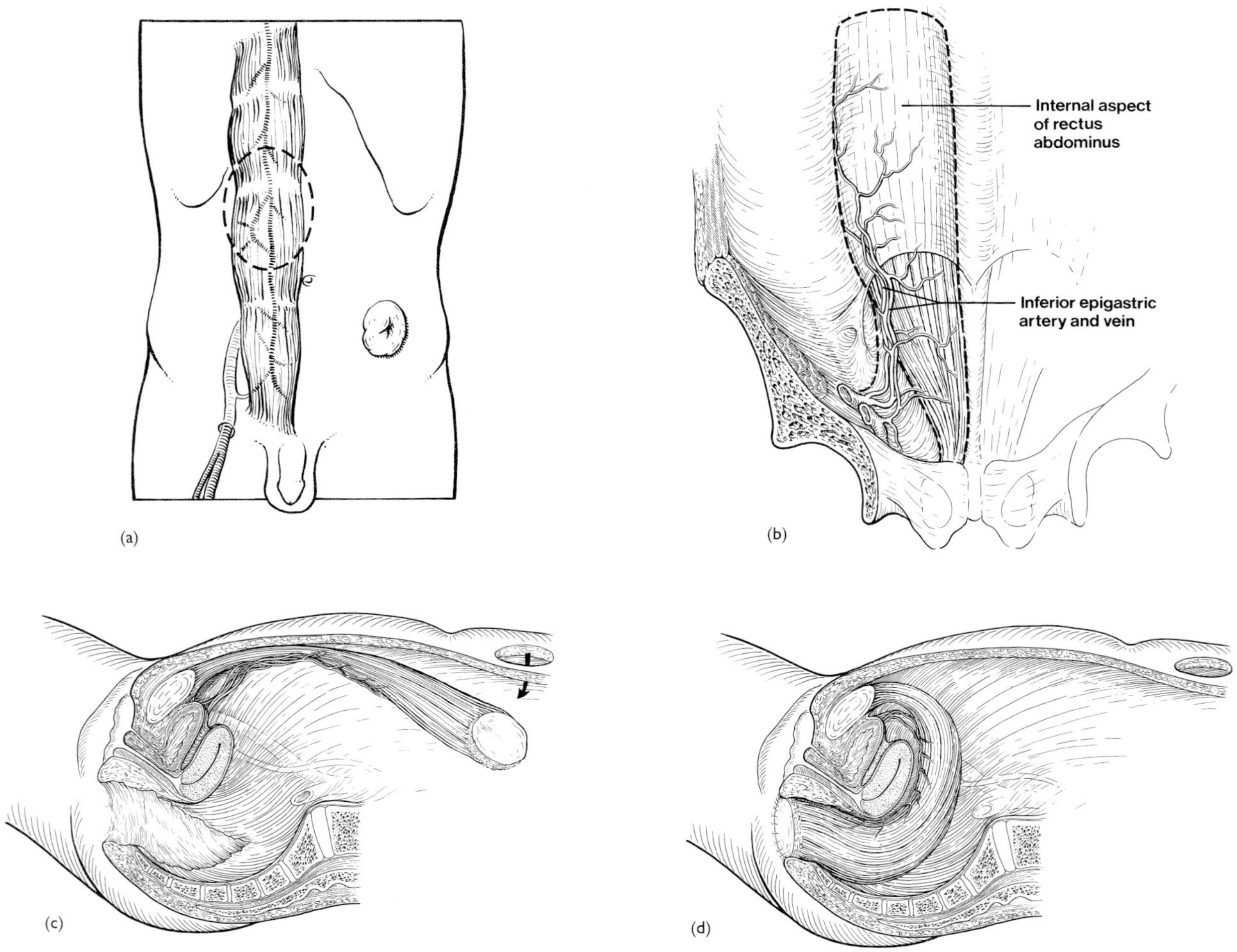

Internal aspect of rectus abdominus

Inferior epigastric artery and vein

(a) (b)

(c) (d)

Figure 10.20a–d Rectus abdominis myocutaneous flap. (a) A disc of skin is elevated on the rectus abdominis, which receives its blood supply via the inferior epigastric artery. (b) Detail of the blood supply to the rectus abdominis. (c) The myocutaneous flap has been cut on the rectus abdominis supplied by the inferior epigastric vessels. (d) The myocutaneous flap is now delivered through the pelvis, on to the perineum; the wound is then closed by primary suture, usually over redivac drains.

We have used this method of closing the pelvic and perineal defects after excising a persistent perineal sinus on a few occasions. Others have now also reported a successful outcome with the rectus flap (Young et al, 1988; Roe and Mortensen, 1989; Skene et al, 1990; Brough and Schofield, 1991). Our results with this procedure are not completely successful. We recorded skin loss in two of seven cases and a persistent though much smaller sinus in three.

Other muscle flaps

The rectus femoris and biceps femoris muscles have been used, but as they serve important locomotor functions they are no longer advocated for closure of a large perineal defect (Hurwitz, 1980; Mathes and Mahai, 1982). The same argument applies to the semimembranosus when used to fill a perineal defect. However, Mann and Springhall (1986) reported five cases where complete healing was achieved by distal division of the semimembranosus rerouted into the perineum without any apparent locomotor deficit. The muscle is more bulky than the gracilis but a myocutaneous flap is rarely feasible.

Closure of vaginoperineal fistula

A vaginoperineal fistula usually consists of a perineal sinus of variable length and a communication with the vagina. Treatment involves excision of the perineal sinus including its apex and either closing the perineum primarily with sutures over suction drains or filling a large defect with gracilis muscle. The communication with the vagina can then be excised and the defect closed with a vaginal advancement flap. If gracilis is rerouted to fill a defect, then the vaginal defect may heal without the need for a flap.

TECHNIQUE OF EXCISION AND ROTATION OF A MYOCUTANEOUS FLAP

General considerations

Position of the patient

The lithotomy position is preferable if a gracilis or semimembranosus flap is being used. The prone jack-knife position must be used for the gluteal flaps. Access to the abdomen and perineum is needed for the rectus abdominis myocutaneous reconstruction and omentoplasty.

Excision of the sinus

The perineal sinus should be excised as widely as possible so that there is no residual fibrous tissue (see Figure 10.12). It may be necessary to excise the coccyx and the lower two bodies of the sacrum, but this should only be used if it improves the prospect of completely excising the sinus. A head-light and a deep-bladed self-retaining retractor are essential. If the sinus is very long, a rectus flap is being used, or if omentoplasty is planned, a synchronous combined abdominoperineal excision is necessary. Long, curved Kocher retractors are invaluable and a suction diathermy unit is useful if bleeding is encountered near the apex of the cavity. Great care is needed when removing the most proximal aspect of the sinus to avoid damage to the small bowel, ureters, bladder, urethra, seminal vesicles or vagina. It is sometimes helpful to insert a probe into the full length of the sinus so that the apex can be felt during excision. Haemostasis should be meticulous after excision of the sinus. If this cannot be achieved, the cavity can be packed before proceeding with a delayed myocutaneous flap 5–7 days later (Leahy and Peel, 1984).

Specific myocutaneous flaps

Gracilis

An ellipse of skin 10 cm broad and 25 cm long is marked just posterior to a line joining the pubic tubercle and the semi-tendinosus tendon at the knee (see Figure 10.17). The skin ellipse is mobilized with the superficial fascia, the gracilis muscle is identified but not disturbed. The adductor longus is then identified medially and the fascia overlying it is divided, revealing the neurovascular pedicle as it emerges from the adductor longus, between the adductor brevis and magnus. The fascia over the adductor magnus is raised with the gracilis and overlying skin. In order to avoid separating the skin from the muscle, a few temporary sutures can be placed between them. The gracilis muscle is then divided at the distal end of the skin flap and the skin is cut, leaving the flap free, apart from its attachment to the neurovascular pedicle and the proximal gracilis muscle. The subcutaneous tissues between the leg wound and the perineum are opened to form a wide tunnel for the flap. The myocutaneous flap is then passed through the tunnel with great care so as to avoid shearing the skin and the vascular pedicle (see Figure 18.14a,b). The donor site can usually be closed over suction drainage. The flap is then sutured into position on the perineum over low-pressure suction drainage to keep any remaining dead space closed. If skin viability is doubtful, preservation of skin should be abandoned and the proximal portion of the gracilis used alone to close the perineal defect. If the perineal skin cannot be

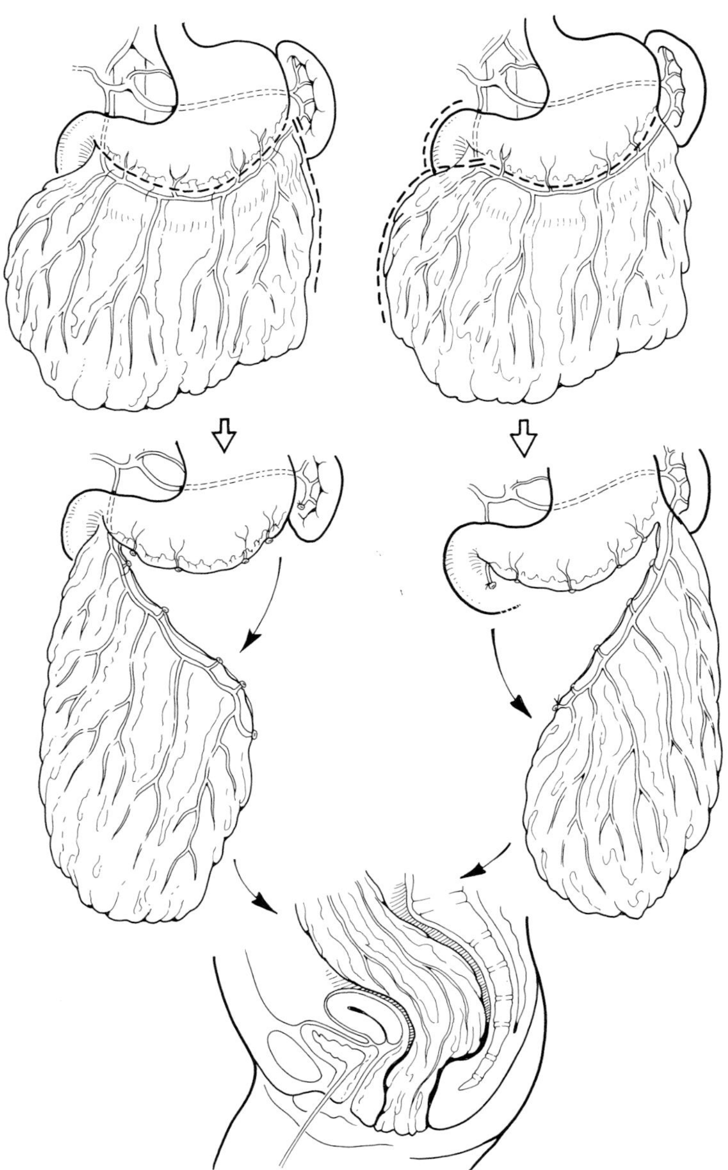

Figure 10.21 Excision and omentoplasty for persistent perineal sinus. This is particularly appropriate in Crohn's disease where the rectus muscle may already have been damaged because of multiple stoma sites. The omentum may be based on the right gastroepiploic artery, in which case the left gastroepiploic close to the short gastric vessels is divided and the left side of the omentum is mobilized in order to bring the apex down to the perineum. In some situations, better length may be obtained by basing the omentum on the left gastroepiploic artery and dividing the right gastroepiploic under the second part of the duodenum, particularly if omentum is adherent under the liver which can then be mobilized from that site to be delivered and on to the perineum.

used to provide skin cover, the area may be covered with Vaseline gauze to allow skin grafting later.

Gluteus maximus

The principle of the flap is that the skin of the lower gluteal region and posterior thigh with the gluteus maximus and tensor fascia lata are elevated as an axial flap based on the inferior gluteal artery (see Figure 10.19a) and with the posterior cutaneous nerve of the thigh to provide the flap with sensation. The flap can be elevated from the inferior border of the piriformis muscle to within 8 cm of the popliteal fossa.

Elevation of two flaps may be used, one with attached skin, the other as muscle alone. Dissection of the flaps commences distally with early identification and preservation of the posterior cutaneous nerve of the thigh on the undersurface of the fascia lata. With the myocutaneous component a narrow segment of the inferior and medial aspects of the gluteus maximus is included with the skin. The flap is elevated just proximal to the ischial tuberosity, leaving the cruciate anastomosis intact. A subcutaneous tunnel is dissected medial to the distal border of each gluteus maximus and extended through the ischiorectal space into the perineum (see Figure 10.19b). The flaps are drawn through each tunnel to fill the cavity so as to close the perineal wound. The muscle alone is placed in the apex of the cavity while the myocutaneous component is used to close the skin defect. A suture should be placed to secure the proximal flap as close to the apex of the cavity as possible. The wounds are then closed over suction drains.

Rectus abdominis

The rectus abdominis myocutaneous flap can be used only if one side of the abdominal wall can be excised with a viable muscle flap without a stoma nearby. In practice it can be used opposite the stoma provided the muscle on that side has not been damaged by repeated laparotomy or a stoma. The abdomen is opened and a synchronous combined excision of the rectum or the perineal sinus is completed. This process may be difficult and if so, it is wise to tape both ureters and the internal iliac vessels. Excision of the sinus leaves an extensive cavity in the pelvis and perineum and haemostasis must be meticulous. A disc of skin slightly larger than the perineal defect is cut over one or other rectus muscle 3–4 cm below the costal margin (Figure 10.20a). The subcutaneous tissue is divided with the skin to the rectus. The segment of rectus above the flap is divided, ligating the superior epigastric vessels (Figure 10.20b). The inferior epigastric vessels are then dissected free, dividing branches or tributaries which do not supply the inferior aspect of the rectus muscle. An adequate length of vascular pedicle is needed to rotate the skin disc and underlying muscle through the pelvis on to the perineum (Figure 10.20c). The defect in the rectus sheath is closed over suction drainage and the skin flap is sutured to the perineal skin over suction drainage with the muscle filling the dead space above (Figure 10.20d).

Omental grafts to fill a perineal sinus

In patients with a stoma it is preferable to avoid damaging the opposite rectus muscle for filling the defect after excision of the perineal sinus. Increasingly, therefore, we use omentum based on the left or right gastroepiploic arcade to fill the defect (Figure 10.21). The omentum is delivered through the pelvis on to the perineum. Redundant omentum can be excised a week later. We have achieved successful healing in five of six Crohn's perineal sinuses using this method.

Postoperative management and complications

Postoperative management

The patient is gradually mobilized after 3–4 days. The intravenous infusion is continued until the stoma is working satisfactorily. The drains may be removed as soon as the amount of fluid decreases to less than 10 mL a day and is no longer blood-stained. The sutures should remain *in situ* for 12–14 days.

Postoperative complications

Damage to the small bowel, bladder or ureter resulting in a fistula to the perineal wound are the most feared complications; however, they are remarkably rare. Bleeding may occur from presacral veins or radiation vasculitis. A haematoma may encourage sepsis, and we therefore advise leaving suction drains *in situ* until they are almost dry. We proceed to a two-stage operation if there is any doubt about the adequacy of haemostasis. Ischaemic necrosis of the skin should be identified early and the skin excised so that the viability of the underlying muscle is not jeopardized. If there are any signs of sepsis, sutures should be removed and adequate drainage established. If the skin has to be removed and the underlying muscle remains viable, later skin grafting is often successful if healing by secondary intention is unsatisfactory.

REFERENCES

Achauer BM, Turpin IM & Furnas DL (1983) Gluteal thigh flap in reconstruction of complex pelvic wounds. *Arch Surg* **118**: 18–22.

Alpsan K, Singh A & Ahmad A (1980) Clinical comparison of perineal wound management. *Dis Colon Rectum* **23**: 564–566.

Altemeier WA, Cuthbertson CR, Alexander JW, Suturins D & Bossert J (1974) Primary closure and healing of the perineal wound in abdominoperineal resection of the rectum for carcinoma. *Am J Surg* **127**: 215–219.

Ambrose NS & Alexander-Williams J (1988) Appraisal of a tissue glue in the treatment of persistent perineal sinus. *Br J Surg* **75**: 484–485.

Anderson R & Turnbull RB Jr (1976) Grafting the unhealed perineal wound after coloproctectomy for Crohn's disease. *Arch Surg* **111**: 335–338.

Aubrey DA, Morgan WP, Jenkins N & Harvey J (1984) Treatment of the perineal wound after proctectomy by intermittent irrigation. *Arch Surg* **119**: 1141–1144.

Baek S, Greenstein A, McElhinney J & Aufses AH (1981) The gracilis myocutaneous flap for persistent perineal sinus after proctocolectomy. *Surg Gynecol Obstet* **153**: 713–716.

Bartholdson L & Hulten L (1975) Repair of persistent perineal sinuses by means of a pedicle flap of muscular gracilis. *Scand J Plast Reconstr Surg* **9**: 74–76.

Baudot P, Keighley MRB & Alexander-Williams J (1980) Perineal wound healing after proctectomy for carcinoma and inflammatory disease. *Br J Surg* **67**: 275–276.

Bernstein LH, Frank MS, Brandt LJ & Boley SJ (1980) Healing of perineal Crohn's disease with metronidazole. *Gastroenterology* **79**: 357–365.

Broader JH, Lasselink BA, Oates GD & Alexander-Williams J (1974) Management of the pelvic space after proctectomy. *Br J Surg* **61**: 94–97.

Brough WA & Schofield PF (1991) The value of the rectus abdominis myocutaneous flap in the treatment of complex perineal fistula. *Dis Colon Rectum* **34**: 148–150.

Bruhn HD, Christophers E, Pohl J & Schoel G (1980) Regulation der Fibrobastenproliferation durch Fibrinogen/Fibrin, Fibronectin and Faktor XIII. In Schimpf K (ed.) *Fibrinogen, Fibrin and Fibrin Glue*, pp 217–226. Stuttgart: Schattauer.

Campos RR, Ayllon JG, Paricio PP et al (1992) Management of the perineal wound following abdominoperineal resection: prospective study of three methods. *Br J Surg* **79**: 29–31.

Cohen BE & Ryan JA (1979) Gracilis muscle flap for closure of the persistent perineal sinus. *Surg Gynecol Obstet* **148**: 33–35.

Corman ML, Veidenheimer MC, Collet JA & Ross VH (1978) Perineal wound healing after proctectomy for IBD. *Dis Colon Rectum* **21**: 155–159.

Crile G & Robert AD (1950) Primary closure of the posterior wound after combined abdominoperineal resection for cancer of the rectum. *Cleve Clin Q* **17**: 5–8.

Eftaiha M & Abcarian H (1978) Management of perineal wounds after proctocolectomy: a retrospective study of 50 cases in which treatment by the open technique was used. *Dis Colon Rectum* **21**: 287–291.

Elliot MS & Todd IP (1985) Primary suture of the perineal wound using constant suction and irrigation following rectal excision for IBD. *Ann R Coll Surg Engl* **67**: 6–7.

Erdmann MWH & Waterhouse N (1995) The transpelvic rectus abdominis flap: its use in the reconstruction of extensive perineal defects. *Ann R Coll Surg Engl* **77**: 229–232.

Ferrari BT & DenBesten L (1980) The prevention and treatment of the persistent perineal sinus. *World J Surg* **4**: 167–172.

Graham JB (1965) Vaginal fistulas following radiotherapy. *Surg Gynecol Obstet* **120**: 1019–1030.

Harper PH, Truelove SC, Lee ECG, Kettlewell MGW & Jewell DP (1983) Split ileostomy and ileocolostomy for Crohn's disease of the colon and ulcerative colitis: a 20-year survey. *Gut* **24**: 106–113.

Hulten L, Kewenter J, Knuttson U & Olbe L (1971) Primary closure of perineal wound after proctocolectomy or rectal incision. *Acta Chir Scand* **137**: 467–469.

Hurwitz DJ (1980) Closure of a large defect of the pelvic cavity by an extended compound myocutaneous flap based on the inferior gluteal artery. *Br J Plast Surg* **33**: 256–261.

Hurwitz DJ & Zwiebel PC (1985) Gluteal thigh flap repair of chronic perineal wounds. *Am J Surg* **150**: 386–391.

Hurwitz DJ, Swartz WM & Mathes SJ (1980) The gluteal thigh flap: a reliable sensate flap for the closure of buttock and perineal wounds. *Plast Reconstr Surg* **68**: 521–530.

Inglemann-Sundberg A (1960) Pathogenesis and operative treatment of urinary fistulas in irradiated tissue. In Youssef AF (ed.) *Gynecological Urology*, pp 263–279. Springfield, IL: CC Thomas.

Irvin TT & Goligher JC (1975) A controlled clinical trial of three different methods of perineal wound management following excision of the rectum. *Br J Surg* **62**: 287–291.

Irving AD & Lyall MH (1984) Perineal healing after panproctocolectomy for IBD. *J R Coll Surg Edinb* **29**: 313–315.

Jalan KN, Smith AN, Ruckley CV, Falconer CWA & Prescott RJ (1969) Perineal wound healing in ulcerative colitis. *Br J Surg* **56**: 749–753.

Johnston GW (1979) The results of vaginoplasty in excision of the rectum. *Br J Surg* **66**: 628–629.

Kasper R (1984) Persistent perineal sinus. *Surg Clin North Am* **64**: 761–768.

Keighley MRB & Allan RN (1988) Management of perianal Crohn's disease. *World J Surg* **12**: 198–202.

Keighley MRB & Burdon DW (1979) *Antimicrobial Prophylaxis in Surgery*. Tunbridge Wells: Pitman Medical.

Korelitz BI & Present DH (1985) Favourable effect of 6-mercaptopurine on fistula of Crohn's disease. *Dig Dis Sci* **30**: 58–64.

Kirkegaard P & Madsen PV (1983) Perineal sinus after removal of rectum: occlusion with fibrin adhesions. *Am J Surg* **145**: 791–794.

Kronberg O, Krahoft J, Backer O et al (1974) Early complications following operations for cancer of the rectum and anus. *Dis Colon Rectum* **17**: 741–749.

Labanter HP (1980) The gracilis muscle flap and musculocutaneous flap in the repair of perineal and ischial defects. *Br J Plast Surg* **33**: 95–98.

Leahy AL & Peel ALG (1984) A polythene pack for perineal wounds. *Br J Surg* **71**: 277.

Lees V & Everett WG (1991) Management of the chronic perineal sinus: not a problem to sit on. *Ann R Coll Surg Engl* **73**: 58–63.

Leicester RJ, Ritchie JK, Wadsworth J, Thompson JPS & Handley TR (1984) Sexual function and perineal wound healing after intersphincteric excision of the rectum for IBD. *Dis Colon Rectum* **27**: 244–248.

Lieberman RC & Feldman S (1984) Primary closure of the perineal wound with closed continuous transabdominal pelvic irrigation after rectal incision. *Dis Colon Rectum* **27**: 526–528.

Linares L, Moteira LF, Andrews H et al (1988) Natural history and treatment of anorectal strictures complicating Crohn's disease. *Br J Surg* **75**: 653–656.

Lubbers E-JC (1982) Healing of the perineal wound after proctectomy for non-malignant conditions. *Dis Colon Rectum* **25**: 351–357.

Macfie J & McMahon MJ (1980) The management of the open perineal wound using a foam elastomer dressing: a prospective clinical trial. *Br J Surg* **67**: 85–89.

McGraw JB, Massey FM, Shanklin KD et al (1976) Vaginal reconstructions with gracilis myocutaneous flaps. *Plast Reconstr Surg* **58**: 176–179.

Manjoney DL, Koplewitz MJ & Abrams JS (1983) Factors influencing perineal wound healing after proctectomy. *Am J Surg* **145**: 183–189.

Mann CV & Springhall R (1986) Use of a muscle graft for unhealed perineal sinus. *Br J Surg* **76**: 1000–1001.

Markowitz J, Rosa J, Grancher K et al (1990) Long-term 6-mercaptopurine treatment in adolescents with Crohn's diasease. *Gastroenterology* **99**: 1347–1351.

Marks CG, Leighton M, Ritchie JK & Hawley PR (1976) Primary suture of the perineal wound following rectal incision for adenocarcinoma. *Br J Surg* **63**: 322–326.

Marti M-C, Roche B & Gumener RG (1994) Skin cover of perineal defects using V–Y flaps. *Int J Colorect Dis* **9**: 163–164.

Maruyama Y, Nakajima H & Kodaira S (1980) Primary reconstruction of perineal defect with bilobed myocutaneous flap. *Br J Plast Surg* **33**: 440–447.

Mathes SJ & Mahai F (1982) *Clinical Application for Muscle and Musculocutaneous Flaps*. St Louis: CV Mosby.

Oakley JR, Fazio VW, Jagelman DG et al (1985) Management of the perineal wound after rectal incision for UC. *Dis Colon Rectum* **28**: 885–888.

Oates GD & Alexander-Williams J (1970) Primary closure of the perineal wound in excision of the rectum. *Proc R Soc Med* (Suppl) **63**: 128.

Orticochea M (1972) The musculocutaneous flap method: an intermediate and heroic substitute for the method of delay. *Br J Plast Surg* **25**: 106–110.

Ritchie JK & Lockhart-Mummery HE (1973) Non-restorative surgery in the treatment of Crohn's disease of the large bowel. *Gut* **14**: 263–269.

Roe AM & Mortensen NJMcC (1989) Perineal reconstruction with rectus abdominis flap after resection of anal carcinoma in Crohn's disease. *J R Coll Soc Med* **52**: 369–370.

Ruckley CV, Smith AN & Balfour TW (1970) Perineal closure by omental graft. *Surg Gynecol Obstet* **131**: 300–302.

Ryan JA Jr (1984) Gracilis muscle flap for the persistent perineal sinus of IBD. *Am J Surg* **148**: 64–70.

Saha SK (1983) Care of perineal wound in abdominoperineal resection. *J R Coll Surg Engl* **28**: 324–327.

Saha SK & Robinson AF (1976) A study of perineal wound healing after abdominoperineal resection. *Br J Surg* **63**: 555–558.

Scammell B & Keighley MRB (1986) Delayed perineal wound healing after proctectomy for Crohn's colitis. *Br J Surg* **73**: 150–152.

Schofield PF (1970) Care of the perineal wound after excision of the rectum. *J R Coll Surg Edinb* **15**: 287–289.

Schwab RM & Kelly KA (1974) Primary closure of perineal wound after proctectomy. *Mayo Clin Proc* **49**: 176–179.

Seckel BR, Schoetz DJ & Coller JA (1985) Skin grafts for circumferential coverage of perianal wounds. *Surg Clin North Am* **65**: 365–371.

Se-min Baek, Greenstein A, McEllinney AJ & Anfses AH (1981) The gracilis myocutaneous flap for persistent perineal sinus after proctocolectomy. *Surg Gynecol Obstet* **153**: 713–716.

Shaw A & Futrell JW (1978) Cure of chronic perineal sinus with gluteus maximus flap. *Surg Gynecol Obstet* **147**: 417–420.

Shukla HA & Hughes LE (1984) The rectus abdominis flap for perineal wounds. *Ann R Coll Surg Engl* **66**: 337–339.

Silen W & Glotzer DJ (1974) The prevention and treatment of the persistent perineal sinus. *Surgery* **75**: 535–542.

Skene AI, Gault DT, Woodhouse CRJ et al (1990) Perineal, vulval and vaginoperineal reconstruction using the rectus abdominis myocutaneous flap. *Br J Surg* **77**: 635–637.

Smith EJ, Sparberg M & Poticha SM (1978) Late occurrence of perineal wound abscess years after total colectomy. *Am J Surg* **135**: 626–629.

Solomon MJ, Atkinson K, Quinn MJ, Eyers AA & Glenn DC (1996) Gracilis myocutaneous flap to reconstruct large perineal defects. *Int J Colorect Dis* **11**: 49–51.

Stanek G, Bosch P & Leber P (1980) Uber die Keimvermehrung in einem Fibrinklebesystem in vergleich zu Blut und das Lyseverhalten mit ohne Faktor XIII. In Schimpf K (ed.) *Fibrinogen, Fibrin and Fibrin Glue*, pp 239–241. Stuttgart: Schattauer.

Strahan J, Wilson W & McMechan E (1967) A review of surgically treated UC. *Ir J Med Sci* **494**: 83–88.

Talbot RW, Ritchie JK & Northover JMA (1989) Conservative proctocolectomy: a dubious option in ulcerative colitis. *Br J Surg* **76**: 738–739.

Terranova O, Sandei F, Rubuffat C, Maruotti R & Pezzuoli G (1979) Management of the perineal wound after rectal incision for neoplastic disease: a controlled clinical trial. *Dis Colon Rectum* **22**: 228–233.

Tolstedt GE, Bell JW & Harkins HN (1961) Chronic perineal sinus following total colectomy for UC. *Am J Surg* **101**: 50–54.

Tompkins RG & Warshaw AL (1985) Improved management of the perineal wound after proctectomy. *Ann Surg* **202**: 760–765.

Turowiski G, Schaadt M, Barthels M, Diehl V & Poliwoda H (1980) Unterschiedlicher Einfluss von Fibrinogen und Faktor XIII auf das Nachstum von Primar und Kulturfibroblasten. In Schimpf K (ed.) *Fibrinogen, Fibrin and Fibrin Glue*, pp 227–237. Stuttgart: Schattauer.

Walton P & Mallik RF (1975) Management of the perineal wound after excision of rectum. *J R Coll Surg Edinb* **20**: 251–254.

Ward MWN, Morgan BG & Clark CG (1982) Treatment of persistent perineal sinus with vaginal fistulas following proctocolectomy for Crohn's disease. *Br J Surg* **69**: 228–229.

Warshaw AL, Ottinger LW & Bartlett MK (1977) Primary perineal closure after proctocolectomy for IBD: prevention of the persistent perineal sinus. *Am J Surg* **133**: 414–419.

Watts JMcK, deDombal FT & Goligher JC (1966) Long-term complications and prognosis following major surgery for UC. *Br J Surg* **53**: 1014–1023.

Williams NS, Nasmyth DG, Jones D & Smith AH (1986) Defunctioning stomas: a prospective controlled trial comparing loop ileostomy with loop transverse colostomy. *Br J Surg* **73**: 566–570.

Winslet MC, Andrews H, Alexander-Williams J, Allan RN & Keighley MRB (1987) Faecal diversion in the management of Crohn's disease. *Gut* **28**: A1344.

Winslet MC, Alexander-Williams J & Keighley MRB (1990) Conservative proctocolectomy with low transection of the anorectum is a poor alternative to conventional proctocolectomy in inflammatory bowel disease. *Int J Colorectal Dis* **5**: 117–119.

Winslet MC, Drolc Z, Allan A & Keighley MRB (1991) Assessment of the defunctioning efficiency of the loop ileostomy. *Dis Colon Rectum* **34**: 699–703.

Wood RAB, Williams RHP & Hughes LE (1977) Foam elastomer dressing in the management of open granulating wounds: experience with 250 patients. *Br J Surg* **64**: 554–557.

Young MRA, Small JO, Leonard AG & McKelvey STD (1988) Rectus abdominis muscle flap for persistent perineal sinus. *Br J Surg* **75**: 1228.

11

IMPAIRED SEXUAL FUNCTION AFTER RECTAL SURGERY

Impaired sexual function has been focused mainly upon the risk of impotence in males after rectal excision for inflammatory bowel disease. Fortunately this is relatively uncommon; it is influenced by age and the technique of rectal excision (Goligher, 1983). Less emphasis has been placed on the problems of impotence and impaired sexual performance in men after rectal surgery for cancer; furthermore, the data are difficult to interpret as preoperative performance has often not been recorded (Bernstein and Bernstein, 1966; Davis and Jelenko, 1975; Williams and Slack, 1980). The problems of sexual dysfunction in women have received even less attention. Despite this, dyspareunia, impaired sexual function and altered body image seem to be common (Stahlgren and Ferguson, 1959; Watts et al, 1966); fertility and pregnancy are also influenced by rectal surgery.

Until recently little was known about the impact of a stoma on sexual function. In the past, few patients having a stoma constructed were counselled preoperatively about sexual activity and expectations. With the introduction of reservoir ileostomy, restorative proctocolectomy and low sphincter-saving resection for cancer, the impact of a stoma on sexual function has been of greater interest to investigators.

ASSESSMENT OF THE PROBLEM

Sexual function

Men

Male impotence has been defined as the failure to sustain an erection allowing normal ejaculation with satisfactory orgasm. However, as most of those who have discussed the problem with patients realize, the problem is not as simple as this. An article by Leicester et al (1984) highlights the complexity of this issue. They undertook a survey of patients from St Mark's Hospital who had undergone intersphincteric excision of the rectum. In the first place they discovered they were able to survey only a propor-

Table 11.1 Analysis of the extent of sexual difficulties after intersphincteric rectal excision.

Sexual problem	*Transient*	*Permanent*
*Men (n = 23)**		
Pain during erection	3	2
Loss of libido	2	2
Pain from perineal wound	1	0
Absent erection	0	0
Impaired erection	2	4
Difficulty of penetration	2	2
Difficulty maintaining erection	2	4
Premature ejaculation	3	1
Failure of ejaculation	1	1
Retrograde ejaculation	0	0
Lack of orgasm	0	1
Impaired orgasm	1	3
Impaired urinary control	1	1
Stoma-related problems	1	2
Women (n = 25)†		
Perineal discomfort	2	5
Loss of satisfaction	0	5
Stress incontinence	0	1
Urinary urgency	0	1
Uterine prolapse	0	2
Lack of orgasm	0	0
Impaired orgasm	1	1
Stoma-related problems	1	1

* No. with transient problem = 7 (30%); with permanent problem = 6 (26%).
† No. with transient problem = 3 (12%); with permanent problem = 5 (20%).
From Leicester et al (1984).

tion of these patients (just under half). It then became apparent that this information could not simply be gleaned by questionnaire, but that both the patient and partner had to be carefully and tactfully interviewed. These authors soon realized that there were many problems, other than the failure of ejaculation, that might be influenced by operation – such as size, stiffness and duration of tumescence. The survey demonstrated that although there were many patients with minor difficulties, none had been rendered impotent (Table 11.1). The problem was therefore more complicated than the issue of impotence alone (Williams and Johnston, 1983; Dozois, 1985).

Few papers on this subject discuss libido; stoma-related sexual problems are rarely addressed; disturbances of micturition in relation to intercourse are usually ignored; and orgasm is discreetly omitted from many surveys. Erection may be present but inadequately sustained, painful or intermittently impaired. There may be difficulty in penetration. Similarly, the problem of sympathetic denervation is not just one of failure of ejaculation but may include retrograde ejaculation, intermittent failure or premature emission (Devlin et al, 1971; Morrow, 1976; Morgan, 1982).

Assessment of impaired sexual fuction must also take into account preoperative sexual performance. Even in younger patients with inflammatory bowel disease, there may be a disturbance of function sometimes related to medication (Bauer et al, 1983). However, in older patients with malignancy the incidence of preoperative impotence can be remarkably high (Williams and Slack, 1980; Kinn and Ohman, 1986); and, even if it is not, many older patients are sexually inactive. Thus, sexual activity may be impaired by age, disease and poor general health. The last two factors are also particularly pertinent in patients with inflammatory bowel disease, and many authors report improved sexual activity after proctocolectomy, rather than the reverse, suggesting that these factors are usually corrected by operation (Burnham et al, 1977; Brooke, 1983).

Impairment of sexual function may be transient. May (1966) reported that 11 of 46 male patients had some impairment of sexual function early after rectal excision, but only three patients were completely impotent 1 year after operation and all had achieved normal function after 2 years. These observations are a salutory reminder that nerve regeneration may occur and that general health, confidence and psychological factors play a crucial role in these functions (Gruner et al, 1977).

Women

It is surprising how frequently in the past women have been excluded from an assessment of sexual function after rectal surgery (Oresland et al, 1994; Bambrick et al, 1996). Dyspareunia is now a recognized complication of proctectomy, particularly if there is impairment of perineal wound healing, perineal sepsis or a sinus. There are, however, other reasons for impaired sexual function (Table 11.2), such as a tight introitus, vaginoperineal fistula, uterine prolapse or a displaced uterus following rectal excision (Harrison and McDonagh, 1950; Watts et al, 1966; Entman and Wilson, 1982).

Assessment of sexual function in women should include pain, discharge and vaginal dryness during intercourse. Other factors should be explored such as pleasure, fulfilment, orgasm, and urinary complications during coitus, as well as stomal-related dysfunction. Dyspareunia may have been present before the operation. Gruner et al (1977) remind us that nearly 30% of patients with severe proctitis suffer from dyspareunia. Petter et al (1977) rightly stress the emotional and psychological factors among women with dyspareunia.

Table 11.2 Sexual problems after rectal excision for inflammatory bowel disease.

Women (*n* = 67)	
5 Mechanical factors (7%):	1 Painful perineal sinus 1 Vaginal stenosis 1 Dyspareunia 1 Urinary incontinence 1 Fear of dislodging bag
Men (*n* = 41)	
11 Impaired sexual function (27%):	7 Permanent failure of erection 2 Temporary failure of erection 2 Failure of ejaculation

From Watts et al (1966).

Table 11.4 Influence of age on impaired sexual function after abdominoperineal excision.

	Age (years)		
Change in function	41–48 (*n* = 7)	49–57 (*n* = 9)	58–65 (*n* = 9)
No sexual disturbance	5	3	1
Erectile impotence	1	2	4
Partial erectile failure	1	3	3
Ejaculatory failure	0	2	3

From Danzi et al (1983).

Factors influencing sexual performance

Age

Sexual function is related to age in normal subjects (Kinsey, 1948; Finkle et al, 1959; Davis and Jelenko, 1975; Corman et al, 1978; Yeager and van Heerden, 1980) as well as in those who have an ileostomy for inflammatory bowel disease and in patients with malignancy (Burnham et al, 1977; Danzi et al, 1983). In an assessment of patients from the Ileostomy Association of Great Britain, Burnham et al (1977) found complete or partial impotence in only 5% of patients under 25 years of age, in 10% aged 26–35 years, in 33% aged 36–45 years and in 53% over 46 years of age (Table 11.3). Similarly, Danzi and colleagues, investigating patients with carcinoma of the rectum treated by abdominoperineal excision, reported disturbance in sexual function in only two of seven patients aged 41–48 (29%), in six of nine patients aged 49–57 years (67%), but in all except one of nine aged 58–65 years (89%) (Table 11.4).

Malignant disease

The influence of advanced malignancy is evident in many functions as well as sexual activity. Radiotherapy and chemotherapy may decrease libido, and radiation-induced perineal discomfort may make intercourse impossible for many weeks. The influence of tumour stage, size and site on the incidence of impaired male sexual function has also been assessed (Deizonne et al, 1982; Frego et al, 1982). Kinn and Ohman (1986) concluded that impotence was unrelated to Dukes' classification and the extent of lymph node involvement (La Monica et al, 1985). Balslev and Harling (1983) also suggested that male impotence was unrelated to tumour size and location.

Inflammatory bowel disease

The overall incidence of male sexual impairment after surgery for inflammatory bowel disease is lower than that after surgery for malignant disease, probably because these patients represent a younger age group and there is a preference where possible for the more conservative perimuscular or intersphincteric rectal excision (Lee and Dowling,

Table 11.3 Changes in sexual function after proctectomy in men.

			Age (years)			
Change in function	*Before* (*n* = 118)	*After* (*n* = 118)	<25 (*n* = 20)	26–35 (*n* = 41)	36–45 (*n* = 27)	>46 (*n* = 30)
Complete erectile impotence	1? (1%)	6 (5%)	0	0	1	5
Partial erectile impotence	3*	13	1	4	8	11
Ejaculatory impotence	1	10	0	10	0	0
Ejaculatory impotence only	1	4	0	4	0	0
Ejaculation poorly maintained	6†	22	0	4	8	10
Total with dysfunction	11 (9%)	45 (38%)	1	10	14	20

? Improved afterwards?
* Two improved afterwards.
† Five improved.
From Burnham et al (1977).

1972; Lyttle and Parks, 1977). However, conservative proctocolectomy is not always possible in Crohn's colitis, particularly when this is complicated by perirectal fistula, stricture and chronic anorectal sepsis (Lockhart-Mummery and Ritchie, 1983).

Chronic ill-health, anaemia, protein-calorie malnutrition and sepsis which is so common in inflammatory bowel disease may be responsible for reduced libido, impaired performance and abstinence (Moody et al, 1992). Nilsson et al (1981) record reduced or absent sexual activity in 6 of 29 (21%) female patients before colectomy and in 4 of 13 (31%) male patients. After conventional proctocolectomy there was a small improvement in sexual activity in men but not in women. These authors ascribe the lack of improvement to construction of a conventional ileostomy which was attended by its own sexual problems (Roy et al, 1970; Ritchie, 1972; Bone and Sorensen, 1974). In our experience, we usually find that sexual performance is improved after conservative and restorative proctocolectomy, particularly in women.

Marital status

Clearly the level of understanding, concern and sensitivity of a patient's sexual partner plays a critical role in the adjustment and rehabilitation of a person's life after stoma construction. Generally, married couples share their problems, are less demanding and have a more realistic understanding of sexual expectations than couples who cohabit. Keltikangas-Jarvinen et al (1984) found that ileostomy patients having a proctocolectomy needed the support of their partner more than colostomy patients with malignancy.

Psychological factors

Since sexual intercourse is such a personal and expressive activity, it is hardly surprising that psychological factors are major determinants of function. Emotional stress, anxiety, guilt, depression, obsession and perception of an altered body image through having a stoma are factors which play an important role in sexual performance (Dyk and Sutherland, 1956; Engel, 1958; Orbach and Tallent, 1965; Fischer and Cleveland, 1967; Druss et al, 1968; Lennenberg, 1971; Kolb, 1975; Morrow, 1976; Gruner et al, 1977).

Fertility

Men

In patients with inflammatory bowel disease, infertility has in the past been related to disordered spermatogenesis from sulphasalazine therapy (Toth, 1979). With the wider use of 5-aminosalicylic acid compounds, male infertility has become less common.

Rectal excision itself may reduce fertility because of impaired emission – particularly retrograde ejaculation – and penetration following operative damage to the sympathetic and parasympathetic supply to the prostate, bladder, sphincter vessicae, seminal vesicles and corpora cavernosa (Goligher, 1951; Walsh and Schlegel, 1988).

Women

Although Willoughby and Truelove (1980) provided excellent data on the fertility of women with ulcerative colitis, there are few data regarding fertility after rectal excision. Gopal et al (1985) found that 66 patients with an ileostomy (mainly for colitis) achieved 82 successful pregnancies, suggesting that fertility is normal in many patients. However, Daly and Brooke (1967) reported that 10 of 62 women who had had a proctocolectomy for colitis were infertile. All of those investigated were found to have tubal occlusion. Even more worrying was the report of Roy et al (1970) who found that only 20 of 497 patients became pregnant after proctocolectomy.

There may be some impairment of fertility after reservoir ileostomy and restorative proctocolectomy, probably from tubal occlusion. Metcalf et al (1986) report that six of eight patients became pregnant after ileoanal anastomosis, four of whom delivered vaginally, and that 10 of 12 patients conceived after Koch pouch construction. The larger current database of women having children after restorative proctocolectomy suggests that infertility may be increased but that most patients wishing a vaginal delivery have a relatively trouble-free pregnancy and delivery (Juhasz et al, 1995; see Chapter 49).

STRUCTURAL AND FUNCTIONAL CONSIDERATIONS

Anatomy

Textbooks of anatomy do not emphasize the surgically important aspects of the autonomic innervation to the pelvis. However, the anatomy is quite simple and the nerves can be readily visualized at laparoscopy and laparotomy, provided the patient is not too fat.

Sympathetic nerves

Figure 11.1 is a stylized drawing of the anatomical arrangement. The sympathetic outflow derived from the white rami of T1–L2 form a series of ganglia consisting of the sympathetic chain just medial to the origin of the psoas muscle. The sympathetic chain lies beside the aorta on the left and the vena cava on the right. Fibres from the sympathetic chain either pass under the iliac vessels to enter the pelvic plexus or form a plexus on the surface of the aorta behind the root of the mesentery (the preaortic plexus). Fibres from the preaortic plexus follow the visceral blood supply to the gut or the iliac and renal vessels.

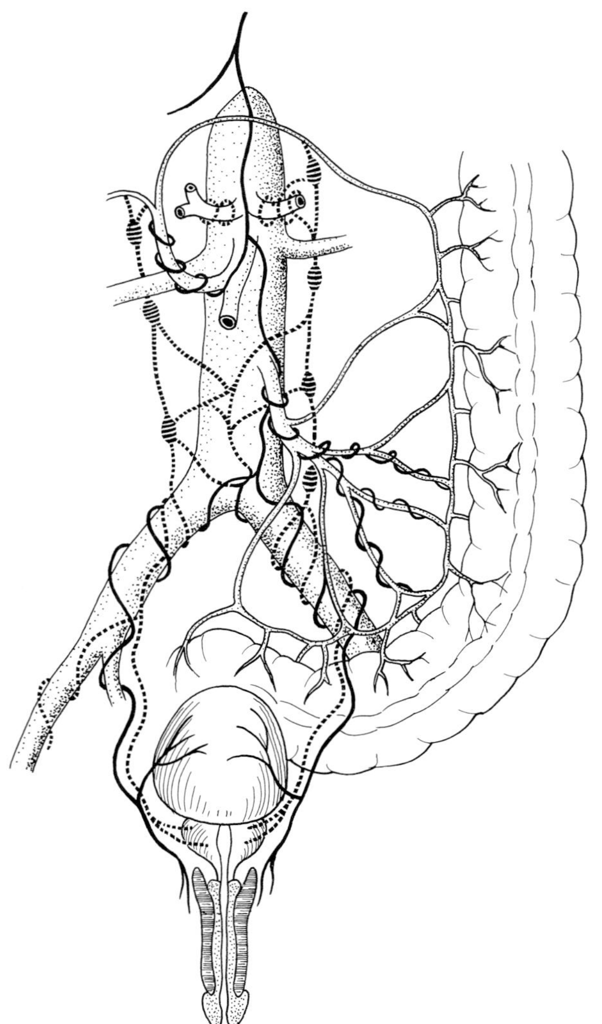

Figure 11.1 The anatomical arrangement of the sympathetic (dotted line) and the parasympathetic (solid line) innervation to the rectum, bladder, seminal vesicles and penis.

As far as the sympathetic supply to the bladder, rectum and genital organs is concerned, the outflow is from the T12–L2 nerve roots, which enter the hypogastric plexus below the aortic bifurcation and form two condensations of nerve fibres just medial to the iliac vessels; these are referred to, rather euphemistically, as the presacral nerves. These fibres lie behind the endopelvic fascia, cross the iliac vessels running laterally just behind the mesorectum to the side wall of the pelvis and enter the viscera with their blood supply or join the nervi erigentes. The sympathetic supply to the rectum follows the middle rectal artery in the lateral ligaments. The sympathetics supplying the uterus and vagina run with the uterine artery in the base of the broad ligaments and the uterosacral ligaments. The sympathetic supply to the bladder follows branches of the internal iliac artery, which supply the detrusor muscle, the sphincter vesicae and, in the male, the smooth muscle surrounding the prostate and seminal vesicles.

Parasympathetic nerves

The parasympathetic outflow is best appreciated in a lateral view of the pelvis (Figure 11.2). The nervi erigentes are formed by the second, third and fourth sacral nerve roots as they emerge from the sacral foramina. The nerves run anterolaterally from the sacrum to the side wall of the pelvis. The parasympathetics lie behind the endopelvic fascia and pass forwards over the origin of the ischiococcygeus and iliococcygeus muscles, where they join the pelvic plexus. With the sympathetic nerves they supply the rectum, the internal sphincter, the base of the bladder, the uterus, cervix and vagina in the female, or the prostate, seminal vesicles and the corpora cavernosa in the male. The supply to the corpora cavernosum is via the deep artery of the penis from the internal pudendal artery. The parasympathetic supply is either direct to the organ of innervation through the endopelvic fascia or with the arterial supply, as described for the sympathetic innerva-

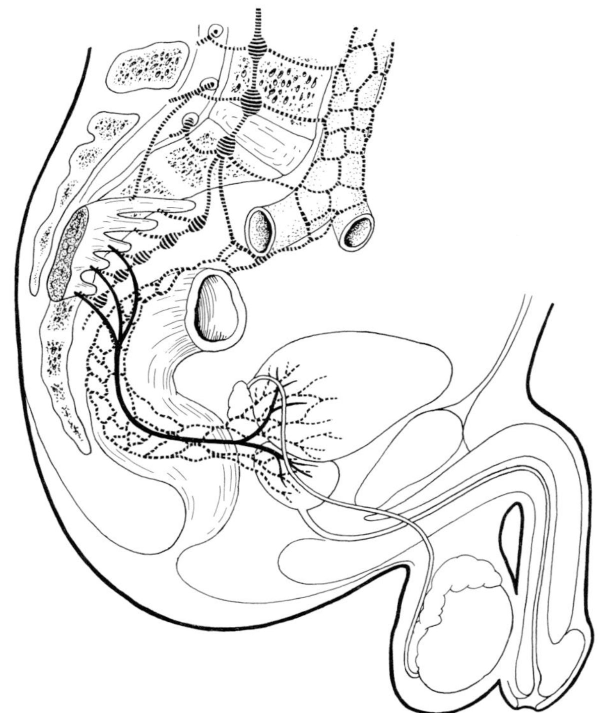

Figure 11.2 The parasympathetic outflow (solid line) and innervation of the bladder and sexual organs is best appreciated in a lateral view of the pelvis. The nervi erigentes can be seen supplying the bladder, seminal vesicles and prostate. The sympathetic fibres (dotted line) are also demonstrated running with the nervi erigentes.

tion (middle rectal, uterine and vesical vessels). Some parasympathetic fibres join the presacral nerves to gain access to the visceral arteries (in particular the inferior mesenteric artery) to supply the sigmoid and upper rectum.

Physiology

The sympathetic nerves supply vasoconstrictor fibres to the pelvic viscera, the lower limb and the vascular supply to the gut and genitalia. The sympathetics entering the bladder through the endopelvic fascia from the side wall of the pelvis are inhibitory to the detrusor muscle but cause contraction of the sphincter vesicae, thereby preventing retrograde flow of semen (Figures 11.1 and 11.2). The sympathetic nerves also supply smooth muscle which surrounds the seminal vesicles and the prostate and infiltrates the prostatic septa. They also supply the smooth muscle surrounding the prostatic urethra and ejaculatory ducts in order to allow ejaculation to clear stored semen in the seminal vesicles and to direct the flow into the urethra. The sympathetic supply not only allows emission of semen, but their vasoconstrictor role also allows detumescence.

Parasympathetic fibres cause vasodilatation of the dorsal artery of the penis which supplies the corpora cavernosa, thereby allowing erection by facilitating both venous congestion and an increased arterial supply to the corpora (Clyne et al, 1982). A similar mechanism is present in the female, in whom the parasympathetic innervation is responsible for venous engorgement of the vagina and secretion from the squamous epithelium. Parasympathetic activity results in contraction of the detrusor and inhibition of the sphincter vesicae as well as the internal anal sphincter. Motor fibres also supply the bulbocavernosus and ischiocavernosus muscles at the root of the penis which causes semen to be propelled down the penile urethra during ejaculation (Figure 11.3).

Erection is initiated by sensory and physical stimuli. In women, cerebral control and peripheral sensory nerve stimuli – particularly in the perineum – play a more critical role than the autonomic nervous

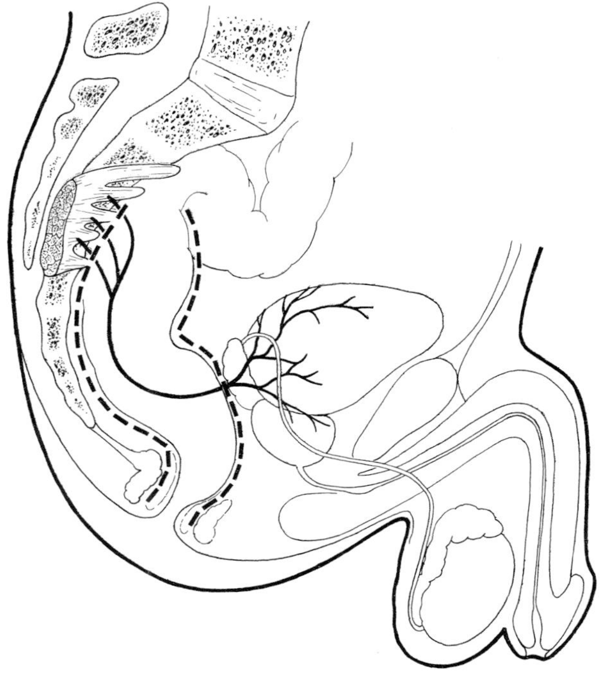

Figure 11.3 The plane of dissection during intersphincteric excision of the rectum (dotted line). Keeping well behind the prostate anteriorly and in front of the presacral fascia, damage to the parasympathetic nerves (solid line) should not be encountered.

system (Williams et al, 1951; Weinstein and Roberts, 1977). Sensory perineal stimuli are mediated by the pudendal nerves. The psychic factors and sensory awareness, in combination with some parasympathetic activity, are responsible for vaginal secretion and orgasm.

Site of damage to the pelvic autonomic nerves

Some damage may occur to the autonomic innervation of the pelvic viscera whenever a pelvic organ is being mobilized. However, even after cystectomy, sexual activity is not always impaired (Bergman et al, 1979; Walsh and Schlegel, 1988). Fortunately, many fibres contribute to the pelvic plexus, and it is only where these neural elements coalesce, as in the presacral nerves, or at their origin, as in the case of the nervi erigentes, that surgical damage is likely to result in serious functional disorders.

Bauer and others (1983) maintain that there are four sites in the pelvis where serious damage to the autonomic innervation may occur (Figures 11.4 and 11.5). The most easily preventable site of damage is over the front of the aorta and below the sacral promontory, where the autonomic plexuses lie on each side of the midline as they enter the sacral hollow. Damage is most frequently encountered in this area during radical high ligation of the inferior mesenteric artery for malignancy (Heald and Leicester, 1981) or in the initial retrorectal discretion to enter the presacral space at the pelvic brim.

The second site for damage is where the nervi erigentes join the pelvic plexus on the side wall of the pelvis, just lateral to the lateral ligaments of the rectum and posterolateral to the bladder. They may be damaged by wide ligation of the lateral ligaments during dissection of the ureters down to the base of the bladder, during division of the lateral ligaments of the uterus during hysterectomy, or when the internal iliac vessels are exposed, as in radical pelvic lymphadenectomy.

The third site and perhaps the most common source of damage is between the sacrum and Waldeyer's fascia where the origin of the pelvic

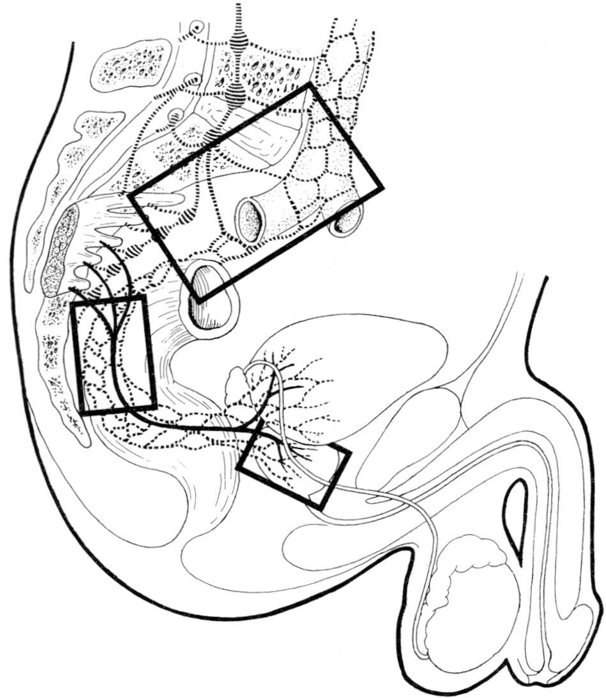

Figure 11.4 Three sites in the pelvis where damage to the autonomic innervation may occur during rectal dissection. The lumbar nerves may be damaged on entering the pelvis. The nervi erigentes may be damaged during lateral dissection of the rectum, and the parasympathetic innervation to the seminal vesicles may be damaged if Denonvilliers' fascia is breached during anterior rectal mobilization. Solid line, parasympathic supply; dotted line, sympathetic supply.

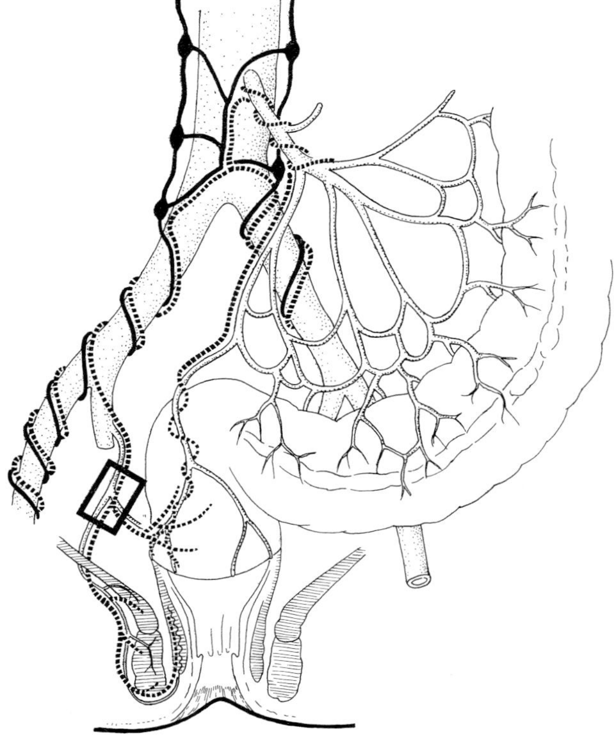

Figure 11.5 Autonomic innervation of the pelvis may be interrupted during radical pelvic clearance, particularly where the internal iliac artery is stripped of its lymph nodes. Solid line, parasympathetic supply; dotted line, sympathetic supply.

nerves may be torn. This plane is rarely entered by the abdominal surgeon since the mesorectum is not adhered to the presacral fascia and the posterior plane is easily seen to the level of the pelvic floor. Furthermore, the surgeon will be anxious not to damage the presacral veins. Damage to the pelvic nerves is usually inflicted by the perineal surgeon as a result of stripping Waldeyer's fascia from the sacrum. Unless the fascia of Waldeyer is deliberately opened just above the anorectal junction, so that the veins on the back of the rectum can be seen, the pelvic nerves are at risk of damage.

The fourth site where the innervation to the bladder and ejaculatory mechanism may be damaged is in front of the rectum if Denonvilliers' fascia is breached during anterior mobilization of the rectum. This site of damage should be rare, unless there is an anterior mid-rectal tumour. Provided the surgeon keeps close to the longitudinal fibres of the rectum the nerves should be safe, since the thick fascial plane protects the periprostatic plexus. However, in anterior rectal tumours this plane may have to be deliberately breached in order to achieve complete circumferential tumour margins. In synchronous combined rectal excision for benign disease, the anterior plane should be defined first by the abdominal surgeon in order to prevent any encroachment on to the prostate.

Operative considerations

Malignant disease

The most important consideration in the surgery of malignant disease is to completely eradicate the tumour and its lymphatic drainage with a wide margin of clearance. In the pelvis, the greatest risk of local recurrence is from inadequate lateral or circumferential clearance of the growth (Silverman et al, 1984; Durdey et al, 1986).

The extent of radical clearance will depend on the location of the tumour. Hence, for anteriorly placed lesions 5 cm from the anal verge treated by anterior resection or abdominoperineal excision of the rectum, a deliberate decision should be taken to open Denonvilliers' fascia and remove the posterior aspect or in some cases the whole of the prostate resulting in deliberate excision of the periprostatic nerves. Sometimes the urethral sphincter can be preserved and an ileal cystoplasty constructed. In female patients, the entire posterior vaginal wall will need to be excised. In posteriorly placed tumours, the coccyx and lower sacral bodies may have to be excised in order to achieve tumour clearance, with potential damage to the nervi erigentes. It is usual surgical practice to divide the levator ani at its origin from the side wall of the pelvis in order to achieve maximum pelvic clearance. The ureters may need to be dissected free and the lateral ligaments divided as widely as possible, which may result in nerve damage. The entire mesorectum should be resected with the rectum from the pelvis to clear all lymphatic tissue in front of the sacrum and the aortic bifurcation (Nicholls et al, 1979; Williams et al, 1980). The same approach should be applied to low stapled or sutured restorative procedures in patients with rectal cancer; however, with tumours of the upper third of the rectum treated by 'sphincter-saving resection' (SSR), the wide pelvic dissection is above the levator ani, so there is less risk of nerve damage (Heald and Leicester, 1981).

In view of the extent of the rectal dissection in malignant disease, some impairment of sexual function is common even in young patients (Santangelo et al, 1987; Masui et al, 1996).

Inflammatory bowel disease

Rectal dissection in patients with inflammatory bowel disease is entirely different. Whenever possible the dissection should be kept as close to the rectum as possible. It may be necessary, particularly in Crohn's disease, to remove some of the mesorectum, pelvic floor, sphincters and perineum if there is extensive perirectal fibrosis, sepsis or a fistula. Nevertheless, the overriding consideration in ulcerative colitis and Crohn's disease is to preserve the autonomic innervation to the bladder and genital organs. These are generally young patients, in whom sexual function is extremely important (Moody et al, 1992).

During the perineal aspect of rectal excision, the intersphincteric plane should be used whenever this is feasible; not that preservation of the external sphincters *per se* will minimize denervation of the prostate and seminal vesicles, but this approach prevents any damage to the levator ani. By leaving the levator ani intact there is no fear of damage to the pudendal nerve. Nevertheless, even complete preservation of the puborectalis will not necessarily prevent damage to the pelvic nerves if Waldeyer's fascia is stripped off the sacrum. It is imperative, therefore, that the posterior plane between the levator ani and the rectum be divided from above so that the *posterior plane is defined by the abdominal operator* (Figure 11.6). There are exceptions, and an experienced colorectal surgeon can enter the correct presacral plane by the perineal route provided Waldeyer's fascia is deliberately divided as in the dissection for postanal repair.

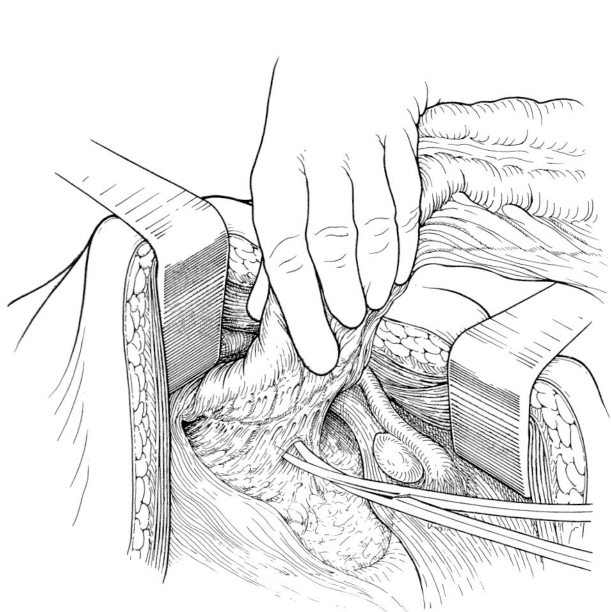

Figure 11.6 Illustration of the importance of the abdominal operator defining the posterior plane during rectal excision.

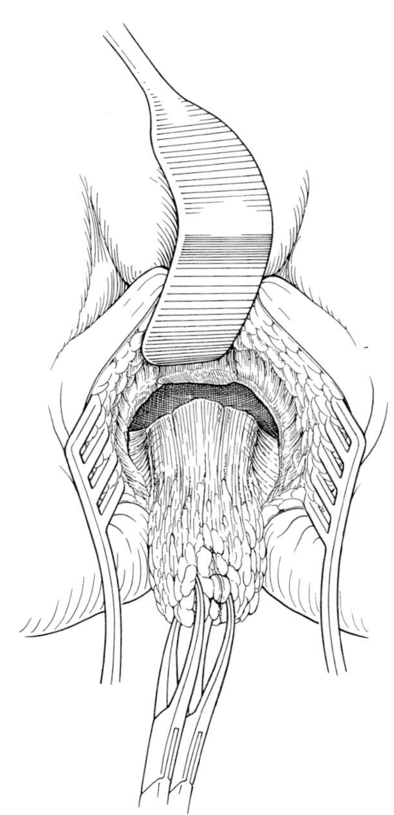

Figure 11.7 Illustration of the importance of the perineal surgeon developing the anterior plane during rectal excision.

If the rectum is being excised as a perineal proctectomy, it is essential to divide Waldeyer's fascia immediately the puborectalis is retracted from the rectum so that the veins on the back of the rectum can be seen. By contrast, the *distal component of the anterior dissection should preferably be undertaken by the perineal surgeon* (Figure 11.7). In this way, particularly if the surgeon keeps strictly in the midline and close to the rectum, the prostate can be dissected off the anterior rectum without fear of damage either to the prostate or to the seminal vesicles which are protected by Denonvilliers' fascia. During rectal excision the abdominal surgeon should keep as close to the anterior aspect bowel as possible. The pelvic peritoneum is divided adjacent to the sides of the rectum and anteriorly well above the prostate. It is probably not necessary to preserve the superior haemorrhoidal artery provided the mesorectum is divided just behind the vessels, since in this way the hypogastric plexus need not be disturbed (Beart, 1986). The lateral ligaments are divided close to the rectum and the whole of the mesorectum is removed with it (Figure 11.8).

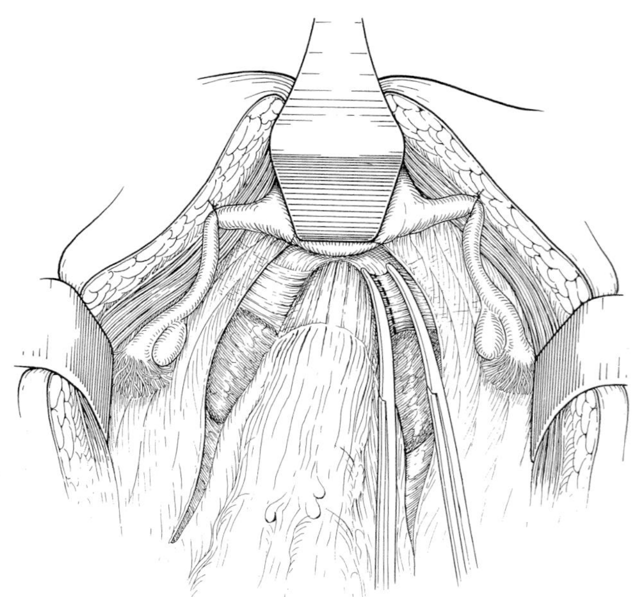

Figure 11.8 Illustration of the importance of dividing the lateral ligaments close to the rectum.

AETIOLOGY

Nerve injury

From the surgeon's point of view, autonomic nerve damage at the base of the bladder, prostate and seminal vesicles is the most important factor in the aetiology of male impotence, particularly as it is potentially avoidable (Santangelo et al, 1987). The avoidance of damage to pelvic autonomic nerves has already been discussed thoroughly in the previous section.

Scar tissue and chronic sepsis

Any residual source of pelvic sepsis or impaired perineal wound healing is likely to give rise to impaired sexual function in women (Tomkins and Warshaw, 1985; Scammell and Keighley, 1986). Prevention includes the avoidance of narrowing the introitus during perineal wound closure, particularly if the posterior vaginal wall has been removed. Any perineal sepsis should be thoroughly drained; metronidazole should be prescribed for patients with chronic perineal sepsis (Bernstein et al, 1980).

Vascular disease

Bilateral occlusion of the internal iliac vessels may be responsible for impotence in elderly patients with peripheral vascular disease (Leriche and Morel, 1948; Sabri and Cotton, 1971; Machledger and Weinstein, 1975; Herman et al, 1978; Queral et al, 1979). Potency is normal if the penile:brachial systolic pressure index is 0.60 or above (Kempczinski, 1979; Nath et al, 1981).

Stoma

A conventional ileostomy or colostomy may create a physical and psychological barrier to satisfactory sexual relationships. The appliance may leak and some partners are upset by noise or odour. The mere presence of an appliance may precipitate a feeling of revulsion. However, these worries and obsessions are generally more common in the patient with the stoma than the partner. Leicester et al (1984) reported that 46% of patients thought that their sexual relationships were impaired because of a stoma, but only 24% of their partners agreed.

Physical problems

Physical problems which are a real embarrassment for the ostomate include dislodgement of the appliance, leakage, noise, smell and discomfort from the plastics used to manufacture the bag and its sealant. Such factors have an impact on sexual activity. Rolstad et al (1983) reported that physical problems with the stoma were encountered in 33% of women and 32% of men with a stoma. Furthermore, it was the appliance and not the stoma, smell or noise which caused the greatest barrier to normal sexual activity. In the report by Nilsson et al (1981) on the influence of conversion to a reservoir ileostomy on sexual activity, physical problems were regularly encountered in 18 of 42 patients (43%) before conversion. Problems included: prolapse with the fear of trauma to the stoma in two; retraction and stenosis causing leakage in seven; and skin excoriation in nine. After construction of a reservoir ileostomy, five patients reported occasional leakage. All except one patient emptied their conventional ileostomy bag and applied a cover to it before intercourse, whereas only 11 patients found the need to intubate the reservoir before coitus, allowing a more spontaneous approach to sexual activity. Burnham et al (1977) reported physical difficulties with the stoma in 10 of 128 men (8%) and in 14 of 175 women (8%) (Table 11.5). A number of patients used some form of garment to disguise the appliance. Some, in addition to emptying the bag, undertook some form of dietary restriction before intercourse. Fears about damage, leakage and displacement were more prevalent among women, whereas men considered the bag to be a hindrance to sexual fulfilment.

Psychological problems

Emotional problems seem to be much more prevalent in the patient with an ileostomy than they are in the partner. Women considered that a stoma made them less attractive and caused them more embarrassment than did the men interviewed in the Ileostomy Association survey (Burnham et al, 1977). Adjectives such as 'unsightly', 'unpleasant' and even 'repulsive' were used by some patients. About 10% of patients considered that their stoma was the cause of marital tension, and 2% blamed the stoma as a cause of divorce. A rather higher rate of stoma-related marital disharmony was reported by Bone and Sorensen (1974). Psychological factors were identified as being responsible for sexual dissatisfaction in 54% of

Table 11.5 Assessment of sexual impairment amongst ileostomates.

	Women	Men
Married after ileostomy	21/175(12)	24/128(19)
Parenthood after ileostomy (<45 years only)	19/148(13)	37/96(38)
Physical problems with stoma during intercourse	14/175(8)	10/128(8)
Emotional problems		
Embarrassment: patient (30%)		
spouse	(8)	(2)
Less attractive: patient (50%)		
spouse	(9)	(6)
Adjectives used: 'unsightly'	37/175(21)	22/128(17)
'unpleasant'	24/175(14)	14/128(11)
'repulsive'	8/175(4)	6/128(5)
Marital breakdown in potent patients	4/175(2)	3/108(2)
Marital tension	21/175(12)	10/128(8)

Values in parentheses are percentages.
From Burnham et al (1977).

women and 45% of men in a North American postal questionnaire (Rolstad et al, 1983).

It is hardly surprising that the creation of an artificial opening on the abdominal wall with a protruding segment of bowel that discharges intestinal contents in an uncontrolled manner into a plastic bag is something of a repugnant device to most patients. Psychologists remind us that sphincter control is an essential component of psychosexual development (Orbach et al, 1957). Control of defecation is fundamental in human socialization. It is not surprising, therefore, that the construction of an ileostomy or a colostomy results in a noticeable adjustment in all levels of personality, apart from the secondary effects of the operation and its convalescence (Dyk and Sutherland, 1956; Morrow, 1976; Wirsching et al, 1975).

Keltikangas-Jarvinen et al (1984) examined the psychological factors related to adaptation after ileostomy and colostomy. There were some obvious differences between the two procedures. Colostomy patients, many of whom had been operated upon for malignant disease, tended to be more hostile (Masui et al, 1996), needing medical support, and were more fearful of the prospect of recurrent disease than ileostomy patients, who needed the support of their immediate family (Le Shan, 1961). Approximately 10% of stoma patients had been suicidal at some stage after operation and many admitted to deep-seated depression (Alexander and Glenn, 1965; Druss et al, 1969). Many more patients expressed a feeling that their body image had been permanently changed after colostomy (44%) than after ileostomy (16%). Ileostomy patients tended to be less anxious and depressed than those with a colostomy. Work capacity (Moody and Maybury, 1996), regarded by many to be an important factor in sexual performance, was impaired in a much greater proportion of patients after colostomy than after ileostomy; however, ileostomy patients, being younger, were more likely to get back to work (Moody and Maybury, 1997). Sexual performance in ileostomy patients was closely correlated with preoperative behaviour and, unlike in patients with a colostomy, decreased frequency of intercourse was uncommon, even though many said the opportunities for sexual expression had been reduced (Moody et al, 1992). Actual sexual activity, as measured by the Heidelberg colostomy questionnaire, was little influenced by ileostomy but greatly impaired in those with a colostomy (Table 11.6).

Table 11.6 Sexual activity (performances/week) before and after construction of a stoma (Heidelberg colostomy questionnaire).

Colostomy		Ileostomy	
Preoperative	*Postoperative*	*Preoperative*	*Postoperative*
0.96	0.31	1.47	1.43
–0.79	–0.47	–0.82	–0.89

From Keltikangas-Jarvinen et al (1984).

Avoidance of a stoma and appliance

Reservoir ileostomy

Construction of a reservoir ileostomy will allow 90% of patients to avoid wearing an appliance (Ecker et al, 1996). However, while it must be acknowledged that elimination of a spout and a bag is a major advantage in young, sexually active individuals who wish to be naked in bed with their partner, the Kock pouch is not a complication-free procedure (Kock, 1983; Kock et al, 1974; Mullen et

Table 11.7 Altered sexual activity before and after conversion to reservoir ileostomy.

	Conventional (*n* = 98)	*Reservoir* (*n* = 56)
No embarrassment	3	37
Uncertainty of leakage	35	6
Inhibited by stoma	19	2
Precautions taken before intercourse	41	11
Sexual activity reduced or absent		
Women	15	1
Men	4	1*

* Impotence after rectal excision.
From Nilsson et al (1981).

al, 1995). Despite this, the influence of a reservoir ileostomy on factors such as embarrassment, inhibition, fear of leakage and actual sexual activity are predictable (Table 11.7). It must be accepted, therefore, that from the sexual point of view the Kock pouch, particularly in young female patients, is a preferred option to conventional ileostomy.

Ileoanal pouch

The attractions of avoiding both an appliance and a stoma are very considerable, but they must be weighed against the possibility of technical failure, prolonged hospital stay, chronic sepsis and the risk of pouch excision (Keighley et al, 1997). Patients must realize that sphincter control may not be absolutely perfect, particularly if there has been some pelvic sepsis or if a mucosectomy has been performed, and that leakage during intercourse is a well-documented complication in a few patients. Episodes of perineal skin excoriation may prove a barrier to normal sexual satisfaction. Nevertheless, the prospect of avoiding a permanent stoma has already had a major impact on sexual function among young patients with ulcerative colitis (Nicholls, 1984; Cohen et al, 1985; Devlin and Plant, 1979). In our Birmingham series, only 3 of 108 males having restorative proctocolectomy reported impairment in sexual function (two with retrograde ejaculation and one with impaired tumescence). In a report from the Mayo Clinic, only 8 of 95 women complained of dyspareunia (Metcalf et al, 1986). Similar results were found at the London Hospital. Dyspareunia, libido and frequency of intercourse were both improved after ileoanal anastomosis (Bambrick et al, 1996).

Counselling

The impact of a stoma can be greatly reduced by careful explanation of its likely effect on sexual activity and performance beforehand. Considerations of sexual function should receive as much attention in young patients as the physical aspects of stoma management (Stevens, 1997; Alexander-Williams, 1997). We found that approximately 15% of our patients did not fully understand the operation of ileostomy beforehand (Phillips et al, 1985) and 18% of ileostomy patients were not informed of the possible sexual problems that might occur after construction (Keltikangas-Jarvinen et al, 1984).

Conception, pregnancy and delivery

Current evidence suggests that marriage rates of patients with an ileostomy are similar to the normal population (Burnham et al, 1977). Children were born to 37 of 96 men under 45 years (39%) in this survey, but to only 16 of 128 women (13%). The latter figure is clearly much lower than the 64% who had children, reported by Stahlgren and Ferguson (1959), but is similar to the conception rate reported from Birmingham by Daly and Brooke (1967). Infertility among women after conventional proctocolectomy was reported in 10 of 62 patients in the Birmingham series; of the four cases that were investigated, all were due to tubal occlusion. Although Metcalf et al (1986) state that reservoir ileostomy and ileoanal anastomosis resulted in minimal impairment of fertility, only 20% became pregnant after Kock pouch construction and only 12% after restorative proctocolectomy. We know of at least six women out of 109 who would like to have conceived and were investigated for infertility after ileoanal anastomosis who were found to have tubal occlusion. This is probably an underestimate of the problem since many women have had some family before restorative proctocolectomy and probably do not wish to seek infertility investigation after pouch construction. Oresland et al (1994) reported bilateral occluded hysterosalpingograms in only 2 of 21 patients, but unilateral occlusion was present in nine.

Although pregnancy is usually uncomplicated in patients who have had a conventional proctocolectomy (Gopal et al, 1985), Hudson (1972) reported ten episodes of intestinal obstruction during 89 pregnancies, with one maternal death. Intestinal obstruction can usually be managed conservatively but early operation must be advised if there is fear of infarction. Apart from intestinal obstruction, stomal prolapse is also reported as an occasional problem during pregnancy (Scudamore et al, 1957; Roy et al, 1970). Furthermore, stomal occlusion, ileostomy dysfunction, retraction and oedema were all more common during pregnancy than beforehand. Spontaneous abortion may be greater in patients with a stoma (Scudamore et al, 1957). Roy et al (1970) reported that 5 of 35 pregnancies in stoma patients resulted in miscarriage. A similar rate (5 of 35) was also reported by Rhodes and Kirsner (1965). An increased incidence of premature labour was also noted by Barwin et al (1974). However, a high miscarriage rate has not been consistently found (Priest et al, 1959; Hudson, 1972; Kretschew, 1972). McEwan (1965) has suggested that iron-deficiency anaemia may be more common and more difficult to control in pregnant patients with a stoma, but it is unclear from this report whether anaemia was confined to patients who still had their diseased bowel *in situ*.

Most patients can deliver vaginally after proctocolectomy, although patients with a perineal sinus may find that this becomes painful during delivery. There are some patients in whom the healed perineal wound has broken down in the early puerperium. The forceps delivery rate is rather higher in ileostomy patients, largely because they seem unable to push out the fetal head, presumably because the pelvic floor is absent in some patients (Hudson, 1972; Gopal et al, 1985). There is no evidence that caesarean section is needed routinely unless surgical treatment is indicated for a prolapsed stoma or intestinal obstruction when the patient is more than 30 weeks pregnant. The 36% caesarean section rate reported by Gopal et al (1985) is not mirrored by the British experience (Hudson, 1972) and may be explained by the rather more liberal attitude to caesarean section in North America compared with Europe. Nevertheless, in a series of women who had undergone proctocolectomy reported by Hudson (1972), caesarean section was used in some patients because they had had a previous caesarean section for fetal distress ($n=11$), because corrective surgery was needed ($n=4$) and in a few cases because of personal preference ($n=10$).

Most patients can deliver vaginally after reservoir ileostomy and following ileoanal anastomosis (Metcalf et al, 1986, Juhasz et al, 1995). However, it is imperative that patients should not be allowed to remain in labour for long periods after restorative proctocolectomy and pouch anal anastomosis for fear of damage to the pelvic floor. Local sphincter damage must be avoided at all costs, so the delivery in such patients must be carefully supervised. If there is any risk of pelvic floor or sphincter damage, the threshold for undertaking a caesarean section must be very low, particularly if there is any predelivery evidence of sphincter impairment. Some units deliberately advise elective caesarean section because of the fear of impaired continence from obstructed labour. We do not subscribe to this view and know of 11 mothers who have had an entirely successful vaginal delivery, leaving only four having a caesarean section, but careful supervision is absolutely essential.

Psychology

The psychological aspects of normal sexual intercourse cannot be dismissed. Support by a partner is crucial to a patient overcoming his or her own fears of a stoma. Patients on a reducing dose of steroids may experience a prolonged period of postoperative depression that may have an adverse effect on sexual function. Patients who have developed a postoperative complication such as sepsis or malnutrition may have a reduced libido. Patience, understanding and support by the partner must be encouraged in the early postoperative period.

There may be long-term psychological debility caused by resentment at having to undergo an operation, or feelings of guilt that, if medical advice had been sought earlier, an operation might not have been necessary. These and other emotional disturbances play an important part in a patient's rehabilitation to normal sexual activity.

INCIDENCE

Incidence in men

Malignant disease

The incidence of permanent impotence in men undergoing an abdominoperineal excision or a low anterior resection is given in Table 11.8. Unfortunately, the numbers of patients in these series are small and not all authors have excluded patients with evidence of preoperative impotence.

The incidence of disordered sexual function after abdominoperineal excision was 43% in the Cleveland Clinic survey, but only 14% were actually impotent (Fazio et al, 1980). Santangelo et al (1987) surveyed men under 60 years: of nine who had an abdominoperineal excision, four were impotent and two suffered from impaired ejaculation. Only one patient in four had minor ejaculatory dysfunction

Table 11.8 Impotence in males after rectal excision for malignant disease.

Authors	*Abdominoperineal excision*	*Anterior resection*
Weinstein and Roberts (1977)	24/24(100)	0/20
Fazio et al (1980)	1/7(14)	0/5
Williams and Slack (1980)	1/5(20)	0/5
Yeager and Van Heerden (1980)	3/20(15)	—
Frego et al (1982)	10/24(42)	—
Balslev and Harling (1983)	20/93(21)	3/17(18)
Danzi et al (1983)	9/26(35)	—
Williams and Johnston (1983)	11/20(55)	5/28*(18)(low)
La Monica et al (1985)	16/20(80)	18/40(45)
Kinn and Ohman (1986)	8/12(66)	8/13(62)
Santangelo et al (1987) (age <60 years)	4/9(44)	4/16(25) 0/4(high) 4/12(33)(low)

*Values in parentheses are percentages.

after high anterior resection, compared with 4 of 12 who were impotent and three who could not ejaculate after low anterior resection. Based on these data, the incidence of impotence appears higher following abdominoperineal excision than anterior resection, but after low anterior resection the incidence is similar.

Contradictory data, however, come from a study by one of us (NSW) which compared patients who had undergone either sphincter-saving resection (SSR) ($n = 40$) or abdominoperineal excision of the rectum (APER) ($n = 38$) for tumours of the lower two-thirds of the rectum (Williams and Johnston, 1983):

- Before SSR, 28 patients (20 male, 8 female) had had an active sex life and 12 patients (9 male, 3 female) were inactive afterwards. Four of the men complained of total erectile impotence and one found it difficult to maintain an erection. Of the 11 men who were sexually active, two complained of difficulty in ejaculation. Thus 6 of 20 men (30%) developed impairment of sexual function after SSR.
- Before APER, 20 patients (17 male, 3 female) had been sexually active and 13 patients (12 male, 1 female) were inactive afterwards. Eight of the men (47%) had complete impotence and three had difficulty in sustaining an erection. One of the five men who was still sexually active was unable to ejaculate. Thus 12 of 18 men (67%) developed impairment of sexual function after APER (cf. SSR $P < 0.06$).

It would therefore appear that although low SSR produces damage to sexual function, presumably as a result of damage to pelvic autonomic nerves, this is less than the damage inflicted by APER when performed for tumours at similar levels in the rectum. One suspects, however, that differences in the data from different centres depend on the degree of local spread of the tumour and the assiduity with which the surgeon attempts to preserve the autonomic pelvic nerves during the operation.

Although anterior resection appears to carry a lower incidence of postoperative sexual disturbance, stapled anastomosis does not seem to differ from hand-sutured reconstruction (Stelzner, 1977; La Monica et al, 1985).

Kinn and Ohman (1986) were unable to correlate the incidence of impotence with the presence of bladder disturbance or abnormal cystometrograms (Watson and Williams, 1952).

Inflammatory bowel disease

The incidence of permanent impotence in men after rectal excision for inflammatory bowel disease is listed in Table 11.9. The frequency of permanent sexual impairment is much less than in patients having a radical resection for cancer. Furthermore, preoperative impairment is less common, despite the fact that sexual performance is influenced adversely by the underlying colitis in a third of patients. The highest incidence of impotence is reported from an early review by Watts et al (1966) in Leeds, at a time when a much wider excision was performed as in the treatment of rectal cancer (Dennis, 1945). Most of the earlier reports indicate a higher incidence of male impotence than the two reviews confined to patients having an intersphincteric excision (Kennedy et al, 1982; Leicester et al, 1984).

Reference is made elsewhere to the lower incidence of male sexual impairment after ileoanal

Table 11.9 Impotence in males after rectal excision for inflammatory bowel disease.

Authors	*Permanent impotence*
Stahlgren and Ferguson (1959)	0/25
Bacon et al (1960)	1/39(2.6)
Donovan and O'Hara (1960)	1/21(4.8)
Van Pronaska and Siderins (1962)	0/79
May (1966)	3/46(6.5)
Watts et al (1966)	7/41(17.1)
Daly and Brooke (1967)	6/100(6.0)
Burnham et al (1977)	6/118(5.1)
Corman et al (1978)	0/76
Fazio et al (1980)	0/9
Nilsson et al (1981)	1/42(2.4)
Bauer et al (1983)	4/135(2.9)
Kennedy et al (1982)*	0/39
Rolstad et al (1983)	1/25(4.0)
Leicester et al (1984)*	0/23
Nicholls (1984)†	0/66
Cohen et al (1985)†	0/82
Dozois (1985)†	0/369
Rothenberger et al (1985)†	0/83

Values in parentheses are percentages.
* Intersphincteric excision.
† Restorative proctocolectomy.

Table 11.10 New sexual problems in ileostomy patients.

Change in function	*Number*
Men	
No rectal excision (n = 42)	
No disturbance	42
Proctectomy (n = 118)	
No disturbance	73
Erectile impotence	6
Partial erectile impotence	12
Difficulty maintaining erection	21
Ejaculation impossible	9
Ejaculation poorly maintained	21
Women	
No rectal excision (n = 57)	
No disturbance	49
Dyspareunia	8
Proctectomy (n = 164)	
No disturbance	110
Dyspareunia	54

From Burnham et al (1977).

pouch anastomosis (Neal et al, 1982). Compared with conventional proctocolectomy, very few cases of impotence have been reported after restorative proctocolectomy in men. However, retrograde ejaculation has been reported in five patients from the literature and in two others from our own series, suggesting that damage to the sympathetic innervation may occur in some patients (Beart, 1986). Nevertheless, this is a remarkable achievement, particularly as preservation of the superior haemorrhoidal vessels is no longer practised by many surgeons when removing the rectum for ulcerative colitis. The incidence of impaired sexual function following perimuscular excision of the rectum or ileoanal pouch anastomosis is almost the same as that reported after subtotal colectomy and ileorectal anastomosis when the contents of the pelvis are not disturbed (Hughes and Russell, 1967; Veidenheimer et al, 1970; Gruner et al, 1975; Jones et al, 1977).

We hope, therefore, that the data collected by Burnham et al (1977) from a cohort of patients belonging to the Ileostomy Association merely represent the legacy of a bygone era (Table 11.10). Their data seem to indicate that the sexual problems in men are usually related to the rectal excision and not to the presence of an ileostomy. Based on the experience with restorative proctocolectomy and intersphincteric excision, the reported 38% incidence of male sexual dysfunction should not be a figure that we need to use when counselling our patients today. The report from the Lahey Clinic (Corman et al, 1978) of no impotence in 76 men following proctocolectomy for inflammatory bowel disease is what can and should now be achieved.

Incidence in women

The problem of impaired sexual function in women is a subject that was almost completely ignored in the surgical literature until the 1980s (Brouillette et al, 1981; Nilsson et al, 1981). Leicester et al (1984) reported permanent sexual difficulties in 20% of female patients and transient problems in a further 12% of women after intersphincteric rectal excision (see Table 11.1). Watts et al (1966) reported a 7% incidence of sexual difficulties after rectal excision for inflammatory bowel disease, most being of a mechanical nature, causing dyspareunia, or related to an appliance. Burnham et al (1977) found that 16% of women with an ileostomy had dyspareunia even though they had not undergone rectal excision. This accords with the observations made by Jones and Orr (1983) and by Gruner et al (1975) that respectively 40% and 50% of their patients complained of dyspareunia after ileorectal anastomosis.

Admittedly, in some female patients symptoms may be associated with severe rectal disease present before the operation, while others may be due to gynaecological or psychological causes. However, in the Ileostomy Association survey undertaken by Burnham et al (Table 11.10), 33% of women who had a proctectomy and an ileostomy complained of dyspareunia. In many patients pain during coitus is due to vaginal stenosis, chronic vaginitis, perineal sepsis, persistent perineal sinus, some degree of uterine prolapse or vaginal dryness.

Metcalf et al (1986) assessed the incidence of sexual dysfunction in women after reservoir ileostomy and ileoanal anastomosis. Compared with the performance before operation, the incidence of dyspareunia fell after both operations, but the reduction was greater after ileoanal anastomosis than after reservoir ileostomy. Frequency of intercourse also rose and only 2% of patients were unable to achieve an orgasm after operation. The Goteborg group reported that sexual arousal was not disturbed by restorative proctocolectomy; 16 out of 20 graded their sexual drive as strong, while five considered that their sexual interest had diminished. Fourteen of 20 patients achieved regular orgasm. Two women had reduced vaginal sensitivity, three had episodes of bowel leakage during orgasm, and five had pain on intercourse. Overall, 19 of 20 women reported that they were content with their sexual life following pouch surgery (Oresland et al, 1994).

ASSESSMENT AND TREATMENT OF SEXUAL PROBLEMS

Psychology

It is often helpful for a stoma care nurse to speak to the patient and partner, preferably in their home environment, so as to evaluate the severity of the problem, evaluate marital harmony and assess the level of understanding and cooperation between the partners (Frizelle and Nelson, 1997). Extramarital relationships may complicate the issue.

Women

Women can sometimes be helped by close consultation between the colorectal surgeon, gynaecologist, psychosexual counsellor or plastic surgical colleagues. A narrowed introitus may be corrected using some form of reconstructive procedure. Patients with a cystocele and a uterine prolapse should be referred to the gynaecologist but, if there is a history of urgency, dribbling or stress incontinence as well, we seek the help of a gynaecologist who has a special interest in urinary incontinence or the expertise of a urologist. The specialty of urogynaecology has now emerged to help women with these particular functional and sexual symptoms.

In these patients, detailed investigations of any functional abnormality by cystometrograms and flow studies are often very valuable. If there is a persistent perineal sinus, serious thought should be given to excising the defect and attempting closure with a myocutaneous flap. Perineorrhaphy is worth considering if the perineal body is deficient. Repair of a vaginoperineal fistula often achieves gratifying results in patients who experience sexual difficulties, discharge and impaired body image as a result of this deformity.

Men

Impotence after pelvic surgery is usually due to neurological or vascular damage. Occasionally a patient with a new stoma may have psychological problems which lead to erectile difficulty, in which case spontaneous nocturnal erections are normally preserved. In practical terms, in the majority of patients there is little point in extensive investigations to try and distinguish between neurological or vascular causes, as the treatment is usually the same. In extremely well-motivated younger men, vascular reconstruction may be considered, but the results are extremely disappointing (Lumley, 1991). If investigations are to be performed (Jevitich, 1981), the best method of looking at the blood supply to the penis is by colour Doppler ultrasound after injection of a vasoactive drug (Desai and Gilbert 1991).

The majority of impotent men are treated (i) by injection of a vasoactive substance into the corpora of the penis, (ii) by a vacuum device, or (iii) by surgical insertion of a penile prosthesis. The vasoactive agent used most commonly is prostaglandin E1 (Porst, 1996). It is a simple matter to teach patients self-injection at home, and following injection a normal erection of variable duration will result. Priapism and penile fibrosis, which have been reported frequently with other vasoactive agents, are rare but can occur. Suction devices (Bodansky, 1994) produce a less normal erection but some men find them preferable to use. Penile prostheses can either be semi-malleable rods which are simple to insert but with which flaccidity is significantly compromised (Moul and McCleod 1986), or inflatable devices which are cosmetically better. The latter consist of fluid-filled cylinders which are inserted into the corpora of the penis, connected to a reservoir in the retropubic space and a pump in the scrotum. When the pump is activated fluid flows from the reservoir into the cylinders, producing an erection. Infection is the biggest complication, but the cosmetic and functional results are very good (Garber, 1994, Lewis, 1995).

Promising results have been obtained in preliminary studies with the oral agent Sildenafil (Viagra) (a selective inhibitor of GMP phosphodiesterase), which causes potentiation of the action of nitric oxide, a potent vasodilator of fundamental importance in the erectile process. The drug has been shown to improve erectile function in men with impotence of varied aetiology (Boolell et al, 1996), and in the future it may be of benefit to impotent men with incomplete neurological or vascular damage.

REFERENCES

Alexander R & Glenn WF (1965) The psychosomatic approach. In Wolman DB (ed) *Handbook of Clinical Psychology*, pp 108–119. New York: McGraw-Hill.

Alexander-Williams J (1997) Counselling of patients with inflammatory bowel disease. In Allen RN, Keighley MRB, Alexander-Williams J & Hawkins C (eds) *Inflammatory Bowel Diseases*, 2nd edn, p 917. London: Churchill Livingstone.

Bacon HE, Bralow SP and Berkley JL (1960) Rehabilitation and long-term survival after colectomy for UC. *JAMA* **172**: 324–328.

Balslev I & Harling H (1983) Sexual dysfunction following operation for carcinoma of the rectum. *Dis Colon Rectum* **26**: 785–788.

Bambrick M, Fazio VW, Hull TL & Georgia P (1996) Sexual function following restorative proctocolectomy in women. *Dis Colon Rectum* **39**: 610–614.

Barwin BW, Harley JM & Wilson W (1974) Ileostomy in pregnancy. *Br J Clin Pract* **20**: 256–258.

Bauer JJ, Galernt IM, Salky B & Kreel I (1983) Sexual dysfunction following proctocolectomy for benign disease of the colon and rectum. *Ann Surg* **197**: 363–367.

Beart R (1986) Burroughs Wellcome's visiting professorial address. London: Royal Society of Medicine.

Bergman B, Nilsson S & Petersen I (1979) The effect on erection and orgasm of cystectomy, prostatectomy and vesiculectomy for cancer of the bladder: a clinical and electromyographic study. *Br J Urol* **51**: 114–120.

Bernstein LH, Frank MS, Brandt LD & Boley SJ (1980) Healing of perineal Crohn's disease with metronidazole. *Gastroenterology* **79**: 357–365.

Bernstein WC & Bernstein EF (1966) Sexual dysfunction following radical surgery for cancer of the rectum. *Dis Colon Rectum* **9**: 328–332.

Bodansky HJ (1994) Treatment of male erectile dysfunction using the active vacuum assist device. *Diabet Med* **11**: 410–412.

Bone J & Sorensen FH (1974) Life with a conventional ileostomy. *Dis Colon Rectum* **17**: 194–199.

Boolell M, Gepi-Attee S, Gingell JC, Allen MJ (1996) Sildenafil, a novel effective oral therapy for male erectile dysfunction. *Br J Urol* **78**: 257–261.

Brooke BN (1983) Indications for emergency and elective surgery. In Allan RN, Keighley MRB, Alexander-Williams J & Hawkins C (eds) *Inflammatory Bowel Diseases*, p 240. London: Churchill Livingstone.

Brouillette JN, Pryor E & Fox TA (1981) Evaluation of sexual dysfunction in the female following rectal resection and intestinal stoma. *Dis Colon Rectum* **24**: 96–102.

Burnham WR, Lennard-Jones JE & Brooke BN (1977) Sexual problems among married ileostomists. *Gut* **18**: 673–677.

Clyne CAC, Hanby A, Jenkins JD & Stuart CJ (1982) Impotence: relevance and assessment in the surgical patient. *Ann R Coll Surg Eng* **64**: 248–254.

Cohen Z, McLeod RS, Stern H, Grant D & Nordgren S (1985) The pelvic pouch and ileoanal anastomosis procedure. *Am J Surg* **150**: 601–607.

Corman ML, Verdenheimer MC & Coller JA (1978) Impotence after proctectomy for inflammatory disease of the bowel. *Dis Colon Rectum* **21**: 418–419.

Daly DW & Brooke BN (1967) Ileostomy and excision of the large intestine for UC. *Lancet* **ii**: 62–64.

Danzi M, Ferulano GP, Abate S & Califani G (1983) Male sexual function after abdominoperineal resection for rectal cancer. *Dis Colon Rectum* **26**: 665–668.

Davis LP & Jelenko C (1975) Sexual function after abdominoperineal resection. *South Med J* **68**: 422–426.

Deizonne B, Baumel H & Domergue J (1982) Les troubles sexuals après amputation abdomino-perineale du rectum. *Ann Chir* **36**: 475–480.

Dennis C (1945) Ileostomy and colectomy in chronic UC. *Surgery* **18**: 435–452.

Desai KM, and Gilbert HG (1991) Noninvasive investigation of penile artery function. In Kirby RS, Carson CC & Webster GD (eds) *Impotence: Diagnosis and Management of Male Erectile Dysfunction*, pp 81–91. Oxford: Butterworth-Heinemann.

Devlin B, Plant JA & Griffin M (1971) Aftermath of surgery for anorectal cancer. *BMJ* **3**: 413–418.

Devlin B & Plant JA (1979) Sexual function in aspects of stoma care. *Br J Sex Med* **6**: 33–37.

Donovan MJ & O'Hara ET (1960) Sexual function following surgery for UC. *N Engl J Med* **262**: 719–720.

Dozois RR (1985) Ileal 'J' pouch – anal anastomosis. *Br J Surg* **72** (Suppl): S80.

Druss RG, O'Connor JF, Purdden JF & Stern LO (1968) Psychologic response to colectomy. *Arch Gen Psychiatr* **18**: 53–59.

Druss RG, O'Connor JF & Stern LO (1969) Psychological response to colectomy. II: Adjustment to a permanent colostomy. *Arch Gen Psychiatr* **20**: 419–427.

Durdey P, Quirke P, Dixon MF & Williams NS (1986) Lateral spread of rectal cancer, the key to local recurrence. *Br J Surg* **73**: A1042.

Dyk RB & Sutherland M (1956) Adaptation of the spouse and other family members to the colostomy patient. *Cancer* **9**: 123–138.

Ecker KW, Hildebrandt U, Haberer M & Feifel G (1996) Biomechanical stabilization of the nipple valve in continent ileostomy. *Br J Surg* **83**: 1582–1585.

Engel GL (1958) Studies of UC: Psychological aspects and their implications for treatment. *Am J Dig Dis* **3**: 315–337.

Entman SS & Wilson G (1982) Conservative coloprotectomy for the sexually active woman. *Surg Gynecol Obstet* **155**: 77–80.

Fazio VW, Fletcher J & Montague D (1980) Prospective study of the effect of resection of the rectum on male sexual function. *World J Surg* **4**: 149–152.

Finkle AL, Moyer TG, Tobenkia W & Karg SJ (1959) Sexual potency in aging males. *JAMA* **170**: 1391–1393.

Fischer S & Cleveland SE (1967) *Body Image and Personality*. New York: Dover.

Frego M, Biasiato R, Ranzato R, Bianchera G, Rampazzo L & D'Amico D (1982) Le disfurzioni sessmali dopa amputazione del retto secondo miles per neoplasia. *Acta Chir Ital* **38**: 525–535.

Frizelle FA & Nelson H (1997) Psychological factors influencing sexual function. In Allan RN, Keighley MRB, Alexander-Williams J & Hawkins C (eds) *Inflammatory Bowel Diseases*, 3rd edn, pp 943–946. London: Churchill Livingstone.

Garber B (1994) Meteor Alpha-1 inflatable penile prosthesis: patient satisfaction and device reliability. *Urology* **43**: 214–217.

Goligher JC (1951) Sexual function after excision of the rectum. *Proc R Soc Med* **44**: 824–827.

Goligher JC (1983) Proctocolectomy and ileostomy for UC. In Allan RN, Keighley MRB, Alexander-Williams J & Hawkins C (eds) *Inflammatory Bowel Diseases*, p 247. London: Churchill Livingstone.

Gopal KA, Amshel AL, Shonberg IL et al (1985) Ostomy and pregnancy. *Dis Colon Rectum* **28**: 912–916.

Gruner OPN, Flatmark A, Nass R et al (1975) Ileorectal anastomosis in UC. Scand J Gastroenterol 10: 641–646.

Gruner OPN, Nass R, Fretheim B & Gjone E (1977) Marital status and sexual adjustment after colectomy: results of 178 patients operated on for UC. *Scand J Gastroenterol* **12**: 193–197.

Harrison JE & McDonagh JE (1950) Hernia of Douglas's pouch and high rectocele. *Am J Obstet Gynecol* **60**: 83–92.

Heald RT & Leicester RJ (1981) The low stapled anastomosis. *Br J Surg* **68**: 333–337.

Herman A, Adar R & Rubenstein Z (1978) Vascular lesions associated with impotence in diabetic and non-diabetic arterial occlusive disease. *Diabetes* **27**: 975–981.

Hudson CN (1972) Ileostomy in pregnancy. *J R Soc Med* **65**: 281–283.

Hughes ESR & Russell IS (1967) Ileorectal anastomosis for UC. *Dis Colon Rectum* **10**: 35–39.

Jevitich MJ (1981) Penile body temperature as screening test for penile arterial obstruction in impotence. *Urology* **17**: 132–135.

Jones PF & Orr G (1983) Colectomy and ileorectal anastomosis. In Allan RN, Keighley RMB, Alexander-Williams J & Hawkins C (eds) *Inflammatory Bowel Diseases*, pp 268–273. London: Churchill Livingstone.

Jones PF, Munro A & Ewan SWB (1977) Colectomy and ileorectal anastomosis for colitis: report on a personal series, with a critical review. *Br J Surg* **64**: 615–623.

Juhasz ES, Fozard B, Dozois RR, Ilstrup DM & Nelson H (1995) Ileal pouch–anal anastomosis function following childbirth: an extended evaluation. *Dis Colon Rectum* **38**: 159–165.

Keighley MRB, Ogunbiyi OA & Korsgen S (1997) Pitfalls and outcome in ileo-anal pouch surgery for ulcerative colitis. *Netherlands J Med*, S23–S27.

Keltikangas-Jarvinen L, Loven E & Moller C (1984) Psychic factors determining the long-term adaptation of colostomy and ileostomy patients. *Psychother Psychosom* **41**: 153–159.

Kempczinski RF (1979) The role of the vascular diagnostic laboratory in the evaluation of male impotence. *Am J Surg* **138**: 278–282.

Kennedy HT, Lee ECG, Claridge G & Truelove SC (1982) The health of subjects living with a permanent ileostomy. *Q J Med* **51**: 341–357.

Kinn A-C & Ohman U (1986) Bladder and sexual function after surgery for rectal cancer. *Dis Colon Rectum* **29**: 43–48.

Kinsey D (1948) *Sexual Behaviour in the Human Male*. Philadelphia: WB Saunders.

Kock NG (1983) Continent ileostomy. In Allan RN, Keighley MRB, Alexander-Williams J & Hawkins C (eds) *Inflammatory Bowel Diseases*, pp 278–280. London: Churchill Livingstone.

Kock NG, Darke N, Kenentes J, Myvold H & Philipson B (1974) The quality of life after proctocolectomy and ileostomy. *Dis Colon Rectum* **17**: 287–292.

Kolb LC (1975) Disturbances of the body image. In Arieti LC (ed.) *American Handbook of Psychiatry*, pp 39–46. New York: Basic Books.

Kretschew KP (1972) *Intestinal Stoma*, pp 281–283. Philadelphia: WB Saunders.

La Monica G, Audisio RA, Tamburini M, Filiberti A & Ventafridda V (1985) Incidence of sexual dysfunction in male patients treated surgically for rectal malignancy. *Dis Colon Rectum* **28**: 937–940.

Lee EC & Dowling BL (1972) Perimuscular excision of the rectum for Crohn's disease and UC. *Br J Surg* **59**: 29–32.

Leicester RJ, Ritchie JK, Wadsworth J, Thomson JPS & Hawley PR (1984) Sexual function and perineal wound healing after intersphincteric excision of the rectum for inflammatory bowel disease. *Dis Colon Rectum* **27**: 244–248.

Lennenberg E (1971) Role of enterostomal therapist and stoma rehabilitation clinics. *Cancer* **28**: 226–229.

Leriche R & Morel A (1948) The syndrome of thrombotic obliteration of the aortic bifurcation. *Ann Surg* **27**: 193–206.

Le Shan L (1961) A basic psychological orientation apparently associated with malignant disease. *Psychiatr Q* **35**: 314–330.

Lewis RW (1995). Long-term results of penile prosthesis implants. *Uro Clin N Am* **22**: 847–856.

Lockhart-Mummery HE & Ritchie JK (1983) In Allan RN, Keighley MRB, Alexander-Williams J & Hawkins C (eds) *Inflammatory Bowel Diseases*, pp 468–480. London: Churchill Livingstone.

Lumley JSP (1991) Arterial revascularization. In Kirby RS, Carson CC, Webster GD (eds) *Impotence: Diagnosis and Management of Male Erectile Dysfunction*, pp 184–192. Oxford: Butterworth-Heinemann.

Lyttle JA & Parks AG (1977) Intersphincteric excision of the rectum. *Br J Surg* **64**: 413–416.

McEwan HP (1965) Pregnancy in patients with surgically treated ulcerative colitis. *J Obstet Gynaecol Br Commonw* **72**: 450–451.

Machledger HI & Weinstein M (1975) Sexual dysfunction following surgical therapy for aorto-iliac disease. *Vasc Surg* **9**: 283–287.

Masui H, Ike H, Yamaguchi S, Oki S & Shimada H (1996) Male sexual function after autonomic nerve-preserving operation for rectal cancer. *Dis Colon Rectum* **39**: 1140–1145.

May RE (1966) Sexual dysfunction following rectal excision for UC. *Br J Surg* **53**: 29–30.

Metcalf AM, Dozois RR & Kelly K (1986) Sexual function in women after proctocolectomy. *Ann Surg* **204**: 624–627.

Moody GA & Mayberry JF (1996) Life insurance and inflammatory bowel disease: is there discrimination against patients? *Int J Colorect Dis* **11**: 276–278.

Moody GA & Mayberry JF (1997) Social consequences of inflammatory bowel disease. In Allan RN, Keighley MRB, Alexander-Williams J & Hawkins C (eds) *Inflammatory Bowel Diseases*, 3rd edn, pp 947–150. London: Churchill Livingstone.

Moody G, Probert CSJ, Srivastava EM, Rhodes J & Mayberry JF (1992). Sexual dysfunction among women with Crohn's disease: a hidden problem. *Digestion* **52**: 179–183.

Morgan RJ (1982) Assessment and treatment of impotence. *J R Soc Med* **75**: 666–669.

Morrow L (1976) Psychological problems following ileostomy and colostomy. *Mt Sinai J Med* **43**: 368–370.

Moul JW & McCleod DG (1986) Experience with the AMS 600 malleable penile prosthesis. *J Urol* **135**: 929–934.

Mullen P, Behrens D, Chalmers T et al (1995) Barnett continent intestinal reservoir: multicenter experience with an alternative to the Brooke ileostomy. *Dis Colon Rectum* **38**: 573–582.

Nath RL, Menzoian J, Kaplan KH et al (1981) The multidisciplinary approach to vasculogenic impotence. *Surgery* **89**: 124–133.

Neal DE, Williams NS & Johnston D (1982) Rectal, bladder and sexual function after mucosal proctectomy with and without a pelvic reservoir for colitis and polyposis. *Br J Surg* **69**: 599–604.

Nicholls J (1984) Restorative proctocolectomy with a three-loop ileal reservoir for UC and familial adenomatous polyposis. *Ann Surg* **199**: 383–388.

Nicholls RJ, Ritchie JK, Wadsworth J et al (1979) Total excision or restorative resection for carcinoma of the middle third of the rectum. *Br J Surg* **66**: 625–627.

Nilsson LO, Kock NG, Kylberg F, Myrvold ME & Palselius I (1981) Sexual adjustment in ileostomy patients before and after conversion to continent ileostomy. *Dis Colon Rectum* **24**: 287–290.

Orbach EC, Bard M & Sutherland AM (1957) Fears and defensive adaptations to the loss of anal sphincter control. *Psychiatr Rev* **44**: 121–175.

Orbach EC & Tallent N (1965) Modifications of perceived body and body concepts. *Arch Gen Psychiatr* **12**: 126–135.

Oresland T, Palmblad S, Ellstrom M et al (1994) Gynaecological and sexual function related to anatominal changes in the female pelvis after restorative proctocolectomy. *Int J Colorect Dis* **9**:77–81.

Petter O, Gruner N, Rerdar N et al (1977) Marital status and sexual adjustment after colectomy. *Scand J Gastroenterol* **12**: 193–197.

Phillips R, Pringle W, Evans C & Keighley MRB (1985) Analysis of a hospital based stomatherapy service. *Ann R Coll Surg Engl* **67**: 37–40.

Porst H (1996). The rationale for prostaglandin E1. *Br J Urol* **155**: 802–805.

Priest FO, Gilchrist RK & Long JS (1959) Pregnancy in the patient with ileostomy and colectomy. *JAMA* **169**: 213–215.

Queral LA, Whitehouse WM, Flinn WR, Zarins CK, Bargan JJ & Yao JSR (1979) Pelvic haemodynamics after aortoiliac reconstruction. *Surgery* **86**: 799–809.

Rhodes JB & Kirsner JB (1965) The early and late course of patients with UC after ileostomy and colectomy. *Surg Gynecol Obstet* **125**: 1303–1314.

Ritchie JK (1972) UC treated by ileostomy and excisional surgery: 15 years' experience at St Mark's Hospital. *Br J Surg* **59**: 345–351.

Rolstad BS, Wilson G & Rotherberger DA (1983) Sexual concerns in the patient with an ileostomy. *Dis Colon Rectum* **26**: 170–171.

Rothenberger DA, Bols JG, Nivatvangs S & Goldberg (1985) The Parks S ileal pouch and anal anastomosis after colectomy and muscosal proctectomy. *Am J Surg* **149**: 390–394.

Roy PH, Sauer WG, Beahrs OH & Farrow GM (1970) Experience with ileostomies: evaluation of long-term rehabilitation in 497 patients. *Am J Surg* **118**: 77–86.

Sabri S & Cotton LT (1971) Sexual function after aorto-iliac reconstruction. *Lancet* **ii**: 1218–1219.

Santangelo ML, Romano G & Sassaroli C (1987) Sexual function after resection for rectal cancer. *Am J Surg* **154**: 502–504.

Scammell B & Keighley MRB (1986) Delayed perineal wound healing after proctectomy for Crohn's colitis. *Br J Surg* **73**: 150–152.

Scudamore HH, Rogers AG, Bargen JA & Bonner EA (1957) Pregnancy after ileostomy for chronic UC. *Gastroenterology* **32**: 295–303.

Silverman SH, Moore J, Thompson H & Keighley MRB (1984) Intraoperative staging of rectal cancer by imprint cytology. *Gut* **25**: A1150.

Stahlgren LH & Ferguson LK (1959) Effects of abdominoperineal resection on sexual function in 60 patients with UC. *Arch Surg* **78**: 604–606.

Stelzner F (1977) Uber Potenztorungen nach Amputation und Kotinerzresektion des Rectums (English abstract). *Zentrabl Chir* **102**: 212–219.

Stevens PJ d'E (1997) Running a stomaltherapy service. In Allan RN, Keighley MRB, Alexander-Williams J & Hawkins C (eds) *Inflammatory Bowel Diseases*, 3rd edn, pp 913–916. London: Churchill Livingstone.

Tomkins RG & Warshaw AL (1985) Improved management of the perineal wound after proctectomy. *Ann Surg* **202**: 760–765.

Toth A (1979) Male infertility due to sulphasalazine. *Lancet* **ii**: 904.

Van Pronaska J & Siderins NJ (1962) The surgical rehabilitation of patients with chronic UC. *Am J Surg* **103**: 42–46.

Veidenheimer MC, Dailey TH & Meissner WA (1970) Ileorectal anastomosis for inflammatory disease of the large bowel. *Am J Surg* **119**: 375–378.

Walsh PC & Schlegal PN (1988) Radical pelvic surgery with preservation of sexual function. *Ann Surg* **208**: 391–400.

Watson PC & Williams DI (1952) The urological complications of excision of the rectum. *Br J Surg* **40**: 19–28.

Watts JM, De Dombal FT & Goligher JC (1966) Long-term complications and prognosis following major surgery for UC. *Br J Surg* **53**: 1014–1022.

Weinstein M & Roberts M (1977) Sexual potency following surgery for rectal cancer: a follow up of 44 patients. *Ann Surg* **185**: 295–300.

Williams DI, Watson PC & Goligher JC (1951) Sexual dysfunction following abdominoperineal resection for carcinoma. *Proc R Soc Med* **44**: 819–828.

Williams JT & Slack WW (1980) A prospective study of sexual function after major colorectal surgery. *Br J Surg* **67**: 772–774.

Williams NS & Johnston D (1983) The quality of life after rectal excision for low rectal cancer. *Br J Surg* **70**: 460–462.

Williams NS, Neal DE & Johnston D (1980) Bladder function after excision of the rectum for low rectal carcinoma. *Gut* **21**: A453–454.

Willoughby CP & Truelove SC (1980) UC and pregnancy. *Gut* **21**: 469–474.

Wirsching M, Druner HU & Herrman G (1975) Results of psychosocial adjustment to long term colostomy. *Psychother Psychosom* **26**: 245–256.

Yeager FS & van Heerden JA (1980) Sexual dysfunction following proctocolectomy and abdominoperineal resection. *Ann Surg* **191**: 169–170.

12

HAEMORRHOIDAL DISEASE

Section I: Causes, natural history and assessment

Haemorrhoids are one of the most common ailments to afflict mankind, but it is impossible to give an accurate figure for their prevalence. Although many patients present with symptomatic disease, many do not and some never have symptoms. Whether such individuals can be considered to have a disease must remain a moot point.

Certainly, vascular cushions within the anal canal do not differ anatomically in normal individuals from those in symptomatic patients. It is therefore probably illogical to talk about the incidence of vascular cushions since they are ubiquitous. Both sexes, all races and all ages have anal cushions. If the cushions are omnipresent then it is only the existence of symptoms that merits classification as a disease.

TERMINOLOGY

The very names that we choose to describe the disease indicate that our assessment is purely subjective and symptom-oriented. The word 'haemorrhoid' is derived from the Greek *haemorrhoides*, meaning flowing of blood (*haem* = blood, *rhoos* = flowing). In the authorized translation of the Holy Bible this is written as 'emerods' (1 Sam 5:9). The word 'pile' comes from the Latin *pila* meaning a pill or ball. To be accurate, we should call the disease 'piles' when the patient complains of a swelling and 'haemorrhoids' when he or she complains of bleeding. What if they have both? In truth, no one who has symptoms that do not include bleeding can be said to have haemorrhoids.

The terms for the disease in use in other languages imply different judgement qualities that further confuse the terminology. Italians, still following the teachings of Galen, refer to *profluvio di sangue*, suggesting an overflow of blood and implying, as do some patients, that such an overflow may be beneficial. Our phlebotomizing predecessors relied on such a belief. The ancient French referred to the *flux d'or* (flow of gold) and the ancient Germans to *goldene ader* (golden veins), implying that proctological symptoms may have been the prerogative of the rich!

In order not to confuse the reader we have chosen to use the term 'haemorrhoidal disease' – while appreciating its limitations – to describe all patients with enlarged anal cushions who complain of symptoms.

ANATOMY, PATHOPHYSIOLOGY AND AETIOLOGY

Beneath the epithelial lining of the anal canal there are rich plexuses of vascular tissue. These serpiginous vessels have been called the 'corpus cavenosi recti'. They connect arteries to veins without intervening capillaries. The vessels are normally interspersed and supported by longitudinal muscle fibres (muscularis submucosae ani) which help to retain the vascular cushions in their position within the upper half of the anal canal. There are three major vascular cushions in the anal canal; one on the left, and an anterior and a posterior one on the right (Figure 12.1). Goligher (1984) stated that two-thirds of the patients requiring treatment for haemorrhoids had three primary cushions, while the remaining third had secondary cushions.

Miles (1939), impressed by the severity of the haemorrhage that occurred if a ligature slipped off a vascular pedicle following haemorrhoidectomy, postulated that each primary pile site was determined by the termination of the right and left main branches of the superior haemorrhoidal artery. The right one was said to divide into an anterior and posterior branch and so the sites of primary haemorrhoids were left or right anterior and right posterior. WHF Thomson (1975), in an injection preparation of the superior rectal arteries in cadavers, failed to substantiate Miles' hypothesis.

Another, even less credible, hypothesis is that the three primary sites are due to a condensation of mesenchyme which represent a continuation into the rectum of three taeniae coli. It has been postulated that the submucosa may be less well supported between these bundles of smooth muscle than it is elsewhere; hence the mucosa prolapses more easily and there is space at these sites for large vascular cushions.

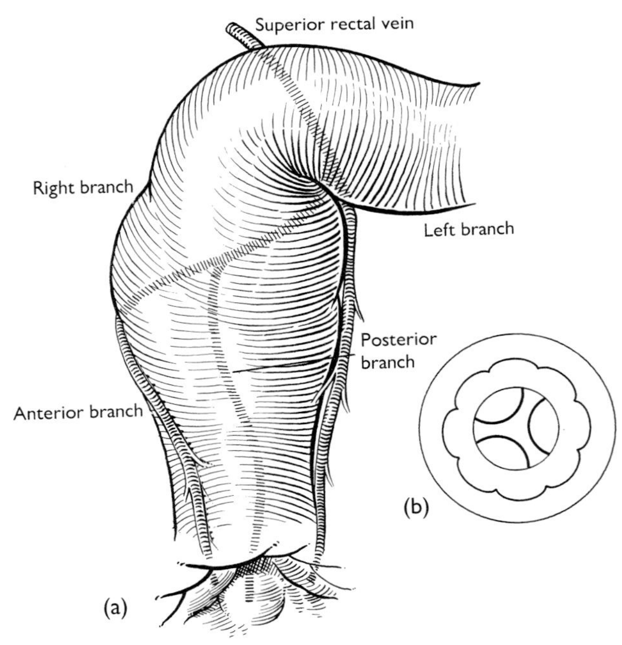

Figure 12.1 (a) Standard anatomical distribution of haemorrhoids according to the branches of the superior rectal vein. (b) At 3, 7 and 11 o'clock as seen through the proctoscope.

Similar, less prominent, vascular channels are found beneath the skin of the outer anal canal. They are not regularly arranged and do not have muscle fibres within the vascular tissue.

The role of the vascular cushions in the process of normal rectal evacuation is incompletely understood, but straining at defecation is obviously important in the development of haemorrhoidal disease. It is readily observed during anoscopy that the cushions rapidly empty and fill. If a patient can prolapse the outer piles on demand, they can be observed to enlarge dramatically and to decongest just as rapidly once they are returned to their normal position within the anal canal. It is postulated that decongestion of haemorrhoids is achieved by rapidly increasing the diameter of the anal canal allowing rapid emptying of 200–300 g of faeces from within the rectum.

At the end of normal defecation, voluntary sphincter contraction returns any residual faecal material from the anal canal to the rectum. It is not necessary for there to be any forced abdominal contraction to evacuate residual anal canal contents. Straining to complete rectal evacuation serves only to congest the vascular cushions, particularly if they are still situated below the zone of sphincter contraction.

The following may be important factors in the aetiology of haemorrhoidal disease.

Venous obstruction

The principal cause of haemorrhoidal disease seems to be congestion and hypertrophy of the internal anal cushions. The cushions congest because (1) they fail to empty rapidly during the act of defecation, (2) they are abnormally mobile, or (3) they are trapped by a tight anal sphincter. When the cushions are congested, they are more likely to bleed and to become oedematous. The oedema causes swelling and stretching of the tissues, and finally hypertrophy.

Failure of the cushions to empty rapidly is an often-postulated but never proven hypothesis to explain the cause of haemorrhoidal disease. Anatomical vascular pathways of venous drainage through the rectal musculature have been demonstrated and it is suggested that a faecal mass impacted in the rectum may compress these veins (Figure 12.2). Furthermore, the act of straining constricts the intermuscular veins by raising intra-abdominal pressure and so impedes the rapid emptying of the cushions. Rapid filling of the cushions can be observed during anoscopy by asking the

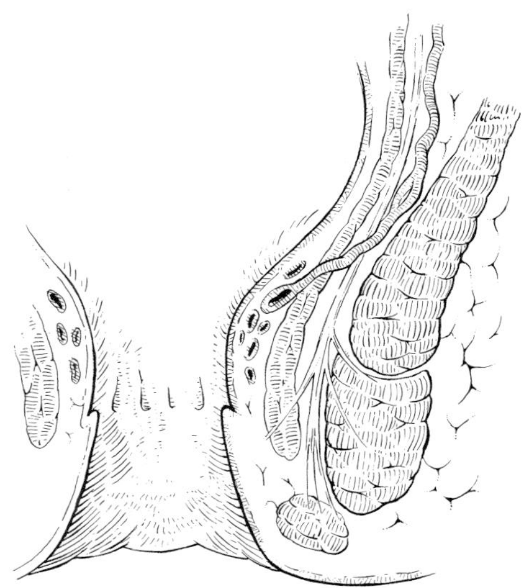

Figure 12.2 Aetiology of haemorrhoids. The internal vascular cushions drain via veins which pass through the circular and longitudinal muscle coats. These veins could become obstructed by a faecal mass.

patient or even a normal subject to strain during examination. Whether the speed of filling and emptying is different in normal asymptomatic individuals from that in those who have or who are prone to develop haemorrhoidal disease is not known. To our knowledge there are no records of attempts to measure these phenomena.

Raised intra-abdominal pressure during pregnancy, from ascites or from a pelvic tumour, or raised portal venous pressure with hepatic cirrhosis, have been postulated as predisposing factors. Jacobs et al (1980) found an incidence of symptomatic internal haemorrhoids in 52 (28%) of 188 patients with known portal hypertension. In another study (Hosking et al, 1989), it was found that haemorrhoids and anorectal varices can coexist in patients with portal hypertension. In the first prospective study of its kind it was found that of 100 patients with cirrhosis, 44% had anorectal varices and 63% had haemorrhoids. The prevalance of anorectal varices differed according to the degree of portal hypertension: it was 19% in cirrhotic patients without portal hypertension and 59% in those who had bled from oesophageal varices. No relationship was found between haemorrhoids and portal hypertension. These authors were of the opinion that the incidence of haemorrhoids in adults was little different from the 50% prevalence claimed in the general population (Buie, 1937). However, the situation in children with portal hypertension seems to be different. In a prospective study, Heaton et al (1993) found that in 60 children with portal hypertension, 33% had haemorrhoids, 35% had anorectal varices and 15% had external anal varices. The patients with extrahepatic disease had a higher incidence of lesions than those with intrahepatic disease. Certainly a 33% incidence of haemorrhoids seems much higher than that expected in a similar group of normal children, although such *comparative* data are not available. Despite this high incidence, Heaton et al (1992) found that only 7% complained of symptoms, and in a similar yet retrospective study the same authors found that 4.7% of 189 children with portal hypertension had symptoms from anorectal varices or haemorrhoids.

During pregnancy the vascular structures of the pelvis and perineum become more prominent. It is not surprising, therefore, that perianal and anorectal venous channels become more evident and more likely to be seen or felt to protrude during defecation. This phenomenon is often termed the 'piles of pregnancy', but it is not necessarily abnormal. It is not known whether nulliparous women are more prone to the symptoms of haemorrhoidal disease than multiparous. Men are twice as likely to have symptoms attributable to haemorrhoidal disease, so that pregnancy alone cannot be considered as the primary aetiological factor.

There is certainly no evidence to support the once perpetuated myth that carcinoma of the rectum predisposes to enlarged anal cushions by obstructing the middle haemorrhoidal veins.

Prolapse of vascular cushions

In the child and healthy adult the submucosal vascular cushions are supported by the pecten band (or, as the French term it, the ligament of Parks) and by the muscularis submucosae. The vascular cushions and the muscularis are normally only loosely attached to the underlying circular muscle. During the act of defecation, as the internal sphincter relaxes, there is an outward rotation of the vascular tissue and the pecten band. This rotation produces parting of the 'lips' of the anorectum (Figure 12.3a–c).

It is probable that some derangement of this natural rotation and return of the anorectum is the fundamental mechanism responsible for haemorrhoidal disease. Some of the factors that disturb the normal eversion and rotation of the anorectum are endocrine, age, constipation and prolonged straining (Jackson and Robertson, 1965).

Elastic tissue in the rectal submucosa, which is

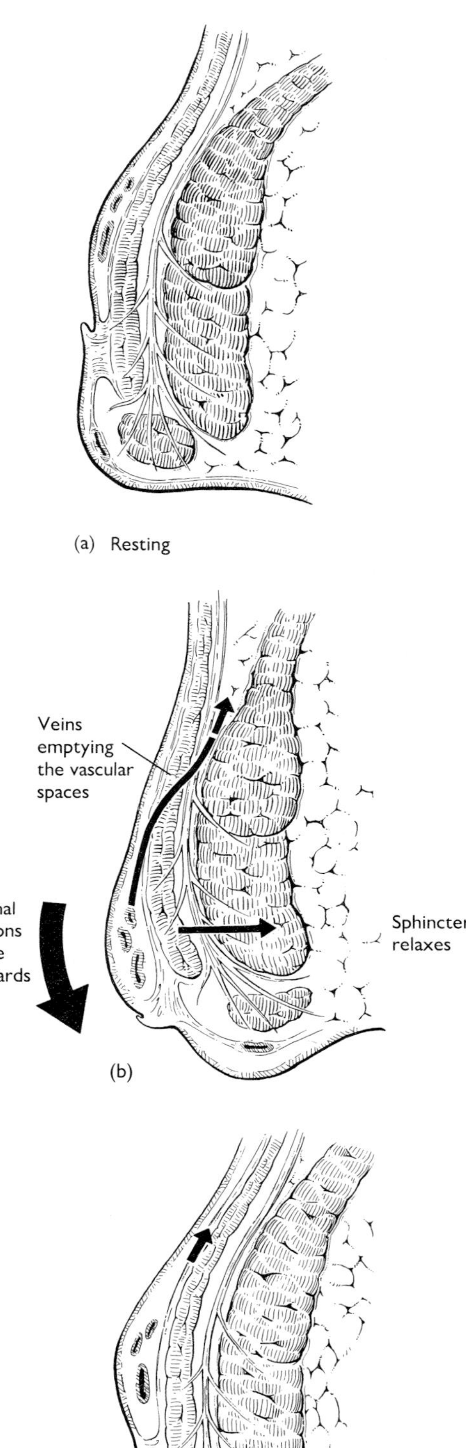

Figure 12.3a–c The effect of normal defecation on the internal vascular cushions.

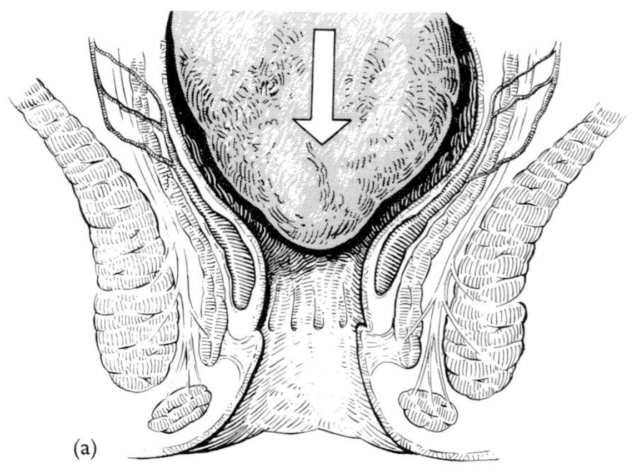

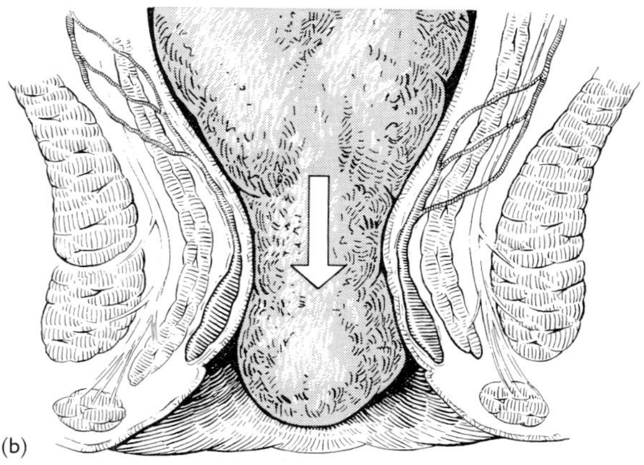

Figure 12.4a,b Aetiology of haemorrhoids. The veins draining the vascular cushions become compressed by a bolus of faeces. The bolus has a shearing effect on the cushions and facilitates their prolapse. Prolonged straining keeps the cushions outside the sphincter, which in turn constricts and congests them.

dense in the newborn, becomes attenuated with age and virtually non-existent in adults with haemorrhoidal disease. This elastic tissue also becomes lax during pregnancy. The efficiency of the muscularis submucosae probably mirrors that of the elastic tissue.

The passage of a hard stool has a shearing effect on the vascular submucosa and facilitates its prolapse from the anal canal. Prolonged straining keeps the vascular cushions outside the lower edge of the internal sphincter, which in turn constricts and congests them (see below) (Figure 12.4a,b).

Heredity

There is no firm evidence of an inherited predisposition to haemorrhoidal disease. A family history is commonly recorded (Acheson, 1960; Gondran, 1976; Brondel and Cleave, 1965), but this is not surprising as diet and defecation habits are usually related to customs and environment, factors that are probably pivotal in the aetiology of haemorrhoidal disease. The argument about hereditary predisposition is not likely to yield any therapeutic or preventive advances and is not worth pursuing.

Geographical and dietary factors

It is a widely held belief that haemorrhoidal disease is the prerogative of Western civilized societies and that it is rare in rural undeveloped countries. First we should consider whether this is true, before we consider why. On what evidence is the increased prevalence in developed countries based? Are patients more likely to complain because medical services are more readily available for non-serious conditions and because proprietary pharmaceutical preparations are more likely to be available for purchase? Is there an increase in anal symptoms due to associated conditions such as pruritus because of less fastidious habits of anal hygiene? These possibilities have a ring of truth. There is no possibility of finding autopsy evidence of haemorrhoidal disease, so the question of relative incidence will not be answered on the evidence of morbid anatomy. The incidence of haemorrhoidal disease is inevitably based on the prevalence of symptoms, since population studies based upon anoscopy are not available. Nevertheless, such respected and careful workers as Burkitt (1972) have stated that haemorrhoidal disease is rare in rural Africa and unknown in primitive communities. He contrasts this with the much higher incidence of anal symptoms in blacks in the USA and in urban Africa. Such opinions cannot be denied. It is possible to speculate further and suggest that the low incidence of haemorrhoidal disease in rural societies is related to the high fibre intake, and that with the adoption of a more 'natural' high-fibre diet in developed countries the incidence will decrease or even disappear. The theory is attractive, and even if it were not true there are other reasons for adopting a high-fibre diet. However, there is no positive or negative evidence from reliable population studies that the incidence of symptoms of haemorrhoidal disease has decreased since the advent of the bran mania of the 1970s; nor is there any evidence from controlled population studies.

If indeed there is a low incidence of haemorrhoidal disease in primitive rural societies, there are factors other than diet that could be cited as important, such as the squatting position for defecation and the lack of social restraint in the timing and location of defecation.

Anal sphincter tone

Measurements of anal sphincter pressures have been made in patients with symptomatic haemorrhoidal disease and compared with those in age- and sex-matched asymptomatic controls. Numerous studies have shown that basal anal pressures are significantly higher in haemorrhoid patients (Hancock and Smith, 1975; Lane and Casula, 1976; Arabi et al, 1977a; Creve and Hubens, 1979; Read et al, 1983; Shafik, 1984; Hiltunen and Matikainen, 1985; Schouten and van Vroonhoven, 1986; Deutsch et al, 1987; Champigneulle et al, 1989; Lin, 1989; Sun et al, 1990, 1992; Farouk et al, 1994). Furthermore, Teramoto et al (1981) in London demonstrated a higher than normal distribution of type I muscle fibres in the external anal sphincter biopsied at haemorrhoidectomy, suggesting a state of tonic contraction of the muscle.

Digital (manual) dilatation of the anus or internal sphincterotomy relieves the anal symptoms and also reduces the resting anal sphincter pressure to the same as that of controls for up to 5 years (Hancock, 1981) (Figure 12.5).

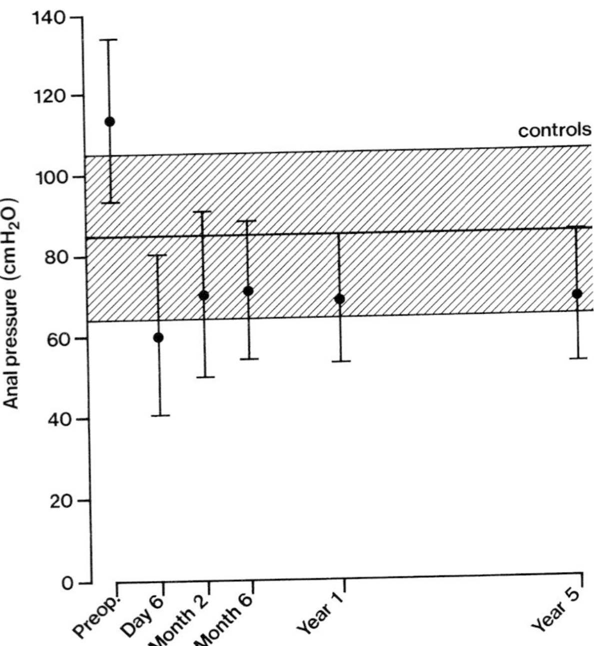

Figure 12.5 Resting anal pressures in haemorrhoidal patients compared with control subjects (shaded area) before and after manual dilatation of the anus. Reproduced with permission from Hancock (1981).

However, it is possibly naive to consider haemorrhoidal disease as a single homogeneous pathophysiological process. In the Birmingham manometric studies (Arabi et al, 1977a), it was proposed that there were two quite different groups of patients with haemorrhoidal disease. The concept of the hypertensive pile patient was introduced on the evidence that just less than half of the haemorrhoidal patients had high anal pressures (greater than ± 2 SD of the mean). These patients tended to be men who presented with non-prolapsing haemorrhoids that bled and caused discomfort. They were recognized clinically as having a tight anal canal. The other patients had anal pressures which were lower than controls: the majority of these patients were women with a rather lax anal canal and haemorrhoids that usually caused symptoms from prolapse; most were multiparous.

Of interest in respect to these manometric findings was a study performed at the Royal London in which ambulant measurements of anorectal pressures and electromyographic (EMG) activity of the external anal sphincter were recorded over a period of 24 hours in patients with prolapsed haemorrhoids and control subjects. Using a probe with microtransducers mounted on it, and surface electrodes, we were able to confirm the findings reported by others using static measurements (Waldron et al, 1989). In addition we demonstrated that haemorrhoidal patients exhibited numerous episodes of spontaneous falls in resting anal pressure which we termed 'sampling reflexes'. These were significantly more common in haemorrhoidal patients than in control subjects (Figure 12.6). It would appear that the greater degree of spontaneous sampling responses in these patients is likely to be due to a normal response of the internal sphincter that allows the anal canal to rid itself of the haemorrhoidal masses. The EMG recordings also showed significantly greater activity in patients than controls. This is perhaps not surprising as the increased external sphincter activity may be an attempt to maintain continence. The chances are that the observed anorectal physiology changes are the effect of the presence of haemorrhoids rather than the cause.

Anal and rectal sensation

Anal electrosensitivity (Roe et al, 1986) and temperature sensation (Miller et al, 1988) are reduced in

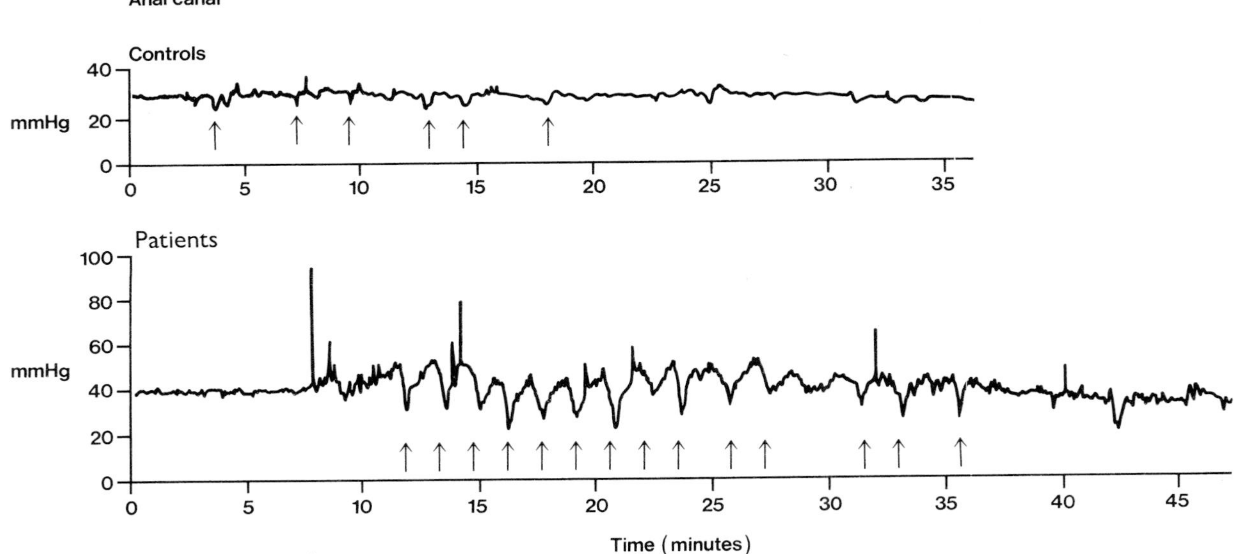

Figure 12.6 Ambulant anal canal pressure. Examples of sampling reflexes in both control subjects and haemorrhoid patients are indicated by arrows. Patients with haemorrhoids have significantly more episodes than controls.

patients with haemorrhoids, the greatest change being in the proximal and mid anal canal, perhaps because of prolapse of less-sensitive rectal mucosa (Read et al, 1983). Rectal sensation to balloon distension does not seem to be affected (Sun et al, 1990).

Defecation habits

Once more, we regret that we can in the main report only folklore, not scientific fact. It is a frequent and reliable observation that many patients with haemorrhoidal disease are those who sit for 10–15 minutes on a comfortable lavatory, taking with them the morning paper or other educational material. Such patients are obsessed by the necessity to have a regular act of defecation and are determined to sit there until they do. They also tend to remain enthroned until the last particle of faeces has been expelled from the anal canal.

If these behavioural factors are commonly associated with haemorrhoidal disease, there is no proof that they are causative or that by abolishing these habits symptoms would be relieved. However, they do form the rationale upon which we advise patients who complain of haemorrhoidal disease to alter their practice of defecation in order to reduce symptoms and the risk of recurrence after outpatient therapy.

However, it should be mentioned that data on the relationship between the incidence of constipation and haemorrhoids has cast doubt on this approach. Thus, Johanson and Sonnenberg (1990) found that in the USA 10 million people complained of haemorrhoids, corresponding to a prevalence of 4.4%. In both sexes, a peak prevalence was noted in the age range 45–65 years, with a subsequent decrease after age 65 years. The development of haemorrhoids before age 20 was unusual. Whites were affected more frequently than blacks, and increased prevalence rates were associated with higher socioeconomic status. This was in contrast to the epidemiology of constipation which demonstrated an exponential increase in prevalence after age 65 years and was more common in blacks and in families with low incomes or low social status. These data thus demonstrated differences in the epidemiological behaviour of haemorrhoids and constipation, and call into question any causality between the two conditions.

EPIDEMIOLOGY

Prevalence

Accurate information on the prevalence of haemorrhoids is difficult to come by. Hospital-based studies are not representative, and community-based studies rely on self-reporting, medical practitioner attendances or admission or operation notes (Loder et al, 1994). The low reported incidence in Africa has already been mentioned. The actual incidence in the West is variable, depending on which method has been used for assessment and what definitions are applied. In the USA, an annual nationwide health questionnaire showed a prevalence, as mentioned above, of 4.4% (Johanson and Sonnenberg, 1990). Similar data are not available in the UK (Loder et al, 1994). A small random sample of men from Inner London revealed a prevalence of 12.3% (Acheson, 1960) compared with a London general practice estimate of 36.4% (Gazet et al, 1970). A North American hospital-based survey found a medical diagnosis of haemorrhoids in 21.6% of patients, and a self-diagnosis in a further 10.9% (Hyams and Philpot, 1970). Hospital-based proctoscopy studies gave prevalences of 86% and 55% (Gazet et al, 1970).

In the USA, 1117 physician visits with haemorrhoids are reported annually per 10 000 population, compared with 1123 visits in England and Wales (Johanson and Sonnenberg, 1991). Annual hospital discharge rates for haemorrhoids per 100 000 population are 47.65 in the USA and 40.69 in England and Wales (Johanson and Sonnenberg, 1991). Haemorrhoidectomy rates in two different surveys in the USA estimated annual rates of 60.4 and 48.65 per 100 000 population (Johanson and Sonnenberg, 1991). The rate in France is 46 per 100 000 population (Johanson and Sonnenberg, 1991). However, there seems to be a falling rate of attendances to medical practitioners and a reduction in hospital discharges and surgical operations in both the USA and in England and Wales. Whether this is a true change in prevalence or a change in health behaviour is uncertain (Nelson, 1991).

Sex incidence

Men seem to suffer from haemorrhoids more than do women. Approximately 60% of hospitalized patients with the condition are men (Ganchrow et al, 1971; Arabi et al, 1977a; Lin, 1989; Walker et al, 1990; Johanson and Sonnenberg, 1991; Bleday et al, 1992; Reis Neto et al, 1992). However, the prevalence in the general population seems to be equal within the limitations of the studies performed (Gazet et al, 1970; Hyams and Philpot, 1970; Johanson and Sonnenberg, 1991).

Age

There is an increasing prevalence with age until the seventh decade, after which there is a slight decline (Hyams and Philpot, 1970; Johanson and Sonnenberg, 1990).

Socioeconomic status and occupation

People in high socioeconomic groups more frequently report haemorrhoids, perhaps reflecting greater awareness and introspection (Acheson, 1960; Hyams and Philpot, 1970; Johanson and Sonnenberg, 1990, 1991). Heavy labourers and people whose occupations require prolonged sitting or standing are alleged to have haemorrhoids more often (Acheson, 1960; Prasad et al, 1976). Although others disagree (Hyams and Philpot, 1970; Brondel and Gondran, 1976), they do accept that such individuals may suffer from more severe symptoms.

Associated conditions

Haemorrhoids may be associated with herniae (Brondel and Gondran, 1976), genitourinary prolapse (Brondel and Gondran, 1976; Heslop, 1987) and prostatism (Akande and Esho, 1989) which is likely to be linked to increased abdominal straining.

SYMPTOMS

Patients with haemorrhoidal disease experience varying degrees of the following symptoms: bleeding, anal swelling, pain, discomfort, discharge, hygiene problems and pruritus. Usually, but not invariably, the larger the cushions and the more they prolapse the more troublesome are the symptoms. However, this is not invariable; young men with a tight anal canal can have severe discomfort and severe bleeding with minimal visible abnormality, while elderly ladies with huge cushions that have mucosa exposed to the exterior may have no complaints.

Bleeding

This is the most common complaint and usually the earliest in the development of the disease. The blood is invariably bright red and is often first noticed on the lavatory paper, particularly after passing a non-bloodstained hard stool. The type of bleeding in haemorrhoidal disease is different from that produced by a rectal neoplasm or ulcerative proctitis, but may be similar to that experienced by patients with fissure-in-ano or even when there is perianal dermatitis with severely macerated skin.

Haemorrhoidal disease can generally be distinguished from these last two conditions by the absence of pain or pruritus.

Later in the development of the disease the bright red bleeding may become profuse, dripping into the pan like a tap or spattering the sides like a jet to mark the end of the act of defecation. This profuse bleeding occurs when the cushions are prolapsed beyond and congested by the sphincter. Such bleeding is pathognomonic of haemorrhoidal disease. Nothing else gives such characteristic pan-spattering except, rarely, a prolapsing low rectal polyp.

Bleeding unrelated to defecation occurs even later in the progression of the disease and may occur continuously as a bright red bloody mucous discharge. This tends to happen particularly in the elderly whose inner vascular cushions, covered with mucous membrane, lie permanently outside the anus. In them, sphincter tone is poor and congestion minimal, so bleeding is rarely profuse.

Younger patients with grossly hypertrophied cushions occasionally prolapse and reduce spontaneously apart from during or after defecation, often at times of physical activity, sporting exertion or ecstasy. The higher anal tone in these sufferers often congests the cushions and so bleeding can be embarrassingly profuse. Such patients are the most prone to bleed enough to become anaemic. However, it should never be assumed that anaemia is caused by haemorrhoidal bleeding alone, even if this seems excessive. Other causes must be sought. If no other sources are identified, treatment of the haemorrhoids should be undertaken. Kluiber and Wolff (1994) recommend that if the haemoglobin level has not been restored by 6 months in such circumstances, efforts to identify an alternative source for the anaemia must be redoubled – advice with which we would wholeheartedly agree.

Prolapse and lumps

Prolapse or lumps protruding through the anus are the real 'piles'. The symptoms of protrusion with spontaneous or self-digital reduction of the mass back into the anal canal is highly characteristic of haemorrhoidal disease. However, it is one that is often misreported by patients in response to history-taking by the doctor. Patients with rectal bleeding diagnose themselves as having 'piles' and expect them to 'come down', for such is popular folklore. Furthermore, the sufferer may misinterpret a perianal vascular channel thrombosis as a prolapsed pile and even, unhappily, try to reduce it. The patient may also interpret oedematous perianal skin tags as prolapsed irreducible piles.

Therefore, a history of lumps prolapsing through the anus should be interpreted with caution, unless the act is witnessed or the patient's story is reliable.

Hypertrophied anal papillae and, rarely, low rectal polyps can prolapse through the anus and, as they can be reduced, are often erroneously diagnosed as prolapsing piles.

Pain and discomfort

Uncomplicated haemorrhoidal disease is usually painless. The presence of severe pain indicates another diagnosis or a complication. Thrombosed prolapsed internal piles (sometimes called 'strangulated') indicate a clinically obvious, very painful complication such as the one that is said to have cost Napoleon Waterloo and the French their Empire. A thrombosed external vascular channel will also be described below. This too is painful and obvious externally. In the absence of such clear external stigmata of thrombosis, acute mind-riveting pain suggests an alternative diagnosis such as fissure, abscess or carcinoma.

Discomfort or a dull pain in the anus after defecation is not uncommon in the presence of congested prolapsed cushions and is characteristically relieved by reduction of the prolapse. Prolapsed cushions in those with low anal canal tone are usually painless.

Discharge, hygiene difficulties and pruritus

A constant mucous discharge from the anus with or without blood-staining is characteristic of patients whose internal cushions, covered with mucous membrane, are constantly prolapsed beyond the anal verge. At best this soils their underclothes, at worst it macerates the skin.

Oedematous or fibrous skin tags may clutter the perianal skin, more commonly with advancing years. Some skin tags are said to be erected in memory of past episodes of complications such as thrombosis within vascular cushions, some bear witness to untidy obstetrical suturing, but most develop *de novo* with the passage of time.

Skin tags mar the once smooth perianal skin that characterizes infancy and, with increasing years, make simple one-wipe hygiene impossible. The lucky ones escape with only soiled underwear, the unlucky suffer pruritus.

NATURAL HISTORY AND COMPLICATIONS

Data on the natural history of untreated haemorrhoidal disease are scanty. We do not know what proportion of people who suffer at some time from bleeding, prolapse, pain or pruritus subsequently have no further trouble or have intermittent minor symptoms or what proportion later have severe complications. We do not know why some patients become progressively worse and develop complications.

Thrombosis and infection of internal vascular cushions

Thrombosis of internal vascular cushions is the most dramatic complication of haemorrhoidal disease and generally the most painful. It usually occurs in those with large piles who have previously experienced a reducible prolapse of the cushions. However, on occasions it can occur as the first manifestation of the disease. We believe that thrombosis occurs only when the cushion is prolapsed and congested by the sphincter. Once thrombosis has occurred, the cushions occasionally return to the anal canal but they are usually so swollen that they remain outside. The gross oedema of the perianal skin may conceal the still-prolapsed cushion at the anus, giving the erroneous impression that the internal component has returned to the anal canal (Figure 12.7a–c). Tissue tension rises within and outside the anal canal and is associated with pain and oedema. Thrombosis can occur in one or all of the primary cushions. The patient is often in so much pain as to prevent sitting, walking or defecation. Depending on the patient's stoicism or sensitivity, strong analgesics may be required.

The oedematous perianal skin is immediately recognizable. If this is parted, and if the patient permits, hard thrombosed cushions can be palpated. They are covered by dark, tense mucous membrane which, after a day or two, may even become necrotic. The condition can be diagnosed simply by inspection after parting the oedematous skin and by external palpation and is unmistakable. It is unnecessary and unjustifiable to attempt internal anal canal palpation or endoscopy. If operative treatment is indicated, as we believe it usually is, anoscopy and rectoscopy or sigmoidoscopy can be performed once the anus or the patient is anaesthetized.

If excision or dilatation is not performed, the natural history of internal cushion thrombosis is one of slow natural resolution. Oedema and inflammatory swelling are maximal for 1–4 days after the thrombosis. Resolution is obvious clinically by 10 days, although it is not usually complete for 4–6 weeks. Even then the enlarged skin tags may remain as a constant memorial to the event. Sometimes there remains a large fibrous polypoid skin tag.

If necrosis of the mucous membrane occurs over the thrombosis, some of the clot may extrude and give symptomatic relief. Rarely does all of it extrude for, as one can observe during emergency haemorrhoidectomy, the clots are present in several non-communicating venous spaces and all cannot be expressed through one incision. Sometimes the epithelial breakdown permits pathogenic bacterial invasion, and gangrene of the cushion has been reported, even extending into the anal canal or rectum. This now seems to be an exceptionally rare event, or if it does occur it responds dramatically to antibiotics. The once-feared serious gangrene and portal pyaemia now fortunately seems relegated to medical history (Lockhart-Mummery and Joshi, 1915; Lockhart-Mummery, 1934; Gabriel, 1948).

Anaemia

Repeated profuse anal bleeding occasionally causes iron-deficiency anaemia, sometimes with haemoglobin levels as low as 4 g/L. It is a greater risk in women before the menopause and in those with blood dyscrasias. With the availability of conservative management for bleeding haemorrhoidal disease, severe anaemia is becoming a rare event as patients are less likely to neglect seeking treatment. The important points to remember are that (1) a haemoglobin estimation is always advisable in anyone complaining of profuse rectal bleeding; (2) anaemia should be corrected before operation when general anaesthesia is employed; and (3) one should always suspect another possible occult cause of intestinal bleeding, such as peptic ulceration or colonic neoplasia. Another source of colonic bleeding should always be considered during the initial examination. In those with anaemia it is advisable to recheck the haemoglobin regularly after the haemorrhoidal disease has been successfully treated to ensure that this cures the anaemia permanently.

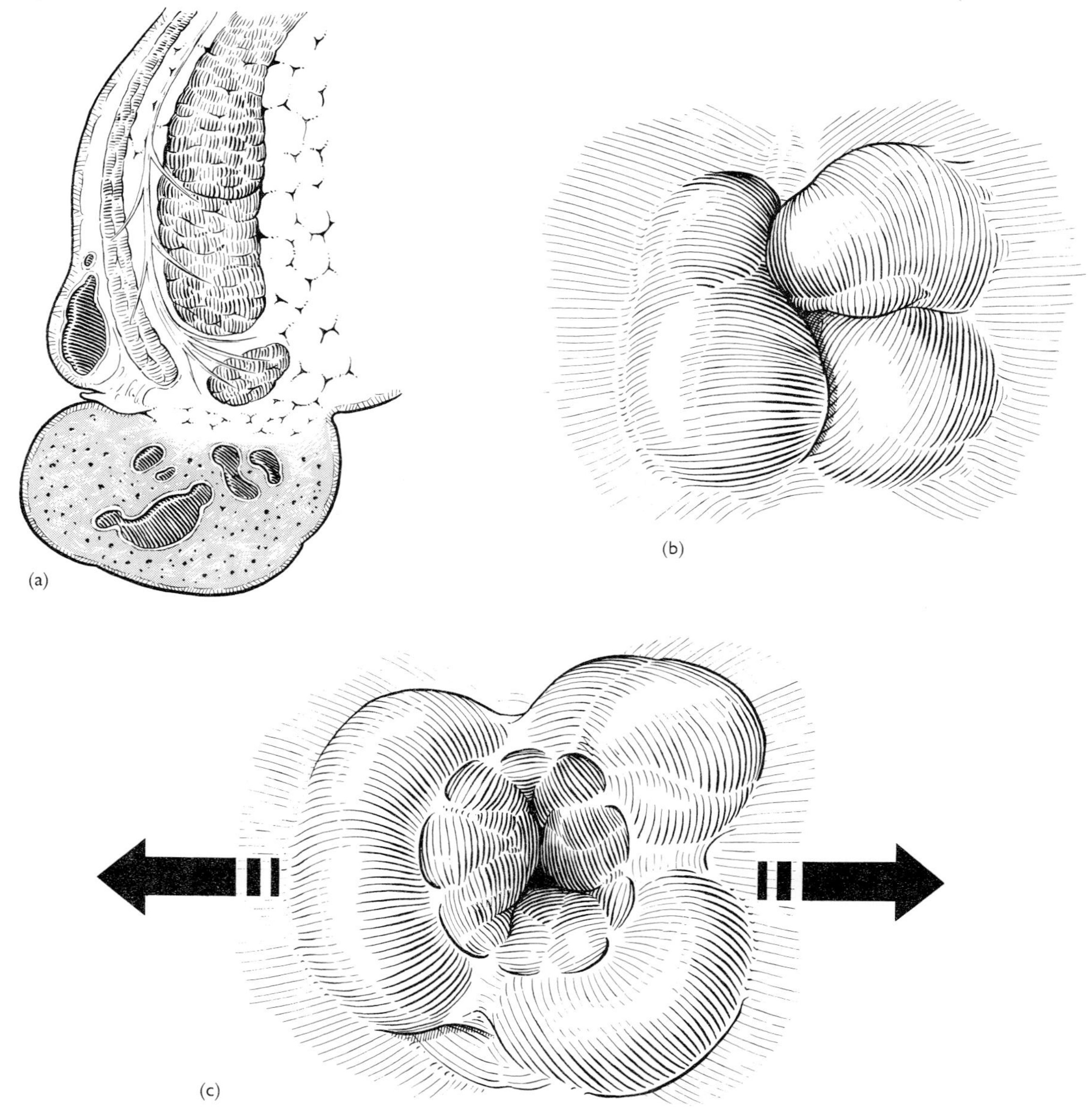

Figure 12.7a–c (a) Sagittal section to show thrombosed internal haemorrhoids. (b) and (c) How thrombosed internal haemorrhoids can be hidden by oedematous skin tags.

Thrombosis of external vascular channels

This is sometimes incorrectly termed 'perianal haematoma'; however, it does not spread in the tissues as does a haematoma due to rupturing of a blood vessel. The thrombosis seems to be intravascular, and Thomson (1982) has shown that the clot has an endothelial lining. It is the tense swelling within the confines of the vascular space that makes the lesion feel hard and smooth and that makes it so painful for the patient. As the thrombosis is in the superficial or external vascular channels, it is not truly part of the spectrum of internal anal cushion disease (Figure 12.8a,b), nor is it necessarily associated with symptomatic or hypertrophied internal cushions. However, it does seem to be a complication that occurs more commonly in those with haemorrhoidal disease than in the normal population. This could be a false impression because the incidence of external vascular channel thrombosis is

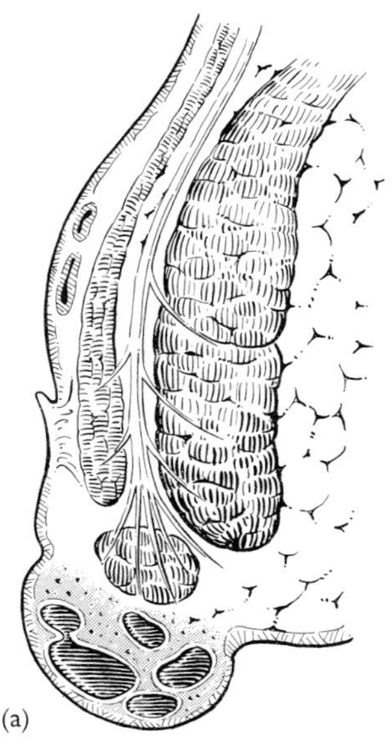

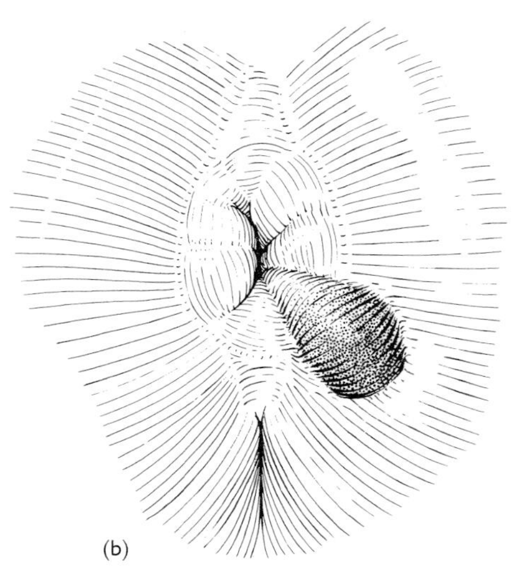

Figure 12.8a–b (a) Sagittal section of thrombosed external pile. (b) Thrombosed external pile as viewed by clinician at anal verge.

often called an 'acute attack of piles' and automatically tends to categorize the patient as a sufferer from haemorrhoidal disease.

The complication is easily recognizable if the anus is inspected and gently palpated. The smooth, hard, tender lump (or lumps) shows blue through the skin, with a variable amount of surrounding oedema. Careful parting of the buttocks shows the lump to be outside and not within the anal canal. It is not necessary to perform a rectal digital examination at this stage, but if one can be performed, with or without anaesthesia, it is clear that the hard clot does not extend up into the internal cushions.

As with thrombosis of the internal cushions, the lesion runs a natural course, usually lasting 5–7 days. It starts with 2–4 days of acute discomfort, then gradual resolution occurs much sooner than with the more serious internal cushion thrombosis. Expectant treatment is usually followed, for often the patient is not seen or referred until resolution has begun or is complete. Management is described later in the chapter.

Perianal dermatitis

This skin complication of haemorrhoidal disease occurs either from maceration due to mucous leakage from permanantly prolapsed cushions, as the consequence of poor hygiene associated with skin tags, or as a sensitivity reaction to locally applied allergenic drugs. Its principal symptom is perianal irritation with occasional bleeding from split skin.

ASSESSMENT OF THE PATIENT

History

The definitive diagnosis of haemorrhoidal disease can be made almost always if a careful history is taken, paying particular attention to the colour and character of the bleeding, the relation of discomfort to defecation, and the unequivocal history of relief from reduction of the prolapse into the anal canal. The importance of detailed assessment by endoscopy in establishing the diagnosis is to exclude the other often more dangerous causes of rectal discharge, prolapse, anal pain and bleeding.

Inspection

Discharge from everted anal canal mucosa in third-degree piles (see below) is readily seen if the patient is examined when comfortable and relaxed in the left lateral position and when he or she can be persuaded to bear down. This manoeuvre will also allow differentiation of true full-thickness rectal prolapse from simple internal cushion prolapse. Alternatively, the patient can be examined in the prone position on a special proctologic table, this being the preferred technique in the USA. A good light, careful inspection and palpation may be required to differentiate haemorrhoidal discharge from a chronic fistula-in-ano or from perianal Crohn's disease.

Palpation

After inspection, palpation is the next important method of assessment. Once again it is important to stress the need for gentleness in palpation for painful anal conditions. The examination must be performed slowly with adequate lubrication; local anaesthesia may be required. In the absence of an episode of thrombosis, acute anal pain is a rare feature of uncomplicated haemorrhoidal disease. Its presence should make one suspect a fissure-in-ano, which is best diagnosed by inspection, an abscess, which should be detected readily by its localized induration, redness and pain, or anal carcinoma, which can be recognized by palpating its hard edge on digital examination. Solitary rectal ulcer may sometimes be identified by palpation.

Endoscopy

Proctoscopy

This will demonstrate the presence of internal vascular cushions and may show them to be bleeding.

The differentiation of causes of rectal or anal bleeding is the most important objective of the assessment. We make no apology for repeating the observation that it is not enough simply to demonstrate that a patient with rectal bleeding has congested internal anal cushions on anoscopy. It does not mean that these have been the cause of bleeding, not even if they are seen to bleed with the trauma of the examination. Other causes of bright red rectal bleeding must be excluded.

Sigmoidoscopy

This will demonstrate the normality of the rectal mucosa and so exclude inflammatory bowel disease. It should also exclude solitary rectal ulcer, mucosal polyps or carcinoma of the rectum.

Bright red rectal bleeding can come from sigmoid neoplasms, so the assessment of rectal bleeding should include *flexible* sigmoidoscopy to 60 cm. This counsel of perfection may not be possible in all circumstances but should be the aim. Full sigmoidoscopy is mandatory whenever there is blood mixed with the stool. In some patients with bright red blood on the toilet paper only, or with characteristic blood spattering after the passage of a normal non-bloody stool, it may be permissible to confine examination to the rectum provided the symptom is cured by treatment.

If there is any doubt whatsoever concerning the diagnosis, the rest of the colon will need investigating, preferably by colonoscopy, or by barium enema if colonoscopy is not readily available.

Ano-rectal physiological measurements

Trials have been conducted to compare different methods of therapy for haemorrhoidal disease, based on whether or not there was a high or low anal canal pressure. The methods of measuring anal pressure are described elsewhere and the results of the trials will be discussed in this chapter when comparing different methods of treatment.

At this stage, all that remains to be said about the methods of assessment is to venture an opinion about the importance of anal pressure measurements in deciding on the form of appropriate treatment for someone with haemorrhoidal disease.

We now believe that manometry and indeed other anorectal physiological studies including anorectal ultrasound have an important role in the assessment of the individual suspected of having an impaired sphincter yet who also requires a haemorrhoidectomy. Such patients are in danger of developing incontinence postoperatively and preoperative physiological assessment will help in decision making and in counselling the patient concerning the risks.

CATEGORIZATION OF DEGREES

It has been traditional to grade haemorrhoidal disease into four degrees, depending on the extent of prolapse. This is to use the term 'piles' in its true meaning.

1. *First-degree piles* (Figure 12.9a) are cushions that do not descend below the dentate line on straining. By this strict definition everyone, even those without symptoms, fits into this category. The definition therefore has to be qualified to include only those individuals with symptoms, usually bleeding.
2. *Second-degree piles* (Figure 12.9b) are cushions that protrude below the dentate line on straining and can be seen at the exterior, only to disappear again immediately straining stops.
3. *Third-degree piles* (Figure 12.9c) are cushions that descend to the exterior on straining or defecation and remain ouside until they are digitally replaced into the anal canal, where they remain until the next bowel movement or possibly the next act of straining.
4. 'Fourth-degree piles' is the term sometimes used to describe mucosal-covered internal cushions that are permanently outside the anal verge and return at once outside when they are replaced. Many regard this simply as a type of third-degree pile.

This staging of piles has only limited value as it refers to one aspect of the disease, prolapse. The severity of the disease can be related as much to the severity of blood loss or the degree of discomfort as to the degree of prolapse. Many elderly people with third- or fourth-degree haemorrhoids have relatively little trouble and may warrant no treatment. Nevertheless, a record of the degree of prolapse may help in assessing the efficacy of particular forms of treatment. For example, we can say with confidence that injection therapy or photocoagulation for haemorrhoidal disease is effective in relieving symptoms in approximately 80% of patients with first- and second-degree piles but in only 20% of those with third-degree piles.

Another serious problem with the grading of prolapse on the basis of one examination is the day-to-day variation in the size of the vascular cushions and their tendency to prolapse. It should be realized that different degrees of prolapse can occur at different times of the menstrual cycle in women, or even at different times of the same day.

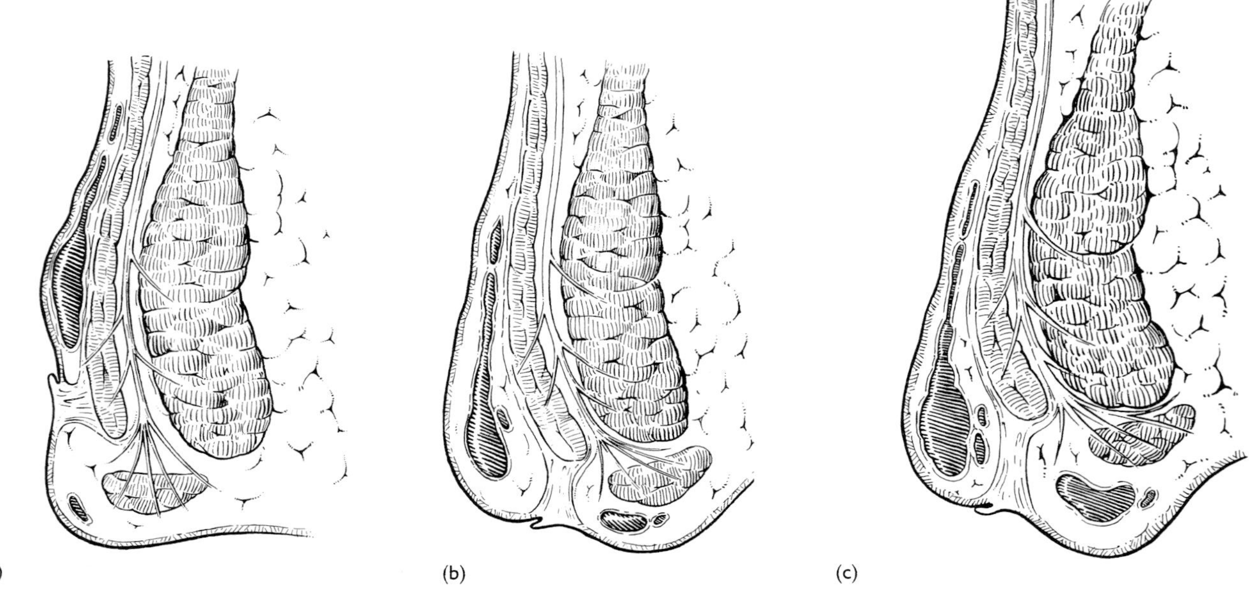

Figure 12.9a–c The three degrees of haemorrhoidal disease: (a) first-degree; (b) second-degree; (c) third-degree.

Section II: History of the management of haemorrhoidal disease

As the art of proctology is based on the study of haemorrhoidal disease, it seems appropriate to trace the history of the development of this cornerstone of our subject.

ANCIENT HISTORY

It seems likely that haemorrhoidal disease is one of the oldest ills known to man. Some would postulate that it was the consequences of man assuming the upright position (Morgagni, 1749).

By the time civilization was sufficiently advanced to consider recording daily events in a form that we can now understand, accounts of haemorrhoidal disease appeared. They were referred to in the writings of the ancient Egyptians, the ancient Greeks and the Hebrews. According to the Edwin Smith Papyrus (1700 BC) the Egyptians appeared to have used the infusion of acacia leaves or of alum as an astringent in the management of anal disorders, although whether these were used primarily for pruritus, condylomata or piles is not clear. Anal disease is referred to in the Code of Hammurabi in Babylon in 2250 BC and in the Papyrus of Eber in about 1500 BC which, like the Edwin Smith Papyrus, concentrates on local polypharmacy for anal disorders.

The inventive genius of the ancient Greeks and their preoccupation with matters anal led to a number of important observations by such as Hippocrates who, in about 400 BC, recommended cautery with a hot iron and simple excision of prolapsing piles. There is some doubt about the authenticity of the Hippocratic treatises but we know that Hippocrates was a great traveller whose journeys took him to Egypt, where he may have learned some of its ancient medical lore.

The ancient Greeks are also recorded as having practised forcible anal dilatation, but once again history is clouded and misinterpretation is rife. Whether forcible anal dilatation was punitive, pleasurable or therapeutic is open to conjecture. By some accounts the Greek habit of ραφινιδοσισ or 'giving radish', apparently practised as a punitive measure, sounds remarkably similar to the forcible manual dilatation championed by Maisonneuvre and later by Lord 2000 or more years later.

The first book of Samuel in the Old Testament also refers to haemorroid disease. When, in recovering the Ark of the Covenant in Gath, the hapless Philistines were sorely punished: 'the hand of the Lord was against the city with a very great destruction: and he smote the men of the city, both small and great, and they had emerods in their secret parts' (1 Sam 5:9); and again when the Ark was moved to Ekron in Northern Philistinia, this city too received the painful proctological curse: 'and the men that died not were smitten with emerods: and the cry of the city went up to heaven' (1 Sam 5:12).

Celsus (25 BC–AD 14) in *De Medicina* refers to ligature of piles with 'a flax thread, a little above where it joins the anus'. He also refers to the necessity to incise the mucosa above the knot to prevent post-operative pain and the advisability of not taking away too much tissue.

In the second century after Christ, Galen – who was a student of the works of Hippocrates – considered that bleeding from the anus was an autotherapeutic form of blood-letting, for had not one of the Aphorisuis of Hippocrates been as follows: 'Haemorrhoids appearing in melancholic and nephaitic affections are favourable.' Many sufferers must have observed then, as now, that symptoms associated with haemorrhoidal disease are often improved after 'a good bleed'. It is not surprising that during the ages when the leech was considered safer than the scalpel, these blood-loving animals were used to decrease perianal congestion. In the galenic era it was also characterized by polypharmacy and superstition. It was suggested that the 'stone of India' worn around the neck, an emerald in the navel or the black leg of a toad in the armpit would check bleeding (Hughes, 1957). However,

Galen was prepared to advise surgery, and in his *Introductis, sen Medicus* states 'we tie a double knot of thread tightly round the base of the haemorrhoid and cut off the thread in two hours'.

Parks, in his classical historical essay 'De haemorrhois' (1955), states that Aetius of Amida in the Byzantine era gave a good description of ligation and excising of piles, as did Paul of Aegina. The method advocated by Aetius was as follows: 'One by one we draw out the haemorrhoids with a volsella, scarify the base and twist it round with the same volsella; then after an interval we fasten a ligature and amputate. The twisting movement combined with the constriction so affects the veins that there is not the least fear of subsequent escape of blood. Our method, then, is to expose the haemorroid, scarify and twist round the base and then hand the volsella to an assistant to hold; we treat the remainder in a similar fashion, drawing them forth with a volsella, scarifying, ligating with tape and handing to an assistant. Then we amputate them in succession beginning with the one that we first drew forth . . . we add a sponge with a thread attached, with the free end lying loose outside. Our judgement is that surgery is the quickest and safest way of getting rid of haemorrhoids'.

The *Susruta Samhita*, the ancient Hindu Sanskrit text, appears to have adopted the method of clamp and cautery: 'A large polypus appearing in a strong person should be clipped off and cauterized with fire. In case of prolapse of the anus, cauterization should be made without the help of any speculum.'

The centre of the medical and cultural world remained in the warm climates of North Africa across to North India where, in the tenth century, El-Zahrawy wrote a 30-volume medical encyclopaedia which was to remain in use for the next 500 years. He described cautery in the treatment of haemorrhoids as the last word in surgical treatment. In about the eleventh century, with the harnessing of fire and domestic architecture, the centre of cultural development started its move northwards to the more enervating climates of middle and northern Europe. It is from here that came the next advances in medical therapy.

MEDIEVAL MEDICINE

Landfrank (Laufrank or Lamfrank), before he worked in Milan, migrated to Paris in AD 1295 and became a great surgical teacher and one of the fathers of French proctology. A year later his *Chirurgie Magna* was written, in which he advocated ligation for piles (ficus). He wrote: 'If it be ficus, that thou mixt know, for it wole be withoute hete and neische, and the cure herof is buit lizt. Thou schalt take a strong threed and knitte there aboute, and every dai thoou schalt streine it more and more, till he falle awei, and then with driying medicyne thou schalt drie it up, or touch hem with an hoot iron that is bettere.' From the French school in Montpellier came Henri de Mondeville (1260–1320), who advised against operating for haemorrhoidal disease, and Guy de Chanliac (1300–1370) who reported the Arabian methods of cauterizing piles.

Montpellier was also the Alma Mater of the father of British proctology, John of Arderne (1306–1390). John of Arderne was first attached to Henry Plantagenet and afterwards to John of Gaunt, with both of whom he travelled widely to Antwerp and throughout France. His precise connection with Laufrank and Montpellier can only be assumed from his writing. He is best known for his brilliant work on fistula-in-ano. There was singularly little development in either the understanding or treatment of haemorrhoidal disease during the Middle Ages. Despite the warning of such masters as John of Arderne, the barber surgeons held sway and treated most sufferers with potions, suction leeches and the occasional lancet.

Another great French military surgeon, Ambrose Pare (1510–1590), who made striking advances in the management of amputations and wounds, had little to offer the sufferers from haemorrhoidal disease apart from comfort that it was beneficial to have a good bleed from time to time. He had no time for surgical treatment: neither had Riverius (1657) who is reputed to have been the first to record the topical applications of nitric acid.

As in Hebrew writings, the anus seems to have been referred to as 'the secret parts', so polite society in the seventeenth century referred discreetly to haemorrhoidal disease as 'Le mal de St Phiacre'.

EIGHTEENTH CENTURY PIONEERS

The galenic hypothesis of therapeutic bleeding was championed by Stahl (1729), who wrote on the management of 'golden veins'. He thought that anal bleeding was nature's safety valve in the plethora of the portal system, while Morgagni (1749) believed that the adoption of the erect posture by man put a high-pressure strain on the lower tributaries of the portal vein, causing them to dilate.

During this century most of the debates were about the relative merits of excision, with its risk of bleeding and stenosis, and ligation, with its risks of gangrene and sepsis.

Lorenz Heister, in his work *Chirurgie* (1739), advised the surgeon treating piles 'to tie up the bleeding tubercles with needle and thread, cutting off those parts which are praeternaturally distended beyond the ligature taking care at the same time to leave a few of the smallest veins open' (presumably to permit free drainage).

In 1774, Jean Louis Petit recognized that it was the stratified epithelial position of the pile that was most sensitive and he observed that if this were incised, the haemorrhoidal plexus could be ligated with much less pain than if it were not. He became the father of subepithelial haemorrhoidectomy.

The great British surgeons of the day, Cheselden, Potts and Hunter, were strangely silent about haemorrhoidal disease.

NINETEENTH CENTURY: THE BIRTH OF PROCTOLOGY

The century began as the last one ended, with a few pioneers making observations at least a century before their time. Samuel Cooper (1809) developed the ideas of Petit, performing submucosal dissection before ligating the base of piles. He claimed that it obviated the risk of stenosis so prevalent after the more conventional simple pile base ligation. Copeland (1810) agreed with Cooper but pronounced the operation technically difficult. It was probably because it was so difficult that the principle lay dormant for over a century before its revival by Calman in 1941. Meanwhile, interest seemed to drift towards non-excisional and conservative methods of management.

Clamp and cautery methods had been in use for many centuries and were revived in 1846 by Cusack from Dublin and von Langenbeck in Germany in 1870 who fitted ivory wings to the clamps for insulation. After a crushing clamp was placed longitudinally along the length of the vascular cushion, the redundant cushion was excised and the tissue coagulated with a hot iron.

In the middle of the nineteenth century the causes of haemorrhoidal disease were being considered. By this time the art of 'pile pondering' had clearly changed from the galenic to Gallic school. No longer were bleeding piles considered beneficial, but harmful. Constipation and straining were implicated as the cause of haemorrhoidal disease. This realization occurred a full hundred years before the bran revolution infiltrated the Western world.

A surprisingly early, anatomically based and physiologically reasoned hypothesis on pile formation by Verneuil (1855) suggested that the superior haemorrhoidal veins were occluded by a faecal bolus where they pass through the musculature of the midrectum, causing anal varicosities. Based on some brilliant anatomical studies, straining at stool was found to be the main cause of the rise in haemorrhoidal vein pressure, by occluding the anastomoses between portal and systemic circulation through the internal sphincter.

While anatomists made academic advances, pragmatic proctologists developed their curative art by empirical strides. The injection treatment of piles began to be developed and practised widely by quacks and legitimate physicians.

Ireland appears to have become the centre for this type of conservative management of haemorrhoidal disease in the nineteenth century. Houston (1843) of Dublin re-introduced the Riverius method of topical nitric acid but it proved rather dangerous.

In 1869, Morgan first treated a patient by injection of persulphate of iron into the congested anal cushions. Colles, also of Dublin, used the method in 1874 but at that time it was not widely adopted in England. Dr Mitchell of Illinois was the pioneer of injection therapy in the USA, using 30% phenol in olive oil. Mitchell (1903) did not publish the formula of his injection material, but sold the secret before he died. As a consequence a large number of unqualified travelling pile doctors spread the image of itinerant commercial proctology so that, until recent years, it has been difficult to eradicate the low public image of colorectal surgery. In 1879, Andrews of Chicago introduced the phenol 'secret' to the medical profession. Then, after a slow start, the injection technique gradually became accepted by the legitimate profession and it was widely practised and recorded in the medical literature (Martin, 1904). At first, the percentage of phenol in the oily base varied from 25% to 95%, but in 1888 Edwards had introduced to Britain a technique of injecting a 10% or 20% solution of phenol in glycerine into the substance of the vascular cushion. The high concentration of phenol used earlier was an effective anaesthetic agent, so despite a low injection site the treatment was not painful.

The history of anal sphincter spasm begins early in the nineteenth century when it was first realized that painful disorders of the anus were associated with a very tight sphincter. At this stage, therapy was directed either towards the gentle stretching of the sphincter or its total surgical division. Copeland (1814) advocated the use of large bougies in overcoming spasm and painful anal conditions as did Salmon (1836).

Once again we have to look to Paris for advances in other methods of conservative management. The early development of physiotherapy and massage of the anus was pioneered by Maisonneuve (1864). The idea of dilatation of the anus came from Fecamier, as early as 1829, in a dissertation presented to the French Academy of Medicine, while in 1864 Maisonneuve described a treatment by manual digital stretching of the anorectum that is remarkably similar to that described by Lord over 100 years later.

Partial division of the sphincter was introduced, also in Paris, by Boyer in 1818. This was the incision of the distal portion of the internal sphincter or the subepithelial narrowing associated with anal fissure and anal stenosis. This superficial sphincterotomy approach was continued by many famous surgeons in France, including Dupuytren (1833). A comparison between anal dilatation and sphincterotomy was reported by Bodenheimer in the United States in 1868. He preferred direct incision of the sphincter and thought that the stretching procedure was dangerous. He referred to the 'mangled, irregular wounds resulting from stretching'. Despite this early enthusiasm for sphincterotomy, we had to wait for another hundred years before interest in internal anal sphincterotomy was revived by Eisenhammer in a series of eloquent writings between the years 1951 and 1971. He became a staunch advocate of this type of approach for most anal ills including haemorrhoids.

By the time Charles Bell wrote in Tidy's *System of Surgery* in 1886, almost every form of therapy known to modern proctology had been tried in the management of haemorrhoidal disease.

An operation that has now largely been abandoned is the total exision of a pile-bearing area with primary suture, advocated by Whitehead (1882). In this an entire tube of mucosa and submucosal vascular tissue was removed with immediate primary suture. Although some surgeons found this technique successful, the breakdown rate of the primary suture at the dentate line was high and secondary haemorrhage common. The subsequent slow healing of the granulating wounds frequently led to such severe stenosis that it resulted in, what became known as, the 'post-Whitehead deformity'. The operation has been largely abandoned in the UK, although in recent decades it has retained some proponents in the USA (McMahon, 1956; Burchell et al, 1967; White et al, 1972). Its ideas survive in a modified form in the Fansler–Anderson operation (1933) described again by Leumeister (1959).

Unfortunately for the bewildered proctologist, many ambiguous anatomical terms were coined in the nineteenth century. Hilton (1877) described the appearance of the lowermost fibres of the internal sphincter, as seen through the perianal skin when stretched tight, as a white line. This is different from the 'pecten' described by Stroud (1896), which is a band of modified skin that lies between the dentate line and Hilton's line. To compound the confusion, 'pecten' is derived from the term 'cock's comb' and is similar to the term dentate (or toothed line), which marks the lower end of the anal columns.

In the nineteenth century the most common surgical management of haemorrhoidal disease was the application of a ligature to the whole of the prolapsed pile, including the skin and the mucous membrane. Needless to say, this was usually a very painful procedure. Salmon, in 1836, introduced the first modification of this technique in Britain, in an attempt to reduce postoperative pain. His method consisted of making a cut with scissors at the mucocutaneous junction and stripping off the mucosal-covered pile above the dentate line and ligating the base in the insensitive area of the mucosa. Salmon wrote very little and his methods, though widely taught in London, were recognized throughout the world only at the beginning of the twentieth century. Allingham and Allingham (1901), also from St Mark's Hospital, reported the first series of haemorrhoidectomies in Great Britain using Salmon's method. In this paper they roundly condemned the Whitehead operation.

TWENTIETH CENTURY: THE ERA OF THE PECTEN BAND

During the early part of the twentieth century most of the English language writings on the subject of operations for haemorrhoidal disease continued to come from surgeons practising at St Mark's Hospital in London. Many of their names are still attached to the techniques. These include Miles (1919), who described the wide V-shaped excision of the perianal skin and division of the pecten band. In 1937, Milligan and colleagues described what was sometimes called the low ligation technique. This later also became associated with the name of Naunton Morgan as the 'Milligan–Morgan haemorrhoidectomy', which became nicknamed the 'smash and grab haemorrhoidectomy' or the 'five-minute job'.

Other modifications of the hemorrhoidectomy operation were those performing a running suture over a clamp applied along the length of the pile (1903). This method later became popular in the USA, being championed by Earl (1911) and Bacon (1949).

The closed haemorrhoidectomy technique stemmed from the submucosal haemorrhoidectomy of Petit (1774) and Cooper (1809) mentioned above. This was popularized by Ferguson at Grand Rapids, Michigan (Ferguson and Heaton, 1959; Ferguson et al, 1971). It is still the technique most commonly used in the USA and in Australia (Failes, 1966).

Anderson (1909) and Cormie and McNair (1959) revived the clamp and cautery method and claimed that it was less painful than excision haemorrhoidectomy. However, as their statements were made before the era of controlled trials, these reports seem to be simply expressions of opinion. As Goligher (1984) observes, this method of clamp and cautery 'seemed to most surgeons a cumbersome way of accomplishing what can be done more easily by simple ligature'. Some might think that the recent emergence of a photocoagulator for internal haemorrhoids has revived the clamp and cautery method but, as will be seen later, the principles are different and rely on mucosal fixation rather than tissue destruction.

Early in the twentieth century conservative proctology began to blossom at the very time that operative treatment by haemorrhoidectomy became so widely practised. Perhaps this was because the then popular techniques of low ligation practised at St Mark's Hospital were so painful. Some of the reasons for the painful nature of haemorrhoidectomy as then practised included the apparently punitive measures of the postoperative greased wide-bore tube tied in the anal canal and the enforced postoperative constipation that lasted until the faeces became very hard. No wonder that some proctologists, and even more patients, embraced with enthusiasm any non-operative measures of mucosal fixation and sphincter stretching that would avoid haemorrhoidectomy.

Fixation by submucosal injection was revived and developed. The technique that was and is most widely used now is that introduced by Blanchard and Alright (Blanchard, 1928). An injection of a weak solution of phenol (5%) in arachis oil is made into the upper aspect of the cushion, aiming to produce not necrosis or thrombosis but submucosal fibrosis to fix the anal cushion in the upper anal canal and prevent it being prolapsed on defecation.

The next method of mucosal fixation to be rediscovered was that of rubber-band ligation. Blaisdell, in a scientific exhibit at the American Medical Association at San Francisco in 1954, first revealed his instrument for the office ligation of internal haemorrhoids using a silk ligature to the insensitive upper aspect or base of the vascular cushion. The instrument was later perfected by Barron (1963), who produced a robust instrument for placing a strong rubber-band to strangulate the base (upper aspect) of the vascular cushion. Several recent modifications of the technique will be described later.

Although cooling with ice has long been used to control the discomfort of acute complications of haemorrhoidal disease, tissue destruction by cold was not possible until the relatively recent development of cryosurgical techniques. Tissue destruction by freezing with liquid nitrogen to –190°C or liquid nitrous oxide to –70°C was first used in oncology and gynaecology and then became a technique in general surgical use. It was applied to the management of haemorrhoids by Fraser and Gill in 1967 and was popularized in the USA by Lewis (Lewis et al, 1969; Lewis, 1973) and in the UK by Lloyd Williams et al (1973). The method will be described in technical detail later.

Infrared photocoagulation, the most recent addition to the proctological armamentarium for mucosal fixation, was used in the management of haemorrhoidal disease following the development of an infrared coagulator by Nath et al (1977). It was popularized in the treatment of haemorrhoidal disease by Neiger (1979) from Bern.

The pecten band or cock's comb is a deposit of fibrous tissue that is found in the subepithelial tissues of the anal canal. Its name implies that it is the same structure as the dentate line but its true anatomical site is not understood clearly by most surgeons.

Miles (1919) describes the pecten and the pecten band as follows: 'The fibrous deposit takes the form of a circular band, varying in thickness and density, completely surrounding the lower part of the anal canal and situated between the mucous membrane of the pecten and the external sphincter muscle. In well-marked instances, the band of fibrous tissue can be distinctly felt and gives an impression to the examining finger such as would be obtained if a rubber umbrella ring had been inserted beneath the skin at the anal margin. I have named this deposit of fibrous tissue in the submucosa of the pecten, the pecten band.'

The pecten band does not exist in the healthy anal canal. It is purely pathological in origin. It is due to passive congestion engendered either by the varicosity of the superior haemorrhoidal veins or possibly in some measure as an impediment to venous return as a result of habitual pressure upon the veins of the rectum induced by the loaded state of the rectum in the chronically constipated. It varies both in thickness and in density in different cases. It limits the expansibility of the anal orifice just as effectively as would a piece of whipcord if tied loosely around the anal canal. In nearly all cases of internal piles, two characteristic symptoms due to the presence of the pecten band manifest themselves, apart from those due to the piles themselves. One of these is difficulty in obtaining complete emptying of the rectum during defecation, and the other is diminished size in the calibre of the faeces passed, the motions being generally voided in short pieces about the size of an ordinary index finger. Both of the symptoms are due solely to the presence of the pecten band and both of them disappear when the band has been divided.

The importance of the pecten band was the cornerstone of recent developments in the management of haemorrhoidal disease. Lord (1968), in his re-introduction of the Maisonneuve procedure, stresses the importance of disrupting this band. Eisenhammer (1951) believes that its division is central to all management of painful anal conditions and its extensive displacement is the key to all disorders of anal laxity. Notarus (1971) divides it in the lateral subcutaneous sphincterotomy that is claimed to cure both painful haemorrhoids and fissure.

It seems likely that haemorrhoidal disease will still plague man in the twenty-first century. It is interesting to conjecture what new discovery or rediscovery will dominate proctological ponderings as we enter the third millenium after Christ and the sixth after haemorrhoidal disease first made its mark on a papyrus.

Section III: Conservative management of haemorrhoidal disease

- Medical management
  - Advice
  - Changing defecation habits
  - Diet manipulation
  - Vasotopic drugs
  - Topical applications
- Invasive therapy (principles of the methods)
  - Mucosal fixation (rationale and mechanism)
  - Injection or sclerotherapy
  - Rubber-band ligation
  - Cryotherapy
  - Photocoagulation
- Bipolar diathermy (BICAP)
- Direct current therapy

A wide variety of treatment is available for haemorrhoidal disease, ranging from advice on diet and bowel habit, through a number of non-operative methods of mucosal fixation and widening of the anus, to a host of different techniques of excision of the internal anal vascular cushions and the external vascular channels. The choice of method depends on the severity and type of the symptoms, on the degree of prolapse, and on the expertise of the operator and equipment available. The art of the practice of proctology is to find the most appropriate match of therapy and disease.

MEDICAL MANAGEMENT

Advice

Advice is best directed at those patients who have only minor symptoms and who have obviously an incorrect diet or hygiene habits. Advice is suitable only for those who are amenable to suggestion and have the intelligence and ability to take it. Whenever possible, it is advisable for the primary physician to try the effect of advice first before referring the patient to a proctologist or moving on to more aggressive treatment, provided of course the correct diagnosis has been made. If the patient's principal complaint is loose stools, itching and smearing of blood on the toilet paper, it is best to begin with advice about a high-fibre diet, avoiding diarrhoeagenic foods or drink, and thorough gentle perianal lavage after defecation. However, we agree with the views of Goligher (1984) who states that the conservative forms of treatment to reduce the degree of prolapse of the anal cushions, such as injection, photocoagulation or band ligation, are so safe and simple that it is seldom justifiable for a proctologist who has been referred a patient with bleeding or prolapse to withhold these forms of treatment until after a trial of the effects of advice alone. Usually injection, coagulation or banding are performed during the investigative anoscopy.

There are exceptions to this rule of initial aggressive therapy. For example, patients in the early weeks of pregnancy or with complicating medical conditions such as blood dyscrasias should be treated as conservatively as possible.

Changing defecation habits

If the patient is obviously infringing the rules of common sense it is reasonable to try to correct an error of bowel habit alone. The three errors of bowel habit that seem to be most prevalent in patients with haemorrhoidal disease are: (1) insistence on having at least one bowel movement daily, come what may; (2) neglect of the first urge to defecate in the morning because it is not convenient to do so; and (3) insistence on trying to pass the last portion of stool from the rectum or anal canal in the belief that, if it is not passed, discomfort will persist all day.

We always take a detailed defecation history from patients and advise them about the disadvantages of any habits that we consider unwise. To aid their memory we also give them a printed list of instructions about a high-fibre diet and defecation habits.

Diet manipulation

Manipulation of the diet and the addition of bulking agents seem to be a logical first line of therapy. The simplest way to achieve a bulky stool is to change to a high-fibre diet; however, a change of diet requires strong motivation and few patients adhere to such advice for long and then only as a token gesture of willingness to please their doctor. Most doctors find it easier to prescribe a simple bulk-forming addition to the patient's normal diet. Many doctors recommend bran with little advice about how and when to take it, while most patients try to eat it heaped on breakfast cereals. It is not surprising that they find it too uninteresting to persist for long. If the patient finds bran unpalatable or unacceptable, doctors usually prescribe sterculia, ispaghula husk, psyllium seed extract and methylcellulose in a variety of pharmaceutical guises, some easier to take than others. It is important to consider the acceptability of these preparations and to find one that the patient positively likes to take. The doctor should try taking them before prescribing them for patients.

Results of trials

When Broader et al (1974) assessed the effect of a bulking agent compared with that of a placebo in 40 patients with haemorrhoidal disease in a prospective randomized trial, they found a slight but insignificant advantage for sterculia (Normacol) over a starch placebo. They recorded the patient's assessment of their bowel habit in 100 consecutive patients attending a rectal clinic with symptomatic haemorrhoidal disease. Only 9% of patients with symptomatic haemorrhoidal disease considered that they were constipated. Furthermore, 30% of patients who took sterculia did not like taking it because it was difficult to swallow or made them feel bloated. Over 50% stopped taking sterculia after the end of the trial, an observation that highlights the problems associated with advice about diet or the prescription of bulk aperients. It is important to choose a palatable preparation that will enjoy a high patient compliance.

In a later, similar study from Wales (Webster et al, 1978) 53 patients were studied in a double-blind crossover trial. They found a similar incidence to Broader et al (1974) of patients who considered that they were constipated before the trial (11%). Although they found no significant difference in the incidence of symptoms in the patients on ispaghula husk (Fybogel) and those on placebo, a significantly greater number of those treated actively reported greater ease and increased frequency of defecation.

A third study from Denmark (Moesgaard et al, 1982) in a double-blind crossover trial of five patients, comparing psyllium seed (Vi-Siblin) with a lactose placebo, found a significantly greater reduction in pain and bleeding in those under active treatment. Furthermore, they claimed that the beneficial effect was still recognizable 3 months later. Nevertheless, the authors concluded that the possible primary role of high-fibre diet in the control of first- and second-degree haemorrhoidal disease was not proven. As other simple, safe treatments such as injection or photocoagulation are significantly more effective (Keighley et al, 1979), these latter techniques should usually be the proctologist's first choice.

Vasotopic drugs

The oral administration of vasotopic drugs has received wide advertisment in continental Europe and Asia but little objective study. Hydroxyethylrutosides have been suggested as they are thought to have some benefit in treating varicose ulceration and oedema of the lower limbs; they are supposed to reduce oedema and anti-inflammatory swelling.

Topical applications

As symptoms associated with haemorrhoidal disease are so common and as only a small proportion of such patients reach a proctological clinic or even the primary physician, it is obvious that most patients go untreated or treat themselves, usually with local applications. The efficacy of local applications has rarely been assessed critically, but anecdotal evidence suggests that they do produce some symptomatic relief. Most of the preparations used contain several ingredients, including topical anaesthetics, steroids and antiseptics. Examples include Anusol, Xyloproct and Proctofoam. There seems to be no rationale for giving an antiseptic or an antibiotic. Although topical anaesthetics may give temporary relief of discomfort they can provoke skin hypersensitivity. There is no evidence that, in relieving irritation, topical steroid therapy is any better than a local anaesthetic alone, or that any of these preparations are better than a simple soft paraffin application. Soft paraffin is frequently used by sufferers for self-medication and probably works by lubricating the swollen cushions or skin tags so that they do not rub together during walking or movement. Astringent or hygroscopic agents are often used, presumably in an attempt to reduce tissue oedema. Perhaps the most common topical agent used in the USA is Preparation H. This is alleged to contain shark liver oil and a 'skin respiratory factor' of unknown formulation which is alleged to improve wound healing (Corman, 1993). Subramanyam et al (1984) created rectal ulcers by performing rectal biopsies on volunteers, and determined the speed of healing using Preparation H suppositories compared with placebo. Although it was claimed that Preparation H produced more rapid and complete healing than the placebo, the number of individuals included in the study was too small to reach statistical significance. Thus, most of these agents may produce symptomatic relief, but it is highly unlikely that any can reduce the size of haemorrhoids.

INVASIVE THERAPY (PRINCIPLES OF THE METHODS)

The history of the treatment of haemorrhoidal disease has traced the parallel development of three broad methods of invasive treatment, each one related to a hypothesis about the cause of the symptoms. These principles are: (1) prevention of prolapse by fixation; (2) prevention of congestion or impedance of venous return by stretching or by dividing the internal sphincter; and (3) excision of the engorged internal vascular cushions.

Some methods, such as freezing, combine the principle of mucosal fixation and tissue destruction; nevertheless, the classification into the three types of treatment is convenient.

Although the three different methods of treatment of haemorrhoidal disease are classified to fit in with the different theories of causation, it must be emphasized that the origin of their use was not logical. It was not based on the discovery of the cause of haemorrhoidal disease; rather the reverse, the treatment usually began in an entirely empirical way. For example, maximal anal dilatation was rediscovered by Lord, almost by accident, and when it was thought to be successful a hypothesis of causation was constructed to explain how or why the treatment might work.

Mucosal fixation (rationale and mechanism)

The mucosa and the submucosal vascular cushions can be fixed to the underlying muscle coat by creating submucosal fibrosis or full-thickness ulceration. The fibrosis or scarring prevents or minimizes prolapse of the cushions through or into the anal canal during defecation.

Methods of fixation include: (1) ligation or suture; (2) injection of an irritant sclerosant; and (3) creating an ulcer by strangulation, burning or freezing. As all methods have a place in the conservative management of haemorrhoids, the techniques are described in detail, together with their results.

How it works

In the normal subject and in the patient with haemorrhoidal disease, the mucosa and muscularis mucosae of the lower rectum and upper anal canal are only loosely adherent to the underlying circular muscle coat and can easily be prolapsed into the lower anal canal. This laxity and ability of the mucosa to prolapse can be observed during the operation of haemorrhoidectomy, particularly when performed in the lithotomy position. The rationale of mucosal fixation is an attempt to abolish or diminish this laxity. This is done to prevent the submucosal vascular cushions prolapsing into or through the anal canal during defecation.

The principal methods of mucosal fixation are: (1) to suture it in position with non-absorbable material; (2) to produce submucosal fibrosis with an irritant sclerosant; or (3) to produce a full-thickness ulcer of the mucosa, which, during healing, will fix the mucosa to the underlying muscle.

Histological studies

There have been a few histological studies on the effect of mucosal fixation, particularly following submucosal injection. Dukes was one of the first to study these changes by serial histological examination of the mucosa following injections of 10% phenol in glycerine and in water (Anderson and Dukes, 1924). The injections produced oedema with infiltration of leucocytes, red blood cells and mononuclear cells. There was also a proliferation of fibroblasts, while later changes included intravascular thrombosis. These early studies are not necessarily relevant to the modern techniques of injection using a less concentrated solution of phenol in oil. Newer sclerosants produce less extravasation of red blood cells, but there is still a cellular response with multinucleated giant cells, histiocytes, lymphocytes and eosinophils around the globules of fat (Graham-Stewart, 1962).

Two or three weeks after injection there is a pronounced fibrocytic response, often associated with palpable mucosal thickening.

Following photocoagulation, rubber-band ligation and cryotherapy, full-thickness mucosal necrosis occurs, producing a typical inflammatory reaction at the edge of the necrosis with healing by granulation tissue and fibrosis. These methods also produce a palpably thickened fibrotic area after 2–3 weeks. There are no recorded observations of venous or arterial thrombosis occurring anywhere other than in the base of the ulcer, so it is unlikely that any of these methods produce a major vascular change in the engorged anal cushion. The effect of agents employed to achieve mucosal fixation are quite dissimilar to those used for injection or cautery of varicose veins, which are claimed to produce intravascular thrombosis.

The degree of thickening and fibrosis depends on the method used. It is probably least after photocoagulation and greatest after large-volume injections or a large area of cryodestruction. Six to 12 weeks later there is often a fibrotic submucosal constriction ring due to submucosal fibrosis that persists indefinitely.

Logistics

As all the mucosal fixation methods tend to be used as office or outpatient procedures, they are usually performed at the time of the patient's first visit to the coloproctologist. They are employed after preliminary proctosigmoidoscopy has established the diagnosis, having excluded a neoplasm or inflammatory bowel disease. In most instances the treatment is applied through the proctoscope that was used for the final diagnostic assessment of the anal canal.

Injection or sclerotherapy

The technique of injection will be described in detail.

Equipment

Until quite recently in the UK the most commonly employed apparatus was still the time-honoured Gabriel syringe and needles (Figure 12.10). However, these have been rapidly replaced by the

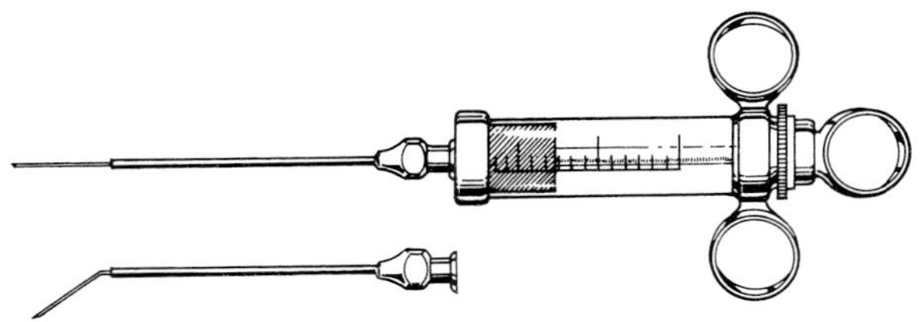

Figure 12.10 Gabriel syringe and needles.

purpose-designed disposable syringes and needles. The particular advantages of the traditional glass syringe and needle were that they were comfortable for the operator and the syringe did not shoot the needle off the end like a dart. It requires considerable force to inject a viscous solution of phenol in oil, and therefore a conventional disposable plastic syringe is uncomfortable for the operator. Furthermore the force exerted by the syringe is likely to dislodge the needle unless there is a mechanism to lock it to the syringe; in addition, phenol denatures conventional plastic. The other advantage of the Gabriel syringe was the design of the shaft of the needle with a bevelled buffer that ensured that the tip of the needle could be inserted for only 1–2 cm, so reducing the risk of placing the injection too deeply into, or even through, the muscle into adjacent structures such as the prostate, as may occur with an unprotected and ungraduated needle. These advantages of the Gabriel syringe are now incorporated into disposable syringes made of phenol-resistant material with three-finger control and a Luer-Lok device to prevent the needle becoming forced off.

The 5% phenol in almond or arachis oil is self-sterilizing and can be kept in a non-sterile condition in a glass jar. Goligher (1984) states that 'in large rectal outpatient clinics where phenol injection is the principal form of therapy and when 15 mL of the solution may be used for each patient, up to 500 mL of the solution may be used during the course of a clinic'. Therefore, he advocates using a wide-necked jar into which the syringe can be dipped for refilling. It is difficult to see how this technique can be justified, even on the grounds of economy. If after attending a rectal clinic a patient were to develop infective hepatitis or acquired immune deficiency syndrome (AIDS), it might be difficult to resist litigation. Proctologists should now use sterilized glass ampoules, despite the extra expense.

Hughes (1957) claimed that 2 mL injections were as good as 5 mL injections and advocated a disposable standard 2 mL syringe and a 2 mL ampoule of phenol in oil for each cushion. The modern technique is to use a disposable 10 mL Luer-Lock syringe, a special needle and a 10 mL ampoule, and to inject 3 mL into the base of each vascular cushion.

Although 5% phenol in almond or arachis oil is the most common injection agent used in the UK, a quinuride solution containing 2.4% of anhydrous quinine-urea, with a pH adjusted to 2.6, is commonly used in the USA. Although no comparative trials have been made, it appears to have a similar effect to phenol in oil and produces submucosal fibrosis rather than obliteration of blood vessels.

Preparation and position of the patient

Although many authors state that submucosal injections can be performed on all patients who attend for the first time with symptoms of haemorrhoidal disease, others advocate the prescription of an oral or rectal cathartic before the patient attends the clinic. Our view is that the presence of some faecal material in the rectum is no contraindication to performing sclerotherapy or any of the other forms of mucosal fixation. It is unwise, however, to perform such a manoeuvre in the face of gross faecal impaction. All patients with a relatively empty rectum can be treated safely at the first attendance. Attempted bowel preparation that has been inadequate often results in a watery stool which makes the procedure more difficult than it would have been with no preparation.

The patient can be treated in the left lateral position, in the knee–chest position or on a special proctology table. In our opinion the least uncomfortable for the patient is the left lateral position, although to inject the right posterior anal cushion does require some agility on the part of the operator. These manoeuvres are often traumatic to the operator's neck so, if this is a problem, he or she may be advised to invest in a special proctology table or to disregard their patients' embarrassment and place them in the knee–chest position.

Technique

An oblique-ended illuminated proctoscope is passed through the anal canal into the rectum, and the obturator removed (Figure 12.11a). If faeces then enter the end of the proctoscope and obscure the view, these are best removed by pushing a ball of cotton wool through the proctoscope and leaving it in position in the rectum. Even two or three balls of wool will not cause the patient any difficulty in subsequent evacuation.

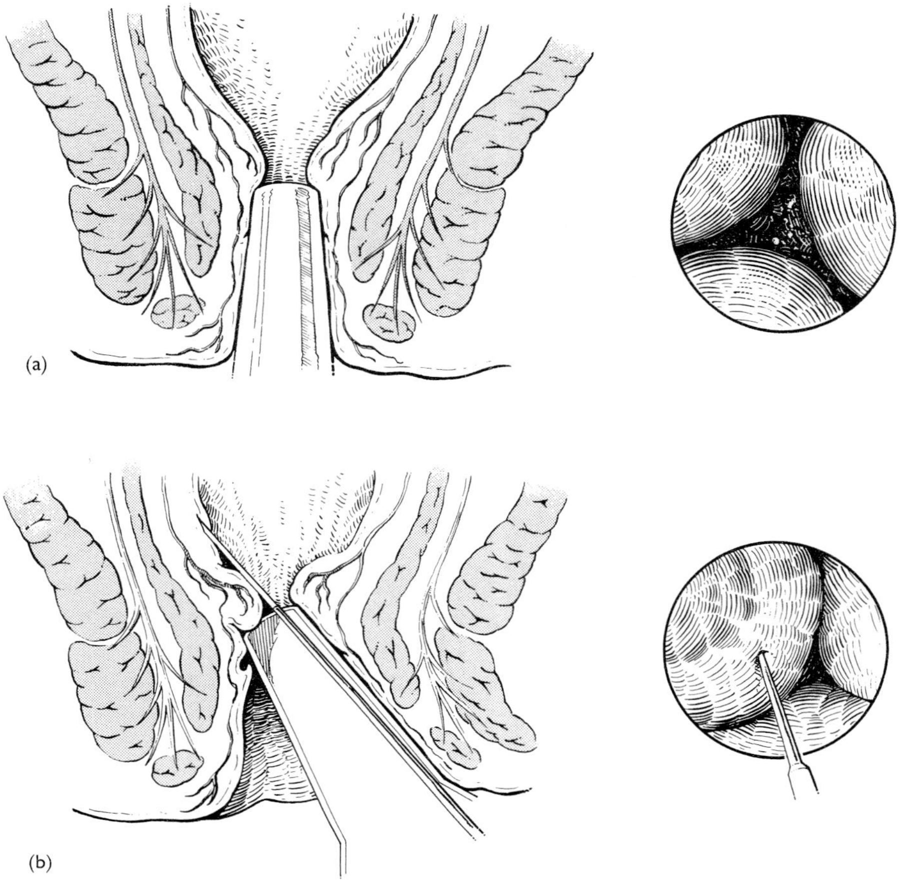

Figure 12.11a,b Technique of injecting haemorrhoids (see text).

Once the mucosa of the rectal ampulla is visible the proctoscope is withdrawn until the mucosa closes over the mouth of the 'scope, indicating the upper end of the anal canal. At this point the mucosa still looks like normal large bowel mucosa. Goligher (1984) recommends that, because the right posterior pile is always the most difficult to inject, it should be injected first. There seems to be merit in this suggestion.

On withdrawing the instrument slightly, the reddish mucosa changes to the purplish mucosa indicating engorged underlying vascular cushions. This is the base of the cushion that will require treatment. The 'scope is then withdrawn further until the pecten line is reached to give an indication of the distance between that line and the base of the cushion (see Figure 12.11). The sclerosant-containing syringe is then held in the operator's dominant hand and the handle of the proctoscope is held with the other hand. The 'scope is then manipulated until the junction between the pink and purple mucosa is positioned over the mouth of the 'scope, indicating the base of the cushion. The needle of the syringe is then introduced obliquely through the mucosa for approximately 1 cm (Figure 12.11b).

Some authorities have stated that the solution can be inadvertently injected directly into a haemorrhoidal vein and that this causes immediate transient pain in the upper abdomen or precordium and the patient may notice an unpleasant taste in the mouth. Although no long-term sequelae are reported (Mann et al, 1988), some operators advocate withdrawing the plunger of the syringe to make sure that the needle is not in the vein. We have attempted this manoeuvre many times but have never been able to withdraw blood through the needle, and so conclude that it is very unusual and perhaps impossible to put the needle directly into a blood vessel in an anal vascular cushion.

A very small quantity of the sclerosant is then

injected, while observing the patient's response. The procedure should be entirely painless. If the patient is aware of discomfort as the solution is injected, it indicates that the needle is either too close to the anal verge, or too deep; the injection should be stopped until the needle is repositioned. If the injection cannot be given painlessly, it should not be given at all. Usually there is no discomfort, and so 3–5 mL is injected beneath the mucosa to produce an obvious swelling. If the injection is too superficial a totally avascular 'bleb' is raised, as with an intradermal injection. This is not ideal and may result in sloughing of the mucosa; if such a bleb appears, the injection should be stopped. If there is no swelling of the mucosa as the solution is injected, it may indicate that the needle has gone through a fold of mucosa and out the other side so that the injection is being made into the lumen of the rectum (Figure 12.12). This may be obvious from the sudden appearance of a lot of oil in the lumen; however, inevitably some oil leaks back into the lumen from the puncture wound. With experience it is soon obvious when an injection is being placed at the right depth.

The needle is withdrawn and the manoeuvre repeated in the right anterior and right posterior positions. It is unwise to inject more than 5 mL of the solution into the base of each cushion. If more is used the submucosal oily injection is likely to track circumferentially round the submucosal plane; this we believe may be the cause of stenotic rings that are found in the upper anorectum. In the past when we misguidedly used manual dilatation for internal haemorrhoids, we encountered many such firm fibrous bands and observed that these were usually in patients who had had previous treatment of their haemorrhoidal disease, usually by injection but sometimes by rubber-band ligation.

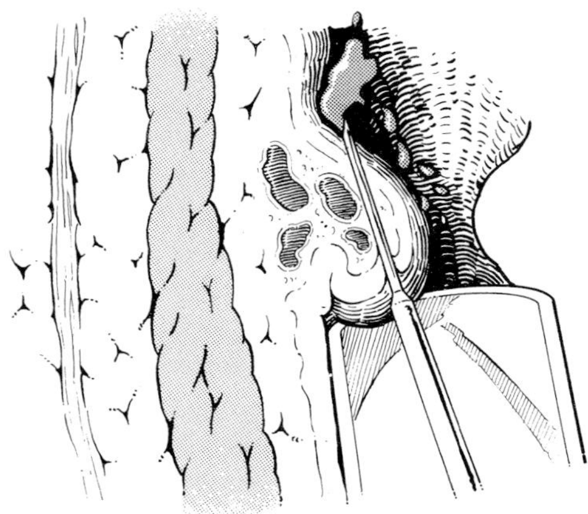

Figure 12.12 Incorrect technique of haemorrhoid injection. The needle has passed through the fold of mucosa overlying the haemorrhoid and the injection is being made into the rectal lumen.

Particular care should be taken when injecting near the midline anteriorly because of the proximity of the prostate and the urethra in the male and the vagina in the female. Fortunately it is rarely necessary to have to inject in the midline because there is rarely a base of a vascular cushion at that site. If there is bleeding from the mucosa when the needle is withdrawn, another cotton-wool ball placed in this position as the proctoscope is withdrawn almost invariably stops the bleeding. On the rare occasions when it does not, a rubber-band ligation may be performed at the injection site.

When injections are being repeated, particularly months or years after the first injection, it may be difficult to distend the submucous space because of the previous fibrosis. Under these circumstances it may be unwise to persist with re-injection but rather to employ an alternative method such as photocoagulation or cryotherapy.

Complications

These include pain from a badly sited injection or from submucosal extravasation, haemorrhage from the puncture point and, very rarely, lower urinary tract sepsis and even impotence in the male from a grossly misplaced injection (Bullock, 1997). A tight encircling submucosal band may occur months or years later from the fibrosis, particularly if there has been radial extravasation. A pronounced inflammatory response to the injected oil (the so-called oleogranuloma) very rarely may occur. Bacteraemia has been reported in 8% of patients undergoing sclerotherapy (Adami et al, 1981). Although none of these patients developed septicaemia, it is recommended that patients at risk (e.g. those with valvular heart disease) should be given prophylactic antibiotic therapy.

Aftercare

No special treatment or precautions are usually required and the patient may return directly to normal activities. However, if there has been discomfort, it is advisable for the patient to rest for the remainder of the day. The injection itself should be painless, but the patient should be warned that a dull perineal ache may occur after a while. This is thought to be due to the phenol in oil tracking down beneath the mucosa towards the sensitive epithelial area. Usually a mild analgesic is sufficient to control this discomfort, but the patient should be warned to lie down with the feet elevated if the pain is anything other than minor.

Patients who feel some discomfort in the anal canal may misinterpret this as the urge to defecate. For this reason injection should not be performed if the rectum is full. If the rectum is empty the patient should be advised to disregard the call for defecation until the next day. In constipated patients it is advisable to make sure that they have a bowel softening agent (e.g. Dulcolax) or bulking agent (e.g. methylcellulose) to ensure easy defecation. The patient should be advised not to strain during defecation and to be sure to replace immediately any mucosal prolapse that might occur during or afterwards. As in all patients having conservative treatment of haemorrhoids, constipation, hard stools and straining should be avoided during the whole treatment period; hence a high-fibre diet and bulking agents are advised indefinitely unless the patient already has a tendency to frequent loose or bulky stools.

Results

In the fifth edition of his textbook *Surgery of the Anus, Rectum and Colon*, Goligher (1984) states 'considering how extensively injection therapy has been used for haemorrhoids, it is disappointing to discover how few worthwhile studies have been made of the late results of treatment. In extenuation of this unsatisfactory state of affairs it must be admitted that it is far more difficult to maintain an efficient follow-up on patients who have received outpatient treatment for haemorrhoids than on those who have undergone a major operation.' In the years since this was written there have been few other reliable long-term results of injection therapy.

We agree with Goligher's condemnation of the limited value of collective reviews such as that by Kilbourne (1934), when over 25 000 patients were reported to have had injection sclerotherapy with a recurrence rate of 15%. This survey was based on a questionnaire to a large number of proctologists who were quoting their results, often from memory and usually with bias.

Milligan (1939, 1943) claimed to have a 5-year follow-up of almost 100% on 200 patients treated by injection at St Mark's Hospital. At 5 years almost all of them considered themselves to be cured, although 15% had needed further treatment during the 5 years. He claimed that 31% of the patients in the series with third-degree piles were cured by injection. This claim, unsubstantiated by other observers who have tried injection sclerotherapy for third-degree haemorrhoids, throws some doubt on the validity of Milligan's figures compiled at a time when objectivity was not an important criteria in the assessment of the results of favoured therapy.

Cheng et al (1981) reported 30 patients 1 year after injection therapy, seven (23%) of whom were either no better or worse. In a similar study, Sim et al (1981) reported a 1-year follow-up on 24 out of 26 patients who had been treated by injection sclerotherapy as part of a controlled trial. Six of their 24 patients were either little improved or worse as a result of treatment. The principal cause of failure in the patients treated by injection was the development of prolapse of the pile in six patients who had not had prolapse before treatment began.

Greca et al (1981), also as part of a comparative trial with rubber-band ligation, reported on the 1-year follow-up of 33 out of 43 patients initially treated by injection. This was a disappointingly poor follow-up response and tended to negate the validity of any conclusions from this study. Nevertheless, 10 of the 33 patients (30%) considered that they were no better or worse 1 year after injection. Most of the failures in this study were in patients with third-degree haemorrhoids who were probably inappropriately chosen for injections.

Santos et al (1993) treated 189 patients with a large dose (3×5 mL) phenol injection and reviewed their results after 4 years. Fifty-three patients (28%) were cured, 26 (12.7%) were improved, 35 (18.5%) remained unchanged, 59 (31.2%) deteriorated and 16 (8.5%) required surgical intervention. They concluded that large-dose single-session sclerotherapy provided only short-term benefits in the majority of patients with symptomatic haemorrhoids.

Khoury et al (1985) performed a randomized trial comparing single with multiple injection treatments. One hundred and two consecutive patients who had not improved with conservative medical treatment and who had first- or second-degree haemorrhoids were randomized. At 3 months, 89.9% of the whole group were either cured or improved of their symptoms and this result was maintained for 12 months after injection. However, there was no difference in the degree of improvement between the two treatment regimens. In the study reported by Khoury et al (1985), neither of the groups were compared with a control group receiving medical therapy alone. Senapati and Nicholls (1988) have performed such a study, although the number randomized (43) was small. One group received bulk laxatives and injection therapy and the other received bulk laxatives alone. After 6 months no significant difference in symptoms could be demonstrated.

From these conflicting data it is difficult to give a precise figure on the expectation of cure from injection and it is more likely that the results are dependent on the extent of the haemorrhoidal disease, rather than on the skill of the operator or the particular technique of injection. It is possible that many patients treated by injection could have experienced equally good results if they had been given simple dietary advice and no injections, as indicated by Senapati and Nicholls (1988). Nevertheless, it seems likely that if injection is used in the management of first- or second-degree piles, particularly those in which bleeding is the principal symptom, more than 70% of the patients will be quite satisfied with the result of treatment and most of those who are not satisfied will need additional treatment within the first few months. Considering the safety and the simplicity of injection for haemorrhoidal disease, these results are difficult to better and a strong case can still be made for using injection as the first line of treatment for minor degrees of haemorrhoidal disease.

Numerous trials have compared injections with other techniques to achieve mucosal fixation. To prevent repetition, the comparisons will be made when each of the other therapeutic options are discussed.

Surveillance

If the patient is rendered asymptomatic by the injection, which is usually the case for first- and some second-degree haemorrhoids, there is no need for a follow-up visit. The patient's and the doctor's time can be saved by asking the patient to return only if complications occur or symptoms persist or recur. It is never easy to inject again within a few weeks, yet we find it surprising that, in many clinics in many parts of the world, the patients are asked to return for review 1 month after injection. In our opinion, there is no point in review within 3 months and then only if the symptoms persist.

One of the common dilemmas that occurs is when the patient has rectal bleeding, for which no cause other than 'internal haemorrhoids' can be found on examination, sigmoidoscopy and even sometimes on barium enema or colonoscopy. As everyone has vascular cushions it is easy to assume that these are responsible for the bleeding. It is therefore important to be sure that the injection has stopped the bleeding because of the possibility of there being an overlooked mucosal lesion higher in the bowel. For this reason, it is very important to impress on patients the need for them to return for review even for the slightest rectal bleeding, and particularly either if the blood is on the stool rather than on the paper or is dark in colour.

Rubber-band ligation

Principle

The principle of rubber-band ligation appears to be similar to that of submucosal injection. It produces fixation of the mucosa but does so by causing ulceration rather than a simple submucosal inflammatory reaction.

Equipment

A number of instruments have been devised to apply a small rubber-band or O-ring tightly around a tongue of mucosa that has been pulled into the barrel of the applicator. This band produces ischaemic necrosis, with sloughing of the mucosa and ulceration. The original Barron ligator was the instrument most frequently used until the suction band equipment became available (Barron, 1963).

The apparatus comprises a long shaft that can be introduced through a proctoscope (Figure 12.13). It contains within it a rod which activates the inner of the two concentric drums at the working end of the instrument. Proximally there is a handle which is squeezed to advance the outer drum so as to release the rubber ring. The rubber O-rings are 2–3 mm diameter and are small sections of black rubber tubing. The tube is supplied almost completely divided so that simple finger pressure will detach each ring individually. The rubber-bands are stretched over a loading cone from which they are pushed on to the

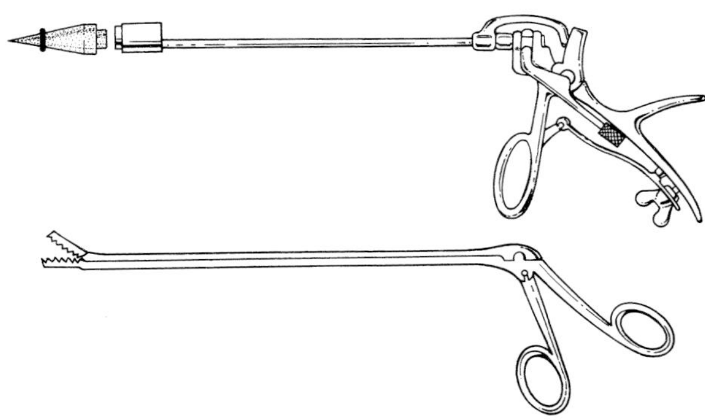

Figure 12.13 Barron banding equipment.

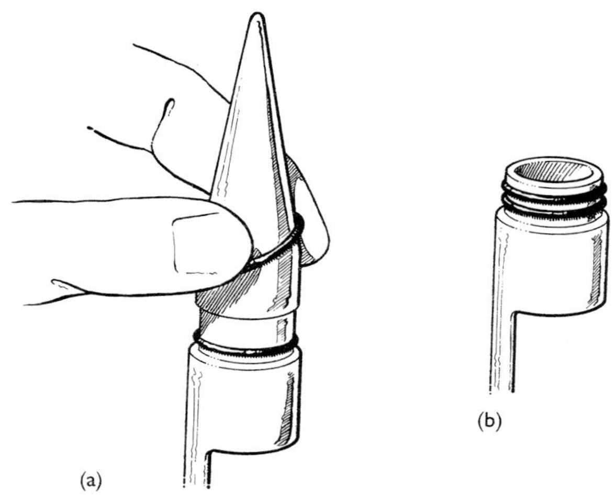

Figure 12.14a,b Loading of elastic bands on Barron applicator.

11 mm inner drum of the instrument (Figure 12.14a,b). Better strangulation of the mucosa appears to occur if two bands are used rather than one. The shaft and drums of the instrument are interchangeable so that a number of shafts can be prepared in advance and interchanged on to the same handle. However, the mechanism of changing the handle is not very simple or swift and some people prefer to reload rubber-bands on to the same instrument if more than one pile is being ligated. This reloading procedure may not be aesthetically desirable if the cylinder becomes contaminated with faeces and may not be necessary anyway (Dodi, 1992).

Another simpler and cheaper form of the Barron ligator is the McGiveny ligator (Figure 12.15) which consists of a short metal cylinder on a long handle

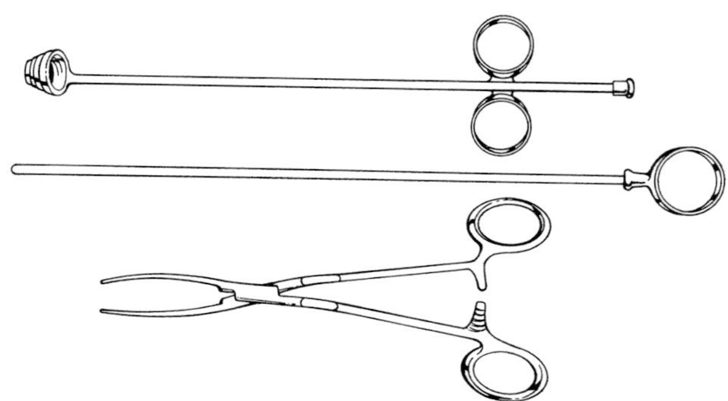

Figure 12.15 McGiveny banding equipment.

with a small groove at the end, over which a single band is stretched using a conical loading cone. A small central rod passes down the hollow shaft of the instrument and dislodges the rubber-band from the end of the metal ring.

Some people attempt to put two rubber-bands on the end of the McGiveny ring, but we have found this manoeuvre difficult; the apparatus seems to work more easily with one ring. We have used both the McGiveny and the Barron instruments for many years, treating several hundred patients. Most of our staff find the Barron instrument more positive and reliable but there are some who prefer the McGiveny.

To obviate the need for an assistant to hold the proctoscope during ligation, a number of ingenious devices have been produced to make it a one-handed procedure. Van Hoorn (1972) described a 1.8 cm proctoscope that has a large rubber-band stretched over its tip. When the vascular cushion is identified and grasped with the forceps, it is pulled into the lumen of the proctoscope; the handle is then squeezed and the rubber ring strangles its contents (Figure 12.16). The disadvantage of this ligator is that it requires large, expensive rubber rings and there is the danger of pulling too much of the vascular cushion into the ligator and so causing pain and resulting in the development of a large ulcer. Also, the special proctoscope gives a poorer view of the anal canal than does the conventional proctoscope; it requires some adjustment and experience to use. We have not had sufficient experience with this ligator to condemn it but are not attracted to the concept.

There is less theoretical disadvantage to another device, produced by Thomson (1980), which is a modified McGiveny applicator fitted within a metal cylinder which fits precisely inside a standard cylindrical Naunton–Morgan proctoscope. The ligator is activated and the rubber-bands pushed off the end by a thumbplate situated at the entrance to the proctoscope (Figure 12.17). It is a practical device and uses the conventional sizes of rubber rings. Another one-handed ligator uses suction to pull sufficient mucosa into the cylinder for it to be ligated (Schofield et al, 1984). Other suction ligators include the Lurz Goltner and McGown devices (McGown, Pembroke Pincs, FL). In our clinic we now prefer to use the suction banding equipment with a lightweight portable suction device. The bands are mounted over Perspex cones to screw-on applicators, so that if only one ligator is available two or three applicators can be charged with bands if two or three bands are to be applied (Figure 12.18). Several other makes of rubber-ring

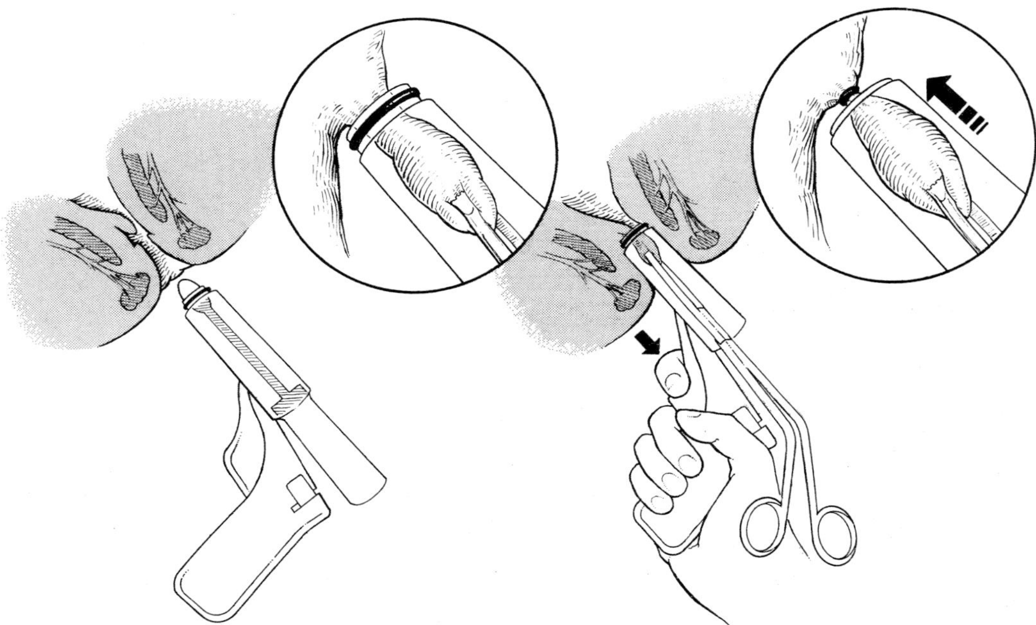

Figure 12.16 Banding equipment, designed by Van Hoorn (1972), which obviates the need for two hands.

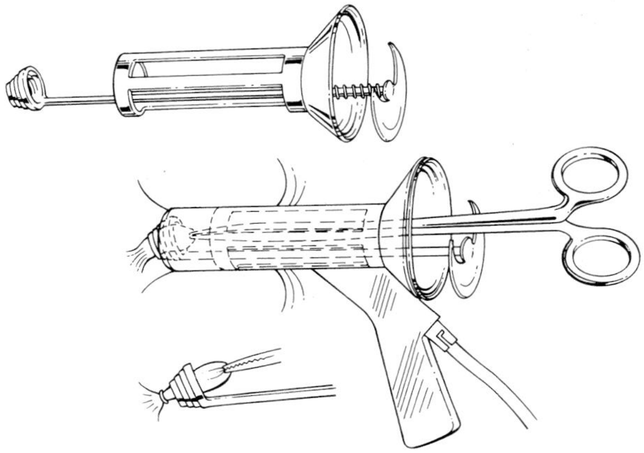

Figure 12.17 Banding equipment designed by Thomson (1980).

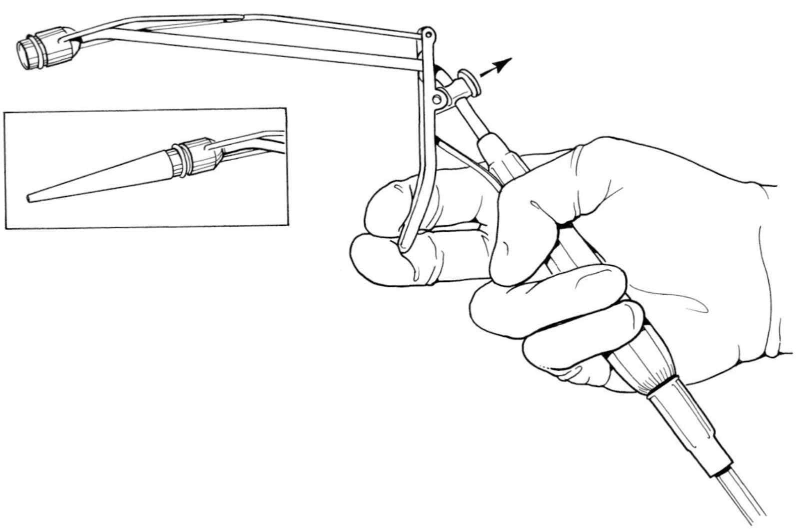

Figure 12.18 Suction band applicator. Suction is applied by placing the thumb over the button (marked by the arrow), the lever is advanced and the band applied to the mucosa adherent to the instrument.

ligation apparatus are available, including the robust but cumbersome Preston 'gun' and a precariously complex multiaction machine popular in France.

Preparation and position of the patient

As with injection, no special bowel preparation is required, but treatment should not proceed until the bowel is emptied if there is gross faecal impaction.

The position on the couch is the same as for injection, but as the Barron instrument requires the operator to use both hands, an assistant is required to hold the proctoscope in position. This of course is not necessary using the suction band apparatus. When the patient is in the left lateral position, the operator sits with the patient's anus at eye level.

Technique

The proctoscope is passed through the anal canal into the rectum. Many surgeons prefer to use an oblique-ended or grooved proctoscope to allow the whole of the internal cushion to prolapse into the lumen so that it is easy to recognize the base (upper limit) of the cushion. As the base of each cushion is ligated it is important to have observed carefully the whole of the engorged cushion and the dentate line. In our opinion many operators, and even many of those who write descriptions of the technique, tend to apply the rubber-band too close to the dentate line. Although there is normally no sensory innervation above this level, a rubber-band ligation applied within 1 cm of the dentate line often causes discomfort. The base of the cushion usually lies 1.5–2 cm above the dentate line and here the mucosal tissue can be grasped with the forceps and pulled into the cylinder of the ligator without causing the patient discomfort.

Once the site for the ligation is determined, the forceps are passed through the cylinder of the ligator and the mucosa is gripped firmly and pulled gently (Figure 12.19a). If this causes the patient discomfort, the ligation should not be performed at this site and the mucosa should be grasped again a little higher up, away from the dentate line. If grasping causes no pain then gentle traction downwards on the forceps and upward pressure with the cylinder fill the cylinder with mucosa and underlying vascular tissue (Figure 12.19b). The handle is then squeezed and the two rubber-bands slip off the inner cylinder to strangulate approximately 1 cm diameter of tissue (Figure 12.19c). Using the suction band technique, the proctoscope is passed first to identify the distribution of the piles. The instrument is then reintroduced so that the suction band applicator is applied to the mucosa above the cushion. Suction is applied by placing the index finger over the suction orifice and the rubber-band is advanced over the cartridge to enclose the neck of the anal mucosa which has been sucked into the instrument (see Figure 12.18).

Barron (1963) recommended that only one ligation should be performed at each session and that subsequent ligations should be performed at

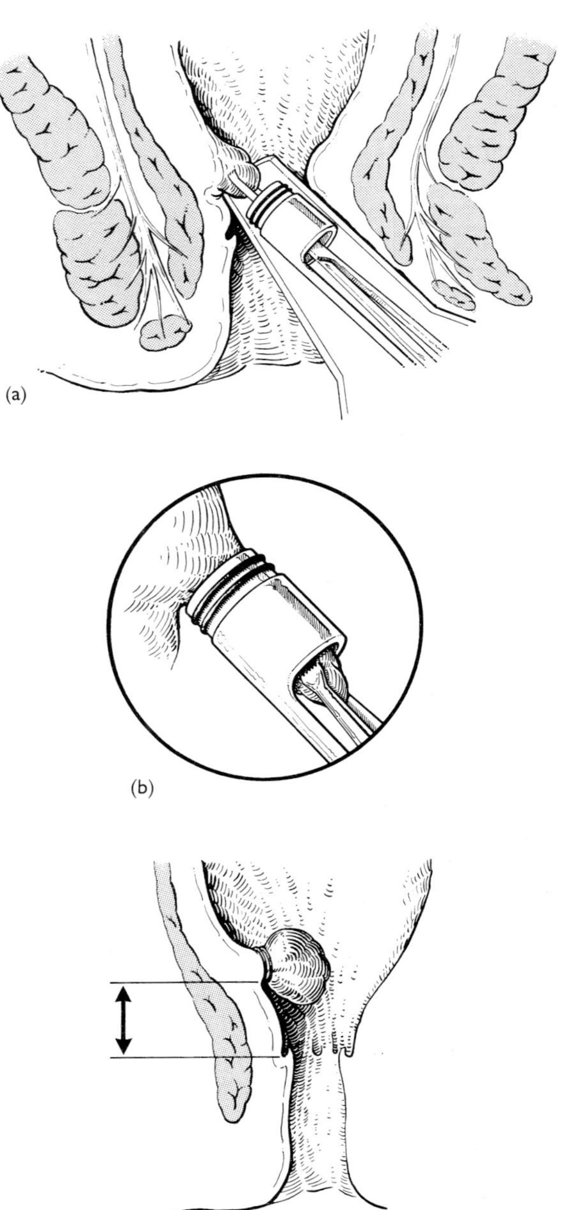

Figure 12.19a–c Technique of applying bands to the base of the pile using Barron equipment.

3-weekly intervals. However, we have found that it is possible to perform two or three ligations at the initial diagnostic attendance. This is obviously economical in time and money and it may be that the first diagnostic and therapeutic consultation is the only visit required. Many people who have described the technique have advocated multiple ligations (Bartizal and Slosberger, 1977; Murie et al, 1980; Cheng et al, 1981; Khubchandani 1983, Goligher, 1984)

Additional procedures after ligation include injection of local anaesthetic or phenol into the strangulated tissue, or freezing of the ligated portion. Despite claims by advocates we can see no theoretical advantage in further complicating the simple ligation technique.

Complications

Pain

The most common complication of rubber-band ligation is pain at the time, or a few moments after, the ligation. This is usually mild, lasts only for an hour or two and is usually controlled by paracetamol. Occasionally there is severe pain at the time of ligation. We used to treat such patients conservatively with analgesics and rest, but now we remove the rubber-band immediately and revert to treatment with photocoagulation. One of the difficulties is the removal of the rubber-band, which is usually rapidly and firmly fixed by oedema of the strangulated mucosa. The rubber-band cannot be pulled off easily and attempts to do so make the patient even more uncomfortable. We have found that the best method is to grasp the strangulated mucosa with the forceps and attempt to rotate it so that the rubber-band, or at least the constricting groove, is seen clearly. Then a small triangular bladed knife is used to cut directly at the centre of the base of the ligated tissue until the band snaps and the mucosa returns to normal colour. Sometimes this manoeuvre can be performed without significant haemorrhage, but occasionally the knife cut produces moderately profuse bleeding. The bleeding usually stops within a minute or two with gentle pressure with a cotton wool ball. On some occasions we have found it useful to have a photocoagulator available to coagulate the bleeding point. Alternatively, the band can be removed by interposing the end of conventional disposable suture-removal scissors or the application of a crochet hook. These techniques are said to produce less bleeding (Corman, 1993). Not infrequently, a general anaesthetic is required to remove the band if outpatient manoeuvres fail.

Even if the patient experiences no discomfort as the rubber-band is 'fired' to strangulate the tissue, a few moments later when they stand up from the couch they may feel sick and faint, and feel they need to open their bowels. If the sufferer lies down for a few minutes the sensation usually passes; if it does not, he or she is given two paracetamol tablets and a glass of water.

Some degree of discomfort occurs in about 20% of patients who have rubber-band ligation, and is severe in about 3%. We believe that now using our advised technique of ligating 1.5–2 cm above the dentate line (Figure 12.19c), post-treatment pain has been virtually abolished. However, a moderate degree of discomfort is more common after this procedure than it is after injection or photocoagulation.

Bleeding

Rubber-band ligation causes tissue necrosis. When the tissue separates, the plane of cleavage between the dead and live tissue is vascular granulation tissue that frequently bleeds. Sometimes there is a small arteriole at the line of separation which can cause moderately severe bleeding. Severe bleeding can necessitate admission and transfusion in about 0.5–1% of patients.

Pelvic cellulitis

In 1980, O'Hara reported the first case of fatal clostridial infection resulting from banding haemorrhoids. Since then, sporadic reports of a similar problem have appeared in the literature, not all of which, thankfully, have resulted in death. The most alarming report was in 1985 by Russell and Donohue (1985), who described four men between 34 and 54 years of age who developed this complication and died. It would appear that earlier recognition and aggressive antibiotic treatment can result in resolution (Scarpa et al, 1988), but the key to the problem is prevention. Measures suggested include screening patients for possible immunodeficiency, rectal washouts prior to banding, prophylactic oral antibiotics and the use of meticulous technique (McGirney, 1981; Katchian, 1982, 1985). Despite this advice, the fear of pelvic cellulitis has recently inhibited some colorectal surgeons from using the technique.

Aftercare and surveillance

It is advisable to give the patient a printed list of instructions about postoperative management. Patients usually forget the details of verbal instructions and often need to refresh their memory.

If aching pain makes the patient uncomfortable but does not interfere with normal activity, simple analgesics are all that are needed and the patient is advised to rest, preferably with the feet elevated. Sitting in a warm bath is also comforting. The patient is advised to avoid alcohol and not to attempt to defecate until the following day. They are also advised to avoid vigorous activity, alcohol and dietary excesses until there are no abnormal sensations, even after defecation.

If there is fever, malaise, urinary hesitancy or retention, or increasing local discomfort after the second post-banding day, the possibility of pelvic cellulitis must be considered and the patient should return to the surgeon for advice.

Patients are also warned of the possibility of secondary haemorrhage when the necrotic tissue sloughs in 7–14 days. They are instructed to lie down and rest if this occurs and to return to the clinic or contact the doctor who performed the ligation if one or more voluminous bloody stools are passed.

Results

Many of the results reported following rubber-band ligation are clouded by the fact that the series are relatively small and appear to indicate the early experience of different clinics in this technique, usually before it has been refined. Furthermore, it is evident that in many published reports the clinicians concerned have not learnt to apply the rubber-band higher above the dentate line than they were accustomed to inject the cushions with phenol in oil.

In Goligher's group's early experience (Clark et al, 1967) they produced such severe pain in some patients that it was necessary to prescribe pethidine for a night or two after the procedure. Other surgeons first adopting the technique of rubber-band ligation have had similar experiences and abandoned the method. In one of the first objective reports of the results of rubber-band ligation for haemorrhoids by Carden (1970), a success rate of greater than 80% was reported.

Within a controlled trial, 24 Birmingham patients had rubber-band ligation in 1971 and were assessed by interview or questionnaire 10 and 34 weeks after treatment (mean 23 weeks). Fourteen of the 24 patients (58%) had no symptoms, the other ten were improved but still had residual symptoms. However, 33% of the patients had pain or discomfort lasting for longer than 2 days. By 1977, the Birmingham group had improved their technique and in the next reported trial (Arabi et al, 1977b) pain was reported in only 5 of 51 patients allocated to rubber-band ligation in a trial comparing rubber-band ligation with lateral sphincterotomy. Forty-five of the 51 patients were assessed at 6 months, at which time eight (18%) were either no better or worse.

In another randomized prospective trial from Glasgow, Murie et al (1980) treated 51 patients by rubber-band ligation, 43 of whom were available for assessment at 1 year. Thirty-one were judged as having an excellent result, seven were moderately successful, none were worse and only five (12%) had no improvement. Their results with rubber-band ligation for third-degree haemorrhoids were better than in many of the other series. Nineteen of 27 patients with third-degree haemorrhoids (70%) had no prolapse at 1 year. However, they found that pain was a significant problem after rubber-band ligation (15 had pain for more than 48 hours) but, unlike some of the other workers, they ligated all three primary sites at a single outpatient visit. At the end of their trial comparing rubber-band ligation and haemorrhoidectomy, they concluded that, for second- and third-degree haemorrhoids, rubber-band ligation should be considered as the first line of treatment.

One of the largest series of rubber-band ligation was that reported by Bartizal and Slosberger (1977). They retrospectively reviewed 670 patients who underwent a total of 3208 rubber-band ligations. Mild to moderate discomfort occurred in 32 (4.8%) of their patients, while pain severe enough to limit activity occurred in only four (0.6%). Nine patients (1%) had severe bleeding, two of whom required readmission to hospital. A similar incidence of complications occurred in Bat et al's (1993) study of 512 patients treated in Israel over a 7-year period. However, Hardwick and Durdey (1994) in a group of 50 patients treated by rubber-band ligation and assessed for pain by linear analogue score found that pain was more frequent than previously acknowledged.

In an attempt to determine whether there was any difference between single or multiple rubber-band ligations with respect to the symptoms produced by the procedure, Khubchandani (1983) randomly allocated 100 consecutive patients to one, two or three ligations at one session. He found no statistical difference in the morbidity or complications resulting from multiple ligations as compared with one ligation. Mild discomfort occurred in 28%, 32% and 39% of those having one, two or three ligations respectively. More severe pain requiring administration of analgesics occurred in 28%, 5% and 23% respectively in the one-, two- and three-ligation groups. He concluded that two or three rubber-band ligations can be performed quite safely at one session without increasing the risk of discomfort or complications. Poon et al (1986) performed a similar prospective randomized study and came to the same conclusions. Lee et al (1994) reached similar conclusions from a retrospective study. At the end of Khubchandani's paper he stressed his belief that the site of the ligation should be at least 1 cm proximal to the dentate line. He also said that the amount of ligated tissue should produce a volume of strangulated tissue no larger than 1 cm diameter. Like us, he stressed that if the vascular tissue appears to be sensitive when it is grasped with the traction forceps the ligation should be abandoned. This seems to us to be a very obvious rule, but one that is, we suspect, disregarded in some of the series where the incidence of discomfort is high.

Another long-term study, previously quoted, in which rubber-band ligation was compared with injection was that performed by Sim et al (1981). They reported a 3-year follow-up in 18 patients treated by rubber-band ligation. Eleven of the patients considered the result excellent, five thought it was moderately successful, none were worse, and only 2 (11%) thought there was little improvement.

In 1980, Wrobleski et al reviewed the records of 266 patients who had undergone rubber-ring ligation for haemorrhoidal disease. The minimum follow-up was 36 months, with a mean of 60 months. Eighty per cent of patients considered themselves to be improved and 69% were totally free of symptoms. Haemorrhoidectomy had been required in 7.5%. Although they found that there were no more complications if they used multiple ligations, they found that those patients who had had a single band applied did just as well as those with two or more ligations. However, they did not state, as seems likely, that the patients who had one band probably had less severe haemorrhoidal disease than those who had three. In a long-term review of the results of rubber-band ligation, Steinberg et al (1975) performed a questionnaire follow-up of 147 patients at a mean of 4.8 years after rubber-band ligation. One hundred and twenty-five patients responded to the questionnaire, although 89% of the patients were either cured or satisfied with the results of treatment, only 44% were totally symptom-free. Further conservative treatment such as rubber-band ligation or dilatation had been required in 12% but only three patients (2%) required a haemorrhoidectomy.

Although these series are not strictly comparable for severity of symptoms or size of haemorrhoids, there is a fairly good uniformity in the overall results of clinical assessment. Therefore, surgeons or clinics using rubber-band ligation as their principal form of treatment for all types of haemorrhoidal disease can feel reasonably confident that, provided they place the rubber-band so that it is at least 1 cm above the dentate line, they should have less than a 3% incidence of severe pain, a 1% incidence of secondary haemorrhage and have 80% or more of their patients well satisfied with the results of treatment for more than 3 years after the procedure. Those who do not learn to site the rubber-bands correctly may join the distinguished ranks of those who have tried the procedure and abandoned it.

Comparisons with other forms of treatment

In a series comparing haemorrhoidectomy, anal dilatation, rubber-band ligation and cryotherapy, Lewis et al (1983) randomly allocated into four groups 112 patients with prolapsing haemorrhoids, all of whom had failed to respond to injections of phenol in oil and required manual replacement after defecation. Of the 30 patients treated by rubber-band ligation, 28 were available for review: 24 of them had required further treatment, including haemorrhoidectomy in 12, anal dilatation in three and injection in nine. It seems that the poor results experienced in this trial were probably because they were selecting only severe degrees of haemorrhoidal disease in patients who had already failed injection treatment and were now considered only suitable for haemorrhoidectomy. However, when the Birmingham group compared rubber-band ligation with injection therapy in patients who had not previously had treatment, the two forms of therapies were found to be almost comparable (Table 12.1). However, when rubber-band ligation was compared with cryosurgery, band ligation was shown to be significantly more effective (Keighley et al, 1979). Moreover, when rubber-band ligation was compared with photocoagulation,

Table 12.1 Randomized trial to compare rubber-band ligation with injection therapy.

	Rubber-band ligation (*n* = 39)	*Injection therapy* (*n* = 43)
Results at 12 months		
Asymptomatic	13	15
Improved	5	8
No better	4	4
Additional therapy	6	6
Lost to follow-up	11	10

From Greca et al (1981).

band ligation was marginally more effective, especially for third-degree haemorrhoids (Ambrose et al, 1983).

Cryotherapy

Principles

When tissue freezes and intracellular water crystallizes, cell membranes are destroyed and tissue death occurs. Tissue freezes and becomes solid at –20°C. Permanent destruction of tissue occurs at –22°C. Rewarming of frozen tissue usually takes 2–3 minutes and immediately after rewarming the frozen tissue looks like normal tissue, but within 15 minutes oedema and increased vascularity occur in the frozen tissues. Within 6 hours there is a microscopical difference between frozen and unfrozen cells. Within 24 hours there is infarction and thrombosis in the area that has been frozen, and in the next 24 hours the tissue becomes necrotic and there is diffuse serous discharge. Sloughing with separation of the frozen from the undamaged tissue takes 10–14 days.

Freezing also destroys nerve endings and immediately induces anaesthesia, so that cellular destruction by freezing is painless, as is frostbite due to atmospheric cold exposure. However, the oedema that occurs on rewarming and the swelling of the adjacent surviving cells causes an increase in tissue tension and is painful.

Cold destruction of tissue by liquid carbon dioxide or liquid nitrogen has long been used by dermatologists to treat skin lesions. These spray techniques are impractical in proctology. Improvement in refrigeration techniques led to the development of closed probes in which either liquid nitrogen or liquid nitrous oxide was allowed to vaporize. Liquid nitrogen boils at –196°C and liquid nitrous oxide boils at –90°C, giving probe tip temperatures of approximately –180°C and –70°C respectively. The liquid nitrogen probes are expensive to manufacture. Simpler, self-contained liquid nitrogen probes are available but are too cumbersome for freezing haemorrhoids, although they do have a place in treating rectal tumours. Therefore, most of the experience in cryosurgery for haemorrhoidal disease has been gained with the use of the liquid nitrous oxide probe. The only advantage of the much more expensive liquid nitrogen is the rapidity with which an 'ice ball' of tissue forms after applying the probe. The lower temperature confers no other advantage. Nitrous oxide is administered from a standard cylinder at a pressure above 40 kgf/cm^2 (3.92×10^6 Pa).

Equipment

The essential item is a liquid nitrous oxide cryoprobe, a gas cylinder and an oblique ended or fenestrated anoscope. Most of our initial experience with this method was with the Spembly cryoprobe. The introduction of essentially the same apparatus by Keymed had a few advantages, including slightly more rapid freezing and defrosting and the ability to hold the tip temperature without continually running gas through the instrument. All probes now have the ability to attach the apparatus to a nitrous oxide scavenging system to prevent prolonged exposure of the gas to the operator and staff. Another reliable apparatus is the Downe Frigitonics CN73 which many experienced operators prefer to other makes. It has the advantage of a very light handle, as the operating switch is on the cylinder head and the trigger is for rewarming only. A variety of exchangeable tips are available, but the long flat or rounded probe is generally best for treating anal vascular cushions.

Preparation and position of the patient

Most advocates of this method initially performed it on the unanaesthetized outpatient. However, it has since become clear that local or general anaesthesia is needed for most patients, and this obviously negates some of the potential advantages of the method of conservative management. Some authors state that nervous patients may be frightened by the initial cold sensation and some of these surgeons have advocated the use of intravenous tranquillizers and have designed special non-heat-conducting anoscopes. In our opinion cryosurgery, if used at all, should be used only for destruction of internal insensitive tissues and is not the best choice for a nervous patient or one with a tight anal canal.

A plastic, grooved proctoscope is the most practical because of poor thermal conduction, but to use a disposable anoscope increases the already high cost of the procedure.

No special bowel preparation is required apart from ensuring that the rectum is not grossly loaded with faeces. As with the other forms of conservative treatment, it is relatively easy and most convenient to perform the treatment in the left lateral position. It must be remembered that to obtain adequate freezing of the tissue twice in each of the three primary cushion sites may take 20–25 minutes. Such a time is very uncomfortable for the patient in the lithotomy or knee–chest position. It may also become very uncomfortable for the operating surgeon if the patient is in the left lateral position.

The procedure is a two-handed technique, with the dominant hand holding the cryoprobe handle and the other hand holding and positioning the proctoscope. In the left lateral position it is helpful to have the patient retract the upper buttock with a hand.

Technique

The fenestrated or bivalve speculum is rotated to expose each of the three primary anal cushions in turn. The application of a generous amount of lubricating jelly when the proctoscope is passed ensures that there is moist contact between the tip of the probe and the anal cushion. The probe is laid along the length of the cushion that is to be frozen and gently pressed laterally while the trigger is squeezed and the nitrous oxide evaporates in the tip (Figure 12.20). The tip of the probe almost immediately becomes frosted and adherent to the surface of the mucous membrane. Gradually an increasing margin of tissue around the edge of the probe turns white: after 2–3 minutes this reaches a maximum width of about 6–7 mm. With the Keymed probe the holding switch is depressed so that the temperature is kept constant and the gas flow minimal. This is continued for 3 minutes. As the probe is switched off, the automatic rewarming device quickly defrosts the tip, which will fall away from the frozen tissue of the cushion. The tissue gradually thaws and resumes an appearance identical to the initial state.

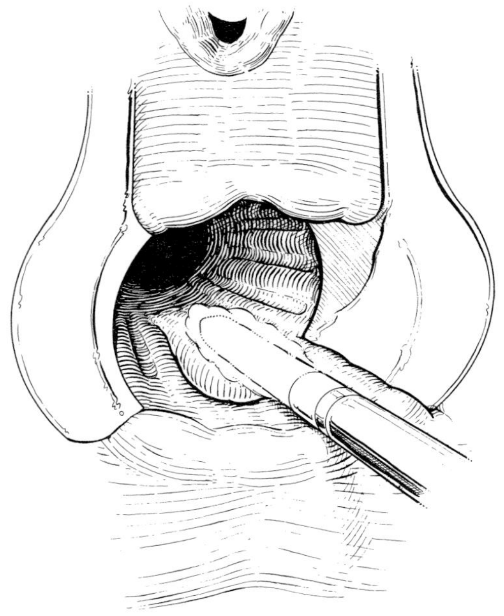

Figure 12.20 Application of a cryoprobe to haemorrhoidal tissue.

Whittaker (1975) also indicated that repeated freezing results in greater tissue destruction than a single freeze and suggested that this was due to large intercellular ice crystals forming at the second episode of freezing. Therefore, most proponents of this technique advise a second application of freezing to the same cushion after a period of 5–10 minutes thawing (Kaufman, 1976).

Goligher (1976), finding that it took a long time to freeze an adequate bulk of the vascular cushion, advocated laying two cryoprobe tips, one on either side of the bulging cushion. While this technique undoubtedly speeds up the process, it doubles the cost of the equipment and is therefore impractical. There is also a danger of causing circumferencial freezing if all three primary cushions are treated. This could result in anal stenosis.

Goligher, presumably realizing the impracticability of the double tip, described a clamp, rather like a hair curling iron, that compressed the vascular cushion against the side of the cryoprobe to increase the size of the tissue frozen (Goligher, 1976). We presume that this ingenious idea was soon abandoned because he omitted any mention of the lateral compression clamp in the detailed description in the fifth edition of his textbook (Goligher, 1984).

Berry and D'Costa (1978) described the technique of moulding the vascular cushion round the probe using a well-lubricated finger. They presumably had no trouble with the finger becoming adherent to the pile mass!

Complications

Pain

Most authors who have described the technique of cryosurgery indicate that general anaesthesia was needed for some patients, or a complete infrahaemorrhoidal block with 20 mL of a 0.5% solution of bupivacaine with adrenaline in others. However, even the infrahaemorrhoidal block is said not to make the area completely insensitive. Furthermore, in our experience the application of the local anaesthetic itself can cause the patient some distress. Many authors describe performing the procedure under diazepam sedation.

We can only conclude from this, and from what we observed from our own small experience with the nitrous oxide cryoprobe, that cryodestruction is not the painless procedure that many of its proponents claim it to be. Without anaesthesia it is suitable only for tissue destruction of the insensitive areas above the dentate line and is indicated only in a small number of patients.

Discharge

One of the striking features of cryodestruction is the profuse serous discharge that tends to occur between the second and tenth day after treatment. This is particularly marked if cryodestruction has been continued exterior to the dentate line. Patients frequently have to wear a dressing that keeps the pile from becoming soaked and makes the skin sore. For this reason cryosurgery for any external component is contraindicated.

Bleeding

Bleeding immediately after cryodestruction is extremely uncommon but, as with any other method of tissue destruction, secondary haemorrhage can occur when the dead tissue separates. Kaufman (1978) reported a 10% incidence of minor bleeding and a 1% incidence of severe secondary haemorrhage requiring admission and transfusion. This is an incidence about equal to that experienced after rubber-band ligation and only slightly less than that experienced after haemorrhoidectomy.

As after any anal procedure, a small proportion of patients experience difficulty with micturition, particularly men with pending prostatic problems.

Aftercare and surveillance

Patients are usually advised to remain off work for 1 week, or until all the discharge has ceased. Constipation does not appear to have been a problem in any of the series reported, but it is presumably advisable to prescribe a regular bland bulk-forming aperient with an appropriate stool softener if there is a tendency towards hard stools. A hot bath or bidet twice a day is a comfort to the patient but does not decrease the time of convalescence.

As it takes a long time for the effects of cryodestruction to subside there is no point in a follow-up review before 8 weeks. As following the other methods of conservative management, there is no virtue in surveillance of asymptomatic patients.

Results

Kaufman stated that all patients were improved after cryosurgery and that three-quarters of his 300 patients were completely cured, although the range of follow-up was only from 6 months to 3 years. Southam (1983) stated that 85% of his patients were completely satisfied at 1 month, and that at 6 months all the 104 patients that he treated appeared to consider that the treatment was completely successful. Berry and D'Costa (1978) insisted that they had cured 35 of 36 patients treated in a follow-up of 9–18 months.

Smith et al (1979) performed an ingenious trial to compare haemorrhoidectomy with cryodestruction to one or other side of the anal canal, determined by random allocation. Somewhat to our surprise, they found that patients could indicate clearly which half of the anal canal was more uncomfortable than the other. Possibly because of logistical difficulties, only 26 patients were included in this study. They concluded that the site of excision and primary suture (haemorrhoidectomy) healed faster than the cryodestruction side. Furthermore, cryodestruction resulted in more frequent residual haemorrhoids and more frequent adjacent thrombosis. Cryodestruction often left large skin tags and, in one patient, because of difficulty in grading the depth of destruction, the internal sphincter was irreparably damaged.

Lewis et al (1983) treated 25 patients with cryotherapy for large prolapsing third-degree haemorrhoids that would otherwise have been treated by haemorrhoidectomy. They all had cryotherapy and one of them suffered from a secondary haemorrhage requiring transfusion, while 5 of the 25 patients later required haemorrhoidectomy for residual piles. They concluded, therefore, that cryosurgery was unsuitable for this group of patients.

Another series from York by O'Callaghan et al (1982) recorded the results in 97 patients with third-degree haemorrhoids treated by cryosurgical destruction and compared them with those of 99 patients treated by an open haemorrhoidectomy. They found that cryodestruction gave equally good results to haemorrhoidectomy, with fewer complications, less time in hospital and less time off work. However, although they indicated that all their patients were suffering from large prolapsing haemorrhoids that would otherwise have been considered for haemorrhoidectomy, their outpatient grading was that 36% were either first- or second-degree piles and only 61% were third-degree.

Goligher's (1976) report was less enthusiastic, possibly because of the higher degree of objectivity or because the cases treated were more advanced. He attempted treatment on 68 patients who were on a waiting list, initially having been advised to have haemorrhoidectomy; he considered that adequate destruction of vascular tissues was obtained in 50 of these 68. He found that 50 of his patients were able to return immediately to their normal activities. Out of a total of 68 patients, only 38 considered they were very pleased with the result, 18 were reasonably satisfied and 12 were disappointed because of continuation of symptoms.

Our own experience is similar to that of Goligher's. We find that cryodestruction is a painful procedure, frequently associated with a profuse discharge and at least a week off work; only about 50% of patients are well satisfied with the treatment. In terms of morbidity and time off work it is slightly better than haemorrhoidectomy, but the long-term results are less predictable. It appears to be considerably less complication-free than does rubber-band ligation or photocoagulation, and we no longer practise the technique. If the literature is anything to judge by, most other coloproctologists agree with our view, as there have been very few publications on the subject in the last five years.

Comparisons with other forms of outpatient treatment

Keighley et al (1979) compared rubber-band ligation with liquid nitrous oxide cryotherapy using a group allocated to a high-fibre diet as a control. Cryotherapy gave results that were no better than diet alone, whereas rubber-band ligation was significantly more effective at controlling symptoms (Table 12.2).

Table 12.2 Randomized trial in haemorrhoid patients with low resting anal pressures.

	Rubber-band ligation (*n* = 35)	*Cryotherapy* (*n* = 36)	*High fibre diet* (*n* = 37)
Complications			
Bleeding	2	3	0
Pain	5	4	0
Abscess	1	0	0
Discharge	0	2	0
Results at 12 months			
Asymptomatic	16	4	4
Improved	7	10	5
No better	3	7	10
Other treatment	2	11	13
Lost to follow-up	7	4	5

From Keighley et al (1979).

Photocoagulation

Principles

A more recent method in the conservative armamentarium for the management of internal haemorrhoids is infrared photocoagulation. Infrared coagulation was developed by Nath et al (1977) for coagulating bleeding points, avoiding the adherence to tissues normally experienced by coagulation diathermy. The technology (Redfield Corp, Montvale, NJ) includes infrared radiation generated by a tungsten–halogen lamp which is focused on to the tissue from a gold-plated reflector housing through a specially made polymer tubing using technology similar to laser devices (Milsom, 1992). This method was adapted to the elective treatment of haemorrhoidal disease by Neiger (1979). He usually employed a 1.5 s pulse of infrared irradiation to give a tissue temperature of 100°C and producing an area of coagulated protein 3 mm diameter and 3 mm deep. The burnt tissue reacts in exactly the same way as does tissue killed by freezing (cryotherapy) or by strangulation (rubber-band ligation). A tissue response occurs in the plane between dead and living tissue. After about 10–14 days the dead tissue separates, leaving a granulation-lined ulcer. The rate of re-epithelialization varies with the size of the ulcer but is usually complete in 4 weeks.

Equipment

The source of the infrared radiation is a 15 V Woolfram halogen lamp with a gold-plated reflector which focuses the rays through a quartz light shaft to the side of the mucosa through a proctoscope (Figure 12.21a). Covering the tip of the probe is a polymer cap which prevents adherence of the probe to the tissues (Figure 12.21b). The supply unit has a timing device which allows a variable duration of radiation. There are two instruments on the market, one from Germany (Lumatec, Munich) and the other from the USA (Redfield Corp, Montvale, NJ).

An angled or fenestrated proctoscope can be used. Unlike with cryosurgery there is very little radiation of energy because the time of exposure is very brief; a non-heat-conducting anoscope is therefore unnecessary.

Preparation and position of the patient

All patients, except those who are grossly constipated, can be treated at the initial diagnostic

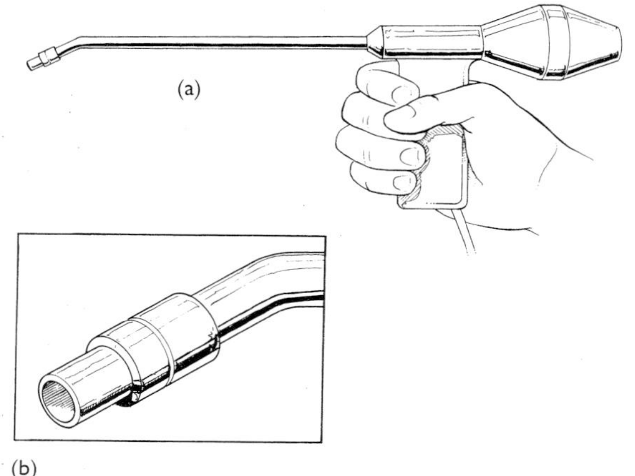

Figure 12.21a,b (a) Infrared photocoagulation equipment. (b) Close-up of tip of photocoagulator.

session. The technique can be performed in the left lateral lithotomy or knee–chest position as the duration of therapy is usually less than 2 minutes.

Technique

The positioning of the angled proctoscope is exactly as described for injection or rubber-band ligation (see above). As the base of the vascular cushion bulges into the end or side of the proctoscope, the probe tip is pressed directly on to the mucosa and the trigger pulled. The pulse of irradiation is automatically timed. It is important that the tip is in complete contact with the mucosa; if it is not the probe does not adhere. If there is not total tip contact, intervening mucus or bowel contents will be burnt and will adhere to and burn a hole in the polymer tip.

On removing the tip from the mucosa the small coagulated area is immediately obvious. Up to six coagulations can be performed at the base of each haemorrhoid; we usually employ three. The whole procedure at the base of each pile takes less than 30 seconds to complete. Because the brightness of the light during infrared radiation causes lack of accommodation of the operator's eye, it is prudent for the operator to close the eye momentarily when the trigger is pulled.

Complications

There seem to be fewer complications after photocoagulation than after any of the previously mentioned treatments. The duration of the radiation limits the destruction to 3 mm, so deeper structures are unlikely to be damaged. Dennison et al (1990) performed the procedure in 51 patients; three developed anal fissures after treatment and no other complications were noted after a median follow-up of 8 months.

Pain

Transient discomfort during application of the probe is common but sustained pain is unusual. Photocoagulation is probably the least pain-provoking of any of the conservative methods of management. It is not necessary to perform any form of regional anaesthesia, nor is it usually necessary to give the patient an oral analgesic afterwards. If the patient experiences persistent discomfort it is because the site chosen is too close to the anal verge and a deeper site should be chosen for the next coagulation. All the three primary cushion sites can be treated at the first session.

Bleeding

Because the damaged tissue is only superficial, the incidence and severity of secondary bleeding seems to be much less than it is after cryosurgery or rubber-band ligation. So far, after several hundred episodes of photocoagulation, we have not had a patient who required admission to hospital or transfusion for secondary haemorrhage. No episodes of urinary retention or infection have been observed. No stenosis has been yet encountered.

Aftercare and surveillance

Because of the low incidence of side-effects little advice or aftercare seems to be needed; however, we still give patients the same instructions as those given after rubber-band ligation.

Results

Long-term studies are not yet available for this method. Leicester et al (1981) reported a 3-month follow-up, at which time 21 of 25 patients were either symptom-free or improved. Only one patient experienced pain and six had experience of bleeding after the treatment. No other side-effects were reported and all ulcers were fully healed by 6 weeks.

Comparisons with other forms of outpatient treatment

Ambrose et al (1983) treated patients by photocoag-

Table 12.3 Randomized trial to compare photocoagulation with rubber-band ligation.

	Photocoagulation (*n* = 140)	*Rubber-band ligation* (*n* = 115)
Results at 12 months		
Asymptomatic	34	33
Improved	30	26
No better	26	20
Repeated treatment	22	6
Other treatment	14	5
Lost to follow-up	14	25

From Ambrose et al (1983).

ulation as part of a randomized trial comparing the technique with rubber-band ligation. All but one of them had either first-degree (26%) or second-degree (74%) haemorrhoids. Photocoagulation was associated with significantly fewer side-effects than was rubber-band ligation, but the clinical results of photocoagulation were similar to those of rubber-band ligation (Table 12.3).

Templeton et al (1983) performed a similar comparative trial in Belfast with random allocation between photocoagulation and rubber-band ligation. They treated 66 patients by infrared coagulation and found a satisfactory outcome in 85% of their patients. There were fewer complications following photocoagulation than after rubber-band ligation and they concluded, as we did, that photocoagulation is simple, fast and effective and has a higher patient acceptability than rubber-band ligation, but is not quite as effective.

However, Weinstein et al (1987) noted a slightly different result in their prospective randomized trial of band ligation and infrared photocoagulation. A significantly better result at 1 month and at 6 months was achieved by banding. There was no difference with respect to pain, although banding was associated with two complications – thrombosed haemorrhoids and delayed bleeding. In addition, Reis Neto et al (1992) found in another randomized controlled trial comparing rubber-band ligation with infrared coagulation that, although coagulation was more effective in controlling bleeding, it was more painful and caused the most serious complications (Table 12.4).

We subsequently compared photocoagulation with injection therapy in another randomized trial (Table 12.5) and found that fewer patients needed additional therapy after injection than after photocoagulation (Ambrose et al, 1983).

We have tried photocoagulation in some patients with third-degree haemorrhoids without curing the symptoms. Thus, photocoagulation seems to be most useful in dealing with first- and second-degree haemorrhoids.

Table 12.4 Complications in a randomized trial of rubber-band ligation compared with photocoagulation at 30 days.

	Photocoagulation (*n* = 80)	*Rubber-band ligation* (*n* = 84)
Moderate or severe pain	69 (86%)	57 (68%)
Pain during defecation	52 (65%)	34 (40%)
Bleeding		
Severe	3 (4%)	1 (1.2%)
Minor	10 (13%)	11 (13%)

From Reis Neto et al (1992).

Table 12.5 Randomized trial to compare photocoagulation with injection therapy.

	Photocoagulation (*n* = 80)	*Injection* (*n* = 63)
Results at 12 months		
Asymptomatic	22	16
Improved	21	15
No better	9	11
Repeated therapy	7	1
Other treatment	12	6
Lost to follow-up	9	14

From Ambrose et al (1983).

BIPOLAR DIATHERMY (BICAP)

With recent advances in endoscopic diathermy techniques, it is perhaps not surprising that some surgeons and physicians have used this methodology to treat patients with haemorrhoids. The technique is designed to produce tissue destruction, ulceration and fibrosis by the local application of heat. The disposable Circon ACMI BICAP (Stanford, CT) haemorrhoid probe uses bipolar RF current to coagulate the blood vessels. Current is passed through the tissue as it travels between adjacent electrodes located at the tip of the probe. Because the current path is short, its advantage over other methods is that the depth of penetration is limited even after multiple applications.

Technique

Using a disposable non-conductive anoscope, the side of the probe is applied directly and firmly to the haemorrhoid above the dentate line. The generator is used on the infinity setting and is activated by a foot switch. A white coagulum approximately 3 mm in depth is produced. All haemorrhoids are treated in one session, and no local anaesthetic is required.

Bipolar diathermy has been compared with rubber-band ligation and found to be technically simpler, producing equally good results in the majority of patients (Griffith et al, 1987). The technique has been compared in a randomized trial with infrared photocoagulation (Dennison et al, 1990) and was found to be equally effective. The technique has also been compared with the Ultroid (see below). We have as yet had no experience with this procedure.

DIRECT CURRENT THERAPY

This technique utilizes a monopolar low-voltage instrument that includes a generator unit, an attachable handle, single-use sterile probes, a grounding pad and a non-conductive anoscope (Ultroid Microvasive, Boston, MA). The probe is placed on to and then into the haemorrhoid. An electrical current up to 16 mA is then passed through the probe. The manufacturer maintains that the mode of action of this device is not thermal but is a consequence of sodium hydroxide production at the negative electrode. Unfortunately, the probe has to be applied to each haemorrhoid for a period of 10 minutes, and this seems to be a major disadvantage. Nevertheless, there have been encouraging reports of its use.

Norman et al (1989) treated 120 patients with complete success and no complications, an amazing result when one considers that 83 patients had third- or fourth-degree haemorrhoids. Zinberg et al (1989) claimed good results in 85% of patients with third-degree haemorrhoids. Both Dennison et al (1990) and Hinton and Morris (1990) found the technique to be effective in randomized studies compared with infrared coagulation and BICAP. However, we believe that this technique is unlikely to gain popularity because of the time required to apply the probe and the fact that equally effective techniques are available. Indeed, a recent prospective randomized study comparing the Ultroid technique with injection sclerotherapy has confirmed our suspicions. Varma et al (1991) in their study of 51 patients concluded that injection sclerotherapy was preferable because it was quicker, less tedious and a more comfortable procedure (Table 12.6).

Table 12.6 Results of randomized trial comparing direct coagulation therapy (the Ultroid) with injection sclerotherapy.

	Sclerotherapy (*n* = 28)	*Coagulation* (*n* = 23)	*P*
Number of sites treated per patient	3 (1–3)	2 (1–3)	<0.001
Treatment time per patient (min)	2 (0.5–5)	12 (5–21)	<0.001
Subjective tolerance score (patient)	1 (1–2)	1 (1–3)	>0.05
Subjective tolerance score (surgeon)	1 (1–1)	2 (1–2)	<0.001
Subjective assessment of results by patient	2 (0–2)	2 (0–2)	>0.5

The values are medians, with range in parenthesis.
From Varma et al (1991).

Section IV: Operative treatment of haemorrhoidal disease

OVERCOMING ANAL CANAL FIBROSIS OR ANAL HYPERTENSION

Rationale

The age-old remedy of stretching the anus was revived by French surgeons early in the nineteenth century when Boyer introduced sphincteric division, later popularized in Britain by Benjamin Brody and the Allinghams. In 1838, Recamier re-introduced the concept of anal dilatation, refined and publicized by Maisonneuve in 1849. Over a hundred years ago the controversy as to whether forcible anal dilatation was preferable to sphincter division attracted just as much attention as it has in the recent past. In those days rhetoric appeared to have more influence than controlled trials. In 1868, Bodenheimer of the USA said that he 'prefered incision to the mangled irregular wounds resulting from stretching'.

Early sphincter division had been haphazard and often too enthusiastic, resulting in a high incidence of incontinence. It was Miles (1919) who introduced a more precise concept when he described the 'pecten band' and popularized the operation, pectenotomy. In this procedure a firm palpable band just beneath the anoderm is incised, causing immediate relaxation of the stenosis at the level of the pecten band. There has been much controversy about the exact anatomical location of the pecten band and a complete failure to demonstrate it convincingly on histological sections (Figure 12.22). It seems most likely that what is described as the pecten band is the lowermost fibres of the involuntary internal sphincter where it is attached to the longitudinal fibres. It appears that this lower edge is rolled inwards towards the anoderm, so giving the obvious band that can be felt and even seen just beneath the surface when the anus of the anaesthetized patient is stretched with a bivalve speculum or with fingers (Eisenhammer, 1953).

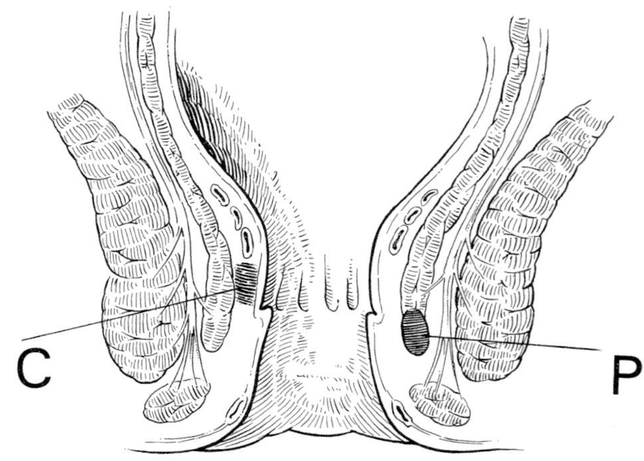

Figure 12.22 Diagram to illustrate pecten band (P), according to Miles (1919) and constricting band (C), according to Eisenhammer (1953).

The modern era of stenosis-relieving procedures dates from the classical series of papers by Eisenhammer (1951) of South Africa who introduced the term 'internal anal sphincterotomy', which he advocated for all forms of what he described as 'chronic internal anal sphincteric contracture'. He introduced a procedure of internal anal sphincterotomy plus what he called 'free dilatation', purposefully coined to contrast with the procedure that he termed, somewhat disparagingly, the 'forcible stretch' procedure. In 1974, Eisenhammer wrote 'it is difficult to comprehend why a surgeon should have to resort to digital manual tearing of a contractured internal anal sphincter to an uncontrolled extent to overcome this pathological problem when the simple definitive operation of dividing a portion of the muscle as an office procedure, under local anaesthesia, on an ambulant regime is obviously the ideal method'.

In addition to the pecten band, there are often higher constriction bands that can be felt in the anorectum when a patient with an anal fissure or painful haemorrhoidal disease has the anal canal stretched digitally. Lord (1969) stresses the importance of breaking down these higher constricting bands, although once again their precise anatomical definition was not clear. We have observed them frequently in patients who have had previous phenol injection or rubber-band ligation, but these are probably iatrogenic fibrous bands. Eisenhammer (1974) described them as merely contractured internal sphincter muscle fibres that assume undue prominence on stretching.

In an attempt to find histological evidence of fibrotic bands encircling the anorectum, Ortiz et al (1978) identified the circular bands of the anorectum demonstrated by stretching with a bivalve speculum. The bands were marked with a silver clip and a 0.5 cm^2 full-thickness biopsy was taken from the band. Investigation performed in five patients having a haemorrhoidectomy failed to show any evidence of connective tissue bands or fibrosis. They concluded that the histological study proved that the tight structures were hypertrophied muscle fibres.

Tightness of the anorectum, with the pecten and other bands constricting the anal canal, is said to be a condition found in many young patients with haemorrhoidal disease and almost all patients with a fissure-in-ano. From the evidence cited above it appears that the anal canal tightness in haemorrhoidal disease is largely caused by muscle spasm and not by tight bands.

Arabi et al (1977b) performed a prospective study of 145 patients with haemorrhoidal disease in whom resting anal canal pressures were compared with 78 age and sex-matched controls. In symptomatic haemorrhoidal disease the mean maximal resting pressure in the anal canal was 106 ± 40 compared with 88 ± 34 cmH_2O in controls. They found that high anal canal pressures were particularly prevalent and significantly different from controls only in the young male patients (Figure 12.23). Similar findings were reported by Hancock and Smith (1975).

Thus there is an alternative hypothesis to the constricting band theory – namely, that in some patients haemorrhoidal symptoms, particularly bleeding and discomfort, are caused by anal canal hypertension. It is generally believed that these high resting anal canal pressures are caused by internal anal sphincter overactivity as evidenced by ultraslow wave (Hancock, 1976) activity. Furthermore, sustained reduction in anal pressure, abolition of ultraslow waves and long-term symptomatic improvement has been reported by Hancock and Smith (1975) following anal dilatation (Hancock, 1981) and by ourselves after anal stretch and internal sphincterotomy (Keighley et al, 1979). An alternative theory, which has merit, is the concept that high resting anal pressures are due to hypertensive anal cushions (Sun et al, 1990) since anal pressures

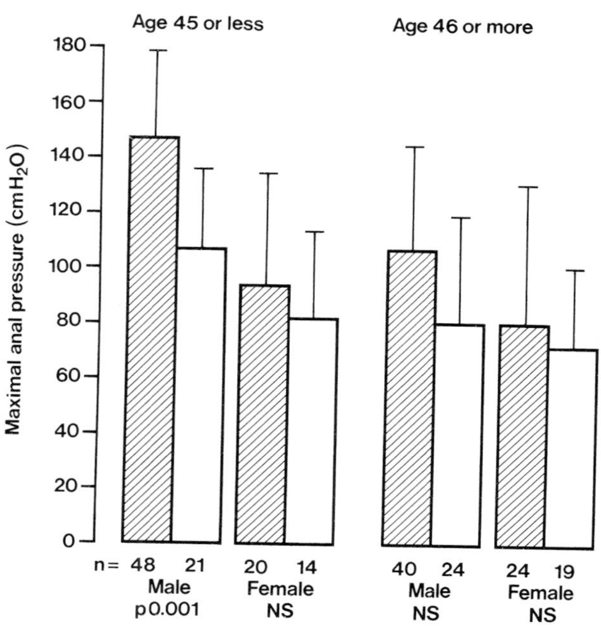

Figure 12.23 Maximal anal pressures in patients with haemorrhoids (▨) compared with age- and sex-matched control subjects (□). NS, not significant.

are normalized after haemorrhoidectomy (Read et al, 1982). However, one suspects that during haemorrhoidectomy there is some stretching of the anorectal ring resulting in reduced internal sphincter activity. Nevertheless recent direct evidence of hypertension in the anal cushions of haemorrhoid patients argues for a dual role of these cushions on the internal sphincter in the pathogenesis of symptomatic haemorrhoids (Sun et al, 1992).

Anal stretch procedure

Because of early experience with incontinence produced by the eight-finger forcible dilatation popularized by Lord (1969), and because we have had to perform operations to correct incontinence on patients who have been treated elsewhere by forcible dilatation, we have abandoned anal dilatation, sometimes called the 'Lord procedure', for patients with piles. In our view, anal dilatation should never be used in multiparous females and should never be repeated, even in men.

Since anal dilatation is not now recommended for treatment of haemorrhoids and as the procedure has been described in detail for the treatment of anal fissure (where it may still have a place), a repeat description is not provided in this chapter.

Results

Lord (1977) reported that he and his colleagues had used the procedure in over 300 patients over 7 years and claimed that no patient who had been cured of symptoms by the procedure had subsequently returned requiring a haemorrhoidectomy.

Hood and Alexander-Williams (1971) performed a randomized controlled trial comparing the anal stretch procedure with rubber-band ligation. This small trial, with only 23 patients having dilatation, showed that only seven (30%) were completely relieved of their symptoms by anal stretch and four (17%) had no improvement. No patients suffered incontinence, but five of the 23 patients still had frequent bleeding, six had frequent prolapse and two continued to complain of pain.

Ortiz et al (1978), in a randomized trial comparing anal stretch with a standard haemorrhoidectomy, treated 30 patients by anal stretch using the method of dilatation advocated by Lord. They also measured anal pressures before and after the procedure. Three of their patients had some impairment of continence preoperatively. After anal stretch, nine became incontinent of flatus but none had faecal incontinence. They found that 6 months after the anal stretch procedure anal pressures were unchanged from their preoperative values. The percentage of patients with flatus incontinence after anal stretch was similar to that reported by other authors and varied from 16% to 25%. Ortiz and associates felt that these poor results from the Lord procedure were not due to the fact that they omitted the postoperative self-dilatation regimen recommended by Lord, because their bad results were characterized by incontinence and pruritus. They believed that these symptoms would probably have been made worse and not improved by the postoperative dilatation. They concluded that forced anal dilatation had no pathophysiological basis, and they could not recommend it over haemorrhoidectomy.

An important longitudinal follow-up study with anal pressure measurement was conducted by Hancock (1981). He performed a prospective study in 48 patients treated by the anal stretch procedure and followed them meticulously for at least 5 years. At 5 years, 31 of his 48 patients (65%) remained symptom-free and cured of their haemorrhoids. Many patients had paired anal pressure measurements. He reported that there was an almost 50% reduction in resting pressure 6 days after dilatation. Two months later the mean anal pressure remained lower than normal. At 5–6 years later, the mean (SD) pressure of the 35 patients examined was 69.8 (16.2) cmH_2O, which was still significantly below the mean pressure of the 40 controls which was 85.0 (20.5) cmH_2O ($P < 0.001$) (see Figure 12.5).

Vellacott and Hardcastle (1980) recorded anal pressures 2 cm from the anal verge under resting conditions in 40 patients 4 and 3 months after maximal anal dilatation according to the method of Lord. Twenty of their patients were treated by post-stretch self-dilatation with the large anal dilator and 20 patients merely had maximal anal dilatation alone. The 20 patients who used bulk aperients as well as the large dilatator had a reduction of anal pressure from 123 ± 34 to 79 ± 31 cmH_2O. In the group who had a bulk laxative alone, the anal pressures fell from 119 ± 34 to 73 ± 26 cmH_2O three months after operation. The difference between the two groups was not significant. They concluded that anal dilatation significantly reduced resting anal pressure but that the use of the postoperative anal dilatator did not improve the results and was an unpleasant and unnecessary imposition upon the patients.

A prospective trial of maximal anal dilatation using Lord's method was reported by Lewis et al (1983). They had selected a group of 112 patients with prolapsing haemorrhoids who had been considered candidates for haemorrhoidectomy.

Thirty-one of these were allocated for treatment by anal dilatation. Long-term follow-up was between 6 months and 5 years. Two patients were lost to follow-up; six patients were completely symptom-free and 25 considered that they were improved; five had required treatment by haemorrhoidectomy and two by injection; three were reported as being incontinent of flatus.

Goligher (1984) was no more enthusiastic about the anal stretch procedure than was Eisenhammer. His own personal experience of manual dilatation was relatively small. In a series of only 28 patients with large haemorrhoids, he reported post-treatment incontinence and haemorrhoidal prolapse in four patients. MacIntyre and Balfour (1972) assessed 51 patients 1 year after maximal anal dilatation. They found that 80% were symptom-free, although 44% still had anal skin tags. Eleven patients (22%) complained of occasional incontinence of flatus and as many as 18 (35%) complained of occasional incontinence of faeces.

Sames (1972) treated 149 patients with haemorrhoidal disease by the anal stretch procedure. His overall impression was that the results were mostly very satisfactory: none reported permanent faecal incontinence and there were only a few cases of temporary incontinence. However, he observed, as have most surgeons, that there is little difference in the appearance of the anal canal on proctoscopy before and after treatment.

A much higher incidence of incontinence was reported by K. Fussell (personal communication cited in Goligher, 1984), who found that 4 of 11 patients treated by the Lord stretch procedure were rendered incontinent. Bates (1972) also reported two elderly patients who developed a complete rectal prolapse after dilatation. McCaffrey (1975) found that 40% of 50 patients developed some incontinence of flatus or mucus for between 4 and 26 days. Furthermore, four of these 50 patients subsequently required a haemorrhoidectomy. Sandilands et al (1981) reported that haemorrhoidectomy or similar treatment was required in 9% of 109 patients followed up for a long time after the anal stretch procedure. Walls and Ruckley (1976) reported an even higher incidence of haemorrhoidectomy after anal dilatation, where 19% of 100 patients continued to complain of prolapsing haemorrhoids requiring excision.

Complications

Bleeding and bruising

Severe bleeding is rare. Many patients develop subcutaneous bruising of varying extent around the anus. Occasionally a large painful submucosal haematoma occurs, but it is relatively uncommon for a patient to have to stay in hospital because of this. Fortunately the appearance of a large haematoma does not appear to be associated with poor results.

Splitting of skin

Splitting of the skin and deeper structures occurs quite commonly during anal dilatation. Lord (1977) stated that he had experience of five patients in whom there was a split of the skin, mucosa and apparently of the sphincter. Splits usually involve the posterior quadrant. In one patient it was complicated by a severe cellulitis of the buttocks. Lord advocated keeping patients in hospital for observation if a split occurred, but did not advise suturing the sphincter as a primary procedure.

Prolapse

Mucosal prolapse may occur in the early weeks after anal stretching. Lord (1977) claimed that this usually subsided during the course of the post-dilatation regime.

Incontinence

This is the most feared and serious complication of maximal dilatation. In a review article, Lord (1983) stated that patients often had transient incontinence of flatus for a few days, occasionally persisting for some weeks. Patients who have a very tight anus before the procedure may have a feeling of insecurity of the sphincter mechanism and may need some sphincter exercises for a few weeks. He claimed that midline posterior splitting causing a 'keyhole' deformity of the anus was very rare and could be avoided by good technique, particularly by ensuring that the strain of the dilatation was placed laterally rather than in the midline posteriorly. There is now anatomical evidence, based on anal ultrasonography, that anal dilatation may permanently disrupt the internal anal sphincter. Despite Lord's optimism, the overwhelming evidence is that up to 10% of patients may be permanently rendered incontinent of flatus or faeces when the eight-finger dilatation is used in the treatment of haemorrhoids and fissure. In view of the medicolegal implications of iatrogenic incontinence and the availability of other effective forms of therapy which do not threaten continence, most surgeons in the UK and North America have abandoned this method of elective therapy.

Conclusion

Our considered opinion is that the anal stretch procedure should not be used for elective treatment of patients with haemorrhoids because of the risk of incontinence.

Internal sphincterotomy

Internal sphincterotomy has been used in a selected group of patients with haemorrhoids who had high resting anal pressures (Schouten and van Vroonhaven, 1986). The operation is usually performed as a subcutaneous technique using a cataract knife under local or general anaesthesia; alternatively, an open internal sphincterotomy may be performed.

Internal sphincterotomy was used only in carefully selected patients since prolapse could be made worse and transient incontinence could occur. Perianal haematoma was also a recognized complication, particularly in patients with haemorrhoids. In Birmingham we found that internal sphincterotomy was therapeutically effective only in young patients with first- or second-degree haemorrhoids who complained of anal discomfort and bleeding (Arabi et al, 1977b).

We subsequently compared anal dilatation, lateral subcutaneous sphincterotomy and high-fibre diet for patients with anal hypertension. This randomized trial left us in no doubt that anal dilatation was far superior to internal sphincterotomy in these patients (Keighley et al, 1979) (Table 12.7). However, since both operations may be complicated by permanent incontinence, sphincterotomy and anal dilatation have been abandoned by both of us.

Table 12.7 Randomized trial in patients with haemorrhoids with high resting anal pressure.

	Anal dilatation (*n* = 37)	*Sphincterotomy* (*n* = 34)	*High fibre diet* (*n* =37)
Complications			
Bleeding	4	1	0
Prolapse	2	0	0
Incontinence	1	1	0
Results at 12 months			
Asymptomatic	11	6	5
Improved	14	6	5
No better	5	12	13
Other treatment	4	9	14
Lost to follow-up	3	1	0

From Keighley et al (1979).

SUTURE

Farag (1978) revived an ancient technique, under the presumptive titles of 'a new technique' and 'a new approach', when he advocated suture of what he described as the perforating veins at the base of the vascular cushion. Wanas likened these veins to those with high-pressure leaks associated with incompetent perforating veins of the lower leg. Although this operation was practised by a few enthusiasts, it now seems to have been entirely abandoned.

HAEMORRHOIDECTOMY (INCLUDING DAY-CASE PROCEDURES)

Many techniques carrying various eponyms have been described for haemorrhoidectomy. There are two basic varieties, open and closed, depending on whether or not the anorectal mucosa and perineal skin are closed after the haemorrhoids have been excised and ligated. Generally, and certainly until recently, the open techniques have been more popular in the UK, but closed haemorrhoidectomy is more popular in North America.

Closed haemorrhoidectomy

When Ferguson and Heaton developed the closed haemorrhoidectomy technique, which they reported in 1959, they were seeking to avoid or minimize some of the then common disadvantages of open haemorrhoidectomy. They had three principal objectives: (1) to remove as much vascular tissue as possible without sacrificing anoderm; (2) to minimize postoperative serous discharge by prompt healing with the immediate lining of the anal canal with stratified squamous epithelium (anoderm); and (3) to prevent the stenosis that may complicate healing of large raw wounds by granulation tissue.

They felt that the closed technique, relying as it did on the known ability of the anal epithelium to heal rapidly despite its microbial rich environment, would result in less postoperative discomfort, minimal inpatient and virtually no outpatient care, no loss of continence and no need for subsequent anal dilatation.

Most colorectal surgeons, at least in the USA, believe that these goals are achieved. The technique is the one most widely practised in the USA today.

Patient selection and preparation

Indications

We believe that more than 90% of patients suffering from haemorrhoidal disease can be managed without operation. However, when operative treatment is indicated, it is our opinion that the closed haemorrhoidectomy technique can be used for almost all patients. The principal indications for operation are excessive bleeding, uncontrolled with rubber-band ligation, severe prolapse or pain and symptomatic haemorrhoids in patients who have other anorectal diseases requiring operation. Relative contraindications to performing closed haemorrhoidectomy include the presence of Crohn's disease, portal hypertension, leukaemia, lymphoma or a bleeding diathesis (Ferguson and Heaton, 1959). Since the complication rate for haemorrhoidectomy in patients with Crohn's disease is high (Buls and Goldberg, 1978), the authors do not recommend closed haemorrhoidectomy in this situation. However, patients with ulcerative colitis may occasionally be treated with closed haemorrhoidectomy provided that restorative proctocolectomy is unlikely to be an option in the future. Patients with portal hypertension can sometimes undergo closed haemorrhoidectomy, but we generally prefer rubber-band ligation. Patients with leukaemia or lymphoma are at high risk of infection following any haemorrhoidectomy because of the compromised status of their immune systems. However, should a patient with leukaemia or lymphoma present with acute strangulated haemorrhoids, we believe that the best course in this group is an open haemorrhoidectomy.

Another special case in which closed haemorrhoidectomy is appropriate is for immediately postpartum prolapsed piles. However, postpartum haemorrhoidal disease and haemorrhoidal diseases associated with pregnancy can usually be managed conservatively. Occasionally, during delivery, prolapse and thrombosis of haemorrhoids can occur; these, in our view, are best treated by immediate closed haemorrhoidectomy (Schottler et al, 1973).

Closed haemorrhoidectomy can also be combined with other anorectal procedures with no increase in morbidity (Jeffery et al, 1977).

Preparation

The evaluation of the patient is the same as that for any patient with haemorrhoids and has already been described in Section I.

Preoperative counselling of the patient includes a thorough explanation of the procedure. Patients should be aware that, even with the closed technique, complete healing may not occur for several weeks.

Patients are admitted on the day of operation. This saves significantly in time and costs and does not compromise the proper preoperative evaluation and preparation of the patient. Preparation consists of a single disposable phosphate enema on the evening before and another enema about 1 hour before operation. Patients with severely symptomatic haemorrhoids should be spared the enemas. No perineal shaving is performed and no other laxative or antibiotic is given. Ideally, the patient should be taking a bulk agent preoperatively as part of the conservative management of the disease. There is no other restriction or addition to the patient's diet.

Anaesthesia

Closed haemorrhoidectomy can be performed under any type of anaesthesia. The local anaesthetic of choice is bupivacaine (0.23%) with 1:200 000 adrenaline. An initial injection of lignocaine can be used if the patient is to receive no other anaesthesia as this minimizes the discomfort during injection of bupivacaine and adrenaline.

Should the patient prefer a regional anaesthetic, either a caudal block or a spinal anaesthetic may be employed. Should regional anaesthesia be used, the authors still use bupivacaine with adrenaline locally, to minimize local bleeding and to provide a useful adjunct for postoperative pain relief. The use of an epidural morphine solution may be beneficial in providing long-term postoperative pain relief.

Even if general anaesthesia is preferred it is advisable also to use bupivacaine with adrenaline to supplement analgesia postoperatively and to reduce bleeding.

Technique and equipment

In the operating room the patient is placed in the prone jack-knife position. This position utilizes a roll beneath the iliac crest as well as two rolls beneath the thorax to provide proper support. In general, when caudal or spinal anaesthesia is chosen, it is induced before positioning the patient. If local anaesthesia is preferred, this is administered after the patient is positioned.

Adhesive tape is used to retract the buttocks laterally and to expose completely the anal verge. When a slight head-down tilt is added, an excellent view of the anus and anal canal is obtained (Figure 12.24). A fibreoptic headlight improves the view even further. The area is simply painted with a colloidal iodine solution. Shaving the perineum causes postoperative discomfort and does nothing to facilitate the operative procedure.

Ferguson initially described his procedure with the patient in the left lateral decubitus position (Ferguson and Heaton, 1959), a position since used successfully by him and his associates. However, we agree with Corman's opinion that the lateral position is awkward for the assistant (Corman, 1984).

When the patient is positioned and draped, bupivacaine with adrenaline is injected into the perirectal spaces through a single puncture on each side of the anus. The operator uses a fan technique to thoroughly infiltrate the perirectal spaces and around the anal canal (Figure 12.25). The anal canal is then thoroughly examined with the Pratt bivalve speculum (Figure 12.26), which allows the surgeon to judge in which quadrants haemorrhoidectomy will be required as well as to inspect the anal canal for any additional pathology. Although a three-quadrant haemorrhoidectomy involving the right posterior, right anterior and left lateral regions is most common, this is by no means the rule. Each patient must be examined individually and only the excess haemorrhoidal tissue is removed. The haemorrhoidal tissue can be easily displayed by passing a swab into the anal canal. On withdrawal the principal haemorrhoidal cushions prolapse and are immediately visible. We aim to preserve as much as possible of the unique skin of the anal canal, the anoderm.

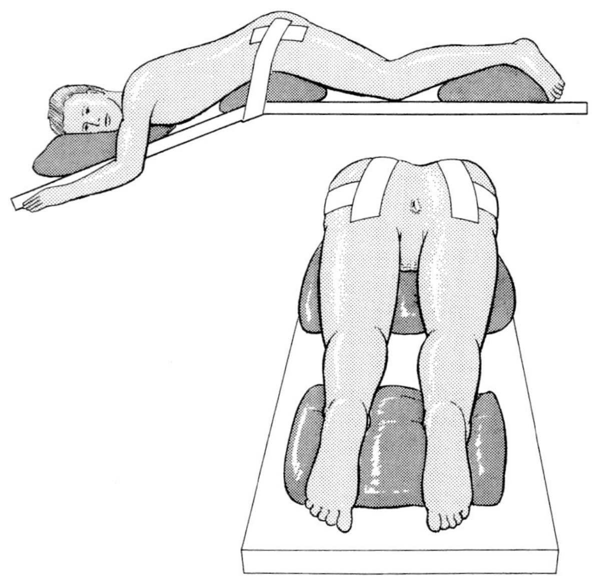

Figure 12.24 Prone jack-knife position for closed haemorrhoidectomy.

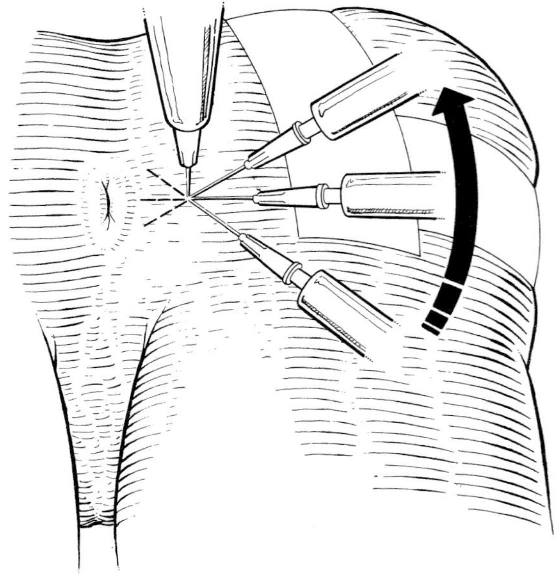

Figure 12.25 Infiltration of perianal and perirectal tissues with bupivacaine and adrenaline solution.

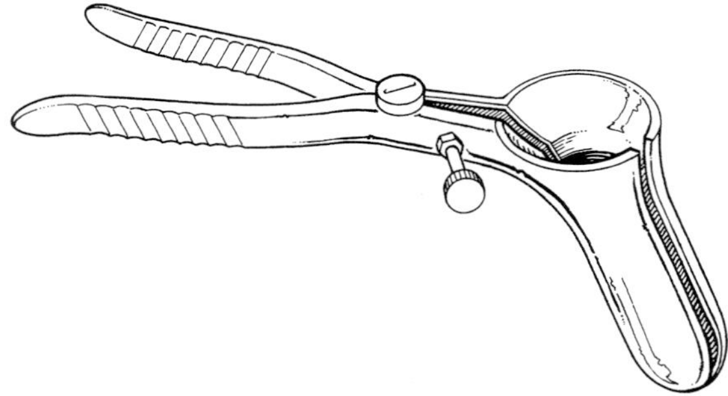

Figure 12.26 A Pratt bivalve speculum.

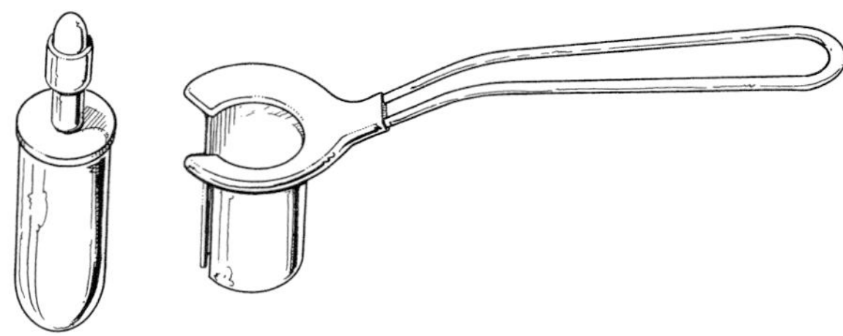

Figure 12.27 The Fansler anoscope.

It is also necessary to inspect the rectal mucosa above the haemorrhoidal tissues since a degree of rectal mucosal prolapse is often a component of symptomatic haemorrhoidal disease. Insertion of the Pratt bivalve anoscope also allows the surgeon to judge whether there is significant anal stenosis present, which may also contribute to symptomatic haemorrhoidal disease. The Pratt bivalve speculum may be used throughout this procedure and is the preferred instrument in the elderly patient. It avoids undue stretching of the internal sphincter and the possible complications of postoperative incontinence. However, after inspection with the bivalve speculum we usually prefer to replace this with the Fansler operating anoscope (Figure 12.27). The Fansler anoscope has a constant diameter of 3.5 cm. This aids in the prevention of excessive excision of anal epithelium and maintains a constant diameter of the anal canal, which helps to prevent anal stenosis.

The Fansler anoscope is positioned so that the operating channel is in line with the redundant haemorrhoidal tissue. The skin tag or anal epithelium adjacent to the haemorrhoidal tissue is grasped with a pair of Aliss forceps and retracted towards the centre of the anal canal. Metzenbaum scissors with their curve towards the anal canal are then used to incise beneath the tissue forceps from the perianal skin upward along the haemorrhoidal tissue, while pressing firmly with the belly of the scissors to buttress them against the internal sphincter (Figure 12.28). This manoeuvre prevents incision of either the external or the internal sphincter. Usually the most prominent region of haemorrhoidal tissue is excised first to minimize subsequent loss of anoderm. We neither use a clamp nor place an apical or crown suture into the pile. Bleeding submucosal vessels are controlled with cautery (Figure 12.29).

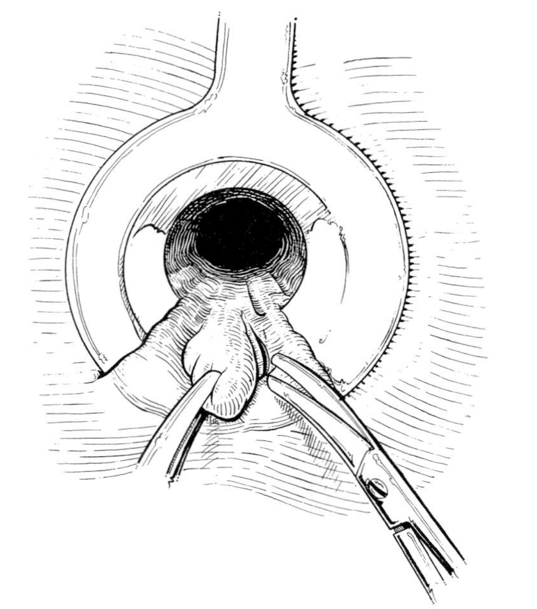

Figure 12.28 Closed haemorrhoidectomy. Two incisions are made upwards from the anal skin on each side of the haemorrhoidal tissue.

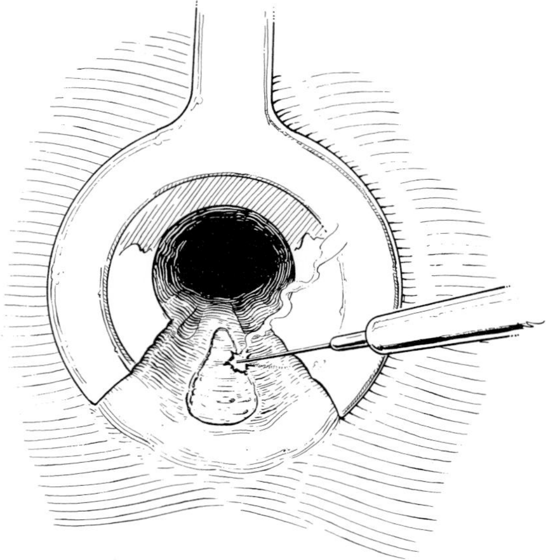

Figure 12.29 Control of bleeding using diathermy after the bulk of haemorrhoidal tissue has been removed.

Following initial excision of the haemorrhoidal cushion, further tissue is filleted from underneath the divided mucosa, leaving the internal sphincter muscle bare. Additionally, vascular tissue beneath the anoderm on each side of the incisions is inverted and trimmed to minimize the chance of recurrence (Figure 12.30). After complete excision of the redundant haemorrhoidal tissue to a point above the internal sphincter, the wound is closed using a running 3/0 chromic suture on a taper-cut needle. Stitching is begun at the apex to fix the rectal mucosa to the underlying submucosa and muscle and to help prevent further rectal mucosal prolapse (Figure 12.31). This is not a haemostatic apical stitch. The wound is closed with a running suture along its entire length, including the extra-anal wounds. We use a chromic catgut suture. However, after performing a study comparing a polyglycolic acid suture and catgut, Khubchandani concluded that the polyglycolic acid suture caused less pain and fewer complications than catgut (Khubchandani et al, 1974). During closure, small bites of the internal sphincter can be included in order to fix the anoderm to the anal canal.

After the first wound has been closed, the anal canal is again inspected and further areas for haemorrhoidectomy are selected in order of decreasing tissue redundancy. By beginning with the largest mass of haemorrhoidal tissue and proceeding to the smallest, it can often be seen that after two or three areas have been excised, no further treatment is indicated where initially there appeared to be obvious haemorrhoidal tissue.

Often, symptomatic skin tags may be excised in the same incision. Occasionally, if there is a large skin tag which does not overlie the axis of the haemorrhoidal tissue, it may be excised transversely and the wound closed with small interrupted absorbable sutures. Should two or three regions be excised and a smaller amount of haemorrhoidal tissue remain, this may be excised simply using a scalpel to incise over the haemorrhoidal tissue and then trim from beneath the anodermal flaps with the Metzenbaum scissors. After excision of the subanodermal haemorrhoidal plexus, the wound is closed completely with an absorbable suture. At the end of the procedure, all the suture lines are inspected again using the Pratt bivalve speculum. Should any bleeding be present, a simple figure-of-eight stitch in the region of the bleeding will control it. The anal canal and anal region are cleaned thoroughly but no packing or dressing is applied.

Although the prone jack-knife position may be uncomfortable for the awake patient, we think it is superior to the lithotomy position because of the superb view of the anal canal it affords and the ease with which an assistant can view the operation. If there is bleeding the blood flows by gravity into the rectum and does not obscure the operative field, as may occur in the lithotomy or left lateral decubitus position.

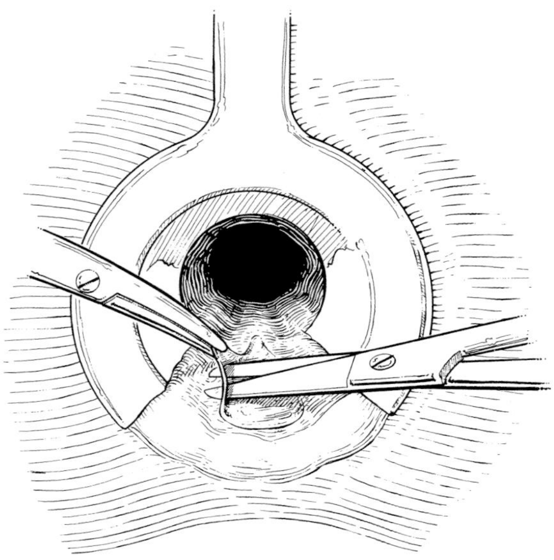

Figure 12.30 Additional vascular tissue beneath the anoderm on each side of the incisions is removed.

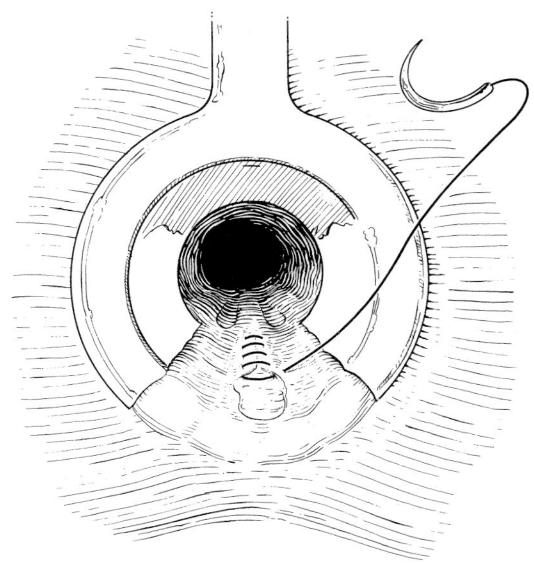

Figure 12.31 The defect in the anal canal mucosa is closed.

Technique

Using a disposable non-conductive anoscope, the side of the probe is applied directly and firmly to the haemorrhoid above the dentate line. The generator is used on the infinity setting and is activated by a foot switch. A white coagulum approximately 3 mm in depth is produced. All haemorrhoids are treated in one session, and no local anaesthetic is required.

Bipolar diathermy has been compared with rubber-band ligation and found to be technically simpler, producing equally good results in the majority of patients (Griffith et al, 1987). The technique has been compared in a randomized trial with infrared photocoagulation (Dennison et al, 1990) and was found to be equally effective. The technique has also been compared with the Ultroid (see below). We have as yet had no experience with this procedure.

DIRECT CURRENT THERAPY

This technique utilizes a monopolar low-voltage instrument that includes a generator unit, an attachable handle, single-use sterile probes, a grounding pad and a non-conductive anoscope (Ultroid Microvasive, Boston, MA). The probe is placed on to and then into the haemorrhoid. An electrical current up to 16 mA is then passed through the probe. The manufacturer maintains that the mode of action of this device is not thermal but is a consequence of sodium hydroxide production at the negative electrode. Unfortunately, the probe has to be applied to each haemorrhoid for a period of 10 minutes, and this seems to be a major disadvantage. Nevertheless, there have been encouraging reports of its use.

Norman et al (1989) treated 120 patients with complete success and no complications, an amazing result when one considers that 83 patients had third- or fourth-degree haemorrhoids. Zinberg et al (1989) claimed good results in 85% of patients with third-degree haemorrhoids. Both Dennison et al (1990) and Hinton and Morris (1990) found the technique to be effective in randomized studies compared with infrared coagulation and BICAP. However, we believe that this technique is unlikely to gain popularity because of the time required to apply the probe and the fact that equally effective techniques are available. Indeed, a recent prospective randomized study comparing the Ultroid technique with injection sclerotherapy has confirmed our suspicions. Varma et al (1991) in their study of 51 patients concluded that injection sclerotherapy was preferable because it was quicker, less tedious and a more comfortable procedure (Table 12.6).

Table 12.6 Results of randomized trial comparing direct coagulation therapy (the Ultroid) with injection sclerotherapy.

	Sclerotherapy (*n* = 28)	*Coagulation* (*n* = 23)	*P*
Number of sites treated per patient	3 (1–3)	2 (1–3)	<0.001
Treatment time per patient (min)	2 (0.5–5)	12 (5–21)	<0.001
Subjective tolerance score (patient)	1 (1–2)	1 (1–3)	>0.05
Subjective tolerance score (surgeon)	1 (1–1)	2 (1–2)	<0.001
Subjective assessment of results by patient	2 (0–2)	2 (0–2)	>0.5

The values are medians, with range in parenthesis.
From Varma et al (1991).

Section IV: Operative treatment of haemorrhoidal disease

OVERCOMING ANAL CANAL FIBROSIS OR ANAL HYPERTENSION

Rationale

The age-old remedy of stretching the anus was revived by French surgeons early in the nineteenth century when Boyer introduced sphincteric division, later popularized in Britain by Benjamin Brody and the Allinghams. In 1838, Recamier re-introduced the concept of anal dilatation, refined and publicized by Maisonneuve in 1849. Over a hundred years ago the controversy as to whether forcible anal dilatation was preferable to sphincter division attracted just as much attention as it has in the recent past. In those days rhetoric appeared to have more influence than controlled trials. In 1868, Bodenheimer of the USA said that he 'prefered incision to the mangled irregular wounds resulting from stretching'.

Early sphincter division had been haphazard and often too enthusiastic, resulting in a high incidence of incontinence. It was Miles (1919) who introduced a more precise concept when he described the 'pecten band' and popularized the operation, pectenotomy. In this procedure a firm palpable band just beneath the anoderm is incised, causing immediate relaxation of the stenosis at the level of the pecten band. There has been much controversy about the exact anatomical location of the pecten band and a complete failure to demonstrate it convincingly on histological sections (Figure 12.22). It seems most likely that what is described as the pecten band is the lowermost fibres of the involuntary internal sphincter where it is attached to the longitudinal fibres. It appears that this lower edge is rolled inwards towards the anoderm, so giving the obvious band that can be felt and even seen just beneath the surface when the anus of the anaesthetized patient is stretched with a bivalve speculum or with fingers (Eisenhammer, 1953).

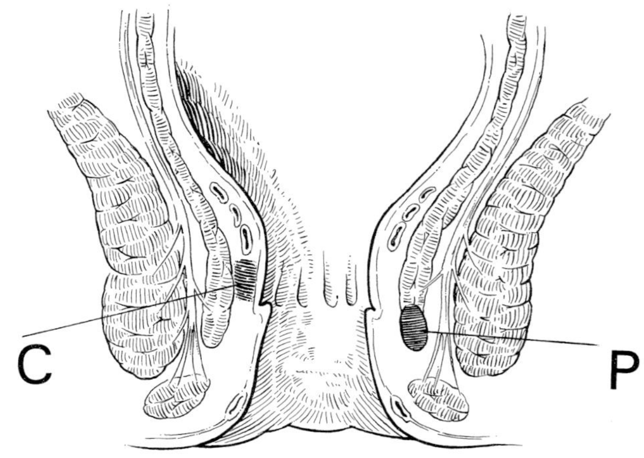

Figure 12.22 Diagram to illustrate pecten band (P), according to Miles (1919) and constricting band (C), according to Eisenhammer (1953).

Variations of technique

Several minor points of our technique differ from those originally described by Ferguson and others who pioneered closed haemorrhoidectomy. Ferguson employed the left lateral position and used Hill–Ferguson anal retractors. Khubchandani also uses a Hill–Ferguson retractor, although he prefers the prone jack-knife position. Both of these surgeons describe the technique of isolating the pedicle and suture ligation. We feel this step is not essential.

Adjuvant sphincterotomy

Khubchandani always performs a superficial sphincterotomy except in patients at risk of incontinence, such as those who are old or have a patulous anus, whereas Ferguson did not employ sphincterotomy routinely. We perform sphincterotomy at operation only if there is evidence of anal stenosis. This is usually determined by the inability to insert the Fansler anoscope. We agree with Khubchandani that sphincterotomy should not be performed in the elderly; in these patients we use only the Pratt bivalve anoscope to avoid undue stretching of the internal sphincter.

Marsupialization

Another variant of the closed haemorrhoidectomy technique is described by Ruiz-Moreno (1977). His closed haemorrhoidectomy is identical to our own except that the external wound is marsupialized rather than closed primarily. He also uses the Parks anal retractor and performs most of the operations in the lithotomy position. He describes no particular rationale for marsupializing the external wounds, although presumably this may reduce the incidence of infection. Ruiz-Moreno's technique is similar to the operation of submucous haemorrhoidectomy described by Sir Alan Parks (Parks, 1956). In fact, Parks did not perform a true closed haemorrhoidectomy, in that part of the rectal mucosa and perianal skin were left open. In Birmingham, we adhere to the technique described by Ferguson and Heaton. However, in order to avoid a knot lying under the anal skin, we use a subcuticular technique to close the skin and the continuous stitch is then taken back on itself so that the knot is inside the anal canal where it is less likely to cause discomfort.

Submucosal haemorrhoidectomy

The Parks haemorrhoidectomy is a closed technique which is used by some in the UK. The operation is performed entirely within the anal canal with the aid of a Parks self-retaining bivalve speculum which exposes the anal canal throughout its length. The submucous and subcutaneous tissues overlying the pile are then infiltrated with local anaesthetic and a weak adrenaline solution. A longitudinal inverted racket-shaped incision is made with scissors in the mucosal covering of the haemorrhoid; the 'handle' is placed in the anorectal mucosa and the circular portion over the skin of the anal canal and perianal region. Mucocutaneous flaps are raised on either side, paying particular attention to divide the mucosal suspensory ligament. Starting from below, the pile is dissected off the sphincter muscles to the upper end of the anal canal, where the slender pedicle is transfixed and ligated and the rest of the pile is excised. The flaps fall back more or less accurately on to the raw surface covering most of it, except for the lower portion which extends out into the perianal region where a small open wound remains. One or two catgut sutures may be used to approximate the flaps and fix them to the internal anal sphincter.

The advantages claimed for submucosal haemorrhoidectomy are the same as those claimed for other closed haemorrhoidectomy techniques.

Postoperative care and follow-up

Throughout the operative procedure we keep intravenous fluid administration to the minimum – ideally 100 mL or less. This helps prevent one of the most common complications of haemorrhoidectomy, namely postoperative urinary retention. Similarly, if the patient is awake and alert, the intravenous fluids are discontinued in the recovery room. If the patient is at increased risk of developing urinary retention, having given a history of nocturia, hesitancy or urgency, oral fluids are also limited after operation.

Patients are started on a regular high-fibre diet with additional psyllium seed. Sitz baths are taken at the patient's discretion. Narcotic analgesics are given on demand and may be necessary for the first 24–48 h. However, after the patient leaves hospital non-narcotic analgesics should be used to avoid constipation. With proper use of bulking agents, the first bowel movement need not be the dreaded event that most patients seem to fear. If the patient has not had a bowel movement by the third postoperative day, a prepackaged phosphate enema is administered. We feel that it is desirable, but not absolutely essential, for the patient to have a bowel movement before leaving hospital. The patient is instructed in the importance of a high dietary fibre intake to prevent further anorectal problems. A rectal examination is not performed before discharge; it adds nothing but discomfort for the patient.

The first postoperative visit, usually the only visit necessary, is scheduled for 3–4 weeks later. With increasing pressure to perform day-care surgery in patients with adequate support services at home, we now offer day-care closed haemorrhoidectomy to well-motivated patients who have no evidence of coexisting medical disorders.

Results

The early results of haemorrhoidectomy are difficult to access and there are few good postoperative comparative trials. The principal criterion of success early after operation is freedom from discomfort. In an early report of closed haemorrhoidectomy by Failes (1966), 21 of 24 patients had experienced pain of sufficient severity to require one or two injections of morphine on the day of operation and one at the time of the first bowel movement, whereas Ganchrow et al (1971) reported that over half of their patients required either no analgesic or only one or two injections of morphine. This has not been shown to be significantly less than following open haemorrhoidectomy although there are few comparative trials.

The long-term follow-up for closed haemorrhoidectomy in Ferguson's series was reported by Ganchrow et al (1971). Of the original 2038 patients, 1018 replied to 5-year follow-up questionnaires. Of those who replied, 95% felt that their symptoms were relieved, 88% felt that they had had satisfactory bowel movements since their operation, and 72% had experienced no further anorectal complaints during the 5 years of follow-up. Itching was the most common complaint mentioned by the patients after 5 years. Other associated anorectal diseases found during the 5-year follow-up included fissure-in-ano in 2.65%, anal stenosis in 1.18%, perianal abscess in 0.64%, rectal polyp in 0.49%, fistula-in-ano in 0.25%, residual haemorrhoidal disease requiring excision in 0.15%, and colon cancer in 0.05%. There is no record of what happened to the other 1020 who did not respond to the questionnaire.

McConnell and Khubchandani (1983) also reported their follow-up of 441 patients following closed haemorrhoidectomy with local anaesthesia. All patients had had a three-quadrant haemorrhoidectomy; in addition 36% had an internal sphincterotomy performed at the same time. After 1 to 7 years, 7.5% had required further treatment for residual haemorrhoidal problems, including one haemorrhoidectomy, and 7.7% developed additional anorectal or colonic pathology, including polyps in 2.9% and fissures in 1.6%. Two carcinomas were found during follow-up. Of the patients contacted for follow-up, 93% were satisfied with the result.

There are three studies with significant numbers of patients which describe complications following closed haemorrhoidectomy (Ganchrow et al, 1971; Buls and Goldberg, 1978; McConnell and Khubchandani, 1983).

McConnell and Khubchandani (1983) reported five early postoperative complications, including wound dehiscence in 2.6%, bleeding in 1.4%, faecal impaction in 0.3%, urinary retention in 0.2% and one pneumothorax. They specifically examined the incidence of postoperative flatus or faecal incontinence. In their study, 12.9% of patients had one or more of these problems. Only three patients had prolonged problems and only one had to wear a pad to prevent soiling.

In their study of 2038 cases, Ganchrow and others reported: minimal bleeding in 1.96%, bleeding requiring suture ligation in 1.32%, cystitis in 0.44%, abscess in 0.2%, and pneumonia in 0.1%. They recorded no instance of anal incontinence. Although they did not report urinary retention as a complication, they used bladder catheterization in 32% of patients. No instance of infection was reported.

Goldberg et al (1980) in Minneapolis reported the incidence of postoperative complications from 500 consecutive haemorrhoidectomies. They found that 10% had acute urinary retention, 4% had bleeding and 6% had skin tags. Anal stenosis occurred in only 1%, fistula-in-ano in 0.4%, anal fissure in 0.2%, incontinence in 0.4%, faecal impaction in 0.4% and thrombosed external haemorrhoids in 0.2%. None developed an abscess. Re-operation was required in 1.25% of the patients with postoperative bleeding. Thus, from the three studies, there was an overall general postoperative complication rate of about 5%, most of which were minor. There are still no large controlled trials to compare the complication rate of open haemorrhoidectomy with closed haemorrhoidectomy.

Conclusions

Those surgeons who have a large experience with closed haemorrhoidectomy – that is those who have performed at least 100 or more of these operations – find the technique to be relatively simple, safe and reliable. The operation can be applied to almost every situation in which the operation of haemorrhoidectomy is indicated. Unfortunately there are inadequate controlled trials to allow us to make an impartial judgement about the relative merits of open and closed haemorrhoidectomy. Most surgeons who pioneered closed haemorrhoidectomy undertook open haemorrhoidectomy during their surgical training and were instructed in open haemorrhoidectomy as the optimum form of treatment. Most of these colorectal surgeons have usually abandoned the open method because they found that it produced a lot of pain, required difficult and painful postoperative nursing and resulted in some late sequelae, particularly stenosis. These surgeons turned to closed haemorrhoidectomy because they felt it caused less pain, primary healing of the wound occurred sufficiently frequently to make postoperative nursing easier, and because they did not encounter postoperative stenosis following this operation. The fear of infection which might have prevented some surgeons from performing a closed haemorrhoidectomy has been proved to be groundless in a large number of patients reported by several authorities (Ganchrow et al, 1971; Khubchandani et al, 1974; Buls and Goldberg, 1978; McConnell and Khubchandani, 1983). There is never a need for postoperative anal dilatation, as there is in some patients after open haemorrhoidectomy. These advantages seem obvious to the surgeon who has adopted and perfected closed haemorrhoidectomy; some feel that they are so obvious that it is not necessary to put the procedure to a comparative trial with open haemorrhoidectomy, and we are surprised that the overwhelming majority of colorectal surgeons in the UK still practice open haemorrhoidectomy.

Open haemorrhoidectomy

The open technique, which is still widely practised in the UK, is based on the procedure originally described by Milligan and associates in 1937, and is usually referred to as the Milligan–Morgan operation. The operation is usually performed under general anaesthesia, but spinal anaesthesia can be used. More recently, with the vogue for ambulant haemorrhoidectomy, anaesthesia has been obtained by pudendal nerve block and intravenous sedation. Preoperative preparation is as described in Section I.

Technique

The patient is placed in the lithotomy position with the buttocks projecting well beyond the end of the table; the anal region is cleaned and draped in the usual way.

Although infiltration was not described in Milligan and colleagues' original paper, we normally infiltrate the subcutaneous tissues of the immediate perianal region with a 1:300 000 adrenaline–saline solution (Figure 12.32). This assists in haemostasis and helps in the isolation of the haemorrhoid pedicle.

The skin-covered component of each of the main piles is seized with artery forceps and retracted outwards (Figure 12.33). This has the effect of causing the lower poles of the mucosal-covered component of the haemorrhoid to protrude to a varying extent, depending on the size of haemorrhoidal tissue.

The purple anal mucosal component of each pile is now grasped in another artery forceps and drawn

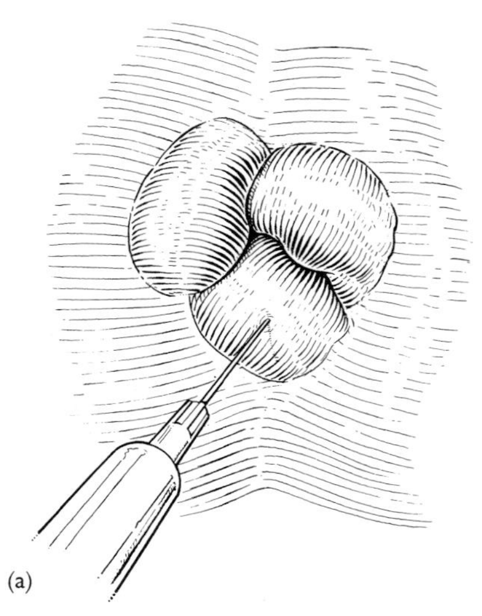

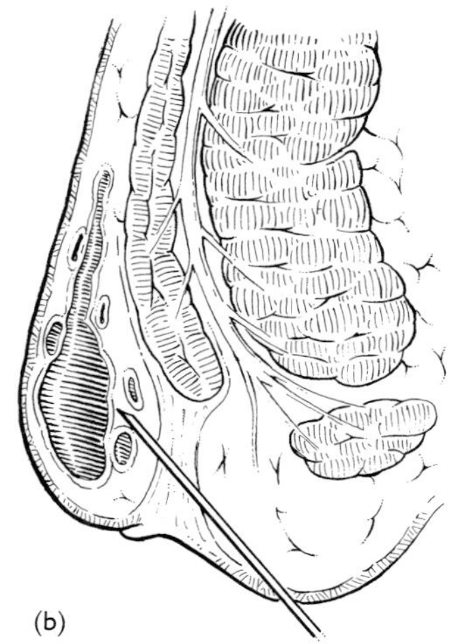

Figure 12.32a,b Infiltration of (a) perianal skin and (b) anal submucosa with 1:300 000 adrenaline–saline solution.

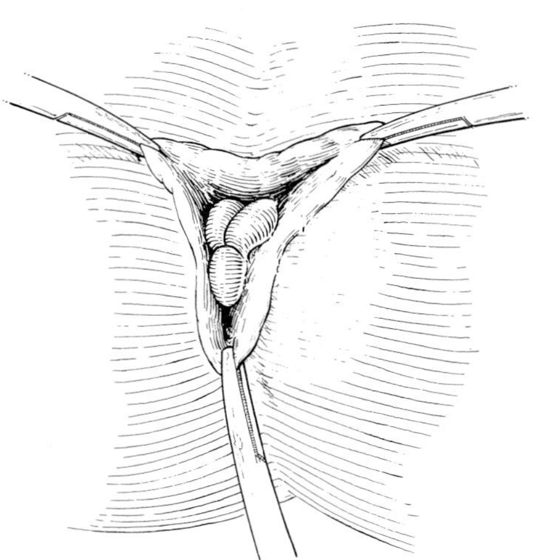

Figure 12.33 Open haemorrhoidectomy. The skin over each of the main haemorrhoids is grasped with artery forceps and is retracted.

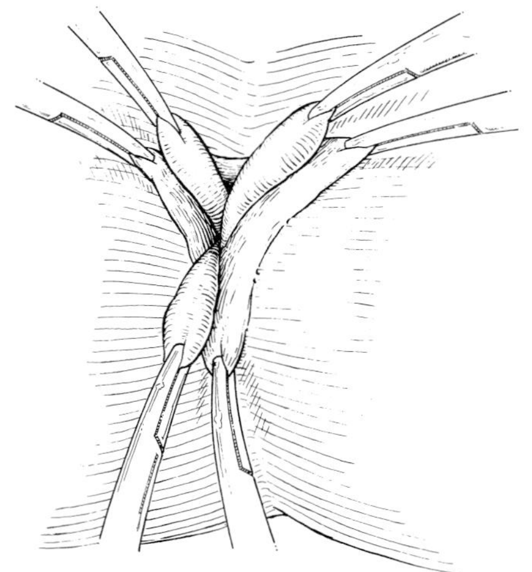

Figure 12.34 The apex of the mucosa over each haemorrhoid is grasped with a second artery forceps and retracted outwards.

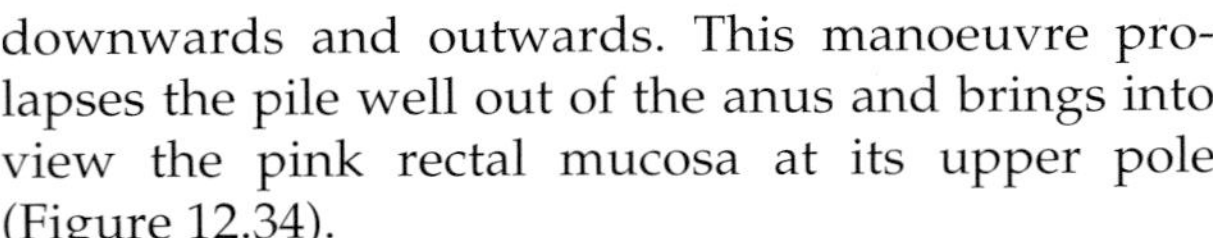

downwards and outwards. This manoeuvre prolapses the pile well out of the anus and brings into view the pink rectal mucosa at its upper pole (Figure 12.34).

The traction of the three haemorrhoids is maintained until pink rectal mucosa shows not only at the upper part of the piles but also on the mucosal folds running between the piles. This indicates that the piles have been drawn down to their maximum extent so that the ligatures can be applied at their upper poles rather than in the middle.

The two forceps attached to the patient's left lateral pile are taken in the palm of the operator's left hand and drawn downwards and to the patient's right, while the extended index finger of the operator's left hand is used to stabilize the inner aspect of the pile and to withdraw it outwards. In this way the upper pole of the pile is exposed during dissection. The operator then makes a V-shaped incision in the anal and perianal skin, as shown in Figure 12.35, with a pair of blunt scissors. The limbs of the V cross the mucocutaneous junction but do not extend into the mucosa; the point of the V should lie 2.5–3 cm away from the anal verge (Figure 12.35). If the tip of the surgeon's left index finger is pressed firmly against the end of the scissors as the V-shaped incision is being made, the lower edge of the internal sphincter is exposed so that it can be preserved while the venous plexus is dissected from it. If the forceps holding the skin component of the haemorrhoid are displaced inwards towards the lumen of the anus, the outer raw surface of the pile will be exposed. Longitudinal strands of fascia and muscle may be seen entering the venous plexus from the region immediately internal to the inferior margin of the internal sphincter. These strands are termed the 'muscularis submucosae ani'. In the classic operation described by Milligan these are not divided, and the only further dissection of the pile consists of making a slight nick in the mucosa above and below to narrow the mucosal pedicle before applying the ligature.

However, we, like many other colorectal surgeons, prefer to free the haemorrhoidal venous

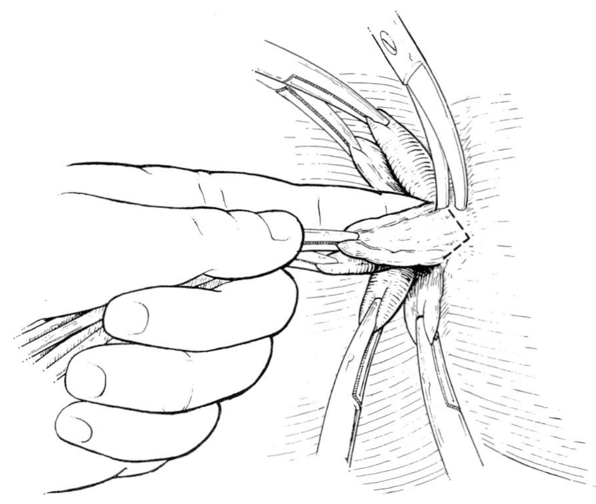

Figure 12.35 A V-shaped incision is made over the anoderm at the base of the haemorrhoid.

plexus further by dissecting it off the internal sphincter for a distance of 1.5–2.0 cm (Figure 12.36). This dissection involves further traction on the forceps downwards and medially, and division of the fibres which contribute to the muscularis submucosae ani. Care must be taken not to injure the internal anal sphincter, which should be visualized throughout the dissection (Figure 12.37). Before division of the fibres, we normally diathermize them to ensure secure haemostasis (Figure 12.38). As the dissection proceeds upwards, the underlying mucosa must be divided on each side of the pedicle. The mucosal incisions should converge towards the apex of the pedicle in order to avoid leaving a broad bulky mucosal pedicle.

The apex of the pedicle is then transfixed with a 0 or 1/0 chromic catgut suture on a round-bodied needle (Figure 12.39). Some prefer to transfix with a non-absorbable suture such as Chinese silk. The ligature over the pedicle is then tied and the forceps on the mucosal aspect of the haemorrhoid is removed and applied to the ends of the ligature. The left pile is thus isolated, held by one pair of forceps on the perianal skin with a second pair on the transfixed pedicle. Retraction of the pile laterally and the ligature medially allows the surgeon to view the apex of the pile to ensure that the transfixion is secure. The isolated haemorrhoid is then excised with scissors a few millimetres below the apical ligature, while the transfixion suture remains clamped and left long for further inspection at the end of the operation (Figure 12.40).

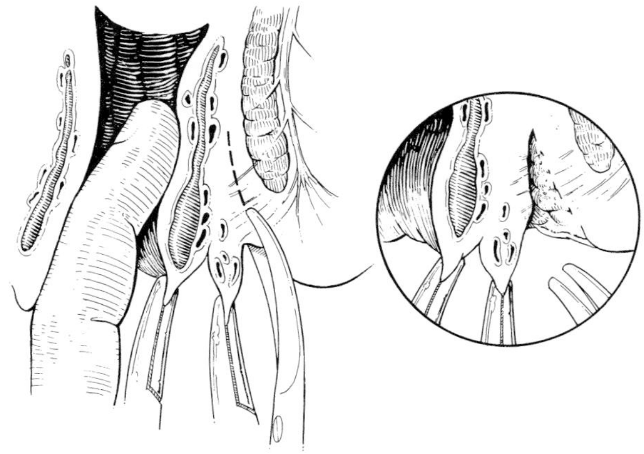

Figure 12.36 The haemorrhoid mass is dissected off the internal sphincter for a distance of 1.5–2.0 cm.

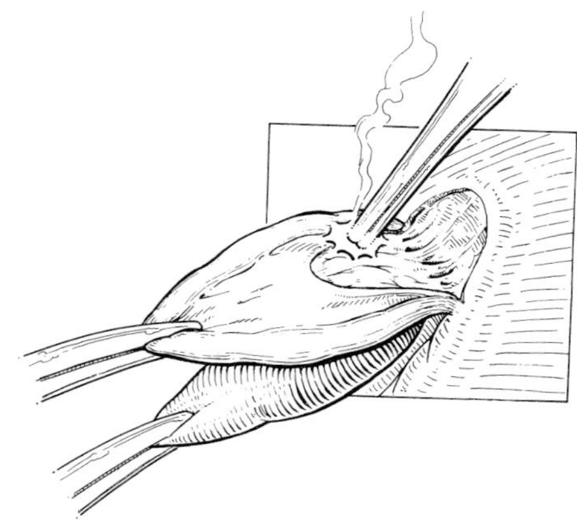

Figure 12.38 Diathermy and dissection of the fibres of the muscularis submucosae ani.

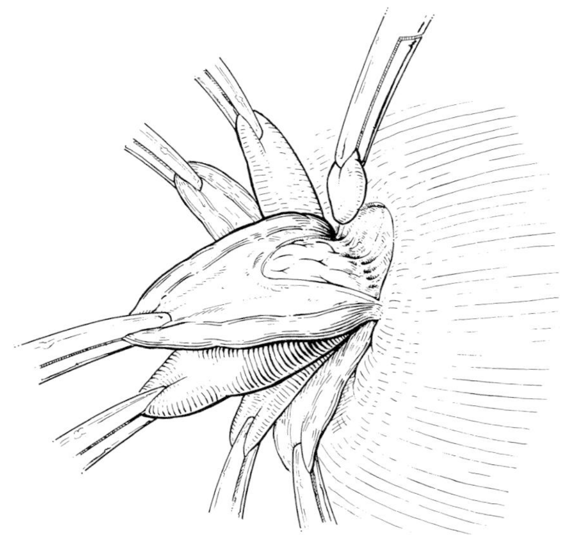

Figure 12.37 The dissection of the haemorrhoidal tissue from the internal sphincter may be aided by a 'peanut'.

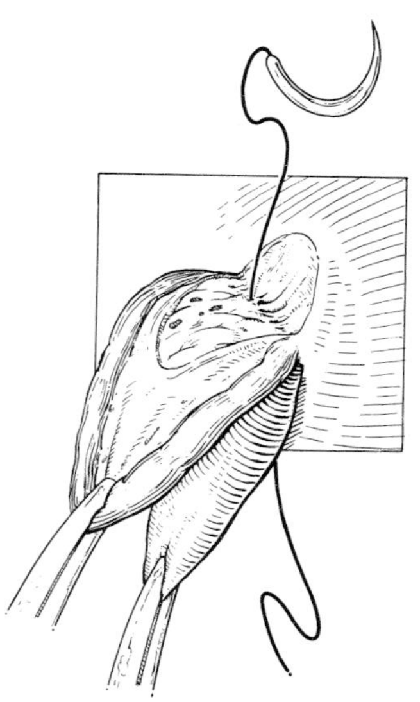

Figure 12.39 Transfixion of the base of the haemorrhoid.

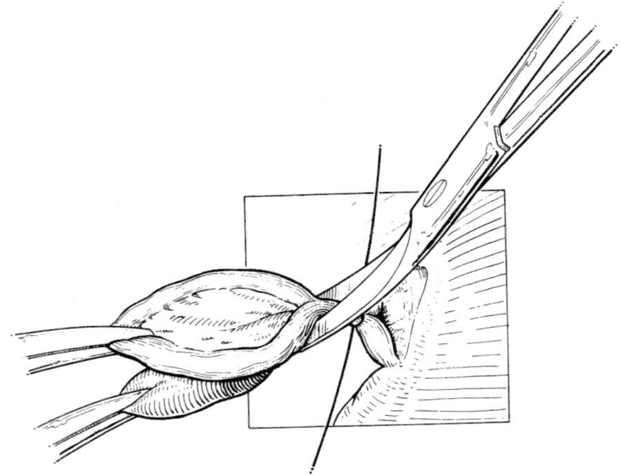

Figure 12.40 Excision of the haemorrhoid after transfixion and ligature of its base.

Attention is then directed to the right posterior or right anterior pile. We prefer to tackle the right posterior haemorrhoid next, since bleeding from it does not obscure the right anterior haemorrhoid whereas the opposite is not true. The procedure is repeated in exactly the same manner for each of these positions, but the pile forceps are held in the surgeon's right hand and retracted to the patient's left, while the scissor dissection must be performed by the left hand. It is essential that in making the skin incisions the surgeon ensures that there is an intact bridge of skin and mucosa between each excised haemorrhoid (Figure 12.41).

At the end of the procedure a Parks or Eisenhammer retractor is inserted into the anal canal and with traction on the transfixion ligatures, the surgeon then ensures that the pedicles are secure and that an adequate bridge of skin and mucosa exist between each of the wounds. The transfixion ligatures are then divided and the skin wounds are trimmed if they appear ragged, leaving three pear-shaped raw areas (Figure 12.42).

We usually dress the wound by tucking three squares of paraffin wax-impregnated gauze into the anal canal, so that they lie on each raw area. These are then covered with dry gauze and wool, and held in place by a T-bandage.

Sometimes, in addition to the three primary haemorrhoids, there exists one or more accessory piles. These may, with care, be incorporated into the excision of one of the main piles. However, if there is any chance that a mucosal bridge is likely to be compromised, it is better either to leave the accessory pile and inject it with sclerosant agent at the end of the procedure, or preferably fillet the mucosal bridge of its vascular elements by scissor dissection from either side, leaving the skin and mucosa intact.

An associated anal fissure can be dealt with by a coexisting internal sphincterotomy, although extreme caution must be exercised in the older patient with a potentially weak anal sphincter. It may indeed be safer in such circumstances to perform no additional procedure but treat the patient postoperatively with 0.2% glyceryl trinitrate ointment.

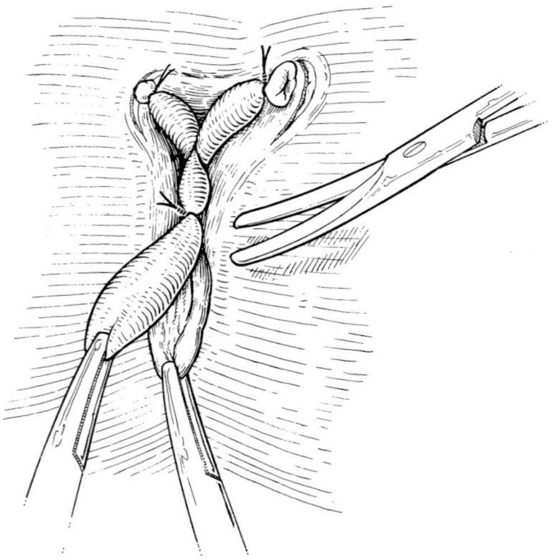

Figure 12.41 Excision of inferior 7 o'clock haemorrhoid after ensuring the retention of skin and mucosal bridges.

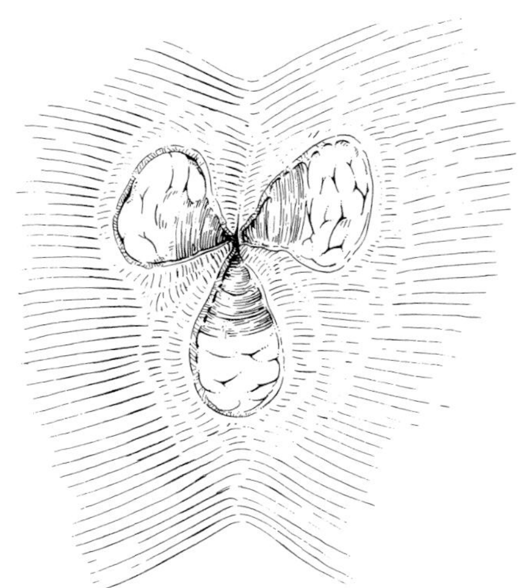

Figure 12.42 The three pear-shaped wounds which remain after open haemorrhoidectomy.

Variations of technique: addition of sphincterotomy or anal stretch

On the assumption that the pain experienced after haemorrhoidectomy is due to spasm of the anal sphincter, there has been a vogue for performing either adjuvant manual dilatation (Watts et al, 1964; Goligher et al, 1969) or sphincterotomy (Eisenhammer 1969, 1974; Asfar et al, 1988). Critical evaluation of anal dilatation has not substantiated any benefit from this addition (Watts et al, 1964; Goligher et al, 1969) and because of the inherent risks to continence we do not recommend this practice. The same may be said of sphincterotomy, but Asfar et al (1988) reported that both an internal and external sphincterotomy was beneficial. We have considerable anxiety in recommending adjuvant sphincterotomy for the reasons already stated.

Postoperative management

The wound needs little attention in the early postoperative period. We usually advise changing the gauze swabs and wool daily until the first bowel action has occurred, the underlying dressing remaining undisturbed. To encourage a relatively gentle first bowel action, we normally prescribe Milpar 10 mL twice a day, together with Fibogel. Non-constipating, non-narcotic analgesics are prescribed liberally. Pain is not usually marked after the first 2–3 days except when the patient has a bowel action. This can vary considerably from patient to patient. Effective relief can often be obtained by immersion in a hot bath immediately after defecation. It was usual practice to detain the patient in hospital until a bowel action had occurred. However, we, like others, discharge our patients within 2–3 days of operation, irrespective of whether or not they have opened their bowels. If when they are about to leave hospital they still have not had a bowel action, we normally prescribe a phosphate enema, which usually produces the desired effect. This policy has not resulted in any greater morbidity compared with the expectant regimen. Patients are reviewed 1 month after discharge, when a rectal examination is performed to ensure that there is no stenosis. If any narrowing is found, we recommend the use of an anal dilator each day.

Day-case haemorrhoidectomy

In certain institutions, particularly in the USA and increasingly in the UK, haemorrhoidectomy is being performed on a day-case basis. Such a technique may be limited because of the need to provide parenteral analgesia. Various new techniques to control pain by means other than parenteral analgesia are being used for day-case haemorrhoidectomy. Thus, Goldstein et al (1993) recommend the use of a subcutaneous morphine pump. O'Donovan et al (1994) reported that Toradol (ketaraloz tromethamine, Syntex Labs, Palo Alto, CA), a new non-steroidal analgesic, was effective in the ambulatory situation. We entirely concur and now use liberal amounts of local anaesthetic and a diclofenec (voltarol) suppository at the end of the operation with oral voltarol and ranitidine with lactulose and Fybogel to take home.

Results

There are few long-term studies on the results of Milligan–Morgan haemorrhoidectomy. Most authors have assessed their patients after 3 or at the most 6 months. It is therefore difficult to be confident about the true recurrence rate. Bennett et al (1963), in their long-term follow-up study, found that recurrence of symptoms occurred in 5% of cases. Murie et al (1980) followed up patients for 42 months; their findings are most illuminating. Of 38 patients who complained of bleeding preoperatively, one (3%) did not improve at all, and five (12%), although improved, still continued to bleed.

Table 12.8 Long-term results of haemorrhoidectomy.

Authors	*n*	*Length of follow-up*	*Patients completely or largely satisfied (%)*
Cormie and McNair (1959)	60	Several years	95
Soderlund (1962)	100	6–7 years	99
Bennett et al (1963)	138	Several years	93
Chant et al (1972)	24	6–7 months	100
Anscombe et al (1974)	50	6 months	98
Jones and Schofield (1974)	100	Several years	95
Murie et al (1980)	41	42 months	95
Cheng et al (1981)	30	1 year	95

Two of 29 patients (6.9%) who had third-degree haemorrhoids preoperatively still had symptoms of prolapse after 42 months.

Despite these treatment failures and the minor degree of soiling which some patients report, over 90% when questioned are satisfied with their operation (Table 12.8).

Whitehead haemorrhoidectomy

We mention this technique for completeness but believe that nowadays it should be avoided when there are better alternatives. The operation involves the circumferential excision of the haemorrhoids and often the anoderm with anchoring of perianal skin and rectal mucosa to a region at or above the previous dentate line (Whitehead, 1882). Many surgeons misinterpreted Whitehead's original operation and sutured the rectal mucosa directly to the anal skin. This often resulted in a mucosal ectropion, the so-called wet anus or Whitehead's deformity. Although various authors have described successful series using a modified technique (Barrios and Khubchandani, 1979; Wolff and Culp, 1988; Khubchandani, 1984), the late complication rates are in the region of 10–13% (Khubchandani, 1984), particularly stenosis and incontinence, and suggest that this is not a technique to be used routinely. Even when the patient has severe circumferential prolapse of haemorrhoids, we would recommend four-pile haemorrhoidectomy as opposed to the Whitehead operation. Indeed, in a randomized trial comparing these two techniques, Seow-Choen and Low (1995) demonstrated that the four-pile haemorrhoidectomy is preferable. Twenty-eight patients with circumferential prolapse were randomized to the two operations, and at 6 months superior results were reported in patients having a four-pile haemorrhoidectomy, even though skin tags were more frequent.

Laser haemorrhoidectomy

The laser has recently been used to perform haemorrhoidectomy either to destroy the haemorrhoidal tissue or to aid in the dissection of the haemorrhoid as part of an open or closed haemorrhoidectomy. Both Nd–Yag and CO_2 lasers have been used. Because laser light is invisible, the operator and attendants must wear goggles to protect the eyes. A red pilot light provided by a low-power laser permits focusing of the therapeutic beam. When used as a destructive tool, the laser beam is aimed directly on to the surface of the pile until the area is covered by a white membrane. Many practitioners now seem to prefer the CO_2 laser because of its predictable biological effects, minimal damage to adjacent normal tissue, good haemostasis and precision (Iwagaki et al, 1989). Some have used a Nd–Yag laser for internal haemorrhoids and a CO_2 laser for external haemorrhoids (Wang et al, 1991).

Results

Several prospective controlled trials comparing laser haemorrhoidectomy with conventional techniques have been reported. Thus, Wang et al (1991) compared Nd–Yag laser haemorrhoidectomy with the closed Ferguson technique in 88 patients. Both the use of narcotic analgesics and the incidence of postoperative acute retention of urine were significantly less with the laser. However, Nicholson and Halleran (1990) found no difference between sapphire-tip Nd–Yag laser haemorrhoidectomy compared with a closed procedure when used for third- or fourth-degree haemorrhoids, and similar results were reported by Sengapore et al (1993). Leff (1992) performed a prospective study that assessed haemorrhoidectomy by means of a CO_2 laser (170 patients) compared with conventional closed haemorrhoidectomy in 56 patients, and observed no differences with respect to pain, wound healing or complications. However, this was not a truly randomized study. Chia et al (1995) in a small study did prospectively randomize 28 patients between CO_2 laser haemorrhoidectomy and conventional Milligan–Morgan open haemorrhoidectomy; there were 14 patients in each arm. The only significant difference was a greater use of analgesics in the conventional group. This study was complemented by pre- and postoperative anorectal physiology measurements, and no significant difference was discernible.

It is still too early to say whether laser haemorrhoidectomy is more beneficial than conventional techniques. There are too few prospective randomized trials to support its routine use. One suspects its costs will outweigh its benefits, but time will tell.

Diathermy haemorrhoidectomy

Instead of using scissor dissection, a Milligan–Morgan haemorrhoidectomy can be achieved using diathermy. It is claimed that blood loss and postoperative pain are less using this technique (Sharif et al, 1991; Lentini et al, 1990). However, in a small randomized study comparing the two methods, Andrews et al (1993) found that there was no significant advantage for the diathermy technique. The authors did conclude, though, that they preferred to use the diathermy technique as it reduced primary haemorrhage. On the other hand, Seow-Choen et al (1992) in their randomized trial between the conventional scissor technique and the diathermy method ($n = 49$) found that diathermy was faster, caused less bleeding and was less painful.

Complications of open and closed haemorrhoidectomy

Although some of the complications of the closed technique were discussed earlier, it is convenient to summarize the problems at this point.

Anal stenosis

The management of anal stenosis is dealt with later in this section.

Pain

The degree of pain after haemorrhoidectomy is considered by many to be the main reason why patients resist the operation. It is not surprising, therefore, that surgeons have modified the technique with the aim of reducing postoperative pain. Various studies, particularly by Goligher and his colleagues, attempted to assess the influence of various modifications to the operation on the severity of postoperative pain. The open technique (Milligan–Morgan operation) was compared with a closed technique (the submucosal haemorrhoidectomy of Parks) (Watts et al, 1964, 1965) but no significant difference in pain scores could be detected between the groups. The addition of a four-finger anal dilatation to the operation (a technique which we would not recommend) also made no difference to the amount of pain experienced by the patients (Goligher et al, 1969). In a more recent study, Roe et al (1987) from Bristol compared the submucosal excision technique ($n = 18$) with the Milligan–Morgan operation ($n = 22$) and found no difference in postoperative pain, as measured by linear analogue scores, between the two groups. Similarly, Ho et al (1997) in a small randomized controlled trial of open ($n = 34$) versus closed ($n = 33$) haemorrhoidectomy found no difference in pain scores between the two groups. Surprisingly, however, wound healing was faster and more reliable using the open technique compared with the closed technique (Table 12.9). These data are contrary to the view of Parks (1956) and Singh and Lal (1975). However, neither of these groups attempted to measure pain objectively.

It is evident from these various studies that pain experienced after haemorrhoidectomy is extremely patient-dependent. Various suggestions have been made as to its cause. Ligation of sensitive epithelium below the dentate line in the course of the excision ligation operation was considered by some to be the main cause, and that is why the submucosal technique was advocated. However, the study by Roe et al (1987) casts doubt on the theory

Table 12.9 Pain after open and closed haemorrhoidectomy

	Open haemorrhoidectomy (n = 34)	*Closed haemorrhoidectomy (n = 33)*	*P*
Postoperative score during first 24 h	5 (1–8)	5 (2–8)	1
Maximum postoperative pain score	5 (3–9)	6 (2–8)	0.6
Pain score at first postoperative bowel movement	4 (0–9)	4 (0–8)	0.3
Ketoprofen requirement (100 mg tablets)	4 (1–12)	2 (2–12)	0.4
Pethidine requirement (1 mg/kg bodyweight i.m.)	0 (0–3)	0.5 (0–3)	0.3

Values are medians (range). Pain scores 0 no pain; 10 worst pain ever experienced. Chi-squared test showed no significant differences between the two groups.
From Ho et al (1997).

since no benefit was observed in terms of pain relief when open haemorrhoidectomy was compared with the closed submucosal technique. Spasm of the sphincter may be a factor, and this was the rationale for performing adjuvant anal dilatation or interal sphincterotomy (Eisenhammer, 1951, 1974); but, as we report, these manoeuvres seem to have had little, if any, impact on the severity or duration of postoperative pain and indeed may be dangerous. The most plausible cause for pain is the exposed raw areas of anal canal that are inevitable after the open operation. The reason why there is no apparent pain relief after the closed technique described by Parks is that there is still an open wound below the dentate line following this operation (Watts et al, 1964). Here, indeed, is the most powerful argument for the Ferguson–Heaton (1959) closed haemorrhoidectomy, and the one so powerfully used by its protagonists. Without exception, those clinicians who favour primary suture of the operative wounds claim significantly less postoperative pain than after the Milligan–Morgan operation.

Acute retention of urine

As with all painful perineal procedures, acute retention of urine may be a problem after haemorrhoidectomy. Both Jones and Schofield (1974) and Goligher (1984) reported that 8% of patients developed acute retention after the Milligan–Morgan technique. Apart from pain, numerous other factors are thought to be responsible. These include spinal anaesthesia, high ligation of the haemorrhoidal pedicle, rough handling of tissue, numerous sutures, fluid overload, rectal packing, tight bulky dressings, anticholinergics and narcotics.

The importance of limiting fluid intake perioperatively has been highlighted by several authors (Bailey and Ferguson, 1976; Scoma, 1976; Hoff et al, 1994). Thus, Bailey and Ferguson (1976) in a prospective randomized controlled trial found that if fluid was markedly restricted the catheterization rate was only 3.5%, compared with 14.9% when unlimited fluids were allowed. Although Gottesman et al (1989) found that 10 mg of urecholine (bethanechol chloride) given subcutaneously may prevent acute retention, such prophylaxis has not become popular. Prophylactic and adrenergic blockade and tranquillizers have been shown to be ineffective (Gottesman et al, 1989; Cataldo and Sengapore, 1991).

Pain and fluid load seem to be the main factors leading to acute retention, and attention should focus on them.

Reactionary or secondary haemorrhage

Reactionary haemorrhage is due to bleeding, either from the main vascular pedicle as a result of a slipped ligature or to a small bleeding point in one of the external anal wounds. It usually occurs soon after the patient returns to the ward or later that evening. With meticulous technique, it is rare for the ligature on the main pedicle to slip. Often the bleeding is no more than a gentle ooze, which can usually be stopped by external pressure. However, it is wise to remember that bleeding from the pedicle into the rectum can occur and remain undetected for some time. Thus, if there is any doubt as to where the bleeding is coming from, and the patient is haemodynamically unstable, he or she should, after appropriate resuscitation, be returned to the operating theatre and be examined under general anaesthesia. The rectum should be irrigated with sterile saline, and the bleeding point detected and secured if possible. Often after the evacuation of clot no bleeding source is evident. The incidence of reactionary haemorrhage seems to be about 1% after open haemorrhoidectomy (Goligher, 1984).

Secondary haemorrhage from sepsis is more serious, for bleeding invariably occurs into the rectum and remains undetected; hence the degree of blood loss can be considerable. Bleeding either involves the main pedicle and results in its erosion or is from the open infected anal wounds. The incidence of secondary haemorrhage ranges from 1.2% to 4% after the Milligan–Morgan technique (Jones and Schofield, 1974; Thomson, 1978; Goligher, 1984). Secondary haemorrhage usually takes place between the seventh and tenth postoperative days, and now that patients are discharged within a few days of operation, or earlier, it invariably takes place at home. The patient may notice a trickle of altered dark blood from the anus, but more commonly has an urge to defecate and passes large amounts of fluid and clotted blood. If undetected, there may be rapid cardiovascular decompression with circulatory collapse. The patient and family doctor must be aware of this complication, which can almost always be confirmed by a rectal examination. Some dark blood may be evident oozing from the anal canal. Digital examination will reveal the presence of soft clots, and after withdrawal some blood may seep away at the same time. The passage of a narrow-bore proctoscope, as recommended by Goligher (1984), should be confirmatory, but rarely will this be possible in the patient's home. Not only will the general practitioner not usually possess such an instrument and appropriate light source, but 1 week after the operation the patient will usually not be able to tolerate the examination. The patient will need to be transferred urgently to hospital and resuscitated if necessary. In the hospital, arrangements will need to be made to examine the patient under anaesthetic.

The patient is placed in the lithotomy or jack-knife position and a bivalve speculum is inserted. Any clot should then be removed by a combination of swabs and irrigation with saline. It should then be possible to observe the bleeding point, which can be under-run using chromic catgut or a Vicryl suture on a small half-circle or 5/8 needle. If this cannot be performed easily or the surgeon is not satisfied with the result, a large Foley catheter or, better still, a condom mounted on a length of Perspex tubing can be passed into the rectum, its balloon inflated and traction exerted so that it compresses the bleeding point. Alternatively, the anorectum can be packed tightly with ribbon gauze. The catheter, condom or pack should remain *in situ* for 48 hours. A blood transfusion is usually required, and antibiotics and a stool softener should be prescribed.

Anal fissure

Anal fissure is a rare complication which may result from a failure of one of the haemorrhoidectomy sites to heal adequately. It may occur in the midline, posteriorly or anteriorly in connection with the right posterior or right anterior haemorrhoid wounds. If it is found that either of these wounds is failing to heal completely and a fissure is developing despite proper attention to baths and irrigation, it is recommended that a sphincter stretch or internal sphincterotomy should be performed (Goligher, 1984). This advice may be satisfactory in young male patients, but caution must be exercised in the older multiparous patients, who may have a deficient pelvic floor, since early intervention of this kind may result in permanent incontinence. It is wise in such cases to wait for some months to determine if a stretch or sphincterotomy is really necessary. Often it is not, and the wound eventually heals, provided the stools are kept soft.

Abscess or fistula formation

Since the Milligan–Morgan technique leaves behind large, wide external wounds, abscess or fistula should not develop provided postoperative care is adequate. Occasionally, if the wounds are narrow, their edges may become adherent and pus may pocket below them. If this occurs, the wound should be reshaped under general anaesthesia. This complication is not mentioned in any of the papers on excision ligation haemorrhoidectomy, so one assumes that the incidence is very low indeed. The problem is more likely to occur after closed haemorrhoidectomy, and it is interesting to note that abscess and fistula were rarely recorded after closed haemorrhoidectomy (Goldberg et al, 1980). However, whether this incidence is less than that after open operation is not known.

Formation of skin tags

Oedema in the perianal skin adjacent to haemorrhoidectomy wounds may result in skin tags, which initially can be quite painful. To prevent the formation of skin tags, all bare wounds should, if possible, be trimmed at operation to leave flat open wounds. However, this is not always possible. A firm dressing and T-bandage might prevent the development of oedema, but this eventually abates and the skin either returns to a normal appearance or fibrosis results in the formation of a skin tag. Skin tags are rarely painful; they may occasionally bleed and, more commonly, they impair anal cleanliness and encourage pruritus. Some patients may find them an aesthetic problem! The incidence of skin tags after operation is difficult to determine but is reported to occur in 4% of patients after excision ligation (Jones and Schofield, 1974). It might be expected that the closed technique would produce no skin tags, but Goldberg et al (1980) describe an incidence of 6%.

Pseudopolyps and epidermal cysts

Occasionally, a foreign-body reaction occurs at the site of the ligated pedicles, which results in the formation of a pseudopolyp of granulation tissue (Gaskin and Childer, 1963; Gehamy and Weakley, 1974). These can be excised if they cause symptoms. Rarely, several months after haemorrhoidectomy, inclusion epidermal cysts may develop in the anal canal. Their formation has been attributed to retention of keratin elements, hair follicles or exfoliated squamous epithelium in the wounds (Gaskin and Childer, 1963). They can be excised if they cause symptoms.

Incontinence

Anal leakage or soiling is common during the early postoperative period, but frank incontinence of liquid and stool is rare. After 6 weeks to 2 months, most patients with imperfect continence regain full control. There does not appear to be any difference in the incidence of transient incontinence between the open and closed techniques. Thus, Roe et al (1987), in their controlled trial comparing submucosal haemorrhoidectomy (partially closed technique) (18 patients) and excision ligation (22 patients), found that 50% of their patients, equally divided between the two groups, complained of soiling in the early postoperative period, but only two in each group complained of frank incontinence. These minor disturbances of continence had resolved in all patients by 6 weeks. At 6 months, Jones and Schofield (1974) found that only one of 100 patients still had any impairment of continence after excision and ligation. By contrast, Bennett et al (1963) reported on the long-term results of haemorrhoidectomy and found that, overall, 26% of patients had minor defects of anal control: 9% had impaired control of flatus, 6% had impaired control of faeces and 17% had occasional soiling of their underclothes. We suspect that many of these patients had had an anal dilatation at the time of haemorrhoidectomy, since this practice was very much in vogue in the 1950s. It has been suggested that another cause for defects of continence after haemorrhoidectomy is the loss of anal canal sensation due to removal of sensory-bearing anal canal epithelium and replacement by scar tissue. It might be expected, therefore, that the closed technique would be superior to the open technique in this respect. Roe et al (1987) found that sensation as measured by mucosal electrosensitivity was impaired after open haemorrhoidectomy, but not so after the submucosal operation. Despite this objective difference, there was no apparent long-term impairment of continence in either group, suggesting that excision of part of the sensory-bearing area cannot be identified as a cause of incontinence in these patients.

Various authors (Read et al, 1982; Mortensen et al, 1987; Roe et al, 1987) have found that haemorrhoidectomy produces a significant but transient reduction in anal canal pressures. Whether this contributes to impaired continence in the early postoperative convalescence is speculative but plausible. One theory is that the presence of large vascular cushions in patients with haemorrhoidal disease causes reflex contraction of the internal and external anal sphincters. Thus, the preoperative anal canal pressures are higher than normal. After haemorrhoidectomy, there is no reflex contraction and the pressure falls to more normal levels. Certainly, the postoperative sphincter pressures are not significantly different from control subjects. It is likely, however, that the decrease in pressures after haemorrhoidectomy signifies some damage to the internal sphincter mechanism during the operation but full recovery usually occurs afterwards.

Management of anal stenosis

Provided adequate mucosal bridges are retained after the excision ligation of haemorrhoids, this complication should be rare. Watts found that none of Goligher's patients developed stenosis such that it was impossible to perform a rectal examination after the operation (Watts et al, 1964). Furthermore, none of his patients required a secondary procedure to correct an anal stenosis. Jones and Schofield (1974) found that 6 of 100 patients undergoing the Milligan–Morgan operation suffered from anal narrowing, five of whom responded to short-term anal dilatation. However, one patient did require an operation to correct the stenosis. Goligher felt that those cases that he had treated by submucosal excision had less anal stenosis than those treated by excision ligation, but this was not supported by careful follow-up data. The incidence of anal stenosis reported by Goldberg, Walker and colleagues using the closed technique was 1%, but we are not told if any of these required re-operation.

If there is any evidence of anal narrowing due to fibrosis at the first outpatient visit, we recommend that the patient use an anal dilator twice daily. A bulk laxative should also be prescribed. If the stricture cannot easily be dilated, consideration will have to be given to performing an anoplasty. However, in our experience anal stenosis of this severity is often accompanied by damage to the underlying sphincter mechanism, and there may be associated incontinence. Therefore, careful assessment, including anorectal physiology and anal ultrasound is required.

Anoplasty is a procedure whereby perianal skin is moved to cover a defect in the anal canal (Corman, 1993). This defect is usually the result of an operative procedure such as excision of a portion or all of the mucosa covering the anal canal, haemorrhoidectomy, excision of an anal fissure, or excision of a lesion in the anal canal. Unfortunately, anal stenosis from 'radical' haemorrhoidectomy still seems to be the most common indication for anoplasty. Of 212 patients with anal stenosis treated by Milsom and Mazier (1986), 88% had previously undergone haemorrhoidectomy.

An anoplasty should be considered for an anal stenosis if medical treatment by laxatives, suppositories, dilatation and enemas has failed.

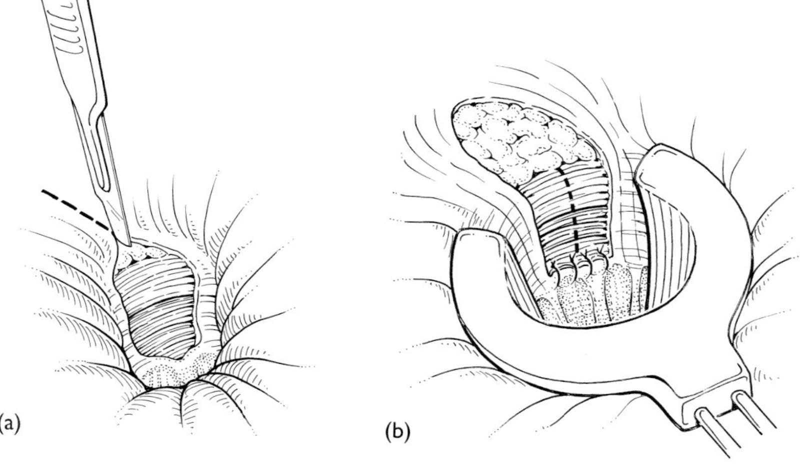

Figure 12.43a,b Treatment of anal stricture by excision of eschar and sphincterotomy. The stricture is first lysed (a) to permit the insertion of a retractor (b). The rectal mucosa is then sutured to the underlying internal anal sphincter prior to a sphincterotomy.

Excision of the eschar and sphincterotomy, which is not a true anoplasty, is a long-established technique for minor anal stenosis. It involves lysis and excision of the eschar, transverse suture of the rectal mucosa to the underlying internal sphincter, and sphincterotomy (Figure 12.43). There are several reports commending the procedure (Pope, 1959; Malgieri, 1961; Turrell and Gerlent, 1969; Shropshear, 1971), but we have no experience of the operation. From the literature it seems likely that it should be performed only when there is mild stenosis, and when sufficient skin bridges remain. The patients we encounter with anal stenosis following haemorrhoidectomy rarely fall into this category.

Anoplasty for mild or moderate stenosis

An advancement flap of the Y–V configuration can be used when only a section of the anoderm is scarred.

Technique

This is performed in the prone jack-knife position or the Lloyd Davies position, depending on the site of the stricture. The strictured area is incised. An internal anal sphincterotomy may or may not be performed depending on continence. A full-thickness flap of skin is elevated over the stricture usually in the posterior midline (Figure 12.44). A 29 mm

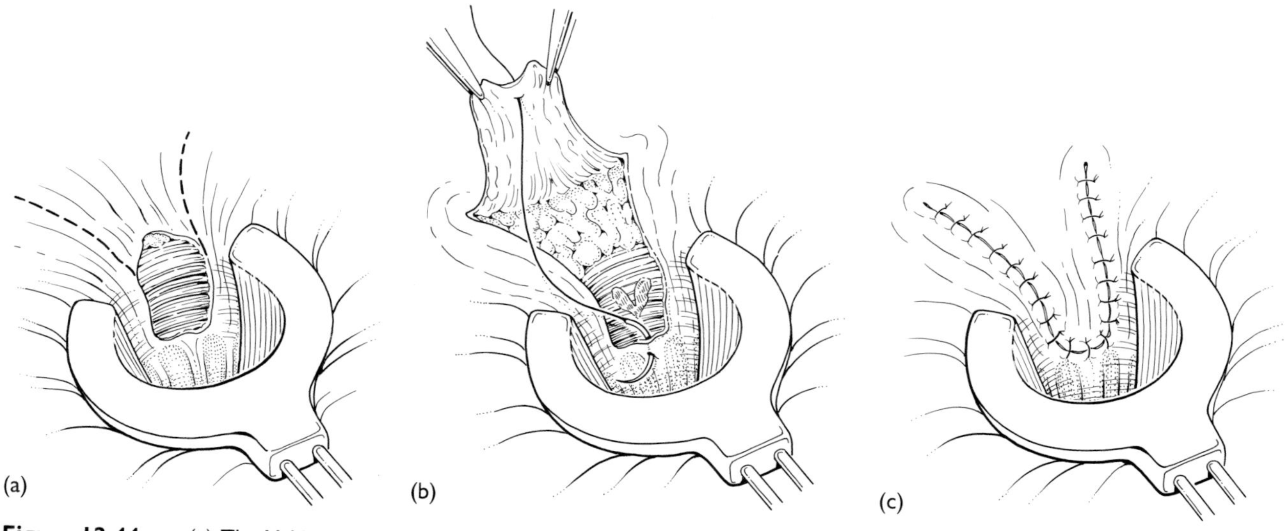

Figure 12.44a–c (a) The Y–V advancement flap. The area of stenosis is excised around the circumference of the anal margin. The dotted lines show the skin incisions for the flap. (b) The flap is elevated and (c) advanced to be sutured to the rectal mucosa and perianal skin.

Hill–Ferguson retractor or Eisenhammer retractor is kept in place for the whole operation to maintain the adequacy of the lumen. The incisions are extended radially for 5–8 cm. It is essential that the pedicle of the flap be broad to ensure its blood supply is maintained. Once the flap has been raised, it is advanced to overlay the defect created by incision of the scar. The apex of the flap is sutured to the apex of the cut rectal mucosa, taking a bite of the underlying internal sphincter. The sides of the flap are then sutured to the rectal mucosa again, taking bites of the underlying internal sphincter. Long-term absorbable sutures such as Vicryl or Maxon are used for this. The external aspect of the wounds may be left open if tension would be produced by closure, or the entire wound can be closed primarily.

The Y–V anoplasty is suitable for strictures which involve 25% of the anal canal circumference, and are ideal for use in strictures associated with an anal fissure. Similarly, a V–Y or island flap anoplasty can be used. The island flap anoplasty, particularly if used bilaterally, can be employed for a stenosis which involves a moderate amount of the circumference, say 25–50%. The technique is illustrated in Figure 12.45. If bilateral flaps are to be used, it is usual to create these from the right and left lateral areas (Figure 12.46).

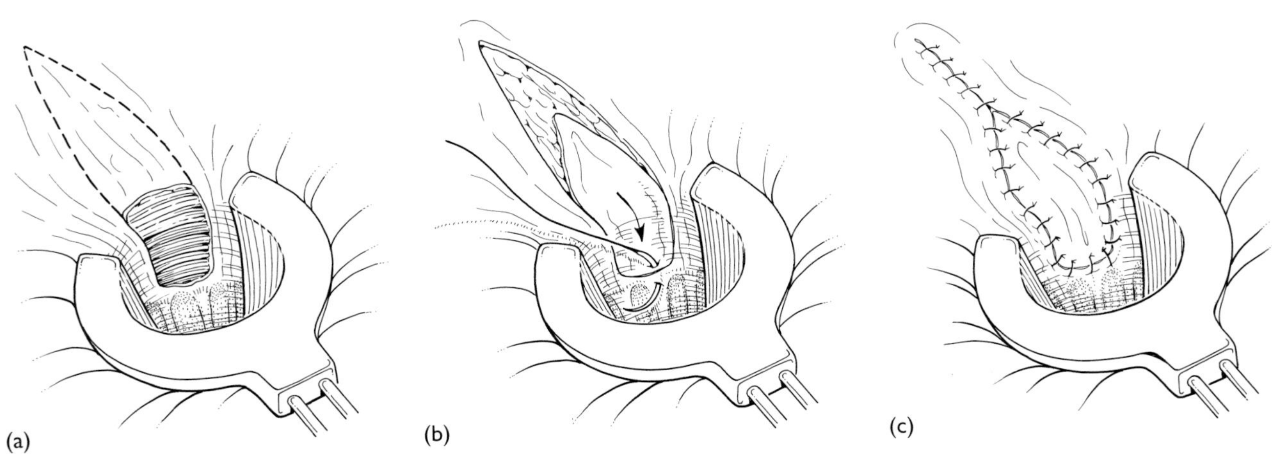

Figure 12.45a–c (a) V–Y or island flap anoplasty. (b) The skin flap is mobilized and advanced. (c) Primary closure is completed.

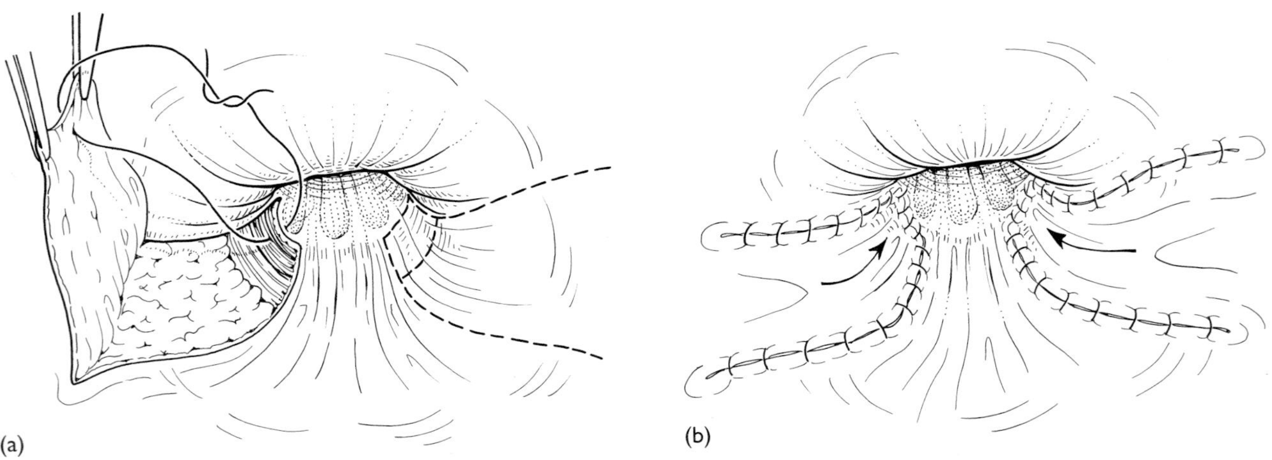

Figure 12.46a,b Bilateral advancement flaps used for moderate stenosis.

Postoperative management

The patient is kept in hospital for 3–5 days and intravenous antibiotics are continued. The bowels are confined by a combination of codeine and loperamide for the period of hospital stay. Bulk agents and gentle laxatives are then given to promote evacuation.

Anoplasty for severe stenosis

If more than 50% of the anal orifice is stenosed, it is necessary to perform a rotation flap. This is the usual situation if a Whitehead haemorrhoidectomy has been performed. It is also a useful procedure to perform if a mucosal ectropion accompanies the stenosis. Rotation flaps are superior to advancement flaps for covering large skin defects as viability and tension on the suture lines are less likely to be problems. Apart from severe stenosis after haemorrhoidectomy, a rotation flap is useful in dealing with a 'keyhole' deformity that may result after excision of an anal fissure or fistula (Figure 12.47).

Technique

The patient is placed in the supine or the jack-knife position. In most instances a single rotation flap will be sufficient. If, for instance, the technique is used for a 'keyhole' deformity, the latter is first excised. The proposed skin incision for the flap is then marked on the perianal skin as depicted in Figure 12.47a. The flap is then elevated by sharp dissection, rotated to cover the defect, and sutured into place with long-term absorbable sutures (Figure 12.47b,c).

For a circumferential anal stenosis as may occur after a Whitehead operation, a bilateral rotation flap (S-plasty) is required (Ferguson, 1959) (Figure 12.48). This procedure commences by incision of the anal canal posteriorly. The lower portion of the internal sphincter may or may not be divided. The anal canal is further incised upwards to allow the insertion of an appropriate retractor. All scar tissue and associated ectropion are excised down to the sphincter musculature, then cephalad to the dentate line. A full-thickness flap is then elevated. The incision for this is commenced in the midline

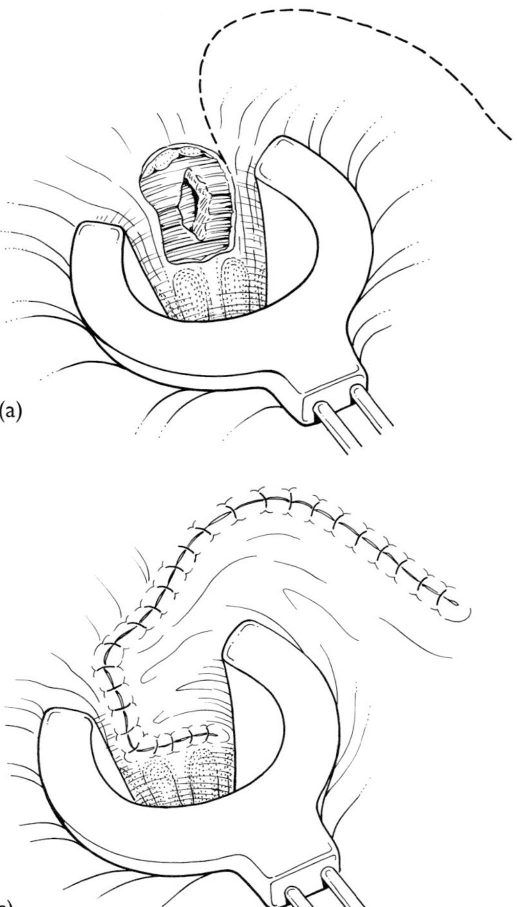

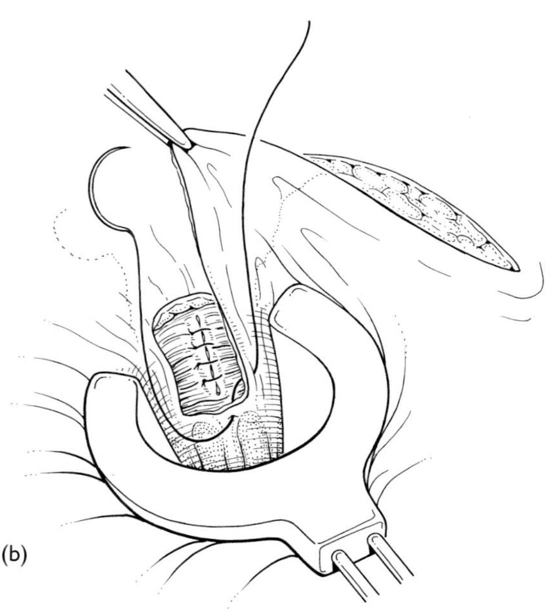

Figure 12.47a–c Rotation flap anoplasty when used for keyhole deformity. (a) The scar is excised. The dotted line indicates the incision to be used for the creation of the flap. (b) The skin flap is mobilized and rotated medially. (c) The wound is closed primarily.

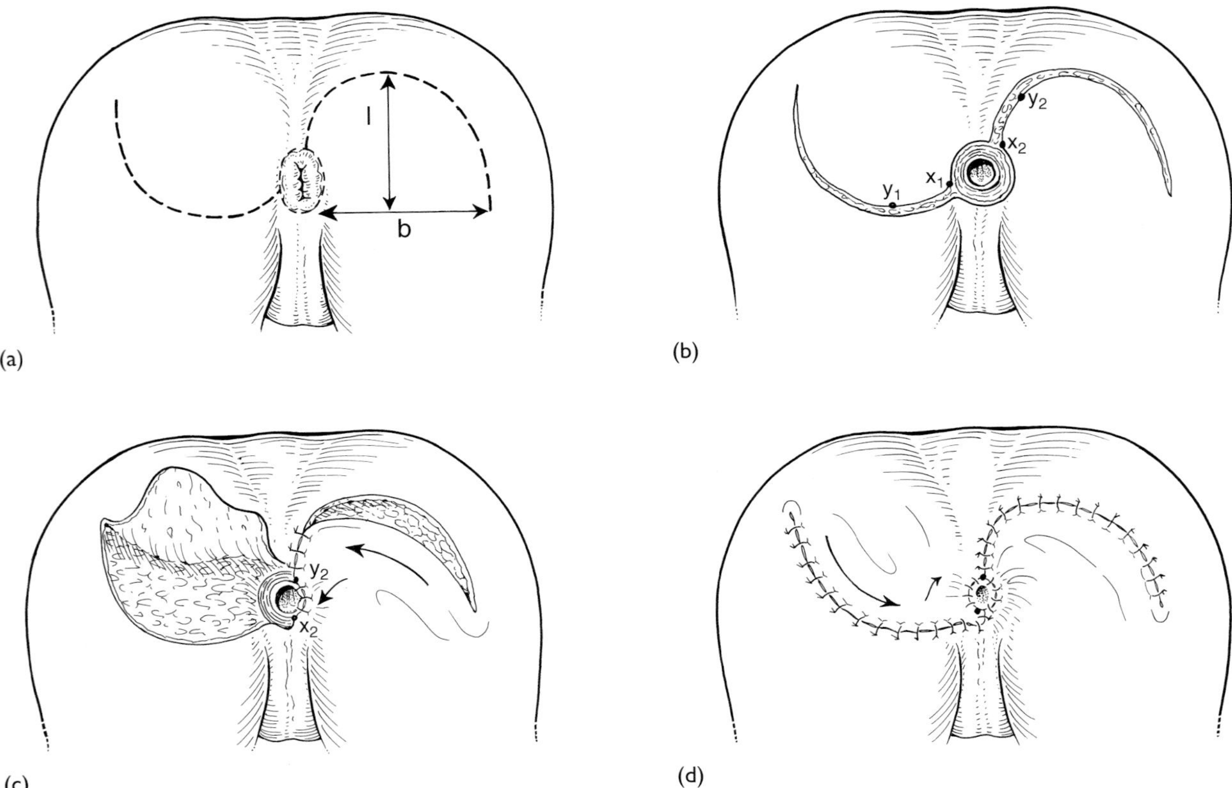

Figure 12.48a–d S-anoplasty for severe anal stenosis. (a) Excision of all scar tissue is performed and the incision lines for the skin flaps are as shown. The length (l) of the flap should be greater than the base (b). The flaps are rotated and sutured to the rectal mucosa and underlying internal sphincter.

posteriorly and carried laterally in a curvilinear fashion for 8–10 cm. A longer length can be obtained by incising further laterally and eventually medially. The flap needs to be thick with sufficient underlying subcutaneous tissue to ensure its viability. A similar incision is then performed on the opposite side and a second flap is raised in an identical fashion. Haemostasis is obtained by careful diathermy and the skin flaps are then rotated into position and sutured to the rectal mucosa and underlying internal sphincter using interrupted sutures. The wounds created by rotation of the flaps are also closed with running sutures. However, if there is tension the peripheral part of the wounds may be left open laterally.

Postoperative management

The bowels are confined as before and antibiotics continued for 5 days. The patient is encouraged not to lie or sit on the flaps in the first few postoperative days. If a haematoma or abscess forms below the flap, this can be released by insertion of a haemostat between the sutures to achieve evacuation of the collection.

Unfortunately, severe stenosis often signifies that the underlying sphincter mechanism has been damaged. The degree to which this has occurred dictates the degree of incontinence that might result after anoplasty. Invariably, even if the sphincter has been only minimally affected, patients will complain of leakage of flatus, mucus and sometimes faeces following the procedure. This may well improve with time. However, if the sphincter was severely deficient beforehand, the operation will not correct incontinence, and indeed may exacerbate it. Preoperative anorectal physiology studies may help to determine the likelihood of such an outcome and may be useful for selection, but they are not infallible. Thus, all patients undergoing such procedures must be warned of the risks of incontinence.

Results

There are few detailed studies of the various anoplasty techniques in the literature. Those that are reported generally extol their virtue. Thus, Sarner (1969) reported 21 patients who underwent one to four advancement flaps for anal stenosis and found that 'adequate relief was achieved in all cases'. Others were equally impressed (Malgieri, 1961; Rand, 1969; Gingold and Arvantis, 1986; Milsom and Mazier, 1986; Rosen, 1988). Similarly, Ferguson (1959) and Ott and Zinberg (1982) had equally gratifying results with rotation flaps. Pearl et al (1990) treated 20 patients by means of a U- or diamond-shaped island flap anoplasty. There were two failures, neither of which were attributable to lack of viability of the flaps.

In our own hands we have found that both advancement flaps and rotation flaps can often deal with the stenosis, but the result may be marred by incontinence. It is the underlying sphincter defect which in our view governs the final outcome and selection of patients is critical. If incontinence exists beforehand, or if physiology and imaging suggests a severely deficient sphincter, a sphincter repair or neosphincter procedure may need to be planned as part of the operation.

COMPARISON OF FORMS OF TREATMENT

There are several ways to treat haemorrhoids and different techniques have their proponents. It is difficult, on reading the literature, to reach a conclusion concerning the best method of therapy for a particular group of patients. In recent years there have been attempts to compare methods of therapy for haemorrhoids using controlled clinical trials, and such studies are to be commended. However, their results are often somewhat confusing. This is usually because follow-up has been too short and the severity of the haemorrhoid or the principal symptom of complaint has not been analysed.

Rubber-band ligation compared with injection therapy

Cheng et al (1981) recorded excellent results in 29 of 30 patients treated by rubber-band ligation, but only 23 of 30 patients benefited after injection therapy. By contrast, Greca et al (1981) reported excellent or satisfactory results in only 18 of 28 patients 1 year after banding, compared with 23 of 33 patients treated by injections. Dercker et al (1973) also compared rubber-band ligation with injection therapy, and found that banding was superior, but both were inferior to haemorrhoidectomy.

Rubber-band ligation compared with cryotherapy

Banding has also been compared with cryosurgery (Keighley et al, 1979; Lewis et al, 1983). Lewis' report found no real difference between the techniques when treating third-degree haemorrhoids. We, on the other hand, found rubber-band ligation to be superior to cryotherapy.

Rubber-band ligation compared with photocoagulation

Weinstein et al (1987) compared rubber-band ligation with photocoagulation and found no significant difference between them, as did Templeton et al (1983). In our study, rubber-band ligation gave rather better long-term results (Ambrose et al, 1983).

Photocoagulation compared with injection therapy

Ambrose et al (1983) found no difference between photocoagulation compared with sclerotherapy in first- and second-degree haemorrhoids. However, Walker et al (1990) found that photocoagulation was superior to both sclerotherapy and banding in patients with non-prolapsing haemorrhoids. Although no significant difference between these three methods was found in patients with prolapsing haemorrhoids, patients treated with photocoagulation tended to have a recurrence more often than those treated by banding or injection.

Rubber-band ligation compared with anal dilatation

Various studies (Hood and Alexander-Williams, 1971; Cheng et al, 1981) have demonstrated that rubber-band ligation is as effective as manual dilatation in controlling symptoms, with the added advantages that rubber-band ligation spares the patient an anaesthetic and eliminates the risk of incontinence.

Rubber-band ligation compared with haemorrhoidectomy

Haemorrhoidectomy has also been compared with conservative therapies. Thus, both Cheng et al (1981) and Murie et al (1980) found that rubber-band ligation was as successful as haemorrhoidectomy. However, Murie et al (1980) found that haemorrhoidectomy was more successful in dealing with haemorrhoids which required digital replacement than was rubber-band ligation. Jones and Schofield (1974) also found no difference between rubber-band ligation and haemorrhoidectomy.

Cryotherapy compared with haemorrhoidectomy

Smith et al (1979) found that haemorrhoidectomy was twice as acceptable to patients as cryosurgery. On the other hand, a retrospective study performed by O'Callaghan et al (1982) suggested that cryosurgery was just as effective as haemorrhoidectomy, and both techniques were equally acceptable to patients. They even suggested that cryosurgery produced fewer complications than haemorrhoidectomy. So much for non-randomized comparisons! Our clinical experience indicates to us that the morbidity of an open haemorrhoidectomy is significantly less than that of cryotherapy.

Meta-analysis studies

MacRae and McLeod (1997) analysed 18 prospective trials of haemorrhoidal treatment. Haemorrhoidectomy was found to be significantly more effective than manual dilatation, and associated with less need for further therapy. There was no significant difference in complications, but more pain was associated with haemorrhoidectomy. Patients who underwent haemorrhoidectomy had a better response to treatment than did patients who were treated with rubber-band ligation, although complications were greater, as was pain. Rubber-band ligation was better than sclerotherapy in response to treatment for all grades of haemorrhoids, with no difference in complication rates. Patients treated with sclerotherapy or infrared coagulation were more likely to require further therapy than those with rubber-band ligation, although pain was greater after rubber-band ligation. The authors concluded that rubber-band ligation should be recommended as the initial mode of therapy for first-, second- and third-degree haemorrhoids. Although haemorrhoidectomy showed better response rates, it was associated with more complications, and they advised that it should be used only when rubber-band ligation fails.

Conclusions and authors' viewpoint

It is often difficult for the individual surgeon to determine the optimum treatment regimen for haemorrhoids because much of the information is contradictory and lacks objectivity. The problem is further compounded by the pressure on the medical profession to avoid inpatient therapy, and therefore anything other than day-care surgery. The regimen we follow is based on available trial data of our own and on clinical experience with meticulous follow-up in a rectal clinic. Nevertheless, we are constantly looking for new approaches, but we believe that these should not be incorporated into the regimen until they have been thoroughly evaluated. Treatment depends not only on the symptoms and extent of the prolapse but also on the patient to be treated. Thus, haemorrhoidectomy in a 130 kg male patient with large gluteal folds is a daunting prospect, and such a patient, even if he suffers from prolapsing piles, may best be served by some form of conservative therapy.

All our patients are advised to avoid straining during defecation and to take a high-fibre diet, if necessary supplementing it with a bulk laxative such as Fibogel. For those patients with first-degree or early second-degree haemorrhoids who present principally with bleeding, we use sclerotherapy at the Royal London and suction band ligation in Birmingham. If the symptoms recur, another injection or application with the band ligator is used. If prolapse is the main symptom, and the patient has second-degree or third-degree haemorrhoids or if bleeding recurs after injections or photocoagulation, we use rubber-band ligation. Although we are concerned about reports of fatal pelvic cellulitis, this has not yet occurred in our practice. We believe that patients should be warned about prolonged discomfort, bleeding or fever, and should understand that they can be reviewed within the same week if they become symptomatic. This serious complication should not arise if such a protocol is followed. In our view, cryosurgery has failed to find a place in the outpatient treatment of haemorrhoids; the continued mucous discharge and swelling makes it an unattractive form of therapy.

Although we accept that manual dilatation may cure symptoms in certain patients who might otherwise require an operation, the risks of incontinence after an uncontrolled stretch make this option unacceptable and we no longer perform the procedure. We perform haemorrhoidectomy only when conservative measures have failed.

The choice of either closed or open haemorrhoidectomy is likely to remain controversial until a satisfactory randomized controlled comparison has been performed. As far as the comparison between submucosal haemorrhoidectomy and the open operation is concerned, both have been shown objectively to produce similar results. However, since we have found the closed technique more anatomically and aesthetically acceptable, we have usually uniformly adopted this North American approach.

MANAGEMENT OF PROLAPSED THROMBOSED INTERNAL HAEMORRHOIDS

Prolapsed thrombosed haemorrhoids cause intense anal pain. They are an ugly sight, there is usually one irreducible purplish haemorrhoid which has prolapsed and is associated with an oedematous skin tag. Medical therapy of this extremely painful condition consists of adequate analgesia until spontaneous resolution occurs; the disease itself enforces rest. Time-dishonoured measures such as the topical application of crushed ice or high elevation of the foot of the bed (Gabriel, 1948; Aird, 1957) may produce minimal symptomatic improvement.

The inadequacy of conservative therapy is well-illustrated by a study performed by Grace and Creed (1975). Of 117 patients with prolapsed thrombosed piles treated with ice-packs and elevation of the foot of the bed, 92 were successfully followed up: 80 (87%) continued to have symptoms, 58 of prolapse, 51 of bleeding and 39 of both these symptoms. While we have so much better surgical therapy to offer, there seems little point in employing these unsuccessful conservative measures. Similarly, we condemn the use of anti-inflammatory drugs.

Active measures are indicated if the complication is referred for appropriate proctological consultation before the fifth post-thrombosis day, when natural resolution has begun to occur.

The choice is between digital dilatation of the anus or emergency haemorrhoidectomy. Either can be performed under local or general anaesthesia. The former can be either by local tissue infiltration or by caudal epidural anaesthesia.

Digital dilatation of the anus is simple to perform with little inconvenience to the patient. If it works, the patient is symptom-free at once and fit to leave hospital on the next day. The disadvantages of the method are that it may not be effective (in our experience in about 45% of patients), that large cushions may remain prolapsed or, worst of all, that forcible dilatation may induce incontinence. As discussed elsewhere, the risk of incontinence is reported to be about 10%, but is devastating for those few in whom it occurs.

Fifty-five patients suffering from acute thrombosed internal haemorrhoids were treated by anal dilatation; the first 41 patients had a short general anaesthetic, while the last 14 had their operation under caudal anaesthesia (Lord, 1972). It was claimed that all except one patient were quickly and completely relieved of their pain. By 3 months after treatment proctoscopy showed a normal or near-normal anal canal. Only one patient had persistent prolapse requiring treatment by rubber-band ligation. Only one patient developed transient incontinence of flatus. There were no other complications and this author concluded that anal dilatation was the optimum treatment for acute thrombosed internal haemorrhoids.

The reported disadvantages of, or objections to, emergency operative excision are that: (1) the operative field is prone to infection with the outside possibility of portal pyaemia; (2) because of the gross oedema, more tissue will be excised than is necessary, resulting in stenosis; (3) less tissue will be excised than is necessary, and so residual tags or recurrent piles result; and (4) it was not necessary to excise the cushions in the first place, simple dilatation would have sufficed. While the last objection may be valid, particularly in patients who have never suffered from prolapse before, the other three objections are invalid, providing reasonable care is taken during the operation, the operator is sufficiently experienced and prophylactic antibiotics are employed. Indeed, it is our experience, shared with many others, that emergency haemorrhoidectomy for thrombosis gives maximal relief to the patient and maximal satisfaction to the surgeon. The oedematous tissues make dissection simple and the patient is so pleased to be relieved of the agony of the acute phase of the thrombosis that the minor postoperative discomfort of the excision is tolerated with equanimity.

The technique of operation is similar to that described previously in detail under elective open haemorrhoidectomy, but with certain important additional manoeuvres. Whether or not general anaesthesia is used, it is advisable to infiltrate the perianal and submucosal areas with a long-acting local anaesthetic with adrenaline. In the young patient with an active anal sphincter, the anus is stretched slowly and gently with four fingers to disperse the oedema and allow the cushions to return within the anal canal. If 5 minutes is taken over this manoeuvre, it is surprising how much the swelling will subside, particularly if the patient is in the prone jack-knife position. The perianal skin quickly contracts and the operative field resembles that during an elective haemorrhoidectomy, except that the oedema has produced separation of tissue planes and dissection is easier. It is not necessary to sacrifice more than the minimum of anoderm, but a generous excision of skin can be made, particularly when there are large skin tags.

The results of emergency haemorrhoidectomy for thrombosed piles are good. Mazier (1973), who favours the closed technique, operated on 400 patients with prolapse and thrombosis. Complications were said to be virtually no more frequent than after the same operation performed electively. Others have also found the operative approach to be equally effective (Smith, 1967; Hansen and Jorgensen, 1975). Eu et al (1994) from Singapore recently compared 204 patients with acutely prolapsed thrombosed haemorrhoids treated by emergency haemorrhoidectomy with 500 patients treated by elective haemorrhoidectomy. They found no differences between the two groups with regard to postoperative morbidity and long-term results. However, it is important to realize the dangers of resecting too much anoderm; the 8% of anal strictures in Tinckler and Baratham's (1964) series is testament to this. If the operator is concerned about excising too much tissue, it is quite reasonable to excise only the most prominent haemorrhoid at the emergency operation. Heald and Gudgeon (1986) have shown that such a limited procedure dramatically improves symptoms and the patient may not even require further elective surgery. Indeed, these authors treated 20 patients in this way and after 2 years none of them had a major recurrence of symptoms, and only five required injection therapy during follow-up.

Over the last 10 years in Birmingham, 42 patients have been treated: 17 by maximal anal dilatation and 25 by emergency haemorrhoidectomy. Although the dilatation achieved immediate pain relief, the prolapsed haemorrhoids continued to discharge and nine subsequently needed a haemorrhoidectomy. The findings at the Royal London have been similar. Emergency haemorrhoidectomy for acute thrombosed internal haemorrhoids is a remarkably easy, low-morbidity procedure. Most patients are discharged home 3 days after admission, which is comparable to the convalescence needed after anal stretch. Since such a high proportion of these patients require haemorrhoidectomy anyway, our philosophy is to proceed with definitive therapy at the time of the emergency while avoiding the risks of iatrogenic incontinence.

MANAGEMENT OF HAEMORRHOIDS IN SPECIAL CIRCUMSTANCES

Pregnancy

Haemorrhoidal disease can develop for the first time during pregnancy or become exacerbated by the presence of the gravid uterus. There is often increased constipation, and increased venous compression in the pelvis. Conservative measures should be used if at all possible as symptoms usually rapidly resolve postpartum. Thus, patients should be advised about diet and be prescribed laxatives and topical agents. However, if prolapse and thrombosis occur, there is no clear-cut answer as to whether surgery should be employed. It is our view that the decision has to be based on the symptoms of each individual patient. If intervention is required, we would favour a surgical approach as opposed to an anal stretch. The reason for this is the increased risk of incontinence in a patient whose sphincter is already under jeopardy from the pregnancy and subsequent birth trauma.

A haemorrhoidectomy can be performed using intravenous sedation and local anaesthesia provided the pregnancy is otherwise uncomplicated. It is advised by some that the left decubitus position is used in the second and third trimesters (Milsom, 1992). Saleeby et al (1991) performed a haemorrhoidectomy on 25 pregnant women, all but 3 in the third trimester. The closed technique was performed under local anaesthetic. All patients experienced relief of their symptoms within 24 hours of the operation. There was only one instance of postoperative haemorrhage, and there were no other maternal or fetal complications.

If the prolapse and thrombosis occur during delivery, there are some who would recommend haemorrhoidectomy immediately postpartum, and good results have been reported (Schottler et al, 1973). Although we have little experience of haemorrhoidectomy in such circumstances, we would generally advise a conservative approach since the perineum is usually very oedematous postpartum, making an operative manoeuvre difficult and risking incontinence.

Inflammatory bowel disease

Exacerbation of haemorrhoidal disease is not uncommon in patients with inflammatory bowel disease. Jeffery et al (1977) conducted a retrospective study on 42 patients with ulcerative colitis and 20 with Crohn's disease who were treated for haemorrhoids between 1935 and 1975 by both surgical and conservative measures. The complication rate in Crohn's disease was higher (11 complications after 26 courses of treatment) compared with that in ulcerative colitis (four complications after 58 courses of treatment). One patient in 42 with ulcerative colitis and 6 out of the 20 with Crohn's disease required rectal excision for complications apparently related to haemorrhoidectomy.

One might conclude that treatment of haemorrhoids is relatively safe for patients with ulcerative colitis, but hazardous for those with Crohn's disease. We would agree with this general philosophy; however, we err on the side of conservatism in both diseases. Although we are more willing to perform a haemorrhoidectomy in patients with ulcerative colitis, we prefer to do this when rectal inflammation is in remission, and when it is unlikely that a pouch procedure will be considered in the future.

Immunocompromised states

Drug therapy

Patients who are receiving immunosuppressive therapy such as steroids, chemotherapeutic agents or antirejection drugs, and who develop haemorrhoidal disease, should be treated as conservatively as possible. If surgery becomes necessary, appropriate precautions should be taken to prevent sepsis and necrosis of wounds. Thus, a complete bowel preparation should be used and antibiotic prophylaxis should be continued for 5 days.

Leukaemia or lymphoma

Patients with these diseases may present with anorectal symptoms and be labelled as having haemorrhoids. It is essential that the patient be examined carefully, if necessary, under general anaesthesia, to establish the diagnosis. Some of these patients may have lesions, which, although resembling haemorrhoids, are in fact lymphomatous or leukaemic infiltrations. In such circumstances, only a biopsy should be contemplated (Vanheuverzwyn et al, 1980; Barnes et al, 1984).

If haemorrhoids are diagnosed they should be treated conservatively. Surgery should be performed only when the haematological disorder is quiescent, and then only using small excisions for prolapsed haemorrhoids and the same prophylactic measures as discussed above.

Patients who are HIV-positive

This subject is covered extensively in Chapter 68.

MANAGEMENT OF THROMBOSED EXTERNAL VASCULAR CHANNELS (OR EXTERNAL PLEXUS HAEMATOMA)

A thrombosed external vascular channel consists of a localized pea-sized subcutaneous swelling which is hard and tender. There is no internal component and minimal perianal swelling. Expectant treatment is usually relied upon as the patient often presents several days after the thrombosis has occurred and the natural history of the condition is one of complete resolution over 5–7 days. It is an advantage if the patient can be put to bed for several days, although in practice this is often difficult. Frequent hot baths are useful, but analgesia is important and should be provided freely. A mild laxative should also be prescribed. Within a few days the pain will usually subside and the patient may return to non-strenuous work. Sometimes the pain does not subside, or the patient has so much discomfort on presentation that conservative treatment is not acceptable. In such circumstances an operation may be required, although we have found that this is rarely necessary.

Operation consists of evacuation of the clot, which can be performed under a short general anaesthetic or under local anaesthesia. A short radial incision is made over the swelling, and the underlying clot is evacuated by squeezing it out between finger and thumb. The wound is left open, and the patient encouraged to take regular warm baths over the following few days.

HYPERTROPHIED ANAL PAPILLOMA OR FIBROSED ANAL POLYP

Anal papillae are fine-pointed projections at the extreme upper end of the anal canal skin at the mucocutaneous junction. They are seen in 50–60% of patients examined (Goligher, 1984). They are usually small and asymptomatic. Occasionally they may hypertrophy, becoming elongated and

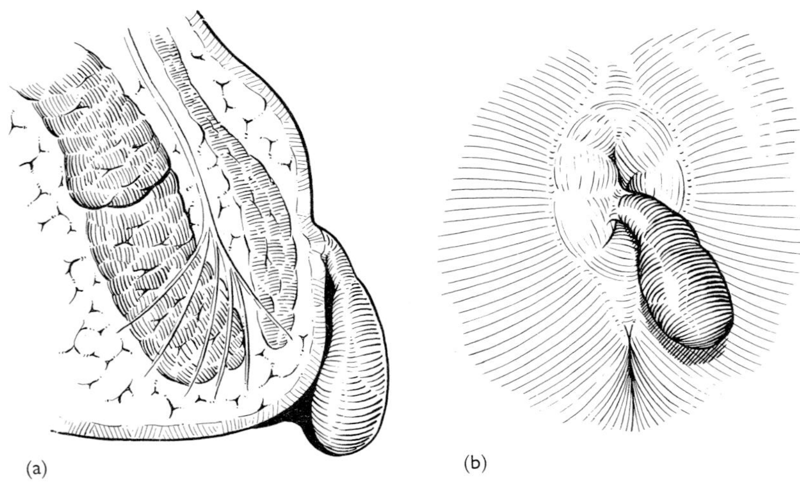

Figure 12.49a,b Fibrosed external anal polyp.

fibrosed. In such circumstances they often acquire a rounded expanded tip and look more polypoidal (Figure 12.49). They may remain asymptomatic or, more often, prolapse on defecation, causing the patient to think that he or she has haemorrhoids. Sometimes they may bleed and occasionally we have seen them prolapse and become strangulated.

The diagnosis of a fibrosed anal polyp can usually be made, on digital examination and on proctoscopy, from its position and appearance. The head usually has a whitish, smooth appearance, resembling anal skin. Occasionally, an oedematous rectal polyp may mimic a fibrous anal polyp and if there is any doubt it should be removed for histological examination. Apart from this situation, the lesion needs to be removed only if it is causing symptoms. This can be done easily through a bivalve speculum after first transfixing and ligating the base.

REFERENCES

Acheson RM (1960) Haemorrhoids in the adult male: a small epidemiological study. *Guys Hosp Rep* **109**: 184–195.

Adami B, Eckardt VF, Suermann RB, Karbach U & Ewe K (1981) Bacteremia after proctoscopy and hemorrhoid injection sclerotherapy. *Dis Colon Rectum* **24**: 273–276.

Aird I (1957) *A Comparison in Surgical Studies*, 2nd edn. Edinburgh: Livingstone.

Akande B & Esho JO (1989) Relationship between haemorrhoids and prostatism: results of a prospective study. *Eur Urol* **16**: 333–334.

Allingham W & Allingham HW (1901) *The Diagnosis and Treatment of Diseases of the Rectum*, 7th edn. London: Baillière.

Ambrose NS, Morris D, Alexander-Williams J & Keighley MRB (1983) A randomised trial of photocoagulation or injection sclerotherapy for the treatment of first- and second-degree haemorrhoids. *Dis Colon Rectum* **28**: 238–240.

Anderson HG (1909) The after results of the operative treatment of haemorrhoids. *BMJ* **2**: 1276.

Anderson HG & Dukes C (1924) The treatment of haemorrhoids by submucous injection of chemicals. *BMJ* **2**: 100.

Andrews BT, Layer GT, Jackson BT & Nicholls RJ (1993) Randomized trial comparing diathermy hemorrhoidectomy with the scissor dissection Milligan–Morgan operation. *Dis Colon Rectum* **36**: 580–583.

Andrews E (1879) The treatment of haemorrhoids by injection. *Med Rec* **15**: 451.

Anscombe AR, Hancock BD & Humphreys WV (1974) A clinical trial of the treatment of haemorrhoids by operation and the Lord procedure. *Lancet* **ii**: 250.

Arabi Y, Alexander-Williams J & Keighley MRB (1977a) Anal pressures in haemorrhoids and anal fissure. *Am J Surg* **134**: 608.

Arabi Y, Gatehouse D, Alexander-Williams J & Keighley MR (1977b) Rubber-band ligation or lateral subcutaneous sphincterotomy for treatment of haemorrhoids. *Br J Surg* **64**: 737–740.

Asfar SK, Juma TA & Ala-Edeen T (1988) Haemorrhoidectomy and sphincterotomy: a prospective study comparing the effectiveness of anal stretch and sphincterotomy in relieving pain after haemorrhoidectomy. *Dis Colon Rectum* **31**: 181–185.

Bacon HE (1949) *The Anus, Rectum and Sigmoid Colon*, 3rd edn. Philadelphia: Lippincott.

Bailey HIR & Ferguson JA (1976) Prevention of urinary retention by fluid restriction following anorectal operations. *Dis Colon Rectum* **19**: 250–255.

Barnes SG, Sattler FR & Ballard JO (1984) Perirectal infections in acute leukemia. *Ann Intern Med* **100**: 515–518.

Barrios G & Khubchandani M (1979) Whitehead operation revisited. *Dis Colon Rectum* **22**: 330–333.

Barron J (1963) Office ligation of internal haemorrhoids. *Am J Surg* **195**: 563.

Bartizal J & Slosberger PA (1977) An alternative to haemorrhoidectomy. *Arch Surg* **112**: 534.

Bat L, Melzer E, Koler M, Dreznick Z & Shemesh E (1993)

Complications of rubber-band ligation of symptomatic internal haemorrhoids. *Dis Colon Rectum* **36**: 287–290.

Bates T (1972) Rectal prolapse after anorectal dilatation in the elderly. *BMJ* **2**: 505.

Bennett RC, Friedman MHW & Goligher JC(1963) The late results of haemorrhoidectomy by ligature and excision. *BMJ* **2**: 216.

Berry AR & D'Costa EFD (1978) The treatment of haemorrhoids by cryosurgery. *J R Coll Surg Edinb* **23**: 37–39.

Blanchard CE (1928) *Textbook of Ambulant Proctology*, p. 134. Youngstown, OH: Medical Success Press.

Bleday R, Pena JP, Rothenberger DA, Goldberg SM & Buls JG (1992) Symptomatic haemorrhoids: current incidence and complications of operative therapy. *Dis Colon Rectum* **35**: 477–481.

Bodenheimer W (1868) *Practical Observations on the Aetiology, Pathology, Diagnosis and Treatment of Anal Fissure*, New York: W Wood.

Broader JH, Gunn IF & Alexander-Williams J (1974) Evaluation of a bulk forming evacuant in the management of haemorrhoids. *Br J Surg* **61**: 142.

Brondel H & Gondran M (1976) Facteurs prèdisposants lies à l'hérédité et à la profession dans la maladie hemorrhoidaire. *Arch Franc Malad l'Appar Dig* **65**: 541–550.

Buie LA (1937) *Practical Proctology*, 2nd edn. Springfield, IL: CC Thomas.

Bullock N (1997) Impotence after sclerotherapy of haemorrhoids. *BMJ* **314**: 419.

Buls JG & Goldberg SM (1978) Modern management of haemorrhoids. *Surg Clin North Am* **58**: 469–478.

Burchell MC, Thow GB & Manson RR (1967) A modified Whitehead haemorrhoidectomy. *Dis Colon Rectum* **19**: 225.

Burkitt D (1972) Varicose veins, deep vein thrombosis and haemorrhoids: epidemiology and suggested aetiology. *BMJ* **2**: 556.

Carden ABG (1970) Dilatation treatment of haemorrhoids. *Med J Aust* **1**: 437.

Cataldo PA & Sengapore AJ (1991) Does alpha sympathetic blockade prevent urinary retention following anorectal surgery? *Dis Colon Rectum* **34**: 1113.

Champigneulle B, Dieterling P, Bigard MA & Gaucher P (1989) Etude prospective de la fonction sphincterienne anale avant et après hemorrhoidectomie. *Gastroenterol Clin Biol* **13**: 452–456.

Chant ADB, May A & Wilken BJ (1972) Haemorrhoidectomy versus manual dilatation of the anus. *Lancet* **ii**: 398.

Cheng FCY, Shum DWP & Ong GB (1981) The treatment of second-degree haemorrhoids by injection, rubber-band ligation, maximal anal dilatation and haemorrhoidectomy: a prospective clinical trial. *Aust J Surg* **51**: 458.

Chia YW, Darzi A, Speakman CTM et al (1995) CO_2 laser haemorrhoidectomy: does it alter anorectal function or decrease pain compared to conventional haemorrhoidectomy. *Int J Colorect Dis* **10**: 22–24.

Clark CG, Giles G & Goligher JC (1967) Results of conservative treatment of internal haemorrhoids. *BMJ* **2**: 12.

Cleave TL (1965) A new conception on the causation, prevention and arrest of varicose veins, varicocele and hemorrhoids. *Am J Proctol* **16**: 35–42.

Cooper S (1809) *A Dictionary of Practical Surgery*. London: Longman.

Corman ML (1984) *Hemorrhoids in Colon and Rectal Surgery*. Phildelphia: Lippincott.

Corman ML (1993) *Hemorrhoids in Colon and Rectal Surgery*, 3rd edn, p 60. Philadelphia: Lippincott.

Cormie J & McNair RJ (1959) The results of haemorrhoidectomy. *Scot Med J* **4**: 571.

Creve U & Hubens A (1979) The effect of Lord's procedure on anal pressure. *Dis Colon Rectum* **22**: 483–485.

Cusack JW (1846) *Dublin Q J Med Sci* **2**: 562.

Dennison A, Whiston BM, Rooney S et al (1990) A randomised comparison of infrared photocoagulation with bipolar diathermy for the outpatient treatment of haemorrhoids. *Dis Colon Rectum* **33**: 32–35.

Dercker H, Hjorth M, Norryd L & Tranberg KG (1973) Comparison of results obtained with different methods of treatment of internal haemorrhoids. *Acta Chir Scand* **139**: 742.

Deutsch AA, Moshkovitz M, Nudelman I, Dinari G & Reiss R (1987) Anal pressure measurements in the study of haemorrhoid aetiology and their relation to treatment. *Dis Colon Rectum* **30**: 855–857.

Dodi G (1992) Multiple rubber band ligation after one loading of instrument. *Int J Colorectal Dis* **7**: 112.

Earl ST (1911) *Diseases of the Anus, Rectum and Sigmoid*. Philadelphia: Lippincott.

Edwards FS (1888) The treatment of piles by injection. *BMJ* **2**: 815.

Eisenhammer S (1951) The surgical correction of internal anal (sphincteric) contracture. *S Afr Med J* **25**: 486–487.

Eisenhammer S (1953) The internal anal sphincter. *S Afr Med J* **27**: 266.

Eisenhammer S (1969) Proper principles and practices in the sugical management of haemorrhoids. *Dis Colon Rectum* **12**: 288.

Eisenhammer S (1974) Internal anal sphincterotomy plus free dilatation versus anal stretch with special criticism of the anal stretch procedure for haemorrhoids: the recommended modern approach to haemorrhoid treatment. *Dis Colon Rectum* **17**: 493.

Eu KW, Seow Choen F & Goh HS (1994) Comparison of emergency and elective haemorrhoidectomy. *Br J Surg* **81**: 308–310.

Failes D (1966) Primary suture of the operative wounds after haemorrhoidectomy. *Aust J Surg* **36**: 63.

Fansler WA & Anderson JK (1933) A plastic operation for certain types of haemorrhoids. *JAMA* **101**: 1064–1066.

Farag AE (1978) Pile suture: a new technique for the treatment of haemorrhoids. *Br J Surg* **65**: 293–295.

Farouk R, Duthie GS, MacGregor AB & Bartolo DC (1994) Sustained internal sphincter hypertonia in patients with chronic anal fissure. *Dis Colon Rectum* **37**: 424–429.

Ferguson JA (1959) Repair of Whitehead deformity of the anus. *Surg Gynecol Obstet* **108**: 115–116.

Ferguson JA & Heaton JR (1959) Closed hemorrhoidectomy. *Dis Colon Rectum* **2**: 176.

Ferguson JA, Mazier WP, Ganchrow MI & Friend WG (1971) The closed technique of hemorrhoidectomy. *Surgery* **70**: 480–484.

Fraser J & Gill W (1967) Observations on ultrafrozen tissue. *Br J Surg* **54**: 770.

Gabriel WB (1948) *The Principles and Practice of Rectal Surgery*, 4th edn. London: HK Lewis.

Ganchrow MI, Mazier WP, Friend WG & Ferguson JA (1971) Hemorrhoidectomy revisited: a computer analysis of 2038 cases. *Dis Colon Rectum* **14**: 128–133.

Gaskin ER & Childer MD (1963) Increased granuloma formation from absorbable sutures. *JAMA* **185**: 212–214.

Gazet JC, Redding W & Rickett JW (1970) The prevalence of haemorrhoids. A preliminary survey. *Proc R Soc Med* **63** Suppl: 78–80.

Gehamy RA & Weakley FL (1974) Internal hemorrhoidectomy by elastic ligation. *Dis Colon Rectum* **17**: 347–353.

Gingold BS & Arvantis M (1986) Y–V anoplasty for treatment of anal stricure. *Surg Gynecol Obstet* **162**: 241–245.

Goldberg SM, Gordon PH & Nivatvongs S (1980) Hemorrhoids. In *Essentials of Anorectal Surgery*. Philadelphia: Lippincott.

Goldstein ET, Williamson PR & Larach SW (1993) Subcutaneous morphine pump for postoperative hemorrhoidectomy pain management. *Dis Colon Rectum* **36**: 439–446.

Goligher JC (1976) Cryosurgery for hemorrhoids. *Dis Colon Rectum* **19**: 223.

Goligher JC (1984) *Surgery of the Anus, Rectum and Colon*, 5th edn. London: Baillière Tindall.

Goligher JC, Graham NG, Clark CG, De Dombal FT & Giles G (1969) The value of stretching the anal sphincters in the relief of post-haemorrhoidectomy pain. *Br J Surg* **56**: 859.

Gottesman L, Milsom JW & Mazier WP (1989) The use of anxiolytic and parasympathomimetic agents in the treatment of postoperative urinary retention following anorectal surgery: a prospective randomized double-blind study. *Dis Colon Rectum* **32**: 867–870.

Grace RH & Creed A (1975) Prolapsing thrombosed haemorrhoids: outcome of conservative management. *BMJ* **2**: 354.

Graham-Stewart CW (1962) Injection treatment of haemorrhoids. *BMJ* **1**: 213.

Greca F, Hares MM, Nevah E et al (1981) A randomised trial to compare rubber-band ligation with phenol injection for treatment of haemorrhoids. *Br J Surg* **68**: 250.

Griffith CD, Morris DL, Wherry DC & Hardcastle JD (1987) Outpatient treatment of haemorrhoids: a randomised trial comparing contact bipolar diathermy with rubber-band ligation. *Coloproctology* **6**: 322–334.

Hancock BD (1976) Internal sphincter and the nature of haemorrhoids. *Gut* **18**: 651–656.

Hancock BD (1981) Lord's procedure for haemorrhoids: a prospective anal pressure study. *Br J Surg* **68**: 729–730.

Hancock BD & Smith K (1975) The internal anal sphincter and Lord's procedure for haemorrhoids. *Br J Surg* **62**: 833–836.

Hansen JB & Jorgensen SJ (1975) Radical emergency operation for prolapsed and strangulated haemorrhoids. *Acta Chir Scand* **141**: 810–812.

Hardwick RH, Durdey P (1994) Should rubber-band ligation of haemorrhoids be performed at the initial outpatient visit? *Ann R Coll Surg Engl* **76**: 185–187.

Heald RJ & Gudgeon AM (1986) Limited haemorrhoidectomy in the treatment of acute strangulated haemorrhoids. *Br J Surg* **73**: 1002.

Heaton ND, Davenport M & Howard ER (1992) Symptomatic haemorrhoids and anorectal varices in children with portal hypertension. *J Paediatr Surg* **22**: 833–835.

Heaton ND, Davenport M & Howard ER (1993) Incidence of haemorrhoids and anorectal varices in children with portal hypertension. *Br J Surg* **80**: 616–618.

Heslop JH (1987) Piles and rectoceles. *Aust N Z J Surg* **57**: 935–938.

Hilton J (1877) *On Rest and Pain*, 2nd edn. WHA Jacobson, London: Bell.

Hiltunen KM & Matikainen M (1985) Anal manometric findings in symptomatic haemorrhoids. *Dis Colon Rectum* **18**: 807–809.

Hinton CP & Morris DL (1990) A randomized trial comparing direct current therapy and bipolar diathermy in the outpatient treatment of third-degree haemorrhoids. *Dis Colon Rectum* **33**: 931–935.

Ho Y-H, Seow-Choen F, Tan M & Leong AFPK (1997) Randomized controlled trial of open and closed haemorrhoidectomy. *Br J Surg* **84**: 1729–1730.

Hoff SD, Bailey HR, Butts DR et al (1994) Ambulatory surgical hemorrhoidectomy: a solution to postoperative urinary retention? *Dis Colon Rectum* **37**: 1242–1244.

Hood TR & Alexander-Williams J (1971) Anal dilatation versus rubber-band ligation for internal hemorrhoids: methods of treatment in out patients. *Am J Surg* **122**: 545–548.

Hosking SW, Smart HL, Johnson AG et al (1989) Anorectal varices, haemorrhoids and portal hypertension. *Lancet* **i**: 349–352.

Hughes ESR (1957) *Surgery of the Anus, Anal Canal and Rectum*, pp 2, 129. Edinburgh: Livingstone.

Hyams L & Philpot J (1970) An epidemiological investigation of haemorrhoids. *Am J Proct* **21**: 177–193.

Iwagaki H, Higuchi Y, Fuchimoto S & Orita K (1989) The laser treatment of haemorrhoids: results of a study on 1816 patients. *Jpn J Surg* **19**: 658–661.

Jackson CC & Robertson E (1965) Etiologic aspects of haemorrhoidal disease. *Dis Colon Rectum* **8**: 185–189.

Jacobs DM, Rubrick MP, Onstad GR et al (1980) The relationship of hemorrhoids to portal hypertension. *Dis Colon Rectum* **23**: 567.

Jeffery PJ, Ritchie JL & Parks AG (1977) Treatment of haemorrhoids in patients with inflammatory bowel disease. *Lancet* **i**: 1084–1085.

Johanson JF & Sonnenberg A (1990) The prevalence of hemorrhoids and chronic constipation: an epidemiologic study. *Gastroenterology* **98**: 380–386.

Johanson JF & Sonnenberg A (1991) Temporal changes in the occurrence of haemorrhoids in the United States and England. *Dis Colon Rectum* **34**: 585–591.

Jones CB & Schofield PF (1974) A comparative study of the methods of treatment for haemorrhoids. *Proc R Soc Med* **67**: 51–53.

Katchian A (1982) Hemorrhoidal banding (letter). *Dis Colon Rectum* **25**: 392–393.

Katchian A (1985) Rubber-band ligation (letter). *Dis Colon Rectum* **28**: 759.

Kaufman HD (1976) Outpatient treatment of haemorrhoids. *Br J Surg* **63**: 462–463.

Kaufman HD (1978) Haemorroids: an 'outpatient package'. *J R Coll Surg Edinb* **23**: 40–43.

Keighley MRB, Buchmann P, Minervium S, Arabi Y & Alexander-Williams J (1979) Prospective trials of minor surgical procedures and high fibre diet for haemorrhoids. *BMJ* **2**: 967–969.

Khoury GA, Lake SP, Lewis MCA & Lewis AAM (1985) A randomised trial to compare single with multiple phenol injection treatment for haemorrhoids. *Br J Surg* **72**: 741–742.

Khubchandani IT (1983) A randomised comparison of single and multiple rubber-band ligations. *Dis Colon Rectum* **26**: 705–708

Khubchandani IT, Trimpi HD & Sheets JA (1974) Evaluation of polyglycolic acid suture vs catgut in closed hemorrhoidectomy with local anesthesia. *South Med J* **67**: 1504–1506.

Khubchandani M (1984) Results of Whitehead operation. *Dis Colon Rectum* **27**: 730–735.

Kilbourne NJ (1934) Internal haemorrhoids: comparative value of treatment by operative and by injection methods. *Ann Surg* **90**: 600.

Kluiber RM & Wolff BG (1994) Evaluation of anemia caused by hemorrhoidal bleeding. *Dis Colon Rectum* **37**: 1006–1007

Lane RHS & Casula G (1976) Anal pressure before and after haemorrhoidectomy. *Br J Surg* **63**: 158 (abstract).

Lee HH, Spencer RJ & Beart RW Jr (1994) Multiple hemorrhoidal bandings in a single session. *Dis Colon Rectum* **37**: 37–41

Leicester RJ, Nicholls RJ & Mann CV (1981) Infrared coagulation: a new treatment for hemorrhoids. *Dis Colon Rectum* **24**: 602.

Leff EI (1992) Haemorrhoidectomy: laser vs non-laser. Outpatient experience. *Dis Colon Rectum* **35**(8): 743–746.

Lentini J, Leveroni JT & Aure C (1990) Twenty-five years' experience with the high-frequency transistorised loop with special reference to haemorrhoidectomy without suture. *Coloproctology* **4**: 239–249

Lewis AAM, Rogers HS & Leighton M (1983) Trial of maximal anal dilatation and elastic band ligation as alterations to haemorrhoidectomy in the treatment of large prolapsing haemorrhoids. *Br J Surg* **70**: 54–56.

Lewis MI (1973) Diverse methods of managing hemorrhoids: cryohemorrhoidectomy. *Dis Colon Rectum* **16**: 175.

Lewis MI, De La Cruz T, Gazxzaniga D & Ball TI (1969) Cryosurgical hemorrhoidectomy: preliminary report. *Dis Colon Rectum* **12**: 371.

Lin J-K (1989) Anal manometric studies in hemorrhoids and anal fissures. *Dis Colon Rectum* **32**: 839–842.

Lloyd Williams K, Haq IU & Elem B (1973) Cryodestruction of haemorrhoids. *BMJ* **1**: 666.

Lockhart-Mummery JP (1934) *Diseases of the Rectum and Colon*, 2nd edn. London: Baillière.

Lockhart-Mummery JP & Joshi MK (1915) Death from strangulated internal haemorrhoids. *Lancet* **i**: 332.

Loder PB, Kamm MA, Nicholls RJ & Phillips RKS (1994) Haemorrhoids: pathology, pathophysiology and aetiology. *Br J Surg* **81**: 946–954

Lord PH (1968) A new regime for the treatment of haemorrhoids. *Proc R Soc Med* **61**: 935.

Lord PH (1969) A day-case procedure for the cure of third-degree haemorrhoids. *Br J Surg* **56**: 747.

Lord PH (1972) A new approach to haemorrhoids. *Prog Surg* **10**: 109–124.

Lord PH (1977) Approach to the treatment of anorectal disease with special reference to hemorrhoids. In Nyhus LM (ed) *Surgery Annual 1977*, vol 9, p. 195. New York: Appleton-Century Crofts.

Lord PH (1983) Maximal anal dilatation. In Todd IP & Fielding LP (eds) *Rob & Smith's Operative Surgery; Alimentary Tract and Abdominal Wall; Colon, Rectum and Anus*, 4th edn.

McCaffrey J (1975) Lord treatment of haemorrhoids: four-year follow-up of 50 patients. *Lancet* **i**: 133.

McConnell JC & Khubchandani IT (1983) Long-term follow-up of closed haemorrhoidectomy. *Dis Colon Rectum* **26**: 797–799.

McGirney J (1981) Haemorrhoidal banding (letter). *Dis Colon Rectum* **24**: 577.

McMahon WA (1956) Anoplasty: complications and final results. *Am J Surg* **92**: 739.

MacIntyre IMC & Balfour TW (1972) Results of the Lord non-operative treatment for haemorrhoids. *Lancet* **i**: 1094.

MacRae HM & McLeod RS (1997) Comparison of haemorrhoidal treatments: a meta-analysis. *Can J Surg* **40**: 14–17

Maisonneuve JG (1849) Du traitement de la fissure à l'anus par la dilatation forcée. *Gaz Hop* (series 3) **1**: 220.

Maisonneuve JG (1864) Clinique chirurgical. *Paris F Savy* **2**: 200.

Malgieri JA (1961) Anoplasty to correct anal stricture. *Dis Colon Rectum* **4**: 289–293.

Mann CV, Motson R & Clifton M (1988) The immediate response to injection therapy for first-degree haemorrhoids. *J R Soc Med* **81**: 146–148.

Martin CF (1904) The injection treatment of internal hemorrhoids. *Am Med* **8**: 365.

Mazier WP (1973) Emergency hemorrhoidectomy: a worthwhile procedure. *Dis Colon Rectum* **16**: 200.

Miles WE (1919) Observations upon internal piles. *Surg Gynecol Obstet* **29**: 496.

Miles WE (1939) *Rectal Surgery*. London: Cassell.

Miller R, Bartolo DCC, Roe A, Cervero F & Mortensen NJMcC (1988) Anal sensation and the continence mechanism. *Dis Colon Rectum* **31**: 433–438.

Milligan ETC (1939) Haemorrhoids. *BMJ* **2**: 412.

Milligan ETC (1943) The treatment of haemorrhoids in recruits. *Med Press Circular* **210**: 84.

Milligan ETC, Morgan C, Naughton Jones LF & Office RR (1937) Surgical anatomy of the anal canal and the operative treatment of haemorrhoids. *Lancet* **ii**: 1119.

Milsom JW (1992) Haemorrhoidal disease. In Beck DE & Wexner SD (eds) *Fundamentals of Anorectal Surgery*, pp 192–214. New York: McGraw-Hill.

Milsom JW & Mazier WP (1986) Classification and management of post-surgical anal stenosis. *Surg Gynaecol Obstet* **163**: 60–64

Mitchell AB (1903) A simple method of operating on piles. *BMJ* **1**: 482–483.

Moesgaard F, Nielson ML, Hansen JB & Knudson JT (1982) High fibre reduces bleeding and pain in patients with hemorrhoids. *Dis Colon Rectum* **25**: 454–456.

Morgagni JG (1729) *Adv Anat* **6**: 111.

Morgagni D (1749) Seats and causes of disease. Letter 32 Article 10. Translated by Benjamin Alexander 1769 2: 105. London: Millar.

Mortensen PE, Olsen J, Pedersen IK & Christiansen J (1987) A randomised study on hemorrhoidectomy combined with anal dilatation. *Dis Colon Rectum* **30**: 755–757.

Murie JA, Mackenzie I & Sim AJW (1980) Comparison of rubber-band ligation and haemorrhoidectomy for second and third-degree haemorrhoids: a prospective clinical trial. *Br J Surg* **67**: 786.

Nath G, Kreitmaier A, Kiefhaber P et al (1977) Neue Infrarotkoagulationsmethode. Verhandlungsband des 3 Kongresses der Deutscher Gesellschaft fur Gastroenterologie, 1976, Munich. Erlangen: Perimed.

Neiger A (1979) Haemorrhoids in everyday practice. *Proctology* **2**: 22.

Nelson RL (1991) Temporal changes in the occurrence of hemorrhoids in the United States and England. *Dis Colon Rectum* **34**: 591–593.

Nicholson J & Halleran D (1990) Laser haemorrhoidectomy: a prospective randomised trial. Presented at the American Society of Colon and Rectal Surgeons 87th Annual Convention, 12–17 June, Anaheim, California, 1988 (unpublished).

Norman DA, Newton R & Nicholas GU (1989) Direct current electrotherapy of internal haemorrhoids: an effective, safe and painless outpatient approach. *Am J Gastroenterol* **84**: 482–486.

Notarus MJ (1971) The treatment of anal fissure by later subcutaneous internal sphincterotomy: a technique and results. *Br J Surg* **58**: 96–160.

O'Callaghan JD, Matheson TS & Hall R (1982) Inpatient treatment of prolapsing piles: cryosurgery versus Milligan–Morgan haemorrhoidectomy. *Br J Surg* **69**: 157–159.

O'Donovan S, Ferrara A, Larach S, Williamson P (1994) Intraoperative use of Toradol facilitates outpatient hemorrhoidectomy. *Dis Colon Rectum* **37**: 793–799.

O'Hara VS (1980) Fatal clostridial infection following haemorrhoidal banding. *Dis Colon Rectum* **23**: 570–571.

Ortiz H, Marti J, Jaurrieta E et al (1978) Lord's procedure: a critical study of its basic principle. *Br J Surg* **65**: 281–286.

Ott C & Zinberg J (1982) anoplasty for anal stricture. *Dis Colon Rectum* **25**: 809–813

Parks AG (1955) De haemorrhois. *Guy's Hosp Rep* **104**: 135.

Parks AG (1956) The surgical treatment of haemorrhoids. *Br J Surg* **43**: 337–351.

Parks AG (1962) Haemorrhoids. *Practitioner* **189**: 309–316

Pearl RK, Hooks VH, Abcarian H et al (1990) Island flap anoplasty for the treatment of anal stricture and mucosal ectropian. *Dis Colon Rectum* **33**: 581–585.

Petit JI (1774) *Traite des Maladies Chirurgicales et des Opérations qui leur Conviennent*, vol. 2, p. 137. Paris: T-F Didot.

Poon CP, Chu KW, Lau WY et al (1986) Conventional vs triple rubber-band ligation for haemorrhoids and prospective randomised trial. *Dis Colon Rectum* **29**: 836–839.

Pope CE (1959) An anorectal plastic operation for fissure and stenosis and its surgical principles. *Surg Gynaecol Obstet* **108**: 249–253.

Prasad GC, Prakash V, Tandon AK & Deshpande PJ (1976) Studies on etiopathogenesis of haemorrhoids. *Am J Proctol* **27**: 33–41.

Rand AA (1969) The sliding skin-flap operation for haemorrhoids: a modification of the Whitehead procedure. *Dis Colon Rectum* **12**: 265–269.

Recamier JC (1838) Extension massage et percussion cadéncee dans le traitement des contractures musculaires. *Rev Med Fr E Strang* **1**: 74.

Read MG, Read NW, Haynes WG et al (1982) A prospective study of the effect of haemorrhoidectomy on sphincter function and faecal continence. *Br J Surg* **69**: 396.

Read NW, Bartolo DCC, Read MG et al (1983) Differences in anorectal manometry between patients with haemorrhoids and patients with decending perineum syndrome: implications for management. *Br J Surg* **70**: 656–659.

Reis Neto JA, Quilici FA, Cordeiro F & Reis JA Jr (1992) Ambulatory treatment of haemorrhoids: a prospective random trial. *Coloproctology* **6**: 342–347.

Roe AM, Bartolo DCC & Mortensen NJMcC (1986) New method for assessment of anal sensation in various anorectal disorders. *Br J Surg* **73**: 310–312.

Roe AM, Bartolo DCC, Vellacott KD, Lock Edmunds J & Mortensen NJ McC (1987) Submucosal versus ligation excision haemorrhoidectomy: a comparison of anal sensation, and sphincter manometry and postoperative pain and function. *Br J Surg* **74**: 948–951.

Rosen L (1988) Anoplasty. *Surg Clin North Am* **68**: 1441–1444

Ruiz-Moreno F (1977) Hemorrhoidectomy – how I do it: semiclosed technique. *Dis Colon Rectum* **20**: 177–182.

Russell TR & Donohue JH (1985) Hemorrhoidal banding: a warning. *Dis Colon Rectum* **28**: 291–293.

Saleeby RG, Rosen L, Stasik SJ et al (1991) Haemorrhoidectomy during pregnancy: risk or relief. *Dis Colon Rectum* **34**: 260–261

Salmon F (1836) *Practical Essay on Stricture of the Rectum*, 4th edn. London: Whittaker, Treacher & Arnot.

Sames CP (1972) Experiences of Lord's procedure for the treatment of haemorrhoids. *Proc R Soc Med* **65**: 782.

Sandilands DGD, Schofield PF & Sykes PA (1981) Lord's procedure for the treatment of haemorrhoids: a long-term follow up. *J R Coll Surg Edinb* **26**: 298.

Santos G, Novell JR, Khoury G, Winslet MC & Lewis AAM (1993) Long-term results of large-dose, single-session phenol injection sclerotherapy for hemorrhoids. *Dis Colon Rectum* **36**: 958–961.

Sarner JB (1969) Plastic relief of anal stenosis. *Dis Colon Rectum* **12**: 277–280.

Scarpa FJ, Hillis W & Sabetta JR (1988) Pelvic cellulitis: a life-threatening complication of hemorrhoidal banding. *Surgery* **103**: 383–385.

Schofield PF, Cunliffe WJ & Hulton N (1984) Elastic band ligation of haemoroids: a new applicator. *Br J Surg* **71**: 212.

Schottler JL, Balcos EG & Goldberg SM (1973) Postpartum hemorrhoidectomy. *Dis Colon Rectum* **16**: 395–396.

Schouten WR & van Vroonhaven TJ (1986) Lateral internal sphincterotomy in the treatment of haemorrhoids: a clinical and manometric study. *Dis Colon Rectum* **29**: 869–872.

Scoma JA (1976) Haemorrhoidectomy without urinary retention and catheterization. *Conn Med* **40**: 751–753.

Senapati A & Nicholls RJ (1988) A randomised trial to compare the results of injection sclerotherapy with a bulk laxative alone in the treatment of bleeding haemorrhoids. *Int J Colorect Dis* **3**: 124–126.

Sengapore A, Mazier P, Luchtefeld MA, Mackeigan JM & Wengert T (1993) Treatment of advanced haemorrhoidal disease: a prospective randomised comparison of cold scalpel vs contact Nd:Yag laser. *Dis Colon Rectum* **36**: 1042–1049.

Seow-Choen F, Ho Y-H, Ang H-G & Goh H-S (1992) Prospective randomized trial comparing pain and clinical function after conventional scissors excision/ligation vs diathermy excision without ligation for symptomatic prolapsed hemorrhoids. *Dis Colon Rectum* **35**: 1165–1169

Seow-Choen F & Low HC (1995) Prospective randomized study of radical versus four piles haemorrhoidectomy for symptomatic large circumferential prolapsed piles. *Br J Surg* **82**: 188–189.

Shafik A (1984) The pathogenesis of haemorrhoids and their treatment by anorectal handotomy. *J Clin Gastroenterol* **6**: 129–137.

Sharif H, Lee L & Alexander-Williams J (1991) How I do it: diathermy haemorrhoidectomy. *Int J Colorect Dis* **6**: 217–219

Shropshear G (1971) Posterior and anterior anal proctotomy: a simplified technic for postoperative anal stenosis. *Dis Colon Rectum* **14**: 62–65

Sim AJW, Murie JA & Mackenzie I (1981) A comparison of rubber-band ligation and sclerosant injection for first and second degree haemorrhoids. *Acta Chir Scand* **147**: 717–720.

Singh J & Lal P (1975) Submucous haemorrhoidectomy versus low ligation excision. *J Ind Med Assoc* **64**: 111–114.

Smith LE, Goodreau JJ & Fouty WJ (1979) Operative hemorrhoidectomy versus cryodestruction. *Dis Colon Rectum* **22**: 10.

Smith M (1967) Early operation for acute haemorrhoids. *Br J Surg* **54**: 141.

Soderlund S (1962) Results of haemorrhoidectomy according to Milligan: a follow-up study of 100 patients. *Acta Chir Scand* **124**: 444.

Southam JA (1983) Haemorrhoids treated by cryotherapy: a critical analysis. *Ann R Coll Surg Engl* **65**: 237–239.

Steinberg DM, Liegois H & Alexander-Williams J (1975) Long-term review of the results of rubber-band ligation of haemorrhoids. *Br J Surg* **62**: 144.

Stroud BB (1896) On the anatomy of the anus. *Ann Surg* **24**: 1.

Subramanyam K, Patterson M & Gourley WK (1984) Effects of Preparation H on wound healing in the rectum of man. *Dig Dis Sci* **29**: 829–834.

Sun WM, Read NW & Shorthouse AJ (1990) Hypertensive anal cushions as a cause of the high anal canal pressures in patients with haemorrhoids. *Br J Surg* **77**: 458–462.

Sun WM, Peck RJ, Shorthouse AJ & Read NW (1992) Haemorrhoids are associated with hypertrophy of the internal anal sphincter but with hypertension of the anal cushions. *Br J Surg* **79**: 592–594.

Templeton JL, Spence RAJ, Kennedy TL et al (1983) Comparison of infrared coagulation and rubber-band ligation for first and second degree haemorrhoids: a randomised prospective clinical trial. *BMJ* **286**: 1387.

Teramoto R, Parks AG & Swash M (1981) Hypertrophy of the external anal sphincter in haemorrhoids: a histometric study. *Gut* **22**: 45.

Thomson JPS (1978) Haemorrhoids and fissure. *Br J Hosp Med* **20**: 600–609.

Thomson WHF (1975) The nature of haemorrhoids. *Br J Surg* **62**: 542.

Thomson WHF (1980) The one-man bander: a new instrument for elastic ligation of piles. *Lancet* **ii**: 1006.

Thomson WHF (1982) The nature of perianal haematoma. *Lancet* **ii**: 467.

Tinckler LF & Baratham G (1964) Immediate haemorrhoidectomy for prolapsed piles. *Lancet* **ii**: 1145.

Turrell R & Gerlent IM (1969) Anal stenosis. In Turrell R (ed) *Diseases of the Colon and Anorectum*, Vol 2, 2nd edn, pp 1051–1056. Philadelphia: WB Saunders.

Vanheuverzwyn R, Delannoy A, Michaux JL et al (1980) Anal lesions in hematologic diseases. *Dis Colon Rectum* **23**: 310–312.

Van Hoorn M (1972) The haemorrhoidal ligating proctoscope. In Maratka Z & Sekta J (eds) *Urgent Endoscopy of Digestive and Abdominal Diseases*. Basel: Karger.

Varma JS, Chung SCS & Li AKC (1991) Prospective randomised comparison of current coagulation and injection sclerotherapy for the outpatient treatment of haemorrhoids. *Int J Colorect Dis* **6**: 42–45.

Vellacott KD & Harcastle JD (1980) Is continued anal dilatation necessary after a Lord's procedure for haemorrhoids? *Br J Surg* **67**: 658.

Waldon DJ, Kumar D, Hallam RI & Williams NS (1989) Prolonged ambulant assessment of anorectal function in patients with prolapsing haemorrhoids. *Dis Colon Rectum* **32**: 968–974.

Walker AJ, Leicester RJ, Nicholls RJ & Mann CV (1990) A prospective study of infrared coagulation injection and rubber-band ligation in the treatment of haemorrhoids. *Int J Colorect Dis* **5**: 113–116.

Walls ADF & Ruckley CV (1976) A five-year follow-up of Lord's dilatation for haemorrhoids. *Lancet* **i**: 1212.

Wang JY, Chang-Chien CR, Chen Js, Lai CR & Tang RP (1991) The role of lasers in haemorrhoidectomy. *Dis Colon Rectum* **34**: 78–82.

Watts JM, Bennett RC, Duthie HL & Goligher JC (1964) Healing and pain after different forms of haemorrhoidectomy. *Br J Surg* **51**: 88.

Watts JM, Bennett RC, Duthie HL & Goligher JC (1965) Pain after hemorrhoidectomy. *Surg Gynecol Obstet* **120**: 1037–1042.

Webster DJT, Gough DCS & Craven JL (1978) The use of bulky evacuant in patients with haemorrhoids. *Br J Surg* **65**: 291.

Weinstein SJ, Rypins EB, Houck J & Thrower S (1987) Single session treatment for bleeding haemorrhoids. *Surg Gynecol Obstet* **165**: 479–482.

White JE, Syphax B & Funderburk WW (1972) A modification of the Whitehead hemorrhoidectomy. *Surg Gynecol Obstet* **134**: 103.

Whitehead W (1882) Surgical treatment of haemorrhoids. *BMJ* **1**: 149.

Whittaker DK (1975) Observations on ice crystals in tissue subjected to repeat freezing. *Proc R Soc Med* **68**: 603–605.

Wolff BG & Culp CE (1988) The Whitehead haemorrhoidectomy: an unjustly maligned procedure. *Dis Colon Rectum* **31**: 587–590.

Wrobleski DE, Corman ML, Veidenheimer MC et al (1980) Long-term evaluation of rubber-band ligation in hemorrhoidal disease. *Dis Colon Rectum* **23**: 478.

Zinberg SS, Stern DH, Furman DS & Wittles JM (1989) A personal experience in comparing three non-operative techniques for treating internal haemorrhoids. *Am J Gastroenterol* **84**: 488.

13
FISSURE-IN-ANO

Anal fissure is a common disorder which may cause symptoms at any age. The usual clinical presentation is of intense anal pain made worse by attempted defecation. Painful defecation is commonly accompanied by the passage of small amounts of blood. Acute anal fissure may resolve spontaneously. Most acute fissures will heal using topical application of steroid or local anaesthetic preparations or with topical nitric oxide donors such as glyceryl trinitrate or isosorbide dinitrate. If the fissure becomes chronic or does not respond to pharmacological manipulation by nitrate compounds, and symptoms persist, surgical treatment by sphincterotomy is advised, under local or general anaesthesia as a day case. Secondary fissure from disorders such as Crohn's disease, tuberculosis, previous anal operations, AIDS, syphilis, leucoplakia, reticulosis, leukaemia and anal malignancy should be considered if the presentation is atypical or if the fissure persists despite conventional therapy.

AETIOLOGY

Children

In infants, anal fissure is usually associated with constipation and may be precipitated by a change in diet. It is postulated that epithelial damage occurs when a faecal bolus impinges on the posterior anal canal below the dentate line. The mucosa at this site is tethered to the internal anal sphincter, and because of the normal configuration of the anorectal angle this area is particularly prone to injury.

Adults

Frequently there are no discernible factors which predispose adults to anal fissure (Lund and Scholefield, 1996a). Childbirth is a recognized factor in some women: Martin (1953) reported that acute anal fissure occurred in association with recent childbirth in 11% of patients; Gough and Lewis (1983) reported that postpartum fissures were more frequently anterior. Pressure from the fetal head on the relatively unsupported anterior anal canal may be one reason for the apparent increased rate of anterior fissures after vaginal delivery. An alternative theory is that previous perineal trauma leads to scarring and tethering of the anterior anal canal, thus rendering it more susceptible to trauma in a subsequent vaginal delivery. However, postpartum fissures are comparatively uncommon, being reported by Lock and Thomson (1977) in only 3% of patients, and by ourselves in only 9% (Table 13.1.)

Table 13.1 Anal fissure: presenting features.

	Lock and Thomson (1977) (*n* = 188)	*Birmingham series* (*n* = 355)
Symptoms (%)		
Pain	87	82
Bleeding	82	74
Pruritus	44	14
Anal swelling	29	32
Discharge	7	4
Bowel habit (%)		
Constipation	14	24
Diarrhoea	4	7
Pathogenesis (%)		
Postpartum	3	9
Previous anal disease	26*	32†
Duration		
Length of history (weeks)	11	21

* Fissure 22%; haemorrhoids 3%; fistula 1%.
† Fissure 14%; haemorrhoids 18%; abscess 2%; fistula 4%.

Alteration in bowel habit is said to be a common predisposing factor in both sexes. As in children, it is suggested that the passage of hard faeces results in direct trauma to the posterior aspect of the anal canal (Lund and Scholefield, 1996a). Although an episode of constipation is sometimes forthcoming from the history before the onset of anal pain, McDonald et al (1983) identified a preceding episode of constipation in only 25% of their patients. Unquestionably, constipation commonly occurs as a consequence of the anal fissure because the patient is afraid to defecate.

Once an anal fissure develops, there is usually excessive activity of the internal anal sphincter (Sumfest et al, 1989) and high resting anal pressures, which perpetuate the condition (Hancock, 1977; Cerdan et al, 1982; McNamara et al, 1990). Such sphincter spasm is responsible for a vicious circle of anal pain, fear of defecation, and passage of hard stools which stimulates further internal sphincter activity (Dodi et al, 1986; Gibbons and Read, 1986). Breaking this cycle by anal dilatation, by topical application of nitrate compounds or by internal sphincterotomy is the basis of modern therapy for anal fissure (García-Aguilar et al, 1996; Lund et al, 1996; Schouten et al, 1996a; Watson et al, 1996; Williams et al, 1996).

Diarrhoea is also recognized as a predisposing factor and was identified in 4% of the patients treated at St Mark's Hospital (Lock and Thomson, 1977) and in 7% of our own patients (Table 13.1).

Previous anal disease is a recognized cause of fissure in 26-32% of patients. In some cases there is a history of a previous fissure that has been treated successfully in the past but which has recurred. In others there is a history of previous haemorrhoidectomy, and in such cases it is possible that postoperative tethering of the anal mucosa, stenosis or deformity lead to an increasing susceptibility to fissure, particularly if complicated by constipation (Lund and Scholefield, 1996a). The same mechanism may be responsible for posterior fissures reported after successful surgical drainage of an intersphincteric abscess (Lock and Thomson, 1977).

PATHOGENESIS

Anal fissure is associated with increased internal anal sphincter activity as evidenced by high anal canal resting pressure and ultra slow waves which are abolished by internal sphincterotomy (Hancock, 1977; Melange et al, 1992; Xynos et al, 1993; Horvath et al, 1995; Arabi et al, 1997). This increased anal hypertonia is most evident in the posterior aspect of the anal canal (Keck et al, 1995), a finding now confirmed by vector manometry (Williams et al, 1995). Farouk et al (1994) showed that there was incoordination of anorectal pressures in anal fissure. Whereas rises in rectal pressure normally generate inhibition of internal anal sphincter activity, in anal fissure these spontaneous increases in rectal pressure are often not accompanied by a sampling reflex. The anal hypertonia is probably generated by sympathetic overactivity, by failure of alpha blockade or beta-adrenergic receptor agonists (Regadas

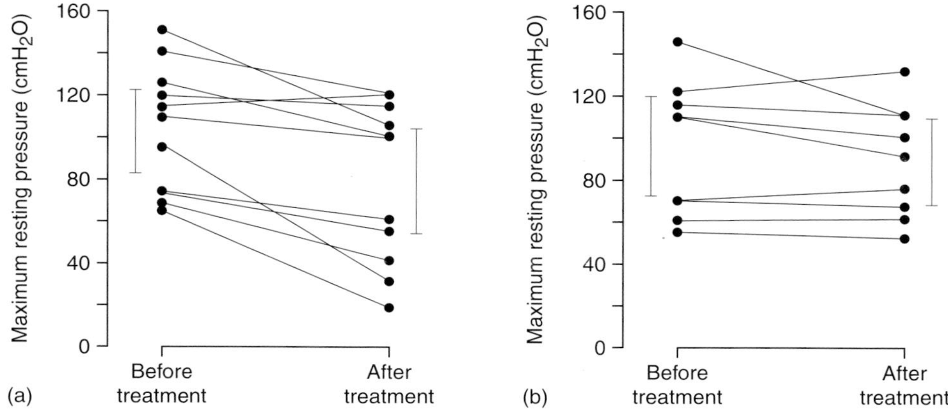

Figure 13.1a–b The impact on maximum anal resting pressure (a) 20 minutes after the application of a 0.2% glyceryl trinitrate ointment, compared with (b) placebo. Bars are 95% confidence intervals: $P = 0.0024$ (pressure before versus pressure after application of ointment; $P = 0.033$ (change in pressure after application of ointment versus change in placebo group); Student's *t*-test (Loder et al, 1994).

et al, 1993). In anal fissure there is supersensitivity of internal anal sphincter relaxation with isoproterenol. Neuronal proliferation may be responsible for the pain in chronic anal fissures (Hörsch et al, 1998).

Another pathway for internal anal sphincter relaxation is the inhibitory neurotransmitter, nitric oxide (O'Kelly et al, 1993; Rattan and Chakder, 1992; Rattan et al, 1992). Although several other substances, such as the calcium-channel blocker nifedipine, decrease anal pressure (Chrysos et al, 1996), none has yet found clinical application (Neri et al, 1988; Enck et al, 1989). The discovery of the nitric oxide pathway presents a new avenue for manipulation of anal pressure and thus potential therapy for anal fissure. Loder et al (1994) reported that glyceryl trinitrate, a nitric oxide donor applied as a 0.2% ointment, caused a 27% decrease in anal pressure (Figure 13.1). Later studies have described healing of fissures with the topical application of glyceryl trinitrate or isosorbide dinitrate (Lund et al, 1996; Schouten et al, 1996a; Watson et al, 1996; see Table 13.8). Localized hypertonia in the posterior anal canal may explain the spasm and pain noted in patients with a fissure, but it did not really provide a hypothesis for causation until Schouten and his group (1994) demonstrated a close correlation between anal pressure and impaired anal blood flow (Figure 13.2). These authors also showed that perfusion of the anoderm in the posterior midline was impaired (Figure 13.3), and was particularly low at the base of the fissure. They concluded, therefore, that anal fissures are ischaemic ulcers.

This accords with postmortem angiographic

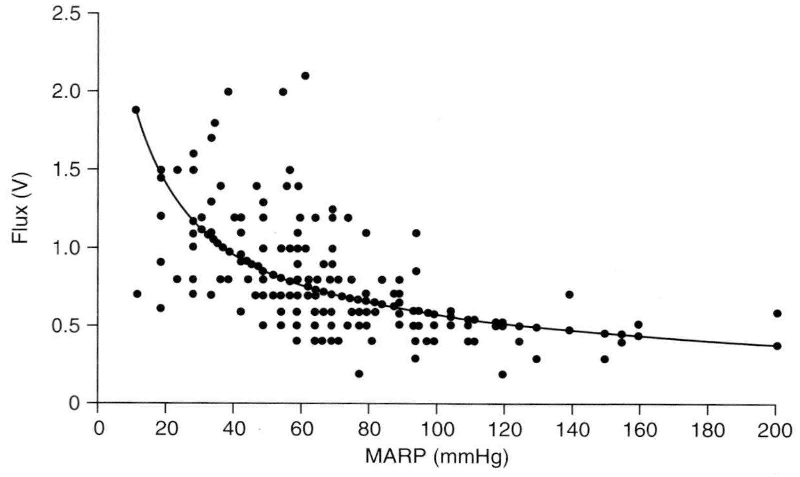

Figure 13.2 The relationship between maximum resting anal pressure (MRAP) and anodermal blood flow expressed as flux (volts) (Schouten et al, 1994).

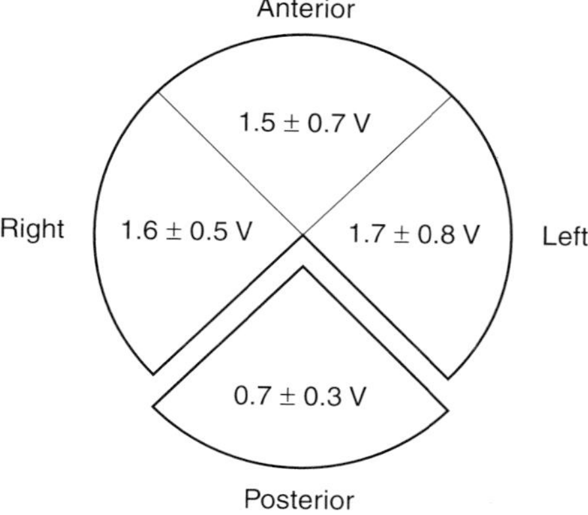

Figure 13.3 Anodermal blood flow, expressed as flux (V), in all quadrants of the anal canal (Schouten et al, 1994).

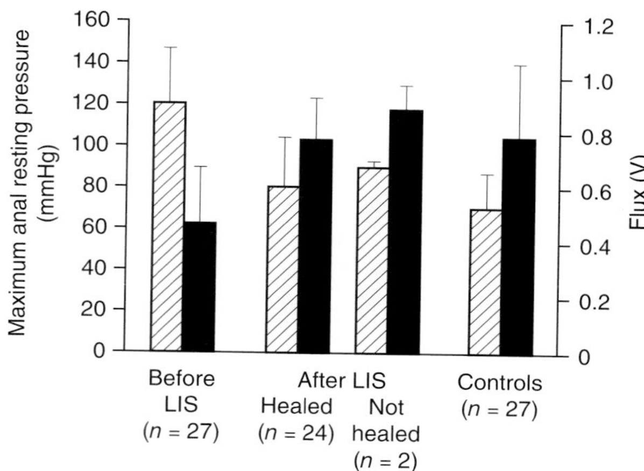

Figure 13.4 The impact of lateral internal sphincterotomy (LIS) in patients with fissures: maximum anal resting pressure (▨) and anodermal blood flow (■), expressed as flux (V); controls are also shown. Values are means and standard deviations (Schouten et al, 1996b).

studies which showed a paucity of branches in the inferior rectal artery in the posterior aspect of the anal canal (Klosterhalfen et al, 1989). Furthermore, raised internal sphincter activity reduces the perfusion index of these small vessels and is probably responsible for the pathogenesis of the anal fissure (Gibbons and Read, 1986). Subsequent studies have shown that when internal sphincterotomy achieves fissure healing, there is an increased blood flow and reduced anal resting pressure (Schouten et al, 1996a) (Figure 13.4).

Hence present data strongly suggest that anal fissures are ischaemic ulcers associated with localized anal hypertonia which may be effectively treated with pharmacological or surgical methods that reduce anal pressure, thereby increasing local blood flow, allowing the ischaemic ulcer to heal (Lund and Scholefield, 1996a).

PATHOLOGY

Primary fissure

A primary anal fissure is a benign superficial ulcer in the anal canal. Typically it is boat-shaped and the transverse fibres of the internal sphincter can usually be seen in its base. A primary fissure involves only the anal mucosa below the dentate line. If it extends more proximally, it is almost certainly secondary to some other disorder. A primary fissure is therefore usually about 1 cm in length and overlies only the lower third of the internal sphincter. At its lower end there may be a tag of oedematous skin. This tag is known as a 'sentinel' pile – sentinel because it guards the fissure. Primary fissures may be acute or chronic (Crapp and Alexander-Williams, 1975).

Acute primary anal fissure

An acute fissure is superficial and the base is formed by loose connective tissue; commonly the transverse fibres of the internal sphincter are not seen. A sentinel pile may not be present and there is rarely a hypertrophied anal papilla (chronic fissure). The edges of the ulcer are sharply demarcated and there is no induration, sepsis, oedema or cavitation. Acute fissures often heal spontaneously and they occur commonly in children, young adults and in the puerperium. The results of surgical treatment are more successful in acute fissure (Frezza et al, 1992). If healing does not occur and symptoms persist, acute fissures invariably become chronic.

Chronic primary anal fissure

Any patient with persistent symptoms for more than a few weeks usually has a chronic fissure. The edges of a chronic fissure are indurated and sometimes undermined; the internal sphincter is usually easily visible at the base. Later the ulcer becomes wider and the external aspect becomes oedematous owing to lymphatic obstruction. If the disorder persists there may be cavitation of the lower aspect of the fissure or undermining from sepsis in the intersphincteric plane. Progressive oedema gives rise to the characteristic skin tag and a hypertrophied anal papilla at the inner margin on the dentate line (Lund and Scholefield, 1996a). Sepsis may complicate the pathology, spreading upwards as a submucous or intersphincteric abscess or downwards to form a perianal abscess beneath the skin tag. Persistent perianal abscess may give rise to a superficial fistula running from the lower border of the fissure underneath the skin tag to emerge just behind it. This 'fissure–fistula' is comparatively rare, being observed in only 4% of our patients. The association of an intersphincteric or submucous abscess is also uncommon, being present in only 2% of our patients.

Secondary fissure

Secondary fissures are those that arise in association with some other pathology such as Crohn's disease, anal tuberculosis, AIDS or a previous anal operation (Grewal et al, 1994). Fissures complicating Crohn's disease and tuberculosis are often painless; they may be complicated by a fistula-in-ano and perianal sepsis. The fissure of Crohn's disease is often a cavitating ulcer with extensive local destruction and sepsis (Hughes, 1977). Secondary fissures tend to be progressive, become chronic and rarely heal with conservative or surgical therapy.

AGE AND INCIDENCE

A fissure-in-ano may occur at any age (Shub et al, 1978) but is most common between the second and fourth decades (Gough and Lewis, 1983; McDonald et al, 1983; Pernikoff et al, 1994) (Table 13.2). A review from St Mark's Hospital of 1712 new patients attending an outpatient clinic over 6 months revealed that 190 patients had an anal fissure (11.1%). The age and sex ranges are shown in Figure 13.5 (Lock and Thomson, 1977). The frequency of anal fissure in our own rectal clinic in Birmingham is 9%.

Table 13.2 Anal fissure: relation to age and sex.

	Lock and Thomson (1977) (*n* = 188)	*Shub et al (1978)* (*n* = 393)	*Gough and Lewis (1983)* (*n* = 82)	*McDonald et al (1983)* (*n* = 81)	*Birmingham series* (*n* = 355)
Age (years): mean	38	NR	36	39	36
Age (years): range	11 months–72	16 months–83	NR	17–74	16–72
Men (%)	58	53	52	49	57
Women (%)	42	47	48	51	43

NR, not recorded.

CLINICAL FEATURES

Children

Children with an anal fissure characteristically scream with pain during defecation, which is often associated with passing small amounts of bright-red blood. Most of these children have constipation, but it is often difficult to know whether this is the cause or the effect of the anal fissure. Anal fissure is one of the most common causes of rectal bleeding in infants. The diagnosis can usually be made by inspection since the perianal skin is puckered by an overactive sphincter, there is usually a small skin tag, and the child will object violently to any attempt at rectal examination.

Adults

History

The principal symptoms in adults are anal pain, bright-red bleeding, perianal swelling and, occasionally, mucous discharge. The pain is acute and is felt in the anal canal during and after defecation. There may be a sensation of tearing during defecation. A dull ache is usually experienced for 3–4 hours after defecation. Constipation soon complicates the clinical picture and aggravates symptoms. Pain may become chronic and intermittent.

Although pain is the most dominant symptom,

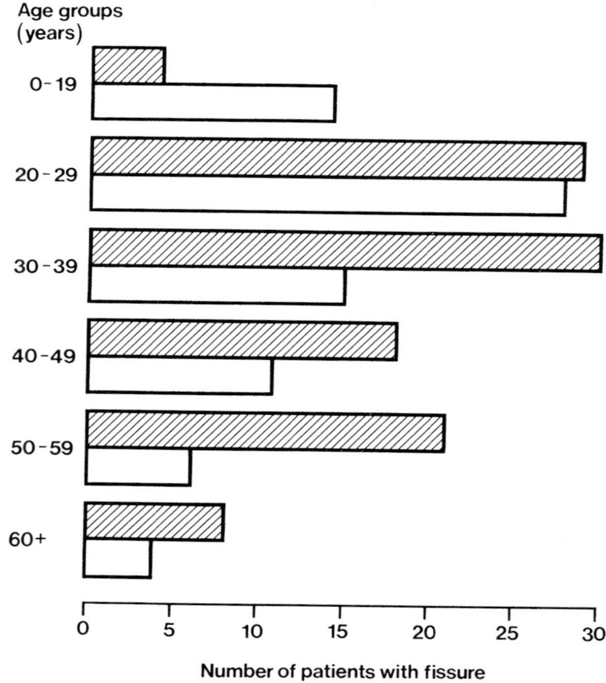

Figure 13.5 Age and sex incidence of fissure-in-ano. ▨, males; □, females (Lock and Thomson, 1977).

rectal bleeding occurs in 74–86% of patients (see Table 13.1). Characteristically, bleeding is only small in amount, is bright red and occurs only during straining or defecation. Profuse blood loss is rare.

Swelling and discharge are characteristic of chronic fissure, which may be complicated by pruritis ani and perianal excoriation. Discharge may indicate an intersphincteric abscess or a fissure–fistula.

Examination

In most patients it is possible to make a diagnosis of anal fissure by inspection alone. The patient is usually anxious and may be in pain; also, patients are naturally fearful of having a rectal examination and the perianal skin is usually puckered by spasm of the internal and external anal sphincters and tightly held buttocks. A recent study reported that sublingual administration of 0.4 mg of glyceryl trinitrate made it possible to perform a rectal examination in 13 of 16 acute fissure patients in whom rectal examination had been quite impossible beforehand (Larpent et al, 1996). This is further evidence of the role of nitric oxide and internal sphincter hypertonia in acute anal fissure.

Inspection

Despite excessive sphincter activity, it is usually possible to see a small skin tag as well as a small amount of discharge or blood on the perineum. If the patient is reassured, it is usually possible to part the buttocks gently. This manoeuvre may be facilitated by smearing some local anaesthetic jelly around the anal margin. It is quite wrong to attempt a rectal examination or proctoscopy at this stage, unless sublingual glyceryl trinitrate has been administered a minute or two beforehand. Since the lesion lies below the dentate line, gentle traction on the lateral margins of the perineum nearly always reveals a fissure if one is present (Figure 13.6).

Palpation

Only after careful inspection has failed to reveal a fissure should the surgeon attempt a rectal examination. Rectal examination can be achieved, some-

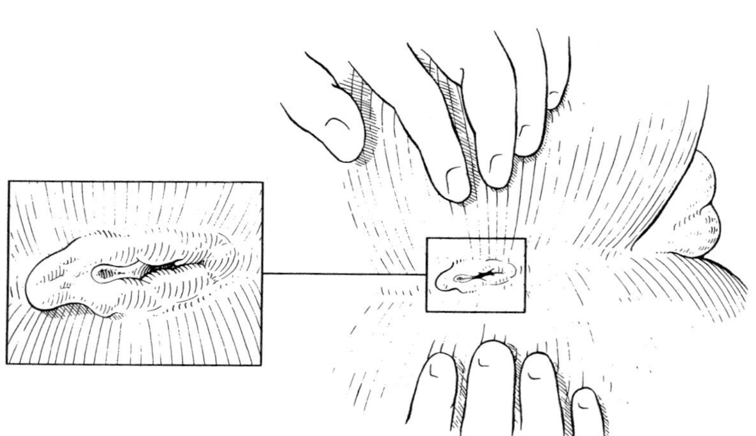

Figure 13.6 The appearance of an anal fissure. If the buttocks are gently parted, the presence of an anal fissure can usually be detected as an ulcer of variable depth associated with a skin tag and an anal papilla. There is usually excessive activity of the anal sphincter.

times without too much pain, by introducing the finger well away from the usual fissure site. Intense spasm of the sphincters is usually a prominent feature (Table 13.3). The fissure may be felt as an irregular, painful depression near the anal margin. Examination directly over the fissure is usually exquisitely painful. In chronic fissures, rectal examination is often comparatively painless and a palpable abnormality is common.

If it is initially obvious that a rectal examination is going to be too painful for the patient , it should be abandoned in favour of examination under anaesthesia or after sublingual glyceryl trinitrate.

Table 13.3 Anal fissure: frequency (%) of different physical signs.

Physical sign	*Lock and Thomson (1977)* (*n* = 188)	*Birmingham series* (*n* = 355)
Anal spasm	69	78
Sentinal tag	38	68
Hypertrophied papilla	16	25
Fissure/fistula	6	6
Intersphincteric abscess	2	4
Haemorrhoids	15	38
Anal stenosis	0	2

Table 13.4 Anal fissure: occurrence (%) at different sites.

Site	*Lock and Thomson (1977)* (*n* = 188)	*Shub et al (1978)* (*n* = 393)	*Gough and Lewis (1983)* (*n* = 97)	*McDonald et al (1983)* (*n* = 81)	*Birmingham series* (*n* = 355)
Anterior	14	27	12	7	7
Posterior	75	66	82	88	89
Both	8	7	2	1	2
Lateral	3	0	3	4	2

Proctoscopy

Proctoscopy is sometimes quite impossible with conventional adult instruments in acute anal fissure. However, a well-lubricated infant sigmoidoscope may allow inspection of the lower rectal mucosa and the anal canal so that any coexisting pathology can be recognized (Lock and Thomson, 1977). If proctoscopy and sigmoidoscopy are painful, the examination should be deferred and performed under general or local anaesthetic prior to definitive treatment.

Associated pathology may be identified during rectal examination and proctoscopy. Haemorrhoids are present in up to a third of patients. Hypertrophied anal papilla are seen in approximately 20% of patients; and a fistula, sometimes with an intersphincteric abscess, may be observed in 5–6% of cases. Anal stenosis is present in 2–3% of patients (Shub et al, 1978; Marby et al, 1979; Abcarian, 1980; Lewis et al, 1988).

Site of fissure

The site of an anal fissure can usually be determined by inspection and confirmed during proctoscopy. Over two-thirds of fissures are single and most lie posteriorly (Table 13.4). In our own experience, 89% were found to be posterior and only 7% were sited anteriorly; 2% occurred at both sites and 2% were lateral. The proportion of anterior fissures is much higher in female patients, being 21% compared with only 9% in the male population (Lock and Thomson, 1977).

Sigmoidoscopy

The proportion of patients with abnormalities on sigmoidoscopy depends on the length of rectum which can be viewed and the number of patients having an endoscopy. We found an abnormality on sigmoidoscopy in 11% of patients with a fissure (Table 13.5). These abnormalities included distal proctitis, metaplastic adenomatous polyps, anal condylomata, Crohn's disease and anal tuberculosis.

Table 13.5 Abnormalities found on sigmoidoscopy.

Abnormality	*Lock and Thomson (1977)*	*Birmingham series*
Total	8/168 (5%)	31/294 (11%)
Distal proctitis	1	10
Adenoma	2	4
Condylomata	1	5
Melanosis coli	1	0
Metaplastic polyps	2	6
Crohn's disease	0	5
Tuberculosis	0	1

OTHER INVESTIGATIONS AND DIFFERENTIAL DIAGNOSIS

Investigations

If an adequate assessment has not been possible in the outpatient clinic, it is necessary to examine the patient by palpation, proctoscopy and sigmoidoscopy under general or local anaesthesia or after sublingual trinitrate, before treatment is commenced. Barium enema or colonoscopy are not usually indicated unless there is strong evidence of some other primary pathology such as Crohn's disease, ulcerative colitis, amoebic colitis or a colorectal neoplasm. Various microbiological, antibody or complement fixation studies may be indicated if an infective cause is suspected (see below).

Differential diagnosis

A small proportion of fissures are secondary to other pathology such as syphilis, AIDS, tuberculosis, Crohn's disease, ulcerative colitis, anal stenosis or previous operations on the anal canal. Such disorders can often be excluded by the history or examination. There are a variety of disorders which may mimic a fissure. Perianal sepsis complicating leukaemia in neutropenic patients can masquerade as an anal fissure (Grewal et al, 1994). Other malignant disorders, such as squamous cell carcinoma, basal cell carcinoma and adenocarcinoma of the lower third of the rectum when complicated by sepsis, may be confused with a fissure. Similar symptoms may be present in Paget's disease of the anus, intersphincteric abscess, proctalgia fugax, thrombosed external plexus haematoma and pruritus ani. All these conditions are described elsewhere, but the principal diagnostic features of the more important disorders are described here.

Crohn's disease

Anal fissures in Crohn's disease are usually painless (Sweeney et al, 1988). Sepsis around the fissure is common and there is often a prominent skin tag. A Crohn's fissure is often broader than a primary fissure and penetrates locally with destruction of the anal sphincters, causing a cavitating ulcer. The fissure may be situated laterally and there may be more than one. Associated fistula, abscess and stenosis are frequent. Proctitis is relatively uncommon. Lewis et al (1988) reported that 5 of 21 patients with unhealed anal fissures after sphincterotomy later proved to have Crohn's disease. Any unhealed fissure should alert the clinician to the possibility of Crohn's disease.

Ulcerative colitis

Typically, perianal disease is associated with Crohn's disease rather than ulcerative colitis. However, fissure may complicate relapse of colitis. The fissure is usually extremely painful and commonly becomes infected. Remission of the colitis is usually associated with healing of the fissure. Unlike with Crohn's disease, skin tags and other perianal disorders are uncommon.

Tuberculous anal fissures

A fissure in anal tuberculosis is often indistinguishable from a simple primary fissure. Tuberculous fissures rarely heal with conventional therapy and frequently progress to form an ulcer with undermined edges. Destruction of sphincter muscle may follow, resulting in multiple anal fistulas. Sigmoidoscopy is usually normal and a diagnosis is established only by culture and the demonstration of acid-fast bacilli.

Syphilitic fissures

A primary chancre may resemble a fissure but it is usually painless and rapidly becomes indurated, with associated inguinal lymphadenopathy. There are often two fissures that lie opposite each other around the circumference of the anal margin. If a fissure is in any way unusual in appearance, or painless, a sample of discharge should be examined for spirochaetes by dark ground illumination. Secondary anal condylomata may be associated with painful fissures; the diagnosis is usually suspected by appearance and confirmed by a positive Wassermann reaction.

Intersphincteric abscess

If a fissure cannot be seen when the anal canal is examined under anaesthetic and there is a reliable history of intense anal pain, the possibility of an intersphincteric abscess must always be borne in mind. Diagnosis can often be made only by exploring the intersphincteric plane over the area of maximum tenderness.

Anal malignancy

Any malignancy invading the anal canal will give rise to intense anal pain on defecation, often associated with some bleeding. The tumour can sometimes be seen emerging from the anal canal and may be mistaken for an anal skin tag. However, rectal examination and biopsy are usually diagnostic. The common tumours to present in this way include lymphoma, squamous or basal cell cancer, adenocarcinoma or cloacogenic malignancy.

Pruritus ani

Fissures may be associated with pruritus. Conversely, idiopathic pruritus may be complicated by fissuring of the skin, which is tender, macerated and moist. Fissures occurring as a result of pruritus are often multiple, and superficial; they tend to radiate from the anal margins, involving only the perineal skin, not the anal canal.

AIDS

Homosexuals, drug abusers and other 'at risk' groups may develop a chronic anal fissure as a consequence of local trauma, impaired mucosal resistance and anorectal sepsis and chronic intestinal infections. Often these fissures are associated with anorectal sepsis.

Proctalgia fugax

There are many patients with symptoms characteristic of an anal fissure who have an apparently normal anal canal. If a fissure is strongly suspected, the examination should be repeated at a later date and preferably under anaesthetic, since it might have been missed at the initial examination. If the patient has no haemorrhoids, and provided an intersphincteric abscess has been excluded, proctalgia fugax is often the presumed diagnosis. The patient may complain of additional bizarre symptoms such as low back pain, disordered defecation, shooting pain down the legs and a history of paraesthesia. It is dangerous to label such patients as having proctalgia fugax until the clinician is absolutely certain that there is no underlying pathology by repeated examination; proctalgia fugax is a diagnosis of exclusion. Equally it is dangerous to treat patients with anal pain and no evidence of a fissure by anal dilatation or sphincterotomy.

PHYSIOLOGICAL CHANGES

Patients with an anal fissure, particularly those with an acute fissure, have significantly higher resting anal canal pressures than control subjects (Arabi et al, 1977), owing to the overactivity of the internal anal sphincter which it is commonly associated with transient or sustained ultra-slow waves (Hancock, 1977) (Figure 13.7). Many other investigators have now confirmed that resting anal canal pressures are increased in anal fissure (Kuypers, 1983; Gibbons and Read, 1986; Melange et al, 1992; Prohn and Bonner, 1995). Abcarian et al (1982) and Northmann and Schuster (1974) reported an abnormal rectoanal inhibitory reflex in a high proportion of patients with anal fissure. Cerdan et al (1982) observed not only an increase in the resting anal pressures but a longer high-pressure zone in fissure patients, which could be entirely abolished by internal sphincterotomy.

We found that increased resting anal pressure could be significantly reduced, both by lateral subcutaneous sphincterotomy and by anal dilatation (Marby et al, 1979; see also Hancock, 1977). Failure to reduce the resting anal pressures was associated with persistent symptoms (Gatehouse et al, 1978). The percentage reduction in anal pressure after treatment is variable, being as great as 50% in the report by Chowcat et al (1986). In our experience the fall in resting pressure was of the order of 20–30%. Like Olsen et al (1987), we reported that the reduction in resting pressure

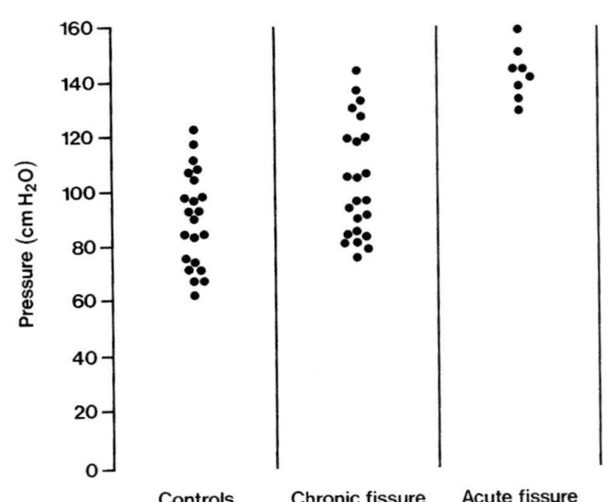

Figure 13.7 Resting anal canal pressures in patients with acute and chronic anal fissure, compared with controls.

was greater following anal dilatation than after lateral subcutaneous sphincterotomy (Table 13.6). Boulos and Araujo (1984) reported a similar reduction in anal pressure following open and closed sphincterotomy. In most series this fall in resting pressure is sustained.

Ultra-slow-wave activity (Figure 13.8) was observed by Hancock (1977) in 10 of 12 patients with an anal fissure, compared with 2 of 40 controls. We have occasionally observed irregular spikes of involuntary external sphincter activity, particularly in patients with an acute anal fissure. These abnormal motility patterns are usually abolished by anal dilatation or sphincterotomy.

Table 13.6 Influence of treatment on anal pressures.

Treatment	*Mean anal pressure* (cmH_2O)			
		After treatment		
	Before treatment	*1 month*	*4 months*	*12 months*
Anal dilatation (*n* = 63)	129	105	104	115
Lateral subcutaneous sphincterotomy:				
Local anaesthesia (*n* = 65)	120	111	107	111
General anaesthesia (*n* = 69)	124	104	107	110
Open sphincterotomy (*n* = 32)	132	94	99	104

Data from Birmingham series.

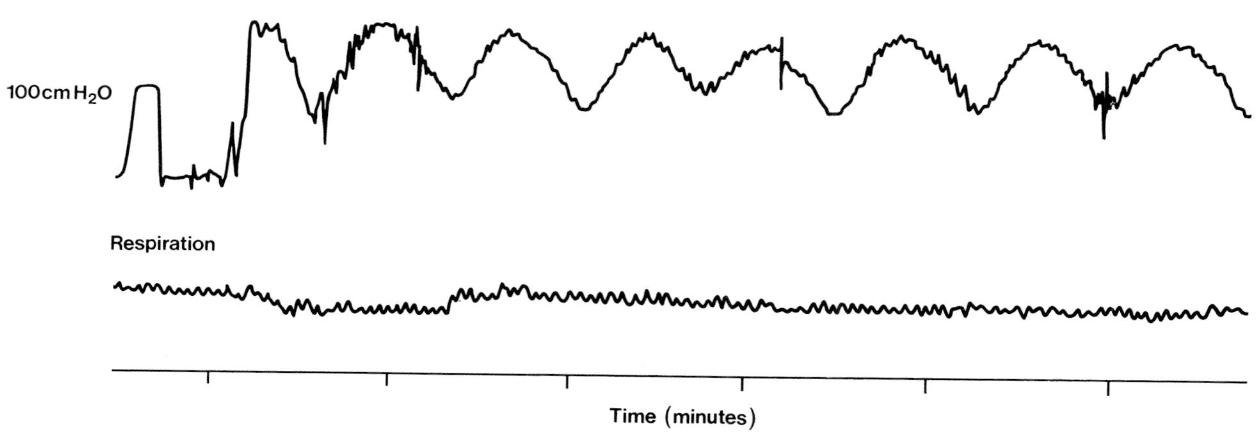

Figure 13.8 Resting anal canal pressures in patients with fissure-in-ano. Ultra-slow-wave activity is commonly demonstrated during a prolonged manometric study.

NATURAL HISTORY

Up to 70% of acute anal fissures resolve spontaneously; if not, they progress to form a chronic fissure. Left untreated, some fissures recur over months or years. Once a chronic fissure has developed, the chances of spontaneous resolution falls to 20–30%, but healing is now often recorded in patients waiting for elective treatment. Thus a fissure may heal, remain static, progress to a fissure–fistula or become complicated by an abscess. The notable exceptions are fissures associated with Crohn's disease where up to 80% may heal without any treatment, and as many are painless they can be ignored unless there is severe rectal disease (Buchmann et al, 1980). Sweeney et al (1988) also reported that 69% of acute fissures in patients with Crohn's disease healed during medical therapy of the bowel disease.

MEDICAL TREATMENT

Nearly 90% of acute anal fissures will heal using conservative measures alone (Frezza et al, 1992). By contrast, only 40% of chronic fissures are likely to heal by conservative therapy.

Bulk laxatives

Most patients either have long-standing constipation or have recently become constipated as a result of the fissure. Thus a bulk laxative such as methylcellulose, ispaghula or sterculia with a mild laxative such as bisacodyl or docusate sodium (Dioctyl), should be prescribed.

Symptomatic treatment

Excessive use of toilet paper should be avoided and patients should be advised to take regular baths and showers or to sit on a bidet after defecation. Hot baths provide symptomatic benefit but have no influence on anal pressures (Pinho et al, 1993). Any local preparations which might cause an allergy should be avoided. Clothing which increases the risk of perspiration around the anus, such as Nylon underwear, should be avoided. Patients should be encouraged to take a high-fibre diet to promote the passage of a soft but bulky stool which then acts as a natural dilator.

Topical steroids and local anaesthetic agents

Application of local, non-steroidal preparations may control pain and promote healing. Local opiate preparations, or silver nitrate or icthammol preparations, have been used as topical agents with symptomatic benefit (Gabriel, 1939).

Local anaesthetic agents may provide symptomatic benefit, particularly in acute fissure-in-ano, but allergy can occur in 2% of patients (Rodkey, 1973; Alexander, 1975). Steroid preparations may be used to reduce inflammation and promote spontaneous healing. Proctosedyl (containing cinchocain and hydrocortisone) with Soframycin may achieve 80% healing within 3 weeks in patients with an acute fissure (General Practitioner Group, 1970). However, high remission rates have been reported by Jensen (1986), using local anaesthetic agents, topical steroids and control of constipation.

Fries and Reitz (1964) found that approximately half of their patients treated by local anaesthetic agents and bulk laxatives were relieved of their symptoms. Lock and Thomson (1977) reported that a similar proportion (54%) were initially rendered asymptomatic but long-term follow-up indicated that healing was maintained in only half. Factors found to be associated with a poor long-term outcome following conservative therapy were the presence of a skin tag and a fibrous anal polyp. Operation was eventually required in 72% of patients with a tag, compared with only 42% without. Similarly, operative treatment became necessary in 84% of patients with an anal polyp, compared with only 48% without. Jensen (1987) found that 1-year recurrence rates were significantly less among patients who continued to take 15 g bran daily (16%) compared with those taking 7.5 g (60%) or no added fibre (68%) (Figure 13.9).

Anal dilators

Some clinicians still use an anal dilator as part of the conservative treatment of anal fissure. However, many patients find self-dilatation painful and dis-

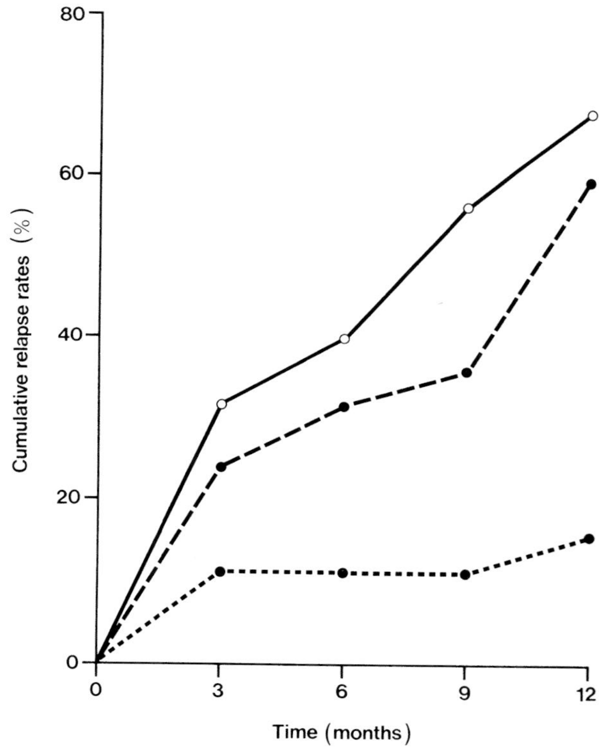

Figure 13.9 Cumulative relapse rate and the influence of oral bran supplements. This study demonstrates that bran in a dose of 15 g/day was associated with a significantly lower recurrence rate. ——, placebo (n = 25); – – –, 7.5 g bran/day (n = 25); - - -, 15 g bran/day (n = 25) (Jensen, 1987).

tasteful and compliance is probably poor. Two trials have evaluated the role of an anal dilator in the conservative treatment of anal fissure (Gough and Lewis, 1983; McDonald et al, 1983). In both trials, patients were randomly allocated to either dilator and lignocaine or to lignocaine alone. McDonald et al (1983) reported healing rates at 6 months of 60% and 52% respectively (Table 13.7). Gough and Lewis (1983) found that 44% and 42% had healed by a month. Hence, both groups concluded that addition of an anal dilator to a regimen of conservative therapy was unnecessary.

Sclerotherapy or botulinum toxin

Sclerotherapy using sodium tetradecyl sulphate after local anaesthetic infiltration has been reported to give healing rates of over 80% (Antebi et al, 1985) but may be complicated by abscess. Although the results appear to be superior to conservative management without sclerotherapy (Shub et al, 1978), we do not recommend sclerotherapy for fissure.

Another novel approach has been the use of botulinum toxin with some reported success (Jost and Schimrigk, 1994). Botulinum toxin achieved healing in three of five cases and achieved a 23% reduction in resting anal pressure (Mason et al, 1996). Jost (1997) reported that 78 of 100 patients were rendered pain-free after injection of botulinum toxin. There was immediate healing in 83% and prolonged healing in 79%. Transient faecal incontinence occurred in seven cases. At the moment there are insufficient data to support this method of treatment.

Topical nitrate preparations

The most recent advance in conservative treatment has been the use of pharmacological agents to reduce anal sphincter hypertonia. Short-term healing has been reported with isoproterenol, but the use of nitric oxide donors to reduce internal anal sphincter activity and resting anal pressures has received greater interest (Loder et al, 1994; Banerjee, 1997). A number of studies using different nitric preparations have been reported and are summarized in Table 13.8. In general most of these investigations report encouraging healing rates, but in most studies some patients have been troubled by headache.

One of the problems with topical therapy is that of prescribing the optimal dose since a standard dose may not be pharmacologically active. Watson et al (1996) used a dose which achieved a 25% reduction in resting anal pressure. If the preparation is a cream it is difficult to record how much of a particular concentration is applied; Lund and Scholefield (1997) used 0.5 g of 0.2% cream. Another issue is that of tachyphylaxis, where increasing doses are needed to provide a sustained reduction in internal anal sphincter activity.

The present position is that pharmacological manipulation is novel, and interesting, but dose and delivery must be quantified (Kennedy et al, 1996; Lund and Scholefield, 1996) and newer, more stable, agents explored. Long-term results are needed, but provided drug-induced headache is rare, this method of conservative therapy may have an important role in the future. Schouten and colleagues, using 1% isosorbide dinitrate, found that all their patients suffered minor headache for the first 48 hours, but that this did not persist and 34 patients were able to continue GTN for 12 weeks when therapy had not achieved healing in the first 6 or 9 weeks. None of their patients withdrew because of headache; 41% were healed at 6 weeks, 65% at 9 weeks and 88% at 12 weeks. All patients experienced complete disappearance of acute anal

Table 13.7 Results of conservative therapy (% healing rates).

Authors	*Salt baths Diet Suppositories*	*Dilator and lignocaine*	*Lignocaine alone*
McDonald et al (1983)			
Healed at 6 weeks	—	68	61
Healed at 6 months	—	60	52
Gough and Lewis (1983)			
Healed at 1 month	—	44	42
Shub et al (1978)			
Healed at 5 years	44	—	—
Lock and Thomson (1977)*			
Healed at 4–8 weeks	54	—	—
Healed at 4 years	28	—	—

* Poor results if tag or polyp present.

Table 13.8 Results of topical nitrate application for anal fissure.

Author	*n*	*Dose*	*Headache*	*Healing*
Watson et al (1996)	19	Minimal dose of GTN to reduce MAP by 25%	2	9/15 at 6 weeks (6 sphincterotomy)
Lund et al (1996)	21	0.2% GTN	4	11/21 at 4 weeks 18/21 at 6 weeks
Schouten et al (1996a)	34	1% isosorbide dinitrate	All initially	14/34 at 6 weeks* 22/34 at 9 weeks 30/34 at 12 weeks†
Bacher et al (1997)	20	Nitroglycerine	4	12/20 at 2 weeks 16/20 at 4 weeks
Lund and Scholefield (1997)	39	0.2% GTN 0.5 g	8	14/39 at 4 weeks 33/39 at 6 weeks‡
Oettlé (1997) (randomized trial)	12 12	GTN crushed tablets Sphincterotomy		10/12 at 22 months§ 12/12 at 22 months

* Fissure pain disappeared at 10 days in 34/34.
†Two patients went on to sphincterotomy, two to island advancement.
‡ Five fissures recorded; four healed with repeat GTN.
§ Two fissures persisted and were treated by sphincterotomy.

pain within 10 days of commencing therapy. Only 4 of 34 patients thus required surgical therapy by sphincterotomy or island advancement flap.

The experience with glyceryl trinitrate is similar. Watson et al (1996) reported that 60% had healed at 6 weeks, but 4 of 21 suffered from troublesome headaches; however none of these patients required sugical treatment. Most authors suggest that nitrates should be re-applied if the fissure does not heal initially. Indeed, Lund and Scholefield (1997) achieved healing in four of five recurrent fissures.

Bacher et al (1997) found that nitroglycerine was significantly more effective than local anaesthetic cream. Oettlé (1997) from South Africa reported the outcome of a small randomized trial, in which at a mean follow-up of 22 months there was healing in 10 of 12 patients using GTN compared with all 12 patients having sphincterotomy. He concludes that GTN should now be the first-line treatment since it could avoid the morbidity of incontinence after internal sphincterotomy (Hananel and Gordon, 1997).

In view of the potential morbidity from incontinence following sphincterotomy, the role of pharmacological agents is likely to assume greater prominence in the future.

SURGICAL TREATMENT

The aim of surgical treatment is to reduce the activity of the internal anal sphincter (Kuypers, 1983; Gibbons and Read, 1986; Hiltunen & Matikainen, 1986; Lund & Scholefield, 1996b) or to cover the anal ulcer by well-vascularized skin so as to allow healing of the ischaemic fissure. There are two types of surgical procedure used for the treatment of chronic fissure-in-ano. The first are operations to reduce anal hypertonia by dilatation or internal sphincterotomy (Frezza et al, 1992; Nielson et al, 1993). The second approach – which has only recently gained acceptance particularly for patients at risk from iatrogenic incontinence – is to excise the fissure and cover the defect with some form of skin flap (Angelchick et al, 1993; Leong and Seow-Choen, 1995; Nyam et al, 1995).

Historical considerations

Anal dilatation has been used for over a century and was recommended for treatment by Graham-Stewart et al (1961), Watts et al (1964), Lord (1968) and Hancock (1977). Anal dilatation is a simple procedure but requires a short but deep intravenous anaesthetic; hence it is usually performed in hospital as a day-stay procedure. One of the reasons why anal dilatation has fallen into disrepute is that forceful dilatation may impair continence permanently. Controlled dilatation is said to achieve healing rates of 93% without incontinence (Sohn et al, 1992), but we have grave reservations about the advisability of anal dilatation because of the risk of incontinence (Nielson et al, 1993).

Internal sphincterotomy has also been performed for well over 50 years but many of the earlier writers failed to appreciate that the divided muscle was the internal sphincter (Miles, 1936). Internal anal sphincterotomy was popularized by Eisenhammer (1951), who described an open posterior approach during which the fissure was also excised. The posterior technique was widely adopted in the UK and the USA (Morgan and Thompson, 1956; Tzu-Chi-Hsu and MacKeigan, 1984; Gingold, 1987) but this operation has fallen into disfavour because the fissures may take several weeks to heal (Bennett and Goligher, 1962). Furthermore, a persistent keyhole deformity may be produced which can be very difficult to treat surgically (Mazier, 1985). The posterior scar tends to create a gutter which is often associated with incontinence of mucus and flatus and also causes troublesome faecal soiling (Hardy, 1967; Walker et al, 1985). Posterior fissurectomy carries a 37% risk of at least sporadic impairment in continence and persistent soiling (Melange et al, 1992). The practice of excising the entire fissure had been abandoned since excision is unnecessary provided the internal sphincter is adequately divided. However, excision may again have a place if island advancement flaps are used for treatment of chronic fissures where there might be a risk of incontinence after sphincterotomy (Sentovich et al, 1996; Farouk et al, 1997). Nevertheless, fissurectomy may be attended by a higher incidence of abscess and stenosis, as well as impaired continence (Bode et al, 1984; Tzu-Chi-Hsu and MacKeigan, 1984). Hence sphincterotomy is now used at a site away from the fissure, usually through a lateral approach either as an open operation or a subcutaneous closed technique (Kortbeek et al, 1992).

Hughes (1953) reported satisfactory results if the fissure was excised and followed by immediate application of a split skin graft. However, this is an extensive procedure with no quarantee of the graft 'taking' for what is usually a simple problem. Alternative and simpler techniques to cover the defect after excision are now practised. The most widely used is the island advancement flap (Nyam et al, 1995; Leong and Seow-Choen, 1995), but other procedures may be more applicable, particularly the Y–V advancement flap, the rotational advancement flap and mucosal advancement techniques (Angelchik et al, 1993). We believe that these techniques are still best reserved for cases of recurrent fissure after a previous anal dilatation or sphincterotomy or in patients with a deficient sphincter where there might be a risk of iatrogenic incontinence. These procedures are also applicable to cases of fissure occurring secondary to anal skin loss, for instance following haemorrhoidectomy complicated by anal stenosis (see Chapter 12) (Pope, 1959; Ferguson, 1975; Tzu-Chi-Hsu and MacKeigan, 1984).

Posterior internal sphincterotomy has now been almost entirely superseded by the lateral approach, either as an open operation or as a closed subcutaneous technique; only these operations will therefore be described in detail.

Lateral internal sphincterotomy avoids a keyhole deformity and the fissure usually heals extremely quickly. The operation may involve a single division of the internal sphincter or multiple radial sections. It may be performed under local anaesthesia using local infiltration, caudal anaesthesia or the epidural route. Using local infiltration, the operation can be performed in the office (Gingold, 1987) or outpatient department (Magee and Thompson, 1966). The concept of immediate therapy using local anaesthetic after consultation and diagnosis is extremely attractive (Ray et al, 1974). However, the results of clinical trials have now persuaded us that local anaesthesia is inferior to a short general anaesthetic for internal sphincterotomy (Marby et al, 1979; Keighley et al, 1981; Weaver et al, 1987). Furthermore, in view of the risk of iatrogenic incontinence we believe that in future the first approach will be topical application of a nitrate preparation.

Most surgeons in the UK still perform either a subcutaneous or open lateral sphincterotomy under general anaesthesia. However, in Europe and North America there are some strong advocates (Rudd, 1975; Abcarian, 1980; Ravikumar et al, 1982) for the subcutaneous and open technique as an outpatient procedure under local anaesthesia. Furthermore, the proponents of this operation report excellent results (Millar, 1971; Notaras, 1971).

Anal dilatation

Case selection

Before advising anal dilatation it is important to exclude factors which might increase the risk of incontinence, such as women with obstetric injuries, previous anal surgery, or neurological disorders. Indeed, many would now take the view that anal dilatation should be used only sparingly – certainly not more than once and probably only in men and nullipara.

Counselling

The risk of flatus incontinence and occasional faecal incontinence should be explained. Patients should be told that the skin tag (if present) will not be removed because it usually disappears once the fissure has healed.

Technique

No bowel preparation is required and patients are usually admitted to a day ward. After anaesthesia, the patient is placed in the left lateral position (although the lithotomy position can be used) with the knees and hips well flexed and with the buttocks a short distance over the edge of the anaesthetic trolley (Figure 13.10a). A sigmoidoscopy is performed unless this has been possible beforehand. The index finger of the right hand is inserted into the anorectum, cautiously followed by the index finger of the left hand. An assistant should hold the patient with the hips and knees well flexed since dilatation often causes the patient to straighten out, making access to the perineum difficult.

The two index fingers should be gently parted in the lateral and anteroposterior plane, then circumferentially around the anus so that the fibres of the internal sphincter may be gently broken radially. Two fingers of each hand can now be inserted and the manoeuvre repeated (Figure 13.10b). Constricting bands may be felt to give way as the anus is progressively dilated. Three fingers of each hand can now be introduced and traction applied in a similar manner (Figure 13.10c). However, most coloproctologists now believe that an eight-finger dilatation is dangerous, and we never advise more than a maximum of four fingers for dilatation. Lestar et al (1987) have described an ingenious

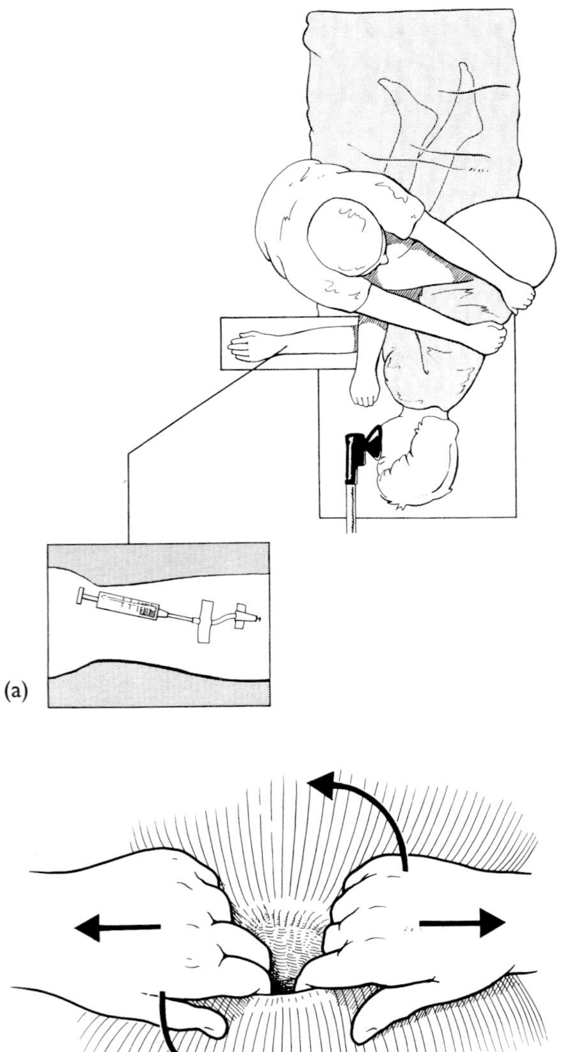

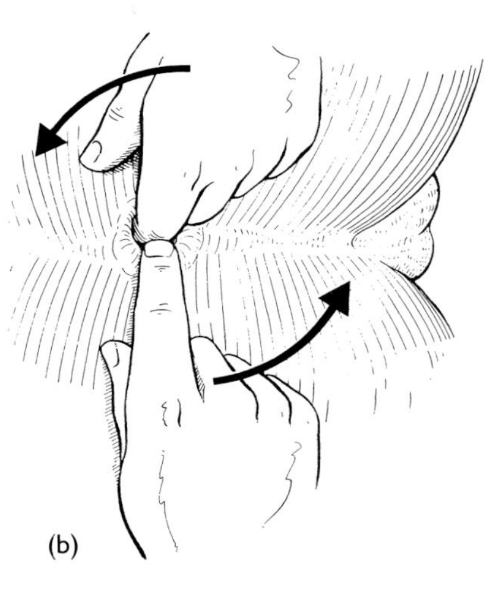

Figure 13.10a–c Anal dilatation. (a) The patient is placed in the left lateral position and is anaesthetized with the knees and hips flexed. Venous access is important for the anaesthetist; a nurse steadies the patient. (b) Two fingers are inserted gently into the anal canal. The canal is dilated using a circumferential sweeping movement. (c) Eventually, using this circumferential sweeping manoeuvre, it is possible to insert three or possibly four fingers into the anal canal.

method of avoiding excessive sphincter dilatation by tying a non-elastic ligature around the surgeon's finger, the length of the ligature depending on the risk of precipitating incontinence – being short (10–12 cm) in multiparous and long (16–18 cm) in young men with high anal pressure.

After dilatation a sponge may be inserted into the anal canal to prevent haematoma. The sponge, liberally smeared with either a lubricating gel or chlorhexidine solution, should be mounted on large sponge-holding forceps of the type illustrated in Figure 13.12b and inserted into the anal canal. If these purpose-designed sponge-holding forceps are used, the blades can be disengaged, released and withdrawn, leaving the sponge in position.

The patient should remain in the left lateral position. The sponge is removed after about one hour. If this is painful, an opiate analgesic may be given. The patient can usually be discharged from hospital after 3–4 h, with a supply of analgesic such as paracetamol which will not cause constipation. We also provide sterculia or ispaghula granules and some local anaesthetic cream which can be applied if required. Although Lord (1968) advises regular postoperative dilatation, we find that patients usually consider this manoeuvre distasteful and the compliance rate is low. Furthermore, fissures heal so quickly after anal dilatation (Marby et al, 1979) that the use of an anal dilator seems unnecessary.

Complications

Side-effects of anal dilatation include bleeding, haematoma, anal discomfort, incontinence of flatus, occasionally temporary liquid stool incontinence and retention of urine. If the patient has coexisting haemorrhoids, anal dilatation may precipitate their prolapse, but this is usually painless (Watts et al, 1964). Bacteraemia, a known complication of anorectal surgery and even rectal examination (Hoffman et al, 1978; Tandberg and Reed, 1978; Sykes et al, 1983), may occur after anal dilatation. Goldman et al (1986) report bacteraemia in 8% of patients and therefore advise that prophylactic antibiotics should be given to all patients with valvular disease or prosthetic implants.

We monitored complications of anal dilatation in 136 patients with anal fissure and reported no cases of urinary retention, but nine patients bled after operation and four developed haematoma. Only one patient developed temporary incontinence of faeces and none of the procedures were complicated by severe anal pain. Prolapse of haemorrhoids occurred in three patients. The overall healing rate at 1 year was 92%. Transient incontinence was reported in over 30% by Watts et al (1964). Permanent incontinence is the most serious complication and may occur in over 10% of patients (Nielsen et al, 1993). The incidence of incontinence varies considerably and must depend on the extent of the dilatation and the amount of force used. However, permanent incontinence must now be recognized as a complication of the operation which must be explained to patients if it is to be used for treatment of anal fissure.

If the patient has a diligent general practitioner, follow-up by the surgeon is probably unnecessary. If the hospital is keeping an audit of results, a follow-up visit at 6 weeks and a final appointment 12 months later is probably adequate.

We do not use an anal dilator postoperatively.

Open internal sphincterotomy

Case selection and counselling

Sphincterotomy is not advised in patients with a risk of incontinence, particularly women with obstetric trauma, anyone who has had a previous anal operation, or anyone with low anal canal pressure (Prohn and Bonner, 1995). In view of the data on incontinence after sphincterotomy from Minneapolis (García-Aguilar et al, 1996), all patients should be informed of this risk before treatment. Recent data also suggest that the length of the sphincterotomy has a direct association with the risk of incontinence, and that the extent of the smooth muscle division should be tailored to the clinical situation (Littlejohn and Newstead, 1997; García-Aguilar et al, 1998).

Technique

Open sphincterotomy is usually performed under general anaesthetic as a day procedure; alternatively, regional or topical local anaesthesia can be used. A disposable phosphate enema is usually ordered to empty the rectum before operation. The operation may be performed in the left lateral, lithotomy or jack-knife position. In practice, most European surgeons use the lithotomy position, placing the legs in stirrups, whereas in North America the prone jack-knife position is preferred. If local anaesthesia is used it is advisable to establish venous access so that midazolam or pethidine can also be administered if there is undue pain or anxiety during the operation. It is also advisable to smear some local anaesthetic lignocaine jelly around the fissure and to infiltrate around the fissure as well as at the operation site. If a general anaesthetic is used it is preferable to avoid muscle relaxants and to employ a light inhalational anaesthetic so as to facilitate identification of the intersphincteric plane. Sigmoidoscopy is advised if this has not been performed earlier.

Most surgeons, including ourselves, prefer a 3 cm lateral circumferential intra-anal incision to approach the internal sphincter (Parks, 1967; Oh, 1978), although Ray et al (1974) use a radial incision. The left half of the perianal skin is shaved before the operation and a Parks self-retaining retractor is inserted with the blades in the 6 and 12 o'clock positions (Figure 13.11a). The intermuscular depression between the internal and external sphincters is defined by palpation, and 30 mL of a 1:200 000 solution of adrenaline with 0.25% bupivacaine is infiltrated into the intersphincteric and submucosal plane proximally as far as the dentate line. A 2–3 cm lateral circumferential incision is made over the skin at the site of infiltration. The mucosa of the lower anal canal is freed from the underlying internal sphincter as far as the dentate line by scissor dissec-

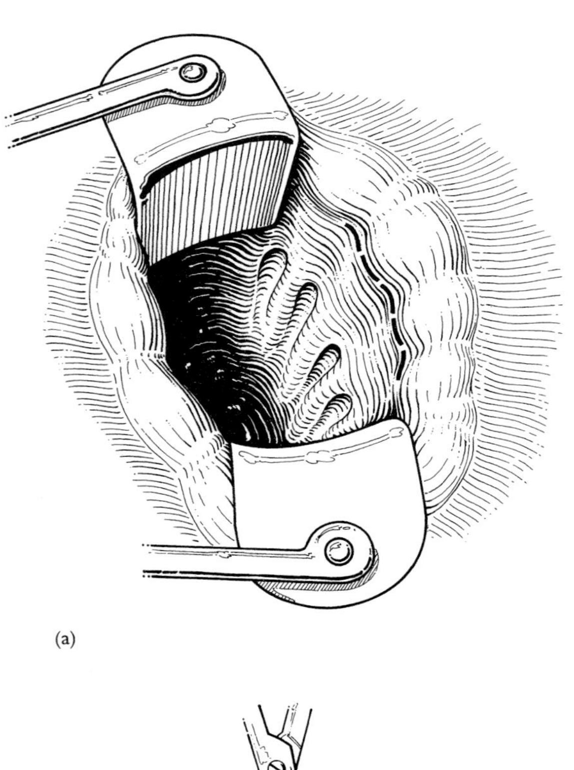

(a)

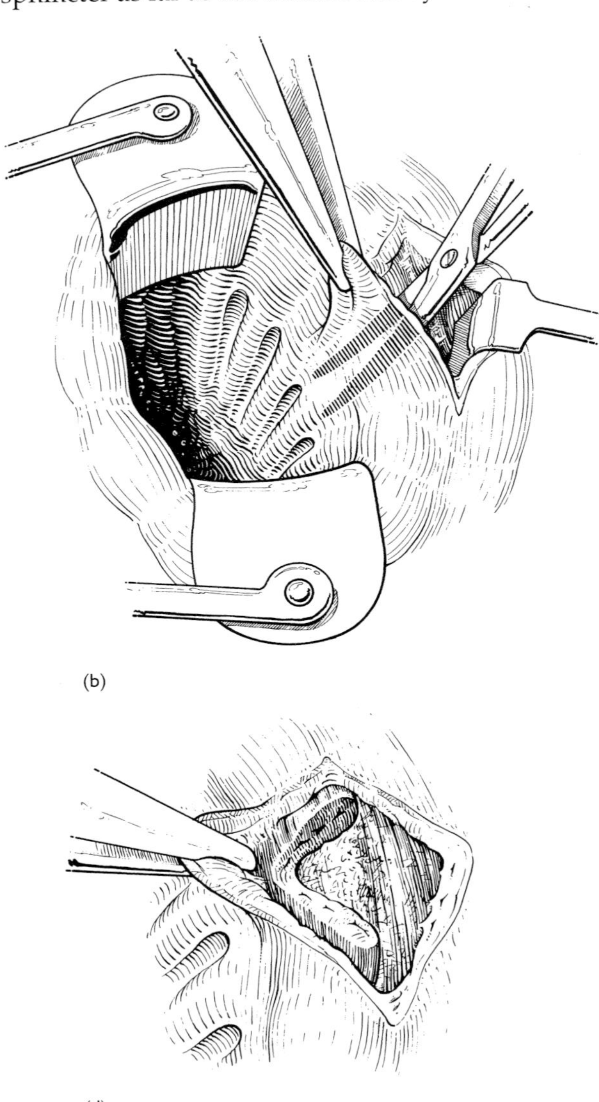

(b)

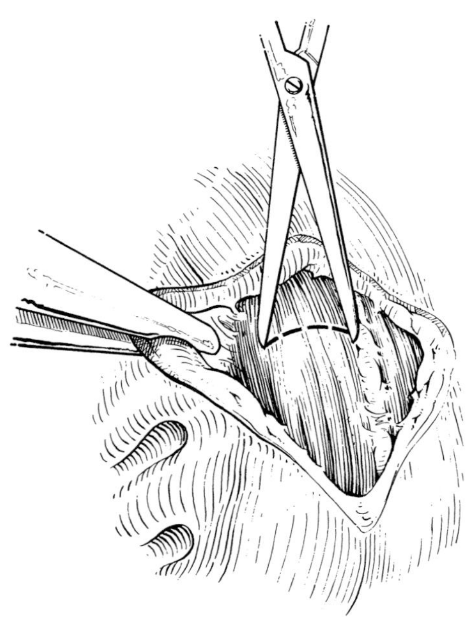

(c)

(d)

Figure 13.11a–d Open internal sphincterotomy. (a) An intra-anal incision is placed just inside the cutaneous margin of the anal canal at the site of the intersphincteric groove. (b) The mucosa of the anal canal is dissected from the internal anal sphincter. The intersphincteric space is then exposed. (c) Once the internal sphincter has been carefully dissected from the mucosa and the external sphincter, it is divided. (d) It is usual to divide only the lower half of the internal anal sphincter.

tion (Figure 13.11b). Care should be taken not to buttonhole the anal mucosa. The intersphincteric plane is then opened using scissor dissection, thus isolating the internal sphincter which is then divided with scissors up to but not above the dentate line (Figure 13.11c). After sphincterotomy, the fibres of the internal sphincter will have retracted circumferentially, leaving the external sphincter visible (Figure 13.11d). All visible bleeding points are secured and the skin wound either left open or sutured. In the open operation, tamponade by an anal sponge is usually not necessary.

Patients are prescribed bulk laxatives and non-constipating analgesics after the operation.

Haematoma and a low-lying fistula-in-ano have been reported but they are rare (Bailey et al, 1978). Apart from occasional urinary retention, delayed healing, bleeding, pain, pruritis ani, discharge and perianal abscess, there are no other specific complications (Walker et al, 1985). Minor complications may be marginally more common following open rather than closed sphincterotomy.

Complications

Internal sphincterotomy results in complete healing of the fissure in 92–100% of patients (Bailey et al, 1978; Lewis et al, 1988; Pernikoff et al, 1994; Lock and Thomson, 1997). Temporary incontinence of flatus and of liquids was reported by Leong et al (1994) in up to 9% but usually resolved 2–3 months after operation. Permanent incontinence has been reported in 5–6% (Walker et al, 1985; Lewis et al, 1988). However, García-Aguilar et al (1996) report

(a)

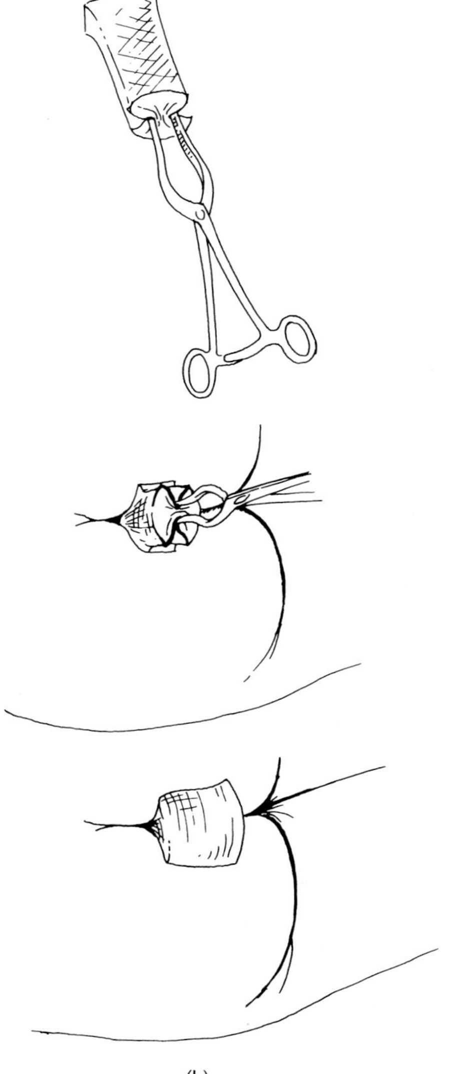

(b)

Figure 13.12a–b Lateral subcutaneous sphincterotomy under local anaesthetic. (a) The intersphincteric plane is infiltrated using lignocaine with a 1:300 000 solution of adrenaline. The perianal skin is similarly infiltrated with the same solution. With the index finger of the left hand in the anal canal, a fine cataract knife with a beaver blade is inserted in the 3 o'clock position in the intersphincteric plane. The blade is introduced, lying parallel to the fibres of the internal sphincter. It is then rotated through 90 degrees and the internal sphincter is divided. (b) In order to prevent a haematoma, anal tamponade is achieved with a sponge placed within the anal canal, using sponge-holding forceps.

persistent flatus incontinence in 30%, soiling in 27% and episodes of true incontinence in 12%. This incidence of incontinence was higher with open than with subcutaneous sphincterotomy.

In the light of these reports, even open sphincterotomy should not now be undertaken without warning patients of the risks, and not until pharmacological agents have been thoroughly explored. It could even be argued that island advancement techniques should be tried first in fissures unhealed by conservative treatment.

Closed lateral subcutaneous sphincterotomy

Case selection and counselling

The remarks above concerning open sphincterotomy are equally applicable to the closed technique. There is a definite risk of incontinence, particularly in patients who have had a previous anal operation, the elderly or those who have a history of obstetric trauma. Patients must be told of this risk before operation.

Rationale

The advantage of subcutaneous sphincterotomy compared with open sphincterotomy is that there is no incision, so there is less postoperative pain and a more rapid return to full activity. The operation can readily be performed in the office or in the outpatient department under local anaesthesia. Furthermore there is a lower incidence of incontinence compared with open sphincterotomy (García-Aguilar et al, 1996).

No bowel preparation is required. It is almost always possible to perform the procedure under local anaesthesia. If a general anaesthetic is preferred the patient is admitted to a day unit. We usually perform the operation in the lithotomy position, when using general anaesthetic, but it is less embarrassing and more comfortable for the patient if the left lateral position may be used for local anaesthetic techniques.

Technique with local anaesthesia

The patient is placed in the left lateral position with the buttocks well over the side of the couch. A tube of local anaesthetic cream, a syringe containing 40 mL of 0.25% xylocaine and a cataract knife are required. After smearing some local anaesthetic cream over the fissure, the index finger of the left hand is placed into the anal canal and a liberal amount of lignocaine solution is infiltrated into the intersphincteric plane at the 3 o'clock position as well as behind the fissure (Figure 13.12a). Pressure is then applied to disperse the local anaesthetic. The intersphincteric plane is seen as a gutter just beyond the anal verge (Figure 13.13a,b). The cataract knife is first inserted into the intersphincteric groove with the blade lying parallel to the fibres of the internal sphincter as far as the dentate line (Figure 13.13c). The knife is then rotated through 90 degrees with the blade at right-angles to the internal sphincter, facing inwards towards the anal mucosa (Figure 13.13d). The blade is now advanced towards the index finger, taking care not to breach the mucosa. During this manoeuvre the fibres of the internal sphincter will be felt to give way (Figure 13.13e). The knife is now removed and a V-shaped defect will be felt. If the procedure has not achieved a palpable deficiency, the operation may need to be repeated on the opposite side of the anal canal. A foam sponge may be inserted so as to minimize postoperative haematoma (see Figure 13.12b).

We prefer to divide the internal sphincter from the intersphincteric plane inwards towards the mucosa, as described by Hoffman and Goligher (1970). Notaras (1969) prefers to place the blade in the submucosal plane and to divide the internal sphincter laterally, but it is conceivable that by using this technique there is less control over the amount of external sphincter that may be divided.

Comment on local anaesthetic sphincterotomy

We used to perform all lateral subcutaneous sphincterotomy procedures under local anaesthesia. Unfortunately, there was a high recurrence rate of 50% compared with 17% after lateral subcutaneous sphincterotomy under general anaesthesia (Marby et al, 1979). Indeed the results were found to be much better when the operation was performed under general anaesthesia (Keighley et al, 1981); in our experience the results of sphincterotomy under general anaesthesia were the same as those achieved by anal dilatation (Weaver et al, 1987). As a result of our own clinical trials we have abandoned outpatient sphincterotomy under local anaesthetic but accept that the procedure has given excellent results when performed under local anaesthetic in other centres (Millar, 1971; Notaras, 1971). Such centres have found that their patients can usually return to work the day after the operation. Postoperative management following lateral subcutaneous sphincterotomy under local anaesthesia is the same as for anal

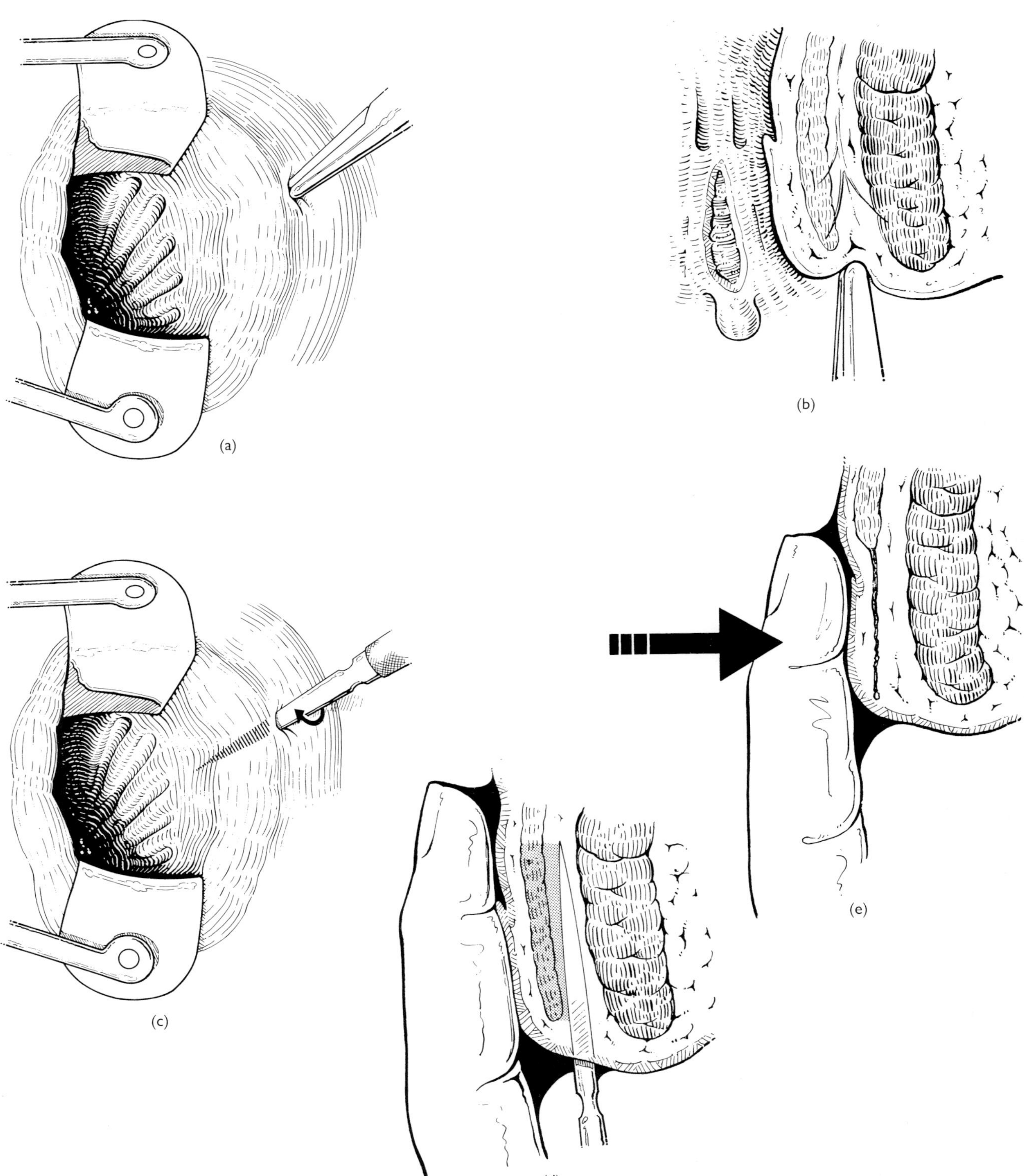

Figure 13.13a–e Lateral subcutaneous sphincterotomy under general anaesthetic. (a) The intersphincteric groove is identified. This lies just inside the anal canal. (b) This shows the intersphincteric groove in a coronal section of the anal canal. (c) A fine cataract knife is inserted in the intersphincteric plane with the knife lying parallel to the fibres of the internal anal sphincter. The blade is then rotated through 90 degrees. (d) The lower fibres of the internal anal sphincter are divided. A finger is placed in the anal canal to ensure that the mucosa is not breached. (e) At the completion of the procedure a defect will be palpable in the internal anal sphincter. Haemostasis is secured using sponge tamponade.

dilatation and consists of using bulk laxatives and non-constipating analgesics. The use of an anal dilator seems to be unnecessary.

Technique with general anaesthesia

The technique of lateral sphincterotomy under general anaesthesia is initially identical to that performed under local anaesthesia and is illustrated in Figure 13.13a–e.

General anaesthesia increases the scope of treatment and allows additional procedures to be more easily carried out. Thus, if a large skin tag is present it may be excised. A light general anaesthetic is desirable in order that anal tone is preserved so as to define the intersphincteric plane before making the incision. If there is a fissure–fistula this can also be laid open (Figure 13.14). There is no evidence that performing internal sphincterotomy with other procedures increases morbidity (Leong et al, 1994). Do not be tempted to divide the internal sphincter at this site since the fistula is usually superficial to the internal sphincter and division is likely to result in a gutter deformity which may be complicated by soiling and incontinence.

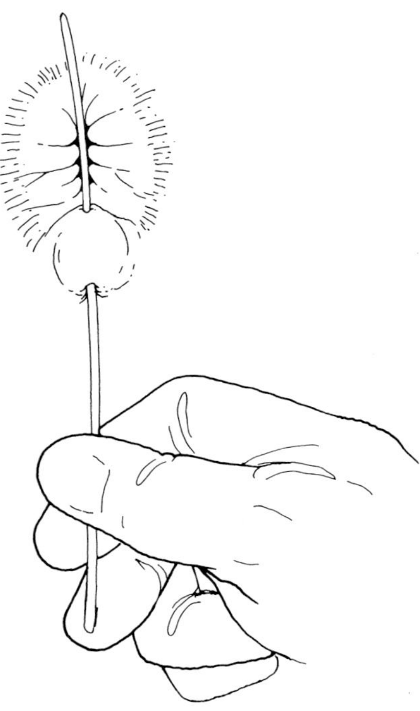

Figure 13.14 Treatment of a fissure–fistula. Occasionally a fistula-in-ano is complicated by a low-lying fistula associated with a skin tag. Under these circumstances the fissure is treated in the usual way and the fistula track is laid open over a fistula probe.

Complications

There are few postoperative complications following subcutaneous sphincterotomy performed under either local or general anaesthesia (Hoffmann and Goligher, 1970; Millar, 1971; Notaras, 1971; Oh, 1978; Lewis et al, 1988; Leong et al, 1994). Haematoma has been reported to occur in 4–6% of cases , abscess in 1–2% and fistula-in-ano in 0.5–1%.

Most patients can go home on the same day and are advised to take non-constipating analgesics and a bulk laxative. However, incontinence is a recognized complication, transient incontinence occurring in 9–14% and permanent incontinence in 6–7%; but a report from Minneapolis suggests that permanent incontinence may be much higher (García-Aguilar et al, 1996). Hence, this method of treatment should not be undertaken unless patients are counselled and the potential morbidity explained.

Results of treatment

The clinical results of anal dilatation, lateral open sphincterotomy and lateral subcutaneous sphincterotomy under local or general anaesthetic are listed in Table 13.9. These are results from non-randomized studies and varying criteria have been used to define recurrence and complications. In particular, the quality and duration of follow-up differs markedly. The anatomical effectiveness of sphincterotomy can be checked by ultrasonography; small defects are associated with a greater risk of recurrence (García-Granero et al, 1998).

Recurrence rates

The recurrence rate following anal dilatation may be as high as 16% (Watts et al, 1964). Comparisons suggest a higher recurrence rate following anal dilatation than sphincterotomy (Collopy and Ryan, 1979; Jensen et al, 1984). Open sphincterotomy has a recurrence rate from 0% to 8% (Lock and Thomson, 1977; Bailey et al, 1978; Lewis et al, 1988) and lateral subcutaneous sphincterotomy under local or general anaesthetic has a rate of only 2–3% (Millar, 1971; Notarus, 1971; Oh, 1978). Lewis et al (1988) compared open sphincterotomy with lateral subcutaneous sphincterotomy: persistent fissure was more common in patients who had an open sphincterotomy than closed sphincterotomy (8% and 5% respectively).

The incidence of complications following all procedures is generally low and comparable. In our own randomized trials, the complication rates at 1 year were as shown in Table 13.10.

Table 13.9 Results of therapy.

Result	Open sphincterotomy			Anal dilatation	Lateral subcutaneous sphincterotomy				
					GA	LA			
	Lock and Thomson (1977) (*n* = 82)	*Bailey et al (1978)* (*n* = 418)	*Lewis et al (1988)* (*n* = 103)	*Watts et al (1964)* (*n* = 90)	*Oh (1978)* (*n* = 200)	*Hoffman and Goligher (1970)* (*n* = 99)	*Millar (1971)* (*n* = 99)	*Notaras (1971)* (*n* = 82)	*Lewis et al (1988)* (*n* = 247)
Recurrence (%)	0	8	8	16	2	3	0	2	5
Complications (%)									
Incontinence of faeces	0	2	6	28	3	12	3	10	7
Bleeding or haematoma	1	1	1	0	4	22	6	0	0
Fistula	0	1	0	0	0.5	1	1	0	0
Abscess	0	0	2	0	2	1	1	0	2
Prolapsed haemorrhoids	0	0	0	1	0	2	1	10	0
Urinary retention	1	0.2	0	0	0	0	0	0	0

GA, general anaesthesia; LA, local anaesthesia.

Table 13.10 Results of randomized controlled trials from the Birmingham series.

	Anal dilatation		Lateral subcutaneous sphincterotomy			
			Local anaesthesia		General anaesthesia	
	A (*n* = 63)	B (*n* = 78)	C (*n* = 78)	D (*n* = 34)	E (*n* = 37)	F (*n* = 48)
Recurrences at 1 year (%)	5	6	17	50	8	5
Complications (%)						
Bleeding	0	9	1	3	3	0
Haematoma	0	0	5	6	0	2
Fistula	0	0	1	0	0	0
Faecal incontinence	0	0	0	3	0	2
Pain	0	0	0	6	6	0

Trials: A versus F (Weaver et al, 1987); B versus C (Marby et al, 1979); D versus E (Keighley et al, 1981).

Incontinence

Faecal and flatus incontinence following sphincterotomy in Leeds was graded and compared with defects in continence among 100 normal subjects (Table 13.11).

Some degree of impaired continence was observed in 11% of the normal subjects, compared with an almost identical figure following lateral subcutaneous sphincterotomy (12%). In contrast, the incidence of impaired continence was much higher after open posterior sphincterotomy (34%) (Melange et al, 1992) and after anal dilatation (31%) (Watts et al, 1964). There was a 2% incidence of abscess in both groups. Lewis et al (1988) found that transient incontinence was more common after open than lateral subcutaneous sphincterotomy, being 14% and 9% respectively, but long-term incontinence was similar (6% and 7%).

Nielsen et al (1993) performed anal ultrasonography in patients after anal dilatation. Eleven of 18 continent patients had sphincter defects (10 internal, 2 external) and both incontinent patients had diffuse defects in the internal sphincter. Given the ultrasonographic findings, they were surprised that more were not incontinent. Similar studies were performed by Sultan et al (1994) before and after open sphincterotomy. All apart from one patient had an obvious defect postoperatively. Incontinence was recorded in three, two of whom had preoperative evidence of postobstetric external

Table 13.11 Comparison of impaired continence.

	n	*Impaired flatus*	*Impaired control of faeces*	*Soiling*	*One or more defects*
Normals	100	10 (10)	3 (3)	2 (2)	11 (11)
Anal dilatation	90	12 (13)	2 (2)	20 (22)	28 (31)
Posterior open sphincterotomy	127	24 (19)	11 (9)	28 (22)	43 (34)
Lateral subcutaneous sphincterotomy	99	6 (6)	1 (1)	7 (7)	12 (12)

Values in parentheses are percentages.
From Watts et al (1964) and Hoffman and Goligher (1970).

Table 13.12 Incontinence after operation for anal fissure

Authors	*Operation*	*n*	*Flatus*	*Liquid*	*Solid*	*Soiling*
Leong et al (1994)	IS	57	9t	0	0	0
Sultan et al (1994)	OIS	15	3ns	0	0	0
Pernikoff et al (1994)	IS	50	14p	2p	2p	22p
Nielson et al (1993)	MDA	32	4	0	0	2
Selvaggi et al (1992)	SIC	56	3t	0	0	2t
Melange et al (1992)	PF	76	13	8	0	7

Operations: OIS, open internal sphincterotomy; IS, open and closed sphincterotomy; SIS, subcutaneous closed sphincterotomy; MDA, manual dilatation of anus; PF, post-fissurectomy. t, transient; p, persistent; ns, not stated.

sphincter injury. The extent of internal sphincter division was greater than expected in females. Thus great care should be exercised regarding the extent of sphincterotomy in women, especially in the presence of previous obstetric trauma.

Admittedly many patients suffered only transient incontinence, particularly after internal sphincterotomy (Selvaggi et al, 1992; Leong et al, 1994; Pernikoff et al, 1994). Permanent incontinence is reported, though it appears to be more common after anal dilatation than sphincterotomy (12% and 3% respectively) (Nielson et al, 1993; Pernikoff et al, 1994) (Table 13.12).

A recent retrospective study based on postal questionnaires from Minneapolis (Table 13.13) may be criticized owing to a rather poor response rate; however it clearly identifies the extent of the permanent morbidity rate from impaired continence (García-Aguilar et al, 1996). Permanent difficulty in controlling gas was reported in 30% of patients after open sphincterotomy and in 24% after subcutaneous sphincterotomy. Soiling of underclothes was reported in 27% after open sphincterotomy compared with 16% after subcutaneous sphincterotomy. Accidental bowel movements were reported by 12% of patients after open sphincterotomy and in 3% after subcutaneous sphincterotomy. These frightening results imply that any operation carries a risk of incontinence but it seems to be worse after open rather than closed sphincterotomy. Clearly, therefore, patients need to be warned about this risk, particularly as inadvertent injury to the external sphincter can occur (Farouk et al, 1997). Given the risk of permanent incontinence, it is likely that pharmacological manipulation is likely to play a greater therapeutic role in the future.

Table 13.13 Non-randomized comparison between open sphincterotomy and closed subcutaneous sphincterotomy (postal questionnaire).

Feature	*Open*	*Closed subcutaneous*
Questionnaires sent	521	343
Questionnaires returned	324	225
Persistent symptoms	3.4%	5.3%
Recurrence of fissure requiring re-operation	3.4%	4.0%
Permanent difficulty controlling gas	30.3%	23.6%
Soiling of underclothes	26.7%	16.1%
Accidental bowel movements	11.8%	3.1%
Dissatisfied or very dissatisfied	10.1%	7.5%

From García-Aguilar et al (1996).

Randomized trials of anal dilatation or sphincterotomy

We have performed three randomized trials to compare anal dilatation with lateral subcutaneous sphincterotomy under either local or general anaesthesia (see Table 13.10). We found that lateral subcutaneous sphincterotomy under general anaesthetic gave results which were comparable to those after anal dilatation. A recurrence rate of 5% or 8%, and a 0% or 2% incidence of incontinence, was found after sphincterotomy, compared with recurrence in 5% and 6%, and no incontinence, after anal dilatation. The incidence of bleeding, haematoma, fistula and pain did not differ significantly between the groups.

Boulos and Araujo (1984) compared subcutaneous with open sphincterotomy. There were no recurrent fissures and the speed of pain relief was comparable in the groups. Bruising was more common in the subcutaneous than in the open operation group; transient impaired control of flatus was similar. However, all operations were performed under general anaesthetic and tamponade was not used. Olsen et al (1987) also compared anal dilatation with lateral subcutaneous sphincterotomy. The numbers were small but recurrence was recorded in three of ten patients after anal dilatation and in only one of ten following sphincterotomy. Two patients in each group had transient incontinence.

Kortbeek et al (1992) reported a randomized trial of open versus subcutaneous sphincterotomy in 112 patients. Complication rates were 7% and 9% respectively, hospital stay was marginally longer for open sphincterotomy (2.3 days versus 1.7 days)

Table 13.14 Randomized controlled trial comparing open sphincterotomy and closed subcutaneous sphincterotomy.

Feature	*Open (n = 54)*	*Closed subcutaneous (n = 58)*
Complications		
Bleeding	1	3
Urinary retention	2	1
Cellulitis	1	0
Thrombosed haemorrhoid	0	1
Totals	4 (7.4%)	5 (8.6%)
Postoperative pain score (lower = less pain)		
Day 1	5.7	3.3
Day 2	5.3	2.6
Day 3	4.2	2.3
Hospital stay (days)	2.3 ± 0.1	1.7 ± 0.2
Healing	94.4%	96.6%

From Kortbeek et al (1992).

Table 13.15 Open lateral internal sphincterotomy randomized to general or localized anaesthetic.

Feature	*General anaesthetic* (*n* = 30)	*Local anaesthetic* (*n* = 26)
Impaired continence at 1 month		
Flatus	3	3
Soiling	3	2
Impaired continence at 12 months		
Soiling	1	0
Postoperative abscess	1	0

From Selvaggi et al (1992).

and healing rates were 94% and 97%. The authors concluded that subcutaneous sphincterotomy gave less discomfort and a shorter stay while providing results which were at least as good as the open procedure (Table 13.14).

Selvaggi et al (1992) compared subcutaneous sphincterotomy under local or general anaesthesia and reported identical results, thus suggesting that local anaesthesia was an acceptable method in compliant patients (Table 13.15).

Advancement flaps

The concept of excising a chronic fissure and covering the defect with a flap of skin or an island of skin and subcutaneous tissue is attractive since there should be no risk of incontinence and a reasonable prospect of healing, particularly if one believes that these are ischaemic ulcers and that skin flaps provide improved blood supply (see Figure 12.45a–c).

Nyam et al (1995) reported the results of island advancement flaps in 21 patients with recurrent fissures with low resting anal pressures who were thus at risk of incontinence from conventional therapy, particularly as anal ultrasonography had demonstrated sphincteric defects in 15. All flaps healed primarily with preservation of sensation. Perfect continence was monitored in all patients, there were no complications, and all fissures healed with minimal discomfort. Subsequently, Leong and Seow-Cheon (1995) performed a randomized trial in 40 patients to compare open sphincterotomy with anal advancement flap. No patients developed incontinence. Hospital stay was comparable but operating time was slightly (5 minutes) longer for the anal advancement flap. One patient developed an abscess after sphincterotomy, there were no complications after advancement flap. However, fissures healed in all 20 patients after sphincterotomy, compared with only 17 of 20 following advancement flap (Table 13.16).

Certainly, island advancement deserves more careful scrutiny in the treatment of anal fissure, particularly in patients with low resting anal pressures who might be at increased risk of incontinence after conventional sphincterotomy (see Figure 12.44a–c). Anoplasty has, of course, a well-recognized role in patients with anal stenosis following a fissurectomy or haemorrhoidectomy (Neelakandan, 1996). Many different types of skin flap have been described, such as the double buttock flap (see Figure 12.45a–d), but this subject is described fully in the chapter devoted to haemorrhoidectomy (Chapter 12).

Table 13.16 Randomized trial comparing open internal sphincterotomy (OIS) with anal advancement flap (AAF) for chronic fissure-in-ano.

Feature	*OIS* (*n* = 20)	*AAF* (*n* = 20)
Operation time (minutes)	5 (5–10)	10 (5–20)
Hospital stay (days)	2 (2–2)	2 (2–3)
Healing of fissure	20/20	17/20
Postoperative incontinence	0	0
Complications	1 abscess	0

From Leong and Seow-Choen (1995).

Millar DM (1971) Subcutaneous lateral internal anal sphincterotomy for anal fissure. *Br J Surg* **58**: 737–739.

Morgan CN & Thompson HR (1956) Surgical anatomy of the anal canal with special reference to the surgical importance of the internal sphincter and conjoint longitudinal muscle. *Ann R Coll Surg Engl* **19**: 88–93.

Neelakandan B (1996) Double Y–V plasty for postsurgical anal stricture. *Br J Surg* **83**: 1599.

Nielson MB, Rasmussen OO, Pedersen JF & Christiansen J (1993) Risk of sphincter damage and anal incontinence after anal dilatation for fissure-in-ano: an endosonographic study. *Dis Colon Rectum* **36**: 677–680.

Neri M, Marzio L, De Angelis C, Peiramico A, Mezzeti A & Cuccurullo F (1988) Effect of ketanserin, a selective antiserotoninergic drug, on human anal canal pressure. *Int J Colorect Dis* **3**: 219–221.

Northmann BJ & Schuster MM (1974) Internal anal sphincter derangement with anal fissures. *Gastroenterology* **67**: 216–220.

Notaras M (1969) Lateral subcutaneous sphincterotomy for anal fissure: a new technique. *Proc R Soc Med* **62**: 713.

Notaras MJ (1971) The treatment of anal fissure by lateral subcutaneous internal sphincterotomy: a technique and results. *Br J Surg* **58**: 96–100.

Nyam DCNK, Wilson RG, Stewart KJ, Farouk R & Bartolo DCC (1995) Island advancement flaps in the management of anal fissures. *Br J Surg* **82**: 326–328.

Oettlé GJ (1997) Glyceryl trinitrate vs sphincterotomy for treatment of chronic fissure-in-ano: a randomized, controlled trial. *Dis Colon Rectum* **40**: 1318–1320.

Oh C (1978) A modified technique for lateral internal sphincterotomy. *Surg Gynecol Obstet* **146**: 623–625.

O'Kelly T, Brading A & Mortensen N (1993) Nerve-mediated relaxation of the human internal anal sphincter: the role of nitric oxide. *Gut* **34**: 689–693.

Olsen J, Mortensen PE, Petersen IL & Christiansen J (1987) Anal sphincter function after treatment of fissure-in-ano by lateral subcutaneous sphincterotomy versus anal dilatation. *Int J Colorect Dis* **2**: 155–157.

Parks AG (1967) The management of fissure-in-ano. *Hosp Med* **1**: 737–739.

Pernikoff BJ, Eisenstat TE, Rubin RJ, Oliver GC & Salvati EP (1994) Reappraisal of partial lateral internal sphincterotomy. *Dis Colon Rectum* **37**: 1291–1295.

Pinho M, Correa JCO, Furtado A & Ramos JR (1993) Do hot baths promote anal sphincter relaxation? *Dis Colon Rectum* **36**: 273–274.

Pope CE (1959) An anorectal plastic operation for fissure and stenosis and its surgical principle. *Surg Gynecol Obstet* **108**: 249–253.

Prohn P & Bonner C (1995) Is manometry essential for surgery of chronic fissure-in-ano? *Dis Colon Rectum* **38**: 735–738.

Rattan S & Chakder S (1992) Role of nitric oxide as a mediator of internal anal sphincter relaxation. *Am J Physiol* **262**: G107–112.

Rattan S, Sarkar A & Chakder S (1992) Nitric oxide pathway in recto-anal inhibitory reflex of opossum internal anal sphincter. *Gastroenterology* **103**: 43–50.

Ravikumar TS, Sridhar S & Rao RN (1982) Subcutaneous lateral sphincterotomy for chronic fissure-in-ano. *Dis Colon Rectum* **25**: 789–801.

Ray JE, Penfold JCB, Garthright JB Jr & Robinson SH (1974) Lateral subcutaneous internal anal sphincterotomy for anal fissure. *Dis Colon Rectum* **17**: 139–144.

Regadas FSP, Batista LKdeO, Albuquerque JLA & Capaz FR (1993) Pharmacological study of the internal anal sphincter in patients with chronic anal fissure. *Br J Surg* **80**: 799–801.

Rodkey CV (1973) Office treatment of rectal and anal disease. *JAMA* **223**: 676–683.

Rudd WW (1975) Lateral subcutaneous internal sphincterotomy for chronic anal fissure: an outpatient procedure. *Dis Colon Rectum* **18**: 319–323.

Schouten WR, Briel JW & Auwerda JJA (1994) Relationship between anal pressure and anodermal blood flow. *Dis Colon Rectum* **37**: 664–669.

Schouten WR, Briel JW, Boerma MO et al (1996a) Pathophysiological aspects and clinical outcome of intra-anal application of isosorbide dinitrate in patients with chronic anal fissure. *Gut* **39**: 465–469.

Schouten WR, Briel JW, Auwerda JJA & De Graaf EJR (1996b) Ischaemic nature of anal fissure. *Br J Surg* **83**: 63–65.

Selvaggi F, Scotto di Carlo E, Silvestri A, Notaroberto A & Festa L (1992) A prospective study of lateral subcutaneous sphincterotomy under general or local anaesthesia for the treatment of anal fissure. *Coloproctology* **14**: 348–350.

Sentovich SM, Falk PM, Christensen MA et al (1996) Operative results of House advancement anoplasty. *Br J Surg* **83**: 1242–1244.

Shub HA, Salvati EP & Rubin RJ (1978) Conservative treatment of anal fissure: an unselected retrospective and continuous study. *Dis Colon Rectum* **21**: 582–583.

Sohn N, Eisenberg M, Weinstein MA, Lugo RN & Alder J (1992) Precise anorectal sphincter dilatation: its role in the therapy of anal fissures. *Dis Colon Rectum* **35**: 322–327.

Sultan AH, Kamm MA, Nicholls RJ & Bartram CI (1994) Prospective study of the extent of internal anal sphincter division during lateral sphincterotomy. *Dis Colon Rectum* **37**: 1031–1033.

Sumfest JM, Brown AC & Rozwadowski JV (1989) Histopathology of the internal anal sphincter in chronic anal fissure. *Dis Colon Rectum* **32**: 680–683.

Sweeney JL, Ritchie JK & Nicholls RJ (1988) Anal fissure in Crohn's disease. *Br J Surg* **75**: 56–57.

Sykes PA, Jones DM & Ostick G (1983) Bacteraemia during anorectal surgery. *J R Coll Surg Edinb* **25**: 178–181.

Tandberg D & Reed WP (1978) Blood cultures following rectal examination. *JAMA* **239**: 1789.

Tzu-Chi-Hsu & MacKeigan JM (1984) Surgical treatment of chronic anal fissure: a retrospective study of 1753 cases. *Dis Colon Rectum* **27**: 474–478.

Walker WA, Rothenberger DA & Goldberg SM (1985) Morbidity of internal sphincterotomy for anal fissure and stenosis. *Dis Colon Rectum* **28**: 832–835.

Watson SJ, Kamm MA, Nicholls RJ & Phillips RKS (1996) Topical glyceryl trinitrate in the treatment of chronic anal fissure. *Br J Surg* **83**: 771–775.

Watts J McK, Bennett RC & Goligher JC (1964) Stretching of anal sphincters in treatment of fissure-in-ano. *BMJ* **2**: 342–343.

Weaver RM, Ambrose NS, Alexander-Williams J & Keighley MRB (1987) Manual dilatation of the anus versus lateral subcutaneous sphincterotomy in the treatment of chronic fissure-in-ano: results of a prospective randomized clinical trial. *Dis Colon Rectum* **30**: 420–423.

Williams N, Scott NA & Irving MH (1995) Effect of lateral sphincterotomy on internal anal sphincter function. *Dis Colon Rectum* **38**: 700–704.

Williams N, Scott NA & Irving MH (1996) Does lateral sphincterotomy affect external anal sphincter function? *Res Surg* **8**: 36–39.

Xynos E, Tzortzinis A, Chrysos E, Tzovaras G & Vassilakis JS (1993) Anal manometry in patients with fissure-in-ano before and after internal sphincterotomy. *Int J Colorect Dis* **8**: 125–128.

14 HIDRADENITIS SUPPURATIVA

Hidradenitis suppurativa is a chronic inflammatory disorder affecting the apocrine glands. The principal sites of the disease are the axillae, perineum, inguinal region, external genitalia and the anal canal. The importance of hidradenitis suppurativa is that it may mimic perianal abscess, anal fistula or Crohn's disease but, unlike these other conditions, successful treatment depends on wide surgical ablation.

AETIOLOGY AND PATHOPHYSIOLOGY

Apocrine disorder

Hidradenitis suppurativa was first described by Velpeau (1839) but Verneuil (1854) recognized that it was a disorder of sweat glands. It is now realized that hidradenitis principally affects the apocrine and not the eccrine sweat glands. Eccrine sweating occurs from the feet and hands, is confined to the dermis and is independent of hair follicles. By contrast, apocrine glands occur in the axilla, groin, anogenital region, the areola and submammary fold, the periumbilical region, the external auditory meatus, the scalp and some areas of the face (Bell and Ellis, 1978; Morgan and Hughes, 1979). The apocrine glands pierce the dermis entering the subcutaneous tissues and are usually associated with hair follicles. Apocrine glands become active only after puberty; their secretions are thick and malodorous, whereas eccrine sweat glands secrete saline. The distribution of apocrine glands varies between individuals and can be determined reliably only by chemical mapping (Morgan and Hughes, 1979).

Morgan and Hughes undertook a histological survey to determine the distribution and density of the apocrine glands in hidradenitis suppurativa. These glands are simple coiled tubular structures; they are situated principally in the dermis but may extend into the subcutaneous fat to a depth of 5 mm below the skin surface (Montagna and Parakkal, 1974). No significant difference in the number or size of apocrine glands was found in patients with hidradenitis suppurativa compared with normal subjects. Apocrine sweating is adrenergically controlled but there is doubt as to the exact mechanism by which the catecholamines reach the glands. Hurley and Shelley (1960) suggested that the first phase of secretion consists of sweat production within the apocrine tubule and the second phase is the expulsion of these secretions to the surface by contraction of myoepithelial cells surrounding the tubules.

Hormonal factors

There is now substantial evidence that hidradenitis suppurativa may be associated with an underlying endocrine disorder (Mortimer et al, 1986b; Harrison et al, 1988). Support for this theory is based on the fact that the onset of disease usually coincides with puberty (Greeley, 1951; Shelley and Cahn, 1955). Androgens are associated with increased keratinization of the skin, a factor which may predispose to keratin occlusion of the apocrine ducts (Brunsting, 1952; Kroepfli, 1976). Hidradenitis is modified by pregnancy (Cornbleet, 1952; Anderson and Dockerty, 1958; Harrison, 1964) and may become active premenstrually (Chalfant and Nance, 1970). Exacerbation of hidradenitis may be associated with hormone administration (Sulzberger, 1941) and increased androgen secretion secondary to Cushing's syndrome (Wile and Curtis, 1948). There is a well-recognized association between hidradenitis and acne, particularly in men: Block (1931) found that 43% of men with hidradenitis suffered from acne. Acne is associated with hormonal imbalance: elevated levels of circulating androgens, hyperprolactinaemia and reduced levels of sex hormone binding globulin (Darley et al, 1982).

Harrison et al (1985) from Cardiff investigated 13 women with hidradenitis who had a history of premenstrual exacerbation of their disease. A comprehensive hormone profile indicated that the only changes (compared with controls) were raised levels of prolactin and testosterone in a small proportion of patients. Elevated levels of prolactin and thyrotrophin were also demonstrated after administration of combined thyrotrophin releasing factor and gonadotrophin releasing hormone (Figure 14.1a,b). There was no significant difference in the basal levels of oestrogen, progesterone, testosterone, dihydroepiandrosterone and thyroxine. It was suggested that the exaggerated prolactin response in women with hidradenitis suppurativa might be due to the release of stored prolactin from

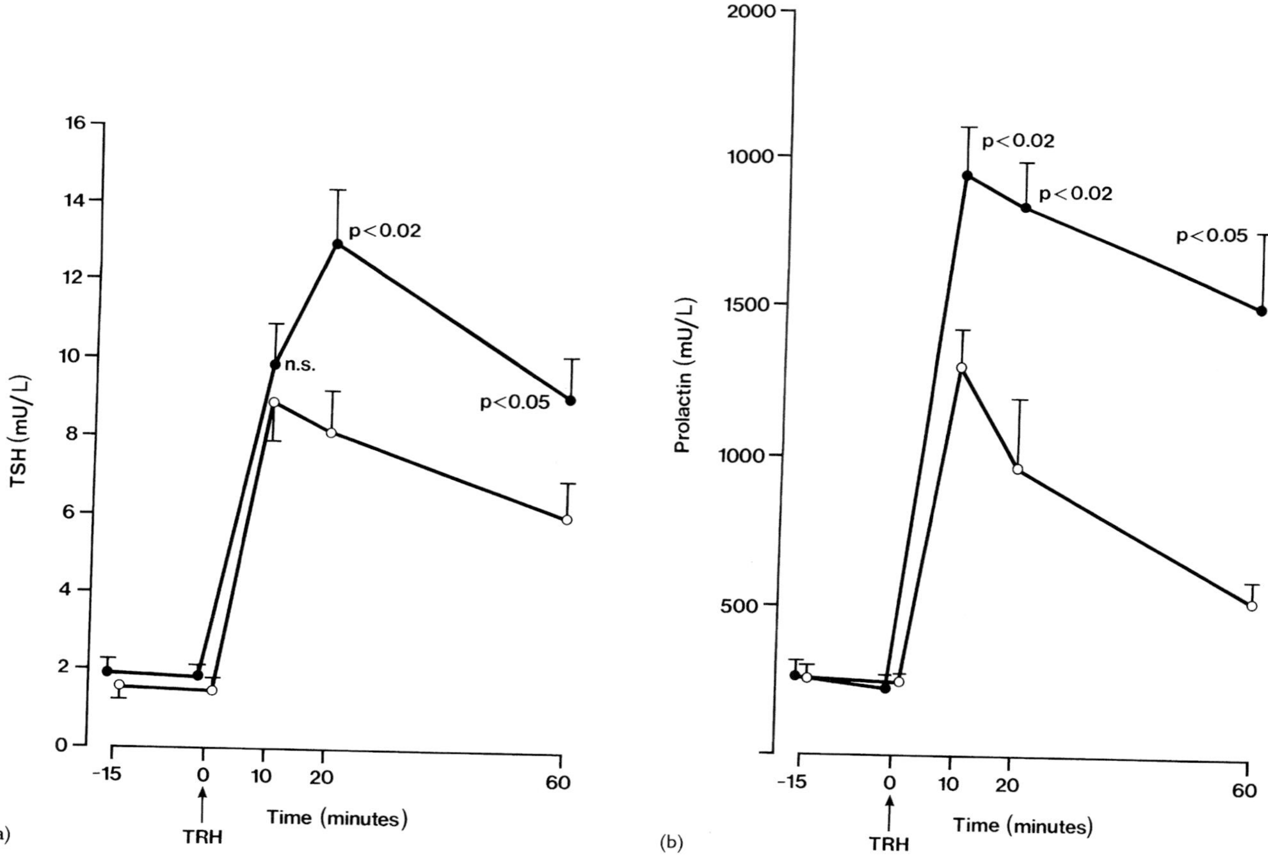

Figure 14.1a,b Endocrine abnormalities in hidradenitis. (a) Thyroid-stimulating hormone (TSH) levels in patients with hidradenitis (•—•; *n* = 13) compared with controls (o—o; *n* = 9). TRH, thyrotrophin-releasing hormone; n.s., not significant. (b) Prolactin levels in hidradenitis compared with controls.

increased oestrogen activity, rather than to a primary defect in the hypothalamo-pituitary axis (Miller et al, 1977; Peillon et al, 1982). Subsequent studies have suggested that the absence of premenstrual exacerbation is associated with raised androgens and reduced progesterone levels, which may be due to peripheral conversion in obese patients (Harrison et al, 1988).

The disordered keratinization in hidradenitis may reflect androgen excess, due either to primary androgen secretion by the gonads and adrenals or to elevated levels of circulating free hormones. Apocrine glands are a rich source of 5α-reductase which is capable of converting testosterone to its active form, 5α-dihydrotestosterone (Hay and Hodgkins, 1978). Apocrine sweat has also been shown to contain dihydroepiandrosterone sulphate which stimulates sebaceous activity (Labows et al, 1979).

Obesity seems to be an aetiological factor, being more prevalent in both males and females with hidradenitis than in normal subjects (Masson, 1969).

Bacterial proliferation secondary to obstruction

Ductal occlusion by keratin plugging is an important factor in the pathogenesis of the hidradenitis, resulting in duct dilatation, sweat retention, periductal leucocyte reaction and bacterial overgrowth (Shelley and Cahn, 1955). Obstruction and infection encourage ectasia of the apocrine gland. The organisms commonly isolated in hidradenitis (Thornton and Abcarian, 1978) are listed in Table 14.1. Staphylococci and aerobic Gram-negative bacteria are most frequent, but the obligate anaerobes are also common, in both the axilla and the perineum (Leacy et al, 1979; Brenner and Lookingbill, 1980). *Streptococcus milleri* may be an important pathogen (Highet et al, 1980).

Table 14.1 Results of wound culture in cases of patients with hidradenitis suppurativa.

Results	%
No growth (*n* = 50)	48
Positive growth (*n* = 54)	52
Staphylococcus epidermidis	44
Escherichia coli	19
α-Streptococcus	15
Others (including mixed flora)	22

Evidence that occlusion of apocrine glands is an important factor in the pathogenesis of hidradenitis emanates from studies in volunteers whose glands were deliberately occluded by tape (Shelley and Cahn, 1955). Occlusion for 6 months resulted in duct dilatation, bacterial proliferation, dermal cellulitis and destruction of glandular units resulting in fibrosis.

Secondary hidradenitis suppurativa occurs in Fox–Fordyce disease, a condition in which apocrine glands become occluded by mucin. Hidradenitis also occurs in acanthosis nigricans (Stone, 1976) as a result of pore occlusion by hyperkeratosis.

Other associated disorders

Other conditions which may be associated with hidradenitis suppurativa include diabetes mellitus (Chapman, 1972), hypercholesterolaemia (Adams and Haisten, 1972), interstitial keratitis (Bergeron and Stone, 1967) and anaemia (Tennant et al, 1968). Although Dvorak et al (1977) showed no evidence of impaired host defence mechanisms in hidradenitis, Bell and Ellis (1978) reported a high incidence of allergy and atopy.

INCIDENCE

The overall incidence of hidradenitis is unknown, since the disease is often misdiagnosed as pilonidal sinus, fistula-in-ano or a skin infection. However, Fitzimmons et al (1985) suggested an incidence of 1 in 300. The disorder is more common in women than men (Tachau, 1939; Wynn Williams, 1953; Pollock et al, 1972; Bell and Ellis, 1978) and may be more common in Negro races than Caucasians (Ching and Stahlgren, 1965; Thornton and Abcarian, 1978).

There is overwhelming evidence that hidradenitis begins only at puberty, and most patients present with the disease in their second to fourth decade (Greeley, 1951; Masson, 1969). Thornton and Abcarian (1978) reported that 78% of patients with the disease were under the age of 31 when they first presented.

PATHOLOGY

Hidradenitis is characterized by chronic fibrosis and progressive destruction of the skin architecture with multiple painful discharging sinuses on hair-bearing skin. Apocrine ducts become occluded with keratin, causing proximal dilatation of the glands, bacterial proliferation and a periductal and dermal cellulitis (Figure 14.2). Secondary infection causes fibrosis which destroys the glandular unit. Destroyed apocrine glands coalesce to form subcutaneous abscesses which discharge through more than one site, resulting in extensive subcutaneous sinuses which rarely heal without intervention.

The histopathology of hidradenitis is usually non-specific and excision specimens often merely demonstrate a thickened dermis associated with a chronic inflammatory cell infiltrate, granulation tissue, giant cells and subcutaneous abscesses. Differentiation from perianal Crohn's disease may be difficult and both conditions may coexist. The presence of coexisting disease in the axilla (61%) or groin (48%) is highly suggestive of hidradenitis (Broadwater et al, 1982).

Very rarely, squamous cell carcinoma is reported in patients with long-standing hidradenitis (Jackman, 1959; Donsky and Mendelson, 1964; Thornton and Abcarian, 1978; Pérez-Diaz et al, 1995).

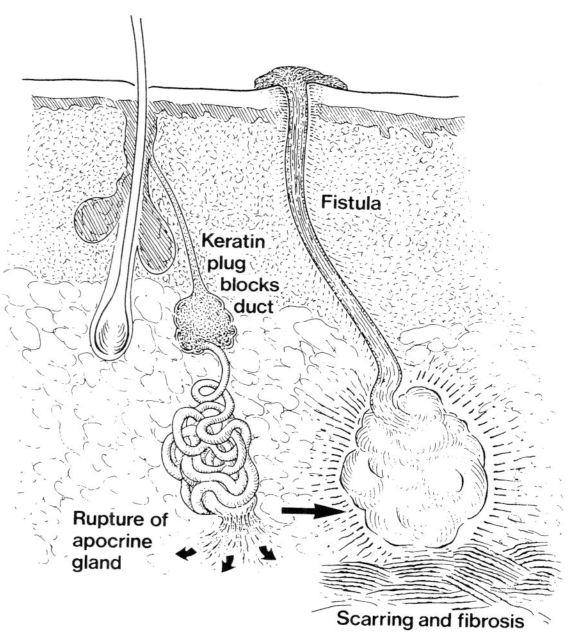

Figure 14.2 The pathology of hidradenitis suppurativa. Blocked apocrine glands and rupture of the glandular tissue is followed by scarring and fibrosis, and eventual fistula formation to the skin.

CLINICAL PRESENTATION

General features

The first sign of the disease is usually the presence of skin sepsis which mimics boils or furuncles. Characteristically, these lesions discharge a small amount of thin offensive fluid, as opposed to pus. Furthermore, the lesions fail to heal, leaving chronic multiple sinuses which intermittently discharge and become secondarily infected, leading to dense fibrosis and scarring. Repeated sepsis results in disfigurement due to painful, offensive, discharging lesions which are socially disabling. Subcutaneous tunnelling involving extensive areas of skin is common, particularly in the perineum, anal regions and groins. Extensive fibrosis may limit movement at the groin flexures.

The disorder is characterized by remission and relapse. Initially the subcutaneous nodules may appear to heal or may discharge and resolve completely for 2–3 years, only later to flare either at the same site or from satellite nodules. Previously uninvolved apocrine glands may also become involved.

There is a particularly aggressive form of hidradenitis known as the 'follicular occlusum tetrad'. This comprises hidradenitis suppurativa, perifolliculitis capitis, nodular cystic acne vulgaris and pilonidal sinus. This condition is rare but may result in severe anorectal sepsis.

Anal disease

Most patients with anal disease have multiple tracks; the perineal lesions may be extensive, with involvement of the scrotum, groin, presacral area and buttocks with extensive fibrosis. Usually there is extensive scarring around the anus. Many patients give a history of having had a previous operation for 'fistula'. Only the distal third of the anal canal is involved. All of the 30 cases reported by Culp (1983) were below the dentate line; none involved the internal anal sphincter or the intermuscular tissues, a feature which distinguishes the disorder from fistula-in-ano.

The typical clinical features are of painful, malodorous discharge and recurrent sepsis with extensive perianal and buttock fibrosis. Extensive fibrosis of the anal canal is rare but is reported.

DIFFERENTIAL DIAGNOSIS

Anal hidradenitis must be distinguished from perianal sepsis and anorectal fistulas (Jackman, 1942; McColl, 1967; Chrabot et al, 1983; Culp, 1983). Anorectal fistulas usually arise from the dentate line, while in hidradenitis there is no abnormality at this site since the apocrine glands are located superficially to this region and in other sites (Hill, 1957). Tracks formed by hidradenitis do not penetrate the internal anal sphincter. Hidradenitis must be distinguished from perianal Crohn's disease, but both disorders may coexist. If there is doubt about the possibility of regional enteritis, sigmoidoscopy biopsy and radiological assessment of the intestinal tract are advisable (Wiltz et al, 1990).

If the sinuses track towards the presacral region they may mimic pilonidal sinus. Early lesions may be difficult to distinguish from skin infections, particularly boils and carbuncles (Cook and Devlin, 1985). The possibility of tuberculosis, lymphogranuloma venereum and granuloma inguinale should always be borne in mind.

CONSERVATIVE TREATMENT

Antibiotic therapy

Long-term antibiotic therapy has been advocated on the basis that many patients with acne obtain benefit from prolonged exposure to fusidic acid, tetracycline and penicillins, but there is no evidence that antibiotic therapy alters the natural history of hidradenitis suppurativa. Most authors consider that long-term antibiotic therapy is unrewarding (Culp, 1983; Harrison et al, 1987), a view to which we subscribe.

Hormone therapy

Alteration of the hormone environment has been explored on the basis that the disease starts at puberty and is associated with premenstrual exacerbation in over 50% of women. Testosterone was advocated (Cornbleet, 1952) but has unacceptable side-effects. A trial to compare ethinyl oestradiol (50 μg) and cyproterone acetate (50 mg) with ethinyl oestradiol (50 μg) and norgestrel (500 μg) resulted in a high recurrence rate in both groups with no significant difference between them (Mortimer et al, 1986a).

Other drug therapy

It has been claimed, but never proven, that vitamin A derivatives might be beneficial in patients with hidradenitis (Leyden et al, 1983). Hydrocortisone had its advocates but it exacerbates acne and is no longer used (Danto, 1958). A depilatory dose of radiotherapy has been tried (Zeligman, 1965) but now abandoned because of its potential dangers.

SURGICAL TREATMENT

Minimal surgery

Injection

Injection of the track with phenol has been used successfully in a few patients with relatively quiescent disease, but multiple treatment sessions are usually necessary and long-term results are poor.

Cryotherapy

Cryotherapy may be appropriate for small areas of relatively inactive disease, but the recurrence rate may be unacceptably high in the long term (Dalrymple and Monaghan, 1987).

Incision and drainage

Incision and drainage of purulent foci does not control the risk of repeated sepsis from the underlying sinus tracks and is an ineffective method of therapy (Barron, 1970). Recurrence rates as high as 83% have been reported using this technique alone (Broadwater et al, 1982).

Deroofing

Deroofing of the tracks alone has its advocates (Brown et al, 1986). Using a malleable probe the sinus openings are explored under local or general anaesthesia and hydrogen peroxide is injected into the sinus. It is important not to create false passages. The entire roof of each tract is then cut away, leaving the floor exposed. In severe cases, repeated sessions may be necessary to lay open all the tracks, and in lesions near the anus a proximal stoma is occasionally desirable (Ching and Stahlgren, 1965).

Excisional surgery

Local excision

Local excision of the sinus track is widely used by surgeons who wish to avoid the morbidity of *en bloc* excision of the entire apocrine glandular region. The concept of minimal excisional surgery would be attractive if long-term recurrence rates were low. Unfortunately in many reports duration and quality of follow-up is unspecified (Armstrong et al, 1965; Pollock et al, 1972; Shaughnessy et al, 1972; Vickers, 1975; O'Brien et al, 1976). Recurrence rates up to 56% are reported from the use of simple local excision alone (Anderson and Dockerty, 1958; Watson, 1985). Knaysi et al (1968) reported a 22% recurrence rate after limited excision, compared with none after wide ablative resection. The factors which seem to be responsible for recurrence after operations for hidradenitis have been critically assessed (Harrison et al, 1988). Low recurrence rates were reported in patients with perianal (nil) and axillary disease (3%) but recurrence was much higher in patients with involvement of the inguinoperineal (37%) and submammary areas (50%). Factors associated with high local recurrence rates are inadequate primary excision, obesity, excessive skin maceration and chronic skin sepsis. Harrison and colleagues therefore argue for a policy of wide ablative excision because of the risks of local recurrence with minimal surgical procedures. However, it is worth noting that 25% of the recurrences are due to disease developing at a new anatomical site.

Wide ablative excision

Wide ablative excision alone is now strongly advised by most authorities for the treatment of hidradenitis suppurativa (Figure 14.3a,b). Morgan and Hughes (1979) suggest preoperative mapping of the apocrine glands to achieve a 2-cm margin of clearance, thereby completely removing all potential areas of locally recurrent disease (Morgan et al, 1983; Harrison et al, 1987).

The technique for mapping is as follows. Eccrine

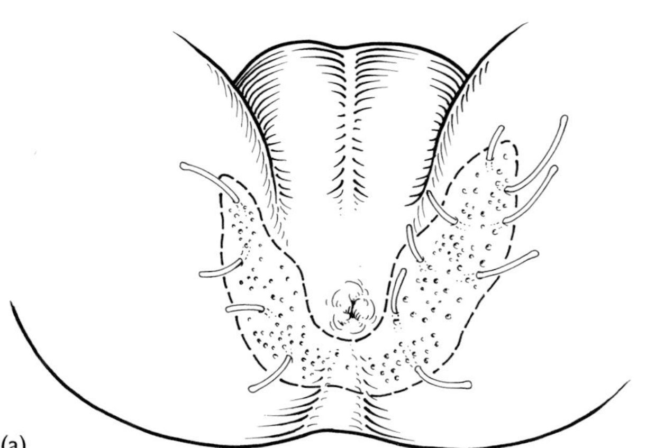

(a)

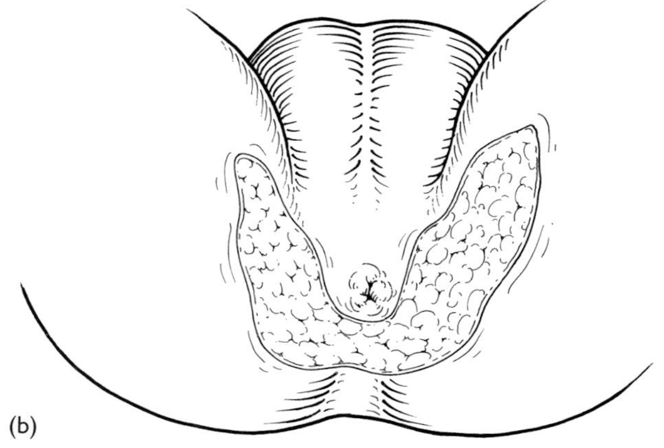

(b)

Figure 14.3a,b Wide ablative excision. (a) Hidradenitis suppurativa results in very superficial sinuses which interconnect. If they continue to suppurate, wide excision of the skin and the subcutaneous tissue of the affected area resolves the sepsis. (b) Wounds are left open to granulate; frequently they heal rapidly.

secretion is first blocked by atropine (1.2 mg i.v.), after which oxytocin (2 units i.v.) is given to stimulate the myoepithelial cells around the apocrine glands. Apocrine secretions can be identified by the iodine–starch method; iodine is applied to the area of study and also to the palm of the hand, which, because of its numerous eccrine glands, acts as a control to ensure that sweating has been abolished by atropine. When the test areas are dry, a mixture containing 75 g of fine starch powder in 100 mL castor oil is applied. Black spots indicate apocrine sweating, which can usually be seen around the base of hair follicles.

Once mapping has been performed, the entire sinus-bearing area and the adjacent apocrine glandular region is removed, leaving healthy subcutaneous tissue. The large denuded area of the perineum and inguinoscrotal region is initially managed by packs soaked in proflavine in liquid paraffin to encourage healthy granulation tissue. The defect may then be allowed to heal by granulation, in which case the raw areas may be covered by Silastic foam (Wood and Hughes, 1975; Wood et al, 1977) on the second or third day after excision.

Wide ablative excision is associated with considerable morbidity and prolonged hospital stay. Hospital stay for such extensive procedures ranges from 11 to 26 days and complete healing takes 6–14 weeks (Morgan et al, 1980).

Morbidity may be reduced by using caudal or spinal anaesthesia to encourage early mobilization. Thornton and Abcarian (1978) used this technique and reported a mean hospital stay of only 7.2 days, and 65% of their patients were discharged from hospital within 5 days. Mean healing times for small defects (2×2 cm) was 3.5 weeks; larger ones took between 5 and 7 weeks to heal but the recurrence rate was only 4%. There is now strong support for wide surgical excision (Conway et al, 1952; Chalfant and Nance, 1970; Shaughnessy et al, 1972), and the principle of leaving the defect open to granulate (Masson, 1969; Lettermann and Schurter, 1974; Vickers, 1975). Local recurrence rates are said to be very low following these extensive procedures (Knaysi et al, 1968; Harrison et al, 1987).

Methods of closing the defect

In view of the morbidity associated with delayed healing by granulation alone (Ariyan and Krizek, 1976), a variety of methods for closing the defect have been advocated by some surgical units.

Primary closure

Primary closure of the defect may be feasible in patients having conservative excision (Jackman and McQuarrie, 1949; Anderson and Perry, 1975; Tasche et al, 1975; Bell and Ellis, 1978). While there are no data on recurrence rates using this technique, one suspects that these are high unless the disease is well localized and inactive; furthermore, lesions are often flat and extensive, making primary closure impossible (Watson, 1985).

Rotation or pedicle flaps

Rotation or pedicle flaps have been used as a method of closing large defects once healthy granulation tissue becomes established (Paletta, 1963; Barron, 1970). Although the techniques are frequently reported (Harrison, 1964; O'Brien et al, 1976) there is little information on recurrence rates (Masson, 1969; Lettermann and Schurter, 1974) apart from the 19% rate reported by Watson (1985).

Split skin grafting

Split skin grafting has been used to cover wide defects created by surgical excision (Conway et al, 1952; Ching and Stahlgren, 1965; Knaysi et al, 1968; Ward et al, 1974; Anderson and Perry, 1975; Hartwell, 1975). However, complete take of the graft is uncommon because of the high risk of sepsis, particularly on the perineum (Brunsting, 1952). Skin grafts are also associated with the morbidity of the donor site. The failure rate of grafting, defined as less than a 50% take, was reported to be 45% by Harrison et al (1987). However, recurrence rates are less, being of the order of 13% (Broadwater et al, 1982; Watson, 1985).

Morgan et al (1983) undertook a controlled trial in patients with bilateral axillary hidradenitis to compare primary excision and skin grafting with application of Silastic foam. Patients preferred the Silastic foam to skin grafting because of earlier mobilization with the Silastic foam and the avoidance of a painful donor site. The median time to healing was 7 weeks following grafting, compared with 12 weeks when the wound was allowed to heal by granulation tissue.

Skin grafting in the perineum is associated with a higher failure rate than at other sites because of the risk of sepsis. Most authorities are of the opinion that skin grafting is not advisable for the majority of patients with perianal or perineal disease.

Specific surgical considerations for perianal hidradenitis

The principles of surgical treatment may need to be modified for the management of anal disease. Fortunately, recurrence rates seem to be low. Culp (1983) reported no recurrence in 27 patients treated by wide excision and followed up for between 1 and 7 years. Similarly, Harrison et al (1987) reported no recurrence after excision of anal hidradenitis. We therefore favour superficial excision of the entire diseased area but have found that a defunctioning colostomy may be needed if the disease is extensive. Skin grafts are not advised as they rarely take on the perineum (Chalfant and Nance, 1970; Ward et al, 1974; Hartwell, 1975).

Occasionally, operations for perineal hidradenitis may be complicated by gas gangrene and synergistic infection or cellulitis; hence antibiotic cover is always advised (Stone and Martin, 1972; Himal et al, 1974; Burbrick and Hitchcock, 1979).

CONCLUSIONS AND RECOMMENDATIONS

Patients should be informed of the need for meticulous hygiene, control of obesity and avoidance of long-term antibiotics. Wide excision and healing by granulation tissue is usually advised, but in some cases a joint approach with a plastic surgeon is needed to achieve long-term control of sepsis.

REFERENCES

Adams JD & Haisten AS (1972) Perianal hidradenitis suppurativa. *Surg Clin North Am* **52**: 467–472.

Anderson DK & Perry AW (1975) Axillary hidradenitis. *Arch Surg* **110**: 9–72.

Anderson MJ & Dockerty MB (1958) Perianal hidradenitis suppurativa: a clinical and pathological study. *Dis Colon Rectum* **1**: 23–31.

Ariyan S & Krizek TJ (1976) Hidradenitis suppurativa of the groin treated by excision and spontaneous healing. *Plast Reconstr Surg* **58**: 44.

Armstrong DP, Pietrell KL, Giblin TR et al (1965) Axillary hidradenitis suppurativa. *Plast Reconstr Surg* **36**: 200–206.

Barron J (1970) The surgical treatment of perianal hidradenitis suppurativa. *Dis Colon Rectum* **13**: 441–443.

Bell BA & Ellis H (1978) Hidradenitis suppurativa. *J R Soc Med* **71**: 511–515.

Bergeron JR & Stone OJ (1967) Interstitial keratitis associated with hidradenitis suppurativa. *Arch Dermatol* **96**: 473–475.

Block B (1931) Metabolism, endocrine glands and skin diseases with special reference to acne vulgaris and xanthoma. *Br J Dermatol* **43**: 61–87.

Brenner DE & Lookingbill DP (1980) Anaerobic micro-organisms in chronic suppurative hidradenitis. *Lancet* **ii**: 921–922.

Broadwater JR, Bryant RL, Petrino RA et al (1982) Advanced hidradenitis suppurativa. *Am J Surg* **144**: 668–670.

Brown SCW, Kazzazi N & Lord PH (1986) Surgical treatment of perineal hidradenitis suppurativa with special reference to recognition of the perianal form. *Br J Surg* **73**: 978–980.

Brunsting HA (1952) Hidradenitis and other variants of acne. *Arch Dermatol Syph* **65**: 303–315.

Burbrick MP & Hitchcock CR (1979) Necrotising anorectal and perineal infections. *Surgery* **68**: 655–661.

Chalfant WP & Nance FC (1970) Hidradenitis suppurativa of the perineum: treatment by radical excision. *Am Surg* **36**: 331–334.

Chapman J (1972) The surgical treatment of hidradenitis suppurativa. *J Natl Med Ass* **64**: 328–330.

Ching CC & Stahlgren LH (1965) Clinical review of hidradenitis suppurativa: management of cases with severe perianal involvement. *Dis Colon Rectum* **8**: 349–352.

Chrabot CM, Prasad NL & Abcarian H (1983) Recurrent anorectal abscesses. *Dis Colon Rectum* **26**: 105–108.

Conway H, Start RB, Climo S, Weeter JC & Garcia FA (1952) The surgical treatment of chronic hidradenitis suppurativa. *Surg Gynecol Obstet* **95**: 455–464.

Cook PJ & Devlin HB (1985) Boils, carbuncles and hidradenitis suppurativa. In *Surgery* (Medical Education Ltd: Int. Series): 440–442.

Cornbleet T (1952) Testosterone for apocrine diseases: hidradenitis, Fox–Fordyce diseases. *Arch Dermatol Syph* **65**: 549–552.

Culp CE (1983) Chronic hidradenitis suppurativa of the anal canal. *Dis Colon Rectum* **26**: 669–676.

Dalrymple JC & Monaghan JM (1987) Treatment of hidradenitis suppurativa with the carbon dioxide laser. *Br J Surg* **74**: 420.

Danto JL (1958) Preliminary and short report. Preliminary studies on the effect of hydrocortisone on hidradenitis suppurativa. *J Invest Dermatol* **31**: 299–300.

Darley CR, Kirby JD, Besser GM, Munro DD, Edwards CR & Rees LH (1982) Circulating testosterone, sex hormone binding globulin and prolactin in women with late onset or persistent acne vulgaris. *Br J Dermatol* **106**: 517–522.

Donsky HJ & Mendelson CG (1964) Squamous cell carcinoma as a complication of hidradenitis suppurativa. *Arch Dermatol* **90**: 488–491.

Dvorak VC, Root RK & McGregor RR (1977) Host defence mechanisms in hidradenitis suppurativa. *Arch Dermatol* **113**: 450–453.

Fitzimmons JS, Guilbert PR & Fitzimmons EM (1985) Evidence of genetic factors in hidradenitis suppurativa. *Br J Dermatol* **113**: 1–8.

Greeley PW (1951) Plastic surgical treatment of chronic suppurativa hidradenitis. *Plast Reconstr Surg* **7**: 143–146.

Harrison BJ, Kumar S, Read GF et al (1985) Hidradenitis

suppurativa: evidence for an endocrine abnormality. *Br J Surg* **72**: 1002–1004.

Harrison BJ, Mudge M & Hughes LE (1987) Recurrence after surgical treatment of hidradenitis suppurativa. *BMJ* **294**: 487–489.

Harrison BJ, Read GF & Hughes LE (1988) Endocrine basis for the clinical presentation of hidradenitis suppurativa. *Br J Surg* **75**: 972–975.

Harrison SH (1964) Axillary hidradenitis. *Br J Plast Surg* **17**: 95–98.

Hartwell SW (1975) Surgical treatment of hidradenitis suppurativa. *Surg Clin North Am* **55**: 1107–1109.

Hay JB & Hodgkins MB (1978) Distribution of androgen metabolising enzymes in isolated tissue of human forehead and axillary skin. *Endocrinology* **79**: 29–39.

Highet AS, Warren RE, Staughton RCD & Roberts SOB (1980) *Streptococcus milleri* causing treatable infection in perineal hidradenitis suppurativa. *Br J Dermatol* **103**: 375–378.

Hill JR (1957) Abscesses and sinuses in the perianal region: differential diagnosis and treatment. *Tex State J Med* **53**: 316–319.

Himal HS, McLean APH & Duff JH (1974) Gas gangrene of the scrotum and perineum. *Surg Gynecol Obstet* **139**: 176–178.

Hurley HJ & Shelley WB (1960) *The Human Apocrine Sweat Glands in Health and Disease*, pp 28, 30, 42. Springfield, IL: CC Thomas.

Jackman RJ (1942) Hidradenitis suppurativa and the treatment of its perianal manifestations. *Am J Dig Dis* **9**: 220–222.

Jackman RJ (1959) Hidradenitis suppurativa: diagnosis and surgical management of perianal manifestations. *Proc R Soc Med* **52** (Suppl): 110–112.

Jackman RJ & McQuarrie HB (1949) Hidradenitis suppurativa: its confusion with pilonidal disease and anal fistula. *Am J Surg* **77**: 349–351.

Knaysi GA, Cosman B & Crikelair GF (1968) Hidradenitis suppurativa. *JAMA* **203**: 73–76.

Kroepfli P (1976) Untersuchungen zur Wirkung der Vitamin-A-Saure bei experimentell augeloster Follikelkeratose. *Dermatologica* **153**: 88–95.

Labows JN, Preti G, Hoelzle E, Leyden T & Kugman A (1979) Steroid analysis of human apocrine secretion. *Steroids* **34**: 249–258.

Leacy RD, Eykyn SJ, Phillips I, Corrin B & Taylor EA (1979) Anaerobic axillary abscess. *BMJ* **2**: 5–7.

Lettermann G & Schurter M (1974) Surgical treatment of hyperhidrosis and chronic hidradenitis suppurativa. *J Invest Dermatol* **63**: 174–182.

Leyden JJ, McGinley FJ & Webster GF (1983) Isotretinoin treatment of acne and related disorders. *J Am Acad Dermatol* **9**: 637–641.

McColl I (1967) The comparative anatomy and pathology of anal glands. *Ann R Coll Surg Engl* **40**: 36–67.

Masson JK (1969) Surgical treatment of hidradenitis suppurativa. *Surg Clin North Am* **49**: 1043–1052.

Miller WL, Knight MM & Gorski J (1977) Estrogen action *in vitro*: regulation of thyroid stimulating and other pituitary hormones in cell culture. *Endocrinology* **101**: 1455–1460.

Montagna W & Parakkal PF (1974) *The Structure and Function of Skin*, 3rd edn. New York: Academic Press.

Morgan WP & Hughes LE (1979) The distribution, size and density of the apocrine glands in hidradenitis suppurativa. *Br J Surg* **66**: 853–856.

Morgan WP, Harding KG, Richardson G & Hughes LE (1980) The use of Silastic foam dressing in the treatment of advanced hidradenitis suppurativa. *Br J Surg* **67**: 277–280.

Morgan WP, Harding KG & Hughes LE (1983) A comparison of skin grafting and healing by granulation, following axillary excision for hidradenitis suppurativa. *Ann R Coll Surg Engl* **65**: 235–236.

Mortimer PS, Dawber PR, Gales MA & Moore RA (1986a) A double-blind controlled crossover trial of cyproterone acetate in females with hidradenitis suppurativa. *Br J Dermatol* **115**: 263–268.

Mortimer PS, Dawber PR, Gales MA & Moore RA (1986b) Mediation of hidradenitis suppurativa by androgens. *BMJ* **292**: 245–258.

O'Brien J, Wysocki J & Arastasi G (1976) Limberg flap coverage for axillary defects resulting from excision of hidradenitis suppurativa. *Plast Reconstr Surg* **58**: 354–358.

Paletta FX (1963) Hidradenitis suppurativa: pathological study and use of skin flaps. *Plast Reconstr Surg* **31**: 307–315.

Peillon F, Vincens M, Cesselin F, Doursmith R & Mowszowicz I (1982) Exaggerated prolactin response of thyrotrophin releasing hormone in women with anovulatory cycles: possible role of endogenous oestrogens and effect of bromocriptine. *Fertil Steril* **37**: 530–535.

Pérez-Diaz O, Calvo-Serrano M, Mártinez-Hijosa E et al (1995) Squamous cell carcinoma complicating perianal hidradenitis suppurativa. *Int J Colorect Dis* **10**: 225–228.

Pollock WJ, Virnelli FR & Ryan RF (1972) Axillary hidradenitis suppurativa: a simple and effective surgical technique. *Plast Reconstr Surg* **49**: 22–27.

Shaughnessy DM, Greminger RR, Margolis IB et al (1972) Hidradenitis suppurativa: a plea for early operative treatment. *JAMA* **222**: 320–321.

Shelley WB & Cahn MM (1955) The pathogenesis of hidradenitis suppurativa in man: experimental and histological observations. *Arch Dermatol* **52**: 562–565.

Stone HH & Martin JD Jr (1972) Synergistic necrotising cellulitis. *Ann Surg* **175**: 702–710.

Stone OJ (1976) Hidradenitis suppurativa following acanthosis nigricans. *Arch Dermatol* **112**: 1142–1144.

Sulzberger MB (1941) Cited in discussion by Ludy JB & Drant P (1941) Hidradenitis suppurativa, papulonecrotic tuberculid and bromoderma. *Arch Dermatol Syph* **44**: 494.

Tachau P (1939) Abscesses of sweat glands in adults. *Arch Dermatol Syph* **40**: 595–600.

Tasche C, Angelata I & Jayaram B (1975) Surgical treatment of hidradenitis suppurativa of the axilla. *Plast Reconstr Surg* **55**: 559–562.

Tennant F, Bergeron JR, Stone OJ & Mullins JF (1968) Anaemia associated with hidradenitis suppurativa. *Arch Dermatol* **98**: 138–140.

Thornton JP & Abcarian H (1978) Surgical treatment of perianal and perineal hidradenitis suppurativa. *Dis Colon Rectum* **21**: 573–577.

Velpeau A (1839) In *Dictionnaire de Médecine: un Répertoir Général des Sciences Médicales sous le Rapport Théorique et Practique*, 2nd edn. Vol. 2, p. 91; vol. 3, p. 304; vol. 19, p. 1. Bechet Jeune.

Verneuil AS (1854) Etude sur les tumeurs de la peau: de quelque maladies des glandes sudoripares. *Arch Gen Med* **94**: 693.

Vickers MA Jr (1975) Operative management of chronic hidradenitis suppurativa of the scrotum and perineum. *J Urol* **114**: 414–416.

Ward JN, Washio H & David HS (1974) Hidradenitis suppurativa of the scrotum and perineum. *Urology* **4**: 463.

Watson JD (1985) Hidradenitis suppurativa: a clinical review. *Br J Plast Surg* **38**: 567–569.

Wile UJ & Curtis AC (1948) Cushing's syndrome with hidradenitis suppurativa. *Arch Dermatol Syph* **58**: 746–747.

Wiltz O, Schoetz DJ Jr, Murray JJ et al (1990) Perianal hidradenitis suppurativa: the Lakey clinic experience. *Dis Colon Rectum* **33**: 731–734.

Wood RAB & Hughes LE (1975) Silicone foam sponge for pilonidal sinus: a new technique for dressing open granulating wounds. *BMJ* **3**: 131–133.

Wood RAB, Williams RHP & Hughes LE (1977) Foam elastomer dressing in the management of open granulating wounds: experience with 250 patients. *Br J Surg* **64**: 554–557.

Wynn-Williams D (1953) Surgical treatment of suppurativa hidradenitis. *Br J Plast Surg* **6**: 231–237.

Zeligman I (1965) Temporary X-ray epilation therapy of chronic axillary hidradenitis suppurativa. *Arch Dermatol* **92**: 690–694.

15 ANORECTAL ABSCESS

Acute anorectal sepsis is a common surgical emergency: in the UK many patients with simple perianal and ischiorectal abscess are assessed and treated in accident and emergency departments; in North America drainage is often performed as an office procedure after initial consultation. There is a 15–47% incidence of recurrent abscess and subsequent fistula-in-ano after surgical drainage. Despite this we generally prefer drainage alone as the primary treatment as fistulotomy may compromise continence. Early drainage is important as the condition may be complicated by necrotizing fasciitis. Anorectal sepsis may be a manifestation of underlying colorectal disease, such as Crohn's disease, ulcerative colitis and neoplasms of the rectum, or may complicate trauma or specific infections. Anorectal sepsis is more prevalent if host defence mechanisms are impaired, as in AIDS, malignant disease, diabetes mellitus and blood dyscrasias or as a result of drug therapy.

AETIOLOGY

Primary anorectal abscess

Anorectal abscesses occur either as a complication of an anal gland infection (cryptoglandular) or from a skin infection. Cryptoglandular infections often result in a chronic intersphincteric collection, which may drain down through the perineum, extend upwards into the supralevator compartment or spread across the sphincter into the ischiorectal fossa (Eisenhammer, 1956, 1961; Parks, 1961). Cryptoglandular infections are caused by intestinal organisms and are invariably associated with an internal opening. Consequently drainage often results in the creation of a fistula between the skin and the anal mucosa at the dentate line. Alternatively, anorectal sepsis may be caused by an infected boil, furuncle or carbuncle around the anal canal. These skin infections are usually staphylococcal in origin and are not usually associated with an internal communication at the dentate line; hence drainage does not result in a fistula (Buchan and Grace, 1973). It has been suggested that cultures of pus from an anorectal abscess may identify which collections are cryptoglandular in origin (Grace et al, 1982; Whitehead et al, 1982). Sometimes perianal infection may be due to obstruction of an apocrine gland and, if so, there may be signs of hidradenitis elsewhere.

Cryptoglandular origin

Anal glands lie between the internal and the external anal sphincters; they communicate with the anal mucosa by ducts which arise from the anal valves at the dentate line (Kratzer, 1950; Granet, 1954). The ducts may terminate in the submucosa or ramify in the internal anal sphincter, but they usually communicate with an anal gland or other ducts in the intersphincteric plane (Figure 15.1). Some acini of the anal glands may run up or down the intersphincteric plane, but they do not normally penetrate the external sphincter as they are visceral, not somatic, structures (Thomson and Parks, 1979). Most individuals have six glands, the majority lie in the submucosa and they rarely penetrate the external sphincter (Seow-Choen and Ho, 1994). Eisenhammer (1978) proposed that the majority of anorectal infections arise from an infected anal gland, resulting in a chronic intersphincteric abscess. The intersphincteric sepsis may: (1) spread cephalad to form a high intersphincteric abscess; (2) spread caudally, resulting in a perianal abscess; (3) spread towards the anal canal, forming a submucous abscess; or (4) penetrate the external sphincter, resulting in an ischiorectal abscess (Figure 15.2).

Proof of Eisenhammer's theory relies on the frequency with which an internal opening can be detected in patients with an anorectal abscess (Nesselrod, 1949), and the incidence of anal fistula following surgical drainage alone (Eisenhammer, 1961, 1964). Unfortunately, neither of these observations necessarily reliably identifies the frequency of an internal communication with the anal canal. Considerable experience is required, by massage of pus and inspection of the anal papilla in patients presenting with an acute anorectal abscess, to demonstrate an associated fistula. Retrospective evaluation of the cryptoglandular origin of anorectal abscess by recording the incidence of subsequent fistulas is also unreliable because in some patients the internal opening may become occluded by debris or fibrosis (Ramanujam et al, 1984). Hence, not all patients having a drainage procedure alone for an abscess arising from an infection of an anal gland will progress to form an anal fistula (Barwood et al, 1996).

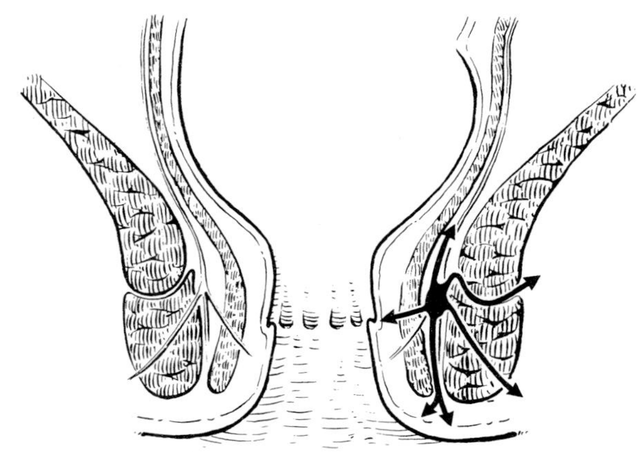

Figure 15.2 The spread of anorectal sepsis. An infected anal gland in the intersphincteric plane may spread: (1) downwards towards the perineum; (2) upwards into the supralevator space; (3) through the external anal sphincter, either to the perianal region, or to the ischiorectal fossa; or (4) internally into the anal canal along the duct to the dentate line.

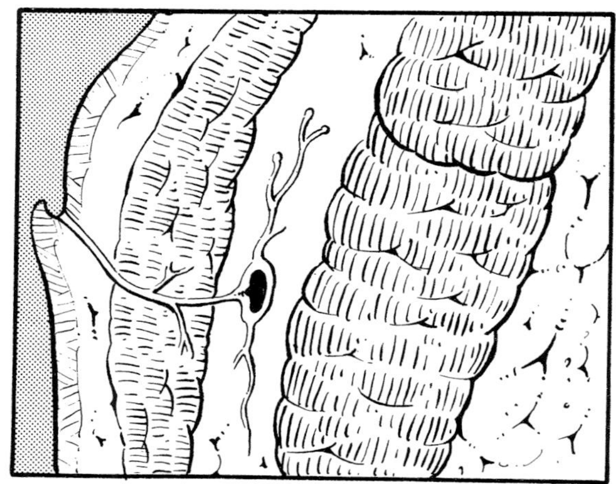

Figure 15.1 Anal glands lie in the intersphincteric space. Their ducts ramify caudally cephalad within the intersphincteric plane. Glandular tissue is connected to the anal epithelium through ducts which open at the dentate line.

Evidence of an internal opening in cryptoglandular anorectal sepsis

From the foregoing remarks it is perhaps not surprising that evidence of an internal opening at the time of initial surgical assessment and drainage is variable. Goligher et al (1967) examined the anal canal of 28 patients under anaesthesia with a bivalve speculum (Table 15.1). Even after pressure over the abscess and gentle probing, a demonstrable communication with the anal canal was found in

Table 15.1 Incidence of internal opening in patients having drainage of an anorectal abscess.

Authors	*n*	*Internal opening (%)*
Goligher et al (1967)	28	15
Buchan and Grace (1973)	133	39
Kovalcik (1979)	181	25
Whitehead et al (1982)	72	44
Ramanujam et al (1984)	1023	35
Eykyn and Grace (1986)	80	66

Table 15.2 Frequency of internal opening according to the site of the abscess.

Site	*No. of openings*	*No. with fistula*
Perianal	437 (43)	151 (35)
Ischiorectal	233 (23)	59 (25)
Intersphincteric	219 (21)	104 (47)
Supralevator	75 (7)	32 (43)
Submucous	59 (6)	9 (15)

Values in parentheses are percentages.
From Ramanujam et al (1984).

only five patients (15%), each of whom had a perianal abscess; none of the eight patients with an ischiorectal abscess had such a communication. Even after internal sphincterotomy, evidence of an underlying intersphincteric abscess was identified in only eight patients (seven with a perianal and one with an ischiorectal abscess). An internal opening was identified in approximately a third of the patients reported by Parks (1961) and a similar proportion was reported by Abcarian (1976), but a somewhat higher incidence was recorded by McElwain et al (1975). Whitehead et al (1982) reported an internal opening in only 32 of 72 patients (44%) with an anorectal abscess and, in common with other series, the incidence of fistula was higher in patients with a perianal abscess (46%) than in those with an ischiorectal abscess (39%). Approximately half of the internal openings were identified at the initial examination under anaesthetic (EUA), the rest being observed at a second EUA 7–10 days later. A similar retrospective survey by Buchan and Grace (1973) identified an internal opening in 52 of 133 patients (39%). Two-thirds of these openings were identified at the time of the initial anaesthetic and only 13 at the second EUA 10 days later.

By contrast, Eisenhammer (1978) states that a fistula could be detected in 90% of cases but details of the patients are lacking in his papers and it is not clear how these internal openings were identified. Eisenhammer's theory is supported by the prospective study of Eykyn and Grace (1986), in which they report that 66% of 80 patients had evidence of an internal opening.

The highest incidence of fistula complicating anorectal sepsis seems to be in patients with intersphincteric and supralevator abscesses (Ramanujam et al, 1984) (Table 15.2).

Among children, an underlying fistula was found more often in the first 2 years of life than in early childhood (Piazza and Radhakrishnan, 1990).

Incidence of fistula after drainage of anorectal sepsis

The incidence of a fistula-in-ano being found after drainage of an anorectal abscess alone, without any attempt to identify an internal opening, is variable. Vasilevsky and Gordon (1984) reported that 31 of 117 patients (26%) having drainage alone subsequently developed a fistula. In our own experience, the incidence of fistula after drainage was only 5% and was higher in perianal than ischiorectal abscess (Winslett et al, 1988). Most authors report a 5–15% incidence of fistula after drainage of anorectal sepsis, the frequency varying with the site of the abscess (Read and Abcarian, 1979; Prasad et al, 1981).

Chrabot et al (1983) studied 97 patients with anorectal sepsis; 32 cases were due to infection in an apocrine gland. Most of the remaining patients had evidence of an underlying fistula: in all 30 patients with an intersphincteric collection, in 13 of 19 with an ischiorectal abscess, in 5 of 12 with a perianal abscess, and in 4 of 7 with a supralevator abscess. Recurrent fistula and sepsis is common in horseshoe abscess (Held et al, 1986).

Skin origin: furuncles, boils and infected apocrine glands

There is probably no communication with the anal canal in a third of patients with anorectal sepsis. These perianal infections are due to sepsis arising from either apocrine glands or hair follicles (Chrabot et al, 1983) and are usually staphylococcal in origin (Eykyn and Grace, 1986). Under these circumstances, further examination under anaesthesia is probably unnecessary. The overall frequency with which skin organisms are recovered from patients with anorectal sepsis ranges from 15% to 25% (Ellis, 1960; Wilson, 1964; Buchan and Grace, 1973; Page and Freeman, 1977).

Secondary anorectal abscess

Specific infections

Perianal abscesses are occasionally caused by a specific micro-organism, the most frequent of which is tuberculosis. Any patient presenting for the first time with anorectal sepsis in association with a fissure, induration or anal stenosis, particularly if the patient has AIDS, is a recent immigrant or is on steroids, should alert the clinician to the possibility of tuberculosis (Bode et al, 1982). In such cases biopsy of the cavity and guinea-pig inoculation for culture would be advised. Atypical tuberculoid reaction in biopsy material may make distinction between acid-fast disease and syphilis, leprosy or Crohn's disease quite difficult (Lowe, 1985). Tuberculosis is also occasionally responsible for recurrent anorectal sepsis (Chrabot et al, 1983).

Other specific infections include legionella (Arnow et al, 1983), actinomycosis, amoebiasis, nocardiasis, schistosomiasis and a variety of fungal infections, which may occasionally present as perianal sepsis. Threadworms may be responsible for perianal sepsis owing to the gravid female threadworm discharging eggs from the anal mucosa to produce granulomas at ectopic sites (Chandrasoma and Mendis, 1977; Vafai and Mohit, 1983; Mortensen and Thomson, 1984; Abercrombie and George, 1992).

Underlying disease

Anorectal sepsis may occur as a complication of specific colorectal disorders or from generalized diseases such as diabetes, AIDS and tuberculosis. The underlying conditions encountered in our Birmingham series are shown in Table 16.3. In AIDS, which is frequently associated with sepsis and local tissue destruction, there may also be features of cryptosporidium infection, giardiasis, and recurrent atypical systemic infections.

Table 15.3 Incidence of underlying disease in 233 cases of anorectal abscess in a Birmingham survey.

Disease	*Number*
Crohn's disease	9
Diabetes mellitus	6
Infective diarrhoea	3
Rectal carcinoma	2
Villous adenoma	2
Sickle cell disease	1
Ulcerative colitis	1

From Winslett et al (1988).

Colorectal disease

Inflammatory bowel disease

The most common coloproctological disorder complicated by sepsis is Crohn's disease (Grace et al, 1982; Winslett et al, 1988). Any anatomical site may be involved, but supralevator abscesses are more frequent in Crohn's disease than in the non-Crohn's population. Less common is the association between perianal sepsis and ulcerative colitis (Kovalcik, 1979). In Crohn's disease, skin tags, anal fissures or ulcers, anal stenosis, chronic perineal induration, long-standing anorectal fistula and rectal involvement (Hughes, 1977) may also be present and any one of these features should alert the surgeon to the possibility of regional enteritis (see Chapter 58).

Colorectal neoplasms

In most series there are a few patients in whom anorectal sepsis may be the first presenting feature of a rectal carcinoma (Bode et al, 1982; Grace et al, 1982). Nelson et al (1985) reviewed the presentation of 15 patients with a carcinoma associated with perianal sepsis. In nine, the carcinoma itself presented as a perianal abscess. In this group the prognosis was very poor and the presence of sepsis was merely a manifestation of advanced local disease: five of the nine patients died within a few months of presentation. In the six remaining patients the carcinoma was an incidental finding and the prognosis was much better. Although the majority of tumours were adenocarcinomas there were three squamous cell tumours.

There are three main groups of adenocarcinoma associated with anorectal sepsis. The first are rectal carcinomas which extend widely into the perianal tissues and outgrow their blood supply, resulting in necrosis and sepsis. These are associated with a poor prognosis and occur predominantly in the elderly. It is therefore important to biopsy any suspicious perianal abscess in elderly patients and to perform a careful examination under anaesthetic. The second category are those tumours which occur in association with an anal fistula. These are often slow-growing (Cabrera et al, 1966; Getz et al, 1981). In some of these cases there is a tumour situated proximally in the rectum and it has been suggested that tumour cells may be seeded into the fistula (Dukes and Galvin, 1956). Some of these tumours represent malignant change in a congenital reduplication and some epidermoid carcinomas arise from anal glands (Lee et al, 1981; Zaren et al, 1983).

Finally, there are those rare tumours which are associated with hidradenitis and arise from apocrine glands (Thornton and Abcarian, 1978) (see Chapter 14). Other malignant tumours associated with anorectal sepsis include carcinoids (Grace et al, 1982) and primary lymphoma of the anorectum (Steele et al, 1985).

Anorectal trauma

Other potential causes of perianal sepsis include local trauma, penetration from foreign bodies inserted into the rectum, and objects passing through the bowel, such as chicken and fish bones (Thomson and Parks, 1979). Occasionally repeated enemas may be complicated by sepsis owing to local trauma (Thomson and Parks, 1979).

Perianal disorders

There are a variety of perianal disorders, or their treatment, which may also become complicated by sepsis. These include ruptured anal haematoma, thrombosed haemorrhoids and anal fissure. Perianal sepsis may also complicate haemorrhoidectomy, injection or rubber-band ligation.

Other pelvic disorders

Conditions which may be responsible for supralevator (pelvic) abscess include salpingitis, Crohn's or diverticular disease, large bowel carcinoma, penetrating injuries, orthopaedic conditions, urological disorders and the complications of acute appendicitis.

Generalized disease

Pancytopenia

Patients with certain blood dyscrasias, those receiving chemotherapy, and those with an immunocompromised state, such as patients receiving drugs to control rejection after transplantation, may develop a rather unusual form of perianal sepsis (Abercrombie and George, 1992; Cohen et al, 1996). Features consist of perineal pain, fever and a tense, fluctuant swelling, often without any evidence of pus. These infections frequently complicate acute leukaemia, thrombocytopenia and other neutropenic states (Bevans et al, 1973; Hanley, 1978; Whitehead et al, 1982; Vasilevsky and Gordon, 1984). If there is a tender perianal swelling without pus, the surgeon should take a biopsy and examine the peripheral blood film (Slater, 1984). Approximately 3% of patients with leukaemia present with anorectal sepsis (Walsh and Stickley, 1934; Blank, 1955). Drainage of these lesions is usually not advised. Treatment should include the use of broad-spectrum bactericidal antibiotics, as well as tackling the underlying haematological disorder (Sehdev et al, 1973). Perianal abscess may be a presenting feature of chronic granulomatous disease but, in these patients, drainage is usually advised (Mulholland et al, 1983).

Diabetes

Any patient with anorectal sepsis may have occult or established diabetes mellitus. Indeed, this may be the first presenting feature of diabetes. Large series have reported that 2–20% of patients with anorectal sepsis are diabetics (Bevans et al, 1973; Kovalcik, 1979; Prasad et al, 1981; Grace et al, 1982; Whitehead et al, 1982; Ramanujam et al, 1984). Abcarian and Eftaiha (1983) reported that 30% of patients with severe anorectal sepsis associated with necrotizing fasciitis were diabetics.

AIDS

Severe perianal sepsis causing marked tissue destruction may be one of the initial presenting features of AIDS. In AIDS patients, recurrent sepsis and failure to respond to conventional therapy is a common feature. Furthermore, metastatic sepsis and severe necrotizing gangrene is now a well-recognized complication particularly in AIDS patients with low CD4 counts (Consten et al, 1996).

Therapeutic agents

Agents causing pancytopenia have already been referred to. Steroids probably also increase the risk of anorectal sepsis, as do other drugs which interfere with normal cellular and humoral defence mechanisms.

Other diseases

Other general disorders associated with anorectal sepsis include hypertension, heart disease, obesity and chronic alcoholism (Bode et al, 1982).

MICROBIOLOGY

Three studies (Grace et al, 1982; Whitehead et al, 1982; Eykyn and Grace, 1986) have shown that skin organisms, principally *Staphylococcus aureus*, are indicative of abscesses which are rarely associated with an underlying fistula. The prospective study by Eykyn and Grace (1986) is undoubtedly the most informative, since all of the patients described had both an initial examination under anaesthetic and a further examination 1 week later, by an experienced surgeon, to detect the presence of a fistula. This clinical assessment was complemented by an extremely comprehensive microbiological survey. The significant microbiological findings are summarized in Table 15.4. Gut-specific anaerobes and *Escherichia coli* were identified significantly more frequently in patients with a fistula than in the remaining patients. By contrast, there were only nine isolates of *Staph. aureus*, eight in patients without fistula and only one (very few colonies present) in the remaining case.

It has been suggested that the identification of skin organisms at the time of drainage of an anorectal abscess makes further evaluation under anaesthetic unnecessary. If, on the other hand, a gut-specific anaerobe is identified and an internal opening has not been found, careful follow-up would be advised since there is a risk that the patient may develop a fistula-in-ano during follow-up. Grace et al (1982) reported no recurrences in the 35 patients in whom a skin organism was cultured, compared with ten recurrent episodes of sepsis or fistula in the 52 patients in whom intestinal pathogens were identified.

The specificity of cultures in defining an underlying fistula was challenged by Lunniss and Phillips (1994) in a study to compare abscess cultures with a surgical search for sepsis in the intersphincteric space in 22 patients with acute anorectal sepsis. The presence of intersphinteric sepsis had a sensitivity and specificity of 100% of an underlying fistula, whereas cultures of gut-related organisms had a sensitivity of 100% but a specificity of only 80%.

Table 15.4 Microbiological differences between abscesses associated with an internal opening compared with those having no fistula.

Finding	*Fistula*	*No fistula*	*P*
Anaerobes isolated	49 (92)	8 (30)	<0.0001
E. coli cultured	45 (85)	5 (18)	<0.0001
Staph. aureus cultured	1 (2)	8 (30)	0.00012
Gut-specific bacteroides	47 (89)	5 (18)	<0.0001
Not gut-specific anaerobes	2 (4)	17 (63)	<0.0001
Gut-specific anaerobes + aerobes	45 (85)	4 (15)	<0.0001

Values in parentheses are percentages.
From Eykyn and Grace (1986).

INCIDENCE

Data on the incidence of anorectal sepsis in the UK are not available. A hospital inpatient enquiry serving a population of 300 000 in 1964–65 reported 5000–6000 admissions per year from anorectal sepsis (Buchan and Grace, 1973). Anorectal sepsis is three times more common in men than women (Hill, 1967). The peak age of presentation is in the third or fourth decade (Vasilevsky and Gordon, 1984) (Figure 15.3). The higher incidence of anorectal sepsis in men has been attributed to occupation, distribution of hair, increased sweating and poor anal hygiene.

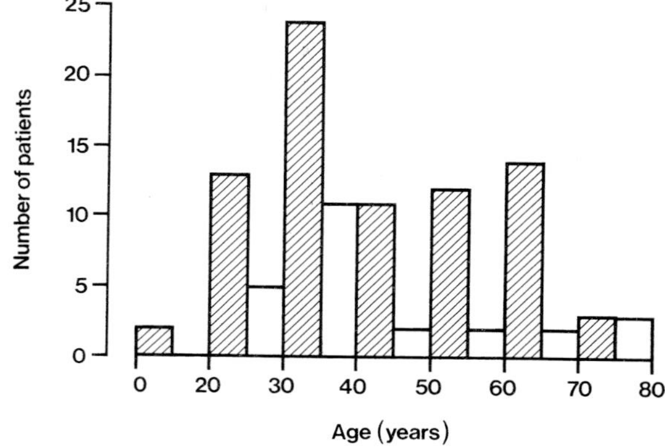

Figure 15.3 Age and sex of patients presenting with anorectal abscess. ▨, male; □, female.

PATHOGENESIS AND SPREAD

It is thought that all cryptoglandular abscesses start from an intersphincteric abscess following infection in an anal gland. In the majority of cases the infective process extends downwards towards the perianal region and the conjoint longitudinal muscle prevents any lateral extension through the external anal sphincter. In a few cases the infective process advances cranially, resulting in a high intermuscular abscess or even a supralevator abscess. The infection may, however, advance towards the lumen of the anal canal along the track of the anal duct, resulting in a submucous abscess. The pathogenesis of ischiorectal abscess is less well-defined. In some patients the intermuscular collection extends laterally through the conjointed longitudinal muscle and through the lower fibres of the external anal sphincter into the ischiorectal fossa. In others, the infection extends caudally in the intermuscular plane and then around the lower border of the external anal sphincter into the ischiorectal fossa. In a few patients a supralevator abscess may burst through the fibres of the puborectalis into the ischiorectal fossa. Finally, the ischiorectal fossa may become infected following an episode of septicaemia from a distant focus (Figure 15.4).

Once the abscess has become localized to a specific anatomical site, further extension may take place around the anal canal. Circumferential spread is particularly common in the ischiorectal fossa (Figure 15.5). The large potential space of the ischiorectal fossa may accommodate considerable volumes of pus, and extension from one side to the other across the midline posteriorly results in the typical horseshoe abscess (Held et al, 1986). Circumanal spread may also occur in patients with an intermuscular abscess (Eisenhammer, 1961) and, occasionally, in perianal abscesses as well.

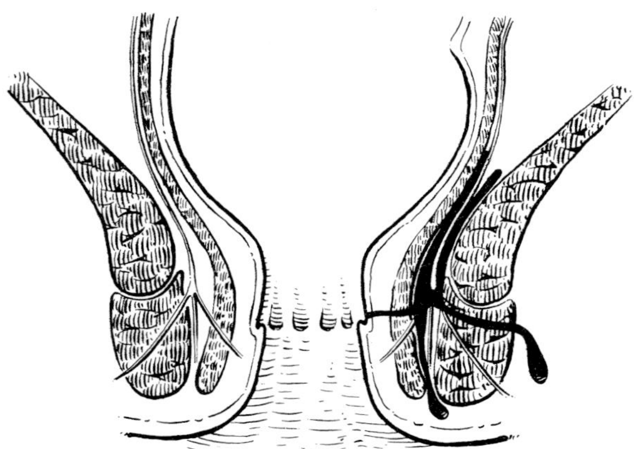

Figure 15.4 The spread of anal gland infection. The anal gland lies in the intersphincteric space: infection may spread: (1) upwards into the supralevator or extrarectal space; (2) laterally through the external anal sphincter into the ischiorectal fossa; or (3) downwards through the intersphincteric plane to form a perianal abscess.

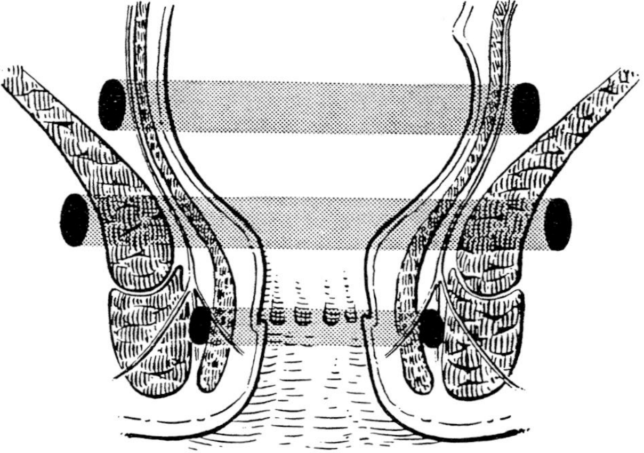

Figure 15.5 Circumferential spread of perianal sepsis. Intersphincteric collections, ischiorectal abscesses and supralevator abscesses may all spread circumferentially around the rectum to infect the same region on the opposite side.

PATHOLOGY

An abscess in the perianal region results from bacterial infection of the loose areolar tissue around an anal gland. There is often extensive tissue damage and necrosis. Enzymes capable of breaking down protein molecules are released from pus, resulting in osmotically active particles which attract fluid into the infective process. Spontaneous discharge of pus is prevented by histiocytes, platelets and fibroblasts, which stimulate the formation of a fibrous capsule, localizing the infective process. Granulation tissue also helps to localize the infective process. The presence of osmosis from protein breakdown and chemotaxis results in considerable tension within the abscess, causing necrosis and small vessel thrombosis.

Histologically, there is a pus-filled cavity surrounded by granulation tissue and fibrosis. There are often focal aggregates of histiocytes forming foreign-body granulomas in the surrounding inflammatory reaction. New blood vessels, some of which are occluded by fibrin thrombi, are seen in the periphery. The peripheral tissues are compressed and there may be areas of focal necrosis.

CLASSIFICATION AND ANATOMICAL SITE

Anorectal sepsis is classified according to its anatomical site: the most common are perianal and ischiorectal. Since it is almost impossible to distinguish a perianal abscess from a low intermuscular abscess, these will be considered together. A high intermuscular abscess is relatively rare and extension to form a suprasphincteric abscess is also uncommon. In our experience most suprasphincteric abscesses are secondary to pelvic rather than anal pathology. High supralevator abscesses may be subdivided into retrorectal, rectovesical, pelvirectal and retroperitoneal. Unlike some groups, we recognize the submucous abscess as an extension through the original track of the anal gland to the submucosal plane of the anus (Figure 15.6). Some authorities subdivide the intersphincteric abscess into superficial and deep postanal and superficial and deep anterior anal collections (Goldberg et al, 1980).

The usual distribution of anorectal sepsis is shown in Table 15.5. Perianal abscess is the most common, followed by ischiorectal abscess. The incidence of intersphincteric abscess is variable and has not been recorded in a number of retrospective studies. Our own clinical impression is that eventual localization into the intersphincteric plane is rare, being found in only 5% (Winslett et al, 1988). However, we recognize that intersphincteric collections are frequently an important source of sepsis. The localization of abscesses in patients with recurrent sepsis is, however, quite different, with a much higher incidence of intersphincteric abscess.

Localization of abscesses around the anal canal is also variable. Thomson and Parks (1979) indicated that 66% of abscesses were located in the posterior quadrant, 22% were anterior and only 11% were sited laterally (2% on the right and 9% on the left). Ramanujam et al (1984) recorded 53% as posterior, 35% as lateral and only 12% as anterior. However, Vasilevsky and Gordon (1984), in their review of patients with recurrent anorectal sepsis, recorded only four posterior horseshoe abscesses and a much higher incidence of laterally placed collections.

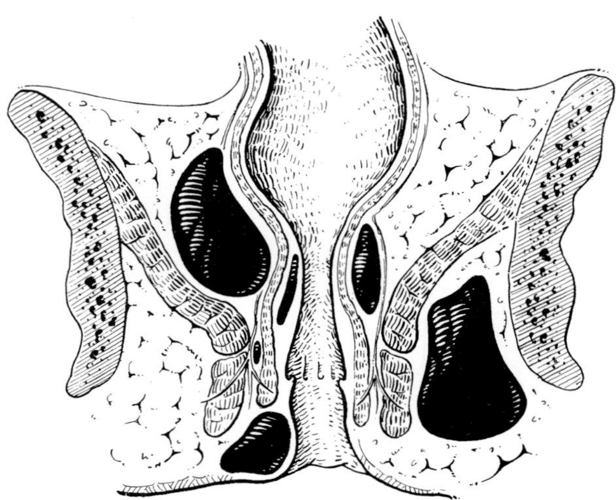

Figure 15.6 Classification of anorectal sepsis. The following anatomical sites are recognized: supralevator abscess; low or high intersphincteric abscess; submucosal abscess; perianal abscess; ischiorectal abscess.

Table 15.5 Frequency (%) of sites of anorectal sepsis.

Authors	*n*	*Perianal*	*Ischiorectal*	*Intersphincteric*	*Submucous*	*Supralevator*
Initial abscess						
Grace et al (1982)	165	75	30	—	5	—
Whitehead et al (1982)	135	84	16	—	—	—
Ramanujam et al (1984)	1023	43	22	21	6	7
Winslett et al (1988)	233	62	24	5	2	7
Recurrent abscess						
Chrabot et al (1983)	97	18	28	44	0	10
Vasilevsky and Gordon (1984)	117	19	61	18	0	2

NATURAL HISTORY

Recurrent sepsis and fistula is a prominent feature of anorectal sepsis unless initial surgical treatment is adequate. In a few patients, anorectal sepsis may progress if not treated adequately to spreading extraperitoneal cellulitis which can be fatal, particularly in diabetic or immunocompromised patients (Badrinath et al, 1994). Some authorities claim a high recurrence if a coexisting fistula is not identified and treated at the time of the initial surgical drainage. Recurrent abscess or fistula was reported in 65% of patients when the abscess was merely drained, whereas 31% had a recurrent abscess when fistulotomy was performed at the time of drainage (Ramanujam et al, 1984). By contrast, recurrence occurred in only 3% of patients managed initially by drainage alone, followed later by a staged fistulotomy. Recurrence has been attributed to: (1) failure to identify an internal opening; (2) inadequate assessment of the extent of the abscess, resulting in incomplete drainage; (3) spontaneous rupture of the abscess so that a proper examination under anaesthetic was never performed; and (4) the presence of an underlying disorder, such as Crohn's disease, AIDS or tuberculosis (Chrabot et al, 1983).

From the foregoing remarks it is not surprising that a high proportion of patients with anorectal sepsis have a history of previous surgery (Fielding and Berry, 1992). Grace et al (1982) recorded a previous drainage procedure, usually at the same site, in 41% of their patients. Previous sepsis was recorded in 27% of the patients seen by Vasilevsky and Gordon (1984) in Montreal. There may be a history of multiple episodes of discharge or repeated surgical drainage, as illustrated by Chrabot's study where 24% of patients had three or more drainage procedures and 14% had at least five.

The risk of recurrent abscess and fistula is very variable. Buchan and Grace (1983) reported a recurrent abscess or fistula in 27% of cases. However, laying open of an associated fistula at the time of draining the acute abscess did not necessarily guarantee a low incidence of recurrent sepsis (Table 15.6). This is in marked contrast to the observations made from Cook County Hospital (Table 15.7), where the overall recurrence rate was so low that it seemed to matter very little whether a fistulotomy was performed at the initial drainage procedure. One wonders if these patients were carefully followed up since the hospital caters for an itinerant population and the rate of recurrent fistula is very much lower than in most other reports.

In some patients, anorectal sepsis will resolve completely without surgical intervention. Most patients who give a history of spontaneous discharge with no further symptoms probably have an anal furuncle which is not cryptoglandular in origin. Chrabot et al (1983) found that in 64 patients with anorectal sepsis 11 spontaneously resolved. However, in 15 other patients in whom the abscess spontaneously ruptured, sepsis recurred at the same site. Apparent resolution is therefore not always associated with long-term cure and follow-up is mandatory if the reliable recurrence rates are to be recorded.

Table 15.6 Risk of recurrent abscess and fistula according to the method of treatment.

Treatment	*n*	*Recurrent abscess*	*Recurrent fistula*
Fistula found at the time of drainage	39	9 (23)	5 (13)
Fistula found at 2nd EUA	13	0	1 (8)
No fistula found at either examination	81	13 (16)	9 (11)
Not examined for a fistula	46	5 (11)	7 (15)

Values in parentheses are percentages.
From Buchan and Grace (1973).

Table 15.7 Risk of recurrent abscess and fistula according to the method of treatment.

Treatment	*n*	*Recurrence*
Unroofing only	688	25 (4)
Drainage and laying open of fistula	323	6 (2)
Secondary fistulotomy	32	1 (3)

Values in parentheses are percentages.
From Ramanujam et al (1984).

CLINICAL FEATURES

Approximately 20–40% of patients give a history of a previous episode of anorectal sepsis which has spontaneously discharged or required surgical drainage. In children the presentation and microbiology is similar but there is a higher incidence of primary pathology such as agranulocytosis, infectious disease, Crohn's disease or threadworms (Abercrombie and George, 1992).

Perianal abscess

Pain, swelling and localized tenderness are the hallmarks of a perianal abscess. Pain is often throbbing in nature and aggravated by coughing, sitting and defecation. The skin over the abscess is erythematous and swollen and the collection of pus is well-localized around the skin of the anal verge. Perianal abscess is rarely complicated by constitutional disturbance. The swelling is usually ovoid, tender and fluctuant. Digital examination is very painful but there is no evidence of intrarectal swelling. In our experience, circumanal extension of a perianal abscess is uncommon and most cavities are posterior or lateral. Sometimes a perianal abscess bursts spontaneously, with relief of pain and disappearance of the swelling.

Ischiorectal abscess

Clinical features of ischiorectal abscess are less well defined. Fever is more common and associated with constitutional disturbance. The swelling is much more diffuse, and tends to involve the entire perianal region. Examination reveals a vague area of swelling beside the rectum but bulging into the anal canal is unusual. Bilateral involvement to form a horseshoe abscess occurs by posterior spread into the ischiorectal fossa of the opposite side. There may be considerable tissue necrosis due to pus under tension in the relatively avascular ischiorectal space. Sometimes a collection high in the ischiorectal fossa may be associated with no clinical signs at all. These high collections are commonly due to an extension of a supralevator abscess and there may be signs of a pelvic abscess (see below).

Intersphincteric and submucosal abscesses

Intersphincteric abscess is usually associated with no visible evidence of sepsis. Patients present with perineal pain and fever. In some cases there is a history of spontaneous discharge with the passage of foul-smelling pus through the anus. Digital examination is very painful and may be possible only under an anaesthetic. There is usually a diffuse swelling confined to one sector of the upper anal canal but circumanal extension may result in an extensive intersphincteric collection which is poorly localized. There may be an associated submucosal abscess owing to pus tracking towards the anal canal along an anal gland; however, this is usually small, involving less than one-third of the circumference of the anus.

Supralevator abscess

Supralevator abscess either arises as an upward extension of an intersphincteric collection or represents a true pelvic abscess due to conditions such as appendicitis, salpingitis, diverticulitis, Crohn's disease, malignancy or a ruptured pelvic viscus. There is usually a mass high up in the pelvis, identifiable by bimanual rectal or vaginal examination. Supralevator abscess is dealt with fully later in this chapter.

INVESTIGATIONS, DIAGNOSIS AND DIFFERENTIAL DIAGNOSIS

In our opinion all patients presenting with anorectal sepsis need a careful examination, including proctosigmoidoscopy, under general anaesthetic. This is not uniformally accepted, especially in North America where anorectal abscesses are often treated as an 'office procedure' under local anaesthetic (Kovalcik, 1979). Nevertheless, thorough assessment of the extent and location of the sepsis can be achieved by local or spinal anaesthetic techniques, although caudal anaesthesia is usually contraindicated because of the risk of meningeal infection. Thorough assessment is important, both to identify the presence of an internal opening and to ascertain the extent of the infective process, particularly any supralevator or intersphincteric component.

Gentle pressure over the abscess during speculum examination of the anal canal should help ascertain if there is an internal opening into the anal canal. Some authorities, principally Eisenhammer (1978), believe that a curved Ferguson probe should be used in the search for an internal opening, but even the use of a soft malleable blunt probe may be associated with the formation of a false passage, particularly in the presence of acute sepsis. We believe that a soft ureteric catheter is probably safer for identifying an internal opening in some patients. Injection of methylene blue into the abscess may be used as a means of identifying a connection with the anal glands, but the technique is not entirely satisfactory in acute sepsis.

We support the policy of culturing pus at the time of drainage, particularly if an internal opening cannot be identified (Grace et al, 1982). If *Staph. aureus* is identified, a second EUA is probably unnecessary since the chance of a missed internal opening is then remote. If, on the other hand, cultures reveal *E. coli*, *Proteus* spp., *Klebsiella* spp. or gut-specific bacteriodes, there is a strong possibility of a fistula (Table 15.8). Under these circumstances, a second EUA 7–10 days after drainage may be worthwhile since 31% of the fistulas associated with an anorectal abscess can be identified at this second examination.

Anorectal ultrasound (Beynon et al, 1986) has been used for defining the precise location of anorectal abscesses and may be used as an alternative to fistulography (Ani and Logundoye, 1979). After using a 7 MHz probe in 22 patients, Law et al (1989) claimed that ultrasonography will reliably identify an intersphincteric abscess and the internal opening of an associated fistula. However, endoanal ultrasonography lacks the ability to image beyond the external sphincter, and therefore cannot reliably identify a perianal, ischiorectal or supralevator abscess. Certainly, Cataldo et al (1993) found that intrarectal ultrasound often failed to image the internal opening of a coexisting fistula, and furthermore the anatomy of the abscess in relation to the external sphincter was often inadequately displayed. MRI is reported to be very effective for identifying the anatomical site of sepsis (Zbar et al, 1996: see Chapter 2). Indeed, many of us now believe that MRI is the investigation of choice in all complex anorectal sepsis to delineate the precise anatomy of the sepsis.

Table 15.8 Organisms isolated from anorectal sepsis.

	Fistula	*No fistula*
Staph. aureus	1	8
Str. milleri	22	1
Other streptococci	18	9
E. coli	45	5
Proteus spp.	12	0
Klebsiella spp.	6	0
Gut-specific bacteroides	62	5
Other bacteroides	63	49

Adapted from Eykyn and Grace (1986).

Differential diagnosis

Anorectal sepsis must be distinguished from other potentially painful infective conditions of the anorectum and perineum, particularly anal fissure, a thrombosed haemorrhoid, Bartholin's abscess, hidradenitis suppurativa and periurethral abscess. Malignancy and inflammatory bowel disease may mimic anorectal sepsis. Specific infections should also be excluded, particularly tuberculosis, fungal infections, schistosomiasis, amoebiasis, leprosy, syphilis, gonorrhoea and AIDS.

TREATMENT

Principles

Antibiotic therapy

Antibiotic treatment alone probably has no influence on the natural history of anorectal abscess unless this complicates pancytopenia. Exposure to antibiotics was shown to have no influence on the organisms recovered at the time of drainage (Eykyn and Grace, 1986). More importantly, antibiotics may delay surgical treatment. Antibiotics are sometimes prescribed in the hope that a small abscess will resolve; however this treatment may allow the abscess to expand into a huge collection associated with extensive tissue necrosis, which may be complicated by synergistic gangrene of the entire perineum (Brightmore, 1972; Marks et al, 1973; Lichtenstein et al, 1978). If the abscess discharges spontaneously there is a high incidence of recurrent abscess or fistula (Chrabot et al, 1983).

Antibiotics may be used during surgical drainage in order to avoid an episode of septicaemia and they are definitely advised in patients with valvular disease of the heart or those with a prosthetic implant. They are also advised in patients who require extensive surgical debridement for synergistic infection of the perineum, and in diabetics.

Primary closure or drainage with or without antibiotic therapy

There was a vogue in the UK for treating any abscess presenting in an accident and emergency department by incision, curettage and primary suture under antibiotic cover (Ellis, 1951, 1970; Benson and Goodman, 1970; Page, 1974; Jones and Wilson, 1976). The argument for this policy is that primary healing is common, further dressings are unnecessary and morbidity is low, provided there is no internal opening (Jones and Wilson, 1976; Stewart et al, 1985). Many patients can therefore return to work earlier following primary suture than after conventional drainage. However, McFie and Harvey (1977) showed that antibiotics did not influence healing times (incision, curettage and primary suture: 9.3 days with antibiotics and 8.8 days without; drainage alone: 9.8 days with antibiotics and 9.3 days without). They also showed that there was a higher recurrence rate after primary suture than after drainage alone. Leaper et al (1976) compared primary suture against drainage alone in 219 patients with anorectal abscess in whom there was no internal opening (Table 15.9). Although healing times were shorter using primary suture, there was a high recurrence rate in both groups, suggesting that there might well have been an unidentified internal opening in some of these patients.

Simms et al (1982) in Birmingham showed that healing time was significantly longer (8.9 days) following drainage and primary suture than following drainage alone (7.8 days). Furthermore, 35% of wounds broke down after primary closure despite the use of antibiotics. Thus we have abandoned primary suture for anorectal sepsis; furthermore, we do not advise curettage or the use of drainage tubes for fear of creating a high fistula, and merely teach that simple drainage alone without extensive skin excision is all that is necessary (Figure 15.7).

Table 15.9 Comparison of incision, curettage and primary suture against drainage alone for anorectal abscess.

	Primary suture (*n* = 110)	*Drainage* (*n* = 109)
Healing (days)	10	35
Off work (days)	8	31
Recurrence		
3 months	3	10
12 months	8	23
After 12 months	8	26

From Leaper et al (1976).

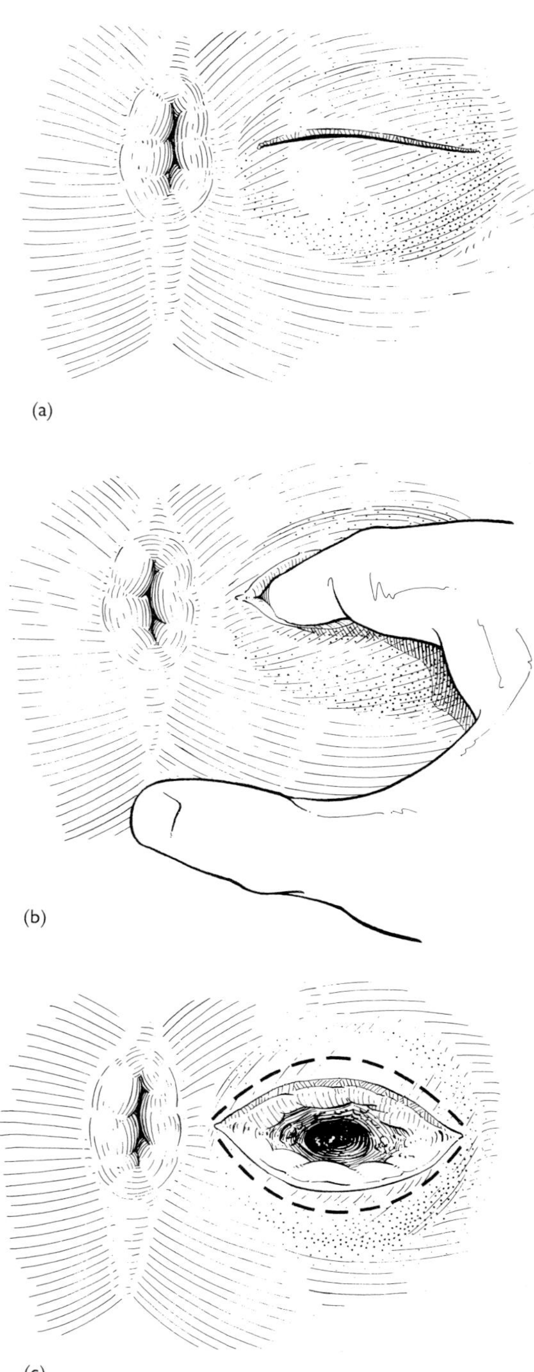

Figure 15.7a–c Drainage of a perianal abscess. (a) An incision is made over the perianal swelling. (b) A finger is inserted into the abscess cavity to break down all loculi. (c) An ellipse of skin is excised around the drainage site to facilitate discharge of all purulent material.

Drainage alone or synchronous fistulotomy

There is still a wide difference of opinion as to the desirability of immediate fistulotomy if an internal opening is identified. Some surgeons take the view that the abscess should be merely drained under general or local anaesthetic (Thomson and Parks, 1979; Goldberg et al, 1980). The argument in favour of this policy is that the incidence of fistula is low and that division of muscle (both the internal and possibly the external anal sphincter) in the presence of established sepsis may lead to excessive sphincter loss and impaired continence. It is argued that if a fistula does develop there is less potential sphincter loss if the track is laid open or excised as an elective procedure (Ramanujam et al, 1984). The counter-argument is that the incidence of fistula and recurrent abscess following drainage alone is high and that synchronous fistulotomy avoids a second admission to hospital. Some claim that laying open a fistula at the time of drainage prevents fibrosis and the gutter deformity which may complicate later fistulotomy. Another aspect of the argument is that cryptoglandular infections are usually secondary to an intersphincteric abscess and that division of the internal anal sphincter allows more efficient drainage and a lower risk of recurrence (Eisenhammer, 1961).

An essential consideration in this debate relates to the experience of the surgeon (Hanley, 1985). Few would disagree that identification of an internal fistula and synchronous fistulotomy should be performed by experienced personnel only. Such difficulties are illustrated by Eykyn and Grace (1986), who found that 5 of 35 fistulas identified at the initial examination were high and were therefore managed by the use of a seton. Furthermore, in this series four patients with a fistula had evidence of Crohn's disease. Even at the second examination under anaesthetic, 4 of 16 fistulas were suprasphincteric or extrasphincteric. Thus we would argue that the inexperienced surgeon should merely drain the abscess, preferably avoiding any attempted curettage. Some authorities advise immediate drainage alone, followed by elective examination under general or spinal anaesthetic 24 hours later by an experienced surgeon to identify and treat the associated fistula if present (Chrabot et al, 1983). An alternative policy proposed by Hanley (1985) is that the fistula should be identified at the initial examination under anaesthetic, that no attempt should be made to lay open the fistula but that a seton should be inserted along the track. The reasons for this policy are that it may be difficult to distinguish a high from a low fistula by using a seton, the sphincter is not divided, and the presence of the seton identifies the fistula track when it requires definitive treatment later. The chances of finding an internal opening is much lower if the abscess is ischiorectal (25%) or perianal (34%) than if it is an intersphincteric (47%) or supralevator abscess (42%) (Tables 15.10 and 15.11).

An important randomized trial compared drainage and immediate fistulotomy against drainage alone (Schouten and Vroonhaven, 1991). The recurrent sepsis rates were 3% and 41% respectively. A high proportion in the drainage-alone group required secondary surgery. However, incontinence was reported in 39% treated by synchronous drainage and fistulotomy compared with 21% following drainage alone. The Singapore group put this question to the test using a prospective randomized trial in which 45 patients with a simple perianal abscess and a coexisting fistula were randomized to drainage alone or drainage and fistulotomy (Tang et al, 1996). The results are shown in Table 15.12. Three of 21 patients having drainage alone developed recurrent anorectal sepsis requiring another operation, compared with none of 24 patients having fistulotomy at the time of drainage. Furthermore, there were no patients with impaired continence in the drainage and fistulotomy group, compared with one patient with flatus incontinence in the drainage-alone group.

A later study, also from Singapore, compared drainage alone with primary fistulotomy (Ho et al, 1997). A fistula was discovered in 24 of 28 patients

Table 15.10 Incidence of fistula-in-ano according to the site of sepsis.

Site of sepsis	*n*	*Fistula*
Perianal	437	151 (34)
Ischiorectal	233	59 (25)
Intersphincteric	219	104 (47)
Supralevator	75	32 (42)
Submucous or intermuscular	59	9 (15)

Values in parentheses are percentages.
From Ramanujam et al (1984).

Table 15.11 Drainage for recurrent sepsis.

Site of sepsis	*n*	*Fistula*
Perianal	12	5 (42)
Ischiorectal	19	13 (68)
Intersphincteric	30	30 (100)
Supralevator	7	4 (57)

Values in parentheses are percentages.
From Chrabot et al (1983).

Table 15.12 Prospective randomized trials of drainage alone versus drainage and fistulotomy for acute perianal abscess.

	Drainage alone	*Drainage plus fistulotomy*
Tang et al (1996)	($n=21$)	($n=24$)
Type of fistula		
Subcutaneous	1	1
Low intersphincteric	13	9
Low trans-sphincteric	7	14
Hospital stay (days)	3 (2–15)	3 (2–23)
Recurrent abscess or fistula	3	0
Incontinence		
Flatus	1	0
Liquid stool	0	0
Solid stool	0	0
Ho et al (1997)	($n=28$)	($n=24$)
Recurrent fistula	7	0
Incontinence	0	0

and laid open at the initial operation. Not surprisingly, 7 of 28 patients in the drainage group developed a fistula later. There was no incontinence in either group. We are surprised how often a fistula was discovered and believe that this policy should be considered only in low fistulas with minimal sepsis and tissue damage.

The authors' policy

We would accept that in experienced hands, particularly in a patient with an uncomplicated anorectal abscess, identification of an internal opening can safely be accompanied by insertion of a seton or synchronous fistulotomy if the track is superficial and there is minimal sepsis. However, we believe that extensive deroofing or excision of a fistula (Lockhart-Mummery, 1975) is dangerous in the presence of acute florid sepsis with tissue destruction (Eisenhammer, 1956). If anorectal sepsis is being managed by inexperienced accident and emergency staff or surgeons in training, we would advise drainage of pus followed by a careful examination under anaesthetic by a senior person 7–10 days later when the results of the cultures are available. On account of the high incidence of fistula in patients with an intersphincteric and a suprasphincteric abscess, and the need to divide the internal sphincter to allow proper drainage, we would usually advise early sphincterotomy and fistulotomy by an experienced colorectal surgeon for these rarer and more complicated abscesses (Hanley, 1978; Read and Abcarian, 1979; Thomson and Parks, 1979).

Management of specific abscesses

Perianal abscess

A careful examination under anaesthetic, using antibiotic cover to prevent an episode of bacteraemia, should be performed by an experienced colorectal surgeon. If an internal opening is found we advise that this should be laid open at the time of drainage by dividing the internal sphincter below the dentate line and leaving the entire cavity open (Figure 15.8b). We do not subscribe to attempted probing for a fistula after drainage of an abscess,

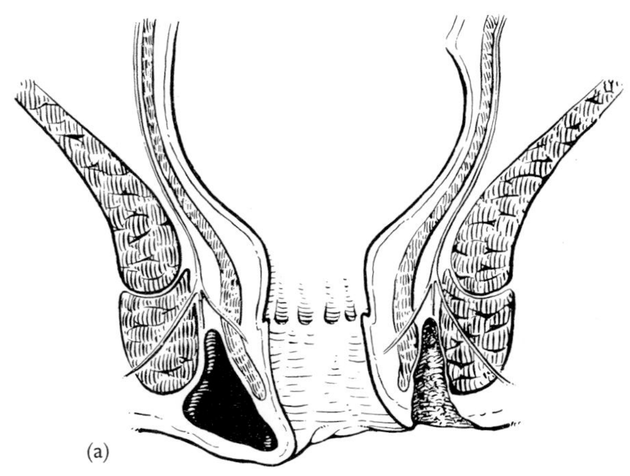

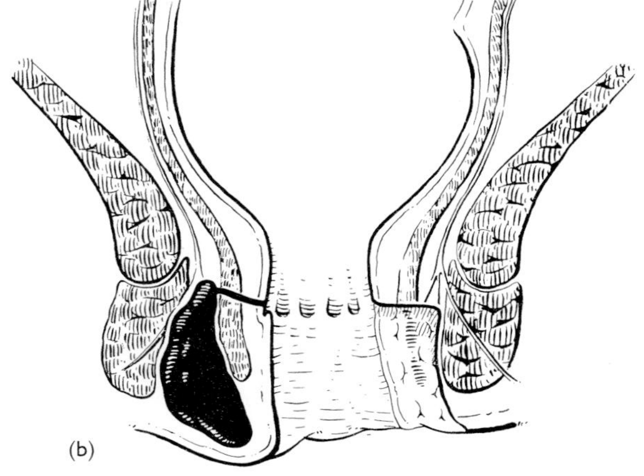

Figure 15.8a–b (a) On the left is a perianal abscess. On the right is the treatment thereof. Treatment of a perianal abscess consists of excising a disc of skin over the abscess and curetting the cavity. (b) On the left is a perianal abscess. On the right is shown our preferred method of treatment: excision of the lower fibres of the internal anal sphincter and the abscess cavity.

since this is likely to create a false passage. If probing is to be used it should be performed only by an experienced surgeon with a soft catheter or a curved malleable probe through the anal crypt towards the abscess. Identification of an internal opening can usually be achieved by gentle pressure over the abscess during inspection of the anal canal with a Sims speculum. If the surgeon is inexperienced or if no internal opening is found, the abscess should simply be drained by incising the skin over the most prominent area of the abscess, pus is sent for culture, the index finger is gently introduced into the cavity, the skin edges are trimmed and a dressing applied (Figure 15.8a). If the cultures grow a faecal organism, a second EUA by an experienced person should be arranged 7–10 days later. If a fistula is found it should be laid open, provided the anatomy of the track can be accurately defined; if not, a seton should be inserted.

Ischiorectal abscess

The overriding consideration in ischiorectal abscess is early drainage of pus since there is a large potential space with a high risk of progression to a horseshoe abscess (Held et al, 1986) or even synergistic necrotizing infection (Flanigan et al, 1978; Jamieson et al, 1984). The presence of a horseshoe extension should be excluded by careful assessment under anaesthesia. Most horseshoe extensions extend posteriorly across the midline and a high proportion are associated with a posterior midline trans-sphincteric fistula. If the abscess is unilateral, a single drainage site is then established over the site of maximal swelling (Figure 15.9). The pus is sent for culture. Curettage should be avoided for fear of creating a suprasphincteric extension or even a high fistula. The index finger is gently inserted to determine if there is any posterior extension across the midline. If a bilateral abscess is found, pus must be drained from both buttocks. If faecal organisms are identified, a second EUA is advised when the acute infection has largely resolved, usually 2–3 weeks later, to determine if there is a trans-sphincteric fistula, a suprasphincteric extension or even an extrasphincteric or suprasphincteric fistula (Figure 15.10).

A low trans-sphincteric fistula can be laid open at the time of drainage, but if a high fistula is identified it is wiser in our view to place a seton along the track to facilitate secondary exploration at a later stage. The lowest incidence of recurrent sepsis in patients with an ischiorectal abscess and horseshoe extension was reported in patients treated by incision counter-drainage and either fistulotomy or seton division of the fistula track (Held et al, 1986).

Intersphincteric abscess

Examination under anaesthesia will reveal an internal opening in almost half of these patients. If an internal opening is not laid open at the time of initial drainage, an EUA at a later date is advised if faecal organisms are identified. The intersphincteric abscess may extend around the anal canal and above the sphincter. Adequate dependent drainage should be obtained and, to do so, an internal sphinc-

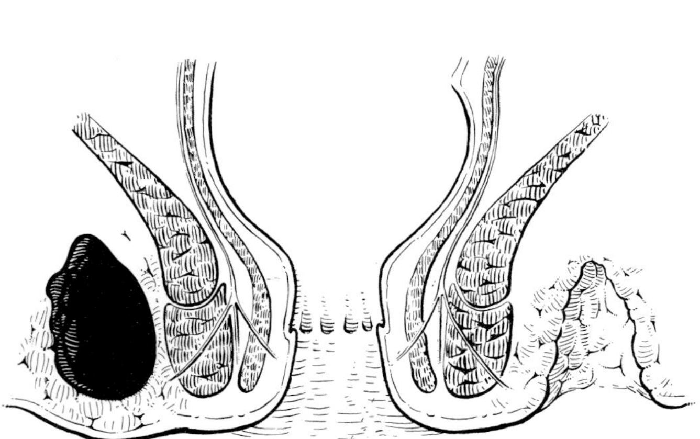

Figure 15.9 Drainage of an ischiorectal abscess. On the left is an ischiorectal abscess. On the right the abscess has been completely excised, leaving a large disc of skin to facilitate further drainage.

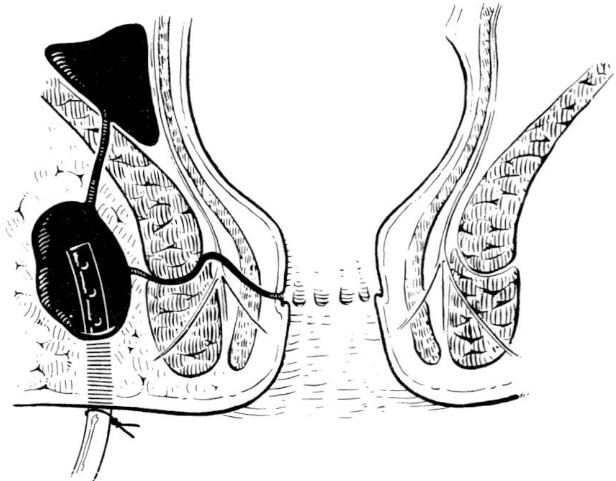

Figure 15.10 Ischiorectal abscess associated with a high blind track and a supralevator abscess. There is also a communication with the dentate line through the duct of the anal gland. Drainage of this abscess in the conventional manner will inevitably lead to a fistula-in-ano.

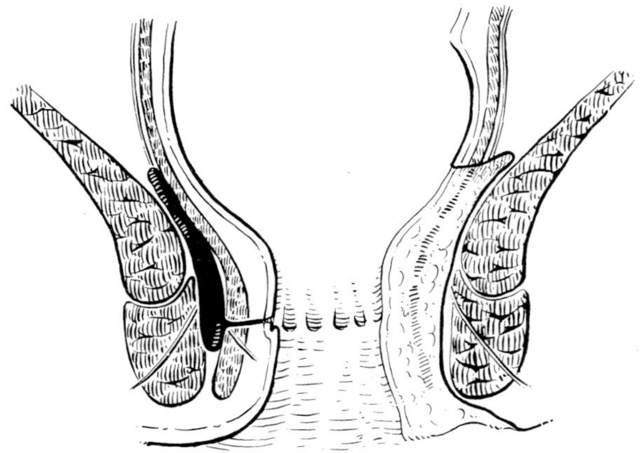

Figure 15.11 Drainage of an intersphincteric abscess. On the left is an intersphincteric abscess. On the right is shown the preferred method of drainage: laying open the abscess cavity and excising the internal anal sphincter.

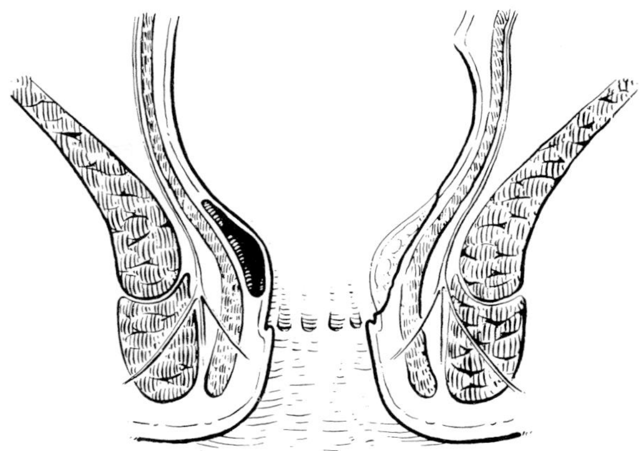

Figure 15.12 Drainage of a submucosal abscess. On the left is a submucosal abscess at the anorectal junction. On the right is shown the optimum treatment: excising the mucosa overlying the abscess, leaving the internal anal sphincter intact.

terectomy should be performed by excising a strip of internal sphincter. This manoeuvre reduces the chance of a recurrent abscess which, in our experience, is common if synchronous sphincterotomy is omitted. A gentle anal dilatation is also advised in male patients since excessive external sphincter activity may prevent adequate drainage (Figure 15.11). In our view a second EUA is always advisable for patients with an intersphincteric abscess, even if an internal sphincterotomy has been performed initially, because there is a risk of early recurrent abscess.

Submucosal abscess

Submucosal abscess alone seems to be an uncommon form of anorectal sepsis. A submucosal abscess should be drained internally by excising the mucosa over the bulging abscess (Figure 15.12). Commonly the abscess is actually found to be part of an intermuscular abscess. If there is no internal opening the abscess may be treated by excising the mucosa (Figure 15.13). If an internal opening is present a long internal sphincterectomy is advised.

Suprasphincteric component of an intersphincteric or ischiorectal abscess (see supralevator abscess)

If the suprasphincteric abscess is an extension of an intersphincteric abscess it should be treated by drainage into the anal canal (Figure 15.13), with a sphincterectomy if there is an internal opening (see Figure 15.11). This abscess should never be drained through the perineum. Conversely, if the abscess is an upward extension of an ischiorectal abscess it must be drained through the perineum, and never through the anus or else an extrasphincteric fistula will have been created (see Figure 15.10) (see supralevator abscess).

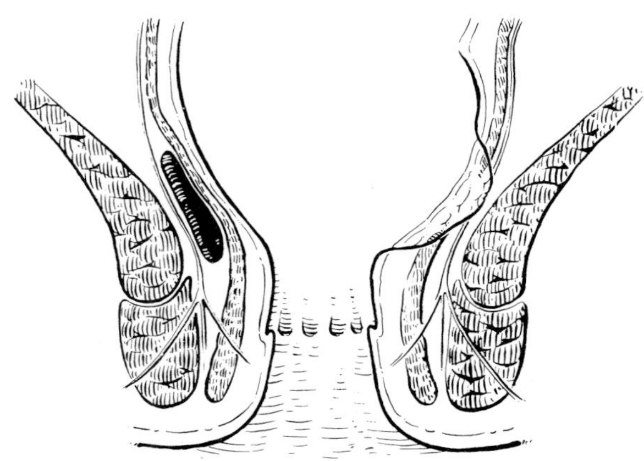

Figure 15.13 Drainage of a high intersphincteric abscess. On the left is a high intersphincteric abscess. On the right is the preferred treatment: excising the mucosa and internal anal sphincter adjacent to the abscess.

Complications

Synergistic gangrene

Necrotizing infection secondary to anorectal abscess is fortunately rare. It is more common in patients with an ischiorectal abscess but the diagnosis is often delayed (Davis et al, 1980). Predisposing conditions include diabetes, obesity, chronic ill-health, steroid therapy and chemotherapy for malignant disease (Bode et al, 1982; Badrinath et al, 1994). Complications resulting from the necrotizing fasciitis around the anus include gas gangrene, sterility, faecal incontinence, recurrent anorectal fistula and septicaemia. Treatment involves wide excision of all necrotic material in the perineum, extensive surgical drainage, antibiotic therapy and nutritional support; a proximal stoma is often necessary.

Recurrence

Recurrence has already been discussed; it invariably indicates that there is a persistent unrecognized anorectal fistula or some underlying disorder, such as hidradenitis suppurativa, Crohn's disease, tuberculosis, AIDS or a missed carcinoma.

Free-floating perineum

Occasionally an extensive horseshoe abscess which presents late or in immunocompromised patients may result in extensive circumferential sepsis around the anorectum. The condition may be complicated by synergistic gangrene. Huge volumes of pus occupy the ischiorectal fossa and anterior triangle. Treatment is by extensive debridement, multiple counter-drainage incisions and a proximal stoma.

Neutropenic patients

Occasionally patients with haematological disease or those receiving chemotherapy with neutropenia present with anal pain. Examination must exclude a fissure or haemorrhoids which should be managed conservatively. Abscess and fistulas often present with pain and swelling but there is very little pus. Treatment should include aggressive intravenous antibiotic therapy directed against *E. coli*, *Bacteroides* spp. and *Pseudomonas aeruginosa*. Early drainage in non-responding patients is usually advised, particularly in those with evidence of an abscess when examined under anaesthesia, or by anorectal ultrasound or MRI. Despite early drainage in septicaemic patients, this group have a high mortality. Close collaboration with microbiologists and haematologists is essential (Vanheuverzwyn et al, 1980; Shaked et al, 1986; Carlson et al, 1988; Barnes et al, 1994; Grewal et al, 1994).

SUPRALEVATOR ABSCESS

Aetiology

A supralevator abscess (Figures 15.14 and 15.15) may be due to pelvic pathology, such as diverticular disease, salpingitis, Crohn's disease, appendicitis, malignancy of the large bowel or foreign-body trauma. Sometimes a supralevator abscess occurs secondary to an intersphincteric cryptoglandular anal gland infection. Appropriate treatment (Figure 15.16) is crucial since ill-advised drainage may be responsible for creating a high fistula-in-ano.

Pathogenesis

It is important to define very carefully the anatomy of any suprasphincteric abscess originating from a cryptoglandular infection. These abscesses may develop in one of two ways (Parks et al, 1976). The infection may track upwards from an intersphincteric abscess, in which case there may or may not be a lower perianal communication. Alternatively, the

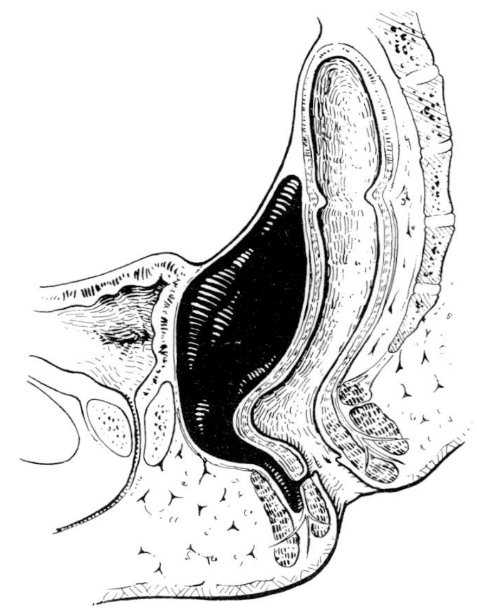

Figure 15.14 An anterior pelvic abscess. There is a large abscess cavity behind the bladder and the prostate and in front of the anorectum.

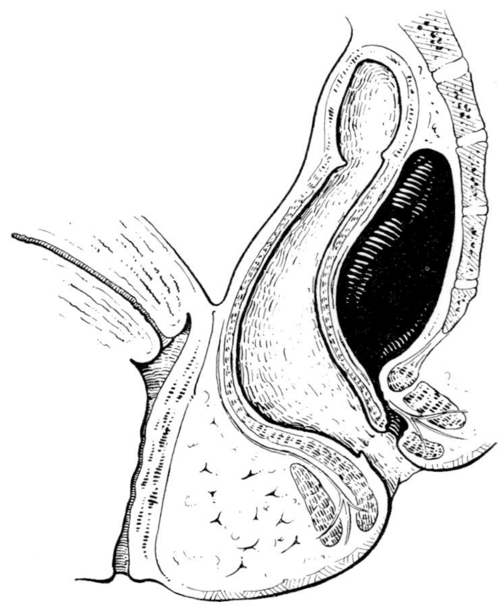

Figure 15.15 Posterior pelvic abscess. There is a large abscess cavity lying in the presacral space behind the rectum.

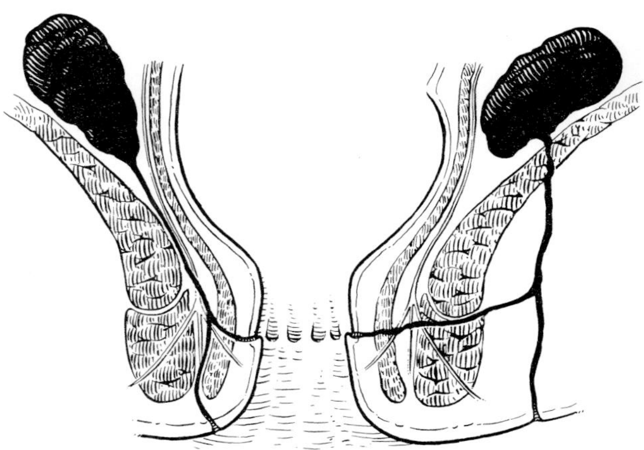

Figure 15.17 Supralevator abscess. On the left is a supralevator abscess which has arisen from an intersphincteric fistula-in-ano. On the right is a supralevator abscess, formed as the result of a high blind track, complicating a trans-sphincteric fistula-in-ano.

collection may be associated with an ischiorectal abscess and a trans-sphincteric fistula (Figure 15.17). The ischiorectal abscess may burst through the levator plate into the suprasphincteric or pararectal space. The upward extension of an ischiorectal abscess is commonly iatrogenic following overenthusiastic curettage by an inexperienced surgeon. Under these circumstances it is very easy to penetrate the levator ani or, even worse, to damage the rectal wall and create either a supralevator sinus or, more seriously, an extrasphincteric fistula.

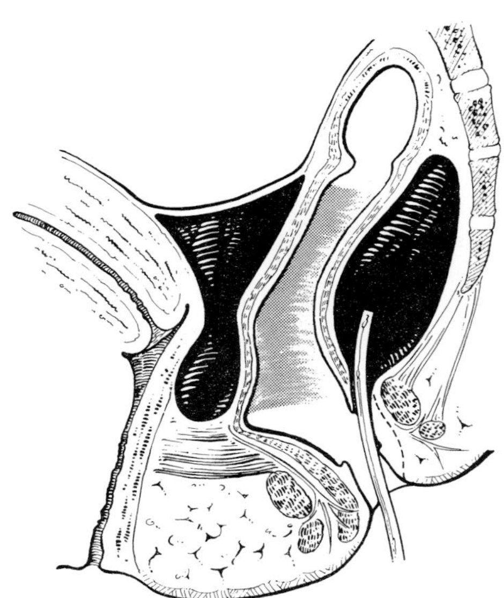

Figure 15.16 Intrarectal drainage of a pelvic abscess. The pelvic abscess has been identified, and a pair of Roberts' artery forceps have been advanced into the abscess cavity through the posterior rectal wall. A soft drainage tube is then inserted into the abscess cavity.

Clinical presentation

There is often considerable delay in diagnosis since clinical symptoms may be minimal, apart from fever, perineal discomfort and urinary tract symptoms. Furthermore, there are usually no external signs of an anorectal infection. One of the dangers of supralevator abscess is that it may expand extensively before a diagnosis is achieved (Hanley, 1979). Rupture of the abscess into the rectum causes a chronic high intersphincteric fistula. The abscess may spread circumferentially and almost surround the rectum before a correct diagnosis is made. Rupture of a high supralevator intersphincteric abscess into the ischiorectal fossa over the puborectalis, if followed by surgical drainage through the ischiorectal fossa, results in a suprasphincteric fistula. Spread to the thigh or buttocks may also occur if pus tracks through the greater sciatic foramen or the obturator foramen.

Treatment

Intersphincteric variety

If a supralevator abscess is secondary to an intersphincteric fistula, the abscess must be drained into the rectum, together with division of most of the internal anal sphincter (Figure 15.18). If this type of abscess is treated by drainage through the perineum, an extrasphincteric fistula is an almost inevitable consequence.

Ischiorectal variety

If a supralevator abscess is due to an upward extension of a trans-sphincteric fistula complicating an ischiorectal abscess, it should never be drained into the rectum since this will amost invariably create an extrasphincteric fistula (Figure 15.18). In these cases a supralevator abscess must be treated by dependent perineal drainage through the ischiorectal fossa. At a later stage the lower fibres of the external sphincter may be laid open to treat the trans-sphincteric fistula.

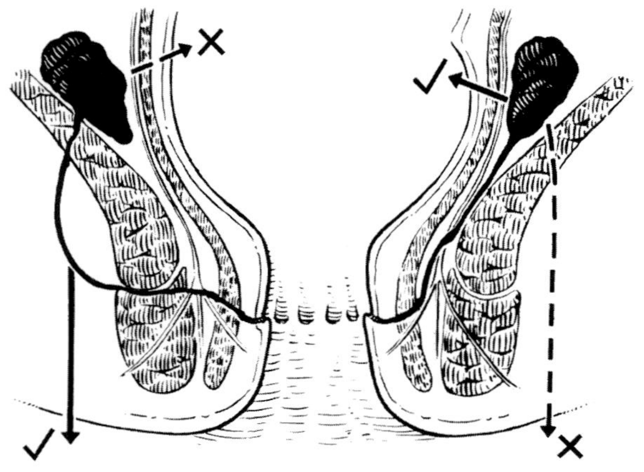

Figure 15.18 Principles of drainage of a supralevator abscess. On the left is a supralevator abscess caused by a trans-sphincteric fistula. This must be drained through the perineum, as in the management of an ischiorectal abscess. On the right is a supralevator abscess complicating an intersphincteric infection. Under these circumstances drainage must be into the rectum above the sphincters; it should never be through the perineum. Incorrect drainage will inevitably lead to a high fistula-in-ano.

Horseshoe extension

If there is a suprasphincteric horseshoe extension around the upper surface of the levator ani, drainage by conventional techniques is often inadequate (Parks and Stitz, 1976). In these patients, the only satisfactory approach, irrespective of a trans-sphincteric component, is to divide all the muscles attached to the coccyx, thereby allowing the visceral structures (principally the puborectalis and iliococcygeus) to ride forwards. This manoeuvre has no harmful effect on the sphincter mechanism since the sphincter ring and puborectalis itself are not disturbed. A postanal extrasphincteric approach is usually needed to achieve division of the pubococcygeus and ischiococcygeus so as to provide adequate drainage of the ischiorectal component as well as releasing pus from the supralevator compartment of the postanal space.

True pelvic abscess

If the suprasphincteric abscess is a complication of pelvic pathology, management depends upon the site of the abscess and the underlying pathology. If the abscess is secondary to a continuing source of sepsis, such as malignancy of the large bowel or Crohn's disease, the primary disease process will need to be excised as well as draining the pus. If the primary process is likely to resolve, as in an abscess complicating diverticular disease, salpingitis, appendicitis or after a previous colorectal procedure, initial drainage alone will usually suffice. Drainage can be achieved into the rectum or into the vagina. If the abscess is very large a drainage tube or preferably a soft Foley or Malecot catheter, left *in situ* for a few days, can be used to facilitate irrigation. Even though there may be pelvic pathology, it is wise to ascertain that the abscess is not cryptoglandular in origin. If it is, a search should be made for a potential opening into the anal canal.

REFERENCES

Abcarian H (1976) Acute suppurations of the anorectum. In Nyhns LM (ed) *Surgery Annual*, Vol. 8, p. 305. New York: Appleton–Century–Crofts.

Abcarian H & Eftaiha M (1983) Floating free-standing anus: a complication of massive anorectal infection. *Dis Colon Rect* **26**: 516–521.

Abercrombie JF & George BD (1992) Perianal abscess in children. *Ann R Coll Surg Engl* **74**: 385–386.

Ani AN & Logundoye SB (1979) Radiological evaluation of anal fistulae: a prospective study of fistulograms. *Clin Radiol* **30**: 21–24.

Arnow PM, Boyko EJ & Friedmann EL (1983) Perirectal abscess

caused by *Legionella pneumophila* and mixed anaerobic bacteria. *Ann Intern Med* **98**: 184–185.

Badrinath K, Jairam N & Ravi HR (1994) Spreading extraperitoneal cellulitis following perirectal sepsis. *Br J Surg* **81**: 297–298.

Barnes SG, Sattler FR & Ballard JO (1994) Perirectal infections in acute leukaemia: improved survival after incision and debridement. *Ann Intern Med* **100**: 515–518.

Barwood N, Clarke G, Levitt S & Levitt M (1996) Fistula-in-ano: a prospective study of 107 patients. *Int J Colorect Dis* **11**: 134.

Benson EA & Goodman MA (1970) Incision with primary suture in the treatment of acute puerperal breast abscess. *Br J Surg* **57**: 55–58.

Bevans DW, Westbrook KC, Thompson BW & Caldwell FT (1973) Perirectal abscess: a potentially fatal illness. *Am J Surg* **126**: 765–768.

Beynon J, Mortensen NJMcC, Foy DMA, Channer JL, Virjee J & Goddard P (1986) Endorectal sonography: laboratory and clinical experience in Bristol. *Int J Colorect Dis* **1**: 212–215.

Blank WA (1955) Anorectal complications in leukaemia. *Am J Surg* **90**: 738–741.

Bode WE, Ramos R & Page CP (1982) Invasive necrotising infection secondary to anorectal abscess. *Dis Colon Rectum* **25**: 416–419.

Brightmore T (1972) Perianal gas-producing infection of non-clostridial origin. *Br J Surg* **59**: 109–116.

Buchan R & Grace RH (1973) Anorectal suppuration: the results of treatment and the factors influencing the recurrence rate. *Br J Surg* **60**: 537–540.

Cabrera A, Tsukada Y & Pickren JW (1966) Adenocarcinomas of the anal canal and perianal tissues. *Ann Surg* **64**: 152–156.

Carlson FW, Ferguson CM & Amerson JR (1988) Perianal infections in acute leukaemia. *Am Surg* **54**: 693–695.

Cataldo PA, Senagore A & Luchtefeld MA (1993) Intrarectal ultrasound in the evaluation of perirectal abscesses. *Dis Colon Rectum* **36**: 554–558.

Chandrasoma PT & Mendis KM (1977) *Enterobius vermicularis* in anal sepsis. *Am J Trop Med Hyg* **26**: 644–649.

Chrabot CM, Prasad ML & Abcarian H (1983) Recurrent anorectal abscesses. *Dis Colon Rectum* **26**: 105–108.

Cohen JS, Paz IB, O'Donnell MR & Ellenhorn JDI (1996) Treatment of perianal infection following bone marrow transplantation. *Dis Colon Rectum* **39**: 981–985.

Consten ECJ, Slors JFM, Danner SA et al (1996) Severe complications of perianal sepsis in patients with human immunodeficiency virus. *Br J Surg* **83**: 778–780.

Davis JC, Dunn JM & Heimbach RD (1980) Indications for hyperbaric oxygen therapy. *Tex Med* **76**: 44–47.

Dukes CE & Galvin C (1956) Colloid carcinoma arising within fistulae in the anorectal region. *Ann R Coll Surg Engl* **18**: 246–261.

Eisenhammer S (1956) The internal anal sphincter and the anorectal abscess. *Surg Gynecol Obstet* **103**: 501–506.

Eisenhammer S (1961) The anorectal and anovulval fistulous abscess. *Surg Gynecol Obstet* **113**: 519–520.

Eisenhammer S (1964) Long-tract anteroposterior intermuscular fistula. *Dis Colon Rectum* **7**: 438–440.

Eisenhammer S (1978) The final evaluation and classification of the surgical treatment of the primary anorectal cryptoglandular intermuscular (intersphincteric) fistulous abscess and fistula. *Dis Colon Rectum* **21**: 237–254.

Ellis M (1951) Use of penicillin and sulphonamides in the treatment of suppuration. *Lancet* **i**: 774–775.

Ellis M (1960) Incision and primary suture of abscesses of the anal region. *Proc R Soc Med* **53**: 652–653.

Ellis M (1970) *The Casualty Officer's Handbook*, Vol. 3. London: Butterworth.

Eykyn SN & Grace RH (1986) The relevance of microbiology in the management of anorectal sepsis. *Ann R Coll Surg Engl* **68**: 237–239.

Fielding MA & Berry AR (1992) Management of perianal sepsis in a district general hospital. *J R Coll Surg Edinb* **37**: 232–234.

Flanigan RC, Kursh DE, McDougal WS & Persky L (1978) Synergistic gangrene of the scrotum and penis secondary to colorectal diseases. *J Urol* **119**: 369–371.

Getz SB, Ough YD, Patterson RB et al (1981) Mucinous adenocarcinoma developing in chronic anal fistula. *Dis Colon Rectum* **24**: 562–566.

Goldberg SM, Gordon PH & Nivatvong S (1980) *Essentials of Anorectal Surgery*. Philadelphia: Lippincott.

Goligher JC, Ellis M & Pissidis AG (1967) A critique of anal glandular infection in the aetiology and treatment of idiopathic anorectal abscesses and fistulas. *Br J Surg* **54**: 977–983.

Grace RH, Harper IA & Thompson RG (1982) Anorectal sepsis: microbiology in relation to fistula-in-ano. *Br J Surg* **69**: 401–403.

Granet E (1954) *Manual of Proctology*. Chicago: YearBook Medical.

Grewal H, Guillem JG, Quan SHQ, Enker WE & Cohen AM (1994) Anorectal disease in neutropenic leukemic patients. *Dis Colon Rectum* **37**: 1095–1099.

Hanley PH (1978) Anorectal abscess fistula. *Surg Clin North Am* **58**: 487–503.

Hanley PH (1979) Anorectal supralevator abscess–fistula-in-ano. *Surg Gynecol Obstet* **148**: 899–904.

Hanley PH (1985) Reflections on anorectal abscess fistula. *Dis Colon Rectum* **28**: 528–533.

Held D, Khubchandani J, Sheets J et al (1986) Management of anorectal horseshoe abscess and fistula. *Dis Colon Rectum* **29**: 793–797.

Hill JR (1967) Fistulas and fistulous abscesses in the anorectal region: personal experience in management. *Dis Colon Rectum* **10**: 421–434.

Ho Y-H, Tan M, Chui C-H et al (1997) Randomized controlled trial of primary fistulotomy with drainage alone for perianal abscesses. *Dis Colon Rectum* **40**: 1435–1438.

Hughes LE (1977) Surgical pathology and management of anorectal Crohn's disease. *J R Soc Med* **71**: 644–651.

Jamieson NV, Everett WG & Bullock KN (1984) Delayed recognition of an intersphincteric abscess as the underlying cause of Fournier's scrotal gangrene. *Ann R Coll Surg Engl* **66**: 434–435.

Jones NAG & Wilson DH (1976) The treatment of acute abscesses by incision, curettage and primary suture under antibiotic cover. *Br J Surg* **63**: 499–501.

Kovalcik PJ (1979) Anorectal abscess. *Surg Gynecol Obstet* **149**: 884–886.

Kratzer GL (1950) Anal ducts and their clinical significance. *Am J Surg* **79**: 34–39.

Law PJ, Talbot RW, Bartram CI & Northover JMA (1989) Anal endosonography in the evaluation of perianal sepsis and fistula-in-ano. *Br J Surg* **76**: 752–755.

Leaper DJ, Page RE, Rosenburg IL, Wilson DH & Goligher JC (1976) A controlled study comparing the conventional treatment of idiopathic anorectal abscess with that of incision, curettage and primary suture under systemic antibiotic cover. *Dis Colon Rectum* **19**: 46–50.

Lee SH, Zucker M & Sato T (1981) Primary adenocarcinoma of an anal gland with secondary perianal fistulas. *Hum Pathol* **12**: 1034–1036.

Lichtenstein D, Stavorovsky M & Irge D (1978) Fournier's gangrene complicating perianal abscess: report of two cases. *Dis Colon Rectum* **21**: 377–379.

Lockhart-Mummery HE (1975) Symposium: Anorectal problems. Treatment of abscesses. *Dis Colon Rectum* **18**: 650–651.

Lowe D (1985) Abscesses, sinuses and fistulas. In *Surgery* (Medical Education Ltd: Int. Series): 436–439.

Lunniss PJ & Phillips RKS (1994) Surgical assessment of acute anorectal sepsis is a better predictor of fistula than microbiological analysis. *Br J Surg* **81**: 368–369.

McElwain JE, Maclean D, Alexander RM, Hoexter B & Guthrie JF (1975) Anorectal problem: experience with primary fistulotomy for anorectal abscess, a report of 1000 cases. *Dis Colon Rectum* **18**: 646–649.

McFie J & Harvey J (1977) The treatment of acute superficial abscesses: a prospective clinical trial. *Br J Surg* **64**: 264–266.

Marks G, Chase WV & Mervine TB (1973) The fatal potential of fistula-in-ano with abscess: analysis of 11 deaths. *Dis Colon Rectum* **16**: 224–230.

Mortensen NJ & Thomson JP (1984) Perianal abscess due to *Enterobius vermicularis*. *Dis Colon Rectum* **27**: 677–678.

Mulholland MW, Delaney JP & Simmons RL (1983) Gastrointestinal complications of chronic granulomatous disease: surgical implications. *Surgery* **94**: 569–575.

Nelson RL, Prasad ML & Abcarian H (1985) Anal carcinoma presenting as a perirectal abscess or fistula. *Arch Surg* **120**: 632–635.

Nesselrod JP (1949) Anal canal and rectum. In Christopher F (ed) *A Textbook of Surgery*, 5th edn, p. 1092. Philadelphia: Saunders.

Page RE (1974) Treatment of axillary abscesses by incision and primary suture under antibiotic cover. *Br J Surg* **61**: 493–494.

Page RE & Freeman R (1977) Superifical sepsis: the antibiotic of choice for blind treatment. *Br J Surg* **64**: 281–284.

Parks AG (1961) Pathogenesis and treatment of fistula-in-ano. *BMJ* **1**: 463–469.

Parks AG & Stitz RW (1976) Symposium: Fistula-in-ano. The treatment of high fistula-in-ano. *Dis Colon Rectum* **19**: 487–499.

Parks AG, Gordon PH & Hardcastle JD (1976) A classification of fistula-in-ano. *Br J Surg* **63**: 1–12.

Piazza DJ & Radhakrishnan J (1990) Perianal abscess and fistula-in-ano in children. *Dis Colon Rectum* **33**: 1014–1016.

Prasad ML, Read DR & Abcarian H (1981) Supralevator abscess: diagnosis and treatment. *Dis Colon Rectum* **24**: 456–461.

Ramanujam PS, Prasad ML, Abcarian H & Tan AB (1984) Perianal abscesses and fistulas: a study of 1023 patients. *Dis Colon Rectum* **27**: 593–597.

Read DR & Abcarian H (1979) A prospective survey of 474 patients with anorectal abscess. *Dis Colon Rectum* **22**: 566–568.

Schouten WR & Vroonhoven TJMV van (1991) Treatment of anorectal abscess with or without primary fistulectomy. *Dis Colon Rectum* **34**: 60–63.

Sehdev MK, Dowling MD, Seal SH & Stearns MW (1973) Perianal and anorectal complications in leukaemia. *Cancer* **31**: 149–152.

Seow-Choen F & Ho JMS (1994) Histoanatomy of anal glands. *Dis Colon Rectum* **37**: 1215–1218.

Shaked AA, Shinar E & Freund H (1986) Managing the granulocytopenic patient with acute perianal inflammatory disease. *Am J Surg* **152**: 510–512.

Simms MH, Curran F, Johnson RA et al (1982) Treatment of acute abscess in the casualty department. *BMJ* **284**: 1827–1829.

Slater DN (1984) Perianal abscess: 'Have I excluded leukaemia?' *BMJ* **289**: 1682.

Steele RJC, Eremin O, Krajewski AS & Ritchie GL (1985) Primary lymphoma of the anal canal presenting as perianal suppuration. *BMJ* **291**: 311.

Stewart MPM, Laing MR & Krukowski ZH (1985) Treatment of acute abscesses by incision, curettage and primary suture without antibiotics: a controlled clinical trial. *Br J Surg* **72**: 66–67.

Tang GL, Chew SP & Seow-Choen F (1996) Prospective randomized trial of drainage alone vs. drainage and fistulotomy for acute perianal abscesses with proven internal opening. *Dis Colon Rectum* **39**: 1415–1417.

Thomson JPS & Parks AG (1979) Anal abscess and fistulas. *Br J Hosp Med* **21**: 413–425.

Thornton JP & Abcarian H (1978) Surgical treatment of perianal and perineal hidradenitis suppurativa. *Dis Colon Rectum* **21**: 573–577.

Vafai M & Mohit P (1983) Granuloma of the anal canal due to *Enterobius vermicularis*: report of a case. *Dis Colon Rectum* **26**: 349–350.

Vanheuverzwyn R, Delannoy A, Michaux JL & Dive C (1980) Anal lesions in hematologic diseases. *Dis Colon Rectum* **23**: 310–312.

Vasilevsky C-A & Gordon PH (1984) The incidence of recurrent abscesses or fistula-in-ano following anorectal suppuration. *Dis Colon Rectum* **27**: 126–130.

Walsh G & Stickley CS (1934) Acute leukaemia with primary symptoms in the rectum. *South Med J* **96**: 684–689.

Whitehead SM, Leach RD, Eykyn SJ & Phillips I (1982) The aetiology of perirectal sepsis. *Br J Surg* **3**: 166–168.

Wilson DH (1964) The late results of anorectal abscess treated by incision, curettage and primary suture under antibiotic cover. *Br J Surg* **51**: 828–831.

Winslett MC, Allan A & Ambrose NS (1988) Anorectal sepsis as a presentation of occult rectal and systemic disease. *Dis Colon Rectum* **31**: 597–600.

Zaren HA, Delone FX & Lerner HJ (1983) Carcinoma of the anal gland: case report and review of the literature. *J Surg Oncol* **28**: 250–254.

Zbar A, DeSouza N, Puni R, Bydder G & Kmiot W (1996) Magnetic resonance imaging (MRI) of anal sphincter sepsis with an internal coil. *Int J Colorect Dis* **11**: 135–139.

16
ANORECTAL FISTULA

A fistula-in-ano is a granulating track between the anorectum and the perineum. (Fistula literally translated from the Latin means a pipe or a reed.) A fistula may consist of primary and secondary tracks. Sometimes these tracks become occluded and a sinus remains.

Many fistulas are low-lying, consisting of a single straight track from the skin to the anal canal, merely traversing the lower fibres of the internal anal sphincter. The majority of such fistulas can, therefore, be managed by simply laying open the track (fistulotomy) with a good prospect of cure and with no impairment of continence. However, the same cannot be said for fistulas which traverse the external sphincter, particularly if they have been associated with a previous ischiorectal abscess. Some of these fistulas are complex, with secondary pararectal or supralevator tracks (Seow-Choen and Nicholls, 1992). Laying open of such fistulas causes serious and often permanent impaired continence. There is growing evidence that even division of the internal anal sphincter, leaving the puborectalis and external sphincter undisturbed, may cause impaired continence after successful elimination of the fistula (Lunnis et al, 1994b). Nevertheless, unless all the secondary tracks are also attended to, there is a risk of recurrent sepsis and fistulation (García-Aguilar et al, 1996). These conflicting objectives pose a real challenge for the colorectal surgeon; on the one hand recurrent sepsis and fistulation must be avoided, while on the other, continence must be preserved.

Possibly in no other field of anorectal surgery is appropriate treatment so critical (Seow-Choen and Nicholls, 1992; Phillips and Lunniss, 1996a,b). The potential for incurring life-long morbidity may be greater than in any other sphere of large bowel surgery. Once even partial sphincter division is complicated by perirectal fibrosis and resulting in a gutter deformity, later reconstructive surgery rarely resolves the imperfections of continence, particularly soiling. Thus, fistulas-in-ano have an unenviable reputation for recurrence and compromised continence. There are few procedures in surgery where the outcome is so greatly influenced by the experience and judgement of the surgeon (van Tets and Kuijpers, 1994).

HISTORICAL CONSIDERATIONS

Treatment of fistula-in-ano was described by Hippocrates in 460 BC (Sainio, 1996). Adams (1849) in his translations for the Sydenham Society describes the use of 'a stalk of fresh garlic' as a means of examining the track of a fistula. These fistulas were thought to complicate infection or 'tubercles' which had a tendency to spread to 'the softer parts'. Fistulas were thought to be exacerbated by local trauma, particularly horse riding and rowing.

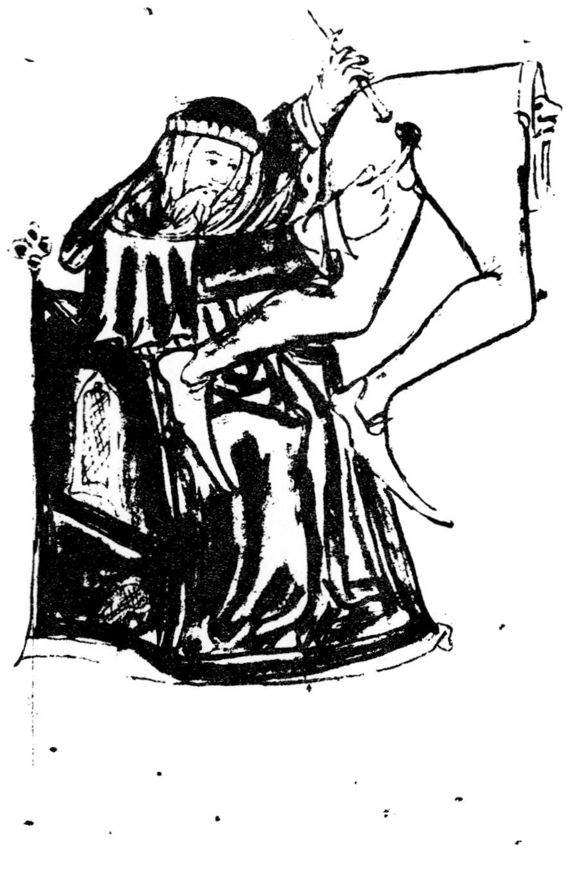

Figure 16.1 John of Arderne passes a flexible probe and feels for the internal opening of a fistula-in-ano. Reproduced with permission from the British Library.

Hippocrates was remarkably advanced in his treatment philosophy. Early drainage was advised 'even before matter is fully formed'. The use of a seton and fistulotomy is also described. Hippocrates advised the use of a strip of linen 'smeared with the caustic juice of euphorbia' to act as a seton, an approach later adopted by ancient physicians and named the Kshara Sutra thread (Deshpande and Sharma, 1973).

Celsus advised using a probe: 'put a probe into the fistula to see where it goes and how deeply it reaches, also whether it is moist or rather dry' (Milne, 1907). The value of palpation in the assessment of anal fistulas was stressed by Paulus Aeginetta, who also believed that the finger-nail was a useful instrument to curette the track (Adams, 1846). Instruments used for treating anal fistulas were unearthed at Pompeii (Gordon-Watson, 1934). In the Middle Ages fistulotomy was widely practised and was described by John of Arderne (Kirkup, 1985) (Figure 16.1). Probes included well-lubricated swine bristle or bronze olivary probes (Woodall, 1617). Percival Pott (1765) advocated laying open anal fistulas and emphasized the importance of packing the wound. In Paris, Felix experimented among prisoners before successfully treating an anal fistula in Louis XIV, an achievement that provided him with an estate, a title and an honorarium of such magnitude that he was able to establish five chairs in Surgery (Garrison, 1921).

Frederick Salmon, founder of St Mark's Hospital over 150 years ago, established the principles for treating fistula-in-ano which are widely used throughout the world today. Indeed, it was the recognition that some surgeons should take a special interest in anal fistulas that was responsible for creating proctology as a specialist surgical discipline.

AETIOLOGY AND PATHOGENESIS

Anal gland theory

Most fistulas occur after drainage of a previous anorectal abscess, but not all abscesses are complicated by a fistula (Henrichsen and Christiansen, 1986) and not all patients with a fistula give a history of previous sepsis (Marks and Ritchie, 1977). Even abscesses caused by faecal anaerobes do not all result in fistulas (Grace et al, 1982). Despite this observation, there is overwhelming evidence that the majority of anal fistulas are associated with sepsis in the intersphincteric plane caused by an infected anal gland (Thomson and Parks, 1979). Some abscesses are quite small and may burst into the anal canal without the patient being aware that there has been any previous episode of perianal infection (Seow-Choen et al, 1992). We and others (Adams and Kovalcik, 1981) found that approximately 70% of patients with an anal fistula had a previous history of anorectal sepsis (Shouler et al, 1986). However, in other reports, the proportion of patients having a history of sepsis is much lower (Hanley, 1979; Khubchandani, 1984).

A chronic abscess is frequently encountered if a careful search of the intersphincteric plane is made during exploration of an anal fistula (Eisenhammer, 1953; Steltzner, 1959; Seow-Choen et al, 1992). Over 90% of fistulas have a major component which is situated in the intersphincteric plane which may extend above the levator ani, into the deep postanal space (Eisenhammer, 1956; Parks et al, 1976; Vasilevsky and Gordon, 1984; Hardcastle, 1985; Lilius, 1986). If a chronic intersphincteric abscess is not adequately drained, particularly in patients with a high intersphincteric fistula, there is a risk of a recurrent fistula sepsis (Hill et al, 1943; Eisenhammer, 1958; Parks, 1961; Nicholls et al, 1990).

The anal glands, eight or more in number, lie in the submucosa, internal sphincter and intermuscular plane (Chiari, 1878; Herrmann and Desfosses, 1980), but they do not traverse the longitudinal muscle fibres or the external anal sphincter since, developmentally, they are visceral and not somatic structures. The glands are flask-shaped and their ducts are lined by modified stratified transitional epithelium (Figure 16.2). The glands are most abundant posteriorly and in the lower anal canal (Bremer, 1930; Tucker and Hellwig, 1934). Most of the glandular tissue is in the lower third of the internal anal sphincter. The glands help to lubricate the anal mucosa by secreting mucus into the anal crypts (Chiari, 1878). These glandular structures are surrounded by aggregates of lymphoid tissue, which explain why anal glands often become involved by tuberculosis and Crohn's disease (Parks and Morson, 1962).

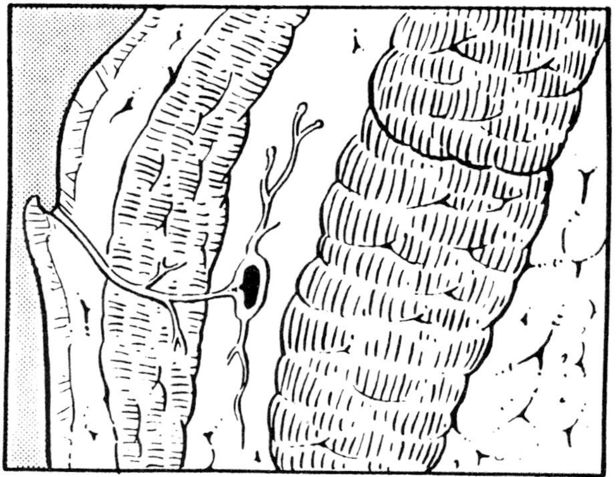

Figure 16.2 Anatomy of an anal gland.

There are two types of anal gland. The first lie completely within the submucosa. The second consist of branched tubules which pierce the muscular layers of the anal canal and are called intermuscular glands, of which there are between six and eight. These intermuscular glands may extend cephalad (Hill et al, 1949). Ductal openings of anal intermuscular glands are distributed equally around the circumference of the anal canal (Parks, 1963).

We and others believe that once an anal gland becomes infected a small abscess is formed in the intersphincteric plane which either spontaneously resolves or ruptures into the anal canal (Eisenhammer, 1956). Some episodes of infection are so minor that the patient is unaware of having had any anal sepsis. In other cases there is no apparent internal opening to the anal canal because the infective process stimulates an area of fibrosis which occludes the duct, a situation which predisposes to a chronic abscess cavity. Spread of sepsis is usually caudal towards the perineum along the fibroelastic septa of the perianal region (Figure 16.3) (Seow-Choen, 1996). Less commonly the infective process spreads upwards (Hanley, 1978), resulting in a high intersphincteric or supralevator abscess (Eisenhammer, 1951). Lateral spread may be via a long fibroelastic septum passing directly through the external sphincter or via the venous plexus to the ischiorectal fossa. Occasionally lateral spread may occur over the top of the puborectalis to enter the ischiorectal fossa by penetrating the levator ani. Alternatively, the abscess may discharge medially along its duct to resolve spontaneously.

Once an abscess is drained or spontaneously discharges it forms a potential fistula. If the track becomes epithelialized the fistula persists (Lunniss et al, 1995b).

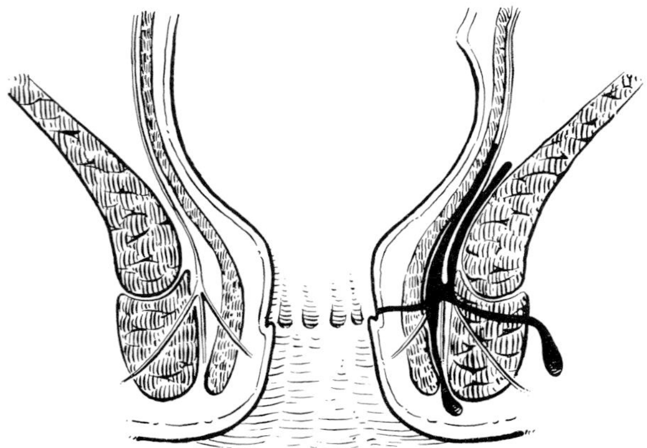

Figure 16.3 The spread of anal gland infection. The anal gland lies in the intersphincteric space: infection may spread (1) upwards into the supralevator or extrarectal space, (2) laterally through the external anal sphincter into the ischiorectal fossa, or (3) downwards through the intersphincteric plane to form a perianal abscess.

Other causes of fistula-in-ano

Although there is overwhelming evidence that most fistulas are due to a pyogenic infection in the anal glands or their associated lymphatics (Parks, 1963; Stirnemann and Halter, 1970; Roschke and Krause, 1983), there are a number of other causes.

Congenital fistulas

Anorectal cryptoglandular fistulas have been reported in early infancy (Duhamel, 1975; Fitzgerald et al, 1985; Shafer et al, 1987; Brem et al, 1989) and in some cases the tracks are lined by columnar or transitional epithelium, suggesting that they might have a congenital or developmental origin (Pople and Ralphs, 1988). Occasionally an intersphincteric, retrorectal or pelvic dermoid may present as a fistula: however, they do not communicate with the anorectum, only with the cyst if it has burst, become secondarily infected or accidentally opened during exploration of an 'abscess' (Mortensen, 1996).

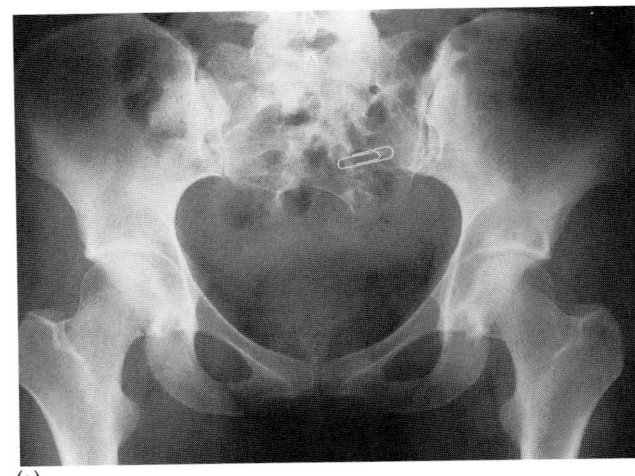

(a)

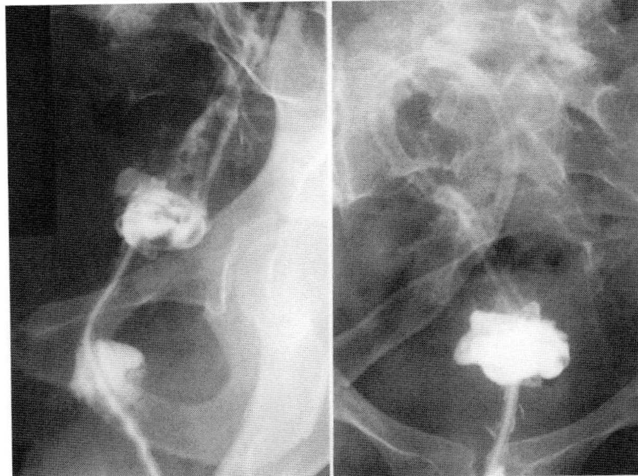

(b)

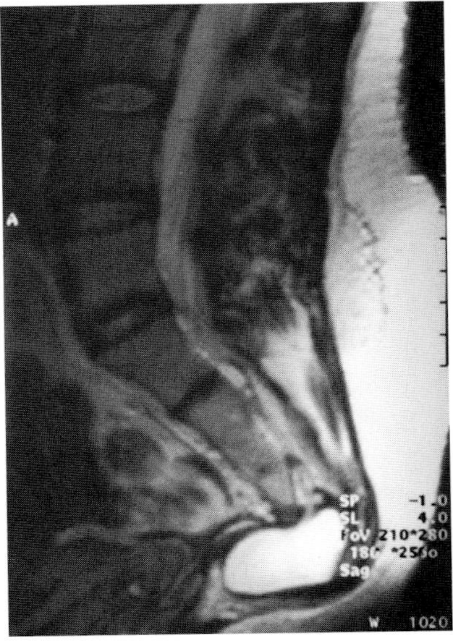

(c)

Figure 16.4a–c Sacrococcygeal cyst. (a) Plain radiograph showing the typical scimitar sign in the lower sacrum (just below the paper-clip). (b) Fistulogram showing communication with the anal canal and presacral dimple. (c) MRI in the same patient, showing coexisting meningocele.

Fistulas may also occur following operations for congenital disorders, such as from anal anastomosis after pull-through procedures for anorectal agenesis or Hirschprung's disease.

Congenital fistulas may arise as a remnant of the medullary canal in spina bifida; they present at birth and discharge cerebrospinal fluid. Infection of a sacrococcygeal teratoma or dermoid cyst may cause an anorectal fistula (Pye and Bundell, 1987). Sinuses may be present in children with complete obstruction from imperforate anus, and anorectal fistulas may present at birth in anorectal agenesis. Occasionally, complex fistulas in adults may be due to connections with embryological rests, such as non-communicating meningocele (Figure 16.4). Rectal reduplication is a rare cause of persistent perianal fistula (La Quaglia et al, 1990). These duplications may be on or in the rectal wall and may communicate with the rectum or be a closed sac.

Pelvic sepsis

Rarely, pelvic sepsis may result in a chronic supralevator abscess which may either spread caudally in the intermuscular space to emerge in the perineum, resulting in a high intersphincteric fistula (Figure 16.5), or may burst through the levator ani, presenting as an atypical ischiorectal abscess and resulting in an extrasphincteric fistula (Parks et al, 1976). The usual causes include appendicitis, salpingitis, diverticular disease, inflammatory bowel disease or a pelvic neoplasm (Fillipini, 1969; Martini, 1970).

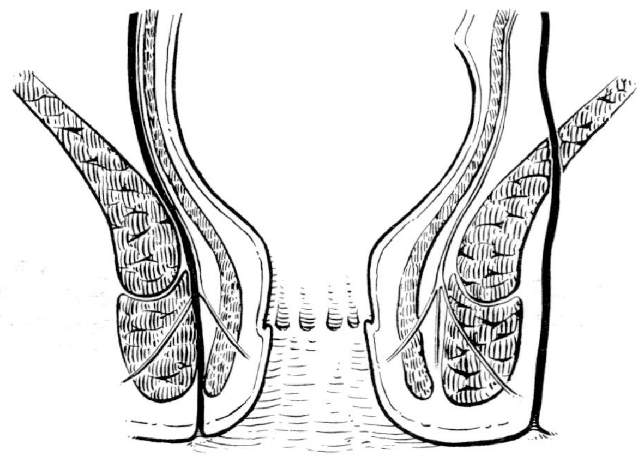

Figure 16.5 An anorectal fistula may arise from pelvic pathology associated with a pelvic abscess. Under these circumstances pus may drain through the intersphincteric plane, or may drain as an extrasphincteric fistula.

Perineal injuries

Fistulas around the anal canal may complicate penetrating perineal injuries due to blunt trauma, stabbings, blast injuries from mines or gunshot wounds sustained as a result of civil or military conflict. Occasionally, ingested foreign bodies, such as fish or chicken bones, may penetrate the rectum. Impalement injury after falling astride a sharp object or as a result of a road traffic accident may result in a high anorectal fistula. The possibility of coexisting urethral trauma should always be considered in these injuries (Stelzner, 1981).

Anal disorders

Fissure

Fissure-in-ano may be complicated by a short superficial fistula running from the base of the fissure to the hypertrophied anal papilla (Roschke, 1964). These are almost always mildine and represent approximately 7% of all anorectal fistulas (Marks and Ritchie, 1977) (see Chapter 13).

Hidradentitis

Hidradenitis suppurativa may also present in the anal canal as a superficial fistula. These fistulas are usually submucous or subcutaneous and are due to obstructed, infected apocrine glands. There is an extreme form of hidradenitis, which can produce multiple and high anal fistulas known as follicular occlusum tetrad. In some parts of Europe the term 'pyoderma fistulans' is used to describe this entity (Krauspe and Stelzner, 1962; Bohme, 1964). It is possible that some of the 56 subcutaneous fistulas described by Marks and Ritchie (1977) were apocrine in origin. This disorder is described in Chapter 14.

Haemorrhoids

Sepsis complicating a thrombosed perianal venous plexus may result in a subcutaneous or submucous fistula.

Operations for anal disease

Operations for anal disorders may result in a chronic infective process which later develops into a fistula. Classically this may occur after sclerotherapy for haemorrhoids. Fistulas occasionally complicate internal sphincterotomy or closed haemorrhoidectomy (Parks and Stitz, 1976).

Inflammatory bowel disease

Crohn's disease

The features typical of perianal Crohn's disease are recurrent abscess, fistulas, skin tags, ulcers and strictures (Crohn, 1960; Cornes and Stecher, 1961; Lockhart-Mummery, 1972; Fisher et al, 1976; Pearl et al, 1993). When we analysed 202 of our own cases of Crohn's disease in some detail, we found that a high proportion of fistulas were extrasphincteric or high trans-sphincteric lesions (Keighley and Allan, 1986). These fistulas are more common in large bowel disease, particularly with rectal involvement, than in ileocaecal disease (Higgins and Allan, 1980; Ambrose et al, 1984; Scammell et al, 1987). Fistulas are often associated with oedematous skin tags and rather indurated perianal skin; in women, they may be confused with Bartholin's gland sepsis (Cripps and Northover, 1998). They are commonly multiple with high blind tracks and the internal opening is above the anorectal ring. However, these unsightly lesions often give rise to minimal symptoms and should be treated with caution (see Chapter 58).

Ulcerative colitis

The presence of perianal disease does not exclude ulcerative colitis. Perianal lesions were identified in 7% of our patients with ulcerative colitis. The most common lesions are fistulas, fissures and abscesses (Buchan and Grace, 1973). However, the presence of perianal fistulas in a diagnosis of ulcerative colitis should arouse suspicion; many cases have now been reclassified as indeterminate colitis or Crohn's disease (see Chapter 49).

Tuberculosis

Although tuberculosis sometimes presents for the first time with a perianal fissure or fistula-in-ano, this is now uncommon among the non-immigrant population (Logan, 1969). Tuberculous anal fistulas are much less common today than they were earlier in the twentieth century (Melchior, 1910; Buie et al, 1939; Jackman and Buie, 1946). Even in Africa, tuberculous fistulas are becoming less common (Eisenhammer, 1978). Ani and Solanke (1976) in Nigeria reported only four (5%) tuberculous fistulas in their series of 82 patients with intestinal tuberculosis, and a similar incidence was reported in an endemic area of tuberculosis from Nigeria (Ajayi et al, 1974). Tuberculous anal fistulas are still evident in over 15% of anorectal fistulas found in India (Shukla et al, 1988). There are no specific clinical features and the diagnosis can be established only by histopathological examination of the fistula. The identification of epitheloid giant cells is much more reliable than the presence of acid-fast bacilli. It is prudent to send any suspicious lesion for guinea-pig culture and biopsy in order to exclude tuberculosis. Latent infection may develop in patients receiving immunosuppressive therapy (Furstenberg, 1965). Chest radiographs are often normal or show only a previously healed focus. The Mantoux reaction is almost always positive. Most cases are presumed to be of bovine origin.

Actinomycosis

Actinomycosis should not be forgotten as a cause of an indurated perineum with multiple fistulas. Actinomycosis may even complicate an anal fistula (Alvarado-Cerna and Bracho-Riquelme, 1994). These lesions will heal completely with appropriate antimicrobial therapy (see Chapter 69).

Sexually transmitted diseases

Anal fistulas may occur as an incidental finding in association with sexually transmitted disease. In the case of AIDS, syphilis and lymphogranuloma venereum, the disorder itself may cause perianal sepsis, which is occasionally complicated by a fistula (Germer, 1970; Pearl et al, 1993). All patients who present with a fistula and a history of a recent sexually transmitted infection, or those who admit to being homosexuals, should be screened for gonorrhoea, syphilis, hepatitis, *Chlamydia* and herpes simplex. They should be counselled by the STD team and should be offered testing for HIV (see Chapter 68).

Malignancy

Anal fistula may be the first presenting feature of an underlying anorectal tumour such as squamous cloacogenic adenocarcinoma and anal glandular malignancy (Taniguchi et al, 1996). Isbister (1995) in his audit identified 2 of 88 fistulas which were secondary to malignancy. Some malignancies may arise in a chronic fistula-in-ano. We have seen three such cases in patients with long-standing fistulas in Crohn's disease. Other authors have reported carcinoma in anal fistulas not necessarily complicating inflammatory bowel disease (Welch and Finlay, 1987; Jensen et al, 1988; Onerheim, 1988).

Predisposing factors

In a case–control study, Jensen (1988) found that patients with anal fistulas consumed more white bread, less wholemeal bread and less raw fruit and vegetables than controls. Jensen also showed (1987) that a high-fibre diet protected against recurrence following surgical therapy. Poor anal hygiene is considered to be an important factor in recurrence (Abcarian et al, 1987).

DIFFERENTIAL DIAGNOSIS

Apart from tuberculosis, hidradenitis, actinomycosis, inflammatory bowel disease, fissure and sexually transmitted disorders, any of which may cause an anal fistula, there are other conditions that should be considered in the differential diagnosis.

Pilonidal sinus should not cause confusion provided the characteristic tuft of hair can be seen emerging from the sinus. However, some pilonidal sinuses may lie very close to the anal verge and in some cases confusion may exist between the two disorders.

A more important distinction is the differentiation between a chronic abscess and a perirectal dermoid cyst or a sacrococcygeal teratoma. If these lesions are inadvertently opened, total excision may prove difficult and a sacrococcygeal fistula may develop, which often defies surgical excision.

Other disorders which need to be distinguished from an anal fistula include a periurethral fistula and a chronically infected Bartholin's gland. It is important to exclude an anorectal fistula in patients with pruritus ani. Sometimes a low rectal carcinoma may present as an anorectal abscess complicated by a fistula. Alternatively, a carcinoma may arise in a long-standing anal fistula (Isbister, 1995). Heidenreich et al (1986) reviewed 131 such cases from the literature. Most of these tumours were colloid carcinomas or adenocarcinomas, but a variety of cell types were described, notably squamous cell and basal cell carcinomas (Stockman and Young, 1953). Kline et al (1964) reported that 44% of cancers arising in a fistula-in-ano were colloid in nature, 34% were squamous and 25% were adenocarcinomas. Most of these tumours were inoperable and had spread widely into the perineum, buttocks and inguinal lymphatics when they eventually presented clinically.

INCIDENCE

Anorectal fistula is a condition which is seen relatively commonly in general surgical practice. Our own audit records 57 fistula operations in a period of four years.

Shields (1937) reported that 0.18% of the population of Staten Island (USA) presented with anal fistula or abscess. The proportion of overall admissions to hospital for anorectal sepsis was 0.56% in Taiwan (Wang et al, 1980) and 0.69% in New York (Buda, 1941). In a colorectal surgical service, anorectal fistulas represented approximately 10% of the overall workload (Raghavaiah, 1976; Marks and Ritchie, 1977; Ferguson and Houston, 1978).

There is a male dominance in almost every reported series (Adams and Kovalcik, 1981). The male:female ratio in a 5-year review of 793 patients at St Mark's Hospital was 4.6:1 (Marks and Ritchie, 1977). A similar ratio was reported from our own unit (Shouler et al, 1986). In Nigeria the male dominance is 8:1 (Ani and Solanke, 1976). This male dominance is not attributable to any demonstrable difference in hormone levels in patients with anal fistula (Lunnis et al, 1995a).

Most patients with an anal fistula present in the third or fourth decade of life (Figure 16.6) and anal fistulas are uncommon after the age of 60

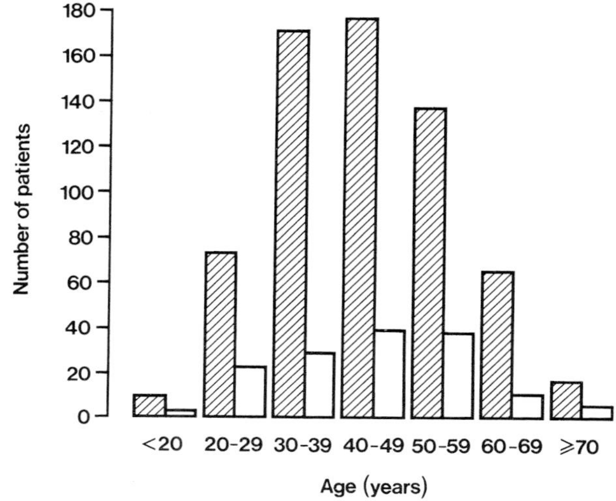

Figure 16.6 Age and sex distribution of fistula-in-ano: ▨, male; □, female.

years (Vasilevsky and Gordon 1984; Bruhl, 1986).

The distribution of anal fistula in Alan Parks' personal series were as follows: intersphincteric in 45%, trans-sphincteric in 30%, suprasphincteric in 20% and extrasphincteric in 5%. This distribution is biased by the nature of his special referral practice. Vasilevsky and Gordon (1984), serving a general community in Montreal, report a distribution which would be more typical of the experience of most other colorectal surgeons: intersphincteric in 3%, trans-sphincteric in 53%, suprasphincteric in 1%; there were no extrasphincteric fistulas (Table 16.1).

There is some difference in the distribution of simple fistulas. The distribution of fistulas reported from the unit in Minnesota by García-Aguilar et al (1996) was as follows: intersphincteric 48%, trans-sphincteric 29%, extrasphincteric 1.6%, and unclassified 20%. Indeed in non-specialized centres, the incidence of high anal fistula is low. Isbister (1995) encountered none in 88 patients. These types of fistula not surprisingly presented in different ways. The history was longer, previous operations for fistula or abscess were more frequent, and horseshoe extensions or lateral or multiple external openings were more common among patients with the more complex trans-sphincteric, suprasphincteric and extrasphincteric fistulas than in those with simple fistula (Table 16.2).

Table 16.1 Classification of fistulas.

	Marks and Ritchie (1977)	*Vasilevsky and Gordon (1984)*	
126 Superficial:	Subcutaneous 54		
	Fissure/fistula 56		
	Postoperative 16		
430 Intersphincteric:	Simple 394	67	56
	Extension upwards 33		9
	Rectal opening 3		2
164 Trans-sphincteric:	Simple 56	85	66
	High ischiorectal extension 87		19
	Supralevator extension 21		
26 Suprasphincteric:	Simple 5	5	3
	With ischiorectal fossa extension 1		0
	Supralevator extension 20		2
23 Extrasphincteric		0	
17 Multiple		6	
7 Unclassified		0	

CLINICAL PRESENTATION

The hallmark of a fistula-in-ano is of an anal discharge preceded by episodes of pain and perianal swelling that either spontaneously discharges or requires surgical drainage. Commonly there is a history of repeated episodes of perianal sepsis (Figure 16.7). Vasilevsky and Gordon (1984) recorded a history of discharge in 65%, anal pain in 34%, a recurrent perianal swelling in 34% and bleeding in 12%. Associated fissure-in-ano was recorded in 14% of their patients. Many patients also have haemorrhoids. A history of pruritus ani is also common. In our own series, a history of pain and discharge was recorded in over 70% of patients (Shouler et al, 1986).

Inspection of the perianal region will usually demonstrate an external opening associated with some perianal excoriation. There may be scars fol-

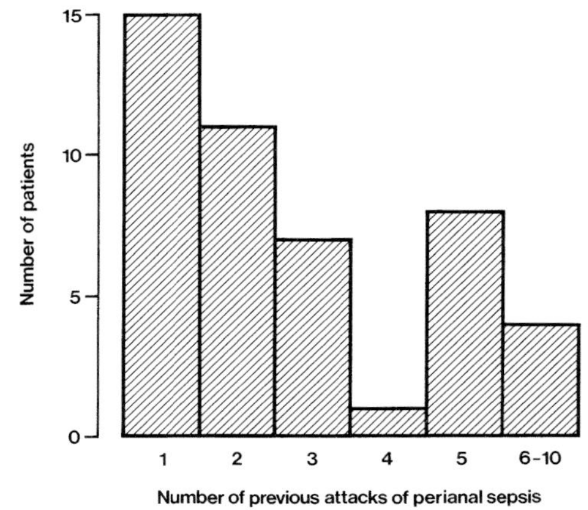

Figure 16.7 The number of previous attacks of perianal sepsis in patients with fistula-in-ano.

Table 16.2 Comparison between four major types of fistula.

	History >1 year	*Previous operation*	*Previous abscess drainage*	*Previous abscess spontaneously discharged*	*Abscess at operation*	*Horseshoe extension*	*Site of internal opening*				
							Anterior	*Lateral*	*Posterior*	*Multiple*	*None*
Intersphincteric	39	7	16	13	28	1 (all intersphincteric)	15	14	45	3	22
Trans-sphincteric	55	34	59	8	28	28 (40/47 ischiorectal)	5	36	17	10	32
Suprasphincteric	66	39	58	15	38	42 (equally distributed between intersphincteric, ischiorectal and supralevator)	12	36	4	24	24
Extrasphincteric	70	39	35	13	17	13 (2/3 supralevator)	9	34	9	13	26

All values are percentages.
From Marks and Ritchie (1977).

lowing previous surgical drainage. Many complex fistulas drain laterally (Marks and Ritchie, 1977), and in 9% of patients there may be evidence of a horseshoe fistula with multiple external openings that usually drain into the midline posteriorly. Palpation usually reveals an intra-anal swelling if there is still a chronic intersphincteric abscess. The fistula track may be easily palpable owing to fibrosis and induration surrounding the track. If there has been extensive previous surgery there may be stenosis and scarring of the anorectum with a gutter deformity. Absence of an external opening should not be taken as evidence that there is no fistula; we found no external evidence of a fistulous opening in 16% of our patients (Shouler et al, 1986).

ANATOMY AND THE SPREAD OF ANORECTAL SEPSIS

It is impossible to classify anal fistulas without a working knowledge of the anatomy of the anorectum, together with an understanding of the relationship of the pelvic floor to these structures (Shafik, 1979).

The muscles of the pelvic floor are arranged in the form of two cylinders, one within the other (Figure 16.8a). The inner tube is visceral and the outer somatic. The inner cylinder is the terminal portion of the gut and consists of mucosa surrounded by submucosa and the expanded circular muscle which forms the internal anal sphincter. Outside the internal anal sphincter and rectal circular muscle is the longitudinal muscle of the large bowel which is largely fibrous around the anus and which separates the visceral and somatic tubes. In its caudal extremity this longitudinal muscle (sometimes called the longitudinal conjoined septum) splits into separate raphes (fibroelastic septa) dividing the external sphincter into bundles around the anus. Infection and fistulas often track along these raphes from the intersphincteric plane to the perianal region or to the ischiorectal fossa. The muscles and anal mucosa of the visceral tube are supplied by the pelvic autonomic nerve plexus. The anal glands are part of the visceral component of the anus.

The outer, somatic cylinder consists of the external sphincter and the puborectalis, which is deficient anteriorly. The puborectalis consists of the inner fibres of the levator ani, the rest of which is formed by the pubococcygeus, the iliococcygeus arising from the white line over the obturator internus, and the ischiococcygeus. The levator ani forms a diaphragm which, apart from its anterior deficiency, separates the pelvis from the perineum. The somatic tube is supplied by the pudendal nerve and a branch from S4. The inner sling of the puborectalis is continuous with the external sphincter posteriorly and laterally and together they are responsible for the voluntary component of continence.

There is a potential space (known as the intersphincteric space) filled with loose areolar tissue, lymphatics and a few blood vessels which separates the visceral and the somatic cylinders. Many of the anal glands lie in this plane and infection readily tracks up and down the intersphincteric space but is discouraged from medial or lateral spread by the longitudinal septum and the internal anal sphincter.

Adjacent to the anorectum are two other important paravisceral compartments which are relatively avascular and contain only loose connective tissue (Figure 16.8b). These compartments readily accommodate spreading anorectal infection from a variety of routes.

Above is the supralevator space, known as the deep post anal space when it is behind the anorectum. The lateral supralevator space is confined by the rectum medially, the peritoneum above, the side walls of the pelvis and iliopsoas laterally and the levator diaphragm below. This space may become infected from above by a retroperitoneal portion of the colon and rectum or by extension of a psoas abscess from the kidney, duodenum, lumbar vertebrae or para-aortic lymphatics. The supralevator space may become infected from below by extension upwards through the intersphincteric plane or by penetration through the levator diaphragm from the ischiorectal fossa.

The lower pararectal space is the ischiorectal fossa, which is confined by the levator ani and sphincters medially, the ischium and obturator internus laterally, the sloping pelvic diaphragm above and the skin of the buttocks below. The ischiorectal fossa extends a considerable distance cranially and its apex lies adjacent to the middle third of the rectum. It may be quite difficult to distinguish the lower aspect of the lateral supralevator compartment from the ischiorectal fossa. The ischiorectal fossa may become infected through the external sphincter from the intersphincteric plane, from the perineum or from the supralevator space through the levator diaphragm.

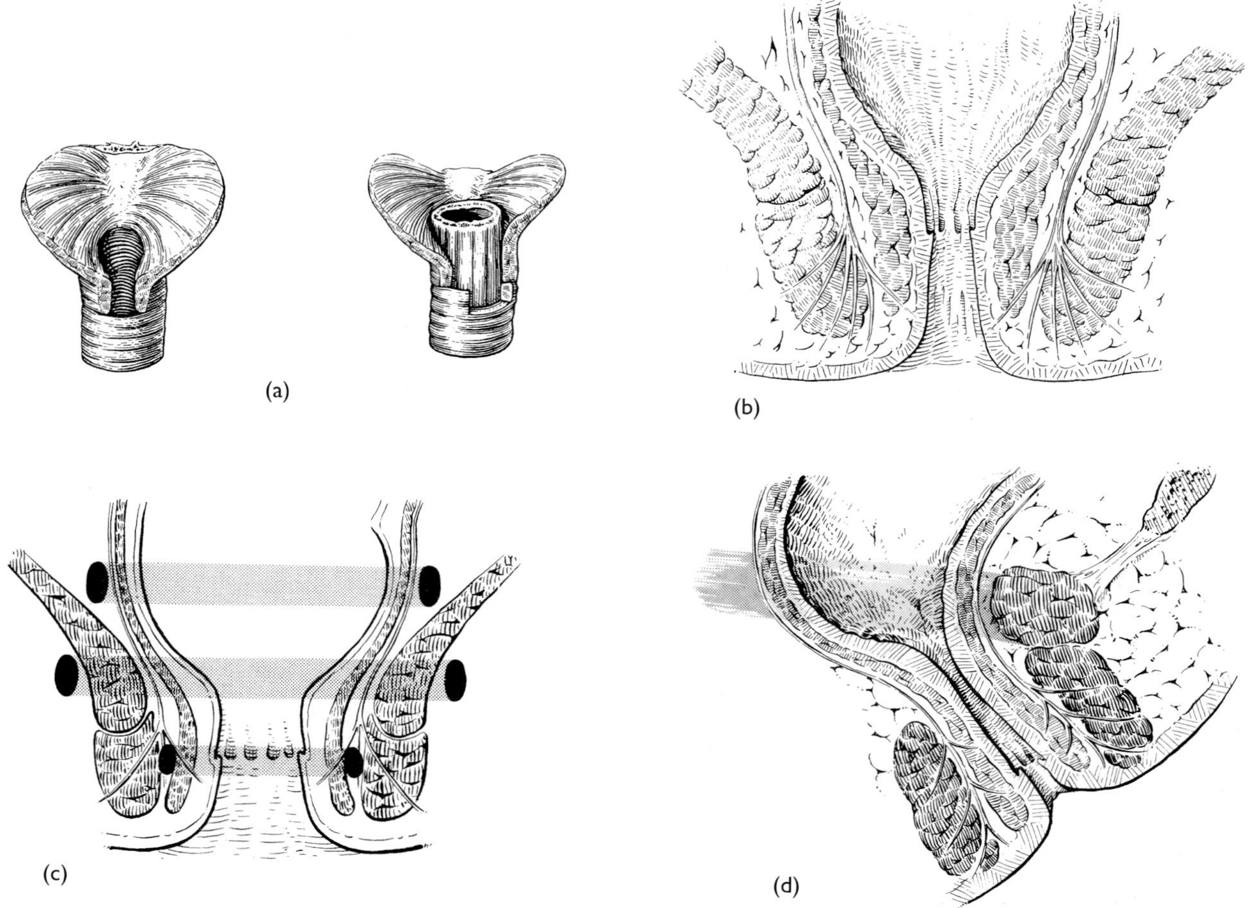

Figure 16.8a–d The anatomy of the pelvic floor and anal sphincters. (a) The outer, somatic muscular tube consists of the levator ani and the external anal sphincter. The inner, smooth muscle or visceral tube consists of the circular and longitudinal muscles of the rectum and anal canal. The circular muscles around the anal canal form the internal anal sphincter. (b) Coronal view of the anorectum showing the distribution of the internal anal sphincter, the longitudinal conjoined ligament, the external sphincter and the puborectalis. (c) Circumferential spread of anorectal infection. (d) A sagittal section of the anorectum demonstrating the normal anatomy, particularly the puborectalis and the external anal sphincter.

It can be readily appreciated that infection in any of these three potential spaces (supralevator space, ischiorectal fossa and intersphincteric space) may track circumferentially as well as in the vertical plane. Hence, infection in the intersphincteric space may surround the anus (Figure 16.8c). An abscess in the ischiorectal fossa may extend through the retrosphincteric space of Courtney to the opposite side, forming a horseshoe abscess that may extend forwards as far as the urogenital triangle (Held et al, 1986). Likewise, any fistula will take a similar course. The supralevator compartment may also communicate around the rectum. Thus the surgeon must assess the anatomy of a fistula in the coronal, sagittal and circumferential planes (Figure 16.8d).

CLASSIFICATION

Readers are often confused by the apparent extraordinary complexity of fistula classifications devised by modern authors (Parks et al, 1976; Hardcastle, 1985, Sainio and Husa, 1995; Marks, 1996). Furthermore, there is no uniformly accepted classification for anal fistula (Abcarian et al, 1987). We make no attempt to modify these excellent descriptions but would advise that any classification should consider both the position of the primary track, in the vertical and horizontal planes, and the secondary track (or extension), also in both planes (Marks and Ritchie, 1977).

Most earlier classifications describe the course of fistula merely in relation to the external sphincter (Milligan and Morgan, 1934). Low fistulas were those that opened into the anal canal at the level of the pectinate line; they could be subdivided into submucous, subcutaneous or trans-sphincteric. All other fistulas were classified as high. Goligher (1975) modified this classification, recognizing that some trans-sphincteric fistulas entered below the puborectalis into the upper anal canal, while the remainder were either supralevator or infralevator. Thompson (1962) classified anal fistulas as simple or complex: complex referring to high fistulas or those that involved at least 75% of the circumference of the anorectum. Developing the concept of a primary intersphincteric origin for anorectal fistulas, Steltzner (1959) classified them as intersphincteric, trans-sphincteric or extrasphincteric. This classification was subsequently modified by Parks et al (1976) to include the suprasphincteric fistula and to incorporate a description of the secondary track and circumferential spread. This classification has now been widely accepted by most authors (Sumikoshi et al, 1974; Steltzner, 1981; Gordon, 1984).

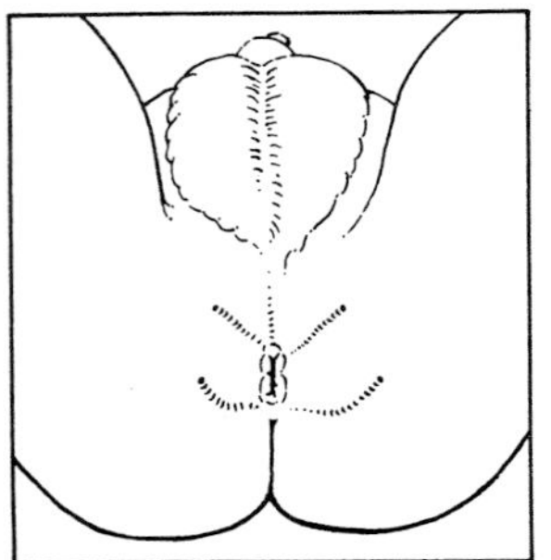

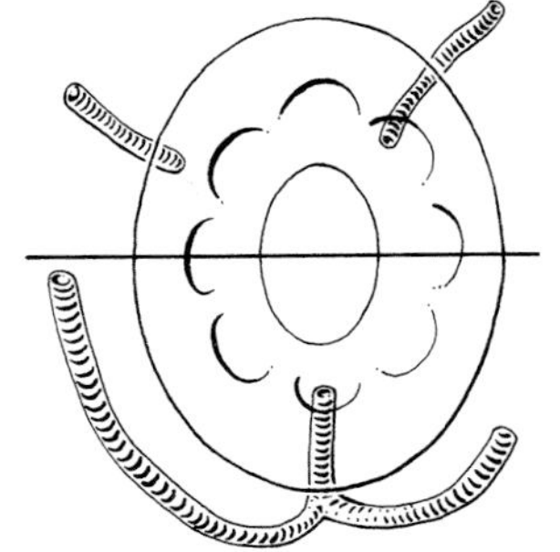

Figure 16.9 Goodsall's rule. Fistulas appearing above a horizontal line drawn through the centre of the anal canal, with the patient in the lithotomy position, usually drain directly into the anal canal. Fistulas lying below this horizontal line usually drain into the midline posteriorly.

Horizontal tracks

Goodsall (1900) stated that fistulas that have an external opening ventral to a horizontal line drawn transversely across the midpoint of the anus in the lithotomy position (Figure 16.9) drain directly into the anus at the dentate line. However, those with an external opening dorsal to the transverse anal line take a curved course to reach the posterior wall of the anal canal in the midline.

Though the majority of fistulas probably conform to Goodsall's rule, there are many exceptions. The frequency of these exceptions was reported by Cirocco and Reilly (1992). Overall, 90% of dorsal (posterior) fistulas obeyed Goodsall's rule, being 87% in men and 97% in women; whereas only 49% of ventral (anterior) fistulas obeyed the rule, being 57% in men but only 31% in women (Table 16.3). Posteriorly, the principal exceptions are very low anal fistulas, which may follow a direct course. Anterior horseshoe fistulas occur despite Goodsall's rule. Aluwihare (1983) in Sri Lanka identified 111 horseshoe fistulas, 35 of which were anterior. Although this experience represents a personal interest by the author, a high proportion of these anterior horseshoe tracks were in patients with recurrent fistulas and almost all the external openings lay more than 2.5 cm from the anal verge. Posterior horseshoe fistulas are often associated with numerous external openings, particularly when the fistula lies in the ischiorectal fossa (Held et al, 1986).

Assessment of circumferential spread must therefore take into consideration the sites of the internal and external opening and the plane of spread, which may be either intersphincteric, ischiorectal or supralevator. Marks and Ritchie

Table 16.3 The predictive accuracy of Goodsall's rule.

Anterior

Accuracy 49%

Male 57% Female 31%

Posterior

Accuracy 90%

Male 57% Female 31%

From Cirocco and Reilly (1992).

(1977) found a horseshoe component in 9% of their anorectal fistulas. Circumferential spread was most common in the ischiorectal fossa secondary to trans-sphincteric fistula. Circumferential spread in the intersphincteric plane may be associated with all types of fistula. Circumferential horseshoe extensions were the least common in suprasphincteric or extrasphincteric fistulas.

The distribution of the internal opening from a series reported from St Mark's Hospital is shown in Figure 16.10 (Marks and Ritchie, 1977). In our own series (Shouler et al, 1986) we found that over 50% of the internal openings were posterior, which probably reflects our high incidence of trans-sphincteric fistulas.

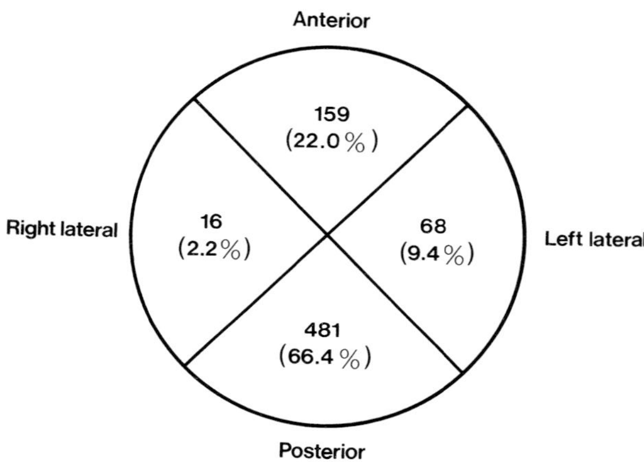

Figure 16.10 Site of internal opening in fistula-in-ano.

Vertical tracks

Vertical tracks can be simply classified as *intersphincteric* if the track lies between the internal and external anal sphincters or *trans-sphincteric* if the track crosses the external anal sphincter on its path from the anus to the perineum (Figure 16.11). Two other groups exist. *Suprasphincteric* fistulas are an interesting group which start in the intersphincteric plane and extend upwards into the supralevator compartment, where they can break through the levator diaphragm into the ischiorectal fossa, discharging into the perineum. *Extrasphincteric* fistulas are those commonly referred to as high fistulas which enter the rectum outside the anorectal ring.

Subdivisions of fistula

Parks et al (1976) subdivided intersphincteric fistulas into seven categories. This may at first seem rather daunting, but what they really describe is the direction of the primary track (up or down), whether there is an associated secondary track and, if so, its direction (up or down), whether the primary or secondary track ends blindly or whether either are associated with an abscess.

All fistulas arise from an infected anal gland, so there is always a potential opening into the anal canal at the dentate line but, in some cases, this may have become occluded by fibrosis. The fistula may spread up or down and may drain either into the perineum below or into the rectum above. Similarly, the exit sites may also become occluded and, if so, there is a tendency to form a secondary abscess.

Intersphincteric fistula

Simple (Figure 16.11a)

The simple intersphincteric fistula has its internal opening at the dentate line. The track passes through the internal sphincter to the site of the infected anal gland and hence downwards in the intersphincteric plane to emerge in the perianal region.

Simple with closed external opening and abscess (Figure 16.11b)

If drainage of a simple track is inadequate or the external opening becomes occluded, recurrent perianal abscess will develop until the fistula is laid open.

High blind track (Figure 16.11c)

A secondary track runs upwards in the intersphincteric plane to the pararectal region but does not enter the rectum and is not associated with an abscess.

High track entering the rectum (Figure 16.11d)

A secondary track extends upwards in the intersphincteric plane and enters the rectum.

High track and a supralevator abscess (Figure 16.11e)

The secondary track passes upwards and ends in a supralevator abscess. It is important to recognize the intersphincteric component of this abscess since treatment involves laying open the entire fistula by dividing the internal sphincter and draining the abscess into the rectum. Any attempt to drain the abscess through the perineum will result in a suprasphincteric fistula.

High blind track and supralevator abscess without a perianal opening (Figure 16.11f)

The lower intersphincteric component of the fistula may be absent. Hence the track runs upwards from the dentate line to the abscess in the intersphincteric plane. These abscesses drain inefficiently because of the continued activity of the internal anal sphincter. There may be a horseshoe component.

High track entering the rectum without a perianal opening (Figure 16.11g)

A long, high, intersphincteric fistula is found which has no external opening.

(a) (b)

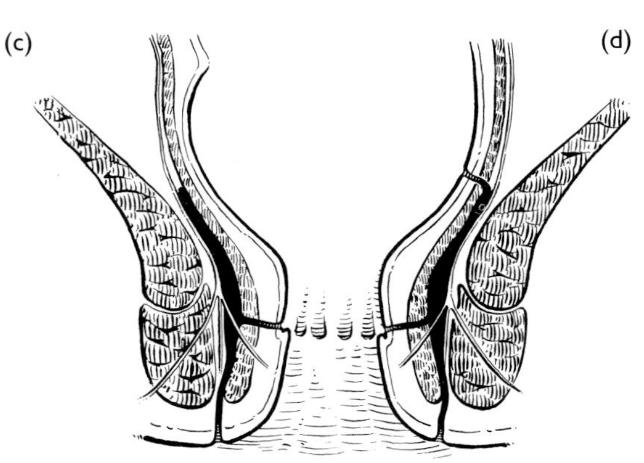

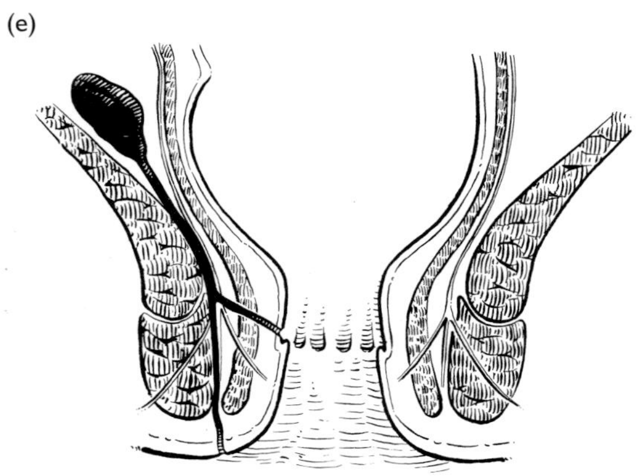

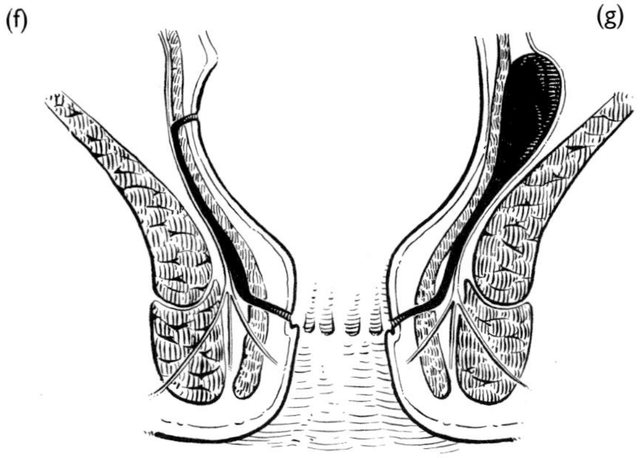

Figure 16.11a–g Intersphincteric fistula. (a) A simple intersphincteric fistula running from the dentate line to the lower border of the anal canal. (b) A simple fistula complicated with a small perianal abscess and a closed external opening. (c) An intersphincteric fistula with a high blind track in the intersphincteric plane. (d) An intersphincteric fistula with a high blind track which opens into the rectum. (e) An intersphincteric fistula with a high blind track complicated by a supralevator abscess. (f) An intersphincteric fistula with a closed distal end, a high intersphincteric track, and an extrarectal abscess. (g) A high intersphincteric fistula with a closed distal end opening into the rectum.

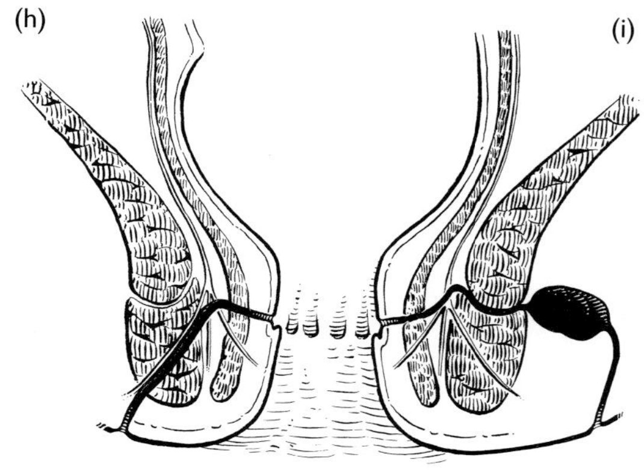

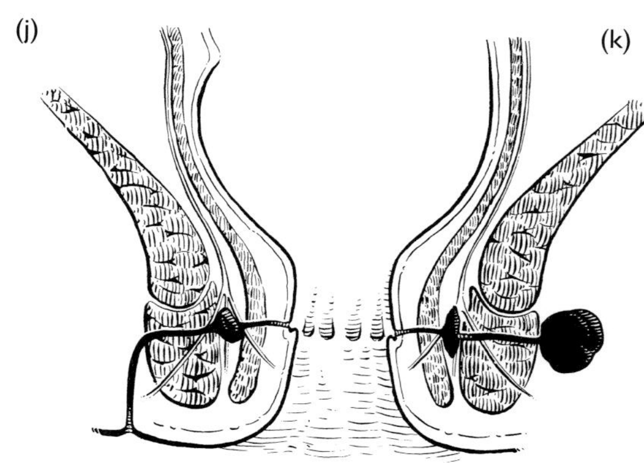

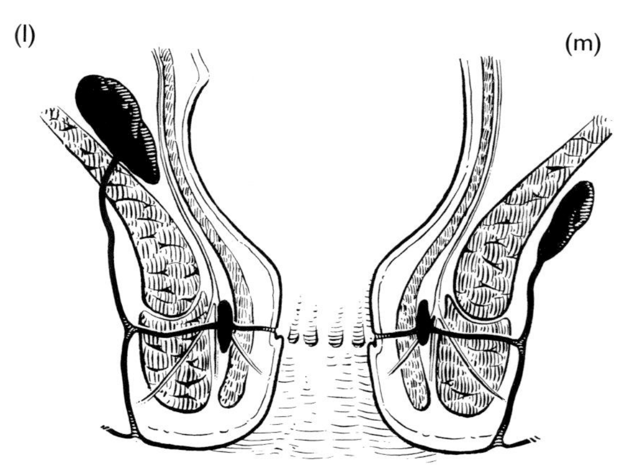

Figure 16.11h–m Trans-sphincteric fistula. (h) A low lying trans-sphincteric fistula. (i) Mid trans-sphincteric fistula, associated with an ischiorectal abscess. (j) Trans-sphincteric fistula with an intersphincteric abscess. (k) Trans-sphincteric fistula with a closed distal end complicated by an ischiorectal and an intersphincteric abscess. (l) Trans-sphincteric fistula complicated by a high blind track and a high ischiorectal abscess. (m) Trans-sphincteric fistula complicated by a high blind track culminating in a supralevator abscess.

Trans-sphincteric fistula

Simple (Figure 16.11h–j)

The uncomplicated trans-sphincteric fistula is not a homogeneous entity. The fistulous track may enter the anal canal at a high or a low level. The track itself may pierce the lower fibres of the external sphincter at the point where one of the fibrous septa traverses the muscle (low trans-sphincteric). Alternatively, the track may follow one of the venous channels directly through the external sphincter opposite its internal opening at the pectinate line to enter the ischiorectal fossa, discharging into the buttock (mid trans-sphincteric). Finally, the track which pierces the external sphincter may pass dangerously close to the anorectal ring before it enters the ischiorectal fossa and the perineum (high trans-sphincteric).

Without perianal opening and recurrent abscess (Figure 16.11k)

Sometimes the exit track becomes occluded, but if the external opening remains closed a recurrent ischiorectal abscess is inevitable.

High blind track (Figure 16.11l)

This is a common and potentially dangerous situation. The secondary track may be iatrogenic following enthusiastic curettage of an ischiorectal abscess during drainage. Alternatively, it may represent inadequate drainage from the apex of the ischiorectal fossa which, in some cases, may be due to a supralevator component. Instead of the track running straight from the anal canal through the sphincters to the perineum, a secondary track runs up to the apex of the ischiorectal fossa and, in some cases, it may extend above the levator ani. The danger of this fistula is that an externally placed probe will tend to follow the secondary track and the inexperienced surgeon may push the probe into the rectum, thus creating an extrasphincteric fistula. Hence it is always advisable to pass probes retrogradely, first searching for the internal opening, which provides the clue to the correct assessment of the fistula.

The technique of fistulectomy has much to recommend it in these complex fistulas with secondary tracks because no muscle is divided and the secondary track may be accurately defined.

High blind track with a supralevator abscess (Figure 16.11m)

This is another potentially dangerous situation unless the primary trans-sphincteric fistula and the secondary translevator track are accurately identified. If the supralevator abscess is incorrectly assumed to be due to an intersphincteric fistula and drained into the rectum, the surgeon will have created an extrasphincteric fistula (see Chapter 15).

Suprasphincteric fistula

Simple (Figure 16.11n)

Suprasphincteric fistulas are more common than most people generally appreciate and they are amenable to conservative surgical treatment. Most fistulas are due to a supralevator abscess complicating an intersphincteric fistula that bursts through the levator ani into the ischiorectal fossa to discharge into the perineum. The fistula track starts in the intersphincteric plane and loops over the puborectalis and external sphincter complex.

With supralevator extension and abscess (Figure 16.11o)

The presence of a supralevator abscess merely reinforces the common aetiology of this fistula. The supralevator collection often spreads around the anorectum and there is commonly a high horseshoe component.

Extrasphincteric fistula (Figure 16.11p,q)

It must be admitted that the majority of extrasphincteric fistulas are iatrogenic, but fortunately they are rare. In the experience of Abcarian and colleagues they occurred in fewer than 3% of patients admitted to a specialist centre (Abcarian et al, 1987). If there is no history of surgical interference, most extrasphincteric fistulas are due to a pelvic abscess caused by rectal or gynaecological disease which has penetrated the pelvic diaphragm and discharged through the buttock. This is a particularly common situation in Crohn's disease or following penetrating injuries (Abcarian et al, 1987).

Unfortunately, most of the remaining extrasphincteric fistulas are due to over-enthusiastic drainage of an ischiorectal abscess, when the rectal wall is inadvertently damaged (Figure 16.11p), or as a result of rectal injuries, surgical damage to the rectum, drainage of a supralevator abscess secondary to a trans-sphincteric fistula into the rectum, or the passage of a probe through a high secondary track complicating a trans-sphincteric fistula (Figure 16.11q).

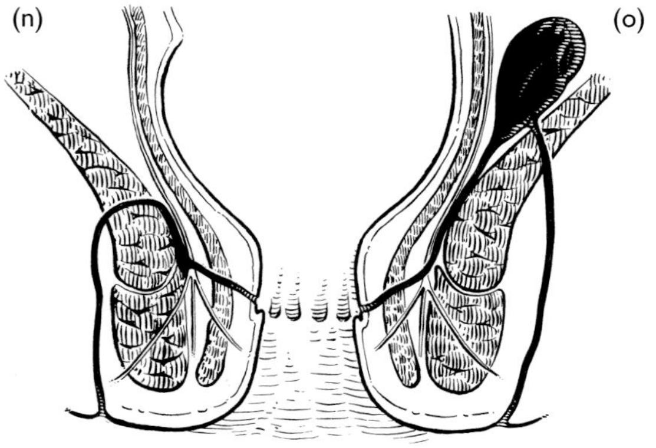

Figure 16.11n–o Suprasphincteric fistula. (n) Simple suprasphincteric fistula. (o) Suprasphincteric fistula complicated by a suprasphincteric abscess.

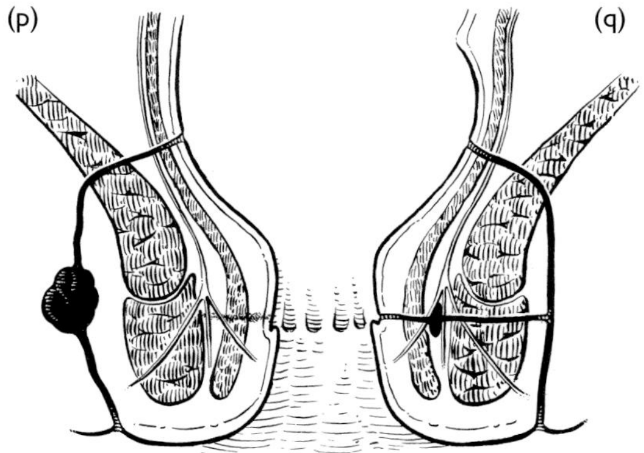

Figure 16.11p–q Extrasphincteric fistula.
(p) Extrasphincteric fistula due to iatrogenic damage to the rectum during drainage of an ischiorectal abscess.
(q) Extrasphincteric fistula complicating a trans-sphincteric fistula due to iatrogenic damage.

ASSESSMENT

Clinical assessment

We believe that a great deal of information concerning the anatomy of anorectal fistulas can be made from clinical assessment alone, sometimes necessitating examination under anaesthesia. Careful inspection of the perineum will identify any external openings, but even in simple, low trans-sphincteric and intersphincteric fistulas there may be no visible opening on the skin and a careful proctoscopic examination is essential. Use of a proctoscope in which a sector of the circumference has been cut away, as in the Welch Allyn instruments, may provide better inspection of the anal valves so as to display the characteristic bead of pus emerging from the internal opening of a fistula. Alternatively, a bivalve speculum may be used but this often proves unsatisfactory in unanaesthetized patients.

Palpation of the perineum will not only identify evidence of any associated chronic perianal or ischiorectal abscess, but frequently defines the direction of the track by the characteristic induration produced by the fistula (Figure 16.12a), associated with the discharge of pus at the external opening (Seow-Choen and Phillips, 1991). Under anaesthesia the direction of the track can often be visualized and the internal opening defined by grasping the external opening with a pair of tissue forceps and applying traction to it.

Digital examination is, of course, essential, both to detect any evidence of an intersphincteric or supralevator abscess and to feel for induration, which will provide a sure guide to the course of the fistula track (Figure 16.12b). Rectal examination may identify the internal opening and will also alert the clinician to the presence of a fibrotic stricture at the anorectal ring or a gutter deformity from previous operations. Rectal examination will act as a crude guide to the tone of the internal anal sphincter and the contractile potential of the external sphincter and puborectalis (Nicholls, 1996).

It is always wise to keep in mind the possibility, even if rare, that there may be two independent fistulas, particularly when there are two or three external openings (Gordon, 1984). The mucosal pattern of the rectum and the sigmoid should be inspected during sigmoidoscopy and, if there is any possibility of inflammatory bowel disease, a biopsy should be obtained. If the fistula is recurrent, tuberculosis should be considered, particularly in the immigrant population, and material should be sent for biopsy and culture. A fistula may be secondary to pelvic pathology, so a careful bimanual or vaginal examination is essential (Parks and Gordon, 1976).

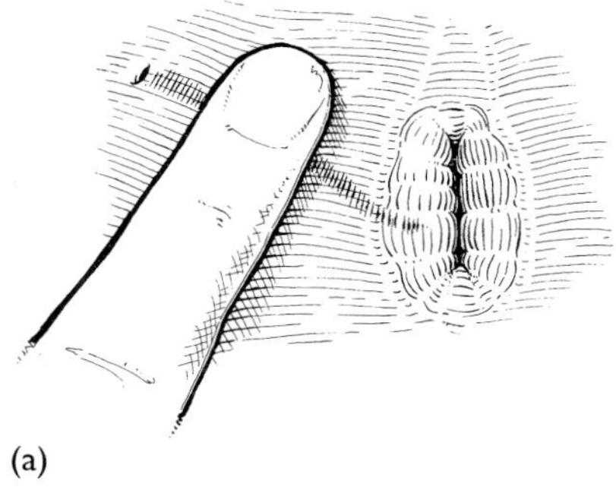

(a)

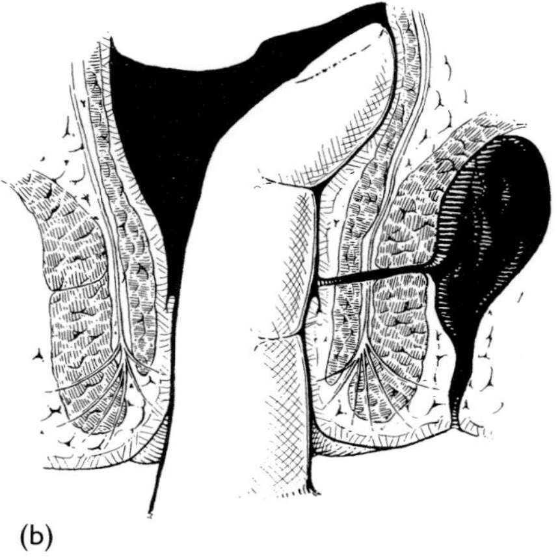

(b)

Figure 16.12a,b Assessment of an anorectal fistula. (a) Palpation around the perineum usually reveals some induration around the fistula track. (b) Rectal examination also identifies areas of induration and coexisting anorectal sepsis.

The accuracy of clinical assessment was checked prospectively by Seow-Choen and Phillips (1991). When the final diagnosis of the primary track was compared with the consultants' and trainees' clinical assessments, the overall accuracies were respectively 85% and 70% (Table 16.4).

Table 16.4 Accuracy of digital assessment in determining the type of primary track.

Primary tracks	*Operative findings*	*Consultants*	*Trainees*
Intersphincteric	12	10	10
Trans-sphincteric	14	14	10
Suprasphincteric	0	0	0
Extrasphincteric	4	1	0
Superficial	4	4	4

From Seow-Choen and Phillips (1991).

Anorectal physiology

Some readers will consider that preoperative manometry is merely the province of the academic. We think not. A small proportion of patients have impairment of continence before ever undergoing surgical treatment (Shouler et al, 1986). Incontinence may be due to pudendal neuropathy, to previous anal operations or to ageing. In patients with a trans-sphincteric fistula it is important to tailor the type of surgical procedure to the patient's sphincter function (Christensen et al, 1986).

Anal manometry will provide information on internal and external sphincter function (Bennett and Duthie, 1964). Since 85% of resting anal pressure is the result of internal sphincter activity (Frenckner and von Euler, 1975), resting pressure provides a useful guide as to how much of the internal anal sphincter can be safely divided (Bennett and Duthie, 1965; Marby et al, 1979). Voluntary contraction provides a measurable assessment of external sphincter and puborectalis activity (Duthie and Watts, 1965). This parameter should help to identify those patients in whom continence is threatened merely by laying open a trans-sphincteric fistula (Bennett, 1962).

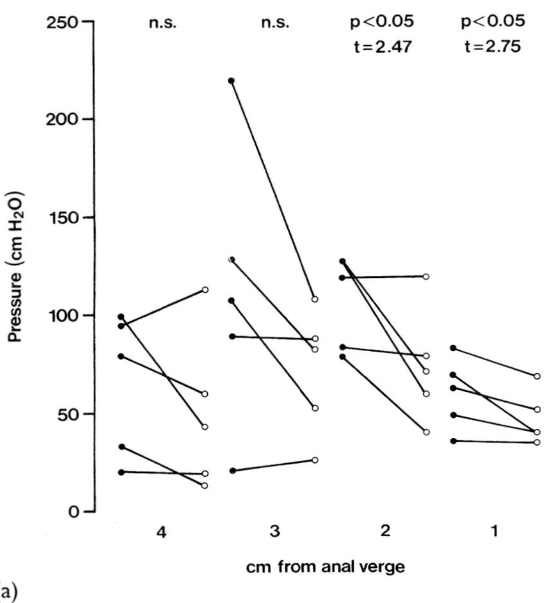

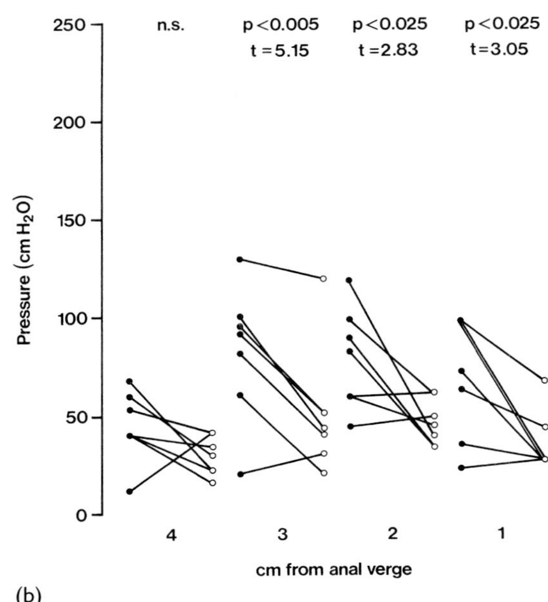

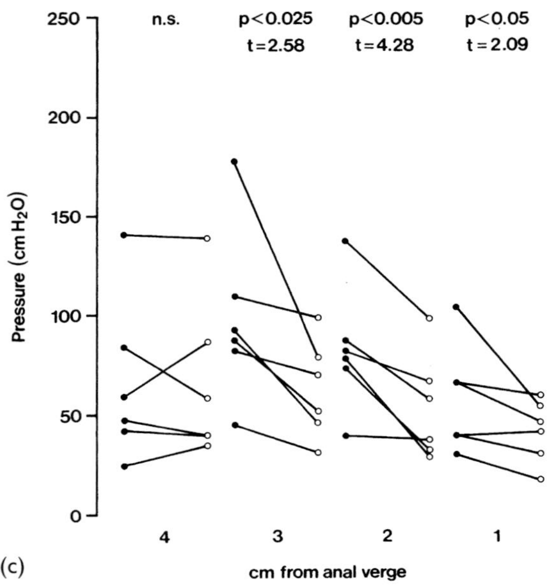

Figure 16.13a–c Anal canal before and after treatment. (a) Resting anal pressures before (●) and after (○) laying open an intersphincteric fistula. Changes in anal pressure have been correlated with the distance of the fistula track from the anal verge. n.s., not significant. (b) Resting anal canal pressures before (●) and after (○) treatment of a trans-sphincteric fistula. The data have been analysed according to the distance of the external opening of the fistula from the anal verge. n.s., not significant. (c) Resting anal canal pressures before (●) and after (○) treatment of a suprasphincteric fistula, according to the site of the fistula from the anal verge. n.s., not significant.

Unfortunately, conventional manometry alone will not identify defects of continence which result from a posterior deformity in the anal canal (Lilius, 1986). Any patient who has had a previous operation, obstetric trauma or a history of soiling should be investigated by the saline infusion test (Tudor and Keighley, 1986), pudendal nerve conduction, anorectal sensation and anal ultrasonography (Lunniss et al, 1994a). Vectormanometry is probably less helpful than transanal ultrasonography in identifying gutter defects.

We and others have shown that treatment of anal fistula has a profound influence on anal sphincter pressures and that this correlates well with the clinical defects of continence (Belliveau et al, 1983; Christensen et al, 1986; Tudor, 1986). Belliveau and colleagues studied 47 fistula patients, but only 18 of these had paired studies preoperatively and postoperatively (Figure 16.13a–c). Division of the lower half of the internal anal sphincter for treatment of simple intersphincteric fistula resulted in a significant fall in resting pressure 1–2 cm from the anal verge, but only one of 12 patients had any impairment of continence afterwards (Table 16.5). More alarming was the fall in resting pressures to less than 50% of the preoperative values in patients having a trans-sphincteric fistulotomy. Defects in continence were recorded in 4 of 7 patients in whom the fistula track was laid open, compared with only 2 of 11 patients in whom the track was cored out and the muscle preserved (Parks, 1961). Somewhat surprisingly, there was a similar significant fall in pressure in patients with suprasphincteric fistulas treated by application of a seton, but only one of nine of these patients had any impairment of continence.

We undertook a more comprehensive assessment of 11 patients before and after fistulotomy for low trans-sphincteric fistula. Patients therefore acted as their own controls and were followed up for a year (Table 16.6). There was a transient fall in resting

Table 16.5 Changes in anal manometry after operation for fistula-in-ano.

	Resting pressure (cmH_2O)	*Voluntary contraction* (cmH_2O)	*No. with impaired control of flatus or liquid stool*
Intersphincteric (n = 12)	107.6 ± 33.5	172.1 ± 55.0	1
Trans-sphincteric			
External sphincteric cut (n = 7)	47.8 ± 17.8*	61.8 ± 34.0†	4
No sphincter division (n = 11)	81.1 ± 20.1*	152.0 ± 54.0	2
Suprasphincteric treated with seton (n = 9)	85.7 ± 32.3	148.2 ± 68.7	1
Controls (n = 8)	99.5 ± 26.1	157.0 ± 45.6	0

* $P < 0.05$.
† $P < 0.005$.
From Belliveau et al (1983).

Table 16.6 Manometric study in 11 patients having fistulotomy for uncomplicated mid- or low-zone trans-sphincteric fistula-in-ano.

		Postoperative			
	Preoperative	*1 month*	*3 months*	*6 months*	*12 months*
Anal manometry					
Maximal resting anal pressure (cmH_2O)	114 ±23	86* ±17	93† ±24	99 ±30	107 ±36
Maximal squeeze anal pressure (cmH_2O)	295 ±49	204* ±54	223† ±91	220† ±59	227† ±62
Saline infusion test					
Volume of first leak (ml)	647 ±34	325* ±31	349† ±39	502† ±47	497† ±61
Residual volume (ml)	1438 ±49	1205* ±94	1267† ±104	1305† ±69	1362† ±104
Clinical evidence of soiling or impaired continence					
Soiling	1	6	5	4	4
Incontinence of flatus	0	5	3	2	1
Incontinence of liquid faeces	0	3	1	1	1
Incontinence of solid stool	0	1	0	0	0

* $P < 0.01$.
† $P < 0.05$.
From Tudor and Keighley (1986).

Table 16.7 Influence of dividing the external sphincter after insertion of a seton for high trans-sphincteric fistula.

	Length of high pressure zone (mm)		*Maximal resting anal pressure* (mmHg)		*Maximum anal squeeze pressure* (mmHg)	
	Patient	*Controls*	*Patient*	*Controls*	*Patient*	*Controls*
Males	33.4	29.0	43.5	60.0	168.5	160
Females	22.7	27.5	29.4	45.5	69*	100

* $P < 0.01$.
From Christensen et al (1986).

anal pressure lasting 3 months but a persistent reduction in squeeze pressures which continued throughout the period of follow-up. This was associated with significant impairment in the patients' ability to prevent liquids from leaking, a phenomenon which closely correlated with a history of soiling and the development of a gutter deformity.

Similar unpaired observations were made in patients treated by insertion of a seton (Christensen et al, 1986). This study demonstrated that the only impairment of sphincter function was to the voluntary component, being confined to women who had a high anterior fistula laid open after the insertion of a seton (Table 16.7).

Examination under anaesthesia

In many patients, examination in the office or the outpatient department may be difficult since chronic sepsis makes thorough examination painful. Attempted passage of probes in the consultation suite should, in our view, not be attempted for fear of creating a high fistula; in any case most patients find the experience singularly unpleasant (Dunphy and Pikula, 1955; Hawley, 1975). Detailed examination of the anal canal should therefore be deferred until the time of operation and surgical treatment. A light general anaesthetic is preferred without the use of a muscle relaxant so that the sphincter complex can be properly assessed by palpation. It is only under these circumstances that we would advise the passage of probes to define the anatomy of the track. This examination also allows the clinician to perform a proper pelvic examination and the opportunity to identify any collections of pus which might merit drainage before treating the fistula.

Identifying the fistula track

Careful palpation will almost always identify areas of induration around the fistula. The internal opening can often be felt. Furthermore, pressure over the indurated area may be associated with the discharge of pus through the internal and external openings. Traction on the external orifice will often define the internal opening and the course of the track. In difficult cases other methods of identification are available.

Saline irrigation

Passage of probes may cause more damage than the surgical procedure itself. We commend the technique, described by Gingold (1983), in which a fine angiocatheter is placed just inside the external opening, which is either occluded with a finger or a purse-string suture to allow injection of saline along the track. Insertion of a Sims speculum enables the surgeon to examine the dentate line carefully. Gentle injection of saline usually defines the internal opening so that a probe can be passed retrogradely, allowing the anal portion of the fistula to be identified. After this the rest of the track can be defined and laid open if this appears to be the best option (Figure 16.14a–d).

Methylene blue

We prefer saline or hydrogen peroxide to methylene blue as the latter is usually messy and a great deal more than the fistula itself is stained during the process. If methylene blue is used, and we accept that the technique may be valuable in selected cases, a very dilute solution ensures adequate staining for identification purposes. We find that the use of methylene blue is helpful in patients with multiple external openings, in patients with a supralevator abscess, and whenever a high secondary track is suspected.

Probing the track

It is essential that the surgeon has an adequate choice of probes available. This author prefers a soft, blunt-ended copper, or preferably silver, probe with an eye

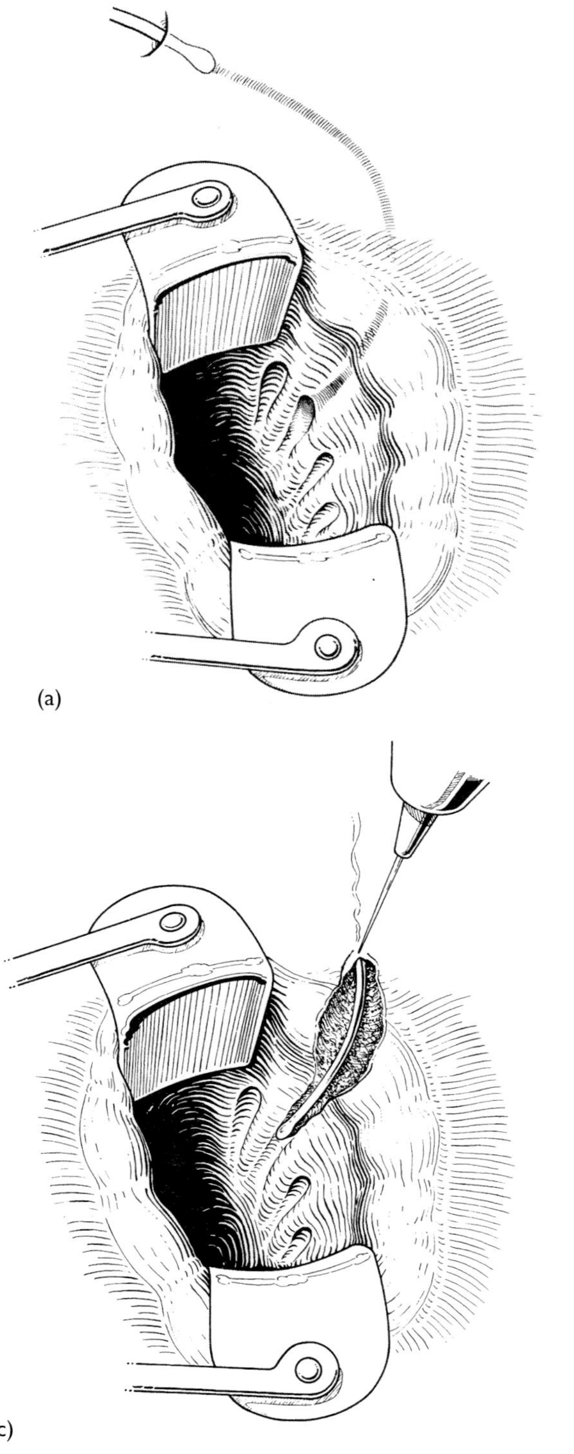

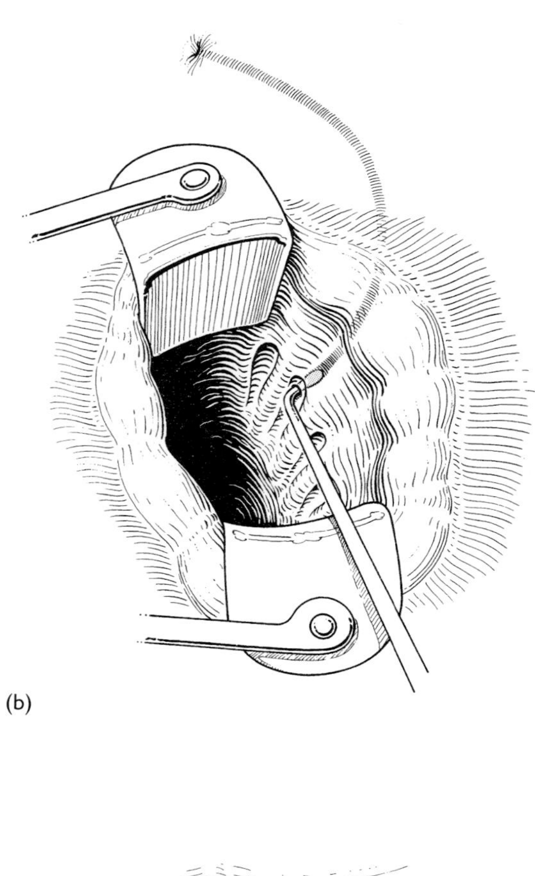

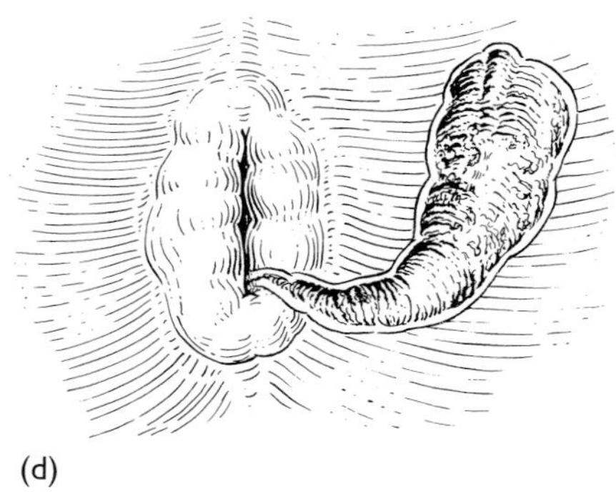

Figure 16.14a–d Laying open of a low lying trans-sphincteric fistula. (a) A soft angiocatheter is inserted through the external component of the fistula into the anal canal. (b) If there is difficulty in identifying the external opening, the internal opening may be probed. (c) Having identified the fistula track, the superficial component of the fistula is laid open by diathermy over the fistula probe. (d) Completed fistulotomy.

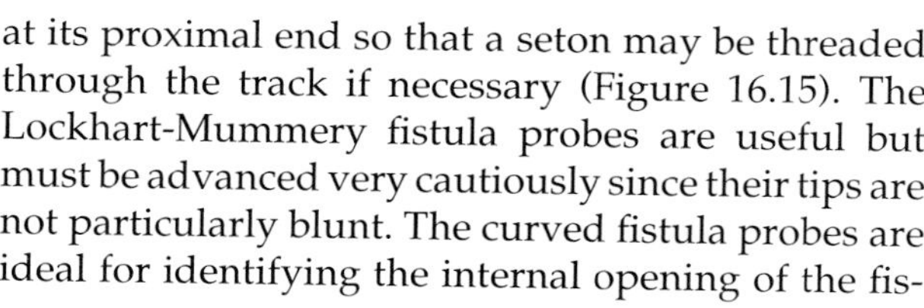

at its proximal end so that a seton may be threaded through the track if necessary (Figure 16.15). The Lockhart-Mummery fistula probes are useful but must be advanced very cautiously since their tips are not particularly blunt. The curved fistula probes are ideal for identifying the internal opening of the fistula so that it can be dilated to allow placement of a malleable probe from the internal to the external opening. Lacrimal probes may also be helpful in certain circumstances but they must be used with the utmost care since their relatively fine points may easily penetrate tissues and create false passages.

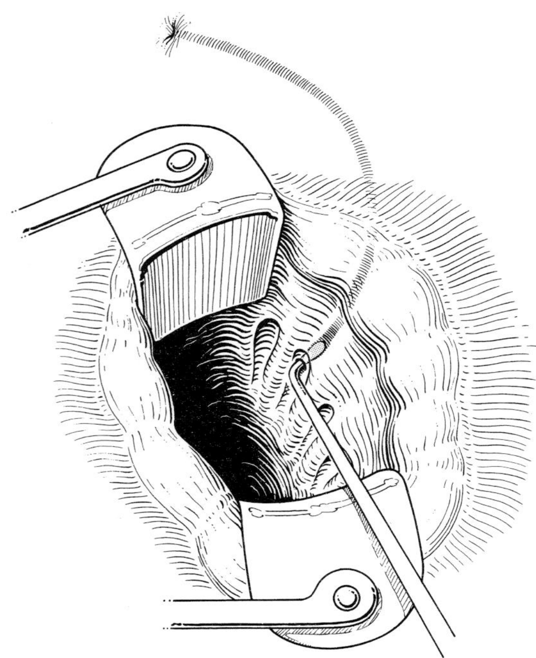

Figure 16.15 Retrograde probing of an anal fistula.

In our opinion, a probe should not be advanced from the perineum into the anal canal unless the probe lies almost parallel to the skin so that its tip can be seen advancing under the skin's surface. Alternatively a probe may be advanced with a finger in the rectum, but do not push! Prograde passage of probes following a course greater than 20 degrees from the perianal skin should be deferred for fear of creating a false passage (Figure 16.16), however confident the surgeon may be that the track is low-lying and simple.

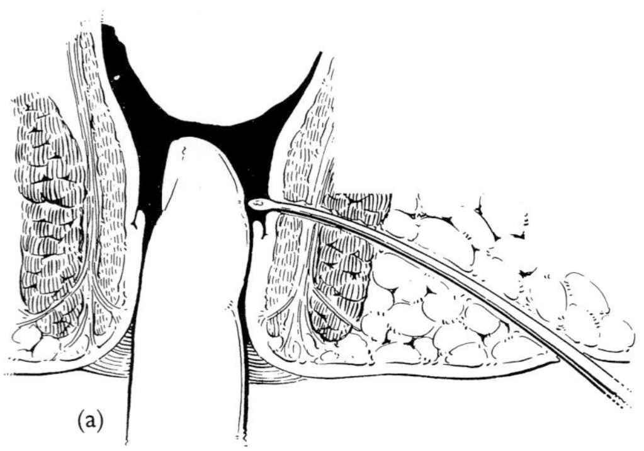

Figure 16.16 Prograde probing of an anal fistula with the examining finger in the anal canal.

Any probe passed progradely that follows a course parallel to the anal canal is either in a secondary track from a trans-sphincteric fistula, in which case 'pushing' will create an extrasphincteric fistula, or a long intersphincteric fistula (Figure 16.17).

We are firmly convinced that it is much safer to pass a probe retrogradely and to mark the fistula with a nylon thread or a silicone rubber seton if there is any doubt whatsoever about the course of the fistula track (see Figure 16.14).

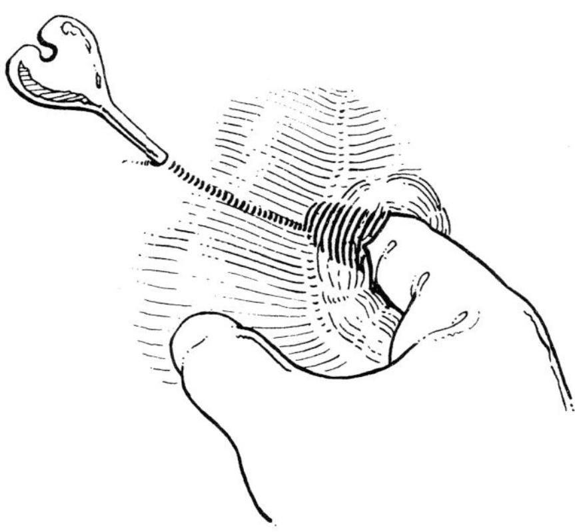

Figure 16.17 Any probe passed progradely that follows a course parallel to the anal canal is either in a secondary track from a trans-sphincteric fistula, in which case 'pushing' will create an extrasphincteric fistula, or a long intersphincteric fistula.

Surgical exploration of the intersphincteric plane

Whenever an intersphincteric component is suspected it may be prudent to explore the intersphincteric plane at the site of the internal opening. This approach may be used if faced with a horseshoe fistula, particularly when no internal opening can be detected in the midline posteriorly. Using a self-retaining speculum, the area adjacent to the suspected internal opening is infiltrated with 1:300 000 adrenaline–saline solution. An elipse of mucosa is raised to expose the internal sphincter, which is dissected free distally to define its lower border before the intersphincteric space is opened to drain any sepsis. The entire intersphincteric space should be inspected to exclude the presence of a high intersphincteric track.

Fistulography

Fistulograms are not widely used in the UK (Ani and Solanke, 1976), although we cannot understand why this is so (Goldberg et al, 1980; Kuijpers, 1982). Certainly, for complex fistulas, particularly those where repeated exploration has failed to define the course of the track, we have found the technique to be reliable and informative, but it is not commonly needed (Parks and Gordon, 1976). Figure 16.18 shows a complex horseshoe fistula.

Injection of contrast medium into abscess cavities as a means of identifying the presence and course of an associated fistula was found to be unreliable by Henrichsen and Christiansen (1986); late fistulas developed in eight patients despite negative radiography. Kuijpers and Schulpen (1985) assessed the accuracy of preoperative fistulography in 25 patients who had a complex fistula (high anal opening or horseshoe extension). The internal opening was correctly identified by fistulography in only five patients (20%), and there were two false-positive findings in the four patients with no internal opening. An internal opening into the rectum was outlined in only one of six patients with an extrasphincteric fistula, and there were two false-positive findings in the remaining 19. High extensions were identified in 9 of 16 patients (56%) but there was one false-positive finding in the remainder. Horseshoe extensions were demonstrated in only four of the six patients. These authors claimed that fistulography was inaccurate and potentially dangerous since, if the result of the examination had been acted upon, there would have been a real risk of iatrogenic damage (Kuijpers and van Tets, 1996).

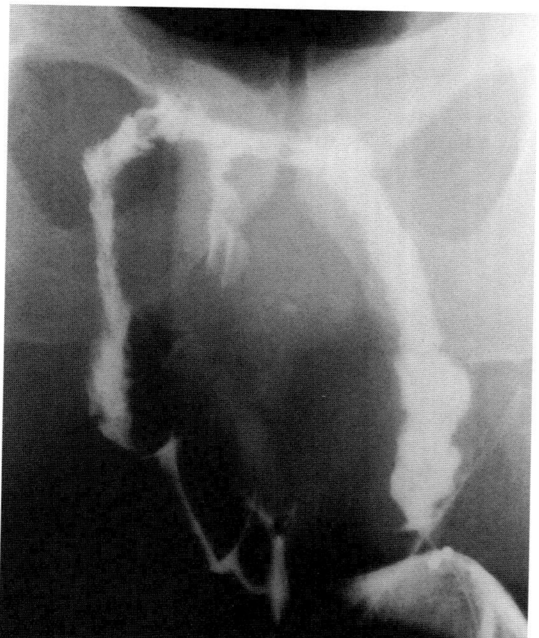

Figure 16.18 Fistulas may be demonstrated by inserting dye through the external opening of the fistula to see their anatomical pathway to the anorectum. This radiograph demonstrates a complex horseshoe fistula.

Transanal and intrarectal ultrasonography

Assessment by ultrasound may require anal and rectal ultrasound as well as echoendoscopy.

Examination may require the use of both 7 and 10 mHz probes. The technique will help to define the internal opening (Figure 16.19), and the presence of sepsis in the intersphincteric plane and sometimes in the deep postanal space. Additionally, defects in the sphincters are identified which may influence the management of anterior fistulas in women. Although some transphincteric fistulas can be visualized, the perineal component of anal fistulas cannot be seen in most patients. Anal ultrasonography therefore gives more information about the sphincters than the anatomy of the fistula. Lunniss et al (1994a) at St Marks, where they have access to ultrasound and magnetic resonance imaging, state that of the two, MRI provides more information on the anatomy of the fistula (see below). Schratter-Sehn et al (1992) found that transrectal ultrasound was more accurate than CT scans in anorectal Crohn's fistulas.

Thus anatomical definition is poor beyond the internal sphincter by anal ultrasound and MRI appears to be more informative (Lunniss and Sultan, 1996). Furthermore, intersphincteric collections do seem to be overdiagnosed by transrectal ultrasound; certainly this was true among the 22 patients investigated by Law et al (1989).

Magnetic resonance imaging

MRI is now regarded as the investigation of choice to define complex anorectal sepsis and fistulas (Figure 16.20a–e) (Scholefield et al, 1997). It is claimed by Lunniss et al (1992, 1994a) to provide 100% accuracy in defining the presence of a fistula and the site of extensions and is 85% accurate in locating the anatomy of the primary track. MRI scanning was particularly useful in patients with doubtful fistulas. It correctly identified sepsis without fistulas, scar tissue alone and blind tracks with no internal opening, thereby preventing

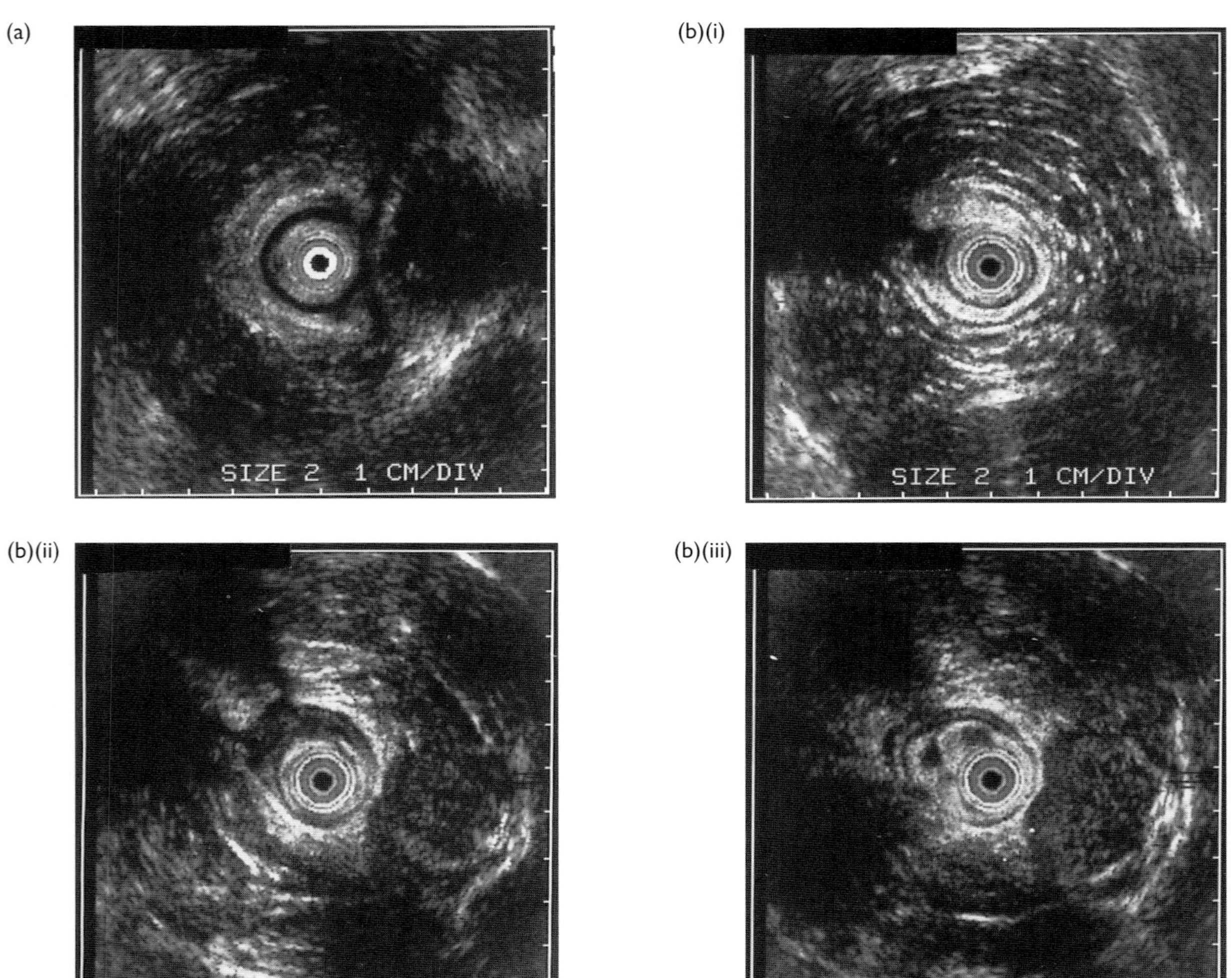

Figure 16.19a,b Ultrasound scans of anorectal fistula in two patients. (a) Anterior anovulval bilateral fistulas opening superficially into the 12 o'clock section of the anal canal, in Crohn's disease. (b)(i)–(iii) Horseshoe fistula with external openings at 5 and 8 o'clock entering into the anal canal in the midline posteriorly, forming a deep postanal abscess.

unnecessary surgical exploration (Lunniss and Sultan, 1996). MRI was also particularly useful in defining horseshoe fistulas but missed 5 of 26 internal openings because imaging of the intersphincteric space is not as good as with anal ultrasound.

Our own experience of MRI appeared to be encouraging when vigorous criteria were applied and when a single dedicated radiologist was involved. However, the overall impression after our initial audit was somewhat disappointing and we have some reservations whether routine MRI is really justified and cost-effective unless one is faced with a recurrent complex case.

TREATMENT

Principles

Preoperative preparation

Although it is quite impossible to assess an anal fistula if stool is present in the lower rectum, a full mechanical bowel preparation is rarely necessary. We admit the patient on the day of operation since the procedures are regarded as 'dirty' and they are usually placed near the end of the operating list (or, if simple, on a day-case list). Two glycerine suppositories are administered before admission and a disposable enema is given on arrival at the hospital.

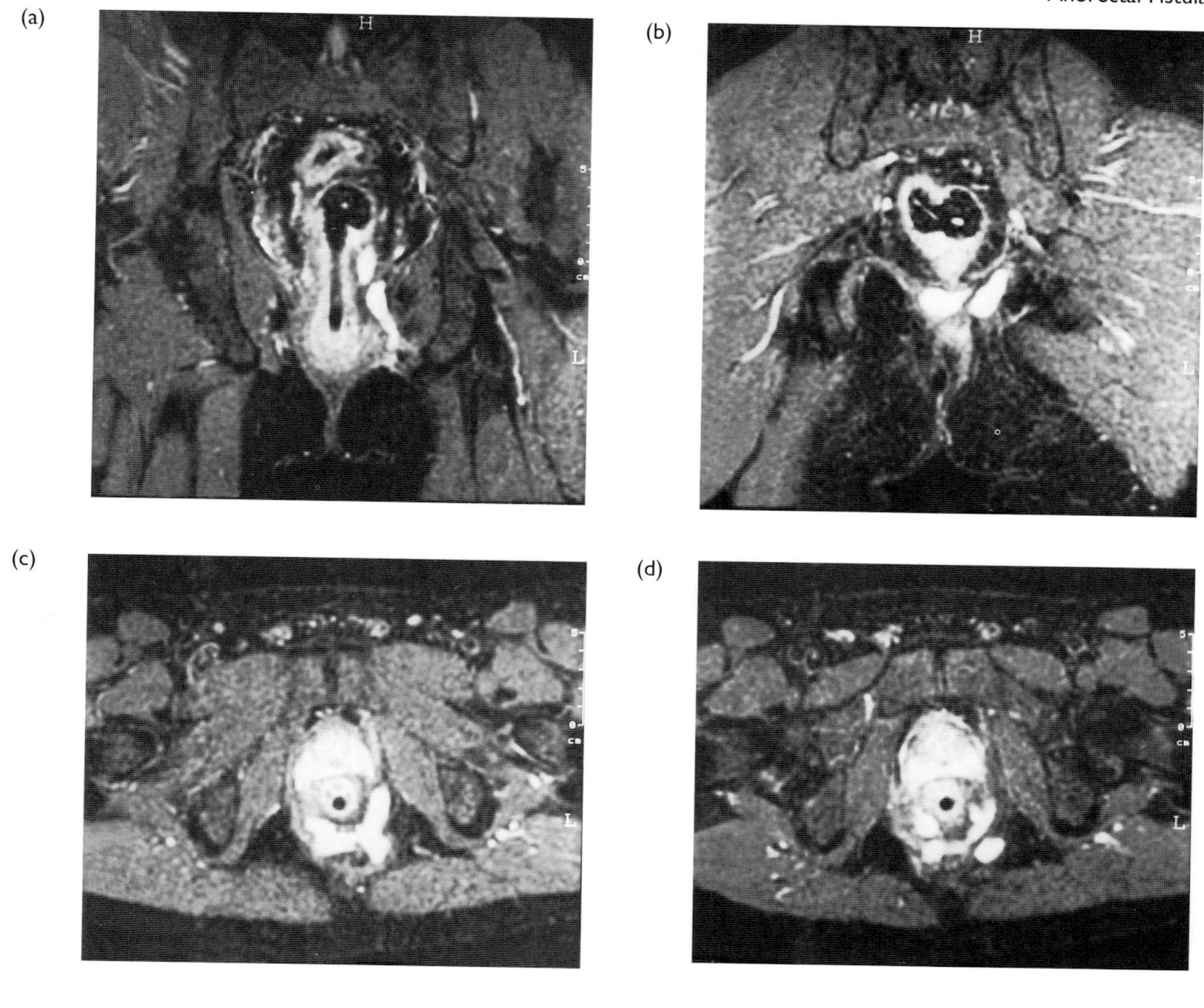

Figure 16.20a–e MRI scans. (a) An MRI scan stir sequence coronal section, the plane passing through the mid anal canal. There is an inert catheter within the anorectum. There is a wide fistula track passing through the left ischiorectal fossa with supralevator extension. The track ends blindly several centimetres above the skin of the buttock. (b) Posterior coronal scan showing a high posterior intersphincteric collection and an abscess high in the left ischiorectal fossa displacing the levator plate cephalad. (c) Axial scan showing a high intermuscular horseshoe collection with the track crossing the external sphincter/puborectalis junction to reach the left ischiorectal fossa. (d) Axial scan above the anorectal junction showing an intermuscular horseshoe abscess and a pararectal extension. (e) Axial scan at the level of the seminal vescicles showing cephalad extension of the intermuscular and pararectal sepsis. All scans courtesy of Dr Peter J Lunniss.

Anaesthesia

Although there is a swing towards performing anal operations using local anaesthetic techniques, particularly in North America (Denecke et al, 1986), we do not advise this method of anaesthesia for anal fistulas. We argue that general anaesthesia is preferable since the duration of the operation is variable, and extensive exploration may be needed to define the track. Similarly, epidural or even caudal anaesthesia is, in our opinion, contraindicated for fistula-in-ano because the sphincters and pelvic floor are rendered completely flaccid. We therefore advise a light general anaesthetic to facilitate accurate identification of the anorectal ring in relation to the fistula.

Position and instruments

In the UK most surgeons prefer the lithotomy position, largely out of habit and training. Certainly for posterior fistulas, where intra-anal exploration and internal sphincterotomy may be needed, the lithotomy position allows better access. However, the prone jack-knife position, which is the preferred approach in North America and is now increasingly practised by European surgeons, affords improved access for anterior fistulas, particularly if they are extrasphincteric, when some form of mucosal advancement technique might be desirable. We prefer the prone position for most anorectal fistula operations. A headlamp is essential if any intra-anal procedures are necessary. It is an advantage, when the lithotomy position is used, if a tray is available under the buttocks for the placement of instruments.

If the fistula is to be excised, haemostasis must be impeccable and a weak adrenaline–saline solution is used to infiltrate the submucosal and intersphincteric planes. A self-retaining intra-anal speculum and a wide selection of fistula probes should also be available. If bleeding is encountered during excision of the fistula track, the cavity may be packed with a gauze swab soaked in adrenaline.

Timing of the operation

We do not subscribe to the view that a fistula track should always be identified and laid open at the time of draining an anorectal abscess. In a recent randomized trial, Schouten and van Vroonhoven (1991) showed that primary fistulectomy during drainage of an anorectal abscess led to increased functional disturbance compared with fistulectomy as a second-stage procedure. We agree with these conclusions despite claims to the contrary (Piazza and Radhakrishnan, 1990; Fucini, 1991). Conversely we do not explore all quiescent fistulas; if there has been no discharge for more than 6 weeks we often arrange to reassess the patient at a later date or simply confine the procedure to a careful examination under anaesthetic unless an obvious fistula is demonstrated.

Treatment of the principal categories of fistula

The principles of treatment are quite simply to define the anatomy of the fistula track and any secondary extensions, to drain any coexisting pus, and then to provide definitive treatment by laying open (fistulotomy), excision or placement of a seton through the fistula track if it enters below the anorectal ring. If, on the other hand, the fistula lies outside the somatic cylinder and above the anorectal ring, the fistula track should be excised or defined with a seton and the defect in the gut closed. A detailed comparison of excision, seton fistulotomy or laying open of the track will follow, together with an evaluation of available methods of treating complex fistulas. Here we shall establish the principles of treatment and list available surgical options (Gordon, 1985).

The increased morbidity for patients with suprasphincteric and extrasphincteric fistulas was amply highlighted in the report by Parks and Stitz (1976). Duration of hospital stay was three times longer in patients with a complex fistula compared with those with an intersphincteric fistula, and the mean number of anaesthetics per patient exceeded five for individuals with a suprasphincteric or extrasphincteric fistula. Furthermore, healing time was at least as long in patients with complex suprasphincteric and extrasphincteric fistulas (Table 16.8). Interestingly, the morbidity from impaired continence of treating trans-sphincteric fistulas was almost as high as in the other, more complex groups with tracks entering above the anorectal ring (Seow-Choen and Phillips, 1991).

Table 16.8 Duration of hospital stay, time to healing and number of assessments under anaesthetic for patients with a high internal opening.

	Intersphincteric (*n* = 33)	*Trans-sphincteric* (*n* = 40)	*Suprasphincteric* (*n* = 55)	*Extrasphincteric* (*n* = 20)
No. of anaesthetics	2.0	4.5	5.5	5.4
Average inpatient stay (days)	20	45	60	65
Average no. of admissions	1.3	1.9	2.0	2.9
Average healing time (months)	4.9	4.6	8.2	8.8

From Parks and Stitz (1976).

Treatment of the intersphincteric type

Intersphincteric fistulas can be readily treated with minimal morbidity or complication by merely laying open the fistula track into the anal canal. Parks et al (1976) advise excision of part of the internal sphincter and the loose areolar tissue of the intersphincteric plane in order to remove all the potentially infected glandular tissue (Dodi, in Abcarian et al, 1987). Unlike with trans-sphincteric fistulas, there seems to be very little evidence that division of the internal sphincter compromises continence.

Simple low track (Figure 16.21a)

The fistula is laid open or excised and in so doing the internal sphincter is divided or partially excised.

High blind track (Figure 16.21b)

Treatment involves dividing the internal sphincter to the full height of the blind tract. Failure to identify the upper extension may predispose to recurrence.

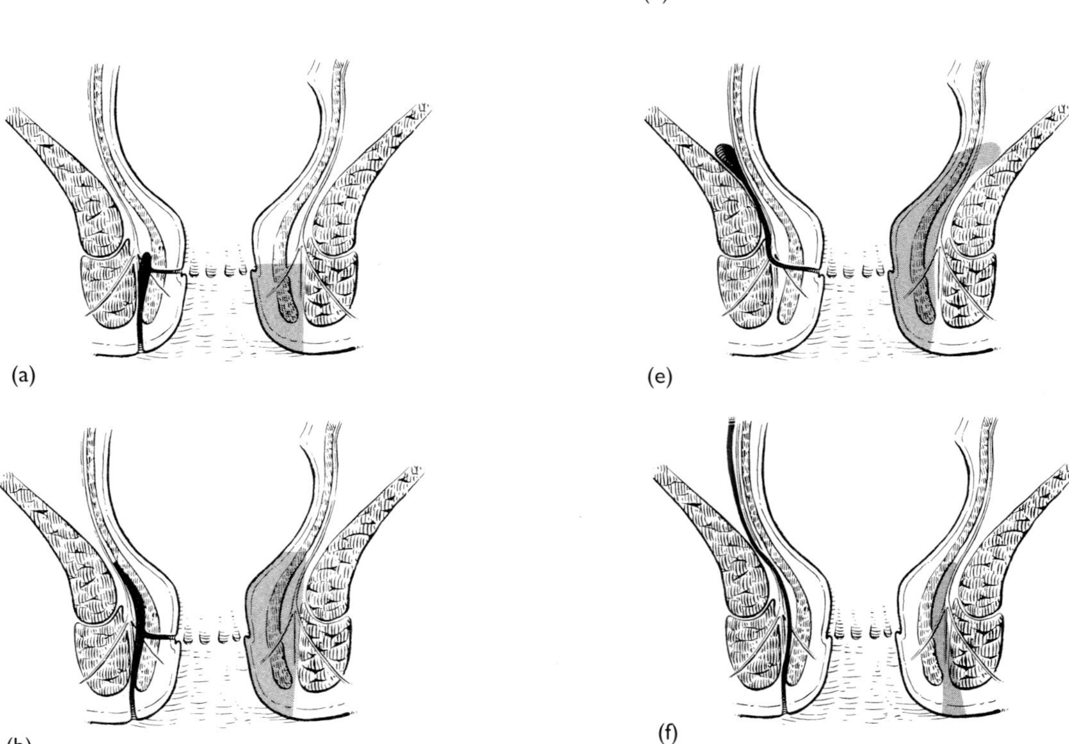

Figure 16.21a–f Treatment of intersphincteric fistula. (a) Simple low intersphincteric fistula treated by excision of the lower fibres of the internal sphincter and the anal mucosa. (b) Intersphincteric fistula with a high blind track being treated by extended internal sphincterotomy and excision of the anal mucosa. (c) Intersphincteric fistula with a high opening into the rectum. The entire fistula track has been laid open, dividing the internal anal sphincter. (d) Intersphincteric fistula with a high track without a perineal opening is managed by excising the whole of the internal anal sphincter, and laying open the entire intersphincteric space. (e) Intersphincteric fistula with a high track and an abscess is also treated by extended sphincterotomy with excision of the anorectal mucosa. (f) Intersphincteric fistula due to a source in the pelvis. The lower component of the fistula track is laid open and the pelvic sepsis is dealt with after any primary pelvic pathology has been excluded.

High track opening into the rectum (Figure 16.21c)

This fistula may alarm the surgeon when a probe is passed along it since the internal opening is well above the anorectal ring. However, if the intersphincteric plane is explored, the true anatomical site of the track will become apparent and the entire fistula can be excised or laid open with impunity.

High track with a perineal opening (Figure 16.21d)

This relatively uncommon fistula often causes confusion. A bead of pus emerges through the anal crypt and a probe only passes upwards. In this case, the correct treatment is to excise the lower fibres of the internal sphincter as well as the fistula, since failure to eradicate the glandular tissue predisposes to recurrence.

High track with supralevator abscess (Figure 16.21e)

This abscess must never be drained through the perineum if there is a track running upward in the intersphincteric plane, since drainage through the perineum will simply result in a suprasphincteric fistula. Treatment consists of internal sphincterotomy and drainage into the anorectum internally (Eisenhammer, 1978).

Secondary to pelvic disease (Figure 16.21f)

If there is a track lying in the intersphincteric plane which occurs secondary to pelvic disease, the underlying disease should be eradicated by resection and the pelvic sepsis should be drained at the same time. The intersphincteric component merely requires gentle curettage and insertion of a drain.

Treatment of the trans-sphincteric type

Coloproctologists have learned to be more cautious in the treatment of trans-sphincteric fistulas. The functional results after successful conventional fistula surgery are inferior to those observed in patients with all other types of fistula, including the rare suprasphincteric and extrasphincteric fistula, as well as the intersphincteric type (Table 16.9). In particular, soiling is more common. Belliveau et al (1983) not only reported impairment of sphincter function after fistulotomy, but also showed that there was a difference between patients managed by preserving the external anal sphincter compared with patients having the more conventional fistulotomy. However, in a non-randomized comparison (Abcarian et al, 1987) and in a randomized trial (Christensen et al, 1986), the benefits of preserving the external sphincter were not really confirmed. Indeed, recent evidence suggests that internal sphincter preservation in trans-sphincteric fistulas is much more important than was previously recognized (Lunniss et al, 1994b) (Table 16.10).

There are four principal techniques for the management of mid or high trans-sphincteric fistula. The first is fistulotomy, still the most widely practised technique. Here the track is merely laid open; since the fistula does not lie above the external sphincter or traverse the puborectalis, faecal incontinence is rare, but minor defects of control and soiling are reported in almost a third of patients (Abcarian et al, 1987).

The second method is seton fistulotomy. An inert material such as Prolene, rubber or (preferably) Silastic is passed through the fistula and tied tight so that the sphincters are divided slowly over 1–4 weeks, in the belief that fibrosis occurs during division of the lower fibres of the sphincter, thereby preserving function (Eisenhammer, 1966; Hamilton, 1975; Kuijpers, 1984, Lentner and Wienert, 1996; Williams et al, 1991a; McCourtney and Finlay, 1995; Pearl et al, 1993). In some series, the functional results of seton fistulotomy differed little from initially laying open the track (Ramanujam et al, 1983) and recurrence rates may be high (Abcarian et al, 1987). Recent results, however, suggest much lower recurrence rates and variable rates of impaired continence (Christensen et al, 1986; McCourtney and Finlay, 1996; Lentner and Weiner, 1996). Our own data indicate a high recurrence rate but a low incidence of incontinence.

Table 16.9 Postoperative function following treatment of fistulas with a high internal opening.

	Intersphincteric (*n* = 30)	*Trans-sphincteric* (*n* = 36)	*Suprasphincteric* (*n* = 55)	*Extrasphincteric* (*n* = 18)
Normal controls	25	24	45	13
Difficulty controlling flatus or soiling	5	12	9	3
	17%	33%	16%	17%
Faecal incontinence	0	0	1	2

From Parks and Stitz (1976).

Table 16.10 Factors influencing continence after anal fistula surgery.

	Resting anal pressure		
	Before	*After*	*Impaired continence*
Division of internal sphincter only (22)	66	44	11
Division of internal and part of external sphincter (15)	68	28	8

From Lunniss et al (1994b).

The third approach is to excise the fistula track only (Parks, 1961; Hawley, 1975) so that the lower part of the external sphincter, and if possible the internal sphincter, are preserved and the anal defect closed either directly (Roschke and Krause, 1983; Mann and Clifton, 1985; Matos et al, 1993) or by an advancement flap of the anorectum (Wedell et al, 1987; Ozuner et al, 1996; Lewis et al, 1995). Advancement flaps are now becoming quite popular and a recent development has been the use of perianal skin (Del Pino et al, 1996). Alternatively, a labial fat pad advancement known as the Martius technique may be suitable in women (see Chapter 65).

A fourth approach, used exclusively for high fistulas, has been laying open and total sphincter reconstruction, usually with a covering stoma (Christiansen and Ronholt, 1995).

Uncomplicated (Figure 16.21g)

Fortunately, most trans-sphincteric fistulas cross at a low level so that laying open the fistula results in division of only the lower portion of the internal and external anal sphincter. If the track crosses at a higher level the track itself may be excised, and the internal defect closed. Alternatively, a seton may be inserted.

High blind track (Figure 16.21h)

This is a potentially dangerous fistula, particularly if complicated by a supralevator abscess fed by the high blind track. The abscess should never be opened into the rectum or else an extrasphincteric fistula will result. It is crucial, therefore, to identify the trans-sphincteric component. The primary and secondary track should be excised, or laid open. It is not always necessary to divide the lower fibres of the external sphincter, particularly if a seton is used for the primary track. The danger of this particular fistula is that probing may result in iatrogenic damage to the rectum.

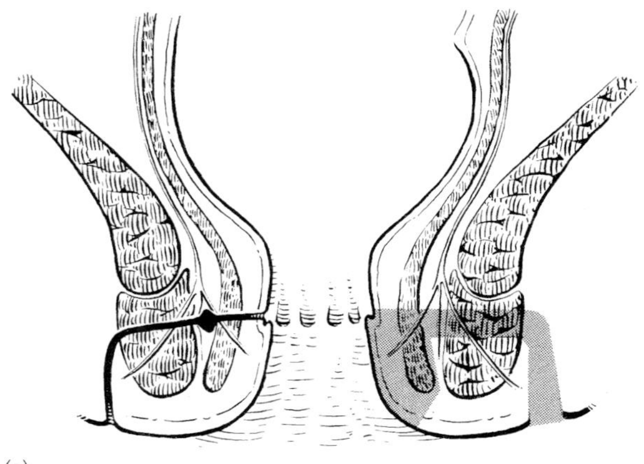

(g)

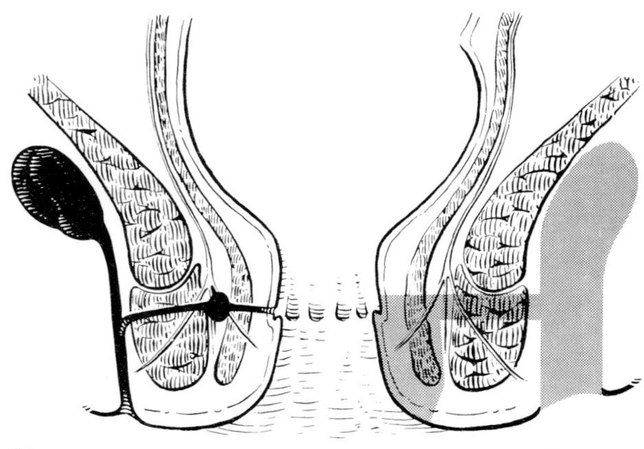

(h)

Figure 16.21g,h Treatment of trans-sphincteric fistula. (g) Simple trans-sphincteric fistula treated by excision of the fistula track and excision of the lower aspect of the internal anal sphincter. (h) Trans-sphincteric fistula with a high blind track managed by coring out the fistula, excision of the internal anal sphincter and drainage of the ischiorectal fossa.

Treatment of the suprasphincteric type

These fistulas are usually due to an intersphincteric track with a blind upper component, complicated by an abscess which bursts or, more commonly, is drained through the levator ani into the ischiorectal fossa.

Uncomplicated (Figure 16.21i)

Once the fistula track is correctly identified, the track lying lateral to the external sphincter is resected and the defect in the levator ani closed so that the fistula is converted into its original intersphincteric component. The residual fistula can then be laid open as a secondary procedure. The use of a seton is not generally advised for these fistulas. Another approach is to excise the track, using a mucosal advancement procedure to close the internal opening.

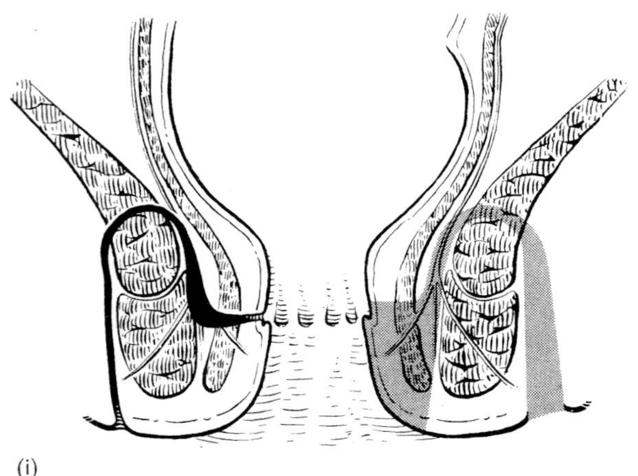

Figure 16.21i Treatment of suprasphincteric fistula. (i) Suprasphincteric fistula treated by excision of the fistula track.

High blind track

The blind track is nearly always associated with a supralevator abscess. Treatment is along the lines described above for the uncomplicated variety but the abscess requires wide drainage into the rectum.

Treatment of the extrasphincteric type (Figure 16.21j–l)

Extrasphincteric fistulas are usually man-made, associated with rectal trauma, complicate inflammatory bowel disease or occur secondary to pelvic sepsis. Multiple fistulas complicating Crohn's disease, particularly if associated with rectal stricture, may eventually require rectal excision. Most non-Crohn's extrasphincteric fistulas can be treated successfully by excision of the fistula and closure of the rectal defect using an anorectal advancement technique (Elting, 1912; McElwain et al, 1975; Oh, 1983; Athanasiadis et al, 1994; Lewis et al, 1995; Ozuner et al, 1996). These operations have traditionally been covered by a proximal stoma. Rather than using a loop sigmoid colostomy, we now prefer to divide the sigmoid colon, oversew the distal bowel end and raise the proximal limb as an end colostomy. This method allows complete defunction of the distal bowel. Furthermore the end stoma is easier to manage and is associated with fewer complications than a loop colostomy. Restoration of intestinal continuity can usually be performed easily using a peristomal technique, provided that the distal limb is merely dropped back at the site of the end colostomy. With improved bowel preparation, antibiotic cover and increased experience with intra-anal procedures, use of a colostomy is not necessarily mandatory in all cases of extrasphincteric fistula.

Secondary to anorectal sepsis (Figure 16.21k)

Some extrasphincteric fistulas cannot be treated successfully without a colostomy, but this is not necessary in all cases, particularly with iatrogenic fistulas when an advancement flap is feasible (Gordon, 1976, 1981). The original trans-sphincteric fistula should be managed as already described, by excision or seton fistulotomy (Walfisch et al, 1997) or by laying open if it is very low. In the past a seton was used for these high iatrogenic fistulas, but today successful treatment can often be achieved by excision of the fistula and closure of the rectal defect, either by direct suture (Parks and Stitz, 1976; Lewis, 1986) or preferably by anorectal advancement flap (Goldberg et al, 1980; Aquilar et al, 1985; García-Aguilar et al, 1996), as in the treatment of rectovaginal fistula (Gallagher and Scarborough, 1962; Hilsabeck, 1989).

Secondary to trauma (Figure 16.21l)

Treatment will involve removal of any foreign body that may be present, debridement of any devitalized tissue, and construction of a proximal stoma if this was not performed immediately after the injury. If debridement and drainage of sepsis have been adequate, these fistulas may heal without any further intervention. If the fistula persists, we prefer to close the defect with an advancement flap if the sphincters are intact or by complete sphincter repair if there is a substantial defect.

Secondary to pelvic sepsis

Any fistula complicating pelvic sepsis should heal by the eradication of the source of infection in the pelvis, by resecting the source of the sepsis and the provision of adequate drainage through the ischiorectal fossa if necessary.

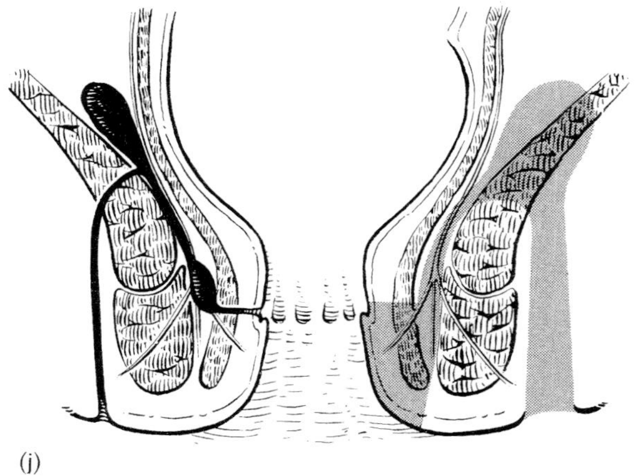

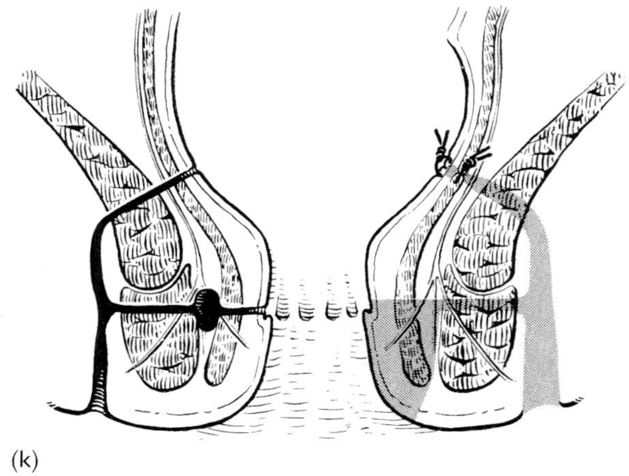

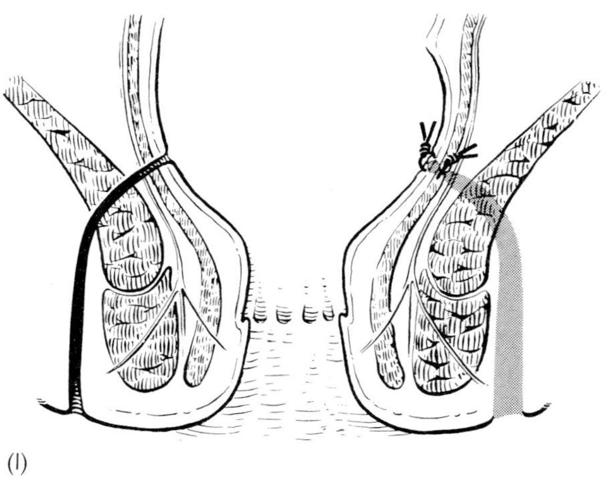

Figure 16.21j–l Treatment of extrasphincteric fistula.
(j) Extrasphincteric fistula complicated by suprasphincteric abscess, managed by extensive fistula excision, drainage and internal sphincterotomy. (k) Extrasphincteric fistula treated by excision of the fistula track and mucosal advancement.
(l) Extrasphincteric fistula treated by excision of the external component and mucosal advancement.

Treatment of horseshoe fistula

Intersphincteric fistulas

Circumferential spread of sepsis in the intersphincteric plane is usually limited and adequate clearance and drainage merely requires excision rather than division of the lower aspect of the internal sphincter.

Suprasphincteric and extrasphincteric fistulas

Circumferential spread of sepsis in the suprasphincteric plane usually only complicates suprasphincteric or extrasphincteric fistulas. Adequate drainage can be achieved by a long internal sphincterotomy for suprasphincteric fistulas. Elimination of circumferential spread in extrasphincteric fistulas necessitates either the use of loose setons or mushroom catheters in the suprasphincteric space or, in the case of collections in the deep postanal space, dislocating the levator ani from the coccyx.

Transphincteric fistulas

Much the most common horseshoe fistula is the posterior extrasphincteric communication complicating an ischiorectal abscess in patients with a trans-sphincteric fistula. Three or four external

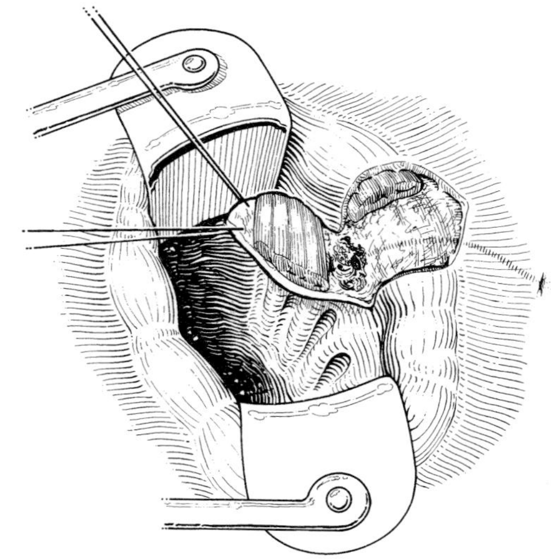

Figure 16.22 Exploring the intersphincteric plane. An incision is made in the intersphincteric groove. The intersphincteric plane is opened with a pair of scissors and a disc of anal mucosa with the lower fibres of the internal anal sphincter is excised to allow drainage of chronic intersphincteric sepsis.

openings may communicate by their common internal opening in the midline posteriorly at the level of the dentate line through the internal part of the external sphincter. There may be technical difficulties in identifying the internal opening. If this is the case, the intersphincteric plane should first be explored in the midline posteriorly to detect whether there is chronic intersphincteric sepsis or a collection in the deep postanal space, and to identify the defect in the external sphincter (Figure 16.22).

There are four approaches to these complex trans-sphincteric fistulas. The first and the most traditional treatment involves laying open all the tracks, identifying the trans-sphincteric midline entry site and laying this open as well (Figure 16.23a). There may be extensive anterior prolongations, which extend to the urogenital triangle, and traditionally these are also laid widely open (Figure 16.23b). There are two major drawbacks to this approach. The first is that these wounds take a long time to heal and, secondly, continence may be compromised by creating a gutter owing to retraction of the partially divided internal and external sphincter. Van Tets and Kuijpers (1994) found that this type of fistula was the one most commonly associated with impaired continence.

The second and more conservative approach involves a partial fistulectomy confined to the internal opening or T-shaped portion of the fistula track so that the intersphincteric and trans-sphincteric components only are laid open and the side tracks merely curetted (Hanley, 1979)

The third approach is to perform a fistulectomy so that the primary trans-sphincteric fistula and all the secondary extensions are excised. Any defect in the muscle may be closed by direct suture, or the internal defect dealt with by an advancement flap (Athanasiadis et al, 1994).

The fourth approach is to use a seton for the posterior trans-sphincteric opening and either to lay open or excise the lateral horsehoe side tracks (Lewis, 1986; Lenter and Wienert, 1996).

Special care must be taken in the management of the rare anterior horseshoe fistula in women. There is no support from the puborectalis, there may have been previous anterior postobstetric sphincter damage, and division of the external sphincter will result in incontinence. Many authorities therefore recommend the use of a seton for such lesions (Hanley, 1978) or the use of advancement flaps to preserve function.

Special considerations in patients with Crohn's disease (see Chapter 58)

We reported spontaneous healing in over two-thirds of perianal fistula complicating Crohn's disease without definitive surgical treatment other than drainage of pus (Buchmann et al, 1980). We take the view that if there is any doubt about the possibility of Crohn's disease, no attempt should be made to treat the fistula along conventional lines, particularly if the rectum is involved (Allan and Keighley, 1988). In our experience there is a high risk of incontinence (50%), even following treatment of low trans-sphincteric fistula, and only one of 12 surgically treated fistulas complicating Crohn's disease healed (Keighley and Allan, 1986). Indeed, there is a high proctectomy rate for patients with fistulas complicating Crohn's disease (Baker and Milton-Thompson, 1974; Alexander-Williams and Buchmann, 1980; Marks et al, 1981).

However, this conservative view is not subscribed to by all surgeons, who claim high healing rates for low anal fistulas in Crohn's patients with a normal anorectum on sigmoidoscopy (Sohn et al, 1980; Hobbis and Schofield, 1982; Wolff et al, 1985; Bernard et al, 1986). A study by Morrison et al (1989) reports healing in 30 of 32 carefully selected patients with fistulas in Crohn's disease when the rectum was judged to be normal. Most were treated by application of a seton or a fistulotomy, usually without a covering colostomy. Bayer and Gordon (1994) reported successful healing in 20 of 28 cases, but eight had severe impairment of continence. Many fistulas took a long time to heal, and five patients required eventual proctectomy. Faucheron et al (1996) in Paris report the outcome in 41 patients managed by loose seton. In 18 patients the seton was removed, eight of whom developed a recurrent fistula, requiring another seton in three, a fistulotomy in three and a proctocolectomy in one. In seven patients a definitive fistulotomy was performed, one of whom required a proctocolectomy. Two patients required a definitive proctocolectomy. In 11 of the patients the loose seton had not been removed. The overall incidence of incontinence was 12% (Figure 16.24).

The anorectal advancement technique is not always possible, especially if there is rectal involvement, and the results do not appear to be very good in Crohn's patients (Jones et al, 1987). In view of the risks of iatrogenic sphincter damage, we are loath to change our somewhat conservative philosophy for the management of anorectal fistula in Crohn's

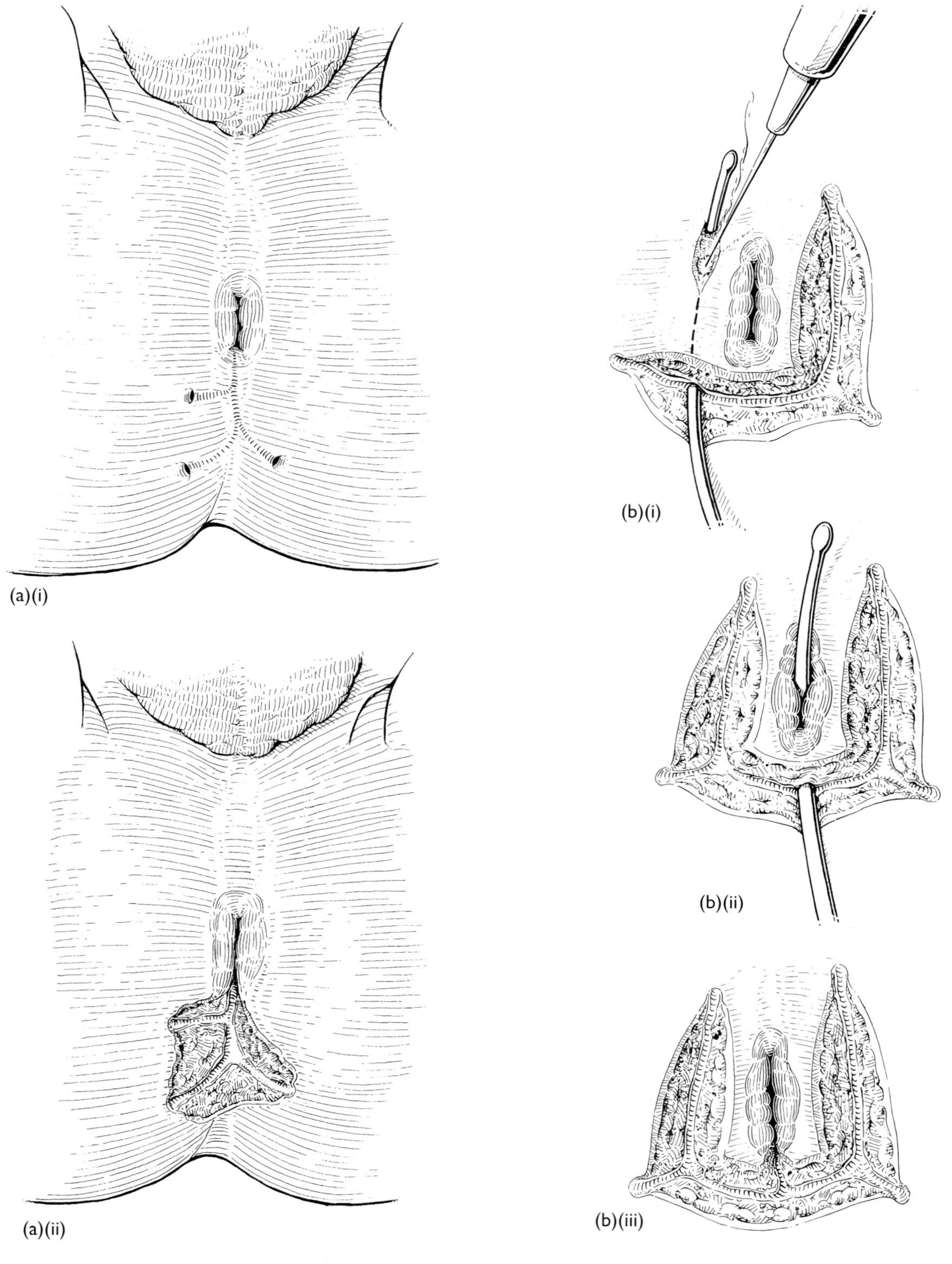

Figure 16.23a,b Laying open a low trans-sphincteric fistula. (a)(i) Three external openings are shown posterior to the anal verge. (a)(ii) Illustrates the fistula track having been laid open with minimal division of sphincter muscle. (b)(i) Laying open of a complex trans-sphincteric fistula over fistula probe. There is an anterior horseshoe extension which is being laid open. (b)(ii) The internal component of the fistula has been identified with a fistula probe. (b)(iii) The internal component has been laid open with minimal division of the sphincter muscles.

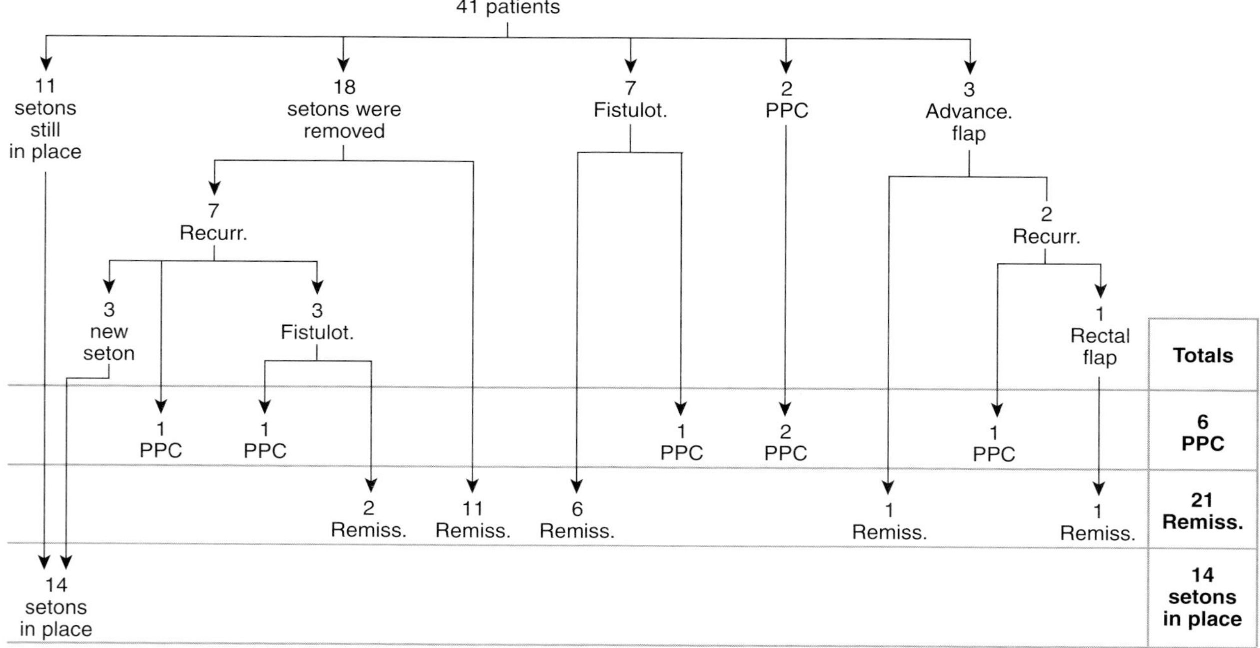

Figure 16.24 Outcome of the use of setons in fistulas complicating Crohn's disease (Faucheron et al, 1996).

disease, but we do accept the role of loose setons for control of local sepsis and faecal diversion in some patients (see Chapter 57).

Management after fistula surgery

Many patients who have extensive fistulas excised or laid open have large cavities around the anus which may easily become infected, with the consequent risk of further muscle loss, and recurrent sepsis and fistula formation. Wounds are deliberately conical so that the defect granulates and heals from within outwards, thereby preventing the pocketing of pus. These open wounds must be properly managed as most patients are encouraged to return home early after operation. Patients should receive proper instruction before discharge regarding the management of their wounds. District nursing services may be unreliable, or unavailable. In our opinion, it is far better to teach the patient and their partner to manage the wound themselves rather than relying on nursing services.

Initially cavities may be filled with a loose dressing soaked in proflavine, hypochlorite solution or eusol, with liquid paraffin to prevent it from adhering to the wound. These dressings to fill the cavity can usually be dispensed with within a week.

Baths are encouraged almost immediately after operation and patients are instructed to direct a shower hose over the granulating area two or three times a day to ensure it is kept clean. This simple expedient is much less messy, less costly in nursing

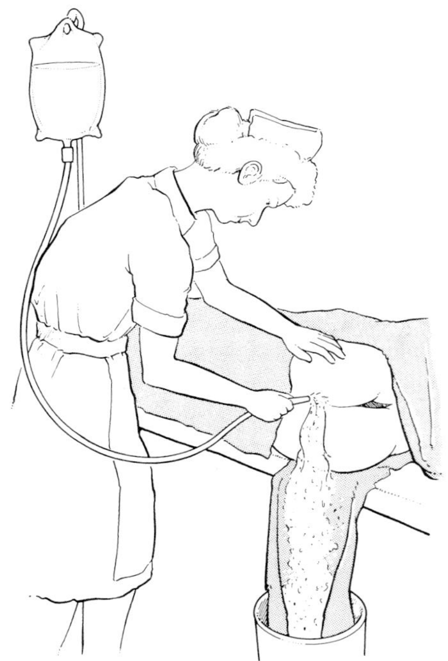

Figure 16.25 Irrigating open anal fistula wounds.

time and more efficient than the time-honoured method of packing or irrigation over a rubber sheet using a nozzle and tubing attached to a douche can (Figure 16.25). We instruct patients to use a bidet. If there is no bidet, regular baths or, better still, a baby bath or tub with some added Milton allows the buttocks and perineum to be regularly irrigated. Application of a soft dry dressing and a regular change of underwear provide adequate hygiene, allow patients to return to work and encourage healthy granulating tissue.

It is crucial that someone, usually the colorectal nurse, inspects the wound regularly to ensure that wounds are clean and granulating satisfactorily and that there is no pocketing of pus or skin bridging.

Overall outcome of treatment

Recurrence rates for treatment of 'low' fistula are given in Tables 16.11 and 16.12. In most reports the recurrence rate is less than 10% and may be slightly lower following excision compared with fistulotomy. Recurrence rates are much lower using a seton (Table 16.13a,b). In a non-randomized comparison of management in trans-sphincteric fistula, an 18% recurrence rate was reported for seton division compared with 57% for fistulotomy (Abcarian et al, 1987). Numbers of recurrences following surgical excision of 'high' fistula-in-ano are too small for comment but early results suggest that recurrence is low (Table 16.14).

Table 16.11 Results of anal fistula surgery.

Classification	Intersphincteric	180
	Trans-sphincteric	108
	Suprasphincteric	6
	Extrasphincteric	6
	Unclassified	75
Treatment	Fistulotomy	300
	Seton	63
	Advancement flap	3
	Other	9
Outcome	Recurrence	31 (8%)
	Incontinence	45 (12%)

From García-Aguilar et al (1996).

Surprisingly, Marks and Ritchie (1977) failed to demonstrate a widely differing incidence of continence according to the type of anal fistula (Table 16.15). What they did show was that approximately a third of patients complain of soiling after successful treatment and that almost one in ten has to wear a pad indefinitely after operation. Fortunately, true faecal incontinence is rare, but impaired control of gas or liquids occurred in about one in five patients following complete clearance of the fistula track. The St Mark's experience is mirrored by many other reports for 'low' fistulas (Table 16.16). Apart from the report by Denecke et al (1986) and that of our own group (Shouler et al, 1986), soiling still occurred in over 24%. True faecal incontinence is variable, ranging from nil to 26%. The present record for more conservative methods of treating extrasphincteric fistulas is more encouraging and holds real promise for a more successful outcome for fistula surgery in the future.

Table 16.12 Recurrence after treatment of fistula-in-ano (most reports confined to low fistulas).

Authors	*n*	*Method*	*Recurrence*
Bennett (1962)	108	Lay open	2 (2)
Hill (1967)	626	Lay open	6 (1.0)
Mazier (1971)	1000	Lay open	39 (3.9)
Ani and Solanke (1976)	82	Lay open	14 (17)*
Parks and Stitz (1976)	16	Lay open	1 (6.3)
	15	Internal sphincterotomy and curettage only	5 (33)
Adams and Kovalcik (1981)	53	Lay open	5 (9)
	80	Excision	0
Kuijpers (1982)	51	Lay open	2 (4)
Gingold (1983)	74	Lay open	1 (1.3)
Khubchandani (1984)	68	Excision	4 (5.8)
	69	Internal sphincterotomy and curettage only	0
Vasilevsky and Gordon (1984)	160	Excision	10 (6.3)
Kronborg (1985)	26	Lay open	3 (11)
Denecke et al (1986)	57	Lay open	0
Lilius (1986)	150	Lay open	8 (5.5)
Shouler et al (1986)	115	Lay open	8 (6.9)

Values in parentheses are percentages.
* Stenosis in nine.

Table 16.13a Results of treating high fistulas with a seton and division.

Authors	*n*	*Recurrence*	*Flatus incontinence*	*Faecal incontinence*	*Soiling*
Parks and Stitz (1976)	57	1	9	1	9
Ramanujam et al (1983)	45	0	1	0	0
Culp (1984)	20	NS	NS	2	1
Kuijpers (1984)	10	0	NS	1	6
Christensen et al (1986)	21	0	13	3	8
Williams et al (1991a)	13	0	7	1	NS
Pearl et al (1993)	89	3	NS	3	NS
Lentner and Wienert (1996)	108	4	NS	1	NS
McCourtney and Finlay (1996)	27	1	2	1	NS

NS, not stated.

Table 16.13b Results of seton fistulotomy.

	n	*Healing time*	*Recurrence*	*Incontinence*	
				Major	*Minor*
Two stage fistulotomy	24	11	2	1	13
Cutting seton	13	16	0	1	7
Short term drainage seton	14	10	2	1	5
Long term drainage seton	23	Not applicable	9	0	6

From Williams et al (1991b).

Table 16.14 Results of surgical treatment of high fistulas.

Author	*n*	*Method*	*Recurrence*	*Faecal incontinence*	*Minor defects of incontinence*
Parks and Stitz (1976)	18	Closure with wire ± rotation flaps	2	2	3
Oh (1983)	15	Mucosal advancement	2	0	0
Kuflerberg et al (1984)	5	Excision, closure and gentamicin beads	0	0	0
Aquilar et al (1985)	189	Mucosal advancement	3	0	13
Mann and Clifton (1985)	5	Re-routing	0	0	0
Lewis (1986)	18	Fistulectomy plus primary closure of defect	1	NS	NS
Matos et al (1993)	13	Core out and excise fistula	4	NS	NS
Christiansen and Ronholt (1995)	14	Total excision and sphincter repair	2	0	3
McCourtney and Finlay (1996)	18	Seton	1	0	0

NS, not stated.

Table 16.15 Functional results of operations for fistula-in-ano in 203 patients.

	Soiling	*Pad needed*	*Flatus incontinence*	*Loose stool incontinence*	*Solid stool incontinence*
Intersphincteric with high extension (*n* = 33)	30	9	24	9	7
Simple trans-sphincteric (*n* = 44)	30	11	23	18	7
Complex trans-sphincteric (high extension) (*n* = 85)	31	9	30	21	1
Suprasphincteric (*n* = 22)	41	9	14	14	5
Extrasphincteric (*n* = 19)	31	5	21	16	0

All values are percentages.
From Marks and Ritchie (1977).

Table 16.16 Percentage incontinence after treatment of low fistula-in-ano.

Author	*n*	*Faecal incontinence*	*Flatus incontinence*	*Soiling*
Bennett (1962)	129	12	16	24
Parks and Stitz (1976)	66	26	0	26
Marks and Ritchie (1977)	204	17	25	31
Vasilevsky and Gordon (1984)	151	1	3	NS
Kronborg (1985)	47	0	10	NS
Denecke et al (1986)	57	17	5	7
Shouler et al (1986)	115	2	2	12

NS, not stated.

COMMON SURGICAL TECHNIQUES AND THEIR OUTCOME

Fistulotomy

Laying open techniques are widely practised for superficial fistulas entering low down in the anus and traversing only the lower fibres of the external sphincter muscles (Shafik et al, 1994). Once the course of the fistula has been accurately located, a blunt probe director is passed along the track into the anus (Figure 16.26a(i)). The roof of the track is laid open using a scalpel blade or a cutting diathermy current (Figure 16.26a(ii)). Healthy granulating tissue should be present throughout the length of the fistula track. Normally the fistula is curetted if there is any concern about the aetiology, and material is sent for culture and histology (Figure 16.26a(iii)). The wound edges are excised to encourage healing from below (Figure 16.26b). Haemostasis is secured and a dressing is applied to the wound. Alternatively, the fistula track may be excised after the track has been laid open. The disadvantages of this approach are that the wound is deeper, there is a greater risk of excising sphincter muscle, and healing may be delayed. Healing can be accelerated by marsupialization (Ho et al, 1998). Furthermore the material obtained for histological examination is generally poor and blind tracks may be missed.

When Shouler et al (1986) reviewed our Birmingham results, 96 of 115 patients had a deroofing procedure: none developed faecal incontinence, ten experienced soiling, and only one patient complained of temporary incontinence of flatus. Patients were off work for only 17 days and had usually been discharged from hospital within 24 hours of operation. However, there were seven recurrences (8%). Others have found that the time off work and healing takes longer (Bennett, 1962; Kuijpers, 1982).

A high recurrence rate of 17% was reported by Ani and Solanke (1976) using fistulotomy, whereas Vasilevsky and Gordon (1984) in Montreal had only ten recurrences (6%) and fewer than 3% had any impairment of continence following deroofing procedures. Similarly Sangwan et al (1994) used fistulotomy in 461 of 503 patients with a recurrence rate of 6.5%. However, Denecke et al (1986), using fistulotomy in 57 patients with low-lying fistulas, found that although there were no recurrences, three patients (5%) became incontinent and four suffered severe urgency of defecation. Van Tets and Kuijpers (1994) reported defects in continence among 27% of 267 patients who were fully continent before operation. The majority of these patients had been treated by laying open of the track, and factors associated with a high risk of incontinence were high fistulas, lateral extensions and posterior internal opening. When Isbister (1995) examined his own audit of fistulotomy in 88 patients, there were only two recurrences (2%). None of the patients was rendered incontinent, but four turned out to have Crohn's disease and two were found to have malignancy. Fistulotomy is still the most common method of treatment. García-Aguilar et al (1996) used fistulotomy in 300 of 375 patients, their overall results being as outlined in Table 16.17. The recurrence rates in other published reports following fistulotomy are shown in Table 16.12.

Fistulectomy

A careful preoperative assessment is required to determine the anatomy of the fistula, but the passage of probes is not mandatory; indeed, one of the arguments for performing fistulectomy is that false passages are not created by probing the track

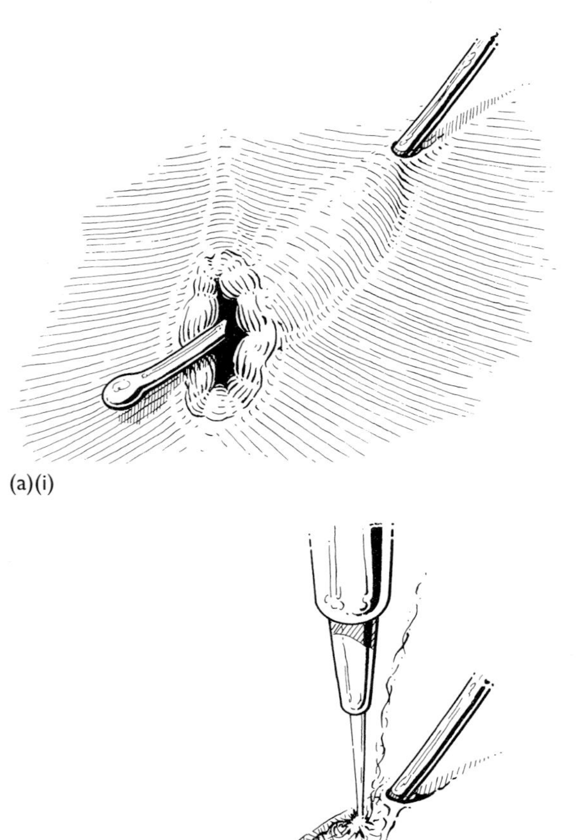

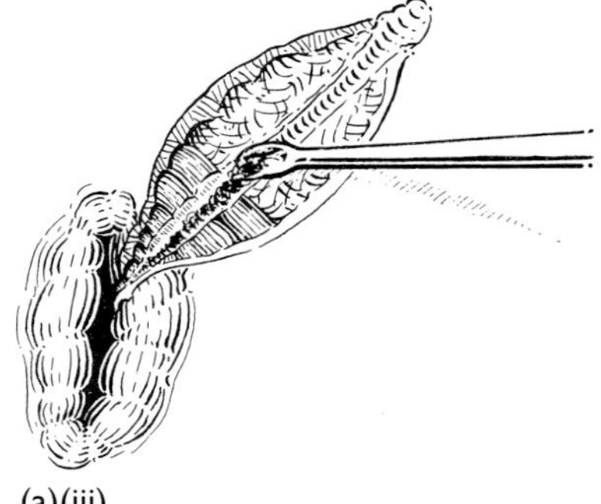

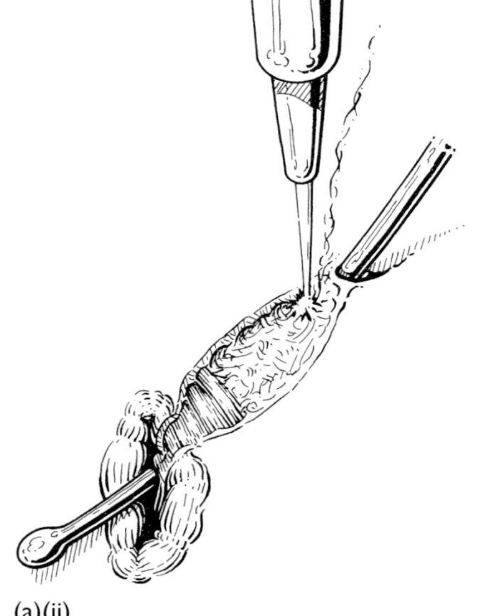

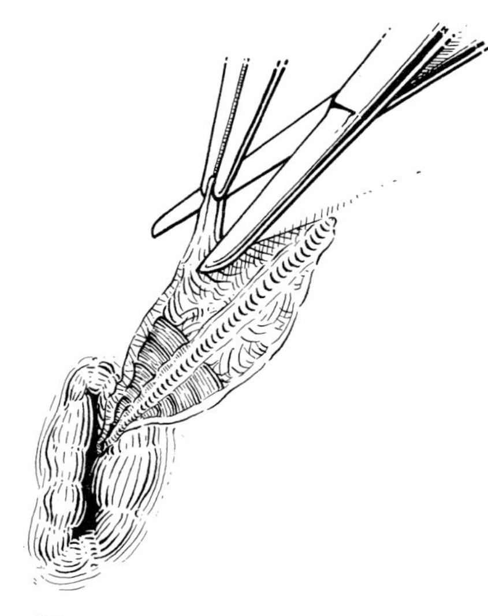

Figure 16.26a,b Laying open and curettage of a low trans-sphincteric fistula in ano. (a)(i) The fistula track has been identified with a fistula probe. (a)(ii) The skin has been divided over the fistula probe and the subcutaneous fat is being divided. (a)(iii) As only superficial fibres of the external anal sphincter lie superficial to the fistula track, the entire fistula is laid open and the fistula track is curetted. (b) The skin margins of the fistulotomy are freshened to facilitate drainage.

Table 16.17 Recent results of fistulotomy.

Author	*n*	*Recurrence*	*Flatus incontinence*	*Faecal incontinence*	*Soiling*
Sangwan et al (1994)	461	30	NS	NS	NS
Isbister et al (1995)	88	2	0	0	0
García-Aguilar et al (1996)	300	24	40	11	NS

NS, not stated.

(Figure 16.27). The external opening is grasped with tissue forceps or stay sutures. It is advisable to commence the dissection posteriorly if the lithotomy position is used, since bleeding from anterior wounds may compromise assessment around a more posterior field. After dividing the skin around the external opening, the tissues around the fistula should be infiltrated with a weak adrenaline–saline solution to reduce bleeding. Haemostasis must be meticulous throughout the operation. Only in this way can the appearance of granulation tissue in the wound be transected with certainty, indicating that a side track, or the fistula itself, has been divided.

After dividing the skin, fine scissors are used to core out the surrounding tissue, leaving the granulating track and its surrounding fibrous tissue, which is withdrawn by gentle traction (Figure 16.27a). If a side track is inadvertently divided, it is advisable to trace the secondary extension before proceeding further with the main fistula (Figure 16.27b). Blind tracks may extend up or even through the ischiorectal fossa and may be difficult to trace to their extremity unless an assistant retracts the surrounding tissues. In this way the peripheral components of the fistula can be precisely defined and the granulation tissue excised. As the dissection proceeds towards the anus, sufficient overlying skin and fascia must be divided to gain access to the sphincter, but the dissection should stop well short of the anal margin unless all the tracks have been traced to their origins. This manoeuvre allows the precise relationship of the fistula to the sphincter to be identified. A decision can then be made as to how best to proceed, depending upon the course of the track and the site of the internal opening. If there is any uncertainty, a flap of mucosa and internal sphincter may be raised around the internal opening at the anal verge to display the anatomy and if necessary allow closure of the defect by advancement flap to preserve the muscles of continence. No striated muscle should be divided until the precise anatomy has been displayed.

If the fistula occupies a low trans-sphincteric position, the overlying external anal sphincter may be divided without compromising continence (Figure 16.27c). If a tunnel is left after coring out the fistula, this may be laid open once it has been established how much sphincter can safely be divided (Figure 16.27d). If, on the other hand, it proves to be a mid or high trans-sphincteric fistula, or the patient is elderly, or there is a history of obstetric trauma, or preoperative manometry indicates poor anal function, the fistula track can merely be cored out from the muscle and then either (1) re-routed into the intersphincteric plane (Mann and Clifton, 1985), or (2) excised, leaving the defect in the sphincter to heal by secondary intention; alternatively it may be closed by suture (Figure 16.27e–g) or closed by raising an advancement flap (discussed below – see Figure 16.30).

The coring out technique is particularly useful for suprasphincteric fistula, the intersphincteric portion of which may be left *in situ* once the defect in the levator is closed; the fistula may then be removed or laid open as a secondary procedure. If the track is extrasphincteric it may be completely excised, leaving only a small defect in the levator ani and rectal wall which may be closed either (1) by direct suture of the levator, rectal muscle and mucosa (Figure 16.27f,g), or (2) obliquely, to prevent two suture lines from overlying each other, using the anorectal flap technique (see Figure 16.31). If, on the other hand, the track is horseshoe in configuration, a rotation flap may be more convenient (Parks and Stitz, 1976). These procedures are described later in detail, but a temporary colostomy will usually be required, particularly in the case of a recurrent fistula (Seow-Choen and Phillips, 1991).

One of the great advantages of fistulectomy is that no muscle is divided until the precise anatomical relationship of the track to the sphincters is ascertained with confidence (Matos et al, 1993). If doubt still exists, the fistula may be dissected out as it penetrates the muscle without jeopardizing function. An additional advantage is that material is available for histology (Lawson, 1970; Mazier, 1971; Adams and Kovalcik, 1981). However, the procedure is tedious and most surgeons do not think that the time devoted to the technique is justified, particularly in the management of simple intersphincteric or low trans-sphincteric fistula.

Adams and Kovalcik (1981) compared the results of fistulectomy with those of fistulotomy. Only one patient developed minor incontinence to liquids after fistulotomy but there were five recurrences. Defects in continence and recurrence did not occur in the patients treated by excision of the fistula track (see Table 16.12). Kronborg (1985) undertook a trial to compare laying open with excision (Table 16.18). Unfortunately, the number of patients in this study was rather small which makes interpretation difficult. However, the time taken to healing was significantly shorter using fistulotomy. There were five recurrences after fistulotomy: three treated by fistulotomy and two by excision. Flatus incontinence was the only reported defect, occurring in one patient after laying open the fistula compared with three patients after excision. Kronborg (1985) concluded that there was no advantage to be gained from the more tedious practice of excision and

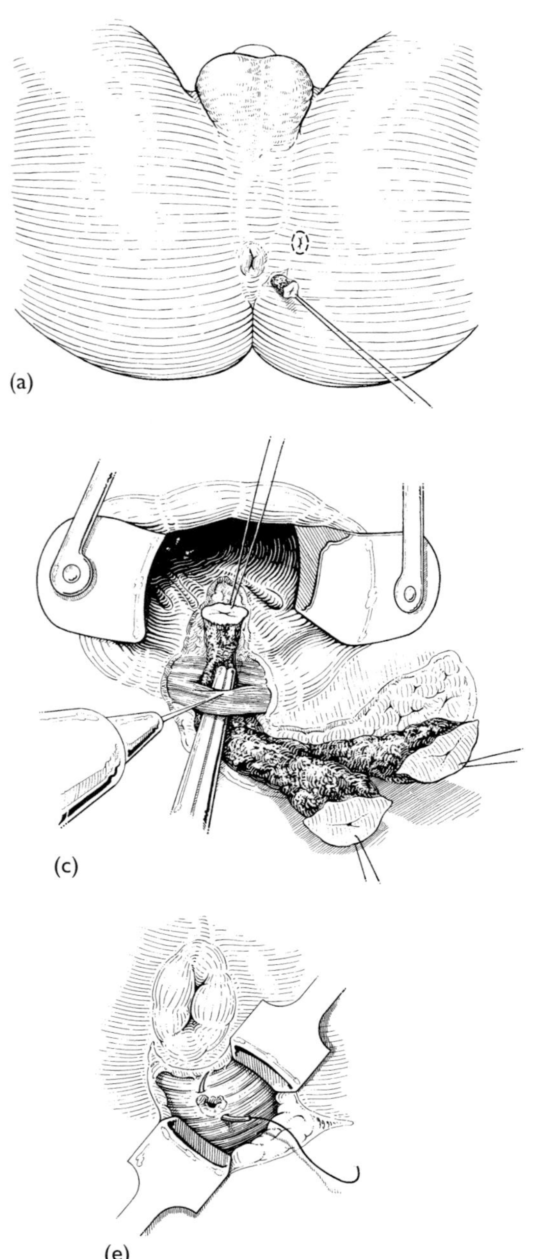

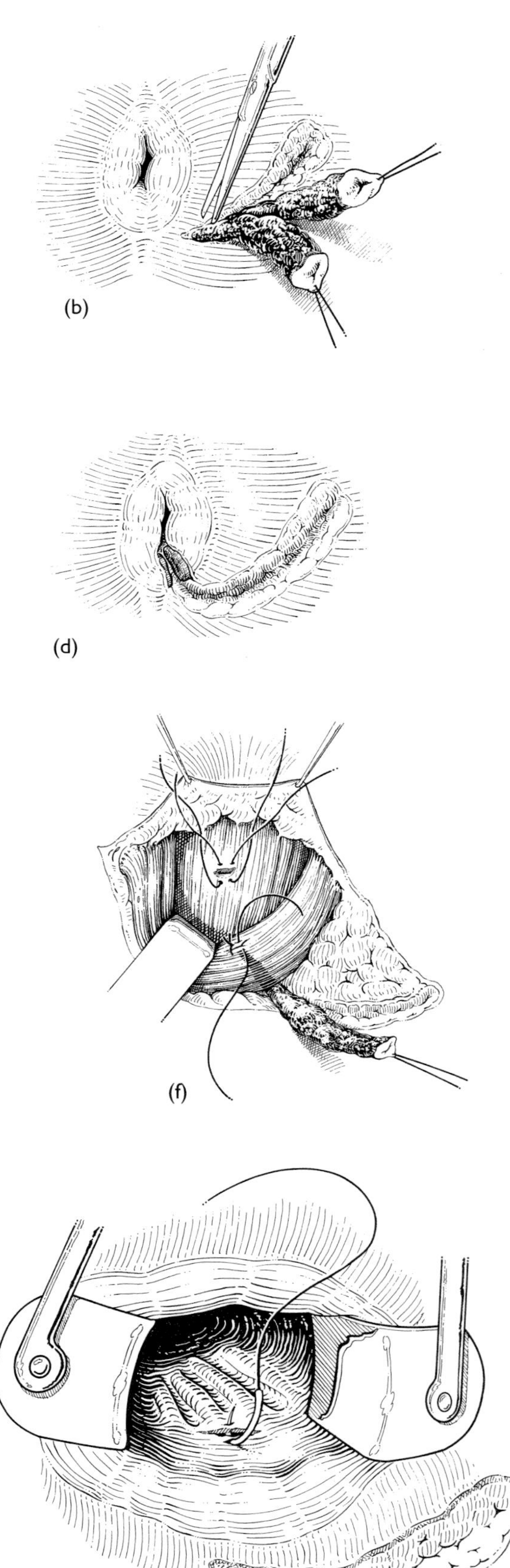

Figure 16.27a–g Fistulectomy. (a) Two anal openings are seen. A small elipse of skin is excised around the fistulas. Traction is applied with a stay suture through the fistula. (b) The fistula tracks are carefully dissected out by a combination of skin division and scissor excisions of perianal fat. (c) The internal component of the fistula is identified. As this is a low trans-sphincteric fistula the external sphincter is divided and the entire fistula track is cored out. (d) Completion of a low-lying fistulotomy. (e) If laying open of the fistula involves division of a large component of the external anal sphincter, the internal opening of the fistula can be closed. (f) The defect in the anorectum may also be closed separately leaving only the external component of the fistula, which is excised. (g) Completion of conservation fistulotomy is achieved by filleting out the internal component of the fistula with closure of the mucosal defect.

recommended that simple low anal fistulas should be laid open and not excised. Matos et al (1993) reported the results of fistulectomy in 13 patients; only seven were successful, two required further surgery and four failed.

Table 16.18 Randomized trial to compare fistulotomy with excision.

	Fistulotomy (*n* = 26)	*Excision* (*n* = 21)
Time to healing (days)	34 (7–850)	41 (26–116)
Surgical revision before healing	3	2
Recurrent fistula or abscess		
At 6 months	2	2
At 22 months	3	2
Flatus incontinence	1	3

From Kronborg (1985).

The principles of fistulectomy as established by Parks (1961) are illustrated in Figure 16.27. The fistula is excised, a longitudinal segment of the internal sphincter overlying the fistula is excised, the fistula itself is cored out and the defect is closed (Thomson and Ross, 1989; Kennedy and Zegerra, 1990). An alternative technique is to use an anorectal flap by excising the internal opening transversely and making two diverging longitudinal incisions from the excision site up into the rectum so that rectal wall can be used to close the defect (see below – Figure 16.30). Khubchandani (1984) compared the techniques of laying open with excision alone (Table 16.19). Hospital stay was similar but four recurrences were recorded in the lay-open group compared with none in those having fistulectomy. The only patient with impaired continence was in the fistulectomy group. These results are far better than those reported by Parks and Stitz (1976), where 5 of 15 patients developed recurrence after fistulectomy.

A variation on this principle is excision of the fistula track and closure of the mucosa and internal sphincter through an intersphincteric approach. This is an attractive concept; Lunniss and Phillips (1996) reported a successful outcome in 7 of 13 patients, all of whom had undergone previously unsuccessful operations.

Use of setons

The seton has been used for the treatment of anal fistula for at least 25 centuries (Rangabashyam, 1996; Goldberg and García-Aguilar, 1996). One potential source of confusion within the literature on the use of setons is that surgeons use them for different purposes (Williams et al, 1991a). Setons may be used to drain pus, to mark a fistula track, to allow staged division, or to deliberately cut through the sphincters (Hertel, 1954; Hess and Daum, 1959; Gabriel, 1963; Eisenhammer, 1966; Hamilton, 1975; Lentner and Wienert, 1996; McCourtney and Finlay, 1996).

Few would argue against the use of setons as a method of marking a fistula track – this is their first main use. They may therefore aid identification of the track during excision (Aluwihare et al, 1973). Indeed, during excision of a fistula a single thread, with a bead on the end to act as a means of traction, may be passed along the track during excision of a trans-sphincteric fistula (Figure 16.28a).

A second role of a seton is merely to act as a drain (Lunniss and Thomson, 1996), in the belief that control of sepsis may sometimes achieve spontaneous healing (Parks and Stitz, 1976). This is especially true in Crohn's disease where conventional surgical treatment may be contraindicated for fear of non-healing or incontinence (Faucheron et al, 1996). Likewise in cryptoglandular fistula the loose seton may be used simply to drain pus prior to definitive treatment. If setons are just used for drainage and

Table 16.19 Comparison of excision and sphincter division with excision and sphincter preservation.

	Excision and sphincter division (lay open) (*n* = 68)	*Excision and sphincter preservation (fistulectomy)* (*n* = 69)
Postoperative hospital stay (days)	3.4	3.7
Complications	8	7
Urinary retention	2	2
Bleeding	1	1
Recurrent abscess	1	2
Recurrent fistula	4	0
Incontinence	1	0
Thromboembolism	0	1

From Khubchandani (1984).

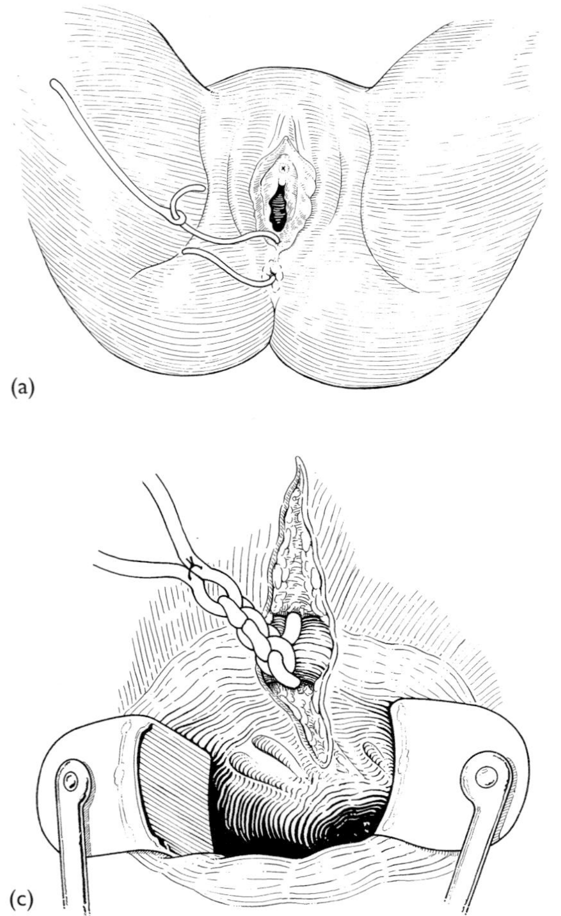

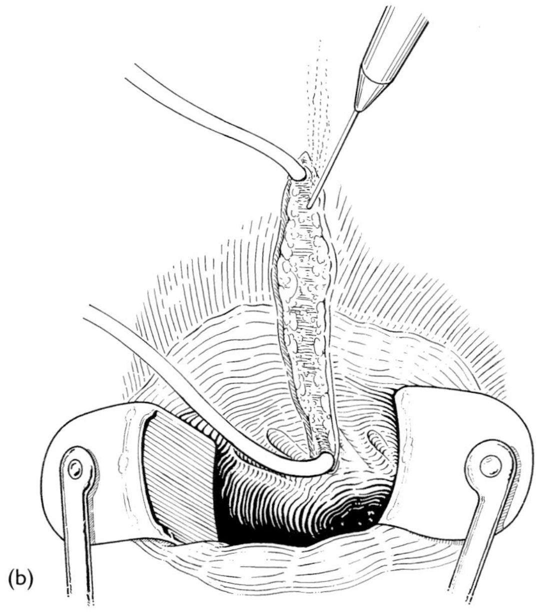

Figure 16.28a–c Seton fistulotomy. (a) A loose seton has been applied through the fistula track to act as a drain. (b) The fistula track having been identified, a rubber seton tube is placed around the track, excising the skin, and the mucosa of the anal canal overlying the fistula. (c) The rubber seton is tied as tightly as possible. It may have to be re-inserted if it has not cut through the sphincter muscle, and a repeat examination under anaesthetic is arranged.

then removed without definitive surgery, 43% persist. Abcarian et al (1987) reported that when the residual fistula was eventually laid open a third of patients developed impairment of continence.

A third approach is to tie a seton loosely around the fistula track to stimulate fibrosis. It is thus argued that 4–6 weeks later the intervening muscle can be divided with impunity because the fibrous reaction prevents retraction of the cut ends (Thomson and Parks, 1979; Gordon, 1985) (Figure 16.28b). However, careful analysis of the functional results has shown that there is no difference between delayed division of sphincter muscle after application of a seton compared with fistulotomy as an initial procedure. This approach may prolong therapy because of repeated operations and hospital admissions (Marks and Ritchie, 1977).

A fourth approach is to use a tight seton to strangulate the isolated sphincters lying within the seton so that they are slowly transected. This technique has sometimes involved repeated tightening of the seton, as in the rubber-band method advocated by Hanley (1978). However, Culp (1984) tied a seton, composed of a narrow Penrose drain, so tightly initially that the average time to achieve sphincter division was 13 days (Figure 16.28c). Various materials are used for tight seton fistulotomy, such as Prolene, silk or rubber, but we prefer Silastic and tie about six knots, the lower of which is secured by a silk stitch.

Christensen et al (1986) reviewed the results of treatment in 23 patients with a high trans-sphincteric fistula using a seton that was tightened every other day. The functional results were surprisingly disappointing. Thirteen patients (62%) complained of temporary incontinence of flatus; soiling was recorded in eight patients and three became frankly incontinent of faeces. However, none had a recurrence. Nevertheless, manometric studies by these authors and others demonstrated considerable impairment of function if the sphincters are divided by a tight seton (Belliveau et al, 1983). Lentner and Wienert (1996) reported their long-term results of seton fistulotomy for trans-sphincteric and inter-

Table 16.20 Results of seton fistulotomy.

	n	*Incontinence*	*Recurrence*
Complex anorectal fistula	65	3	2
Anterior fistula in women	24	0	1
Complex Crohn's fistula	21	Drainage only	
Complex AIDS fistula	3	Drainage only	
Fistula with massive sepsis	3	2	0

From Pearl et al (1993).

sphincteric fistulas. These authors deliberately tightened the seton slowly over an average of 55 weeks per patient; the treatment was entirely on an outpatient basis, only 3.7% relapsed and incontinence was reported in 0.9%. McCourtney and Finley (1996) reported 18 cryptoglandular non-Crohn's anorectal fistulas treated with a cutting seton; 17 healed and there was no incontinence. Pearl et al (1993) reported that only 3 of 65 complex anorectal fistulas recurred and only three developed incontinence; they used a seton in 24 anterior fistulas in women with only one recurrence, and none became incontinent (Table 16.20).

Although incontinence after the use of a seton is not as frequent as with some other methods of treatment (see Table 16.13a), there seems little doubt that their use does not completely protect against incontinence to the extent that was originally hoped (García-Aguilar et al, 1998; Hämäläinen and Sainio, 1997). Indeed, it could be argued that the fibrosis stimulated by the use of a seton increases the risk of a gutter deformity developing postoperatively if the sphincter needs to be divided later. We recently audited our results of seton fistulotomy within the context of our overall experience of non-Crohn's anorectal fistulas in Birmingham. Almost all simple intersphincteric fistulas had been treated by simple fistulotomy (95%); in contrast, seton fistulotomy was almost exclusively confined to trans-sphincteric (76%), suprasphincteric (10%) and extrasphincteric fistulas. Deliberate repeat application or tightening of the seton was used in 14 of 38 patients, sometimes more than once. The recurrent fistula rate was disappointingly high (42%), but only one patient developed any severe impairment of continence requiring sphincter repair.

There is one situation in which the use of a seton is regarded as optimum treatment (Williams et al, 1991a), namely among female patients with a high anterior trans-sphincteric fistula (Culp, 1984). However, many would now prefer fistulectomy and advancement flap or even a direct division and sphincter repair in this situation (Christiansen and Ronholt, 1995). A second situation where setons have been advised is for suprasphincteric or extrasphincteric fistulas (Kuijpers, 1984). On the other hand, it is precisely in these groups that the worst results are reported (Vasilevsky and Gordon, 1984; Christensen et al, 1986). Our current view is that most suprasphincteric and extrasphincteric fistulas are best managed by excision and advancement flaps provided all sepsis has been adequately drained.

The results of seton treatment in Minneapolis are displayed in Table 16.13b. In this series the cutting seton has been compared with short- and long-term seton drainage (Williams et al, 1991b). We believe that the cutting seton is the optimum treatment of most high trans-sphincteric fistulas despite some of the functional results reported in the literature (Figure 17.29a–d).

Repair by laying open and direct suture of the sphincter defect

Excellent exposure of both the visceral and somatic defects can be obtained by opening the intersphincteric plane and mobilizing the rectum forward in the posterior quadrant. Defects can be repaired by direct suture of the external sphincter and puborectalis complex posteriorly and then by closure of the smooth muscle wall of the rectum anteriorly (Changyul, 1983). The mucosa is more conveniently sutured later by insertion of an intra-anal speculum to ensure complete inversion of the mucosal edges.

The disadvantage of this approach is that the three suture lines lie directly one upon the other and, should any sepsis occur in the intersphincteric plane, there is a substantial risk that the repair may break down (Ferguson and Houston, 1978). Parks and Stitz (1976) advised the use of wire for repair and reported two recurrences in 18 patients, but Lewis (1986) found equally good results using Vicryl. These fistulas are, of course, uncommon and surgical experience is limited, but the recurrence rate is gratifyingly low and defects in continence seem to be infrequent (see Table 16.14). Christiansen and Ronholt (1995) reported their results in 14 patients: there were two recurrences and three had minor defects in continence.

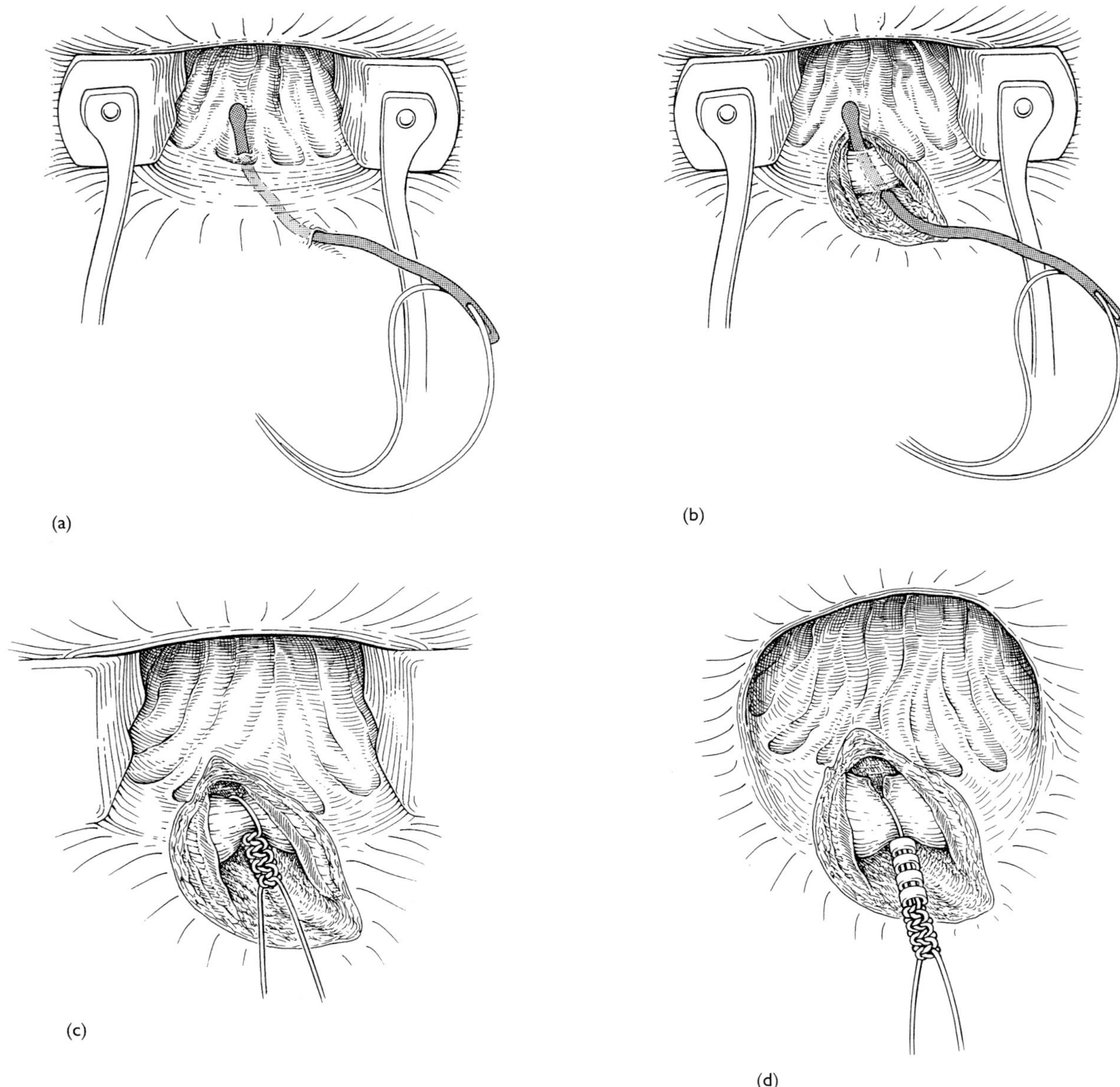

Figure 16.29a–d The cutting seton. (a) A soft malleable probe has been advanced gently through the fistula track. (b) All skin, fat, internal sphincter and anal mucosa between the internal and external components of the fistula overlying the probe are divided leaving only the external sphincter, and in some cases puborectalis, to be encircled by the seton. A soft rubber vascular 'sloop' is threaded through the eye of the malleable fistula probe which is then threaded through the remaining component of the fistula track. (c) The rubber seton is tied tightly using a series of knots and the ends of the rubber tubing are left long. (d) When the patient returns to the clinic about a week later, if the seton has not already cut through the sphincter, a series of rubber-bands is applied beyond the knots to tighten the seton around the muscle. This process may be repeated until the muscle is completely divided.

Kuflerberg et al (1984) successfully treated five patients by excision and direct suture of the defect, but they incorporated gentamicin polymethylmethacrylate copolymer beads into the wound to prevent sepsis, since the patients did not have a protecting stoma.

Some surgeons advised that a protective colostomy should be raised whenever fistula surgery involved repair of the anal sphincters. A stoma is often already present in patients who have developed traumatic or iatrogenic fistulas, since construction of a proximal defunctioning colostomy is the usual initial therapy. However, there is now a growing feeling among the more experienced authorities that surgical defunction is not always necessary, particularly if the bowel has been adequately prepared and the patient maintained on intravenous fluids for 7–10 days after operation (Goldberg et al, 1980). Proximal decompression is therefore usually reserved for patients with recurrent extrasphincteric fistula, preferably using an end colostomy as already described.

Anorectal advancement flap

Encouraged by the success of advancement flaps for the treatment of rectovaginal fistulas, Oh (1983), Aquilar et al (1985) and Hilsabeck (1989) reported the results of an identical procedure for extrasphincteric fistula-in-ano. Results were so spectacular and conventional therapy so disappointing for high trans-sphincteric fistulas that Aquilar and colleagues extended the use of this procedure to include all 'high' fistulas and reported a series of 189 patients. This approach is now considered the treatment of choice for extrasphincteric, suprasphincteric and some high trans-sphincteric fistulas (Jones et al, 1987; Wedell et al, 1987; Reznick and Bailey, 1988; Shemesh et al, 1988; Lewis and Bartolo, 1990; Athanasiadis et al, 1994; Lewis et al, 1995; Ozuner et al, 1996; Kreis et al, 1998; Miller and Finan, 1998).

The principle of the operation is to remove that portion of the fistula lying outside the sphincters and pelvic floor (Finan, 1996) (Figure 16.30a). An anorectal flap is then developed, with its base sited cranially (Figure 16.30b). The deeper aspect of the fistula track is excised (Figure 16.30c). The defect in the levator ani is closed in suprasphincteric or extrasphincteric fistula and the defect in the sphincter is closed in trans-sphincteric fistulas. The internal opening is then excised by resecting the lower portion of the flap (Figure 16.30d). To provide an oblique repair, the mucosa and internal sphincter are mobilized and sutured below the defect in the levator ani for high fistulas and below the defect in the sphincters for trans-sphincteric fistulas (Figure 16.30e). A covering colostomy is not usually constructed.

A standard bowel preparation is used on the day before operation and a stoma site is marked in case it is needed. A general anaesthetic is administered, the patient is catheterized and a single dose of antibiotic is given intravenously. If the fistula has an anterior internal opening, the prone jack-knife position is used to provide adequate access to the internal opening. Conversely, we prefer the lithotomy position for the more usual posterior internal opening. The course of the track must be carefully identified by dissection, with probes or with a seton. The extrasphincteric portion of the track is dissected out, particular attention being paid to identify any potential side tracks entering the lower anal canal at the dentate line through the external sphincter. The external track should be excised as a cone-shaped defect with its base on the perineum, tapering to a point as the track passes through the levator ani into the rectum.

A bivalved anal retractor provides access to the internal opening, but if the fistula opens posteriorly visualization may be quite difficult, particularly if it is just above the shelf created by the puborectalis sling. A small elliptical incision is made transversely above and below the internal opening through the entire thickness of the anorectal wall. Traction is applied to the external portion of the fistula track and the intermuscular portion of the fistula is excised in continuity.

The perineal wound is packed and the defect in the levator ani (for suprasphincteric or extrasphincteric fistulas) and rectal muscle (for extrasphincteric fistulas) are identified with stay sutures. Likewise the defect in the external sphincter is identified (for trans-sphincteric fistulas). A flap of anorectal wall (mucosa and internal sphincter) is then raised by enlarging the transverse mucosal defect slightly and cutting two diverging longitudinal flaps, approximately 4 cm long, at the ends of the transverse incision, the base being uppermost (Figure 16.30b). The deep aspect of the fistula is excised (Figure 16.30c).

The defects in the levator ani, wall of the rectum and anal sphincter (depending on the type of fistula) are then closed with interrupted absorbable sutures (Figure 16.30d). The internal opening is excised by removing the lower margin of the flap. The remaining flap is then advanced distally and approximated to the lower cut edge with absorbable sutures (Figure 16.30e). Further illustrations of the technique are provided in Figure 16.31.

Aquilar et al (1985) and more recently Del Pino et al (1996) and Robertson and Mangione (1998) used a similar technique but advanced a perianal flap into the anal canal. Aquilar and colleagues reported an 8% incidence of soiling and stenosis and minor incontinence of flatus in 7% (see Table 16.14). Their results are exceptional, with only 3 of 189 patients (2%) developing a recurrence. In contrast, Del Pino and colleagues reported one recurrence in eight patients with non-Crohn's fistulas.

We prefer to avoid extending the perineal inci-

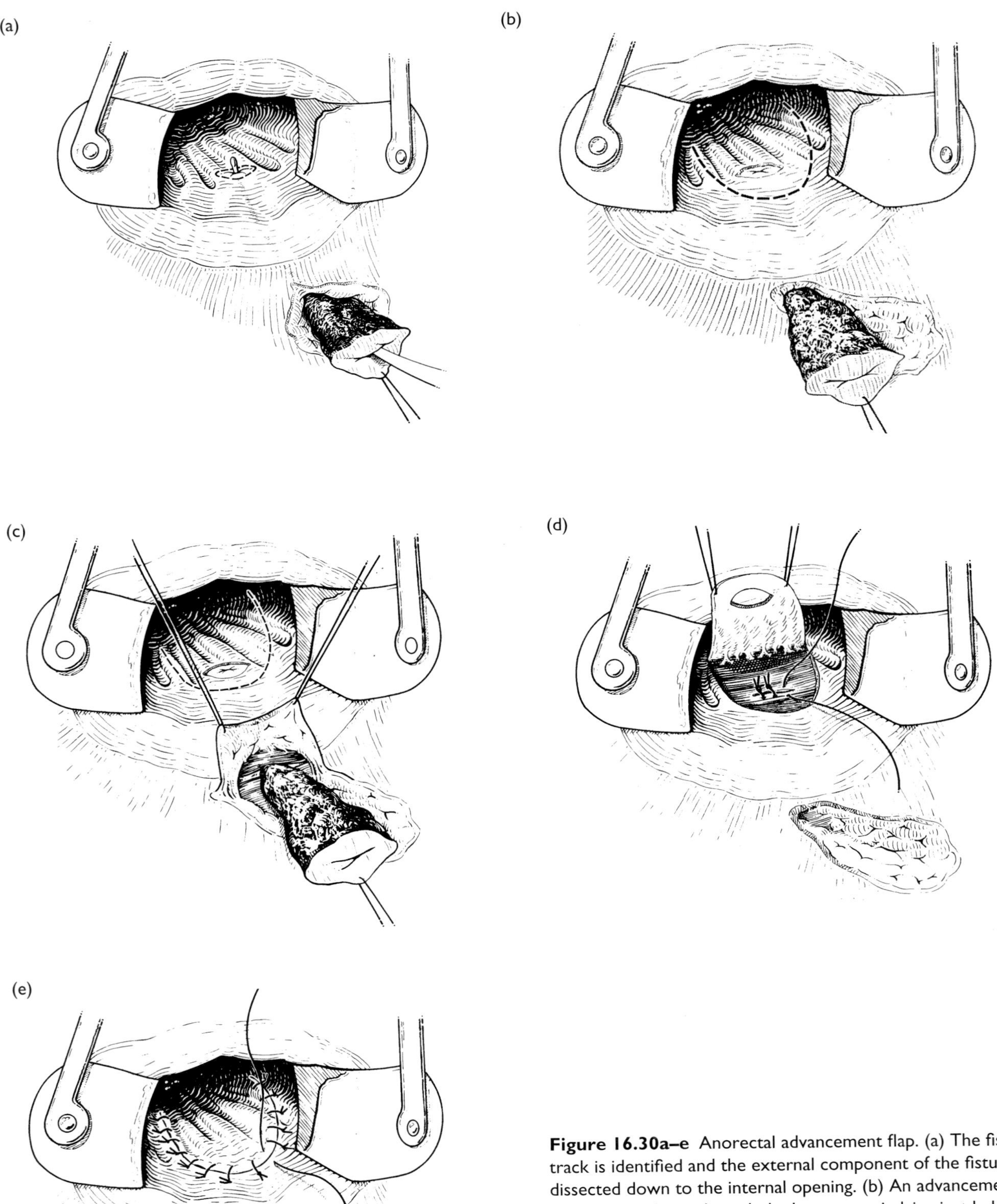

Figure 16.30a–e Anorectal advancement flap. (a) The fistula track is identified and the external component of the fistula is dissected down to the internal opening. (b) An advancement flap is cut in the anal canal, the lower margin lying just below the internal opening, with both lateral extensions diverging from one another across the anal columns. (c) The fistula is excised. (d) The defect in the internal anal sphincter is closed. The internal opening in the flap is excised and the rectal advancement flap is mobilized. (e) The rectal advancement flap is then sutured to the anal mucosa.

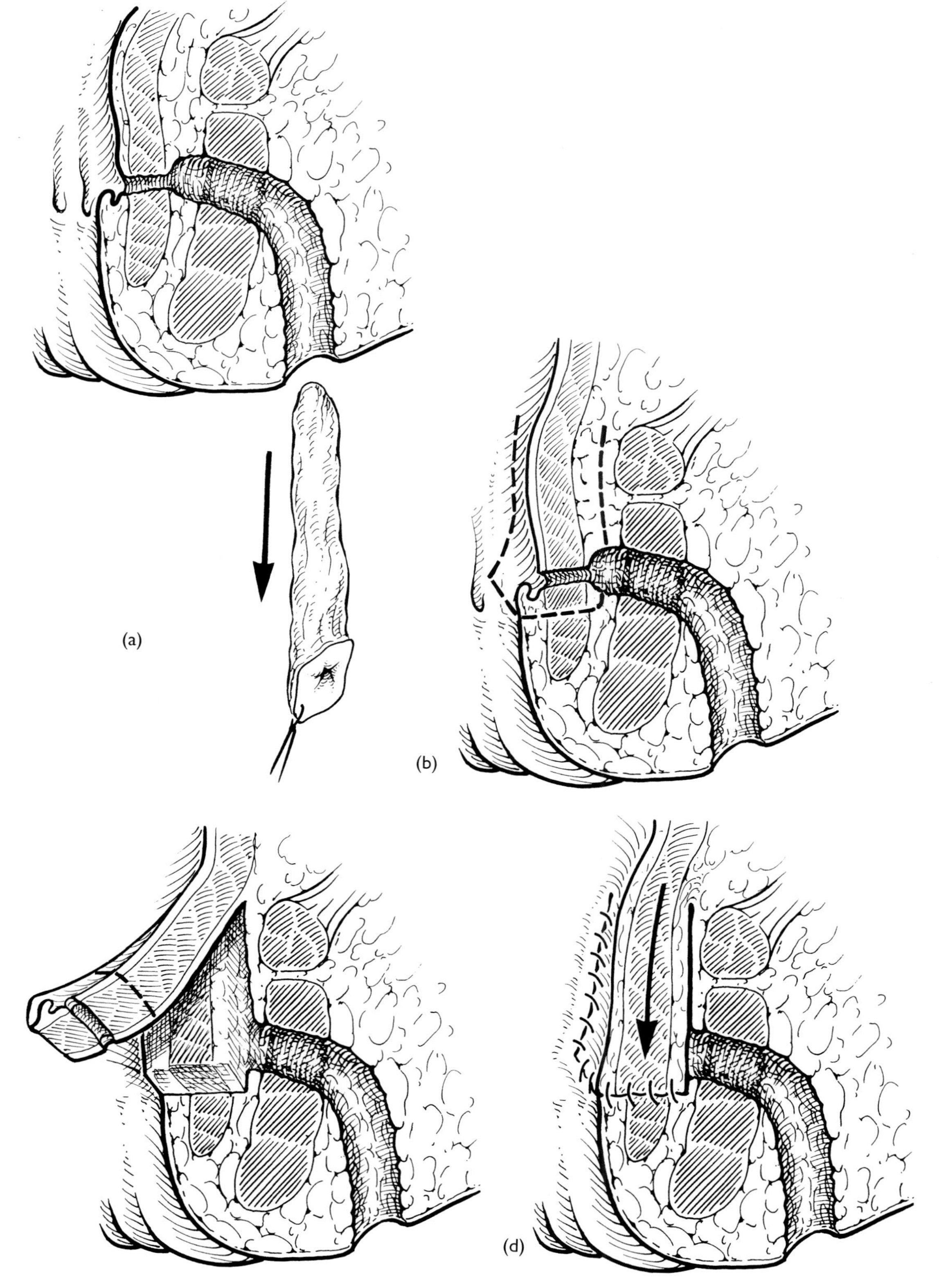

Figure 16.31a–d Further details of the advancement flap technique. (a) The fistula track is excised from the external opening to the intersphincteric plane. (b) The flap, incorporating the internal opening, is raised along with full-thickness internal sphincter. (c) The raised flap, with line marking the level of division to excise the internal opening. (d) The advancement flap is sutured to a site distal to the excised internal opening (Nicholls, 1996).

sion into the anal canal because we believe it may be responsible for an area of fibrosis, resulting in an anal deformity which may be associated with soiling.

Wedell et al (1987) reported satisfactory results in 29 of 30 patients treated by advancement flap. However, Jones et al (1987) reported a success rate of only 57% when this technique was used in anal fistula complicating Crohn's disease. Similarly Ozuner et al (1996) found a recurrence rate of 32% when this technique was used in Crohn's disease.

Recent experience with non-Crohn's fistulas treated by anorectal advancement is very variable. Ozuner et al (1996) from the Cleveland Clinic reported a recurrence rate of 31% when advancement flaps were used in 19 patients with cryptoglandular infections. Athanasiadis et al (1994), in a series of 224 patients, reported an 11% recurrence rate for trans-sphincteric fistulas and 20% for suprasphincteric fistulas managed in this way, with impaired continence in 21% with a trans-sphincteric and 43% with a suprasphincteric fistula. In contrast, Lewis et al (1995) reported no recurrences and no patients with incontinence after advancement flap with very little change in resting or squeeze pressure after therapy. The overall outcome of advancement flaps is summarized in Table 16.21.

Table 16.21 Results of anorectal advancement flaps (non-Crohn's).

Author	*n*	*Recurrence*	*Flatus incontinence*	*Faecal incontinence*	*Soiling*
Aquilar et al (1985)	189	3	13	0	NS
Wedell et al (1987)	27	0	3	0	NS
Shemesh et al (1988)	8	1	0	0	0
Lewis et al (1995)	11	1	0	0	NS
Ozuner et al (1996)	19	6	NS	NS	NS

NS, not stated.

RECOMMENDATIONS OF THE AUTHORS

We recommend a very thorough assessment of all anorectal fistulas and excision of almost all fistula tracks so that lateral extensions and high tracks can be identified accurately. We then remove the extrasphincteric component of the fistula and define the site at which the track traverses or bypasses the sphincters. Intersphincteric fistulas are excised and the tracks laid open. In contrast, most trans-sphincteric fistulas are managed using a cutting Silastic seton which is tightened in the outpatient clinic by application of rubber-bands or replacement of a new seton in theatre (see Figure 16.29a–d). Increasingly we use the advancement flap for anterior fistulas in postpartum patients and for suprasphincteric and extrasphincteric anorectal fistulas.

REFERENCES

Abcarian H, Dodi G, Girona J et al (1987) Symposium: Fistula-in-ano. *Int J Colorect Dis* **2**: 51–71.

Adams D & Kovalcik PJ (1981) Fistula-in-ano. *Surg Gynecol Obstet* **153**: 731–732.

Adams F (1846) Paulus Aeginetta: The Seven Books, Vol. 2, p. 399 (translation). London: Sydenham Society.

Adams F (1849) The Genuine Works of Hippocrates, Vol. II: On fistulae, pp 13–822. London: Sydenham Society.

Ajayi OO, Barigo OG & Nnamdi K (1974) Anal fistulas in a tropical population. *Dis Colon Rectum* **17**: 55–60.

Alexander-Williams J & Buchmann P (1980) Perianal Crohn's disease. *World J Surg* **4**: 203–208.

Allan A & Keighley MRB (1988) Management of perianal Crohn's disease. *World J Surg* **12**: 198–202.

Aluwihare APR (1983) Anterior horseshoe fistulas. *Ann R Coll Surg Engl* **65**: 121–122.

Aluwihare APR, Jayaratre SS & Panagamuwa B (1973) Perianal abscess. *Proc Ceylon Ass Adv Sci* **1**: 52.

Alvarado-Cerna R & Bracho-Riquelme R (1994) Perianal actinomycosis: a complication of a fistula-in-ano. *Dis Colon Rectum* **37**: 378–380.

Ambrose NS, Keighley MRB, Alexander-Williams J & Allan RN (1984) Clinical impact of colectomy and ileorectal anastomosis in the management of Crohn's disease. *Gut* **25**: 223–227.

Ani AN & Solanke TF (1976) Anal fistula: a review of 82 cases. *Dis Colon Rectum* **9**: 51–55.

Aquilar PS, Plasencia G, Hardy TG Jr, Hardman RF & Stewart WRC (1985) Mucosal advancement in the treatment of anal fistula. *Dis Colon Rectum* **28**: 496–498.

Athanasiadis S, Kohler A & Nafe M (1994) Treatment of high anal fistulae by primary occlusion of the internal istium, drainage of the intersphincteric space, and mucosa advancement flap. *Int J Colorect Dis* **9**: 153–157.

Baker WM & Milton-Thompson GJ (1974) Management of anal fistula in Crohn's disease. *Proc R Soc Med* **67**: 8–9.

Bayer I & Gordon PH (1994) Selected operative management of fistula-in-ano in Crohn's disease. *Dis Colon Rectum* **37**: 760–765.

Belliveau P, Thomson JPS & Parks AG (1983) Fistula-in-ano: a manometric study. *Dis Colon Rectum* **26**: 152–154.

Bennett RC (1962) A review of the results of orthodox treatment for anal fistulae. *Proc R Soc Med* **55**: 756–757.

Bennett RC & Duthie HL (1964) The functional importance of the internal anal sphincter. *Br J Surg* **51**: 355–357.

Bennett RC & Duthie HL (1965) Pressure and sensation in the anal canal after minor anorectal procedures. *Dis Colon Rectum* **8**: 131–136.

Bernard B, Morgan S & Tasse D (1986) Selective surgical management of Crohn's disease of the anus. *Can J Surg* **29**: 318–321.

Bohme H (1964) Die pyodermia fistulans significa. *Dtsch Med Wochenschr* **26**: 1265–1267.

Brem H, Guttman FM, Laberge JM & Doody D (1989) Congenital anal fistula with normal anus. *J Paediatr Surg* **24**: 183–185.

Bremer JL (1930) *Textbook of Histology*, 4th edn, pp 289–290. Philadelphia: Blackiston.

Bruhl S (1986) Perianal fistulae. Part A: Survey. *Coloproctology* **8**: 109–114.

Buchan R & Grace RH (1973) Anorectal suppuration: the results of treatment of the factors influencing the recurrence rate. *Br J Surg* **60**: 537–540.

Buchmann P, Keighley MRB, Alexander-Williams J, Allan RN & Thompson H (1980) The natural history of perianal Crohn's disease. *Am J Surg* **140**: 642–644.

Buda AM (1941) General considerations of fistula-in-ano: the role of foreign bodies as causative factors. *Am J Surg* **54**: 384–387.

Buie LA, Smith ND & Jackman RJ (1939) The role of tuberculosis in the anal fistula. *Surg Gynecol Obstet* **68**: 191–195.

Changyul O (1983) Management of high recurrent anal fistula. *Surgery* **93**: 330–332.

Chiari H (1878) Uber nalen divertikel der recthumschteimhant und ihre beziehung zu den anal fisteln. *Wien Med Press* **19**: 1482–1483.

Christensen A, Nilas L & Christiansen J (1986) Treatment of trans-sphincteric anal fistulas by the seton technique. *Dis Colon Rectum* **29**: 454–455.

Christiansen J & Ronholt C (1995) Treatment of recurrent high anal fistula by total excision and primary sphincter reconstruction. *Int J Colorect Dis* **10**: 207–209.

Cirocco WC & Reilly JC (1992) Challenging the predictive accuracy of Goodall's rule for anal fistulas. *Dis Colon Rectum* **35**: 537–542.

Cornes JS & Stecher M (1961) Primary Crohn's disease of the colon and rectum. *Gut* **2**: 189–201.

Cripps NPJ & Northover JMA (1998) Anovestibular fistula to Bartholin's gland. *Br J Surg* **85**: 659-661.

Crohn BB (1960) Rectal complications of inflammation of the small and large bowel. *Dis Colon Rectum* **3**: 99–102.

Culp CE (1984) Use of penrose drains to treat certain anal fistulas: a primary operation seton. *Mayo Clin Proc* **59**: 613–617.

Del Pino A, Nelson RL, Pearl RK & Abcarian H (1996) Island flap anoplasty for treatment of transsphincteric fistula-in-ano. *Dis Colon Rectum* **39**: 224–226.

Denecke H, Demmel N & Heberer G (1986) Operative procedure and results in anal fistulas. Presented at the World Congress of Gastroenterology, São Paolo.

Deshpande PJ & Sharma KR (1973) Treatment of fistula-in-ano by a new technique: review of follow-up of 200 cases. *Am J Proctol* **24**: 49–60.

Duhamel J (1975) Anal fistulae in childhood. *Am J Proctol* **26**: 40–43.

Dunphy JE & Pikula J (1955) Fact and fancy about fistula-in-ano. *Surg Clin North Am* **35**: 1469–1477.

Duthie HL & Watts JM (1965) Contribution of the external anal sphincter to the pressure zone in the anal canal. *Gut* **6**: 64–68.

Eisenhammer S (1951) The surgical correction of chronic internal anal (sphincteric) contraction. *S Afr Med J* **25**: 486–490.

Eisenhammer S (1953) The internal anal sphincter: its surgical importance. *S Afr Med J* **27**: 266–270.

Eisenhammer S (1956) The internal anal sphincter and the anorectal abscess. *Surg Gynecol Obstet* **103**: 501–506.

Eisenhammer S (1958) A new approach to the anorectal fistulous abscess based on the high intermuscular lesion. *Surg Gynecol Obstet* **106**: 595–599.

Eisenhammer S (1966) The anorectal fistulous abscess and fistula. *Dis Colon Rectum* **9**: 91–106.

Eisenhammer S (1978) The final evaluation and classification of the surgical treatment of the primary anorectal cryptoglandular intermuscular (intersphincteric) fistulous abscess and fistula. *Dis Colon Rectum* **21**: 237–254.

Elting AW (1912) The treatment of fistula-in-ano with special reference to the Whitehead operation. *Ann Surg* **56**: 744–752.

Faucheron J L, Saint-Marc O, Guibert L & Parc R (1996) Long-term seton drainage for high anal fistulas in Crohn's disease: a sphincter-saving operation? *Dis Colon Rectum* **39**: 208–211.

Ferguson EF & Houston CH (1978) Iatrogenic supralevator fistula. *S Afr Med J* **71**: 490–495.

Fillipini L (1969) Die Divertikulitis des Dickdarms. *Internist* **10**: 275.

Finan PJ (1996) Management by advancement flap technique. In Phillips RKS & Lunniss PJ (eds) *Anal Fistula*, pp 107–114. London: Chapman & Hall.

Fisher J, Martz F & Calkins WG (1976) Colonic perforation in Crohn's disease. *Gastroenterology* **71**: 835–838.

Fitzgerald RJ, Harding B & Ryan W (1985) Fistula-in-ano in childhood: a congenital aetiology. *J Ped Surg* **20**: 80–81.

Frenckner B & von Euler C (1975) Influence of pudendal block on the function of anal sphincter. *Gut* **16**: 482–489.

Fucini C (1991) One-stage treatment of anal abscesses and fistulas: a clinical appraisal on the basis of two different classifications. *Int J Colorect Dis* **6**: 12–16.

Furstenberg H (1965) Die Fistelkrankheit. *Praxis* **54**: 945–947.

Gabriel WB (1963) *The Principles and Practice of Rectal Surgery*, 5th edn, pp 739. Springfield, IL: CC Thomas.

Gallagher DM & Scarborough RA (1962) Repair of low rectovaginal fistula. *Dis Colon Rectum* **5**: 193–195.

García-Aguilar J, Belmonte C, Wong WD, Goldberg SM & Madoff RD (1996) Anal fistula surgery: factors associated with recurrence and incontinence. *Dis Colon Rectum* **39**: 723–729.

García-Aguilar, Belmonte C, Wong DW, Goldberg SM & Madoff RD (1998) Cutting seton *versus* two-stage seton fistulotomy in the surgical management of high anal fistula. *Br J Surg* **85**: 243–245.

Garrison FH (1921) *An Introduction to the History of Medicine*. Philadelphia: WB Saunders.

Germer WD (1970) Infektiose und invasive Erkrankungen. In Gross R, Jahn D & Scholmerich P (eds) *Lehrbuch der Inneren Medizine*, 2nd edn, p. 54, Stuttgart: Schattauer.

Gingold BS (1983) Reducing the recurrence risk of fistula-in-ano. *Surg Gynecol Obstet* **156**: 661–662.

Goldberg SM & García-Aguilar J (1996) The cutting seton. In Phillips RKS & Lunniss PJ (eds) *Anal Fistula*. London: Chapman & Hall.

Goldberg SM, Gordon PH & Nivatvongs S (1980) *Essentials of Anorectal Surgery*, p. 106. Philadelphia: Lippincott.

Goligher JC (1975) *Surgery of the Anus, Rectum and Colon*, 3rd edn, pp 210. London: Baillière Tindall.

Goodsall DH (1900) In Goodsall DH & Miles WE (eds) *Diseases of the Anus and Rectum, Pt I*. London: Longman.

Gordon PH (1976) The chemically defined diet and anorectal procedures. *Can J Surg* **19**: 511–513.

Gordon PH (1981) The operative treatment of fistula-in-ano. *Coloproctology* **3**: 195–199.

Gordon PH (1984) Complicated fistulae. *Coloproctology* **6**: 334–337.

Gordon PH (1985) Management of fistula-in-ano. *Ann R Coll Surg Engl* **58** (Suppl): 10–14.

Gordon-Watson C (1934) Progress in rectal surgery. *St Barts Hosp J* **41**: 104.

Grace RH, Harper IA & Thompson RG (1982) Anorectal sepsis: microbiology in relation to fistula-in-ano. *Br J Surg* **69**: 401–403.

Hämäläinen K-PJ, Sainio AP (1997) Cutting seton for anal fistulas: high risk of minor control defects. *Dis Colon Rectum* **40**: 1443–1447.

Hamilton H (1975) Symposium: The deep postanal space. *Dis Colon Rectum* **18**: 642–645.

Hanley PH (1978) Rubber band seton in the management of abscess–anal fistula. *Ann Surg* **187**: 435–437.

Hanley PH (1979) Anorectal supralevator abscess–fistula-in-ano. *Surg Gynecol Obstet* **148**: 899–904.

Hardcastle JD (1985) The classification of fistula-in-ano. *Ann R Coll Surg Engl* **58** (Suppl): 6–9.

Hawley PR (1975) Anorectal fistula. *Clin Gastroenterol* **4**: 635–649.

Heidenreich A, Collarini HA & Paladino AM (1986) Cancer in anal fistulas. *Dis Colon Rectum* **29**: 371–376.

Held D, Khubchandani J, Sheets J et al (1986) Management of anorectal horseshoe abscess and fistula. *Dis Colon Rectum* **29**: 793–797.

Henrichsen S & Christiansen J (1986) Incidence of fistula-in-ano complicating anorectal sepsis: a prospective study. *Br J Surg* **73**: 371–372.

Herrmann G & Desfosses L (1980) Sur la muquese de la région cloacale du rectum. *Compes Rend Acad Sci* (III) **90**: 1301–1302.

Hertel E (1954) Zur schrittweisen spaltung der anal fisteln mittels einer schraubenshlinge. *Chirurg* **25**: 16–18.

Hess H & Daum R (1959) Die Behandlung der anal Fisteln mit dem Drahtzugverfahren. *Chirurg* **30**: 355–358.

Higgins CS & Allan RN (1980) Crohn's disease of the distal ileum. *Gut* **21**: 933–940.

Hill JR (1967) Fistulas and fistulous abscesses in the anorectal region: personal experience in management. *Dis Colon Rectum* **10**: 421–434.

Hill MR, Shryock EH & Rebell FG (1943) Role of the anal glands in the pathogenesis of anorectal disease. *JAMA* **121**: 742–746.

Hill MR, Small CS, Hunt GM & Richards LJ (1949) Development of anal ducts and glands with reference to the pathogenesis of anorectal disease. *Arch Pathol* **47**: 350–360.

Hilsabeck JR (1989) Transanal advancement of the anterior rectal wall for vaginal fistulas involving the lower rectum. *Dis Colon Rectum* **13**: 236–241.

Ho YH, Tan M, Leong AFPK & Seow-Choen F (1998) Marsupialization of fistulotomy wounds improves healing: a randomized controlled trial. *Br J Surg* **85**: 105–107.

Hobbis JH & Schofield PF (1982) Management of perianal Crohn's disease. *J R Soc Med* **75**: 414–417.

Isbister WH (1995) Fistula-in-ano: a surgical audit. *Int J Colorect Dis* **10**: 94–96.

Jackman RJ & Buie LA (1946) Tuberculosis and anal fistula. *JAMA* **130**: 630–632.

Jensen SL (1987) Maintenance therapy with unprocessed bran in the prevention of acute anal fissure recurrence. *J R Soc Med* **80**: 296–298.

Jensen SL (1988) Diet and other risk factors in fissure-in-ano: prospective case control study. *Dis Colon Rectum* **31**: 770–773.

Jensen SL, Shokough-Amiri MH, Hagen K et al (1988) Adenocarcinoma of the anal ducts: a series of 21 cases. *Dis Colon Rectum* **31**: 267–272.

Jones IT, Fazio VW & Jagelman DG (1987) The use of transanal rectal advancement flaps in the management of fistulas involving the anorectum. *Dis Colon Rectum* **30**: 919–929.

Keighley MRB & Allan RN (1986) Dangers of surgical treatment for perianal Crohn's disease. *Dig Dis Sci* **31**: 531S.

Kennedy HL & Zegerra JP (1990) Fistulotomy without external sphincter division for high anal fistulae. *Br J Surg* **77**: 898–901.

Khubchandani M (1984) Comparison of results of treatment of fistula-in-ano. *J R Soc Med* **77**: 369–371.

Kirkup J (1985) The history and evolution of surgical instruments. IV: Probes and their allies. *Ann R Coll Surg Engl* **67**: 56–60.

Kline RJ, Spencer RJ & Harrison EG Jr (1964) Carcinoma associated with fistula-in-ano. *Arch Surg* **89**: 989–994.

Krauspe C & Stelzner F (1962) Pyodermia fistulans sinifica. *Chirurg* **33**: 534–538.

Kreis ME, Jehle EC, Ohlemann M, Becker HD & Starlinger MJ (1998) Functional results after transanal rectal advancement flap repair of trans-sphincteric fistula. *Br J Surg* **85**: 240–242.

Kronborg O (1985) To lay open or excise a fistula-in-ano: a randomized trial. *Br J Surg* **72**: 970.

Kuflerberg A, Zer M & Robinson S (1984) The use of PMMA beads in recurrent high anal fistula: a preliminary report. *World J Surg* **8**: 970–974.

Kuijpers HC & van Tets WF (1996) Fistolography. In Phillips RKS & Lunniss PJ (eds) *Anal Fistula*, pp 53–58. London: Chapman & Hall.

Kuijpers JH (1982) Diagnosis and treatment of fistula-in-ano. *Neth J Surg* **34**: 147–152.

Kuijpers JHC (1984) Use of the seton in the treatment of extrasphincteric anal fistula. *Dis Colon Rectum* **27**: 109–110.

Kuijpers JHC & Schulpen T (1985) Fistulography for fistula-in-ano. Is it useful? *Dis Colon Rectum* **28**: 103–104.

Law PJ, Talbot RW, Bartram CI & Northover JMA (1989) Anal endosonography in the evaluation of perianal sepsis and fistula-in-ano. *Br J Surg* **76**: 752–755.

Lawson TC (1970) Current concepts of surgical treatment of anorectal fistula. *S Afr Med J* **63**: 708–710.

La Quaglia MP, Feins N, Erakus A & Hendren A (1990) Rectal duplications. *J Paediatr Surg* **25**: 980–984.

Lentner A & Wienert V (1996) Long-term indwelling setons for low trans-sphincteric and intersphincteric anal fistulas: experience with 108 cases. *Dis Colon Rectum* **39**: 1097–1101.

Lewis A (1986) Excision of fistula-in-ano. *Int J Colorectal Dis* **1**: 265–267.

Lewis P & Bartolo DCC (1990) Treatment of trans-sphincteric fistulae by full thickness anorectal advancement flaps. *Br J Surg* **77**: 1187–1189.

Lewis WG, Finan PJ, Holdsworth PJ, Sagar PM & Stephenson BM (1995) Clinical results and manometric studies after rectal flap advancement for intralevator trans-sphincteric fistula-in-ano. *Int J Colorect Dis* **10**: 189–192.

Lilius HG (1986) Investigation of human foetal anal ducts and intramuscular glands and a clinical study of 150 patients. *Acta Chir Scand* **383** (Suppl): 1–88.

Lockhart-Mummery HE (1972) Crohn's disease of the large bowel. *Br J Surg* **59**: 823–826.

Logan VSCD (1969) Anorectal tuberculosis. *Proc R Soc Med* **62**: 1227–1230.

Lunniss PJ & Phillips RKS (1996) The intersphincteric approach. In Phillips RKS & Lunniss PJ (eds) *Anal Fistula*, p 115–122. London: Chapman & Hall.

Lunniss PJ & Sultan AH (1996) Magnetic resonance imaging (MRI) and endosonography (AES). In Phillips RKS & Lunniss PJ (eds) *Anal Fistula*, pp 59–68. London: Chapman & Hall.

Lunniss PJ & Thomson JPS (1996) The loose seton. In Phillips RKS & Lunniss PJ (eds) *Anal Fistula*, pp 87–94. London: Chapman & Hall.

Lunniss PJ, Armstrong P, Barker PG et al (1992) Magnetic resonance imaging (MRI) of anal fistulae. *Lancet* **340**: 394–396.

Lunniss PJ, Barker PG, Sultan AH et al (1994a) Magnetic resonance imaging of fistula-in-ano. *Dis Colon Rectum* **37**: 708–718.

Lunniss PJ, Kamm MA & Phillips RKS (1994b) Factors affecting continence after surgery for anal fistula. *Br J Surg* **81**: 1382–1385.

Lunniss PJ, Jenkins PJ, Besser GM, Perry LA & Phillips RKS (1995a) Gender differences in incidence of idiopathic fistula-in-ano are not explained by circulating sex hormones. *Int J Colorectal Dis* **10**: 25–28.

Lunniss PJ, Sheffield JP, Talbot IC, Thomson JPS & Phillips RKS (1995b) Persistence of idiopathic anal fistula may be related to epithelialization. *Br J Surg* **82**: 32–33.

McCourtney JS & Finlay IG (1995) Setons in the surgical management of fistula-in-ano. *Br J Surg* **82**: 448–452.

McCourtney JS & Finlay IG (1996) Cutting seton without preliminary internal sphincterotomy in management of complex high fistula-in-ano. *Dis Colon Rectum* **39**: 55–58.

McElwain JW, MacLean MD, Alexander-Williams RM, Hoexter B & Guthrie JF (1975) Anorectal problems: experience with primary fistulectomy for anorectal abscess, a report of 1000 cases. *Dis Colon Rectum* **18**: 646–649.

Mann CV & Clifton MA (1985) Rerouting of the track for the treatment of high anal and anorectal fistula. *Br J Surg* **72**: 134–137.

Marby M, Alexander-Williams J & Buchmann P et al (1979) A randomized controlled trial to compare anal dilatation with lateral subcutaneous sphincterotomy for anal fissure. *Dis Colon Rectum* **22**: 308–311.

Marks CG (1996) Classification. In Phillips RKS & Lunniss PJ (eds) *Anal Fistula*, pp 23–46. London: Chapman & Hall.

Marks CG & Ritchie JK (1977) Anal fistulas at St Mark's Hospital. *Br J Surg* **64**: 84–91.

Marks CG, Ritchie JK & Lockhart-Mummery HE (1981) Anal fistulas in Crohn's disease. *Br J Surg* **68**: 525–527.

Martini GA (1970) Erkrankungen des Dun- und Dickdarmes. In: Gross R, Jahn D & Scholmerich P (eds) *Lehrbuch der Inneren Medizin*, 2nd edn, p. 495. Stuttgart: Schattauer.

Matos D, Lunniss PJ & Phillips RKS (1993) Total sphincter conversation in high fistula-in-ano: results of a new approach. *Br J Surg* **80**: 802–804.

Mazier WP (1971) The treatment and care of anal fistulas: a study of 1000 patients. *Dis Colon Rectum* **14**: 134–144.

Melchior E (1910) Beitrage zur Pathologie und Therapie der Fistula ani. *Bruns Beitr Klin Chir* **70**: 745.

Miller GV & Finan PJ (1998) Flap advancement and core fistulectomy for complex rectal fistula. *Br J Surg* **85**: 108–110.

Milligan ETC & Morgan CN (1934) Surgical anatomy of the anal canal with special reference to anorectal fistulae. *Lancet* **ii**: 1150–1156, 1213–1217.

Milne JS (1907) *Surgical Instruments in Greek and Roman Times*, pp 16. Oxford: Clarendon Press.

Morrison JG, Gathright JB, Ray JE et al (1989) Surgical management of anorectal fistulas in Crohn's disease. *Dis Colon Rectum* **32**: 492–496.

Mortensen N (1996) Other conditions. In Phillips RKS & Lunniss PJ (eds) *Anal Fistula*, p 169. London: Chapman & Hall.

Nicholls G, Heaton ND & Lewis AM (1990) Use of bacteriology in anorectal sepsis as an indicator of anal fistula: experience in a district general hospital. *J R Soc Med* **83**: 625–626.

Nicholls RJ (1996) Clinical assessment. In Phillips RKS & Lunniss PJ (eds) *Anal Fistula*, pp 47–52. London: Chapman & Hall.

Oh C (1983) Management of high recurrent anal fistula. *Surgery* **93**: 330–332.

Onerheim RM (1988) A case of perianal mucinous adenocarcinoma arising in a fistula-in-ano: a clue to the early pathologic diagnosis. *Am J Clin Pathol* **89**: 809–812.

Ozuner G, Hull TL, Cartmill J & Fazio VW (1996) Long-term analysis of the use of transanal rectal advancement flaps for complicated anorectal/vaginal fistulas. *Dis Colon Rectum* **39**: 10–14.

Parks AG (1961) The pathogenesis and treatment of fistula-in-ano. *BMJ* **1**: 463–469.

Parks AG (1963) Aetiology and surgical treatment of fistula-in-ano. *Dis Colon Rectum* **6**: 17–22.

Parks AG & Gordon PH (1976) Perineal fistula of intra-abdominal or intrapelvic origin simulating fistula-in-ano: report of seven cases. *Dis Colon Rectum* **19**: 500–506.

Parks AG & Morson BC (1962) The pathogenesis of fistula-in-ano. *Proc R Soc Med* **55**: 751–754.

Parks AG & Stitz RW (1976) The treatment of high fistula-in-ano. *Dis Colon Rectum* **19**: 487–499.

Parks AG, Gordon PH & Hardcastle JC (1976) A classification of fistula-in-ano. *Br J Surg* **63**: 1–12.

Pearl RK, Andrews JR, Orsay CP et al (1993) Role of the seton in the management of anorectal fistulas. *Dis Colon Rectum* **36**: 573–579.

Phillips RKS and Lunniss PJ (1996a) Surgical evaluation and management. In Phillips RKS & Lunniss PJ (eds) *Anal Fistula*. London: Chapman & Hall.

Phillips RKS & Lunniss PJ (1996b) Approach to the difficult fistula. In Phillips RKS & Lunniss PJ (eds) *Anal Fistula*. London: Chapman & Hall.

Piazza DJ & Radhakrishnan J (1990) Perianal abscess and fistula-in-ano in children. *Dis Colon Rectum* **33**: 1014–1016.

Pople IK & Ralphs DNL (1988) An aetiology for fistula-in-ano. *Br J Surg* **75**: 904.

Pott P (1765) *Remarks on the Disease, Commonly Called a Fistula-in-Ano*, pp 115. London: Hawes, Clarke & Collins.

Pye G & Bundell JW (1987) Sacrococcygeal teratoma masquerading as fistula-in-ano. *J R Soc Med* **80**: 251–252.

Raghavaiah NV (1976) Anal fistula in India. *Int Surg* **61**: 243–245.

Ramanujam PS, Prasad L & Abcarian H (1983) The role of seton in fistulotomy of the anus. *Surg Gynecol Obstet* **157**: 419–422.

Rangabashyam N (1996) Management by chemical seton. In Phillips RKS and Lunniss PJ (eds) *Anal Fistula*, pp 103–106. London: Chapman & Hall.

Reznick RK & Bailey HB (1988) Closure of the internal opening for treatment of complex fistula-in-ano. *Dis Colon Rectum* **31**: 116–118.

Robertson WG & Mangione JS (1998) Cutaneous advancement flap closure: alternative method for treatment of complicated anal fistulas. *Dis Colon Rectum* **41**: 884–887.

Roschke W (1964) Das perianale Hamaton und die perianale Spontanthrombose. *Chirurg* **35**: 467–470.

Roschke W & Krause H (1983) *Die proktologische Sprechstunde*, 5th edn, pp 176–184. Munich: Urban & Schwarzenberg.

Sainio P (1996) Epidemiology. In Phillips RKS & Lunniss PJ (eds) *Anal Fistula*, pp 1–12. London: Chapman & Hall.

Sainio P & Husa A (1995) Fistula-in-ano: clinical features and long-term results of surgery in 199 adults. *Acta Chir Scand* **151**: 169–176.

Sangwan, YP, Rosen L, Riether RD et al (1994) Is simple fistula-in-ano simple? *Dis Colon Rectum* **37**: 885–889.

Scammell BE, Andrews H, Allan RN, Alexander-Williams J & Keighley MRB (1987) Results of proctocolectomy for Crohn's disease. *Br J Surg* **74**: 671–674.

Scholefield JH, Borg DP, Armitage NCM & Wastie ML (1997) Magnetic resonance imaging in the management of fistula in ano. *Int J Colorect Dis* **12**: 276–279.

Schouten WR & van Vroonhoven TJMV (1991) Treatment of an anorectal abscess with or without primary fistulectomy: results of a prospective randomized trial. *Dis Colon Rectum* **34**: 60–63.

Schratter-Sehn AU, Lochs H, Vogelsang H et al (1992) Comparison of transrectal ultrasonography and computed tomography in the diagnosis of periano-rectal fistulas in patients with Crohn's disease. *Gastroenterology* **102**: A691.

Seow-Choen F (1996) Relation of abscess to fistula. In Phillips RKS & Lunniss PJ (eds) *Anal Fistula*, pp 13–24. London: Chapman & Hall.

Seow-Choen F & Nicholls RJ (1992) Anal fistula. *Br J Surg* **79**: 197–205.

Seow-Choen F & Phillips RKS (1991) Insights gained from the management of problematical anal fistulae at St Mark's Hospital, 1984–88. *Br J Surg* **78**: 539–541.

Seow-Choen F, Hay AJ, Heard S & Phillips RKS (1992) Bacteriology of anal fistulae. *Br J Surg* **79**: 27–28.

Shafer AD, McGlone TP & Flanagan RA (1987) Abnormal crypts of Morgagni: the cause of perianal abscess and fistula-in-ano. *J Paediatr Surg* **22**: 203–204.

Shafik A (1979) A new concept of the anatomy of the anal sphincter mechanism and the physiology of defecation. *Dis Colon Rectum* **22**: 408–414.

Shafik A, Wahab EA, Olfat ES & Khalil A (1994) Anorectal fistulae: results of treatment with cauterization. *Dig Surg* **11**: 16–19.

Shemesh EI, Kodner IJ, Fry RD & Neufeld DM (1988) Endorectal sliding flap repair of complicated anterior anoperineal fistulas. *Dis Colon Rectum* **31**: 22–24.

Shields RM (1937) Anorectal fistula. *Surg Clin N Am* **17**: 279–295.

Shouler PJ, Grimley RP, Keighley MRB & Alexander-Williams J (1986) Fistula-in-ano is usually simple to manage surgically. *Int J Colorect Dis* **1**: 113–115.

Shukla HS, Gupta SC, Singh G & Singh PA (1988) Tubercular fistula-in-ano. *Br J Surg* **75**: 38–39.

Sohn N, Korelitz BI & Weinstein MA (1980) Anorectal Crohn's disease: definitive surgery for fistulas and recurrent abscess. *Am J Surg* **139**: 394–397.

Steltzner F (1959) *Die anorectalen Fisteln*. Berlin: Springer.

Steltzner F (1981) *Die anorektalen Fisteln*, 3rd edn. Berlin: Springer.

Stirnemann H & Halter F (1970) *Erkrankungen von Rektum und Analkanal*, 3rd edn Bern: Huber.

Stockman JM & Young VT (1953) Carcinoma associated with anorectal fistula. *Am J Surg* **86**: 560–561.

Sumikoshi Y, Takano M, Okada M, Kiratuka J & Sato S (1974) New classification of fistulas and its application to the operations. *Am J Proctol* **25**: 72–78.

Taniguchi S, Yamanari H, Inada K et al (1996) Adenocarcinoma in the anal canal associated with a fistula: report of a case. *Surg Today, Jpn J Surg* **26**: 707–710.

Thompson HR (1962) The orthodox conception of fistula-in-ano and its treatment. *Proc R Soc Med* **55**: 754–756.

Thomson JPS & Parks AG (1979) Anal abscesses and fistulas. *Br J Hosp Med* **21**: 413–425.

Thomson JPS & Ross AHMcL (1989) Can the external anal sphincter be preserved in the treatment of trans-sphincteric fistula-in-ano? *Int J Colorect Dis* **4**: 247–250.

Tucker CC & Hellwig GG (1934) Histopathology of the anal crypts. *Surg Gynecol Obstet* **58**: 145–149.

Tudor RG (1986) The morbidity and mortality of complicated diverticular disease. MD thesis, University of Birmingham.

Tudor RG & Keighley MRB (1986) Impaired sphincter function after fistulotomy for low fistula-in-ano. *Br J Surg* **73**: 1042.

van Tets WF & Kuijpers JC (1994) Continence disorders after fistulotomy. *Dis Colon Rectum* **37**: 1194–1197.

Vasilevsky C-A & Gordon PH (1984) Results of treatment of fistula-in-ano. *Dis Colon Rectum* **28**: 225–231.

Walfisch S, Menachem Y & Koretz M (1997) Double seton: a new modified approach to high transsphincteric anal fistula. *Dis Colon Rectum* **40**: 731–732.

Wang F, Hsu H & Yang S (1980) Anal fistula and abscess: review of 518 cases. *Southeast Asian J Surg* **3**: 9–15.

Wedell J, Meier zu Eissen P, Banzhaf G & Kleine L (1987) Sliding flap advancement for the treatment of high level fistulae. *Br J Surg* **74**: 390–391.

Welch GH & Finlay IG (1987) Neoplastic transformation in longstanding fistula-in-ano. *Postgrad Med J* **63**: 503–504.

Williams JG, MacLeod CA, Rothenberger DA & Goldberg SM (1991a) Seton treatment of high anal fistulae. *Br J Surg* **78**: 1159–1161.

Williams JG, Rothenberger DA, Nemer FD & Goldberg SM (1991b) Fistula-in-ano in Crohn's disease: results of aggressive surgical treatment. *Dis Colon Rectum* **34**: 378–384.

Wolff BG, Culp CE, Beart RW, Ilstrup DM & Ready RL (1985) Anorectal Crohn's disease: a longterm perspective. *Dis Colon Rectum* **28**: 709–711.

Woodall J (1617) *The Surgeon's Mate*, p 12. London: Lisle.

17
PILONIDAL SINUS

Pilonidal sinus is a chronic inflammatory condition associated with hair. Most pilonidal sinuses occur in the postanal region but they may be found in the axilla, the groins, the interdigital web of the hands or feet and on the occiput. Pilonidal sinus is generally regarded as an acquired disorder, although the pits through which hairs enter the subcutaneous tissue may be congenital. The acquired aetiology of pilonidal sinus is supported by its occurrence in perineal wounds and amputation stumps.

Pilonidal sinus is rare before the age of 15 years and never occurs before puberty. It is more common in men than women, and is rarely active in persons over the age of 40. Indeed, pilonidal sinus is usually a self-limiting disorder. Complications include abscess, recurrent sepsis, time lost from work and chronic disability usually following failed surgical treatment.

Although there are many surgical procedures that can be used with success in the treatment of this condition, late recurrence even ten years after surgical treatment is now well recognized; in some instances, surgical treatment is associated with more morbidity than the disease itself. For these reasons emphasis is placed on conservative management with minimal surgical intervention.

PATHOLOGY

Pilonidal sinus is a chronic inflammatory disorder consisting of a midline pit sited behind the anal canal between the buttocks (Søndenaa and Pollard, 1992). It is often associated with lateral secondary tracks, which usually emerge cephalad and away from it (Figure 17.1). Occasionally, the secondary track may emerge caudal to the midline pit, or the track may be perianal, often with intersphincteric, trans-sphincteric or subcutaneous communications (Weston and Schlachter, 1963; Wilson et al, 1971; Walsh and Mann, 1983; Taylor and Hughes 1984; Ortiz et al, 1987).

The orifice of the primary track is lined with stratified squamous epithelium and extends cranially for 2–4 cm, to end in either a blind cavity or an orifice. Apart from the orifice, most of the track is lined with granulation tissue; and in the majority of cases loose hairs lie free within the sinus. Their roots lie cephalad and their ends usually emerge from the orifice. The midline pits consist of indentations of skin containing keratin plugs and debris. They may be isolated or connected to the primary pilonidal sinus.

Midline fibrous bands prevent penetration from the sinus to the sacrum, so septic complications track laterally to form secondary tracks which discharge to the skin surface. The orifice of secondary tracks is not lined with skin but with granulation tissue only. No hair follicles, sebaceous or sweat glands are found in the walls of secondary tracks which are lined by chronic inflammatory cells, often with a foreign-body giant cell reaction.

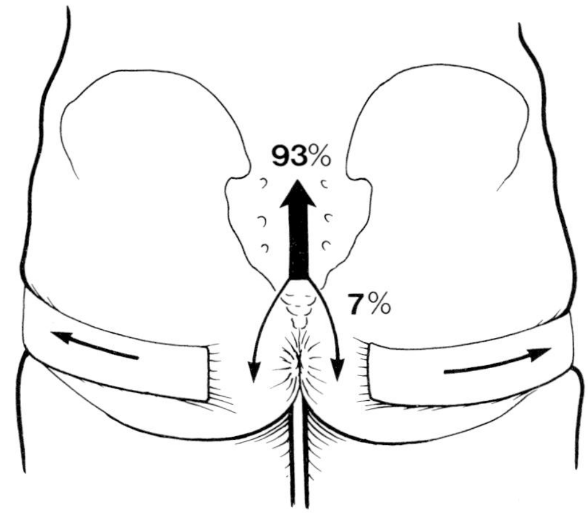

Figure 17.1 Direction of pilonidal sinuses. In 93% of cases the sinus runs cranially from the skin pit.

AETIOLOGY AND PATHOGENESIS

Congenital hypothesis

For many years the congenital hypothesis was accepted and numerous theories were proposed (Fox, 1935; Kooistra, 1942; Patey and Scarff, 1946; Ewing, 1947; Gabriel, 1963; Lord and Millar, 1965). These theories all suggested that there was a pre-existing epithelial lined track in the midline of the natal cleft formed by squamous epithelium. The origin of this track was thought to be a caudal remnant of the medullary canal, attraction dermoid or an inclusion dermoid.

Medullary canal theory

It was suggested that caudal remnants of the medullary canal persist in the sacrococcygeal region and that these form small cysts which later rupture, causing a blind-ended sinus in the midline. If this theory were correct, these cysts would be lined by cuboidal and not, as is the case, by squamous epithelium. The theory is therefore untenable and cannot explain pilonidal sinus in the axilla, in the interdigital clefts, within wounds and in the groins.

Traction dermoid theory

It has been suggested that skin might sometimes be invaginated in a cephalad direction into a subcutaneous position when the tail bud retracts during development. Epithelial lined sinuses with a fibrous band attached to the coccyx would remain asymptomatic unless loose hair was forced inwards and sepsis supervened. Against this theory is the fact that presacral dimpling is uncommon in children and that a pilonidal sinus is not lined by squamous epithelium throughout its extent. Haworth and Zachary (1955) examined 500 children and identified a presacral sinus or dimpling in only 14; these tracks appeared to be quite different histologically from the epithelial orifice of a pilonidal sinus. Furthermore, a pilonidal sinus is not connected to the coccyx by a fibrous band. It seems unlikely, therefore, that this is a tenable theory.

Inclusion dermoid theory

Sequestration of epithelial rests results in dermoid cysts, which may subsequently become cystic or infected. These lesions are almost always in the midline and may occur in the presacral region, intersphincteric plane or in the pelvis; they are lined by squamous epithelium and may contain subcutaneous material, hair and other vestigial structures, depending upon the degree of differentiation of the epithelial element. They are always present, although not necessarily clinically evident, at birth. This is not, however, an acceptable theory for the pathogenesis of pilonidal sinus, since a pilonidal sinus is never found at birth, cysts are rare, and the epithelial lining is found only at the orifice.

Acquired hypothesis

An acquired theory is now widely accepted as the principal cause for pilonidal sinus (Brearley, 1955; Weale, 1964; Notaras, 1970; Bascom, 1980; Golz et al, 1980). The strongest arguments in favour of an acquired hypothesis are the occupational incidence of pilonidal sinus in barbers and jeep drivers (Casberg, 1949; Currie et al, 1953; Oldfield, 1956; Karydakis, 1973; Clothier and Haywood, 1984) and their propensity to recur, especially after radical surgical ablation. Furthermore, these recurrences are superficial so it is unlikely that missed, deep extensions can be implicated as their cause (Healy and Hoffert, 1955; Hamilton et al, 1963; McCaughan, 1965; Thomas, 1968). Finally, there is evidence of pilonidal sinus formation in incisions remote from the perianal area, such as in amputation stumps, in the umbilicus and in perineal wounds (Smith, 1948; Shoesmith, 1953; Gillis, 1954; Clery and Clery, 1963; Thorlakson, 1966; Calapinto, 1977).

The mainstay of an acquired theory rests on the presence of shed hairs within the sinus (Søndenaa and Pollard, 1992). Hair is found in almost 90% of all patients having surgical treatment, although they are reported to occur less frequently by pathologists (Buie and Curtiss, 1952; Brearley, 1955; Lord and Millar, 1965; Golz et al, 1980). Although shed hairs are common (Bascom, 1983), hair follicles are virtually never found in the depths of a pilonidal sinus (Dwight and Maloy, 1953; Raffman, 1959). The hairs are detached, but the theory that the cut ends migrate towards the opening of a sinus and subsequently fracture is also disproved by the fact that the root of the hair is usually found in the depths of the sinus with the free edge protruding from the pit (Weale, 1964) (Figure 17.2). Examination of the hair usually indicates that they have scales on their surface which act as barbs, so if the roots are introduced into a small epithelial pit, movement of the buttocks will encourage migration away from the tip towards the root. In this way hair shed from the head or the perineum drills its way into the subcutaneous tissue (Williams, 1955). Frictional resistance against the scales on the hair and repeated local trauma, as occurs in jeep drivers, helps to encourage penetration and subsequent drilling by the roots (Brearley, 1955; Patey and Williams, 1956; Zimmerman, 1984).

The main stumbling block to the acquired theory centres around how the roots of hair are capable of penetrating normal skin. Admittedly, there are some patients, but not many, with a pre-existing history of perianal excoriation from self-induced trauma (Søndenaa et al, 1995a). This occurs particularly in males with excessive hyperhidrosis and poor anal hygiene who have a macerated skin. The theory of primary implantation is probably acceptable in barbers, since the interdigital web space becomes softened and traumatized owing to repeated immersion in water. Moreover, there are pits adjacent to the umbilicus or in a healing wound which allow implantation. However, an acquired theory as the sole cause of pilonidal sinus seems unlikely in the majority, since in a few patients hair follicles can be seen at the entrance to the pits (Bascom, 1983) and very long hairs may be present, which are presumably from the head, as they are much longer than either pubic or perianal hair.

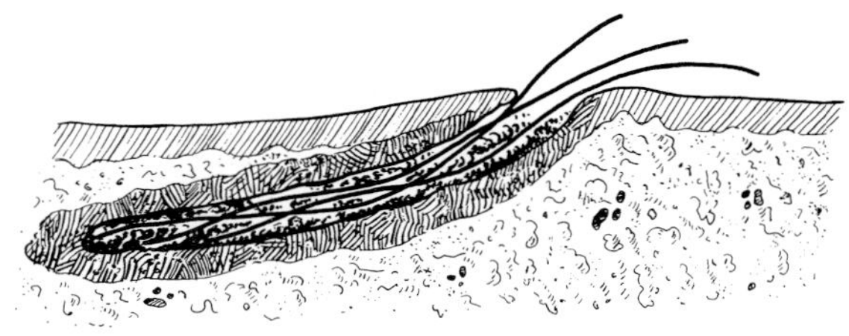

Figure 17.2 Pathology of pilonidal sinus. A cross-section through a pilonidal sinus; cranial is to the left, caudal is to the right. The sinus track is lined with chronic granulation tissue, epithelial debris and hair. The sinus track lies in the subcutaneous tissues.

Combined congenital and acquired hypothesis

We believe that it is unlikely that postanal pilonidal sinus is entirely an acquired condition. Asymptomatic and uncomplicated postanal pits are found in children and adults. These pits may be single or multiple, they are probably congenital traction pits (Lord, 1975), and are confined to the epithelium. Hair follicles may be found in these pits and the hair may subsequently become detached and drill into the subcutaneous plane (Jones, 1992). We believe that it is more likely that shed hairs from the head, back or perineum become implanted into the pits, where they subsequently drill cranially (Hueston, 1953). Once in the subcutaneous tissues, hair causes a foreign-body giant cell reaction, epithelial debris and sebaceous material collect and an abscess may develop which cannot point in the midline because of presacral fibrous septa. Lateral secondary tracts are thus formed. Changes in skin, sebaceous glands and gluteal muscle with puberty may predispose to the increased risk of further drilling and secondary sepsis after adolescence (Palmer, 1959; Patey, 1969).

INCIDENCE

The true incidence of pilonidal sinus is unknown, but Mansoory and Dickson (1982) state that over 70 000 patients with the disorder were admitted to non-government hospitals in the USA in 1973. In 1985, more than 7000 patients were admitted to hospital in England and Wales for treatment of pilonidal sinus. A Norwegian study calculated an incidence of 25 per 100 000 inhabitants, a family history was recorded in 38% of patients, 37% were overweight, and local trauma was reported in 34% (Søndenaa et al, 1995a).

Age

The average age of onset is 21 years (Kooistra, 1942), but the mean age of hospital admission is 25 years. In Søndenaa et al's study (1995a), the mean age was less for women (19 years) than for men (21 years). Few patients present for the first time under the age of 17 years, and it is exceedingly rare over the age of 45 years (Figure 17.3a). We and others believe that pilonidal sinus is a self-limiting disorder and that it burns itself out in middle age (Hopping, 1954; Bascom, 1987).

Sex

Pilonidal sinus is more common in men than in women (Figure 17.3b), the proportion of males varying from 63% to 79% (Eftaiha and Abcarian, 1977; Farringer and Pickens, 1978; Rainsbury and Southam, 1982; Guyuron et al, 1983).

Race

The condition is probably universal but may be less common in Afro-Caribbeans. Although fair-skinned races and individuals with soft, fair hair were thought to be exempt from developing pilonidal sinus, they are not. The disorder does, however, seem to be more common in individuals with dark, stiff hair or patients with auburn hair.

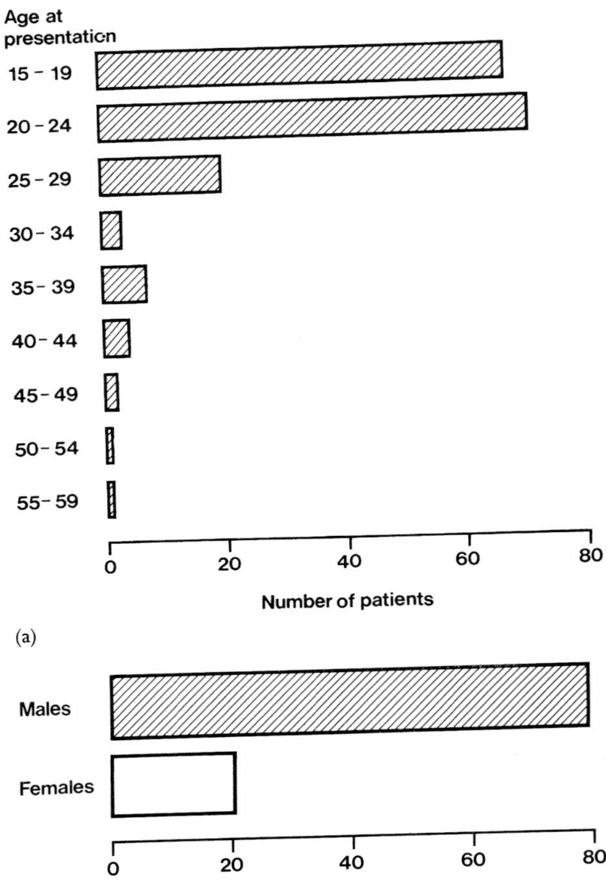

Figure 17.3a,b Age and sex of pilonidal sinus. (a) Age at presentation. The majority of pilonidal sinuses present before the age of 30 years (Eftaiha and Abcarian, 1977). (b) The majority of pilonidal sinuses are identified in men (80%) (Guyuron et al, 1983).

CLINICAL PRESENTATION

Pilonidal sinus may be an incidental finding, it may give rise to recurrent episodes of chronic sepsis and sometimes presents with an acute pilonidal abscess. Pilonidal sinus may also present as a recurrent sinus after surgical treatment, a condition Lord (1984) would prefer to term 'postoperative ulcer with hair'.

Asymptomatic

The typical appearance is of one or more minute midline pits in the presacral area, approximately 5 cm behind the anus. These pits may or may not contain hair, they are painless and may never give rise to symptoms. This is not an uncommon finding in older patients, some of whom may have had minor sepsis but have never sought medical advice, while others have experienced no symptoms at all. Eftaiha and Abcarian (1977) report that 11% of the cases seen at the Cook County Hospital in Chicago were quiescent or identified as an incidental finding.

Chronic sepsis

A high proportion of patients present with low-grade chronic symptoms consisting of discomfort on sitting or repeated discharge from the secondary tract. Occasionally they suffer repeated acute episodes of sepsis requiring drainage. Sometimes an abscess may burst spontaneously.

Examination identifies the tell-tale midline pit, often with secondary tracks which may lie close together or be widely separated by long indurated communications in the subcutaneous tissue. The orifices are lined by prominent granulation tissue and may discharge seropurulent material when pressure is applied over the tracks. Although 80% of these secondary tracks are cranial to the pit, some proceed towards the anus (Notaras, 1970). The primary pit has a characteristic smooth edge over its dorsal surface, and there may be a tuft of loose hair projecting from the orifice. Pus rarely discharges from the midline pit.

Acute abscess

A tender, red, indurated swelling, usually to one side of the midline but near the natal cleft overlying the sacrum, is typical of a pilonidal abscess. Midline pits with or without hair will be visible; they are often the only evidence that this is a pilonidal abscess.

Acute pilonidal abscess often discharges spontaneously, thereby forming a secondary track. Some patients require surgical drainage bcause of a painful abscess or discharge from an incompletely draining abscess. Acute abscess is a common presentation in urban and deprived communities (Eftaiha and Abcarian, 1977).

MICROBIOLOGY

Acute abscess

Staphylococcus aureus and *epidermidis* predominate in acute pilonidal abscess, but mixed anaerobes may be present which are likely to be resistant to cloxacillin (Søndenaa et al, 1995b).

Chronic pilonidal sinus

The contents of the sinus were sterile in 50% of patients requiring operation for pilonidal sinus in a Norwegian study (Søndenaa et al, 1995b). Rainsbury and Southam (1982) reported their

Table 17.1 Preoperative cultures in pilonidal sinus ($n = 98$).

Aerobes	
Staph. epidermidis	8
Staph. aureus	3
Streptococcus spp.	5
Enterococcus	1
Diphtheroids	2
E. coli	2
Proteus	2
Anaerobes	
Mixed flora	24
Peptostreptococcus	4
Micro-aerophilic streptococcus	1
Bacteroides fragilis	11
Others	3

From Søndenaa et al (1995b).

findings in quiescent disease and recovered anaerobes in most patients (usually in a mixed culture); staphylococci were uncommon and aerobic Gram-negatives included *E. coli*, *Proteus* spp., and *Pseudomonas* spp. Streptococci were present occasionally. The Norwegian group obtained preoperative cultures from 98 patients, and positive cultures, predominantly anaerobes and staphylococci, were recovered from 49 (Table 17.1). Preoperative bacterial isolates did not appear to correlate with postoperative sepsis, but the incidence of postoperative sepsis was very high (43%). Two antibiotic studies suggested that re-operation for wound complications was lower (6%) when cloxacillin had been used preoperatively, whereas cefoxitin use proved virtually no different from no antibiotic cover (16% and 15% respectively). Conversely, 13% developed recurrence when cloxacillin had been used whereas no recurrences were reported in those given cefoxitin or no antibiotic (Søndenaa et al, 1995b). These data imply that antibiotics may reduce the risk of wound infection if primary closure is used but they have no influence on recurrence rates.

DIFFERENTIAL DIAGNOSIS

Hidradenitis suppurativa

Hidradenitis suppurativa may be confused with an acutely inflamed pilonidal sinus, but there are many features which should make the distinction easy. Unlike pilonidal sinus, hidradenitis does not confine itself to the natal cleft, is more common in women than in men, and is rarely self-limiting. On physical examination, the midline of the natal cleft is never involved, the sinuses do not contain hair, the tracks are more superficial, and multiple sinuses are found throughout the perineum. The presence of sepsis in the axilla or groins may support the diagnosis of hidradenitis in a doubtful case. However, hidradenitis and pilonidal sinus may coexist (Anderson and Dockerty, 1958).

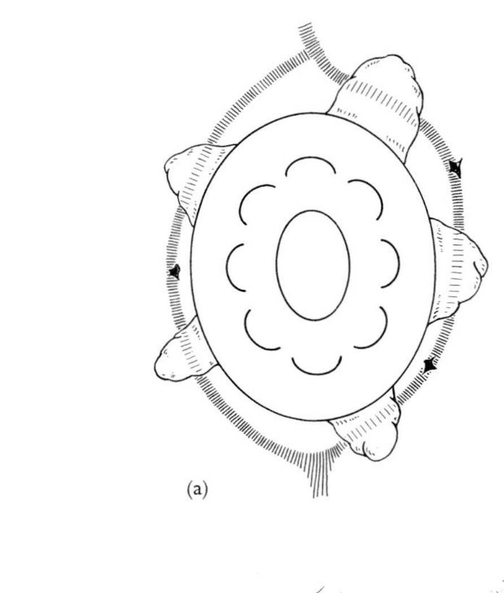

Fistula-in-ano

In a few patients it may be exceedingly difficult to distinguish fistula-in-ano from pilonidal sinus, particularly if the secondary tracks emerge caudal to a minute midline pit. Vallance (1982) reported four cases of pilonidal sinus which presented as perianal abscess or an apparent fistula. Lord (1984) also described cases of pilonidal sinus tracking around the perianal region (Figure 17.4). Walsh and Mann (1983) found hair-containing perianal sinuses and hair in extrasphincteric or trans-sphincteric fistulas with an intersphincteric component (Figure 17.5). However, these patients had all had previous perianal surgery and they might have acquired secondary inclusion sinuses from previous operations. Indeed, true endoanal pilonidal sinus seems to be exceedingly rare (Weston and Schlachter, 1963; Wilson et al, 1971; Ortiz et al, 1987).

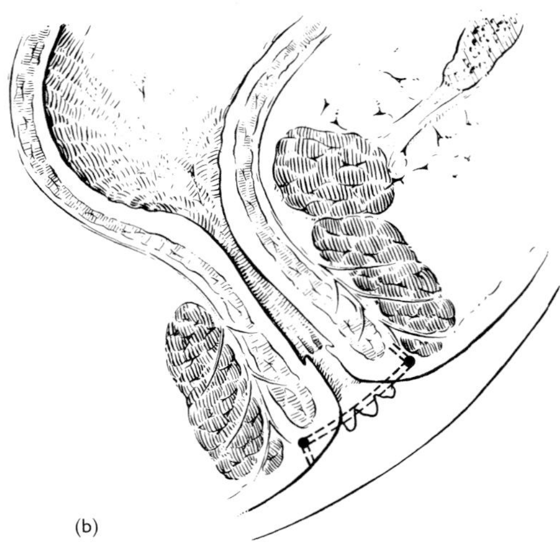

Figure 17.4a,b Perianal pilonidal sinus: 7% of pilonidal sinuses occur around the anal canal. (a) The circumferential track of a perianal pilonidal sinus is shown. (b) A sagittal section indicating the anatomical site of a perianal pilonidal sinus. Note that it is extremely superficial, and lies below the intersphincteric groove.

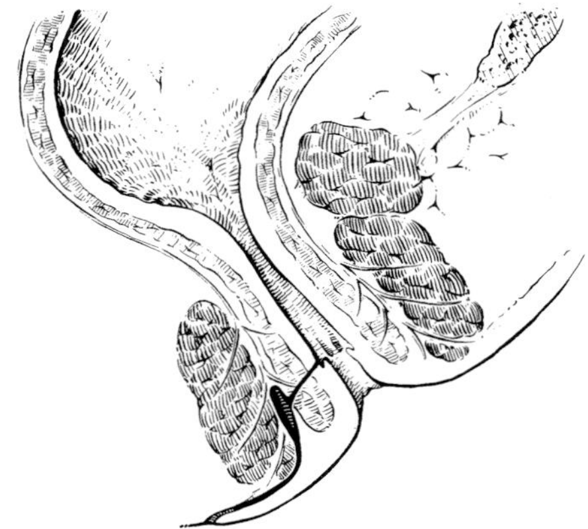

Figure 17.5 Fistula-in-ano associated with an intersphincteric circumferential pilonidal sinus. In some instances a pilonidal sinus may be complicated by an anal gland infection, and may therefore communicate with the intersphincteric glandular tissue and the anal canal; these are very rare.

Congenital abnormalities

A saccrococcygeal sinus is a vestigial remnant of the medullary canal. These sinuses track towards the sacrum and the coccyx. They may be continuous with the sacral canal and the central canal of the spinal cord. If there is a communication with the spinal cord, they are usually present at birth and may be associated with spina bifida and meningocele. There is a high mortality rate associated with communicating sinuses because of the risk of meningitis.

Presacral sinuses or dimples have already been referred to as examples of traction dermoids. Inclusion dermoids also occur at this site and may become infected to form a sinus. Large sacrococcygeal teratomas are easily recognized at birth; smaller teratomas may not be so obvious and may present later if they become infected.

COMPLICATIONS

The most common complications are acute and chronic infection. Malignant change can occur but is exceedingly rare (Matt, 1958). Most malignancies in pilonidal sinus are squamous cell carcinomas (Goodall, 1961), but occasionally basal cell carcinoma and sweat gland adenocarcinoma may occur. Malignancy presents either as an indurated lesion or as an incidental finding on histological examination of the resected specimen. Despite this, nodal metastases are common and the 5-year survival is only 61% (Philipsen et al, 1981). Many patients develop local recurrence after surgical excision.

NATURAL HISTORY

Clothier and Haywood (1984) studied the natural history of pilonidal sinus among 42 military hospital personnel. The disorder was clinically active only between the ages of 17 and 45 years (Figure 17.6). Normal progress of the disease was one of chronic remission and relapse; activity appeared to be greatest in the second decade. Many patients over 30 years, treated by drainage alone, had no further symptoms and did not require excisional surgery. In those who underwent ablative surgery, 45% had a recurrence. These authors had to admit that pilonidal sinus was often made worse by surgical therapy. It has therefore been suggested that, like acne, this is a self-limiting disease (Goodall, 1975). Hence, drainage of the abscess and minimal surgery for quiescent disease is advised (Ortiz et al, 1977; Armstrong and Barcia, 1994).

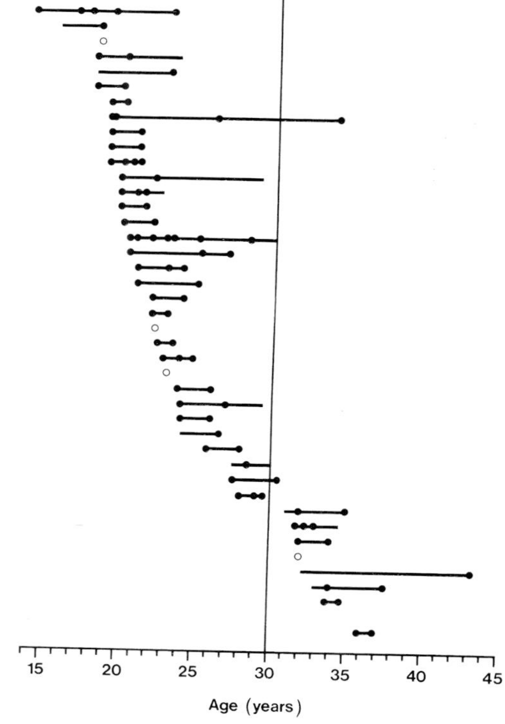

Figure 17.6 Natural history of pilonidal sinus. The horizontal lines represent pilonidal disease; operations are illustrated by the closed circles; open circles represent cases in whom the history is less than 3 weeks. Note that in many cases the sinus spontaneously resolves without surgical treatment (Clothier and Haywood, 1984).

EMERGENCY TREATMENT OF ABSCESS

Pilonidal abscess is usually treated merely by drainage under local, regional or general anaesthesia (Eftaiha and Abcarian, 1977). In compliant patients, local infiltration (Figure 17.7), with or without sedation, is sufficient to lance an abscess and achieve immediate drainage; otherwise general anaesthesia should be used. These abscesses are rarely multilocular so it is usually unnecessary to curette the cavity. A small ellipse of skin is excised, the contents evacuated and the cavity is packed (Hanley, 1980).

The policy in some centres is to drain the abscess as a day procedure and arrange readmission 2–3 weeks later for definitive excision of the pilonidal area, and instruction of open wound management. Patients are taught to manage their own wounds and ensure that the area is shaved by a friend or relative (Eftaiha and Abcarian, 1977). When this policy was applied at the Cook County Hospital there were few complications (acute retention in 3%), patients were discharged from hospital at 48 hours, and only one of 175 developed a recurrent sinus (Eftaiha and Abcarian, 1977).

An alternative approach is to excise the entire pilonidal area as an emergency procedure, but this policy may result in infection and a very large wound. Moreover, the precise anatomy of the pilonidal area may be difficult to define and a 60% recurrence rate is not unusual (Clothier and Haywood, 1984).

Drainage alone in patients over 30 years old may be a definitive procedure. In Jensen and Harling's series (1988), a policy of drainage alone achieved healing in 58% of patients and only 27% required definitive treatment of the underlying pilonidal sinus. It is our policy to incise and drain all acute pilonidal abscesses and to offer definitive surgery only if a sinus remains after 3–6 months. Matter et al (1995) in Israel compared drainage alone with excision for acute abscess. Recurrence rates were 55% and 41% respectively, but time off work was halved in the drainage-alone group (Table 17.2).

Table 17.2 Comparison of excision and drainage alone for pilonidal abscess.

	Excision ($n = 29$)	*Drainage alone* ($n = 29$)
Recurrence	12 (41%)	16 (55%)
Hospital stay (days)	4 (2–8)	3 (0–12)
Time off work (days)	14 (3–60)	7 (3–30)
Time to healing (days)	30 (15–70)	30 (10–60)

Medians and ranges.
From Matter et al (1995).

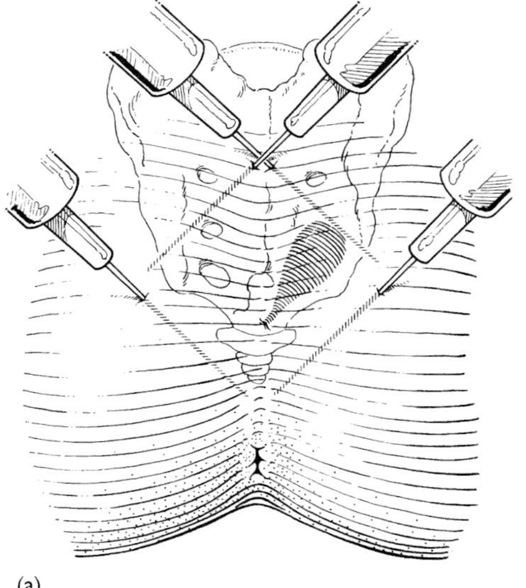

(a)

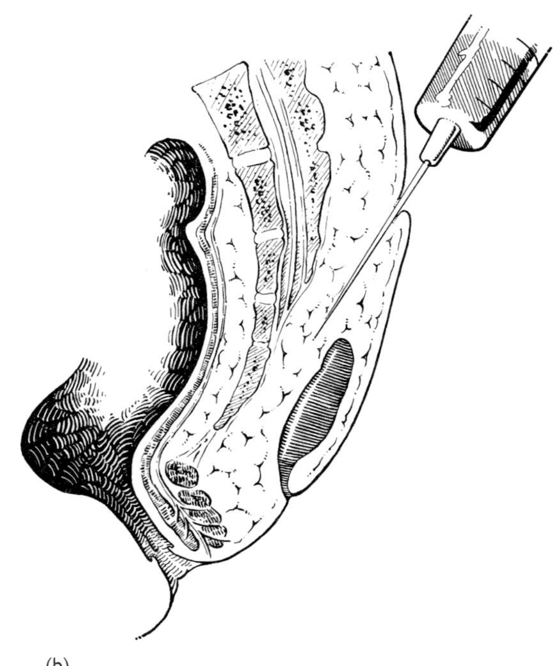

(b)

Figure 17.7a,b Local infiltration for local anaesthetic excision of pilonidal sinus. (a) As a pilonidal sinus lies only in the subcutaneous tissues local anaesthetic may be infiltrated, both in the midline by needles placed laterally, and laterally by needles placed medially. (b) Infiltration of local anaesthetic must also be deep to the pilonidal sinus, adjacent to the presacral fascia.

ELECTIVE TREATMENT

Treatment consists of either conservative measures or ablative surgery. Although surgical excision may be associated with healing rates of 80–100%, there are some patients in whom this form of treatment may be associated with a very high morbidity, owing to delayed healing, time lost from employment, and recurrent disease. Clothier and Haywood (1984) reported a recurrence rate of 38% for excision alone. Furthermore, recurrence may occur many years after surgical treatment (Notaras, 1970).

In view of the morbidity associated with ablative surgery, conservative treatment has many attractions, particularly for a condition which is probably self-limiting anyway. It is noteworthy, too, that patients with pilonidal sinus are notoriously poor at attending follow-up appointments. Personal hygiene often leaves much to be desired. Indeed, Edwards (1977) reported that only 40% of patients attended for review, and only those who were diligent enough to attend actually achieved good results. Much of the literature on surgical therapy for pilonidal sinus is based upon short-term follow-up. One suspects that the true recurrence rates are far higher than the literature suggests (Guyuron et al, 1983).

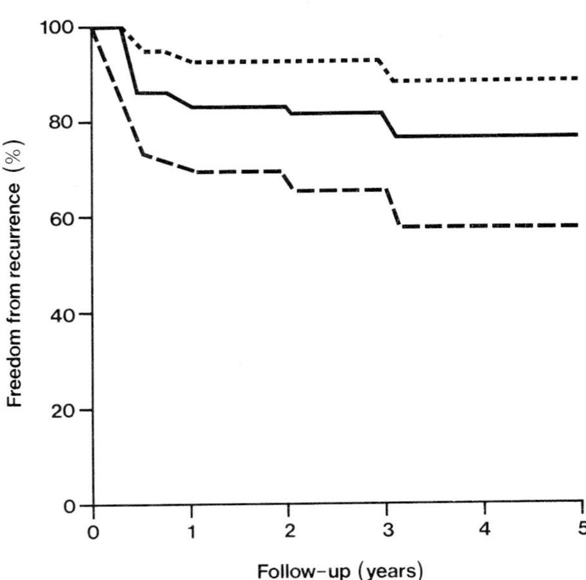

Figure 17.8 Freedom from recurrence in pilonidal disease. Recurrence rates were difficult to assess in incomplete attenders. The true incidence of recurrence can only be assessed among patients who are prepared to attend regularly for follow-up (Edwards, 1977). ——, overall ($n = 102$); - - - -, complete attenders ($n = 62$); — —, incomplete attenders ($n = 40$).

Conservative surgery

Excision of midline pits and clearing of tracks

Lord and Millar (1965) were the first to propose minimal surgery. They described excision of the midline pit under local anaesthesia, the secondary tracks being dilated so that hair within them could be removed by a fine Nylon brush. Edwards (1977) provided a 5-year appraisal of this technique. The recurrence rate in the 62 regular attenders was only 11%, compared with 43% in the remainder who defaulted (Figure 17.8). Since one of the most important aspects of surgical treatment is to prevent entry of hair into an excision site, it is hardly surprising that defaulters had such poor results. The median duration of time off work was only 10 days and the median healing time was 39 days. Advocates of this approach insist that the area must be kept clean and the skin shaved weekly until the excision scars are healed, so as to prevent recurrence. In Lord's own words: 'the excision of the pits and the clearing of the tracks is relatively simple and straightforward. The vital and more difficult part of the treatment is to ensure that healing is not delayed by hairs growing into the wound from surrounding skin ... one hair can spoil it!' (Lord, 1984).

Technique

The patient is placed in the left lateral position and the presacral area is examined with a good light to identify the pits, which are then marked by an indelible pen. All lateral sinuses and indurated tracks are marked as well. Mapping out of the pilonidal sinuses is important since they may become invisible once the local anaesthetic agent is injected subcutaneously. The proposed incisions should be confined to a 1 cm circle around the lateral sinus opening and a 2.5 × 1 cm ellipse around the pits. Multiple excisions may be needed if there are multiple pits (Figure 17.9), and long incisions should be avoided.

Local anaesthetic solution is infiltrated around the pits and the lateral openings, taking care to inject deep to the sinus to achieve adequate anaesthesia. Lord used 0.5% lignocaine with 1:200 000 adrenaline. Using a pointed scalpel blade, the skin and subcutaneous tissue around the pits is excised but the excision is not deepened as far as the presacral fascia. It is an advantage to disect the lower side first so that the rest of the incision is not obscured by bleeding from above. The pits are then grasped in a toothed forceps and, using short pointed scissors, the base is cut free so that a boat-shaped piece of tissue is removed. Any lateral track issuing from the side of the specimen will be identified by the granulation tissue within it.

All lateral tracks are dilated with sinus forceps and the hair within them is removed with a small wire brush. A small disc of skin from the orifice of the lateral sinus is then excised, using the fine scalpel blade, to ensure good drainage. Aftercare involves regular shaving and baths until the excision sites have completely healed.

(a)

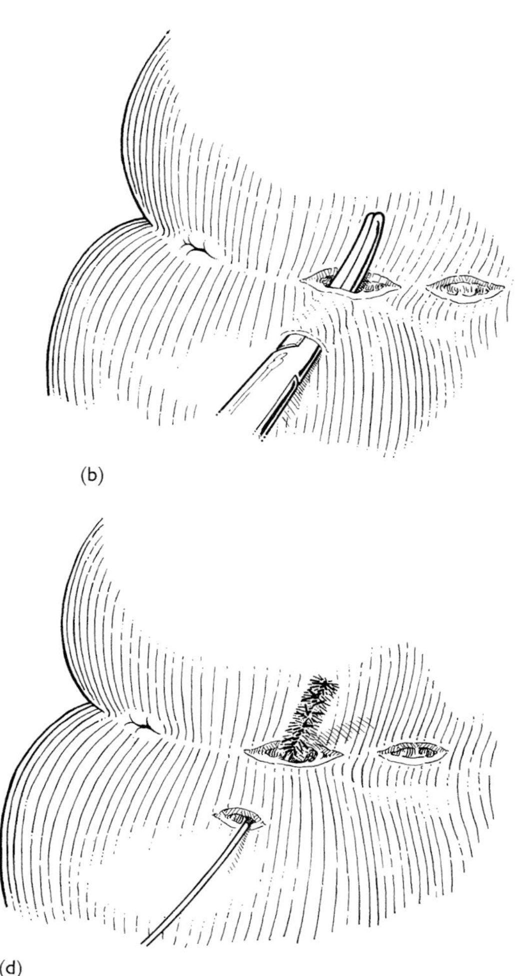

(b)

(c)

(d)

(e)

Figure 17.9a–e Excision of midline sinuses and their lateral tracks. (a) An incision is placed around the midline pits and any lateral extensions. (b) The lateral extensions are first cleared by inserting a pair of artery forceps between the two incisions to remove all granulation tissue. (c) Alternatively, the lateral aspect of the pilonidal sinus may be excised, as in fistula-in-ano. (d) In order to ensure that all granulation tissue and hair has been recovered from the lateral tract, a fine wire brush may be placed between the two incisions after excising the primary midline disease. (e) Completion of the operation. The midline disease has been completely excised. The lateral tracts have been removed, and the perianal hair is shaved from the incision sites.

Table 17.3 Comparison of excision with an open wound and Lord's technique for chronic pilonidal sinus.

	Excision and open wound ($n = 21$)	*Lord's technique* ($n = 21$)
Recurrence	6 (28%)	6 (28%)
Hospital stay (days)	5 (1–14)	4 (1–7)
Time off work (days)	15 (3–35)	7 (2–20) *
Time to healing (days)	30 (10–20)	14 (7–60)†

Medians and ranges. *$P < 0.002$; † $P < 0.001$.
From Matter et al (1995).

The Israel group (Matter et al, 1995) compared Lord's technique with excision and open wound management. Recurrence rates were identical but time off work and healing time was significantly shorter with Lord's technique (Table 17.3), suggesting that minimal surgery may not influence success rates but it certainly minimizes morbidity.

Follicle removal

Bascom (1983) believes that a pilonidal sinus is due to rupture of a midline hair follicle in a pit. Once any concomitant abscess has been drained, the central pit is excised. If there is a lateral sinus, the central pit is excised and the lateral sinus curetted. Review of 161 patients indicated that healing was achieved after a mean of 3 weeks and that the recurrence rate was only 16%.

Cryosurgery

Following acceptance of conservative treatment for pilonidal sinus (Abramson, 1970; Dortan, 1970; Broadrick et al, 1971; Sebrechts and Anderson, 1971), Gage and Dutta (1977) investigated cryosurgery for treatment of 29 patients with relatively quiescent pilonidal sinus. The procedure was performed under local anaesthesia. After adequate infiltration of all side tracks and the central pits, the entire ramifications of the sinus were laid open by scalpel or cautery. After gentle curettage to remove excess granulation tissue, liquid nitrogen spray was applied to the exposed tracks, using a single freeze–thaw cycle to avoid freezing the presacral fascia. The hospital stay ranged from 2 to 5 days and healing was achieved in 3–36 weeks. The reported recurrence rate was 3%. Similar results were also reported by O'Connor (1979).

Despite these apparently good results, cryosurgery is now rarely used for this condition.

Phenol injection

Phenol injection has been used since the 1960s but the procedure has not gained wide popularity (Maurice and Greenwood, 1964). Most surgeons use pure phenol, which is painful; the technique is therefore usually performed under general anaesthesia (Shorey, 1975). In order to protect the surrounding skin, a liberal application of petroleum jelly is smeared over the area. The midline pits are gently dilated with a probe and, using a blunt nose coned needle, the phenol solution is introduced into the sinus. The phenol is then expressed down the secondary tracks and compressed, so that by repeated application a 3 minute exposure to the sclerosing agent is achieved.

The recurrence rate reported by Shorey (1975) was 19%, being largely confined to patients with active disease. A rather different picture emerges from a report by Hegge et al (1987). Phenol injection was confined to patients whose disease persisted despite shaving or drainage of acute abscess. Only 1–5 mL of an 80% solution of phenol was injected into the sinuses as an outpatient procedure. The procedure took approximately 15 minutes and was tolerated well without complications such as skin burns, fat necrosis or severe pain. The procedure was repeated at 4–6 weekly intervals where necessary. Half of the patients needed only one treatment; 12% had five or more injections; 43 patients were followed up for a mean of 3 years and only three developed a recurrence (6%).

The Erlangen group, however, reported quite a different outcome (Schneider et al, 1994). Using 80% phenol, healing was achieved in only 60%, took a mean of 6 weeks and 50 of 45 patients developed an abscess. They concluded that phenol has no place in therapy.

Laying open tracks

If the acquired theory of pilonidal sinus is true, then the most attractive and logical form of therapy, which might be attended by minimal morbidity, is to lay open the sinus tracks. All of the tracks must be identified, either by probes or by injection with a weak solution of methylene blue. If there are blind lateral sinuses the skin will need to be opened over the extremity of the lateral opening.

The problem with laying open the tracks is the very high recurrence rate (67%) reported by some authors (Clothier and Haywood, 1984), but this is not universal and there are some reports of recurrence in less than 10% (Ortiz et al, 1977; McLaren, 1984), despite a long hospital stay and a mean

Table 17.4 Results of surgical treatment by laying open tracks.

	n	*Recurrence*	*Wound breakdown*	*Reoperation*	*Hospital stay (days)*	*Healing time*
Abscess						
Incision and drainage	42	23 (54)	0	17 (40)	15	6 weeks
Chronic sinus with cellulitis						
Incision and curettage	18	2 (11)	0	2 (11)	29	6 weeks
Excision and packing	34	3 (9)	0	3 (9)	21	7 weeks
Chronic uninfected sinus						
Excision and primary suture	41	5 (12)	5 (12)	8 (20)	14	11 days
Excision and partial suture	22	0	1 (5)	0	20	20 days

Values in parentheses are percentages.
From McLaren (1984).

healing time of 6 weeks (Table 17.4). Results of laying open the tracks are comparable to excision and marsupialization. The advantage of the laying-open procedure compared with excision is that it can be performed under local anaesthesia. Notaras (1970) found that laying-open of the sinus tracks was associated with a shorter hospital stay than was excision, but a longer period of healing, with a recurrence rate of 13% (Table 17.5).

Technique

The patient is placed in the left lateral position and the midline pit is infiltrated with a local anaesthetic solution to allow the pit to be dilated sufficiently to permit the passage of a probe into the various secondary tracks (Figure 17.10). If a blind track is discovered without a skin opening, the blind end should be opened using a fine blade, after infiltration with a local anaesthetic solution. Once the tracks have all been defined the overlying skin is infiltrated with local anaesthetic. If the local anaesthetic is placed in the tissues earlier, the tracks may be difficult to define and the infiltration is not then applied to the optimum sites. We prefer to lay open the sinus tracks using a cutting diathermy to minimize blood loss. Once all the tracks have been laid open they are gently curetted

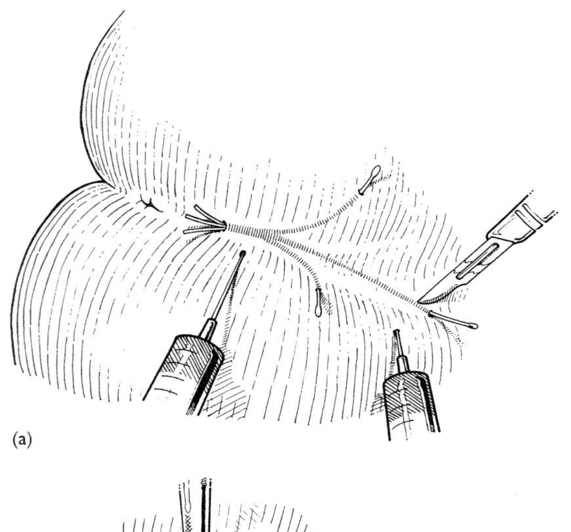

(a)

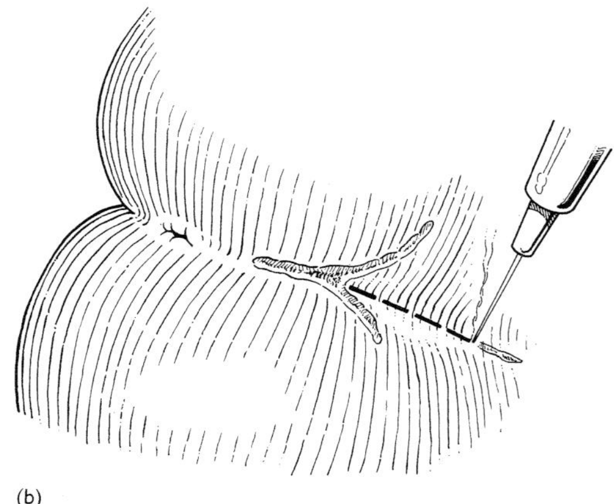

(b)

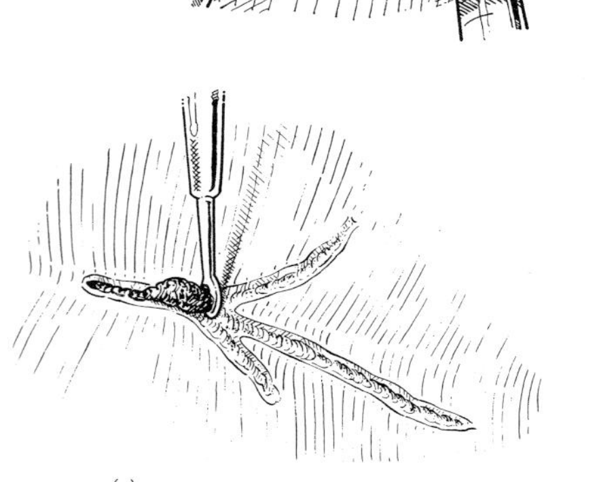

(c)

Figure 17.10a–c Laying open of multiple pilonidal sinus tracks. (a) Separate flexible olivery bougies are passed from the central pit along lateral or midline tracks. Local anaesthetic is infiltrated around the tracks and deep to them. (b) The skin overlying each track is divided either by sharp scalpel dissection, or using a diathermy. (c) The granulation tissue within the tracks is curetted and all hair and epithelial debris removed.

Table 17.5 Results of various surgical treatments.

Authors	n	Hospital stay (days)	Disability period (days)	Recurrence (%)
Lay open only				
Notaras (1970)	45	17	49	13
Edwards (1977) (excision of pits only)	102	NR	39	24
Ortiz et al (1977)	14	NR	39	7
Bascom (1983) (excision of follicle only)	161	NR	21	16
Senapati and Thompson (1996) (excision of midline pits, lateral drainage)	161	DC	NR	10
Excision and lay open				
Palumbo et al (1951)	113	17	NR	22
Healy and Hoffert (1955)	47	26	NR	17
Notaras (1970)	41	26	44	13
Sood et al (1975)	28	16	67	0
Wood and Hughes (1975)	72	10	84	14
(with foam elastomer)	40	6	44	0
Fuzun et al (1994)	45	2	17	0
Matter et al (1995)	21	5	15	28
Søndenaa et al (1995c)	60	NR	NR	5
Spivak et al (1996)	47	DC	NR	13
Excision and marsupialization				
MacFee (1942)	147	14	69	13
Abramson (1970)	159	NR	NR	7
Cavanagh et al (1979)	26	NR	NR	8
Spivak et al (1996)	26	1	NR	4
Excision and primary closure				
Goodall (1961)	126	17	NR	38
Gabriel (1963)	89	14	NR	4
Hamilton et al (1963)	393	12	17	26
McCaughan (1965)	1080	23	NR	26
Cherry (1968)	202	11	12	8
Notaras (1970)	43	16	NR	9
Karydakis (1973) (lateral incision)	754	8	NR	1
Wood and Hughes (1975)	26	9	NR	46
Rainsbury and Southam (1982)	72	13	NR	5
Fuzun et al (1994)	46	5	11	4
Khaira and Brown (1995)	46	1	21	17
Søndenaa et al (1995c)	60	NR	NR	10
Spivak et al (1996)	56	DC	NR	11
Kitchen (1996) (lateral wound)	141	4	NR	4
Excision and Z-plasty				
Monro and McDermott (1965)	20	21	NR	0
Middleton (1968)	30	16	NR	10
Sood et al (1975)	23	12	1	0
Mansoory and Dickson (1982)	120	12	NR	2
Excision and rhomboid flap				
Azab et al (1984)	30	10	NR	3
Gwynn (1986)	20	11	NR	5
Chavez et al (1988)	14	NR	NR	7
Manterola et al (1991)	25	4	14	0
Galizia et al (1995)	22	4	8	0
Excision and split skin graft				
Boger and Pinkham (1951)	25	28	NR	0
Rupnick (1958)	39	26	NR	3
Guyuron et al (1983)	58	10	28	5

NR, no results; DC, day case.

and packed with gauze soaked in an antiseptic solution. Aftercare involves regular shaving, dressings and baths.

We no longer recommend laying open and prefer the Lord or Bascom approach if conservative therapy is advised.

Bascom's operation

One serious disadvantage of conventional excision and either open wound management or primary closure is that midline wounds in the natal cleft may not heal owing to shearing forces from the buttocks. Thus wounds that avoid the midline are thought to be more likely to heal (Karydakis, 1973; Mann and Springall, 1987). Bascom (1980, 1983, 1987) described a technique of excising the midline pits with drainage of the abscess or curettage of the cavity and transposing the sinus away from the midline through a lateral incision which is left open for drainage.

Technique

Operations are performed under local anaesthetic as day-case procedures, in either the prone or left lateral position. All midline pits are excised together with a small amount of surrounding tissue (Figure 17.11a). These pits communicate with the midline sinus or abscess. A longitudinal lateral incision is made so as to explore the sinus, which is opened to remove all pus, granulation tissue and hair with a currette (Figure 17.11b). A 'release' incision is then made below the pilonidal cavity to divide the fibrous tissue connection with the sacrum. This incision is extended across the midline so that the fibro-fatty base can be raised as a flap from the opposite buttock and sutured to the bridge of skin between the midline pits and the lateral drainage wound. Bascom now no longer sutures the fibro-fatty flap and merely performs the 'release' incision. The lateral drainage wound is left open but the midline pit excisions are closed (Figure 17.11c). The patients are

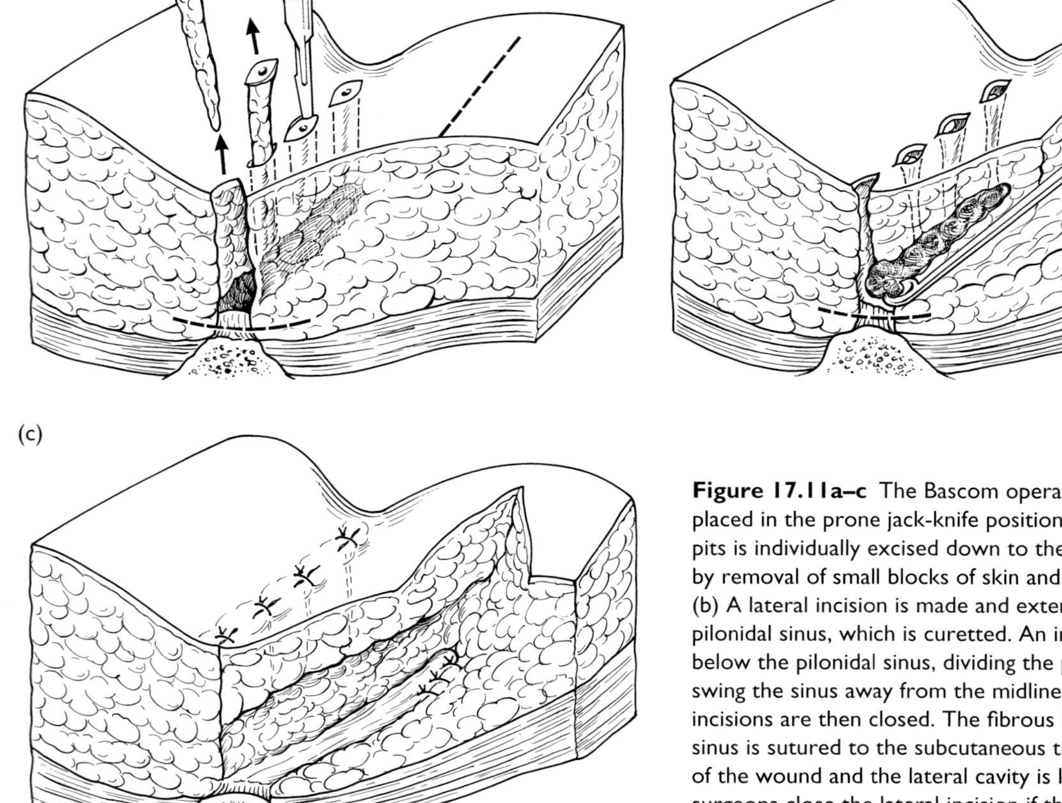

Figure 17.11a–c The Bascom operation. The patient is placed in the prone jack-knife position. (a) Each of the midline pits is individually excised down to the presacral sinus cavity by removal of small blocks of skin and subcutaneous tissue. (b) A lateral incision is made and extended down to the pilonidal sinus, which is curetted. An incision is then made below the pilonidal sinus, dividing the presacral fascia so as to swing the sinus away from the midline. (c) The midline pit incisions are then closed. The fibrous base of the pilonidal sinus is sutured to the subcutaneous tissue on the medial side of the wound and the lateral cavity is left open. Some surgeons close the lateral incision if there is no coexisting sepsis.

instructed in changing their own dressing. We have now modified this original description by closing the lateral wound in non-infected cases.

Senapati and Thompson (1996) reported their experience of the Bascom procedure in 161 patients. Most patients had returned to their normal activities within 2 days of operation. Eight had postoperative bleeding which stopped spontaneously. Six developed postoperative abscess requiring re-opening of the lateral wound. One midline wound failed to heal. Mean healing time of the lateral wound was 4 weeks. Sixteen patients (10%) of the 133 who could be contacted for follow-up developed a recurrent pilonidal sinus requiring a second Bascom procedure (Bascom, 1987). Bascom himself describes a 16% recurrence rate with this approach (Bascom, 1983).

We have some experience with the procedure which is certainly feasible as a day-case operation and causes very little morbidity. It is useful for the infected pilonidal sinus, but it remains to be seen if this is superior to excision and primary closure of quiescent pilonidal sinus.

Preventive measures after conservative surgery

Conservative surgery relies upon the need to prevent the growth of hair over the pilonidal area while the excision site is healing. Shaving is still the most effective way of preventing recurrence and should be undertaken at least weekly by the patient's relatives or close friends. Attention to hygiene is essential and Goodall (1975) believes that the perineal region should be scrubbed. Depilatory creams are less effective than shaving and are expensive and may be allergenic. Electrolysis has been tried and abandoned.

There was a vogue for radiotherapy to prevent hair growth: small doses merely arrest growth and unacceptably high doses are needed to achieve permanent control. In view of the risk of iatrogenic malignancy, radiotherapy as an adjuvant to surgical excision is not recommended.

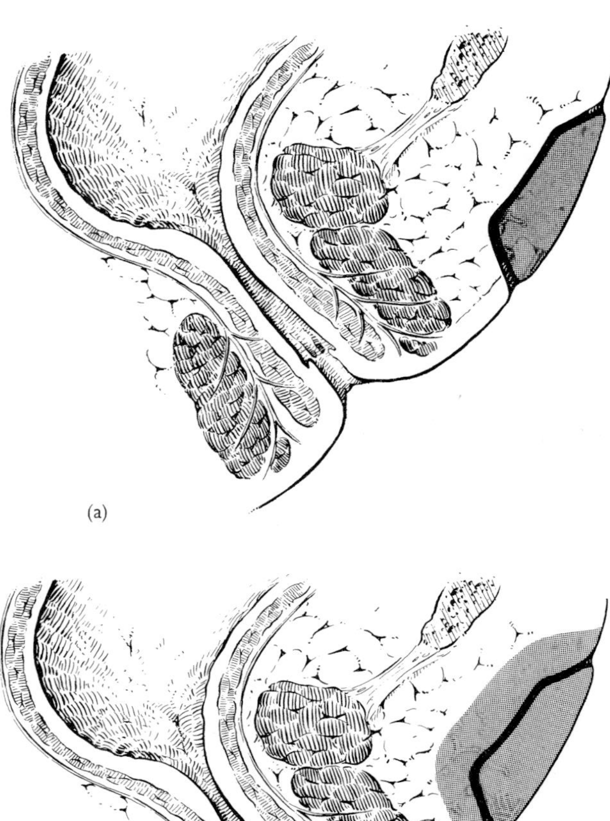

Figure 17.12a,b Excision of pilonidal sinus. It may be preferable to excise all the pilonidal material rather than laying open the sinus tracks. (a) The principle of laying open a pilonidal sinus merely by excising the skin over it. (b) The principle of excision whereby the sinus track itself and the subcutaneous tissues beneath it are excised.

Radical excision

Despite the theoretical advantages of minimal surgery, excision is still the most widely practised form of surgical treatment today. The sinus may simply be excised to its base (Figure 17.12a) or the entire sinus is removed (Figure 17.12b). What happens after excision is a matter of great debate. The defect may be left open to granulate, it may be partly closed by a technique of marsupialization, or it may be sutured, either by primary closure or by some form of flap. Sometimes the defect may be closed by primary or secondary skin grafting.

The usual practice of excision is to define the extent of the pilonidal area by probes or methylene blue injection so that the entire area can be excised as completely as possible. We have abandoned the use of methylene blue since it often extrudes into normal tissue, making delineation of the tracks imprecise. In order to avoid a wide area of excision, some surgeons deliberately remove only a

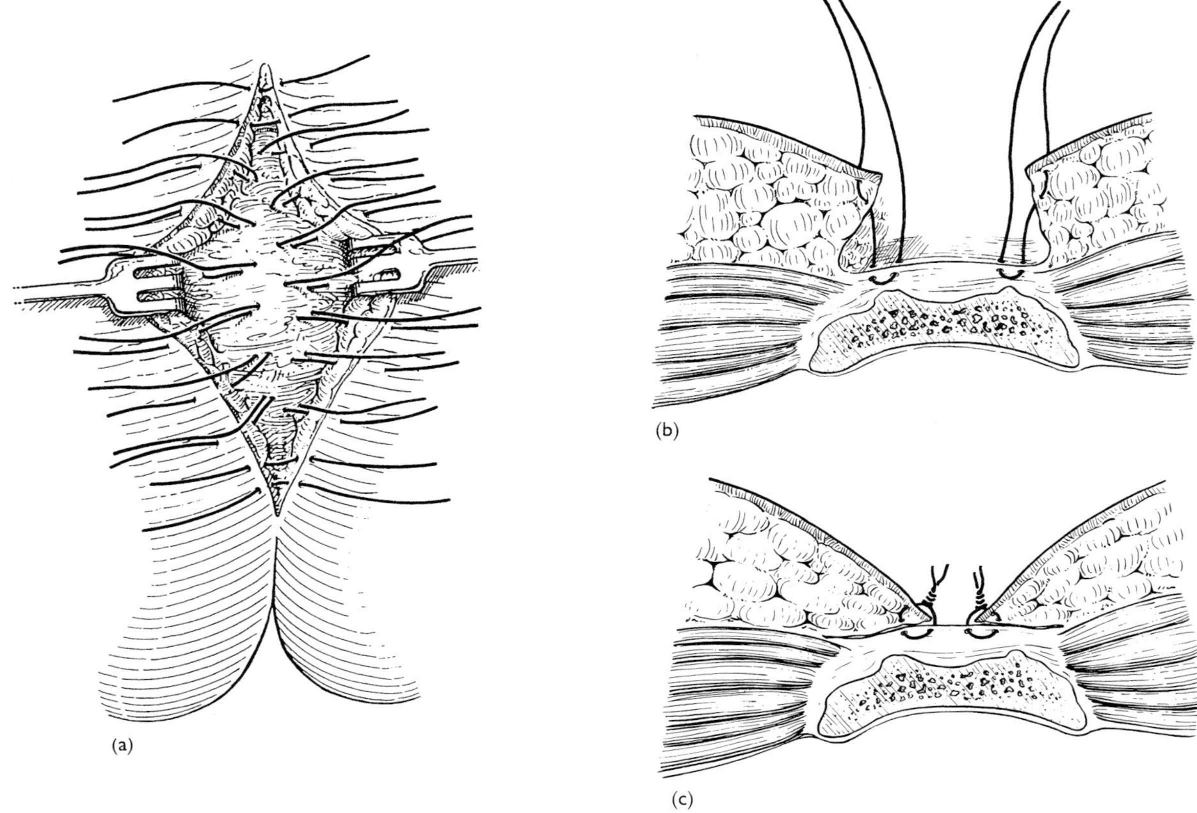

Figure 17.13a–c Excision and marsupialization of a pilonidal sinus. (a) The pilonidal sinus has been excised with exposure of the presacral fascia. This large defect can be closed by marsupialization whereby the skin is sutured down to the presacral fascia. (b) The principles of the operation, which leaves a defect in the midline, but allows epithelialization over the presacral fascia. (c) The completed operation once the lateral sutures have been tied.

tongue of lateral skin containing a sinus if the secondary track emerges over the buttocks. Most surgeons keep the area of skin loss as small as possible (MacFee, 1942) and deliberately undermine the edges, a practice which is particularly appropriate if the defect is to be partly closed by marsupialization (Figure 17.13a–c)

Technique

Excision may be performed under general or regional anaesthesia. Antibiotic cover is advised but the persistent use of antibiotics is not recommended (Marks et al, 1985). It is rarely possible to excise the area using local anaesthesia unless it is very small. The operation may be performed with the patient in the left lateral position, particularly if the defect is to be left open (Figure 17.14). On the other hand, the prone jack-knife position is recommended if the excision is extensive, if primary closure or marsupialization is planned, if surgery is for recurrent disease where skin or gluteal flaps are planned, or if a Thiersch graft is to be applied. The advantage of the lateral position is that anaesthesia is easier, with less respiratory embarrassment, and the procedure can be accomplished more rapidly.

The entire pilonidal area is excised with a blade or cutting diathermy. It is unwise to excise the presacral fascia since it is rarely penetrated by the pilonidal sinus and excision often results in considerable blood loss. Haemostasis must be meticulous, particularly if the defect is to be closed.

Excision and healing by granulation

There is a high incidence of breakdown after primary suture in the presence of sepsis or if the patient is obese. Under these circumstances healing by secondary intention is preferred to primary suture; this policy is more appropriate in hirsute men (Gabriel, 1963); however, partial closure by marsupialization may be appropriate. The defect is

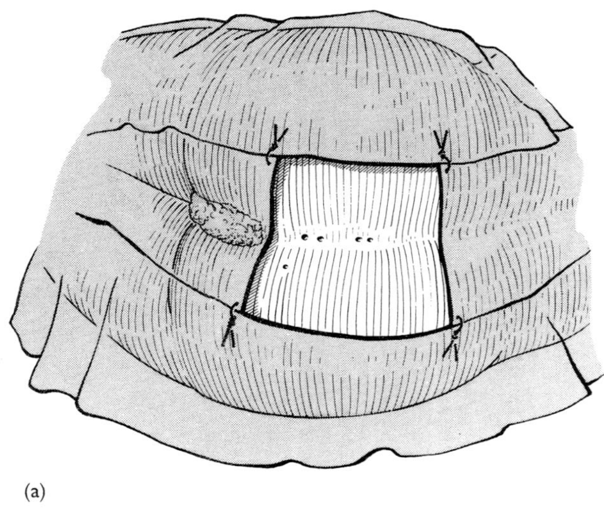

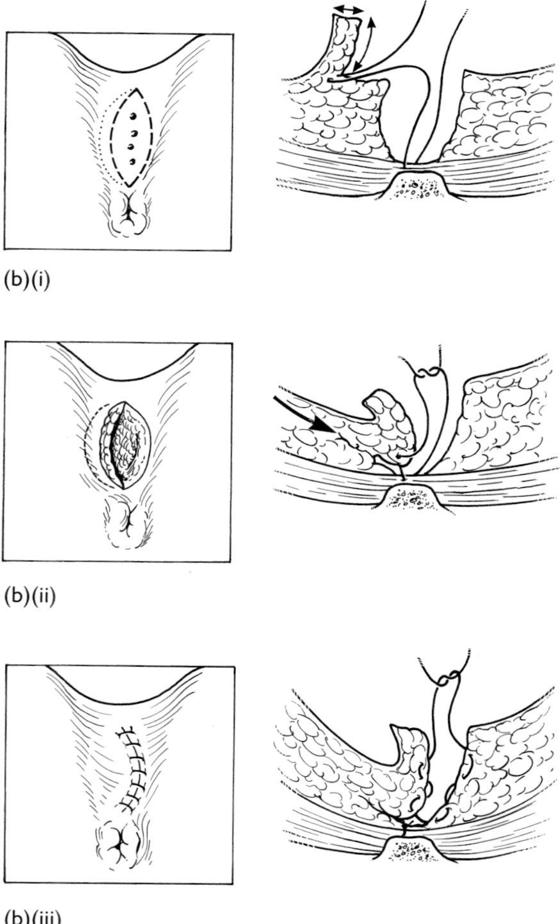

Figure 17.14a,b Excision and primary closure of pilonidal sinus. (a) The patient is placed in the left lateral position. A sponge is placed over the anus and the towels are sutured into position. (b)(i)–(iii) The Karydakis flap. A bi-concaved incision based to one side of the midline cleft is made which incorporates the primary opening and the whole of the pilonidal tract with any secondary openings that may be present. The skin and pilonidal sinus is excised. The medial flap of skin and subcutaneous tissue is mobilized to achieve primary closure. The deep tissues are exposed and the skin is sutured.

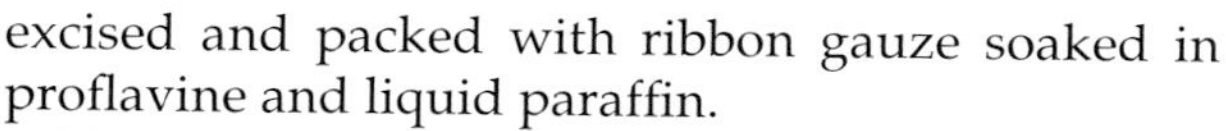

excised and packed with ribbon gauze soaked in proflavine and liquid paraffin.

Notaras (1970) compared the results of primary suture against excision alone; these are retrospective data and it is probable that there was some selection in the treatments provided. The mean hospital stay was 16 days for primary suture, compared with 26 days for excision alone. Mean time to complete healing was 12 days for primary closure, compared with 70 days in those patients whose wounds were left open. However, many patients with granulating wounds returned to work before healing was achieved and the mean time off work was only 6 weeks for primary suture, compared with 8 weeks in those whose wounds were left to granulate. Two recent randomized trials to compare leaving wounds open or primary suture both seem to show that recurrence rates are lower in the open management group with a higher rate of infection after primary suture (Fuzen et al, 1994; Søndenaa et al, 1995c). These results are summarized in Table 17.6.

We believe that wounds should probably be left open if they are infected whereas quiescent disease in non-obese patients can probably be safely closed using perioperative antibiotic cover. The main disadvantage of leaving these wounds open is that they may take a long time to heal (Cherry, 1968). Wood and Hughes (1975) advocate filling the cavity with

Table 17.6 Randomized trials of open versus primary wound closure.

	Open	*Primary closure*
Fuzun et al (1994)	(*n* = 45)	(*n* = 46)
Hospital stay (days)	2.4	4.7
Return to work (days)	17.6	10.7
Postoperative infection (%)	1.8	3.6
Recurrence (%)	0	4.4
Søndenaa et al (1995c)	(*n* = 60)	(*n* = 60)
Postoperative infection (%)	30	13
Recurrence (%)	5	10

elastomer foam to encourage early mobilization, facilitate local hygiene and achieve earlier healing.

Elastomer foam method

The elastomer is reconstituted by adding 10 mL of silicone elastomer (Dow Corning) to 0.6 mL of the catalyst. The mixture is poured into the granulating wound while the skin edges are held apart. The mixture expands and sets into a soft pliable foam in about two minutes. Before the foam is inserted, we usually advise a short period (2–3 days) of packing with gauze until all bleeding has stopped and granulation tissue is beginning to form. The patient has often been discharged from hospital by this stage and the foam is then inserted by the district nurse. It is secured in position by surgical adhesive tape (Micropore). The patient is then instructed to remove the foam twice daily, wash it in water and soak it in chlorhexidine while taking a bath to keep the area clean. The sponge is replaced, once the skin around the cavity has been dried, and is secured by tape, as before. The sponge must be remodelled at approximately weekly intervals, both because as the cavity contracts it no longer fits snugly into the defect, and because after this time it tends to disintegrate. After about 4–6 weeks, the cavity is so small that the sponge will no longer fit and a small dry dressing is applied to the residual area of granulation tissue.

The results of excision and laying open are listed in Table 17.5. Recurrence rates vary from nil to 28%. Hospital stay is much longer than modern surgical practice will justify and most patients will now be discharged on the day of operation or 3–5 days later; the period of disability seems to vary between 7 and 17 weeks (Palumbo et al, 1951; Healy and Hoffert, 1955; Notaras, 1970; Sood et al, 1975; Wood and Hughes, 1975; Fuzun et al, 1994; Søndenaa et al, 1995c; Matter et al, 1995; Spivak et al, 1996).

Excision and marsupialization

The concept of suturing the skin edges of the excised defect to the margins of the cavity or the presacral fascia is not new (MacFee, 1942) and is still practised by some (Goodall, 1961; Abramson, 1970). The reported recurrence rate is 7% (Goodall, 1961; Abramson, 1970; Cavanagh et al, 1979). Hospital stay is shorter than when the entire cavity is packed and the period of disability is also reduced. Spivak et al (1996) in a non-randomized comparison reported lower recurrence rates with marsupialization than with primary closure or leaving the wound open (see Table 17.5).

Technique

The pilonidal sinus is excised with the patient in the prone or left lateral position. It is important to conserve skin and undermine the subcutaneous tissue. Once haemostasis has been achieved the skin edges are approximated to the presacral fascia using a series of interrupted sutures which are not tied until all have been placed (see Figure 17.13). The residual defect is then packed and the dressing held in position by tying the ends of the sutures over the packing.

Excision and primary closure

One problem with primary closure is that unless the cavity is completely obliterated the wound will break down and healing rates will be longer than excision alone. Another problem with primary suture is that although primary healing may appear to have been successful, a small area of breakdown may subsequently emerge and form a recurrent sinus. Complete primary healing is achieved in between 51% and 92% of patients (Holm and Hulten, 1970; Lamke et al, 1974; Rainsbury and Southam, 1982; Zimmerman, 1984) (Table 17.7). Delayed healing does not appear to be related to the extent of the pilonidal sinus, the age of the patient or the presence of organisms in the excised specimen.

The mean duration of hospital stay ranges from day-case procedures to 23 days; but disability, particularly if primary healing is achieved, is substantially less than if the defect is left open to granulate (Goodall, 1961; Gabriel, 1963; Hamilton et al, 1963; McCaughan, 1965; Cherry, 1968; Notaras, 1970; Karydakis, 1973; Wood and Hughes, 1975; Rainsbury and Southam, 1982; Clothier and Haywood, 1984; Fuzun et al, 1994; Khaira and Brown, 1995; Spivak et al, 1996; Søndenaa et al, 1995c). Recurrence rates after primary closure vary between 1% and 38% (see Table 17.5), but late recur-

Table 17.7 Cumulative rate of wound healing after excision and primary closure.

Complete healing (months)	*No. of patients*	*%*
1	37	51
2	55	76
3	58	82
4	63	88
5	65	90
6	66	92

From Rainsbury and Southam (1982).

Table 17.8 Results of a randomized trial of therapy.

	n	Healed without further surgery	Healed after revisional surgery	Recurrent sinuses			Never healed
				Early	3 months	Late	
Excision and packing	33	29 (64)	2 (66)	1	0	4	0
Excision and suture	33	29 (14)	3 (22)	0	4	4	1
Excision, suture and clindamycin	33	30 (11)	1 (11)	3	3	3	0

Values in parentheses are median time to healing (days).
From Kronborg et al (1985).

rence may occur in up to 20% of patients (Close, 1955; Gabriel, 1963; Foss, 1970). Notaras (1970) recorded a 10% recurrence rate at 1 year but a further 8% recurred up to 10 years after the original operation.

Ninety-nine patients with a quiescent pilonidal sinus (Kronborg et al, 1985) were randomly allocated to excision alone, excision and primary suture, or excision and primary suture under antibiotic cover (Table 17.8). Healing after primary suture occurred in 90% and was the same irrespective of antibiotic cover, but healing took longer after excision and open wound management. Recurrences were fewer following excision alone (15%) compared with primary suture (24%), many of which occurred late after the original excision. Similar trends in favour of lower recurrence rates with open wound management were recorded in the two recent trials by Søndenaa et al (1995c) and Fuzun et al (1994).

Technique

Primary suture may be performed in the prone jackknife position or in the left lateral position. We advise short-term, broad-spectrum antibiotic cover if this technique is used. Local anaesthesia may be feasible (Zimmerman, 1984) if the sinuses are small but it is not appropriate where excision involves a large defect.

The defect should not be sutured under tension and haemostasis should be meticulous. It is imperative to obliterate the cavity by taking deep through-and-through bites of skin and subcutaneous tissue which incorporate the presacral fascia. A second vertical mattress suture is used to approximate the skin and superficial tissue (see Figure 17.14). It is our practice to leave at least two small suction drains in the depths of the cavity and to suture a tightly rolled gauze dressing over the incision to provide some external pressure in an attempt to obliterate the potential space.

Patients are encouraged to mobilize early; the suction drains are removed after 48–72 h, depending on the amount of drainage, and the sutures are removed 7–10 days after operation, after which the patient can be discharged from hospital.

An alternative technique described by Karydakis (Kitchen, 1996), and in our view an important advance in the primary closure technique, is that of avoiding a wound in the midline cleft. The principle of the *Karydakis flap* is excision of the pilonidal sinus using a vertical eccentric elliptical incision, undercutting the medial tuck skin flap with primary closure of the defect leaving a lateral wound. Karydakis' results were spectacular, with a recurrence rate of just 1% in a series of 754. The cynics have been reassured, however, by a recent independent report of results in 141 patients with a recurrence rate of 4%. The operation gave good results even in patients with recurrent pilonidal sinus. It is also possible to modify the procedure in patients with lateral tracks to leave a small T-shaped wound (Kitchen, 1996). An asymmetrical biconcave incision is made over a secondary opening or to one side of the midline. An ellipse of skin is excised such that the medial edge crosses the midline (see Figure 17.14b(i)) to encompass the primary pit. The entire pilonidal sinus is excised. The medial side of the wound is then undercut for a distance of about 2 cm to produce a thick flap (see Figure 17.14b(ii)). The defect is then closed using absorbable sutures to close the defect over a suction drain to obliterate any dead space (see Figure 17.14b(iii)).

Another method of reconstruction is to approximate the medial aspect of the gluteal muscles over the presacral fascia as a method of closing the dead space (Farringer and Pickens, 1978). After excision of the sinus, the fascia over the medial aspect of the gluteus maximus is incised and a pad of muscle with its fascia is sutured over the sacrum (Figure 17.15). Primary healing has been reported in 89% of patients. It may be unnecessary to use the gluteal muscles, and a D-shaped excision may facilitate primary closure, a procedure which is reported to give results which are almost identical to those achieved with a gluteal flap (Mann and Springall, 1987) (Figure 17.16).

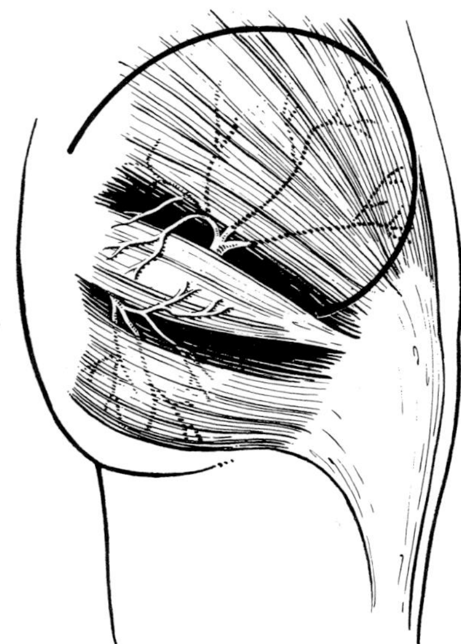

Figure 17.15 Gluteus maximus myocutaneous flap. If there is a large defect in the pilonidal area after wide excision, a myocutaneous flap, such as the gluteus flap, may be used to achieve primary closure.

Closure by Z-plasty

The aim of Z-plasty is to avoid a midline scar. The technique is feasible only if complete removal of the pilonidal sinus can be achieved through a narrow excision (Monro and McDermott, 1965). Most series report only small numbers of patients (Middleton, 1968; Sood et al, 1975). Mansoory and Dickson (1982) used the Z-plasty technique in 120 carefully selected patients and only one recurrence was reported.

The pilonidal sinus is excised through a narrow segment of skin. Two incisions which are three-quarters the length of the excision site are then made 30 degrees from the midline. The apex of each skin fold is rotated towards the opposite defect and sutured over suction drains (Figure 17.17). The aim of this procedure is to avoid any midline dead space by taking the skin closure away from the gluteal fold. The reported recurrence rates of this operation are low (see Table 17.5).

Suture using the rhomboid flap and others

Five reports claim that the rhomboid flap achieves primary closure even when the excision has been wide (Azab et al, 1984; Gwynn, 1986; Chavez et al, 1988; Manterola et al, 1991; Galizia et al, 1995). An oblique, inverted, V-shaped incision is made over

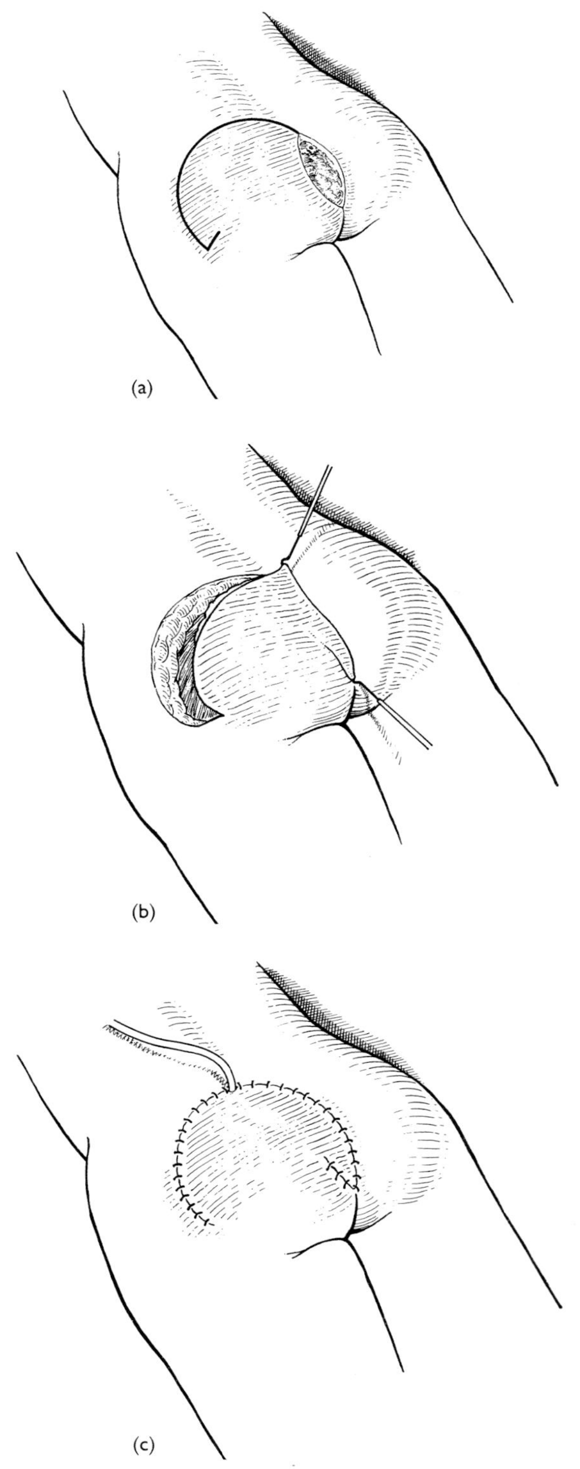

Figure 17.16a–c Details of the rotational gluteal flap. (a) The skin incision around the myocutaneous flap once the pilonidal disease has been fully excised. (b) The myocutaneous flap being rotated medially to close the pilonidal defect. (c) Completed closure of the defect over a closed suction drain.

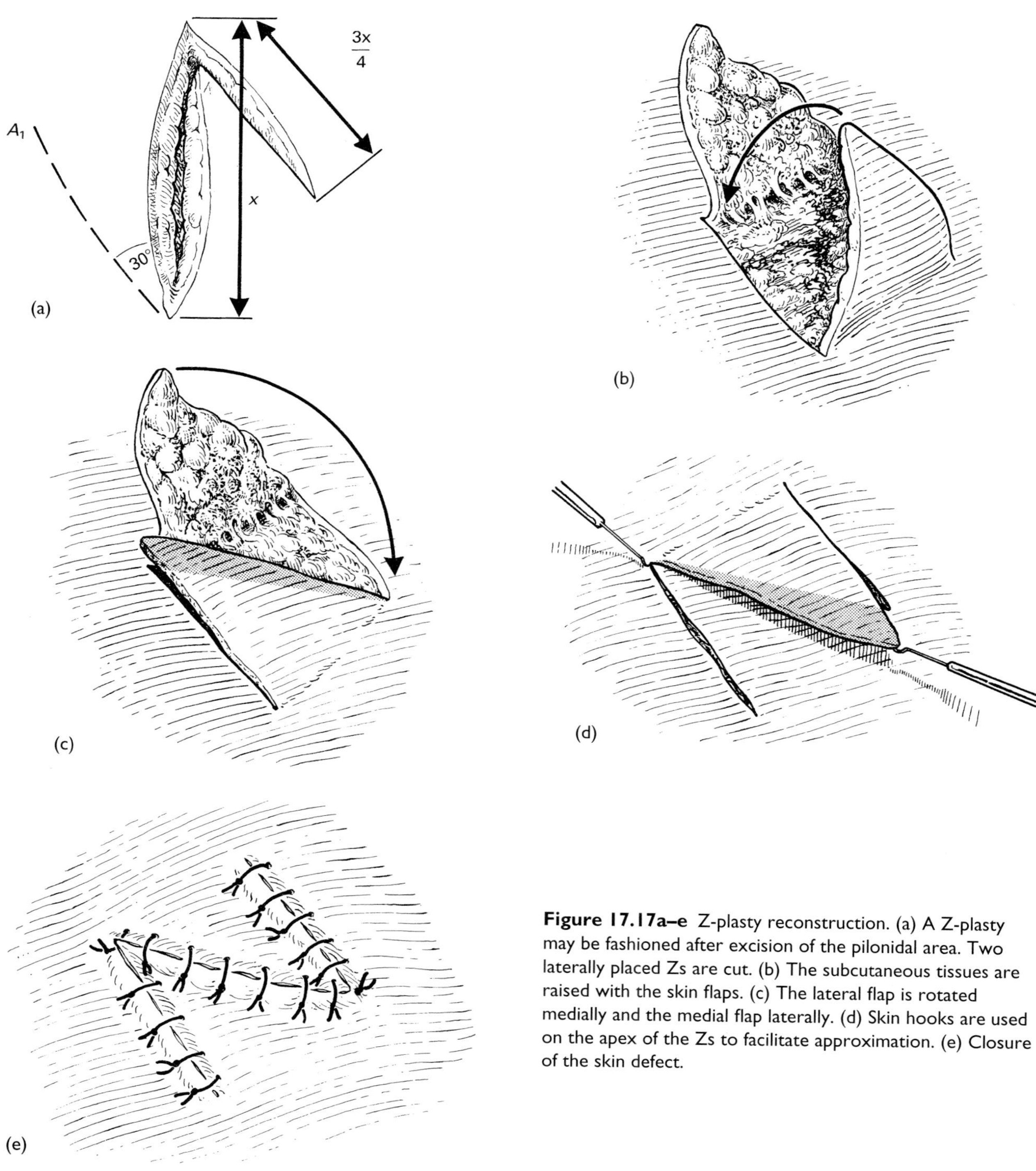

Figure 17.17a–e Z-plasty reconstruction. (a) A Z-plasty may be fashioned after excision of the pilonidal area. Two laterally placed Zs are cut. (b) The subcutaneous tissues are raised with the skin flaps. (c) The lateral flap is rotated medially and the medial flap laterally. (d) Skin hooks are used on the apex of the Zs to facilitate approximation. (e) Closure of the skin defect.

one or other buttock so that the medial incision bisects the extended line of the posterolateral edge of the excision with the transverse extremity of the defect (Figure 17.18). This reconstruction flattens the natal cleft, prevents any macerating action of the buttocks and eliminates any midline dead space. Recurrence rates appear to be low (see Table 17.5).

Myocutaneous flap and other procedures

The gluteus maximus myocutaneous flap, based upon the superior gluteal vessels and nerve, has been used for decubitus ulcers (Minami et al, 1977; Baek et al, 1980) and may be used for recurrent pilonidal sinus (Pérez-Gurri et al, 1984). The skin, subcutaneous tissues and gluteus maximus are divided and rotated medially to close the defect (see Figure 17.15).

Another procedure for closing large defects involves rotating a flap of skin and subcutaneous tissue only from the buttock. The width of the flap should be no less than half the length of its free edge (Hirschowitz et al, 1970; Fishbein and Handelsman, 1979). A V–Y flap is also described to close large pilonidal defects and is illustrated in Figure 17.19 (Khatri et al, 1994).

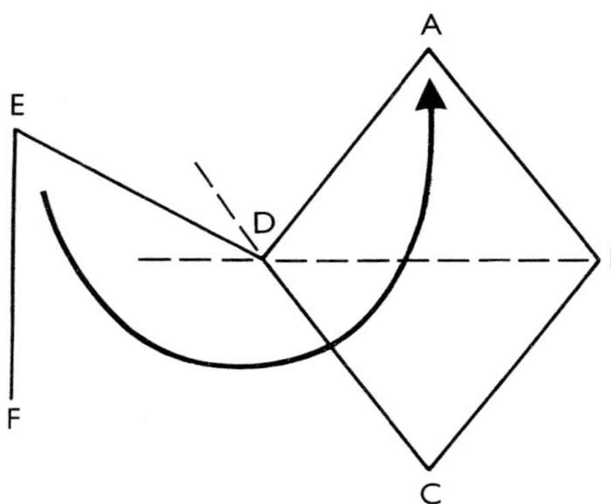

Figure 17.18 The principle of a rhomboid flap for closure of a wide pilonidal sinus. A rhomboid is cut for excision of the disease, and a lateral extension, marked D–E and E–F, is also cut so that the laterally placed V can be rotated into the defect as shown.

Excision and split skin grafting

Skin grafts may be used as a primary procedure at the time of excision, or they may be placed on an excision site which is granulating satisfactorily. Primary grafting in an attempt to ablate recurrent disease may be appropriate for large defects. Results of secondary grafting are rather disappointing, since split skin may not take on rapidly contracting granulation tissue. In many cases the defect will probably heal more quickly at this stage without grafting.

Primary skin grafting has been used by a few enthusiasts, usually for recurrent disease, with good results (Boger and Pinkham, 1951; Rupnick, 1958). Guyuron et al (1983) reported a median hospital stay of 10 days, a period off work of only 5 weeks, and only five recurrences in 58 patients (see Table 17.5).

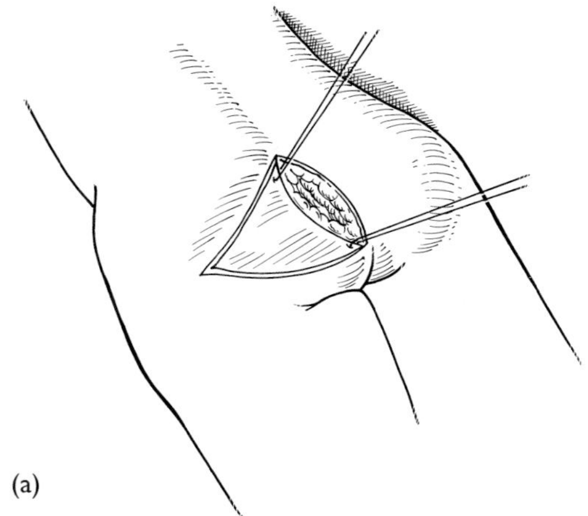

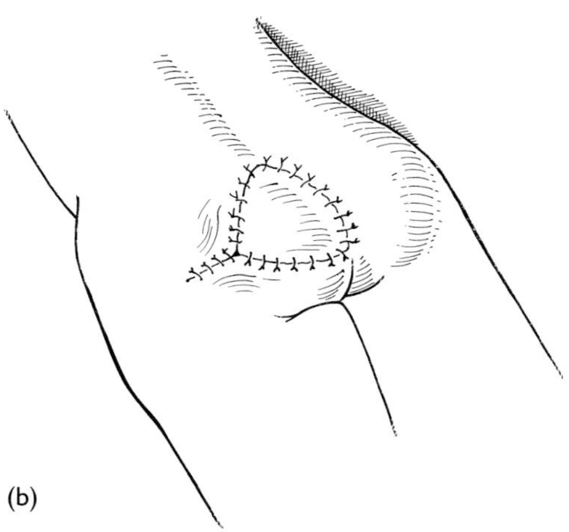

Figure 17.19a,b A V–Y-plasty for reconstruction after pilonidal sinus excision. (a) The entire pilonidal sinus is excised. A long lateral V incision is made and skin mobilized to achieve primary closure using a Y-plasty. (b) After the operation.

CONCLUSIONS AND RECOMMENDATIONS

We make no apologies for stressing the role of conservative management in pilonidal sinus since it is a self-limiting disease in which treatment may inflict far more morbidity than the disease itself. The importance of anal hygiene and judicious shaving cannot be overemphasized. As can be seen, the elective treatment of pilonidal sinus is varied and outcome depends a great deal on the diligence of the patient in keeping the area clean and free of hair. Different surgeons will have fixed views as to optimum treatment. It is therefore a matter of opinion as to which procedure is favoured. In our view, acute pilonidal abscess should be managed by drainage alone. For most patients with an inactive pilonidal sinus, some form of minimal surgery is usually successful, provided local depilatory measures and hygiene are strictly adhered to. We prefer excision of midline pits and clearing of the tracks using the Lord or Bascom approach. If conservative surgery is unsuccessful, excision and primary closure leaving a wound away from the midline is preferred if the disease is quiescent. For infected sinus treatment we prefer excision and open wound management rather than major reconstructive methods.

REFERENCES

Abramson DJ (1970) An open semi primary closure operation for pilonidal sinuses, using local anaesthesia. *Dis Colon Rectum* **13**: 215–219.

Anderson MJ Jr & Dockerty MB (1958) Perianal hidradenitis suppurativa: a clinical and pathologic study. *Dis Colon Rectum* **1**: 23–31.

Armstrong JH & Barcia PJ (1994) Pilonidal sinus disese: the conservative approach. *Arch Surg* **129**: 914–919.

Azab ASC, Kamal MS, Saat RA, Abou al Atta KA & Ali NA (1984) Radical cure for pilonidal sinus by a transposition rhomboid flap. *Br J Surg* **71**: 154–155.

Baek LSM, Williams GD, McElhinney AJ & Simon BE (1980) A gluteus maximus myocutaneous island flap for the repair of a sacral decubitus ulcer. *Ann Plast Surg* **5**: 471–476.

Bascom JU (1980) Pilonidal disease: origin from follicles of hairs and results of follicle removal as treatment. *Surgery* **87**: 567–572.

Bascom JU (1983) Pilonidal disease: long-term results of follicle removal. *Dis Colon Rectum* **26**: 800–807.

Bascom JU (1987) Repeat pilonidal operations. *Am J Surg* **154**: 118–122.

Boger EV & Pinkham EW Jr (1951) Primary split-skin graft in treatment of pilonidal cysts. *US Armed Forces Med J* **2**: 1733–1736.

Brearley R (1955) Pilonidal sinus; a new theory of origin. *Br J Surg* **43**: 62–67.

Broadrick GL, Ehrlich FE & Kramer SG (1971) Simplified treatment of pilonidal disease on an outpatient basis. *Surgery* **70**: 630–637.

Buie LA & Curtiss RK (1952) Pilonidal disease. *Surg Clin North Am* **32**: 1247–1259.

Calapinto ND (1977) Umbilical pilonidal sinus. *Br J Surg* **64**: 494–495.

Casberg MA (1949) Infected pilonidal cysts and sinuses. *Bull US Army Med Dept* **9**: 493–496.

Cavanagh CR, Schnug GE, Girvin GW & McGonigle DJ (1979) Definitive marsupialization of the acute pilonidal abscess. *Am Surg* **36**: 650–651.

Chavez C, Raffo A & Larenas P (1988) Quista sacrocoxigeo: un tratamiento quirurgico definitivo y sus fundamentos fisiopatalogicos. *Cuader Chil Cirug* **32**: 285–288.

Cherry JK (1968) Primary closure of pilonidal sinus. *Surg Gynecol Obstet* **126**: 1263–1269.

Clery AP & Clery AB (1963) Pilonidal disease of the umbilicus. *Br J Surg* **50**: 666–668.

Close AS (1955) Pilonidal cysts: an analysis of surgical failures. *Ann Surg* **141**: 523–526.

Clothier PR & Haywood IR (1984) The natural history of the post anal (pilonidal) sinus. *Ann R Coll Surg Engl* **66**: 201–203.

Currie AR, Gibson T & Goodall AL (1953) Interdigital sinuses of barber's hands. *Br J Surg* **41**: 278–286.

Dortan HE (1970) Conservative treatment of pilonidal disease. *Am Surg* **36**: 349.

Dwight R & Maloy K (1953) Pilonidal sinus, experience with 449 cases. *N Engl J Med* **249**: 926.

Edwards MH (1977) Pilonidal sinus: a 5-year appraisal of the Millar–Lord treatment. *Br J Surg* **64**: 867–868.

Eftaiha M & Abcarian H (1977) The dilemma of pilonidal disease: surgical treatment. *Dis Colon Rectum* **20**: 279–286.

Ewing MR (1947) Hair-bearing sinus. *Lancet* **i**: 427.

Farringer JL & Pickens DR (1978) Pilonidal cyst: an operative approach. *Am J Surg* **135**: 262–264.

Fishbein RH & Handelsman JC (1979) A method for primary reconstruction following radical excision of sacrococcygeal pilonidal disease. *Ann Surg* **190**: 231–235.

Foss MVL (1970) Pilonidal sinus: excision and closure. *Proc R Soc Med* **63**: 752.

Fox SL (1935) The origin of pilonidal sinus, with an analysis of its comparative anatomy and histogenesis. *Surg Gynecol Obstet* **60**: 137–149.

Fuzun M, Bakir H, Soylu M et al (1994) Which technique for treatment of pilonidal sinus – open or closed? *Dis Colon Rectum* **37**: 1148–1150.

Gabriel WB (1963) *Principles and Practice of Rectal Surgery*, 5th edn. London: HK Lewis.

Gage AA & Dutta P (1977) Cryosurgery for pilonidal disease. *Am J Surg* **133**: 249–254.

Galizia G, Lieto E, Castellano P et al (1995) Radical treatment of pilonidal disease with Dufourmentel's technique. *Int J Surg Sci* **2**: 207–211.

Gillis L (1954) Infected traumatic epidermoid cysts: the result of rubbing by an artificial limb. *Proc R Soc Med* **47**: 9.

Golz A, Argov S & Barzilai A (1980) Pilonidal sinus disease: comparison among various methods of treatment and a survey of 160 patients. *Curr Surg* **37**: 77–85.

Goodall P (1961) The aetiology and treatment of pilonidal sinus. *Br J Surg* **49**: 212–218.

Goodall P (1975) Management of pilonidal sinus. *Proc R Soc Med* **68**: 675.

Guyuron B, Dinner MI & Dowden RV (1983) Excision and grafting in treatment of recurrent pilonidal sinus disease. *Surg Gynecol Obstet* **156**: 201–204.

Gwynn BR (1986) Use of the rhomboid flap in pilonidal sinus. *Ann R Coll Surg Engl* **68**: 40–41.

Hamilton JE, Stephens G & Claugus EC (1963) Pilonidal sinus: excision and primary closure. *Surgery* **54**: 597–603.

Hanley PH (1980) Acute pilonidal abscess. *Surg Gynecol Obstet* **150**: 9–11.

Haworth JC & Zachary RB (1955) Congenital dermal sinus in children: their relation to pilonidal sinuses. *Lancet* **ii**: 101–114.

Healy MJ & Hoffert PW (1955) Pilonidal sinus and cyst. *Surg Clin North Am* **35**: 1497–1502.

Hegge HGJ, Vos GA, Patka P & Hoitsma HFW (1987) Treatment of complicated or infected pilonidal sinus disease by local application of phenol. *Surgery* **102**: 52–54.

Hirshowitz B, Mahler D & Kaufmann-Friedmann K (1970) Treatment of pilonidal sinus. *Surg Gynecol Obstet* **131**: 119–122.

Holm J & Hulten L (1970) Simple primary closure of pilonidal sinus. *Acta Chir Scand* **136**: 537–540.

Hopping RA (1954) Pilonidal disease. *Am J Surg* **88**: 780–788.

Hueston JT (1953) The aetiology of the pilonidal sinus. *Br J Surg* **41**: 307–311.

Jensen SL & Harling H (1988) Prognosis after simple incision and drainage for a first-episode acute pilonidal abscess. *Br J Surg* **75**: 60–61.

Jones DJ (1992) Pilonidal sinus. *BMJ* **305**: 410–412.

Karydakis GE (1973) New approach to the problem of pilonidal sinus. *Lancet* **ii**: 1414–1415.

Kharia HS & Brown JH (1995) Excision and primary suture of pilonidal sinus. *Ann R Coll Surg Engl* **77**: 242–244.

Khatri VP, Espinosa MH & Amin AK (1994) Management of recurrent pilonidal sinus by simple V–Y fasciocutaneous flap. *Dis Colon Rectum* **37**: 1232–1235.

Kitchen PRB (1996) Pilonidal sinus: experience with the Karydakis flap. *Br J Surg* **83**: 1452–1455.

Kooistra HP (1942) Pilonidal sinuses: a review of the literature and report of 350 cases. *Am J Surg* **55**: 3–17.

Kronborg O, Christensen K & Zimmermann-Nielsen C (1985) Chronic pilonidal disease: a randomized trial with a complete 3-year follow-up. *Br J Surg* **72**: 303–304.

Lamke LO, Larsson J & Nylen B (1974) Results of different types of operation for pilonidal sinus. *Acta Chir Scand* **140**: 321–324.

Lord PH (1975) Anorectal problems: etiology of pilonidal sinus. *Dis Colon Rectum* **18**: 661–664.

Lord PH (1984) *Presidential Address: Pilonidal Sinus*. London: Royal Society of Medicine.

Lord PH & Millar DM (1965) Pilonidal sinus: a simple treatment. *Br J Surg* **52**: 292–300.

McCaughan JS (1965) The results of surgical treatment of pilonidal cysts. *Surg Gynecol Obstet* **121**: 316–318.

MacFee WF (1942) Pilonidal cysts and sinuses: a method of wound closure. *Ann Surg* **116**: 687–699.

McLaren CA (1984) Partial closure and other techniques in pilonidal surgery: an assessment of 157 cases. *Br J Surg* **71**: 561–562.

Mann CV & Springall (1987) 'D' excision for sacrococcygeal pilonidal sinus disease. *J R Soc Med* **80**: 292–295.

Mansoory A & Dickson D (1982) Z-plasty for treatment of disease of the pilonidal sinus. *Surg Gynecol Obstet* **155**: 409–411.

Manterola C, Barroso M, Araya JC & Fonseca L (1991) Pilonidal disease: 25 cases treated by the Dufourmentel technique. *Dis Colon Rectum* **34**: 649–652.

Marks J, Harding KG, Hughes LE & Ribeiro CD (1985) Pilonidal sinus excision: healing by open granulation. *Br J Surg* **72**: 637–640.

Matt JG (1958) Carcinomatous degeneration of pilonidal cysts. *Dis Colon Rectum* **1**: 353–355.

Matter I, Kunin J, Schein M & Eldar S (1995) Total excision versus non-resectional methods in the treatment of acute and chronic pilonidal disease. *Br J Surg* **82**: 752–753.

Maurice BA & Greenwood RK (1964) A conservative treatment of pilonidal sinus. *Br J Surg* **51**: 510–512.

Middleton MD (1968) Treatment of pilonidal sinus by Z-plasty. *Br J Surg* **55**: 516–518.

Minami RT, Mills R & Pardoe R (1977) Gluteus maximus myocutaneous flaps for the repair of pressure sores. *Plast Reconstr Surg* **60**: 242–249.

Monro RS & McDermott FT (1965) The elimination of casual factors in pilonidal sinus treated by Z-plasty. *Br J Surg* **52**: 177–179.

Notaras MJ (1970) A review of three popular methods of treatment of postanal (pilonidal) sinus disease. *Br J Surg* **57**: 886–890.

O'Connor JJ (1979) Surgery plus freezing as a technique for treating pilonidal disease. *Dis Colon Rectum* **22**: 306–307.

Oldfield MC (1956) A barber's interdigital pilonidal sinus. *Lancet* **ii**: 1244–1245.

Ortiz HH, Marti J & Stiges A (1977) Pilonidal sinus: a claim for simple track incision. *Dis Colon Rectum* **20**: 325–328.

Ortiz H, Marti J, DeMiguel M, Carmona A & Cabanas IP (1987) Hair-containing lesions within the anal canal. *Int J Colorect Dis* **2**: 153–154.

Palmer WH (1959) Pilonidal disease: a new concept of pathogenesis. *Dis Colon Rectum* **2**: 301–303.

Palumbo LT, Larimore OM & Katz IA (1951) Pilonidal cysts and sinuses: a statistical review. *Arch Surg* **63**: 852–857.

Patey DH (1969) A reappraisal of the acquired theory of sacrococcygeal pilonidal sinus and an assessment of its influence on surgical practice. *Br J Surg* **56**: 463–466.

Patey DH & Scarff RW (1946) Pathology of postanal pilonidal sinus: its bearing on treatment. *Lancet* **ii**: 484.

Patey DH & Williams ELS (1956) Pilonidal sinus of the umbilicus. *Lancet* **ii**: 281–282.

Pérez-Gurri JA, Temple WJ & Ketcham AS (1984) Gluteus maximus myocutaneous flap for the treatment of recalcitrant pilonidal disease. *Dis Colon Rectum* **27**: 262–264.

Philipsen SJ, Gray G, Goldsmith E et al (1981) Carcinoma arising in pilonidal sinuses. *Ann Surg* **193**: 506–512.

Raffman RH (1959) A re-evaluation of the pathogenesis of pilonidal sinus. *Ann Surg* **150**: 895–898.

Rainsbury RM & Southam JA (1982) Radical surgery for pilonidal sinus. *Ann R Coll Surg Engl* **64**: 339–341.

Rupnick EJ (1958) Primary split skin grafting for treatment of large pilonidal cysts. *US Armed Forces Med J Q* **9**: 957–964.

Schneider IHF, Thaler K & Kockerling F (1994) Treatment of pilonidal sinuses by phenol injections. *Int J Colorect Dis* **9**: 200–202.

Sebrechts TH & Anderson JP (1971) Common sense in the treatment of pilonidal disease. *Dis Colon Rectum* **14**: 57–61.

Senapati A & Thompson MR (1996) The outpatient management of pilonidal sinus: Bascom's operation. Presented at Royal Society of Medicine, unpublished.

Shoesmith JH (1953) Pilonidal sinus in an above-knee amputation stump. *Lancet* **ii**: 378–379.

Shorey BA (1975) Pilonidal sinus treated by phenol injection. *Br J Surg* **62**: 407–408.

Smith TE (1948) Anterior or perineal pilonidal cysts. *JAMA 136*: 973–975.

Søndenaa K & Pollard ML (1992) Histology of chronic pilonidal sinus. *APMIS* **103**: 267–272.

Søndenaa K, Andersen E, Nesvik I & Søreide JA (1995a) Patient characteristics and symptoms in chronic pilonidal sinus disease. *Int J Colorect Dis* **10**: 39–42.

Søndenaa K, Nesvik I, Andersen E, Natås O & Søreide JA (1995b) Bacteriology and complications of chronic pilonidal sinus treated with excision and primary suture. *Int J Colorect Dis* **10**: 161–166.

Søndenaa K, Nesvik I, Andersen E & Søreide JA (1995c) Recurrence rate of chronic pilonidal sinus. *Eur J Surg*.

Sood SC, Green JR & Parui R (1975) Results of various operations for sacrococcygeal pilonidal disease. *Plast Reconstr Surg* **56**: 559–566.

Spivak H, Brooks VL, Nussbaum M & Friedman I (1996) Treatment of chronic pilonidal disease. *Dis Colon Rectum* **39**: 1136–1139.

Taylor BA & Hughes LE (1984) Circumferential perianal pilonidal sinuses. *Dis Colon Rectum* **27**: 120–122.

Thomas D (1968) Pilonidal sinus: a review of the literature and a report of 100 cases. *Med J Aust* **2**: 184–188.

Thorlakson RN (1966) Pilonidal sinus of the umbilicus. *Br J Surg* **53**: 76–78.

Vallance S (1982) Pilonidal fistulas mimicking fistulas-in-ano. *Br J Surg* **69**: 161–162.

Walsh TH & Mann CV (1983) Pilonidal sinuses of the anal canal. *Br J Surg* **70**: 23–24.

Weale FE (1964) A comparison of barber's and postanal pilonidal sinuses. *Br J Surg* **51**: 513–516.

Weston SD & Schlachter IS (1963) Pilonidal cyst of the anal canal. *Dis Colon Rectum* **6**: 139–141.

Williams ES (1955) Quoted by Patey DH & Scarff RW. In Pilonidal sinus. *Lancet* **i**: 772.

Wilson E, Failes DG & Killingback M (1971) Pilonidal sinuses of the anal canal. *Dis Colon Rectum* **14**: 468–470.

Wood RAB & Hughes LE (1975) Silicone foam sponge for pilonidal sinus: a new technique for dressing open granulating wounds. *BMJ* **4**: 131–133.

Zimmerman CE (1984) Outpatient excision and primary closure of pilonidal cysts and sinuses: long-term follow-up. *Am J Surg* **148**: 658–659.

18

PERIANAL WARTS

Condylomata acuminata are caused by up to 60 different strains of the human papillomavirus (HPV). Types 6 and 11 are typically associated with benign disease whereas types 16 and 18 are more likely to lead to invasive squamous cell carcinoma. The disorder is invariably sexually transmitted. The high proportion of male patients affected suggests that perianal warts are often acquired as a result of homosexual contact with an infected partner, but heterosexual acquisition is also frequent. However, not all condylomata are acquired by sexual contact; the virus may persist in skin and can be transmitted by hands.

Perianal lesions are often inadequately eradicated by local topical therapy and there is a high risk of recurrence after all forms of treatment. In many cases recurrence may be due to reinfection. Diathermy excision has been the mainstay of surgical treatment, but scissor excision is associated with a lower incidence of scarring and stenosis in extensive lesions. Combination therapy with adjuvant topical interferon and surgery may be advised for recurrent and extensive warts. Interferon should be avoided in HIV-positive patients; in this group, topical 5FU combined with surgery might be a better alternative.

HPV types 16 and 18 are associated with cervical and anal intra-epithelial neoplasia which may progress to invasive squamous cell carcinoma, particularly in homosexual and heterosexual men, with HIV patients being particularly at risk. Such high-risk patients need careful surveillance.

AETIOLOGY AND PREDISPOSING FACTORS

Human papillomavirus (HPV)

The human papillomavirus which causes perianal warts (Billingham and Lewis, 1982) is biochemically, antigenically and immunologically distinct from verruca vulgaris, the virus responsible for the common wart. HPV 1 and 4 are associated with plantar warts and HPV 2 is usually responsible for verruca vulgaris. In contrast, genital warts are caused by HPV 6 and 11 (80%), HPV 2 (18%), and HPV 16 and 18 (2%) (Frasier, 1994; Cohen et al, 1990). For years it has been known that warts can be transmitted by a cell-free filtrate (Lewis and Wheeler, 1967). Later electron microscopic studies reported by Oriel and Almeida (1970) indicated that intracellular virus particles and inclusion bodies were present in 13 of 25 patients with anogenital warts. The incubation period for HPV is 1–6 months and the virus of condylomata acuminata is difficult to eradicate.

There are more than 60 types of HPV (deVilliers, 1989). Those associated with anal condylomata are usually types 6, 11 and 2. Types 6 and 11 are typically associated with benign disease (Duggan et al, 1989; Langenberg et al, 1993). Types 16 and 18 are far less common but these are associated with cervical cancer (Lorinez et al, 1987) and invasive squamous cell carcinoma of the anus and perianal region.

Accuracy of DNA typing is dependent on the method used. A single virus type is not always present; in fact, mixed infections were reported in 42% when material from condylomata, dysplasia and squamous cell carcinoma were examined (Duggan et al, 1989). Furthermore, sequential biopsies found different types on different days in 50/63 patients, so the HPV type may vary on different occasions. Thus, finding type 6 or 11 does not ensure a low risk of malignancy and emphasizes the importance of completely clearing these infections, as well as ensuring adequate follow-up.

Transmission

The disease is spread principally by intercourse from subjects carrying the virus in the urethra, vagina or anorectum. The task of tracing all contacts, particularly in promiscuous homosexual men, may be impossible. Another mechanism of infection is that the virus lies dormant on the mucosa of the anorectum and may result in the formation of anal warts only following local trauma which allows the virus access to the tissues (Young, 1964). Against this theory is the evidence that warts rarely, if ever, complicate other surgical operations or disorders like fissure or fistula which are associated with tissue damage.

With increasing exposure of children to sexual abuse, sexually transmitted condyloma acuminata are becoming more prevalent in children – quite apart from the risk of transmission at birth from an infected birth canal, transplacental spread or by infected hands (Stumpf, 1980; Raimer, 1992; Budayr et al, 1996). There are a few patients who are not sexually active who acquire perianal warts from hand-borne transmission.

Recurrence and reinfection

The high recurrence of genital warts after therapy is caused by many factors. Repeated inoculation from continued sexual contact is one of the most common reasons for recurrence (Greene, 1992). HPV has a long incubation period and the virus may lie dormant in the skin for a considerable length of time, especially in thick keratinized hair-bearing areas which may be resistant to topical therapy and which are not in close proximity to lymphatics (Hatch, 1991). HPV in pilosebaceous appendages may cause reinfection from hair shafts and sweat glands. Also there may be missed lesions causing a reservoir of infection, as in the anal canal.

AIDS

Condylomata acuminata is sexually transmitted and although perianal warts may be seen in heterosexual men and women, it is now becoming particularly common among promiscuous homosexual men (Marino, 1964; Waugh, 1972; Sohn and Robilotti, 1977). Of the 80 patients with perianal warts reported by Oriel (1971), 72 were men and 95% admitted to homosexual practices. Similarly, a high proportion of women with the disease admit to having had anal intercourse (Abcarian and Sharon, 1982). Condylomata acuminata are a frequent feature among HIV-positive and AIDS patients. In a study of 97 men with AIDS, 54% had HIV infection (Palefsky et al, 1990). There is evidence in these patients of malignant transformation to AIN (intraepithelial neoplasia) in 15% which may progress to carcinoma-in-situ and invasive anogenital squamous cell carcinoma, often at an early age (Burns and van Goidsenhoven, 1970; Daling et al, 1982; Croxson et al, 1984; Longo et al, 1986; Bradshaw et al, 1992).

Transplant recipients

Immunocompromised patients in general have a higher incidence of condylomata acuminata and anogenital neoplasia than the general population (Sillman and Sedlis, 1991). Genital warts are reported to affect 43% of renal transplant recipients. Furthermore the increased survival of transplant patients increases the risk of recurrence and dysplastic premalignant lesions (Palefsky, 1991).

Coexisting disease

A history of associated sexually transmitted disease is extremely common. Abcarian and Sharon (1982) reported that 75% of their patients in Chicago had attended STD clinics for treatment of other warts or sexually transmitted diseases such as gonorrhoea, Chlamydia, herpes or Cryptosporidium, and some had syphilis (Table 18.1). A similar pattern of coexisting disease was observed in Copenhagen (Jensen, 1985). Of the 185 men with anal condylomata in Chicago (Abcarian and Sharon, 1982), 74 had antibodies to hepatitis A or B, 20 had parasitic infections and 14 had enteropathogens associated with the gay bowel syndrome (Table 18.2). A more recent survey of such individuals would undoubtedly have recovered many with the HIV virus and other pathogens associated with sexually transmitted diseases, such as Chlamydia, herpes simplex, Gardnerella and cryptosporidia (Andrews et al, 1986).

Table 18.1 History of sexually transmitted disease in 200 patients with anal condylomata acuminata.

Type	*No. of patients*
Gonococcal urethritis	35
Gonococcal proctitis	24
Penile syphilitic chancre	5
Anal syphilitic chancre	4
Scrotal chancre	1
Pelvic inflammatory disease	1
Genital herpes	5*

* Four men, one woman.
From Abcarian and Sharon (1982).

Table 18.2 History of communicable disease in 185 men with anal condylomata acuminatum.

Type	*No. of patients*
Hepatitis (A or B)	74
Parasitic disease (amoebiasis, giardiasis)	20
Shigellosis	14
Scabies	9
Phthiriasis	4

From Abcarian and Sharon (1982).

INCIDENCE

The incidence of anal condylomata is increasing (Sohn and Robilotti, 1977). It is the most common sexually transmitted disease (Bradshaw et al, 1992) and now represents a serious public health problem with one million new cases seen yearly (Department of Health and Social Security, 1979; Centers for Disease Control, 1986). Many more patients with anal lesions are now being referred directly to STD clinics, particularly as both general practitioners and the public are becoming more concerned with tracing contacts and identifying individuals who may be at risk of carrying the AIDS virus. AIDS patients and those receiving immunosuppression following transplantation are particularly susceptible to anogenital warts (van Driel et al, 1996).

Males are more commonly affected than women: the ratio varies in the literature, from 9.2:1 to 3:1 (Powell et al, 1970; Swerdlow and Salvati, 1971; Abcarian and Sharon, 1982; Jensen, 1985).

Condylomata acuminata affect people who are most sexually active and the majority of patients are 20–30 years of age (Table 18.3). Some children are now acquiring infection at birth or from sexual abuse (Budayr et al, 1996).

Table 18.3 Age distribution of patients with condylomata acuminatum.

Age (years)	*Men*	*Women*
<20	3	2
20–30	92	3
30–40	76	6
40–50	10	2
50–60	3	2
>60	1	0
Total	185	15

APPEARANCE AND SITES OF CONDYLOMATA

Warts may be discrete or multiple; they are usually elevated pink vegetative excrescences in the anal canal and on the surrounding perianal skin. Large lesions may coalesce to form polypoidal pedunculated or sessile masses which become hypertrophic with surface keratinization. Lesions tend to be moist and easily traumatized, resulting in perianal bleeding.

Table 18.4 Distribution of lesions.

	Number		
	Podophyllin	Surgical excision	Total
Perianal alone	4 (13)	6 (20)	10 (17)
Perianal plus:			
Anal canal	12 (40)	10 (33)	22 (37)
Anal canal, genitalia	5 (17)	6 (20)	11 (18)
Anal canal, genitalia, rectum	1 (3)	0	1 (2)
Genitalia	6 (20)	5 (17)	11 (18)
Rectum	2 (7)	3 (10)	5 (9)

Values in parentheses are percentages.
From Jensen (1985).

Warts often involve the anal canal but most authorities suggest that rectal involvement is uncommon (Corman, 1984). However, Jensen (1985) records involvement above the dentate line in 5 of 60 patients (9%) (Table 18.4). Warts are commonly located elsewhere, in particular on the penis, vulva, scrotum, vagina and urethra (Abcarian and Sharon, 1982). Other sites of involvement include the hands, feet and face (Table 18.5).

Table 18.5 Warts associated with anal and perianal condylomata.

Location	Men	Women
Plantar	4	0
Hands	2	1
Facial	3	0
Urethral	4	3
Penile	12	—
Scrotal	12	—
Vulva	—	7
Vaginal	—	5

From Abcarian and Sharon (1982).

CLINICAL FEATURES

Patients usually complain of pruritus ani and swellings that bleed during defecation. Pain may be a feature and vaginal discharge is common in women (Table 18.6). Many patients will already have been treated for anogenital condylomata (Table 18.7). The duration of history is variable but most patients seek advice and treatment within 4–12 weeks. Occasionally warts will regress spontaneously (Pyrhonen and Johansson, 1975; Williams et al, 1976; LeBlanc et al, 1985; Kirby, 1988).

Table 18.6 Presenting symptoms.

Symptom	Podophyllin	Surgical excision	Total
Feeling of lumps	26	27	53 (88)
Anal itching or discharge	21	23	44 (73)
Bleeding	11	13	24 (40)
Pain or discomfort	6	8	14 (23)
Vaginal discharge	2	1	3 (20)

Values in parentheses are percentages.
From Jensen (1985).

Table 18.7 Methods of prior treatment in 80 patients with recurrent anal condylomata acuminata.

Type of therapy*	No. of patients
Podophyllin	75
Single surgical excision	44
Multiple surgical excisions	26
Outpatient fulguration	17
Acid compounds	11
Cryotherapy	6

*Many patients were treated with multiple treatment modalities.

HISTOLOGY AND MALIGNANT CHANGE

Histologically, condylomata acuminata are squamous papillomas. The principal microscopic features are papillomatosis, hyperkeratinization, acanthosis and the presence of clear cells within the acanthotic epithelium. Normally, maturation, polarity and mild atypia is evident in the epithelium. If the lesions have been recently treated by podophyllin, enlarged cells become prominent, with a pale basophilic cytoplasm, dispersed chromatin and large perinuclear and paranuclear vacuolization. Sometimes, eosinophilic cells with pyknotic nuclei or other nuclear alterations are seen after podophyllin treatment. These histological features are temporary and will regress completely within a few days of discontinuing treatment (Prasad and Abcarian, 1980). Kovi et al (1974) reported aggregates of uniform spherical particles in the nuclei of anal condylomata.

Giant condylomata may become locally invasive without penetrating lymphatics or blood vessels and are known as Buschke–Lowenstein tumours (Buschke and Lowenstein, 1925; Macharek and Weakley, 1960; Khoblich and Failing, 1967). They invade surrounding structures, such as the sacrum, coccyx, buttocks or even the abdominal wall (Judge, 1969; Shah and Hertz, 1972; Abcarian et al, 1976; Alexander and Kaminsky, 1979; Elliot et al, 1979). Sometimes they may undergo frank malignant change (Prasad and Abcarian, 1980; Lee et al, 1981) and, if so, treatment may fail to control the destruction of local structures, particularly the meninges, rectum and perineum, resulting in fatal sepsis (Shah and Hertz, 1972). In a review of 42 cases, the recurrence rate was 66% and malignant transformation occurred in 56% (Chu et al, 1994). This tumour is associated with HPV types 6 and 11.

Squamous metaplasia and *in situ* change has been recognized for many years in anal condylomata, even of short duration, in young men (Konketzny, 1914; Grisson and Delvaneo, 1915; Siegal, 1962). Some of these lesions become frankly malignant and result in invasive squamous cell carcinoma (Friedberg and Serlin, 1963; Sturm et al, 1975). One variant is Bowenoid papulosis or carcinoma-in-situ usually associated with HPV type 16 or 18 (Greene, 1992). Prasad and Abcarian (1980) reported six patients in their series of 330 (1.8%) with malignant change; two had giant condylomata, and frank malignant invasion had developed in four. Many more cases of invasive carcinoma have since been identified, particularly in homosexuals, immunocompromised patients and those with AIDS (Congilosi and Madoff, 1995).

Papillomavirus has considerable malignant potential (Syverton, 1952). Ejeckam et al (1983) showed that the virus-induced Shope papilloma in rabbits underwent malignant change in 25% of animals. Longo et al (1986) reported a patient with a 15-month history of anal warts in whom *in situ* malignant change was identified in the surgical excision specimen. Thirteen similar cases have been reported (Oriel and Whimster, 1971; Fitzgerald and Hamit, 1974; Kovi et al, 1974; Croxson et al, 1984; LeBlanc et al, 1985). Ten of the 13 recorded cases were homosexuals, five had AIDS, there was a further patient with a Kaposi sarcoma, and one patient had been treated for a lymphoma.

Immunological factors are thought to play an important role in the malignant potential of this virus-induced cancer (Pyrhonen and Johansson, 1975). Longo et al (1986) suggested that a similar malignant potential occurred in Bowen's disease and Paget's disease of the anus (Scoma and Levy, 1975; Williams et al, 1976). The natural history of AIDS patients with warts who develop carcinoma-in-situ differs from the non-AIDS group. Those with the HIV virus seem to progress rapidly from warts to *in situ* change. By contrast, a long history of recurrent warts over many years is recorded in patients who are not AIDS sufferers but who develop malignant change. Furthermore, the recent increase in malignant change in perianal warts and the rising prevalence of AIDS in some societies seems more than coincidence.

Dysplasia should not be confused with the changes which occur following local therapy. Severe atypia and loss of polarity is rare following topical treatment, whereas the changes occurring after podophyllin are usually transitory. Once malignant cells invade the stroma the diagnosis of malignant transformation should not be in doubt and these lesions should be treated as any other squamous cell carcinoma of the region (Sawyers, 1972; Buroker et al, 1976, 1977; Cummings et al, 1982). The intranuclear virus particles commonly present in benign condylomata were not observed by Prasad and Abcarian (1980) in lesions undergoing malignant change.

It appears, therefore, that there are two distinct potential malignant processes in condylomata acuminata. The giant condylomata of Buschke and Lowenstein is malignant from inception and probably represents a locally agressive variant of squamous cell carcinoma. In contrast, the carcinoma-in-situ seen in long-standing perianal warts is not normally a malignant process but represents, like Bowen's disease and possibly Paget's disease, a cutaneous manifestation of a lesion which is predisposed to develop cancer (Sigurgeirsson et al, 1991). This malignant transformation is accelerated by viral and immunological factors. Hence immunocompromised or AIDS patients have a greater risk of rapid malignant change. Likewise, whereas HPV 6 and 11 have low oncogenicity, HPV 16 and 18 may induce high-grade genital intra-epithelial neoplasia and eventual malignancy (Reid and Lorencz, 1991).

Malignant change has also been recorded in vulval warts (Charlewood and Shippel, 1953; Rhatigan and Saffos, 1977) and penile warts (Moriame, 1950; Rhatigan et al, 1971; Sigurgeirsson et al, 1991).

The association between anal warts, homosexual behaviour and anal cancer is now recognized, and is similar to the link between cervical cancer and its associations with human papillomavirus. A half of patients with anal cancer have HPV type 16 and 18 DNA incorporated into the genome of their tumour cells (Scholefield et al, 1991), but there is a great variation in the prevelance of HPV 16 associated anal cancer throughout the world (Northfield, 1991). Some patients with genital warts have evidence of intra-epithelial neoplasia (AIN), which is a recognized premalignant entity. A study of 210 homosexual and bisexual men revealed evidence of intra-epithelia neoplasia in 35%, and anal warts and HIV were independent risk factors for AIN (Carter et al, 1995). There is growing support for the view that the increasing incidence of genital HPV infection will ultimately lead to an increased incidence of anal cancer (Jones and James, 1992). A study of 53 anal carcinomas revealed that 18 were associated with HPV; DNA studies showed principally HPV 6 and 11 in perianal cancers and HPV 16 and 18 in anal cancer (Ramanujam et al, 1996). However, there are no long-term studies to confirm or refute the hypothesis that AIN in anal warts, especially in HIV patients, actually progresses to anal cancer (Morgan et al, 1994).

INVESTIGATIONS AND DIFFERENTIAL DIAGNOSIS

Investigations

A search should be made for sexual contacts. The risk of reinfection must be clearly explained. Other sexually transmitted infections, particularly AIDS, hepatitis, gonorrhoea, lymphogranuloma venereum and syphilis, should be excluded by serology and bacterial culture. These patients should also be screened to exclude Chlamydia, herpes simplex and specific enteropathogens.

A thorough clinical assessment should include a search for oral, vaginal, urethral, vesical as well as penile and scrotal warts. Patients should have a colposcopy to exclude CIN3 or VIN3 as well as a routine speculum exam to search for vaginal warts. A proctosigmoidoscopy should be performed to exclude anorectal warts and, since the urethra may also be involved, cystourethroscopy is advised. Biopsies of suspicious lesions should be taken to exclude carcinoma-in-situ.

Differential diagnosis

The only disorders likely to be confused with anal condylomata are condylomata lata of secondary syphilis and squamous cell carcinoma.

Condylomata lata are smoother and rather flatter than condylomata acuminata and there may be other signs of syphillis such as a maculopapular rash or snail track ulcers. In condylomata lata there is induration and the weeping mass contains numerous spirochaetes which can easily be seen under the microscope by dark-ground illumination of smears taken from the lesion. Serology at this stage is also always positive.

Squamous cell carcinoma may begin as a polypoidal mass emerging from the anus and can be quite difficult to distinguish macroscopically from anal condylomata. With time, the lesions ulcerate and invade surrounding structures and are associated with lymphatic and eventually disseminated metastatic disease. Differentiation between anal condylomata and malignancy may be possible only by total local excision.

CONSERVATIVE TREATMENT AND SEXUAL COUNSELLING

Conservative topical therapy is usually commenced in the STD clinic, by the general practitioner or even by the patients themselves (see Table 18.7). Topical applications consist primarily of chemical and antimitotic agents. Immunotherapy and interferon and may have a role but should probably be avoided in AIDS patients and transplant recipients.

One of the most common reasons for early recurrence of warts after successful initial treatment (Thomson and Grace, 1978) is reinfection caused by further sexual intercourse with the same or a new partner carrying the virus. Hence Jensen (1985) stressed the importance not only of examining all partners but explaining to patients the risks of treatment failure if they continue their promiscuous habits. Patients are strongly advised to refrain from sexual intercourse during the treatment period. Advice concerning abstinence is often ignored. Patients should be told to wear a contraceptive sheath during intercourse and for 4 months after completion of treatment. Sexual partners should be traced and offered treatment if anal condylomata are present.

Chemical agents

Podophyllin

Podophyllin is a resin extract from the root of the May apple plant. The active agent podophyllotoxin is antimitotic. It remains the most widely used topical chemical agent and has been used with variable success for at least 50 years (Kaplan, 1942; Marks, 1947). Podophyllin may be applied in a solution of liquid paraffin or in benzoin tincture, as either a 10% or 20% concentration (Culp and Kaplan, 1944). Recently, purified podophyllotoxin emulsions of 0.25% and 0.5% have become available for therapy, which can be self-administered (Wang et al, 1994; Syed et al, 1994). Simmons (1981) compared treatment with 10% and 25% solutions of conventional podophyllotoxin but found that only approximately 25% of lesions completely disappeared, despite repeated applications over 3 months. Podophyllin may cause skin irritation and must be applied with great care; it cannot be used in the anal canal. Reported complications of podophyllin include severe necrosis, scarring and fistula-in-ano (Congilosi and Madoff, 1995). From this point of view, preparations of purified podophyllotoxin are an advantage and may be more effective than podophyllin (Bonnez et al, 1994).

Conventional podophyllin is applied to the warts with cotton-wool swabs on a stick. The solution is allowed a contact time of between 5 and 10 minutes, after which it is washed off. The process is repeated weekly for up to 3 months. In contrast, purified podophyllotoxin can be self-administered to perianal lesions and applied locally in the clinic to anal lesions. However, many clinicians advise surgical excision of intra-anal condylomata (Table 18.8).

Table 18.8 Results of a trial to compare podophyllin with surgical excision.

	Podophyllin (*n* = 30)	*Excision* (*n* = 30)
Initial treatment failure	7 (23)	2 (7)
Mean number of treatments	5	1
Recurrence at 1 year of those initially cleared	17/25 (68)	8/28 (29)
Side-effects		
Severe pain	3	4
Moderate pain	3	12
Mild pain	4	9
Bleeding	4	11
Soiling	4	0

Values in parentheses are percentages.
From Jensen (1985).

Caustic acids

Topical trichloroacetic or bichloracetic acid (Fowler's solution – bismuth sodium, triglycollamate 3%, achromycin and bichloracetic acid) has been advocated by Swerdlow and Salvati (1971). These components cause tissue sloughing but are much less expensive than podophyllin. The solutions require neutralization by sodium bicarbonate. At least four applications are needed and the recurrence rate is approximately 25% – which is similar to that reported with podophyllin. A combination of podophyllin and trichloroacetic acid gave recurrence rates which were the same as podophyllin alone (Gabriel and Thin, 1983). Finally, ammoniated mercury has been used by Grace et al (1967).

Chemotherapeutic agents

Chloroquine was applied to warts with some success by Murphy and Petty (1965), and later colchicine was found to eradicate some urethral warts (Gigax and Robinson, 1971). Attention then focused on treatment with antimitotic drugs, such as topical thiotepa (Cheng and Veenema, 1965;

Halverstadt and Parry, 1969) and 5-fluorouracil (Nel and Fourie, 1973; Wallin, 1977). Bleomycin is both an antibiotic as well as an antitumour agent (Umezawa, 1965; Mishima and Matunaka, 1972) and, apart from pneumonitis and occasional idiosyncracy, has remarkably few side-effects, particularly when used topically. Shumack and Haddock (1979) used topical injections of bleomycin for warts and reported no skin necrosis. Figuero and Gennaro (1980) treated ten patients by injecting 0.1 mL of a solution containing 1 mg/mL bleomycin into the base of all lesions every 3–4 weeks over a variable period and achieved complete healing in seven.

Prolonged use of 5FU will result in erosive dermatitis. Topical 5FU has been used for vaginal or urethral warts with a 68% response rate without recurrence at 6–12 months, but in one report none of the perianal warts completely disappeared with 5FU (Pride, 1990). The greatest value of 5FU may be to prevent recurrence after successful eradication, especially in immunocompromised patients (Krebs, 1991; King, 1992). Topical 5FU has not been approved by the FDA (Food and Drug Administration) in the USA for treatment of genital warts.

Immunotherapy

The concept of vaccinating patients against their own virus is interesting (Biberstein, 1944; Kirby, 1988), but Powell et al (1970) argued that the virus responsible for condylomata acuminata was a surface agent and unlikely to stimulate a humoral antibody response. Using autogenous vaccine, remission was reported in 28 of 35 patients (Powell et al, 1970). Immunotherapy was later advocated by Abcarian and colleagues (Abcarian et al, 1976; Abcarian and Sharon, 1977). Patients were admitted to hospital for 48 hours so that at least 5 g of tissue could be excised. After washing, the tissue was suspended in tissue culture medium containing antibiotics and homogenized. The homogenate was frozen and thawed four times prior to centrifugation. The supernatant was pasteurized by heating to 56°C, centrigued at 4°C, cultured to ensure sterility and stored for repeated inoculation. Immunization was achieved by six-weekly 0.5 mL injections into the deltoid muscle.

Abcarian and Sharon (1982) reported the results of treatment in 200 patients with a mean follow-up of 46 months. There were no adverse reactions. Total disappearance of the lesions around the anus was achieved in 84% of patients; furthermore, associated genital lesions usually disappeared as well, but condylomata on the face, hands and feet were unaffected. Improvement was achieved in a further 22 patients and half of the failures achieved complete clearance after a further course of autovaccination. Results in patients with recurrent disease did not differ from patients presenting with anal condylomata for the first time (Table 18.9). However, the vaccine was not effective in HIV-positive patients. In recent years vaccination has fallen into disuse because of concerns about HIV status, but immunotherapy may have a role in the treatment of giant condylomata.

Wiltz et al (1995) compared recurrence rates of excision alone, bichloroacetic acid, podophyllin, interferon A or excision followed by twice-weekly autogenous condylomata acuminata vaccination for 10 weeks. The combined surgery and vaccination group had a recurrence rate of only 4.6% compared with 50% for surgery along (Table 18.10).

Table 18.9 Results of immunotherapy in 200 patients with anal condylomata acuminata.

Patient group	*n*	*Complete clearance*	*Partial improvement*	*No response*
Primary	120	101 (84.2)	13 (10.8)	6 (5)
Recurrent	80	66 (82.5)	10 (12.5)	4 (5)
Total	200	167 (83.5)	23 (11.5)	10 (5)

Values in parentheses are percentages.

Table 18.10 Recurrence rates following treatment by various methods.

Method	*n*	*Recurrence (%)*
Surgery alone	20	50
Bichloroacetic acid	10	50
Podophyllin	5	85
Interferon	5	85
Surgical incision and vaccination	43	4.6

From Wiltz et al (1995).

Interferon

Interferons are proteins with antiviral, antitumour and immunomodulatory actions which can restore natural killer cell activity (Cauda et al, 1987). Interferons alpha and gamma are available for clinical use and were found to be effective in plantar warts. Interferon may be used for topical intra-incisional and systemic therapy (Trofatter, 1991).

Side-effects of interferon include viral syndrome, gastrointestinal complaints, leukopenia, thrombocytopenia and abnormal liver function. Interferon should not be used in patients with cardiac or renal failure (Browder et al, 1992). Tolerance appears to develop to viral syndrome, and non-steroidal anti-inflammatory agents often provide effective therapy.

Topical interferon

While topical therapy minimizes side-effects, two randomized controlled trials demonstrated no advantage over placebo cream. Thus at the moment topical therapy is not advised as a primary treatment (Vesterinen et al, 1984; Kraus and Stone, 1990).

Intra-incisional interferon

Large doses may be given directly to an area of disease without inducing side-effects. Clearance rates of 47–62% have been reported, but recurrence rates range from 20% to 40%. High costs and repeated therapy make this an unattractive mode of treatment unless the conylomata are resistant to all other forms of therapy (Browder et al, 1992; Welander et al, 1990). Current recommendations are to inject 1×10^6 IU under no more than five lesions, three times a week for no more than 8 weeks.

Systemic interferon

Systemic interferon is most useful for treating large or multiple lesions which are difficult to inject. There is a high rate of side-effects and variable response rates.

Adjuvant therapy with interferon

Adjuvant systemic interferon may reduce recurrence rates compared with surgery or laser ablation, but there is usually a high incidence of side-effects (Eron et al, 1986; Condylomata International Collaborative Study Group, 1993).

Adjuvant topical therapy appears to have a real place in current management. A randomized study of intralesional interferon given after surgical excision or fulguration showed a reduced recurrence rate from 39% to 12% at a mean follow-up of 3.8 months (Table 18.11). Likewise a retrospective comparison of intralesional interferon and fulguration showed that adjuvant interferon reduced recurrence rates at 13 weeks from 35% to 18% (Vance and Davis, 1990). Similarly, podophyllin with intra-incisional interferon achieved a response rate of 67%, compared with 42% with podophyllin alone (Douglas et al, 1990).

Table 18.11 Recurrence in intra-incisional prospective randomized trial of topical adjuvant interferon.

Method	*n*	*Recurrence (%)*
Surgery, interferon and diathermy	25	12
Surgery, saliva and diathermy	18	39

From Fleshner and Freilich (1994).

SURGICAL TREATMENT

The mainstay of surgical therapy has been the application of physical agents such as diathermy, cryotherapy, laser and ultrasonic destruction in addition to simple surgical excision. Excision is now assuming greater importance following the recognition of early malignant transformation.

Physical agents

Cryotherapy

Cryotherapy can be applied using nitrous oxide (Graber et al, 1967) or liquid nitrogen (Hall, 1960; Lyall, 1966; Nahra et al, 1969), but most of the earlier methods of application were crude and resulted in considerable discomfort together with destruction of adjacent tissues and discharge. More sophisticated instruments, with interchangeable heads that can be selected according to the volume of tissue requiring therapy, are now available (Simmons et al, 1981). There are a number of advocates of cryotherapy because treatment is painless, but satisfactory clinical data on the results are lacking and treatment requires careful control of the depth and width of therapy (Savin, 1975; Ghosh, 1977; O'Connor, 1979). One trial showed an advantage of cryotherapy over topical trichloracetic acid in terms of both recurrence and side-effects (Godley et al, 1987). Freezing is, however, non-standardized and difficult to quantify for individual lesions, and discharge following therapy is often considerable. Most small lesions can be cleared with cryotherapy, but recurrence occurs in approximately 20% of patients over the following 6 months. We have now largely abandoned the technique.

Laser destruction

Laser therapy may be used for the treatment of anal condylomata. Billingham and Lewis (1982) conducted a trial to compare the carbon dioxide laser with diathermy excision. One half of the perianal region was treated by laser and the other by electrocoagulation. Recurrences were more common on the side treated by laser and the patients experienced more postoperative pain on that side. Another study compared the CO_2 laser with diathermy (Duus et al, 1985). No significant differences were found in the recurrence rate, pain, healing time or scarring. At 6 months, the cure rate for refractory warts was 36% in the cautery group and 43% in the laser group. In view of the high cost of laser equipment and the risks of fumes in HIV patients, which must be removed by vacuum, we believe laser has yet to find a place for routine therapy (Sawchuck et al, 1989).

Diathermy

Diathermy excision or contact destruction is probably used more widely than any other mode of treatment. It is remarkable, therefore, how little information is available on the immediate and long-term results of treatment (Simmons et al, 1981). Diathermy excision may be performed under local or general anaesthesia. Our policy is to use a local anaesthetic if there are numerous discrete pedunculated lesions confined to the perianal skin with no anal involvement. General anaesthesia is employed for large confluent condylomata with a wide base or when the anal canal is involved.

We use a very fine-tipped diathermy probe and a 1% lignocaine solution with adrenaline to raise the lesion from the surrounding skin. As much skin as possible is preserved so that only the pedicle of the wart is divided. For very small lesions, the tip of the wart may be grasped with fine tissue forceps and application of the diathermy literally explodes the lesion, leaving a small white scar on the pedicle. Excessive skin loss must be avoided as this may lead to scarring and stenosis at the anal margin. We reviewed our results and found that complete initial clearance of the warts was achieved in 37 of 41 cases, but that condylomata recurred in 9 of 37 patients (24%) who were initially cleared of their lesions (Andrews et al, 1986). None of our patients developed stenosis or excessive perianal scarring. Jensen (1985) reported a similar recurrence rate of 29% at one year.

Surgical excision

Scissor excision

It has been argued that diathermy excision may be associated with excessive skin loss and potential scarring from fibrosis around the diathermied skin bridges, particularly in patients with extensive anal condylomata. Thomson and Grace (1978) therefore described the method of scissor excision. This technique may be performed under local or general anaesthesia. The base of the warts are infiltrated with a 1:300 000 solution of adrenaline (Figure 18.1a), both as a means of minimizing blood loss and to lift the papilliferous lesion from the surrounding normal skin. Using a fine pair of scissors and dissecting forceps, each lesion is excised from its base (Figure 18.1b,c). This rather painstaking procedure leaves minimal epithelial defects, which tend to approximate as the adrenaline solution disperses (Figure 18.1d). It is advisable to start treatment at the most dependent site so that bleeding does not obscure visualization of the remaining lesions. Similarly, lesions in the anal canal should be excised after infiltration with a weak adrenaline solution (Figure 18.1e,f). When excision is complete, an adrenaline-soaked pressure dressing is applied. Diathermy coagulation is not used.

Thomson and Grace (1978) reported their results in 75 patients: postoperative bleeding occurred in four patients; despite eradication of the condylomata, 42% developed recurrence during follow-up. Two randomized trials showed that scissor excision is preferable to conservative treatment with podophyllin (Jensen, 1985; Khawaja, 1989). Although diathermy may give lower recurrence rates than scissor excision, because of the risk of fumes in HIV-positive patients we believe that scissor excision is preferrable in these high-risk patients.

Wide excision

Wide surgical excision is advised in patients with giant anal condylomata or for lesions with histological evidence of *in situ* malignant change (Gingrass

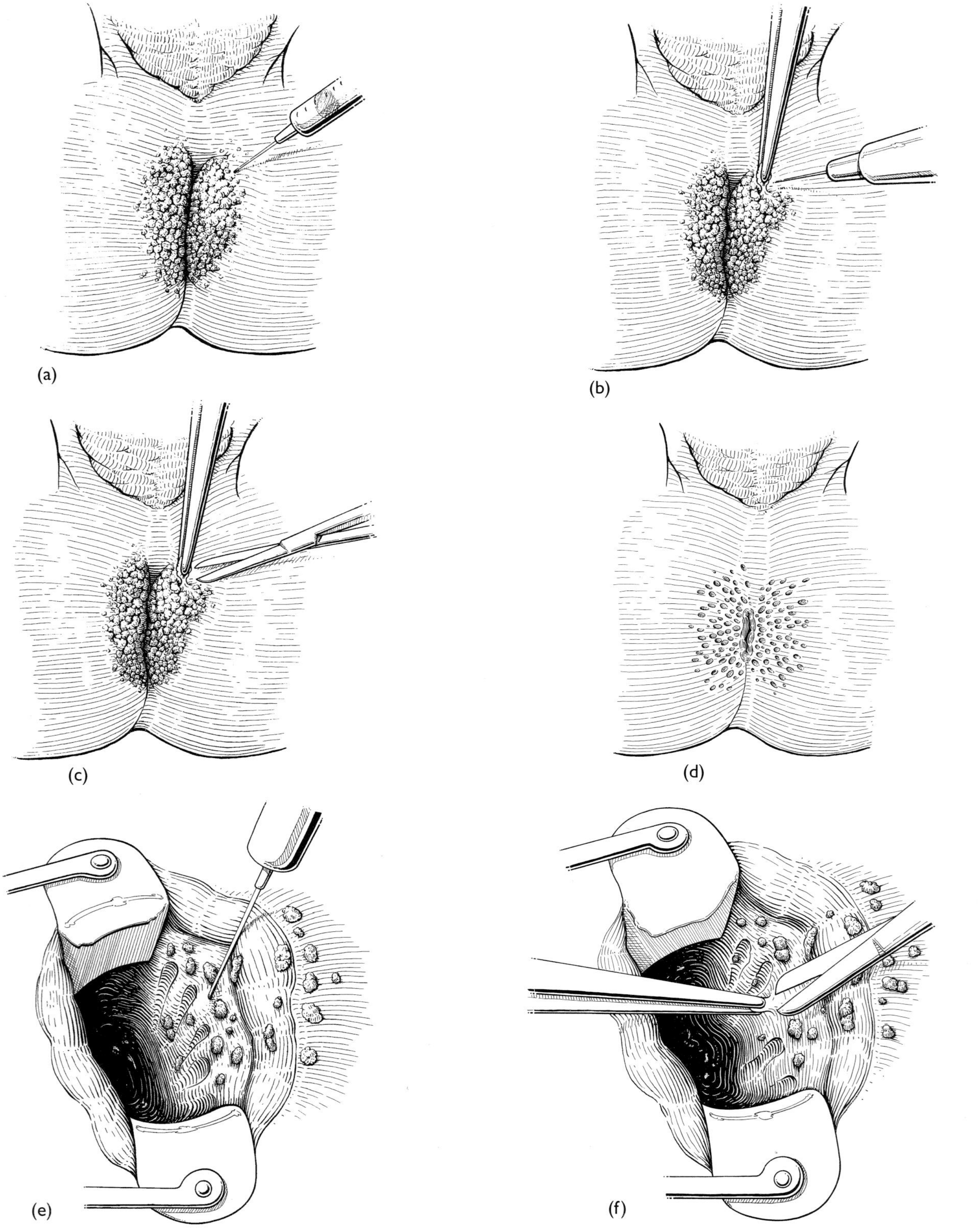

(a)

(b)

(c)

(d)

(e)

(f)

Figure 18.1a–f Scissor excision of anal condylomata. (a) Infiltration of 1:300 000 adrenaline solution under the perianal component of the warts. (b,c) Each wart is being elevated from the remainder of the skin and the pedicle excised with scissors. (d) The completed scissor excision of perianal warts. (e) A patient with intra-anal and perianal warts. The intra-anal warts are first treated by infiltration of the submucosa under each condylomatous mass. (f) Each wart is elevated from the anal mucosa and the base excised with scissors.

et al, 1978; Prasad and Abcarian, 1980; Croxson et al, 1984). These patients must be followed up carefully.

If there is evidence of squamous cell carcinoma, wide excision, or preferably radiotherapy with chemotherapy, is feasible for small lesions not invading the sphincters. In locally advanced lesions, response to radiotherapy and chemotherapy is so spectacular that traditional abdominoperineal excisions may not be needed (Buroker et al, 1976, 1977; Corman and Haggitt, 1977; Welch and Malt, 1977; Madden et al, 1981; Nigro et al, 1981) (see Chapter 34).

Surgical or diathermy excision versus podophyllin therapy

There is some debate as to which of the two most common forms of treatment should be offered as the initial therapy.

Jensen (1985) performed a randomized trial to compare the use of 25% podophyllin in benzoin tincture weekly for 6 weeks against scissor excision using the technique described by Thomson and Grace (1978). Surgical excision was usually performed under local anaesthesia and if very large lesions were encountered they were deliberately managed as two-stage procedures. Patients were followed for at least a year after treatment (Figure 18.2). There was a progressive increase in recurrence rate with time, and this was significantly less at all time points after excision compared with podophyllin therapy. Initial treatment failures were also more common (see Table 18.8). The mean number of attendances for treatment was five in the podophyllin group compared with one in the surgical group, but postoperative pain was more common after surgical excision. Hence, surgical excision required fewer visits and was associated with a lower rate of recurrence.

Khawaja (1989) compared 25% podophyllin with scissor excision in a randomized trial. At 6 weeks, 79% had cleared with podophyllin compared with 89% after excision. A median of four applications were needed in the podophyllin group, whereas surgical treatment was completed in one session in 16 of the patients managed by scissor excision. In the surgical group, 11 experienced pain compared with only 5 of 19 patients treated by podophyllin. There were no complications of burns, stenosis or scarring in either group. At 42 weeks the cumulative probability of recurrence was 60% with podophyllin but only 19% following scissor excision. Similar disappointing results have now been reported by others using podophyllin (Halverstadt and Parry, 1969; Gigax and Robinson, 1971).

Treatment in immunocompromised patients

Immunocompromised patients have a greater risk of condylomata acuminata, recurrent warts and anogenital neoplasia than the general population. Genital warts affect 43% of transplant recipients and 30% of HIV-positive patients (Sillman and Sedlis, 1991; Puy-Montbrun et al, 1992). These warts are also more aggressive, recur earlier and are more frequently dysplastic (Palefsky, 1991). Recurrence rates after surgical excision may exceed 50% (Gottesman et al, 1990).

Podophyllin may make interpretation of dysplastic lesions difficult and should probably be avoided in high-risk patients. Diathermy or laser surgery should be used with caution in HIV-positive patients because of the risk of dispersal of viral particles of HIV, HPV and hepatitis; thus some extraction facility must be used or excision should be with scissors.

Reduced recurrence when treating immunodeficient patients may be achieved with adjuvant topical 5FU (Krebs, 1991). In contrast, the role of interferon is uncertain because of the risk of an increase in transplant rejection as well as side-effects such as leukopenia, virus syndrome and thrombocytopenia (Eron et al, 1986; Kovarik et al, 1988).

Follow-up must be diligent in this group because of the risk of recurrence and anal cancer.

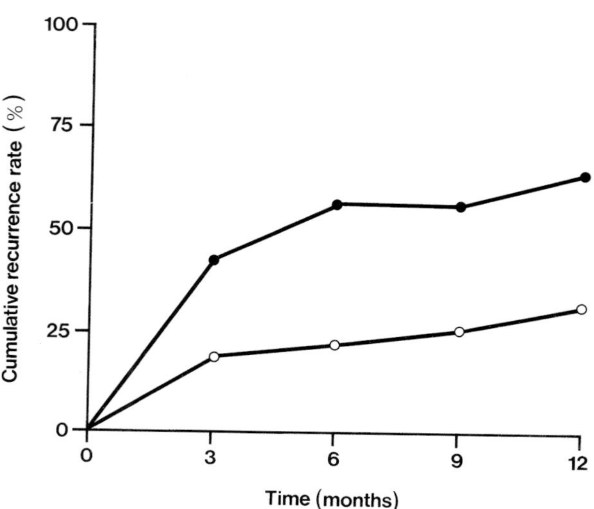

Figure 18.2 Cumulative recurrence rates for treatment of perianal warts (●, podophyllin application; ○, radial surgical excision). From Jensen (1985).

SUMMARY OF AUTHORS' POLICY

We believe that surgical excision is superior to podophyllin therapy for most patients with extensive perianal warts but accept that podophyllin is an appropriate first-line treatment for small lesions in patients presenting to STD clinics.

Adjuvant treatment with interferon would be advised in patients with recurrent perianal condylomata who are not immunocompromised and who do not have the HIV virus. In contrast, scissor excision alone is probably safest in HIV-positive patients where adjuvant interferon may be unsafe and where diathermy or laser treatment is likely to cause dispersal of the HIV virus. All potentially malignant lesions should be kept under careful scrutiny.

REFERENCES

Abcarian H & Sharon N (1977) The effectiveness of immunotherapy in the treatment of anal condylomata acuminata. *J Surg Res* **22**: 231–236.

Abcarian H & Sharon N (1982) Long-term effectiveness of the immunotherapy of anal condyloma acuminatum. *Dis Colon Rectum* **25**: 648–651.

Abcarian H, Smith D & Sharon N (1976) The immunotherapy of anal condyloma acuminatum. *Dis Colon Rectum* **19**: 237–244.

Alexander RB & Kaminsky DB (1979) Giant condyloma acuminatum (Buschke–Lowenstein tumor) of the anus: case report and review of the literature. *Dis Colon Rectum* **21**: 561–565.

Andrews HA, Wyke J, Rat T et al (1986) Sexually transmitted disease: a new hazard for the gastroenterologist? *Gut* **27**: A1259.

Biberstein H (1944) Immunization therapy of warts. *Arch Dermatol* **50**: 12–22.

Billingham RP & Lewis FG (1982) Laser versus electrical cautery in the treatment of condylomata acuminata of the anus. *Surg Gynecol Obstet* **155**: 865–867.

Bonnez W, Elswich RK Jr, Bailey-Farchione A et al (1994) Efficacy and safety of 0.5 per cent podofilox solution in the treatment and suppression of anogenital warts. Am J Med **96**: 420–425.

Bradshaw BR, Nuovo GJ, DiConstanzo D & Cohen SR (1992) Human papillomavirus type 16 in a homosexual man. *Arch Dermatol* **128**: 949–952.

Browder JF, Araujo OE, Myer NA & Flowers FP (1992) The interferons and their use in condyloma acuminata. *Ann Pharmacother* **26**: 42–45.

Budayr M, Ankney RN & Moore RA (1996) Condyloma acuminata in infants and children: a survey of colon and rectal surgery. *Dis Colon Rectum* **39**: 1112–1115.

Burns FJ & van Goidsenhoven GE (1970) Condylomata acuminata of the rectum with associated malignancy. *Proc R Soc Med* **63** (Suppl): 119.

Buroker T, Nigro N, Correa J et al (1976) Combination preoperative radiation and chemotherapy in adenocarcinoma of the rectum. *Dis Colon Rectum* **19**: 660–663.

Buroker TR, Nigro N, Bradley G et al (1977) Combined therapy for cancer of the anal canal: a follow-up report. *Dis Colon Rectum* **20**: 677–678.

Buschke A & Lowenstein L (1925) Uber carcinomahnliche Condylomata acuminata des Penis. *Klin Wochenschr* **4**: 1726.

Carter PS, De Ruiter A, Whatrup C et al (1995) Human immunodeficiency virus infection and genital warts as risk factors for anal intraepithelial neoplasia in homosexual men. *Br J Surg* **82**: 473–474.

Cauda R, Tyring SK, Grossi CE et al (1987) Patients with condyloma acuminatum exhibit decreased interleukin-2 and interferon gamma production and depressed natural killer activity. *J Clin Immunol* **7**: 304–311.

Centers for Disease Control (1986) Condylomata acuminatum, 1966–83. *MMWR* **33**: 81.

Charlewood GP & Shippel S (1953) Vulval condyloma acuminata as a premalignant lesion in the Bantu. *S Afr Med J* **27**: 149–151.

Cheng SF & Veenema RJ (1965) Topical application of thiotepa to penile and urethral tumours. *J Urol* **94**: 259–262.

Chu QD, Vezeridis MP, Libbey NP & Wanebo HJ (1994) Giant condyloma acuminatum (Buschke–Lowenstein tumour) of the anorectal and perianal regions: analysis of 42 cases. *Dis Colon Rectum* **37**: 950–957.

Cohen BA, Honig P & Androphy E (1990) Anogenital warts in children. *Arch Dermatol* **126**: 1575–1580.

Condylomata International Collaborative Study Group (1993) Randomized placebo-controlled double-blind combined therapy with laser surgery and systemic interferon alpha 2a in the treatment of anogenital condylomata acuminatum. *J Infect Dis* **167**: 824–829.

Congilosi SM & Madoff RD (1995) Current therapy for recurrent and extensive anal warts. *Dis Colon Rectum* **38**: 1101–1107.

Corman ML (1984) *Colon and Rectal Surgery*, pp 211–214. Philadelphia: Lippincott.

Corman ML & Haggitt RC (1977) Carcinoma of the anal canal. *Surg Gynecol Obstet* **145**: 674–676.

Croxson T, Chabon AB, Rorat E & Brash IM (1984) Intraepithelial carcinoma of the anus in homosexual men. *Dis Colon Rectum* **24**: 325–330.

Culp OS & Kaplan IW (1944) Condylomata acuminata: two hundred cases treated with podophyllin. *Ann Surg* **120**: 251–256.

Cummings BJ, Thomas GM, Keane TJ et al (1982) Primary radiation therapy in the treatment of anal canal carcinoma. *Dis Colon Rectum* **25**: 778–782.

Daling JR, Weiss NS, Klopfenstein LL et al (1982) Correlates of homosexual behaviour and the incidence of anal cancer. *JAMA* **247**: 1988–1990.

Department of Health and Social Security (1979) Sexually transmitted diseases. In *On the State of Public Health: Annual Report of the Chief Medical Officer of the Department of Health and Social Security for the Year 1978*, pp 1–65. London: HMSO.

deVilliers EM (1989) Heterogeneity of the human papillomavirus group. *J Virol* **63**: 4898–4903.

Douglas JM, Eron LJ, Judson FN et al (1990) A randomized trial of combination therapy with intralesional interferon alpha 2b and podophyllin versus podophyllin alone for the therapy of anogenital warts. *J Infect Dis* **162**: 52–59.

van Driel WJ, Ressing ME, Brandt RMP et al (1996) The current status of therapeutic HPV vaccine. *Ann Med* **28**: 471–477.

Duggan MA, Boras VF, Inoue M, McGregor SE & Robertson DI (1989) Human papillomavirus DNA determination of anal condylomata, dysplasias, and squamous carcinomas with *in situ* hybridization. *Am J Clin Pathol* **92**: 16–21.

Duus BR, Philipsen T, Christensen JD, Lundvall F & Sondergaard J (1985) Refractory condylomata acuminata: a controlled clinical trial of a carbon dioxide laser versus conventional surgical treatment. *Genitourin Med* **61**: 59–61.

Ejeckam GC, Idikio HA, Nayak V & Gardiner JP (1983) Malignant transformation in an anal condyloma acuminatum. *Can J Surg* **26**: 170–173.

Elliot MS, Werner ID, Immelman EJ & Harrison AC (1979) Giant condyloma (Buschke–Lowenstein tumor) of the anorectum. *Dis Colon Rectum* **22**: 497–500.

Eron LG, Judson F, Tucker S et al (1986) Interferon therapy for condylomata acuminata. *N Engl J Med* **315**: 1059–1064.

Figuero S & Gennaro AR (1980) Intralesional bleomycin injection in treatment of condyloma acuminatum. *Dis Colon Rectum* **23**: 550–551.

Fitzgerald DM & Hamit HF (1974) The variable significance of condylomata acuminata. *Ann Surg* **179**: 328–331.

Fleshner PR & Freilich MI (1994) Adjuvant interferon for anal condyloma: a prospective, randomized trial. *Dis Colon Rectum* **37**: 1255–1259.

Frasier LD (1994) Human papillomavirus infections in children. *Pediatr Ann* **23**: 354–360.

Friedberg MJ & Serlin O (1963) Condyloma acuminatum: its association with malignancy. *Dis Colon Rectum* **6**: 352–355.

Gabriel G & Thin RN (1983) Treatment of anogenital warts: comparison of trichloracetic acid and podophyllin versus podophyllin alone. *Br J Vener Dis* **59**: 124–126.

Ghosh AK (1977) Cryosurgery of genital warts in cases in which podophyllin treatment failed or was contraindicated. *Br J Vener Dis* **53**: 49.

Gigax JH & Robinson JR (1971) The successful treatment of intraurethral condylomata acuminata with colchicine. *J Urol* **105**: 809–811.

Gingrass PJ, Burrick MP, Hitchcok CR et al (1978) Anorectal verrucose carcinoma: report of two cases. *Dis Colon Rectum* **21**: 120.

Godley MJ, Bradbeer CS, Gellan M & Thin RN (1987) Cryotherapy compared with trichloracetic acid in treating genital warts. *Genitourin Med* **63**: 390–392.

Gottesman LG, Miles AJ & Milson JW et al (1990) The management of anorectal disease in HIV-positive patients (symposium). *Int J Colorect Dis* **5**: 61–72.

Graber EQ, Barber HR & O'Rourke JJ (1967) Simple surgical treatment of condyloma acuminatum of the vulva. *Obstet Gynecol* **29**: 247–250.

Grace DA, Ochsner JA, McLain CR & Smith JP (1967) Vulvar condylomata acuminata in prepubertal females. *JAMA* **201**: 151–152.

Greene I (1992) Therapy for genital warts. *Dermatol Clin* **10**: 253–267.

Grisson O & Delvaneo E (1915) Monstroser Tumour der Genitalgegend. *Dermatol Wochenschr* **60**: 89–109.

Hall AF (1960) Advantages and limitations of liquid nitrogen in the therapy of skin lesions. *Arch Dermatol* **82**: 9–16.

Halverstadt DB & Parry WL (1969) Thiotepa in the management of intraurethral condylomata acuminata. *J Urol* **101**: 729–732.

Hatch KD (1991) Vulvovaginal human papillomavirus infections: clinical implications and management. *Am J Obstet Gynecol* **165**: 1183–1188.

Jensen SL (1985) Comparison of podophyllin application with simple surgical excision in clearance and recurrence of perianal condylomata acuminata. *Lancet* **ii**: 1146–1148.

Jones DJ & James RD (1992) Anal cancer. *BMJ* **305**: 169–171.

Judge JR (1969) Giant condyloma acuminatum involving vulva and rectum. *Arch Pathol* **88**: 46–48.

Kaplan HL (1942) Condylomata acuminata. *N Orl Med Surg J* **94**: 388.

Khawaja HT (1989) Podophyllin versus scissor excision in the treatment of perianal condylomata acuminata: a prospective study. *Br J Surg* **76**: 1067–1068.

Khoblich R & Failing JF Jr (1967) Giant condyloma acuminatum (Buschke–Lowenstein tumour) of the rectum. *Am J Clin Pathol* **48**: 389–395.

King AR (1992) Genital warts therapy. *Semin Dermatol* **11**: 247–255.

Kirby P (1988) Interferon and genital warts: much potential mode of progress. *JAMA* **259**: 570–572.

Konketzny GE (1914) Uber einen ungewohnlichen Penistumor. *MMW* **61**: 905.

Kovarik J, Mayer G, Polanka E et al (1988) Adverse effect of low-dose prophylactic human recombinant leukocyte interferon alpha treatment in renal transplant recipients. *Transplantation* **45**: 402–405.

Kovi J, Tillman RL & Lee Shi (1974) Malignant transformation of condyloma acuminatum: a light microscopic and ultrastructural study. *Am J Clin Pathol* **61**: 702–710.

Kraus SJ & Stone KM (1990) Management of genital infection caused by human papillomavirus. *Rev Inf Dis* **12**: S620–632.

Krebs HB (1991) Treatment of genital condylomata with topical 5-fluorouracil. *Dermatol Clin* **9**: 333–341.

Langenberg A, Cone RW, McDougall J, Kiviat N & Corey L (1993) Dual infection with human papillomavirus in a population with overt genital condylomas. *J Am Acad Dermatol* **28**: 434–442.

LeBlanc KA, Cole P, Grafton W & Goldman LI (1985) Perianal squamous cell carcinoma in situ. *Surg Rounds* **8**: 72–76.

Lee SH, McGregor DH & Kuziez MN (1981) Malignant transformation of perianal condyloma acuminatum: a case report with review of literature. *Dis Colon Rectum* **24**: 462–467.

Lewis GM & Wheeler CE Jr (1967) *Practical Dermatology*, 3rd edn, p 679. Philadelphia: WB Saunders.

Longo WE, Ballantyne GH, Gerald WL & Modlin IM (1986) Squamous cell carcinoma in situ in condyloma acuminatum. *Dis Colon Rectum* **29**: 503–506.

Lorinez AT, Temple GF, Kurman RJ, Jenson AB & Lancaster WD (1987) Oncogenic association of specific human papillomavirus types with cervical neoplasia. *J Natl Cancer Inst* **79**: 671–677.

Lyall A (1966) Management of warts. *BMJ* **2**: 1576–1579.

Macharek GF & Weakley DR (1960) Giant condylomata acuminata of Buschke and Lowenstein. *Arch Dermatol* **82**: 41–47.

Madden MV, Elliot MS, Both JBC & Louw JH (1981) The management of anal carcinoma. *Br J Surg* **68**: 287–289.

Marino AW Jr (1964) Proctologic lesions observed in male homosexuals. *Dis Colon Rectum* **7**: 121–128.

Marks MM (1947) Condylomata acuminata: podophyllin in compound tincture of benzoin, an improvement in technic of treatment. *J Mt Sinai Med Assoc* **14**: 749.

Mishima Y & Matunaka M (1972) Effect of bleomycin on benign and malignant cutaneous tumours. *Acta Dermatol Venerol (Stockh)* **52**: 211–215.

Morgan AR, Miles AJ & Wastell C (1994) Anal warts and squamous carcinoma-in-situ of the anal canal. *J R Soc Med* **87**: 15.

Moriame B (1950) Transformation maligne de végétation vénérienne de la verge. *Arch Belg Dermatol Syph* **6**: 175.

Murphy JC & Petty S (1965) Cloroquine treatment of warts: a double-blind clinical study. *Rocky Mt Med J* **62**: 25–26.

Nahra KS, Moschella SL & Swinton NW Sr (1969) Condyloma acuminatum treated with liquid nitrogen: report of five cases. *Dis Colon Rectum* **12**: 125–128.

Nel WS & Fourie ED (1973) Immunotherapy and 5% topical 5-flourouracil ointment in the treatment of condylomata acuminata. *S Afr Med J* **47**: 45–49.

Nigro ND, Vaitkevicius VK, Buroker T et al (1981) Combined therapy for cancer of anal canal. *Dis Colon Rectum* **24**: 73–75.

Northfield JMA (1991) Editorial: Epidermoid cancer of the anus – the surgeon retreats. *J R Soc Med* **84**: 389–390.

O'Connor JJ (1979) Perianal and anal condylomata (correspondence). *Proc R Soc Med* **72**: 232.

Oriel JD (1971) Anal warts and anal coitus. *Br J Vener Dis* **47**: 373–376.

Oriel JD & Almeida JE (1970) Demonstration of virus particles in human genital warts. *Br J Vener Dis* **46**: 37–42.

Oriel JD & Whimster IW (1971) Carcinoma in situ associated with virus-containing anal warts. *Br J Dermatol* **84**: 71–73.

Palefsky JM (1991) Human papillomavirus-associated anogenital neoplasia and other solid tumours in human immunodeficiency virus-infected individuals. *Curr Opin Oncol* **3**: 881–885.

Palefsky JM, Gonzales J, Greenblatt RM, Ahn DK & Hollander H (1990) Anal intraepithelial neoplasia and anal papillomavirus infection among homosexual males with group IV HIV disease. *JAMA* **163**: 1911–1916.

Powell LC Jr, Pollard M & Jinkins JL Sr (1970) Treatment of condyloma acuminata by autogenous vaccine. *South Med J* **63**: 203–205.

Prasad ML & Abcarian H (1980) Malignant potential of perianal condyloma acuminatum. *Dis Colon Rectum* **23**: 191–197.

Pride GL (1990) Treatment of large lower genital tract condylomata acuminata with topical 5-fluorouracil. *J Reprod Med* **35**: 384–387.

Puy-Montbrun T, Denis J, Ganansia R et al (1992) Anorectal lesions in human immunodeficiency virus-infected patients. *Int J Colorect Dis* **7**: 26–30.

Pyrhonen S & Johansson E (1975) Regression of warts: an immunological study. *Lancet* **i**: 592–595.

Raimer SS (1992) Family violence, child abuse, and anogenital warts. *Arch Dermatol* **128**: 842–844.

Ramanujam PS, Venkatesh KS, Co Barnett T & Fietz MJ (1996) Study of human papillomavirus infection in patients with anal squamous carcinoma. *Dis Colon Rectum* **39**: 37–39.

Reid R & Lorincz AT (1991) Should family physicians test for human papillomavirus infection? *J Fam Pract* **32**: 183–188.

Rhatigan RM & Saffos RO (1977) Condyloma acuminatum and squamous carcinoma of the vulva. *South Med J* **70**: 591–594.

Rhatigan RM, Jiminez S & Chopskie EJ (1971) Condyloma acuminatum and carcinoma of the penis. *South Med J* **65**: 423–428.

Savin S (1975) The role of cryosurgery in management of anorectal disease: preliminary report on results. *Dis Colon Rectum* **18**: 292–297.

Sawchuck WS, Weber PJ, Lowy DR & Dzubow LM (1989) Infectious papillomavirus in the vapor of warts treated with carbon dioxide laser or electrocoagulation: detection and protection. *J Am Acad Dermatol* **21**: 41–49.

Sawyers JL (1972) Squamous cell cancer of the perianus and anus. *Surg Clin North Am* **52**: 935–941.

Scholefield JH, Kerr IB, Shepherd NA et al (1991) Human papillomavirus type 16 DNA in anal cancers from six different countries. *Gut* **32**: 674–676.

Scoma JA & Levy EI (1975) Bowen's disease of the anus: report of two cases. *Dis Colon Rectum* **18**: 137–140.

Shah IC & Hertz RE (1972) Giant condyloma acuminatum of the anorectum: report of two cases. *Dis Colon Rectum* **15**: 207–210.

Shumack PH & Haddock MJ (1979) Bleomycin: an effective treatment for warts. *Aust J Dermatol* **20**: 41–42.

Siegal A (1962) Malignant transformation of condyloma acuminatum: review of the literature and report of a case. *Am J Surg* **103**: 613–617.

Sigurgeirsson B, Lindelof B & Eklund G (1991) Condylomata acuminata and risk of cancer: an epidemiological study. *BMJ* **303**: 341–344.

Sillman FH & Sedlis A (1991) Anogenital papillomavirus infection and neoplasia in immunodeficient women: an update. *Dermatol Clin* **9**: 353–369.

Simmons PD (1981) Podophyllin 10% and 25% in the treatment of anogenital warts. *Br J Vener Dis* **57**: 208–209.

Simmons PD, Langlet F & Thin RNT (1981) Cryotherapy versus electrocautery in the treatment of genital warts. *Br J Vener Dis* **57**: 273–274.

Sohn N & Robilotti JG Jr (1977) The gay bowel syndrome: a review of colonic and rectal conditions in 200 male homosexuals. *Am J Gastroenterol* **67**: 478–484.

Stumpf PG (1980) Increasing occurrence of condylomata acuminata in premenarchal children. *Obstet Gynecol* **56**: 262–264.

Sturm JT, Christenson CE, Uecker JH et al (1975) Squamous-cell carcinoma of the anus arising in a giant condyloma acuminatum: report of a case. *Dis Colon Rectum* **18**: 147–151.

Swerdlow DB & Salvati EP (1971) Condyloma acuminatum. *Dis Colon Rectum* **14**: 226–231.

Syed TA, Lundin S & Ahmad SA (1994) Topical 0.3 percent and 0.5 percent podophyllotoxin cream for self-treatment of condylomata acuminata in women: a placebo-controlled, double-blind study. *Dermatology* **189**: 142–145.

Syverton JT (1952) The pathogenesis of the rabbit papilloma-to-carcinoma sequence. *Ann NY Acad Sci* **54**: 1126–1140.

Thomson JPS & Grace RH (1978) The treatment of perianal and anal condylomata: a new operative technique *J R Soc Med* **71**: 180–185.

Trofatter KF (1991) Interferon treatment of anogenital human papillomavirus related diseases. *Dermatol Clin* **9**: 343–351.

Umezawa H (1965) Bleomycin and other antitumour antibiotics of high molecular weight. *Antimicrob Agents Chemother* **28**: 1079–1085.

Vance JC & Davis D (1990) Interferon alpha-2b injections used as an adjuvant therapy to carbon dioxide laser vaporization of recalcitrant anogenital condylomata acuminata. *J Invest Dermatol* **95**: S146–148.

Vesterinen E, Meyer B, Cantell K & Purola E (1984) Topical treatment of flat vaginal condyloma with human leukocyte interferon. *Obstet Gynecol* **64**: 535–538.

Wallin J (1977) 5-Fluorouracil in the treatment of penile and urethal condylomata acuminata. *Br J Vener Dis* **53**: 240–243.

Wang B, Wang B & Shao Y (1994) A primary clinical trial of genital warts treated with domestic highly purified podophyllotoxin. *Chung Kuo I Hsueh Ko Hsueh Yuan Hsueh Pao* **16**: 122–125.

Waugh M (1972) Condylomata acuminata. *BMJ* **2**: 527–528.

Welander CE, Homesley HD, Smiles KA & Peets EA (1990) Intralesional interferon alfa-2b for the treatment of genital warts. *Am J Obstet Gynecol* **162**: 348–354.

Welch JP & Malt RA (1977) Appraisal of the treatment of carcinoma of the anus and anal canal. *Surg Gynecol Obstet* **145**: 837–841.
Williams SL, Rogers LW & Quan SH (1976) Perianal Paget's disease: report of 7 cases. *Dis Colon Rectum* **19**: 30–40.
Wiltz OH, Torregrosa M & Wiltz O (1995) Autogenous vaccine: the best therapy for perianal condyloma acuminata? *Dis Colon Rectum* **38**: 838–841.
Young HM (1964) Viral warts in the anorectum possibly precluding rectal cancer. *Surgery* **55**: 367.

19 PRURITUS ANI

Pruritus ani is a common and often disabling symptom. Disorders responsible for pruritus include a variety of anal conditions, allergy, skin disease, bacterial, fungal or viral infections, diabetes, inflammatory bowel disease, gynaecological disorders and psychological conditions. However, in the majority of patients the condition is idiopathic and the pathophysiology is poorly understood. Perianal irritation is mediated by stimulation of cutaneous sensory nerve endings, resulting in excessive scratching and consequent damage to the perianal skin. Excessive perianal soiling and moisture also play an important part in producing pruritus. Treatment is directed at improving anal hygiene and treating any underlying disorder. Some patients with idiopathic pruritus cannot be cured because they continue to traumatize the perianal skin by uncontrolled anal scratching.

INCIDENCE AND NATURAL HISTORY

Overall incidence

There are no reliable data on the incidence of pruritus ani. The incidence is difficult to document because patients may find symptoms hard to talk about or may regard them as being so unimportant that they do not report them to their doctor (Jones, 1992). In an attempt to assess the occurrence of pruritus ani in Birmingham, we distributed questionnaires to patients attending hospital outpatient departments for the treatment of complaints not associated with the alimentary tract. The response revealed that 45% of individuals had suffered from some perianal irritation within the 5 years prior to answering the questionnaire. This implies that the complaint is probably widespread.

Age and sex incidence

We found that individuals were more commonly troubled by pruritus in the second and third decade but all ages may suffer. Men have a higher incidence than women but both sexes are frequently affected (Bowyer and McColl, 1966; Daniel et al, 1994).

Natural history

Pruritus ani is commonly an intermittent complaint of mild severity in which exacerbations may be associated with stress, diet, environmental changes or relapse of a predisposing cause. Occasionally pruritus can become very severe, particularly in highly strung individuals who may even become suicidal. However, in most patients there are remissions and relapses and it is therefore important to adopt a confident and positive attitude with patients during consultation.

PREDISPOSING FACTORS

Pruritus ani may be conveniently subdivided into either (1) a secondary disorder caused by a specific pathological mechanism, or (2) a primary condition which is idiopathic. Patients in whom pruritus is a secondary phenomenon are a much easier group to treat because attention to the underlying problem will often alleviate symptoms.

Anorectal disorders

Primary disorders which may cause intense perianal irritation include haemorrhoids, fissure, fistula, chronic anorectal sepsis, proctitis or proctocolitis, skin tags, anal warts, hidradenitis, anal and/or rectal prolapse, and some rectal tumours, especially villous adenoma, anorectal polyps, and rectal or anal carcinoma (Murie et al, 1981).

Hypersensitivity

Patients with pruritus ani may give a history of cutaneous hypersensitivity reactions or atopy. Hypersensitivity may be induced by topically applied ointments or suppositories for the treatment of anal fissure, haemorrhoids or pruritus. Such preparations often contain a mixture of antibiotic, steroid and local anaesthetic in a greasy base. This combination of drugs is particularly prone to produce skin sensitivity, especially in susceptible individuals (Fisher, 1976, 1980; Fisher and Brancaccio, 1979). Allergy is also commonly observed in response to applications of local anaesthetics, particularly lignocaine (Alexander, 1975). Consequently, although these preparations are frequently applied for the treatment of pruritus ani, they may potentiate rather than alleviate symptoms. For this reason, withdrawal of all topical agents is an absolute prerequisite for the treatment of pruritus. Nevertheless, certain astringent lotions known to be associated with a low incidence of hypersensitivity may subsequently be used (Allenby et al, 1993). Contact dermatitis from contraceptive sheaths can occur in patients practising anoreceptive intercourse. Men sensitive to rubber should be informed that non-rubber condoms are available (e.g. Fourex (Schmidt) and Lambskin (Youngs Rubber)).

Primary skin disease

Primary skin disease which involves the perianal region may occasionally cause pruritus ani, but this is not common. Usually there is evidence of the dermatological lesion at other sites; for example, psoriasis of the perianal skin may be accompanied by the same lesion at the elbows, wrists or ankles. Besides psoriasis, lichen planus, lichen simplex, eczema and leucoplakia may also cause pruritus ani.

Bacterial infections

Specific bacterial pathogens may cause pruritus ani. Anal syphilis usually produces an acutely painful chancre but it can cause intense perianal irritation. Serological tests for syphilis, such as the treponema immobilization test (TPI) and the fluorescent treponemal antibody test (FTA), provide confirmation of the diagnosis. A rare but frequently discussed cause of pruritus ani is *Corynebacterium minutissimum* (Bowyer and McColl, 1966). This organism is responsible for a condition known as erythrasma, characterized by red scaly patches occurring in the axillae and groins and sometimes confined to the perianal region (Smith et al, 1982). Diagnosis of erythrasma is made by examination of the skin under ultraviolet light because porphyrin produced by *C. minutissimum* exhibits a characteristic pink fluorescence under ultraviolet light. Anal tuberculosis may cause pruritus and is more likely to occur in recent immigrants from Asia, diabetics and those who are immunosuppressed.

Other bacterial diseases which should be excluded in patients with discharging lesions around the anus are impetigo, furuncles or carbuncles from staphylococci or *Pseudomonas* spp. Pruritus ani may also occur secondary to a urinary tract infection.

Fungal infections

Invasion of the skin by yeasts may occur if there has been damage by trauma, hypersensitivity reactions, steroids or when the colonic microflora is altered following the use of broad-spectrum antibiotics (Winner and Hurley, 1964; Ambrose et al, 1985). *Candida albicans* is a common saprophyte in the skin. Infected skin rapidly becomes hyperaemic, macerated with white plaques and pruritus ani then develops in the macerated areas (Pirone et al, 1992). The diagnosis of perianal candidiasis can be made by observing the typical pseudomycelia from scrapings of the perianal skin with a scalpel blade and subsequently smearing the blade on a glass slide for microscopic analysis. *C. albicans* may also invade the skin as a secondary pathogen, particularly in immunosuppressed patients receiving steroids, antimetabolites, azathioprine, cyclosporin, or as a complication of diabetes, a gynaecological disorder or advanced malignancy. Whenever *C. albicans* is isolated in women it is wise to test the urine for glucose and for candida in the urine and vagina. Monilial vulvitis is often associated with pruritus ani in diabetic patients.

Other fungal infections of perianal skin are uncommon but should be excluded. These infections often affect only one side of the perianal margin. The diagnosis is confirmed by taking skin scrapings and microscopy. Occasionally ringworm, usually tinea cruris but occasionally *Epidermophyton floccosum* and *Trichophyton rubrum* or *T. mentagrophytes*, may cause pruritus ani and is characterized by an extensive erythematous lesion with a scaly edge in the groins.

Viral infections

Condylomata acuminata may be responsible for pruritus ani. Warts are circumanal and often involve the anus as well as the genitalia. These virus-induced lesions are spread by direct contact (Sohn and Robilotti, 1977). The irritating discharge from warts frequently causes pruritus ani. Other viral causes of pruritus ani include anogenital herpes simplex and occasionally molluscum contagiosum. In herpes, a sore, reddened macule develops into a vesicle which ruptures (Jeansson and Molin, 1970; Chang, 1977). Inguinal lymphadenopathy is common and there may be a history of anoreceptive intercourse. Molluscum contagiosum is characterized by umbilicated papules which may involve any site (Brown and Weinberger, 1974; Felman and Nikitas, 1980).

Parasites

The most common cause of pruritus in children is threadworms (*Enterobius vermicularis*). Threadworms are much less common as a cause of pruritus ani in adults. Typically more than one member of a family complains of intense perianal irritation at night. The condition is more prevalent where there is poor hygiene or overcrowding. The worms infest the large bowel. The fertilized female emerges from the anus and lays her eggs on the perianal skin. This causes irritation, contamination of the hands and transmission through food or direct contact. Diagnosis can be made by demonstrating ova from a strip of sellotape placed on the anal region in the morning before bathing or defecation.

Other parasitic infestations which may cause pruritus ani include scabies (*Sarcoptes scabiei*) and pediculosis pubis.

Predisposing medical disorders

Diarrhoea

Diarrhoea from any cause can predispose to pruritus ani because it is difficult to clean the perianal skin when liquid faeces pass through the anal sphincters. For this reason inflammatory bowel disease may cause pruritus from frequent loose stools and sphincter damage, and anal skin tags make hygiene difficult. Patients after restorative proctocolectomy also frequently complain of pruritus despite complete continence. Pruritus may be associated with other psychosomatic disorders, especially chronic perineal pain and the irritable bowel syndrome (Jones, 1992).

Anal soiling

Anal soiling or seepage may cause pruritus, since the perianal skin cannot be kept completely clean. This is a common problem after operation for anal fissure, fistula or haemorrhoids, owing to a defect or scar in the anal canal (Murie et al, 1981).

Diabetes

Diabetes mellitus is frequently associated with pruritus ani, particularly when it is undiagnosed or poorly controlled. Furthermore, diabetes may cause pruritus ani on account of its association with perianal candidiasis.

Sexually transmitted disease

In the homosexual community, particularly in those with AIDS, a variety of bacterial, viral or fungal infections, commonly termed the 'gay bowel syndrome', may give rise to pruritus ani; examples include herpes simplex, lymphogranuloma venereum, molluscum contagiosum, shigellosis, Campylobacter, Cryptosporidium, Chlamydia, amoebiasis, giardiasis, *Enterobius vermicularis*, candidiasis, tuberculosis, strongyloides, Salmonella, Yersinia, scabies, gonorrhoea, syphilis, viral hepatitis and condylomata acuminata. Anorectal trauma, proctitis, anal disease and progressive neuropathy involving the sphincters make these subjects particularly susceptible to pruritus (Sohn and Robilotti, 1977; Fisher, 1980, Robertson et al, 1980; McMillan and Lee, 1981; McMillan et al, 1983; Robbins et al, 1983; William 1983; Welch et al, 1984).

Psychological causes

Very few cases of pruritus are a direct result of psychological disease, but many patients have an exacerbation of pruritus as a consquence of emotional stress. Primary psychological disorders associated with pruritis ani include dermatitis artefacta, neurotic excoriation, parasitophobia, senile pruritus and localized neurodermatitis.

IDIOPATHIC PRURITUS ANI

Unfortunately, despite thorough screening for specific causes, most cases of pruritus ani appear to be idiopathic.

Anal seepage

Anorectal physiological assessments have been used to study patients with long-standing idiopathic pruritus ani (Eyars and Thomson, 1979; Allan et al, 1987). In a Birmingham study, 32 patients with pruritus ani were compared with 20 controls. Rectal and anal sensation, as well as resting and squeeze anal sphincter pressures, were similar in the two groups (Figure 19.1). However, patients with pruritus ani leaked saline at lower volumes than controls (Haynes and Read, 1982) (Figure 19.2). These findings suggest that increased seepage of fluid through the anal sphincters may be of importance in idiopathic pruritus ani. The patients were also asked to

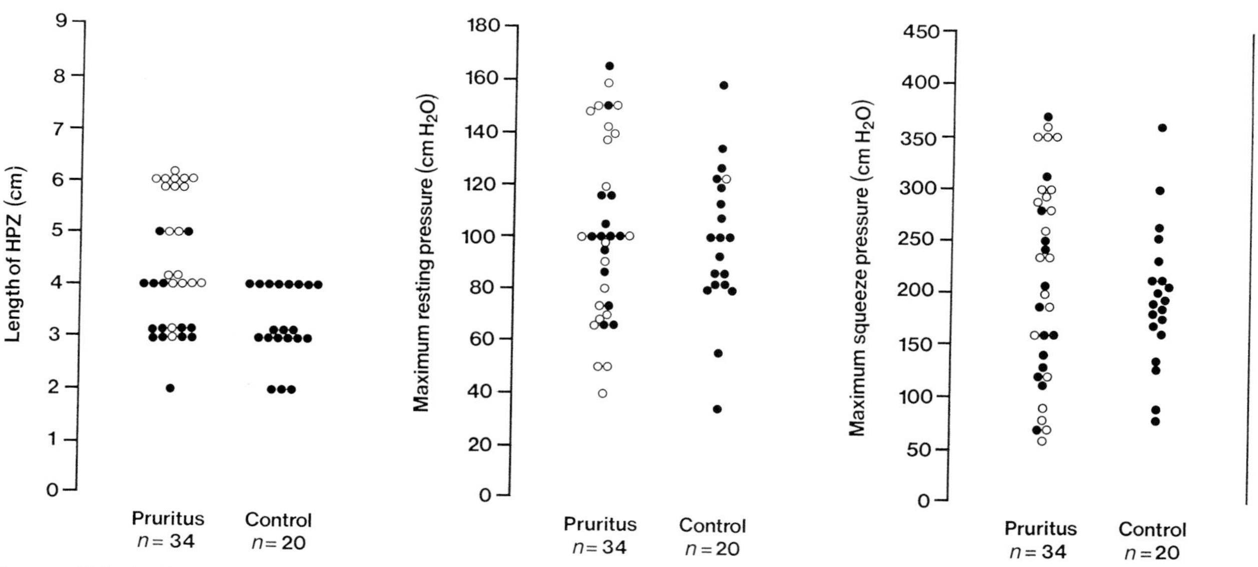

Figure 19.1 Anal manometry in pruritis ani patients: the length of the high-pressure zone (HPZ), maximum resting pressure, and squeeze pressure in patients with pruritis compared with controls. The pruritis group are subdivided into those with coexisting anal disease (○) and those without (●) (Allan et al, 1987).

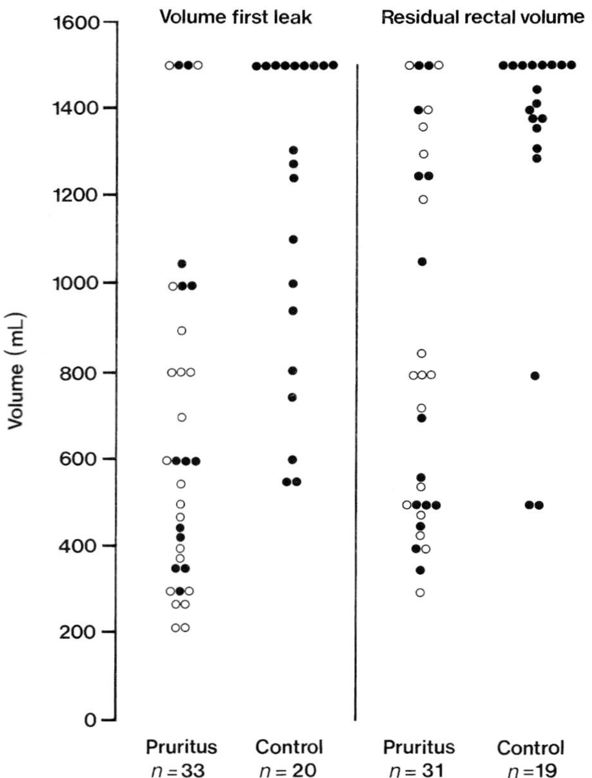

Figure 19.2 Saline infusion test in patients with pruritis ani compared with age- and sex-matched controls. Two parameters are used: the volume of first leak, shown on the left, and residual rectal volume after infusing 1.5 L of saline into the rectal ampulla. The pruritis group are subdivided into those with coexisting anal disease (○) and those without (●) (Allan et al, 1987).

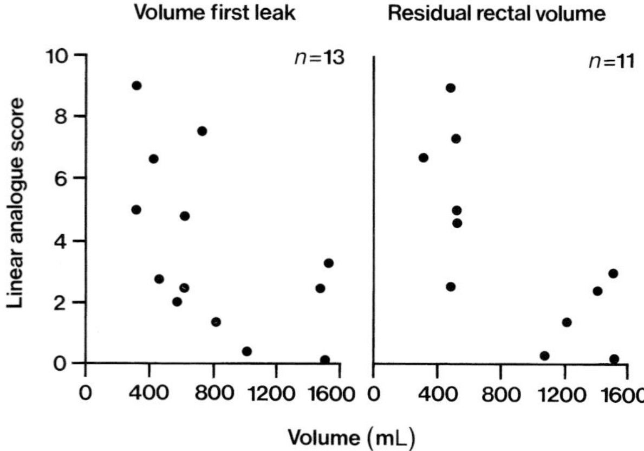

Figure 19.3 The relationship between symptoms and the results of the saline infusion test in Figure 19.2. Symptoms are based on a linear analogue score. Note that patients with high scores had early leakage of saline (Allan et al, 1987).

score the severity of their pruritus ani on a linear analogue scale, when symptoms were found to correlate well with the extent of the fluid leak (Figure 19.3). The leak may be due to a deficiency in the function of the internal anal sphincter (Eyars and Thompson, 1979). Patients with pruritus ani who had coexisting anal disease (mainly haemorrhoids) did not suffer from excessive fluid leakage. This suggests that the existence of anal pathology is not the sole cause of pruritus ani.

We found that the degree of internal anal sphincter relaxation in response to rectal distension was far greater in patients with pruritus compared with controls (Figure 19.4). Thus the exaggerated rectoanal inhibitory reflex was found only in those patients without coexisting anal disease (Figure 19.5).

Farouk et al (1994) confirmed our findings in some elegant ambulatory measurements. These showed no difference between idiopathic pruritis ani and controls with respect to resting anal and maximum squeeze pressures, internal anal EMG frequency, the number of internal sphincter relaxations and pudendal nerve latency. However, in pruritis ani patients, there was a significantly greater rise in intrarectal pressures during rectal distension, and internal sphincter relaxation was greater and significantly more prolonged (Table 19.1).

On the basis of these findings it is postulated that there is an exaggerated rectoanal inhibitory reflex in primary pruritis ani which results in increased leakage of faecal fluid through the anal canal, accounting for the irritation in pruritus ani. Some leakage, however, may be caused by coexisting anal pathology, probably as a result of increased mucus production or by an interference with the mucosal closure of the anal canal (Allan et al, 1987).

Table 19.1 Pressure changes and duration of daytime transient internal sphincter relaxations.

Feature	*Controls*	*Patients*
Rise in rectal pressure (cmH_2O)	18 (11–37)	29 (18–60)
Fall in anal pressure (cmH_2O)	29 (21–43)	39 (15–52)
Duration (s)	8 (5–12)	29 (18–55)

From Farouk et al (1994).

Colonic bacterial flora

Various bacterial enzymes such as enterobacterial endopeptidases are known to cause itching (Keele, 1957; Shelley and Arthur, 1957). When we examined

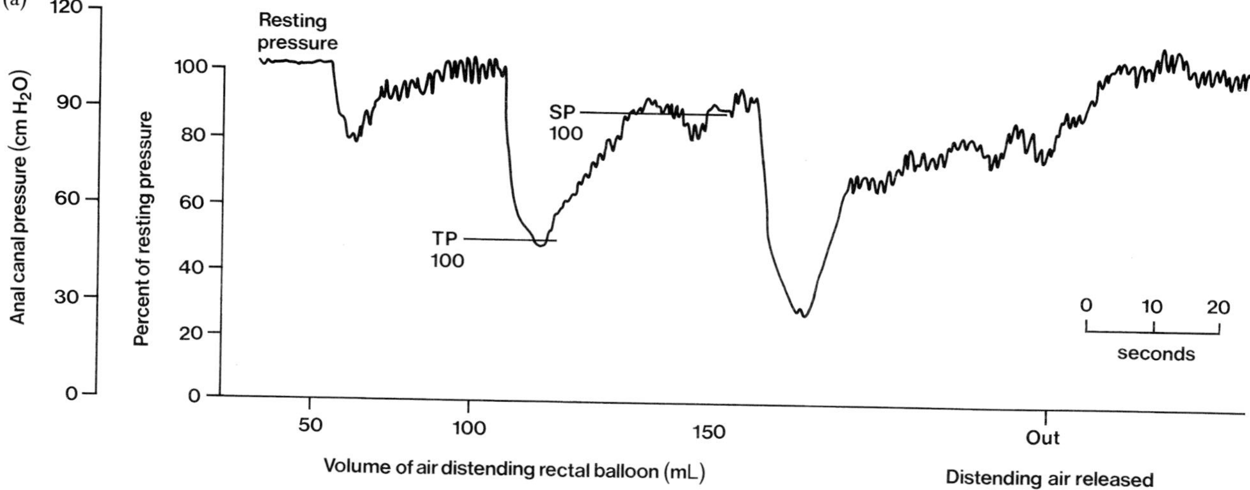

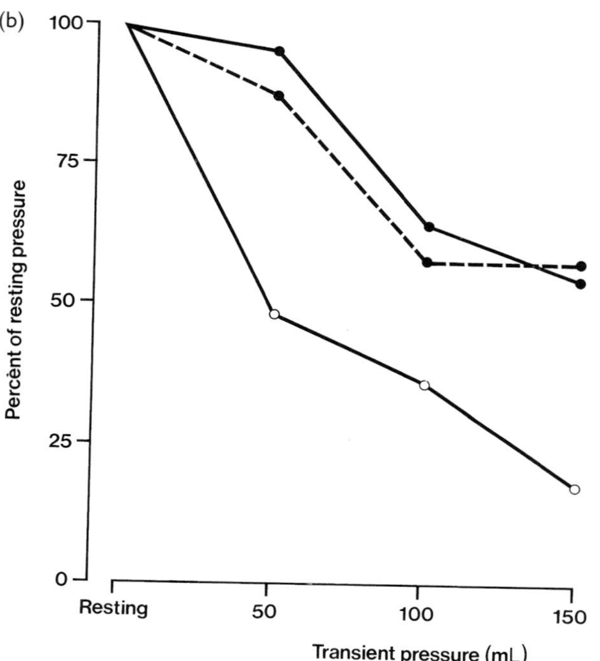

Fgure 19.4a,b The rectoanal inhibitory reflex in pruritis ani. (a) Typical trace of resting anal canal pressure following distension of a rectal balloon with 50, 100 and 150 mL of air. TP, trough pressure; SP, stable pressure. (b) Percentage fall in resting anal pressure after the introduction of 50, 100 and 150 mL of air into a rectal balloon, for patients with the condition and for age- and sex-matched controls. The pruritis group are subdivided into those with coexisting anal disease (top line, *n* = 25) and those without (bottom line, *n* = 15). Controls (*n* = 6) are shown by the broken line (Eyars and Thomson, 1979).

the faecal flora of patients with pruritus ani it did not differ from that of controls (Silverman et al, 1989).

Mycotic flora

Dodi et al (1985) examined the mycotic flora in patients with pruritus, with or without anorectal disease, and in those without pruritus, subdivided according to the anorectal disease. *C. albicans* was equally distributed in all four groups. The total incidence of mycoses was significantly greater (52%) in patients with pruritus than in those without (26%) The presence of dermatophytes was always associated with pruritus ani.

Diet

Patients with pruritus ani may become asymptomatic on withdrawal of specific dietary constituents (Brooks, 1969; Friend, 1976). These include coffee, tea, beer, chocolate and tomatoes. However, as pruritus ani shows a strong tendency to relapse or remit in any one individual, these findings are difficult to interpret.

Psychological factors

Psychological factors are often considered to be important in the pathogenesis of pruritus ani. Certainly, many such patients appear to be of a neurotic disposition. In an attempt to investigate this possibility, Smith et al (1982) studied 25 patients using the Minnesota Multiphasic Personality Inventory to assess their psychological status. Using this test they were unable to find statistically significant deviations from a normal population.

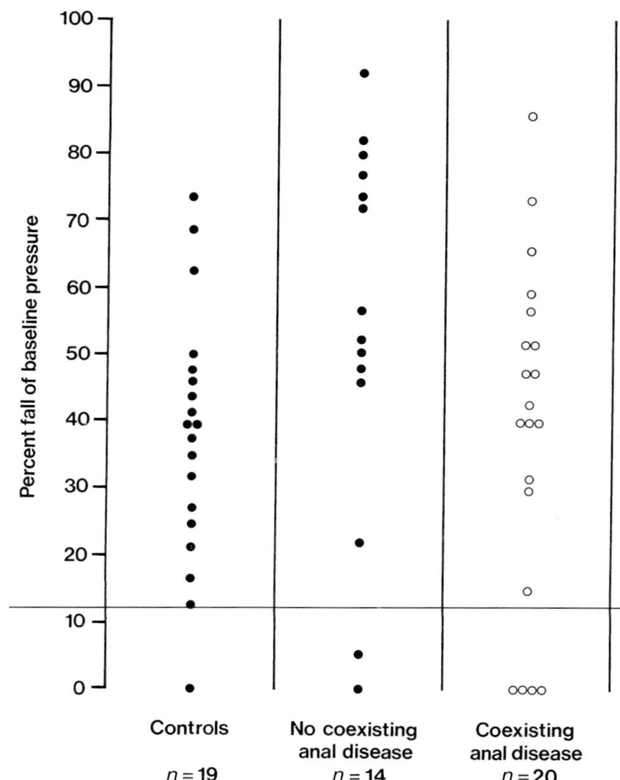

Figure 19.5 Percentage reduction in basal pressure following the introduction of 50 mL of saline into a rectal balloon, for patients with pruritis ani and age- and sex-matched controls. The pruritis group are subdivided into those with coexisting anal disease and those without (Allan et al, 1987).

CLINICAL ASSESSMENT

Clinical assessment of a patient with pruritus ani must include a careful history to assess the duration of symptoms, their severity and natural history. A history of any potential predisposing pathology should be sought; for example, skin disorders, perianal infection, diabetes mellitus, gynaecological disorders, or inflammatory bowel disease. Details of any change in the type of underwear may be of importance, since hypersensitivity and excessive moisture may develop with certain materials such as Nylon. Hypersensitivity may result from the use of certain types of toilet paper and topical preparations. A history of previous anal surgery should be recorded. Symptoms suggestive of underlying anorectal disease should also be sought, particularly pain, bleeding, discharge, altered bowel habit or prolapse. A psychiatric history and a brief assessment of personality would be wise. A history of anoreceptive intercourse may be informative.

Clinical examination must include a detailed inspection of the perianal region followed by proctoscopy and sigmoidoscopy. A careful search should be made for evidence of any localized or general dermatological disease, so the examination must include inspection of the elbows, knees, hands and flexures. The fingers should be examined for signs of fungal infection or coexisting hypersensitivity to lotions applied to the perianal skin and for evidence of faecal material under the nails as evidence of excessive scratching (Alexander-Williams, 1983).

The perianal skin must be examined. This is sometimes red and inflamed. Scratch marks on the skin indicate that the patient has exacerbated symptoms by this activity. Obvious perianal disease, such as condylomata acuminata, skin tags or the external orifice of a fistula, may be visible. A small portable ultraviolet light can be used to exclude the presence of *Corynebacterium minutissimum*. The examination involves scraping the skin for mycelia using a small scalpel blade. The blade is then placed in a receiver and sent for microscopic examination. Retraction of the buttocks may reveal further perianal pathology, such as haemorrhoids, mucosal prolapse, perianal haematoma, fissure in ano, skin tags or evidence of inflammatory bowel disease. By asking the patient to strain, a rectal prolapse may be demonstrated. Rigid sigmoidoscopy and proctoscopy are next performed to exclude coexisting anorectal disease. Examination is completed by stool culture for enteric pathogens, including ova, cysts and parasites. Serological tests for syphilis and HIV may also be arranged at this stage.

TREATMENT

Once the patient has been examined it may be possible to identify a predisposing cause for the pruritus ani, or the surgeon may consider that the patient has idiopathic pruritus ani. In either case it is wise to tell the patient at an early stage that the complaint tends to behave in a remitting and relapsing manner. It should also be pointed out that the surgeon cannot guarantee a cure but that he or she will provide support and offer advice about diet and anal hygiene.

Treatment when a predisposing cause is identified

Systemic disease

If the history reveals underlying systemic disease, then this should be treated. Certain disorders such as diabetes mellitus, sexually transmitted disease, a severe allergy, a generalized dermatological condition, gynaecological disease or a severe psychiatric disorder are best managed jointly with the appropriate specialist.

Local allergy

If the history reveals the use of topical agents applied to the perianal skin, these should be withdrawn. Many cases of pruritus ani are secondary to hypersensitivity induced by local applications, especially if steroids, antibiotics or local anaesthetics have been used.

Anal disease

Appropriate treatment for coexisting haemorrhoids, fissure, warts, fistula or ulcers should be instituted. It is always advisable to treat any underlying disorder first before embarking on therapy for the pruritus ani but patients should be told that the symptoms of pruritus may not always disappear even though the anal disorder has been treated successfully (Pirone et al, 1992).

Anal fistula

Anal fistula, for example, can be a rewarding disease to treat if discharge from the fistula is the primary cause of pruritus.

Haemorrhoids

Permanently prolapsed third-degree internal haemorrhoids causing continuous mucous leakage warrant definitive treatment provided care is taken not to damage the internal sphincter. Rubber-band ligation is often effective, but sometimes a haemorrhoidectomy is required. A trial designed to assess the impact of treatment for haemorrhoids on coexisting pruritus ani was reported from Glasgow (Murie et al, 1981). Eighty-two patients with uncomplicated, prolapsing haemorrhoids were studied before and after successful treatment by either haemorrhoidectomy or rubber-band ligation. Forty-one of these patients with haemorrhoids complained of pruritus ani before treatment and this was reduced to 18 patients after treatment. In this prospective study both haemorrhoidectomy and rubber-band ligation reduced the incidence of pruritus ani. These encouraging results have not been mirrored by everyone. Our experience seems to imply that symptoms of perianal irritation or discharge were only improved in one-third of patients having outpatient therapy for piles (Keighley et al, 1979; Greca et al, 1981).

Anal fissure

It may be a difficult decision to treat a chronic anal fissure associated with pruritus ani particularly if the internal sphincter may be damaged. When patients present with pain, the fissure should be treated initially by pharmacological agents. Dilatation of the anus should be avoided since this may precipitate incontinence of liquid faeces or mucus, thereby exacerbating pruritus. If glyceryl trinitrate or other nitric oxide donors fail, a skin advancement flap would be preferred to sphincterotomy (see Chapter 13).

Skin tags

Sometimes anal skin tags are thought to exacerbate pruritus by making anal hygiene difficult.

Improvement in anal hygiene or control of diarrhoea may itself diminish the size of large oedematous skin tags. Jensen (1988) undertook a randomized trial of excising skin tags or adopting an expectant policy for this group of patients. He found that 67% were asymptomatic after excision, compared with 55% of those receiving no therapy. He concluded that excision of hypertrophied anal skin is not justified. We support his conclusions in most patients unless the tags are large and persist despite conservative therapy. Thus it is probably worth avoiding excision of skin tags, at least until a trial of improved anal hygiene has been thoroughly explored. If tags are excised it is important to avoid creating a skin furrow.

Anal incontinence

Anal incontinence due to iatrogenic sphincter damage or parturition injury frequently predisposes to pruritus ani because of faecal soiling or mucous leakage. Pelvic floor or sphincter repair is not advised for the treatment of pruritus. Pruritus ani often persists despite improvement in continence after surgery (Yoshioka and Keighley, 1989). On the other hand, if pruritus is associated with a sphincter deficiency and a gutter deformity, successful repair frequently controls soiling and may improve the associated pruritus. We do not think there is any role for isolated internal anal sphincter repair for pruritis ani.

Bacterial infections

Syphilis should be treated with penicillin. Gonorrhoea may be associated with resistant strains of *Neisseria* and therapy should be closely monitored by the microbiology department. Tuberculosis should be treated with triple therapy until the results of culture and their sensitivities are known. *Corynebacterium minutissimum* should be treated with topical sodium fusidate ointment (2%) applied to the perianal skin every 6 hours. If this is ineffective, oral erythromycin 0.5 g 6-hourly for 10 days should be tried.

Fungal infections

Microbiological reports will not be available until some days after initial consultation with the patient. Isolation of *Candida* is common in patients who do not have pruritus, so most clinicians advise on therapy according to the clinical presentation. Obvious candidial infection is usually treated by topical nystatin cream (100 000 units/g) applied to the perianal skin four times daily. If there is no response, topical miconazole or ketoconazole should be tried. Primary fungal infections of the perianal skin with *Trychophyton rubrum* are treated with oral griseofulvin 125 mg 8-hourly until the patient is asymptomatic. Ringworm can be treated by clotrimazole, tolnaftate, haloprogin or miconazole cream.

Viral infections

Anal warts can be treated by topical application of a 25% suspension of podophyllin in compound benzoin tincture. The tincture makes the suspension very sticky and therefore it is less likely to run off the warts on to adjacent normal skin. The suspension is best applied with a cotton-wool bud mounted on a stick while the buttocks are held apart for 5 minutes. Culp and Kaplan (1944) reported that 82% achieved a complete cure with one application and another 15% cleared up completely with a second application. Others have failed to produce such good results and many cases of condylomata acuminata are very resistant to treatment with podophyllin (see Chapter 18). Such cases require surgical destruction with diathermy or excision after infiltrating the anal canal and perianal skin with 1:300 000 adrenaline in saline (Thomson and Grace, 1978). Warts in the genital region may also be treated by topical or systemic acyclovir (Corey et al, 1982; Mendal et al, 1982). Unfortunately, condylomata acuminata show a strong tendency to recur. Perhaps the most promising form of treatment for anal warts is by autogenous vaccine prepared from excised material that is then administered back to the patient by subcutaneous injection (0.5 mL) each week for 6 weeks (Abcarian et al, 1976).

There is no specific therapy for herpes simplex apart from drying agents, such as alcohol or zinc sulphate. If there is no response, topical or systemic acyclovir may be used.

Molluscum contagiosum is treated by excision, by application of 25% trichloracetic acid, or by liquid nitrogen destruction.

Parasites

Scabies is treated using benzyl benzoate. Pediculosis infestations usually respond to dichlorodiphenyltrichloroethane (DDT) powder or benzyl benzoate. Piperazine is the most effective therapy for threadworm. A single dose is given and repeated 2 weeks later. An alternative therapy for threadworm is an oxyuricide; this treatment stains the stool red. It is advisable to treat all other members of the household.

Treatment of idiopathic cases

Most cases of pruritus ani are idiopathic and these are more difficult to treat. Frequently these cases are associated with degenerative changes in the internal anal sphincter which have a characteristic appearance on anal ultrasonography.

Anal hygiene

The importance of adequate perianal cleanliness cannot be overemphasized in the treatment of idiopathic pruritus ani. Individuals who pay attention to careful perianal hygiene seldom suffer from this condition. In the sixteenth century Rebelars' character Gargantua charged his father Grangousier a puncheon of Breton wine for advice on perianal cleanliness. After trying various implements for postdefecation cleansing, including an attorney's hat and a gentlewoman's velvet mask, Gargantua concluded that there was 'none so comforting as the neck of a goose, that is well downed, if you hold her neck betwixt your legs' (Rebelars, 1952). Sadly, in contemporary society such methods would be unacceptable as well as expensive! Currently a bidet is ideal. This allows the perianal skin to be washed with tepid water and blotted with cotton-wool after defecation (Banov, 1971). For patients who do not have the use of a bidet, a large plastic bowl is adequate. When washing facilities are not available, moist tissues can be used; they are available in sachets that can be easily carried in the pocket. After washing, the anal skin should be clean and completely dry. When the skin is very sore, gentle drying of the skin with a hair-dryer is effective. Once the skin is dry it should be kept dry, and loose-fitting cotton underwear is advisable.

Patients should be told that irritants such as toilet paper must be avoided: cleansing with water is the only way to control the habit of rubbing the anal region with many sheets of paper. Repeated use of paper may damage the epithelium, allowing bacteria to enter the skin. Some toilet paper is allergenic (Keith et al, 1969).

It is advisable to make the patient understand the cause of pruritis ani and the rationale of treatment. One should emphasize that the condition frequently recurs if scratching persists. If there is a desire to scratch, the anal region should be washed. As patients often do not remember all they are told during the initial consultation, we give them a copy of our 'ten rules' for pruritus sufferers (Table 19.2).

Many patients find that their symptoms respond to simple, improved perianal hygiene as outlined above, but for patients who scratch the perianal skin

Table 19.2 The ten rules for patients with pruritus ani.

1. *Keep the area clean by washing*, after every bowel action and night and morning. The nightly bath is particularly important if you itch at night. A bidet is ideal but sitting in the bath or a large bowl of water is a good substitute. Make sure that all the small particles of motion are removed from the skin crevices around the anus.
2. *Avoid rubbing with a bar of soap*, or a rough flannel. Soap remaining in the skin crevices can be very irritating. A few suds in the water and the finger tips or cotton wool are all that are needed.
3. *If you are away from home* or good toilet facilities when you have to pass a motion, use medicated wipes which provide better, gentler cleaning than hard paper.
4. *Keep the area dry*. Dab the skin dry gently with a towel or very soft paper. Do not rub. A hair dryer is the gentlest way of drying thoroughly.
5. *Avoid excessive moisture*. Never leave a wet dressing on the anal skin. Wear cotton underwear, never nylon. Avoid any firm foundation garment that presses the buttocks together. The free circulation of air will prevent moisture accumulating. A loose skirt is better than tight jeans. Avoid tights, use stockings or crutchless tights.
6. *After drying gently* keep a thin pledget of cotton wool dusted with powder against the anus inside the pants. The pledget should be about twice as large as a 50p piece and should be changed each time you wash.
7. *Avoid perfumed talcum powder*: this tends to collect into small solid lumps in the skin crevices and the perfume may cause allergy. ZeaSORB or other special drying powders are better. Baby powder may be tolerated but it is not ideal. Use ZeaSORB to dust the cotton wool pledget.
8. *Avoid ointments and creams* unless specifically prescribed by a specialist. Any greasy preparation tends to keep the skin soggy, which is what we are trying to avoid. Many preparations are hyperallergenic and should be avoided. Lotions may be prescribed in the acute stage of the condition and usually applied after cleaning, before drying. Silver nitrate or magenta paint lotions are often helpful but should not be used without medical advice.
9. *Keep the bowels regular* and smooth with plenty of roughage in the diet. Some dietary items cause irritation or loose motions in some people, avoid anything that does this to you. Do not sit and strain for many minutes when passing a motion, take more roughage if necessary.
10. *As the condition improves*, gradually reduce the strict regimen described here, but remember the principles of keeping the area clean and dry and avoid damage to skin by rubbing or medication. If the condition recurs, as it may from time to time, start the routine again at once until the irritation is controlled.

during the night, chlorpheniramine maleate (4 mg orally), which acts as both a systemic antipruritic and a sedative, may be useful on retiring to bed.

Antidiarrhoeals

If the pruritus is potentiated by loose stools in the absence of an underlying disorder, oral antidiarrhoeal drugs such as codeine phosphate may help alleviate the patient's symptoms. Bulking agents may also be useful if patients pass loose sloppy stools. Ispaghula, sterculia or methylcellulose may improve the patient's symptoms. Coarse bran may not be as useful because fine particles of the bran excreted in the stool can adhere to the skin furrows of the perianal region and are difficult to clean away.

Topical applications

Local application of antiseptics, local anaesthetics and antibiotics are generally not recommended because of the danger of allergy, but they may sometimes prove efficacious (Allenby et al, 1993). In contrast, astringent lotions have a place if perianal dermatitis causes the skin to become moist and ulcerated. One of the most widely used astringents is a very dilute aqueous solution of silver nitrate. This is safe and effective but has the disadvantage of staining clothes and fingers.

We carried out a randomized prospective crossover trial of three widely used local applications for pruritus ani. These were aluminium acetate solution (5%), crotamiton (Eurax Lotion) (10%), and a bland cream which acted as the control. Thirty-seven patients were treated with these lotions and were assessed using a linear analogue scale before and at 2 weeks after treatment with each agent. We were unable to demonstrate any significant reduction in symptoms with the use of any of these lotions. No one preparation appeared to be superior to the rest.

Local surgical therapy

Anaesthetic solutions injected into the perianal skin have been used for treatment of pruritus ani (Gabril, 1929). However, the technique can cause severe skin necrosis and is not recommended. Other operative procedures used to treat pruritus ani in the past have included undermining of the perianal skin (Bacon, 1949). The rationale of this procedure is to divide the sensory nerve supply of the perianal area. Unfortunately, sepsis and separation of the wound may occur and the control of symptoms is frequently disappointing. We do not recommend this approach. We do not believe that excision of anal skin ridges or skin tags is advisable unless the patient no longer scratches and has carefully followed advice concerning anal hygiene. If a skin lesion prevents adequate cleaning, excision may then be justified.

REFERENCES

Abcarian H, Smith D & Sharon N (1976) The immunotherapy of anal condylomata acuminata. *Dis Colon Rectum* **19**: 237–239.

Alexander S (1975) Dermatological aspects of anorectal disease. *Clin Gastroenterol* **4**: 651–657.

Alexander-Williams J (1983) Pruritus ani. *BMJ* **287**: 159–160.

Allan A, Ambrose NS, Silverman S & Keighley MRB (1987) Physiological study of pruritus ani. *Br J Surg* **74**: 576–579.

Allenby CF, Johnstone RS, Chatfield S, Pike LC & Tidy G (1993) Perinal: a new no-touch spray to relieve the symptoms of pruritis ani. *Int J Colorect Dis* **8**: 184–187.

Ambrose NS, Johnson M, Burdon DW & Keighley MRB (1985) The influence of single-dose intravenous antibiotics on faecal flora and emergence of *Clostridium difficile*. *J Antimicrob Chemother* **15**: 319–326.

Bacon HE (1949) *Anus, Rectum and Sigmoid Colon*, 3rd edn, vol. 1. Philadelphia: Lippincott.

Banov L (1971) The prophylactic value of anal hygiene. *South Med J* **64**: 1521–1523.

Bowyer A & McColl I (1966) The role of erythrasma in pruritus ani. *Lancet* **ii**: 572–573.

Brooks LH (1969) Further studies of the management of pruritus ani. *Dis Colon Rectum* **93**: 193–195.

Brown ST & Weinberger J (1974) Molluscum contagiosum: sexually transmitted disease in 17 cases. *J Am Vener Dis Assoc* **1**: 35–38.

Chang TW (1977) Genital herpes and type 1 herpes virus hominis. *JAMA* **238**: 155–158.

Corey L, Nahmias AJ, Guinan ME et al (1982) A trial of topical acyclovir in genital herpes simplex virus infections. *N Engl J Med* **306**: 1313–1319.

Culp OS & Kaplan IW (1944) Condylomata acuminata: two hundred cases treated with podophyllin. *Ann Surg* **120**: 251–255.

Daniel GL, Longo WE & Vernava AM (1994) Pruritis ani: causes and concerns. *Dis Colon Rectum* **37**: 670–674.

Detrano SJ (1984) Cryotherapy for chronic specific pruritus ani. *J Dermatol Surg Oncol* **10**: 483–484.

Dodi G, Pirone E, Bettin A et al (1985) The microflora in proctological patients with and without pruritus ani. *Br J Surg* **72**: 967–969.

Eyars AE & Thomson JPS (1979) Pruritus ani: is anal sphincter dysfunction important in aetiology? *BMJ* **2**: 1549–1551.

Farouk R, Duthie GS, Pryde A & Bartolo DCC (1994) Abnormal transient internal sphincter relaxation in idiopathic pruritis ani: physiological evidence from ambulatory monitoring. *Br J Surg* **81**: 603–606.

Felman YM & Nikitas JA (1980) Genital molluscum contagiosum. *Cutis* **26**: 28–32.

Fisher AA (1976) Antihistamine dermatitis. *Cutis* **18**: 329–336.

Fisher AA (1980) Allergic reaction to topical (surface) anaesthetics. *Cutis* **25**: 584–625.

Fisher AA & Brancaccio RR (1979) Allergic contact sensitivity to propylene glycol in a lubricant jelly. *Arch Dermatol* **115**: 1451.

Friend WG (1976) The cause of idiopathic pruritus ani. *Dis Colon Rectum* **20**: 40–42.

Gabril WB (1929) Treatment of pruritus ani and anal fissure: the use of anaesthetic solutions in oil. *BMJ* **1**: 1070–1072.

Greca F, Hares MM, Nevah E, Alexander-Williams J & Keighley MRB (1981) A randomized trial to compare rubber band ligation with phenol injection for treatment of haemorrhoids. *Br J Surg* **68**: 250–252.

Haynes WG & Read NW (1982) Anorectal activity in man during rectal infusion of saline: a dynamic assessment of the anal continence mechanism. *J Physiol* **330**: 45–56.

Jeansson S & Molin L (1970) Genital herpes virus hominis infections: a venereal disease? *Lancet* **i**: 1064.

Jensen SL (1988) A randomized trial of simple excision of nonspecific hypertrophied anal papillae versus expectant management in patients with chronic pruritus ani. *Ann R Coll Surg Engl* **70**: 348–349.

Jones DJ (1992) Pruritis ani: ABC of colorectal diseases. *BMJ* **305**: 575–577.

Keele CA (1957) Chemical causes of pain and itch. *Proc R Soc Med* **50**: 477–484.

Keighley MRB, Alexander-Williams J, Buchmann P, Minervini S & Arabi Y (1979) Prospective trials of minor surgical procedures and high fibre diet for haemorrhoids. *BMJ* **2**: 967–969.

Keith L, Reich W & Bush IM (1969) Toilet paper dermatitis. *JAMA* **209**: 269.

McMillan A & Lee TD (1981) Sigmoidoscopic and microscopic appearance of the rectal mucosa in homosexual men. *Gut* **22**: 1035–1041.

McMillan A, Gilmour HM, Slatford K & McNeillage GLC (1983) Proctitis in homosexual men. *Br J Vener Dis* **59**: 260–264.

Mendal A, Adler MW, Sutherland S et al (1982) Intravenous acyclovir treatment for primary genital herpes. *Lancet* **1**: 697–700.

Murie JA, Sim AJW & MacKenzie I (1981) The importance of pain, pruritus and soiling as symptoms of haemorrhoids and their response to haemorrhoidectomy or rubber band ligation. *Br J Surg* **68**: 247–249.

Pirone E, Infantine A, Masin A et al (1992) Can proctological procedures resolve perianal pruritus and mycosis? A prospective study of 23 cases. *Int J Colorect Dis* **7**: 18–20.

Rebelars F (1952) Gargantua and Pantagruel (translated by Thomas Urquhart and Peter Molteux). *Great Books of the Western World*, vol. 24, pp 16–18. Chicago: Encylopedia Britannica.

Robbins RD, Sohn N & Weinstein MA (1983) Colorectal view of venereal disease. *NY State J Med* **94**: 323–326.

Robertson DHH, McMillan A & Young M (1980) *Clinical Practice in Sexually Transmissible Disease*. Tunbridge Wells: Pitman Medical.

Shelley WB & Arthur RP (1957) The neurohistology and neurophysiology of the itch sensation in man. *Arch Dermatol* **76**: 296–323.

Silverman SH, Youngs DJ, Allan A, Ambrose S & Keighley MRB (1989) The faecal microflora in pruritus ani. *Dis Colon Rectum* **32**: 416–468.

Smith LE, Henrichs D & McCullah RD (1982) Prospective studies in the aetiology and treatment of pruritus ani. *Dis Colon Rectum* **25**: 358–363.

Sohn N & Robilotti JG (1977) The gay bowel syndrome: a review of colonic and rectal conditions in 200 male homosexuals. *Am J Gastroenterol* **67**: 478–481.

Thomson JPS & Grace RH (1978) The treatment of perianal and anal condylomata acuminata: a new operative technique. *J R Soc Med* **71**: 180–181.

Welch K, Finkbeiner W, Alpers CE et al (1984) Autopsy findings in the acquired immune deficiency syndrome. *JAMA* **252**: 1152–1159.

William DC (1983) The gay bowel syndrome: differential diagnosis and management of anorectal and intestinal disease in homosexual man. In McCormack WM (ed) *Diagnosis and Treatment of Sexually Transmitted Diseases*, pp. 194–209. Boston: Wright.

Winner HJ & Hurley R (1964) *Candida albicans*. London: Churchill Livingstone.

Yoshioka K & Keighley MRB (1989) Critical assessment of the quality of continence after post anal repair for faecal incontinence. *Br J Surg* **76**: 1054–1057.

20

FAECAL INCONTINENCE

Faecal incontinence is now recognized as a common and distressing symptom with many causes, the commonest of which is cerebral degeneration. Faecal incontinence often occurs with urinary incontinence and is reported in 20% of patients in elderly care institutions. In surgical practice, post-obstetric sphincter injury and/or pudendal neuropathy is the cause most commonly referred for assessment and treatment. Ultrasound evidence of sphincter defects is reported in 30% of primigravidae, but clinical evidence of incontinence is evident in only 13% in the first 6 weeks after vaginal delivery and in 4% in the first 2 years after childbirth. Only 3% of these sphincter defects are clinically recognized by obstetric staff. Non-neuropathic sphincter defects resulting in incontinence occur after anal surgery, particularly fistulotomy (see Chapter 16), sphincterotomy (Chapter 13), haemorrhoidectomy and anal dilatation (Chapter 12). Other causes include neurological disorders, diabetes, demyelinating disease, cauda equina defects and autonomic neuropathy. Anorectal malformations frequently present in adult life with impaired continence, usually associated with colonic inertia and impaired evacuation. Persistent incontinence may occur in 15–25% of patients after successful correction of a rectal prolapse (Chapter 23). Colorectal disease or sphincter-preserving operations for colorectal disease may be complicated by imperfect continence.

Incontinence may be caused by anatomical defects in the internal sphincter resulting in low resting anal pressure, but there is often some other defect as well. External sphincter defects result in urgency and poor voluntary squeeze pressures; often internal and external sphincter defects occur in combination. The worst prognosis is in patients with neuropathic incontinence caused by impaired conduction in the pudendal nerves or sacral outflow resulting in progressive denervation of the striated sphincter and pelvic floor with anaesthesia of the anorectum. Neuropathy is frequently associated with perineal descent which complicates impaired rectal evacuation and straining. This form of pelvic floor failure increases in incidence with age and results in progressive deteriorating continence which can be difficult to treat.

Women in particular are often embarrassed about their symptoms; they may become reclusive, being confined to their homes, afraid to visit their neighbours, friends and even family, having lost all feeling of self-respect, which may result in psychological morbidity. Many of these patients feel unable to discuss their symptoms with the medical profession, feeling unclean, misunderstood and isolated.

Treatment options cannot be offered without counselling, comprehensive patient information and thorough physiological and psychological assessment. Conservative management may be sufficient using sphincter strengthening regimes, biofeedback, enemas and intermittent use of an anal occlusive device. Surgical treatment of pelvic floor failure may be disappointing, but in well-selected patients, some form of pelvic floor repair can achieve continence in 40–50% of patients. Sphincter repair for isolated defects achieves excellent results, but patients should be warned that results are less predictable if there is coexisting pelvic floor neuropathy. Muscle transposition has a small place in a few patients with persistant incontinence after pelvic floor repair and in extensive sphincter trauma. The place of the electrically stimulated gracilis transposition will be thoroughly reviewed in this chapter as will the early results of the implantable artificial sphincter. Some patients with impaired evacuation may need access for antegrade colonic irrigation. Others will consider that their quality of life is better with a stoma. Usually this requires rectal excision and an end colostomy that can be irrigated. Some, particularly younger patients, decide to have a reservoir ileostomy rather than colostomy irrigation.

DEFINITIONS

The severity and frequency of incontinence together with its impact on quality of life needs to be recorded (Elliot et al, 1987; Pescatori et al, 1992). The most widely used scoring system separately scores the frequency of solid, liquid and flatus incontinence as well as the use of pads and the impact on quality of life (Oliveira et al, 1996). This 20-point score is described in Table 20.1 and certainly allows comparison of outcome in different centres (Yoshioka et al, 1997). Unfortunately, it does not separate passive incontinence from urgency and has no assessment of soiling, which should be classified on its own (Engel et al, 1995). The St Marks group applied this classification and reported 66 patients with passive incontinence alone, 42 with urgency alone, 38 with passive and urge incontinence and 5 with soiling. A more elaborate score uses a linear analogue scale and documents specific effects of incontinence on quality of life (Schuster et al, 1994).

Incontinence may be 'passive', resulting in the

Table 20.1 Continence grading scale.

Type of incontinence	*Frequency* Never	Less than once a month	Less than once a week/once or more a month	Less than once a day/once or more a week	More than once a day
Solid	0	1	2	3	4
Liquid	0	1	2	3	4
Gas	0	1	2	3	4
Requires pad	0	1	2	3	4
Lifestyle alteration	0	1	2	3	4

From Oliveira et al (1996).

Table 20.2 Types of faecal incontinence (*n* = 151).

	Passive incontinence alone (*n* = 66)	*Urge incontinence alone* (*n* = 42)
Age	55.9 ± 15.5	42.4 ± 14.7
Max resting pressure	50.7 ± 23.3	68.8 ± 31.0
Max voluntary component	72.3 ± 55.3	42.0 ± 33.7
IAS defect only	23	1
EAS defect only	12	10
EAS + IAS defects	14	20
Both normal	17	11

From Engel et al (1995).

passage of faeces without the patient being aware of it (Engel et al, 1995). Passive incontinence is more frequent in the elderly and is a common feature of rectal prolapse, senile incontinence or neuropathic faecal incontinence. The physiological data suggest that a greater proportion have internal sphincter defects, low resting pressures and sensory loss (Table 20.2). These patients also have abnormal rectoanal inhibition with spontaneous relaxation and rectal contraction (Farouk et al, 1993, 1994; Speakman and Kamm, 1993; Goes et al, 1995; Buntzen et al, 1995; Speakman et al, 1995; Gee et al, 1995; Pucciani et al, 1997). Urgency is characterized by patients being aware of, but being unable to prevent, the passage of faeces. This type of incontinence typifies those individuals with a pelvic floor or sphincter injury with normal neuromuscular innervation. These patients frequently have external sphincter defects and reduced voluntary contraction. Often the pelvic floor musculature cannot sustain an acute anorectal angle (Hill et al, 1994a; Gee and Durdey; 1995; Hajivassiliou et al, 1996).

Urgency refers to patients who must defecate immediately, otherwise incontinence may occur if toilet facilities are not available. This type of incontinence is common in patients with a narrow or inflamed rectum such as patients with inflammatory bowel disease or radiation proctitis. Patients may only be incontinent to liquids or flatus. Some patients may be incontinent of mucus as in villous adenoma, haemorrhoids, rectal prolapse, a Whitehead deformity or an inflammatory process in the rectum. The frequency of incontinence in relation to the consistency of stool should be recorded (Womack et al, 1986; Miller et al, 1988c). The patient should be asked if they need to wear a sanitary towel or a small pledget of cottonwool in the natal cleft. Further enquiry should discover if these measures are for security or whether they become soiled.

Soiling should be distinguished from faecal incontinence (Felt-Bersma et al, 1989). Soiling usually indicates that the anal canal is deformed from scarring or that there is a solid faecal mass in the rectum (Read and Abouzekry, 1986), as in megarectum or anorectal agenesis (Hassink et al, 1993; Stewart et al, 1994). Patients with soiling from anal deformity are usually continent but leak small amounts of faecal material which causes excoriation and perianal discomfort.

An assessment of bowel habit is essential. Some patients with incontinence have intermittent diarrhoea, there may be underlying diverticular disease, irritable bowel syndrome or even inflammable bowel disease (Read et al, 1984). Others will be found to be constipated or to suffer from impaired rectal evacuation, resulting in repeated straining and perineal descent (Moore-Gillon, 1984; Bruck et al, 1988; Lubowski et al, 1988a; Skomorowska et al, 1988; Mackie and Parks, 1989). A questionnaire (Table 20.3) has been proposed to standardize information amongst patients with incontinence but it is doubtful whether this will be widely used (Schuster et al, 1994). Incontinence is a highly complex disorder of anorectal perception, evacuation and retention, hence the need for clear definitions if treatments are to be comprehensively compared.

A high proportion of patients with soiling are men. Physiologically there is dyssynergy of rectal sensation and anal relaxation. Frequently the rectoanal inhibitory reflex is excessively deep or exquisitely sensitive to rectal distension or there may be spontaneous bursts of internal sphincter inhibition and rectal contraction (Farouk et al, 1994; Hoffmann et al, 1995; Goes et al, 1995). Many of the patients with soiling have an asymmetric high-pressure zone on vector manometry (Braun et al, 1994) and there may be excessive fibrosis in the anal canal (Sultan et al, 1994a) from previous anal surgery. Men with soiling tend to have a long high-pressure zone and higher resting and squeeze pressures than incontinent patients (Table 20.4). Over two-thirds have had previous anal surgery (Sentovich et al, 1995).

Table 20.3 Incontinence questionnaire (as proposed by the World Congress of Gastroenterology Working Party, Rome, 1991).

QUESTIONNAIRE

We need to assess the severity of your symptoms. Please answer the following questions on a scale of 0–10 in which 0 = no problem and 10 = the most severe it has ever been.

Before / After treatment

1 (a) When you pass stool do you have any warning?
Always plenty of warning 0 ______ No warning at all 10 ☐ ☐

(b) Can you distinguish between gas and solid stool?
Always distinguish 0 ______ Never distinguish 10 ☐ ☐

2 If you have loss of bowel control for gas, answer the following questions. If this is not a problem write 0 to all the questions. If the question does not apply to you do not write anything.

(a) How frequently does it occur?
Never 0 ______ Less than once a month ______ Less than once a week ______ Every day ______ Many times a day 10 ☐ ☐

(b) How much 'gas' do you leak?
None 0 ______ A lot 10 ☐ ☐

(c) How bad is the problem?
None 0 ______ A terrible problem 10 ☐ ☐

(d) How much does it interfere with your social life?
Never 0 ______ A great deal 10 ☐ ☐

(e) How much does it interfere with your work situation?
Never 0 ______ Had to stop working 10 ☐ ☐

(f) How much does it interfere with your sexual relations?
Never 0 ______ Stopped intercourse 10 ☐ ☐

3 If you have loss of bowel control for liquids, answer the following questions. If this is not a problem write 0 to all the questions. If the question does not apply to you do not write anything.

(a) How frequently does it occur?
Never 0 ______ Less than once a month ______ Less than once a week ______ Every day ______ Many times a day 10 ☐ ☐

(b) How much liquid do you leak?
None 0 ______ A lot 10 ☐ ☐

(c) How bad is the problem?
None 0 ______ A terrible problem 10 ☐ ☐

(d) How much does it interfere with your social life?
Never 0 ______ A great deal 10 ☐ ☐

(e) How much does it interfere with your work situation?
Never 0 ______ Had to stop working 10 ☐ ☐

(f) How much does it interfere with your sexual relations?
Never 0 ______ Stopped intercourse 10 ☐ ☐

Table 20.3 *Continued*

4 If you have a loss of bowel control for solid stool, answer the following questions. If this is not a problem write 0. If the question does not apply to you do not write anything.

(a) How frequently does it occur?

Never 0	Less than once a month	Less than once a week	Every day	Many times a day 10	☐	☐

(b) How much solid stool do you leak?

None 0 ________ A lot 10 ☐ ☐

(c) How bad is the problem?

None 0 ________ A terrible problem 10 ☐ ☐

(d) How much does it interfere with your social life?

Never 0 ________ A great deal 10 ☐ ☐

(e) How much does it interfere with your work situation?

Never 0 ________ Had to stop working 10 ☐ ☐

(f) How much does it interfere with your sexual relations?

Never 0 ________ Stopped intercourse 10 ☐ ☐

Table 20.4 Results of anal manometry in men with soiling (leakers) and incontinent patients.

	Normal (n = 20)	*Leaker* (n = 14)	*Incontinent* (n = 11)
Resting manometry			
Mean maximum pressure (cmH_2O)	102	82*	59†
Sphincter length (cm)	3.48	3.96*	3.00*
Squeezing manometry			
Mean maximum pressure (cmH_2O)	196	161*	97†
Sphincter length (cm)	4.20	4.29	3.77

*$P < 0.05$ compared with normal men.
*$P < 0.005$ compared with normal men.
From Sentovich et al (1995).

PHYSIOLOGICAL CONSIDERATIONS

The anal canal is normally closed at rest and during sleep. The moist mucosal surfaces of the anal canal are in close proximity due to constant activity of the internal and external anal sphincters, the puborectalis (Wheatley et al, 1977; Lestar et al, 1989) and the surface properties of the anal cushions.

Anal cushions

There is both direct and circumstantial evidence that the anal cushions play an important role in keeping the anal canal closed (Haas et al, 1984). Haemorrhoidectomy may be complicated by anal soiling even in the presence of normal sphincter pressures (Bennett et al, 1963; Bruck et al, 1988) and normal anal ultrasonography. Furthermore, patients with prominent anal cushions tend to have high anal sphincter pressures (Hancock and Smith, 1975; Arabi et al, 1977). Anal cushions tend to hold the mucosa in apposition by their surface secretory function. The cushions themselves are easily distensible, being filled with wide channel blood vessels (Thomson, 1975). Anal cushions are compressed by high sphincter pressures but expand to keep the anal canal closed when anal pressures fall. Gibbons et al (1986a) measured anal sphincter pressures and compliance using probes of different diameter. Wide channel probes gave higher values for resting and squeeze pressures than did smaller probes.

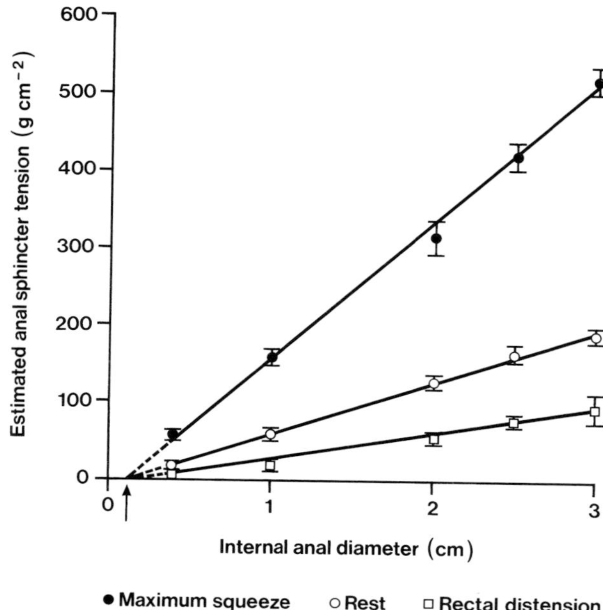

Figure 20.1 The anal canal is open at zero tension. The estimated anal sphincter tension is plotted against the internal anal sphincter diameter from measurements at rest (○), maximum pelvic floor contraction (●), and during rectal distension (□). If the data points are expressed in a linear fashion, the anus is likely to be opened at zero tension.

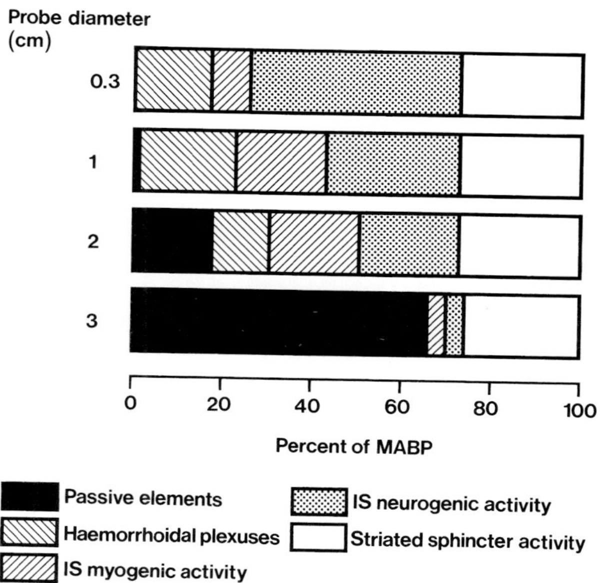

Figure 20.2 Components of resting anal pressure. The percentage components of the maximum resting anal basal pressure (MABP) are plotted according to probe diameter. IS, internal sphincter.

When tension within the anal canal was plotted against probe diameter, the anus was theoretically open at zero tension (Caro et al, 1978) (Figure 20.1). Since all patients were continent, some other factor must operate to prevent leakage. It is proposed that the distensible vascular anal cushions fulfil this function (Gibbons et al, 1986a; Lestar et al, 1989).

Internal sphincter

The internal anal sphincter is the expanded distal segment of the circular smooth muscle of the gut. The muscle exhibits continuous activity which is both under autonomic control and locally innervated by an intermyenteric plexus (since activity can be blocked by circular rectal myotomy) (Kamm et al, 1989). The internal sphincter provides the most important component of resting anal pressure when the anal canal is closed (Figure 20.2). The activity of the smooth muscle component is completely inhibited by rectal distension: the rectoanal inhibitory reflex (Lestar et al, 1989). This reflex is mediated through the enteric nervous system by nitric oxide, synthesized by L-arginine and catalysed by nitric oxide synthase. Nitric oxide donors such as glyceryl trinitrate or diltiazem have been shown to inhibit internal sphincter activity (Stebbing et al, 1995, 1997; Davies et al, 1995; O'Kelly, 1996; Luman et al, 1997).

Indirect evidence of impaired internal sphincter activity in faecal incontinence is largely based on manometry. Impaired resting anal pressure is common amongst patients with faecal incontinence (Wald and Turugunthla, 1984; Hiltunen, 1985; Loening-Baucke and Anuras, 1985; Yoshioka et al, 1987a; Rogers et al, 1988a; Pedersen and Christiansen, 1989; Penninckx et al, 1989; Farouk et al, 1993, 1994; Goes et al, 1995; Hoffman et al, 1995; Pucciani et al, 1997) (Figure 20.3). Snooks et al (1984c) studied ten patients with faecal incontinence after anal dilatation. Eight displayed evidence of impaired internal anal sphincter dysfunction with extremely low resting pressures. Incontinence in association with gross perineal descent is not associated with increased fibre density in the puborectalis but there is significant reduction in resting pressures compared with patients with perineal descent who are continent (33 versus 78 cmH_2O) (Womack et al, 1986). Impairment of internal sphincter function in incontinence has received insufficient attention until recently (Duthie and Watts, 1965; Swash et al, 1988; Lestar et al, 1989; Klosterhalfen et al,

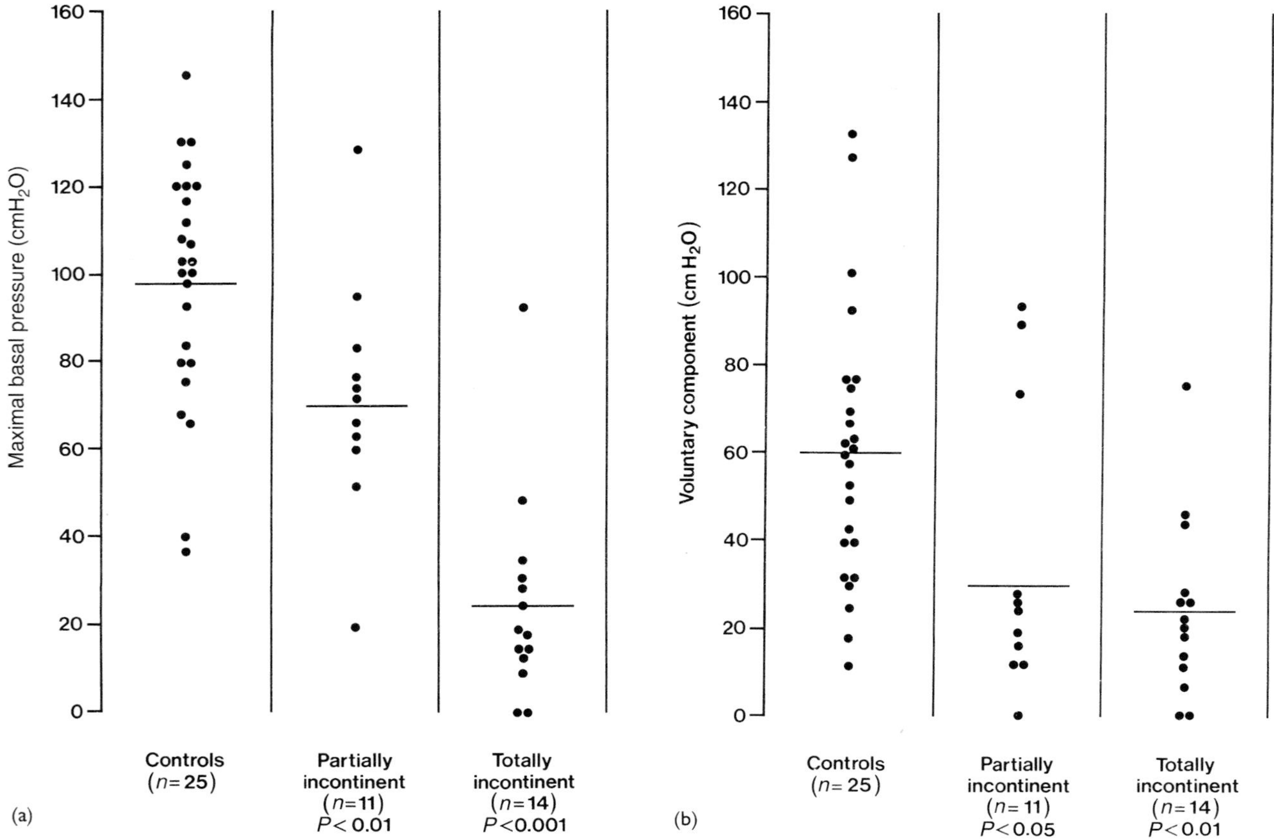

Figure 20.3a,b Anal manometry in faecal incontinence. (a) Maximum resting anal canal pressure (cmH_2O) in patients with partial faecal incontinence and total faecal incontinence compared with controls. (b) The voluntary component of squeeze pressure in patients with partial faecal incontinence and total incontinence compared with controls.

1990; Speakman et al, 1990; Sun et al, 1990a; Burnett and Bartram, 1991) and the potential role of pharmacological agents such as octreatide in improving function deserves more attention than it has previously received (Guitierrez and Shah, 1975; Schiller et al, 1982; Enck et al, 1989b; Speakman and Kamm, 1991; Speakman et al, 1991; Rasmussen et al, 1996).

The internal anal sphincter is essential as a means for allowing rectal contents to come into contact with the sensitive anal mucosa during the rectoanal inhibitory (sampling) reflex (Schuster et al, 1965). Involuntary inhibition of internal sphincter activity following rectal distension may be impaired in idiopathic incontinence. However, the internal anal sphincter may be so deficient in patients with faecal incontinence that the rectoanal inhibitory reflex cannot be elicited at all (Bannister et al, 1989). Although Loening-Baucke and Anuras (1985) showed no reduction in resting pressure, threshold or amplitude of the rectoanal inhibitory reflex with age, the numbers studied were small. Most other groups (NW Read et al, 1979; Matheson and Keighley, 1981) have recorded a progressive fall in resting pressure after the age of 60 years, indicating progressive degeneration in internal sphincter function with age (Klosterhalfen et al, 1990; Kuijpers and Scheuer, 1990; Eckardt and Elmer, 1991).

Ultrastructural changes in the internal sphincter are also frequently observed in idiopathic faecal incontinence, with loss of smooth muscle cells, stretching of elastic tissue, increased collagen deposition and disruption of smooth muscle cells (Swash et al, 1988).

Defects in the internal sphincter can be observed using anal ultrasonography in incontinence (Pittman et al, 1990; Burnett and Bartram, 1991; Speakman et al, 1991). Internal sphincter defects are observed after previous sphincterotomy, haemorrhoidectomy, sphincterotomy, fistulotomy and very commonly in obstetric injuries (Deen et al, 1993b; Tjandra et al, 1993; Emblem et al, 1994; Falk et al, 1994; Farouk and Bartolo, 1994; Solomon et al, 1994).

The internal anal sphincter also increases in width with increasing age due to progressive fibrosis. The collagen content of the internal anal sphincter in incontinent patients is significantly higher than in controls (Speakman et al, 1995). The width of the internal anal sphincter on anal ultrasonography is inversely correlated with resting anal canal pressures.

Direct measurement of internal anal sphincter activity is now achievable using fine needle electromyography. Ambulatory measurements made from ultrasonographically guided needle electrodes display a variety of patterns in incontinence (Sorensen et al, 1994). These include gross impairment of electrical activity, episodes of spontaneous inhibition or exaggerated rectoanal inhibition (Farouk et al, 1993, 1994; Goes et al, 1995).

Clinically, defects in the internal sphincter in the absence of neuropathy and with an intact external sphincter rarely lead to incontinence, but soiling may be evident and flatus control may be defective. When there is a defect in the internal and external sphincters, urge incontinence is usually present. If there is a defect in the internal sphincter and pudendal or spinal neuropathy, even in the presence of an intact striated sphincter, passive incontinence is likely. Thus, defects in the internal sphincter in a woman with a history of a difficult delivery or who chronically strains is likely to be symptomatic (Swash, 1993).

Innervation of the internal sphincter

The internal sphincter has a dual autonomic innervation (Burleigh, 1983). The sympathetic (L1 and L2) fibres via the hypogastric nerves are excitatory and the parasympathetic (S2–S4) innervation through the pelvic nerves is inhibitory. Internal sphincter activity is almost completely abolished by damage to the parasympathetic nerves, as occurs in lesions affecting the sacral outflow (Gunterberg et al, 1976). Conversely, resting anal canal pressures are only slightly reduced in patients with complete cervical or dorsal cord compression (Denny-Brown and Robertson, 1935) and in patients receiving muscle relaxants or after pudendal nerve block (Frenckner and Von Euler, 1975). The internal sphincter is devoid of ganglion cells (Frenckner and Ihre, 1976b; Carlstedt et al, 1988) and intrinsic nerve cell perikarya are absent in the autonomic plexus of the distal smooth muscle wall of the anal canal. Although ganglion cells are absent, there are many nerve fibres associated with high concentrations of the sympathetic neurotransmitter noradrenaline (Baumgarten et al, 1971).

Studies in patients having spinal anaesthesia (T6–T12), caudal anaesthesia (S1–S5) and pudendal nerve block (S2–S4) indicate that resting anal tone is maintained even though the external sphincter is paralysed (Frenckner and Von Euler, 1975; Frenckner and Ihre, 1976b). Normally there is tonic excitatory sympathetic discharge within the internal sphincter which keeps the anal canal closed. This is abolished by spinal anaesthesia, resulting in a 50% fall in anal canal pressure. Anal tone, particularly anal pressure response to bladder distension is abolished by epidural anaesthesia (Buntzen et al, 1995). There is also pharmacological evidence that internal sphincter tone is caused by continuous sympathetic activity, since infusion of noradrenaline increases tone which may be blocked by α-adrenoreceptor antagonists such as phentolamine and phenoxybenzamine (Guitierrez and Shah, 1975). Isoprenaline is inhibitory and may be blocked by β-adrenoreceptor antagonists such as propranolol. Phenylephrine also increases anal sphincter tone in normals and incontinent patients and may have a role in treatment (Carapeti et al, 1998).

Defects in the innervation of the internal anal sphincter in some patients with faecal incontinence is probable (Speakman et al, 1992) and may occur in association with defects in rectal sensation (Speakman and Kamm, 1993).

Pharmacological studies have indicated that in addition to the classical adrenergic and non-cholinergic elements, some innervation is non-adrenergic and cholinergic in nature. Neuropeptides play an important role in neural control of gastrointestinal motility. Several neuropeptides have been found in the internal anal sphincter such as vasoactive intestinal peptide (VIP), neuropeptide-y (NPY), galanin, calcitonin gene-related peptide (CGRP) and substance P. However, Speakman et al (1993) failed to demonstrate any changes in these among patients with faecal incontinence.

Rectoanal inhibitory reflex

If small increments of air are introduced into the rectum there is a transient rise followed by a profound fall in resting anal canal pressure. This is known as the rectoanal inhibitory or sampling reflex. A similar phenomenon, observed by ambulatory recordings, occurs spontaneously (Miller et al, 1988a; Kumar et al, 1989; Farouk et al, 1994). The precise configuration of the reflex depends upon the recording site (Schuster et al, 1965). A fall in resting pressure is observed in the upper anal canal (internal sphincter), whereas a rise in pressure after rectal distension is often seen in the lower anal canal (external anal sphincter) (Duthie and Bennett, 1963; Duthie, 1971; Bartolo, 1984). Recordings in the rectum show a contractile response to rectal distension that is mediated by a spinal reflex (Penninckx et al, 1989). The character of the reflex is also influenced by the distending volume, an internal sphincter response being observed alone with small volumes and a superimposed external anal sphincter response observed with larger volumes (Meunier and Mollard, 1977). The amplitude and duration of the reflex is also modified by the distending volumes and the nature of the distension (Parks et al, 1962; Schuster et al, 1965; Arhan et al, 1972; Ihre, 1974; Haynes and Read, 1982; Read et al, 1983b) (Figure 20.4).

Spontaneous rectoanal inhibitory reflexes seen during ambulatory recordings last between 10 and 30 seconds and tend to be more prolonged at night. The reflex is important for initiating and controlling defecation. Relaxation of the internal sphincter allows the faecal bolus to enter the sensitive epithelium of the midanal canal (anal transition zone). Once the bolus is recognized, the external sphincter and puborectalis either relax, allowing normal defecation or, if this is socially unacceptable, the pelvic floor and sphincters contract, forcing faecal material back into the rectum from the anal canal, which returns to its closed position. The rectoanal inhibitory reflex is preserved after high cord compression, resection of the rectum if the anal transition zone is retained, spinal anaesthesia and pudendal nerve block, and following administration of muscle relaxants (Duthie, 1971; Frenckner and Ihre, 1976b; Lane and Parks, 1977; Read and Bannister, 1985). It has been suggested therefore that relaxation of the internal anal sphincter is probably mediated by the intrinsic intramural plexus since re-innervation may be observed after ileoanal anastomosis (Kmiot and Keighley, 1990) and the response is blocked by low rectal myotomy (Kamm et al, 1989). Spontaneous internal sphincter relaxation occurs in normals and in patients with idiopathic faecal incontinence, but the fall in pressure and its duration is greater in incontinence (Sun et al, 1990a). Furthermore, in incontinence there may be episodes of spontaneous rectal contraction (Farouk et al, 1994; Goes et al, 1995). Spontaneous restoration of the anorectal pressure gradient is defective in some incontinent patients, implying a disordered sampling reflex possibly due to sensory loss (Roe et al, 1986). The threshold for the rectoanal inhibition is higher in incontinent patients (Miller et al, 1988b).

There is now substantial evidence that the rectoanal inhibitory reflex is mediated by non-adrenergic non-cholinergic fibres which innervate the circular rectal smooth muscle and internal sphincter from the rectal myenteric ganglia. These nerve fibres contain nitric oxide synthase which facilitates nitric oxide release from L-arginine (O'Kelly et al, 1993), resulting in smooth muscle relaxation. The reaction is dependent on several cofactors such as calcium, calmodulin and nicotinamide adenine dinucleotide phosphate (NADPH) (Stebbing et al, 1996). Nitric oxide is soluble, diffuses rapidly and has a short half-life, being inactivated by the formation of NO_3 after contact with the superoxide anion $^{\cdot}O_2^-$. Smooth muscle relaxation can be mimicked by application of nitric oxide from an exogenous source such as glyceryl trinitrate or diltiazem which has been used for chemical sphincterotomy in anal fissure (see Chapter 13). Nitric oxide scavengers could theoretically play a role in augmenting internal sphincter activity in the medical treatment of incontinence (Davies et al, 1995; O'Kelly, 1996; Stebbing et al, 1997). Recent work suggests that phenylephrine may have a role in this setting. In Hirschsprung's disease, where the rectoanal inhibitory reflex is absent, nitric oxide synthase-containing nerves are absent in the aganglionic non-relaxing segment of the gut (O'Kelly et al, 1994a,b).

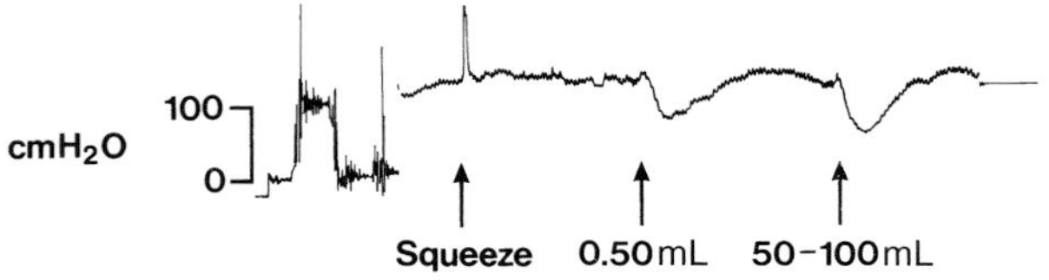

Figure 20.4 The rectoanal inhibitory reflex. A resting anal canal pressure profile is shown at the highest resting pressure within the anal canal. A response to maximum squeeze of the pelvic floor muscles is shown, with the subsequent fall in resting pressure following introduction of 50 mL, and later 100 mL of air into a rectal balloon.

External sphincter and puborectalis

Voluntary control of continence is provided principally by the striated muscle complex of the puborectalis and the external anal sphincter. It seems likely that the rest of the pelvic diaphragm (pubococcygeus, ischiococcygeus and iliococcygeus) plays a more supportive role in dividing the pelvis from the perineum. Although there has been some controversy about innervation of the striated muscles of continence (Stelzner, 1960) there now seems to be little doubt (Stelzner, 1960; Williams and Warwick, 1973; Percy et al, 1981; Wunderlich and

Swash, 1983; Kiff and Swash, 1984a,b; Snooks and Swash, 1984a; Snooks et al, 1985c) that the external anal sphincter is supplied by the pudendal nerve and that the puborectalis receives its innervation directly from the sacral outflow through branches from S3 and S4 (Swash, 1993).

Innervation of the striated muscles

The pudendal nerve arises from the anterior primary rami of the second, third and fourth sacral spinal nerves; it supplies the peripheral aspects of the deep surface of the levator ani and the external anal sphincter, as well as providing sensory fibres to the anal canal and perineum (Swash and Snooks, 1985). The perineal branch of the pudendal nerve supplies the perineum, the posterior urethra and the periurethral striated sphincter (Beersiek et al, 1979; Gosling, 1979; Snooks and Swash, 1984a,b).

Evidence for a dual nerve supply to the muscles of continence is provided by transcutaneous stimulation of the spinal cord and cauda equina. Stimulation at the vertebral level of L1 is associated with a rapid response in the puborectalis that can be demonstrated by electromyographic electrodes in the muscle. This rapid response is due to the muscle's direct innervation through S4. Recording electrodes in the external sphincter or mounted on a catheter to detect motor activity in the urethral striated sphincter show much greater delay than in the puborectalis because of the longer conduction time through the pudendal nerve. Measurement of pudendal nerve terminal motor latency and direct stimulation of the nerve (Jost and Schimrigk, 1994) provides further evidence that the pudendal nerve does not supply the puborectalis since there is no response following pudendal nerve stimulation in this muscle (Figure 20.5a). Idiopathic faecal incontinence is associated with a delay in the spinal latency to the external sphincter

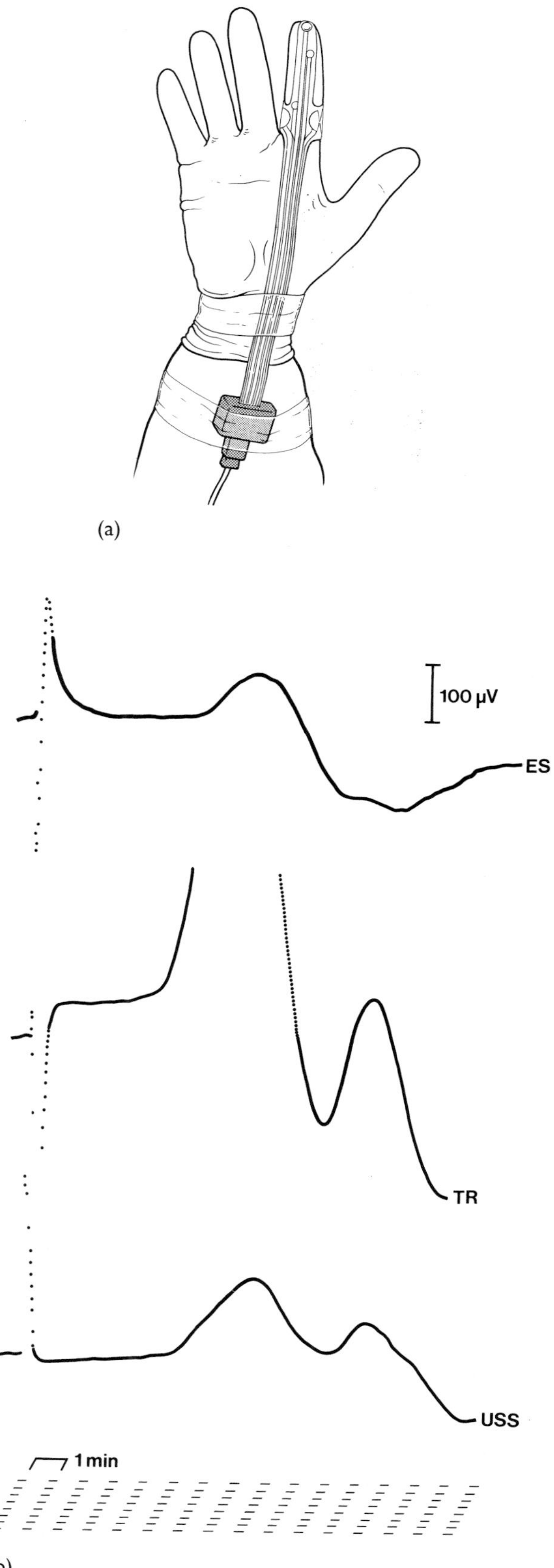

Figure 20.5a,b Measurement of pudendal nerve terminal motor latency. (a) Disposable glove with a stimulating probe at the tip of the index finger (stimulation is achieved by palpation around the ischial spine as the pudendal nerve runs around it). The evoked response in the external anal sphincter can be recorded in the more proximal recording device in order to measure terminal motor latency.
(b) Recordings in the external anal sphincter (ES), puborectalis (PR) and urethral striated sphincter (USS) in a normal subject after spinal stimulation at the L1 level. Latency to the response in the external anal sphincter is longer than that to the puborectalis muscle, reflecting a shorter conduction path to the puborectalis. The latency to the urethral striated sphincter muscle is similar to that of the external anal sphincter muscle.

Table 20.5 Spinal stimulation studies.

		Spinal latency (ms)		
	n	*Puborectalis*	*External anal sphincter*	*Urethral striated sphincter*
Control	21	4.8	5.5	4.9
Anorectal incontinence	23	6.0	6.3	—
Double incontinence	17	—	—	6.9

From Snooks and Swash (1986).

Table 20.6 Pudendal and perineal nerve terminal motor latencies (NTML).

	n	*Pudendal NTML* (ms)	*Perineal NTML* (ms)
Control	21	1.9	2.4
Anorectal incontinence	23	2.3	3.3
Double incontinence	17	2.6	4.1

From Snooks and Swash (1986).

but not the puborectalis (Snooks and Swash, 1986). Furthermore, the pudendal nerve terminal motor latency is increased (Sangwan et al, 1996a; Pfeifer et al, 1997), indicating that in most patients the delay in conduction is confined to the terminal portion of the nerve (Vernava et al, 1993; Roig et al, 1995). If patients suffer from both faecal and urinary incontinence there is a significant delay in spinal latency to the urethral striated sphincter and prolongation of the perineal nerve terminal motor latency, as well (Tables 20.5 and 20.6).

The puborectalis and external sphincter muscles both display continuous tonic motor activity at rest. In this way the resting tone of the internal sphincter around the anal canal is reinforced by the external sphincter and puborectalis. However, there are morphological differences in these muscles, in the composition of type 1 and type 2 fibres, in their fibre size and in their susceptibility to denervation (Parks et al, 1977; Swash, 1985a,b,c,d). Furthermore, these muscles have different embryological origins (Wendell-Smith, 1967; Kerremans, 1969; Lawson, 1974a,b; Wood, 1985).

Upper motor neurone damage by cervical or dorsal cord compression abolishes voluntary control of defecation but the anal reflexes are preserved. Under these circumstances most patients become constipated and reflex rectal evacuation can often be achieved by self-administered enemas. There is good resting anal tone and the rectoanal inhibitory reflex is usually preserved; indeed it may be deeper and last longer than in normal subjects (Denny-Brown and Robertson, 1935; Varma and Stephens, 1972; Frenckner, 1975; Duthie, 1979).

Cauda equina lesions produce a more variable picture. If, as in the case of a central prolapsed disc, the entire sacral outflow is compressed, the anus is patulous, the perineum is anaesthetic and there is retention of urine and no voluntary control over defecation. In long-standing lesions involving the cauda equina or in patients with meningomyelocele, resting anal pressures are low and there is no voluntary component (Meunier and Mollard, 1977). Similar manometric findings are found in patients after low spinal anaesthesia or bilateral pudendal nerve block (Frenckner and von Euler, 1975; Frenckner and Ihre, 1976a,b). The rectum is often large and compliant but shows little contractile activity in response to rectal distension (White et al, 1940). Rectal sensation is blunted and is appreciated as abdominal and not perineal discomfort. Sometimes the rectoanal inhibitory reflex is preserved but there is no reflex contraction of the external anal sphincter.

Gross perineal descent may occur in cauda equina lesions (Butler, 1954). Most patients with extensive lower motor neurone lesions are incontinent. However, Andreoli et al (1986) reported only a small reduction in resting and squeeze anal pressure in unilateral sacral lesions. Furthermore, resting rectal, anal and perineal sensation was preserved, as well as the anocutaneous and rectoanal inhibitory reflexes. On the other hand, bilateral sacral lesions result in loss of motor and sensory function, rendering patients completely incontinent (Gunterberg et al, 1976).

It is possible to identify the level of spinal cord or cauda equina damage by transcutaneous spinal cord stimulation at distances between the following vertebral levels: C6, L1 and L4. Normal values are shown in Table 20.7. It is also possible to modulate sphincter and bowel function for potential therapeutic benefit in incontinent patients after spinal trauma (Chia et al, 1996; Krogh et al, 1997).

Table 20.7 Transcervicolumbar spinal latencies and conduction velocities: controls.

	Latency to puborectalis (ms)	*Conduction velocity* (ms)
C6	11.0 ± 1.5	C6–L1 = 67.4 ± 9.1
L1	5.3 ± 0.5	L1–L4 = 57.9 ± 10.3
L4	3.8 ± 0.6	

From Henry and Swash (1985).

External sphincter

The striated muscle fibres of the external sphincter surround the internal sphincter. Voluntary contraction is accompanied by rapid recruitment and high anal pressures are achieved in normal subjects. Similar contractile pressures are recorded after coughing and may prove a better assessment of maximal sphincter recruitment than squeeze pressures (Meagher et al, 1993) (Figure 20.5b).

External sphincter function cannot be sustained and there is rapid fatigue, hence it usually merely provides a final control mechanism if faecal material enters the upper anal canal.

Shafik (1975) has suggested that the external sphincter functions as two slings. A centre sling is attached to the anococcygeal raphe posteriorly and loops around the anterior anorectum to provide an opposite force to that of the puborectalis (Shafik, 1985). He describes the lowest fibres of the external sphincter as a posterior sling with anterior attachment to the perineal body (Shafik, 1984). In practice, the sphincter does not seem to be so clearly divided into these components, but the concept of three opposing slings explains the circumferential differential in pressure within the anal canal (Taylor et al, 1984; Perry et al, 1990; Roberts et al, 1990). High anal pressures are prominent posteriorly in the upper anal canal, while the highest caudal pressures are observed anteriorly (Gibbons et al, 1986a,b; Perry et al, 1990) (Figure 20.6a).

It used to be felt that neuropathy affecting the external sphincters was less common than denervation of the puborectalis in idiopathic incontinence. However, chronic straining at stool and prolonged labour results in the pudendal nerve becoming stretched, causing delayed conduction and increased fibre density in the external sphincter following attempted reinnervation in response to axonal degeneration (Parks et al, 1977; Neill et al, 1981; Henry et al, 1982; Kiff and Swash, 1984a; Kiff et al, 1984; Lubowski et al, 1988a). Despite an early report suggesting a poor correlation between pudendal nerve latency and perineal descent, there is now substantial evidence that the degree of perineal descent has a direct correlation with pudendal nerve latency (Jones et al, 1987; Ho and Goh, 1995) (Figure 20.6b). This progressive denervation from straining becomes more common with increasing age (Figure 20.6c).

Apart from external sphincter damage, trauma to the puborectalis by the fetal head used to be regarded as the most important cause of incontinence (Sunderland, 1978; Henry et al, 1982). On the other hand, Snooks et al (1984d) have provided evidence of pudendal neuropathy, persistent perineal descent and external sphincter damage after vaginal deliveries. Damage usually occurs with the first delivery but is particularly common in multiparous women who have large babies needing forceps deliveries, who are in the second stage of labour for a long time, or who have sustained a third-degree tear (Snooks et al, 1986). Thus difficult vaginal deliveries may result in impaired rectal evacuation from denervation of the pelvic floor, which may also impair anorectal sensory awareness of a faecal bolus (Gee et al, 1995). These patients may become constipated (MacArthur et al, 1997) or more commonly, they have a feeling of incomplete evacuation which results in chronic staining. Repeated straining in these women causes further pudendal nerve damage from a stretch injury. Subsequent vaginal deliveries frequently cause further damage to the pudendal nerves. Initially, this may not be severe enough to cause faecal incontinence and there may be a poor correlation at this stage between the extent of neuropathy and the severity of incontinence (Infantino et al, 1995). However, with time and progressive straining, coupled with the impact of the menopause on striated muscle function, denervation leads to clinical impairment of continence and pelvic floor failure (Donnelly et al, 1996).

Hill et al (1994a) undertook a long-term study of 21 women with neuropathic faecal incontinence treated conservatively. They found that 12 patients became more incontinent, 8 remained unchanged and one woman with early postpartum damage improved. Mean maximal resting pressure remained unchanged, maximal squeeze pressure fell from 48 cmH_2O to 30 cmH_2O and pudendal nerve latency increased from 2.15 ms to 2.40 ms. The data on the natural history of denervation shed a good deal of light on events after vaginal delivery. It seems that some women develop immediate incontinence caused by third-degree tears that are inadequately repaired, that break down or that are unrecognized (Sultan et al, 1993a,d, 1994a,c; Sorensen et al, 1993; Henriksen et al, 1994; Walsh et al, 1996; Wynne et al, 1996). The majority of women do not sustain a complete sphincter disruption and their incontinence is transient, but they sustain a pudendal neuropathy resulting in altered anorectal sensory awareness and impaired rectal emptying leading to straining. Subsequent vaginal deliveries increase the risk of damage (Ryhammer et al, 1995). Over time and with a changed hormonal environment, repeated straining leads to progressive neuropathy and incontinence due to denervation of anorectal mucosa and the external anal sphincter, which may not be correctable by surgical repair (Thorpe et al, 1995).

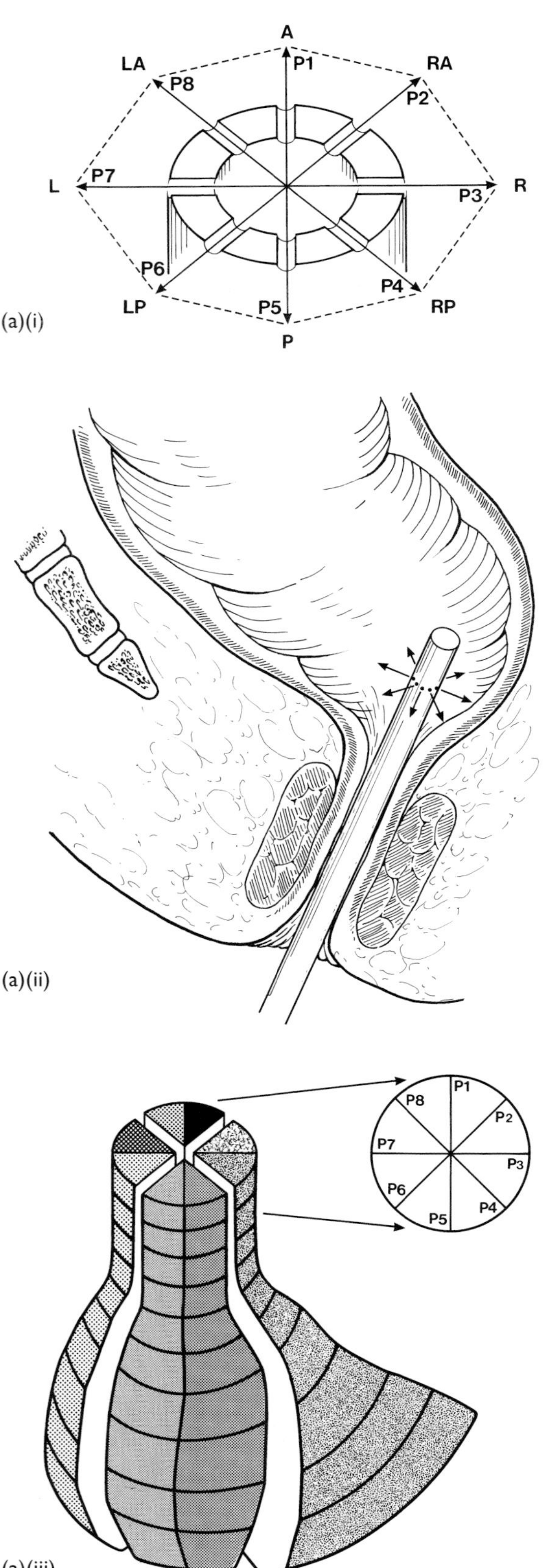

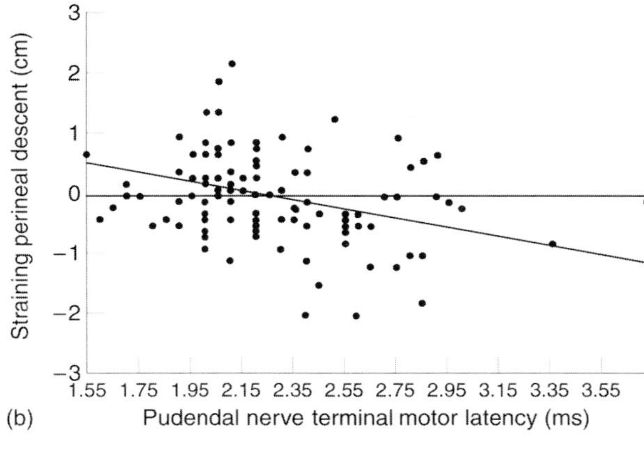

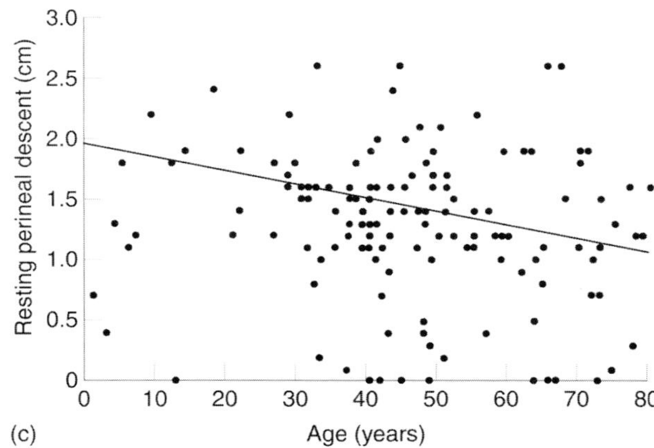

Figure 20.6a–c Measurement of anal pressure. (a) Vector diagram of anal pressures. (i) The catheter and pressure diagram from eight side-holes, located at a specific distance from the anal verge. A, anterior; P, posterior; L, left; R, right. (ii) The station pull-out device with the anal manometry probe placed in the rectum, with the eight side-ports illustrated. (iii) An eight quadratic wedge of the pressure vectogram. The area of the polygon is a reflection of the net pressure at a specific level in the anal canal. The pressure vector volume at a specific level is the area multiplied by the distance between stations. The length of each arrow represents the magnitude of the pressure. (b) Relationship between pudendal nerve motor terminal latency and straining perineal descent ($R^2 = 0.08$; $r = -0.283$; $P < 0.01$).
(c) Relationship between age and resting perineal descent ($R^2 = 0.09$; $r = -0.301$; $P < 0.01$). (b) and (c) From Ho and Goh (1995).

Anocutaneous reflex

The anocutaneous reflex is evoked by stroking the perianal skin, which causes a transient contraction of the external anal sphincter. The reflex can be confirmed manometrically or electromyographically by a rise in anal pressure or increased electrical activity in the external sphincter in response to the cutaneous stimulus. The reflex tests the integrity of the pudendal nerve and sacral plexus and may be absent in faecal incontinence. 'Anal reflex' latency was proposed as a test of pudendal nerve function (Henry et al, 1982). Increased latency was reported in faecal incontinence (Henry et al, 1980). There is, in fact, a long and a short response (Pedersen et al, 1978). The short response is abolished by epidural anaesthesia (Pedersen et al, 1982) but is unlikely to be a reflex (Henry and Swash, 1978) since it is not increased in faecal incontinence (Bartolo et al, 1983b) and is probably due to direct stimulation of the recording electrode (Marsden et al, 1978; Stalberg and Trontelj, 1979; Wright et al, 1985). The long response is a true spinal cord reflex but because it has a wide range of values in normal subjects is of little value in assessing pudendal nerve function (Wright et al, 1985).

Puborectalis

Posteriorly, the external sphincter is continuous with the fibres of the puborectalis which form the inner component of the levator ani (Figure 20.7). The levator ani may be divided into three parts. The inner fibres consist of the puborectalis which acts as a sling around the anorectum (Lawson, 1974a,b). The remaining parts include the ischiococcygeus and the iliococcygeus (Figure 20.8). The posterior interdigitating fibres form the anococcygeal raphe. The puborectalis sling used to be considered crucial for continence by maintaining an acute angle between the posterior aspect of the rectum and the anal canal (Tagart, 1966; Hajivassiliou et al, 1996). The puborectalis was thought by some to act as a flutter valve (Parks et al, 1962, 1966; Kerremans, 1969), the anorectal angle becoming more acute with increasing intra-abdominal pressure, thereby securing continence during coughing, sneezing, micturition and straining (Parks, 1975). However, during the last decade the importance of the anorectal angle in maintaining continence has been questioned (Pennickx et al, 1990) on the grounds that (1) the anterior aspect of the rectum is rarely in apposition with the anal canal; (2) the anorectal angle is made more obtuse by rectopexy, which frequently restores continence; and (3) postanal repair frequently restores continence without having any influence on the anorectal angle (Womack et al, 1988; Yoshioka et al, 1988; Miller et al, 1989; Pinho and Keighley, 1990).

The upper part of the external sphincter is histologically similar to that of the puborectalis (Beersiek et al, 1979). This puboanal sphincter is quite differ-

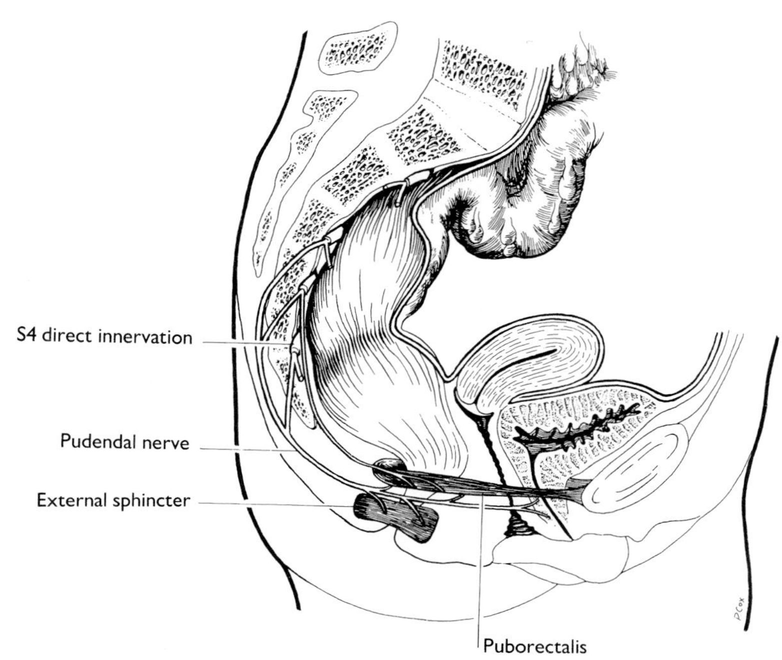

Figure 20.7 A sagittal section of the pelvis to illustrate the innervation of the sphincters and puborectalis. The puborectalis and external anal sphincter are largely supplied by the pudendal nerve, but a separate direct innervation from S4 supplies the puborectalis sling.

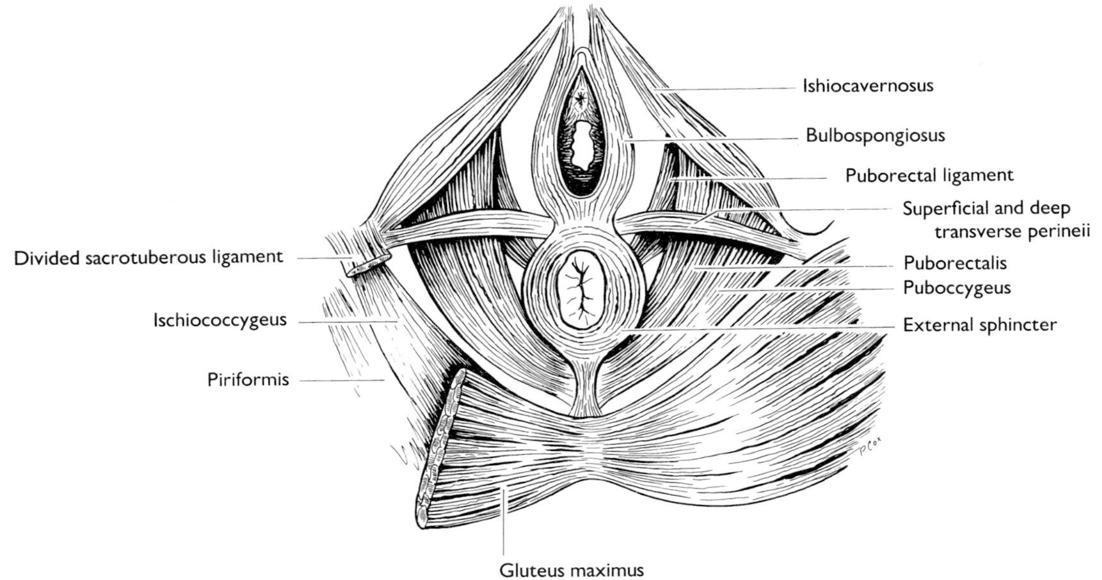

Figure 20.8 The levator ani viewed from the perineum. The components of the pelvic floor muscle are shown, in particular the puborectalis and pubococcygeus lying immediately above the external anal sphincter. The puborectal ligament is also shown, together with the superficial and deep transverse perineii.

ent from the rest of the levator ani and the external sphincter (Schuster, 1975).

Anorectal sensation

Rectal sensation

Although the rectal mucosa is insensitive to painful stimuli (Duthie and Bennett, 1963), distension is appreciated. The smallest distending volume first recognized by the patient is between 20 and 40 mL. Increasing volumes in the rectum give rise to a transient desire to defecate and with even larger volumes there is a feeling of urgency followed by a constant desire to defecate (Farthing and Lennard-Jones, 1978).

Afferent sensory fibres from the rectum are conveyed through the sacral parasympathetics (Bennett, 1972; Williams et al, 1996). Sensation of rectal distension may also be mediated by efferent fibres of the sacral plexus and the pudendal nerve, since the sensation of rectal filling is preserved after ileoanal and coloanal anastomosis even though the rectum has been removed (Parks and Stuart, 1973; Lane and Parks, 1977; Williams et al, 1980). Bilateral sacral denervation results in reduced sensory awareness to rectal distension as well as impaired discrimination between solids and liquids (Gunterberg et al, 1976). It is probable that distension is widely recognized throughout the gastrointestinal tract and innervated by local myenteric connections linked to the usual autonomic pathways.

Most of the present evidence indicates that rectal sensation is not usually impaired in faecal incontinence (Rogers et al, 1988a,d; Yoshioka et al, 1988; Ferguson et al, 1989; Holmberg et al, 1995; Meagher et al, 1996), even though the sampling reflex may be defective (Miller et al, 1988b; Farouk et al, 1993, 1994). There are, however, some patients in whom the threshold for rectal sensation is increased (Lubowski and Nicholls, 1988; Sun et al, 1990b) (Figure 20.9), suggesting that there is a visceral sensory abnormality in neurogenic faecal incontinence (Speakman and Kamm, 1993). Buser and Miner (1986) also reported delayed recognition of rectal distension in 13 of 46 patients with incontinence. These changes were often associated with urgency and soiling but could be reversed by biofeedback (Whitehead et al, 1981).

Rectal sensation may sometimes be impaired in diabetics with faecal incontinence (Cerulli et al, 1979; Goldberg et al, 1980; Wald and Turugunthla, 1984; Pintor et al, 1994) but the majority of diabetics have normal appreciation of rectal distension (Rogers et al, 1988b). The changes in diabetic patients with or without faecal incontinence are shown in Table 20.8.

Table 20.8 Results of anorectal physiology investigation and statistical evaluation in group A (diabetic incontinent patients), group B (diabetic neuropathic patients) and in controls of group C (Birmingham).

	Group A *Diabetic incontinent*	*Group B* *Diabetic no incontinence*	*Group C* *Controls*		*P<*
Anal resting pressure (mmHg)	56.6 ± 14	59.9 ± 15	53.2 ± 17	A vs B	ns
				A vs C	ns
				B vs C	ns
Maximum squeeze pressure (mmHg)	105 ± 30	115 ± 34	129 ± 23	A vs B	ns
				A vs C	0.025
				B vs C	ns
Squeeze pressure duration (s)	7.0 ± 4.7	15.7 ± 6.7	17 ± 5.7	A vs B	0.0005
				A vs C	0.0005
				A vs C	ns
PNTML (pudendal nerve terminal motor latency) (ms)	3.64 ± 1.40	2.37 ± 0.52	1.82 ± 0.46	A vs B	0.005
				A vs C	0.0005
				B vs C	0.005
Fullness threshold (mL)	71.4 ± 46	45 ± 11	42 ± 10	A vs B	0.025
				A vs C	0.05
				B vs C	ns
Desire to defecate threshold (mL)	124 ± 52	74 ± 18	77 ± 10	A vs B	0.005
				A vs C	0.005
				B vs C	ns
Maximum tolerated volume threshold (mL)	157 ± 41	129 ± 41	112 ± 22	A vs B	0.05
				A vs C	0.005
				B vs C	ns

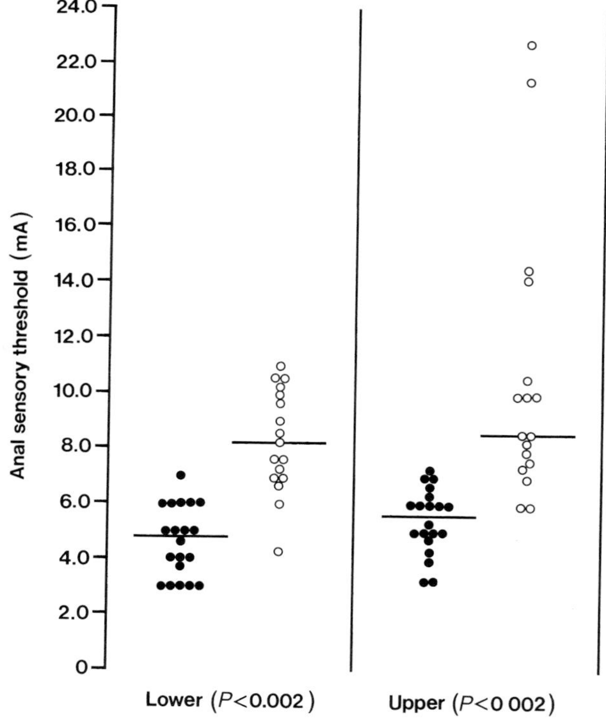

Figure 20.9 Anal sensation in incontinence. Anal sensory threshold is measured by mucosal electrosensitivity. Values in the lower half of the anal canal are shown on the left, and in the upper half of the anal canal on the right. Patients with incontinence (●) have significantly lower threshold sensation than normal subjects (○).

Anal sensation

The anal canal is supplied with numerous sensory nerve endings. Painful stimuli can be appreciated in the distal third of the anal canal, although light touch and temperature are best felt in the zone just above the anal valves (the anal transition zone) (Duthie and Gairns, 1960). The pudendal nerve and the sacral plexus convey sensory nerve fibres from the perianal region and anal canal (Warwick and Williams, 1973; Lawson, 1974a). In pudendal neuropathy from perineal descent, the large-diameter sensory axons are damaged early in the course of the natural history of this form of incontinence (Gee et al, 1995). Sensation in the upper anal canal is thought to be conveyed by parasympathetic fibres through the S2 and S3 nerve roots (Last, 1978), discrimination being mediated by the free nerve endings present in the anal transition zone (Kantner, 1957). However, excision of this zone does not impair the ability to discriminate liquids from solids (Yoshioka and Keighley, 1987). Furthermore, anal stimuli resulting in cortical evoked potentials are still preserved after coloanal anastomosis (Sedgwick, 1982).

Anal sensation can be assessed objectively by measuring mucosal electrosensitivity (Kiesswetter, 1977; Powell and Feneley, 1980). Roe et al (1986) showed that threshold anal sensation was impaired in the upper and lower zones of the anal canal in patients with idiopathic incontinence compared with controls (Figure 20.9). This finding has now been confirmed by many others (Hancke and Schurholz, 1987; Miller et al, 1988d; Rogers et al, 1988a; Sun et al, 1992). Felt-Bersma et al (1997) reported impaired anal sensation using mucosal electrosensitivity in patients with faecal incontinence, soiling, constipation, haemorrhoids, mucosal prolapse, anal deformity, rectal prolapse, sphincter defects and following a variety of anal surgical procedures.

Temperature sensation (Miller et al, 1987) is a highly specialized sensory modality which may be responsible for distinguishing liquids from gas (Dyke, 1986; Vierck et al, 1986; Rogers et al, 1988d).

Anal sensation may be impaired in diabetics with faecal incontinence (Rogers et al, 1988b). Although local anaesthetics are effective in the anal canal, they do not cause incontinence and have no influence on resting anal pressures (Read and Read, 1982).

FACTORS INFLUENCING NORMAL CONTINENCE

Factors that are important in maintaining continence include: the consistency of the stool, the capacity of the rectum, the preservation of a normal sampling reflex, an anorectal pressure gradient, normal anorectal sensation, normal resting anal tone, resistance to opening, and an intact innervated striated muscle at the anorectum formed by the puborectalis and external anal sphincter. Many of these factors have already been considered.

The consistency of the stool is important. There are some patients who are only incontinent if the contents of the rectum are liquid (Read et al, 1984). Many patients with idiopathic faecal incontinence have diarrhoea and some patients have features of the irritable bowel syndrome. Unheralded episodes of fluid faeces entering the rectum at speed often defy the normal motor activity of the pelvic floor and the external anal sphincters (Brook, 1991). These patients tend to have a poor result from conventional surgical therapy. Resting sigmoid pressures and sigmoid motility index are higher in patients with idiopathic faecal incontinence compared with normal subjects (Table 20.9). Thus patients with the irritable bowel syndrome frequently present with faecal incontinence even though they may be nulliparous and have an intact internal and external anal sphincter. These patients are very difficult to treat as they have an unpredictable bowel habit when the anorectal pressure gradient is overcome by incoordinated rectal contractions.

The capacity and compliance of the rectum is important in the control of defecation. Reduced capacity is associated with urgency, frequency and occasional incontinence (Buchmann et al, 1980). Impaired continence is now recognized as a consequence of repeated straining in patients with perineal descent (Womack et al, 1986, Gee et al, 1995; Ho and Goh, 1995). Maintenance of normal continence thus depends on the interaction between several factors (Duthie, 1971; Parks, 1975; Swash, 1980, 1982a,b).

Table 20.9 Changes in anorectal function in faecal incontinence (mean values) (Birmingham data).

	Incontinent	*Normals*
Maximum resting anal pressure (cmH_2O)	58	87
Maximum squeeze pressure (cmH_2O)	120	193
Rectoanal inhibitory reflex present (%)	31	100
Anocutaneous reflex present (%)	47	100
Threshold rectal sensation (mL)	42	29
Maximum volume retained (mL)	268	>400
Basal sigmoid pressure (cmH_2O)	44	27
Motility index	680	320
Transit markers passed in 5 days (%)	76	75
Resting anorectal angle (°)	123	88
Pelvic floor descent rest (cm)	+2.2	−0.4
Pelvic floor descent straining (cm)	+0.6	−4.3
Anal sensation (threshold: midzone)	13.7	5.3
Rectal emptying: % passed in 1 min	75	75
Saline infusion: volume of first leak (mL)	180	960
Pudendal nerve terminal motor latency (ms)	2.4	2.0
Fibre density in puborectalis	1.7	1.4

AETIOLOGY AND INCIDENCE

Overview

The principal causes of faecal incontinence are outlined in Table 20.10. In surgical practice the commonest causes referred for investigation and possible operation are women with obstetric trauma, which may be caused by sphincter disruption (Henriksen et al, 1994), pudendal nerve neuropathy, surgical injury to the sphincters following operations on the anal canal and faecal impaction (Schoetz, 1985; Keighley, 1991; Swash, 1993) (Tables 20.11 and 20.12). A high proportion of women with obstetric tears have abnormal perineal descent and pudendal neuropathy. Some women give a long history of straining, from impaired anorectal sensory awareness and disordered rectal evacuation in association with incontinence. Rectal prolapse (Setti-Carraro and Nicholls, 1994), rectal intussusception (Lazorthes et al, 1998) or mucosal prolapse (Mathai and Seo-Choen, 1995) is associated with faecal incontinence. Incontinence occurs in 70% of patients with rectal prolapse. Impaired rectal compliance with or without sphincter insufficiency is frequently responsible for urgency after coloanal anastomosis (Otto et al, 1996), radiation and inflammatory proctitis.

Table 20.10 Principal causes of faecal incontinence.

A. Congenital
- Hirschsprung's disease
- Anorectal agenesis

B. Acquired
1. Trauma
   - Perineal trauma
   - Sphincter injury
     - Postoperative
     - Postpartum
2. Rectovaginal fistula
   - Trauma
   - Inflammatory
   - Malignant
3. Inflammatory disease
   - Crohn's disease
   - Ulcerative colitis
4. Functional disease
   - Irritable bowel syndrome
   - Rectal prolapse
   - Megarectum
5. Malignant disease
   - Villous adenoma
   - Colorectal carcinoma
6. Postirradiation
   - Proctitis
7. Postoperative (after colorectal or anal surgery)
8. Neurological disease
   - Diabetic neuropathy
   - Demyelinating multiple sclerosis
   - Inflammatory arachnoiditis
   - Cauda equina lesions
     - Spina bifida
     - Central prolapse disc
     - Trauma
     - Postoperative
   - Pudendal neuropathy
     - Parturition injury
     - Perineal descent
   - Other peripheral and central lesions
   - Neurofibromatosis
   - Degenerative
     - Cerebrovascular accident
     - Dementia

The entity of ischaemic proctitis is now recognized by some as a cause of incontinence (Cohen et al, 1986; Schmidt, 1986). Neurological causes of incontinence may be due to cerebral degeneration (Peet et al, 1995), upper motor neurone lesions, lower motor neurone lesions, peripheral nerve lesions from the sacral outflow or pudendal nerve or from demyelinating disorders (Waldron et al, 1993). In children, meningocele, Hirschsprung's disease, anorectal atresia or surgical treatment of teratomas may result in incontinence (Schier et al, 1986; Ackroyd and Nour, 1994; Hassink et al, 1996). Mixed motor and sensory loss may also be responsible for incontinence in diabetes mellitus, particularly if there is diarrhoea and an autonomic neuropathy (Cohen et al, 1986; Rogers et al, 1988b, Pintor et al, 1994).

Traumatic injury to the sphincters may be acquired from road traffic accidents, impalement injury, anoreceptive intercourse, foreign bodies or surgical operations. Sexual trauma is increasingly recognized as a cause of incontinence in North America and Europe (Fang et al, 1984; Critchlow et al, 1985; Christiansen and Pedersen, 1987).

Normal sphincters, abnormal rectum

The underlying disorders in patients who gave a history of liquid or solid faecal incontinence between 1975 and 1980 in Birmingham are shown in Table 20.11. The most common pathologies were carcinoma of the rectum, inflammatory bowel disease, rectal prolapse and previous colorectal operations. The postoperative group, however, rarely complained of persistent incontinence unless there was a rectal stricture (Rasmussen et al, 1990). Furthermore, in most postoperative patients the incontinence was only transient and usually confined to the first year after operation. A few patients developed incontinence later because of an exacerbation of proctitis after a previous colectomy and ileorectal anastomosis for inflammatory bowel disease. Surprisingly, there were only a few patients

Table 20.11 Underlying diagnosis in 341 patients with incontinence seen in Birmingham between 1975 and 1980.

Diagnosis	*Number*
Carcinoma of the rectum	104
Inflammatory bowel disease	70
37 Crohn's disease	
21 Ulcerative colitis	
10 Diverticular disease	
2 Radiation proctitis	
Rectal prolapse	40
Previous colorectal operation	32
14 Ileorectal anastomosis for inflammatory bowel disease	
12 Low anterior resection	
6 Coloanal anastomosis	
Descending perineum syndrome	22
Previous operation on the anal canal	20
Bolus obstruction	16
Villous adenoma	14
Neurological	5
Obstetric trauma	5
Repeated self-dilatation	4
Imperforate anus	3
Trauma following road accidents	3
Cause unknown	8

Table 20.12 Aetiology of incontinence of 334 patients being considered for surgical treatment between 1978 and 1990. (Patients with malignancy, active ulcerative colitis and rectal prolapse excluded) (Birmingham).

Obstetric trauma alone	122
100 Neuropathic faecal incontinence	
22 Sphincter injury	
Surgical trauma	57
24 Laying open fistula-in-ano	
20 Anal dilatation (some had other anal procedures as well)	
6 Subcutaneous sphincterotomy	
5 Haemorrhoidectomy	
2 Excision of a fissure	
Descending perineum syndrome alone	36
Neurological	32
8 Diabetes mellitus	
6 Meningomyelocele	
4 Central prolapsed disc	
3 Multiple sclerosis	
3 Sacral involvement in a pelvic neoplasm	
2 AIDS	
2 Arachnoiditis	
2 Metastases in dorsal or cervical spine	
2 Von Recklinghausen's disease	
Previous successful rectopexy but persistent incontinence	25
Imperforate anus*	22
Idiopathic pelvic floor neuropathy	15
Megarectum	6
Repeated self-dilatation	6
Trauma following road accident	5
Unknown	8

*Eight had an ectopic anus.

who presented with incontinence due to bolus obstruction but most had a megarectum (Chapter 22). Other principal causes of incontinence included the descending perineum syndrome, previous operations on the anal canal, obstetric trauma, congenital malformations and neurological disorders.

Normal rectum, abnormal sphincters

The patients in Birmingham with incontinence without underlying malignancy, inflammatory bowel disease or rectal prolapse are listed in Table 20.12. The principal underlying causes for incontinence were surgical trauma, perineal descent, pelvic floor neuropathy, persistent incontinence after a successful rectopexy, obstetric damage, congenital anomalies and neurological disorders. One of the largest groups of patients developing incontinence were those who had had a previous operation on the anal canal, such as anal dilatation, sphincterotomy, fistula operations, haemorrhoidectomy or excision of a fissure-in-ano (JG Williams et al, 1991). The relative proportion of post-traumatic causes of incontinence differs markedly between men and women (Engel et al, 1995) (Table 20.13).

Table 20.13 Types of faecal incontinence (n = 151)

	Female (n = 129)	*Male* (n = 22)
Factors that patients ascribed to causation:		
Obstetric	39	–
Haemorrhoidectomy	3	5
Fistulotomy	5	3
Lateral sphincterotomy	4	2
Vaginal hysterectomy	4	–
Rectal prolapse	6	3
Others	12	4
None	56	4

From Engel et al (1995).

Incidence

The incidence of incontinence is uncertain both because there are few unselected epidemiological studies (Enck et al, 1991) and because many patients are reluctant to volunteer information concerning impaired continence to the profession. However, a recent study reported a prevalence figure of 5% for solid stool incontinence and 20% have some problem with flatus or liquid stool continence (Giebel et al, 1998).

Persistent defects of continence in the adult population born with Hirschsprung's disease or anorectal agenesis is rare. As a referral centre for a regional population of just over 5 million, we see perhaps one or two new cases each year. Perineal trauma is often managed locally but we encounter on average two cases a year from our local catchment of 500 000 people.

Postobstetric damage is far more common than has been recognized in the past. Ultrasonographic studies have identified that 30% of primigravidae have some defect in the sphincters which persists (Sultan et al, 1993a–c, 1994a,b). Fortunately, most of these injuries are incomplete and do not cause any defect in continence. Unfortunately, clinical detection underestimates the problem and only 1.9–2.2% of women were recognized as having sustained a sphincter defect and only 1% were identified as having third-degree tears (Henriksen et al, 1994). Prospective studies reported that 13% of primigravidae and 23% of multigravidae had some defect of continence in the first 6 weeks after childbirth (Sultan et al, 1993a). Our own study based on interview of 906 mothers up to 2 years after childbirth identified 4% with new symptoms of impaired continence (MacArthur et al, 1997). Long-term studies are needed to identify the proportion of mothers who become incontinent after the menopause from pudendal neuropathy and sphincter injury. In our referral practice the 1996 audit indicated that we had seen 45 patients in that year with incontinence from childbirth injuries, of whom 9 had a sphincter repair, 3 repair of a rectovaginal fistula, 5 had some form of pelvic floor repair, 4 had had a muscle transposition and 6 had a stoma. The remainder were all managed conservatively.

The incidence of incontinence after anorectal surgery is reviewed elsewhere but the global figures from the literature report solid or liquid faecal incontinence (not gas) in 12% after open sphincterotomy (Garcia-Aguilar et al, 1996), 27% after fistulotomy (van Tets and Kuijpers, 1994), 6% after haemorrhoidectomy (Bennett et al, 1963) and 10% after anal dilatation (Nielsen et al, 1993). In terms of our referral practice, in 1996 we saw 12 patients with iatrogenic incontinence, of whom 8 had surgical treatment.

Rectal prolapse is associated with faecal incontinence in 55–80% of patients depending on their age at presentation. Abdominal rectopexy restores continence in 60–75% of patients. Many of those with persistent incontinence are pleased that their prolapse has been successfully controlled and elderly patients are quite content to wear a pad, hence in our experience the call for surgical intervention is low. Furthermore, in our experience, unlike those at St Marks (Setti-Carraro and Nicholls, 1994), the results of pelvic floor repair in elderly patients who have had a prolapse operation previously are poor. Thus in 1996, although we operated on 20 patients with prolapse, only one pelvic floor repair was performed for postrectopexy incontinence.

The commonest cause of bowel incontinence is senile dementia, where it often coexists with urinary incontinence (Cardozo and Khullar, 1994). Indeed, urinary incontinence is much more prevalent than bowel incontinence at all ages in women. The epidemiological data from a Leicestershire Survey reported that the prevalence of urinary incontinence was 22.7%, faecal incontinence was 3.1% and double incontinence to faeces and urine 17.7% (Peet et al, 1995).

Congenital anomalies

Frequently, patients with low forms of anorectal agenesis have little impairment in continence following early successful surgical treatment (Ide Smith et al, 1978; de Vries, 1984; Templeton and O'Neill, 1986; Ackroyd and Nour, 1994; Hassink et al, 1996) (see Chapter 72). Patients with a high defect and agenesis affecting the pelvic diaphragm and genital tract, resulting in a rectovaginal or rectourethral fistula, are usually incontinent (Templeton and O'Neill, 1986), even if an attempt has been made to refashion the anal canal using a pull-through procedure (Santulli et al, 1965; Taylor et al, 1973; Nixon, 1984). Most of the patients are initially managed by constructing a colostomy (McGill et al, 1978). The outcome of subsequent reconstruction by abdominoanal, sacroperineal or posterior sagittal anorectoplasty is often poor not only because of sphincter and pelvic floor dysfunction but also because of colonic inertia, poor rectal evacuation and bolus obstruction. Hence some patients prefer to accept a well-sited stoma than life with an incontinent perineal opening (Cywes et al, 1971; Stephens and Smith, 1971; Pena, 1985; Brain and Keily, 1989).

Both of us have been involved in the management of a number of adults with high anorectal defects. Some eventually settled for a colostomy but some with strictures have been improved by anorectoplasty and some with incontinence do surprisingly well with non-stimulated gracilis transposition. Others may require resection of the inert neorectum and anorectal reconstruction, which may need augmenting with a muscle transposition and even with a continent colonic irrigation system.

By contrast, low defects have a much better prognosis (Iwai et al, 1979; Hassink et al, 1993). Anoplasty is usually advised for anovaginal or anovestibular fistula (Nixon, 1984). Some surgeons, however, advocate mobilizing the distal anorectum and rerouting it posteriorly through the sphincters, with synchronous repair of the perineal body (Santulli et al, 1965). Kiesewetter and Chang (1977) undertook 24 such operations in children and reported good results in 22.

It is unusual to encounter this problem in adults since most defects have been corrected at birth. Eighteen patients with an ectopic anus lying immediately behind the vulva or scrotum have been seen in Birmingham. Almost all had had a corrective operation early in life, in which the anal canal had been fashioned anterior to the external sphincters, and all patients were incontinent (Pena, 1983). In 11 patients, surgical rerouting of the anal canal through the sphincters was performed, which restored continence to 9 cases (Keighley, 1986). Katz et al (1978) undertook a survey of American colorectal surgeons and identified 29 such cases (Table 20.14). Not all were incontinent, three had a rectovaginal fistula and severe soiling was a prominent symptom. Ten of these patients had an ectopic anal orifice which was managed successfully by a rerouting procedure. The results and technique of rerouting the anal canal are presented later in this chapter.

Table 20.14 Imperforate anus and ectopic orifices in 29 patients aged 15–68 years.

	Number
Presentation	
Soiling	12
Incontinence	8
Abnormal bowel habit	5
Rectovaginal fistula	3
Associated findings	
Rectovaginal fistula	9
Other congenital anomaly	4
Surgical treatment	
None	10
Reroute anal canal	10
Anoplasty	2
Repair of rectovaginal fistula	4
Others	3

From Katz et al (1978).

Trauma to the sphincters

The most common cause of sphincter damage is the result of operations for fistula-in-ano and third-degree obstetric tears; nevertheless, some patients may sustain injury from other causes.

Occasionally, severe sphincter injury may be seen following pelvic trauma. All patients with this injury seen by us have been young males who have been involved in major traffic accidents. All had sustained a fractured pelvis and many had evidence of urethral trauma as well. They were initially managed by immediate colostomy.

Parks collected a remarkable series of patients with sphincter injuries, mostly resulting from military combat but some caused by obstetric tears or previous operative intervention (Motson et al, 1983).

The majority of patients with sphincter damage have low basal and squeeze pressures and a gaping deficiency in the anorectal ring which can be defined by examination under anaesthesia and now by anal ultrasound, usually under anaesthesia. In our experience, a high proportion of patients with perineal trauma managed by immediate colostomy do not need a repair and are continent when the stoma is closed. On the other hand, large persistent sphincter defects do require repair. In a few an anal advancement flap is necessary to close a fistula to the urethra. The results of repairs in this group are usually satisfactory and the stoma can be closed 2–3 months later (Nikiteas et al, 1996).

Trauma to the sphincters may also occur following repeated anorectal dilatation. This may be associated with loss of anal sensitivity and reduced anal tone, resulting in faecal soiling. A reduction in anal pressure is evident in homosexuals practising anoreceptive intercourse (Miles et al, 1990). Similar damage may occur from the passage of a variety of objects into the rectum.

As already highlighted, many women with third-degree tears have evidence of a pudendal neuropathy as well as a gaping deficiency in the external anal sphincter ring (Browning and Motson, 1984; Fang et al, 1984).

Iatrogenic incontinence after anal operations

Incontinence from previous operations on the anal canal remains a common occurrence. Although obstetricians take pride of place in the causation of iatrogenic incontinence, childbirth injuries are influenced by the patient and the fetus, whereas the surgeon must accept blame for incontinence following anal operations. Much of the blame relates to patient selection, particularly with respect to post-dilatation incontinence. We find that the two procedures carrying the greatest risk of iatrogenic incontinence are maximal anal dilatation and fistulotomy. In view of the risks of impaired continence after fistula operations, we believe that these procedures should never be delegated to unsupervised junior resident staff and that setons should be used more widely, particularly as the incidence of incontinence after their use is low (Hasegawa and Keighley, 1998).

Some of the patients being considered for anal operations already have some impairment of anal continence preoperatively with evidence of perineal descent, a weak internal sphincter or pudendal neuropathy. For obvious legal reasons these symptoms and functional abnormalities must be recorded and patients must be warned about the risks of impaired continence after operation.

Sphincterotomy

Open internal anal sphincterotomy is now recognized as causing incontinence in 12% of cases (Bennett and Duthie, 1964; Marby et al, 1979) and patients must be appraised of this risk beforehand (Garcia-Aguilar et al, 1996; Boulos and Arauje, 1984). For this reason nitric oxide donors, particularly glyceryl trinitrate, should be used as first-line therapy. Sphincterotomy should be used sparingly and some form of island advancement flap would be preferred, particularly in women and where preoperative investigation indicates low resting pressures, sphincter defects or long pudendal nerve latencies.

Haemorrhoidectomy

A deficiency in the internal or external anal sphincters may occur following haemorrhoidectomy. This deficiency is usually caused by excising part of the internal sphincter and is made worse in some cases by splitting of the internal and external sphincter if combined with an anal dilatation. Although the incidence of incontinence is reported to be 6% following haemorrhoidectomy (Bennett et al, 1963), it is still a well-recognized hazard, particularly if the procedure results in a Whitehead deformity, which is often associated with mucus leakage as well as soiling (Bannister et al, 1987).

Read et al (1982) conducted a prospective study to determine the incidence and causes of incontinence after haemorrhoidectomy. Unfortunately, a number of their patients had an anal dilatation as well. Nevertheless, there was a 10% incidence of minor incontinence and a quarter of their patients had impaired anorectal function after operation. Felt-Bersma et al (1989) found that haemorrhoidectomy was the most common cause of soiling. Furthermore, a high proportion of patients requiring haemorrhoidectomy had evidence of exaggerated perineal descent, pudendal nerve conduction defects and increased fibre density before operation.

Operations for fistula-in-ano

One of the largest groups of patients to develop iatrogenic incontinence are those who have had an operation for fistula-in-ano. The majority of these patients have undergone partial or complete division of the sphincter. Incontinence is a recognized hazard of operation for high fistula-in-ano, but these are rare (Parks et al, 1976). The majority of patients with incontinence after fistula surgery have had multiple operations for trans-sphincteric fistula and many have had perioperative sepsis. Soiling is a prominent feature in patients after fistula operations. Manometric studies have demonstrated that although anal canal pressures may not be affected by fistulotomy, leakage of saline persists in a high proportion of patients, even following low trans-sphincteric division of the external sphincter. Most patients with persistent incontinence after fistula operations are treated by sphincter repair (Keighley and Fielding, 1983; Nikiteas et al, 1996). A few of these patients are subsequently identified as having Crohn's disease (see Chapter 16).

Anal dilatation

Anal dilatation is a frequent cause of incontinence, particularly amongst multiparous women with perineal descent and low resting anal pressures having a forceful eight-finger dilatation (Lord, 1968; MacDonald et al, 1992; Nielsen et al, 1992). Forceful dilatation of the external sphincter and puborectalis results in a profound and persistent fall in anal canal pressures (Hancock and Smith, 1975; Marby et al, 1979; Snooks et al, 1984c). If a patient has a weak pelvic floor, perineal descent or pudendal neuropathy before the operation, or if anal dilatation is repeated, particularly if there is no anal canal pathology, there is a considerable risk of subsequent incontinence (Matheson and Keighley, 1981; Henry, 1983; Keighley, 1987a; MacDonald et al, 1992). Anal dilatation results in severe damage to the internal anal sphincter on anal ultrasonography (Speakman et al, 1991).

MacIntyre and Balfour (1977) reported incontinence within a week of anal dilatation in 10 of 55 patients; it persisted in four. Long-term incontinence after forceful dilatation by the technique advocated by Lord (1975) may occur in up to 20% of patients (MacIntyre and Balfour, 1977). Snooks et al (1984c) studied ten patients who developed incontinence after anal dilatation. Seven had haemorrhoids, two had had a fissure and one patient had a stretch for an anal fissure after a previous haemorrhoidectomy. Some of these patients had had repeated dilatation and doubt was expressed about the evidence for anal pathology in two patients who had undergone an anal dilatation for anal pain. Eight of the patients had reduced resting anal pressures of less than 40 cmH_2O, three patients had low squeeze pressures, and fibre density in the external sphincter was abnormal in four. Many patients being considered for anal dilatation have abnormal perineal descent on straining (Ambrose and Keighley, 1986).

Many now believe that anal dilatation should be outlawed, whereas others still believe it has a role in treatment (Thomson et al, 1998). In our opinion, it should never be used in parous women, particularly if they have a lax anal canal, prolonged pudendal nerve conduction and abnormal perineal descent (see Chapters 12 and 13).

Excision of fissure

Soiling is a well-recognized complication of posterior sphincterotomy or excision of an anal fissure. This is due to a gutter deformity from excising the posterior aspect of the internal anal sphincter with the fissure.

Obstetric trauma

Patients with postobstetric faecal incontinence are one of the most common groups to be referred for investigation and treatment. Incontinence is directly related to parturition injuries as pregnancy itself has no impact on sphincter morphology or function (Sultan et al, 1993d). Usually there is a history of a difficult vaginal delivery, long second stage of labour, cephalopelvic disproportion, forceps delivery or a perineal tear (MacArthur et al, 1991). Only about a third have ultrasound evidence of a completely or partially severed sphincter. The remainder have low resting and squeeze anal canal pressures, impaired anal sensation, an abnormal rectoanal inhibitory reflex, excessive perineal descent and pudendal neuropathy.

Aetiology

Read et al (1984) examined a group of 34 women with incontinence and found that 16 had had a protracted labour and 15 had sustained a perineal tear. Many of these patients were incontinent to liquids only, and there was a high incidence of underlying irritable bowel syndrome (Table 20.15). Hence structural defects in the sphincter often coexist with a motility defect in the colon.

Table 20.15 Findings in 34 women with incontinence of faeces.

Finding	*Number*
Vaginal delivery	28
16 Protracted labour	
15 Perineal tears	
Incontinent of liquids and solids	15
10 Leaked at least once a day	
Incontinent of liquids alone	19
7 Leaked at least once a day	
Diarrhoea	22
Irritable bowel syndrome	13
Diverticular disease	4

From Read et al (1984).

Anal manometry, anal sensation, pudendal nerve latency and perineal descent

A series of important studies have emerged concerning the changes in anal pressure, perineal descent and pudendal nerve terminal motor latency before and after childbirth. Comparisons have been made between vaginal delivery and caesarean section, together with an assessment of the impact of parity, duration of labour and forceps delivery on these parameters (Snooks et al, 1984d, 1985b, 1986).

These studies demonstrated an immediate fall in resting and squeeze anal canal pressure confined to women having vaginal delivery. The first delivery caused a permanent lowering of resting pressure which was protected by caesarean section (Wynne et al, 1996). Patients after vaginal delivery also had

Table 20.16 Results 48–72 hours after delivery.

		Perineal descent		*Anorectal pressure*	
	PNTML (ms)	*Rest* (cm)	*Strain* (cm)	*Rest* (cmH_2O)	*Contraction* (cmH_2O)
Vaginal delivery	2.21	+0.44	−1.02	63.5	57.9
Caesarean section	1.98	+1.12	+0.48	74.0	73.0
Controls	1.94	+1.66	+0.79	71.6	104.7

PNTML, pudendal nerve terminal motor latency.
From Snooks et al (1984d).

increased perineal descent and prolonged pudendal nerve terminal motor latency compared with controls (Table 20.16). When comparisons were made between the changes 48–72 hours after childbirth and at 2 months, perineal descent persisted in women after vaginal delivery irrespective of whether or not they had a forceps delivery (Figure 20.10). Although pudendal nerve latency recovered at 2 months in most patients after vaginal delivery, multigravid patients having a forceps delivery had a persistent conduction defect (Table 20.17; Figure 20.11). Mean fibre density also remained abnormal 2 months after vaginal delivery (Figure 20.12).

We believe that the cause of idiopathic faecal incontinence in most female patients is obstetric in origin (Parks et al, 1977; Kiff and Swash, 1984a,b; Snooks et al, 1985c; Beevors et al, 1991). Further evidence of obstetric damage affecting the pudendal nerve after vaginal delivery is provided by impairment of anal canal sensation, particularly after prolonged labour and forceps delivery, in multiparous patients (Cornes et al, 1991). Furthermore, there is a relationship between the extent of perineal descent and anal mucosal electrosensitivity (Gee et al, 1995).

Table 20.17 Changes in pudendal nerve terminal motor latency (ms).

	48–72 hours	*2 months*
Vaginal delivery		
Primipara	2.06	1.96
Multipara	2.24*	1.95
Forceps delivery		
Primipara	2.27*	1.96
Multipara	2.37*	2.30*
Caesarean section		
Primipara	2.08	1.97
Multipara	1.83	1.89

*Significantly different from controls.

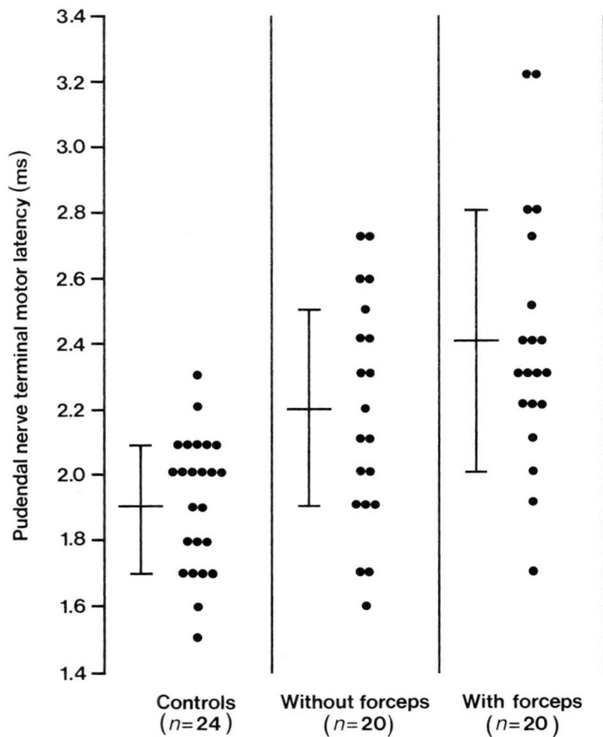

Figure 20.11 Pudendal nerve terminal motor latency 48–72 h after delivery in multiparous women, delivered with or without forceps, compared with controls.

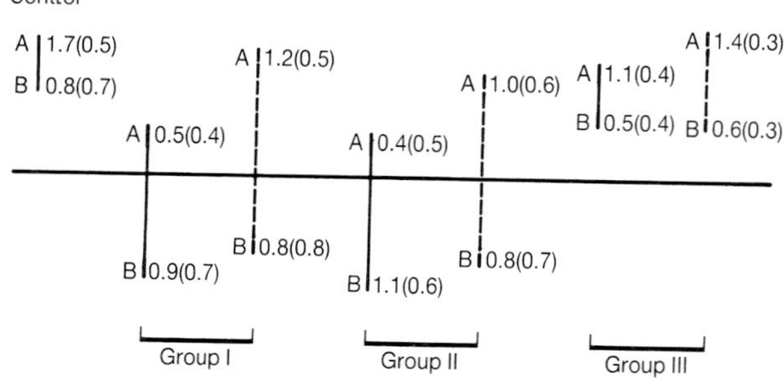

Figure 20.10 Perineal position in relation to the plane of the ischial tuberosity. A, Results at rest; B, values on straining. On the left are controls. Group I refers to patients having a vaginal delivery. The solid line represents perineal descent 48–72 h after delivery; the dotted line indicates the results 2 months after delivery. Group II represents patients who have had a forceps delivery. Group III represents patients delivered by caesarean section.

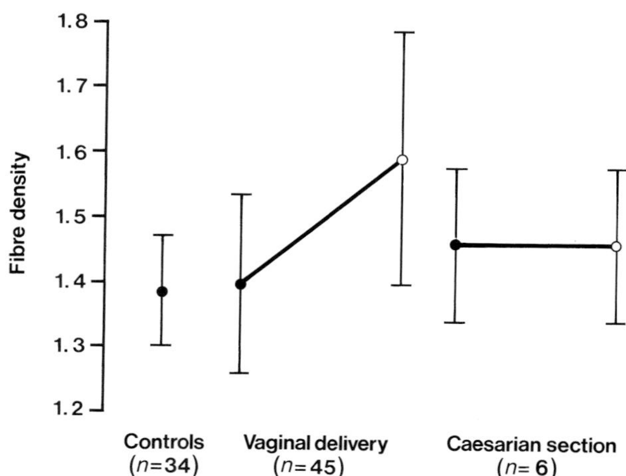

Figure 20.12 Fibre density of the external and sphincter muscle before (●) and after (○) vaginal delivery or caesarean section.

Factors particularly associated with incontinence are parity (most damage usually occurs with the first delivery), birthweight, duration of the second stage of labour, forceps delivery and third-degree tear. Direct evidence now indicates that pudendal neuropathy due to vaginal delivery persists and may worsen with time (Snooks et al, 1990). Perineal descent is certainly progressive with time after obstetric trauma and correlates with increasing pudendal neuropathy. Multiple vaginal deliveries also increase the risk of urinary and faecal incontinence, even in the absence of a sphincter tear (Ryhammer et al, 1995).

Anal sphincter morphology

Sultan et al (1993a) studied 202 consecutive women before and after childbirth using anal ultrasonography and functional measurements. Ten of 79 primiparous women (13%) were incontinent 6 weeks after delivery and 28 (35%) had a sphincter defect on endosonography which persisted in all 22 women who agreed to be restudied 6 months later. By contrast 11 of 48 multiparous women (23%) had anal incontinence or urgency: of these 19 (40%) had a sphincter defect before delivery and 21 (44%) afterwards. None of the 23 women who had elective caesarean section had a new sphincter defect. Sphincter defects were seen in 8 of 10 women having forceps delivery but in none of 5 who had a vacuum extraction. Internal sphincter defects were associated with low resting anal pressure, and external sphincter defects caused a fall in the squeeze anal pressures. Sphincter defects correlated closely with incontinence after childbirth.

Ultrasound must attempt to distinguish partial from full-thickness injury. Partial-thickness defects are seen in only one slice across the anal canal, they are common and do not always result in incontinence, whereas full-thickness defects occur throughout the anal canal and are invariably symptomatic (Tjandra et al, 1993; Falk et al, 1994; Sultan et al, 1994c) and may be visualized by vaginal endosonography (Sultan et al, 1994c). Sorensen et al (1993) reported that among 38 women with rupture of the anal sphincter after childbirth, 19 were complete injuries (9 incontinent), 14 were partial (4 incontinent) and 5 were superficial (1 incontinent). Perry et al (1990) studied the anal vector profile by eight-channel manometry and found that the vectosymmetry index was abnormal in over half of all women having an episiotomy, suggesting that there were many women with a latent subclinical sphincter injury after vaginal delivery.

Third-degree tears

Third-degree tears were reported by Sultan et al (1994a) to occur in less than 0.5% of vaginal deliveries. We found an incidence of 0.4% and were surprised to find that not all are responsible for faecal incontinence (MacArthur et al, 1997). Factors associated with complete sphincter disruption were forceps delivery, primiparous delivery, birthweight exceeding 4 kg and occipito-posterior position. Bowel incontinence occurred in 47% of those with third-degree tears and 85% had complete sphincter defects on ultrasonography. Vacuum extraction was associated with fewer third-degree tears than forceps. Episiotomy did not protect and primary repair was indicated in most women. Walsh et al (1996) reported a similar incidence (0.56%) and also confirmed the risk to primigravidae mothers with high birthweight infants, and the risk following forceps delivery. By contrast, Henriksen et al (1994) reported third-degree tears in 1% of deliveries.

Third-degree tears, unlike partial sphincter defects, are relatively uncommon and badly managed. Many could be prevented by more rigorous selection criteria for vaginal delivery. They are likely to be missed unless the perineum is carefully examined by a senior obstetrician with a colorectal surgeon. Primary repair should be performed in a fully equipped operating theatre by an obstetrician and a colorectal surgeon. A protecting stoma might be advisable if laxatives cannot be tolerated. Postpartum faecal impaction must be prevented and thorough follow-up offered.

Sorensen et al (1993), like ourselves, found that vacuum extraction did not protect from third-degree tears and advised caesarean section for large fetal head circumference and prolonged second stage in primigravidae.

The management of third-degree tears complicated by recto- or anovaginal fistula is addressed in Chapter 65. However, as these women all have a sphincter defect as well as a fistula, repair will only restore continence if any closure method (advancement flap or mucosal reconstruction) is combined with a sphincter repair and a levatorplasty (Khanduja et al, 1994; Londono-Schimmer et al, 1994; Engel et al, 1994; Watson and Phillips, 1995; Mazier et al, 1995).

Incidence

A survey of 25 000 women having a vaginal delivery indicated that only 1040 (5%) had had an episiotomy or had sustained a third-degree tear. Of these, 41 developed faecal incontinence and 31 a rectovaginal fistula (Venkatesh et al, 1989). Obstetricians reported an incidence of a partial sphincter defect in 2.2% and a third-degree tear in 1%, which seems to be a gross underestimate (Henriksen et al, 1994). The true incidence of faecal incontinence amongst women having vaginal delivery is largely unknown (Jacobs et al, 1990). Sleep and Grant (1987) in a trial of pelvic floor exercises reported that 3% of 1609 women experienced 'occasional faecal loss' 3 months after delivery. Sultan et al (1993a) found that 10% of 127 women developed flatus or faecal incontinence 6 weeks after vaginal delivery.

When we studied the incidence of bowel incontinence after childbirth, we interviewed 906 women who replied to a questionnaire (760 symptomatic and 146 non-symptomatic). In total, 55 women (6.1%) reported passive incontinence or urgency of whom 36 (4%) had never had incontinence before the delivery (MacArthur et al, 1997) (Table 20.18).

Table 20.18 Bowel incontinence after childbirth (*n* = 906).

Bowel incontinence reported at interview		55 (6.1%)
Bowel incontinence for the first time		36 (4.0%)
Passive incontinence	7	
Urgency often with passive incontinence	32	
Soiling often with passive incontinence	13	
Previous incontinence		19 (2.1%)
Previous obstetric injury	7	
Inflammatory bowel disease	3	
Irritable bowel syndrome	7	
Others	2	

From MacArthur et al (1997).

Table 20.19 Obstetric factors of significance in new incontinence after childbirth.

	36 new incontinence	*847 never incontinent*
Forceps delivery	8 (22.2%)	102 (12.0%)
Vacuum extraction	4 (11.1%)	14 (1.6%)

None of the 63 patients having elective caesarean section became incontinent.

Other non-significant factors include:
- Emergency caesarean section
- Parity
- Age of mother
- Method of induction of labour
- Episiotomy
- First- or second-degree tears
- Duration of labour
- Fetal presentation
- Birthweight
- Head circumference
- Duration of gestation
- Epidural anaesthesia

From MacArthur et al (1997).

The majority developed incontinence within 2 weeks of delivery, and in 22 (61%) incontinence persisted when interviewed 10 months later (MacArthur et al, 1997). Only 5 women (14%) consulted their doctor about incontinence; 11 thought the problem might resolve, 5 were too embarrassed, 8 did not think it was bad enough to trouble the doctor, and 5 thought it was all part of having a baby. Two did not think that the doctor could do anything about it anyway! We also examined obstetric risk factors (Table 20.19). The only two significant factors were forceps delivery and vacuum extraction.

Prevention

It is thought by many that early episiotomy might minimize the rate of third-degree tear, and possibly pelvic floor and sphincter damage (Donald, 1979; House, 1981; Kitzinger and Walters, 1981; Flood, 1982; Zander, 1982). A trial comparing patients randomly allocated to a restrictive or liberal policy of episiotomy gave episiotomy rates of 10 and 51% respectively (Sleep et al, 1984). There was no evidence from this study that the incidence of incontinence or third-degree tears was influenced by the more liberal policy. A randomized trial also compared vaginal delivery in the squatting or semi-recumbent positions (Gardosi et al, 1989). Forceps deliveries were halved using the squatting position and duration of second stage was only 31 minutes compared with 45 minutes, but the incidence of labial tears was higher. Most obstetricians seem opposed to the introduction of the squatting position for vaginal deliveries. In view of the rising rate of litigation surrounding obstetric-induced faecal incontinence, it is likely that the caesarean section rate will rise in the UK as it has in North America.

Corman (1985a), in his experience of 28 women requiring sphincter reconstruction for third-degree tears, makes the point that in some women the anus is congenitally ectopic, lying 1–2 cm in front of the sphincter ring, and that some of these women also have an anovaginal or rectovaginal fistula. He is convinced that this is not an acquired defect from a totally deficient perineal body and feels that these cases should be identified before delivery and offered caesarean section. Many believe that women must now be counselled about the risks of sphincter injury and bowel incontinence after childbirth. They should be told that 30% will have an observable defect in the sphincter after their first vaginal delivery and that this can be prevented by caesarean section. They should be told that the risk of bowel incontinence in the first 6 weeks after a first delivery is 13% and that 6% will continue to be incontinent for at least 2 years. They should understand the severity of this morbidity from women who have experienced these distressing events and their impact on body image, sexual relations and self-esteem (Anonymous, 1994). They should then be told the risks of caesarean section so that they are then able to make a choice after the consultation as to the preferred method of childbirth (Swash, 1993; MacArthur et al, 1993; Bick, 1994; Sultan et al, 1993a,b; Kamm, 1994). Freedom of choice for mothers wishing to avoid obstetric damage by caesarean section is now being promulgated by women obstetricians (Amu et al, 1998; Paterson-Brown, 1998; *The Times*, 1998).

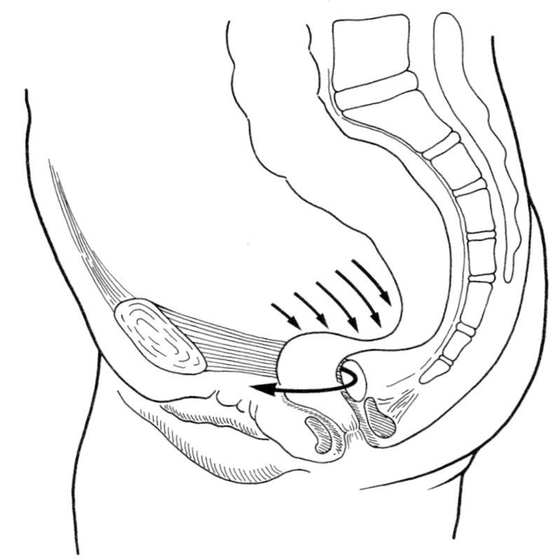

Figure 20.13 The flap valve mechanism of the anorectal angle. The valve is closed by the intra-abdominal pressure (small arrowheads), acting against the pull of the puborectalis muscle (large arrow).

Idiopathic pelvic floor neuropathy (neuropathic faecal incontinence)

In many patients it is difficult to be certain of the precise aetiology of faecal incontinence. The majority of patients are women and most are multiparous. In many patients there is a history of a prolonged labour, difficult vaginal delivery and a perineal tear. Frequently patients also give a history of having some difficulty in defecation, particularly evacuation, consequently they have to strain. Examination usually fails to identify other predisposing factors, such as faecal impaction, a rectal prolapse, a deficiency in the sphincter ring, gross neurological damage, a congenital anomaly or a gutter deformity in the anus. In such cases it may be very difficult to be certain that the cause is obstetric, hence we would prefer to acknowledge this difficulty and use the term idiopathic or neurogenic faecal incontinence. In so doing, we fully acknowledge that in many of these patients the cause is a combination of obstetric damage and perineal descent. (Thorpe et al, 1995; Ho and Goh, 1995).

Aetiology

Formerly, most clinicians assumed that the principal cause of idiopathic incontinence was a neuropathy affecting the pelvic floor muscles, particularly the puborectalis. Evidence was based upon histological features of muscle damage and attempted reinnervation of the puborectalis from biopsies obtained during postanal repair (Parks et al, 1977; Beersiek et al, 1979; Parks and Swash, 1979; Neill et al, 1981). It was suggested that the brunt of the neuropathic process occurred in the puborectalis, resulting in a deficient anorectal angle, which was thought to be important in maintaining a flap or flutter valve (Figure 20.13). There is now substantial evidence that the external anal sphincter is as important as the puborectalis sling in idiopathic faecal incontinence (Kiff and Swash, 1984b; Snooks et al, 1985b) and that it is the external sphincter and the anal transition zone that becomes denervated in pudendal neuropathy complicating perineal descent (Vernava et al, 1993; Gee et al, 1995; Infantino et al, 1995).

Flap or flutter valve theory

It was postulated that the mucosa of the anterior rectal wall closed off the upper anal canal during episodes of increased intra-abdominal pressure. A valve was thought to result from the anterior rectal wall being in contact with the posterior sling of the puborectalis, a mechanism that clearly depends on maintaining an acute anorectal angle (Parks et al, 1962, 1966; Parks, 1975) by the tonic activity of the puborectalis (Phillips and Edwards, 1965; Tagart, 1966; Kerremans, 1969; Duthie, 1971).

The flutter valve theory (Phillips and Edwards, 1965), based upon fairly primitive radiological techniques, suggested that the anorectal angle remained closed due to intra-abdominal pressure exerted above the pelvic diaphragm. The theory was supported by manometric evidence of higher forces in the posterior and proximal portions of the anal canal (Collins et al, 1967). Videoproctography with simultaneous measurement of anorectal pressures and electrical activity in the external sphincter and puborectalis (Read et al, 1983b; Bartolo et al, 1986a) showed that the anterior wall of the rectum was always separated from the puborectalis sling, even during a Valsalva manoeuvre. The Valsalva manoeuvre was associated with a profound increase in rectal and anal pressures, but increased puborectalis and external sphincter activity always maintained anal canal pressures which were higher than those in the rectum. During these events no contrast leaked from the rectum despite the anorectal junction never having actually closed. It seems likely, therefore, that continence is preserved by the activity of both the external anal sphincter (Bartolo et al, 1983c,d; Snooks et al, 1985b) and the puborectalis (Kerremans, 1969; Varma and Stephens, 1972).

The anorectal angle in itself seems to be unimportant since there is no improvement following postanal repair, even among patients who are rendered continent (Bartolo et al, 1983c; Yoshioka et al, 1988). Continence during coughing and episodes of increased intra-abdominal pressure is largely due to the closing action of the external sphincters. If a flap valve really existed this mechanism would result in obstructed defecation since the anterior rectal wall would be forced into the upper anal canal (Bartolo et al, 1985, 1986b; Bartolo and Roe, 1986). It is suggested that the puborectalis acts as a sphincter and not as a flap valve. During rest, the anal canal is kept closed and continence is maintained by the anal cushions and internal sphincter, reinforced by the tonic activity of the external anal sphincter and the puborectalis (Gowers, 1877; Bennett and Duthie, 1964; Duthie and Watts, 1965; Thomson, 1975; Read et al, 1984; Gibbons et al, 1986a).

Denervated muscle

There is histochemical evidence of nerve damage resulting from denervation and attempted reinnervation of the external anal sphincter and, to a lesser extent, the puborectalis. The levator ani is also severely affected in this process (Parks et al, 1977; Beersiek et al, 1979; Parks and Swash, 1979; Neill et al, 1981).

As in all striated muscle, there are type 1 and type 2 fibres. The external anal sphincter and puborectalis muscles display type 1 fibre predominance. This is characteristic of muscles with tonic postural function (Johnson et al, 1973). Although type 1 fibre predominance may occur in neuromuscular disorders (Duibowitz and Brooke, 1973), there is no evidence for this in patients with idiopathic faecal incontinence. Type 1 fibres depend on oxidative metabolic pathways and are capable of sustained contraction (Burke et al, 1971). Both the external sphincter and puborectalis muscles are in a state of continuous partial activity, even during sleep (Floyd and Wells, 1953; Porter, 1962).

Table 20.20 Histometric abnormalities in pelvic floor muscles in faecal incontinence.

Muscle	*Fibre type*	*Increase in diameter (%)*	*Type I fibre predominance (%)*	
			Control	*Incontinence*
External sphincter	Type I	36	78	85
	Type 2	54		
Puborectalis	Type I	132	75	82
	Type 2	135		
Levator ani	Type I	21	69	68
	Type 2	61		

From Henry and Swash (1985).

Detailed comparisons have been made between the histological changes in the external anal sphincter, puborectalis and levator ani of incontinent patients and normal subjects. The results of a histometric analysis are shown in Table 20.20. The principal quantitative changes are an increase in type 1 fibres in the muscles of continence, with muscle fibre hypertrophy in the puborectalis (Edgerton, 1970, Schwartz et al, 1976; Swash and Schwartz, 1977).

Biopsies may show a few scattered striated muscle fibres embedded in fibrous tissue or fat (Figure 20.14) and fibre-type grouping where type 1 and type 2 fibres have regrouped, being innervated by a single axon (Figure 20.15). Scattered rod bodies derived from Z-band material are found in about 30% of puborectalis biopsies (Engel, 1971; Swash and Schwartz, 1984).

Innervation

A neuropathy affecting the external anal sphincter and the puborectalis occurs in idiopathic incontinence, as evidenced by fibre-type grouping and increased fibre density (Parks et al, 1977; Beersiek et al, 1979; Neill and Swash, 1980; Neill et al, 1981). Two theories have been advanced for this nerve damage. The first is that there may be a traumatic injury to the sacral nerves and direct trauma to the pelvic floor and puborectalis by the fetal head during vaginal delivery (Snooks et al, 1984d). The second is that degenerative changes in the external sphincter occur secondary to perineal descent, causing a traction injury in the pudendal nerve (Parks et al, 1977; Henry et al, 1982). The second mechanism

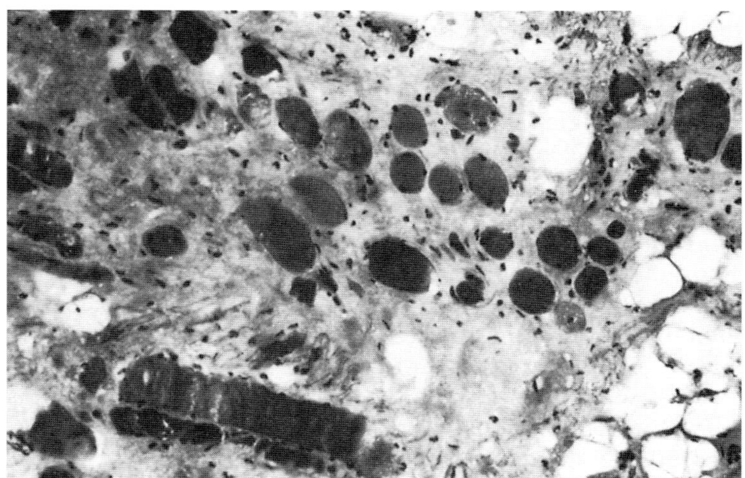

Figure 20.14 The external anal sphincter muscle in idiopathic neuropathic faecal incontinence. Note that there is marked fibrosis and fat replacement with hypertrophy of the few remaining muscle fibres. From Henry and Swash (1992). Reproduced with permission from Butterworth-Heinemann Ltd.

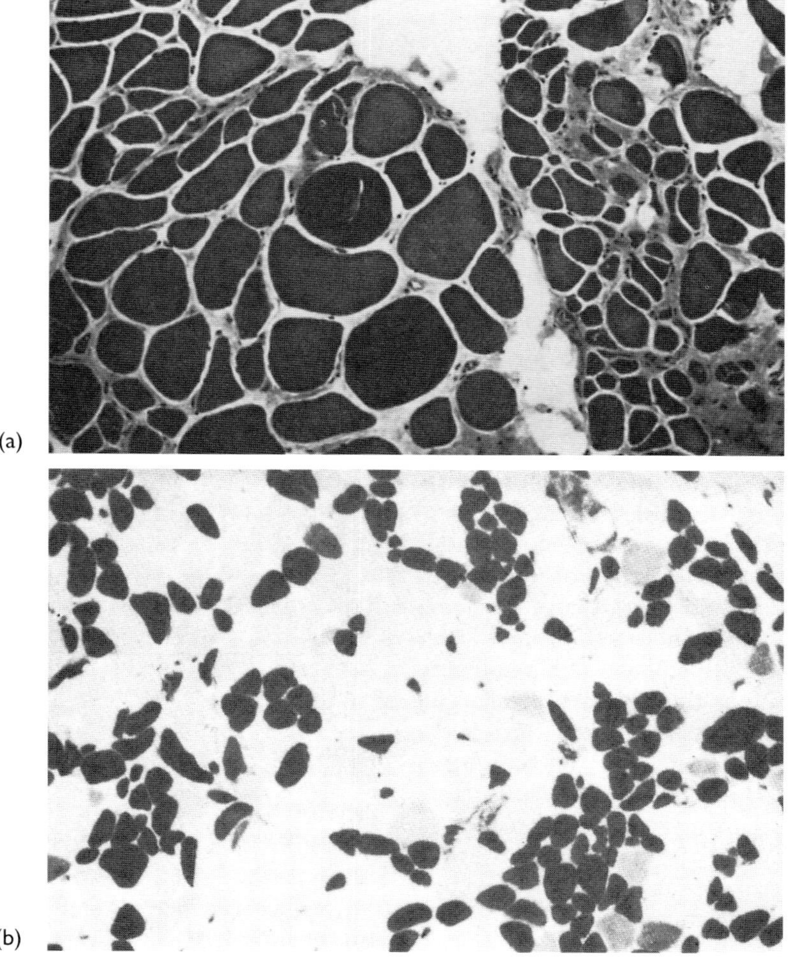

Figure 20.15a,b Fibre type in neuropathic faecal incontinence. (a) External anal sphincter biopsy in incontinence. The dark type I fibres are grouped suggestive of denervation with subsequent re-innervation. (b) Control biopsy. Note that the small dark type I fibres are intermingled in a mosaic distribution with the paler type 2 fibres. From Henry and Swash (1992). Reproduced with permission from Butterworth-Heinemann Ltd.

explains the impaired function in the periurethral striated sphincter in those women with faecal and urinary incontinence (Snooks and Swash, 1984a,b; Snooks et al, 1984a). Damage to the external anal sphincter may also occur centrally due to a cauda equina lesion. It may be impossible to separate these aetiologies completely since obstetric damage may result in a weak pelvic floor, resulting in increased perineal descent which later denervates the external sphincter (Snooks et al, 1985a,c). This would explain the defects in fibre density, both in the puborectalis and the external anal sphincter, as well as the increased pudendal and perineal nerve terminal motor latency of idiopathic faecal incontinence (Swash, 1982a,b; Kiff and Swash, 1984a,b; Snooks et al, 1985a,c).

There is now substantial evidence of a conduction defect in the terminal portion of the pudendal nerve in idiopathic faecal incontinence with loss of the fast conducting axons (Swash and Schwartz, 1981) due to a traction injury to the pudendal nerve (Jones et al, 1987; Ho and Goh, 1995). Abnormal descent of the perineum during straining is usually of the order of 2–3 cm (Oettle et al, 1985; Ambrose and Keighley, 1986; Bartolo et al, 1986c; Snooks et al, 1986; Jones et al, 1987, Jorge et al, 1993). The terminal portion of the pudendal nerve in the adult is approximately 9 cm in length. Hence a stretching force of 20–30% is usually exerted on the nerve. Since irreversible damage develops when nerves are stretched as little as 12%, it is likely that stretching is the mechanism responsible for the terminal motor conduction defect in idiopathic incontinence (Sunderland, 1978).

Kiff and Swash (1984a,b) showed prolongation of the pudendal nerve terminal motor latency associated with an increased mean fibre density in the external sphincter. This was associated with significantly low resting and squeeze anal pressures (Table 20.21). Snooks et al (1985b) showed that fibre density was increased in both the external sphincter and the puborectalis. They also showed that there was a conduction defect to both the external sphincter and puborectalis after transcutaneous spinal cord stimulation at the L1 level. The end-result of pudendal neuropathy is a short anal canal, low anal pressures, delayed conduction, increased fibre density and anal anaesthesia (Rogers et al, 1988a) (Table 20.22). Furthermore, longitudinal studies have shown that pudendal neuropathy progresses with time (Hill et al, 1994b).

Reference has already been made to the presence of a proximal motor defect in some patients with idiopathic incontinence. Snooks et al (1985c) showed, by transcutaneous stimulation at two sites (L1 and L4), that there was delayed conduction in the cord or cauda equina in 23% of their incontinent patients (Figure 20.16). They also showed a close correlation between latency in the terminal portion of the pudendal nerve and the spinal latency to the external anal sphincter (Figure 20.17).

We and others believe that idiopathic faecal incontinence is multifactorial in origin (Swash et al, 1985). Most patients have a neuropathy affecting the puborectalis and external sphincter but commonly the levator ani, periurethral striated sphincter and internal anal sphincter are also affected. Many of these patients have delayed conduction in the cauda equina as well as in the terminal branches of the pudendal nerve. The proximal component may be due to spinal stenosis, spondylosis or a disc lesion (Snooks et al, 1985c) causing a nerve root defect.

Table 20.21 Abnormalities in idiopathic faecal incontinence.

	Incontinent	*Controls*
Length of high-pressure zone (cm)	2.7	4.0
Maximal resting anal pressure (cmH_2O)	39	80
Maximum squeeze pressure (cmH_2O)	48	120
Mean integrated EMG activity (µV/s)		
Puborectalis	28	71
External sphincter	31	67
Mean fibre density: external sphincter	1.8	1.5
PNTML: right side (ms)	3.2	2.0
left side (ms)	3.0	1.9

PNTML, pudendal nerve terminal motor latency.
From Kiff and Swash (1984b).

Table 20.22 Combined sensory and motor deficit in faecal incontinence (medians only given).

	Faecal incontinence (*n* = 11)	*Controls* (*n* = 9)
Anal canal length (cm)	3	4
Squeeze pressure (cmH_2O)	60	150
Resting pressure (cmH_2O)	40	100
Right PNTML (ms)	2.4	2.0
Fibre density	1.73	1.38
Mucosal electrosensitivity: upper (mA)	18.4	5.3
middle (mA)	10.1	3.7
lower (mA)	8.9	4.4
Threshold rectal sensation (mL)	95	80
Urgency volume (mL)	125	125
Maximum tolerated volume (mL)	150	150

PNTML, pudendal nerve terminal motor latency.
From Rogers et al (1988a).

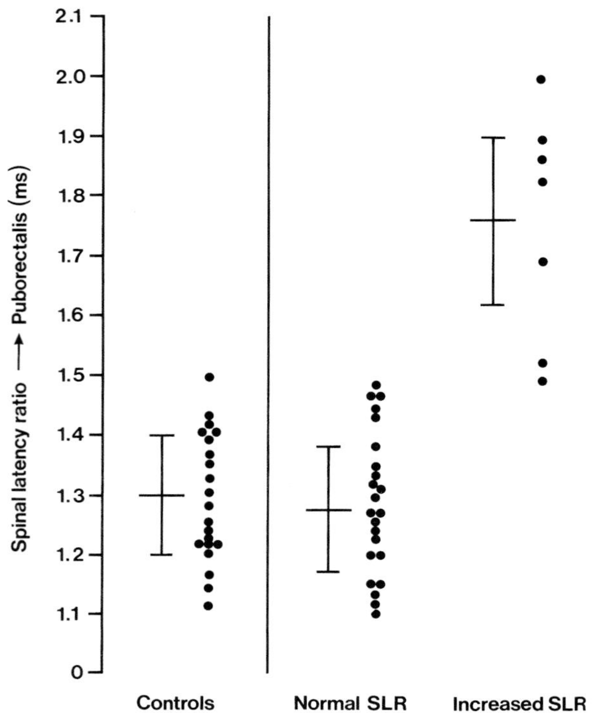

Figure 20.16 Distribution of spinal latency ratio (SLR) in the puborectalis muscle in control subjects and in patients with idiopathic anorectal incontinence. Those with a normal spinal latency are shown in the centre; those with increased spinal latency ratios are on the right.

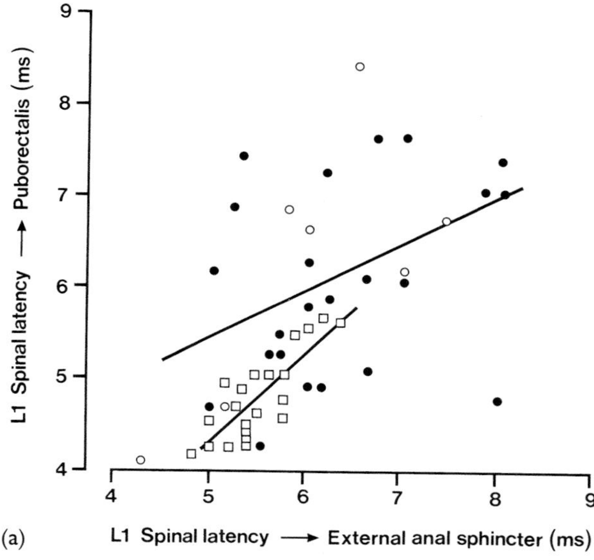

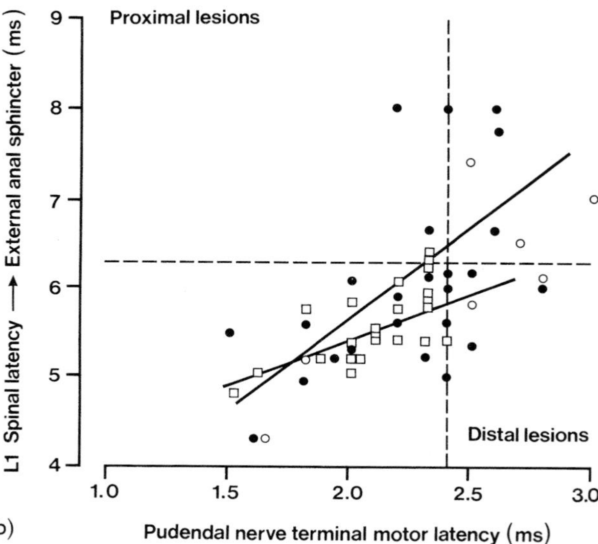

Figure 20.17a,b Motor latency in faecal incontinence. (a) Correlation of spinal latencies to the puborectalis and external anal sphincter muscles in control subjects (□; $r = 0.82$, $P < 0.001$) compared with patients with faecal incontinence (●, normal SLR ($r = 0.46$, $P < 0.05$); ○, increased SLR). (b) Correlation of spinal latencies to the external anal sphincter muscle and the pudendal nerve terminal motor latencies. Control subjects are shown in the open squares ($r = 0.6$, $P < 0.001$); patients with idiopathic faecal incontinence are shown in the circles (●, normal SLR ($r = 0.6$, $P < 0.001$); ○, increased SLR).

Neurological disorders

Most colorectal surgeons are unlikely to encounter many patients who have a neurological cause for incontinence, apart from those with pelvic floor neuropathy. Nevertheless, it is important to be aware of central and peripheral neurological lesions that may give rise to incontinence, since some patients are amenable to surgical treatment.

Patients with an upper motor neurone lesion generally cope with their bowels remarkably well. They have no sensation in the buttocks but anal tone is well preserved (Frenckner, 1975). These patients can defecate by the use of repeated enemas and their main disability is that of constipation because of incomplete evacuation and colonic inertia rather than incontinence.

Faecal incontinence is a much greater problem in patients with a lower motor neurone lesion affecting the sacral outflow (MacDonagh et al, 1992).

Common causes include meningocele, surgical treatment of teratomas, chordomas, cauda equina compression, arachnoiditis and tumours of the sacrum or sacral outflow (Schier et al, 1986). There is loss of anal tone because the external and internal anal sphincters are paralysed, and there is no awareness of faecal leakage because the entire perineum is anaesthetic. Patients with an acute central prolapsed disc usually have a distended bladder, the anus is patulous, there is buttock anaesthesia and the anal reflex is absent. These patients require urgent spinal cord decompression.

Various peripheral neuropathies may be associated with faecal incontinence, such as diabetes mellitus, multiple neurofibromatosis with tumours occupying the sacral foramina and multiple sclerosis (Waldron et al, 1993). We have found that in the last group palliative pelvic floor repair may be helpful in the short term, but most patients eventually require a stoma because they have evacuatory problems as well as incontinence.

Diabetic patients with incontinence are of interest: the majority have diarrhoea and are usually only incontinent to liquids. All patients reported by Schiller et al (1982) had an autonomic neuropathy, as evidenced by a history of urinary incontinence, sweat disturbance, impotence and orthostatic hypotension. Over half had a peripheral neuropathy and steatorrhoea was present in one-third. Incontinent diabetics were found to have low resting anal canal pressures but squeeze pressures were normal. These patients were unable to retain large volumes of liquid in the rectum and were incontinent of solid spheres. It appears that the internal sphincter is often abnormal in such patients (Phillips and Edwards, 1965).

Incontinence in diabetics is often associated with urgency as well as diarrhoea, due to the autonomic neuropathy affecting the whole of the gastrointestinal tract (Wald, 1985). Faecal incontinence in most diabetics appears to be intermittent and associated with a variety of physiological abnormalities (Rogers et al, 1988b). Wald and Turugunthla (1984) found that incontinent diabetics had impaired rectal threshold sensation, and Erckenbrecht et al (1984) observed a delayed response of the external sphincter to rectal distension in diabetics. Both abnormalities were improved by biofeedback (Wald, 1981). Schiller et al (1982) found that resting pressures were lower in diabetic patients with changes in the rectoanal inhibitory reflex. Both Rogers et al (1988b) and Pintor et al (1994) found defects in sensation, resting anal pressures, fibre density and in pudendal nerve terminal motor latency.

Faecal impaction

Aetiology and incidence

Faecal impaction as a cause of incontinence is usually confined to geriatric patients (Stokes and Motta, 1982; Irvine, 1986; Barrett, 1992) or patients with megarectum (Stewart et al, 1994). Younger patients with megarectum or severe anismus may become incontinent if they develop bolus obstruction in the rectum (Johnston and Gibson, 1960). However, the problem of faecal impaction is unquestionably more common in the elderly and complicates general debility, inactivity and confusional states, as well as depression or drug therapy used for psychiatric illness at all ages (Ehrentheil and Wells, 1955; Watkins and Oliver, 1965; Exton-Smith, 1973; Banks and Marks, 1977; Read, 1983). In some patients, incontinence associated with faecal impaction is made worse by administration of laxatives since the faecal bolus remains in the rectum and the laxatives merely encourage liquid faecal material to leak around the obstructing scybala (Fabris and Robino, 1971; Gurll and Steer, 1975). Once the obstructing mass has been delivered from the rectum, laxatives are valuable in preventing relapse (Brocklehurst and Khan, 1969).

Geboes and Bossaert (1977) reported that faecal impaction was the reason for admission to a geriatric unit in 18% of acutely ill patients and in 27% with chronic symptoms. Read et al (1985) reported that 42% of patients admitted to a geriatric unit had faecal impaction. Patients with faecal impaction have a much higher intake of laxatives and drugs which are capable of causing constipation than do patients of the same age and sex without rectal disorders (Read et al, 1985).

Pathogenesis

Leakage of mucus and liquids around a solid faecal bolus may be due to stretching of the sphincters by the faecal mass (Exton-Smith, 1973). On the other hand, overflow incontinence may be due to reflex inhibition of internal sphincter tone caused by rectal distension (Schuster et al, 1963). There is some evidence that rectal sensory awareness is impaired in patients with faecal impaction but, as this may not recover after treatment, rectal anaesthesia is more likely to be the cause rather than the result of impaction (Smith, 1968; Newman and Freeman, 1974; Meunier et al, 1976; Molnar et al, 1983; Wald, 1983). Apart from impaired rectal sensation, some patients may have reduced rectal contraction in response to distension (Banks and Marks, 1977). Indeed, the normal gastrocolic reflex may be absent and the syndrome may be exacerbated by increased water absorption from the colon (Exton-Smith, 1973).

In a detailed physiological study, Read and Abouzekry (1986) showed that there was no impairment of resting or squeeze pressures and increased perineal descent in impacted patients. However, the volume which would initiate the sampling reflex was lower in impacted patients. Rectal sensation and perineal sensation were also impaired (Table 20.23) and the anorectal angle was more obtuse. Initiation of rectal contraction required much higher volumes in patients with faecal impaction and there was impairment of rectal evacuation (Read et al, 1985). Some patients with faecal impaction also have pudendal neuropathy (Percy et al, 1982).

Barrett et al (1989) compared the clinical presentation of faecal incontinence without bolus obstruction with faecal impaction in geriatric patients. Patients with faecal impaction were more mentally alert, urinary incontinence was less common and they were more mobile. Pudendal nerve terminal motor latency was increased, resting pressures were higher and the rectoanal inhibitory reflex was usually preserved (Table 20.24).

Geriatric faecal incontinence

Faecal incontinence is one of the most unpleasant consequences of failing mental and physical health in old age. It is distressing for the sufferer and unpleasant for those who care for such patients (Keighley, 1983). Many geriatric patients with faecal incontinence are senile, immobile and have urinary incontinence as well. There tend to be two groups of patients in the geriatric population: those with faecal impaction, already considered, whilst the remainder have an empty rectum and a rather patulous anus. The prevalence of faecal incontinence in

Table 20.23 Abnormalities in elderly patients with faecal impaction compared with controls.

	Impacted patients (*n* = 55)	*Elderly controls* (*n* = 36)	*P*
Anal pressures (cmH_2O)			
Highest resting	69 ± 5	65 ± 5	NS
Highest squeeze	156 ± 13	171 ± 15	NS
Rectoanal inhibitory reflex			
Volume initiating reflex	17 ± 4	26 ± 4	$P<0.05$
Rectal sensation (mL)			
Highest volume causing no sensation	100 (0–950)	0 (0–150)	$P<0.001$
Highest volume causing constant sensation	225 (0–950)	100 (0–200)	$P<0.01$
Anorectal angle (°)			
Rest	119 ± 3	92 ± 3	$P<0.001$
Squeeze	113 ± 4	93 ± 3	$P<0.001$
Strain	130 ± 4	106 ± 3	$P<0.001$

NS, not significant. Values are ± SEM; numbers in parentheses show ranges.
From Read and Abouzekry (1986).

Table 20.24 Faecal incontinence in geriatic patients.

	Geriatric patients		
	Faecal incontinence	*Faecal impaction*	*Controls*
Mean age (years)	80	76	77
Faecal impaction (%)	69	100	0
Urinary incontinence (%)	84	47	16
Dementia (%)	59	33	16
Mental status score	4.5	9.7	9.8
Other neurological disease (%)	43	53	36
Immobile (%)	64	26	13
Resting pressure (cmH_2O)	55	84	74
Squeeze pressure (cmH_2O)	37	44	51
PNTML (ms)	2.0	2.2	2.1
RAI present (%)	53	89	82

PNTML, pudendal nerve terminal motor latency; RAI, rectoanal inhibitory reflex.
From Barrett et al (1989).

geriatric institutions is at least 10% (Swash, 1985a) if not substantially higher, 20% being quoted by Peet et al (1995).

Until quite recently faecal incontinence was regarded as being almost inevitable in geriatric institutions, the main problem being ignorance. A controlled trial of regular enemas and lactulose for patients with faecal impaction and codeine with twice weekly enemas for those with neuropathic incontinence achieved restoration of continence in two-thirds of the treated group, whereas most of the controls remained incontinent (Tobin and Brocklehurst, 1986). Patients with faecal impaction did better than those with neuropathic incontinence and the success rate among well-motivated patients using these simple conservative measures was 89%.

It is rarely necessary to consider a stoma for the management of faecal incontinence in the elderly unless there is inflammatory bowel disease or a damaged sphincter.

Disorders associated with faecal incontinence

Some of the disorders that may be associated with faecal incontinence have already been referred to; those encountered by us are listed in Table 20.25. Many of these patients have an abnormal bowel habit (Read et al, 1984). Patients with the descending perineum syndrome may have difficulty in opening their bowels and incontinence. Diarrhoea is commonly associated with faecal incontinence and may be present even in patients with sphincter injuries. There is a high incidence of underlying diverticular disease, particularly in patients with a pelvic floor neuropathy. The irritable bowel syndrome may be common and may compromise a weak pelvic floor due to abnormal motility patterns in the sigmoid colon (see Chapter 25).

Table 20.25 Associated disorders in 212 patients with faecal incontinence (Birmingham series).

Disorder	*Number*
Irritable bowel syndrome	54
Severe diarrhoea	39
Mucosal prolapse	24
Diverticular disease	21
Vaginal prolapse	14
Solitary rectal ulcer	7
Urinary incontinence	6
Crohn's disease (quiescent)	4
Megacolon	2

Solitary ulcer and mucosal prolapse (Mathai and Seo-Choen, 1995) may occur in relation to the descending perineum syndrome. Some patients also have a vaginal prolapse, and some are doubly incontinent of urine and faeces.

The possibility of underlying inflammatory bowel disease must never be forgotten. Some patients with sphincter damage eventually prove to have Crohn's disease.

Descending perineum syndrome

Definition

This abnormality is a common feature in our incontinent practice. Patients are defined as having the descending perineum syndrome if the anocutaneous junction descends by more than 3 cm in relation to the ischial tuberosity during a maximum straining effort. Measurement of perineal descent may be performed using a modified form of the perineometer described by Henry et al (1982). The syndrome may also be defined radiologically by videoproctography (Jorge et al, 1993). Normally the anorectal junction should lie above the pubococcygeal line (a line drawn between the lower margin of the symphysis pubis and the tip of the coccyx). In patients with the descending perineum syndrome the anorectal junction lies below this line and descends even further during straining (Figure 20.18). Oettle et al (1985) showed that the perineometer underestimated the degree of perineal descent by 59% when compared with the radiological method (Figure 20.19). The mean descent assessed by the perineometer was only 1.2 cm, compared with a figure of 2.9 cm derived from lateral radiographs of the pelvis. The perineometer takes no account of anal canal shortening during straining.

Perineal descent was observed in many of our patients who had no other cause for incontinence. In our experience descent was unrelated to age but increased stepwise in women according to the number of vaginal deliveries (Ambrose and Keighley, 1986). However, perineal descent was also observed in 26% of patients who had become incontinent after previous anal operations (especially after anal dilatation), in 72% of patients with persistent incontinence after rectopexy and in 64% of patients who had sustained obstetric trauma. Four of 24 patients with marked perineal descent became incontinent after laying open a fistula-in-ano and none of these had evidence of severe sphincter damage. Furthermore, nine of 16 patients who developed incontinence after anal dilatation also had evidence of perineal descent during straining. Similarly, two of five patients who had had a previous haemorrhoidectomy had evidence of perineal descent; both had undergone anal dilatation at the time of their haemorrhoidectomy. It seems unlikely, therefore, that a high proportion of patients who develop incontinence after colorectal operations have evidence of perineal descent beforehand. These patients, even if not incontinent when first seen, have a weak pelvic floor and are liable to become incontinent if the anorectal ring is damaged, for instance, following forceful dilatation of the anus (Parks et al, 1966; Henry et al, 1982; Bartolo et al, 1983c,d; Pinho et al, 1990).

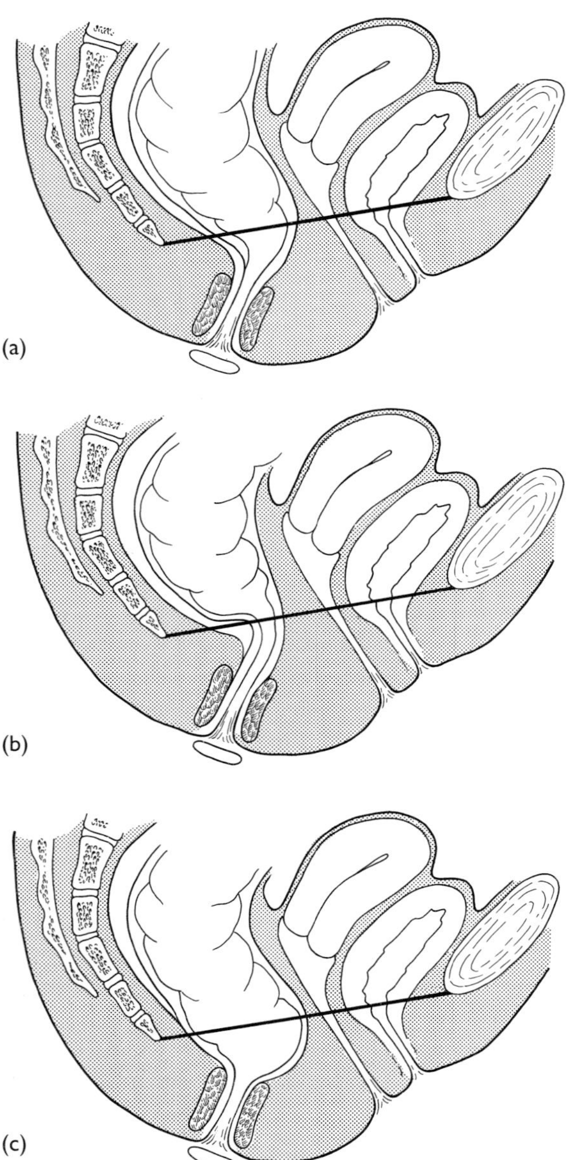

Figure 20.18a–c Videoproctographic evidence of perineal descent. (a) The position of the anorectal angle in faecal incontinence. Note that the anorectal angle lies below the pubococcygeal line, and that the anal canal is short. Furthermore, the anorectal angle is obtuse. (b) The response to a maximum pelvic floor contraction. Movement of the pelvic floor is poor. The anorectal angle only just rises above the pubococcygeal line, and the anorectal angle remains relatively obtuse. (c) The changes with attempted defecation. Here the perineum descends considerably below the pubococcygeal line. The anorectal angle also descends towards the perineum.

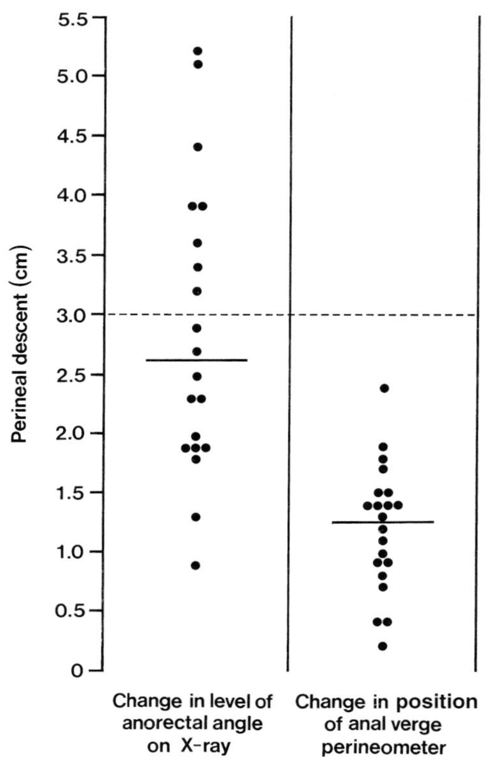

Figure 20.19 A comparison in the measurement of perineal descent by perineometer and videoproctography. It will be seen that the perineometer grossly underestimates the extent of perineal descent.

Clinical features

In our series of 36 patients with abnormal perineal descent, 20 had an anterior mucosal prolapse; 19 patients gave a long history of straining and previous difficulty in defecation; 14 patients also had a history of rectal bleeding and were shown to have first- or second-degree haemorrhoids on proctoscopy. The classical symptoms of rectal fullness caused by an anterior mucosal prolapse was described in only three of our patients. Mucus discharge was troublesome in six patients and three had severe pruritus ani (Table 20.26). A solitary rec-

Table 20.26 Clinical findings in 36 patients with the descending perineum syndrome and incontinence.

Finding	*Number*
Anterior mucosal prolapse	20
Repeated straining	19
Incomplete rectal evacuation	18
Bleeding	14
Solitary rectal ulcer	7
Mucous discharge	6
Perineal pain	5
Pruritus ani	3
Rectal fullness	3

tal ulcer was also present in seven of these patients, and five of them complained of a dull aching sensation in the perineum, particularly during straining and sitting.

Aetiology

There is convincing evidence that the pelvic floor muscles become progressively neuropathic following years of constant straining during defecation (Ho and Goh, 1995). This weakness in the pelvic floor results in descent of the whole pelvic diaphragm (Parks et al, 1977).

There is histological and histochemical evidence of a neuropathy, principally affecting the puborectalis and the external anal sphincter (Swash, 1980, 1985b,d) as described in idiopathic pelvic floor neuropathy (Beersiek et al, 1979).

Concentric needle electromyography shows that there are abnormalities in the motor unit potential difference. Single-fibre electromyography indicates that fibre density is greatly increased in incontinent patients with the descending perineum syndrome (Stalberg and Trontelj, 1979; Swash and Schwartz, 1981), suggesting that there is marked collateral reinnervation of the damaged muscles (Neill and Swash, 1980). Perineal descent is associated with a neuropathy that is much more prominent in the distribution of the pudendal nerve (Henry et al, 1982; Kiff et al, 1984), as witnessed by increased fibre density in the external anal sphincter (Neill et al, 1981; Kiff and Swash, 1984a,b).

Perineal descent is more common in women, not only because of parturition injury but because constipation and outlet obstruction is more common in females, with a higher proportion straining during defecation (Connell et al, 1965; Wyman et al, 1978; Drossman et al, 1982; Moore-Gillon, 1984).

Snooks et al (1985b) found that fibre density was abnormal much more frequently in the external anal sphincter (60%) as compared with the puborectalis (25%) (Figure 20.20). Half of their patients had delayed pudendal nerve terminal motor latency (Figure 20.21) and some had evidence of an increased spinal latency to both voluntary muscles of continence. However, these abnormalities were less severe than those observed in patients with neuropathic faecal incontinence. Jones et al (1987) showed that there was a direct correlation between the extent of the perineal descent during straining and the pudendal nerve terminal motor latency (Figure 20.22). Lubowski et al (1988a,b) measured pudendal nerve terminal motor latency before, during and after straining. The conduction time increased significantly during straining and recovered over 4 minutes. These changes correlated with the degree of perineal descent and the position of the perineum at rest, suggesting that perineal descent causes pudendal nerve damage. These findings have recently been challenged from work in the USA where no correlation was found between perineal descent and pudendal nerve terminal motor

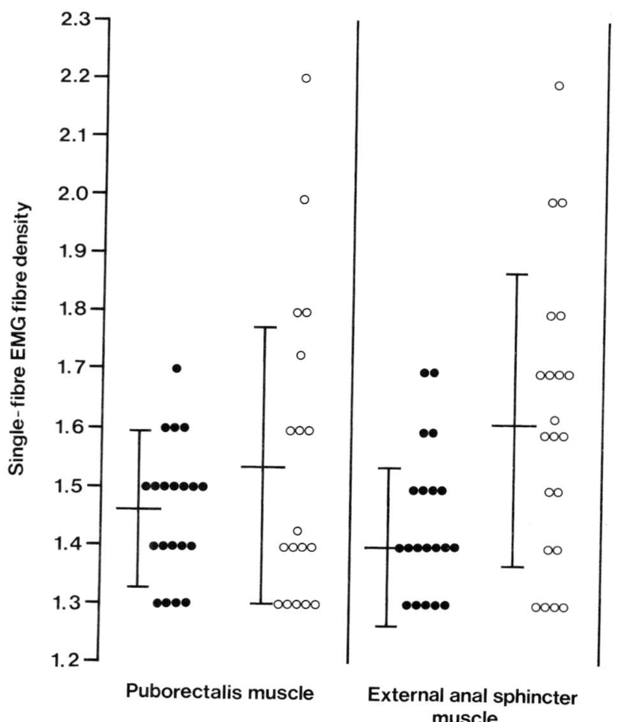

Figure 20.20 Incontinence is often associated with chronic straining. These data show fibre density in the puborectalis and external anal sphincter muscle in normal subjects (●) and patients with chronic straining (○). EMG, electromyographic.

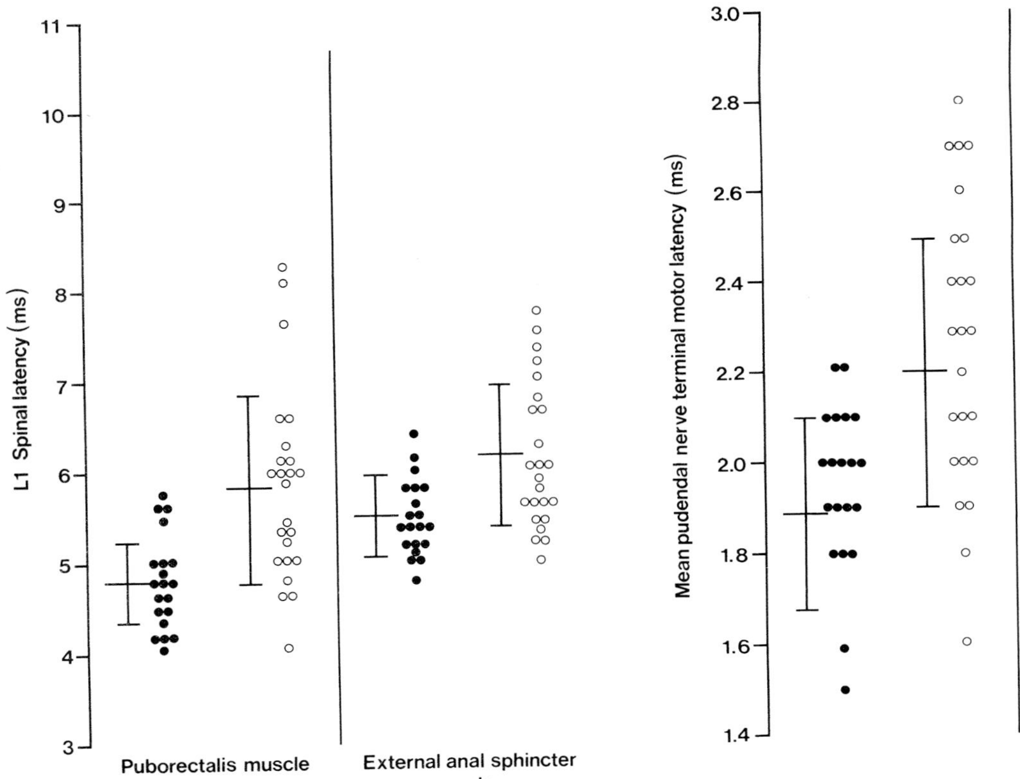

Figure 20.21 Spinal latency in the puborectalis and external and sphincter muscle in patients with chronic perineal descent (○) compared with controls (●). Changes in the mean pudendal nerve terminal motor latency in patients with chronic descent (○) and controls (●) is also shown.

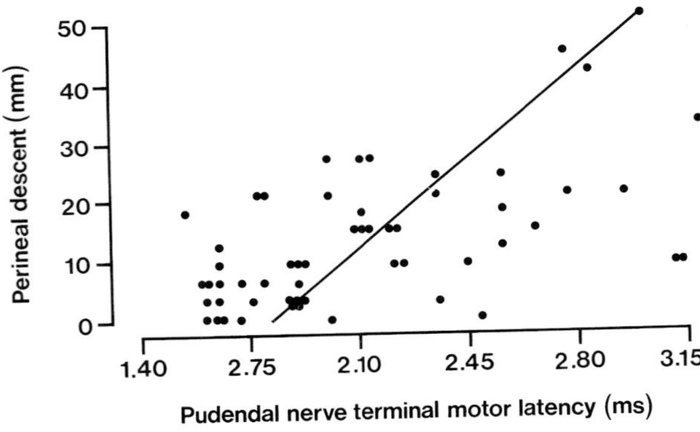

Figure 20.22 The relationship between perineal descent and pudendal nerve terminal motor latency.

latencies (Jorge et al, 1993). The Singapore group, however, support Jones et al (1987) and confirm a direct correlation between perineal descent and pudendal nerve latency (Ho and Goh, 1995).

Bartolo and colleagues (Bartolo et al, 1983c,d; Read et al, 1984) pointed out that perineal descent can occur in both sexes. However, continence was compromised much more commonly in women than men (Read et al, 1984; Bartolo et al, 1985; Read and Bannister, 1985). Bartolo et al (1985) studied motor unit potential duration in males and females with perineal descent. Perineal descent was associated with external sphincter damage in both sexes but puborectalis motor unit potential duration was only abnormal in the women (Figure 20.23). These data emphasize the obstetric aetiology in perineal descent; indeed, there is some evidence that prolonged vaginal delivery may be responsible for impaired rectal evacuation, perineal descent and subsequent incontinence. Womack et al (1986) suggested that the incontinence associated with the descending perineum syndrome was not necessarily due to puborectalis denervation but to impaired rectal compliance and deficient internal sphincter activity as well.

Thus prolonged straining and perineal descent impairs external anal sphincter function largely due to a conduction defect in the terminal portion of the pudendal nerve. Women are much more susceptible to incontinence than men because the puborectalis has already been compromised by childbirth injury

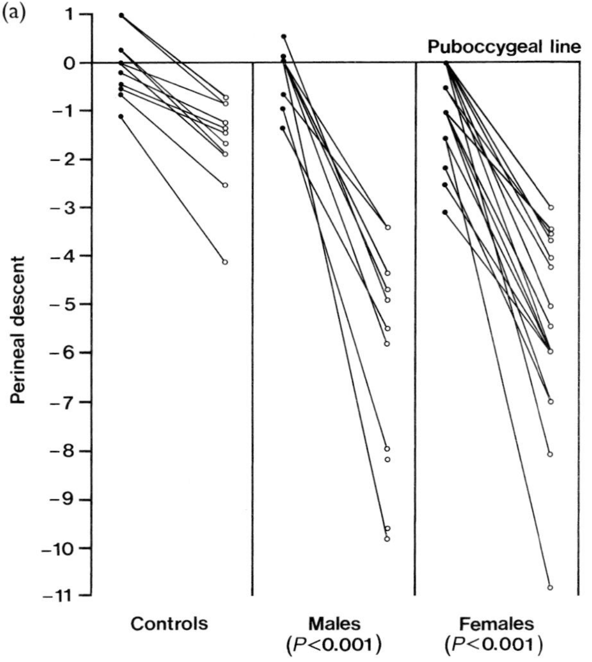

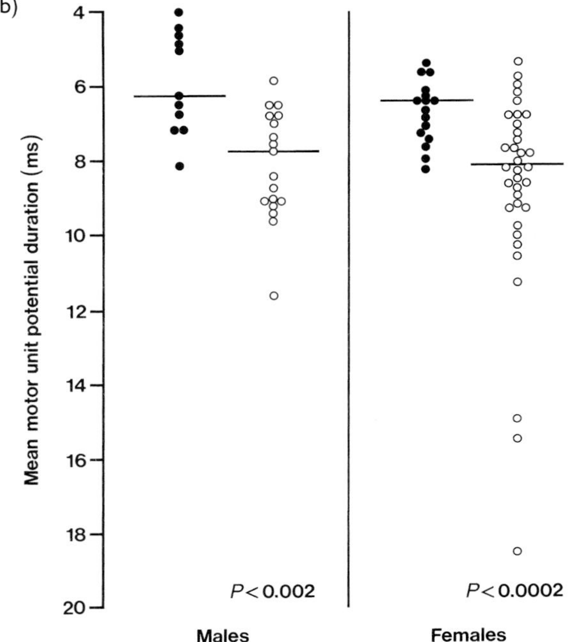

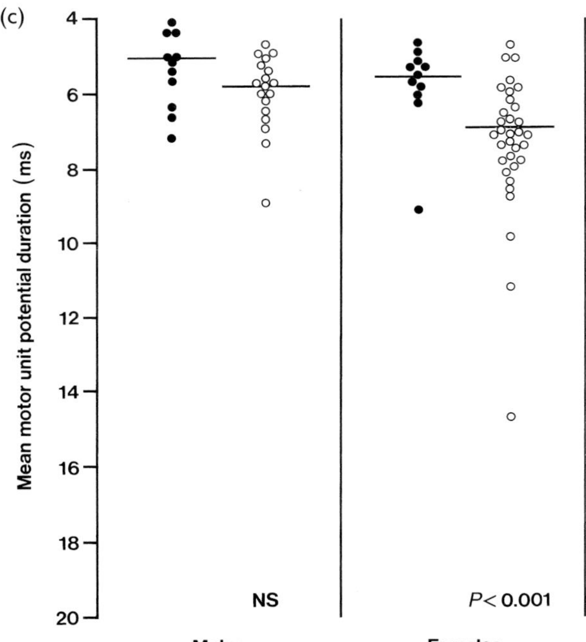

Figure 20.23a–c Changes in anorectal physiology in individuals with a history of chronic straining at stool. (a) The extent of descent of the anorectal angle is shown in relation to the pubococcygeal line in controls, and in male and female patients with perineal descent. ●, Rest; ○, strain.
(b) Scattergram of external and sphincter mean motor unit potential duration in male and female patients (○) compared with controls (●). (c) Scattergram of puborectalis mean motor unit potential duration in male and female patients (○) with chronic perineal descent compared with controls (●). NS, not significant.

Natural history

Surprisingly little is known about the natural history of perineal descent. Many of these patients are not incontinent despite severe pelvic floor failure. Only 13 of 29 patients had faecal incontinence in a report by Mackie and Parks (1989). There is now circumstantial evidence among individuals with an anterior mucosal prolapse that if patients with perineal descent continue to strain, 30% become incontinent and 20% develop a rectal prolapse over 10 years (Allen-Mersh et al, 1987) (Figure 20.24).

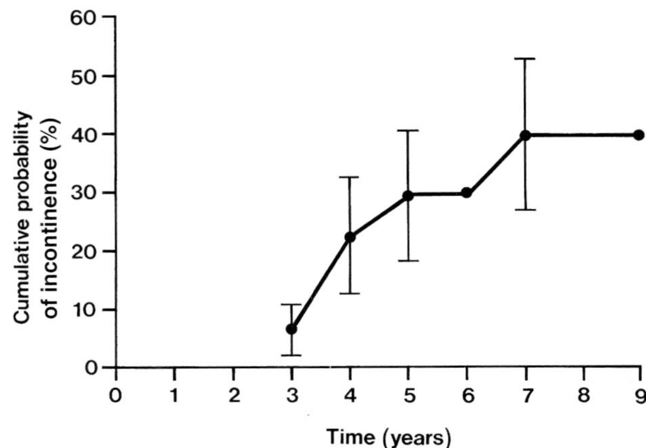

Figure 20.24 Cumulative probability that a patient with anterior mucosal prolapse associated with clinically diagnosed perineal descent will develop sphincter laxity and incontinence over 10 years.

Persistent incontinence after rectopexy

A high proportion of patients with faecal incontinence and a full-thickness rectal prolapse exhibit clinical evidence of perineal descent. Rectopexy alone controls the incontinence in approximately 50–70% of patients (see Chapter 23). There are three possible reasons for the restoration of continence by rectopexy. The first is that the pelvic floor neuropathy is reversible once the prolapsing bowel is controlled. The second is that the incontinence is largely due to a sensory failure, leaving the patient unable to distinguish faeces from descent of the prolapse. The third reason is that the rectal prolapse no longer stretches the puborectalis and sphincters. Nevertheless, there are some patients in whom incontinence persists; these are patients with a short anal canal, severe perineal descent and poor sphincter function (Yoshioka and Keighley, 1989).

Twenty-five patients with persistent incontinence after rectopexy, 15 of whom had perineal descent in excess of 3 cm, were treated in Birmingham by postanal repair. Biopsies showed that the puborectalis and external sphincter had changes compatible with neuropathy and attempted reinnervation (Parks et al, 1977). The manometric findings did not differ from those in patients with the descending perineum syndrome or with neuropathic faecal incontinence (Keighley et al, 1980; Neill et al, 1981). Unfortunately, in our experience the results of postanal repair in these particular patients is poor. Better results were reported by Setti-Carraro and Nichols (1994).

CLINICAL FEATURES AND DIFFERENTIAL DIAGNOSIS

Symptoms

A thorough history is essential in assessing patients with faecal incontinence. Specific enquiry about continence among patients attending a proctology clinic or in those with known bowel disease is the only way in which the true incidence of incontinence can be discovered. The degree, severity and frequency of incontinence should be sought, particularly whether incontinence is to liquids only or to solids as well and whether the problem is one of sphincter control or a lack of awareness, or both. The history should include details of stool consistency, frequency of defecation and enquiry into the possibility of steatorrhoea. True incontinence should be distinguished from soiling and urgency. Soiling is much more common in men with high resting anal pressures (Parellada et al, 1998). Symptoms associated with the irritable bowel syndrome or diverticular disease should be noted. It may be possible to establish from the history whether there is a full-thickness rectal prolapse. The history may also identify impaired rectal evacuation, an anterior mucosal prolapse or the descending perineum syndrome.

A history of incontinence of urine and evidence of a vaginal or uterine prolapse should be sought. A sexual history should be obtained and the possibility of homosexual behaviour or specific disease should be considered. Male patients may be impotent if the incontinence is due to diabetes. A history of neurological symptoms is essential. Previous anorectal trauma should be noted. A careful obstetric history should always be taken, noting previous difficult vaginal deliveries, perineal tears or evacuation difficulties. All previous operations on the anorectum should be recorded, particularly anal dilatation, sphincterotomy, operations for fistula-in-ano and haemorrhoidectomy. Previous gynaecological operations should be recorded, together with a history of large or small bowel resections. A comprehensive drug history must be included.

An incontinence score helps to quantify the degree of incontinence and its social impact (Pescatori et al, 1992; Oliveira et al, 1996). It is helpful to distinguish passive incontinence where there is no awareness of defecation, caused by internal sphincter abnormalities in older patients, from urge incontinence associated with striated muscle injury (Hill et al, 1994a; Engel et al, 1995; Gee and Durdey, 1995).

Examination

The urine should be tested to exclude diabetes mellitus. After examination of the abdomen a neurological assessment of the lumbosacral segment is advised, noting the presence of knee and ankle jerks and sensation around the buttocks. The anocutaneous reflex should be tested and the patient should be asked to bear down so as to assess the degree of perineal descent, mucosal prolapse and to exclude a full-thickness rectal prolapse. The perineum is inspected for evidence of scarring, fistula, skin tags, a patulous anus or skin excoriation.

Rectal examination should assess the degree of resting anal tone, as well as the influence of voluntary contraction on sphincter activity and movement of the puborectalis during contraction. Some patients do not seem to know what to do when asked to squeeze. Some authors believe that the educated digit can accurately assess the activity of the sphincters at rest and after voluntary contraction (Orrom et al, 1990a). We do not agree: apart from patients with an obviously patulous anus, digital examination, in our experience, is a poor predictor of anal canal pressure (Arabi et al, 1977). Eckardt and Kanzler (1993) reported a poor correlation between clinical assessment of resting and squeeze anal tone and resting and squeeze pressures, but they admitted that a well-educated finger could detect most sphincter injuries that justified repair.

The perineal body should be assessed and a vaginal examination performed to detect a rectocele, complete uterine prolapse or any other gynaecological pathology. If one can discreetly examine the underclothes or a sanitary towel, useful information may be gained regarding the degree of soiling or incontinence. Examination is incomplete without a thorough proctoscopy to exclude haemorrhoids, fissure, fistula or abscess. Sigmoidoscopy should also be performed to exclude malignant disease, villous adenoma, inflammatory bowel disease, polyps, solitary rectal ulcer or proctitis.

INVESTIGATION

Radiology

If there is any suspicion of a neurological lesion, radiography of the chest, pelvis, sacrum and spine is advised so as to exclude bony destruction, osteolytic or osteoporotic secondaries and soft tissue tumour swelling, as in fibrosarcoma or neurofibroma. The disc spaces should be examined as well as the intervertebral and sacral foramina. It is not the province of a colorectal surgeon to be ordering invasive investigations such as myelography before a neurologist is consulted but computed tomography (CT) and magnetic resonance imaging (MRI) may be extremely helpful in defining soft tissue swellings in patients with incontinence in whom an underlying neurological or intestinal pathology is suspected.

It is difficult to know how often contrast radiology is justified for patients with faecal incontinence. We certainly do not advise a barium enema in all patients with the descending perineum syndrome and rarely feel that contrast enemas are justified in elderly incontinent patients with a full-thickness rectal prolapse. We have encountered only one colorectal cancer in over 200 patients treated for rectal prolapse. The decision to order a barium enema and a small bowel meal largely depends upon clinical assessment and sigmoidoscopic findings. If there is any suspicion of a tumour, then a flexible sigmoidoscopy or colonoscopy and, if necessary, a barium enema would be advised. If there is a serious possibility of underlying inflammatory bowel disease (for instance in a patient with an area of proctitis or a complicated anal fistula or rather oedematous skin tags), a full radiological examination of the gut with colonoscopy is desirable.

Special investigations of continence

Special investigations of continence are not always needed in order to decide upon the most appropriate form of surgical treatment but they are desirable if the cause of incontinence is to be accurately determined (Karulf et al, 1991; Wexner et al, 1992; Andromanakos et al, 1996). Furthermore, measurements of anal function are helpful in evaluating the response to conservative or surgical treatment (O'Kelly and MacMortensen, 1992; Keating et al, 1997). Anyone with a special interest in the problem of incontinence is likely to want to assess the degree and quality of physiological malfunction (see Table 20.9). Perhaps the most useful aspect of preoperative physiological assessments is their ability to predict the outcome of surgical treatment (Parks, 1992; Rasmussen et al, 1992; Nikiteas et al, 1996; Korsgen et al, 1997).

Anal manometry and reflexes

Anal manometry

Anal canal pressures may be measured using solid-state microtransducers, open-ended continuously perfused catheters and closed water- or air-filled balloon probes. Duthie (1971) implied that perfusion and closed balloon techniques were comparable. This is not the case. The pressures recorded from perfused catheters depend upon the rate of perfusion and they tend to be lower than those of balloon probes (Pinho et al, 1991) (Figure 20.25a,b). There is a short lag phase when recording squeeze pressures using perfused catheters (Hill et al, 1960; Duthie and Watts, 1965; Ihre, 1974; Schuster, 1975;

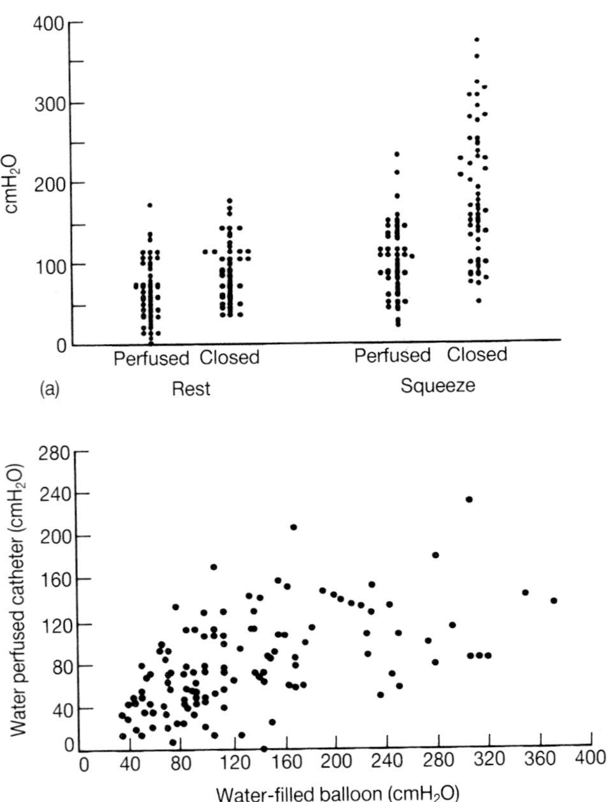

Figure 20.25a,b A comparison between perfused catheters and closed, water-filled balloon probe for measurement of anal pressure. (a) The perfused and closed methods for measuring rest and squeeze and canal pressures; $P < 0.02$. (b) Correlation between the two parameters, which indicates that the water perfused catheter technique provides lower values than the closed water-filled balloon probe.

Hancock, 1976). There is a close correlation between the diameter of the recording balloon and anal pressure: bigger balloons record higher pressures (Duthie et al, 1970; Guitierrez et al, 1975; Gibbons et al, 1986b) for both resting and squeeze pressures (Figure 20.26). Tip transducers are expensive but they were thought on theoretical grounds to be more accurate than a recording device attached to a transducer. Unfortunately, results are not reproducible (Ten Cate Hoedemaker, 1987) and vary with radial position (Miller et al, 1988a). Recent renewed interest has been centred on air-filled balloons, provided the dead space can be reduced by occluding the lumen and volume under the bell of the transducer. Miller et al (1988a) have showed that air balloons more accurately record rapid changes in pressure but results are lower than those of water-filled balloons. Publications should therefore specify which methods of recording have been used, the position of the patient and the normal values recorded (Johnson et al, 1990; Meshkinpour et al, 1997). Clinicians should be advised to choose a system and to continue with it rather than changing from one type to another, so that comparisons can be made before and after treatment and during follow-up (Hancock, 1976; Keighley et al, 1989; Favetta et al, 1996).

A typical trace in a patient with incontinence is shown in Figure 20.26. In almost all groups of incontinent patients the resting and squeeze pressures are significantly lower than in normal subjects (NW Read et al, 1979, 1984; Hiltunen, 1985; Delechenaut et al, 1992; Favetta et al, 1996; Andromanakos et al, 1996). Patients who are incontinent to liquids and solids have lower squeeze pressures than those who are incontinent to liquids alone (Read et al, 1984). The length of the high-pressure zone is also shorter in incontinent patients than in normal subjects and

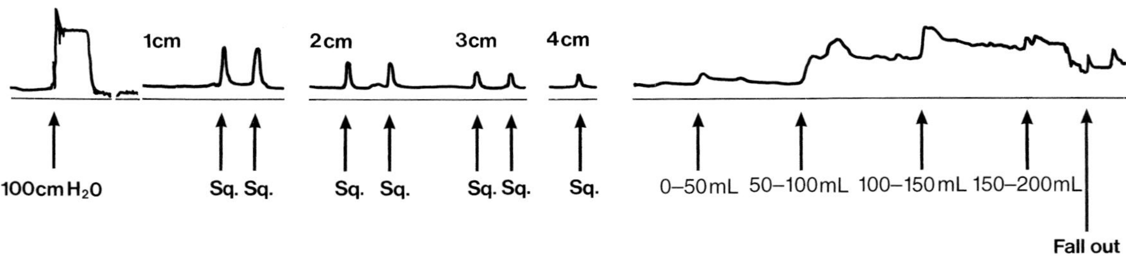

Figure 20.26 A typical anal pressure profile in faecal incontinence. On the left is shown the standardization to 100 cmH_2O. Recordings are obtained 1, 2, 3 and 4 cm from the anal verge. The basal pressures are shown, and the response to a maximum squeeze and strain effort are indicated. On the right is the response in resting anal pressure, recorded 1 cm from the anal verge, in response to 50-mL increments of air in a rectal balloon. The rectoanal inhibitory reflex is absent, and the balloon falls out after 200 mL of air have been introduced into it.

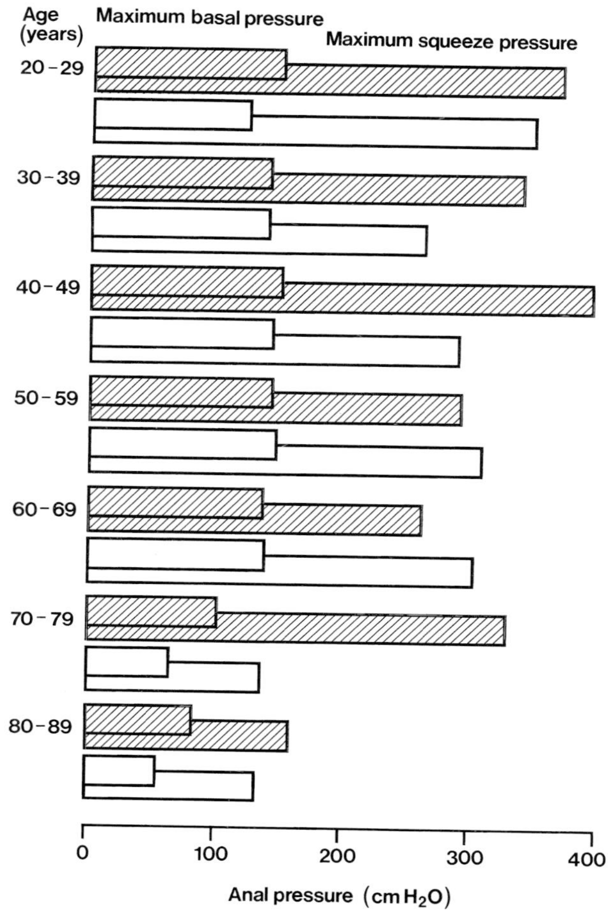

Figure 20.27 Changes in resting and squeeze anal canal pressure with age. Note that resting and squeeze pressures fall in both sexes after the age of 80, and in women over the age of 70. ▨, Men; □, women.

is shorter in women than men (Nivatvongs et al, 1981). Anal pressures remain remarkably stable throughout life but begin to fall after the age of 60 (Matheson and Keighley, 1981; Bannister et al, 1987). Hence, for statistical analysis patients must be matched with controls of the same age and sex (Figure 20.27) (Coller, 1987). Pressures tend to be lower in female patients than in male subjects (Enck et al, 1989a; Laurberg and Swash, 1989; Orrom et al, 1990b; Cali et al, 1992).

Vectormanometry assesses the forces within the anal canal and identifies defects seen as low-pressure zones (Braun et al, 1994; Williams et al, 1995). However, vectormanometry has now been largely superseded by anal ultrasonography (Yang and Wexner, 1994).

Anocutaneous reflex

The anocutaneous reflex is elicited by stroking the perianal skin and recording the external sphincter contraction that follows (Bartolo et al, 1983a,b). The measurement of latency in the anocutaneous reflex is spurious and is no longer used in assessment of pudendal nerve function (Henry and Swash, 1978; Henry et al, 1980; Bartolo et al, 1983b; Wright et al, 1985).

Rectoanal inhibitory reflex

The rectoanal inhibitory reflex can be assessed by placing a soft balloon in the rectum and recording the anal pressure at the site of maximal basal pressure. There should be a profound fall in anal pressure after introducing 50 mL of air in a rectal balloon (Aaronson and Nixon, 1972). The sampling reflex may also be detected as spontaneous episodes of sphincter inhibition during ambulatory manometry (Farouk et al, 1993, 1994). In some incontinent patients the anocutaneous and sampling reflex may be absent (Binnie et al, 1990).

Anal sensation

Anal sensation is measured using mucosal electrosensitivity and is impaired in most patients with faecal incontinence (Roe et al, 1986; Miller et al, 1987; Rogers et al, 1988a). Some authors have questioned the validity of this test (Felt-Bersma et al, 1997) but it correlates with age, anal manometry, single-fibre EMG and perineal discent (Gee and Durdey, 1995).

Rectal manometry and emptying

Rectal pressures may be measured by perfused catheters or by compliance studies with an air- or water-filled rectal balloon using continuous infusion or by incremental volumes (Akervall et al, 1989). Rectal contractions may be induced by infusion of air or water (Scharli and Kiesewetter, 1970). Three responses may be observed: low-amplitude contractions, high-amplitude contractions and propagated contractions (Whitehead et al, 1980). There may be impaired distensibility of the rectum in some patients with perineal descent and incontinence. Furthermore, there may be incoordination of the rectoanal inhibitory reflex (Pucciani et al, 1997) or spontaneous rectal contractions creating a rectoanal pressure gradient (Goes et al, 1995; Farouk et al, 1994). Rectal emptying may be impaired (see Evacuation protography).

Rectal sensation

Rectal sensation may be assessed by infusing fluid or distending a rectal balloon with air or using electrical mucosal stimulation (Speakmann and Kamm, 1993; Meagher et al, 1996). Three volume parameters are recorded: (1) the 'threshold volume', when the patient is first aware of a desire to defecate; (2) the volume associated with a constant desire to defecate, termed 'constant sensation'; (3) the 'maximum tolerated volume' (Hoffmann et al, 1995). In incontinent patients the balloon often falls out before the maximum tolerated volume is reached. The rectal sensation to distension and to electrical stimulation is impaired in incontinent patients (Speakmann and Kamm, 1993) and compliance may also be reduced (Holmberg et al, 1995).

Tests of continence

Tests of liquid continence can be assessed by perfusing saline at body temperature through a fine-bore rectal tube over approximately 25–30 minutes using a simple roller pump. Simultaneous monitoring of anal and rectal pressures identifies episodes of reflex anal or rectal contractions (NW Read et al, 1979). With the patient seated on a commode the volume infused when the first leak occurs is recorded. In normal subjects this volume is in excess of 1.5 L but in incontinent patients leakage usually starts after infusion of between 250 and 600 mL, the volume being less in patients who are incontinent of liquids only (Read et al, 1984) (Table 20.27). The other measurement commonly used is the total volume retained in the rectum; this is the difference between the volume infused (1.5 L) and the volume passed during the test. In normal subjects the entire volume is retained; in incontinent patients the volume retained ranges from 500 mL to 1000 mL, depending upon the degree of incontinence (NW Read et al, 1979, 1983a).

Tests of solid continence can be performed by measuring the traction required to displace varying sizes of spheres inserted into the rectum. For most practical purposes a sphere measuring 1.8 cm in diameter is generally used. The weight necessary to pull the sphere through the anus at rest and after voluntary sphincter contraction is recorded. In normal subjects the weights necessary to displace a 1.8-cm sphere with the sphincter relaxed and contracted have mean values of 685 and 1065 g respectively. In incontinent patients the mean values were 530 and 790 g respectively (NW Read et al, 1979).

Perineal descent

Measurement of perineal descent can be made using the perineometer (Henry et al, 1982; Ambrose and Keighley, 1986) (Figure 20.28) or by video-proctography (Jorge et al, 1993). In normal subjects the perineum usually lies 2.5 cm deep to the tuberosity and descends less than 1.5 cm. In patients with perineal descent the resting position is only slightly lower than normal but during straining descent is usually well beyond the tuberosity and exceeds 3 cm. Although this technique underestimates the degree of descent because changes in anal length cannot be measured, compared with a

Table 20.27 Comparison between patients incontinent to solids or liquids.

	Solids + liquids (*n* = 15)	*Liquids only* (*n* = 19)	*Controls* (*n* = 18)
Maximum basal pressure (cmH_2O)	43 ± 5	54 ± 5	83 ± 7
Maximum squeeze pressure (cmH_2O)	90 ± 10	124 ± 12	192 ± 19
Saline infusion test			
Volume first leak (mL)	383 ± 114	415 ± 100	1500
Total volume held (mL)	720 ± 106	861 ± 85	1500
Anorectal angle (°)			
Rest	114 ± 4	117 ± 5	92 ± 3
Squeeze	108 ± 5	112 ± 6	91 ± 4
Strain	127 ± 5	126 ± 5	109 ± 7
Perineal descent (cm)			
Rest	2.3 ± 0.4	1.5 ± 0.5	0.3 ± 0.2
Strain	5.2 ± 0.5	4.3 ± 0.6	1.9 ± 0.6

From Read et al (1984).

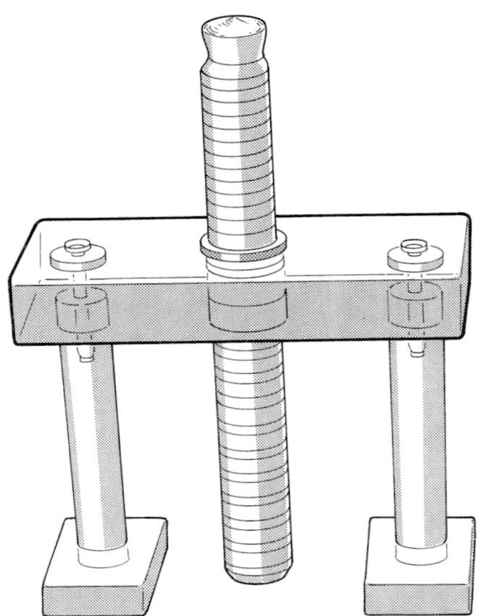

Figure 20.28 Perineometer for assessment of perineal descent. The lateral pylons are placed on the ischial tuberosity and the central mobile spindle rests on the anal verge. Changes in the position of the perineum during straining can thereby be recorded.

radiological assessment the procedure is non-invasive and clinically useful (Bartolo et al, 1983d; Oettle et al, 1985). Patients with gross perineal descent at rest have limited movement on straining (Skomorowska et al, 1988).

Electromyography

Electromyography in patients with incontinence can be used in six ways (Wexner et al, 1991b). The first is merely to record electrical activity in the muscles of continence during anorectal function, such as during videoproctography (Womack et al, 1985; Bartolo et al, 1986c; Pinho et al, 1991; Thorpe et al, 1995). The electromyographic trace should be integrated and continuously recorded in conjunction with other assessments of motor function. Fine barbed electrode wires (0.13 mm) are inserted through a hypodermic needle after anaesthetizing the skin with lignocaine jelly; this is well tolerated and almost painless (Read et al, 1983b).

The second function is to determine whether there is any electromyographic evidence of inappropriate puborectalis contractions during attempted defecation (Snooks et al, 1985a; Shouler and Keighley, 1986) or impaired recruitment or evidence of denervation (Infantino et al, 1995).

The third function is that of sphincter mapping (Tjandra et al, 1993). This used to be useful in patients with an ectopic anus, congenital anomalies and after disruption of the sphincter ring following a third-degree obstetric trauma or fistulotomy (Archibald and Goldsmith, 1967; Chantraine, 1973; Kiff, 1983; Kiff et al, 1984). Mapping of the sphincter may be very painful if there is scar tissue and the procedure has now been completely superseded by endoluminal ultrasonography and magnetic resonance imaging (Tjandra et al, 1993; Emblem et al, 1994).

Fourthly, electromyography may be used to assess the degree of denervation by measurement of the fibre density and evidence of conduction defects by nerve latency (Jost and Schimrigk, 1994; Pfeifer et al, 1997) (Figure 20.29).

Fifthly, surface electromyography may provide a measure of striated muscle function which may be utilized in biofeedback retraining (Pinho et al, 1991; Sorensen et al, 1991).

Finally, internal anal sphincter electromyography may be used to evaluate smooth muscle function (Farouk et al, 1994; Sorensen et al, 1994).

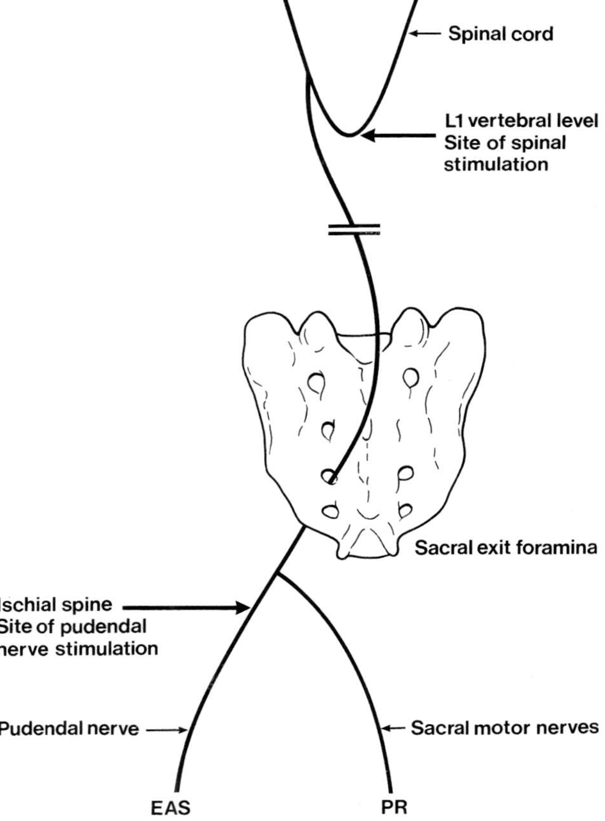

Figure 20.29 Sites of stimulation: conus medullaris (spinal stimulation) and ischial spine (transrectal pudendal nerve stimulation). EAS, external anal sphincter; PR, puborectalis.

Motor unit potential duration

Motor unit potential duration may be prolonged, particularly in partially denervated muscle where there has been attempted reinnervation. It is measured using a concentric needle electrode inserted without anaesthesia into the external anal sphincter and then advanced into the puborectalis. Twenty motor unit potentials are recorded from each of four sites. The advantage of this technique over measurement of fibre density is that it is less painful and less subject to bias (Bartolo et al, 1986c). The disadvantage is that individual muscle fibre action potentials cannot usually be recognized reliably within the motor unit action potential (Swash, 1985c).

Fibre density

Single-muscle fibre action potentials can only be recorded extracellularly using an electrode with a small leading off surface. The cannula of the electrode is used as a reference electrode with a separate surface ground electrode. This technique records only one or two single-muscle fibre potentials within the limited area of uptake of the electrode. The recordings are made with a trigger delay, hence potentials are derived from a single motor unit. The advantage of single-fibre electromyography is that fibre density can be measured; this provides a quantitative assessment of the number of muscle fibres belonging to a single motor unit. It is therefore an index of attempted reinnervation with fibre-type grouping. Fibre density is normally less than 1.5 but it increases with age (Neill and Swash, 1980). Potentials must be greater than 100 mV and 20 consecutive recordings of sufficient clarity must be used to determine fibre density. Fibre density is increased in idiopathic incontinence because there are more fibres within the uptake area of the electrode innervated by an individual axon or its branches.

The neuromuscular jitter (variability in interval between two successive components of a multicomponent motor unit) may also be used as a parameter of nerve damage. It is a measure of end-plate function (Davis et al, 1983).

Pudendal or perineal nerve terminal motor latency

Stimulation of the pudendal nerve as it crosses the ischial spine while recording the evoked potential in the external anal or urethral sphincter (Jost and Schimrigk, 1994) is achieved by specifically designed fingerstalls (Neill and Swash, 1980) which are now available as disposable items (Rogers et al, 1988c). Recordings are made from both sides of the pelvis as pudendal nerve damage may be asymmetrical in some patients (Lubowski et al, 1988b; Pfeifer et al, 1997). Pudendal nerve terminal motor latency is prolonged in idiopathic faecal incontinence and perineal nerve terminal latency is also abnormal in patients with double incontinence (Kiff and Swash, 1984a; Snooks et al, 1984a; Vernava et al, 1993; Roig et al, 1995). Pudendal nerve terminal motor latency, fibre density and perineal descent increase with age (Laurberg and Swash, 1989; Vernava et al, 1992) (Figures 20.30–20.32).

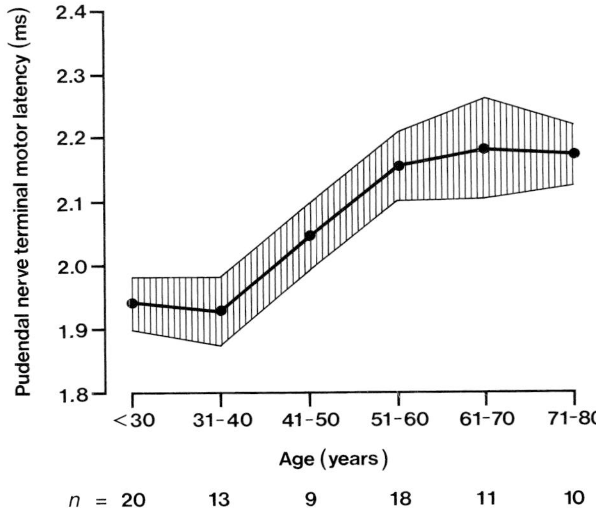

Figure 20.30 Pudendal nerve terminal motor latency changes with increasing age. There is an increase in the motor latency at about the fifth decade.

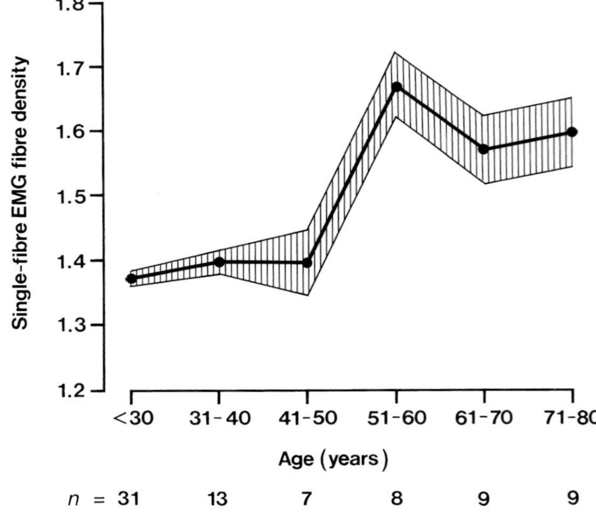

Figure 20.31 Single-fibre electromyographic (EMG) density measurements correlated with age. The fibre density increases after the fifth decade.

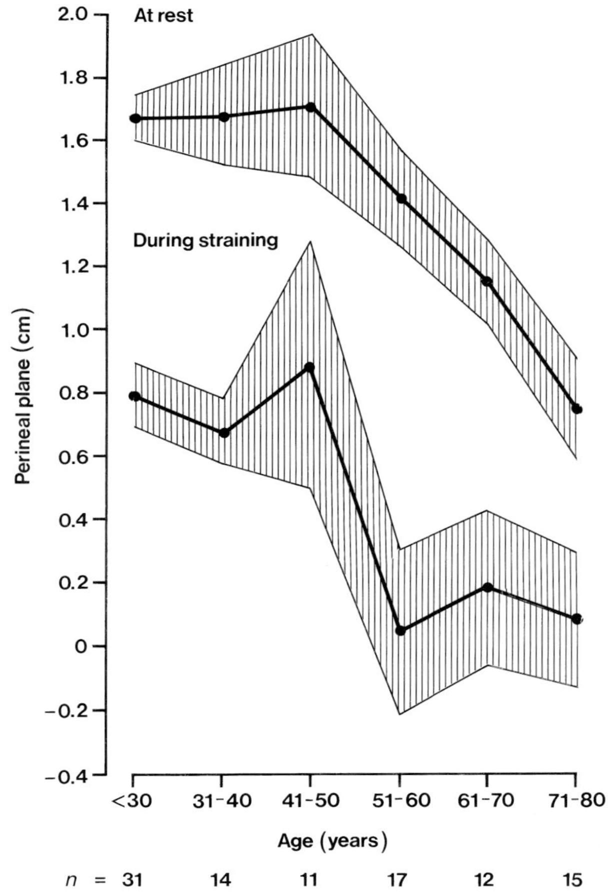

Figure 20.32 Perineal descent measurements related to age. Both the at rest and during straining measurements are lower after the fifth decade.

Pudendal latency is increased in patients with long-standing constipation and perineal descent, even unilateral pudendal nerve conduction defects imply pudendal neuropathy and occur in patients with pelvic floor disorders (Ho and Goh, 1995; Sangwan et al, 1996a,b). The test is reliable and is a useful predictor of outcome (Rieger et al, 1997b; Tetzschner et al, 1997; Chen et al, 1998).

Transcutaneous spinal latency

Transcutaneous electrical stimulation of the spinal cord or cauda equina allows identification of conduction defects in the cord, cauda equina and motor nerve roots (Merton et al, 1982). If transcutaneous stimulation is used in conjunction with pudendal nerve terminal motor latency it is possible to determine whether the conduction defect is in the terminal portion of the nerve or in the cauda equina.

Transcutaneous stimulation may be performed at C6 (thoracic outflow in the spinal cord), L1 (terminal portion of the spinal cord) or at the L4 vertebral level (cauda equina). In this way cord defects can be distinguished from cauda equina lesions (Snooks and Swash, 1985). The ratio of the L1 latency over the L4 latency is known as the spinal latency ratio (Snooks and Swash, 1984a). This was found to be prolonged in some patients with faecal incontinence, indicating the presence of a cauda equina conduction defect (Snooks et al, 1985c).

Cortical conduction studies

Electrical stimulation of the motor cortex to determine the conduction time of evoked potentials in the sphincters is now possible in conscious subjects (Merton et al, 1982). These techniques have not been widely used in pelvic floor disorders, although they have in other neurological disease (Cowan et al, 1984; Dick et al, 1984).

Evacuation proctography

Preston et al (1984) described a method of assessing anorectal function which was less cumbersome than conventional barium enema: 100–150 cm of dilute barium suspension was placed into a rectal balloon mounted on a fine catheter. The technique was devised particularly for patients with constipation in order to assess if they were capable of passing the balloon.

Conventional contrast radiology and balloon proctograms have now been completely superseded by combined dynamic imaging with or without simultaneous physiological monitoring (Womack et al, 1985) (Figure 20.33). The balloon proctography system described by Lahr et al (1986) provides a poor physiological assessment compared with videoproctography because contrast material is confined to a piece of Paul tubing and the method of manometry is unreliable (Lahr et al, 1988; Keighley et al, 1989). The principle of videoproctography is based upon the descriptions by Mahieu and others (Mahieu et al, 1984a,b; Bartolo et al, 1985; Womack et al, 1985). No bowel preparation is used. A known quantity of contrast material mixed with cellulose having the consistency of faeces is introduced through a wide-bore tube or a pistol injector. A radio-opaque paste is used to mark the anal canal. A surface marker is fixed to the symphysis pubis and a flexible marker to the perineal skin midway between the symphysis pubis and the coccyx. Simultaneous manometry and electromyography may be included. The

(a)

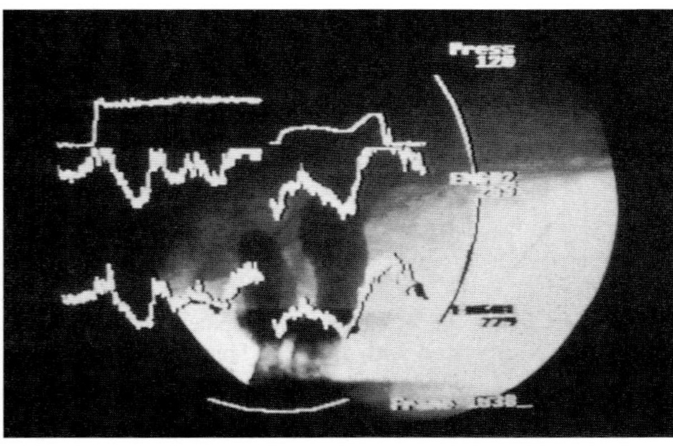

(b)

(c)

Figure 20.33a–c Dynamic videoproctography with simultaneous rectal and anal manometry and puborectalis EMG measurements. (a) The situation at rest. (b) Changes with attempted rectal evacuation: the anorectal angle widens, the intrarectal pressure rises, and there is inhibition of the anal sphincter. (c) A patient with an intrarectal intussusception: an inappropriate contraction of the puborectalis and external anal sphincter is demonstrated. At the tip of the intussusception there was a solitary ulcer.

patient is placed on a Perspex commode and seated on a water-filled tyre.

Examinations are performed in the seated position with lateral screening and the facility for radiography if needed (Oya et al, 1994). Pelvic floor movement with or without manometry and electromyographic activity are monitored at rest, during maximal pelvic floor contraction and during attempted defecation over 1 minute. The degree of perineal and pelvic floor descent is calculated from video recordings related to the pubococcygeal line, which is traced over frozen frames. The anorectal angle and anal canal length can be calculated from a computer-determined centroid of the rectal image during rest and maximal pelvic floor contraction and during defecation (Figure 20.34a,b).

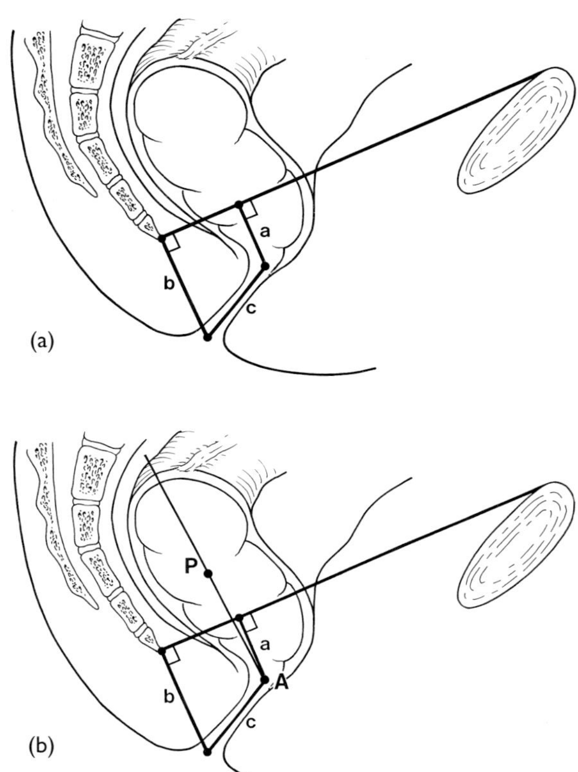

Figure 20.34a,b Measurement during videoproctography. (a) A lateral radiograph. The pubococcygeal line has been drawn. a = the distance between the anorectal angle and the pubococcygeal line, and represents the pelvic floor descent; b = the distance between the pubococcygeal line and the perineum, and represents perineal descent; c = the length of the anal canal. (b) This drawing includes the centroid. The centroid is the centrepoint (P) of the rectal image, such that a line between it and the anorectal angle (A) bisects the rectal image into two equal areas. It may be used for measurement of the anorectal angle.

Measurement of angles is more reliable using the centroid than the postrectal line (Yoshioka et al, 1991; Thorpe et al, 1995). However, the reliability of measuring the anorectal angle has been questioned (Jorge et al, 1992b). Topographical abnormalities, such as rectal deformity, strictures, rectocele, intussusception, rectal prolapse and abnormal pelvic floor movement are recorded. The amount of contrast material evacuated in 1 minute is measured to assess the efficiency of rectal emptying (Versluis et al, 1995). Faecal incontinence is usually associated with a short anal canal, perineal descent, an obtuse anorectal angle and leakage of contrast. In some patients an open upper anal canal and rectocele are present during pelvic floor contraction. In some, rectal evacuation is impaired.

The technique of videoproctography can be combined with cystometrography and is particularly useful in assessment of patients with faecal and urinary incontinence. Such a combined technique can also include simultaneous physiological measurement including manometric monitoring of the rectum and bladder, electromyography of the puborectalis, as well as investigating the changes in the rectum and bladder during filling and emptying (Thorpe et al, 1995). We used this technique to study 12 women with idiopathic faecal incontinence. Eight of them were demonstrated to have genuine stress incontinence of urine. In seven of these eight patients, the severity of their urinary incontinence was shown to be of type 2a or greater, indicating that pelvic floor dysfunction may be the causal factor of both their rectal and urinary incontinence.

Sigmoid manometry and transit studies

Sigmoid motility

Assessment of sigmoid motility disturbance usually involves manometry rather than studies of electromyographic activity (Taylor et al, 1978). Four-channel continuously perfused catheters with side openings placed at 10, 15, 20 and 25 cm from the anal verge have been used, being inserted during sigmoidoscopy (Taylor et al, 1984). The

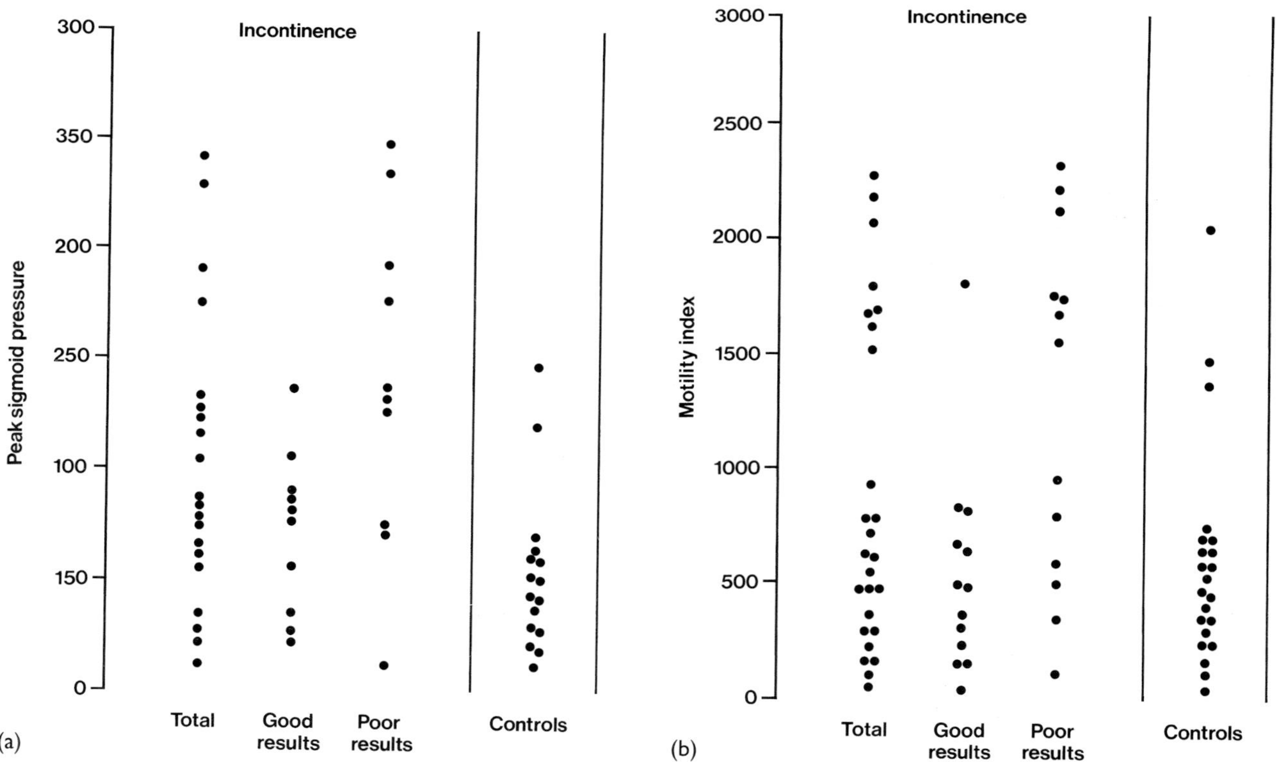

Figure 20.35a,b Motility index and peak sigmoid pressures in faecal incontinence, related to the outcome of postanal repair. (a) Peak sigmoid pressures in incontinence, compared with controls. Those with a poor result had significantly higher peak sigmoid pressures than those who obtained a good result. (b) Motility index in incontinence, compared with controls. Patients obtaining a poor result after postanal repair tended to have a higher motility index than those with a satisfactory outcome.

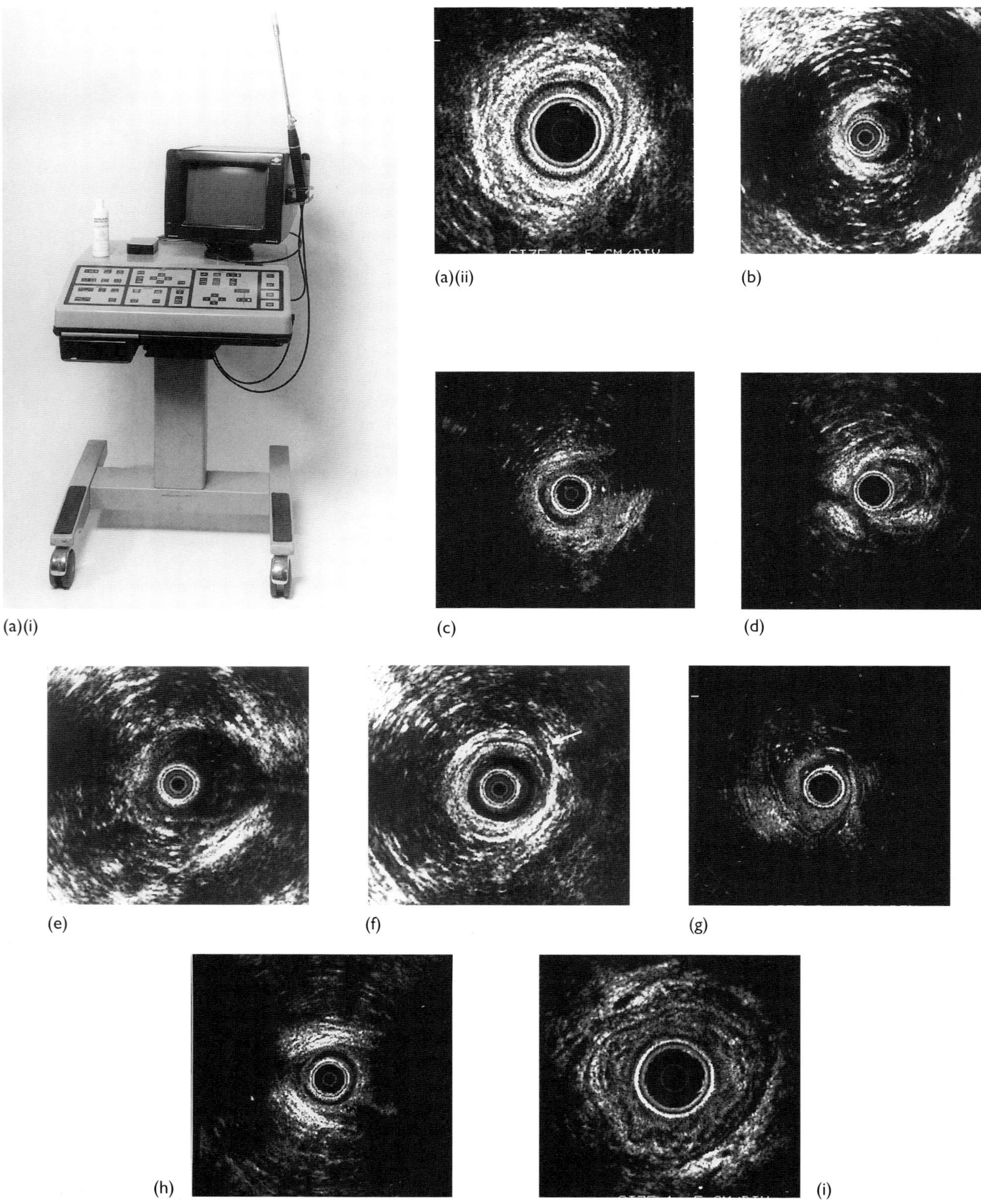

(a)(i) (a)(ii) (b) (c) (d) (e) (f) (g) (h) (i)

Figure 20.36a–i Anal ultrasonography. The ultrasound views are orientated with the posterior plane in the nine o'clock position. (a) (i) Ultrasound apparatus and (ii) normal appearances. (b) Defects in the internal anal sphincter from previous surgical treatment. (c) Anterior sphincter injury from third-degree obstetric tear. (d) Complex posterior anal fistula: trans-sphincteric track. (e) Ectopic anus. (f) Postoperative after sphincter repair. (g) Abscess and trans-sphincteric fistula. (h) Chronic anterior anal fissure. (i) Full-thickness rectal prolapse: patulous anus, atrophic internal sphincter.

catheters are strapped to the buttock and continuous recordings can be obtained over 3–4 hours. More recently, ambulatory techniques have been used (Kumar et al, 1989). Episodes of spontaneous high-pressure activity have been observed in incontinent patients, particularly in younger female subjects with the irritable bowel syndrome and perineal descent. Peak basal sigmoid pressures and sigmoid motility index were significantly higher among incontinent patients than controls (Keighley and Shouler, 1984). We have subsequently shown that a high sigmoid motility index identifies a group of patients who do badly following postanal repair (Figure 20.35a,b).

Transit studies

Studies of colonic transit are rarely abnormal in incontinent patients but transit is sometimes delayed in younger patients with prolapse and incontinence (Keighley and Shouler, 1984).

Anorectal ultrasound

The morphology of the internal anal sphincter and most of the external anal sphincter, the puborectalis and the rectovaginal septum can be displayed with remarkable clarity using endoanal ultrasonography (Law and Bartram, 1989). We use this investigation as the method of choice (Deen et al, 1993a) to display any defects in the internal and external anal sphincters, to exclude any evidence of active cryptoglandular infection as well as assessing the function of the striated sphincters and puborectalis (Mortensen, 1992; Falk et al, 1994; Farouk and Bartolo, 1994; Sultan et al, 1994a,c; Eckardt et al, 1994; Rieger et al, 1996). We and others have found an excellent correlation between anal ultrasound imaging and defects in the internal and external sphincter as displayed during surgical dissection (Deen et al, 1993b; Sultan et al, 1993b,d).

Anal ultrasonography is performed using a Bruel and Kjaer (Nrum, Denmark) ultrasound scanner (Type 1846) with a rectal endoprobe (Type 1850) and a 7-mHz transducer (Solomon et al, 1994). The transducer is covered by a sonolucent plastic cone of 1.7 cm external diameter filled with degassed water for acoustic coupling. The examination is performed with the patient in the left lateral position; serial images are taken at rest and during a maximum squeeze effort at the anorectal junction and in three zones (upper, mid, lower) of the anal canal (Tjandra et al, 1992).

The internal and external anal sphincters can be measured directly from a hard copy using calipers (Law et al, 1990; Burnett and Bartram, 1991).

Examples of anal ultrasonography are shown in Figure 20.36. Normal appearances are displayed in Figure 20.36a(ii). Defects in the internal sphincter are evident from a break in the ring of sphincter deep to the submucosa (Figure 20.36b). A deficiency in the external sphincter and its circumferential extent can be displayed (Figure 20.36c); such sphincter damage may be associated with a weak puborectalis sling which is found to be relatively inert on dynamic assessment. Anal ultrasound can also display the site of fistulas (Figure 20.36d), the external sphincter in ectopic anus (Figure 20.36e) and to monitor the results of sphincter repair (Figure 20.36f).

Anal sphincter imaging in faecal incontinence using anal ultrasonography has largely replaced the more invasive technique of electromyography (Felt-Bersma et al, 1992; Sentovich et al, 1997) and provides anatomical definition of injuries to the internal and external sphincters which are of proven value in planning restorative surgery (Cuesta et al, 1992). Imaging has also been of benefit in assessing the results of sphincter repair (Nielsen et al, 1992). Persistant incontinence after sphincter repair is most frequently due to breakdown or disruption of the repair which can be easily identified by endoluminal ultrasound (Deen et al, 1993c; Nielsen et al, 1994; Felt-Bersma et al, 1995, 1996; Ternent et al, 1997).

Magnetic resonance imaging

Conventional MRI may be helpful in identifying and localizing anorectal sepsis. However, the definition provided in the anal canal is not sufficiently sensitive for MRI to be applicable in assessing small tumours, localized sepsis or sphincter injury. Intrarectal coils have the potential for providing much greater information of the sphincters and pelvic floor. deSouza et al (1995) demonstrated sphincter defects and intersphincteric sepsis using this method of imaging. More refinements are likely and the potential for high-quality imaging is considerable, particularly with the development of the endoluminal MRI coil.

PREVENTION OF INCONTINENCE

It is evident that many patients suffer from iatrogenic incontinence which should be preventable. Obstetric injuries could be avoided by a more rigorous selection of patients with cephalopelvic disproportion for elective caesarean section, by preventing a prolonged second stage of labour and by performing an episiotomy whenever the sphincters are liable to be damaged by the fetal head (Cook and Mortensen, 1998).

In view of the long-term morbidity of obstetric injuries and the risks of litigation, a far higher level of supervision is needed during labour, especially in primigravida. The threshold for caesarean section should be low, forceps should be replaced, where possible, by ventouse suction. If a tear has occurred, the perineum must be assessed carefully by an expert and repairs undertaken in proper theatre facilities by fully trained personnel. Postobstetric bowel management is likely to avoid pelvic floor disorders from impaired evacuation.

Anal dilatation or sphincterotomy should never be performed if there is evidence of perineal descent, particularly in multiparous women. Both should be avoided in elderly patients and anybody with underlying inflammatory bowel disease or a previous history of incontinence and neither should be repeated in a patient unless absolutely necessary. Medical sphincterotomy should be used whenever tolerated in the treatment of fissure-in-ano. Most patients with non-infected perianal Crohn's disease should be managed conservatively but early drainage of sepsis is essential in order to preserve anorectal function. Setons or advancement flaps should be used whenever a fistula-in-ano involves a substantial component of the striated component of the anal sphincters.

CONSERVATIVE TREATMENT

Control of bowel habit

A high proportion of patients with faecal incontinence have diarrhoea, which may or may not be associated with colicky left iliac fossa pain. The diarrhoea is usually intermittent but greatly exacerbates the frequency of faecal leakage. First-line treatment in all patients with a history of diarrhoea is therefore to try simple constipating agents, such as codeine phosphate or loperamide (MG Read et al, 1979) although the results may be disappointing if there is coexisting irritable bowel syndrome. Loperamide is particularly useful if the diarrhoea is due to excessive small intestinal motility or previous small bowel resection. It reduces stool weight, frequency, urgency and incontinence by retarding transit and it stimulates anal sphincter function (Ruppin, 1987; Goke et al, 1992). If there is excessive intestinal hurry associated with colic then a small dose of diphenoxylate hydrochloride with atropine (Lomotil) may be helpful. Excessive dosage with Lomotil should be avoided as it may cause a dry mouth, tachycardia and nystagmus. Other preparations such as kaolin may be of benefit and should be considered if first-line drugs fail. It is not advisable, however, to prescribe agents containing morphine or opium if prolonged treatment is contemplated. Bulking agents, such as ispaghula (Isogel) or methylcellulose may improve the consistency of a liquid stool. Alternative bulking agents include sterculia (Inolaxine) or ceratonia with starch (Arobon).

In patients with the irritable bowel syndrome and a hypertonic sigmoid colon associated with colic and diarrhoea, treatment with peppermint oil, dicyclomine hydrochloride (Merbentyl), propanthelene bromide or mepenzolate may be helpful. The aim of therapy is to try to achieve passage of one or two well-formed stools a day (Schoetz, 1985). We reported our initial results of conservative therapy using antidiarrhoeal agents alone in 39 patients with severe faecal incontinence who were being assessed for surgical treatment (Keighley and Fielding, 1983). Treatment with antidiarrhoeal agents restored continence in only six cases (15%). Although this may seem to be a poor response to therapy it nevertheless identified for us a small group of patients in whom surgical treatment was unnecessary.

Dietary advice may help some patients; clearly, irritant and highly spiced foods causing diarrhoea should be avoided. Avoidance of coffee, beer, dairy products and citrus fruits is also advocated by Cohen et al (1986).

Keeping the rectum empty

There is one sure way of preventing or controlling incontinence and that is by ensuring that the rectum contains no faecal material. Some patients with incontinence therefore use suppositories or even disposable enemas to achieve this. Glycerine suppositories or an irritant suppository, such as bisacodyl (Dulcolax), may be helpful but they rarely achieve complete clearance of the rectum. Disposable phosphate enemas are of course more efficient but there is less patient compliance and the procedure may be messy (Iwama et al, 1989). There are a variety of small volume enemas which may be self-administered: proprietary preparations include Micralax and Relaxit which are both based upon the laxative effect of sodium citrate. However, our experience with both preparations has been disappointing. There is substantial evidence that twice-weekly enemas and a mild laxative may completely control incontinence from faecal impaction but the results in elderly with neuropathic incontinence is less encouraging (Tobin and Brocklehurst, 1986).

Some patients who wish to avoid surgery or a stoma are willing to use high-volume enemas on a regular basis in order to keep the rectum empty (Dick et al, 1996). The success of this approach is largely determined by motivation. There are, of course, obvious difficulties in incontinent patients of achieving a seal around the anus to prevent leakage (Shandling and Gilmour, 1987). However, a number of patients born with anorectal agenesis or Hirschsprung's disease treated by pull-through operations prefer this to more surgery. Some of the best results are in patients with soiling rather than frank incontinence. Briel et al (1997) reported on the results of using a colostomy irrigation set (see Figure 9.24) after the first bowel action in the morning or in the evening for those whose sleep was disturbed. Washouts took from 10–90 minutes and were used from 2 times a week to twice a day depending on control. In the 22 out of 32 of those who persisted with irrigation 92% with soiling obtained benefit compared with 60% with faecal incontinence. An alternative is antegrade irrigation either using an appendicostomy tube (Mitrofanoff, 1980; Malone et al, 1990; Squire et al, 1993; Griffiths and Malone, 1995; Yamamoto et al, 1996) or a caecal flap conduit (Kiely et al, 1994). At the Royal London Hospital we have described a continent colonic conduit for the management of severe constipation (see Figures 21.23 to 21.31) (Maw et al, 1997a). This has obvious application not only for evacuatory disorders (Maw et al, 1996) but also as a means of helping patients with incontinence complicating anorectal malformation (Maw et al, 1997b).

Pharmacological methods

Pharmacological augmentation in internal sphincter failure may be a therapeutic option in the future (Siproudhis et al, 1998). Knowledge of the non-adrenergic and non-cholinergic transmitters responsible for internal sphicter inhibition should lead to the development of nitric oxide antagonists.

Alternatively, stimulation of the internal sphincter using the cholinergic pathways with agents such as octreotide should provide further opportunities for the non-surgical management of faecal incontinence (Rasmussen et al, 1996). Agents such as phenylephrine may well be useful in this context (Carapeti et al, 1998).

Biofeedback and sphincter exercises

If patients are only occasionally incontinent it is worthwhile considering sphincter exercises or biofeedback (Patankar et al, 1997a,b). External electrical treatment, pelvic floor exercises and biofeedback is also helpful for patients who seem to have forgotton how to contract the pelvic floor and in those, such as diabetics, with a sensory disorder (Wald, 1981; Buser and Miner, 1986). In order to re-educate patients to use their pelvic floor muscles we use manometry, videoproctographic playback or surface electromyographic recordings to reinforce pelvic floor and sphincter exercises. Because sensory awareness is critical, patients are taught to contract their pelvic floor and sphincter at threshold volumes. Patient cooperation is greatly improved by admitting patients for 48 hours for a period of intensive therapy and instruction on matters such as diet, an exercise programme, drugs and enemas. Using a surface electromyographic anal probe, patients are taught to contract the sphincters and levator ani in response to rectal distension. They then take the apparatus home and are reviewed after 6–8 weeks of outpatient therapy (Figure 20.37). MacLeod (1979) recommended this form of retraining only when there are some remaining intact anal sphincter fibres. He used a device in which electrical impulses generated by the active muscles were fed back to the patient in the form of audible or visible signals. Muscle contraction was triggered by an impulse delivered and recorded through an anal plug. MacLeod (1983) then reported his results in 50 patients with a variety of causes of anal incontinence (Table 20.28). The group in whom treatment was most successful were patients with faecal

Table 20.28 Results reported using biofeedback.

	n	*Good response*	*Poor response*
McLeod (1983)			
Fistula laid open	18	13	5
Haemorrhoidectomy	14	13	1
Multiple operations	4	2	2
Idiopathic	3	3	0
Local excision of squamous carcinoma	3	1	2
Neurological	3	1	2
Rectal prolapse	3	1	2
Radiation	2	2	0
Total	50	36 (72%)	
Keighley and Fielding (1983)			
Idiopathic	13	3	10
Rectal prolapse	10	1	9
Fistula laid open	6	3	3
Anal dilatation	4	3	1
Diabetes	3	1	2
Total	36	11 (30%)	

soiling after a haemorrhoidectomy. Another group that seemed to respond well were patients with partial sphincter damage after fistula operations. Results in patients with neuropathic faecal incontinence or after colorectal resection was poor. In his experience outpatient therapy was just as successful as admitting patients to hospital (MacLeod, 1987).

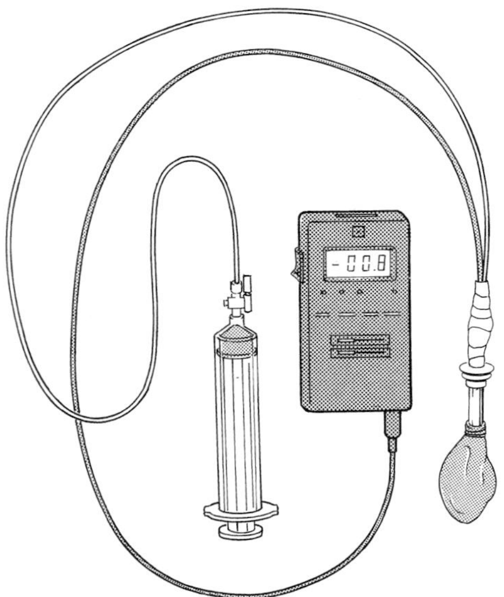

Figure 20.37 Biofeedback apparatus. A simple device for pelvic floor retraining and sphincter strengthening exercises. A probe containing a balloon is placed in the rectum. The probe also contains a surface EMG, which lies inside the anal canal. The EMG is connected to a digital display unit. The balloon is connected to a 50-mL syringe. Inflation of the balloon should be followed by pelvic floor contraction, and increased electrical activity on the EMG visual display.

We first used the apparatus devised by Hopkinson and Lightwood (1966) for stimulating the pelvic floor and external anal sphincter. The equipment (Figure 20.38) consists of a dumbbell-shaped Perspex plug containing two parallel electrodes placed 1 cm apart and connected to a portable tetanizing current generator. This is a battery-operated device which delivers an asymmetrical biphasic pulse of 0–8 V every 1–3 seconds. Patients are instructed to insert the device for 10 minutes twice daily for a month while attending physiotherapy. When we first analysed our results for all patients with incontinence they were inferior to those reported by MacLeod (1987). However, there was a large number of patients with rectal prolapse and neuropathic incontinence in our group. Results in the postoperative group were much better and 60% reported a good response to therapy. There was also a significant improvement in anal squeeze pressures after 1 month's therapy (Table 20.29). We found improved results using a surface electromyographic probe with a hand-held display but results were better if we admitted patients for initial therapy.

Diabetic patients with sensory impairment having passive incontinence may be improved by a biofeedback technique which utilizes the sampling reflex (Binnie et al, 1990). The patient is seated so that the recording trace is visible, a rectal balloon is distended until sensation is eventually perceived and the inhibitory reflex is observed by the patient. The procedure is repeated using lower volumes and the patient is told when the rectal balloon is distended if it cannot be felt. It is usually possible to reduce sensory threshold by biofeedback (Figure 20.39).

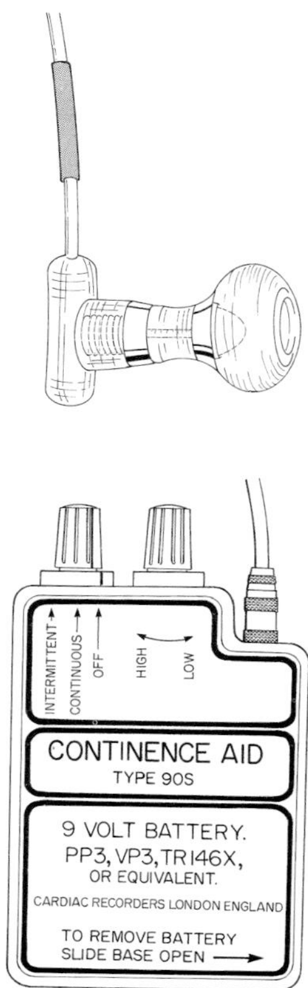

Figure 20.38 Continence aid. A plug with surface EMG probes is placed inside the anal canal. A stimulus is applied to the surface probes, which can be felt by the patient. Patients should be taught to contract their pelvic floor muscles as the current is applied.

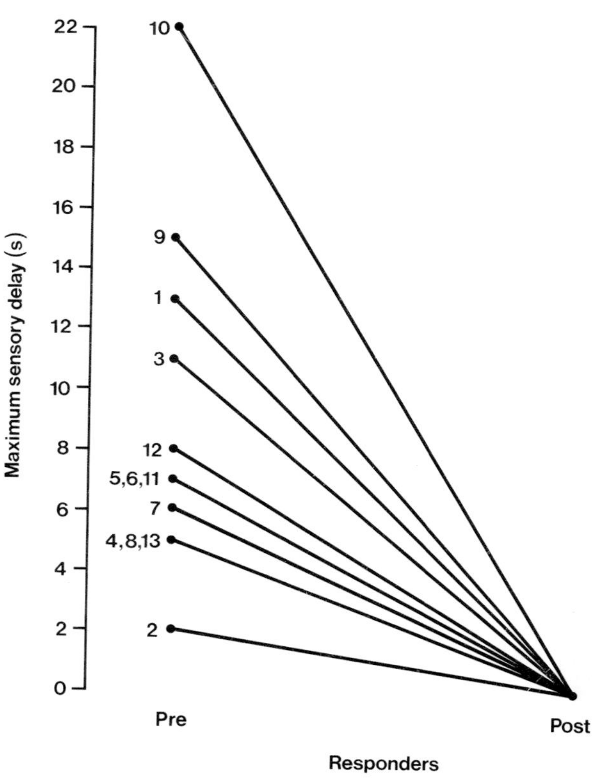

Figure 20.39 Time from rectal balloon distension to conscious rectal sensation before and after biofeedback retraining in 13 patients with faecal incontinence and sensory delay.

Table 20.29 Influence of treatment on anal pressures (cmH_2O) (Birmingham).

		Resting pressure		*Maximum squeeze pressure*	
	n	*Before*	*After*	*Before*	*After*
Physiotherapy	35	61 ± 7	67 ± 7	124 ± 10*	140 ± 11
Postanal repair	67	63 ± 6*	72 ± 5	136 ± 9	138 ± 8
Sphincter repair	29	72 ± 3	77 ± 6	94 ± 10†	164 ± 14

Values are mean ± SEM.
* $P < 0.05$.
† $P < 0.01$.

Once the sensory threshold is less than 20 mL, patients are taught to contract their sphincters as soon as the inhibitory reflex is seen or the distension is felt. To overcome selection bias, the technique of forced choice may be used, in which the patient has to decide whether rectal distension is real or false (Penninckx et al, 1989). Provided the sensory threshold can be reduced to 20 mL or less, results of biofeedback for sensory deficits are excellent (Schuster, 1977; Whitehead et al, 1980; Jensen and Lowry, 1992).

Motor defects respond even better, particularly if there is partial sphincter loss or a neuromuscular defect in the external sphincter (Schuster, 1966; Alva et al, 1967; Engel et al, 1974; Cerulli et al, 1979; MacLeod, 1987; Pescatori et al, 1991). These authors report that 60–70% of their patients were greatly improved using this technique but results in spinal cord lesions are more disappointing. Recent results of studies using biofeedback and pelvic floor exercises are set out in Table 20.30. The outcome is variable. The group from Nijmegen (Scheuer et al, 1994;

Table 20.30 Results of biofeedback for faecal incontinence.

	Number	Comments	Completely continent	Improved but not completely continent	No better
Arhan et al (1994)	47	Children (congenital or faecal impaction)		23	24
Enck et al (1994)	18	Long term results	3	7	8
Keck et al (1994)	15	Various aetiologies	4	7	4
Scheuer et al (1994)	10	Neurogenic incontinence	0	2	8
Guillemot et al (1994)	24	Various aetiologies		No absolute figures available	
Sangwan et al (1995)	28	(same group as Keck et al)	13	8	7
van Tets et al (1996)	12	(same group as Scheuer et al)	0	0	12
Patankar et al (1997a)	72	Incomplete follow-up in 13		50	9
Rieger et al (1997a)	30	Pelvic floor exercises	8	20	2

van Tets et al, 1996) report very disappointing results whereas at the Lahey Clinic (Keck et al, 1994; Sangwan et al, 1995) 70% of patients were improved and some have been rendered completely continent. Some studies claiming 85% improvement do not have complete follow-up (Patankar et al, 1997a). Most studies in adults fail to identify groups who will benefit, thus age, cause of incontinence, severity of symptoms and preoperative physiology failed to identify a group that might benefit (Rieger et al, 1997a). Almost all studies report reduced threshold sensation with increased resting and squeeze pressures after biofeedback (Keck et al, 1994; Scheuer et al, 1994; Guillemot et al, 1994).

Biofeedback may also have a role for treatment in children with soiling complicating faecal impaction or in anorectal agenesis (Arhan et al, 1994). Ho et al (1996) from Singapore and Taiwan report improvement in defecation frequency and improved continence after four biofeedback sessions among patients with incontinence after anterior resection or total colectomy. The only study providing long-term results (Enck et al, 1994) seems to indicate that initial improvement is sustained with time but this is not a universal finding (Loening-Baucke, 1990; Guillemot et al, 1994; Perozo et al, 1997).

Our own experience with biofeedback indicates that results are largely governed by patient motivation, the thin, well turned out person who exhibits a high degree of personal hygiene, who is psychologically stable and who is not involved with litigation frequently responds well to biofeedback. Furthermore, if they continue to exercise they usually maintain their improvement (Korsgen, 1995).

Other non-surgical methods which need greater research are physical occlusive devices such as the continence plug (Christiansen and Roed-Petersen, 1993).

SURGICAL TREATMENT

The range of surgical treatments for faecal incontinence has widened considerably in the last decade. Procedures include some form of pelvic floor repair, sphincter repair, muscle transposition with or without electrical stimulation of the nerve or muscle (Baeten et al, 1995; Wexner et al, 1996a) and the artificial anal sphincter (Lehur et al, 1996; Wong et al, 1996). If these techniques fail, some patients will elect to have a permanent stoma and if that is the case, in our experience, most will require anorectal excision since mucus discharge from the defunctioned rectum in incontinent patients is often intolerable (Keighley, 1991).

Anterior and posterior reefing procedures

Reefing procedures involve plication of the anterior and/or posterior fibres of the external anal sphincter (Figures 20.40 and 20.41).

These operations are now largely historical and although they may be used with anoplasty for stenosis or deformity of the anus, the procedure has largely been superseded by pelvic floor repair (Stricker et al, 1988).

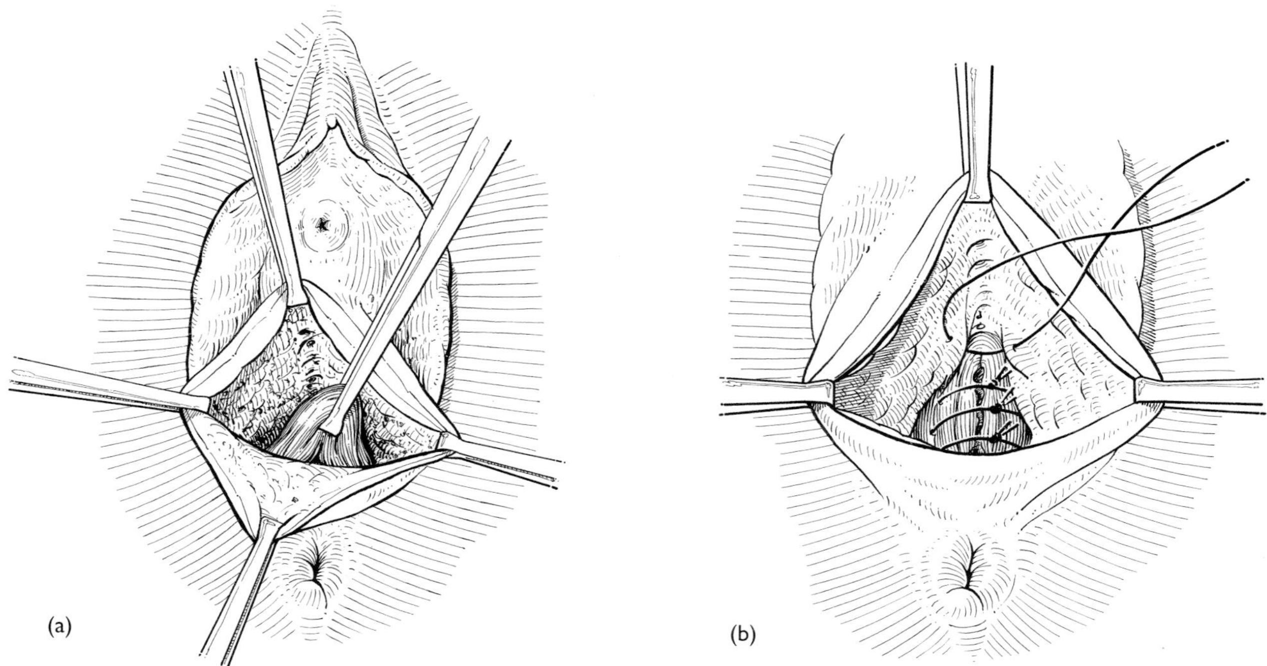

Figure 20.40a,b Anterior sphincter reefing procedure. (a) The patient is placed in the lithotomy position. A transverse incision is used. The external anal sphincter is dissected from the perineal body and from the internal anal sphincter. (b) The apex of the external sphincter is retracted anteriorly and a series of sutures are placed between both limbs of the sphincter as a plication procedure.

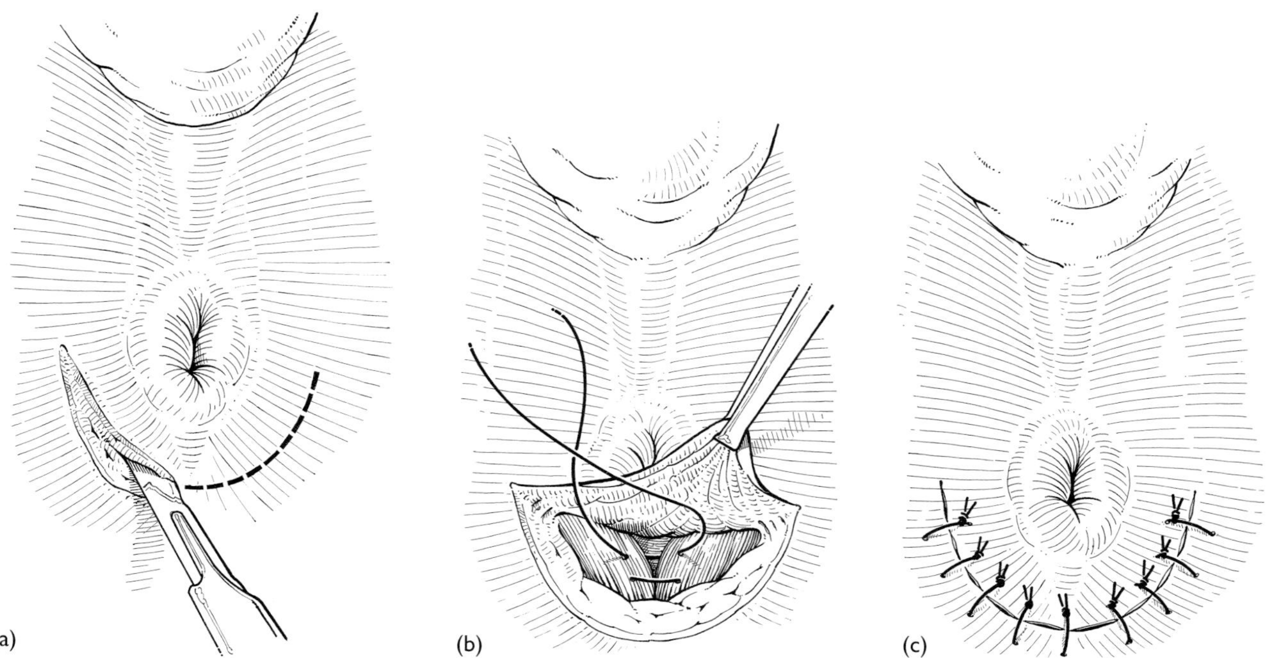

Figure 20.41a–c Posterior sphincter reefing procedure. (a) The patient is placed in the lithotomy position. A circular incision is made just behind the external anal sphincter. (b) The anterior skin flap is raised, and the external anal sphincter is dissected from the skin and the internal anal sphincter. The sphincter apex is then retracted posteriorly and a series of sutures reef the two limbs of the external anal sphincter. (c) Completion of the operation with closure of the skin defect.

Postanal repair

Postanal repair is an operation that was originally designed to restore an obtuse anorectal angle and to elongate the functional length of the anal canal (Penninckx, 1992). Evidence now suggests that it has no influence on the anorectal angle. In order to approximate the inner fibres of the puborectalis the operation must be performed within the pelvis, either from above or below. Access from above is poor and the operation is now exclusively performed from the perineum. Perineal approaches to the puborectalis include the posterior precoccygeal exposure and the intersphincteric approach. Most surgeons now use the intersphincteric approach since the sacrum prevents adequate exposure to the inner fibres of the pelvic diaphragm. Although Parks believed that the lithotomy position was optimum (Parks, 1974), the prone jack-knife position is widely used in North America (Nichols, 1982; Schoetz, 1985).

The principle of the operation is to expose the pubococcygeus, puborectalis and ischiococcygeus through the intersphincteric plane and to approximate these muscles posteriorly with the posterior fibres of the external sphincter (Keighley, 1987b). The operation increases the length of the high-pressure zone in the anal canal (Womack et al, 1988; Yoshioka et al, 1988). Browning and Parks (1983) and later Scheuer et al (1989) showed that there was a significant improvement in resting and squeeze anal canal pressures following operation. However, neither of these authors were able to confirm these observations, nor did they report any significant improvement in resting and squeeze anal canal pressures (see Table 20.29) or in the anorectal angle (Womack et al, 1988; Yoshioka and Keighley, 1989).

We found that incontinent patients undergoing postanal repair had significantly low resting and squeeze pressures, impaired anal sensation, obtuse anorectal angles, a short high-pressure zone, early leakage during the saline infusion test, and poor pelvic floor movements. Only the length of the high-pressure zone was improved by operation (Table 20.31). Predictors of poor outcome are presented in Table 20.32.

Table 20.31 Results before and after postanal repair compared with age- and sex-matched controls.

	Controls (n = 19)	Postanal repair (n = 19) Before	Postanal repair (n = 19) After
Maximum resting anal pressure (cmH_2O)	108.3 ($P<0.001$)	49.7	47.3
Maximum squeeze anal pressure (cmH_2O)	138.6 ($P<0.001$)	77.2	68.1
Threshold anal sensation (mA)	5.3 ($P<0.01$)	13.7	14.4
Resting anorectal angle (°)	118.2 ($P<0.01$)	130.2	132.4
Maximum squeeze angle (°)	104.3 ($P<0.01$)	119.4	114.7
Length of high-pressure zone (cm)	4.6 ($P<0.05$)	3.2 ($P<0.05$)	4.0
Compliance (mL/cmH_2O)	14.5	13.1	13.1
Rectal emptying (%/mm)	75	75	42
Saline infusion test: volume first leak (mL)	800 ($P<0.01$)	180	174
Pelvic floor descent at rest (cm)	3.3 ($P<0.05$)	6.3	6.1
Pelvic floor descent during straining (cm)	4.9 ($P<0.05$)	7.2	7.1

Table 20.32 Positive predictive parameters of poor outcome (median values).

	Improved	*Not improved*
Anal pressures (cmH_2O)		
Rest	50	29
Squeeze	90	38
Pelvic floor descent (cm)		
Rest	4.6	7.6
Strain	6.5	10.3
Perineal descent (cm)		
Rest	7.9	10.2
Strain	8.2	10.2
Anal canal length (cm)	4.3	2.9

Results

The clinical results of postanal repair are set out in Table 20.33 (Browning et al, 1983; Keighley, 1984; Henry and Simson, 1985; Habr-Gamma et al, 1986; Yoshioka and Keighley, 1989; Scheuer et al, 1989; Jameson et al, 1994; Setti-Carraro et al, 1994).

Habr-Gamma et al (1986) reported that only 48% of their patients become completely continent of solids and liquids and that 38% were continent of solids only. We initially reported that 63% of patients achieved complete continence of faeces (Keighley, 1984). Browning et al (1983) indicated that as many as 74% of patients were completely continent of liquids and solids, complete continence being achieved in 91% of men and 71% of women.

These early enthusiastic results were not reproduced when functional outcome was assessed critically by independent observers in patients followed up some years after the operation. Henry and Simson (1985) found that only 56% of patients having postanal repair were rendered completely continent of solids and liquids and results were worse in patients with neuropathic faecal incontinence. Furthermore, 30% were not improved at all. Likewise long-term results indicate deteriorating function over time with only 30% remaining continent when reviewed 5–8 years after operation (Jameson et al, 1994; Setti-Carraro et al, 1994).

We critically assessed our own results in 124 patients operated upon over 10 years (Yoshioka et al, 1988). Although 71% of the 84 individuals followed up for more than 3 years still felt improved, objective assessment of the quality of continence indicated otherwise (Table 20.34). Continued soiling was recorded in 63% of patients, pads were still worn in 55% and only 34% were completely continent of liquids, solids and flatus.

Results of postanal repair do not appear to be influenced by age but a poor functional outcome was reported in patients with perineal descent, mucosal or full-thickness rectal prolapse, and intractable pruritus ani, perineal pain or solitary rectal ulcer and neuropathic incontinence (Henry and Simson, 1985). Prolonged pudendal nerve latency was a predictor of poor outcome (Setti-Carraro et al, 1994). It has been suggested that progressive neurological damage to the pelvic floor muscles is responsible for poor functional outcome (Laurberg et al, 1990).

Table 20.33 Results of postanal repair.

	n	*Continent of solids and liquids*	*Continent of solids only*	*No better*
Browning and Parks (1983)	140	104	17	19
Henry and Simson (1985)	129	72	18	39
Habr-Gamma et al (1986)	42	22	17	3
Yoshioka and Keighley (1989) (long term)	116	40	66	10
Scheuer et al (1989)	39	18	9	12
Jameson et al (1994) (long term)	38	10	9	17
Setti Carraro et al (1994)	34	9	21	4

Table 20.34 Quality of continence after postanal repair (*n* = 124): 1976–1986.

Follow-up >3 years	84
Still improved	60 (71)
Soiling	53 (63)
Pads worn	46 (55)
Completely continent of faeces and flatus	29 (34)

Values in parentheses are percentages.

Table 20.35 Physiological parameters associated with a poor outcome after postanal repair.

	Failed postanal repair		
	Preoperative	*Postoperative*	*Controls*
Mean maximum resting pressure (cmH_2O)	31.2	27.6	80.0
Mean maximum squeeze pressure (cmH_2O)	79.2	64.3	201.0
Mean fibre density	1.9	2.0	1.5
Pudendal nerve terminal motor latency (ms)	2.6	3.0	1.9

From Snooks et al (1984b).

Snooks et al (1984b) and later Jameson et al (1994) showed that patients who were not improved by postanal repair had low resting anal canal pressures, high fibre density and prolonged pudendal nerve terminal motor latencies compared with controls (Table 20.35). None of these parameters was improved by operation. Rainey et al (1990) found that patients with mild incontinence did badly.

We found that the following parameters were of prognostic significance: resting and squeeze pressures, length of the high-pressure zone, volume of first leakage during saline infusion and pelvic floor descent at rest and during straining (Yoshioka et al, 1988). Unlike Browning, we found that the results in men were very disappointing and no longer recommend the operation in male patients (Table 20.36). Scott et al (1990) found that anal pressures could not reliably predict outcome.

We have encountered few specific postoperative complications other than haematoma in 21% of our 124 patients, and a small area of skin necrosis in the centre of the anterior skin flap, in 25%. Ischaemia over the apex of the anterior wound was more common when a V-shaped incision and thin anterior skin flaps were used. Since adopting a transverse incision this complication is now rare. Wound infection was reported in 11%. Rectal damage was sustained in 10% but only two out of the 12 developed a fistula, both being successfully managed by an advancement flap. We do not believe that it is usually necessary to construct a defunctioning colostomy. Henry and Simson (1985), in their 242 patients, reported wound sepsis in 15%, wound dehiscence in 2% and fistula in 2%; there were no deaths.

The operation is technically more difficult if patients have had a previous rectopexy and in our experience the results are poor in this group.

Table 20.36 Results of postanal repair.

	Browning et al (1983)	*Keighley (1984)*
Women (n)	117	81
Continent of solids and liquid	83 (71)	54 (67)
Continent of solids only	16 (13)	17 (21)
No better	18 (16)	10 (12)
Men (n)	22	8
Continent of solids and liquid	20 (91)	2 (25)
Continent of solids only	1 (5)	2 (25)
No better	1 (5)	4 (50)

Values in parentheses are percentages.

Technique

The operation is performed under general anaesthesia with the patient in the lithotomy position using a deep Trendelenburg tilt. A wedge or sandbag should be placed underneath the buttocks so that the tip of the coccyx can be easily palpated (Figure 20.42a). Alternatively, the prone jack-knife position may be used and this has now become our preferred approach. The patient should have had a thorough preoperative mechanical bowel preparation and short-term antibiotic cover. The patient is catheterized.

The operation site is infiltrated with local anaesthetic and a week adrenaline solution. A curved posterior incision is used, at least 4 cm behind the anus. A thick anterior skin flap is raised, using tissue forceps, until the posterior fibres of the external anal sphincter are visualized (Figure 20.42b). The inner fibres of the external anal sphincter ring are then defined and retracted posteriorly. The next phase of the operation is to develop the intersphincteric plane; as the dissection proceeds deeper, the rectum is retracted anteriorly with a small Kocher's retractor. At first it may be quite difficult to place a wide retractor in front of the rectum but as the plane is developed and the perineal aspect of the levator ani becomes visible a wider Kocher's retractor can be used. The rectum is displaced anteriorly and Waldeyer's fascia divided transversely (Figure 20.42c). If Waldeyer's fascia is not completely divided the rectum cannot be adequately mobilized from the sacrum and the levator ani will not be fully exposed. Furthermore, there will be insufficient space available between the two limbs of the puborectalis to achieve an adequate repair.

The repair may be performed in two layers, or as a mass closure. Using a layered closure, first the puborectalis is sutured, then the ischiococcygeus and pubococcygeus as a second layer. We prefer a mass closure technique taking all layers of the pelvic diaphragm. All of the sutures are placed and clipped before being tied (Figure 20.42d). We use 2/0 Prolene sutures, starting posteriorly with the sphincter muscle and working forwards. The knots are placed on the deeper aspect of the repair. By rotating the Kocher's retractor from side to side it is possible to take bites of the pelvic floor muscles on either side of the rectum. It is impossible to tie the most anteriorly placed sutures if the wide Kocher's retractor is left *in situ*; hence this is replaced by a pair of curved artery forceps (Figure 20.42e). A second layer of sutures may be used to buttress the deeper layer.

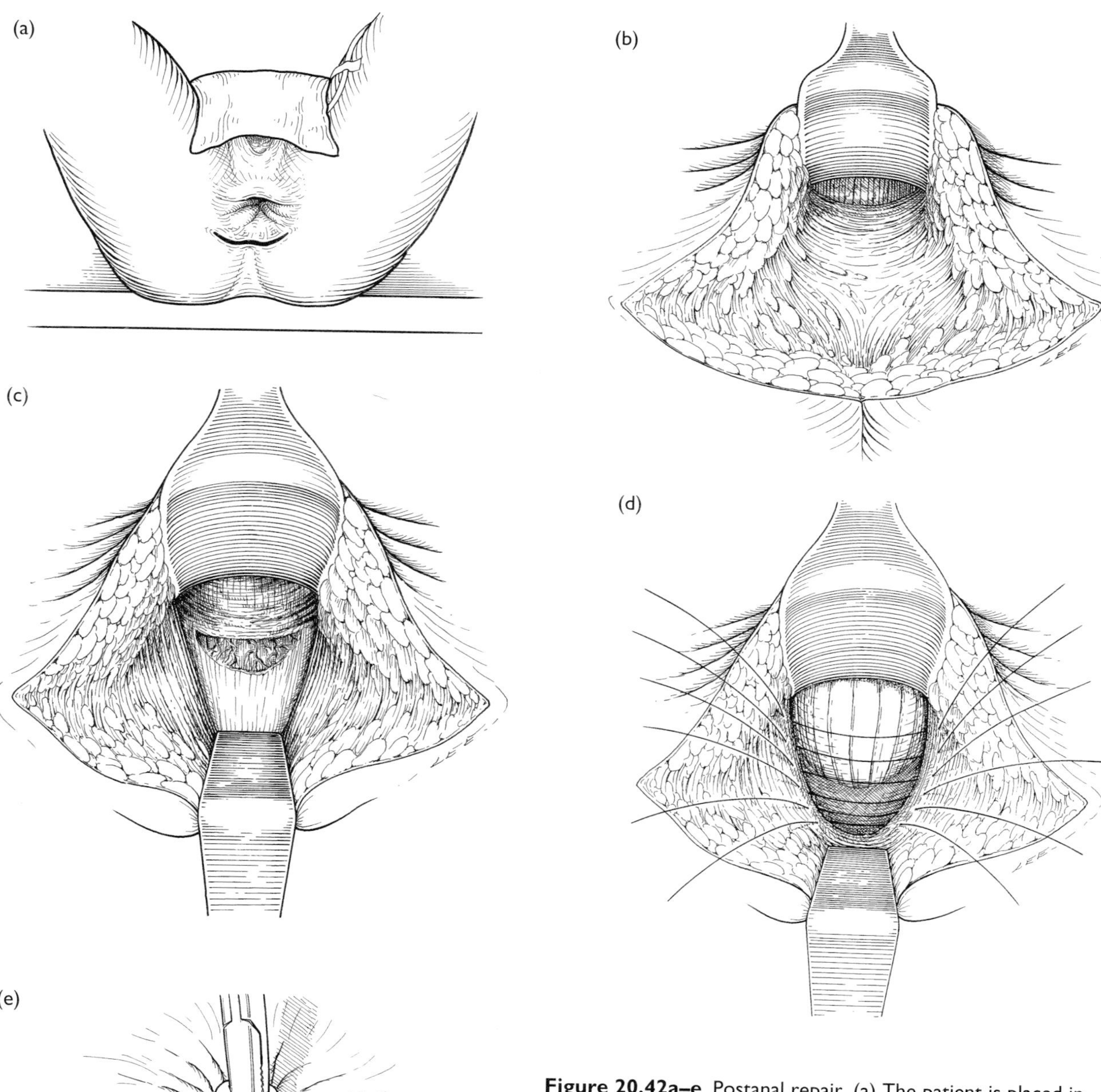

(e)

Figure 20.42a–e Postanal repair. (a) The patient is placed in the lithotomy position and catheterized. A curved postanal incision is made 3 cm behind the anal verge at the level of the tip of the coccyx. (b) The anterior skin flap is raised, and the external anal sphincter muscle can be seen adjacent to the anal verge. The external anal sphincter is dissected from the internal sphincter and the intersphincteric plane is opened. (c) With an anterior retractor displacing the rectum anteriorly and a posterior rectractor inside the external sphincter, Waldeyer's fascia can be visualized and incised transversely. The rectum can then be gently mobilized by finger dissection off the sacrum, and the anterior rectractor replaced to lift the rectum away from the pelvic floor muscles. (d) The repair. Mass sutures are placed through the entire medial limbs of the puborectalis and ischiococcygeus sling. None of the sutures are tied until the anterior retractor is removed. (e) The anterior rectractor is replaced by a curved artery forceps to hold the skin away from the muscle and the sutures are tied.

The operation is completed by placing two suction drains into the space behind the rectum. The skin is closed transversely with Prolene.

Patients should be warned that they will not gain continence immediately after postanal repair; indeed, incontinence is quite a common postoperative complication. Early incontinence may be due to pain. Continence may also be compromised because of postoperative diarrhoea or the deliberate use of laxatives to avoid postoperative constipation. The urinary catheter can usually be removed on the third postoperative day and patients should be mobilized early. Early baths should be encouraged. Patients should not be allowed to strain in the early postoperative period. It is advisable therefore to prescribe a bulk laxative. Continence is usually achieved by 6–8 weeks but sometimes it can take longer. We advise postoperative pelvic floor exercises as we believe that these facilitate rehabilitation. Poor results are associated with progressive denervation, particularly in patients who strain (Gee and Durdey, 1997).

Anterior levatorplasty and external sphincter plication

As a consequence of the relatively poor results of postanal repair and the observation of a rectocele during videoproctography in 70–90% of patients with idiopathic faecal incontinence (Figure 20.43), we and others have explored an anterior rather than a posterior pelvic floor repair (Osterberg et al, 1996), particularly if there is a deficient perineal body, in women with postobstetric neurogenic faecal incontinence.

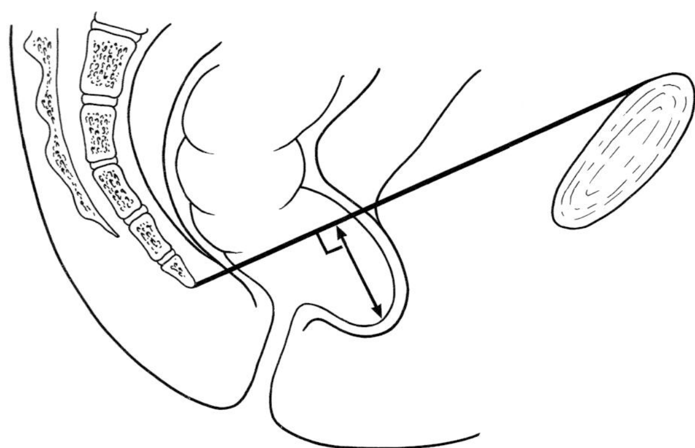

Figure 20.43 Videoproctographic evidence of rectocele. Many patients with faecal incontinence have evidence of a rectocele during straining.

Results

Miller et al (1989) reported the results of anterior sphincter plication with levatorplasty in 30 patients: 14 with neurogenic incontinence and third-degree tears and 16 with idiopathic faecal incontinence. Continence to solids and liquids was achieved in 71% of those with third-degree tears and in 62% of patients with idiopathic incontinence (Table 20.37). In Birmingham we have used this approach both in combination with postanal repair and as an isolated procedure for faecal incontinence (Pinho et al, 1990). Osterberg et al (1996) followed 54 women with obstetric trauma for a median of 8.5 years, reporting good results in 74%. However, in 31 with idiopathic incontinence only 45% were satisfactory. Good results were associated with a cloacal defect and youth. Preoperative severity of symptoms or length of follow-up had no impact on outcome.

Table 20.37 Anterior sphincter plication and anterior levatorplasty.

	Traumatic sphincter injury (n = 14)	*Idiopathic faecal incontinence* (n = 16)
Continent of solids and liquids	10	10
Continent of solids only	3	3
No better	1	3

From Miller et al (1989).

Technique

After bowel preparation and antibiotic cover the patient is anaesthetized and placed in the lithotomy or jack-knife position. We now prefer the prone jack-knife position. A urethral catheter is inserted. A headlamp is advised. A curved transverse incision is placed immediately behind the introitus (Figure 20.44a). The rectovaginal septum is dissected to the level of the posterior fornix by keeping immediately behind the vaginal epithelium. There is often considerable bleeding from vaginal veins and this must be controlled by diathermy. The skin over the perineal body and anal verge is grasped so as to dissect out the external sphincter; a tape is placed underneath the muscle (Figure 20.44b). The two limbs of the levator ani are identified in front of the sphincter. A series of Prolene sutures are placed from behind, working forwards (Figure 20.44c) to plicate the external anal sphincter (Figure 20.44d) and the anterior fibres of the levator ani (Figure 20.44e). The sutures are left long and not tied until the repair is

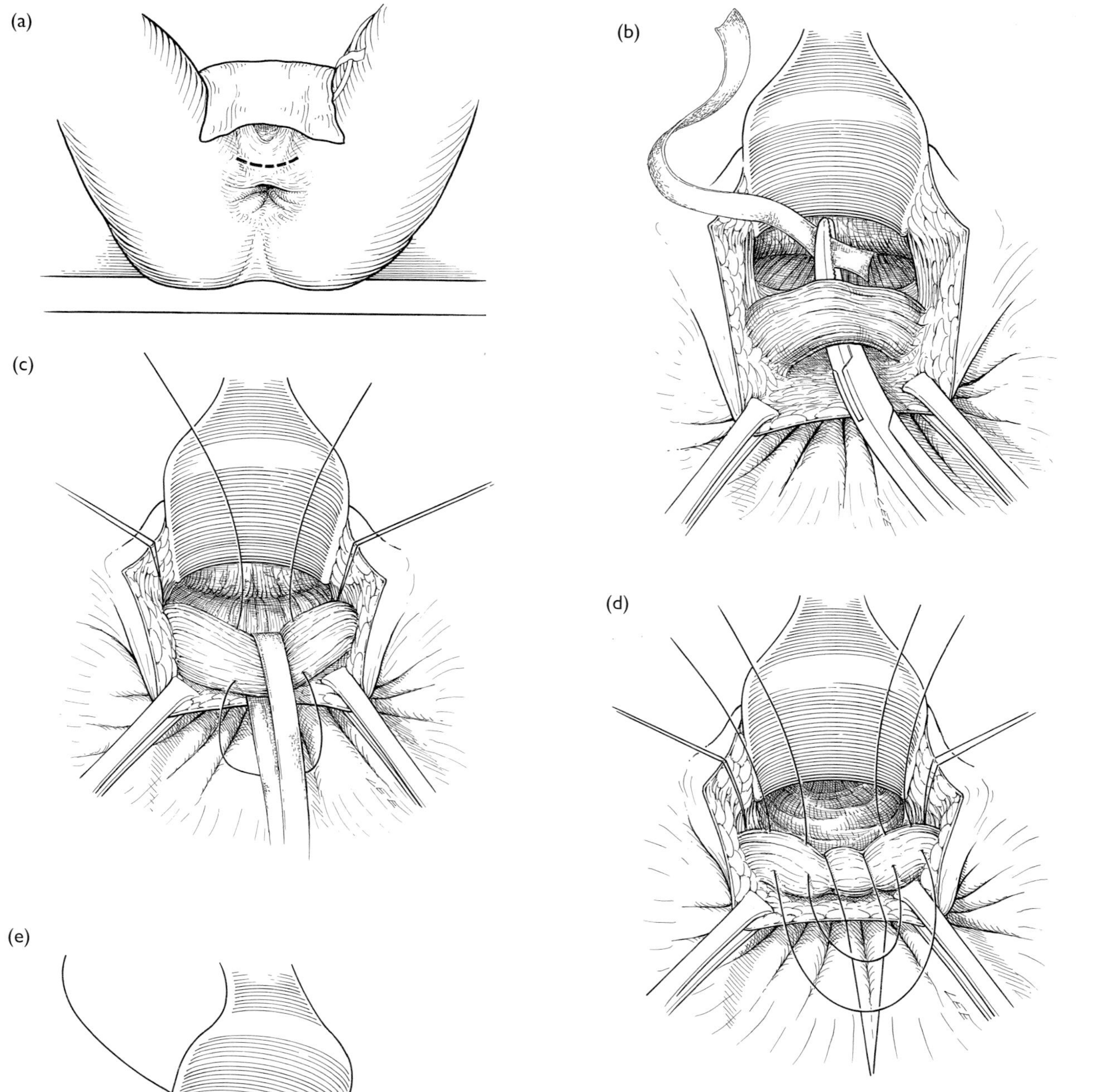

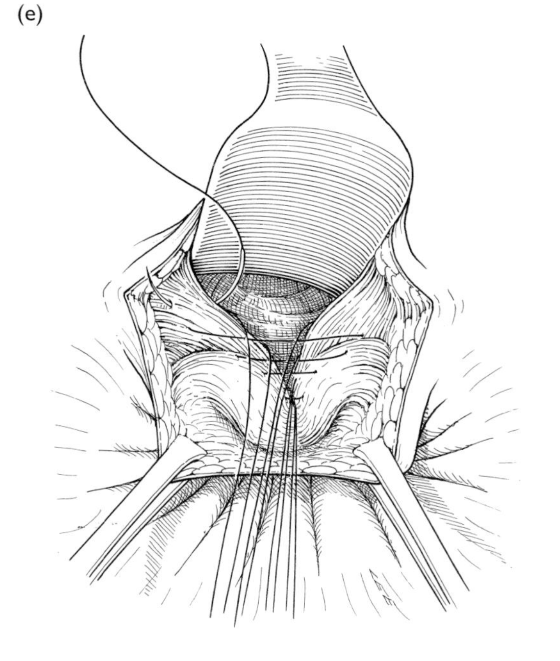

(a)

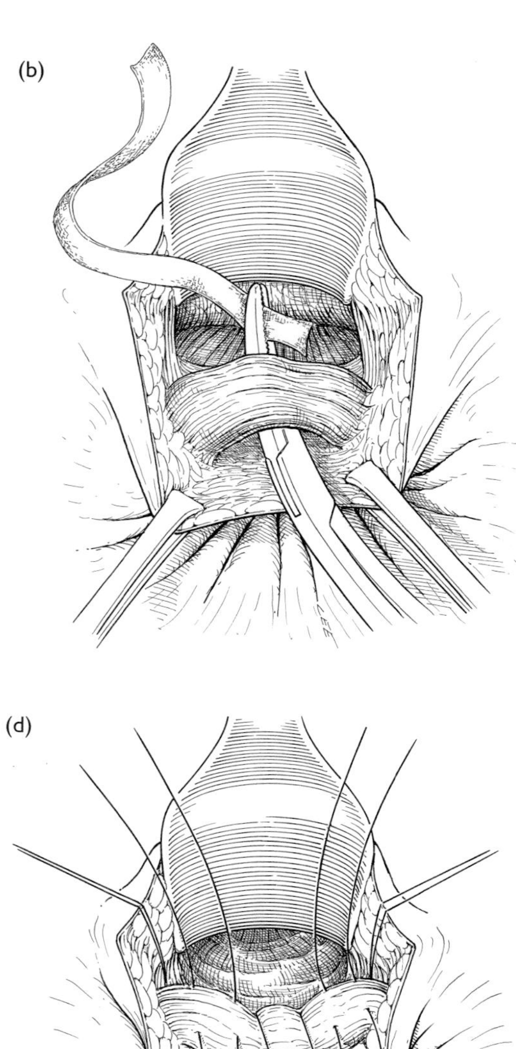

(c)

(e)

Figure 20.44a–f Anterior levatorplasty. (a) The patient is placed in the lithotomy position and catheterized. A transverse incision is made 2 cm in front of the anterior anal border, between the anus and posterior vaginal fourchette. (b) The external anal sphincter is dissected from the internal sphincter, and a soft tape is placed underneath it for posterior retraction. (c) The entire rectovaginal septum is opened so that the levator muscle can be seen on either side of the rectum and vagina. A series of interrupted sutures are placed through the external anal sphincter to plicate it. (d) The external anal sphincter plication is completed and stay sutures are placed through the levators on either side. (e) By rotation of the anterior retractor, the anterior fibres of the puborectalis can be identified. These are then plicated so as to oppose the pelvic floor in the midline anteriorly. *(continued overleaf)*

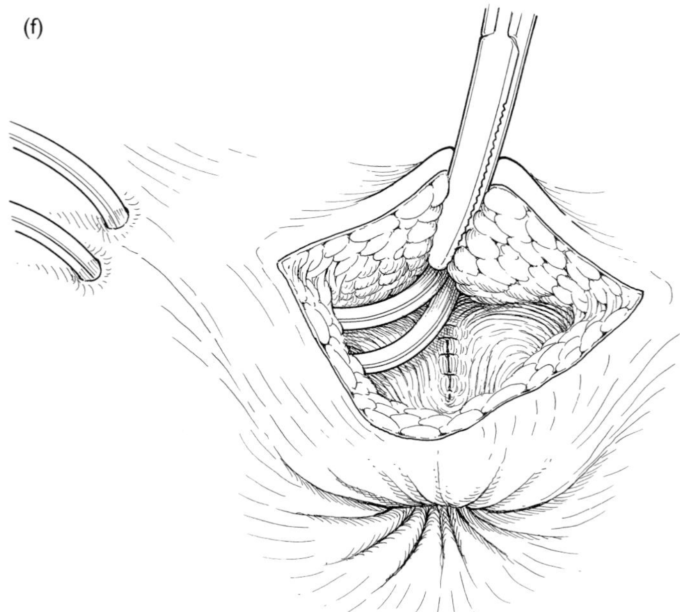

Figure 20.44a–f *(continued)* (f) The anterior retractor is removed. A curved artery forcep is placed anteriorly to retract the skin. Two Redivac drains are placed in the rectovaginal septum, and the sutures are tied.

complete. It is most important to ensure that the levator sutures do not incorporate the vagina. The knots are placed on the deeper aspect of the muscle. Two closed suction drains are inserted in front of the repair. The repair approximates the pelvic floor muscles across the midline without tension once the retractors are removed (Figure 20.44f). A covering stoma is not used. If the rectum is inadvertently opened during dissection of the rectovaginal septum, a Parks' retractor should be inserted into the anorectum and the mucosal defect closed with a continuous Vicryl suture. Excessive retraction with the Parks' blades should be avoided as resting pressures and internal anal sphincter function can be compromised (van Tets et al, 1997). The dissection and repair should then be completed in the usual way, possibly substituting Dexon for Prolene if there is a lot of faecal contamination.

Postoperative management is as for postanal repair; some patients are troubled by dyspareunia for the first few weeks after leaving hospital. Occasionally Prolene sutures may work their way out or become very superficial and may have to be removed.

Total pelvic floor repair

Anterior levatorplasty with sphincter plication has been used by ourselves and others (Engel et al, 1994) in patients who have had a rather disappointing result following a postanal repair (Keighley, 1991) with improvement in 42% (Pinho et al, 1991) (Figure 20.45). Christiansen and Skomorowska (1987) used this approach and reported improvement in six of eight patients who had had persistent incontinence after postanal repair. The anterior component was performed as a pelvic procedure in six and as a perineal levatorplasty in two. The combination of anterior levatorplasty with postanal repair is termed total pelvic floor repair.

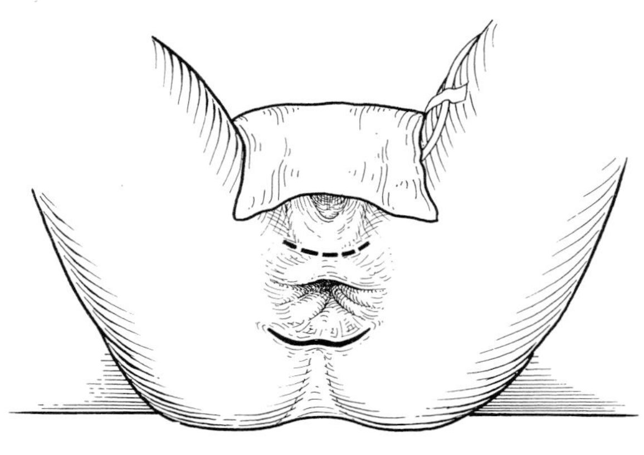

Figure 20.45 Total pelvic floor repair. Total pelvic floor repair involves a combination of postanal repair with anterior sphincter plication and anterior levatorplasty.

Results

The early results of synchronous total pelvic floor repair has been encouraging with 55% continent to solids and liquids (Pinho and Keighley, 1990; Oya et al, 1991). The results appeared to be superior to a historical series of 47 patients having a postanal repair alone (Table 20.38). Pelvic floor repair increased the length of the anal canal, corrected the degree of pelvic floor descent at rest and during straining and eliminated the rectocele in 70% but had no influence on anal pressures or the anorectal angle (Pinho et al, 1992).

We undertook a randomized trial with 12 patients in each group to compare postanal repair, anterior levatorplasty with sphincter plication and total pelvic floor repair. Results at 2 years indicated that total pelvic floor repair was significantly more effective in restoring continence than either anterior or posterior repair (Table 20.39). Furthermore, the quality of life and social well-being was significantly improved after total pelvic floor repair compared with either of the other component procedures.

We have now reviewed the long-term results (18–78 months) of total pelvic floor repair in 75 women with postobstetric neuropathic faecal incontinence without a localized sphincter injury (Korsgen et al, 1997). Sixty-six women were traced, of whom 6 required re-operation for persistant incontinence, involving a stoma in 4 and a graciloplasty in 2. There was a significant improvement in incontinence score. Daily incontinence fell from 73% to 23%. However, only 14% were rendered completely continent. Those with marked improvement were socially more active than those with little or no improvement. Anal manometry, anorectal sensation or pudendal nerve latency did not predict outcome, whereas perineal descent, obesity or a history of straining were associated with poor results. Patients with coexisting symptoms of irritable bowel syndrome also fared badly. Social activity remained compromised despite pelvic floor repair in many patients.

We have also tried to examine the role of internal anal sphincter plication to explore whether this improves the results of pelvic floor repair. In a small randomized study (Deen et al, 1995) adjuvant internal sphincter plication proved no clinical benefit and resulted in a fall in anal pressures. We therefore concluded that internal sphincter plication was not advised in pelvic floor repair. Interestingly, Morgan et al (1997) reported that rotation island or advancement anoplasty frequently improved internal sphincter deficiency, whereas direct internal anal sphincter repair produced no symptomatic improvement at all.

Table 20.38 Results of total pelvic floor repair (Birmingham).

	Synchronous (n = 22)		*Staged* (n = 14)		*Previous postanal repair* (n = 47)	
	Preop.	*Postop.*	*Preop.*	*Postop.*	*Preop.*	*Postop.*
Continent of solids, liquids and flatus	0	9 (41)	0	2 (14)	0	2 (4)
Continent of solids and liquids	0	12 (55)	0	6 (43)	0	6 (13)
Continent of solids	3	21 (95)	3	13 (93)	7	29 (62)
Still incontinent	–	1 (4)	–	1 (7)	–	19 (40)

Values in parentheses are percentages.

Table 20.39 Results of randomized trial.

	Complete continence of solids and fluids		*Continent score > 3.5*		
	6 months	*24 months*	*Preop.*	*6 months*	*24 months*
Total pelvic floor repair (*n* = 12)	9	8	12	3	2
Anterior levatorplasty and sphincter plication (*n* = 12)	4	4	12	8	8
Postanal report (*n* = 12)	4	5	12	8	7

From Deen et al (1993c).
Values are mean ± SD.
* $P < 0.05$.
† $P < 0.01$.

Technique

The procedure begins as a postanal repair followed by the anterior dissection of the rectovaginal septum. Placement of sutures should be delayed until the entire mobilization is complete. The repair begins posteriorly and finishes with the anterior sphincter plication and levatorplasty (Pinho and Keighley, 1990). The effect of the operation is to repair a hernia in the levator ani, close and elongate the upper anal canal and provide support anteriorly, thereby controlling any rectocele which may be present (Figure 20.46a).

Sphincter repair

Most colorectal surgeons take the view that sphincter repair usually gives extremely good functional results (Browning and Motson, 1983; Oliveira et al, 1996) provided that the repair does not become infected or breaks down (Browning and Motson, 1984; Engel et al, 1994; Felt-Bersma et al, 1996; Ternent et al, 1997), and provided there is no evidence of neuropathy (Motson, 1985; Yoshioka and Keighley, 1989; Sangwan et al, 1996a,b). Sphincter reconstruction is the procedure of choice for complete or partial damage to the external anal sphincter, but recent evidence indicates that the results of repair for sphincter defects complicating obstetric trauma, as opposed to fistulotomy injury or trauma, are not as good as the literature suggests (Londono-Schimmer et al, 1994; Simmang et al, 1994; Nikiteas et al, 1996; Sitzler and Thomson, 1996). The defect in the external sphincter is usually visible but can be confirmed by ultrasonography, which has now replaced electromyography as it is less painful and more informative (Law et al, 1990; Tjandra et al, 1993; Emblem et al, 1994; Nielsen et al, 1994; Bartram and Sultan, 1995; Rieger et al, 1996).

A defunctioning proximal colostomy is still sometimes advised (Keighley and Fielding, 1983; Sitzler and Thomson, 1996) if there is a high risk of sepsis due to previous anal operations, poor mechanical bowel preparation, a large defect, previous sphincter repair, possible Crohn's disease or gross obesity. Nevertheless, a covering stoma is rarely considered if there is a small defect following obstetric damage and where the mechanical bowel preparation is satisfactory, since restricting oral intake will discourage bowel movements in the first week after operation, thereby reducing the risk of sepsis after which laxatives are prescribed to prevent impaction, minimizing soiling and subsequent sepsis.

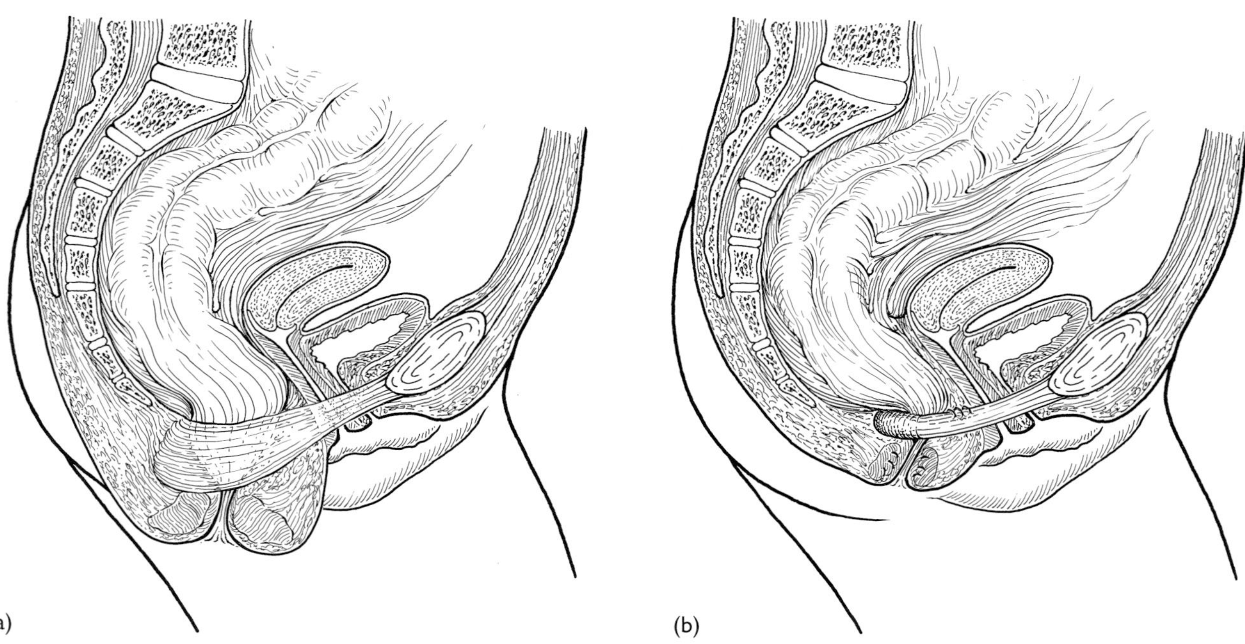

Figure 20.46a,b The influence of total pelvic floor repair on pelvic anatomy. (a) A sagittal section in a patient with faecal incontinence. Note the lax puborectalis muscle, the perineal descent, the obtuse anorectal angle and the short anal canal. (b) The results of total pelvic floor repair. The anorectal angle has been restored. The anal canal length has been elongated. The anterior aspect of the pelvic floor has been repaired to act as a buttress against the postanal repair.

Results

Browning and Motson (1984) reported the outcome in 97 patients treated at St Mark's Hospital. Only 13 of these were women with obstetric injury, the majority of patients having sustained sphincter damage from fistula operations or anorectal trauma. The low incidence of obstetric damage probably explains in part their excellent results, with 78% of patients being rendered completely continent of liquids and solids following sphincter reconstruction. These authors freely admit that the results were poor among women having sustained obstetric tears. Fang et al (1984) from Minneapolis reported their results in 79 patients. Despite the fact that 43 of their patients had sustained third-degree tears, with only seven having traumatic injuries, 55% were rendered completely continent of flatus and of both liquid and solid stool. This group did not use a defunctioning stoma.

A summary of outcome reported in the literature is given in Table 20.40. Most series report that two-thirds of all patients were rendered completely continent of solids and liquids after operation. Londono-Schimmer et al (1994), reporting the St Mark's Hospital experience, showed that only 50% had good or excellent results, 25% considered that the outcome of terms of function was poor and 9% had a permanent stoma. Poor results were more common in the obstetric injuries and other iatrogenic causes as compared with fistula defects (Engel et al, 1997) or trauma (Figure 20.46b). Poor results are also observed in women with coexisting irritable bowel syndrome (Donelly et al, 1998; Harraf et al, 1998). Furthermore, preoperative evidence of pudendal neuropathy was associated with worse results. Sangwan et al (1996a,b) also Simmang et al (1994) reported poor results in both unilateral and bilateral neuropathy. By contrast, Engel and Brummelkamp (1994), studying only the postobstetric injuries from St Mark's, showed that pudendal neuropathy did not affect prognosis, which accords with our own findings too (Nikiteas et al, 1996). Age is not necessarily associated with a poor outcome, though our data disputed this. Oliveira et al (1996) from the Florida Cleveland experience, Engel et al (1994) from St Mark's as well as Simmang et al (1994) from St Louis report good results even in elderly patients after sphincter repair. The clear message from most reports in this decade is that some sphincter repairs do fail, usually from breakdown in the repair which is easily identified by postoperative ultrasonography. Furthermore, repeat repair may restore continence (Sitzler and Thomson, 1996; Nikiteas et al, 1996; Oliveira et al, 1996).

Variation in technique

Most authorities advise that the entire scarred area of the sphincter be preserved so as to facilitate a flap-over repair, since sutures are less likely to tear out from fibrous tissue rather than healthy muscle (Loygue and Dubois, 1964; Parks and McPartlin,

Table 20.40 Results of sphincter repair.

	Continent of solids and liquids	*Continent of solids only*	*No better ± stoma*
Hagihara and Griffen (1976)	6	0	1
Slade et al (1977)	16	13	1
Castro and Pittman (1978)	8	9	2
Rudd et al (1982)	18	3	0
Keighley and Fielding (1983)	24	6	4
Fang et al (1984)	44	24	7
Browning and Motson (1984)	65	13	7
Pezim et al (1987)	10	23	7
Christiansen and Pederson (1987)	15	7	1
Fleshman et al (1991a)	28	24	3
Londono-Schimmer et al (1994)	47	24	23
Simmang et al (1994)	31	10	1
Engel et al (1994)	42	9	2
Oliveira et al (1996)	39	5	1
Sangwan et al (1996b)	9	4	2
Sitzler and Thomson (1996)	23	2	6
Nikiteas et al (1996)	19	9	14
Felt-Bersma et al (1996)	6	6	6
Ternent et al (1997)	6	2	6

1971; Castro and Pittman, 1978; Corman, 1980; Rudd et al, 1982; Wexner et al, 1991a). End-to-end repair is generally considered to be inferior to the flap-over technique (Blaisdell, 1940) but Arnaud et al (1991) dispute this opinion. Fang et al (1984) do not believe that the external sphincter should be dissected free from the internal sphincter. They also found that results did not depend upon the site of the injury around the anus and that a rectovaginal fistula was not a contraindication to the operation. Indeed the results of sphincter repair if needed in rectovaginal fistula are very gratifying, with 80–90% rendered continent (Khanduja et al, 1994; Mazier et al, 1995; Watson and Phillips, 1995). Surprisingly few authors stress the importance of preserving the anal mucosa and preventing its retraction so as to avoid a postoperative stricture (Motson, 1985). If there is insufficient length in the external anal sphincter the option of suturing the external sphincters to the puborectalis, as described by Christiansen and Pedersen (1987), should be considered (Figure 20.47).

If the results are poor due to postoperative sepsis and breakdown of the repair, repeat repair may be successful (Yoshioka and Keighley, 1989; Engel et al, 1994; Sitzler and Thomson, 1996). Likewise, a poor result may follow repair of a third-degree tear, due to perianal sepsis and breakdown of the repair or as a result of an inexperienced obstetrician. Under these circumstances repeat repair is certainly worth while and may be combined with a pelvic floor repair (Gledhill and Waterfall, 1984). We found that five of the seven patients who had a poor result following sphincter repair had had third-degree obstetric tears with evidence of neuropathy (Yoshioka and Keighley, 1989). The varying incidence of third-degree tears or neuropathy are factors responsible for the differing success rates reported following sphincter repair (Motson, 1985).

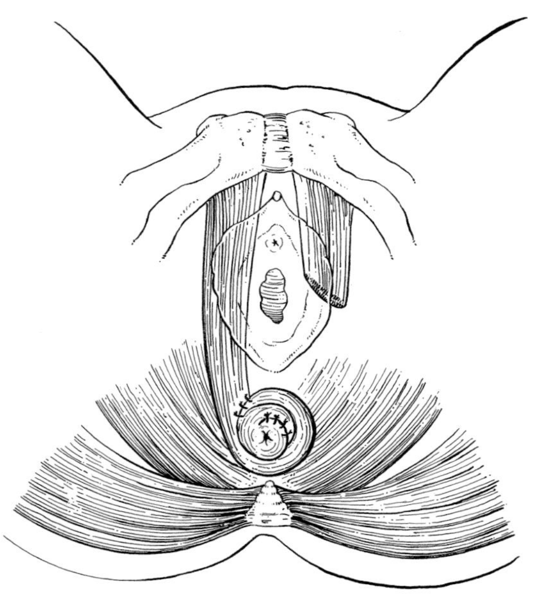

Figure 20.47 Puborectalis plication. If the external anal sphincter has been completely destroyed it is possible to utilize the puborectalis as a circular muscle sling around the anal canal. One limb of the puborectalis is divided anteriorly in the rectovaginal septum. It is then plicated around the puborectalis of the opposite side.

If there is a deficient perineal body after sphincter repair, or if there has been excessive skin loss because of severe perineal sepsis, some form of rotation skin flap might be advised. The Lahey Clinic group advise using a cruciate incision over the perineal body which is reconstructed as a double Z-plasty (Figure 20.48). We were once very enthusiastic about this technique, but there is a high incidence of skin loss from necrosis of the corners. We have now completely abandonded the Z plasty and, like the Cleveland group in Florida, use a circum-anal incision and leave part of these wounds open (Oliveira et al, 1996).

Many patients with third-degree tears have both a sphincter defect and a pelvic floor neuropathy and in such patients sphincter repair should probably be combined with a postanal repair (Browning et al, 1988). Browning et al (1988) reported the outcome of seven patients with a sphincter and pelvic floor disorder treated by direct sphincter repair and postanal repair. All had a covering colostomy and although eventually all were continent of solids, they leaked liquids and had troublesome urgency. In most postobstetric injuries, there is a deficient perineal body and rectocele as well as the sphincter injury. Certainly in our practice we dissect the whole of the rectovaginal septum so as to incorporate an anterior levatorplasty with the spincter repair.

Browning and Motson (1984) reported a high incidence of postoperative fistula (7), stricture (16) and sinus (16), which they subsequently attributed to the use of wire for the repair. Most surgeons now prefer absorbable materials.

Diverting stoma

A diverting proximal colostomy is now largely reserved: (1) for patients who already have a stoma following perineal trauma; (2) where the risk of sepsis is high, such as in patients requiring re-operations, poor bowel preparation, the obese, diabetics,

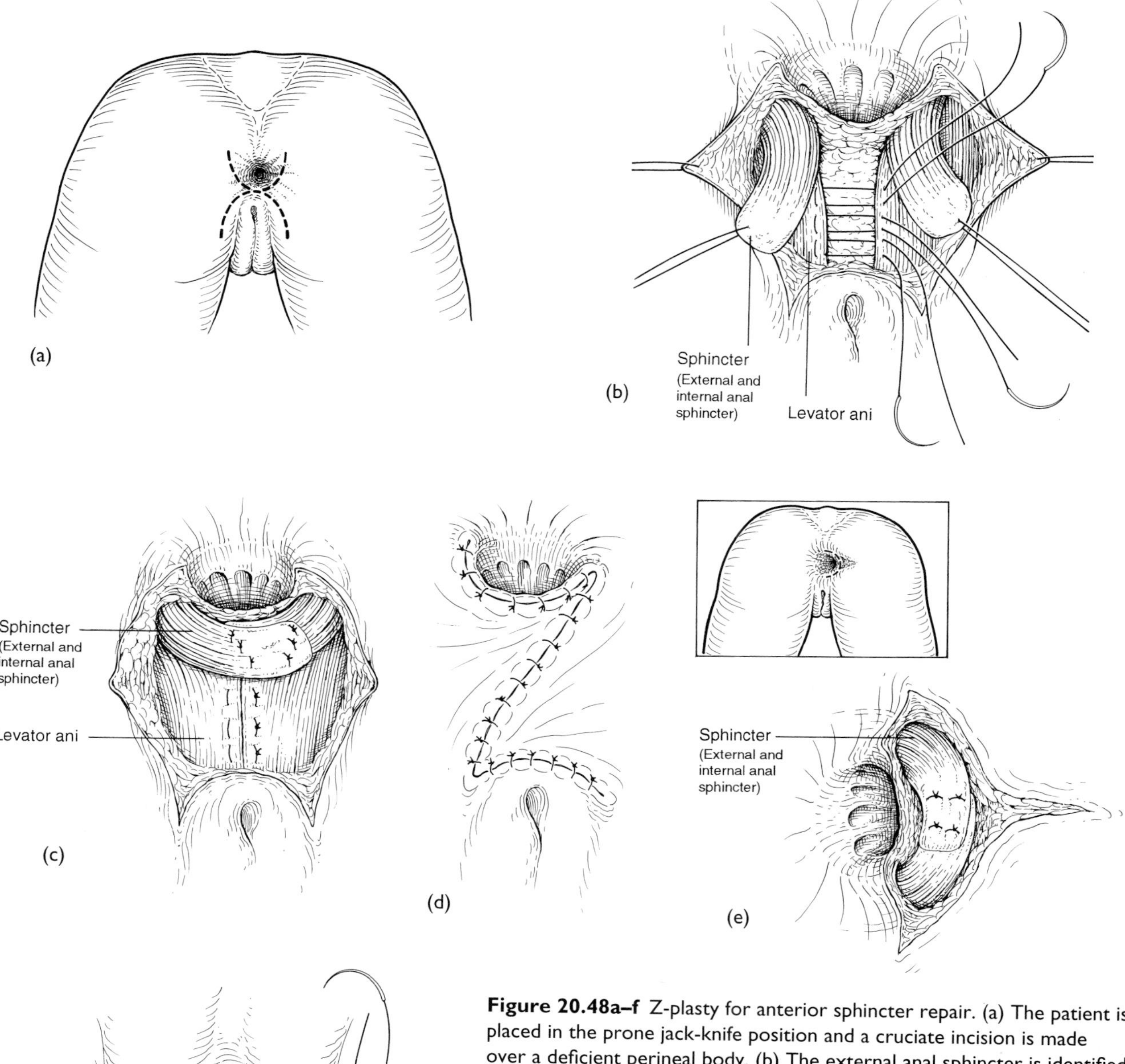

Figure 20.48a–f Z-plasty for anterior sphincter repair. (a) The patient is placed in the prone jack-knife position and a cruciate incision is made over a deficient perineal body. (b) The external anal sphincter is identified and dissected on either side. The rectovaginal septum is also separated to define the levators on either side. (c) A flap-over repair of the anterior sphincter muscles is performed using the scar tissue to buttress the repair and a levatorplasty undertaken. (d) The wound is closed as a Z-plasty to increase the space between the posterior vaginal wall and the anal canal. (We often no longer advise the Z-plasty closure.) (e) Sphincter repair for lateral fistulotomy injury. The patient has been placed in the prone jack-knife position. A circumanal incision is made centred on the site of scarring. The sphincter on either side of the scar tissue is mobilized. A flap-over repair completes the operation. The wound is generally left open. (f) Repair of a post-traumatic injury affecting the anterior anorectum. The patient has been placed in the lithotomy position. The rectal wall as well as the levators and the sphincter are identified and mobilized. The defect in the rectal wall is closed and levatorplasty is then performed followed by a flap-over sphincter repair. The wound is often left open. Frequently there is already a proximal colostomy.

extensive sphincter deficiency, or where there has been a previous failed repair; (3) in combined sphincter and pelvic floor deficiency; and (4) where there is an associated rectovaginal fistula. Some authors do not think that a proximal stoma is ever needed (Fang et al, 1984).

The question of a routine diverting stoma is a complex one, particularly as recent data derived from a randomized trial in this unit seem to show some real benefit. Our study, admittedly small, showed that postoperative faecal impaction and secondary breakdown was less common with a stoma (Table 20.41). Furthermore, the long-term functional results were better in those patients who had had a stoma (Table 20.42). Certainly we found that women who had been incontinent from an obstetric injury often welcomed the thought of a covering stoma, despite having to face two operations, because they were fearful of continued incontinence or impaction while the muscle repair was healing. In economic terms, avoidance of a stoma is desirable provided, of course, that it does not compromise long-term continence. Our current practice is to council all patients, warning them that if there are technical difficulties, if the repair is tight, if there has been poor rectal evacuation or if this is their second attempted repair they probably should have a covering stoma. If the patient is determined to avoid a stoma, we warn them that they will be given fluids by an intravenous infusion for a week, after which they may be incontinent because laxatives will be prescribed to prevent faecal impaction in the first 2–3 weeks. Quite a few patients in our experience elect to have a defunctioning stoma which is constructed through an abdominal trephine or via a laparoscopic approach.

Our own experience of sphincter repair is that results are generally favourable in patients who

Table 20.41 Complications of sphincter repair (randomized trial).

	Covering stoma (*n* = 14)	*No covering stoma* (*n* = 17)
Complications of repair		
Breakdown of repair	0	2
Wound sepsis	5	4
Faecal impaction	0	3
Readmission with complications	0	2
Complications of stoma		
Prolapsed stoma	0	–
Ischaemic stoma	0	–
Parastomal hernia	1	–
Readmission with complications	0	–
Complications of closing stoma		
Intestinal obstruction	1	–
Enterocutaneous fistula	1	–
Hernia	3	–
Readmission with complications	2	–
Hospital stay (days) (mean ± SD)	8.4 ± 2.5 + 7.1 ± 2.4	8.5 ± 3.6

Table 20.42 Functional results of sphincter repair.

	Functional score					
	Covering stoma (*n* = 14)			*No covering stoma* (*n* = 17)		
Randomized trial	*Preop.*	*Postop.*	*P-value*	*Preop.*	*Postop.*	*P-value*
Overall incontinence score	13.7	5.6	< 0.001	13.6	9.7	< 0.02
Solid stool continence	2.2	0.8	< 0.01	1.9	1.2	NS
Liquid stool continence	2.6	1.1	< 0.02	2.5	1.5	NS
Gas continence	3.1	1.5	< 0.01	3.4	2.7	NS
Having to use pads	2.7	1.1	< 0.02	2.6	1.9	NS
Lifestyle	3.1	1.0	< 0.001	3.2	2.0	NS
Stool frequency per 24 hours	2.9	3.1		2.5	1.9	
Impaired evacuation	6	3		6	6	
Urgency of defecation	14	3		17	13	
Soiling	12	4		15	9	

have sustained perineal trauma. Indeed in those patients with fractures of the pelvis and anorectal trauma managed by immedate colostomy, 40% recover sufficiently to make sphincter repair unnecessary. Those requiring repair often need attention to urethral injuries, sometimes involving fistulas to the rectum; the rectal injury may require repair as well as the sphincter. The stoma is left *in situ* until the repair or fistula has healed and most regain full continence.

We found that there was a sex difference in terms of the outcome following repair of postfistulotomy defects. Successful repair of defects in women with previous obstetric trauma did not always restore continence. Persistent soiling was a feature in some patients in both sexes. Repeat sphincter repair following breakdown from sepsis gave good results in 2 out of 2 such cases. The most disappointing results in our experience were in women with postobstetric sphincter defects, where only 59% achieved liquid and solid continence. Factors associated with a poor outcome were obesity, age over 50 years and perineal descent (Nikiteas et al, 1996). We would therefore now counsel this group some of whom are advised to have a covering stoma (Yoshioka et al, 1997).

We and others have shown that sphincter repair is followed by very considerable improvement in squeeze anal canal pressures, from 94 to 164 cmH_2O (see Table 20.29) (Fleshman et al, 1991b; Wexner et al, 1991a; Oliveria et al, 1996). Likewise there is an increase in the length of the high-pressure zone and restoration of the ultrasound defect on repeat imaging (Engel et al, 1994; Felt-Bersma et al, 1996; Ternent et al, 1997).

Technique

Efficient bowel preparation and short-term systemic antibiotic cover is used. Patients are catheterized and the operation is performed under a general anaesthetic. The position of the patient depends upon the site of the sphincter damage. For tears in the posterior or posterolateral fibres of the sphincter we prefer the patient in the prone jack-knife position with the buttocks strapped apart (Figure 20.49a). The incision is placed to one side of the midline, avoiding the tip of the coccyx. For improved access, the lower fibres of the gluteus maximus may be divided and a self-retaining retractor is placed at either end of the wound. It is unnecessary to open the anorectum, unless there has been previous rectal trauma, and all anal mucosa should be preserved. The pelvic floor may be left intact or may be repaired at the same time.

For anterior or anterolateral injuries the lithotomy position is usually preferred by surgeons in the UK (Figure 20.49b). However, many units in North America as well as this author prefers the prone jack-knife position for both anterior and posterior injuries (Figure 20.49c). If an extensive anterior levatorplasty is needed, the lithotomy position may provide better access.

The procedure starts by making a circumanal incision so as to dissect off the mucosa of the anal canal from the inner aspect of the scarred sphincter. (Figure 20.49d). The mucosa is inadequately supported at this point and there may be some mucosal prolapse. The mucosa is often tethered to the underlying scar tissue but the mucosa should be completely freed from the internal sphincter and surrounding fibrosis. By lifting the perianal skin, undamaged sphincter should then be identified lateral to the scar, which is dissected free (Figure 20.49e). A tape is then passed underneath the external anal sphincter at the site of the damaged segment (Figure 20.49f). Care must be taken not to stray too far laterally because the nerve supply to the external anal sphincter enters the muscle at this point. A nerve stimulator may be used to identify the terminal portion of the pudendal nerve if excessive lateral dissection is needed. Once the mucosa has been completely dissected from the scar tissue the fibrous remnant of the sphincter is divided. In our experience damage is usually confined to a third or a quarter of the circumference of the sphincter. Once the scar has been divided, the lateral aspect of the healthy muscle is dissected further to allow free overlap of about 1.5 cm. Before repairing the sphincter, the entire rectovaginal septum is mobilized to the level of the pelvic peritoneum so as to expose the levator ani on either side of the vagina as in anterior levatorplasty. The levators and perineal body are repaired prior to the double-breasted sphincteroplasty (Figure 20.49g).

The repair is performed using two layers of interrupted 2/0 Prolene sutures. The cut end of the deeper aspect of the scar is sutured to the deeper aspect of the muscle (Figure 20.49h) and the superficial aspect of the scar to the superficial aspect of the muscle. None of the sutures are tied until all have been accurately placed. It is most important to avoid repairing the muscle too tightly. When the sphincter repair is complete the mucosa is sutured with catgut to the skin edge over the sphincter repair so as to avoid retraction of the anal mucosa (Figure 21.49i). The centre section of the wound is left open for drainage.

If the repair is tight, or if there has been contamination or if there are risk factors such as obesity, diabetes or previous failed repair, a loop left iliac fossa colostomy is raised.

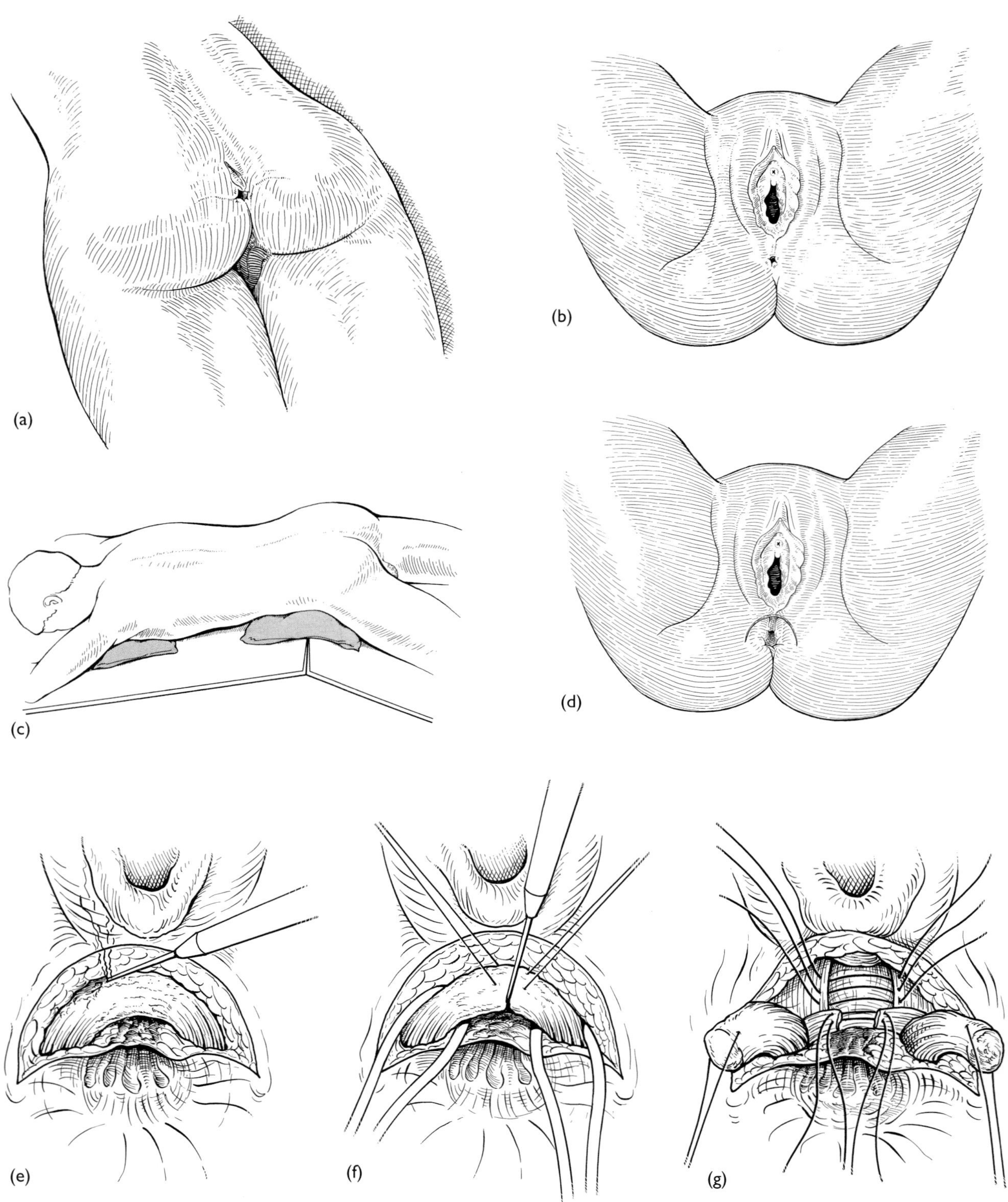

Figure 20.49a–g Sphincter repair. (a) The prone jack-knife position is used for posterior injuries. (b) The patient may be placed in the lithotomy position for repair of anterior sphincter deficiencies. (c) Alternatively the patient is placed in the prone jack-knife position. (d) A circumanal incision is made based on the clinically defined sphincter defect. The mucosa is dissected off the anal canal. Healthy sphincter is identified lateral to the defect. (e) Scissor or diathermy dissection of the sphincter achieves mobilization to healthy muscle. (f) Tapes are placed under the healthy sphincter to act as retractors so that the mucosa can be dissected away. The central scar tissue is divided. (g) The rectovaginal septum is then thoroughly mobilized so as to identify the transverse perinei and the levators on either side of the vagina.

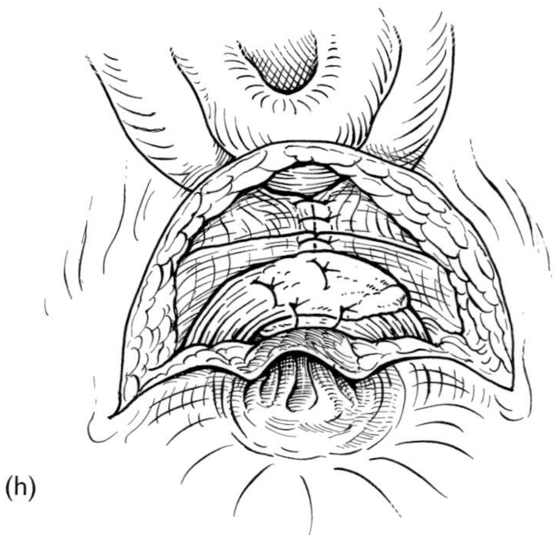

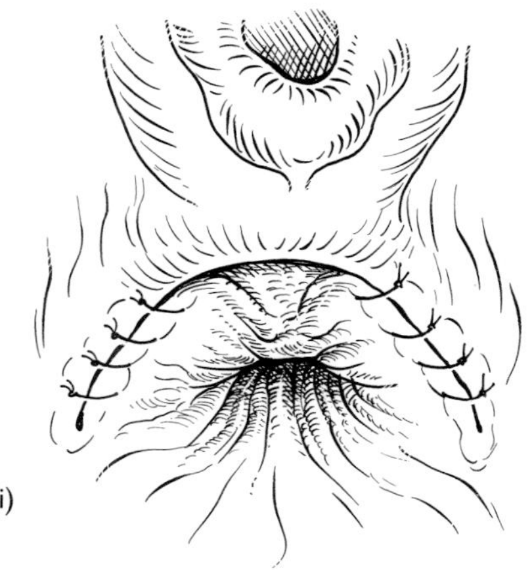

Figure 20.49h,i (h) A levatorplasty is performed and the transverse perinei muscles are approximated in the midline followed by a flap-over sphincter repair. (i) The mucosa is sutured back to the divided skin but the anterior aspect of the wound is left open for drainage purposes.

Rerouting procedures for ectopic anus

Anorectal malformations usually demand some form of immediate surgical treatment at birth. High defects involving the pelvic floor are often associated with rectourethral or rectovaginal fistula and are best managed by construction of a diverting sigmoid colostomy (McGill et al, 1978). Low defects, by contrast, have a much better prognosis and some form of a cutback anoplasty is often advised for anovaginal or anovestibular fistulas (Nixon, 1984). It is unusual in adult colorectal practice to encounter patients with an ecotopic anus because most are corrected at birth or during childhood (Kerremans et al, 1974).

We reported 14 patients with an ectopic anus lying immediately behind the vulva or the scrotum, all of whom presented with incontinence (Keighley, 1986). Assessment of the defect requires careful rectal and vaginal examination to exclude a rectovaginal fistula. In male patients it is wise to perform a cystourethroscopy to exclude a rectourethral communication. Sigmoidoscopy should be performed to exclude any underlying bowel disease. Videoproctographic assessment of the anatomy of the rectum in relation to the pelvic floor, vagina and perineum is also advised. If there is a history of constipation, assessment of intestinal transit by marker studies and sigmoid motility is strongly advised. Perhaps the most important investigation is electromyography, not of the pelvic floor but to detect the site and the function of the external anal sphincter. This should be marked before operation. The site of the true external sphincter may sometimes be apparent by skin movement approximately 2 cm anterior to the tip of the coccyx during pelvic floor contraction.

Ten patients in our series were women and four were men. A proximal stoma was present prior to the rerouting procedure in only two. Two patients, both with a history of constipation, had a poor functional result following the rerouting procedure; one now has a reservoir ileostomy, the other a conventional colostomy. One female adolescent patient developed retraction of the rerouted anus due to early dehiscence of the skin sutures and a stricture developed. This was subsequently successfully corrected by an abdominoanal pull-through procedure with completely satisfactory functional results. One male patient developed a transient rectourethral fistula which resolved spontaneously after catheter drainage. Long-term results indicated that 12 of 14 patients were rendered completely continent by the operation but a stoma was subsequently needed in two because of incapacitating constipation. None developed strictures.

Technique

Preoperative bowel preparation must be thorough because some patients tend to be constipated. Every effort should be made to clear faecal residue from the bowel. The patient is anaesthetized, placed in the lithotomy position and catheterized.

A single dose of intravenous antibiotic is given. The first manoeuvre is to excise a disc of skin over the previously located external anal sphincter ring, which has been marked preoperatively. Careful dissection should identify the circular fibres of the external anal sphincter. The centre of the sphincter ring is then opened using a fine pair of dissecting scissors. It is imperative to stay precisely in the midline and not to divide any muscle fibres. The centre of the sphincter muscle should then be dissected over a distance of about 5 cm and a small swab introduced within the sphincter ring to control any bleeding (Figure 20.50a). Attention is now focused on mobilization of the ectopic anorectum. The anus (or more precisely the rectum) is usually patulous and close to the posterior margin of the vulva or the base of the scrotum. There is usually considerable bleeding from small vessels. The ectopic anus must be mobilized, with the utmost care, well above the pelvic floor muscle over a distance of at least 8–10 cm so that the anorectum can be brought through the sphincter ring without being under any tension (Figure 20.50b). Dissection will be close to the posterior margin of the vagina in women and the prostate and urethra in men. These structures will be densely adherent to the anorectum if there has been a previous rectovaginal or rectourethral fistula. Although the anterior aspect of the dissection will have to be kept close to the anorectum, it is wise to avoid a plane that is too close to the bowel posterolaterally in order not to impair the blood supply to the mobilized anorectum. Mobilization of the anorectum must be to the level of the cervix in women and above the prostate in men.

During rectal mobilization the fibres of both lateral limbs of the puborectalis are usually easily identified as they proceed forwards on either side of the vagina and posteriorly around the mobilized external anal sphincter. The inner fibres of the levator ani must be carefully distinguished from the external anal sphincter if the perineum is to be successfully repaired. At this point, two linen tapes are passed from the anterior to the posterior incision through the sphincter ring (Figure 20.50c). It is usually necessary to dilate the space inside the sphincter ring in order to allow passage of the anorectum into the perineum. Two stay sutures are then placed on the free edge of the mobilized anorectum, which is gently eased through the sphincter ring to its correct anatomical position (Figure 20.50d–f). The tapes are then removed and the anal canal is carefully sutured to the perianal skin. A series of Prolene sutures may also be used to approximate the levator ani across the midline to restore the perineal body (Figure 20.50g). Access to the levator ani may be compromised through the small anterior incision, in which case the anterior incision should

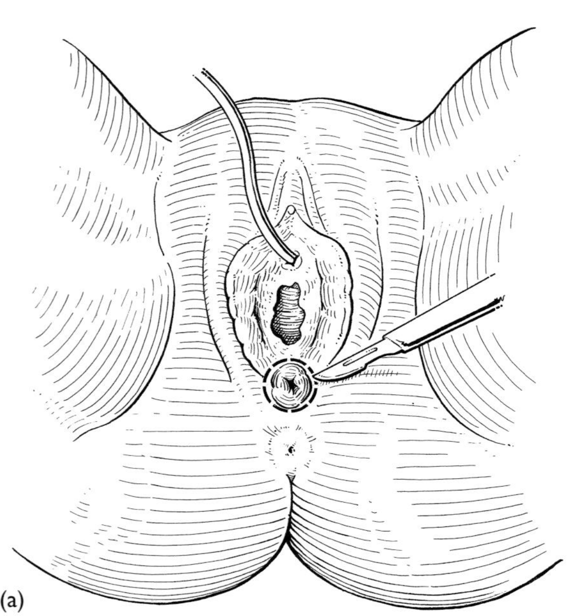

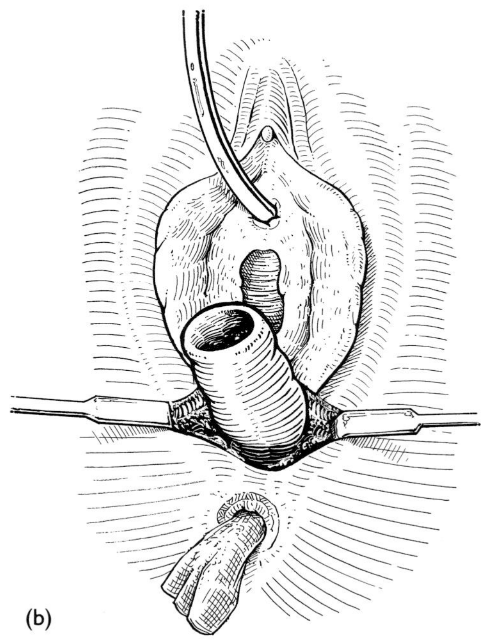

Figure 20.50a,b Rerouting of the anal canal. (a) The anal canal lies in the posterior fourchette of the vulva. The site of the external anal sphincters has already been identified by electromyography and the skin overlying the external anal sphincters has been marked. (b) The anorectum is dissected from its abnormal anterior position in the vulva and a tunnel is created inside the sphincter ring.

be extended posteriorly towards the rerouted anus. Two suction drains are placed inside the levator ani and the skin of the anterior defect is closed longitudinally so as to increase the distance of the rerouted anus from the vagina.

Patients should not be allowed to become constipated postoperatively. A bulk laxative should therefore be administered when oral intake is resumed. In order to ensure that the rerouted anorectum does not retract, removal of the perineal sutures should be delayed until complete maturation has been achieved.

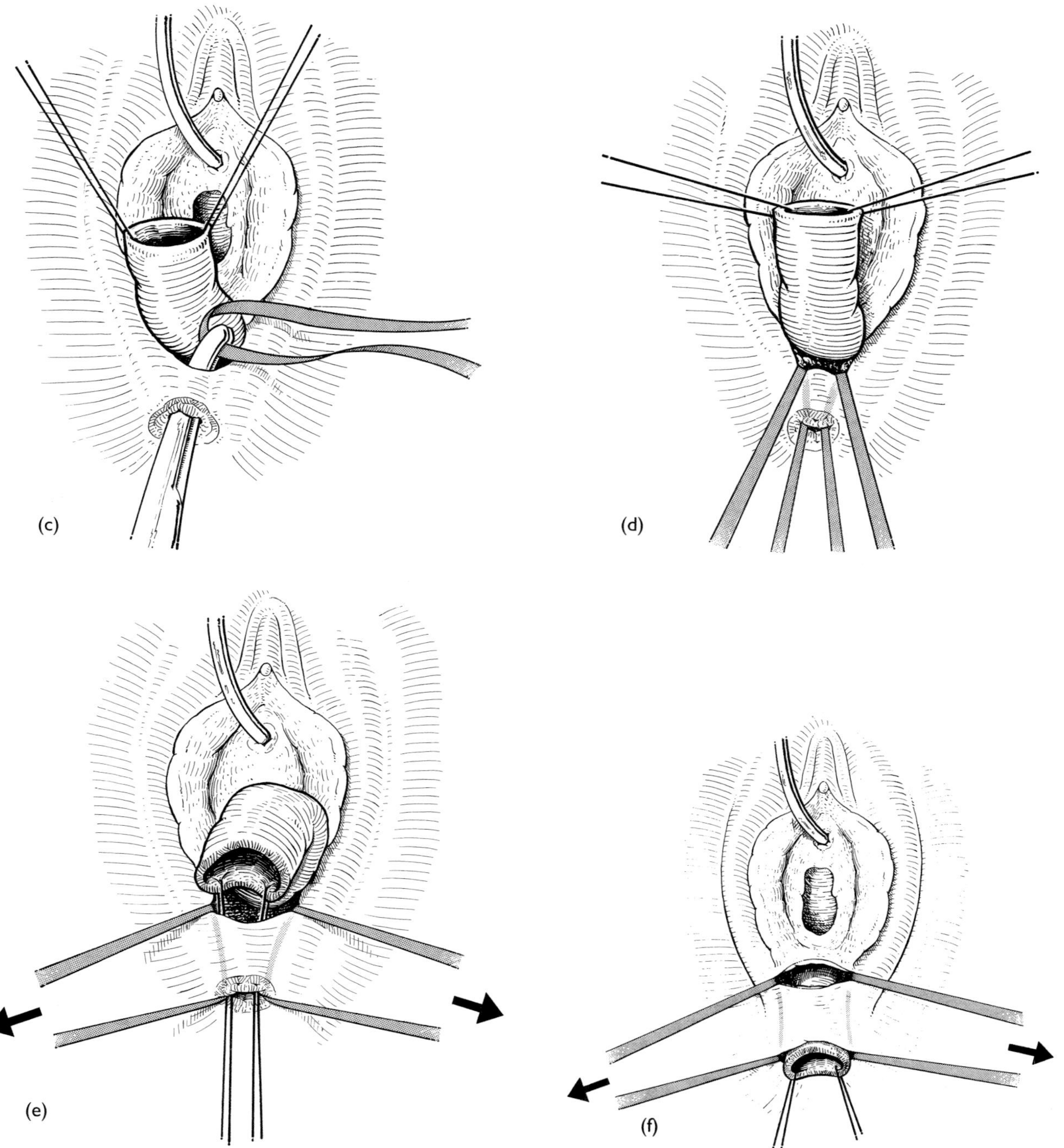

Figure 20.50c–f (c) A tunnel is developed through the external anal sphincters to meet the anterior dissection of the anorectum. (d) The fully mobilized anorectum is now gently delivered through the anal sphincters. (e) Delivery of the mobilized anorectum through the sphincters. Note that quite extensive anterior dissection is necessary to achieve the rerouting manoeuvre without the anal canal being under tension. (f) The anorectum has been rerouted and will be sutured to the anal verge.

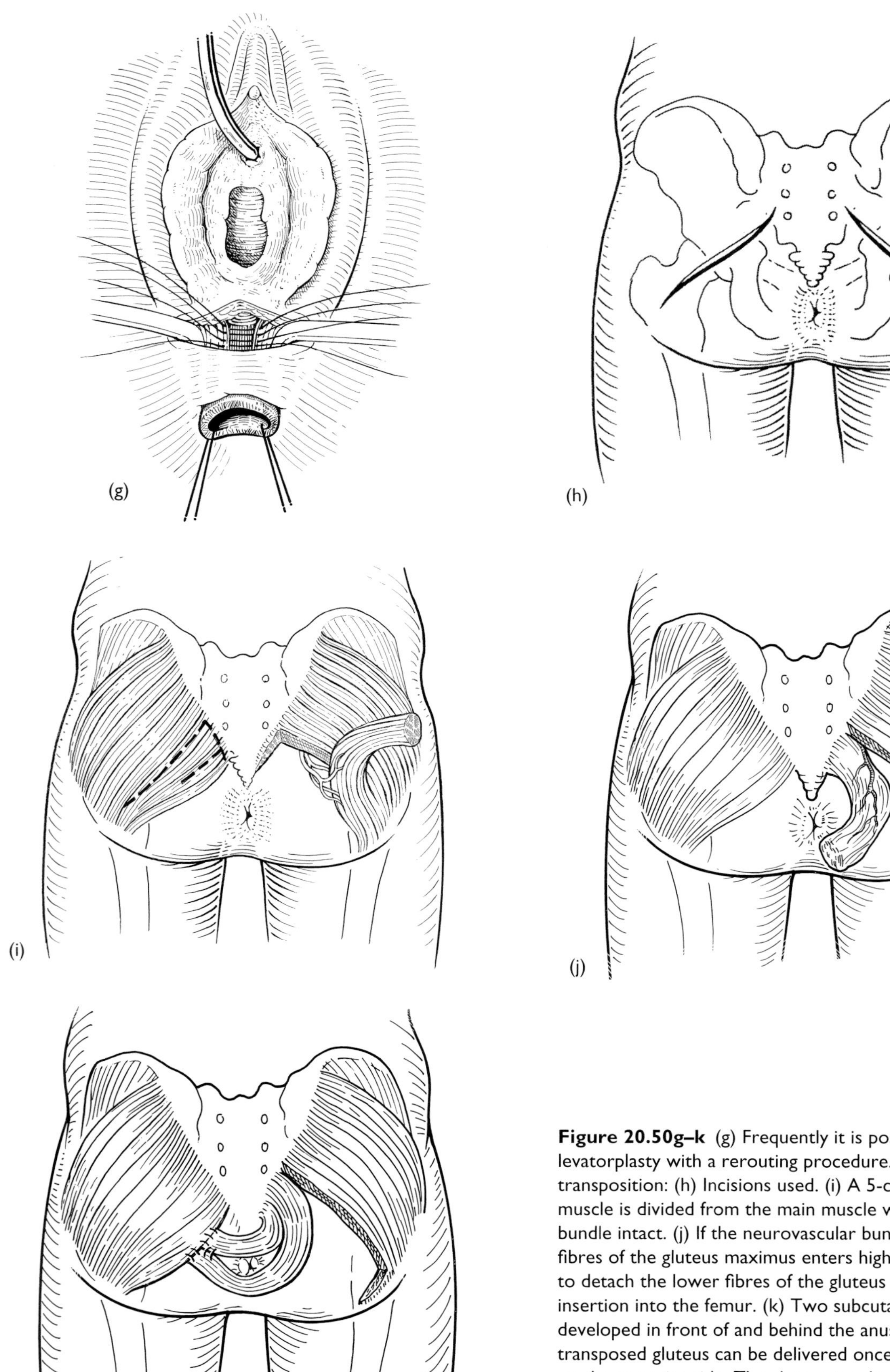

Figure 20.50g–k (g) Frequently it is possible to include a levatorplasty with a rerouting procedure. Gluteus maximus transposition: (h) Incisions used. (i) A 5-cm-wide strip of muscle is divided from the main muscle with its neurovascular bundle intact. (j) If the neurovascular bundle to the lower fibres of the gluteus maximus enters high up it may be wiser to detach the lower fibres of the gluteus maximus from their insertion into the femur. (k) Two subcutaneous tunnels are developed in front of and behind the anus so that the transposed gluteus can be delivered once split to the gluteus on the opposite side. The gluteus is split without damaging the blood supply to either limb so that the end of the muscle can be sutured to the opposite gluteus and to each other.

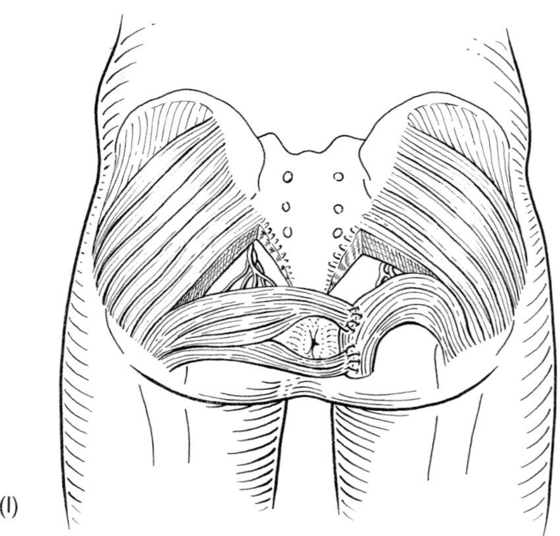

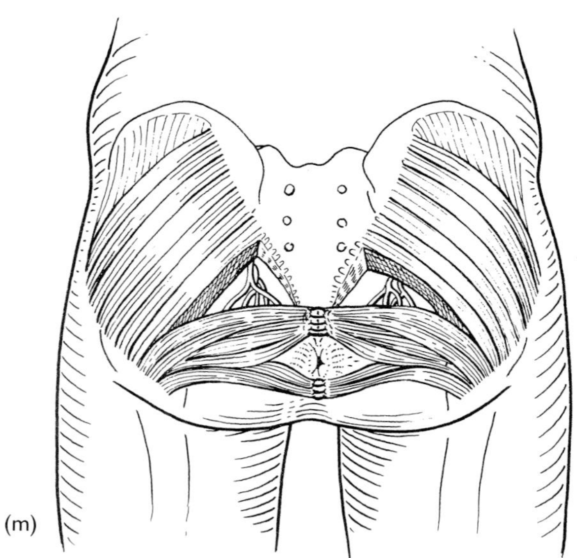

Figure 20.50l,m (l,m) Alternative configurations.

Muscle transposition

Various muscles have been used to augment the failing anal sphincter and the pelvic floor. A free smooth muscle collar from the sigmoid colon may be placed around the colon after pull-through operations but there is little, if any, evidence of objective improvement, despite enthusiastic reports of the operation (Chittenden, 1930; Stone and McLanahan, 1941; von Rapport, 1952; Dittertov and Grim, 1983; Schmidt, 1986).

Non-stimulated striated muscle has also been used to provide improved sphincter function. The transposed gracilis is the most widely used pedicle muscle graft and will be described. However, other transposition procedures have been employed using muscles such as the gluteus maximus, the fascia lata, sartorius and adductor longus but few reports provide clinical follow-up on more than a very small number of patients. The puborectalis muscle has been used to buttress a damaged external anal sphincter by using one limb to encircle the anus (see Figure 20.47). The clinical results of this novel approach have not been reported (Christiansen and Pedersen, 1987).

Gluteoplasty

There is renewed interest in gluteal flaps based upon preliminary encouraging reports from Chicago (Pearl et al, 1991) and Madrid (Devesa et al, 1992). Devesa et al (1992) report restoration of continence in 6 out of 10 patients after gluteus maximus transposition. Unilateral gluteus transposition was shown to be effective in two patients with severe sphincter loss following perineal trauma (Enriquez-Navascues and Devesa-Mugica, 1994). The results of bilateral gluteoplasty involving suture of the two split muscles across the midline was reported by Devesa et al (1997). Twenty patients were treated with this technique: 7 developed wound sepsis, 2 developed anal stenosis and 2 required late tightening of the muscle. The functional results indicate that 6 were fully continent (35%), a further 4 were improved (24%) and 7 (41%) had poor results.

We have undertaken a small randomized trial of unilateral gluteoplasty compared with pelvic floor repair for postobstetric incontinence (Yoshioka et al, 1997). There was less morbidity with pelvic floor repair but functional results were equivalent (Table 20.43). We believe, therefore, that gluteoplasty should be held in reserve when pelvic floor repair fails in patients wanting another surgical intervention who are unsuitable for electrically stimulated gracioplasty.

Technique

The patient is placed in the prone jack-knife position with the buttocks and anus exposed and a urethral catheter is passed. Two mirror-image incisions are made on each side of the buttocks from the border

Table 20.43 Results of randomized trial comparing total pelvic floor repair and gluteus maximus transposition.

	Total pelvic floor repair (*n* = 12)			*Gluteus maximus transposition* (*n* = 12)		
	Preop.	*Postop.*	*P-value*	*Preop.*	*Postop.*	*P-value*
Bowel habit (mean, times/day)	3.4 ± 1.5	2.8 ± 1.3	n.s.*	3.6 ± 1.0	3.0 ± 0.9	n.s.*
Poor evacuation	7	4	P = 0.0736#	6	2	P = 0.2207#
Urgency	11	6	P = 0.0724#	11	8	P = 0.3711#
Soiling	12	7	P = 0.2482#	11	7	P = 0.1336#
Incontinence						
Total	13.1 ± 2.7	6.6 ± 4.5	P = 0.004	13.8 ± 3.8	7.7 ± 6.1	P = 0.033
Solid	2.0 ± 0.8	0.8 ± 0.9	P = 0.061	2.5 ± 0.9	1.3 ± 1.5	P = 0.087
Liquid	2.7 ± 0.5	1.4 ± 0.9	P = 0.049	3.0 ± 0.6	1.6 ± 1.3	P = 0.045
Gas	3.0 ± 0.6	1.9 ± 1.2	P = 0.025	3.3 ± 0.6	1.8 ± 1.1	P = 0.105
Pad	2.8 ± 1.1	1.3 ± 1.3	P = 0.015	2.3 ± 1.1	1.2 ± 1.5	P = 0.019
Lifestyle	2.8 ± 0.8	1.2 ± 1.2	P = 0.007	2.9 ± 0.9	1.8 ± 1.2	P = 0.022

From Yoshioka et al (1998).
* Paired *t*-test.
\# McNemar test.

of the mid-sacrum towards the acetabulum. The lower fibres of the gluteus maximus are dissected free, preserving the neurovascular bundle, and a Nylon tape is placed under the muscle. Usually the sacral and coccygeal origin of the gluteus maximus is detached with its aponeurosis (Figure 20.50g,h). On the other hand, the configuration of the neurovascular bundle may favour dividing the femoral attachment (Figure 20.50i). Two stay sutures are placed through the aponeurotic tissue, for traction, and a 5-cm-wide strip of muscle is divided parallel with the muscle bundles. The neurovascular pedicle of the inferior half of the muscle is found entering its deep surface, after leaving the pelvis via the greater sciatic foramen. A nerve stimulator is used to check the contractability of the muscle. We used to make two mirror-image curved para-anal incisions lateral to the anus, approximately 2 cm from the anal orifice (Figure 20.50g) but we now rarely find this necessary. Two subcutaneous tunnels are created, in front of and behind the anus from one gluteus to the other.

Usually only one muscle is split parallel with its fibres (Figure 20.50j) to achieve a length necessary to reach the contralateral side where the anterior and posterior muscular strips are sutured together and independently to the undivided opposite muscle with 20 PDS (Figure 20.50k). The resulting effect is a thick muscular ring surrounding the anus without tension on the sutures but sufficiently tight to maintain it closed under basal conditions. Two drains are placed, one on each side, from the anus to above and lateral to the parasacral wounds.

The alternative methods of reconstruction involve a bilateral split for end-to-end anastomosis or a unilateral split to a mobilized segment of the contralateral muscle (Figure 20.50l and 20.50m).

Unstimulated gracilis transposition

When the external anal sphincter is partially damaged, some form of repair is usually possible. However, repair may not always be feasible if a substantial part of the external sphincter has been lost from trauma, prolonged disuse or denervation Under these circumstances, surgical reconstruction with the innervated gracilis muscle may be used to create an artificial sphincter (Pickrell et al, 1952, 1955; Corman, 1983). This operation has only been recommended where attempts at direct repair have been unsuccessful or where the sphincter has been destroyed by trauma. The operation was first described by Pickrell et al (1952) and usually reserved for children with congenital high imperforate anus (Pickrell et al, 1955). It has also been used for rectal prolapse (Atri, 1980). The principal indication for graciloplasty seems to be for patients with incontinence in whom all other methods of repair have failed or where the sphincter has been destroyed by trauma or synergistic gangrene (McGregor, 1965; Lewis, 1972; Nieves et al, 1975 Corman, 1979; Ben-Hur et al, 1980).

Results

The best results have been in patients who have sustained extensive perineal trauma (Corman, 1980) or those with congenital anomalies (Kiesewetter and Turner, 1963). The results of operation (Table 20.44) are very variable. Some excellent results have now

Table 20.44 Results of gracilis sling procedures.

	n	*Continent of solids and liquids*	*Continent of solids only*	*No better*
Lequit et al (1985)	10	4	5	1
Corman (1985b)	22	8	10	4
Simonson et al (1976)*	22	17	2	3
Yoshioka and Keighley (1989)	6	0	0	6
Wang et al (1988)	5	4	0	1
Christiansen et al (1990)	13†	6	4	2
Faucheron et al (1994)	22	1	18	3
Kumar et al (1995)	10	9	0	1
Sielezneff et al (1996)	8	5	3	0

* Perineal colostomy and gracilis sling procedure.
† One death from sepsis.

been reported by Corman (1985b), among patients followed up for more than 5 years, and by Wang et al (1988). Lequit et al (1985) report improvement in 9 of 10 patients with normal basal pressures (60 cmH_2O) or where squeeze pressures exceed 100 cmH_2O, but poor results in patients with low anal pressures. The best results were recorded in patients with congenital defects or traumatic lesions, but results were poor in patients with obstetric injury and iatrogenic incontinence following anal operations. In Birmingham we reported the results of eight graciloplasty procedures; all six patients who had had previously unsuccessful postanal repairs or sphincter repairs had a poor outcome and now have a colostomy (Yoshioka et al, 1988). By contrast, we have experienced a definite improvement in 6 of 9 young patients with congenital defects treated by graciloplasty.

It is difficult to know how a gracilis transplant achieves a functional result. Some believe that it merely acts as an inert encircling band, others that it actively contracts to close the anal canal (Christiansen et al, 1990), and a few believe that it can be trained to respond to rectal distension (Lequit et al, 1985). In a few cases the procedure has been performed alone to restore continence in patients given a perineal colostomy after a previous abdominoperineal excision of the rectum (Simonson et al, 1976). Current evidence suggests that the operation is usually unlikely to be beneficial unless the muscle is converted from a fast-twitch to a fatigue-resistant muscle by electrical stimulation (Magovern et al, 1986; Hallan et al, 1989; Williams et al, 1990a). However, further reports have appeared indicating that the non-stimulated graciloplasty may restore continence, particularly in trauma and anal atresia (Faucheron et al, 1994; Sielezneff et al, 1996). One paper proposes bilateral gracioplasty with restoration of continence in 9 of 10 patients (Kumar et al, 1995), however, the long-term results are less spectacular.

The great advantage of the non-stimulated wrap is that the muscle can be fitted with muscle or nerve electrodes in the future for electrostimulation (Konsten et al, 1993; Faucheron et al, 1994; George et al, 1993, Seccia et al, 1994; Shatari et al, 1995, Baeten et al, 1995; Geerdes et al, 1996; Ratani et al, 1997; Mander et al, 1997a,b). An alternative strategy for the future, however, is to transpose the pudendal nerve to innervate a skeletal muscle so as to convert a fast twitch muscle to sphincter (Sato and Konishi, 1996; Congilosi et al, 1997; Sato et al, 1997). Nerve transposition at the moment is experimental and its clinical application speculative but it may be a worthwhile development in the future.

Technique of unstimulated graciloplasty

Good mechanical bowel preparation and perioperative antibiotic prophylaxis is essential. The patient is catheterized and placed in the lithotomy position to expose the thigh as well as the anus. We find it easier to place the leg in the Allan stirrups so that the medial aspect of the knee is easily visible (Simonson et al, 1976; Castro and Pittman, 1978; Corman, 1980). It is imperative to drape the whole of the leg since this may have to be taken out of the stirrups or adducted in them at the close of the operation. The buttocks should be placed well over the end of the table so that the tip of the coccyx is easily palpable. The entire perineum and adductor compartment of the leg should be cleaned with antiseptic skin preparation. We usually use the right gracilis muscle placed anticlockwise around the anal canal and sutured to the left ischial tuberosity. If a previous right graciloplasty has been performed, or the use of the left gracilis muscle is preferred for any other reasons, then this will be inserted in a counterclockwise

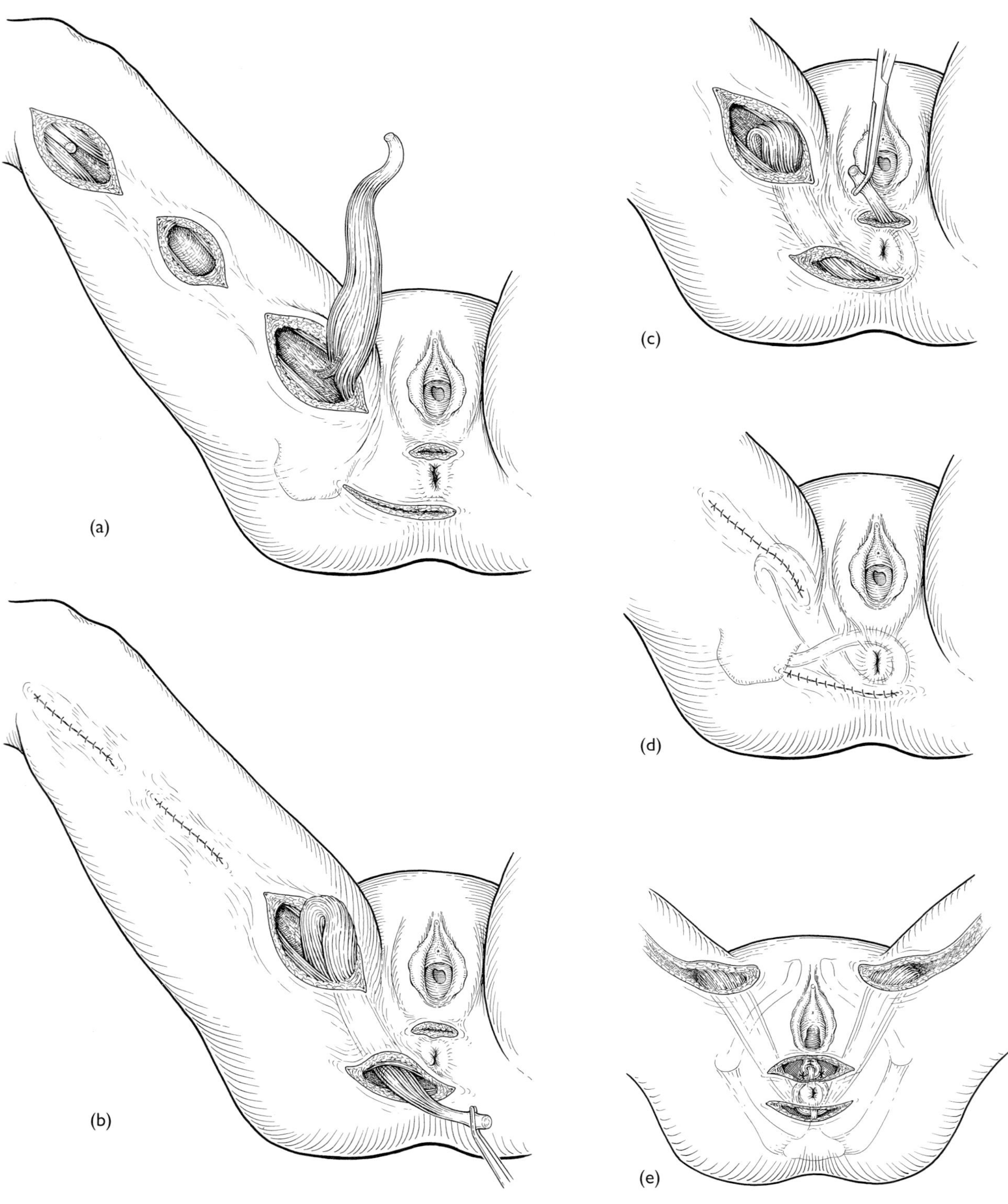

Figure 20.51a–e Graciloplasty. (a) A series of thigh incisions is used to identify and mobilize the gracilis muscle. Great care must be taken proximally not to damage the neurovascular bundle which enters the deep aspect of the muscle in the proximal third of the thigh. The tendon's insertion to the medial aspect of the tibia is divided. (b) A tunnel is developed around the anal canal and the tendon of the gracilis muscle is gently delivered around the anal canal to create a posterior sling. (c) The gracilis muscle has been rerouted behind the sphincter. (d) The tendon of the gracilis is sutured to the ischial tuberosity with ethibond; and the skin sutures have been closed. (e) Double graciloplasty: both tendons are routed around the anus and sutured to each other.

manner and sutured to the right ischial tuberosity (alpha loop).

Two or three incisions are usually needed to mobilize the gracilis muscle. A proximal incision is used to expose the neurovascular bundle which lies close to the muscle's origin, embedded in its medial aspect (Figure 20.51a). A tape is placed around the muscle so that no further damage can be incurred by the terminal fibres of the anterior branch of the obturator nerve supplying the gracilis. The entire muscle should be gently freed distally using blunt dissection inside its investing layer of fascia. The gracilis tendon is only visualized after retracting the tendon of sartorius upwards at its insertion into the upper medial aspect of the tibia. The gracilis tendon is then divided as close to its fan-like insertion as possible and the muscle, after full mobilization, is delivered through the most proximal incision in the thigh. The two distal incisions may then be closed (Figure 20.51b).

Two small transverse incisions are placed anterior and posterior to the anus about 1 cm from the anal margin. These incisions must not divide the anterior and posterior anococcygeal and anoperineal raphae since it is preferable to develop the tunnel beneath these superficial fibrous slings, thereby ensuring that the muscle is placed deeply in the perineum around the deficient external anal sphincter. A wide tunnel is developed between the proximal thigh incision and the incision in the posterior perianal region so that the muscle may be drawn through to the perianal region (Figure 20.51c). Two further tunnels are then constructed around the external anal sphincter on either side of the anal canal beneath the anterior and posterior raphae and between the two perianal incisions. The gracilis tendon is then passed anticlockwise if the right gracilis muscle is used and clockwise if the left gracilis muscle is preferred. The tendon and muscle are placed beneath the anterior and posterior raphae around the anus and then underneath its muscle belly, prior to attachment to the ischial tuberosity. Adduction may be necessary in order to suture the tendon to the ischial tuberosity at the correct tension. Once tension has been taken off the proximal component of the muscle, the tendon can be pulled round the sphincter and under itself anteriorly to allow suture to the ipsilateral ischial tuberosity (Figure 20.51d).

We have explored the double graciloplasty which provides a viable muscle buttress around the anus without having to suture the tendon to the ischial tuberosity. Both gracilus muscles and tendons are mobilized as described. Both tendons encircle the anus under the anterior and posterior raphe (Figure 20.51e), and the two tendons are sutured to one another anteriorly. In our view this seems to achieve a more secure method of fixation than by suture to the ischial tuberosity but there are two leg wounds which most patients would prefer to avoid.

Electrostimulated gracilis transposition

Historical development

Electrostimulation of the gracilis for 2–3 months using a pulse generator with its electrode on or near the neurovascular bundle (Figure 20.52a) will convert a fast twitch to a slow twitch muscle, which has far greater resistance to fatigue (Salmons, 1980; Salmons and Hendriksson, 1981). In our original description of the operation the position of the electrode was adjusted until a point with the lowest contraction threshold was found; the electrode was then sutured into position in the muscle (Figure 20.52b). The wires were routed to a receiver placed subcutaneously over ribs 8–9 in the midclavicular line (Figure 20.52b). The rerouting of the gracilis tendon and muscle was as already described and a covering stoma was raised.

Electrical stimulation was started 4 weeks after the operation, using an external stimulator to activate the receiver, but subsequently a totally implantable stimulator was used. Once there was evidence of reduced fusion frequency and increased duration of tetany, usually after stimulation for 6–8 weeks, the stoma was closed. Defecation was achieved by discontinuing external activation of the generator in response to a call to stool. Defecation was deferred by increasing the power of the stimulator. Normally the stimulator was set at a subtetanic frequency to maintain resting anal tone.

At the Royal London we initially reported the use of transposed gracilis with prolonged neuromuscular stimulation in six patients with faecal incontinence: two failed postanal repairs, two unsatisfactory ileoanal pouches, one incontinent patient after ileorectal anastomosis and an incontinent patient with hidradenitis (Williams et al, 1990a). Despite a covering stoma all developed local sepsis; three patients achieved continence. The same principle was used to construct a neorectum and a neosphincter after proctocolectomy (Williams et al, 1989) and after abdominoperineal excision of the rectum (Williams et al, 1990b). In Italy, Cavina et al (1990) also used electrical stimulation to achieve an improved result when transposing the gracilis muscle to form a neoanal sphincter as part of a total reconstruction after abdominoperineal excision of the rectum. The Italian experience included 47 patients: in two the colon became ischaemic, but

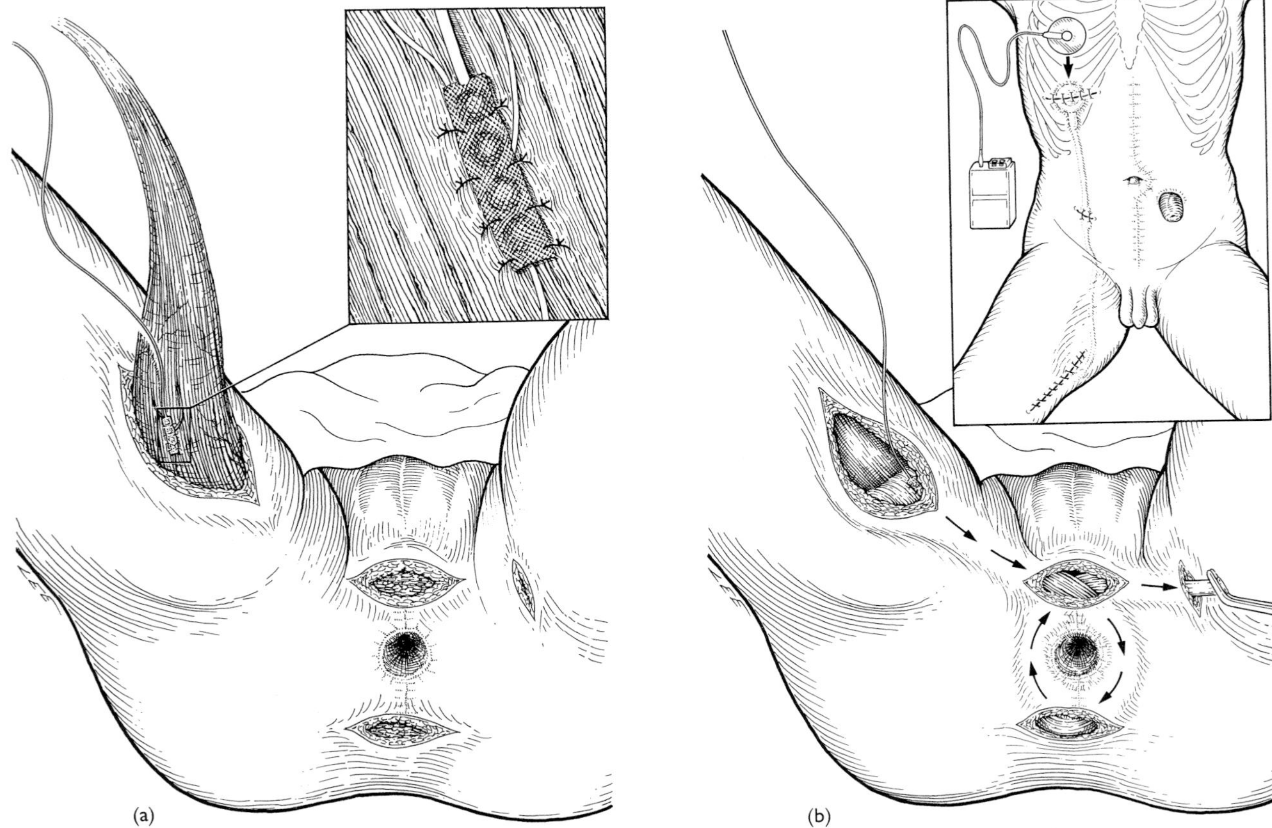

Figure 20.52a,b Electrically stimulated gracilis neosphincter: the original technique. (a) An electrode for electrical stimulation was sutured to the proximal gracilis muscle near the neuromuscular bundle. (b) The gracilis muscle was rerouted around the anal canal. The stimulation was triggered by an external pulse generator which activated a receiving device under the costal margin.

65% attained good function. This was somewhat surprising since the electrical stimulation in this series was provided through exteriorized wires and was performed during short periods for several weeks postoperatively, after which the wires were removed (Cavina et al, 1990). Such a technique would not have led to conversion from fast twitch to slow twitch muscle, which is the principle of our technique. In order to achieve conversion it is essential that the electrical stimulation continues indefinitely (Baeten et al, 1991; NS Williams et al, 1991).

Since our initial report on this technique we have modified the procedure in several important ways. In order to prevent ischaemic necrosis of the muscle and severe perineal sepsis, we divided the blood supply to the distal part of the gracilis several weeks before transposition, i.e. the delay procedure. We believed at the time that such a manoeùvre would allow rudimentary communicating vessels to open up between the segmental blood supply, ensuring subsequent viability of the transposed muscle. Although using this modification, only one of 22 patients developed ischaemic necrosis, compared with 5 of 11 who had previously not undergone the modification ($P<0.05$), we now believe that this manoeuvre may not be necessary. We positioned the electrode on the main nerve to the gracilis, as opposed to its peripheral branches. This ensured reliable en masse contraction of the muscle. A totally implantable stimulator was also used, which allowed continuous stimulation, and was less of an encumbrance for the patient. It could be programmed by radiotelemetry and turned on and off by the patient using a magnet. Using these modifications, we constructed an electrically stimulated neosphincter in 23 patients with faecal incontinence as well as ten patients as part of a total reconstruction after abdominoperineal excision of the rectum. Sixteen of the patients with incontinence had functioning neosphincters. All were improved and most had acceptable, although not perfect continence. The patients selected for the procedure were those in whom a conventional operation to correct their incontinence had either failed or was contraindi cated and in whom a colostomy was the only other option (Williams, 1992).

Further experience has allowed us to streamline the procedure. We now have a technique which produces consistent results and is described below. Since other groups have demonstrated that transposition of the gracilis without earlier division of the distal blood supply does not result in ischaemia, we have abandoned the initial delay procedure.

Electrically stimulated gracilis neoanal sphincter

Indications

The neosphincter can be used for several types of patients:

1. Incontinent patients who have a deficient anal sphincter mechanism as a result of trauma or neurogenic damage. These patients have an intact rectum and anal canal and construction of a neosphincter is indicated if a conventional operation, such as postanal repair, has failed or is contraindicated.
2. Some patients with anorectal agenesis. Those who have had an unsuccessful pull-through procedure and in whom electromyographic mapping indicates the absence of any functioning anal sphincter, thus ruling out a rerouting procedure.
3. Some patients who have undergone an abdominoperineal excision of the rectum (APER) for cancer. Suitable patients must have no evidence of local recurrence or distant metastases. The colon will first need to be brought down to the perineum and sutured to the perineal skin several weeks before neosphincter construction. Similarly, patients who have low rectal cancer and are about to undergo APER may be considered for the procedure. In such individuals, the colon will be sutured to the perineal skin at the time of the resection.

When the electrically stimulated neosphincter is used as described for patients in categories 2 and 3, we often combine it with a conduit procedure. Using the conduit to irrigate the distal colon in an antegrade fashion facilitates 'neorectal' evacuation (see pp 737–746, Chapter 21). Such a combination is termed total anorectal reconstruction (TAR).

Contraindications

1. Damaged gracilis muscle. In practice, this includes patients with spina bifida, and those with generalized neurological diseases such as multiple sclerosis. Similarly, patients with myopathic disease affecting the limb muscles are unsuitable for the procedure. If there is any doubt about gracilis muscle function, it should be tested by electromyography.
2. Disseminated malignant disease or local pelvic recurrence.
3. Lack of sufficient manual dexterity to use the hand-held telemetry equipment which controls the electrical stimulator.
4. Persistent perineal sepsis or Crohn's disease.
5. A cardiac pacemaker *in situ*.

Preoperative preparation

Counselling

This is a most important part of the preparation where the procedure must be fully explained. It must be stressed that there are at least two stages to the procedures and sometimes three, and that a leg wound will result. The latter is an important consideration, particularly for women. The pros and cons of the procedure versus a permanent colostomy must be discussed, and it must be made clear that success cannot be guaranteed. The prospective patient should meet a patient of similar age and sex who has had the procedure for a similar indication. The patient should be shown the stimulator and hand-held controlling device and be provided with appropriate literature. They must then be given sufficient time to make a decision and encouraged to return for further discussion.

Marking the site of the stimulator and covering stoma

Having made the decision to undergo the operation, a site is chosen where the stimulator is to be implanted. Usually this is in a subcutaneous pocket in the upper quadrant of the abdomen. This will be on the left side if the covering stoma is to be on the right. Once chosen, the site must be marked with indelible ink. Similarly, the stoma care nurse must site the position for the covering stoma. In those patients in whom a colonic pull-through procedure is not to be performed, either a loop ileostomy in the right iliac fossa or transverse colostomy can be used. In those who are to have a colonic pull-through, a loop ileostomy is essential.

Anaesthesia

It is imperative that the anaesthetist uses no muscle relaxants during implantation of the electrode on the nerve to the gracilis. If muscle relaxants are used, they will make it impossible to observe muscle contraction during nerve stimulation.

The operation

The operation described here is for incontinent patients with an intact anorectum but deficient anal sphincter.

Stage 1: Transposition of gracilis muscle; implantation of electrode and neurostimulator; construction of covering stoma

The patient is placed in the modified Lloyd Davies position on the operating table. If the covering stoma is to be eventually sited on the right side of the patient's abdomen, the left gracilis muscle is chosen for mobilization.

A longitudinal incision is made on the innermost aspect of the thigh along a line from the medial femoral condyle towards the inferior pubic ramus, commencing approximately 2 cm proximal to the femoral condyle. At its most proximal part, the incision is curved in the direction of the anterior superior iliac spine.

The gracilis muscle is mobilized in its distal half by division and ligation of the two or three distal vessels that supply it on its lateral surface (Figure 20.53a). The intervening and overlying areolar tissue is also cleared from the muscle.

The tendon of the gracilis muscle is traced down to its insertion in the tibia. The tendon is divided with strong scissors as close to its insertion as possible. It is also necessary to separate the gracilis tendon from the sartorius. Once the tendon has been divided, it is clamped in a small artery forceps which is then used as a retractor. By exerting traction in a proximal direction, the muscle can be mobilized upwards towards the main vascular pedicle. Further peripheral vessels are divided and ligated. All areolar tissue overlying the muscle and binding it to the deeper muscles is divided. The main vascular pedicle is identified entering the lateral border of the gracilis, usually at the junction of the proximal and distal two-thirds of the muscle. The pedicle consists of an artery and two venae commitantes. Once identified, the vascular pedicle is carefully cleared of areolar tissue and freed up to its point of exit beneath the adductor longus. Further careful dissection of the blood supply which is a branch of the obturator artery, should continue at this point, since it is the mobility of the proximal blood supply which limits the degree of muscle that can be transposed. The blood supply can be mobilized virtually to its origin, and time doing this is time well spent as it will allow complete encirclement of the anal canal by muscle as opposed to tendon when it comes to the transposition. The peripheral branches of the nerve to gracilis lying above the main vascular pedicle can be identified using a nerve stimulator which helps to ensure their preservation (Figure 20.53b).

Mobilization of the muscle continues proximally by dividing the areolar tissue overlying its medial surface of the upper third up to its origin from the lower half of the body of the pubis and the inferior pubic ramus. The main nerve to the gracilis is then sought by entering the plane between the adductor longus and adductor brevis muscles approximately 3 cm proximal to the main vascular bundle.

The main nerve is a continuation of the anterior branch of the obturator nerve. It traverses the superior surface of the adductor brevis muscle in a lateral to medial direction. In its upper part, it gives off a branch to the adductor brevis and then emerges from beneath the medial border of the overlying adductor longus to split into several branches which enter the upper part of the lateral border of the gracilis muscle. By exerting downward traction on the upper part of the gracilis, the main nerve is put on the stretch. Identification of the nerve is confirmed by stimulation with a disposable nerve stimulator (set at 0.5 V) and observing an en masse contraction of the gracilis muscle. The areolar tissue on either side of the nerve binding it to the adductor brevis muscle is cleared. The tissue overlying the nerve is left undisturbed, and the site for electrode implantation is selected distal to the branch to the adductor brevis but proximal to the main nerve division into its peripheral branches.

A 2-cm incision is then made in the upper quadrant of the abdomen at a point which will in the future mark the lower part of the subcutaneous pocket in which the stimulator will be placed. Another 2-cm incision is then made approximately 5 cm above the mid-inguinal point. Both incisions are made on the side on which the muscle has been mobilized. A long artery forceps (Lloyd Davies type) is then passed subcutaneously from the lower incision to emerge to the upper incision (Figure 20.53c). The subcutaneous track is enlarged by opening and closing the jaws of the artery forceps. The tip of the electrode plate (Medtronic) is then grasped in the jaws of the forceps and the plate and the lead are then drawn downwards to emerge through the lower incision. The forceps is then passed from the upper end of the thigh wound under the adductor longus muscle in the plane between it and the adductor brevis, and is tunnelled subcutaneously until its tip emerges through the

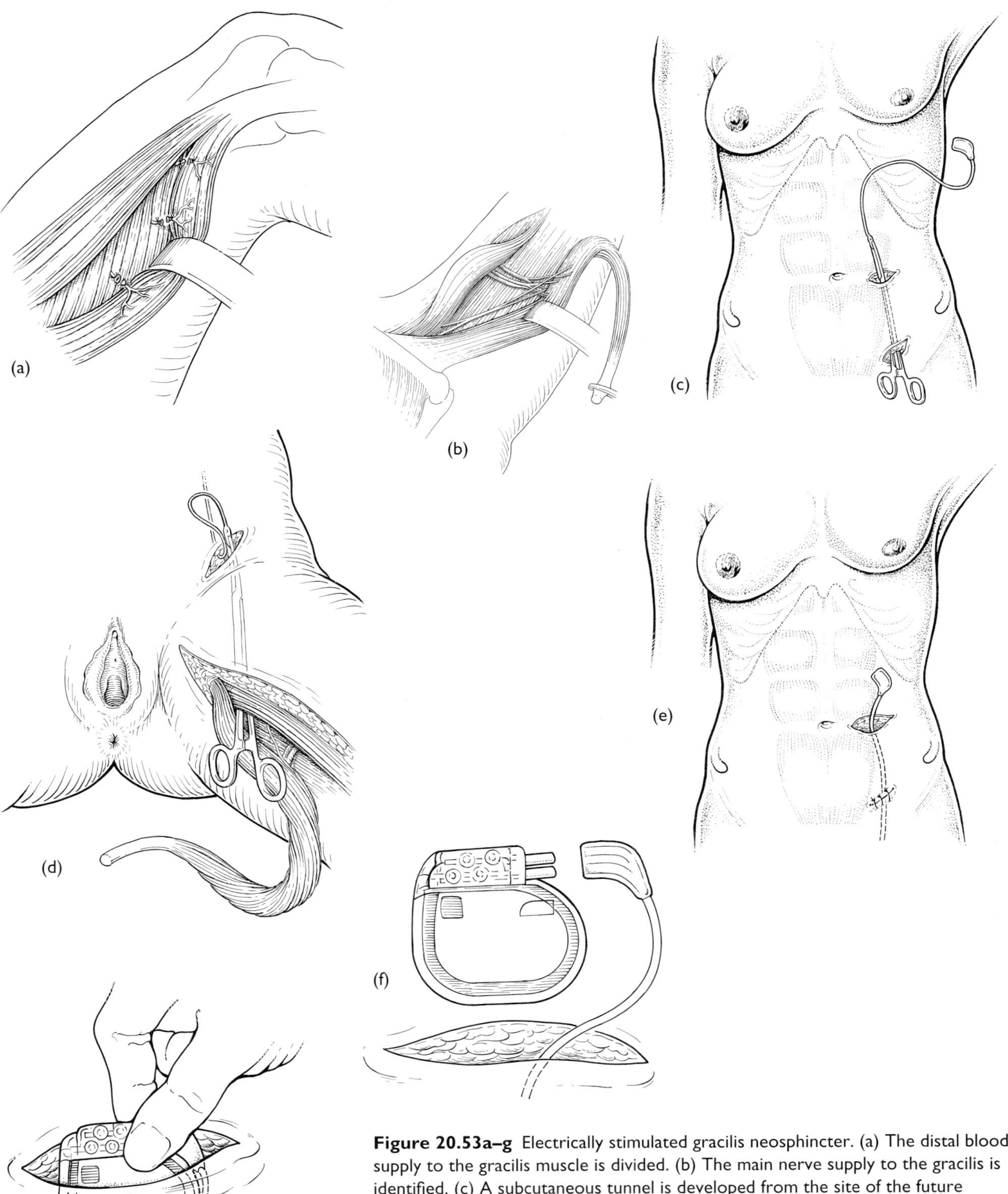

Figure 20.53a–g Electrically stimulated gracilis neosphincter. (a) The distal blood supply to the gracilis muscle is divided. (b) The main nerve supply to the gracilis is identified. (c) A subcutaneous tunnel is developed from the site of the future pocket for the stimulator and the small groin incision. (d) A further tunnel is created by pushing the Lloyd Davies forceps below the adductor longus to emerge through the groin incision. By this means, the electrode plate is delivered into the thigh wound for subsequent suture onto the main nerve to the gracilis. (e) A subcutaneous pocket is created in the upper abdomen. (f) The lead is connected to the stimulator by pushing the pins into the sockets and the screws are tightened. (g) The stimulator is placed in the pocket with the excess lead behind it.

skin incision above the inguinal ligament. The subsequent track which has been created is enlarged. Once again, the tip of the electrode plate is grasped in the jaws of the artery forceps and gently brought down through the subcutaneous tunnel, so that it emerges parallel to the main nerve (Figure 20.53d).

If it is decided to implant the stimulator at this time, the upper abdominal incision is enlarged transversely to approximately 5 cm in length, and is deepened to create a subcutaneous pocket large enough to take the stimulator (Medtronic Inc., Minnesota, USA) (Figure 20.53e–g).

If it is decided not to implant the stimulator, the proximal connector of the lead is placed in a silastic sheath and buried in a small subcutaneous pocket ready for implantation at a later date. The latter manoeuvre is performed on occasions when the surgeon is concerned that sepsis may be a problem postoperatively and obviates the risk of losing an expensive stimulator.

The electrode plate is then sutured over the main nerve in its long axis (Figure 20.54). The plate has pre-cut holes for non-absorbable sutures. The sutures should all be placed first before they are tied. Six interrupted 3.0 non-absorbable silk sutures are used on a round-bodied needle. Each suture passes through the hole on the periphery of the electrode plate, then through the underlying adductor brevis muscle, taking care not to damage the nerve, and back through the plate, so that when tied the knot lies on the superior surface of the plate. Once the position of the electrode is correct, all the sutures are tied. The position of the electrode plate is then checked by connecting the lead to a Grass stimulator. The voltage is gradually increased until an en masse contraction of the gracilis is achieved; the threshold for this contraction is usually approximately 0.5 V. If the stimulator is to be implanted, the two pins of the electrode lead are pushed into their respective connection ports on the stimulator and the screws are screwed down to make contact with the pins.

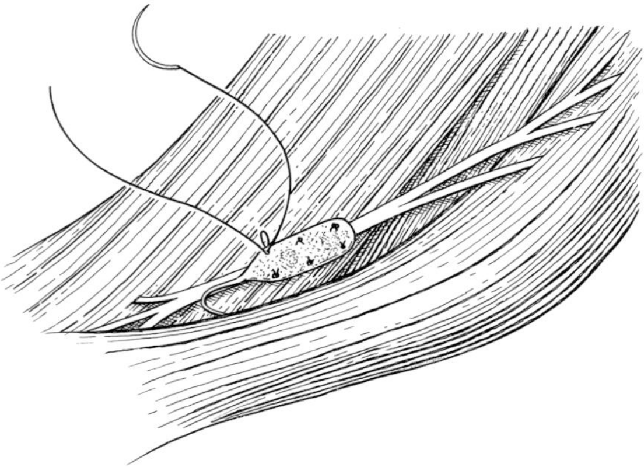

Figure 20.54 The electrode is sutured over the main nerve in its long axis.

The implant, which has been turned off with the radiotelemetry programming unit, is placed in the subcutaneous pocket, ensuring that any redundant lead is placed behind the implant (Figure 20.53g). The transverse skin wound is closed with subcuticular Prolene.

The small wound above the groin is next closed, after first ensuring that a loop of excess lead no less than 1.5 cm in diameter is left in a small subcutaneous pocket at this point. This will relieve strain on the system and provide for patient growth and mobility. Transposition of the gracilis muscle around the anal canal is achieved using two curvilinear incisions approximately 3 cm from the right and left margins of the anal verge. A circumferential subcutaneous tunnel around the anal canal and external to any remaining external anal sphincter is created. This is deepened to ensure that it can easily accommodate the gracilis muscle when it is transposed. The skin bridges anteriorly and posteriorly are preserved. Care must be exercised in creating the space anteriorly between the anterior wall of the anorectum and the posterior vaginal wall in the female. In many of these patients, there is often considerable scarring in this region. This dissection is aided by infiltration of the plane with a weak solution of adrenaline in saline (1 in 300 000).

By gentle dissection with scissors, the plane is opened sufficiently to allow the insertion of a Jacques catheter which can then be used to retract the anorectum downwards and allow the plane to be further dissected under direct vision (Figure 20.55a). An incision is then made in the skin crease between the thigh and the buttock on the side of the muscle to be transposed. Through this incision, a tunnel is created into the thigh to emerge adjacent to the upper part of the mobilized gracilis. It is necessary in creating this tunnel to divide Scarpa's fascia with scissors. The tunnel needs to be at least three finger breadths wide. A similar tunnel is then created from this incision to that on the lateral side of the anal verge.

Using Roberts forceps attached to the free tendon of the gracilis, the muscle is brought into the perineum through the tunnel, ensuring that the muscle is not twisted (Figure 20.55b). The muscle should be brought round the anal canal in a gamma configuration. A small incision is made over the contralateral ischial tuberosity. The incision is deepened down to bone, and three interrupted O-Ethibond sutures are attached to the underlying periosteum. The sutures are left long and clipped with the needles attached. The gracilis muscle is transposed in an anticlockwise or clockwise direction depending on the side used, and its tendon is brought out through the incision overlying the ischial tuberosity (Figure 20.55c).

The ipsilateral leg is then adducted to the midline, and the muscle pulled through its tunnels so that it fits snugly around the anal canal. In order to prevent the transposition from being too tight, we normally leave a Hegar dilator size 14 within the anal canal. The tendon of the gracilis is then sutured to the ischial tuberosity (Figure 20.55c).

Once positioned, the stimulator is turned on at the threshold voltage to ensure that contraction of

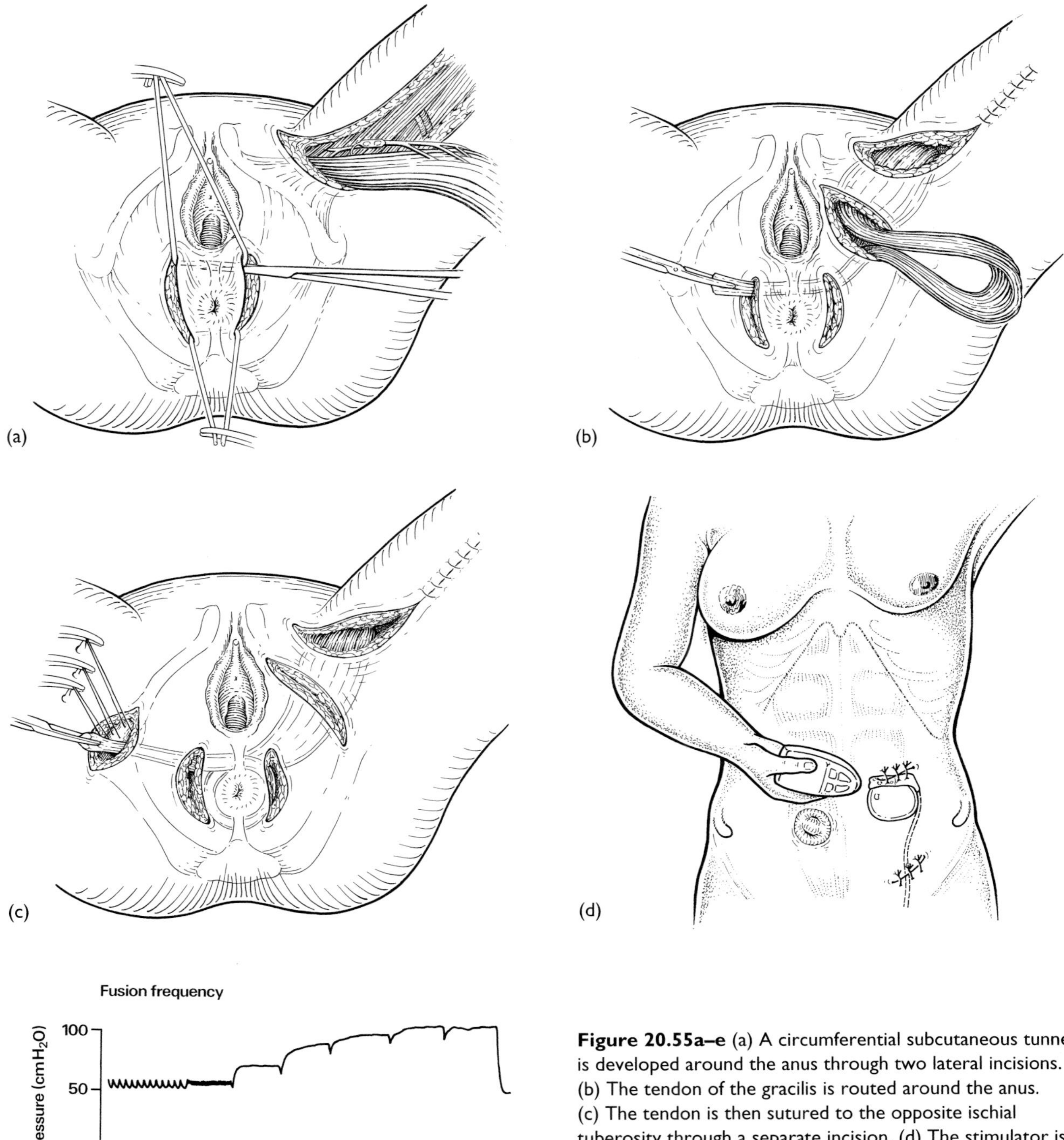

Figure 20.55a–e (a) A circumferential subcutaneous tunnel is developed around the anus through two lateral incisions. (b) The tendon of the gracilis is routed around the anus. (c) The tendon is then sutured to the opposite ischial tuberosity through a separate incision. (d) The stimulator is turned on with the hand-held telemetry device. (e) Fused contraction as frequency of stimulation is increased.

the gracilis occurs and occlusion of the anal orifice is achieved (Figure 20.55d). All wounds are closed after first spraying them with Tribiotic spray. Subcuticular Prolene is used for the leg wound and interrupted 20 Vicryl for the perineal skin wounds.

A covering loop stoma is then constructed. We usually use a loop ileostomy sited in the right iliac fossa and often perform the operation laparoscopically if there has been no previous abdominal surgery.

Postoperative regimen

The patient is nursed with the legs together for the first 3 days and is then encouraged to mobilize. Oral fluids are started after flatus has been passed. Long-term electrical stimulation commences on the 10th day, provided all wounds are healing satisfactorily. The stimulator is programmed using the programming unit. The 'training' protocol at present is as shown in Table 20.45.

After 8 weeks, some conversion of 'fast' to 'slow' twitch muscle should have occurred which can be demonstrated by anorectal manometry using a microtransducer. With the probe positioned in the anal canal at the site of the neosphincter, the frequency of stimulation can gradually be increased until a smooth (fused) contraction takes place (Figure 20.55e). The minimum frequency which produces such a tetanic contraction is known as the tetanic fusion frequency (TFF). Immediately postoperatively, TFF is usually 25 pulses per second. After 8 weeks, it invariably decreases to 10–15 pulses per second. When this reduction has occurred, the off time can be reduced to zero, so the stimulator is working in continuous mode, and the neosphincter is also contracting continuously, so occluding the anal canal.

At this point, the patient is admitted for Stage 2, that is, closure of the covering stoma. After closure of the stoma, the patient should be instructed on how to turn the stimulator off or on using the hand-held telemetry equipment. This equipment also allows the patient to increase the voltage of stimulation up to a level predetermined by the surgeon.

Initially, there may be problems in rectal evacuation which frequently occur in patients who previously 'strained' before they developed incontinence. No doubt the straining was to some extent responsible for their incontinence, but when continence is improved, their 'old' habits may return. It is essential in such cases to institute a suppository regimen as soon as possible. If patients lack the sensation of impending evacuation, they should be encouraged to try to evacuate every 6–8 hours initially, gradually increasing the interval, depending on the results of such a regimen. If the problem remains severe such patients may require a colonic conduit procedure.

Table 20.45 Postoperative 'training' protocol for electrically stimulated gracilis neoanal sphincter.

	Weeks				
	1 & 2	*3 & 4*	*5 & 6*	*7 & 8*	*>8*
Pulse width (μs)	210	210	210	210	210
Frequency (Hz)	12	12	12	12	12
On time (s)	2	2	2	2	4
Off time (s)	6	4	2	1	1

Electrically stimulated neosphincter in patients with anorectal agenesis

Patients with anorectal agenesis invariably undergo some form of pull-through procedure in early childhood. The techniques and results are detailed in Chapter 72. A proportion of these patients reach adolescence and early adulthood with poor function; many have had to revert to a colostomy. They are usually classified as being incontinent. However, this incontinence results not only because they have a deficient or absent sphincteric apparatus, but because of other deficiencies of anorectal function. Thus, they lack normal anorectal sensation, they have no reservoir capable of storing faeces, the normal anorectal reflexes are absent and they are unable to evacuate satisfactorily. Even if the sphincter can be replaced satisfactorily, the other deficiencies mar the result. Thus, of the nine patients who had previously undergone pull-through procedures for anorectal agenesis on whom we performed an electrically stimulated neoanal sphincter, only four had reasonable function, and evacuation still remained a problem in these patients (Williams et al, 1991).

As a consequence, in this group of patients we have modified our approach. In those patients who have had a pull-through procedure for anorectal agenesis and in whom evacuation has been a problem in addition to incontinence, we now combine the operation of the electrically stimulated neosphincter with a colonic conduit procedure (see pp 737–746, Chapter 21). Such a combination allows evacuation to be achieved by antegrade colonic lavage, and the neosphincter maintains continence in between irrigation. Such an approach removes the need for a permanent colostomy and hopefully restores continence to a group of young patients at a crucial time in their lives.

This combined procedure is performed in two stages. The first stage consists of construction of the electrically stimulated neosphincter, as described previously, although the stimulator is usually not inserted at this stage. The conduit is constructed from the proximal transverse colon using the technique described in detail in Chapter 21. Briefly, the ascending colon is transected approximately 10 cm from the ileocaecal junction. An enterotomy is made 15 cm distal to the transection in the transverse colon. A 5-cm valve is constructed by intussuscepting the proximal colon so that it emerges through the enterotomy. The valve is stabilized using three rows of interrupted ethibond sutures, and between these, three rows of staples delivered via a GIA instrument without the blade are inserted. The valve is placed back within the colonic lumen and the enterotomy is closed. The base of the valve is stabilized using a row of interrupted 2.0 Maxon sutures inserted circumferentially between the serosa of the valve and the serosa of the colon. The afferent limb of the conduit proximal to the valve is narrowed using the GIA to the calibre of a size 14 silastic urinary catheter inserted through it and through the valve. The afferent limb of the conduit is exteriorized in the right iliac fossa, preferably below the 'bikini' line. Exteriorization is performed using a skin flap to prevent stenosis, and the conduit orifice is sutured circumferential to the skin so that it lies a few millimetres below the surface.

Gastrointestinal continuity is then established by anastomosing the transected proximal ascending colon end to side, with the transverse colon approximately 10 cm distal to the valve. A loop ileostomy is next constructed as close as possible to the ileocaecal junction.

Two to three weeks after this procedure, the stimulator is inserted, and training of the gracilis neosphincter commences as an outpatient procedure. The silastic catheter is normally removed 4–6 weeks later, provided a gastrografin contrast study shows no evidence of leakage. The patient is next taught to intubate the conduit with a catheter and to irrigate the distal colon in an antegrade direction using 1–2 L of tepid tapwater. At an appropriate time, normally 2–3 months after the initial procedure, the loop ileostomy is closed.

The patient initially intubates the conduit on a daily basis, and after turning off the stimulator so as to relax the neosphincter, irrigates the colon to produce evacuation. The subsequent frequency of irrigation depends on the individual patient, but it is important for the patient to irrigate sufficiently often to prevent impaction.

Alternative technique of electrical stimulation

The technique of stimulation described above is direct stimulation of the main nerve to the gracilis. An alternative technique described by Baeten et al (1988) is intramuscular stimulation. In this technique the gracilis is transposed around the anal canal in a similar manner to that described previously. Implantation of the stimulation equipment is performed at least 6 weeks after the transposition. The site of lowest threshold for stimulation of the transposed gracilis is first localized using transcutaneous stimulation in the medial part of the upper thigh. An incision is made at this site, and the gracilis muscle is exposed. An intramuscular flexible coil wire of platinum iridium is introduced into the muscle as an anode (Model 4300 Medtronic Kerkrode, The Netherlands) about 4 cm distant to the obturator nerve towards the anus (Geerdes, 1996). With the introduction of a similar electrode, the optimal position for the cathode is determined during electrical stimulation (as close as possible to the intramuscular branches of the nerve). This electrode is then pulled transversely through the muscle perpendicular to the muscle fibres, and fixed to the epimysium. The length of the bare surface of the electrode can be adjusted to the diameter of the muscle. Subsequently, the leads are tunnelled subcutaneously to a pocket in the lower abdominal wall and connected to an Itrel™ pulse generator (Model 7424 Medtronic Kerkrode, The Netherlands).

The training programme for the muscle is similar to that previously described for the neural technique of stimulation.

The advantages of intramuscular stimulation are thought to be stability of the electrode and no damage to the nerve to the gracilis, which is believed to be a problem with direct neural stimulation. The advantages of neural stimulation are en masse contraction of the muscle, and thus enhanced function and more complete conversion of the type 2 fibres to type 1 fibres. A lower threshold of contraction is also more likely, and hence the longevity of the stimulator will be increased. Interestingly, after 26 weeks of stimulation the average threshold of stimulation using intramuscular stimulation was just less than 3 V (Baeten et al, 1995). Using neural stimulation over an equivalent period resulted in an average stimulation threshold of 1.5 V. However, the only way to determine which is the superior method of stimulation is to perform a randomized controlled trial, and this remains to be done.

Results

Incontinent patients with a deficient anal sphincter alone

Twenty patients who were incontinent because of a deficient anal sphincter underwent an electrically stimulated neoanal sphincter in our initial study (Williams et al, 1991). Each of these patients had previously undergone a conventional surgical procedure for their incontinence. When assessed a mean of 6 months postoperatively, 12 patients had functioning neosphincters and all of these patients had noted an improvement in function (Table 20.46). When assessed, one patient was still in the process of training, one patient died 7 months postoperatively from a myocardial infarction, and in six the operation had been unsuccessful. Five of the failures occurred early on in our experience: four were due to muscle necrosis with associated sepsis and one due to inability to cope with the external apparatus. The physiological results in this group of patients are illustrated in Table 20.47 and show that the electrically stimulated neosphincter provided the patient with a mean functioning resting pressure of 62 cmH_2O ($P<0.05$).

Wexner et al (1996b) used the same protocol as ourselves, and despite a considerable morbidity, presumably due to the learning curve, had a 60% success rate in their first 14 patients. They also demonstrated that the average mean squeeze pressure increased from 43 mmHg prior to surgery to 151 mmHg after the operation ($P<0.01$). They concluded that despite a steep learning curve, the stimulated gracilis operation is a viable operation for selected patients with severe incontinence.

As a result of our initial findings in 1993, we commenced a prospective multicentre trial using neural stimulation (Mander et al, 1997b). This trial included most of those patients from the Cleveland Clinic in Florida described above by Wexner et al (1996b). In addition, a further five centres were included in addition to our own. Sixty-four patients were entered into the trial, and their demographic details are summarized in Table 20.48. Most ($n=48$) had undergone at least one previous operation to restore continence for a variety of aetiologies. Obstetric trauma ($n=19$), iatrogenic trauma ($n=11$), pudendal neuropathy ($n=10$), anal atresia ($n=7$), neurological damage ($n=6$), trauma ($n=6$), miscellaneous ($n=5$). The operation was usually performed in three stages with most ($n=54$) undergoing a delay procedure. The stimulators used were all purpose designed (NICE Inc, Florida, USA), but were the first generation. The complications that occurred after each stage are listed in Table 20.49.

At the time of review (1996), nine patients had not had their stoma closed, two had died from unrelated causes, two had failed for technical reasons and five were awaiting closure. Of the 55 patients whose stoma had been closed for one month, 44 (77%) had a good functional result and 11 had a poor functional result. Two of the latter were still

Table 20.46 Electrically stimulated neosphincter – functional outcome at 6 months follow-up (n = 12).

Continence category*	No. of patients	
	Preop.	*Postop.*
1	0	0
2	0	9
3	0	3
4	4	0
5	8	0

*1 = Continent to solids, liquids and flatus. 2 = Continent to solids and liquids but not flatus. 3 = Continent to solids but occasional episodes of liquid incontinence. 4 = Occasional episodes of incontinence of solids and frequent episodes of incontinence of liquids. 5 = Frequent episodes of incontinence of solids and liquids.

Table 20.47 Electrically stimulated neosphincter – anal and neoanal canal pressures (n = 12).

	Pressure (cmH_2O)
Preop. MBP	38 (25–60)
NP_{Off}	35 (29–42.5)
$NP_{Functioning}$	62 (49–75)
Preop. MAP	58 (33–90.5)
NP_{Max}	105 (69–124)

Values are medians with range in parentheses.
MBP, maximum basal pressure; MAP, maximum achieved pressure; NP_{Off}, neosphincter off pressure; $NP_{Functioning}$, functioning neosphincter pressure; NP_{Max}, maximum neosphincter pressure.

Table 20.48 Multicentre trial of electrically stimulated gracilis neosphincter – demographics.

No. of patients	64
Cleveland Clinic, Florida	15
Royal Infirmary of Edinburgh	13
The Royal London Hospital, Whitechapel	12
St George's Hospital, Sydney	8
Sahgren's Hospital, Gothenburg	7
University of Naples	5
Queen Elizabeth Hospital, Birmingham	4
Male/female	17/47
Age (years)	44.5 (15–76)
Follow-up (months)	16 (2–45)

Table 20.49 Multicentre trial of electrically stimulated gracilis neosphincter – postoperative complications.

Stage 1	
(Delay + defunctioning stoma)	
Saphenous nerve palsy	4
Mild lymphoedema	3
Mild wound infection	4
Parastomal hernia	1
Ileostomy fistula	1
Stage 2/3	
Leg wound sepsis	4
Perineal sepsis	
Mild	6
Moderate	5
Severe	3
Stimulator sepsis	3
DVT	3
Neuropraxia	3

incontinent, but nine had severe evacuatory difficulties. When all patients were assessed, there was a mean reduction in continence scores from 18.5 to 6 ($P<0.05$) (Jorge and Wexner, 1993) (Figure 20.56). There was also a significant increase in maximum sphincter pressures (Figure 20.57). At a median of 10 months follow-up (range 1–35 months) a good functional result was maintained in 29 patients (56%). Most of the subsequent failures were due to hardware complications, including plate migration and battery depletion. There were 27 recorded depletions in 21 patients and a median length of battery life of 11 months.

The following conclusions can thus be drawn from this study. Our preliminary results were reproduced in a multicentre setting with an initial good result being achieved in 70% of patients. This initial good result was negated by hardware deficiencies in a number of patients. Evacuatory difficulties were a major problem in 20% of patients. As a consequence of these findings we are now using a more reliable stimulator, which has been suitably modified (Medtronic Inc, USA). Patients are counselled that evacuatory problems may occur after neosphincter construction, particularly if they have previously had such problems. In the latter group we also warn that a conduit procedure may subsequently be required.

Baeten et al (1995) described their results using intramuscular stimulation in 1995. They use the terms 'dynamic graciloplasty' to describe their technique. Between 1986 and 1994, 52 patients (37 women, 15 men) were treated by dynamic graciloplasty. The causes of faecal incontinence were anal atresia ($n=12$), perineal trauma ($n=24$), cauda equina syndrome ($n=2$) and pudendal nerve lesions ($n=14$). Thus, 40 patients were equivalent to those we describe above and can be classified as incontinent patients due to a deficient anal sphincter alone. Most of these patients had undergone one or more unsuccessful incontinence operation (Table 20.50); 32 of these 40 patients (80%) were judged to

Figure 20.56 Multicentre neosphincter trial. Continence scores at one month following stoma closure.

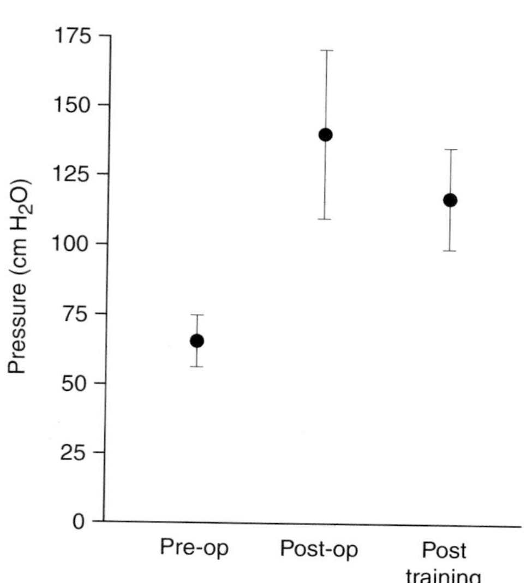

Figure 20.57 Multicentre neosphincter trial. Maximum sphincter pressures one month following stoma closure.

Table 20.50 Characteristics of the patients with severe faecal incontinence before dynamic graciloplasty, according to the cause of incontinence.

	Trauma	*Cauda lesion*	*Pudendopathy*
No. of patients	24 (46.2)	2 (3.8)	14 (26.9)
Age (years)	48 ± 11.0	44 ± 30.4	52 ± 10.2
Male sex – no. (%)	4 (7.7)	1 (1.9)	2 (3.8)
Duration of incontinence (years)	11 ± 11.6	13 ± 13.4	14 ± 11.7
No. with previous procedure			
Colostomy	3	0	1
Graciloplasty	1	0	1
Surgery	16	0	11
Biofeedback	7	0	5
Rectal sensibility (mL)	35 ± 14.3	100 ± 70.7	40 ± 19.3
Rectal capacity (mL)	150 ± 78.3	–	130 + 46.8

From Baeten et al (1995).

have had a successful result approximately 2 years after surgery. Success was assessed not only by incontinence scores but also by a variety of quality of life scores performed by an independent research worker. Compared with a permanent stoma, there are financial advantages too (Adang et al, 1998). The physiology data were also similar to our own, as were the morbidity data, although despite the absence of a 'delay' procedure, ischaemic necrosis of the gracilis did not appear to be a problem. However, the authors stressed the steep learning curve of the procedure, and in a separate article (Geerdes et al, 1996) they described in detail the complications that may occur and their management.

Problems may be categorized as technical, infective or physiological. They include failure of the distal part of the muscle to contract, which may be due to ischaemia, too tight a wrap which may cause stenosis and emptying difficulties or worse erosion of the muscle or tendon into the anal canal. An increased threshold of stimulation due to fibrosis may occur over time. We contend that this is more likely with intramuscular stimulation as opposed to neural stimulation. However, it can also be due to electrode displacement or fracture of electrode leads. Pain may be experienced in the transposed and stimulated gracilis muscle or in the knee, around the anal canal and over the neurostimulator or lead. Muscular pain may be caused by muscle fatigue. This can be reduced by decreasing the stimulating amplitude or frequency and restarting intermittent stimulation to retrain the muscle. If pain is only experienced when the stimulator is switched on, stimulation of sensory nerves through an open circuit is possible. Such pain is often felt in the knee. Pain over the stimulator pocket or the lead is often due to infection, or local tissue or skin irritation. Irritation over the pocket is treated by repositioning the stimulator in a deeper pocket.

Once infection has affected the hardware, antibiotics are rarely successful and removal is usually required. However, with the use of prophylactic systemic and local antibiotics, this should not be a major problem.

The functional outcome may be marred by difficulties in rectal evacuation, which is not related to anal stenosis (Rosen et al, 1998). The most likely reason for this problem is an underlying rectal sensory abnormality, which may not be as obvious preoperatively. As previously explained, this is a major problem in patients with anorectal atresia.

It should be noted that most patients treated worldwide by an electrically stimulated gracilis neosphincter have been difficult to deal with. Most have had multiple operations previously, and their only other option has been a permanent colostomy. It is expected that the complication rate will decrease if patients can be treated at an earlier stage.

Incontinent patients following pull-through procedures for anorectal atresia

The results of the electrically stimulated gracilis neosphincter in this group of patients is inferior to that of those patients described above who retain their rectum and anal canal. Not only do atresia patients lack the correct anatomical arrangement, but as a consequence their physiological defects are more profound. Thus, of our original nine patients with anorectal agenesis, four only retained their neosphincter and all complained of severe problems with anorectal function, particularly impairment of rectal evacuation. Interestingly, the only other group with a comparable experience to our own (Baeten et al, 1995) describe only 6 of 12 atresia patients (50%) successfully treated by dynamic graciloplasty. Similar problems with evacuation were experienced in this group, despite an absence of anal stenosis.

Since difficulty in evacuation has been the main problem after neosphincter formation in patients with anorectal agenesis, we have recently combined the technique with a conduit procedure when indicated. So far, nine patients have been treated with this combination, and after approximately a mean of 12 months follow-up, none have had to revert to a stoma. A variety of conduits may be used for this purpose (Krogh and Laurberg, 1998; Shankar et al, 1998).

Implantable materials

Dacron sling

The Dacron sling described by Labrow et al (1980) did not differ in principle from the Silastic rings used for the treatment of rectal prolapse (Jackman et al, 1980). A strip of Silastic sheet measuring approximately 1.5 cm in width was placed subcutaneously to encircle the anal canal. The Dacron-impregnated Silastic material was said to offer the mechanical advantage of elasticity in its longitudinal axis, thereby allowing some dilatation of the anal canal for the passage of the faecal bolus. The operation was performed with the patient in the prone or supine position. Incisions were made over both ischiorectal fossae (Figure 20.58a). A tunnel was developed posteriorly by division of the anococcygeal raphe (Figure 20.58b), which was then completed anteriorly to a depth of about 4 cm (Figure 20.58c). A 1.5–2.0-cm strip of the material was placed through the tunnel (Figure 20.58d), without twisting the sheet, so that it encircled the anus (Figure 20.58e). The appropriate tension on the Dacron sheet was tested using the tip of the index finger in the anus. When the optimum tension was determined, the two ends (Figure 20.58f) were secured using the TA 30 or GIA stapler (Figure 20.58g).

Horn et al (1985) reviewed the results among 16 patients operated upon at the Lahey Clinic. Three patients developed postoperative urinary retention and the operation site became infected, causing skin erosion necessitating removal and reinsertion of the sling. One patient died of an intercurrent illness, leaving only 15 for follow-up. Three patients were reported to be continent of liquids and solids, four were only continent of solids, five had severe leakage and three were absolute failures. Labrow et al (1980) reported good results in 50% of their patients. Stricker et al (1988), however, indicated that only 6 of 14 patients were improved by this procedure. The procedure now seems to have become obsolete and, because there are better alternatives, it cannot be recommended.

Magnetic occlusion device

Schier et al (1986) used a magnetic ring placed in the perianal region around a pull-through procedure in children with neuropathic incontinence but only 9 of 25 patients achieved acceptable results and sepsis was a common complication. This technique is now of historical interest only.

Implantable artificial sphincter

Artificial sphincter implants have been used for urinary incontinence for many years. The prosthesis has undergone various modifications and the cumulative risk of mechanical failure with the AMS 800, which is the latest model used for urinary incontinence, is less than 5% after 2.5 years (Hald, 1986). The principal elements of the device are an inflatable cuff with a pressure-regulating balloon and a pump. The urinary device was modified so that the cuff was placed around the anus, the balloon lay extraperitoneally near the bladder, and the pump or control assembly was in the scrotum (Figure 20.59). Christiansen and Lorentzen (1987) originally reported a successful outcome with this device in a man with neurogenic faecal incontinence. In a subsequent report using the same device, Christiansen and Spars (1992) performed the operation in 12 patients. In two patients severe infection ensued, and the device had to be explanted. Of the remaining patients, seven were described as having normal continence and three had episodic incontinence for gas and liquid.

Lehur et al (1996) implanted the AMS 800 device in 14 consecutive patients (Lehur et al, 1996) between 1989 and 1995. After a median of 20 months follow-up, three devices had to be removed because of erosion, sepsis or pain. Rupture of the cuff occurred in another patient and needed replacement. In two further patients the position of the control pump in the scrotum needed repositioning. Of the 10 patients with an activated sphincter for more than 4 months, nine had normal continence for solid or liquid stools and one patient remained incontinent. Wong et al (1996) reported similar results.

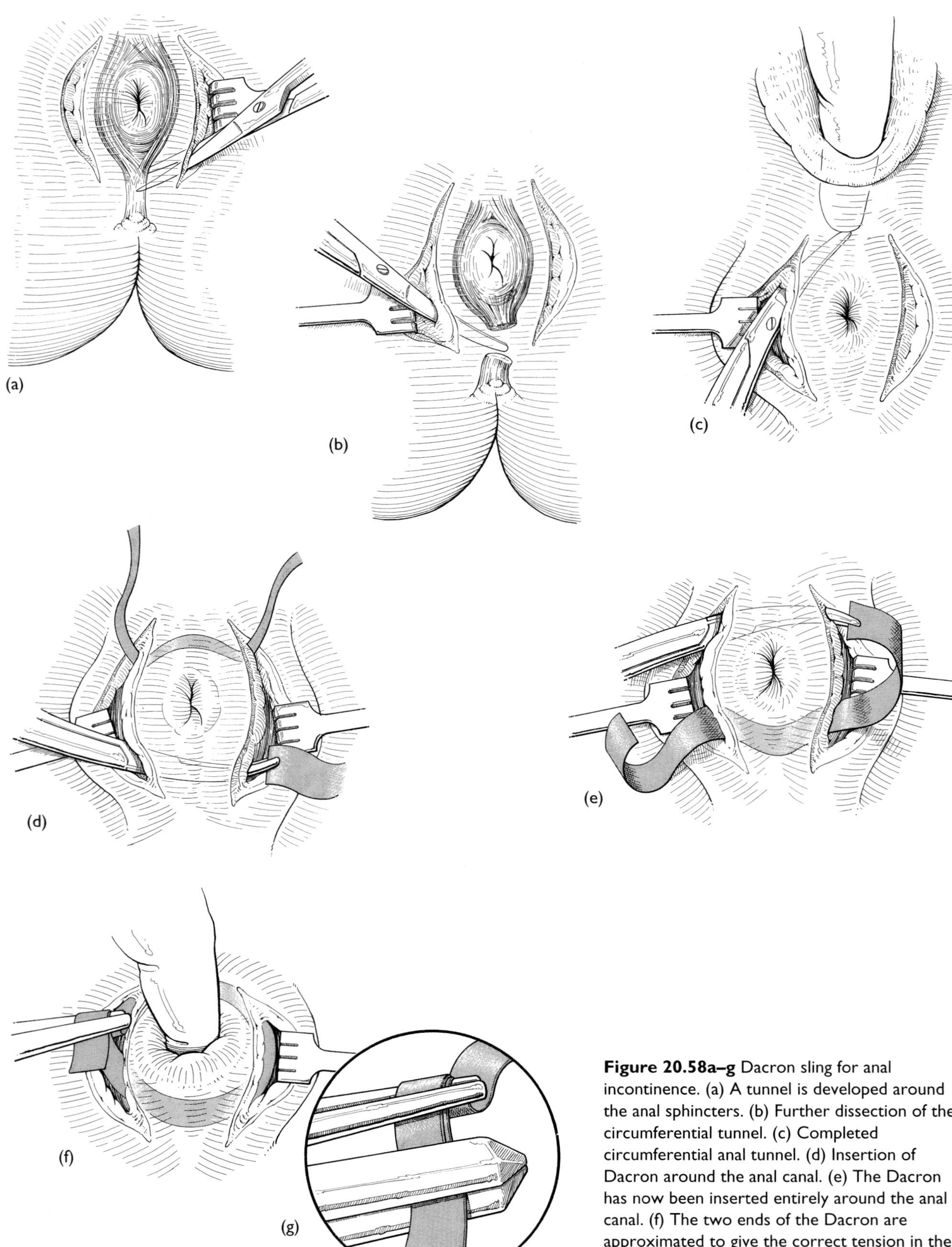

Figure 20.58a–g Dacron sling for anal incontinence. (a) A tunnel is developed around the anal sphincters. (b) Further dissection of the circumferential tunnel. (c) Completed circumferential anal tunnel. (d) Insertion of Dacron around the anal canal. (e) The Dacron has now been inserted entirely around the anal canal. (f) The two ends of the Dacron are approximated to give the correct tension in the anal canal. (g) The two ends of the Dacron are approximated with staples.

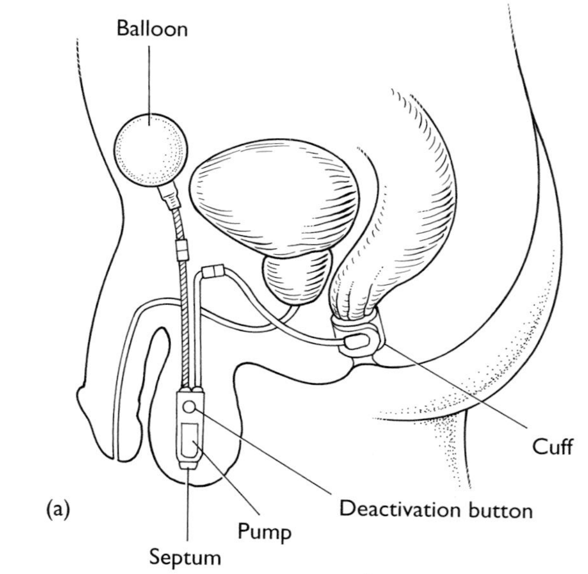

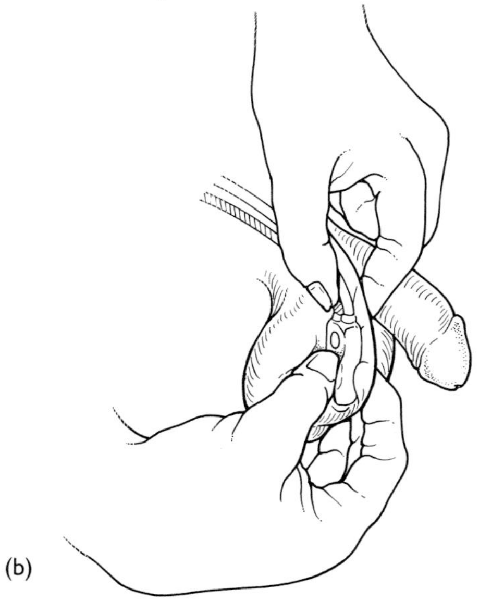

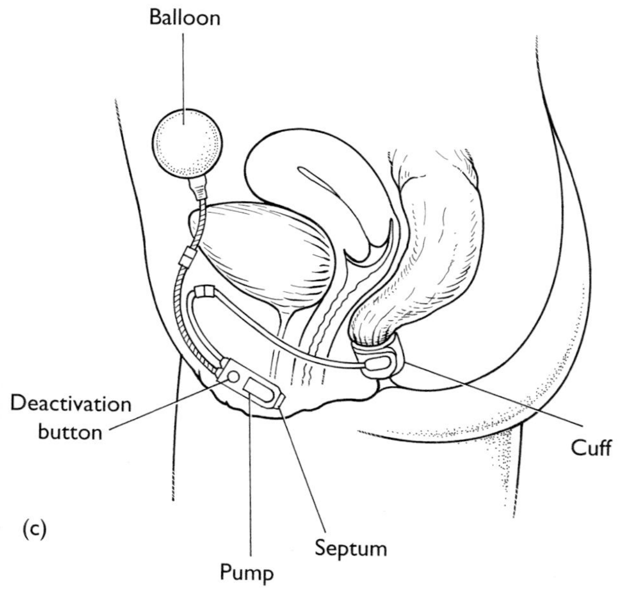

Balloon
Cuff
Deactivation button
Pump
Septum
(a)

(b)

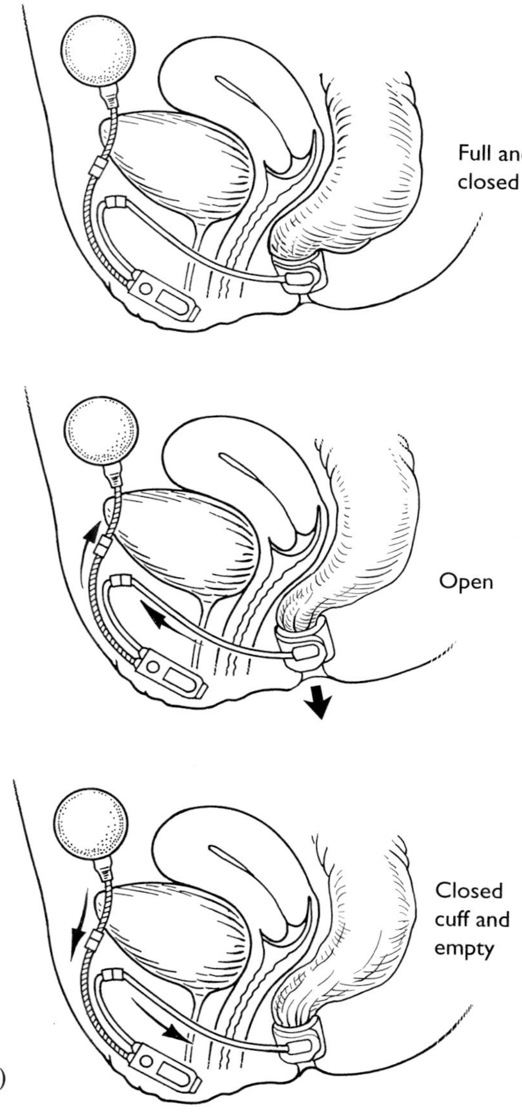

Balloon
Deactivation button
Cuff
Pump
Septum
(c)

Full and closed
Open
Closed cuff and empty
(d)

Figure 20.59a–d Artificial bowel sphincter. (a) A cuff is placed around the anal canal. An inflatable pump control assembly is placed in the scrotum and the balloon reservoir under the symphysis pubis. (b) The pump in males is placed in the scrotum. To open the cuff to defecate, the pump must be squeezed and released several times. (c) The same arrangement is used in women but the pump is placed in the labia. (d) When the cuff is closed the stool stays in the rectum. When the pump is repeatedly squeezed (in the labia in women) the cuff opens and the bowel can empty. Fluid then automatically returns to the cuff which again closes around the anal canal.

The urinary device has now been modified specifically for use in anal incontinence, and is known as the ABS[R] Artificial Bowel Sphincter (Pfizer-American Medical Systems P-AMS, Minneapolis, MN, USA). The modifications include larger cuffs, a reinforced cuff closing system which is more resistant to straining effort, a deactivation button on the control pump, which allows the cuff to be left deflated for a prolonged period of time without surgery, an access port located at the end of the pump, which allows fluid to be added to the system without additional surgery (Michot et al, 1997).

It is too early to determine how effective this modified device will be. However, we remain somewhat sceptical about its long-term future. Not only is there the risk of sepsis, but any foreign body applied so close to the rectum and anal canal is likely eventually to erode through into the bowel lumen. Nevertheless, the experience by the group in Nantes (Lehur et al, 1998) and from St Marks (Vaizey et al, 1998) suggest that the artificial bowel sphincter may be an important therapeutic advance for the treatment of faecal incontinence.

Intestinal stoma

There are some patients who remain incontinent despite repeated surgical endeavour and who eventually accept an intestinal stoma. In many of these patients there is a sense of relief that they now have some control over faecal evacuation, even though this may be at the expense of having to wear an appliance. Some patients have such appalling anal function when first seen that an intestinal stoma is advised as definitive treatment. Other patients only accept an intestinal stoma when all other endeavours have failed. We prefer an end colostomy, provided there is no colonic motility disorder, so that patients may have the option of managing their stoma by irrigation. Under these circumstances the upper rectum is oversewn and an end colostomy raised through a small trephine in the left rectus muscle. Some of these patients continue to have troublesome incontinence of mucus from the rectal stump, and may require a proctectomy. A few patients prefer an ileostomy to an end colostomy, largely due to problems of odour attending a colostomy, and some of these opt to have a reservoir ileostomy.

REFERENCES

Aaronson I & Nixon HH (1972) A clinical evaluation of anorectal pressure studies in the diagnosis of Hirschsprung's disease. *Gut* **13**: 138–146.

Ackroyd R & Nour S (1994) Long-term faecal continence in infants born with anorectal malformations. *J R Soc Med* **87**: 695–696.

Adang EMM, Engel GL, Rutten FFH, Geerdes BP & Baeten CGMI (1998) Cost-effectiveness of dynamic graciloplasty in patients with fecal incontinence. *Dis Colon Rectum* **41**: 725–734.

Akervall S, Fasth S, Nordgren S, Oresland T & Hulten L (1989) Rectal reservoir and sensory function studied by graded isobaric distension in normal man. *Gut* **30**: 496–502.

Allen-Mersh TG, Henry MM & Nicholls RJ (1987) Natural history of anterior mucosal prolapse. *Br J Surg* **74**: 679–682.

Alva J, Mendeloff AI & Schuster MM (1967) Reflex and electromyographic abnormalities associated with faecal incontinence. *Gastroenterology* **53**: 101.

Ambrose S & Keighley MRB (1986) Outpatient measurement of perineal descent. *Ann R Coll Surg Engl* **67**: 306–308.

Amu O, Rajendran S & Bolaji II (1998) Maternal choice alone should not determine method of delivery. *BMJ* **317**: 463–464.

Andreoli F, Ballon F, Bigotti A et al (1986) Anorectal continence and bladder function. Effects of major sacral resection. *Dis Colon Rectum* **29**: 647–652.

Andromanakos N, Deen KI, Grant EA & Keighley MRB (1996) Anorectal physiology in the assessment and management of patients with faecal incontinence. *Hellenic J Gastroenterol* **9**: 151–154.

Anonymous (1994) *BMJ* **309**: 815–816.

Arabi Y, Alexander-Williams J & Keighley MRB (1977) Anal pressure in haemorrhoids and anal fissure. *Am J Surg* **134**: 608–610.

Archibald KC & Goldsmith EJ (1967) Sphincteric electromyography. *Arch Phys Med Rehabil* **48**: 2349–2352.

Arhan P, Faverdin C & Thouvenot J (1972) Anorectal motility in sick children. *Scand J Gastroenterol* **7**: 309–314.

Arhan P, Faverdin C, Devroede G et al (1994) Biofeedback re-education of faecal continence in children. *Int J Colorectal Dis* **9**: 128–133.

Arnaud A, Sarles JC, Sielezneff I, Orsoni P & Joly A (1991) Sphincter repair without overlapping for fecal incontinence. *Dis Colon Rectum* **34**: 744–747.

Atri SB (1980) The treatment of complete rectal prolapse by graciloplasty. *Br J Surg* **67**: 431–432.

Baeten C, Spaans F & Fluks A (1988) An implanted neuromuscular stimulator for faecal incontinence following previously implanted gracilis muscle. *Dis Colon Rectum* **31**: 134–137.

Baeten CGM, Konsten J, Spaans F et al (1991) Dynamic graciloplasty for treatment of faecal incontinence. *Lancet* **338**: 1163–1165.

Baeten CGMI, Geerdes BP, Adang EMM et al (1995) Anal dynamic graciloplasty in the treatment of intractable fecal incontinence. *N Engl J Med* **332**: 1600–1605.

Banks S & Marks IN (1977) The aetiology, diagnosis and treatment of constipation and diarrhoea in geriatric patients. *S Afr Med J* **51**: 409–414.

Bannister JJ, Abouzekry L & Read NW (1987) Effect of aging on anorectal function. *Gut* **28**: 353–357.

Bannister JJ, Read NW, Donnelly TC & Sun WM (1989) External

and internal anal sphincter responses to rectal distension in normal subjects and in patients with idiopathic faecal incontinence. *Br J Surg* **76**: 617–621.

Barrett JA (1992) Colorectal disorders in elderly people. *BMJ* **305**: 764–766.

Barrett JA, Brocklehurst JC, Kiff ES, Ferguson G & Faragher EB (1989) Anal function in geriatric patients with faecal incontinence. *Gut* **30**: 1244–1251.

Bartolo DCC (1984) Anorectal function in incontinence. MS thesis. London: University of London.

Bartolo DCC & Roe AM (1986) Obstructed defaecation. *Br J Hosp Med* **35**: 228–236.

Bartolo DCC, Jarratt JA & Read NW (1983a) The use of conventional electromyography to assess external and sphincter neuropathy in man. *J Neurol Neurosurg Psychiatry* **46**: 115–118.

Bartolo DCC, Jarratt JA & Read NW (1983b) The cutaneo-anal reflex: a useful index of neuropathy. *Br J Surg* **70**: 660–663.

Bartolo DCC, Jarratt JA, Read MG, Donnelly TC & Read NW (1983c) The role of partial denervation of the puborectalis in idiopathic faecal incontinence. *Br J Surg* **70**: 664–667.

Bartolo DCC, Read NW, Jarratt JA, Read MG, Donnelly TC & Johnson AG (1983d) Differences in anal sphincter function and clinical presentation in patients with pelvic floor descent. *Gastroenterology* **85**: 68–75.

Bartolo DCC, Roe AM, Virjee J & Mortensen NJMcC (1985) Evacuation proctography in obstructed defaecation and rectal intussusception. *Br J Surg* **72** (Suppl): 111–116.

Bartolo DCC, Roe AM, Locke-Edmunds JC & Mortensen NJMcC (1986a) Flap-valve theory of anorectal continence. *Br J Surg* **73**: 1012–1014.

Bartolo DCC, Roe AM, Locke-Edmunds JC & Mortensen NJMcC (1986b) Rectal intussusception. The commonest abnormality in the descending perineum syndrome. *Gut* **27**: A624.

Bartolo DCC, Roe AM & Mortensen NJMcCC (1986c) The relationship between perineal descent and denervation of the puborectalis in continent patients. *Int J Colorectal Dis* **1**: 91–95.

Bartram A & Sultan AH (1995) Anal endosonography in faecal incontinence. *Gut* **37**: 4–6.

Baumgarten HC, Holstein AF & Stelzner F (1971) Differences in the innervation of the large intestine and internal anal sphincter in mammals and humans. *Verh Anat Ges* **66**: 43–47.

Beersiek F, Parks AG & Swash M (1979) Pathogenesis of anorectal incontinence: a histometric study of the anal sphincter musculature. *J Neurol Sci* **42**: 111–127.

Beevors MA, Lubowski DZ, King DW & Carlton MA (1991) Pudendal nerve function in women with symptomatic utero-vaginal prolapse. *Int J Colorectal Dis* **6**: 24–28.

Ben-Hur N, Gilai A, Golan J, Sagher U & Isaac M (1980) Reconstruction of the anal sphincter by gracilis muscle transfer: the value of electromyography in the preoperative assessment and postoperative management of the patient. *Br J Plast Surg* **33**: 681–690.

Bennett RC (1972) Sensory receptors of the anorectum. *Aust NZ J Surg* **42**: 42–45.

Bennett RC & Duthie DL (1964) The functional importance of the internal anal sphincter. *Br J Surg* **51**: 355–357.

Bennett RC, Freidman MHW & Goligher JC (1963) Late results of haemorrhoidectomy by ligature and excision. *BMJ* **2**: 216–219.

Bick DE (1994) Characterisation of long-term postpartum morbidity. Thesis, Medical School, University of Birmingham.

Binnie NR, Kawimbe BM, Papachrysostomou M & Smith AN (1990) Use of the pudendo-anal reflex in the treatment of neurogenic faecal incontinence. *Gut* **31**: 1051–1055.

Blaisdell PC (1940) Repair of the incontinent sphincter arc. *Surg Gynecol Obstet* **70**: 692–697.

Boulos BP & Arauje JGC (1984) Adequate internal sphincterotomy for chronic anal fissure: subcutaneous or open technique? *Br J Surg* **71**: 360–362.

Brain AJL & Keily EM (1989) Posterior sagittal anorectoplasty for reoperation in children with anorectal malformations. *Br J Surg* **76**: 57–59.

Braun JC, Treutner KH, Dreuw B, Klimaszewski M & Schumpelick V (1994) Vectormanometry for differential diagnosis of fecal incontinence. *Dis Colon Rectum* **37**: 989–996.

Briel JW, Schouten WR, Vlot EA, Smits S & Van Kessel I (1997) Clinical value of colonic irrigation in patients with continence disturbance. *Dis Colon Rectum* **40**: 802–805.

Brocklehurst JC & Khan MY (1969) A study of faecal stasis in old age and the use of Dorbanex in its prevention. *Gerontol Clin* **11**: 293–300.

Brook A (1991) Bowel distress and emotional conflict. *J R Soc Med* **84**: 39–42.

Browning GGP & Motson RW (1983) Results of Parks' operation for faecal incontinence after anal sphincter injury. *BMJ* **286**: 1873–1875.

Browning GGP & Motson RW (1984) Anal sphincter injury. Management and results of Parks sphincter repair. *Ann Surg* **199**: 351–356.

Browning GGP & Parks AG (1983) Postanal repair for neuropathic faecal incontinence: correlation of clinical results and anal canal pressures. *Br J Surg* **70**: 101–104.

Browning GGP, Rutter KPR, Motson RW & Neill ME (1983) Postanal repair for idiopathic faecal incontinence. In Sir Alan Parks Memorial Symposium. *Ann R Coll Surg Engl* **65** (Suppl): 30–33.

Browning GGP, Henry MM & Motson RW (1988) Combined sphincter repair and postanal repair for the treatment of complicated injuries to the anal sphincters. *Ann R Coll Surg Engl* **70**: 58–59.

Bruck CE, Lubowski DZ & King DW (1988) Do patients with haemorrhoids have pelvic floor denervation? *Int J Colorectal Dis* **3**: 210–214.

Buchmann P, Mogg GAG, Alexander-Williams J, Allan RN & Keighley MRB (1980) Relationship of proctitis and rectal capacity in Crohn's disease. *Gut* **21**: 137–140.

Buntzen S, Nordgren S, Delbro D & Hulten L (1995) Anal and rectal motility responses to distension of the urinary bladder in man. *Int J Colorectal Dis* **10**: 148–151.

Burke RE, Levine ON, Zajac FE, Tsairis P & Engel WK (1971) Mammalian motor units: physiological/histochemical correlation in three fibre types in cat gastrocnemius muscle. *Science* **174**: 709–712.

Burleigh DE (1983) The internal anal sphincter. In Sir Alan Parks Memorial Symposium. *Ann R Coll Surg Engl* **65** (Suppl): 25–26.

Burnett SJD & Bartram CI (1991) Endosonographic variations in the normal internal and sphincter. *Int J Colorectal Dis* **6**: 2–4.

Buser WD & Miner PBJr (1986) Delayed rectal sensation with fecal incontinence. *Gastroenterology* **91**: 1186–1191.

Butler ECB (1954) Complete rectal prolapse following removal of tumours of the cauda equina. *Proc R Soc Med* **47**: 521–522.

Cali R, Blatchford GJ, Perry RE, Pitsch RM, Thorson AG & Christensen MA (1992) Normal variation in anorectal manometry. *Dis Colon Rectum* **35**: 1161–1164.

Carapeti E, Kamm MA, Evans BE & Phillips R (1998) Topical phenylephrine increases anal sphincter resting pressure – a possible treatment for faecal incontinence. Paper presented at the Royal Society for Medicine, London, 25 February 1998.

Cardozo L & Khullar V (1994) Urinary incontinence in adult women. *Prescribers J* **34**: 134–141.

Carlstedt A, Nordgren S, Fasth S, Appelgren L & Julten L (1988) Sympathetic nervous influence on the internal anal sphincter and rectum in man. *Int J Colorectal Dis* **3**: 90–95.

Caro CG, Pedley TJ, Schroter RC & Seed WA (1978) *The Mechanics of the Circulation*. Oxford: Oxford University Press.

Carpentier A & Chachques JC (1985) Myocardial substitution with a stimulated skeletal muscle: first successful clinical case. *Lancet* **i**: 1267.

Castro AF & Pittman RE (1978) Repair of the incontinent sphincter. *Dis Colon Rectum* **21**: 183–187.

Cavina E, Seccia M, Evangelista G et al (1990) Perineal colostomy and electrostimulated gracilis neosphincter after abdomino-perineal resection of the colon and anorectum: a surgical experience and follow-up study in 47 cases. *Int J Colorectal Dis* **5**: 6–11.

Cerulli MA, Nikoomanesh P & Schuster MM (1979) Progress in biofeedback conditioning for faecal incontinence. *Gastroenterology* **76**: 742–746.

Chantraine A (1973) EMG examination of the anal and urethral sphincters. In Desmedt JE (ed.) *New Developments in Electromyography and Clinical Neurophysiology*, Vol. 2, pp 421–432.

Chen AS-H, Luchtefeld MA, Senagore AJ, MacKeigan JM & Hoyt C (1998) Pudendal nerve latency: does it predict outcome of anal sphincter repair? *Dis Colon Rectum* **41**: 1005–1009.

Chia YW, Lee TKY, Kour KH & Tan ES (1996) Microchip implants on the anterior sacral roots in patients with spinal trauma: does it improve bowel function? *Dis Colon Rectum* **39**: 690–694.

Chittenden AS (1930) Reconstruction of anal sphincter by muscle slips from the glutei. *Ann Surg* **92**: 152–154.

Christiansen J & Lorentzen M (1987) Implantation of artificial sphincter for anal incontinence. *Lancet* **i**: 244–245.

Christiansen J & Pedersen IK (1987) Traumatic anal incontinence: results of surgical repair. *Dis Colon Rectum* **30**: 189–191.

Christiansen J & Roed-Petersen K (1993) Clinical assessment of the anal continence plug. *Dis Colon Rectum* **36**: 740–742.

Christiansen J & Skomorowska E (1987) Persisting incontinence after postanal repair treated by anterior perineoplasty. *Int J Colorectal Dis* **2**: 9–11.

Christiansen J & Sparso B (1992) Treatment of anal incontinence by an implantable prosthetic anal sphincter. *Ann Surg* **214**: 383–386.

Christiansen J, Sorensen M & Rasmussen OO (1990) Gracilis muscle transposition for faecal incontinence. *Br J Surg* **77**: 1039–1040.

Cohen M, Rosen L, Khubchandari I, Sheets J, Stasik J & Riether R (1986) Rationale for medical or surgical therapy in anal incontinence. *Dis Colon Rectum* **29**: 120–122.

Coller JA (1987) Clinical application of anorectal manometry. *Gastroenterol Clin North Am* **16**: 17–33.

Collins CD, Duthie HL, Shelley T & Whittaker GE (1967) Force in the anal canal and anal continence. *Gut* **8**: 354–360.

Congilosi SM, Johnson DRE, Medot M et al (1997) Experimental model of pudendal nerve innervation of a skeletal muscle neosphincter for faecal incontinence. *Br J Surg* **84**: 1269–1273.

Connell AM, Hilton C, Irving G, Lennard-Jones JE & Miesiewicz JJ (1965) Variation of bowel habit in two population studies. *BMJ* **2**: 1095–1099.

Cook TA & Mortensen NJMcC (1998) Management of faecal incontinence following obstetric injury. *Br J Surg* **88**: 293–299.

Corman ML (1979) Management of faecal incontinence by gracilis muscle transposition. *Dis Colon Rectum* **22**: 290–292.

Corman ML (1980) Follow up evaluation of gracilis muscle transposition for fecal incontinence. *Dis Colon Rectum* **23**: 552–555.

Corman ML (1983) The management of anal incontinence. *Surg Clin North Am* **63**: 177–192.

Corman ML (1985a) Anal incontinence following obstetrical injury. *Dis Colon Rectum* **28**: 86–89.

Corman ML (1985b) Gracilis muscle transposition for anal incontinence: late results. *Br J Surg* **72** (Suppl): S21.

Cornes H, Bartolo DCC & Stirrat GM (1991) Changes in anal canal sensation after childbirth. *Br J Surg* **78**: 74–77.

Cowan JMA, Rothwell JC, Dick JPR, Thompson PD, Day BL & Marsden CD (1984) Abnormalities in central motor pathway conduction in multiple sclerosis. *Lancet* **ii**: 304–307.

Critchlow JF, Houliham MJ, Landolt CC & Weinsterin ME (1985) Primary sphincter repair in anorectal trauma. *Dis Colon Rectum* **28**: 945–947.

Cuesta MA, Meijer S, Derksen EJ, Boutkan H & Meuwissen SGM (1992) Anal sphincter imaging in fecal incontinence using endosonography. *Dis Colon Rectum* **35**: 59–63.

Cywes S, Cremin BJ & Louw JH (1971) Assessment of continence after treatment for anorectal agenesis: a clinical and radiological correlation. *J Pediatr Surg* **6**: 132–137.

Davies MG, Fulton GJ, Hagen OP (1995) Clinical biology of nitric oxide. *Br J Surg* **82**: 1598–1610.

Davis GR, Brown IT, Schwartz MS & Swash M (1983) A dedicated microcomputer-based instrument for internal analysis of multicomponent waveforms in single fibre EMG. *Electroencephalogr Clin Neurophysiol* **56**: 110–113.

Deen KI, Kumar D, Williams JG, Olliff J & Keighley MRB (1993a) The prevalence of anal sphincter defects in faecal incontinence: a prospective endosonic study. *Gut* **34**: 685–688.

Deen KI, Kumar D, Williams JG, Olliff J & Keighley MRB (1993b) Anal sphincter defects: correlation between endoanal ultrasound and surgery. *Ann Surg* **281**: 201–205.

Deen KI, Oya M, Ortiz J & Keighley MRB (1993c) Randomized trial comparing three forms of pelvic floor repair for neuropathic faecal incontinence. *Br J Surg* **80**: 794–798.

Deen KI, Williams JG, Kumar D & Keighley MRB (1993d) Anal sphincter surgery for faecal incontinence: the role of endosonography. *Colo-proctology* **6**: 352–355.

Deen KI, Kumar D, Williams JG, Chir M, Grant EAA & Keighley MRB (1995) Randomized trial of internal anal sphincter plication with pelvic floor repair for neuropathic fecal incontinence. *Dis Colon Rectum* **38**: 14–18.

Delechenaut P, Leroi AM, Weber J, Touchais JY, Czernichow P & Denis PH (1992) Relationship between clinical symptoms of anal incontinence and the results of anorectal manometry. *Dis Colon Rectum* **35**: 847–849.

Denny-Brown D & Robertson EG (1935) An investigation of the nervous control of defaecation. *Brain* **58**: 256–310.

deSouza NM, Kmiot WA, Puni R et al (1995) High resolution magnetic resonance imaging of the anal sphincter using an internal coil. *Gut* **37**: 284–287.

Devesa JM, Vicente E, Enriquez JM et al (1992) Total fecal incontinence – a new method of gluteus maximus transportation: preliminary results and report of previous experience with similar procedures. *Dis Colon Rectum* **35**: 339–349.

Devesa JM, Fernandez JM, Gallego BR, Vicente E, Nuno J & Enriquez JM (1997) Bilateral gluteoplasty for fecal incontinence. *Dis Colon Rectum* **40**: 883–888.

De Vries PA (1984) The surgery of anorectal anomalies. Reoperation for fecal incontinence. *Curr Probl Surg* **21**: 59–60.

Dick AC, McCallion WA, Brown S & Boston VE (1996) Antegrade colonic enemas. *Br J Surg* **83**: 642–643.

Dick JPR, Cowan JMA, Day BL et al (1984) The corticomotorneurone connection is normal in Parkinson's disease. *Nature* **310**: 407–409.

Dittertov L & Grim M (1983) Puborektalisersatz durch modrfizierte grazilispfastik. In Hofman V & Kapherr S (eds) *Anorektale Fehlbildungen*, pp 127–129. Stuttgart: Gustav Fischer.

Donald I (1979) *Practical Obstetric Problems*, p 817. London: Lloyd-Luke.

Donnelly VS, O'Connell PR & O'Herlihy C (1996) The effect of HRT on anorectal function in postmenopausal women with faecal incontinence – a preliminary study. Paper presented at the 8th International Congress on Menopause, 3–7 November, Sydney, Australia.

Donnelly VS, O'Herlihy C, Campbell DM & O'Connell PR (1998) Postpartum fecal incontinence is more common in women with irritable bowel syndrome. *Dis Colon Rectum* **41**: 586–589.

Drossman DA, Sandler RS, McKee DC & Lovitz AJ (1982) Bowel patterns among subjects not seeking health care. Use of a questionnaire to identify a population with bowel dysfunction. *Gastroenterology* **83**: 529–534.

Duibowitz V & Brooke MH (1973) *Muscle Biopsy: A Modern Approach*. London: WB Saunders.

Duthie HL (1971) Progress report: anal continence. *Gut* **12**: 844–852.

Duthie HL (1979) The anorectal region. In *Scientific Basis of Gastroenterology*, pp 477–484. Edinburgh: Churchill Livingstone.

Duthie HL & Bennett RC (1963) The relationship of sensation in the anal canal to functional anal sphincter: a possible factor in anal continence. *Gut* **4**: 179–182.

Duthie HL & Gairns FW (1960) Sensory nerve endings and sensation in the anal region of man. *Br J Surg* **47**: 585–595.

Duthie HL & Watts JM (1965) Contribution of the external anal sphincter to the pressure zone in the anal canal. *Gut* **6**: 64–68.

Duthie HL, Kwong NK & Brown B (1970) Adaptability of the anal canal to distension. *Br J Surg* **57**: 388 (Abstract).

Dyke PJ (1986) Detection thresholds of cutaneous sensations in health and disease in man. In Yaksh TL (ed.) *Spinal Afferent Processing*, pp 345–362. New York: Plenum Press.

Eckardt VF & Elmer T (1991) Reliability of anal pressure measurements. *Dis Colon Rectum* **34**: 72–77.

Eckardt VF & Kanzler G (1993) How reliable is digital examination for the evaluation of anal sphincter tone? *Int J Colorectal Dis* **8**: 95–97.

Eckardt VF, Jung B, Fischer B, Lierse W (1994) Anal endosonography in healthy subjects and patients with idiopathic fecal incontinence. *Dis Colon Rectum* **37**: 235–242.

Edgerton VR (1970) Morphology and histochemistry of the soleus muscle for normal and exercised rats. *Am J Anat* **127**: 81–87.

Ehrentheil OF & Wells EP (1955) Megacolon in psychotic patients: a clinical entity. *Gastroenterology* **29**: 285–290.

Elliot MS, Hancke E, Henry MM et al (1987) Faecal incontinence (symposium). *Int J Colorectal Dis* **3**: 173–186.

Emblem R, Dhaenens G, Stien R, Morkrid L, Aasen AO & Bergan A (1994) The importance of anal endosonography in the evaluation of idiopathic fecal incontinence. *Dis Colon Rectum* **37**: 42–48.

Enck P, Kuhlbusch R, Lubke H, Frieling T & Erckenbrecht JF (1989a) Age and sex and anorectal manometry in incontinence. *Dis Colon Rectum* **32**: 1026–1030.

Enck P, Arping G, Engle S, Bielefeldt K & Erckenbrecht JF (1989b) Effects of cisapride on ano-rectal sphincter function. *Aliment Pharmacol Ther* **3**: 539–545.

Enck P, Bielefeldt K, Rathmann W, Purrmann J, Tschope D & Erckenbrecht JF (1991) Epidemiology of faecal incontinence in selected patients groups. *Int J Colorectal Dis* **6**: 143–146.

Enck P, Daublin G, Lubke HJ & Strohmeyer G (1994) Long-term efficacy of biofeedback training for fecal incontinence. *Dis Colon Rectum* **37**: 997–1001.

Engel AF & Brummelkamp WH (1994) Secondary surgery after failed postanal or anterior sphincter repair. *Int J Colorectal Dis* **9**: 187–190.

Engel AF, Kamm MA, Sultan AH, Bartram CI & Nicholls RJ (1994) Anterior anal sphincter repair in patients with obstetric trauma. *Br J Surg* **81**: 1231–1234.

Engel AF, Kamm MA, Bartra CI & Nicholls RJ (1995) Relationship of symptoms in faecal incontinence to specific sphincter abnormalities. *Int J Colorectal Dis* **10**: 152–155.

Engel AF, Lunniss PJ, Kamm MA & Phillips RKS (1997) Sphincteroplasty for incontinence after surgery for idiopathic fistula in ano. *Int J Colorectal Dis* **12**: 323–325.

Engel BT, Nikoomanesh P & Schuster MM (1974) Operant conditioning of rectosphincteric response in the treatment of fecal incontinence. *N Engl J Med* **290**: 646–649.

Engel WK (1971) Ragged red fibres in ophthalmoplegia syndromes and their differential diagnosis. In *Proceedings of the 2nd International Congress on Muscle Diseases, Perth*, p 237. Amsterdam: Excerpta Medica.

Enriquez-Navascues JM & Devesa-Mugica JM (1994) Traumatic anal incontinence. Role of unilateral gluteus maximus transposition supplementing and supporting direct anal sphincteroplasty. *Dis Colon Rectum* **37**: 766–769.

Erckenbrecht JF, Winter HJ, Cimir I, Berger H, Berges W & Weinbeck M (1984) Is incontinence in diabetes mellitus due to diabetic autonomous neuropathy? In Roman C (ed.) *Gastrointestinal Motility*, pp 483–484. London: MTP Press.

Exton-Smith AN (1973) Constipation in geriatrics. In Jones FA & Goddings GW (eds) *Management of Constipation*, pp 156–175. Oxford: Blackwell Scientific.

Fabris F & Robino A (1971) Diarrhoea and constipation in the aged. *G Gerontol* **19**: 200–219.

Falk PM, Blatchford GJ, Cali RL, Christensen MA & Thorson AG (1994) Transanal ultrasound and manometry in the evaluation of fecal incontinence. *Dis Colon Rectum* **37**: 468–472.

Fang DT, Nivatvongs S, Vermeulen FD, Herman FN, Goldberg SM & Rotherberger DA (1984) Overlapping sphincteroplasty for acquired anal incontinence. *Dis Colon Rectum* **27**: 720–722.

Farouk R & Bartolo DCC (1994) The use of endoluminal ultrasound in the assessment of paitents with faecal incontinence. *J R Coll Surg Edinb* **39**: 312–318.

Farouk R, Duthie GS, Pryde A, McGregor AB & Bartolo DCC (1993) Internal anal sphincter dysfunction in neurogenic faecal incontinence. *Br J Surg* **80**: 259–261.

Farouk R, Duthie GS, MacGregor AB & Bartolo DCC (1994) Evidence of electromechanical dissociation of the internal anal sphincter in idiopathic fecal incontinence. *Dis Colon Rectum* **37**: 595–601.

Farthing MJG & Lennard-Jones JE (1978) Sensibility of the rectum to distension and the anorectal distension reflex in ulcerative colitis. *Gut* **19**: 64–69.

Faucheron JL, Hannoun L, Thome C & Parc R (1994) Is fecal continence improved by nonstimulated gracilis muscle transposition. *Dis Colon Rectum* **37**: 979–983.

Favetta U, Amato A, Interisano A & Pescatori M (1996) Clinical, manometric and sonographic assessment of the anal sphincters. *Int J Colorectal Dis* **11**: 163–166.

Felt-Bersma RJF, Janssen JJWM, Klinkenberg-Knol EC, Hoitsma

HFW & Meuwissen SGM (1989) Soiling: anorectal function and results of treatment. *Int J Colorectal Dis* **4**: 37–40.

Felt-Bersma RJF, Cuesta MA, Koorevaar M et al (1992) Anal endosonography: relationship with anal manometry and neurophysiologic tests. *Dis Colon Rectum* **35**: 944–949.

Felt-Bersma RJF, van Baren R, Koorevaar M, Strijers RL & Cuesta MA (1995) Unsuspected sphincter defects shown by anal endosonography after anorectal surgery. *Dis Colon Rectum* **38**: 249–253.

Felt-Bersma RJF, Cuesta MA & Koorevaar M (1996) Anal sphincter repair improves anorectal function and endosonographic image. *Dis Colon Rectum* **39**: 878–885.

Felt-Bersma RJF, Poen AC, Cuesta MA & Meuwissen SGM (1997) Anal sensitivity test: what does it measure and do we need it? *Dis Colon Rectum* **40**: 811–816.

Ferguson GH, Redford J, Barrett JA & Kiff ES (1989) The appreciation of rectal distension in fecal incontinence. *Dis Colon Rectum* **32**: 964–967.

Fleshman JW, Peters WR, Shemesh EI, Fry RD & Kodner IJ (1991a) Anal sphincter reconstruction: anterior overlapping muscle repair. *Dis Colon Rectum* **34**: 739–743.

Fleshman JW, Dreznick Z, Fry RD & Kodner IJ (1991b) Anal sphincter repair for obstetric injury: manometric evaluation of functional results. *Dis Colon Rectum* **34**: 1061–1067.

Flood C (1982) The real reason for performing episiotomies. *World Med* **6**: 51.

Floyd WF & Walls EW (1953) Electromyography of the sphincter ani extremus in man. *J Physiol (Lond)* **122**: 599–609.

Frenckner B (1975) Function of the anal sphincters in spinal man. *Gut* **16**: 638–644.

Frenckner B & Ihre T (1976a) Function of the anal sphincters in patients with intussusception of the rectum. *Gut* **17**: 147–151.

Frenckner B & Ihre T (1976b) Influence of autonomic nerves on the internal anal sphincter in man. *Gut* **17**: 306–312.

Frenckner B & Von Euler C (1975) Influence of pudendal block of the function of the anal sphincters. *Gut* **16**: 482–489.

Garcia-Aguilar J, Belmonte C, Wong WD, Loury AC & Maddoff RD (1996) Open vs closed sphincterotomy for chronic anal fissure. *Dis Colon Rectum* **39**: 440–443.

Gardosi J, Hutson N & Lynch CB (1989) Randomised, controlled trial of squatting in the second stage of labour. *Lancet* **ii**: 74.

Geboes K & Bossaert H (1977) Gastrointestinal disorders in old age. *Age Ageing* **6**: 197–200.

Gee AS & Durdey P (1995) Urge incontinence of faeces is a marker of severe external anal sphincter dysfunction. *Br J Surg* **82**: 1179–1182.

Gee AS & Durdey P (1997) Preoperative increase in neuromuscular jitter and outcome following surgery for faecal incontinence. *Br J Surg* **84**: 1265–1268.

Gee AS, Mills A & Durdey P (1995) What is the relationship between perineal descent and anal mucosal electrosensitivity? *Dis Colon Rectum* **38**: 419–423.

Geerdes BP, Heineman E, Konsten J, Soeters PB & Baeten CGMI (1996) Dynamic graciloplasty. Complications and management. *Dis Colon Rectum* **39**: 912–917.

George BD, Williams NS, Patel J, Swash M & Watkins ES (1993) Physiological and histochemical adaptation of the electrically stimulated gracilis muscle to neoanal sphincter function. *Br J Surg* **80**: 1342–1346.

Gibbons CP, Trowbridge EA, Bannister JJ & Read NW (1986a) Role of anal cushions in maintaining continence. *Lancet* **i**: 886–888.

Gibbons CP, Bannister JJ, Trowbridge EA & Read NW (1986b) An analysis of anal sphincter pressure and anal compliance in normal subjects. *Int J Colorectal Dis* **1**: 231–237.

Giebel GD, Lefering R, Troidl H & Blöchl H (1998) Prevalence of fecal incontinence: what can be expected. *Int J Colorect Dis* **13**: 73–77.

Gledhill T & Waterfall WE (1984) Postanal repair to restore fecal continence after failed sphincteroplasty. *Can J Surg* **27**: 256–257.

Goes RN, Simons AJ, Masri L & Beart RW (1995) Gradient of pressure and time between proximal anal canal and high-pressure zone during internal anal sphincter relaxation. *Dis Colon Rectum* **38**: 1043–1046.

Goke M, Ewe K, Donner K & Meyer zum Buschenfelde (1992) Influence of loperamide and loperamide oxide on the anal sphincter. *Dis Colon Rectum* **35**: 857–861.

Goldberg DA, Hodges K, Hersh T & Jinich H (1980) Biofeedback therapy for fecal incontinence. *Am J Gastroenterol* **74**: 342–345.

Gosling J (1979) The structure of the bladder and urethra in relation to function. *Urol Clin N Am* **6**: 31–38.

Gowers WR (1877) The autonomic action of the sphincter ani. *Proc R Soc* **26**: 77–84.

Griffiths DM & Malone PS (1995) The Malone antegrade continence enema. *J Pediatr Surg* **30**: 68–71.

Guillemot F, Bouche B, Gower-Rousseau C et al (1994) Biofeedback for the treatment of fecal incontinence. Long-term clinical results. *Dis Colon Rectum* **38**: 393–397.

Guitierrez JG & Shah AN (1975) Autonomic control of the internal anal sphincter in man. In Van Trappen G (ed.) *Fifth International Symposium of Gastrointestinal Motility*, pp 363–373. Leuven: Typoff Press.

Guitierrez JG, Oliai A & Chey WY (1975) Manometric profile of the internal anal sphincter in man. *Gastroenterology* **68**: 907 (Abstract).

Gunterberg B, Kewenter J, Petersen I & Stener B (1976) Anorectal function after major resections of the sacrum with bilateral or unilateral sacrifice of sacral nerves. *Br J Surg* **63**: 546–554.

Gurll N & Steer M (1975) Diagnostic and therapeutic considerations for fecal impaction. *Dis Colon Rectum* **18**: 507–511.

Haas P, Fox TA & Haas GP (1984) The pathogenesis of haemorrhoids. *Dis Colon Rectum* **27**: 442–450.

Habr-Gamma A, Alves PA, da Silva C, Sousa AHJr, Femenias Vieira MJ & Brunetti-Neto C (1986) Treatment of faecal incontinence by postanal repair. *Coloproctology* **8**: 244–246.

Hagihara PF & Griffen WO (1976) Delayed correction of anal incontinence due to anal sphincteral injury. *Arch Surg* **111**: 63–66.

Hajivassiliou CA, Carter KB & Finlay IG (1996) Anorectal angle enhances faecal continence. *Br J Surg* **83**: 53–56.

Hald T (1986) Artificial sphincter. *World J Urol* **4**: 41–44.

Hallan RI, Williams NS, Pilot M-A, Grahn MF, Koeze TH & Watkins ES (1989) Converted striated muscle neosphincter: a canine model. *Br J Surg* **76**: 635 (Abstract).

Hancke E & Schurholz M (1987) Impaired rectal sensation in idiopathic faecal incontinence. *Int J Colorectal Dis* **2**: 146–148.

Hancock BD (1976) Measurement of anal pressure and motility. *Gut* **17**: 645–657.

Hancock BD & Smith K (1975) The internal anal sphincter and Lord's procedure for haemorrhoids. *Br J Surg* **62**: 833–836.

Harraf F, Schmulson M, Saba L et al (1998) Subtypes of constipation predominant irritable bowel syndrome based on rectal perception. *Gut* **43**: 388–394.

Hasegawa H & Keighley MRB (1998) An audit of seton fistulotomy. Paper presented at the West Midlands Surgical Society, May, Birmingham.

Hassink EA, Rieu PN, Severijnen RS, Staak FH & Festen C (1993) Are adults content or continent after repair for high anal atresia? *Ann Surg* **218**: 196–200.

Hassink EA, Rieu PN, Severijnen RS, Brugman-Boezeman AT & Festen C (1996) Adults born with high anorectal atresia – how do they manage? *Dis Colon Rectum* **39**: 695–699.

Haynes WG & Read NW (1982) Anorectal activity in man during rectal infusion of saline: a dynamic assessment of the anal continence mechanism. *J Physiol* **330**: 45–46.

Henriksen TB, Bek KM, Hedegaard M & Secher NJ (1994) Methods and consequences of changes in the use of episiotomy. *BMJ* **309**: 1255–1258.

Henry MM (1983) The descending perineum syndrome. In Sir Alan Parks Memorial Symposium. *Ann R Coll Surg Engl* **65** (Suppl): 24–25.

Henry MM & Simson JNL (1985) Results of postanal repair: a retrospective study. *Br J Surg* 72 (Suppl): S17–S19.

Henry MM & Swash M (1978) Assessment of pelvic floor disorders and incontinence by electrophysiological recording of the anal reflex. *Lancet* **i**: 1290–1291.

Henry MM & Swash M (1985) *Coloproctology and the Pelvic Floor*, 1st edn. London: Butterworth.

Henry MM & Swash M (1992) *Coloproctology and the Pelvic Floor*, 2nd edn, pp 176–177. London: Butterworth-Heinemann.

Henry MM, Parks AG & Swash M (1980) The anal reflex in idiopathic faecal incontinence: an electrophysiological study. *Br J Surg* **67**: 781–783.

Henry MM, Parks AG & Swash M (1982) The pelvic floor musculature in the descending perineum syndrome. *Br J Surg* **69**: 470–472.

Hill J, Corson RJ, Brandon H, Redford J, Faragher EB & Kiff ES (1994a) History and examination in the assessment of patients with idiopathic fecal incontinence. *Dis Colon Rectum* **37**: 473–477.

Hill J, Mumtaz A & Kiff ES (1994b) Pudendal neuropathy in patients with idiopathic faecal incontinence progresses with time. *Br J Surg* **81**: 1492–1949.

Hill JR, Kelley ML, Schlegel JF & Code CF (1960) Pressure profile of the rectum and anus of healthy persons. *Dis Colon Rectum* **3**: 203–209.

Hiltunen K-M (1985) Anal manometric findings in patients with anal incontinence. *Dis Colon Rectum* **28**: 925–928.

Ho YH, Chiang JM, Tan M & Low JY (1996) Biofeedback therapy for excessive stool frequency and incontinence following anterior resection or total colectomy. *Dis Colon Rectum* **39**: 1289–1292.

Ho YH & Goh HS (1995) The neurophysiological significance of perineal descent. *Int J Colorectal Dis* **10**: 107–111.

Hoffmann BA, Timmcke AE, Gathright JB, Hicks TC, Opelka FG & Beck DE (1995) Fecal seepage and soiling: a problem of rectal sensation. *Dis Colon Rectum* **38**: 746–748.

Holmberg A, Graf W, Osterberg A & Pahlman L (1995) Anorectal manovolumetry in the diagnosis of fecal incontinence. *Dis Colon Rectum* **38**: 502–508.

Hopkinson BR & Hardman J (1973) Silicone rubber perianal suture for rectal prolapse. *Proc R Soc Med* **66**: 1095–1098.

Hopkinson BR & Lightwood R (1966) Electrical treatment of anal incontinence. *Lancet* **i**: 344–351.

Horn HR, Schoetz DJ Jr, Coller JA & Viedenheimer MC (1985) Sphincter repair with a silastic sling for anal incontinence and rectal procidentia. *Dis Colon Rectum* **28**: 868–872.

House MJ (1981) To do or not to do episiotomy. In Kitzinger S (ed.) *Episiotomy: Physical and Emotional Aspects*, pp 6–12. London: National Childbirth Trust.

Infantino A, Melega E, Negrin P, Masin A, Carino S & Lise M (1995) Striated anal sphincter electromyography in idiopathic fecal incontinence. *Dis Colon Rectum* **38**: 27–31.

Ide Smith E, Tunnell WP & Rainey Williams G (1978) A clinical evaluation of the surgical treatment of anorectal malformations (imperforate anus). *Ann Surg* **187**: 583–592.

Ihre T (1974) Studies on anal function in continent and incontinent patients. *Scand J Gastroenterol* **25**: 1–64.

Irvine RE (1986) Faecal incontinence is not inevitable. *BMJ* **292**: 1618–1619.

Iwai N, Ogita S, Kida M et al (1979) A clinical and manometric correlation for assessment of postoperative continence in imperforate anus. *J Paediatr Surg* **14**: 538–543.

Iwama T, Imajo M, Yaegashi K & Mishima Y (1989) Self washout method for defecational complaints following low anterior rectal resection. *Jpn J Surg* **19**: 251–253.

Jackman FR, Francis JN & Hopkinson BR (1980) Silicone rubber band treatment of rectal prolapse. *Ann R Coll Surg Engl* **62**: 386–387.

Jacobs PPM, Scheuer M, Kuijpers JH & Vingerhoets MH (1990) Obstetric fecal incontinence: role of pelvic floor denervation and results of delayed sphincter repair. *Dis Colon Rectum* **33**: 494–497.

Jameson JS, Speakman CTM, Darzi A, Chia YW & Henry MM (1994) Audit of postanal repair in the treatment of fecal incontinence. *Dis Colon Rectum* **37**: 369–372.

Jensen LL & Lowry AC (1992) Biofeedback for anal incontinence: what is the mechanism of success? *Dis Colon Rectum* **35**: 11.

Johnson GP, Pemberton JH, Ness J, Samson M & Zinsmeister AR (1990) Transducer manometry and the effect of body position on anal canal pressures. *Dis Colon Rectum* **33**: 469–475.

Johnson MA, Polgar J, Weightman D & Appleton D (1973) Data on the distribution of the fibre types in thirty-six human muscles: an autopsy study. *J Neurol Sci* **18**: 111–129.

Johnston ID & Gibson JB (1960) Megacolon and volvulus in psychotics. *Br J Surg* **47**: 394–395.

Jones PN, Lubowski DZ, Swash M & Henry MM (1987) Relation between perineal descent and pudendal nerve damage in idiopathic faecal incontinence. *Int J Colorectal Dis* **2**: 93–95.

Jorge JM & Wexner SD (1993) Aetiology and management of faecal incontinence. *Dis Colon Rectum* **36**: 77–97.

Jorge JMN, Wexner SD, Ehrenpreis E, Nogueras JJ & Jagelman DG (1992a) Does perianal descent correlate with pudendal neuropathy. *Dis Colon Rectum* **35**: 11–12.

Jorge JMN, Wexner SD, Marchetti F, Rosato GO, Sullivan ML & Jagelman DG (1992b) How reliable are currently available methods of measuring the anorectal angle. *Dis Colon Rectum* **35**: 332–338.

Jorge JMN, Wexner SD, Ehrenpreis ED, Nogueras JJ & Jagelman DG (1993) Does perineal descent correlate with pudendal neuropathy? *Dis Colon Rectum* **36**: 475–483.

Jost WH & Schimrigk K (1994) Magnetic stimulation of the pudendal nerve. *Dis Colon Rectum* **37**: 697–699.

Kamm MA (1994) Obstetric damage and faecal incontinence. *Lancet* **344**: 730–733.

Kamm MA, Lennard-Jones JE & Nicholls RJ (1989) Evaluation of the intrinsic innervation of the internal anal sphincter using electrical stimulation. *Gut* **30**: 935–938.

Kantner M (1957) Neue morphologische Ergerbrisse uber die peripherischen Nervenausbreitungen und ihre deutung. *Acta Anat* **31**: 397–425.

Karulf RE, Coller JA, Dartolo DCC et al (1991) Anorectal physiology testing. *Dis Colon Rectum* **34**: 464–468.

Katz LD, Zinkin LD, Stonesifer GL & Rosin JD (1978) Imperforate anus and ectopic orifices in adult patients. *Dis Colon Rectum* **21**: 633–635.

Keating JP, Stewart PJ, Eyers AA, Warner D & Bokey EL (1997) Are special investigations of value in the management of patients with fecal incontinence? *Dis Colon Rectum* **40**: 896–897.

Keck Jo, Staniunas RJ, Coller JA et al (1994) Biofeedback training is useful in fecal incontinence but disappointing in constipation. *Dis Colon Rectum* **37**: 1271–1276.

Keighley MRB (1983) Management of faecal incontinence in the elderly. *Geriatr Med Today* **2**: 45–61.

Keighley MRB (1984) Postanal repair of faecal incontinence. *J R Soc Med* **77**: 285–288.

Keighley MRB (1986) Re-routing procedures for ectopic anus in the adult. *Br J Surg* **73**: 974–977.

Keighley MRB (1987a) Iatrogenic incontinence. In Gooszen HG, Ten Cate Hoedemaker HO, Weterman IT & Keighley MRB (eds) *Disordered Defaecation*, pp 125–132. Dordrecht: Martinus Nijhoff.

Keighley MRB (1987b) Postanal repair. *Int J Colorectal Dis* **2**: 236–239.

Keighley MRB (1991) Results of surgery in idiopathic faecal incontinence. *S Afr J Surg* **29**: 87–93.

Keighley MRB & Fielding JWL (1983) Management of faecal incontinence and results of surgical treatment. *Br J Surg* **70**: 463–468.

Keighley MRB & Shouler PJ (1984) Abnormalities of colonic function in patients with rectal prolapse and faecal incontinence. *Br J Surg* **71**: 892–895.

Keighley MRB, Makuria T, Alexander-Williams J & Arabi Y (1980) Clinical and manometric evaluation of rectal prolapse and incontinence. *Br J Surg* **67**: 54–56.

Keighley MRB, Henry MM, Bartolo DCC & Mortensen NJMcC (1989) Anorectal physiology measurement: report of a working party. *Br J Surg* **76**: 356–357.

Kerremans R (1969) *Morphological and Physiological Aspects of Anal Continence and Defaecation*. Brussels: Editions Arsica.

Kerremans RPJ, Penninckx FMA & Beckers JPV (1974) Function evaluation of ectopic anus and its surgical consequences. *Am J Dis Child* **128**: 811–814.

Khanduja KS, Yamashita HJ, Wise WE, Aguilar PS & Hartmann RF (1994) Delayed repair of obstetric injuries of the anorectum and vagina. *Dis Colon Rectum* **37**: 344–349.

Kiely EM, Ade-Ajayi N & Wheeler RA (1994) Caecal flap conduit for antegrade continence enemas. *Br J Surg* **81**: 1215.

Kiesswetter H (1977) Mucosal sensory threshold of urinary bladder and urethra measured electrically. *Urol Int* **32**: 437–448.

Kiesewetter WB & Chang JH (1977) Imperforate anus: a five to thirty year follow-up perspective. *Prog Pediatr Surg* **10**: 111–120.

Kiesewetter WB & Turner CR (1963) Continence after surgery for imperforate anus. A critical analysis and preliminary experience with the sacroperineal pull-through. *Ann Surg* **158**: 498–512.

Kiff ES (1983) The clinical use of anorectal physiology studies. In Sir Alan Parks Memorial Symposium. *Ann R Coll Surg Engl* **65** (Suppl): 132–134.

Kiff ES & Swash M (1984a) Normal proximal and delayed distal conduction in the pudendal nerves of patients with idiopathic (neurogenic) faecal incontinence. *J Neurol Neurosurg Psychiatr* **47**: 820–823.

Kiff ES & Swash M (1984b) Slowed conduction in the pudendal nerves in idiopathic (neurogenic) faecal incontinence. *Br J Surg* **71**: 614–616.

Kiff ES, Barnes P & Swash M (1984) Evidence of pudendal neuropathy in patients with perineal descent and chronic straining at stool. *Gut* **25**: 1279–1282.

Kitzinger S & Walters R (1981) *Some Women's Experiences of Episiotomy*. London: National Childbirth Trust.

Kmiot WA & Keighley MRB (1990) Surgical options in ulcerative colitis: the role of ileoanal anastomosis. In Allan RN, Keighley MRB, Alexander-Williams J & Hawkins C (eds) *Inflammatory Bowel Diseases*, 2nd edn, pp 445–458. Edinburgh: Churchill Livingstone.

Klosterhalfen B, Offner F, Topf N, Vogel P & Mittermayer C (1990) Sclerosis of the internal anal sphincter: a process of aging. *Dis Colon Rectum* **33**: 606–609.

Konsten J, Baeten CG, Spaans F, Havenith MG & Soeters PB (1993) Follow-up of anal dynamic graciloplasty for fecal continence. *World J Surg* **17**: 404–409.

Korsgen S (1995) Functional outcome after restorative proctocolectomy for ulcerative colitis. Thesis, University of Birmingham.

Korsgen S, Deen KI & Keighley MRB (1997) Long-term results of total pelvic floor repair for postobstetric fecal incontinence. *Dis Colon Rectum* **40**: 835–839.

Krogh K & Laurberg S (1998) Malone antegrade continence enema for faecal incontinence and constipation in adults. *Br J Surg* **85**: 974–977.

Krogh K, Nielsen J, Djurhuus JC, Mosdal C, Sabroe S & Laurberg S (1997) Colorectal function in patients with spinal cord lesions. *Dis Colon Rectum* **40**: 1233–1239.

Kuijpers HC & Scheuer M (1990) Disorders of impaired fecal control. *Dis Colon Rectum* **33**: 207–211.

Kumar D, Williams NS, Waldron D & Wingate DL (1989) Prolonged manometric recording of anorectal motor activity in ambulant human subjects: evidence of periodic activity. *Gut* **30**: 1007–1011.

Kumar D, Hutchinson R & Grant E (1995) Bilateral gracilis neosphincter construction for treatment of faecal incontinence. *Br J Surg* **82**: 1645–1647.

Labrow S, Rubin RJ, Hoexter B & Salvati E (1980) Perineal repair of rectal procidentia with an elastic fabric sling. *Dis Colon Rectum* **23**: 467–469.

Lahr CJ, Rotherberger DA, Jensen LL & Goldberg SM (1986) Balloon topography: a simple method of evaluating anal function. *Dis Colon Rectum* **29**: 1–5.

Lahr CJ, Cherry DA, Jensen LL & Rotherberger DA (1988) Balloon sphincterography. Clinical findings after 200 patients. *Dis Colon Rectum* **31**: 347–351.

Lane RHS & Parks AG (1977) Function of the anal sphincters following coloanal anastomosis. *Br J Surg* **64**: 596–599.

Last RJ (1978) *Anatomy: Regional and Applied*, 6th edn. London: Churchill Livingstone.

Laurberg S & Swash M (1989) Effects of aging on the anorectal sphincters and their innervation. *Dis Colon Rectum* **32**: 737–742.

Laurberg S, Swash M & Henry MM (1990) Effect of postanal repair on progress of neurogenic damage to the pelvic floor. *Br J Surg* **77**: 519–522.

Law PJ & Bartram CI (1989) Anal endosonography: technique and normal anatomy. *Gastrointest Radiol* **14**: 349–353.

Law PJ, Kamm MA & Bartram CI (1990) A comparison between electromyography and anal endosonography in mapping external anal sphincter defects. *Dis Colon Rectum* **33**: 370–373.

Lawson JON (1974a) Pelvic anatomy. I. Pelvic floor muscles. *Ann R Coll Surg Engl* **54**: 244–252.

Lawson JON (1974b) Pelvic anatomy. II. Anal canal and associated sphincters. *Ann R Coll Surg Engl* **54**: 280–300.

Lazorthes F, Gamagami R, Cabarrot P & Muhammad S (1998) Is rectal intussusception a cause of idiopathic incontinence? *Dis Colon Rectum* **41**: 602–605.

Lehur PA, Michot F, Denis P et al (1996) Results of artificial sphincter in severe anal incontinence. Report of 14 consecutive implantations. *Dis Colon Rectum* **39**: 1352–1355

Lehur PA, Glemain P, Bruley des Varannes S, Buzelin JM & Leborgne J (1998) Outcome of patients with an implanted artificial anal sphincter for severe faecal incontinence. *Int J Colorect Dis* **13**: 88–92.

Lequit R Jr, van Baal JG & Brummelkamp WH (1985) Gracilis muscle transposition in the treatment of fecal incontinence: long-term follow-up and evaluation of anal pressure recordings. *Dis Colon Rectum* **28**: 1–4.

Lestar B, Penninckx F & Kerremans RP (1989) The composition of anal basal pressure. An *in vivo* and *in vitro* study in man. *Int J Colorectal Dis* **4**: 118–122.

Lewis MI (1972) Gracilis-muscle transplant for the correction of anal incontinence: report of a case. *Dis Colon Rectum* **15**: 292–298.

Loening-Baucke V (1990) Efficacy of biofeedback training in improving faecal incontinence and anorectal physiologic function. *Gut* **31**: 1395–1402.

Loening-Baucke V & Anuras S (1985) Effects of age and sex on anorectal manometry. *Am J Gastroenterol* **80**: 50–53.

Londono-Schimmer EE, Garcia-Duperly R, Nicholls RJ, Ritchie JK, Hawley PR & Thomson JPS (1994) Overlapping anal sphincter repair for faecal incontinence due to sphincter trauma: five year follow-up functional results. *Int J Colorectal Dis* **9**: 110–113.

Lord PH (1968) A new regime for the treatment of haemorrhoids. *Proc R Soc Med* **61**: 935.

Lord PH (1975) Conservative management of haemorrhoids. *Clin Gastroenterol* **4**: 601–608.

Loygue G & Dubois F (1964) Surgical treatment of anal incontinence. *Am J Proctol* **15**: 361–374.

Lubowski DZ & Nicholls RJ (1988) Faecal incontinence associated with reduced pelvic sensation. *Br J Surg* **75**: 1086–1088.

Lubowski DZ, Swash M, Nicholls RJ & Henry MM (1988a) Increase in pudendal nerve terminal motor latency with defaecation straining. *Br J Surg* **75**: 1095–1097.

Lubowski DZ, Jones PN, Swash M & Henry MM (1988b) Asymmetrical pudendal nerve damage in pelvic floor disorders. *Int J Colorectal Dis* **3**: 158–160.

Luman W, Pryde A, Heading RC & Palmer KR (1997) Topical glyceryl trinitrate relaxes the sphincter of Oddi. *Gut* **40**: 541–543.

MacArthur C, Lewis M & Knox EG (1991) Health and childbirth. *Br J Obstet Gynaecol* **98**: 1193–1204.

MacArthur C, Lewis M & Bick DE (1993) Stress incontinence after childbirth: predictors, persistence, impact and medical consultation. *Br J Midwifery* **5**: 207–215.

MacArthur C, Bick DE & Keighley MRB (1997) Faecal incontinence after childbirth. *Br J Obstet Gynaecol* **104**: 46–50.

MacDonald A, Smith A, McNeill AD & Finlay IG (1992) Manual dilatation of the anus. *Br J Surg* **79**: 1381–1382.

MacDonagh R, Sun WM, Thomas DG, Smallwood R & Read NW (1992) Anorectal function in patients with complete supraconal spinal cord lesions. *Gut* **33**: 1532–1538.

McGill CW, Polk HC & Canty TG (1978) The clinical basis for a simplified classification of anorectal agenesis. *Surg Gynecol Obstet* **146**: 177–181.

McGregor RA (1965) Gracilis muscle transplant in anal incontinence. *Dis Colon Rectum* **8**: 141–143.

MacIntyre IMC & Balfour TW (1977) Results of the Lord non-operative treatment for haemorrhoids. *Lancet* **i**: 1094.

Mackie EJ & Parks TG (1989) Clinical features in patients with excessive perineal descent. *J R Coll Surg Edinb* **34**: 88.

MacLeod JH (1979) Biofeedback in the management of partial anal incontinence. A preliminary report. *Dis Colon Rectum* **22**: 169–171.

MacLeod JH (1983) Biofeedback in the management of partial anal incontinence. *Dis Colon Rectum* **26**: 244–246.

MacLeod JH (1987) Management of anal incontinence by biofeedback. *Gastroenterology* **93**: 291–294.

Magovern GJ, Park SB, Magovern GJ et al (1986) Latissimus dorsi as a functioning synchronously paced muscle component in the region of a left ventricular aneurysm. *Ann Thorac Surg* **41**: 116.

Mahieu P, Pringot J & Bodart P (1984a) Defecography: I. Description of a new procedure and results in normal patients. *Gastrointest Radiol* **9**: 247–251.

Mahieu P, Pringot J & Bodart P (1984b) Defecography: II. Contribution to the diagnosis of defecation disorders. *Gastrointest Radiol* **9**: 253–261.

Malone PS, Ransley PG & Kiely EM (1990) Preliminary report: the antegrade continence enema. *Lancet* **336**: 1217–1218.

Mander BJ, Wexner BJ, Wexner SD et al (1997a) Preliminary results of a multicentre trial of the dynamic graciloplasty in faecal incontinence. *Int J Colorectal Dis* **111**: 114.

Mander BJ, Wexner SD, Williams NS et al (1997b) The electrically stimulated gracilis neoanal sphincter. Preliminary results of a multicentre trial. *Br J Surg* **84** (Suppl 1): 39.

Marby M, Alexander-Williams J, Buchmann P et al (1979) A randomized controlled trial to compare anal dilatation with lateral subcutaneous sphincterotomy for anal fissure. *Dis Colon Rectum* **22**: 308–311.

Marsden CD, Merton PA & Norton HB (1978) The latency of the anal reflex. *J Neurol Neurosurg Psychiatr* **41**: 813–818.

Matheson DM & Keighley MRB (1981) Manometric evaluation of rectal prolapse and faecal incontinence. *Gut* **22**: 126–129.

Mathai V, Seo-Choen F (1995) Anterior rectal mucosal prolapse: an easily treated cause of anorectal symptoms. *Br J Surg* **82**: 752–753.

Maw A, Eccersley AJ & Williams NS (1997a) The continent colonic conduit for faecal incontinence and rectal evacuatory disorders. *Gut* **40** (Suppl 1): A55.

Maw A, Eccersley AJ, Ratani RS & Williams NS (1997b) The colonic conduit as a treatment for incontinence after pull through procedures in ano-rectal malformation. *Int J Colorectal Dis* **50**: 129.

Maw A, Hughes F, Doherty A, Stuchfield B & Williams NS (1996) The continent colonic conduit for the treatment of evacuatory disorders of the colon and rectum. *Int J Colorectal Dis* **11**: 140.

Mazier WP, Senagore AJ & Schiesel EC (1995) Operative repair of anovaginal and rectovaginal fistulas. *Dis Colon Rectum* **38**: 4–6.

Meagher AP, Lubowski DZ & King DW (1993) The cough response of the anal sphincter. *Int J Colorectal Dis* **8**: 217–219.

Meagher AP, Kennedy ML & Lubowski DZ (1996) Rectal mucosal electrosensitivy – what is being tested? *Int J Colorectal Dis* **11**: 29–33.

Merton PA, Moreton HB, Hill DK & Marsden CD (1982) Scope of a technique for electrical stimulation of human brain, spinal cord and muscle. *Lancet* **ii**: 597–600.

Meshkinpour H, Movahedi H & Welgan P (1997) Clinical value of anorectal manometry index in neurogenic fecal incontinence. *Dis Colon Rectum* **40**: 457–461.

Meunier P & Mollard P (1977) Control of the internal anal sphincter (manometric study with human subjects). *Pflugers Arch Ges Physiol Mensch Tiere* **350**: 233–239.

Meunier P, Mollard P & Marachal J-M (1976) Physiology of megarectum: the association of megarectum with encopresis. *Gut* **17**: 224–227.

Michot F, Lehur PA & Forestier F (1997) Artificial anal sphincter. *Semin Colon Rectal Surg* **8**: 1–6.

Miles AJ, Allen-Mersh TG & Westel C (1990) The damaging and cumulative effect of anoreceptive intercourse on internal anal sphincter function. Paper presented at the Association of Surgeons of Great Britain and Ireland, April 1990, Harrogate.

Miller R, Bartolo DCC, Cervero F & Mortensen NJMcC (1987) Anorectal temperature sensation: a comparison of normal and incontinent patients. *Br J Surg* **74**: 511–515.

Miller R, Bartolo DCC, Roe AM & Mortensen NJMcC (1988a) Assessment of microtransducers in anorectal manometry. *Br J Surg* **75**: 40–43.

Miller R, Bartolo DCC, Cervero F & Mortensen NJMcC (1988b) Anorectal sampling: a comparison of normal and incontinent patients. *Br J Surg* **75**: 44–47.

Miller R, Bartolo DCC, Locke-Edmunds JC & Mortensen NJMcC (1988c) Prospective study of conservative and operative treatment for faecal incontinence. *Br J Surg* **75**: 101–105.

Miller R, Bartolo DC, Roe A, Cervero F & Mortensen NJ (1988d) Anal sensation and the continence mechanism. *Dis Colon Rectum* **31**: 433–438.

Miller R, Orrom WJ, Cornes H, Duthie G & Bartolo DCC (1989) Anterior sphincter plication and levatorplasty in the treatment of faecal incontinence. *Br J Surg* **76**: 1058–1060.

Mitrofanoff P (1980) Cystostomie continente trans-appendiculare dans le traitement des vessies neurologiques. *Chir Pediatr* **21**: 297–305.

Molnar T, Taitz LS, Unwin OM & Wales JKH (1983) Anorectal manometry results in defaecation disorders. *Arch Dis Child* **58**: 257–261.

Moore-Gillon V (1984) Constipation: what does the patient mean? *J R Soc Med* **77**: 108–110.

Morgan R, Patel B, Beynon J & Carr ND (1997) Surgical management of anorectal incontinence due to internal and anal sphincter deficiency. *Br J Surg* **84**: 226–230.

Mortensen N (1992) Rectal and anal endosonography. *Gut* **33**: 148–149.

Motson RW (1985) Sphincter injuries: indications for, and results of repair. *Br J Surg* **72** (Suppl): S19–S21.

Motson RW, McPartlin JF & Browning GGP (1983) Anal sphincter injury. In Sir Alan Parks Memorial Symposium. *Ann R Coll Surg Engl* **65** (Suppl): 33–35.

Neill ME & Swash M (1980) Increased motor unit fibre density in the external anal sphincter muscle in anorectal incontinence: a single fibre EMG study. *J Neurol Neurosurg Psychiatry* **43**: 343–347.

Neill ME, Parks AG & Swash M (1981) Physiological studies of the pelvic floor in idiopathic faecal incontinence and rectal prolapse. *Br J Surg* **68**: 531–536.

Newman HF & Freeman J (1974) Physiologic factors affecting defaecation sensation. *J Am Geriatr Soc* **22**: 553–554.

Nichols DH (1982) Retrorectal levatorplasty for anal and perineal prolapse. *Surg Gynaecol Obstet* **154**: 251–254.

Nielsen MB, Hauge C, Rasmussen OO, Pedersen JF & Christiansen J (1992) Anal endosonographic findings in the follow-up of primarily sutured sphincteric ruptures. *Br J Surg* **79**: 104–106.

Nielsen MB, Rasmussen OO, Pedersen JF & Christiansen J (1993) Risk of sphincter damage and anal incontinence after anal dilatation for fissure-in-ano. An endosonographic study. *Dis Colon Rectum*: **36**: 677–680.

Nielsen MB, Dammegaard L & Pedersen JF (1994) Endosonographic assessment of the anal sphincter after surgical reconstruction. *Dis Colon Rectum* **37**: 434–438.

Nieves PM, Valles TG, Aranguren G & Maldonado D (1975) Gracilis muscle transplant for correction of traumatic anal incontinence: report of a case. *Dis Colon Rectum* **18**: 349–354.

Nikiteas N, Korsgen S, Kumar D & Keighley MRB (1996) An audit of sphincter repair; factors associated with poor outcome. *Dis Colon Rectum* **39**: 1164–1170.

Nivatvongs S, Stern HS & Fryd DS (1981) The length of the anal canal. *Dis Colon Rectum* **67**: 216–220.

Nixon HH (1984) Review of anorectal anomalies. *J R Soc Med* **77** (Suppl 3): 27–29.

Oettle GJ, Roe AM, Bartolo DCC & Mortensen NJMcC (1985) What is the best way of measuring perineal descent? A comparison of radiographic and clinical methods. *Br J Surg* **72**: 999–1001.

O'Kelly TJ (1996) Nerves that say NO: a new perspective on the human rectoanal inhibitory reflex. *Ann R Coll Surg Engl* **78**: 31–38.

O'Kelly TJ & MacMortensen NJ (1992) Tests of anorectal function. *Br J Surg* **79**: 988–989.

O'Kelly T, Brading A & Mortensen N (1993) Nerve mediated relaxation of the human internal anal sphincter: the role of nitric oxide. *Gut* **34**: 689–693.

O'Kelly TJ, Davies J, Tam P, Mortensen MJMcC & Brading AFB (1994a) Abnormalities of nitric oxide producing neurones in Hirschsprung's disease: morphology and implications. *J Pediatr Surg* **29**: 294–299.

O'Kelly TJ, Davies J, Mortensen MJMcC & Brading AFB (1994b) The distribution of nitric oxide synthase containing neurones in the human rectal myenteric plexus and anal canal; morphological evidence that nitric oxide mediates the rectoanal inhibitory reflex. *Dis Colon Rectum* **37**: 350–357.

Oliveira L, Pfeifer J & Wexner SD (1996) Physiological and clinical outcome of anterior sphincteroplasty. *Br J Surg* **83**: 502–505.

Orrom WJ, Wong WD, Rothenberger DA & Jensen RN (1990a) Evaluation of an air-filled microballoon and mini-transducer in the clinical practice of anorectal manometry. *Dis Colon Rectum* **33**: 594–597.

Orrom WJ, Williams JG, Rothenberger DA & Wong WD (1990b) Portable anorectal manometry. *Br J Surg* **77**: 876–877.

Osterberg A, Graf W, Holmberg A, Pahlman L, Ljung A & Hakelius L (1996) Long-term results of anterior levatorplasty for fecal incontinence. *Dis Colon Rectum* **39**: 671–675.

Otto IC, Ito K, Ye C, Hibi K, Kasai Y, Akiyama S & Takagi H (1996) Causes of rectal incontinence after sphincter-preserving operations for rectal cancer. *Dis Colon Rectum* **39**: 1423–1427.

Oya M, Ortiz J, Chatapadyhay G, Grant E & Keighley MRB (1991) Total pelvic floor repair is the operation of choice for neuropathic faecal incontinence. *Br J Surg* **78**: 1491–1497.

Oya M, Ortiz J, Grant EA, Chattopadhyay G, Asprer J & Keighley MRB (1994) A video proctographic assessment of the changes in pelvic floor function following three forms of repair for post-obstetric neuropathic faecal incontinence. *Dig Surg* **11**: 20–24.

Parellada CM, Miller AS, Williamson MER & Johnston D (1998) Paradoxical high anal resting pressures in men with idiopathic faecal seepage. *Dis Colon Rectum* **41**: 593–597.

Parks AG (1974) Royal Society of Medicine, Section of Proctology: Meeting 27 November 1974. President's address. Anorectal incontinence. *Proc R Soc Med* **68**: 681–690.

Parks AG (1975) Anorectal incontinence. *Proc R Soc Med* **68**: 681–690.

Parks AG & McPartlin JF (1971) Late repair of injuries of the anal sphincter. *Proc R Soc Med* **64**: 1187–1189.

Parks AG & Stuart AE (1973) The management of villous tumours of the large bowel. *Br J Surg* **60**: 688–695.

Parks AG & Swash M (1979) Denervation of the anal sphincter causing idiopathic anorectal incontinence. *J R Coll Surg Edinb* **24**: 94–96.

Parks AG, Porter NH & Melzack J (1962) Experimental study of the reflex mechanism controlling the muscles of the pelvic floor. *Dis Colon Rectum* **5**: 407–414.

Parks AG, Porter NH & Hardcastle J (1966) The syndrome of the descending perineum. *Proc R Soc Med* **59**: 477–482.
Parks AG, Gordon PH & Hardcastle JD (1976) A classification of fistula-in-ano. *Br J Surg* **63**: 1–12.
Parks AG, Swash M & Urich H (1977) Sphincter denervation in anorectal incontinence and rectal prolapse. *Gut* **18**: 656–665.
Parks TG (1992) The usefulness of tests in anorectal disease. World J Surg **16**: 804–810.
Patankar SK, Ferrara A, Larach SW et al (1997a) Electromyographic assessment of biofeedback training for fecal incontinence and chronic constipation. *Dis Colon Rectum* **40**: 907–911.
Patankar SK, Ferrara A, Levy JR, Larach SW, Williamson PR & Perozo SE (1997b) Biofeedback in colorectal practice. *Dis Colon Rectum* **40**: 827–831.
Paterson-Brown S (1998) Should doctors perform an elective caesarean section on request? Yes, as long as the woman is fully informed. *BMJ* **317**: 462–463.
Pearl RK, Prasad ML, Nelson RL, Orsay CP & Abcarian H (1991) Bilateral gluteus maximus transposition for anal incontinence. *Dis Colon Rectum* **34**: 478–481.
Pedersen E, Harving H, Klemar B & Torring J (1978) Human anal reflexes. *J Neurol Neurosurg Psychiatry* **41**: 813–881.
Pedersen E, Klemar B, Schroder HDAA & Torring J (1982) Anal sphincter response after perianal electrical stimulation. *J Neurol Neurosurg Psychiatry* **45**: 770–773.
Pedersen IK & Christiansen J (1989) A study of the physiological variation in anal manometry. *Br J Surg* **76**: 69–71.
Peet SM, Castleden CM & McGrother CW (1995) Prevalence of urinary and faecal incontinence in hospitals and residential and nursing homes for older people. *BMJ* **311**: 1063–1064.
Pena A (1983) Posterior sagittal anorectoplasty as a secondary operation for the treatment of fecal incontinence. *J Pediatr Surg* **18**: 762–773.
Pena A (1985) Surgical treatment of high imperforate anus. *World J Surg* **9**: 236–243.
Penninckx F (1992) Faecal incontinence: indications for repairing the anal sphincter. *World J Surg* **16**: 820–825.
Penninckx FM, Lestar B & Kerremans RP (1989) A new balloon-retaining test for evaluation of anorectal function in incontinent patients. *Dis Colon Rectum* **32**: 202–205.
Penninckx F, Debruyne C, Lestar B & Kerremans R (1990) Observer variation in the radiological measurement of the anorectal angle. *Int J Colorectal Dis* **5**: 94–97.
Percy JP, Neill ME, Swash M & Parks AG (1981) Electrophysiological study of motor nerve supply of the pelvic floor. *Lancet* **i**: 16–17.
Percy JP, Neill ME, Kandia TK & Swash MA (1982) A neurogenic factor in faecal incontinence in the elderly. *Age Ageing* **11**: 175–179.
Perozo SE, Ferrara A, Patankar SK, Larach SW & Williamson PP (1997) Biofeedback with home trainer programme is effective for both incontinence and pelvic floor dysfunction. *Techniques Coloproctol* **5**: 6–9.
Perry RE, Blatchford GJ, Christensen MA, Thorson AG & Attwood SEA (1990) Manometric diagnosis of anal sphincter injuries. *Am J Surg* **159**: 112.
Pescatori M, Pavesio R, Anastasio G & Daini S (1991) Transanal electrostimulation for fecal incontinence: clinical, psychologic and manometric prospective study. *Dis Colon Rectum* **34**: 540–545.
Pescatori M, Anastasio G, Bottini C & Mentasti A (1992) New grading and scoring for anal incontinence: evaluation of 335 patients. *Dis Colon Rectum* **35**: 482–487.
Pezim ME, Spencer RJ, Stanhope CR, Beart RW Jr, Ready RL & Ilustrup DM (1987) Sphincter repair for fecal incontinence after obstetrical or iatrogenic injury. *Dis Colon Rectum* **30**: 521–525.
Pfeifer J, Salanga VD, Agachan F, Wiss EG & Wexner SD (1997) Variation in pudendal nerve terminal motor latency according to disease. *Dis Colon Rectum* **40**: 79–83.
Phillips SF & Edwards DAW (1965) Some aspects of anal continence and defaecation. *Gut* **6**: 396–405.
Pickrell KL, Broadbent TR, Masters FW & Metzger JT (1952) Construction of a rectal sphincter and restoration of anal continence by transplanting the gracilis muscle. *Ann Surg* **135**: 853–862.
Pickrell KL, Georgiade N, Maguire C & Crawford H (1955) Correction of rectal incontinence. *Trans Am Proctol Soc* **54**: 721–726.
Pinho M & Keighley MRB (1990) Results of surgery for idiopathic faecal incontinence. *Ann Med* **22**: 426–447.
Pinho M, Yoshioka K, Ortiz J, Oya M & Keighley MRB (1990) The effect of age on pelvic floor dynamics. *Int J Colorectal Dis* **5**: 207–208.
Pinho M, Hosie K, Bielecki K & Keighley MRB (1991) Assessment of noninvasive intraanal electromyography to evaluate sphincter function. *Dis Colon Rectum* **34**: 69–71.
Pinho M, Ortiz J, Oya M, Panagamuwa B, Asperer J & Keighley MRB (1992) Total pelvic floor repair for the treatment of neuropathic fecal incontinence. *Am J Surg* **163**: 340–343.
Pintor MP, Zara GP, Falletto E, Monge L, Demattei M, Carta Q & Masenti E (1994) Pudendal neuropathy in diabetic patients with faecal incontinence. *Int J Colorectal Dis* **9**: 105–109.
Pittman JS, Benson JT & Sumners JE (1990) Physiologic evaluation of the anorectum. *Dis Colon Rectum* **33**: 476–478.
Porter NH (1962) A physiological study of the pelvic floor in rectal prolapse. *Ann R Coll Surg Engl* **31**: 379–401.
Powell PH & Feneley RCL (1980) The role of urethral sensation in clinical urology. *Br J Urol* **52**: 539–541.
Preston DM, Lennard-Jones PE & Thomas BM (1984) The balloon proctogram. *Br J Surg* **71**: 29–32.
Pucciani F, Bologna A, Rottoli ML, Cianchi F & Cortesini C (1997) Idiopathic faecal incontinence and internal anal sphincter dysfunction: role of the rectoanal inhibitory reflex. *Techniques Coloproctol* **5**: 14–18.
Rainey JB, Donaldson DR & Thomson JPS (1990) Postanal repair: which patients derive most benefit. *J R Coll Surg Edinb* **35**: 101–105.
Rasmussen O, Christensen B, Sorensen M, Tetzschner T & Christiansen J (1990) Rectal compliance in the assessment of patients with fecal incontinence. *Dis Colon Rectum* **33**: 650–653.
Rasmussen OO, Sorensen M, Tetzchner T & Christiansen J (1992) Dynamic anal manometry: physiological variations and pathophysiological findings in fecal incontinence. *Gastroenterology* **103**: 103–113.
Rasmussen OO, Hansen CR, Zhu BW & Christiansen J (1996) Effect of octreotide on anal pressure and rectal compliance. *Dis Colon Rectum* **39**: 624–627.
Ratani RS, Yazaki E, Scott M, Pilot MA & Williams NS (1997) Electrically stimulated smooth muscle neosphincter. *Br J Surg* **84**: 1286–1289.
Read MG & Read NW (1982) Role of anorectal sensation in preserving continence. *Gut* **23**: 345–347.
Read MG, Read NW & Duthie HL (1979) Effect of loperamide on anal sphincter function in patients with diarrhoea. *Gut* **20**: A942.
Read MG, Read NW, Haynes WG, Donnelly TC & Johnson AG (1982) A prospective study of the effect of haemorrhoidectomy on sphincter function and faecal incontinence. *Br J Surg* **69**: 396–398.

Read NW (1983) Drug induced constipation. *Mims Magazine* 19–21.

Read NW & Abouzekry L (1986) Why do patients with faecal impaction have faecal incontinence? *Gut* **27**: 283–287.

Read NW & Bannister JT (1985) Anorectal manometry: techniques in health and disease. In Henry MM & Swash M (eds) *Coloproctology and the Pelvic Floor*, pp 65–87. London: Butterworth.

Read NW, Harford WV, Schmulen AC, Read MG, Santa Ana C & Fordtran JS (1979) A clinical study of patients with faecal incontinence and diarrhoea. *Gastroenterology* **76**: 747–756.

Read NW, Haynes WG, Bartolo DCC et al (1983a) Use of anorectal manometry during rectal infusion of saline to investigate sphincter function in incontinent patients. *Gastroenterology* **85**: 105–113.

Read NW, Bartolo DCC, Read MG, Hall J, Haynes WG & Johnson AG (1983b) Differences in anorectal manometry between patients with haemorrhoids and patients with descending perineum syndrome: implications for management. *Br J Surg* **70**: 656–659.

Read NW, Bartolo DCC & Read MG (1984) Differences in anal function in patients with incontinence to solids and in patients with incontinence to liquids. *Br J Surg* **71**: 39–42.

Read NW, Abouzekry L, Read MG, Howell P, Ottwell D & Donnelly TC (1985) Anorectal function in elderly patients with fecal impaction. *Gastroenterology* **89**: 959–966.

Rieger NA, Sweeney JL, Hoffmann DC, Young JF & Hunter A (1996) Investigation of fecal incontinence with endoanal ultrasound. *Dis Colon Rectum* **39**: 860–864.

Rieger NA, Wattchow DA, Sarre RG et al (1997a) Prospective trial of pelvic floor retraining in patients with fecal incontinence. *Dis Colon Rectum* **40**: 821–826.

Rieger NA, Sarre RG, Saccone GTP, Schloithe AC & Wattchow DA (1997b) *Int J Colorect Dis* **12**: 303–307.

Roberts PL, Coller JA, Schoetz DJ & Veidenheimer MC (1990) Manometric assessment of patients with obstetric injuries and fecal incontinence. *Dis Colon Rectum* **33**: 16–20.

Roe AM, Bartolo DCC & Mortensen NJMcC (1986) New method for assessment of anal sensation in various anorectal disorders. *Br J Surg* **73**: 310–312.

Rogers J, Henry MM & Misiewicz JJ (1988a) Combined sensory and motor deficit in primary neuropathic faecal incontinence. *Gut* **29**: 5–9.

Rogers J, Levy DM, Henry MM & Misiewicz JJ (1988b) Pelvic floor neuropathy: a comparative study of diabetes mellitus and idiopathic faecal incontinence. *Gut* **29**: 756–761.

Rogers J, Henry MM & Misiewicz JJ (1988c) Disposable pudendal nerve stimulator: evaluation of the standard instrument and new device. *Gut* **29**: 1131–1133.

Rogers J, Hayward MP, Henry MM & Misiewicz JJ (1988d) Temperature gradient between the rectum and the anal canal: evidence against the role of temperature sensation as a sensory modality in the anal canal of normal subjects. *Br J Surg* **25**: 1083–1085.

Roig JV, Villoslada C, Lledo S et al (1995) Prevalence of pudendal neuropathy in fecal incontinence. *Dis Colon Rectum* **38**: 952–958.

Rosen HR, Novi G, Zoech G, Feil W, Urbarz C & Schiessel R (1998) Restoration of anal sphincter function by single-stage dynamic graciloplasty with a modified (split sling) technique. *Am J Surg* **175**: 187–193.

Rudd WH, Sullivan ES, Corman ML, Devroede G & Schuster MM (1982) Anal incontinence (symposium). *Dis Colon Rectum* **25**: 90–107.

Ruppin H (1987) Review: Loperamide – a potent antidiarrhoeal drug with actions along the alimentary tract. *Aliment Pharmacol Ther* **1**: 179–190.

Ryhammer AM, Bek KM & Laurberg S (1995) Multiple vaginal deliveries increase the risk of permanent incontinence of flatus and urine in normal premenopausal women. *Dis Colon Rectum* **38**: 1206–1209.

Salmons S (1980) Functional adaptation in skeletal muscle. *Neurol Sci* **3**: 134–137.

Salmons SS & Henriksson J (1981) The adaptive response of skeletal muscle to increased use. *Muscle Nerve* **4**: 94–105.

Sangwan YP, Coller JA, Barrett RC, Roberts PL, Murray JJ & Schoetz DJ (1995) Can manometric parameters predict response to biofeedback therapy in fecal incontinence? *Dis Colon Rectum* **38**: 1021–1025.

Sangwan YP, Coller JA, Barrett RC, Murray JJ, Roberts PL & Schoetz DJ (1996a) Unilateral pudendal neuropathy. *Dis Colon Rectum* **39**: 249–251.

Sangwan YP, Coller JA, Barrett RC et al (1996b) Unilateral pudendal neuropathy. Impact on outcome of anal sphincter repair. *Dis Colon Rectum* **39**: 686–689.

Santulli TV, Schullinger JH & Armoury RA (1965) Malformations of the anus and rectum. *Surg Clin North Am* **45**: 1253–1271.

Sato T & Konishi F (1996) Functional perineal colostomy with pudendal nerve anastomosis following anorectal resection: An experimental study. *Surgery* **119**: 641–651.

Sato T, Konishi F & Kanazawa K (1997) Functional perineal colostomy with pudendal nerve anastomosis following anorectal resection: a cadaver operation study on a new procedure. *Surgery* **121**: 569–574.

Scharli AF & Kiesewetter WB (1970) Defaecation and continence: some new concepts. *Dis Colon Rectum* **13**: 81–107.

Scheuer M, Kuijpers HC & Jacobs PP (1989) Postanal repair restores anatomy rather than function. *Dis Colon Rectum* **32**: 960–963.

Scheuer M, Kuijpers HC & Bleijenber G (1994) Effect of electrostimulation on sphincter function in neurogenic fecal continence. *Dis Colon Rectum* **37**: 590–594.

Schier F, Schneiger W & Willital GH (1986) Anal incontinence in childhood: psychosocial development after sacral sphincter replacement. *Coloproctology* **8**: 115–118.

Schiller LR, Santa Ana CA, Schulen AC et al (1982) Pathogenesis of fecal incontinence in diabetes mellitus: evidence for internal-anal-sphincter dysfunction. *N Engl J Med* **307**: 1666–1671.

Schmidt E (1986) Surgery for anal incontinence. *Coloproctology* **8**: 218–222.

Schoetz DJ Jr (1985) Operative therapy for anal incontinence. *Surg Clin North Am* **65**: 35–65.

Schuster MM (1966) Clinical significance of motor disturbances of the enterocolonic segment. *Am J Dig Dis* **2**: 320.

Schuster MM (1975) The riddle of the sphincters. *Gastroenterology* **69**: 249–262.

Schuster MM (1977) Biofeedback treatment for gastrointestinal disorders. *Med Clin North Am* **61**: 907–912.

Schuster MM, Hendrix TR & Mendeloff AI (1963) The internal sphincter response. Manometric studies on its normal physiology, normal pathways and alteration in bowel disease. *J Clin Invest* **42**: 196–207.

Schuster MM, Hookman P, Hendrix TR & Mendeloff AI (1965) Simultaneous manometric recording of internal and external anal sphincter reflexes. *Bull Johns Hopkins Hosp* **116**: 79–88.

Schuster MM, Corazziari E, Erckenbrecht J, Ihre T & Keighley MRB (1994) Faecal incontinence. *Gastroenterology Int* **7**: 1–12.

Schwartz MS, Sargeant MK & Swash M (1976) Longitudinal fibre splitting in neurogenic muscular disorders: its relation to the pathogenesis of 'myopathic' change. *Brain* **99**: 617–636.

Scott ADN, Henry MM & Phillips RKS (1990) Clinical

assessment and anorectal manometry before postanal repair: failure to predict outcome. *Br J Surg* **77**: 628–629.
Seccia M, Menconi C, Balestri R & Cavina E (1994) Study protocols and functional results in 86 electrostimulated graciloplasties. *Dis Colon Rectum* **37**: 897–904.
Sedgwick EM (1982) Clinical application of the spinal and cortical somatosensory evoked potentials. *Amsterdam Excerpta Medica* 207–214.
Sentovich SM, Rivela LJ, Blatchford GJ, Christensen MA & Thorson AG (1995) Patterns of male fecal incontinence. *Dis Colon Rectum* **38**: 281–285.
Sentovich SM, Blatchford GJ, Rivela LJ, Lin K, Thorson AG & Christensen MA (1997) Diagnosing anal sphincter injury with transanal ultrasound and manometry. *Dis Colon Rectum* **40**: 1430–1434.
Setti-Carraro P & Nicholls RJ (1994) Postanal repair for faecal incontinence persisting after rectopexy. *Br J Surg* **81**: 305–307.
Setti-Carraro P, Kamm MA & Nicholls RJ (1994) Long-term results of postanal repair for neurogenic faecal incontinence. *Br J Surg* **81**: 140–144.
Shafik A (1975) A new concept of the anatomy of the anal sphincter mechanism and the physiology of defaecation. The external sphincter: a triple loop system. *Invest Urol* **12**: 412–419.
Shafik A (1984) Pelvic double-sphincteric control complex. Theory of pelvic organ continence with clinical application. *Urology* **23**: 611–618.
Shafik A (1985) A new concept of the anatomy of the anal sphincter. Mechanism and the physiology of defaecation. *Coloproctology* **7**: 107–112.
Shandling B & Gilmour RF (1987) The enema continence catheter in spina bifida: successful bowel management. *J Pediatr Surg* **22**: 271–273.
Shankar KR, Losty PD, Kenny SE et al (1998) Functional results following the antegrade continence enema procedure. *Br J Surg* **85**: 980–982.
Shatari T, Teramoto T, Kitajima M & Minamitant H (1995) Conversion of the rabbit gracilis muscle for transposition as a neoanal sphincter by electrical stimulation. *Surg Today* **25**: 233–236.
Shouler P & Keighley MRB (1986) Changes in colorectal function in severe idiopathic chronic constipation. *Gastroenterology* **90**: 414–420.
Sielezneff, Bauer S, Bulgar JC & Sarles JC (1996) Gracilis muscle transposition in the treatment of faecal incontinence. *J Colorectal Dis* **11**: 15–18.
Simmang C, Birbaum EH, Kodner IJ, Fry RD & Fleshman JW (1994) Anal sphincter reconstruction in the elderly: does advancing age affect outcome? *Dis Colon Rectum* **37**: 1065–1069.
Simonson OS, Stolf NAG, Aun F, Raia A & Habra-Gama A (1976) Rectal sphincter reconstruction in perineal colostomies after abdominoperineal resection for cancer. *Br J Surg* **63**: 389–391.
Siproudhis L, Bellissant E, Juguet F, Allain H, Bretagne J-F & Gosselin M (1998) Effects of cholinergic agents on anorectal physiology. *Aliment Pharmacol Ther* **12**: 747–754.
Sitzler PJ & Thomson JPS (1996) Overlap repair of damaged anal sphincter. *Dis Colon Rectum* **39**: 1356–1360.
Skomorowska E, Hegedus V & Christiansen J (1988) Evaluation of perineal descent by defaecography. *Int J Colorectal Dis* **3**: 191–194.
Slade MS, Goldberg SM, Schottler JL et al (1977) Sphincteroplasty for acquired anal incontinence. *Dis Colon Rectum* **20**: 33–35.
Sleep J & Grant A (1987) Pelvic floor exercises in postnatal care. *Midwifery* **3**: 158–164.
Sleep J, Grant A, Gracia J, Elbourne D, Spencer J & Chalmers J (1984) West Berkshire perineal management trial. *BMJ* **289**: 587–590.
Smith B (1968) Effects of irritant purgatives on the myenteric plexus in man and mouse. *Gut* **9**: 139–143.
Snooks SJ & Swash M (1984a) Perineal nerve and transcutaneous spinal stimulation: new methods for investigation of the urethral striated sphincter musculature. *Br J Urol* **56**: 406–409.
Snooks SJ & Swash M (1984b) Abnormalities of the innervation of the urethral striated sphincter musculature in incontinence. *Br J Urol* **56**: 401–405.
Snooks SJ & Swash M (1985) Motor conduction velocity in the human spinal cord: slowed conduction in multiple sclerosis and radiation myelopathy. *J Neurol Neurosurg Psychiatry* **48**: 1135–1139.
Snooks SJ & Swash M (1986) The innervation of the muscles of continence. *Ann R Coll Surg Engl* **68**: 45–49.
Snooks SJ, Barnes PRH & Swash M (1984a) Damage to the innervation of the voluntary anal and periurethral sphincter musculature in incontinence: an electrophysiological study. *J Neurol Neurosurg Psychiatry* **47**: 1269–1273.
Snooks SJ, Swash M & Henry M (1984b) Electrophysiologic and manometric assessment of failed postanal repair for anorectal incontinence. *Dis Colon Rectum* **27**: 733–736.
Snooks S, Henry MM & Swash M (1984c) Faecal incontinence after anal dilatation. *Br J Surg* **71**: 617–618.
Snooks SJ, Setchell M, Swash M & Henry MM (1984d) Injury to innervation of pelvic floor sphincter musculature in childbirth. *Lancet* **ii**: 546–550.
Snooks SJ, Barnes PRH, Swash M & Henry MM (1985a) Damage to the innervation of the pelvic floor musculature in chronic constipation. *Gastroenterology* **89**: 977–981.
Snooks SJ, Henry MM & Swash M (1985b) Anorectal incontinence and rectal prolapse: differential assessment of the innervation to puborectalis and external anal sphincter muscles. *Gut* **26**: 470–476.
Snooks SJ, Swash M & Henry MM (1985c) Abnormalities in central and peripheral nerve conduction in patients with anorectal incontinence. *J R Soc Med* **78**: 294–300.
Snooks SJ, Swash M, Henry MM & Setchell M (1986) Risk factors in childbirth causing damage to the pelvic floor innervation. *Int J Colorectal Dis* **1**: 20–24.
Snooks SJ, Swash M, Mathers SE & Henry MM (1990) Effect of vaginal delivery on the pelvic floor: a 5-year follow-up. *Br J Surg* **77**: 1358–1360.
Solomon MJ, McLeod RS, Cohen EK, Simons MK & Wilson S (1994) Reliability and validity studies of endoluminal ultrasonography for anorectal disorders. *Dis Colon Rectum* **37**: 546–551.
Sorensen M, Tetzschner T, Rasmussen O & Christiansen J (1991) Relation between electromyography and anal manometry of the external anal sphincter. *Gut* **32**: 1031–1034.
Sorensen M, Tetzschner, Rasmussen, Bjarnesen J & Christiansen J (1993) Sphincter rupture in childbirth. *Br J Surg* **80**: 392–394.
Sorensen M, Nielsen MB, Pedersen JF & Christiansen J (1994) Electromyography of the internal anal sphincter performed under endosonographic guidance. *Dis Colon Rectum* **37**: 138–143.
Speakman CTM & Kamm MA (1991) The internal anal sphincter: new insights into faecal incontinence. *Gut* **32**: 345–346.
Speakman CTM & Kamm MA (1993) Abnormal visceral autonomic innervation in neurogenic faecal incontinence. *Gut* **34**: 215–221.

Speakman CTM, Hoyle CHV, Kamm MA, Henry MM, Nicholls RJ & Burnstock G (1990) Adrenergic control of the internal anal sphincter is abnormal in patients with idiopathic faecal incontinence. *Br J Surg* **77**: 1342–1344.

Speakman CTM, Burnett SJD, Kamm MA & Bartram CI (1991) Sphincter injury after anal dilatation demonstrated by anal endosonography. *Br J Surg* **78**: 1429–1430.

Speakman CTM, Hoyle CHV, Kamm MA, Henry MM, Nicholls RJ & Burnstock G (1992) Decreased sensitivity of muscarinic but not 5-hydroxytryptamine receptors of the internal anal sphincter in neurogenic faecal incontinence. *Br J Surg* **79**: 829–832.

Speakman CTM, Hoyle CHV, Kamm MA, Henry MM, Nicholls RJ & Burnstock G (1993) Neuropeptides in the internal anal sphincter in neurogenic faecal incontinence. *Int J Colorectal Dis* **8**: 201–205.

Speakman CTM, Hoyle CHV, Kamm MA et al (1995) Abnormal internal anal sphincter fibrosis and elasticity in fecal incontinence. *Dis Colon Rectum* **38**: 407–410.

Squire R, Kiely EM, Carr B, Ransley PG & Duffy PG (1993) The clinical application of the Malone antegrade colonic enema. *J Pediatr Surg* **28**: 1012–1015.

Stalberg E & Trontelj V (1979) *Single Fibre Electromyography*. Old Woking: Mirvalle Press.

Stebbing JF, Brading AF & Mortensen NJMcC (1995) Nitrergic inhibitory innervation of porcine rectal circular smooth muscle. *Br J Surg* **82**: 1183–1187.

Stebbing JF, Brading AF & Mortensen NJMcC (1996) Nitrergic innervation and relaxant response of rectal circular smooth muscle. *Dis Colon Rectum* **39**: 294–299.

Stebbing JF, Brading AF, Mortensen NJMcC (1997) Role of nitric oxide in relation of the longitudinal layer of rectal smooth muscle. *Dis Colon Rectum* **40**: 706–710.

Stelzner F (1960) Uber die Anatomie des analen sphincterorgans wie die der chirurg sieht. *Z Anat Entwicklungsgeschamte* **121**: 525–535.

Stephens FD & Smith ED (1971) *Ano-Rectal Malformations in Children*, pp 373–377. Chicago: Year Book Medical.

Stewart J, Kumar D & Keighley MRB (1994) Results of anal or low rectal anastomosis and pouch construction for megarectum and megacolon. *Br J Surg* **81**: 1051–1053.

Stokes SA & Motta GJ (1982) The geriatric patient. In Broadwell DC & Jackson BS (eds) *Principles of Ostomy Care*, pp 545–562. London: Mosby.

Stone HB & McLanahan S (1941) Results with the fascia plastic operation for anal incontinence. *Ann Surg* **31**: 73–77.

Stricker JW, Schoetz DJ Jr., Coller JA & Veidenheimer MC (1988) Surgical correction of anal incontinence. *Dis Colon Rectum* **31**: 533–540.

Sultan AH, Kamm MA, Hudson CN, Thomas JM & Bartram CI (1993a) Anal-sphincter disruption during vaginal delivery. *N Engl J Med* **329**: 1905–1911.

Sultan AH, Kamm MA, Hudson CN & Bartram CI (1993b) Effect of pregnancy on anal sphincter morphology and function. *Int J Colorectal Dis* **8**: 206–209.

Sultan AH, Kamm MA, Bartram CI & Hudson CN (1993c) Anal sphincter trauma during instrumental delivery. *Int J Gynaecol Obstet* **43**: 263–270.

Sultan AH, Nicholls RJ, Kamm MA, Hudson CN, Beynon J & Bartram CI (1993d) Anal endosonography and correlation with in vitro and in vivo anatomy. *Br J Surg* **80**: 508–511.

Sultan AH, Kamm MA, Talbot IC, Nicholls RJ & Bartram CI (1994a) Anal endosonography for identifying external sphincter defects confirmed histologically. *Br J Surg* **81**: 463–465.

Sultan AH, Kamm MA, Hudson CN & Bartram CI (1994b) Third degree obstetric anal sphincter tears: risk factors and outcome of primary repair. *BMJ* **308**; 887–891.

Sultan AH, Loder PB, Bartram CI, Kamm MA & Hudson CN (1994c) Vaginal endosonography. New approach to image the undisturbed anal sphincter. *Dis Colon Rectum* **37**: 1296–1299.

Sun WM, Read NW, Miner PB, Kerrigan DD & Donnelly TC (1990a) The role of transient internal sphincter relaxation in faecal incontinence? *Int J Colorectal Dis* **5**: 31–36.

Sun WM, Read NW & Miner PB (1990b) Relation between rectal sensation and anal function in normal subjects and patients with faecal incontinence. *Gut* **31**: 1056–1061.

Sun WM, Donnelly TC & Read NW (1992) Utility of a combined test of anorectal manometry, electromyography, and sensation in determining the mechanism of 'idiopathic' faecal incontinence. *Gut* **33**: 807–813.

Sunderland S (1978) *Nerves and Nerve Injuries*, 2nd edn, pp 82–86. Edinburgh: Churchill Livingstone.

Swash M (1993) Childbirth is responsible for most cases. *BMJ* **307**: 636–637.

Swash M (1980) Idiopathic faecal incontinence: histopathological evidence on pathogenesis. In Wright R (ed.) *Recent Advances in Gastrointestinal Pathology*, pp 71–89. London: WB Saunders.

Swash M (1982a) The neuropathy of idiopathic faecal incontinence. In Smith WT & Cavanagh JB (eds) *Recent Advances in Neuropathology, Vol. 2*. Edinburgh: Churchill Livingstone.

Swash M (1982b) Early and late components of the human anal reflex. *J Neurol Neurosurg Psychiatry* **45**: 767–769.

Swash M (1985a) New concepts in incontinence. *BMJ* **290**: 4–5.

Swash M (1985b) Histopathology of the pelvic floor muscles. In Henry MM & Swash M (eds) *Coloproctology and the Pelvic Floor*, pp 129–150. London: Butterworth.

Swash M (1985c) Anorectal incontinence: electrophysiological tests. *Br J Surg* **72** (Suppl): S14.

Swash M (1985d) Pathophysiology of idiopathic (neurogenic) faecal incontinence. In Sir Alan Parks Memorial Symposium. *Ann R Coll Surg Engl* **65** (Suppl): 22–23.

Swash M & Schwartz MS (1977) Implications of longitudinal fibre in neurogenic and myopathic disorders. *J Neurol Neurosurg Psychiatry* **40**: 1152–1159.

Swash M & Schwartz MS (1981) *Neuromuscular Disease: A Practical Approach to Diagnosis and Management*. New York: Springer.

Swash M & Schwartz MS (1984) *Muscle Biopsy Pathology*. London: Chapman & Hall.

Swash M & Snooks SJ (1985) Electromyography in pelvic floor disorders. In Henry MM & Swash M (eds) *Coloproctology and the Pelvic Floor*, pp 86–103. London: Butterworth.

Swash M, Snooks JJ & Henry MM (1985) Unifying concept of pelvic floor disorders and incontinence. *J R Soc Med* **78**: 906–911.

Swash M, Gray A, Lubowski DZ & Nicholls RJ (1988) Ultrastructural changes in internal anal sphincter in neurogenic faecal incontinence. *Gut* **29**: 1692–1698.

Tagart REB (1966) The anal canal and rectum, their varying relationship and its effect on anal continence. *Dis Colon Rectum* **9**: 449–452.

Taylor BM, Beart RW & Phillips SF (1984) Longitudinal and radial variations in pressure in the human anal sphincter. *Gastroenterology* **86**: 693–697.

Taylor I, Duthie HL & Zachary RB (1973) Anal continence following surgery for imperforate anus. *J Pediatr Surg* **8**: 497–503.

Taylor I, Darby C & Hammond P (1978) Comparison of rectosigmoid myoelectric activity in the irritable colon during relapses and remissions. *Gut* **19**: A457.

Templeton JM & O'Neill JA Jr (1986) Anorectal malformations. In Welsh KJ, Randolph JG, Ravitch MM et al (eds) *Pediatric Surgery*, 4th edn, pp 1022–1035. Chicago: Year Book Medical.

Ten Cate Hoedemaker HO (1987) Anatomy of the anorectum. In Gooszen HG, Ten Cate Hoedemaker HO, Weterman IT & Keighley MRB (eds) *Disordered Defaecation*, pp 3–16. Dordrecht: Martinus Nijhoff.

Ternent CA, Shashidharan M, Blatchford GJ, Christensen MA, Thorson AG & Sentovich SM (1997) Transanal ultrasound and anorectal physiology findings affecting continence after sphincteroplasty. *Dis Colon Rectum* **40**: 462–467.

Tetzschner T, Sørensen M, Rasmussen O, Lose G & Christiansen J (1997) Reliability of pudendal nerve terminal motor latency. *Int J Colorect Dis* **12**: 280–284.

The Times (1998) Doctors call for right to choose Caesarean birth. 14 August.

Thomson WHF (1975) The nature of haemorrhoids. *Br J Surg* **62**: 542–552.

Thomson WH, Cooke SG & Strugnell NA (1998) A study of controlled digital dilation of the anus in the treatment of chronic anal fissure. *Abstracts of the Association of Coloproctology of Great Britain and Ireland Annual Meeting, St Helier, 29 June–1 July*. Oxford: Blackwell Science.

Thorpe AC, Roberts JP, Williams NS, Blandy JP & Badenoch DF (1995) Pelvic floor physiology in women with faecal incontinence and urinary symptoms. *Br J Surg* **82**: 173–176.

Tjandra JJ, Milsom JW, Stolfi VM et al (1992) Endoluminal ultrasound defines anatomy of the anal canal and pelvic floor. *Dis Colon Rectum* **35**: 465–470.

Tjandra JJ, Milsom JW, Schroeder T, Fazio VW (1993) Endoluminal ultrasound is preferable to electromyography in mapping anal sphincteric defects. *Dis Colon Rectum* **36**: 689–692.

Tobin GW & Brocklehurst JC (1986) Faecal incontinence in residential homes for the elderly: prevalence, aetiology and management. *Age Ageing* **15**: 41–46.

Vaizey CJ, Kamm MA, Gold DM, Bartram CI, Halligan S & Nicholls RJ (1998) Clinical, physiological, and radiological study of a new purpose-designed artificial bowel sphincter. *Lancet* **352**: 105–108.

van Tets WF & Kuijpers JC (1994) Continence disorders after fistulotomy. *Dis Colon Rectum* **37**: 1194–1197.

van Tets WF, Kuijpers JHC & Bleijenberg G (1996) Biofeedback treatment is ineffective in neurogenic fecal incontinence. *Dis Colon Rectum* **39**: 992–994.

van Tets WF, Kuijpers JHC, Mollen R & Goor H (1997) Influence of Parks' anal retractor on anal sphincter pressures. *Dis Colon Rectum* **40**: 1042–1045.

Varma KK & Stephens FD (1972) Neurovascular reflexes of anal continence. *Aust NZ J Surg* **41**: 236–272.

Venkatesh KS, Ramanujam PS, Larson DM & Haywood MA (1989) Anorectal complications of vaginal delivery. *Dis Colon Rectum* **32**: 1039–1041.

Vernava AM III, Longo WE & Daniel GL (1992) Pudendal neuropathy and the importance of EMG evaluation of fecal incontinence. *Dis Colon Rectum* **35**: 11.

Vernava AM, Longo WE & Daniel GL (1993) Pudendal neuropathy and the importance of EMG evaluation of fecal incontinence. *Dis Colon Rectum* **36**: 23–27.

Versluis PJ, Konsten J, Geerdes B, Baeten CGMI & Oei KTK (1995) Defecographic evaluation of dynamic graciloplasty for fecal incontinence. *Dis Colon Rectum* **38**: 468–473.

Vierck CJ, Greenspan JD, Ritz LA & Yeomans DC (1986) The spinal pathways contributing to the ascending conduction and descending modulation of pain sensation and reactions. In Yaksh TL (ed.) *Spinal Afferent Processing*, pp 142–147. New York: Plenum Press.

von Rapport E (1952) Plasticher ersatz des museulus sphincter ani. *Zentralbl Chir* **77**: 579–581.

Wald A (1981) Biofeedback therapy for faecal incontinence. *Ann Intern Med* **95**: 146–149.

Wald A (1983) Biofeedback for neurogenic faecal incontinent rectal sensation is a determinant of outcome. *J Paediatr Gastroenterol Nutr* **2**: 302–306.

Wald A (1985) Diabetes-associated fecal incontinence in the geriatric patient. *Geriatr Med Today* **4**: 40–48.

Wald A & Turugunthla AK (1984) Anorectal sensorimotor dysfunction in fecal incontinence and diabetes mellitus. *N Engl J Med* **310**: 1282–1287.

Waldron DJ, Horgan PG, Patel FR, Maguire R & Given HF (1993) Multiple sclerosis: Assessment of colonic and anorectal function in the presence of faecal incontinence. *Int J Colorectal Dis* **8**: 220–224.

Walsh CJ, Mooney EF, Upton GJ & Motson RW (1996) Incidence of third-degree perineal tears in labour and outcome after primary repair. *Br J Surg* **83**: 218–221.

Wang JY, Lai CR, Chen JS, Lin Se, Chang-Chien CR & Fan HA (1988) Gracilis muscle transposition for anal incontinence: a report of five cases. *Southeast Asian J Surg* **11**: 89–92.

Warwick R & Williams PL (eds) (1973) *Gray's Anatomy*, 35th edn. Edinburgh: Longmans.

Watkins GA & Oliver GA (1965) Giant megacolon in the insane: further observations in patients treated with subtotal colectomy. *Gastroenterology* **48**: 718–727.

Watson SJ & Phillips RKS (1995) Non-inflammatory rectovaginal fistula. *Br J Surg* **82**: 1641–1643.

Wendell-Smith CP (1967) Studies on the morphology of the pelvic floor. PhD thesis, p 305. London: University of London.

Wexner SD, Marchetti F & Jagelman DG (1991a) The role of sphincteroplasty for fecal incontinence re-evaluated: a prospective physiologic and functional review. *Dis Colon Rectum* **34**: 22–30.

Wexner SD, Marchetti F, Salanga VD, Corredor C & Jagelman DG (1991b) Neurophysiologic assessment of the anal sphincters. *Dis Colon Rectum* **34**: 606–612.

Wexner SD, Jorge JMN, Nogueras JJ & Jagelman DG (1992) Physiological assessment of colorectal functional disorders: use or abuse of technology? *Dis Colon Rectum* **35**: 11–12.

Wexner SD, Gonzalez-Padron A, Rius J et al (1996a) Stimulated gracilis neosphincter operation: initial experience, pitfalls, and complications. *Dis Colon Rectum* **39**: 958–964.

Wexner SD, Gonzalez-Padron A, Teoh T-A & Moon HK (1996b) The stimulated gracilis neosphincter for faecal incontinence. A new use for an old concept. *Plast Reconstr Surg* **98**: 693-699.

Wheatley IC, Hardy KJ & Dent J (1977) Anal pressure studies in spinal patients. *Gut* **18**: 488–490.

White JC, Verlot MG & Ehrentheil O (1940) Neurogenic disturbances of the colon and their investigation by the colonmetrogram. *Ann Surg* **112**: 1042–1057.

Whitehead WE, Engel BT & Schuster MM (1980) Irritable bowel syndrome: physiological and psychological differences between diarrhoea-predominant and constipation-predominant patients. *Dig Dis Sci* **5**: 404–413.

Whitehead WE, Orr WC, Engel BT & Schuster MM (1981) External anal sphincter response to rectal distension: learned response or reflex. *Psychophysiology* **19**: 57–62.

Williams JG, Wong WD, Jensen L, Rothenberger DA & Goldberg SM (1991) Incontinence and rectal prolapse: a prospective manometric study. *Dis Colon Rectum* **34**: 209–216.

Williams N, Barlow J, Hobson A, Scott N, Irving M (1995) Manometric asymmetry in the anal canal in controls and patients with fecal incontinence. *Dis Colon Rectum* **38**: 1275–1280.

Williams NG, Price R & Johnston D (1980) The long term effect of sphincter preserving operations for rectal carcinoma on function of the anal sphincter in man. *Br J Surg* **67**: 203–208.

Williams NS (1992) Anorectal reconstruction. *Br J Surg* **79**: 733–734.

Williams NS, Hallan RI, Koeze TH & Watkins ES (1989) Construction of a neorectum and neoanal sphincter following previous proctocolectomy. *Br J Surg* **76**: 1191–1194.

Williams NS, Hallan RI, Koeze TH, Pilot MA & Watkins ES (1990a) Construction of a neoanal sphincter by transposition of the gracilis muscle and prolonged neuromuscular stimulation for the treatment of faecal incontinence. *Ann R Coll Surg Engl* **72**: 108–113.

Williams NS, Hallam RI, Koeze TH & Watkins ES (1990b) Restoration of gastrointestinal continuity and continence after abdomino-perineal excision of the rectum arising in an electrically stimulated neoanal sphincter. *Dis Colon Rectum* **33**: 561–565.

Williams NS, Patel J, George BD, Hallan RI & Watkins ES (1991) Development of an electrically stimulated neoanal sphincter. *Lancet* **338**: 1166–1169.

Williams NS, Corry DG, Abercrombie JF & Powell J (1996) Transposition of the anorectum to the abdominal wall. *Br J Surg* **83**: 1739–1740.

Williams PL & Warwick R (1973) *Functional Neuroanatomy of Man*. Edinburgh: Churchill Livingstone.

Womack NR, Williams NS, Holmfield JH, Morrison JFB & Simpkins KD (1985) New method for dynamic assessment of anorectal function in constipation. *Br J Surg* **72**: 994–998.

Womack NR, Morrison JFB & Williams NS (1986) The role of pelvic floor denervation in the aetiology of idiopathic faecal incontinence. *Br J Surg* **73**: 404–407.

Womack NR, Morrison JFB & Williams NS (1988) Prospective study of the effects of postanal repair in neurogenic faecal incontinence. *Br J Surg* **75**: 48–52.

Wong WD, Jensen LL, Bartolo DCC, Rothenberger DA (1996) Artificial anal sphincter. *Dis Colon Rectum* **39**: 1345–1351.

Wood B (1985) Anatomy of the anal sphincters and pelvic floor. In Henry MM & Swash M (eds) *Coloproctology and the Pelvic Floor*, pp 3–21. London: Butterworths.

Wright AL, Williams NS, Gibson JS, Neal DE & Morrison JFB (1985) Electrically evoked activity in the human external anal sphincter. *Br J Surg* **72**: 38–41.

Wunderlich M & Swash M (1983) The overlapping innervation of the two sides of the external anal sphincter by the pudendal nerves. *J Neurol Sci* **59**: 97–109.

Wyman JB, Heaton KW, Manning AP & Wicks ACB (1978) Variability of colonic function in healthy subjects. *Gut* **19**: 146–150.

Wynne JM, Myles JL, Jones I et al (1996) Disturbed anal sphincter function following vaginal delivery. *Gut* **39**: 120–124.

Yamamoto T, Kubo H & Honzumi M (1996) Fecal incontinence successfully managed by antegrade continence enema in children: a report of two cases. *Surg Today* **26**: 1024–1028.

Yang YK & Wexner SD (1994) Anal pressure vectography is of no apparent benefit for sphincter evaluation. *Int J Colorectal Dis* **9**: 92–95.

Yoshioka K & Keighley MRB (1987) Physiological parameter should dictate the surgical management of longstanding idiopathic chronic constipation. *Gut* **28**: A1362.

Yoshioka K & Keighley MRB (1988) Clinical and manometric assessment of gracilis muscle transplant for fecal incontinence. *Dis Colon Rectum* **31**: 767–769.

Yoshioka K & Keighley MRB (1989) Critical assessment of the quality of continence after postanal repair for faecal incontinence. *Br J Surg* **76**: 1054–1057.

Yoshioka K, Hyland G & Keighley MRB (1987a) Clinical and physiological evaluation of postanal repair. *Gut* **28**: A1362.

Yoshioka K, Poxon V & Keighley MRB (1987b) Does the position of the patient influence the results of anorectal manometry? *Gut* **28**: A1362.

Yoshioka K, Hyland G & Keighley MRB (1988) Physiological changes after postanal repair and parameters predicting outcome. *Br J Surg* **75**: 1220–1224.

Yoshioka K, Pinho M, Ortiz J, Oya M, Hyland G & Keighley MRB (1991) How reliable is measurement of the anorectal angle by videoproctography? *Dis Colon Rectum* **34**: 1010–1013.

Yoshioka K, Ogunbiyi OA & Keighley MRB (1997) Randomized trial of faecal diversion in sphincter repair. *Gut* **40**: A55.

Yoshioka K, Ogunbiyi OA & Keighley MRB (1998) Comparison of total pelvic floor repair (TPFR) or gluteus maximus transposition (GMT) for faecal incontinence. *Dis Colon Rectum* (in press).

Zander L (1982) Episiotomy: has familiarity bred contempt? *J R Coll Gen Pract* **32**: 400–401.

21 CONSTIPATION

Surgeons are sometimes asked to see constipated patients because a physician has exhausted the available medical therapeutic options without relief of symptoms. These patients require careful clinical and physiological assessment (Kumar, 1992). Many of them have a personality disorder. They are frequently demanding, dissatisfied and unhappy and need help, but most are unsuitable for operative treatment. Others may have a predisposing cause which has been overlooked; only a few will justify surgical assessment. Any underlying endocrine, metabolic, neurological, intestinal or drug-induced cause must be excluded. Abnormal myenteric nerves and ganglia may occur in adults and should be identified by biopsy and special staining techniques. Megacolon or megarectum should be excluded by barium enema.

Cases of idiopathic chronic constipation may be classified into three groups: (1) total or partial colonic inertia, for which subtotal colectomy and caecorectal or ileorectal anastomosis may occasionally be considered; (2) outlet obstruction, or anismus which might be resolved in children by pelvic floor or internal sphincter myectomy or in adults by biofeedback; and (3) a combination of colonic inertia and anismus. All three groups often have coexisting features of irritable bowel syndrome. Selected patients in all groups may also be treated by a procedure which allows colonic irrigation in a distal direction to achieve evacuation (antegrade colonic enema).

DEFINITIONS

The frequency of defecation varies widely, so much so that it is difficult to define what is normal. Furthermore, the word 'constipation' has different meanings for different people (Talley et al, 1993; Koch et al, 1997). The term may imply that stools are too hard, too difficult to evacuate, too infrequent, too bulky or even too small. These symptoms are difficult to quantify (Berman et al, 1990).

Stool frequency is the easiest parameter to measure. However, patients tend to exaggerate the problems and it is wise to ask them to record meticulously the number of bowel movements over a period of 4–6 weeks. Stool consistency, rather than frequency, correlates with colonic transit time (Degen and Phillips, 1996). If one suspects the patient of being an unreliable witness it may be worth admitting them to a metabolic unit for faecal collections (Eaton-Smith et al, 1974) and dietary assessment to substantiate the problem. Most studies of stool frequency indicate that the majority of women pass on average three stools per week, compared with men who have an average of five bowel movements per week (Connell et al, 1965; Rendtorff and Kashgarian, 1967; Martelli et al, 1978b). Women tend to pass harder stools than men (Degen and Phillips, 1996). The data in normals do not seem to vary according to whether they are compiled by questionnaire or stool collections. It is tacitly assumed that these subjects are normal. However, it should be remembered that 6% of all subjects have the irritable bowel syndrome, 1% of the population have constipation, defined as the passage of two stools per week, and 29% take laxatives (Lennard-Jones, 1985; Kamm, 1987).

The symptom of incomplete evacuation is unreliable since rectal sensation is extremely variable and the rectum can accommodate itself to a wide range of stool volumes before a desire to defecate is appreciated (Edwards and Beck, 1971; Ihre, 1974). Straining and a feeling of impaired evacuation are non-specific of outlet obstruction whereas rectal pain and digital manoeuvres are usually indicative of evacuatory disorders (Koch et al, 1997). Anismus, if one accepts the term (Schouten et al, 1997), can be defined as straining for more than 25% of the time taken to defecate (Kamm, 1987). Alternatively, it can be defined by EMG and evacuatory proctography (Roberts et al, 1992).

Impaired colonic transit may be associated with infrequent defecation, abdominal bloating and abdominal pain but all of these symptoms are non-specific and probably suggest a panintestinal motility disorder (Agachan et al, 1996; Gorard et al, 1996; Degen and Phillips, 1996). Delayed colonic transit may be entirely secondary to impaired rectal evacuation. Stool weight varies from 35 to 220 g per stool. There are wide geographical variations, the weight being much greater in rural Africa than in Westernized civilizations (Glober et al, 1977). Age also exerts an influence on stool weight, which tends to decrease with advancing age (Colon and Jacob, 1977).

In a survey, 350 patients with a mean age of 37 years attending a non-gastroenterological outpatient clinic were asked in a questionnaire: 'What do you mean by constipation'; 48% of replies implied infrequent defecation, but only 22% used terms like 'pain' or 'difficulty with defecation'. Only 38% said they were never constipated. The proportion taking laxatives was 32% of women and 16% of men; 81% of laxatives were not prescribed but were bought over the counter. Of the responders, 25% (no age or sex difference) expressed belief in the benefits of regular purgation even in the presence of a normal bowel frequency (Moore-Gillon, 1984).

Concern over bowel function appears to be part of the heritage of the English-speaking world. In the then best-selling book of the early 1900s *The Royal Road to Health* (Tyrell, 1907) the colon was referred to as 'the human cesspool'. Even today some individuals regard colonic lavage in much the same light as a visit to the sauna, and in the past Arbuthnot-Lane (1908) encouraged surgeons to perform a colectomy for almost any ailment in the belief that the colon was a source of potent toxins.

AETIOLOGY

Congenital

Constipation may be congenital due to absent ganglia in the distal colon, rectum or anus. Occasionally this may involve the stomach, duodenum and the whole or part of the small bowel, which in the past has been uniformly incompatible with life until extended myotomy-myectomy was developed (Ziegler et al, 1993). Hirschsprung's disease is discussed in Chapter 73. Other congenital disorders resulting in 'constipation' include hypoganglionosis and hyperganglionosis (Howard, 1984), spina bifida, meningocele (Thorpe et al, 1994), von Recklinghausen's disease and neonatal spinal cord or sacral tumours. Not all cases of megacolon and megarectum are due to congenital loss of autonomic ganglia: most result from long-standing chronic constipation, previous surgery for anorectal agenesis and Hirschsprung's disease, and drug therapy (see Chapter 22). Hereditary proctalgia fugax has been proposed to be associated with hypertrophy and hypertonia of the internal anal sphincter (Kamm et al, 1991b; Celik et al, 1995). A family history may be evident in slow transit constipation and was present in 22 of 33 patients (Knowles et al, 1998), sometimes involving identical twins or family members with Hirschsprung's disease.

Acquired constipation in children

Acquired constipation which is not due to an aganglionic segment of the colon, rectum or anal canal often commences in childhood. The prevalence of constipation in children varies from 3–16% (Loening-Baucke, 1993). One of the principal symptoms is soiling due to overflow incontinence around a solid faecal bolus (Silverberg, 1984). Other symptoms include painful bowel movements, stool withholding manoeuvres and infrequent bowel movements. Many of these children have behavioural problems and complex social backgrounds. There is a high incidence of sexual abuse, parental discord or psychopathology (Leroi et al, 1995). They often have abnormal rectoanal physiology with a shallow rectoanal inhibitory reflex indicative of a failure of the internal sphincter to relax (Loening-Baucke, 1984). Impaired sensory awareness in the rectum is reported (Kubota et al, 1997). Features of encopretic constipated children are raised rectal pressures during defecation due to sphincter spasm, impaired rectal sensation and a disordered rectoanal inhibitory reflex (Sutphen et al, 1997). There is sometimes a family history of functional bowel disorders. However, investigations should exclude anorectal malformations, strictures and neurogenic or metabolic causes (Heij et al, 1990).

About half to two-thirds of the children with soiling will improve with magnesium salts, high-fibre diet and bowel retraining (Loening-Baucke, 1993). Those who do not improve with these conservative measures can be identified by evidence of a failure to expel a balloon containing 100 mL of fluid from the rectum (Loening-Baucke, 1989). Parameters of rectal sensation, anal manometry or barium enema are unhelpful in predicting the outcome of conservative therapy (Meunier et al, 1984). The value of genetic markers as a means of tracing patients with the potential of developing constipation is being explored (Gottlieb and Schuster, 1986).

Segmental dilatation of the colon is a rare cause of constipation in infants (Etzioni et al, 1980).

Acquired constipation in adults

Acquired constipation in adults is much more common in women than in men (Gattuso and Kamm, 1993). It usually presents in adolescents (MacDonald et al, 1993a) and in the second and third decades, but there is often a history of bowel disturbance from childhood. Constipation is a common problem in the elderly. Acquired constipation may be due to pelvic operations or a variety of disorders (Table 21.1), including endocrine, gynaecological, neurological or metabolic disease, drugs and poisons. However, a large proportion of younger patients do not have any detectable predisposing cause. These individuals have a high prevalence of previous sexual abuse (40%) and many exhibit features of hypochondriasis, depression and hysteria (Heymen et al, 1993; Leroi et al, 1995).

Idiopathic constipation

Idiopathic constipation is a diagnosis which is made by exclusion of all other organic causes of altered bowel habit. There may be a positive family history. Typically the colon is of normal length and diameter on barium enema and of normal appearance on colonoscopy. However, there may be areas of melanosis coli (Holstock et al, 1970) and the colon may be extremely long in some patients with colonic inertia. The rectoanal inhibitory reflex is preserved (Poisson and Devroede, 1983) and there are ganglia in the colon, rectum and anal canal (Preston, 1985). It is proposed that there are five groups of patients with idiopathic constipation:

1. those with colonic inertia (Watier et al, 1979; Read et al, 1986) who have delayed transit through the whole of the colon (Hinton et al, 1969; Cummings et al, 1976);
2. those who have an area of segmentation causing delayed transit in a segment of the colon alone (Meunier et al, 1979b; Arhan et al, 1981; Orr and Robinson, 1981; Metcalf et al, 1987);
3. those with outlet obstruction, sometimes termed anismus, caused by inappropriate

Table 21.1 Specific disorders complicated by constipation.

Endocrine
Glucagonoma
Hypercalcaemia
Hyperparathyroidism
Milk alkali syndrome
Hypothyroidism
Panhypopituitary syndromes
Phaeochromocytoma
Pregnancy
Poisons
Arsenic
Lead
Mercury
Phosphorus
Neurological
Central neurological disorders
Tumours
Trauma
Cerebrovascular
Disseminated sclerosis
Parkinson's disease
Peripheral disorders
von Recklinghausen's disease
Autonomic neuropathy
Multiple endocrine neoplasia
Tabes dorsalis
Metabolic
Amyloid
Diabetes
Hypokalaemia
Porphyria
Hypercalcaemia
Uraemia
Bowel disorders
Obstruction
Diverticular disease
Carcinoma
Volvulus
Aganglionosis, hypoganglionosis
Chagas' disease
Chronic intestinal obstruction
Megacolon
Postobstetric
Psychogenic
Anxiety
Depression
Obsessional personality
Sexual abuse, rape
Anorexia nervosa, bulimia, eating disorders

contraction of the pelvic floor, obstruction associated with a sigmoidocele, faecal trapping in a rectocele, rectal obstruction by a rectal intussusception or a functional obstruction due to a hypertonic internal anal sphincter (Wasserman, 1964; Martelli et al, 1978a);

4. those with outlet obstruction and colonic inertia; and
5. individuals without any of these abnormalities who are often severely disturbed psychologically and who may be litigenous.

In the group with idiopathic slow transit constipation or colonic inertia, colectomy specimens often reveal degeneration of the autonomic plexus in the colon which principally affects the argyrophil neurones; it is not known, however, whether this degeneration is congenital or acquired (Misiewicz, 1975; Smith et al, 1977; Ford et al, 1996). Using a range of quantitative sensory automic tests, we have recently demonstrated that a population of patients with 'idiopathic' slow transit constipation (STC) have evidence of a small fibre peripheral neuropathy. In this study 33 STC patients were studied. None had an abnormality on neurological examination or nerve conduction studies; 15 had abnormalities on qualitative tests and 11 of these had reduced reflex sweating in the presence of normal sweat gland responses (Figure 21.1a); 12 of the 33 patients had small fibre dysfunction with significant elevation of thermal thresholds (Figure 21.1b). These findings were similar to those recorded in nine diabetic patients with gastrointestinal symptoms (Knowles et al, 1998).

In our experience, many patients with idiopathic slow transit constipation have evidence of both colonic inertia and outlet obstruction (Keighley and Shouler, 1984; Henry, 1989). Koch et al (1997) found that 59% had outlet obstruction, 27% had colonic inertia, 16% had both and 8% had no demonstrable abnormality.

Gut regulatory peptides that appear to influence colonic motility include gastrin, pancreatic polypeptide, motilin, glucagon, vasoactive intestinal polypeptide (VIP) and peptide histidine methionine (Kock et al, 1967; Calam et al, 1983; Preston et al, 1983b; Koch et al, 1988). The intramural distribution of VIP, substance P, somatostatin and neuropeptide Y varies widely in the large bowel (Ferri et al, 1988). Increased VIP levels are thought to be responsible for some of the motility disturbance in diverticular disease. In idiopathic constipation reduced levels of VIP were found in the bowel wall, but mucosal content of VIP was normal (Milner et al, 1990). Levels of substance P and neuropeptide Y were unaltered in constipation, and levels of calcitonin gene-related peptide and motilin may also be reduced (Dolk et al, 1990a).

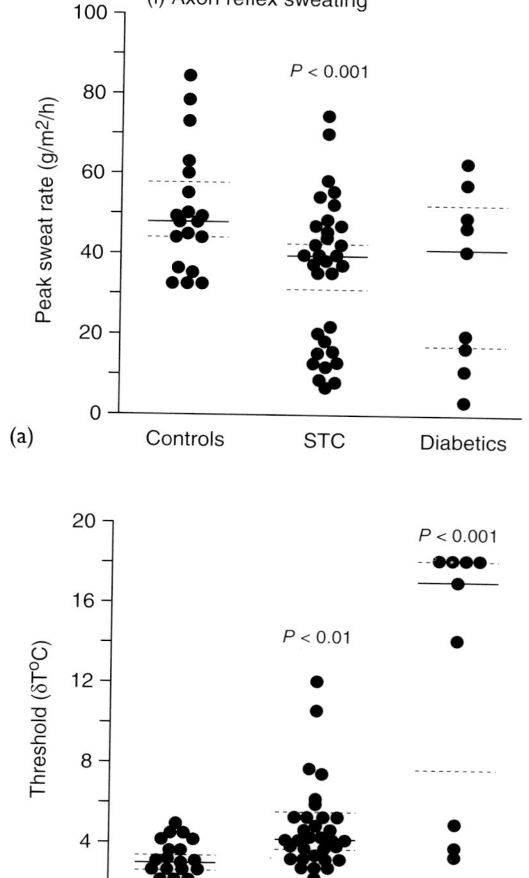

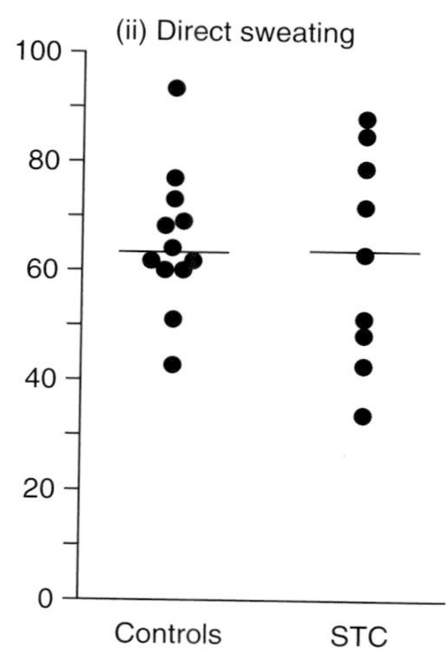

Figure 21.1 (a) Comparison of peak rates of axon reflex sweating (nicotinic injection) and direct sweating (methacholine injection) in slow transit constipation (STC) patients, diabetics and controls. Note the significant reduction in axon reflex sweating in the STC group in the presence of normal intrinsic sweat gland function. (b) Comparison of warm sensory thresholds in controls, STC patients and diabetics. Although less marked than in diabetics, note the elevation of threshold in some STC cases. Values are medians and 95% confidence intervals. *P* values: Kruskall–Wallis One-Way ANOVA – Dunn's test comparing each group with controls. From Knowles et al (1998).

Endocrine and gynaecological causes

The most important endocrine disorders to exclude in constipation are myxoedema, hypercalcaemia from primary or secondary hyperparathyroidism or the milk alkali syndrome, hyperphosphataemia and phaeochromocytoma. Other endocrine causes which should be considered are glucagonoma, hypopituitary syndromes and ovarian secretory tumours.

Although some patients become more constipated during pregnancy (Winship, 1975; Lawson et al, 1985), others find that their bowel habit is improved (Turnbull et al, 1989). Changes in bowel habit frequently occur with the menstrual cycle and some constipated patients even develop diarrhoea just before menstruating (Rees and Rhodes, 1976; Wald et al, 1981). Preston et al (1983c) reported that patients with slow transit constipation were more likely to have irregular periods, galactorrhoea, ovarian cysts and breast disease and had greater difficulty in becoming pregnant than age-matched controls (Preston, 1985). Initial studies in patients with constipation suggested that they had raised levels of prolactin (569 μmol/L) compared with controls (176 μmol/L) and those with the irritable bowel syndrome (189 μmol/L). These investigators also found that patients with slow transit constipation had low urinary oestrogen excretion and low plasma oestradiol concentrations. They concluded, therefore, that in some cases, constipation is associated with disordered ovarian function. However, Kamm et al (1989b) found no difference in total transit times or frequency of evacuation when ovulating women were studied during the follicular and luteal phases of the cycle. Similarly, Turnbull et al (1989) showed no changes in orocaecal transit during the menstrual cycle. Nor were there differences in the findings on pelvic ultrasound between constipated women and normal subjects (Kamm et al, 1989a).

Patients with severe idiopathic constipation are almost exclusively women of reproductive age. Although levels of sex hormone binding globulin, luteinizing hormone and follicle-stimulating hormone were normal, there was a constant reduction of steroid hormones: oestradiol, cortisol and testosterone in the luteal and follicular phases, and progesterone, 17-hydroxyprogesterone, androstenedione and dehydroepiandrosterone in the follicular phase (Kamm et al, 1991a).

Neurological causes

Autonomic neuropathy may be congenital or acquired (Fukai and Fukuda, 1985). The congenital variety manifests itself as Hirschsprung's disease (Lefebvre et al, 1984; Silverberg, 1984; Earlam, 1985; Starling et al, 1986) and is discussed in Chapter 73. Acquired loss of myenteric nerves may occur in Chagas' disease, multiple sclerosis, scleroderma, diabetes, amyloid disease, advanced malignancy, Crohn's disease and with certain medications (Howard, 1984; Pfeifer et al, 1996). Drug-induced myenteric damage occurs following prolonged medication with anticholinergics, tricyclic or tetracyclic compounds, the anthraquinones, bisacodyl, chlorpromazine, mepacrine and the alkaloids such as vincristine (Smith, 1968, 1972, 1973; Howard et al, 1984).

Loss of myenteric nerves results in a functional proximal obstruction, sometimes with dilatation and altered peristalsis. There is impaired relaxation in the aganglionic segment. Autonomic neuropathy may be either patchy, as in diabetes, or confined to a short segment of the anus. It may involve a variable length of the left colon or the whole of the large bowel (Howard, 1984). Myenteric loss is much less common in the small bowel (Furness and Costa, 1980, 1987). Chronic laxative abuse is associated with changes in the autonomic plexus of the colon which are best displayed by silver stains. The most frequent findings are a loss of the argyrophilic neurones and axons with enlarged nuclei (Krishnamurthy et al, 1985).

Peripheral neurological disorders rarely result in constipation, and incontinence is much more common in patients with cauda equina lesion, sacral meningioma and von Recklinghausen's disease (Read, 1987). High cord compression results in reduced colonic activity, whereas low cord transection may cause increased colonic motility, especially in the sigmoid (Connell et al, 1963). Traumatic constipation is a term used by Devroede et al (1979) to describe patients who cannot defecate normally after damage to the sacral segments of the cord or the nervi erigentes. In these patients incontinence is also a feature. Colonic transit is prolonged, rectal pressures are low, and the anal canal is spastic with an exaggerated distension reflex. Constipation is common in upper motor neurone lesions after spinal cord injury. Menardo et al (1987) reported that slow transit is usually confined to the left colon and rectum, probably as a result of interruption of the parasympathetic innervation to the large bowel. In paraplegics with faecal incontinence the rectum is sometimes filled by a huge faecolith.

Constipation is a common feature in patients who have had a previous cerebrovascular accident and intellectual impairment or depression. It is a common feature in multi-infarct dementia. The brain is a potent inhibitor of colonic function. As a result psychological factors may act as a primary cause, and constipation is common in severe depression. In generalized cerebrovascular disease constipation may be associated with impaired mobility, diet and medication (Kamm, 1987). Parkinson's disease, or therapy to control the extrapyramidal manifestations of the disease (Lennard-Jones, 1985), is frequently associated with constipation.

Demyelinating disorders such as multiple sclerosis are associated with constipation in 40% of patients. Likewise posterior column degeneration from tabes dorsalis may be associated with constipation as well as urinary symptoms. Investigation in severe cases indicates somatic and visceral neuropathy with abnormal spinal cord conduction and cystometrograms as well as absent postprandial colonic motility (Glick et al, 1982).

Localized damage to the autonomic supply of the bladder and rectum may be responsible for constipation after pelvic surgery, especially following cystectomy, rectopexy or hysterectomy (Bannister et al, 1988; Taylor et al, 1989). Constipation is particularly common after hysterectomy (van Dam et al, 1997) which may result from disturbed autonomic innervation of the hindgut (Smith et al, 1990). Constipation may be associated with pudendal neuropathy in 24% of patients. It is more common in elderly patients and in those with outlet obstruction (Vaccaro et al, 1994, 1995a). Some patients therefore may suffer from constipation from outlet obstruction which may be associated with incontinence.

Metabolic causes

Most diabetic patients with an autonomic neuropathy complain of incontinence but a few suffer from constipation (Battle et al, 1989). Other metabolic disorders associated with constipation are porphyria, hypercalcaemia from hyperparathyroidism, uraemia and amyloid disease.

Bowel disorders

Certain obstructive bowel diseases, such as carcinoma, volvulus, hernia, benign strictures, pseudo-obstruction, polyps, adhesions or endometriosis, may be responsible for chronic constipation (Nehme, 1984; Read, 1987).

Chronic intestinal pseudoobstruction (CIP) results in intestinal obstruction causing constipation without a mechanical blockage. It is rare. If the colon is the primary site, constipation and colonic dilatation are the usual forms of presentation. Usually sporadic, one third of cases are familial: autosomal recessive or dominant and sex linked. CIP is either caused by a visceral neuropathy or a visceral myopathy, abnormalities occur in smooth muscle actin and mitochondria (Milla, 1991; Smith et al, 1992; Lowsky et al, 1993). Apart from constipation, pain and malnutrition are major management problems which require a multidisciplinary team consisting of gastroenterologist, surgeon, nutritionalist, pain management consultants and a psychologist.

It is likely that all patients with chronic idiopathic constipation suffer from the irritable bowel syndrome and that the disordered colonic motility or rectal emptying represent one end of the spectrum of this disorder. Certainly, coexisting disordered gastric emptying and small bowel transit are now well recognized (Panagamuwa et al, 1994; MacDonald et al, 1997). Likewise, bladder symptoms and biliary dyskinesia are also evident in some of these constipated patients (Bannister et al, 1988; MacDonald et al, 1991, 1993a,b).

It must also be recognized that childbirth can have a profound impact on colorectal function. Prolonged labour and difficult or assisted delivery may not only cause incontinence from pelvic floor injury, pudendal neuropathy and sphincter damage but many of these women suffer from evacuatory disorders as well, resulting in constipation with or without faecal incontinence. In some women, the evacuatory failure dominates the clinical picture, while in others incontinence is the principal distressing complaint. Nevertheless, both components usually coexist, making surgical treatment frequently unsuccessful (Snooks et al, 1990).

Other colorectal disorders which are commonly associated with constipation include rectal prolapse and solitary rectal ulcer. It is difficult to know whether the disordered bowel habit is responsible for, or secondary to, the underlying pathology. However, even after successful treatment of a rectal prolapse, persisting constipation, particularly among the younger age group, may become more incapacitating than the original prolapse. In patients with the solitary rectal ulcer syndrome constipation commonly persists even when the ulcer is no longer visible.

There are certain painful anal conditions which may cause constipation from the fear of defecating. If prompt attention is not given to these disorders a vicious circle develops whereby pain results in retention of faeces and hard scybala form in the rectum, which increases the discomfort of attempted defecation. It has been suggested that many young adults with chronic constipation may have had an undiagnosed painful fissure in early life. Sadly, by the time these patients are referred to the profession only 43% recover with magnesium salts, diet and bowel retraining (Leoning-Baucke, 1989). Apart from fissure, thrombosed haemorrhoids and perianal abscess may have a similar influence on bowel function. Diverticular disease may also be associated with constipation, and paradoxically it is surprisingly common for patients with distal ulcerative colitis to be constipated. It might be thought that the two conditions would be mutually exclusive, however gross faecal loading on the right side of the colon in patients with a distal ulcerative proctitis is common. Sometimes ulcerative proctitis may be ischaemic in origin as a consequence of pressure from hard faeces resulting from constipation.

Psychogenic factors

Constipation is common in patients with anxiety and depression (Gorard et al, 1996). It is a prominent feature of anorexia nervosa, bulimia and other eating disorders, as well as sleep disorders, fatigue and decreased sexual drive (Heymen et al, 1993). Many of these patients are dissatisfied, demanding and are often deeply unhappy. They may be attention seekers, and can manipulate the medical profession (Preston, 1985). Frequently the medication of patients with anxiety and depression further exacerbates the constipation (Gorard et al 1994).

Psychogenic causes of constipation may stem from sex abuse or childhood feelings of disgust at normal defecation (Leroi et al, 1995), and a sense of rebellion against their environment, gaining satisfaction from retained faeces in the rectum. In the elderly, constipation may be associated with depression, cerebral deterioration and blunted awareness.

Constipated patients often lie about the use of laxatives and the history of their bowel habit may be unreliable (Hinton and Lennard-Jones, 1968). Not infrequently they fail to cooperate during physiological assessment (Pinho et al, 1991a; Karlbom et al, 1995). We found that constipated individuals being admitted for operation had higher depression scores than controls. Psychological screening tests were also capable of identifying patients who were unlikely to be improved by surgical treatment; such as those with high anxiety and depression scores (Fisher et al, 1988) (Figures 21.2 and 21.3). Heymen et al (1993) from the Florida Cleveland Clinic found that the Minnesota Multiphasic Personality Inventory (MMPI) was a valuable tool for assessing the psychological function of patients with constipation. It revealed a somatization type of defensive structure in the psychological function of patients with levator spasm and colonic inertia which could aid in the selection of persons unsuitable for surgical intervention.

Drug-induced causes and poisons

A variety of medications may cause constipation; some of these are listed in Table 21.2. Codeine and other opiates are widely prescribed in proprietary preparations for headache and menorrhagia. This might explain the higher frequency of constipation among women. Anticholinergic drugs, antihistamines, certain anticonvulsants or calcium- and aluminium-containing antacids constipate. Antidepressants must always be considered since many patients have a history of depression, which itself may be associated with constipation and which may be made worse by drugs such as the monoamine oxidase inhibitors, tricyclic compounds or the phenothiazines (Gorard et al, 1994). Many clinicians investigate such patients without taking a full drug history and have even considered a colectomy, only to discover a few months later that the bowel habit has returned to normal because the patient's therapy for depression has been discontinued. Iron supplements, drugs causing hypocalcaemia and antimitotic agents for malignant disease may also cause constipation.

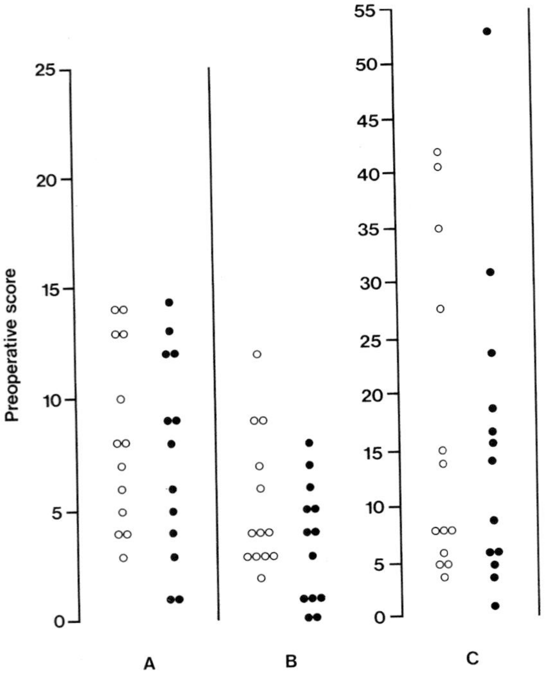

Figure 21.2 Psychiatric screening to predict surgical outcome. Preoperative scores in constipated patients (○), who were improved by operation, compared with controls (●). A, Hospital anxiety and depression (HAD) scale: anxiety scores; B, HAD scale: depression scores; C, general health questionnaire scores.

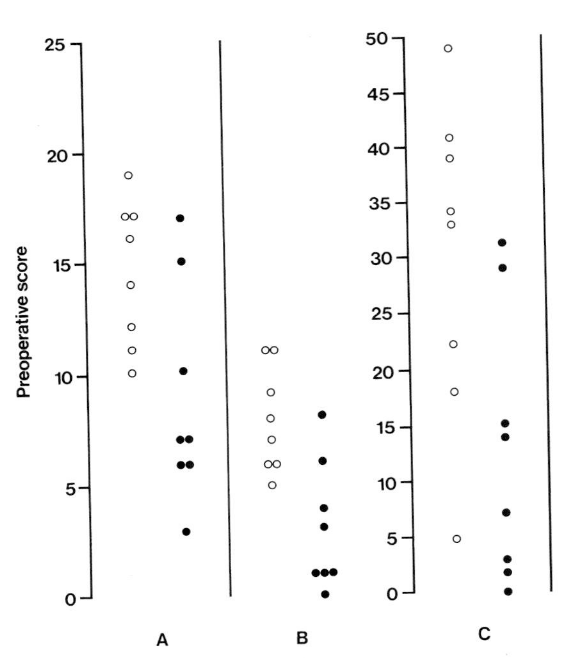

Figure 21.3 Psychiatric screening to predict surgical outcome. Preoperative scores in constipated patients (○), who were not improved by operation compared with controls (●). A, HAD scale: anxiety scores; B, HAD scale: depression scores; C, general health questionnaire.

Table 21.2 Drugs causing constipation.

Anaesthetic agents
Analgesics
Anticholinergics
Antacids: calcium and aluminium compounds
Anticonvulsants
Antidepressive agents, e.g. monoamine oxidase inhibitors
phenothiazines
tricyclic compounds
Antihistamines
Barium sulphate
Bismuth
Diuretics: especially if associated with hypokalaemia
Drugs for treatment of Parkinson's disease
Ganglion blocking agents
Haematinics, e.g. iron
Hypotensives
Long-standing laxatives
Muscle relaxants
Opiates: codeine, dihydrocodeine
Oral contraceptives
Psychotrophic drugs

The chronic use of laxatives is an important drug-induced cause of constipation. There is growing evidence that young people who have been encouraged to take laxatives as children, with the idea that they should keep the colon clean, develop damage to the myenteric plexus of the colon (Krishnamurthy et al, 1985). Eventually the colon can no longer respond to stimulant laxatives such as bisacodyl, senna or cascara (Preston and Lennard-Jones, 1982), it becomes inert and may even dilate (Sladen, 1972). Hence after years of frequent and vigorous laxative abuse spontaneous defecation may be seriously impaired (Pennington, 1985). Consequently the dose of laxatives is increased, which may result in episodic diarrhoea and potassium depletion, further aggravating the syndrome (Cooke, 1977). Some laxatives, particularly the anthracene compounds, cause chronic inflammatory changes in the rectal mucosa (Meisel et al, 1977) or melanosis coli (Badiali et al, 1985).

Chronic constipation may be caused by lead, mercury, arsenic and phosphorus poisoning.

Dietary factors and other general lifestyle factors

The relationship between dietary fibre and bowel habit has been recognized for years. Stool bulk and frequency are closely associated with the intake of dietary fibre (Brodribb, 1977) but with the growing use of convenience foods, dietary fibre intake has decreased and constipation has become more prevalent. Transit time is also closely correlated with dietary fibre (Harvey et al, 1973; Payler et al, 1975; Ornstein et al, 1981). Furthermore, dietary fibre increases stool weight and its water content (Cummings et al, 1978). Individual variations in stool output in response to dietary fibre are as much related to personality as they are to diet (Tucker et al, 1981). There is also a strong placebo effect of fibre supplements (Devroede, 1975); indeed, increased fibre intake may exacerbate symptoms, particularly those of pain and abdominal distension (Bateman and Smith, 1988).

Constipation may be aggravated by lack of exercise or inadequate fluid intake or it may be occupational. Frequent voluntary suppression of the urge to defecate may eventually lead to constipation. Inadequate fluid intake removes the stimulus of repeated gastric distension which stimulates intestinal activity. Stool water content, and hence consistency, is related to the state of hydration, hence increasing oral fluids is one of the essential lines of conservative therapy. The mineral content of the water supply is another factor since water from limestone sources tends to constipate, whereas water from acid soil often has a mild laxative effect. The sedentary or bedridden patient is more troubled by constipation because colonic motor activity is reduced during periods of impaired physical activity.

Previous surgical operations

Some patients develop long-standing constipation after various surgical operations. The incidence of previous surgical procedures in constipated patients compared with controls reported by Preston and Lennard-Jones (1986) is listed in Table 21.3.

Hysterectomy is sometimes complicated both by constipation and impaired bladder function (Roe et al, 1988; Parys et al, 1989). Taylor et al (1990) in a case control study compared the bowel habit of 91 posthysterectomy women with paired controls. Constipation and urinary frequency were significantly more common in the patients who had had a hysterectomy. Oophorectomy (unilateral or bilateral) had no effect on bowel habit, suggesting local autonomic damage to pelvic viscera rather

Table 21.3 Previous surgical procedures in slow transit constipation.

	Controls		*Patients*
Appendicectomy	12	*	28
Colectomy for constipation	0		8
Hysterectomy	2	*	12
Ovarian cystectomy	2	*	14
Non-abdominal	28		24

*Significant differences ($P < 0.05$).
From Preston and Lennard-Jones (1986).

than a hormonal aetiology. Another study found that 31% of patients with normal bowel habit developed severe constipation after hysterectomy which was unrelated to the type of hysterectomy but more common in younger women (van Dam et al, 1997). However, hysterectomy is a major life event and there are no epidemiological studies to confirm that it predisposes to constipation. A similar mechanism may be responsible for constipation after rectopexy and cystectomy (Broden et al, 1988) but in many patients with rectal prolapse there is abnormal colonic transit before rectopexy (Dolk et al, 1990b).

PREVALENCE AND INCIDENCE

In the UK, constipation, defined as the passage of fewer than two stools per week, is present in less than 1% of the population, but nearly 30% of the population take regular laxatives (Connell et al, 1965). In North America over 4 million people are estimated to suffer from constipation and it is regarded as the most common digestive complaint. The prevalence is 2%: laxatives are prescribed for 2 million individuals every year. There are 92 000 annual hospital admissions of patients with constipation (Figure 21.4). The incidence increases with age, particularly among women (Figure 21.5) and it is more common among low income groups (Figure 21.6a) (Sonnenberg and Koch, 1989). A study from the Olmsted County, Minnesota (Talley et al, 1993) identified a 19% prevalence of functional constipation and 11% prevalance of outlet delay. Outlet delay but not functional constipation was more common in women (Figure 21.6b); furthermore, there was an overlap between both groups and the irritable bowel syndrome (Figure 21.6c).

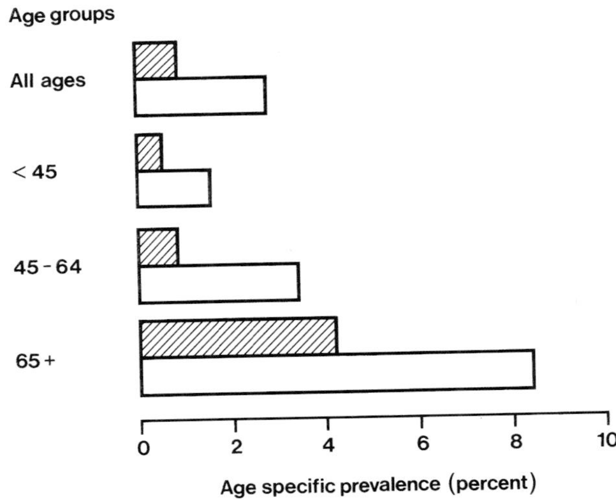

Figure 21.5 Age-specific prevalence of constipation, examined with respect to sex and race. The prevalence shown represents the average of figures derived between 1982 and 1985. ▨, Male; □, female.

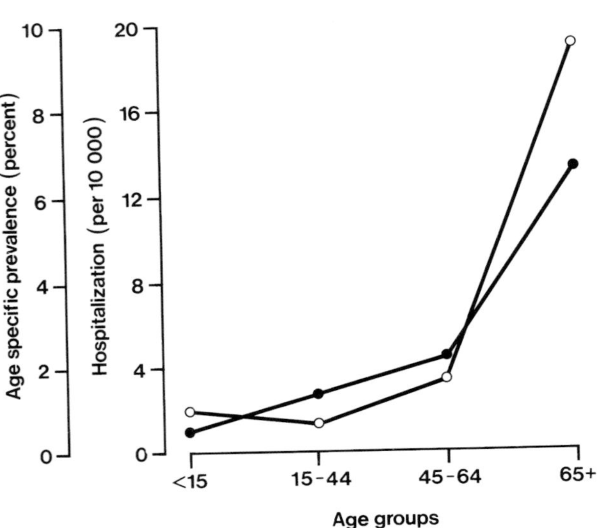

Figure 21.4 Age-specific prevalence of constipation. ●, Overall prevalence; ○, prevalence among patients admitted to hospital.

Chronic constipation often runs in families. For instance, when one of two twins is constipated the chance of the second being constipated as well is four times greater if they are monozygotic. The genetic predisposition to constipation increases when a parent or sibling is affected (Bakwin and Davidson, 1971). Furthermore, the diseases associated with constipation may also be familial (Faulk et al, 1978).

The higher incidence of constipation in women may be hormonal. Typically idiopathic chronic constipation occurs in young women: 20% give a history of symptoms starting before the age of 5 years whilst most of the remainder date the onset of symptoms from the menarche (Preston, 1985). If constipation is a complication of diverticular disease or the irritable bowel syndrome it tends to become more evident later in life (Thompson and Heaton, 1980). Constipation secondary to cerebrovascular disease or rectal ischaemia occurs in the elderly (Klein, 1982).

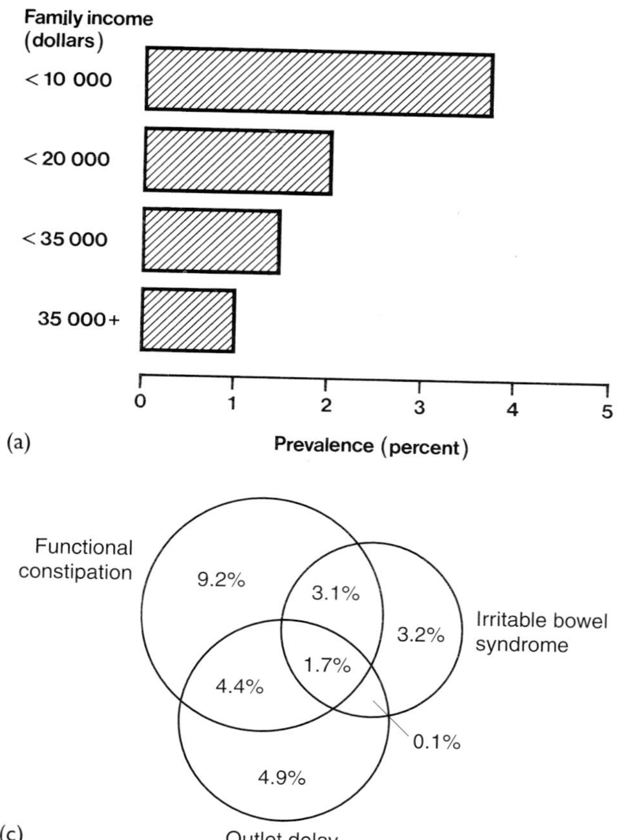

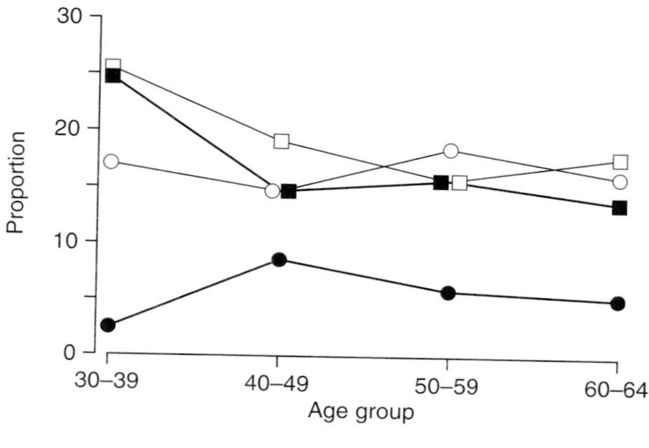

Figure 21.6 (a) Prevalence of constipation by annual income (US dollars) of the head of the family. Prevalence represents data obtained between 1982 and 1985. (b) Prevalence of constipation (functional constipation and outlet delay) according to age and sex. Functional constipation: ■, male; □, female. Outlet delay: ●, male; ○, female. (c) Overlap between functional constipation, outlet delay and irritable bowel syndrome. (b) and (c) From Talley et al (1993).

PATHOPHYSIOLOGY OF IDIOPATHIC CHRONIC CONSTIPATION

Broadly speaking, chronic idiopathic constipation can be subdivided into three groups based upon a variety of physiological studies (Table 21.4). These are: (1) anismus or outlet obstruction, levator spasm or rectal inertia, (2) colonic delay and (3) a combination of both. In all three the irritable bowel syndrome frequently coexists. Some would argue that all three groups are merely a manifestation of irritable bowel syndrome (Talley et al, 1993).

Table 21.4 Classification of 198 patients with chronic constipation (1983–1990: Birmingham).

Associated pathology (*n* = 113)	*Number*	*Idiopathic* (*n* = 85)	*Number*
Previous pelvic surgery*	46	Colonic inertia (delayed transit or no response to bisacodyl)	45
Hysterectomy	34	Outlet obstruction (could not pass a 100-mL balloon or EMG evidence of increased puborectalis activity on attempted defecation)	69
Uterine prolapse repair	17		
Rectopexy	16		
Oophorectomy or other gynaecological procedures	10		
Ventrosuspension	4		
Cystectomy	3		
Rectal prolapse	22		
Megacolon or megarectum	16		
Solitary rectal ulcer	16		
Spinal cord lesion	6		
Meningocele	3		
Ectopia vesicae	2		
Myxoedema	2		

*Many had had more than one operation.

Outlet obstruction

In outlet obstruction or anismus (Watier et al, 1979; Park et al, 1996). Patients have difficulty in rectal evacuation either from failure of the puborectalis muscle and external sphincter to relax during attempted defecation, or due to a hypertonic internal sphincter (Ger et al, 1993). Alternatively, evacuatory disorders may be due to failure of coordinated rectal contraction. In many patients rectal pressures are insufficient to achieve rectal evacuation either because of poor rectal contraction or increased sphincter pressures (Halligan et al, 1995). Passage of contrast during videoproctography, balloon evacuation or isotopic evacuation studies is impaired (Hutchinson et al, 1993; Papachrystostomou et al, 1993), often in association with perineal descent and a failure of the anorectal angle to unlock during straining (Keighley and Shouler, 1984; Johansson et al, 1985; Kuijpers and Bleijenberg, 1985; Womack et al, 1985; Turnbull et al, 1986; Barnes and Lennard-Jones, 1988; Bartolo et al, 1988; Pinho et al, 1991a; Piloni et al, 1997).

The principal features of outlet obstruction are poor pelvic floor movements on attempted defecation, impaired rectal evacuation (Grotz et al, 1993), failure of the external sphincter and puborectalis to relax on attempted defecation (Read et al, 1986) or hypertonia of the internal anal sphincter (Kamm et al, 1991b). At the Royal London Hospital, dynamic integrated proctography is used to diagnose anismus. In a study comparing 70 constipated patients with 20 controls, anismus was defined as (1) demonstration of puborectalis EMG recruitment >50%; (2) evidence of an adequate level of intrarectal pressure during straining (>50 cmH_2O); and (3) presence of defective evacuation (Roberts et al, 1992). Most patients with anismus have a normal rectoanal inhibitory reflex, normal rectal sensation and normal or increased resting anal pressures. Sometimes radio-opaque markers are retained in the rectum alone or in the rectosigmoid or left colon as well (Kuijpers et al, 1986). Sometimes there is coexisting distal colonic inertia (Shouler and Keighley, 1986). Indeed current views propose that many patients with colonic inertia have a primary evacuatory disorder and that the colonic changes are all secondary to rectal dysfunction (Karlbom et al, 1995).

The whole issue of paradoxical sphincter or pelvic floor contraction during attempted defecation has been thoroughly assessed by Voderholzer et al (1997) in Munich. They found that paradoxical contraction was present in 41% of constipated patients. However, when they assessed oroanal and rectosigmoid transit times, they found delay in all of the constipated group, irrespective of paradoxical contraction. They even proposed that paradoxical contraction was a laboratory artefact induced by trying to perform functional studies during the normally private act of defecation. In agreement with this, Schouten et al (1997) in Rotterdam demonstrated paradoxical pelvic floor contraction in incontinent patients and in normals. They therefore stated that anismus is not exclusively found in constipation and so doubted its significance. However, we take the opposite view, believing that impaired rectal evacuation is almost ubiquitous in constipation but that its cause is protean such as poor rectal pressure from impaired contraction, puborectalis spasm, failure of external sphincter relaxation or internal sphincter hypertrophy. We also agree with Karlbom et al (1995) that in most patients colonic inertia is probably secondary to impaired rectal evacuation (Papachrystostomou et al, 1993, 1994).

The failure of rectal evacuation (MacDonald et al, 1993b) is not confined to solids or compressible balloons but can include liquids (Turnbull et al, 1986; Halligan et al, 1994; Mellgren et al, 1994a,c; Alstrup et al, 1997). Videoproctography with or without simultaneous peritonography (Bremmer et al, 1995; Sentovich et al, 1995) often demonstrates perineal descent, an incomplete rectal prolapse or an anterior mucosal prolapse that appears to obstruct defecation, an enterocele or a rectocele (Kerremans, 1968a,b; Bartolo et al, 1985; Johansson et al, 1985; Womack et al, 1985; Jones et al, 1998). These changes are associated with two life events: the first being constipation in childhood leading to straining which becomes a life-long functional behavioural disorder, the second is childbirth. Obstetric trauma and impaired evacuation similarly may result in life-long straining. Both groups develop perineal descent, progressive pudendal neuropathy and anal anaesthesia (Speakman et al, 1993; Broens et al, 1994; Engel and Kamm, 1994; Solana et al, 1996) (Figure 21.7a). Electrophysiological studies not only demonstrate failure of inhibition in the pelvic floor and external sphincter during defecation (Jones et al, 1987) but also conduction defects to these muscles (Bartolo et al, 1985; Vaccaro et al, 1994). Some patients have impaired rectal sensation (Shouler and Keighley, 1986; Varma et al, 1988) (Figure 21.7b). Others have evidence of increased internal sphincter activity on attempted defecation and at rest (Meunier et al, 1984), with a shallow rectoanal inhibitory reflex; these internal sphincter abnormalities are more common in children (Loening-Baucke, 1984).

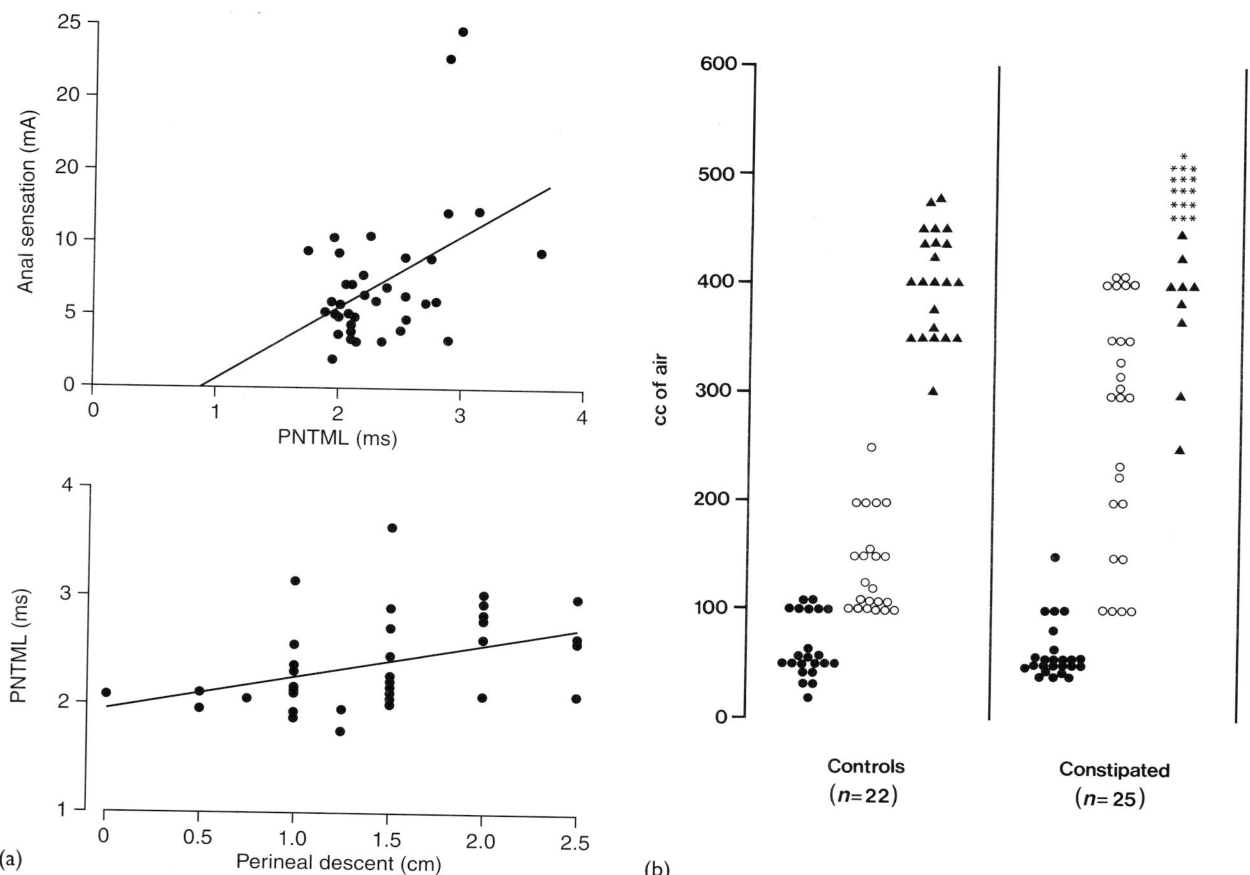

Figure 21.7 (a) Correlation between anal sensation and pudendal nerve terminal motor latency (PNTML) and between PNTML and perineal descent. From Engel and Kamm (1994). (b) Rectal sensation (cc of air) in controls and in constipated patients. ●, Threshold volumes; ○, constant sensation; ▲, maximum tolerated volume; *, maximum tolerated volumes in excess of 450 cc (unrecordable).

Colonic inertia

Constipation may be due to colonic inertia or a failure of the bowel to propel its contents in an orderly prograde manner. This disorder of colonic motility may be confined to a segment of the colon or the rectum or to the whole of the large bowel (Arhan et al, 1981; Poisson and Devroede, 1983; Metcalf et al, 1987). Colonic inertia is usually identified by the delay in the excretion or passage of radio-opaque markers, isotopic scans or a failure of the colon to respond to a stimulant (Hinton et al, 1969; Ducrotte et al, 1986; Krevsky et al, 1986; Preston and Lennard-Jones, 1986; Roe et al, 1986b; Shouler and Keighley, 1986; Bassotti et al, 1988; Varma et al, 1988). In colonic inertia not only is orocaecal transit delayed but gastric emptying is also delayed and small bowel motility is deranged (Bannister et al, 1986; Panagamuwa et al, 1994; MacDonald et al, 1997). Usually, patients with chronic idiopathic constipation have evidence of both colonic inertia and outlet obstruction, but it is usual for one aspect of the dual abnormality to dominate the clinical problem (Keighley and Shouler, 1984; Barnes and Lennard-Jones, 1985; Ducrotte et al, 1986; Kuijpers et al, 1986; Roe et al, 1986a,b).

The majority of patients with idiopathic constipation have coexisting irritable bowel syndrome in which constipation predominates in a symptom complex including: dyspepsia, abdominal distension, backache, headache, menstrual disturbance and bladder symptoms.

Taylor et al (1989), in a case control study, found that patients who had had a hysterectomy had a decreased frequency of defecation and used more laxatives than controls (Table 21.5).

Many of these patients also had urinary frequency (Varma, 1992). Urological abnormalities

Table 21.5 Case control study of the impact of hysterectomy on bowel function.

	Bowels open <4 times/week	*Laxatives taken >2 times/week*
Hysterectomy	14	16
Controls	6	7

From Taylor et al (1989).

such as an increase in the threshold micturition volume and bladder capacity and an acontractile bladder are found in a variable proportion of patients with chronic constipation (Bannister et al, 1988; Varma and Smith, 1988; Kerrigan et al, 1989).

Colonic inertia is identified by delayed passage of transit markers; however, a single bolus ingestion of radio-opaque pellets with a radiograph 4–5 days later is a very crude assessment of delayed transit in constipated patients (Hinton et al, 1969). Improved assessment can be made by repeated ingestion of markers until a steady state is reached, when a plain radiograph will identify segmental delay (Metcalf et al, 1987; van der Sijp et al, 1993; Notghi et al, 1994). In view of the recognition of segmental colonic stasis, we recommend that transit marker studies should be used for screening only and that radioisotopic examination provides more useful therapeutic information (Krevsky et al, 1986; Roberts et al, 1988; Hutchinson et al, 1995; Lubowski et al, 1995; Notghi et al, 1995).

Colonic inertia may also be identified by rectosigmoid manometry or myoelectrical activity (Shafik, 1995). Resting and postprandial motor activity is reduced (Pezim et al, 1993), with few mass contractions (Ferrara et al, 1994), and there is a poor response to stimulant laxatives such as bisacodyl (Preston and Lennard-Jones, 1986; Roe et al, 1986b; Shouler and Keighley, 1986; Bassotti et al, 1988; Wegman et al, 1989).

In colonic inertia, evidence now indicates that colonic smooth muscle is hypersensitive to cholinergic stimulation, suggesting a smooth muscle myopathy (Slater et al, 1997). In addition, these patients have alterations in the neural composition of the colonic myenteric plexus, indicative of impaired innervation of colonic smooth muscle (Park et al, 1995). In view of the family history, a genetic basis for the small fibre neuropathy, as in Hirschspring's disease, is worth pursuing.

PATHOLOGICAL FINDINGS

Some patients with constipation have a congenital or acquired disorder of the myenteric plexus of the colon (Tanner et al, 1976). The normal myenteric plexus contains ganglia connected by a network of nerve trunks. Parasympathetic cholinergic fibres are excitatory, whilst the noradrenergic sympathetic fibres inhibit motor activity. Each ganglion contains argyrophil and non-argyrophil neurones, the former being responsible for coordinating peristalsis. If a sufficient number of these argyrophil neurones are congenitally absent or destroyed, peristalsis is impaired.

Histological examination of colectomy specimens using routine stains is normal among patients with idiopathic slow transit constipation. Using silver stains, there is evidence of degeneration of the argyrophil cells, abnormal neurones, broken axons and debris in the autonomic plexus (Smith et al, 1977). Schwannosis is also a feature. In some patients the changes are consistent with acquired damage from purgatives. Some specimens exhibit features of chronic non-specific inflammatory change. Krishnamurthy et al (1985) found that the most common features were loss of axons and argyrophilic neurones. Some patients have evidence of melanosis coli but this is not uniform and is not diagnostic of laxative abuse, although it is more common in patients taking anthraquinones. The mucosa has a dark brown colour due to deposits of free and bound lipofuscin in the lamina propria (Badiali et al, 1985). Using immunohistochemistry, the myenteric plexus showed an increase in supporting tissues with increased immunoreactive nerve fibres. These findings suggest an abnormality in the innervation of the circular muscle which becomes atrophied in constipation (Park et al, 1995). Similarly the response of the circular muscle to cholinergic stimulation is abnormal (Slater et al, 1997).

CLINICAL PRESENTATION

History

Patients with constipation usually complain of infrequent defecation but the history may be unreliable. Furthermore, symptoms may be episodic (Agachan et al, 1996). The duration of constipation may be variable: it should be established whether it has been present from birth, occurred during childhood or began later in life, particularly with the menarche or after any emotional experience, a severe illness or surgical operation. Some women have features of anorexia nervosa, bulimia or other eating disorders. Predisposing factors which should be sought include a drug history and a history of psychiatric disease or psychological disturbance. Sometimes there has been sexual abuse (Leroi et al, 1995) or rape including anal intercourse. Passage of hard stools is almost universal and over 90% of patients also complain of difficulty in evacuating faecal contents as well as an infrequent bowel habit (Table 21.6). Passage of bulky faeces which may obstruct defecation and cause rectal bleeding is also quite common. Abdominal symptoms include pain, distension with bloating, nausea, occasionally vomiting and audible borborygmi. If there is gross faecal impaction there may be a history of overflow incontinence. Episodic diarrhoea and constipation with abdominal distension, pain, heartburn, nausea, mucus discharge, flatulent dyspepsia and anal pain with incontinence is also reported, particularly in patients with the irritable bowel syndrome. However, symptoms are non-specific and rarely distinguish colonic inertia from anismus (Figure 21.8) (Koch et al, 1997).

In female patients, a detailed obstetric and gynaecological history is relevant and in both sexes a history of previous operation should be recorded. There is evidently an increased incidence of epilepsy and Raynaud's phenomenon (Preston, 1985) in patients with idiopathic constipation. Preston and Lennard-Jones (1986) reported that the majority of patients with slow transit constipation passed one stool a week with laxatives. Fibre intake was normal. There was usually impaired sensation of rectal fullness before defecation and a high proportion needed to use digital pressure to assist defecation. All were women and most gave a history of painful irregular periods. There was an increased rate of ovarian cystectomy, hysterectomy and division of adhesions. Hesitancy of micturition, cold hands and blackouts were common.

Constipated patients often appear to have a rather neurotic or obsessional personality and many seem dissatisfied. It is difficult in such individuals to know which came first. There may be overt features of anxiety or depression.

Many constipated patients of long standing have a personality disorder which is not recognized as a psychiatric illness and does not fall into a specific pattern of disease. Many are highly intelligent, rather intense individuals who are very demanding and unhappy, wanting an urgent solution to a long-standing problem. Furthermore, they are poor witnesses and are manipulative. They have often visited many different clinicians and they usually refuse to accept psychological or psychiatric help if some emotional disturbance or personality disorder seems apparent. Even worse are patients with

Table 21.6 Symptoms/signs of constipation.

Symptom/sign	%
Hard stools	98
Difficulty of evacuation	92
Abdominal pain	82
Large size of stool	80
Obstruction of toilets	66
Rectal bleeding	64
Abdominal distension	60
Faecal impaction	50
Digital extraction of faeces	48
Episodic diarrhoea	44
Incontinence	40
Poor appetite	38
Nausea	35
Abdominal mass	27
Passage of pelleted stools	25
Vomiting	22
Abdominal tenderness	17
Audible borborygmi	10

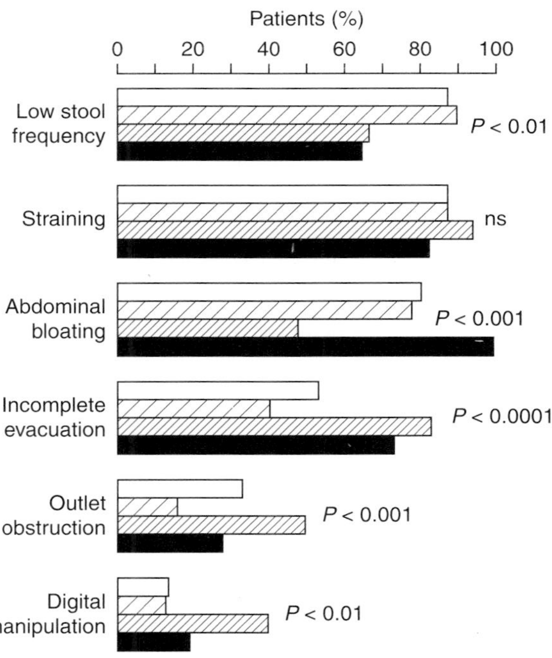

Figure 21.8 Prevalence of symptoms with respect to outcome of functional diagnostic work-up. □, No abnormal finding (n = 15); ▨, slow transit (n = 52); ▨, disordered defecation (n = 112); ■, both (n = 11). From Koch et al (1997).

eating disorders, particularly anorexia, since they almost always refuse to accept that there is any psychological disturbance and somatosize all their symptoms to the gastrointestinal tract, particularly the colon and the rectum. Many of these patients hide underlying eating or sexual disorders or emotional problems.

Clinical examination

Signs of underlying endocrine, neurological or metabolic disorders should be sought and the urine should be tested to exclude diabetes and porphyria. There may be abdominal tenderness with some distension, and palpable faeces may be felt throughout the colon. On rectal inspection the anus may be patulous, especially if there is a neurological cause or faecal impaction is present. Perianal anaesthesia is further evidence of a neurological disorder. An abnormal sweat test suggests subclinical autonomic neuropathy (Altomare et al, 1992). The anocutaneous reflex may be absent and there may be evidence of perineal descent. Rectal examination often reveals normal anal tone at rest but poor pelvic floor movements on contraction (Pinho et al, 1991a). There may be hypertonia of the anal canal. Gross faecal impaction is uncommon except in the elderly. Indeed the rectum is usually empty. A rectal prolapse should be sought. Sigmoidoscopy will exclude ulcerative proctitis, solitary ulcer, rectal intussusception, a neoplasm, rectal stricture, and gross anal disorders such as fissure, haemorrhoids or chronic anorectal abscess. There may be melanosis coli.

Faecal impaction

Faecal impaction may be defined as a mass of solid faecal material which completely fills and distends the rectum and cannot be passed by the patient. It is more common in the elderly and in disabled subjects who have been immobilized for a long time. It is also more common in children with severe constipation and adolescents who have had operations for anorectal agenesis or Hirschsprung's disease or who have acquired megarectum. Impaction may complicate codeine therapy and is seen in patients who have no rectal sensation as a result of paraplegia or spina bifida. The principal symptoms are not constipation but soiling, diarrhoea, rectal discomfort, lower abdominal pain, rectal fullness, nausea, anorexia and tenesmus. Urinary retention is a common complication; rarely stercoral ulceration may cause faecal peritonitis. Soiling is due to liquid faeces leaking around the solid faecal mass and the constant inhibition of the internal sphincter due to persistent distension of the rectum.

Patients with faecal impaction have impaired rectal sensation, reduced rectal compliance, impaired colonic and rectal motility, an inability to retain a balloon being distended in the rectum, but anal canal length and anal pressures are normal (Varma et al, 1988). If impaction is complicated by megarectum, anal canal length is reduced, there is more profound rectal sensory loss but compliance is increased.

Natural history

If there is no identifiable correctable underlying cause, constipation tends to be progressive. In idiopathic constipation patients find that despite dietary advice they cannot manage without laxatives. With time the dose of laxatives has to be increased to achieve spontaneous defecation, leading to progressive colonic damage. Sometimes a megacolon or megarectum develops. Megacolon is more common in patients with colonic inertia than with outlet obstruction (Lane and Todd, 1977). Megacolon may also complicate long-standing faecal impaction (Porter, 1961).

Some patients with an underlying emotional problem or with features of the irritable bowel syndrome improve spontaneously. Such patients will often admit that there were psychological problems which have now resolved, a dominating relative who has now moved away, or a time of personal stress or guilt which has passed. Such information indicates that operative treatment of the non-dilated colon or rectum must never be entertained lightly, even in the presence of demonstrable physiological abnormalities, particularly if there is any suspicion of an underlying stress-related factor. Reference has already been made to the poor outcome among depressed or anxious patients having surgical treatment (Fisher et al, 1988).

Complications

Various complications of constipation, such as urinary retention, stercoral ulceration and faecal incontinence, have already been referred to. Stercoral ulceration and perforation are more common in the sigmoid colon than the rectum and are a more frequent occurrence in the elderly (Huttenen et al, 1975; Shatila and Ackerman, 1977; Gekas and

Schuster, 1981). Other problems include recurrent urinary tract infections from incomplete voiding of the bladder (Neuman et al, 1973). Three case control studies have established a link between cancer of the large bowel and constipation, particularly in women (Higginson, 1966; Bjelke, 1974). This increased cancer risk seems more closely related to stool weight than to transit times (Report from the International Agency for Research on Cancer Intestinal Microecology Group, 1977).

INVESTIGATIONS

Before describing the available investigations in these difficult and often demanding patients, it would be well to take stock and decide how fruitful the proposed investigations are likely to be. It must be acknowledged that you can rarely tell a patient that investigations are a waste of time, surgery has nothing to offer and then show them the door! On the other hand, we all work under financial constraints and neither government health care budgets nor insurance company policies will continue to fund all that the medical profession may desire in terms of exhaustive investigations. Rantis et al (1997) reported the value of the standard 'work up' for patients at the Florida Cleveland Clinic being investigated for constipation. They found that all patients were investigated by barium enema or colonoscopy in order to exclude organic pathology, of which 84% were normal. All patients had a transit marker study in which only 25% were abnormal. Fifty-one percent had defecography of which 46% were abnormal. Seventy-four per cent had manometry but an abnormality was discovered in only 14%. Only 36% had a rectal biopsy but only one (6%) was abnormal. The average cost of investigations was US$2750 (range $1150–4792). Overall, $140 368 was expended on 51 patients, of whom only 23% benefited. Exhaustive tests are costly and their benefits are unclear.

Sigmoidoscopy

Sigmoidoscopy will identify solitary ulcer, proctitis and most obstructing lesions, as well as allowing inspection of the anal canal to exclude any predisposing anal pathology.

Barium enema

Further assessment should include a barium enema. Not only is a barium enema helpful in excluding other colorectal disease, such as diverticulitis, ulcerative colitis, endometriosis and carcinoma, but it may provide evidence of a megacolon or megarectum (Lennard-Jones, 1985). Preston et al (1982a) assessed the transverse diameter of the right, transverse and sigmoid colon in patients with megacolon and found a wide range of values, thereby placing some doubt on the reliability of barium enema for establishing megacolon. Although the length of the sigmoid colon is greater in constipated patients than in normal subjects, there are no specific diagnostic features of idiopathic constipation and most radiologists are unable to distinguish constipated from non-constipated subjects (Partiquin et al, 1978). Increased colonic length was reported in nine of 24 (37%) patients with constipation, and in four individuals (17%) the width of the colon was increased (Krishnamurthy et al, 1985).

Barium enema cannot be used to diagnose short segment Hirschsprung's disease.

Rectal biopsy

It is clearly important to exclude Hirschsprung's disease in adults with constipation. Typically, anorectal aganglionosis presents at birth or in early life. Sometimes short segment Hirschsprung's disease presents in adults but we are becoming increasingly sceptical about the existence of this condition since absence of ganglia is normal in the anal transitional zone. Nevertheless, we believe that a full-thickness rectal biopsy should be performed in dilating disease since it is the only way of excluding an aganglionic segment. The biopsy should be taken under general anaesthetic. A longitudinal strip of submucosa and muscle is excised over a distance of 3–6 cm from the anal verge (Pinho et al, 1991b). The biopsy must be above the dentate line since, as explained above, the zone immediately adjacent to this site normally contains very few ganglion cells anyway.

Anal manometry

Resting and maximum squeeze pressures may be normal in idiopathic constipated patients but a few have increased resting internal sphincter activity (Kamm, 1987) and in some there is evidence of sphincter denervation. Martelli et al (1978b) found that the upper anal canal pressures were unstable and often associated with ultra-slow waves (Hancock, 1976). In contrast to Hirschsprung's disease, Orr and Robinson (1981) reported that the rectoanal inhibitory reflex was always present in chronic idiopathic constipation. The rectoanal inhibitory reflex is usually absent in all forms of Hirschsprung's disease and is therefore said to be diagnostic of the condition (Haddad and Devroede-Bertrand, 1981) unless the segment is extremely short. The specificity and sensitivity of the rectoanal inhibitory reflex has however been questioned. In Birmingham we found that 8 of 25 patients with idiopathic constipation had no rectoanal inhibitory reflex despite the presence of normal ganglion cells on full-thickness rectal biopsy. Furthermore, a few patients with an aganglionic segment had an inhibitory response (Shouler and Keighley, 1986). The threshold for the rectoanal inhibitory reflex may be increased in constipation (Meunier et al, 1979b). Anorectal manometry is probably not the investigation of choice to identify the paradoxical puborectalis syndrome (Ger et al, 1993).

Rectal sensation, compliance, rectal contraction

Rectal sensation and rectal sensory evoked potential are known to be impaired in patients with a megarectum; it is also abnormal in children and adults with idiopathic constipation (Meunier et al, 1979a; Speakman et al, 1993; Solana et al, 1996). We found that although threshold pressures did not differ from controls, constant sensation volumes were above the normal range in 15 constipated patients (60%) (Shouler and Keighley, 1986) and the maximum tolerated volume was unrecordable in 16 (64%).

Compliance is often normal unless there is proctitis or a solitary ulcer, in which case it is reduced. There may be episodes of high-pressure waves in the rectum in response to rectal distension (Bannister et al, 1986). However, more usually rectal pressures are low and often fail to exceed anal pressures which may be abnormally high (MacDonald et al, 1993b; Karlbom et al, 1995; Halligan et al, 1995). In megarectum compliance is increased and there is virtually no motor activity in the rectum (Varma and Smith, 1986, 1988; Varma et al, 1988).

Colonic motility

Colonic pressure studies should be performed over long periods preferably using ambulatory techniques with simultaneous traces in the ileum, right, left, sigmoid colon and rectum (Kumar and Gustavsson, 1988). Investigation is technically difficult in constipated patients but preinvestigation purgation makes interpretation of the basal activity impossible. Stimulation may be with a variety of agents such as neostigmine, laxatives or food. Three parameters are usually analysed: mean amplitude of pressure waves, percentage of activity and motility index (Parks and Connell, 1969). In constipation the principal colonic motor disorder consists of exaggerated segmentation and absent mass movement, which delays the transit of faecal material through the colon (Choudhoury et al, 1976; Bassotti et al, 1988; Meunier et al, 1984; Ferrara et al, 1994). Preston and Lennard-Jones (1982) suggested that patients complaining of idiopathic constipation could be divided into two groups: (1) those with the irritable bowel syndrome who have normal gut transit and pain from hypersegmentation; and (2) those with slow transit and a hypomotile sigmoid colon. Meunier et al (1979b) found that there was marked variability in the motility pattern of the sigmoid colon in constipated patients at rest, after neostigmine and following a meal. We found that, with the exception of four patients with hyperactive pressures (16%), basal sigmoid pressures in constipated patients were similar to controls (Figure 21.9). However, there was a marked difference in the response to bisacodyl, there being only two non-responders in our control group (10%) compared with 13 in our constipated group (52%). In view of the complexity of ambulatory 24-hour intestinal motility studies (Bassotti et al, 1993), Rogers and Misiewicz (1989) developed software for a fully automated computer analysis of colonic motility which compares well with manual systems (Figure 21.10).

Transit

An objective assessment of propulsive activity can be obtained by transit studies (Figure 21.11). It is claimed that colonic transit studies are not compromised by anismus (Miller et al, 1991) but this must be challenged since most authorities are now of the view that colonic inertia is often secondary to anismus (MacDonald et al, 1997). Some transit markers have laxative properties (Tomlin

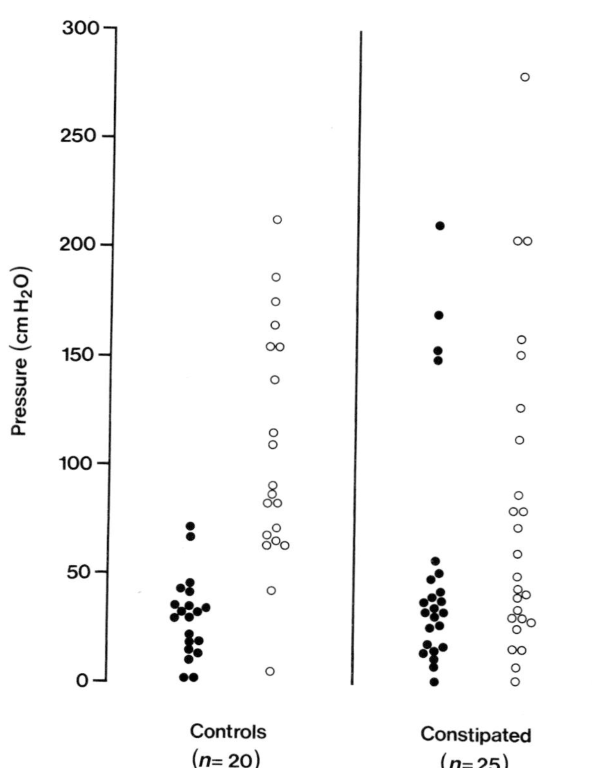

Figure 21.9 Peak sigmoid pressures (cmH_2O) at rest (●, maximal basal pressures) and after intrarectal bisacodyl (○, maximum stimulated pressures), in controls and in constipated patients.

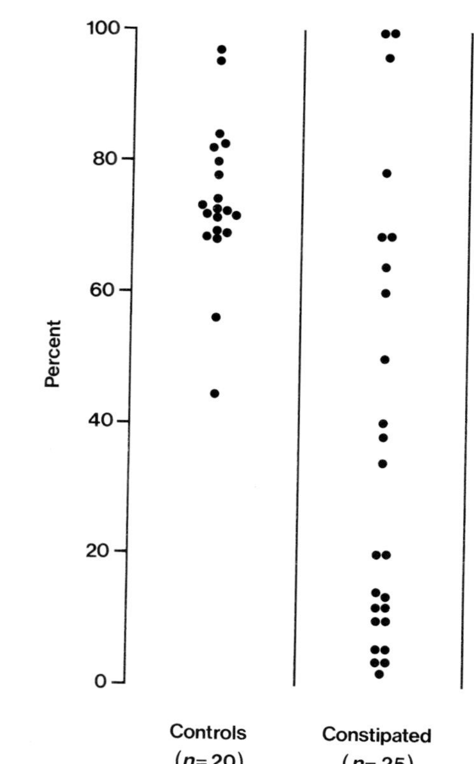

Figure 21.11 Transit times in constipated patients compared with controls. The percentage of markers passed at 5 days is shown for both groups.

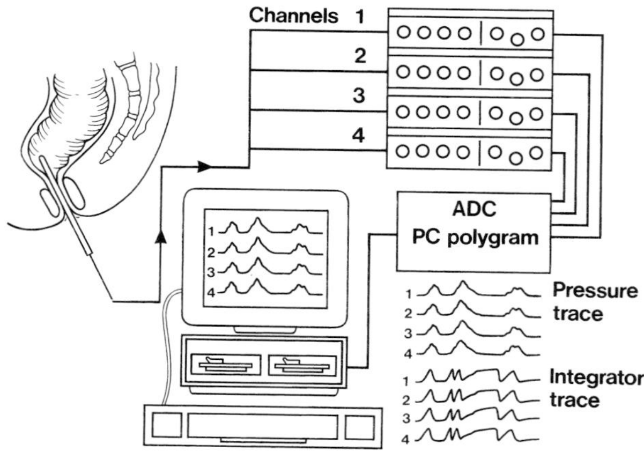

Figure 21.10 Synchronous recording of manometric data from the rectum, sigmoid and anal canal on a polygraph and computer.

and Read, 1988; Gilmore, 1990). Furthermore, some patients with diarrhoea are, in fact, constipated when assessed by marker studies (Cummings et al, 1976; McLean et al, 1992).

Poisson and Devroede (1983) administered 20 radio-opaque markers to patients taking a normal diet without laxatives. Although stools may be X-rayed, these investigators found that more information could be obtained by serial daily abdominal radiographs for one week, so that the number of markers in the right, left and rectosigmoid area could be assessed. Results in normal adults and children are shown in Table 21.7.

Metcalf et al (1987) reported a simple method of assessing segmental colonic transit using three different shapes of markers (Figure 21.12). More precise information on segmental transit can be obtained by colonic scintigraphy (Stivland et al, 1991; Kamm et al, 1992; Lubowski et al, 1995). This is capable of demonstrating segments of the colon with impaired motility, which might identify patients in whom segmental resection is justified (Krevsky et al, 1986; Picon et al, 1992; Hutchinson et al, 1995; Notghi et al, 1994, 1995; van der Sijp et al, 1993) (Figure 21.13).

Table 21.7 Number of markers in different segments of the large bowel in healthy subjects who ingested 20 markers while eating a high-residue diet.

	Days after ingestion							
	1	*2*	*3*	*4*	*5*	*6*	*7*	*Mean transit time (hours)*
Children								
Total colon	20	13	7	4	0	0	0	62
Right colon	14	1	0	0	0	0	0	18
Left colon	12	4	0	0	0	0	0	20
Rectosigmoid	20	12	7	5	0	0	0	34
Adults								
Total colon	20	20	18	10	5	3	0	93
Right colon	20	10	4	1	0	0	0	38
Left colon	15	11	8	4	3	1	0	37
Rectosigmoid	9	12	10	7	3	1	0	34

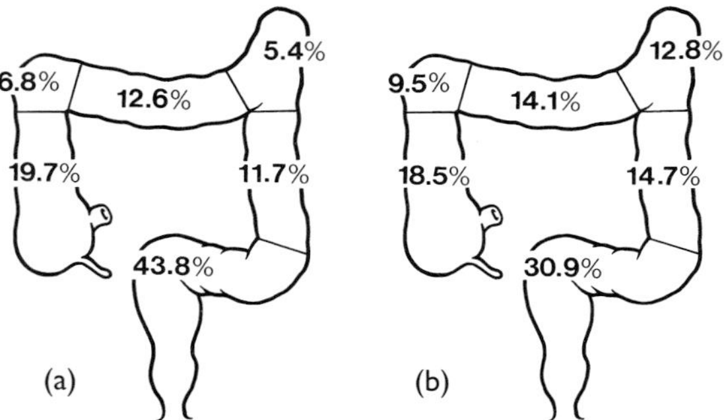

Figure 21.12 Proportion of total colonic transit time spent in the caecum and ascending colon, hepatic flexure, transverse colon, splenic flexure, descending colon, sigmoid colon and rectum in 73 normal subjects, separately analysed for (a) men (mean colonic transit = 30.7 ± 3.0 hours) and (b) women (mean colonic transit = 38.8 ± 2.9 hours).

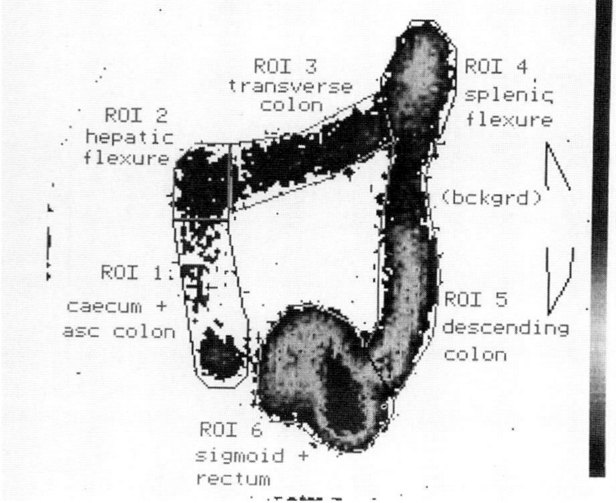

Figure 21.13 Colonic scintigram, with regions of interest: caecum and ascending colon, hepatic flexure, transverse colon, splenic flexure, descending colon and rectum and sigmoid, corrected for background activity.

Electromyography

Sigmoid myoelectrical activity (Taylor et al, 1975; Wegman et al, 1989) is increased in patients whose constipation is due to diverticular disease or the irritable bowel syndrome (Snape et al, 1976; Bueno et al, 1980). Frieri et al (1983) indicated that myoelectrical activity was increased in slow transit constipation and proposed that increased segmentation was responsible for slowing colonic transit.

Electromyography of the puborectalis and external sphincter may identify inappropriate activity during attempted defecation (Lubowski et al, 1992). Usually these muscles become electrically silent during straining; failure to relax or increased activity is a feature of anismus or outlet obstruction (Turnbull et al, 1986). However, many now feel that because needle electromyography is so painful and the test is untrue to the normal process of having a bowel movement, a diagnosis of anismus using this technique is invalid (Schouten et al, 1997). Single-fibre electromyography may indicate attempted reinnervation following repeated stretch of the pudendal nerve from straining. Similarly, conduction studies may identify prolonged latency in the terminal portion of the pudendal nerve (Bartolo et al, 1985; Preston, 1985; Vaccaro et al, 1995b).

Evacuation proctography

The balloon proctogram provided a simple way of evaluating the relationship of the rectal ampulla to the anal canal and pelvis, the anorectal angle and the degree of perineal descent and efficiency of rectal evacuation (Preston et al, 1982a; Barnes and Lennard-Jones, 1985). Balloon proctography has been almost completely superseded by videoproctography for measuring anorectal angles, the length of the anal canal and pelvic floor movements (Pinho et al, 1991a), as well as perineal descent, identifying a mucosal prolapse, rectocele, sigmoidocele, intussusception, an unrecognized rectal prolapse, and assessing rectal emptying (Kerremans, 1968b; Johansson et al, 1985; Lesaffer and Milo, 1988; Pinho et al, 1991a; Yoshioka et al, 1991). Videoproctography may be performed simultaneously with anorectal manometry and electromyographic recordings of the sphincters and pelvic floor (Muzzio et al, 1984; Womack et al, 1985; Roe et al, 1986b; Lestar et al, 1989; Thorpe et al, 1993). A careful audit of the videoproctographic findings in normals indicates that there is a wide range of values for the anorectal angle and pelvic floor descent at rest during contraction and during straining. Furthermore, 81% of healthy women have a rectocele and up to 50% of normal subjects have an intussusception (Shorvon et al, 1989). The importance of videoproctography is the identification of the physiological abnormalities in outlet obstruction so that those which are amenable to correction can be treated (Roberts et al, 1992).

Conventional defecography identifies intussusception, rectocele, rectal prolapse, sigmoidocele as well as evaluating emptying patterns, perineal descent and pelvic floor movement during defecography (Halligan et al, 1994; Mellgren et al, 1994a; Papachrystostomou et al, 1994; Alstrup et al; 1997; Piloni et al, 1997; Jones et al, 1998). In outlet obstruction, the pelvic floor either remains almost stationary during straining or there is marked perineal descent. Pezim et al (1993) at the Mayo Clinic made an important observation. They described a group of patients with an immobile perineum associated with impaired evacuation, very little change in the anorectal angle and minimal descent of the perineum. They found that this group, which incidentally could be identified clinically by descent of the perineum of less than 1 cm, were a very unrewarding group who seemed to do badly whatever treatment was tried. We agree.

Addition of contrast in the peritoneal cavity provides greater information if enterocele is suspected (Sentovich et al, 1995; Bremmer et al, 1995) (Figure 21.14). Sometimes, it is necessary to introduce contrast with air into the sigmoid colon or to image the small bowel in order to distinguish a sigmoidocele from a peritoneocele with small bowel within it. Vaginal contrast may help if obstructed defecation is associated with a vaginal vault prolapse. Furthermore, intravenous contrast to delineate the bladder or an associated cystogram may be appropriate if there is a coexisting cystocele (Thorpe et al,

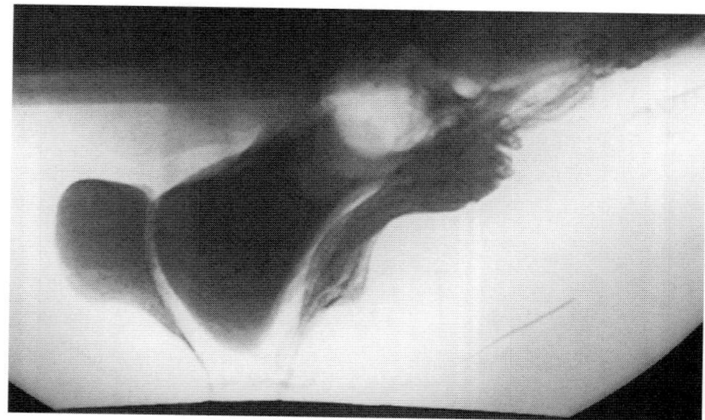

Figure 21.14 Evacuatory proctography. Contrast in the peritoneal cavity demonstrating a sigmoidocele.

1993). At the Royal London Hospital, we have performed simultaneous dynamic electromyographic proctography and cystometography in a group of patients with chronic constipation (n = 16). By this investigation, 10 of these were shown also to have obstructed micturition, eight of whom exhibited an inappropriate contraction of the puborectalis during micturition. In some patients in whom a large rectocele was demonstrated, the rectocele was shown to distort the urethra sufficiently to obstruct micturition (Thorpe et al, 1993) (Figure 21.15). Hutchinson et al (1993) have developed scintographic defecography both to quantify rectal emptying and to define pathology with a technique

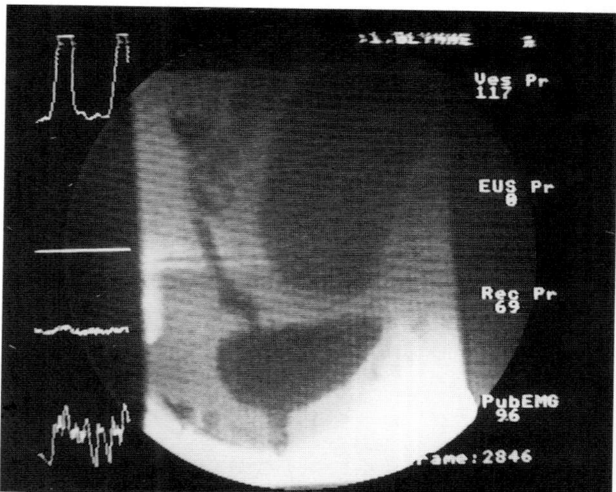

Figure 21.15 Combined dynamic proctography and cystometography in a patient with paradoxical contraction of the puborectalis and a rectocele. The intravesical pressure (trace 1) is grossly raised during attempted micturition and paradoxical recruitment of the puborectalis (trace 4) occurs. The large rectocele is largest during defecation and advances in an anterior direction, causing the bladder neck and urethra to become angulated and obstructing bladder emptying.

requiring far less radiation to young women than conventional videoproctography (Figures 21.16 and 21.17). Alternatively, isotopic imaging of the colon can be performed with later assessment during defecation (Lubowski et al, 1995) (Figure 21.18a,b). A new and potentially exciting imaging technique is that of soft endorectal and vaginal MRI to provide simultaneous sagittal, coronal and axial images of the pelvic viscera and the pelvic floor. This technique identified a number of abnormalities in obstructed defecation when conventional proctography was normal (Healy et al, 1997).

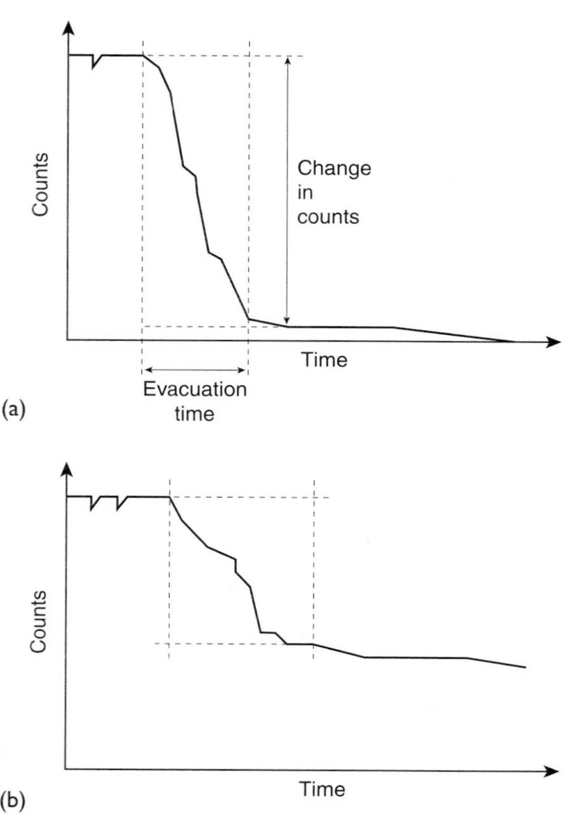

Figure 21.16 Isotopic rectal emptying in (a) a normal patient and (b) a constipated patient. From Hutchinson et al (1993).

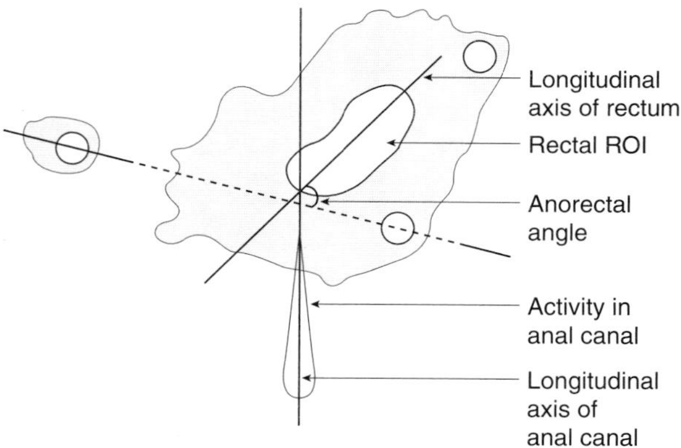

Figure 21.17 Measurement of anorectal angle with isotopic defecography. From Hutchinson et al (1993).

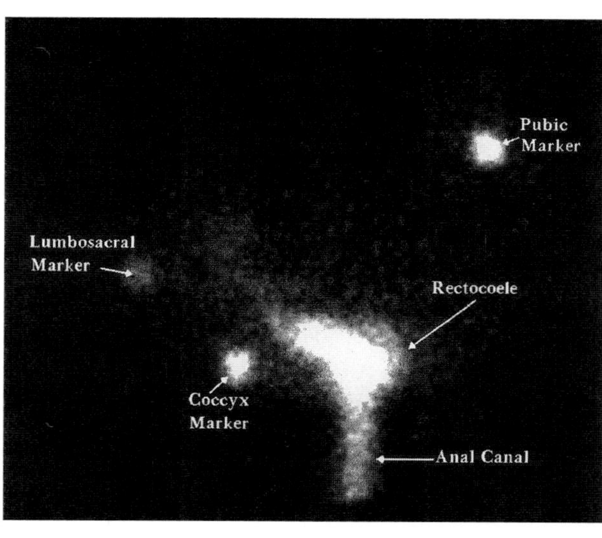

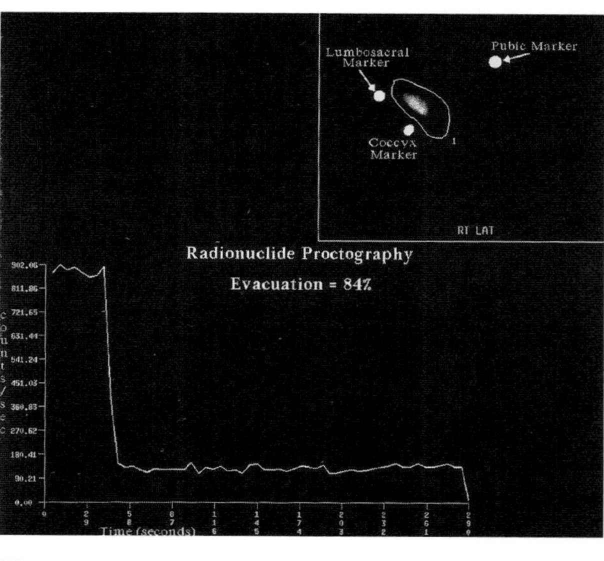

Figure 21.18 Defecogram showing (a) normal emptying of the rectum; (b) rectal emptying with a rectocele.

DIFFERENTIAL DIAGNOSIS

Some of the principal disorders to be considered in the differential diagnosis of constipation are listed in Table 21.8.

Table 21.8 Differential diagnosis of idiopathic constipation.

Other gastrointestinal diseases	Solitary rectal ulcer
Cystic fibrosis	Strictures
Duodenal stenosis	Ulcerative or ischaemic proctitis
Gastric cancer	Neurological colonic disease
Sprue	Chagas' disease
Colonic disorders	Colonic hypoganglionosis
Colorectal cancer	Hirschsprung's disease
Diverticular disease	Megacolon and megarectum
Irritable bowel syndrome	Anal disorders
Pseudo-obstruction	Anal fissure
Rectal prolapse	Anal stenosis
Segmental dilatation of the colon	Anorectal abscess
Sigmoid volvulus	Thrombosed haemorrhoids

NON-SURGICAL TREATMENT

General measures and diet

Part of the therapy of idiopathic constipation involves reassuring the patient that there is no serious underlying bowel disorder and explaining that emotional stress and hormonal factors play an important part in exacerbation of symptoms. Therapy depends upon attempted correction of the underlying physiological, psychological and social factors that may be responsible for the symptoms. Laxatives will almost certainly have to be prescribed and we no longer believe that prolonged use should be avoided. Indeed, control of bowel frequency with laxatives seems a more fruitful avenue for treatment than surgery. Patients should be reassured that it is not harmful to have only two or three bowel actions per week.

Patients should be encouraged to take regular physical exercise and to drink plenty of fluids. In the past, a high-fibre diet or bulking agents were prescribed but most patients find increased intake of dietary fibre and bulk laxatives exacerbate symptoms of abdominal pain, bloating, nausea and flatulence. Patients should avoid excessive straining at stool. Stimulant suppositories are sometimes helpful, especially in an attempt to establish reflex defecation.

Medical therapy: laxatives, suppositories and enemas

Laxatives

Most laxatives stimulate mucosal ion secretion in the small bowel and produce an increased fluid load to the ileocaecal region. There is a net accumulation of fluid and electrolytes in the lumen of the colon resulting in increased faecal water excretion (Binder, 1977). Most compounds act as stool softeners in small doses but in excessive doses they act as cathartics, causing abdominal colic and diarrhoea with excessive fluid and electrolyte loss.

Saline cathartics

Saline cathartics act as a consequence of their osmotic properties: component ions are not completely absorbed from the small bowel, hence an increased fluid and electrolyte load is presented to the colon. Such compounds include magnesium sulphate, magnesium hydroxide, magnesium citrate, sodium phosphate and sodium sulphate. Most of these agents act within 3 hours but they must be taken with large volumes of fluid, both to prevent dehydration and to maximize the laxative effect. Sodium picosulphate is widely used for barium enema and colonoscopy preparation and is remarkably effective, even in the most constipated patients, but it must be used in conjunction with a high fluid load (Takada et al, 1993).

Contact cathartics

These agents act both by interfering with electrolyte transport and by increasing the propulsive activity of the bowel when applied directly to the colonic mucosa. They take longer to act than saline cathartics and their maximum effect is usually 6 hours after ingestion. The principal compounds in this group are phenolphthalein, bisacodyl, the anthraquinones, senna, cascara and danthron (Dorbanex).

Castor oil

Castor oil is hydrolysed by pancreatic lipase into its active form, ricinoleic acid. The effect on the small and large bowel is similar to that of bile acids. There is a net secretion of sodium and water. Both castor oil and bile acids cause inflammatory changes to the mucosa of the colon and rectum. Dioctyl has a similar mode of action but it is less active than castor oil; its principal disadvantage is that it may be hepatotoxic.

Osmotic agents

Lactulose is a semisynthetic disaccharide which is not hydrolysed by intestinal enzymes. It acts as an osmotic cathartic and retains water and electrolytes in the lumen of the gut. Further metabolism of this unabsorbed sugar is achieved by colonic bacteria which release organic acids; these acids then act as laxatives. Lactulose, however, causes marked abdominal distension and many patients with constipation soon become intolerant to it. Other osmotic agents include mannitol, sorbitol and polyethylene glycol. Lactulose, which is now widely used in Britain, is probably less effective than senna in elderly patients (Passmore et al, 1993).

Mineral oil

Liquid paraffin is indigestible and tasteless; it lubricates the stool but unfortunately it often leaks around a solid faecal bolus, causing incontinence. It may be associated with respiratory complications and can impair absorption of fat-soluble compounds such as fat-soluble vitamins; it is therefore not recommended.

Other agents

Prostaglandin analogues may be used in patients with mild dyspepsia and constipation, but they are limited because of their side-effects (Roarty et al, 1997). The prokinetic cisapride (Ueda et al, 1994) also may be useful in patients with gastro-oesophageal reflux, duodenogastric reflux and constipation. At a dose of 20 mg b.d. the frequency of defecation is increased and laxative intake may be reduced (Muller-Lissner et al, 1987). Erythromycin is a prokinetic agent (Minocha et al, 1995) but has no effect on distal colonic motility (Jameson et al, 1992). Similarly, vancomycin was thought to be potentially effective but Celik et al (1994) reported disappointing results. Erythromycin should not be used with cisapride. Psyllium is often effective in chronic idiopathic constipation (Ashraf et al, 1995). Trimebutin and meleate (Modulon or Debridat) was proposed for treatment but Schang et al (1993) reported disappointing results.

Suppositories

Suppositories have a rapid onset of action and may be helpful in establishing reflex defecation for bowel retraining. However, glycerine suppositories are rarely effective in constipated patients and suppositories containing a surface laxative, such as bisacodyl, or a saline cathartic, such as sodium acid phosphate, are more likely to achieve a response.

Enemas

Enemas may be the only way for patients with constipation to achieve defecation. The proprietary mini enemas containing sodium citrate are rarely effective in patients with chronic constipation. Disposable phosphate enemas are more reliable. Fleet sodium phosphate enemas are easier to administer and may be more effective. Some patients find that the only way to achieve rectal evacuation is by twice-weekly soap and water enemas, usually given by themselves or a relative. The role of antegrade enemas (Hill et al, 1994; Williams et al, 1994) is discussed later. Colonic lavage using the same technique as in colostomy irrigation is often effective if patients will tolerate the technique (see Chapter 9).

A policy for laxative treatment in constipation

First-line therapy includes bulking agents and dietary advice; compounds like ispaghula, sterculia and methylcellulose should be tried. Stimulant laxatives are best avoided where possible since compounds like bisacodyl and senna cause colic and tolerance occurs with prolonged administration. Most clinicians therefore advise using magnesium sulphate, magnesium citrate or sodium phosphate. Lactulose is best avoided because it causes abdominal distension.

Treatment of faecal impaction

Faecal impaction should be excluded in any patient with a history of chronic constipation. Although it is sometimes possible to disimpact patients by the use of mineral oil, magnesium salts and repeated enemas, the process is unpleasant and the problem is often incompletely resolved. Some clinicians feel that manual evacuation under a general anaesthetic is never necessary. This, in our view, is unrealistic. Patients with gross impaction suffer from a vicious cycle and the only way to resolve matters in some is physically to extract the faecal mass which is obstructing the anorectum.

Biofeedback retraining

So disappointing are results of surgical therapy for outlet obstruction and idiopathic slow transit constipation that many coloproctologists have actively explored retraining the sphincter and pelvic floor to relax in response to rectal distension and attempted defecation (Fleshman et al, 1992). Particularly is this so, when many cases of colonic inertia seem merely to represent back pressure from disordered rectal evacuation (McLeod, 1983). Only recently have there been reports with adequate follow-up in patients with anismus to assess the role of this method of treatment in constipation (Kawimbe et al, 1991; Lestar et al, 1991; Fleshman et al, 1992; Rieger et al, 1997; Karlbom et al, 1997).

We have developed a hand-held digital display unit connected to an anal probe with a rectal balloon. On the anal probe are radially placed surface electromyographic sensors from which impulses are integrated and displayed numerically. An audible signal is also generated from the anal probe. Patients are assessed in the outpatients department and taught to relax the anal canal on attempted defecation and in response to rectal distension. The apparatus is loaned to the patient who is asked to continue the exercises at home, both with and without the apparatus.

Lowery et al (1983) claimed that biofeedback was frequently successful in children with encopresis. Van Baal et al (1984) used this technique in children with an abnormal rectoanal inhibitory reflex. Weber et al (1987) reported that 15 of 26 adults and children with an impaired rectoanal inhibitory reflex were improved with biofeedback. However, Fleshman et al (1992) found that few of their patients obtained long-term benefit. Kawimbe et al (1991) reported that clinical benefit persisted for a mean of 6 months only. Lestar et al (1991) found that 11 of 16 patients were immediately improved and nine obtained continued benefit for at least a year. Encouraging reports have been documented by some (Turnbull and Ritvo, 1992; Karlbom et al, 1997); others, however, report a very disappointing outcome (Rieger et al, 1997). Results in children have been unsatisfactory too, with only a third obtaining long-term benefit (Loening-Baucke, 1991).

Papachrystostomou and Smith (1994) in Edinburgh used biofeedback in 22 patients with obstructive defecation. Clinically, 29% became completely asymptomatic and 57% were improved. Objectively, biofeedback significantly increased the defecation rate, the opening of the anorectal angle (more obtuse) during defecation and the extent of pelvic floor movement. It also reduced EMG voltage in the external sphincter during defecation and improved rectal sensation. Park et al (1996) at the Florida Cleveland Clinic suggested that there were two groups of patients: those with a flattened anorectal angle and a closed anal canal who rarely improved (25% only) and those with puborectalis indentation and a narrow angle who usually benefited (86%).

Koutsomanis et al (1995) at St Marks performed a randomized crossover trial to test the importance of visual display on the outcome of biofeedback for constipation. Results were just as successful without the visual display, indicating that biofeedback can be delivered successfully without a lot of expensive apparatus. There was a significant reduction in the time spent straining and in anorectal pain. A small study from Sweden showed no difference when EMG and manometry feedback was compared: 6 of 26 could not tolerate treatment, in the remainder bowel function and abdominal pain improved in 75% (Glia et al, 1997). A large cohort of 194 surprisingly old (median age: 71 years) patients was reported from the Florida Cleveland Clinic (Gilliland et al, 1997). Only 35% achieved a successful outcome. Results were not influenced by age, sex or duration of symptoms, but they were greatly influenced by patient motivation. When patients were willing to attend for five or more sessions, 63% were improved. Thus, biofeedback probably has a role, but the outcome is likely to depend on the personality of the therapist and the willingness of the patient to be helped. Indeed, many now consider that this treatment is a form of psychotherapy for a behavioural disorder.

SURGICAL TREATMENT

Until relatively recently there were few reports of surgical treatment involving sufficient numbers of patients or with adequate follow-up to evaluate the place of surgical therapy in chronic constipation (Pfeifer et al, 1996; Nyam et al, 1997). In the past, many reports on surgical treatment have combined patients with Hirschsprung's disease, megacolon and idiopathic constipation (Lynn and Van Heerden, 1975; Lane and Todd, 1977; McCready and Beart, 1979; Hughes et al, 1981). Some surgeons hold the view that surgical treatment should never be contemplated even when the patient has already been seen by an experienced gastroenterologist and has incapacitating symptoms (Todd, 1985; Henry, 1989). Our view is that operation should never be undertaken lightly and is never justified unless conservative therapy has been fully explored. There should be no psychological contraindications to operation (Hasegawa et al, 1998) and patients must have been comprehensively screened to exclude a primary metabolic or neurological disorder. Symptoms should be attributable to the underlying colorectal motility disorder and a clear correctable physiological defect should have been detected before operation.

Treatment is dictated by the two major defects in motility: outlet obstruction may be managed by measures designed to produce relaxation of the pelvic floor, and colonic inertia may be managed by some form of surgical resection. Colonic inertia and outlet obstruction often coexist, hence the relative importance of each component has to be carefully assessed (MacDonald et al, 1991; Miller et al, 1991).

Outlet obstruction

Impaired rectal evacuation is difficult to treat successfully in adults. In children with internal sphincter hypertonia, response to treatment by anal dilatation or anorectal myectomy is much more promising. A variety of therapeutic options have been explored in adults but so far few have achieved long-term benefit.

Anal dilatation

There have been a few reports suggesting that anal dilatation may have a role in therapy. Anal dilatation seems to be particularly indicated in children with soiling complicating chronic constipation and high anal pressures (Loening-Baucke, 1984; Meunier et al, 1984). It is possible that some of these children had an anal fissure in the past (Clayden and Lawson, 1976). Taylor et al (1980) describe seven patients with a hypotonic anal canal associated with adult megacolon who were treated by anal dilatation. All apparently improved and none required further surgical treatment. Freeman (1984) used anal dilatation in 28 children: 8 had no further soiling and required no more laxatives, in 14 the soiling was controlled but laxatives were still needed and only 6 did not respond. In a randomized trial we found that controlled anal dilatation was inferior to anorectal myectomy in the treatment of adult constipation (Yoshioka and Keighley, 1987a), whereas in children the results appear to be comparable (Freeman, 1984).

Maria et al (1997) reported on the outcome of self-dilatation with dilators for 30 minutes daily over 3 months. They found that the frequency of bowel movements improved, and that the use of laxatives and enemas fell after treatment. They consider that this method of therapy could be used with effect in the majority of patients.

We are now very dubious about anal dilatation, particularly in outlet obstruction, as it may precipitate incontinence in a potentially litigenous patient group.

Anorectal myectomy

This operation (for details see Chapter 22) involves excising a 1–2-cm-wide strip of internal sphincter and rectal circular muscle throughout the anal canal and lower third of the rectum (Figure 21.19). Anorectal myectomy has been used with effect in children with short segment Hirschsprung's disease and in some children with constipation (Bentley,

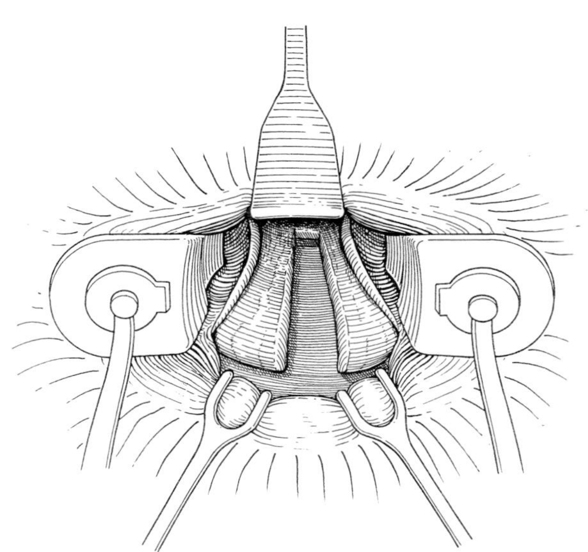

Figure 21.19 Anorectal myectomy. The internal anal sphincter has been dissected from the anorectal mucosa and from the external anal sphincter. A longitudinal segment of internal anal sphincter and rectal circular muscle has been excised.

1966; Thomas et al, 1970). Freeman (1984) reported that 14 of 16 children were improved, although 10 still continued to use laxatives (Table 21.9). The results in children seem to be promising and argue strongly for the existence of internal sphincter hyperactivity as a cause of constipation. However, the results of operation in patients over the age of 10 years seem to be far from satisfactory (Martelli et al, 1978a; Pinho et al, 1991b).

We first reported the results of this technique in 29 patients with outlet obstruction, eight of whom had evidence of short segment Hirschsprung's disease. An early follow-up indicated that 62% were improved but that benefit was confined to patients in whom the operation achieved a fall in resting anal pressures. A subsequent trial indicated that anorectal myectomy was superior to controlled anal dilatation and that the operation not only reduced anal pressures but was associated with objective improvement in rectal evacuation. The best results appeared to be in patients with normal colonic transit and a short history (Yoshioka and Keighley, 1987b). However, clinical evidence of deterioration led us to review 63 patients who had undergone the procedure and who had been followed up for a mean of 30 months. Spontaneous rectal evacuation was achieved in only 17% and 10% suffered mild incontinence, albeit transient in most cases (Pinho et al, 1991b). As a result we no longer recommend this therapy.

Partial division of the puborectalis

Partial division of the posterior fibres of the puborectalis sling might be considered a reasonable approach for patients in whom the muscle will not relax during defecation. The procedure was described by Wasserman (1964). Wallace and Madden (1969) used it in 69 patients (55 adults and 14 children) but no critical appraisal of the results was provided. We used a similar procedure, dividing the inner fibres of the puborectalis on either side of the midline, in seven patients, but only one was improved (Keighley and Shouler, 1984). Kamm et al (1988a) used lateral division in 15 patients with outlet obstruction but only three improved; benefit was only recorded in one of three patients with megarectum. Furthermore, three patients had minor incontinence. Posterior division of the puborectalis was also associated with disappointing results and iatrogenic morbidity, only two of nine were improved and five had some postoperative incontinence (Barnes et al, 1985).

Botulinum A toxin

As a result of disappointment with surgical division of the puborectalis local injection of *Clostridium botulinum* A toxin has been used by us in an attempt to partially paralyse the muscle. Symptoms were improved in the short term in seven patients with reduced anorectal pressures and an increased anorectal angle on straining. Four of the original

Table 21.9 Postoperative results of anal dilatation and anorectecal myectomy in children with soiling from constipation.

	n	*No soiling; no laxatives*	*No soiling; still taking laxatives*	*No better*
Anal dilatation	28	8	14	6
Anorectal myectomy	16	4	10	2
Failed anal dilatation, subsequent anorectal myectomy	5	4	0	1
Anal dilatation for fissure	12	10	0	2

seven patients experienced medium-term benefit, but required repeat injection at approximately 3-monthly intervals (Hallan et al, 1988). At the present time, none of the original seven patients continue with this therapy.

Joo et al (1996) from the Cleveland Clinic (Florida) reported the use of botulinum A toxin in four patients who failed to improve with biofeedback. There was no morbidity and two achieved longstanding benefit.

Sphincter displacement

Buchmann et al (1997) described a method of fixing the posterior component of the puborectalis and the sphincter to the sacrum and the ischial tuberosities to prevent constant closure of the anorectal junction. In a series of 26 patients, 85% were considerably improved.

Other treatments

Obturator internus autotransplantation to hold the anal canal open has also been proposed (Farag et al, 1993).

Rectocele repair

Repair of a rectocele for impaired rectal evacuation is a worthwhile form of treatment in properly selected cases (Siproudhis et al, 1993; Delemarre et al, 1994; Infantino et al, 1995; Halligan and Bartram, 1995; Murthy et al, 1996; Pucciani et al, 1996). Surgical correction should, where possible, be confined to patients in whom defecation becomes physically obstructed by the rectocele, such as in those having to digitate to achieve rectal evacuation. Perhaps the most rewarding group are those who find that it is necessary to push the rectocele backwards by inserting a finger into the vagina and applying pressure to the posterior vaginal wall (Block, 1986). This group seem to have a better outcome as compared with those who either apply perineal pressure or who need to digitate rectally (Karlbom et al, 1996). Most patients with rectoceles associated with obstructed defecation have had a previous hysterectomy. Those needing enemas were reported to be a group in whom symptoms were not always improved. Likewise, patients whose principal symptom is pain do badly.

Barium trapping in the rectocele on defecography seems to be associated with good results after rectocele repair, provided that the defect is low in the septum, whereas patients with prolonged colonic transit times have a disappointing outcome (Mellgren et al, 1995). The size of the rectocele probably has less bearing on the outcome (van Dam et al, 1996), although Karlbom et al (1996) found that patients with rectoceles having a large area had a poor result after repair. Similarly, Delemarre et al (1994) reported better results in patients with smaller rectoceles.

The results of rectocele repair in terms of improving rectal evacuation so that digitation was no longer necessary, bowel frequency increased and, in some cases, laxatives were no longer needed, are shown in Table 21.10. Murthy et al (1996) only operated on 32 of 132 patients with outlet obstruction and a palpable rectocele. They preferred to confine operation to patients who needed to digitate and those with barium trapping.

The majority of surgeons use an endorectal technique for repair (Khubchandani et al, 1983; Sehapayak, 1985). In the endoanal repair (usually performed in the pro-jack-knife position), a flap of mucosa is raised off the rectal circular muscle to expose the rectal wall over a distance of between 6 cm and 10 cm above the dentate line. The rectal muscle is plicated, usually with a series of vertically placed sutures and to obliterate the bulge (Figure 21.20a–e). The redundant mucosa is excised and the defect is closed (Sarles et al, 1989). Some surgeons

Table 21.10 Results of rectocele repair in terms of improved rectal evacuation.

	n	*Improved (no further digitation, increased bowel frequency)*
Khubchandani et al (1983)	59	37 (63)
Siproudhis et al (1993)	26	20 (77)
Janssen and van Dijke (1994)	76	38 (50)
Mellgren et al (1995)	25	13 (52)
van Dam et al (1996)	75	53 (71)
Murthy et al (1996)	35	32 (92)
Karlbom et al (1996)	34	27 (79)
Khubchandani et al (1997)	105	86 (82)

Values in parenthesis are percentages.

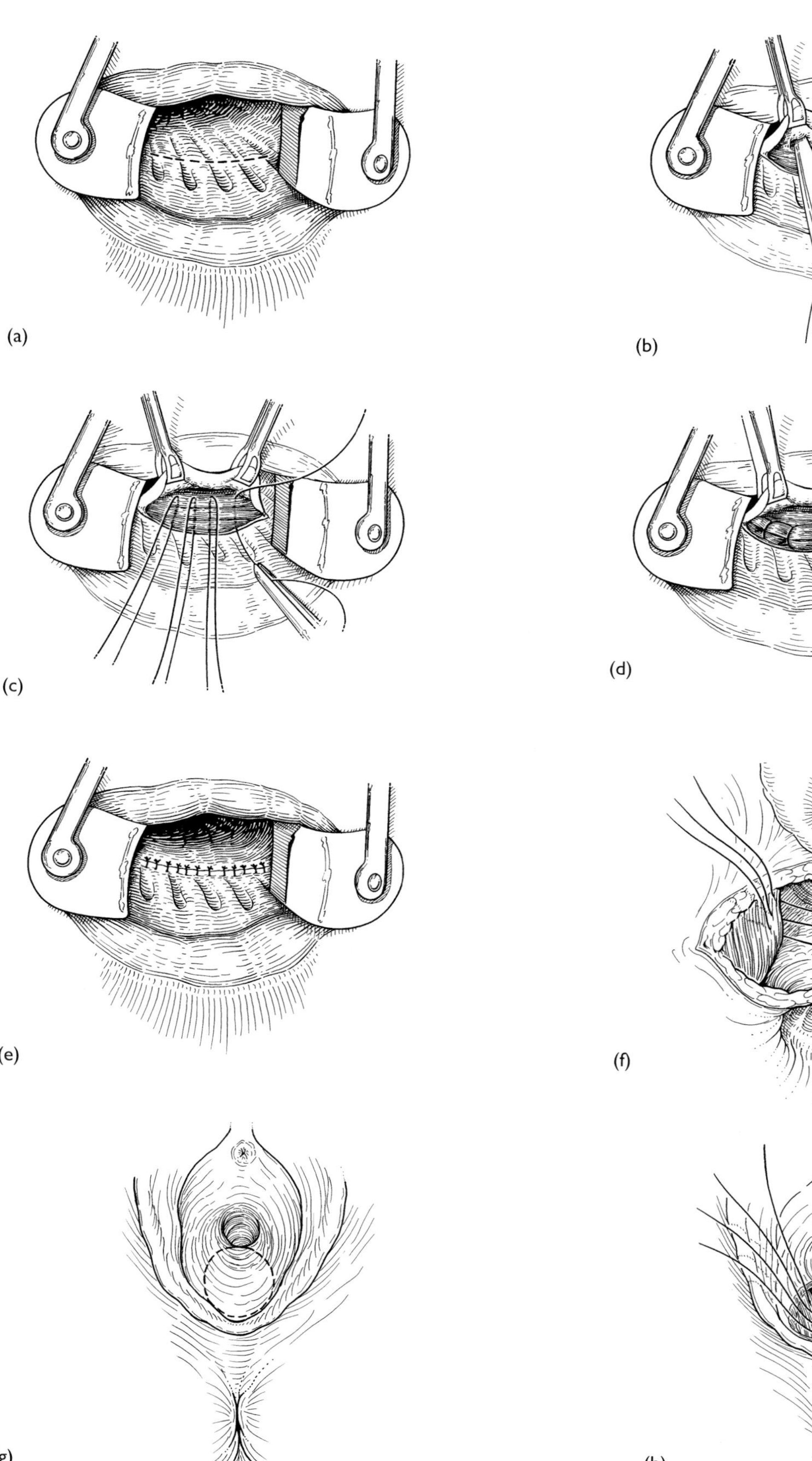
(a)
(b)
(c)
(d)
(e)
(f)
(g)
(h)

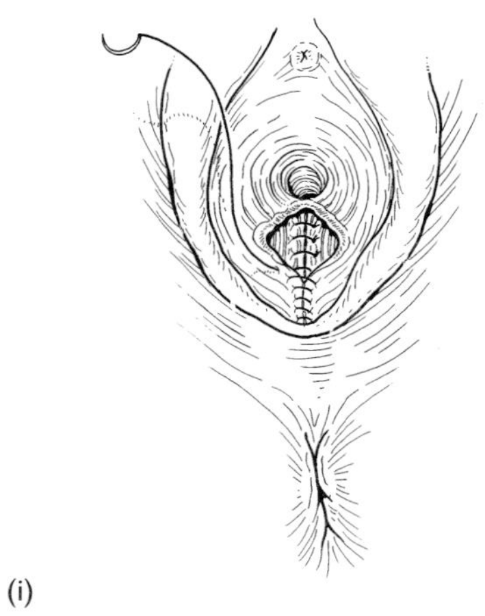

(i)

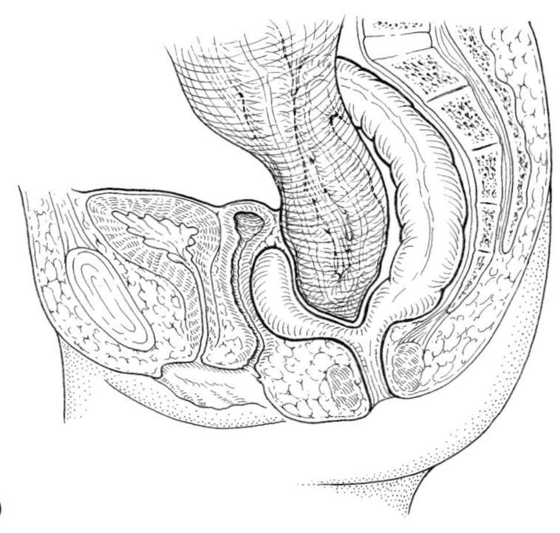

(j)

Figure 21.20a–j Endorectal repair of rectocele. (a) The patient is placed in the prone jack-knife position with the buttocks strapped apart. The anal mucosa is incised transversely 1 cm above the dentate line. (b) The anorectal mucosa is dissected from the internal anal sphincter and the rectal circular muscle to a height of 10 cm. (c) The rectal muscular layer is concertinaed together with 3/0 polyglycolic acid sutures. (d) The sutures in the rectal circular muscle have been tied. (e) The anorectal mucosa is being approximated to the cut edge of the anal canal. (f) Perineal approach to rectocele repair. Transverse incision is made over the perineal body. The rectovaginal septum is completely mobilized. A standard levatorplasty completes the procedure. (g) An ellipse of vaginal epithelium is excised. (h) The levators on either side of the vagina are identified and approximated. (i) The vaginal epithelium is closed after excising a large disk overlying the rectocele. (j) Sigmoidocele. The appearances of a sigmoidocele are illustrated. There is a very deep rectovaginal pouch. Usually the patient has already had a hysterectomy. The sigmoid apex, creating an obstruction at the anorectal angle resulting in a small rectocele. Correction is by excision of the sigmoid colon and rectopexy with or without repair of the rectocele.

prefer to plicate the rectal muscular wall with horizontal mattress sutures (Murthy et al, 1996).

We have approached the rectocele in the same manner as described in Chapter 20 for anterior levatorplasty. Using a transverse perineal incision the whole of the rectovaginal septum is exposed, separating each structure in order to demonstrate the levator ani, which is plicated with a series of horizontal mattress sutures (Figure 21.20f). Parker and Phillips (1993) have proposed using Marlex Mesh to repair the defect through the perineal approach.

The gynaecologists repair these by posterior colporrhaphy. They excise the vaginal skin, dissecting out the levators on either side of the defect and repairing the pelvic floor, after which the vaginal epithelium is closed (Figure 21.20g–i).

The long-term results vary from centre to centre. Endorectal repair appears to give the best results, but the numbers in most series are small. The rectocele is certainly reduced in size by operation and rectal emptying appears to be improved in those patients studied by defecography before and after repair.

An attempt should be made to divide rectocele into subgroups. The high or wide septal defects often associated with sigmoidocele and vaginal descent probably require resection rectopexy, vaginal or colposuspension and elimination of the deep Douglas pouch (Figure 21.20j). The wide rectocele associated with a cystocele probably should be treated by anterior and posterior colpography (Figure 21.20g–i). Only the narrow-necked, low rectocele associated with barium trapping or digitation should be treated by the colorectal surgeon using a transanal or a perineal approach (Figure 21.20i–f).

Our own experience of rectocele repairs bears out the comments made by others concerning patient selection. Obese patients, those who habitually strain, rectoceles with a wide septal defect, patients with pelvic pain and individuals with high expectations do not usually do well. Emptying may be improved, but many continue to strain and some still complain of fullness and pain. Provided patients understand that the objective is improved rectal emptying, usually without having to digitate, as opposed to being completely asymptomatic, the operation is worth undertaking.

Sigmoidocele

Occasionally a sigmoid loop may prolapse through the pouch of Douglas, causing obstructed defecation. In our experience of videoproctography for outlet obstruction, sigmoidocele has been seen in only a handful of radiographs. Jorge et al (1994) from the Cleveland Clinic (Florida) reported sigmoidocele in 24 of 289 examinations for constipation. Sigmoidocele can usually be diagnosed clinically by feeling hard scyballa in the bowel within a vaginal bulge which is not a straightforward rectocele (Figure 21.20j). Sigmoidoceles are more common in women, especially after hysterectomy. Mellgren et al (1994c) found that they were frequently associated with rectal intussusception (55%) or a rectal prolapse (38%).

Sigmoidocele is usually confirmed by videoproctography, preferrably after introducing contrast and air into the sigmoid colon rather than to the rectum alone. Peritoneal and small bowel contrast helps to identify the anatomy (see Figure 21.14).

Surgical treatment usually involves rectopexy and resection of the lower descending colon, the prolapsed sigmoid and the upper rectum as an extended resection rectopexy with colposuspension and obliteration of the Pouch of Douglas (Mellgren et al, 1994b; Jorge et al, 1994).

Incomplete rectal intussusception

Perhaps the most controversial subject is the role of rectopexy for incomplete rectal intussusception. The demonstration of a rectal intussusception by defecography is regarded by most people as a normal finding and, therefore, of no pathological significance (Johansson et al, 1985). Furthermore, repeated evacuation proctography may fail to identify this abnormality on a second examination, thus questioning the reliability of radiographic diagnosis. Certainly, all patients with incomplete rectal intussusception seem to spend a great deal of the time on the lavatory straining. The straining is considered to be the cause and most patients are told to stop, explaining that the act of straining has become a behavioural disorder.

If the intussusception progresses to a full-thickness prolapse, then surgical treatment seems justified (see Chapter 23). If the intussusception is responsible for rectal ulceration, surgery may also be acceptable, particularly if the solitary ulcer causes recurrent bleeding (see Chapter 24). However, the role of rectopexy for incomplete intussusception causing obstructive defecation is much more complex. By straining, these patients have caused an intussusception which may obstruct defecation. Thus, a vicious circle is created, leading to more straining which exacerbates the condition (Figure 21.21).

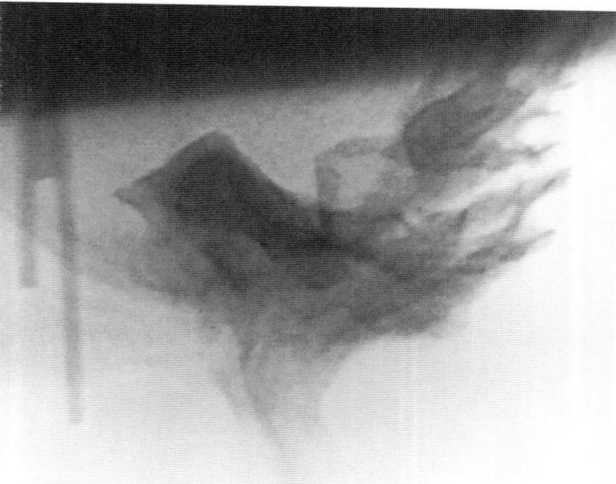

Figure 21.21 Incomplete rectal intussusception. A defecating proctogram which demonstrates marked perineal descent and an incomplete rectal intussusception.

Unfortunately, rectopexy often makes symptoms worse in these patients (Orrom et al, 1991). Our view is that these patients must be counselled very carefully. Some intussusceptions do seem to obstruct the passage of stool through the rectum. If rectopexy is offered, patients should be warned that symptoms may persist, despite correction of the anatomical defect. These patients should also understand that they must give up their life-long habit of straining.

Segmental colonic resection

Great care is necessary in selecting patients with constipation for a bowel resection because it is irreversible. Thus a preliminary stoma may be advisable in some patients to see if symptoms are improved. If a localized segment of bowel with delayed transit can be defined, it might be attractive to confine resection to the segment involved, thereby avoiding the potential morbidity of subtotal colectomy; particularly diarrhoea and incontinence. In practice, the results of segmental resection have been generally disappointing (McCready and Beart, 1979; Hughes et al, 1981; Preston et al, 1982b; Gasslander et al, 1987; Hasegawa et al, 1999; Kamm

Table 21.11 Results of colectomy for slow transit constipation.

	Segmental colectomy (*n* = 13)	*Subtotal colectomy* (*n* = 48)
Further operation	8 (62%)	17 (35%)
Eventual stoma	2 (15%)	12 (25%)
After first operation		
Grade 1	3 (23%)	22 (46%)
2	1	9
3	9	16
4 Faliure	0 9 (69%)	1 17 (35%)
Final		
Grade 1	5 (38%)	24 (50%)
2	4	12
3	2	0
4 Failure	2 4 (31%)	12 12 (25%)

From Hasegawa et al (1999).

et al, 1991c). The one possible exception is patients who have already had a vagotomy, gastrectomy or small bowel resection or elderly patients with intractable constipation.

With increasing use of scintigraphic methods, patients with localized colonic inertia can be identified and segmental resection may be justified, although the results of this policy still seem disappointing (De Graaf et al, 1996; Hasegawa et al, 1999). In the Birmingham series, segmental colectomy gave a much higher re-operation rate than subtotal colectomy for recurrent constipation, but faecal incontinence was not encountered (Table 21.11).

Subtotal colectomy

In our view, surgical resection should never be undertaken lightly in chronic constipation, even though delayed transit and hypomotility are demonstrated by colonic motility studies (Henry, 1989; Yoshioka and Keighley, 1989; Pemberton et al, 1991; Nyam et al, 1997).

Many patients complain of symptoms other than constipation, such as abdominal bloating and pain, which are not necessarily relieved by normalizing bowel frequency (Wexner et al, 1991; Pfeifer et al, 1996). Kamm et al (1988b) reported persistent abdominal pain and bloating in many patients after operation (Table 22.12). In 1989 we found that distension persisted in 82% of patients after colectomy and ileorectal anastomosis, although persistent pain was reported in only 39% (Yoshioka and Keighley, 1989). Ten of the 44 patients reported by Kamm et al (1988b) required psychiatric treatment; likewise 5 of our 40 patients needed psychological therapy. Some patients unpredictably developed diarrhoea (38% in the St Mark's series), and 14% became incontinent (Kamm et al, 1988b). Some patients develop recurrent constipation after resection and anastomosis, despite a patent anastomosis, necessitating further surgery (Walsh et al, 1987; Yoshioka and Keighley,

Table 21.12 Early results (%) of subtotal colectomy for severe idiopathic chronic constipation in 44 women with a normal diameter colon.

	Before operation	*After operation*
Abdominal pain	98	71
Abdominal bloating	95	45
Straining on defecation	95	33
Laxatives	88	30
Incontinence	0	14

From Kamm et al (1988b).

1989). Furthermore, adhesive obstruction appears to be particularly common, ranging from 0% to 50% (average 12%), following resection for constipation (Hughes et al, 1981; Preston et al, 1982b; Leon et al, 1987; Akervall et al, 1988; Pena et al, 1992).

Motility abnormalities in the stomach and small bowel may be one cause of failure and persistent symptoms after subtotal colectomy. The results of subtotal colectomy may be marginally better using a caecorectal rather than an ileorectal anastomosis. The only problem with a caecorectal anastomosis is that dilatation of the caecum may occur later. In older patients, ileosigmoid anastomosis may cause less troublesome diarrhoea than ileorectal anastomosis, but in younger individuals recurrent constipation is common after ileosigmoid anastomosis (Table 21.13). The St Mark's group found that failure to expel a 50-mL water balloon was associated with poor results after subtotal colectomy and concluded that the balloon expulsion test was of predictive value when subtotal colectomy was being considered for slow transit constipation.

The outcome of subtotal colectomy is influenced by psychological parameters (Fisher et al, 1988). Patients with high HAD scores due to anxiety and depression do badly. Also patients with coexisting colonic inertia and outlet obstruction have a very poor outcome, as do patients with documented psychiatric disorders (Hasegawa et al, 1998) (Tables 21.14 and 21.15). There is also a real risk of precipitating incontinence if an anorectal myectomy or puborectalis division has been performed prior to subtotal colectomy in an attempt to correct anismus. Postpartum injuries also increase the risk of incontinence after subtotal colectomy. Therefore, if a patient has both outlet obstruction and colonic inertia, only non-invasive therapy should be explored for the impaired rectal evacuation unless a colonic conduit is contemplated. After subtotal colectomy there is not only a high incidence of adhesive obstruction: 18% (Kamm et al, 1988b); 30% (Hughes et al, 1981); 24% (Walsh et al, 1987), but also a high proportion of patients who finish up with a stoma: 14% (Kamm et al, 1988b); 24% (Walsh et al, 1987); 15% (Yoshioka and Keighley, 1989); 24% (Hasegawa et al, 1999). Occasionally we have had to convert a non-functioning ileorectal anastomosis to an ileoanal pouch for a few women refusing a stoma who have developed recurrent constipation (Hosie et al, 1990). We are not enthusiastic about this approach since 50% over 10 years have continued symptoms and psychological instability resulting in pouch excision.

The results from the literature in terms of bowel habit seem amazingly good (Table 21.13). However, Lubowski et al (1996) in Sydney report that 52% had

Table 21.13 Results of subtotal colectomy for chronic constipation.

	n	*Normal bowel habit*
Subtotal colectomy + caecorectal anastomosis		
Goligher (1984)	10	6
Ryan and Oakley (1985)	21	18
Kamm et al (1988b)	20	14
Yoshioka and Keighley (1989)	5	3
Subtotal colectomy + ileosigmoid anastomosis		
Belliveau et al (1982)	37	34
Klatt (1983)	9	9
Subtotal colectomy + ileorectal anastomosis		
McCready and Beart (1979)	6	6
Hughes et al (1981)	17	5
Walsh et al (1987)	21	12
Akervall et al (1988)	12	8
Kamm et al (1988b)	24	7
Yoshioka and Keighley (1989)	34	24
Pemberton et al (1991)	38	38
Wexner et al (1991)	16	16
Stabile et al (1991)	11	11
Takahashi et al (1994)	38	26
Piccirillo et al (1995)	54	52
Redmond et al (1995)	34	30
Pluta et al (1996)	24	17
Lubowski et al (1996)	59	47
Nyam et al (1997)	74	72
Hasegawa et al (1998)	76	32

Table 21.14 Results of operation in patients with psychological problems.

	Psychological (*n* = 10)	*Non-psychological* (*n* = 51)	
Subtotal colectomy	10 (100%)	38 (74%)	NS
Segmental colectomy	0	13 (26%)	
Number with impaired evacuation	8 (80%)	25 (49%)	
Total no. of operations (mean SD)	5.3 (3.5)	1.6 (1.2)	*P* = 0.009
Total hospital stay (days) (mean SD)	59.5 (44.7)	22.8 (21.5)	*P* = 0.029
Total no. of admissions (mean SD)	6.1 (4.1)	2.2 (2.2)	*P* = 0.015
Eventual stoma	7 (70%)	7 (14%)	*P* = 0.0005
Final assessment			
Satisfactory	2 (20%)	27 (53%)	NS
Improvement	1	15	
Poor } Failure	0 } 7 (70%)	2 } 9 (18%)	*P* = 0.002
Stoma }	7 }	7 }	

From Hasegawa et al (1999).

Table 21.15 Results of colectomy for impaired emptying and slow transit.

	Slow transit + impaired emptying (*n* = 33)	*Slow transit alone* (*n* = 28)	
Subtotal colectomy/segmental colectomy	25/8	23/5	
Final assessment			
Satisfactory	11 (33%)	18 (64%)	*P* = 0.031
Improvement	9 (27%)	7 (25%)	
Poor } Failure	2 } 13 (39%)	0 } 3 (11%)	*P* = 0.025
Stoma }	11 }	3 }	

From Hasegawa et al (1999).

persistent abdominal pain, 6 of 59 patients became incontinent and 10% needed to take antidiarrhoeal medication. Similar experience has been reported by others (Pluta et al, 1996; Pfeifer et al, 1996).

We have recently reviewed our long-term results in 61 patients referred to the Birmingham Unit, where the median follow-up since colectomy was 7 years. The majority had a subtotal colectomy (48 cases) but some initially had a partial colectomy (13 cases). Sixteen (26%) required more than one operation and re-operation was more common after segmental colectomy (62%) than after subtotal colectomy (33%). Only 29 (47%) were eventually satisfied, despite a mean number of 2.2 operations. Fourteen patients (23%) finally had a stoma. Results in 10 patients with documented psychological disturbance were significantly worse than the rest (Table 21.14). The failure rate was also significantly greater in patients with outlet obstruction (39%) than those with colonic inertia alone (11%). These results indicate that the long-term outcome following subtotal colectomy is much worse than most reports suggest. However, about two-thirds of the psychologically stable patients without anismus have good long-term function. Patients should, therefore, be counselled about the failure rate, the risk of incontinence and the high stoma rate. Those with impaired rectal evacuation or with a psychological illness are unsuitable for operation. Details of the operation can be found in Chapter 22, pp 782–786.

Restorative proctocolectomy

Restorative proctocolectomy may have a place in the management of patients with megacolon and megarectum (see Chapter 22) but the results for pouch surgery for colonic inertia are often poor and we would generally not recommend this approach. It must be said, however, that most patients press for a rectal excision without a permanent stoma if a previous subtotal colectomy and ileorectal anastomosis has been unsuccessful because of recurrent constipation. Nevertheless, the recurrent constipation is almost always caused by impaired rectal evacuation, so it is hardly surprising that pouch surgery usually fails.

When we looked at restorative proctocolectomy in megabowel, the results were remarkably good (Stewart et al, 1994). However, the same cannot be said for patients with colonic inertia (Hosie et al, 1990). In our long-term review (Hasegawa et al, 1999), eight patients had a restorative proctocolectomy, of whom six have now required further surgery for continued symptoms and dissatisfaction. Three of these patients had a Koch pouch, all of whom became dissatisfied, despite five revision operations, and all have now had their reservoir ileostomy excised.

From time to time, surgeons may be driven to revising a subtotal colectomy for a restorative proctocolectomy because of continued abdominal distension, pain and poor evacuation. It is sometimes impossible to refuse another operation which avoids a permanent stoma but patients must be told that the long-term results are very poor. Nevertheless, in our latest long-term review of this group (Bain and Keighley, 1999), half still have a functioning pouch and are pleased not to have a stoma.

Stoma

The thought of a stoma is usually completely unacceptable in patients seeking treatment for constipation. However, in some it might be justified to consider a trial of loop ileostomy if slow transit coexists with outlet obstruction and the principal symptom is pain, abdominal distension as well as infrequent defecation. In some of our patients, the quality of life has been so greatly improved that no further surgical treatment is advised. Those that have subsequently undergone colectomy have sometimes been disappointed and they should, where possible, be persuaded to keep their stoma. In some patients an end or loop ileostomy is used after failed subtotal colectomy and ileorectal anastomosis, particularly if there is incontinence.

In some centres colostomy is advocated rather than ileostomy (van der Sijp et al, 1993), but in our view a colostomy has rarely been satisfactory for slow transit constipation. In these manipulative patients complex procedures such as a reservoir ileostomy has in our experience been nothing short of a complete disaster, with disappointed patients who have a very high rate of nipple valve failure and dissatisfaction.

Antegrade colonic enema (ACE)

The term antegrade colonic enema is used for the construction of a catheterizable conduit into the proximal colon through which enemas or irrigation fluid can be administered in a distal direction to achieve colonic and rectal evacuation. The appendix has been used most frequently, particularly in children. Indeed, irrigation of the colon via an appendicostomy was first described by Dalby in 1894 and numerous subsequent papers in the early 1900s reported its use for patients with colitis (Weir, 1902; Moynihan, 1903; Hutchinson, 1905; Stanmore Bishop, 1905).

Keetley (1905a) seems to have been the first to describe the technique for use in patients with constipation. In 1905 he reported successfully creating an appendicostomy in a 15-year-old girl who had always been constipated, through which colonic irrigations were performed. He also recommended this operation for patients with 'mucous; colitis, amoebic dysentery and ileocaecal intussusception (Keetley, 1905b). However, the technique was used relatively infrequently over subsequent years, perhaps because faecal leakage was prone to occur.

In 1980, Mitrofanoff reported the use of the appendix to create a continent catheterizable cystostomy in patients who had impaired bladder emptying. The appendix was isolated on its vascular pedicle, tunnelled submucosally into the bladder and brought out onto the abdominal wall to a funnel of skin, facilitating catheterization through a continent stoma. This technique became established in urological surgery both for the native bladder and in conjunction with enteric pouches commonly used in urinary diversion (Mitchell, 1986; Weingarten and Cromie, 1988).

Malone et al (1990) adopted the Mitrofanoff procedure for the treatment of chronically constipated or faecally incontinent children, and his procedure was termed the ACE (antegrade colonic enema) procedure. The ACE procedure is accomplished by isolating the appendix from the caecum on its vascular pedicle. The appendix is reversed, and its distal end amputated before re-implantation in a non-refluxing fashion into the caecum. The distal end of the appendix is anastomosed to the mucosal opening in the caecum by means of absorbable sutures. The appendix is placed in the submucosal tunnel and the seromuscular layers of the caecum are closed over it, thus creating a non-refluxing channel (Figure 21.22). The proximal end of the

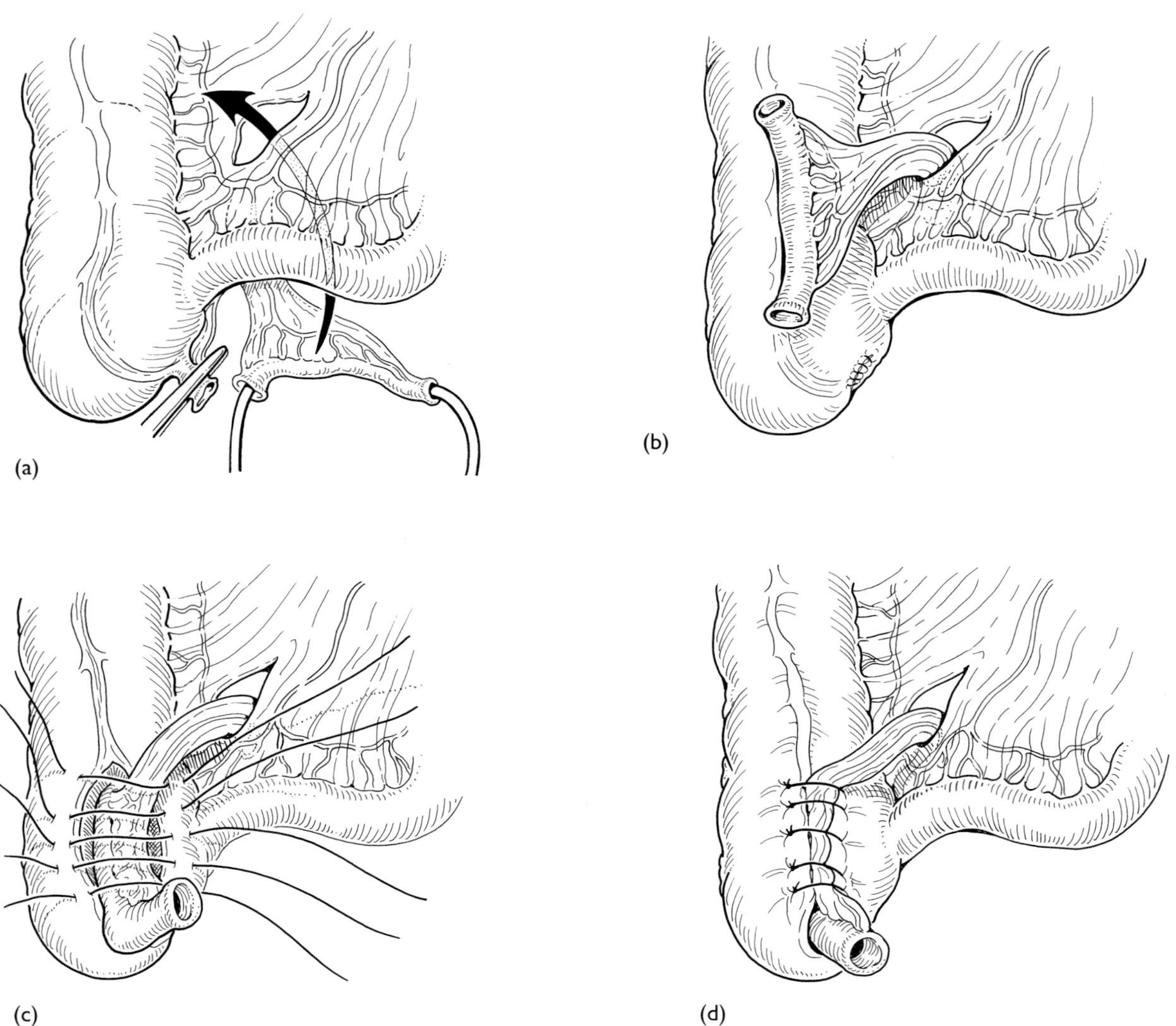

Figure 21.22a–d Appendicostomy for ACE. (a) The mesoappendix is preserved and (b) the appendix is relocated through the mesentery along the caecum in an antiperistaltic fashion (c). The appendix is laid within a submucosal space, its distal end is amputated, and this is then anastomosed to the caecum (d). The seromuscular layer is closed over the enterocaecostomy without compromising the mesenteric vascular pedicle. The proximal end of the appendix is exteriorized. From Tsang and Dudley (1995).

appendix with a cuff of caecum is exteriorized in the right iliac fossa. The caecum is anchored to the anterior abdominal wall, with no kinking of the appendix. The stoma is fashioned by means of a broad-based lateral skin flap that is made into a tube and anastomosed to the cuff of the caecum. This flap serves to bury the appendix and minimizes discharge onto the abdominal wall. The resulting non-refluxing continent stoma provides access to the proximal colon by way of a narrow catheterizable channel. The patient catheterizes the appendicostomy on a regular basis and antegrade colonic irrigation is performed.

In 1991, Wheeler and Malone described 13 patients aged between 3 and 18 years in whom the procedure had been performed. Three patients suffered from intractable chronic idiopathic constipation and the remaining 10 from a combination of constipation and faecal incontinence secondary to a variety of causes. Follow-up ranged from one to 20 months. The time taken to achieve colonic emptying varied from 20 to 30 minutes. Two patients experienced minor leakage of rectal fluid, but the other 11 remained completely clean between enemas, given at an interval that varied between 48 and 72 hours. The procedure successfully achieved colonic emptying in each case, but one patient developed severe stomal stenosis which required repeated dilatations and subsequently revision. No other complications were reported at that time. Since then, Malone and colleagues have updated their data and others have reported successful application of the technique in children (Squire et al, 1993; Toogood et al, 1995; Dick et al, 1996; Ellsworth et al, 1996). However, stomal stenosis seems to be a particular problem which may require revision.

We initially considered the use of a reversed appendicostomy to conduct antegrade colonic irrigation in constipated adult patients. One female patient underwent this procedure, but was unable to catheterize the appendix with a sufficiently large calibre catheter through which effective irrigation could be performed. Furthermore, the appendix is not always available or is stenosed in adults. For these reasons we devised the continent colonic conduit to treat selected patients with rectal evacuatory disorders who had not responded to conservative measures. Initially, we placed the conduit in the sigmoid colon (Williams et al, 1994) (Figure 21.23) in such patients, but have subsequently modified the procedure by placing it in the transverse colon (Hughes and Williams, 1995a) (Figure 21.24). We have also widened the application of the technique to treat selected patients with slow transit constipation, since it is less radical and less unpredictable than colectomy and ileorectal anastomosis.

Continent colonic conduit

Indications and preoperative assessment

A colonic conduit may be considered for all patients with slow colonic transit as an alternative to colectomy and ileorectal anastomosis or stoma formation. It is also appropriate for patients with a rectal evacuatory disorder such as anismus, when conservative measures have failed and a stoma is being considered. We have also used the procedure for selected patients with faecal incontinence in whom difficulty in rectal evacuation is a predominant symptom. Patients must undergo extensive counselling by both the surgeon and colorectal nurse specialist. A psychological opinion is often necessary. Discussion must include not only the complications of the operation, but the fact that it might fail and the patient might have to resort to a permanent stoma. Patients must understand the need to intubate the colon through an aperture on their abdominal wall on a regular basis. Ideally, they should meet a patient who has previously undergone the procedure, and be encouraged to watch a video of a patient using the irrigation equipment. This rigorous assessment and counselling are essential, and are intended to try to select highly motivated patients who have a positive mental attitude.

Patients undergo vigorous bowel preparation. The site of the conduit aperture is determined in

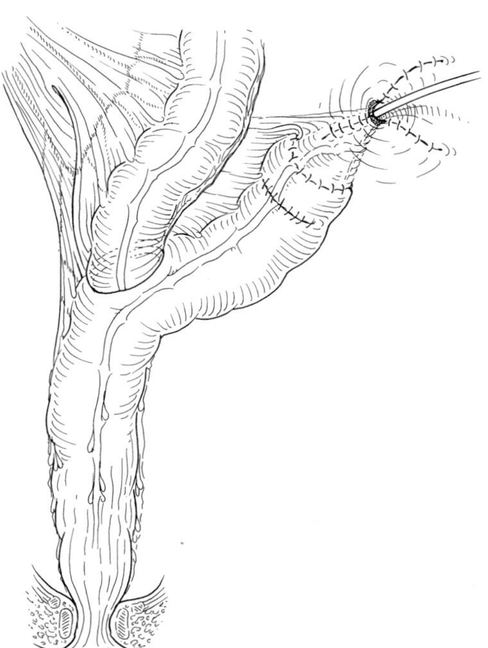

Figure 21.23 Sigmoid colonic conduit.

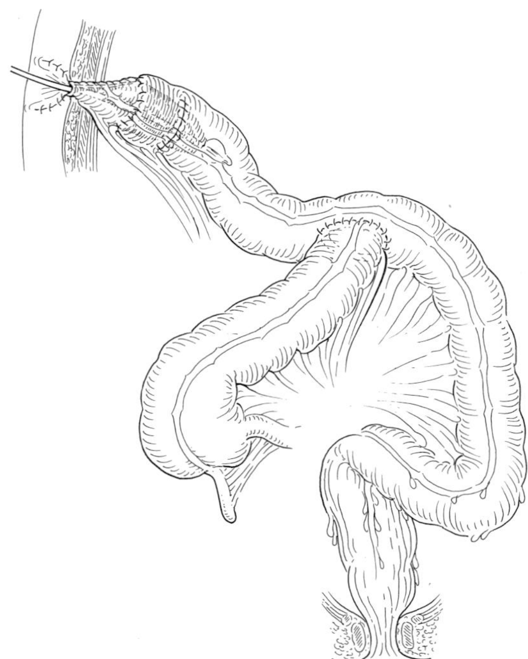

Figure 21.24 Transverse colonic conduit.

consultation with the colorectal nurse specialist and is marked with an indelible marker on the abdominal wall. Prophylactic antibiotics are given at induction of general anaesthesia, and are continued for two doses following the operation.

Operative procedure

The patient is positioned supine on the operating table, and a urinary catheter and nasogastric tube are inserted. A midline incision is performed, and the caecum, ascending colon, hepatic flexure and proximal half of the transverse colon are mobilized. The site for conduit formation (usually the hepatic flexure) is marked by the placement of Babcock forceps and distally from here, a 15-cm segment of the colon is measured out (Figure 21.25). The greater omentum is removed from this length of colon, and in cases where the mesocolon is particularly bulky, the peritoneal leaves are reflected and excess fat is removed, taking particular care to avoid damaging the mesenteric vessels. These manoeuvres allow the intussusception of the colon during formation of the valve. The ascending colon is transected approximately 15 cm from the ileocaecal junction, and 15 cm distally a 2-cm colotomy is made. A Babcock forceps is passed through the colotomy towards the blind end of the transected colon and the full thickness of the colon is grasped 5 cm from the transection line. The bowel is intussuscepted through the transverse colon to create the valve which is stabilized using a combination of non-absorbable sutures (Ethibond, Ethicon Ltd) and staples. The sutures are placed in three rows of three at the two o'clock, six o'clock and ten o'clock positions (Figure 21.26). Between these are placed three rows of staples using a stapler (TA 55 Multifire (staple height 4.8 mm), Autusuture Ltd), from the cartridge of which the pin has been removed. The valve is made a minimum of 5 cm long to prevent reflux of irrigant fluid and colonic contents onto the abdominal wall.

A size 14 silastic Foley catheter is inserted from the open end of the colon through the valve and the balloon inflated. Two non-absorbable purse-string sutures are placed around the apex of the valve, and these are tightened carefully around the catheter, leaving a gap of approximately 1 cm. It is important to leave this space around the catheter if conduit intubation is not to be impeded. The distal part of the catheter is positioned to lie in the lumen of the transverse colon beyond the colotomy and the valve is introduced back into the transverse colon. The colotomy is then closed with a continuous Maxon suture. As a further precaution against deintussusception, the base of the valve is secured from its external aspect to the afferent limb of the conduit using circumferentially placed interrupted sutures. The afferent limb of the conduit is narrowed using a stapler, the excess bowel trimmed off and the staple line oversewn (Figures 21.27 and 21.28).

Intestinal continuity is restored, joining the ascending colon to the distal transverse colon with an end-to-side colocolic anastomosis. The site for this is chosen distally to the conduit so that the conduit is able to reach to the abdominal wall and form a stoma without tension. At the aperture site, skin flaps are marked out on the abdominal wall. An 'inverted wine glass' shape is used with a broad-based lateral flap (Figure 21.29). The flap is

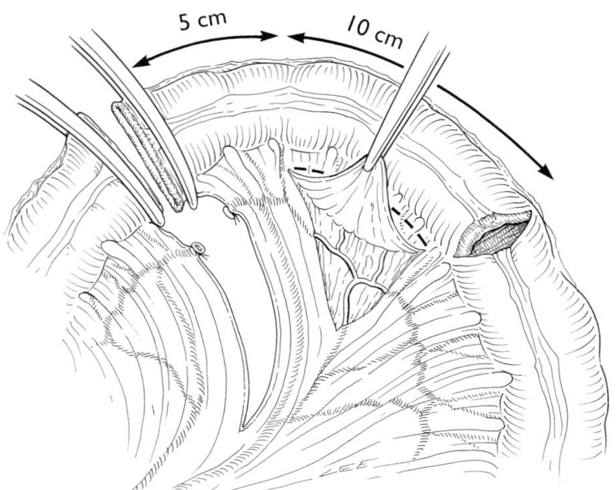

Figure 21.25 Removal of the omentum, debulking of the mesocolon and formation of a transverse colotomy 15 cm from the point of colonic transection at the hepatic flexure.

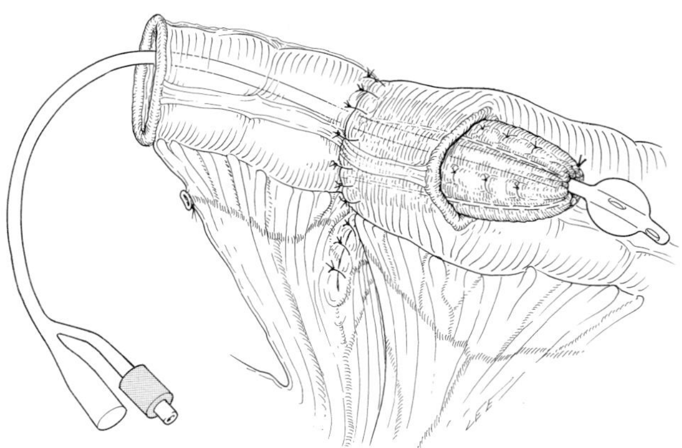

Figure 21.26 Formation of the conduit valve by intussusception and valve stabilization with sutures and staples.

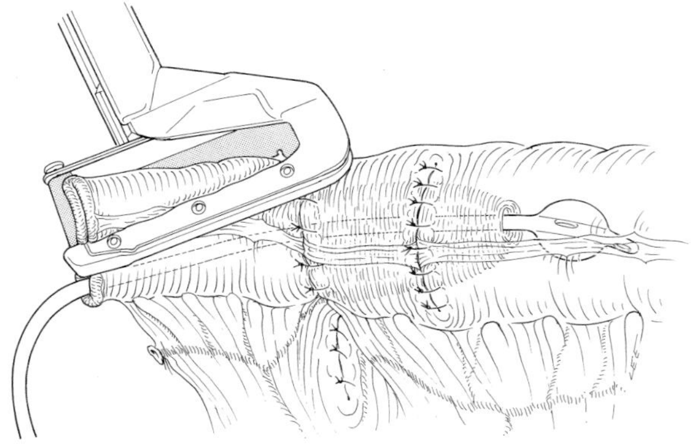

Figure 21.27 Narrowing of the afferent limb of the conduit by stapling.

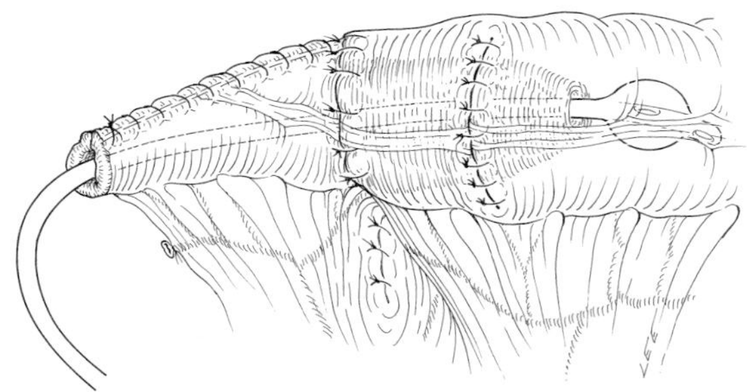

Figure 21.28 Appearance of the afferent limb of the conduit after narrowing.

fashioned, leaving sufficient bulk of subcutaneous fat to maintain its vascularity. This helps to prevent stenosis of the conduit aperture. The catheter and conduit are passed through the abdominal wall without tension. A small 'V'-shaped piece is excised from the conduit wall and the conduit entrance is sutured to the lateral skin flap (Figure 21.30). The arms of the skin flap are then sutured to the conduit entrance, leaving the entrance slightly recessed (Figures 21.31 and 21.32). This provides a good cosmetic appearance, minimizes mucous leakage and allows easy passage of the catheter into the conduit. The abdomen is closed and the catheter firmly sutured to the abdominal wall to prevent it from being dislodged.

Between 7 and 10 days after the operation a gastrografin contrast study is performed via the catheter to check the integrity of the valve and the colonic anastomosis. If there is no leak, irrigation with warm tapwater at approximately 35°C is performed via the catheter. The volumes are gradually increased each day until satisfactory colonic evacuation is achieved. The irrigation solution is delivered via a specialized giving set (Coloplast) that has a controllable valve which allows the rate of fluid

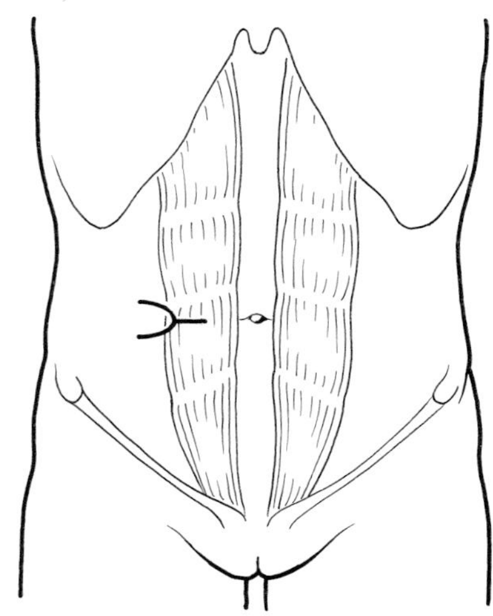

Figure 21.29 Inverted 'wine-glass' shape and positioning of the abdominal wall skin flaps for a transverse colonic conduit.

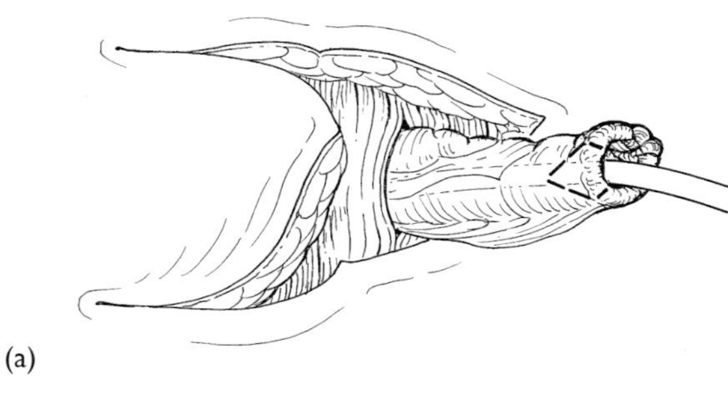

(a)

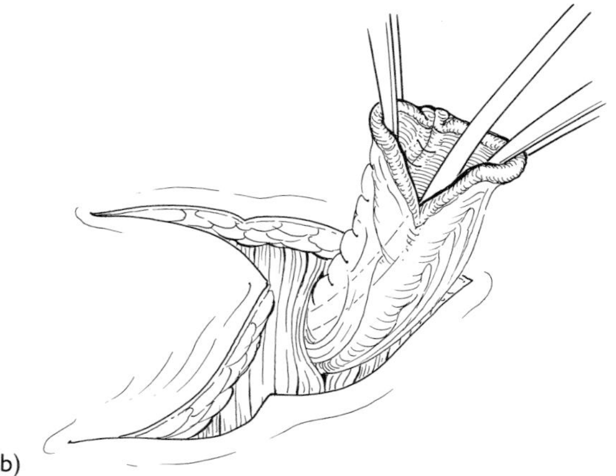

(b)

Figure 21.30a,b Excision of a V-shaped segment from the tip of the afferent limb of the conduit.

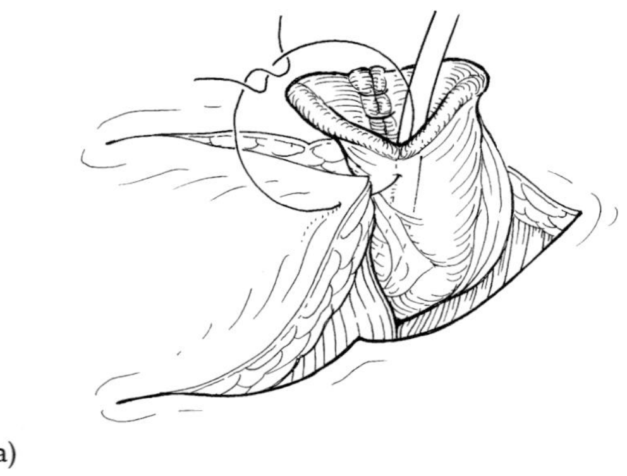

(a)

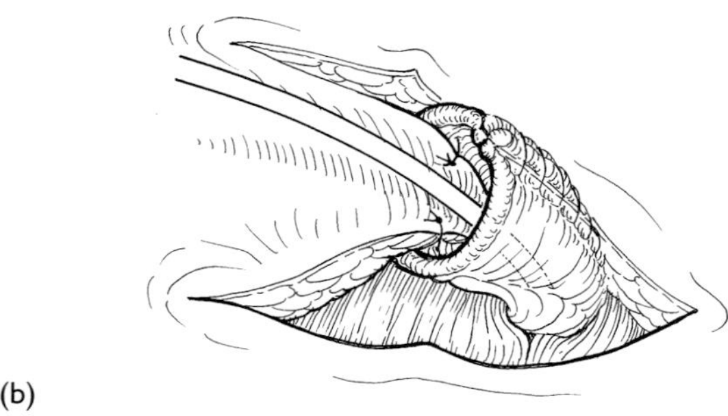

(b)

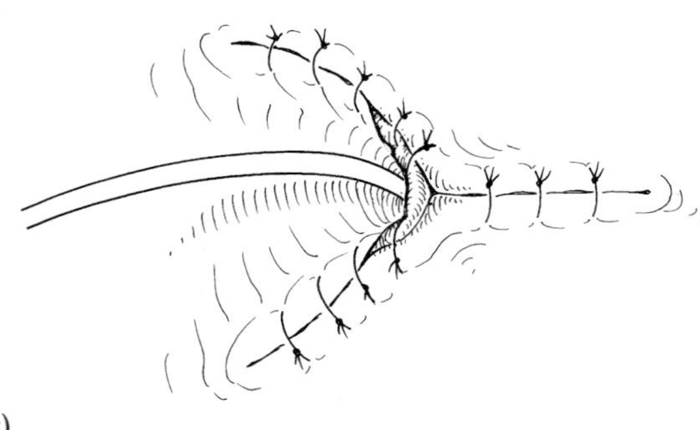

(c)

Figure 21.31a–c Formation of the conduit entrance.

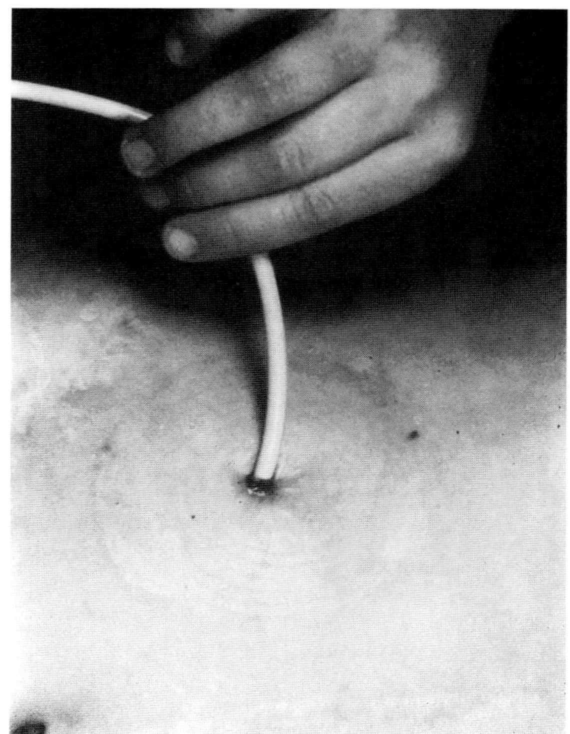

Figure 21.32 Final appearance of the conduit entrance.

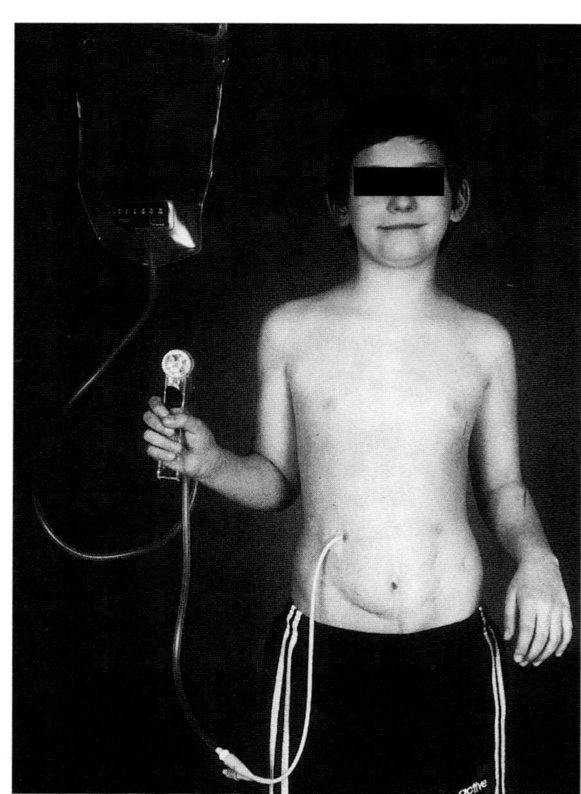

Figure 21.33 A 10-year-old boy with high anorectal atresia and poor function after a previous pull-through procedure treated with a transverse colonic conduit. The irrigation apparatus is shown.

flow into the conduit catheter to be regulated (Figure 21.33). The patient is discharged when able to irrigate alone.

Postoperative course

At home the patient experiments with various irrigation regimens, self-adjusting the volumes and frequency until they have devised a protocol which gives them acceptable evacuation and continence. Most patients use tapwater as the irrigant solution without problems, but others prefer to use a saline solution. Some may need to irrigate more than once daily, and some require the use of a phosphate enema given through the catheter beforehand. Patients are seen for follow-up at approximately 4 weeks. The catheter is removed and the patient taught to self-intubate the conduit with the largest catheter size that easily passes through the valve. If possible, patients use a size 22 catheter, but Foley catheters above 12F seem to suffice equally well.

The catheter is then left out between irrigations. The valve is usually continent to faeces, but may not always be so to flatus, and the stoma may produce a small amount of mucus. To prevent soiling of the clothes and potential social embarrassment, most patients wear a gauze pad or small specially designed 'cap' containing a charcoal filter over the conduit entrance. These lie flush and are not visible under the patient's clothes. Patients are seen regularly in the outpatient clinic and periodically have measurements of blood electrolytes to ensure no biochemical disturbances result from the irrigation.

After a few months, patients are discharged from regular clinic visits, but are given telephone access to members of the department with experience of the technique and to the colorectal nurse specialist, so that they can discuss problems at any time. Regular follow-up questionnaires about their continence and quality of life are sent so that patients' long-term progress can be monitored.

Patients, results and complications

The Cleveland Clinic score was used for the assessment of continence in all patients (Jorge and Wexner, 1993).

Sigmoid conduits

Sigmoid conduits were constructed in 12 women suffering from severe constipation, median age at surgery being 36.5 years (range 26–52). All patients had rectal evacuatory disorders due to paradoxical pelvic floor contraction (anismus) or developing following pelvic or anorectal surgery. In addition, four patients had slow colonic transit demonstrable on marker studies or scintigraphy. In four patients there was significant faecal soiling or incontinence as well as constipation (Table 21.16). In one patient suffering both incontinence and constipation following a haemorrhoidectomy, an electrically stimulated gracilis neosphincter (ESGN) was initially formed. This improved her incontinence, but because of persistent evacuatory problems a sigmoid conduit was subsequently added.

Median follow-up to date is 18 months (range 4–55 months). Eight patients (67%) had their conduits removed. In one patient fat necrosis of the mesentery developed around the conduit valve in the immediate postoperative period. In seven patients rectal evacuation was demonstrable with conduit irrigation, but abdominal bloating and pain, which was present preoperatively, persisted. Despite removing the conduit and performing an ileorectal anastomosis ($n = 4$), all seven patients continued to complain of unremitting abdominal or pelvic pain.

Four patients (33%) retain their conduit, stool frequency increasing from a median of 0.75 per week (range 0.3–7 per week) preoperatively to a median of 7 per week (range 4–14 per week) postoperatively. For patients with incontinence as a feature,

Table 21.16 Aetiology and symptomatology of patients undergoing sigmoid conduit construction.

Patient	*Slow transit*	*Evacuatory disorder after pelvic or anorectal surgery *†*	*Anismus*	*Constipation*	*Combined constipation and incontinence*
1	+	+		+	
2		+	+	+	
3		+			+
4	+		+		+
5		+		+	
6		+		+	
7			+	+	
8			+	+	
9		+	+		+
10	+		+	+	
11		+	+		+
12	+	+	+	+	
Total	4	8	8	8	4

*Hysterectomy, rectopexy or haemorrhoidectomy.
†Some patients developed anismus after pelvic or anorectal surgery.

continence scores improved from a median of 13.6 (range 11–16) preoperatively to a median of 8 (range 4–12) postoperatively. Patients irrigated with a mean of 2 L of warmed tapwater daily, or in one case every 48 hours, the whole process taking less than 10 minutes to complete. Serial monitoring of blood biochemistry showed no abnormalities due to irrigation in either sigmoid or transverse conduit patients.

Transverse conduits

Twenty-seven transverse colonic conduits were constructed in 12 male and 15 female patients. Median age at surgery was 30 years (range 8–74 years). Twenty-four patients had faecal incontinence as their major symptom, two-thirds also sufferred from constipation due to disordered rectal evacuation. Two patients with rectal evacuatory disorders and one patient with slow colonic transit had severe constipation, but no incontinence. The underlying diagnoses are as shown in Table 21.17. Ten patients with high anorectal atresia and one patient with Hirschsprung's disease had pull-through procedures as neonates, but had poor functional results, and one patient had a coloperineal anastomosis and a transverse conduit constructed as the first stage of her planned total anorectal reconstruction following abdominoperineal excision of the rectum.

Fifteen patients had an electrically stimulated gracilis neosphincter (ESGN) constructed in addition to a transverse conduit, in eight of whom the ESGN was performed as the primary incontinence procedure. In two cases the ESGN functioned well until hardware complications developed. In another patient a perineal wound infection caused the sutures anchoring the gracilis muscle to the contralateral ischial tuberosity to become detached. In five patients incontinence improved with dynamic graciloplasty, but the persistence of preoperative evacuatory difficulties necessitated the addition of a conduit. In six patients simultaneous conduit and neosphincter formation were performed.

One patient was lost to review, and follow-up to date or excision of the conduit is a median of 22 months (range 6–48 months). Of the evaluable cases ($n = 26$), all other failures occurred shortly after conduit construction and six conduits (23%) have been excised for a variety of reasons. These included leakage from conduit entrance ($n = 1$), persistent abdominal pain ($n = 2$) and psychological problems ($n = 3$).

Twenty patients (77%), 2 with isolated constipation, 4 with isolated incontinence and 13 with combined symptoms, retain their transverse conduits. For patients with constipation, stool frequency increased from a median of 3 per week (range 1–7 per week) preoperatively to a median of 7 per week at 21 months after the operation ($P = 0.03$: Wilcoxon matched-pairs signed rank test) (Figure 21.34). For patients with faecal incontinence, Cleveland Clinic scores improved from a median of 19 (range 6–20) preoperatively to a median of 7 (range 5–13) at 21 months following the operation ($P = 0.007$: Wilcoxon) (Figure 21.35). Almost all the improvement occurred within the first 3 months ($P = 0.0004$: Wilcoxon) and, despite fluctuations in individual patient scores after this time, statistically significant improvements persisted at all follow-up assessments. Patients irrigate with a mean of 1.2 L (range 0.75–2 L) of warm tapwater a mean of 0.94 times per day (range 0.1–1.6 per day). Eight patients experienced mild abdominal cramps or dizziness when they began irrigation, but this was transient, lasting only 2–3 weeks. The conduits are mostly continent, although there is occasional mucus discharge or flatus incontinence from the conduit entrance in four patients which is managed by the wearing of a small 'cap'. One conduit is persistently incontinent of liquid faeces and the patient is awaiting revision.

A subgroup of 10 patients were prospectively

Table 21.17 Underlying aetiology in transverse colonic conduit patients.

Aetiology	*Constipated*	*Incontinent*	*Combined constipation and incontinence*
High anorectal atresia		4	6
Hirschsprung's disease			1
Williams–Noonan syndrome			1
Pelvic fracture		2	2
Slow transit	1		
Posthysterectomy or rectopexy	1	1	3
Obstetric trauma			3
Anismus postspinal injury	1		
Abdominal perineal excision of the rectum		1	
Total	3	8	16

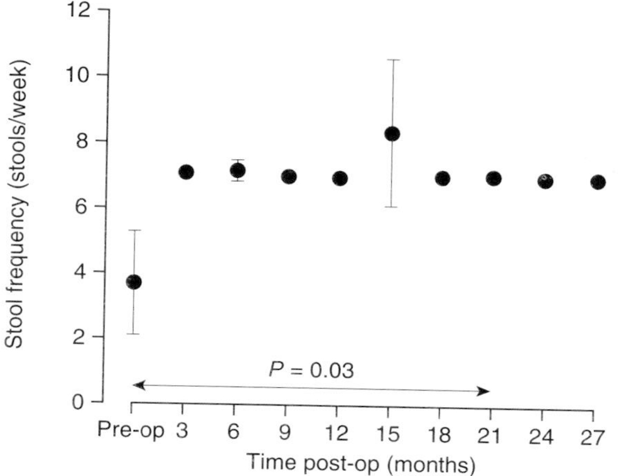

Figure 21.34 The effect of the transverse colonic conduit upon stool frequency in constipated patients and patients with combined constipation and incontinence. *P* value: Wilcoxon matched-pairs signed rank test.

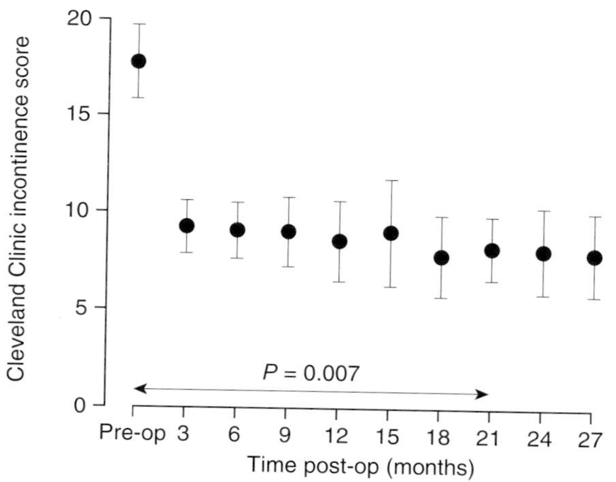

Figure 21.35 The effect of the transverse colonic conduit upon continence scores in patients with faecal incontinence and combined incontinence and constipation. *P* value: Wilcoxon matched-pairs signed rank test.

evaluated as to the effects of the transverse conduit on their quality of life. Assessments were made using the Nottingham Health Profile (Hunt et al, 1981, 1985), and Hospital Anxiety and Depression Scale (Snaith and Zigmond, 1983). Although not statistically significant because of small numbers, there were trends towards increased energy and decreased social isolation. Patients were also assessed with a direct questioning of objective scoring system (The Royal London Hospital (RLH) Score) in which patients self-select five areas of their life that they consider to be particularly affected by their bowel problems. Each dimension is marked on a visual linear analogue scale from 1 to 10 according to severity and a total out of 50 is derived (50 = profound effect; 0 = no effect). The RLH score showed a marked improvement in most cases, patients being more confident and having greater self-esteem. A repeated theme throughout was that patients found they were able to participate in physical sports such as swimming, and that they could travel on public transport or spend whole days without the constant fear of incontinence.

Other techniques of ACE

Other attempts have been made to produce a continent catheterizable conduit into the caecum so as to achieve distal colonic irrigation. Kiely et al (1994) described a tubularized distally based caecal or colonic flap. The flap was tubularized with a two-layered closure over an 8F silicone tube. The caecum was re-approximated with a two-layered closure and imbricated around the tubularized caecal flap. This technique was used in four children, two of whom developed stomal stenosis. Sheldon et al (1997) reported on the ACE in ten patients with faecal incontinence due to severe congenital malformation. Eight of these patients had a tubularized segment of ileum constructed to form the conduit, the remaining two had a Malone appendicostomy. Six achieved complete continence and four continued to soil occasionally. Pseudomembranous colitis occurred in one patient and persistent ileus in two.

Marsh and Kiff (1996) described using the ileocaecal segment as a conduit, the ileocaecal valve theoretically providing continence (Figure 21.36). A

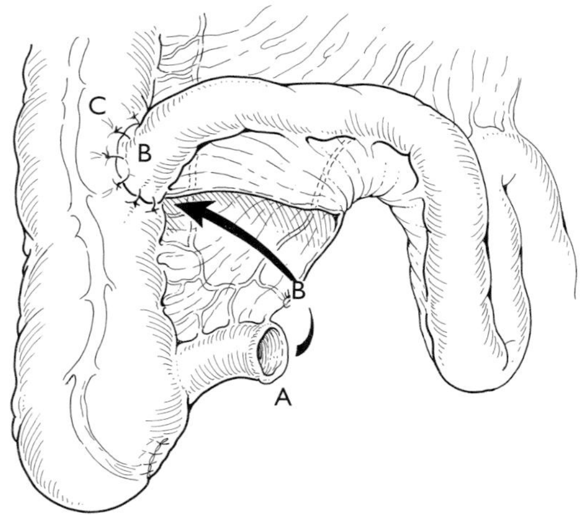

Figure 21.36 Ileocaecostomy. The proximal terminal ileum (B) is anastomosed to the ascending colon (C). The distal terminal ileum (A) is exteriorized as the ileocaecostomy.

right iliac fossa grid iron incision was made and the caecum, appendix and terminal ileum were delivered into the wound. Appendicectomy was performed. The terminal ileum was divided between clamps 5–7 cm proximal to the ileocaecal junction, and intestinal continuity was restored with an ileocolic anastomosis. The distal terminal ileum was delivered via a separate stab incision through the lower abdominal wall as an ileocaecostomy. An antimesenteric full-thickness V-shaped segment was excised from the terminal ileum before mucocutaneous suture to give the ileocaecostomy entrance a smaller diameter.

The theoretical risk of an incompetent ileocaecal valve may allow reflux from the valve, and the removal of the ileocaecal valve from the circuit may exacerbate incontinence if used for its treatment. Nevertheless, Marsh and Kiff (1996) used this technique in seven patients and only one patient experienced significant leakage after irrigation. However, the length of follow-up was not specified.

Shandling et al (1996) have piloted the use of a percutaneously inserted caecostomy tube with a retention loop. The tube was placed using local anaesthetic under X-ray and ultrasound screening. They have now treated more than five patients, claiming resolution of soiling in all (Chait et al, 1996, 1997). Their technique has now been adopted using a gastrostomy button (Mickey-Medical Innovations, Draper, Utah, USA) or Carpak button (Wheeling, Illinois, USA) or a specially designed low-profile 'trapdoor' catheter (Cook, Illinois) in place of the caecostomy tube. The trapdoor catheter has a coiling mechanism retaining it in the caecum. It is also flexibly extendable so that it will traverse an abdominal wall of any thickness.

Kalidasan et al (1997) operated on seven children using a button. In their series, the caecum was exposed through a Lanz incision in the right iliac fossa and mobilized as necessary. The button caecostomy device was inserted and exteriorized through the Lanz incision. Similarly Fukunaga et al (1996) used a Bard gastrostomy button (Bard International Products, Tewksburg, MA, USA) in a similar way in two children and one adult. The vogue now is to use the percutaneous techique. However, in each of these reports, follow-up has been short, and such a technique in adults is not, in our opinion, a long-term solution.

Conclusions

Our experience with the transverse colonic conduit for incontinence when associated with a rectal evacuatory disorder is encouraging with overall 20 of 26 (77%) of conduits remaining *in situ* and benefiting patients in terms of improved continence scores and quality of life. Some of these patients also have an electrically stimulated gracilis neosphincter and the relative benefit of each procedure is difficult to discern; suffice it to say that the combination of techniques seems to be particularly effective.

For patients with a rectal evacuation disorder alone, we would no longer recommend the placement of the conduit in the sigmoid colon; the optimal site is the transverse colon. However, even when the conduit is constructed at this site, the procedure is less successful when performed for constipation alone. In such patients, only 7 of 15 cases (46%) still have their conduits in place. While it is true that some were removed for postoperative morbidity, most were removed because of failure to improve symptoms. All these patients were women with persistent abdominal pain and bloating or rectal and perineal pain, which was not improved by the surgery. Despite excision of the conduit and formation of a stoma, these symptoms persisted.

Our own results in patients with constipation seem less favourable than some published series of ACE techniques. However, most of these studies included predominantly children. Our experience is similar to the other few series which consist primarily of adult patients. Thus, Lehur et al (1997) reported the outcome in 12 patients with slow colonic transit, seven of whom had concomitant faecal incontinence. Constipation was improved in 80% of patients retaining their appendicostomy or caecal tube, and faecal incontinence was improved in all. Two patients had stoma formation, but symptoms of abdominal pain and bloating only improved in 55% of patients. These results underline the importance of careful selection of constipated patients for operative intervention. Some of these patients have autonomic neuropathy and abnormal motility affecting the small bowel or other regions of the gastrointestinal tract. It is wise to perform oesophageal and small bowel motility studies routinely before contemplating surgery. Other patients seem to have marked psychological and emotional problems, and these patients should be identified before surgery, preferably with the help of a psychologist.

All the operative procedures described for ACE, apart from the 'gastrostomy button techniques', have one predominant complication, namely stomal stenosis resulting in difficulty in intubation (Table 21.18).

Stenosis rates range between 0 and 50%, but in the larger series with longer follow-up the range seems

Table 21.18 Stomal complications in published series of operative ACE procedures.

Reference	*n*	*ACE procedure*	*Intubation difficulty or stomal stenosis*	*Treatment*
Malone et al (1990)*	5	A	1 (20)	Dilatation
Wheeler and Malone (1991)*	13	A	1 (8)	Revision
Squire et al (1993)†	25	A, B, C, D	5 (20)	Dilatation 3 Revision 2
Borzi and Gough (1993)	2	L	0	
Williams et al (1994)	10	E	1 (10)	Revision
Kiely et al (1994)†	6	C	2 (33)	Revision
Hill et al (1994)	6	B, C, J	3 (50)	Revision
Griffiths and Malone (1995)*	21	A, B, C	5 (21)	Dilatation
Roberts et al (1995)*	8	A, C	3 (38)	Dilatation 2 Revision 1
Kiely et al (1995)†	27	B, C	6 (22)	Dilatation or revision
Toogood et al (1995)	10	A, C	4 (40)	Dilatation
Koyle et al (1995)§	22	A, B, C, G	3 (15)	Revision
Hughes and Williams (1995b)	9	F	0	
Stock and Hanna (1996)	4	B	0	
Dick et al (1996)	13	B, C	13 (38)	Revision
Ellsworth et al (1996)#	18	A, B, C, D	5 (28)	Dilatation 3 Revision 2
Marsh and Kiff (1996)	7	H	0	
Waxman et al (1996)§	23	A, B, C, D, G, I, J	3 (13)	Unknown
Yamamoto et al (1996)	2	B, C	0	
Mor et al (1997)	18	A, B, C, D	7 (39)	Catheter-in-situ 3 Revision 2
Teichman et al (1997)	2	B	0	
Webb et al (1997)#	10	B, J	0	
Goepel et al (1997)	10	K	0	
Gerharz et al (1997)	1	K	0	
Lehur et al (1997)	12	A, B, C	Unknown	
Sheldon et al (1997)	10	A, D	0	

A, Reversed appendicostomy; B, orthotopic appendicostomy; C, tubularized caecal or colonic flap; D, tubularized ileal flap; E, sigmoid colonic conduit; F, transverse colonic conduit; G, ureter; H, ileocaecostomy, I, tube or button caecostomy; J, laparoscopic orthotopic appendicostomy; K, reversed, orthotopic Mainz type appendicostomy; L, pedicled gastric tube.

Values in parentheses are percentages.

* † # § May be duplication of some patients across studies.

to be between 10% and 40%. This complication is a particular problem with the reversed appendicostomy and tubularized ileal flap, perhaps because their vascularity is the most compromised. When stenosis does occur after the appendicostomy procedure, it usually requires intermittent dilatation under anaesthetic or revisional surgery. For some patients this is the reason for failure to use the ACE and their conversion to a stoma. For others, construction of a new ACE is necessary. Entrance stenosis has occurred in only two patients with a colonic conduit (5%), but it has not been a major problem and has not been the cause of long-term failure.

With all these procedures, a proportion of patients may have some reflux of faeces, liquid stool or flatus onto the abdominal wall. There is no method which entirely guarantees against this, although we would maintain that a colonic conduit is superior in this regard to a caecal, ileal or colonic flap. If reflux remains a particular problem, a balloon catheter or gastrostomy button can be placed through the irrigant channel and drawn backwards against the continence mechanism. The catheter can then be left indwelling.

There might also be a small amount of mucous discharge from the conduit aperture. This can usually be managed by wearing a purpose-designed 'cap'. This cannot be seen under the clothes and has a charcoal filter that has the added benefit of neutralizing any odour should there be retrograde leakage of faeces or flatus.

In many reports, phosphate enemas, either alone or in combination, are used for irrigation purposes, and these may cause abdominal colic. Hyperphosphataemia and other metabolic disturbances are other potential problems. As a result we have advised the use of normal warmed tapwater for the irrigation. It is generally sufficient, and biochemical monitoring has failed to show any deleterious effect (Williams et al, 1994). Some patients do require phosphate enemas which are diluted and given mixed with or before the tapwater irrigation. Because of toxicity, we advise that phosphate enema administration should not be repeated until evacuation has occurred.

Antegrade colonic irrigation, although not problem-free, is successful in treating faecal incontinence and constipation. The technique is particularly useful for combined constipation and faecal incontinence as the mechanical effect of achieving a completely clean colon and rectum addresses both these problems. Antegrade colonic irrigation is far superior to retrograde enemas. It is more effective with fewer accidents, it is aesthetically more pleasing because there is less mess and the entire procedure can be performed with greater independence on the part of the patient. Wearing pads can be reduced and frequently abandoned.

Of the techniques available, we would favour the transverse colonic conduit as achieving all the aims of the procedure in the adult patient. Whereas an appendicostomy can be very successful in a child, it is usually of insufficient calibre to allow the intubation of the colon by a catheter of sufficient diameter to produce adequate flow rates for the irrigant in adult patients. In addition, the appendix is often absent or obliterated in the adult, and stenosis of the aperture on the abdominal wall is a frequent complication. It should also be remembered that children will eventually grow into adults, and we are already having to convert some older teenagers from an appendicostomy to a colonic conduit. Ileal and caecal flaps are also prone to stenosis of the aperture, and one suspects that reflux is a more common problem, as there is no mechanism to prevent it.

The method of ileocaecostomy described by Marsh and Kiff (1996), which uses the ileocaecal valve as a continence mechanism, has superficial attractions. However, we have certain reservations about this technique. First, not all ileocaecal valves are continent. In addition, removal of the ileocaecal valve from the circuit means there is no immediate barrier to the reflux of irrigant fluid into the terminal ileum. This is known to cause abdominal cramps and pain and may increase the chances of the rapid absorption of any enema fluid and development of toxic side-effects such as phosphate poisoning. Although Marsh and Kiff did not use it for incontinence, if used for this purpose, the incontinence may be exacerbated because intestinal transit will be hastened due to the absence of the ileocaecal valve. For one patient in whom we revised a conduit to an ileocaecostomy, we certainly found that incontinence has become worse: he has to irrigate at least three times daily to remain clean.

The use of a percutaneously inserted caecostomy tube also has certain superficial attractions. The procedure can be done under local anaesthetic with X-ray guidance and ultrasound screening. However, complications, including abdominal wall cellulitis, tube placement in the terminal ileum, tube dislodgement and prolonged ileus may all occur (Shandling et al, 1996; Chait et al, 1996, 1997; Fukunaga et al, 1996; Kalidasan et al, 1997). The technique as yet has not been performed in adults, and the concern must be that leaving a foreign body implanted in the colon for a long period will lead to erosion and other septic problems. Nevertheless, it may be useful as an initial procedure to select which patients may benefit in the long term from a colonic conduit.

A colonic conduit procedure can dramatically improve the quality of life of some patients with severe constipation, particularly when associated with incontinence. It also has a role to play in patients with incontinence either alone or together with a neosphincter. For those patients with slow transit constipation plus or minus a rectal evacuation disorder or those with a rectal evacuation disorder alone, great care must be exercised in selection. Patients must realize that their symptoms of abdominal pain and bloating may not be improved, despite their frequency in bowel action being increased. Nevertheless, with these provisos, the technique can be beneficial even in this group of patients, and has the advantage of not precluding the formation of a stoma or a colectomy and ileorectal anastomosis at a later date.

REFERENCES

Agachan F, Chen T, Pfeifer J, Reissman P & Wexner SD (1996) A constipation scoring system to simplify evaluation and management of constipated patients. *Dis Colon Rectum* **39**: 681–685.

Akervall S, Fasth S, Nordgren S, Oresland T & Hulten L (1988) The functional results after colectomy and ileorectal anastomosis for severe constipation (Arbuthnot Lane's disease) as related to rectal sensory function. *Int J Colorectal Dis* **3**: 96–101.

Alstrup N, Ronholt C, Fu C, Rasmussen O, Sorensen M &

Christiansen J (1997) Viscous fluid expulsion in the evaluation of the constipated patient. *Dis Colon Rectum* **40**: 580–583.

Altomare D, Pilot M-A, Scott M et al (1992) Detection of subclinical autonomic neuropathy in constipated patients using a sweat test. *Gut* **33**: 1539–1543.

Arbuthnot-Lane WA (1908) The operative treatment of chronic constipation. *BMJ (Clin Res)* **I**: 126–130.

Arhan P, Devroede G, Jehannin B et al (1981) Segmental colonic transit time. *Dis Colon Rectum* **24**: 625–629.

Ashraf W, Park F, Lof J & Quigley EMM (1995) Effects of psyllium therapy on stool characteristics, colon transit and anorectal function in chronic idiopathic constipation. *Aliment Pharmacol Ther* **9**: 639–647.

Badiali D, Marcheggiano A, Pallone F et al (1985) Melanosis of the rectum in patients with chronic constipation. *Dis Colon Rectum* **28**: 241–245.

Bain I & Keighley MRB (1999) The long term results of pouch surgery for constipation. (in press).

Bakwin H & Davidson M (1971) Constipation in twins. *Am J Dis Child* **121**: 179–181.

Bannister JJ, Timms JM, Barfield LJ, Donnelly TC & Read NW (1986) Physiological studies in young women with chronic constipation. *Int J Colorectal Dis* **1**: 175–182.

Bannister JJ, Lawrence WT, Smith A, Thomas DG & Read NW (1988) Urological abnormalities in young women with severe constipation. *Gut* **29**: 17–20.

Barnes PRH & Lennard-Jones JE (1985) Balloon expulsion from the rectum in constipation of different types. *Gut* **26**: 1049–1052.

Barnes PRH & Lennard-Jones JE (1988) Function of the striated anal sphincter during straining in control subjects and constipated patients with a radiologically normal rectum or idiopathic megacolon. *Int J Colorectal Dis* **3**: 207–209.

Barnes PRH, Hawley PR, Preston DM & Lennard-Jones JE (1985) Experience of posterior division of the puborectalis muscle in the management of chronic constipation. *Br J Surg* **72**: 475–477.

Bartolo, DCC, Roe AM, Virjee J & Mortensen NJMcC (1985) Evacuation proctography in obstructed defaecation and rectal intussusception. *Br J Surg* (Suppl) **72**: S111–S116.

Bartolo DCC, Roe AM, Virjee J, Mortensen NJMcC & Locke-Edmunds JC (1988) An analysis of rectal morphology in obstructed defaecation. *Int J Colorectal Dis* **3**: 17–22.

Bassotti G, Gaburri M, Imbimbo BP et al (1988) Colonic mass movements in idiopathic chronic constipation. *Gut* **29**: 1173–1179.

Bassotti G, Crowell MD & Whitehead WE (1993) Contractile activity of the human colon: lessons from 24 hour studies. *Gut* **34**: 129–133.

Bateman DN & Smith JM (1988) A policy for laxatives. *BMJ* **297**: 1420–1421.

Battle WM, Snape WJ Jr, Alavi A, Cohen S & Braunstein S (1989) Colonic dysfunction in diabetes mellitus. *Gastroenterology* **79**: 1217–1221.

Belliveau P, Goldberg SM, Rothenberger DA & Nivatvongs S (1982) Idiopathic acquired megacolon: the value of subtotal colectomy. *Dis Colon Rectum* **25**: 118–121.

Bentley JFR (1966) Posterior excisional anorectal myotomy in management of chronic faecal accumulation. *Arch Dis Child* **41**: 144–147.

Berman IR, Manning DH & Harris MS (1990) Streamlining the management of defecation disorders. *Dis Colon Rectum* **33**: 778–785.

Binder HJ (1977) Pharmacology of laxatives. *Ann Rev Pharmacol Toxicol* **17**: 355–367.

Bjelke E (1974) Epidemiologic studies of cancer of the stomach, colon and rectum. *Scand J Gastroenterol* **9** (Suppl): 31.

Block IR (1986) Transrectal repair of rectocele using obliterative suture. *Dis Colon Rectum* **29**: 707–711.

Borzi P & Gough DC (1993) Pedicled gastric tube as a catheterising conduit. *Eur Urol* **24**; 103–105.

Bremmer S, Ahlback S-O, Uden R & Mellgren A (1995) Simultaneous defecography and peritoneography in defecation disorders. *Dis Colon Rectum* **38**: 969–973.

Broden G, Dolk A & Holmstrom B (1988) Evacuation difficulties and other characteristics of rectal function associated with procidentia and the Ripstein operation. *Dis Colon Rectum* **31**: 283–286.

Brodribb AJM (1977) Treatment of symptomatic diverticular disease with a high fibre diet. *Lancet* **i**: 664.

Broens PMA, Penninckx FM, Lestar B & Kerremans RP (1994) The trigger for rectal filling sensation. *Int J Colorectal Dis* **9**: 1–4.

Buchmann P, Bruhin R, Sartoretti Ch & De Lorenzi D (1997) Sphincteropexy: a new operation to cure outlet obstruction in adults. *Dig Surg* **14**: 413–418.

Bueno L, Fioramonti J, Ruckesbusch Y et al (1980) Evaluation of colonic myelectric activity in health and functional disorders. *Gut* **21**: 480–485.

Calam J, Unwin RJ & Peart WS (1983) Neurotensin stimulates defaecation in man. *Lancet* **i**: 737–738.

Celik AF, Tomlin J & Read NW (1994) The effect of oral vancomycin on chronic idiopathic constipation. *Aliment Pharmacol Ther* **9**: 63–68.

Celik AF, Katsinelos P, Read NW, Khan MI & Donnelly TC (1995) Hereditary proctalgia fugax and constipation: report of a second family. *Gut* **36**: 581–584.

Chait PG, Connoly BL, Shandling B et al (1996) Percutaneous cecostomy and low profile button placement in the treatment of children with fecal incontinence. *Radiology* **201**: 1005.

Chait PG, Shandling B, Richards HM et al (1997) Fecal incontinence in children: treatment with percutaneous cecostomy tube placement – a prospective study. *Radiology* **203**: 621–624.

Choudhoury AR, Dinoso VP & Lorber SH (1976) Characterization of a hyperactive segment at the rectosigmoid junction. *Gastroenterology* **71**: 584–588.

Clayden GS & Lawson JON (1976) Investigation and management of longstanding chronic constipation in childhood. *Arch Dis Child* **51**: 918–923.

Colon AR & Jacob LH (1977) Defecation patterns in American infants and children. *Clin Pediatr (Philadelphia)* **16**: 999–1000.

Connell AM, Frankel H & Guttmann L (1963) The motility of the pelvic colon following complete lesions of the spinal cord. *Paraplegia* **1**: 98–115.

Connell AM, Hilton C, Irvine G, Lennard-Jones JE & Misiewicz JJ (1965) Variation of bowel habit in two population samples. *BMJ* **2**: 1095–1099.

Cooke WT (1977) Laxative abuse. *Clin Gastroenterol* **6**: 659–673.

Cummings JH, Jenkins DJA & Wiggins HS (1976) Measurement of the mean transit time of dietary residue through the human gut. *Gut* **17**: 210–218.

Cummings JH, Southgate DAT, Branch W, Houston H, Jenkins DJA & James WPT (1978) Colonic response to dietary fibre from carrot, cabbage, apple, bran and guar gum. *Lancet* **i**: 5–8.

Dalby SW (1894) Opening the caecum for intestinal obstruction (Report of the Medical Society of London). *BMJ* (17 November): 112.

De Graaf EJR, Gilberts ECAM & Schouten WR (1996) Role of segmental colonic transit time studies to select patients with slow transit constipation for partial left-sided or subtotal colectomy. *Br J Surg* **83**: 648–651.

Degen LP & Phillips SF (1996) How well does stool form reflect colonic transit? *Gut* **39**: 109–113.

Delemarre JBVM, Kruyt RH, Doornbos J et al (1994) Anterior rectocele: assessment with radiographic defecography, dynamic magnetic resonance imaging, and physical examination. *Dis Colon Rectum* **37**: 249–259.

Devroede G (1975) Roving critic. In Reilly RW & Kirsner JB (eds) *Fiber Deficiency and Colonic Disorders*, pp 120–123. New York: Plenum Press.

Devroede G, Arhan P, Duguay C et al (1979) Traumatic constipation. *Gastroenterology* **77**: 1258–1267.

Dick AC, McCallion WA, Brown S et al (1996) Antegrade colonic enemas. *Br J Surg* **83**: 642–643.

Dolk A, Broden G, Holmstrom B, Johansson C & Schultzberg M (1990a) Slow transit chronic constipation (Arbuthnot Lane's disease). An immunohistochemical study of neuropeptide-containing nerves in resected specimens from the large bowel. *Int J Colorectal Dis* **5**: 181–187.

Dolk A, Broden G, Holmstrom B, Johansson C & Nilsson BY (1990b) Slow transit of the colon associated with severe constipation after the Ripstein operation: a clinical and physiologic study. *Dis Colon Rectum* **33**: 786–790.

Ducrotte P, Rodomanski B, Weber J et al (1986) Colonic transit time of radiopaque markers and rectoanal manometry in patients complaining of constipation. *Dis Colon Rectum* **29**: 630–634.

Earlam R (1985) A vascular cause for Hirschsprung's disease. *Gastroenterology* **88**: 1274–1279.

Eaton-Smith AN, Bendall MJ & Kent F (1974) A new technique for measuring the consistency of faeces: a report on its application to the assessment of Senokot therapy in the elderly. *Age Ageing* **4**: 58–62.

Edwards DAW & Beck ER (1971) Movement of radiopacified feces during defecation. *Am J Dig Dis* **16**: 709–711.

Ellsworth PI, Webb HW, Crump JM et al (1996) The Malone antegrade colonic enema enhances the quality of life in children undergoing urological incontinence procedures. *J Urol* **4**: 1416–1418.

Engel AF & Kamm MA (1994) The acute effect of straining on pelvic floor neurological function. *Int J Colorectal Dis* **9**: 8–12.

Etzioni A, Benderly A & Bar-Maor JA (1980) Segmental dilatation of the colon, another cause of chronic constipation. *Dis Colon Rectum* **23**: 580–582.

Farag A, Gadallah NA & El-Shereif EMBM (1993) Obturator internus muscle autotransplantation: a new concept for the treatment of obstructive constipation. *Eur Surg Res* **25**: 341–347.

Faulk DL, Anuras S, Gardner GD, Mitros FA, Summers RWW & Christensen J (1978) A familial visceral myopathy. *Ann Intern Med* **89**: 600–606.

Ferrara A, Pemberton JH, Grotz RL & Hanson RB (1994) Prolonged ambulatory recording of anorectal motility in patients with slow-transit constipation. *Am J Surg* **67**: 73–79.

Ferri GL, Adrian TE, Allen JM et al (1988) Intramural distribution of regulatory peptides in the sigmoid-recto-anal region of the human gut. *Gut* **29**: 762–768.

Fisher SE, Breckon K, Andrews HA & Keighley MRB (1988) Psychiatric screening for patients with faecal incontinence or chronic constipation referred for surgical treatment. *Br J Surg* **76**: 352–355.

Fleshman JW, Dreznik Z, Meyer K, Fry RD, Carney R & Kodner IJ (1992) Outpatient protocol for biofeedback therapy of pelvic floor outlet obstruction. *Dis Colon Rectum* **35**: 1–7.

Ford MJ, Camilleri M, Joyner MJ & Hanson RB (1996) Autonomic control of colonic tone and the cold pressor test. *Gut* **39**: 125–129.

Freeman NV (1984) Intractable constipation in children treated by forceful anal stretch or anorectal myectomy: preliminary communication. *J R Soc Med* **77** (Suppl 3): 6–8.

Frieri G, Parisi F, Corazziari E & Caprilli R (1983) Colonic electromyography in chronic constipation. *Gastroenterology* **84**: 737–740.

Fukai K & Fukuda H (1985) Nerves in the colon: discovery and rediscovery. *Gastroenterology* **89**: 222–223.

Fukunaga K, Kimura K, Lawrence JP, Soper RT & Phearman LA (1996) Button device for antegrade enema in the treatment of incontinence and constipation. *J Paediatr Surg* **31**: 1038–1039.

Furness JB & Costa M (1980) Types of nerves in the enteric nervous system. *Neuroscience* **5**: 1–20.

Furness JB & Costa M (1987) *The Enteric Nervous System*. Edinburgh: Churchill Livingstone.

Gasslander T, Larsson J & Wetterfors J (1987) Experience of surgical treatment of chronic idiopathic constipation. *Acta Chir Scand* **153**: 553–555.

Gattuso JM & Kamm MA (1993) Review article: the management of constipation in adults. *Aliment Pharmacol Ther* **7**: 487–500.

Gekas P & Schuster MH (1981) Stercoral perforation of the colon: case report and review of the literature. *Gastroenterology* **80**: 1054–1058.

Ger G-C, Wexner SD, Jorge MN & Salanga VD (1993) Anorectal manometry in the diagnosis of paradoxical puborectalis syndrome. *Dis Colon Rectum* **36**: 816–825.

Gerharz EW, Vik V, Webb G et al (1997) The in situ appendix in the Malone antegrade continence enema procedure for faecal incontinence. *br J Urol* **79**: 985–986.

Gilliland R, Heymen S, Altomare DF, Park UC, Vickers D & Wexner SD (1997) Outcome and predictors of success of biofeedback for constipation. *Br J Surg* **84**: 1123–1126.

Gilmore IT (1990) Orocaecal transit time in health and disease. *Gut* **31**: 250–251.

Glia A, Gylin M, Gullberg K & Lindberg G (1997) Biofeedback retraining in patients with functional constipation and paradoxical puborectalis contraction. *Dis Colon Rectum* **40**: 889–895.

Glick ME, Meshkinpour H, Haldeman S, Bhatia NN & Bradley WE (1982) Colonic dysfunction in multiple sclerosis. *Gastroenterology* **83**: 1002–1007.

Glober GA, Nomura A, Kamiyama S, Shimada A & Abba BC (1977) Bowel transit time and stool weight in populations with different colon-cancer risks. *Lancet* **ii**: 110–111.

Goepel M, Sperling H, Stöhrer M et al (1997) Management of neurogenic fecal incontinence in myelodysplastic children by a modified continent appendiceal stoma and antegrade colonic enema. *Urology* **49**: 758–761.

Goligher JC (1984) In *Diseases of the Anus, Colon and Rectum*, 5th edn. London: Baillière Tindall.

Gorard DA, Libby GW & Farthing MJG (1994) Influence of antidepressants on whole gut and orocaecal transit times in health and irritable bowel syndrome. *Aliment Pharmacol Ther* **8**: 159–166.

Gorard DA, Gomborone JE, Libby GW & Farthing MJG (1996) Intestinal transit in anxiety and depression. *Gut* **39**: 551–555.

Gottlieb SH & Schuster M (1986) Dermatolglyphic (fingerprint) evidence for a congenital syndrome of early onset constipation and abdominal pain. *Gastroenterology* **91**: 428–432.

Griffiths DM & Malone (1995) The Malone antegrade continence enema. *J Pediatr Surg* **30**: 68–71.

Grotz RL, Pemberton JH, Levin KE, Bell AM & Hanson RB (1993) Rectal wall contractility in healthy subjects and in patients with chronic severe constipation. *Ann Surg* **218**: 761–768.

Haddad H & Devroede-Bertrand G (1981) Large bowel motility disorders. *Med Clin North Am* **65**: 1377–1396.

Hallan RI, Melling J, Womack NR, Williams NS, Waldron DJ & Morrison JFB (1988) Treatment of anismus in intractable constipation with botulinum A toxin. *Lancet* **ii**: 714–717.

Halligan S & Bartram CI (1995) Is barium trapping in rectoceles significant? *Dis Colon Rectum* **38**: 764–768.

Halligan S, McGee S & Bartram CI (1994) Quantification of evacuation proctography. *Dis Colon Rectum* **37**: 1151–1154.

Halligan S, Thomas J & Bartram C (1995) Intrarectal pressures and balloon expulsion related to evacuation proctography. *Gut* **37**: 100–104.

Hancock BD (1976) Measurement of anal pressure and motility. *Gut* **17**: 645–657.

Harvey RF, Pomare EW & Heaton K (1973) Effects of increased dietary fibre on intestinal transit. *Lancet* **i**: 1278–1280.

Hasegawa H, Fatah C, Radley S & Keighley MRB (1999) Long term results of colorectal resection for chronic constipation. To be published in Vol 3, 1999, *Colorectal Disease*.

Heij HA, Morrman-Voestermans CGM, Vos A & Kneepkens CMF (1990) Triad of anorectal stenosis, sacral anomaly and presacral mass: a remediable cause of severe constipation. *Br J Surg* **77**: 102–104.

Healy JC, Halligan S, Reznek RH et al (1997) Magnetic resonance imaging of the pelvic foor in patients with obstructed defaecation. *Br J Surg* **84**: 1555–1558.

Henry MM (1989) Surgery for constipation. *BMJ* **298**: 346.

Heymen S, Wexner SD & Gulledge AD (1993) MMPI assessment of patients with functional bowel disorders. *Dis Colon Rectum* **36**: 593–596.

Higginson J (1966) Etiological factors in gastrointestinal cancer in man. *J Natl Cancer Inst* **37**: 527–545.

Hill J, Stott S & MacLennan I (1994) Antegrade enemas for the treatment of severe idiopathic constipation. *Br J Surg* **81**: 1490–1491.

Hinton JM & Lennard-Jones JE (1968) Constipation: definition and classification. *Postgrad Med J* **44**: 720–723.

Hinton JM, Lennard-Jones JE & Young AC (1969) A new method for studying gut transit times using radio-opaque markers. *Gut* **10**: 842–847.

Holstock DJ, Misiewicz JJ, Smith T & Rowlands EN (1970) Propulsion mass movements in the human colon and its relationship to meals and somatic activity. *Gut* **11**: 91–99.

Hosie K, Kmiot W & Keighley MRB (1990) Functional bowel disorders: further indications for restorative proctocolectomy. Paper presented at the British Society of Gastroenterology, Dublin Meeting, 1989, p 47.

Howard ER (1984) Muscle innervation of the gut: structure and pathology. *J R Soc Med* **77**: 905.

Howard ER, Garrett JR & Kidd A (1984) Constipation and congenital disorders of the myenteric plexus. *J R Soc Med* **77** (Suppl 3): 13–19.

Hughes SF & Williams NS (1995a) Continent colonic conduit for the treatment of faecal incontinence associated with disordered evacuation. *Br J Surg* **82**: 1318–1320.

Hughes SF & Williams NS (1995b) Antegrade enemas for the treatment of severe idiopathic constipation (Letter; comment). *Br J Surg* **82**: 567.

Hughes ES, McDermott FT, Johnson WR & Polglase AL (1981) Surgery for constipation. *Aust N Z J Surg* **51**: 144–148.

Hunt SM, McKenna SP, McEwen J, Williams J & Papp E (1981) The Nottingham Health Profile: Subjective health status and medical consultations. *Soc Sci Med* **15A**: 221–229.

Hunt SM, McEwan J & McKenna SP (1985) Measuring health status: a new tool for clinicians and epidemiologists. *J Roy Coll of General Practitioners* **35**: 185–189.

Hutchinson Jnr (1905) The value of the vermiform appendix in the treatment of ulcerative and membranous colitis. *BMJ* (13 May): 1039.

Hutchinson R, Mostafa AB, Grant EA et al (1993) Scintigraphic defecography: quantitative and dynamic assessment of anorectal function. *Dis Colon Rectum* **36**: 1132–1138.

Hutchinson R, Notghi A, Smith NB, Harding LK & Kumar D (1995) Scintigraphic measurement of ileocaecal transit in irritable bowel syndrome and chronic idiopathic constipation. *Gut* **36**: 585–589.

Huttenen R, Heikkinen E & Larmi TK (1975) Stercoraceous and idiopathic perforations of the colon. *Surg Gynecol Obstet* **140**: 756–760.

Ihre T (1974) Studies on anal function in continent and incontinent patients. *Scand J Gastroenterol* **9** (Suppl 25): 1–64.

Infantino A, Masin A, Melega E, Dodi G & Lise M (1995) Does surgery resolve outlet obstruction from rectocele? *Int J Colorectal Dis* **10**: 97–100.

Jameson JS, Rogers J, Misiewicz JJ, Raimundo AH & Henry MM (1992) Irritable bowel syndrome. *Aliment Pharmacol Ther* **6**: 589–595.

Janssen LWM & van Dijke CF (1994) Selection criteria for anterior rectal wall repair in symptomatic rectocele and anterior rectal wall prolapse. *Dis Colon Rectum* **37**: 1100–1107.

Johansson C, Ihre T & Ahlback SO (1985) Disturbances in the defecation mechanism with special reference to intussusception of the rectum (internal procidentia). *Dis Colon Rectum* **28**: 920–924.

Jones HJS, Blake H & Swift RI (1998) A prostpective audit of the usefulness of evacuating proctography. *Ann R Coll Surg Engl* **80**: 40–45.

Jones PN, Lubowski DZ, Swash M & Henry MM (1987) Is paradoxical contraction of puborectalis muscle of functional importance? *Dis Colon Rectum* **30**: 667–670.

Joo JS, Agachan F, Wolff B, Nogueras JJ & Wexner SD (1996) Initial North American experience with botulinum toxin type A for treatment of anismus. *Dis Colon Rectum* **39**: 1107–1111.

Jorge JM & Wexner SD (1993) Aetiology and management of faecal incontinence. *Dis Colon Rectum* **36**: 77–97.

Jorge JMN, Yang YK & Wexner SD (1994) Incidence and clinical significance of sigmoidoceles as determined by a new classification system. *Dis Colon Rectum* **37**: 1112–1117.

Kalidasan V, Elgabroun MA & Giuney EJ (1997) Button caecostomy in the management of faecal incontinence. *Br J Surg* **84**: 694.

Kamm MA (1987) The surgical treatment of severe idiopathic constipation. *Int J Colorectal Dis* **2**: 229–235.

Kamm MA, Hawley PR & Lennard-Jones JE (1988a) Lateral division of the puborectalis muscle in the management of severe constipation. *Br J Surg* **75**: 661–663.

Kamm MA, Hawley PR & Lennard-Jones JE (1988b) Outcome of colectomy for severe idiopathic constipation. *Gut* **29**: 969–973.

Kamm MA, McLean A, Farthing MJG & Lennard-Jones JE (1989a) Ultrasonography shows no abnormality of pelvic structures in women with severe idiopathic constipation. *Gut* **30**: 1241–1243.

Kamm MA, Farthing MJG & Lennard-Jones JE (1989b) Bowel function and transit rate during the menstrual cycle. *Gut* **30**: 605–608.

Kamm MA, Hoyle CVH, Burleigh DE, Law PJ, Swash M & Martin JE (1991a) Hereditary internal anal sphincter myopathy causing proctalgia fugax and constipation. A new identified condition. *Gastroenterology* **100**: 805–810.

Kamm MA, van der Sijp JR, Hawley PR, Phillps RK & Lennard-Jones JE (1991b) Left hemicolectomy with rectal excision for severe idiopathic constipation. *Int J Colorectal Dis* **6**: 49–51.

Kamm MA, Farthing MJG, Lennard-Jones JE, Perry LA & Chard T (1991c) Steroid hormone abnormalities in women with severe idiopathic constipation. *Gut* **32**: 80–84.

Kamm MA, Sijp JRM van der & Lennard-Jones JE (1992) Observations of the characteristics of stimulated defaecation in severe idiopathic constipation. *Int J Colorectal Dis* **7**: 197–201.

Karlbom U, Pahlman L, Nilsson S & Graf W (1995) Relationships between defecographic findings, rectal emptying and colonic transit time in constipated patients. *Gut* **36**: 907–912.

Karlbom U, Graf W, Nilsson S & Pahlman L (1996) Does surgical repair of a rectocele improve rectal emptying? *Dis Colon Rectum* **39**: 1296–1302.

Karlbom U, Hållden, M, Eeg-Olofsson KE, Påhlman L & Graf W (1997) Results of biofeedback inconstipated patients. A prospective study. *Dis Colon Rectum* **40**: 1149–1155.

Kawimbe BM, Papachrysostomou NR, Binnie CN & Smith AN (1991) Outlet obstruction constipation (anismus) managed by biofeedback. *Gut* **32**: 1175–1179.

Keetley CB (1905a) The surgical treatment of chronic constipation. (Correspondence). *BMJ* (17 June): 1358.

Keetley CB (1905b) Report of the Annual Meeting of the Surgical Section of the BMA. *Lancet* (12 August): 453.

Keighley MRB & Shouler P (1984) Outlet syndrome: is there a surgical option? *J R Soc Med* **77**: 559–563.

Kerremans R (1968a) Radiocinematografie van de ano-rectale streek. *Overdruk Tijdschr Gastroenterol* **11**: 81–91.

Kerremans R (1968b) Radio-cinematographic examination of the rectum and the anal canal in cases of rectal constipation. *Acta Gastroenterol Belg* **31**: 561–570.

Kerrigan DD, Lucas, MG, Sun WM, Donnelly TC & Read NW (1989) Idiopathic constipation associated with impaired urethrovesical and sacral reflex function. *Br J Surg* **76**: 748–751.

Khubchandani IT, Sheets JA, Stasik JJ & Hakki AR (1983) Endorectal repair of rectocele. *Dis Colon Rectum* **26**: 792–796.

Khubchandani IT, Clancy JP, Rosen L, Riether RD & Stasik JJ (1997) Endorectal repair of rectocele revisited. *Br J Surg* **84**: 89–91.

Kiely EM, Ade-Ajayi N & Wheeler RA (1994) Caecal flap conduit for antegrade continence enemas. *Br J Surg* **81**: 1215.

Kiely EM, Ade-Ajayi N & Wheeler RA (1995) Antegrade continence enemas in the management of intractable faecal incontinence. *J R Soc Med* **88**: 103P–104P.

Klatt GR (1983) Role of subtotal colectomy in the treatment of incapacitating constipation. *Am J Surg* **145**: 623–625.

Klein H (1982) Constipation and fecal impaction. *Med Clin North Am* **66**: 1135–1141.

Knowles CH, Scott MA, Wellmer A et al (1998) Idiopathic slow transit constipation: a sensory and autonomic neuropathy linked to Hirschsprung's disease? *Gut* (in press).

Koch A, Voderholzer WA, Klausr AG & Muller-Lissner S (1997) Symptoms in chronic constipation. *Dis Colon Rectum* **40**: 902–906.

Koch TR, Carney JA, Go L & Go VLW (1988) Idiopathic chronic constipation is associated with decreased colonic vasoactive intestinal peptide. *Gastroenterology* **94**: 300–310.

Kock NG, Darle N & Dotevall G (1967) Inhibition of intestinal motility in man by glucagon given intraportally. *Gastroenterology* **53**: 88–92.

Koutsomanis D, Lennard-Jones JE, Roy AJ & Kamm MA (1995) Controlled randomised trial of visual biofeedback versus muscle training without a visual display for intractable constipation. *Gut* **37**: 95–99.

Koyle MA, Kaji DM, Duque M et al (1995) The Malone antegrade continence enema for neurogenic and structural fecal incontinence and constipation. *J Urol* **2**: 759–761.

Krevsky B, Malmud LS, D'Ercole F, Maurer AH & Fisher RS (1986) Colonic transit scintigraphy: a physiologic approach to the quantitative measurement of colonic transit in humans. *Gastroenterology* **91**: 1002–1012.

Krishnamurthy S, Schuffler MD, Rohrmann CA & Pope CE (1985) Severe idiopathic constipation is associated with a distinctive abnormality of the colonic myenteric plexus. *Gastroenterology* **88**: 26–34.

Kubota M, Suita S & Kamimura T (1997) Abnormalities in visceral evoked potentials from the anal canal in children with chronic constipation. *Surg Today Jpn J Surg* **27**: 632–637.

Kuijpers HC & Bleijenberg G (1985) The spastic pelvic floor syndrome. A cause of constipation. *Dis Colon Rectum* **28**: 669–672.

Kuijpers HC, Bleijenberg G & de Morree H (1986) The spastic pelvic floor syndrome. Large bowel outlet obstruction caused by pelvic floor dysfunction: a radiological study. *Int J Colorectal Dis* **1**: 44–48.

Kumar D (1992) Symposium on constipation. *Int J Colorectal Dis* **7**: 47–67.

Kumar D & Gustavsson S (1988) *Gastrointestinal System: Motility Disorders*. Chichester: Wiley.

Lane RHS & Todd IP (1977) Idiopathic megacolon: a review of 42 cases. *Br J Surg* **64**: 305–310.

Lawson M, Keru F & Everson GT (1985) Gastrointestinal transit time in human pregnancy: prolongation in the second and third trimesters followed by postpartum normalization. *Gastroenterology* **89**: 996–999.

Lefebvre MP, Leape LL, Pohl DA, Safaii H & Grand RJ (1984) Total colonic aganglionosis initially diagnosed in an adolescent. *Gastroenterology* **87**: 1364–1366.

Lehur PA, de Kerviler B, Rouyer J et al (1997) Intractable constipation in adults: value of antegrade colonic enemas. *Int J Colorectal Dis* **12**: 121 (A19) (Abstract).

Lennard-Jones JE (1985) Pathophysiology of constipation. *Br J Surg* **72**(Suppl): S7–13.

Leon SH, Krishnamurthy S & Shuffler MD (1987) Subtotal colectomy for severe idiopathic constipation. *Dig Dis Sci* **32**: 1249–1254.

Leroi AM, Bernier C, Watier A et al (1995) Prevalence of sexual abuse amongst patients with functional disorders of the lower gastrointestinal tract. *Int J Colorectal Dis* **10**: 200–206.

Lesaffer L & Milo R (1988) Descending perineum syndrome: control defecogram with a 'perineum device', perspective in prevention and conservative therapy. *JBR-BTR* **71**: 709–712.

Lestar B, Penninckx FM & Kerremans RP (1989) Defecometry: a new method for determining the parameters of rectal evacuation. *Dis Colon Rectum* **32**: 197–201.

Lestar B, Penninckx FM & Kerremans RP (1991) Biofeedback defaecation training for anismus. *Int J Colorectal Dis* **6**: 202–207.

Loening-Baucke V (1984) Abnormal rectoanal function in children recovered from chronic constipation and encopresis. *Gastroenterology* **87**: 1299–1304.

Loening-Baucke V (1989) Factors determining outcome in children with chronic constipation. *Gut* **30**: 999–1006.

Loening-Baucke V (1991) Persistence of chronic constipation in children after biofeedback treatment. *Dig Dis Sci* **36**: 153–160.

Loening-Baucke V (1993) Constipation in early childhood: patient characteristics, treatment and longterm follow up. *Gut* **34**: 1400–1404.

Lowery SP, Srour JW, Whitehead WE & Schuster MM (1983) Bowel training as treatment of functional encopresis: long term follow up. *Gastroenterology* **84**: 1234.

Lowsky R, Davidson G, Wilman S, Jeejeebhoy KN & Hegele RV (1993) Familial visceral myopathy associated with a mitochondrial myopathy. *Gut* **34**: 279–283.

Lubowski DZ, King DW & Finlay IG (1992) Electromyography of the pubococcygeus muscles in patients with obstructed defaecation. *Int J Colorectal Dis* **7**: 184–187.

Lubowski DZ, Meagher AP, Smart RC & Butler SP (1995) Scintigraphic assessment of colonic function during defaecation. *Int J Colorectal Dis* **10**: 91–93.

Lubowski DZ, Chen FC, Kennedy ML & King DW (1996) Results of colectomy for severe slow transit constipation. *Dis Colon Rectum* **39**: 23–29.

Lynn HB & Van Heerden JA (1975) Rectal myectomy in Hirschsprung's disease. A decade of experience. *Arch Surg* **10**: 991–994.

McCready RA & Beart RW Jr (1979) The surgical treatment of incapacitating constipation associated with idiopathic megacolon. *Mayo Clin Proc* **54**: 779–783.

MacDonald A, Shearer M, Paterson PJ & Finlay IG (1991) Relationship between outlet obstruction constipation and obstructed urinary flow. *Br J Surg* **78**: 693–695.

MacDonald A, Baxter JN & Finlay IG (1993a) Idiopathic slow-transit constipation. *Br J Surg* **80**: 1107–1111.

MacDonald A, Paterson PJ, Baxter JN & Finlay IG (1993b) Relationship between intra-abdominal and intrarectal pressure in the proctometrogram. *Br J Surg* **80**: 1070–1071.

MacDonald A, Baxter JN, Bessent RG, Gray HW & Finlay IG (1997) Gastric emptying in patients with constipation following childbirth and due to idiopathic slow transit. *Br J Surg* **84**: 1141–1143.

McLean RG, Smart RC, Lubowski DZ, King DW, Barbagallo S & Talley NA (1992) Oral colon transit scintigraphy using indium-III DTPA: variability in healthy subjects. *Int J Colorectal Dis* **7**: 173–176.

McLeod JH (1983) Biofeedback in the management of partial anal incontinence. *Dis Colon Rectum* **26**: 244–246.

Malone PS, Ransley PG & Kiely EM (1990) Preliminary report: the antegrade continence enema. *Lancet* **336**: 1217–1218.

Maria G, Anastasio G, Brisinda G & Civello IM (1997) Treatment with puborectalis syndrome with progressive anal dilatation. *Dis Colon Rectum* **40**: 89–91.

Marsh PJ & Kiff ES (1996) Ileocaecostomy: an alternative surgical procedure for antegrade colonic enema. *Br J Surg* **83**: 507–508.

Martelli H, Devroede G, Arhan P & Duguay C (1978a) Mechanisms of idiopathic constipation: outlet obstruction. *Gastroenterology* **75**: 623–631.

Martelli H, Devroede G, Arhan P et al (1978b) Some parameters of large bowel motility in normal man. *Gastroenterology* **75**: 612–618.

Meisel JL, Bergman D, Graney D et al (1977) Human rectal mucosa: proctoscopic and morphological changes caused by laxatives. *Gastroenterology* **72**: 1274–1279.

Mellgren A, Bremmer S, Johansson C et al (1994a) Defecography: results of investigations in 2,816 patients. *Dis Colon Rectum* **37**: 1133–1141.

Mellgren A, Dolk A, Johansson C, Bremmer S, Anzen B & Holmstrom B (1994b) Enterocele is correctable using the ripstein rectopexy. *Dis Colon Rectum* **37**: 800–804.

Mellgren A, Johansson C, Dolk A et al (1994c) Enterocele demonstrated by defaecography is associated with other pelvic floor disorders. *Int J Colorectal Dis* **9**: 121–124.

Mellgren A, Anzen B & Nilsson B-Y et al (1995) Results of rectocele repair. *Dis Colon Rectum* **38**: 7–13.

Menardo G, Bausano G, Corazziari E et al (1987) Large bowel transit in paraplegic patients. *Dis Colon Rectum* **30**: 924–928.

Metcalf AM, Phillips SF, Zinsmeister AR, MacCarty RL, Beart RW & Wolff BG (1987) Simplified assessment of segmental colonic transit. *Gastroenterology* **92**: 40–47.

Meunier P, Marechal J & Jaubert de Beaujeu M (1979a) Rectoanal pressures and rectal sensitivity studies in chronic childhood constipation. *Gastroenterology* **77**: 330–336.

Meunier P, Rochas A & Lambert R (1979b) Motor activity of the sigmoid colon in chronic constipation: comparative study with normal subjects. *Gut* **20**: 1095–1101.

Meunier P, Louis D & de Beauje MJ (1984) Physiologic investigation of primary chronic constipation in children: comparison with the barium enema study. *Gastroenterology* **87**: 1351–1357.

Milla PJ (1991) Chronic intestinal pseudoobstruction. In Kamm MA & Lennard-Jones JE (eds) *Gastrointestinal Transit*, pp 57–170. Peterfield: Wrightson Biomedical.

Miller R, Duthie GS, Bartolo DCC, Roe AM, Locke-Edmunds J & Mortensen MJMcC (1991) Anismus in patients with normal and slow transit constipation. *Br J Surg* **78**: 690–692.

Milner P, Crowe R, Kamm MA, Lennard-Jones JE & Burnstock G (1990) Vasoactive intestinal polypeptide levels in sigmoid colon in idiopathic constipation and diverticular disease. *Gastroenterology* **99**: 666–675.

Minocha A, Katragadda R, Rahal PS & Ries A (1995) Erythromycin shortens orocaecal transit time in diabetic male subjects: a double-blind placebo-controlled study. *Aliment Pharmacol Ther* **9**: 529–533.

Misiewicz JJ (1975) Colonic motility. *Gut* **16**: 311–314.

Mitchell ME (1986) Use of bowel in undiversion. *Urol Clin North Am* **13**: 349–358.

Mitrofanoff P (1980) Cystomie continente trans-appendiculaire dans le traitment des vessies neurologiques [Trans-appendicular continent cystostomy in the management of the neurogenic bladder]. *Chir Pediatr* **21**: 297–305.

Moore-Gillon V (1984) Constipation: What does the patient mean? *J R Soc Med* **77**: 108–110.

Mor Y, Quinn FMJ, Carr B et al (1997) Combined Mitrofanoff and antegrade continence enema procedures for urinary and fecal incontinence. *J Urol* **158**: 192–195.

Moynihan BGA (1903) A brief experience in abdominal surgery. *Lancet* (21 November): 1429–1430.

Muller-Lissner SA and the Bavarian Constipation Group (1987) Treatment of chronic constipation with cisapride and placebo. *Gut* **28**: 1033–1038.

Murthy VK, Orkin BA, Smith LE & Glassman LM (1996) Excellent outcome using selective criteria for rectocele repair. *Dis Colon Rectum* **39**: 374–378.

Muzzio PC, Pomerri F, Locatelli R, del Borrello M & Pittarello F (1984) Defecographic and tonometric aspects in idiopathic anorectal constipation. *J Belge Radiol/Belgisch Tijdschr Radiol* **67**: 87–91.

Nehme AE (1984) Constipation: an uncommon etiology. *Dis Colon Rectum* **27**: 819–821.

Neuman PZ, deDomenico IJ & Nogrady MB (1973) Constipation and urinary tract infection. *Pediatrics* **52**: 241–245.

Notghi A, Hutchinson R, Kumar D, Smith NB & Harding LK (1994) Simplified method for the measurement of segmental colonic transit time. *Gut* **35**: 976–981.

Notghi A, Mills A, Hutchinson R, Kumar D & Harding LH (1995) Reporting simplified colonic transit studies using radionuclides: clinician friendly report. *Gut* **36**: 274–275.

Nyam DCNK, Pemberton JH, Ilstrup DM & Rath DM (1997) Long-term results of surgery for chronic constipation. *Dis Colon Rectum* **40**: 273–279.

Ornstein MH, Littlewood ER, Baird IM, Fowler J, North WRS & Cox AG (1981) Are fibre supplements really necessary in diverticular disease of the colon? A controlled clinical trial. *BMJ* **282**: 1353–1356.

Orr WC & Robinson MG (1981) Motor activity of the rectosigmoid in patients with chronic constipation. *Gastroenterology* **80**: 1244.

Orrom WJ, Bartolo DCC, Miller R, Mortensen NJMcC & Roe AM (1991) Rectopexy is an ineffective treatment for obstructed defecation. *Dis Colon Rectum* **34**: 41–46.

Panagamuwa B, Kumar D, Ortiz P & Keighley MRB (1994) Motor abnormalities in the terminal ileum of patients with chronic idiopathic constipation. *Br J Surg* **81**: 1685–1688.

Papachrystostomou M & Smith AN (1994) Effects of biofeedback on obstructive defecation – reconditioning of the defecation reflex? *Gut* **35**: 252–256.

Papachrystostomou M, Stevenson AJM, Ferrington C, Merrick MV & Smith AN (1993) Evaluation of isotope proctography in constipated subjects. *J Colorectal Dis* **8**: 18–22.

Papachrystostomou M, Smith AN & Merrick MV (1994) Obstructive defaecation and slow transit constipation: the proctographic parameters. *Int J Colorectal Dis* **9**: 115–120.

Park HJ, Kamm MA, Abbasi AM & Talbot IC (1995) Immunohistochemical study of the colonic muscle and innervation in idiopathic chronic constipation. *Dis Colon Rectum* **38**: 509–513.

Park UC, Choi SK, Piccirillo MF, Verzaro R & Wexner SD (1996) Patterns of anismus and the relation to biofeedback therapy. *Dis Colon Rectum* **39**: 768–773.

Parker MC & Phillips RKS (1993) Repair of rectocele using Marlex mesh. *Ann R Coll Surg Engl* **75**: 193–194.

Parks TG & Connell AM (1969) Motility studies in diverticular disease of the colon. *Gut* **10**: 534–542.

Partiquin H, Mortelli H & Devroede G (1978) Barium enema in chronic constipation: is it meaningful? *Gastroenterology* **75**: 619–622.

Parys BT, Haylen BT, Hutton JL & Parson KF (1989) The effects of simple hysterectomy on vesicourethral function. *Br J Urol* **64**: 694–699.

Passmore AP, Wilson-Davies K, Stoker C & Scott ME (1993) Chronic constipation in long-stay elderly patients: a comparison of lactulose and a senna-fibre combination. *BMJ* **307**: 769–771.

Payler DK, Pomare EW, Heaton KW & Harvey RF (1975) The effect of wheat bran on intestinal transit. *Gut* **16**: 209–213.

Pemberton JH, Rath DM & Ilstrup DM (1991) Evaluation and surgical treatment of severe chronic constipation. *Ann Surg* **214**: 403–413.

Pena JP, Heine JA, Wnog WD, Christienson CE & Balcos EG (1992) Subtotal colectomy for constipation – a long term follow up study. *Dis Colon Rectum* **35**: 19 (Abstract).

Pennington CR (1985) Laxative abuse in the elderly. *Geriatr Med Today* **4**: 65–69.

Pezim ME, Pemberton JH, Levin KE, Litchy WJ & Phillips SF (1993) Parameters of anorectal and colonic motility in health and in severe constipation. *Dis Colon Rectum* **36**: 484–491.

Pfeifer J, Agachan F & Wexner SD (1996) Surgery for constipation. *Dis Colon Rectum* **39**: 444–460.

Piccirillo MF, Reissman P, Carnavos R & Wexner SD (1995) Colectomy as treatment for constipation in selected patients. *Br J Surg* **82**: 898–901.

Picon L, Lemann M, Flowie B, Rambaud J-C, Rain J-D & Jian R (1992) Right and left colonic transit after eating assessed by a dual isotopic technique in healthy humans. *Gastroenterology* **103**: 80–85.

Piloni V, Bassotti G, Fioravanti P, Amadio L & Montesi A (1997) Dynamic imaging of the normal pelvic floor. *Int J Colorectal Dis* **12**: 246–253.

Pinho M, Yoshioka K & Keighley MRB (1991a) Are pelvic floor movements abnormal in disordered defecation? *Dis Colon Rectum* **34**: 1117–1119.

Pinho M, Yoshioka K & Keighley MRB (1991b) Long term results of anorectal myectomy for chronic constipation. *Br J Surg* **76**: 1163–1164.

Pluta H, Bowes KL & Jewell LD (1996) Long-term results of total abdominal colectomy for chronic idiopathic constipation. *Dis Colon Rectum* **39**: 160–166.

Poisson J & Devroede G (1983) Severe chronic constipation as a surgical problem. *Surg Clin North Am* **63**: 193–217.

Porter NH (1961) Megacolon: a physiological study. *Proc R Soc Med* **54**: 1043–1047.

Preston DM (1985) Arbuthnot Lane's disease: chronic intestinal stasis. *Br J Surg* **72**(Suppl): S8–S10.

Preston DM & Lennard-Jones JE (1982) Does failure of bisacodyl-induced colonic peristalsis indicate intrinsic nerve damage? *Gut* **23**: A891.

Preston DM & Lennard-Jones JE (1986) Severe chronic constipation of young women: idiopathic slow transit constipation? *Gut* **27**: 41–48.

Preston DM, Lennard-Jones JE & Parks AG (1982a) Balloon proctogram: a new technique for the study of disorders of defaecation. *Gut* **23**: A437.

Preston DM, Hawley PR & Lennard-Jones JE (1982b) Results of colectomy for slow transit constipation. *Gut* **23**: A903.

Preston DM, Barnes PRH & Lennard-Jones JE (1983a) Proctometrogram: does it have a role in the evaluation of adults with chronic constipation? *Gut* **24**: A1010–1011.

Preston DM, Adrian TE, Lennard-Jones JE & Bloom SR (1983b) Impaired gastrin release in chronic constipation. *Gut* **24**: A481.

Preston DM, Rees LH & Lennard-Jones JE (1983c) Gynaecological disorders and hyperprolactinaemia in chronic constipation. *Gut* **24**: A480.

Pucciani F, Rottoli RL, Bologna A et al (1996) Anterior rectocele and anorectal dysfunction. *Int J Colorectal Dis* **11**: 1–9.

Rantis PC, Vernava AM, Daniel GL & Longo WE (1997) Chronic constipation – is the work-up worth the cost? *Dis Colon Rectum* **40**: 280–286.

Read NW (1987) Constipation. *Surgery (Medicine Group)* **1**: 1160–1163.

Read NW, Timms JM, Barfield LJ, Donnelly TC & Bannister JJ (1986) Impairment of defecation in young women with severe constipation. *Gastroenterology* **90**: 53–60.

Redmond JM, Smith GW, Barofsky I, Ratych RE, Goldsborough DC & Schuster M (1995) Physiological tests to predict long-term outcome of total abdominal colectomy for intractable constipation. *Am J Gastroenterol* **90**: 748–753.

Rees WDW & Rhodes J (1976) Altered bowel habit and menstruation. *Lancet* **ii**: 475–477.

Rendtorff RC & Kashgarian M (1967) Stool patterns of healthy adult males. *Dis Colon Rectum* **10**: 222–228.

Report from the International Agency for Research on Cancer Intestinal Microecology Group (1977) Dietary fibre, transit time, faecal bacteria, steroids and colon cancer in two Scandinavian populations. *Lancet* **ii**: 207–211.

Rieger NA, Wattchow DA, Sarre RG et al (1997) Prospective study of biofeedback for treatment of constipation. *Dis Colon Rectum* **40**: 1143–1148.

Roarty TP, Weber F, Soykan I & McCallum RW (1997) Misoprostol in the treatment of chronic refractory constipation: results of a long-term open label trial. *Aliment Pharmacol Ther* **11**: 1059–1066.

Roberts DP, Waldron DW, Newell M, Garvie PN & Williams NS (1988) Comparison of radioopaque marker and radioisotopic assessment of whole bowel transit time in constipated patients. *Gut* **29**: A441.

Roberts JP, Womack NR, Hallan RI, Thorpe AC & Williams NS (1992) Evidence for dynamic integrated proctography to redefine anismus. *Br J Surg* **79**: 1213–1215.

Roberts JP, Moon S & Malone PS (1995) Treatment of neuropathic urinary and faecal incontinence with synchronous bladder reconstruction and the antegrade continence enema procedure. *Br J Urol* **75**: 386–389.

Roe AM, Bartolo DCC & Mortensen NJMcC (1986a) Techniques in evacuation proctography in the diagnosis of intractable constipation and related disorders. *J R Soc Med* **79**: 331–333.

Roe AM, Bartolo DCC & Mortensen NJMcC (1986b) Diagnosis and surgical management of intractable constipation. *Br J Surg* **73**: 854–861.

Roe AM, Bartolo DCC & Mortensen NJMcC (1988) Slow transit constipation. Comparison between patients with and without previous hysterectomy. *Dig Dis Sci* **33**: 1159–1163.

Rogers J & Misiewicz JJ (1989) Fully automated computer analysis of intracolonic pressures. *Gut* **30**: 642–649.

Ryan JA & Oakley WC (1985) Cecoproctostomy. *Am J Surg* **149**: 636–639.

Sarles JC, Arnaud A, Selezneff I & Oliver S (1989) Endo-rectal repair of rectocele. *Int J Colorectal Dis* **4**: 167–171.

Schang JC, Devroede G & Pilote M (1993) Effects of trimebutine on colonic function in patients with chronic idiopathic constipation: evidence for the need of a physiologic rather than clinical selection. *Dis Colon Rectum* **36**: 330–336.

Schouten WR, Briel JW, Auwerda JJA et al (1997) Anismus: fact or fiction? *Dis Colon Rectum* **40**: 1033–1041.

Sehapayak S (1985) Transrectal repair of rectocele: an extended armamentarium of colorectal surgeons. A report of 355 cases. *Dis Colon Rectum* **28**: 422–433.

Sentovich SM, Rivela LJ, Thorson AG, Christensen MA & Blatchford GJ (1995) Simultaneous dynamic proctography and peritoneography for pelvic floor disorder. *Dis Colon Rectum* **38**: 912–915.

Shafik A (1995) Electrorectography in chronic constipation. *World J Surg* **19**: 772–775.

Shandling B, Chait PG & Richards HF (1996) Percutaneous cecostomy: a new technique in the management of fecal incontinence. *J Pediatr Surg* **4**: 534–537.

Shatila AH & Ackerman NB (1977) Stercoraceous ulcerations and perforations of the colon: report of cases and survey of the literature. *Dis Colon Rectum* **20**: 524–527.

Sheldon CA, Minevich E, Wacksman J et al (1997) Role of the antegrade continence enema in the management of the most debilitating childhood recto-urogenital anomalies. *J Urol* **158**: 1277–1279.

Shorvon PJ, McHugh S, Diamant NE, Somers S & Stevenson GW (1989) Defecography in normal volunteers: results and implications. *Gut* **30**: 1737–1749.

Shouler P & Keighley MRB (1986) Changes in colorectal function in severe idiopathic chronic constipation. *Gastroenterology* **90**: 414–420.

Silverberg M (1984) Constipation in children. *Curr Concepts Gastroenterol* **86**: 14–22.

Siproudhis L, Dautreme S, Ropert A et al (1993) Dyschezia and rectocele – a marriage of convenience? *Dis Colon Rectum* **36**: 1030–1036.

Sladen GE (1972) Effects of chronic purgative abuse. *Proc R Soc Med* **65**: 288–290.

Slater BJ, Varma JS & Gillespie JI (1997) Abnormalities in the contractile properties of colonic smooth muscle in idiopathic slow transit constipation. *Br J Surg* **84**: 181–184.

Smith AN, Varma JS, Binnie NR & Papachrysostomou M (1990) Disordered colorectal motility in intractable constipation following hysterectomy. *Br J Surg* **77**: 1361–1366.

Smith B (1968) Effects of irritant purgatives on the myenteric plexus in man and the mouse. *Gut* **9**: 139–143.

Smith B (1972) Pathology of cathartic colon. *Proc R Soc Med* **65**: 288.

Smith B (1973) Pathologic changes in the colon produced by anthraquinone purgatives. *Dis Colon Rectum* **16**: 455–458.

Smith B, Grace RH & Todd IP (1977) Organic constipation in adults. *Br J Surg* **64**: 313–314.

Smith V, Lake BD, Kamm MA & Nicholls RJ (1992) Intestinal pseudo-obstruction with deficient smooth muscle alpha-actin. *Histopathology* **21**: 535–542.

Snaith RP & Zigmond AS (1983) The Hospital Anxiety and Depression Scale. *Acta Psychiatrica Scandinavica* **67**: 361–370.

Snape WJ, Carlson GM & Cohen S (1976) Colonic myoelectric activity in the irritable bowel syndrome. *Gastroenterology* **70**: 326–330.

Snooks SJ, Swah M, Mathers SE & Henry MM (1990) Effect of vaginal delivery on the pelvic floor: a five year follow-up. *Br J Surg* **77**: 1358–1360.

Solana A, Roig JV, Villoslada C, Hinojosa J & Lledo S (1996) Anorectal sensitivity in patients with obstructed defaecation. *Int J Colorectal Dis* **11**: 65–70.

Sonnenberg A & Koch TR (1989) Epidemiology of constipation in the United States. *Dis Colon Rectum* **32**: 1–8.

Speakman CTM, Kamm MA & Swash M (1993) Rectal sensory evoked potentials: an assessment of their clinical value. *Int J Colorectal Dis* **8**: 23–28.

Squire R, Kiely EM, Carr B et al (1993) The clinical application of the Malone antegrade colonic enema. *J Pediatr Surg* **28**: 1012–1015.

Stabile G, Kamm MA, Hawley PR & Lennard-Jones JE (1991) Colectomy for idiopathic megarectum and megacolon. *Gut* **32**: 1538–1540.

Stewart J, Kumar D & Keighley MR (1994) Results of anal low rectal anastomosis and pouch construction for megarectum and megacolon. *Br J Surg* **81**: 1051–1053.

Stanmore Bishop E (1905) Report of a meeting of the Manchester Medical Society. *BMJ* (18 March): 598.

Starling JR, Croom RD III & Thomas CG Jr (1986) Hirschsprung's disease in young adults. *Am J Surg* **151**: 104–109.

Stivland T, Camilleri M, Vassallo M et al (1991) Scintigraphic measurement of regional gut transit in idiopathic constipation. *Gastroenterology* **101**: 107–115.

Stock JA & Hanna MK (1996) Appendiceal cecoplication: a modification of the Malone antegrade colonic enema procedure. *Tech Urol* **2**: 40–42.

Sutphen J, Borowitz S, Ling W, Cox DJ & Kovatchev B (1997) Anorectal manometric examination in encopretic-constipated children. *Dis Colon Rectum* **40**: 1051–1055.

Takada H, Hioki K, Ambrose NS, Alexander-Williams J & Keighley MRB (1993) Potentially explosive colonic gas is not eliminated by successful mechanical bowel preparation. *Dig Surg* **10**: 20–23.

Takahashi T, Fitzgerald SD & Pemberton JH (1994) Evaluation and treatment of constipation. *Rev Gastroenterol Mex* **59**: 133–138.

Talley NJ, Weaver AL, Zinsmeister AR & Melton J (1993)

Functional constipation and outlet delay: a population-based study. *Gastroenterology* **105**: 781–790.
Tanner MS, Smith B & Lloyd JK (1976) Functional intestinal obstruction due to deficiency of argyrophil neurones in the myenteric plexus. *Arch Dis Child* **51**: 837–841.
Taylor I, Duthie HL, Smallwood R & Linkens D (1975) Large bowel myoelectrical activity in man. *Gut* **16**: 808–814.
Taylor I, Hammond P & Darby C (1980) An assessment of anorectal motility in the management of adult megacolon. *Br J Surg* **67**: 754–756.
Taylor T, Smith AN & Fulton PM (1989) Effect of hysterectomy on bowel function. *BMJ* **299**: 300–301.
Taylor T, Smith AN & Fulton M (1990) Effects of hysterectomy on bowel and bladder function. *Int J Colorectal Dis* **5**: 228–231.
Teichman JMH, Rogenes VJ & Barber DB (1997) The Malone antegrade continence enema combined with urinary diversion in adult neurogenic patients. Early results. *Urology* **49**: 963–967.
Thomas CG, Bream CA & DeConninck P (1970) Posterior sphincterotomy and rectal myotomy in the management of Hirschsprung's disease. *Ann Surg* **171**: 796–809.
Thompson WS & Heaton KW (1980) Functional bowel disorders in apparently healthy people. *Gastroenterology* **79**: 283–288.
Thorpe AC, Williams NS, Badenoch DF, Blandy JP & Grahn MF (1993) Simultaneous dynamic electromyographic proctography and cystometrography. *Br J Surg* **80**: 115–120.
Thorpe AC, Evans RE & Williams NS (1994) Constipation and spina bifida occulta: is there an association? *J R Coll Surg Edinb* **39**: 221–224.
Todd IP (1985) Constipation: results of surgical treatment. *Br J Surg* **72**(Suppl): S12–S13.
Tomlin J & Read NW (1988) Laxative properties of indigestible plastic particles. *BMJ* **297**: 1175–1176.
Toogood GJ, Bryant PA & Dudley NE (1995) Control of faecal incontinence using the Malone antegrade continence enema procedure: a critical appraisal. *Pediatr Surg Int* **10**: 37–39.
Tsang TM & Dudley NE (1995) Surgical detail of the Malone antegrade continence enema procedure. *Pediatr Surg Int* **10**: 33–36.
Tucker DM, Sandstead HH, Logan GM Jr et al (1981) Dietary fiber and personality factors as determinants of stool output. *Gastroenterology* **81**: 879–883.
Turnbull GK & Ritvo PG (1992) Anal sphincter biofeedback relaxation treatment for women with intractable constipation symptoms. *Dis Colon Rectum* **35**: 530–536.
Turnbull GK, Lennard-Jones JE & Bartram CI (1986) Failure of rectal expulsion as a cause of constipation: why fibre and laxatives sometimes fail. *Lancet* **i**: 767–769.
Turnbull GK, Thompson DG, Day S, Martin J, Walker E & Lennard-Jones JE (1989) Relationships between symptoms, menstrual cycle and orocaecal transit in normal and constipated women. *Gut* **30**: 30–34.
Tyrell CA (1907) *The Royal Road to Health*, 45th edn. New York: Tyrell's Hygienic Institute.
Ueda S, Iishi H, Tatsuta M, Oda K & Osaka S (1994) Addition of cisapride shortens colonoscopy preparation with lavage in elderly patients. *Aliment Pharmacol* **8**: 209–214.
Vaccaro CA, Cheong CMO, Wexner SD, Salanga VD, Phillips RC & Hanson MR (1994) Role of pudendal nerve terminal motor latency assessment in constipated patients. *Dis Colon Rectum* **37**: 1250–1254.
Vaccaro CA, Cheong DMO, Wexner SD et al (1995a) Pudendal neuropathy in evacuatory disorders. *Dis Colon Rectum* **38**: 166–171.
Vaccaro CA, Wexner SD, Teoh T-A, Choi SK, Cheong DMA & Salanaga VD (1995b) Pudendal neuropathy is not related to physiologic pelvic outlet obstruction. *Dis Colon Rectum* **38**: 630–634.
van Baal JG, Leguit P Jr & Brummelkamp WH (1984) Relaxation biofeedback conditioning as treatment of a disturbed defecation reflex: report of a case. *Dis Colon Rectum* **27**: 187–189.
van Dam JH, Schouten WR, Ginai AZ, Huisman WM & Hop WCJ (1996) The impact of anismus on the clinical outcome of rectocele repair. *Int J Colorectal Dis* **11**: 238–242.
van Dam JH, Gosselink MJ, Drogendijk AC, Hop WCJ & Schouten WR (1997) Changes in bowel function after hysterectomy. *Dis Colon Rectum* **40**: 1432–1437.
van der Sijp JRM, Kamm MA, Nightingale JMD et al (1993) Radioisotope determination of regional colonic transit in severe constipation: comparison with radio opaque markers. *Gut* **34**: 402–408.
Varma JS (1992) Autonomic influences on colorectal motility and pelvic surgery. *World J Surg* **16**: 811–819.
Varma JS & Smith AN (1986) Reproducibility of the proctometrogram. *Gut* **27**: 288–292.
Varma JS & Smith AN (1988) Neurophysiological dysfunction in young women with intractable constipation. *Gut* **29**: 963–968.
Varma JS, Bradnock J, Smith RG & Smith AN (1988) Constipation in the elderly: a physiologic study. *Dis Colon Rectum* **31**: 111–115.
Voderholzer WA, Neuhaus DA, Klauser AG, Tzavella K, Muller-Lissner SA & Schindlbeck NE (1997) Paradoxical sphincter contraction is rarely indicative of anismus. *Gut* **41**: 258–262.
Wald A, Van Thiel DH, Hoechstetter L et al (1981) Gastrointestinal transit: the effect of the menstrual cycle. *Gastroenterology* **80**: 1497–1500.
Wallace WC & Madden WM (1969) Partial puborectalis resection: a new surgical technic for anorectal dysfunction. *South Med J* **62**: 1123–1126.
Walsh PV, Peebles-Brown DA & Watkinson G (1987) Colectomy for slow transit constipation. *Ann R Coll Surg Engl* **69**: 71–75.
Wasserman IF (1964) Puborectalis syndrome. Rectal stenosis due to anorectal spasm. *Dis Colon Rectum* **7**: 87–97.
Watier A, Devroede G, Duguay C, Duranceau A, Arhan P & Toppercar A (1979) Mechanisms of idiopathic constipation: colonic inertia. *Gastroenterology* **76**: 1267.
Waxman SW, Koyle MA, Johnstone M et al (1996) Applications and modifications of the Malone antegrade continence enema (MACE) with coincidental urinary tract reconstruction. *J Urol* **155**: 485A, Abstract 698.
Webb HW, Barraza MA & Crump JM (1997) Laparoscopic appendicostomy for management of fecal incontinence. *J Paediatr Surg* **32**: 457–458.
Weber J, Ducrotte P, Touchai JY, Roussignol C & Denis P (1987) Biofeedback training for constipation in adults and children. *Dis Colon Rectum* **30**: 844–846.
Wegman EA, Aniss AM, Bolit TD, Davis AE & Gandevia SC (1989) Human rectosigmoid electromyography: a new approach and some pitfalls. *J R Soc Med* **82**: 88–90.
Weingarten JL & Cromie WJ (1988) The Mitrofanoff principle: an alternative form of continent urinary diversion. *J Urol* **140**: 1529–1531.
Weir RF (1902) *New York Medical Record* (9 August): 201.
Wexner SD, Daniel N & Jagelman DG (1991) Colectomy for constipation: physiologic investigation is the key to success. *Dis Colon Rectum* **34**: 851–856.
Wheeler RA & Malone PS (1991) Use of the appendix in reconstructive surgery: a case against incidental appendicectomy. *Br J Surg* **78**: 1283–1285.
Williams NS, Hughes SF & Stuchfield B (1994) Continent colonic

conduit for rectal evacuation in severe constipation. *Lancet* **343**: 1321–1324.

Winship DH (1975) Gastrointestinal disease. In Burrow GN & Ferris TF (eds) *Medical Complications During Pregnancy,* pp 275–350. Philadelphia: WB Saunders.

Womack NR, Williams NS, Holmfield JHM, Morrison JFB & Simpkins KC (1985) New method for the dynamic assessment of anorectal function in constipation. *Br J Surg* **72**: 994–998.

Yamamoto T, Kubo H & Honzumi M (1996) Fecal incontinence successfully managed by antegrade continence enema in children: a report of two cases. *Surg Today* **26**: 1024–1028.

Yoshioka K & Keighley MRB (1987a) Randomized trial comparing anorectal myectomy and controlled anal dilatation for outlet obstruction. *Br J Surg* **74**: 1125–1129.

Yoshioka K & Keighley MRB (1987b) Anorectal myectomy for outlet obstruction. *Br J Surg* **74**: 373–376.

Yoshioka K & Keighley MRB (1989) Clinical results of colectomy for severe constipation. *Br J Surg* **76**: 600–604.

Yoshioka K, Matsui Y, Yamada O et al (1991) Physiologic and anatomic assessment of patients with rectocele. *Dis Colon Rectum* **34**: 704–708.

Ziegler MM, Royal RE, Brandt J, Drasnin J & Martin LW (1993) Extended myectomy-myotomy: a therapeutic alternative for total intestinal aganglionosis. *Ann Surg* **28**: 504–511.

22

ADULT MEGACOLON AND MEGARECTUM

A number of different disorders may cause large bowel dilatation associated with severe constipation. In children, the predominant cause is Hirschsprung's disease, diagnosis of which is confirmed by manometry and from anorectal myectomy specimens showing absent ganglia with thick nerves (Robertson and Kernohan, 1938; Fairgreave, 1963; Lawson and Nixon, 1967; Aronson and Nixon, 1972; Udassin et al, 1983). Hirschsprung's disease can occasionally occur in adolescence (Todd, 1977) but most cases of adult megabowel do not have neonatal obstruction.

Unlike Hirschsprung's disease, which is usually confined to male infants, both sexes are affected in idiopathic megacolon or megarectum. Symptoms usually start in early or late childhood and the brunt of the disease primarily affects the rectum, and colon changes usually occur as a secondary phenomenon (Stewart et al, 1994; Kim et al, 1995; Gattuso et al, 1996a,b,c, 1997; Gattuso and Kamm, 1997). Other disorders responsible for adult megabowel include chronic idiopathic intestinal pseudo-obstruction, recurrent volvulus and recurrent degenerative disorders, often associated with neurological disease or long-term psychotropic drug therapy affecting the intrinsic innervation of the colon and rectum (Palmer and McBirnie, 1967; Krishnamurthy et al, 1985; Stabile et al, 1992a,b; Crowe et al, 1992; Boeckxstaens et al, 1993; Keef et al, 1993).

In contrast to the well-defined histological abnormalities in Hirschsprung's disease and chronic primary intestinal pseudo-obstruction, the pathological basis underlying idiopathic megacolon or megarectum are largely unknown (Gattuso et al, 1997). Idiopathic megacolon and megarectum usually presents in adolescence with soiling and incontinence secondary to faecal impaction in a megarectum. A few patients have had surgery in childhood for anorectal agenesis or Hirschsprung's disease. Treatment usually involves rectal resection by the Duhamel procedure or rectal excision and coloanal anastomosis; subtotal colectomy is of use for megacolon alone and restorative proctocolectomy for megacolon and megarectum.

ADULT HIRSCHSPRUNG'S DISEASE

There are now serious doubts as to whether Hirschsprung's disease occurs in adults, but because there is a substantial literature on the role of surgery for adult Hirschprung's disease, this entity is included here.

Aetiology

Hirschsprung's disease is characterized by congenital absence of ganglion cells in Auerbach's plexus (Cameron, 1928; Tiffin et al, 1940; Whitehouse and Kernohan, 1948). The diseased segment is variable in length but usually terminates 1–2 cm above the dentate line. The proximal limit of the aganglionic bowel ranges from the descending colon to the rectum. Two groups are recognized: those with disease confined to the rectosigmoid junction (30%) and those extending for a variable length into the left colon (Lorenzo et al, 1985). Occasionally, aganglionosis may involve the entire large bowel (Boley, 1984; Lefebvre et al, 1984), and there are a few reported cases in which the entire small and large bowel are involved (Furness and Costa, 1980, 1987). In a small number of cases the aganglionic segment may be no more than 1 or 2 cm in length. Such cases are difficult to diagnose because they do not present in the usual manner but with constipation and faecal soiling. It should be appreciated that ganglion cells are normally sparse in the submucosa 2 cm above the dentate line, which may lead to further diagnostic confusion.

Total loss of neurones in the segment above the anal transition zone causes a functional obstruction in the aganglionic bowel and the segment becomes spastic (Shuster et al, 1970). As a consequence, the proximal bowel becomes hypertrophied and dilated in an attempt to overcome this functional obstruction. Earlam (1985) reported both absent ganglion cells and thickened arterioles in Hirschsprung's disease with fibroblast transformation of smooth muscles and therefore proposed an ischaemic aetiology in a third of patients.

The majority of cases of Hirschsprung's disease are thought, however, to be due to a failure of migration of the neuroblasts from the myenteric plexus and the condition may seem to be familial. The *Ret* gene has been found to be mutated in up to 40% of children with this disorder (Robertson et al, 1997). Furthermore, mutations have also been identified in the *Endr-B* gene (endothelium receptor B). Despite the absence of ganglia there are no pharmacological reasons for spasticity since the sensitivity to acetylcholine, noradrenaline, isoprenaline and histamine are normal. There is a normal contractile response to bethanechol and pilocarpine and normal inhibition to serotonin (Penninckx and Kerremans, 1975b).

Incidence

Hirschsprung's disease is uncommon in adult life and most are cases that have been missed in childhood (San Filippo et al, 1972; Swenson et al, 1973; Lynn and Van Heerden, 1975). Metzgar et al (1978) reported 69 patients, presenting for the first time and over the age of 10 years, from a series of 536 patients. The mean age of presentation in patients over 10 years was 21 (range: 10–59 years) (McCready and Beart, 1980). Barnes et al (1986) described 29 patients who presented at 10 years of age or over, of whom only 19 were men. There is often a family history, hence there is a higher incidence of the disease among affected families than in the population at large (Luukkonen et al, 1990).

Pathological features

Typical disease

There is gross dilatation of the proximal non-affected colon while the aganglionic segment is narrow and acts as a functional obstruction. Typically, the affected bowel (usually the rectum and a variable segment of proximal bowel) has no ganglia in the myenteric plexus and there are hypertrophied nerves (Figure 22.1). Complete absence of ganglia is the only way to establish the diagnosis beyond doubt. Garrett and Howard (1981) described a variant of Hirschsprung's disease in which the numbers of ganglion cells were reduced (hypoganglionosis). This also causes chronic constipation and should be distinguished from Hirschsprung's disease. There is also a condition with increased numbers of ganglion cells which may be associated with difficulty in defecation (hyperganglionosis) (Howard et al, 1982).

In normal subjects, the anal transition zone contains very few or even no ganglia for up to 2 cm above the dentate line (Aldridge and Campbell, 1968; Weinberg, 1970). Furthermore, this zone of reduced or absent ganglia increases with age. The

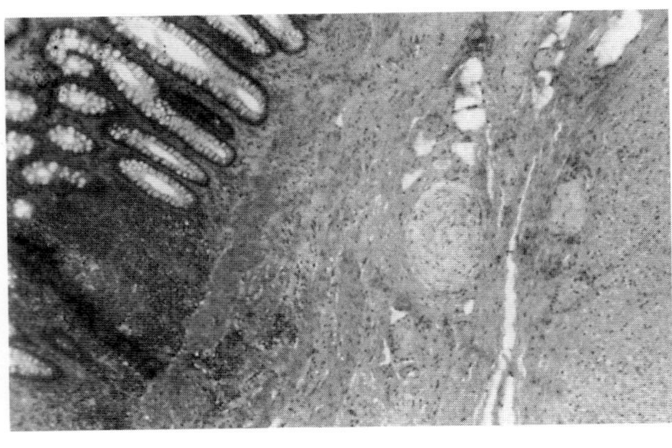

(a)

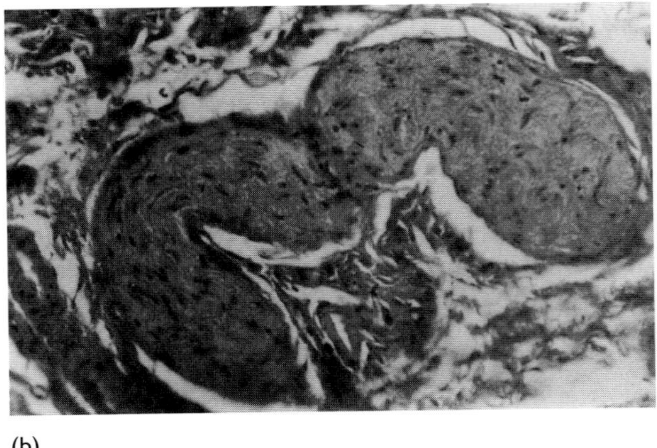

(b)

Figure 22.1 Histopathology of Hirschsprung's disease. Two high-power photomicrographs which demonstrate thick nerves and absent ganglia typical of Hirschsprung's disease.

normal distribution of ganglia is not known in patients over the age of 15 years. Hence there are problems in interpreting full-thickness anorectal biopsies in suspected adult onset disease. The dilemma is further increased since a mild form of the disorder may go unrecognized during childhood and only present with troublesome symptoms in adult life (Fairgreave, 1963; Stone et al, 1965).

Mean acetylcholinesterase activity is increased in rectal biopsy specimens from the aganglionic segment of Hirschsprung's disease. This is probably due to the larger numbers of nerve fibres. The adrenergic innervation of the aganglionic segment is associated with tissue concentrations of acetylcholinesterase which are two or three times greater than those found in the normal anorectal segment (Gannon et al, 1969; Garrett et al, 1969; Meier-Ruge et al, 1972; Dale et al, 1979). Fluorescent adrenergic nerves are also found in association with aganglionic tissue. Neurones containing 5-hydroxytryptamine are also absent in Hirschsprung's disease and there are low concentrations of vasoactive intestinal peptide (VIP) and substance P in the affected segment of the bowel (Tafuri et al, 1974; Rogawski et al, 1978; Dupont et al, 1980; Freund et al, 1981).

In Hirschsprung's disease there are large regional differences in the distribution of autonomic ganglia and neurotransmitters. Garrett and Howard (1981) describe four regions: (1) the most proximal ganglionic segment of the bowel, in which acetylcholinesterase staining is normal; (2) the distal area of ganglionic bowel, usually the anal transition zone, which contains only a few small ganglia and a sparse distribution of nerves in the circular muscle; (3) the proximal segment of aganglionic bowel, which contains positive acetylcholinesterase nerve trunks but no ganglia in the intermuscular zone, and has fewer nerves than normal in the circular muscle; (4) the distal aganglionic bowel, which contains much larger nerves in the intermuscular zone and in the circular muscle than those at any other level. Furthermore, they stain more strongly for acetylcholinesterase.

Electron microscopy shows that the ganglionic tissue is devoid of collagen and the ganglion cells are unsupported. Putative neuroeffector sites with axons containing vesicles are seen in close proximity to the muscle cells. It is apparent that the nerves entering the aganglionic segment of bowel would normally have been destined for ganglia, but in the absence of ganglion cells such nerves pass into the muscle layers and create abnormal neuroeffector junctions with smooth muscle cells.

The severity of symptoms appears to correlate with the histopathological findings. It is probable that acetylcholinesterase released by these nerves accentuates the uncoordinated contraction of the muscle in the distal bowel, creating a functional obstruction. Failure of the internal sphincter to relax in response to rectal distension exacerbates the obstruction. Disordered motor activity present in the distal aganglionic segment further increases the obstruction, the severity of which is related to the number of acetylcholinesterase-positive nerves present in the circular muscle layer. A study from the Netherlands using two monoclonal antineurofilament antibodies revealed that all tissue sections from the colon affected by Hirschsprung's disease showed heavy staining of hyperplastic axon bundles, which was not seen in normals or in patients with other colorectal disorders (Kluck et al, 1984).

Short and ultra-short segment disease

In short segment Hirschsprung's disease the aganglionic segment only extends for a distance of 2 or 3 cm from the area normally occupied by ganglia (i.e. 2 cm above the dentate line). Male preponderance is less marked than in the more typical form of the disease.

Ultra-short segmental disease is now thought to be due to a very short aganglionic segment in the upper anal canal previously labelled as anal achalasia (Devroede, 1983).

Clinical features

It may seem remarkable that Hirschsprung's disease should persist undiagnosed into adult life but this diagnosis must be considered in patients with intractable constipation (Luukkonen et al, 1990). McCready and Beart (1980) described 50 cases presenting in adult life at the Mayo Clinic between 1950 and 1978. Todd (1977) reported 35 cases seen at St Mark's Hospital between 1954 and 1976. Madsen (1964) reported nine adults from a total of 157 patients with aganglionic disease in a series from Denmark. Barnes et al (1986) reported 22 individuals born with neonatal disease requiring revisional surgery as adults, and a further 29 with adult onset disease. Adult-onset Hirschsprung's disease may affect women and Elliot and Todd (1985) reported that only 26 of 39 patients were men.

In adult patients the principal symptoms are constipation and abdominal distension in approximately two-thirds of cases and severe lower abdominal colic in one-third, the symptoms often commencing in childhood. Soiling, faecal impaction and urinary symptoms are rare. Most patients require laxatives and only one in four is able to defecate without the aid of repeated enemas. Additional symptoms in adult life include anorexia, vomiting, lassitude, weight loss and tiredness. There may be explosive borborygmi. If there is gross abdominal distension there may be cardiac or respiratory embarrassment (Metzgar et al, 1978).

In patients with short or ultra-short Hirschsprung's disease the clinical features may be less typical. Abdominal distension and therefore cardiorespiratory symptoms are rare. There may be a history of incontinence or soiling. Chronic constipation is common, with features of outlet obstruction, and evidence of megarectum is variable.

Investigations

Radiological

A plain radiograph of the abdomen, or even a chest radiograph, may alert the clinician to the possibility of Hirschsprung's disease. Colonic dilatation with a cut-off point in the descending colon or rectosigmoid is typical of an aganglionic segment (Figure 22.2). A barium enema is usually diagnostic in the common form of the disease. Typically, there is a megacolon and a cone-shaped transitional zone leading into a narrow segment, which may be best displayed on a lateral radiograph of the pelvis. The site of the narrow segment is variable (Starling et al, 1986). Gross faecal retention may be evident in the proximal dilated colon (Figure 22.3). The typical narrow segment was only seen in 11 of 26 adults with Hirschsprung's disease (Elliot and Todd, 1985). A narrow rectum is therefore not always found in adult Hirschsprung's disease (Horovitz and Baier, 1974; Taylor, 1984).

In short or ultra-short segment Hirschsprung's disease the barium enema may be completely normal, or there may be delayed colonic transit and impaired rectal evacuation.

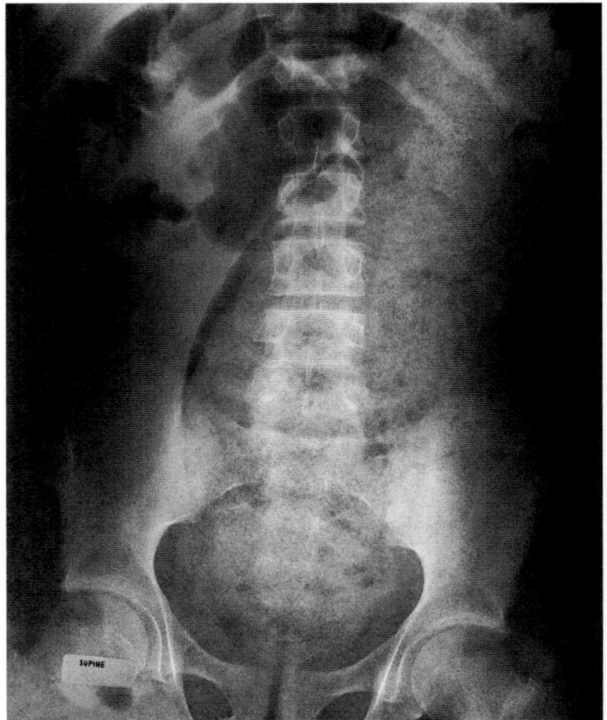

Figure 22.2 Plain abdominal radiograph in Hirschsprung's disease, demonstrating gross megarectum full of solid faecal material.

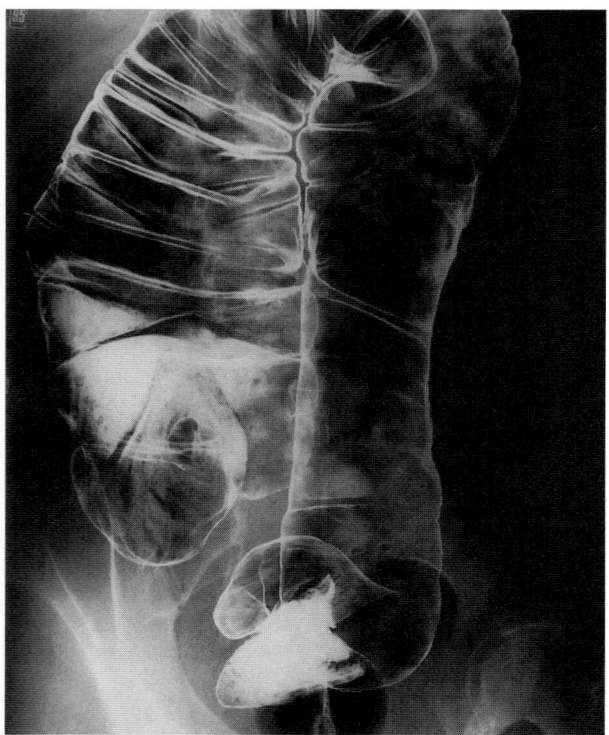

Figure 22.3 Barium enema examination in adult Hirschsprung's disease (mild case). The barium enema demonstrates colonic dilatation and a stricture at the anorectal junction.

Anal manometry

Absence of the rectoanal inhibitory reflex is regarded as diagnostic of Hirschsprung's disease but it is sometimes absent in adult megacolon without an aganglionic segment, as well as in rectal prolapse, faecal incontinence and idiopathic constipation. Absence of the rectoanal inhibitory reflex in Hirschsprung's disease is independent of the proximal extent of the aganglionic bowel (Lawson and Nixon, 1967; Schuster et al, 1968; Arhan et al, 1972). However, the rectoanal inhibitory reflex may be present in short segment disease (Penninckx and Kerremans, 1975a; Barnes et al, 1986; Yoshioka and Keighley, 1987) (Table 22.1). Not only is the rectoanal inhibitory reflex absent in Hirschsprung's disease but when a balloon distends the rectal ampulla pressure within is much greater than in normal subjects, hence the rectum is unable to accommodate faeces within it and will not dilate in response to a wave of peristalsis (Figure 22.4). Measurement of rectal pressure in response to rectal distension may be used to evaluate prognosis and the need for an operation (Arhan et al, 1979).

Faverdin et al (1981) found that a high proportion (41%) of patients with Hirschsprung's disease had ultra-slow waves and that the rectoanal inhibitory reflex was sometimes masked by faecal impaction (Figure 22.5). By contrast, Penninckx and Kerremans (1975a) reported that anal pressures were normal in Hirschsprung's disease and that ultra-slow waves, unlike idiopathic megarectum, were rare.

Biopsy

In view of the preceding comments it is essential to provide the pathologist with full-thickness biopsies or an anorectal myectomy specimen if Hirschsprung's disease, particularly the ultra-short variety, is suspected. Mucosal biopsies are only reliable if histochemical stains for acetylcholinesterase or acid phosphatase are available. Full-thickness biopsy specimens should therefore be taken from different levels or as a strip, as in anorectal myectomy. The only way to obtain a satisfactory biopsy is by excising a full-thickness segment of the rectal wall at different levels or as a strip. The only problem in using anorectal myectomy for diagnosis and possible therapy is the small risk of incontinence. However, the technique of anorectal myectomy may be the only way to make the diagnosis of short segment Hirschsprung's disease (Table 22.1).

Staining for acetylcholinesterase, acid phosphatase, catecholamines and non-specific esterase may help in the diagnosis (Garrett and Howard, 1981). The real advantage of histochemical methods

Table 22.1 Hirschsprung's disease: classification and characteristics.

Type	*Aganglionosis*	*Rectal biopsy*	*Rectoanal inhibitory reflex*	*Barium enema*
Classic disease	Above the anorectal junction	Aganglionosis	Absent	Narrow segment on lateral films of rectum
Short segment disease	Stops around the anorectal junction	Aganglionosis	Absent	Normal
Ultra-short segment disease	Limited to anal canal	Unreliable	May be present	Normal

From Poisson and Devroede (1983).

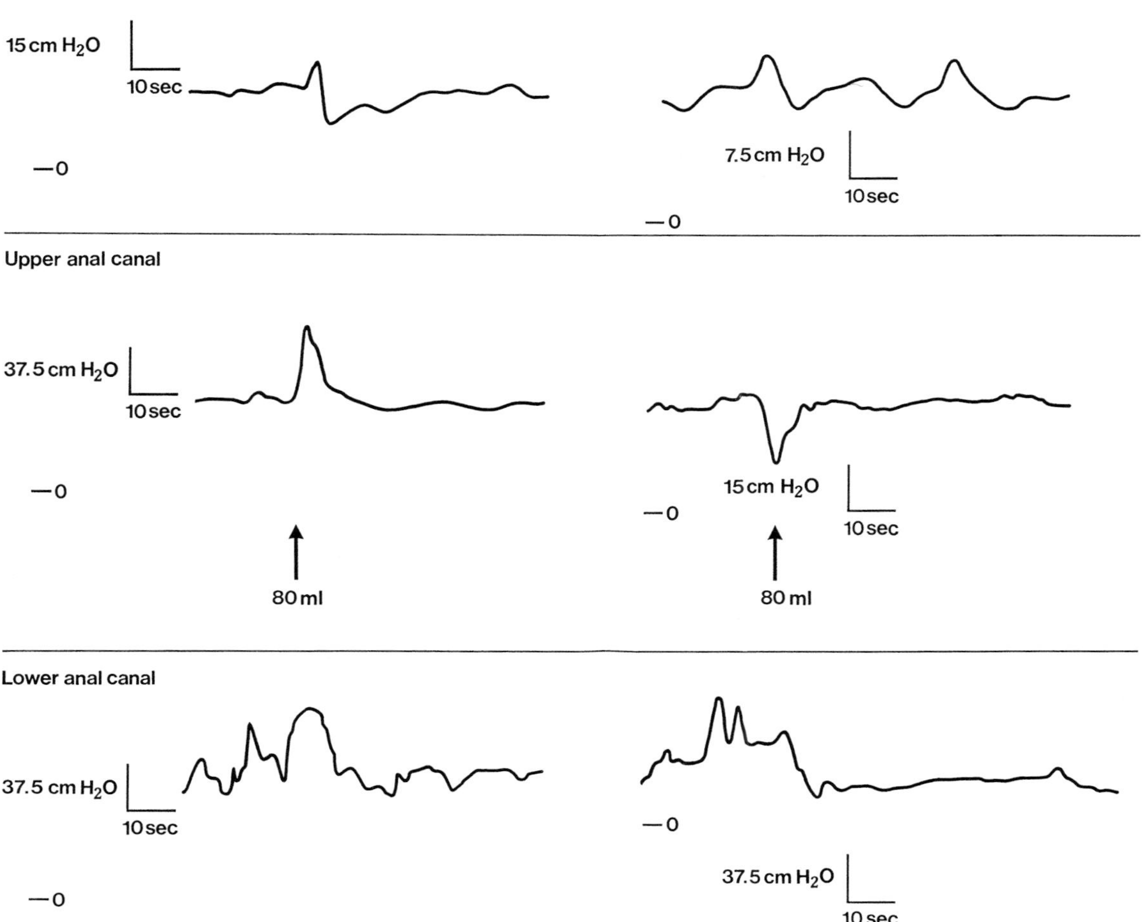

Figure 22.4 Rectoanal inhibitory reflex in Hirschsprung's disease. Simultaneous recordings are obtained from the rectal ampulla and from the upper and lower end of the anal canal (note the difference in scale). The response to the introduction of 80 mL of air into a rectal catheter is compared in Hirschsprung's disease (left-hand trace) and normal subjects (right-hand trace).

is that that diagnosis can be made from mucosal biopsies, which avoids the need for an invasive biopsy technique requiring general anaesthesia. Howard et al (1982) consider that the single most helpful histochemical procedure for establishing the diagnosis of Hirschsprung's disease is staining for acid phosphatase because this gives a clear pictorial display of the intermyenteric ganglia. The diagnosis may be missed if based upon random suction or punch biopsy taken from the midrectum and above.

Differential diagnosis

The differential diagnosis includes Chagas' disease, hypoganglionosis and hyperganglionosis, idiopathic megacolon and chronic idiopathic intestinal pseudo-obstruction.

Surgical treatment

General considerations

There are few reports of the results of operation for adult Hirschsprung's disease. Frequently, clinical series span a long period, in which many different surgical procedures have been used. Operations which produce satisfactory results in children are not necessarily the procedures of choice in adults. One of the largest adult series is of 50 patients managed at the Mayo Clinic between 1950 and 1978

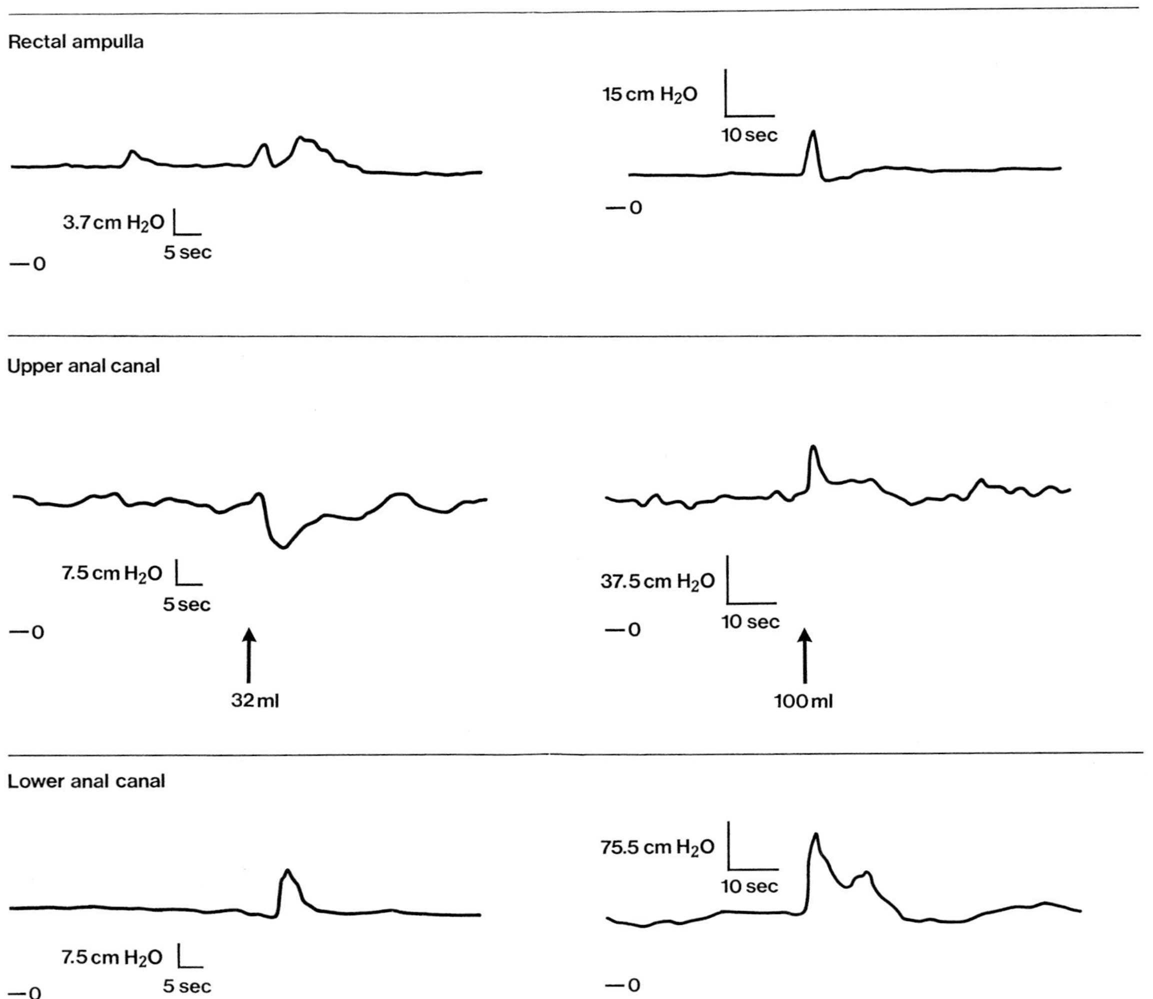

Figure 22.5 Rectoanal inhibitory reflex in Hirschsprung's disease. The response to different volumes of air in a rectal catheter is demonstrated using simultaneous recordings from the rectal ampulla and the upper and lower end of the anal canal.

(McCready and Beart, 1980). The results are summarized in Table 22.2.

The best functional results seem to have been achieved by the Soave procedure, the Duhamel operation and subtotal colectomy. The Swenson operation was accompanied by a high incidence of complications; nevertheless, 14 of 16 patients eventually achieved a satisfactory functional outcome. Anterior resection was associated with an operative death, and one of the five remaining patients had a poor functional result. Results of anorectal myectomy have been disappointing, satisfactory function being achieved in only seven of 13 patients. Somewhat surprisingly, subtotal colectomy was associated with an apparently satisfactory outcome even though a part of the aganglionic segment was not removed. The retained aganglionic rectum was associated with at least two complications attributed to a persistent functional obstruction in the rectum.

Others suggest, however, that both anterior resection and subtotal colectomy give indifferent results (Rosin et al, 1950; Jennings, 1967). Hamdy and Scobie (1984) suggest that combined anterior resection and anorectal myectomy may be beneficial, but the view of most authorities is that the aganglionic segment should be totally removed or bypassed using the Duhamel procedure (Fairgreave, 1963; State, 1963; Todd, 1977; Elliot and Todd, 1985; Natsikas and Sbarounis, 1987). The Duhamel procedure may require a covering stoma for decompression, or the proximal colon may be delivered

Table 22.2 Results of surgical treatment for adult Hirschsprung's disease.

Operation	*n*	*Good result*	*Complications*
Soave procedure	3	3	Leak + fistula Cuff abscess
Duhamel procedure	4	4	Urinary retention
Swenson procedure	16	14	Abscess (3) Stricture Impotent + urinary retention Impotent + haematoma + leak
Anorectal myectomy	13	7	Haematoma
Anterior resection	6	4	Death from leak
Subtotal colectomy and ileorectal anastomosis	7	7	Pelvic abscess Faecal fistula
Other procedure	1		

From McCready and Beart (1980).

through the rectal stump as a perineal colostomy. Kim et al (1995) report the results of 11 patients treated by the Duhamel operation. Two developed fistula-in-ano at the anastomotic site. They therefore indicated that a covering stoma is sometimes necessary. The functional results in this Korean series were excellent.

Barnes et al (1986) report excellent results in 17 of 20 patients with adult onset Hirschsprung's disease treated by the Duhamel operation, compared with a satisfactory outcome in 7 of 11 patients following the Soave sleeve resection and coloanal anastomosis. A review of 39 patients treated by the Duhamel technique provided evidence of satisfactory bowel function in 36 patients, without mortality, and only six required a defunctioning stoma.

A review of the literature suggests that the Duhamel procedure, the Soave operation, Swenson's operation and anorectal myectomy (Table 22.3) are the procedures that have been used most widely for the management of adult Hirschsprung's disease, hence further description of surgical treatment will be confined to these options.

Soave operation

The Soave procedure involves resection of as much of the aganglionic segment as possible, then stripping the mucosa from the retained rectal stump (Soave, 1964). The operation is now usually performed as a one-stage procedure by anastomosing the ganglionic colon to the anal canal inside a sleeve of anorectal muscular tube (Boley, 1968). The coloanal anastomosis is performed using an intra-anal technique. The disadvantage of the operation for the treatment of Hirschsprung's disease is that an aganglionic segment of rectal muscular tube is left *in situ* even though the mucosal disease may have been excised. Despite

Table 22.3 Review of results of four surgical procedures for adult Hirschsprung's disease.

Operation	*n*	*Good result*	*Complications*
Soave endorectal procedure	16	9	Impotence (2) Soiling (4)
Swenson procedure	37	33	Rectovaginal fistula (1) Impotence (2) Abscess (3) Dehiscence (3)
Duhamel procedure	53	47	Soiling (2) Dehiscence (3)
Anorectal myectomy	30	15	Haematoma (1) Repeated myectomy (1) Anterior resection needed (3)

From Metzgar et al (1978), McCready and Beart (1980), Hamdy and Scobie (1984), Elliot and Todd (1985), Barnes et al (1986) and Natsikas and Sbarounis (1987).

these theoretical objections, the results of this procedure in adult patients have been quite encouraging.

San Filippo et al (1972) reported on the use of the Soave operation in 18 patients, although most were children and there was a high incidence of complications, including anastomotic leaks (17%) and late strictures (11%). In their study the Soave operation gave better results than the Swenson operation or the Duhamel procedure. Two further isolated reports indicate that the Soave operation was associated with good functional results in adult patients (McGavity and Cody, 1974). Care must be taken to avoid damaging the pelvic nerves at the pelvic brim, but a close rectal dissection inside the superior haemorrhoidal pedicle is probably unnecessary and the mesorectum can be removed as in restorative proctocolectomy.

Surgical procedure

It is important to have an accurate assessment of the length of the aganglionic segment preoperatively. Many of these patients have an established stoma, either in the sigmoid or transverse colon, before operation. It is therefore wise to obtain biopsies from the anorectum and from the stoma preoperatively. If there are ganglia in the rectum there is no need for operative biopsies since the length of the aganglionic segment is known. If there are ganglia in a sigmoid colostomy despite an aganglionic rectum, no operative biopsies will be needed and it is advisable to use the bowel proximal to the stoma for coloanal anastomosis. The need for operative biopsy arises when the upper rectum is aganglionic and the patient has a transverse colostomy or if the patient has no stoma at all. Under these circumstances most surgeons would wish to retain the colostomy for decompression and to define the site of normal ganglia in the left colon so that this can be used for the anastomosis. One can usually judge the length of the aganglionic segment preoperatively by barium enema but operative submucosal biopsies are necessary to confirm this.

If the patient has no stoma, mechanical preparation is often quite difficult and may have to be extended over 2 or 3 days. We usually find that if patients are maintained on a liquid diet and sodium picosulphate is given, followed by a rectal washout, mechanical preparation is usually satisfactory. However, the quality of preparation should be carefully checked and, if inadequate, further measures will need to be taken. If there is a stoma a standard preparation of the proximal colon is performed, together with a distal colostomy washout.

Operation should be performed under general anaesthesia, the patient being placed in the Lloyd Davies position, catheterized and with a sandbag placed under the buttocks. The whole perineum should lie well beyond the end of the operating table. Subcutaneous heparin and compression stockings or leg bags are advised with perioperative antimicrobial prophylaxis. If the patient has no stoma, a site for a transverse colostomy or a loop ileostomy should have been marked preoperatively.

The abdomen is opened using a long midline incision. The proximal extent of the bowel for resection and anastomosis is selected and, if necessary, confirmed by immediate biopsy by taking a submucosal disc measuring 1 cm × 1 cm (Figure 22.6a). If the results of frozen section biopsy are required, some other aspect of the operation can usually be performed while waiting for these results. The entire left colon and splenic flexure can be mobilized, carefully preserving the vascular arcades between the territory of the middle colic artery and the upper left colonic vessels. If a sigmoid colostomy is present, this can be detached from the skin and anterior abdominal wall, any colonic contents being contained by applying tapes around the bowel above and below the stoma (Figure 22.6b).

By this stage the precise length of the aganglionic segment should be known and the colon can be transected through a zone known to contain ganglia. The proximal end of the divided colon should be protected by placing a finger of a glove over the Potts' clamp or by stapling the divided bowel. The distal large bowel (usually the descending colon, sigmoid and rectum) is mobilized, taking care not to damage the pelvic autonomic plexus. The vascular supply to the sigmoid colon is divided but the superior haemorrhoidal vessels are preserved. Distal mobilization continues down to the pelvic peritoneum, which is divided close to the rectum.

At this point opinion differs, one viewpoint is that further dissection of the rectum in the pelvis should be avoided to prevent damage to the autonomic nerves. If this view is held, the rectal muscular wall is divided at this point around the circumference of the bowel and a plane developed between the muscle coat and the mucosa of the entire rectum. To facilitate this manoeuvre, a weak adrenaline solution can be used to develop the submucosal plane so that troublesome bleeding can be prevented. It is preferable not to divide the rectum but to use the mucosal attachment as a convenient retractor so that this submucosal plane can be opened around the circumference of the rectum. Sometimes this is impossible and the rectum will have to be divided. Tissue forceps are then applied to the cut edges of the rectal mucosa and the submucosal plane

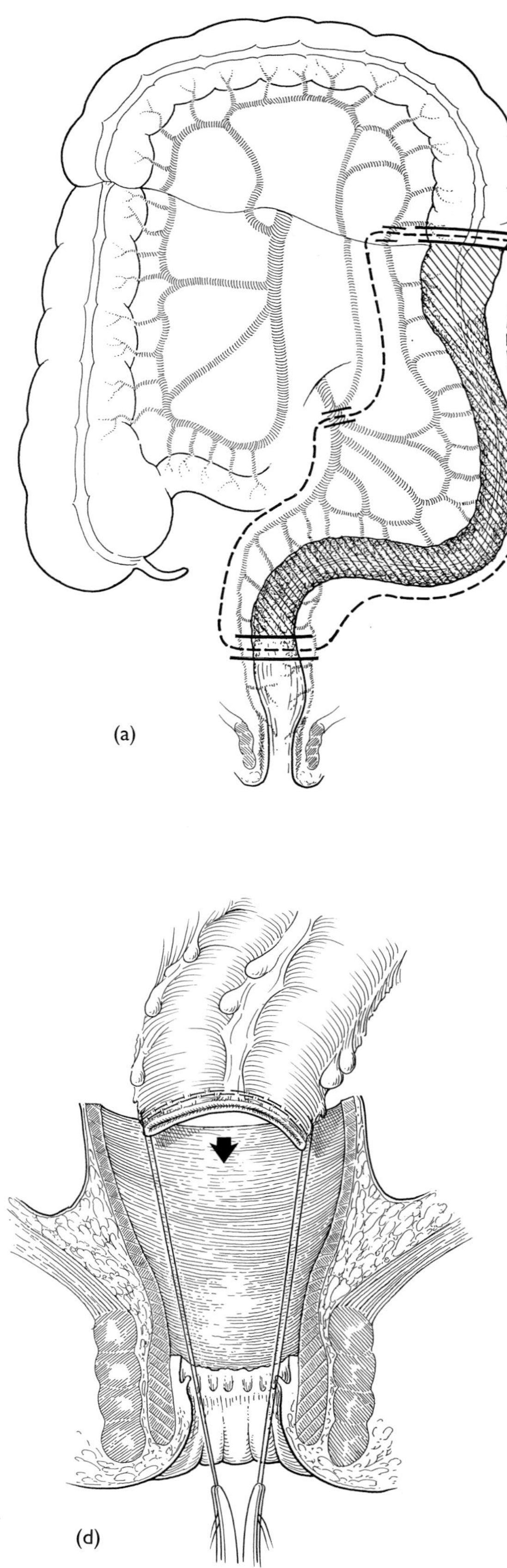

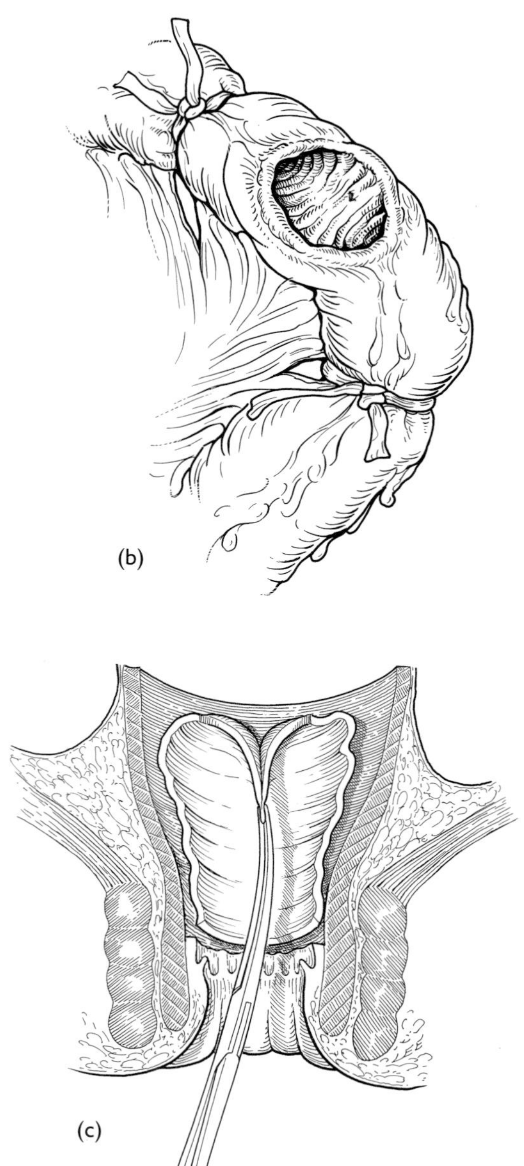

Figure 22.6a–d The Soave operation. (a) The extent of resection depends upon the length of the aganglionic segment. In the diagram, the aganglionic segment commences in the descending colon and continues down into the anorectum. The resection therefore involves excision of the entire aganglionic segment down to the pelvic floor, as well as approximately 5 cm of normally innervated colon beyond the splenic flexure. (b) If there is a proximal colostomy it is convenient to isolate the bowel on either side of it with tapes in order to minimize contamination. (c) The rectum has been transected at the pelvic floor and the rectal mucosa of the residual rectal stump is excised to just above the dentate line, leaving a rectal muscular sleeve. (d) The proximal innervated colon has been transected with staples to minimize faecal contamination. Two stay sutures have been applied to the cut end of the colon, which is being delivered through the rectal muscular tube to the perianal skin. (*Continued*)

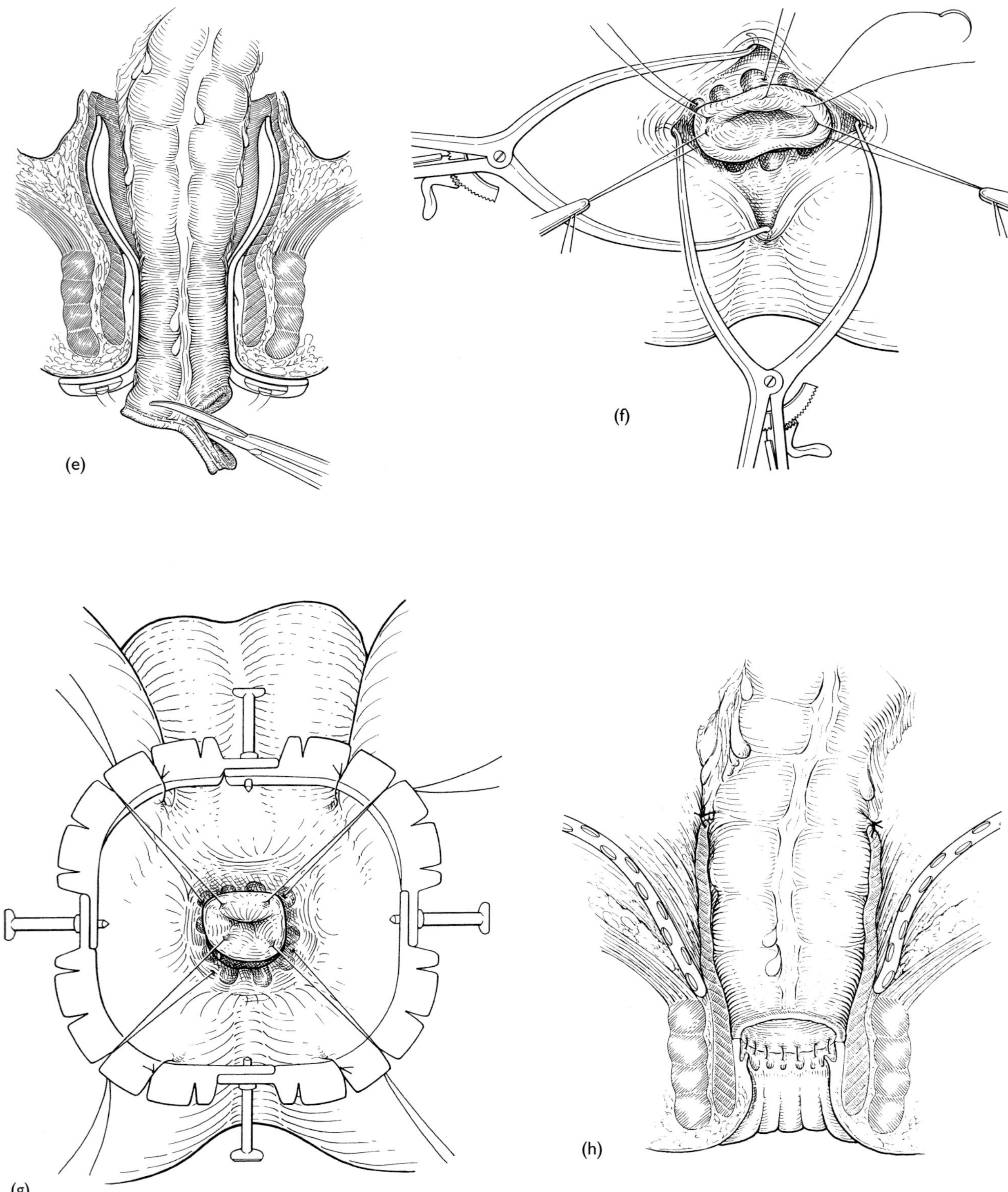

Figure 22.6e–h (e) A Park's retractor has been inserted into the anorectum and the staple line is being excised from the proximal colon. (f) The coloanal anastomosis may be fashioned with two Gelpi retractors set at right-angles to one another. This helps to efface the anus and allow direct coloanal anastomosis under vision. (g) An alternative method of coloanal anastomosis is with the use of a Lone star retractor. (h) The Soave procedure completed: sutured end to end straight coloanal anastomosis in a rectal sleeve.

developed in the same way. The aim of the dissection is to strip the entire mucosa from the rectal muscular tube. It is usually possible to continue this mucosal excision to within 5 cm of the anal verge, at which point the remaining mucosal excision will be performed from below. We prefer not to evert the mucosal tube through the anal canal, as described by Coran and Weintraub (1976), since we believe that this technique compromises anal function.

The procedure described above is tedious and often results in a muscular tube which is frayed and somewhat avascular. We now prefer to divide the superior rectal vessels and continue the rectal dissection down to the pelvic floor just behind the mesorectum. If the dissection is kept close to the rectum, damage to the autonomic plexus should not occur. The dissection can be taken down to the levator ani and at this point the rectum can be divided and the entire mucosal excision performed from below (Figure 22.6c).

Perineal mucosal protectomy can only be performed satisfactorily with the use of the self-retaining anorectal retractor. The mucosal excision is started after prior infiltration of a weak adrenaline solution in the submucosal plane. The anal mucosa is divided transversely just above the dentate line around its circumference. The cut edges of the anal mucosa are held by a series of clips. A pair of Gelpi retractors is then inserted between the internal sphincter and the mucosa. With the index finger of the left hand inside the rectum grasping the clips of the mucosa it is possible to proceed with the mucosal excision well up into the rectum. The lower part of the mucosal excision is the most difficult because of the close attachment of the mucosa to the internal sphincter at this point. This is also the area where bleeding is most troublesome. Once the rectum is reached, the mucosal excision is much easier and a curved Kocher's retractor provides good access to the limit of the transected rectum. The mucosa can now be removed, usually as an intact cylinder, and a gauze pack soaked in adrenaline inserted into the rectum to control any residual bleeding.

Attention must now be directed to the proximal colon. The inferior mesenteric artery should be divided about 2 cm from its origin on the aorta so as to avoid damaging the sympathetic nerves; the inferior mesenteric vein is then divided under the pancreas as it joins the splenic vein. The entire left colon is mobilized with the splenic flexure and its cut end is delivered into the pelvis to assess whether there is an adequate length for anastomosis to the anal canal without tension. Two stay sutures are placed on the proximal colon. After reinserting the self-retaining anal retractor the stay sutures are passed through the rectal sleeve and out through the anal canal (Figure 22.6d). The proximal colon is drawn through the sleeve so that an anastomosis can be performed using a peranal technique. If the end of the colon has been closed with staples the staple line is excised (Figure 22.6e). Before commencing the anastomoses it is wise to pass two suction drains into the sleeve and out through the anal canal, since their placement at a later stage in the operation is difficult. A temporary protecting colostomy, caecostomy or ileostomy is usually advised if a stoma is not already present. One operator can be conveniently fashioning the stoma while the anastomosis is being performed by the other.

The endoanal anastomosis is performed in a manner similar to that described for coloanal anastomosis in carcinoma of the rectum. Two self-retaining anal Gelpi retractors are used at right-angles to each other or a Parks' retractor with the blades in the two lateral positions. A series of interrupted 2/0 Vicryl sutures are used (on a 25-mm needle) to anastomose the anal mucosa and internal sphincter to the full thickness of the ganglionic colon. Approximately 10–12 sutures are placed at the upper and lower aspects of the circumference of the anus and then tied. The Parks' retractor is withdrawn and reinserted inside the colon with the blades overlying the area of the suture line. Completion of the anastomosis is achieved by placing 8–10 sutures between the descending colon and the anal canal over the lateral quadrants (Figure 22.6f,g). If Gelpi retractors or the Lone star retractor is used they do not need to be readjusted during the anastomosis. Two suction drains are placed by the abdominal surgeon so that they lie in the sleeve between the rectal muscular tube and the descending colon. Two further suction drains are placed in the pelvis if necessary (Figure 22.6h).

Provided a defunctioning colostomy or ileostomy has been raised the abdominal wall can be closed. If the operation takes more than 4 hours it is advisable to give a second dose of antibiotic during the procedure. The protecting stoma should not be opened until the abdominal skin incision has been sutured. An immediate mucocutaneous suture with Prolene for the stoma completes the operation.

Patients will need to be maintained on an intravenous infusion for 3–4 days until bowel sounds have returned and flatus is appearing through the stoma. Mobilization is encouraged as early as possible and the patient can begin to take food after 3–4 days. The catheter can usually be removed at this time, as can the closed suction drains. It is a good idea to encourage early reuse of the sphincter muscles by physiotherapy and pelvic floor exercises.

The stoma sutures can be removed 5–6 days after operation and the skin sutures at 10 days. Provided the patient is confident with the management of the stoma, they can usually be discharged from hospital soon after the stoma is functioning.

Apart from sepsis, another feared complication is that of bleeding into the sleeve from inadequate haemostasis after mucosal excision. If this occurs, the best plan is to return the patient to theatre, to pack the anastomosis site with ribbon gauze soaked in proflavine and to insert two further suction drains between the suture lines. This is much easier for the patient to tolerate than balloon tamponade (McCourtney et al, 1996). One of the more troublesome sources of infection is within the sleeve. This may sometimes require drainage by removing one of the coloanal sutures. However, serious pelvic sepsis is rarely a problem since the operation site is protected by a defunctioning stoma.

The patient may be seen once or twice after the operation and is usually readmitted 3–4 months later for closure of the stoma. It is important that the coloanal anastomosis be carefully assessed before closure to exclude any continuing sepsis, to be certain that there is no stricture and to assess the function of the anal sphincters, preferably by manometry. After closure of the stoma, the patient should be followed up so that bowel function can be assessed.

Swenson operation

Swenson and Bill (1948) proposed a different method for the treatment of congenital megacolon. This involved a complete anorectal resection with coloanal anastomosis. The technique involves eversion of the anal canal and secondary anastomosis after pulling the descending colon through the anal sphincters and delaying the anastomosis until the blood supply to the descending colon is known to be satisfactory. This two-stage operation is now merely historical.

In 1975 Swenson et al reported their 25-year results. Seventy-one of their 282 patients were over the age of 10 years. There was a moderate incidence of complications which included anastomotic breakdown in 5%, rectal stricture in 6% and 4% required a colostomy. Serious sepsis occurred in 3% of patients. Despite these complications the long-term results were quite good. By contrast, the Mayo Clinic experience of this operation indicated that results were far from satisfactory (McCready and Beart, 1980). Six of the 17 patients had serious complications, and impotence was reported in two. Three of their patients required colostomies because of anastomotic breakdown and two required secondary operation because of poor functional results.

We have no experience with this procedure, having relied upon the Soave procedure or the Duhamel operation for the management of adult Hirschsprung's disease. Results with the Swenson operation seem to be unsatisfactory even in experienced hands (Clausen and Davis, 1963). The operation carries the risk of imperfect continence due to anorectal eversion and for these reasons we do not propose to describe the procedure in detail.

Duhamel procedure

The Duhamel operation was introduced (Duhamel, 1960) to overcome three important disadvantages of all previous operations: (1) to avoid impotence by completely eliminating a pelvic dissection; (2) to minimize the complications of an end-to-end anastomosis since leakage was common, particularly when attempting immediate anastomosis of the dilated proximal colon to the anal canal; and (3) to preserve the anterior aganglionic rectum to establish a reservoir to accommode faecal material before defecation.

The original procedure required modification to avoid stool becoming sequestrated in the anterior aganglionic rectal pouch. Furthermore, stenosis of the side-to-side colorectal anastomosis tended to produce a spur between the lumen of both viscera (Soper and Miller, 1968). The aganglionic segment tended to progressively dilate and balloon forward. Secondary surgical procedures to remove more of the aganglionic rectum and to excise the spur resulted in improved functional results in all five patients reported by San Filippo et al (1972) in whom this form of reoperation was advised.

Todd's experience (1977) of the Duhamel procedure has been encouraging, with no serious postoperative complications. From his extensive personal experience he believes that this is the operation of choice for adult Hirschsprung's disease. The overall results of this procedure are generally good, and with the increasing use of stapling devices the operation is quicker to perform and less demanding. Furthermore, it is not necessary to retain very much of the anterior rectum (Gordon, 1983). Satisfactory results have also been reported by Louw (1961) and Ehrenpreis et al (1966). Natsikas and Sbarounis (1987) found that it was wise to use a covering or preliminary stoma if the proximal bowel was dilated. Elliot and Todd (1985) reported results in 39 patients without mortality: 13% developed a dehiscence but all except three patients were continent at follow-up, with a bowel habit of at least three stools per week. We have encountered one stricture which was easily resolved by restapling the spur (Figure 22.7a,b).

Surgical procedure

The original operation consisted of rectal mobilization and transection of the rectal stump with excision of all of the aganglionic bowel except for the low rectum. A posterior end-to-side colorectal anastomosis was then constructed using conventional suture techniques and the spur between the colon and rectum then crushed with a clamp, which was left *in situ* through the anus until it had sloughed.

Gordon (1983) described the operation using stapling devices for the entire reconstruction. Such a technique seems logical and potentially much safer than the conventional suture technique.

Preparation of the patient and assessment of the length of aganglionic segment to be excised is precisely the same as already described for the Soave procedure. The patient is placed supine in the Lloyd Davies position, catheterized and given antibiotics. The left colon and sigmoid colon are mobilized through a midline laparotomy incision. The left colon is transected at a point convenient for anastomosis and through a ganglionic segment of the colon (Figure 22.7c). A Prolene purse-string suture is placed around the proximal colon. A Potts' clamp, which acts as a useful retractor, is placed on the distal cut end of the colon. The rectum is carefully mobilized and the superior haemorrhoidal vessels preserved. Dissection should proceed down to the levator ani and a tunnel then developed between the posterior aspect of the rectum and the puborectalis sling (Figure 22.7d). At this point the assistant inserts a circular (CEEA) stapling gun into the anorectum. The surgeon then guides the cartridge holder backwards by lifting the handle of the instrument upwards, so that the ring of the head of the gun can be seen just above the puborectalis sling at the back of the lower third of the rectum (Figure 22.7e). The central pin is then advanced through the back of the rectum, removed and the proximal ganglionic bowel with the anvil is secured within it through a purse string. The proximal colon is then

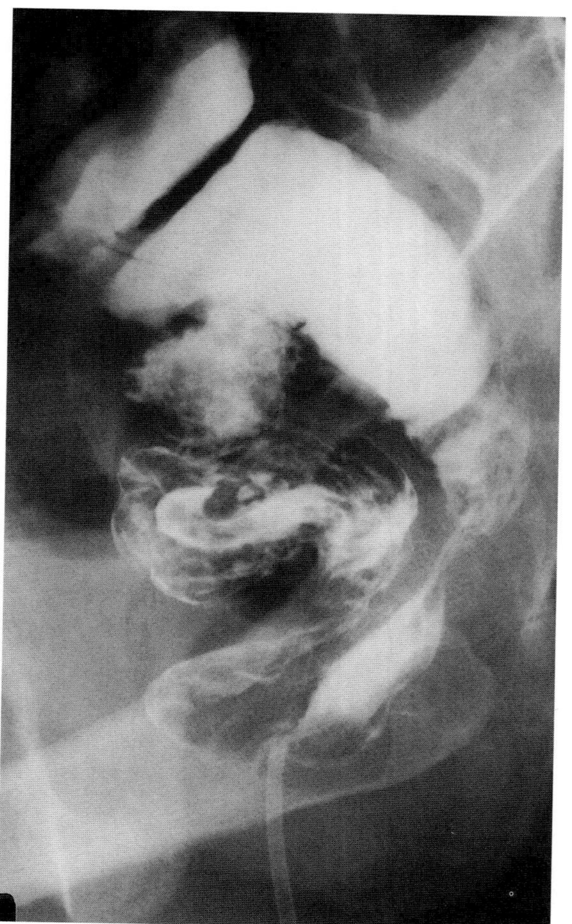

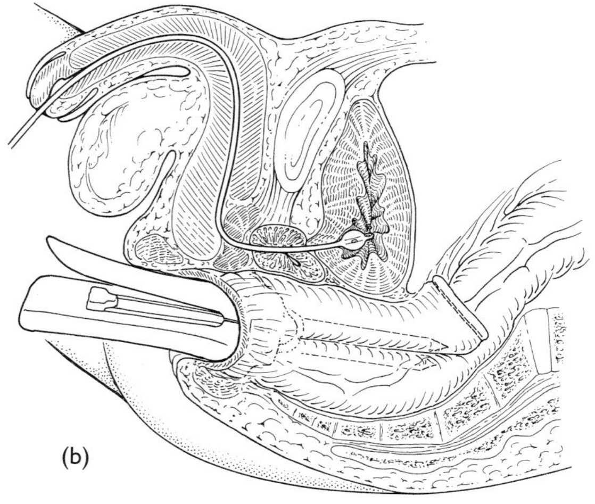

Figure 22.7a,b Post Duhamel stricture. (a) A stricture after a Duhamel procedure which was managed by stapled division of the spur (see b). (b) The spur between the back of the rectum and the anterior aspect of the colon is divided with a long linear staple cutter, preferably at least 90 mm. *(Continued)*

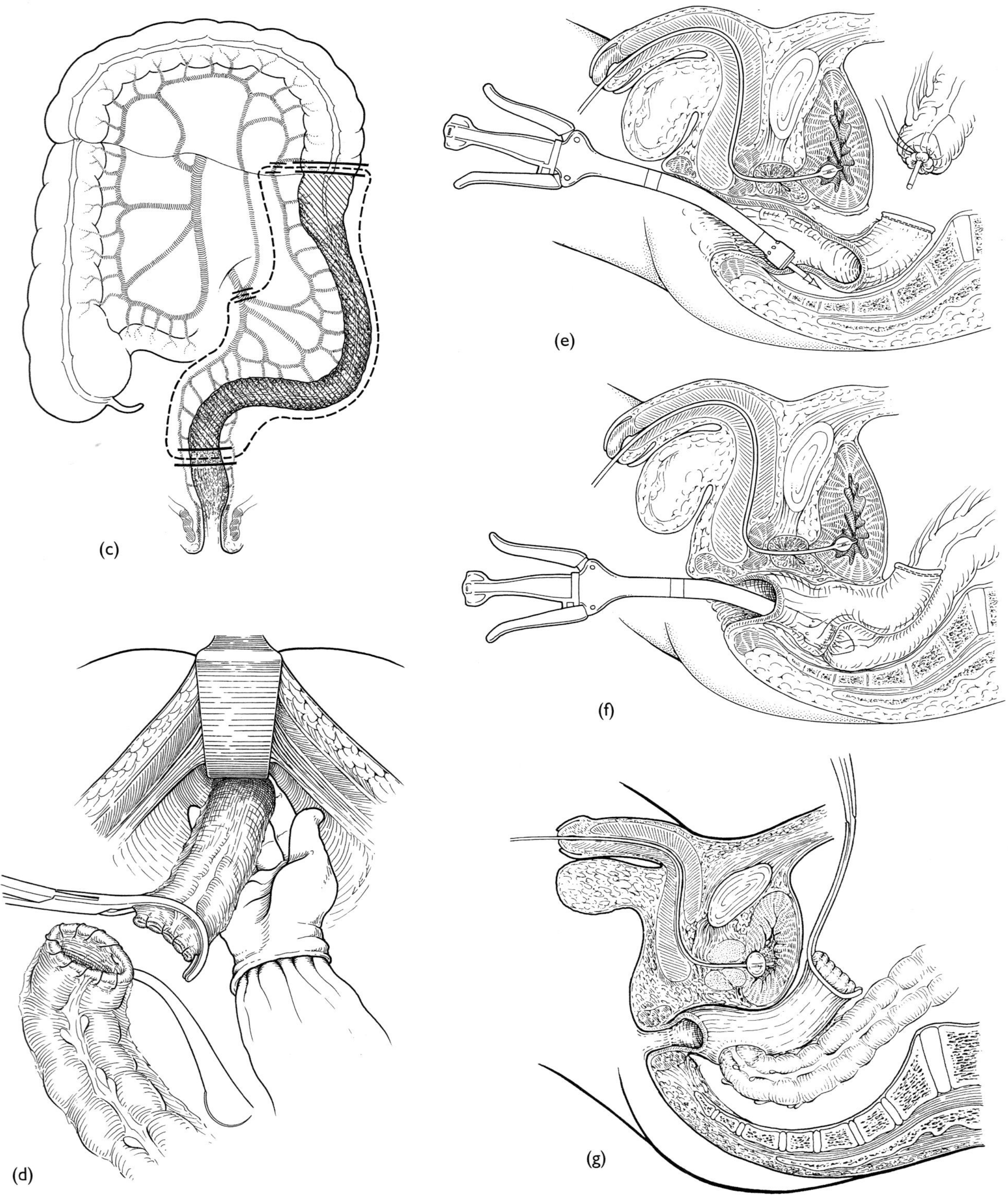

Figure 22.7c–g Duhamel procedure. (c) The aganglionic segment is excised together with approximately 5 cm of normally innervated proximal colon. The distal transection line is at the level of the pelvic brim. (d) The denervated rectal stump is mobilized down to the tip of the coccyx. A purse-string whip stitch is placed around the distal end of the innervated colon. (e) The upper rectum has been transected with a TL 55. A premium CEA is introduced into the low rectal ampulla. The pin in the cartridge holder is advanced through the back of the rectum. The anvil is placed into the proximal colon with a purse-string suture. (f) A stapled end-to-side colorectal anastomosis is achieved with the circular stapling device. (g) If the linear staple cutter has been too short to achieve a complete side-to-side anastomosis, a second enterotomy may need to be made to complete the anastomosis. (*Continued*)

guided down so that the anvil pin is pushed into the receiver in the cartridge holder (Figure 22.7f). The circular stapling device is then closed and fired. The tilting anvil facilitates atraumatic removal of the circular stapling device, thus completing the end-to-side colorectal anastomosis (Figure 22.7g).

The side-to-side anastomosis between the posterior rectum and the descending colon must now be constructed using the GIA 90 or TLC 75 stapler. The GIA or TLC is introduced from below through the completed circular staple ring (Figure 22.7h). A line of staples is used to construct the lower anastomosis. If this is not long enough to achieve a satisfactory functional result, and this is usually the case if the regular GIA 50 or TLC 50 is used, then a second row of staples should be introduced, where possible from below. This may not be possible, in which case the abdominal surgeon must make two small enterotomies in the colon and rectum approximately 10 cm above the lower line of the staples

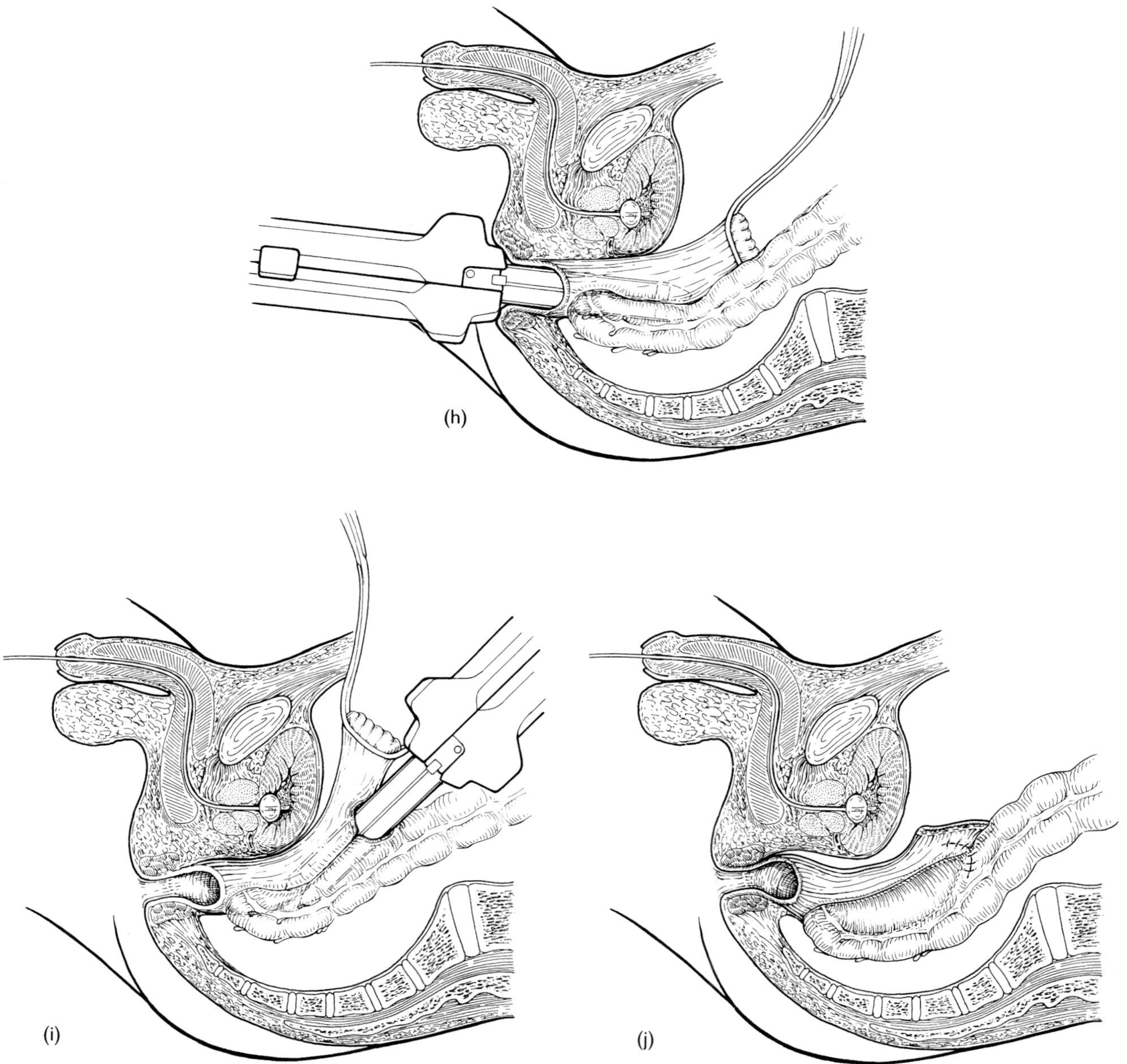

Figure 22.7h–i (h) The spur is being stapled and divided using a linear staple cutter. The lower aspect of the stapled anastomosis is performed through the stapled colorectal anastomosis. (i) The upper aspect of the side-to-side anastomosis is performed through a separate rectotomy and colotomy as shown. (j) The rectotomy and colotomy is closed, which completes the operation.

(Figure 22.7i). A second stapler is then inserted pointing downwards to the end of the lower row of staples. The two enterotomies must now be closed (Figure 22.7j).

The lower anastomosis should be carefully inspected and palpated. If there appears to be a large spur between the colon and the rectum, the intervening tissue can be grasped with tissue forceps and excised by application of a third line of staples, using the GIA instrument from below (see Figure 27.6).

The entire reconstruction can be tested under water by filling the pelvis and injecting 50 mL of air into the anus from below. Any air leakage should be easily defined and any defect oversewn. Using this technique, Gordon (1983) does not believe that a proximal defunctioning stoma is necessary provided bowel preparation is impeccable. Postoperative management is similar to the Soave procedure but because there is no proximal stoma, the period of intravenous fluid support is usually rather longer and food is restricted until the passage of flatus is well established.

There are no specific postoperative complications; indeed, clinical progress is usually remarkably straightforward. Most patients can leave hospital after 10–12 days. Regular review of the functional results is advised.

Anorectal myectomy

This operation was first introduced for the treatment of Hirschsprung's disease in 1966 by Lynn. He proposed that excising a segment of anorectal smooth muscle might be of value in three groups of patients: (1) those with aganglionosis involving only a short segment of the anorectum; (2) patients with residual symptoms after treatment for aganglionic megacolon by low anterior resection; and (3) those who have had a poor functional result following a pull-through procedure. Five of the eight patients over the age of 10 years treated by this procedure had a good result when Lynn and van Heerden reviewed their results in 1975. All patients in whom ganglion cells could be identified in the upper end of the myectomy specimen were asymptomatic following this operation. Lee and Koh (1977), however, reported disappointing results in two of three patients, although both were thought to have a longer than anticipated aganglionic segment. The Mayo Clinic experience was also disappointing, with only seven of 13 patients achieving a satisfactory result (McCready and Beart, 1980). Ganglia were present in the proximal segments of the myectomy specimen in two of the five patients who were considered to be treatment failures. This implies that the success of the operation is not always guaranteed by excising smooth muscle up to the ganglionic bowel.

In our opinion, anorectal myectomy is a diagnostic procedure which may be of therapeutic value in short segment Hirschsprung's disease but can be complicated by impaired continence (Yoshioka and Keighley, 1987; Pinho et al, 1989). Generally the operation is simple, complications are few and in some patients no further surgical procedure is required (Nissan et al, 1971).

Surgical procedure

Standard bowel preparation and single-dose antibiotic cover is advised. Although the operation may be performed using a caudal or spinal anaesthetic, it is much easier to gain access to the anorectal smooth muscle with the patient under general anaesthesia and with some muscle relaxation so that a self-retaining retractor can be placed inside the anorectal ring to keep the sphincter dilated. Urinary catheterization and anticoagulants are not used.

The patient is placed in the lithotomy position with a sandbag under the buttocks. A headlamp is advised. A Parks' self-retaining anal retractor is inserted into the anal canal. A 20-mL syringe containing saline or a 1:300 000 solution of adrenaline in saline is used to infiltrate the submucosal and intersphincteric planes in the midline posteriorly (Figure 22.8a). A transverse incision is made 2 cm above the dentate line from 4 o'clock to 8 o'clock. The mucosa of the anal canal is then raised off the fibres of the internal sphincter, and subsequently the circular fibres of the rectal muscle, using scissors and a pair of fine dissecting forceps for a distance of 10 cm (Figure 22.8b); haemorrhage is controlled by diathermy. The dissection should proceed well into the rectal ampulla (Figure 22.8c), hence adequate exposure and retraction are essential. At this point the third blade of the anal retractor is placed under the mobilized mucosa.

Once the submucosal plane has been developed, the lower margin of the internal sphincter must be defined by dissecting the lower anal mucosa off the smooth muscle (Figure 22.8c). This allows a second plane to be developed between the internal and external sphincters using scissor dissection which must be extended well beyond the anorectal ring into the rectum (Figure 22.8d). A strip of the internal sphincter and rectal smooth muscle approximately 1 cm wide is then excised (Figure 22.8e) as high as is possible into the rectum (Figure 22.8f). Haemostasis should then be carefully secured and the specimen

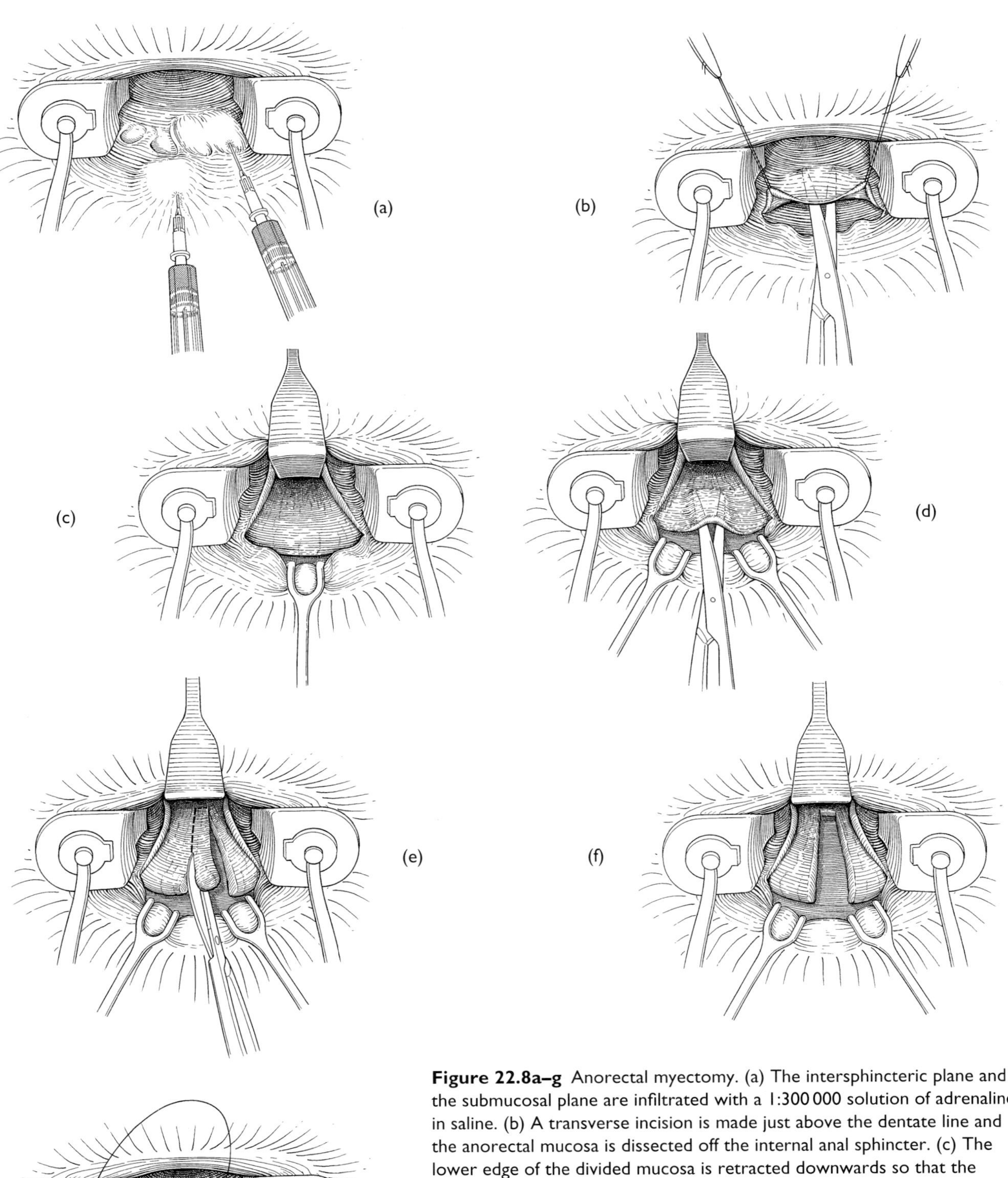

Figure 22.8a–g Anorectal myectomy. (a) The intersphincteric plane and the submucosal plane are infiltrated with a 1:300 000 solution of adrenaline in saline. (b) A transverse incision is made just above the dentate line and the anorectal mucosa is dissected off the internal anal sphincter. (c) The lower edge of the divided mucosa is retracted downwards so that the lower aspect of the internal anal sphincter can be seen. A Kocher's retractor is placed underneath the mobilized anorectal mucosa. Alternatively, the third blade of a Park's retractor may be used. (d) The intersphincteric plane is developed so that the internal anal sphincter and the rectal circular muscle is dissected free in the posterior midline. (e) A longitudinal strip of internal anal sphincter and rectal circular muscle is excised over a distance of 8–10 cm. (f) Completed anorectal myectomy. (g) After haemostasis the anal mucosal incision is closed with a running catgut or Vicryl suture.

orientated for subsequent histological examination. The mucosal defect should be closed to achieve haemostasis (Figure 22.8g).

A sponge or Vaseline gauze pack may be left in the anorectum for the first few hours after operation to prevent local bleeding. There are no specific aspects to postoperative management apart from the avoidance of faecal impaction by laxatives, if this is necessary. Patients are usually allowed home the same day provided there is no bleeding. Patients are seen 2–3 weeks later to review their progress and the results of histological examination.

ADULT IDIOPATHIC MEGACOLON AND MEGARECTUM

Adult megacolon is idiopathic and may be the end-result of long-standing chronic constipation. Until recently this entity was not fully recognized as being distinct from Hirschsprung's disease. Indeed we believe that short and ultra-short segment Hirschsprung's disease is probably a form of idiopathic megabowel which can only be reliably distinguished from Hirschsprung's disease by a full-thickness rectal biopsy, since an absent rectoanal inhibitory reflex is not necessarily diagnostic of aganglionosis. Conservative treatment with faecal disimpaction and laxatives is sometimes successful but surgical treatment is often indicated (Watkins, 1966). Anal dilatation, sphincterotomy or anorectal myectomy may be tried in patients with high resting anal canal pressures but rarely achieves lasting benefit if there is a megarectum, and can compromise continence. Subtotal colectomy and caecorectal or ileorectal anastomosis give good results if the dilating disease is confined to the colon. If dilatation is confined to the rectum alone, some form of rectal excision or bypass is preferable, either using the Duhamel operation or preferably by total rectosigmoid excision and coloanal anastomosis. If, as is sometimes the case, the entire large bowel is dilated and non-functioning, restorative proctocolectomy and ileoanal anastomosis may be the best surgical option, provided sphincter function is adequate.

Aetiology

Idiopathic megacolon and megarectum is a rare disorder of uncertain aetiology. We recognize that there is a group of patients with primary dilating disease who are usually referred in adolescence or early adult life. Most patients have prolonged constipation (Belliveau et al, 1982) and are found to have a congenital or acquired degenerative abnormality in the autonomic plexus of the large bowel (Smith, 1968). We used to be of the opinion that these patients did not have Hirschsprung's disease and that the brunt of the disease usually occurred in the rectum with proximal extension to the rest of the colon in time (Stewart et al, 1994). Recent studies, however, have suggested disordered innervation of the longitudinal muscle (Gattuso et al, 1996a) resulting in thickening of the longitudinal compared with the circular muscle of the rectum (Gattuso et al, 1997). In our experience, some of these patients have had long-standing cerebral degeneration: hydrocephalus, birth trauma or ischaemic disease. Others have epilepsy or are on long-term psychiatric medication. A few have had surgery for anorectal agenesis at birth. In some patients dilatation of the bladder and ureters is found. In patients with dilating disease confined to the colon, there is often a history of repeated caecal and sigmoid volvulus.

Others have a different experience of this disorder. Thus Barnes et al (1986) at St Marks Hospital describes two groups: (1) those with symptoms which commence in childhood, who do badly after surgical resection; and (2) those who first present in adult life and are usually improved by subtotal colectomy and either ileorectal or caecorectal anastomosis if the dilated segment does not involve the rectum.

There may be associated disorders such as imperforate anus or a funnel anus (Jarvinen and Rintala, 1985). Megarectum is more likely to occur if there is long-standing faecal impaction. By contrast, megacolon is more prevalent if the segment of colonic stasis is above the rectosigmoid junction.

Recently, Gattuso and Kamm (1997) described the clinical features of idiopathic megarectum and megacolon and, like ourselves, recognized three main groups: (1) those with dilating disease confined to the rectum and sigmoid (n = 22); (2) those with dilating disease which did not involve the rectum being confined to the colon (n = 18); and (3) those with megarectum and megacolon (n = 23).

Incidence

Idiopathic megarectum and megacolon is rare: we reported 34 cases in 1994 (Stewart et al, 1994) and

Table 22.4 Results of surgical treatment in 34 patients.

		Previous operation			Results				
Reconstruction after resection	*n*	*Total*	*Anal surgery*	*Previous resection*	*Continent*	*Soiling*	*Constipation*	*Incontinent*	*Dissatisfied (pouch excised)*
Megarectum with or without megasigmoid									
Straight colodistal rectal anastomosis	8	1	0	0	6 (1 still has a loop ileostomy)	0	1 (underwent loop ileostomy)	0	1
Straight coloanal anastomosis	2	0	0	0	2	0	0	0	0
Coloanal anastomosis with colonic J pouch	8	1	1*	0	6	1 (underwent loop ileostomy)	1 (underwent restorative procto-colectomy)	0	1
Megacolon only									
Ileorectal anastomosis	1	0	0	0	1	0	0	0	0
Megacolon and megarectum									
Loop ileostomy alone	1	0	0	0	0	–	–	–	–
Restorative proctocolectomy and J pouch–ileoanal anastomosis	14	11	2*	9 (all for previous megacolon or volvulus)	12	1	0	1 (underwent graciloplasty)	4

*One patient with anorectal agenesis in each case. One patient died.
From Stewart et al (1994).

have treated six more since (Table 22.4). Barnes et al (1986) reported 134 patients seen over 15 years but 51 of these patients had Hirschsprung's disease. However, Gattuso and Kamm (1997) went through all their records at St Marks and decided that only 63 were genuine cases seen between 1969 and 1991. Goligher reports a personal experience of only 18 cases in his entire surgical career (Goligher, 1984). Unlike idiopathic constipation, which is much more common in women, and Hirschsprung's disease, which is more common in males, the sex incidence is almost equal (Lane and Todd, 1977; Barnes et al, 1986). The majority of patients with acquired megarectum or megacolon present under the age of 30 years (Taylor, 1984) and a family history is rare.

Pathology

The macroscopic pathology is poorly described in megarectum and megacolon. The colon is thick walled as well as grossly dilated. The rectal findings are quite unique, there is always a faecaloma in the megarectum and the pararectal veins are enormously dilated. The wall of the rectum is very thickened, largely due to hypertrophy of the longitudinal fibres, and there is no normal 'waist' between the rectal ampulla and the anal canal. The dilated rectum continues imperceptably into a wide, short anus. The mucosa usually looks normal but may be ulcerated from the faecal impaction. These macroscopic findings are quite important to the surgeon. The wall of the anorectum is normally too thick to enable the circular stapling devices to achieve a coloanal anastomosis. However, if the anorectal wall is almost completely divided by diathermy down to the mucosa it is then, and only then, possible to transect the anorectum with a linear stapler such as the TL 55 so that a double-stapled anastomosis is then achievable (see Figures 22.18a,b).

Colectomy specimens examined by conventional histopathological techniques have in the past revealed normal ganglion cells and, unlike Hirschsprung's disease, there is no evidence of hypertrophied nerve bundles and absent ganglia (Garrett and Howard, 1981). Using silver stains, most excision specimens show degeneration of the argyrophil cells, as described in patients with idiopathic chronic constipation. Indeed, until recently the neuropathological changes of both disorders seemed to be almost indistinguishable. Unlike Hirschsprung's disease, ganglia are present throughout the large bowel and there are no cholinergic nerves demonstrable by histochemical staining for acetylcholinesterase (Meier-Ruge et al, 1972).

Gattuso et al (1996a) undertook a detailed immunohistochemical study to examine the enteric innervation in five resection specimens from idiopathic megarectum and megacolon. They investigated innervation using cytochemical staining for protein gene product 9.5 (PGP9.5), S100 protein, vasoactive intestinal polypeptide (VIP), calcitonin gene-related peptide (CGRP) and NADP diaphorase. Compared with control specimens, patients with megabowel showed hypertrophy of the muscularis mucosa and the muscularis externa. Immunoreactivity to PGP9.5 and S100 protein was normal. There was a decrease in the density of innervation to the longitudinal muscle in rectal tissue with fewer VIP- and NADP diaphorase-containing nerves. In the muscularis mucosa and lamina propria of rectal samples in patients with megarectum, VIP immunoreactivity was higher and more NADPH diaphorase-containing nerves were seen. CGRP-immunoreactive nerve fibres were only observed in the myenteric plexus and no CGRP-immunoreactive cell bodies were seen. Thus there appeared to be an increase in VIP and nitric oxide nerve fibres in the lamina propria and muscularis mucosa but a decrease in the longitudinal rectal muscle in megarectum.

Routine pathology also showed significant thickening of the muscularis mucosa, circular muscle and longitudinal muscle in idiopathic megarectum. This thickening was relatively greater in the longitudinal than the circular muscle. Also fibrosis was more common in longitudinal muscle (58%) compared with circular muscle (38%) and muscularis mucosa (29%). Furthermore, the density of neural tissue in the longitudinal muscle seemed to be reduced in megarectum (Gattuso et al, 1997).

Clinical presentation

It is sometimes very difficult to distinguish idiopathic megacolon or megarectum from Hirschsprung's disease on clinical grounds. This is further complicated in the adult literature by reports that contain both groups of patients.

A useful clinical account of idiopathic megacolon and megarectum is by Barnes et al (1986). In this paper 29 patients with adult-onset Hirschsprung's disease are included for comparison. All of the adults with an aganglionic segment complained of constipation, usually from birth, requiring enemas to achieve defecation. In this group, abdominal pain and distension were common and the rectum was usually empty. The remaining 65 patients had normal rectal biopsies and were classified as having idiopathic megacolon, even though the rectoanal inhibitory reflex was abnormal in seven of 41 patients (17%). In 35 patients the constipation commenced in childhood and in this group soiling was present in 28 and was invariably associated with faecal impaction and a palpable abdominal mass (Figure 22.9). Six of this group were socially or psychologically disturbed and two were mentally retarded. The remaining 30 patients with idiopathic megacolon presented for the first time in adult life, although they had been constipated for many years before; seven had spurious diarrhoea. Abdominal pain and swelling was common (Figure 22.10) but only nine had soiling with faecal impaction. Eleven of these patients had had previous surgical treatment (rectopexy or large bowel resection). Two suffered from epilepsy, two had psychological disorders

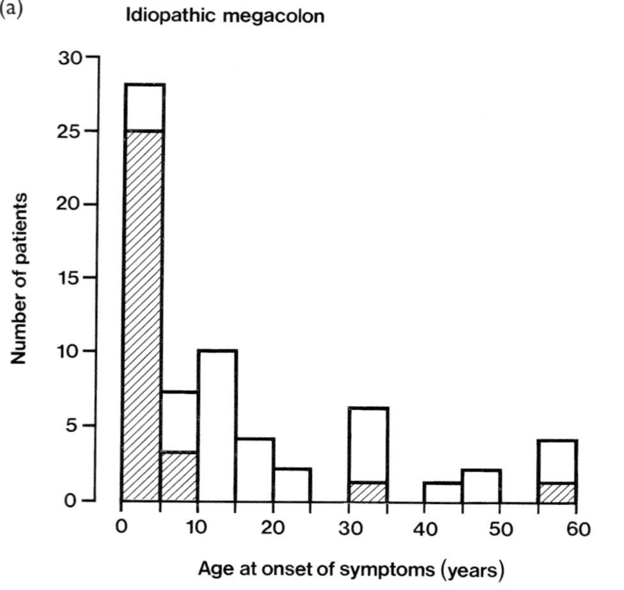

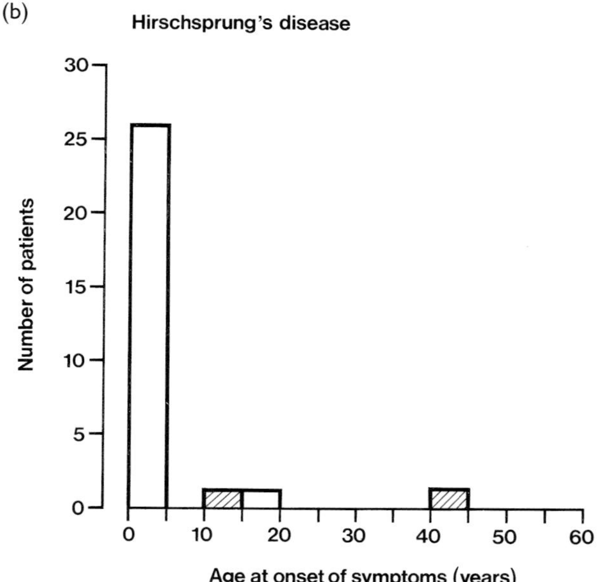

Figure 22.9a,b Age of onset of symptoms in idiopathic megacolon and Hirschsprung's disease. (a) Idiopathic megacolon: age at onset of symptoms. ▨, Patients with a history of faecal soiling; □, patients without soiling. (b) Hirschsprung's disease: the age at onset of symptoms, ▨, Patients presenting with faecal soiling; □, patients without soiling.

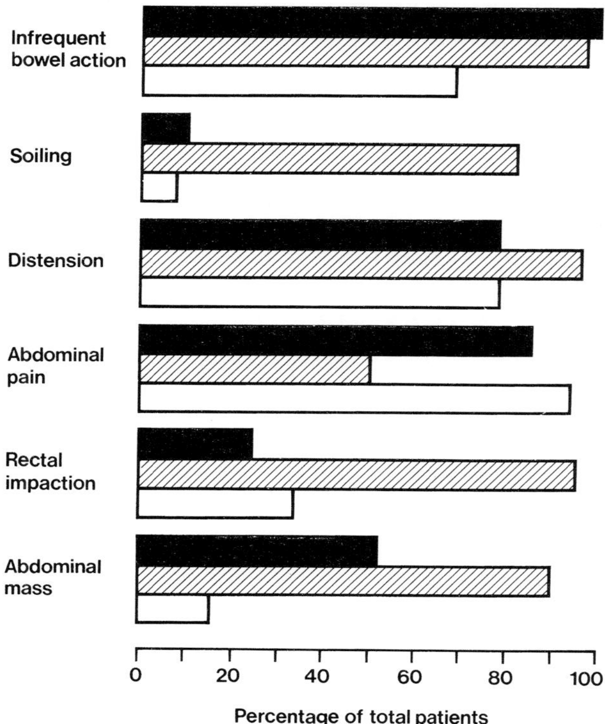

Figure 22.10 Clinical features in patients with megacolon of different types. ■, Adult Hirschsprung's disease; ▨, childhood-onset megacolon; □, adult megacolon.

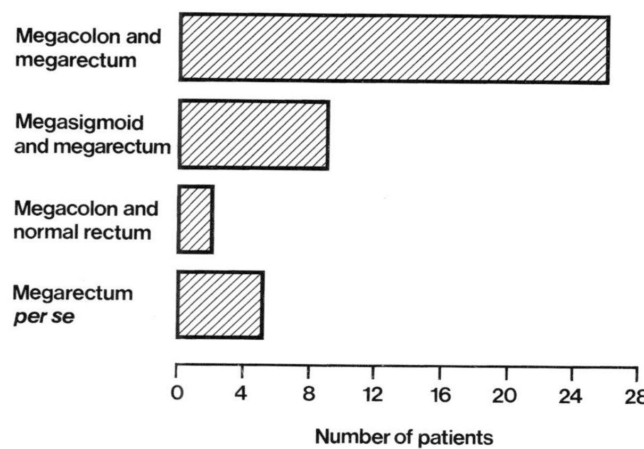

Figure 22.11 The relative distribution of megacolon and megarectum in 42 patients described by Lane and Todd (1977).

and were on tranquillizers and three were of low intelligence.

Idiopathic megacolon may exist without a megarectum, but in some of these patients rectal function is impaired and secondary megarectum may develop later although usually megacolon remains as a distinct colonic entity (Figure 22.11). In some patients megacolon and megarectum may coexist. In others the initial presentation is of a dilated rectum and sigmoid only; however, in this group the proximal colon may not function normally and, if surgical treatment is directed to the dilated segment only, later dilatation or stasis in the proximal bowel may occur. If the megacolon is confined to the sigmoid the patient may present with an atypical sigmoid volvulus. However the rest of the colon is usually functionally abnormal and further resection is commonly required if the volvulus is merely treated by sigmoid colectomy alone (Kune, 1966).

Lane and Todd (1977) describe 42 patients with megacolon or megarectum, none of whom had Hirschsprung's disease. All patients presented with constipation but in 13 (31%) incontinence was also a feature. Abdominal pain and distension were common, provided the patients did not have a megarectum (Table 22.5). Unlike patients with chronic constipation, none of these patients had urinary tract symptoms. A large proportion of patients with megarectum were mentally subnormal, posing special problems with regard to medical and surgical management; furthermore, patients with gross faecal impaction also had a lax anal canal and tended to soil.

Gattuso and Kamm (1997) described the clinical presentation of 63 patients who they felt definitely did not have Hirschsprung's disease. They classified them into three groups: idiopathic megarectum, idiopathic megacolon and megarectum, and megacolon alone. The megacolon group was significantly older than those with megarectum, 82% of whom became symptomatic under the age of 10 years. Six of 18 with megacolon had a volvulus. Bowel habit was variable, faecal incontinence was always associated with faecal impaction in the rectum and occurred in 77% of patients with megarectum and in 57% of patients with a megarectum and

Table 22.5 Clinical presentation of megacolon.

Constipation	42/42
Abdominal pain	21/42
Incontinence	13/42
Abdominal distension	12/42
Mentally retarded	7/42
Lax anus	3/42
Urinary symptoms	0/42

From Lane and Todd (1977).

a megacolon. Abdominal distension was present in 60% and abdominal pain in 40%. Mental retardation and psychiatric illness was more common in patients with megarectum than in those with megacolon.

These authors then studied the clinical presentation of 29 patients (7 women) seen prospectively: 22 had a megarectum alone, 6 had megacolon alone and one had both. Again, megacolon patients were older than the others. The symptoms differed strikingly between megarectum and megacolon. Faecal impaction was present in all 22 megarectum patients, 17 of whom had had previous manual disimpaction under general anaesthesia. In the megarectum patients, abdominal pain and distension was usually associated with faecal impaction and relieved by bowel evacuation. Symptoms in megacolon were variable. Five of 22 patients with megarectum were mentally retarded and one had severe autism and another had manic depression.

Investigations

Plain radiograph

Evidence of a megacolon and megarectum can often be obtained from a plain abdominal radiograph. Plain X-ray may identify spina bifida occulta: 2 of 18 with megarectum and 2 of 3 with megacolon had this defect in the lumbosacral outflow. In a few patients the diagnosis can be assumed from a chest radiograph, which may demonstrate bilateral elevation of the diaphragm with a gas-filled colon below (Taylor et al, 1980). In these circumstances it is imperative to exclude organic colonic obstruction. We found that a plain abdominal X-ray provides almost more information than any other test and it is totally noninvasive. It clearly identifies the faecaloma in megarectum and usually demonstrates if the proximal colon is full of faecal residue and if it is dilated.

Contrast studies

A diagnosis of megacolon or megarectum can only be reliably made by barium enema. Nevertheless, barium enema does not provide a reproducible method of assessing the diameter of the colon since this is dependent upon the use of relaxants and the amount of air insufflation used during the investigation. Lane and Todd (1977) did not even attempt to use bowel preparation prior to barium enema but merely delineated the wall of the colon by a dilute barium solution or by Gastrografin. If a single-contrast technique is used, gross dilatation is usually visible on initial screening. If this is the case, great care must be taken to avoid overfilling the colon with barium, since this may prove extremely difficult to remove despite washouts and enemas.

Even using a standardized technique, measurement of colonic diameter is non-specific and only gross dilatation can be diagnosed with confidence (Partiquin et al, 1978). Lane and Todd (1977) were able to classify the radiological findings of their patients into four groups (Figure 22.11). The majority had a megacolon and a megarectum (69%); 21% had a megasigmoid and a megarectum; isolated dilatation of the colon or rectum was rare. Barium enema is an important means of excluding Hirschsprung's disease since in this disorder the ganglionic rectum is typically narrow and the proximal colon dilated. However, these radiological features may not always be present, particularly in short segment or ultra-short segment disease (Taylor, 1984; Barnes et al, 1986). Barium enema will also exclude an obstructing lesion, which must always be considered in the differential diagnosis of this disorder (Figure 22.12a). Upper gastrointestinal contrast studies were normal with no evidence of duodenal dilatation in any of the patients studied prospectively by Gattuso and Kamm (1997). Isotope transit studies, however, identified impaired gastric emptying in 6 of 10 patients with megarectum, small bowel transit was normal and colonic delay occurred in the dilated bowel. Abdominal bloating did not correlate with delayed gastric emptying (Gattuso et al, 1996b).

Sigmoidoscopy and colonoscopy

In megarectum, the sigmoidoscope is said to enter a huge capacious rectum (Figure 22.12b), although in many patients with a megarectum it is impossible to use endoscopy because of gross faecal impaction. If the patient has been well prepared, sigmoidoscopy will give a good indication of whether a megarectum is present, although it rarely provides accurate information on the capacity, distensibility or diameter of the rectum. Colonoscopy, in our experience, is equally unreliable, particularly as large volumes of air are needed to distend the colon.

Rectal biopsy

An aganglionic segment can only be confidently excluded by excising a full thickness of rectal wall at several sites from the anal verge. Ganglia are normally sparse or even absent in the 2-cm zone above the dentate line. Hence the lowest biopsy should be

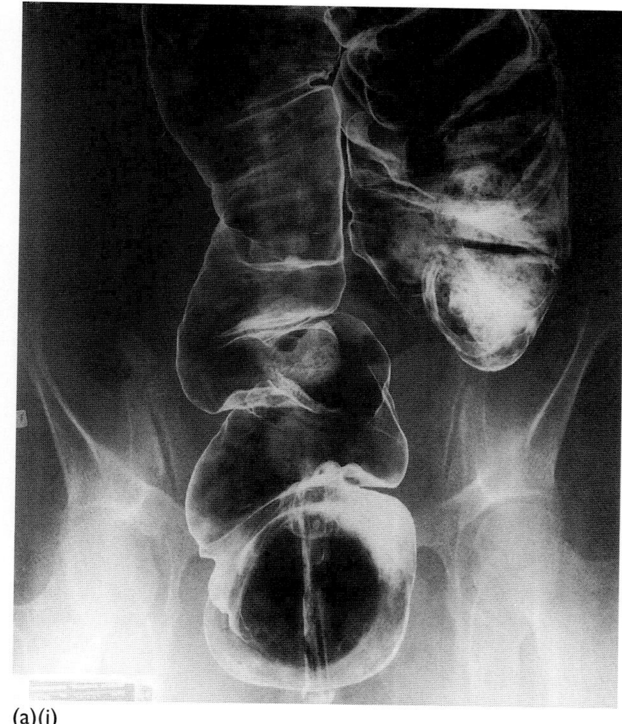

(a)(i)

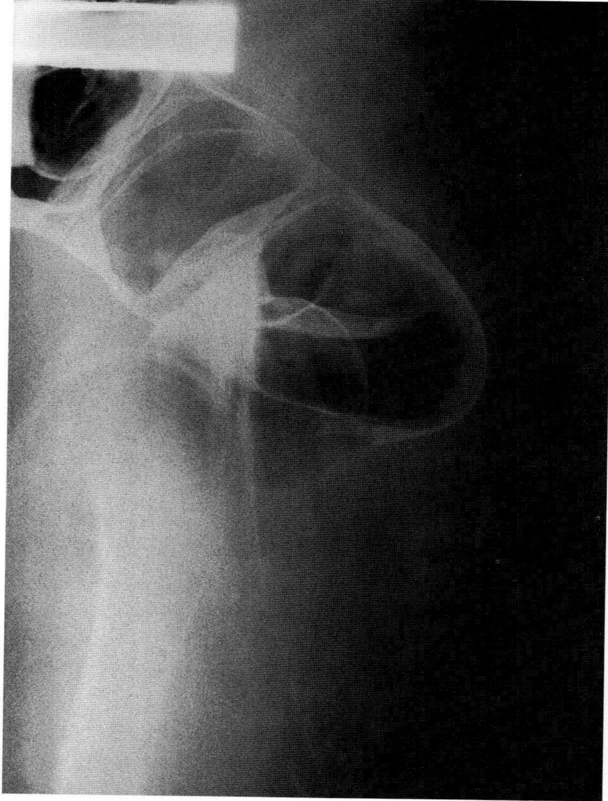

(a)(ii)

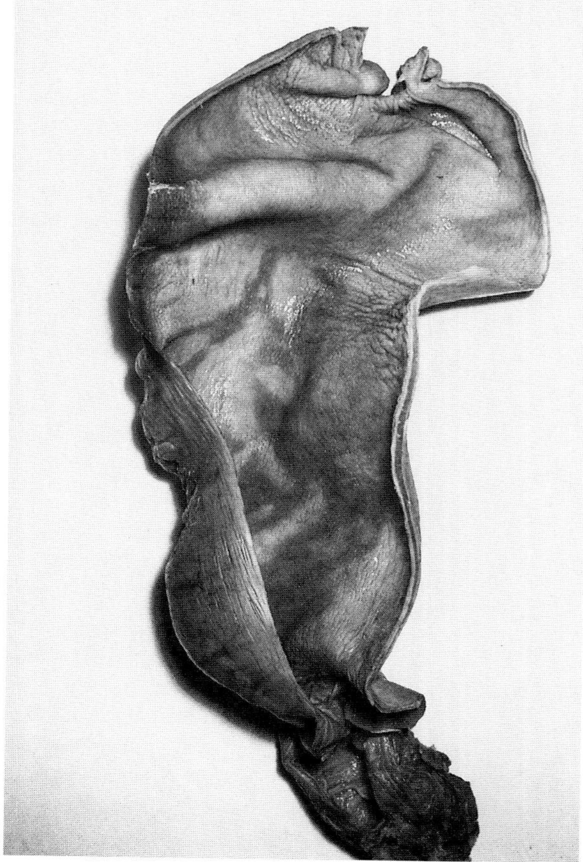

(b)

Figure 22.12a,b Radiographic and pathological features of megacolon and megarectum. (a) A barium enema examination demonstrating a stenosis at the anorectal junction (anteroposterior and lateral views). (b) Gross pathology of megacolon: excision specimens of an adult with a megarectum and a megasigmoid.

no less than 4 cm above the anal verge in adults. We recommend biopsies at 12, 8 and 4 cm. The procedure must be performed under a general anaesthetic and the defect closed with sutures. An alternative approach is to remove an 8-cm strip of internal sphincter and circular muscle of the rectum by performing an anorectal myectomy (Yoshioka and Keighley, 1987) but there is a risk of incontinence, particularly as sphincter function is compromised anyway (Gattuso et al, 1996b), hence open biopsies are preferred. Mucosal biopsies stained for anticholinesterase provide a reliable alternative method of diagnosing conventional Hirschsprung's disease but, as previously explained, cannot exclude the ultra-short segment variety.

Some patients with idiopathic megacolon may exhibit either hypoganglionosis or hyperganglionosis. A diagnosis of hypoganglionosis is made if there are just a few scattered intermyenteric ganglion cells in the anorectal biopsy; the ganglia are fewer and smaller than normal. Hyperganglionosis is extremely rare but histochemical stains show extensive ganglionic tissue in the intermyenteric zone of the submucosa. This disorder may be present in the entire large bowel (Howard et al, 1982).

Rectoanal inhibitory reflex

The rectoanal inibitory reflex has been used as a means of excluding Hirschsprung's disease, since its absence in children closely correlates with an aganglionic segment (Lawson and Nixon, 1967). In adults, however, this reflex may be absent in a variety of disorders, such as idiopathic constipation, rectal prolapse and anorectal incontinence. Barnes et al (1986) found that the reflex was present in one patient with Hirschsprung's disease and was absent in seven of 41 with idiopathic megarectum. Taylor (1984) reported the absence of the reflex in four of 23 patients with idiopathic megarectum. Gattuso and Kamm (1997) found that the rectoanal inhibitory reflex was present in 14 of 22 patients with megarectum and in 5 of 6 with megacolon.

Anal pressures

Resting anal pressures are frequently raised in idiopathic megacolon and ultra-short waves are common (Barnes et al, 1986). Taylor et al (1980) reported that 7 of 15 patients with idiopathic megarectum had persistently raised resting anal canal pressures (Figure 22.13), which led them to advise repeated anal dilatation as a means of treatment. By contrast, Gattuso and Kamm (1997) reported that maximum resting anal pressures were lower than normal in 12 of 22 patients with megarectum but there was no evidence of abnormal perineal descent.

Rectal sensation

Appreciation of distension within the rectum is impaired in megarectum (Faverdin et al, 1981; Luukkonen et al, 1990). Taylor et al (1980) found that threshold volumes were substantially greater in patients with megacolon compared with normals. In our experience, rectal sensation appears to be grossly impaired compared with normal subjects. By contrast, Lane and Todd (1977) found that impaired rectal sensation was present in only half of their patients. Gattuso and Kamm (1997) reported that rectal sensation was absent in five patients with megarectum; however, peranal sensation was normal in all patients.

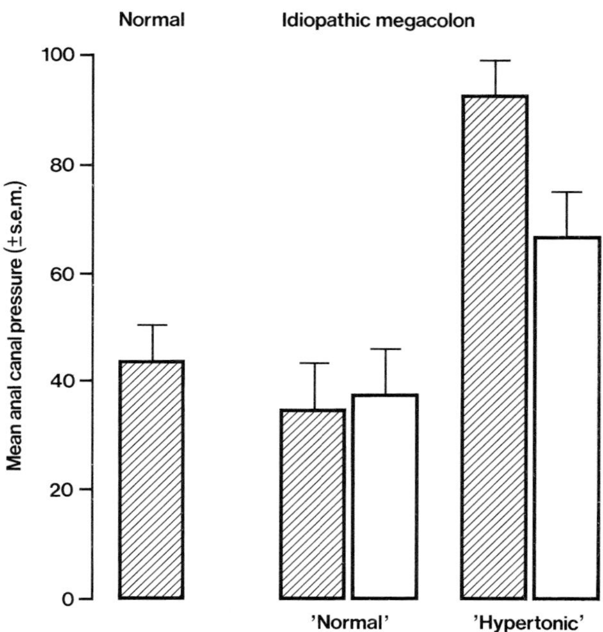

Figure 22.13 Anal manometry in idiopathic megacolon compared with normal patients. Mean resting anal canal pressures (cmH_2O) are shown. Two subgroups of patients with idiopathic megacolon are recognized: those with normal anal canal pressures and those with a hypertonic anal sphincter. ▨, Initial findings; □, after 15 months follow-up.

Electromyography

Patients with idiopathic megarectum often have paradoxical contraction of the puborectalis and external sphincter during straining (Barnes et al, 1986). Gattuso and Kamm (1997) found this to be the case in half of the patients with megarectum. However, pudendal nerve latency was normal in all their prospectively studied patients.

Rectal evacuation studies

Using a simulated stool of paste, impaired rectal evacuation was recorded in all except one patient with a megarectum compared with only 2 of 6 with megacolon (Gattuso and Kamm, 1997).

Differential diagnosis

Hirschsprung's disease and Chagas' disease need to be excluded in adults with a megarectum. Other causes of autonomic neuropathy, such as lead poisoning, diabetes, cauda equina lesions and long-standing drug therapy (Prout, 1984), should also be excluded. A distal obstructing lesion, such as a carcinoma, Crohn's disease, ischaemic stricture or volvulus, may masquerade as megarectum or megacolon. Impaired neuronal innervation to the hind-gut may be associated with congenital megacolon. Garrett and Howard (1981) described hypoganglionosis and hyperganglionosis in the anorectum, which must be distinguished from Hirschsprung's disease and which can involve the colon as well (Pescatori et al, 1986). Chronic intestinal pseudo-obstruction usually, but not always, involves the small bowel. Most patients have had life-long intestinal obstructive symptoms and a laparotomy has nearly always been performed. The diagnosis is confirmed by biopsy or resection specimens.

Conservative treatment

Medical treatment by laxatives, repeated rectal washouts and enemas may control constipation, but it is usually necessary to disimpact the rectum by manual evacuation under a general anaesthetic before conservative therapy can be started. After clearing the rectum, bowel habit may become manageable by repeated laxatives. A word of caution, however, needs to be made concerning faecal disimpaction. The procedure can have a permanent damaging effect on the sphincter. This can be identified by anal ultrasonography and was reported in 9 of 14 patients who had had a previous disimpaction. Since low resting anal pressures are frequently observed in megarectum patients anyway, extreme care is needed when advising patients to have a faecal disimpaction under general anaesthesia (Gattuso et al, 1996c).

In some patients constipation is successfully controlled using bisacodyl suppositories. Medical therapy gives the best results in patients whose symptoms commence in childhood with soiling and faecal impaction. Lane and Todd (1977) were able to report improvement by conservative therapy alone in 17 of 35 patients. The group in whom conservative therapy seemed to be most effective were those with a megasigmoid and megarectum (Figure 22.14).

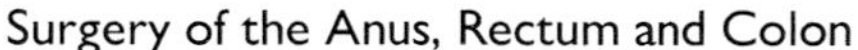

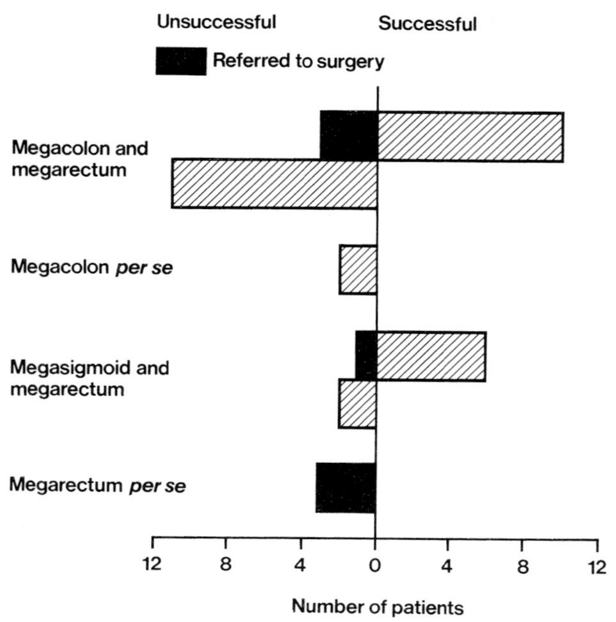

Figure 22.14 The results of conservative treatment for megacolon and megarectum in the 42 patients described by Lane and Todd (1977).

Surgical treatment

Conservative surgical therapy

Anal dilatation or sphincterotomy

Anal dilatation has been used in patients with idiopathic megarectum and appears to be beneficial among those with high resting anal pressures and ultra-slow waves (Taylor, 1984). For the reasons already stated it should not be used in patients with low anal pressure.

Internal sphincterotomy has been used in a few patients with anal hypertension, but comprehensive follow-up data for this mode of therapy are lacking and we would not recommend it.

Anorectal myectomy

The long-term results of anorectal myectomy for patients with chronic constipation and in a small number with megarectum are most disappointing and there is a small risk of incontinence (Pinho et al, 1989). We do not recommend this procedure and if aganglionosis is to be excluded, multiple rectal biopsies would be preferred.

Resection

Resection was required in over half of the patients reported from St Mark's Hospital (Lane and Todd,

1977; Gattuso and Kamm, 1997). The more radical resections were generally associated with the best results. None of the 34 patients having a sigmoid resection alone had a satisfactory outcome. Only eight patients had a subtotal colectomy, using caecorectal anastomosis in five and an ileorectal anastomosis in three. The results of caecorectal anastomosis were marginally better than ileorectal anastomosis. A few patients had episodic incontinence after ileorectal anastomosis but this was not reported after caecorectal anastomosis. After caecorectal anastomosis some patients needed to continue intermittent laxative therapy.

Barnes et al (1986) reported that subtotal colectomy and caecorectal or ileorectal anastomosis resulted in a successful outcome in 11 of 16 patients with adult-onset idiopathic megacolon and megarectum. On the other hand, only two of four patients with childhood-onset idiopathic megacolon were improved by subtotal colectomy. The results in one patient after the Soave procedure were poor but two were improved by the Duhamel operation. Belliveau et al (1982) reported good results following subtotal colectomy and ileorectal anastomosis even though some patients had neuropsychiatric disorders. The data on resection for chronic constipation also imply that any procedure short of subtotal colectomy is unlikely to control symptoms. We believe that nothing other than a total colectomy is suitable for megacolon, provided the rectum is normal.

Patients with a megarectum pose a special problem. In such patients faecal stasis in the rectum often persists despite an ileorectal anastomosis. If there is no dilatation of the proximal colon one approach, and the one that we support, is to perform a low anterior resection or even a total rectal excision, as in the Soave procedure, leaving only the anal stump and performing a coloanal anastomosis. Some patients with an apparently normal left colon might be best treated in the same way as those with Hirschsprung's disease, by the Swenson or, preferably, the Duhamel procedure (Stabile et al, 1991). This option is particularly suited to patients with a patulous anus from chronic faecal impaction. In our experience, however, the proximal colon rarely functions normally and some, more radical resection is often advisable, provided that the anal sphincter is normal.

If there is gross dilatation of the rectum and colon then there is, we believe, a place for a restorative proctocolectomy and pouch anal anastomosis (Hosie et al, 1990). A similar approach incorporating a segment of colon for the pouch was described by Boley (1984), but the functional outcome is likely to be comparable, if not better, using restorative proctocolectomy. Restorative proctocolectomy is rarely performed as a primary procedure unless there is gross megacolon or megarectum.

Our experience among patients with idiopathic megacolon and megarectum is summarized in Table 22.4. Megacolon alone is best treated by subtotal colectomy. Megarectum alone can be successfully treated by excision of the rectum and sigmoid with coloanal anastomosis. We used to use a colonic pouch but no longer advise this since the colonic pouch may also dilate with time. Megarectum with a megacolon should be managed by restorative proctocolectomy, as anything less is commonly complicated by recurrent constipation. However, restorative proctocolectomy may result in incontinence, particularly if it is used in patients with a patulous anus with very low resting anal pressures.

The role of a stoma should never be ignored in these patients. If there is gross dilatation of the colon and rectum and a patulous anus, a loop ileostomy alone may be the best treatment. It is obviously preferred to a colostomy. If the problem is one of rectal dilatation alone, either a loop colostomy or an end colostomy oversewing the rectal stump might be considered. However, in view of the risk of subsequent colonic inertia, we still prefer an ileostomy for megarectum, even though a colostomy affords the patient an opportunity to be taught colostomy irrigation. Nevertheless, colonic irrigation is not something that these patients generally accept.

Subtotal colectomy

It is usually much more difficult to prepare the bowel in patients with a megacolon and megarectum than in patients with chronic constipation alone. Manual evacuation is damaging to the sphincters and even afterwards, despite laxatives and enemas, it may not be possible or wise to remove a faecaloma. It is our policy, therefore, not even to attempt bowel preparation in many of these patients but, at operation, to milk the solid faecal bolus from the rectum into the colon which is to be resected and to perform on-table rectal washout.

Surgical procedure

All patients are given perioperative antibiotic cover and preoperative subcutaneous heparin. Subtotal colectomy is performed with the patient in the supine position. A long midline incision is used. After a careful laparotomy to exclude any other pathology the small bowel is protected by large wet mops. Colonic mobilization is usually started on the right side by dividing the lateral peritoneum and the peritoneal attachments between the hepatic flexure and the undersurface of the right lobe of the liver, taking care not to damage the duodenum. The omentum is preserved by dissecting between the transverse mesocolon with the middle colic vessels and the rest of the omentum. The middle colic vessels are ligated in two or three pedicles quite close to the bowel. Before mobilizing the splenic flexure we recommend dividing the peritoneum on the lateral side of the left colon. The sigmoid colon is mobilized from the ovarian vessels and the left ureter. The assistant then places a retractor under the left subcostal region to expose the splenic flexure. The peritoneum over the splenic flexure is divided, taking care not to enter the perinephric fascia, and the splenic flexure is delivered into the wound. The colonic vessels may be ligated close to the bowel, taking the upper and lower left colic and middle colic vessels. The sigmoid vessels are usually divided in two or three bunches in the sigmoid mesocolon, preserving the superior haemorrhoidal vessels. The sigmoid mesocolon is divided at the rectosigmoid junction to reach the mesenteric attachment of the bowel.

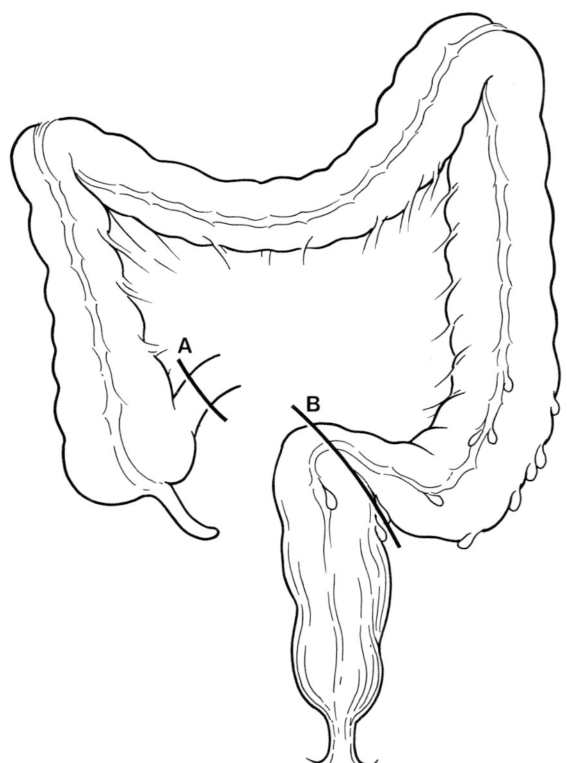

Figure 22.15 Subtotal colectomy and ileorectal anastomosis. The ileum is transected just proximal to the caecum. The rectum is usually transected at the pelvic brim, provided that there is no evidence of megarectum.

If there is any palpable faecal residue this should be milked out of the rectum into the segment to be resected. A curved non-crushing clamp may then be applied to the rectum to facilitate a rectal washout.

At this point a decision must be made as to whether or not to resect the caecum and perform an ileorectal anastomosis (Figure 22.15) or to preserve the caecum and use a caecorectal anastomosis for reconstruction.

Subtotal colectomy and caecorectal anastomosis

If the caecum is to be preserved it is usual to retain 5–7 cm of the right colon, dividing the mesentery up to attachment to the bowel (Figure 22.16a) and ligating any remaining vessels between the ileocolic artery and the middle colic vessels. Crushing bowel clamps are then applied at the site selected for resection where the mesentery has been divided and a non-crushing clamp is applied to the caecum (Figure 22.16b). The colon is then removed. It is usual to remove the appendix at this stage, burying the stump with a purse-string suture. The anastomosis often lies best if the caecum is rotated so that the terminal ileum enters from the right. An end-to-end anastomosis is then performed with a single layer of continuous extra mucosal PDS or by the functional end-to-end stapling technique. Any defect in the mesentery is closed (Figure 22.16c,d).

Subtotal colectomy and ileorectal anastomosis

If the caecum is to be resected with the colon, the caecum, appendix and terminal ileum are mobilized by dividing the lateral peritoneum and the inferior peritoneal attachments to the terminal ileum (Figure 22.17a). The vessels running to the caecum from the ileocolic artery are ligated to the site at which the mesentery of the terminal ileum is to be divided. As much of the terminal ileum is preserved as possible. Crushing bowel clamps are applied to the site selected for resection and a non-crushing clamp is applied across the proximal ileum (Figure 22.17b). The colon is removed and an ileorectal anastomosis is constructed. The anastomosis may be either end-to-end or end-to-side. A single-layer end-to-end anastomosis is constructed using continuous extramucosal PDS sutures (Figure 22.17c) or an end-to-side anastomosis is fashioned by oversewing the cut edge of the terminal ileum with continuous Vicryl or with staples. The antimesenteric border of the terminal ileum is then opened longitudinally (Figure 22.17d) and the anastomosis completed as a single- or two-layer technique (Figure 22.17e). Any defect in the mesentery is then closed with an absorbable suture. Many surgeons today prefer to staple the ileum side to side with the rectum resecting the colon and closing the enterotomy at the same time, thereby creating a stapled functional end-to-end anastomosis (Figure 22.17f).

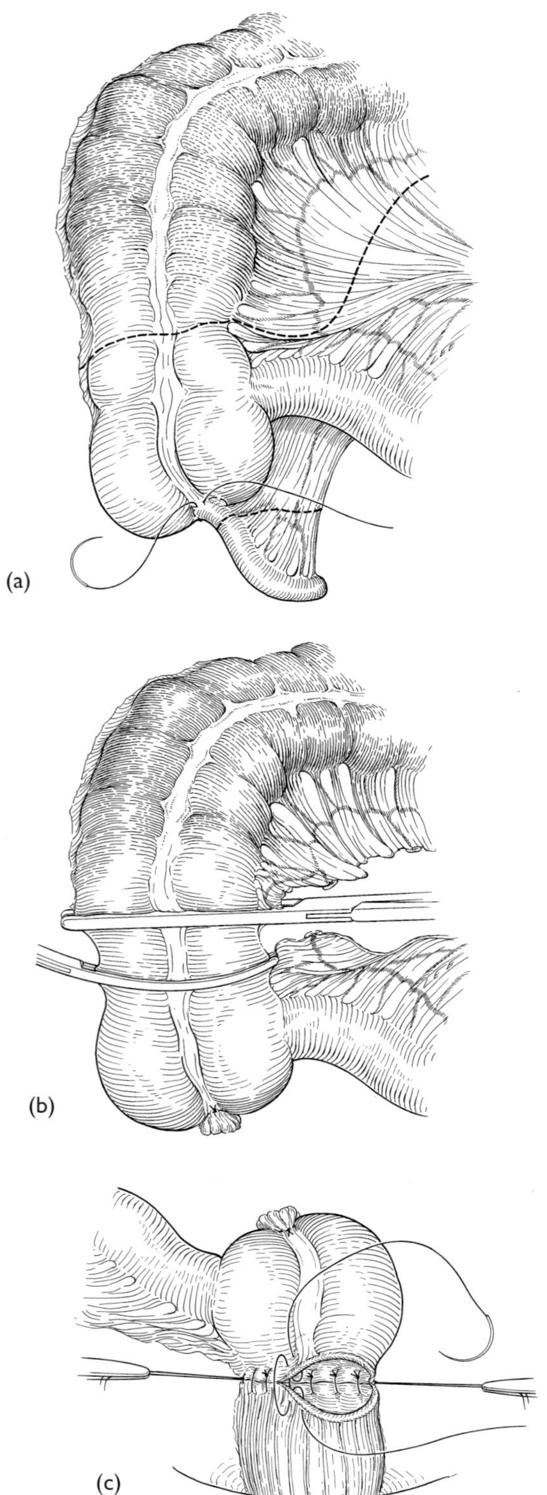

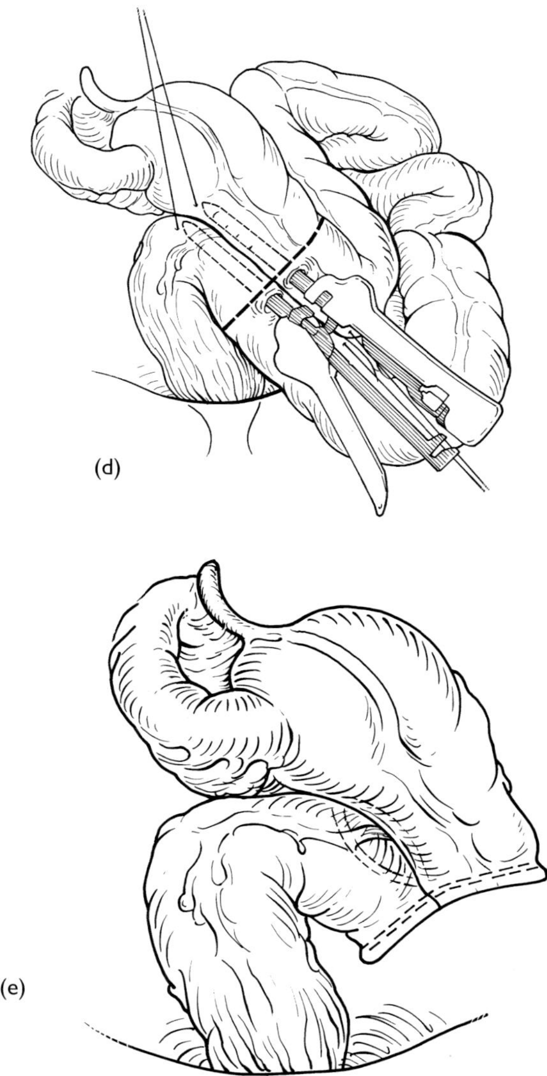

Figure 22.16a–e Subtotal colectomy and caecorectal anastomosis. (a) The level of transection of the ascending colon. The bowel is divided just above the caecum and the appendix is removed. (b) Having divided the mesentery, the upper pole of the caecum is transected. (c) A single-layer caecorectal anastomosis is being completed. (d) An alternative method of performing a caecorectal anastomosis is using the functional end-to-end stapled anastomosis. Having completely mobilized the colon and the upper rectum, two enterotomies are made in the lower sigmoid and mid-ascending colon to create a side-to-side anastomosis. (e) The anastomosis is completed by transecting the ascending colon and rectum beyond the two enterotomies which closes the two bowel ends and resects the specimen.

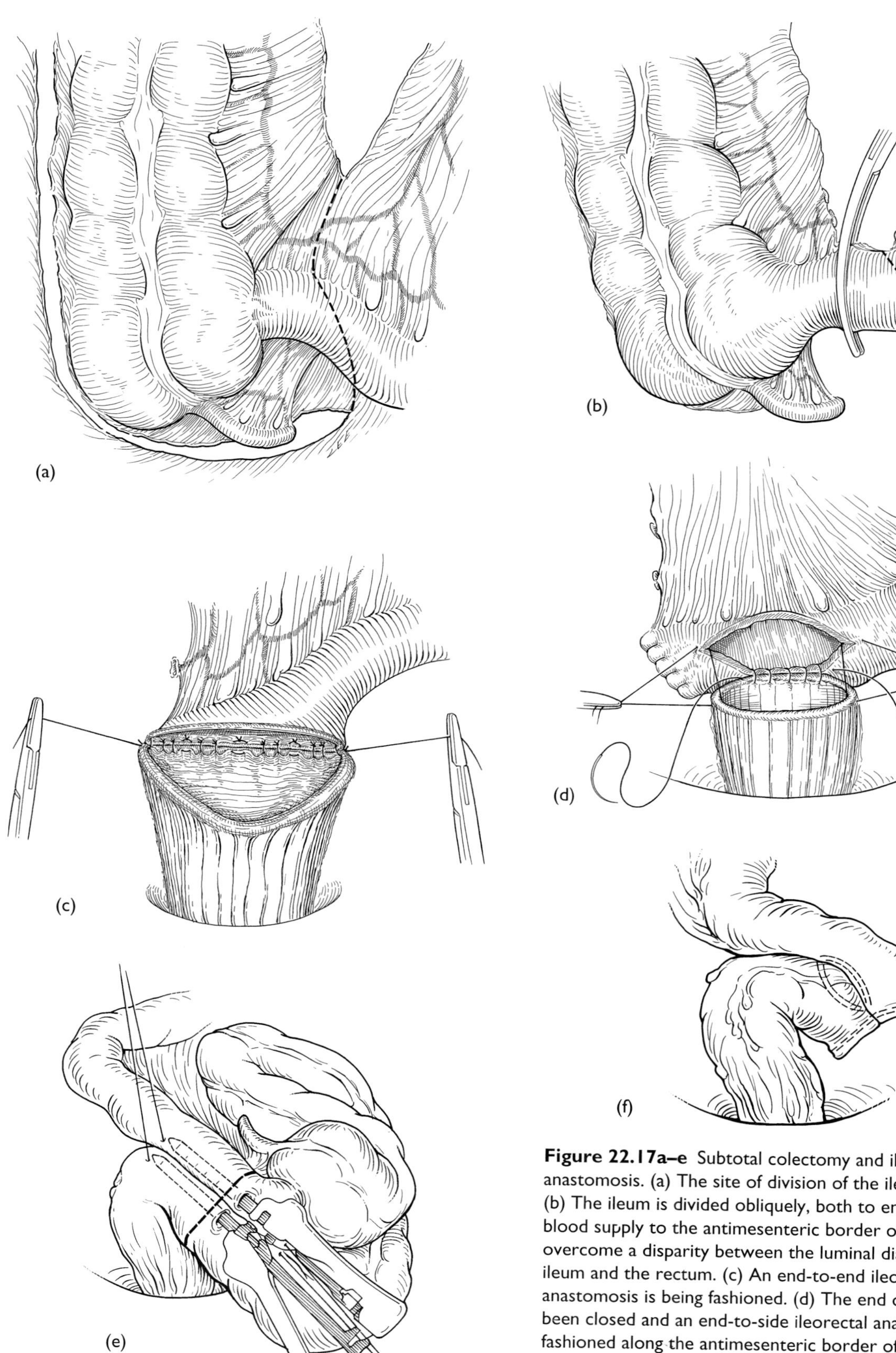

Figure 22.17a–e Subtotal colectomy and ileorectal anastomosis. (a) The site of division of the ileal mesentery. (b) The ileum is divided obliquely, both to ensure an adequate blood supply to the antimesenteric border of the ileum and to overcome a disparity between the luminal diameter of the ileum and the rectum. (c) An end-to-end ileorectal anastomosis is being fashioned. (d) The end of the ileum has been closed and an end-to-side ileorectal anastomosis is being fashioned along the antimesenteric border of the ileum. Alternatively a stapled technique may be used. (e) Stapled ileorectal anastomosis. (f) Completed anastomosis.

The patient is encouraged to mobilize early after operation. The bladder catheter can usually be removed 48 hours after operation and free fluids allowed as soon as bowel sounds return. Bowels are usually opened 4–6 days after operation and early postoperative diarrhoea is to be expected. It is therefore frequently necessary to prescribe codeine, loperamide or kaolin. Most patients can safely be discharged from hospital 8–10 days after operation. Patients should be warned that the diarrhoea is likely to persist for 6–10 weeks; thereafter it frequently slowly declines to between two and four bowel movements per day after 4 or 5 months. The first postoperative assessment is usually made 4–6 weeks after operation, and depending upon clinical progress thereafter.

Rectosigmoid excision and coloanal anastomosis

Patients with a megarectum but with an apparently normal colon proximal to the descending colon may be treated by excision of the entire rectum and sigmoid colon (Kusunoki et al, 1991). The normal calibre descending or transverse colon may either be anastomosed to the anal canal as a straight coloanal procedure or with a colonic pouch (Stabile et al, 1992b; Pelissier et al, 1992). We have reported 18 patients having resection for a megarectum and a megasigmoid; only eight had a coloanal pouch procedure, six of whom have had excellent functional results but two developed recurrent constipation resulting in restorative proctocolectomy in one and a defunctioning stoma in another (Stewart et al, 1994). Some of these patients have impaired colonic motility despite a macroscopically normal colon, while others developed colonic inertia some years later. This operation would not be advised unless the dilated bowel is confined to the rectum and provided there is normal colonic motor activity (Lewis et al, 1992).

A colonic pouch is no longer advised in megarectum (Figure 22.18i) because patients have impaired rectal evacuation anyway and late dilatation of the pouch has now been seen in two of our cases. The ten remaining cases that we reported having resection for megarectum were treated by colorectal excision and either very low colodistal rectal anastomosis or straight coloanal anastomosis. Of these, eight have had excellent results and are fully continent. Our current practice, therefore, is to use a straight coloanal anastomosis (see Figure 22.6e,h). Originally we believed, owing to the thickness of the anal wall, that all these reconstructions

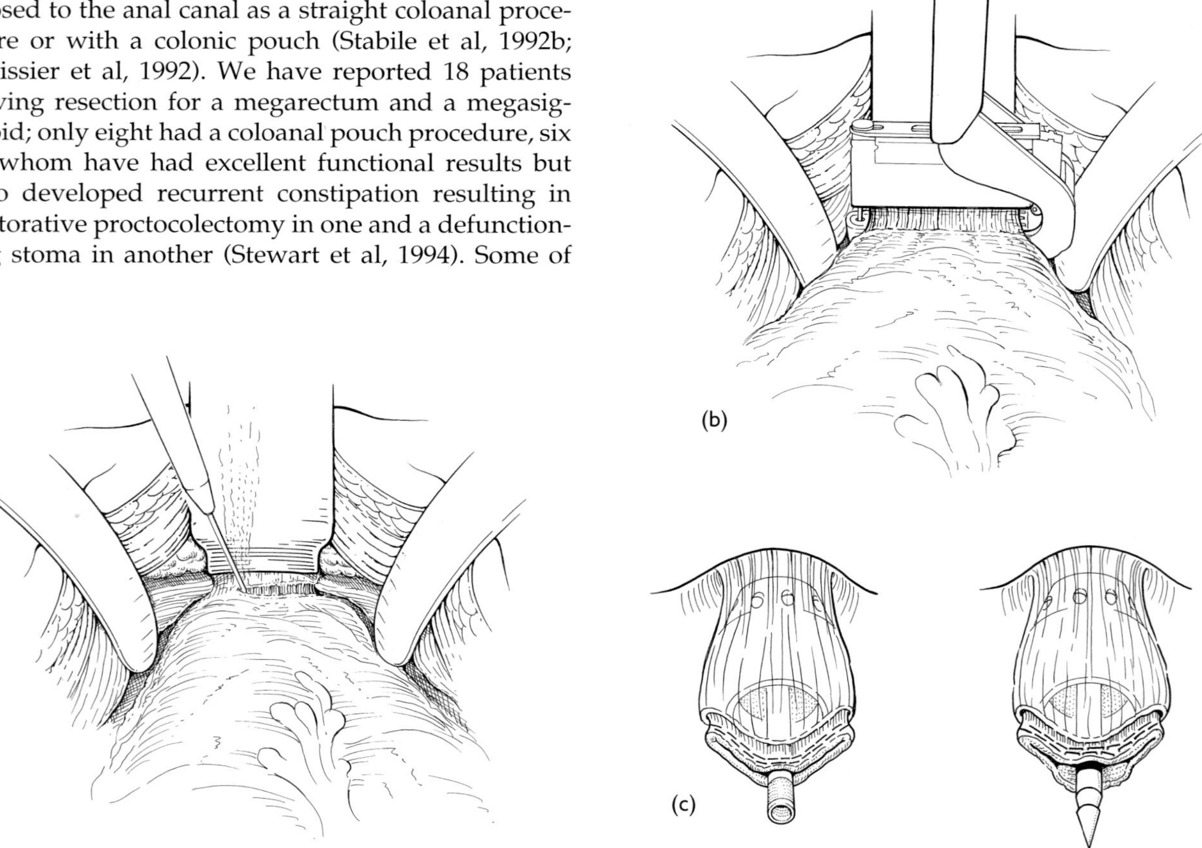

Figure 22.18a–l Stapled coloanal anastomosis for megarectum. It is often impossible to perform a stapled coloanal or colo-low rectal anastomosis because the bowel wall is so thickened. If the faecaloma is milked back into the resection specimen, it is possible to diathermy the wall of the anorectum almost down to the mucosa (b) so that a TL 30 or TL 55 can then be applied (c). *(Continued)*

had to be performed by hand suture using a peranal technique. Now we discover that stapling is possible by dividing most of the anal or low rectal longitudinal muscle with diathermy (Figure 22.18a) almost down to the mucosa so that the bowel can then be transected with the linear stapler (TL 55 or TL 30) (Figure 22.18b) and a double-stapled end-to-end coloanal anastomosis fashioned, using the circular stapling device. However, extreme care is needed not to push the cartridge holder too forcibly against the stapled transected anorectum or else the thin residual bowel wall will split (Figure 22.18c) and a hand-sutured method will then be necessary (see Figure 22.6e).

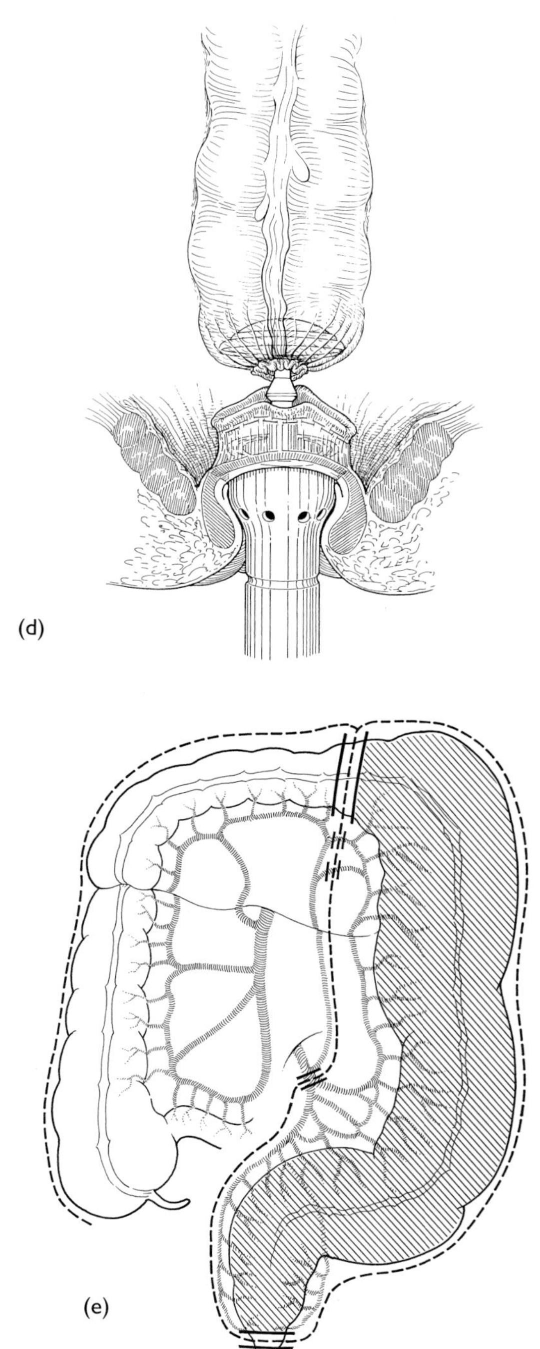

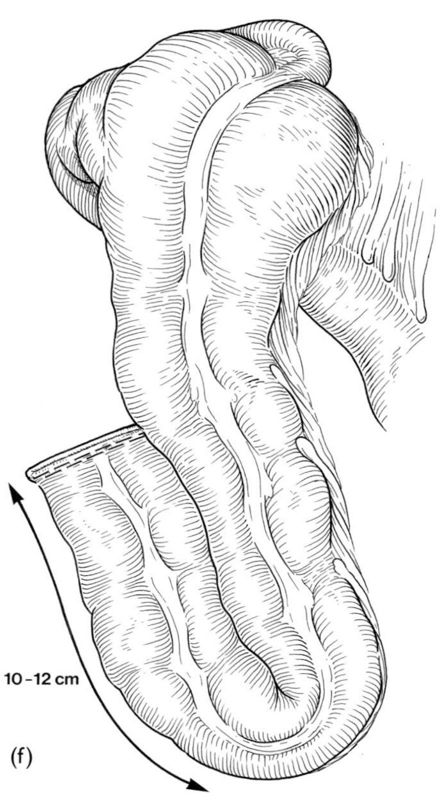

Figure 22.18a–l (*Continued*) Great care must then be exercised when the circular stapler is introduced into the anorectum because the transected staple line is very thin. If excessive force is applied to push the circular stapling device towards the pelvis, the staple line may split (d). Provided the abdominal surgeon controls the cartridge holder of the circular stapling device, a successful straight coloanal or colo-low distal rectal anastomosis can be achieved. We believe that for megabowel a straight coloanal anstomosis is now preferred to the pouch coloanal anastomosis as illustrated in Figure 22.18d. Rectosigmoid excision for megacolon and megarectum. Rectal excision with a variable amount of proximal colon and coloanal anastomosis with colonic J pouch. (e) The extent of colorectal excision: the entire area of dilated colon and rectum is resected down to the level of the dentate line. The marginal artery is carefully preserved so that the proximal colon has an adequate blood supply for restoration of intestinal continuity. (f) The hepatic flexure has been mobilized. The end of the colon has been closed using a linear staple cutter. Two 10-cm limbs of colon are being prepared for the construction of a colonic J pouch. (*Continued*)

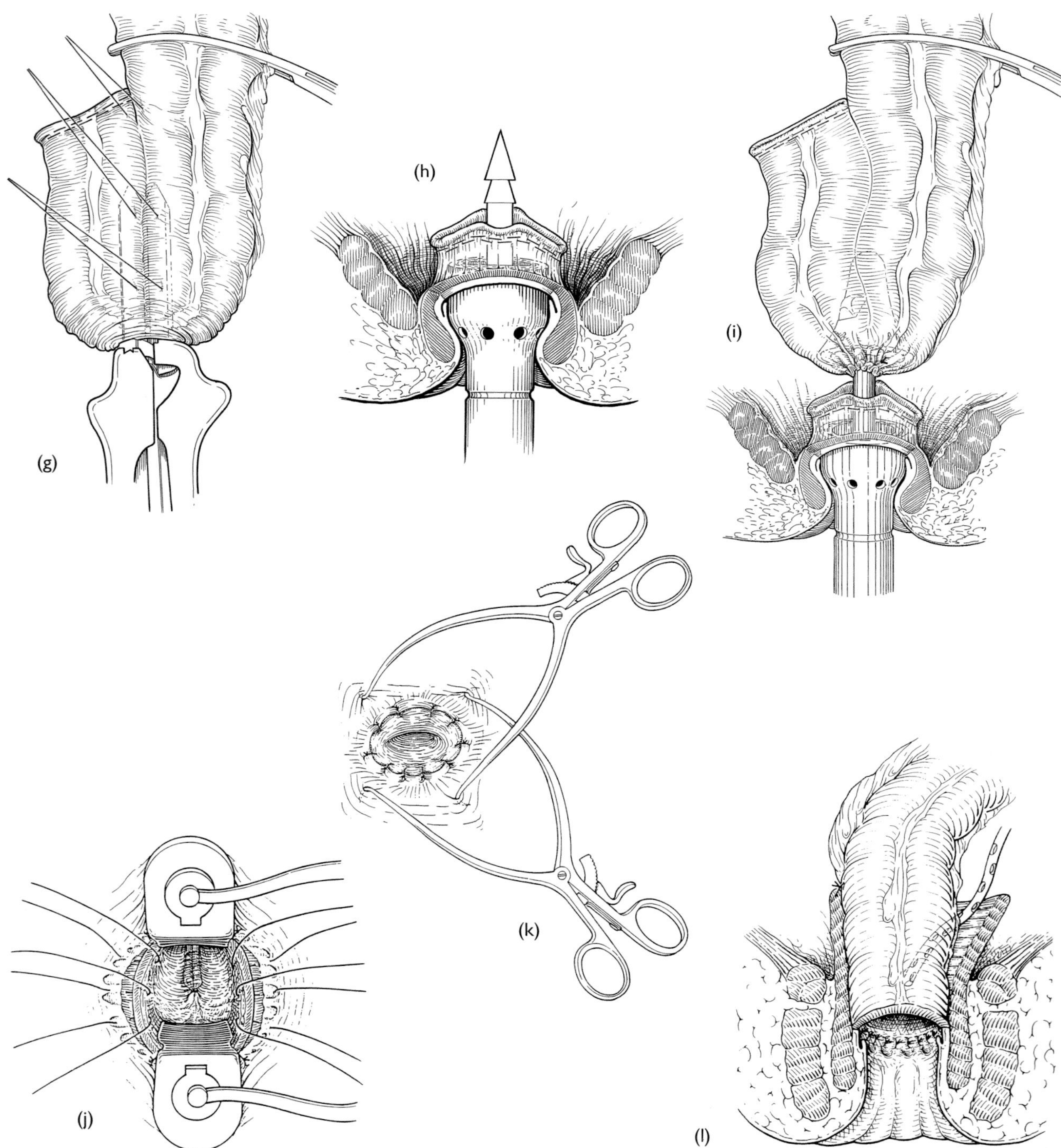

Figure 22.18a–l (*Continued*) If a colonic pouch is being used the following apply: (g) Three stay sutures have been placed between the two limbs of the colon to facilitate pouch construction. A distal apical colotomy is made and a linear staple cutter is advanced between the two walls of the colon to achieve a side-to-side colocolonic anastomosis. (h) The anorectal junction is transected using a linear staple device, either the TL 30 or the TA 30. A double staple coloanal anastomosis is performed with the circular stapling device, with a detachable anvil; the central spindle is advanced with the spike through the centre of the transected anal staple line. (i) The anvil is placed inside the colonic pouch and the apical purse-string suture is tied. The circular staple device is closed, the gun is fired, and the coloanal anastomosis is completed. (j) In some patients it is impossible to perform a stapled coloanal anastomosis, on account of the width of the anorectum in megarectum. Under these circumstances the anorectum is transected with scissors, and a sutured coloanal anastomosis is performed using the apex of the colonic J pouch. (k) A pair of Gelpi retractors may be used to facilitate a sutured coloanal anastomosis. (l) The completed handsewn anastomosis.

Surgical procedure

The patient is placed in the Lloyd Davies position, catheterized and given short-term antibiotic cover. Access to the perineum is essential and the buttocks should be placed well over the end of the operating table. The perineal procedure is facilitated by the use of a perineal tray and a headlamp is essential. A long midline incision is used for access. The usual findings are of an enormously dilated rectum with some enlargement of the sigmoid; sometimes the bladder is also dilated, in association with megaureters. The proximal colon is normal in diameter; the anus is often quite patulous, especially if there has been faecal impaction. Under these circumstances bowel preparation may be impossible and faecal disimpaction is contraindicated, hence the faecaloma must be milked into the segment being resected at the time of operation.

The splenic flexure is taken down and the rectum is mobilized just behind the superior rectal vessels, taking care not to damage the pelvic nerves at the pelvic brim. The inferior mesenteric artery is ligated before its first branch but some distance from the preaortic sympathetic plexus (Figure 22.18e). The superior mesenteric vein is ligated as it enters the splenic vein. The left colonic arcades are preserved. The rectal dissection is often difficult and bloody owing to the large rectal veins and the size of the rectum. Dissection should proceed down to the low rectum at the level of the levator ani. The anal canal may be very dilated, in which case conventional staple transection usually fails because the anorectum is so thick. If this is the case the anal canal is merely divided and a sutured coloanal anastomosis is fashioned. The proximal colon may be divided by staples to minimize contamination, but it is usually necessary to perform an on-table lavage in order to clear the proximal faecal residue before an anastomosis is fashioned. Once the colonic lavage is completed, the distal few centimetres of the colon is transected and either a purse-string is inserted for a stapled anastomosis or the colon is transected with staples to minimize contamination during delivery of the colon to the perineum for a sutured anastomosis.

The blood supply to the descending colon is usually based on the middle colic vessels and the marginal arcade (Figure 22.18e). If sufficient left colon can be mobilized to allow construction of a reservoir colonic pouch (Figure 22.18f), two lengths of colon (6 cm × 6 cm) are held together by stay sutures to allow pouch construction with the TLC 75 or GIA 90 stapler (Figure 22.18i). However, we no longer advise this for dilating disease and prefer a straight coloanal anastomosis. If the anorectum has been successfully closed by stapled transection after partial division of the rectal wall or a purse-string suture, the colodistal rectal or coloanal anastomosis may be completed with the premium EEA stapling device. If it has been impossible to cross-staple the anus or insert a perianal purse-string, or if the transected anorectum has split, a sutured coloanal anastomosis is used (see Figure 22.18d,j,k).

We usually advise a covering ileostomy even when on-table assessment of the anastomosis indicates that it is intact.

We believe the operation has a real place for patients who have reasonable anal sphincter function and in whom the dilated bowel is confined to the rectum and sigmoid when the rest of the large bowel is normal. One late complication is a high anorectal stricture. If this persists it can be resolved by a transrectal approach in the prone position by an anorectal strictureplasty (Figure 22.19).

Restorative proctocolectomy

If the dilated large bowel involves the rectum and the entire colon, we now consider that restorative proctocolectomy may be the optimum initial form of therapy, provided sphincter function is satisfactory. We have reported our experience of this approach in 15 patients with megacolon and megarectum. Five had an initial restorative proctocolectomy, while the remaining ten had had a variety of procedures before: one had had a previous coloanal pouch procedure with recurrent constipation and two had had a subtotal colectomy and ileorectal anastomosis with later development of a megarectum. The remaining seven had had various operations for volvulus. In all except two patients the functional results were acceptable (Stewart et al, 1994).

Brown and Shorthouse (1997) report two cases treated by restorative proctocolectomy who had poor anal function but in whom sphincter recovery occurred once the faecaloma had been eliminated, resulting in a successful outcome.

The techniques of restorative proctocolectomy are discussed elsewhere (see Chapter 49). In megacolon and megarectum the rectal excision may be difficult and bleeding from dilated rectal veins can be considerable. Furthermore, stapled transection of the anus is rarely possible, owing to the very thick anorectal wall, unless the anorectal longitudinal muscle is divided almost down the mucosa. There is also a danger that too much anus may be excised because the anorectal junction is poorly defined and the anus dilated. We believe that a stapled ileoanal anastomosis is frequently inappropriate in these

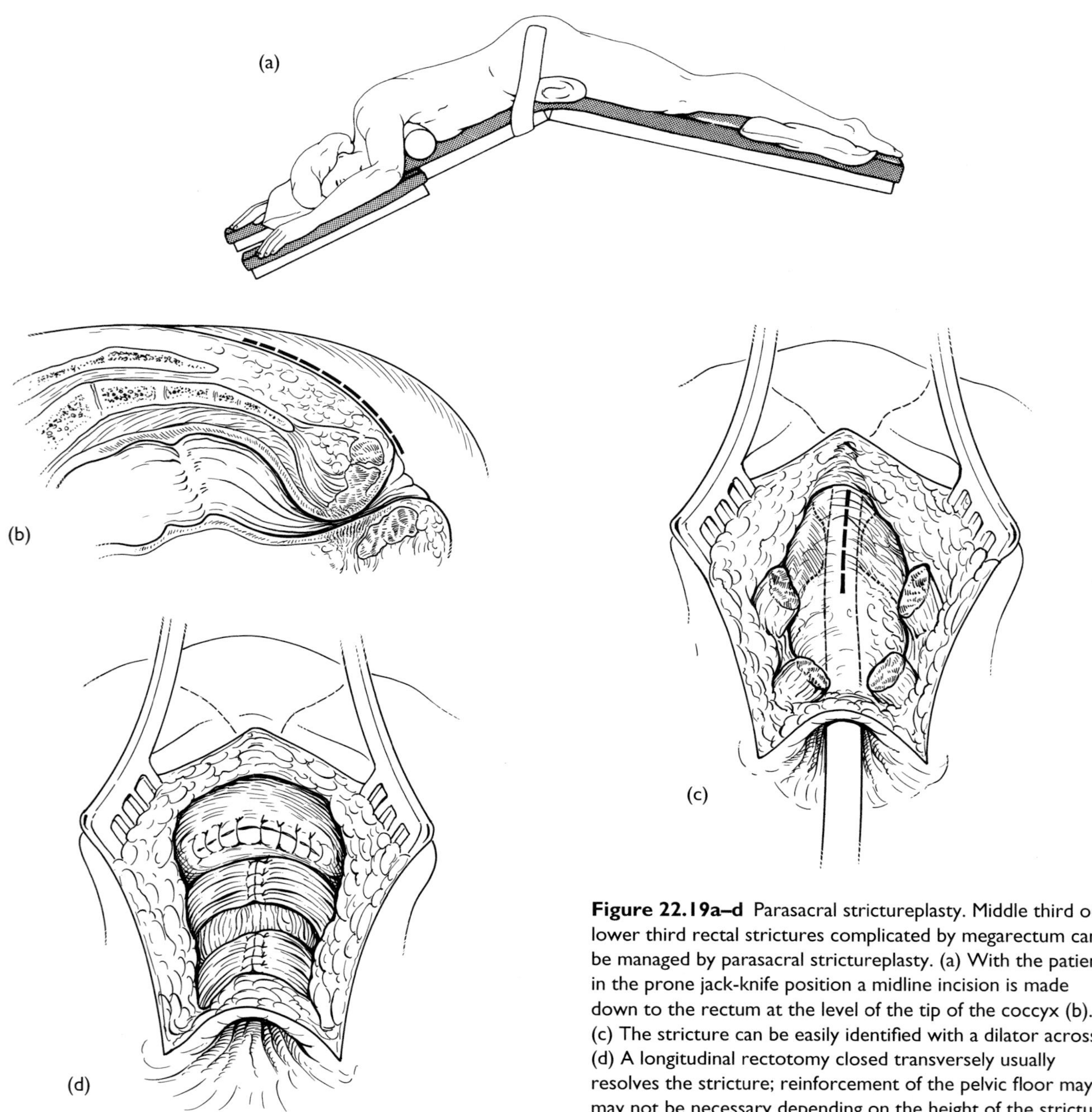

Figure 22.19a–d Parasacral strictureplasty. Middle third or lower third rectal strictures complicated by megarectum can be managed by parasacral strictureplasty. (a) With the patient in the prone jack-knife position a midline incision is made down to the rectum at the level of the tip of the coccyx (b). (c) The stricture can be easily identified with a dilator across it. (d) A longitudinal rectotomy closed transversely usually resolves the stricture; reinforcement of the pelvic floor may or may not be necessary depending on the height of the stricture.

patients and therefore advise scissor division of the anorectum with sutured ileoanal anastomosis, leaving a short anorectal cuff (Figure 22.20). For this reason, most patients have a proximal temporary defunctioning ileostomy with restoration of intestinal continuity after 6–8 weeks.

Permanent stoma

Occasionally a permanent stoma may be necessary for adult megacolon and megarectum. This option must be considered as a method of initial therapy, or if reconstructive surgery fails or is contraindicated or if the patient prefers to have a stoma rather than a reconstruction (Stabile et al, 1992a). Only one of our patients elected to have a stoma as her initial and definitive operation; she is entirely satisfied with her choice, having preferred not to have her covering stoma closed. The seven other patients with a stoma have required one because of poor functional results (Stewart et al, 1994).

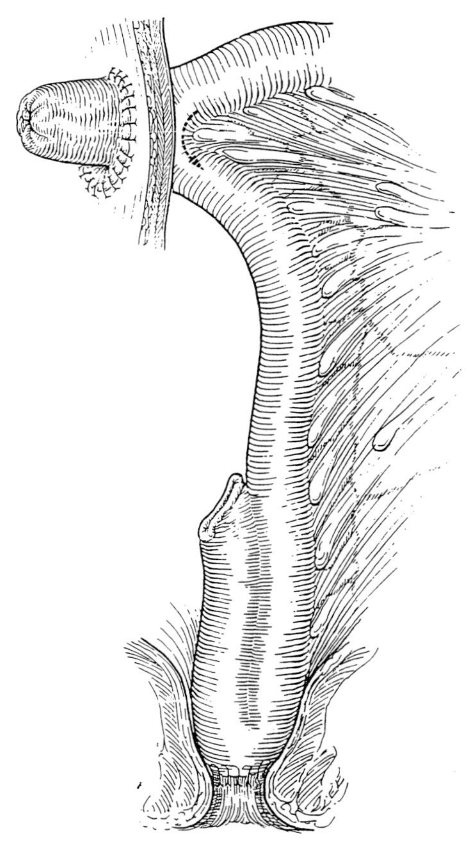

Figure 22.20 Restorative proctocolectomy using a J pouch ileoanal anastomosis is occasionally used for megacolon and megarectum. Under these circumstances a sutured ileoanal anastomosis is probably necessary because staple transection of the anus is not possible owing to the thickness of the gut wall; a covering ileostomy is usually advised.

REFERENCES

Aldridge RT & Campbell PE (1968) Ganglion cell distribution in the normal rectum and anal canal. A basis for the diagnosis of Hirschsprung's disease by anorectal biopsy. *J Pediatr Surg* **3**: 475.

Arhan P, Faverdin C & Thouvenot J (1972) Anorectal motility in sick children. *Scand J Gastroenterol* **7**: 309–314.

Arhan P, Persoz B, Faverdin C, Revillon Y & Pellerin D (1979) Le coefficient d'elasticite de la paroi rectale (CEPR): un test pronostic de la maladie de Hirschsprung. *Chir Pediatr* **20**: 185–191.

Aronson I & Nixon HH (1972) A clinical evaluation of anorectal pressure studies in the diagnosis of Hirschsprung's disease. *Gut* **13**: 138–146.

Barnes PRH, Lennard-Jones JE, Hawley PR & Todd IP (1986) Hirschsprung's disease and idiopathic megacolon in adults and adolescents. *Gut* **27**: 534–541.

Belliveau P, Goldberg SM, Rothenberger DA & Nivatvongs S (1982) Idiopathic acquired megacolon: the value of subtotal colectomy. *Dis Colon Rectum* **25**: 118–121.

Boeckxstaens GE, Pelkmans PA, Herman AG & Maercke YMV (1993) Involvement of nitric oxide in the inhibitory innervation of the human isolated colon. *Gastroenterology* **104**: 690–697.

Boley SJ (1968) An endorectal pull-through operation with primary anastomosis for Hirschsprung's disease. *Surg Gynecol Obstet* **127**: 353–362.

Boley SJ (1984) A new operative approach to total aganglionosis of the colon. *Surg Gynecol Obstet* **159**: 481–484.

Brown SR & Shorthouse AJ (1997) Restorative proctocolectomy for idiopathic megarectum: Postoperative recovery of hypotonic anal sphincters: Report of two cases. *Dis Colon Rectum* **40**: 625–627.

Cameron JAM (1928) On aetiology of Hirschsprung's disease. *Arch Dis Child* **3**: 210.

Clausen EG & Davis VG (1963) Early and late complications of the Swenson pull-through operation for Hirschsprung's disease. *Am J Surg* **106**: 372–376.

Coran AG & Weintraub WH (1976) Modification of the endorectal procedure for Hirschsprung's disease. *Surg Gynecol Obstet* **143**: 277–282.

Crowe R, Kamm MA, Burnstock G & Lennard-Jones JE (1992) Peptide-containing neurons in different regions of the submucous plexus of human sigmoid colon. *Gastroenterology* **102**: 461–467.

Dale G, Bonham JR, Lowdon P, Wagget J, Rangecroft L & Scott DJ (1979) Diagnostic value of rectal mucosal acetylcholinesterase levels in Hirschsprung's disease. *Lancet* **i**: 347–349.

Devroede G (1983) Constipation: mechanisms and management. In Slesinger MH & Fordtran JS (eds) *Gastrointestinal Disease*, 3rd edn, pp 288–308. Philadelphia: WB Saunders.

Duhamel B (1960) A new operation for the treatment of Hirschsprung's disease. *Arch Dis Child* **35**: 38–39.

Dupont C, Navarro J, Chenut B & Rosselin G (1980) Modifications of VIP intestinal content associated with abnormal nervous myenteric plexus: a biologic feature of chronic intestinal obstruction. *J Pediatr* **96**: 1037–1039.

Earlam R (1985) A vascular cause for Hirschsprung's disease. *Gastroenterology* **88**: 1274–1279.

Ehrenpreis T, Livaditis A & Okmian L (1966) Results of Duhamel's operation for Hirschsprung's disease. *J Paediatr Surg* **1**: 40–46.

Elliot MS & Todd IP (1985) Adult Hirschsprung's disease: results of the Duhamel procedure. *Br J Surg* **72**: 884–885.

Fairgreave J (1963) Hirschsprung's disease in the adult. *Br J Surg* **50**: 506–514.

Faverdin C, Dornic C, Arhan P et al (1981) Quantitative analysis of anorectal pressures in Hirschsprung's disease. *Dis Colon Rectum* **24**: 422–427.

Freund HR, Humphrey CS & Fischer JE (1981) Reduced tissue content of vasoactive intestinal peptide in aganglionic colon of Hirschsprung's disease. *Am J Surg* **141**: 243–246.

Furness JB & Costa M (1980) Types of nerves in the enteric nervous system. *Neuroscience* **5**: 1–20.

Furness JB & Costa M (1987) *The Enteric Nervous System*. Edinburgh: Churchill Livingstone.

Gannon BJ, Noblet HR & Burnstock G (1969) Adrenergic innervation of bowel in Hirschsprung's disease. *BMJ* **2**: 187–191.

Garrett JR & Howard ER (1981) Myenteric plexus of the hind-gut: developmental abnormalities in humans and experimental studies. *Ciba Found Symp* **83**: 326–354.

Garrett JR, Howard ER & Nixon HH (1969) Autonomic nerves in rectum and colon in Hirschsprung's disease. A cholinesterase and catecholamine histochemical study. *Arch Dis Child* **44**: 406–409.

Gattuso JM & Kamm MA (1997) Clinical features of idiopathic megarectum and idiopathic megacolon. *Gut* **41**: 93–99.

Gattuso JM, Hoyle CHV, Milner P, Kamm MA & Burnstock G (1996a) Enteric innervation in idiopathic megarectum and megacolon. *Int J Colorectal Dis* **11**: 264–271.

Gattuso JM, Kamm MA, Morris G & Britton KE (1996b) Gastrointestinal transit in patients with idiopathic megarectum. *Dis Colon Rectum* **39**: 1044–1050.

Gattuso JM, Kamm MA, Halligan SM & Bartram CI (1996c) The anal sphincter in idiopathic megarectum. *Dis Colon Rectum* **39**: 435–439.

Gattuso JM, Kamm MA & Talbot IC (1997) Pathology of idiopathic megarectum and megacolon. *Gut* **41**: 252–257.

Goligher JC (1984) In *Diseases of the Anus, Colon and Rectum*, 5th edn, pp 340–341. London: Baillière Tindall.

Gordon PH (1983) An improved technique for the Duhamel operation using the EEA stapler. *Dis Colon Rectum* **26**: 690–692.

Hamdy MH & Scobie WG (1984) Anorectal myectomy in adult Hirschsprung's disease: a report of six cases. *Br J Surg* **71**: 611–613.

Horovitz IL & Baier I (1974) An unusual case of aganglionic megacolon. *Dis Colon Rectum* **17**: 249.

Hosie KB, Kmiot WA & Keighley MRB (1990) Constipation: another indication for restorative proctocolectomy. *Br J Surg* **77**: 801–802.

Howard ER, Garrett JR & Kidd A (1982) Congenital neuronal disorders of the hind-gut: the value of anorectal biopsies. *Scand J Gastroenterol* **17**: 151–153.

Jarvinen HJ & Rintala R (1985) Funnel anus and megacolon in an adult. *Dis Colon Rectum* **28**: 957–959.

Jennings PJ (1967) Megarectum and megacolon in adolescents and young adults. Results of treatment at St Mark's Hospital. *Proc R Soc Med* **60**: 805–806.

Keef KD, Du C, Ward SM, McGregor B & Sanders KM (1993) Enteric inhibitory neural regulation of human colonic circular muscle: role of nitric oxide. *Gastroenterology* **105**: 1009–1016.

Kim CY, Park J-G, Park KW, Park KJ, Cho MH & Kim WK (1995) Adult Hirschsprung's disease: Results of the Duhamel's procedure. *Int J Colorectal Dis* **10**: 156–160.

Kluck P, Muijen GNP, Kamp AWM et al (1984) Hirschsprung's disease studied with monoclonal antineurofilament antibodies on tissue sections. *Lancet* **i**: 652–653.

Krishnamurthy S, Schuffler MD, Rohrmann CA & Pope CE (1985) Severe idiopathic constipation is associated with a distinctive abnormality of the colonic myenteric plexus. *Gastroenterology* **88**: 26–34.

Kune GA (1966) Megacolon in adults. *Br J Surg* **53**: 199–205.

Kusunoki M, Shoji Y, Yanagi H et al (1991) Function after abdominal rectal resection and colonic J pouch-anal anastomosis. *Br J Surg* **78**: 1434–1438.

Lane RHS & Todd IP (1977) Idiopathic megacolon: a review of 42 cases. *Br J Surg* **64**: 305–310.

Lawson JON & Nixon HH (1967) Anal canal pressure in the diagnosis of Hirschsprung's disease. *J Paediatr Surg* **2**: 544–552.

Lee YK & Koh YB (1977) Anorectal excision myomectomy for distal short segment Hirschsprung's disease. *Am J Proctol* **28**: 52–58.

Lefebvre MP, Leape LL, Pohl DA, Safaii H & Grand RJ (1984) Total colonic aganglionosis initially diagnosed in an adolescent. *Gastroenterology* **87**: 1364–1366.

Lewis WG, Holdsworth PJ, Stephenson BM, Finan PJ & Johnston D (1992) Role of the rectum in the physiological and clinical results of coloanal and colorectal anastomosis after anterior resection for rectal carcinoma. *Br J Surg* **79**: 1082–1086.

Lorenzo MD, Yazbech S & Brochu P (1985) Aganglionosis of the entire bowel: four new cases and review of the literature. *Br J Surg* **72**: 657–658.

Louw JH (1961) The Duhamel type operation for Hirschsprung's disease. *S Afr Med J* **35**: 1033–1036.

Luukkonen P, Heikkinen M, Huikuri K & Harvinen H (1990) Adult Hirschsprung's disease: clinical features and functional outcome after surgery. *Dis Colon Rectum* **33**: 65–69.

Lynn HB (1966) Rectal myectomy for aganglionic megacolon. *Mayo Clin Proc* **41**: 289–296.

Lynn HB & van Heerden JA (1975) Rectal myectomy in Hirschsprung's disease: a decade of experience. *Arch Surg* **110**: 991–993.

McCourtney JS, Hussain N & Mackenzie I (1996) Balloon tamponade for control of massive presacral haemorrhage. *Br J Surg* **83**: 222.

McCready RA & Beart RW (1980) Adult Hirschsprung's disease. Results of surgical treatment in the Mayo Clinic. *Dis Colon Rectum* **23**: 401–407.

McGavity WC & Cody JE (1974) Complications of Hirschsprung's disease in adults. *Am J Gastroenterol* **61**: 390–393.

Madsen CM (1964) *Hirschsprung's Disease: Congenital Intestinal Aganglionosis*, p 245. Copenhagen: Munksgaard.

Meier-Ruge W, Lutterbek PM, Herzog B, Morger R, Moser R & Scharli A (1972) Acetylcholinesterase activity in suction biopsies of the rectum in the diagnosis of Hirschsprung's disease. *J Paediatr Surg* **7**: 11–15.

Metzgar PP, Alvear DT, Arnold GC & Stoner RR (1978) Hirschsprung's disease in adults: report of a case and review of the literature. *Dis Colon Rectum* **21**: 113–117.

Natsikas NB & Sbarounis CN (1987) Adult Hirschsprung's disease: an experience with the Duhamel–Martin procedure with special reference to obstructed patients. *Dis Colon Rectum* **30**: 204–206.

Nissan S, Barr-Maor JA & Levy E (1971) Anorectal myectomy in the treatment of short segment Hirschsprung's disease and idiopathic megacolon. *J Paediatr Surg* **6**: 738–741.

Palmer JA & McBirnie JE (1967) Atonic megacolon. *Can J Surg* **10**: 15–20.

Partiquin H, Martelli H & Devroede G (1978) Barium enema in chronic constipation: is it meaningful? *Gastroenterology* **75**: 619–624.

Pelissier EP, Blum D, Bachour A & Bosset JF (1992) Stapled coloanal anastomosis with reservoir procedure. *Am J Surg* **163**: 435.

Penninckx FM & Kerremans R (1975a) Evaluation of anorectal motility and rectoanal reflex in Hirschsprung's disease and functional constipation. *Acta Paediatr Scand* **148**: 47–51.

Penninckx F & Kerremans R (1975b) Pharmacological characteristics of the ganglionic and aganglionic colon in Hirschsprung's disease. *Life Sci* **17**: 1387–1394.

Pescatori M, Mattana C & Castiglioni GC (1986) Adult megacolon due to total hypoganglionosis. *Br J Surg* **73**: 765.

Pinho M, Yoshioka K & Keighley MRB (1989) Long term results of anorectal myectomy for chronic constipation. *Br J Surg* **76**: 1163–1164.

Poisson J & Devroede G (1983) Severe chronic constipation as a surgical problem. *Surg Clin North Am* **63**: 193–217.

Prout BJ (1984) Constipation. *Gastroenterol Pract* 17–24.

Robertson HE & Kernohan JW (1938) The myenteric plexus in congenital megacolon. *Proc Staff Meetings Mayo Clin* **13**: 123–125.

Robertson K, Mason I & Halls I (1997) Hirschspring's disease: genetic mutations in mice and men. *Gut* **41**: 436–441.

Rogawski MA, Goodrich JT, Gershon MD & Touloukian RJ (1978) Hirschsprung's disease: absence of serotonergic neurons in the aganglionic colon. *J Paediatr Surg* **13**: 608–609.

Rosin JD, Bargen JA & Waugh JM (1950) Congenital megacolon of a man 54 years of age. Report of a case. *Mayo Clin Proc* **25**: 710.

San Filippo JA, Allen JE & Jewett TC (1972) Definitive surgical management of Hirschsprung's disease. *Arch Surg* **105**: 245–247.

Schuster MM, Tobon F, Reid NCRW & Talbert JL (1968) Nonsurgical test for the diagnosis of Hirschsprung's disease. *N Engl J Med* **278**: 188–194.

Shuster G, Kim IC & Barbero GJ (1970) Rectal motility patterns in infants and children with aganglionic megacolon. *Am J Dis Child* **119**: 494–499.

Smith SB (1968) Effect of irritant purgatives on the myenteric plexus in man and the mouse. *Gut* **9**: 139–142.

Soave F (1964) Hirschsprung's disease: a new surgical technique. *Arch Dis Child* **39**: 116–119.

Soper RT & Miller FE (1968) Congenital aganglionic megacolon (Hirschsprung's disease): diagnosis, management and complications. *Arch Surg* **96**: 554–561.

Stabile G, Kamm PR, Hawley PR & Lennard-Jones JE (1991) Results of the Duhamel operation in the treatment of idiopathic megarectum and megacolon. *Br J Surg* **78**: 661–663.

Stabile G, Kamm MA, Hawley PR & Lennard-Jones JE (1992a) Results of stoma formation for idiopathic megarectum and megacolon. *Int J Colorect Dis* **7**: 82–84.

Stabile G, Kamm MA, Phillips RKS, Hawley PR & Lennard-Jones JE (1992b) Partial colectomy and coloanal anastomosis for idiopathic megarectum and megacolon. *Dis Colon Rectum* **35**: 158–162.

Starling JR, Croom RD III & Thomas CG Jr (1986) Hirschsprung's disease in young adults. *Am J Surg* **151**: 104–109.

State D (1963) Segmental colon resection in the treatment of congenital megacolon (Hirschsprung's disease). *Am J Surg* **105**: 93–98.

Stewart J, Kumar D & Keighley MRB (1994) Results of anal or low rectal anastomosis and pouch construction for megarectum and megacolon. *Br J Surg* **81**: 1051–1053.

Stone WD, Hendrix TR & Schuster MM (1965) Aganglionosis of the entire colon in an adolescent. *Gastroenterology* **48**: 636.

Swenson O & Bill AH (1948) Resection of rectum and rectosigmoid with preservation of the sphincter for benign spastic lesions producing megacolon: an experimental study. *Surgery* **24**: 212–220.

Swenson O, Sherman JO & Fisher JH (1973) Diagnosis of congenital megacolon: an analysis of 501 patients. *J Paediatr Surg* **8**: 587–593.

Swenson O, Sherman JO, Fisher JH & Cohen E (1975) The treatment and postoperative complications of congenital megacolon. 25 year follow up. *Ann Surg* **182**: 266–272.

Tafuri WL, Maria TA, Pitella JEH, Bogliolo L, Hial W & Diniz CR (1974) An electron microscope study of the Auerbach's plexus and determination of substance P of the colon in Hirschsprung's disease. *Virchows Arch [A]* **362**: 41–49.

Taylor I (1984) Assessment of anorectal motility measurements in the management of adult megacolon. *Clin Gastroenterol* **51**: 61–68.

Taylor I, Hammond P & Darby C (1980) An assessment of anorectal motility in the management of adult megacolon. *Br J Surg* **67**: 754–756.

Tiffin ME, Chander LR & Faber JH (1940) Localized absence of myenteric plexus in congenital megacolon. *Am J Dis Child* **59**: 1071–1073.

Todd IP (1977) Adult Hirschsprung's disease. *Br J Surg* **64**: 311–312.

Udassin R, Nissan PJ, Lerrnau O & Hod G (1983) The mild form of Hirschsprung's disease (short segment). *Ann Surg* **194**: 767–770.

Watkins GL (1966) Operative treatment of acquired megacolon in adults. *Arch Surg* **93**: 620–624.

Weinberg AG (1970) The anorectal myenteric plexus: its relation to hypoganglionosis of the colon. *Am J Clin Pathol* **54**: 637–639.

Whitehouse FR & Kernohan JW (1948) Myenteric plexus in congenital megacolon. Study of eleven cases. *Arch Intern Med* **82**: 75.

Yoshioka K & Keighley MRB (1987) Anorectal myectomy for outlet obstruction. *Br J Surg* **74**: 373–376.

23
RECTAL PROLAPSE

Rectal prolapse is a distressing condition that is associated with faecal incontinence in 50–70% of patients (Andrews and Jones, 1992). Incontinence is particularly prevalent in elderly patients (Stenchever, 1984). The prolapse itself is socially embarrassing, especially if it descends during normal social activities. Bleeding and mucous discharge are common symptoms. Women are principally affected; when men develop a prolapse there is usually some underlying predisposing factor. Young patients invariably give a history of straining at stool for many years.

Rectal prolapse appears to be a true intussusception of the rectum through the sphincters. It is associated with a deep rectovaginal or rectovesical peritoneal pouch, lax lateral ligaments and loss of attachment of the rectum to the sacrum; consequently genital prolapse is common and urinary incontinence may coexist (Hudson, 1988). There is marked perineal descent and the anus may be patulous. The pelvic floor becomes stretched and a traction neuropathy frequently affects the pudendal nerve.

CHILDREN WITH RECTAL PROLAPSE

Rectal prolapse is relatively uncommon in children but when it occurs there is usually some predisposing factor. It is essentially a self-limiting condition that rarely requires surgical treatment.

Predisposing conditions

Rectal prolapse often occurs in children with chronic respiratory disease such as cystic fibrosis. Stern et al (1982) reported rectal prolapse in 112 of 605 patients with cystic fibrosis (18%). In a third of children the prolapse preceded the diagnosis. Kulczycki and Shwachman (1958) reported a 28% incidence of prolapse in cystic fibrosis. Malnutrition appears to be a predisposing factor, especially when it occurs in association with diarrhoeal disorders such as amoebiasis, giardiasis and worms (Soriano et al, 1966; Taynor and Michener, 1966; Narasanagi, 1973; Nwako, 1975; Bhandari and Ameta, 1977). Malnutrition is a particularly important predisposing factor in Africa and India due, it is thought, to a lack of rectal support from the perirectal fat. A high incidence of prolapse was observed in Rwanda among children in refugee camps (Chaloner et al, 1996). It has also been suggested that children are more susceptible than adults to rectal prolapse because the rectal mucosa is more lax owing to the lack of attachment to the muscularis (Santulli, 1983). Other anatomical factors which may predispose to prolapse in children are the straight course of the rectum, the flat sacrum and the lack of support from the levators and endopelvic fascia.

Incidence

Rectal prolapse is most common in children under the age of 3 years and is most frequent in the first year of life. At this age, and because the mucosa is lax, mucosal prolapse is more common than full-thickness prolapse. In most studies, the sex incidence is equal (Datta and Das, 1977; Corman, 1985).

Symptoms and signs

A child may appear to be straining and in pain; there may be some blood and mucus on the nappy. Attacks of screaming may suggest abdominal colic and constipation. Mucosal protrusion or a complete rectal prolapse may be seen on straining. The sphincter may be lax. Often there will be evidence of an underlying cause such as cystic fibrosis or malnutrition. Sometimes, if the child has been straining excessively, a fissure-in-ano may develop, which may be visible on anal inspection.

It may be difficult to distinguish a full-thickness rectal prolapse from an ileocolic or colocolic intussusception. An intussusception commonly has a polyp at its apex. If the protrusion is an intussusception which arises in the ileum or colon there is a sulcus between the intussusception and the anal canal. A prolapse must also be distinguished from a polyp or haemorrhoids.

Treatment

Conservative treatment is usually successful in the management of children with a rectal prolapse and this is the policy we advise. As the child grows, so the support around the rectum develops. This was the rationale behind strapping the buttocks together to maintain the rectum in its normal position. Children with severe malnutrition may require nutritional support as well as replacement of the prolapse.

Treatment of prolapse in children is to control any associated respiratory disease, prevent constipation by the use of bulk laxatives and to encourage the proper use of the chamber-pot. The child should not be allowed to sit for longer than it is necessary to pass urine.

If, despite strapping the buttocks, restoring nutrition and the use of stool softeners, the prolapse is not controlled, injection sclerotherapy is advised (Kay and Zachary, 1970). The sclerosing fluid may be phenol in almond oil, although 70% alcohol or 30% saline is preferable at this age. Injection may be given through the anal canal or through the perianal skin adjacent to the levator ani into the ischiorectal fossa. The child must be sedated for this procedure and there is a small risk of perianal or ischiorectal abscess following injection (Corman, 1985), particularly if more than 35 mL of sclerosant is used. Datta and Das (1977) reported an 83% cure rate in 30 patients after one injection; in the patients in whom the prolapse persisted, repeated injection invariably controlled the prolapse. Malyshev and Gulin (1973) reported a 96% success rate with 70% alcohol in 353 children.

Surgical treatment is rarely needed in children because so many respond to conservative therapy. Excision of the mucosal prolapse has been used but is not recommended because of the risk of creating a segment of unsupported mucosa at the anal verge. An anal encircling suture may be used as a temporary expedient. Narasanagi (1973) reported one failure from breakage in three children treated in this way. By contrast, Groff and Nagaraj (1990) point out that an encircling suture generally controls the prolapse satisfactorily and can often be removed at a later date. Other surgical procedures which are described include: linear cauterization of the anorectum (Hight et al, 1982); packing of the

Table 23.1 Results of therapy for rectal prolapse in children.

	Number	*Cure (%)*
Sclerosing injections		
Kay and Zachary (1970)	51	100*
Malyshev and Gulin (1973)	353	96*
Datta and Das (1977)	30	83*
Anal encircling procedure		
Narasanagi (1973)	30	97*
Groff and Nagaraj (1990)	10	100*
Presacral packing		
Nwako (1975)	100	100*
Linear cauterization		
Hight et al (1982)	73	97*
Rectopexy		
Ashcroft et al (1977)	4	100*
Chino and Thomas (1984)	4	100*

* Needed replacing in two.

presacral space with gauze or Gelfoam; trans-sacral rectopexy with excision of the pelvic peritoneal pouch and levatorplasty; transcoccygeal rectopexy with pelvic floor repair (Ashcroft et al, 1977; Chino and Thomas, 1984); and perineal rectopexy (Heald, 1926). However, the preferred procedure if an encircling suture fails is perineal proctosigmoidoscopy (Nash, 1972).

The results of surgical treatment are summarized in Table 23.1. Hight et al (1982) somewhat surprisingly found that only 29 of 102 children responded to conservative measures; the remaining 73 underwent linear cautery of the anorectum, with a successful outcome in 71.

If surgical treatment is needed we would advise an encircling perianal suture as a temporary measure in an attempt to stabilize the rectum adjacent to the sacrum. If after removal of the suture the rectal prolapse recurs, we would remove the redundant rectosigmoid, repair the pelvic floor and obliterate the pouch of Douglas by rectosigmoidectomy.

ADULT RECTAL PROLAPSE

Aetiology

There is some debate as to whether rectal prolapse is due to a sliding hernia, an intussusception or a combination of both. Alexis Moscowitz, in 1912, described rectal prolapse as a sliding hernia and on that basis attempted to establish sound anatomical principles for treatment. Thus he advised repair of the levator hiatus and obliteration of the deep peritoneal cul-de-sac in combination with amputation of the prolapse. Sadly this policy was attended by a high recurrence rate of 48% and thus cast doubt on the sliding hernia theory (Porter, 1962).

Cineradiographic studies by Broden and Snellman (1968), later confirmed by defecography, demonstrated that rectal prolapse was not a sliding hernia but an intussusception and that the anatomical abnormalities were the result of the prolapse rather than its cause (Thauerkauf et al, 1970; Womack et al, 1987; Broden et al, 1988a,b; Yoshioka et al, 1989a). These secondary anatomical abnormalities include the peritoneal cul-de-sac, diastasis of the levators, stretching and denervation of the anal sphincters, a redundant rectosigmoid, loss of the horizontal position of the rectum with attenuation of its sacral and pelvic attachments, loss of support to the uterus and bladder and perineal descent. The relative importance of these factors will be briefly examined since the consequences of a complete rectal intussusception differ according to any coexisting functional disorder and the age of the patient.

Intussusception

The intussusception theory was propounded following cineradiological studies of patients attempting evacuation of barium which had been instilled into the rectum (Broden and Snellman, 1968). In patients with a rectal prolapse the apex of a circumferential intussusception was observed 6–8 cm from the anal verge (Devadhar, 1965). The anterior and posterior wall of the prolapse was of equal length. Sometimes the prolapse was incomplete, particularly in young patients with a history of rectal pain, tenesmus, bleeding and mucous discharge (White et al, 1980). Incomplete intussusception may be difficult to diagnose clinically since the pelvic floor may be normal if perineal descent is not excessive and the anal canal is not lax. With the introduction of videoproctography, incomplete intussusception may be readily visualized as an unfolding of the upper rectum into the anal canal or low rectal ampulla. However, intussusception is a frequent observation even among asymptomatic individuals, hence the significance of this radiological appearance is open to doubt (Hoffman et al, 1984; Berman et al, 1987).

The significance of incomplete rectal intussusception has also been questioned by Mellgren et al (1997) who, using repeated defecography, found that a rectal intussusception was not observed at the second examination in 38 of 41 patients. Furthermore, only one of these patients went on to develop a complete rectal prolapse. Thus, although intussusception is the most plausible theory in the pathogenesis of prolapse, intussusception itself is of uncertain significance. Furthermore, the results of rectopexy in incontinent patients with intussusception are poor (Briel et al, 1997).

In complete rectal prolapse the intussusception continues through the anus and everts on to the perineum (Womack et al, 1987). It has been suggested that incomplete intussusception may be associated with inappropriate contraction of the pelvic floor during defecation, causing a syndrome which may be characterized by ulceration of the anterior anorectum (Rutter and Riddell, 1975). By contrast, complete rectal prolapse is usually associated with a weak pelvic floor and the entire anorectal wall everts through the anal sphincters. The intussusception theory can also be confirmed by applying radio-opaque clips to the four quadrants of the rectal mucosa 6 and 10 cm from the anal verge. Radiographic screening during attempted defecation demonstrates that the clips descend and eventually appear on the perineum or within the anal canal (Pantanowitz and Levine, 1975).

The reason why rectopexy is such a successful treatment for rectal prolapse as compared with rectosigmoidectomy is that the rectum, once fixed to the sacrum, can no longer intussuscept (Blatchford et al, 1989), and provided the material used to fix the rectum to the sacrum does not become detached, the prolapse does not recur (Hool et al, 1997).

Sliding hernia

It used to be thought that complete rectal prolapse was a true sliding hernia, allowing the rectum to prolapse through a weak pelvic floor as a consequence of the long mobile anterior peritoneal reflection (Moscowitz, 1912). If this were true one would expect the anterior aspect of the prolapse to be longer or to precede the rest of the prolapse. However, when a prolapse emerges during straining this is a circumferential phenomenon with the apex at the centre of the completely prolapsed bowel. It is more likely that the long anterior rectovaginal peritoneal pouch is secondary to repeated intussusception. If a rectal prolapse is due to a sliding hernia of the pelvic peritoneum it is difficult to understand why posterior rectopexy would prevent recurrent prolapse. Furthermore, the failure of rectosigmoidectomy to control prolapse is further evidence in favour of a continued intussusception, despite obliteration of the sliding hernia (Friedman et al, 1983).

Pelvic floor deficiency

Most patients, particularly the elderly, with a complete rectal prolapse also have a weak pelvic floor. It was once thought that a deficiency in the levator ani was the primary abnormality in this condition. However, there are some patients with rectal prolapse in whom pelvic floor function is normal (Keighley et al, 1980; Neill et al, 1981; Keighley and Shouler, 1984; Snooks et al, 1985). These include young male patients, some young females who are continent and most elderly nulliparous women. In complete intussusception there may be electromyographic evidence of an overactive pelvic floor and external anal sphincter (Womack et al, 1987). On the other hand, pelvic floor failure is evident in many patients, particularly those in whom faecal incontinence accompanies the prolapse (Agachan et al, 1997). These incontinent patients have low anal canal pressures at rest and during attempted pelvic floor contraction (Penninckx et al, 1978; Hiltunen et al, 1986; Sun et al, 1989; Metcalf and Loening-Baucke, 1988; Hamalainen et al, 1996). This abnormality is associated with delayed pudendal nerve conduction time (Parks et al, 1977; Agachan et al, 1997) and a wide anorectal angle (Parks et al, 1966). In patients with a rectal prolapse and associated incontinence there is a neuropathy of the pelvic floor and external sphincter which is probably due to repeated straining during defecation. The pelvic floor and sphincter abnormality may be reversible, since incontinence improves in approximately 70% of patients following procedures which are merely designed to control the intussusception (Keighley et al, 1983; Tjandra et al, 1993; Schultz et al, 1996; Tolwinski et al, 1997). The above findings suggest, therefore, that in most patients the deficiency is not the cause but the result of the prolapse. Conceivably pelvic floor weakness may be responsible for prolapse in paraplegia or in cauda equina lesions, such as in spina bifida (Nash, 1972).

Associated abnormalities

Apart from the peritoneal cul-de-sac and lax ligamentous attachments of the rectum to the pelvis by the endopelvic fascia, particularly the lateral ligaments, other secondary anatomical features are common in rectal prolapse (Figure 23.1a). Uterine descent is frequent, particularly in the elderly. Many patients with rectal prolapse give a history of vaginal or abdominal hysterectomy or a colporrhaphy. In a study from Edinburgh, eight of 50 female patients with a rectal prolapse had a uterine prolapse, 20 had had a hysterectomy and 12 had had some form of colporrhaphy (Vongsangnak et al, 1985a). Loygue et al (1984) reported that 54 of 200 female patients with rectal prolapse had an associated genital prolapse. Urinary incontinence as well as faecal incontinence may coexist. The urinary incontinence is often associated with a cystocele. Nine of the 30 women in Edinburgh who had bowel incontinence, also suffered from urinary incontinence (Vongsangnak et al, 1985a).

The anorectal angle is significantly more obtuse in patients with rectal prolapse compared with control subjects, in fact a straight anorectum is highly suggestive of a prolapse that may have been missed clinically. The anal canal is shorter than in normal people and there is usually some descent of the perineum and pelvic floor at rest (Yoshioka et al, 1989a). Pelvic floor movements during a maximum squeeze effort are often remarkably vigorous, even in the elderly, with elevation of the pelvic floor and reduction in the anorectal angle. During straining, videoproctography not only reveals the intussusception and emergence of the prolapse, but there is marked perineal descent.

The sigmoid colon is often redundant if there is associated colonic stasis and may contribute to a sigmoidocele which not infrequently occurs with a prolapse (see Chapter 21).

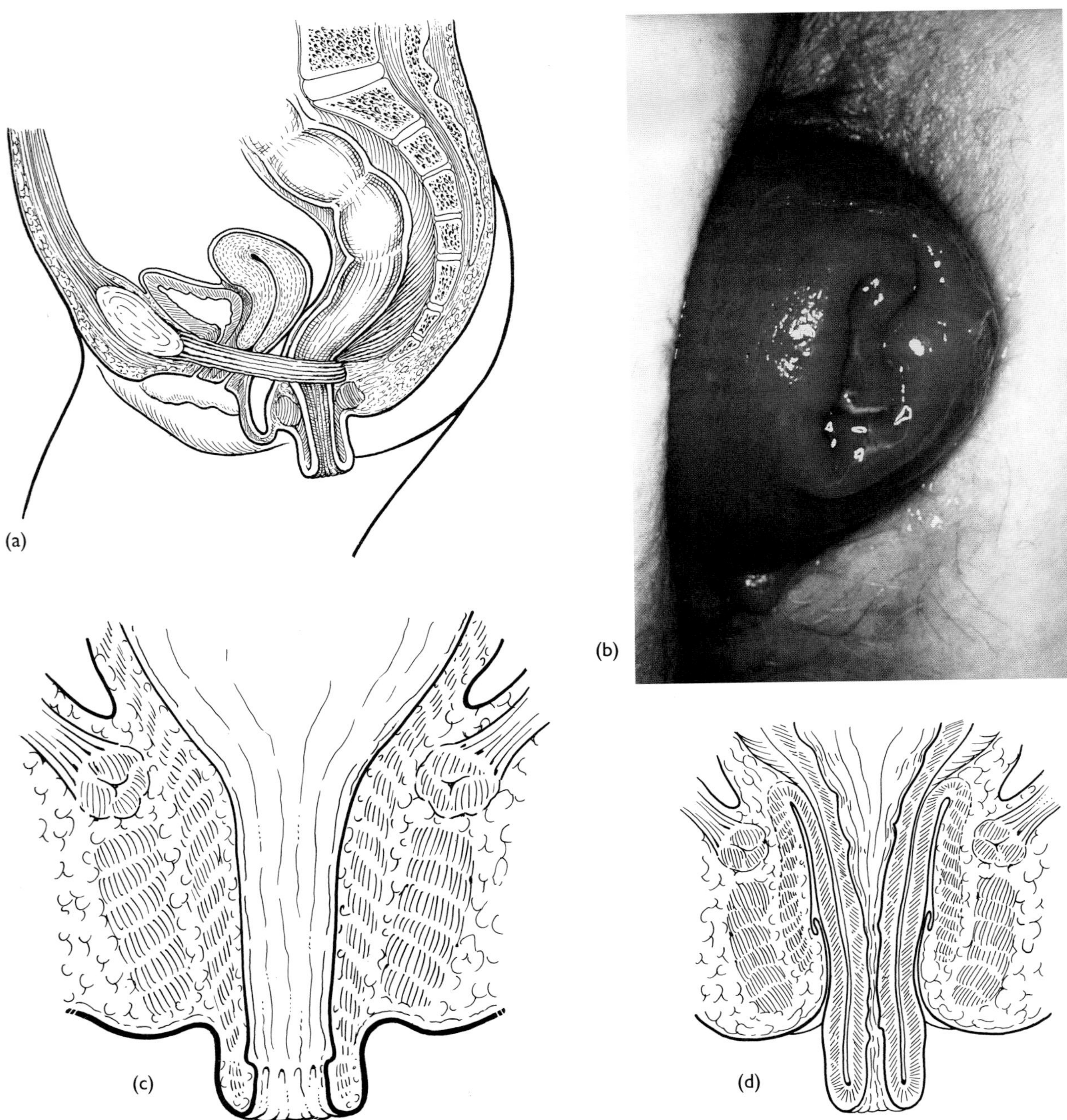

Figure 23.1a–d Pathophysiological abnormalities in rectal prolapse. (a) Sagittal section of the pelvis, indicating the gross anatomical defects in rectal prolapse. Note the long rectovaginal pouch, the uterine and vaginal descent, the lax pelvic floor, the attenuated lateral ligaments, the obtuse anorectal angle and the weak external anal sphincter. (b) Macroscopic features of a full-thickness rectal prolapse. Note that this is a circumferential prolapse with a more prominent anterior component due to the rectovaginal pouch, which descends with the prolapse. (c,d) It is important to differentiate a circumferential mucosal prolapse (c) from a complete intussusception of the rectum through the anal canal (d). Circumferential mucosal prolapse may be amenable to treatment by the Délorme's procedure.

Incidence

Sex, age and parity

Women

There is a higher incidence of prolapse in women than in men and this is particularly correlated with age (Table 23.2). Thus over 50% of female patients with prolapse are over the age of 70 years (Loygue et al, 1984). Rectal prolapse is not confined to the multiparous, a third of elderly patients with prolapse are unmarried and have had no children (Mortensen et al, 1984; Watts et al, 1985). Of 120 consecutive patients with rectal prolapse seen in Birmingham between 1976 and 1984, 40 (33%) were nulliparous, of whom 87% were over the age of 60 years. Although the overall incidence of incontinence in our series of women was 64%, in nulliparous women it was only 22%, compared with 85% in women who had had a vaginal delivery. Incontinence was not, however, confined to the elderly, indeed there is a distinct group of young women, some with eating disorders, who usually have a life-long history of straining with prolapse in whom the bowel dysmotility is the dominant feature (Malik et al, 1997).

Men

Men are much less likely to suffer from rectal prolapse than women (Huber et al, 1995). There have been only 17 men in our series of 269 patients with rectal prolapse and only three presented over the age of 50 years. Seven were from overseas: one was a Nigerian student, two were Jamaican and four were from Egypt. The remaining ten British subjects included two from psychiatric units, four young patients who habitually strained and two who were referred from prison and had been on hunger strike; only two seemed normal. All the male patients with rectal prolapse had normal pelvic floor function and only two gave a history of incontinence. One patient developed a prolapse following repeated manual bladder compression to facilitate voiding after a traumatic paraplegia. These findings are similar to those at the London Hospital and other institutions in the UK. In contrast, rectal prolapse is common in young men in Egypt and is associated with schistosomiasis and amoebic dysentery (Abou-Enein, 1978).

Predisposing factors

Senile dementia

It used to be taught that many patients with rectal prolapse were mentally defective or senile (Altemeier et al, 1971). Vongsangnak et al (1985a) reported that 53% of patients with rectal prolapse had a mental illness. We accept that many patients are very old and infirm but true senile dementia was evident in only a few of our patients. We do not therefore support the notion that dementia is a predisposing factor.

Straining

In some male patients and most younger women there is a long history of straining and some have an associated solitary rectal ulcer. Indeed, seven of the 17 men in the Birmingham series had a solitary ulcer as well as a prolapse.

Schistosomiasis and amoebiasis

Both of these disorders may coexist with rectal prolapse.

Table 23.2 Female patients seen in Birmingham between 1976 and 1984.

Age (years)	*Total no.*	*No. with incontinence*	*Nulliparous*	*No. with incontinence*	*Multiparous*	*No. with incontinence*
Total	120	77 (64)	40	9 (22)	80	68 (85)
10–19	1	0	1	0	0	0
20–29	4	3	1	0	3	3
30–39	2	0	0	—	2	0
40–49	7	4	1	0	6	4
50–59	17	10	2	0	15	10
60–69	26	19	8	1	18	18
70–79	38	24	14	3	24	21
80–89	24	17	12	5	12	12
90–100	1	0	1	0	0	0

Values in parentheses are percentages.

Neurological disorders

Neurological disorders may predispose to rectal prolapse in either sex. Although rectal prolapse is rare in demyelinating disorders and upper motor neurone disease, prolapse is a problem in some cauda equina lesions, particularly in some children with spina bifida (Nash, 1972). Under these circumstances there is usually disordered colonic motility and rectal inertia.

Vaginal delivery

Most nulliparous patients who develop a rectal prolapse have a normal pelvic floor and the prolapse is a true intussusception (Thauerkauf et al, 1970). By contrast, multiparous patients have a higher incidence of incontinence and have a lax pelvic floor as well as an intussusception (Anderson et al, 1981). Many give a history of obstetric trauma or even a previous anal dilatation (Bates, 1972). These patients constitute a group with low anal sphincter pressures and an obtuse anorectal angle (Table 23.3). Pudendal nerve terminal motor latency is prolonged and the physiological defect is identical to that in patients with neuropathic faecal incontinence (Henry et al, 1982; Keighley and Shouler, 1984; Hamalainen et al, 1996).

Constipation

Some patients with rectal prolapse give a long history of constipation. These are principally younger individuals who have no associated history of incontinence, but constipation is probably more common preoperatively than is generally realized (Scaglia et al, 1994). These patients, as well as those with a solitary rectal ulcer or an incomplete intussusception, have disordered rectal emptying (Yoshioka et al, 1989a). Colonic transit is often delayed in rectal prolapse; sometimes this is secondary to anismus. We believe that this represents a distinct group in whom the prolapse is secondary to gross colonic inertia. In these patients the Minneapolis group recommend that subtotal colectomy should be combined with rectopexy (Watts et al, 1985).

Hypermotile sigmoid colon

There are a group of patients with the irritable bowel syndrome and a hypermotile sigmoid colon who have a rectal prolapse, usually with faecal incontinence (Table 23.3). Like a similar group with neuropathic incontinence, episodes of incontinence coincide with unpredictable episodes of colicky abdominal pain and diarrhoea (Keighley and Shouler, 1984). These patients may continue to have symptoms despite surgical treatment because the underlying motility defect persists, resulting in episodic diarrhoea and incontinence.

Others

Systemic sclerosis may be associated with prolapse. The functional prognosis is poor because of sphincter involvement and a low compliance rectum (Leighton et al, 1993).

Symptoms

The typical symptoms in rectal prolapse are: prolapse, mucous discharge, occasional bleeding, and either some diarrhoea or, conversely, severe constipation with or without a history of straining.

Patients usually give a history of incomplete evacuation in association with the prolapse. Frank incontinence of liquids, mucus or even solids is evident in some patients. Diarrhoea and urgency

Table 23.3 Coloanal function in rectal prolapse compared with faecal incontinence.

	Prolapse alone			*Prolapse + incontinence*			*Incontinence alone*		
	Patients		*Controls*	*Patients*		*Controls*	*Patients*		*Controls*
Maximum resting anal pressure	46		74	34	*	72	50	*	84
Maximum squeeze pressure	218		194	89	*	170	100	*	176
Rectoanal inhibitory reflex absent	4		0	8	*	0	11	*	0
Resting anorectal angle	89		74	132	*	82	123	*	88
Motility index	505		630	750	*	260	680	*	320
Peak sigmoid pressure	44		36	43		27	34		24
Contrast passed in 1 min (%) (videoproctogram)	80		75	91		81	94		78
Markers passed in 5 days (%)	55	*	82	68		72	72		78

* Significant difference.
From Keighley and Shouler (1984).

is common and there may be associated proctitis or the irritable bowel syndrome.

The principal complaint in patients with a rectal prolapse is of the prolapse itself. Although incontinence occurs in 50–80% of patients (Kupfer and Goligher, 1970; Penfold and Hawley, 1972; Keighley et al, 1983), as far as the patient is concerned this is a secondary problem. Indeed, in a number of patients, usually elderly, in whom rectopexy has cured the prolapse but with continued incontinence, no further treatment is considered because the principal symptom has been controlled. Many elderly patients are so pleased that the prolapse is cured that occasional leakage of mucus and faeces is accepted. These elderly patients do not object to wearing a pad.

Despite the prolapse, incontinence may be the dominant clinical presentation in some women. These patients often have a weak internal anal sphincter (Spencer, 1984; Hiltunen et al, 1986; Metcalf and Loening-Baucke, 1988) as well as a pudendal nerve conduction defect resulting in increased fibre density in the external sphincter. The pelvic floor is also neuropathic in some patients, while in others there may be a loss of normal rectal sensation and patients seem no longer able to distinguish faeces from descent of the prolapse. By contrast, in some patients the rectum is irritable and contracts vigorously in response to rectal distension; these patients often have diarrhoea (Sun et al, 1989).

The prolapse may bleed from trauma or as a result of venous mucosal congestion due to straining, impaired rectal evacuation or true constipation. A prolapse invariably secretes large quantities of mucus. Mucous discharge is a prominent symptom, and may cause perianal excoriation.

Patients with an incomplete intussusception or occult prolapse give a history of impaired rectal evacuation, tenesmus, rectal pain, mucous discharge and bleeding. The diagnosis is made by videoproctography in patients with the typical symptom complex (Ihre and Seligson, 1975; Mellgren et al, 1997) and may be associated with a solitary ulcer.

Signs

The diagnosis of overt rectal prolapse may be missed unless the patient overcomes his or her embarrassment and forcibly strains down when being examined in the left lateral position (Figure 23.1b). It may be necessary to ask the patient to bear down in the squatting position or even to sit on the lavatory in order to demonstrate the prolapse. A patient may be incorrectly labelled as having idiopathic faecal incontinence, before it becomes apparent that this is secondary to a prolapse which has been missed through failure to examine the patient while forcibly straining. It is also important in our view to distinguish a circumferential mucosal prolapse from a complete procidentia which involves all layers of the bowel wall. In mucosal prolapse a plication operation such as the Délorme's procedure may be ideal, whereas in a complete prolapse a rectopexy is a more appropriate procedure (Figure 23.1c,d).

Table 23.4 Associated disorders in 120 female patients seen in Birmingham (1976–1984).

Disorder	*Number*
Patulous anus	78
Incontinence of faeces	77
Perineal descent	66
Uterine prolapse, cystocele or rectocele	54
Severe constipation	24
Diarrhoea	18
Incontinence of urine	9
Colorectal polyps	7
Solitary rectal ulcer	5
Villous adenoma	2
Paraplegia	1

A high proportion of patients have marked perineal descent at rest or during straining (Table 23.4). The anal canal is always patulous; in fact if the anus is not patulous, the diagnosis should be seriously questioned. It is important to examine the vagina in these patients as there is often either a complete procidentia, cystocele or rectocele. The rectovaginal septum is often atrophic and the perineal body deficient and scarred. Rectal examination reveals an almost straight anorectum, with loss of the normal anorectal angle due to a lax puborectalis. The sphincters are weak and attempted contraction often evokes a rather feeble response (Figure 23.1a). Indeed the patulous anus will often admit three or four fingers quite easily. Sometimes, a rectal prolapse may become incarcerated and require urgent perineal excision (Ramanujam and Venkatesh, 1992; Tjandra et al, 1993).

Investigations

It used to be argued that investigations were quite unnecessary apart from a sigmoidoscopy to exclude an intussuscepting polyp or neoplasm in elderly patients with rectal prolapse. Although barium enema or colonoscopy ensures that gross pathology elsewhere in the anorectum is not missed, one wonders whether such examinations are necessary in patients living in residential homes for the elderly, whose principal concern is the prolapse that falls out every time they go to the toilet or get up.

The question of investigation is much more pertinent in younger patients who may have an underlying functional bowel disorder. Barium enema is generally unnecessary unless the clinician suspects underlying inflammatory bowel disease, polyps or malignant disease. Sigmoidoscopy is always necessary to exclude a solitary ulcer, polyps or mucosal disease. In these patients there may be a primary functional abnormality which has either been responsible for the prolapse or which may identify a group in whom the surgical treatment should be modified. If a solitary ulcer is present or if there is a history of constipation, a videoproctogram provides important anatomical information, allows assessment of pelvic floor movement and the efficiency of rectal emptying. Videoproctography and anorectal physiology may predict whether continence will be restored after rectopexy (Yoshioka et al, 1989a). Colonic transit studies may highlight patients who might benefit from a sigmoid resection or a subtotal colectomy in addition to rectopexy.

Colonic motility studies may identify patients with a hypermotile colon in whom episodic diarrhoea is likely to persist. Anal manometry and nerve conduction studies might indicate patients in whom a synchronous pelvic floor repair is indicated. Extended videoproctography with contrast in the sigmoid may identify those patients with a coexisting sigmoidocele in whom synchronous sigmoidectomy would be advised.

In view of the overwhelming evidence that the rectal prolapse is easily cured but that the function of the bowel may well deteriorate after operation (Loygue et al, 1984; Schlinkert et al, 1985; Watts et al, 1985; Holmstrom et al, 1986b; Mann and Hoffman, 1988; Yoshioka et al, 1989b), it behoves us to select a procedure which will best correct the functional disturbances as well as curing the prolapse.

Sigmoidoscopy

Distal proctitis is a common finding in patients with rectal prolapse and does not signify that there is underlying inflammatory bowel disease. The inflammatory change in the rectal mucosa usually resolves once the prolapse is controlled. The characteristic sigmoidoscopic findings if proctitis is present is a segmental abnormality commencing at the anal verge which stops quite abruptly at 10–12 cm. The mucosa is diffusely inflamed and there is contact bleeding. The histological changes are nonspecific. Biopsies reveal submucosal haemorrhage, a chronic inflammatory infiltrate and obliteration of the lamina propria by fibrosis. There may be superficial mucosal ulceration, irregularity of the crypts and depletion of goblet cells. In some patients there may be features of the solitary rectal ulcer syndrome.

Barium enema

This is probably the least useful investigation and is advised only if there is serious doubt about the underlying diagnosis or coexisting pathology.

Videoproctography

In view of the ability to freeze video frames and to reduce the screening time to 15–20 seconds, this investigation has moved from being a research tool to an investigation which could improve the functional results of treatment (Preston et al, 1984). An obtuse anorectal angle, a short anal canal and excessive pelvic floor descent at rest or on straining indicates a group of patients who are likely to remain incontinent after rectopexy (Yoshioka et al, 1989a) (Table 23.5). It is uncertain whether the addition of a pelvic floor repair will reduce the number of patients with persistent incontinence. Impaired rectal emptying and poor pelvic floor movements might signify a group of patients who may have persistent constipation. Videoproctography may

Table 23.5 Factors predicting return of continence after rectopexy.

	Continence improved (*n* = 6)	*Incontinence persisted* (*n* = 3)
Volume of first leak (cm³)	80 (40–300)	30 (10–40)
Anorectal angle (rest) (degrees)	115 (109–134)	147 (121–151)
Pelvic floor descent (straining) (cm)	2.0 (0.9–4.3)	4.8 (3.8–6.8)
Anal canal length (rest) (cm)	3.7 (3.6–6.2)	2.3 (1.2–3.1)

From Yoshioka et al (1989a).

identify an incomplete intussusception which is common in solitary rectal ulcer but which may occur in asymptomatic individuals (Shorvon et al, 1989). The results of rectopexy in solitary ulcer and incomplete intussusception are generally disappointing and are discussed in Chapters 21 and 24.

Physiological investigations

These investigations are rarely performed routinely, but they may help in selecting the best operation, particularly in young patients and in those with continuing functional disturbance after surgical correction of the prolapse.

Anal manometry

Resting anal pressures and maximum squeeze pressures (Figure 23.2) are much lower in patients with prolapse who are incontinent. The internal anal sphincter, as well as the striated muscle, is impaired in rectal prolapse (Hancock, 1976; Keighley et al, 1983; Hiltunen et al, 1986) (Table 23.6). Furthermore, preoperative anal pressures are of predictive value in identifying patients who are likely to remain incontinent after rectopexy (Table 23.7).

Saline infusion test

Tests of fluid continence (Read et al, 1979) indicate that patients with rectal prolapse invariably leak saline at much smaller volumes than normal individuals (Metcalf and Loening-Baucke, 1988).

Rectal sensation and compliance

Rectal sensation is usually normal in patients with prolapse but intraluminal distension may result in abnormal rectal contractions, suggesting that the mucosa is irritable (Sun et al, 1989). This observation is frequently associated with proctitis and solitary rectal ulceration. Maximum tolerated volumes tend to be low in patients who are also incontinent (Figure 23.2). Rectal compliance is reduced in prolapse.

Table 23.6 Preoperative anal canal pressures in 98 patients with rectal prolapse (Birmingham data).

	Continent (n = 38)	*Incontinent* (n = 60)	*Controls* (n = 40)
Maximum basal pressure (cmH_2O)	63.7 ± 21 SD $P < 0.01$	28.3 ± 11 SD $P < 0.01$	78.3 ± 28 SD
Maximum squeeze pressure (cmH_2O)	159 ± 43 SD $P < 0.01$	78.4 ± 24 SD $P < 0.001$	179 ± 39 SD

Table 23.7 Predictive value of preoperative pressures in 60 incontinent patients with rectal prolapse (Birmingham data).

	Became continent (n = 38)	*Remained incontinent* (n = 22)
Maximum basal pressure (cmH_2O)	38.2 ± 14 SD	19.8 ± 9 SD $P < 0.05$
Maximum squeeze pressure (cmH_2O)	89.3 ± 31 SD	65.2 ± 22 SD $P < 0.05$

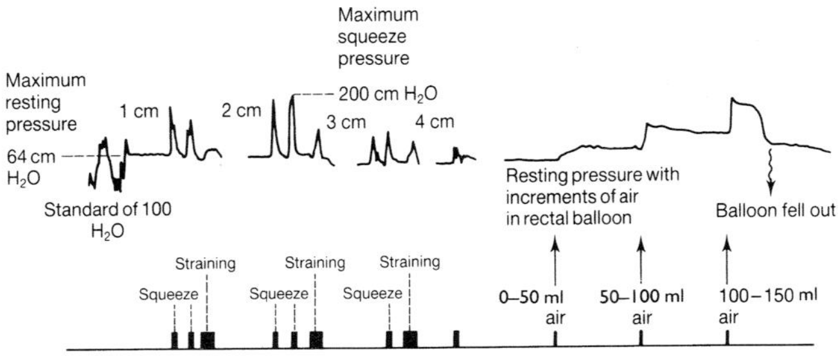

Figure 23.2 Anal manometry in a patient with rectal prolapse and incontinence. On the left the probe has been standardized. Resting, squeeze and straining anal canal pressures are recorded at 1, 2, 3 and 4 cm from the anal verge. Further recordings are obtained at 1 cm from the anal verge after incremental 50-mL volumes of air are introduced into a rectal balloon. Note that the rectoanal inhibitory reflex is absent and that the balloon fell out after the insertion of 150 mL of air.

Anal reflexes

The rectoanal inhibitory reflex and the anocutaneous reflex are absent in a high proportion of patients with rectal prolapse. The rectoanal inhibitory reflex may be absent because resting pressures are so low, while absence of the cutaneous reflex suggests a pudendal neuropathy.

Electromyography and nerve conduction

Single-fibre electromyography of the external sphincter and puborectalis in incontinent prolapse patients provides evidence of nerve damage and attempted reinnervation. Concentric needle electrodes in the sphincter and pelvic floor demonstrate reduced spontaneous action potentials, which are often bifid or biphasic. Pudendal nerve terminal motor latency is prolonged in incontinent patients (Parks et al, 1977; Kiff et al, 1984).

Colonic function studies

Colonic transit times may be greatly prolonged in constipated subjects with rectal prolapse. In all other groups colonic transit is normal. Similarly, resting sigmoid pressures are low in constipated subjects and there is no response to intrarectal bisacodyl (Preston and Lennard-Jones, 1982). Transit studies and colonic manometry may be helpful in identifying patients in whom segmental or subtotal colectomy would be indicated to eliminate postoperative constipation, which may occur despite successful control of the prolapse. Ambulatory studies should help to identify patients with frequent rectal contractions in the presence of low anal pressure in whom episodic diarrhoea and incontinence might be a problem later. However, Farouk et al (1994) found that rectopexy frequently overcame this pressure gradient.

Differential diagnosis

Mucosal prolapse

Mucosal prolapse is not an intussusception and should be distinguished from a complete rectal prolapse by careful examination during straining (Allen-Mersh et al, 1989) (Figure 23.1c,d). There is marked perineal descent at rest in about 20% of patients with mucosal prolapse, and one-third give a history of straining. Bleeding (56%), pain (32%) and constipation (47%) are prominent features especially in women. In complete prolapse persistent straining reveals a circumferential ring of mucosa which quite suddenly gives way to a complete eversion of the rectum through a patulous anus. The prolapse then remains visible until the patient either draws it in by some form of pelvic floor manoeuvre or pushes it back. By contrast, a mucosal prolapse is usually anterior, but it may be circumferential; it is rarely associated with a patulous anus and it never remains prolapsed after the patient has stopped straining. Anterior mucosal prolapse may be associated with the descending perineal syndrome. The natural history of anterior prolapse is that it remains static in 89% of patients. However, in a small proportion who develop perineal descent, 30% become incontinent and one in five of these patients eventually develop an overt rectal prolapse (Allen-Mersh et al, 1989).

Sphincter and pelvic floor deficiency

Patients who are incontinent from a defect in the external sphincter often have a visible area of mucosa overlying the sphincter deficiency. The mucosa is only visible at the site of the sphincter deficiency but may descend for 1–2 cm on straining. The diagnosis can be easily distinguished from a complete prolapse by rectal examination, when a gutter in the sphincter will be readily felt. Idiopathic incontinence may be difficult to differentiate from rectal prolapse if the patient is too embarrassed to strain during clinical examination.

Haemorrhoids

Sometimes it may be difficult to distinguish haemorrhoids from a complete rectal prolapse. Mucous discharge, bleeding, prolapse and perineal descent are prominent features of both disorders. Squamous metaplasia over an area of prolapse is virtually diagnostic of piles. Straining will reveal a progressive downward displacement of two or three haemorrhoids with an area of intervening normal sphincter, as compared with the circumferential mushrooming of a rectal prolapse. Straining during proctoscopy should also help to distinguish prolapsing piles from a complete rectal prolapse. The two disorders rarely coexist.

Polypoidal tumours

Adenomatous polyps or a villous adenoma at the apex of an intussusception should be easily distinguished from a rectal prolapse by sigmoidoscopy. Usually these tumours will be easily visible on the apex of an intussusception during straining.

Proctitis

Distal proctitis is commonly associated with a prolapse. If a prolapse cannot be demonstrated and there is no perineal descent an alternative cause for proctitis must be sought.

Solitary ulcer

Solitary rectal ulcer may occur in association with an overt rectal prolapse but this is relatively uncommon since the surrounding fibrosis usually fixes the anterior mucosa to the surrounding structures and prevents prolapse. Solitary ulcer is much more commonly associated with an incomplete intussusception of the rectum and the results of rectopexy when there is a coexisting intussusception are poor (van Tets and Kuijpers, 1995). If a rectal ulcer is observed it must be biopsied in order to exclude a carcinoma and cultured to exclude specific infections.

Psychological disorders

There are some patients with overt rectal prolapse who also give a history of perineal pain, disordered bowel function, anxiety and depression. Some with coexisting eating disorders develop a prolapse from malnutrition. These patients may be under the care of psychiatrists and may never see a surgeon. Patients with a rectal prolapse, or rectal intussusception and a solitary ulcer, may have underlying psychological disorders. Psychogeriatric disease may be seen in patients from elderly care homes with a prolapse. It must be remembered that failure to demonstrate a prolapse on routine clinical examination is quite common and if patients give a history of prolapse it is quite wrong to label them as being neurotic until they have been repeatedly examined, preferably after straining in the squatting position or during proctography.

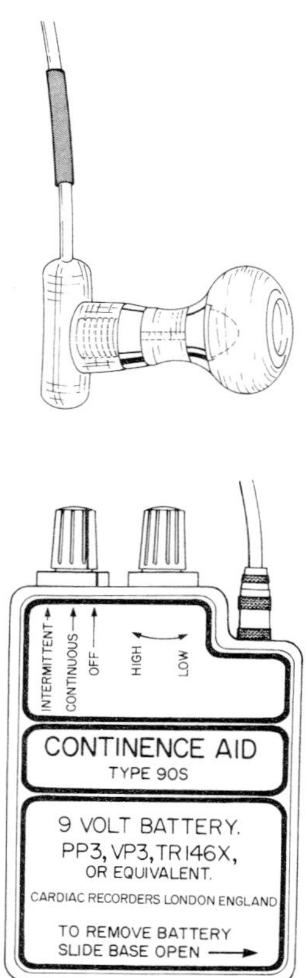

Figure 23.3 Continence aid to provide an electrical stimulus to the external sphincter and the pelvic floor muscles. This device is generally unsatisfactory in the treatment of rectal prolapse.

Conservative management

Conservative management is rarely successful as a means of controlling a rectal prolapse. However, attempts to re-educate younger patients to defecate without straining are often helpful because some early recurrences after operation may be due to repeated straining before perirectal fibrosis has fixed the rectum to surrounding structures.

In constipated patients it is worthwhile trying to establish a normal bowel habit by dietary advice and the use of a gentle laxative. Some elderly incontinent patients have quite forgotten how to contract the pelvic floor. Pelvic floor exercises and biofeedback retraining may help such patients to become continent after rectopexy. Although anal devices which deliver an electrical stimulus have been devised for the treatment of rectal prolapse (Figure 23.3) (Hopkinson and Lightwood, 1966), it has never, in our experience, controlled the rectal prolapse itself (Hopkinson and Hardman, 1973) but it may help those with persistent incontinence after rectopexy. Hamalainen et al (1996) found that biofeedback was of very little value in patients with low basal pressures who remained incontinent after successful surgical control of the prolapse.

Surgical management

Principles

It used to be thought that the principal aim of operation was the control of the prolapse; however current evidence suggests that the correction of any associated functional bowel disturbance is equally important to patients (Kuijpers, 1992). Patients with a prolapse may become afraid to go out because of fear that the prolapse may come down. They are also too embarrassed to participate in social functions for fear of incontinence. Some elderly patients do not want to seek medical advice, either because of the fear of an operation and the fact they may end up with a colostomy or from ignorance that surgical treatment can usually control the problem.

The aim of treatment is twofold: (1) to control the prolapse and (2) to restore continence and prevent constipation from impaired evacuation. The surgeon must first select an operation which is associated with minimal morbidity and mortality, bearing in mind the patient's age and infirmity, and which will guarantee that the prolapse can be controlled. Secondly, he or she should take into account the patient's expectation of the likely functional result. Hence, a perineal rectosigmoidectomy with a recognized 20% recurrence rate may be most appropriate for an elderly patient with a short life expectancy whose principal concern is the prolapse and who is likely to die from other conditions in the next two years. A combined rectopexy with pelvic floor repair may be desirable in younger incontinent patients, whereas a rectopexy and partial or subtotal colectomy may be appropriate in patients in whom there is established slow transit constipation. Likewise, the Délorme's procedure may be the best treatment option for a small circumferential partial-thickness rectal prolapse.

The principal methods available for treatment of rectal prolapse will be described, with special reference to mortality, recurrence rates, complications and functional outcome. Emphasis will be placed on procedures which have given good results in our hands. A large proportion of patients with rectal prolapse are elderly, live in institutions which care for the aged, many of whom are likely to die of coexisting disease within 2 or 3 years of operation. Follow-up from reported series is therefore often incomplete and the true incidence of recurrence or residual disorders of defecation are poorly documented. Recurrence rates may be very optimistic if follow-up is less than 5 years, since Tjandra et al (1993) reported that a third of recurrences occurred 3–14 years after treatment.

A variety of procedures are available for the treatment of rectal prolapse. These may be usefully classified into: perianal suture, plication, excision, pelvic floor repair, exclusion, rectopexy and resection. These procedures are usually performed through either an abdominal or perineal approach. Some procedures may be combined.

Operative findings

The striking feature in most women with rectal prolapse is the long anterior peritoneal pouch which extends over the rectum to the level of the pelvic floor and the anorectal junction before returning anteriorly over the back of the vagina, thence to cover the uterus. This deep peritoneal pouch is not always seen in male patients (see Figure 23.1).

The rectum is extremely mobile, and the mesorectum is attenuated and provides little support to the rectum. Similarly, the lateral ligaments are almost completely deficient and sometimes the middle rectal vessels are non-existent. As a result the retrorectal space is very wide, hence posterior and lateral dissection is extremely easy and relatively bloodless. The pelvic floor is also atrophic, particularly the puborectalis sling and the rectovaginal septum. The perineal body is commonly deficient. The remainder of the large bowel is usually normal apart from a mobile redundant sigmoid colon.

Perineal operations

Encircling procedures

The attractions of perianal suture techniques or placement of inert support collars around the anus are that the procedure does not threaten life, it may be repeated and a major operation is avoided. If these procedures had been successful no one would have explored abdominal operations. The encircling devices which have been used include wire, Silastic bands, silicone implantable collars or muscle (Table 23.8). Procedures that use synthetic material are rarely employed by the modern colorectal surgeon and are included here for the sake of completeness.

Wire (Figure 23.4)

The problems encountered with Thiersch wire included infection, inadequate control of the prolapse because the wire is tied too loosely, extrusion of the wire through the skin, fracture or faecal impaction because the wire is tied too tightly. The prolapse usually recurs once the wire is removed (Porter, 1962) except in children when malnutrition has been corrected. Vongsangnak et al (1985b) reviewed the results of treatment by Thiersch wire in 25 patients. A total of 62 procedures were required in an attempt to control these prolapses and a number of patients eventually required a rectopexy. Complications occurred in 59% and

Table 23.8 Result of treatment: perianal suture.

Authors	*n*	*Mortality*	*Recurrent prolapse*	*Comments*
Porter (1962): wire	82	0	54 (67)	Breakage 18; too tight 7
Vongsangnak et al (1985b): wire	25/62†	0	24 (39)	Breakage 8; cut out 4; sepsis 12; faecal impaction 9
Baker (1970): nylon	62	0	14 (22)	Cut out 11; infection 7
Jackman et al (1980)*: silicone rubber	44	0	8 (18)	Infection 5; constipation 4; fracture 4
Hunt et al (1985): silastic rings	41	0	6 (15)	Sepsis 7; cut out 8; fracture 3
Sainio et al (1991b): mesh	14	0	2 (15)	No sepsis or breakage but impaction in 3
Ladha et al (1985): Angelchick	8	1	0	Sepsis 1
Khanduja et al (1988): modified Angelchick	16	0	0	Breakage 3; erosion 1; sepsis 2
Atri (1980): gracilis muscle	15	0	NS	Poor follow-up

Values in parentheses are percentages.
* Updated by Earnshaw and Hopkinson (1987).
† No. of procedures: analysed in 25 patients.
NS, not stated.

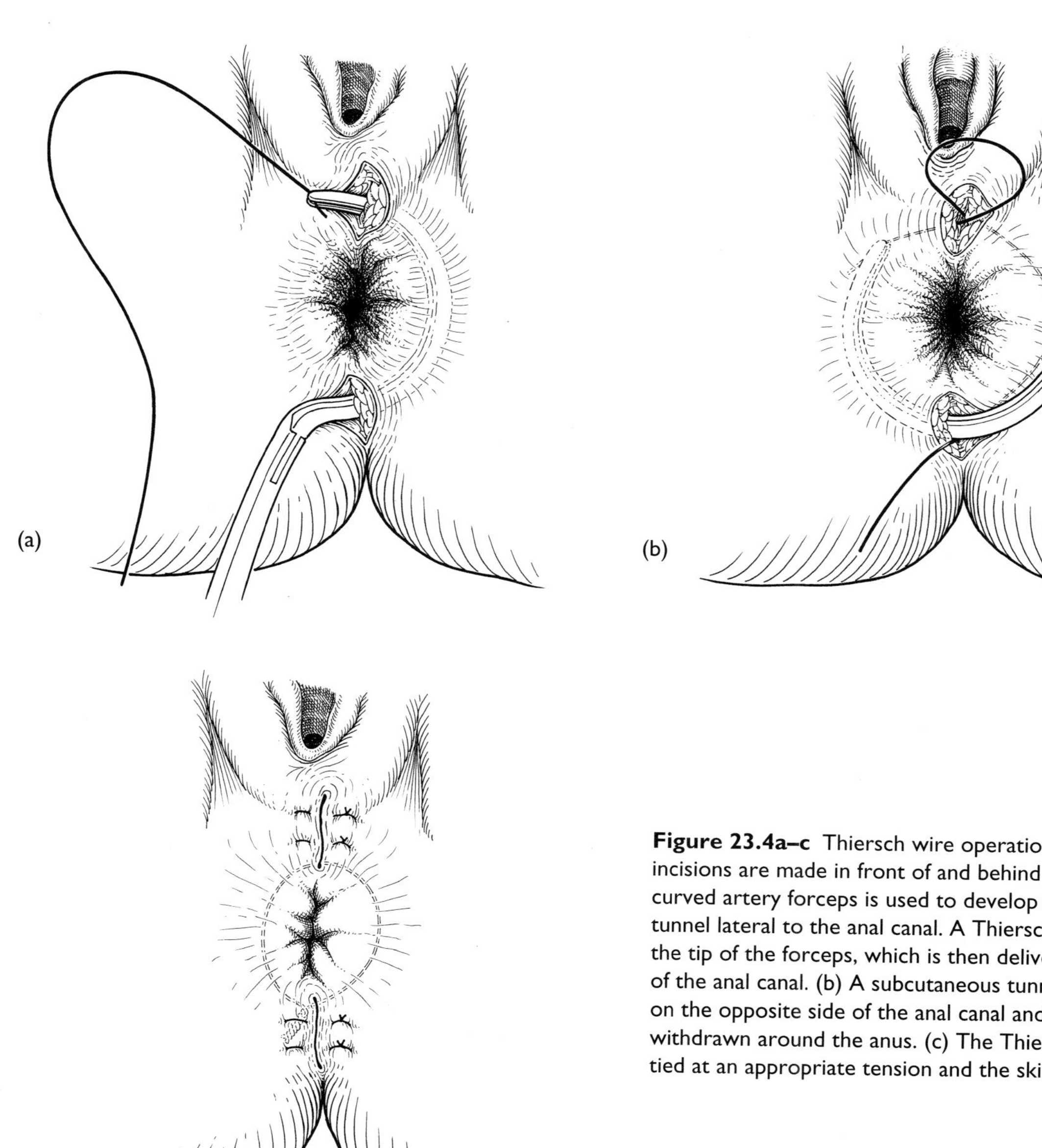

Figure 23.4a–c Thiersch wire operation. (a) Two small incisions are made in front of and behind the anal canal. A curved artery forceps is used to develop a subcutaneous tunnel lateral to the anal canal. A Thiersch wire is grasped by the tip of the forceps, which is then delivered around one half of the anal canal. (b) A subcutaneous tunnel is now developed on the opposite side of the anal canal and the Thiersch wire is withdrawn around the anus. (c) The Thiersch wire has been tied at an appropriate tension and the skin incision closed.

included: breakage of the wire (13%), fracture (7%), sepsis (20%) and faecal impaction (15%). Recurrence of prolapse occurred in 39%. Patients were in hospital for a mean of 9 days, which does not seem to be any less than for an abdominal procedure. Hence we concur with these authors that the use of Thiersch wire to control a rectal prolapse is now obsolete and should no longer be inflicted on elderly patients.

Other encircling materials

Nylon has been used as an alternative to wire (Baker, 1970) and was reported as having a much lower rate of recurrence (22%) than that in Porter's review (1962) of the Thiersch wire procedure (67%). The problem with Nylon is its inelasticity, which results in the creation of a rigid bar around the anal canal. The concept of using silicone rubber as an alternative to wire or Nylon is more attractive. Silicone rubber is inert and will stretch. Jackman et al (1980) reported encouraging results but problems still persist due to sepsis and the difficulty in assessing the correct tension of the Silastic rings (Earnshaw and Hopkinson, 1987). Silastic has been used as an alternative to silicone (Hunt et al, 1985). Polypropylene mesh has also been used in elderly debilitated patients and was not associated with sepsis (Sainio et al, 1991b).

For the insertion of silicone rubber perianal bands, the patient is placed in the lithotomy or prone jack-knife position and the skin is prepared in the usual manner. It is usually unnecessary for the patient to have a general anaesthetic. The procedure may be performed under a caudal or spinal anaesthetic. Alternatively, local infiltration using a large volume (60 mL) of a dilute solution of bupivacaine hydrochloride (0.25%) may be used. On account of the dangers of infection around the foreign material, single-dose antibiotic prophylaxis is advised.

A small incision is made posteriorly just behind the sphincter and a second, similar incision anteriorly. With the index finger of the left hand in the anus and with a length of silicone rubber tubing mounted on a large aneurysm needle, the silicone rubber is threaded around the sphincter at the desired height, first around the left side of the anterior skin incision (Figure 23.5a). At this point the rubber is withdrawn from the aneurysm needle. The empty needle is then passed around the right side of the anal canal through the anterior skin incision. The end of the rubber is then attached to the aneurysm needle, which is withdrawn from its original site posteriorly (Figure 23.5b). Both limbs of the rubber are then pulled posteriorly and the desired tension judged by clipping the tubing (Figure 23.5c). Once the correct length has been determined, the two lengths of silicone rubber are sutured together using 4/0 Prolene (Figure 23.5d). The ends are then cut and the ring retracts around the anus. The skin incisions are closed with Prolene.

More than one band of silicone rubber may be used. It has been suggested that one should be placed above the levator ani and two around the anal canal. This technique may be of benefit to patients who refuse definitive surgical therapy. Hunt et al (1985) prefer to use two oblique incisions, apply 1–4 rings and use a cable gun applicator to secure the two ends of Silastic tubing (which they prefer to silicone).

Prosthetic collars

A logical development of encircling sutures has been the use of a silicone Angelchik collar, as described in the treatment of gastro-oesophageal reflux. Ladha et al (1985) describe eight poor-risk patients treated by this method: one died early after operation and one patient's prosthesis had to be removed because of sepsis, but in the remainder the prolapse was satisfactorily controlled.

Khanduja et al (1988) used a similar prosthesis on 16 patients. There were no deaths. Three prostheses broke, one eroded through the rectal wall and two more became infected. It is unlikely that these devices have any advantage over silicone or Silastic tubing and they are much more expensive.

Muscle

The gracilis muscle may be used as an alternative to a perianal suture, with (NS Williams et al, 1991) or without (Atri, 1980) electrical stimulation. A similar approach is used and described for the treatment of faecal incontinence (see Chapter 20).

Mucosal reduction procedures

Délorme's procedure

Unlike an abdominal plication operation (Devadhar, 1965), perineal plication of a rectal prolapse, usually known as the Délorme's procedure, has gained in popularity, particularly for elderly high-risk patients with coexisting diseases (Nay and Blair, 1972; Uhlig and Sullivan, 1979; Christiansen and Kirkegaard, 1981; Gundersen et al, 1985; Monson et al, 1986; Houry et al, 1987; Abulafi et al, 1990; Oliver et al, 1994; Senapati et al, 1994; Tobin

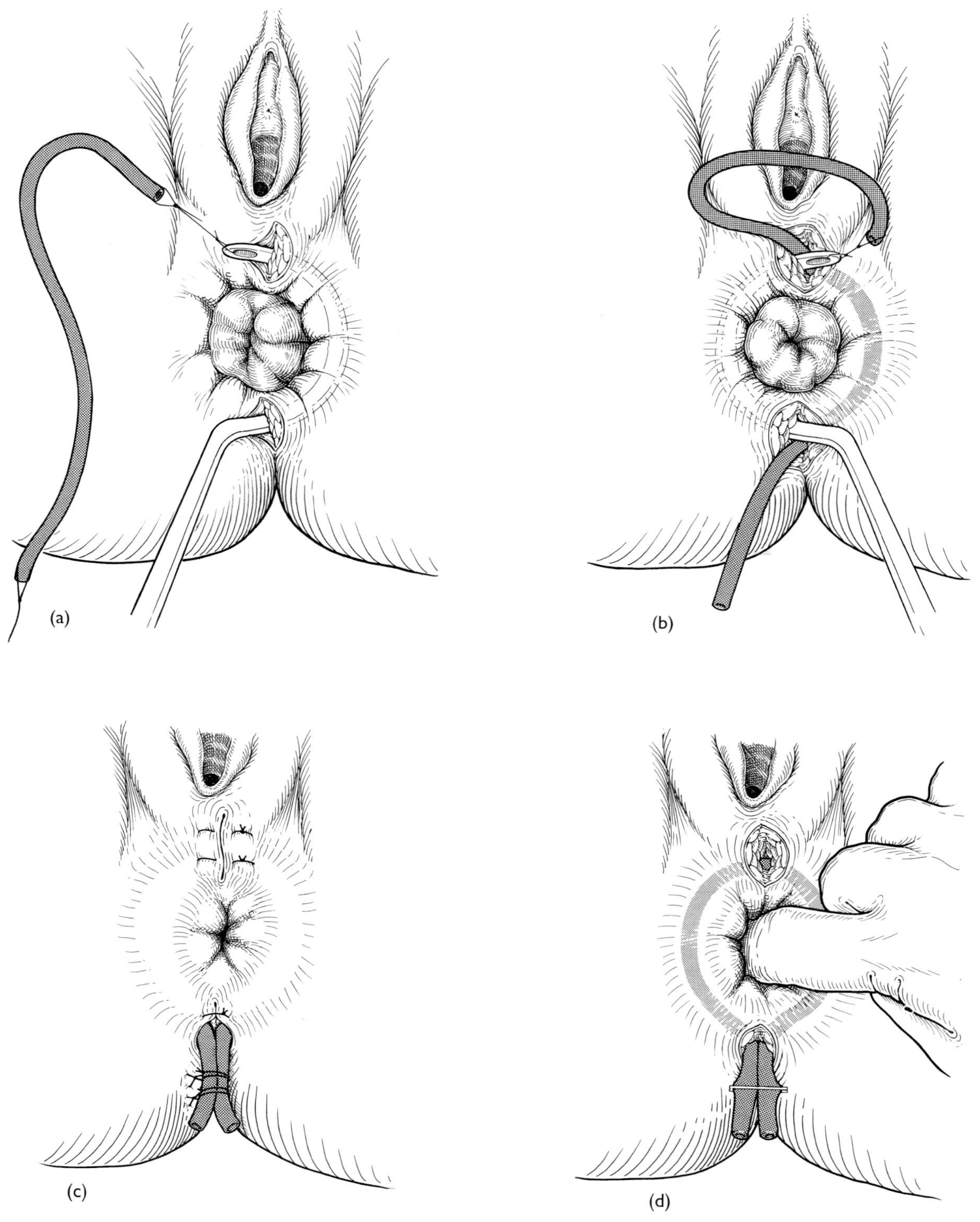

Figure 23.5a–d Perianal encirclement using Silastic wire for the treatment of rectal prolapse. (a) Two incisions are made in front of and behind the anal canal. A tunnel is developed to one side of the anal canal and a Silastic ring is routed around one half of the anal canal. (b) The Silastic sling is now introduced around the opposite side of the anal canal and the prolapse is reduced. (c) The Silastic loop is tightened until an appropriate tension is reached and the limbs are sutured together. (d) The two limbs may be stapled together; completion of the procedure prior to returning the ends of the Silastic loop into the subcutaneous tunnel.

and Scott, 1994; Plusa et al, 1995; Lechaux et al, 1995). The advantages of this operation are that it does not involve a bowel resection, it is performed entirely via the perineum (Ejaife and Elias, 1977), only one death has been reported and the recurrence rate is moderately low (Table 23.9).

For the Délorme's procedure, the patient is placed in the lithotomy position with a steep Trendelenburg tilt, or in the prone jack-knife position, and is catheterized because of the risk of incontinence or voiding difficulties after operation. The bowel is prolapsed to its maximum extent, as in rectosigmoidectomy and is held with tissue forceps or stay sutures (Figure 23.6a). A 1:300 000 solution of adrenaline is infiltrated in the submucosal plane to facilitate mucosal excision and to reduce the amount of bleeding. The mucosa is circumferentially divided around the prolapse just beyond the anal verge at the dentate line, using a cutting diathermy, and the numerous submucosal vessels are secured either by ligature or diathermy (Figure 23.6b). The mucosa is stripped off the underlying bowel wall to the apex of the prolapse and is then excised from inside the prolapse as far as is possible. A series of longitudinally placed PDS, Vicryl or Prolene sutures are used to plicate the prolapse by taking approximately four bites of the rectal muscle from the prolapsed bowel (Figure 23.6c). When all the 4–6 longitudinal sutures have been placed they are tied (Figure 23.6c). It is possible in some patients to repair the pelvic floor muscles outside the prolapse once it has been plicated (Figure 23.6d). The mucosa inside the anus is then sutured to the cut edge of the dentate line using interrupted or continuous sutures (Figure 23.6e). It is important to check at the end of the operation that there is no stricturing of the anorectal junction by digital examination.

The operation is extremely safe since it can be performed under local anaesthesia and it does not involve an anastomosis. Furthermore, the procedure can be repeated if a recurrence occurs later (Monson et al, 1986). Late deaths from coexisting disease are common, hence long-term follow-up is rarely achievable. The main source of morbidity is from bleeding (Gundersen et al, 1985), or occasionally late stenosis may develop (Houry et al, 1987). Incontinence is frequently improved and late problems from poor evacuation are uncommon. Senapati et al (1994) report that incontinence was improved in 46% of their 32 patients, in none was constipation made worse and there were no deaths, but 4 (12.5%) developed recurrence. Plusa et al (1995) examined the physiological changes after the Délorme's operation and reported that there was no adverse affect on anal manometry or rectal emptying and that anorectal sensation was improved. Tobin and Scott (1994) reported no deaths in a series of 49 operations, which was remarkable, given the

Table 23.9 Results of treatment: plication.

Authors	*Procedure*	*n*	*Mortality*	*Recurrent prolapse*	*Comments*
Devadhar (1965)	Abdominal	28	0	0	
Nay and Blair (1972)	Délorme's	30	0	3 (10)	
Uhlig and Sullivan (1979)	Délorme's	44	0	3 (7)	
Christiansen and Kirkegaard (1981)	Délorme's	30	0	2 (6)	
Gundersen et al (1985)	Délorme's	18	0	1 (5)	Haemorrhage 2
Monson et al (1986)	Délorme's	27	0	2 (7)	
Houry et al (1987)	Délorme's	18	0	3 (16)	Rectal stenosis 1
Abulafi et al (1990)	Délorme's	22	0	1 (5)	
Muto et al (1984)	Gant–Miwa	11	0	2 (18)	
Tobin and Scott (1994)	Délorme's	49	0	11/43 (26)	Poor results in elderly demented patients. Repeat Délorme's worth while
Senapati et al (1994)	Délorme's	32	0	4 (12.5)	Short operating time; many had had previous operations for prolapse. None had worse constipation; incontinence improved in 46%
Oliver et al (1994)	Délorme's	40	1 (0.5%)	9 (22)	Minor complications in 25%; well tolerated in debilitated patients
Lechaux et al (1995)	Délorme's and pelvic floor repair	85	1 (1.2)	11 (13.5)	Recurrence 22% in elderly; 5% in younger patients
Plusa et al (1995)	Délorme's	19	0	?	Improved sensation

Values in parentheses are percentages.

very old age group of the series. However, there were 11 recurrences in the 43 who could be followed up (26%). Most of the recurrences occurred in frail demented elderly patients, whereas recurrence was much less common in younger patients. Oliver et al (1994) reported one death from a series of 40 but there were 9 recurrences (22%). Lechaux et al (1995) combined pelvic floor repair with a standard Délorme's operation in 85 patients. There was one death and 11 recurrences (13.5%). The recurrence rate was 22% in the very old, compared with 5% in younger patients. Some data indicated that the Délorme's operation gave inferior results to rectosigmoidectomy (Finlay and Aitchison, 1991), particularly when rectosigmoidectomy was combined with a pelvic floor repair (Agachan et al, 1996). We

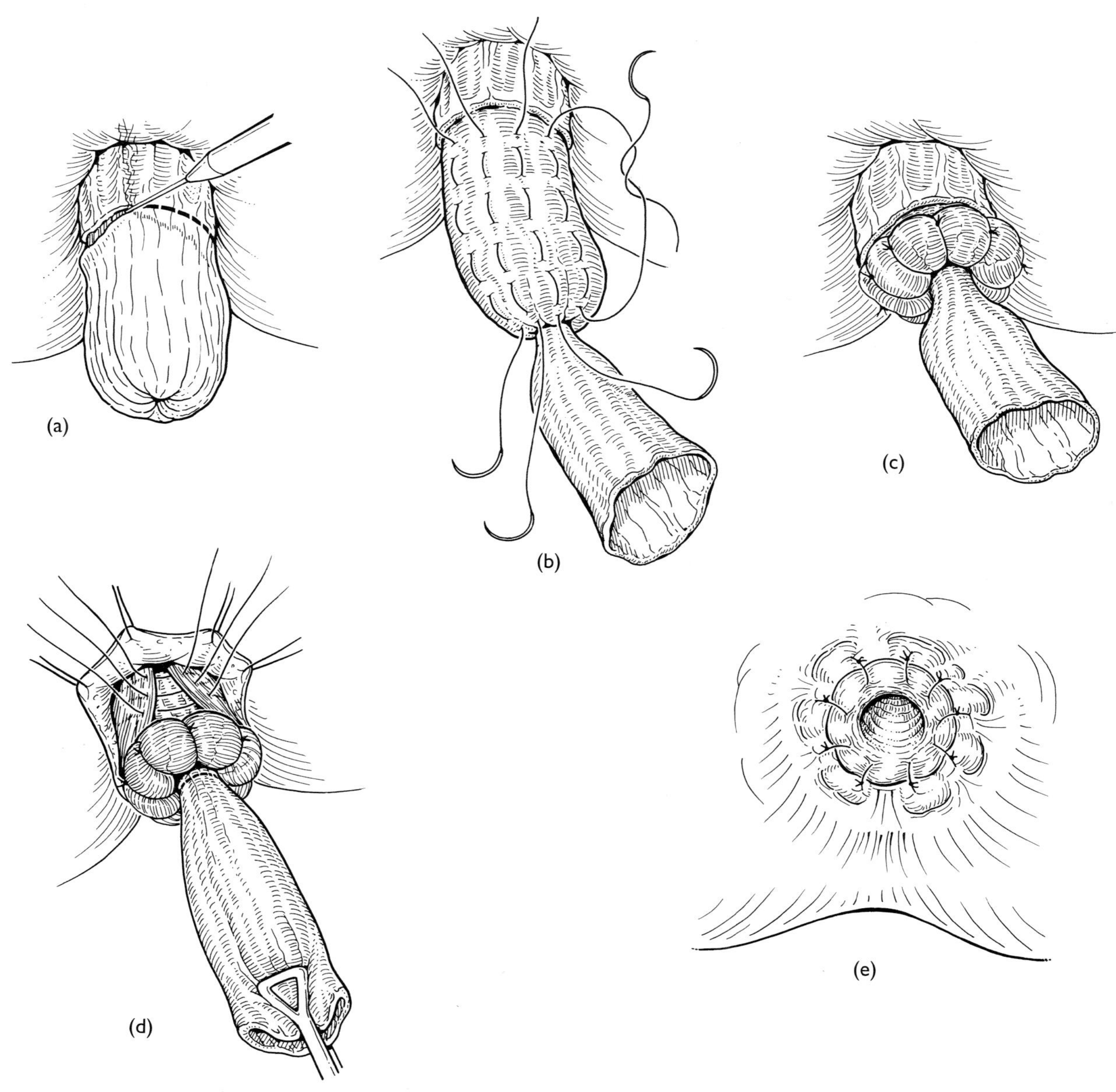

Figure 23.6a–e The Délorme's operation. (a) The prolapse is everted. The mucosa and bowel wall is divided at the level of the dentate line. The entire outer wall of the prolapse is stripped from the circular muscle layer until the apex of the prolapse. (b) A series of absorbable sutures are used to plicate the rectal bowel wall. Six to eight sutures are placed so as to concertina the bowel wall and thus reduce the residual prolapse. (c) The sutures are now tied. (d) A pelvic floor repair may be performed at the same time and the mucosa of the prolapse is excised from within the bowel. (e) The operation is completed by direct mucosa-to-mucosa suture between the inner aspect of the reduced prolapse and the dentate line.

believe that the operation is a useful method of surgical treatment in patients unfit for rectopexy and it can be repeated if recurrence should develop later (Tobin and Scott, 1994).

Gant–Miwa plication

A somewhat different approach to the Délorme's operation is that of mucosal reduction and multiple rectal plication. This option, known as the Gant–Miwa plication, is widely used in parts of Europe and Japan (Arakawa, 1979).

The rectal prolapse is delivered on to the perineum; local anaesthetic may be infiltrated under the mucosa. A tag of mucosa is lifted off the muscle layers and ligated by suture. This simple manoeuvre is repeated so that 20–30 tags are created over the surface of the entire prolapse. The prolapse is replaced (Muto et al, 1984) and the tags eventually disappear over a period of 4 months. Recurrence rates are said to be less than 10%, but unreported observations from Japan suggest that the recurrence rate is much higher.

Rectosigmoidectomy

Rectosigmoidectomy has been used extensively to excise the prolapse, to obliterate the deep peritoneal pouch and, where necessary, to repair the pelvic floor muscles in elderly patients deemed unfit for a major abdominal procedure, since the anastomosis is at the dentate line and a laparotomy is avoided (Altemeier et al, 1952, 1971; Altemeier, 1972). The operation is associated with low morbidity and provides access for synchronous pelvic floor repair (Finlay and Aitchison, 1991). Recurrence rates vary considerably from 3 to 43%, but incontinence may persist due partly to the loss of a rectal reservoir as well as some impairment in resting sphincter activity (Williams et al, 1992; Johansen et al, 1993; Deen et al, 1994).

The operation of rectosigmoidectomy may be performed either in the exaggerated lithotomy position or in the prone jack-knife position, usually under general anaesthesia. Some surgeons use spinal or epidural anaesthesia, while others prefer their patients to be fully relaxed and asleep. The patient should be catheterized. The prolapse must be everted on to the perineum by grasping the rectum through the anal canal with three pairs of Allis tissue forceps (Figure 23.7a). An incision is then made with a cutting diathermy current to excise the anterior aspect of the prolapse (Figure 23.7b), dividing the muscle layer of the rectum at a more peripheral site than the mucosa (Figure 23.7c). The submucosal vessels should be ligated or secured by diathermy. Two stay sutures may be placed on the lateral aspect of the cut edge of the rectum to prevent it slipping back into the anal canal and to act as markers.

The next phase is to withdraw the rectum as far as possible on to the perineum (Figure 23.7d). The anterior rectovaginal peritoneal pouch is then seen and the peritoneum divided over the anterior and lateral aspect of the prolapse (Figure 23.7e) and its proximal edge is grasped with two fine stay sutures. It should then be possible to withdraw the entire rectum and most of the sigmoid colon through the peritoneal sac of the sliding hernia (Figure 23.7f,g). The sigmoid mesentery is divided between clips, the vessels ligated by transfixion suture and the bowel partially divided (Figure 23.7h,i). The anterior aspect of the pelvic floor may also be exposed and sutures placed on both sides for repair when the bowel has been fully mobilized (Figure 23.7j). The prolapse is then lifted up to expose the posterior component and the anorectal junction is divided using diathermy (Figure 23.7k). The entire rectal wall is mobilized and Waldeyer's fascia is transected as in the dissection for postanal repair to expose the puborectalis and levators (Figure 23.7l). The mesorectum is then divided.

At this point and before bowel is completely transected, the anterior and posterior levatorplasty sutures are tied. They must not be too tight or else there will be a stricture above the coloanal anastomosis. The sigmoid is now transected with diathermy and the distal sigmoid may be closed with staples (Figure 23.7m). The operation is completed by anastomosing the proximal sigmoid colon to the anal canal as an intra-anal coloanal anastomosis (Figure 23.7n). It is important not to obstruct the bowel by placing too many sutures across the pelvic floor, a sufficient space must be left to accommodate the bowel above the coloanal anastomosis.

In Britain the operation of rectosigmoidectomy is rarely performed because the rate of recurrent prolapse was reported to be very high (Table 23.10). Despite the disappointment expressed by some clinicians who have used the procedure but reported high recurrence rates (Porter, 1962; Thauerkauf et al, 1970; Friedman et al, 1983), Altemeier et al (1971), Gopal et al (1984) and Prasad et al (1986) report excellent results when the procedure is combined with repair of the pelvic floor. Improvement in continence was spectacular in the report by Prasad et al (1986) when the pelvic floor was also repaired. The combined approach may be useful in children with persistent prolapse despite conservative therapy, or where the prolapse cannot

Table 23.10 Results of treatment: rectosigmoidectomy.

Authors	*Additional procedure*	*n*	*Mortality*	*Recurrent prolapse*	*Comments*
Porter (1962)		110	1	64 (58)	
Altemeier et al (1971)	+ Anterior pelvic floor repair	106	0	3 (3)	Abscess 4
Friedman et al (1983)	+ Anterior pelvic floor repair	27	0	12 (44)	
Gopal et al (1984)	+ Anterior pelvic floor repair	18	0	1 (5)	Mucosal prolapse 2
Thauerkauf et al (1970)	+ Pelvic floor repair	34	0	13 (38)	
Finlay and Aitchison (1991)	+ Pelvic floor repair	17	1	1 (5)	All elderly patients Poor reservoir function 3
Prasad et al (1986)	+ Rectopexy + posterior and anterior pelvic floor repair; 4 coloanal anastomosis	25	0	NS	
Ramanujam et al (1994)	+ Pelvic floor repair	72	0	4 (5.5)	Anastomotic leaks 2
Johansen et al (1993)		20	1	0	Improved continence in 90%

Values in parentheses are percentages.
NS, not stated.

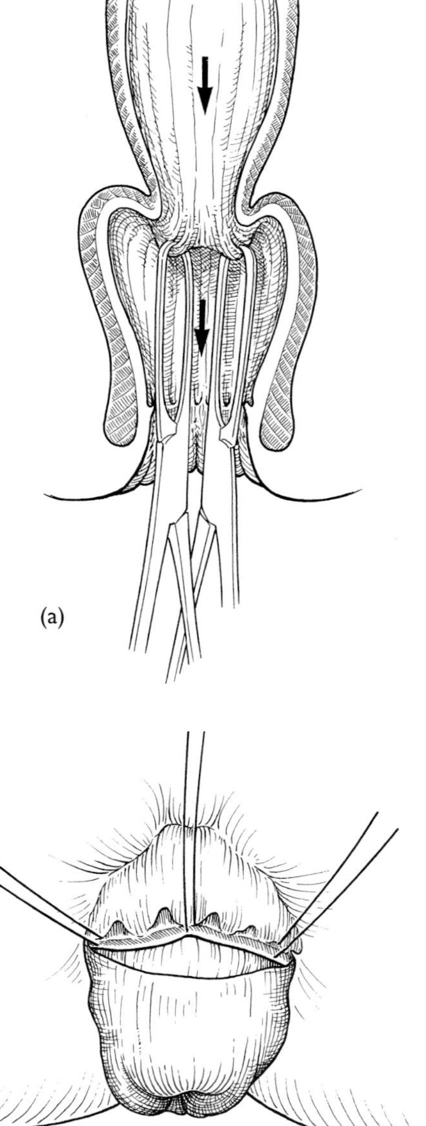

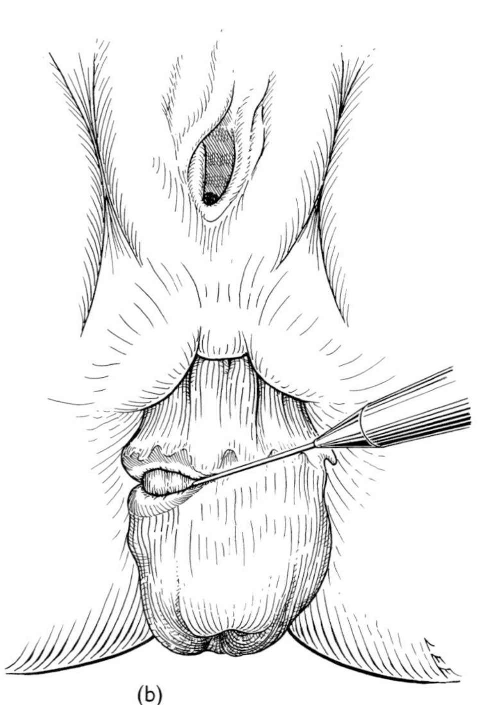

Figure 23.7a–n Perineal rectosigmoidectomy (lithotomy position). (a) The rectal prolapse is delivered on to the perineum. (b) A transverse incision is made anteriorly to divide the mucosa at the dentate line. (c) The anterior wall of the rectal prolapse is also divided. *(Continued)*

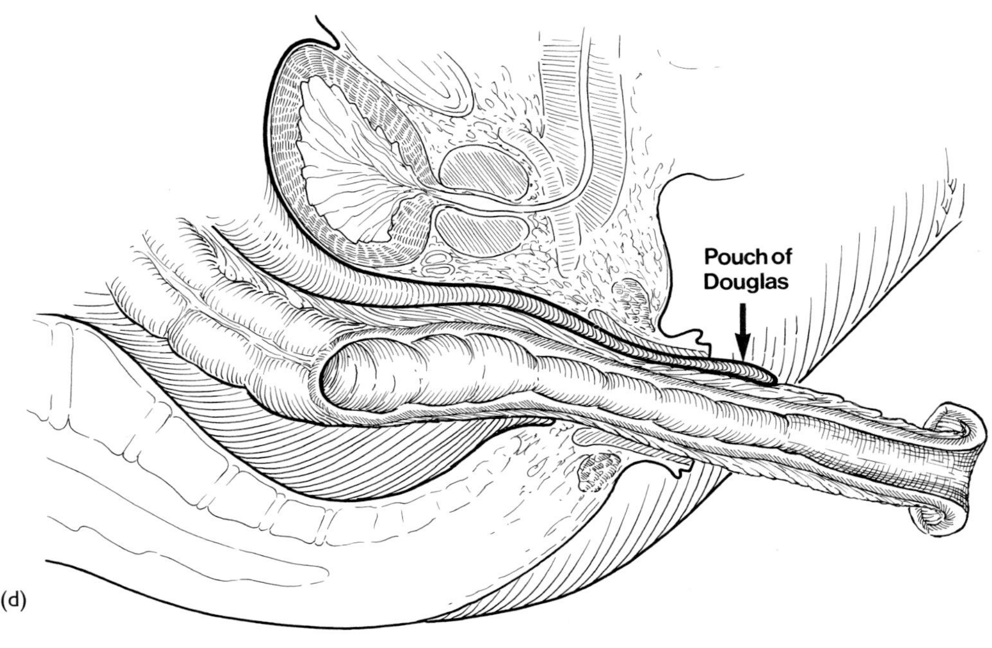

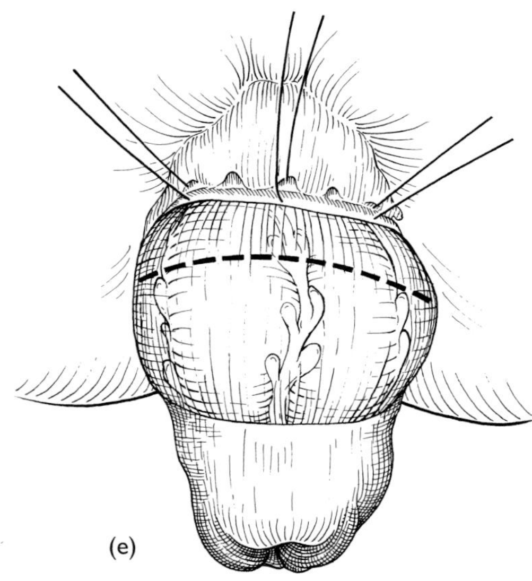

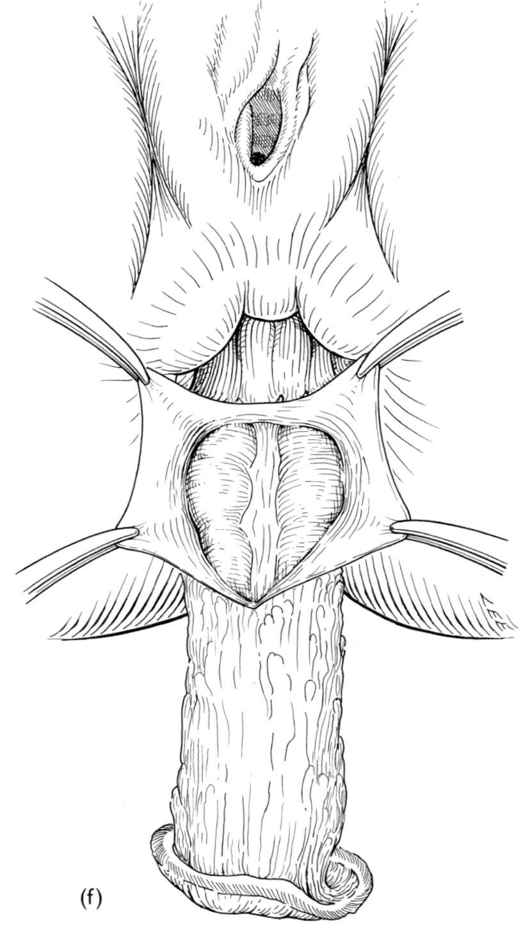

Figure 23.7a–n (*Continued*) (d) Once the anterior wall has been divided, the rectovaginal pouch will be easily seen. (e) The peritoneal coat should be opened transversely. (f) The sigmoid colon is now exposed. (*Continued*)

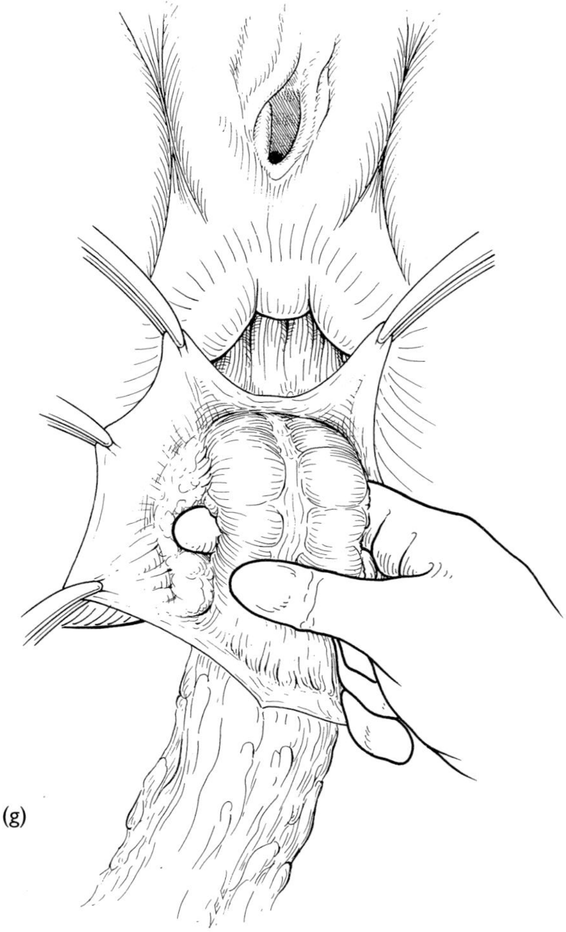

(g)

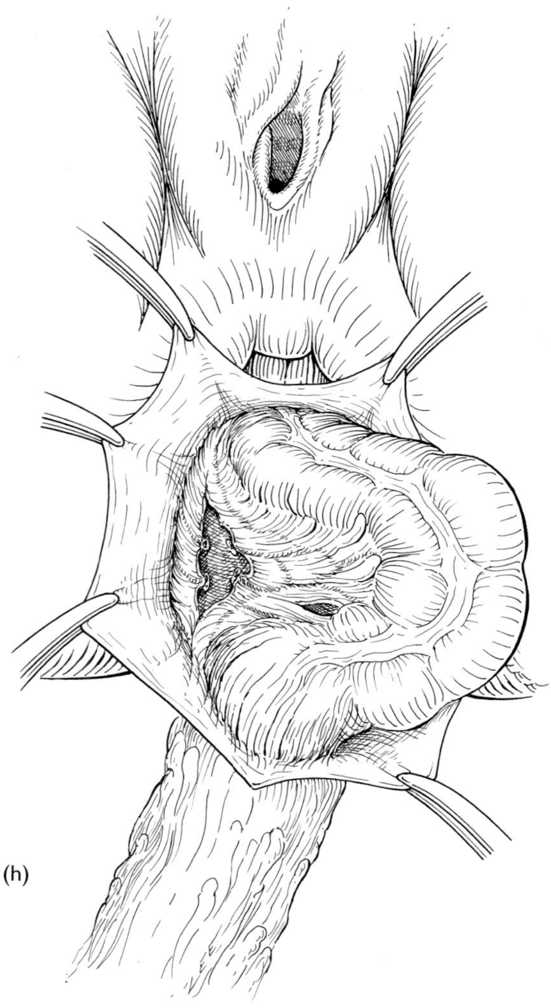

(h)

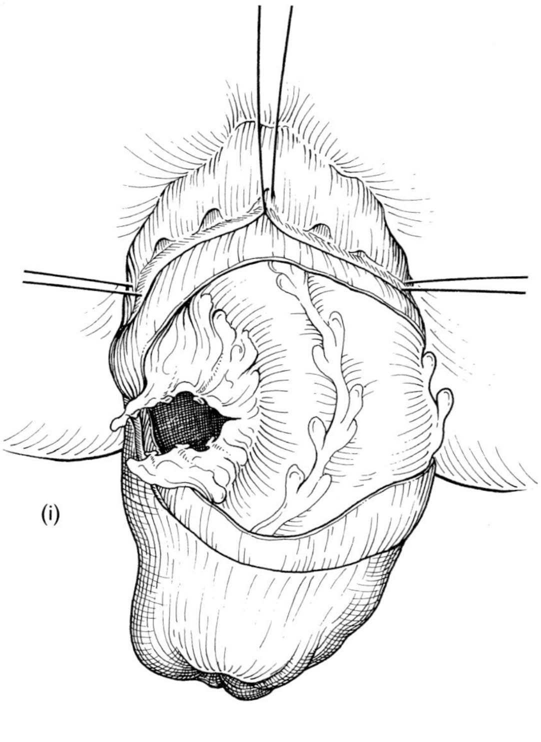

(i)

Figure 23.7a–n (*Continued*) (g) The sigmoid colon can now be drawn down through the divided peritoneal pouch. (h) The vessels in the sigmoid mesentery are divided and ligated. (i) The same appearances in a smaller prolapse. (*Continued*)

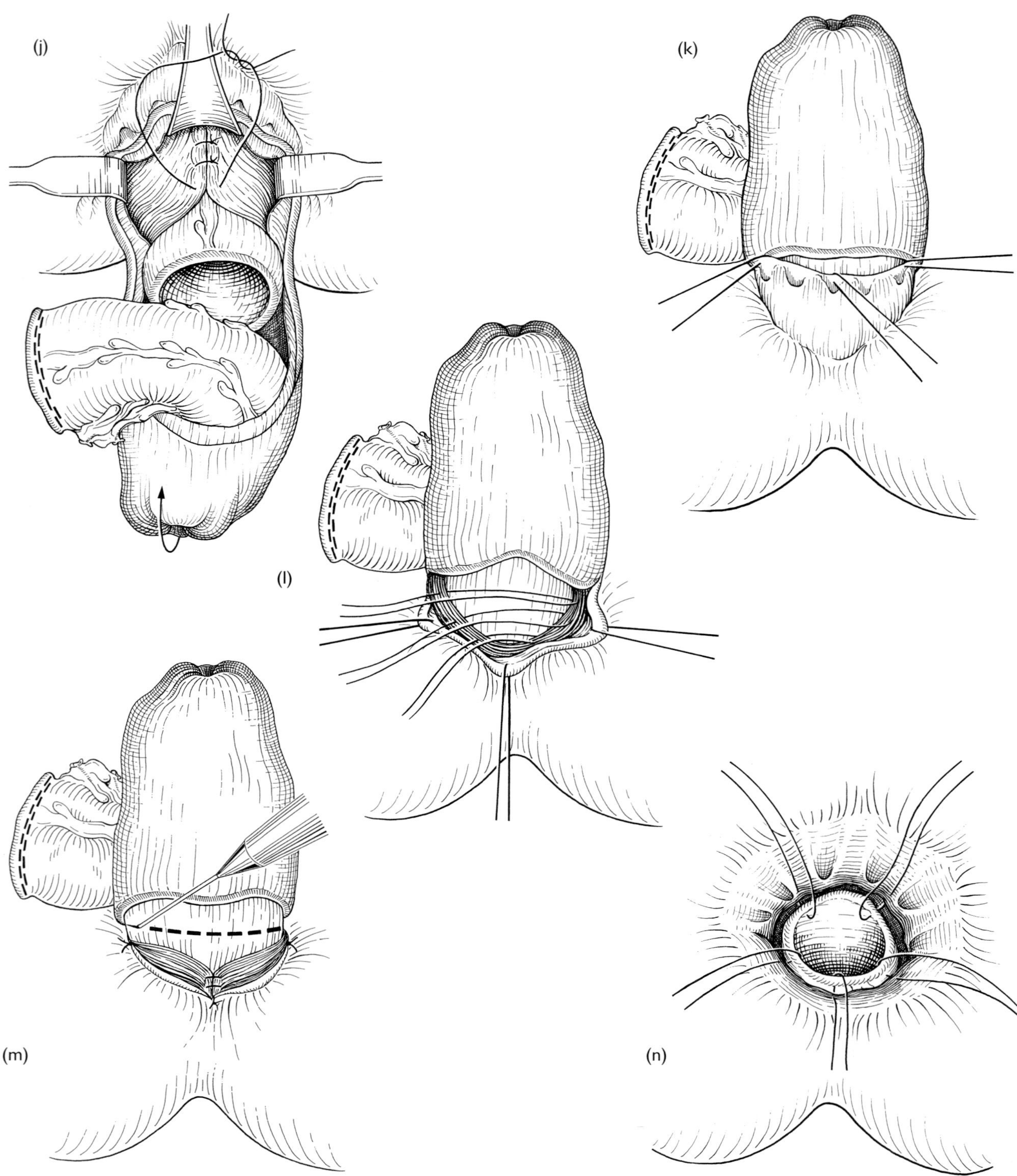

Figure 23.7a–n (*Continued*) (j) While the sigmoid colon is pulled in a downward direction, the anterior fibres of the levator ani can usually be easily identified and plicated. The proximal end of the sigmoid colon is then transected. (k) The rectal prolapse is now elevated upwards to expose the posterior aspect of the prolapse. The mucosa and rectal wall of the posterior component of the prolapse is then divided. (l) The mesorectum is exposed and the posterior component of the puborectalis sling can be seen lying quite superficially and may be repaired. (m) The mesorectum is then divided and ligated between arterial clamps, and the entire rectal prolapse with the sigmoid colon is excised. (n) The two divided ends of bowel are now anastomosed using a suture technique.

Table 23.11 Results of randomized controlled trials of treatment for rectal prolapse in elderly patients (Birmingham).

	Perineal rectosigmoidectomy (*n* = 10)	*Resection rectopexy* (*n* = 10)
Deaths	0	0
Anastomotic leaks	0	0
Recurrent prolapse/ mucosal prolapse	1/2	0/2
Soiling	6	2
Defecation frequency (bowel movements per day)	3 (1–6)	1 (1–3)

From Deen et al (1994).

be reduced. Johansen et al (1993) reported no recurrences following 20 perineal rectosigmoidectomies and pelvic floor repair; furthermore, incontinence was improved in 90%. Likewise, Ramanujam et al (1994) reported only four recurrences in 72 patients (5.5%). There were no deaths but the coloanal anastomoses broke down in two patients, one of whom required a colostomy.

Increasingly surgeons are using rectosigmoidectomy with total pelvic floor repair for elderly patients with rectal prolapse. A retrospective review reported 37% recurrence with the Délorme's operation, 12% with rectosigmoidectomy alone and 4% when combined with pelvic floor repair (Agachan et al, 1996). Thus, with pelvic floor repair, results are good and the risks of dehiscence of the coloanal anastomosis is low. The main theoretical objection is that the rectal reservoir is removed and some patients complain of urgency.

We compared perineal rectosigmoidectomy with abdominal rectopexy in a small prospective randomized trial (Deen et al, 1994). The clinical outcome was similar, except that there was one recurrence after rectosigmoidectomy. However, the quality of continence was better after abdominal rectopexy and there was much less urgency. We found that anal pressures and compliance fell after perianal rectosigmoidectomy but these parameters improved or remained the same after abdominal rectopexy (Table 23.11). We had to conclude from this trial that function was superior after resection rectopexy and in view of the higher recurrence rate with rectosigmoidectomy this procedure should probably be reserved for very elderly, frail patients only (Kim et al, 1996).

Pouch perineal rectosigmoidectomy and rectopexy

A new departure from the standard Altemier operation was developed by us in Birmingham as a result of the above trial, which found that perineal rectosigmoidectomy was associated with significant lower resting and squeeze anal pressures, and reduced neorectal capacity compared with abdominal rectopexy. Patients also complained of urgency and soiling due to the weak sphincter and narrow neorectum. Consequently we explored an operation where the length of bowel resected was reduced, thus preserving the sigmoid and the sigmoid mesentery, forming a stapled sigmoid pouch while at the same time fixing the pouch to the presacral fascia and performing a total pelvic floor repair.

We have compared the functional results in seven patients having pouch perineal rectosigmoidectomy with a conventional procedure. Those with a pouch had less soiling and urgency than the conventional group (Yoshioka et al, 1998). Despite small numbers, we do believe that this modification is indicated if rectosigmoidectomy is planned among elderly patients with a short life expectancy (Table 23.12). The patient is placed in the prone jack-knife position with the buttocks strapped apart (Figure 23.8a). We prefer to start with the posterior dissection. The prolapsed rectum is retracted anteriorly over the vulva. The anal canal is divided at the dentate line (Figure 23.8b). The rectorectal plane is

Table 23.12 Results of non-randomized comparison between pouch and straight perineal rectosigmoidectomy.

	Pouch perineal rectosigmoidectomy (*n* = 7)	*Straight perineal rectosigmoidectomy* (*n* = 7)
Hospital stay (days)	11.7 ± 4.9	8.9 ± 2.6
Breakdown of anastomosis	1	0
Recurrent prolapse	0	3
Function: preop–postop		
Constipation	1–2	1–10
Incontinence	6–2	6–6
Urgency	5–3	6–6
Soiling	6–2	6–6

From Yoshioka et al (1998).

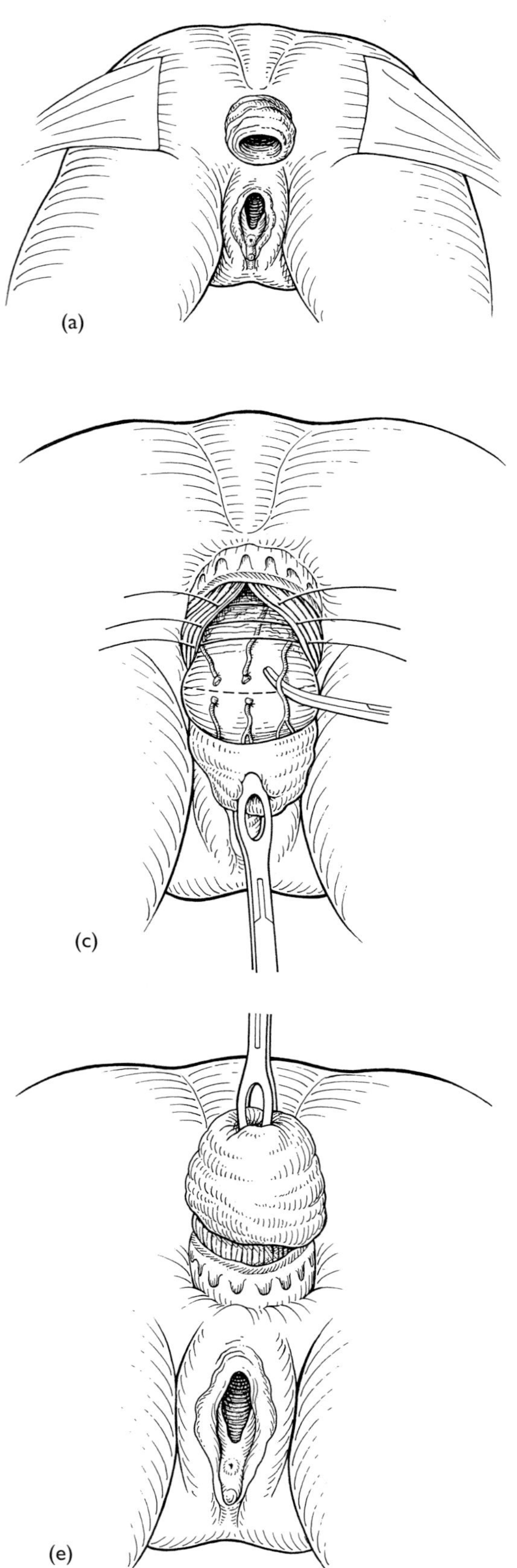

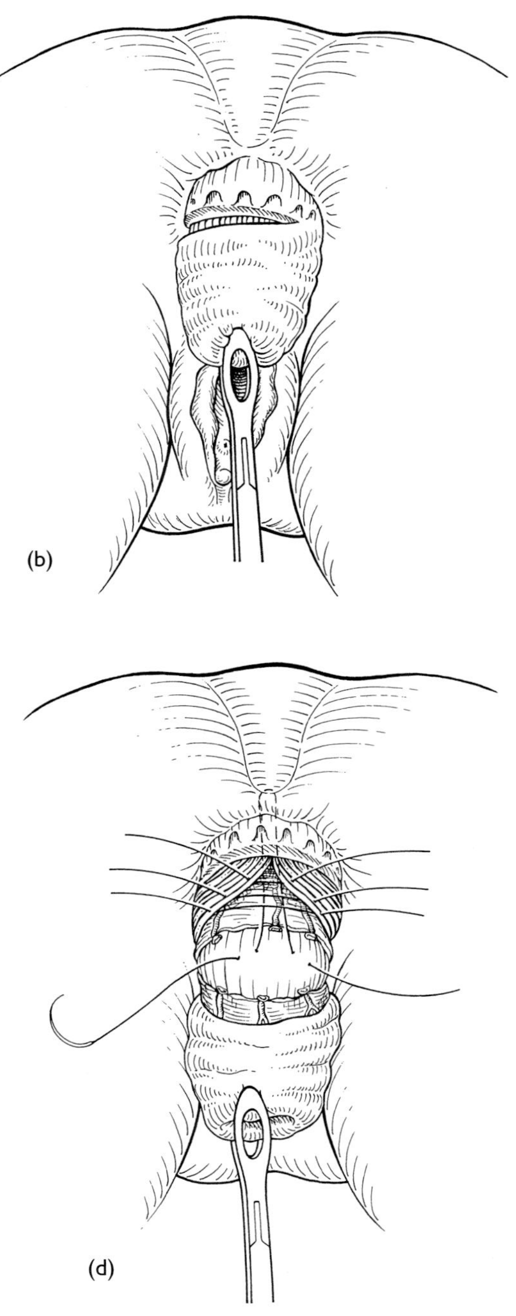

Figure 23.8a–l Pouch perineal rectopexy and rectosigmoidectomy (prone jack-knife position). (a) The prolapse has been delivered on to the perineum. (b) The posterior wall of the prolapse is divided. (c) The mesorectum is exposed, the vessels are ligated and the posterior sling of the puborectalis is being repaired. (d) A rectopexy suture is placed in the upper rectum to the sacrum. (e) The anterior wall of the rectum is divided. (*Continued*)

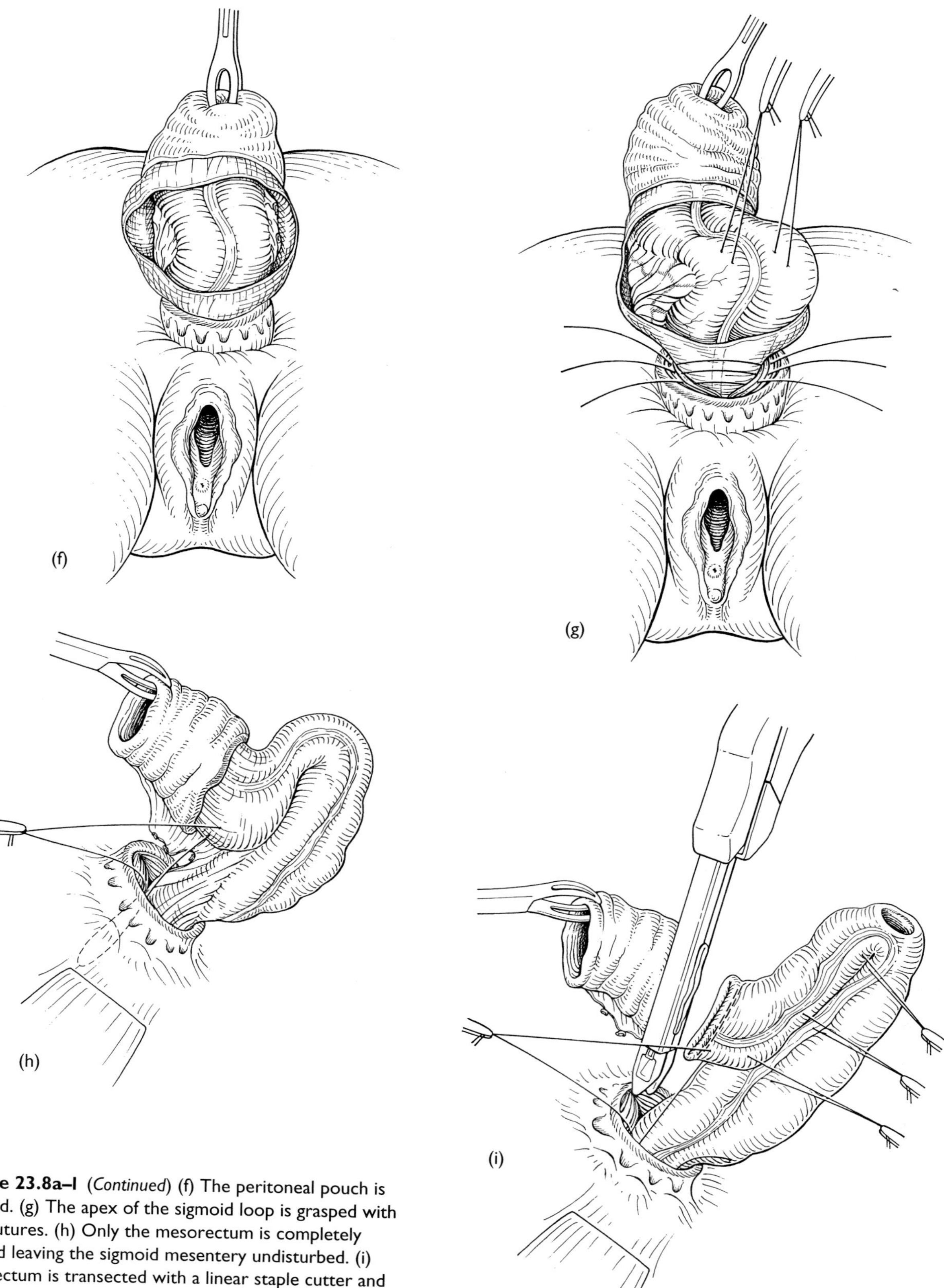

Figure 23.8a–l (*Continued*) (f) The peritoneal pouch is opened. (g) The apex of the sigmoid loop is grasped with stay sutures. (h) Only the mesorectum is completely divided leaving the sigmoid mesentery undisturbed. (i) The rectum is transected with a linear staple cutter and an enterotomy is placed at the apex of the sigmoid. (*Continued*)

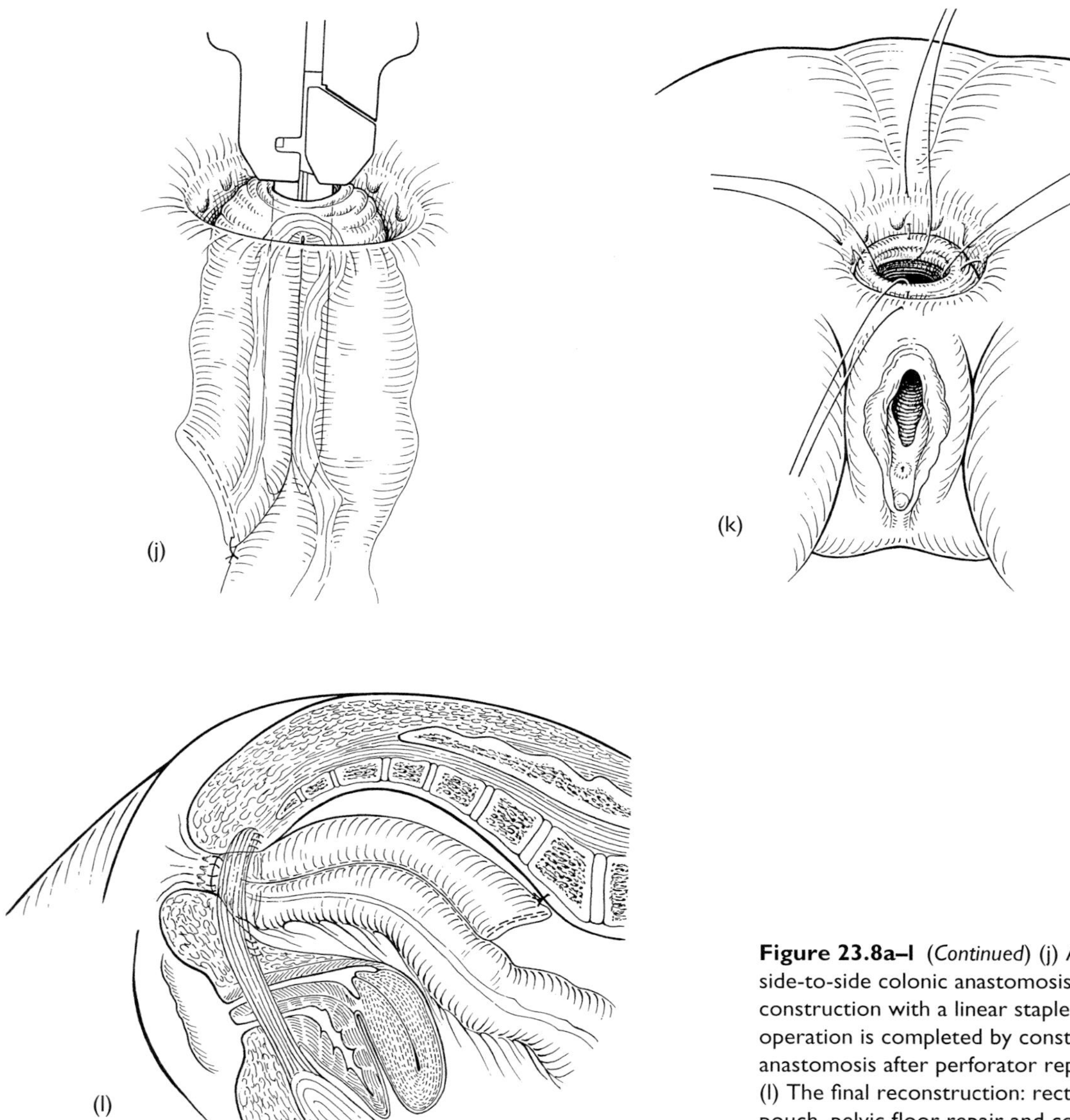

Figure 23.8a–l (*Continued*) (j) A stapled side-to-side colonic anastomosis is used for pouch construction with a linear staple cutter. (k) The operation is completed by constructing a coloanal anastomosis after perforator repair (not shown). (l) The final reconstruction: rectopexy, colonic J pouch, pelvic floor repair and coloanal anastomosis.

developed after dividing Waldeyer's fascia and the pelvic floor is easily seen, further dissection is continued over the presacral fascia as far as the promontory. A series of 0 Prolene sutures are placed between the two limbs of the puborectalis (Figure 23.8c). The mesorectum is then divided between clips and tied, leaving the longitudinal fibres of the rectum exposed. It is essential at this stage to place at least one, preferably two, sutures between the proximal rectum and the presacral fascia as a form of 'rectopexy'. These sutures are left long and not tied until the pouch has been constructed (Figure 23.8d). The prolapse is now retracted posteriorly to expose the anterior aspect of the prolapse so that the anal canal can be divided at the dentate line (Figure 23.8e). The rectovaginal pouch containing the sigmoid colon then bulges into the wound, and the peritoneum is divided so as to deliver the sigmoid into the wound (Figure 23.8f). The apex of the sigmoid loop is identified with stay sutures, but the sigmoid mesentery with the blood supply is carefully preserved. At this stage a series of interrupted sutures can be placed between the anterior leaves of the levator ani as an anterior levatorplasty (Figure 23.8g).

When seen from the side, the prolapse has been

delivered and its vessels divided prior to amputation at the level of the upper rectum. Sutures have been placed in the pelvic floor for repair and a 'pexy' suture fixes the neorectum to the presacral fascia; the blood supply to the sigmoid loop is preserved (Figure 23.8h). The next step is to amputate the prolapse at the upper rectum just distal to the 'pexy' using a linear staple cutter (PLC 75 or GIA 70). A series of stay sutures are then placed on the antimesenteric border of the sigmoid and an apical enterotomy is opened at the site of the proposed coloanal anastomosis (Figure 23.8i). The side-to-side colonic pouch is then constructed with a linear staple cutter (PLC 75 or GIA 70) (Figure 23.8j), the stay sutures are removed, the pouch is replaced in the pelvis and the 'pexy' suture is tied. It is then essential to check that the pelvic floor repair is not too tight since it must not compromise the capacity or the blood supply of the pouch. Once this is done the pelvic floor sutures may be tied. The end-to-side coloanal anastomosis is performed with interrupted 3/0 Vicryl sutures (Figure 23.8k). The completed reconstruction is shown in Figure 23.8l.

Pelvic floor repair alone

The concept of using a pelvic floor repair alone for the correction of rectal prolapse is based upon the belief that the rectal prolapse occurs secondary to a weakness in the pelvic diaphragm. Few now believe this to be the case, since pelvic floor repair alone fails to correct the prolapse. Even abdominal pelvic floor repair after rectal mobilization is associated with disappointing results (Table 23.13), and the results of perineal repairs are even worse.

Parks (1975) reported a 50% recurrence rate using postanal repair for rectal prolapse. Only by combining postanal repair with a perineal rectopexy has the control of prolapse become acceptable (Rogers and Jeffery, 1987). Reconstructing the pelvic floor with fascia lata is an interesting new approach with good results in a small, 20-patient series (El-Sibai et al, 1997).

Perineal rectopexy

Rectopexy is usually achieved after abdominal mobilization of the rectum but this may not be the ideal approach in high-risk patients. Rectal fixation to the sacrum can be achieved by the perineal route after posterior mobilization of the rectum, as in the operation of postanal repair. Mobilization is relatively straightforward but fixation can be more difficult. The mesorectum may be sutured to the presacral fascia (Thomas, 1975) or fixed by intervening material such as Teflon (Wyatt, 1981) or polyvinyl alcohol sponge (Rogers and Jeffery, 1987). Perineal rectopexy is usually combined with a postanal repair. The results of perineal rectopexy are difficult to assess since the numbers of patients reported are generally small (Table 23.14) and the additional procedures (pelvic floor repair or rectosigmoidectomy) make interpretation difficult (Hagihara and Griffen, 1975; Woods and DeCosse, 1976; Nichols, 1982).

Perineal rectopexy is usually performed in the lithotomy position. Access to the pelvic floor is gained via the intersphincteric plane after full posterior mobilization of the rectum. Thomas (1975), on the other hand, approached the rectum with the patient in the prone jack-knife position, using the trans-sacral route and excising the tip of the coccyx. The mobilized rectum is then fixed to the sacrum with non-absorbable sutures and the operation completed by repairing the deficient puborectalis behind the rectum. Perineal rectopexy is certainly

Table 23.13 Results of treatment: pelvic floor repair.

Authors	*Procedure*	*n*	*Mortality*	*Recurrent prolapse*	*Comments*
Snellman (1961)	Abdominal anterior repair	42	0	4 (10)	
Porter (1962)	Abdominal anterior repair	46	0	23 (50)	
Kupfer and Goligher (1970)	Abdominal posterior repair	63	1	5 (8)	Mucosal prolapse 8
Klaaborg et al (1985)	Abdominal posterior repair	23	0	3 (13)	
Hughes and Gleadell (1962)	Abdominoperineal anterior and posterior repair	84	1	5 (6)	Two surgeons
Parks (1975)	Perineal: postanal repair	18	0	9 (50)	
Rogers and Jeffery (1987)	Perineal: postanal repair + perineal rectopexy	24	0	1 (4)	
El-Sibai et al (1997)	Puborectal sling with fascia lata	20	0	0	

Values in parentheses are percentages.

Table 23.14 Results of treatment: rectopexy.

Procedure and authors	*n*	*Mortality*	*Recurrent prolapse*	*Comments*
Abdominal/anterior rectopexy				
Ripstein operation				
Gordon and Hoexter (1978 review)	1111	4 (0.3)	26 (2)	Faecal impaction 14; stricture 20
Morgan (1980)	64	2 (1.6)	2 (3)	Stenosis
Launer et al (1982)	54	0	4 (7)	Stricture 9
Holmstrom et al (1986b)	108	3 (2.8)	5 (4)	Stricture 4
Tjandra et al (1993)	142	1 (0.1)	10 (8)	A third of recurrences 3–14 years post-op
Abdominal/posterior rectopexy				
Teflon				
Jurgeleit et al (1975)	55	0	4 (7)	
Eisenstat et al (1979)	30	0	0	
Lescher et al (1979)	88	0	2 (2)	Stricture 2
Kuijpers and Morree (1988)	30	0	0	
Nylon strip				
Loygue et al (1984)	275	2 (0.7)	12 (4.3)	
Polypropylene (Marlex)				
Notarus (1979)	32	0	0	
Romero-Torres (1979)	24	1	0	
Hilsabeck (1981)	17	0	0	
Keighley et al (1983)	100	0	0	
Ivalon				
Penfold and Hawley (1972)	101	0	3 (3)	Mucosal prolapse 31; sepsis 2
Naughton Morgan et al (1972)	150	4 (2.6)	3 (2)	Mucosal prolapse 12
Anderson et al (1981)	40	1 (2.5)	1 (2.5)	Infection 2
Atkinson and Taylor (1984)	40	0	4 (10)	Mucosal prolapse 12; faecal impaction 1
Anderson et al (1984)	42	0	1 (2)	Pelvic sepsis 1; mucosal prolapse 4
Boulos et al (1984)*	32	0	5 (16)	
Vongsangnak et al (1985a)	53	0	0	Mucosal prolapse 3
Mann and Hoffman (1988) (extended rectopexy)	66	0	0	Mucosal prolapse 6
McCue and Thomson (1991)	53	0	2 (4)	Infection 2; impaction 2
Suture only				
Loygue et al (1971)	146	2 (1.3)	5 (3)	
Carter (1983)	32	0	0	
Goligher (1984)	52	0	1 (2)	
Graham et al (1984)	23	1 (4.3)	0	
Blatchford et al (1989)	42	0	2 (5)	
Keighley (unpublished)	27	0	0	
Sayfan et al (1997)	19	0	0	37% with mild constipation but 68% constipated preoperatively
Lyophylized dura				
Schwemmel and Hunger (1973)	62	0	5 (8)	Sepsis 2
Absorbable mesh				
Araat and Pircher (1988)	62	0	4 (7)	
Wire slings				
Soliman (1994)	28	0	0	
Polypropylene (Marlex) + vaginal suspension				
Barham & Collopy (1993)	24	0	0	Useful for coexisting vault prolapse
Perineal posterior rectopexy				
Teflon				
Wyatt (1981)	22	0	1 (4)	Mucosal prolapse 3
Suture + PAR				
Thomas (1975)	44	0	0	Mucosal sepsis 4
+ Rectosigmoidectomy + PAR				
Prasad et al (1986)	25	0	NS	
Ivalon + PAR				
Rogers and Jeffery (1987)	24	0	1 (4)	

Values in parentheses are percentages. PAR, postanal repair; NS, not stated. * Young patients only.

an attractive alternative for poor-risk patients. The great advantage of the approach is that the rectopexy can easily be combined with postanal repair.

Perineal rectopexy and postanal repair

The patient is placed in the lithotomy position in a steep Trendelenburg tilt with a sandbag under the buttocks. Alternatively, the operation may be performed in the prone jack-knife position. A curved postanal incision is made approximately 6 cm behind the anus (Figure 23.9a) after infiltration of the subcutaneous tissues and the intersphincteric plane with 1:300 000 adrenaline solution. The intersphincteric plane is opened and the rectum mobilized anteriorly using a curved Kocher's retractor (Keighley and Fielding, 1983). Waldeyer's fascia is divided (Figure 23.9b) so that the rectum can be completely mobilized posteriorly as far as the sacral promontory (Figure 23.9c). Using copper malleable retractors it is feasible to place three or four 0 Prolene sutures from the mesorectum to the sacrum in the midline. The fixed rectum is then retracted anteriorly to facilitate a pelvic floor repair (Figure 23.9d,e), using PDS or Prolene as described for postanal repair. The wounds are then closed with Prolene over two suction drains (Figure 23.9f).

Conclusions

In our opinion, perineal operations are inferior to rectopexy or resection, however, they do have a role in elderly patients deemed unfit for a major laparotomy. The simpliest operation is the Délorme's procedure but the recurrence rate is high, especially in debilitated patients. Nevertheless, the Délorme's operation can be repeated if a prolapse recurs. Perineal rectosigmoidectomy is a bigger operation but potentially with a lower recurrence rate than the Délorme's procedure, it should certainly include a pelvic floor repair, and function may be improved by constructing a colonic pouch. If the patient is fit enough and life expectancy is likely to be greater than 5 years, an abdominal approach would be preferred.

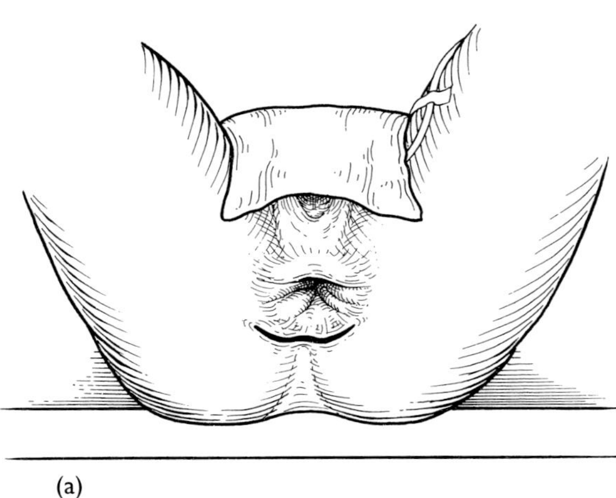

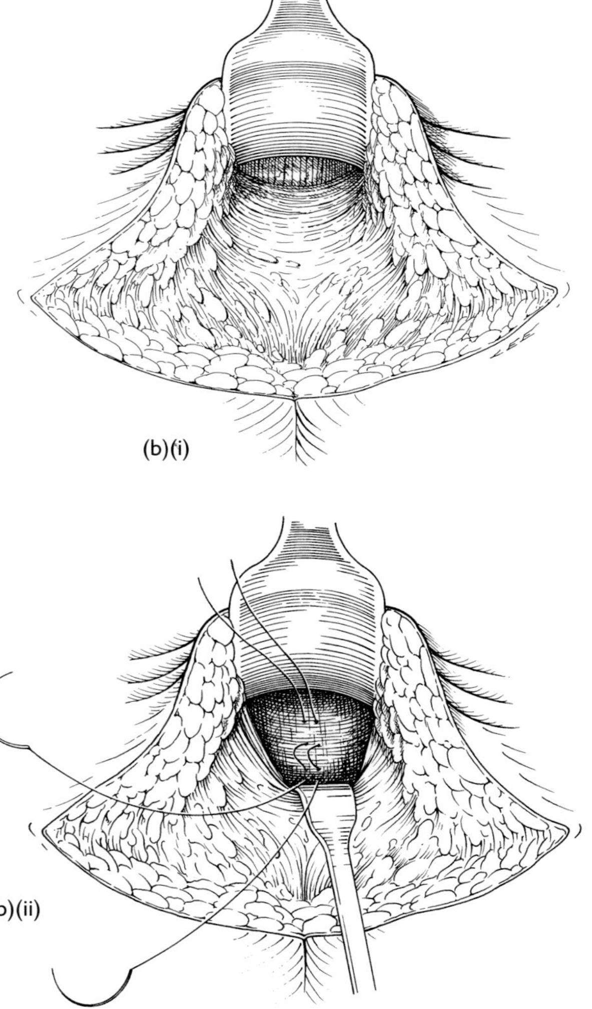

Figure 23.9a–f Perineal rectopexy. (a) The patient is placed in the Lloyd Davies position and a transverse incision is made 3 cm behind the anal verge, as in postanal repair. (b) (i) The anterior skin flap is raised and the external anal sphincter is identified. The intersphincteric plane is developed and the rectum is mobilized anteriorly after dividing Waldeyer's fascia. Anterior rectal mobilization can be achieved by gentle blunt dissection from the presacral fascia. (ii) Once the rectum has been fully mobilized anteriorly, and with posterior traction on the puborectalis sling, a series of interrupted sutures are placed between the mesorectum and the presacral fascia. (*Continued*)

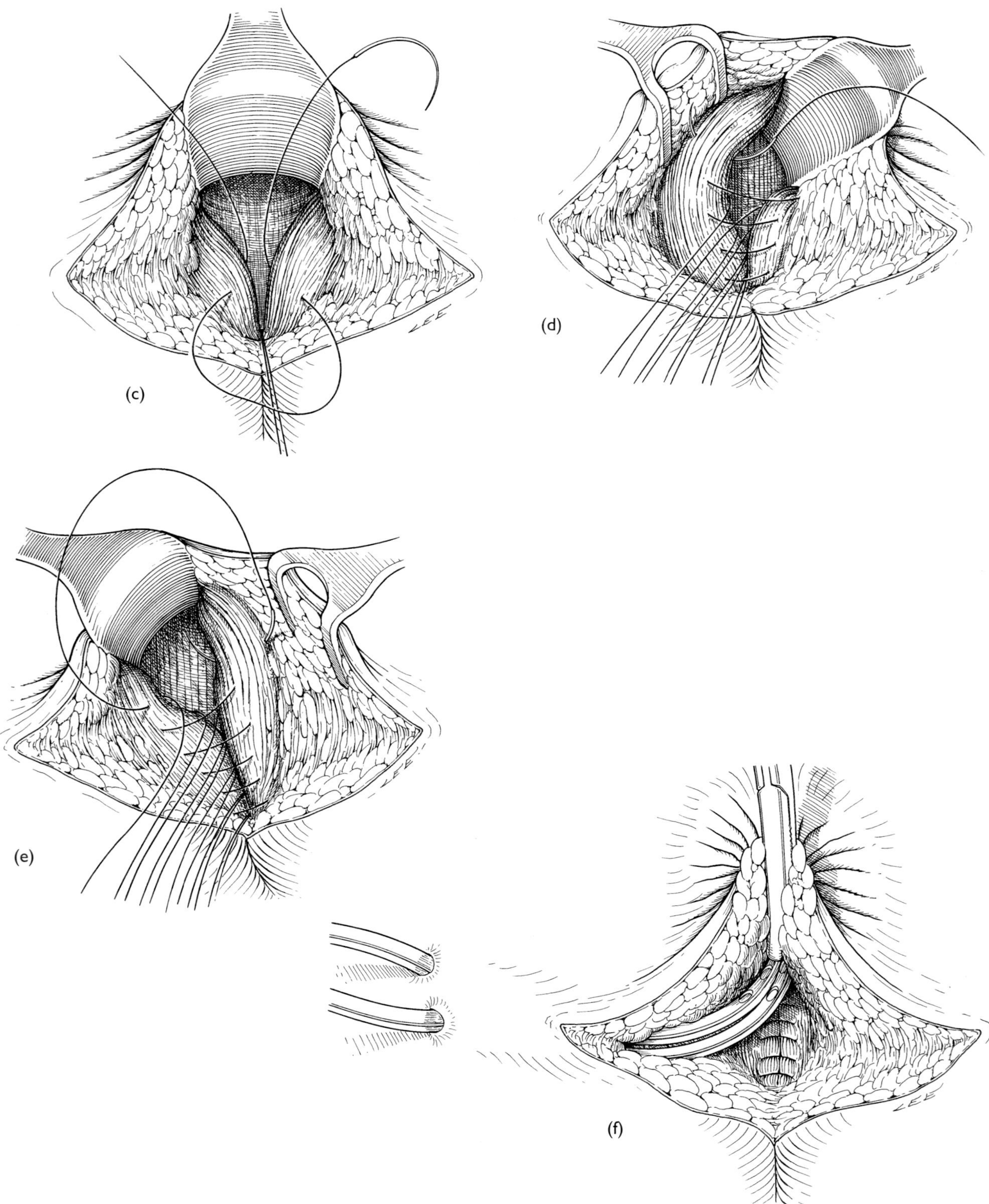

Figure 23.9a–f (*Continued*) (c) The commencement of the postanal repair after sutured rectopexy. (d) Placement of the posterior sutures for the postanal repair. (e) Rotation of the anterior retractor facilitates the placement of the anterior sutures through the puborectalis sling. (f) The anterior retractor has been removed. A cholecystectomy forceps is inserted into the presacral space to retract the skin. The sutures of the postanal repair are tied, and two closed suction drains are placed in the presacral space.

Abdominal procedures

The overall results of abdominal operations are generally superior to perineal procedures in younger, fit patients with a rectal prolapse (Table 23.14). The abdominal approach is more logical if one believes that the rectal prolapse is due to a poorly supported rectum which intussuscepts through the pelvic floor. Using the abdominal approach the rectum can be fully mobilized and fixed in a way that would not allow an intussusception to occur; simultaneously the peritoneal sliding hernia can be obliterated, the pelvic floor repaired and any coexisting resection may be performed if indicated. Associated anatomical defects, such as a deficient urethrovesical angle, uterine or vaginal descent, may also be corrected (Mann and Hoffman, 1988) at the same time (Barham and Collopy, 1993).

In some circumstances it may be optimum to combine an abdominal with a perineal procedure. It is certainly easier to repair the pelvic floor and to correct a rectocele from below. Hence Hughes and Gleadell (1962) undertook a combined abdomino-perineal approach for prolapse.

Abdominal procedures may involve exclusion procedures, pelvic floor repair, anterior or posterior rectopexy to fix the rectum, resection alone or resection with rectopexy. Each of these options will be examined. However, mortality is slightly higher after an abdominal compared with a perineal procedure and it is therefore essential to consider risk factors as well as cure of the prolapse. Furthermore, correction of any coexisting functional bowel disorder is an important consideration in patients with a long life expectancy who will not want to exchange cure of the prolapse by life-long poor bowel function.

Sigmoid exclusion procedure (Table 23.15)

Lahaut's operation

In this procedure the rectum is mobilized fully in the pelvis and the rectosigmoid is sutured to the posterior rectus sheath, while the sigmoid is extraperitonealized behind the rectus muscle. Mortensen et al (1984) reviewed the results of this operation when carried out in 33 patients in the Bristol area. There were no recurrent prolapses, and in 11 of 12 patients continence improved; however, two patients developed faecal impaction, one developed a faecal fistula which was probably ischaemic in origin, and a further patient developed obstruction.

We have no experience of this operation but believe that its morbidity is substantially higher than that of simple rectopexy.

Extraperitonealization of the sigmoid

Instead of placing the rectosigmoid in the posterior rectus sheath it may be positioned in a tunnel fashioned from the posterior parietal peritoneum above the pelvic brim. The results of this approach were reported from a survey of 32 patients. Only one patient developed a recurrence; subsequent bowel function was not referred to (Ananthakrishnan et al, 1988). Recently, Tolwinski et al (1997) reported 41 patients treated in this way, with one death and one recurrence, but 24% have persistent constipation.

Pelvic floor repair via the abdomen

Few surgeons now rely on pelvic floor repair alone for the treatment of rectal prolapse (Graham, 1942). When the operation is performed via the abdomen the failure rate lies between 6 and 50% (see Table 23.13). Most surgeons who at one time relied upon pelvic floor repair changed to abdominal rectopexy (Goligher, 1984). Repair of the pelvic floor through the abdomen is difficult; access, even in a wide female pelvis, is poor and the muscles are thin and attenuated and hold sutures poorly.

The abdominal operation involves full anterior and posterior mobilization of the rectum. Originally the puborectalis was repaired in front of the rectum (Graham et al, 1984). Latterly, most surgeons have repaired the entire pelvic floor behind the rectum

Table 23.15 Results of treatment: sigmoid exclusion procedures.

Procedure and authors	*n*	*Mortality*	*Recurrent prolapse*	*Comments*
Lahaut's operation				
Mortensen et al (1984)	33	1 (3)	1 (3)	Fistula 1; faecal impaction 2; obstruction 1
Extraperitonealization of sigmoid				
Ananthakrishnan et al (1988)	32	0	1 (3)	
Tolwinski et al (1997)	41	1 (2)	1 (3.4)	24% constipation rate, only 1 person still incontinent

Values in parentheses are percentages.

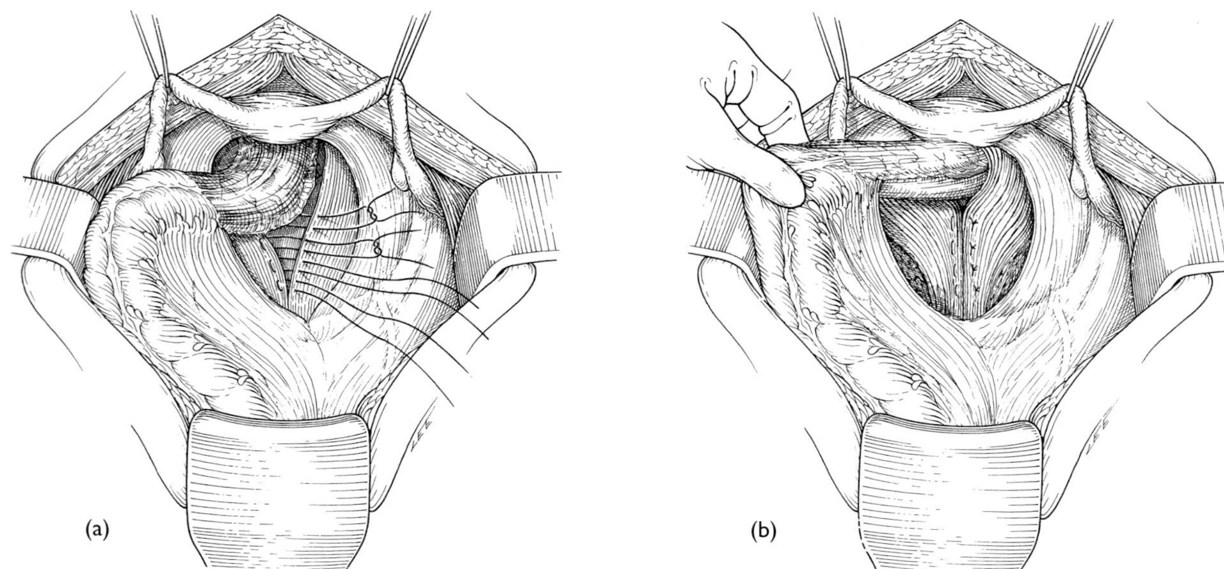

Figure 23.10a,b Ruscoe–Graham pelvic floor repair. (a) The pelvic peritoneum is divided on the lateral and anterior aspects of the rectum. The rectum is mobilized behind the superior haemorrhoidal vessels down to the tip of the coccyx. The lateral ligaments are divided. The inner fibres of the puborectalis sling can then be seen from above, and a series of interrupted sutures are used to repair the pelvic floor. (b) The completed posterior pelvic floor repair.

(Figure 23.10a,b). The pelvic floor may also be repaired as a combined abdominal and perineal procedure. Hughes describes an operation involving a gynaecologist: sutures being placed through the pelvic floor by the abdominal surgeon and then withdrawn to the perineal operation site so that the perineal aspect of the pelvic floor is included with each suture (Hughes and Gleadell, 1962). In our experience it is much easier to repair a pelvic floor deficiency from below than from above (Snellman, 1961).

Porter (1962) reviewed a collective series of 46 patients who had undergone pelvic floor repair alone: 50% developed a recurrent prolapse. It is likely that these data are unrepresentative since three later independent studies report recurrences of only 8–13% (Snellman, 1961; Kupfer and Goligher, 1970; Klaaborg et al, 1985). In the most recent report of this technique, two-thirds of incontinent patients regained continence, but one-third became constipated after pelvic floor repair (Klaaborg et al, 1985).

Rectopexy (see Table 23.14)

Most surgeons today believe that rectopexy has become the operation of choice for control of rectal prolapse even in elderly patients (Kirkman, 1975; Wise et al, 1991). If it is believed that a rectal prolapse is due to an intussusception (Wedell et al, 1980), fixation of the mobilized rectum in the pelvis will resolve the problem. This concept is now supported by the literature since the recurrence rate following rectopexy, irrespective of the method of fixation, is usually less than 2% (Table 23.14). Furthermore, continence is restored in 60–80% of patients treated by rectopexy alone and there is a significant rise in anal pressures (Hiltunen and Matikainen, 1992). The only questions which now need to be answered are: how should the rectum be fixed (foreign material or sutures) and when should the operation be combined with colonic resection or pelvic floor repair?

Anterior rectopexy

The Ripstein operation was one of the earlier methods of rectopexy (Ripstein, 1965, 1969, 1972). The principle behind the operation is full mobilization of the rectum, which is then fixed to the sacral promontory by means of a sling of material (polypropylene, Teflon or even fascia) so that the rectum is tethered anteriorly and along its sides to the sacrum (Figure 23.11) (Launer et al, 1982). The problem with anterior fixation is that the front of the rectum is encircled by the foreign body and if an

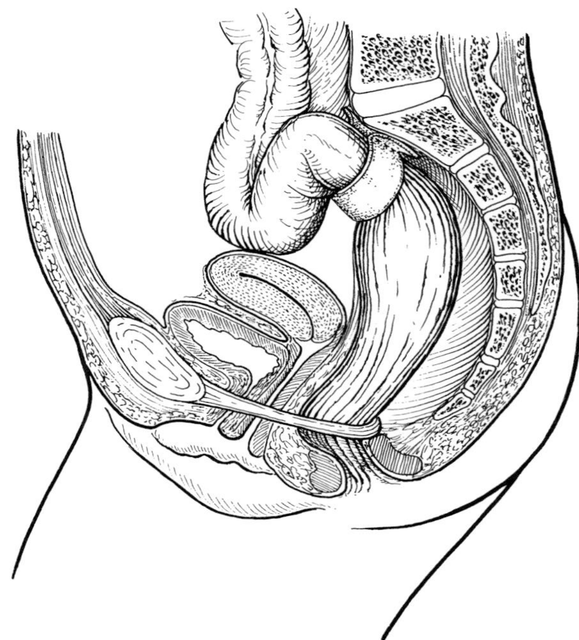

Figure 23.11 Anterior rectopexy. A variety of foreign materials may be used to fix the rectum to the sacrum after full mobilization. A collar of material thus encircles the upper rectum. The treatment is frequently complicated by stenosis at the rectopexy site.

intense fibrous reaction develops the rectum becomes constricted (Ahlbaack et al, 1979). Occasionally a stenosis develops, leading to incapacitating constipation, sometimes necessitating reoperation.

Gordon and Hoexter (1978), in a postal review, received replies from surgeons treating over 1000 cases of rectal prolapse by the Ripstein procedure. Although this survey seemed to underestimate the true incidence of complications, faecal impaction was reported in 14 cases (7%) and a tight fibrous rectal stricture occurred in 20 patients. It is hardly surprising that a collar of mesh surrounding the anterolateral aspects of the rectum and attached posteriorly to the sacrum causes a high incidence of stricture (McCue and Thomson, 1991). Launer et al (1982), in a personal series, reported strictures in 17% of patients postoperatively. Morgan (1980), using Teflon around the front of the rectum, reported stenosis in one of six cases. Surprisingly, however, a review of over 100 Ripstein operations reported recurrence in 4% and a stricture in only 3% (Holmstrom et al, 1986b). Continence improved in 72%, however, constipation became more common and rose from 27% before rectopexy to 43% afterwards.

Tjandra et al (1993) at the Ohio Cleveland Clinic reported 142 Ripstein operations. There was one death and 10 recurrences (8%). A third of the recurrences occurred 3–14 years after the operation, emphasizing the importance of adequate follow-up if the true recurrence rates are to be documented. Scaglia et al (1994) report that if the Ripstein rectopexy preserves the lateral ligaments, there is no difficulty with rectal evacuation. If, on the other hand, the lateral ligaments are divided, the threshold for rectal sensation rises and constipation is more common.

Posterior rectopexy

The advantages of posterior rectopexy is that only the posterior aspect of the rectum is fixed to the sacrum, usually by means of a synthetic mesh (Ihre, 1972). The mesh is attached to the sacrum and thence to the lateral aspect of the rectum by suturing the divided lateral attachments of the rectum to the sides of the mesh, leaving a space posteriorly (see Figure 23.13). This procedure causes no anterior restriction and allows the rectum to distend during defecation (Efron, 1977). Today, most surgeons have dispensed with mesh and merely suture the mesorectum to the presacral fascia.

There is wide divergence of opinion regarding additional corrective surgery. Some surgeons advocate restoring the rectovaginal septum, excising and closing the anterior rectovaginal peritoneal pouch, reinforcing the lateral ligaments and even repairing the levator ani (Mann and Hoffman, 1988). We have not found any of these additional procedures necessary during abdominal rectopexy. Indeed, the operation is kept as simple as possible, dividing only the lateral peritoneum and restricting rectal mobilization to a complete posterior dissection to the tip of the coccyx and dividing the lateral ligaments.

The type of foreign material is, we suspect, the least important consideration. Indeed, foreign materials are rarely used today. Teflon, polypropylene (Marlex), polyvinyl alcohol sponge and Gore-Tex are the materials which have been used most widely in the past. Teflon is rather soft but holds sutures well (Jurgeleit et al, 1975; Eisenstat et al, 1979; Lescher et al, 1979; Kuijpers and Morree, 1988). Polypropylene is stiffer and seems to be more inert (Notarus, 1979; Greene, 1983). We have never encountered sepsis around this material and no cases of sepsis have been reported in the literature (Romero-Torres, 1979; Hilsabeck, 1981). Polyvinyl alcohol sponge seems to be the least attractive material to use: it becomes very soft when wet, it holds sutures poorly, and there is a considerable risk of infection developing around this material (Naughton-Morgan et al, 1972; Penfold and Hawley, 1972; Anderson et al, 1981, 1984; Atkinson and Taylor, 1984; Boulos et al, 1984; Vonsangnak et al, 1985a; Mann and Hoffman, 1988). Furthermore, we have ten patients in our own series who were referred from other centres with a recurrent prolapse after rectopexy using polyvinyl alcohol sponge. When these patients were re-operated upon the sponge was found encased in fibrous tissue in the pelvis, often loosely attached to the rectum but no longer in proximity to the sacrum. If a patient strains in the early postoperative period there is, we believe, a real risk that the sutures will tear from the mesh.

Another alternative to conventional materials such as polypropylene, Teflon, Ivalon or even Nylon strips (Loygue et al, 1984) is to use absorbable meshes made with polyglycolic acid or polygalactone. Araat and Pircher (1988) reported 62 rectopexies performed using absorbable mesh; there was a 7% recurrence rate but no patient developed pelvic sepsis. Gore-Tex is a material which seems to be associated with a low rate of sepsis.

Athanasiadis et al (1996) reviewed their results of rectopexy using Ivalon, Vicryl or Gore-Tex. One hundred and forty-five had a concomitant resection and 77 did not. There were three recurrences only, and all occurred in the rectopexy alone group. Infection of the implant occurred in four patients (Table 23.16) and was more common in the resection group. No infections were reported with Gore-Tex, one with Vicryl mesh and three with Ivalon.

There have been encouraging reports of posterior rectopexy using sutures alone to attach the rectum to the presacral fascia (Loygue et al, 1971; Carter, 1983; Goligher, 1984; Graham et al, 1984; Watts et al, 1985). In Birmingham, we have adopted the sutured rectopexy since 1988 as a consequence of combining rectopexy with a sigmoid colectomy (Sayfan et al, 1990) and the recurrence rate has remained less than 2%. In London we have used the same technique to correct all rectal prolapses since 1986 with a similar low recurrence rate. We merely mobilize the rectum to the pelvic floor and attach it to the sacrum using a series of Prolene, PDS or Ethibond sutures through the mesorectum and the periosteum of the sacrum in the midline.

The standard posterior rectopexy should probably be modified for male patients. There is a small risk of rendering such patients impotent. Care should therefore be exercised in preserving the presacral nerves and avoiding damage anteriorly to Denonvilliers' fascia. It has been suggested that at least one lateral ligament should be preserved, since the lateral pararectal tissues carry parasympathetic fibres which run with the middle rectal vessels to the male genitalia and are important in maintaining normal ejaculatory function (Abou-Enein, 1978). However, such a policy seems unnecessary since sexual function is unimpaired after restorative proctocolectomy, despite division of both lateral ligaments. Preservation of the lateral ligaments was assessed by Speakman et al (1991) in a randomized trial. It was associated with significantly less constipation but a much higher recurrence rate (Table 23.17). In a non-randomized comparison, Scaglia et al (1994) found identical results, namely that preserving the lateral ligaments reduces the risk of constipation.

Table 23.16 Rates of infected implants using different materials in mesh rectopexy.

	Resection		*Non-resection*		
Mesh material	*n*	*Number infected*	*n*	*Number infected*	*Total % infected*
Ivalon	54	2 (37)	33	1 (3.0)	3.4
Vicryl	84	1 (1.2)	25	0	0.9
Gore-Tex	7	0	19	0	0
Totals	145	3 (2)	77	1 (1.3)	

Numbers in parentheses are percentages.
From Athanasiadis et al (1996).

Table 23.17 Impact of preserving the lateral ligaments in Marlex posterior rectopexy.

	Lateral ligaments divided (*n* = 12)		*Lateral ligaments preserved* (*n* = 14)	
	Preoperative	*Postoperative*	*Preoperative*	*Postoperative*
Continence score	3	2	4	2
Time straining (%)	54	54	12	56
No. constipated	6	7	3	10
Rectal prolapse	12	0	14	6

From Speakman et al (1991).

Surgical procedure: abdominal rectopexy alone

Preoperative bowel preparation is important to prevent constipation and straining after operation. This is one of the few rectal operations in which the Lloyd Davies position is not essential, and therefore the supine position is preferred by some. However, others like ourselves feel that the Lloyd Davies position does afford better access. A general anaesthetic is generally used but some elderly patients in our series have had their operations performed under a spinal or epidural anaesthetic. It is our policy to give single-dose perioperative antibiotic cover.

A low midline incision is generally used, but in younger women, a transverse incision is often preferred and does not compromise rectal mobilization. The small bowel is retracted from the pelvis and retained in the upper abdomen by abdominal packs. The patient is placed in a steep head-down Trendelenburg tilt. The rectum is mobilized by dividing the pelvic peritoneum on both sides of the rectum. As these patients have a long rectovaginal or rectovesical pouch, division of the anterior peritoneum is not considered necessary (Figure 23.12a). The presacral space is opened immediately behind the superior haemorrhoidal vessels and the rectum is mobilized posteriorly as far as the tip of the coccyx; the attenuated lateral ligaments are then divided (Figure 23.12b). The rectum is pulled straight and fixed, either by suture to a small rectangular piece of Marlex mesh (polypropylene) attached to the sacrum (Figure 23.12c) or by interrupted sutures alone to the presacral fascia. In Marlex rectopexy four interrupted prolene sutures are inserted in the midline on or below the sacral promontory (Figure 23.12d) and through the polypropylene mesh, leaving two free margins (Figure 23.12e). The free margins are sutured to the divided lateral ligaments of the rectum. Mesh is never allowed to completely encircle the rectum and at least the anterior half of the rectal circumference is left free.

In sutured rectopexy the prolene sutures are merely placed through the presacral fascia, as described, and then through the mesorectum in the midline thereby, avoiding the superior haemorrhoidal vessels which have divided at this point into two branches away from the midline (Figure 23.13a). We believe that it is safer to place the sutures in the midline of the sacrum since there is less risk of damage to the presacral veins or the pelvic nerves (Figure 23.13b). If massive bleeding does occur from presacral veins, the use of sterilized drawing pins through the bleeding point into the sacrum seems to be a valuable method of control (Lucarotti et al, 1991; Stolfi et al, 1992). No attempt is

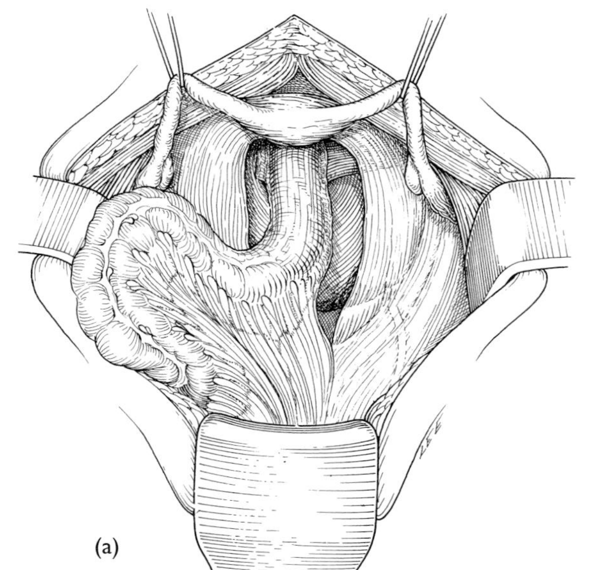
(a)

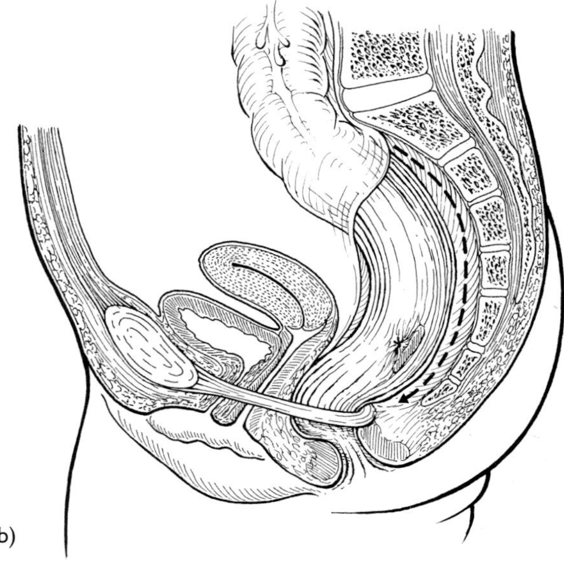
(b)

Figure 23.12a–e Posterior polypropylene rectopexy. (a) A midline incision is made. The peritoneum over the lateral aspects of the sigmoid is mobilized. The peritoneum on the lateral aspects of the rectum is divided, but the anterior peritoneum in the rectovaginal pouch is not divided. A retrorectal dissection proceeds behind the superior haemorrhoidal vessels to the tip of the coccyx, and the lateral ligaments are divided. (b) The extent of the posterior dissection and the divided lateral ligaments. *(Continued)*

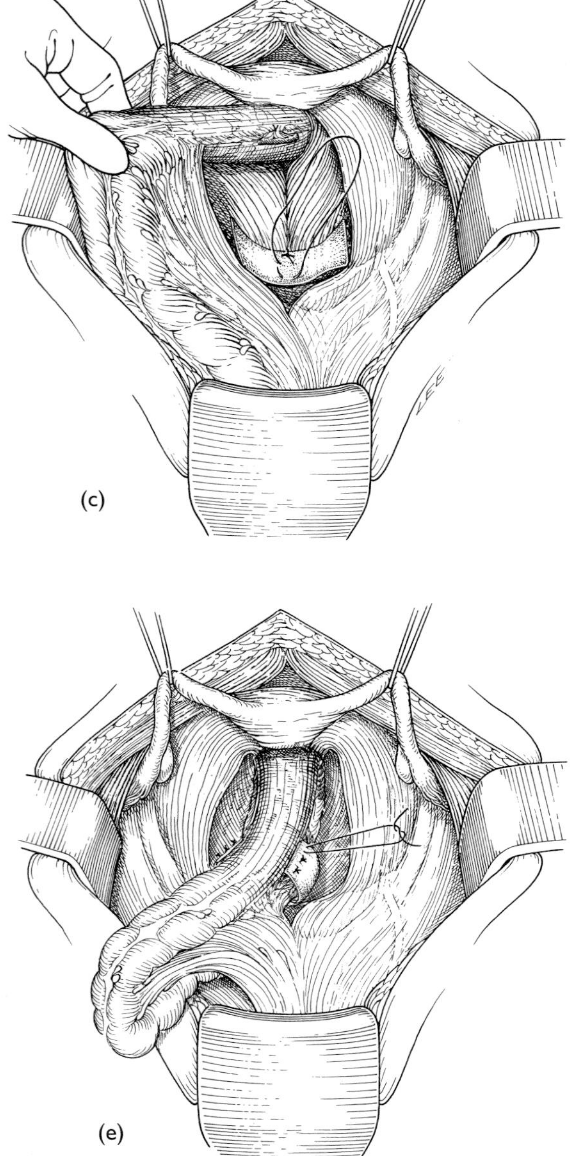

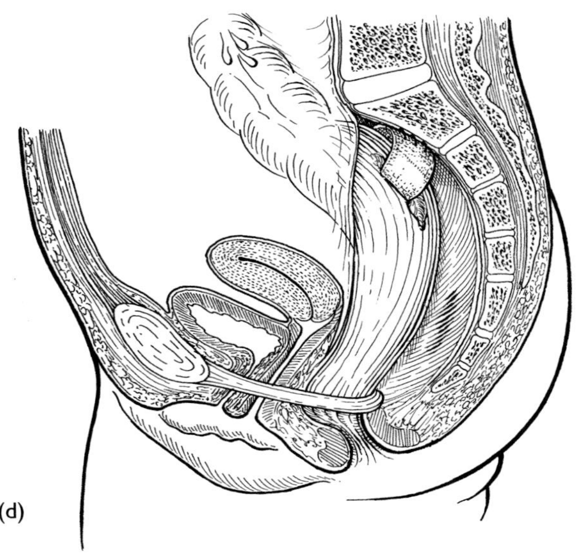

Figure 23.12a–e (*Continued*) (c) A rectangular strip of polypropylene mesh measuring 3.5 x 2.0 cm is cut. Three interrupted Prolene sutures secure the centre of the polypropylene mesh to the presacral fascia. It is essential that these sutures be placed in the midline, otherwise the presacral veins may be damaged. (d) This sagittal view shows the fully mobilized rectum and the polypropylene mesh sutured to the presacral fascia, with the lateral aspects of the mesh attached to the divided lateral ligaments. (e) The completed posterior rectopexy. Note that the lateral edges of the polypropylene mesh lie loosely attached to the divided lateral ligaments, and the anterior aspect of the rectum is free.

made to suture the pelvic peritoneum, and the abdomen is closed in the usual way after placing two suction drains in the pelvis.

Until quite recently Ivalon (polyvinyl alcohol sponge) posterior rectopexy was the most widely practised operation in Britain (Wells, 1959; Ellis, 1966). Mortality is uncommon and the recurrence rate ranges from nil to 8%. Boulos et al (1984) highlight the poor functional outcome in young patients as well as reporting a 25% recurrence rate. Ivalon rectopexy should probably be avoided in younger patients because many are likely to need further surgery. Unlike the Ripstein operation, faecal impaction from rectal stenosis is rare (Atkinson and Taylor, 1984). Perhaps the real reason why there has been a move away from Ivalon is the risk of sepsis around this particular foreign body (Penfold and Hawley, 1972; Lake et al, 1984; Wedell et al, 1987; Athanasiadis et al, 1996).

Ross and Thomson (1989) describe the management of eight patients who developed chronic pelvic sepsis after Ivalon rectopexy (the Wells' operation). Sepsis invariably developed within 3 months and presented with pelvic pain, vaginal or anal discharge, intermittent fever and diarrhoea. In five of these patients it had been possible to remove the

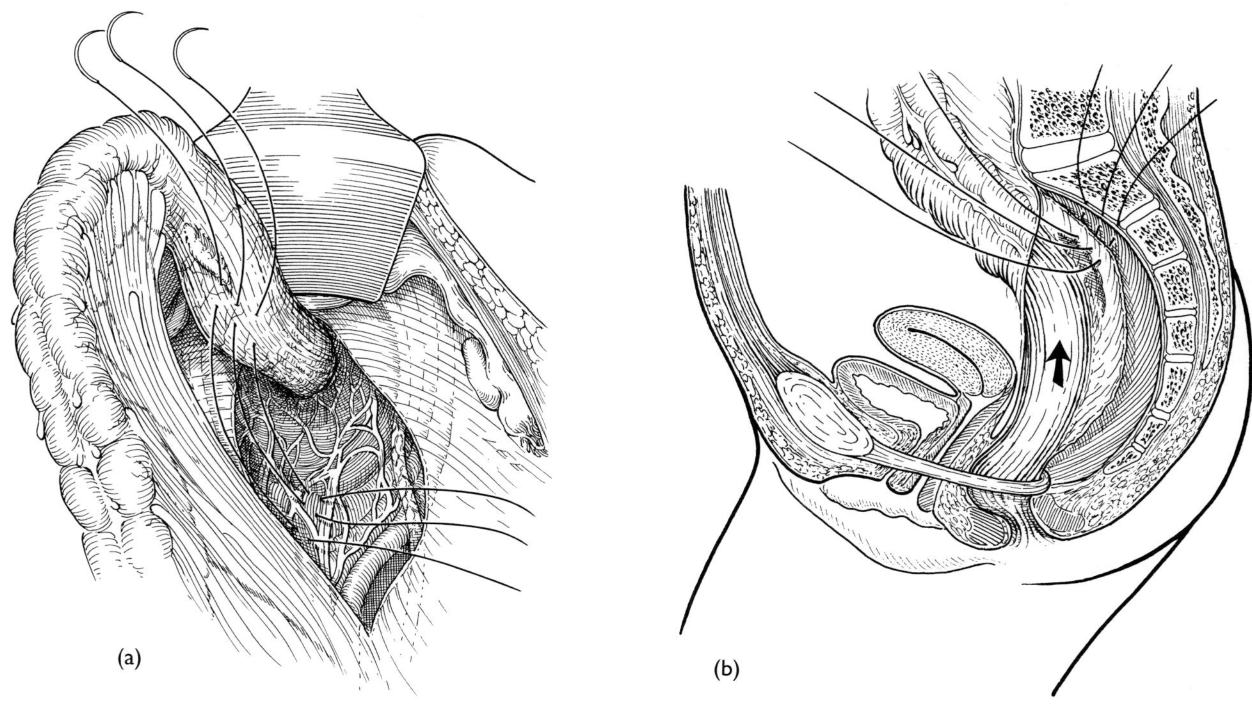

Figure 23.13a,b Sutured rectopexy. (a) The rectum has been fully mobilized down to the tip of the coccyx and the lateral ligaments have been divided. A series of three interrupted sutures are placed between the presacral fascia and the mesorectum, with the rectum forcibly retracted upwards out of the pelvis. (b) Sagittal section of the mobilized rectum being attached to the presacral fascia by a series of interrupted sutures.

infected material per vaginam or per rectum without incurring morbidity or recurrence. They advise against the use of Ivalon when the bowel is damaged at operation or if there is a risk of pelvic haematoma.

The incidence of functional bowel disturbance after Ivalon rectopexy seems to be comparable with other methods of posterior rectopexy. Approximately 25% of incontinent patients remain incontinent of solids, and almost half remain incontinent of liquids despite successful rectopexy (Anderson et al, 1984). The incidence of constipation after Ivalon rectopexy increases from 29 to 47% (Mann and Hoffman, 1988; McCue and Thomson, 1991). Alternative foreign materials include: polypropylene mesh (Marlex), Gore-Tex (Soliman, 1994), lyophilized dura (Schwemmel and Hunger, 1973), strips of Nylon (Loygue et al, 1984) and Teflon (Kuijpers and Morree, 1988).

In an attempt to dispense with a foreign body, with the attendant risk of sepsis, Araat and Pircher (1988) reported their experience using absorbable mesh (Vinyl or Dexon). None of the 62 patients treated in this way developed pelvic sepsis but four (7%) had a recurrence. One case of sepsis was reported in 109 patients having a Vicryl mesh rectopexy (Athanasiadis et al, 1996).

In the 1980s, there was a move away from Ivalon because of the risks of sepsis and also it was felt that constipation was a real problem with Ivalon. A number of centres reported the results of Marlex rectopexy. The morbidity and recurrence rate was remarkably low (Table 23.14). We reviewed the outcome of 165 cases (Yoshioka et al, 1989b). Only ten were men, 39 had had previous operations for prolapse that had failed, there were no deaths, no infection occurred around the mesh and minor morbidity occurred in 22%. Follow-up was achieved in 135 of the patients: 22 had died in 2 years and in eight the follow-up was too short. Only two recurrences were identified (1.5%) but there were seven mucosal prolapses, all of which were controlled by rubber band ligation. Incontinence fell from 58% to 16% but constipation rose from 24% to 44%. There was a small rise in resting anal pressure after operation but compliance fell somewhat, saline continence improved but percentage rectal emptying fell from 83% to 58% (Yoshioka et al, 1989b) (Table 23.18).

The persistent incontinence did not usually

Table 23.18 Physiological abnormalities in rectal prolapse and influence of rectopexy.

	Controls (*n* = 15)		Rectal prolapse (*n* = 12)	
			Preoperative	*Postoperative*
Maximum resting anal pressure (cmH_2O)	86 (53–113)	*	50 (21–80)	57 (18–80)
Maximum squeeze pressure (cmH_2O)	129 (60–171)	*	79 (33–121)	82 (30–110)
Absent rectoanal inhibitory reflex	0	*	4	4
Increased EMG activity in puborectalis on attempted defecation	2		2	2
Compliance (cmH_2O/ml)	13.1 (6.0–26)	*	9.18 (4.3–20)	7.89 (5.4–16)
Volume of saline first leaked (cm^3)	800 (80–1500)	*	60 (5–1500)	120 (30–1500)
Anorectal angle (rest) (°)	112 (85–134)	*	124 (109–151)	126 (100–154)
Rectal emptying (%)	75 (0–100)		83 (42–100)*	58 (0–100)

Values in parentheses are ranges.
*Significant differences.

trouble very old patients who were quite happy that their prolapse was controlled. A few with persistent incontinence underwent postanal repair, but the results were very poor and we rarely now advise further surgical treatment for persistent incontinence. The persistent or new constipation was a bigger problem and has led to some patients having a colonic resection at a later date but the results of these were often rather disappointing.

On the basis of these data, we felt that an alternative to Marlex rectopexy such as fixation by suture alone should be explored. Fortunately, the issue has been clarified by a prospect randomized trial from the Royal Free Hospital London (Novell et al, 1994). The results are reproduced in Table 23.19. Sutured rectopexy alone was associated with fewer complications, a lower incidence of late postoperative incontinence and a lower incidence of constipation. There were two recurrences, one in each group. On the basis of these data, we believe that Ivalon and all varieties of mesh should no longer be stocked in the operating theatre since sutures are just as effective and functional results are better.

Table 23.19 Randomized trial of sponge versus sutured rectopexy (no resections).

	Ivalon sponge (*n* = 31)	*Sutured alone* (*n* = 32)
Hospital stay (days)	14 (8–52)	14 (8–50)
Mortality	0	0
Complications	6 (19%)	3 (9%)
Recurrent prolapse	1 (3%)	1 (3%)
Late postoperative incontinence	6/10	2/10
Postop constipation	15 (48%)	10 (31%)

From Novell et al (1994).

Most authors use non-absorbable sutures (Nylon or Prolene) but some have now changed to absorbable materials such as PDS. Loygue et al (1971) have the largest series of 146 patients, with a 3% recurrence rate. For some reason they have changed their policy of sutured rectopexy to the use of Nylon strips (Loygue et al, 1984). Many other surgeons, including ourselves, have adopted their original suggestion using sutured rectopexy, having become disenchanted with conventional Nylon or Marlex rectopexy (Efron, 1977; Carter, 1983; Goligher, 1984; Graham et al, 1984) principally because it allows a resection to be performed at the same time without the risk of sepsis if mesh is used (Athanasiadis et al, 1996). Recurrence rates following sutured rectopexy are very low and the procedure can be safely combined with a colonic resection (Sayfan et al, 1990).

Sayfan et al (1997) in Israel has subsequently reported results of 19 sutured rectopexy procedures alone. Constipation fell from 68% to 37% but in almost all cases the constipation was only mild. He therefore believes that addition of a resection is not always necessary.

The real problem after abdominal rectopexy is not that of persistent incontinence despite successful control of the prolapse but of persistent or acquired constipation (Speakman et al, 1991; Madden et al, 1992; Tjandra et al, 1993).

Resection alone

Perhaps the most controversial method of treating rectal prolapse involving a laparotomy is that of sigmoid or partial rectal resection alone without concomitant rectopexy. The Mayo Clinic have used high anterior resection for at least a decade and

Table 23.20 Results of treatment: resection.

Procedure and authors	*n*	*Mortality*	*Recurrent prolapse*	*Comments*
Anterior resection				
Muir (1962)	50	1 (2)	0	Mucosal prolapse common
Thauerkauf et al (1970)	62	3 (4)	3 (4)	
Review (from Thauerkauf)	202	7 (3.5)	4 (2)	
Schlinkert et al (1985)	113	1 (1)	8 (7)	Anaesthetic complication 8; stricture 2
High resection	52	1 (2)	3/27* (11)	Morbidity 10 (19)
Low anterior resection	29	0	2/24* (9)	Morbidity 22 (76)
Sigmoid resection + rectopexy				
Watts et al (1985)	138	0	2 (1.4)	Anastomotic leaks 5
Huber et al (1995)	42	0	0	7% complication rate; constipation 43–26%; incontinence 67–23%

Values in parentheses are percentages.
*Not all patients followed up.

continue to believe that this is the optimum approach, despite the popularity of rectopexy elsewhere (Schlinkert et al, 1985). Muir (1962) was the original protagonist and reported no recurrence in 50 patients having an anterior resection. Thauerkauf et al (1970) reported three recurrences in 62 patients, and in their literature review found a mortality of 3.5% and a recurrence rate of 2%.

The problem with resection alone is the potentially fatal complication of anastomotic dehiscence and the fear that some patients may develop incontinence (Table 23.20). Schlinkert et al (1985) reported that incontinence was improved in 23 (20%), remained the same in 13 (11%) but became worse in ten (9%). Continence after resection alone is inferior to rectopexy. Perhaps the strongest argument against a resection is the increased potential morbidity from sepsis (anastomotic leakage, pelvic abscess, septicaemia, wound infection) which occurred in 52% of patients after low anterior resection, compared with 19% after high anterior resection. Initially after resection the recurrence rate was low but it gradually increases with time and was found to be greater at 10 years after high anterior resection than it was with low anterior resection: being 14 and 9% respectively (Schlinkert et al, 1985). These data further emphasize the importance of long follow-up if true recurrence rates are required.

In view of the cumulative increased recurrence rate after anterior resection and the risk of anastomotic leak, most surgeons now believe that a sigmoid resection should be combined with rectopexy in fit patients requiring long-term avoidance of constipation and a low risk of recurrence.

Resection rectopexy

The concept of combined rectopexy and sigmoid resection is not new (Figure 23.14) and was initially advocated by Frykman and Goldberg (1969). When Watts et al (1985) reviewed their results of surgery for rectal prolapse in the University of Minnesota, 138 had had the Frykman–Goldberg procedure. Five anastomotic leaks were reported (4%), with recurrent prolapse in only two (1.4%). Continence was improved in all except one patient, constipation

Table 23.21 Resection with rectopexy compared with rectopexy alone.

Preoperative status and outcome	*Marlex rectopexy alone (n = 16)*	*Rectopexy with sigmoidectomy (n = 13)*
Incontinent before operation	12	9
Unchanged or worse	3	3
Continence restored	9	6
Constipated before operation	3	5
Unchanged or worse	3	1
Constipation improved	0	4
Normal bowel habit before operation	13	8
Unchanged	9	8
Became constipated	4	0

From Sayfan et al (1990).

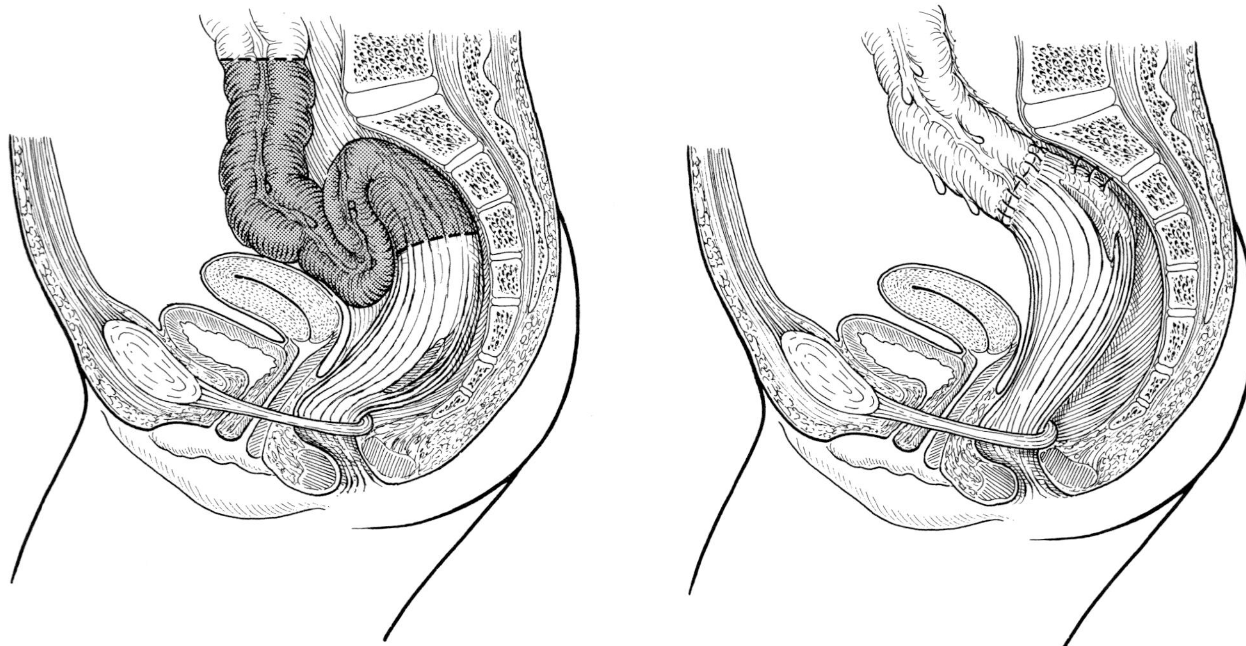

Figure 23.14a,b Rectopexy and sigmoidectomy. (a) At the completion of a rectopexy there may be a long redundant segment of sigmoid colon, which may angulate into the pelvis from the rectopexy site. It is now our practice to excise this redundant sigmoid colon during rectopexy. The sites of sigmoid transection are shown. (b) The completed sutured rectopexy and sutured colorectal anastomosis after sigmoidectomy.

was improved in 56%, remained the same in 35% and was worse in 9%. Huber et al (1995) reported the results of resection rectopexy in 42 patients without mortality and without recurrence. Incontinence fell from 67% to 23% and constipation fell from 43% to 26% (Table 23.19).

We have compared resection rectopexy with Marlex rectopexy alone (Table 23.21). No patient developed a recurrent prolapse, there were no anastomotic leaks, incontinence was not increased by performing a resection and none developed constipation for the first time when resection was combined with rectopexy (Sayfan et al, 1990). These and other data (Table 23.22) suggest that, in selected younger patients who have or who are likely to develop constipation, resection with rectopexy is likely to result in superior functional results (Luukkonen et al, 1992). When Duthie and Bartolo (1992) compared resection rectopexy with sutured or mesh rectopexy, no major differences emerged apart from the higher incidence of constipation after the use of Ivalon alone.

Table 23.22 Continence and constipation after rectopexy and alternative procedures.

	Incontinent				*Constipated*			
Authors	*Same*	*Improved*	*Restored*	*Operation*	*Same*	*Improved*	*Worse*	*Precipitated*
Broden et al (1988b) (*n* = 15)	30	70	—	Ripstein	NS	NS	NS	NS
Broden et al (1988b) (*n* = 15)	—	—	—	Ripstein	20	NS	NS	NS
Holmstrom et al (1986a) (*n* = 108)	28	72	NS	Ripstein	27	NS	NS	43
Mortensen et al (1984) (*n* = 34)	8	92	NS	Lahaut	NS	NS	NS	6
Klaaborg et al (1985) (*n* = 23)	25	75	NS	Roscoe Graham	27	NS	NS	30
Schlinkert et al (1985) (*n* = 113)*	28	50	—	Anterior resection	NS	NS	NS	NS
Watts et al (1985) (*n* = 138)	40	60	—	Rectopexy + sigmoid colectomy	35	56	9	—
Mann and Hoffman (1988) (*n* = 66)	26	34	38	Ivalon	29	NS	NS	47
Yoshioka et al (1989b) (*n* = 135)	16	12	72	Ivalon	24	—	22	18
Sayfan et al (1990) (*n* = 13)	23	—	77	Sutured and sigmoid colectomy	8	31	—	—

Values are percentages.
*22% rendered incontinent or incontinence worse after operation.
NS, not stated.

Tjandra et al (1993) reviewed the functional outcome of the Ripstein rectopexy compared with resection rectopexy at the Cleveland Clinic, Ohio. Results were comparable in terms of improved continence, but constipation was much less common after resection rectopexy (Table 23.23).

Table 23.23 Functional outcome: rectopexy versus resection rectopexy.

	Constipation		*Incontinence*	
	Preop.	*Postop.*	*Preop.*	*Postop.*
Rectopexy (n = 129)	47 (36)	42 (33)	48 (37)	25 (19)
Resection rectopexy (n = 18)	12 (67)	2 (11)	5 (28)	3 (17)

Values in parentheses are percentages.
From Tjandra et al (1993).

Table 23.24 Randomized trial: extent of resection in resection rectopexy.

	Sigmoidectomy (n = 13)	*Left hemicolectomy* (n = 12)
Deaths	0	2
Recurrence	2	0
Severe bleeding	0	1
Function: pre- and postop:		
Constipation	4–1	4–1
Incontinence	10–1	7–3
Urgency	7–4	8–6
Soiling	9–5	7–4

From Yoshioka et al (1998).

The extent of resection, we suspect, depends largely on preoperative symptoms. In a small randomized study to compare sigmoidectomy with left hemicolectomy, no major functional advantages of left hemicolectomy emerged (Table 23.24).

The two immediate perioperative deaths were entirely due to coexisting ischaemic heart disease and cannot be attributable to the operative procedure.

Laparoscopic rectopexy with or without resection

Inevitably, the instrument manufacturers, entrepreneureal surgeons and the public, driven by the media, have explored the role of laparoscopic techniques for the treatment of rectal prolapse (Vassilakis et al, 1997). In fact, laparoscopic surgery may have a role in the selective management of rectal prolapse (Figure 23.15). We have certainly used it for patients wishing to avoid a wound, where a wound is contraindicated on psychiatric grounds (self-mutilation syndromes) and where perineal rectosigmoidectomy is unsuitable.

The problem is whether in performing a laparoscopic procedure, therapy is compromised. Laparoscopic rectopexy is not difficult, but can the rectum be pulled up sufficiently well to achieve appropriate fixation and is the fixation good enough? Although laparoscopic rectopexy takes longer to perform than open rectopexy (Solomon and Eyers, 1996), the time difference is not great and the hospital stay is reduced (Table 23.25). However, the operating time for laparoscopic resection rectopexy (Baker et al, 1995) is at least twice as long as

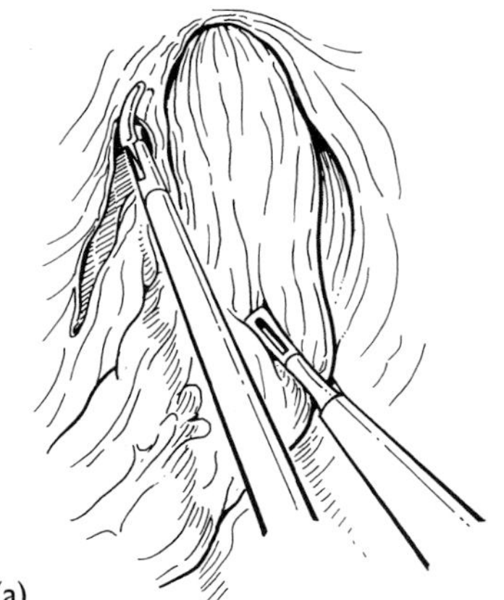
(a)

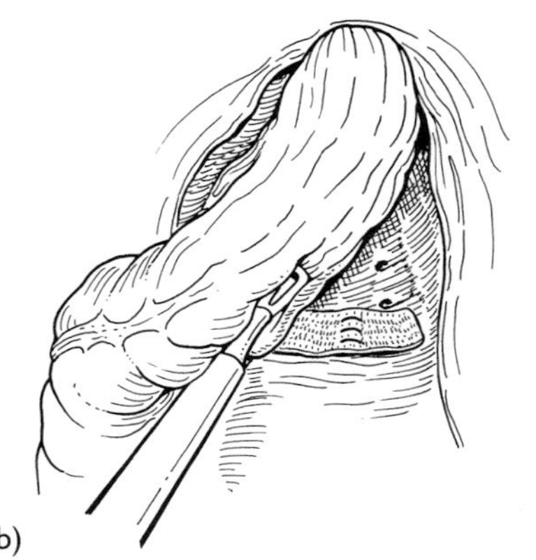
(b)

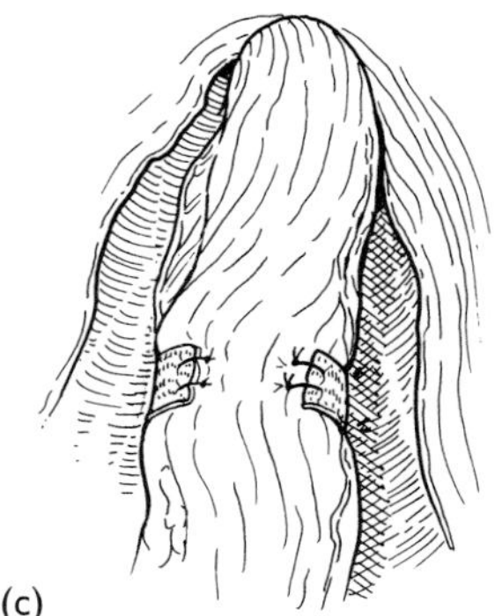
(c)

Figure 23.15 Laparoscopic rectopexy. The rectum is mobilized using scissors and diathermy. The entire retrorectal plane is developed. The rectum is pulled upwards with Babcock forceps. Mesh is then stapled to the presacral fascia and the divided lateral ligaments are attached to the sides of the mesh.

that of open resection rectopexy and although hospital stay is reduced, the cost benefit for laparoscopic resection rectopexy is likely to be minimal (Table 23.26). Thus, will surgeons be driven to performing an operation such as rectopexy alone which gives inferior results to resection rectopexy, just in the quest of avoiding a scar?

Table 23.25 Rectopexy alone (Marlex mesh).

	Laparoscopic (*n* = 21)	*Abdominal* *(historical)* (*n* = 21)
Operating time (min)	198 (90–280)	130 (90–185)
Postoperative solids by mouth (days)	2.7 (1–5)	5.8 (4–8)
Postoperative hospital stay (days)	6.3 (4–12)	11.0 (6–42)
30-day mortality	0	1
30-day morbidity	4	6
Haematoma	3	–
Pseudomembranous colitis	1	–
Deep venous thrombosis	–	1
Dehiscence	–	1
Ileus	–	3
Chest infection	–	1
Early recurrence	0 (very short follow-up)	0

From Solomon and Eyers (1996).

Table 23.26 Resection rectopexy.

	Laparoscopic (*n* = 8)	*Abdominal* (*n* = 10)
Blood loss (estimated)	184 ± 31	285 ± 35
Operation time (min)	177 ± 23	86 ± 8
Hospital stay (hours)	95 ± 16.7	183 ± 8.9
Time to passage of flatus	2.8 ± 1.9	3.9 ± 1.1
Oral intake	2.8 ± 1.9	4.5 ± 0.7
Recurrences	not stated	not stated

From Baker et al (1995).

It is far too early to know about recurrence rates. There are some series which suggest that none have been identified so far (Baker et al, 1995; Stitz and Lumley, 1996) but Monson (1996) reported two recurrences from the 68 laparoscopic rectopexy procedures undertaken in Hull. Hainsworth and Bartolo (1996) showed little difference between laparoscopic and open rectopexy other than that the laparoscopic operation took twice as long and that constipation was more common after the laparoscopic procedure. Thus, it is likely that laparoscopic rectopexy may have a role, provided it is safe, provided recurrence rates do not prove to be higher and provided a resection is not indicated. However, a randomized controlled trial must be performed before it is introduced as accepted practice into colorectal surgery.

Management of recurrent rectal prolapse

Specialist centres at least and other units will inevitably be faced with patients referred who have had previous failed procedures. In the past, many recurrences were due to inadequate control by encircling wire or silicone tubes. Now we are beginning to see more cases after the Délorme's procedure or rectosigmoidectomy (Fengler et al, 1997; Hool et al, 1997). We have certainly encountered recurrences after Ivalon sponge rectopexy, either because the sponge is still attached to the rectum but has worked loose from the sacrum or because the mesh has parted company with the bowel (Table 23.27).

Repeated abdominal procedures are demanding, so there is much to be said for re-doing the Délorme's operation if it has failed or even for using it if a perineal rectosigmoidectomy has failed, especially in elderly debilitated patients (Tobin and Scott, 1994; Senapati et al, 1994).

Table 23.27 Recurrent rectal prolapse.

	Original operation			*Final operation (some patients more than one)*		
	Hool et al (1997)	*Fengler et al (1997)*	*Own series*	*Hool et al (1997)*	*Fengler et al (1997)*	*Own series*
Anal encircling	3	2	26	2	1	–
Délorme's procedure	1	1	7	–	1	–
Perineal rectosigmoidectomy	5	10	3	2	7	2
Rectopexy	12	–	13*	19	3	8
Resection rectopexy	2	–	–	3	2	37
Anterior resection	1	1	2	3	–	3
Total	23	14	50	29	14	50

*Two laparoscopic.

However, in younger patients, especially those in whom rectopexy has failed because of continued straining, will inevitably require another repeated pelvic dissection. Under these circumstances, time must be set aside for what is often a demanding operation. The ureters will have to have been carefully identified. Great care is needed not to damage the presacral veins and iatrogenic damage to the rectum will need to be excluded by on-table air insufflation if the rectum is to be retained. Usually we perform a repeat rectopexy with a sigmoidectomy or a left hemicolectomy in these cases. Occasionally, it is wiser to resect the rectum and sigmoid, performing a low colorectal or even sometimes a coloanal anastomosis. In such cases a covering stoma is often advised.

Physiological changes after operation

When we undertook a detailed physiological study in patients with rectal prolapse we found that resting pressures, squeeze pressures, compliance, saline continence and the anorectal angle were all significantly impaired compared with controls. However, studies before and after rectopexy (Table 23.25) indicated that none of these abnormalities was corrected by a Marlex rectopexy (Yoshioka et al, 1989b). By contrast, Broden et al (1988a) and Farouk et al (1992) recorded an improvement in resting pressures after rectopexy, particularly the abnormal rectoanal pressure gradient (Farouk et al, 1994), as did Sainio et al (1991a) and Holmstrom et al (1986a). There is now substantial evidence that rectal evacuation and colonic transit may become impaired after rectopexy alone (Broden et al, 1988b; Sayfan et al, 1990; Scaglia et al, 1994).

We and others found that low resting pressures, excessive perineal descent and a short anal canal identified a group in whom incontinence was likely to persist after rectopexy (Agachan et al, 1997). Sainio et al (1991a) found that anal pressures were of no predictive value and that surgical treatment need not be modified in patients with low resting pressures. Conversely, JG Williams et al (1991) showed that resting pressures below 50 mmHg were associated with persistent incontinence and suggested that these patients should be considered for a synchronous pelvic floor repair.

Rational choice of surgical therapy

We believe that the optimum surgical procedure for rectal prolapse must now take account of the age, sex and general health of the patient as well as any coexisting functional bowel disorder which is present or may develop after operation (Madden et al, 1992). In elderly patients unfit to withstand a major abdominal procedure, we believe that pouch rectosigmoidectomy with pelvic floor repair and rectopexy carried out via the perineum or the Délorme's procedure might be the most appropriate surgical treatment. Results of these options are superior to any encircling procedure around the anus. Of these options, we now prefer pouch perineal rectosigmoidectomy with pelvic floor repair for poor risk patients but we do accept that the Délorme's operation has a place for treatment of this group.

In patients who are not constipated and are fit enough to withstand a laparotomy, we still believe that a posterior sutured resection (sigmoidectomy) rectopexy is the optimum treatment for control of the prolapse and avoidance of iatrogenic constipation. In young patients with severe constipation and demonstrable colonic inertia, subtotal colectomy might, in certain circumstances, be combined with rectopexy; however, if rectal emptying is impaired, the prognosis is likely to be poor. Most patients with incontinence will improve by resection rectopexy alone but a few with low resting anal pressures, a very obtuse anorectal angle and marked perineal descent deserve combined resection rectopexy and pelvic floor repair.

REFERENCES

Abou-Enein A (1978) Prolapse of the rectum in young men: treatment with a modified Roscoe Graham operation. *Dis Colon Rectum* **22**: 117–119.

Abulafi AM, Sherman IW, Fiddian RV & Rothwell-Jackson RL (1990) Délorme's operation for rectal prolapse. *Ann R Coll Surg Engl* **72**: 382–385.

Agachan F. Nogueras JJ & Wexner SD (1996) The comparison of three perineal procedures for the treatment of rectal prolapse (RP). *Int J Colorect Dis* **11**: 138.

Agachan F, Pfeifer J, Reissman P, Weiss EG, Nogueras JJ & Wexner SD (1997) Anorectal physiology in the rectal prolapse patient. *Techniques Coloproctol* **5**: 1–5.

Ahlbaack S, Broden B, Broden G, Ewerth S & Holmstrom B (1979) Rectal anatomy following Ripstein's operation for prolapse studied by cineradiography. *Dis Colon Rectum* **22**: 333–339.

Allen-Mersh TG, Henry MM & Nicholls RJ (1989) Natural history of anterior mucosal prolapse. *Br J Surg* **74**: 679–682.

Altemeier WA (1972) One stage perineal surgery for complete rectal prolapse. *Hosp Pract* **7**: 102–108.

Altemeier WA, Ginsefi J & Hoxworth P (1952) Treatment of extensive prolapse of the rectum in aged or debilitated patients. *Arch Surg* **65**: 72–80.

Altemeier WA, Culbertson WR, Schowengerdt C & Hunt J (1971) Nineteen years' experience with the one-stage perineal repair of rectal prolapse. *Ann Surg* **6**: 993–1001.

Ananthakrishnan N, Parkash S & Sridher K (1988) Retroperitoneal colopexy for adult procidentia, a new procedure. *Dis Colon Rectum* **31**: 104–106.

Anderson JR, Kinninmonth AWG & Smith AR (1981) Polyvinyl alcohol sponge rectopexy for complete rectal prolapse. *J R Coll Surg Engl* **26**: 292–294.

Anderson JR, Wilson BG & Parks TG (1984) Complete rectal prolapse: the results of Ivalon sponge rectopexy. *Postgrad Med J* **60**: 411–414.

Andrews NJ & Jones DJ (1992) Rectal prolapse and associated conditions. *BMJ* **305**: 243–245.

Araat M & Pircher W (1988) Absorbable mesh in the treatment of rectal prolapse. *Int J Colorectal Dis* **3**: 141–143.

Arakawa K (1979) Procidentia of the rectum in Japan. *J Jpn Soc Coloproctol* 224–229.

Ashcroft KW, Amoury RA & Holder TM (1977) Levator repair and posterior suspension for rectal prolapse. *J Paediatr Surg* **12**: 241–245.

Athanasiadis S, Weyand G, Heiligers J, Heumuller L & Bathelmes L (1996) The risk of infection of three synthetic materials used in rectopexy with or without colonic resection for rectal prolapse. *Int J Colorect Dis* **11**: 42–44.

Atkinson KG & Taylor DC (1984) Wells procedure for complete rectal prolapse: a ten year experience. *Dis Colon Rectum* **27**: 96–98.

Atri SP (1980) The treatment of complete rectal prolapse by graciloplasty. *Br J Surg* **67**: 431–432.

Baker R, Senagore AJ & Luchtefeld MA (1995) Laparoscopic-assisted vs. open resection; rectopexy offers excellent results. *Dis Colon Rectum* **38**: 199–201.

Baker WNW (1970) Results of using monofilament nylon in Thiersch's operation for rectal prolapse. *Br J Surg* **57**: 37–39.

Barham K & Collopy BT (1993) Post hysterectomy rectal and vaginal prolapse, a commonly overlooked problem. *Aust NZ J Obstet Gynaecol* **33**: 300.

Bates T (1972) Rectal prolapse after anorectal dilatation in the elderly. *BMJ* **2**: 505.

Berman IR, Harris MS & Leggett JT (1987) Rectal reservoir reduction procedures for internal rectal prolapse. *Dis Colon Rectum* **30**: 765–771.

Bhandari B & Ameta DK (1977) Etiology of prolapse rectum in children with special reference to amoebiasis. *Indian J Paediatr* **14**: 635–637.

Blatchford GJ, Perry RE, Thorson AG & Christensen MA (1989) Rectopexy without resection for rectal prolapse. *Am J Surg* **158**: 574–576.

Boulos PB, Stryker SJ & Nicholls RJ (1984) The long term results of polyvinyl alcohol (Ivalon) sponge for rectal prolapse in young patients. *Br J Surg* **71**: 213–214.

Briel JW, Schouten WR & Boerma MP (1997) Long-term results of suture rectopexy in patients with fecal incontinence associated with incomplete rectal prolapse. *Dis Colon Rectum* **40**: 1228–1232.

Broden B & Snellman B (1968) Procidentia of the rectum studied with cineradiography: a contribution to the discussion of consecutive mechanism. *Dis Colon Rectum* **11**: 330–347.

Broden G, Dolk A & Holmstrom B (1988a) Recovery of the internal anal sphincter following rectopexy: a possible explanation for continence improvement. *Int J Colorectal Dis* **3**: 23–28.

Broden G, Dolk A & Holmstrom B (1988b) Evacuation difficulties and other characteristics of rectal function associated with procidentia and the Ripstein operation. *Dis Colon Rectum* **31**: 283–286.

Carter AE (1983) Rectosacral suture fixation for complete rectal prolapse in the elderly, the frail and the demented. *Br J Surg* **70**: 522–523.

Chaloner EJ, Duckett J & Lewin J (1996) Paediatric rectal prolapse in Rwanda. *J R Soc Med* **90**: 688–689.

Chino ES & Thomas CG Jr (1984) Transsacral approach to repair of rectal prolapse in children. *Am Surg* **50**: 70–75.

Christiansen J & Kirkegaard P (1981) Délorme's operation for complete rectal prolapse. *Br J Surg* **68**: 537–538.

Corman ML (1985) Rectal prolapse in children. *Dis Colon Rectum* **28**: 535–539.

Datta BN & Das AK (1977) Treatment of prolapsed rectum in children with injections of sclerosing agents. *J Indian Med Assoc* **69**: 275–276.

Deen KI, Grant E, Billingham C & Keighley MRB (1994) Abdominal resection rectopexy with pelvic floor repair versus perineal rectosigmoidectomy and pelvic floor repair for full-thickness rectal prolapse. *Br J Surg* **81**: 302–304.

Devadhar DSC (1965) A new concept of mechanism and treatment of rectal procidentia. *Dis Colon Rectum* **8**: 75–81.

Duthie GS & Bartolo DCC (1992) Abdominal rectopexy for rectal prolapse: a comparison of techniques. *Br J Surg* **79**: 107–113.

Earnshaw TJ & Hopkinson BR (1987) Late results of silicone rubber perianal suture for rectal prolapse. *Dis Colon Rectum* **30**: 86–88.

Efron G (1977) A simple method of posterior rectopexy for rectal procidentia. *Surg Gynecol Obstet* **145**: 75–76.

Eisenstat TE, Rubin RJ & Salvati EP (1979) Surgical treatment of complete rectal prolapse. *Dis Colon Rectum* **22**: 522–523.

Ejaife JA & Elias EG (1977) Délorme's repair for rectal prolapse. *Surg Gynecol Obstet* **144**: 757–758.

El-Sibai O, Badawi M & Abbas MA (1997) Puborectoplasty in the treatment of complete rectal prolapse. *Dig Surg* **14**: 34–38.

Ellis H (1966) The polyvinyl sponge wrap operation for rectal prolapse. *Br J Surg* **53**: 675–676.

Farouk R, Duthie GS, Bartolo DCC & MacGregor AB (1992) Restoration of continence following rectopexy for rectal prolapse and recovery of the internal and sphincter electromyogram. *Br J Surg* **79**: 439–440.

Farouk R, Duthie GS, MacGregor AB & Bartolo DCC (1994) Rectoanal inhibition and incontinence in patients with rectal prolapse. *Br J Surg* **81**: 743–746.

Fengler SA, Pearl RK, Prasad ML et al (1997) Management of recurrent rectal prolapse. *Dis Colon Rectum* **40**: 832–834.

Finlay IG & Aitchison M (1991) Perineal excision of the rectum for prolapse in the elderly. *Br J Surg* **78**: 687–689.

Friedman R, Muggia-Sulum M & Freund HR (1983) Experience with the one stage perineal repair of rectal prolapse. *Dis Colon Rectum* **26**: 789–791.

Frykman HM & Goldberg SM (1969) The surgical treatment of rectal procidentia. *Surg Gynecol Obstet* **129**: 1225–1230.

Goligher JC (1984) In *Surgery of the Anus, Rectum and Colon*, 5th edn, pp 267–279. London: Baillière Tindall.

Gopal KA, Amshel AL, Shonberg IL & Eftaiha M (1984) Rectal prolapse in elderly and debilitated patients: experience with the Altemeier procedure. *Dis Colon Rectum* **27**: 376–381.

Gordon PH & Hoexter B (1978) Complications of the Ripstein procedure. *Dis Colon Rectum* **21**: 277–280.

Graham RR (1942) The operative repair of massive rectal prolapse. *Ann Surg* **115**: 1007–1012.

Graham W, Clegg JF & Taylor V (1984) Complete rectal prolapse repair by a simple technique. *Ann R Coll Surg Engl* **66**: 87–89.

Greene FL (1983) Repair of rectal prolapse using a puborectal sling procedure. *Arch Surg* **118**: 398–401.
Groff DB & Nagaraj HS (1990) Rectal prolapse in infants and children. *Am J Surg* **160**: 531–532.
Gundersen AL, Cogbill TH & Landercasper J (1985) Reappraisal of Délorme's procedure for rectal prolapse. *Dis Colon Rectum* **28**: 721–724.
Hagihara PF & Griffen WO (1975) Transsacral repair of rectal prolapse. *Arch Surg* **110**: 343–344.
Hainsworth PJ & Bartolo DCC (1996) Outcome after laparoscopic and open resection rectopexy. *Int J Colorectal Dis* **11**: 155.
Hamalainen K-PJ, Raivio P, Antila S, Palmu A & Mecklin J-P (1996) Biofeedback therapy in rectal prolapse patients. *Dis Colon Rectum* **39**: 262–265.
Hancock BD (1976) Measurement of anal pressure and motility. *Gut* **17**: 645–651.
Heald CL (1926) A simple bloodless operation for anorectal prolapse in children. *Surg Gynecol Obstet* **42**: 840–841.
Henry MM, Parks AG & Swash M (1982) The pelvic floor musculature in the descending perineum syndrome. *Br J Surg* **69**: 470–472.
Hight DW, Hertzler JH, Philippart AI & Benson CD (1982) Linear cauterisation for the treatment of rectal prolapse in infants and children. *Surg Gynecol Obstet* **154**: 400–402.
Hilsabeck JR (1981) Transabdominal posterior proctopexy using an inverted T of synthetic material. *Arch Surg* **116**: 41–44.
Hiltunen KM & Matikainen M (1992) Improvement of continence after abdominal rectopexy for rectal prolapse. *Int J Colorectal Dis* **7**: 8–10.
Hiltunen KM, Matikainen M, Auvinen O & Hietanen P (1986) Clinical and manometric evaluation of anal sphincter function in patients with rectal prolapse. *Am J Surg* **151**: 489–492.
Hoffman MJ, Kodner JJ & Fry RD (1984) Internal intussusception of the rectum: diagnosis and surgical management. *Dis Colon Rectum* **27**: 435–441.
Holmstrom B, Broden G, Dolk A & Frenckner B (1986a) Increased anal resting pressure following the Ripstein operation: a contribution to continence? *Dis Colon Rectum* **29**: 485–487.
Holmstrom B, Broden G & Dolk A (1986b) Results of the Ripstein operation in the treatment of rectal prolapse and internal rectal procidentia. *Dis Colon Rectum* **29**: 845–848.
Hool GR, Hull TL & Fazio VW (1997) Surgical treatment of recurrent complete rectal prolapse. *Dis Colon Rectum* **40**: 270–272.
Hopkinson BR & Hardman J (1973) Silicone rubber perianal suture for rectal prolapse. *Proc R Soc Med* **66**: 1095–1098.
Hopkinson BR & Lightwood R (1966) Electrical treatment of anal incontinence. *Lancet* **i**: 297–298.
Houry S, Lechaux JP, Huguier M & Molkhou JM (1987) Treatment of rectal prolapse by Délorme operation. *Int J Colorectal Dis* **2**: 149–152.
Huber FT, Stein H & Siewert JR (1995) Functional results after treatment of rectal prolapse with rectopexy and sigmoid resection. *World J Surg* **19**: 138–143.
Hudson CN (1988) Female genital prolapse and pelvic floor deficiency. *Int J Colorectal Dis* **3**: 181–185.
Hughes ESR & Gleadell LW (1962) Abdominoperineal repair of complete prolapse of the rectum. *Proc R Soc Med* **55**: 1077–1080.
Hunt TM, Fraser IA & Maybury I (1985) Treatment of rectal prolapse by sphincteric support using silastic rods. *Br J Surg* **72**: 491–492.
Ihre T (1972) Internal procidentia of the rectum: treatment and results. *Scand J Gastroenterol* **7**: 643–646.
Ihre T & Seligson U (1975) Intussusception of the rectum – internal procidentia. Treatment and results in 90 patients. *Scand J Gastroenterol* **18**: 391–396.
Jackman FR, Francis JN & Hopkinson BR (1980) Silicone rubber band treatment of rectal prolapse. *Ann R Coll Surg Engl* **62**: 385–387.
Johansen OB, Wesner SD, Daniel N, Nogueras JJ & Jagelman DG (1993) Perineal rectosigmoidectomy in the elderly. *Dis Colon Rectum* **36**: 767–772.
Jurgeleit HC, Corman ML, Coller JA & Veidenheimer MC (1975) Procidentia of the rectum: Teflon sling repair of rectal prolapse. Lahey Clinic experience. *Dis Colon Rectum* **18**: 464–467.
Kay NR & Zachary RB (1970) The treatment of rectal prolapse in children with injections of 30 per cent saline solutions. *J Paediatr Surg* **5**: 334–337.
Keighley MRB & Fielding JWL (1983) Management of faecal incontinence and results of surgical treatment. *Br J Surg* **70**: 463–468.
Keighley MRB & Shouler PJ (1984) Abnormalities of colonic function in patients with rectal prolapse and faecal incontinence. *Br J Surg* **71**: 892–895.
Keighley MRB, Makuria T, Alexander-Williams J & Arabi Y (1980) Clinical and manometric evaluation of rectal prolapse and incontinence. *Br J Surg* **67**: 54–56.
Keighley MRB, Fielding JWL & Alexander-Williams J (1983) Results of Marlex mesh abdominal rectopexy for rectal prolapse in 100 consecutive patients. *Br J Surg* **70**: 229–232.
Khanduja KS, Hardy TG, Aguilav PS et al (1988) A new silicone prosthesis in the modified Thiersch operation. *Dis Colon Rectum* **31**: 380–383.
Kiff ES, Barnes PRH & Swash M (1984) Evidence of pudendal neuropathy in patients with perineal descent and chronic straining at stool. *Gut* **25**: 1279–1282.
Kirkman NF (1975) Procidentia of the rectum. Results of abdominal rectopexy in the elderly. *Dis Colon Rectum* **18**: 470–472.
Kim D-S, Wong WD, Lowry AC, Goldberg SM & Madoff RD (1996) Complete rectal prolapse – evolution of management and results. *Int J Colorectal Dis* **11**: 136.
Klaaborg KE, Qvist N & Kongburg O (1985) Rectal prolapse and anal incontinence treated with a modified Roscoe Graham operation. *Dis Colon Rectum* **28**: 582–584.
Kuijpers HC (1992) Treatment of complete rectal prolapse: to narrow, to wrap, to suspend, to fix, to encircle, to plicate or to resect? *World J Surg* **16**: 826–830.
Kuijpers JHC & Morree H de (1988) Towards a selection of the most appropriate procedure in the treatment of complete rectal prolapse. *Dis Colon Rectum* **31**: 355–357.
Kulczycki LL & Shwachman H (1958) Studies in cystic fibrosis of the pancreas: occurrence of rectal prolapse. *N Engl J Med* **259**: 409–412.
Kupfer CA & Goligher JC (1970) One hundred consecutive cases of complete rectal prolapse of the rectum treated by operation. *Br J Surg* **57**: 481–487.
Ladha A, Lee P & Berger P (1985) Use of Angelchik anti-reflux prosthesis for repair of total rectal prolapse in elderly patients. *Dis Colon Rectum* **28**: 5–7.
Lake SP, Hancock BD & Lewis AAM (1984) Management of pelvic sepsis after Ivalon rectopexy. *Dis Colon Rectum* **27**: 589–590.
Launer DP, Fazio VW, Weakley FL, Turnbull RB, Jagelman DG & Lavery IC (1982) The Ripstein procedure: a 16 year experience. *Dis Colon Rectum* **25**: 41–45.
Lechaux JP, Lechaux D & Perez M (1995) Results of Délorme's procedure for rectal prolapse. *Dis Colon Rectum* **38**: 301–307.

Leighton JA, Valdovinos MA, Pemberton JH, Rath DM & Camilleri M (1993) Anorectal dysfunction and rectal prolapse in progressive systemic sclerosis. *Dis Colon Rectum* **36**: 182–185.

Lescher TJ, Corman ML, Coller J & Veidenheimer MC (1979) Management of late complications of Teflon sling repair for rectal prolapse. *Dis Colon Rectum* **23**: 445–467.

Loygue J, Huguier M, Malafosse M & Biotois H (1971) Complete prolapse of the rectum. A report on 140 cases treated by rectopexy. *Br J Surg* **58**: 847–848.

Loygue J, Nordlinger B, Malafosse M, Huguet C & Parc R (1984) Rectopexy to the promontory for the treatment of rectal prolapse: report of 257 cases. *Dis Colon Rectum* **27**: 356–359.

Lucarotti ME, Armstrong CP & Bartolo DCC (1991) Control of presacral bleeding in rectal surgery. *Ann R Coll Surg Engl* **73**: 289–290.

Luukkonen P, Mikkonen V & Jarvinen H (1992) Abdominal rectopexy with sigmoidectomy vs. rectopexy alone for rectal prolapse: A prospective, randomized study. *Int J Colorectal Dis* **7**: 219–222.

McCue JL & Thomson JPS (1991) Clinical and functional results of abdominal rectopexy for complete rectal prolapse. *Br J Surg* **78**: 921–923.

Madden MV, Kamm MA & Santhanam AN (1992) Abdominal rectopexy for complete prolapse: prospective study evaluating changes in symptoms and anorectal function. *Dis Colon Rectum* **35**: 48–55.

Malik M, Stratton J & Sweeney, W Brian (1997) Rectal prolapse associated with bulimia nervosa. *Dis Colon Rectum* **40**: 1382–1385.

Malyshev YI & Gulin VA (1973) Our experience with the treatment of rectal prolapse in infants and children. *Surg Gynecol Obstet* **24**: 470–472.

Mann CV & Hoffman C (1988) Complete rectal prolapse: the anatomical and functional results of treatment by an extended abdominal rectopexy. *Br J Surg* **75**: 34–37.

Mellgren A, Schultz I, Johansson C & Dolk A (1997) Internal rectal intussusception seldom develops into total rectal prolapse. *Dis Colon Rectum* **40**: 817–820.

Metcalf AM & Loening-Baucke V (1988) Anorectal function and defaecation dynamics in patients with rectal prolapse. *Am J Surg* **155**: 206–210.

Monson J (1996) Management of rectal prolapse. Paper presented at the American, British and Australian Associations of Colorectal Surgery Tripartite Meeting, London.

Monson JRT, Jones NAG, Vowden P & Brennan TG (1986) Délorme's operation: the first choice in complete rectal prolapse? *Ann R Coll Surg Engl* **68**: 143–145.

Morgan B (1980) The Teflon sling operation (Ripstein) for repair of complete rectal prolapse. *Aust N Z J Surg* **50**: 121–123.

Mortensen NJ McC, Vellacott KD & Wilson MG (1984) Lahaut's operation for rectal prolapse. *Ann R Coll Surg Engl* **66**: 17–18.

Moscowitz AV (1912) The pathogenesis and anatomy and care of prolapse of the rectum. *Surg Gynecol Obstet* **15**: 7–21.

Muir EG (1962) The surgical treatment of rectal prolapse in the adult. *Proc R Soc Med* **55**: 105–109.

Muto T, Konishi F, Kamiya J, Sawada T, Sugihara K & Morioka Y (1984) Gant-Miwa technique (mucosal plication of prolapsed rectum) with Thiersch operation in the treatment of rectal prolapse. *Coloproctology* **6**: 310–314.

Narasanagi SS (1973) Rectal prolapse in children. *J Indian Med Assoc* **62**: 378–380.

Nash DF (1972) Bowel management in spina bifida patients. *Proc R Soc Med* **65**: 70–71.

Naughton Morgan C, Porter NH & Kugman DJ (1972) Ivalon (polyvinyl alcohol) sponge in the repair of complete rectal prolapse. *Br J Surg* **59**: 846–848.

Nay HR & Blair CR (1972) Perineal surgical repair of rectal prolapse. *Am J Surg* **123**: 577–579.

Neill ME, Parks AG & Swash M (1981) Physiological studies of the anal sphincter musculature in faecal incontinence and rectal prolapse. *Br J Surg* **68**: 531–536.

Nichols DH (1982) Retrorectal levatorplasty for anal and perineal prolapse. *Surg Gynecol Obstet* **154**: 251–254.

Notarus MJ (1979) A technique of abdominal repair for rectal prolapse. *Proctology* **1**: 35–37.

Novell JR, Osborne MJ, Winslet MC & Lewis AAM (1994) Prospective randomized trial of Ivalon sponge versus sutured rectopexy for full-thickness rectal prolapse. *Br J Surg* **81**: 904–906.

Nwako F (1975) Rectal prolapse in Nigerian children. *Int Surg* **60**: 284–285.

Oliver GC, Vachon D, Eisenstat TE, Rubin RJ & Salvati EP (1994) Délorme's procedure for complete rectal prolapse in severely debilitated patients. *Dis Colon Rectum* **37**: 461–467.

Pantanowitz D & Levine E (1975) The mechanism of rectal prolapse. *S Afr J Surg* **13**: 53–56.

Parks AG (1975) Anorectal incontinence. *Proc R Soc Med* **68**: 681–690.

Parks AG, Porter NH & Hardcastle J (1966) The syndrome of the descending perineum. *Proc R Soc Med* **59**: 477–479.

Parks AG, Swash M & Urich H (1977) Sphincter denervation in anorectal incontinence and rectal prolapse. *Gut* **18**: 656–659.

Penfold JCB & Hawley PR (1972) Experiences of Ivalon-sponge implant for complete rectal prolapse at St Mark's Hospital, 1960–1970. *Br J Surg* **59**: 846–848.

Penninckx F, Kerremans R & Beckers J (1978) Evaluation manometrique et myographique de la continence anale en cas de prolapsus rectal. *Ann Gastroenterol Hepatol* **14**: 305–311.

Plusa SM, Charig JA, Balaji V, Watts A & Thompson MR (1995) Physiological changes after Délorme's procedure for full-thickness rectal prolapse. *Br J Surg* **82**: 1475–1478.

Porter NH (1962) Collective results of operation for rectal prolapse. *Proc R Soc Med* **55**: 1087–1091.

Prasad ML, Pearl RK, Abcarian H, Orsay C & Nelson R (1986) Perineal proctectomy, posterior rectopexy and postanal levator repair for the treatment of rectal prolapse. *Dis Colon Rectum* **29**: 541–552.

Preston DM & Lennard-Jones JE (1982) Does failure of bisacodyl induced colonic peristalsis indicate intrinsic nerve damage? *Gut* **23**: A891.

Preston DM, Lennard-Jones JE & Thomas BM (1984) The balloon proctogram. *Br J Surg* **71**: 29–32.

Ramanujam P & Venkatesh KS (1992) Management of acute incarcerated rectal prolapse. *Dis Colon Rectum* **35**: 1154–1156.

Ramanujam PS, Venkatesh KS & Fietz MJ (1994) Perineal excision of rectal procidentia in elderly high-risk patients. *Dis Colon Rectum* **37**: 1027–1030.

Read NW, Harford WV, Schmulen AC, Read MG, Santa Ana C & Fordtran JS (1979) A clinical study of patients with faecal incontinence and diarrhoea. *Gastroenterology* **76**: 747–756.

Ripstein CB (1965) Surgical care of massive rectal prolapse. *Dis Colon Rectum* **8**: 34–38.

Ripstein CB (1969) A simple effective operation for rectal prolapse. *Postgrad Med J* **45**: 201–204.

Ripstein CB (1972) Procidentia: definitive corrective surgery. *Dis Colon Rectum* **15**: 334–336.

Rogers J & Jeffery PJ (1987) Post anal repair and intersphincteric Ivalon sponge rectopexy for the treatment of rectal prolapse. *Br J Surg* **74**: 384–386.

Romero-Torres R (1979) Sacrofixation with Marlex mesh in

massive prolapse of the rectum. *Surg Gynecol Obstet* **149**: 709–711.
Ross AH & Thomson JPS (1989) Management of infection after prosthetic abdominal rectopexy (Wells' procedure). *Br J Surg* **76**: 610–612.
Rutter KRP & Riddell RH (1975) The solitary rectal ulcer syndrome of the rectum. *Clin Gastroenterol* **4**: 505–509.
Sainio AP, Voutilainen PE & Husa AI (1991a) Recovery of anal sphincter function following transabdominal repair of rectal prolapse: cause of improved continence? *Dis Colon Rectum* **34**: 816–821.
Sainio AP, Halme LE & Husa AI (1991b) Anal encirclement with polypropylene mesh for rectal prolapse and incontinence. *Dis Colon Rectum* **34**: 905–908.
Santulli TV (1983) Rectal prolapse in children. In Rudolph AM & Hoffman JI (eds) *Paediatrics*, 17th edn, pp 990–991. Norwalk, CT: Appleton-Century-Crofts.
Sayfan J, Pinho M, Alexander-Williams J & Keighley MRB (1990) Sutured posterior abdominal rectopexy with sigmoidectomy compared with Marlex rectopexy for rectal prolapse. *Br J Surg* **77**: 143–145.
Sayfan J, Koltun L & Orda R (1997) Constipation in rectal prolapse – the key to choosing the appropriate rectopexy. *Techniques Coloproctol* **5**: 38–41.
Scaglia M, Fasth S, Hallgren T, Nordgren S, Oresland T & Hulten L (1994) Abdominal rectopexy for rectal prolapse; influence of surgical technique on function outcome. *Dis Colon Rectum* **37**: 805–813.
Schlinkert RT, Beart RW, Wolf BG & Pemberton JH (1985) Anterior resection for complete rectal prolapse. *Dis Colon Rectum* **28**: 409–412.
Schultz I, Mellgren A, Dolk A, Johansson C & Holmstrom B (1996) Continence is improved after the Ripstein rectopexy; different mechanisms in rectal prolapse and rectal intussusception? *Dis Colon Rectum* **39**: 300–306.
Schwemmel K & Hunger J (1973) Der ano-rektale Prolaps. *Dtsch Med Wochenschr* **98**: 1125–1129.
Senapati A, Nicholls RJ, Thomson JPS & Phillips RKS (1994) Results of Délorme's procedure for rectal prolapse. *Dis Colon Rectum* **37**: 456–460.
Shorvon PJ, McHugh S, Diamant NE, Somers S & Stevenson GW (1989) Defecography in normal volunteers: results and implications. *Gut* **30**: 1737–1749.
Snellman B (1961) Pelvic floor repair for rectal prolapse. *Dis Colon Rectum* **4**: 199–202.
Snooks SJ, Nicholls RJ, Henry MM & Swash M (1985) Electrophysiological and manometric assessment of the pelvic floor in the solitary rectal ulcer syndrome. *Br J Surg* **72**: 131–133.
Soliman SM (1994) Triple suspension rectopexy for complete rectal prolapse. *Ann R Coll Surg Engl* **76**: 115–116.
Solomon MJ & Eyers AA (1996) Laparoscopic rectopexy using mesh fixation with a spiked chromium staple. *Dis Colon Rectum* **39**: 279–284.
Soriano LR, del Mundo F & Naguit-Sim L (1966) Rectal prolapse in children with trichariasis. *J Philippine Med Assoc* **42**: 843–848.
Speakman CTM, Madden MV, Nicholls RJ & Kamm MA (1991) Lateral ligament division during rectopexy causes constipation but prevents recurrence: results of a prospective randomized study. *Br J Surg* **78**: 1431–1433.
Spencer RJ (1984) Manometric studies in rectal prolapse. *Dis Colon Rectum* **27**: 523–525.
Stenchever MA (1984) Management of genital prolapse in the geriatric patient. *Ger Med Today* **3**: 75–78.
Stern RC, Izant RJ Jr, Boat TF, Wood RE, Mathews LW & Doershuk CF (1982) Treatment and prognosis of rectal prolapse in cystic fibrosis. *Gastroenterology* **82**: 707–710.
Stitz RW & Lumley JW (1996) Laparoscopic colorectal surgery for cancer 1996. *Int J Colorectal Dis* **107**: 139.
Stolfi VM, Milsom JW, Lavery IC, Oakley JR, Church JM & Fazio VW (1992) Newly designed occluder pin for presacral hemorrhage. *Dis Colon Rectum* **35**: 166–169.
Sun WM, Read NW, Carmel Donelly T, Bannister JJ & Shorthouse AJ (1989) A common pathophysiology for full thickness rectal prolapse and solitary rectal ulcer. *Br J Surg* **76**: 290–295.
Taynor LA & Michener WM (1966) Rectal procidentia – a rare complication of ulcerative colitis; report of 2 cases in children. *Cleveland Clin Q* **33**: 115–117.
Thauerkauf FJ, Beahrs OH & Hill JR (1970) Rectal prolapse: causation and surgical treatment. *Ann Surg* **171**: 819–835.
Thomas CG (1975) Procidentia of the rectum. Transsacral repair. *Dis Colon Rectum* **18**: 473–477.
Tjandra JJ, Fazio VW, Church JM, Milsom JW, Oakley JR & Lavery IC (1993) Ripstein procedure is an effective treatment for rectal prolapse without constipation. *Dis Colon Rectum* **36**: 501–507.
Tobin SA & Scott IHK (1994) Délorme operation for rectal prolapse. *Br J Surg* **81**: 1681–1684.
Tolwinski W, Dadan H, Zalewski B & Okulczyk B (1997) Surgical treatment of complete rectal prolapse by the Moore procedure – short and long term results. *Dig Surg* **14**: 409–412.
Uhlig BE & Sullivan ES (1979) The modified Délorme operation: its place in surgical treatment for massive rectal prolapse. *Dis Colon Rectum* **22**: 513–514.
van Tets WF & Kuijpers JHC (1995) Internal rectal intussusception – fact or fancy? *Dis Colon Rectum* **38**: 1080–1083.
Vassilakis JS, Chalkiadakis G, Zoras OJ & Xynos E (1997) Laparoscopically assisted excision rectopexy for rectal prolapse. *Techniques Coloproctol* **1**: 68–72.
Vongsangnak V, Varma JS, Watters D & Smith AN (1985a) Clinical, manometric and surgical aspects of complete prolapse of the rectum. *J R Coll Surg Edinb* **30**: 251–254.
Vongsangnak V, Varma JS & Smith AN (1985b) Reappraisal of Thiersch's operation for complete rectal prolapse. *J R Coll Surg Edinb* **30**: 185–187.
Watts JD, Rothenberger DA, Buls JG, Goldberg SM & Nivatvongs S (1985) The management of procidentia: 30 years experience. *Dis Colon Rectum* **28**: 96–102.
Wedell J, Neier P & Fiedler R (1980) A new concept for the management of rectal prolapse. *Am J Surg* **139**: 723–725.
Wedell J, Schlageter M, Meier zu Eissen P, Banzhaf G, Castrup W & Van Calker H (1987) Die Problematic der Pelvinen Sepsis nach Rectopexie mittels Kunstoff und ihre Behandlung. *Chirurg* **58**: 423–427.
Wells C (1959) New operation for rectal prolapse. *Proc R Soc Med* **52**: 602–604.
White CM, Findlay JM & Price JJ (1980) The occult rectal prolapse syndrome. *Br J Surg* **67**: 528–530.
Williams JG, Wong WD, Jensen L, Rothenberger DA & Goldberg SM (1991) Incontinence and rectal prolapse: a prospective manometric study. *Dis Colon Rectum* **34**: 209–216.
Williams JG, Rothenberger DA, Madoff RD & Goldberg SM (1992) Treatment of rectal prolapse in the elderly by perineal rectosigmoidectomy. *Dis Colon Rectum* **35**: 830–834.
Williams NS, Patel J, George BD, Hallam RI & Watkins ES (1991) Development of an electrically stimulated neoanal sphincter. *Lancet* **338**: 1166–1169.

Wise WE Jr, Padmanabhan A, Meesig DM, Arnold MW, Aguilar PS & Stewart WRC (1991) Abdominal colon and rectal operations in the elderly. *Dis Colon Rectum* **34**: 959–963.

Womack NR, Williams NS, Holmfield HJM & Morrison JFB (1987) Pressure and prolapse: the cause of solitary rectal ulcer. *Gut* **28**: 1228–1233.

Woods JH & DeCosse JJ (1976) A parasacral approach to rectal prolapse. *Arch Surg* **111**: 914–915.

Wyatt AP (1981) Perineal rectopexy for rectal prolapse. *Br J Surg* **68**: 717–719.

Yoshioka K, Hyland G & Keighley MRB (1989a) Anorectal function after abdominal rectopexy: parameters of predictive value in identifying return of continence. *Br J Surg* **76**: 64–68.

Yoshioka K, Heyen F & Keighley MRB (1989b) Functional results after posterior abdominal rectopexy for rectal prolapse. *Dis Colon Rectum* **32**: 835–838.

Yoshioka K, Ogunbiyi OA & Keighley MRB (1998) Pouch perineal rectosigmoidectomy gives better functional results than conventional rectosigmoidectomy in elderly patients with rectal prolapse. *Br J Surg* **85**: 1525–1526.

24

SOLITARY RECTAL ULCER SYNDROME

The solitary rectal ulcer syndrome describes a symptom complex consisting of rectal bleeding, mucous discharge, tenesmus, perineal or abdominal pain, a feeling of obstructed defecation, incomplete evacuation and some alteration in bowel habit (Martin et al, 1984). Close questioning reveals that almost all patients strain at stool and visit the lavatory up to 20 times a day because of a sense of wanting to open their bowels when frequently they pass nothing. They feel there is something in the rectum which needs to be passed and strain for several hours a day in an abortive attempt to defecate (Kang et al, 1995). Some of these patients have a complete rectal prolapse. Many more are now known to have an incomplete intussusception, perineal descent and impaired rectal evacuation on defecography. An ulcer may be present, usually on the anterior rectal wall 6–10 cm from the anal verge, but the absence of an ulcer does not exclude the diagnosis, since some patients merely have an erythematous area. Others have submucosal cysts with multiple ulcers or polypoidal lesions in the low rectum.

The mechanism of this obscure disorder is probably multifactorial; some patients cannot relax their puborectalis muscle during defecation, many develop an intussusception, the tip of which may become ischaemic (Lonsdale, 1993). Those patients who have an overactive external sphincter generate high intrarectal pressures, which may cause mucosal ulceration from venous congestion and damage.

Biopsy of the ulcerated or polypoidal area reveals a typical histological appearance of mucosal ulceration, epithelial hyperplasia, crypt distortion and a reversal in the sulphomucin:sialomucin ratio. In the lamina propria there is fibromuscular obliteration of vessels, inflammation and telangiectasia with profound submucosal fibrosis and a thickened muscularis mucosa (Tjandra et al, 1993).

Most forms of therapy are unsuccessful unless the patients can be taught not to strain.

AETIOLOGY

The aetiology of solitary rectal ulcer is unknown (Snooks et al, 1985; Johansson et al, 1992) but is almost certainly the result of a variety of factors, which are discussed below (Tjandra et al, 1992).

Anterior mucosal prolapse and pelvic floor disorder

Most patients with the solitary ulcer syndrome give a history of chronic straining, tenesmus and incomplete defecation (Tjandra et al, 1992). Some patients may spend more than 2 hours a day sitting on the lavatory on up to 20 occasions because of an urge to defecate, when in fact the rectum is empty (Nicholls and Simson, 1986). Rutter and Riddell (1975) have suggested that this sensation is due to an anterior mucosal prolapse which develops following many years of straining during defecation, a feature also commonly observed in the descending perineum syndrome (Parks et al, 1966). Indeed, because many patients with solitary rectal ulcer strain, they have marked perineal descent at rest and during attempted defecation (Pescatori et al, 1985; Kang et al, 1995). The anterior prolapse is felt by the patient as something in the rectum that needs to be passed. The patient consequently attempts to defecate by straining, which is both abortive and causes further prolapse of the rectal mucosa.

Descent of the anterior mucosal prolapse may also result in, or be associated with, reflex contraction of the pelvic floor, an inappropriate response since the pelvic floor should relax as part of normal defecation. Evidence for inappropriate pelvic floor contraction is based on electromyographic and videoproctographic studies (Halligan et al, 1995b). There are some patients who have electromyographic evidence of hyperactivity of the puborectalis both at rest and during straining (Rutter, 1974). One theory is that the inappropriate contraction of the puborectalis muscle results in trauma to the mucosal prolapse, thereby rendering its tip ischaemic (Figures 24.1–24.3) (Johansson et al, 1992; Siproudhis et al, 1992). Ischaemia results in fibromuscular obliteration of the lamina propria and the formation of an ulcer. Once the ulcer has developed, a vicious circle is established whereby the ulcer itself gives rise to a further desire to defecate. More

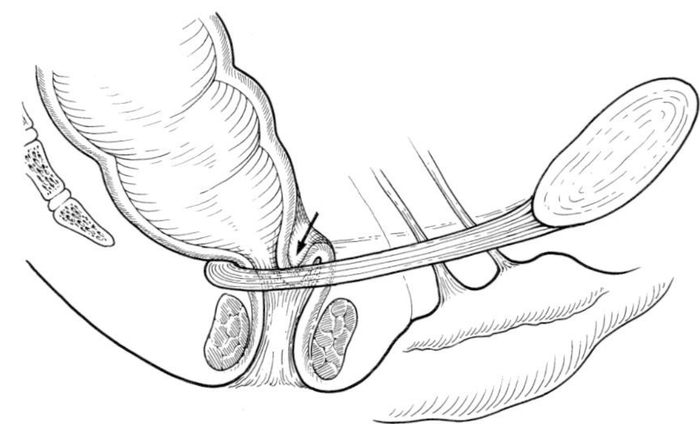

Figure 24.1 Mechanism of anterior prolapse and solitary rectal ulcer.

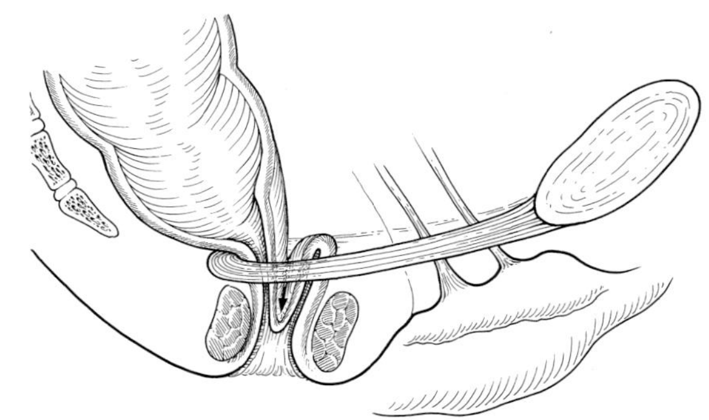

Figure 24.2 Mechanism of solitary rectal ulcer in incomplete intussusception.

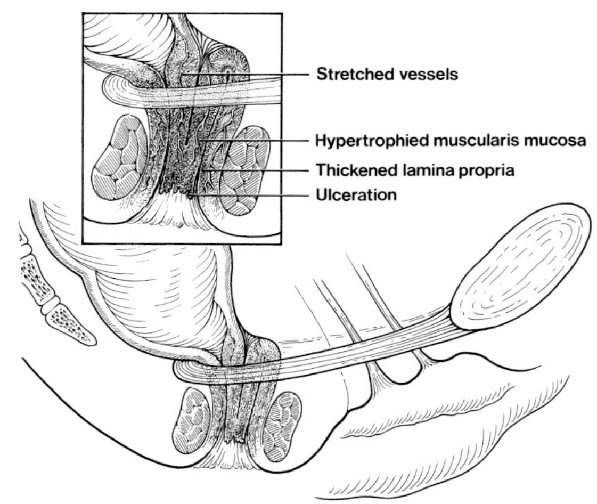

Figure 24.3 Mechanism of solitary rectal ulcer.

Table 24.1 Proctographic findings in solitary rectal ulcer.

Finding	*Number*
Kuijpers et al (1986) (n = 19)	
Internal intussusception and funnel anorectum	12
Spastic puborectalis with an acute anorectal angle	5
Anterior mucosal prolapse	1
Normal appearances	1
Womack et al (1987) (n = 18)	
Rectal invagination	15
2 Anterior wall prolapse	
8 Intra-anal intussusception	
5 Full thickness prolapse	
Unable to void	2
Rectocele	1

trauma is inflicted on the anterior aspect of the anorectum and the ulcer becomes self-perpetuating.

Videoproctographic appearances may, in some patients, demonstrate a persistently closed anorectal angle during defecation, despite perineal descent. However, this observation is relatively uncommon, being reported in only 5 of 19 patients in a study from Holland (Kuijpers et al, 1986) (Table 24.1) and in as few as 4 of 43 patients in a similar study from Belgium (Mahieu, 1986). The combination of an anterior mucosal prolapse and inappropriate activity of the puborectalis could explain the common finding of an ulcer situated at the anorectal junction 4–7 cm from the anal verge on the anterior aspect of the rectum. However, anterior mucosal prolapse is not the only abnormality seen on proctography and inappropriate puborectalis contraction is not confined to patients with the solitary rectal ulcer syndrome (Shouler and Keighley, 1986). At the Royal London, puborectalis dysfunction was a fairly infrequent finding in solitary rectal ulcer (Womack et al, 1987). Similarly, Snooks et al (1985) recorded increased electrical activity in the puborectalis during straining in only half of their patients. In Birmingham we were able to demonstrate abnormal contraction of the pelvic floor on attempted defecation in only 4 of 16 patients, despite the fact that an anterior mucosal prolapse was present in one-third of them (Keighley and Shouler, 1984a).

Overt prolapse or occult intussusception of the rectum

Some patients with solitary rectal ulcer have an overt rectal prolapse which can sometimes only be demonstrated by straining in the squatting position (White et al, 1980). It has been assumed that in the bulk of patients the ulcer develops as a result of trauma to the apex of the prolapse, either by the patient attempting to reduce the prolapse digitally or by contraction of the external canal sphincter when the prolapse emerges from the anus. The incidence of overt rectal prolapse ranges from 6% to 39% (Table 24.2) and depends on how assiduously the investigators have looked for it. An overt rectal prolapse may be the end-result of an occult intussusception but the natural history of incomplete intussusception is variable. Some authors report that repeat defecography frequently fails to demonstrate incomplete intussusception, whereas others suggest that they may progress to full-thickness prolapse (see Chapter 23).

As a result of videoproctography a substantial proportion of patients with solitary rectal ulcer have been shown to have an occult intussusception (Ihre, 1972; Lewis et al, 1977; Feczko et al, 1980) (Figure 24.4). At the Royal London Hospital, 94% of patients with solitary rectal ulcer were found to have either an intussusception on videoproctography or overt rectal prolapse. Kang et al (1995) from St Mark's reported on 52 patients: 24 had no intussusception or prolapse, 14 had intussusception alone and 14 had a full-thickness prolapse. Why patients with an occult intussusception develop a solitary rectal ulcer is not clear. Unlike patients with overt rectal prolapse, those with an occult intussusception usually have no electromyographic or histological evi-

Table 24.2 Age, site and associated prolapse in solitary rectal ulcer.

							Prolapse		
Authors	*Mean age (years)*	*Male*	*Ulcer*	*Single*	*Anterior*	*Polyp*	*Mucosal*	*Incomplete*	*Complete*
Madigan and Morson (1969)	32	48	100	71	38	0	*	*	16
Martin et al (1981)	31	35	57	67	33	25	18	39	34
Ford et al (1983)	34	42	67	47	67	10	12	7	25
Keighley and Shouler (1984a)	32	27	91	88	70	10	33	6	18
Stuart (1984)	34	40	100	*	*	0	*	17	55
Britto et al (1987)	51	70	100	80	40	0	*	*	*

Values are percentages.
* Not recorded.

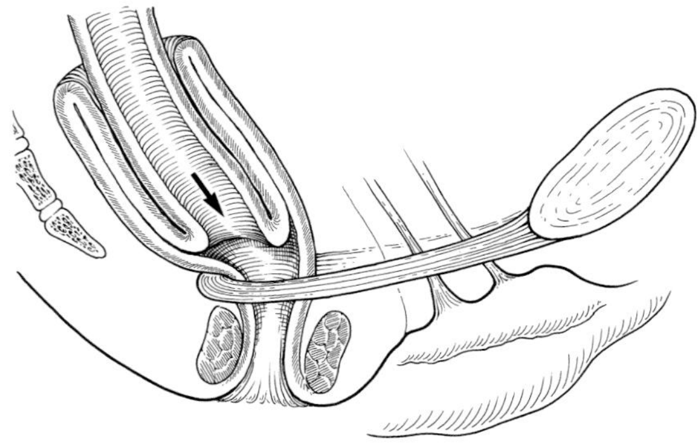

Figure 24.4 Incomplete intussusception in solitary ulcer.

dence of pelvic floor neuropathy, despite the presence of perineal descent. Anal resting pressures are higher than in patients with a complete prolapse but lower than the group with neither prolapse nor intussusception (Kang et al, 1995). In some patients, particularly those with an ulcer, there is electromyographic evidence of increased external anal sphincter activity during defecation resulting in high voiding pressures. This creates rectal hypertension adjacent to the intussuscepting rectum which could be responsible for the ulcer.

Alternatively, the presence of the intussusception initiates a desire to defecate but, as the rectum is empty and there is nothing to pass, there is a tendency to strain, often quite violently, resulting in the tip of the intussuscepted rectum becoming congested, ischaemic and subsequently ulcerated (see Figure 24.3). In effect, these patients try to pass their own rectum. This hypothesis could certainly explain the aetiology of ulcers situated higher in the rectum. It would also explain why a few patients without overt rectal prolapse respond to rectopexy (Schweiger and Alexander-Williams, 1977). Occult intussusception now appears to be the most common radiographic feature found during videoproctography in the solitary rectal ulcer syndrome (Womack et al, 1987). Kuijpers et al (1986) identified an intussusception in 12 of 19 patients (see Table 24.1). Mahieu (1986) observed an intussusception in 34 of 43 patients: 19 were external prolapses, 10 were intra-anal and 5 intrarectal. In Birmingham we found an intussusception in 14 of 21 patients with a solitary rectal ulcer who did not have a complete rectal prolapse. Using sigmoidoscopy, Martin et al (1981) identified an occult prolapse in only 14% of their patients (Figure 24.5).

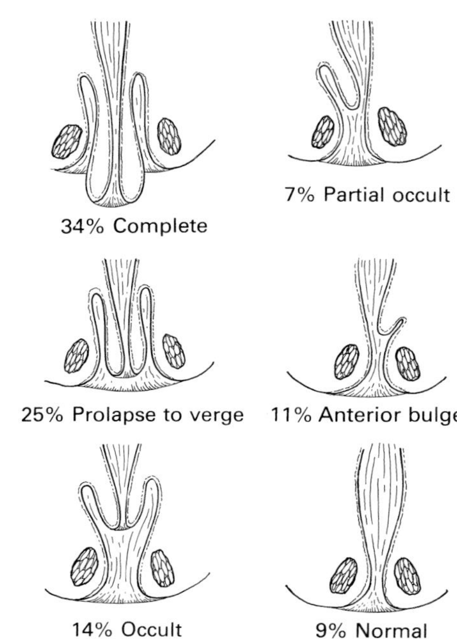

Figure 24.5 Underlying rectal abnormality in solitary rectal ulcers. From Martin et al (1981).

Other causes

There are other theories which have been proposed for the pathogenesis of solitary rectal ulcer syndrome. These may be mere speculation, and if they are responsible for the syndrome of the solitary ulcer they are relatively uncommon. It is important to distinguish causes of ulceration from causes of the syndrome. For instance, radiation or ergotamine suppositories may cause rectal ulcers but patients do not have the symptom complex associated with this disorder (Potel et al, 1985; Levine, 1987).

Ischaemia

Local ischaemia occurring at the apex of an intussusception or an anterior rectal prolapse may be important in the pathogenesis of solitary ulcer, as previously described (Devroede et al, 1973; Martin et al, 1981, Lonsdale, 1993; Kang et al, 1996). Devroede et al (1982) described 36 patients with rectal pain, bleeding and tenesmus in whom faecal incontinence was prominent. They claimed that the ulceration and fibrosis were due to a steal syndrome from the haemorrhoidal to the iliac vessels in three of their patients.

Rectal digitation

Thompson and Hill (1980) propose that solitary ulcers may be traumatic, as a result of rectal digitation. Some of these patients are unable to achieve rectal evacuation unless they apply pressure over the posterior vault of the vagina or digitally extract faecal material. As the rectum is empty these manoeuvres merely result in local trauma to the rectum. Against this theory is that anoreceptive homosexuals do not develop rectal ulcers, nor do patients with outlet obstruction who digitate (Keighley and Shouler, 1984b). It also fails to explain why many paraplegic patients or those with chronic constipation who also find that digital extraction of faecal contents is necessary do not inevitably develop a solitary rectal ulcer. Digitation is recorded among 51–73% of patients with the solitary ulcer syndrome.

Other causes of trauma

Some patients with solitary rectal ulcer obtain sexual arousal from the passage of various objects into the rectum. This practice is difficult to identify from a patient's history. Other patients deliberately inflict rectal injury upon themselves as a form of attention seeking. Sexual abuse may be responsible.

Other theories

Other possible causes of solitary rectal ulcer include inflammatory bowel disease and a variety of drugs, such as antibiotics, antimetabolites and certain suppository preparations.

INCIDENCE

Solitary rectal ulcer is a relatively infrequent condition. However, there is an impression that with the introduction of defecography and with increased awareness of the condition, the diagnosis is being made more frequently.

Age

The solitary rectal ulcer syndrome can occur at almost any age (Tjandra et al, 1993). It is characteristically persistent and may have been present for many years before being diagnosed (Ford et al, 1983; Saul and Sollenberger, 1985) but symptoms seem to be most prominent in the second and third decades (Figure 24.6). The mean age of initial diagnosis is remarkably constant in the UK, being 31–51 years (Haskel and Rovner, 1965; Madigan and Morson, 1969; Martin et al, 1981; Ford et al, 1983) (see Table 24.2). Most patients, however, have symptoms for a mean of 4 years before the diagnosis is finally established. Delay in diagnosis was a prominent feature of the Cleveland Clinic experience (Tjandra et al, 1993). This disorder seems to be uncommon under the age of 10 years but may persist until at least 70 years (Goodall and Sinclair, 1957; Howard et al, 1971; Tedesco et al, 1976; Kennedy et al, 1977; Boulay et al, 1983).

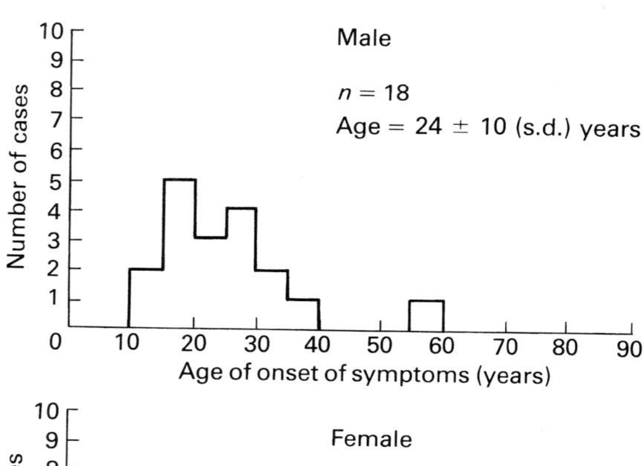

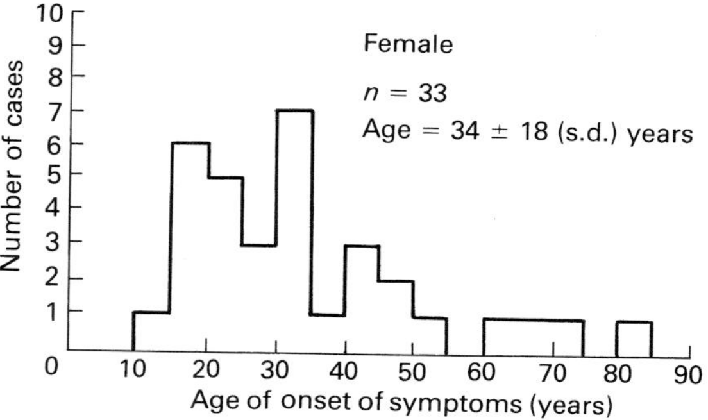

Figure 24.6 Age and sex in solitary rectal ulcer.

Sex

Unlike rectal prolapse, which occurs almost exclusively in women, solitary ulcer effects both sexes; the proportion of males is very variable, ranging from 27% to 70%, but in most series the female:male ratio is 3:1 (Madigan, 1964; Stuart, 1984; Levine, 1987).

Family history

There is no known increased incidence of solitary ulcer within families.

Social history

Solitary ulcer affects patients of all social strata and there are no known occupational factors in its pathogenesis.

CLINICAL FEATURES

Symptoms

The principal symptoms of the solitary rectal ulcer syndrome are rectal bleeding, mucous discharge, rectal pain and a feeling of obstructed defecation (Table 24.3).

Bleeding is characteristically bright red and in small amounts, occurring principally during straining on defecation (Madigan, 1964; Rowland et al, 1976; Stuart, 1984). However, solitary rectal ulcer may be responsible for massive rectal bleeding, necessitating repeated blood transfusions and sometimes surgical intervention (Delaney and Hitch, 1974; Alborti-Florr et al, 1985; Barbier et al, 1985). Two patients in our current series of 41 have presented in this way, but chronic rectal bleeding was common and has been one of the most frequent presenting symptoms. Bleeding is presumably due to trauma, mucosal congestion or ischaemia.

Mucous discharge is thought to be due to the anterior prolapse, incomplete intussusception or complete rectal prolapse and this symptom rarely disappears unless the prolapse itself is controlled.

Symptoms were said to be trivial in 18% of the Northern Ireland series, troublesome in 53% and disabling in 29% (Martin et al, 1981). At the Royal London (Womack et al, 1987) we found that symptoms differed according to the presence or absence of a visible ulcer (Table 24.4).

Bleeding, pain, straining, tenesmus, difficulty with defecation and self-digitation were more common among patients with an ulcer.

Bowel habit

Alteration in bowel habit is common in patients with this syndrome. The majority (51–84%) give a history of straining (Kumar et al, 1992). The most frequent disorder of bowel habit is an almost constant desire to defecate, which tends to be abortive. When closely questioned, patients often state that they go to the toilet in an attempt to defecate 10–20 times a day. True constipation (the passage of infrequent, hard stools) is present in 14–64% of patients (Table 24.5). Diarrhoea tends to be less common, occurring in 15–86%.

Anal incontinence may be present but is much more prevalent when solitary ulcers are associated with a complete prolapse (Kang et al, 1995). Incontinence is reported to occur in between 12 and 57% of patients. It may be the result of pudendal

Table 24.4 Symptoms according to the presence or absence of ulceration.

	Ulceration (*n* = 11)	*No ulceration* (*n* = 7)
Bleeding	100	71
Pain	91	28
Straining	82	43
Difficulty initiating defecation	82	28
Tenesmus	73	57
Self-digitation	73	43
Aware of a prolapse	45	14

Values are percentages.
From Womack et al (1987).

Table 24.3 Principal symptoms.

	Madigan and Morson (1969)	*Martin et al (1981)*	*Ford et al (1983)*	*Keighley and Shouler (1984a)*	*Meka et al (1984)*	*Mahieu (1986)*	*Britto et al (1987)*
Rectal bleeding	91	98	97	89	67	88	80
Mucous discharge	68	96	97	45	42	79	45
Tenesmus	24	93	62	42	22	86	30
Pain	42	47	*	36	28	60	25

Values are percentages.
* Not recorded.

Table 24.5 Bowel habit.

	Martin et al (1981)	*Ford et al (1983)*	*Keighley and Shouler (1984a)*	*Mahieu (1986)*
Difficulty of rectal evacuation	90	70	61	33
Anal incontinence	57	*	21	12
Rectal digitation	51	73	52	21
Straining	51	70	84	49
Constipation	49	22	64	14
Diarrhoea	20	42	15	86
Variable	4	22	9	*
Normal bowel habit	27	12	22	*

Values are percentages.
* Not recorded.

neuropathy associated with perineal descent from straining.

Personality

Some patients with this syndrome have a personality disorder, while in others there may be a history of sexual trauma, child abuse or overdominating parents (Jalan et al, 1970; Gadd, 1979). Many are introspective or neurotic. The majority of patients are obsessional about their bowels. The failure of most forms of medical and surgical therapy only serves to enhance the emotional and psychological features of this syndrome. It is difficult to know whether patients have a primary personality disorder or whether these features are secondary to a life dominated by repeated visits to the lavatory and a condition that is poorly understood by the medical profession and which is rarely cured.

Signs

Examination of the abdomen is usually normal but the sigmoid colon may be palpable due to faecal residue within it. Inspection of the anal canal and perineum is usually normal and, unlike rectal prolapse, the anus is rarely patulous unless there is a coexisting prolapse. Long-standing straining is commonly associated with marked perineal descent at rest and on attempted defecation. A small anterior mucosal prolapse is commonly visible. There may be indirect evidence of faecal incontinence such as perianal excoriation or soiling of underclothes. The patient must be asked to strain down, if necessary in the squatting position, so as to exclude a full-thickness rectal prolapse.

Rectal examination is generally painful, the external sphincter often being in spasm. Deep rectal examination is usually impossible. The rectal mucosa commonly feels oedematous and there may be an ulcer or polypoidal lesion palpable on the anterior wall of the rectum. There is often some induration around the ulcer and the mucosal folds may feel thickened. It may be quite impossible to feel the ulcer on account of the severity of pain.

PATHOLOGY

Macroscopic appearances

A typical solitary rectal ulcer varies in size from 1 to 5 cm^2; it is shallow and associated with a grey-white slough. There is often considerable surrounding oedema associated with an area of diffuse fibrosis, resulting in a thickened rectal wall (Kang et al, 1996), a localized mass or even a segment of rectal stenosis. In some cases the fibrous reaction is less prominent and there may be multiple ulcers or polypoidal projections around an area of granularity and localized proctitis. The ulcers may be round, oval, linear, serpiginous or stellate. There may be adjacent cysts or pseudopolyps, and in some cases there may be no ulcer but a friable cauliflower-shaped mass (Epstein et al, 1960; Black et al, 1972; Mulder and Te Velde, 1974; Franzin et al, 1982) or an area of distal proctitis. Most solitary rectal ulcers can be readily distinguished from malignant ulcers because they are punched out, shallow and without rolled edges.

Site

Solitary rectal ulcers classically occur on the anterior wall of the anorectum opposite the puborectalis sling, 5–8 cm from the anal verge (Figure 24.7). Current evidence, however, indicates that the location of these ulcers may be more variable and there are some patients with the syndrome who have no ulceration at all. The term 'solitary' is thus inappropriate, since only 47–88% are in fact single. It is also apparent from sigmoidoscopic examination and colonoscopy that ulcers may be present anywhere from 3 to 17 cm from the anal verge (Husa et al, 1978; Hershfield et al, 1984). Similar ulcers may be identified elsewhere in the colon or on the apex of a stoma. Although 38–70% of ulcers are found on the anterior aspect of the anorectum, they may be found in a lateral or posterior position in a varying proportion of patients (Madigan and Morson, 1969; Martin et al, 1981; Keighley and Shouler, 1984a) (Figure 24.8).

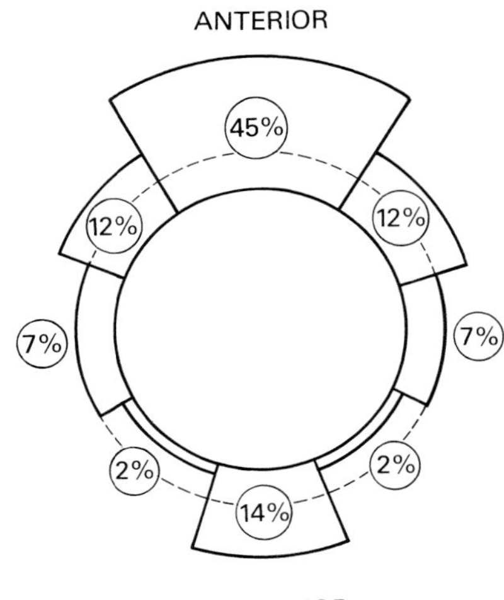

Figure 24.8 Radial distribution of solitary rectal ulcer.

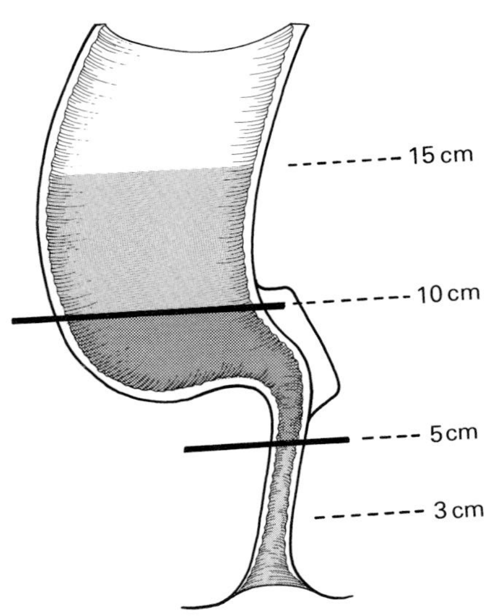

Figure 24.7 Usual site of solitary rectal ulcer.

Table 24.6 Histology of solitary ulcer (37 biopsy specimens).

Histology	%
Fibrous obliteration of the lamina propria	100
Disorientation of muscle fibres	100
Mucosal erosion and ulceration	54
Cystic changes	22
Villous pattern	15

From Ford et al (1983).

Histological features

The term 'solitary rectal ulcer' and 'colitis cystica profunda' are essentially synonymous. The lamina propria is replaced by collagen and there is fibromuscular replacement of the mucosa (Levine, 1987) in both disorders. There is intense fibrosis and a predominance of sialomucins. In addition, muscle fibres are seen splaying out into the lamina propria. There is hypertrophy of the muscularis mucosa and distorted crypts. The epithelium is hyperplastic and there may be displacement of mucous glands deep to the muscularis mucosa, responsible for the appearances and for the term 'colitis cystica profunda'. The frequency of these findings from 37 consecutive biopsies is shown on Table 24.6. Sometimes there are additional non-specific features such as

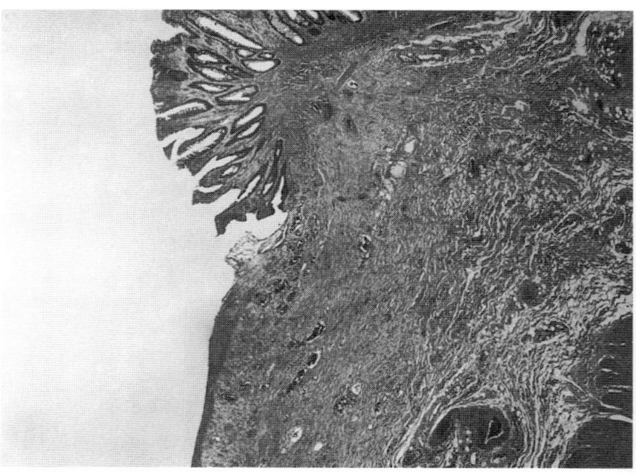

Figure 24.9 Histopathology of solitary ulcer.

Table 24.7 Biopsy appearances of solitary ulcer (46 biopsies).

Appearance	%
Mucosal change	100
Ulceration (50%)	
Epithelial hyperplasia (65%)	
Transitional mucosa (56%)	
Crypt distortion (76%)	
Reversal in sulpho:sialomucin ratio (100%)	
Changes in lamina propria	100
Fibromuscular obliteration (100%)	
Inflammatory infiltrate (39%)	
Telangiectasia (65%)	
Thickened muscularis mucosa	74
Submucosal fibrosis	70

From Britto et al (1987).

regenerating epithelium, granulation tissue surrounding the ulcer and a polymorph or eosinophilic exudate (Figure 24.9). Britto et al (1987) reported on the histopathology of this disorder as seen in India (Table 24.7). The histological features invariably present were fibromuscular obliteration of the lamina propria and reversal of the sulphomucin:sialomucin ratio. Ulceration was evident in only half of the biopsies. In some there was epithelial hyperplasia and changes in the mucosal morphology. Even submucosal fibrosis was observed in only 70%. However, lamina propria fibrosis is a useful feature for distinguishing solitary ulcer from Crohn's disease (Levine et al, 1986). Localized colitis cystic profunda is characterized by submucosal cysts. The cyst epithelium may be columnar, cuboidal or a flattened epithelium. Sometimes the cyst epithelium disappears altogether, leaving lakes of mucus within the submucosa. In solitary ulcer these cysts are always accompanied by replacement of the lamina propria with collagen and disorientated smooth muscle cells (Goodall and Sinclair, 1957). Kang et al (1996) found increased thickness of the muscularis propria and inner circular muscle compared with rectal prolapse. Other features included decussation of the muscular layers and nodular induration.

INVESTIGATIONS

Sigmoidoscopy

Sigmoidoscopy may be impossible because of pain, but the diagnosis is usually established by endoscopy. The most common finding is an indurated ulcerated lesion, usually on the anterior rectal wall 5–7 cm from the anal verge. Characteristically the ulcer is shallow, of variable size and shape and covered by a white or grey slough. It is frequently surrounded by a patch of erythema and oedema. There may be contact bleeding from the ulcer or the surrounding mucosa. Alternatively there may be no ulcer, merely an area of granular mucosa, single or multiple polypoidal lesions or multiple ulcers (Thomson et al, 1981). Sometimes the ulcer is complicated by rectal stenosis. Asking the patient to strain down during sigmoidoscopy may reveal an occult intussusception, but the only way of accurately identifying an intussusception is by videoproctography.

Barium enema

Contrast enema examination may help to distinguish a solitary ulcer from malignancy or inflammatory bowel disease. Mahieu (1986) reported the barium enema findings in 33 patients (Table 24.8).

Table 24.8 Radiographic features of solitary rectal ulcer syndrome.

Finding	%
Barium enema (*n* = 33)	
Thickened rectal folds	79
Rectal spasm	73
Ulceration	48
Nodular folds (pseudopolyp, pseudotumour)	27
Granularity	6
Rectal stricture	6
Proctography (*n* = 43)	
Rectal intussusception	79
Full rectal prolapse (44%)	
Intra-anal intussusception (23%)	
Intrarectal intussusception (12%)	
Puborectalis dysfunction	9
Rectocele	5
Unable to evacuate at all	2

From Mahieu (1986).

There was an abnormality in all patients, particularly thickened rectal mucosal folds, but ulceration was identified in less than half.

Videoproctography

A voiding proctogram is the best method of demonstrating an intussusception or anterior mucosal prolapse. Associated inappropriate contraction of the pelvic floor during voiding may also be suspected if the anorectal angle remains acute despite perineal descent. However, to be sure of such a diagnosis, simultaneous electromyography of the pelvic floor is required. Videoproctography will also provide objective assessment of rectal emptying and will demonstrate the morphology of the rectum, movement of the pelvic floor and the extent of perineal descent. Halligan et al (1995b) reported that evacuation time was more prolonged in solitary ulcer but 19 of their 23 patients had a prolapse: internal in 12 and complete in 7 which may have influenced emptying.

Anal ultrasonography

Endosonography demonstrates sphincter defects in some patients and fragmentation of the internal sphincter in others. The internal anal sphincter and occasionally the external anal sphincter diameters were increased in solitary ulcer, suggesting degeneration of the former and overactivity of the latter (Halligan et al, 1995a) (Figure 24.10). Rectal wall thickening is also demonstrated near the site of the ulcer (Van Outryve et al, 1993).

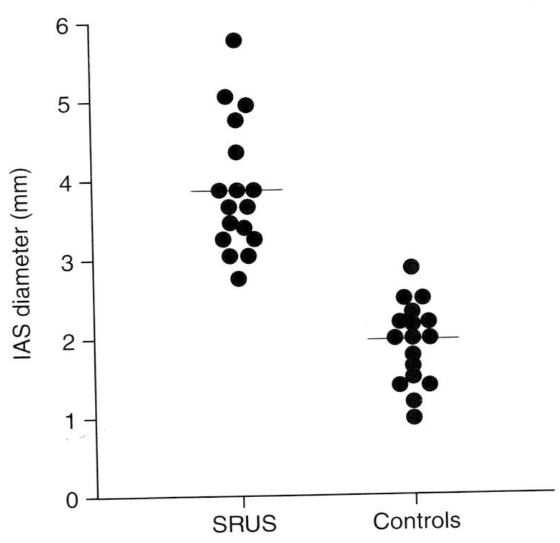

Figure 24.10 Internal anal sphincter (IAS) diameter in patients with solitary rectal ulcer syndrome (SRUS), compared with asymptomatic subjects. From Halligan et al (1995a).

PHYSIOLOGICAL ABNORMALITIES

We studied 16 patients with solitary ulcer and compared them with a group of age- and sex-matched subjects. Resting and squeeze anal pressures in ulcer patients did not differ from those found in the controls (Figure 24.11). Despite this finding, three patients with a painful ulcer had irregular spikes of involuntary external sphincter activity at rest (Figure 24.12) and one patient developed ultra-slow wave activity after straining (Figure 24.13). Initial rectal sensation (threshold volume) was normal in the rectal ulcer patients and the mean volume required to produce a constant rectal sensation was also similar. However, three patients had hyperactive external sphincter complexes after rectal distension which was associated with considerable rectal pain. There was a significant difference in the maximum tolerated volume in the ulcer patients compared with that in the controls (Figure 24.14). The maximum tolerated volume was less than 200 mL in half of the ulcer patients, compared with none in the controls. The rectoanal inhibitory reflex was absent in 6 of 16 patients. Only 4 of 16 patients had electromyographic evidence of inappropriate puborectalis contraction on attempted defecation (Figure 24.15).

These physiological changes are unlikely to represent a primary abnormality since most of the mano-

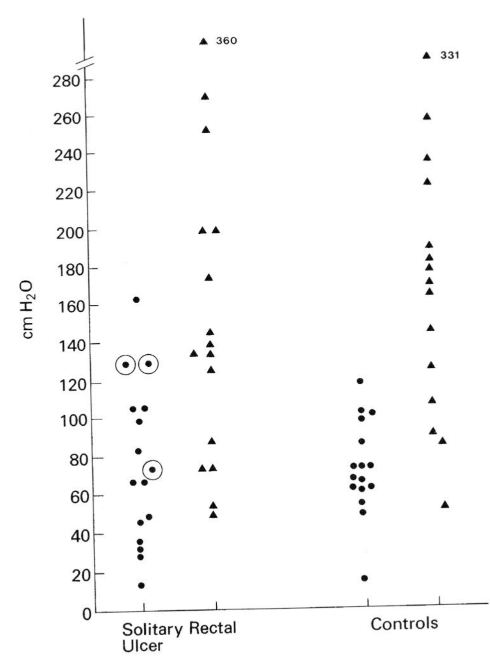

Figure 24.11 Anal pressures in solitary rectal ulcer. •, Maximum anal pressure; ⊙, resting external sphincter hyperactivity; ▲, maximum squeeze pressure.

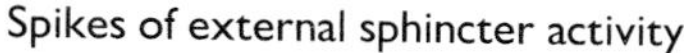

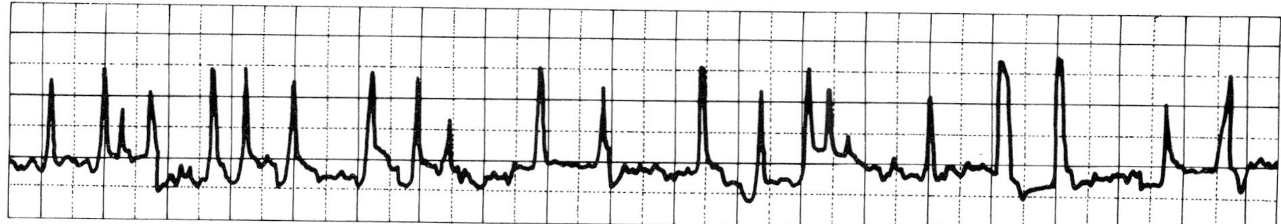

Figure 24.12 Tracing of resting anal canal pressures showing spikes of external sphincter activity at rest.

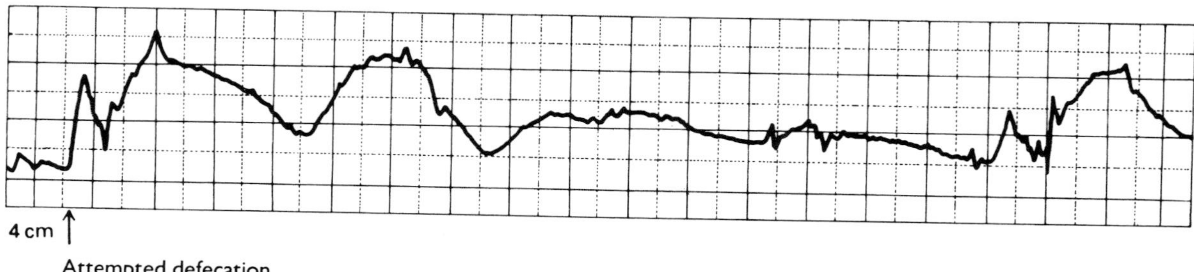

Figure 24.13 Tracing of anal canal pressures at rest with the response to straining showing ultra-slow wave activity.

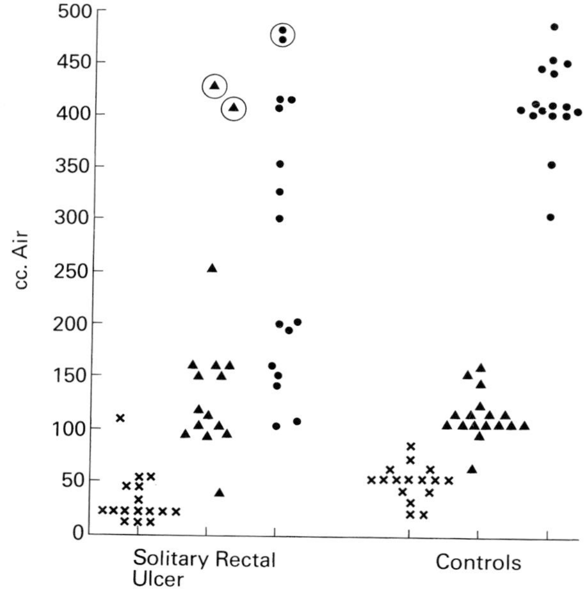

Figure 24.14 Results of rectal sensation in patients with solitary rectal ulcer compared with controls. ×, Threshold sensation; ▲, constant sensation; Ⓐ, megacolon; •, maximum tolerated volume; ⦿, unrecordable.

metric and sensory changes are likely to occur with a painful lesion at the anorectal junction.

There are other studies that shed light on the physiological abnormalities in this syndrome. Pescatori et al (1985) confirmed the exaggerated perineal descent in these patients and also showed that resting and squeeze pressures were reduced in half of them. They also observed an absent rectoanal inhibitory reflex, an obtuse anorectal angle in patients with incomplete prolapse, as well as denervation of the external anal sphincter in some patients.

Snooks et al (1985) compared 20 solitary ulcer patients with controls. Although resting anal pressures were similar, the maximum squeeze pressure was reduced in the ulcer patients (Table 24.9). As might be expected from the degree of perineal descent, there was evidence of delayed pudendal nerve conduction and external anal sphincter denervation, as witnessed by increased fibre density.

At the Royal London we performed a videoproctographic study using simultaneous intrarectal manometry with a telemetry capsule and electromyographic recordings from the puborectalis and external anal sphincter in 18 patients (Womack et al, 1989). All except one patient who voided had an intussusception (two anterior rectal wall prolapses, eight incomplete intussusceptions and five complete prolapses). Two patients could not void. Ulceration was associated with high intrarectal pressures induced by increased external sphincter activity. Kang et al (1995) proposed that there were three distinct groups with solitary ulcer: those without an intussusception; those without a prolapse

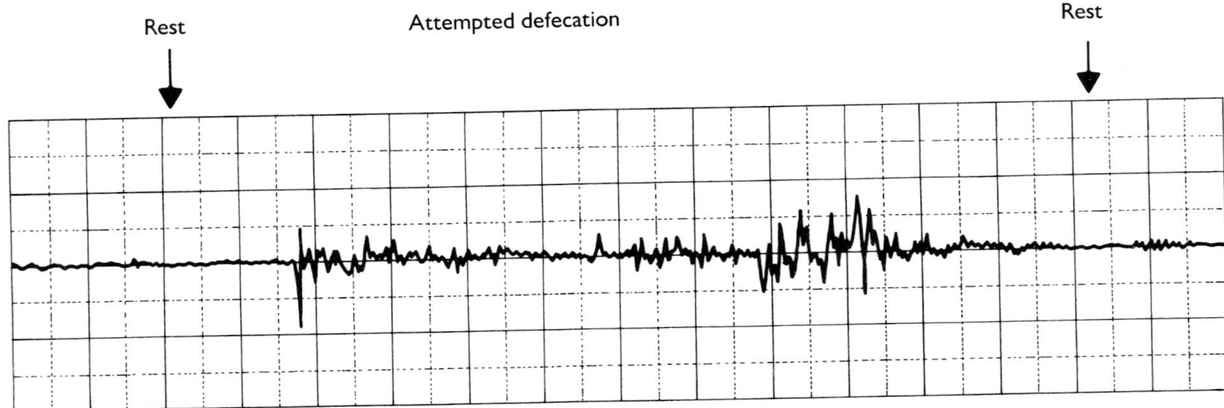

Figure 24.15 Increased EMG activity in the puborectalis on straining.

Table 24.9 Physiological changes in solitary rectal ulcer.

	Patients (n = 20)	*Controls* (n = 20)
Resting anal pressure (cmH_2O)	64 (20–100)	68 (50–96)
Maximum voluntary contraction pressure (cmH_2O)	73 (20–200)	108 (40–200)
Paradoxical puborectalis contraction on straining	10	0
External sphincter: fibre density	1.73 (±0.33)	1.4 (±0.13)
Pudendal nerve terminal motor latency (ms)	2.3 (±0.3)	1.9 (±0.2)
Perineal position (+above, −below ischial tuberosity, cm)		
Rest	+1.3 (±0.3)	+2.5 (±0.6)
Strain	−1.5 (±1.0)	+0.9 (±1.0)

Values in parentheses are ranges or standard deviations.
From Snooks et al (1985).

(both groups had high resting and squeeze pressures, but reduced anal and rectal sensation); and those with coexisting prolapse (this group had low resting and squeeze pressures).

DIFFERENTIAL DIAGNOSIS

It is essential to distinguish a solitary ulcer from a carcinoma of the rectum. The relative youth of some patients must never be used as an excuse not to biopsy, on the grounds that malignancy is unlikely. Malignant disease may occur in the young and is frequently misdiagnosed for months because the diagnosis is not seriously entertained. The medicolegal implications of performing an abdominoperineal excision for an ulcer which proves to be a benign solitary rectal ulcer are considerable!

Apart from malignancy, solitary ulcers should be distinguished from gonococcal proctitis by biopsy, serology and microbiological examination. Similar investigations are required to exclude gumma or other manifestations of syphilis, chlamydial proctitis or lymphogranuloma venereum. If the lesion is polypoidal, the differential diagnosis will include a benign polyp or a villous adenoma.

In some patients with proctitis the possibility of inflammatory bowel disease or traumatic proctitis should be excluded by biopsy and contrast radiology. Disorders which must be excluded in an atypical case are listed in Table 24.10. Apart from inflammatory bowel disease and benign or malignant neoplasms, specific chronic infections should also be excluded.

Table 24.10 Differential diagnosis.

Inflammatory bowel disease
Crohn's disease
Ischaemic proctitis
Ulcerative proctitis
Neoplasms
Adenocarcinoma
Benign adenomatous polyps
Carcinoid
Leiomyosarcoma
Lymphoma
Melanoma
Villous adenoma
Infections
Actinomycosis
Amoebiasis
Herpes
Lymphogranuloma venereum
Schistosomiasis
Syphilis
Iatrogenic
Drugs: 5-fluorouracil, contraceptives, aminophylline suppositories
Pseudomembranous colitis
Radiation proctitis
Others
Anal duct cysts
Endometriosis
Lymphangiectasia
Lymphoid polyps
Myoepithelial hamartoma
Pneumatosis intestinalis
Stercoral and traumatic ulcer
Submucosal foreign body
Submucosal haemorrhage

From Levine (1987).

NATURAL HISTORY

Remarkably little is known about the natural history of this disorder except that the majority of patients give a long history of symptoms. A high proportion of solitary ulcers are resistant to therapy and seem to alter very little throughout a period of follow-up (Madigan and Morson, 1969). A few heal for a while then recur. Ford et al (1983) report that although lesions often did not heal, they frequently changed in appearance from single to multiple and from ulcers to proliferative lesions. Some patients have typical symptoms but no ulcer is visible on endoscopy (Thompson and Hill, 1980; Womack et al, 1987). Some of these patients develop ulcers while others do not. In our experience there are a few patients whose ulcers heal spontaneously, but symptoms usually persist despite therapy.

TREATMENT

Conservative

The mainstay of conservative therapy is to try to stop patients from spending hours on the lavatory attempting to defecate by straining. 'Rapid reflex' defecation can sometimes be achieved by the use of an irritant suppository or a phosphate enema. Some clinicians prefer to rely on a high-fibre diet and to teach patients that they must avoid sitting on the lavatory for more than one minute. Brandt-Gradel et al (1984) gave 21 patients 30–40 g of fibre per day and told them to stop straining: three remained

Table 24.11 Conservative treatment (avoidance of straining plus high fibre diet) in 21 patients.

	Symptoms	*Ulcer healing*
No change	3	6
Short-term improvement	14	0
Long-term improvement	4	15

From Brandt-Gradel et al (1984).

unimproved, and although the remaining 18 were improved this was transient in 14. Nevertheless 15 of the 21 ulcers healed (Table 24.11). Martin also claims improvement in 70% of patients after treatment with bulk laxatives (Martin et al, 1981).

Biofeedback may have a place in management if there is obstructed defecation (Binnie et al, 1992). The role of biofeedback may be considerable, but like treatment for incontinence and anismus the results very much depend on the compliance of the patient and their attitude to treatment (Vaizey et al, 1997). Those individuals who are eager to help themselves and are slightly obsessional do well, particularly if they control the habit of sitting on the lavatory every time they have a 'call' to stool. Biofeedback should certainly be offered; in our experience about 30% are improved and a few appear to be 'cured' of their condition.

Topical and systemic therapy

The use of topical steroids cannot be recommended on current evidence since healing is rare (Martin et al, 1981). Oral sulphasalazine has been used but healing is unusual (Table 24.12). Sucralfate retention enemas provided long-term cure in five of six patients (Zargar et al, 1991). We have used metronidazole in a small number of patients with ulcers resistant to other forms of therapy but none have healed.

Table 24.12 Results of therapy.

	Response (%)
Bulk laxatives	70
Steroids (locally)	12
Sulphasalazine	10
Local excision	0
Rectopexy	83

From Martin et al (1981).

Surgical

Local excision

Local excision of a solitary rectal ulcer is a difficult procedure. It may be performed as a transanal or trans-sphincteric operation, as described for the local treatment of rectal carcinoma. Although local excision is sometimes feasible it often results in a distorted narrow rectum which may form a stricture, and symptoms invariably persist. Despite this, Ford et al (1983) report complete remission in 5 of 16 patients having a local excision. We have no personal experience of this form of therapy but we have some patients referred with an ulcer despite previous local excision.

Excision of mucosal prolapse

In the past it has been suggested that if an anterior mucosal prolapse is present in association with a solitary rectal ulcer it should be treated either by excision or injection sclerotherapy, on the grounds that if the prolapse is eliminated the sensation of obstructed defecation might be removed. In practice, local treatment of the mucosal prolapse does nothing to alter the fundamental underlying disorder, the anterior prolapse inevitably recurs and symptoms persist.

Internal sphincterectomy and anorectal myectomy

It has been suggested that excision of a strip of the internal sphincter might correct existing anismus (Poisson and Devroede, 1983). We have tried this approach in a few patients but have abandoned sphincterectomy because the functional disorder has usually persisted. Anorectal myectomy has also been used but the long-term results of this procedure in patients with anismus were very disappointing (Pinho et al, 1989) and there is a risk of incontinence.

Division of the puborectalis

If the cause of solitary ulcer is due to inappropriate contraction of the pelvic floor during attempted defecation (Rutter and Riddell, 1975; Dough and Wright, 1981), it might seem logical to try to treat these patients by partial division of the innermost fibres of the puborectalis sling (Kamm et al, 1988). Wasserman (1964) used a similar approach in four patients with excellent results. A much larger series has been reported by Wallace and Madden (1969), in which 72 consecutive patients underwent a similar procedure to divide the internal fibres of the puborectalis. However, the majority of the patients had chronic constipation and not the solitary rectal ulcer syndrome. Nevertheless, some patients were improved and none developed faecal incontinence.

We have tried this procedure in six patients who had electromyographic evidence of abnormal pelvic floor contraction during straining. None of the patients became incontinent. In one patient the results of therapy were quite spectacular. However, in the remaining five cases no improvement was achieved and we would no longer recommend this procedure for the treatment of this syndrome.

Anal dilatation

It could be argued that anal dilatation should be considered for treatment of this syndrome on the basis that intrarectal hypertension might be relieved. However, almost all of these patients have marked perineal descent and evidence of pudendal neuropathy, hence anal dilatation might precipitate incontinence and, in our view, should be avoided.

Rectopexy

Rectopexy has been advocated for the treatment of the solitary rectal ulcer syndrome on the grounds that a high proportion of patients have an incomplete or full-thickness rectal prolapse. Most of the encouraging results following rectopexy are either in patients whose ulcer is associated with a full-thickness prolapse or where the follow-up is very short (Madigan, 1964). Martin et al (1981) reported that five of six patients with a solitary ulcer and a full-thickness prolapse treated by rectopexy had no further symptoms. Schweiger and Alexander-Williams (1977) reported improvement in symptoms among 12 patients seen in Ehlangen and Birmingham treated by rectopexy. However, the follow-up in these patients was short and many of the Birmingham patients developed recurrent symptoms. A review of 14 patients in Birmingham treated more recently by rectopexy was less encouraging (Table 24.13) and only seven patients were improved by rectopexy (50%). The results of rectopexy largely depended on whether there was a complete rectal prolapse: five of six ulcers healed when a full-thickness rectal prolapse was evident, compared with healing in only two of eight patients who had an internal intussusception. Furthermore, symptoms related to impaired defecation persisted in all these patients, presumably because they continued to strain.

The results of rectopexy alone for rectal intussusception have been uniformly unsatisfactory (Kruyt et al, 1990; McCue and Thomson, 1990). A few ulcers have healed but, almost without exception, symptoms have persisted (Hoffman et al, 1984; Holmstrom et al, 1986; Christiansen et al, 1992).

For this reason the experience of Nicholls and Simson (1986) in the treatment of 14 patients with the solitary rectal ulcer syndrome without overt rectal prolapse is surprising. The type of rectopexy described by them for the treatment of solitary rectal ulcer differs in many respects from the conventional procedure for rectal prolapse. The rectum is mobilized anteriorly as well as posteriorly down to the anal canal. A long sheet of polypropylene mesh is placed posteriorly and sutured to the sacrum and the rectum; in addition, a second mesh sling is placed anteriorly. The excess pelvic peritoneum is excised and closed above the rectopexy. There were two failures after this operation. Of the 12 who improved, two developed constipation. Bleeding was controlled in all patients. Only one patient continued to complain of mucous discharge and three patients stopped straining. The mean time spent on the lavatory fell from 146 to 15 minutes and the number of visits to the lavatory fell from 87 to 34. The authors admit that the follow-up is short but this is the only paper to suggest that rectopexy may have a role in controlling symptoms in patients with solitary ulcers who do not also exhibit a complete prolapse.

In the study by Sitzler et al (1996), results of rectopexy were best if there was a coexisting prolapse and poor among those with incontinence and obstructed defecation.

Table 24.13 Results of therapy.

	n	*Asymptomatic*	*Ulcer healed*
Spontaneous healing: asymptomatic	8	8	6
Dietary advice and retraining	33	2	9
Rectopexy	14	0	7
Full thickness prolapse	6	0	5
Incomplete intussusception	8	0	2
Abdominoperineal excision	1	1	Excised
Coloanal sleeve resection	1	0	0
Anterior resection	1	0	0
Colostomy	2	2	0

From Keighley and Shouler (1984a; updated).

Low anterior resection

A few patients with intractable symptoms or bleeding after unsuccessful rectopexy have been treated by low anterior resection with excision of the ulcer and stapled coloanal anastomosis. A variant of low anterior resection involves excision of all mucosa to the dentate line and a low coloanal intra-anal anastomosis. Guy and Ham (1988) report a successful outcome using this approach. In Birmingham we have used total rectal excision with or without a colonic pouch and coloanal anastomosis in eight patients; six have been substantially improved even though minor symptoms persist, and one is now known to have developed solitary ulcers in the colonic pouch.

Colostomy

Colostomy has been used as a last resort for patients with incapacitating tenesmus, bleeding and mucous discharge (Stavorovsky et al, 1977). Unfortunately, although bleeding may stop, most other symptoms are not alleviated. We have known of at least five patients in whom colostomy has been used when all other procedures have failed. In all five, symptoms have persisted despite the colostomy; none of these patients will accept the prospect of a stoma in the long term and most have insisted that it be reversed. Other authors have had a similar experience (Kennedy et al, 1977; Ford et al, 1983). Colostomy has been used as a temporary measure in patients with massive rectal bleeding from a solitary ulcer, and although the ulcer may not heal, patients usually stop straining and consequently the bleeding no longer continues (Stavorovsky et al, 1977).

Abdominoperineal excision

Abdominoperineal excision of the rectum is clearly a last resort and an operation that is never undertaken lightly in patients with a benign condition of unknown aetiology. Despite this the operation may have to be entertained in a very carefully selected group, if the patient will accept a permanent colostomy. This is certainly an option if rectal excision and sphincter-saving procedures fail. It may also have to be used for continued massive bleeding, but where possible the sphincters should be preserved in case bowel continuity can be restored at a later date.

Other procedures

The Délorme's operation, multiple ligation of the intussuscepting mucosa as an intra-anal procedure (Gant–Miwa procedure) or staple reduction have all been advocated but the functional results are usually disappointing (Berman et al, 1985).

AUTHORS' VIEW ON SURGICAL TREATMENT

We believe that surgical treatment should never be undertaken lightly for a condition which is essentially due to repeated chronic straining. To date, the only published effective treatment seems to be by abdominal rectopexy. Our own experience suggests that abdominal rectopexy is only justified for patients with a complete rectal prolapse. Furthermore, if there is evidence of delayed colonic transit, rectopexy with sigmoid colectomy might be more appropriate than rectopexy alone. The long-term results of rectopexy for incomplete intussusception are so poor and the presence of an incomplete intussusception so common that we cannot recommend rectopexy for ulcers associated with an internal intussusception. However, we do accept that there are occasional exceptions in stable well-motivated patients in whom the intussusception obstructs rectal evacuation. For patients with repeated bleeding long-term benefit can be achieved by total rectal excision and coloanal anastomosis or abdomino-perineal excision.

REFERENCES

Alborti-Florr JJ, Halters S & Dunn GD (1985) Solitary rectal ulcer as a cause of massive lower gastrointestinal bleeding. *Gastrointest Endosc* **31**: 53–54.

Barbier P, Luder P, Triller J, Ruchti Ch, Hassler H & Stafford A (1985) Colonic haemorrhage from a solitary minute ulcer. *Gastroenterology* **88**: 1065–1068.

Berman IR, Manning DH & Dudley Wright K (1985) Anatomic specificity in the diagnosis and treatment of internal rectal prolapse. *Dis Colon Rectum* **28**: 816–826.

Binnie NR, Papachrysostomou M, Clare N & Smith AN (1992) Solitary rectal cancer: the place of biofeedback and surgery in the treatment of the syndrome. *World J Surg* **16**: 836–840.

Black HC, Gardner WA & Weidner MG (1972) Localised colitis

cystica profunda, a benign lesion simulating malignancy. *Am Surg* **38**: 237–239.

Boulay CED, Fairbrother J & Isaacson PG (1983) Mucosal prolapse syndrome: a unifying concept for solitary ulcer syndrome and related disorders. *J Clin Pathol* **36**: 1264–1268.

Brandt-Gradel V, Huibregtse K & Tytgat GNJ (1984) Treatment of solitary rectal ulcer syndrome with high fibre diet and abstention of straining at defaecation. *Dig Dis Sci* **29**: 1005–1008.

Britto E, Borges AM, Swaroop VS, Jagannath P & DeSouza LJ (1987) Solitary rectal ulcer: 20 cases seen in an oncology centre. *Dis Colon Rectum* **30**: 381–386.

Christiansen J, Zhu B-W, Rasmussen O & Sorensen M (1992) Internal rectal intussusception: results of surgical repair. *Dis Colon Rectum* **35**: 1026–1029.

Delaney H & Hitch WS (1974) Solitary rectal ulcer: a cause of life-threatening haemorrhage. *Surgery* **76**: 830–832.

Devroede G, Beaudry R, Haddad H et al (1973) Discrete ulcerations of the rectum and sigmoid. *Am J Dig Dis* **18**: 695–702.

Devroede G, Vobecky S, Mosse S et al (1982) Ischaemic faecal incontinence and rectal angina. *Gastroenterology* **83**: 970–980.

Dough JH & Wright FF (1981) Acute and chronic benign ulcers of the rectum. *Surg Gynecol Obstet* **153**: 398–402.

Epstein SE, Ascari WQ, Ablow RC, Seaman WB & Lattes R (1960) Colitis cystica profunda. *Am J Clin Pathol* **45**: 186–201.

Feczko PJ, O'Connell DJ, Riddell RH & Frank PH (1980) Solitary rectal ulcer syndrome: radiological manifestations. *Am J Roentgenol* **35**: 499–506.

Ford MJ, Anderson JR, Gilmour HM, Holt S, Sircus W & Heading RC (1983) Clinical spectrum of 'solitary ulcer' of the rectum. *Gastroenterology* **84**: 1533–1540.

Franzin G, Dina R, Scarpa A & Fratton A (1982) The evolution of the solitary ulcer of the rectum: an endoscopic and histopathological study. *Endoscopy* **14**: 131–134.

Gadd A (1979) Benign idiopathic recurrent rectal ulceration. *Scand J Gastroenterol* **14** (Suppl 54): 111–113.

Goodall HB & Sinclair ISR (1957) Colitis cystica profunda. *J Pathol Bacteriol* **73**: 33–42.

Guy PJ & Ham M (1988) Colitis cystic profunda of the rectum treatment by mucosal sleeve resection and coloanal pull through. *Br J Surg* **75**: 289.

Halligan S, Sultan A, Rottenberg G & Bartram CI (1995a) Endosonography of the anal sphincters in solitary rectal ulcer syndrome. *Int J Colorectal Dis* **10**: 79–82.

Halligan S, Nicholls RJ & Bartram CI (1995b) Proctographic changes after rectopexy for solitary rectal ulcer syndrome and preoperative predictive factors for a successful outcome. *Br J Surg* **82**: 314–317.

Haskell B & Rovner H (1965) Solitary ulcer of the rectum. *Dis Colon Rectum* **8**: 333–336.

Hershfield NB, Langevin JE & Kelly JK (1984) Endoscopic and histological features of the solitary rectal ulcer syndrome. *Gastrointest Endosc* **30**: 162–163.

Hoffman MJ, Kodner IJ & Fry RD (1984) Internal intussusception of the rectum. Diagnosis and surgical management. *Dis Colon Rectum* **27**: 435–441.

Holmstrom B, Broden G & Dolk A (1986) Results of the Ripstein operation in the treatment of rectal prolapse and internal procidentia. *Dis Colon Rectum* **29**: 845–848.

Howard RJ, Mannax SJ, Eusebio EB, Shea MA & Goldberg SM (1971) Colitis cystica profunda. *Surgery* **69**: 306–308.

Husa A, Santavirta S & Makinen J (1978) Colitis cystic profunda. *Ann Chir Gynaecol* **67**: 25–26.

Ihre T (1972) Internal procidentia of the rectum: treatment and results. *Scand J Gastroenterol* **7**: 643–646.

Jalan KN, Brunt PW, Maclean N et al (1970) Benign solitary ulcer of the rectum: a report of 5 cases. *Scand J Gastroenterol* **5**: 143–147.

Johansson C, Nilsson BY, Mellgren A, Dolk A & Holmstrom B (1992) Paradoxical sphincter reaction and associated colorectal disorders. *Int J Colorectal Dis* **7**: 89–94.

Kamm MA, Hawley PR & Lennard-Jones JE (1988) Lateral division of the puborectalis muscle in the management of severe constipation. *Br J Surg* **75**: 661–663.

Kang YS, Kamm MA & Nicholls RJ (1995) Solitary rectal ulcer and complete rectal prolapse: one condition or two? *Int J Colorectal Dis* **10**: 87–90.

Kang YS, Kamm MA, Engel AF & Talbot IC (1996). Pathology of the rectal wall in solitary rectal ulcer syndrome and complete rectal prolapse. *Gut* **38**: 785–790.

Keighley MRB & Shouler P (1984a) Clinical and manometric features of the solitary rectal ulcer syndrome. *Dis Colon Rectum* **27**: 507–512.

Keighley MRB & Shouler P (1984b) Outlet obstruction: is there a surgical option? *J R Soc Med* **77**: 559–563.

Kennedy DK, Hughes ESR & Masterton JP (1977) The natural history of benign ulcer of the rectum. *Surg Gynecol Obstet* **144**: 718–720.

Kruyt RH, Delemarre JBVM, Gooszen HG & Vogel HF (1990) Selection of patients with internal intussusception of the rectum for posterior rectopexy. *Br J Surg* **77**: 1183–1184.

Kuijpers HC, Schreve RH & Hoedemaker TC (1986) Diagnosis of functional disorders of defaecation causing the solitary rectal ulcer syndrome. *Dis Colon Rectum* **29**: 128–129.

Kumar D, Bartolo DCC, Devroede G et al (1992). Symposium on constipation. *Int J Colorect Dis* **7**: 47–67.

Levine DS (1987) Solitary rectal ulcer syndrome and localised colitis cystica profunda, analogous syndromes caused by rectal prolapse. *Gastroenterology* **92**: 243–253.

Levine DS, Surawicz CM, Ajer TN & Rubbin CE (1986) Demonstration of mucosal fibrosis differentiates solitary rectal ulcer syndrome from idiopathic inflammatory bowel disease. *Clin Res* **34**: 30A.

Lewis FW, Mahoney MP & Heffernan CK (1977) The solitary ulcer syndrome of the rectum: radiological features. *Br J Radiol* **50**: 227–228.

Lonsdale RN (1993) Microvascular abnormalities in the mucosal prolapse syndrome. *Gut* **34**: 106–109.

McCue JL & Thomson JPS (1990) Rectopexy for internal rectal intussusception. *Br J Surg* **77**: 632–634.

Madigan MR (1964) Solitary ulcer of the rectum. *Proc R Soc Med* **57**: 403–404.

Madigan MR & Morson BC (1969) Solitary ulcer of the rectum. *Gut* **10**: 871–881.

Mahieu PHG (1986) Barium enema and defaecography in the diagnosis and evaluation of the solitary rectal ulcer syndrome. *Int J Colorectal Dis* **1**: 85–90.

Martin CJ, Parks TG & Biggard JD (1981) Solitary rectal ulcer syndrome in Northern Ireland 1971–1980. *Br J Surg* **68**: 744–747.

Martin JK, Culp CE & Welland LH (1984) Colitis cystica profunda. *Dis Colon Rectum* **27**: 153–156.

Meka R, Trinkl W, Sassaris M & Hunter F (1984) Colitis cystica profunda. *Curr Concepts Gastroenterol* **6**: 18–20.

Mulder H & Te Velde J (1974) Colitis cystica profunda: pseudotumours in the rectum. *Radiol Clin Biol* **43**: 529–539.

Nicholls RJ & Simson JNL (1986) Anterior posterior rectopexy in the treatment of the solitary ulcer syndrome without overt prolapse. *Br J Surg* **78**: 222–224.

Parks AG, Porter NH & Hardcastle J (1966) The syndrome of the descending perineum. *Proc R Soc Med* **59**: 477–482.

Pescatori M, Marta G, Mattana C, Vulpio C & Vecchio F (1985) Clinical picture and pelvic floor physiology in the solitary rectal ulcer syndrome. *Dis Colon Rectum* **28**: 862–867.

Pinho M, Yoshioka K & Keighley MRB (1989) Long term results of anorectal myectomy for chronic constipation. *Br J Surg* **76**: 1163–1164.

Poisson J & Devroede C (1983) Severe chronic constipation as a surgical problem. *Gastroenterology* **63**: 192–217.

Potel F, Bogomotetz WV & Fenzy A (1985) Syndrome du prolapsus magneux anorectal: un concept modernet unitaire de l'ulcere solitaire due rectum et lesions du meme type. *Gastroenterol Clin Biol* **9**: 561–563.

Rowland R, Hecker R, Willing R et al (1976) Solitary ulcer of the rectum. A report of 15 cases. *Med J Aust* **1** (Suppl): 21–23.

Rutter KRP (1974) Electromyographic changes in certain pelvic floor abnormalities. *Proc R Soc Med* **67**: 53–56.

Rutter KRP & Riddell RH (1975) The solitary ulcer syndrome of the rectum. *Clin Gastroenterol* **4**: 505–530.

Saul SH & Sollenberger LC (1985) Solitary rectal ulcer syndrome: its clinical and pathological underdiagnosis. *Am J Surg Pathol* **9**: 411–412.

Schweiger M & Alexander-Williams J (1977) Solitary ulcer syndrome of the rectum. Its association with occult rectal prolapse. *Lancet* **i**: 170–171.

Shouler P & Keighley MRB (1986) Changes in colorectal function in severe idiopathic constipation. *Gastroenterology* **90**: 414–420.

Sitzler PG, Nicholls RJ & Kamm MA (1996) Surgery for solitary rectal ulcer syndrome. *Int J Colorectal Dis* **11**: 136.

Siproudhis L, Ropert A, Lucas J et al (1992) Defecatory disorders, anorectal and pelvic floor dysfunction: a polygamy? Radiologic and manometric studies in 41 patients. *Int J Colorectal Dis* **7**: 102–107.

Snooks SJ, Nicholls RJ, Henry MM & Swash M (1985) Electrophysiological and manometric assessment of the pelvic floor in the solitary rectal ulcer syndrome. *Br J Surg* **72**: 131–133.

Stavorovsky M, Weintroub S, Patan J & Rozen P (1977) Successful treatment of a benign solitary rectal ulcer by temporary diverting sigmoidostomy: report of a case. *Dis Colon Rectum* **20**: 347–350.

Stuart M (1984) Proctitis cystica profunda: incidence, aetiology and treatment. *Dis Colon Rectum* **24**: 153–156.

Tedesco FJ, Sumner HW & Kassens WD (1976) Colitis cystica profunda. *Am J Gastroenterol* **65**: 339–343.

Thompson H & Hill D (1980) Solitary rectal ulcer: always a self-induced condition? *Br J Surg* **67**: 784–785.

Thomson G, Clark A, Handyside J & Gillespie G (1981) Solitary ulcer of the rectum – or is it? A report of 6 cases. *Br J Surg* **68**: 21–24.

Tjandra JJ, Fazio VW, Church JM et al (1992) Clinical conundrum of solitary rectal ulcer. *Dis Colon Rectum* **35**: 227–234.

Tjandra JJ, Fazio VW, Petras RE et al (1993) Clinical and pathologic factors associated with delayed diagnosis in solitary rectal ulcer syndrome. *Dis Colon Rectum* **36**: 146–153.

Vaizey CJ, Toy AJ & Kamm MA (1997) Prospective evaluation of the treatment of solitary rectal ulcer syndrome with biofeedback. *Gut* **41**: 817–820.

Van Outryve MJ, Pelckmans PA, Fierens H & Van Maercke YM (1993) Transrectal ultrasound study of the pathogenesis of solitary rectal ulcer syndrome. *Gut* **24**: 1422–1426.

Wallace WC & Madden WM (1969) Partial puborectalis resection. *South Med J* **62**: 1123–1129.

Wasserman IF (1964) Puborectalis syndrome. *Dis Colon Rectum* **7**: 87–92.

White CM, Findlay JM & Price JJ (1980) The occult rectal prolapse syndrome. *Br J Surg* **67**: 528–530.

Womack NR, Williams NS, Holmfield JHM & Morrison JFB (1987) Anorectal function in the solitary rectal ulcer syndrome. *Dis Colon Rectum* **30**: 319–323.

Womack NR, Williams NS, Holmfield JHM & Morrison JFB (1989) Pressure and prolapse: the cause of solitary rectal ulceration. *Gut* **28**: 1225–1233.

Zargar SA, Khuroo MS & Mahajan R (1991) Sucralfate retention enemas in solitary rectal ulcer. *Dis Colon Rectum* **34**: 455–457.

toms. Similar findings have also been reported by others (Drossman et al, 1982; Whitehead et al, 1982). Manning et al (1978) suggest that the frequency of these symptoms is greater in patients with the irritable bowel syndrome than in those with organic disease. Approximately 37% of patients with constipation have the irritable bowel syndrome (Probert et al, 1994).

Harvey et al (1983) investigated the prevalence of the irritable bowel syndrome among a group of 1000 patients attending a medical gastroenterological clinic. They found that 44.9% had features of the spastic colon syndrome (Table 25.4). The irritable bowel syndrome was found to be the cause of non-specific abdominal pain in patients admitted through casualty for observation in 27% of women and in 19% of men (Doshi and Heaton, 1994). It is a common cause of symptoms after hysterectomy (Heaton et al, 1993). Jones and Lydiard (1992) reported a 22% prevalence figure which spanned all ages. Thompson and Heaton (1980) found that only 20% of patients with the irritable bowel syndrome ever sought medical advice. Eastwood et al (1987) indicate that 30–40% of all patients attending gastrointestinal outpatient departments have features of the syndrome. Medical consultation may be precipitated by the worry of serious underlying disease, the availability of free health care, screening programmes or propaganda stressing the importance of health check-ups. Repeated consultations by several different physician groups is a common phenomenon and one which may generate unrealistic expectations.

Table 25.4 Diagnosis in 1000 patients attending a medical gastrointestinal clinic with a frequency of more than 20/100.

Organic		*Non-organic*	
Peptic ulcer	197	Irritable bowel syndrome (pain, altered bowel habit)	449
Gastro-oesophageal reflux	188	Painless diarrhoea	107
Inflammatory bowel disease	168	Endoscopy negative dyspepsia	77
Gallstones	48	Depression and abdominal pain	50
Carcinoma of the colon	28	Painless constipation	39
Coeliac disease	26	Habit disorders	34
Cirrhosis of the liver	21	Anxiety with gut symptoms	24
Infective diarrhoea	21		

From Harvey et al (1983).

AGE AND SEX INCIDENCE

Intestinal symptoms in the absence of organic disease may present at any age (Hahn et al, 1997a). Chaudhary and Truelove (1962) observed that the majority of patients were aged between 20 and 60 years. Waller and Misiewicz (1969) found that most patients were under 40 years of age. Many patients have a long history, usually exceeding 10 years. Paediatricians also recognize that functional diarrhoea or constipation with abdominal pain may occur in children from the age of 1 year (Davidson and Wasserman, 1966). It is unclear, however, whether children progress to the adult syndromes or whether symptoms in children improve with age (Stone and Barbero, 1970; Dimson, 1971). It is potentially dangerous to label elderly patients as having the irritable bowel syndrome without thorough examination, since organic disorders of the large bowel are much more prevalent in the elderly.

Women more commonly present with functional bowel disorders than men (Goulston, 1972a). The ratio of women to men is about 2:1 (Harvey et al, 1983). In children, the sexes are equally affected. The incidence by age and sex is set out in Table 25.5.

Table 25.5 Prevalence and consultation rates by age for the irritable bowel syndrome.

	20–29		*30–39*		*40–49*		*50–59*		*60–69*		*70–79*		*>80*	
	Men	*Women*	*Men*	*Women*	*Men*	*Women*	*Men*	*Women*	*Men*	*Women*	*Men*	*Women*	*Men*	*Women*
No. of questionnaires returned	89	92	120	137	150	161	142	130	153	140	106	116	25	59
No. (%) with symptoms of the irritable bowel syndrome	26 (29)	25 (27)	34 (28)	43 (31)	26 (17)	48 (30)	14 (10)	29 (22)	25 (16)	24 (17)	17 (16)	23 (20)	5 (20)	11 (19)
No (%) with the irritable bowel syndrome consulting GP	5 (19)	9 (36)	12 (35)	12 (28)	7 (27)	13 (27)	2 (14)	10 (34)	10 (40)	11 (46)	6 (35)	9 (39)	2 (40)	9 (82)

From Jones and Lydiard (1992).

SYMPTOMS

Over 70% of patients with the irritable bowel syndrome can be diagnosed from the history alone (Harvey et al, 1987). Symptoms are usually long-standing and there may be a family history in 30% of patients. A history of high caffeine consumption, smoking and frequent time off work due to minor illnesses is common. Diffuse symptoms are common, especially backache, fatigue, urinary and gynaecological symptoms, headache, nausea, dysphagia and abdominal complaints (Thompson and Heaton, 1980). Symptoms such as weight loss, anaemia and recent change in bowel habit with altered blood in the stool suggesting malignancy of the large bowel are uncommon. The principal symptoms are of abdominal pain relieved by defecation, loose, frequent stools associated with pain, abdominal distension, the passage of mucus and incomplete evacuation after defecation (Oettle and Heaton, 1987). The number of symptoms may alert clinicians to the diagnosis since patients with the irritable bowel syndrome usually have four or five symptoms, whereas multiple symptoms are unusual in organic disease (Manning et al, 1978). There is also a high incidence of proctalgia fugax in patients with the irritable bowel syndrome (Thompson and Heaton, 1980).

Pain is variable in severity, from mild discomfort to an intensity comparable to renal colic. Pain may be in the lower abdomen or in the left iliac fossa, its location is commonly variable. Pain in the right iliac fossa after meals seems to be associated with food arriving in the caecum, as measured using the hydrogen breath test (Cann et al, 1983b). In some patients, ileocaecal emptying appears to be impaired (Trotman and Price, 1986). Cook et al (1987) found that pain was better tolerated in patients with irritable bowel syndrome than in normal individuals. Pain is usually colicky but it may be constant and is frequently associated with abdominal distension and flatulence.

The characteristic alteration in bowel habit consists of intermittent episodes of diarrhoea or constipation associated with the passage of hard, pelleted stools. Symptoms were found to be unrelated to alteration in intestinal transit, stool weight or consistency (Oettle and Heaton, 1987). Patients often have a feeling of incomplete rectal evacuation (Hunt, 1957; Oettle and Heaton, 1986). Diarrhoea may also be accompanied by urgency, particularly in the mornings, and with relief of abdominal pain. Diarrhoea in the irritable bowel syndrome is rarely associated with the passage of blood, although 10% of patients have concomitant haemorrhoids (Waller and Misiewicz, 1969). Patients with diarrhoea have a rectum which is hypersensitive to rectal distension; this is not evident in those with constipation (Prior et al, 1990b). A history of abdominal pain, distension, straining and scybala was more common in the irritable bowel syndrome than in inflammatory bowel disease or peptic ulcer (Thompson, 1984a).

Other non-specific symptoms include loss of concentration, depression, anxiety, loss of libido, increased fatigue, altered affect and sleep disturbance (Hislop, 1971). A social history sometimes reveals marital disharmony or recent stress from emotional or financial problems (Mendeloff et al, 1968). Many patients, particularly women, admit to not being able to cope with stress (Johnsen et al, 1986). Sexual dysfunction is more common in irritable bowel than in peptic ulcer or inflammatory bowel disease (Thompson, 1984b). Other, non-specific symptoms include urinary frequency, nocturia, back pain, an unpleasant and often metallic taste in the mouth, and dyspareunia (Whorwell et al, 1986b). Patient-perceived severity is not related to a severity score or to psychological factors but it has an impact on quality of life. Thus, if patients can be reassured, quality of life may be improved considerably (Hahn et al, 1997b).

CLINICAL EXAMINATION

Examination is usually normal, although the patient is often tense and anxious. Examination of the abdomen is commonly made more difficult because the patient cannot relax. The sigmoid colon may be palpable and there may be pain on rectal examination. Fielding (1981) reported that pain elicited by tapping the posterior rectal mucosa was significantly more common in patients with the irritable bowel syndrome compared with controls (70% versus 5% respectively). The presence of audible gas during palpation of the right iliac fossa from a distended caecum is present in approximately one-third of patients, especially when diarrhoea is a predominant symptom.

Previous operations are common and include appendicectomy, hysterectomy, uterine suspension, removal of a normal gallbladder or laparotomy for adhesions; thus abdominal scars are common (Goulston, 1972a; Fielding, 1981; Prior et al, 1992). Sigmoidoscopy is mandatory for diagnosis. Patients should be told that sigmoidoscopy will exclude any serious rectal pathology. The presence of a normal rectum offers considerable reassurance, even if a colonoscopy or barium enema needs to be performed at a later date. The presence of a normal rectum is a great reassurance, for even if pathology is demonstrated elsewhere in the large bowel, patients can be told that a permanent colostomy will not be necessary.

PATHOPHYSIOLOGY

Motility

There is a widespread motility disorder involving smooth muscle not only of the large bowel but of the small intestine, bladder, gastro-oesophageal junction and the gallbladder (Kumar and Wingate, 1985; Preston et al, 1985; Whorwell et al, 1986a; Sciarretta et al, 1987; Smart and Atkinson, 1987). Whorwell et al (1981) reported that patients had lower oesophageal sphincter pressures than controls; furthermore, increased abdominal pressure caused gastro-oesophageal reflux. Smart and Atkinson (1987) demonstrated an abnormal response to insulin-induced hypoglycaemia, a poor protective response to increased abdominal pressure and abnormalities of pulse with respiration, suggesting a diffuse disorder of autonomic function.

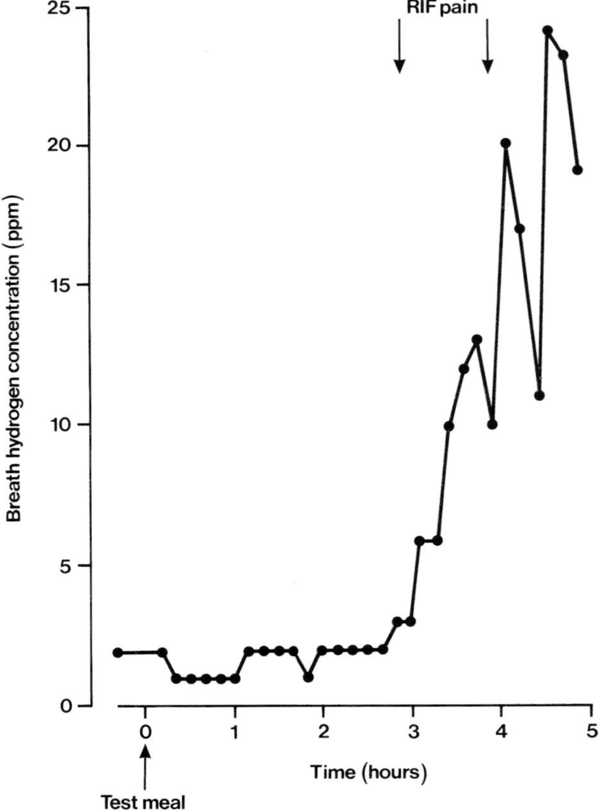

Figure 25.1 Breath hydrogen profile in the irritable bowel syndrome. Peak breath hydrogen concentrations and the appearance of the meal in the colon is associated with typical symptoms. RIF pain, right iliac fossa pain.

Cann et al (1983b) failed to demonstrate any change in the rate of gastric emptying but small bowel transit was abnormal, as measured by the hydrogen breath test (Figure 25.1). The rise in breath hydrogen associated with entry of unabsorbed carbohydrate residues into the colon may accompany the onset of pain in the right iliac fossa. Small bowel transit times (Thompson et al, 1979) were significantly shorter than those of controls in patients with abdominal pain but not in those with constipation (Figure 25.2). Kumar and Wingate (1985) reported spontaneous and stress-evoked irregular contractile activity in the small bowel, especially in men with the irritable bowel syndrome. Abnormal small bowel activity involves the jejunum as well as the ileum and may occur at night; propulsive waves coincide with episodes of abdominal pain (Kellow and Phillips, 1987). Dysmotility of the duodenum and jejunum was observed in irritable bowel syndrome, but reduced orocaecal transit did not correlate well with diarrhoea (Gorard et al, 1994).

Whole gut transit varies according to symptoms (Cann et al, 1983b): in patients with diarrhoea, whole gut transit times are shorter than those in controls, whereas in constipated patients, whole gut transit times are delayed (Table 25.6). Delayed transit is often associated with abdominal distension, bloating and pain which is relieved by defecation (Marcus and Heaton, 1987). Motility disturbance is very variable and is more common in psychoneurotic patients (Creed, 1994).

Sigmoid motility is increased in constipated patients but reduced in those with the irritable bowel syndrome having diarrhoea (Chaudhary and Truelove, 1961; Connell, 1962). However, motility studies in the sigmoid colon have provided conflicting results, depending on the manometric methods, bowel preparation used and the clinical subgroups

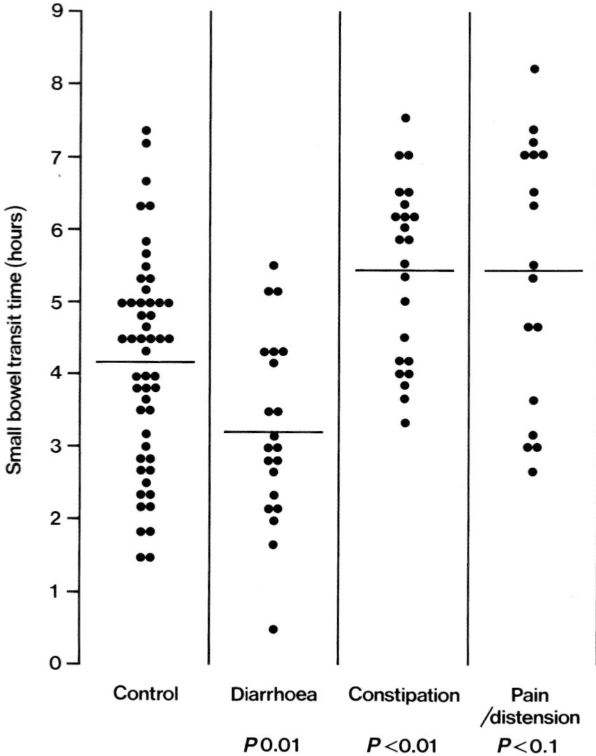

Figure 25.2 Small bowel transit time in three groups of patients with the irritable bowel syndrome, compared with controls. Those with constipation or with pain and distension had significantly longer small bowel transit times than those with diarrhoea.

studied. Hence patients with diarrhoea and abdominal pain had a hyperactive sigmoid colon, particularly after luminal distension and after food (Connell et al, 1965; Holdstock et al, 1969; Whitehead et al, 1980; Trotman and Misiewicz, 1988; Rogers et al, 1989). Painless diarrhoea was associated with migrating long spike bursts throughout the colon, especially after food.

Sensory parameters

Balloon distension of the rectum reproduced some of the symptoms of the irritable bowel syndrome, particularly in patients with pain, urgency and abdominal distension (Ritchie, 1973). Swarbrick et al (1980) showed that balloon distension of the colon in 29 of 48 patients was associated with pain characteristic of their disease, often at distant sites. Ritchie (1977) indicated that balloon distension caused no symptoms in asymptomatic diverticular disease but resulted in pain among those with symptomatic diverticular disease. This and other evidence suggests that symptoms in uncomplicated diverticular disease are probably due to the irritable colon syndrome and unrelated to radiographic diverticulosis on barium enema (Thompson et al, 1982). Increased sensitivity in the anorectum is associated with excessive motor reflex activity in the rectum, which may explain the symptoms of pain before defecation (Camilleri and Choi, 1997).

Myoelectrical activity

Two types of slow wave activity are present in the rectosigmoid. The major component has a frequency of 6–12 cycles per minute (Figure 25.3a) but there is a second, less obvious, component with a frequency of 3 cycles per minute (Snape et al, 1976) (Figure 25.3b). The 3-cycles/minute pattern at rest seems to be characteristic of the irritable bowel syndrome (Snape et al, 1977) and persists even when patients become asymptomatic (Taylor et al, 1978a). Taylor et al (1978b) showed that the 3-cycles/minute activity occurred in 50% of patients with the irritable bowel syndrome compared with only 14% of patients with diarrhoea from organic disease (Figure 25.4). The short spike bursts appear to

Table 25.6 Transit measurements in normal volunteers and patients with irritable bowel syndrome.

	Irritable bowel syndrome			
	Control	*Diarrhoea*	*Constipation*	*Pain*
Gastric emptying (+0.5 h)				
Females	1.6	1.6	1.8	1.4
Males	1.3	1.3	—	—
Small bowel transit time (h)	4.2	3.3*	5.4*	5.4*
Whole gut transit (50% markers: h)	54	35*	87*	61
Daily stool weight (g)				
Females	112	128	61*	86
Males	166	230*	—	—

*Significantly different from controls $P < 0.05$.
From Cann et al (1983b).

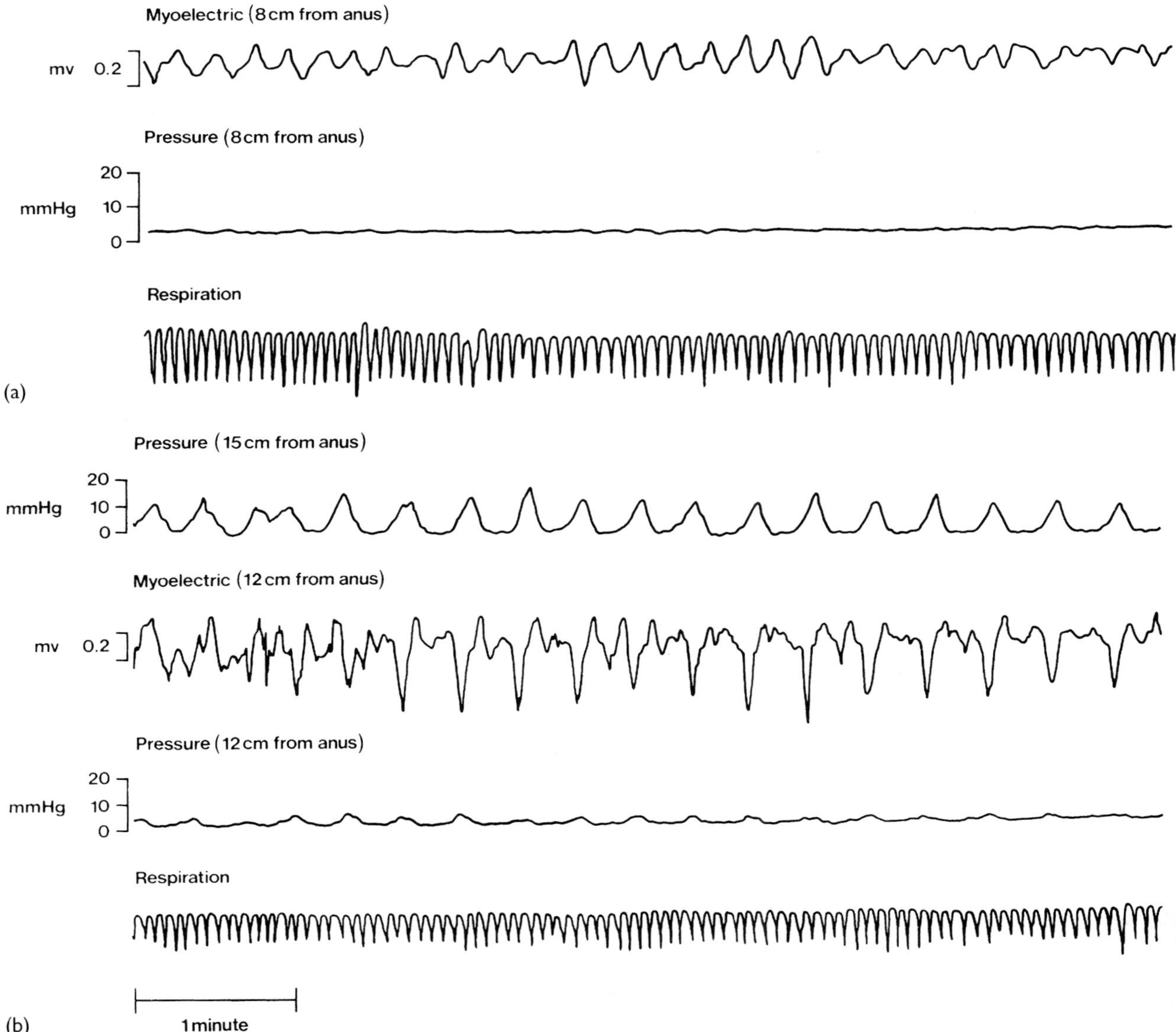

Figure 25.3a,b Colorectal manometry and myoelectrical activity in the irritable bowel syndrome. (a) Simultaneous myoelectrical activity and manometry 8 cm from the anal verge in a normal subject. (b) Manometric and myoelectrical data in a patient with the irritable bowel syndrome during an episode of colicky abdominal pain. From Snape et al (1976).

originate from circular smooth muscle fibres and correlate with episodes of abdominal pain (Bueno et al, 1980; Frexinos et al, 1987). The 3-cycles/minute contractile activity increased after administration of cholecystokinin and pentagastrin (Figure 25.5) in patients with the irritable bowel syndrome but not in normal subjects (Snape et al, 1976). This pattern was also observed in psychoneurotic patients without intestinal symptoms (Latimer et al, 1981).

Recently, studies have become less costly and less invasive using isotopic techniques which define areas of rapid or delayed transit.

Neuroendocrine abnormalities (Stivland et al, 1991)

The possible relationship between the irritable bowel syndrome and the motor response to cholecystokinin has already been referred to (Harvey and Read, 1973). A variety of endocrine abnormalities were identified by Preston et al (1985); increased pancreatic polypeptide levels were found in many patients provided they did not suffer from constipation, in which case impaired release of motilin and

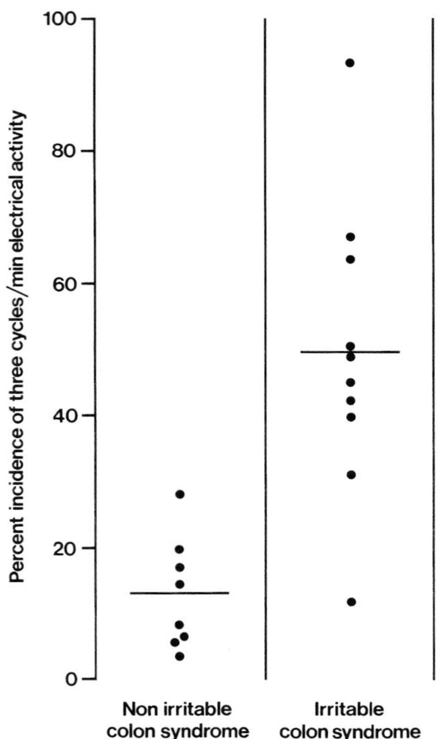

Figure 25.4 The percentage incidence of 3-cycles/minute electrical activity in the irritable colon syndrome compared with normal controls.

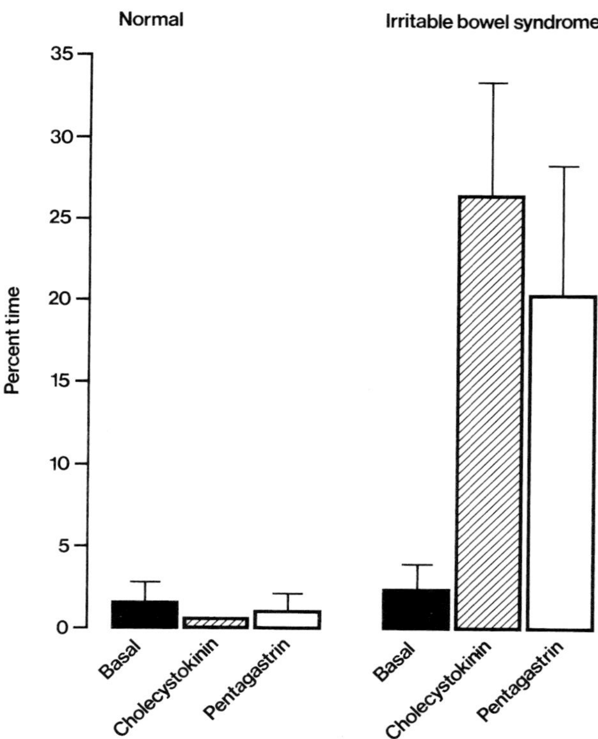

Figure 25.5 Percentage of total recording time occupied by 3 cycles/minute of colonic contractions for the 10-minute period after cholecystokinin or pentagastrin administration in normal subjects and in patients with the irritable bowel syndrome. From Snape et al (1977).

gastrin was evident (Vantrappen et al, 1979). An earlier study suggested, however, that fasting and postprandial gut hormone levels were normal in the irritable bowel syndrome (Besterman et al, 1981). Although constipation may be caused by hypothyroidism or hyperparathyroidism and diarrhoea from thyrotoxicosis, carcinoid tumours, glucogonoma, medullary carcinoma of the thyroid or pancreatic islet cell tumours, none seem likely to be implicated in the irritable bowel syndrome. Adrenal medullary activity is increased in patients with diarrhoea and the irritable bowel syndrome and there may be increased sensitivity to parasympathomimetic drugs (Wright and Das, 1969).

AETIOLOGY

The irritable bowel syndrome appears to be due to a diffuse disorder of smooth muscle function but the underlying mechanisms for initiating this acquired disorder are unknown. Two possible mechanisms are altered bowel sensitivity and psychosocial factors. Other theories include infective diarrhoea and diet.

Infective diarrhoea

Irregularity of bowel habit and abdominal pain commonly persists in patients after an attack of infective enteritis even when repeated stool cultures fail to demonstrate evidence of an enteropathogen (Neal et al, 1997). Chaudhary and Truelove (1962) reported that approximately a quarter of patients with irritable bowel dated the onset of symptoms with an attack of dysentery, but a microbiological aetiology was lacking (Connell et al, 1964).

Lactose intolerance

Lactose malabsorption causes diarrhoea, abdominal pain and distension which are often indistinguishable from the irritable bowel syndrome. Symptoms are precipitated by consuming milk products and there is reduced lactase activity in the jejunal mucosa. Weser et al (1965) studied 27 symptomatic subjects and identified 13 with reduced lactase activity from jejunal biopsies associated with flat lactose tolerance curves. Gudmand-Hoyer et al (1973) identified flat lactose tolerance curves in 20 of 98 patients with the irritable bowel syndrome. However, the incidence of lactose intolerance in the normal population is probably similar to that reported in the irritable bowel syndrome (Pena and Truelove, 1972).

Treatment of patients by dietary exclusion and food challenge indicates that food intolerance is very common in this syndrome and that dairy products are frequently responsible for symptoms (Nanda et al, 1989). Malabsoption of fructose or sorbitol has also been implicated, but the proportion of individuals with malabsorption in irritable bowel syndrome does not appear to differ from that in the normal population (Hyams, 1983; Rumessen and Gudmand-Hoyer, 1988). Bile acid malabsorption has also been implicated by some (Oddson et al, 1978).

Food allergy

Intolerance to food may be a factor in the aetiology of the irritable bowel syndrome (Nanda et al, 1989). Intolerance to wheat, dairy products, beverages and citrus fruits was found in 14 of 21 patients (Bentley et al, 1983). Food allergens are potential causative agents, and a trial of dietary exclusions showed improvement in 72 of 91 patients over 15 months (Nanda et al, 1989).

Rectal prostaglandin E_2 levels rose after eating food products which were associated with onset of diarrhoea (Jones et al, 1982). Most luminal factors probably aggravate underlying irritable bowel syndrome rather than being the intrinsic cause.

Diet

Gastrocolic reflex

Many patients with the irritable bowel syndrome complain of postprandial pain which is associated with exaggerated sigmoid pressures (Holdstock et al, 1969) and increased myoelectrical activity in response to food (Snape et al, 1978). Fat intake is often responsible for the exaggerated postprandial sigmoid motility disorder in the irritable bowel syndrome (Wright et al, 1980) and may be inhibited by ingestion of protein or amino acids. Inhibition of postprandial activity was observed with anticholinergic agents, suggesting that a neurohumoral factor may be responsible for this reflex (Snape et al, 1979).

Fibre

The irritable bowel syndrome may be due to lack of dietary fibre (Burkitt et al, 1972); hence bran has been used successfully in the long-term control of symptoms (Harvey et al, 1987; Prior and Whorwell, 1987). However, fibre may make certain symptoms worse, particularly abdominal distension (Thompson, 1984a). Furthermore, response is better in men than in women and in those with constipation, particularly if the history is short (Harvey et al, 1987).

Drugs

Certain drugs may precipitate symptoms; these include antacids, antibiotics, analgesics, diuretics, laxatives and β-blockers (Read et al, 1980).

PSYCHOGENIC FACTORS

The interplay between psychogenic factors and the irritable bowel syndrome has received much attention (Whitehead et al, 1992). Psychological symptoms include: somatization, anxiety, phobia and paranoia. Patients with this syndrome seem less able to cope with stress and there is a higher incidence of depression, especially among women (Johnsen et al, 1986). Interestingly, an increased incidence of the disorder was recorded near the end of World War II (Peters and Bargen, 1944). Stress has been a feature in many adult patients (Waller and Misiewicz, 1969) and it is also identified in children with this disorder (Stone and Barbero, 1970). Nailbiting is common (Heaton and Mountford, 1992). Although stress is often responsible for exacerbating symptoms it cannot always be implicated as the sole cause of disease (Welch et al, 1985). Nevertheless, there is a high incidence of psychiatric disorder, especially depression, in these patients (Rose et al, 1986). Marital disharmony, dyspareunia and sexual dissatisfaction are more common than in patients with inflammatory bowel disease or peptic ulceration (Ford et al, 1982; Creed and Guthrie, 1987).

The role of physical and sexual abuse in the development of irritable bowel syndrome is controversial. Patients with the irritable bowel syndrome are probably more neurotic, anxious and depressed than the normal population (Ford et al, 1987). However, studies which have attempted to assess these symptoms in the irritable bowel syndrome are flawed since (a) the assessment of psychiatric symptom scores have not been validated, (b) the classification of the irritable bowel syndrome has often been imprecise and (c) selective populations have been used for study (Mendeloff et al, 1970; Hislop, 1971; Creed and Guthrie, 1987). Indeed, Whitehead et al (1980) reported that in patients with painful diarrhoea the incidence of psychopathology was not increased and could not be correlated with the severity of symptoms.

Severe underlying psychological disturbance is associated with a poor prognosis (Creed and Guthrie, 1987) and is often manifest by disordered close personal relationships and a failure to respond to stress or to cope with threatening situations (Creed et al, 1988). Increased psychopathology (Creed and Guthrie, 1987) is particularly evident in patients who seek medical advice (Sandler et al, 1984); conversely the incidence is much less in patients with the irritable bowel syndrome who do not consult the medical profession.

INVESTIGATIONS

Both from the point of view of the patient and the surgeon the most important consideration is the exclusion of serious pathology. Some clinicians have argued against exhaustive investigation on the grounds that patients become introverted, and that symptoms are aggravated. Considerable clinical judgement is therefore required to decide whether patients should have the sort of investigations recommended by the Sheffield group (Table 25.7) or whether history, clinical examination and flexible sigmoidoscopy is sufficient to exclude left colonic cancer and inflammatory bowel disease. It is said that patients with non-organic disease can usually be detected when first interviewed (Thompson, 1984a,b). Under these circumstances it is now our practice in young patients without a history of bowel disease to advise a flexible sigmoidoscopy and a barium enema if necessary so that patients can be reassured that there is no serious organic pathology. More extensive investigations are expensive and are only undertaken if there has been no response to medical therapy or a change in the symptom pattern during long-term follow-up (Wells et al, 1997).

Table 25.7 Screening investigations.

Full blood count + erythrocyte sedimentation rate
Plasma urea/electrolytes/calcium
Liver function tests
Rectal biopsy
Stool microscopy + culture
Barium meal + follow-through
Barium enema
Thyroid function tests
Fecal fat excretion
Serum folate + vitamin B_{12}
Schilling test
[^{14}C]glycocholate breath test
Lactose tolerance tests
Urinary 5-hydroxyindoleacetic acid

From Cann et al (1983b).

It must be remembered that organic pathology in the pelvis may give rise to intestinal symptoms and that a gynaecological, orthopaedic and urological assessment may be indicated in some patients.

DIFFERENTIAL DIAGNOSIS

Disorders other than colorectal carcinoma and inflammatory bowel disease which require exclusion are endocrine pathology, upper gastrointestinal disease, pancreaticobiliary disorders and serious psychiatric disease. Endocrine disorders to be excluded include disturbed thyroid function, hyperparathyroidism, carcinoid tumours, adrenocortical and medullary tumours, islet cell tumours, glucogonoma and medullary carcinoma of the thyroid. Chronic pancreatitis, gallstones, pancreatic carcinoma or biliary dyskinesia may be difficult to distinguish from the irritable bowel syndrome and they may require investigation by ultrasonography, cholecystography, cholecystokinin provocation tests, endoscopic retrograde cholangiopancreatography (ERCP) and CT scanning. Upper gastrointestinal disease such as gastro-oesophageal reflux, peptic ulcer, gastric carcinoma and Crohn's disease can be excluded by endoscopy and barium follow-through examination.

MEDICAL TREATMENT

General

The management of the irritable bowel syndrome requires much time, patience and insight into the patient's personality and lifestyle. Once the patient has been reassured that there is no organic pathology, most surgeons will refer the patient back to their primary care physician or seek the advice of an understanding gastro-enterologist. For this reason we do not propose to deal exhaustively with medical therapy, but recognize that some of these patients have established a relationship with a surgeon and will wish to remain under that person's surveillance.

The natural history of the irritable bowel syndrome is one of repeated episodes of intestinal symptoms, often precipitated by emotional stress, which are interspersed with periods of complete relief of symptoms. Holmes and Salter (1982) reviewed 77 patients who were diagnosed as having the irritable bowel syndrome 6 years earlier to assess the prognosis of this disorder. Forty-four of their patients remained symptomatic; hence the authors concluded that the irritable bowel syndrome was a chronic relapsing condition which was rarely cured. Harvey et al (1987) take a more optimistic view, and report an 85% short-term response to high-fibre diet and bulking agents, with 68% of patients remaining symptom free after 5 years.

Placebo

Scrutiny of the available placebo control trials suggests that approximately one-third of patients with the irritable bowel syndrome improve on placebo therapy (Moriarty, 1992). The implication is that no potentially harmful therapy should be advised unless it is substantially better than a placebo. Furthermore, considerable therapeutic benefit is to be derived from the physician–patient encounter alone. Factors of importance in the doctor–patient interview are the reassurance that there is no serious underlying disorder and an understanding by the patient that someone is interested in his or her problem. Satisfactory explanation by the doctor of the psychophysiological cause of symptoms is also important (Creed and Guthrie, 1987; Harding et al, 1997).

Bran

There is not much evidence to support the use of bran alone in the irritable bowel syndrome. Bran has been shown to improve symptoms in uncomplicated diverticular disease but such symptoms are probably due to the irritable bowel rather than the radiological abnormality seen in the sigmoid colon (Brodribb, 1977). Although Lucey et al (1987) showed the symptomatic advantage of bran over placebo, present evidence suggests that bran therapy should be confined to patients whose principal symptom is constipation. Although some studies show benefit with bran, most suggest that symptoms are made worse by bran or high-fibre intake (Soltoff et al, 1976; Manning et al, 1977; Cann et al, 1984; Snook and Shepherd, 1994).

Diet

A diet low in fat and with a high protein content may improve symptoms. If there is any evidence of lactase deficiency, elimination of milk products should be explored. Dietary challenge may identify other foods, particularly cereal products, which aggravate symptoms and these should be avoided within reason (Nanda et al, 1989). There is a real danger in using elimination diets of making the patient introspective and a balance will have to be struck between selective dietary intake and dietary obsession.

Drugs

Ispaghula alone in a dose of 20–30 g has been shown to increase stool weight and improve symptoms in the irritable bowel syndrome (Kumar et al, 1987). Ispaghula gave results which were superior to placebo therapy but did not control abdominal pain or bloating (Prior and Whorwell, 1987).

Results from drug trials seem to imply that a combination of agents provides significantly greater symptomatic improvement than single agents alone (Goulston, 1972b; Ritchie and Truelove, 1980). Neither tranquillizers alone nor antidepressants in normal doses are usually of benefit in the irritable bowel syndrome (Clouse et al, 1994). Furthermore, anticholinergic agents by themselves are not associated with significant improvement (Ivey, 1975; Page and Dirnberger, 1981). The only patients in whom antispasmodics appear to be beneficial are those with postprandial pain, but there is a high incidence of side-effects (Page and Dirnberger, 1981).

In view of the disturbance of intestinal transit in the irritable bowel syndrome, agents known to enhance gastric emptying and small bowel transit, such as the peripheral dopamine antagonist domperidone, might be considered advantageous (Fielding, 1982). However, Cann et al (1983a) were unable to demonstrate any clinical benefit with this agent.

Combination therapy using bulking agents (either ispaghula or bran), psychotropic drugs (lorazepam or Motival) and smooth muscle relaxants (hyoscine or mebeverine) were compared by Ritchie and Truelove (1980). The best results were recorded using a combination of ispaghula, Motival and mebeverine.

The calcium antagonist nicardipine inhibits postprandial motility and intraluminal pressure and may therefore have a place in the treatment of the irritable bowel syndrome (Prior et al, 1987). Calcium channel blockers may play a role in reducing colonic motility (Maxton and Whorwell, 1990). Calcium polycarbophil may have a role in treatment (Toskes et al, 1993). Medical treatment of irritable bowel syndrome should probably be directed to motility disorders or altered visceral sensation (Figure 25.6). Antimuscarinic agents, serotoninergic antagonists, alpha 2 adrenergic agents or somatostatin analogues may be directed at abnormal motility.

Poynard et al (1994) undertook a meta-analysis of smooth muscle relaxants in the irritable bowel syndrome and reported that the following were effective in controlling colic and better than a placebo: cimetropium bromide, pinaverium bromide, trimebutine, octilium bromide and mebeverine. Peppermint oils and hyoscine were less effective (Table 25.8). Evans et al (1996) reported that mebeverine normalizes disordered motility and improves symptoms. Maxton et al (1996) explored the role of 5-hydroxytryptamine antagonists, particularly ondansetron, which reduced bowel frequency.

Drugs modulating afferent gut receptors and having an influence on psychosocial factors include tricyclics, selective serotonin uptake inhibitors, serotoninergic antagonists, kappa opioid antagonists, alpha 2 adrenergic agents and somatostatin analogues. Low-dose antidepressants have been shown to be effective (Figure 25.7).

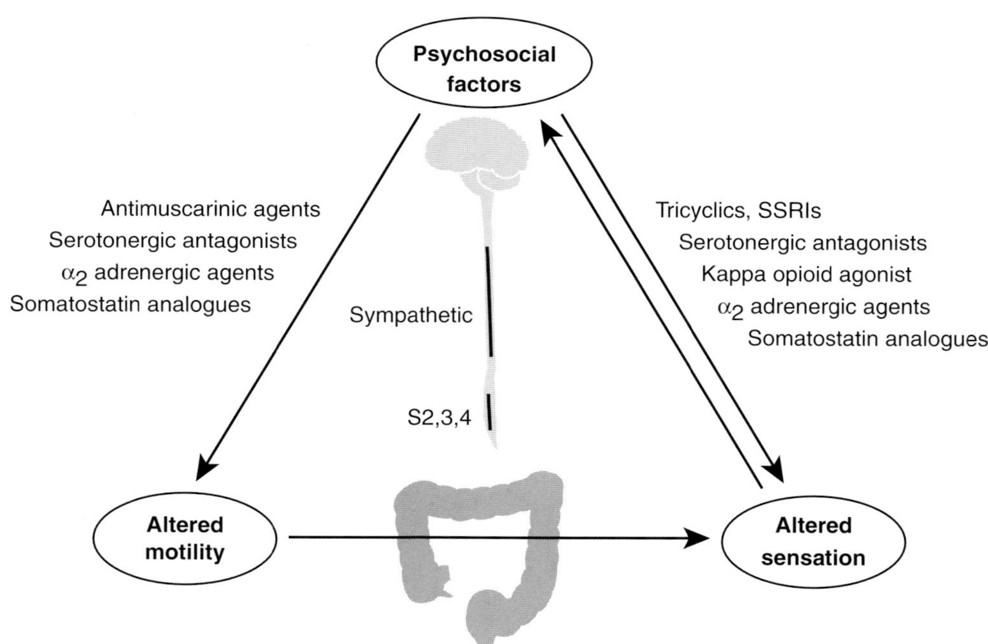

Figure 25.6 Potential new pharmacological agents in the treatment of irritable bowel syndrome, based on experimental studies performed in healthy subjects, or in patients with the syndrome. From Camilleri and Choi (1997).

Table 25.8 Efficacy of anticholinergics/antispasmodics in the treatment of the irritable bowel syndrome.

				Abdominal pain			*Overall assessment*				
		n	*Duration (weeks)*	*Drug (%)*	*Placebo (%)*	*P*	*Drug (%)*	*Placebo (%)*	*P*	*Side-effects (%)*	*References*
Mebeverine	PG	40	16	23	28	NS				None	Kruis et al (1986)
	XO	24	8	83	33	< 0.05	83	33	< 0.05	None	Tasman-Jones (1973)
	XO	60	2	71	22	< 0.001	71	25	≤ 0.001	10	Capurso et al (1984)
	PG	36	8				81	55	< 0.01		Berthelot & Centonze (1981)
Peppermint oil	XO	29	2				83	17	<0.001		Dew et al (1995)
	XO	41	2				39	52	NS	24	Nash et al (1986)
	XO	18	9				50	13	< 0.01		Rees et al (1979)
Octylonium	XO	60	2	73	22	< 0.001	71	25	≤ 0.001	10	Capurso et al (1984)
Prifinium	XO	18	3				78	33	< 0.01		Pial & Mazzacca (1979)
Trimebutine	XO	20	4	60	20	< 0.01					Moshal & Herron (1979)
	PG	30	24	75	66	NS	62	68	NS		Fielding (1980)
Cimetropium	PG	35	24				89	69	< 0.05		Dobrilla et al (1990)
	PG	15	24	80	28	< 0.05					Pial et al 1987
	PG	48	24	87	16	< 0.01	87	24	< 0.01	48	Centonze et al (1988)
Dicyclomine	PG	49	2	56	41	< 0.05	84	53	< 0.01		Page & Dirnberger (1981)
Hyoscine	PG	182	4				76	64	< 0.001		Schafer & Ewe (1990)

PG, parallel group; XO, cross-over.
From Camilleri and Choi (1997).

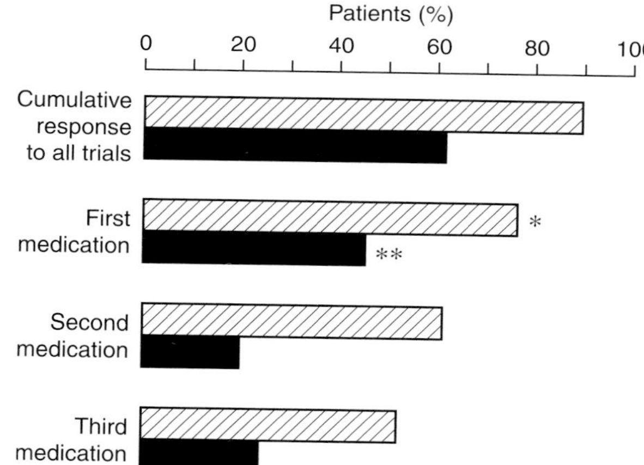

Figure 25.7 Percentage of patients assessed as having improvement (hatched) or complete remission (black) of irritable bowel syndrome during antidepressant treatment (n = 138). *$P < 0.05$; **$P < 0.01$. From Clouse et al (1994).

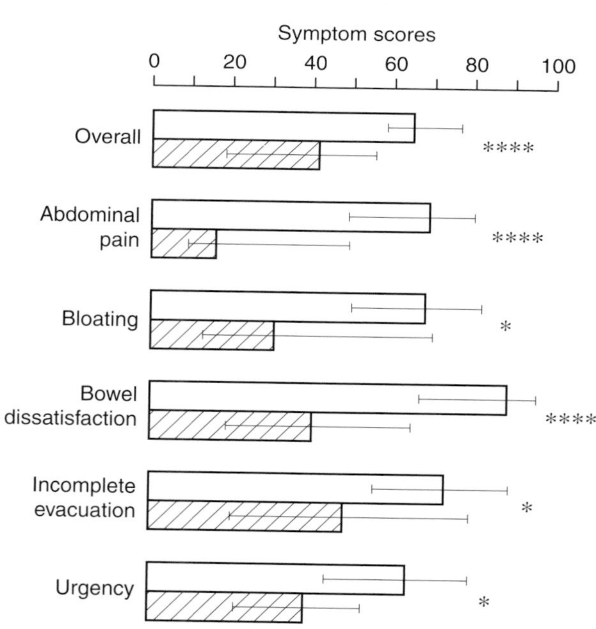

Figure 25.8 Comparison of the classical symptoms of the irritable bowel syndrome in patients after hypnotherapy (white), with controls (hatched). Results expressed as median and interquartile range. ****$P < 0.0001$; *$P < 0.05$. From Houghton et al (1996).

Psychotherapy and hypnotherapy

Swedlund et al (1983) reported the results of psychotherapy in 101 patients with the irritable bowel syndrome given standard medical therapy with bulking agents, anticholinergic drugs, antacids and mild tranquillizers. These patients were randomly allocated to receive psychotherapy (10 sessions of 1 hour each over 3 months) or no psychotherapy. Although there was an improvement in the psychotherapy group this difference only became evident after 1 year. Patients in the psychotherapy group seemed to have learned more effectively how to cope with their symptoms and lifestyle than the controls. Harvey et al (1989) reported sustained improvement in 20 of 33 patients treated by hypnotherapy. Hypnotherapy may be associated with objective changes in anorectal physiology (Prior et al, 1990a).

Houghton et al (1996) reported that hypnotherapy reduced abdominal pain, bloating, nausea, flatulence, urinary symptoms, bowel habit, lethargy, backache and dyspareunia (Figure 25.8). It also improved mood, focus of control, wellbeing, work attitude and less time was lost from work. These results appear to be sustained during follow-up.

Surgical considerations

Most surgeons would not operate for the irritable bowel syndrome alone but recognize that many patients with disorders of defecation also have features of the syndrome. Careful evaluation is thus emphasized for all patients with incontinence, rectal prolapse, solitary ulcer constipation and inflammatory bowel disease to determine the prominence of the irritable bowel syndrome in these clinical disorders.

REFERENCES

Aggarwal A, Cutts SF, Abell TL et al (1994) Predominant symptoms in irritable bowel syndrome correlate with specific autonomic nervous system abnormalities. *Gastroenterology* **106**: 945–950.

Agreus L, Svardsudd K, Nyren O et al (1994) The epidemiology of abdominal symptoms: prevalence and demographic characteristics in a Swedish adult population. *Scand J Gastroenterol* **29**: 102–109.

Bentley SJ, Pearson DJ & Rix KJ (1983) Food hypersensitivity in irritable bowel syndrome. *Lancet* **ii**: 296–298.

Berthelot J & Centonze M (1981) Etude contrôllée en double aveugle Duspatalin (Mébévérine) contre placebo, dans le traitement du côlon irritable. *Gaz Med Fr* **88**: 2343.

Besterman HS, Sarson DL, Ramband JC, Stewart JS, Guerin S & Bloom SR (1981) Gut hormone responses in the irritable bowel syndrome. *Digestion* **21**: 219–224.

Bi-zhen W & Qi-ying P (1988) Functional bowel disorders in apparently healthy Chinese people. *Chin J Epidemiol* **9**: 345–349.

Brodribb AJM (1977) Treatment of symptomatic diverticular disease with a high fibre diet. *Lancet* **i**: 664–666.

Bueno L, Fioramonti J, Ruckebusch Y, Frexinos J & Coulom P (1980) Evaluation of colonic myoelectrical activity in health and functional disorders. *Gut* **21**: 480–485.

Burkitt DP, Walker ARP & Painter NS (1972) Effect of dietary fibre on stools and transit times and its role in the causation of disease. *Lancet* **ii**: 1408–1412.

Camilleri M & Choi MG (1997) Review article: irritable bowel syndrome. *Aliment Pharmacol Ther* **11**: 3–15.

Cann PA, Read NW & Holdsworth CD (1983a) Oral domperidone: double blind comparison with placebo in irritable bowel syndrome. *Gut* **24**: 1135–1140.

Cann PA, Read NW, Brown C, Hobson N & Holdsworth CD (1983b) Irritable bowel syndrome: relationship of disorders in the transit of a single solid meal to symptom patterns. *Gut* **24**: 405–411.

Cann PA, Read NW & Holdsworth CD (1984) What is the benefit of coarse wheat bran in patients with irritable bowel syndrome? *Gut* **25**: 168–173.

Capurso L, Koch M, Tarquini M et al (1984) The irritable syndrome: A cross-over study of octilonium bromide, mebeverine and placebo. *Clin Trials J* **21**: 285–291.

Centonze V, Imbimbo BP, Campanozzi F et al (1988) Oral cimetropium bromide, a new antimuscarinic drug, for long-term treatment of irritable bowel syndrome. *Am J Gastroenterol* **83**: 1262–1266.

Chaudhary NA & Truelove SC (1961) Human colonic motility. A comparative study of normal subjects, patients with ulcerative colitis and patients with irritable bowel syndrome. I. Resting patterns of motility. II. The effect of Prostigmin. III. Effects of emotions. *Gastroenterology* **40**: 1–89.

Chaudhary NA & Truelove SC (1962) The irritable colon syndrome. A study of the clinical features, predisposing causes and prognosis in 130 cases. *Q J Med* **31**: 307–312.

Christensen J (1992). Pathophysiology of the irritable bowel syndrome. *Lancet* **340**: 1444–1447.

Clouse RE, Lustman PJ, Geisman RA & Alpers DR (1994) Antidepressant therapy in 138 patients with irritable bowel syndrome: a five year clinical experience. *Aliment Pharmacol Ther* **8**: 409–416.

Connell AM (1962) The motility of the pelvic colon. II. Paradoxical motility in diarrhoea and constipation. *Gut* **3**: 342–348.

Connell AM, Gaafer M, Hassanein MA & Khayal MA (1964) Motility of the pelvic colon. III. Motility responses in patients with symptoms following amoebic dysentery. *Gut* **5**: 443–448.

Connell AM, Jones FA & Rowlands EN (1965) Motility of the pelvic colon. IV. Abdominal pain associated with colonic hypermotility after meals. *Gut* **6**: 105–112.

Cook IJ, van Eeden A & Collins SM (1987) Patients with irritable bowel syndrome have greater pain tolerance than normal subjects. *Gastroenterology* **93**: 727–733.

Creed F (1994) Psychological treatment is essential for some. *BMJ* **309**: 1647.

Creed F & Guthrie E (1987) Psychological factors in the irritable bowel syndrome. *Gut* **28**: 1307–1318.

Creed F, Craig T & Farmer R (1988) Functional abdominal pain, psychiatric illness, and life events. *Gut* **29**: 235–242.

Davidson M & Wasserman R (1966) The irritable colon of childhood: chronic non-specific diarrhoea syndrome. *J Pediatr* **69**: 1027–1032.

Dew MJ, Evans BK & Rhodes J (1995) Peppermint oil for the irritable bowel syndrome: a multicentre trial. *Br J Clin Pract* **38**: 394.

Dimson SB (1971) Transit time related to clinical findings in children with recurrent abdominal pain. *Paediatrics* **47**: 666–669.

Dobrilla G, Imbimbo BP, Piazzi L & Bensi G (1990) Longterm treatment of irritable bowel syndrome with cimetropium bromide: a double-blind placebo-controlled trial. *Gut* **31**: 355–358.

Doshi M & Heaton KW (1994) Irritable bowel syndrome in patients discharged from surgical wards with non-specific abdominal pain. *Br J Surg* **81**: 1216–1218.

Drossman DA, Sandler RS, McKee DC & Lovitz AJ (1982) Bowel dysfunction among subjects not seeking health care. *Gastroenterology* **83**: 529–534.

Drossman DA, Li Z, Andruzzi E et al (1993) U.S. householder survey of functional gastrointestinal disorders. *Dig Dis Sci* **38**: 1569–1580.

Eastwood MA, Eastwood J & Ford MJ (1987) The irritable bowel syndrome: a disease or a response? *J R Soc Med* **80**: 219–222.

Evans PR, Bakk YT & Kellow JE (1996). Mebeverine alters small bowel motility in irritable bowel syndrome. *Aliment Pharmacol Ther* **10**: 787–793.

Fielding JF (1980) Double-blind trial of trimebutine in the irritable bowel syndrome. *Ir Med J* **73**: 377–379.

Fielding JF (1981) The diagnostic sensitivity of physical signs in the irritable bowel syndrome. *J Irish Med Assoc* **74**: 143–144.

Fielding JF (1982) Domperidone treatment in the irritable bowel syndrome. *Digestion* **23**: 125–127.

Ford MJ, Eastwood J & Eastwood MA (1982) The irritable bowel syndrome: soma and psyche. *Psychol Med* **12**: 705–707.

Ford MJ, Miller PMcC, Eastwood J & Eastwood MA (1987) Life events, psychiatric illness and the irritable bowel syndrome. *Gut* **28**: 160–165.

Francis CY, Morris J & Whorwell PJ (1997) The irritable bowel severity scoring system: a simple method of monitoring irritable bowel syndrome and its progress. *Aliment Pharmacol Ther* **11**: 395–402.

Frexinos J, Fioramonti J & Bueno L (1987) Colonic myoelectrical activity in IBS painless diarrhoea. *Gut* **28**: 1613–1618.

Gorard DA, Libby GW & Farthing (1994) Ambulatory small intestinal motility in 'diarrhoea' predominant irritable bowel syndrome. *Gut* **35**: 203–210.

Goulston K (1972a) Clinical diagnosis of the irritable colon syndrome. *Med J Aust* **1**: 1122–1125.

Goulston K (1972b) Drug usage in the irritable colon syndrome. *Med J Aust* **1**: 1126–1127.

Gudmand-Hoyer E, Rus P & Wulff HR (1973) The significance of lactose malabsorption in the irritable colon syndrome. *Scand J Gastroenterol* **8**: 273–277.

Hahn BA, Kirchdoerfer LJ, Fullerton S & Mayer E (1997a) Evaluation of a new quality of life questionnaire for patients with irritable bowel syndrome. *Aliment Pharmacol Ther* **11**: 547–552.

Hahn BA, Kirchdoerfer LJ, Fullerton S & Mayer E (1997b) Patient perceived severity of irritable bowel syndrome in relation to symptoms, health resource utilization and quality of life. *Aliment Pharmacol Ther* **11**: 553–559.

Harding JP, Hamm LR, Ehsanullah RSB et al (1997) use of a novel electronic data collection system in multicenter studies of irritable bowel syndrome. *Aliment Pharmacol Ther* **11**: 1073–1076.

Harvey RF & Read AE (1973) Effect of cholecystokinin on colonic motility and symptoms in patients with the irritable bowel syndrome. *Lancet* **i**: 1–3.

Harvey RF, Salih SY & Read AE (1983) Organic and functional disorders in 2000 gastroenterology outpatients. *Lancet* **ii**: 623–634.

Harvey RF, Mauad EC & Brown AM (1987) Prognosis in the irritable bowel syndrome: a 5-year prospective study. *Lancet* **i**: 963–969.

Harvey RF, Hinton RA, Gunary RM & Barry RE (1989) Individual and group hypnotherapy in treatment of refractory irritable bowel syndrome. *Lancet* **ii**: 424–429.

Heaton KW (1983) Irritable bowel syndrome: still in search of its identity. *BMJ* **287**: 852–853.

Heaton KW & Mountford RA (1992) Nail-biting in the population and its relationship to irritable bowel syndrome. *J R Soc Med* **85**: 457.

Heaton KW, Ghosh S & Braddon FEM (1991) How bad are the symptoms and bowel dysfunction of patients with the irritable bowel syndrome? A prospective, controlled study with emphasis on stool form. *Gut* **32**: 73–79.

Heaton KW, Parker D & Cripps H (1993) Bowel function and irritable bowel symptoms after hysterectomy and cholecystectomy – a population based study. *Gut* **34**: 1108–1111.

Hislop IG (1971) Psychological significance of the irritable colon syndrome. *Gut* **12**: 452–459.

Holdstock DJ, Misiewicz JJ & Walker SL (1969) Observations on the mechanism of abdominal pain. *Gut* **10**: 19–31.

Holmes KM & Salter RH (1982) Irritable bowel syndrome – a safe diagnosis? *BMJ* **285**: 1533–1534.

Houghton LA, Heyman DJ & Whorwell PJ (1996) Symptomatology, quality of life and economic features of irritable bowel syndrome – the effect of hypnotherapy. *Aliment Pharmacol Ther* **10**: 91–95.

Hunt T (1957) The spastic colon. *Practitioner* **179**: 561–579.

Hyams JS (1983) Sorbitol intolerance: an unappreciated cause of functional gastrointestnal complaints. *Gastroenterology* **84**: 30–33.

Ivey KJ (1975) Are anticholinergics of use in the irritable colon syndrome? *Gastroenterology* **68**: 1300–1307.

Johnsen R, Jacobsen BK & Forde OH (1986) Associations between symptoms of irritable colon and psychological and social conditions and lifestyle. *BMJ* **292**: 1633–1639.

Jones R & Lydiard S (1992) Irritable bowel syndrome in the general population. *BMJ* **304**: 87–90.

Jones VA, McLaughlin P, Shorthouse M & Workman E (1982) Food intolerance: a major factor in the pathogenesis of the irritable bowel syndrome. *Lancet* **ii**: 1115–1117.

Kay L, Jorgensen T & Jensen KH (1994) The epidemiology of irritable bowel syndrome in a random population: prevalence, incidence, natural history and risk factors. *J Intern Med* **236**: 23–30.

Kellow JE & Phillips SF (1987) Altered small bowel motility in irritable bowel syndrome is correlated with symptoms. *Gastroenterology* **92**: 1885–1893.

Kruis W, Weinsierl M, Schussler P & Holl J (1986) Comparison of the therapeutic effect of wheat bran, mebeverine and placebo in patients with the irritable bowel syndrome. *Digestion* **34**: 196–201.

Kumar A, Kumar N, Vij JC, Sarin SK & Anand BS (1987) Optimum dosage of ispaghula husk in patients with irritable bowel syndrome: correlation of symptom relief with gut transit time and stool weight. *Gut* **28**: 150–155.

Kumar D & Wingate DL (1985) The irritable bowel syndrome: a paroxysmal motor disorder. *Lancet* **i**: 973–980.

Latimer P, Sarna S, Campbell D, Latimer M, Waterfall W & Daniel EE (1981) Colonic motor and myoelectrical activity: a comparative study of normal subjects, psychoneurotic patients and patients with the irritable bowel syndrome. *Gastroenterology* **80**: 893–901.

Longstreth GF & Wolde-Tsadik G (1993) Irritable bowel-type symptoms in HMO examinees. *Dig Dis Sci* **38**: 1581–1589.

Lucey MR, Clark ML, Lowndes J & Dawson AM (1987) Is bran efficacious in irritable bowel syndrome? A double blind placebo controlled crossover study. *Gut* **28**: 221–225.

Manning AP, Heaton KW, Harvey RF & Uglow P (1977) Wheat fibre and the irritable bowel syndrome. *Lancet* **ii**: 417–418.

Manning AP, Thompson WG, Heaton KW & Morris AF (1978) Towards positive diagnosis of the irritable bowel. *BMJ* **2**: 653–654.

Marcus SN & Heaton KW (1987) Irritable bowel-type symptoms in spontaneous and induced constipation. *Gut* **28**: 156–159.

Massarrat S, Saberi-Firoozi M, Soleimani A et al (1995) Peptic ulcer disease, irritable bowel syndrome and constipation in two populations in Iran. *Eur J Gastroenterol Hepatol* **7**: 427–433.

Maxton DG & Whorwell PJ (1990) Effect of intra-colonic nicardipine on colonic motility in irritable bowel syndrome. *Aliment Pharmacol Ther* **4**: 305–308.

Maxton DG, Morris J & Whorwell PJ (1996) Selective 5-hydroxytryptamine antagonism: a role in irritable bowel syndrome and functional dyspepsia? *Aliment Pharmacol Ther* **10**: 595–599.

Mendeloff AI, Monk M, Siegel CI & Lilienfield A (1968) Comparison of characteristics of patients with ulcerative colitis and with irritable colon in metropolitan Baltimore 1960–1964. *Gastroenterology* **54**: 1257.

Mendeloff AI, Monk M, Siegel CI & Lilienfield A (1970) Illness experiences and life stresses in patients with irritable colon and ulcerative colitis. *N Engl J Med* **282**: 14–17.

Moriarty KJ (1992) The irritable bowel syndrome. *BMJ* **304**: 1166–1169.

Moshal MG & Herron M (1979) A clinical trial of trimedbutine (Mebutin) in spastic colon. *J Int Med Res* **7**: 231–234.

Nanda R, James R, Smith H, Dudley CRK & Jewell DP (1989) Food intolerance and the irritable bowel syndrome. *Gut* **30**: 1098–1104.

Nash P, Gould SR & Bernardo DE (1986) Peppermint oil does not relieve the pain of irritable bowel syndrome. *Br J Clin Pract* **40**: 292–293.

Neal KR, Hebden J & Spiller R (1997) Prevalence of gastrointestinal symptoms six months after bacterial gastroenteritis and risk factors for development of the irritable bowel syndrome: postal survey of patients. *BMJ* **314**: 779–782.

Oddson E, Rask-Madsen J & Krag E (1978) A secretory epithelium of the small intestine with increased sensitivity to bile acids in irritable bowel syndrome associated with diarrhoea. *Scand J Gastroenterol* **13**: 409–416.

Oettle GJ & Heaton KW (1986) 'Rectal dissatisfaction' in the irritable bowel syndrome. A manometric and radiological study. *Int J Colorectal Dis* **1**: 183–185.

Oettle GJ & Heaton KW (1987) Is there a relationship between symptoms of the irritable bowel syndrome and objective measurements of large bowel function? A longitudinal study. *Gut* **28**: 146–149.

Page JG & Dirnberger GM (1981) Treatment of the irritable colon syndrome with bentyl (dicyclomine hydrochloride). *J Clin Gastroenterol* **3**: 153–156.

Pena AS & Truelove SC (1972) Hypolactasia and the irritable colon syndrome. *Scand J Gastroenterol* **7**: 1257–1263.

Peters GA & Bargen JE (1944) The irritable bowel syndrome. *Gastroenterology* **3**: 399–410.

Pial G & Mazzacca G (1979) Prifinium bromide in the treatment of the irritable colon syndrome. *Gastroenterology* **77**: 500–502.

Pial G, Visconti M, Imbimbo B et al (1987) Long-term treatment of irritable bowel syndrome with cimetropium bromide, a new antimuscarinic compound. *Curr Ther Res* **41**: 967–977.

Poynard T, Naveau S, Mory B & Chaput JC (1994) Meta-analysis of smooth muscle relaxants in the treatment of irritable bowel syndrome. *Aliment Pharmacol Ther* **8**: 499–510.

Preston DM, Adrian TE, Christofides ND, Lennard-Jones JE & Bloom SR (1985) Positive correlation between symptoms and circulating motilin, pancreatic polypeptide and gastrin concentrations in functional bowel disorders. *Gut* **26**: 1059–1064.

Prior A & Whorwell PJ (1987) Double blind study of ispaghula in irritable bowel syndrome. *Gut* **28**: 1510–1513.

Prior A, Harris SR & Whorwell PJ (1987) Reduction of colonic motility by intravenous nicardipine in irritable bowel syndrome. *Gut* **28**: 1609–1612.

Prior A, Colgan SM & Whorwell PJ (1990a) Changes in rectal sensitivity after hypnotherapy in patients with irritable bowel syndrome. *Gut* **31**: 896–898.

Prior A, Maxton DG & Whorwell PJ (1990b) Anorectal manometry in irritable bowel syndrome: differences between diarrhoea and constipation predominant subjects. *Gut* **31**: 458–462.

Prior A, Stanley KM, Smith ARB & Read NW (1992) Relation between hysterectomy and the irritable bowel: a prospective study. *Gut* **33**: 814–817.

Probert CSJ, Emmett PM, Cripps HA & Heaton KW (1994) Evidence for the ambiguity of the term constipation: the role of irritable bowel syndrome. *Gut* **35**: 1455–1458.

Read NW, Krejs GJ, Read MG, Santa Ana CA, Morawsky G & Fortrand JS (1980) Chronic diarrhoea of unknown origin. *Gastroenterology* **78**: 264–271.

Rees WD, Evans BK & Rhodes J (1979) Treating irritable bowel syndrome with peppermint oil. *Br Med J* **2**: 835–836.

Ritchie J (1973) Pain from distension of the pelvic colon by inflating a balloon in the irritable colon syndrome. *Gut* **6**: 105–112.

Ritchie J (1977) Similarity of bowel distension characteristics in the irritable colon syndrome and diverticulosis. *Gut* **18**: A990.

Ritchie J & Truelove SC (1980) Comparison of various treatments for irritable bowel syndrome. *BMJ* **281**: 1317–1319.

Rogers J, Henry MM & Misiewicz JJ (1989) Increased segmental activity and intraluminal pressures in the sigmoid colon of patients with the irritable bowel syndrome. *Gut* **30**: 634–641.

Rose JDR, Troughton AH, Harvey JS & Smith PM (1986) Depression and functional bowel disorders in gastrointestinal outpatients. *Gut* **27**: 1025–1028.

Rumessen JJ & Gudmand-Hoyer E (1988) Functional bowel disease: malabsorption and abdominal distress after ingestion of fructose, sorbitol and fructose–sorbitol mixtures. *Gastroenterology* **95**: 694–700.

Sandler RS, Drossman DA, Nathan HP & McKee DC (1984) Symptom complaints and health care seeking behaviour in subjects with bowel dysfunction. *Gastroenterology* **87**: 314–318.

Schafer E & Ewe K (1990) Efficacy and toleration of Buscopan plus buscopan, paracetamol and placebo in ambulatory patients with IBS. *Fortschr Med* **108**: 488–492.

Schlemper RJ, van der Werf SDJ, Vandenbroucke JP, Biemond I & Lamers CB (1993) Peptic ulcer, non-ulcer dyspepsia and irritable bowel syndrome in The Netherlands and Japan. *Scand J Gastroenterol* **28**: 33–41.

Sciarretta G, Fagioli G, Furno A et al (1987) [^{75}Se]HCAT test in the detection of bile acid malabsorption in functional diarrhoea and its correlation with small bowel transit. *Gut* **28**: 970–975.

Smart HL & Atkinson M (1987) Abnormal vagal function in irritable bowel syndrome. *Lancet* **ii**: 475–478.

Snape WJ, Carlson GM & Cohen S (1976) Colonic myoelectric activity in the irritable bowel syndrome. *Gastroenterology* **70**: 326–330.

Snape WJ, Carlson GM, Matarazzo SA & Cohen S (1977) Evidence that abnormal myoelectrical activity produces colonic motor dysfunction in the irritable bowel syndrome. *Gastroenterology* **72**: 383–387.

Snape WJ, Matarazzo SA & Cohen (1978) Effect of eating and gastrointestinal hormones on human colonic myoelectrical and motor activity. *Gastroenterology* **75**: 373–378.

Snape WJ, Wright SH, Cohen S & Battle WM (1979) The gastrocolonic response: evidence for a neural mechanism – neural versus hormonal mediation. *Gastroenterology* **77**: 1235–1240.

Snook J & Shepherd HA (1994) Bran supplementation in the treatment of irritable bowel syndrome. *Aliment Pharmacol Ther* **8**: 511–514.

Soltoff JI, Gudmand-Hoyer E, Kreg B, Kristensen E & Wolff HR (1976) A double blind trial of wheat bran on symptoms of irritable bowel syndrome. *Lancet* **1**: 270–272.

Spiller RC (1994) Irritable bowel or irritable mind? Medical treatment works for those with clear diagnosis. *BMJ* **309**: 1646–1647.

Stivland T, Camilleri M, Vassallo M, et al (1991) Scintigraphic measurement of regional gut transit in idiopathic constipation. *Gastroenterology* **101**: 107–115.

Stone RT & Barbero GJ (1970) Recurrent abdominal pain in childhood. *Paediatrics* **45**: 732–733.

Swarbrick EDT, Hegarty JE, Bat L, Williams CB & Dawson AM (1980) Site of pain from the irritable bowel. *Lancet* **ii**: 443–446.

Swedlund J, Sjodin I, Otto Ottosson J-O & Dotevall G (1983) Controlled study of psychotherapy in irritable bowel syndrome. *Lancet* **ii**: 589–592.

Talley NJ, Zinsmeister AR, Van Dyke C & Melton LJ (1991) Epidemiology of colonic symptoms and the irritable bowel syndrome. *Gastroenterology* **101**: 927–934.

Tasman-Jones C (1973) Mebeverine in patients with the irritable colon syndrome: double blind study. *N Z Med J* **77**: 232–235.

Taub E, Cuevas JL, Cook EW, Crowell M & Whitehead WE (1995) Irritable bowel syndrome defined by factor analysis: gender and race comparisons. *Dig Dis Sci* **40**: 2647–2655.

Taylor I, Darby C & Hammond P (1978a) Comparison of recto-sigmoid myoelectrical activity in the irritable colon syndrome during relapses and remissions. *Gut* **19**: 923–929.

Taylor I, Darby C, Hammond P & Basu P (1978b) Is there a myoelectrical abnormality in the irritable colon syndrome? *Gut* **19**: 391–395.

Thompson WG (1984a) The irritable bowel. *Gut* **25**: 305–320.

Thompson WG (1984b) Gastrointestinal symptoms in the irritable bowel compared with peptic ulcer and inflammatory bowel disease. *Gut* **25**: 1089–1092.

Thompson WG & Heaton KW (1980) Functional bowel disorders in apparently healthy people. *Gastroenterology* **79**: 283–288.

Thompson WG, Laidlow JM & Wingate DL (1979) Abnormal small bowel motility demonstrated by radiotelemetry in a patient with irritable colon. *Lancet* **ii**: 1321–1323.

Thompson WG, Patel DG, Tao H & Nair R (1982) Does uncomplicated diverticular disease cause symptoms? *Dig Dis Sci* **27**: 605–608.

Thompson WG, Dotevall G, Drossman DA, Heaton KW & Kruis W (1989) Irritable bowel syndrome: guidelines for the diagnosis. *Aliment Pharmacol Ther* **11**: 3–15.

Toskes PP, Connery KL & Ritchey TW (1993) Calcium polycarbophil compared with placebo in irritable bowel syndrome. *Aliment Pharmacol Ther* **7**: 87–92.

Trotman IF & Misiewicz JJ (1988) Sigmoid motility in diverticular disease and the irritable bowel syndrome. *Gut* **29**: 218–222.

Trotman IF & Price CC (1986) Bloated irritable syndrome defined by dynamic [^{99m}Tc] bran scan. *Lancet* **i**: 364–365.

Vantrappen F, Janssens J, Peeters TL, Bloom SR, Christofides ND & Hellemans J (1979) Motilin and the interdigestive migrating motor complex in man. *Dig Dis Sci* **24**: 497–500.

Waller SL & Misiewicz JJ (1969) Prognosis in the irritable bowel syndrome. A prospective study. *Lancet* **ii**: 753–759.

Weber FH, McCallum RW (1992) Clinical approaches to irritable bowel syndrome. *Lancet* **340**: 1447–1452.

Welch GW, Hillman LC & Pomare EW (1985) Psychoneurotic symptomatology in the irritable bowel syndrome: a study of reporters and non-reporters. *BMJ* **291**: 1382–1384.

Wells NEJ, Hahn BA & Whorwell PJ (1997) Clinical economics review: irritable bowel syndrome. *Aliment Pharmacol Ther* **11**: 1019–1030.

Weser E, Rubin W, Ross L & Sieisenger MH (1965) Lactase deficiency in patients with the 'irritable colon syndrome'. *N Engl J Med* **273**: 1070.

Whitehead WE, Engel BT & Schuster MM (1980) Irritable bowel syndrome. Physiological and psychological differences between diarrhoea-predominant and constipation-predominant patients. *Dig Dis Sci* **25**: 404–413.

Whitehead WE, Winget C, Fedaravicius AS, Wooley S & Blackwell B (1982) Learned illness behaviour in patients with irritable bowel syndrome and peptic ulcer. *Dig Dis Sci* **27**: 202–208.

Whitehead WE, Crowell MD, Robinson JC, Heller BR & Schuster MM (1992) Effects of stressful life events on bowel symptoms: subjects with irritable bowel syndrome compared with subjects without bowel dysfunction. *Gut* **33**: 825–830.

Whorwell PPJ, Clouter C & Smith CL (1981) Oesophageal motility in the irritable bowel syndrome. *BMJ* **282**: 1101–1103.

Whorwell PJ, Lupton EW, Erduran D & Wilson K (1986a) Bladder smooth muscle dysfunction in patients with irritable bowel syndrome. *Gut* **27**: 1014–1017.

Whorwell PJ, McCallum M, Creed FH & Roberts CT (1986b) Non-colonic features of irritable bowel syndrome. *Gut* **27**: 37–40.

Wright JT & Das AK (1969) Excretion of 4-hydroxy-3-methoxy mandelic acid in cases of ulcerative colitis and diarrhoea of nervous origin. *Gut* **10**: 628–630.

Wright SH, Snape WJ, Battle W, Cohen S & London RL (1980) Effect of dietary components on gastrocolonic response. *Am J Physiol* **238**: 228–232.

Zuckerman MJ, Guerra LG, Foland JA, Drossman DA & Gregory G (1990) Comparison of bowel patterns in Hispanics and whites. *Gastroenterology* **98**: A403 (Abstract).

26

CHRONIC IDIOPATHIC PERINEAL PAIN

There is a group of patients with rather ill-defined symptoms of pelvic pain in which no physical abnormality can be detected, yet patients complain of severe, often unremitting perineal or rectal discomfort for which treatment often offers little prospect of cure. There are usually strong underlying psychiatric and emotional factors which, although not necessarily causal, complicate and compromise medical management. Such patients often present to rectal clinics because they are thought to have anal pathology, particularly fissures, haemorrhoids, chronic anorectal sepsis or proctitis. Some are referred from other specialists, particularly urologists who no longer think that the symptoms are due to prostatitis, or orthopaedic surgeons who find no abnormality on radiographs of the lumbar spine and coccyx. Gynaecologists may also refer patients because of perineal pain which has the characteristics of a rectal rather than a vaginal origin. Occasionally these patients have already been seen by a neurologist or a psychiatrist. Patients are commonly referred from gastroenterologists after investigation of motility disorders and many of these patients have underlying irritable bowel syndrome and chronic constipation (Bleijenberg and Kuijpers, 1987). Some of these patients self refer or get passed on to colorectal surgeons because other specialists have been unable to improve their symptoms.

The surgeon should be wary about treating these patients unless a definitive abnormality which can account for the symptoms is identified. Some patients complain of anal pain, or more usually deep perineal pain and have no demonstrable abnormality, yet they undergo an empirical anal stretch which may be repeated. Not only are many patients not improved by the therapy but some are left with serious complications, particularly incontinence. Another danger with this group of patients is to give them a 'label' without thoroughly excluding organic pathology, such as malignancy.

CLINICAL SYNDROMES

There are said to be three principal groups of syndromes: proctalgia fugax, coccygodynia and chronic idiopathic anal pain. However, these divisions may be artificial. Even if these three do prove to be due to different pathophysiological mechanisms, the underlying natural history, emotional overtones, methods of investigation and clinical approach are comparable (Ger et al, 1993).

Proctalgia fugax or the levator syndrome

Proctalgia fugax was first described by Thaysen (1953) and is a relatively well-defined syndrome of obscure causation. It is found more commonly among young men (Thompson, 1979) and may regress spontaneously in later life (Abrahams, 1935).

Patients complain of a sudden onset of severe anal, rectal or perineal pain which is usually self-limiting and which rarely lasts more than 30 minutes (Ewing, 1953; Ibrahim, 1961). They state that the pain occurs in spasms and is relieved by hip flexion. These symptoms may be more common among the medical profession (Penny, 1970) and other professional groups such as teachers.

Thompson (1984) found that symptoms were often associated with mucous discharge and abdominal distension. Approximately two-thirds of patients complain of pain during the day, and only a third report that pain is precipitated by defecation. In 90% of cases the pain is localized to the anus and exacerbations occasionally occur after intercourse (Thompson, 1981).

The term 'levator syndrome' is probably synonymous with proctalgia fugax. It has been applied to patients who have pain that may be reproduced by palpating the lateral aspect of the pelvic floor and relieved by levator massage (Grant et al, 1975). The term is used more widely in North America where the syndrome appears to be more common in women than men (Hull et al, 1993); furthermore, symptoms are often worse at night, frequently waking the patient from sleep (Corman, 1984).

Coccygodynia

This group of symptoms consists of severe rectal and perineal pain, localized to the sacrum and coccyx and often made worse by sitting down. It is usually described as a continuous burning sensation or dull ache with acute exacerbations. Radiation of pain to the buttocks and thighs is common. The condition was first described by Simpson (1859), who recognized that it was more common in women. Thiele (1936) found that surgical treatment was usually ineffective and that the results of coccygectomy were particularly unrewarding (Thiele, 1950). In a series of 324 patients, 85% were women and most were in their fifth or sixth decade (Thiele, 1963).

Chronic idiopathic anal pain

This entity is even more obscure than those already described. Although Neill and Swash (1982) admit that a high proportion of these patients are emotionally labile, with features of depression, anxiety and neuroticism, they believe that a collective term to describe these individuals is useful. Todd (1985) also recognizes this syndrome, which is characterized by pelvic, perineal or anorectal pain associated with a feeling of something obstructing the rectum. Female patients often describe the pain as a bearing down discomfort, like labour pains, or the feeling of something often described as a ball obstructing the anorectum. There may be a history of tenesmus; discomfort is usually maximal when standing still and is relieved by lying down. It has been suggested that symptoms might be due to an incomplete intussusception of the rectum, but proctograms are usually normal. Even if an intussusception is demonstrated, it may not be responsible for symptoms since this may be a normal phenomenon.

In the study reported by Neill and Swash (1982), 35 patients with symptoms compatible with the syndrome were exhaustively investigated. These investigations failed to identify any demonstrable pathology; 57% gave a history of previous pelvic surgery. Operations included hysterectomy, vaginal repair and various anal operations, particularly haemorrhoidectomy, pelvic floor repair, rectopexy and anal dilatation. Some patients also gave a history of laminectomy. Eleven per cent had had a previous myelogram and 37% gave a history of sciatica. Some women attributed the onset of symptoms to a difficult delivery. In our own experience some of these patients are seeking compensation for perineal tears and minor faecal incontinence.

Postproctectomy syndrome

Similar symptoms may occur after abdominoperineal excision of the rectum. The patient complains of pain which is described as an uncomfortable sensation, as if the rectum and anal canal were still present. This syndrome has been termed 'phantom rectum' and is akin to 'phantom limb', which occurs after amputation. Sometimes perineal pain after abdominoperineal excision of the rectum is attributed to a perineal hernia, which is common, and only occasionally is repair justified for persistent pain, small bowel obstruction or urinary symptoms (Beck et al, 1987).

INCIDENCE

The only data on the incidence of these syndromes are from a study by Thompson (1979), who interviewed 301 healthy subjects in the UK. He found that 41 of them (14%) had features which, on direct enquiry, were compatible with one of these syndromes. Manning et al (1978), together with a number of other observers, considered that proctalgia fugax was commonly associated with the irritable bowel syndrome (Bensande, 1965; Thompson, 1979). To explore this hypothesis further, Thompson (1984) interviewed 50 patients labelled as having the irritable bowel syndrome with a history of abdominal pain and altered bowel habit in whom extensive intestinal investigations were normal. In addition, he studied 49 patients with peptic ulcer disease and 49 with radiographic features of inflammatory bowel disease (Table 26.1). Proctalgia fugax was significantly more common in patients with the irritable bowel syndrome, but when his analysis was confined to females no significant difference emerged.

Table 26.1 Proctalgia fugax: incidence.

	All patients			*Females*		
	n	*Proctalgia fugax*	*P*	*n*	*Proctalgia fugax*	*P*
Irritable bowel syndrome	50	25 (50)	<0.05	39	22 (56)	NS
Peptic ulcer disease	49	10 (20)	<0.05	15	8 (53)	NS
Inflammatory bowel disease	49	14 (29)	NS	26	11 (42)	NS

Values in parentheses are percentages.
NS, not significant.

PREDISPOSING FACTORS

Reference has already been made to the fact that many of these patients are emotionally labile, or psychologically disturbed. Some have a history of psychiatric disorders, and are often taking a variety of drugs (Granet, 1954). It must be admitted, however, that although many patients have sought a psychiatric opinion before referral, treatment with tricyclic antidepressants, benzodiazepines, phenothiazines and analgesics often fails to relieve symptoms. In many patients there are overt symptoms of depression, with insomnia and disruption of family life. Some patients describe abnormal or unfulfilled sexual behaviour. In women, the disorder seems to intensify when the husband retires and spends long hours at home without meaningful occupation. Pain is used by some as a means towards invalidity benefit or attention seeking. However, psychiatric advice is usually unrewarding.

There may be a genuine fear of malignant disease, sexually transmitted infection or colitis. There is a constant fear by some that the condition will eventually necessitate the construction of a stoma. Although reassurance is an important aspect of management, symptoms usually persist.

Straining is undoubtedly an important component to the symptom complex in some patients. However, this practice is so deeply ingrained in many patients that no amount of retraining and biofeedback seems to have long-term benefit. The predisposing factors reported from the Florida Cleveland Clinic are outlined in Table 26.2 (Ger et al, 1993).

Table 26.2 Factors associated with chronic intractable rectal pain (n = 60).

Associated factors	*No. of patients*	*Percentage*
Constipation or dyschezia	34	57
Previous pelvic surgery	26	43
Previous anal surgery	19	32
Anxiety depression	15	25
Irritable bowel syndrome	6	10
Prior spinal surgery	5	8

From Ger et al (1993).

Table 26.3 Types of anal and perineal pain.

Disorder	*Mean age at onset*	*Sex predominance*	*Nature of pain*	*Site*	*Radiation*	*Time of onset*	*Aggravating factors*	*Relieving factors*	*Associated features*
Proctalgia fugax	Young adults	M	Sudden crescendo, lasts minutes, stops spontaneously	Upper anal canal, constant site	Nil	Mostly at night	Anxiety	Stretching anus, flexing thighs	Tense introspective personality; 'irritable bowel' syndrome
Coccygodynia	Adults	F	Continuous vague ache with exacerbations	Lower sacrum, perineum and anal canal	Thighs and coccyx	Any time during the day	Sitting posture?, defecation, trauma to coccyx?	—	Tender spots in sacrococcygeal region, levator muscle spasm
Descending perineum syndrome	Any age?	F	Constant heavy dull perineal ache, sometimes with sharp pain	Perineum and anal canal	Nil, possibly to lower abdomen	Usually late in day	Standing, walking, after defecation	Lying down	Irregular bowel habit, straining at stool
Chronic idiopathic anal pain	58 years	F	Continuous dull throbbing, burning likened to a ball in the anal canal, intermittent or continuous	Mid anal canal, well localized, and may be unilateral	Sacrum, thighs, lower abdomen, anterior perineum and vagina	Any time, usually late in the day	Sitting	Lying down	Pelvic or spinal surgery, myelography, perineal descent

CLINICAL PRESENTATION AND EXAMINATION FINDINGS

The cardinal feature of all these syndromes is that clinical examination is normal. It is imperative, however, that clinical examination should be thorough. Assessment must include a neurological examination, paying particular attention to the lumbosacral plexus. Although pelvic examination is, of course, essential, it is also important to assess the function of the sphincters and pelvic floor. The perineum must be carefully inspected at rest and after straining (Parks et al, 1966; Henry et al, 1982; Ambrose and Keighley, 1985). A detailed proctosigmoidoscopy is essential to exclude pathology in the anal canal and rectum. The cardinal clinical features of the syndromes which constitute chronic idiopathic perineal pain are listed in Table 26.3.

INVESTIGATIONS AND PHYSIOLOGICAL ABNORMALITIES

An occult rectal prolapse must be excluded by careful inspection during sigmoidoscopy and by videoproctography while straining. The results of defecography in the Cleveland Clinic series are outlined in Table 26.4. A complete endoscopic or radiological examination of the intestinal tract is usually important to positively exclude organic pathology, particularly as perineal symptoms are often accompanied by symptoms of flatulent dyspepsia, heartburn and altered bowel habit (Thompson and Heaton, 1980). Special investigations include electromyography of the pelvic floor to detect any evidence of partial denervation of the puborectalis or conduction defects of the pudendal nerve (Hardcastle and Parks, 1970). Resting electromyography may detect bursts of striated muscle activity during episodes of pain (Douthwaite, 1962). Neill and Swash (1982) recorded increased fibre density in 11 of 24 patients studied by single-fibre electromyography. Translumbar stimulation at the L1–L4 vertebral levels may reproduce the pain. Motility and sensory studies of the anorectum and sigmoid colon will exclude sensory impairment, evidence of aganglionosis, indirect evidence of pudendal nerve damage and evidence of increased motility in the rectosigmoid. Harvey (1979) recorded high-pressure waves during episodes of pain in patients with proctalgia fugax. There is often a major abnormality of the anal smooth muscles (Eckardt et al, 1996). Assessment of perineal descent should be made clinically and confirmed if necessary by videoproctography (Henry, 1985).

Table 26.4 Cinedefecography findings in chronic rectal pain (n = 40).

Finding	*No. of patients*	*Percentage*
Rectocele	21	40
Increased perineal descent	15	30
Non-relaxing puborectalis	12	24
Incomplete intussusception	9	18

From Ger et al (1993).

If there is any impairment of straight leg raising or pain on dorsiflexion of the foot during hip flexion a thorough radiological assessment of the lumbar spine, sacroiliac joints and hips is indicated. Careful examination of the sacral foramina should help to exclude a neurofibroma, and high-quality radiographs of the coccyx should identify any bony abnormality which might be responsible for pain, particularly Paget's disease, osseous metastases or localized osteoporosis. However, even though Boisson et al (1966) proposed that fibrosis around the sacral nerve roots might be responsible for symptoms, we do not think that myelograms or radiculograms should be undertaken lightly. Invasive procedures often make symptoms worse and may lead to iatrogenic complications. If the spinal cord or nerve roots are thought to be implicated, magnetic resonance imaging is the preferred investigation.

DIFFERENTIAL DIAGNOSIS

It is essential that there is no underlying organic disease. Anal conditions which may mimic chronic idiopathic perineal pain include chronic anal fissures, small unsuspected intersphincteric or supralevator abscesses, thrombosed haemorrhoids or a cavernous haemangioma in the anorectum. Neurological disorders must be excluded, particularly intradural or extradural compression of the cauda equina, demyelinating disorders, neurofibromata or pelvic lymphoma. Even peripheral nerve lesions may masquerade as proctalgia fugax. Colorectal cancer, intussuscepting polyps, rectal prolapse, solitary ulcer and proctocolitis should be excluded by sigmoidoscopy. Perineal hernia should be excluded by CT (So et al, 1997).

The fear or presence of sexually transmitted disease often has considerable psychological overtones which are sometimes expressed as bizarre perineal symptoms. These disorders should be excluded by appropriate serology, biopsies and swabs from the anorectum, vagina and urethra. Gynaecological disorders, particularly bacterial and fungal vaginitis, endometriosis, ovarian tumours and cyclical hormonal dysfunction, may be responsible for chronic perineal pain. Prostatitis, prostatic calculi and bladder neoplasm may present with low-grade constant perineal discomfort.

There is a long list of iatrogenic causes of perineal pain which should also be excluded. These include chronic radiation damage to the pelvis, neurosurgical and orthopaedic operations on the pelvis, operations on the anal canal and childbirth injuries. It is absolutely essential to exclude malignancy, particularly after previous pelvic surgery. One of the greatest errors is to label a person neurotic when the root cause is a recurrence of malignancy in the pelvis after previous radical surgery, often combined with chemoradiation therapy.

CLINICAL MANAGEMENT

Probably the most important step is to exclude organic disease, preferably using non-invasive methods. These problems cannot possibly be handled in a busy outpatient clinic. A patient with chronic idiopathic perineal pain needs a period of time during which he or she receives the clinician's undivided attention. After a thorough history and a detailed clinical examination all the previous radiographs should be reviewed. Simple anorectal physiological studies will also help to reassure a patient that there is no functional disorder. During these investigations and during conversations it is possible to piece together a picture of the patient's home life, sexual orientation, possible fear of assault, previous trauma, guilt and a genuine concern of undetected malignant disease. If all the investigations, including videoproctography, are normal then the patient should be reassured, not that there is nothing the matter but that there is no serious underlying disease, so that they can come to accept that their problems are a nuisance rather than a disease.

Certain specific therapies have been tried but none are usually successful; indeed, surgical treatment in particular can often make matters worse. This is certainly true of coccygectomy as well as rectopexy for radiological evidence of intussusception. Sacral rhizotomy is an unrewarding exercise; only six of 24 patients treated by Albrektsson (1981) in this way were improved, and 25% developed complications from the procedure. In our experience one should never be persuaded to do another anal dilatation in a patient with a normal anal canal, particularly if there are signs of perineal descent, since there is a real risk of iatrogenic incontinence, carrying medicolegal overtones.

Less invasive methods of therapy that are usually completely ineffective include glyceryl trinitrate, salt baths, pelvic floor exercises, levator massage, percutaneous vibration and biofeedback. Topical steroids and local anaesthetic preparations may be tried but their success is usually short lived. Sohn et al (1982) used high-voltage electrogalvanic stimulation in 80 patients with proctalgia fugax. This group reported excellent results without recurrence of pain in 69% of patients during a follow-up of at least 1 year. They postulated that treatment achieves motor neurone suppression and causes muscle fatigue in the levator ani. These observations need to be reproduced by others. Treatment by this method is contraindicated in pregnancy and in patients who have cardiac pacemakers.

Hull et al (1993) reported that electrogalvanic stimulation improved 19% of patients but that in 57% there was no relief. Biofeedback has been used and short-term follow-up suggests that patients often derive considerable benefit (Grimaud et al, 1991). Ger et al (1993) found that biofeedback was the most effective method of treatment, with benefit in 43% (Table 26.5). In case clinicians pressurized to do something for these patients may be tempted to explore the potential of pudendal nerve block, we would remind readers that Neill and Swash (1982) failed to achieve any benefit with this form of therapy. Non-steroidal anti-inflammatory drugs may have some benefit, but continued exposure to narcotic analgesics is not advised, both because of their constipating effect and the risk of addiction.

If there is a history of chronic constipation, bulking agents or stimulant suppositories may improve bowel habit and afford some symptomatic improvement.

Table 26.5 Results of treatment in chronic rectal pain (n = 38).

	Excellent	*Good*	*Poor*
Electrogalvanic stimulation (n = 29)	2 (7)	9 (31)	18 (62)
Biofeedback (n = 14)	2 (14)	4 (29)	8 (57)
Steroid caudal block (n = 11)	0	2 (18)	9 (82)

Values in parentheses are percentages.
From Ger et al (1993).

Finally, these syndromes are difficult to manage and the clinician must apply tact, patience and sympathy in dealing with patients. It should always be remembered that although no obvious cause for the patient's symptoms is present, this does not mean that one does not exist.

REFERENCES

Abrahams A (1935) Proctalgia fugax. *Lancet* **ii**: 444.

Albrektsson B (1981) Sacral rhizotomy in cases of anococcygeal pain: a follow up of 24 cases. *Acta Orthop Scand* **52**: 187–190.

Ambrose MS & Keighley MRB (1985) Outpatient measurement of perineal descent. *Ann R Coll Surg Engl* **67**: 306–308.

Beck DE, Fazio FW, Jagelman DG, Lavery IC & McGonagle BA (1987) Postoperative perineal hernia. *Dis Colon Rectum* **30**: 21–24.

Bensande A (1965) Proctalgies fugaces. *Acta Gastroenterol Belg* **28**: 594–604.

Bleijenberg G & Kuijpers HC (1987) Treatment of the spastic pelvic floor syndrome with biofeedback. *Dis Colon Rectum* **30**: 108–111.

Boisson J, Debbasch L & Bensande A (1966) Les algies anorectales essentielles. *Arch Fr Mal App Dig* **55**: 3–24.

Corman ML (1984) *Colon and Rectal Surgery*, pp 733–734. Philadelphia: JB Lippincott.

Douthwaite AH (1962) Proctalgia fugax. *BMJ* **2**: 164–165.

Eckardt VF, Dodt O, Kanzler G & Bernhard G (1996) Anorectal function and morphology in patients with sporadic proctalgia fugax. *Dis Colon Rectum* **39**: 755–762.

Ewing MR (1953) Proctalgia fugax. *BMJ* **1**: 1083–1085.

Ger GC, Wexner SD, Jorge MN et al (1993). Evaluation and treatment of chronic intractable rectal pain – a frustrating endeavor. *Dis Colon Rectum* **36**: 139–145.

Granet E (1954) *Manual of Proctology*. Chicago: Year Book Publishers.

Grant SR, Salvati EP & Rubin RJ (1975) Levator syndrome: an analysis of 316 cases. *Dis Colon Rectum* **18**: 161–163.

Grimaud J-C, Bouvier M, Naudy B, Guien C & Salducci J (1991) Manometric and radiologic investigations and biofeedback treatment of chronic idiopathic anal pain. *Dis Colon Rectum* **34**: 690–695.

Hardcastle JD & Parks AG (1970) A study of anal incontinence and some principles of surgical treatment. *Proc R Soc Med* **63**: 116–118.

Harvey RF (1979) Colonic motility in proctalgia fugax. *Lancet* **ii**: 713–714.

Henry MM (1985) Descending perineum syndrome. In Henry MM & Swash M (eds) *Coloproctology and the Pelvic Floor*, pp 299–302. London: Butterworth.

Henry MM, Parks AG & Swash M (1982) The pelvic floor musculature in the descending perineum syndrome. *Br J Surg* **69**: 470–472.

Hull TL, Milsom JW, Church J, Oakley J, Lavery I & Fazio V (1993) Electrogalvanic stimulation for levator syndrome: How effective is it in the long term? *Dis Colon Rectum* **36**: 731–733.

Ibrahim H (1961) Proctalgia fugax. *Gut* **2**: 137–140.

Manning AP, Thompson WG, Heaton KW et al (1978) Towards positive diagnosis of the irritable bowel. *BMJ* **2**: 653–654.

Neill ME & Swash M (1982) Chronic perianal pain: an unsolved problem. *J R Soc Med* **75**: 96–101.

Parks AG, Porter NH & Hardcastle JD (1966) The syndrome of the descending perineum. *Proc R Soc Med* **59**: 477–482.

Penny RW (1970) The doctor's disease: proctalgia fugax. *Practitioner* **204**: 843–845.

Simpson JY (1859) Clinical lectures on the diseases of women. Lecture XVII. On coccygodynia and the diseases and deformities of the coccyx. *Med Times Gaz* **40**: 1–7.

So JB-y, Palmer MT & Shellito PC (1997) Postoperative perineal hernia. *Dis Colon Rectum* **40**: 954–957.

Sohn N, Weinstein MA & Robbins RD (1982) The levator syndrome and its treatment with high-voltage electrogalvanic stimulation. *Am J Surg* **144**: 580–582.

Thaysen ThEH (1953) Proctalgia fugax: a little known form of pain in the rectum. *Lancet* **ii**: 243–246.

Thiele GH (1936) Tonic spasm of the levator ani, coccygeus and piriformis muscles: its relationship to coccygodynia and pain in the region of the hip and down the leg. *Trans Am Procol Soc* **37**: 145–155.

Thiele GH (1950) Coccygodynia: the mechanism of its production and its relationship to anorectal disease. *Am J Surg* **79**: 110–116.

Thiele GH (1963) Coccygodynia: cause and treatment. *Dis Colon Rectum* **6**: 422–434.

Thompson WG (1979) *The Irritable Gut*, pp 125–130. Baltimore: University Park Press.

Thompson WG (1981) Proctalgia fugax. *Dig Dis Sci* **26**: 1121–1124.

Thompson WG (1984) Proctalgia fugax in patients with the irritable bowel, peptic ulcer or inflammatory bowel disease. *Am J Gastroenterol* **79**: 450–452.

Thompson WG & Heaton KW (1980) Proctalgia fugax. *J R Coll Physicians Lond* **14**: 247–248.

Todd IP (1985) Clinical evaluation of the pelvic floor. In Henry MM & Swash M (eds) *Coloproctology and the Pelvic Floor*, pp 187–188. London: Butterworth.

27

MOLECULAR BIOLOGY OF COLORECTAL CANCER

There is now substantial evidence supporting the concept that the accumulation of genetic changes within a cell leads to the development of neoplastic transformation. Thus the phenotype of the cell and its function or dysfunction is regulated by its genotype at any one time. However, it has become increasingly recognized that epigenetic alterations within cells are also important determinants of the final phenotype. Nowhere is the elucidation of these molecular events better illustrated than in colorectal cancer.

There are good reasons why this particular malignancy, together with recent advances in molecular biology techniques, has served as a paradigm for the genetic description of tumorigenesis. Firstly, colorectal cancer is an extremely common tumour and its evolution is staged through a relatively consistent series of pathological precursors (the adenoma–carcinoma sequence). Secondly, the cancer and its precursors can be sampled easily by colonoscopy, yielding material for molecular analysis. Finally, there are two distinct syndromes in which individuals display a marked predisposition to the development of colorectal cancer. The genetic lesions in FAP (familial adenomatous polyposis) and HNPCC (hereditary non-polyposis colorectal cancer) are now well delineated and their study has contributed enormously to our understanding of the molecular pathology of sporadic colorectal cancer.

CANCER GENES

The development of cancer represents the culmination of a highly complex process whereby environmental, dietary and hereditary factors, acting either alone or in combination, cause structural changes in vital regulatory genes leading to cellular dysfunction. In cancer this is manifested by cellular resistance to normal homeostatic signals, inappropriate cell proliferation, and the acquisition of an invasive phenotype with metastasis of the tumour and ultimately the death of the patient.

The notion that genetic alterations may underlie the basis of cancer is not a new concept. Evidence supporting this hypothesis has accrued over the last few decades from familial, epidemiological and cytogenetic studies. However, it is only with the advent of powerful molecular biology techniques in the last decade to identify somatic and inherited mutations in cancers that direct evidence has been provided for this genetic basis. In essence, cancer results from mutations in at least three different types of genes: oncogenes, tumour suppressor genes, and DNA mismatch repair genes (reviewed in Bishop, 1991; Marshall, 1991; Weinberg, 1991; Ponder, 1992; Bodmer, 1994; Chung and Rustgi, 1995).

Oncogenes

Oncogenes are mutated versions of the normal regulatory cellular genes called proto-oncogenes. They were originally identified in avian and rodent oncogenic viruses. It has become apparent that the genetic sequences responsible for oncogenic transformation are in fact segments of normal DNA within the viral genome but are aberrantly expressed. Most proto-oncogenes function in a positive manner to regulate cell proliferation, and mutations within these genes enhance or activate their cellular function leading to uncontrolled cell proliferation. Oncogenes display a dominant mode of function in that a mutation in one allele is sufficient to exert their cellular effect despite the expression of a normal functioning or 'wild-type' protein from the remaining allele.

Over 70 oncogenes have been identified, and many of them are expressed in different types of tumour. One of the best studied oncogenes is the *ras* family. The *ras* family encode proteins related to G proteins, which are membrane-bound and involved in signal transduction pathways within the cell. K-*ras* is located on the long arm of chromosome 12 (12q) and contains point mutations in 40–50% of colorectal cancers. Activation of other oncogenes has been detected in colorectal cancer, including c-*myc*, *src* and tyrosine kinase. Kinases are enzymes that catalyse the phosphorylation of tyrosine residues within proteins. The process of phosphorylation is a recurring biochemical theme in cancer biology. Phosphorylation of a tyrosine residue can critically alter the biochemical activity of the protein molecule, which in turn can have a significant downstream effect on cell behaviour.

Tumour suppressor genes

These are, again, normal cellular genes which function in the maintenance of cell homeostasis. These gene products repress cell proliferation and promote cell differentiation. This group displays a recessive mode of action as both alleles have to be inactivated by mutation or gene loss before they lose their function. Inactivation of tumour suppressor genes can occur either by inherited or by somatic mutations and lead to loss of control of cell proliferation and tumour formation. This is not the case in mutations occurring in proto-oncogenes, which are all somatic in nature and not inherited (see below in hereditary cancer).

The retinoblastoma gene (Rb) was the first tumour suppressor gene to be isolated. Its tumour suppressor function is dramatically demonstrated by the finding that the introduction of a normal Rb gene into an Rb-negative cell abrogates *in vivo* tumorigenicity of an otherwise tumorigenic cell line (Marshall, 1991). Among the best studied tumour suppressor genes involved in colorectal cancer are the adenomatous polyposis coli (APC) gene located on chromosome 5q and p53 on 17p. The cellular functions of the APC protein are not completely clear, although evidence indicates that it has an important role in cell-to-cell signalling and modulating early cell differentiation (see below).

DNA mismatch repair genes and microsatellite instability

The process of DNA mismatch repair has been studied and characterized in most detail in prokaryotic cells such as the bacteria *E. coli*. In bacteria these genes encode for enzymes that recognize and repair mispaired bases during DNA replication.

Additionally, this system identifies and rectifies small deletions or insertions on one strand of the DNA helix. These genes are highly conserved throughout evolutionary history; thus there is a totally analogous system present in human (eukaryotic) cells and homologous mismatch repair genes have now been identified in eukaryotes. Dysfunction of these gene products manifests itself by a phenomenon known as 'microsatellite instability' (MI).

Segments of non-coding regions of DNA within genes (protein-coding regions within DNA account for only approximately 3% of the human genome) contain highly repetitive sequences of DNA known as 'DNA repeats'. The most common repeat is $(A)_n$ followed by $(CA)_n$, where $n = 10–60$. As these regions do not encode for proteins, variations within them are inconsequential and well-tolerated throughout evolution. This has enhanced genetic diversity within these regions which are unique to a particular individual and are fixed for life. Their pattern can be found in any nucleated cell obtained from a particular person and form the basis of DNA finger-printing. One class of these repeats is known as 'microsatellites', which are composed of repetitive DNA sequences of one to six bases. Instability within microsatellites is revealed by either an increase or a decrease in the number of bases within the repeat. This is detected by a corresponding increase or decrease in the size of the microsatellite as detected by amplification of these sequences using the polymerase chain reaction (PCR) (Figure 27.1). DNA mismatch repair and HNPCC are discussed in detail below (reviewed in Chung and Rustgi, 1995; Eshelman and Markowitz, 1995).

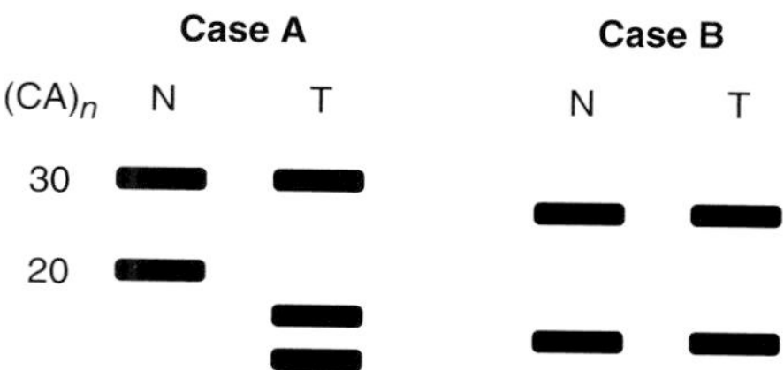

Figure 27.1 Microsatellite instability in colorectal cancer: analysis of the $(CA)_n$ microsatellite locus in two patients. In case A, normal colonic tissue (N) displays a heterogenous pattern with $(CA)_n$ repeat lengths of 30 and 20. The two alleles here represent inherited maternal and paternal copies. Analysis of tumour (T) from case A reveals microsatellite instability in one of the alleles with $(CA)_n$ repeat lengths of 19 and 18. In case B, the same allele pattern of $(CA)_n$ repeats is seen in both normal and tumour tissues.

MECHANISMS OF ACTIVATION AND INACTIVATION OF ONCOGENES AND TUMOUR SUPPRESSOR GENES

The most common mechanisms of activation of oncogenes or inactivation of tumour suppressor genes is by point mutation or deletions. However, the pattern of changes differs between the classes of gene, as do the subsequent effects on gene function, and this is discussed below. A point mutation is the substitution of one base-pair of DNA for another with a corresponding single amino acid change. The new protein will be identical to the wild-type apart from a single amino acid (a mis-sense mutation). This simple change may have a number of functional effects on the protein it encodes for, depending on the position of the mutation and the new amino acid. For instance, the mutated sequence may encode for the signal for termination of translation (stop codon) causing premature truncation of the protein, rendering it non-functional. Alternatively, DNA deletion (ranging from a single base-pair to part or all of a gene or to part of a chromosome) can occur in tumour cells. A large deletion will remove and inactivate all the genes contained in it. Small DNA deletions that remove mRNA occurring in a multiple of three base-pairs will result in the absence of those amino acids from the final protein sequence. Clearly, the consequences of this will depend upon the functional role of this segment in the wild-type protein. However, if the deleted segment in the mRNA is not a multiple of three base-pairs, then this introduces a frame shift into the reading sequence of the DNA. The most common effect of such frame shifts is truncation of the protein as a premature stop codon is introduced which terminates translation.

Activating mutations in human oncogenes are exemplified by the *ras* family. Under normal circumstances the proteins encoded by the *ras* family of oncogenes alternate between an activated and a deactivated state, but the mutated protein is maintained in a permanent state of activation. This is due to point mutations at only three amino acids. All of these mutations are mis-sense in that they allow the translation of a full-length *ras* protein. Interestingly, these mutations are restricted to just three codons of the *ras* protein (a triplet of nucleotides encoding for one amino acid), 12, 13 and 61. In contrast, inactivation of a tumour suppressor gene requires an independent mutation in both alleles of that gene and there are differences in the type of structural alteration between the first and second of these 'hits'. The first of the inactivating mutations is generally confined to the gene itself or the DNA immediately adjacent to the gene. These mutations can be missense, non-sense (encoding for a stop codon in translation) or deletions which can be in frame or cause frame shifts to the reading sequence of the DNA. For example, APC mutations are commonly non-sense and produce a truncated gene product. The mutation inactivating the second allele of a tumour suppressor gene is probably due to an error of mitosis and tends to cause loss of a large segment of the chromosome in which the gene is located.

The structural differences between the two inactivating mutations in tumour suppressor genes has been of considerable use in their detection and localization. Within a polymorphic area of the genome (where there are small differences in the DNA sequence between individuals) it is possible to visualize both parental copies of the region independently using a DNA probe (using Southern blotting). If one copy has been lost during malignant transformation, this is detected as a loss of heterozygosity (i.e. a reduction from two visible bands to one) (Figure 27.2). As the second mutation is so large, a probe located some distance away from the gene can still reveal this loss. Thus by performing these studies with polymorphic probes on DNA extracted from matched tumour and normal tissue from an individual, it is possible to detect loss of a particular tumour suppressor gene and its approximate location. Indeed, this technique proved very effective in delineating the genetic lesions involved in colorectal tumorigenesis (see below).

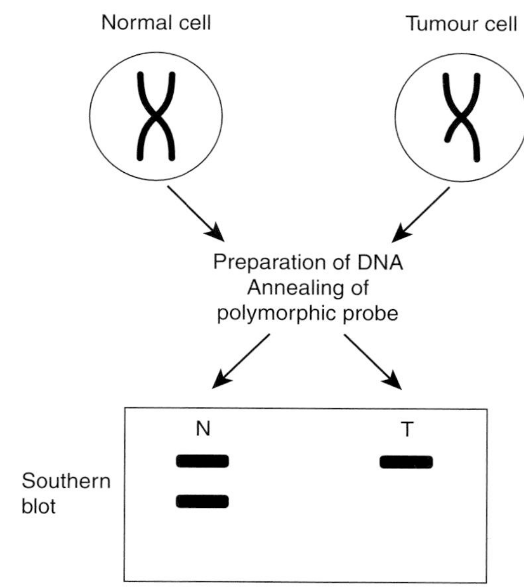

Figure 27.2 Southern blot analysis revealing loss of heterozygosity in a tumour. In tumour cells (T) there has been partial chromosomal deletion resulting in loss of one copy of the tumour suppressor gene allele. In contrast, in normal tissue (N) both parental copies are retained and two bands are visualized.

CELL CYCLE CONTROL, APOPTOSIS, AGEING AND CANCER

The cell cycle

Many of the cancer genes described in this chapter either have a direct effect on the regulation of the cell cycle (i.e. the events necessary for cellular duplication) or impinge on the process by involvement in other crucial intracellular signalling pathways. Thus a description of the events involved in the cell cycle and its control is important in the context of the effect of a loss of normal gene function in neoplasia.

In its simplest form, the cell cycle can be considered to involve four stages: a DNA synthesis phase (S phase) and a mitosis/nuclear division (M phase), each separated by gaps (G_1 and G_2) (Figure 27.3). These occur in a cyclical manner in tissues with rapid cell turnover. The ultimate aim of cell replication is the generation of two identical daughter cells both with an intact genomic structure. Not surprisingly, this process is highly complex and involves the integration and transduction of many different signals from the extracellular microenvironment to the cell nucleus. The importance of the molecules within these signalling pathways is highlighted by their evolutionary conservation from the simplest organisms such as yeast and bacteria, through other invertebrates, to mammals, and finally to humans.

Progression through the cell cycle is controlled at key 'checkpoints' (Figure 27.3) where decisions as to whether or not to proceed with cell replication have to be made before another cycle is initiated. These

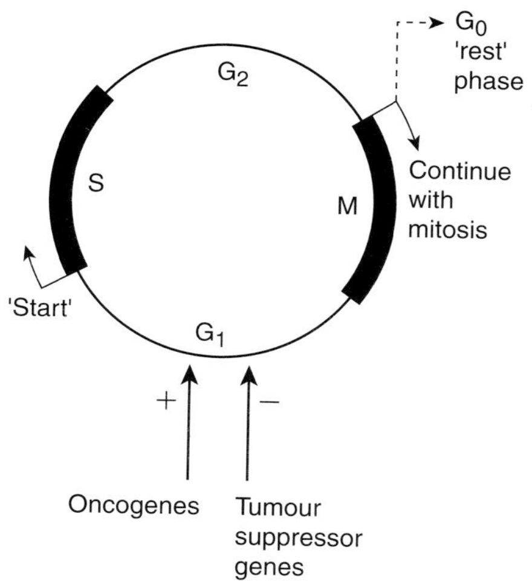

Figure 27.3 The cell cycle: schematic showing the positive action of oncogenes (uncontrolled cell proliferation) and the negative action of tumour suppressor genes (arrest of cell proliferation).

checkpoints are at G_1/S and G_2/M. The first of these checkpoints (G_1/S) is known as the 'start' and passage through this point usually results in completion of the cell cycle and the production of two daughter cells. The second occurs immediately prior to mitosis (G_2/M). Cells are able to arrest the cycle at this point for a prolonged period of time and can 'rest' in G_0. This cycle is intimately linked with a number of other regulatory processes: DNA repair, cellular differentiation, cell senescence and programmed cell death (apoptosis). If a cell is unable to respond appropriately to external stimuli, arrest of the cell cycle will occur to allow repair of damaged DNA. Alternatively, if it is does not undergo apoptotic death, a cell progeny with abnormal DNA and an unstable genome will result.

Apoptosis

Apoptosis differs from necrotic cell death in that it is a highly regulated and active process in which cells undergo programmed cell death under the control of specific cytoplasmic proteins (Wylie, 1980). Uncontrolled cell proliferation has always been recognized as a central feature of neoplasia, but recently it has become apparent that impaired apoptosis is equally as important during tumorigenesis. The DNA of cells undergoing apoptosis is cleaved into multiples of 180 base-pairs and this is manifested by the detection of a characteristic DNA ladder pattern on an agarose gel (Vaux and Strasser, 1996). Apoptosis is a normal physiological process occurring during embryogenesis, ageing and during general defence by eliminating damaged cells. This process is necessary for tissue homeostasis by maintaining the balance between cell division and death. It also acts as a general defence mechanism by eliminating effete cells and probably has a role in ageing.

During neoplasia the balance between cell proliferation and cell death is disturbed. This is reflected in tissues by a net growth advantage which may also be associated with an increased life-span of the cells affected. Both of these processes aid in the clonal selection and outgrowth of a cell population in which other genetic alterations drive the transformation further towards the malignant phenotype (McDonnell, 1993). There is a gradual decrease in the fraction of apoptotic cells during the progression from normal epithelium, through adenoma formation to carcinoma (Bedi et al, 1995). The molecular mechanisms involved in inducing apoptosis are not entirely clear, but are distributed through a number of key regulatory cellular pathways. DNA damage, either due to ionizing radiation or to mutagen exposure, results in an increase in the expression of p53 which activates apoptosis (see below). The decreased apoptosis index observed in colorectal cancer is likely to be linked to mutational inactivation of the APC and p53, and other undiscovered genes. Certainly, transfer of a functional p53 gene into human colorectal cancer cells does induce apoptosis (Shaw et al, 1992). However, p53 mutations are generally detected once carcinoma formation has occurred (see below). Dysfunction of the APC gene is of more importance in the initiation of tumorigenesis, partly through its own role in maintaining cell number homeostasis, but also by activating apoptotic pathways. Again expression of functional APC into colorectal tumour cells lacking the gene product does result in apoptosis (Morin et al, 1996).

There is at least one known human gene that encodes for a protein that inhibits apoptosis, and that is Bcl-2 (Vaux et al, 1992; Hengartner and Horvita, 1994). In normal colorectal epithelium, expression of Bcl-2 is confined to the rapidly dividing cells at the base of the crypt. During malignant progression this area of expression increases upwards towards the apex of the crypt, so that in carcinoma all crypt cells express Bcl-2. This pattern of Bcl-2 activity is closely matched by the apoptosis index within the same crypts which decreases during colorectal tumorigenesis. These findings indicate that over-expression of Bcl-2 is an early event during malignant transformation of the epithelium, and that, together with other early molecular alterations (e.g. APC mutations), loss of apoptosis may facilitate tumour initiation (Giardello et al, 1995).

Cell senescence and telomerase

The integrity of chromosomes during cell division is maintained by specialized DNA sequences at each end, called telomeres. However, DNA replication is confined to the intrachromosomal DNA and the telomeres progressively shorten during successive rounds of cell division by somatic cells (Harley et al, 1990). Only germ cells and somatic cells can maintain telomeres owing to the action of telomerase, an enzyme whose expression is confined to these cell types. This is consistent with the replication function of these cells throughout life. Progressive shortening of telomeres beyond a critical length probably signals cell cycle arrest and activates the senescence pathways during ageing.

Not surprisingly, recent evidence suggests that a disturbance of this process is implicated in neoplasia. Inappropriate expression of telomerase has been observed in 80–90% of human cancers and can immortalize somatic cells (NW Kim et al, 1994; Haber, 1995; Morin, 1996). During colorectal tumorigenesis, the majority of adenomas do not express telomerase, while invasive cancers possess this activity (Li et al, 1996).

HISTORICAL REVIEW OF THE GENETIC BASIS OF CANCER

Epidemiological studies revealing the familial clustering of some cancers (including colorectal cancer) suggested that cancer may be inherited and therefore possess a genetic basis (Hansen and Cavenee, 1987). However, other explanations for these observations were possible, and in many of the families studied the cancers appeared to arise as sporadic malignancies in isolated individuals. Indeed, even in HNPCC which was suspected to be an inheritable disorder for many decades, confounding factors such as chance population clusterings and the effect of environmental factors on gene penetrance (complete gene penetrance exists when 100% of individuals harbouring a predisposing mutation develop the disease) and phenocopies (individuals within families with the same disease but not the same causative mutation) served to hinder the identification of the genetic lesions responsible for the disease.

Rous (1911) provided the first direct evidence of a genetic basis in cancer by demonstrating that a cell-free filtrate from a chicken sarcoma was able to induce sarcoma in chickens. His studies also yielded compelling evidence for the role of viruses in tumorigenesis. Indeed, some 60 years after his original observations further studies have revealed that the v-*src*, a transduced cellular gene, is responsible for the oncogenicity of the Rous sarcoma virus (Stehlin et al, 1976). A significant advance in elucidating the genetic basis of cancer was made by Weinberg and his colleagues who provided good evidence for the positive roles of oncogenes in the malignant transformation of benign cells (Shih et al, 1981; Bernstein and Weinberg, 1985). They demonstrated that cultured murine fibroblasts acquired a malignant phenotype following the introduction of DNA from human cancer cells (Shih et al, 1981). Moreover, this group also showed that DNA from metastatic human tumour cells could induce metastasis of these otherwise non-metastasizing murine cells (Bernstein and Weinberg, 1985).

In contrast, the earliest evidence for the existence of tumour suppressor genes emerged through experiments in which tumour cells and normal cells were fused. The resultant hybrids were found to be non-tumorigenic (Harris, 1988). These results suggested that genetic material within the normal cells possessed the ability to modulate the behaviour of malignant cells. The accurate identification of tumour suppressor genes was facilitated by later studies involving transfer of specific, single chromosomes which resulted in the abrogation of the malignant phenotype of many different types of tumour cells (Stanbridge and Cavenee, 1989).

Further evidence for the existence of tumour suppressor genes was provided by Knudson and his seminal studies on the genetics and natural history of retinoblastoma. Knudson suggested that the differences in the natural history and epidemiology of retinoblastoma in sporadic and inherited cases could be explained by a ‘two-mutation’ model (Knudson, 1971). In inherited retinoblastoma, one inactivating mutation is already present in the germ line and therefore all somatic cells in this individual will contain this mutation. A second somatic mutation is required in an already predisposed retinoblast, and this accounts for the observation that inherited retinoblastoma is often bilateral and multifocal. Conversely, sporadic retinoblastoma requires two somatic mutations in one retinal cell causing unilateral and unifocal tumours. Subsequent studies of retinoblastoma confirmed that the Rb1 gene was located on the long arm of chromosome 13 (13q) and that this gene was indeed inactivated in the inherited condition (Stanbridge and Cavenee, 1989). The molecular genetic studies of the retinoblastoma were significant as they illustrated how a combination of germline (i.e. *inherited*) and somatic (i.e. *acquired*) mutations contributed to tumour development.

CLONALITY AND TUMOUR INITIATION BY SOMATIC MUTATION

Clonality is a fundamental characteristic of all human cancers. Studies investigating the inactivation of the X chromosome support this concept. Random inactivation of one copy of the X chromosome occurs at an early developmental stage in all the cells of a female fetus. All subsequent daughter cells inherit the same specific X inactivation from parental cells and this pattern can be determined. Colorectal adenomas (and hence carcinomas) arise from the clonal expansion of a small number of cells that have originated from a single intestinal crypt cell (Fearon et al, 1987). All these cells exhibit the same genetic change that initially conferred a growth advantage in the parent cell, while further genetic lesions accumulate in subsequent daughter cells, each providing further growth advantages. In contrast, normal colonic mucosa is polyclonal in origin. Tumour cell clonality does not imply homogeneity, as tumours can exhibit a monoclonal composition but diversify in a number of unrelated ways. Indirect evidence for tumour cell clonality is further provided by the very techniques used to detect somatic genetic changes in DNA extracted from tumour cells. These techniques typically require at least 30–50% of all the tumour cells to harbour the mutation under investigation. Thus this implies their presence in a large population of cells occurring as a result of clonal selection and subsequent expansion (Kern, 1993).

The seminal studies of Vogelstein and others have demonstrated that the histopathological transition of the adenoma–carcinoma sequence in patients with colorectal cancer is associated with an accumulation of genetic events (mutations in the classes of genes described above) that confers a significant growth advantage to a clonal population of cells (Fearon and Vogelstein, 1990). These genetic changes tend to correlate with progression through the adenoma–carcinoma sequence through a relatively consistent order of events (Figure 27.4).

An implication of this model is that any clonal somatic genetic alteration detected in invasive cancers should logically have major biological importance in having conferred significant growth advantage(s) to the tumour cells. Mathematical modelling of age-dependent tumour incidence suggests that at least five or six somatic genetic alterations are necessary for the development of the final colorectal cancer phenotype (Peto, 1977). Moreover, the accumulation of these genetic events in colorectal epithelium requires several years, even decades, and this is broadly consistent with the typical age of patients diagnosed with (sporadic) colorectal cancer.

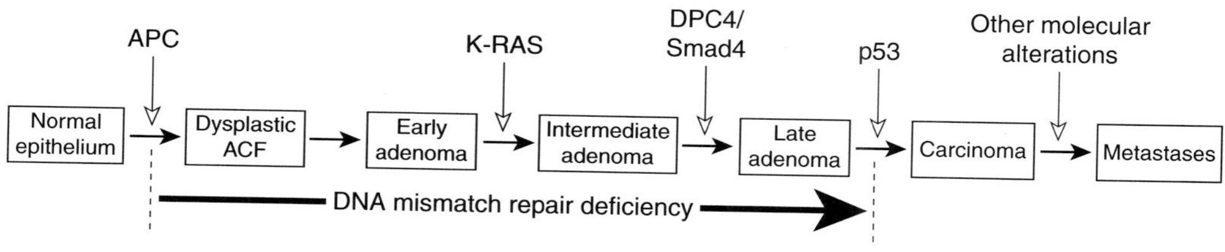

Figure 27.4 A molecular description of colorectal tumorigenesis (see text).

TUMOUR PROGRESSION: SOMATIC MUTATIONS IN ONCOGENES AND TUMOUR SUPPRESSOR GENES

The morphological stages of colorectal tumorigenesis from normal epithelium include aberrant crypt foci, adenoma, and finally carcinoma. Each of these morphological stages will be discussed in the context of the typical molecular lesions observed. However, it is possible to make two general comments about these genetic events. Firstly, passage along each stage of this morphological progression is associated with the acquisition of increasing numbers of genetic alterations. Secondly, the temporal pattern of some of these genetic alterations implies that they may have a pivotal role in the initiation or progression of malignant transformation.

Aberrant crypt foci (ACF)

These lesions were first identified in 1987 after methylene blue staining of whole-mount preparations of colonic mucosa from carcinogen-treated rodents (Bird, 1987; McLellan and Bird; 1988). Aberrant crypts are two to three times larger than a normal crypt and are microscopically elevated from the surrounding mucosa. Similar lesions have now been described in grossly normal human colorectal mucosa (Pretlow et al, 1991). These human ACF have many features in common with carcinogen-induced lesions in rodents. In particular, they occur with greater frequency in individuals at increased risk of colorectal cancer, display a spectrum of cellular architecture from near normal to dysplasia (Pretlow et al, 1991; Ronucci et al, 1991), and contain cells with mutated DNA (Jen et al, 1994; AJ Smith et al, 1994; Yamashita et al, 1995; Heinen et al, 1996).

ACF may well represent the earliest discernible precursor of colorectal cancer in humans and precede the development of an adenoma. This is supported by studies of the molecular lesions within ACF which have cast light on the important initiating genetic alterations in colorectal tumorigenesis. For instance, microsatellite instability is known to occur in ACF, indicating that mutations in DNA mismatch repair genes are early somatic events in colorectal tumorigenesis (Heinen et al, 1996). However, of crucial importance, it appears that a mutation in the APC gene has to occur before the cells within ACF display a dysplastic picture. In contrast, K-*ras* mutations are not associated with dysplastic ACF. Thus if a *ras* gene mutation is the first genetic event, a non-dysplastic ACF will develop with no capacity for further malignant progression. Indeed, cells with *ras* mutations are very common (Pretlow et al, 1993), but these cells are not dysplastic in the absence of an APC mutation and probably regress through apoptotic cell death (Shpitz et al, 1996). Conversely, an APC mutation occurring first will lead to the development of a dyplastic lesion which, driven by the accumulation of other genetic events, will progress further (Jen et, 1994; A J Smith et al, 1994).

The APC gene product has emerged as having a vital role in maintaining normal cellular architecture and function in the colorectal epithelium. Germline mutations in this gene are responsible for the syndrome of FAP (see below). The importance of this gene is underscored by the observation that, after its identification, somatic APC mutations were found to occur in the great majority of sporadic colorectal cancers (Miyoshi et al, 1992; Powell et al, 1992). In such instances the mutations were identical to those observed in FAP patients, with over 90% of them resulting in inactivation of the gene by causing premature truncation of the transcript (Miyoshi et al, 1992; Powell et al, 1992).

Kinzler and Vogelstein (1996) have recently proposed that APC acts as a molecular 'gatekeeper' of colonic epithelial cell proliferation and that its inactivation is necessary before net cellular proliferation occurs. A gatekeeper gene functions by maintaining constant numbers within the rapidly renewing cell populations of the colorectal epithelium. In this model, a mutated gatekeeper gene results in an irreversible imbalance of cell division over cell attrition, while mutations in other genes (e.g. *ras*) with an intact gatekeeper gene do not lead to any over growth disturbance. Certainly, the biological relevance of the gatekeeper model for APC is supported by the findings of studies examining the effects of molecular lesions in ACF that have been outlined above (Jen et al, 1994; AJ Smith et al, 1994). These studies suggest that it is not merely the accumulation of genetic events, but also their order, that can determine the capacity to initiate the neoplastic process. It has also emerged that not all genes that can effect cell growth are necessarily able to initiate neoplasia. Interestingly, expression of a wild-type (i.e. functional APC protein) in colorectal cells containing mutated APC induces apoptotic death of these cells (Morin et al, 1996). This would suggest that APC may be able to initiate or control cell death. The pivotal role of the APC gene is likely to be tissue-specific, as although it is expressed ubiquitously, it probably only has a gatekeeper function in the colorectal epithelium. This suggests that components of the luminal microenvironment may well be able to modulate APC activity in colorectal epithelial cells.

The mechanism by which the APC gene product exerts such a fundamental influence on the control of cell proliferation in colorectal epithelium is not entirely clear. The protein localizes to the basolateral membrane of colorectal epithelial cells with increasing expression as the cells mature and migrate up to the apex of the crypt (KJ Smith et al, 1993; Miyashiro et al, 1995). It is known that the wild-type APC gene product associates with the microtubule cytoskeleton and that this association is dependent upon the carboxy-terminal of the protein (Munemitsu et al, 1994; KJ Smith et al, 1994). The vast majority of APC mutations lead to truncated proteins lacking this carboxy-terminal structure (Powell et al, 1992), preventing this interaction. The APC gene encodes for a large protein of 2843 amino acids with no strong homology to proteins of known function. However, the identification of proteins that interact with APC has yielded some intriguing clues as to its mode of function. The most important insight into its function comes from the finding that APC interacts with β-catenin (Rubinfeld et al, 1993; Su et al, 1993b). Catenins are cytoplasmic proteins that are essential for cadherin-dependent cell-to-cell adhesion in epithelia (Kemler, 1993). Moreover, a quantitative or qualitative down-regulation of intercellular cohesion is an early and pivotal event during cancer progression (Dorudi and Hart, 1993). The APC gene contains β-catenin binding sites (Rubinfeld et al, 1996) which are modulated by phosphorylation, but mutant APC lacks part of the protein sequence necessary for catenin binding.

The β-catenin connection directs APC to two vital areas of cell function, the first being cellular adhesion, and here APC may be able to modulate cell-to-cell adhesion through its gatekeeper function. In this context, it is possible that APC has a downstream role in communicating the adhesion status between cells, thus connecting the cadherin–catenin axis to other components involved in cell-to-cell signalling. The second process links APC and β-catenin directly to an important intracellular signalling pathway (wnt), a discovery originally made in invertebrate experimental systems (Gumbiner, 1995). This link is further strengthened by the recent finding that APC/β-catenin is associated with another component of this pathway, a protein kinase called GSK3-β (Rubinfeld et al, 1996).

Given these observations and the biological consequences of APC inactivation in neoplasia, it is likely that the APC gene product is able to integrate extracellular signals and transduce them to the nucleus via β-catenin and related proteins. The emerging picture is of APC as a master molecule within intracellular signalling pathways with the ability to control cell proliferation and early differentiation (Figure 27.5). Even with the information available, it is not at all surprising to see why APC

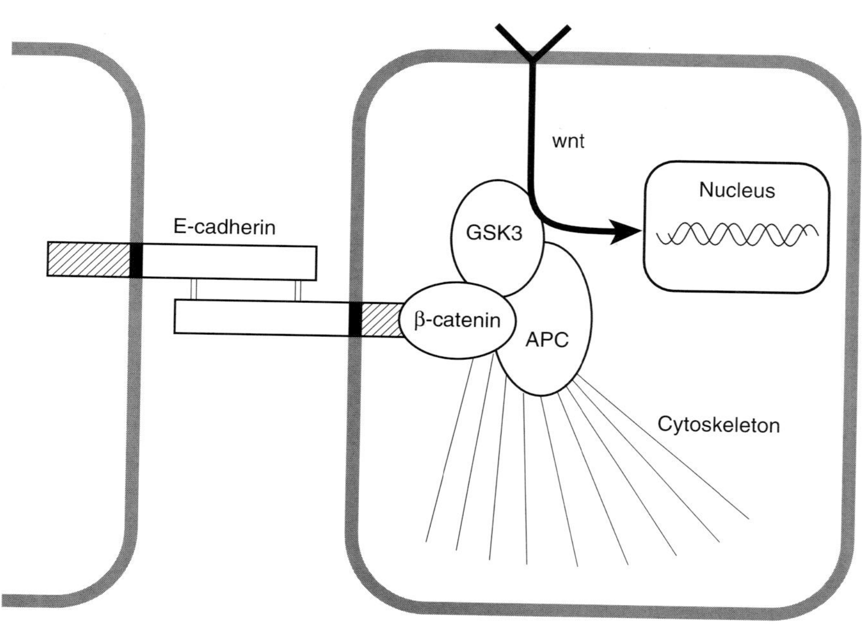

Figure 27.5 APC and its intracellular interactions. APC is linked to two vital processes of intracellular function. Firstly, its association with β-catenin may allow modulation of cell adhesion and intercellular signalling. Secondly, the GSK3 kinase and its integration with β-catenin and APC links this complex to an important intracellular signalling pathway (wnt).

dysfunction will have such a fundamental effect on cell behaviour at a very early stage in malignant transformation.

Interestingly, these findings still do not shed any light on the tissue specificity of the APC gene dysfunction in colorectal epithelial cells. However, an important lesson to emerge from this work is the realization that the complex signalling pathways in human tumorigenesis can be understood only by using the powerful experimental systems found in invertebrates and eukaryotes. This will become apparent again in the discussion of HNPCC below, where it will be seen how a convergence of human linkage analysis and experimental studies in nonhuman systems provided such crucial information in the elucidation of one of the most important mechanisms of colorectal tumorigenesis.

Adenoma and cancer formation

Adenomas are often categorized as early (type I), intermediate (type II) or late (type III) on the basis of their size, the amount of villous architecture and the extent of dysplasia. This is a useful classification when considering the accumulation of genetic alterations during progressive malignant transformation of the colorectal epithelium. As discussed earlier, APC gene mutations occur in ACF which are now considered to be the earliest discernible precursor of colorectal cancer. Certainly, mutated APC is a common finding in early adenomas as small as 5 mm in patients without polyposis (Vogelstein et al, 1988). Mutations in the K-*ras* gene can be detected in 50% of intermediate adenomas (>1 cm) and in 50% of colorectal cancers (Bos et al, 1987; Forrester et al, 1987). Adenomas less than 1 cm diameter are thought not to have a significant risk of malignant progression, and interestingly *ras* mutations are identified in only approximately 10% of lesions this size. However, *ras* mutations are more frequent in adenomas with high-grade dysplasia (Miyaki et al, 1990). These findings are consistent with the hypothesis that *ras* mutations do not initiate malignant transformation but are among the genetic alterations necessary to drive the progression of colorectal tumorigenesis.

Ras proteins are part of a large superfamily of regulatory proteins called guanosine triphosphates that control numerous cellular processes. As alluded to before, they play a pivotal role in modulating signals between cell surface receptors and the nucleus. The evolutionary importance of these proteins is underscored by the observation that *ras* homologues are present even in lower organisms. Three *ras* oncogenes have been identified in mammals (H-*ras*, K-*ras* and N-*ras*). However, of the three mutant proteins, only K-*ras* has been observed with significant frequency in colorectal tumours. Unusually in cancer molecular biology, K-*ras* demonstrates a distinct mutational 'hotspot' since single base substitutions within codons 12 or 13 account for 90% of the K-*ras* mutations detected in colorectal neoplasms. This does increase the ease of detection of *ras* mutations, compared with assessing allelic alterations in other oncogenes and tumour suppressor genes. These mutations maintain the K-*ras* protein in a continuously active state, resulting in constant activation of downstream signalling pathways that control cellular proliferation and differentiation (Boguski and McCormick, 1993).

Allelic losses within chromosomes 17p and 18q are common events in colorectal tumours. Not surprisingly, these regions were suspected to contain tumour suppressor genes (Vogelstein et al, 1988, 1989). Loss of heterozygosity (LOH) on chromosome 18q occurs as a relatively late event in colorectal tumorigenesis and can be detected in approximately 70% of cancers, 50% of late (type III) adenomas, and only infrequently (10%) in earlier adenomas. The minimal common deletion unit on 18q is centred around locus 18q21, and a candidate tumour suppressor gene called DCC (deleted in colorectal cancer) was cloned from this region (Fearon et al, 1990). This gene encodes for a protein with very close homology to a large family of cell adhesion molecules. However, despite the known role of cell adhesion dysfunction in cancer biology (Edelman, 1988), the importance of this gene product in colorectal tumorigenesis has been questioned recently. Although the expression of DCC is absent or greatly reduced in the majority of colorectal cancer cell lines studied (Fearon et al, 1990), specific allelic alteration of the DCC gene is a rare finding in colorectal cancers (Cho et al, 1994). Similarly, transfer of a normal copy of chromosome 18 into human colorectal cancer lines does abrogate their tumorigenicity, but specific transfer of the DCC gene itself does not affect the biology of these cells *in vivo*.

All of these findings indicate that loss of DCC is unlikely to have a causal role in colorectal tumorigenesis. Recent studies of transgenic mice lacking the murine homologue of DCC (called Dcc) have revealed that these animals have normal intestines and do not display an increased incidence of colonic tumours (Fazeli et al, 1997). However, inactivation of murine DCC did result in death of the animals shortly after birth, but this was due to failure of development of the nervous system. Interestingly, a recent finding has revealed that human DCC has significant sequence homology to a receptor protein originally identified in invertebrates that is responsible for guiding developing axons during early morphogenesis.

The 18q21 region is large enough to contain other candidate tumour suppressor genes. A candidate tumour suppressor gene called DPC (deleted in pancreatic cancer) located at 18q21 has recently been identified (Hahn et al, 1996). This gene is homologous to Smad4 and encodes for a transcription factor that mediates signal transduction in the TGFβ (transforming growth factor) pathway (Eppert et al, 1996). Inactivation of DPC4/Smad4 by mutation has been identified in a small proportion of colorectal cancers (MacGrogan et al, 1997). DPC4/Smad4 has very significant sequence homology to the MAD family of genes mediating signal transduction of TGFβ originally identified in invertebrates (Riggins et al, 1996). TGFβ signalling results in growth inhibition in epithelial tissues (Massague, 1990). The importance of inactivation of this signalling pathway in colorectal cancer was recently highlighted by the finding that the gene for the TGFβ type II receptor (TGFβ RII) is mutated in the majority of patients with HNPCC (see below) and in those patients with sporadic cancer displaying the replication error phenotype (Markowitz et al, 1995; Parsons et al, 1995). A recurring theme in the elucidation of the molecular pathogenesis of colorectal cancer is the enormous insights gained from studies of hereditary colorectal cancer. For instance, the importance of the TGFβ pathway in the regulation of cell proliferation in colonic epithelium has only emerged through intensive investigation of HNPCC. Additional candidate tumour suppressor genes on chromosome 18 have now been cloned and mutations within them may represent other targets for TGFβ inactivation in colorectal tumorigenesis (Thiagalingam et al, 1996).

Allelic loss of the short arm of chromosome 17 occurs in more than 75% of colorectal cancers, but LOH on 17p is an uncommon event in adenomas (Vogelstein et al, 1988; Baker et al, 1989). Indeed, LOH on 17p is rare even in large adenomas with high-grade dysplasia, containing foci of cancer. The importance of allelic loss on chromosome 17p in late colorectal tumorigenesis is underscored by the frequent observation that this genetic lesion is associated with progression from adenoma to carcinoma (Vogelstein et al, 1988). The common deletion unit in this region contained the p53 gene (called p53 as it is a 53 kDa protein), and it rapidly became apparent that 17p allelic loss targeted p53 as the major, if not the sole, tumour suppressor gene in this region (reviewed in Lane and Benchimol, 1990; Levine et al, 1991). Most p53 mutations lead to the production of a protein with a prolonged half-life that can be detected by immunohistochemistry, as the wild-type gene product is not normally detectable. It has now become clear that p53 is the most frequently mutated gene in all human cancers and it has emerged as having a central role in malignant transformation (Hollstein et al, 1991).

The p53 gene product is a nuclear phosphoprotein and is a transcription factor binding specific DNA sequences, activating the transcription of downstream genes (Kern et al, 1991). An important downstream target for p53 binding is the p21 protein (identical to WAF1, Cip1 and Sdi1). WAF1 is a cell cycle regulatory protein and has a pivotal role in driving and controlling the cell cycle. The importance of the p53 protein in tumour suppression is seen in the cell's response to DNA damage sustained, for instance, as a result of environmental exposure to mutagens or ionizing radiation. DNA damage induces over-expression of p53 which transactivates the p21 gene leading to cell cycle arrest (reviewed in Hartwell and Kastan, 1994). This arrest typically occurs between the G_1 and S phases of the cell cycle (see Figure 27.3), allowing repair of the damaged DNA through activation of DNA repair enzymes. However, if the cellular damage sustained is too great, then apoptotic death will occur, preventing proliferation of a cell containing mutated DNA. Thus any abrogation of p53 function by mutational inactivation will allow unchecked cell cycle progression after DNA damage and the appearance of a neoplastic cell population.

The molecular basis underlying the selection of mutated p53 occurring only in the final stages of colorectal tumorigenesis remains unknown. Interestingly, in the Li–Fraumeni syndrome, in which individuals have germline p53 mutations, the risk of developing colorectal cancer is not increased (Makin et al, 1990). Certainly, it appears that p53 mutations are not rate-limiting lesions necessary for the initiation of colorectal tumorigenesis. The cancer spectrum (typically breast, sarcoma and brain) of individuals with the Li–Fraumeni syndrome suggest that in colorectal cells the effects of p53 dysfunction are abrogated by the expression of other genes. Thus the growth pathways controlled by p53 may well have much greater redundancy in colorectal cells through the expression of other tissue-specific gene products. Inactivation of these p53-modifying genes may well be necessary before the manifestations of p53 loss become apparent by altered cellular phenotype.

Limitations of a genetic model for colorectal tumorigenesis

The intensive studies of the last decade have produced important data concerning the molecular pathogenesis of sporadic colorectal cancer. In particular, the genetic alterations identified to date, together with their relative timing and frequency during colorectal cancer progression, have provided data for an attractive model for tumour development (Fearon and Vogelstein, 1990).

However, this model does have limitations. Undoubtedly, additional oncogenes and tumour suppressor genes contributing to colorectal tumorigenesis remain to be discovered. Moreover, approximately 40% of colorectal cancers contain three of the four common genetic alterations (i.e. *ras* mutations, and allelic loss of 5q, 18q and 17p), while about 40% of cancers possess any two of the four and only 10% contain all four of these genetic lesions (Fearon and Vogelstein, 1990).

Importantly, this model does not encompass other key phenotypic changes associated with malignant transformation, such as growth factor expression, angiogenesis and adhesion molecule activity. These and many other features of neoplasia are influenced strongly by epigenetic alterations that are extremely difficult to assess, but have a role in tumorigenesis as important as any of the genetic or allelic changes described above.

Epigenetic alterations during colorectal cancer progression

Epigenetic alterations modify the phenotype of a cell without any changes to the genotype. Chromosome stability, gene expression and post-translational modification of protein are all levels of epigenetic modulation that can have a direct role in oncogenesis. Arguably, the most relevant in colorectal tumorigenesis is DNA methylation, with both hypo- and hyper-methylation contributing to tumour progression. The presence of a methyl group in cytosine residues in DNA plays an important role in the regulation of gene transcription (Jones and Buckley, 1990; Tate and Bird, 1993; Verdine, 1994). DNA methylation of gene promoters can lead to suppression of transcription, either through the direct effects of methylation on transcription factors or by binding of repressor proteins to the methylated DNA (Tate and Bird, 1993).

Significant loss of methylation occurs very early on in colorectal tumorigenesis with hypomethylation observed in type I adenomas when compared with normal mucosa within the same specimen (Goelz et al, 1985; Feinberg et al, 1988). Hypomethylation in DNA is associated with increased gene expression and may contribute to the activation of oncogenes during early tumorigenesis (Ferguson et al, 1995). Additionally, it has been suggested that hypomethylated DNA in premalignant cells is more susceptible to mutagenesis, perhaps as a result of less tight chromatin packing and therefore enhanced carcinogen access (Jones and Buckley, 1990). Hypermethylation of cytosine residues in promoter regions of genes results in down-regulation of transcription and may represent a mechanism whereby tumour suppressor genes are inactivated without structural alteration to the gene. Interestingly, alterations in the level of DNA methyltransferase, the enzyme responsible for cytosine methylation, has been observed even in normal large bowel epithelium of patients with colorectal cancer (El-Deiry et al, 1991).

The importance of gene expression and methylation status has recently been elegantly highlighted in sporadic colorectal cancers with microsatellite instability. Hypermethylation of the *hMLH1* promoter is a common finding in the majority of replication-error positive sporadic colorectal cancers and this is associated with loss of *hMLH1* protein expression (Herman et al, 1998). Such methylation has even been detected in microsatellite stable tumours and those unstable cancers with known mutations of a DNA mismatch repair gene. Human colorectal cancer cell lines with microsatellite instability also frequently demonstrate hypermethylation (Herman et al, 1998). Moreover, chemical reversal of this methylation resulted in re-expression of *hMLH1* protein and restoration of DNA mismatch repair function. These pivotal findings demonstrate the significance of epigenetic modulation of gene expression in eukaryotic cells and reveal that epigenetic mechanisms may prove to be just as important as genetic alterations in the emergence of the malignant phenotype in colorectal cancer.

HEREDITARY CANCER SYNDROMES

Somatic cells are not the only targets for gene mutations. Mutations can occur in ova and spermatocytes and these can be transmitted via the germline, resulting in an inherited cancer syndrome. Both FAP and HNPCC are examples of such genetic lesions. However, only mutations in tumour suppressor genes are known to be transmitted in this way. Oncogenes are not responsible for inherited cancer syndromes as presumably their dominant mode of action is incompatible with normal embryonic development. If an individual inherits a mutation in one allele of a tumour suppressor gene from one parent, then every cell in the body will be heterozygous for that mutation. In a predisposed tissue, this leads to a high risk of at least one cell acquiring a mutation in the remaining allele needed for full inactivation of that gene, and subsequent cancer development at a relatively young age. Thus according to Knudson's two-hit hypothesis (described above), two mutations are required for tumour development (reviewed in Knudson, 1993). The first is already transmitted via the germline and is responsible for the cancer predisposition, while the second is acquired in later life.

Knudson originally proposed his two-mutation model to explain the development of retinoblastoma (Knudson, 1971). His hypothesis at the time was based on observations on the age of onset and multiplicity of tumours in either the inherited or sporadic forms of retinoblastoma. In inherited cases every retinoblast already contained a mutated allele, and thus retinoblastoma arose after a second somatic mutation in the remaining allele in an already predisposed cell. Independent inactivation of the remaining allele in several retinoblasts results in multifocal tumours, often occurring bilaterally. In contrast, in the sporadic disease two inactivating somatic mutations were required in the same retinoblast before a tumour developed. Thus sporadic retinoblastoma tends to occur at a later age, and is generally unilateral and single (Figure 27.6).

It is important to appreciate that the germline mutation is recessive at the cellular level as both alleles need to be inactivated to produce the phenotype. However, hereditary retinoblastoma is transmitted as an autosomal dominant trait because of the very high likelihood of a second somatic mutation inactivating the remaining allele in at least one retinoblast. This model of inactivation of tumour suppressor genes after germline mutations has subsequently been proven to be correct and is certainly operational for FAP.

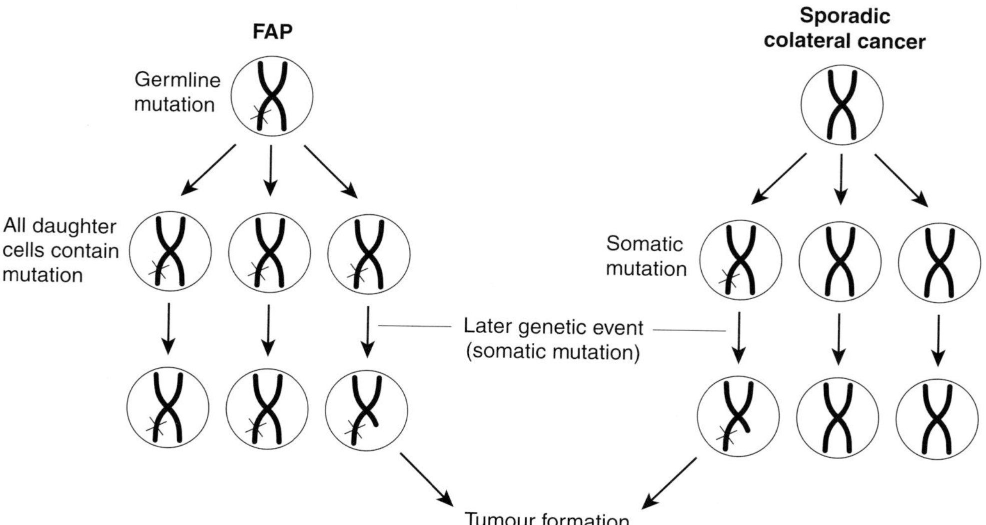

Figure 27.6 The Knudson 'two-hit' hypothesis in FAP and sporadic colorectal cancer.

HEREDITARY COLORECTAL CANCER

Inheritance of a single mutated gene can lead to a marked predisposition to colorectal cancer characterized by two different syndromes, familial adenomatous polyposis (FAP) and hereditary non-polyposis colorectal cancer (HNPCC). Indeed, epidemiological evidence indicates that up to 15% of colorectal cancers occur as in a dominantly inherited pattern (Houlston et al, 1992).

Familial adenomatous polyposis (FAP)

FAP accounts for fewer than 1% of all patients with colorectal cancer and is typified by the development of hundreds of thousands of adenomas during the second and third decades of life. These occur predominantly in the large bowel, but adenomas are also common in the upper gastrointestinal tract. Untreated, the large numbers of adenomas almost always guarantees the development of carcinoma. FAP can be regarded as a generalized growth disorder because extracolonic manifestations of the disease are observed frequently, including retinal lesions, osteomas, and desmoid tumours. Some of these non-colonic features characterize a number of eponymous syndromes which are discussed elsewhere in this volume.

Although the disease has long been recognized, the molecular pathogenesis of FAP has become clear only recently. Herrera et al (1986) reported the presence of a deletion of chromosome 5q in a patient with FAP. Genetic linkage studies subsequently localized the adenomatous polyposis coli (APC) gene to chromosome 5q21 (Bodmer et al, 1987; Leppert et al, 1987). Using positional cloning techniques, the gene was rapidly cloned and sequenced and its causal role in FAP was confirmed by the demonstration of cosegregation of mutant APC alleles in affected families (Groden et al, 1991; Joslyn et al, 1991; Kinzler et al, 1991; Nishisho et al, 1991). It appears that, as in hereditary retinoblastoma, initiation of adenoma formation in FAP requires a somatic mutation in the remaining wild-type allele inherited from the unaffected parent. Studies in both humans and in a murine model of FAP (the murine homologue of APC is mutated in the multiple intestinal neoplasia (Min) mouse) have now confirmed that the rate-limiting step for adenoma formation is inactivation of the remaining functional allele (Ichii et al, 1992; Levy et al, 1994; Luongo et al, 1994). These observations provide strong evidence for Knudson's two-hit hypothesis that was originally expounded to explain tumour development in retinoblastoma. The structure and the function of the APC gene have already been discussed in the context of sporadic colorectal cancer.

Genotype and phenotype in FAP

Remarkably, the clinical features of FAP patients are not uniform despite the consistent finding that almost all the identified mutations within the gene result in C-terminal truncation of the protein. This is due to the differential phenotypic effect of mutational location within the APC gene, but additionally, there is evidence that epigenetic and environmental influences are significant. For instance, the presence of retinal lesions (congenital hypertrophy of the retinal pigment epithelium, CHRPE) is associated with truncating mutations in exon 9 between codons 463 and 1387 (Olschwang et al, 1993), while truncating mutations at another site (between codons 1403 and 1578) are associated with frequent extracolonic features such as desmoid tumours and osteomas, but not CHRPE (Davies et al, 1995). Mutational site also modulates the colonic manifestations of FAP. An attenuated form of the disease in which patients develop only a relatively small number of polyps is a frequent characteristic of truncating mutations up to codon 157 (Spirio et al, 1993). However, mutations further along the gene, between codons 1250 and 1464, are associated with a more aggressive phenotype with very large polyp numbers (Nagase and Nakamura, 1993).

These latter observations are consistent with the putative mode of interaction of the APC protein as normal APC molecules are thought to act as homodimers (i.e. two identical protein chains linked together). Moreover, there is evidence that mutant APC protein can inactivate wild-type protein by binding with it (Su et al, 1993a). A very truncated protein, resulting from proximal mutations, is probably incapable of interacting with the wild-type protein, leading to a mild phenotype; whereas a near full-length mutant protein, produced by very distal mutations, will bind and inactivate wild-type protein and result in a more aggressive form of the disease.

Determining the mutational profile of patients with FAP may well have some important applications in their clinical management. If it is possible to predict with some accuracy the phenotype of the disease, then the precise form of surgery offered to patients can be chosen. For example, patients with aggressive disease, including significant rectal involvement, may be best treated by proctocolectomy which may be restorative. Conversely, total colectomy with an ileorectal anastomosis is an appropriate option in individuals with attenuated FAP and relative rectal sparing. Further delineation of the phenotypic effects of different APC mutations will be of great therapeutic value and currently this is an area of intense study.

Environmental factors

Environmental and epigenetic factors must also be important modifiers of the FAP phenotype as patients with identical truncating mutations can still develop different clinical features of the disease. For instance, indistinguishable truncating mutations will give rise to Gardener's syndrome (mandibular osteomas and desmoid tumours) in some, but not in all, patients with FAP (Nishisho et al, 1991). Elucidating the precise mechanisms of environmental and epigenetic modulation of the FAP phenotype is an extraordinarily complex process. While the inheritance of germline mutations in patients with FAP predisposes them to colorectal cancer, other genetic alterations are required before carcinoma develops. The consequences of these additional mutations will in turn be affected by environmental factors and the genes themselves are under the influence of other modifying genes. Thus the molecular pathways in a multigenetic disorder such as colorectal cancer, albeit after tumour initiation due to a single germline mutation, becomes overwhelmingly complex. This is quite unlike the genotype–phenotype relationship of a classical monogenetic disorder such as cystic fibrosis, where a single genetic lesion always leads to the development of the same disease state in a reproducible manner.

The precise components of the luminal environment that modulate the FAP phenotype in the presence of identical genotypes are not clear. Diet is an obvious target for environmental modulation of phenotype, given the association between dietary factors and colorectal cancer. While human diets are so complex that ascribing a particular component of the diet as the culpable factor for this modulation is a very difficult task, studies of the Min (multiple intestinal neoplasia) mouse have provided some intriguing clues to this problem. These mice develop multiple intestinal adenomas due to a truncating mutation of the murine homologue of the APC gene. The number of polyps varies quite dramatically between the different inbred strains harbouring this mutation. Linkage studies have revealed that a single locus, MOM1 (modifier of Min) on chromosome 4 accounts for many of these phenotypic differences (Dietrich et al, 1993).

A strong candidate MOM1 gene, encoding for a secreted phospholipase, has subsequently been cloned from this site (MacPhee et al, 1995). The finding that the MOM1 gene encodes for a phospholipase is illuminating given the known association between the lipid content of the diet and colorectal cancer. Additionally, it is now known that nonsteroidal anti-inflammatory drugs (NSAIDS) can prevent or even cause regression of colorectal adenomas in both humans and mice (Giardello et al, 1993; Boolbol et al, 1996). NSAIDS inhibit the enzyme cyclooxygenase that is responsible for metabolizing the lipid arachidonic acid. Thus, the Min mouse model provides a striking example of how phenotype can be altered by the action of modifier genes which are themselves subject to modulation by components of the luminal environment.

Hereditary non-polyposis colorectal cancer (HNPCC, or the Lynch syndrome)

HNPCC is an autosomal dominant genetic disorder in which individuals have a high risk of developing cancer. The term 'non-polyposis' merely distinguishes the syndrome from FAP. Synchronous adenomatous polyps are a common feature of HNPCC, but the disease is not characterized by the presence of hundreds of adenomas as in FAP. HNPCC has long been suspected to have an inherited basis, but only became fully characterized in the 1980s and 1990s through intensive studies of familial kindreds by clinical epidemiologists (Lynch et al, 1996).

Typically, individuals with HNPCC develop colorectal cancer at an average age of 45 years. Patients with HNPCC account for 2–5% of all patients with colorectal cancer. However, the stringent fulfilling criteria used for HNPCC were originally implemented to identify kindreds for genetic analysis (Vasen et al, 1991). Therefore the real prevalence of HNPCC is likely to be significantly underestimated if these criteria are rigidly enforced. Indeed, evidence is accruing that an inherited susceptibility is a more common functional component in the development of colorectal cancer than was previously recognized (Cannon-Albright et al, 1988; Hall et al, 1994, 1996).

Delineation of the genetic pathogenesis of HNPCC represents an extremely productive convergence of a number of disciplines, from tumour and molecular biologists to yeast geneticists. Detailed linkage analysis of large kindreds from North America, Europe and New Zealand using microsatellite markers provided the first significant line of investigation. These efforts yielded two loci on chromosomes 2p16 and 3p21 at which there was tight linkage in affected families (Lindblom et al, 1993; Pelkomaki et al, 1993). A new phenomenon became apparent during the course of these LOH studies. Rather than the classical deletion of one allele normally seen in tumour tissue, additional new alleles could be distinguished from alleles in DNA extracted from normal colon (Aaltonen et al, 1993; Ionov et al, 1993; Thibodeau et al, 1993). The differences in the size of these bands were quite small and usually occurred in multiples of 2–5 base-pairs. These alterations were found to occur in regions containing short nucleotide repeats, called 'microsatellites'. The instability observed in these microsatellites arose as a result of differences in the number of these mono-, di-, or tri-nucleotide DNA repeats between tumour tissue and normal colon, and was termed 'microsatellite instability' (MI) or 'replication error phenotype' (RER). Further examination of paired tumour and normal colon samples from patients with HNPCC revealed that the RER phenotype was present in most of the tumours from HNPCC patients, but was an infrequent occurrence in sporadic cancers. Interestingly, RER positivity in sporadic colorectal cancers was found to be a particular feature of proximal tumours (i.e. proximal to the splenic flexure), which is a characteristic of HNPCC. These findings were rapidly confirmed by other groups and it became evident that the RER phenotype was a constant feature of a small subset of many other solid cancers (reviewed in Meltzer, 1995).

This pattern of quite subtle allelic alteration did not fit the classical tumour suppressor gene paradigm in which mutation occurs in one allele with deletion of the other, manifested by LOH. Additionally, further linkage analysis had revealed linkage to a number of different loci on different chromosomes in the pedigrees studied (Peltomaki et al, 1993). The discovery of the genes responsible for the RER phenotype was facilitated by some extraordinarily intuitive observations by biologists studying replication fidelity in prokaryotes. These investigators recognized that the pattern of microsatellite instability found in human colorectal cancers was similar to that observed in bacteria and yeast containing mutations in the *mutS* and *mutL* genes encoding for DNA mismatch repair enzymes (Strand et al, 1993). Moreover, it was suggested that germline mutations in human homologues of *mutS* and *mutL* may account for the syndrome of HNPCC (Strand et al, 1993). These keen insights into the putative molecular basis of HNPCC stimulated an intense search for human homologues of prokaryotic DNA mismatch repair genes, culminating in the identification of five candidate human genes (reviewed in Marra and Boland, 1995).

The notion that a *mutS* homologue may be involved in the pathogenesis of HNPCC, at least in the type linked to chromosome 2, was strengthened considerably by the finding that one (*hMSH2*) was located on chromosome 2p (Fishel et al, 1993). However, direct evidence of a causal association between DNA mismatch repair gene dysfunction and HNPCC was then provided by the identification of germline mutations in *hMSH2* and in *mutL* homologues in HNPCC families (Leach et al, 1993; Marra and Boland, 1995). Experimental studies have also produced strong supporting evidence for the role of *mutS* and *mutL* homologues in HNPCC. For example, RER-positive tumour extracts are deficient in mismatch repair activity *in vitro* (Umar et al, 1994). Furthermore, transfer of a human chromosome containing a normal copy of *hMLH1* into a human colorectal cancer cell line with an *hMLH1* mutation abrogated the RER phenotype and restored mismatch repair activity (Koi et al, 1994). Germline mutations in four human DNA mismatch repair genes (*hMSH2, hMLH1, hPMS1* and *hPMS2*) are now thought to account for the great majority of HNPCC families (Kinzler and Vogelstein, 1996). It is expected that other genes will be discovered that account for other HNPCC kindreds not harbouring mutations in the genes described above.

Microsatellite instability and cancer formation

The rate of spontaneous mutations in expressed genes in tumour cells that exhibit the RER phenotype and have mismatch repair deficiency is significantly higher than in normal cells (Battacharyya et al, 1994; Eshelman et al, 1995). Colorectal cancer cell lines deficient in mismatch repair activity accumulate several types of mutations, including large deletions and loss of complete exons (Battacharyya et al, 1994; Eshelman et al, 1995). Moreover, these alterations are not just restricted to DNA microsatellite sequences. This global mutator phenotype results in considerable genetic instability and provides a mechanism for accelerated tumour development in patients with HNPCC by generating the multiple mutations necessary for tumorigenesis.

The discovery of DNA mismatch repair genes has raised the possibility that an alternative pathway for tumour development exists in HNPCC and those sporadic colorectal cancers exhibiting microsatellite instability. Indeed, there is some evidence to support this notion. The tumour suppressor gene paradigm characterized by LOH is rarely observed in

HNPCC. Rather, allelic loss occurs by point mutations causing premature protein truncation and frame shifts in the DNA reading sequence (Konishi et al, 1996). Moreover, an accumulation of mutations in the tumour suppressor genes and oncogenes (APC, K-*ras* and p53) commonly seen in sporadic colorectal cancer tumorigenesis occur less frequently in HNPCC (Konishi et al, 1996). However, this inverse relationship between the presence of microsatellite instability and the absence of mutations in APC, K-*ras* and p53 is not a constant phenomenon (Huang et al, 1996). Certainly, it appears that colorectal cancers without microsatellite instability lose approximately 25% of randomly chosen alleles, but RER-positive tumours lose none (Aaltonen et al, 1993). Thus it is conceivable that there are at least two pathways for the multiple genetic alterations required for colorectal tumorigenesis: subtle alterations due to deficient DNA mismatch repair occurring in HNPCC and a small proportion of sporadic cancers, with gross allelic loss being responsible for the great majority.

Apart from mutations in mismatch repair genes, colorectal tumours with microsatellite instability contain other genetic alterations that do not appear to be present in sporadic RER-negative cancers. Colorectal cancers are generally insensitive to the epithelial proliferation-suppressing effect of the cytokine TGFβ. In RER-positive cancers this is almost always due to frameshift mutations in a ten-adenine repeat microsatellite sequence embedded in the coding region of the TGFβ RII gene (Markowitz et al, 1995). Similarly, mutations have also been identified in an eight-guanine repeat in the insulin-like growth factor II receptor (IGFIIR) (Souza et al, 1996). The significance of this latter finding is underscored by the observation that soluble IGFIIR is involved in the secretion and full activation of the TGFβ pathway (Souza et al, 1996). Additionally, colorectal cancers with microsatellite instability often contain defects in HLA locus genes which may allow them to escape immune surveillance.

Some 12–15% of all patients with sporadic colorectal cancers also exhibit the RER phenotype, but mutations in the known human mismatch repair genes account for only a proportion of these cases, while in the remainder the molecular basis of the microsatellite instability is yet to be defined. Additionally, 40–50% of colorectal cancers arising in very young patients (under 35 years), in whom a hereditary component is likely, lack microsatellite instability (Liu et al, 1995). All of these RER-positive tumours share many clinicopathological features found in cancers seen in HNPCC patients (H Kim et al, 1994). In particular, there is a predominance of right-sided tumours, and the histological picture of poor differentiation, abundant mucin production and a pronounced host lymphocytic infiltrate is common in both HNPCC and RER-positive sporadic cancers (H Kim et al, 1994).

A population-based Finnish study has revealed that patients with germline mutations of *hMLH1* do demonstrate a stage-for-stage survival benefit compared with individuals with microsatellite stable sporadic cancers (Sankila et al, 1996). Arguably, the mutator phenotype of RER-positive tumours might generate many potential tumour neoantigens eliciting a specific antigen-driven immune response against the tumour cells. The florid host response seen in RER-positive colorectal cancers may account for this survival advantage, but currently there is no evidence to indicate that this pronounced lymphocytic infiltrate is necessarily a reflection of a specific antitumour immune response. Additionally, the survival benefit seen in this Finnish study may be related to other unidentified molecular effects of these *hMLH1* mutations. Notwithstanding these considerations, other small non-population-based studies have demonstrated a survival benefit for patients with RER-positive colorectal cancers (Lothe et al, 1993; Thibodeau et al, 1993). Certainly, uncorrected defective DNA replication in these microsatellite-unstable tumours may lead to an accumulation of mutations in critical genes whose subsequent dysfunction leads to cell death.

Comparison of FAP and HNPCC

Kinzler and Vogelstein have recently suggested that FAP is a disease of tumour initiation, while HNPCC is one of tumour progression (Kinzler and

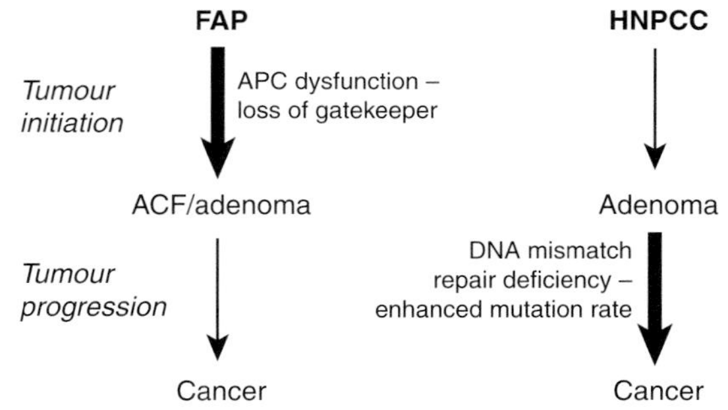

Figure 27.7 Comparison of FAP and HNPCC. FAP is a disorder of accelerated tumour initiation as a result of loss of the gatekeeper function of the APC gene. In HNPCC, DNA mismatch repair deficiency leads to an enhanced mutation rate and accelerated tumour progression, but the rate of tumour initiation is not increased.

Vogelstein, 1996). According to this hypothesis, in FAP the gatekeeper mechanism is defective resulting in the formation of huge numbers of adenomas; however, sufficient additional mutations in other oncogenes and tumour suppressor genes accumulate in at least one of these adenomas, leading to cancer progression. In contrast, in HNPCC the rate of adenoma formation is the same as that in the general population, but defective DNA mismatch repair allows the rapid accumulation of mutations in oncogenes and tumour suppressor genes, with accelerated tumour progression. Interestingly, in both of these inherited colorectal syndromes the median age of tumour diagnosis is similar at 42 years, some 25 years earlier than the median age of sporadic colorectal cancer patients (Figure 27.7).

CLINICAL IMPLICATIONS OF THE GENETIC BASIS OF COLORECTAL CANCER

The huge advances made in elucidating the molecular pathogenesis of both sporadic and hereditary colorectal cancer have potentially far-reaching clinical implications. However, the application of these genetic findings into routine clinical practice is hampered both by technical issues and by problems in the interpretation of the results obtained. Broadly, there are three areas of clinical management where the genetic alterations found in colorectal cancers may have useful application.

Genetic testing for hereditary colorectal cancer

Clearly, the development of a genetic technique for making a firm diagnosis of a hereditary colorectal cancer syndrome is of great importance to affected patients and their families. Despite the identification of some of the causative genes, genetic testing in this context is not in routine clinical use. The genes are either very large (as in APC) or multiple (DNA mismatch repair genes). Moreover, in both FAP and HNPCC, there are no mutational hot-spot regions. Several techniques have been employed to detect alterations in these genes, including direct DNA sequencing, heteroduplex analysis and SSCP or single-stranded chain polymorphism (reviewed in Luce et al, 1996). However, each of these techniques has its specific limitations; in particular, they are either quite insensitive or are appropriate only for examining small segments of DNA.

Notwithstanding these limitations, the use of *in vitro* transcription translation assays is able to detect mutations in approximately 85% of FAP and 50–60% of HNPCC kindreds. The development of this technique is aided by the knowledge that virtually all APC mutations, and at least 50% of those occurring in HNPCC, result in the production of a truncated protein. The gene transcript is amplified and subsequently transcribed and translated in an *in vitro* system. In the presence of a mutation, protein truncation will then be revealed by altered electrophoretic mobility of the reaction products, with the truncated protein migrating faster than the full-length gene product. For example, an individual who is heterozygous for such a mutation will show two bands, a shortened polypeptide generated from the mutated allele and a full-length protein from the wild-type allele. Such tests have now been developed for FAP (Powell et al, 1992; van der Luijt et al, 1994) and HNPCC (Liu et al, 1996).

There are still considerable problems that need to be overcome before these tests can be offered routinely to patients. Firstly, they do not detect all FAP and HNPCC kindreds. Secondly, the validity of a negative result cannot be guaranteed as this may be due either to the relative insensitivity of the technique or to the presence of a mutation that simply is not detected by the test. Finally, genetic testing for these conditions, which with appropriate management are essentially non-lethal, has significant ethical considerations. For instance, should prenatal testing be offered? These issues underscore the importance of conducting any such testing under the auspices of a family cancer clinic with significant input from trained genetic counsellors who can address the medical and psychological questions with patients and their families. Nonetheless, the potential value of these techniques should not be underestimated as they may obviate the need for repeated examination of family members who do not harbour a kindred-specific mutation.

Early detection of colorectal cancer

Curative interventions for colorectal cancer depend upon early detection of the tumour. In colorectal cancer the only genetic targets that can be realistically exploited for early detection strategies are K-*ras* mutations and, perhaps, a few cluster regions in the p53 gene. As stated previously, the presence of a mutational hot-spot at codon 12 in the K-*ras* gene allows detection of allelic alteration with relative ease, compared with analysis of the APC gene which would be a daunting task. The initial strategy used in colorectal cancer patients examined paired primary tumours and stool samples (Sidransky et al, 1992). DNA was extracted and purified from the stool samples and then examined for the presence of *ras* mutations by using PCR to amplify the small amounts of target DNA followed by a *ras* plaque hybridization assay. This study revealed that eight of nine patients with a K-*ras* mutation in their primary tumours also exhibited similar *ras* mutations in stool DNA from exfoliated tumour cells. Patients without a *ras* mutation in their cancers and those without cancer demonstrated a negative test. Since then other investigators have confirmed these findings in patients with colorectal cancer (Tobi et al, 1994). While these techniques are experimentally feasible, they are not appropriate for translation into routine clinical practice.

Staging and prognostic stratification

Conventional histopathological staging provides a static description of the anatomical extent of tumour spread within a surgical specimen. Currently, such tumour staging, when performed accurately, gives the best guide to the prognosis of patients who have undergone putatively curative colorectal cancer resection. The limitations of conventional staging are highlighted by the considerable prognostic heterogeneity of patients within a given tumour stage. For instance, not all patients with lymph node-negative cancers are cured of their disease. Conversely, treatment failure is not a uniform outcome in patients with Dukes' stage C tumours. More precise stratification of prognostic groups assumes importance with the emerging evidence of the clinical value of adjuvant chemotherapy regimens (Salz and Kelsen, 1997).

Can the knowledge of the molecular alterations during colorectal tumorigenesis aid in this problem? Molecular techniques have been used both to study primary colorectal cancers in an attempt to identify clinically useful prognostic alterations, and to enhance conventional tumour staging by examining lymph nodes for the presence of genetically detected metastases. The former line of investigation has been extensively reviewed by Gryfe et al (1997). In summary, no firm conclusions can be drawn from these studies which have investigated the prognostic significance of many of the common genetic alterations observed in colorectal cancers. Careful prospective studies with appropriate statistical analysis are needed to determine if the presence or absence of any of these genetic alterations are independent prognostic indicators. Some limited data are available on the genetic staging of colorectal cancer. The presence of mutations in the K-*ras* and p53 genes has been used in this context. A study by Hayashi et al (1995) demonstrated that the presence of these specific genetic alterations in the lymph nodes of colorectal cancers assessed as tumour-free by conventional histopathology is associated with reduced survival. The obvious implication of this is that these mutations are contained in occult lymph node micrometastases not detected by histology. However, K-*ras* mutations are present in only 40–50% of colorectal cancers, and mutations in the p53 gene, while a more frequent finding in colorectal carcinoma, are not confined to a single site. Therefore, genetic diagnosis of lymph node metastasis in colorectal cancer will require analysis of a panel of genes and/or several sites within target genes.

These problems will limit the translation of such techniques to routine clinicopathological use for the foreseeable future. New technology based on attaching DNA oligonucleotides to a microchip for parallel hybridization will increase our ability to analyse simultaneously several mutated genes (Wallace, 1997). However, by themselves these novel technologies will not translate into improved patient outcome unless corresponding advances are made in adjuvant treatment modalities for patients with colorectal cancer.

CONCLUSION

Our understanding of the molecular pathogenesis of colorectal cancer increased at a phenomenal rate in the 1990s. Delineation of the genetic basis of hereditary colorectal cancer syndromes, together with the use of powerful prokaryotic experimental systems, has underpinned many of the new insights made in the tumorigenesis of sporadic bowel carcinoma. Genetic screening is becoming available for members of families with high risk, but their use requires caution and, certainly, should be conducted under the auspices of a family cancer clinic. The translation of other molecular techniques into the clinical management of patients with colorectal malignancy needs further evaluation.

REFERENCES

Aaltonen LA, Pelkomaki P, Leach FS *et al* (1993) Clues to the pathogenesis of familial colorectal cancer. *Science* **260**: 812–816.

Baker SJ, Fearon ER, Nigro JM *et al* (1989) Chromosome 17 deletions and p53 mutations in colorectal carcinomas. *Science* **244**: 217–221.

Battacharyya NP, Skandalis A, Ganesh A, Groden J & Meuth M (1994) Mutator phenotypes in human colorectal carcinoma cell lines. *Proc Natl Acad Sci USA* **91**: 6319–6323.

Bedi A, Pasricha PJ, Akhtar AJ *et al* (1995) Inhibition of apoptosis during development of colorectal cancer. *Cancer Res* **55**: 1811–1816.

Bernstein SC, Weinberg RA (1985) Expression of the metastatic phenotype in cells transfected with human metastatic tumour DNA. *Proc Natl Acad Sci USA* **82**: 1726–1730.

Bird RP (1987) Observation and quantification of aberrant crypts in the murine colon treated with a colon carcinogen: preliminary findings. *Cancer Lett* **37**: 147–151.

Bishop JM (1991) Molecular themes in oncogenesis. *Cell* **64**: 235–248.

Bodmer WF (1994) Cancer genetics. *Br Med Bull* **50**: 517–526.

Bodmer WF, Bailey C, Bodmer J et al (1987) Localisation of the gene for familial adenomatous polyposis on chromosome 5. *Nature* **328**: 614–616.

Boguski MS & McCormick F (1993) Proteins regulating *Ras* and its relatives. *Nature* **366**: 643–654.

Boolbol SK, Dannenberg AJ, Chadurn A et al (1996) Cyclooxygenase-2 overexpression and tumour formation are blocked by sulindac in a murine model of familial adenomatous polyposis. *Cancer Res* **56**: 2556–2560.

Bos JL, Fearon ER, Hamilton SR *et al* (1987) Prevalence of *ras* gene mutations in human colorectal cancer. *Nature* **327**: 293–297.

Cannon-Albright LA, Skolnick MH, Bishop DT, Lee RG, Burt RW (1988) Common inheritance of susceptibility to colonic adenomatous polyps and colorectal cancers. *N Engl J Med* **319**: 533–537.

Cho KR, Oliner JD, Simons JW *et al* (1994) The DCC gene: structural analysis and mutations in colorectal carcinomas. *Genomics* **19**: 525–531.

Chung DC & Rustgi AK (1995) DNA mismatch repair and cancer. *Gastroenterology* **109**: 1685–1699.

Davies D, Armstrong J, Thakker N *et al* (1995) Severe Gardner syndrome in families with mutations restricted to a specific region of the APC gene. *Am J Hum Genet* **57**: 1151–1158.

Dietrich WF, Lander ES, Smith JS *et al* (1993) Genetic identification of Mom-1, a major modifier locus affecting Min-induced intestinal neoplasia in the mouse. *Cell* **75**: 631–639.

Dorudi S & Hart IR (1993) Mechanisms underlying invasion and metastasis. *Curr Opin Oncol* **5**: 130–135.

Edelman GM (1988) Morphoregulatory molecules. *Biochemistry* **27**: 3533–3543.

El-Deiry WAS, Nelkin BD, Celano P *et al* (1991) High expression of the DNA methyltransferase gene characterizes human neoplastic cells and progression stages of colon cancer. *Proc Natl Acad Sci USA* **88**: 3470–3474.

Eppert K, Scherer SW, Ozcelik H *et al* (1996) MADR2 maps to 18q21 and encodes a TGF-β-regulated mad-related protein that is functionally mutated in colorectal carcinoma. *Cell* **86**: 543–552.

Eshelman JR, Lang EZ, Bowerfind GK *et al* (1995) Increased mutation rate at the hprt locus accompanies microsatellite instability in colon cancer. *Oncogene* **10**: 33–37.

Eshelman JR & Markowitz SD (1995) Microsatellite instability in inherited and sporadic neoplasms. *Current Opin Oncol* **7**: 83–89.

Fazeli A *et al* (1997) Phenotype of mice lacking functional Dcc. *Nature* **386**: 798–804.

Fearon ER & Vogelstein B (1990) A genetic model for colorectal tumorigenesis. *Cell* **61**: 759–767.

Fearon ER, Hamilton SR & Vogelstein B (1987) Clonal analysis of human colorectal tumours. *Science* **238**: 193–197.

Fearon ER, Cho KR, Nigro JM *et al* (1990) Identification of a chromosome 18q gene that is altered in colorectal cancers. *Science* **247**: 49–56.

Feinberg AP, Gehrke CW, Kuo KC & Ehrlich M (1988) Reduced genomic 5-methylcytosine content in human colonic neoplasia. *Cancer Res* **48**: 1159–1161.

Ferguson AT, Lapidus RG, Baylin SB & Davidson NE (1995) Demethylation of the estrogen receptor gene in estrogen receptor-negative breast cancer cells can reactivate estrogen receptor gene expression. *Cancer Res* **55**: 2279–2283.

Fishel R, Lescoe MK, Rao MR *et al* (1993) The human mutator gene homolog *MSH2* and its association with hereditary nonpolyposis colon cancer. *Cell* **75**: 1027–1038.

Forrester K, Almoguera C, Han K, Grizzle WE & Perucho M (1987) Detection of high incidence of K-*ras* oncogenes during human colon tumorigenesis. *Nature* **327**: 298–303.

Giardello FM, Hamilton SR, Krush AJ *et al* (1993) Treatment of colonic and rectal adenomas with sulindac in familial adenomatous polyposis. *N Engl J Med* **328**: 1313–1316.

Giardello FM, Zehnbauer BA, Hamilton SR & Jones RJ (1995) Inhibition of apoptosis during the development of colorectal cancer. *Cancer Res* **55**: 1811–1816.

Goelz SE, Vogelstein B, Hamilton SR & Feinberg AP (1985) Hypomethylation of DNA from benign and malignant human colon neoplasms. *Science* **228**: 187–190.

Groden J, Thliveris A, Samowitz W *et al* (1991) Identification and characterization of the familial adenomatous polyposis coli gene. *Cell* **66**: 589–600.

Gryfe R, Swallow C, Bapat B *et al* (1997) Molecular biology of colorectal cancer. *Curr Probl Cancer* **21**: 233–300.

Gumbiner BM (1995) Signal transduction of β-catenin. *Curr Opin Cell Biol* **7**:634–640.

Haber DA (1995) Telomeres, cancer, and immortality. *N Engl J Med* **332**: 955–956.

Hahn SA, Schutte M, Hoque AT *et al.* (1996) DPC4, a candidate tumor suppressor gene at human chromosome 18q21.1. *Science* **271**: 350–353.

Hall NR, Bishop DT, Stephenson BM & Finan PJ (1996) Hereditary susceptibility to colorectal cancer. Relatives of early onset cases are particularly at risk. *Dis Colon Rectum* **39**: 739–743.

Hall NR, Finan PJ, Ward B, Turner G & Bishop DT (1994) Genetic susceptibility to colorectal cancer in patients under 45 years of age. *Br J Surg* **81**: 1485–1489.

Hansen MF & Cavenee WK (1987) Genetics of cancer predisposition. *Cancer Res* **47**: 5518–5527.

Harley CB, Futcher AB & Greider CW (1990) Telomeres shorten during ageing of human fibroblasts. *Nature* **345**: 458–460.

Harris H (1988) The analysis of malignancy by cell fusion: the position in 1988. *Cancer Res* **48**: 3302–3306.

Hartwell LH & Kastan M (1994) Cell cycle control and cancer. *Science* **266**: 1821–1828.

Hayashi N *et al* (1995) Genetic diagnosis of lymph-node metastasis in colorectal cancer. *Lancet* **345**: 1257–1259.

Heinen CD, Shivapurkar N, Tang Z, Groden J & Alabaster O (1996) Microsatellite instability in aberrant crypt foci from human colons. *Cancer Res* **56**: 5339–5341.

Hengartner MO & Horvita HR (1994) Prevention of programmed cell death in *Caenorhabditis elegans* by human Bcl-2. *Cell* **76**: 665–676.

Herman JG, Umar A, Polyak K *et al* (1998) Incidence and functional consequences of *hMLH1* promoter hypermethylation in colorectal cancer. *Proc Natl Acad Sci USA* **95**: 6870–6875.

Herrera L, Kakati S, Gibas L, Pietrzak E & Sandberg A (1986) Gardner syndrome in a man with an interstitial deletion of 5q. *Am J Med Genet* **25**: 473–476.

Hollstein M, Sidransky D, Vogelstein B & Harris CC (1991) p53 mutations in human cancers. *Science* **253**: 49–53.

Houlston RS, Collins A, Slack J & Morton NE (1992) Dominant genes for colorectal cancer are not rare. *Ann Hum Genet* **56**: 99–103.

Huang J, Papadopoulos N, McKinley AJ *et al* (1996) APC mutations in colorectal tumors with mismatch repair deficiency. *Proc Natl Acad Sci USA* **93**: 9049–9054.

Ichii S, Horii A, Nakatsuru S *et al* (1992) Inactivation of both APC alleles in an early stage of colon adenomas in a patient with familial adenomatous polyposis (FAP). *Hum Mol Genet* **1**: 387–390.

Ionov Y, Peinado MA, Malkhosyan S, Shibata D & Perucho M (1993) Ubiquitous somatic mutations in simple repeated sequences reveal a new mechanism for colonic carcinogenesis. *Nature* **363**: 558–561.

Jen J, Powell SM, Papadopoulos N *et al* (1994) Molecular determinants of dysplasia in colorectal lesions. *Cancer Res* **54**: 5523–5526.

Jones PA & Buckley JD (1990) The role of DNA methylation in cancer. *Adv Cancer Res* **54**: 1–23.

Joslyn G, Carlson M, Thliveris A *et al* (1991) Identification of deletion mutations and three new genes at the familial poylposis locus. *Cell* **66**: 601–613.

Kemler R (1993) From cadherins to catenins: cytoplasmic protein interactions and regulation of cell adhesion. *Trends Genet* **9**: 317–321.

Kern SE (1993) Clonality: more than just a tumour progression model. *J Natl Cancer Inst* **85**: 1020–1021.

Kern SE, Kinzler KW, Bruskin A *et al* (1991) Identification of p53 as a sequence-specific DNA binding protein. *Science* **252**: 1708–1711.

Kim H, Jen J, Vogelstein B & Hamilton SR (1994) Clinical and pathological characteristics of sporadic colorectal carcinomas with DNA replication errors in microsatellite sequences. *Am J Pathol* **145**: 148–156.

Kim NW, Piatyszek MA, Prowse KR *et al* (1994) Specific association of human telomerase activity with immortal cells and cancer. *Science* **266**: 2100–2015.

Kinzler KW, Nilbert MC, Su L-K *et al* (1991) Identification of FAP locus genes from chromosome 5q21. *Science* **253**: 661–665.

Kinzler KW & Vogelstein B (1996) Lessons from hereditary colorectal cancer. *Cell* **87**: 159–170.

Knudson AG (1971) Mutation and cancer: statistical study of retinoblastoma. *Proc Natl Acad Sci USA* **68**: 820–882.

Knudson AG (1993) Antioncogenes in human cancer. *Proc Natl Acad Sci USA* **90**: 10914–10921.

Koi M, Umar A, Chauhan DP *et al* (1994) Human chromosome 3 corrects mismatch repair deficiency and microsatellite instability and reduces *N*-methyl-*N*′-nitro-*N*-nitrosoguanidine tolerance in colon tumour cells with homozygous *hMLH1* mutation. *Cancer Res* **54**: 4308–4312.

Konishi M, Kikuchi-Yanoshita R, Tanaka K *et al* (1996) Molecular nature of colon tumors in hereditary nonpolyposis colon cancer, familial polyposis, and sporadic colon cancer. *Gastroenterology* **111**: 307–317.

Lane DP & Benchimol S (1990) p53: oncogene or antioncogene? *Genes Dev* **4**: 1–8.

Leach FS, Nicolaides NC, Papadopoulos N *et al* (1993) Mutations of a mutS homolog in hereditary nonpolyposis colorectal cancer. *Cell* **75**: 1215–1225.

Leppert M, Dobbs M, Scambler P *et al* (1987) The gene for familial adenomatous polyposis maps to the long arm of chromosome 5. *Science* **238**: 1411–1413.

Levine AJ, Momand J & Finlay CA (1991) The p53 tumour suppressor gene. *Nature* **351**: 453–456.

Levy DB, Smith KJ, Beazerp-Barclay Y *et al* (1994) Inactivation of both APC alleles in human and mouse tumours. *Cancer Res* **54**: 5953–5958.

Li ZH, Salovaara R, Aaltonen LA & Shibata D (1996) Telomerase activity is commonly detected in hereditary nonpolyposis colorectal cancers. *Am J Pathol* **148**: 1075–1079.

Lindblom A, Tannergard P, Werelius B & Nordenskjold M (1993) Genetic mapping of a second locus predisposing to hereditary non-polyposis colon cancer. *Nat Genet* **5**: 279–282.

Liu B, Farrington SM, Petersen GM *et al* (1995) Genetic instability occurs in the majority of young patients with colorectal cancer. *Nat Med* **1**: 348–352.

Liu B, Parsons R, Papadopoulos N *et al* (1996) Analysis of mismatch repair genes in hereditary non-polyposis cancer patients. *Nat Med* **2**: 169–174.

Lothe RA, Peltomaki P, Meling GI *et al* (1993) Genomic instability in colorectal cancer: relationship to clinicopathological variables and family history. *Cancer Res* **53**: 5849–5852.

Luce MC, Binnie CG, Cayouette MC & Kam-Morgan LNW (1996) Identification of DNA mismatch repair gene mutations in hereditary nonpolyposis colon cancer patients. *Int J Cancer* **69**: 50–52.

Luongo C, Moser AR, Gledhill S & Dove WF (1994) Loss of Apc^+ in intestinal adenomas from Min mice. *Cancer Res* **54**: 5947–5952.

Lynch HT, Smyrk T & Lynch JF (1996) Overview of natural history, pathology, molecular genetics and management of HNPCC (Lynch syndrome). *Int J Cancer* **69**: 38–43.

MacGrogan D, Pegram M, Slamon D & Bookstein R (1997) Comparative mutational analysis of DPC4 (Smad4) in prostatic and colorectal carcinomas. *Oncogene* **15**: 1111–1114.

MacPhee M, Chepenik K & Liddell R (1995) The secretory phospholipase A2 gene is a candidate for the Mom1 locus, a major modifier of ApcMin-induced intestinal neoplasia. *Cell* **81**: 957–966.

Makin D, Li FP, Strong LC et al (1990) Germ line p53 mutations in a familial syndrome of breast cancer, sarcomas, and other neoplasms. *Science* **250**: 1233–1237.

Markowitz S, Wang J, Myeroff L *et al* (1995) Inactivation of the type II TGF-beta receptor in colon cancer cells with microsatellite instability. *Science* **268**: 1336–1338.

Marra G & Boland C (1995) Hereditary nonpolyposis colorectal cancer: the syndrome, the genes, and historical perspectives. *J Natl Cancer Inst* **87**: 1114–1125.

Marshall CJ (1991) Tumor suppressor genes. *Cell* **64**: 313–326.

Massague J (1990) The transforming growth factor-β family. *Ann Rev Cell Biol* **6**: 597–641.

McDonnell TJ (1993) Cell division versus cell death: a functional model of multistep neoplasia. *Mol Carcinog* **8**: 209–213.

McLellan EA & Bird RP (1988) Aberrant crypts: potential preneoplastic lesions in the murine colon. *Cancer Res* **48**: 6187–6192.

Meltzer SJ (1995) Dr Strange DNA, or how I learned to stop cloning and love the computer. *Gastroenterology* **109**: 611–614.

Miyaki M, Seki M, Okamoto M *et al* (1990) Genetic changes and histopathological types in colorectal tumors from patients with familial adenomatous poylposis. *Cancer Res* **50**: 7166–7173.

Miyashiro I, Senda T, Matsumine A *et al* (1995) Subcellular localization of the APC protein: immunoelectron microscopy study of the association of the APC protein with catenin. *Oncogene* **11**: 89–96.

Miyoshi Y, Nagase H, Ando H *et a*l (1992) Somatic mutations of the APC gene in colorectal tumors: mutation cluster region in the APC gene. *Hum Mol Genet* **1**: 229–233.

Morin GB (1996) Telomere integrity and cancer. *J Natl Cancer Inst* **88**: 1095–1096.

Morin PJ, Vogelstein B & Kinzler KW (1996) Apoptosis and APC in colorectal tumorigenesis. *Proc Natl Acad Sci USA* **93**: 7950–7954.

Munemitsu S, Souza B, Muller O *et al* (1994) The APC gene product associates with microtubules *in vivo* and promotes their assembly *in vitro*. *Cancer Res* **54**: 3676–3681.

Nagase H & Nakamura Y (1993) Mutations of the APC (adenomatous polyposis coli) gene. *Hum Mutat* **2**: 425–434.

Nishisho I, Nakamura Y, Miyoshi Y *et al* (1991) Mutations of chromosome 5q21 genes in FAP and colorectal cancer patients. *Science* **253**: 665–669.

Olschwang S, Tiret A, Laurent-Puig P *et al* (1993) Restriction of ocular fundus lesions to a specific subgroup of APC mutations in adenomatous polyposis coli patients. *Cell* **75**: 959–968.

Parsons R, Myeroff L, Liu B *et al* (1995) Microsatellite instability and mutations of the transforming growth factor beta type II receptor gene in colorectal cancer. *Cancer Res* **55**: 5548–5550.

Pelkomaki P, Aaltonen LA, Sistonen P *et al* (1993) Genetic mapping of a locus predisposing to human colorectal cancer. *Science* **260**: 810–812.

Peto R (1977) Epidemiology, multistage models, and short-term mutagenesis tests. In *Origins of Human Cancer*, pp 1403–1428. Cold Spring Harbor, NY: Cold Spring Harbor Laboratory.

Ponder BA (1992) Molecular genetics of cancer. *BMJ* **304**: 1234–1236.

Powell SM, Zilz N, Beazer-Barclay Y *et al* (1992) APC mutations occur early during colorectal tumorigenesis. *Nature* **359**: 235–237.

Pretlow TP, Barrow BJ, Ashton WS *et al* (1991) Aberrant crypts: putative preneoplastic foci in human colonic mucosa. *Cancer Res* **22**: 287–294.

Pretlow TP, Brasitus TA, Fulton NC *et al* (1993) K-*ras* mutations in putative preneoplastic lesions in human colon. *J Natl Cancer Inst* **85**: 2004–2007.

Riggins GJ, Thiagalingam S, Rozenblum E *et al* (1996) Mad-related genes in the human. *Nat Genet* **13**: 347–349.

Ronucci L, Stamp D, Medline A, Cullen JB & Bruce WR (1991) Identification and quantification of aberrant crypt foci and microadenomas in the human colon. *Human Pathol* **22**: 287–294.

Rous P (1911) A sarcoma of the fowl transmissable by an agent separable from the tumour cells. *J Exp Med* **13**: 397–411.

Rubinfeld B, Souza B, Albert I *et al* (1993) Association of the APC gene product with beta-catenin. *Science* **262**: 1731–1734.

Rubinfeld B, Albert I, Porfiri E *et al* (1996) Binding of GSK3-beta to the APC-beta-catenin complex and regulation of complex assembly. *Science* **272**: 1023–1025.

Salz LB & Kelsen DP (1997) Adjuvant treatment of colorectal cancer. *Ann Rev Med* **48**: 191–202.

Sankila R, Aaltonen LA, Jarvinen HJ *et al* (1996) Better survival rates in patients with MLH1-associated hereditary colorectal cancer. *Gastroenterology* **110**: 682–687.

Shaw P, Bovey R, Tardy S *et al* (1992) Induction of apoptosis by wild-type p53 in a human colon tumor-derived cell line. *Proc Natl Acad Sci USA* **89**: 4495–4499.

Shih C, Padhy LC, Murray M & Weinberg RA (1981) Transforming genes of carcinomas and neuroblastomas introduced into mouse fibroblasts. *Nature* **290**: 261–264.

Shpitz BHK, Medline A, Bruce WR *et al* (1996) Natural history of aberrant crypt foci. *Dis Colon Rectum* **39**: 763–767.

Sidransky D, Tokino T, Hamilton SR *et al* (1992) Identification of *ras* oncogene mutations in the stool of patients with curable colorectal tumor. *Science* **256**: 102–105.

Smith AJ, Stern HS, Penner M *et al* (1994) Somatic *APC* and K-*ras* codon 12 mutations in aberrant crypt foci from human colons. *Cancer Res* **54**: 5527–5530.

Smith KJ, Johnson KA, Bryan YM *et al* (1993) The APC gene product in normal and tumour cells. *Proc Natl Acad Sci USA* **90**: 2846–2850.

Smith KJ, Levy DB, Maupin P *et al* (1994) Wild-type but not mutant APC associates with the microtubule cytoskeleton. *Cancer Res* **54**: 3672–3675.

Souza RE, Appel R, Yin J *et al* (1996) Microsatellite instability in the insulin-like growth factor II receptor gene in gastrointesinal tumours. *Nat Genet* **14**: 255–257.

Spirio L, Oschwang S, Groden J *et al* (1993) Alleles of the APC gene: an attenuated form of familial polyposis. *Cell* **75**: 951–957.

Stanbridge EK & Cavenee WK (1989) Heritable cancer and tumour suppressor genes: a tentative connection. In Weinberg RA (ed) *Oncogenes and the Molecular Origins of Cancer*, pp 281–306. Cold Spring Harbor, NY: Cold Spring Harbor Laboratory.

Stehlin D, Varmus HE, Bishop JM & Vogt PK (1976) DNA related to the transforming gene(s) of avian sarcoma viruses is present in normal avian DNA. *Nature* **260**: 170–173.

Strand M, Prolla TA, Liskay RM & Petes TD (1993) Destabilization of tracts of simple repetitive DNA in yeast by mutations affecting DNA mismatch repair. *Nature* **365**: 274–276.

Su L-K, Johnson KA, Smith KJ *et al* (1993a) Association between wild type and mutant APC gene products. *Cancer Res* **53**: 2728–2731.

Su L-K, Vogelstein B & Kinzler KW (1993b) Association of the APC tumor suppressor protein with catenins. *Science* **262**: 1734–1737.

Tate PH & Bird AP (1993) Effects of DNA methylation on DNA-binding proteins and gene expression. *Curr Opin Genet Dev* **3**: 226–231.

Thiagalingam S, Lengauer C, Leach FS *et al* (1996) Evaluation of candidate tumor suppressor genes on chromosome 18 in colorectal cancers. *Nat Genet* **13**: 343–346.

Thibodeau SN, Bren G & Schaid D (1993) Microsatellite instability in cancer of the proximal colon. *Science* **260**: 816–819.

Tobi M, Luo FC & Ronai Z (1994) Detection of K-*ras* mutation in colonic effluent samples from patients without evidence of colorectal carcinoma. *J Natl Cancer Inst* **86**: 1007–1010.

Umar A, Boyer JC, Thomas DC *et al* (1994) Defective mismatch repair in extracts of colorectal and endometrial cancer cell lines exhibiting microsatellite instability. *J Biol Chem* **269**: 14367–14370.

van der Luijt R, Khan PM, Vasen H *et al* (1994) Rapid detection of translation-terminating mutations at the adenomatous polyposis coli (APC) gene by direct protein truncation test. *Genomics* **20**: 1–4.

Vasen HFA, Mecklin J-P, Meera-Khan PM & Lynch HT (1991) The International Collaborative Group on Hereditary Nonpolyposis Coloretcal Cancer (ICG–HNPCC). *Dis Colon Rectum* **34**: 424–425.

Vaux DL & Strasser A (1996) The molecular biology of apoptosis. *Proc Natl Acad Sci USA* **93**: 2239–2244.

Vaux DL, Weissman IL & Kim SK (1992) *C. elegans* cell survival gene ced-9 encodes a functional homolog of the mammalian proto-oncogene Bcl-2. *Science* **258**:, 1955–1957.

Verdine GL (1994) The flip side of DNA methylation. *Cell* **76**: 197–200.

Vogelstein B, Fearon ER, Hamilton SR *et al* (1988) Genetic alterations during colorectal tumor development. *N Engl J Med* **319**: 525–532.

Vogelstein B, Fearon ER, Kern SE *et al* (1989) Allelotype of colorectal carcinomas. *Science* **244**: 207–211.

Wallace RW (1997) DNA on a chip: serving up the genome for diagnostics and research. *Mol Med Today* **3**: 384–389.

Weinberg RA (1991) Tumor suppressor genes. *Science* **254**: 1138–1145.

Wylie AH (1980) Glucocorticoid-induced thymocyte apoptosis is associated with endogenous endonuclease activation. *Nature* **284**: 555–556.

Yamashita N, Minamoto T, Ochia T, Onda M & Esumi H (1995) Frequent and characteristic K-*ras* activation and absence of p53 protein accumulation in aberrant crypt foci of the colon. *Gastroenterology* **108**: 434–440.

28

POLYPOID DISEASE

The term 'polyp' is merely descriptive of any lesion that is elevated above the mucosal surface of the bowel. The word derives from the Latin *polypus* which means many-footed or (more colloquially) an octopus, which a stalked polyp may resemble. This type of polyp is, however, just one of several different macroscopic types. Thus polyps may be sessile, in which case they are flat with no stalk; or they may be villous, with many fronds wafting free in the bowel lumen, resembling seaweed. Such a macroscopic description is of limited use to the clinician unless a histological term is appended to it. By qualifying the polyp as adenomatous or hamartomatous, for instance, it is possible to appreciate its significance and prognosis.

Polyps can vary in size, shape and behaviour. They may be acquired or inherited, benign or malignant, symptomatic or asymptomatic. They may be single, occur in clusters or occupy virtually all the colonic mucosa. When the latter occurs the term 'polyposis syndrome' is applied. The various syndromes are considered in Chapter 29.

CLASSIFICATION

Although it is frequent practice to equate the term polyp with adenoma, it is essential to realize that, although common, an adenoma is by no means the only histological type of polyp that exists. Table 28.1 divides the various types into two groups: the neoplastic and non-neoplastic. Much of the older literature is confusing since it fails to make this differentiation. Although occasionally neoplastic tissue can be found in non-neoplastic polyps and vice versa, the division holds good for most polyps. Although it may be possible to differentiate certain types of polyps by their naked-eye appearance (e.g. a large villous adenoma), the only sure means of identification is a biopsy and a detailed histological report from an experienced pathologist. This is particularly important in the interpretation of dysplasia and malignant transformation.

Table 28.1 Polypoid disease.

Neoplastic
- Single:
  1. Adenoma (tubular, tubulovillous, villous)
  2. Carcinoid
  3. Connective tissue polyp (fibroma, lipoma, leiomyoma, lymphoid)
- Multiple (see Table 29.1)

Non-neoplastic
- Hamartoma:
  1. Peutz–Jeghers polyps
  2. Juvenile polyps
- Inflammatory (pseudopolyp):
  e.g. ulcerative colitis, Crohn's disease, dysenteries
- Metaplastic (hyperplastic) polyps

NON-NEOPLASTIC POLYPS

Metaplastic or hyperplastic polyps

Metaplastic or hyperplastic polyps are usually minute (2–5 mm diameter), plaque-like and the same colour as normal mucous membrane. They are invariably present on sigmoidoscopy in the elderly, although they may occur at all ages. They are the most common type of polyp found in the rectum and are four times more common in men than in women (Williams et al, 1980, 1994). In the colon, however, only 10% of small polyps (less than 5 mm diameter) prove to be metaplastic, the vast majority being adenomas (Grundquist et al, 1979; Waye et al, 1980). Epidemiological studies reveal considerable variation in the frequency of metaplastic polyps between populations; they are most common in the West. 'Hyperplastic' is the term that has been applied in the USA ever since the lesion was first described by Westhues (1934). In the UK the preferred term is 'metaplastic' (Morson, 1962), suggesting altered growth rather than abnormal nuclear activity and cellular regeneration (Williams et al, 1980).

The nodules are flat-topped and only rarely pedunculated. On microscopic examination (Figure 28.1) they are made up of elongated tubules which often show cystic dilatation; the lining epithelium appears serrated owing to patchy flattening of its cells and the goblet cells are reduced in numbers (Morson and Dawson, 1990). There may be a slight increase in the round cells in the lamina propria and fragmentation of the muscularis mucosae with some of the fibres extending into the lamina propria. The whole polyp resembles small intestinal epithelium, except that the cells at the base of the

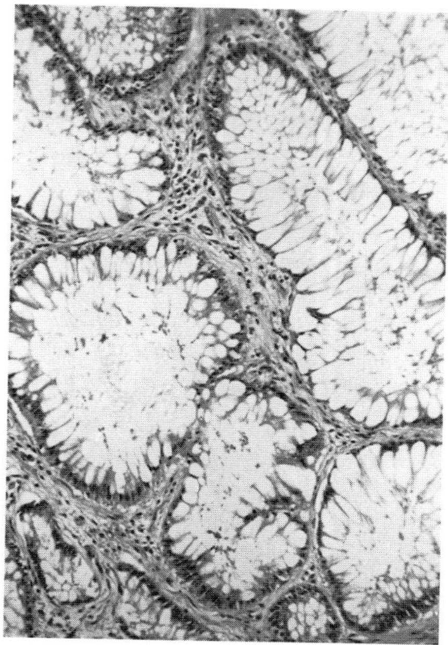

Figure 28.1 Microscopic appearance of metaplastic polyp displaying serrated goblet pattern.

crypts are hyperplastic (hence their American name). They are distinguished, therefore, from the disorderly maturation and dedifferentiation of adenomatous polyps in that maturation is maintained, although its regulation is disturbed. They do not progress (as far as is known) to develop dysplastic or neoplastic changes.

The aetiology is unknown, but migrant Japanese who emigrated to Hawaii showed increased numbers of metaplastic polyps, suggesting that environmental factors are important (Stemmermann and Yatani, 1973). With regard to pathogenesis, it is suggested that the cells forming a metaplastic polyp grow more slowly and have a longer life-span than the adjacent normal mucosal cells (Hayashi et al, 1974). The retained epithelium fails to detach, becoming 'hypermature'. A number of histochemical studies have identified phenotypic alternatives within affected crypts of metaplastic polyps. These include a reduction of O-acetylation of sialomucins in goblet cells (Jass et al, 1984), reduction of immunostaining of colonocytes for IgA (Jass and Faludy, 1985) and the appearance of CEA (Jass et al, 1984), and peanut binding sites (Boland et al, 1982). Most of these changes have also been described in hyperproliferative mucosa and their significance is unclear. Recently, the selective expression by the serrated epithelium of two trefoil peptides, pS2 and hSP, and of epidermal growth factor/urogastrone, all of which are also expressed in gastrointestinal cell lineage that is associated with chronic ulceration, has been described (Hanby et al, 1992). This raises the possibility that metaplastic polyps do consist of a truly metaplastic type of epithelium that is either induced inappropriately in the absence of ulceration or arises as a reparative phenomenon in response to local mucosal damage of indeterminate type (Williams et al, 1994). Although there are some reports suggesting that these polyps are causally associated with carcinoma, there are no hard data to support this contention. The polyps' coexistence with carcinoma probably reflects merely their ubiquity and increased frequency with age. However, there is an alternative view that believes there is more of a relationship between metaplastic polyps and cancer than has previously been realized. The proponents cite as evidence their increased frequency in the distal colon and rectum, and their higher incidence in populations at high risk of developing cancer. They are up to 18 times more frequent in colons bearing colorectal cancer than in age-matched autopsy controls (Eide, 1986) and they frequently form clusters around adenomas and carcinomas in both the proximal and distal large bowel (Cappell and Forde, 1989).

These observations persuaded Jass (1983) to suggest that metaplastic polyps may share some aetiological factors with carcinomas and that they might be regarded as markers of high-risk populations (although of no significance to individuals). However, there is little evidence to refute or support this hypothesis. Indeed, there are two studies in the literature in which patients with distal colorectal metaplastic polyps have been colonoscopically screened for cancer; one has shown an increased risk of adenoma formation, whereas the other has not (Blue et al, 1991; Rex et al, 1992).

Metaplastic polyps are usually asymptomatic, being discovered on routine sigmoidoscopy. Although the vast majority are tiny and insignificant, larger metaplastic polyps are occasionally found in the colon, either semipedunculated or as a sessile mound of shiny tissue, and these may cause clinical features akin to adenomas.

Management

Although it is accepted that metaplastic polyps are innocuous, the question arises whether once seen they should be removed. The nagging suspicion is that even if one is confident on macroscopic examination as to their nature, only histological examination can prove their true identity.

Management is a matter of individual philosophy. Removal of every minute polyp will certainly eliminate the risk of leaving a small adenomatous polyp behind, and may reduce the subsequent risk of carcinoma. However, since metaplastic polyps tend to be multiple, removal may be a time-consuming process with an associated – albeit low – morbidity. Since they recur, frequent follow-up would be necessary, reinforcing or inculcating any neurotic tendency or cancer phobia the patient might possess. It is our belief, therefore, that if the clinician sees one or a group of metaplastic polyps, a representative polyp should be removed and subjected to histological assessment. If the clinical suspicion is confirmed then nothing further is required, and provided there is no other reason for follow-up the patient should be reassured and discharged.

Hamartomatous polyps

A hamartoma is a tumour-like malformation in which the tissues of a particular part of the body are arranged haphazardly, usually with an excess of one or more of its components. The term was coined by Albrecht (1904) to distinguish it from a true neoplastic lesion. The lesion has therefore no tendency toward excessive growth. Its growth is coordinated with that of the surrounding tissue and it stops growing after adolescence (Walter and Israel, 1967). Two types of colorectal polyp fall into this category: the juvenile polyp and the Peutz–Jeghers polyp (Welch and Hedberg, 1975).

Juvenile polyps

As the name suggests, juvenile polyps are most commonly seen in infants and children under 10 years old. They do, however, occur in adults. First described by Verse (1908), the juvenile polyp is differentiated from other polyps by its characteristic macroscopic and microscopic features.

The majority of juvenile polyps are 1–2 cm in diameter and have a smooth surface. There is usually a slender stalk covered with normal colonic mucosa which is continuous with the adjacent lining of the colon; as it extends on to the body of the polyp the epithelium becomes replaced by granulation tissue. Despite this description, 25% of these polyps are sessile (Mazier et al, 1982).

A juvenile polyp can often be simply identified by glancing at the slide prior to examination under the microscope. There is a characteristic pattern of dilated cystic spaces which are filled with mucus. This appearance led some pathologists in the past to refer to them as 'mucus retention cysts' (Roth and Helwig, 1963). On microscopic examination these spaces are lined by columnar secreting epithelial cells (Figure 28.2). The bulk of the polyp, however, is made up of connective tissue infiltrated with acute and chronic inflammatory cells. Eosinophils are particularly prevalent, a finding that has prompted some workers to suggest that juvenile polyps result from an allergic reaction. It is of interest that there is a statistically significant increase in the incidence of allergy in children with juvenile polyps and in the families of these children (Alexander et al, 1970).

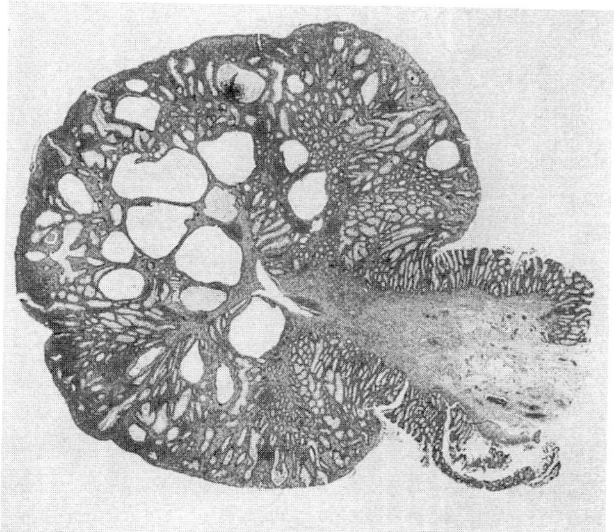

Figure 28.2 Microscopic appearance of a juvenile polyp. Note the cystic dilated glands lined by normal appearing epithelium.

Although it was considered that about 90% of juvenile polyps were to be found within 20 cm of the anal verge (Knox et al, 1960; Mazier et al, 1982), colonoscopic studies have shown that over 50% of children affected have more than one juvenile polyp, and these are distributed evenly throughout the large bowel (Mestre, 1986; Latt et al, 1993; Lehmann and Elitsur, 1996).

These polyps may produce a variety of clinical features. The most common presenting complaint is rectal bleeding followed by prolapse or protrusion of the polyp through the anus. Torsion of the pedicle may occur (about 10% of cases) which results in bleeding and extrusion of the tissue in the faeces. Occasionally a polyp can produce a colonic intussusception with bleeding and symptoms and signs of large bowel obstruction (Roth and Helwig, 1963; Holgersen et al, 1971; Franklin and McSwain, 1972).

In addition to the other common symptoms associated with colon and rectal tumours such as diarrhoea, tenesmus and proctalgia, rectal prolapse has been described (Cabrera et al, 1959).

The majority (70%) of patients present with a few polyps, but 30% have multiple polyps. Rarely there are more than ten polyps present and the patient is then considered to suffer from juvenile polyposis (see later) (McColl et al, 1964; Smilow et al, 1966; Veale et al, 1966, Mestre, 1986).

Polyps within the rectum may be removed by transanal excision or sigmoidoscopic snare and the diagnosis can then be substantiated. Before the advent of colonoscopy it was common practice to leave the more proximally located polyps, if biopsy of rectal or distal sigmoid lesions showed them to be juvenile polyps (Goligher, 1984). The alternative then would have been laparotomy and colotomy. Today these patients should be treated by colonoscopy and polypectomy in the usual manner. Indeed, it has been recommended (Douglas et al, 1980) that colonoscopy should be the first-line investigation in all young patients with rectal bleeding as their main or only symptom. Since the examination is performed under sedation the procedure is more comfortable and less time-consuming than barium enema and allows simultaneous removal of the polyps.

Recurrence of a juvenile polyp is not uncommon and may occur in 10–20% of cases (Horrilleno et al, 1957; Knox et al, 1960; Ko et al, 1995). Despite this risk the juvenile polyp on its own is neither a malignant nor a premalignant lesion and therefore routine follow-up is not recommended (Nugent et al, 1993).

Peutz–Jeghers polyps

Peutz–Jeghers polyps are described later in this chapter.

Inflammatory polyps

Inflammatory polyps may be found as scattered worm-like or thread-like (filiform) tags of essentially normal mucosa in the colon of any patient suffering from a chronic inflammatory disease. In the past they have been referred to as 'pseudopolyps' to distinguish them from neoplastic polyps, but 'inflammatory polyp' is now the preferred term. The diseases in which they most commonly occur are ulcerative colitis, Crohn's disease, amoebiasis, schistosomiasis and occasionally diverticulitis. Although not generally thought of as having an inflammatory aetiology, ischaemic colitis may be associated with these polyps. Inflammatory polyps are the result of ulceration with undermining of adjacent mucosa and the formation of mucosal tags of various shapes and sizes. They are usually not inflamed, although some may show superficial ulceration of the tip with a characteristic covering of white slough. Larger inflammatory polyps may occur which are composed primarily of connective tissue. These polyps themselves do not have a malignant propensity.

Benign lymphoid polyps

Benign lymphoid polyps form part of the spectrum of lymphoid hyperplasia. This condition was first described by Cohnheim (1865) and his term 'gastrointestinal pseudoleukaemia' was used to differentiate it from lymphatic leukaemia. Focal or diffuse hyperplasia tends to occur where lymphoid follicles are prominent; that is, in the terminal ileum, caecum or rectum (Ewing, 1940; Symmers, 1948). When prominent the hyperplasia is referred to as a 'benign lymphoid polyp'.

These polyps are frequently included in the category of inflammatory polyps since lymphoid hyperplasia is thought to occur as a consequence of an immunological process, itself promoted by infection and local inflammation. For this reason pathologists have referred to them as 'anal tonsils' (Morson and Dawson, 1990). However, it should be pointed out that not all authors agree that inflammation is the aetiological factor. Thus it has been suggested that these polyps are congenital malformations or hamartomas (Gruenwald, 1942). This suggestion is supported by the occasional familial incidence (Granet, 1949; Keeling and Beatty, 1956) and the reported association with familial polyposis (Gruenberg and Mackman, 1972; Venkitachalam et al, 1978).

Benign lymphoid polyps are most frequently present in the lower third of the rectum as smooth, round, submucous lesions (Cornes et al, 1961) (Figure 28.3). While the majority are sessile, pedunculated polyps occasionally occur. They are usually single but may number four or five. They are slightly more common in men than in women and although they may occur at any age they more commonly do so in the third and fourth decades (Cornes et al, 1961; Price, 1978; Byrne et al, 1982). Their size may vary from a few millimetres to 3 cm diameter.

Microscopically the polyps are composed of relatively normal lymphoid tissue having a follicular pattern with a clearly defined germinal centre. Sometimes sarcoid-like lesions are seen. They usually lie in the submucosa, covered by an attenuated mucous membrane. Although its surface may be umbilicated, ulceration of the overlying mucosa is not a feature. Involvement of the muscle layers is very rare. This relatively well-organized structure and the absence of invasion of the deep structures

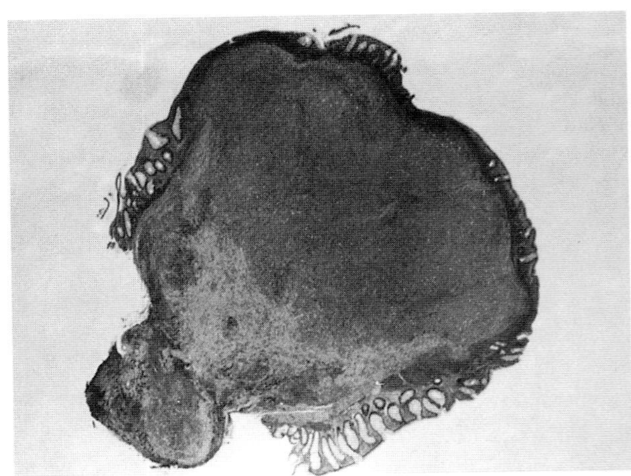

Figure 28.3 Lymphoid polyp in the rectum. The lesion is reactive and not malignant.

differentiate these polyps from malignant lymphoma. They may be asymptomatic or may present with symptoms usually ascribed to polyps (e.g. rectal bleeding, abdominal pain and intussusception). If situated in the anal canal they may cause considerable local anal pain. On double-contrast barium study a fleck of barium in the centre of the polyp is characteristic (Johnson et al, 1978). The polyps frequently regress spontaneously (Morson and Dawson, 1990); nevertheless they should be removed to make the diagnosis and differentiate them from other polyps (Hayes and Burr, 1952; Holtz and Schmidt, 1958; Cornes et al, 1961). As might be expected recurrence is rare, being about 5% (Cornes et al, 1961). Since malignant change does not occur (Stout, 1959; Cornes et al, 1961) there is no urgent need to remove remnants of a partially excised polyp of this type.

NEOPLASTIC POLYPS: ADENOMA

From the clinical point of view adenomas are the most important types of polyps. Not only do they frequently cause symptoms but it is now understood that they are the main precursor of colorectal cancer. The nomenclature in relation to adenomas has, in the past, been confusing, mainly because pathologists and surgeons have classified them in different ways. There is a common belief among surgeons that adenomatous polyps and villous adenomas (or villous papilloma) are entirely separate entities. Histologically, however, they represent either end of the adenoma spectrum. In between there is the intermediate form, the tubulovillous or villoglandular adenoma. All three lesions are thus macroscopic and microscopic variants of one neoplastic process and the word 'adenoma' is applicable to them all.

In order to eliminate confusion with regard to terminology, the World Health Organization (Morson and Sobin, 1976, Jass and Sobin, 1989) recommended a preferred nomenclature based on histology: the adenomatous polyp is termed 'tubular adenoma', villous papilloma becomes 'villous adenoma', and the intermediate type previously known as the villoglandular adenoma becomes the 'tubulovillous adenoma'. It should be realized that these categories are not always clearly distinct and there may be some overlap. It is convenient, however, from a practical point of view to subdivide polyps into adenomas and villous adenomas.

Aetiology

Many of the factors considered to be of aetiological importance in the development of colorectal carcinoma are implicated in the formation of polyps and these are considered in Chapters 27 and 30.

Pathology

Macroscopic appearances

The typical *tubular adenoma* is small, spherical and pedunculated, with a smooth surface broken into lobules by intercommunicating clefts (Figure 28.4). It may be as small as 1 mm diameter or larger than 5 cm. The smaller tumours are more likely to have a smooth contour and the larger ones a lobular pattern. Although often pedunculated they may be sessile. These tumours are often darker in colour than the surrounding mucosa since they are vascular, and haemorrhage frequently occurs within them as a result of trauma. With the smaller lesions this contrast in colour may not be so obvious. In the case of a pedunculated lesion the pedicle is usually 1–3 cm

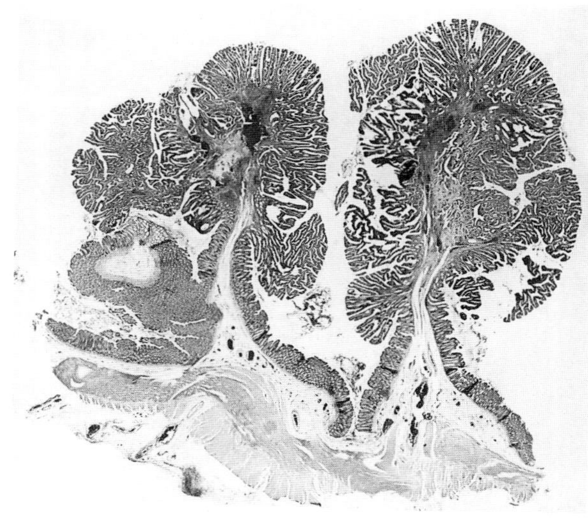

Figure 28.4 Tubular adenoma: low-power microscopic appearance.

in length but may be longer. It is broader at its base and narrow at its junction with the 'head' of the polyp.

It is important to realize that not all adenomas are polypoid in nature. In recent years the flat adenoma has been described (Figure 28.5). *Flat adenomas* are identified endoscopically or grossly by their configuration and have been described as protruding less than the thickness of the mucosa above the surrounding mucosa on histopathological examination. Muto et al (1985) described these lesions as minimally elevated plaque-like lesions measuring less than 10 mm diameter, often with a central depression. In addition, depressed adenomas have been described which are thinner than the surrounding mucosa (Muto et al, 1985; Kuramato et al, 1990; Kobayashi et al, 1992; Hamilton, 1993; Yao et al, 1994).

The *villous adenoma* is usually large and sessile with a shaggy surface made up of numerous fronds resembling seaweed (Figure 28.6). Its consistency is usually soft and its edges are ill-defined. It may be flat or protrude into the bowel lumen. It often extends over a considerable area of the bowel wall, the so-called carpet-like lesion, and is often circumferential. Its colour, like that of a large tubular adenoma, is darker than the surrounding mucosa.

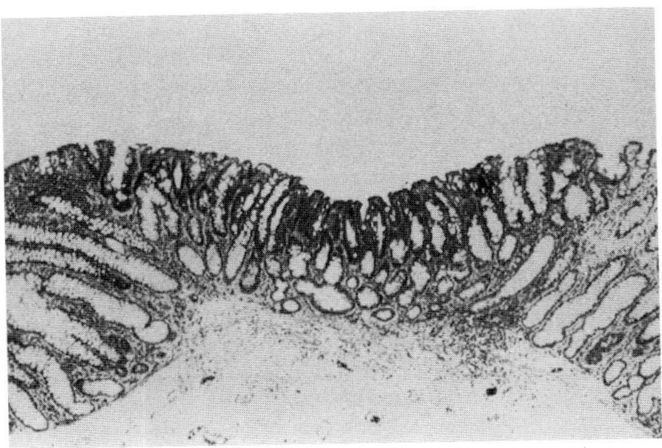

Figure 28.5 Flat tubular adenoma, showing an abrupt transition from non-neoplastic epithelium to adenomatous epithelium. The adenomatous glands have enlarged calibre and the epithelium has scattered residual goblet cells. There is no protrusion of the dysplastic glands above the surrounding mucosal surface. Photo courtesy of Prof. P Quirke, Leeds General Infirmary.

Microscopic appearances

The *tubular adenoma* consists of closely packed epithelial tubules separated by normal lamina propria which grow and branch horizontally to the muscularis mucosae (Day and Morson, 1978) (Figure 28.7). The tubules may branch in a regular or irregular pattern. Focal cystic dilatation of tubules may occur and secondary infection or haemorrhage may be present within the substance of the polyp. In pedunculated polyps the pedicle consists of normal mucosa and submucosa.

The *villous adenoma* consists of a central core of connective tissue which forms numerous delicate, frond-like branches or villi. The epithelial cells which cover the villi and constitute its surface grow vertically towards the bowel lumen. In between the villi the mucosa rests directly on the muscularis mucosae with no intervening connective tissue (Figure 28.8).

The *tubulovillous adenoma* is an intermediate form of adenoma, often having elements of tubular and villous pattern in different degree. More commonly, however, it has a uniform histology with broad, stunted villi, and epithelial tubules similar to those in a tubular adenoma (Morson and Dawson, 1990). The term 'aberrant crypt foci' has

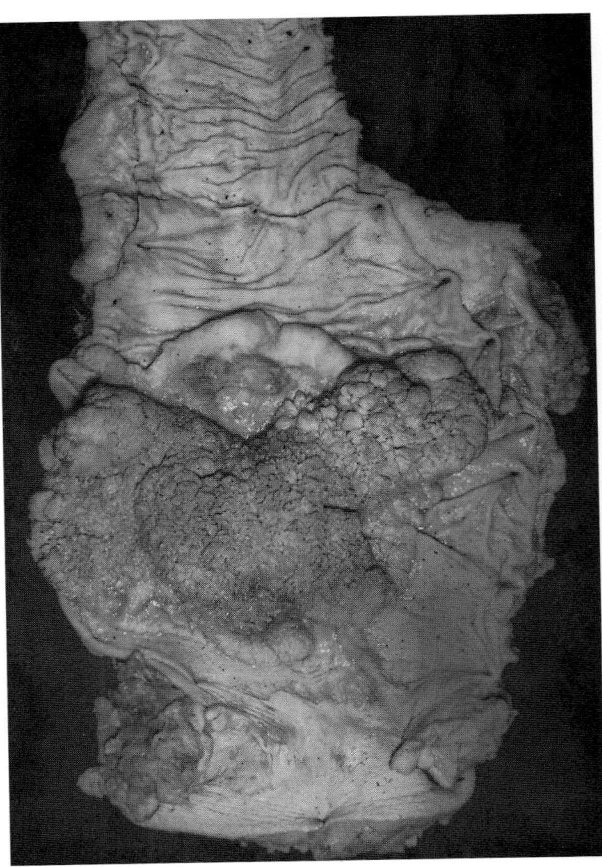

Figure 28.6 Macroscopic appearance of large villous adenoma showing evidence of malignant change.

been coined to describe the very earliest histological change which precedes an adenoma (Pretlow et al, 1992). Such crypt foci are characterized by groups of crypts with enlarged diameter, thickened hypercellular epithelium and altered mucin pattern as visualized by macroscopic or microscopic *en face* examination of colorectal mucosa after staining with methylene blue. However, the histopathology of aberrant crypt foci is variable. Most of these lesions identified in man are not composed of dysplastic epithelium but instead resemble a hyperplastic (metaplastic) polyp with its characteristic serrated glands and epithelium and distended goblet cells (Nucci et al, 1993).

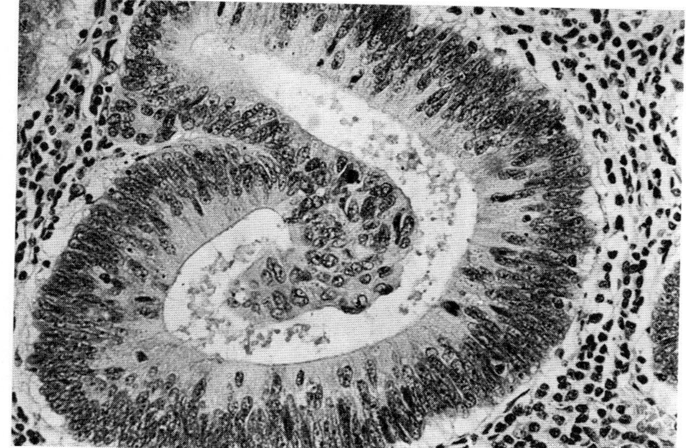

Figure 28.7 Tubular adenoma: high-power microscopic appearance.

The *flat adenoma* consists of an abrupt transition from non-neoplastic epithelium to adenomatous epithelium (see Figure 28.5). The adenomatous glands tend to be distorted and have an increased calibre. The dysplastic glands do not protrude above the surrounding mucosal surface (Muto et al, 1985; Jarmillo et al, 1995; Stolte and Betake, 1995).

Dysplasia

The epithelial cells covering an adenoma are similar no matter whether it is primarily tubular or villous. These cells may be very similar to those constituting normal colorectal mucosa, but often the nuclei are hyperchromatic, pleomorphic and increased in number resulting in a crowded appearance within

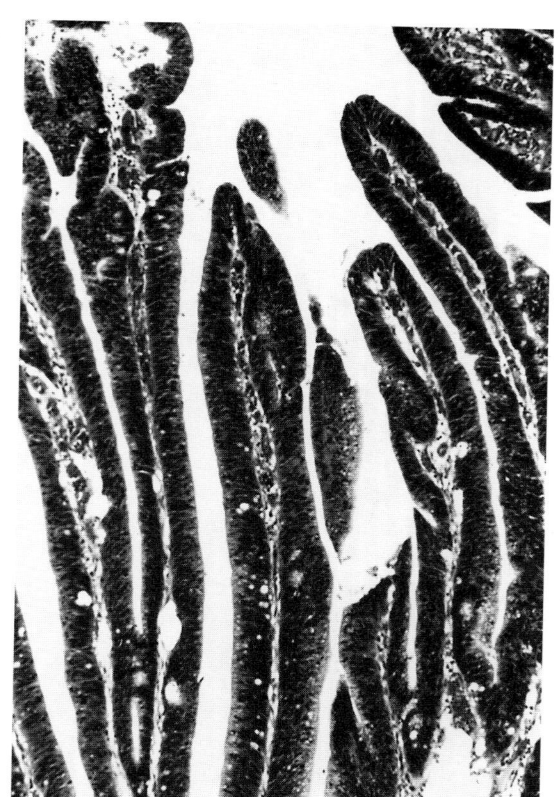

(a)

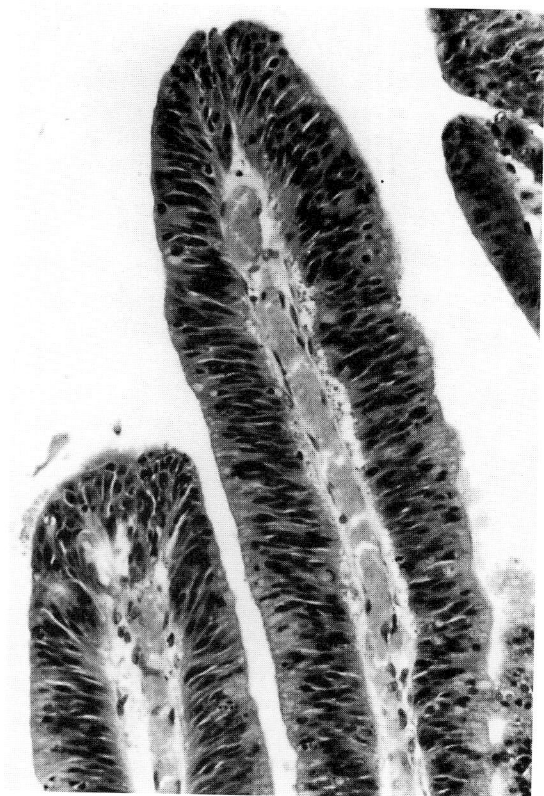

(b)

Figure 28.8a,b Microscopic appearance of villous adenoma. (a) Low power showing delicate villous processes, each with a core of connective tissue. (b) High power showing dysplastic cells, some with mucin production covering a villous process.

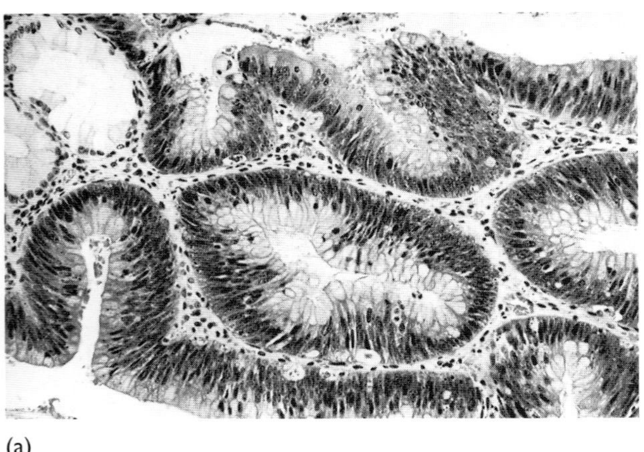

(a)

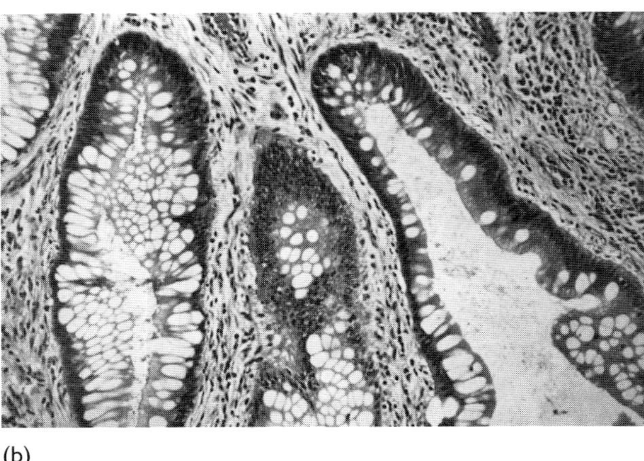

(b)

Figure 28.9a,b (a) Severe dysplasia in tubulovillous adenoma. (b) Mild to moderate dysplasia in tubular adenoma.

the epithelium. As a result there is often diminution or absence of mucus in the protoplasm, although in some villous adenomas it may be actually increased (Gramlich et al, 1988). In addition there may be increased mitotic figures and the cells may form several layers or even masses which, in the case of tubular adenomas, project into the lumen of the tubules or, in the case of villous adenomas, into the connective tissue core. These features of dysplasia or atypia (Figure 28.9) vary in degree, not only in different tumours but also within the same tumour.

Despite this variation, several authors have attempted to grade the degree of dysplasia as mild, moderate or severe on the basis of nuclear changes such as enlargement, pleomorphism, loss of polarity, stratification and an increase in the number of mitotic figures (Potet and Soullard, 1971; Ekelund and Lindstrom, 1974; Kozuka, 1975). Severe dysplasia is regarded by some histopathologists as equivalent to carcinoma-in-situ. It is imperative to draw the distinction between a polyp with carcinoma-in-situ and a true malignant polyp. The latter demonstrates invasion of carcinoma cells through the muscularis mucosae: such a polyp is a true malignant lesion, whereas polyps exhibiting signs of carcinoma-in-situ may be considered to be benign from the clinical standpoint. About 60% of adenomas show only mild epithelial dysplasia, about 30% have moderate dysplasia and the remaining 10% show severe dysplasia. These proportions are generalizations, since the histological changes which are considered to be atypical are subjective. Furthermore, there is variation based on size and histological type. Thus severe dysplasia increases with size and is greatest in the villous variety. Some authors (Ekelund and Lindstrom, 1974) have found that the degree of dysplasia increases the closer the polyp is to the anus or to an associated carcinoma, and is greater in men than in women. Others (Kozuka, 1975) have found an increase with age. Muto et al (1985) have drawn attention to a disproportionately high incidence of severe dysplasia in flat adenomas.

The most important question concerning the dysplasia found in polyps is whether there is a progression through the various grades to frank carcinoma. This concept of the adenoma–carcinoma sequence is discussed in detail in Chapter 27.

Another histological variation apart from epithelial dysplasia that may cause concern for the histopathologist is the presence of benign adenomatous epithelium deep to the muscularis mucosae. This appearance has been described as an 'adenomatous polyp with submucosal cysts' (Frechner, 1973), or as 'epithelial misplacement in adenomatous polyps' (Greene, 1974). A more apt term is probably 'pseudocarcinomatous invasion' (Muto et al, 1973) since this conveys the importance of its correct interpretation. Approximately 2.4% of all adenomatous polyps possess this characteristic (Muto et al, 1973). Gland-like structures are present in the submucosa and they usually show the same degree of dysplasia of the epithelium that overlies the surface of the polyp. Deposits of haemosiderin pigment and areas of recent haemorrhage are frequently present around the submucosal glands. It is suggested that pseudocarcinomatous change is secondary to haemorrhage within the polyp perhaps as a result of torsion of the pedicle. Certainly these changes are more common in large polyps with long pedicles situated in the sigmoid colon which is the most muscular and active part of the colon.

Cell turnover and origin of adenomas

Using tritiated thymidine it has been demonstrated that the surface epithelium of colonic mucosa in healthy humans is replaced by new cells every 4–8 days (Cole and McKalen, 1961; Lipkin et al, 1963; MacDonald et al, 1964). In the normal mucosa cell division is limited to the lower third of the crypts of Lieberkuhn; the dividing cells migrate upwards to reach the surface by the ninth day. As they migrate they become differentiated into mature goblet cells or absorptive cells. Exfoliation of cells is perfectly balanced by cell division and migration. Elias et al (1981) showed that the epithelial surface in adenomatous polyps was increased by up to 226 times and the number of cells up to 370 times. These changes are probably explained by the findings of Lipkin (1974) who showed there were two types of change that could occur in normal mucosa. In phase 1, some cells continued to divide as they migrated to the surface of the mucosa. In phase 2, in addition to continued mitoses, the cells developed properties that prevented them from being shed. The combination of these two phases was thought to result in adenoma formation.

A stathmokinetic assessment of colonic cell turnover in humans can be made by maintaining a mucosal biopsy in organ culture and counting the number of metaphase arrest figures that occur after vincristine administration. This *in vitro* technique has shown that the mucosa adjacent to tubular adenomas and in familial adenomatous polyposis exhibits increased crypt cell production (Barsoum et al, 1992; Hall et al, 1992).

Thus, it has been assumed that an adenomatous polyp develops as a result of excessive proliferation of colonocytes within the base of the crypts. This explanation, though, ignores the role of dying colonocytes which perish by apoptosis (Gavrieli et al, 1992; Hall et al, 1994). Two groups have recently investigated the role of both cell proliferation and cell death in adenomas. Both groups found that, as with Lipkin's classic model, in normal mucosa the proliferating cells were restricted to the lower third of the crypts. However, in adenomas not only was the proliferative activity markedly increased, but the apoptopic activity of the normal crypts was significantly decreased; furthermore, the proliferation predominated at the luminal surface and apoptosis at the base, a complete reversal of the normal pattern (Moss et al, 1996, Sinicrope et al, 1996).

One explanation of these findings is that in adenomas genetic alterations occur preferentially in the cells at the base of the crypt, and that apoptosis eliminates damaged cells. Diminished apoptosis at the luminal end of the crypt may mean that the effort to control the damage has failed there, so the adenoma puckers up and out, commonly as a polypoid lesion (Shiff and Rigas, 1997). Alternatively, the adenomatous polyp grows inwards (Moss et al, 1996), so that proliferating cells migrate towards the base of the crypt. It is believed that the normal crypt grows outwards, so by analogy when apoptosis and proliferation are inverted in the adenomatous crypt the cells of these crypts might migrate in the reverse direction. This is a fascinating concept, but awaits further evidence.

Ultrastructure, chromosome and ploidy abnormalities

In normal colonic mucosa there are four basic cell types: undifferentiated, enterochromaffin, goblet and absorptive cells. Electron microscopy also demonstrates a further four types: three kinds of partially differentiated cells (an intermediate cell, an immature goblet cell and an immature absorptive cell) and a hypermature or exhausted goblet cell. Although each of these cell types is present in adenomas, the relative ratio of mature to immature cells at each level of the crypt is different from that in normal tissue. In normal tissue there is progression from the base, where undifferentiated cells are present, to the surface, where mature absorptive cells and some exhausted goblet cells are in abundance. In adenomas this sequence is absent owing to the failure of cells to differentiate, so that there are more intermediate cells on the surface (Fisher and Sharkey, 1962; Imai et al, 1965; Pittman and Pittman, 1966; Lorenzsonn and Trier, 1968; Kavin et al, 1970; Kaye et al, 1973; Fenoglio et al, 1975).

Chromosome abnormalities were also demonstrated in early studies (Enterline and Arvan, 1967) although these were not universal findings (Messinetti et al, 1968). Enterline and Arvan (1967) demonstrated that trisomy of one or more chromosomes was common. Pseudodiploid sets were also frequent. Furthermore, although individual abnormal chromosomes were rare when atypia was absent, such changes became more frequent as atypia increased. Hyperploidy was also present with dysplasia and was more prevalent with villous lesions. Further studies using flow cytometry which measures more accurately the DNA and RNA content of cells (ploidy studies) demonstrated conflicting results. The incidence of aneuploidy, which indicates abnormal DNA content, varied from 6% to 30% of adenomas (Van den Ingh et al, 1986; Goh and Jass, 1986; Quirke et al, 1986). While the incidence of aneuploidy appeared to be related to increasing size, its link with histological type and dysplasia was less evident.

The development of molecular biological techniques has helped to define more accurately these abnormalities in chromosome structure, and these genetic aspects are discussed in detail in Chapter 27.

Incidence

The true incidence of polyps within the large intestine is difficult to determine. Few studies have been performed on asymptomatic individuals, and where they have, the subjects have usually undergone proctosigmoidoscopic examination only, so that the remaining colon was not visualized. Occasionally in these older studies a barium enema examination was performed, but this invariably used a single-contrast rather than a double-contrast technique. The incidence of polyps in these studies ranged from 2.9% to 11.5% if the subject was investigated on one occasion only (Miller et al, 1950; Wilson et al, 1955). If annual inspection was instituted as was the case in Enquist's series of 7608 patients over the age of 45 years, the rate increased to about 20% (Enquist, 1957). Complete information concerning the histological type of polyps was not available from these older studies.

More accurate data have emerged from double-contrast barium enema and colonoscopy studies. Welin (1967) found benign polyps in 2897 of 24 783 patients (11.7%) studied by double-contrast barium enema. Again, no pathological detail was available. Numerous colonoscopy surveys have been reported, but most patients included were referred for the investigation and therefore had symptoms. Thus, the National Polyp Study, which is the largest prospective study of polyp incidence and recurrence ever mounted, found that of 9112 patients undergoing colonoscopy for a variety of reasons, 2632 (28.9%) had at least one histologically proven adenoma (Winawer et al, 1992). Since symptoms are not always referable to the polyp, the true incidence of polyps among this population is impossible to deduce from the data.

Asymptomatic population studies have been performed to screen for the presence of faecal occult blood. These have demonstrated the incidence of adenomas to be between 0.2% and 1.4% (Lee, 1983; Dybahl et al, 1984; Lallemand et al, 1984, Kewenter et al, 1994; Hardcastle et al, 1996; Kronborg et al, 1996). Once again, however, the data do not necessarily reflect the true incidence of polyps since not all polyps bleed at the time of screening. This point is amply illustrated from several colonoscopic screening studies in asymptomatic patients which have demonstrated adenomas in 30–60% of people at the age of 65 years (Di Sario et al, 1991; Lieberman and Smith 1991; Rex et al, 1991). The prevalence at age 50 years ranges from 11% to 28% in these studies.

It might be expected that the only accurate data would come from autopsy studies. However, studies have demonstrated tremendous variations (from 2.4% to 69%): Dukes (1926) 9.4%; Stewart (1931) 4.2%; Susman (1932) 6%; Lawrence (1936) 2.4%; Mayo and Schlicke (1942) 16%; Atwater and Bargen (1945) 69%; Helwig (1947) 9.5%; Swinton and Haug (1947) 7%; Moore (1960) 27%, and Berge et al (1973) 12.5%. There are several reasons for these differences. Many studies were retrospective in nature and incorporated data based on the observations of a number of investigators (Chapman, 1963). There was lack of uniformity as to the smallest size of polyp to be included. Some of the series included children (Lawrence, 1936) and subjects of different nationalities who are known to have different prevalence rates of colorectal neoplasm (Lawrence, 1936; Helwig, 1947).

More recent prospective autopsy studies carried out in areas where the incidence of colorectal cancer is high confirm the high prevalence rate of adenoma in the general population. Thus A R Williams et al (1982) found one or more adenomas in 73 of 198 men, a prevalence of 36.9%, and in 48 of 167 women, a prevalence of 28.7%.

Wagner et al (1996), in calculating the number of patients needed for a screening study, assessed from the literature that 30% of asymptomatic individuals will have polyps of some kind (including both adenomas and hyperplastic polyps) at age 50 years, and 50% will have polyps at age 65 years. In keeping with cross-sectional data from autopsy studies, polyp incidence after age 65 years was assumed to rise slightly and then decline after the age of 70 years to about 1% a year.

Anatomical distribution

The subjects investigated in clinical and autopsy studies are derived from different populations and there are inevitably discrepancies in the data. Many of the earlier surgical papers which reviewed large numbers of patients (Grinnell and Lane, 1958; Enterline, 1976) claimed that the majority of adenomas occurred in the sigmoid colon and rectum, but since the rest of the colon was not always visualized these data were clearly biased.

More accurate clinical information is now available from colonoscopy studies. Thus Shinya and Wolff (1979) analysed their series of 5786 endoscopically removed adenomas. The largest number of each form of adenoma occurred in the sigmoid colon, followed by the descending colon. In all zones tubular adenomas were most common, followed (in diminishing order) by tubulovillous and villous adenomas. One interesting fact to emerge contrary to previous belief (Spratt et al, 1958; Olsen and Davis, 1969) was that villous adenomas were commonly present above the rectosigmoid region. A similar distribution was also found by Gillespie et al (1979) in 1049 adenomas which were removed from 620 patients, 47.5% of the tumours occurring in the sigmoid colon. Data from a prospective colonoscopy study by Tedesco et al (1980) were similar, as were those from Minopoulos et al (1983), Tripp et al (1987) and Grossman et al (1989), although the numbers were smaller. The distribution of adenomas found in 1867 patients in the National Polyp Study again confirms the data from these smaller studies and is depicted in Table 28.2. The low percentage of rectal polyps in all these studies no doubt reflects the ease with which these lesions can be removed by rigid sigmoidoscopy.

The anatomical distribution in autopsy studies is broadly similar to that reported from colonoscopy studies, but there are differences, particularly when several adenomas are present. In cases with a single adenoma, A R Williams et al (1982) found that a disproportionate number occurred in the proximal 10% and distal 20% of the bowel. Similar findings were obtained by Ekelund (1963) in a microscopic study in Malmo, Sweden. He found 56.1% of solitary adenomas in the sigmoid colon and rectum and 18.8% in the caecum. When cases with more than one adenoma were considered, this site predilection appeared diluted, so that a more even distribution was apparent. Some series (Chapman, 1963; Eide and Stalsberg, 1978; Vatn et al, 1985; Ozick et al, 1995) have also demonstrated a shift in the distribution of adenomas to the right side of the colon in older age groups. This finding is of particular interest since some reports have demonstrated an increase in the incidence of adenocarcinoma in the ascending colon of the elderly (Haenszel and Correa, 1971; de Jong et al, 1972; Snyder et al, 1977), thus providing more circumstantial evidence for the adenoma–carcinoma sequence.

Table 28.2 Distribution of colorectal adenomas by colonoscopy

Site	%
Caecum	8
Ascending colon	9
Hepatic flexure	4
Transverse colon	10
Splenic flexure	4
Descending colon	14
Sigmoid colon	43
Rectum	8

From O'Brien et al (1990).

In summary, it does appear that approximately two-thirds of adenomas occur in the bowel distal to the splenic flexure and one-third occur proximal to this site. This pattern is less pronounced when more than one polyp is present or in elderly patients.

Age and sex incidence

Adenomas can occur at any age but they increase in frequency with advancing years, with higher rates in males at all ages. Thus A R Williams et al (1982) in their autopsy study found a prevalence rate of 20% in men aged below 54 years which rose to 52.4% in men over 75 years. The corresponding rates for women were 14.8% and 32.8%. The overall prevalence was 36.9% for men and 28.7% for women. Various colonoscopy studies also confirm the higher incidence of polyps in men compared with women. The average age of patients in colonoscopy studies is 55–60 years (Gillespie et al, 1979; Minopoulos et al, 1983; Winawer et al, 1992), which is similar to that recorded in one of the largest 'surgical' series reported before the era of endoscopy (Grinnell and Lane, 1958).

Size and histological type

The data from colonoscopy studies are biased with respect to size, since it is common policy in many units not to remove the very small polyps (less than 3 mm diameter), some of which will not be adenomas. Similarly, at the other end of the spectrum, not all large polyps (more than 30 mm) can be removed endoscopically. For these reasons the size of the majority of adenomas from such series ranges between 5 mm and 20 mm diameter (Gillespie et al, 1979; Shinya and Wolff, 1979; Minopoulos et al, 1983; O'Brien et al, 1990). The older surgical series tend to be biased to include lesions whose size is at the upper end of the scale. Thus Grinnell and Lane (1958) found that the average size of 1856 tubular and tubulovillous adenomas from 1335 patients was 12 mm, the range being 2–70 mm. The corresponding figure for villous adenomas was 37 mm, with a range from 5–90 mm.

The overall picture is perhaps more truly represented by autopsy studies which show that the majority (about 85%) of adenomas are less than 10 mm diameter with only 10–15% being larger than this. The larger the size, the greater is the risk of malignancy. Size also tends to increase with age (O'Brien et al, 1990).

The relative proportions of the histological varieties will also vary according to which type of study has been mounted. Since villous adenomas are usually larger than the other types, they will tend to feature more frequently in surgical series and less frequently in data from colonoscopic studies.

The histological allocation of a particular polyp to one or other adenoma type is to some extent subjective. The accuracy of classification will depend on the care with which the polyp is examined and the number of histological sections taken, since if more than 20–25% of villous elements are present the polyp will be termed tubulovillous, whereas with only 15% present it will be called tubular (Morson and Dawson, 1990). Despite these variations, most investigators are agreed that tubular adenomas are the most common histological type (70–80%), tubulovillous are the next most frequent, and villous adenomas are third in frequency.

Incidence of malignant change

It is essential to make the distinction between carcinoma-in-situ (focal carcinoma, intramucosal cancer) and frank invasive carcinoma. For the latter to be present there must be invasion through the muscularis mucosae (Fisher and Turnball, 1952; Grinnell and Lane, 1958) whereas in carcinoma-in-situ this layer is never breached (Figure 28.10).

The overall incidence of malignant change depends on the type of study conducted. The incidence of malignancy reported in polyps removed via the colonoscope is 2.4–5% (Table 28.3). This cannot be the true incidence since not all polyps are retrieved and most that are lost are small. Since the risk of malignancy increases with size of polyp, the incidence of malignancy is perhaps overestimated. The overall incidence of malignancy in colonoscopy series is, however, probably more accurate than the older surgical series which tended to exclude most small polyps. Grinnell and Lane (1958) found an

Table 28.3 Incidence of malignancy in colonoscopically removed adenomata.

Authors	*n*	*Malignant polyps* (%)
Coutsoftides et al (1978)	416	4.3
Nivatvongs and Goldberg (1978)	580	4.0
Gillespie et al (1979)	1047	4.7
Shinya and Wolff (1979)	5786	4.9
Colacchio et al (1981)	729	5.3
Minopoulos et al (1983)	180	4.4
Winawer et al (1991) (National Polyp Study)	3002	4.2
Watanabe et al (1997)	1365	2.4

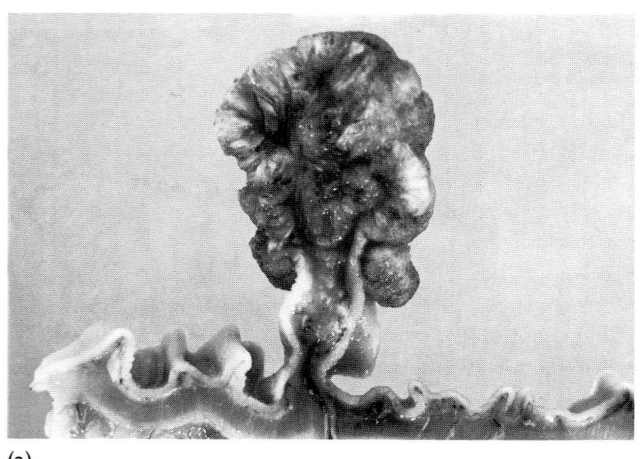

(a)

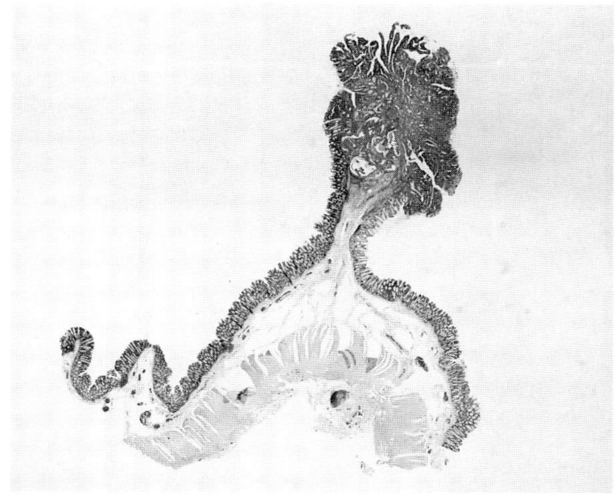

(b)

Figure 28.10a,b Adenomatous polyp with carcinoma extending into stalk – the malignant polyp.

overall incidence of 6.3% in 1856 lesions removed surgically, and in a series of polyps reported by Muto et al (1985) the equivalent percentage was 8%. The results from autopsy studies are in the range 1–2%.

Several important points emerge from more recent studies. They all confirm that the incidence of malignancy increases with increasing size of polyp, a fact that has been recognized for some time (Grinnell and Lane, 1958; Enterline et al, 1962; Muto et al, 1973; Morson and Dawson, 1990; O'Brien et al, 1990). Table 28.4, which is taken from the classic paper by Shinya and Wolff (1979), illustrates the risk of malignancy associated with the size of the polyps that can be removed via the colonoscope. Prior to colonoscopy it was considered that polyps with diameter 1 cm or less could be disregarded as they never became malignant. As can be seen, invasive carcinoma can and does occur in adenomas of all three histological forms in this size range.

The other fact with which all authors seem to agree is the increased risk of malignant change in villous lesions, although this is not so evident in adenomas removed via the colonoscope (see Table 28.4). Since many villous lesions are large and cannot be removed via the endoscope, the surgical series present a more accurate incidence. The incidence of carcinoma arising in villous adenomas treated by surgical excision varies between 11% and 42%. These data are calculated from series consisting of more than 50 patients (Table 28.5).

It is difficult to be sure whether it is the villous nature of the adenomas that confers the greater risk of carcinoma, or whether this is merely a reflection of the size of the lesion.

Spread from a malignant polyp

From a practical point of view it is important to consider the degree of spread that occurs with a

Table 28.4 Size of adenoma related to invasive carcinoma.

	Tubular			*Tubulovillous*			*Villous*		
		Invasive carcinoma			*Invasive carcinoma*			*Invasive carcinoma*	
Size of adenoma (cm)	No.	No.	(%)	No.	No.	(%)	No.	No.	(%)
0.5–0.9	1489	5	(0.3)	132	2	(1.5)	40	1	(2.5)
1.0–1.9	1713	61	(3.6)	776	50	(6.4)	249	14	(5.7)
2.0–2.9	432	28	(6.5)	475	54	(11.4)	100	17	(17.0)
3.0+	91	10	(11.0)	159	24	(15.0)	130	17	(13.1)
Total	3725	104	(2.8)	1542	130	(8.4)	519	49	(9.5)

From Shinya and Wolff (1979).

Table 28.5 Incidence of malignant change in villous adenomata.

Authors	*No. of cases of villous adenoma examined*	*Incidence of invasive carcinoma* (%)
Grinnell and Lane (1958)	216	31.8
Wheat and Ackerman (1958)	50	16.0
Enterline et al (1962)	81	55.0
Southwood (1962)	180	11.7
Bacon and Eisenberg (1971)	261	30.7
Hanley et al (1971)	217	11.0
Quan and Castro (1971)	215	24.0
Orringer and Eggleston (1972)	65	42.0
McCabe et al (1973)	169	28.0
Nivatvongs et al (1973)	72	4.0
Jahadi and Baldwin (1975)	264	18.0
Welch and Welch (1976)	258	29.0
Chiu and Spencer (1978)	331	29.0
Brunetaud et al (1989)	208	5.7
Steele et al (1996)	82*	6.1

* Includes all histological types of adenoma.

'malignant polyp'. Although it may be possible on clinical examination to determine if a large villous adenoma in the rectum is malignant, this is rarely the case with smaller lesions viewed through the endoscope. Endoscopically detected lesions are usually removed before the diagnosis of malignancy is established. The question of the need for more radical treatment such as resection can be resolved only by examining the data on the incidence of lymph node metastases. At present this is a contentious subject, although it is hoped that endoscopic ultrasonography may clarify this dilemma in the future. It is the purpose of this section merely to describe the facts; their implications for management are discussed later.

In order to obtain the data on lymph node involvement, only series in which the malignant polyps were removed by surgical resection can be usefully scrutinized. In units with an aggressive policy towards treatment, usually the polyp is removed endoscopically, the diagnosis of malignancy is then made and resection follows. Many reports do not comment on the time between endoscopy and surgical removal, but presumably this was short and is unlikely to have had an important bearing on spread. Of much greater importance is the indication for surgical excision. Thus in some units (Morson et al, 1984) only those patients in whom the pathologist reported that endoscopic removal was incomplete were advised to have a resection; cases where some element of doubt existed were discussed further and treatment was based upon histological differentiation, age and overall health. In other units (Colacchio et al, 1981) all patients with a malignant polyp seem to have been advised to undergo surgery, but not all did so, either because they refused or were considered high risk. In other series (Cooper, 1983) it is impossible to be certain what proportion of the total cases with malignant polyps underwent resection.

The issue is further complicated by the fact that some authors include only pedunculated polyps in their series, whereas others also include sessile lesions. Furthermore, it is not always clear how many villous lesions were included. It might be considered that the data obtained in the precolonoscopic era, when all malignant polyps were surgically resected, would be of greater value. However, these reports almost exclusively concentrated on rectal lesions. The defects in the various studies no doubt account for the marked differences observed in the incidence of lymph node metastases (Table 28.6). The consensus is, however, that approximately 10% of malignant colorectal polyps that can be resected via the colonoscope may have spread to the lymph nodes at the time the polyp is resected. There are certain pathological characteristics that increase the likelihood of malignant spread: they are sessile polyps, poorly differentiated lesions and vascular and lymphatic invasion.

Most data concerning lymph node metastases in villous adenomas are available from surgical series. Although most of these series predate the colonoscopy era, it appears that almost all the lesions removed would not have been treatable by

Table 28.6 Incidence of lymph node metastases with malignant polyp removed in studies before and after the introduction of colonoscopy.

Authors	*No. of malignant polyps*	*No. (%) with lymph node metastases*
Precolonoscopy era		
Lockhart Mummery and Dukes (1952)	23	7 (23)
Grinnell and Lane (1958)	27	1 (3.7)
Enterline et al (1962)	61	0
Postcolonoscopy era		
Coutsoftides et al (1978)	15	1 (6.6)
Nivatvongs and Goldberg (1978)	23	2 (8.8)
Gillespie et al (1979)	16	0
Shinya and Wolff (1979)	46	1 (2.1)
Colacchio et al (1981)	24	6 (25)
Cooper (1983)	56	5 (8.9)
Webb et al (1985)	10	0
Cranley et al (1986)	38	3 (7.9)
Richards et al (1987)	44	6 (7.5)
Muto et al (1991)	27	1 (3.7)

Table 28.7 Incidence of lymph node metastases in malignant villous adenomata removed surgically.

Authors	*No. excised*	*No. with metastases*
Grinnell and Lane (1958)	52	15 (29)
Enterline et al (1962)	45	13 (29)
Southwood (1962)	12	3 (25)

Numbers in parentheses are percentages.

colonoscopic polypectomy owing to their size. As can be seen in Table 28.7, at least 25% of the malignant villous adenomas removed surgically have lymph node involvement.

Evidence for the adenoma–carcinoma sequence

There is abundant evidence now linking adenoma with carcinoma. Although this evidence used to be virtually entirely circumstantial, there is now molecular genetic data which confirm the sequential development. On the other hand, the belief that all carcinomata commence life as benign adenomas is still contentious. An alternative pathway for the development of colorectal cancer may be via the small flat (non-polypoid) adenomas described by Muto et al (1985). The molecular genetic data which supports the concept for the adenoma carcinoma sequence is reviewed in Chapter 27. The circumstantial evidence is discussed below.

Anatomical distribution

Most authors have found a similar distribution of adenomas and carcinomata within the large bowel, the majority being found in the distal bowel but with a second relatively high incidence in the caecum. A good example was an autopsy study by Ekelund (1963), who found that one-half of his patients had adenomas of the rectum and sigmoid colon and this proportion was only slightly less than those who were found to have a carcinoma. With minor variations, the data from Helwig (1959) and Berge et al (1973) were similar. Most of the colonoscopy studies, as already pointed out, have found the majority of adenomas to be situated distal to the splenic flexure. However, in recent years, some authors have demonstrated a left-to-right shift in the location of colonic carcinoma (Greene, 1983). Coincident with this change of distribution, adenomas seem to have similarly changed in their location, a finding that further supports the link between the two conditions.

Synchronous carcinoma

A large proportion of patients with colorectal carcinoma also have one or more adenomas often adjacent to the tumour. In patients originally diagnosed as having one carcinoma, the incidence of associated adenomas on colonoscopy was 28–30% (Langevin and Nivatvongs, 1984; Maxfield, 1984; Pagana et al, 1984). In 3–7% of lesions there is a second tumour in the large bowel. An associated adenoma was found in 75% of patients with two or more synchronous carcinomata (Heald and Bussey, 1975).

Metachronous carcinoma

Patients with polyps in association with a carcinoma of the colon or rectum are twice as likely to develop a subsequent carcinoma after resection compared with patients who have no polyps at the time of their operation (Bussey et al, 1967). Similarly, Olsen et al (1988) found that patients had an increasing risk of recurrence of polyps with increasing numbers found on initial colonoscopy, and that overall 79% of recurrent polyps showed malignant changes. These findings were confirmed in a similar study from Finland (Kellokumpu and Husa, 1987).

Epidemiological data

Most of the epidemiological data relating to colorectal carcinoma have also been found to apply to adenomas. This topic is discussed elsewhere in this book. Suffice it to say that both conditions are more prevalent in Western society, in which a low-fibre, high-meat diet is common (see Chapter 30).

Age

If adenomas precede carcinomas it might be expected that patients with benign lesions would be younger. This is certainly the case with familial adenomatous polyposis (FAP). A clear difference exists in this condition between the age at which polyps appear and the development of carcinoma in patients who either refused operation or were treated by limited resection, leaving most of the colon still with polyps. Apart from this unique condition, however, most of the data on age have failed to demonstrate a difference between patients with an adenoma and patients with carcinoma (Grinnell and Lane, 1958; Enterline et al, 1962). These findings are usually explained by the fact that patients with carcinoma are symptomatic and the date of onset can be recorded accurately, whereas adenomas are asymptomatic (especially when small) and their time of onset is impossible to record accurately. This explanation seems reasonable, especially in the light of recent studies. Thus data from cancer detection clinics on asymptomatic patients show that patients with adenomas are approximately 8 years younger than patients with carcinoma (Enterline, 1976). Further temporal evidence is provided from colonoscopic follow-up studies, in which the mean age of patients with adenomas was approximately 5 years younger than those with invasive adenocarcinoma, suggesting a temporal relationship, with adenomas developing first (Winawer et al, 1991). Since Morson (1974) estimated that the evolution of the polyp–cancer sequence is approximately 10 years, these newer data add further weight to the argument.

Experimental carcinogens

Most of the experimental carcinogens such as dimethylhydrazine and azoxymethane, used to induce colorectal carcinoma in the laboratory animal, first produce microadenomas which later appear as adenomas and subsequently as invasive adenocarcinoma.

Histological evidence

The proponents of the adenoma–carcinoma sequence have used the finding of contiguous benign adenomatous tissue within a carcinoma as evidence for this hypothesis. Thus, careful histological study of malignant tumours may show all gradations from an adenoma with a microscopic focus of invasive carcinoma to an obvious carcinoma with some residual benign tumour at one edge. Muto et al (1985) found that 278 of 1961 colorectal cancers (14.2%) contained varying proportions of adenomatous tissue, and the three histological variants were equally represented. Colonoscopy studies demonstrating an incidence of carcinoma of 3–4% in apparently benign adenomas provide further evidence of the histological transformation.

Summary

Despite all the circumstantial and molecular genetic evidence, there is still no absolute proof that every adenocarcinoma of the large bowel develops from an adenoma. Nevertheless, there are few gastrointestinal pathologists who doubt that the concept is valid. Perhaps the best evidence for the adenoma–carcinoma sequence comes from attempts to interrupt the natural history by removing adenomas. Thus Gilbertsen (1974) reported on a 25-year follow-up of 18 000 subjects examined at the University of Minnesota cancer prevention clinic. These individuals had routine sigmoidoscopies and any polyps detected were removed. During follow-up only 11 carcinomas were detected in this part of the bowel, although the expected number of carcinomas based on age and distribution of the population would be 75–80. All the lesions detected during follow-up were early cancers and none of the patients died as a result of them. Of great significance also is the fact that in the area beyond the reach of the sigmoidoscope, the same incidence of carcinoma was found as was anticipated on statistical grounds. More recently, the National Polyp Study showed a greater than 75% reduction in the incidence of colorectal cancer compared with control groups of patients (Winawer et al, 1992). Similarly, other colonoscopic studies have shown a reduction in cancer incidence after polypectomy (Murakami et al, 1990; Atkin et al, 1992).

CLINICAL FEATURES OF NEOPLASTIC POLYPS

The symptoms and signs of adenomatous polyps depend to some extent on their size, number, site and degree of villous component. They may remain asymptomatic, as witnessed by their discovery on routine rectal examination or on endoscopic examination in patients with positive faecal occult blood test during a screening programme. Symptoms are not infrequent, however, and include:

1. *Bleeding*. The nature of the blood loss depends on the site of the polyp. The more distal the lesion, the brighter red is the blood. The amount lost is usually relatively small and the bleeding often occurs during defecation. Occasionally a patient presents with symptoms of anaemia due to chronic bleeding. Rarely there is severe haemorrhage.
2. *Diarrhoea and passage of mucus*. Larger polyps are more prone to produce these symptoms from mucus discharge, particularly if the lesions are situated in the rectum and are villous in nature (see below).

3. *Prolapse.* Occasionally a low-lying polyp will prolapse through the anus on straining. The patient often believes this to be prolapsing haemorrhoids, which may of course coexist. Rarely, prolapse may result in ischaemia with autopolypectomy or gangrenous change in the polyp.
4. *Abdominal colic.* This may rarely occur due to colocolic intussusception.

A large villous adenoma situated in the rectum often presents with a characteristic symptom complex (Figure 28.11). The patient complains of tenesmus and the frequent passage of mucus which may be tinged pink owing to slight blood loss. The mucus loss may be so great as to cause incontinence. As time progresses bleeding may become more obvious. Although general health may deteriorate the patient usually remains surprisingly healthy for a time despite the severity of the symptoms. Southwood (1962) and Wheat and Ackerman (1958) have pointed out that weight loss is common and may be due to the chronic fluid and electrolyte loss.

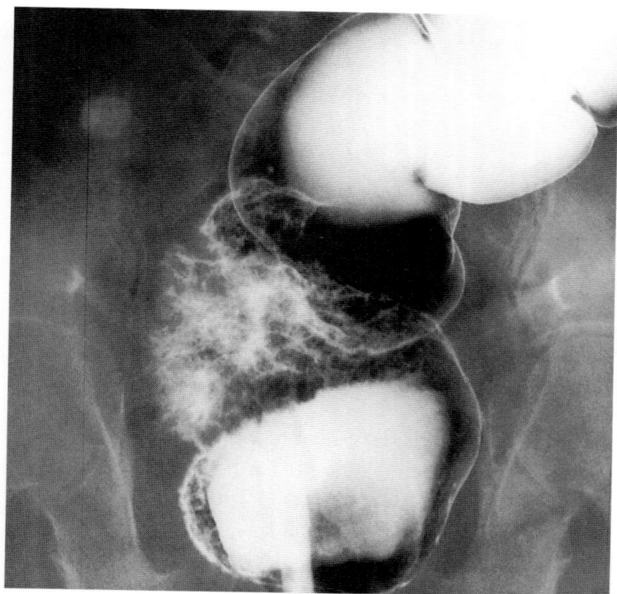

Figure 28.11 A large villous tumour of the rectum extending low down on the right, demonstrated by double-contrast barium enema.

Although the majority of villous adenomas occur in the rectum and sigmoid colon, a third are to be found in a more proximal site. In proximal lesions mucus discharge, incontinence and tenesmus are rare.

Fluid and electrolyte depletion syndrome

McKittrick and Wheelock (1954) were the first to recognize that villous adenomas could lead to serious metabolic disturbance and collapse as a consequence of severe mucous diarrhoea. A year later Fitzgerald (1955) described the first case of this associated syndrome in Britain in a paper entitled 'Extreme fluid and electrolyte loss due to villous papilloma'. Since then numerous cases have been reported, although the syndrome remains relatively rare, occurring in approximately 2% of patients with this type of tumour (Pheils, 1979).

One of the largest series is that of Shnika et al (1961) who collected 18 cases. The patients presented with a variety of symptoms and signs including severe dehydration, lethargy, weakness, oliguria, acidotic breathing, mental confusion and hypotension. Although diarrhoea was common it was not universal. Hypokalaemia and hyponatraemia were common, as were acidosis and uraemia.

Although the composition of the fluid loss from these tumours has been determined, the mechanism for the loss is unclear. Duthie and Atwell (1963) in a classical experiment utilizing isolated loops of colon containing villous adenomas measured bidirectional fluxes of water, sodium and potassium. They demonstrated that there was an increased movement of sodium and water from blood into the bowel lumen (exsorption) while movement in the reverse direction (insorption) was unaffected. Bidirectional flux of potassium was not altered. Lee and Keown (1970) reached the same conclusion by simply comparing the electrolyte concentrations of the fluid loss from these tumours with that lost from normal colon and present in the serum. Such results suggest that the villous adenoma cells function abnormally; hence the fluid loss is not primarily a result of a larger surface area but of abnormally functioning cells. Nevertheless, the area of these carpet lesions is closely related to the extent of electrolyte disturbance.

DIAGNOSIS

Rectal examination

Since a significant number of villous adenomas are situated in the lower rectum, digital examination is often diagnostic. The examination must be done with care, since these tumours are soft and may be difficult to palpate, often being described as 'velvety' in consistency.

Some non-villous adenomas may be felt per rectum. A lesion with a long pedicle may be confused with a hard pellet of faeces, but traction downwards with the finger will invariably establish the diagnosis.

Rigid sigmoidoscopy

The majority of villous adenomas are within the reach of the rigid sigmoidoscope. Southwood (1962) found that in 174 of 180 patients (97%) with a villous adenoma the tumour was within 30 cm of the anal verge. Even with the sigmoidoscope, diagnosis may be difficult since the view is frequently obscured by profuse mucus secretion or blood as a result of abrasion during examination. In addition the sigmoidoscope can easily be advanced past a villous lesion without the tumour being observed. It may also be difficult to determine the exact extent of some of these tumours as their edges may be indistinct; in some cases the lesion tends to 'fade out' into the surrounding mucosa.

A tubular adenoma, be it sessile or polypoid, is more easily recognizable than a villous lesion because it is less likely to bleed or secrete mucus; however, it can be missed if the sigmoidoscope is inserted too rapidly and it behoves the surgeon to take special care to examine the bowel while the instrument is being withdrawn as well as while it is being advanced. Polypoid lesions are more likely to be visualized during withdrawal as they tend to prolapse into the lumen.

Flexible fibre sigmoidoscopy

The flexible sigmoidoscope is being used increasingly by gastrointestinal physicians and surgeons as the first diagnostic procedure for the detection of colonic disease in patients with colorectal symptoms suggestive of a neoplasm. For the detection of polyps it has certain advantages over the rigid instrument. It is possible to negotiate the rectosigmoid junction in nearly all cases. Once through this region most of the sigmoid colon can be visualized and in some patients the scope may be passed to the splenic flexure. Since most polyps lie distal to the splenic flexure (Grinnell and Lane, 1958; Gillespie et al, 1979) it is not surprising that the yield with flexible sigmoidoscopy is about three times as high as with the rigid instrument (Marks et al, 1979; McCallum et al, 1984). The examination is relatively comfortable for the patient and with practice can be performed in about 10 minutes (Marks et al, 1979) without the need for conventional bowel preparation, although we use a phosphate enema just before the examination. If a polyp is seen it can be snared there and then, but because of the risk of explosion in a relatively unprepared bowel, insufflation should be by non-flammable gas such as carbon dioxide. Instrument designs have improved considerably and there are now more simple, robust and less costly sigmoidoscopes which can be reliably used in the outpatient setting (Reynolds et al, 1983). At present we use the rigid instrument initially and only if this is negative do we proceed to flexible sigmoidoscopy. This policy, however, is likely to change now these more robust flexible instruments are becoming available, particularly since they can be more easily sterilized.

Whether or not a polyp is detected by the methods described above, the rest of the colon needs to be visualized. If a polyp has been seen there may be others sited more proximally or there may be a coexisting carcinoma. The incidence of synchronous polyps beyond the reach of the rigid proctoscope and flexible sigmoidoscope is approximately 50% (O'Brien et al, 1990). If a polyp has not been seen it is important to rule out pathology in the rest of the bowel. It used to be debatable whether the next investigation should be double-contrast barium enema or colonoscopy (Durdey et al, 1987). However, virtually all are now agreed that colonoscopy is the next investigation of choice for the reasons discussed below.

There is little doubt that double-contrast barium examination is superior to the single-contrast examination for the detection of polyps (Figure 28.12). C B Williams et al (1982b) showed that whereas 70–80% of polyps more than 1 cm diameter were seen by double-contrast enema, only 50% were detected by single-contrast examination. Although barium enema is cheaper and quicker than colonoscopy (Dodds et al, 1977; Fork, 1983), it has the disadvantage that it is uncomfortable for the patient since the colon is distended while the patient is not sedated. It is relatively inaccurate in the sigmoid colon owing to overlapping folds and because of the frequent presence of diverticular dis-

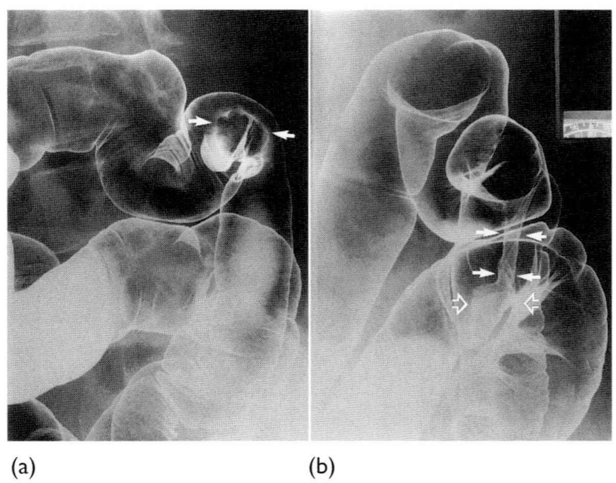

(a) (b)

Figure 28.12a,b (a) Double-contrast barium enema showing polyp in the splenic flexure (arrows). (b) Erect film revealing the long pedicle (arrows). The polyp (arrowheads) is now in the descending colon.

ease, and in the caecum owing to faecal residue (Farrands et al, 1983). It has an appreciable false-positive rate. If a polyp is found it cannot be removed and the colon has to be cleared of barium before polypectomy can be performed (Durdey et al, 1987).

Colonoscopy is more comfortable for the patient since it is performed under sedation, but is slightly more hazardous than radiology. It has the advantage that any polyp detected can be removed. Although the false-positive rate is low there are patients in whom even the most skilled endoscopist cannot negotiate the entire length of the colon, because of fixation or undue mobility (Obrecht et al, 1984; Durdey et al, 1987).

Despite the latter objection, colonoscopy is now regarded as the first-choice diagnostic procedure for the detection of polyps. We investigated 76 consecutive patients with large bowel symptoms by both double-contrast barium enema and colonoscopy (Durdey et al, 1987). Of the 11 patients who were subsequently found to have colonic polyps, only two patients (18%) were correctly diagnosed by barium enema, whereas in ten patients (91%) colonoscopy correctly detected the polyps.

If colonoscopic services are deficient, absent or the patient cannot tolerate the examination, we would recommend the following compromise policy. If flexible sigmoidoscopy proves negative and there is a high index of suspicion, the patient should have a double-contrast barium enema. If that is negative and the patient is now asymptomatic, no further action is required. If the patient continues to have symptoms a colonoscopy must be performed.

Patients in whom a polyp is detected on rigid or flexible sigmoidoscopy must also be advised to have a colonoscopic examination in the first instance, the rationale being that further polyps are likely to be present and will need removal. This is particularly so in patients if the polyp found in the rectum or sigmoid colon is greater than 1 cm diameter, if the polyp has a villous component, or if multiple polyps are present (Atkin et al, 1992). The same policy should be adopted for all patients who are at risk of developing polyps, such as those with a family history of colon cancer or familial adenomatous polyposis.

Flat adenomas

These are usually asymptomatic, being detected only in the course of an endoscopy. This type of polyp is unique in that it is usually small and flat, often with a central depression (Muto et al, 1985). Even on colonoscopy it can be difficult to detect, and the same applies in the resected colorectal specimen. Ninety per cent of flat adenomas are smaller than 1 cm and more than half are less than 5 mm (Muto and Watanabe, 1993). The signficance of flat adenomas is the high incidence of carcinomas which occur at a rate of 5.8% even when the lesions are as small as 2–4 mm, and this rate rapidly rises to 36.4% when the lesions are 9–10 mm (Table 28.8). Approximately 10% of adenomas in the series described by Muto et al (1985) were flat adenomas. They were most frequently located in the left colon

Table 28.8 Size and grade of atypia in flat adenomas.

Size (mm)	*Mild*	*Moderate*	*Severe*	*Total*	*Malignancy rate* (%)
2–4	43	6	3	52	5.8
5–6	31	6	4	41	9.8
7–8	12	6	6	24	25.0
9–10	5	2	4	11	36.4
Totals	91	20	17	128	13.3

From Muto and Watanabe (1993).

and rectum (Muto and Watanabe, 1993). It was thought that flat adenomas occurred only in the Japanese, but they have now been found in studies from Australia, Canada, Europe and the United Kingdom (Muto and Watanabe, 1993; Jarmillo et al, 1995; Stolte and Betake, 1995). The so-called *de novo* carcinomas may well arise from pre-existing flat adenomas through the adenoma–carcinoma sequence (Nivatvongs and Dorudi, 1996). The management of flat adenomas is the same as for sessile adenomas.

Recent molecular analysis of flat adenomas suggests that these superficial lesions are aetiologically distinct from other polypoid tumours (Minamoto et al, 1994), as the mutation rate in the K-*ras* gene was both significantly reduced (16% in flat adenomas compared with 50% in ordinary colorectal adenomas) and did not occur in the same codons.

MANAGEMENT PRINCIPLES

Once a polyp has been visualized it should be removed, since its exact type cannot be determined without histological examination. Exceptions to this rule are pseudopolyps in patients with inflammatory bowel disease, and the minute metaplastic lesions which are so frequent that most clinicians regard them as the rule rather than the exception. In addition the general health and age of the patient and the size of the polyp must be taken into account; it would be folly to pursue the removal of an asymptomatic polyp less then 1 cm diameter in an 80-year-old patient with severe underlying medical problems. However, with modern techniques most polyps can be removed by colonoscopy with minimal risk.

Most polyps within the rectum can be removed using the rigid or flexible sigmoidoscope if small, the operating sigmoidoscope if large and on a pedicle, or by a transanal surgical manoeuvre if large and sessile. The treatment of polyps in a more proximal position has been revolutionized by the introduction of the colonoscope. Over 95% of polyps proximal to the rectum are suitable for colonoscopic polypectomy. Surgical excision should never be entertained without first attempting colonoscopic polypectomy since some lesions that look sessile or malignant on barium enema prove to be on a small stalk endoscopically.

There are few indications for laparotomy and colotomy or resection today. If the polyp is too large to be removed endoscopically or if it has caused an intussusception then a resection may be needed. However, if there is some technical difficulty whereby the endoscopist fails to remove the polyp, we prefer an operative colonoscopy rather than resection or colotomy.

The colonoscope is passed at laparotomy or laparoscopy and with the help of the surgeon the polyp is snared. This manoeuvre allows polypectomy to be performed without opening the bowel and prevents peritoneal contamination. The technique is of particular use when a polyp has to be removed together with another procedure such as cholecystectomy. If, on the other hand, colonoscopic polypectomy is impossible because of the size of the polyp, there may be a case for a resection possibly laparoscopically performed.

TECHNIQUES FOR POLYP REMOVAL

Peranal excision of pedunculated polyp

A large polyp with a long pedicle situated in the lower rectum can often be hooked down through the anal orifice. This manoeuvre may be aided by the introduction of a Park's anal retractor. The base of the pedicle is then transfixed and the polyp plus its stalk is excised leaving 10–15 mm of the stalk distal to the ligature (Figure 28.13). The base should be doubly ligated before excision. In case of a broad pedicle a Goodsall stitch may be utilized for added security (Figure 28.14).

Polypectomy through rigid sigmoidoscope

With the move towards flexible instruments, the technique using a rigid sigmoidoscope is not employed as often as previously. Nevertheless, for lesions less than 10 cm from the anal verge it is ideal. This area tends to be pain-sensitive and is also awkward for fibre endoscopy (C B Williams et al, 1982b). For all but the smaller polyps the manoeuvre should be performed under anaesthesia and an operating sigmoidoscope can be used. There are

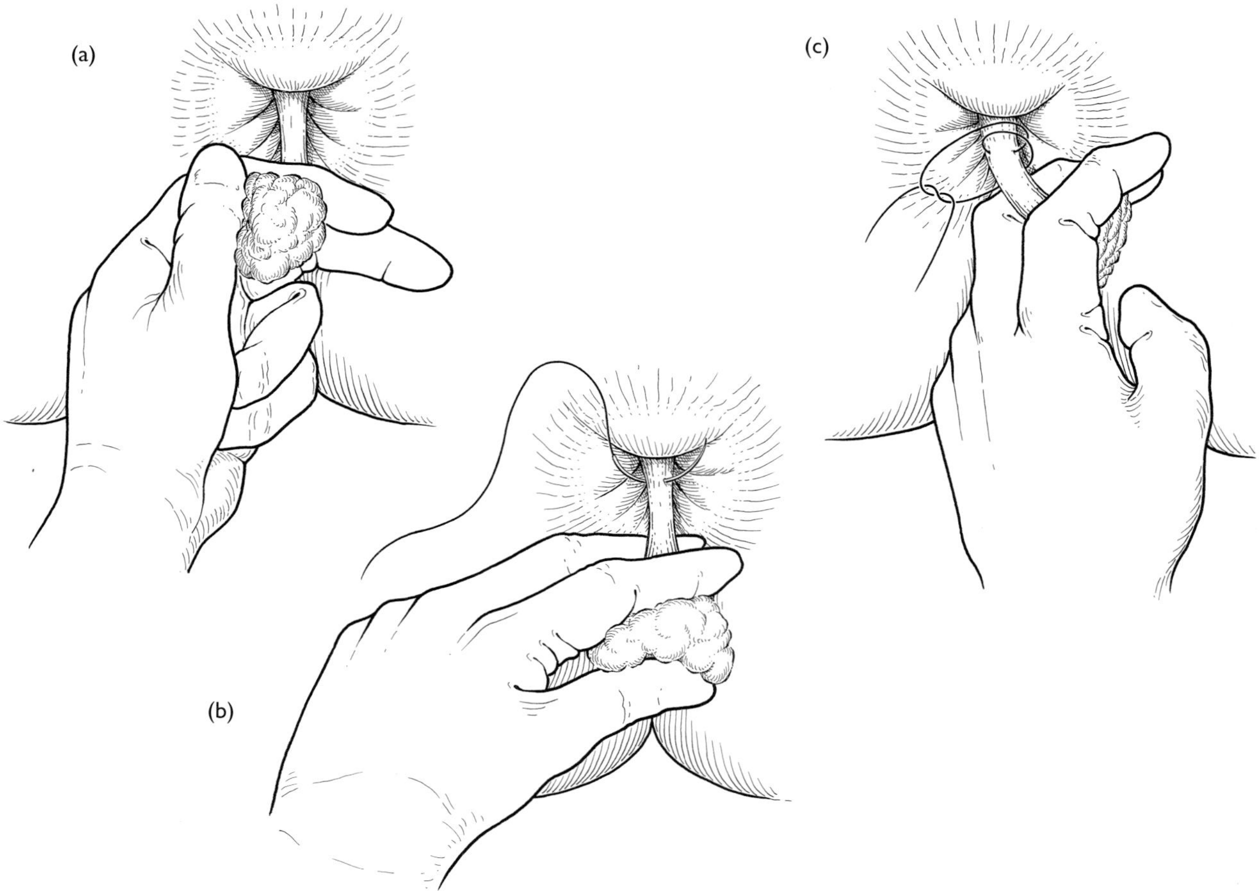

(a)

(c)

(b)

Figure 28.13a–c Peranal excision of a pedunculated rectal polyp. (a) The polyp is hooked down through the anal orifice and its base is transfixed (b), ligated (c) and excised.

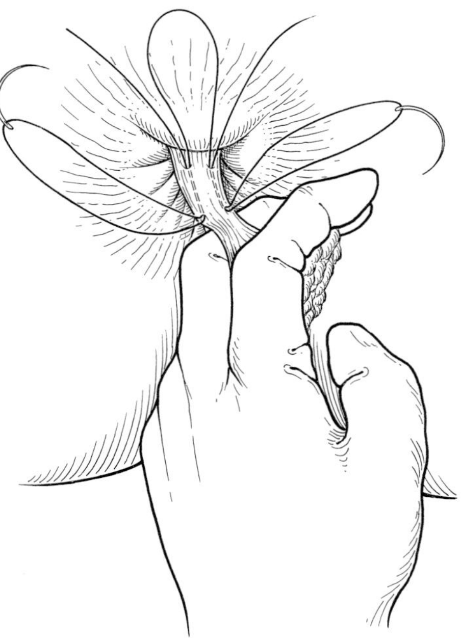

Figure 28.14 Ligation of the base of a broad rectal polyp using a Goodsall stitch.

several types available, of which the Lloyd–Davies sigmoidoscope is the best-known. Various modifications have been made to the instrument so that it can now be used with a fibreoptic light source, and in some cases air insufflation can be maintained while snaring is performed.

Technique

Although general anaesthesia is desirable, the operation can be conducted under spinal or epidural anaesthesia if the patient is unfit. The procedure can be performed in either the left lateral or lithotomy position (we prefer the latter). The operating sigmoidoscope is inserted into the anal canal; because of its broad diameter it may be necessary to dilate the sphincter gently prior to insertion. The obturator is removed in the usual way and the polyp is located. The suction tube is then attached with its distal end projecting from the end of the sigmoidoscope.

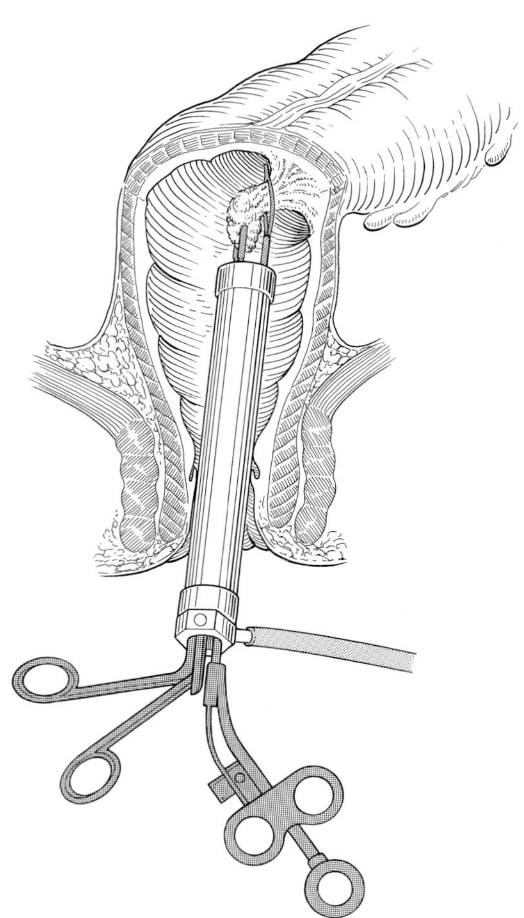

Figure 28.15 Polypectomy via a rigid sigmoidoscopy using the Frankfeldt snare.

For polyps with a pedicle a snare is used (Figure 28.15). This is a rigid instrument with an insulated shaft handle and there are several designs available; the Frankfeldt snare is the one we prefer. Before insertion through the lumen of the scope, the ability of the snare to open and close is checked. It is then attached to the diathermy equipment and an appropriate current is selected to give a slow coagulating effect. The instrument is inserted with the snare closed. On reaching the polyp the snare is opened and manipulated over the head of the polyp so that it lies at the base of the pedicle. The snare is then gradually closed and traction is exerted downwards to ensure that the base of the pedicle is encompassed without tenting the underlying mucosa. The diathermy current is then applied so that it cuts through the base of the polyp until the polyp is detached and becomes free within the bowel lumen. It is then a simple matter to retrieve it with the biopsy forceps. If possible the base that remains should be biopsied so that it can be scrutinized histologically. At the completion of the manoeuvre the wound in the mucosa is checked to ensure that haemostasis is complete.

Sessile polyps can be difficult to remove by the method described. One technique which may be useful is to draw the polyp down through the opened snare using grasping forceps. While moderate traction is exerted the snare is gently closed round the disc of mucosa bearing the polyp. Although there is little risk of perforation in the extraperitoneal part of the rectum, this technique is more dangerous in the intraperitoneal rectum. For this reason many surgeons have preferred to treat sessile polyps with a button electrode or diathermy forceps. The latter are usually long alligator biopsy forceps, the shaft of which is covered by a thin rubber tube. The use of either of these instruments has two disadvantages. First, it is difficult to gauge the amount of tissue destroyed and thus it is impossible to be sure that the procedure has been performed adequately; secondly, it is not possible to retrieve sufficient intact portions of the polyp for accurate histological assessment. Thus for sessile polyps in the upper rectum we have found the flexible sigmoidoscope and snare to be preferable, if a little more tedious. This snare is finer than the Frankfeldt instrument and piecemeal removal is more easily accomplished with less risk.

Complications

The complications of this technique are perforation, haemorrhage and intraluminal gas explosion; they are identical to the complications after colonoscopic polypectomy and are discussed later.

Colonoscopic polypectomy

The technique of passing the colonoscope through the colon has been discussed elsewhere (Chapter 2), so only the important points concerning polypectomy are discussed here.

Instruments

Both single-channel and twin-channel endoscopes of various lengths are available for therapeutic colonoscopy. One advantage of the twin-channel instrument is that one channel can be used for suction or the passage of holding or biopsy forceps, while the other channel may be used for insertion of the snare. The disadvantage of the twin-channel colonoscope is that it is thicker than the single-channel instrument, which makes it less flexible and more painful for the patient. Most units, therefore, use a single-channel endoscope.

A variety of accessory instruments are necessary for polypectomy. They include high-frequency diathermy snares, polyp retrievers, grasping forceps and high-frequency electrosurgical equipment. All instruments should be appropriately insulated. The electrosurgical units are available with widely differing power outputs; this makes it impossible to indicate the power setting that would be applicable to all units. The optional settings should be carefully evaluated with any new equipment before endoscopy by testing the effects on tissue *in vitro*. Prior to polypectomy it is always advisable to check that the snares and grasping forceps open and close satisfactorily before insertion through the instrument. Small sessile polyps may not be easily dealt with using the snare, and in these cases 'hot biopsy' is necessary. The hot biopsy forceps are similar to the biopsy forceps used during the diagnostic procedure, but they are sheathed to provide insulation.

Back-up instruments must be available when a polypectomy is to be performed. There is nothing more frustrating than technical failure when a polyp is identified after a difficult examination.

Technique of snaring

In all patients with a suspected polyp it is essential to try to obtain a colonoscopic examination of the entire colon since more than one polyp is likely to be present and an associated carcinoma needs to be excluded. The polyp can be removed during intubation, but we prefer to perform polypectomy during withdrawal of the instrument if it is felt that the polyp is not in an ideal position for polypectomy when first seen. Prior to snaring, it is important that the assistant ensures that there is good contact between the diathermy plate and the skin of the thigh. An adhesive plate is normally used. When the polyp is first seen a decision must be taken as to whether the lesion is of suitable size for endoscopic polypectomy, and if it is, whether it should be removed whole or piecemeal. It is often technically possible to remove a polyp of 4–5 cm diameter, but if it is thought to be a carcinoma, it makes sense to take multiple biopsies from it and withdraw.

The polyp should be snared only when the colonoscope has been optimally positioned in relation to it and when the instrument shaft is free of tension. Sometimes it may be necessary to move the patient if the best position of the endoscope in relation to the polyp has not been obtained. To ensnare the polyp the tip of the endoscope is usually positioned 2–3 cm distal to the lesion and the snare is passed through the instrument channel. The loop of the snare is then opened in the lumen of the colon and is then placed over the polyp and manoeuvred to the base of the head (Figure 28.16). During this manoeuvre it is useful both to manipulate the tip of the colonoscope and partially open and close the snare, since repeated movements of the snare may cause flexion of the wire loop enabling it to encircle the polyp head. Some examiners use their right hand to control the colonoscope shaft by torque to

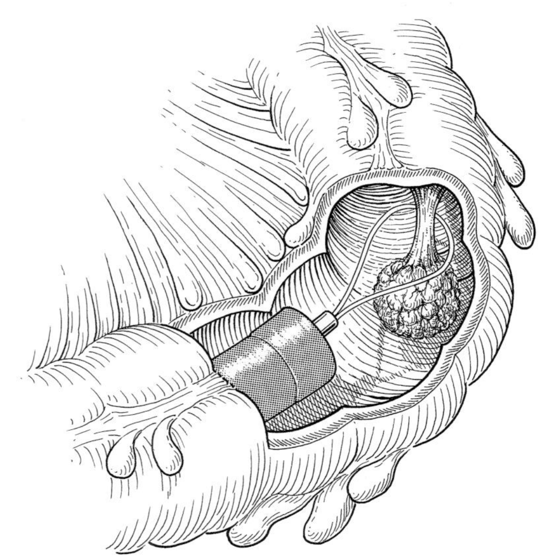

Figure 28.16 Colonoscopic polypectomy. The snare has been passed down the colonoscope, opened, and manoeuvred over the head of the polyp to encircle the pedicle.

the right or left, inserting and withdrawing while the assistant opens and closes the snare (Waye, 1980). Before the loop is closed, the sheath of the snare should be pushed up against the stalk or base of the polyp (Figure 28.17). Failure to do this with the end of the sheath positioned several centimetres away from the polyp often causes the head of the polyp to slip out of the snare when it is closed.

Once the snare is snugly positioned around the base or stalk, the polyp's head becomes livid. The snare should then be withdrawn several centimetres down the colonoscope to pull the polyp away from the colonic wall. This manoeuvre ensures that the polyp has been successfully snared and minimizes thermal damage to the bowel wall. The current is then applied and the snare slowly closed to sever the polyp. When placing a snare over a pedunculated polyp which has a stalk of sufficient length, it is wise to leave a remnant of the stalk so that it can be resnared should postpolypectomy bleeding occur. In the case of a sessile polyp, the lesion is always snared at the base if possible to include 2–3 mm of normal mucosa. After closing the snare, a 'pseudo-stalk' of normal mucosa is formed by pulling the polyp into the lumen (Figure 28.18). Flat polyps can be elevated by saline injection in the submucosa beneath the lesion. This manoeuvre increases the safety of polypectomy and has been useful for colonoscopic resection of lesions previously requiring surgical resection (Inoue et al, 1993).

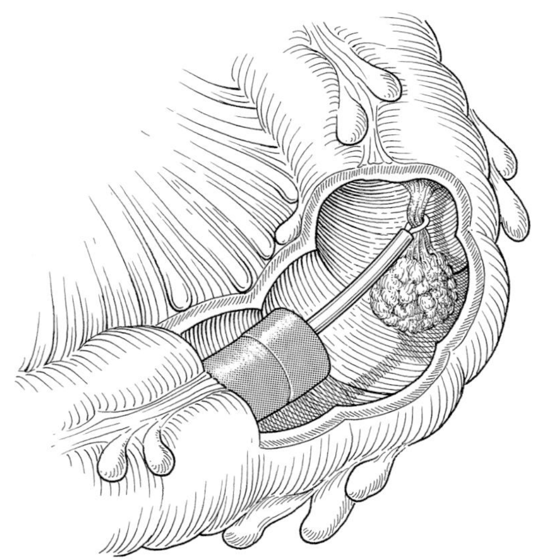

Figure 28.17 The sheath of the snare has been pushed up against the stalk of the polyp and closed around it.

Once the polyp is free and lying in the lumen it should be removed. This can be achieved in one of two ways. Firstly, the grasping forceps can be used (Figure 28.19); these have three prongs which when open can surround most polyps. On closure the polyp is gripped by the prongs and the colonoscope is then withdrawn with the forceps still in position. No attempt is made to withdraw the forceps along the channel of the colonoscope. The second method of retrieval involves the use of suction. If the polyp is small it can be sucked up through the suction channel; if a trap is fitted to that channel the polyp

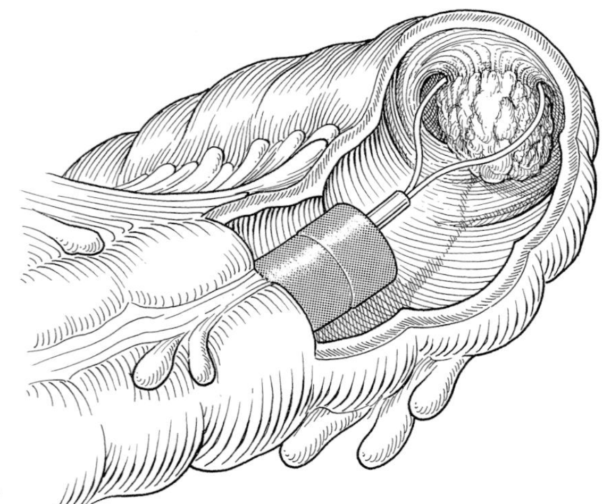

(a)

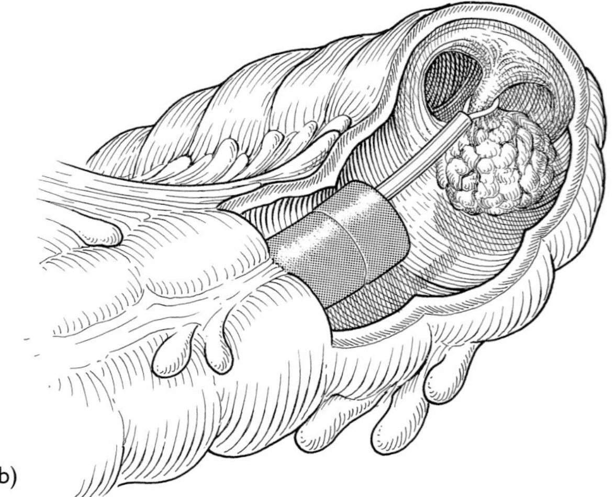

(b)

Figure 28.18a,b Colonoscopy excision of a sessile polyp. (a) The base of the polyp is snared including 2–3 cm of normal mucosa. (b) After closure of the snare, a pseudopolyp of normal mucosa is formed by pulling the polyp into the lumen.

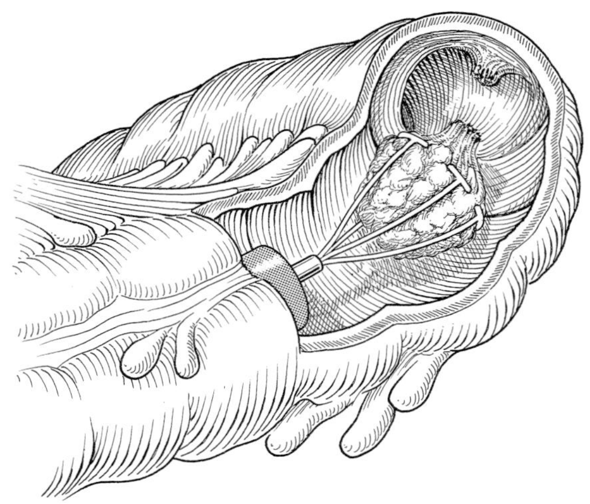

Figure 28.19 Removal of a polyp after its base has been divided by grasping forceps.

can be retrieved. If the polyp is too large to pass through the suction channel, the vacuum can be increased and continuously applied and the endoscope removed altogether with the polyp adherent to its tip.

Large polyps, particularly sessile ones, can often only be removed by piecemeal resection. This technique is performed by placing the snare loop around a portion of the head of the polyp without attempting to encircle the base completely (Figure 28.20). The electrocautery current is applied as the snare is being closed with removal of a portion of the polyp. The resected portion may be large or small depending upon the position of the snare wire. This process is repeated until all the polyp has been resected. The optimal power setting should be selected for each snare application. This particular technique requires considerable skill and experience, for it is easy to induce haemorrhage or perforate the colon. It is also essential to retrieve all parts of the polyp after piecemeal resection to ensure that pathological examination is as complete as possible.

After polypectomy the site of removal should be examined carefully to confirm haemostasis.

Another technique also available for large polyps in the sigmoid colon involves deliberate sigmoidorectal intussusception (Gillespie et al, 1978; Strauss et al, 1978). The polyp is snared using a wire snare without a handle; the loop is tightened around the base of the lesion and the colonoscope is withdrawn leaving the snare in place. Afterwards under general anaesthesia the polyp is drawn down as an intussusception to the anal verge by traction and then excised and the wound sutured. We have no experience with this technique, but it would appear that it is particularly useful for broad-based lesions in the sigmoid colon which are thought to be too large for safe piecemeal resection and where the only alternative is laparotomy.

Several polyps can usually be removed at one session. Retrieval may be difficult and require repeated

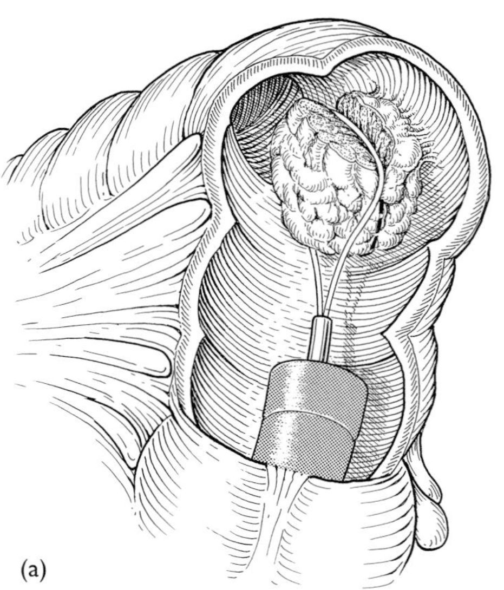

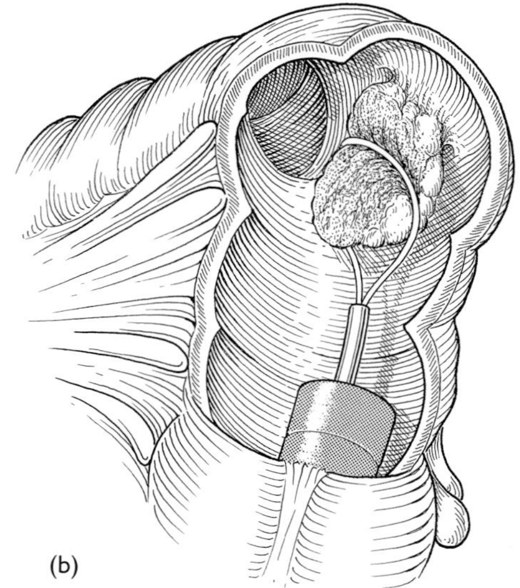

Figure 28.20a,b Piecemeal removal of large sessile polyp using the diathermy snare.

withdrawal of the instrument and reintubation. This is reasonable for three or four polyps, but if there are more it may be necessary to give an enema after the procedure and collect all the fluid returned in the hope of retrieving most polyps.

Hot biopsy forceps technique

This technique (Williams, 1973) involves the use of standard biopsy forceps in an insulated sheath (Figure 28.21). During biopsy, current is applied which passes around the cups of the forceps and coagulates the base of the polyp, while the part of the polyp grasped by the jaws of the forceps is preserved for histological examination. This technique can be used to biopsy and fulgurate polyps up to 6–8 mm diameter. In order to prevent burning the colonic wall, the polyp is grasped by the forceps and by manipulating the scope it is tented away to form a short pseudopedicle. Coagulation is applied for 2–3 seconds and the forceps are then withdrawn after the coagulation effect is seen. If any of the polyp remains it can be retouched with the forceps closed.

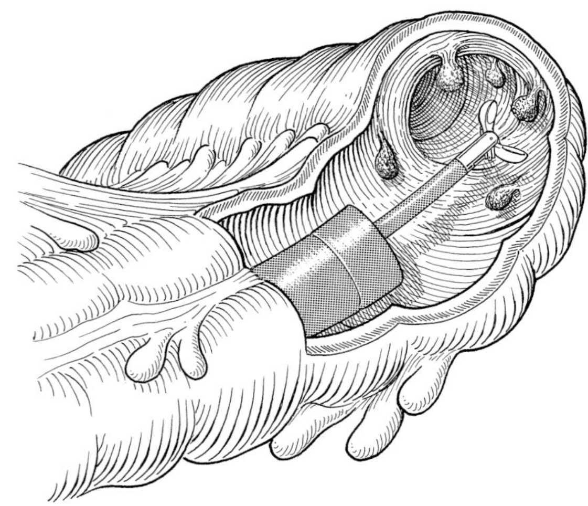

Figure 28.21 Use of hot biopsy forceps to deal with small (6–8 mm) polyps.

Complications of polypectomy

Bleeding, perforation and gas explosion have been the most frequently described complications of colonoscopic polypectomy. In addition there is a condition known as the postpolypectomy syndrome.

Haemorrhage

Bleeding following polypectomy may be primary or reactionary and is rarely secondary. It is usually due to incomplete coagulation of blood vessels in the polyp stalk or base. Several reasons may account for this: the diathermy setting may be too high; the endoscopist may be overambitious and attempt to resect a polyp that is too large; the vessel in the stalk may be larger than the size of stalk suggests; or an underlying coagulation defect may exist. The latter condition should be obvious prior to the procedure, but it is always a good idea for the endoscopist to enquire concerning easy bruising, anticoagulant therapy, etc.

Minor primary haemorrhage is common and usually subsides very quickly. Nivatvongs (1988) found that minor bleeding occurred in 53% of 1576 polypectomies. Major haemorrhage requiring blood transfusion is rare, however. Review of the literature suggests that this problem occurs in about 1–2% of cases (Roseman, 1973; Berci et al, 1974; Geenan et al, 1974; Rogers et al, 1975; Fruhmorgen and Demling, 1979; Williams and Tan, 1979; Nivatvongs, 1988; Habr-Gama and Waye, 1989; Waye et al, 1992; Jentschura et al, 1994). Secondary haemorrhage occurs even less frequently: thus of the 1500 polypectomies performed by Williams and Tan (1979) this complication occurred in only four patients (0.3%) 7–10 days following the procedure.

Treatment of postpolypectomy haemorrhage

Pulsatile severe bleeding, although rare, may arise from a resected polyp stalk. In these circumstances the wisest approach is to continue to sever the polyp grasped within the snare in the usual fashion. After the polyp has been removed, the entire area including surrounding tissue should be resnared and held for several minutes. The snare should then be gently released and the base observed. If bleeding continues the snare should be reapplied, and several episodes of 'snare strangulation' may be needed before haemostasis is achieved. It should be pointed out that it is extremely unwise to apply the electrocautery current to the tissue that has been bunched up in this manner, since perforation may occur.

If the above measure fails, some authors (Carlyle and Goldstein, 1975; Cotton and Williams, 1980) have recommended selective arterial catheterization with vasopressin infusion (see Chapter 62). This technique, in our view, should not be attempted in severe haemorrhage as it often fails and may waste valuable time. A procedure we have found useful is the infusion of large volumes of iced water containing adrenaline through a polyethylene catheter to the bleeding site. An alternative is the electrohydrothermal probe (Matek et al, 1979). This instrument combines irrigation with electrocoagulation. It allows optimal visualization and prevents the electrode sticking to the coagulum, and thus the application of energy to the bleeding site is more accurate. Although we have had no experience with this instrument, others are enthusiastic (Fruhmorgen, 1981).

If the measures discussed above fail and the patient continues to bleed profusely there is no option but to perform a laparotomy. Colotomy and underrunning of the vessel should be performed and localization can be improved if it is necessary by on-table colonoscopy. Such a procedure will have a lower morbidity than colonic resection in these circumstances.

Perforation

This is an uncommon yet serious event occurring in fewer than 1% of diagnostic procedures (Roseman, 1973; Wolff and Shinya, 1973; Berci et al, 1974; Greenen et al, 1975; Rogers et al, 1975; Williams and Tan, 1979; Fruhmorgen, 1981; Waye et al, 1992; Gedebou et al, 1996; Damore et al, 1996; Jentschura et al, 1994; Lo and Beaton, 1994), but up to 3% after therapeutic procedures (Damore et al, 1996). It may result from uncontrolled straightening or rotating manoeuvres prior to polypectomy. Perforation in the region of the polypectomy site may be caused mechanically by the tip of the colonoscope, the forceps, snare or grasper, or may result from tissue necrosis. The patient may not complain of excessive pain at the time of perforation, particularly if heavily sedated. The endoscopist may be aware of this complication only when faced with a view of omentum, spleen or other intra-abdominal organ. Persistent abdominal pain after the sedation has worn off should make the clinician suspicious. The finding of peritonitis on abdominal examination and pneumoperitoneum on straight abdominal radiography will confirm the diagnosis. If the diagnosis is clear, immediate laparotomy with simple suture of the defect is usually required, although selected patients with minimal signs may be managed conservatively, since the colon is often empty and antibiotic therapy can be commenced immediately. In the few patients who present late and in whom a sealed perforation is strongly suspected, some authors have recommended conservative treatment (Smith and Nivatvongs, 1975; Carpio et al, 1989; Christie and Marazzo, 1991; Hall et al, 1991). Such a decision may be considered in the following circumstances: stable condition; late diagnosis; good bowel preparation; pneumoperitoneum not expanding; no evidence of peritonitis; no distal obstruction; improvement with supportive care; absence of underlying pathology.

The choice of therapy must be judged for the individual patient. Laparotomy should be undertaken if the patient shows signs and symptoms of peritonitis. Fever and leucocytosis alone or in combination are not necessarily absolute indications for surgical intervention, but the burden of responsibility falls on the surgeon for unwarranted delay (Corman, 1993). Recently, laparoscopic repair has been reported as a successful means of repairing a perforation caused by the colonoscopy (Chardavoyne and Wise, 1994; Schlinkert and Rasmusson, 1994; Mehdi et al, 1996; Miyahara et al, 1996). This seems a reasonable approach in an otherwise uncomplicated case; but if the signs of perforation are present with faecal contamination, and yet the perforation is not seen on laparosocopy, it is prudent to perform a formal laparotomy. If a conservative regimen is pursued, careful monitoring with daily abdominal radiographs and follow-up with regular ultrasound scanning of the abdomen will be necessary to detect increasing pneumoperitoneum and the presence of an intra-abdominal abscess. Subcutaneous, retroperitoneal and mediastinal emphysema after colonoscopy have been reported as well as pneumoscrotum and pneumothorax (Lezak and Goldhamer, 1974; Yassinger et al, 1978; Fishman and Golman, 1981; Amshel et al, 1982; Schmidt et al, 1986; Goerg and Duber, 1996). These presentations do not necessarily mean free perforation of the colon, and hence are not direct indications for surgical exploration.

Gas explosion

The few intracolonic explosions that have occurred during polypectomy seem to have been in patients prepared using mannitol. This oligosaccharide enjoyed a brief spell of popularity as a bowel preparation for patients undergoing colorectal surgery (Donovan et al, 1980) and barium enema examination (Palmer and Khan, 1979) in addition to colonoscopy (Newstead and Morgan, 1979) before this danger was appreciated. Since mannitol is nonabsorbable, hyperosmolar and not unpleasant to take orally, it was considered the ideal bowel preparation. Unfortunately, it is fermentable by certain bacteria and seems to provide a nutrient for gas-producing organisms (Williams et al, 1979; Keighley et al, 1981). Since a fatal outcome was described from such an explosion in a patient prepared using mannitol (Bigard et al, 1979), we – like many other centres – have abandoned its use, preferring the more conventional preparations described in Chapter 3. There still remains a theoretical risk of explosion from the production of the combustible gases hydrogen and methane, which are liberated by bacterial action of faeces in the normal manner. However, the concentration of these gases in the colon at the time of colonoscopy is only a minute fraction of that required for combustion (Bond and Levitt, 1974; Ragins et al, 1974). Provided electrocoagulation is performed in a bowel that contains little faecal residue, the risk of explosion should remain merely theoretical. Even so, some colonoscopists routinely insufflate the colon with carbon dioxide prior to polypectomy. This technique also has the advantage that carbon dioxide is absorbed faster than air and seems to be more comfortable for the patient (Hussein et al, 1984).

Postpolypectomy syndrome

This rare syndrome which is also seen after forceps biopsy has been described following polypectomy (Sugarbaker et al, 1974; Rogers et al, 1975). The patient complains of abdominal pain and marked distension which is accompanied by a brief period of fever. The symptoms are temporary and usually subside in a day or so. Such a clinical picture suggests a perforation, but straight abdominal radiography shows no intraperitoneal gas. It has been suggested that the cause may be local peritoneal irritation resulting from transmural coagulation (Sugarbaker et al, 1974; Rogers et al, 1975; Cohen and Waye, 1986), but sealed perforation cannot altogether be ruled out despite negative findings on radiography.

Overall mortality rates

The overall mortality from perforation and haemorrhage following polypectomy seems to be about 0.05% (range 0–0.1%) (Roseman, 1973; Wolff and Shinya, 1973; Berci et al, 1974; Geenan et al, 1974; Rogers et al, 1975; Prorock et al, 1977; Schwesinger et al, 1979; Fruhmorgen, 1981; Macrae et al, 1983).

Methods to reduce complications

As discussed above, mannitol should probably not be used for bowel preparation, particularly if polypectomy is likely. If polypectomy is performed after the use of mannitol, insufflation of the colon should be with carbon dioxide. All manoeuvres should be performed under adequate sedation: if the patient is restless, the risks, particularly of perforation, are great. Since the greatest risk of haemorrhage seems to be associated with polyps of 2 cm or more in size, where these are identified on barium enema the patient is best admitted to hospital and preliminary haematological investigations performed. The likelihood of bleeding is minimized by use of a coagulation current only, at a low setting (15–30 watts), and very gentle snare closure to avoid cutting too rapidly (Macrae et al, 1983). Haemorrhage usually occurs immediately and the endoscopist must have sufficient experience to be competent to resnare the stalk. If this fails, blood should be sent for cross-matching and the patient admitted immediately, preferably to a surgical ward. Although most patients will settle with conservative measures, occasionally surgical intervention will be needed to preserve life. Secondary haemorrhage is rare but may occur up to 14 days after polypectomy. All patients should be warned of the possibility and advised to return immediately should bleeding persist or be profuse.

Any patient who complains of persistent abdominal pain after colonoscopic polypectomy should be admitted for observation and an abdominal radiograph obtained to exclude perforation.

Follow-up after polypectomy for adenoma

Up to recently, little information was available concerning the frequency with which polyps recurred after polypectomy so there were no clear guidelines based on natural history as to how often these patients should be followed up. Previous evidence suggested that 20–30% of patients with one polyp at initial colonoscopy would subsequently develop a new lesion, but the time interval was poorly documented. Thus C B Williams et al (1982b) tried to reinvestigate 800 patients who had undergone polypectomy and were considered subsequently to have a 'clean' colon. Only 330 patients were in fact studied at a mean of 3.6 years after the initial procedure. Barium enema and colonoscopy revealed that 1.5% had carcinomas, 8.5% had adenomas greater than 1 cm diameter, and 27% had adenomas less than 1 cm. Olsen et al (1988) found that in 457 patients with one initial polyp the 5-year recurrence rate was 28%, whereas if the patient originally had more than four polyps the rate increased to 59%.

These results emphasize the need for follow-up in most patients, although a sense of proportion needs to be maintained. It seems unnecessary and relatively harsh to subject an elderly patient with one or two small adenomas to regular check colonoscopies. The recommendations in the literature for follow-up frequency of the fit patient with a normal life expectancy used to be variable: thus Theuerkauf (1978) and the American Cancer Society (Winawer, 1980) suggested a complete colonoscopy every 2–3 years, whereas others (Buntain et al, 1972; Welch and Hedberg, 1975) recommended more frequent checks. However, the results of the National Polyp Study from the USA have helped clarify follow-up protocols.

The National Polyp Study was initiated as a multicentre prospective randomized trial designed to assess the appropriate time for follow-up colonoscopy for patients newly diagnosed with adenomas (Winawer et al, 1992, 1993). Patients with inflammatory bowel disease, a previous history of colorectal cancer, familial adenomatous polyposis, a malignant polyp, a sessile adenoma with a base larger than 3 cm or an incomplete colonoscopy (3%) were excluded from the study. Patients were randomized either to two follow-up colonoscopies over 3 years (at 1 year and at 3 years) or to one follow-up colonoscopy at 3 years after the initial colonoscopy. Both groups were offered a follow-up colonoscopy at 6 years. There were 1418 patients randomized into the study from 1980 to 1990. The average age of adenoma diagnosis was 61.2 years. At the initial colonoscopy, over one-third of patients had adenomas more than 1 cm diameter, 43% had two or more adenomas detected, and 10% had adenomas with high-grade dysplasias or invasive carcinomas. At first follow-up, whether at 1 or 3 years, 47% of patients had polyps detected and 29% had adenomas, but only 3% had a pathologically advanced adenoma, defined as an adenoma of more than 1 cm, or with high-grade dysplasia or invasive carcinoma. Additional follow-up findings at 1 and 3 years, and at 3 years for those who also had a 1-year follow-up colonoscopy, are shown in Table 28.9, which shows that even though additional polyps (and adenomas) were detected at follow-up, very few patients had pathologically advanced adenomas detected. With two examinations within 3 years, the percentage of patients with one or more adenomas detected at follow-up increased to 42%; however, the percentage with pathologically advanced adenomas was 3.3% whether two examinations within 3 years or only one examination following initial colonoscopy had been performed (Table 28.10). Thus, the more colonoscopies that are done, the more adenomas are detected. However, patients with pathologically advanced adenomas are detected as well by one examination at 3 years as by two examinations within 3 years. Based on these results, a 3-year follow-up examination can be recommended following the initial colonoscopy provided that the colon was cleared of all identified polyps on initial examination.

The data from the National Polyp Study also

Table 28.9 Findings at follow-up colonoscopy after initial polypectomy in the National Polyp Study.

	First follow-up examination		*Second follow-up examination*
Follow-up finding	*1 year later* (*n* = 545)	*3 years later* (*n* = 428)	*3 years later with examination also at 1 year* (*n* = 338)
Polyps	262 (48.1)	194 (45.3)	131 (38.8)
Adenoma	150 (27.5)	137 (32.0)	73 (21.6)
Histologic type of adenoma			
Tubular	135 (24.8)	117 (27.3)	66 (19.5)
Villous	15 (2.8)	20 (4.7)	7 (2.1)
Size of largest adenoma (cm)			
Small (≤ 0.5)	92 (16.9)	87 (20.3)	55 (16.3)
Medium (0.6–1.0)	46 (8.4)	38 (8.9)	15 (4.4)
Large (> 1.0)	12 (2.2)	12 (2.8)	3 (0.9)
Dysplasia and invasive cancer			
Low-grade dysplasia	147 (27.0)	132 (30.8)	71 (21.0)
High-grade dysplasia	3 (0.6)	3 (0.7)	1 (0.3)
Invasive cancer	0 (0)	2 (0.5)*	1 (0.3)†
Pathologically advanced adenomas‡	14 (2.6)	14 (3.3)	3 (0.9)

Values in parentheses are percentages.
* Dukes' stage A ($T_1N_0M_0$); † Dukes' stage B_1 ($T_2N_0M_0$); ‡ any large adenoma (>1.0 cm) or adenoma with high-grade dysplasia or invasive cancer.
From Winawer et al (1992).

Table 28.10 Comparison of the findings of two colonoscopy follow-up examinations at 1 and 3 years with the findings of one colonoscopy follow-up examination at 3 years in the National Polyp Study.

Follow-up finding	*Follow-up colonoscopy at 1 and 3 years (n = 338)*	*Follow-up colonoscopy at 3 years only* (n = 428)*	*Relative risk (95% c.i.)*	*P value*
Any adenoma detected	141 (41.7)	137 (32.0)	1.3 (1.1–1.6)	0.006
Adenoma with advanced pathologic features†	11 (3.3)‡	14 (3.3)	1.0 (0.5–2.2)	0.99

Values in parentheses are percentages or 95% confidence intervals.
* Reference category. † Any adenoma that was large (> 1.0 cm) or had high-grade dysplasia or invasive cancer.
‡ Values based only on patients who returned for both examinations.
From Winawer et al (1992, 1993).

showed that the findings at the first follow-up colonoscopy were predictive of findings at subsequent examinations. Patients with adenomas detected at the first follow-up colonoscopy had a greater likelihood of having pathologically advanced adenomas at subsequent follow-up examinations than those with no adenomas detected at the first follow-up colonoscopy. These data suggest that a longer wait (e.g. 5 years or more) between re-examinations is reasonable for those with no adenomas at follow-up colonoscopy (Zauber et al, 1996).

A surveillance protocol based primarily on the findings of the National Polyp Study is given in Table 28.11. These recommendations recognize that some people are at lower risk than others for subsequent adenomas and that a follow-up interval longer than that tested in the National Polyp Study may be acceptable. However, the finding that polypectomy intervention can achieve a significant reduction in colorectal cancer incidence suggests that those at higher risk should be followed with colonoscopy. Those identified at higher risk include patients with multiple adenomas, large size of adenomas, age of 60 years or more, and a positive family history of one or more first-degree relatives with colorectal cancer. The surveillance intervals suggested should be suspended for patients exhibiting symptoms (Zauber et al, 1996).

At the Royal London Hospital we see all our polyp patients at least once annually, apart from the old and infirm. At each visit (if they remain asymptomatic) a flexible sigmoidoscopic examination is performed as an outpatient procedure. If clear they go on to have full colonoscopy every third year. If they are symptomatic or if flexible sigmoidoscopy shows a lesion, they proceed to colonoscopy irrespective of whether they were due to have this investigation.

Although the suggested protocol in Table 28.11 seems sensible, we as yet remain unconvinced concerning the longer follow-up period. We have adopted the 3-year regime, but still await data from controlled trials with regard to the 5-year plus follow-up period advocated for those with a normal follow-up colonoscopy. We are concerned that not all colonoscopies will be complete or obtain perfect visualization of the colon. There is thus the risk of leaving behind a polyp which if untreated for such a long time could lead to the development of carcinoma.

Table 28.11 Recommendations for initial and surveillance management of patients with adenomas.*

Initial examination

1 Full colonoscopy for those with one or more adenomas detected.
All polyps detected should be removed and reviewed pathologically.

2 Finding the hyperplastic polyps only without accompanying adenomas in the rectosigmoid does not warrant full colonoscopy even though some patients with right-sided disease will be missed.

Full surveillance examination

1 Follow-up colonoscopy at 3 years for patients at baseline who had multiple adenomas or adenomas of size >0.5 cm or for those with a family history of colorectal cancer.

2 Patients with single small (<0.5 cm) tubular adenomas only and with no family history of colorectal cancer can wait until 5 years after initial colonoscopy for further follow-up.

Subsequent surveillance examinations

1 If an adenoma is detected at the first follow-up colonoscopy, then subsequent follow-up should be scheduled for 3 years.

2 If no adenomas are detected at first follow-up, then further follow-up could be extended to 5 years.

Consideration should be given to issues of co-morbidity and anxiety of the individual patient in recommending follow-up surveillance.

* Patients with sessile adenomas with a base greater than 3 cm or those with malignant polyps are excluded from these recommendations.
From Zauber et al (1996).

Operative removal

In the precolonoscopic era it was common practice to submit the patient to laparotomy if the polyp could not be reached or removed with the operating sigmoidoscope. The procedure most commonly performed if this operation was required was colotomy and polypectomy. This procedure is hardly ever used now, although in certain situations operative intervention is still needed for polyp removal. Thus, if the polyp is inaccessible to the colonoscopist, and is either causing symptoms or greater than 2 cm diameter, operation should be performed if repeated colonoscopy has failed. Similarly, if a polyp is deemed to be too large or sessile for endoscopic removal, surgical resection may be required. It is also necessary when a polyp is only partially removed and histological examination confirms that it is an invasive carcinoma. Certain patients with multiple polyps may also require surgery. The decision to operate requires appraisal of the operative risk together with the risk of leaving the polyp behind. In high-risk cases, especially when the indication for operation is inaccessibility, it is always worth repeating the colonoscopy; a lesion inaccessible on one day may be reached on another, particularly if a more experienced operator performs the procedure or general anaesthesia is used.

The type of operation needed will depend on the indication for performing it. The only indication for colotomy and polypectomy would seem to be a pedunculated polyp less than 2 cm diameter causing symptoms that cannot be removed by operative colonoscopy. All other indications require some form of resection, and in most cases this should be segmental. It has been stated that segmental resection for polyps carries an operative risk of approximately 6–7% compared with that for colotomy and polypectomy of 0.6% (Grinnell and Lane, 1958). These data were generated over 30 years ago, but with modern advances in anaesthesia and antibiotics the operative risk is now much lower; however, this is difficult to prove since with the advent of colonoscopy the number of patients having segmental colectomy is very small and no large series are available for adequate analysis.

Very occasionally colectomy and ileorectal anastomosis may be indicated for multiple polyps other than those that occur in familial adenomatous polyposis. We would perform this operation only for the patient in whom the polyps were impossible to control by colonoscopic removal, either because the polyps were so numerous or because they had frequently recurred.

Management of the patient with a malignant polyp that has been removed via the colonoscope

This problem is one of the most controversial in colorectal surgery. The central issue revolves around the number of patients who have residual disease, particularly in the lymph nodes, after colonoscopic polypectomy. The policy of many groups has been to submit all patients to laparotomy and resection if the histological examination of the polyp shows it to contain invasive carcinoma. As discussed previously, the incidence of lymph node metastases is variable. There are certainly series (Wolff and Shinya, 1975; Gillespie et al, 1979) where operation has not been widely used, and others (Colacchio et al, 1981) in which resection has been required in as many as 25% of patients. The latter data convinced many surgeons that resection is always indicated. St Mark's Hospital, on the other hand, for some time remained stalwarts of a much more conservative management regimen, and supported their policy with the following data (Morson et al, 1984). Of 60 patients with malignant polyps, 46 were treated by polypectomy alone as local excision was judged complete and the invasive carcinoma was well or moderately well-differentiated. None of these patients developed recurrence within the 5-year period of follow-up. The remaining 14 patients underwent surgical resection because of invasive malignancy at the cut end of the stalk or because of a poorly differentiated tumour, and residual tumour was found at the site of the polypectomy in two cases but regional lymph nodes were not involved in any of them. Other authors (Christie, 1984, 1988; De Cosse, 1984) also supported this conservative regimen but usually made the point that it should be applied only to histologically favourable lesions. Of particular interest in this context was the work of Cooper (1983) who attempted to classify the characteristics of malignant polyps that should be treated by surgery. He advocated that long-stalked malignant polyps may be treated by polypectomy alone, except in cases with poorly differentiated carcinoma, or in those with lymphatic invasion of carcinoma at the resection margin. Short-stalked polyps with cancer limited to the head may be treated similarly, but sessile polyps should undergo surgical resection after polypectomy. However, it is now clear from the accumulation of more data that sessile polyps can be treated in a similar manner to pedunculated polyps (Zauber et al, 1996).

The above studies and the data from others have thus helped us to formulate a policy in

Table 28.12 Malignant polyp criteria.

Favourable criteria (surgical resection not required)
Complete endoscopic resection
Carcinoma not poorly differentiated
Absence of vascular or lymphatic invasion
Resection margin free of cancer
Unfavourable criteria (consider surgical resection)
Uncertain endoscopic resection
Carcinoma poorly differentiated
Histologic evidence of vascular or lymphatic invasion
Cancer extends to resection margin

From Zauber et al (1996).

management of patients with malignant polyps (Lipper et al, 1983; Fucini et al, 1986; Nivatvongs et al, 1991; Cooper et al, 1995) that is in broad agreement with other authors (Zauber et al, 1996). Thus, various favourable and unfavourable criteria have been identified, which are summarized in Table 28.12.

Cranley et al (1986), in a review of nine series, showed that the incidence of residual or lymph node associated cancer in cases with favourable criteria was 0.3% and 1.5% for pedunculated and sessile polyps respectively. In contrast, Coverlizza et al (1988) found that patients with malignant polyps with unfavourable criteria had an incidence of lymph node metastases of 8.5% and 14.4% for pedunculated and sessile polyps. The mortality rate from elective colonic resection averages 1–2%, and varies from 0.2% in young healthy patients to more than 5% in elderly patients with significant co-morbidity (Greenburg et al, 1981; Richards et al, 1987). Therefore, we believe that a patient with a malignant polyp and favourable criteria should not usually be referred for surgical resection because the risk of surgery exceeds that of residual cancer. Most good-risk patients with unfavourable criteria should be referred for abdominal surgery unless the polyp is located in the low rectum where local excision might be an acceptable option. Whereas in the main this policy is in agreement with other authors, we should point out that we do not use the degree of histological differentiation as a prognostic indicator; like Langer et al (1984), we have found histological interpretation to be unreliable owing to heterogeneity of the tumour and to interobserver variation between pathologists.

The above advice must be tempered by the realization that the surgical cure rate for cancers with lymph node involvement is significantly less than 100%. Since the risk of lymph node spread is low, even if unfavourable criteria are present, patients at high risk for surgery should probably not have further surgical treatment. Conversely, since there is always a slight risk of lymph node metastases, even when prognostic criteria are favourable, a more radical approach may be justified for a few very young and otherwise healthy patients.

Patients with evidence of residual carcinoma after polypectomy or with sessile malignant polyps that cannot be removed colonoscopically and who are also unfit for surgical resection may be treated by laser therapy. Some groups have used the neodymium–yttrium aluminium garnet (Nd-YAG) laser for this purpose (Mathus-Vliegen and Tytgat, 1986), but at the Royal London Hospital we have used photodynamic therapy. This technique requires the patient to receive haematoporphyrin derivative 48 hours before treatment. The haematoporphyrin derivative subsequently localizes selectively in the neoplastic tissue. The drug, being photosensitive, is activated by red light generated from a dye laser and produces singlet oxygen which is cytotoxic. We have developed a light-delivery system which can be passed through a colonoscope and is able to deliver light at the optimum dosage to the appropriate site (Allardice et al, 1989). As yet we have limited experience in this method of treating colonic polyps, but the patients treated so far have at least had no serious side-effects. Since the haematoporphyrin derivative localizes in the neoplastic tissue, the technique has the theoretical advantage of being more selective and hence safer than conventional laser therapy. It is interesting to note in a series from the Netherlands that 10% of patients with large sessile polyps or with residual malignancy after polypectomy treated by Nd–YAG photocoagulation suffered a major complication (bleeding, perforation or stenosis) (Mathus-Vliegen and Tytgat, 1986).

Follow-up

If a malignant polyp has favourable criteria and no further surgical treatment has been undertaken, a follow-up colonoscopy in 3–6 months to ensure complete resection is recommended if the polyp was either large or sessile, or if it contained a short stalk (Zauber et al, 1996). Any residual irregularity at the polypectomy site should be biopsied. Thereafter, it is recommended that follow-up colonoscopy should be performed at 3 years and if negative every 5 years thereafter (Bond et al, 1993), although we would still favour 3-yearly review.

TREATMENT OF VILLOUS ADENOMA OF THE RECTUM

Villous adenomas of the rectum are often too large and extensive to be removed using the sigmoidoscope or colonoscope and require some form of operative excision. Furthermore, up to a quarter of lesions will be malignant. Malignant change is often missed even when biopsies are reported by an experienced pathologist, because of the problems of sampling error (Taylor et al, 1981). The best form of biopsy is therefore complete removal of the lesion. This can often be accomplished by either the transanal or the trans-sphincteric route. For very extensive or high lesions that cannot be dealt with in this way, some form of anterior resection or coloanal excision will need to be performed.

Apart from the usual preoperative preparation, adequate attention must be paid to the correction of any fluid and electrolyte imbalance. Very occasionally patients will present with the full-blown syndrome of dehydration, hypovolaemia and shock due to profuse mucous diarrhoea. Most of these patients will have extensive carpet lesions occupying most of the rectum. In these circumstances, resuscitation will be necessary before proceeding to surgery. All patients must also undergo full colonoscopy, preferably preoperatively, since the lesions are often accompanied by neoplasms elsewhere within the colon. Thomson et al (1977) found one or more additional tumours in 30 of 121 patients (25%) with sessile villous adenomas of the rectum. Jahadi and Baldwin (1975) found that 32 of their 264 patients (12%) had an associated lesion, and a similar incidence was noted by Adair and Everett (1983) and by Christiansen et al (1979).

Transanal excision including transanal endoscopic microsurgery (TEM)

Many villous adenomas of the lower rectum can be removed intact via the transanal route using the conventional excisional technique, and indeed this is the best method of biopsy. Even if the tumour extends more proximally or is situated higher up, it is sometimes possible to deliver the tumour into the field of operation by intussusception of the proximal bowel (Parks, 1966). The introduction of transanal endoscopic microsurgery (TEM) by Buess et al (1984) has widened the scope of the transanal technique. Using this technique, it is possible to excise much larger and extensive tumours than can be dealt with by the conventional approach.

Conventional technique

The operation may be performed equally easily with the patient in the lithotomy position or the jack-knife position, although the latter may give better exposure to anterior tumours. The anal sphincter is gently dilated to allow the insertion of a suitable anal retractor. We prefer to use the one designed by Parks which is self-retaining and has a third blade which can sometimes further aid exposure. After insertion the lesion is assessed with regard to its extent and position on the rectal wall. The retractor is then adjusted to give maximum exposure. Although the third blade is sometimes useful, it is not always; a right-angled narrow Lane's retractor or a Kocher's retractor is sometimes superior. Since these tumours are friable the view during the procedure is often obscured and therefore good exposure from the outset is essential. With this in mind it is also important to have a second assistant who can remove the smoke and blood throughout the procedure with an efficient sucker. Once the retractor is in place it is useful to pack the lumen of the rectum above the lesion. This has the advantage of preventing any residual faeces intruding into the operating field and it also helps to delineate the upper aspect of the tumour.

The submucosal plane beneath the tumour and around its margins is infiltrated with 10–20 mL of saline and adrenaline 1 in 300 000, depending on size (Figure 28.22). The solution rapidly spreads and the adenoma is lifted off the underlying muscle. To aid repair at the end of the excision, we place stay sutures approximately 1–2 cm away from the edge of the proposed excision margin (Figure 28.23). The needles are left on these sutures so that they can be used to repair the defect after the tumour has been excised. An incision through the rectal mucosa about 1 cm from the edge of the tumour is then made with scissors. Connective tissue within the oedematous submucosa is divided just deep to the mucosa and tumour (Figure 28.24a). The submucosa frequently contains small blood vessels, some of which are easily seen but some are not; it is therefore good practice to electrocoagulate most strands of tissue before division, since even a small amount of blood may obscure the correct plane of dissection (Figures 28.24a,b). Haemostasis should be painstaking throughout the dissection and great care should be exercised in attempting to remove the tumour in one piece. With large lesions it is necessary to remove the retractor and reposition it several times

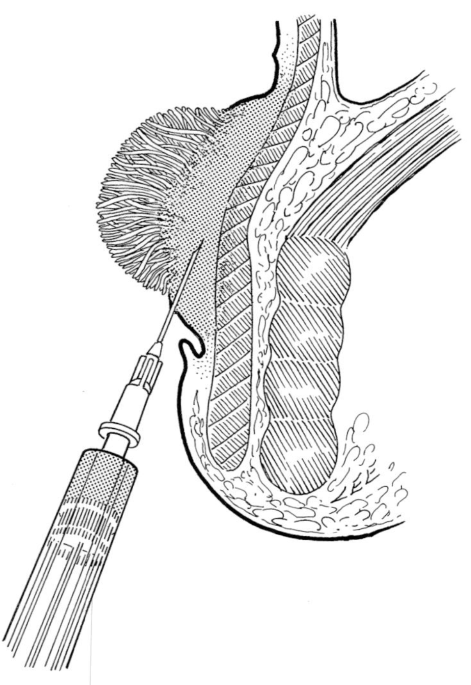

Figure 28.22 Excision of villous adenoma via the transanal route. The submucosal plane beneath and around the margin of the tumour is infiltrated with 1 in 300 000 adrenaline–saline solution.

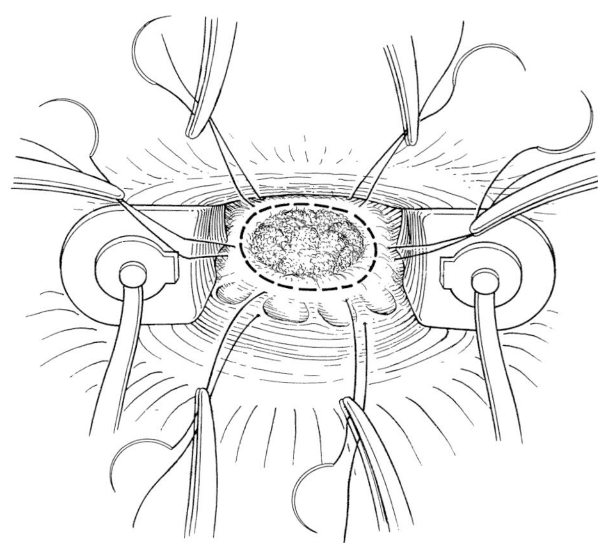

Figure 28.23 Excision of villous adenoma. This shows all the stay sutures in place, the dotted line representing the line of incision through the mucosa.

in order to achieve the best exposure (see below). It may be necessary to inject further amounts of saline and adrenaline which tend to diffuse out from the submucosal plane once the mucosa has been incised.

After removal (Figure 28.24c) the defect is inspected and palpated to determine if there is any evidence of malignant infiltration. Any further haemostasis is also secured. Although it is reasonable to leave small defects to granulate, we prefer to suture the cut mucosa in all but the smallest defects as this secures haemostasis and convalescence seems to be smoother. Closure can easily be accomplished by exerting traction on the stay sutures so that the edges of the defect can be defined. Since the needles have been left on these sutures it is a simple matter to close the defect (Figure 28.24d). With large, circumferential defects in particular (see below) mucosal cover is essential, otherwise fibrosis and stenosis are likely to occur.

After excision and repair of the defect the pack in the upper rectum is removed and replaced by another which fills out the rectum and exerts some compression on its walls, the aim being to prevent haematoma formation.

Conventional transanal excision of extensive circumferential lesions

The technique of removal is almost identical to that described above, with the obvious difference that the whole tumour cannot be exposed at any one time. It is therefore necessary to withdraw the retractor and reinsert it at a different angle in order to excise tumour from the area of rectum not originally seen. Although it is desirable to remove the tumour whole, this is not always possible with an extensive lesion and it may need to be removed in segments. If the upper end of the lesion can be seen transanally during assessment, it should be possible to close the resulting defect by plication of the raw area using intramural sutures (Parks and Stuart, 1973). Commencing at the lower edge of the wound, taking multiple bites of the circular muscles of the rectum until the upper edge is reached (Figure 28.25a), we use 2/0 polyglycolic acid sutures (Dexon) on a small round-bodied needle for this procedure but 2/0 chromic catgut is just as suitable. About ten such sutures are placed around the rectum and when tied they produce a concertina-like effect, drawing the mucosal edges together. The

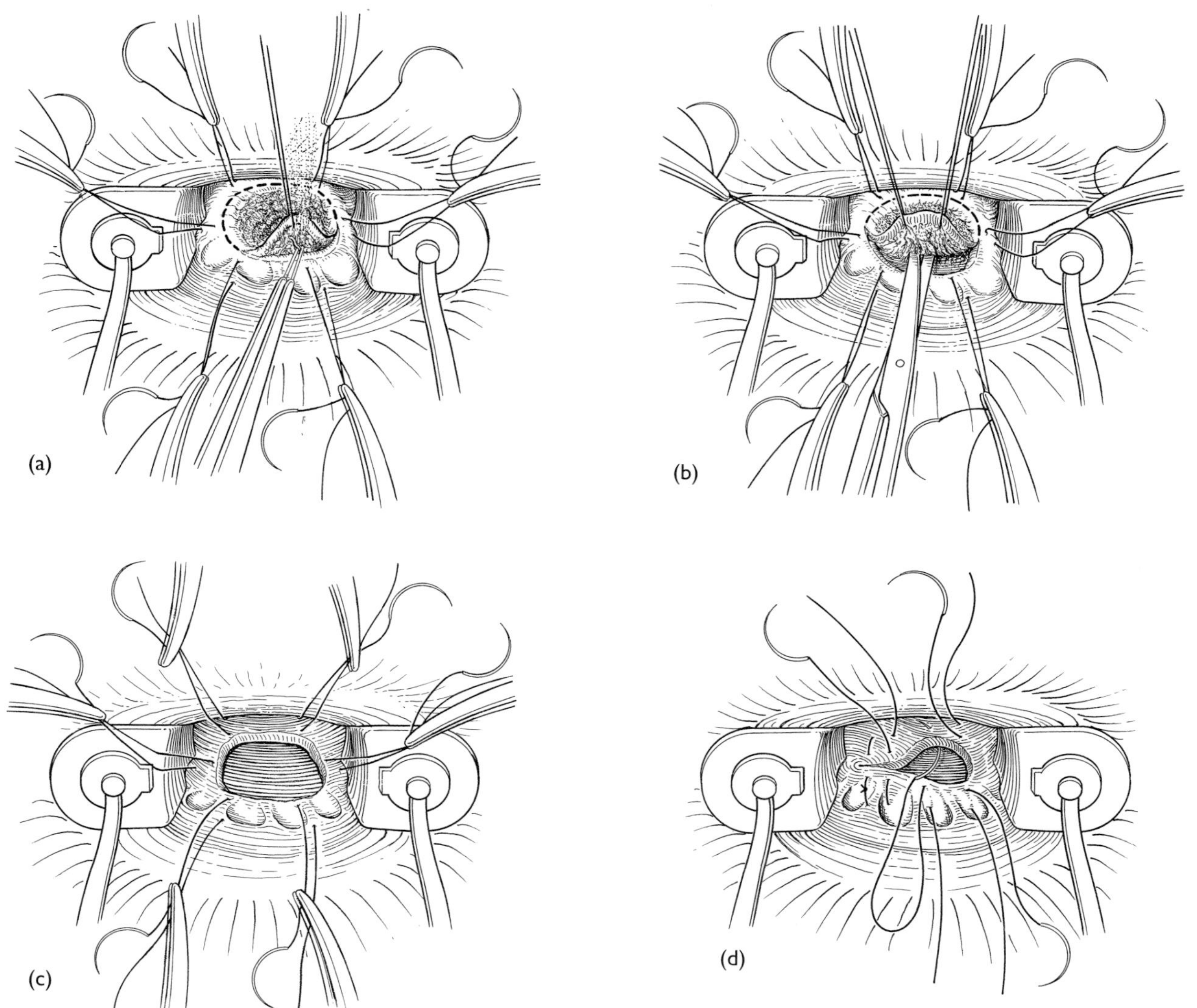

Figure 28.24a–d Transanal excision of villous adenoma. (a) The mucosa has been incised and the submucosal blood vessels are electrocoagulated before division. (b) The lesion is gradually excised using sharp dissection in the submucosal plane. (c) The lesion has been removed entirely, revealing the underlying muscle. (d) The defect in the mucosa–submucosa surface is repaired using the stay sutures.

mucosal edges may then be sutured together provided there is no tension (Figure 28.25b). If this cannot be achieved – a situation that in our experience is very rare – the edges are approximated as much as possible by suturing the mobilized mucosa to the denuded rectal wall, thus leaving a much narrower raw area to granulate.

Parks (1983) suggested that this technique was suitable for circumferential wounds up to 10–12 cm in length. This is not always possible and the feasibility of closing the defect varies with the site of the defect and the build of the patient. If on initial assessment it is considered that the lesion extends proximally too far for repair to be achieved by intra-anal excision alone, rectal excision should be performed using the transanal coloanal pull-through technique, with or without a colonic pouch for reconstruction.

Transanal endoscopic microsurgery (TEM)

TEM was the first endoscopic procedure to be developed for operations in the gastrointestinal tract (Buess, 1996). This development started in 1980, and the first clinical application was in 1983 (Buess et al, 1984, Buess, 1994). The reasons for the approach were the inaccessibility and invasiveness of the posterior approaches, and the limited view

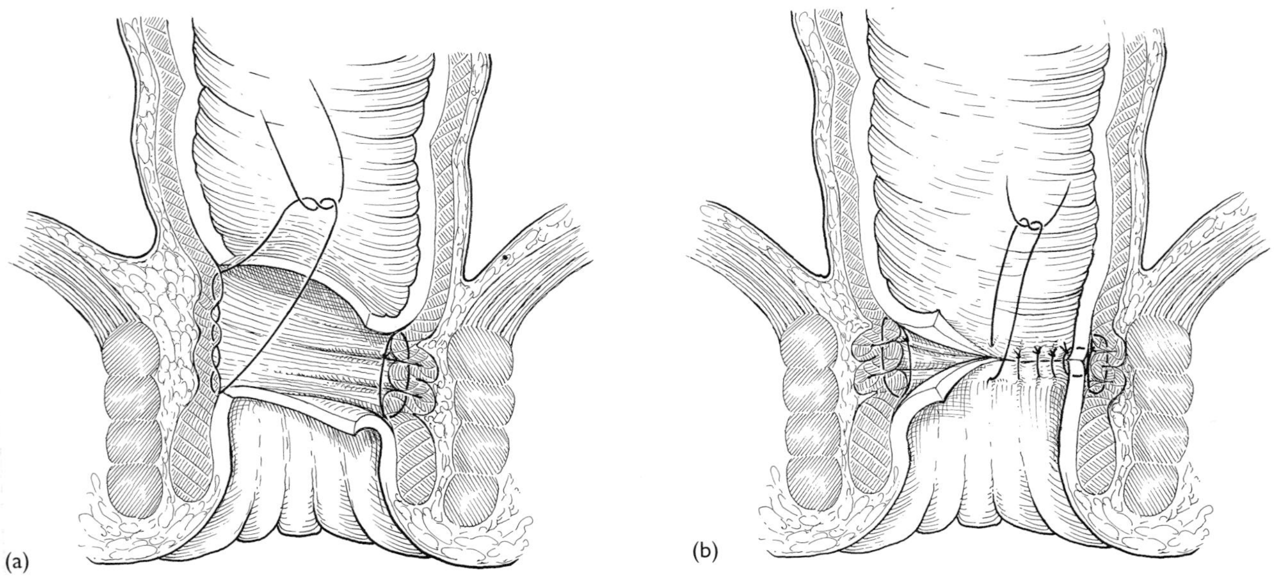

Figure 28.25a,b Closure of the defect after transanal excision of circumferential villous adenoma. (a) The underlying muscle is plicated. (b) Closure of the mucosal defect after plication of the underlying muscle.

given by the conventional transanal approach, resulting in a high recurrence rate of adenomas.

The technique, which is rather complex and costly and needs substantial training, is described in detail in Chapter 32. Briefly, it involves inflating the rectum via a rigid rectoscope of 40 mm diameter. Under constant CO_2 insufflation, the endoscopic view is stable. Via a stereoscopic technique with the operative field magnified, the operator manipulates purpose-designed instruments through the channels of the rectoscope (see Figure 32.90). The tumour is excised by high-frequency diathermy, and the defect in the wall closed by endoscopically controlled continuous suturing. There is, as might be expected, a steep and lengthy learning curve. However, once mastered, we believe that this technique provides substantial benefits for patients with villous adenomas of the rectum which cannot be removed by the conventional transanal technique. Nevertheless, because of the few cases in any institution who are likely to require the technique, it is perhaps prudent to have only a few centres in any one country which specialize in the procedure.

Rectal excision and transanal coloanal pull-through technique for circumferential lesions

The patient should be placed in the modified lithotomy–Trendelenburg position and prepared for laparotomy and anterior resection. The lower part of the tumour is then dissected transanally as far as possible from below upwards in the manner described above. Approximately 6–7 cm of circular muscle is thus denuded. The abdomen is then opened and the rectum is fully mobilized as in anterior resection. The freed distal part of the lesion is then retracted proximally within the rectal lumen by the perineal operator using a gauze pledget to prevent its subsequent transection (Figure 28.26a), and a right-angled or aortic clamp placed across the rectum at a point distal to that reached by the intra-anal submucosal excision. The rectum and sigmoid are then removed leaving a rectal stump which is denuded of mucosa (Figure 28.26b).

Sometimes in more proximal lesions it is easier to resect the tumour entirely from above, removing anal mucosa in continuity with the rectum as in restorative proctocolectomy. The remaining descending and transverse colon is then fully mobilized, taking down the splenic flexure so that its distal end can reach the pelvis. Stay sutures are placed at the corners of the cut descending colon. It is a good plan to transect the descending colon with a stapling instrument to avoid contamination. The perineal operator then passes two long artery forceps through the denuded muscular cuff of the rectum and the surgeon ensures that the correct stay suture is grasped so that rotation of the colon is prevented as it is pulled through the rectal stump (Figure 28.26c). It is a good plan to use stay sutures

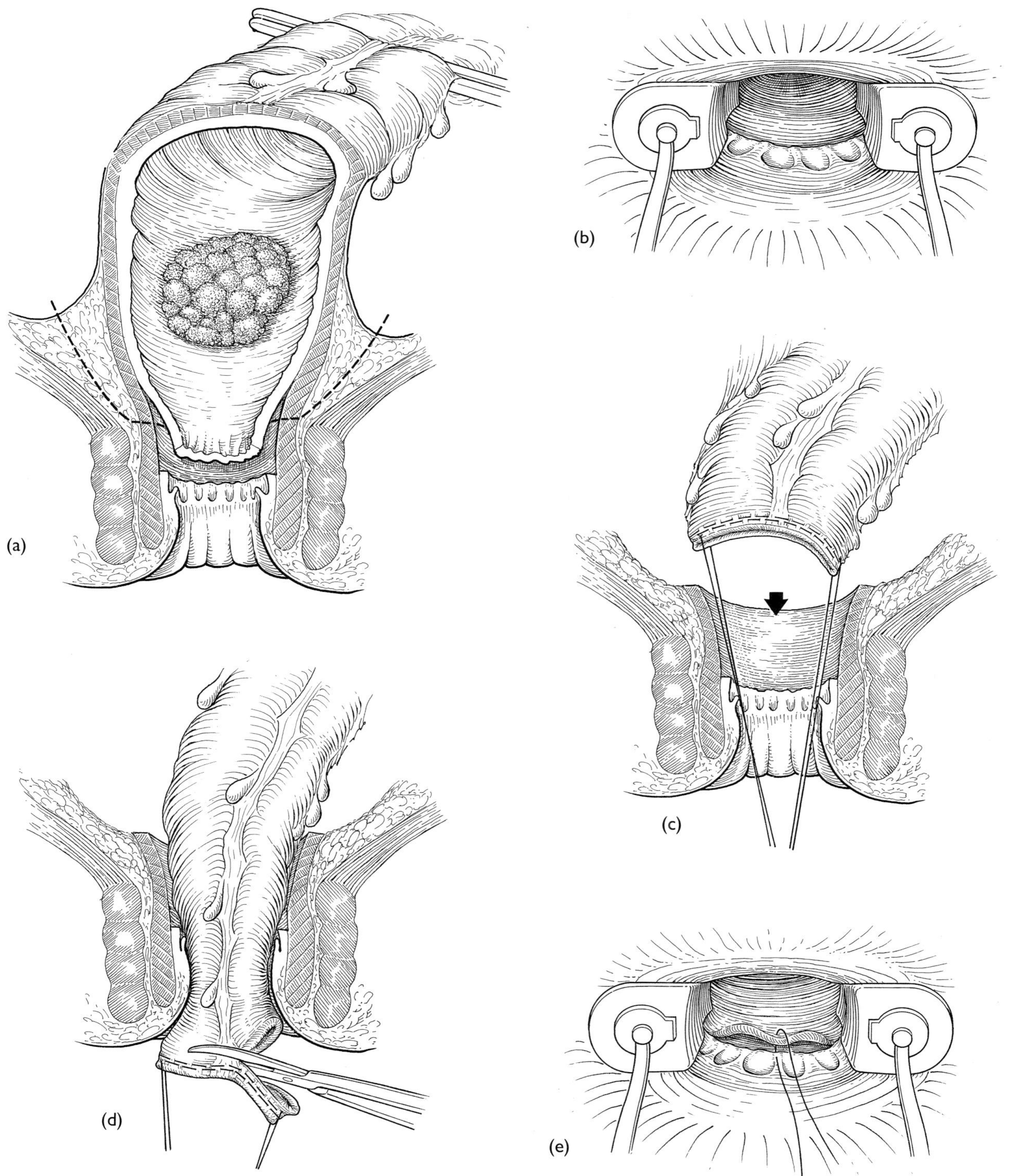

Figure 28.26a–g Transanal coloanal pull-through technique for excision of villous adenoma. (a) The rectal mucosa has been dissected circumferentially via the transanal route. The dotted line represents the line of transection of the rectal muscular cuff and surrounding tissue. (b) View via transanal route of the denuded rectal muscular cuff after the circumferential excision of the rectal mucosa and submucosa. (c) The stapled end of the descending colon is brought down through the denuded muscular cuff via the stay sutures and the correct alignment is ensured. (d) The stapled end of the distal colon is excised. If it is likely that the stay sutures will be sacrificed, two more are positioned more proximally to avoid retraction. (e) Interrupted 2/0 Vicryl or Dexon sutures are placed between the edge of the pulled-through colon and anal mucosa taking a deep bite of the underlying internal sphincter. This is continued circumferentially. (*Continued*)

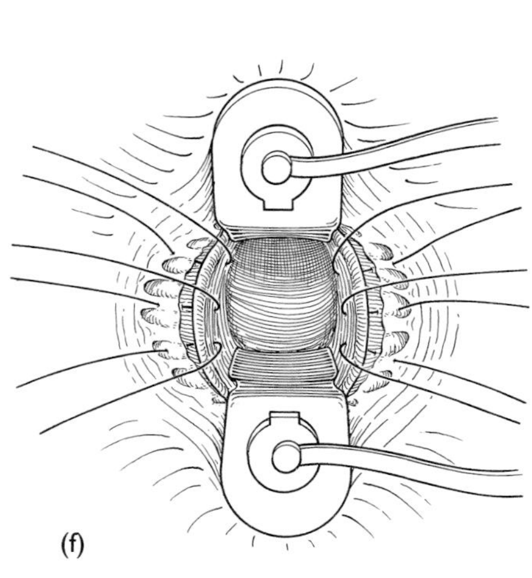

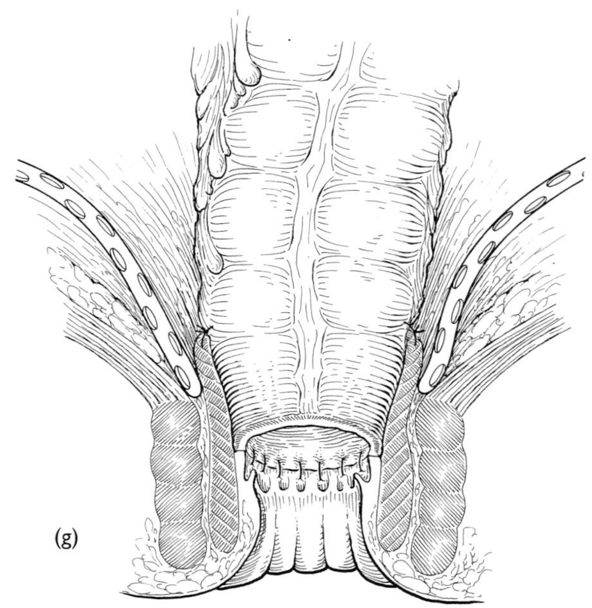

Figure 28.26a–g (*Continued*) (f) until the anastomosis is complete. (g) Transanal coloanal pull-through technique. The anastomosis is complete: note the tacking sutures between the pulled-through colon and the upper edge of rectal muscular cuff. Two suction drains are left down to the pelvis.

of different colours to identify the right and left sides. The perineal operator pulls the colon down to the level of the cut anal mucosa, and checks that there is no excessive tension on the pulled-through colon. If tension is apparent, further mobilization of the colon without damage to the marginal artery within the abdomen is essential. Once the colon comfortably resides within the rectal muscular cuff, the coloanal anastomosis is performed via the transanal route. The stapled end of the pulled-through colon is excised (Figure 28.26d) and stay sutures are replaced at a higher level if necessary to assist traction. The anal retractor is reinserted if possible through the anal sphincter into the colon. This permits direct exposure of the divided end of the colon above and the proximal limits of the anorectal mucosa below. Interrupted 2/0 or 3/0 Dexon or polygalactin (Vicryl) sutures are placed through the edge of the anal mucosa, then deeply through the internal sphincter, and finally through the full thickness of the colon (Figure 28.26e,f). It is best initially to place a suture in each of the four quadrants and then complete the anastomosis by further sutures between them: 12–20 sutures are usually required (Figure 28.26g). After the anastomosis is complete, a few loosely tied tacking sutures are inserted via the abdomen between the upper margin of the rectal muscular cuff and the serosa of the pulled-through colon. Suction drains are inserted between the pulled-through colon and rectal muscle on each side (Figure 28.26g). Sometimes it is possible to perform a low stapled coloanal anastomosis or even a colonic pouch anal anastomosis (see Chapter 32).

A covering stoma is then constructed to defunction the anastomosis. Although it is often possible to perform a covering loop transverse colostomy we prefer a loop ileostomy. There is a slight risk that during construction or subsequent closure of a transverse colostomy the blood supply to the distal colon may be damaged. Since there is always some concern that the pulled-through colon might not have an adequate blood supply, it seems wise to use a proximal ileostomy. Furthermore, our patients find a loop ileostomy significantly easier to manage than a transverse colostomy (Williams et al, 1984).

Trans-sphincteric technique of York Mason

The trans-sphincteric technique was originally described by Bevan (1917) and revived by York Mason (Mason, 1970). The principles are that the anal sphincters and rectal wall are divided in the longitudinal axis of the rectum and its interior is laid open like a book. If the cut layers are accurately sutured together at the end of the procedure, sphincter function is said to be retained when the reconstruction has healed.

Conventionally the approach has been regarded as an alternative technique to transanal excision. In our opinion, however, it is less suitable than transanal resection for excision of circumferential villous adenomas or those that are situated on the posterior wall of the rectum, since these tumours may be transected with the risk of recurrence and sphincter function may be compromised. However, trans-sphincteric excision may be more applicable for anterior or anterolateral lesions 8–12 cm from the anal verge, since these are often too high for endoanal excision and resection can be performed using this approach under direct vision. The trans-sphincteric approach may also be an advantage over conventional transanal excision because the risks of perforation are less for anterior lesions, and the upper limit of certain tumours can be reached more easily than with the transanal approach. We tend to avoid the technique if possible since the functional results are superior and the morbidity is lower using the transanal route. Nevertheless, up to recently we still used the technique in selected cases when it was impossible to remove the lesion by the transanal route. However, since experience has been gained with transanal endoscopic microsurgery (TEM), the transphincteric approach is becoming increasingly obsolete in our institutions. Nevertheless, we describe it here for the sake of completeness and because from time to time it may have a place.

Operative details

The patient is positioned in the jack-knife position with arms extended and hands crossed above the head (Figure 28.27). It is essential that the chest and pelvis are raised and supported to allow the abdominal wall to move freely during respiration. If the patient is obese it is possible to perform the procedure in the lateral position.

The buttocks are strapped apart with adhesive strapping (Figure 28.28a). The anal verge is marked in the midline posteriorly by a pair of stay sutures. The incision is made commencing just to the left of the sacrococcygeal region and passes downwards to end between the two stay sutures at the anal verge (Figure 28.28a). It is useful to infiltrate the subcutaneous tissue and underlying layers with adrenaline and saline solution (1 in 300 000) prior to making the incision. As the incision is deepened the lower fibres of the gluteus maximus come into view in the upper

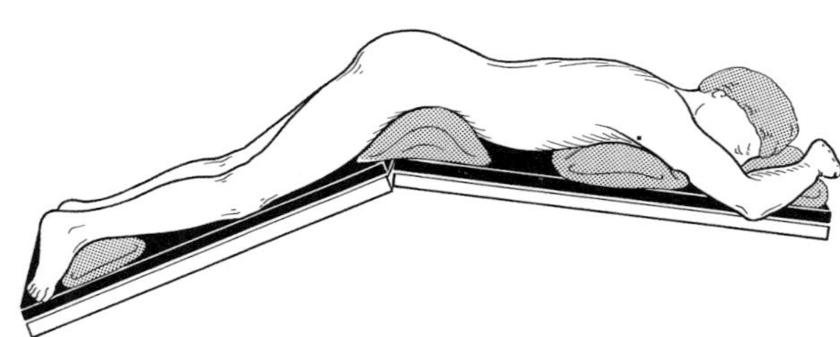

Figure 28.27 Jack-knife position for trans-sphincteric excision of villous adenoma.

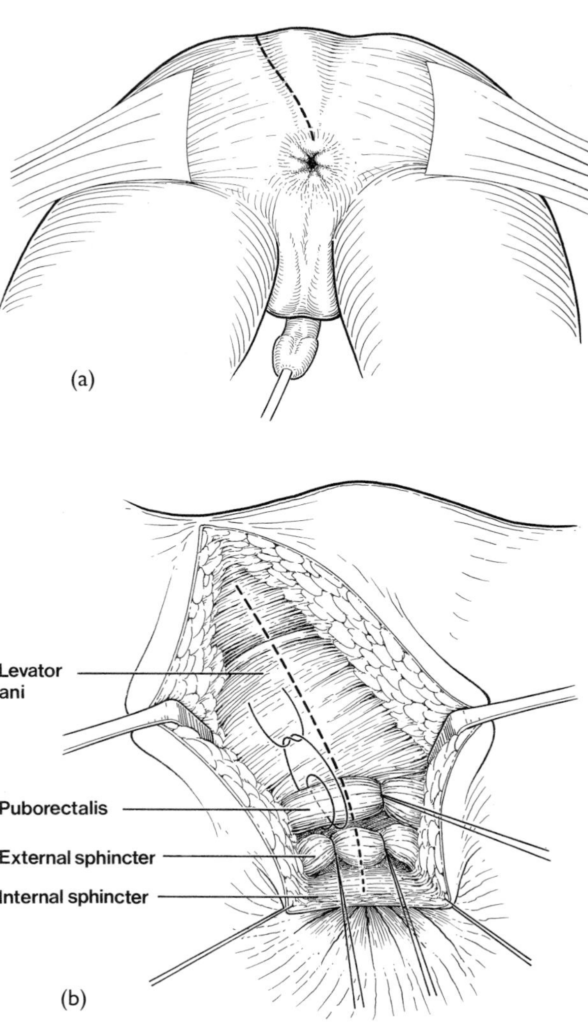

Figure 28.28a,b Trans-sphincteric excision of villous adenoma. (a) The buttocks are strapped apart and the incision lies towards the left of the sacrococcygeal region. (b) The underlying muscles are identified and are ligated and divided in the line of the incision.

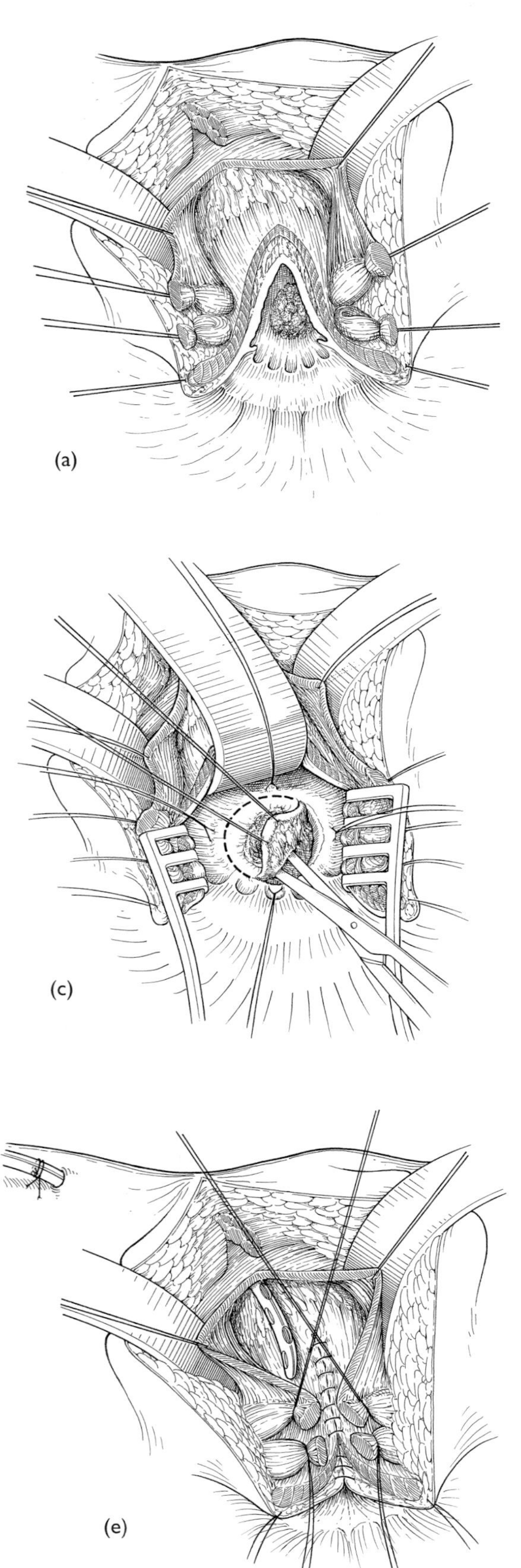

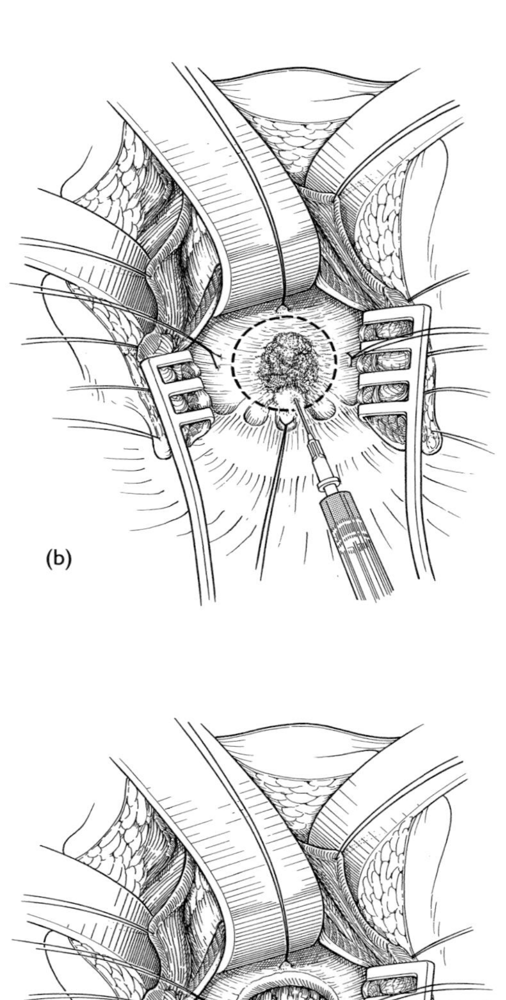

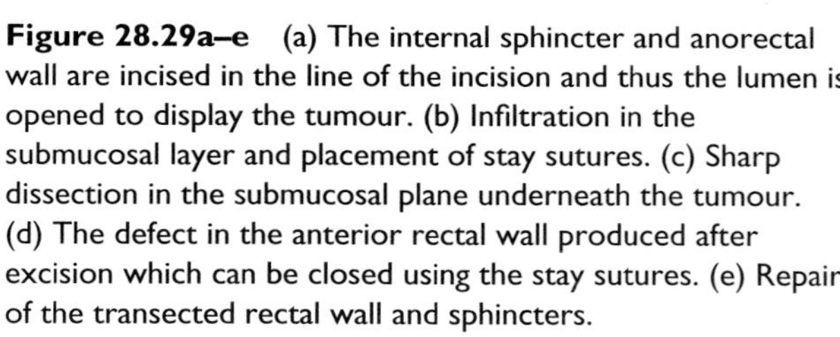

Figure 28.29a–e (a) The internal sphincter and anorectal wall are incised in the line of the incision and thus the lumen is opened to display the tumour. (b) Infiltration in the submucosal layer and placement of stay sutures. (c) Sharp dissection in the submucosal plane underneath the tumour. (d) The defect in the anterior rectal wall produced after excision which can be closed using the stay sutures. (e) Repair of the transected rectal wall and sphincters.

part of the wound and at the lower end the superficial fibres of the external anal sphincter are seen. Between these two landmarks the incision is extended through the ischiorectal fat until the levator ani is visualized (Figure 28.28b). The underlying muscles are then divided in the line of the incision. Prior to division of each muscle, paired identifying sutures are inserted and the incision proceeds between them. This is an essential step since it accurately identifies each muscle layer and allows correct apposition at the end of the procedure. We use differently coloured sutures for each muscle that is divided, since this aids identification during reconstruction of the anatomy. The external sphincter is usually divided between two pairs of sutures; although some think of this muscle as being made up of different anatomical components, these cannot be visualized individually at operation and the muscle should be regarded as one structure. With the patient in the prone jack-knife position the internal sphincter lies distal to the lower end of the external sphincter and can be recognized by its pale colour.

The puborectalis sling is not usually clearly demarcated from the levator ani which is recognizable as a thin sheet of muscle often with fat interspersed between its obliquely arranged fibres. The fibres of the puborectalis are arranged transversely and are more robust. For this reason it is essential that the stay sutures marking the puborectalis are securely tied to avoid them being lost by retraction after division. The anorectal musculature is divided from above down: first the levator ani and puborectalis, then the external anal sphincter, and finally the longitudinal muscle coat of the rectum with the internal sphincter. It is a fruitless exercise to try to dissect between the internal sphincter and the anorectal mucosa; hence the wall of the rectum and anal canal are then finally opened in the line of the skin incision (Figure 28.29a). The anorectal lumen is entered and with suitable retraction the lesion is visualized. The submucosal plane beneath the tumour and its surrounding normal mucosa is infiltrated with adrenaline and saline solution. Stay sutures are then placed circumferentially around the lesion approximately 2 cm away from its edge in normal mucosa (Figure 28.29b). The incision is commenced at least 1 cm from the edge of the tumour and can be made using cutting diathermy. The submucosal plane is entered and vessels transversing it are coagulated prior to their division.

The tumour is excised using scissor dissection (Figure 28.29c,d). The mucosal defect can often be closed primarily using interrupted 2/0 Dexon or Vicryl sutures. If this is not possible the underlying muscle can be plicated and the mucosal gap considerably reduced as previously described for transanal excision. After repair of the defect, the wall of the rectum and internal sphincter is closed with a continuous suture of 2/0 catgut. The external sphincter is then repaired; and finally the puborectalis and levator ani muscles are reconstructed at each stage, making sure that there is correct apposition of each transected layer (Figure 28.29e).

Other trans-sphincteric techniques

For posterior and circumferential lesions, a modified technique has been described that avoids transection of tumour tissue (Jackson and Mason, 1984). In this technique access is gained to the submucosal plane by longitudinal incision through the muscle of the rectal wall; the lumen is not opened. The edges of the divided rectal muscle are held apart to afford clear vision as submucosal dissection proceeds forwards and on either side (Figure 28.30a). Blood vessels transversing the submucosal space are electrocoagulated before division. In the case of a circumferential lesion the dissection continues on both sides until it is complete and a closed mucosal tube containing the tumour is obtained (Figure 28.30b). Any sign of a breach of the muscularis mucosae by tumour suggests that the lesion is malignant, and if this is confirmed on frozen section examination the operation should be abandoned in favour of a more radical procedure.

Once the mucosal tube is free it can be resected – but there is one snag: these tumours are soft and their proximal and distal extent are difficult to determine by palpation from without. It is thus necessary to open the mucosa to ensure that the lines of proposed transection are above and below the limits of tumour extension. After excision of the mucosal tube containing the tumour, the mucosal defect can be completely or partially closed as described for transanal excision.

This technique for a circumferential growth has the potential disadvantage of transecting tumour. Since there is an extensive wound posteriorly there is a theoretical risk of seeding malignant cells. If tumour is inadvertently transected it would seem prudent to irrigate the wound with a cancericidal agent such as 1% cetrimide. Because of this risk and the technical difficulties of the trans-sphincteric exposure, we prefer the transanal route. However, if the transanal route is not possible with either conventional excision or TEM, the trans-sphincteric approach as described may be preferable if the only alternative is sacrifice of the anal sphincter,

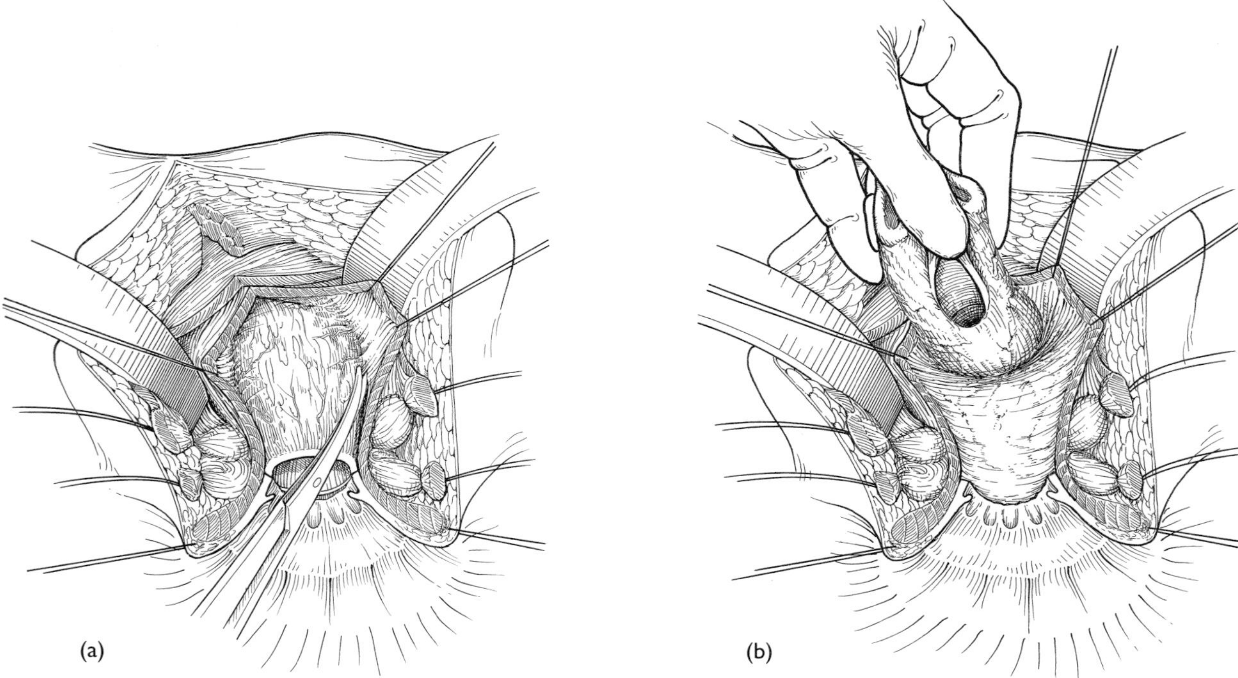

Figure 28.30a,b (a) Modified trans-sphincteric technique for excision of posterior or circumferential lesions. The sphincter muscles have been divided but the rectum has not been entered. The anorectal tube is dissected from its overlying muscles by sharp dissection. (b) For circumferential lesions a mucosal tube containing the tumour is obtained.

although in such patients it is usually possible to perform an abdominotransanal procedure.

Postoperative management

Whichever technique is used, the resected specimen should be carefully pinned out and correctly oriented before fixation so that detailed histological examination can be performed more easily. If a circumferential mucosal defect has been left, it is recommended that regular dilatation should be performed until the exposed muscle has completely epithelialized. The surgeon should perform the dilatation initially and the patient may take over after several weeks if this is possible or necessary. A St Mark's dilator may be used for low lesions, whereas a Hegar's dilator is usually required for those situated more proximally. Inadequate dilatation may result in stricture formation. It is not necessary to await complete epithelialization of the rectum before the covering stoma is closed (Jackson and Mason, 1984). With mucosal reconstruction after excision, these procedures are rarely, if ever, necessary.

Other techniques for removal of villous adenomas of the rectum

Occasionally a small, low-lying lesion can be prolapsed through the anal sphincter and dealt with in a similar manner to that previously described for tubular adenomas, i.e. by transfixion and ligation of an artificial pedicle and transection. Larger lesions can be treated by contact diathermy fulguration. Using a button electrode via the transanal route enables extensive lesions to be treated. This method, however, has certain disadvantages. It is extremely unlikely to destroy the tumour completely. Since the whole tumour is not removed, it is not possible to be certain if it is malignant. Furthermore, several sessions are usually required to gain control. As a primary treatment we have found it in the main unacceptable except for elderly, frail patients whose tumours cannot be removed by transanal excision and who are unable to tolerate a more major resection. It may be useful for the treatment of recurrence following previous excisional surgery provided malignancy has been excluded.

A more refined technique of diathermy is available, which utilizes the principles of closed cysto-diathermy used in transurethral resection of bladder tumours (Ottery et al, 1986; Kelly, 1989; Berry et al, 1990; Kettlewell, 1991; Wetherall et al, 1993). A larger version of the transurethral resectoscope is used; the rectum is first distended with irrigating fluid, then under direct vision the tumour is resected down to muscle with the diathermy loop. Wetherall et al (1993) from Leicester achieved successful clearance in 22 of 23 patients using this technique. The method seems safe and patients' stay in hospital is short. This technique is still in its infancy, but having used it in a few selected cases we believe it to be superior to the technique of button diathermy in poor-risk patients. However, we would not regard it as an alternative to transanal excision and there is a real risk of seeding malignant cells on to the denuded rectum; consequently it is only advised as palliation in high-risk patients.

An alternative technique for treating a large villous adenoma in a patient who is unfit for major resection is photocoagulation using a laser. Brunetaud et al (1989) treated 56 villous adenomas of the rectum using the Nd–YAG laser, and no serious complications occurred apart from late haemorrhage and minor stenosis. Treatment was generally successful, but a mean of six sessions were required for each patient, and one unfortunate individual required 26 laser sessions. Similarly, Hyser and Gau (1996) treated 34 villous adenomas of the colon and rectum; 23 tumours were benign and 11 contained carcinoma-in-situ. The mean age was 70 years and an average of 3.3 treatments were performed for each patient. Five patients (15%) suffered complications of mild stricture (2), self-limited bleeding (2) and small colovaginal fistula (1). Only one tumour which originally contained carcinoma-in-situ recurred during an average of 32 months follow-up. However, Mathus-Vliegen and Tytgat (1991) treated 241 patients with colorectal adenomas using the Nd–Yag laser. Recurrence was common, particularly in large lesions, so the authors concluded that laser therapy for extensive adenomas seemed appropriate only for symptomatic relief (Banerjee et al, 1995).

Photodynamic therapy has been used for villous adenomas (Loh et al, 1994). In 7 of 8 patients treated, the adenomas were eradicated after a median of 12 months. These lesions were in the main in patients

(a)

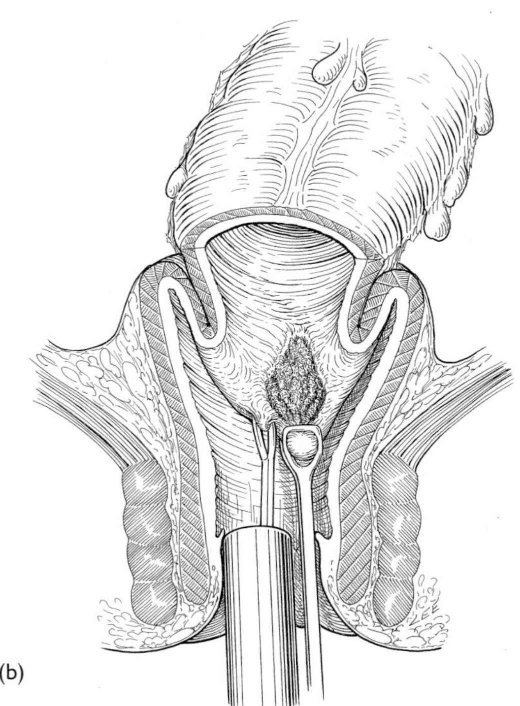

Figure 28.31a,b Removal of high, small rectal villous adenoma by intussusception of the upper rectum using the rigid sigmoidoscope.

who had previously been incompletely treated by Nd–Yag laser. Despite these excellent results with both types of laser therapy, most experts believe such therapy and diathermy can be regarded only as palliative, designed to alleviate symptoms. A significant disadvantage of laser resection and diathermy excision is the problem of pathological interpretation, since the specimen is delivered in separate fragments and accurate orientation is impossible.

Tumours in the upper rectum beyond the reach of the palpating finger usually need to be treated by anterior resection, which should be as radical as if dealing with a carcinoma, since until the lesion has been excised its true nature remains unknown. Occasionally a lesion at this level can be intussuscepted into the lower rectum using the operating sigmoidoscope (Parks, 1983) and removed transanally as previously described. The sigmoidoscope is passed through the parted blades of the anal retractor and advanced to the level of the lesion (Figure 28.31a). The tumour or neighbouring mucosa is grasped by long crocodile forceps, and the sigmoidoscope and forceps are gently withdrawn together causing intussusception of the bowel (Figure 28.31b). The sigmoidoscope is removed over the shaft of the forceps enabling tissue forceps or stay sutures to be applied to the edge of the tumour, which is now situated in the lower rectum or anal canal. Resection then continues as previously described. It should be noted that few tumours are suitable for this manoeuvre and there is a risk of perforation.

Complications

Transanal excision

Conventional transanal excision (Parks' technique) tends to be a relatively safe operation with an operative mortality ranging between nil and 5% (Parks and Stuart, 1973; Welch and Welch, 1976; Thomson et al, 1977; Chiu and Spencer, 1978; Adair and Everett, 1983, Heimann et al, 1992; Whitlow et al, 1996). Both reactionary and secondary haemorrhage may occur in approximately 5% of cases (Adair and Everett, 1983). A similar incidence of perforation is also to be expected. Stricture formation may also occur for a variable period after operation: Thomson (1985) described one stricture after 24 such operations (4.2%), and Adair and Everett (1983) reported one after 22 operations (4.5%). The incidence of all these complications will vary according to the number of circumferential lesions included in each series and the area of bowel wall the lesions occupy in the proximal direction.

Reactionary haemorrhage is usually successfully treated by conservative measures. Packing of the rectum with gauze is usually all that is required; if this fails, balloon tamponade may be successful. Occasionally the patient has to be returned to the operating theatre for evacuation of clot and ligature of the bleeding vessel. A secondary haemorrhage is treated in a similar manner. It should be remembered that intrarectal bleeding of this nature may, like bleeding after haemorrhoidectomy, often remain concealed. Any patient who becomes shocked after the procedure must have a rectal examination performed in order to exclude this complication. A full-thickness perforation usually occurs above the peritoneal reflection and will usually require a laparotomy; this will enable its extent to be assessed more fully than can be achieved via the transanal route, enabling the repair to be more accurate, and allowing the construction of a covering proximal colostomy.

Strictures following this operation can usually be treated by intermittent dilatation.

Complications following TEM are claimed to be lower than with conventional techniques. Buess (1996) records a mortality rate of 0.5% over an 11-year experience which includes many resections for T_1 and T_2 carcinomas. The complications are discussed in detail in Chapter 32; they include haemorrhage, pyrexia, dehiscence of the suture line and temporary incontinence. Buess reported that of 190 adenomas operated on between 1989 and 1993, re-intervention for complications was required in only 3% of patients (Mentges et al, 1994). Salim et al (1994) published a survey covering the experience of 44 clinics in Germany. In 1900 patients, 1411 adenomas and 435 carcinomas were resected. Complications occurred in 6.3% of patients, but only 2.3% required further surgical intervention. The specific problems seen in the learning phase of TEM were analysed by Salim et al (1994) who reported that TEM seemed to be associated with lower complication rates compared with conventional surgical procedures, and that the mortality rate of 0.2% was also lower.

Trans-sphincteric excision

The most prominent complications following trans-sphincteric excision are wound sepsis and faecal fistula. Their exact incidence is difficult to determine from the literature as most series are quite small. Mason (1974) had one fistula in 26 cases (4%) of villous adenoma treated by this technique. Although he recommended a covering colostomy for only the more extensive lesions, our own experience at the Royal London Hospital of two fistulas in seven cases suggests that a stoma should be used for all patients undergoing the procedure. Other workers have also experienced a relatively high incidence of fistula formation (Westbrook et al, 1982). Although Mason's patients had no problems with continence, we and others (Corman, 1984; Thompson and Tucker, 1987; Staimmer, 1994) have not been so fortunate. It is for these reasons that we recommend removal of villous adenomas by the transanal route whenever this is feasible. With the introduction of TEM, we believe that the trans-sphincteric approach will become less attractive, but it may still have a role.

Recurrence following local treatment

Diathermy or excision of villous adenomas via the transanal route using the conventional technique has a recurrence rate that varies between 11.5% and 27% (Southwood, 1962; Quan and Castro, 1971; Jahadi and Baldwin, 1975; Chiu and Spencer, 1978; Adair and Everett, 1983) (Table 28.13).

Christiansen et al (1979) treated 174 patients with villous adenomas of the colon and rectum: 120 had benign lesions, 99 of which were in the rectum and 21 in the colon. The rectal lesions were treated in the main by a transanal technique and the overall recurrence rate of the whole group was 30%. Parks and Stuart (1973) in their original paper described three recurrences after transanal excision of 26 benign rectal tumours; follow-up periods ranged from 6 months to 10 years. The recurrence in one of their patients was malignant despite the original lesion being benign. Heimann et al (1992) treated 46 of 51 patients with villous adenomas by either transanal excision (23) or posterior proctectomy (23), and only two of these patients developed local recurrence.

Table 28.13 Recurrence after transanal excision or diathermy of villous adenoma.

Authors	*n*	*Recurrence*
Southwood (1962)	113	13 (11.5)
Quan and Castro (1971)	72	9 (12.5)
Parks and Stuart (1973)	26*	3 (11.5)
Jahadi and Baldwin (1975)	24*	3 (12)
Thomson et al (1977)	20*	3 (15)
Chiu and Spencer (1978)	26*	7 (27)
Adair and Everett (1983)	40	7 (17.5)

*Excision only.
Numbers in parentheses are percentages.

It is difficult to be sure that a recurrence has arisen *de novo*, since it is very easy to leave a small focus of tumour behind. Many of the so-called recurrences are probably residual tumour which has increased in size. Such a recrudescence is more likely the greater the area of rectal wall that the tumour occupies. Recurrence would be expected to be greater in patients whose tumours showed malignant change. In practice patients with tumours that exhibit malignant infiltration through the muscularis mucosae undergo more radical resection. The fate of patients with tumours exhibiting carcinoma-in-situ (i.e. no invasion through the muscularis mucosae) has been poorly documented in the literature.

Recurrence following trans-sphincteric excision is said to be low. Mason (1974) recorded only two cases in the 26 patients he treated and both were subsequently found to have had an invasive carcinoma as the primary lesion. Since most series are small and follow-up has been limited, it is difficult to ascertain the true recurrence rate in the average colorectal unit. Since the surgeon has more direct vision of the lesion using a trans-sphincteric approach, it might be expected that recurrence would be less than after transanal excision. It is unlikely that this factor alone will convince surgeons to use the trans-sphincteric approach with its higher morbidity.

Since TEM has been performed only relatively recently, there are few data on recurrence. Said and Stippel (1995) reported on 286 cases operated on from 1983 to 1993. All patients had large sessile rectal adenomas (greater than 2 cm diameter). The 1-year and 5-year recurrence rates were respectively 1.2 ± SEM 0.7% and 7.0 ± 1.9%. Steele et al (1996) operated on 77 patients with benign rectal adenomas using TEM. In 70 (91%) excision was complete. After a mean follow-up of 7.4 months (range 0–24 months), four recurrences (5.2%) were detected, three of which occurred in patients who had been operated on for recurrent disease. Buess and Mentges (1992) operated on 229 rectal adenomas between 1983 and 1991 and reported a recurrence rate of 8.7%, 3% at the site of the previous lesion and 5.7% at distant sites within the rectum. Chiavellati et al (1994) reported no recurrences in 24 patients with benign rectal tumours treated by TEM, although follow-up was very short.

AUTHOR'S RECOMMENDATIONS

Many low rectal villous adenomas can be treated successfully by the conventional peranal techniques, particularly if the prone position is used for anterior lesions within approximately 8 cm of the anal verge. For lesions between 5 cm and 10 cm from the anus, the trans-sphincteric approach affords good exposure, but suffers from the risks of wound breakdown with a resulting fistula and poor function. Occasionally it may be indicated, but considerable thought should be given to its use, particularly when the new modality of transanal endoscopic microsurgery is available. The latter has been shown to be successful in the hands of experienced endoscopic surgeons, and seems particularly useful for lesions located more than 8 cm from the anal verge up to about 15 cm. We suspect that in time this technique will be more widely used and the trans-sphincteric approach will become obsolete. Electrodiathermy excision and laser destruction should be reserved for palliation in patients who are unfit for open surgery.

REFERENCES

Adair HM & Everett WG (1983) Villous and tubulovillous adenomas of the large bowel. *J R Coll Surg Edinb* **28**: 318–323.

Albrecht E (1904) *Verch Disch Path Ges* **7**: 153.

Alexander RH, Beckworth JB, Morgan A & Bill AH (1970) Juvenile polyps of the colon and their relation to allergy. *Am J Surg* **120**: 222–225.

Allardice JT, Rowland AC, Williams NS & Swain CP (1989) A new light delivery system for the treatment of obstructing gastrointestinal cancers by photodynamic therapy. *Gastrointest Endosc* **35**: 548–551.

Amshel AL, Shonberg IL & Gopal KA (1982) Retroperitoneal and mediastinal emphysema as a complication of colonoscopy. *Dis Colon Rectum* **25**: 167–168.

Atkin WS, Morson BC & Cuzick J (1992) Long-term risk of colorectal cancer after excision of rectosigmoid adenomas. *N Engl J Med* **326**: 658–662

Atwater JS & Bargen JA (1945) The pathogenesis of intestinal polyps. *Gastroenterology* **45**: 395.

Bacon HE & Eisenberg SQ (1971) Papillary adenoma or villous tumour of the rectum and colon. *Ann Surg* **174**: 1002.

Banerjee AK, Jehle EC, Shorthouse AJ & Buess G (1995) Local excision of rectal tumours. *Br J Surg* **82**: 1165–1173.

Barsoum GH, Hendrickse C, Winslet MC et al (1992) Reduction of mucosal crypt cell proliferation in patients with colorectal adenomatous polyps by dietary calcium supplementation. *Br J Surg* **79**: 481–583.

Berci G, Pannick JF, Schapiro M & Corlin R (1974) Complications of colonoscopy and polypectomy. *Gastroenterology* **67**: 584–585.

Berge T, Ekelund G, Mellner C et al (1973) Carcinoma of the colon and rectum in a defined population: an epidemiological clinical and post mortem investigation of colorectal carcinoma and co-existing benign polyps in Malmo, Sweden. *Acta Chir Scand* **4** (Suppl): 38.

Berry AC, Souser RG, Campbell WB, Mortensen NJMcC & Kettlewell (1990) Endoscopic transanal resection of rectal tumours: a preliminary report of its use. *Br J Surg* **77**: 134–137.

Bertario L, Presciuttini S, Sala P, Rossetti C & Pietroiusti M (1994) Causes of death and postsurgical survival in familial adenomatous polyposis: results from the Italian Registry. *Semin Surg Oncol* **10**: 225–234.

Bevan AD (1917) Carcinoma of the rectum: treatment by local excision. *Surg Clin N Am* **1**: 1233.

Bigard MA, Gaugher P & Lasalle C (1979) Fatal colonic explosion during colonoscopic polypectomy. *Gastroenterology* **77**: 1307.

Blue MG, Sivak MV, Achkar E, Matzen R & Stahl R (1991) Hyperplastic polyps seen at sigmoidoscopy are markers for additional adenomas seen at colonoscopy. *Gastroenterology* **100**: 564–566.

Boland CR, Montgomery CK & Kim YS (1982) A cancer-associated mucin alteration in benign colonic polyps. *Gastroenterology* **82**: 664–672.

Bond JH and the Practice Parameters Committee of the American College of Gastroenterology (1993) Polyp guidelines: diagnosis, treatment and surveillance for patients with non-familial colorectal polyps. *Ann Intern Med* **119**: 836–843

Bond JH Jr & Levitt MD (1974) Factors affecting the concentration of combustible gases in the colon during colonoscopy. *Gastroenterology* **68**: 1445.

Brunetaud JM, Mosquet L, Houcke M et al (1985) Villous adenomas of the rectum: results of endoscopic treatment with argon and Nd:YAG lasers. *Gastroenterology* **89**: 832–837.

Brunetaud JM, Maunoury V, Cochelard D et al (1989) Endoscopic laser treatment for rectosigmoid villous adenoma: factors affecting the results. *Gastroenterology* **97**: 272–277.

Buess GF (1994) Endoluminal rectal surgery (TEM). In Buess G, Cuschieri A & Perisat J (eds) *Operative Manual of Endoscopic Surgery*, Vol 1, pp 303–325. Heidelberg: Springer Verlag.

Buess GF (1996) Local procedures, including endoscopic resection in colorectal cancer. In Williams NS (ed) *Colorectal Cancer*. London: Churchill Livingstone.

Buess GF & Mentges B (1992) Transanal endoscopic microsurgery (TEM). *Minim Invas Ther* **1**: 101–109

Buess G, Hutterer F, Theiss J et al (1984) Das system fur die transanale endoskopische Rektum-operation. *Chirurg* **55**: 677–680

Buntain WL, Remine WH & Farrow GM (1972) Pre-malignancy of polyps of the colon. *Surg Gynecol Obstet* **134**: 499.

Bussey HJR, Wallace MH & Morson BC (1967) Metachronous carcinoma of the large intestine and intestinal polyps. *Proc R Soc Med* **60**: 208.

Byrne WJ, Jimine ZJF, Euler AR & Golladay ES (1982) Lymphoid polyps (focal lymphoid hyperplasia of the colon in children). *Pediatrics* **69**: 598–600.

Cabrera A, Restrepo C & Lega Siccar J (1959) Polyps of the rectum and of the distal portion of the colon. *Rev Lat Amer Anat Path* **3**: 55–68.

Cappell MS & Forde KA (1989) Spatial clustering of multiple hyperplastic, adenomatous and malignant colonic polyps in individual patients. *Dis Colon Rectum* **32**: 641–652.

Carlyle DR & Goldstein HM (1975) Angiographic management of bleeding following transcolonic polypectomy. *Dig Dis* **20**: 1196–1201.

Carpio G, Albu E, Gumbs MA & Gerst PH (1989) Management of colonic perforation after colonoscopy: report of three cases. *Dis Colon Rectum* **32**: 624–626.

Chapman I (1963) Adenomatous polypi of large intestine: incidence and distribution. *Ann Surg* **157**: 223–226.

Chardavoyne R & Wise L (1994) Exploratory laparoscopy for perforation following colonoscopy. *Surg Laparosc Endosc* **4**: 241–243.

Chiavellati L, D'Elia G, Zerilli M, Tremiterra S & Stipa S (1994) Management of large malignant rectal polyps with transanal endoscopic microsurgery. Is there anything better for the patient? *Eur J Surg Oncol* **20**: 658–666.

Chiu YS & Spencer RJ (1978) Villous lesions of the colon. *Dis Colon Rectum* **22**: 493–495.

Christiansen J, Kirkegaard P & Ibsen J (1979) Prognosis after treatment of villous adenomas of the colon and rectum. *Ann Surg* **189**: 404–409.

Christie JP (1984) Malignant colon polyps: cure by colonoscopy or colectomy? *Am J Gastroenterol* **79**: 543–547.

Christie JP (1988) Polypectomy or colectomy? Management of 106 consecutively encountered colorectal polyps. *Ann Surg* **54**: 93–99.

Christie JP & Marrazzo J III (1991) Miniperforation of the colon: not all post-polypectomy perforations require laparotomy. *Dis Colon Rectum* **34**: 132–135.

Cohen LB & Waye JD (1986) Treatment of colonic polyps: practical considerations. *Clin Gastroenterol* **15**: 359–376.

Cohen PR (1991) Association of sebaceous gland tumors and internal malignancy: the Muir–Torre syndrome. *Am J Med* **90**: 606–613.

Cohnheim J (1865) Ein Foll von Pseudoleukamie. *Virchows Arch (Path Anat)* **33**: 451–454.

Colacchio TA, Forde KA & Scantlebury VP (1981) Endoscopic polypectomy: inadequate treatment for invasive colorectal carcinoma. *Ann Surg* **194**: 704–707.

Cole JW & McKalen A (1961) Observations of cell renewal in human rectal mucosa *in vivo* with thymidien-I^{131}. *Gastroenterology* **41**: 122.

Cooper HS (1983) Surgical pathology of endoscopically removed malignant polyps of the colon and rectum. *Am J Surg Pathol* **7**: 613–623.

Cooper HS, Deppisch LM, Gourley WK et al (1995) Endoscopically removed malignant colorectal polyps: clinicopathologic correlations. *Gastroenterology* **108**: 1657–1665.

Corman ML (1984) *Colon and Rectal Surgery*. Philadelphia: Lippincott.

Corman ML (1993) *Colon and Rectal Surgery*. Philadelphia: Lippincott.

Cornes JS, Wallace MH & Morson BC (1961) Benign lymphomas of the rectum and anal canal: a study of 100 cases. *J Pathol Bacteriol* **82**: 371–382.

Cotton PB & Williams CB (1980) *Practical Gastrointestinal Endoscopy*. Oxford: Blackwell Scientific.

Coutsoftides T, Sivak MV, Sanford PB & Jagelman D (1978) Colonoscopy and the management of polyps containing invasive carcinoma. *Ann Surg* **188**: 638–641.

Coverlizza S, Risio M, Ferrari A et al (1989) Colorectal adenomas containing invasive carcinoma: pathologic assessment of lymph node metastatic potential. *Cancer* **64**: 1937–1947.

Cranley JP, Petras RE, Carey WD, Paraod K & Sivak KV (1986) When is endoscopic polypectomy adequate therapy for colonic polyps containing invasive carcinoma? *Gastroenterology* **91**: 419–427.

Damore LJ, Rantis PC & Vernava AM (1996) Colonoscopic perforations: etiology, diagnosis, and management (review). *Dis Colon Rectum* **39**: 1308–1314.

Day DW & Morson BC (1978) Pathology of adenomas. In Morson BD (ed) *The Pathogenesis of Colorectal Cancer*, pp 43–57. Philadelphia: WB Saunders.

De Cosse JJ (1984) Malignant colorectal polyp. *Gut* **25**: 433–436.

De Jong UW, Day NE, Muir CS et al (1972) The distribution of cancer within the large bowel. *Int J Cancer* **10**: 463–477.

Di Sario JA, Foutch PG, Mai HD et al (1991) Prevalence and malignant potential of colorectal polyps in asymptomatic average risk men. *Am J Gastroenterol* **86**: 941–945.

Dickinson AJ, Savage AP, Mortensen NJMcC & Kettlewell MGW (1993) Long-term survival after endoscopic transanal resection of rectal tumours. *Br J Surg* **80**: 1401–1404.

Dodds WJ, Stewart ET & Hogan WJ (1977) Role of colonoscopy and roentgenology in the detection of polypoid colonic lesions. *Am J Dig Dis* **22**: 646–649.

Donovan IA, Arabi Y, Keighley MRB et al (1980) Modification of the physiological disturbances produced by whole gut irrigation by preliminary mannitol administration. *Br J Surg* **67**: 134–137.

Douglas JR, Campbell CA, Salisbury DM et al (1980) Colonoscopic polypectomy in children. *BMJ* **3**: 1386.

Dozois R (1985) St Mark's 150th Centenary Meeting.

Dukes CE (1926) Simple tumours of the large intestine and their relation to cancer. *Br J Surg* **13**: 720.

Durdey P, Weston P & Williams NS (1987) Colonoscopy or barium enema as the first line investigation of colonic disease. *Lancet* **ii**: 549–551.

Duthie HL & Atwell JD (1963) The absorption of water, sodium and potassium in the large intestine with particular reference to the effects of villous papillomas. *Gut* **4**: 373.

Dybahl JH, Haug K, Bakkevold K, Olsen KO & Vetvick K (1984) Screening for occult faecal blood loss in a community by means of Hemoccult II slides and tetramethylbenzidine test. *Scand J Gastroenterol* **19**: 343–349.

Eide TJ (1986) Prevalence and morphologic features of adenomas of the large intestine in individuals with and without colorectal cancer. *Histopathology* **10**: 111–118.

Eide TJ & Stalsberg H (1978) Polyps of the large intestine in Northern Norway. *Cancer* **42**: 2839–2848.

Ekelund G & Lindstrom C (1974) Histopathological analysis of benign polyps in patients with carcinoma of the colon and rectum. *Gut* **15**: 654.

Ekelund G (1963) On cancer and polyps of colon and rectum. *Acta Pathol Microbiol Scand* **59**: 165–170.

Elias H, Hyde DM, Mullens RS & Lambert FC (1981) Colonic adenomas: stereology and growth mechanisms. *Dis Colon Rectum* **24**: 331–342.

Enquist IF (1957) The incidence and significance of polyps of the colon and rectum. *Surgery (St Louis)* **42**: 681.

Enterline HT (1976) Polyps and cancer of the large bowel. *Curr Top Pathol* **63**: 95–141.

Enterline HT & Arvan DA (1967) Chromosome constitution of adenoma and adenocarcinoma of the colon. *Cancer* **20**: 1764.

Enterline HT, Evans GW, Mercado-Lugo R, Miller L & Fitts WT Jr (1962) Malignant potential of adenomas of colon and rectum. *JAMA* **179**: 322–330.

Ewing J (1940) *Neoplastic Diseases: A Treatise on Tumours*, 4th edn. Philadelphia: WB Saunders.

Farrands PA, Vellacott SD, Amar SS et al (1983) Flexible fiberoptic sigmoidoscopy and double contrast barium enema examination in the identification of adenomas and carcinoma of the colon. *Dis Colon Rectum* **26**: 725–727.

Fearon ER & Vogelstein B (1990) A genetic model for colorectal tumorigenesis. *Cell* **61**: 759–767.

Fenoglio CM, Richart RM & Kaye GI (1975) Comparative electron-microscopic features of normal hyperplastic and adenomatous human colonic epithelium. II: Variations in surface architecture found by scanning electron microscopy. *Gastroenterology* **69**: 100.

Fisher ER & Sharkey DA (1962) The ultrastructure of colonic polyps and cancer with special reference to the epithelial inclusion bodies of Leuchtenberger. *Cancer* **15**: 160.

Fisher ER & Turnball RB Jr (1952) Malignant polyps of rectum and sigmoid: therapy based on pathological considerations. *Surg Gynecol Obstet* **94**: 619.

Fishman EK & Golman SM (1981) Pneumoscrotum after colonoscopy. *Urology* **18**: 171–172.

Fitzgerald MG (1955) Extreme fluid and electrolyte loss due to villous papilloma. *BMJ* **1**: 831–832.

Fork FT (1983) Reliability of routine double contrast examination of the large bowel: a prospective study of 259 patients. *Gut* **24**: 672–677.

Franklin R & McSwain B (1972) Juvenile polyps of the colon and rectum. *Ann Surg* **175**: 887–891.

Frechner RE (1973) Adenomatous polyp with submucosal cysts. *Am J Clin Path* **59**: 498.

Fruhmorgen P & Demling L (1979) Complications of diagnostic and therapeutic colonoscopy in the Federal Republic of Germany. *Endoscopy* **11**: 146–150.

Fruhmorgen P (1981) Therapeutic colonoscopy. In Hunt RH & Waye JD (eds) *Colonoscopy*. London: Chapman & Hall.

Fucini C, Wolff BG & Spencer RJ (1986) An appraisal of endoscopic removal of malignant colonic polyps. *Mayo Clin Proc* **61**: 123–126.

Gadson P, McCoy J, Wikstrom AC & Gustafsson JA (1990) Suppression of protein kinase C and the stimulation of glucocorticoid receptor synthesis by dexamethasone in human fibroblasts derived from tumor tissue. *J Cell Biochem* **43**: 185–198.

Gavrieli Y, Sherman Y & Ben-Sasson SA (1992) Identification of programmed cell death *in situ* via specific labeling of nuclear DNA fragmentation. *J Cell Biol* **119**: 1402–1430.

Gedebou TM, Wong RA, Rappaport WD et al (1996) Clinical presentation and management of iatrogenic colon perforations. *Am J Surg* **172**: 454–457.

Geenan JE, Schmidt MG & Hogan WJ (1974) Complications of colonoscopy (abstract). *Gastroenterology* **66**: 812.

Gentry WC Jr, Eskritt NE & Gorlin RJ (1974) Multiple hamartoma syndrome (Cowden's disease). *Arch Dermatol* **109**: 521–525.

Gilbertsen V (1974) Proctosigmoidoscopy and polypectomy in reducing the incidence of rectal cancer. *Cancer* **34**: 936–939.

Gillespie PE, Chambers TJ, Chan KW et al (1979) Colonic adenomas: a colonoscopy survey. *Gut* **20**: 240–245.

Gillespie PE, Nicholls RJ, Thompson JPS & Williams CB (1978) Snare polypectomy by sigmoid–rectal intussusception. *BMJ* **1**: 1395.

Goerg KJ & Duber C (1996) Retroperitoneal, mediastinal and subcutaneous emphysema with pneumothorax after colonoscopy [German] *Dtsch Med Wochenschr*. **121**: 693–696.

Goh HS & Jass JR (1986) DNA content and the adenoma carcinoma sequence in the colorectum. *J Clin Pathol* **39**: 387–392.

Goligher J (1984) *Surgery of the Anus, Rectum and Colon*, 5th edn. London: Baillière Tindall.

Gramlich TL, Hennigar RA & Schulte BA (1988) The incidence and carbohydrate histochemistry of dystrophic goblet cells in colon. *Mod Pathol* **1**: 366–371.

Granet E (1949) Simple lymphomas of the sphincteric rectum in identical twins. *JAMA* **141**: 990–991.

Greenburg AG, Saik RP, Coyle JJ et al (1981) Mortality and gastrointestinal surgery in the aged: elective vs emergency procedures. *Arch Surg* **116**: 788–791.

Greene FJ (1974) Epithelial misplacement in adenomatous polyps of the colon and rectum. *Cancer* **33**: 206.

Greene FL (1983) Distribution of colorectal neoplasms: a left to right shift of polyps and cancer. *Am J Surg* **49**: 62–65.

Greenen JE, Schmitt MG Jr, Wu WC & Hogan WT (1975) Major complications of colonoscopy: bleeding and perforation. *Am J Dig Dis* **20**: 231.

Grinnell RS & Lane N (1958) Benign and malignant adenomatous polyps and papillary adenomas of colon and rectum: an analysis of 1856 tumours in 1335 patients. *Int Abstr Surg* **106**: 519–538.

Grossman S, Milos ML, Tekawa IS & Jewell NP (1989) Colonoscopic screening of persons with suspected risk factors for colon cancer. II: Past history of colorectal neoplasms. *Gastroenterology* **96**: 299–306.

Gruenberg J & Mackman S (1972) Multiple lymphoid polyps in familial polyposis. *Ann Surg* **175**: 552–554.

Gruenwald P (1942) Abnormal accumulation of lymph follicles in the digestive tract. *Am J Med Sci* **203**: 823–829.

Grundquist S, Gabriellson B & Sundelin P (1979) Diminutive colonic polyps: clinical significance and management. *Endoscopy* **11**: 36–42.

Habr-Gama A & Waye JD (1989) Complications and hazards of gastrointestinal endoscopy. *World J Surg* **13**: 193–201.

Haenszel W & Correa P (1971) Cancer of the colon and rectum and adenomatous polyps: a review of epidemiological findings. *Cancer* **28**: 14–24.

Hall C, Dorricott NJ, Donovan IA & Neoptolemos JP (1991) Colon perforation during colonoscopy: surgical versus conservative management. *Br J Surg* **78**: 542–544.

Hall C, Youngs D & Keighley MRB (1992) Crypt cell production rates at various sites around the colon in Wistar rats and humans. *Gut* **33**: 1528–1531.

Hall PA, Coates PJ, Ansari B & Hopwood D (1994) Regulation of cell number in the mammalian gastrointestinal tract: the importance of apoptosis. *J Cell Sci* **107**: 3569–3577.

Hamilton SR (1993) Flat adenomas: what you can't see can hurt you. *Radiology* **187**: 309–310.

Hanby AM, Poulsom R, Singh S et al (1992) Hyperplastic polyps: a cell lineage which both synthesizes and secretes trefoil-peptides and has phenotypic similarity with the ulcer-associated cell lineage. *Am J Pathol* **141**: 663–668.

Hanley PH, Hines MO & Ray JE (1971) Villous tumours: experience with 217 patients. *Ann Surg* **37**: 190.

Hardcastle JD, Chamberlain JO, Robinson MHE et al (1996) Randomised controlled trial of faecal occult blood screening for colorectal cancer. *Lancet* **348**: 1472–1477.

Hayashi T, Yatani R, Apostol J & Stemmerman GN (1974) Pathogenesis of hyperplastic polyps of the colon: a hypothesis based on ultrastructure and *in vitro* kinetics. *Gastroenterology* **66**: 347–356.

Hayes HT & Burr HB (1952) Benign lymphomas of the rectum. *Am J Surg* **84**: 545–550.

Heald RJ & Bussey HJR (1975) Clinical experiences at St Mark's Hospital with multiple synchronous cancers of the colon and rectum. *Dis Colon Rectum* **18**: 6–10.

Heimann TM, Oh C, Steinhagen RM et al (1992) Surgical treatment of tumours of the distal rectum with sphincter preservation. *Ann Surg* **216**: 432–436.

Helwig EB (1947) Evolution of adenomas of large intestine and their relation to carcinoma. *Surg Gynecol Obstet* **84**: 36.

Helwig EB (1959) Adenomas and the pathogenesis of cancer of the colon and rectum. *Dis Colon Rectum* **2**: 5–17.

Herrera L, Isekati S, Gibas L et al (1986) Gardner syndrome in a man with interstitial deletion of 5q. *Am J Med Genet* **25**: 473–476.

Holgersen LO, Miller RE & Zintell HA (1971) Juvenile polyps of the colon. *Surgery* **69**: 288–293.

Holtz F & Schmidt LA (1958) Lymphoid polyps of the rectum and anus. *Surg Gynecol Obstet* **106**: 639–642.

Horrilleno EG, Eckert C & Ackerman LV (1957) Polyps of the rectum and colon in children. *Cancer* **10**: 1210.

Hussein AMS, Bartram CI & Williams CB (1984) Carbon dioxide insufflation for more comfortable colonoscopy. *Gastrointest Endosc* **30**: 68–70.

Hyser MJ & Gau FC (1996) Endoscopic Nd:YAG laser therapy for villous adenomas of the colon and rectum. *Am Surg* **62**: 577–581.

Ichii S, Horii Nakatsuru S et al (1992) Inactivation of both APC alleles in an early stage of colon adenomas in a patient with familial adenomatous polyposis (FAP). *Human Mol Genet* **1**: 387–390.

Imai H, Saito S & Stein AA (1965) Ultrastructure of adenomatous polyps and villous adenomas of the large intestine. *Gastroenterology* **47**: 188.

Inoue H, Takeshita K, Hori H et al (1993) Endoscopic mucosal resection with a cap-fitted panendoscope for esophagus, stomach, and colon mucosal lesions. *Gastrointest Endosc* **39**: 58–62.

Iwama T & Mishima Y (1994) Factors affecting the risk of rectal cancer following rectum preserving surgery in patients with familial adenomatous polyposis. *Dis Colon Rectum* **37**: 1024–1026.

Jackson BT & Mason AY (1984) Trans-sphincteric resection. In Todd IP & Fielding LP (eds) *Rob & Smith's Operative Surgery. Vol. 3: Colon, Rectum and Anus*, pp 366–380. London: Butterworth.

Jahadi MR & Baldwin A (1975) Villous adenomas of the colon and rectum. *Am J Surg* **130**: 729–732.

Jaramillo E, Watanabe M, Slezak P & Rubio C (1995) Flat neoplastic lesions of the colon and rectum detected by high resolution video-endoscopy and chromoscopy. *Gastrointest Endosc* **42**: 114–122.

Jass JR (1983) Relation between metaplastic polyp and carcinoma of the colorectum. *Lancet* **i**: 28–30.

Jass JR & Faludy J (1985) Immunohistochemical demonstration of IgA and secretory component in relation to epithelial cell differentiation in normal colorectal mucosa and metaplastic polyp: a semiquantitative study. *Histochem J* **17**: 373–380.

Jass JR & Sobin LH (eds) (1989) *International Histological Classification of Tumors*. Berlin: Springer.

Jass JR, Filipe MI, Abbas S et al (1984) A morphologic and histochemical study of metaplastic polyps of the colorectum. *Cancer* **53**: 510–515.

Jentschura D, Raute M, Winter J et al (1994) Complications in endoscopy of the lower gastrointestinal tract: therapy and prognosis. *Surg Endosc* **8**: 672–676.

Johnson RC, Bleshman MH & Deford JW (1978) Benign lymphoid hyperplasia manifesting as a caecal mass. *Dis Colon Rectum* **21**: 510–513.

Kavin H, Hamilton DG, Greasley RE, Eckert JD & Zuidema G (1970) Scanning electron microscopy: a new method in the study of rectal mucosa. *Gastroenterology* **59**: 426.

Kaye GI, Fenoglio CM, Pascal PR & Lane N (1973) Comparative electron microscopic features of normal hyperplastic and adenomatous human colonic epithelium: variations in cellular structure relative to the process of epithelial differentiation. *Gastroenterology* **64**: 926.

Keeling WM & Beatty GL (1956) Lymphoid polyps of the rectum: report of three cases in siblings. *Arch Surg* **73**: 753–756.

Keighley MRB, Taylor EQ, Hares MM et al (1981) Influence of oral mannitol preparation on colonic microflora and the risk of explosion during endoscopic diathermy. *Br J Surg* **68**: 554.

Kellokumpu I & Husa A (1987) Colorectal adenomas: morphologic features and the risk of developing adenomas and carcinomas in the colorectum. *Scand J Gastroenterol* **27**: 833–841.

Kelly MJ (1989) Use of the urological resectoscope in benign and malignant rectal lesions: review of 12 cases. *Proc R Soc Med* **82**: 588–590.

Kettlewell MGW (1991) Endoscopic transanal resection for rectal cancer. *Int J Colorect Dis* **6**: 82–83.

Kewenter J, Brevinge H, Engaras B, Haglind E & Ahren C (1994) Results of screening, rescreening and follow-up in a prospective randomised study for detection of colorectal cancer by faecal occult blood testing: results for 68,308 subjects. *Scand J Gastroenterol* **29**: 468–473.

Knox WG, Miller RE, Begg CF & Zintel HA (1960) Juvenile polyps of the colon: a clinicopathologic analysis of 75 polyps in 43 patients. *Surgery (St Louis)* **48**: 201.

Ko FY, Wu TC & Hwang B (1995) Intestinal polyps in children and adolescents: a review of 103 cases. *Acta Paediatr Sin* **36**: 197–202.

Kobayashi M, Watanabe H, Ajioka Y et al (1992) PCNA-positive cell distribution in depressed types of early carcinoma and adenoma of the large intestine. *Gastroenterol Jpn* **27**: 684.

Kozuka S (1975) Premalignancy of the mucosal polyp in the large intestine. I: Histological gradation of the polyp on the basis of epithelial pseudostratification and glandular branching. *Dis Colon Rectum* **18**: 483.

Kronborg O, Fenger C, Olsen J, Jorgensen OD & Sondergaard O (1996) Randomised study of screening for colorectal cancer with faecal occult blood test. *Lancet* **348**: 1467–1471.

Kuramoto S, Ihara O, Sakai S et al (1990) Depressed adenoma in the large intestine: endoscopic features. *Dis Colon Rectum* **33**: 108–112.

Lallemand RC, Vakil PA, Pearson P & Box V (1984) Screening for asymptomatic bowel cancer in general practice. *BMJ* **288**: 31–32.

Langer JC, Cohen Z, Taylor BR et al (1984) Management of patients with polyps containing malignancy removed by colonoscopic polypectomy. *Dis Colon Rectum* **27**: 6–9.

Langevin JM & Nivatvongs A (1984) The true incidence of synchronous cancer of the large bowel. A prospective study. *Am J Surg* **147**: 330–333.

Latt TT, Nicholl R, Domizio P, Walker-Smith JA & Williams CB (1993) Rectal bleeding and polyps. *Arch Dis Child* **69**: 144–147.

Lawrence JC (1936) Gastrointestinal polyps: statistical study of malignancy incidence. *Am J Surg* **31**: 499.

Lee FI (1983) Screening for colorectal cancer in a factory based population with Fecatest. *Br J Cancer* **48**: 843–847.

Lee RO & Keown D (1970) Villous tumours of the rectum associated with severe fluid and electrolyte disturbance. *Br J Surg* **57**: 197–201.

Lehmann CU & Elitsur Y (1996) Juvenile polyps and their distribution in pediatric patients with gastrointestinal bleeding. *W V Med J* **93**: 133–135.

Lezak MB & Goldhamer M (1974) Retroperitoneal emphysema after colonoscopy. *Gastroenterology* **66**: 118–120.

Lieberman D &, Smith FW (1991) Screening for colon malignancy with colonoscopy. *Am J Gastroenterology* **86**: 946–951.

Lipkin M (1974) Phase I and phase II proliferative lesions of colonic epithelial cells in diseases leading to colonic cancer. *Cancer* **34**: 378.

Lipkin M, Bell R & Sherlock P (1963) Cell proliferation kinetics in the gastrointestinal tract of man. I: Cell removal in colon and rectum. *J Clin Invest* **42**: 767.

Lipper S, Kahn LB & Ackerman LV (1983) The significance of microscopic invasive cancer in endoscopically removed polyps of the large bowel. *Cancer* **52**: 1691–1699.

Lo AY & Beaton HL (1994) Selective management of colonoscopic perforations. *J Am Coll Surg* **179**: 333–337.

Lockhart-Mummery HE & Dukes CE (1952) The surgical treatment of malignant rectal polyps. *Lancet* **ii**: 751–755.

Loh CS, Bliss P, Bown SG & Krasner N (1994) Photodynamic therapy for villous adenomas of the colon and rectum. *Endoscopy* **26**: 243–246.

Lorenzsonn V & Trier JS (1968) The fine structure of human rectal mucosa: the epithelial lining of the base of the crypt. *Gastroenterology* **55**: 88.

MacDonald WC, Trier JS & Everett NB (1964) Cell proliferation and migration in the stomach, duodenum and rectum of man: radiographic studies. *Gastroenterology* **46**: 405.

Macrae FA, Tan KG & Williams CB (1983) Towards safer colonoscopy: a report on the complications of 5000 diagnostic or therapeutic colonoscopies. *Gut* **24**: 376–383.

Marks G, Boggs HW, Castro AF et al (1979) Sigmoidoscopic examination with rigid and flexible fiberoptic sigmoidoscopes in the surgeon's office. *Dis Colon Rectum* **22**: 162–168.

Mason AY (1970) Surgical access to the rectum: a trans-sphincteric exposure. *Proc R Soc Med* **65** (Suppl): 1.

Mason AY (1974) Trans-sphincteric surgery of the rectum. *Progr Surg* **13**: 66–69.

Matek W, Fruhmorgen P, Kaduk B et al (1979) Modified electrocoagulation and its possibilities in the control of gastrointestinal bleeding. *Endoscopy* **11**: 253–258.

Mathus-Vliegen EM & Tytgat GN (1986) Laser photocoagulation in the palliation of colorectal malignancies. *Cancer* **57**: 2212–2216.

Mathus-Vliegen EM & Tytgat GN (1991) The potential and limitations of laser photoablation of colorectal adenomas. *Gastrointest Endosc* **37**: 9–17.

Maxfield RG (1984) Colonoscopy as a routine preoperative procedure for carcinoma of the colon. *Am J Surg* **147**: 477–480.

Mayo CW & Schlicke CP (1942) Carcinoma of the colon and rectum: a study of metastases and recurrences. *Surg Gynecol Obstet* **74**: 825.

Mazier PW, Mackeigan JM, Billingham RP & Dingnan RD (1982) Juvenile polyps of the colon and rectum. *Surg Gynecol Obstet* **154**: 829–832.

McCabe SC, McSherry BCK, Sussman EB et al (1973) Villous tumours of the large bowel. *Am J Surg* **126**: 336.

McCallum RW, Meyer CT, Marignani P et al (1984) Flexible sigmoidoscopy: diagnostic yield in 1015 patients. *Am J Gastroenterol* **79**: 433–437.

McColl I, Bussey HJR, Veale AMO & Morson BC (1964) Juvenile polyposis coli. *Proc R Soc Med* **57**: 896.

McKittrick LS & Wheelock FCJ (1954) *Carcinoma of the Colon*, pp 61–63. Springfield, IL: CC Thomas.

Mehdi A, Closset J, Gay F et al (1996) Laparoscopic treatment of a sigmoid perforation after colonoscopy: case report and review of literature. *Surg Endosc* **10**: 666–667.

Mentges B, Buess G, Raestrup H, Manncke K & Becker HD (1994) TEM results of the Tubingen Group. *Endosc Surg Allied Technol* **2**: 247–250.

Messinetti S, Zelli GP, Marcellino LR & Alcini E (1968) Benign and malignant tumours of the gastrointestinal tract: chromosome analysis in study and diagnosis. *Cancer* **21**: 1000.

Mestre J (1986) The changing pattern of juvenile polyps. *Am J Gastroenterol* **81**: 312–314.

Miller CJ, Day E & L'Esperance ES (1950) Value of proctoscopy as routine examination in preventing deaths from cancer of large bowel. *NY State J Med* **50**: 2023.

Minamoto T, Sawaguchi K, Mai M et al (1994) Infrequent K-*ras* activation in superficial-type (flat) colorectal adenomas and adenocarcinomas. *Cancer Res* **54**: 2841–2844.

Minopoulos GL, McIntyre RLE, Lee ECG & Kettlewell MGW (1983) Colonoscopic polypectomy in a regional teaching hospital. *Br J Surg* **70**: 51–53.

Miyahara M, Kitano S, Shimoda K et al (1996) Laparoscopic repair of a colonic perforation sustained during colonoscopy. *Surg Endosc* **10**: 352–353.

Moore JM (1960) The incidence and importance of polyps of the large intestine. *Scott Med J* **5**: 83.

Morson BC (1962) Precancerous lesions of the colon and rectum. *JAMA* **179**: 316–321.

Morson BC (1974) Evaluation of cancer of the colon and rectum. *Cancer* **34**: 845–849.

Morson BC & Dawson MP (1990) *Gastrointestinal Pathology*, 3rd edn. Oxford: Blackwell Scientific.

Morson BC & Sobin LH (1976) *International Histological Classification of Tumours. 15: Histological Typing of Intestinal Tumours*. Geneva: WHO.

Morson BC, Whiteway JE, Jones EA, Macrae FA & Williams CB (1984) Histopathology and prognosis of malignant colorectal polyps treated by endoscopic polypectomy. *Gut* **25**: 437–444.

Moss SF, Liu TC, Petrotos A et al (1996) Inward growth of colonic adenomatous polyps. *Gastroenterology* **111**: 1425–1432.

Murakami R, Tsukuma H, Kanamori S et al (1990) Natural history of colorectal polyps and the effect of polypectomy on occurrence of subsequent cancer. *Int J Cancer* **46**: 159–164.

Muto T & Watanabe T (1993) Flat adenomas and minute carcinomas of the colon and rectum. *Persp in Colon Rectal Surg* **6**: 117–132.

Muto T, Bussey HJR & Morson BC (1973) Pseudocarcinomatous invasion in adenomatous polyps of the colon and rectum. *J Clin Path* **26**: 25.

Muto T, Kamiya J, Sawada T et al (1985) Small 'flat adenoma' of the large bowel with special reference to its clinicopathologic features. *Dis Colon Rectum* **28**: 849–851.

Muto T, Sawada T & Gugihara K (1991) Treatment of carcinoma in adenomas. *World J Surg* **15**: 35–40.

Newstead GL & Morgan BP (1979) Bowel preparation with mannitol. *Med J Austr* **2**: 581.

Nivatvongs S (1988) Complications in colonoscopic polypectomy. *Ann Surg* **54**: 61–63.

Nivatvongs S & Dorudi S (1996) Colorectal polyps and their management. In Williams NS (ed) *Colorectal Cancer*, pp 39–54. London: Churchill Livingstone.

Nivatvongs S & Goldberg SM (1978) Management of patients who have polyps containing invasive carcinoma removed via colonoscope. *Dis Colon Rectum* **21**: 8–11.

Nivatvongs S, Balcos EG, Schottler JL et al (1973) Surgical management of large villous tumours of the rectum. *Dis Colon Rectum* **16**: 508.

Nivatvongs S, Rojanasakul A, Reiman HM et al (1991) The risk of lymph node metastasis in colorectal polyps with invasive adenocarcinoma. *Dis Colon Rectum* **34**: 323–328.

Nucci M, Robinson R & Hamilton SR (1993) Phenotypic characterization of abberant crypt foci in the human colorectum. *Mod Pathol* **6**: 50A.

Nugent KP, Talbot IC, Hodgson SV & Phillips RK (1993) Solitary juvenile polyps: not a marker for subsequent malignancy. *Gastroenterology* **105**: 698–700.

O'Brien MJ, Winawer SJ, Zauber AG et al (1990) The National Polyp Study: Patient and polyp characteristics associated with high-grade dysplasia in colorectal adenomas. *Gastroenterology* **98**: 371–379.

Obrecht WR Jr, Wu WC, Gelfand DW & Ott DJ (1984) The extent of successful colonoscopy: a second assessment using modern equipment. *Gastrointest Radiol* **9**: 161–162.

Olsen HW, Lawrence WA, Snook CW & Mutch WM (1988) Review of recurrent polyps and cancer in 500 patients with initial colonoscopy for polyps. *Dis Colon Rectum* **31**: 222–227.

Olsen RO & Davis WC (1969) Villous adenomas of the colon: benign and malignant. *Arch Surg* **98**: 487.

Orringer MB & Eggleston JC (1972) Papillary (villous) adenomas of the colon and rectum. *Surgery* **62**: 378.

Ottery FD, Bruskewitz RC & Weese JL (1986) Endoscopic transrectal resection on rectal tumours. *Cancer* **57**: 563–566.

Ozick LA, Jacob L, Donelson SS, Agarwal SK & Freeman HP (1995) Distribution of adenomatous polyps in African-Americans. *Am J Gastroenterol* **90**: 758–760.

Pagana TJ, Ledesma EJ, Mittelman A & Nava HR (1984) The use of colonoscopy in the study of synchronous colorectal neoplasms. *Cancer* **53**: 356–359.

Palmer KR & Khan AN (1979) Oral mannitol: a simple and effective bowel preparation for barium enema. *BMJ* **3**: 1038.

Parks AG (1966) Benign tumours of the rectum. In Rob C, Smith R & Morgan CN (eds) *Abdomen of Rectum and Anus: Clinical Surgery*, Vol 10, pp 541–458. London: Butterworth.

Parks AG (1983) Peranal endorectal operative techniques. In Tod IP & Fielding LP (eds) *Rob & Smith's Operative Surgery. Vol 3: Colon, Rectum and Anus*, 4th edn. London: Butterworth.

Parks AG & Stuart AE (1973) The management of villous tumours of the large bowel. *Br J Surg* **60**: 688–695.

Pfeffer L, Lipkin M, Stutman O & Kopelovich L (1976) Growth abnormalities of cultured human skin fibroblasts derived from individuals with hereditary adenomatosis of the colon and rectum. *J Cell Physiol* **89**: 29–38.

Pheils MT (1979) Villous tumours of the rectum. *Dis Colon Rectum* **22**: 406–407.

Pittman FE & Pittman JC (1966) An electron microscopic study of the epithelium of normal human sigmoid colonic mucosa. *Gut* **7**: 644.

Potet F & Soullard J (1971) Polyps of the rectum and colon. *Gut* **12**: 468.

Pretlow TP, O'Riordan MA, Pretlow TG et al (1992) Abberant crypts in human colonic mucosa: putative preneoplastic lesions. *J Cell Biochem Suppl* **16G**: 55–62.

Price AB (1978) Benign lymphoid polyps and inflammatory polyps. In Morson BC (ed) *The Pathogenesis of Colorectal Cancer*, pp 33–42. Philadelphia: WB Saunders.

Prorock JJ, Stahler EJ, Hartzell GW & Sugarman HJ (1977) Surgical management of colonoscopic perforation. *Gastrointest Endosc* **23**: 238.

Quan SHQ & Castro EB (1971) Papillary adenomas (villous tumours): a review of 215 cases. *Dis Colon Rectum* **14**: 267–280.

Quirke P, Fozard JBJ, Dixon MF et al (1986) DNA aneuploidy in colorectal adenomas. *Br J Cancer* **53**: 477–482.

Ragins J, Shinya H & Wolff WI (1974) The explosive potential of colonic gas during colonoscopic electrosurgical polypectomy. *Surg Gynecol Obstet* **138**: 554.

Reale MA, Fearon ER (1994) Molecular genetics of hereditary colorectal cancer. *Haemat Oncol Ann* **2**: 129.

Rex DK, Lehman GA, Hawes RH et al (1991) Screening colonoscopy in asymptomatic average-risk persons with negative faecal occult blood tests. *Gastroenterology* **100**: 64–67.

Rex DK, Smith JJ, Ulbright TM & Lehman GA (1992) Distal colonic hyperplastic polyps do not predict adenomas in asymptomatic average-risk subjects. *Gastroenterology* **102**: 317–319.

Reynolds KR, Armitage NC, Balfour TW et al (1983) Flexible sigmoidoscopy as outpatient procedure. *Lancet* **ii**: 1072.

Richards WO, Webb WA, Morris SJ et al (1987) Patient management after endoscopic removal of the cancerous colon adenoma. *Ann Surg* **205**: 665–672.

Rogers BHG, Silvis E, Nebel OT, Sugawa CL & Mandelstam P (1975) Complications of flexible fiberoptic colonoscopy and polypectomy. *Gastrointest Endosc* **23**: 73–75.

Roseman DM (1973) Report from San Diego. *Gastrointest Endosc* **20**: 36.

Roth SI & Helwig EB (1963) Juvenile polyps of the colon and rectum. *Cancer* **16**: 468.

Said S & Stippel D (1995) Transanal endoscopic microsurgery in large, sessile adenomas of the rectum: a ten-year experience. *Surg Endosc* **9**: 1106–1112.

Salm R, Lampe H, Bustos A & Matern U (1994) Experience with TEM in Germany. *Endosc Surg Allied Technol* **2**: 251–254.

Schlinkert RT & Rasmussen TE (1994) Laparoscopic repair of colonoscopic perforations of the colon. *J Laparoendosc Surg* **4**: 51–54.

Schmidt G, Borsch G & Wegener M (1986) Subcutaneous emphysema and pneumothorax complicating diagnostic colonoscopy. *Dis Colon Rectum* **29**: 136–138.

Schwesinger WH, Levine BA & Ranies R (1979) Complications in colonoscopy. *Surg Gynecol Obstet* **148**: 270–281.

Shiff SJ & Rigas B (1997) Colon adenomatous polyps: do they grow inward? *Lancet* **349**: 1853–1854.

Shinya H & Wolff WI (1979) Morphology, anatomic distribution and cancer potential of colonic polyps: an analysis of 7000 polyps endoscopically removed. *Ann Surg* **190**: 679–683.

Shnika TK, Friedman MHW, Kidd EG & MacKenzie WC (1961) Villous tumours of the rectum and colon characterised by severe fluid and electrolyte loss. *Surg Gynecol Obstet* **112**: 609–612.

Sinicrope FA, Roddey G, McDonnell TJ et al (1996) Increased apoptosis accompanies neoplastic development in the human colorectum. *Clin Cancer Res* **2**: 1999–2006.

Smilow PC, Pryor CA & Swinton NW (1966) Juvenile polyposis coli. *Dis Colon Rectum* **9**: 248.

Smith LE & Nivatvongs J (1975) Fiberoptic colonoscopy: complications of colonoscopy and polypectomy. *Dis Colon Rectum* **19**: 407.

Snyder DN, Heston JF, Meigs JW & Flannery JT (1977) Changes in site distribution of colorectal carcinoma in Connecticut 1940–73. *Am J Dig Dis* **22**: 791–797.

Southwood WFM (1962) Villous tumours of the large intestine: their pathogenesis, symptomatology, diagnosis and management. *Ann R Coll Surg Engl* **30**: 23.

Spirio L, Olschwang S, Groden J & et al (1993) Alleles of the APC gene: an attenuated form of familial polyposis. *Cell* **75**: 951–957.

Spratt JS, Ackerman LV & Mayer CA (1958) Relationship of polyps of the colon to colonic cancer. *Ann Surg* **148**: 682.

Staimmer D (1994) Erge bnisse der lokalen Therapie in der SGKRK-Studie und in Munchen–Neuperlach: In Hermanek & Marzoli (eds) *Lokale Therapie des Rektum Kurzinons*, pp 131–136. Heidelberg: Springer Verlag.

Steele RJC, Hershman MJ, McC Mortensen NJ, Armitage NCM & Scholefield JH (1996) Transanal endoscopic microsurgery: initial experience from three centres in the United Kingdom. *Br J Surg* **83**: 207–210.

Stemmermann GN & Yatani R (1973) Diverticulosis and polyps of the large intestine. *Cancer* **31**: 1260–1270.

Stewart MJ (1931) Precancerous lesions of the alimentary tract. *Lancet* **ii**: 617–619.

Stolte M & Bethke B (1995) Colorectal mini *de novo* carcinoma: a reality in Germany too. *Endoscopy* **27**: 286–290.

Stout AP (1959) Tumours of the colon and rectum (excluding carcinoma and adenoma). In Turell R (ed) *Diseases of the Colon and Anorectum*, p 295. Philadelphia: WB Saunders.

Strauss RJ, Gordon L & Wise L (1978) Colonoscopic prolapse and sigmoidoscopic removal of pedunculated polyps in the sigmoid colon. *Surg Gynecol Obstet* **48**: 439–440.

Sugarbaker PH, Vineyard GC, Lewicki AM et al (1974) Colonoscopy in the management of diseases of the colon and rectum. *Surg Gynecol Obstet* **139**: 341–349.

Susman W (1932) Polypi coli. *J Path Bact* **35**: 29.

Swinton NW & Haug AD (1947) The frequency of precancerous lesions in the rectum and colon. *Lahey Clin Bull* **5**: 84.

Symmers D (1948) Lymphoid disease: Hodgkin's granuloma, giant follicular lymphadenopathy, lymphoid leukaemia, lymphosarcoma and gastrointestinal pseudo leukaemia. *Arch Pathol* **45**: 73–131.

Taylor EW, Thompson H, Oates GD et al (1981) Limitations of biopsy in preoperative assessment of villous papillomas. *Dis Colon Rectum* **24**: 259–261.

Tedesco FJ, Waye SD, Avella JR & Villabos MM (1980) Diagnostic implications of the spatial distribution of colonic mass lesions (polyps and cancers): a prospective colonoscopic study. *Gastrointest Endosc* **26**: 95–97.

Theuerkauf FJ (1978) Rectal and colonic polyp relationships via colonoscopy and fibersigmoidoscopy. *Dis Colon Rectum* **21**: 2–8.

Thompson BW & Tucker WE (1987) Trans-sphincteric approach to lesions of the rectum. *South Med J* **80**: 41–43.

Thomson JPS (1985) St Mark's 150th Centenary Meeting.

Thomson WO, Gillespie G & Blumgart LH (1977) The clinical significance of pneumatosis cystoides intestinalis: a report of five cases. *Br J Surg* **64**: 590–592.

Tonelli F, Valanzano R & Brandi ML (1994) Pharmacologic treatment of desmoid tumors in familial adenomatous polyposis: results of an *in vitro* study. *Surgery* **115**: 473–479.

Tripp MR, Morgan TR, Sampliner RE et al (1987) Synchronous neoplasm in patients with diminutive colorectal adenomas. *Cancer* **60**: 1599–1603.

Van den Ingh HF, Griffoen G & Cornelise CJ (1986) Flow cytometric detection of aneuploidy in colorectal adenomas. *Cancer Res* **45**: 3392–3397.

Vatn MH, Myren J & Serck-Hanssen A (1985) The distribution of polyps in the large intestine. *Ann Gastroenterol Hepatol (Paris)* **21**: 239–245.

Veale AMO, McColl I, Bussey HJR & Morson BC (1966) Juvenile polyposis coli. *J Med Genet* **3**: 5.

Venkitachalam PS, Hirsch E, Elguezabai A & Littman L (1978) Multiple lymphoid polyposis and familial polyposis of the colon: a genetic relationship. *Dis Colon Rectum* **21**: 336–341.

Verse M (1908) Ueber die Histogenese der Schleimhautcarcinome. *Verch Disch Ges Pathol* **12**: 95.

Wagner JL, Tunis S, Brown M, Ching A & Almeida R (1996) Cost-effectiveness of colorectal cancer screening in average-risk adults. In Young G, Rozen P & Levin B (eds) *Prevention and Early Detection of Colorectal Cancer*. London: WB Saunders.

Walter JB & Israel MS (1967) *General Pathology*, 2nd edn. London: Churchill.

Watanabe T (1997) *Colorectal Surgical Course: Management of Malignant Polyps*. Ft Lauderdale: Cleveland Clinic.

Waye JD (1980) *Colonoscopy Techniques, Landmarks and Polypectomy*. Westwood, NJ: Medc.

Waye JD, Frankel A & Braunfield SF (1980) The histopathology of small colon polyps. *Gastrointest Endosc* **26**: 80.

Waye JD, Lewis BS & Yessayan S (1992) Colonoscopy: a prospective report of complications. *J Clin Gastroenterol* **15**: 1–4.

Webb WA, McDaniel L & Jones L (1985) Experience with 1000 colonoscopic polypectomies. *Ann Surg* **201**: 626.

Welch CE & Hedberg SE (1975) *Polypoid Lesions of the Gastrointestinal Tract*, pp 186–199, 2nd edn. Philadelphia: WB Saunders.

Welch JP & Welch CE (1976) Villous adenomas of the colorectum. *Am J Surg* **131**: 185–191.

Welin S (1967) Results of the Malmo technique of colon examination. *JAMA* **199**: 369.

Westbrook KC, Lang NP, Broadwater JR & Thompson BW (1982) Posterior surgical approaches to the rectum. *Ann Surg* **195**: 677–685.

Westhues M (1934) *Die pathologisch: anatomischen Grundlagen der Chirurgie des Rektumkazin ans*. Leipzig: Thieme.

Wetherall AP, Williams NMA & Kelly MJ (1993) Endoscopic transanal resection in the management of patients with sessile rectal adenomas, anastomotic stricture and rectal cancer. *Br J Surg* **80**:788–793.

Wheat MW Jr & Ackerman LV (1958) Villous adenomas of the large intestine. *Ann Surg* **147**: 476.

Whitlow CB, Beck DE & Gathright JB (1996) Surgical excision of large rectal villous adenomas (review). *Surg Oncol Clin N Am* **5**: 723–734.

Williams AR, Balasoorya BAW & Day DW (1982) Polyps and cancer of the large bowel: a necropsy study in Liverpool. *Gut* **23**: 835–842.

Williams CB (1973) Diathermy biopsy: technique for the endoscopic management of small polyps. *Endoscopy* **5**: 215.

Williams CB & Tan G (1979) Complications of colonoscopy and polypectomy. *Gut* **20**: A903.

Williams CB, Bartram CL, Bat L et al (1979) Bowel preparation with mannitol is hazardous. *Gut* **20**: A933.

Williams CB, Goldblatt M & Delaney P (1982a) Top and tail endoscopy and follow-up in Peutz–Jeghers syndrome. *Endoscopy* **14**: 82–84.

Williams CB, Macrae FA & Bartram CI (1982b) A prospective study of diagnostic methods in polyp follow-up. *Endoscopy* **14**: 74–78.

Williams GT (1994) Metaplastic polyposis. In Phillips RKS, Spigelman AD & Thomson JPS (eds) *Familial Adenomatous Polyposis and Other Polypoid Syndromes*, pp 174–186. London: Edward Arnold.

Williams GT, Arthur JF, Bussey HJR & Morson BC (1980) Metaplastic polyps and polyposis. *Histology* **41**: 155–170.

Williams NS, Nasmyth DG, Jones D & Smith AH (1984) Comparison of defunctioning stomas: a prospective controlled trial. *Br J Surg* **71**: 909.

Wilson GS, Dale EH & Brines OA (1955) Symposium on early diagnosis of tumours of rectum and colon: evaluation of polyps detected in 20,847 routine sigmoidoscopic examinations. *Am J Surg* **9**: 834.

Winawer SJ (Chair) (1980) *International Work Group in Colorectal Cancer*. Geneva: WHO.

Winawer SJ, Zauber AG, Stewart E et al (1991) The natural history of colorectal cancer: opportunities for intervention. *Cancer* **67**: 1143–1149.

Winawer SJ, Zauber AG, O'Brien MJ et al (1992) The National Polyp Study Work Group. Design, methods and characteristics of patients with newly diagnosed polyps. *Cancer* **70**: 1236–1245.

Winawer SJ, Zauber AG, Ho MN et al (1993) Prevention of colorectal cancer by colonoscopic polypectomy. *N Engl J Med* **329**: 1977–1981.

Wolff WI & Shinya H (1973) Polypectomy via the fiberoptic colonoscope. *N Engl J Med* **288**: 329.

Wolff WI & Shinya H (1975) Definitive treatment of malignant polyps of the colon. *Ann Surg* **182**: 516.

Wyatt AP (1975) Prolonged symptomatic and radiological remission of colonic gas cysts after oxygen therapy. *Br J Surg* **62**: 837–839.

Yao T, Tada S & Tsuneyoshi M (1994) Colorectal counterpart of gastric depressed adenoma: a comparison with flat and polypoid adenomas with special reference to the development of pericryptal fibroblasts. *Am J Surg Pathol* **18**: 559–568.

Yassinger S, Midgley RC, Cantor DS et al (1978) Retroperitoneal emphysema after colonoscopic polypectomy. *West J Med* **128**: 347–350.

Zauber AG, Bond JH & Winawer SJ (1996) Surveillance of patients with colorectal adenomas or cancer. In Young GP, Rozen P & Levin B (eds) *Prevention and Early Detection of Colorectal Cancer*, pp 195–215. London: WB Saunders.

29

POLYPOSIS SYNDROMES

Polyposis syndromes should be classified according to their histological type. The classification described by Morson (1962) is summarized in Table 29.1. For the surgeon, familial adenomatous polyposis and its variants, Gardner's syndrome and Turcot's syndrome, are the most important, since operative intervention is crucial in order to prevent malignant transformation.

Table 29.1 Classification of polyposis syndromes.

Neoplastic	*Hamartomatous*
Familial adenomatous polyposis	Juvenile polyposis coli
Gardner's syndrome	Peutz–Jeghers syndrome
Turcot's syndrome	Neurofibromatous polyposis
Lymphosarcomatous (lymphomatous) polyposis	Ruvalcaba–Myrhe–Smith syndrome
Leukaemic polyposis	Lipomatous polyposis
Inflammatory	Canada–Cronkhite syndrome
Ulcerative colitis	Cowden's disease
Crohn's disease	*Unclassified*
Other inflammatory polyposis: amoebiasis, schistosomiasis, eosinophilic polyposis, granulomatous polyposis, diffuse histoplasmosis	Metaplastic polyposis
	Pneumatosis cystoides intestinalis

Modified from Morson (1962).

NEOPLASTIC POLYPOSIS

Familial adenomatous polyposis (FAP)

Familial adenomatous polyposis is an inherited disease which is autosomal dominant and in which the colon primarily contains numerous adenomata (Figure 29.1). The disease is due to a mutation of the APC (adenomatous polyposis coli) gene located on the long arm of chromosome 5q21. The term 'familial polyposis coli' used to be applied to the disease, but with the realization that polyps frequently occur elsewhere within the gastrointestinal tract the term 'familial adenomatous polyposis' is now preferred. The syndrome used to be distinguished from that of multiple adenomata by the number of polyps present: if they exceeded 100, familial adenomatous polyposis was considered to be present (Bussey, 1975a). It is now known that there are several types of FAP, most of which are characterized by the presence of thousands of polyps. The condition is usually apparent during youth and the most important feature is that malignancy will invariably supervene, usually before the age of 40 years, if colectomy has not been performed. However, a much rarer variety has been identified which is known as 'attenuated adenomatous polyposis coli' (AAPC) and is characterized by a smaller number of colonic adenomas than is usually seen in typical FAP (Leppert et al, 1990); the average may be only 30. Furthermore, 70% of adenomas in AAPC are located proximal to the splenic flexure, a trait very different from typical FAP. This condition arises from mutations at the proximal end of the APC gene (Spirio et al, 1993). Colonic cancer seems to occur at a slightly older age than typical FAP, with the average age being 50 years.

Two case reports in the middle of the nineteenth century were probably the first descriptions of FAP (Corvisart, 1847; Chargelaigue, 1859). However, it was Cripps (1882) who realized and documented its familial association. There followed a paper by Handford (1890) which showed the malignant propensity of these polyps, and this was later confirmed by Lockhart-Mummery (1925). Since then numerous publications have demonstrated the very high risk of malignancy in these patients.

A variant of the disease, characterized by extra-

(a)

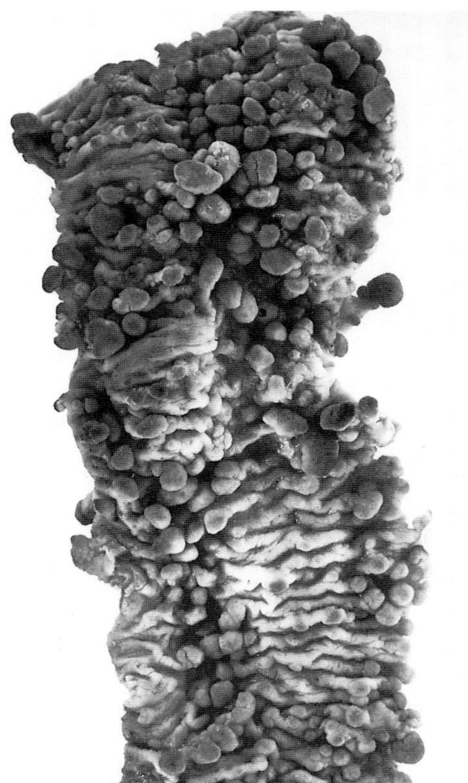

(b)

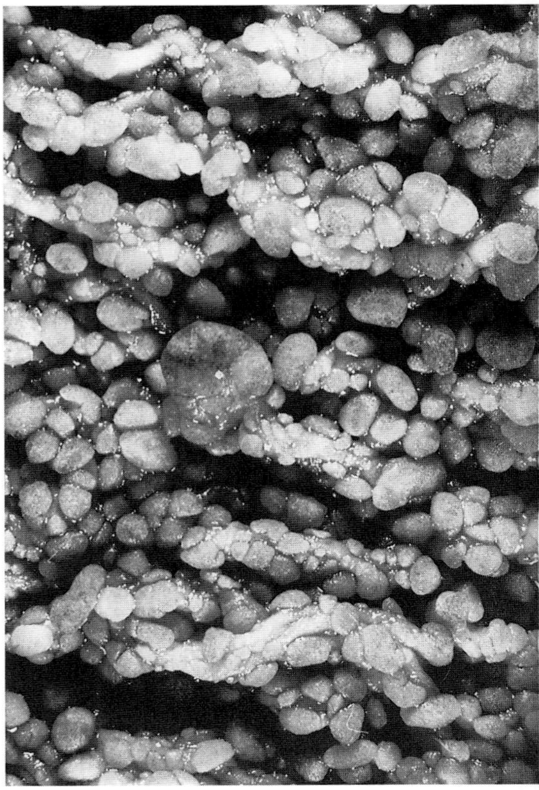

Figure 29.1a,b Colectomy specimen from a patient with familial adenomatous polyposis.

gastrointestinal lesions such as osteomata, cysts and soft tissue tumours, was described by Gardner in the early 1950s (Gardner, 1951; Gardner and Plenk, 1952; Gardner and Richards, 1953). Although he was not the first to describe the condition (Devic and Bussey, 1912; McKittrick et al, 1935), it has subsequently become known as Gardner's syndrome. Yet another variant of the syndrome was described by Turcot et al (1959) and later by others (Camiel et al, 1968; Baughman et al, 1969) and is characterized by malignant tumours of the central nervous system. Sometimes the neurological tumour presents before the polyposis is recognized (Rothman et al, 1975). It is thought that Turcot's syndrome differs from the other syndromes in its method of inheritance. A generation is frequently spared and this is thought by some to be due to variable gene penetrance (Smith and Kern, 1973). Others regard transmission of Turcot's syndrome as an autosomal recessive condition (Erbe, 1976; Itoh et al, 1979).

Genetics of FAP (see also Chapter 27)

Familial adenomatous polyposis and its variants are rare diseases. The basic disease is inherited as an autosomal dominant trait and is thus equally distributed between the sexes. The expression of the genetic defect is at least 80% and may be higher. Considerable progress has been achieved in understanding the genetic basis of the disease. Herrera et al (1986) and others (Augenlicht et al, 1987; Law et al, 1988) noted that there were alterations of gene structure and expression. Bodmer and his associates at the Imperial Cancer Research Foundation found that the primary defect was an allelic deletion of the long arm of chromosome 5 (Bodmer et al, 1987), a finding also observed by other groups (Leppert et al, 1987). Within four years of that discovery, the gene itself was identified and named the APC gene (Burt and Groden, 1993; Smith et al, 1993). It was also ascertained that most FAP families had separate and distinct mutations on the APC gene. However, the unifying feature of these mutations was that they were almost all severe mutations which resulted in truncation of the APC protein. The truncation is caused by the incidental occurrence of a 'stop' translation signal created by the mutation. Single base-pair mutations sometimes change the DNA base-pair triplet from one that codes for an amino acid to one that is a stop signal. More commonly, a one or two base-pair deletion or addition causes a 'frame shift' of the reading triplets, giving rise to an accidental stop triplet somewhere downstream from the mutation. Such mutations are called 'non-sense mutations'. The function of the APC gene probably relates to cell adhesion, as the APC protein attaches to catenin, which in turn attaches to E cadherin (Hamilton et al, 1995; Rubinfeld et al, 1993; Su et al, 1993a). E Cadherin is one of the major proteins involved in cell adhesion complexes. The APC protein also attaches to microtubules, although the significance of this observation is unknown. The APC gene appears to be a tumour suppressor gene. Functionally, this connotation implies that the normal gene function is to inhibit cell growth. A mutated and dysfunctional gene leads to release of growth control. At the molecular level, the term 'tumour suppressor gene' implies that both alleles of a gene must be mutated for function to be entirely lost. Several studies have indeed found that both copies of the APC gene are mutated in some but not all colonic polyps, and malignancies from patients with FAP (Su et al, 1993b; Ichii et al, 1992).

FAP, Garder's syndrome, most Turcot's syndrome families and AAPC all arise from mutations of the APC gene. It was hoped that the discovery of the APC gene would provide a molecular explanation of the difference between FAP and Gardner's syndrome. On the contrary, both conditions were not only found to arise from mutations of the same gene, but the location of the mutations within the APC gene did not distinguish between them. Furthermore, an identical APC mutation was found to give rise to FAP in one family and to Gardner's syndrome in another. Thus, a modifying gene is postulated, but not yet demonstrated as a possible explanation as to why some families exhibit prominent extraintestinal manifestions, while others do not (Burt and Petersen, 1996).

However, there are several specific correlations between the location of the disease causing mutations in the APC gene and certain clinical manifestations. Thus, the ocular signs, congenital hypertrophy of the retinal pigment epithelium (CHRPE) is present when the APC gene is distal to exon 9, but not if the mutation is proximal to that location (Olschwang et al, 1993). A higher density of colonic adenomas is observed when mutations are located in the central portion of exon 15 (Nagase et al, 1992) (Figure 29.2). This higher density was estimated to represent approximately 5000 adenomas in the colon with fully developed polyposis, compared with 1000–2000 adenomas that are generally observed.

As discussed above, mutations at the extreme proximal end of the APC gene give rise to the attenuated adenomatous polyposis coli (AAPC), which exhibits a smaller number (average 30) of colonic

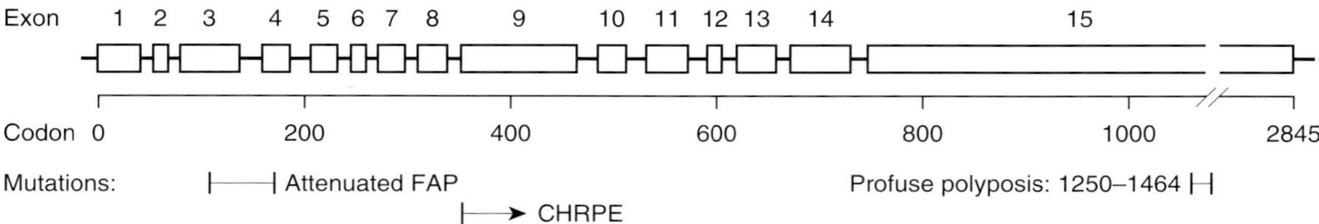

Figure 29.2 The adenomatous polyposis colon (APC) gene. A correlation between the clinical phenotype and location of APC mutations has been noted in profuse-type FAP, congenital hypertrophy of the retinal epithelium (CHRPE), and attenuated familial adenomatous polyposis (APC).

adenomas (Spirio et al, 1993). However, location of the mutation does not appear to be the only determinant of adenoma expression. One investigation described a polyp phenotype that varied between families with an identical APC mutation (Giardiello et al, 1994). Some affected persons had hundreds of colonic adenomas scattered equally throughout the colon, while others had colonic adenomatosis confined mostly to the distal colorectum. Either modifying mutations or environmental factors thus appear to be altering the effect of some disease-causing mutations.

Despite the inherited nature of the disease, in approximately 20% of patients there is no clear family history of the disease and in others it appears to have skipped a generation or two. Although this may be due to the difficulty in obtaining exact information in all cases about family members, it does appear that some cases result from spontaneous mutation of the APC gene (Fraser-Roberts, 1959; Veale, 1965a; Morson and Dawson, 1990).

Incidence and pathology of FAP

The incidence of familial adenomatous polyposis and its variants has been estimated to be between 1 in 7000 and 1 in 10 000 new births (Reed and Neel, 1955; Alm and Licznerski, 1973; Jarvinen, 1992; Rustgi, 1994; Burt, 1995). These estimates are imprecise because the condition is not obvious at birth and in rare instances may sometimes manifest itself only in the fourth or fifth decade.

Although the number of polyps in 'full blown' FAP is usually greater than 100, there may be considerable variation from case to case. For example, Bussey (1975a) found a range of 157 to 3673 with a mean of 981. The polyps also vary in size, but only 1% of them usually exceed 1 cm diameter. There is also variation in shape, with both sessile and pedunculated lesions being present, and in age of onset. The original development of the polyps and their speed of growth in any single patient varies greatly within a family. Of course the timing of surgical intervention in the natural history of the condition will also influence the number of polyps seen. Early detection in the offspring of affected individuals will tend to induce earlier surgical intervention with fewer polyps in the specimen, while late detection will result in the finding of more polyps. The distribution of polyps throughout the colon is of interest. Although all segments are invariably involved there seems to be a predilection for the left side. Up to the time of writing only two cases have been reported in the English literature in which the rectum was spared of the disease (Moertel et al,

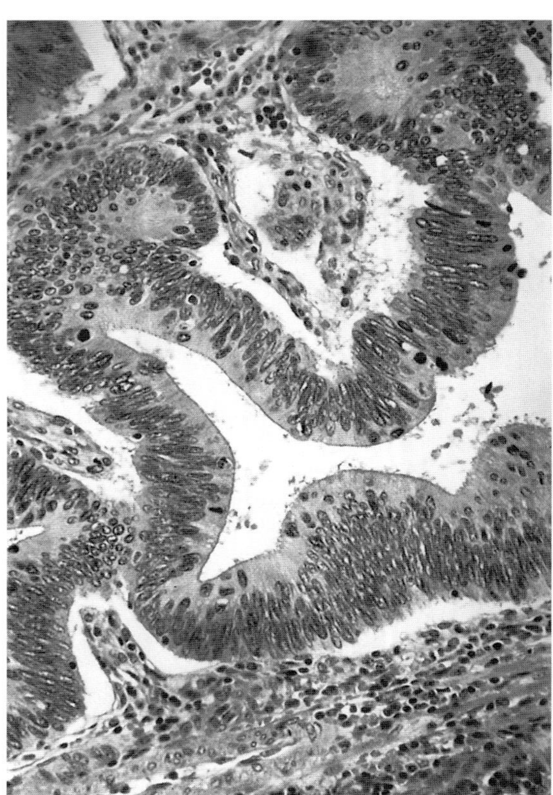

Figure 29.3 Common histological appearance in FAP of adenomatous polyps exhibiting high-grade dysplasia.

1970; Dick et al, 1984). In a few patients there seems to be a lack of polyps in the caecum and right side of the colon.

Histologically the adenomatous polyps seen in this condition are similar to those seen in non-polyposis patients. They are predominantly tubular adenomata but tubulovillous and villous adenomata are also seen.

All tumours are at first non-malignant and most of them remain so, but after an interval of several years carcinoma develops in one or more sites (Figure 29.3). Often the development of symptoms suggests that malignant transformation has occurred. Thus Alm and Licznerski (1973) found that 65% of symptomatic patients had developed malignancy, and Morson and Bussey (1970) noted a similar incidence (67%). These patients tend to develop multiple carcinomas, and in an analysis of 151 surgical specimens, 47.5% had multiple cancers (Bussey, 1975a), one patient having as many as seven.

Extracolonic polyps in FAP

In the past it was considered that polyps situated in parts of the gastrointestinal tract other than the colon were rare. Although there were numerous case reports attesting to their presence in the stomach and duodenum (Gardner and Richards, 1953; McKusick, 1962; Duncan et al, 1968; Hoffman and Goligher, 1971), the overall incidence was considered to be low. With the introduction of endoscopy it soon became clear that the coexistence of stomach and duodenal polyps was more frequent than previously realized, although there does seem to be some geographical variation. Thus, in three Japanese studies the incidence of associated adenomas in the stomach was approximately 36% (Utsunomiya et al, 1974; Ohsato et al, 1977; Watanabe et al, 1978), whereas only six gastric adenomas were diagnosed in 71 patients (8.4%) in three non-Japanese studies (Jarvinen et al, 1983a; Burt et al, 1984; Bulow et al, 1985). There is also, however, a condition termed 'fundic gland polyposis' which is frequently found in patients with FAP. In this condition there are multiple, sessile polyps in the fundus of the stomach, which histologically shows cystic, dilated fundic glands, and are considered to be hamartomas (Watanabe et al, 1978; Burt 1995). The condition was originally described in a Japanese population (Watanabe et al, 1978) but has been found in patients worldwide (Jarvinen et al, 1983a; Burt et al, 1984), and is considered to be present in 50–100% of affected individuals (Burt, 1995). Although for some time fundic gland polyposis was thought to be a specific manifestation of FAP, similar endoscopic and histological findings have been diagnosed in patients without colonic polyposis (Nishiura et al, 1984). The condition does not carry a malignant potential. From a practical standpoint, anyone who is found to have fundic gland polyposis on endoscopy should also have a colonoscopy to exclude FAP.

The incidence of duodenal adenoma seems to be far greater than that of gastric adenoma and is more consistent throughout the world. Initial reports from various countries demonstrated an incidence of 61–100% in series consisting of between 7 and 33 patients (Ushio et al, 1976; Ohsato et al, 1977; Jarvinen et al, 1983a; Burt et al, 1984; Ojerskog et al, 1987). Adenomata of the papilla of Vater were diagnosed in 12 of 24 patients (Iida et al, 1981) and biliary duct adenomas were found (Jarvinen et al, 1983a). Interestingly, there was often histological evidence of adenomatous change without the presence of macroscopic polyp formation (Ranzi et al, 1981; Burt et al, 1984; Bulow et al, 1985).

These retrospective findings led to a series of prospective studies using side-viewing as well as forward-viewing endoscopes. These prospective studies have tended to reveal an even higher incidence of duodenal and periampullary polyps. Thus, the Cleveland Clinic in 1987 found that only 33 of 100 patients had duodenal polyps (Sarre et al, 1987a), whereas Church et al (1992) reported 129 of 147 patients (88%). Similar findings were reported at St Mark's Hospital (Spigelman et al, 1989b, 1994) where duodenal polyps were present in 90% of patients in their prospective study, but in only 49% of their earlier retrospective study. They also found that the periampullary region was abnormal in 90% of patients, with 75% having definite adenomas, while the remaining 15% had either hyperplasia present or occasionally inflammation.

There is a serious risk of malignant change in these gastroduodenal lesions. Jagelman et al (1988) found that the incidence of upper gastrointestinal malignancy was 4.5% in 1255 FAP patients. In a review of 29 cases of periampullary carcinoma in FAP, an average interval of 16 years lapsed between diagnosis of the polyposis and the occurrence of the carcinoma. In addition, synchronous duodenal adenomas had been diagnosed in 50% of these patients at their initial presentation (Sugihara et al, 1982), evidence suggesting that the periampullary carcinomas developed from pre-existent adenomas. The incidence of periampullary cancer in FAP patients with extracolonic manifestation appears to be at least 12% (Bussey, 1975b). Church et al (1992) estimated that the risk of periampullary cancer in FAP patients was 100 times that of the non-polyposis population. Offerhaus et al (1992) from John Hopkins School of Medicine calculated that the relative risk (observed cancers over the number expected in the general population) was 331 for duodenal cancer and 124 for periampullary cancer. There was no excess risk for gastric cancer. However, it is interesing to note that in countries in which gastric cancer is prevalent, patients with FAP have a higher risk of developing this cancer than the normal population. In Korea this risk has been calculated to be seven times that of the non-FAP population (Park et al, 1992), and in Japan to be three times (Iwama et al, 1993).

Jejunal and ileal adenomas have also been found but their true incidence is difficult to determine. Confusion can arise if biopsy material is not obtained. Thus in a prospective study, Watanabe et al (1977) found that 9 of 16 patients had multiple, small polypoid masses in the terminal ileum which turned out to be benign lymphoid polyps. On the other hand, eight patients had true adenomata in the jejunum and three exhibited similar lesions in the ileum. Hamilton et al (1979) found terminal ileal adenomas in nine patients who had undergone previous colectomy and suggested that the occurrence of these lesions was related to the colectomy. Another study (Burt et al, 1984) in which the terminal ileum of nine patients was examined endoscopically showed that six of them had adenomata and three had lymphoid aggregates. Spigelman and Phillips (1994) have estimated that the incidence of jejunal adenomas is 40% and that of ileal adenomas is 10%. However, the malignant potential of these lesions is as yet unknown.

Pancreatico-hepatobiliary tumours in FAP

There have been numerous case reports of biliary tree neoplasms in FAP patients, and it appears that there is a significantly higher risk than for the general population (Walsh et al, 1987; Lees and Hermann, 1981; Jarvinen et al, 1983b). Similarly, there seems to be a particular prevalence for the development of hepatoblastoma (Kingston et al, 1982; Li et al, 1987; Garber et al, 1988; Hughes and Michels, 1991). These tumours tend to occur in childhood and measurement of serum alphafetoprotein may prove useful in diagnosis (Hughes and Michels, 1991; Schneider et al, 1992). Other hepatic tumours which seem to be more frequently found in FAP patients are hepatoma (Veale et al, 1965b) and hepatocellular carcinoma (Zeze et al, 1983; Laferla et al, 1988).

Clinical features of FAP

Familial adenomatous polyposis is characterized by the development of adenomas at about the age of puberty with the subsequent development of cancer during early adulthood. The natural history of the disease is very variable; some reports mention polyps and carcinoma developing in patients before puberty. At the other end of the spectrum there are occasional reports of polyps appearing in patients after the age of 40 years. It is suggested that late onset of polyps demonstrates a low degree of penetrance of the basic genetic defect. In the early stages of the disease there are few symptoms and it is desirable to detect the syndrome in asymptomatic family members when they are routinely screened. Bussey (1975a) suggested that the polyps are often present for 10 years before producing symptoms. Indeed, the development of symptoms is suggestive of malignancy. Bleeding and diarrhoea are the most frequent complaints followed by abdominal pain and mucous discharge. If weight loss, anaemia or intestinal obstruction supervene, a carcinoma is very likely to have developed.

Gardner's syndrome

Originally Gardner's syndrome was described as consisting of cutaneous cysts, osteomata and fibromata in addition to the polyposis. As time has progressed further extracolonic lesions have been described. Gardner's syndrome is a variant of FAP and, as explained previously, is due to the same mutations of the APC gene.

The absolute distinction between FAP and Gardner's syndrome has become somewhat blurred in recent years. For example, when panorex radiography was performed on persons from FAP families without clinically evident extraintestinal growths, up to 90% were found to have osteosclerotic lesions of the maxilla or mandible. Desmoid tumours (see below) and CHRPE lesions, in particular, do not correlate with other extraintestinal lesions and may occur in persons otherwise thought to have FAP (Burt & Petersen, 1996). Most importantly, Gardner's syndrome also arises from mutations of the APC gene. It is expected that genetic studies will soon determine why some families exhibit more prominent extraintestinal lesions than others.

Skin lesions

The cutaneous lesions are variously described as sebaceous cysts, pilar cysts or epidermoid cysts. Leppard (1974) found them histologically to be epidermoid cysts. They occur most commonly on the head, neck and arms, but can be seen on any part of the body. Although these cysts are common in the general population they are very uncommon before puberty. Development of cysts, particularly if epidermoid or multiple, in patients of this age group should alert the clinician to the possibility of FAP (Leppard, 1974; Bussey, 1975b).

Osteoma

The classic locations for osteomata are the mandible and maxilla. Localized thickening of the cortex of long tubular bones is the most common finding in some series (Watne et al, 1975). These bony lesions may be the only extracolonic lesions (Utsunomiya and Nakamura, 1975; Watne et al, 1975). Thus Utsunomiya and Nakamura (1975) surveyed 29 patients with known FAP using pantomography of the maxilla and mandible. They reported a characteristic finding of lesions approximately 3–10 mm in diameter with increased radiological density. This change was found in eight patients with known extracolonic manifestations and in 19 of 21 patients with polyposis and no other extracolonic manifestations. Similar findings were noted by Jarvinen et al (1982) and Iida et al (1981). These bony tumours may be present for many years before the onset of intestinal symptoms (Bussey, 1975b), and in view of the high incidence of these bony abnormalities it was suggested (Schuchardt and Ponsky, 1979) that radiographic surveys might ultimately serve as complementary screening tests for family members at risk. However, genetic testing has made these investigations superfluous.

Periampullary malignant disease

Cabot (1935) was perhaps the first to establish the possible association between periampullary carcinoma and FAP when he described the occurrence of a carcinoma at the ampulla of Vater in a 36-year-old man with FAP. MacDonald et al (1967) confirmed this association and several further case reports subsequently appeared (Melmed and Bouchier, 1972; Schnur et al, 1973). Both Jones and Nance (1977) and Sugihara et al (1982) have reviewed the literature and found that the average age at the time of diagnosis of malignant disease of the ampullary region was 45 years. The average time interval between diagnosis of the polyposis and detection of the duodenal lesion was 15.1 years (Jones and Nance, 1977). Current awareness of duodenal polyps and periampullary lesions, together with increasing expertise in end-viewing and side-viewing endoscopy, should help to reduce this time interval (Church et al, 1992; Spigelman and Phillips, 1994) (see before). Resection of the colon is no protection against periampullary carcinoma; approximately 12% of patients who survived 5 years after colectomy subsequently developed carcinoma of the duodenum, ampulla of Vater or pancreas (Bussey, 1975b).

Bile duct carcinoma

The relationship between duodenal polyps (particularly in the second part of the duodenum), bile duct carcinoma and ampullary cancer brings into focus the possible association between altered bile composition in the pathogenesis both of these tumours and of colonic cancers. We found only a small increase of a minor bile acid (12 oxo-lithocholate) in patients with FAP compared with controls, suggesting that bile acids are unlikely to be implicated in the aetiology of periampullary cancer (Barker et al, 1993).

Thyroid carcinoma

Crail (1949) and Camiel et al (1968) were the first to draw attention to an association between thyroid carcinoma and FAP. Several case reports (Smith and Kern, 1973; Keshgegian and Enterline, 1978; Lee and Mackinnon, 1981) have followed. A study on this subject from St Mark's Hospital (Plail et al, 1985) identified 7 of 449 women (1.6%) with polyposis who developed a carcinoma of the thyroid, but there were no cases in the 524 men studied. The authors calculated that women with FAP had approximately 40–50 times the risk of developing thyroid carcinoma compared with a normal subject. Papillary carcinoma seems to be the most frequent histological type but the association between these pathologies is nevertheless rare. In those patients in whom carcinoma of thyroid has been described it was usual for the thyroid lesion to precede the detection of the polyposis.

Dental abnormalities

Although abnormalities such as impacted supernumerary teeth, unerupted teeth, early cavities and dentigerous cysts (Figure 29.4), have been described in association with Gardner's syndrome (Gardner, 1969), some authors (Jarvinen et al, 1982) have

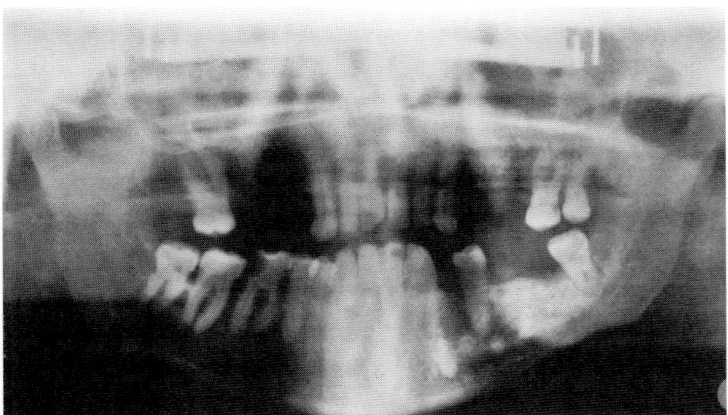

Figure 29.4 Radiograph of jaws showing numerous dental cysts in FAP (Gardner's variant).

found them to be no more common than in the general population.

Congenital hypertrophy of retinal pigment epithelium

There is a very high incidence (87.5–100%) of congenital hypertrophy of the retinal pigment epithelium (CHRPE) in Gardner's syndrome and FAP (Traboulsi et al, 1987; Berk et al, 1988; Lewis et al, 1988; Chapman et al, 1989) (Figure 29.5).

Three kinds of lesions have been detected on ophthalmoscopic examination, and they belong to one of two categories, namely those with or without a halo. The three kinds of pigmented lesions observed are (a) ovoid or round lesions with a dark frame or central pigmentation, (b) ovoid or round simple dark lesions, and (c) spotty or gathered spotty dark lesions (Iwama et al, 1990). Chapman et al (1989) observed CHRPE in all of 40 FAP patients drawn from 25 pedigrees. Traboulsi et al (1987) reported that 90.2% of patients with Gardner's syndrome had CHRPE. Similarly, Berk et al (1988) found that 87.5% of 40 FAP patients had similar lesions. It has also been demonstrated that individuals in the same family of affected patients show similar ocular manifestations (Iwama et al, 1990). Hence ophthalmological examination to detect CHRPE has been used for screening purposes in the past (Morton et al, 1992).

Other associated lesions

The occurrence of extracolonic polyps has been previously discussed and the incidence seems to be particularly high in Gardner's syndrome in contrast to FAP alone. Various case reports have suggested an association between a variety of miscellaneous conditions such as skin pigmentation (Weston and Weiner, 1967), carcinoma of the gallbladder (Burney and Asser, 1970), carcinoid of the small bowel (Heald, 1967), adrenal cancer (Marshall et al, 1967) and transitional cell carcinoma of bladder (Capps et al, 1968).

Desmoid tumours

Gardner considered that the fibrous masses found in the syndrome named after him were the most difficult to classify. It was Smith (1958, 1959) who first termed them 'desmoid tumours'. In a review of the literature he found four prior reports of desmoid tumours associated with colonic polyposis, includ-

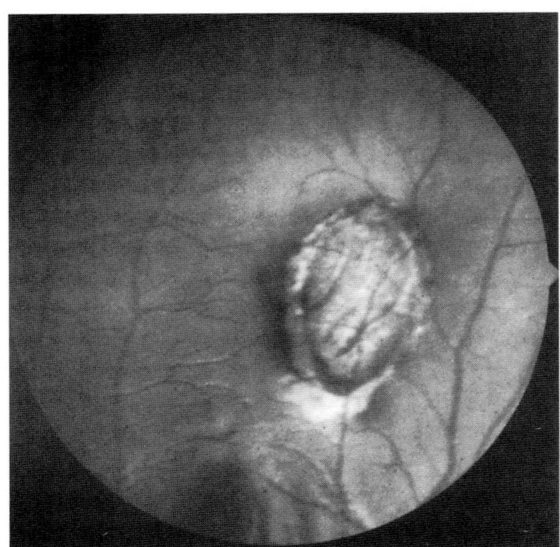

(a)

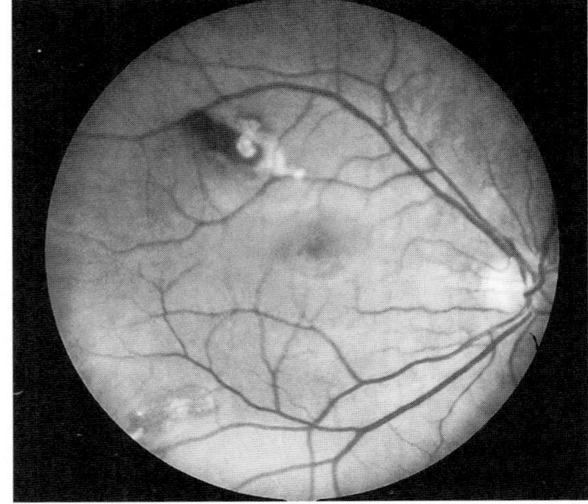

(b)

Figure 29.5a,b Congenital hypertrophy of retinal pigment epithelium in FAP.

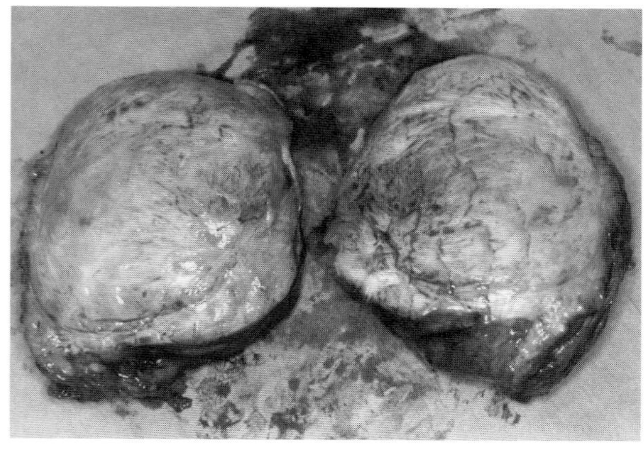

(a)

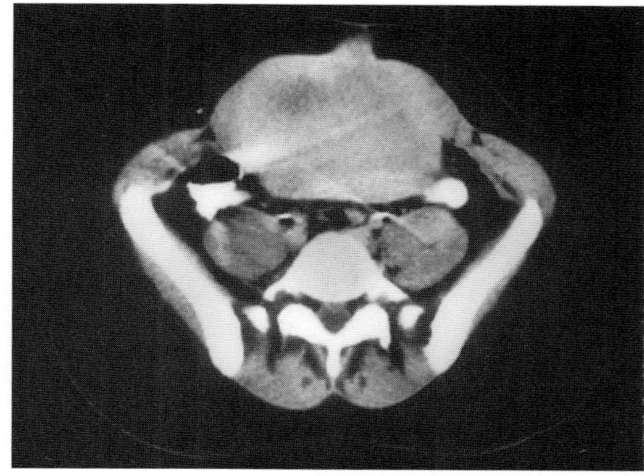

(b)

Figure 29.6a,b (a) Macroscopic appearance of desmoid tumour. (b) CT scan of abdominal wall showing desmoid tumour in a patient with FAP.

ing one of Gardner's original patients. These tumours occur most frequently in the abdominal wall (Figure 29.6) but may be found within the abdomen or pelvis. They may thus be classified according to site into extra-abdominal, abdominal-wall or intra-abdominal (Enzinger et al, 1967). Much has been learned about these tumours in recent years, particularly in relationship to FAP and the subject has been reviewed extensively in an excellent article by Clark and Phillips (1996).

Epidemiology

Desmoid tumours are rare with an incidence of less than 0.1% of all tumours (Pack and Ehlich, 1944; Dahn et al, 1963). However, about 2% of desmoids are FAP-associated, and FAP patients have about a 1000-fold greater risk of developing desmoids than the general population (Gurbuz et al, 1994). Incidences from 3.6% to 13% (Lockhart-Mummery, 1967; Lofti et al, 1989) have been reported from various registries. They have a peak incidence between 28 and 31 years of age (range 5 months to 80 years). Desmoid tumours are a frequent cause of morbidity and mortality in FAP patients and seem to be the second most common cause of death in some series, the first being colorectal cancer (Arvanitis et al, 1990; Iwama et al, 1993; Bertario et al, 1994). Desmoids are particularly renowned for making surgery very difficult in FAP patients, and this factor contributes to their impact on mortality (Penna et al, 1993a,b; Mao et al, 1995).

Aetiology and genetics

It seems that initiation by trauma, steroids and an underlying inherited defect are all involved, but the precise role of each is unknown (Clark and Phillips, 1996).

Between 68% and 86% of intra-abdominal and abdominal-wall desmoids in FAP occur within the first 5 years after abdominal surgery (Richards et al, 1981; Hayry et al, 1982; Jones et al, 1986; Lofti et al, 1989; Penna et al, 1993a; Gurbuz et al, 1994; Rodriguez-Bigas et al, 1994). Intra-abdominal desmoids may be particularly associated with surgical trauma, and in one series only 4% were found at the initial laparotomy (Penna et al, 1993a). On the other hand, only approximately 30% of sporadic abdominal-wall desmoids occur after surgery (Beradi and Canlas, 1973; Hayry et al, 1982). The relationship between desmoids and oestrogens is based mainly on circumstantial evidence. Thus, there is a higher incidence in females of reproductive age and a tendency for them to develop in pregnancy (Pack and Ehlich, 1944; Dahn et al, 1963; Brasfield and Das-Gupta, 1969; Harvey et al, 1979; Kinzbrunner et al, 1983). There have also been reports of regression after the manopause and after oophorectomy (Strode, 1954; Kollevold, 1973; Caldwell, 1976; Reitamo et al, 1982). Oestrogen binding sites have been identified in 25–75% of mixed desmoids (Hayry et al, 1982; Rivadeneyra and Santiago Payan, 1982; Lim et al, 1986). Some desmoid cells grow in culture in response to oestrogen, and this is inhibited by tamoxifen (Farelli et al, 1994).

Greater understanding of the genetic events which occur in FAP has resulted in information relating these events to the formation of desmoids. Some familial clustering of desmoids in patients with FAP has been noted (Gardner and Richards, 1953; Kinzbrunner et al, 1983; Klemmer et al, 1987; Lofti et al, 1989; Kitamura et al, 1991; Berk et al,

1992; Brooks et al, 1992; Eden et al, 1992) and an increased risk of developing desmoids in first-degree relatives has been identified (Gurbuz et al, 1994). These observations thus underline the possible hereditary nature of desmoid development.

Fibroblasts cultured from skin biopsies in patients with FAP show similar defects in the organization of cytoplasmic actin to those of tumour fibroblasts (Pfeffer et al, 1976, Kopelovitch et al, 1977; Rasheed and Gardner, 1981; Kopelovitch, 1984), abnormalities of growth pattern and increased susceptibility to viral transformation. These findings suggest that desmoid tumours are a phenotypic variant of FAP due to abnormal fibroblastic response caused by the effects of the germline mutation.

An important step in the adenoma–carcinoma sequence is a somatic mutation (second hit) in the remaining normal APC gene in the colonic epithelium (Levy et al, 1994; Smith et al, 1994). A clonal deletion of 5q bearing the normal copy of APC has been identified in an intra-abdominal desmoid in FAP (Dangel et al, 1994). Loss of heterozygosity in 5q 21–22 indicating loss of wild-type APC has also been demonstrated (Okamoto et al, 1990; Yoshida et al, 1991). Bridge et al (1992) described frequent clonal chromosomal arrangements, especially 5q deletion in fibroblasts from sporadic and FAP associated desmoids. These and other pieces of evidence suggest that desmoids may result from a 'second-hit' mutation followed by clonal expansion, and therefore are true neoplasms.

Pathology

Seventy per cent of desmoids in FAP are intra-abdominal, 15% occur in the abdominal wall and 15% are extra-abdominal (McAdam and Goligher, 1970; Richards et al, 1981; Jones et al, 1986; Gurbuz et al, 1994). About 80% of intra-abdominal desmoids are in the small bowel mesentery. Other sites include the transverse mesocolon, ligamentum teres and retroperitoneum; multiple sites are involved in 5–38% of cases (McAdam and Goligher, 1970; Reitamo et al, 1986; Burke et al, 1990a,b; Einstein et al, 1991; Gurbuz et al, 1994).

There is a spectrum of macroscopic appearance. In general those of the abdominal wall tend to be well encapsulated with a pearly, whorled appearance on the cut surface (see Figure 29.6a). They may show evidence of cystic degeneration or haemorrhage. Desmoids vary in size from 1 to 30 cm diameter. Mesenteric desmoids and retroperitoneal disease tend to be less well encapsulated and may take the form of dense fibromatosis with indistinct margins. There is no true capsule, and the desmoid grows compressing and infiltrating surrounding tissues such that the infiltrative margin may extend several centimetres beyond the palpable tumour margin. Eventually, small bowel, ureters and mesenteric blood vessels may become encased and obstructed (Clark and Phillips, 1996; Farmer et al, 1994).

Sporadic desmoids tend to grow slowly, but those that occur in FAP tend to be more aggressive (Burke et al, 1990b). Church (1995) has suggested that 10% of intra-abdominal desmoids in FAP regress completely, 29% undergo cycles of growth and resolution, 47% remain stable after diagnosis, and 10% grow rapidly. They do not metastasize.

Microscopically, desmoids consist of mature, highly differentiated fibroblasts in an abundant collagen matrix. Aggregates of lymphocytes are frequently located at the margins. There is a wide range of cellularity, often with acellular areas towards the centre of the tumour, and a dense cellular periphery, which consists of a preponderance of myoblasts (Kiryu et al, 1985; Hasegawa et al, 1990). The constituent cells have ill-defined cytoplasm and pale nuclei, mitoses are rare and nuclear atypia is absent.

Clinical features

Desmoids are often asymptomatic, being discovered incidentally on examination or at laparotomy. They can grow to a considerable size before causing symptoms and may present simply as a mass. In approximately one-third of cases pain is a predominant symptom. Tethering and compression of the small bowel can cause obstruction, and thus cachexia may be a problem. The mesenteric blood vessels may become occluded, resulting in intestinal ischaemia and consequent fistula and sepsis (Waddell, 1975; Keusch and Bauer, 1989; Doi et al, 1993).

Retroperitoneal desmoids in particular may cause ureteric compression, resulting in hydronephrosis and renal failure. Penna et al (1993a) reported that 27% of intra-abdominal desmoids caused hydronephrosis, perforation, impaired pouch function or obstruction requiring laparotomy. Desmoids, when found at laparotomy, may interfere with the planned surgery (Kyle and Keenan, 1992; Penna et al, 1993b).

It is important to realize that some FAP patients may present with a desmoid tumour before they develop colonic polyps. Thus the large bowel must be investigated when a sporadic desmoid is diagnosed and the patient must be followed up accordingly (McAdam and Goligher, 1970; Halata et al, 1989; Lofti et al, 1989).

Investigations

CT is the investigation of choice for demonstrating the presence of intra-abdominal desmoids (Baron and Lee, 1981; Magid et al, 1984, 1988; Einstein et al, 1991; Brooks et al, 1994) (see Figure 29.6b). Early mesenteric lesions appear as ill-defined soft tissue infiltration of mesenteric fat. Later, a mass may be seen, with displacement infiltration, tethering and encasement of small bowel loops. The tumours show mixed attenuation and variable enhancement.

MRI has advantages when investigating extra-abdominal desmoids. Not only does it have multi-planar imaging capabilities, but contrast resolution is superior to that of CT, particularly in the presence of postoperative or radiotherapy changes (Sundaram et al, 1988).

Several radio-isotopes are taken up by desmoids. Tc-99m (V) dimercaptosuccinic acid is taken up more reliably than gallium-97 citrate and has the advantage that scanning can be done hours rather than days after injection. This type of scanning may be useful in follow-up after treatment, as it has a greater sensitivity than CT in the differentiation of residual scarring from active disease (Hardoff et al, 1988; Kobayashi et al, 1994; Hudson et al, 1984). Intravenous urography plays a major role in follow-up of patients with intra-abdominal desmoids because of the high incidence of ureteric involvement, which in the early stages is often asymptomatic (Farmer et al, 1994).

Treatment

Treatment of desmoids is considered in detail later in the chapter.

Turcot's syndrome

Turcot's syndrome is an eponym given to familial polyposis in association with malignant tumours of the central nervous system. The syndrome was originally described by Turcot et al (1959) and was confirmed by others (Camiel et al, 1968; Baughman et al, 1969). Some authors have noted that the neurological condition may declare itself before the polyposis (Rothman et al, 1975).

Turcot's syndrome was thought to be a distinct clinical syndrome, and separate from FAP. However, it has now been demonstrated that most families with a clinical diagnosis of Turcot's syndrome have genetic mutations of the APC gene (Hamilton et al, 1995). Affected persons with brain tumours in these families usually develop medulloblastoma-type tumours. Additional malignancies include anaplastic astrocytomas and ependymonas. A smaller number of families with clinically defined Turcot's syndrome have been found to have mutations on one of the mismatch repair genes, the complex of genes mutated in HNPCC. The most common type of brain tumour in these individuals is glioblastoma multiforme. Although some overlap was observed, the colonic phenotype in families with APC mutations was usually the same as that seen in typical FAP, while that in families with mismatch repair gene mutations was similar to that expected in HNPCC: fewer larger adenomas and frequent multiple primary adenocarcinomas.

Diagnosis of FAP and its variants

Many patients with polyposis are asymptomatic and the diagnosis is often only made during screening of the family of a known patient. Since the rectum is rarely spared, digital examination of the rectum, sigmoidoscopy and biopsy are usually all that is required to confirm the diagnosis. Occasionally a young subject will present with bleeding per rectum and change of bowel habit, and careful questioning will reveal a family history of bowel problems.

The main differential diagnosis in these circumstances is inflammatory bowel disease or lymphoid hyperplasia, but colonoscopy will be diagnostic. Occasionally, when the latter is unavailable, sigmoidoscopy and barium enema should distinguish between these conditions (Figure 29.7). Difficulty might conceivably occur in the few cases where the rectum is spared of disease and the barium enema reveals polypoid disease. In this rare situation the pseudopolyps of ulcerative colitis should be easily distinguished from the true adenomata of FAP, since the latter occur in a haustral colon of normal calibre. In ulcerative colitis the colon is shortened and featureless, and usually exhibits other radiological features of the disease. However, in practice all such patients will nowadays undergo colonoscopy when the appearance of the polyps together with their histological examination will differentiate the condition from other forms of polyposis.

Once the diagnosis has been established, all patients should have a thorough investigation of the rest of the gastrointestinal tract, including upper gastrointestinal endoscopy with a side-viewing scope and a small bowel barium meal to establish the presence of extracolonic neoplasms. As stated,

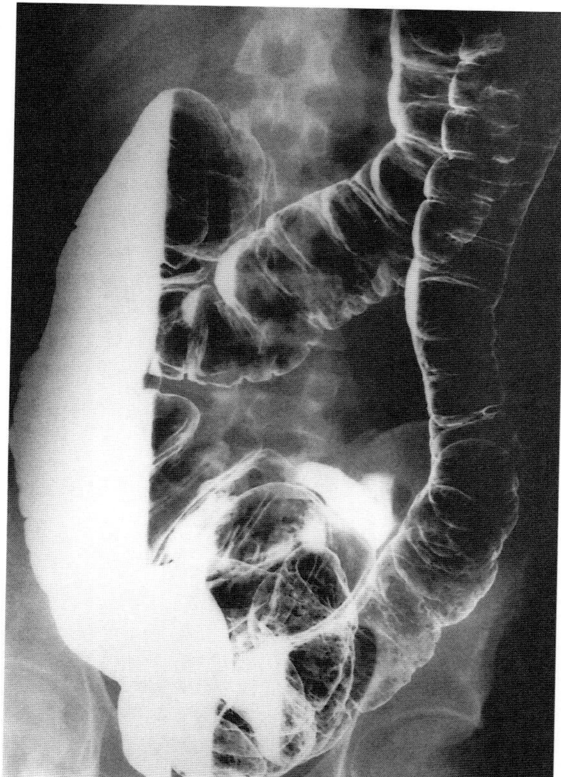

Figure 29.7 Double-contrast barium enema in a patient with FAP.

colonoscopy is essential, not only to confirm the diagnosis, but also to establish if any of the polyps have undergone malignant change (Goligher, 1984). It might be argued that once the diagnosis has been made the patient needs a colectomy anyway and colonoscopy is unnecessary since the findings will not influence management; we do not subscribe to this view, since the diagnosis is usually made during family screening for disease and the patients are likely to be in their early 'teens. Under these circumstances the impact of a major operation on a child's potential educational attainment must be taken into consideration. Surgery is therefore planned either before important school examinations become a hurdle, usually at the age of 13 years, or between school and higher education at 18 years. For this reason a colonoscopic assessment of the size and number of the polyps together with exclusion of malignant change plays an important role in the timing of surgical treatment. If the polyps are large and very numerous we usually favour early colectomy.

If there are no obvious extragastrointestinal manifestations of the other variants of the disease, it is worth performing skull and jaw radiography to determine if oesteomata are present. Similarly a CT scan of the head is worthwhile to eliminate brain tumours which are features of Turcot's syndrome.

In patients who initially just present with extragastrointestinal manifestations, enquiry about bowel habit and family history are essential. This is particularly important with patients who present with the more bizarre features of the disease such as desmoid tumours or multiple sebaceous cysts, especially when the latter occur in young people. A rectal examination and sigmoidoscopy must always be included in the investigation of these patients.

Genetic testing for FAP and its variants

The identification of the APC gene has allowed the development of genetic testing for the diagnosis of FAP. These tests use DNA, which is most often purified from white blood cells obtained at phlebotomy. Three types of tests have been developed: (1) linkage tests, (2) *in vitro* truncated protein testing, and (3) mutation tests.

Linkage testing

In these tests small fragments of polymorphic DNA that lie very near or even within the APC gene are used to track the mutant APC gene in a family. Once a clinical diagnosis has been made in two family members, these DNA markers can be used to make genetic diagnoses in other at-risk family members. DNA markers in and around the APC gene are now of sufficient accuracy that over 95% of individuals in families with known FAP can be diagnosed with greater than 98% accuracy (Petersen et al, 1990; Burt and Groden, 1993).

In vitro *truncated protein (IVTP) testing*

IVTP testing (also called the transcription translation assay) takes advantage of the observation that most disease-causing mutations in FAP result in truncation of the APC gene (Powell et al, 1993). DNA is first amplified in the test-tube by the polymerase chain reaction. It is then processed to RNA by *in vitro* transcription and finally to protein by *in vitro* translation. The protein is then placed on an electrophoretic gel that separates by size. All patients with FAP have two alleles, a normal and a mutated allele. The *in vitro* process described will thus result in APC protein of normal length and a truncated protein. Two bands will be seen if a mutation is present in one of the alleles. If both alleles are normal, both proteins are of identical length and only one band is seen on the electrophoretic gel. This method can detect a mutation in up to 87% of individuals with FAP. However, once a mutation is observed in one family member, the accuracy for other family members approaches 100%.

Mutation testing

This is the optimal test since it directly detects the presence of the mutation in the APC gene (Peterson et al, 1993). Bacterial enzymes known as 'restriction enzymes' cut DNA at a site with a specific base-pair sequence. Once the specific mutation in an FAP family is identified, a restriction enzyme is designed to detect the new base-pair sequence defined by the mutation and make a cut in the DNA at that point.

To perform mutational testing, DNA is first amplified by the polymerase chain reaction, and the specific restriction enzyme is applied. The DNA is then placed on the electrophoretic gel. If no mutation is present, a single band is observed. If one allele is mutated, two bands are seen, one repressing the normal allele and one the mutated allele. Three bands may also be seen depending on the size of the fragments in the mutant allele.

Comparison of the tests

Both linkage testing and IVTP testing are now available for the diagnosis of FAP. Linkage testing costs about 100 dollars per person, whereas IVTP costs approximately 1000 dollars. However, linkage testing requires that a firm clinical diagnosis be made in at least two family members before others can be diagnosed. On the other hand, IVTP can make a diagnosis in an individual patient independent of the family setting. Unfortunately it will diagnose the presence of the mutation in only 87% of families. However, once the mutation has been identified, the test is virtually 100% in the other family members. Direct detection of the mutation is clearly optional, but is made difficult as most FAP families have a different and distinct mutation of the FAP gene. Finding that mutation may be very difficult and at present is limited to only a few research laboratories.

Principles of management of FAP

The principles of management are to treat the patient before a carcinoma develops and to detect the disease in other members of the family.

Screening of family members

It is necessary first to establish a family tree so that all family members at risk can be identified. This may prove a difficult task but help is now available from clinical geneticists. Accurate documentation of two or three generations of a family involves a considerable amount of detection work, but clinical genetic departments are adept at this task and being non-surgical are less of a threat to families who naturally fear that all their relatives may require an operation. This neutral group of professionals are the best people to explain to each family member the risks involved and to combine genetic screening and fundal examination before sigmoidoscopy is necessary. In order to assist in these tasks, several surgical units have set up polyposis registries in collaboration with their geneticist colleagues (see below).

The children of patients with FAP have a 50% chance of developing the disease. Genetic testing should generally not be done before the age of 12 years because of issues of parental bonding, self-image and peer rejection. IVTP testing should first be performed in the affected family member. If testing is positive in that person, it will work with a high degree of accuracy for other family members. If a diagnosis cannot be made with the IVTP method, then linkage testing should be done in that family. Those who test positive should have annual or biannual flexible sigmoidoscopy to determine the emergence of colonic adenomas. Clinical screening should still be done in those who test negative by linkage testing because of the small chance of error with this method. In these individuals, surveillance of the colon should commence at puberty since this will limit the psychological damage associated with repeated examinations. All available data suggest that no case of carcinoma will be missed if colonic surveillance starts at this age.

As stated above, flexible sigmoidoscopy should now be used in preference to rigid sigmoidoscopy as a method of diagnosis when screening for FAP. It allows the distal sigmoid colon to be examined in most cases and thus FAP will not be overlooked in the few patients with rectal sparing. The frequency of repeat examination is empirical; some units have recommended twice-yearly visits for patients up to 40 years old (Bulow, 1991). Most patients will develop polyps before the age of 40 years if they are going to do so, but there are a few who will develop them after this age (Lockhart-Mummery, 1967): hence colonic surveillance should probably continue, albeit less frequently, up to the age of 60 years. Surveillance of the duodenum must also be undertaken using a side-viewing endoscope to detect duodenal polyps and periampullary carcinoma. It is now recommended that this should be performed at least every 3 years once colonic adenomas are detected. However, if prominent lesions are found in the duodenum, yearly endoscopies are recommended (Burt and Petersen, 1996).

Because of the high diagnostic sensitivity and specificity of CHRPE, it is now generally agreed that ophthalmoscopy involving wide-angle fundus photography should be used as a supplementary screening method in unaffected first-degree relatives.

Orthopantomography detection of multiple osteomata in the mandible has also been used as a screening method (Bulow et al, 1986). However, taking into consideration the detection of the FAP gene, the high diagnostic sensitivity of CHRPE and the lower diagnostic sensitivity of pantomography, this method can no longer be recommended as a screening method (Hunt et al, 1993).

Patients frequently seek advice about having children. We believe this is beyond the remit of the surgeon and it is better for geneticists to explain fully the risks of this condition. Information will have to include the risks associated with extraintestinal disease as well as the development of carcinoma in sites other than the colon. Now that the APC gene has been detected, genetic testing makes it possible to estimate the risk for FAP of an unborn child. A chorionic villus sample can be taken by biopsy at 10 weeks of pregnancy and linkage analysis or probing for the mutation (if known for that family) can be performed on the sample. Burn et al (1991) found that in a group of 66 patients (25 affected, 27 spouses and 14 at-risk individuals), approximately 70% would request prenatal testing. However, only 12 patients (18%) would consider termination of pregnancy.

Polyposis registries

To improve the prognosis of polyposis patients, various registries have been established. The first of these was established by Lockhart-Mummery in 1925 at St Mark's Hospital (Bussey, 1975a). Since then national registers have been established in Sweden, Denmark, Norway, Finland, The Netherlands, Poland and Japan (Alm and Licznerski, 1973; Jarvinen et al, 1984; Bulow, 1986; Gedde-Dahl et al, 1989; Krokowicz, 1989; Vasen, 1989; Utsunomiya et al, 1990) and several regional registers have been initiated all over the world (Rhodes et al, 1991; Morton et al, 1993). The impact of the registries on prognosis has been well illustrated by the highly significant difference in incidence of colorectal cancer between offspring probands of individuals with FAP examined as a result of that individual being diagnosed and call-up cases diagnosed as a result of a prophylactic examination (Bulow, 1986; Vasen, 1989; Krush and Giardello, 1990; Neale et al, 1990). For instance, in the Danish study of the diagnosis of FAP, 67% of probands had carcinoma in contrast to only 2% among call-up cases (Bulow, 1991). Furthermore, the Danish figures show a significant improvement in the prognosis of the total group of polyposis patients after the establishment of the registry (Bulow, 1986). In order to improve understanding of the disease, representatives of the major polyposis centres have established an international research forum (Thomson, 1988; Herrera, 1990). This group, established in 1985 and known as the Leeds Castle Polyposis Group, has planned various multicentre studies of both clinical and basic scientific aspects.

Treatment of colonic polyps

Treatment of familial adenomatous polyposis is influenced by the natural history of the disease, which is variable. Although there is evidence that regression of polyps in FAP can be achieved occasionally by long-term non-steroidal anti-inflammatory drugs (NSAIDs), surgery is the mainstay of therapy (Waddell and Loughry, 1983; Waddell et al, 1989; Labayle et al, 1991; Rigau et al, 1991; Giardiello et al, 1993; Nugent et al, 1993a; Spagnesi et al, 1994). If patients are left long enough without a colectomy they will all develop carcinoma. The average age at which symptoms develop is about 20 years and the average age at which carcinoma is detected is 35 years. However, in a number of recorded cases malignant change has taken place at 15–20 years of age (Bussey, 1975a); it therefore seems wise in most patients to proceed to surgical resection before this age. Importantly, it has been shown that despite the development of polyposis registries, with consequent careful screening and follow-up, colonoscopy is not a reliable screening test for malignancy in patients with established polyps. Prophylactic colectomy is therefore strongly indicated (Mills et al, 1997).

The procedure of choice for FAP is the subject of much debate at present, particularly since the advent of restorative proctocolectomy (RPC) (Parks and Nicholls, 1978). The other options are colectomy and ileorectal anastomosis (IRA), proctocolectomy, or colectomy and rectal mucosectomy but without restoration of gastrointestinal continuity.

Conventional panproctocolectomy has the advantage of eliminating all colorectal polyps and virtually eliminating the risk of carcinoma of the large bowel. However, this operation does not protect against ampullary or small bowel malignancy. In addition there is the burden of an ileostomy in a condition where 50% of family members are at risk of disease, and the patient is exposed to the small risk of pelvic nerve damage with resulting bladder and sexual problems. Also there is a perineal wound, which although less likely to break down than after proctocolectomy for inflammatory bowel disease, may leave the patient with a persistent sinus. Intersphincteric excision of the rectum reduces the risk of pelvic nerve injury and rectal mucosectomy eliminates problems with the perineal wound. The risk with a long rectal mucosectomy is that all the diseased mucosa may not be removed and there is then a slight risk of carcinoma developing in any remnant left behind. The overwhelming disadvantage, however, of any procedure that leaves behind a permanent ileostomy is that it is a poor advertisement of treatment for other members of the family. Although a patient with an ileostomy can lead a full and active life, it is hard to convince a young and active family member, who may well be asymptomatic, to undergo such a procedure. It is for this reason that sphincter-saving procedures such as colectomy with ileorectal anastomosis or restorative proctocolectomy have become popular.

The procedure of colectomy and ileorectal anastomosis has the advantage that gastrointestinal continuity is restored and bowel function is reasonable. Its disadvantage is that polyps are left in the rectum with the potential for malignant change. To prevent this unfortunate outcome the patient needs to be followed up regularly to attend to rectal polyps. Repeated endoscopy is needed so that repeated fulguration of residual and newly formed polyps can be performed. Not only can this procedure be uncomfortable, it also requires the patient to return repeatedly for sigmoidoscopic examination. In addition, although it would seem logical, if the adenoma–carcinoma sequence is accepted, that removal of polyps removes the risk of carcinoma, this does not necessarily follow. There is evidence to suggest that carcinoma can develop *de novo* in rectal mucosa not occupied by polyps.

The operation of restorative proctocolectomy has the advantage that the disease is eradicated, gastrointestinal continuity is restored, continence is maintained, and follow-up involving sigmoidoscopy is not necessary in terms of preventing cancer. Although function after RPC appears to be slightly inferior to that after IRA (Table 29.2), there is little to choose between the two operations. Thus, although frequency of defecation and night evacuation are more common after RPC (Madden et al, 1991; Ambroze et al, 1992), other end-points, including anal irritation, dietary restriction, antidiarrhoeal medication, quality of life and continence, are little different. There is less urgency of defecation after RPC (Madden et al, 1991), but one study has reported a higher incidence of night incontinence (Ambroze et al, 1992).

Nevertheless, restorative proctocolectomy is potentially a complex procedure, especially in a fat man, and although mortality is very low, morbidity may be high. Although results are steadily improving the procedure is still developing and the long-term results in FAP are unknown. Further modifications may be desirable before it can be categorically accepted as the operation of first choice for all patients with FAP.

The conventional policy in many units dealing with these patients was to perform a colectomy and ileorectal anastomosis in the first instance, provided

Table 29.2 Complications and function following surgery for familial adenomatous polyposis.

	*St Mark's Hospital, 1977–89**		*Mayo Clinic, 1978–88†*	
	RPC (*n* = 37)	*IRA* (*n* = 62)	*RPC* (*n* = 94)	*IRA* (*n* = 21)
Complication rate (%)	57	21	26	17
Re-laparotomy rate (%)	24	3	5	6
Frequency per 24 h	4.5 (2–15)‡	3 (1–11)‡	5 (2)§	4 (2)§
Urgency (<15 min) (%)	17	50	–	–
No. of night evacuations	43	10	1 (1)§	1 (1) §
Normal continence (%)	60	72	87	83
Fulguration of rectal polyps (%)	–	44	–	61

* Madden et al (1991); † Ambroze et al (1992). There were no deaths in either series. Values are ‡ median (range) and § means (SD). RPC, restorative proctocolectomy; IRA, colectomy with ileorectal anastomosis.
From Setti-Carraro and Nicholls (1996).

patients were likely to be reliable in attending for follow-up. Follow-up at regular 6-month intervals was usually necessary so that rectal polyps if present could be destroyed by fulguration. This policy is changing not only because of the advent of restorative proctocolectomy, but also because of the risk of developing rectal cancer after ileorectal anastomosis. Our view is that today restorative proctocolectomy should usually be the operation of choice to prevent colorectal cancer in FAP. However, most patients will never have experiencd an ileostomy, and, as they are fit, asymptomatic adolescents, the surgical outcome must be fully explained since bowel habit is permanently altered by this operation.

Carcinoma risk after colectomy and ileorectal anastomosis

There is considerable controversy concerning the incidence of carcinoma following colectomy and ileorectal anastomosis. The evidence against ileorectal anastomosis comes mainly from the Mayo Clinic. Moertel et al (1970) found that in 145 patients treated by subtotal colectomy and ileorectal anastomosis there was a continuing risk of rectal cancer, which was 25% at 15 years of follow-up and 59% after 23 years. They found that women were at greater risk than men and that the incidence was markedly increased if the patient had a carcinoma in the resected colon. Another factor with important clinical application was that the risk of carcinoma was considerably reduced if there were fewer than 20 polyps in the rectum compared with patients having more than 100. Some doubt has since been expressed about how many of these patients actually had a true ileorectal anastomosis. It would appear that many underwent an ileosigmoid anastomosis and it is unknown what influence the latter procedure might have had on the outcome, particularly since surveillance following this operation is more difficult than after a true ileorectal anastomosis (Jagelman, 1983).

Fuel for the controversy was further supplied by reports from other centres, notably St Mark's Hospital, which showed a low incidence of carcinoma development. Thus Bussey (1975a) reported a series of 89 patients treated by true ileorectal anastomosis and 6-monthly surveillance. Included in this series were 47 patients followed for 10 years, 27 followed for 15 years and 13 followed for 20 years. Only two patients (2.2%) developed a carcinoma, both of which were Dukes' A lesions, and both patients survived. Schaupp and Volpe (1972) found that only one of 36 patients (3%) developed colorectal cancer; 30 patients had been followed for 10 years and five for 20 years. Similarly, Gingold et al (1979) from the Cleveland Clinic found no case of carcinoma in 25 patients followed for 10–20 years after ileorectal anastomosis for polyposis. Hubbard (1957) found that only one of 17 children (5.8%) developed rectal carcinoma during a mean follow-up of 8 years. The latest data from St Mark's paints a somewhat different picture of 222 patients with FAP treated by subtotal colectomy and ileorectal anastomosis, and followed up for 20 years. Fifty-three have died, of whom 29 developed intestinal malignancy. There are now 24 patients (12%) who are known to have developed a rectal carcinoma (Nugent et al, 1993c). The risk of rectal cancer at St Mark's was greatly influenced by the age at which a subtotal colectomy and IRA was performed. Patients having prophylactic surgery over 35 years of age had a much higher incidence of later cancer in the rectal stump than the younger group. Furthermore, the risk of cancer depended on the length of follow-up. They therefore propose that subtotal colectomy and IRA is still the operation of choice in young patients, but that conversion to RPC may be advised later in life, particularly if rectal polyps are numerous or difficult to clear.

Undeterred by earlier reports from St Marks and other centres, the Mayo Clinic reassessed their data (Bess et al, 1980). After elimination of patients who were found on histological review not to have adenomatous polyps, and of those who had invasive carcinoma of the rectum at the time of colectomy or who died immediately postoperatively, they found that 46 (32%) of 143 patients developed a carcinoma during a median follow-up period of approximately 20 years. Similarly, data from the Japanese Registry showed a 37% risk of developing rectal cancer over a 20-year period (Iwama et al, 1993). Heiskanen and Jarvinen (1997) from the Finnish Registry have demonstrated a 25% risk over 20 years. Multivariate analysis of the Mayo Clinic data showed a highly significant association between the number of rectal polyps present preoperatively and the survival period free from rectal cancer. Once more there was a strong correlation between the presence of cancer in the resected colon and subsequent development of rectal cancer. Since the length of the rectal stump had previously been suggested as the reason for differences between the Mayo Clinic results and those from other centres, this factor was assessed. De Cosse et al (1977) had suggested that there was considerably less risk with an anastomosis sited at least 15 cm distally; Bess et al (1980) analysed their results according to whether the anastomosis was performed above or below this level. The lower anastomosis did not afford better protection from the subsequent development of cancer. Of particular importance was the finding that 24 (52%) of the 46 cancers developed within 10 cm of the anal sphincter. Reservations were expressed about these data since the number of patients with low anastomoses (n = 23) was considerably smaller and the follow-up shorter than those with high anastomoses (n = 80). Indeed, other studies have now shown that patients with a rectal stump longer than 10 cm (Iwama et al, 1993) or 15 cm (Bulow, 1984; Sarre et al, 1987b; De Cosse et al, 1992) are at increased risk.

Genetic factors may also be important. Thus, a type of mutation in the APC gene has been described that is associated with a particularly severe phenotype of FAP (Caspari et al, 1994). Death from colorectal cancer occurred in patients with this mutation about 10 years earlier than in those with other mutations.

Making recommendations from these contradictory data – particularly at a time when restorative proctocolectomy is not fully tested – is clearly difficult. There is no doubt that there is a risk of developing carcinoma after colectomy and ileorectal anastomosis which relates to the number of polyps in the rectum, the age of the patient and the presence of coexisting carcinoma. This may also be related to how much colorectum remains. Genetic factors may also be involved, and in the future will need to be taken into consideration. There may be a geographic difference, with a lower incidence in the UK compared with the USA. Consequently there has been general unease about performing colectomy and ileorectal anastomosis in the USA which has not until recently affected surgeons in the UK to the same degree.

Conclusions and recommendations

The choice between RPC and IRA is governed by the various factors discussed above. However, it should be realized that because rectal cancer after colectomy and IRA is only one cause of death in patients with FAP, RPC will make only a small contribution to the reduction in mortality rate (Setti-Carraro and Nicholls, 1996). Nevertheless, since there is little to choose between the two procedures from a functional point of view, the choice should be based on the perceived risk of developing cancer in the rectum. Those at particular risk include patients over the age of 30 years and those presenting with symptoms or uncontrollable rectal adenomas. Similarly, those patients who present with a non-metastatic colorectal cancer or who have a strong family history of rectal cancer, or in whom long-term follow-up cannot be guaranteed, should have an RPC. On the other hand, those with metastatic cancer and those with desmoid tumours at operation or a family history of such (Ambroze et al, 1992) should undergo IRA. Asymptomatic patients under the age of 30 years with a relatively spared rectum may be offered a colectomy and IRA, provided follow-up is assured. The length of the rectal stump should not exceed 10–15 cm. However, one suspects that as more centres become adept at RPC and the morbidity falls, this operation will become the first-choice procedure for all patients, as it has in our centres.

Technique of colectomy and ileorectal anastomosis (IRA)

Colectomy and ileorectal anastomosis are carried out in virtually an identical fashion to the operation described for ulcerative colitis in Chapter 47. There are, however, a few points that require emphasis when the operation is used to treat patients with polyposis. Particular care must be exercised in mobilizing the distal sigmoid colon and upper rectum to avoid damage to pelvic autonomic nerves. No more than 10–15 cm of distal rectum should be left; hence the anastomosis is sited at the level of the peritoneal reflection. The resulting rectal stump should then provide adequate reservoir function and at the same time allow the rectal mucosa to be easily surveyed by routine outpatient sigmoidoscopy.

The ileum should be divided obliquely between crushing clamps at approximately 7–10 cm from the ileocaecal junction. A soft clamp should be placed proximally on the ileum and the crushing clamp cut off. The lumen of the ileum should then be inspected for the presence of polyps: if polyps are absent the anastomosis can proceed; if they are present, localized to a small segment of the distal ileum and are of moderate size, the involved segment may be resected or the polyps snared; if they are small and infrequent the polyps can be ignored provided their presence is noted. A preoperative small bowel barium meal should assist the decision-making.

The anastomosis may be end-to-end, but if there is considerable discrepancy in lumen size we prefer a side-to-end anastomosis (side of ileum to end of rectum). The anastomosis can be performed in either one or two layers depending on the surgeon's preference.

Results

Mortality and morbidity

Bess et al (1980) reported 11 deaths in 203 patients (5%) and non-fatal complications occurred in 13% of patients. The data from St Mark's Hospital are more reassuring, with a mortality of 1.6% in 174 patients, although morbidity (11%) was similar to that reported by Bess and associates; 11 patients developed intestinal obstruction and five had an anastomotic breakdown (Bussey et al, 1985). Since the pelvis is not dissected, sexual function is not at risk (Jagelman, 1991, Ambroze et al, 1992).

Bowel function and quality of life

These factors were extensively investigated by Alm (1975) over a long period in 48 patients who had undergone colectomy and ileorectal anastomosis for polyposis. All patients were continent. Within 2–3 months of the operation more than 50% of patients had fewer than five stools per 24 hours, after 5 years almost 60% of them had one or two stools per day and none had more than four. Although the stools gradually became more formed their consistency was largely influenced by the patient's diet. Sexual disturbances that could be attributed to the operation were not encountered. All patients were able to return to school, to continue their profession or education, or return to full-time employment by 1–2 months after operation.

These data indicate that excellent functional results may be achieved after this procedure. Other groups also seem to confirm these findings (Table 29.2). However, if the patients need continued fulguration for residual rectal polyps over a long time, bowel function may deteriorate. Presumably this is due to fibrosis within the rectum and a reduction in its distensibility.

Follow-up after IRA

Surveillance should comprise at least an annual examination and should continue for life. If the operation has been performed for patients with numerous polyps, a situation which should now not arise, examination should be performed every 6 months. Sigmoidoscopy should be performed with the aid of a good sucker, and the knee–elbow position may facilitate the procedure since rectal contents are often fluid and require removal. Flexible sigmoidoscopy is proving useful with these patients, especially now it is appreciated that polyps may develop in the ileum. Although examination can be performed in the outpatient clinic with the patient conscious, it is preferable to examine some patients under general anaesthesia; this allows a more comprehensive assessment of the rectal lumen and also enables fulguration of any polyps to be performed at the same time. Patients may not always comply with such a regimen, and if follow-up is becoming a problem conversion to restorative proctocolectomy may be advisable.

Cancer of the rectal remnant is not the main reason for removing the rectum after IRA. In a Scandinavian study of 297 patients, the rectal stump had been removed in 47 patients (15.8%) after 25 years of follow-up (De Cosse, 1992). In 34 (11.4%), the indication was multiple large adenomas, severe dysplasia, stricture and incontinence; in only 13 patients (4.4%) was the indication cancer. Secondary restorative proctocolectomy can be offered to most of these patients unless there is a cancer in the lower rectum, faecal incontinence or intra-abdominal desmoid (Madden et al, 1991; Penna et al, 1993a). The functional results differ only slightly from those of RPC performed as a first operative procedure (Penna et al, 1993a).

In the past, surveillance in these patients was restricted to examination of the rectum. Since we now know that patients can develop extracolonic polyps, upper gastrointestinal endoscopy with a side-viewing scope should also be performed annually. Whether it is necessary to perform a regular small bowel barium meal or ileoscopy remains to be determined.

Spontaneous regression of polyps in the retained rectum

Although long-term regular surveillance is mandatory in patients after ileorectal anastomosis, spontaneous regression is a well-described phenomenon (Hubbard, 1957; Cole and Holden, 1959; Localio, 1962; Shepherd, 1971; Nicholls et al, 1988; Feinberg et al, 1988). Although the mechanism has not been established, some authors feel that a slightly lower pH in the faecal stream passing over the polyps may have an inhibitory effect on polyp growth (Bennett et al, 1953). Regression seems only to occur in patients who have had a true ileorectal anastomosis as opposed to an ileosigmoid anastomosis. It is as well to remember that regression is usually only a temporary phenomenon.

Treatment of recurrent polyps

Medical treatment

There is evidence that regression, occasionally complete, of colorectal and duodenal adenomas can be achieved by long-term use of non-steroidal anti-inflammatory drugs (NSAIDs), both in patients with an intact colon and in those following ileo-rectal anastomosis (Waddell and Loughry, 1983; Waddell et al, 1989, Labayle et al, 1991; Rigau et al, 1991; Giardello et al, 1993, Nugent et al, 1993a, Spagnesi et al, 1994; Heiskanen and Jarvinen, 1997). In two controlled trials (Nugent et al, 1993a; Spagnesi et al, 1994), sulindac seemed to reduce cell proliferation and the number and size of adenomas. Indomethacin, delivered to the rectal remnant after IRA, induced almost complete regression in both number and size of adenomas within 1–3 months (Hirata et al, 1994). Nevertheless, it cannot be assumed that regression of polyps in the rectal remnant removes the risk of rectal cancer (Niv and Fraser, 1994). Sulindac has to be taken on a long-term basis, and we have shown in patients with spontaneous polyps who are at high risk of recurrence that compliance is extremely poor (Taylor et al, 1995).

Thus, although sulindac and other agents may have a role in patients with rectal polyps who have failed to show significant spontaneous regression after IRA, and who are unsuitable for pouch surgery, we are not optimistic that patients will be able to tolerate the therapy. In addition, there are now reports which show that sulindiac does not appear to have any effect on periampullary polyps (Richard et al, 1997).

Surgical treatment

Fulguration of polyps is performed as previously described. Since many polyps may have to be treated on one occasion, treatment may be tedious. If numerous polyps are present it is probably wiser to treat them over several sessions since the risk of perforation may be less. If this is done, some authorities (Goligher, 1984) recommend fulguration from above downwards, otherwise rigidity and narrowing of the fulgarized lower rectum may prevent the large sigmoidoscope from reaching the upper rectum at subsequent sessions to deal with the remaining polyps. A good sucker is also a useful asset.

For a few days following treatment it is quite usual for the patient to complain of lower abdominal pain and the passage of blood and mucus, symptoms that are usually related to a temporary iatrogenic proctitis. Occasionally a brisk secondary haemorrhage may occur. Repeated fulguration may leave the patient with a strictured rectum requiring repeated dilatation; if this proves difficult, rectal excision may have to be considered.

For patients who develop numerous polyps following ileorectal anastomosis which fulguration fails to control, it is wise to consider an alternative manoeuvre. Restorative proctocolectomy should be discussed with the patient. Removal of the rectal mucosa may prove difficult as a result of fibrosis due to repeated diathermy. However, since the operation now usually involves complete rectal excision, only a very short segment of anal mucosa above the dentate line needs to be excised and the problem of rectal fibrosis rarely presents a problem. If restorative proctocolectomy is contraindicated because of poor anal function or ileal polyposis, the entire rectum should be removed and a permanent ileostomy constructed. Rectal excision should be performed either by the intersphincteric technique or entirely through the abdomen leaving the anal sphincter intact. These techniques prevent pelvic nerve damage and limit the morbidity due to a perineal wound.

Technique of restorative proctocolectomy (RPC)

Restorative proctocolectomy is the operation we regard as the procedure of first choice for patients with numerous rectal polyps. The operation is identical to that which we perform for ulcerative colitis but we prefer to excise all the anal mucosa above the dentate line and therefore tend to perform a hand-sewn ileoanal anastomosis as described in Chapter 48. The clinical results of restorative proctocolectomy for FAP are altogether different from an identical procedure in ulcerative colitis. In our experience all patients are fully continent, pouchitis is rare, and the mean frequency of defecation over 24 hours is three times at 6 months and twice at 12 months after operation.

Surveillance of the pouch after restorative proctocolectomy

In recent years, reports of recurrent polyp formation after restorative proctocolectomy have become more frequent (Wolfstein et al, 1982; Myrhoj et al, 1989; Nugent et al, 1993b). In addition, there are reports of polyps forming after end ileostomy (Hamilton et al, 1979), above the anastomosis after ileorectal anastomosis (Iida et al, 1989), and in a continent ileostomy (Stryker et al, 1987). So far, there does not seem to be a higher risk of adenocarcinoma formation after ileal pouch formation, but follow-up is relatively short. Invasive adenocarcinoma has been reported at the ileo-anal anastomosis following RPC (Hoehner and Metcalf, 1994), but this probably arose from residual mucosa following an incomplete rectal mucosectomy. The increased tendency to perform a totally stapled anastomosis just above the dentate line will inevitably leave behind some rectal mucosa which in FAP patients is known to contain microadenomas (Tsunoda et al, 1990; Deen et al, 1994). Such patients are therefore theoretically at greater risk of developing rectal cancer and should be carefully followed up. However, we would strongly encourage that FAP patients should not undergo a stapled anastomosis, but should have a complete mucosectomy of a very short rectal stump and a transanal ileo-anal anastomosis constructed by hand.

Technique of conventional proctocolectomy

Although conventional proctocolectomy is described in detail elsewhere it should be stressed that it is rarely indicated now as the first-line operation for the treatment of FAP. If the rectum has to be removed it is preferable to perform an intersphincteric excision and to retain the anal sphincter in case a pouch is a possible option for the future.

Treatment of extracolonic gastrointestinal polyps

Large multiple polyps localized to the terminal ileum should be treated at the time of surgery. If polyps are detected elsewhere within the small bowel they should if possible be excised through an enterotomy and the patient followed up by regular small bowel enemata or ileoscopy. It is not yet known whether small bowel polyps in FAP become malignant, so their treatment must remain empirical. The same applies to gastric polyps which in our view should be kept under regular endoscopic review, the larger polyps being removed by diathermy excision.

There is no evidence to support total gastrectomy as a prophylactic measure in these patients. Early detection of a malignant periampullary lesion by screening offers the only prospect of long-term survival. There are a few long-term survivors who have had a restorative proctocolectomy and a radical pancreatico-duodenectomy.

Management of desmoid tumours

The treatment of patients with abdominal-wall or extra-abdominal desmoid tumours may be difficult, but surgery is still the mainstay. Radical excision with a margin of healthy tissue around the tumour will usually control these lesions in the short term, but there is a considerable risk of local recurrence and even malignant transformation. Prosthetic material or a myocutaneous flap is often necessary to bridge large fascial defects (Holyoke et al, 1973; Sheridan et al, 1986; Weinstein et al, 1986). Further resection may be feasible and desirable in patients with abdominal wall recurrence. However, not all of these tumours need excision and the small ones may be left with impunity. Generally speaking, desmoids in the abdominal wall should be removed if there is progressive enlargement, if they produce symptoms or if the patient is concerned from the cosmetic point of view; however, there are some who believe that any form of operation may accelerate the growth of these tumours.

Intra-abdominal desmoid tumours are less common. They pose a serious problem because it is difficult to apply the principles of wide *en bloc* resection to them. When the lesions are peripheral in the mesentery, they can be simply excised with or without an accompanying portion of bowel. More commonly, however, these lesions are either in the proximal mesentery intimately involving the blood supply to large segments of bowel, where removal would often entail sacrifice of nearly all of the intestine (Hoover, 1983), or in the pelvis, thereby compromising the viability of the rectum or a pelvic pouch if they are removed. There is a perioperative mortality rate of 10–60%, usually from loss of blood, and a major morbidity rate of 22–60% (Kim et al, 1971; Johnson et al, 1972; Jones et al, 1986; Jarvinen, 1987; Farmer et al, 1994). Recurrence following excision of intra-abdominal desmoids is high, occurring in 65–88% of cases. Most authors recommend that surgery should be avoided for mesenteric desmoids because of the high risk of accelerated growth and recurrence (Lofti et al, 1989; Church, 1995). However, operation may be needed to bypass small bowel obstruction or relieve ureteric obstructions.

It is the impression from the literature that most patients with inoperable intra-abdominal desmoid tumours do badly. Two of the four patients in the series of Naylor et al (1979) died from small bowel obstruction and a third died from coronary artery disease. All of the four patients described by McAdam and Goligher (1970) died from the local effects of intra-abdominal desmoids.

Although there are some favourable short-term reports suggesting that radiotherapy may be beneficial (Ewing, 1940; Pack and Ariel, 1958), others (Cole and Giuss, 1969) have not been so impressed.

Since desmoids are radio-resistant it is difficult to accept that irradiation could serve any useful purpose. Nevertheless, there are reports that when used as an adjuvant therapy after resection, radiation may reduce the risk of recurrence. Recurrence rates of 40–70% after surgery alone have been reported to drop to 20–40% (Rock et al, 1984; Kharsand and Karakousis, 1985). However, intra-abdominal desmoids are even more resistant than those elsewhere to radiotherapy.

An alternative therapy using drugs that affect the metabolism of cyclic AMP was suggested by Waddell (1975) to be effective. A combination of indomethacin and ascorbic acid was shown by Waddell and Gerner (1980) to be successful in the treatment of three patients, while a fourth patient who was resistant to these drugs responded to sulindac (Waddell, 1982).

Since these first reports, there have been others suggesting some benefit from a variety of NSAIDs. However, there are no controlled trials, and the reports tend to be anecdotal. Overall, the results of NSAIDs alone show an objective response rate of about 50% (Waddell, 1983; Klein et al, 1987; Tsukada et al, 1992).

Approximately 40% of desmoids are oestrogen receptor positive, so it has been suggested that tamoxifen and its chlorinated analogue tormifene may prove to be a useful form of therapy in resistant or recurrent disease. Oestrogen receptor blockade restricts RNA synthesis and other transcription of genes involved in tumour growth. However, tamoxifen also has an effect on prostaglandin metabolism and may also act via stromal epithelial interactions (Benson and Baum, 1993) inducing transforming growth factor beta production in stromal fibroblasts which inhibits fibroblast growth *in vitro* (Coletta et al, 1990). Most patients treated with tamoxifen or tormifene have been women, who were often given NSAIDs or other treatments in addition (Kinzbrunner et al, 1983; Klein et al, 1987; Procter et al, 1987; Wilson et al, 1987; Gansar and Krementz, 1988; Eagel et al, 1989; Brooks et al, 1994). The response rate when treating intra-abdominal desmoids seems to be about 50% with anti-oestrogens alone.

Other agents such as theophylline, testolactone chlorothiazide, ascorbic acid and corticosteroids have all been shown to have an effect. Although the reasoning behind using these agents is sound, the data as yet remain unconvincing (Waddell, 1975; Harvey et al, 1979; Gansar and Krementz, 1988; Lofti et al, 1989; Gadson et al, 1990; Umemoto et al, 1991). The same applies to warfarin (Waddell and Kirsch, 1991), interleukin-2 (Seiter and Kemeny, 1993) and interferon alpha (Geurs and Kok, 1993).

Various chemotherapy agents have been used as a last resort in recurrent, irresectable or aggressive desmoid disease. Objective response has been noted with almost all agents including combinations of actinomycin D, cyclophosphamide, vincristine and methotrexate (Hutchinson et al, 1979; Weiss and Lackman, 1991), but there are few cases reported.

The antisarcoma regimen consisting of doxorubicin and dacorbazine seems more promising. Nine cases have been reported with complete regression in four and partial regression in five (Lin et al, 1989; Patel et al, 1993; Hamilton et al, 1996).

The Muir–Torre syndrome

This is not a true polyposis syndrome, but it is convenient to discuss it here since adenomatous colonic polyps are a particular feature.

The syndrome is a rare autosomal dominant condition first described in 1967 in an individual who had multiple benign sebaceous adenomata and kerato-acanthomata of the skin and multiple internal malignancies (large bowel, duodenum and larynx) (Muir et al, 1967). The skin stigmata include sebaceous hyperplasia, adenoma and carcinoma with kerato-acanthoma and basal cell carcinoma. The visceral neoplasms include colonic adenomatous polyps and colonic adenocarcinoma in addition to tumours of the stomach, oesophagus, breast, uterus, ovaries, bladder and larynx, and squamous cell carcinomas of mucous membranes (Grignon et al, 1987). Colorectal neoplasms are the most common, representing approximately 50% of all visceral tumours (Cohen and Kohn, 1991) (Table 29.3).

The condition usually becomes manifest from the fifth decade when multiple skin lesions develop. At this stage, internal malignancies are not usually present, although they often develop later. Intestinal polyps are described in 38% of cases, and as in HNPCC (Lynch II syndrome) the colorectal cancers in this condition are predominantly right-sided (Schwartz et al, 1989) but often multiple. The tumours tend to be low-grade with a good prognosis after resection. Patients with the Muir–Torre syndrome need periodic evaluations for the development of malignancies. Screening for cancer in relatives of individuals with this disorder is clearly essential.

Table 29.3 Sites of malignancy in 120 patients with the Muir–Torre syndrome.

Malignancy	*n*	*Number of cancers*
Colorectal		119
Colon	64	105
Rectum	14	14
Genitourinary		59
Bladder	12	17
Uterus	11	12
Renal pelvis	6	9
Ovary	6	6
Prostate	5	5
Ureter	5	5
Vulva	2	2
Cervix	1	1
Hypernephroma	1	1
Testicle	1	1
Breast	14	14
Haematological		12
Non-Hodgkin's lymphoma	6	6
Chronic lymphocytic leukaemia	3	3
Polycythemia vera	2	2
Hodgkin's lymphoma	1	1
Head and neck		11
Laryngeal	7	7
Inner ear	1	1
Lip	1	1
Parotid	1	1
Tongue	1	1
Small intestine		8
Duodenum	4	6
Ileum	1	1
Jejunum	1	1
Lung	3	3
Gastric	2	2
Melanoma	2	2
Pancreas	2	2
Other		2
Biliary	1	1
Chondrosarcoma	1	1
Unknown	1	1
Totals	120	235

From Cohen and Kohn (1991).

Lymphosarcomatous (lymphomatous) polyposis

In the light of recent changes in the nomenclature relating to lymphomas, the title of this entity should be 'lymphomatous polyposis' which describes the infiltration of Hodgkin's or non-Hodgkin's lymphoma into the mucosa or submucosa of the colon. Radiologically it may simulate familial adenomatous polyposis (Davies et al, 1970) but colonoscopy and biopsy will confirm the diagnosis. The patient may or may not have other stigmata of lymphoma. Treatment and prognosis are those of the underlying condition and the reader is advised to consult the appropriate haematological textbooks for details.

Leukaemia polyposis

Colorectal infiltrations in chronic leukaemia may be multiple and can be mistaken for familial adenomatous polyposis (Bussey, 1975a).

Benign lymphoid polyposis

Benign lymphoid polyposis occupies one end of the spectrum of lymphoid hyperplasia. It is rare and usually occurs in childhood. Although most cases regress spontaneously and undoubtedly represent an exaggerated physiological lymphoid hyperplasia (Louw, 1958), typically around puberty it may become a pathological entity. The condition may be familial (Louw, 1958) or may occur in patients with immunodeficiency diseases (Shaw and Hennigar, 1974). Since it may result from infection it is conveniently classified as a type of inflammatory polyposis.

Macroscopically the mucosa bulges over many grey sessile nodules measuring up to 6 mm in diameter. Microscopically they do not differ from the more focal lesions. It is clearly imperative to differentiate this condition from FAP since the polyps are not premalignant.

Although surgery may be required for complications such as bleeding (Swartley and Stayman, 1962), elective radical surgery (Cosens, 1958; Freeman, 1964; Collins et al, 1966) is unnecessary provided the diagnosis is certain. Similarly, the suggestion that benign lymphoid polyposis should be treated by radiotherapy or chemotherapy (Symmers, 1948; Cosens, 1958; Cornes et al, 1961) is in our opinion unwarranted. Provided the polyps are not causing symptoms these young patients should be managed conservatively. Very often spontaneous regression occurs.

HAMARTOMATOUS POLYPOSIS

Juvenile polyposis

Juvenile polyposis is very rare and has only relatively recently been recognized (McColl et al, 1964; Smilow et al, 1966; Veale et al, 1966). The polyps may involve the large bowel alone or they may occur in conjunction with involvement in other parts of the gastrointestinal tract (McColl et al, 1964; Bussey 1975b). In one-third of cases a familial mode of inheritance is observed, which seems to be an autosomal dominant trait. The familial type is believed to be due to mutations in a protein tyrosine phosphate gene (TPN) but its exact location has still to be determined (Lynch and Lynch, 1998). The cases that are not familial may have other associated congenital abnormalities (McColl et al, 1964; Bussey, 1975b; Erbe, 1976; Morson and Dawson, 1990).

After the first descriptions of the condition it was believed for some time that there was no danger of carcinoma development (Roth and Helwig, 1963; Smilow et al 1966; Sachatello et al, 1970; Romer et al, 1971; Williams et al, 1980). However, further reports have demonstrated that some of the polyps may demonstrate adenomatous features (Kaschula, 1971; Enterline, 1976; Goodman et al, 1979; Ramaswamy et al, 1981; Read and Vose, 1981) with malignant potential. In addition, juvenile polyposis has been reported in families with histories of adenomatous polyposis and colonic carcinoma (Lynch and Krush, 1967; Grigioni et al, 1981), and several instances of separate colonic cancers in patients and relatives of patients with juvenile polyposis have also been documented (Veale et al, 1966; Stemper et al, 1975; Restrepo et al 1978; Grigioni et al, 1981; Rozen and Baratz, 1982). More recently, several studies demonstrated frank malignancy within polyps from these patients (Jarvinen and Franssila, 1984). Murday and Slack (1989) analysed the cumulative risk of colorectal cancer development in 87 patients with juvenile polyposis; they found this to be 68% by 60 years of age. It is for these reasons that juvenile polyposis is now considered to be a premalignant condition akin to adenomatous polyposis. However, there is some controversy concerning management.

Jarvinen and Fransilla (1984) advocate prophylactic colectomy for affected individuals. On the other hand, Giardiello et al (1991) believe that the data do not justify prophylactic colectomy solely for the risk of colorectal cancer, although surgery would be indicated if there were symptoms such as persistent bleeding. In patients not treated by prophylactic colectomy, periodic screening by colonoscopy is essential. There is no agreement on the frequency of screening, but this will be influenced by the number of juvenile polyps and rate of new polyp formation. First-degree relatives should be screened because of the familial nature of the disease and because affected individuals may be symptomatic (Jass, 1994).

The Peutz–Jeghers syndrome

The very rare, usually familial, syndrome of pigmentation of the mouth and other parts of the body together with gastrointestinal polyps was first described by Peutz (1921). Jeghers (1944) later described several patients with the disease. Although it is almost invariably a familial disease transmitted as an autosomal dominant, sporadic cases do occur (Neely and Gillespie, 1967). Recently Jenne et al (1998) mapped the gene responsible for the Peutz–Jeghers syndrome (PJS) to chromosome 19p13.3. PJS is thought to have a frequency about one-tenth that of FAP (Burt et al, 1985).

The most frequent site for polyps is the upper small bowel, but they may occur in the stomach and large bowel (Morson, 1962). There are occasional reports of polyps in other sites besides the gastrointestinal tract (Hafter, 1954). Macroscopically the polyps may be sessile but are more often pedunculated, with short, broad pedicles. The outer surface has a coarse, lobulated pattern not unlike that of an adenomatous polyp but the lobules tend to be larger (Figure 29.8a). The polyps vary in size from a few millimetres to as much as 5 cm diameter. The microscopic appearance is characteristic (Figure 29.8b).

The essential feature is a branching core of muscular tissue derived from the muscularis mucosae, the branches of which become thinner and eventually disappear as they reach the periphery of the polyp. Each branch is covered by histologically normal epithelium. There is no excess of lamina propria as in juvenile polyps, and no nuclear hyperchromatism or glandular irregularity as in a true adenoma. The appearances are thus those of a true hamartoma (Bartholomew and Dahlin, 1957; Rintala, 1959), perhaps produced by an overgrowth of the muscularis mucosae (Morson and Dawson, 1990).

The disease occurs equally in males and females. The age of onset varies but is most common in childhood or adolescence. Not all the features occur concurrently or are present in every case (Bartholomew and Dahlin, 1957). The cutaneous pigmentation often precedes the polyp formation and may

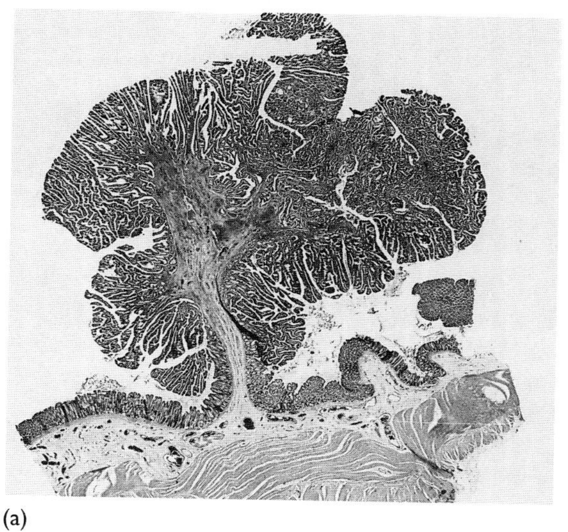

(a)

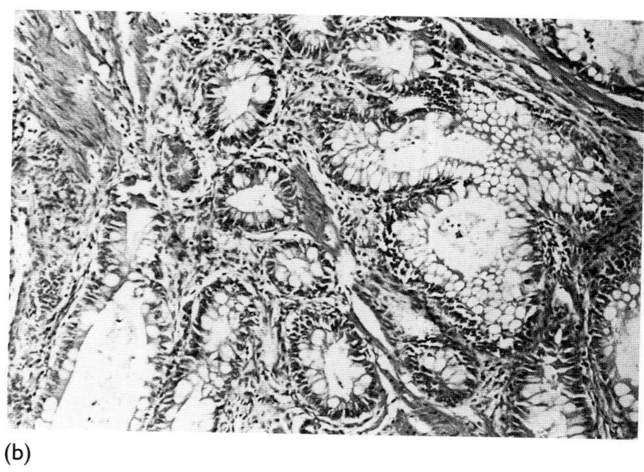

(b)

Figure 29.8a,b (a) Characteristic structure of polyp in Peutz–Jeghers syndrome. (b) Microscopic appearance of polyp in Peutz–Jeghers syndrome, with crypts with goblet cells and Paneth cells associated with interlacing bundles of smooth muscle.

actually disappear after puberty (Welch and Hedburg, 1975). The pigmentation consists of clusters of black or dark brown, freckle-like spots, 1–2 cm diameter, on and around the lips and buccal mucosa. Similar spots may be present on the fingers and toes (Bussey, 1978). The polyps tend to occur in crops in different parts of the bowel rather than simultaneously. The two most common symptoms are abdominal pain and rectal bleeding. The former is characterized by attacks of severe colic which commonly occur shortly after a meal. These are probably related to intermittent intussusception. Less commonly an intussusception produces a full-blown attack of intestinal obstruction which requires surgical intervention. The bleeding may be major or minor, the latter leading to chronic anaemia. Other symptoms common to all polyps such as prolapse per rectum and passage of the polyp following torsion and autoamputation may occur.

There is debate concerning the malignant potential of the polyps in this syndrome. Originally it was believed that there was no risk (Bartholomew and Dahlin, 1957; Dormandy, 1957; Rintala, 1959; Morson, 1962), but several reports have demonstrated malignancy arising in these polyps (Bussey, 1970; Reid, 1974; Utsunomiya et al, 1975; Cochet et al, 1979). These initial reports were confirmed by two large studies involving a total of 103 patients from opposite sides of the Atlantic. Both studies confirmed a high relative risk for both intestinal and extraintestinal malignancy (Giardiello et al, 1987; Spigelman et al, 1989a). In addition, survival was impaired with the risk of mortality from cancer approaching 40% by 40 years of age (Spigelman et al, 1989a). The transformation of some hamartomas into dysplastic (adenomatous) polyps and cancer was also demonstrated (Spigelman et al, 1989a; Perzin and Bridge, 1982; Settaf et al, 1990; Niimi et al, 1991). Malignant tumours may also arise *de novo* or from existing adenomas (Spigelman et al, 1995). There also seems to be an increased risk of extraintestinal malignancy. Gynaecological tumours, especially sex cord tumours of the annular tubules and adenoma malignum of the cervix, seem to be particularly prevalent (Young et al, 1982; Choi et al, 1993; Srivatsa et al, 1994). Feminizing Sertoli cell tumours of the testis, which are otherwise rare, also occur in this syndrome (Wilson et al, 1986), as does bilateral breast cancer (Trau et al, 1982) and pancreatic cancer (Giardiello et al, 1987; Spigelman et al, 1989a).

Management used to be conservative in most centres, surgery being resorted to only when a major complication such as intussusception or massive haemorrhage occurred which failed to respond to conservative therapy. Since most of the small bowel is affected, extensive resection was clearly out of the question. However, with the advent of endoscopy a more aggressive policy has been recommended. Thus, gastroduodenal and colonic polyps are now managed by regular upper and lower endoscopy every two years, with polyps greater than 0.5 cm in size being removed to prevent blood loss, intussusception and malignant change (Williams et al, 1982;

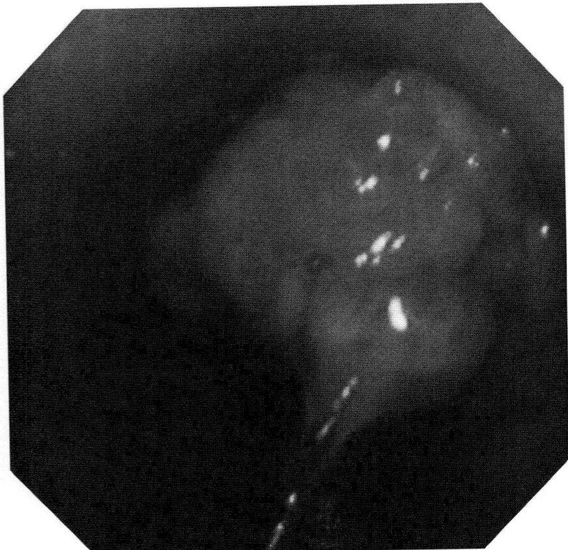

Figure 29.9 Hamartomatous jejunal polyp in a patient with the Peutz–Jegher's syndrome as seen down the enteroscope. Photograph courtesy of Dr C P Swain, Royal London Hospital.

Spigelman and Phillips, 1989). It is also recommended that any small bowel polyp greater than 1.5 cm diameter should be excised at laparotomy (Williams et al, 1982). The rationale of this approach is based not only on the knowledge that malignancy may supervene but that many of the small polyps disappear spontaneously and the tendency to polyp formation declines progressively at 25–30 years of age (Williams, 1984).

The approach of polypectomy through small enterostomies (Utsunomiya et al, 1975) has been improved by the use of peroperative enteroscopy (Mathus-Vliegen and Tytgat, 1985) which increases the yield of polyps and provides an additional and less invasive means for their removal (Spigelman et al, 1990). Small bowel enteroscopy is now being developed for use in the non-operative situation. Such a technique may well revolutionize the care of patients with Peutz–Jegher's syndrome and indeed others with small bowel polyps. At present it is possible to advance these 'scopes at best for only about 100 cm from the first part of the duodenum. Nevertheless, even now this approach may be useful (Figure 29.9).

Generalized juvenile gastrointestinal polyposis

Generalized juvenile gastrointestinal polyposis with multiple juvenile polyps throughout the entire gastrointestinal tract is a rare condition and is thought to be a separate hereditary entity from juvenile polyposis (Sachatello et al, 1970).

The Canada–Cronkhite syndrome

The Canada–Cronkhite syndrome is one of the rare generalized gastrointestinal polypoid syndromes whose components have only recently been classified. The cardinal features are:

1. the presence of multiple hamartomatous polyps of the juvenile (retention) variety (Figure 29.10)
2. ectodermal changes consisting of alopecia, onychodystrophy (Figure 29.11) and hyperpigmentation
3. the absence of a family history of polyposis
4. adult onset
5. the eventual development of diarrhoea and weight loss.

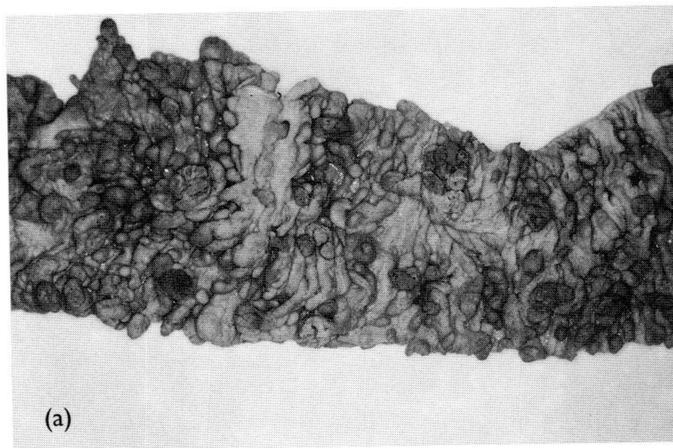

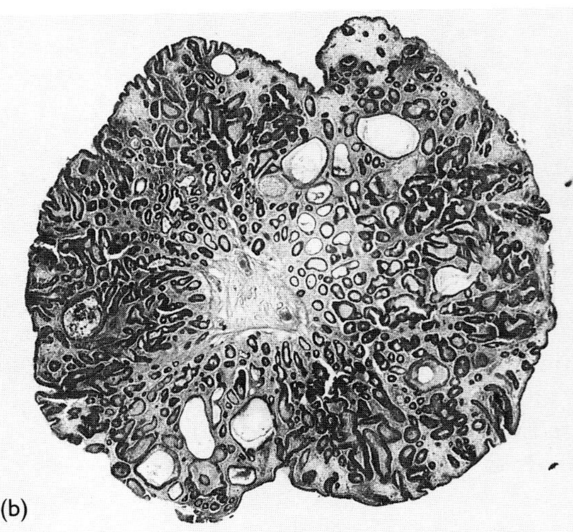

Figure 29.10a,b The Canada–Cronkhite syndrome. (a) Colectomy specimen showing intact and ulcerated polyps. (b) Rectal polyp showing cystic dilatation.

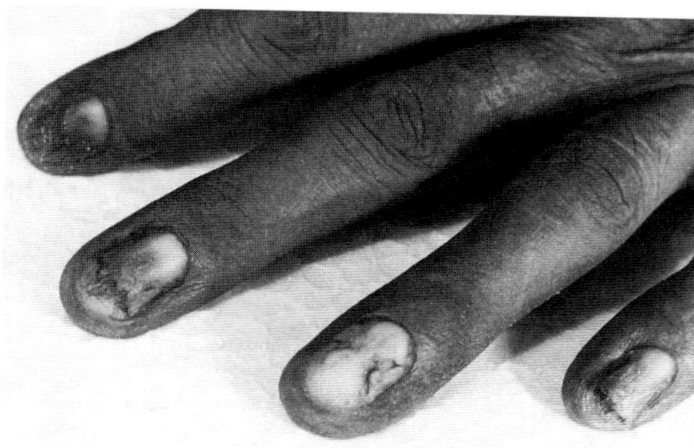

Figure 29.11 Onychodystrophy of the fingernails in the Canada–Cronkhite syndrome.

The coexistence of these clinical and pathological characteristics separates the syndrome from other types of gastrointestinal polyposis.

Cronkhite and Canada described the syndrome in 1955. A further 54 cases were reported in the literature by 1982, and were the subject of an extensive review (Daniel et al, 1982).

The clinical presentation of general lassitude, diarrhoea and weight loss is typical. Loss of taste, dry mouth, vomiting and peripheral paraesthesia are less frequent. Anaemia, oedema and tetany are the result of malabsorption. Hypokalaemia is common. The hyperpigmentation takes the form of brown macular lesions which occur most frequently on the upper limbs, the lower limbs and the face, in that order. The nails are usually dystrophic, fragile and discoloured, and in about one-fifth of patients are absent altogether. The appearance of multiple, rounded filling defects on barium examination is characteristic; in some cases the finding of giant rugal folds in the stomach led to an initial diagnosis of Ménétrier's disease. Indeed a relationship between the Canada–Cronkhite syndrome and Ménétrier's diseases has been suggested by many authors (Martini and Dolle, 1961; Gill and Wilken, 1967; Kindbloom et al, 1977; Rubin et al, 1980). Morphologically the gastric mucosa is similar in both disorders (Gill and Wilken, 1967; Palmer, 1968), and both diseases are associated with a protein-losing enteropathy and symptomatic remissions. However, Ménétrier's disease is confined to the stomach and is not usually associated with ectodermal changes. In the Canada–Cronkhite syndrome the stomach and colon are involved in almost all cases, the duodenum in 75% and the jejunum and ileum in 50%.

The initial belief that this disease is relentlessly progressive and eventually fatal is now known to be incorrect. Long-term survival of up to 18 years with minimal or no symptoms has been recorded in several patients. However, the prognosis is poor in most cases.

Although it was generally assumed that juvenile polyps did not undergo malignant transformation, recent evidence suggests that this is not the case (see above). Single or multiple carcinomas have been found in approximately 13% of cases. It is wise, therefore, to biopsy all polyps greater than 1 cm diameter (Daniel et al, 1982). There are specific reports of gastrointestinal cancer arising in the Canada–Cronkhite syndrome, but the exact relationship is unknown owing to its rarity (Katayama et al, 1985).

Treatment should be supportive in the first instance and should be aggressive, since these patients have been demonstrated to enter prolonged remission. They need fluid and electrolyte correction, nutritional supplementation, correction of anaemia and coagulation defects, and prophylactic peptic ulcer therapy.

Antibiotics seem to have produced remissions in some patients: tetracycline, ampicillin and a combination of trimethoprim with sulphamethoxazole have all been used. They seem particularly useful when bacterial overgrowth is proven or strongly suspected. Steroids have also been claimed to be successful in severely ill patients; however, it is recommended that they should be reserved for carefully selected patients who have failed to respond to all other measures.

Surgery carries a high risk in these usually extremely debilitated patients. Operation is indicated only for treatment of complications such as prolapse, intussusception, obstruction and malignancy, not for symptomatic relief. At present the risk of developing carcinoma is insufficient for prophylactic colectomy to be recommended.

Intestinal ganglioneuromatosis

Intestinal ganglioneuromatosis is defined as a proliferation of ganglion cells, neurites (axons and dendrites) and supporting cells within the gastrointestinal tract (Haggitt and Reid, 1986). Any layer of the gastrointestinal wall may be involved alone or in combination with others. The masses formed by proliferation of neural elements may project into the lumen as polyps, diffuse thickenings of the mucosa, nodular masses within the gut wall, or projections from the serosal surface. Hereditary intestinal ganglioneuromatosis occurs in three different settings: (a) as a component of Von Recklinghausen's disease, (b) in association with multiple endocrine neoplasia type 2b and type 3, and (c) as an isolated abnormality (Hochberg et al, 1974; Carney et al, 1976; Mendelsohn and Diamond, 1984).

Almost all of the reported cases of multiple endocrine neoplasia type 2 have had intestinal tract involvement often predating detection of the endocrine lesions (Carney et al, 1976). Affected individuals may complain of either diarrhoea or constipation. The diarrhoea is presumably due to overproduction of calcitonin, prostaglandins and 5-hydroxytryptamine, whereas the constipation is postulated as being due to overgrowth of ganglion cells secreting vasoactive intestinal polypeptide which is thought to inhibit intestinal motility.

The gastrointestinal tract including the colon may be involved in as many as 25% of patients with Von Recklinghausen's disease. Most lesions in the gut are neurofibromata, but ganglioneuromatosis may be present also (Raszkowski and Hufner, 1971; Hochberg et al, 1974). The polyps can appear in any part of the gastrointestinal tract. Inheritance is autosomal dominant with the gene NFI isolated and sequenced on chromosome 17q. The gene codes for a protein named neurofibromin. The protein bears homology to $p120^{GAP}$, a GTPase activating protein for *ras* oncogene products (McCormick, 1992). Intestinal ganglioneuromatosis has been reported also in families lacking the features of multiple endocrine neoplasia syndrome or Von Recklinghausen's disease (Mendelsohn and Diamond, 1984).

The malignant potential of intestinal ganglioneuromatosis appears to be quite low, but in Von Recklinghausen's disease the neurofibromata in the gut as elsewhere may undergo malignant change (Hochberg et al, 1974).

The Ruvalcaba–Myrhe–Smith syndrome

The Ruvalcaba–Myrhe–Smith syndrome consists of macrocephaly, mental deficiency, an unusual craniofacial appearance, hamartomatous intestinal polyposis and pigmented macules on the shaft and glans of the penis (Ruvalcaba et al, 1980; DiLiberti et al, 1983). The syndrome is thought to be transmitted by an autosomal dominant gene. The polyps which have been described only in the colon and on the tongue are thought to be hamartomas. Some authorities, however, consider this syndrome to be a variant of juvenile polyposis.

Lipomatous polyposis

Multiple submucosal lipomas may occur in the small intestine or colon and eventually cause intussusception or bleeding (Ling et al, 1959). Colonoscopy is usually diagnostic. Since the condition is entirely benign, elective surgery is usually unnecessary.

Cowden's disease

In 1963, Lloyd and Dennis described a patient with multiple anocutaneous hamartomata, fibrocystic disease of the breast, non-toxic goitre, breast cancer and thyroid cancer. Since then other cases have been described and the syndrome has been termed 'Cowden's disease' (Weary et al, 1970; Gentry et al, 1974; Burnett et al, 1975; Siegel, 1975). In 1978, a similar patient was described (Weinstock and Kawanishi, 1978) in whom multiple gastric and rectosigmoid polyps were found. Biopsy of the gastric polyps showed them to be hyperplastic, but the colonic polyps were not examined histologically. Cowden's disease is now thought to be an autosomal dominant disease (Allen et al, 1980).

UNCLASSIFIED POLYPOSIS

Metaplastic polyposis

Multiple metaplastic polyposis is a recently described condition which is rare and difficult to distinguish from adenomatous polyposis (Williams et al, 1980; Williams, 1994). Although it is recognized that metaplastic polyps can be multiple, it is most unusual for them to be sufficiently large and numerous to warrant the term 'polyposis'. Of the 244 patients with metaplastic polyps reviewed by Williams et al (1980), seven patients had more than 50 polyps in their colon and each had been diagnosed clinically as suffering from adenomatous polyposis. The difference is clearly essential since the metaplastic nature of the polyps implies that they have no malignant potential and prophylactic colectomy is unwarranted. Regular follow-up is recommended, however, for although these patients are no more likely to develop adenoma and carcinoma than the general population, the large number of polyps present make such a development difficult to recognize. Since the number of patients is small, regular colonoscopy is feasible.

Pneumatosis cystoides intestinalis

See Chapter 38.

REFERENCES

Allen BS, Fitch MH & Smith JG (1980) Multiple hamartoma syndrome. *J Am Acad Dermatol* **9**: 65–71.

Alm T (1975) Surgical treatment of hereditary adenomatosis of the colon and rectum in Sweden during the last 20 years. *Acta Chir Scand* **141**: 228–237.

Alm T & Licznerski G (1973) The intestinal polyposis. *Clin Gastroenterol* **2**: 577.

Ambroze WL Jr, Dozois RR, Pemberton GH, Beart RW JR & Ilstrup DM (1992) Familial adenomatous polyposis: results following ileal pouch–anal anastomosis and ileorectostomy. *Dis Colon Rectum* **35**: 12–15.

Arvanitis ML, Jagelman DG, Fazio, VW, Lavery IC & McGannon E (1990) Mortality in patients with familial adenomatous polyposis. *Dis Colon Rectum* **33**: 639–642.

Augenlicht LH, Wahrman MZ, Halsey H et al (1987) Expression of cloned sequences in biopsies of human colonic tissue and in colonic carcinoma induced to differentiate in vitro. *Cancer Res* **47**: 6017–6021.

Barker GM, Radley S, Bain I, Davis A, Lawson AM, Keighley MR, Neoptolemos JP (1994) Biliary bile acid profiles in patients with familial adenomatous polyposis before and after colectomy. *Br J Surg* **81**: 441–444.

Baron RL & Lee JK (1981) Mesenteric desmoid tumors: sonographic and computed tomographic appearance. *Radiology* **140**: 777–779.

Bartholomew JG & Dahlin DC (1957) Intestinal polyposis associated with mucocutaneous melanin pigmentation (Peutz–Jeghers syndrome). *Gastroenterology* **34**: 434.

Baughman EA, List CF, Williams JR et al (1969) The glioma polyposis syndrome. *N Engl J Med* **281**: 1345–1346.

Bennett LR, Connon FE, Gouze M & Schenberg MD (1953) Further studies on the effects of small intestinal microsomal fraction upon transplantable tumours. *Proc Soc Exper Biol Med* **82**: 655.

Benson JR & Baum M (1993) Breast cancer, desmoid tumours and familial adenomatous polyposis: a unifying hypothesis. *Lancet* **342**: 848–850.

Beradi RS & Canlas M (1973) Desmoid tumor and laparotomy scars. *Int Surg* **58**: 254–256.

Berk T, Cohen Z, McCleod RS & Parker JA (1988) Congenital hypertrophy of the retinal pigment epithelium as a marker for familial adenomatous polyposis. *Dis Colon Rectum* **31**: 253–257.

Berk T, Cohen Z, McLeod RS & Stern HS (1992) Management of mesenteric desmoid tumours in familial adenomatous polyposis. *Can J Surg* **35**: 393–395.

Bertario L, Presciuttini S, Sala P, Rossetti C & Pietroiusti M (1994) Causes of death and postsurgical survival in familial adenomatous polyposis: results from the Italian Registry. *Semin Surg Oncol* **10**: 225–234.

Bess MA, Adson MA, Elveback LR & Moertel CG (1980) Rectal cancer following colectomy for polyposis. *Arch Surg* **115**: 460–467.

Bodmer WF, Bailey CJ, Bussey HJR et al (1987) Localisation of the gene for familial adenomatous polyposis on chromosome 5 (letter). *Nature* **328**: 614–616.

Brasfield RD & Das-Gupta TK (1969) Desmoid tumors of the anterior abdominal wall. *Surgery* **65**: 241–246.

Bridge JA, Sreekantaiah C, Mouron B et al (1992) Clonal chromosomal abnormalities in desmoid tumors: implications for histopathogenesis. *Cancer* **69**: 430–436.

Brooks AP, Reznek RH, Nugent K et al (1994) CT appearances of desmoid tumours in familial adenomatous polyposis: further observations. *Clin Radiol* **49**: 601–607.

Brooks MD, Ebbs SR, Colletta AA & Baum M (1992) Desmoid tumours treated with triphenylethylenes. *Eur J Cancer* **28A**: 1014–1018.

Bulow S (1984) The risk of developing rectal cancer after colectomy and ileorectal anastomosis in Danish patients with polyposis coli. *Dis Colon Rectum* **27**: 726–729.

Bulow S (1986) Clinical features of familial polyposis coli. *Dis Colon Rectum* **29**: 102–107.

Bulow S (1991) Diagnosis of familial adenomatous polyposis. *World J Surg* **15**: 41–46.

Bulow S, Holm NV, Sondergaard JO, Nitt IN & Tetens G (1986) Mandibular osteomas in unaffected sibs and children of patients with familial polyposis coli. *Scand J Gastroenterol* **21**: 744.

Bulow S, Wauristen DKB, Johansen A, Svendsen LB & Sondergaard JO (1985) Gastroduodenal polyps in familial polyposis coli. *Dis Colon Rectum* **28**: 90–93.

Burke AP, Sobin LH & Shekitka KM (1990a) Mesenteric fibromatosis: a follow-up study. *Arch Pathol Lab Med* **114**: 832–835.

Burke AP, Sobin LH, Shekitka KM, Federspiel BH & Helwig EB (1990b) Intra-abdominal fibromatosis: a pathological analysis of 130 tumours with comparison of clinical subgroups. *Am J Surg Pathol* **14**: 335–341.

Burn J, Chapman P, Delhanty J et al (1991) The UK Northern Region genetic register for familial adenomatous polyposis coli: the use of age of onset, congenital hypertrophy of retinal pigment epithelium and DNA markers in risk calculations. *J Med Genet* **28**: 289–296

Burnett JW, Goldner R & Calton GJ (1975) Cowden's disease. *Br J Dermatol* **93**: 329–336.

Burney B & Asser D (1970) Polyposis coli with adenocarcinoma associated with carcinoma *in situ* of the gall bladder. *Am J Surg* **132**: 100–102.

Burt RW (1995) Polyposis syndromes. In Yamada T, Alpers DH, Owyang C, Powell DW & Silverstein FE (eds) *Textbook of Gastroenterology*, 2nd edn. Philadelphia: JB Lipincott.

Burt RW & Groden J (1993) The genetic and molecular diagnosis of adenomatous polyposis coli. *Gastroenterology* **104**: 1211–1214.

Burt RW & Petersen GW (1996) Familial colorectal cancer: diagnosis and management. In Young G, Rozen P & Levin B (eds) *Prevention and Early Detection of Colorectal Cancer*. London: WB Saunders.

Burt RW, Berenson MM, Lee RG et al (1984) Upper gastrointestinal polyps in Gardner's syndrome. *Gastroenterology* **86**: 295–301.

Burt RW, Bishop DT, Cannon LA et al (1985) Dominant inheritance of adenomatous colonic polyps and colorectal cancer. *N Engl J Med* **312**: 1540–1544.

Bussey HJR (1970) Gastrointestinal polyposis. *Gut* **11**: 970.

Bussey HJR (1975a) *Familial Polyposis Coli*. Baltimore: Johns Hopkins University Press.

Bussey HJR (1975b) Extra colonic lesions associated with polyposis coli. *Proc R Soc Med* **2**: 577–602.

Bussey HJR (1978) Polyposis syndrome. In Morson BC (ed) *The Pathogenesis of Colorectal Cancer*, pp 81–94. Philadelphia: WB Saunders.

Bussey HJR, Eyers AA, Ritchie SM & Thomson JPS (1985) The rectum in adenomatous polyposis: the St Mark's policy. *Br J Surg* **72** (Suppl): 529–531.

Cabot RC (1935) Case records of the Massacchusetts General Hospital. *N Engl J Med* **212**: 263.

Caldwell EH (1976) Desmoid tumor: musculoaponeurotic fibrosis of the abdominal wall. *Surgery* **79**: 104–106.

Camiel MR, Mule JE, Alexander IL & Benninghoff DL (1968) Association of thyroid carcinoma with Gardner's syndrome in siblings. *N Engl J Med* **278**: 1056–1058.

Capps WF, Lewis MI & Gazzaniga DA (1968) Carcinoma of the colon, ampulla of Vater and urinary bladder associated with familial multiple polyposis. *Dis Colon Rectum* **11**: 298.

Carney JA, Go VLW, Sizemore, GW & Hayles AB (1976) Alimentary tract ganglioneuromatosis: major component of the syndrome of multiple endocrine neoplasia, type 2b. *N Engl J Med* **295**: 1287–1291.

Caspari R, Friedl W, Mandl M et al (1994) Familial adenomatous polyposis: mutation of codon 1309 and early onset of colon cancer. *Lancet* **343**: 629–632.

Chapman PD, Church W, Burn J & Gunn A (1989) Congenital hypertrophy of retinal pigment epithelium: a sign of familial adenomatous polyposis. *BMJ* **298**: 353–354.

Chargelaigue A (1859) Des polyps du rectum. Thesis, Paris.

Choi CG, Kim SH, Kim JS et al (1993) Adenoma malignum of the uterine cervix in Peutz–Jeghers syndrome: CT and US features. *J Comput Assist Tomogr* **17**: 819–821.

Church JM (1995) Desmoid tumours in patients with familial adenomatous polyposis. *Sem Colon Rectal Surg* **6**: 29–32.

Church JM, McGannon E, Hull-Boiner S et al (1992) Gastroduodenal polyps in patients with familial adenomatous polyposis. *Dis Colon Rectum* **35**: 1170–1173.

Clark SK & Phillips RKS (1996) Desmoids in familial adenomatous polyposis. *Br J Surg* **83**: 1494–1504.

Cochet B, Carrol J, DesBaillets L et al (1979) Peutz–Jeghers syndrome associated with gastrointestinal carcinoma: report of two cases in a family. *Gut* **20**: 169.

Cohen PR & Kohn SR (1991) Association of sebaceous gland tumors and internal malignancy: the Muir–Torre syndrome. *Am J Med* **90**: 606–613.

Cole JW & Holden WD (1959) Postcolectomy regression of adenomatous polyps of the rectum. *Arch Surg* **79**: 385–392.

Cole NM & Giuss LW (1969) Extra-abdominal desmoid tumours. *Arch Surg* **98**: 530.

Coletta AA, Wakefield LM, Howell FV et al (1990) Anti-oestrogens induce the secretion of active transforming growth factor beta from human fetal fibroblasts. *Br J Cancer* **62**: 405–409.

Collins JD, Falk M & Guibone R (1966) Benign lymphoid polyposis of the colon: case report. *Paediatrics* **38**: 897–899.

Cornes JS, Wallace MH & Morson BC (1961) Benign lymphomas of the rectum and anal canal: a study of 100 cases. *J Pathol Bacteriol* **82**: 371–382.

Corvisart L (1847) Hypertrophie partielle de la muqueuse intestinale. *Bull Soc Anat* **22**: 400.

Cosens CG (1958) Gastrointestinal pseudoleukaemia: a case report. *Ann Surg* **148**: 129–133.

Crail HW (1949) Multiple primary malignancies arising in rectum, brain and thyroid: report of a case. *US Nav Med Bull* **49**: 123.

Cripps WH (1882) Two cases of disseminated polyps of the rectum. *Trans Path Soc Lond* **33**: 165–168.

Cronkhite LW & Canada WJ (1955) Generalised gastrointestinal polyposis: an unusual syndrome of pigmentation, alopecia and onychotrophia. *N Engl J Med* **252**: 1011–1015.

Dahn I, Jonsson N & Lundh G (1963) Desmoid tumours: a series of 33 cases. *Acta Chir Scand* **126**: 305–314.

Dangel A, Meloni AM, Lynch AT & Sandberg AA (1994) Deletion (5q) in a desmoid tumor of a patient with Gardner's syndrome. *Cancer Genet Cytogenet* **78**: 94–98.

Daniel ES, Ludwin SL, Lewis KJ et al (1982) The Cronkhite–Canada syndrome: an analysis of clinical and pathological features and therapy. *Medicine (Balt)* **61**: 293–309.

Davies SW, Scarrow GD & McCauley MB (1970) Multiple lymphomatous polyposis of the gastro-intestinal tract. *Br J Surg* **57**: 125–131.

De Cosse JJ, Adams MD, Kuzama J et al (1975) Effect of ascorbic acid on rectal polyps of patients with familial polyposis. *Surgery* **78**: 608.

De Cosse JJ, Adams MB & Condon RE (1977) Familial polyposis. *Cancer* **39**: 267–273.

De Cosse JJ, Bulow S, Neale K et al (1992) Rectal cancer risk in patients treated for familial adenomatous polyposis. *Br J Surg* **79**: 1372–1375.

Deen KI, Hubscher S, Bain I, Patel R & Keighley MRB (1994) Histological assessment of the distal 'doughnut' in patients undergoing stapled restorative proctocolectomy with high or low anal transection. *Br J Surg* **81**: 900–903.

Devic A & Bussey NM (1912) Un cas de polypose adenomateuse generalisée a tout l'intestine. *Arch Mal App Digest Par* **6**: 278.

Dick JA, Owen, WJ & McColl I (1984) Rectal sparing in familial polyposis coli. *Br J Surg* **71**: 664.

Dickinson AJ, Savage AP, Mortensen NJMcC & Kettlewell MGW (1993) Long-term survival after endoscopic transanal resection of rectal tumours. *Br J Surg* **80**: 1401–1404.

DiLiberti JH, Weleber RG & Budden S (1983) Ruvalcaba–Myre–Smith syndrome: a case with probable autosomal dominant inheritance and additional manifestations. *Am J Med Genet* **15**: 491–495.

Doi K, Iida M, Kohrogi N et al (1993) Large intra-abdominal desmoid tumors in a patient with familial adenomatosis coli: their rapid growth detected by computerized tomography. *Am J Gastroenterol* **88**: 595–598.

Dormandy TL (1957) Gastrointestinal polyposis with mucocutaneous pigmentation. *N Engl J Med* **256**: 1093, 1141, 1186.

Dozois R (1985) St Mark's 150th Centenary Meeting.

Duncan BP, Dohner VA & Priest JH (1968) The Gardner's syndrome: need for early diagnosis. *J Paediatr* **72**: 497.

Eagel BA, Zentler-Munro P & Smith IE (1989) Mesenteric desmoid tumours in Gardner's syndrome: review of medical treatments. *Postgrad Med J* **65**: 497–501.

Eden CG, Breach NM & Goldstraw P (1992) Treatment of desmoid tumours in Gardner's syndrome. *Thorax* **47**: 662–663.

Eide TJ (1986) Prevalence and morphologic features of adenomas of the large intestine in individuals with and without colorectal cancer. *Histopathology* **10**: 111–118.
Einstein DM, Tagliabue JR & Desai RK (1991) Abdominal desmoids: CT findings in 25 patients. *Am J Roentgenol* **157**: 275–279.
Enterline HT (1976) Polyps and cancer of the large bowel. *Curr Top Pathol* **63**: 95–141.
Enzinger FM & Shiraki M (1967) Musculo-aponeurotic fibromatosis of the shoulder girdle (extra-abdominal desmoid). Analysis of 30 cases followed up for 10 or more years. *Cancer* **20**: 1131–1140.
Erbe RW (1976) Inherited gastrointestinal polyposis syndromes. *N Engl J Med* **294**: 1101–1104.
Ewing J (1940) *Neoplastic Diseases: A Treatise on Tumours*, 4th edn. Philadelphia: WB Saunders.
Farmer KCR, Hawley PR & Phillips RKS (1994) Desmoid disease. In Phillips RKS, Spigelman AD & Thomson JPS (eds) *Familial Adenomatous Polyposis and Other Polyposis Syndromes*, pp 128–142. London: Edward Arnold.
Fearon ER & Vogelstein B (1990) A genetic model for colorectal tumorigenesis. *Cell* **61**: 759–767.
Feinberg SM, Jagelman DG, Sarre RG et al (1988) Spontaneous resolution of rectal polyps in patients with familial polyposis following abdominal colectomy and ileorectal anastomosis. *Dis Colon Rectum* **31**: 169–175.
Fraser-Roberts JA (1959) *An Introduction to Medical Genetics*. Oxford: Oxford University Press.
Freeman FJ (1964) Lymphoid hyperplasia and gastrointestinal bleeding in children. *Guthrie Clin Bull* **33**: 175–179.
Gadson P, McCoy J, Wikstrom AC & Gustafsson JA (1990) Suppression of protein kinase C and the stimulation of glucocorticoid receptor synthesis by dexamethasone in human fibroblasts derived from tumor tissue. *J Cell Biochem* **43**: 185–198.
Gansar GF & Krementz ET (1988) Desmoid tumors: experience with new modes of therapy. *South Med J* **81**: 794–796.
Garber JE, Li FP, Kingston JE et al (1988) Hepatoblastoma and familial adenomatous polyposis. *J Natl Cancer Inst* **80**: 1626–1628.
Gardner EJ (1951) A genetic and clinical study of intestinal polyposis, a predisposing factor for carcinoma of the colon and rectum. *Am J Hum Genet* **3**: 167–176.
Gardner EJ (1969) Gardner's syndrome re-evaluated after twenty years. *Proc Utah Acad* **46**: 1–11.
Gardner EJ & Plenk HP (1952) Hereditary pattern for multiple oesteomas in a family group. *Am J Hum Genet* **4**: 31–36.
Gardner EJ & Richards RC (1953) Multiple cutaneous and subcutaneous lesions occurring simultaneously with hereditary polyposis and oesteomatosis. *Am J Hum Genet* **5**: 139.
Gedde-Dahl T, Heim S, Loth ER et al (1989) Polyposeprojektet. *Nord Med* **12**: 104.
Gedebou TM, Wong RA, Rappaport WD et al (1996) Clinical presentation and management of iatrogenic colon perforations. *Am J Surg* **172**: 454–457.
Gentry WC Jr, Eskritt NE & Gorlin RJ (1974) Multiple hamartoma syndrome (Cowden's disease). *Arch Dermatol* **109**: 521–525.
Geurs F & Kok TC (1993) Regression of a great abdominal desmoid tumor with doxorubicin. *J Clin Gastroenterol* **16**: 264–265.
Giardiello FM, Hamilton SR, Kern SE et al (1991) Colorectal neoplasia in juvenile polyposis or juvenile polyps. *Arch Dis Child* **66**: 971–975.
Giardiello FM, Hamilton SR, Krush AJ et al (1993) Treatment of colonic and rectal adenomas with sulindac in familial adenomatous polyposis. *N Engl J Med* **328**: 1313–1316.
Giardiello FM, Krush aJ, Petersen GM et al (1994) Phenotypic variability of familial adenomatous polyposis in 11 unrelated families with identical APC gene mutations. *Gastroenterology* **106**: 1542–1547.
Giardiello FM, Welsh SB, Hamilton SR et al (1987) Increased risk of cancer in the Peutz–Jeghers syndrome. *N Engl J Med* **316**: 1511–1514.
Gill W & Wilken BJ (1967) Diffuse gastrointestinal polyposis associated with hypoproteinaemia. *J R Coll Edinb* **12**: 149.
Gingold BS, Jagelman D & Turnbull RB (1979) Surgical management of familial polyposis and Gardner's syndrome. *Am J Surg* **137**: 54.
Goligher J (1984) *Surgery of the Anus, Rectum and Colon*. London, Baillière Tindall.
Goodman ZD, Yardley JH & Milligan FD (1979) Pathogenesis of colonic polyps in multiple juvenile polyposis: report of a case associated with gastric polyps and carcinoma of the rectum. *Cancer* **43**: 1906–1913.
Grigioni WF, Alampi G, Martinelli G & Piccaluga A (1981) Atypical juvenile polyposis. *Histopathology* **5**: 361–376.
Grignon DJ, Shum DT, Bruckschwaiger O (1987) Transitional cell carcinoma in the Muir–Torre syndrome. *J Urol* **138**: 406–408.
Gurbuz AK, Giardiello FM, Petersen GM et al (1994) Desmoid tumours in familial adenomatous polyposis. *Gut* **35**: 377–381.
Hafter E (1954) Gastrointestinal polyposis mit melanose der hippenund Mundschleinhaut (Peutz–Jeghersches syndrom). *Gastroenterologia* **84**: 341.
Haggitt RC & Reid BJ (1986) Hereditary gastrointestinal polyposis syndromes. *Am J Surg Pathol* **10**: 871–887.
Halata MS, Miller J & Stone RK (1989) Gardner syndrome: early presentation with a desmoid tumor: discovery of multiple colonic polyps. *Clin Pediatr (Phila)* **28**: 538–540.
Hamilton L, Blackstein M, Berk T et al (1996) Chemotherapy for desmoid tumours in association with familial adenomatous polyposis: a report of three cases. *Can J Surg* **39**: 247–252.
Hamilton SR, Bussey HJR, Mendelsohn G et al (1979) Ileal adenomas after colectomy in patients with adenomatous polyposis coli/Gardner's syndrome. *Gastroenterology* **77**: 1252–1257.
Hamilton SR, Liu B, Parsons RE et al (1995) The molecular basis of Turcot's syndrome. *N Engl J Med* **332**: 839–847
Handford H (1890) Disseminated polypi of the large intestine becoming malignant. *Trans Path Soc Lond* **41**: 133.
Hardoff R, Ben-Dov D & Front A (1988) Gallium 67 scintigraphy in the evaluation of Gardner's syndrome. *Cancer* **61**: 2353–2358.
Harvey JC, Quan SH & Fortner JG (1979) Gardner's syndrome complicated by mesenteric desmoid tumors. *Surgery* **85**: 475–477.
Hasegawa T, Hirose T, Kudo E, Abe J & Hizawa K (1990) Cytoskeletal characteristics of myofibroblasts in benign neoplastic and reactive fibroblastic lesions. *Virchows Arch A: Pathol Anat Histopathol* **416**: 375–382.
Hayry P, Reitamo JJ, Totterman S, Hopfner-Hallikainen D & Sivula A (1982) The desmoid tumor. II: Analysis of factors possibly contributing to the etiology and growth behavior. *Am J Clin Pathol* **77**: 674–680.
Heald RJ (1967) Gardner's syndrome in association with two tumours of the ileum. *Proc R Soc Med* **60**: 914–915.
Heiskanen I & Jarvinen HJ (1997) Fate of the rectal stump after colectomy and ileorectal anastomosis for familial adenomatous polyposis. *Int J Colorect Dis* **12**: 9–13.
Herrera L, Kekati S, Gibas L (1986) Gardner syndrome in a man with interstitial deletion of 5q. *Am J Med Genet* **25**: 473–476.
Herrera L (1990) The Leeds Castle Polyposis Group. In Herrera

L (ed) *Familial Adenomatous Polyposis*, pp 155–158. New York: Alan R Liss.

Hirata K, Itoh H & Ohsato K (1994) Regression of rectal polyps by indomethacin suppository in familial adenomatous polyposis: report of two cases. *Dis Colon Rectum* **37**: 943–946.

Ho HC, Burchell S, Morris P & Yu M (1996) Colon perforation, bilateral pneumothoraces, pneumopericardium, pneumomediastinum, and subcutaneous emphysema complicating endoscopic polypectomy: anatomic and management considerations. *Am Surg* **62**: 770–774.

Hochberg FH, Dasilva AB, Galdabini J & Richardson EP (1974) Gastrointestinal involvement in Von Recklinghausen's neurofibromatosis. *Neurology* **24**: 1144–1151.

Hoehner JC & Metcalf AM (1994) Development of invasive adenocarcinoma following colectomy with ileoanal anastomosis for familial polyposis coli. Report of a case. *Dis Colon Rectum* **37**: 824–828.

Hoffmann DC & Goligher JC (1971) Polyposis of the stomach and small intestine in association with familial polyposis coli. *Br J Surg* **58**: 126.

Holyoke ED, Leafstedt S & Douglass H Jr (1973) Desmoid tumors of abdominal wall: wide excision and repair with woven mesh. *NY State J Med* **73**: 2588–2590.

Hoover HC (1983) Surgical aspects of hereditary intestinal polyposis. *Dis Colon Rectum* **26**: 409–412.

Hubbard TB (1957) Familial polyposis of the colon: the fate of the retained rectum after colectomy in children. *Am Surg* **23**: 557–586.

Hudson TM, Vandergriend RA, Springfield DS et al (1984) Aggressive fibromatosis: evaluation by computed tomography and angiography. *Radiology* **150**: 495–501.

Hughes LJ & Michels VV (1991) Risk of hepatoblastoma in familial adenomatous polyposis. *Am J Med Genet* **43**: 1023–1025.

Hunt LM, Robinson M, Hugkulstone CE et al (1994) Congenital hypertrophy of the retinal pigment epithelium and mandibular osteomata as markers in familial colorectal cancer. *Br J Cancer* **70**: 173–176.

Hutchinson RJ, Norris DG & Schnaufer L (1979) Chemotherapy: a successful application in abdominal fibromatosis. *Pediatrics* **63**: 157–159.

Ichii S, Horii Nakatsuru S et al (1992). Inactivation of both APC alleles in an early stage of colon adenomas in a patient with familial adenomatous polyposis (FAP). *Human Mol Genet* **1**: 387–390.

Iida M, Itoh H, Matsui T et al (1989) Ileal adenomas in postcolectomy patients with familial adenomatous polyposis coli/Gardner's syndrome: incidence and endoscopic appearance. *Dis Colon Rectum* **32**: 1034–1038.

Iida M, Yao T, Itoh H, Ohasato K & Watanabe H (1981) Endoscopy features of adenoma of the duodenal papilla in familial polyposis of the colon. *Gastrointest Endosc* **27**: 6–8.

Itoh H, Ohsato K, Yao T et al (1979) Turcot's syndrome and its mode of inheritance. *Gut* **20**: 414–419.

Iwama T & Mishima Y (1994) Factors affecting the risk of rectal cancer following rectum preserving surgery in patients with familial adenomatous polyposis. *Dis Colon Rectum* **37**: 1024–1026.

Iwama T, Mishima Y, Okamoto N & Inou EJ (1990) Association of congenital hypertrophy of the retinal pigment epithelium with familial adenomatous polyposis. *Br J Surg* **77**: 273–276.

Iwama T, Mishima Y & Utsunomiya J (1993) The impact of familial adenomatous polyposis on the tumorigenesis and mortality at the several organs: its rational treatment. *Ann Surg* **217**: 101–108.

Jagelman DG (1983) Familial polyposis coli. *Surg Clin North Am* **63**: 117–128.

Jagelman DG (1991) Choice of operation in familial adenomatous polyposis. *World J Surg* **15**: 47–49.

Jagelman DG, De Cosse JJ & Bussey HJR (1988) Upper gastrointestinal cancer in familial adenomatous polyposis. *Lancet* **i**: 1149–1150.

Jarvinen HJ (1987) Desmoid disease as a part of familial adenomatou polyposis coli. *Act Chir Scand* **153**: 379–383.

Jarvinen HJ (1992) Epidemiology of familial adenomatous polyposis in Finland: impact of family screening on the colorectal cancer rate and survival. *Gut* **33**: 357–360.

Jarvinen HJ & Fransilla KO (1984) Familial juvenile polyposis coli: increased risk of colorectal cancer. *Gut* **25**: 792–800.

Jarvinen HJ, Peltokallio P, Landtman M & Wolff J (1982) Gardner's stigmas in patients with familial adenomatous coli. *Br J Surg* **69**: 718–721.

Jarvinen H, Nyberg M & Peltokallio P (1983a) Upper gastrointestinal tract polyps in familial adenomatosis coli. *Gut* **24**: 333–339.

Jarvinen HJ, Nyberg M & Peltokallio P (1983b) Biliary involvement in familial adenomatous coli. *Dis Colon Rectum* **26**: 525–528.

Jarvinen HJ, Husa A, Aukee S et al (1984) Finnish registry for familial adenomatous coli. *Scand J Gastroenterol* **19**: 941.

Jass JR (1994) Juvenile polyposis. In Phillips RKS, Spigelman AD & Thomson JPS (eds) *Familial Adenomatous Polyposis and Other Polyposis Syndromes*, pp 203–214. London: Edward Arnold.

Jeghers H (1944) Pigmentation of skin. *N Engl J Med* **231**: 88–100.

Jenne DE, Reimann H, Nezu et al (1998) Peutz–Jeghers syndrome is caused by mutations in a novel serine threonine kinase. *Nat Genet* **18**: 38–44.

Johnson JG, Gilbert E, Zimmerman B & Watne AL (1972) Gardner's syndrome: colon cancer and sarcoma. *J Surg Oncol* **4**: 354.

Jones IT, Jagelman DG, Fazio VW et al (1986) Desmoid tumors in familial polyposis coli. *Ann Surg* **204**: 9497.

Jones JR & Nance FC (1977) Periampullary malignancy in Gardner's syndrome. *Ann Surg* **185**: 565.

Kaschula RO (1971) Mixed juvenile adenomatous and intermediate polyposis coli: report of a case. *Dis Colon Rectum* **14**: 368–374.

Katayama Y, Kimura M & Konn M (1985) Cronkhite–Canada syndrome associated with rectal cancer and adenomatous changes in colonic polyps. *Am J Surg Pathol* **9**: 65–71.

Keshgegian AA & Enterline HT (1978) Gardner's syndrome with duodenal adenomas, gastric adenomyoma and thyroid papillary follicular adenoma. *Dis Colon Rectum* **21**: 255–260.

Keusch CF & Bauer J (1989) Mesenteric fibromatosis in Gardner's syndrome. *Mt Sinai J Med* **56**: 318–320.

Khii S, Horii Nakatsuru S et al (1992) Inactivation of both APC alleles in an early stage of colon adenomas in a patient with familial adenomatous polyposis (FAP). *Human Mol Genet* **1**: 387–390

Khorsand J & Karakousis CP (1985) Desmoid tumours and their management. *Am J Surg* **149**: 215–218.

Kim DH, Goldsmith HS, Quan SH & Huvos AG (1971) Intra-abdominal desmoid tumor. *Cancer* **27**: 1041–1045.

Kindbloom LG, Angervall L, Santesson B & Selander S (1977) Cronkhite–Canada syndrome. *Cancer* **39**: 2651.

Kingston JE, Draper GJ & Mann JR (1982) Hepatoblastoma and polyposis coli. *Lancet* **i**: 457.

Kinzbrunner B, Ritter S, Domingo J & Rosenthal CJ (1983) Remission of rapidly growing desmoid tumors after tamoxifen therapy. *Cancer* **52**: 2201–2204.

Kiryu H, Tsuneyoshi M & Enjoji M (1985) Myofibroblasts in fibromatoses: an electron microscopic study. *Acta Pathol Jpn* **35**: 533–547.

Kitamura A, Kanagawa T, Yamada S & Kawai T (1991) Effective chemotherapy for abdominal desmoid tumor in a patient with Gardner's syndrome: report of a case. *Dis Colon Rectum* **34**: 822–826.

Klein WA, Miller HH, Anderson M & De Cosse JJ (1987) The use of indomethacin, sulindac and tamoxifen for the treatment of desmoid tumors associated with familial polyposis. *Cancer* **60**: 2863–2868.

Klemmer S, Pascoe L & De Cosse J (1987) Occurrence of desmoids in patients with familial adenomatous polyposis of the colon. *Am J Med Genet* **28**: 385–392.

Kobayashi H, Sakahara H, Hosono M et al (1994) Soft-tissue tumors: diagnosis with Tc-99m (V) dimercaptosuccinic acid scintigraphy. *Radiology* **190**: 277–280.

Kollevold T (1973) Desmoid tumour and carcinoma mamma in the same patient. *Acta Chir Scand* **139**: 573–576.

Kopelovich L (1984) Skin fibroblasts from humans genetically predisposed to colon cancer are abnormally senstive to SV40. *Cancer Invest* **2**: 333–338.

Kopelovich L, Colom S & Pollack R (1977) Defective organisation of actin in cultured skin fibroblasts from patients with inherited adenocarcinoma. *Proc Natl Acad Sci* **74**: 3019–3022.

Krokowicz P (1989) Management of familial polyposis in Poland. *Proceedings of the Fourth International Symposium on Colorectal Cancer. Hereditary Colorectal Cancer*, Kobe.

Krush AJ & Giardello FM (1990) Development of a genetics registry: hereditary intestinal polyposis and hereditary colon cancer registry at the Johns Hopkins Hospital 1973–88. In Herrera L (ed) *Familial Adenomatous Polyposis*, pp 43–60. New York: Alan R Liss.

Kyle SM & Keenan RA (1992) Mesenteric fibromatosis preventing restorative proctectomy. *Aust NZ J Surg* **62**: 240–241.

Labayle D, Fischer D, Vielh P et al (1991) Sulindac causes regression of rectal polyps in familial adenomatous polyposis. *Gastroenterology* **101**: 635–639.

Laferla G, Kaye SB & Crean GP (1988) Hepatocellular and gastric carcinoma associated with familial polyposis coli. *J Surg Oncol* **38**: 19–21.

Latt TT, Nicholl R, Domizio P, Walker-Smith JA & Williams CB (1993) Rectal bleeding and polyps. *Arch Dis Child* **69**: 144–147.

Law DS, Olschwang S & Monpelat SP (1988) Concerted nonsyntenic allelic loss in human colorectal carcinoma. *Science* **241**: 961–964.

Lee FI & MacKinnon MP (1981) Papillary thyroid carcinoma associated with polyposis coli. *Am J Gastroenterol* **76**: 138–140.

Lees CD & Hermann RE (1981) Familial polyposis coli associated with bile duct cancer. *Am J Surg* **141**: 378–380.

Leppard B (1974) Epidermoid cysts and polyposis coli. *Proc R Soc Med* **67**: 1036–1037.

Leppert M, Dobbs M, Scambler P et al (1987) The gene for familial polyposis coli maps to the long arm of chromosome 5. *Science* **238**: 1411–1412.

Leppert M, Burt R, Hughes JP et al (1990) Genetic analysis of an inherited predisposition to colon cancer in a family with a variable number of adenomatous polyps. *N Engl J Med* **322**: 904–908.

Levy DB, Smith KJ, Beazer-Barclay Y et al (1994) Inactivation of both APC alleles in human and mouse tumors. *Cancer Res* **54**: 5953–5958.

Lewis RA, Crowder WE, Eierman LA, Neussbaum RL & Ferrel RE (1988) The Gardner syndrome: significance of ocular features. *Ophthalmology* **91**: 916–925.

Li FP, Thurber WA, Seddon J & Holmes GE (1987) Hepatoblastoma in families with polyposis coli. *J Am Med Assoc* **257**: 2475–2477.

Lim CL, Walker MJ, Mehta RR & Das-Gupta TK (1986) Estrogen and antiestrogen binding sites in desmoid tumors. *Eur J Cancer Clin Oncol* **22**: 583–587.

Lin BP, Scott GS, Loughman NT & Newland RC (1989) Mesenteric fibromatosis: cytologic, histologic, and ultrastructural findings in a case. *Diagn Cytopathol* **5**: 69–74.

Ling CS, Leagus C & Stahlgren LH (1959) Intestinal lipomatosis. *Surgery* **46**: 1054–1059.

Lloyd KM & Dennis M (1963) Cowden's disease: a possible new symptom complex with multiple system involvement. *Ann Intern Med* **58**: 136–142.

Localio SA (1962) Spontaneous disappearance of rectal polyps following subtotal colectomy and ileoproctostomy for polyposis of the colon. *Am J Surg* **103**: 81–82.

Lockhart-Mummery HE (1967) Intestinal polyposis: the present position. *Proc R Soc Med* **60**: 381.

Lockhart-Mummery JP (1925) Cancer and heredity. *Lancet* **i**: 427–429.

Lotfi AM, Dozois RR, Gordon H et al (1989) Mesenteric fibromatosis complicating familial adenomatous polyposis: predisposing factors and results of treatment. *Int J Colorect Dis* **4**: 30–36.

Louw JH (1958) Polypoid lesions of the large bowel in children with particular reference to benign polyposis. *Paediat Surg* **3**: 195.

Lynch HT & Krush AJ (1967) Hereditary polyposis and adenocarcinoma of the colon. *Gastroenterology* **53**: 517–527.

Lynch HT & Lynch JF (1998) Genetics of colon cancer. *Digestion* **59**: 481–492.

MacDonald JN, Davis WC, Crago HR & Berk AD (1967) Gardner's syndrome and periampullary malignancy. *Am J Surg* **113**: 425.

Madden MV, Neale KF, Nicholls RJ et al (1991) Comparison of morbidity and function after colectomy with ileorectal anastomosis or restorative proctocolectomy for familial adenomatous polyposis. *Br J Surg* **78**: 789–792.

Magid D, Fishman EK, Jones B et al (1984) Desmod tumors in Gardner syndrome: use of computed tomography. *Am J Roentgenol* **142**: 1141–1145.

Magid D, Fishman EK, Wharam M Jr & Siegelman SS (1988) Musculoskeletal desmoid tumors: CT assessment during therapy. *J Comput Assist Tomogr* **12**: 222–226.

Mao C, Huang Y & Howard JM (1995) Carcinoma of the ampulla of Vater and mesenteric fibromatosis (desmoid tumour) associated with Gardner's syndrome: problems in management. *Pancreas* **10**: 239–245.

Marshall WH, Martin FIR & MacKay IR (1967) Gardner's syndrome with adrenal carcinoma. *Aust Ann Med* **16**: 242–244.

Martini GA & Dolle W (1961) Ménétrier-Syndrom Polyadenomatosis des margens mit Eiweissverlust in den Mazen-Darm-Kanal. *Dtsch Med Wschr* **86**: 2524.

Mathus-Vliegen EMH & Tytgat GNJ (1985) Peutz–Jeghers syndrome: clinical presentation and new therapeutic strategy. *Endoscopy* **17**: 102–104.

Mayo CW & Schlicke CP (1942) Carcinoma of the colon and rectum: a study of metastases and recurrences. *Surg Gynecol Obstet* **74**: 825.

McAdam WAF & Goligher JC (1970) The occurrence of desmoids in patients with familial polyposis coli. *Br J Surg* **57**: 618.

McColl I, Bussey HJR, Veale AMO & Morson BC (1964) Juvenile polyposis coli. *Proc R Soc Med* **57**: 896.

McCormick F (1992) Coupling of *ras* p21 signalling and GTP hydrolysis by GTPase activating proteins. *Phil Trans R Soc Lond B* **336** (1276): 43–47.

McKittrick LS, Malory TB & Talbott JH (1935) Case records of the Massachusetts General Hospital. *N Engl J Med* **212**: 263.

McKusick UA (1962) Genetic factors in intestinal polyposis. *JAMA* **182**: 281.

Melmed RN & Bouchier IAD (1972) Duodenal involvement in Gardner's syndrome. *Gut* **13**: 524.

Mendelsohn G & Diamond MP (1984) Familial ganglioneuromatous polyposis of the large bowel: report of a family with associated juvenile polyposis. *Am J Surg Pathol* **8**: 515–520.

Mills SJ, Chapman PD, Burn J & Gunn A (1997) Endoscopic screening and surgery for familial adenomatous polyposis: dangerous delays. *Br J Surg* **84**: 74–77.

Moertel CG, Hill JR & Adson MA (1970) Surgical management of multiple polyposis: the problem of cancer in the retained bowel segment. *Arch Surg* **100**: 521–525.

Morson BC (1962) Precancerous lesions of the colon and rectum. *JAMA* **179**: 316–321.

Morson BC & Bussey HJR (1970) Predisposing causes of intestinal cancer. In Ravitch MM et al (eds) *Current Problems in Surgery*. Chicago: YearBook Medical.

Morson BC & Dawson MP (1990) *Gastrointestinal Pathology*, 3rd edn. Oxford: Blackwell Scientific.

Morton DG, Gibson J, MacDonald F et al (1992) Role of congenital hypertrophy of the retinal pigment epithelium in the predictive diagnosis of familial adenomatous polyposis. *Br J Surg* **79**: 689–693.

Morton DG, MacDonald F, Haydon J et al (1993) Screening practice for familial adenomatous polyposis: the potential for regional registers. *Br J Surg* **80**: 255–258.

Muir E, Yates-Bell A & Barlow K (1967) Multiple primary carcinoma of the colon, duodenum and larynx associated with kerato-acanthomata of the face. *Br J Surg* **54**: 191–195.

Murday V & Slack J (1989) Inherited disorders associated with colorectal cancer. *Cancer Surveys* **8**: 139–157.

Myrhoj T, Bulow S & Mogensen AM (1989) Multiple adenomas in terminal ileum 25 years after restorative proctocolectomy for familial adenomatous polyposis: report of a case. *Dis Colon Rectum* **32**: 618–620.

Nagase H, Miyoshi Y, Horii A et al (1992) Correlation between the location of germline mutations in the APC gene and the number of colorectal polyps in familial adenomatous polyposis patients. *Cancer Res* **52**: 4055–4058

Naylor EW, Gardner EJ & Richards RC (1979) Desmoid tumours and mesenteric fibromatosis in Gardner's syndrome. *Arch Surg* **114**: 1181–1185.

Neale K, Ritchie S & Thompson JPS (1990) Screening of offspring of patients with familial adenomatous polyposis: the St Mark's Hospital Polyposis Register experience. In Herrera L (ed) *Familial Adenomatous Polyposis*, pp 61–66. New York: Alan R Liss.

Neely MG & Gillespie G (1967) Peutz–Jeghers syndrome: sporadic and familial. *Br J Surg* **54**: 378.

Nicholls RJ, Springall RG & Gallager P (1988) Regression of rectal adenomas after colectomy and ileorectal anastomosis for familial adenomatous polyposis. *BMJ* **296**: 1707–1708.

Niimi K, Tomada H, Furusawa M, Hayashi I & Okumura Y (1991) Peutz–Jeghers syndrome associated with adenocarcinoma of the cecum and focal carcinomas in harmartomatous polyps of the colon: a case report. *Jpn J Surg* **21**: 220–223.

Nishiura M, Hirota T, Itabashi M, Ashio K, Yamada T & Oguro Y (1984) A clinical and histopathological study of gastric polyps in familial polyposis coli. *Am J Gastroenterol* **79**: 98–103.

Niv Y & Fraser GM (1994) Adenocarcinoma in the rectal segment in familial polyposis coli is not prevented by sulindac therapy. *Gastroenterology* **107**: 854–857.

Nugent KP, Farmer KCR, Spigelman AD, Williams CB & Phillips RKS (1993a) Randomized controlled trial of the effect of sulindac on duodenal and rectal polyposis and cell proliferation in patients with familial adenomatous polyposis. *Br J Surg* **80**: 1618–1619.

Nugent KP, Spigelman AD, Nicholls RJ et al (1993b) Pouch adenomas in patients with familial adenomatous polyposis. *Br J Surg* **80**: 1620.

Nugent KP, Spigelman AD & Phillips RKS (1995) Colorectal cancer: surgical prophylaxis and chemoprevention [Review}. *Ann R Coll Surg Engl* **77**: 372–376.

Offerhaus GJA, Giardiello FM, Krush AJ et al (1992) The risk of gastrointestinal cancer in familial adenomatous polyposis. *Gastroenterology* **102**: 1980–1982.

Ohsato K, Yao T, Watanabe H, Iida M & Itoh H (1977) Small intestinal involvement in familial polyposis diagnosed by operative intestinal fiberoscopy: a report of four cases. *Dis Colon Rectum* **20**: 414–420.

Ojerskog B, Myrvold LO, Philipson BM & Ahren C (1987) Gastroduodenal and ileal polyps in patients treated surgically for familial polyposis coli with protocolectomy and continent ileostomy. *Acta Chir Scand* **153**: 681–686.

Okamoto M, Sato C, Kohno Y et al (1990) Molecular nature of chromosome 5q loss in colorectal tumors and desmoids from patients with familial adenomatous polyposis. *Hum Genet* **85**: 595–599.

Olschwang S, Tiret A, Laurent-Puig P et al (1993) Restriction of occular fundus lesions to a specific subgroup of APC mutations in adenomatous polyposis coli patients. *Cell* **75**: 959–968.

Pack GT & Ariel IM (1958) *Tumours of the Soft Somatic Tissues*. London: Cassell.

Pack GT & Ehlich HE (1944) Neoplasms of the anterior abdominal wall with special consideration of desmoid tumours: experience with 391 cases and a collective review of the literature. *Int Abstr Surg* **79**: 177–198.

Palmer ED (1968) What Ménétrier really said. *Gastrointest Endosc* **15**: 83.

Park JG, Park KJ, Ahn YO et al (1992) Risk of gastric cancer among Korean familial adenomatous polyposis patients: report of three cases. *Dis Colon Rectum* **35**: 996–998

Parks AG & Nicholls RJ (1978) Proctocolectomy without ileostomy for ulcerative colitis. *BMJ* **2**: 85–88.

Patel SR, Evans HL & Benjamin RS (1993) Combination chemotherapy in adult desmoid tumors. *Cancer* **72**: 3244–3247.

Penna C, Kartheuser A, Parc R et al (1993a) Secondary proctectomy and ileal pouch–anal anastomosis after ileorectal anastomosis for familial adenomatous polyposis. *Br J Surg* **80**: 1621–1623.

Penna C, Tiret E, Parc R et al (1993b) Operation and abdominal desmoid tumors in familial adenomatous polyposis. *Surg Gynecol Obstet* **177**: 263–268.

Perzin KH & Bridge MF (1982) Adenomatous and carcinomatous changes in hamartomatous polyps of the small intestine (Peutz–Jeghers syndrome): report of a case and review of the literature. *Cancer* **49**: 971–983.

Petersen GM, Slack J & Nakamura Y (1990) Screening guidelines and premorbid diagnosis of familial adenomatous polyposis using linkage. *Gastroenterology* **100**: 1658–1664.

Peterson GM, Francomano C, Kinzler K & Nakamura Y (1993) Presymptomatic direct detection of adenomatous polyposis coli (APC) gene mutations in familial adenomatous polyposis. *Human Genet* **91**: 307–311.

Peutz JLA (1921) Very remarkable case of familial polyposis of mucous membrane of intestinal tract and nasopharynx accompanied by peculiar pigmentations of skin and mucous membrane. *Nederl Maandschr V Geneesk* **10**: 134–146.

Pfeffer L, Lipkin M, Stutman O & Kopelovich L (1976) Growth abnormalities of cultured human skin fibroblasts derived from individuals with hereditary adenomatosis of the colon and rectum. *J Cell Physiol* **89**: 29–38.

Plail RO, Glazier G, Thomson JPS & Bussey HJR (1985) Adenomatous polyposis: an association with carcinoma. Frontiers in Colorectal Cancer. St Mark's 150th Anniversary, London.

Powell SM, Petersen GM, Krush AJ et al (1993) Molecular diagnosis of familial adenomatous polyposis. *N Engl J Med* **329**: 1982–1987.

Procter H, Singh L, Baum M & Brinkley D (1987) Response of multicentric desmoid tumours to tamoxifen. *Br J Surg* **74**: 401.

Ramaswamy F, Elhosseinny AA & Tchertkoff V (1981) Juvenile polyposis of the colon with atypical adenomatous changes and carcinoma in situ. *Dis Colon Rectum* **24**: 393–398.

Ranzi T, Castagnone D, Velio P & Polli EE (1981) Gastric and duodenal polyps in familial polyposis coli. *Gut* **22**: 363–373.

Rasheed S & Gardner MB (1981) Growth properties and susceptibility to viral transformation of skin fibroblasts from individuals at high generic risk for colorectal cancer. *J Natl Cancer Inst* **66**: 43–49.

Raszkowski HJ & Hufner RF (1971) Neurofibromatosis of the colon: a unique manifestation of Von Recklinghausen's disease. *Cancer* **27**: 134–142.

Read K & Vose PC (1981) Diffuse juvenile polyposis of the colon: a premalignant condition. *Dis Colon Rectum* **24**: 205–210.

Reale MA & Fearon ER (1994) Molecular genetics of hereditary colorectal cancer. *Haematol Oncol Ann* **2**: 129.

Reed TE & Neel JV (1955) A genetic study of multiple polyposis of the colon (with an appendix deriving a method of eliminating relative fitness). *Am J Hum Genet* **7**: 236.

Reid JD (1974) Intestinal carcinoma in the Peutz–Jeghers syndrome. *JAMA* **170**: 633.

Reitamo JJ, Hayry P, Nykyri E & Saxen E (1982) The desmoid tumour. I: Incidence, sex-, age- and anatomical distribution in the Finnish population. *Am J Clin Pathol* **77**: 665–673.

Reitamo JJ, Scheinin TM & Hayry P (1986) The desmoid syndrome: new aspects in the cause, pathogenesis and treatment of the desmoid tumor. *Am J Surg* **151**: 230–237.

Restrepo C, Moreno J, Duque E et al (1978) Juvenile colonic polyposis in Columbia. *Dis Colon Rectum* **21**: 600–612.

Rhodes M, Chapman PD, Burn J & Gunn A (1991) Role of a regional register for familial adenomatous polyposis: experience in the Northern Region. *Br J Surg* **78**: 451–452

Richard CS, Berk T, Bapat BV et al (1997) Sulindac for periampullary polyps in FAP patients. *Int J Colorecl Dis* **12**: 14–18

Richards RC, Rogers SW & Gardener EJ (1981) Spontaneous mesenteric fibromatosis in Gardner's syndrome. *Cancer* **47**: 597–601.

Rigau J, Pique JM, Rubio E et al (1991) Effects of long-term sulindac therapy on colonic polyposis. *Ann Intern Med* **115**: 952–954.

Rintala A (1959) The histological appearance of gastrointestinal polyps in the Peutz–Jeghers syndrome. *Acta Chir Scand* **117**: 366.

Rivadeneyra J & Santiago-Payan H (1982) The estrogenic receptor in desmoid tumors: preliminary report. *Arch Invest Med (Mex)* **13**: 105–108.

Rock MG, Pritchard DJ, Reiman HM, Soule EH & Brewster RC (1984) Extra-abdominal desmoid tumors. *J Bone Joint Surg (Am)* **66**: 1369–1374.

Rodriguez-Bigas MA, Mahoney MC, Karakousis CP & Petrelli NJ (1994) Desmoid tumors in patients with familial adenomatous polyposis. *Cancer* **74**: 1270–1274.

Romer H, Cotle C & Essenfeld-Yahr R (1971) Behaviour of the rectal juvenile polyps in vitro. *Gut* **12**: 194–199.

Roth SI & Helwig EB (1963) Juvenile polyps of the colon and rectum. *Cancer* **16**: 468.

Rothman D, Su CP & Kendall AB (1975) Dilemma in a case of Turcot's (glioma polyposis) syndrome: report of a case. *Dis Colon Rectum* **18**: 514–515.

Rozen P & Baratz M (1982) Familial juvenile colonic polyposis with associated colon cancer. *Cancer* **49**: 1500–1503.

Rowntree AC, Allardice JT, Woods WW et al (1993) Prospective clinical trial to determine the influence of Sulindac on the formation of recurrent colonic adenomatous polyps. *Br J Surg* **80**: 1477.

Rubin M, Tuthill RJ, Rosato EF & Cohen S (1980) Cronkhite–Canada syndrome: report of an unusual case. *Gastroenterology* **79**: 737.

Rubinfield B, Souza B, Albert I et al (1993) Association of the APC gene product with B catenin. *Science* **262**: 1731–1734

Rustgi AK (1994) Hereditary gastrointestinal polyposis and non-polyposis syndromes. *N Engl J Med* **331**: 1694–1702.

Ruvalcaba RHA, Myrhe J & Smith DW (1980) Sotos syndrome with intestinal polyposis and pigmentary changes of genitalia. *Clin Genet* **18**: 413–416.

Sachatello CR, Pickren CA & Grace JT (1970) Generalized juvenile gastrointestinal polyposis: a hereditary syndrome. *Gastroenterology* **58**: 699–708.

Sarre RG, Frost AG, Jagelman DG et al (1987a) Gastric and duodenal polyps in familial adenomatous polyposis: a prospective study of the nature and prevalence of upper gastrointestinal polyps. *Gut* **28**: 306–314.

Sarre RG, Jagelman DG, Beck GJ et al (1987b) Colectomy with ileorectal anastomosis for familial adenomatous polyposis: the risk of rectal cancer. *Surgery* **101**: 20–26.

Schaupp WC & Volpe PA (1972) Management of diffuse colonic polyposis. *Am J Surg* **124**: 218.

Schneider BL, Haque S, van Hoff J, Touloukian RJ & West AB (1992) Case report: familial adenomatous polyposis following liver transplantation for a virilizing hepatoblastoma. *J Pediatr Gastroenterol Nutrit* **15**: 198–201.

Schnur PL, David E, Brown PW et al (1973) Adenocarcinoma of the duodenum and Gardner's syndrome. *JAMA* **233**: 1229.

Schuchardt WA & Ponsky JL (1979) Familial polyposis and Gardner's syndrome. *Surg Gynecol Obstet* **148**: 97–103.

Schwartz RA, Goldberg DJ, Mahmood F et al (1989) The Muir–Torre syndrome: a disease of sebaceous and colonic neoplasms. *Dermatologica* **178**: 23–28.

Seiter K & Kemeny N (1993) Successful treatment of a desmoid tumor with doxorubicin. *Cancer* **71**: 2242–2244.

Settaf A, Mansori F, Bargash S & Saidi A (1990) Peutz–Jeghers syndrome with carcinomatous degeneration of a duodenal harmatomatous polyp. *Ann Gastroenterol Hepatol (Paris)* **26**: 285–288.

Setti-Carraro P & Nicholls RJ (1996) Choice of prophylactic surgery for the large bowel component of familial adenomatous polyposis. *Br J Surg* **83**: 885–892.

Shaw EB & Hennigar GR (1974) Intestinal lymphoid polyposis. *Am J Clin Path* **61**: 417.

Shepherd A (1971) Familial polyposis of the colon with special reference to regression of rectal polyposis after subtotal colectomy. *Br J Surg* **58**: 85–91.

Sheridan R, D'Avis J, Seyfer AE & Quispe G (1986) Massive abdominal wall desmoid tumor: treatment by resection and abdominal wall reconstruction. *Dis Colon Rectum* **29**: 518–520.

Siegel MJ (1975) Cowden's disease: a report of a case with malignant melanoma. *Cutis* **16**: 258.

Smilow PC, Pryor CA & Swinton NW (1966) Juvenile polyposis coli. *Dis Colon Rectum* **9**: 248.

Smith AJ, Stern S, Penner M et al (1994) Somatic APC and K-*ras* codon 12 mutations in aberrant cryptic foci from human colons. *Cancer Res* **54**: 5527–5530.

Smith KJ, Johnson KA, Bryan TM et al (1993) The APC gene product in normal and tumour cells. *Proc Natl Acad Sci* **90**: 2846–2850.

Smith WG (1958) Multiple polyposis: Gardner's syndrome and desmoid tumours. *Dis Colon Rectum* **1**: 323.

Smith WG (1959) Desmoid tumours in familial multiple polyposis. *Mayo Clin Proc* **34**: 31.

Smith WG & Kern BB (1973) The nature of the mutation in familial multiple polyposis: papillary carcinoma of the thyroid, brain tumours and familial multiple polyposis. *Dis Colon Rectum* **16**: 264–271.

Spagnesi MT, Tonelli F, Dolara P et al (1994) Rectal proliferation and polyp occurrence in patients with familial adenomatous polyposis after sulindac treatment. *Gastroenterology* **106**: 362–366.

Spigelman AD & Phillips RKS (1989) Management of the Peutz–Jeghers patient. *J R Soc Med* **82**: 681.

Spigelman AD & Phillips RKS (1994) The upper gastrointestinal tract. In Phillips RKS, Spigelman AD & Thomson JPS (eds) *Familial Adenomatous Polyposis and Other Polyposis Syndromes*, pp 106–127. London: Edward Arnold.

Spigelman AD, Murday V & Phillips RKS (1989a) Cancer and the Peutz–Jeghers syndrome. *Gut* **30**: 1588–1590.

Spigelman AD, Williams CB, Talbot IC, Domizio P & Phillips RKS (1989b) Upper gastrointestinal cancer in patients with familial adenomatous polyposis. *Lancet* **ii**: 783–785.

Spigelman AD, Thomson JPS & Phillips RKS (1990) Towards decreasing the relaparotomy rate in the Peutz–Jeghers syndrome: the role of peroperative small bowel endoscopy. *J Surg* **77**: 301–302.

Spigelman AD, Arese P, Phillips RKS (1995) Polyposis: the Peutz–Jegher's syndrome. *Br J Surg* **82**: 1311–1314.

Spirio L, Olschwang S, Groden J et al (1993) Alleles of the APC gene: an attenuated form of familial polyposis. *Cell* **75**: 951–957

Srivatsa PJ, Keeney GL & Podratz KC (1994) Disseminated cervical adenoma malignum and bilateral ovarian sex cord tumors with annular tubules associated with Peutz–Jeghers syndrome. *Gynecol Oncol* **53**: 256–264.

Stemper TJ, Kent TH & Summers RW (1975) Juvenile polyposis and gastrointestinal carcinoma: a study of a kindred. *Ann Intern Med* **83**: 639–646.

Strode JE (1954) Desmoid tumours particularly as related to surgical removal. *Ann Surg* **139**: 335–363.

Stryker SJ, Carney JA & Dozois RR (1987) Multiple adenomatous polyps arising in a continent reservoir ileostomy. *Int J Colorect Dis* **2**: 43–45.

Su LK, Johnson KA, Smith K et al (1993a) Association between wild type and mutant APC gene products. *Cancer Res* **53**: 2728–2731.

Su LK, Vogelstein B & Kinzler K (1993b) Association of the APC tumour suppressor proteins with catenins. *Science* **262**: 1734–1737.

Sugihara K, Muto T, Kamiya J et al (1982) Gardner's syndrome associated with periampullary carcinoma, duodenal and gastric adenomatosis. *Dis Colon Rectum* **25**: 766–771.

Sundaram M, McGuire MH & Herbold DR (1988) Magnetic resonance imaging of soft tissue masses: an evaluation of fifty-three histologically proven tumors. *Magn Reson Imaging* **6**: 237–248.

Swartley RN & Stayman JW (1962) Lymphoid hyperplasia of the intestinal tract requiring surgical intervention. *Ann Surg* **155**: 238–240.

Symmers D (1948) Lymphoid disease: Hodgkin's granuloma, giant follicular lymphadenopathy, lymphoid leukaemia, lymphosarcoma and gastrointestinal pseudo leukaemia. *Arch Pathol* **45**: 73–131.

Thomson JPS (1988) Leeds Castle Polyposis Group Meeting. *Dis Colon Rectum* **31**: 613.

Tonelli F, Valanzano R & Brandi ML (1994) Pharmacologic treatment of desmoid tumors in familial adenomatous polyposis: results of an *in vitro* study. *Surgery* **115**: 473–479.

Traboulsi EI, Krush AJ, Gardner EJ et al (1987) Prevalence and importance of pigmented ocular fundus lesions in Gardner's syndrome. *N Engl J Med* **316**: 661–667.

Trau H, Schewach-Millet M, Fisher BK & Tsur H (1982) Peutz–Jeghers syndrome and bilateral breast cancer. *Cancer* **50**: 788–792.

Tsukada K, Church JM, Jagelman DG, Fazio VW & Lavery IC (1991) Systemic cytotoxic chemotherapy and radiation therapy for desmoid in familial adenomatous polyposis. *Dis Colon Rectum* **34**: 1090–1092.

Tsukada K, Church JM, Jagelman DG et al (1992) Noncytotoxic drug therapy for intra-abdominal desmoid tumor in patients with familial adenomatous polyposis. *Dis Colon Rectum* **35**: 29–33.

Tsunoda A, Talbot IC & Nicholls RJ (1990) Incidence of displasia in the anorectal mucosa in patients having restorative proctocolectomy. *Br J Surg* **77**: 506–508.

Turcot J, Depres JP & St Pierre F (1959) Malignant tumours of the central nervous system associated with familial polyposis of the colon. *Dis Colon Rectum* **2**: 465–466.

Umemoto S, Makuuchi H, Amemiya T et al (1991) Intra-abdominal desmoid tumors in familial polyposis coli: a case report of tumor regression by prednisolone therapy. *Dis Colon Rectum* **34**: 89–93.

Ushio K, Sasagawa M, Doi H et al (1976) Lesions associated with familial polyposis coli: studies of lesions of the stomach, duodenum, bones and teeth. *Gastrointest Radiol* **1**: 67–68.

Utsunomiya J & Nakamura T (1975) The occult osteomatous changes in the mandible in patients with familial polyposis coli. *Br J Surg* **62**: 45.

Utsunomiya J, Maki T, Iwama T et al (1974) Gastric lesions of familial polyposis coli. *Cancer* **34**: 745–754.

Utsunomiya J, Gocho H, Miyanga T, Hamaguchi E & Kashimure A (1975) Peutz–Jeghers syndrome: its natural course and management. *Johns Hopkins Med J* **136**: 71–82.

Utsunomiya J, Miki Y, Juroki T & Iwama T (1990) Phenotypic expression of Japanese patients with familial adenomatous polyposis. In Herrera L (ed) *Familial Adenomatous Polyposis*, pp 61–66. New York: Alan R Liss.

Vasen HFA (1989) The value of screening and central registration of familial adenomatous polyposis: a study of 82 families in The Netherlands. In *Screening for Hereditary Tumours* (thesis), p 51. Utrecht: Drukkerij Elink.

Veale AMO (1965a) Intestinal polyposis genetics. In *Laboratory Memoirs*, Vol. 15. Cambridge: Cambridge University Press.

Veale AMO (1965b) Intestinal polyposis. In *Eugenics Laboratory Memoirs*, Vol 40. Cambridge: Cambridge University Press.

Veale AMO, McColl I, Bussey HJR & Morson BC (1966) Juvenile polyposis coli. *J Med Genet* **3**: 5.

Waddell WR (1975) Treatment of intra-abdominal and abdominal-wall desmoid tumours with drugs that affect the metabolism of cyclic 35 adenosine monophosphate. *Ann Surg* **181**: 299.

Waddell WR (1983) Non-steroidal anti-inflammatory drugs and tamoxifen for desmoid tumours and carcinoma of the stomach. *J Surg Oncol* **22**: 197–211.

Waddell WR & Gerner RE (1980) Indomethacin and ascorbate inhibit desmoid tumours. *J Surg Oncol* **15**: 85.

Waddell WR & Kirsch WM (1991) Testolactone, sulindac, warfarin, and vitamin K^1 for unresectable desmoid tumors. *Am J Surg* **161**: 416–421.

Waddell WR & Loughry WR (1983) Sulindac for polyposis of the colon. *J Surg Oncol* **24**: 83–87.

Waddell WR, Ganser GF, Cerise EJ & Loughry WR (1989) Sulindac for polyposis of the colon. *Am J Surg* **157**: 175–179.

Walsh N, Qizilbash A, Banerjee R & Waugh GA (1987) Biliary neoplasia in Gardner's syndrome. *Arch Pathol Lab Med* **111**: 76–77.

Watanabe H, Enjoji M, Yoa T et al (1977) Accompanying gastroenteric lesions in familial adenomatosis coli. *Acta Pathol Jpn* **27**: 823–839.

Watanabe H, Enjoji M, Yao T & Ohasato K (1978) Gastric lesions in familial adenomatous coli, their incidence and histological analysis. *Hum Pathol* **9**: 269–283.

Watne AL, Core SK & Carrier JM (1975) Gardner's syndrome. *Surg Gynecol Obstet* **141**: 53.

Waye JD, Lewis BS & Yessayan S (1992) Colonoscopy: a prospective report of complications. *J Clin Gastroenterol* **15**: 1–4

Weary PE, Gorlin RJ & Gentry WC Jr et al (1970) The multiple hamartoma syndrome (Cowden's disease). *Arch Dermatol* **106**: 682–690.

Weinstein LP, Kovachev D & Chaglassian T (1986) Abdominal wall reconstruction. *Scand J Plast Reconstr Surg* **20**: 109–113.

Weinstock JV & Kawanishi H (1978) Gastrointestinal polyposis with anocutaneous hamartomas (Cowden's disease). *Gastroenterology* **74**: 890–895.

Weiss AJ & Lackman RD (1991) Therapy of desmoid tumors and related neoplasms. *Compr Ther* **17**: 32–34.

Welch CE & Hedberg SE (1975) *Polypoid Lesions of the Gastrointestinal Tract*, 2nd edn, pp 186–199. Philadelphia: WB Saunders.

Weston SD & Weiner M (1967) Familial polyposis associated with a new type of soft tissue lesion (skin pigmentation). *Dis Colon Rectum* **10**: 311.

Williams AR, Balasoorya BAW & Day DW (1982) Polyps and cancer of the large bowel: a necropsy study in Liverpool. *Gut* **23**: 835–842.

Williams CB (1984) Benign tumours. In Bouchier I, Hodgson A & Keighley MRB (eds) *Textbook of Gastroenterology*, pp 823–841. London: Baillière Tindall.

Williams CB & Tan G (1979) Complications of colonoscopy and polypectomy. *Gut* **20**: A903.

Williams GT (1994) Metaplastic polyposis. In Phillips RKS, Spigelman AD & Thomson JPS (eds) *Familial Adenomatous Polyposis and Other Polypoid Syndromes*. London: Edward Arnold.

Williams GT, Arthur JF, Bussey HJR & Morson BC (1980) Metaplastic polyps and polyposis. *Histology* **41**: 155–170.

Wilson AJ, Baum M, Singh L & Kangas L (1987) Antioestrogen therapy of pure mesenchymal tumour. *Lancet* **i**: 508.

Wilson DM, Pitts WC, Hintz RL & Rosenfeld RG (1986) Testicular tumors with Peutz–Jeghers syndrome. *Cancer* **57**: 2238–2240.

Wolfstein IH, Bat L & Neumann G (1982) Regeneration of rectal mucosa and recurrent polyposis coli after total colectomy and ileoanal anastomosis. *Arch Surg* **117**: 1241–1242.

Young RH, Welch WR, Dickersin R & Scully RE (1982) Ovarian sex cord tumour with annular tubules: review of 74 cases including 27 with Peutz–Jeghers syndrome and four with adenoma malignum of the cervix. *Cancer* **50**: 1384–1402.

Zeze F, Ohsato K, Mitani H, Ohkuma R & Koide O (1983) Hepatocellular carcinoma associated with familial polyposis of the colon: report of a case. *Dis Colon Rectum* **26**: 465–468.

30

COLORECTAL CANCER: EPIDEMIOLOGY, AETIOLOGY, PATHOLOGY, STAGING, CLINICAL FEATURES, DIAGNOSIS AND SCREENING

EPIDEMIOLOGY

Malignant disease of the large bowel was responsible for 17 223 deaths in England and Wales in 1990, and 19 000 deaths in the United Kingdom a year later (CRC, 1993). It is now second only to lung cancer as the most common cause of death from malignant disease (OPCS, 1992; CRC 1993).

The situation is similar in the USA where colorectal carcinoma is now the most common solid tumour after skin malignancies. In 1992 in the USA, it was estimated that 156 000 new cases would be diagnosed and 58 300 deaths would occur (Boring et al, 1992). In Australia the number of deaths is approximately 3500 annually, and similarly it is the second most common cause of death from malignant disease (McDermott, 1983).

In each of these countries, despite major fluctuations in the death rates from other cancers, the mortality from colorectal cancer has been maintained at approximately the same level for the last 40 years (Miller, 1983; Stower and Hardcastle, 1985). This remains the case despite a marked improvement in the operability rate.

Geographical distribution

Colorectal carcinoma is not uniformly distributed among all populations. The highest incidences are in western Europe and North America, whereas intermediate rates prevail in eastern Europe (Table 30.1). The lowest rates are seen in Asia, Africa and South America excluding Argentina. However, there is some evidence that the incidence of the disease in Africa is now increasing, probably as a result of improving lifestyle (Iliyasu et al, 1996). The incidence of rectal carcinoma shows less international variation than does that of cancer of the colon. It is of interest that other neoplastic diseases have a similar international distribution; these include carcinoma of breast and prostate (Howell, 1976; Stemmerman, 1979) and adenomatous colorectal polyps (which are obviously of greater significance in the present context). Variations in incidence between countries are much larger than variations within each country. Nevertheless, in high-risk countries there are still notable differences. Thus Blot et al (1976), in a study that examined the incidence of the disease in 3056 counties of the USA, found that the tumour predominated in the north east and was consistently elevated in counties with large populations, high income and high educational levels. Other have also found that the disease occurs more frequently in urban than in rural areas (Clemmesen, 1977; Waterhouse et al, 1976).

Table 30.1 Incidence of colorectal cancer in various countries (per 100 000, age-adjusted to world population).

	Colonic	*Rectal*	*Colorectal*
Nigeria	1.3	1.2	2.5
India	4.6	4.4	9.0
Osaka (Japan)	6.3	6.9	13.2
East Germany	13.6	12.0	25.6
Vas (Hungary)	9.1	11.0	20.1
Connecticut (USA)	30.1	18.2	48.3
Detroit (USA)			
White	26.2	16.0	42.2
Black	24.5	13.8	38.2
Birmingham (UK)	16.5	16.1	32.6
Oxford (UK)	15.7	15.4	31.1
Ayrshire (UK)	16.6	14.0	30.0
Denmark	16.2	16.7	32.9
Finland	7.9	7.7	15.6
New Zealand			
Maori	7.4	4.6	12.0
Non-Maori	23.0	15.4	38.4
Hawaii			
Japanese	22.4	16.3	38.7
Caucasian	23.9	13.5	37.4
Hawaiian	14.1	9.4	23.5

Adapted from Waterhouse et al (1976).

Some of the differences in geographical variation may be due to a failure of detection in areas of low incidence, where techniques for diagnosis are perhaps less sophisticated and patient tolerance of symptoms is high. This explanation, however, probably accounts for only a small part of the variations, and does not explain for example the marked differences in incidence between Denmark and Finland or the low rate recorded in Japan.

Age and sex incidences

The most common decade of life for the development of rectal cancer is 60–69 years and the incidence of the disease tends to increase with advancing age (Goligher, 1941, 1984; Chu et al, 1994). The figures are similar for colon cancer. Much attention has concentrated on the incidence and fate of the disease in younger patients. The reported incidence of the disease in patients below 40 years old varies between 2% and 4% (Coffey and Cardenas, 1964; Falterman et al, 1974; Hsu and Guzman, 1982; Lundy et al, 1983; Pitluk and Poticha, 1983; Umpleby et al, 1984; Marble et al, 1992). The majority of these patients are 20–40 years old; however, since Steiner (1865) reported a case of colon cancer in a 9-year-old boy, sporadic cases have been described in patients under 20 (Fraser, 1938; Saner, 1946; Johnson et al, 1959; Mayo and Pagtalunan, 1963; McCoy and Parks, 1984). It has been stated (Bulow, 1980) that in this younger age group there is a predominance of right-sided lesions in males and left-sided lesions in females, but this has not been substantiated by others (Umpleby et al, 1984).

The sex distribution of colorectal carcinoma overall in England and Wales is approximately equal. The same is true in the USA (Silverberg, 1981) and in Australia (McDermott, 1983). However, these all-inclusive data hide certain differences. When the incidences of carcinoma of colon and rectum are examined separately, certain differences in sex incidence emerge. The ratio between males and females in the UK for carcinoma of the colon is approximately 2 : 3 and for carcinoma of the rectum is approximately 8 : 7. The corresponding USA data are 7 : 9 for colonic cancer and 9 : 5 for rectal cancer (Silverberg, 1981). Similarly, whereas at younger ages the incidence of colorectal cancer between the sexes is similar, in the older ages males tend to predominate (dos Santos Silva and Swerdlow, 1996).

Site distribution

For many years the data on distribution of carcinoma in the colon and rectum have demonstrated a preponderance of lesions in the rectum. Thus of the 14 430 patients who died from colorectal cancer in England and Wales in 1978, 10 381 had carcinoma of the colon and 6049 had carcinoma of the rectum. The statistics from Australia are similar (McDermott et al, 1981).

In the USA a number of reports have been published documenting a change in the anatomical distribution of the disease. The experience of the End Results group of the National Cancer Institute (Axtell and Chiazzi, 1966), as well as that of other tumour registries, was reviewed and the results demonstrated a gradual increase in the ratio of carcinoma of the colon to carcinoma of the rectum between the years 1940 and 1962. These results were confirmed by data from the Connecticut Tumor Registry (Meigs et al, 1977). Other studies from individual institutions have also confirmed this trend (Cady et al, 1974; Rhodes et al, 1977; Morganstern and Lee, 1978; Welch, 1979; Rosato and Marks, 1981). Despite these findings in the USA, the same does not appear to be the case in the UK and Australia (Chapuis et al, 1981; McDermott et al, 1981).

Most authors seem to agree about the distribution of tumours within the colon. Thus, approximately 50% of all colon growths are in the sigmoid, 25% are in the right colon (caecum and ascending colon), and the remaining 25% are in the transverse colon, splenic flexure, descending colon and hepatic flexure, in descending order of frequency (Judd, 1924; Fraser, 1938; Smiddy and Goligher, 1957; McDermott et al, 1981). There is, however, some recent evidence suggesting that although the order of frequency has remained the same, since the late 1960s the relative proportions have changed with a marked shift towards an increase in right colon lesions (Meigs et al, 1977; Rhodes et al, 1977; Slater et al, 1984; Eide, 1986, Loffeld et al, 1996). The distribution of growths within the rectum is difficult to determine because authors who have studied this subject have often used different measurements when dividing the rectum into its upper, middle and lower segments. Another problem has been that most data are based on operative specimens and thus some cases are excluded. The consensus, however, seems to be that, apart from minor variations, rectal cancers are equally distributed between the three segments of the rectum (Dukes, 1940; Goligher, 1941).

Synchronous carcinomas

The criteria used to define synchronous cancers of the large bowel were defined by Warren and Gates (1932). Each tumour must be distinct and the possibility that one is not the metastasis of the other must be excluded. The cancers need not, however, be diagnosed at the same time. Moertel et al (1958) arbitrarily set 6 months as the period during which tumours must be diagnosed to be considered synchronous. The reported incidence of synchronous tumours is variable and the reason probably relates to the degree of assiduity with which the rest of the large bowel is investigated after detection of one neoplasm. This applies particularly to patients who are initially found to have a rectal carcinoma.

The incidence of synchronous carcinoma ranges from 1.5% to 8% (Botsford et al, 1965; Diamente and Bacon, 1966; Devitt et al, 1969; Traviesco et al, 1972; Heald and Bussey, 1975; Reilly et al, 1982; Nottle et al, 1983; Langevin and Nivatvongs, 1984; Passman et al, 1992; Rosen et al, 1992), the higher incidences being found in series in which colonoscopy was employed to assess all patients. Benign polyps have been reported to occur in 12–60% of patients with single carcinomas (Floyd et al, 1966; Reilly et al, 1982) and in 57–86% of patients with synchronous carcinomas (Swinton and Pashley, 1962; Ekelund and Pihl, 1974; Heald and Bussey, 1975; Lasser, 1978; Welch, 1981; Reilly et al, 1982).

Earlier studies emphasized the frequency with which synchronous cancers occurred in the same surgical segments (Moertel et al, 1958; Swinton and Pashley, 1962; Heald and Bussey, 1975; Welch, 1981). Of 261 multiple synchronous primary cancers, Moertel et al (1958) found that 68% were confined to the same surgical specimen. Lasser (1978) found 62 cases of synchronous primary cancer in his series of 1002 patients, an incidence of 6.2%. Although most of the latter were more than 5 cm distant from each other, at least 60% were in the same surgical segment. In the more recent studies which have employed colonoscopy before surgery or within a 6-month period after it, a much higher proportion of tumours were outside the segment of standard resection (Reilly et al, 1982; Langevin and Nivatvongs, 1984). Interestingly, in one study the tumour was missed on double-contrast barium enema in each patient with a synchronous carcinoma (Reilly et al, 1982). These findings therefore reinforce the widely voiced opinion, held also by the present authors, that all patients with a colorectal cancer should undergo total colonoscopy and this should preferably be performed before operation.

The inaccuracy of a barium enema is illustrated by a study of 389 patients in whom 50% of synchronous cancers were not detected on the initial barium study, and the majority of these would not have been included in the planned resection specimen (Barillari et al, 1990). In patients with stenotic lesions which cannot be negotiated by colonoscopy, a full endoscopic examination of the remaining colon should be performed within 6 months of surgical resection.

Patients with synchronous colonic cancers seem to have the same prognosis as patients with solitary carcinomas. Passman et al (1996) found, in an 18-year multi-institutional study of 160 patients with 339 synchronous tumours, that survival was the same as for 4718 patients with solitary cancers on a stage-for-stage basis.

AETIOLOGY

As yet we do not fully comprehend the basic process underlying the development of carcinoma of the large bowel. Nevertheless, great strides have been made towards a more complete understanding, particularly with the advent of molecular biological techniques.

Although there are well-defined genetic syndromes, environmental factors still seem to be highly important. The most cogent evidence for this statement relates to the high incidence of colorectal cancer in 'sophisticated' societies. This is not purely a genetic difference, since migrants moving from low-incidence areas to high-incidence areas are at greater risk of developing the disease. Thus, first- and second-generation Japanese immigrants to Hawaii and California have a higher incidence of

Table 30.2 Exogenous factors possibly involved in colonic carcinogenesis.

Agent	*Origin*	*Effect*	*Presumed stage of action*	*Mechanism*	*Evidence**
Long-chain fatty acids	Dietary fat	Stimulate	Promotion	Cytotoxicity ↑ cell proliferation ↑	+
Bile acids	Endogenous (stimulated by dietary fat)	Stimulate	Promotion	Cytotoxicity ↑→ cell proliferation ↑	+
Diacylglycerol	Dietary fat	Stimulate	Promotion	Protein kinase C activity ↑→ cell proliferation ↑	±
Thermolysed caesin	Dietary protein	Stimulate	Promotion	Promotion	?
Ammonia	Protein (product of fermentation)	Stimulate	?	?	–
Bilirubin/haem	Endogenous/ dietary meat	Stimulate	Promotion	Cytotoxicity ↑ Cell proliferation ↑	± ?
Heterocyclic amines	Cooked meat	Stimulate	Initiation	Genotoxic	±
Fecapentaenes	Colonic bacteria	Stimulate	Initiation	Genotoxic	–
Hydroxyanthraquinones	Herbal laxatives	Stimulate	Initiation	Genotoxic Cell proliferation ↑	± ±
Non-starch polysaccharides	Dietary fibre	Inhibit	Initiation	Adsorption water, carcinogens → exposure (time) ↓	+
Short-chain fatty acids	Dietary fibre, resistant starch	Inhibit	Promotion	Differentiation ↑ Cell proliferation ↓ down-regulation of certain genes	+ ±
Fish oil	Fish in the diet	Inhibit	Promotion	Prostaglandins ↓→ cell proliferation ↓	±
Non-steroidal anti-inflammatory drugs	Drug	Inhibit	Promotion	Prostaglandins ↓→ FAP polyps ↓ Cell proliferation ↓	+
Antioxidants	Diet (vegetables, fruit)	Inhibit	Initiation	Oxygen radicals ↓→ cell damage ↓	±
Vitamin D	Diet, sun exposure	Inhibit	Promotion	Cell proliferation ↓	±

* Evidence: + Reasonably firm evidence for effect in humans, at least on a basis of mechanistic or epidemiologic considerations; ± doubtful effect in humans; – no evidence for effect in humans; ? no data available.
From Kleibeuker et al (1966).

the carcinoma than their compatriots who still reside in Japan (Haenszel and Correa, 1971). Similarly, Puerto Ricans migrating to the USA acquire an increased risk for the disease (Stubbs, 1983); the same is true of Polish migrants moving to the USA and Australia (Staszewski et al, 1971). Also, the incidence of carcinoma among European Jews in Israel is higher than that among Asian and African-born Jews (Modan, 1979).

The influence of factors such as fat, fibre, protein, calcium and other elements of lifestyle such as smoking (Giovannucci et al, 1994a,b; Heineman et al, 1995) probably operate through multiple overlapping pathways which influence the complex milieu of the epithelial cell. This milieu consists of exposure to luminal, local and systemic factors which may vary according to exogenous (environmental) as well as endogenous (e.g. physiological) influences. Environmental factors may influence the molecular events in colorectal cancer in various ways, including: methylation of DNA signal transduction across cell membranes, epithelial interaction with phytochemicals, fermentive production of butyrate and influences on the genome, and epithelial biology cell replication and dietary arylamines and their metabolism. Thus, there is likely to be a complex interaction of genetic and environmental factors in a variety of ways which will modify risk for carcinogenesis in the large bowel (Potter et al, 1993; Potter, 1996).

Since various studies have consistently demonstrated that certain dietary constituents correlate well with geographical variations of the disease, considerable emphasis has been placed on the factors that may be responsible for these differences (Table 30.2).

Dietary factors

Fibre

The most popular dietary theory relates the lack of fibre in the Western diet to the high risk. This hypothesis originated from findings in South African Bantus, who had a low incidence of large bowel cancer and who, owing to their high intake of fibre, produced bulkier stools than their white counterparts. Burkitt (1971) thus popularized the simple yet logical theory that a high fibre intake reduces intestinal transit time and thereby reduces the exposure of the gut mucosa to potential carcinogens. Furthermore, the opportunity for bowel bacteria to produce carcinomas is diminished and as a result of the increased bulk of the stool a dilution effect is produced (Burkitt, 1971). There is substantial indirect evidence to support this theory.

Several case–control studies have shown a negative association between the disease and dietary intake of vegetables and cereal fibre (Howe et al, 1992); the average weight of faeces is heavier in low-risk groups compared with high-risk groups (Stemmerman et al, 1981). Furthermore, higher fibre intake and more rapid intestinal transit have been recorded in low-risk groups (Burkitt, 1971). Despite this supportive evidence, there are criticisms of the concept and other contrary reports which question its validity. Thus in the previously mentioned studies the populations differed in respects other than dietary intake, and these factors might have been responsible for the different incidence of disease. Only one large epidemiological study with adequate control data has demonstrated a low risk for those individuals with a high fibre intake (Modan et al, 1975), whereas several international surveys have been unable to confirm this finding (Drasar and Irving, 1973; Armstrong and Doll, 1975). Experimental studies that have investigated the role of dietary fibre have also produced conflicting evidence. One study failed to demonstrate any protective effect of bran against experimentally induced colon cancer (Cruse et al, 1978).

Thus, although the fibre concept appears attractive in theory and is supported by circumstantial evidence, there is little scientific evidence to confirm its role. However, a prospective controlled trial set up in Australia is attempting to answer whether an increase in fibre and other dietary manipulations can protect against colorectal neoplasia (MacLennan et al, 1995). Although numbers are small and follow-up is relatively short, preliminary data suggest that a combination of fat reduction and a supplement of wheat bran can reduce the incidence of large adenomas. Similar preliminary data come from a prospective controlled trial in Canada (McKeowen-Eyssen et al, 1994).

If fibre is protective against colorectal cancer, this protection may come from phytic acid which is a major constitutent of cereals, pulses and seeds. Phytic acid is an important antioxidant component of fibre which has been demonstrated to have antineoplastic activity in animal models of colorectal cancer (Owen et al, 1996). The various mutagenic events which occur throughout colorectal carcinogenesis, such as loss of heterozygosity in tumour suppressor genes such as APC, MCC, DCC and p53, may be affected by antioxidants (Greenwald et al, 1995a,b).

Animal fat

There is evidence that a diet rich in animal fat, like most Western diets, is also a major risk factor (Potter et al, 1993). The proportion of animal fat in a Western diet is significantly greater than that in the diet of low-risk populations (Wynder and Reddy, 1974). Some nutritional statistics on fat and meat consumption correlate positively with the incidence of colonic cancer (Drasar and Irving, 1973; Armstrong and Doll, 1975; Nigro and Bull, 1987), and case–control studies support the association (Haenszel et al, 1973; Dales et al, 1978). In addition, some authors have found significant changes in tissue n3 and n6 fatty acid status in the mucosa of patients with colorectal adenomas compared with normal controls, thus indicating that these dietary components may participate in the early phases of colorectal carcinogenesis (Fernandez-Banares et al, 1996).

Nevertheless, these views have been challenged. Enstrom (1975) noted that a steady increase in the frequency of beef consumption in the USA from 1940 to 1970 was accompanied by stable or declining rates of incidence and mortality from colorectal disease. No association between fat intake and carcinoma was demonstrated when populations in low-risk Finland and high-risk Denmark were compared (Jensen and MacLennan, 1979). A carefully conducted case–control study performed as part of the Japan–Hawaii cancer study was also unable to confirm an association (Stemmerman, 1979).

The implication of fat as a possible aetiological factor is linked to the concept that the Western diet favours the development of a bacterial flora containing organisms that are capable of degrading bile salts to carcinogens (Nagengast et al, 1995). Since the same type of diet seems to lead to a greater excretion of bile salts in the faeces, the risk may be compounded. Thus Wynder and Reddy demonstrated greater faecal excretion of bile acids and neutral steroids in normal omnivorous people than in groups eating little or no meat (Reddy and Wynder, 1973; Reddy et al, 1974). Furthermore, these authors found greater concentrations of these substances in the faeces of cancer patients than in control subjects (Reddy and Wynder, 1977). Other authors have also found that populations at greater risk of developing carcinoma excrete greater quantities of bile acids than those at less risk (Hill, 1975, 1983; Crowther et al, 1976). Experimental studies have also shown that rats fed either vegetable oil or beef fat and treated with dimethylhydrazine developed more colon tumours than did animals on a control diet (Reddy et al, 1976). In addition, some authors have found a positive association between deoxycholic acid (DCA) in the serum and colorectal adenomas (Bayerdorffer et al, 1994, 1995). Furthermore, this association results from the DCA fraction which is absorbed from the colon.

The bile-salt/bacteria theory gains credence when it is considered that the bile acids have a chemical structure that is similar to carcinogens such as methylcholanthrene. Furthermore, it is known that certain bacteria – particularly *Clostridium paraputrificum* – can dehydrogenate the steroid nucleus, an effect that might be important in the development of compounds with structures similar to known carcinogens. It is therefore of particular interest that some authors (Drasar et al, 1976) have found that *C. paraputrificum* is particularly prevalent in the intestinal flora of high-risk groups. Furthermore, others (Hill et al, 1975) have noted its presence in the faeces of colon cancer patients more often than in control subjects. Hill et al (1971) also noted that the excretion of bile acids is greater and the ratio of anaerobic to aerobic bacteria in faeces is higher in subjects from countries with a high colorectal cancer incidence than in those with a low incidence. Certain anaerobes are more active in the degradation of bile acids and it is found that excreted bile acids are more often degraded in high-incidence populations than in low-incidence ones. It thus appears that bacteria within the large bowel do have an important role in colon carcinogenesis. However, although certain organisms have been identified in high-risk populations, there are no hard data linking a specific bacterium to the development of colorectal carcinoma. Many of the studies involve only small numbers of patients, and any patient may have up to 400 species of bacteria in the gut, making interpretation of results difficult.

It is possible that a component of fats may be responsible for colorectal carcinogenesis; n3 fats inhibit tumour cell proliferation and increased levels are found in colorectal cancer (Imray et al, 1990; Hendrickse, 1991; Hendrickse et al, 1991). The dietary fat theory of carcinogenesis presupposes that diet to a large extent controls the intestinal flora and that a diet with a high content of fat or meat allows bacteria that are particularly prone to produce carcinogens to flourish in the gut. Several studies, however, have examined the faecal flora of people living in the same country but taking different diets and all have failed to show a marked difference in flora. Some authors have tried unsuccessfully to alter faecal flora by dietary manipulation (Drasar and Jenkins, 1976).

Low vegetable intake

The lack of vegetables, in particular those of the cruciferous family such as cabbage, has been put forward as a major dietary cause of colorectal cancer. Bjelke (1973) was the first to draw attention to this possibility when he conducted dietary interviews in patients and control subjects and found that patients with cancer ate significantly fewer vegetables than controls. These findings were consistent in his two studies, one performed in Minnesota and the other in New York, and were corroborated by two separate studies (Modan et al, 1975; Graham et al, 1978).

Further support for the 'vegetable' theory comes from some experimental work. Wattenberg (1971) examined the activity of arylhydrocarbon hydroxylase (AHH) in the colon of rodents. Under normal circumstances this enzyme acts as a metabolic barrier to noxious chemicals. Wattenberg found that several cruciferous vegetables significantly increased the activity of this enzyme. After extraction of the active ingredients (indoles) he demonstrated that feeding these to rats inhibited the activity of carcinogens in the induction of gastrointestinal tumours. He also inhibited tumour formation by feeding either raw or cooked vegetables to his experimental animals.

Other dietary components

Other dietary components have been implicated in the aetiology of colorectal cancer. Several authors (Yudkin 1972; Cleave, 1974) have unconvincingly attempted to relate high sugar intake to the development of carcinoma. Similarly, excessive alcohol consumption has been suggested as a possible risk factor (Breslow and Enstrom, 1974; McMichael and Bonnet, 1981, Glynn et al, 1996), but case–control studies have been unable to confirm this association.

Attention has been focused on micronutrients. Davies and Daly (1984) suggested that a diet depleted of potassium increases the likelihood of polyps undergoing malignant change. Nelson (1984) suggested that the changing pattern of colorectal cancer may be caused by selenium deficiency, exacerbated by increased intakes of zinc and fluoride which are known to antagonize the action of selenium. Giovannucci et al (1995) have reported that there is an increased risk in subjects with a low folate and methionine intake which is particularly marked in those with a high alcohol intake. Calcium depletion may also play a role in colon carcinogenesis (see below).

Bile acids

Apart from the action of bacteria converting bile acids into potential carcinogens, recent evidence suggests that bile acids may also have a direct toxic action on the colonic mucosa which may lead to neoplastic change (Barker et al, 1994). Thus Rainey et al (1984) demonstrated that bile acids when administered per rectum are capable of promoting dimethylhydrazine-induced tumours in experimental rats. Similarly, Wilpart et al (1983) demonstrated that the secondary bile acids, deoxycholic acid and lithocholic acid, are carcinogenic. In view of these findings it is of considerable interest that some authors (Summerton et al, 1983) have found receptors to deoxycholic acid in approximately one-third of colorectal cancers. Others (Turjman et al, 1982) have also found receptors to lithocholic acid in these tumours. Some studies have demonstrated that the direct toxic effects of bile acids may be related to the amount of calcium present in the diet. Thus Wargovich et al (1983) showed that the adverse effects of deoxycholic acid on colonic mucosa could be ameliorated by administering the bile acid in the form of a calcium soap; similar findings were obtained by others (Vahouny et al, 1984).

Newmark et al (1984) attempted to explain these findings by hypothesizing that bile acids and fatty acids are toxic to the colon because they are potent scavengers of calcium. A diet rich in calcium contains sufficient to reach the colon so that all bile acids and fatty acids will be bound by it. Calcium depletion of the mucosa leads to cell desquamation and proliferation and since in these circumstances bile acids remain unbound they are free to cause alterations in cellular DNA, a combination that may lead to neoplastic change. It has also been shown that increased crypt cell production rates in humans may be reversed by calcium supplements (Barsoum and Bhavanandan, 1989; Barsoum et al, 1992a,b; Hall et al, 1992). As a result of these experimental findings, various prospective randomized trials have been commenced to test whether calcium supplementaion in the diet is beneficial (Lipkin and Newmark, 1995). However, early results are not encouraging (Cats et al, 1995).

Previous cholecystectomy

Much has been written to suggest an association between colorectal carcinoma and previous cholecystectomy, but the literature is inconsistent. Vernick and Kuller (1981) found that there was a significant increase in the relative risk of right-sided colon cancer in both sexes following this operation. However, Linos et al (1981) could demonstrate this risk only in women, a finding confirmed in an autopsy study of 864 patients by Allende et al (1984). Allende and associates also suggested that gallbladder disease might be a risk factor and that the risk was increased further by gallbladder surgery. Although some authors (Adami et al, 1983; Blanco et al, 1984) have not been able to demonstrate an association, this might have been related to the fact that their patients had not been followed up for long enough. This was well exemplified by a study carried out by Mannes et al (1984) who investigated 331 patients following cholecystectomy and compared them with a matched control group. They showed no increase in adenoma carriage during the first 10 postoperative years, but a significant increase in carriage occurred in patients who had undergone surgery more than 10 years previously and who were more than 60 years old. Reid et al (1996) attempted a metanalysis of 95 relevant studies in the literature, finding 35 with age- and sex-matched controls that were suitable for such assessment. They concluded that although there was a small observed association between cholecystectomy and colorectal cancer development, this could have resulted from publication bias for positive results or bias within the included studies. If there is indeed a real effect, the risk to an individual is very small.

These data are further supported by a very good autopsy study from Ashford in Kent (Mercer et al, 1995), which was also unable to confirm any association between colorectal cancer and cholecystectomy or between cancer and gallstones.

The adenoma–carcinoma sequence

The relationship betweeen adenomas and carcinomas is discussed fully in Chapter 28, and Chapter 29 covers the association between familial adenomatous polyposis and its related diseases.

Inflammatory diseases

The risk of colorectal cancer in patients with longstanding ulcerative colitis is well appreciated and is discussed extensively in Chapter 44. The relationship between Crohn's colitis and carcinoma has in the past been considered to be more tenuous and controversial; however, data from the three-centre study described in Chapter 52 showed that there was a 6-fold risk of carcinoma in Crohn's colitis.

Although diverticular disease and carcinoma frequently coexist and pose difficulty in identifying a large bowel neoplasm (Stewart, 1931), there is no evidence to link the two disorders. Similarly, although tumour-like granulomas of amoebiasis, tuberculosis or (very rarely) syphilis may be confused with a carcinoma, none of these diseases has been demonstrated to lead to cancer.

Although infection with *Schistosoma mansoni* is a precursor of bladder carcinoma, infestation of the large bowel does not seem to be a precursor of bowel carcinoma (Dimmette et al, 1956; Zaky and Hashem, 1962). On the other hand, there is a suggestion that infection with *S. japonicum* may lead to carcinoma of the large bowel in countries where this organism is endemic (Cheng et al, 1980) (see Chapter 69). In China, for instance, both conditions are common and frequently coexist. In addition, the histological changes that precede the development of malignancy are similar to those in ulcerative colitis. Eradication of the infection reduces the incidence of carcinoma (Cheng et al, 1980, 1981).

Ureterosigmoidostomy

Although the preferred method of urinary diversion today is into an isolated ileal conduit (see Chapter 70), there is a residuum of patients who, with or without total cystectomy, have had both ureters anastomosed to the sigmoid colon. Numerous cases are now reported which show that patients who have had this operation are at increased risk of colorectal carcinoma. The tumours invariably are to be found around the anastomosis and the latent period tends to be not less than 20 years (Urdaneta et al, 1966; Kille and Glick, 1967; Whitaker et al, 1971; Mogg, 1977; Thompson et al, 1979; Harford et al, 1984).

Some investigators (Stewart et al, 1982), using the colonoscope, have demonstrated a high incidence of adenomas in addition to carcinomas in these patients, evidence which supports both the adenoma–carcinoma sequence and the risk of malignancy after ureterosigmoidoscopy. Some authors have also demonstrated that the polyps may be of the juvenile type (Ali et al, 1984; Cipolla and Garcia, 1984) which may also undergo malignant change (Jarvinen and Franssila, 1984). The theory is that chronic infection occurs in the urinary tract and that bacterial *n*-nitrosation occurs in the urine. These *n*-nitroso compounds are potential carcinogens, particularly when applied to intestinal epithelium.

Gastric surgery

Several retrospective studies have identified an increased mortality from colorectal cancer after surgery for peptic ulcer (Ross et al, 1982; Inokuchi et al, 1984; Watt et al, 1984; Bundred et al, 1985; Caygill et al, 1987), although this association remains controversial (Houghton et al, 1987; Toft Gaard, 1987; Kune et al, 1988a). The overall risk appears to be doubled but may vary with the nature of the operation performed. A subgroup analysis reported a 9.5-fold excess risk in female patients treated by Billroth I gastrectomy and an 8-fold excess mortality in females with duodenal ulcer treated by vagotomy (Caygill et al, 1988). If a risk does exist it may be related to altered bile acid metabolism since this has been implicated both after gastrectomy (Watt et al, 1984; Bundred et al, 1985) and after truncal vagotomy (Mullan et al, 1990). Mullan and associates demonstrated that vagotomized individuals developed significantly more colorectal adenomas and cancers compared with a control group, and they also had significantly increased proportions of chenodeoxycholic acid and lithocolic acid and significantly decreased proportions of colic acid in their duodenal bile. Whether peptic ulceration and surgery for it are interlinked with colorectal cancer, however, remains to be determined. The doubled mortality which has been demonstrated was apparent only 15–20 years after gastric surgery. Whether it is worth screening such patients also remains speculative.

Genetic predisposition

Both environmental and genetic factors play a role in colorectal carcinogenesis. Genetic factors are more important than previously realized. Apart from familial adenomatous polyposis (FAP) and its variants, the other major group of patients with a hereditary predisposition to develop large bowel carcinoma are those suffering from hereditary nonpolyposis colon cancer (HNPCC).

The term HNPCC was originally coined to differentiate the condition from FAP (Utsunomiya et al, 1981). The genetic basis of both FAP and HNPCC are considered in detail in Chapters 27 and 29. It should be realized that the genetic abnormalities which have been demonstrated in these conditions may be responsible for some cases of sporadic cancer. Thus, Nishisho et al (1991) have noted that since the phenotypic manifestations of FAP can vary widely, it is likely that some patients with colorectal cancer but without polyposis have inherited mutation of the APC gene. Mutations at the APC locus are a common early somatic event in polyps and cancer (Powell et al, 1992), supporting the idea that for some individuals the first hit is the germline mutation of the gene, and for others it is an early somatic event.

Irradiation

Patients who have received pelvic irradiation seem to be at higher risk of developing rectosigmoid cancer compared with the normal population.

The criteria for classifying a tumour as radiation-induced were established by Black and Ackerman (1965) and have been based on careful pathological study. Thus the carcinoma should show an adequate lead time of 10 or more years between completion of radiotherapy and tumour onset. The radiation exposure should be considerable and the damage to tissue adjacent to the tumour should be severe.

The largest series was reported by Castro et al (1973) who identified 26 patients who had developed a colorectal tumour following irradiation therapy for cancer of the cervix. Over 50% of patients had symptomatic and clinically documented chronic radiation proctocolitis at the site of the subsequent tumour, 69% had a postirradiation interval of more than 10 years, and 58% had histological proof of radiation-related damage affecting the bowel segment. Fifty-eight per cent of the tumours in the irradiated patients were colloid carcinoma and this is a significantly greater proportion than is usually seen in non-irradiated colorectal cancer. Although reports such as this and many others suggest that there is a link between irradiation and colorectal cancer, they do not prove cause and effect; hence it is impossible from these reports to determine whether or not the assembled cases represent an excess above the expected incidence among normal subjects matched for age and sex. Further confusion arises when it is realized that patients with gynaecological malignancy seem to be at greater risk of developing colorectal cancer whether or not they receive radiation (Bailar, 1963; Schoenberg et al, 1969; Schottenfeld et al, 1969; Schoenberg and Christine, 1979).

In order to evaluate the colorectal cancer risk it is necessary to compare the risk in patients with gynaecological cancer treated with radiation with those treated without radiation. Furthermore, the patients need to be matched for age and stage of disease. Because patients with extensive disease are often irradiated, such a study may be difficult to perform. Attempts, however, have been made to assess the risk by comparing the incidence of subsequent colorectal cancer developing after irradiation for benign conditions (e.g. ankylosing spondylitis or menorrhagia) with that expected in the normal population (Palmer and Spratt, 1956; Stander, 1957; Court Brown and Doll, 1965; Smith and Doll, 1976). Sandler and Sandler (1983) after reviewing the literature concluded that the risk of developing colorectal cancer after pelvic irradiation was real and was 1–8 times that for the general population. For patients who received radiotherapy for gynaecological cancer the risk was calculated to be 2.0–3.6 times greater. In view of the 10-year latency period these patients should be screened regularly for colorectal cancer for a considerable period after radiotherapy by endoscopy.

Molecular events and environmental factors

Vogelstein and colleagues (Baker et al, 1989; Vogelstein et al, 1989; Fearon and Vogelstein, 1990; Fearon et al, 1990; Kinzler et al, 1991) have provided extensive evidence that there is an accumulating (but not necessarily linear) series of chromosomal and genetic changes that accompany (and probably play a causal role in) the transition from normal colonic mucosa to metastatic carcinoma (see Chapter 27). The most common changes that were noted were those involving a known oncogene, K-*ras*; loss of heterozygosity on 5q (already known by then to be the site of the APC gene), and loss of heterozygosity on chromosomes 18q and 17p. Changes in DNA methylation seem to be an early step in these genetic changes (Feinberg and Vogelstein, 1983). Certain environmental and dietary factors seem to influence DNA methylation. Thus, chronic deficiency of both methionine and choline results in alterations of DNA methylation and produces tumours in rodents (Hoffman, 1984). More importantly from the human situation, deficiency of folate may have similar effects (Yunis and Soreng, 1984). Animal studies have shown that isothiocyanates found in large amounts in cruciferous vegetables inhibit both carcinogenesis and DNA methylation (Wattenberg, 1977, 1978; Steinmetz and Potter, 1991; Howe et al, 1992).

There is also evidence that dietary factors influence other processes at the molecular level. Thus, fat is an important source of diacyl glycerol which is normally an intracellular messenger leading to protein kinase activation, phosphorylation and cell turnover. Weinstein and associates (Guillem and Weinstein, 1990; Morotomi et al, 1990) have suggested that the interaction of fat, bile acids and bacteria produces excessive intraluminal diacyl glycerol which will mimic and amplify cell replication signals.

The fermentation of fibre results in intraluminal production of volatile fatty acids, particularly butyrate. It has been shown that volatile fatty acids will induce apoptosis in colonic tumour cell lines. This is yet another possible explanation for the lower risk that a diet rich in fermentable fibre may confer (Hague et al, 1993).

It is also possible that dietary constituents could influence both early and late stages of the carcinogenic process via effects on gene expression. For instance, the level of dietary fat has been shown in experimental models to alter both the production of eicosanoids, which in turn can influence DNA synthesis and tumour promotion, and the induction of genes coding for phase I and II metabolizing enzymes (Rosenthal, 1987; Rutten and Flake, 1987; Nicosia and Patrono, 1989; Kim et al, 1990). Further, fasting and refeeding are followed by structured changes in the chromatin at the site of genes involved in metabolic regulation. The degree and kinds of changes are dependent on the amount of fat and protein in the diet (Castro, 1987); this could have a major effect on cell replication rates via endocrine and paracrine mechanisms.

Dietary factors with the capacity for direct DNA damaging effects include arylamines. The transversion and transition mutations seen with high frequency in K-*ras* may be related to the interaction between arylamines and DNA (Beland and Kadlubar, 1985).

Conclusions

There is evidence linking the environmental and physiological factors known to influence colorectal carcinogenesis with the molecular biological changes which have recently been demonstrated. Unfortunately, the picture at present is far from coherent. It is clear that colorectal carcinogenesis is extremely complicated, and will take time to unravel, but there is now genuine optimism that this process will be understood in the near future.

Dietary prevention

Since various dietary factors seem to be implicated in the development of colorectal neoplasia, a variety of prospective studies have been initiated to determine if alteration of diet can prevent the disease developing.

De Cosse et al (1989) conducted a small randomized controlled trial investigating the effect of supplements of fibre and vitamins in patients with FAP who had undergone a colectomy and ileorectal anastomosis. There was no significant reduction in the number or size of adenomas remaining in the rectal stump in the test group compared with controls. However, only 62 patients were entered into the trial, thus making any small difference difficult to determine.

Alberts et al (1990) have set up a trial to investigate the effect of wheat bran supplement on adenoma recurrence in approximately 1400 subjects in Arizona. The European Cancer Prevention (ECP) Organisation have organized a similar study in 800 individuals (Faivre et al, 1990). Other studies in Canada (McKeown-Eyssen et al, 1994) and in the USA (Schatzkin et al, 1990; Rossouw et al, 1995) are ongoing.

One study has recently been reported from Australia. A total of 424 participants were randomized to three groups: a low-fat diet, a 25 g wheat bran supplement, or 20 mg of beta-carotene. Colonoscopy to ascertain adenoma recurrence was performed after 2 and 4 years of follow-up. The investigators concluded that a low-fat diet reduced the occurrence of large adenomas and suggested the effect could be enhanced by the addition of wheat bran to a low-fat diet. These findings need to be confirmed by longer follow-up and larger numbers (Schatzkin, 1996).

Chemoprevention

There is a vogue at present to try to prevent cancer development in a population by giving individuals an agent which interferes with the carcinogenesis pathway. Chemoprevention has been defined as the use of specific chemical compounds to prevent, inhibit or reverse carcinogenesis (Greenwald and Kelloff, 1993; Greenwald et al, 1995a,b; Kelloff et al, 1994, 1995). Since there is now an established pathway of colorectal cancer from adenoma through to metastatic disease, this tumour has particularly been targetted by research workers.

In the broadest sense, chemoprevention encompasses dietary cancer prevention. However, chemoprevention is appropriately defined more strictly in terms of agents used and their administration, and delivery to target sites.

A host of agents have been postulated as possible chemopreventative drugs, and the most promising are listed in Table 30.3, together with their postulated mechanisms of action. Many controlled trials have been set up using some of these agents, but as yet there are no definitive answers as to their efficacy. Since these are by their nature long-term studies, it will take many years before meaningful results will be available. The most promising agents are discussed below.

Several trials using calcium to prevent colorectal adenomas and cancers are in progress (Alberts et al, 1992; Hofstad et al, 1992; Rozen, 1992; Bostick et al, 1993; Faivre et al, 1993; Armitage et al, 1995). Calcium's potential was suggested by epidemiological studies which associated high dietary calcium intake with decreased colonic cancer risk or mortality. The preventative action of calcium relates to its ability to bind free bile acids such as deoxycholic acid which may be carcinogenic. Calcium also decreases total protein kinase C, tyrosine kinase and decarboxylase, all of which are involved in signal transduction pathways that are important in neoplastic development. Calcium has been shown to decrease the proliferation of normal appearing colonic cells from high-risk subjects (e.g. previous colonic neoplasm, familial association) and some early premalignant lesions (e.g. tubular adenoma). Distribution of proliferating cells over the height of the crypt may also be altered especially in individuals with FAP. Treatment with calcium salts decreased total protein kinase C, tyrosine kinase and ornithine decarboxylase (ODC) activities in rat colonic cancer models. ODC activity was also decreased following calcium treatment of patients with adenoma.

Certain non-steroidal anti-inflammatory drugs may also be chemopreventative. NSAIDs reduce inflammation by inhibiting the cyclo-oxygenase activity of prostaglandin (PG) H synthetase. Aspirin in particular is effective as it irreversibly inhibits the enzyme. As a consequence of the inhibition, the formation of prostaglandins is inhibited. Prostaglandins may enhance carcinogenesis by proliferation induction, mutagenesis formation of reactive oxygen species and immune system suppression (Marnett, 1992). Epidemiological evidence suggests that aspirin is associated with a reduced risk of gastrointestinal cancer (Kune et al, 1988b; Rosenberg et al, 1991; Thun et al, 1991, 1992, 1993; Gridley et al, 1993; Suh et al, 1993; Peleg et al, 1994; Schreinemachers and Everson, 1994). Decreased risk for premalignant lesions in the colon has also been associated with aspirin use (Greenberg et al, 1993; Logan et al, 1993; Peleg et al, 1993). Several phase II and III studies have been commenced examining the efficiency of aspirin in chemoprevention.

Other NSAIDs are being investigated, of which

Table 30.3 Possible chemopreventive mechanisms in colorectal cancer.

Agent	*Mechanism*	*Effect in colorectal carcinogenesis*
Calcium	Inhibitis carcinogen uptake (binds bile and fatty acids)	Inhibits proliferation
NSAIDs	Inhibit prostaglandin synthesis Inhibit carcinogen activation (inhibit co-oxidation by PGH synthetase)	Inhibits proliferation, gene mutations and damage (e.g. APC, MSH2, MLH1, MCC, DCC, K-*ras*, p53
Beta-carotene	Converts to vitamin A Antioxidant and free radical scavenging	Inhibits proliferation, promotes differentiation Inhibits proliferation, gene mutations and damage
Folic acid	Inhibits hypomethylation	Inhibits gene mutations and damage Inhibits proliferation (e.g. inhibits over-expression of oncogenes)
Vitamin C	Inhibits carcinogen activation (inhibits *N*-nitrosation)	Inhibits gene mutations and damage
Vitamin E	Antioxidant and free-radical scavenging	Inhibits proliferation, gene mutations and damage
DFMO	Inhibits ODC	Inhibits proliferation
Oltipraz	Carcinogen detoxification (enhance GST activity)	Inhibits gene mutations and damage
Ursodeoxycholic acid	Inhibits bile acid synthesis	Inhibits proliferation
HMG-CoA reductase inhibitors	Inhibits protein isoprenylation Inhibits bile acid synthesis Inhibits cholesterol synthesis	Inhibits proliferation via inhibition of expression of mutated *ras*
Perillyl alcohol	Inhibits protein isoprenylation Inhibits carcinogen activation (inhibits cytochromes P_{450})	Inhibits proliferation via inhibition of expression of mutated *ras* Inhibits gene mutations and damage

APC, adenomatous polyposis coli (gene); DCC, deleted in colonic cancer (gene); DFMO, 2-difluoromethylornithine; GST, glutathione-*S*-transferases; HMG-CoA, 3-hydroxy-3-methylglutaryl coenzyme A; MCC, missing in colonic carcinogenesis (gene); MLH1, MSH2, mutator genes; NSAID, non-steroidal anti-inflammatory drug; ODC, ornithine decarboxylase; PG, prostaglandin.
From Kleibeuker et al (1996).

sulindac appears the most promising. Sulindac's cyclo-oxygenase inhibition is due to its metabolite sulindac sulphide, and this produces a prolonged anti-inflammatory effect. Case studies have demonstrated that it prevents or causes regression of polyps in FAP patients (Waddell et al, 1989; Charneau et al, 1990; Friend, 1990; Earnest et al, 1991; Labayle et al, 1991; Winawer et al, 1991; Schusshein et al, 1993). Three small randomized controlled studies in patients with FAP showed that sulindac seems to reduce the size and frequency of polyps (Nugent et al, 1993; Winde et al, 1993; Spagnesi et al, 1994). However, in a prospective randomized controlled trial in patients with sporadic adenomas treated by sulindac or placebo who underwent colonoscopic polypectomy for their initial lesion, we found no significant differences between the two groups (Rowntree et al, 1993). Furthermore, we found that compliance was difficult even over a relatively short follow-up period of 2 years. In addition, a large percentage of the 700 patients considered for the trial either refused to take part or were considered by the investigators to have contraindications to randomization. These findings underline the difficulties with any chemopreventative programme, particularly one using NSAIDs.

Vitamins may be more easily tolerated and accepted by patients. Beta-carotene is metabolized to retinoid vitamin A. Retinoids in general act as the promotion phase of carcinogenesis by inhibiting proliferation and inducing differentiation. Folic acid is important in maintaining normal cellular methylation and in gene expression. Vitamin C has been shown to inhibit DMH-induced cancer in the rat colon (Reddy et al, 1982; Colacchio and Memoli, 1986; Colacchio et al, 1989). Vitamin E reacts with a variety of oxyradicals and singlet oxygen. Free radicals are implicated in carcinogenesis. Furthermore, vitamin E has also been shown to inhibit DMH-induced carcinogenesis in the mouse (Cook and McNamara, 1980). Thus, there are theoretical reasons and some experimental data which suggest that these vitamins might be chemopreventative, but the results of controlled trials will be necessary to confirm or refute these concepts.

PATHOLOGY

Macroscopic appearances

There are four macroscopic types of colorectal cancer.

1. *Ulcerative cancer* (Figure 30.1) presents as a typical malignant ulcer with raised rolled edges, often with a necrotic base. It may be circular or oval in shape and can occupy more than one quadrant of the bowel circumference. This type of lesion tends to infiltrate the bowel wall deeply and is consequently more likely to perforate than other forms.
2. *Polypoid (cauliflower) cancer* (Figure 30.2) is a proliferative type of lesion which protrudes into the bowel lumen and is not usually associated with infiltration of the bowel wall. It tends to be lobulated, the lobules being of variable size. It is not unusual for part of its surface to ulcerate and as time progresses the surface area of ulceration may increase. Presumably many ulcerated lesions started life as polypoid growths. Polypoid lesions are more common in the caecum and ascending colon.
3. *Annular or stenosing cancer* (Figure 30.3) is a circumferential lesion which varies in extent. Annular lesions tend to have an ulcerated surface. There has been a suggestion (Miles, 1926), based on the natural history of untreated patients, that annular lesions commence as small, discrete ulcers which gradually grow around the bowel wall. Annular lesions can extend for several centimetres in the longitudinal axis of the bowel or they may be very short. The longer lesions tend to occur more frequently in the rectum and the shorter lesions are seen more frequently in the transverse and left colon. The very short lesions typically seen in the sigmoid colon give the impression that the bowel has been constricted by a thread tied tightly around it. This appearance has led to the descriptive term of 'string' carcinoma. This type of lesion is obviously more likely to cause intestinal obstruction than other forms.
4. *Diffusely infiltrative cancer* is usually an extensive lesion which infiltrates the bowel wall often for at least 5–8 cm. It is similar to linitis plastica of the stomach in that the mucosa usually remains

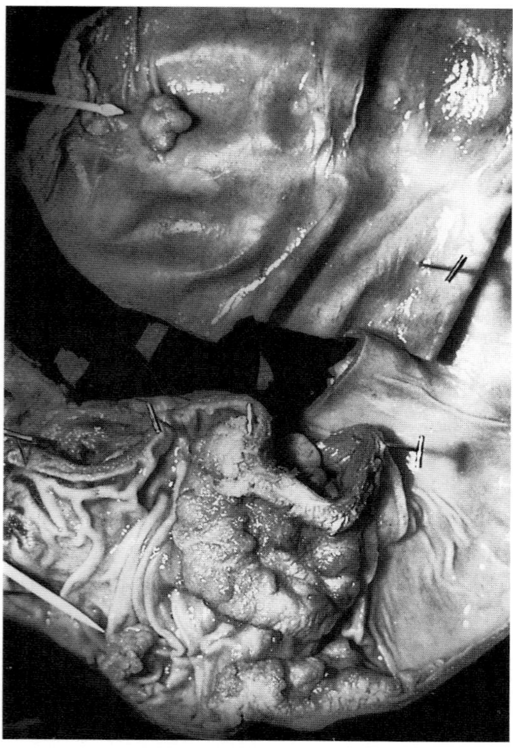

Figure 30.1 An ulcerated stenosing colon carcinoma.

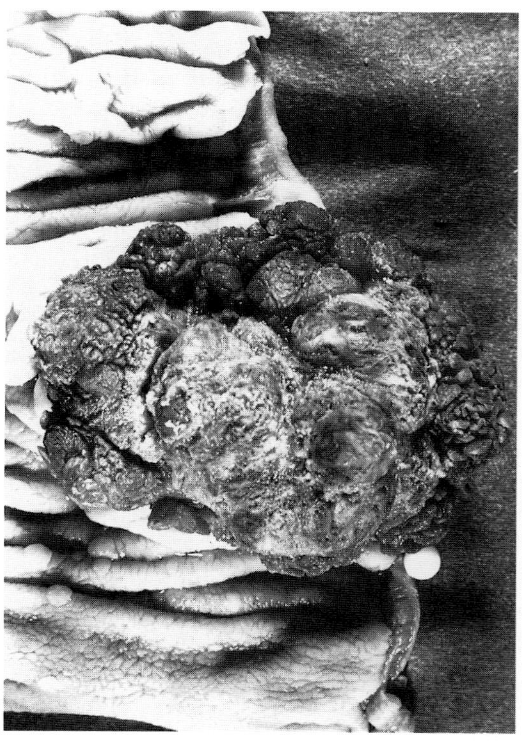

Figure 30.2 A polypoid carcinoma of the sigmoid colon.

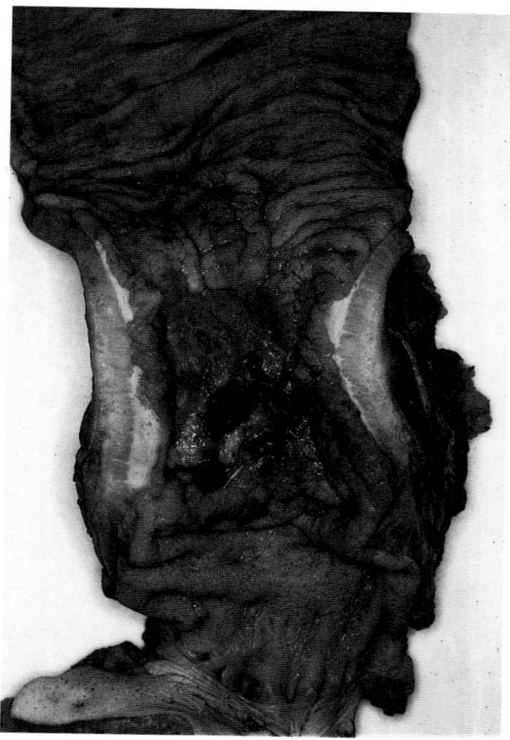

Figure 30.3 An annular or stenosing colorectal carcinoma.

intact over the surface although some part of it eventually becomes ulcerated. It occurs less frequently than the other types.

A *colloid* growth is also described by some authors. The term is applied to a lesion that produces a large amount of mucin and hence has a gelatinous appearance. The structure may be polypoidal or ulcerated and infiltration may or may not be present. It is a moot point therefore whether this lesion should be categorized as a separate entity.

The macroscopic appearance has been related to prognosis by some authors. Ulcerated or infiltrative lesions appear to have a worse prognosis than polypoid lesions (Grinnell, 1939; Coller et al, 1941). Such studies have not, however, considered macroscopic type as the single variable, and it is likely that such differences merely represent differences in local and lymphatic spread in that polypoid lesions tend to grow into the bowel lumen rather than through the wall.

Associated changes in the remaining large intestine

Colorectal cancer may produce macroscopic changes in the rest of the large bowel. Such changes will usually depend on the macroscopic type of the carcinoma: thus a constricting lesion may cause intestinal obstruction and the degree of change observed in the rest of the colon will depend on the length of time the obstruction has been present. If the obstruction is chronic the proximal colon will be dilated and often thickened, owing to hypertrophy of the muscular layer which develops as the colon attempts to push its contents through the obstructive lesion. If obstruction has occurred acutely the distended colon will be thin-walled. Dilatation of the small bowel will be present if the ileocaecal valve becomes incompetent. If obstruction has been present for some time, the inspissated faeces which occupy the colonic lumen may cause mucosal ulceration which eventually may perforate. Such changes are termed 'stercoral ulceration' and result from pressure necrosis. Perforation, however, may not occur only at the site of stercoral ulceration; any part of the dilated proximal colon may be affected, particularly the caecum which may split. In addition the tumour itself may perforate and in this case the perforation may become walled off locally by omentum and small bowel so that a pericolic abscess is present. Alternatively free peritonitis may result.

As discussed in Chapter 28, associated adenomatous polyps are often present in the remaining colon. These may be single or multiple, small or large. Less frequently one or more synchronous carcinomas are present, the incidence in resected specimens being approximately 3% (Goligher et al, 1951).

Microscopic features and tumour grade

Colorectal carcinomas vary in their degree of differentiation not only from tumour to tumour but also from area to area within the same tumour; i.e. they tend to be heterogeneous in their morphology. This makes classification rather subjective and dependent on the number of sections taken from the lesion. Pathologists tend to determine the degree of differentiation by gaining an overall impression. Most have used either a numbering system (1 to 3 or 4) based on that described by Broders (1925), or a series of descriptive terms such as 'well differentiated', 'moderately differentiated', 'poorly differentiated' or 'undifferentiated' (or 'anaplastic'). Dukes (1940), using the numbering system, originally recognized five grades of differentiation but subsequently modified this categorization to four grades so as to agree with the system described by Grinnell (1939). These four categories are as follows.

- *Grade I* (Figure 30.4a) resembles an adenoma, but active epithelial proliferation is present and the malignant component breaches the muscularis mucosae.
- *Grade II* (Figure 30.4b) – the malignant cells are more crowded together but are still arranged in a relatively regular glandular pattern, with the walls of the glands one or two layers thick. The nuclei stain deeply and irregular mitotic figures are not common.
- *Grade III* (Figure 30.4c) describes a range of differentiation. At best the cells are arranged in irregular folded rings usually two or three rows deep around spaces or as solid clumps. Mitotic figures are frequent. At worst the tumours are composed of very anaplastic cells which form sheets with no attempt to form glandular structures.
- *Colloid* or *mucinous* tumours (Figure 30.5) vary in their degree of differentiation, but the one feature they have in common is that they produce an abundant amount of mucin occupying at least 60% of the tumour volume. Mucinous tumours should be classified as such when greater than 50% of the tumour is mucinous (Jass and Sobin, 1989) since they have been reported as having a poorer prognosis.

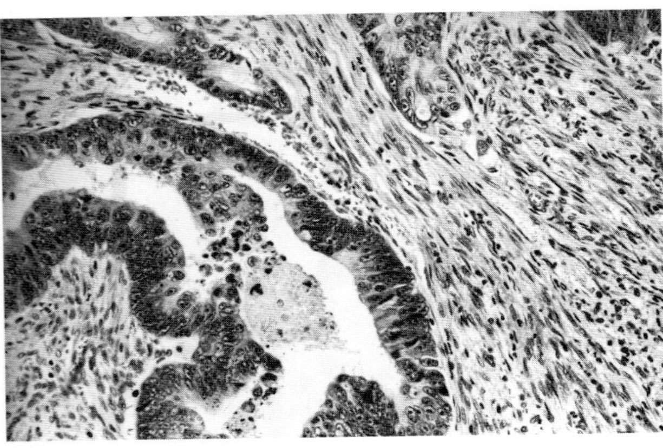
(a)

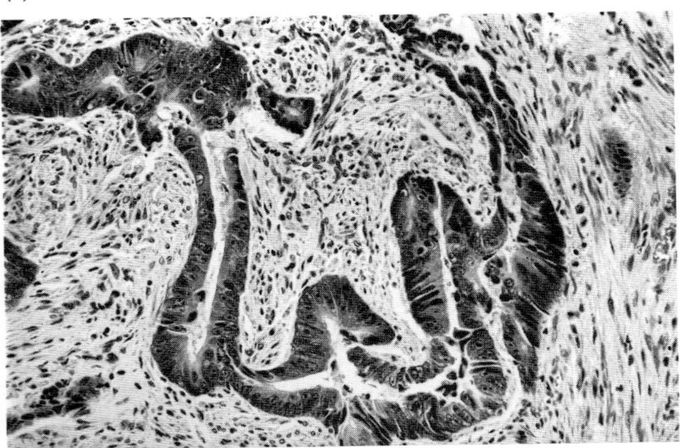
(b)

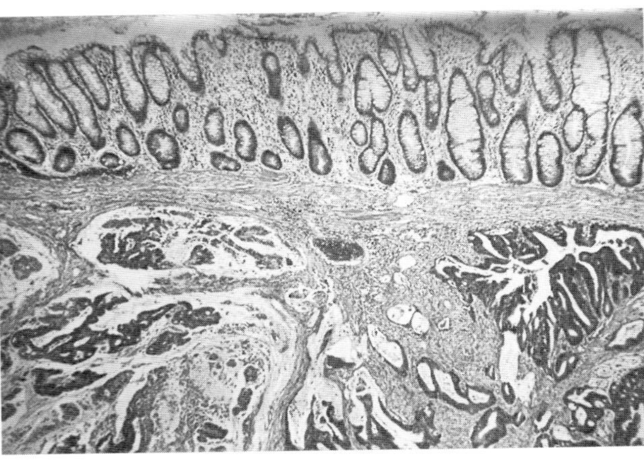
(c)

Figure 30.4a–c Microscopic appearance of colorectal adenocarcinomas. (a) Grade I or well-differentiated lesion. (b) Grade II or moderately differentiated lesion. (c) Grade III or poorly differentiated lesion.

Applying the descriptive grading system to the numerical system, 'well differentiated' refers to grade I, 'moderately differentiated' refers to grade II, and 'poor' or 'anaplastic' refers to grade III, with 'colloid' remaining as a separate group. Alternatively these categories may be referred to as 'low-grade', 'average' or 'high-grade'.

The distribution of these categories of grading varies from series to series because of the subjective nature of grading and the heterogeneity of the tumours. The average distribution seems to be 20% well-differentiated, 60% average differentiation and 20% poorly differentiated (Morson and Dawson, 1990).

The heterogeneous nature of tumours and the interobserver variations in the reporting of histological grade make interpretation difficult. This is

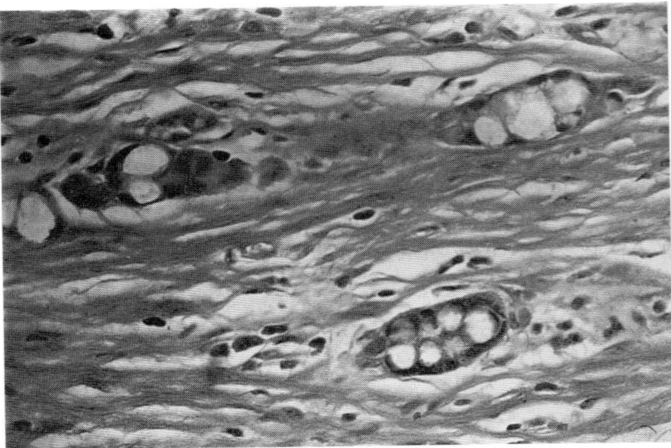

Figure 30.5 Colloid or mucinous adenocarcinoma.

particularly true with respect to the interpretation of biopsies. We found that the accuracy of agreement between the histological grade of one or two biopsies taken from 70 rectal cancers was 56% (Thomas et al, 1983; Williams et al, 1985). This was achieved when one experienced pathologist examined the sections. If the same individual examined multiple deep and superficial biopsies (minimum of five) from the same tumour, agreement was achieved in 86% of cases. However, when the same multiple biopsies were assessed by three independent pathologists, agreement fell to only 44% of cases. This study therefore casts considerable doubt on the use of biopsies to determine the grade of the tumours. Clinical decisions based on such an assessment should be discouraged.

Besides the histological grade of a tumour, other microscopic features may be important in respect to prognosis.

Spratt and Spjut (1976) demonstrated that the character of the tumour margin correlated with survival rate. Cancers with well-circumscribed borders or a mixed margin were associated with a significantly better prognosis than those with a poorly defined tumour border where cancer cells infiltrated normal tissue around the periphery.

Another histological criterion which reflects host–tumour interaction is the presence or absence of inflammatory infiltrates and the identification of lymphocytes within the tumour. Ackerman and Del Regato (1970) found that tumours with a pushing margin surrounded by inflammatory infiltrates of plasma cells and lymphocytes metastasize less frequently than those with no inflammatory infiltrate surrounding them. This infiltrate is thought to be an indication of the patient's antitumour immune response, and is considered by de Mascarel et al (1981) to be more important than the degree of cellular differentiation. Jass et al (1986, 1987) have included the character of the margin (whether pushing or infiltrating) and the inflammatory response, together with the grading features of the tumour, into a staging system (Figure 30.6); infiltrating borders together with a poor inflammatory response have a worse response. Such a staging system has not been widely adopted and at the time of writing has not been tested by other groups in large prospective series (Quirke and Shepherd, 1997).

The DNA content of colorectal cancer cells seems also to be important as far as prognosis is concerned. Using flow cytometry, Wolley et al (1982) were able to divide colorectal tumours into diploid and aneuploid tumours (Figure 30.7a). Patients with the aneuploid tumours had a significantly worse prognosis than patients with diploid tumours

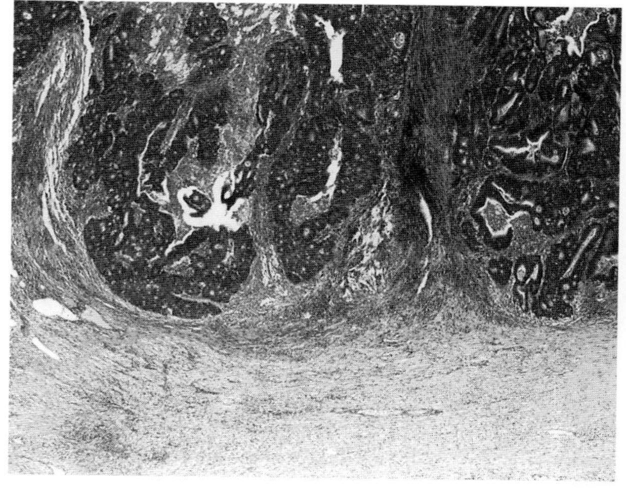

(a)

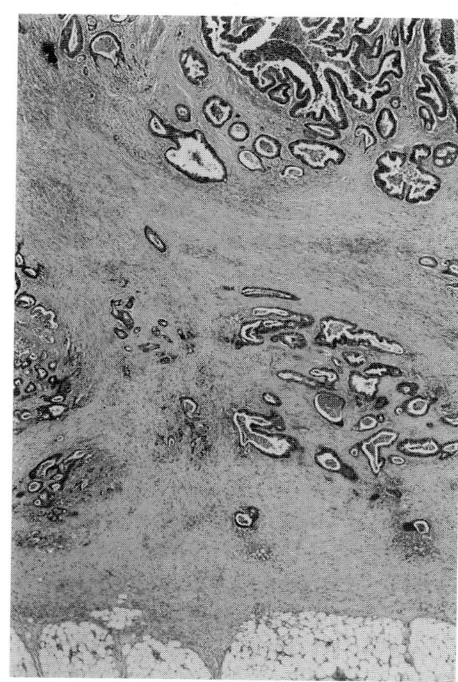

(b)

Figure 30.6a,b (a) Rectal carcinoma with a 'pushing' margin. The lower border of the tumour is well circumscribed. (b) Carcinoma with an 'infiltrating' margin. The lower border is poorly circumscribed and irregular. Courtesy of Dr R Feakins, Royal London Hospital.

(Figure 30.7b). This finding was confirmed in two further studies (Armitage et al, 1985; Kokal et al, 1986). Our own study, which limited investigation to patients with rectal cancer (Quirke et al, 1986), also agreed with the findings of Wolley and associates. In addition, since DNA content is a quantitative assessment, we found that there was a high degree of agreement (96%) between biopsy and

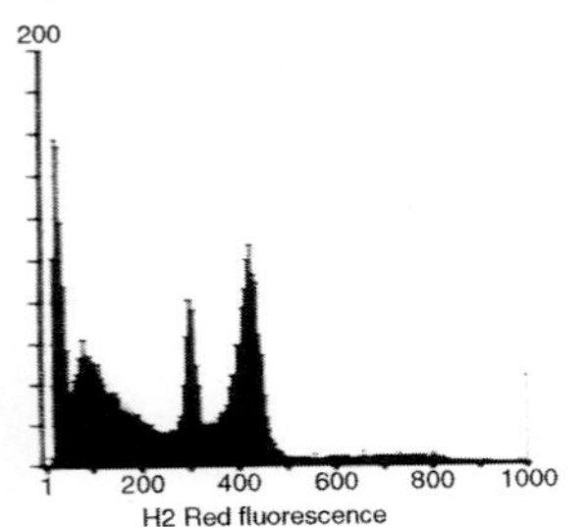

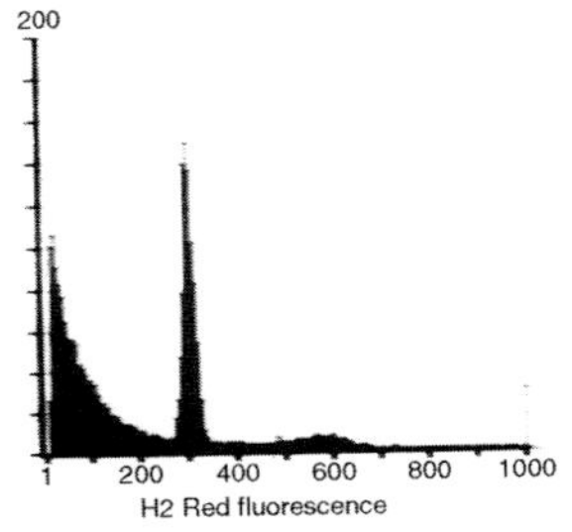

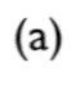

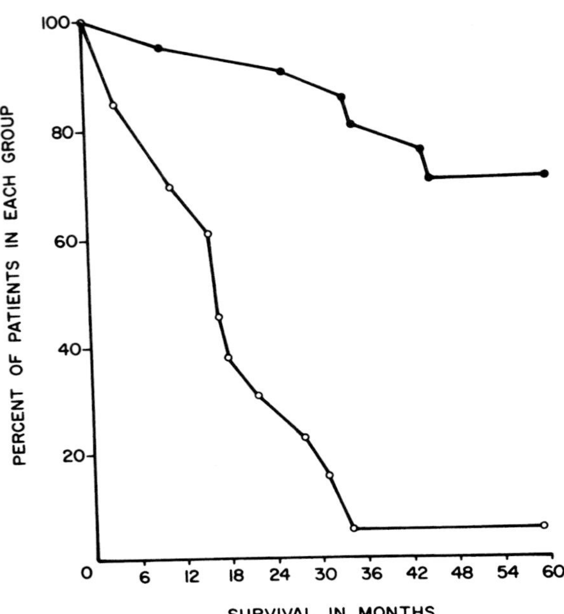

(b)

Figure 30.7a,b Ploidy of colorectal cancers using flow cytometry. (a) A diploid tumour on the right and an aneuploid tumour on the left. (b) Aneuploid tumours (o) were found to have a significantly worse prognosis than diploid tumours (●) (Wolley et al, 1982).

resected specimen when DNA content was measured using flow cytometry.

Since the initial work on ploidy and survival was performed, numerous further studies have been undertaken (Koha et al, 1992; Tsuchiya et al, 1992; Kouri et al, 1993; Foggi and Carbognani 1993; Silvestrini et al, 1993; Yamazoe et al, 1994; Zaras et al, 1994; Chapman et al, 1995; Sanguedolce et al, 1995; Tang et al, 1995; Vijayen et al, 1995; Baretton et al, 1996; Pietra et al, 1996). While most agree that ploidy does have some prognostic value, the balance of opinion is that on its own it is not an independent variable and certainly seems no better than Dukes' staging.

Relationship of pathology and genetics

As illustrated in Chapter 27, the molecular genetics of colorectal carcinogenesis are gradually being understood. Their relationship with the pathological changes are now being unravelled, and this relationship might provide more refined prognostic indicators. The strongest pathological association with molecular alteration is between the mutation of the APC (adenomatous polyposis coli) gene and the development of colorectal epithelial dysplasia (Figure 30.8).

Current data suggest that the APC mutation is the usual initiating event in the adenoma–carcinoma sequence as evidenced by the high prevalence (60%) of APC mutations in small adenomas (Powell et al, 1992) and the evidence of APC mutation in dysplastic aberrant crypt foci (Jen et al, 1994). A similar frequency of APC mutations has also been found in colorectal cancers.

Mutations of codon 12 in the K-*ras* gene occur in sporadic colorectal cancers with a frequency of about 40% (Bell et al, 1991; Laurent-Puig et al, 1992). K-*ras* mutations are seen at similar frequencies in large adenomas, but K-*ras* mutation is an infrequent event in small adenomas (Vogelstein et al, 1988; Scott et al, 1993). This indicates that K-*ras* mutation may be involved in the transition from a small to a large adenoma or may be an initiating event in a small proportion of adenomas which then rapidly progress to larger adenomas (Fearon and Vogelstein, 1990). *Ras* mutations have also been associated with exophytic growth of colorectal cancers (Redston et al, 1995).

Mutations of the p53 gene located at 17p13 occur frequently in colorectal tumours, but infrequently in adenomas (Kikuchi-Yanoshita et al, 1992), and are thus a late, rather than an initiating event, which may accompany the progression from adenoma to carcinoma. The majority of mutations are point mutations and occur in the most conserved regions of the gene (Lothe et al, 1992; Hamelin et al, 1994). Allele loss of the p53 gene is also seen frequently (in up to 75% of cases) in colorectal tumours (Campo et al, 1991; Cawkwell et al, 1994; Iacopetta et al, 1994) but infrequently in adenomas (Kikuchi-Yanoshita et al, 1992). In some studies, p53 mutation (Hamelin et al, 1994) and expression detected by immunohistochemistry (which detects stabilized, i.e. mutant p53) have been found to correlate with poor survival in sporadic colorectal cancer (Sun et al, 1992; Auvinen et al, 1994). We found that in 10 out of 21 sporadic colorectal cancers (48%), abnormal p53 expression was detected using the monoclonal antibiotic Pab 1801 (Taylor et al, 1993). This is similar to the

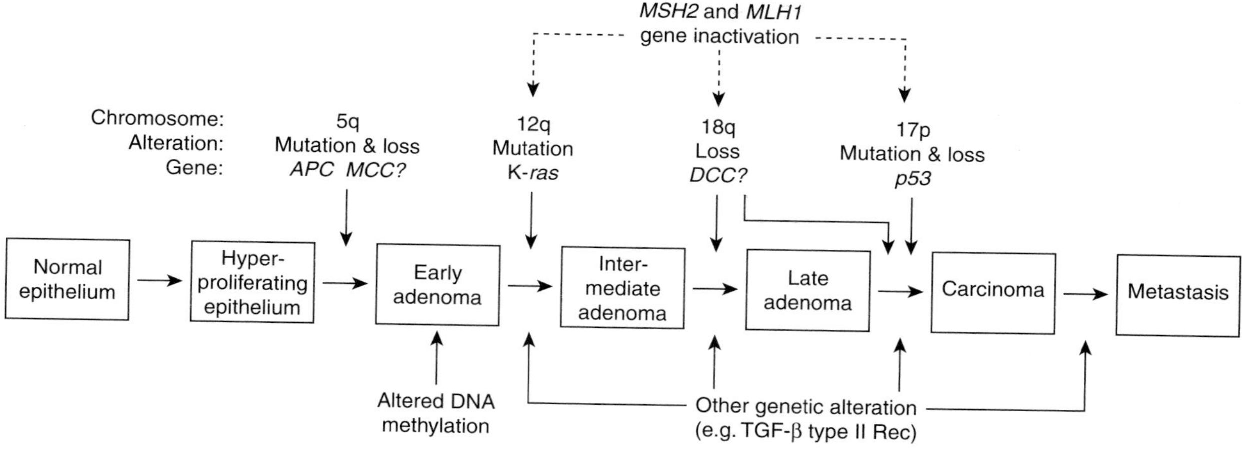

Figure 30.8 Gene defects in colorectal tumorigenesis (Fearon and Vogelstein, 1990).

incidence detected by others (Van den Berg et al, 1989; Scott et al, 1991). However, we were unable to demonstrate that this expression was an independent variable as far as survival was concerned.

The DCC gene at 18q21 is a candidate tumour suppressor gene identified owing to a high frequency of allele loss on 18q (Fearon et al, 1990). Allele loss involving the DCC gene region in colorectal cancer was originally reported to be as frequent as 71% (Fearon et al, 1990). However, using intragenic markers this frequency was found to be substantially lower (29–33%) (Huang et al, 1993; Cawkwell et al, 1994). Allele loss of the DCC gene appears to be a late event in colorectal cancer progression since Ookawa et al (1993) found that the highest frequencies of allele loss were in advanced staged tumours and metastases.

Microsatellite instability has also been described in sporadic adenocarcinomas (Ionov et al, 1993; Thibodeau et al, 1993) and in a few adenomas (Shibata et al, 1994). It is not yet known whether this is due to mutations in the same mismatch repair genes that cause HNPCC, or indeed whether these sporadic cases could in fact be HNPCC cases that were not identified owing to insufficient family data. This idea is supported by the finding that sporadic colorectal cancers with microsatellite instability tend to be found on the right side of the colon (Lothe et al, 1992; Thibodeau et al, 1993) which is a feature of HNPCC. Similarly, these tumours tend to be large in size, are mucinous or poorly differentiated, and have a striking host inflammatory response with desmoplastic and lymphoid aggregates or Crohn's-like lymphoid reaction (Kim et al, 1994). Microsatellite instability appears also to confer a better prognosis (Lothe et al, 1992; Thibodeau et al, 1993).

The role of the putative metastasis suppressor gene NM23 (Steag et al, 1988) is not clear. However, there is some evidence that allele loss, mutation and a relative lowering of RNA and protein expression (in comparison with non-metastatic tumours which show increased expression) are evident only in late-stage tumours associated with metastases (Cohn et al, 1991; Wang et al, 1993; Yamaguchi et al, 1993).

This is a rapidly advancing field, and it is likely that these and other genetic events will help to explain not only the pathogenesis of colorectal neoplasia but also its pathological behaviour.

Spread

Colorectal cancer may spread by one of five routes: (1) direct, (2) lymphatic, (3) venous, (4) transcoelomic, or (5) implantation.

Direct spread

Direct spread may occur in both the transverse plane and the longitudinal plane of the bowel wall. Transverse spread of a small, localized lesion may lead to complete encirclement of the bowel lumen. It has been suggested that such growth is slow: in the upper part of the rectum, for instance, it would take approximately 2 years to complete (Miles, 1926). Intramural, longitudinal spread may occur, but is not as frequent as transverse spread. It may occur in a proximal or distal direction. Only distal spread, however, has been examined in any detail, and in the main such investigation has been confined to rectal tumours; the reason is the need for surgeons to gain adequate distal clearance when performing a rectal excision. This subject is particularly pertinent at the present time with the swing towards sphincter preservation for low rectal cancers.

Handley (1910) was the first to demonstrate that distal intramural spread occurred. He described two cases out of a series of 12 patients in which microscopic permeation of cancer cells occurred in the bowel wall for a considerable distance both proximal and distal to the tumour. The publication of these results provoked considerable controversy which has still not entirely abated. In 1913, Cole found no evidence of permeation beyond the macroscopic edge of the growth in 19 cases. In 1920 and again in 1931, Miles concluded from clinical studies and histological data that this type of spread was always trivial. Westhues (1934) found only one instance of intramural spread in 74 cases and this occurred only in a proximal direction. However, Connell and Rottino (1949) reported that four of nine cases of rectal cancer exhibited distal intramural spread. This startling finding led Quer et al (1953) and Grinnell (1954) to reinvestigate the problem. Their conclusions were that distal intramural spread did sometimes occur and consequently at least 5 cm of macroscopically normal tissue distal to the growth must be removed within the course of a rectal excision if recurrence was to be avoided. Thus was born the '5 cm rule' of distal resection.

Such a generalized rule seems not to be justified, however, when the earlier data are examined in detail. Thus, for instance, although Grinnell found evidence of distal spread in 12% of potentially curative resections, virtually all of these patients had 'advanced tumours of high grade malignancy . . . so advanced that only a palliative resection could be done. Even in curative resections the prognosis for the patient is poor' (Grinnell, 1954). In fact, Grinnell found no survivors among patients with intramural spread although most of these patients were treated by abdominoperineal excision of the rectum (APER). Similarly Penfold (1974) who studied the pathology of 546 abdominoperineal excision specimens found an 8.8% incidence of both intramural and lymphatic downward spread. It is of great interest that no patient in his study with downward spread greater than 1 cm survived for 5 years and most died of their cancer.

The findings from our own study strongly support the view that distal intramural spread greater than 1 cm is uncommon, but when it does occur the patients have tumours that are incurable with the available treatment options (Williams et al, 1983). Thus in 50 abdominoperineal excision specimens in which the tissue distal to the tumour was meticulously examined for the presence of microscopic distal spread (Figure 30.9a), five patients (10%) had spread of more than 1 cm (Figure 30.9b). Each of

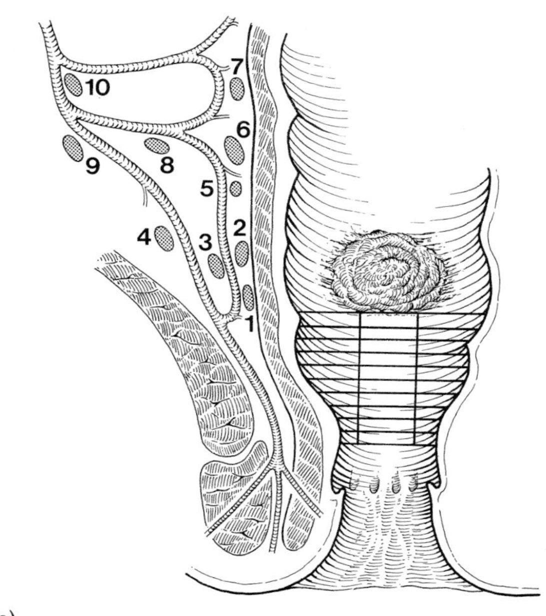

(a)

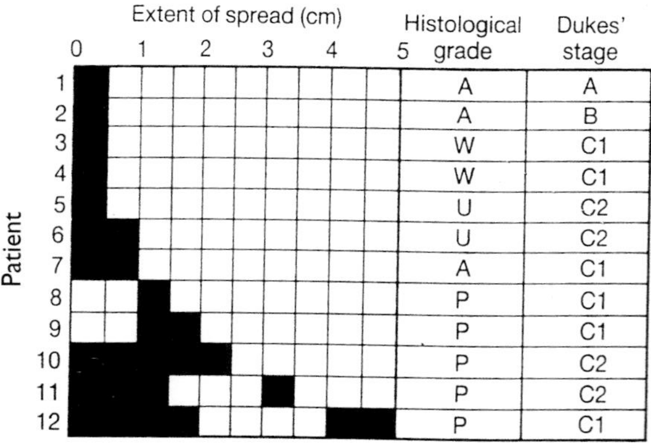

(b)

Figure 30.9a,b Determination of the extent of distal intramural spread. (a) Outline drawing of a rectum removed by abdominoperineal excision showing the position of the carcinoma and lymph nodes. The bowel distal to the tumour was serially sectioned, each transverse strip measuring 5 mm in thickness. Each block was then sectioned at 10 mm intervals and stained for microscopic deposits. (b) Extent of distal intramural spread in 12 APER sections. Only five had spread greater than 1 cm and each of these was Dukes' C, poorly differentiated tumour. A, average differentiation; P, poorly differentiated; U, undifferentiated; W, well differentiated (Williams et al, 1983).

these patients had a poorly differentiated Dukes' C lesion and each was dead or dying from distant metastases within 3 years of operation, despite the fact that the rectal excision had been performed with a minimum of 5 cm of distal clearance. Our study also showed that distal spread most often takes place through lymphatics in the submucosal layer, although the intermuscular, subserous and subfascial layers may be implicated. The lymphatics tend to be the main channel of invasion although the blood vessels may also act as conduits. Intramural spread is invariably continuous, in marked contrast to the pattern of radial spread which is often discontinuous (see later).

The rarity of extensive intramural spread of tumour in patients who undergo potentially curative resections for rectal carcinoma (Table 30.4) was also emphasized by Quer et al (1953) who found distal spread of more than 1.5 cm in only one of 89 resections. Hence these authors recommended a distal margin of clearance of 2.5 cm when the growth was well differentiated or of average differentiation, and 6 cm when the growth was poorly differentiated. Likewise, Black and Waugh (1948) stated 'only 2 cm of normal bowel need be allowed above and below the lesion in order to remove the whole of the primary lesion'.

These views are supported by many authors who have been unable to find a correlation between the extent of the distal margin of resection and the incidence of local recurrence (Baker et al, 1955; Beal and Cornell, 1956; Lofgren et al, 1957; Williams et al, 1966; Copeland et al, 1968; Slanetz et al, 1972; Manson et al, 1976; Wilson and Beahrs, 1976) (Table 30.5). A meticulous follow-up of 556 patients who had undergone low anterior resection for rectal carcinoma at the Mayo Clinic reported by Wilson and Beahrs (1976) found that patients with a 2–3 cm distal margin of resection fared just as well in the long term as did patients with wider margins of clearance. Others, including ourselves (Pollett and Nicholls, 1981; Williams et al, 1983), have confirmed these findings.

The implications of these clinicopathological studies are discussed in depth elsewhere. Suffice it to say here that we believe there is sufficient evidence to reduce the minimum margin of distal clearance of the rectal wall from 5 cm to 2 cm during rectal excision. That is *not* to say that all cases should be resected with this margin. Wherever possible it is probably best to obtain as much clearance as possible. However, if in the course of a rectal excision the taking of 5 cm of distal rectal wall would jeopardize the anal sphincter, we believe that this margin can be safely reduced to 2 cm so that continence can be preserved.

The question of distal spread in the mesorectum is perhaps a different story. Most of the histological studies alluded to above have concentrated on distal intramural spread and not distal spread in the mesorectum. Our own study (Williams et al, 1983) did in fact include this tissue. However, a study by Heald et al (1982) suggested that distal spread

Table 30.4 Distal intramural spread – accumulated data.

Reference	*No. of cases*	*No. with spread*
Clogg (1908)	25	0
Handley (1910)	10	2
Cole (1913)	20	1
Westhues (1934)	74	0
Black and Waugh (1948)	103	4
Quer et al (1953)	91	5
Grinnell (1954)	76	9
Williams et al (1983)	50	12
Total	449	33 (7.4%)
Distal spread exceeding 2 cm		11 (2.5%)

Table 30.5 Comparison of distal margin of clearance, local recurrence and 5-year survival rates.

	Length of clearance (cm)			
Reference	<4	>4	<5	>5
Recurrence				
Deddish & Stearns (1961)	4/62 (6.5%)	4/39 (10%)		
Manson et al (1976)			9/76 (11.8%)	3/30 (10%)
Wilson and Beahrs (1976)			56/400 (14%)	20/156 (13%)
Pollett and Nicholls (1981)			15/232 (6.5%)	8/102 (7.8%)
Williams et al (1983)			7/48 (15%)	3/31 (10%)
Crude 5-year survival rates				
Copeland et al (1968)			46/141 (32.6%)	86/206 (41.8%)
Pollett and Nicholls (1981)			159/232 (68.5%)	71/102 (69.6%)
Williams et al (1983)			33/48 (69%)	18/31 (58%)

greater than 2 cm could occur in the mesorectum, and this might take place when a potentially curative procedure could be performed. This finding was confirmed by Scott et al (1995) who found that, in 20 specimens resected for rectal cancer, four patients had metastatic deposits in the mesorectum distal to the tumour. Heald therefore recommended that all the mesorectum should be removed down to the pelvic floor, but this can be 'shaved off' the wall of the rectum so that the latter can be divided 2 cm below the tumour, if by so doing the sphincter can be spared. Such a manoeuvre is known as 'total mesorectal excision' (TME).

Spread through the bowel wall radially also accompanies circumferential growth. It is classically stated that this type of invasion affects the layers of the bowel sequentially. Thus the tumour first invades the mucosa and then sequentially spreads through the submucosa, the muscle coat and the serosa. If left to its own devices the tumour will then involve the perirectal or pericolic fat or peritoneum. Further spread in this direction involves other structures depending on the site of the tumour.

Radial spread from colonic carcinomas that are situated retroperitoneally will involve structures on the posterior abdominal wall such as the duodenum, ureter, kidney and the iliacus or psoas muscles. Tumours on the anterior wall of the colon may spread to involve the small intestine, stomach or pelvic organs.

Radial spread from a cancer situated on the posterior wall of the rectum may extend through the mesorectum to the fascia of Waldeyer. The latter may act as a deterrent to further spread but invasion through it is not uncommon and in such cases the sacral plexus, sacrum or coccyx may become involved. Anterior spread from a tumour situated below the peritoneal reflection in the male may result in invasion of the prostate, seminal vesicles and bladder. In the female such spread will first penetrate the cervix uteri and posterior vaginal wall, unless the patient has had a hysterectomy, when anterior infiltration may involve the bladder.

Although radial spread is thought to occur in continuity with subsequent serial involvement of each layer of the bowel wall, some studies show that this is not necessarily the case. We meticulously searched for microscopic radial spread in 52 operative rectal excision specimens (Quirke et al, 1986). Slices were taken at 5–10 mm intervals of the whole tumour and the surrounding mesorectum in the transverse plane (Figure 30.10). Then sections 10 mm thick were cut on a sledge microtome and stained with haematoxylin–eosin. Histopathological examination of each section was performed looking for radial invasion of the tumour. Fourteen of the 52 cases (27%) were found to have this form of spread. In eight cases it appeared continuous with the primary neoplasm, whereas in six cases it proved to be discontinuous. The routes of spread varied: in seven of the specimens the spread was macroscopically visible, but in the remaining seven it was present only on microscopic examination (Figure 30.11). The latter findings highlight the difficulty of determining whether a resection has been curative or not. There is no doubt that surgeons overestimate the number of curative procedures they perform when dealing with rectal cancer. Eighty-five per cent of our patients who had undergone resection and who had evidence of radial extension of the tumour developed a local recurrence, compared with only 3% of patients who had no evidence of this form of spread.

These data were confirmed in a much larger prospective study in Leeds in which rectal excision specimens were subjected to a simpler examination of circumferential margin tumour involvement and patients were followed up for 5 years (Quirke and Scott, 1992; Adam et al, 1994). The additional data showed that if the circumferential margin was involved, there was a 12-fold increased risk of local recurrence and a 3-fold increased risk of death. These findings were confirmed by other groups (Ng et al, 1993).

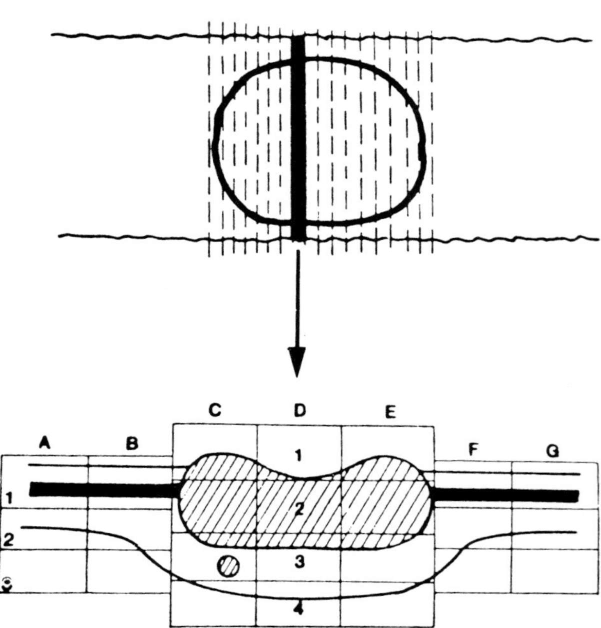

Figure 30.10 Blocks taken in study to investigate the radial spread of rectal cancer (Quirke et al, 1986).

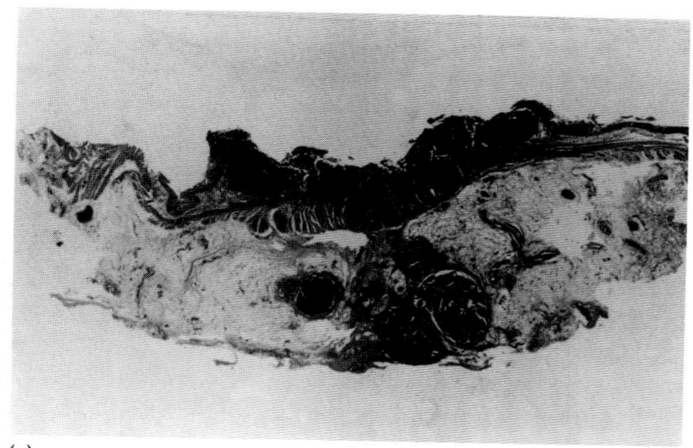

(a)

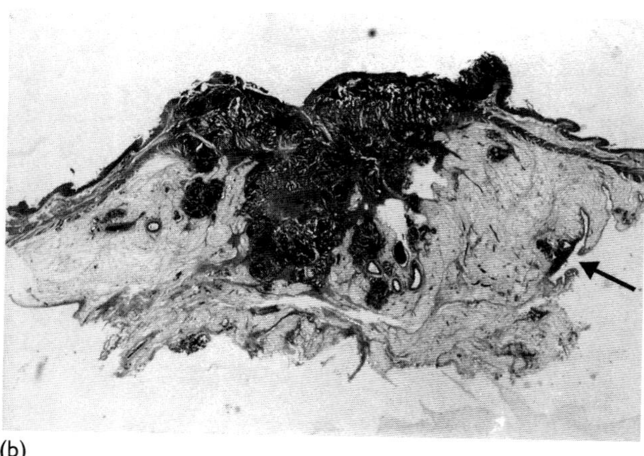

(b)

Figure 30.11a,b (a) Radial spread of rectal cancer up to the lateral margin of excision which was noted macroscopically. (b) Radial spread of rectal cancer to the lateral margin of excision (arrow) which was detected only by microscopic examination of numerous sections.

The findings illustrate clearly that leaving residual disease behind in the pelvis is by far the main reason for the subsequent development of local recurrence after resection for rectal cancer. Another important point to emerge from our original study was that pathologists as well as surgeons underestimate the degree of radial spread. If the conventional method of detecting radial spread was employed, six of 52 specimens (12%) were found to be so affected compared with 14 of 52 (27%) when the multiple section technique was used.

Lymphatic spread

Enlargement of lymph nodes in relation to colorectal carcinoma does not necessarily mean invasion by malignancy. Colorectal carcinoma commonly produces an inflammatory reaction within the nodes draining it. Conversely, microscopic invasion of lymph nodes will not necessarily produce enlargement. These findings have particular relevance to both surgeon and pathologist. The surgeon should never assume the situation is hopeless because the lymph nodes are enlarged.

The pathologist theoretically needs to find and section every node in the excised specimen to be sure of the pathological stage. In practice this is an extremely difficult manoeuvre, but techniques have been developed that improve the yield of nodes. Such techniques are designed to dissolve the fat in the mesentery and are based on those originally developed by Westhues (1930), Monroe (1949), Pickren (1956) and Durkin and Haagensen (1980). Using these techniques Jinnai (1982) has shown that the yield of lymph nodes is increased by approximately 50% compared with conventional methods. It comes as no surprise, therefore, to find that a considerable proportion of patients thought to be free of lymphatic metastases do in fact have microscopic involvement of their nodes. The counsel of perfection for the pathologist should therefore be to examine as many nodes as possible, and it should always be indicated on the report how many are in fact found.

Lymphatic spread in relation to colon cancer

Numerous studies from dissection of post-mortem and operative specimens have helped to delineate the lymphatic pathways along which colon cancer spreads (Clogg, 1908; Rankin, 1933; Coller et al, 1940; Dukes, 1945, 1951; Gilchrist and David, 1947). Although these ideas seem to be basically correct, there is evidence that exceptions are more common than was previously realized.

The commonly accepted wisdom is that the paracolic lymph nodes become involved initially. As the disease advances the glands on the lower main colon vessels are involved and gradually the process extends upwards along these vessels. Eventually, depending on the site of tumour, the glands along the superior haemorrhoidal, inferior mesenteric or superior mesenteric arteries become involved, and when the lesion is particularly advanced invasion of the para-aortic nodes may occur.

Although it was assumed that lymph node invasion was always a gradual progression of involvement, Jinnai (1982) showed that in approximately one-third of cases the disease 'skips' not to the next node but to nodes situated at a higher level. Another generally held belief is that distant metastases occur only when the lymph nodes have been involved. Finlay and McArdle's data show clearly that this belief is false (Finlay et al, 1982). Occult and overt hepatic metastases may be present in the absence of lymph node involvement. Whether lymph node invasion can occur when the primary lesion has not penetrated through to the serosa is a different matter. Few studies are available. Jinnai (1982) examined this point, and in contrast to the findings in rectal cancer he found that lymph node involvement in these circumstances only very rarely occurs. The same issue has been investigated also in patients with 'malignant' polyps. In patients with these lesions the incidence of lymph node metastases is disputed (see Chapter 28), but most authors do agree that microscopic invasion can occur; whether such invasion is clinically important, however, is a different matter.

As the reader will appreciate, the incidence of lymph node involvement in colon carcinoma will vary according to how meticulous the pathologist is in his or her technique. If surgical resection specimens are investigated, the extent of the surgical clearance will also be a limiting factor. Dukes (1951) reported that only 38% of specimens handled by him had lymph node metastases, whereas Jinnai (1982) found that nodes were involved in 60% of his cases.

Lymphatic spread in relation to rectal cancer

The pathways for lymphatic spread of a rectal cancer were initially carefully worked out by Miles (1910, 1926). From his operative and post-mortem studies he concluded that this form of spread occurred in three directions: upwards, lateral and downwards. Upward spread consists of spread along the lymphatics and glands which accompany the superior rectal and inferior mesenteric vessels as they lie in the mesorectum and base of the mesocolon. Further spread upwards from these structures results in invasion of the para-aortic nodes. In Miles' experience lateral spread was relatively common, the lymphatics and nodes in the lateral ligaments being involved initially with spread eventually reaching the nodes around the internal iliac vessels on the pelvic side walls. Downward spread involved the lymphatics of the sphincter ani, the perianal skin and ischiorectal fat. If spread involved tissue around the anal canal, the inguinal nodes might also be affected.

Miles considered that upward dissemination was the most frequent mode of lymphatic spread, but lateral and downward spread also occurred relatively frequently. For this reason he advocated that treatment should be abdominoperineal excision of the rectum, as this was the only procedure that could deal satisfactorily with all three modes of lymphatic spread. This view was accepted for many years but was then challenged by the findings of Dukes (1930), Westhues (1930, 1934), Wood and Wilkie (1933) and Gabriel et al (1935). These authors found that whereas upward spread was common, lateral or downward spread was rare. Downward spread seemed to occur only when the glands along the superior rectal vessels were choked with metastases, allowing retrograde spread to occur. The relative infrequency of lateral and downward lymphatic spread was emphasized by Goligher's study (Goligher et al, 1951) performed in Dukes' laboratory: 1500 abdominoperineal excision specimens were dissected and lymph node involvement below the level of the primary tumour was found in 98 cases (6.5%). In 68 of these specimens the glands lay within 6 mm of the lower margin of the growth, and in only 30 cases (2%) was spread greater than 20 mm. All of these cases had extensive involvement of the nodes around the superior rectal vessels. An even lower incidence of downward lymphatic spread was found by Glover and Waugh (1945). In our own smaller study of distal intramural spread we also looked for extramural, downward lymphatic spread in 50 abdominoperineal excision specimens (Williams et al, 1983). In three cases (6%) a single involved lymph node was found distal to the distal margin of the tumour. In each case, the tumour was poorly differentiated, of Dukes' stage C2, and the involved node was close to the distal margin of resection (respectively 7 mm, 10 mm and 13 mm from it). One of these cases also showed distal intramural spread of 5 cm. This study therefore supports the view that distal lymphatic spread occurs rarely and only when the upward route is extensively involved.

The situation as regards lateral lymphatic spread seems to be somewhat more complex. Virtually all studies performed to date have used operative specimens to assess this form of spread. Since it is not usual to excise the lymph nodes around the internal iliac vessels in either an abdominoperineal excision of the rectum or a sphincter-saving resection, it is likely that such spread has been underestimated. In addition, only lymph node invasion has been sought. It is clear from our own study (Quirke et al, 1986) which examined multiple lateral sections that even in operative specimens invasion of lateral lymphatic channels is more frequent than previously thought. In addition there are data from surgeons who, over the years, have performed a radical lymphadenectomy in which the nodes around the internal iliac vessels were routinely excised.

Involvement of these nodes by tumour seems to depend on whether the growth lies above or below the peritoneal reflection. Thus Sauer and Bacon (1952) found that in 21 cases treated by radical lymphadenectomy in which the growth was extraperitoneal, six had involvement of nodes around the internal iliac vessels. Eleven of their cases with growths above the peritoneal reflection, however, did not have lateral lymphatic involvement. Takahashi and Kajitani (1982) in a much larger series came to similar conclusions; in 507 cases with tumours below the peritoneal reflection, metastases were found in the internal iliac nodes in 83 (16.4%), whereas in 236 cases with growths above the reflection only eight (3.4%) had involved iliac nodes. Both Hojo et al (1982) and Jinnai (1982) agree with these findings.

These studies suggest that whereas wide lateral lymphatic spread occurs with extraperitoneal rectal cancers, it is uncommon in tumours above the peritoneal reflection. It should be remembered that these studies cannot be the final word on the subject since only lymph nodes were sought. If multiple lateral sections were taken from such operative specimens, there is little doubt that more cases would be found to have invasion of lymphatic channels. The crucial question that remains to be answered is whether survival can be improved by more extended lateral clearance. The standard techniques of abdominoperineal excision of the rectum and sphincter-saving resection surprisingly do not seem to differ in the amount of lateral tissue removed (Quirke et al, 1986), so it is perhaps to be expected that survival and local recurrence rates are similar (Williams, 1985) after either procedure. Surgeons who practise extended pelvic lymphadenectomy do claim a benefit, but no controlled trials exist to verify their claims. This subject is discussed more extensively later.

Like lymphatic spread in colonic carcinoma, spread from rectal cancer has been assumed to take place in an orderly fashion from node to node. Discontinuous spread was considered to be unusual. However, when Jinnai (1982) and colleagues used their more careful technique for identifying lymph node involvement, they found that discontinuous spread occurred in over 30% of cases. Unlike the case in colonic tumours, it was also found that nodes could be involved in some rectal tumours which had not already spread through the bowel wall. Thus in 10% of cases in which lymph nodes were involved, the primary tumour had not spread further than the submucosa and in 23.7% of cases the growths had spread to the rectal muscle but had not invaded the perirectal tissues. In the study by Hojo et al (1982), the corresponding data were 17% and 36.2% respectively. These data would appear to have considerable implications for the local treatment of rectal cancer.

From the foregoing it can be seen that the incidence of lymphatic metastases in rectal cancer is impossible to determine with any degree of accuracy unless all nodes are examined. Previous data and the derived correlations and clinical implications must therefore be treated with caution. It would seem that the overall incidence of lymph node involvement using conventional staining techniques in operative specimens is 50–60%. Dukes found an incidence of approximately 50% in his 1000 rectal cancer cases treated by abdominoperineal excision of the rectum, and Jinnai (1982) and colleagues found that 60% of their cases were involved. Neither study, however, included the nodes around the internal iliac vessels.

Genetic detection of lymph node metastases

The above data are derived from studies which used conventional staining techniques to detect metastatic disease in lymph nodes. However, conventional staining techniques may not be sensitive enough. There is now considerable interest in the detection of lymph node invasion using new genetic techniques.

Hayashi et al (1995) used mutant allele specific amplication (MASA) to detect mutations of K-*ras* or p53 in 120 colorectal cancers from patients who had no histologically detectable lymph node metastases at the time of surgery. Somatic mutations were identified by MASA in 71 tumours. They next examined preserved tissues from corresponding regional lymph nodes using MASA to look for the specific mutations found in the primary. Of 37 patients with genetically positive nodes, 27 had developed a tumour recurrence within 5 years of surgery, compared with none of the 34 patients who were MASA-negative.

Others have used reverse transcriptase–polymerase chain reaction (RT–PCR) to detect CEA expression of carcinoma cells in lymph nodes (Mori et al, 1995). They have demonstrated that this method, which detects DNA, is far more sensitive than conventional techniques in revealing micrometastases. PCR has also been used in this way to detect mutations in K-*ras* and the APC gene with similar results (McKinley et al, 1997). Unfortunately, not all tumours express these mutations, and CEA expression is non-specific. We have therefore taken an alternative path and have used RT–PCR to detect cells expressing cytokeratin-20

(CK-20) in the lymph nodes of specimens removed from patients with colorectal cancer (Dorudi et al, 1998). Cytokeratin-20 was chosen since it is expressed selectively by the epithelial cells derived from the large intestine. Therefore, the finding of CK-20 cells in lymph nodes which do not normally contain epithelial cells is indicative of invasion by cancer cells derived from the colorectal cancer. Although immunohistochemical studies using monoclonal antibodies to a variety of epithelial markers have been used by several authors (Greenson et al, 1994; Jeffers et al, 1994), the method we use detects RNA, and thus viable cells; in addition it is far more specific than the other markers previously studied. Using RT–PCR to detect CK-20, we found that in 18 colorectal cancer specimens, four Dukes' stage B patients were found to harbour viable colonic mucosal cells within their lymph nodes. Two of the four Dukes' C patients had additional positive nodes detected (Table 30.6). Thus, this technique and other genetic methods are likely in the future to change previous concepts of staging and perhaps help target the paients who might benefit from adjuvant chemotherapy.

Table 30.6 Genetic diagnosis of lymph node metastases by detection of CK20 RNA.

Case	*Sex/age*	*Stage/site*	*Histo*	*Gen*
1	M/38	B/caecum	0/5	1/5†
2	F/71	C/caecum	12/18	12/18
3	F/73	B/sigmoid	0/8	0/8
4	F/84	B/rectum	0/6	0/6
5	M/69	B/rectum	0/5	1/5†
6	M/73	B/rectum	0/8	0/8
7	M/67	B/caecum	0/8	0/8
8	M/86	B/rectum	0/8	0/8
9	M/42	B/rectum	0/6	0/6
10	F/70	B/rectum	0/16	1/16§
11	F/77	B/rectum	0/9	0/9
12	M/82	B/rectum	0/11	0/11
13	F/76	B/hepatic flexure	0/6	2/6†
14	F/62	B/sigmoid	0/10	0/10
15	F/65	B/rectum	0/8	0/8
16	M/79	C/caecum	15/15	15/15
17	M/55	C/rectum	8/11	9/11
18	F/66	C/sigmoid	3/7	5/7‡

Histo, conventional histopathology; Gen, RT-PCR for CK20.
† Patients restaged by genetic lymph node metastases diagnosis. ‡ Patients in whom additional lymph node metastases diagnosed. § Patient in whom nodal metastasis was diagnosed by Southern blot.
From Dorudi et al (1998).

Blood-borne spread

Colon and rectal tumours may spread via the blood stream to a variety of organs. The most common organ to be involved is the liver, metastases reaching it via the portal vein. The incidence of hepatic metastases depends on the method used to detect them. Palpation of the liver at the time of surgery has been shown to be inaccurate. Thus Goligher (1941) found that in 893 patients with rectal cancer, hepatic metastases were detected by the surgeon in 11.5% of cases. Thirty of the patients who were thought to have normal livers at laparotomy subsequently died in the postoperative period, and at post-mortem in five of them liver metastases were demonstrated to be present.

The accuracy of detection at operation will, however, vary depending on how carefully the liver is assessed. This probably explains why authors such as Cedermark et al (1977) found that 37.1% of their patients had hepatic metastases at laparotomy. In our own series of 70 consecutive rectal cancers, using bimanual palpation of the liver, we found that ten patients (14.2%) had overt metastases (Williams et al, 1985). No matter how carefully the liver is examined at operation, even using operative ultrasonography, the number of metastases will be underestimated. Thus even in the series reported by Cedermark et al (1977) the incidence of liver metastases present at post-mortem in their 456 patients was 48% – approximately 10% more than found at operation. It would also appear that the incidence of liver metastases found at necroscopy depends on the diligence of the pathologist. As explained elsewhere, occult hepatic metastases are demonstrated on serial imaging of the liver in 30% of patients in whom the liver is thought to be clear at the time of surgery (Finlay et al, 1982). These metastases are often not demonstrated on the preoperative scans because they are less than 2 cm diameter. It can be imagined, therefore, how difficult it might be at necroscopy to determine the presence of such small metastases.

The lung is the second most frequent site of blood-borne metastases. It has been estimated from several studies that approximately 10% of all patients with adenocarcinoma of the colon and rectum will develop pulmonary metastases at some time during the course of their disease (McCormack and Attiyeh, 1979). The majority of these patients develop lung lesions as one facet of their generalized disease; however, about 10% (i.e. 1% of the total) will develop metastases in the lungs alone. Schulten et al (1976) followed 185 patients for 4–14 years after curative resection and found that 28 (15.1%) developed pulmonary metastases in which four (2.2%) were solitary.

Other sites to which colorectal carcinoma may infrequently metastasize are the adrenal glands, kidneys, bones and ovary. In the study by Cedermark et al (1977) in which 457 autopsies were performed on patients who died from a primary colorectal cancer, the incidence of metastases in the ovaries was 18.2%, in the adrenal glands 14%, in the brain 8.3% and in the kidney 6.6%. Bacon and Jackson (1953) found that metastases were detected clinically in the bones in 6% and in the brain in 1.3%. The overall incidence of osseous metastases from rectal cancer is said to be higher than for colonic tumours (Buirge, 1941; Abrams, 1950; Besbeas and Stearns, 1978). Of the 765 patients with disseminated carcinoma from the colon and rectum seen at the Memorial Sloan Kettering Cancer Center between 1960 and 1970, the incidence of osseous metastases from rectal carcinoma was 8.9% (32 cases) and from colonic carcinoma was 5.1% (21 cases) (Besbeas and Stearns, 1978).

Venous invasion

In order for a tumour to metastasize, part of it must gain access to the blood stream. If the bowel wall containing a colorectal carcinoma is sectioned, invasion of veins is often demonstrated and presumably this is the route of access into the systemic circulation. It would appear that there is a significant correlation between venous invasion and Dukes' stage, hepatic metastases and survival rates (Talbot et al, 1980; Kotanagi et al, 1995), such that the greater the incidence and degree of venous invasion the worse the prognosis. However, it should be stressed that hepatic metastases can still be present in the absence of venous invasion, and although venous invasion is important from a prognostic point of view, it is not an independent variable (Tsuchiya et al, 1995). The incidence of venous invasion in resected specimens seems to be approximately 50%. Intramural and extramural veins may be involved and as expected the greater the extramural involvement the worse the prognosis. When assessing a resection specimen for venous invasion only, extramural invasion should be counted (Talbot et al, 1980; Quirke and Shepherd 1997). Kotanagi et al (1995) have also demonstrated that venous invasion in metastatic lymph nodes was a particular indicator for the presence of liver metastases.

Release of carcinoma cells into the circulation

Various studies have demonstrated that neoplastic cells from colorectal cancer are frequently released into the circulation (Cole et al, 1954; Moore et al, 1957; Long et al, 1960; Sellwood et al, 1965). The difficulty has been in determining whether these cells are viable and capable of producing distant metastases. Some studies have linked the finding of cells in the blood draining from a colorectal carcinoma with a poor prognosis. Thus Moore and Sako (1959) found cancer cells in 6 of 16 inoperable cancers (37%) but in only 7 of 44 resectable cancers (16%). Other workers remain to be convinced, as they have found on long-term follow-up that the presence of cells in the venous blood draining from a tumour does not influence the development of metastases.

These studies are to be treated with caution since the methodology employed is outdated when compared with current techniques. More refined culture techniques are needed when studying this problem. Specific stains have to be used to distinguish cancer cells from macrophages and fibroblasts. Before viability of the cells can be accepted, the research workers have to demonstrate that the cancer cells can grow either in tissue culture or as implants in an immune deprived animal (i.e. as xenografts). These criteria remain to be fulfilled for cells draining from colorectal tumours. It is for these reasons also that one must remain sceptical about the data that supported the concept of the 'no touch' technique pioneered by Turnbull from the Cleveland Clinic. This technique was developed from the research work carried out by Warren Cole and his colleagues (Cole et al, 1954), which suggested that when tumours were mobilized large numbers of cancer cells capable of seeding were showered into the circulation. Once again, before this concept can be accepted the studies need to be repeated using modern techniques to detect cell viability.

Progress in this field is being made using the new genetic techniques. Our own group have demonstrated that using RT–PCR we could detect circulating CK-20 cells in both the peripheral and mesenteric blood of 8 out of 8 patients with metastatic carcinoma and none in control subjects (Marshall et al, 1997). Since this technique detects RNA, the cells are viable; and since CK-20 is specific for colorectal tissue, it is likely that these cells emanate from the cancer and may be responsible for the metastases.

Transcoelomic spread

Spread within the peritoneal cavity may occur. In the early stages of transcoelomic spread the peritoneum close to the tumour is involved, with small, white, discrete nodules. These plaques can eventually become more widespread with involvement of the omentum as well as the peritoneum. Invariably when the tumour has widely disseminated within the peritoneal cavity, ascites is produced. Cells may also reach the ovaries and produce large secondary deposits known as Krukenberg's tumours.

There is some debate as to how transcoelomic spread occurs. The cells may be carried from the primary tumour via the subperitoneal lymphatics (Miles, 1926). An alternative theory is that viable cells shed from the serosal surface of a tumour which has penetrated through the bowel wall are carried by peritoneal fluid and intestinal movement to be implanted at distant peritoneal sites (Pomeranz and Garlock, 1955). The implantation theory once again depends on whether these shed cells are viable and capable of growth. Several studies are available that demonstrate that malignant cells are present at operation in the peritoneal fluid (Quan, 1959; Moore et al, 1961). However, attempts to grow cells obtained from washings of the peritoneal cavity have invariably been unsuccessful. This situation contrasts sharply with the ease with which cells can be cultured from malignant ascitic fluid. The failure to grow cells from peritoneal washings may be due to the inadequacy of the technology available in the past. Once again these experiments need to be repeated using the criteria already discussed.

The rate of growth of peritoneal metastases has been calculated from serial computed tomographic (CT) measurements. Tumour doubling time varied between 58 days and 74 days (mean 70 days) (Havelaar et al, 1984). This rate is similar to that of metastatic tumour in the liver and retroperitoneal lymph nodes, but much faster than pulmonary metastases (Collins, 1962; Welin et al, 1963).

As would be expected, involvement of the peritoneal surface has a very negative effect on prognosis, even when the involvement is confined locally. Shepherd et al (1995) prospectively assessed the pathological prognostic factors in 209 resections for rectal carcinoma performed between 1988 and 1993. Local peritoneal involvement was detected in 54 cases (25.8%). Multivariate analyses demonstrated that this feature carried an independent prognostic disadvantage for all patients.

Spread by implantation

Peritoneal spread may occur by implantation. There are also other areas where implantation may play a part in the dissemination of a carcinoma. Of interest in this regard is the view that suture line recurrence is caused by the implantation of cells shed from the tumour into the bowel lumen at the time of resection and anastomosis. In certain instances recurrences in the abdominal wound and in previous haemorrhoidectomy scars (Morgan, 1950; Goligher et al, 1951; Killingback et al, 1965) have also been explained by the implantation theory.

The belief that shed neoplastic cells can lodge on raw surfaces created by the surgeon and can grow is, however, a contentious subject, particularly with regard to suture line recurrence. The concept originally arose from Ryall's observation in the early 1900s (Ryall, 1907, 1908). He recorded several cases in which implantation seemed to be the only explanation for recurrence. Several workers have since demonstrated the presence of exfoliated malignant cells in the lumen of bowel being resected for a colorectal cancer (Cole et al, 1954; Rosenberg, 1979). For the implantation theory to hold water the cells need to be viable. Although the animal work of Vink (1954) and Cohn et al (1963) supported the concept, a study by Rosenberg (1979) cast considerable doubt on it. Using trypan blue exclusion, non-specific esterase activity and tritiated thymidine uptake as tests of cell viability, he was unable in the majority of cases to demonstrate that cells shed into the bowel lumen were alive. That is perhaps where the matter might have rested, but for a report by Umpleby and his colleagues from Bristol (Umpleby et al, 1984). They began with the premise that malignant cells could resist staining by trypan blue and that this was not a reliable test for viability. In a series of experiments using sophisticated culture techniques and injecting these shed cells into immune deprived mice, they demonstrated unequivocally that such cells were viable. Whether these cells can implant and grow on a raw surface, however, is still open to debate.

With regard to suture line recurrence, we believe that the vast majority of cases are due to recurrent tumour growing into the lumen from without. It is interesting to note that Umpleby et al (1984) found viable cells in the lumen of the right colon during right hemicolectomy, yet suture line recurrence after this operation is virtually unknown. In our view the reason why suture line recurrence is more common after rectal excision is that residual microscopic disease is more often left behind in the pelvis owing to radial infiltration of the tumour (Quirke et al, 1986); this grows and enters the lumen of the bowel at its weakest point – the anastomosis.

A study in Birmingham showed a highly significant correlation between positive cytology smears from the side wall of the pelvis and local pelvic recurrence, further supporting the view that inadequate lateral excision is the most common cause of local recurrence. It is our belief, however, that true implantation of cancer cells can still occur on the suture line and other raw surfaces, but only rarely. Such a theory would explain why such recurrences may occur after resection of pathologically very early lesions (Morson et al, 1963). Experimental studies also suggest that the type of suture material might influence the chance of anastomotic recurrence. Experiments in mice have shown that the use of protein-based and multifilament sutures are more likely to result in shed colorectal cancer cells adhering to the anastomotic line (Uff and Phillips, 1993).

While implantation appears to be a rare cause for suture line recurrence, it seems prudent to ensure that detached viable cancer cells shed into the lumen of the bowel are destroyed at the time of operation. Various agents such as povidone-iodine and sodium hypochlorite solution seem to be effective in this context, our preference being 1% cetrimide solution.

Implantation as a cause of recurrence distant to the anastomosis has received particular attention recently because of port-site recurrences which have been demonstrated after laparoscopic resection for colorectal cancer and for other abdominal tumours, notably, ovary, stomach and the biliary tract (Nduka et al, 1994). Until the era of laparoscopy, implantation as a cause for recurrence in the abdominal wall was recognized but was considered to be very rare and thought to occur only in patients who had widespread intra-abdominal metastatic disease to start with. Thus, Hughes et al (1983) found that 11 of 1603 patients who underwent resection for colorectal cancer developed wound recurrence, and most of these had disseminated intra-abdominal disease. Reilly et al (1996) studied the incidence of incisional local recurrence in 1711 patients who had undergone a potentially curative resection for a primary tumour. Eleven patients (0.6%) had documented incisional recurrence (nine abdominal wounds, one perineal wound and one stoma wound). Of these 11 patients, two had primary B2 tumours and nine had primary stage C disease. Thus, after conventional operation, the incidence of true implantation recurrence in the wound has been confirmed to be very uncommon.

The incidence after laparoscopic surgery seems to be greater. Although there are no prospective controlled data, most authors have been alarmed by the incidence (Fusco and Paluzzi 1993; Berends et al, 1994; Berman et al, 1995; Jaquet et al, 1995). In a review of the subject, Wexner and Cohen (1995) found a mean incidence of 6.3% (range 1.5–21%) reported in the literature between 1993 and 1995. These occurred 3–26 months after the initial resection (mean 7.2 months) (Table 30.7). These authors also highlighted the case of a patient reported by Wade et al (1994) who underwent laparoscopic cholecystectomy for gallstones. The pathology specimen showed an unsuspected polypoid carcinoma. The patient underwent re-exploration at 21 days and several nodules were found at the umbilical port site. One of these nodules contained a nidus of metastatic gallbladder carcinoma cells. A similar case was recorded by Jacobi et al (1994).

These data and further reports have convinced us that implantation in the abdominal wall can occur after laparoscopy for colorectal cancer. It does seem to be more common than after conventional surgery. However, poor technique must have a bearing on this, as very low rates of port-site recurrence are reported from experienced units in the USA, Australia and Spain (Fielding et al, 1997; Khalili et al, 1998; Lacy et al, 1998). Research studies

Table 30.7 Port-site recurrence after surgery for colorectal carcinoma.

Reference	*Dukes' stage*	*Interval to recurrence (months)*	*Series incidence (%)*
Alexander et al (1993)	C	3	NS
Walsh et al (1993)	C	6	NS
Fusco and Paluzzi (1993)	C	10	NS
Guillou et al (1993)	C	NS	NS
O'Rourke et al (1993)	B	2.5	NS
Stitz* (1993)	D	NS	NS
Cirocco et al (1994)	C	9	NS
Wilson et al (1994)	NS	NS	NS
Nduka et al (1994)	C	3	NS
Prasad et al (1994)	B	6	4
	A	26	–
Berends et al (1994)	B	NS	21
	C	NS	–
	D	NS	–
Lauroy et al (1994)	A	9	NS
Boulez and Herriot (1994)	3–stages NS	NS	3.5
Ramos et al (1994)	C	NS	1.5
	C	NS	–
	C	NS	–
Ngoi* (1994)	B	NS	4.5
Gionnone* (1994)	C	2	NS
Gould* (1994)	NS	4	NS
Newman et al* (1994)	C	6	NS
Cohen and Wexner (1994)	B	3	NS
	B	6	NS
	C	6	NS
	C	9	NS
	C	12	NS
Fingerhut (1995)	A	NS	3.3
	B	NS	–
	B	NS	–
Totals	3A, 8B, 15C, 2D, 5 NS	7.2 (range 3–26)	6.3 (range 1.5–21)

* Personal communication. NS, not stated.
Adapted from Wexner and Cohen (1995).

suggest that the induced pneumoperitoneum aerosolization by CO_2 insufflation and contaminated instruments are important factors in their development (Jones et al, 1995; Bouvy et al, 1996; Hewett et al, 1996). The impact of port-site recurrence on laparoscopic resection of colorectal cancer is discussed elsewhere in greater depth (Chapter 36). However, we believe that the incidence of this complication is sufficiently high for surgeons not to perform the technique outside a prospective controlled trial. We also think that such trials should be conducted only after the phenomenon has been studied further and strategies developed which are likely to combat the problem.

STAGING OF COLORECTAL CANCER

The staging of colorectal cancer for many years depended on the pathologist's assessment of spread obtained from detailed examination of the operative specimen. Dukes' classification was the first to be accepted and was originally used for rectal carcinoma (Dukes, 1930, 1940). By 1932 the classification took the following form (Figure 30.12).

- *Stage A:* growth limited to the wall of the rectum, there being no extension into the extrarectal tissues and no metastases in the lymph nodes.
- *Stage B:* the growth extends through the wall into the extrarectal tissues but the lymph nodes are free from metastases.
- *Stage C:* lymph nodes are involved with the tumour.

By 1935 the importance of proximal lymph node involvement in the resected mesentery became apparent (Gabriel et al, 1935). The stage C classification was modified to reflect this difference: *stage C1* was used to describe cases in which only regional lymph nodes were involved or those in which the upward spread had not reached the point of ligation of blood vessels; *stage C2* was used to describe cases in which lymph node spread reached the proximal point of vascular ligature.

Using this classification in operable rectal cancer, Dukes (1940) found that 15% were stage A, 35% were stage B and 50% were stage C. Approximately two-thirds of the C cases were classified as C1 and the remaining one-third belonged to stage C2. The validity of this staging method was borne out in the 1958 report of Dukes and Bussey, each stage correlating with a significant difference in 5-year survival. In 1939 the original Dukes classification was extended for use in colon cancer as well as rectal cancer (Simpson and Mayo, 1939).

Although the Dukes system was considered by many surgeons and pathologists to be satisfactory, in the USA various modifications were thought to be important. Kirklin et al (1949) and Astler and Coller (1954) offered modifications to Dukes' original classification which attempted to combine the prognostic significance of mural penetration and/or involvement of lymph nodes.

In the system adopted by Kirklin and associates, stage A referred to growths that had not yet penetrated through the muscularis mucosae. These were, in fact, carcinomas-in-situ and were considered by Dukes not to be true invasive carcinomas. Kirklin's group divided stage B into two categories, B1 and B2, according to whether the tumour had penetrated superficially or deeply into the rectal wall. Stage B, however, excluded tumours that had reached the perirectal tissues. Thus their stage B was equivalent to Dukes' stage A.

In the Astler–Coller modification, B1 and B2 represented respectively incomplete and complete penetration of the muscularis propria (or the serosa where present); i.e. the entire bowel wall. Stages C1 and C2 represented involvement of lymph nodes in the absence of (C1) or presence of (C2) mural penetration. Five-year survival data for the Astler–Coller system were stage A (1 patient) 100%; B1 (48 patients) 66.6%; B2 (164 patients) 53.9%; C1 (14 patients) 42.8%; and C2 (125 patients) 22.4%.

These American modifications of the original Dukes stages supported the fact that mural penetration had independent prognostic significance of nodal involvement. However, considerable confusion was and still is created in the literature, as it has not always been appreciated that different studies have used different staging systems. None of these pathological staging classifications, including the Dukes system, took into consideration the presence of distant metastases. In recent years it has been customary to include a stage D category for patients with extensive spread (Turnbull et al, 1967). This category, however, varies in its interpretation. Some reserve it for patients who have only distant metastases, whereas others include those patients who have residual local tumour remaining after excision. The latter is not always supported by pathological proof that the remaining tissue is malignant.

In an attempt to standardize pathological reporting and to provide a more clinicopathological

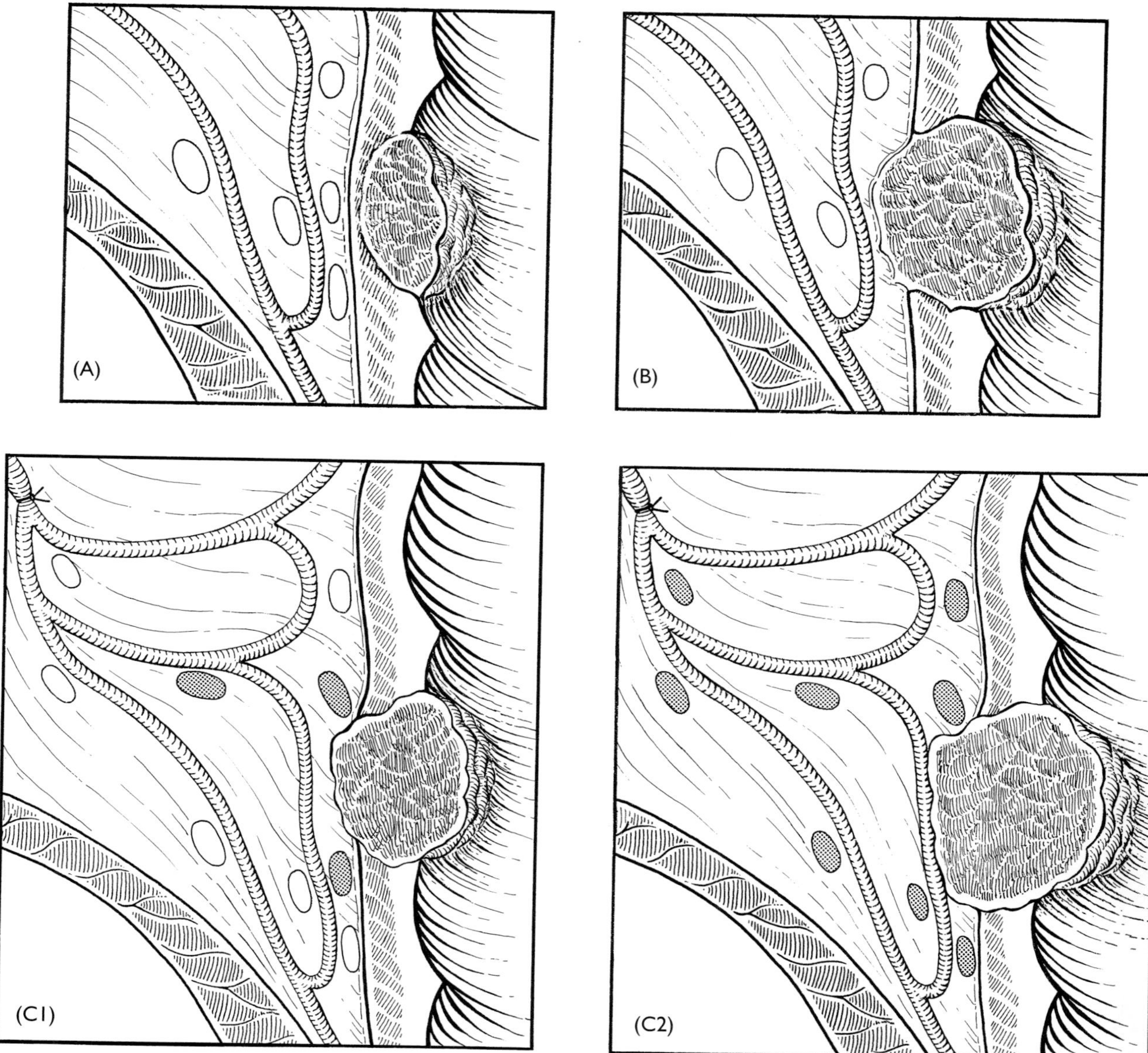

Figure 30.12 Dukes' staging of colorectal cancer.

system, the TNM (tumour, node, metastasis) system was recommended (Beart et al, 1978; Wood et al, 1979). The American Joint Committee Task Force on Colon and Rectum analysed 1826 cases and applied Union Internationale Contre le Cancer (UICC) criteria to them, and confirmed the importance of postsurgical staging. The TNM system provides uniformity for staging both colon and rectal cancer and takes into account the presence of distant metastases. The original TNM system omitted observations such as mural penetration which have prognostic importance. However, in recent years it has been modified to include these factors (Table 30.8). A similar system has also been developed by the Japanese Research Society for Cancer of the Colon and Rectum; this system is even more complex than the TNM, and is based on the system used to stage gastric cancers. It has now been applied to over 5000 patients (Hojo et al, 1982), but because of its complexity it is doubtful whether it will ever be accepted internationally.

In an attempt to retain a simpler system while recognizing the importance of clinical factors, the Australians recommended a clinicopathological

Table 30.8 TNM classification of colorectal carcinoma.

pT	*Microscopic description of depth of primary tumour on pathologic examination*
pT_x	Minimum requirements to assess the primary tumour cannot be met
pT_0	No evidence of primary tumour
pT_{is}	*In situ* carcinoma (intra-epithelial or invasive into muscularis mucosae and/or lamina propria only)
pT_1	Tumour invades through muscularis mucosae into sub-mucosa
pT_2	Tumour invades into but not through muscularis propria
pT_3	Tumour invades through muscularis propria into subserosa or into non-peritonealized pericolonic or perirectal tissue
pT_4	Tumour invades directly into other organs or structures and/or perforates the visceral peritoneum of the specimen
pN	*Regional lymph node status on pathologic examination*
pN_x	Minimum requirements to assess the regional lymph nodes cannot be met
pN_0	No regional lymph node metastasis found
pN_1	Metastasis in 1–3 pericolonic or perirectal lymph nodes
pN_2	Metastasis in four or more pericolonic or perirectal lymph nodes
pN_3	Metastasis in lymph node along the course of a major named vascular trunk [iliocolic; right, middle or left colic; inferior mesenteric; superior rectal (haemorrhoidal); and/or internal iliac arteries but not sigmoid arteries] and/or metastasis in apical lymph node(s) when marked by the surgeon
pM	*Distant metastasis after definitive regional therapy*
pM_x	Minimum requirements to assess distant metastatis cannot be met
pM_0	No distant metastasis found
pM_1	Distant metastasis documented by pathologic examination (including external or common iliac lymph nodes)

Stage groupings	T	N	M
Stage 0	T_{is}	0	0
Stage I	1 or 2	0	0
Stage II	3 or 4	0	0
Stage III	Any	1, 2 or 3	0
Stage IV	Any	Any	1

From Henson et al (1994).

classification (Davis and Newland, 1982). This system formally recognizes the presence of metastases and also includes a special subsection for tumours removed by local excision. The latter consists of category A where the carcinoma is confined to the mucosa, XA where the tumour does not spread beyond the muscularis propria, and XB where the tumour spreads beyond the muscularis propria.

It has become clear in recent years that a staging classification based on pathological features alone is inadequate; the presence of metastases has to be included. The inclusion of a D category makes it imperative that there is uniformity in clinical assessment. Patients categorized as D cases in the past were in the main those who had macroscopic hepatic metastases present at laparotomy. With the introduction of sophisticated imaging techniques, however, hepatic metastases not palpable at operation are more likely to be detected both preoperatively by CT scanning and ultrasonography and peroperatively using the flat liver ultrasound probe. As pointed out previously, patients may be included in the D category if they have local residual disease left after resection; sometimes inclusion in this category is based on the surgeon's impression, without pathological evidence of residual disease. Even if such evidence is sought it may be missed unless a very detailed pathological assessment of the operative specimen is carried out (Quirke et al, 1986). It is clear, therefore, that although clinical features need to be included in the staging of patients with colorectal cancer, there has to be uniformity in how the assessment is carried out. The criteria for the presence of metastatic or residual disease also need to be defined both by the clinician and the pathologist. If uniformity were agreed on an international basis, patients could be split into high-risk subgroups and trials of therapy would be more comparable and hence more meaningful. This approach has been highly successful in the treatment of other neoplasms which had previously proved resistant to treatment.

For these reasons the United Kingdom Coordinating Committee for Cancer Research (UKCCCR) set up a working party with the aim of standardizing the clinicopathological assessment of patients with colorectal cancer. This working party consisted of surgeons, pathologists, radiologists, radiotherapists and statisticians, each with particular expertise in dealing with the disease. The group was also joined by the chairman of the Committee on Clinicopathology Staging of Large Bowel Cancer set up by the American Society of Colon and Rectal Surgeons, the aim being to achieve international agreement of terms and classification. The recommendations of the working party concerning the pathological reporting of colorectal tumours removed at operation were first published in 1988 (Williams et al, 1988) and have since been updated and are summarized in Table 30.9. This is an attempt to obtain uniformity among pathologists, but it must be stressed that these pathological features have to be considered along with standardized clinical and operative findings before a true prognosis can be determined. The recommendations of the working party concerning the clinical and operative findings are summarized below.

Table 30.9 Pathological reporting (recommended by UKCCCR working party on staging of colorectal cancer 1997).

The pathologist should record the following characteristics:

1. *Gross description*
   (a) Distance of upper edge of growth from proximal margin and lower edge of growth from distal margin (cm). State whether fixed or fresh.
   (b) Axial and transverse diameters of growth (cm).
   (c) Circumference of bowel at mid-point of tumour (cm).
   (d) Appearance of tumour (ulcerating, protuberant, diffusely infiltrating, perforated)
2. *Local spread*
   (a) Spread through tissues of bowel wall
      (i) Cannot be assessed (e.g. previous local excision or radiotherapy)
      (ii) Neoplastic process limited to mucosa (this is often reported as severe dysplasia in UK)
      (iii) Limited to submucosa
      (iv) Limited to muscularis propria (external)
      (v) Beyond muscularis propria but not penetrating peritoneum or invading adjacent organs
      (vi) Penetrates peritoneum, and/or
      (vii) Invades adjacent organs.
   (b) Extent of spread beyond bowel wall (mm) and clearance at deep excision margin (mm) to be measured on gross specimen and confirmed histologically.
   (c) Involvement of proximal and distal margins of specimen requires histological confirmation only when the margins are close to the tumour (< 5 cm) or tumour is highly infiltrative)
   (d) State whether tumour excision is complete or incomplete.
3. *Lymphatic spread*
   (a) Number of nodes draining bowel segment harbouring tumours.
   (b) Number of nodes with metastatic cancer.
   (c) Metastasis in apical node (immediately below vessel ligature).
   (d) Extramural tumour deposits apparently not within nodes.
   (e) Lymphatic or perineural permeation (yes/no).
4. *Venous spread*
   Invasion of extramural veins.
5. *Histology*
   (a) Type (adenocarcinoma, mucinous adenocarcinoma, signet ring cell carcinoma, other).
   (b) Differentiation (poor or other).
   (c) Invasive margin (expanding or infiltrating).
   (d) Peritumoral lymphocytes (conspicuous or not).
6. *Other pathology*
   (a) Synchronous carcinoma.
   (b) Adenoma.
   (c) Other.

After all clinicopathological features have been considered, the patient may be categorized as having undergone a procedure that is curative, non-curative, or indeterminate for cure.

Non-curative operations

These are operations in which tumour has been left behind. The procedures should be categorized into two groups:

- *Non-curative owing to the presence of distant metastases*. Whenever possible this must be supported by histological confirmation. The latter proviso may be waived when metastases are convincingly demonstrated on imaging but biopsy is not feasible (e.g. lung metastases detected on chest radiography).
- *Non-curative owing to the presence of residual local disease*. This must be confirmed by histological examination. Included in this category are patients whose operative specimens on histological examination show tumour at any margin of excision.

Curative operations

Curative operations are defined as procedures in which metastases have been excluded by preoperative imaging and the surgeon has removed all tumour, as confirmed by postoperative histological examination of the specimen.

Indeterminate for cure

If there is any doubt the patient should be classified as having an operation which is indeterminate for cure. Procedures during which the specimen has been perforated either spontaneously or operatively should be classified as indeterminate for cure. The definition of 'curative' can be applied only to operations in which the tumour has been resected together with a segment of bowel and its associated area of lymphatic drainage. Procedures in which the tumour is removed by local excision can be classified only as either non-curative or indeterminate.

CLINICAL FEATURES

The mode of presentation of a colorectal cancer depends on several factors. Broadly speaking there are two categories of presentation, acute or emergency, and chronic or elective. When a patient presents electively the site of the tumour will often dictate the symptom complex. Emergency cases present with one of the complications of the carcinoma, which are usually obstruction, perforation or haemorrhage. The proportion of patients who present to the surgeon in one of these two ways depends on the type of practice. Surgeons who work in a private clinic or specialized hospital without an emergency room will see very few acute cases. On the other hand, if the surgeon's practice is in a large National Health Service or community hospital serving a relatively large population, approximately a quarter of cases will present as emergencies. These data were obtained from the records of the Leeds General Infirmary in the 1950s (Goligher and Smiddy, 1957); despite recent emphasis on screening and early diagnosis, the proportion of acute presentations does not seem to have fallen appreciably (N S Williams, 1985, unpublished observations).

In this section, the clinical features of the elective presentation of colorectal cancer are described; acute or emergency presentations are discussed elsewhere (Chapters 60 (Obstruction), 62, 65 and 66 (Forms of perforation)).

Elective presentation of colonic carcinoma

In general, the more distal the lesion the more obstructive are the symptoms. The reason is that the left colon has a narrower calibre than the right and its contents tend to be less fluid. Furthermore, carcinomas on the right side tend to be soft and friable in consistency, whereas those on the left side tend to be scirrhous and annular. These comments are only generalizations and there can be considerable overlap. Usually patients present with clinical features of the primary tumour only, but occasionally they may complain of symptoms relating to metastases and deny any abdominal or gastrointestinal problems. The following are the usual clinical features which may be encountered; however, one or any combination of them may present.

Change in bowel habit

Changed bowel habit is probably the most common symptom, particularly with left-sided lesions. At the onset the complaint is often quite trivial, for instance the frequency of bowel action may increase from once every two days to a daily action. So insidious is the onset of this symptom that the patient frequently disregards it and does not seek medical advice.

As time progresses, however, the problem becomes worse. Either constipation or diarrhoea may be prevalent, but commonly the two conditions alternate. This may be the result of taking either laxatives or constipating agents to alleviate the principal symptom.

Abdominal pain

Pain is not an infrequent complaint. It may vary from a central or lower abdominal colic to a constant deep-seated ache in one quadrant of the abdomen. Colic is more likely to emanate from an obstructing left-sided lesion. Constant pain may indicate local extension and fixity to adjacent organs. Frequently the patient with abdominal colic complains of nausea and abdominal distension. The latter may be alleviated after several days by the passage of loose stool or flatus. This symptom complex is that of chronic large bowel obstruction.

Occasionally the abdominal pain radiates to the back if the patient has a retroperitoneal extension of a tumour from the ascending colon. Lumbar pain may be due to retroperitoneal extension of a tumour in the descending colon.

Bleeding

Bleeding may be obvious or occult. The blood may vary in hue from bright red to black. The more proximal the lesion, the more altered will the blood become. A tumour in the sigmoid or descending colon may produce bright red bleeding of insignificant amount. The patient may well ignore this symptom, or the doctor may be prepared to attribute it to haemorrhoids. It should be emphasized that even if the practitioner finds haemorrhoids on proctoscopy, the patient must have a more thorough investigation of the rest of the colon and rectum.

When occult bleeding occurs the patient usually presents with symptoms of anaemia, such as fatigue or breathlessness. This form of presentation is frequent with lesions of the caecum and right colon, and indeed anaemia may be the only sign of the underlying colorectal neoplasm. The anaemia is hypochromic and microcytic, due to iron deficiency, and its presence in any patient without an obvious cause demands full investigation of the whole of the gastrointestinal tract, paying particular attention to the colon.

Passage of mucus

The passage of mucus is common; it may be separate from the stool or mixed with it. The patient often describes the symptoms as 'passing slime'. Rarely the volume of mucus is profuse, as in patients with a bulky villous lesion. It is highly unusual, however, for such a carcinoma of the colon to cause the syndrome which may occur with rectal villous neoplasms characterized by dehydration and hypokalaemia.

Weight loss

Although weight loss of 1–2 kg may occur, particularly in the presence of abdominal pain, it is an unusual symptom in patients with an uncomplicated colonic cancer. More severe loss of weight is highly suspicious of dissemination. Occasionally a neoplasm of the transverse colon will invade the stomach and produce similar symptoms to that of a primary gastric carcinoma with anorexia, nausea and weight loss.

Abdominal mass

Occasionally the patient may become aware of an abdominal mass, but usually if one is present it is found by the clinician on palpation. Its site within the abdomen depends on the position of the tumour within the colon: thus a caecal lesion is felt in the right lower quadrant, a transverse colon lesion is usually felt in the epigastrium, etc. The mass is usually deeply situated and may be mobile or fixed. Fixity suggests local extension into adjacent organs. If a sigmoid lesion is mobile and prolapses into the pelvis, it may be felt through the rectal wall on rectal examination.

Symptoms related to metastases

Each of the above clinical features emanates usually from the primary growth. In approximately 5% of cases (Corman, 1984), however, the patient may present with symptoms related to metastases only, the primary tumour remaining 'silent'. Bone pain, jaundice, pathological fracture, neurological symptoms, personality changes, thrombophlebitis migrans and skin nodules (particularly at the umbilicus – Sister Joseph's nodule) have all been described as presenting symptoms. Other dermatological problems that may be associated with either a symptomatic or asymptomatic primary colorectal cancer are acanthosis nigricans, dermatomyositis, pemphigoid and pyoderma gangrenosum (Rosato et al, 1969).

Other modes of presentation

Other less common modes of presentation may result from abscess and fistulation. A sigmoid or descending colon lesion may form a fistula into the bladder and produce a colovesical fistula. The symptoms and signs are identical to those when such a fistula is caused by diverticular disease (see Chapter 65). Very occasionally a colocutaneous fistula results from a colonic carcinoma ulcerating through the abdominal wall. Fistulation into other parts of the gastrointestinal tract may occur causing a variety of clinical features. Thus fistula formation between colon and small intestine can occasionally result in a blind loop syndrome and a gastrocolic fistula may result in severe diarrhoea and weight loss.

Elective presentation of rectal carcinoma

Many of the symptoms and signs described above, particularly those ascribed to left-sided lesions, may occur with a rectal carcinoma. Nevertheless, rectal carcinoma tends to be associated with a characteristic symptom complex and because of its distal site it can often be palpated per rectum.

Bleeding is perhaps the most common symptom and is frequently ignored by the patient. It may also be ignored by the patient's medical attendant if rectal bleeding is assumed to be due to 'piles' and the examination is less than adequate. The blood is often red, but not bright red. It may be mixed in with the stool or passed separately, and although small amounts are usual, on occasions the volume may be alarming. Although bleeding may occur alone, bowel habit is invariably altered. The patient frequently has the urge to defecate but on going to the lavatory passes only blood and mucus. Such 'tenesmus' is often most acute in the early morning and occurs as soon as the patient rises from bed. It may continue for the first part of the day and then subside. For this reason this symptom is termed 'morning diarrhoea'. It should be stressed that it is not diarrhoea as such because so often faeculant material is not passed. It should also be stated that this symptom is not always confined to the early morning and may continue throughout the day and even wake the patient during the night.

If the growth is constricting the rectum, abdominal colic may be the main complaint. Local anorectal pain is, however, unusual unless there has been spread to local structures, particularly where a tumour has invaded the sacral plexus posteriorly. If this occurs the patient may feel the most intense discomfort in either the sacral region or in the distribution of one or both sciatic nerves. Pain may also be experienced if the tumour invades downwards and encroaches on the anal canal or perianal skin; this pain is usually aggravated by defecation in a similar manner to an anal fissure.

Invasion of the anal canal and anal sphincter may also lead to incontinence, and invasion of the perineal skin may result in the formation of a fistula-in-ano. Occasionally the tumour is felt by the patient to be protruding through the anal orifice.

Other structures may be invaded and give rise to characteristic symptoms. Thus the bladder or urethra may be involved, with the formation of a recto-urethral or rectovesical fistula. The patient with this complication often complains initially of recurrent dysuria and urinary frequency which may lead to pneumaturia. Spread anteriorly in the female may lead to a rectovaginal fistula or, less commonly, a rectouterine fistula. These fistulas will often result in the passage of mucus and blood per vaginam and occasionally faeces will present. Rarely a rectal tumour may be so locally aggressive that it presents as a large pelvic mass which either compresses or invades pelvic blood vessels and lymphatics and produces unilateral or bilateral leg oedema.

Evaluation

General and abdominal examination

A full clinical examination is clearly essential in all cases of suspected colorectal carcinoma. Not only is the clinician looking for signs that may help to confirm the diagnosis, but also in cases where the diagnosis has already been made it is important to assess the extent of spread and the fitness of the patient for surgical treatment.

Severe cachexia with loss of muscle bulk suggests the presence of metastases. Similarly icterus suggests hepatic secondaries. Skin nodules should be sought, as frequently the patient is unaware of them. Evidence of intra-abdominal metastases may be present on abdominal palpation. Abdominal distension with shifting dullness suggests the presence of ascites secondary to peritoneal seedlings. Irregular hepatic enlargement which is hard suggests hepatic metastases. Liver secondaries have to be extensive before they are usually detected on palpation. We found that none of seven patients with liver secondaries emanating from a rectal carcinoma was detected on routine clinical examination (Williams et al, 1985).

Abdominal distension due to flatus may be present in patients whose growths are responsible for subacute intestinal obstruction. The tumour itself may be palpable; right-sided lesions are stated to be more often palpable than left-sided ones (Goligher, 1984), although this is not the authors' experience. Palpable left-sided lesions can be differentiated from inspissated faeces by the fact that they fail to indent on pressure with the finger.

Carcinomas at the splenic and hepatic flexures may be palpable, but in order for them to be felt the clinician must purposefully perform a bimanual palpation of both loins during full inspiration and expiration. Examination of the inguinal regions for the presence of palpable lymph nodes is useful. Although spread to these nodes is unusual in rectal cancer, if the tumour has invaded distally into the anal canal these nodes may be involved. Supraclavicular lymph nodes may occasionally be enlarged in advanced cases.

After general and abdominal examination it is necessary to proceed with digital examination followed by sigmoidoscopy and either a barium enema or a colonoscopy. It is our belief that provided there are experienced personnel and the facilities available all patients with a possible colorectal cancer should also have a colonoscopy. If digital, sigmoidoscopic and radiological examination are negative and symptoms continue, the possibility of a tumour must still be considered. Even if a lesion is found on one of the initial investigations, full evaluation of the rest of the colon should be performed to exclude the presence of a synchronous tumour.

Digital examination

If a carcinoma is present in a mobile redundant loop of sigmoid colon it may prolapse down into the pouch of Douglas and be palpable extrarectally. Otherwise, a carcinoma of colon will not be felt per rectum unless it produces an intussusception (which is very rare). On the other hand, approximately 75% of carcinomas of the lower two-thirds of the rectum (0–12 cm from the anal verge) should be palpable per rectum (Williams et al, 1985). For diagnostic purposes a rectal examination is usually performed with the patient conscious in the left lateral position and without bowel preparation. At this assessment the site, mobility, depth of invasion, and possible lymph node metastases should be recorded. More information may be gained with the patient anaesthetized after suitable bowel preparation, particularly if the lesion is high or the patient is nervous. It is better to perform all examinations under anaesthesia in the lithotomy position so that a bimanual examination can also be performed to assess fixity to local structures in the pelvis.

As noted in the section on pathology, a rectal carcinoma may take various macroscopic forms, the characteristics of which should be discernible by digital palpation. Thus an early growth may be felt as a disc-like lesion raised like a small plateau with a flat and definite edge. Another type of lesion is the polypoid friable growth which has some areas of induration and ulceration. More typical is the malignant ulcer with raised, everted edges and a deep central crater. Another common variant is the annular lesion. If this type of tumour is situated low in the rectum it is usually easy to confirm that it is annular. However, an annular lesion situated at a higher level may not be so easy to assess. Thus if part of it is at a lower level than the rest, this may be the only region palpable by the finger; consequently this may be wrongly assessed as an ulcerated lesion situated on only one part of the rectal wall. From a diagnostic point of view such an error is irrelevant; on the other hand full evaluation is essential when planning optimal surgical therapy.

The relative position of the tumour to the anorectal ring, the cervix, the prostate or the tip of the coccyx should be ascertained. The size of the lesion should be assessed by measuring the distance from its upper and lower limits to the anal verge, together with the circumferential involvement of the rectum. The degree of fixity should also be evaluated. An early lesion may be mobile on the muscle coat of the rectum; however, it is difficult to be certain on this point and so often one can only detect whether the tumour is free from adjacent structures. If fixity is detected, its degree should be noted. The tumour may become adherent to the prostate, seminal vesicles, bladder, posterior vaginal wall or uterus anteriorly or to the sacrum or coccyx posteriorly. Apart from the tumour fixity, other signs may indicate spread. Thus induration may be felt around the growth due either to submucous spread or to extrarectal spread into the perirectal tissues. Occasionally hard, enlarged pararectal lymph nodes on the back of the rectum can be palpated against the sacrum, or extensive induration may be felt in one or other of the lateral ligaments.

Although all of the above characteristics should be routinely sought, it must be realized that digital examination is a relatively crude examination and too much reliance cannot be placed on it. This is particularly pertinent in the selection of patients for treatment. Thus although a tumour may be felt to be fixed and thus locally invasive, the fixity may be due to inflammation and not malignancy, thereby influencing treatment. In addition there is considerable interobserver error when determining the mobility of a tumour (Nicholls et al, 1982; Williams et al, 1985). We found that the overall accuracy in the detection of malignant fixation in cancers situated 0–12 cm from the anal verge was 63% (Williams et al, 1985). Furthermore, in 17% of cases two observers reported quite different degrees of fixity.

Proctoscopy and sigmoidoscopy

All patients with a palpable rectal carcinoma will need a full evaluation of the colon. However, in the preliminary outpatient clinic it is usually only necessary to establish the diagnosis quickly. This can be done by proctoscopic or sigmoidoscopic biopsy; alternatively, if the tumour is palpable immediate diagnosis may be made by imprint cytology using a spatula or a serrated glove. Once the diagnosis has been confirmed the patient can undergo colonoscopy as an outpatient or be admitted to hospital for endoscopy after bowel preparation just before resection.

If a tumour is not palpable on digital examination, sigmoidoscopy is mandatory. There is still some controversy as to whether the rigid or the flexible sigmoidoscope should be used. The pros and cons have been discussed elsewhere (see Chapter 28). In our view the flexible instrument if available should be used at the first referral outpatient visit every time a tumour is suspected and is not felt or seen using a rigid instrument. The flexible sigmoidoscope has the important advantages that it can be passed to a higher level in the colon and the view is far superior to the rigid instrument. Thus the diagnosis can be established rapidly. Several papers have established the instrument's superior diagnostic yield compared with the rigid sigmoidoscope. McCallum et al (1984) using flexible sigmoidoscopy found an abnormality in 35% of examinations. Eighty-five neoplastic lesions were identified in 78 patients. Adenomas were found in the younger age groups. Among patients over the age of 60 years, 3.3% had carcinomas compared with 0.8% of patients younger than 60 years. Of more importance, over 50% of the neoplastic lesions were detected beyond 20 cm from the anal verge and were unlikely to have been detected using the rigid instrument. Similar results were also published in an audit of 1333 examinations (Armitage and Hardcastle, 1984).

There is still reluctance on the part of some surgeons to accept flexible sigmoidoscopy as a routine outpatient procedure. The instruments are considered to be too expensive and to require a high level of operator skill, and cannot be sterilized as easily as the rigid sigmoidoscopes. While it is true that the flexible instrument is more expensive than the rigid varieties, the greater diagnostic yield is likely to reduce the need for outpatient barium enemas, thereby reducing overall cost. Although a new skill is needed, it is easily acquired particularly since many surgeons now have expertise in upper gastrointestinal endoscopy. Finally, manufacturers are now making instruments that are far more robust than their predecessors and may be easily sterilized.

The sigmoidoscopic appearance of a tumour is characteristic. The examiner usually first notices the raised, everted lower edge of the lesion which appears darker than the normal pale pink mucosa. The tumour is often red or purple. The macroscopic nature of the carcinoma will be noted to be ulcerated, annular or polypoid. Occasionally the instrument can be negotiated past the tumour into the proximal colon but this may cause haemorrhage and is probably unnecessary. Biopsies should be taken from the centre and the periphery of the lesion. Brush cytology may be used with the flexible instrument. The view may be obscured by blood, mucus or faeces, but a satisfactory view can be obtained by using a separate sucker (if the rigid instrument is used) or by suction and washing (with the flexible endoscope). It is prudent to take several biopsies since it is easy for the clinician initially to miss the lesion and to biopsy normal mucosa. The flexible instrument has the disadvantage that the biopsy samples are small, and an experienced pathologist is needed to interpret the slides.

Even though sigmoidoscopy may not reveal a tumour, the presence of blood and mucus in the lumen may raise the suspicion that a neoplasm exists at a more proximal site beyond the reach of the instrument. Such a finding makes further study mandatory. Proctosigmoidoscopy enables the examiner to determine if there is other pathology which may be responsible for the symptoms. It must be emphasized, however, that even if other pathology is present a colorectal cancer cannot be excluded until the rest of the colon has been investigated. We must stress that neither barium enema nor colonoscopy alone are adequate investigations to rule out rectal carcinoma and therefore digital rectal examination and sigmoidoscopy must precede them.

Barium enema examination

Although there has been controversy over the years concerning the relative merits of single- or double-contrast barium examination, it is now accepted that the double-contrast technique is to be preferred.

The tumour may cause a stricture either of a 'string' or 'napkin ring' type. The string type is quite short, usually about 2 cm in length, whereas the napkin ring type is up to 8 cm (Figure 30.13). The longer type of stricture tends to be characteristic. The line of barium in the stenosed part is often slightly eccentric owing to the greater bulk of the tumour in the part of the bowel wall from which it originated. There is 'shouldering' of the growth giving the appearance of an 'apple core' deformity, the latter term being sometimes used for this type of stricture. Carcinomatous strictures can be differentiated from spasm by their constant position, their failure to dilate even after administration of hyoscine butylbromide, and the disruption of the mucosa. These features help to differentiate the lesion from a stricture caused by diverticular disease. It must be pointed out, however, that where there is marked diverticular disease, particularly in the sigmoid colon, it is extremely difficult to rule out an underlying carcinoma.

Apart from diverticular disease, strictures due to other diseases can mimic a neoplastic lesion. Differentiation from Crohn's disease is occasionally a problem, but usually other radiological evidence for this diagnosis is present; e.g. the presence of skip lesions or other strictures, 'cobblestone' appearance of the mucosa, linear ulceration or fissuring, and involvement of the terminal ileum (see Chapter 51). An ischaemic stricture may be mistaken for a carcinoma: characteristically the former has four radiological features, 'thumb-printing', ragged

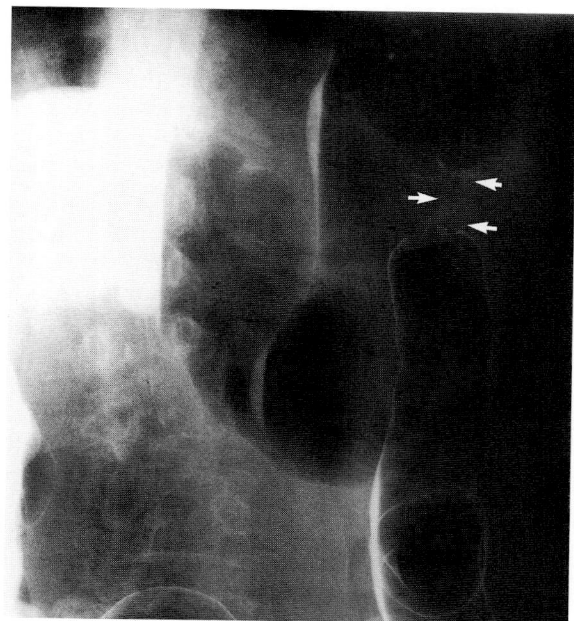

Figure 30.13 Double-contrast barium enema demonstrating a tight annular (napkin ring) carcinoma near the splenic flexure.

'sawtooth' irregularity of the bowel contour, tubular narrowing and sacculation (Boley et al, 1963) (see Chapter 63). Previous radiation, particularly of the pelvis for treatment of gynaecological cancer, may lead to a stricture of the left colon or upper rectum (see Chapter 64); the history will suggest the diagnosis, and radiologically the diseased segment is far more extensive than is the case with a carcinoma. In addition it is rare for such a lesion to exist in isolation – usually loops of small intestine are also involved. Other rare causes of colonic stricture which may occasionally be confused with carcinoma include lymphoma, tuberculosis, amoebiasis, systemic sclerosis, congenital bands (producing a string-like lesion of the ascending colon) and torsion of an appendix epiploica (causes a typical 'signet ring' appearance) (Cummack, 1969).

Apart from a stricture, another radiological abnormality may be that of a large polypoid filling defect (Figure 30.14). If the bowel has been badly prepared a polypoid lesion has to be differentiated from faeces. Usually faecal masses are multiple and move in position when different films are compared. Occasionally an appendix mass or abscess can produce a soft tissue shadow which can mimic a caecal carcinoma. In the case of an abscess the history and clinical examination strongly suggest the diagnosis, and the finding that the shadow contains a loculus of gas with a fluid level in the erect position clinches it. There is usually distortion of the terminal ileum and pelvic colon. An appendix mass may be more difficult to differentiate, but the history and clinical course invariably resolve the dilemma. Rarely an intussusception can mimic a neoplastic filling defect, but in any case in the adult a polyp or carcinoma (Figure 30.14) is the usual cause of this abnormality.

The radiologist's attention is drawn to a stenosing lesion when the retrograde progress of barium is held up. After some time the barium usually passes through the narrowed lumen and outlines the lesion. Occasionally, despite the absence of clinical obstruction, barium will not pass through the tumour. This suggests that intestinal obstruction is imminent and requires the radiologist to inform the surgical team urgently so that the patient can be admitted as an emergency. Such a radiographic finding also suggests that vigorous preoperative bowel preparation should be avoided.

A large lesion is rarely missed on radiological examination. Sources of difficulty are overlapping coils of bowel which obscure the view, poor bowel preparation and extensive diverticular disease. Overlapping is a particular problem in the sigmoid colon and at the splenic flexure, but oblique views should help to clarify the situation. Smaller lesions are more difficult to visualize and can be difficult to exclude even for an experienced radiologist.

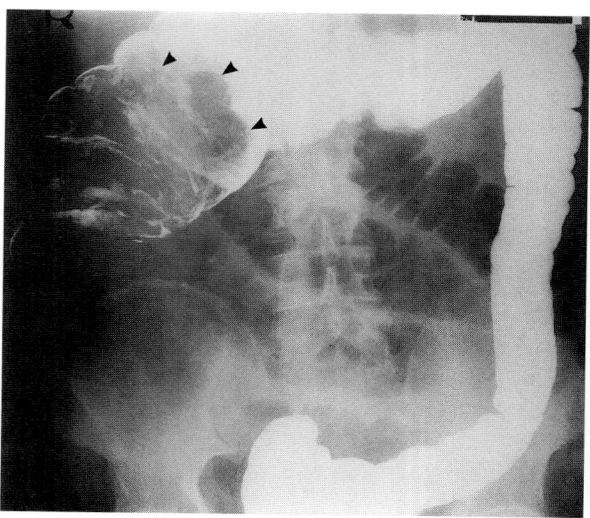

Figure 30.14 Barium enema showing a large polypoid carcinoma of the ascending colon which has intussuscepted into the transverse colon (arrowheads). There is marked gaseous distension of the small bowel indicating small bowel obstruction.

A question frequently raised by radiologists is when is it safe to perform a barium enema examination after a biopsy has been taken? This is of particular importance when dealing with a patient with a rectal carcinoma. The neoplasm has often been biopsied just before a barium enema examination is requested. Some radiologists have in the past refused to do the examination so soon after biopsy on the grounds that there is a risk of barium peritonitis. This problem has been clarified by Harned et al (1982) and Culp and Carlson (1984). Their studies indicate that a delay of at least 7 days is advisable following rectal or colonic biopsy with proctosigmoidoscopic forceps. However, superficial biopsy performed with flexible endoscopic forceps is a safe procedure and no delay is necessary.

Colonoscopy

In many units it is still the policy to perform a double-contrast barium enema if digital examination and proctosigmoidoscopy are normal. If there is still doubt about a possible colonic tumour a colonoscopy will be performed. Even in the most expert hands it is recognized that radiology can be misleading (Brady et al, 1994). Lauer et al (1965) from the Mayo Clinic recorded a false positive rate of 0.8% and a false negative rate of 6.9% in a large series of cases. The errors are usually due to lesions within the caecum or sigmoid colon.

The threshold for performing colonoscopy will clearly depend on the degree of local endoscopic and radiological expertise. It is our view, however, that if a patient requires a barium enema for symptoms suggestive of a neoplasm then colonoscopy is mandatory if the radiological examination is negative. Even if a barium enema shows evidence of diverticular disease but no tumour, there is evidence to suggest that these patients should also have a colonoscopic examination. Thus Boulos et al (1984) reported a series of 65 patients who all had a barium enema followed by colonoscopy. Of the 46 patients in whom the radiograph showed apparently straightforward diverticular disease, eight (17%) had polyps and three (6%) were found to have a carcinoma. These findings have also been confirmed to some extent by Farrands et al (1983) who, although not using full colonoscopy, found that in 84 patients with polyps or cancer submitted to both flexible fibreoptic sigmoidoscopy and double-contrast barium enema there was a miss rate of 25% in the sigmoid colon on barium enema alone, mainly due to coexisting diverticular disease. Obviously the rate of misdiagnosis will vary with individual radiologists. To miss a carcinoma is a tragedy; no matter how skilled the radiologist, errors do occur, and can be avoided if colonoscopy is performed when the barium enema is negative.

There is an increasingly accepted view, to some extent propagated by ourselves (Durdey et al, 1987), that full colonoscopy should be the first investigation following proctosigmoidoscopy, in much the same way that upper gastrointestinal endoscopy has superseded barium meal as the first-line examination for upper gastrointestinal symptoms. Most clinicians believe, however, that this is unwise since they consider that colonoscopy carries significantly more risk than barium enema (Williams et al, 1985). Air leaks are sometimes reported, presumably owing to the high pressure that may be generated by endoscopy, particularly when the tip impinges on the mucosa in a closed loop (Ehrlich et al, 1984; Humphreys et al, 1984). Furthermore a full colonoscopy is not always possible even with modern instrumentation. Even the most skilled operators fail in approximately 10% of patients and the less experienced will naturally be less successful (MacCarty, 1992). Thus Obrecht et al (1984) found that senior residents under supervision managed total endoscopy in only 83% of patients. Despite these misgivings, it is our personal view that as time progresses, more facilities become available and more young surgeons and physicians are trained in colonoscopy, the examination's safety will be improved and its cost-effectiveness will be established. This is not to say that barium enema will become obsolete; indeed each examination will complement the other. In future other less invasive imaging techniques using CT may play a more prominent role.

If the barium enema and subsequent colonoscopy are both negative and the patient still has suspicious symptoms, what should be the next course of action? This will depend to some extent on the confidence that one has in the radiological and colonoscopic examinations. It might be that bowel preparation was poor for one of them, or that the operator was relatively inexperienced. In these circumstances the appropriate procedure should be repeated and the previous fault corrected. If repeat examination is still negative, a CT scan may be helpful (Okoda et al, 1994) and the rest of the gastrointestinal tract should be thoroughly investigated, particularly with a small bowel meal to exclude Crohn's disease of the terminal ileum. If still no cause is found for the patient's symptoms, the surgeon may be forced to perform a laparoscopy with on-table colonoscopy. With the advent of laparoscopy, an exploratory laparotomy is virtually obsolete.

EARLY DIAGNOSIS AND SCREENING

In order to improve the ultimate prognosis of colorectal cancer, it would seem logical to detect it at the earliest possible stage. This involves early diagnosis in symptomatic patients or screening of asymptomatic patients.

There is little question that diagnosis could be speeded up in the case of many patients with symptoms. So often an interval of 6–12 months or even longer elapses between the onset of symptoms and detection of the carcinoma (Holliday and Hardcastle, 1979). There are sceptics, however, who suggest that once symptoms occur the tumour is usually so advanced that its earlier detection and treatment would not change the eventual outcome. It is certainly true that some patients who present with a relatively short history are subsequently found to have widespread metastases. This occurrence has led some experienced colorectal surgeons (Goligher, 1984) to suggest that certain active growths are incurable almost from their onset, their prognosis being dictated by their histopathological characteristics and not by the time of their detection. Although this point of view may have some credence, it fails to take into consideration the now generally accepted adenoma–carcinoma syndrome. There can be little doubt that even if all carcinomas are not derived from adenomas, a certain proportion are. Their evolution takes time, and if the symptoms produced by them or by their precursor adenomas can be agressively investigated their earlier detection and treatment should improve prognosis.

Methods of improving earlier detection in symptomatic patients

There appear to be three areas where there may be a delay in the investigation of symptoms: these can be classified as patient delay, family doctor delay and hospital delay. To accelerate the diagnosis each of these must be dealt with separately.

Patient delay

There are usually two reasons why patients fail to attend their own family medical practitioner when they first develop symptoms. The first is fear, and the second is ignorance as to what their symptoms may represent. It is difficult to determine the percentage of patients who suffer trepidation, and even more difficult to improve their situation. Certainly more widespread public education will counter ignorance, but it is unlikely to have an effect on patients who already suspect the disease they may have but are frightened of doing anything about it.

In a study by Holliday and Hardcastle (1979), 99 of 299 patients with colorectal cancer stated that they were ignorant of the implications of their symptoms and 86 did not regard them as serious. Thirty-one believed their symptoms to be due to a dietary indiscretion alone and only 13 (4.3%) mentioned the possibility of cancer. Thirty per cent of patients with rectal tumours thought they had piles. Education of the public by doctors and the media might improve this state of affairs. Certainly such measures for patients with possible breast cancer led to earlier consultation (Eardley and Wakefield, 1976). Nevertheless, it is necessary to weigh in the balance the risk of inducing neurosis leading to needless consultations, against the benefits of early detection of cancer.

Family doctor delay

The average delay before referral to a surgeon once the patient presents with symptoms to the general practitioner is approximately 14 weeks in the UK (Holliday and Hardcastle, 1979). For patients with a rectal cancer the delay is often attributable to failure to perform a rectal examination. Clearly there is room for improvement and it is the duty of all undergraduate teachers to stress to students that a physical examination is incomplete without a digital rectal examination. Since, however, approximately a third of rectal cancers are not within reach of the examining finger, and since rectal examination cannot diagnose colonic tumours, it is essential that patients with suspicious symptoms be referred to the appropriate specialist even if rectal examination is negative.

Referral to another department is also sometimes the cause of delay. This mistake cannot always be easily rectified as the patient with a colonic carcinoma may complain of symptoms not referrable to the gastrointestinal tract, such as fatigue due to anaemia from a bleeding caecal carcinoma. It is imperative that if this error does occur, the department that initially sees the patient ensures an immediate consultation with the appropriate specialist.

Hospital delay

Once the patient has been referred to hospital, delay may occur in three areas: waiting for an outpatient appointment; outpatient examination and investigation; and delay before inpatient facilities are available for treatment. The total time will depend on local factors. At the Royal London Hospital the average hospital delay is 7–8 weeks and in Birmingham it is similar. The patients are seen within 1.5–2 weeks of referral. There is then a short delay for colonoscopy and biopsy or barium studies if required. A longer delay is usually due to poor-quality barium enemas with false negative reports and the need to perform colonoscopy as well. Once a diagnosis has been made the patient is admitted as soon as possible provided hospital facilities are available. Increasingly colorectal units are offering rapid access 'one stop clinics' to provide a more rapid diagnostic service with investigation where indicated.

Open-access sigmoidoscopy is a method designed to speed referral to hospital. Hence general practitioners, if concerned, can send their patient to have a flexible sigmoidoscopy without formal referral. If the staff in the open-access clinic think the patient merits further investigation despite a negative sigmoidoscopy, this can be arranged. Such an arrangement reduces the waiting time for an outpatient appointment which in certain regions can be considerably longer than the two weeks averaged in our own institutions. Donald et al (1985) demonstrated the value of such an arrangement in Gloucester. During the first three years of its existence their open access clinic saw 1458 patients. A total of 516 abnormalities were found to account for symptoms in 506 patients, a diagnostic rate of 35%. Forty-four benign tumours and 38 malignant tumours were identified. If patients suffered from bleeding and rigid proctosigmoidoscopy showed no cause for it, the patients underwent flexible sigmoidoscopy. Of 41 patients investigated in this way, a cause for the bleeding was found in 32, the most common being a malignant tumour. Other studies (Kalra et al, 1988; Vellacott et al, 1987) have emphasized that the maximum yield from open-access flexible sigmoidoscopy clinics is in patients over 40 years old who present with rectal bleeding and/or diarrhoea. Such data amply illustrate the value of an open-access clinic.

Screening of asymptomatic patients

Screening of colorectal neoplasia may be defined as the efficient application of a relatively simple and inexpensive test to a large number of persons in order to classify asymptomatic people likely or unlikely to have colorectal cancer (Winawer, 1981). Considerable effort is being expended in this direction in the hope that prognosis will be improved by earlier detection and treatment. Before screening of asymptomatic subjects can be accepted, several issues need to be addressed. Is the incidence of the disease sufficiently high to justify the effort and expense of a screening programme? What are the expected benefits and risks? Which are the populations at risk that should be screened? How sensitive and specific are the available screening tests? How sensitive and specific are the diagnostic tests? Is screening cost-effective? What is the patient compliance for screening? (Winawer, 1980).

Incidence

The incidence and mortality from colorectal cancer in northern Europe and the USA is second only to lung cancer. Thus any method that can reduce the incidence of the disease is justified.

Benefits

Although screening is a logical method for improving prognosis, there has up to recently been little evidence that such a programme reduces mortality in the population studied. Most evidence has been circumstantial. Thus it is accepted that the survival rate in patients with localized carcinomas is approximately twice that in patients with non-localized disease, and several groups showed that the 15-year survival rate in asymptomatic patients may be as high as 90% compared with that of patients complaining of symptoms (Hertz, 1980).

Retrospective data from uncontrolled studies were encouraging. Dales et al (1973) reported a study of screening for rectosigmoid cancer which utilized sigmoidoscopy; they demonstrated a small advantage in survival rates for the screened group over the 7-year period of study. A larger and more persuasive study came from the Cancer Detection Centre at the University of Minnesota (Gilbertsen, 1979). Over a 28-year period, 21 150 men and women were examined annually by proctosigmoidoscopy. Twenty-seven adenocarcinomas were found on the first examination and 13 on subsequent examinations. All polyps were removed. The incidence of subsequent cancers was only 15% of the number expected in the same community. Eighty per cent of these cancers were confined to the submucosa. The 5-year survival rate of the 13 patients with adenocarcinomas detected after the start of the survey was 85%. Of the screened patients with a tumour, 22% had metastases compared with 55% of a group of symptomatic patients seen in the University of Minnesota. Of the 27 patients with carcinomas detected at the first examination, 25 were followed up for 5 years. There were 16 survivors (64%), twice the overall 5-year survival rate found in the normal referral practice.

Similar findings were obtained in a collaborative study between the Memorial Sloan Kettering Cancer Center and the Strang Clinic in New York (Sherlock and Winawer, 1977) in which 21 961 subjects were studied by proctosigmoidoscopy and faecal occult blood testing. Most of these subjects were asymptomatic but 7% had minor symptoms. Thirty-two cancers were detected on initial examination and 27 on subsequent examinations. Fifty-nine per cent of the cancers detected on initial examination and 74% of those on subsequent examinations were Dukes' A or B lesions. The 5-year survival rate in this group was 88% and further follow-up indicated that the 15-year survival was maintained at this level.

The optimism of these retrospective studies has now been borne out by the results of several prospective controlled studies which are discussed in more detail later in this chapter. Each of these trials used faecal occult blood as a screening test. Mandel et al (1993) of the Minnesota group were the first to publish mortality figures and found a one-third reduction (from 0.9% to 0.6%) in colorectal cancer mortality in patients randomized to screening. Hardcastle et al (1996) reported the results of the largest occult blood screening programme – over 150 000 subjects followed up for 7.8 years. They found a 15% reduction in colorectal cancer related mortality. Similarly, Kronberg et al (1996) found an 18% reduction in mortality in their screened group.

Despite certain criticisms of these studies which are discussed later, it does now seem beyond doubt that screening can reduce the mortality from colorectal cancer within a population.

The potential benefits of screening must be weighed against the potential risks. The latter depend to a large extent on the method selected for screening. Thus although faecal occult blood testing is without risk, the same is not true for endoscopic methods. There have been no deaths reported in patients who have had surgery as a result of early diagnosis made by positive screening tests (Winawer, 1981).

Patients at risk

Populations at risk from colorectal cancer (Table 30.10) may be classified as average-risk or high-risk groups. The average-risk group may be defined as men and women aged 40 years or over who have no underlying disease, past history or family history that would place them at a higher risk for colorectal cancer. High-risk factors include ulcerative colitis involving the entire colon of more than 7 years' duration, left-sided ulcerative colitis of more than 15 years' duration, a past history of adenoma and colon cancer or female genital cancer (Winawer et al, 1976; Anderson and Romsdahl, 1977; Lynch et al, 1977; Deveroede, 1980). Other individuals who are at high risk are those with a genetic predisposition.

Table 30.10 Patients at risk of colorectal cancer.

Age	Over 40 years in asymptomatic men and women
Associated disease	Ulcerative colitis Crohn's disease Peutz–Jeghers syndrome Familial adenomatous polyposis
Past history	Colon cancer or polyps Female genital or breast cancer
Family history	Juvenile polyps Colon cancer or polyps Familial polyposis syndromes

Adapted from Winawer (1981).

The risk of developing colorectal cancer is closely related to a positive family history (Table 30.11). Much work in recent years has been done to define this group and considerable progress has been made.

At the upper end of the 'genetic risk' spectrum lies the dominantly inherited familial adenomatous polyposis (FAP) syndrome comprising fewer than 0.5% of all colorectal cancers (Mulcahy et al, 1997). Mutations in the adenomatous polyposis coli (APC) gene are responsible for FAP. Hereditary non-polyposis colorectal cancer (HNPCC) accounts for 5–10% of all colorectal cancer (Mulcahy et al, 1997). Whereas FAP results from a mutation of a single gene, HNPCC results from a dominantly inherited alteration within one of four DNA mismatch repair genes that have been identified to date (Table 30.12), which in turn leads to widespread genomic instability. The clinical HNPCC syndrome is defined by the

Table 30.11 Lifetime risk of developing colorectal cancer.

	Risk
More than two first-degree relatives affected (suggests dominant pedigree)	1 in 3
Two first-degree relatives affected	1 in 6
One first-degree relative aged <45 years affected	1 in 10
One first-degree and one second-degree relative affected	1 in 12
One first-degree relative aged >45 years affected	1 in 17
General population	1 in 50

From Lovett (1976).

Table 30.12 Genetic alterations in hereditary and sporadic colorectal cancer.

Condition	Gene location	Percentage of cases showing mutation
Familial adenomatous polyposis	APC (5q21)	100
Hereditary non-polyposis colorectal cancer	hMLH1 (3p21)	30–70
	hMSH2 (2p21–22)	30–50
	hPMS1 (2q31–33)	<10
	hPMS2 (7p22)	<10
Sporadic colorectal cancer	p53 (17p53)	70
	DCC (18q21)	65
	APC (5q21)	60
	K-*ras* (12p12)	50
	NM23 (17q21)	25
	Microsatellite instability	15

From Mulcahy et al (1997).

'Amsterdam criteria' which will require the presence of colorectal cancer in at least three family members spanning two generations with one or more cases diagnosed before 50 years of age (Vasen et al, 1993).

Tumours tend to occur in the right colon and subjects with HNPCC syndrome (Lynch type II) also have increased incidence of gastrointestinal, urinary tract and gynaecological malignancies (Lynch et al, 1993).

Criteria for screening high-risk populations

Screening subjects at very high risk of cancer (i.e. those with a 1 in 2 risk) is the least controversial aspect in the ongoing debate about screening for colorectal cancer. Endoscopic screening, although time-consuming, expensive and potentially hazardous, is justified in these subjects because of its accuracy for neoplasia. Regular sigmoidoscopy starting in adolescence is indicated for subjects in families with FAP. Intermittent gastroduodenoscopy with a side-viewing endoscope is also justified in these cases (Debinski et al, 1995) because of the high incidence of upper gastrointestinal malignancy (Spigelman et al, 1989).

The predominance of right-sided colorectal cancer in subjects with HNPCC syndrome makes total colonoscopy the investigation of choice, and regular examination has been shown to reduce the incidence of cancer in affected families (Jarvinen et al, 1995). The average age at which such patients develop carcinoma seems to be 44 years (Lynch et al, 1993; Jarvinen et al, 1995). Therefore, it is recommended that screening should begin at 25 years, or at least 5 years earlier than the earliest onset of colorectal cancer in the family (Lynch et al, 1993; Vasen et al, 1993). The optimum screening interval is debatable, but colonoscopy every 1–3 years is recommended depending on the presence of neoplasm at the initial endoscopy (Lynch et al, 1993; Vasen et al, 1993; Green et al, 1995; Jarvinen et al, 1995). However, Vasen's group reported a high percentage of cancers presenting between screening procedures (interval cancers) and recommended biennial or annual screening for known gene cancers (Vasen et al, 1995). Because of the risk of extracolonic tumours in HNPCC syndrome, recommendations for screening other systems have recently been suggested by the 1996 international collaborative group on HNPCC (Weber, 1996). These are outlined in Table 30.13.

Screening of other subjects who do not belong to FAP or HNPCC families, yet who have a high genetic risk of developing cancer, is controversial. The data are also sparse. If detection of early cancer and polyps was the only positive screening point, data from small family cancer studies would tentatively support only a policy of regular colonoscopic screening in subjects with a lifetime risk of 1 in 2 (Houlston et al, 1990; Luchtefeld et al, 1991; Carpenter et al, 1995). However, psychological factors come into play. Few experts would deny screening to subjects with two or more first-degree relatives with colorectal cancer. The problem arises in those with one first-degree relative affected. Euchs et al (1994) calculated that subjects with one affected family member had a relative risk of 1.7 times greater than those with a negative family history and suggested recommending that such individuals should undergo colonoscopic screening from the age of 40 years (Burt et al, 1992), especially if the affected family member was under 55 years old at diagnosis (Levin and Murphy, 1992). If such recommendations are to be adopted, this will result in a huge burden for endoscopic services, and it remains to be seen whether such advice will be cost-effective.

The future of screening these high-risk groups is likely to involve genetic testing. Since FAP and HNPCC are associated with germline mutations, it is possible to determine the carrier status of relatives. This will therefore allow those individuals without mutations to be reassessed while concentrating colonoscopic screening on those family members who carry the mutant genes.

Table 30.13 Recommended guidelines for screening subjects with hereditary non-polyposis colorectal cancer syndrome.

Cancer site	*Screening procedure*	*Age at initial screen* (years)	*Interval between screenings* (years)
Colorectal	Colonoscopy	20–25	2
Endometrial or ovarian	Gynaecological exam Transvaginal sonography Measurement of serum marker CA-125	30–35	1–2
Stomach*	Gastroscopy	30–35	1–2
Urinary tract	Sonography Urinary cytology	30–35	1–2

* Only in families at high risk of these cancers.
From Mulcahy et al (1997).

Screening tests for populations at average risk

The ideal screening test should be one that is sensitive enough to detect all the cancers and premalignant tumours without a high false positive rate and with no false negative rate – i.e. high specificity (Farrands and Britton, 1985). The following have all been used as screening tests in asymptomatic patients who were at average risk.

- digital examination of the rectum
- rigid proctosigmoidoscopy
- flexible fibreoptic sigmoidoscopy
- barium enema examination
- tumour markers
- faecal occult blood tests.

Digital examination and rigid proctosigmoidoscopy

Digital rectal examination and rigid proctosigmoidoscopy were used in the Austrian national screening programme for early diagnosis of colorectal cancer. In 20 000 patients studied prospectively, 312 tumours were eventually diagnosed but only 75 (24%) were picked up by the screening methods (Weiss et al, 1977). Other groups claim greater success: thus in patients over 40 years old the detection rate of invasive cancer was 0.12% at the Mayo Clinic (Moertel et al, 1966), 0.13% at the Minnesota Cancer Detection Center (Gilbertsen and Nelms, 1978), and 0.12% at the Strang Institute (Sherlock and Winawer, 1977). The frequency of detection of polyps was much higher, ranging from 3.1% to 12.3%. These studies, however, fail to state the number of missed tumours, and since only 30–40% of all colorectal tumours occur within 25 cm of the anus a substantial proportion must be missed no matter how accurately rigid sigmoidoscopy is carried out. In addition the method is not without risk. Gilbertsen (1974) reported five perforations in 103 000 examinations, and although this is a very small incidence such an occurrence is a serious cause of morbidity in an asymptomatic patient. The cost in both time and money is also excessive. Thus Hertz et al (1960) detected only 0.22% of cancers or one in every 450 examinations, and at the most only six patients were seen per hour.

Flexible sigmoidoscopy

Fibreoptic sigmoidoscopy is now superseding the rigid instrument as a screening device. It has a greater yield, which Vellacott et al (1982) estimated to be approximately three times that of the rigid instrument. Lipshutz et al (1979) screened 200 asymptomatic patients over the age of 40 years with the flexible instrument, and found 53 polyps in 39 patients; 22 of these lesions were greater than 0.5 cm diameter, and more than half were beyond the reach of the conventional rigid sigmoidoscope. Case–control studies show that screening sigmoidoscopy and polypectomy reduces colorectal cancer incidence and mortality due to distal disease in average-risk populations (Aitkin et al, 1992; Newcomb et al, 1992; Selby et al, 1992; Shapiro et al, 1992). The American Cancer Society recommend sigmoidoscopy every 3–5 years for people at average risk and a negative initial examination. However, Rex et al (1994) found no cancers or large (>1 cm) or dysplastic polyps in any patient examined a mean of 3–4 years after a normal flexible sigmoidoscopy, suggesting a longer screening interval is more appropriate.

The disadvantages of the flexible instrument from the screening point of view are that it needs trained staff to perform the examination, and it causes discomfort to the patients, who need to come to hospital for the investigation and usually require a phosphate enema. Despite these potential drawbacks, Atkin et al (1992) have proposed screening by a single flexible sigmoidoscopy between the ages of 55 and 60 years. Their rationale is that the sequence of changes from polyp to cancer is a slow and orderly process taking perhaps 10–25 years to complete. Since colorectal cancer is often diagnosed in the seventh decade, sigmoidoscopy of people in their late 50s would be expected to identify pathologically early lesions. In addition, sigmoidoscopic screening might also indirectly identify a substantial number of proximal neoplasms because large or villiform polyps in the distal large bowel serve as markers of susceptibility for proximal disease (Atkin et al, 1992). Subsequent colonoscopic screening of this relatively small group of patients (estimated at 3–5%) with distal adenomas might be expected to identify up to a third of proximal adenomas or carcinomas. A randomized controlled trial has commenced in the UK to determine if once-only flexible sigmoidoscopy is of benefit in screening a population. Initial data suggested that it is feasible and acceptable to patients (Atkin et al, 1996).

Barium enema

Although barium enema (and even colonoscopy) could theoretically be used for screening asymptomatic patients, the workload, expense and discomfort for the patient make them inappropriate examinations.

Tumour markers

Various serum tumour markers have been sought in an attempt to find a simple screening test for colorectal cancer. Most work has concentrated on the value of serum carcinoembryonic antigen (CEA), but the optimism expressed initially has not been fulfilled. The antigen is non-specific and raised levels have been found in the sera of patients with tumours in a wide range of sites such as lung, stomach or larynx (Bordes et al, 1973), as well as in patients with benign and inflammatory disorders such as ulcerative colitis, Crohn's disease and diverticular disease (Booth et al, 1973). This lack of specificity suggests that serum CEA concentration would be useless as a screening test, and this has been confirmed by two large studies (Costanza et al, 1974; Hansen et al, 1974).

Sialyltransferase in the plasma has been studied as a tumour marker. Although this may be elevated in patients with advanced disease, it is rarely raised in patients with an early lesion. Henderson and Kessel (1977) found that plasma sialyltransferase levels were raised in 18 of 20 patients with metastatic disease but in only 27 of 41 patients with early disease. Similar findings were obtained when galactosyltransferase II (an isoenzyme of galactosyltransferase) was studied as a potential marker for screening (Podolsky et al, 1978).

Faecal occult blood tests

All the tests described above have their defects. A more practical method seems to be the detection of faecal occult blood based on the assumption that polyps and cancers bleed intermittently, and during the last 20 years considerable interest has been shown in screening using this technique.

Van Deen first detected the presence of blood in the faeces in 1864 (Irons and Kirsner, 1965) using gum guaiac as an indicator. The method was modified by Weber in 1893, and the term 'occult bleeding' was first used by Boas in 1901 in connection with the diagnosis of carcinoma of the gastrointestinal tract.

Early work in this field involved using Haemostat (orthotoludine), benzidine and guaiac solutions to detect occult blood. The tests were usually performed on a single stool specimen brought in by the patient who was taking an uncontrolled diet. These tests were abandoned since they proved unreliable, owing to a high percentage of false negative and false positive results (Winawer, 1976). A resurgence in interest occurred in the mid-1960s when Greegor (1967) used guaiac-impregnated slides with a stabilized reagent designed for his patients to use at home; the slides were mailed back to his office. He showed that it was possible to detect carcinomas among asymptomatic patients at risk with reasonable accuracy when they were placed on a high-roughage, meat-free diet, and six smears were obtained. These initial observations were followed by similar studies using the same Haemoccult method in Hawaii by Glober and Pesco (Winawer, 1980), in the USA by Hastings (1974) and by Miller and Knight (1977), and in Germany by Fruhmorgen and Demling (1978) and by Ganauck et al (1984). All of these studies suggested that the test may be useful as a screening method in colorectal cancer. It is not very sensitive, so cancers will be missed if the test is not repeated; but Haemoccult is very specific, so investigations based on a positive test will provide a reasonably high yield of pathology.

Since that time the literature on this subject has become extensive and numerous variations of the test preparation have been described. However, they are all based on the same chemical reactions: the oxidation of a phenolic compound to a quinone structure which in turn changes colour by an intermolecular reaction. Hydrogen peroxide facilitates the oxidation process which is catalysed by a number of naturally occurring peroxidases and catalases including haemoglobin. In the Haemoccult test, which is still the most popular and best studied, gum guaiac is impregnated in a test paper and hydrogen peroxide is provided in a developer solution. The resultant phenolic oxidation of guaiac in the presence of blood yields a blue colour (Irons and Kirsner, 1965; Thornton and Illingworth, 1955). Chemical alteration of haemoglobin as it passes through the gastrointestinal tract can diminish its peroxidase-like activity and render stools negative (Huntsman and Liddell, 1961; Irons and Kirsner, 1965; Burton et al, 1976); this is accelerated by pancreatic juice and trypsin (Bramkamp, 1939; Goulston, 1980). As a consequence, upper gastrointestinal bleeding is less likely to be detected than colonic bleeding, so it decreases the number of positive results from other sources.

Each Haemoccult II slide (SmithKline Diagnostics, Sunningvale, CA, USA) contains two windows of guaiac-impregnated paper, on which the patient smears a small amount of stool with a supplied applicator. This is usually repeated with two subsequent bowel motions, then the three-slide package is returned to the laboratory. Even a single reaction among the six smears is termed a positive test on that patient and further investigation is advised.

Numerous other commercial tests using guaiac are available. They include Faecatest (Labsystem, Oy, Helsinki, Finland), Quick-Cult (Laboratory Diagnostics, Morganville, NJ, USA), FeCult (Gamma Diagnostics, Houston, TX, USA) and Haemoscreen (E. Merck Diagnostica, Darmstadt, Germany). Others – such as Haematest (Miles Labs, Elkhardt, IN, USA) – are based on either orthotolidine or a benzidine derivative (e.g. Hemo-Fec from Med-Kjemi A/s Hon, Norway).

Despite the value of many of the newer agents there is still a problem with their specificity and sensitivity. As a consequence the search for a better technique continues.

A method which depends on electrostatic binding of haemoglobin to a filter has been studied by Graham et al (1984). The faecal filtrate is bound electrostatically to a filter and then washed free of interfering substances. The method is six times more sensitive than Haemoccult but it requires an incubation period and several filtration and washing stages, and thereby loses the simplicity of chemical card tests.

Barrows et al (1978) developed an immunochemical technique for occult blood detection. It was said to be specific for human haemoglobin and therefore was not influenced by foodstuffs, animal haemoglobin, drugs, etc. The authors adapted the technique to a relatively simple filter paper (punch disc) suitable for clinical screening. Immunochemical methods are far more specific than chemical techniques and hence dietary and chemical restrictions for the test are not required; also, the smear remains stable for 30 days. The disadvantages include a 24–48 hour delay between receiving and interpreting the test, and greater technical complexity and cost compared with other available tests. Nevertheless, further validation and clinical testing are clearly required.

Sensitivity and clinical findings of available tests

The guaiac slides are the only type to have been tested extensively. Haemoccult, the most widely used test, has been shown to be positive in 50–60% of patients with proven malignancy (Ribet et al, 1980; Songster et al, 1980; Doran and Hardcastle, 1982; Macrae and St John, 1982; Crowley et al, 1983). There are several reasons for this high *false negative* rate.

Bleeding needs to take place at a rate exceeding 20 mL per day if a Haemoccult test is to be reliably positive (Morris et al, 1976; Stroehlein et al, 1976; Heinrich and Icagic, 1980; Doran and Hardcastle, 1982). Since normal blood loss from the gastrointestinal tract (Riches et al, 1957; Cameron, 1960; Herzog et al, 1982) is about 0.5–2.0 mL per day, losses up to ten times normal may be missed. A rarer technical failure may result from ingestion of vitamin C, since this can inhibit the guaiac reaction (Jaffe et al, 1975; Garrick et al, 1977).

Additionally, tumours do not always bleed. Doran and Hardcastle (1982) documented the large daily fluctuations in bleeding rates from tumours in individual patients. These rates varied between zero and 75 mL per 24 h, a finding corroborated by Macrae and St John (1982). Polyps bleed even less (Herzog et al, 1982; Macrae and St John, 1982) and some authors who have performed colonoscopic studies (Griffith et al, 1981; Crowley et al, 1983) suggest that only ulcerated neoplasms bleed.

Another factor that may account for false negative results is that occult blood is not uniformly distributed in faeces (Rosenfield et al, 1979). Small stool samples can therefore test negative even though blood is readily demonstrable in other portions.

To reduce the number of false negative results, Greegor (1967) advised taking six Haemoccult smears from each subject, representing two separate portions of three consecutive bowel motions, and this regimen is the one now generally accepted.

The *false positive* rate seems to be between 2% and 5% (Simon, 1985) and arises from several causes. The test detects haemoglobin in the stool from any source, whether endogenous (e.g. ulcers, gastritis or haemorrhoids) or exogenous (e.g. meat in the diet). Moreover, certain common foods containing the enzymes peroxidase and catalase can produce false positive results: these include red and white meats, fish, fresh fruit and uncooked vegetables (Thornton and Illingworth, 1955; Illingworth, 1965; Irons and Kirsner, 1965). It is for this reason that Greegor (1967) advised that screened populations should be on a meat-free diet. Although some investigators (Winawer, 1980; Hardcastle, 1987) have adhered to this advice, others have not (Million et al, 1982; Siba, 1983) and this makes comparison of clinical studies difficult. Drugs may also cause problems. Thus iron has been claimed to be a cause of false positive results (Lifton and Kreiser, 1982). Since aspirin and non-steroidal anti-inflammatory agents are well-known mucosal irritants, patients should be advised to stop taking these compounds prior to testing. Although H_2 antagonists such as cimetidine may produce false positive Haemoccult reactions in gastric aspirates (Norfleet et al, 1980; Hauser et al, 1981), this does not appear to be the case in stool specimens (Herzog and Holtermuller, 1981; Norfleet and Rhodes, 1982).

The reported screening studies using Haemoccult blood tests fall into two main categories: uncontrolled and controlled studies. Numerous uncontrolled studies have been described and the results of some selected ones are summarized in Table 30.14. Several points emerge.

The size of the populations screened varied enormously. Compliance was also variable, and only 15–30% of subjects returned their slides. Different dietary advice was given to different groups. The overall positive rate was 2–6% of individuals tested. The predictive value of a positive test for colorectal cancer was only about 5%. Benign colonic polyps were detected in almost all studies; however, the predictive value for the detection of polyps was less than 20%. Most of the positive results were associated with trivial pathology. Overall, most screening programmes revealed colorectal cancer in 0.03–0.2% of all persons initially enrolled (i.e. 3–20 persons of every 100 000 entered). Many authors reported that the detected tumours tended to have an earlier Dukes' staging than might have been expected. However, these uncontrolled studies are liable to several biases which may produce a misleading picture of the efficacy of faecal occult blood testing when used for screening purposes:

- *Lead-time bias* may cause inaccurate measurement of the increase in survival in screen-detected cases. In a patient in whom the time of death due to bowel cancer is not altered by screen-prompted treatment, but in whom treatment was performed early owing to screen detection, the increased period between treatment and death gives a false impression of length of survival.
- *Length bias* refers to the phenomenon of detection of relatively less aggressive tumours by a single screening effort in a population. Individuals in whom the disease is aggressive are less likely to be available for screening compared with those in whom less aggressive disease results in longer survival and hence greater likelihood of being screened. An accumulation of longer survivors in the screened group gives a false impression of improved survival as a result of screening.
- *Selection bias*, in which a population selects itself to be screened, causes screening results to be based on a group of patients who are more health-conscious and motivated to help themselves. This effect has been shown to produce an outcome better than could be expected in the population as a whole.

The only way to minimize the above biases and to obtain some indication of the effect on mortality that might be achieved by mass screening is the use of randomized controlled trials. Such studies have been running over the last two decades and some of these have now been reported. They are:

- in the USA, the University of Minnesota programme set up by Gilbertsen and associates (Gilbertsen, 1979; Gilbertsen et al, 1980a,b; Nivatvongs et al, 1982) and the Sloan Kettering programme under the direction of Winawer and his colleagues (Winawer, 1979, 1980, 1983; Winawer et al, 1977, 1980a,b, 1982)
- in the UK, the Nottingham study directed by Hardcastle (Hardcastle et al, 1986; Hardcastle, 1990)
- in Denmark, the Funen study led by Kronborg (Kronborg et al, 1987, 1989)
- in Sweden, the Goteborg study (Kewenter et al, 1994).

The Minnesotan study involved 46 551 subjects aged over 50 years randomized into one control

Table 30.14 Selected uncontrolled studies of faecal occult blood screening.

Reference	*No. enrolled*	*No. tested (%)*	*Minimum age (yr)*	*Meat-free diet*	*No. of tests*	*No. positive (%)*	*No. of cancers/polyps*	*Predictive values cancers/polyps (%)*	*Enrolled with cancer (%)*
Greegor (1967)	—	278 (—)	'most' 40	Yes	6	24 (8.5)	2/3	8/14	0.72
Hastings (1974)	3450	2625 (76)	None	Yes	3	159 (6.1)	5/—	3/—	0.14
Miller and Knight (1977)	2332	2278 (98)	20	No	3	64 (2.7)	1/7	2/11	0.04
Goodman (1977)	2500	1749 (70)	35	Yes	3	9 (0.5)	—/—	—/—	0
Helfrich et al (1977)	—	8930 (—)	18	No	—	157 (1.8)	3/2	2/1	0.03
Fruhmorgen and Demling (1978)	6007	5016 (84)	40	Yes	3	136 (2.7)	13/83	10/61	0.22
Heeb and Ahlvin (1978)	5740	3956 (69)	—	Yes	3	79 (2.0)	5/5	6/6	0.09
Elwood et al (1978)	11 115	1690 (15)	55	Yes	3	58 (3.4)	2/—	3/—	0.02
Bralow and Kopel (1979)	3798	3008 (79)	40	Yes	—	329 (10.9)	7/11	2/3	0.18
Winchester et al (1980)	54 101	14 074 (26)	—	Yes	6	617 (4.4)	30/40	5/7	0.06
Kurnick et al (1980)	—	5420 (—)	—	No	4	120 (2.2)	9/—	8/—	0.17
Gnauck (1980)	—	16 100 (—)	45	—	—	531 (3.3)	75/106	14/20	0.47
Schwartz et al (1980)	—	3 480 000 (—)	30	—	—	38 030 (1.1) 4262	332/—	8/—	0.01
Larkin (1980)	5840	5565 (95)	—	Yes	3	780 (14.0)	4/6	1/1	0.07
Chambers and Morgan (1980)	2500	1156 (46)	40	No	3	68 (5.9)	3/10	4/15	0.16
Stuart et al (1981)	6574	4498 (68)	None	—	1	234 (5.2)	13/31	6/13	0.20
Farrands et al (1981)	8925	2439 (27)	40	No	3	124 (5.1)	4/8	3/6	0.04
Million et al (1982)	5812	1646 (28)	40	No	6	37 (2.3)	2/5	5/16	0.03
Sontag et al (1983)	13 522	2964 (22)	40	Yes	6	135 (4.6)	14/44	10/33	0.10
Hardcastle et al (1983)	9807	3613 (37)	45	Yes	3	77 (2.1)	12/27	16/35	0.12
Siba (1983)	—	3791 (—)	45	No	6	97 (2.6)	6/18	6/19	0.16
Habba and Doyle (1983)	2143	1628 (76)	40	No	6	37 (2.3)	5/6	14/16	0.23

Modified from Simon (1985).

group and two experimental groups. The latter were tested for occult bleeding every 1 or 2 years respectively using Haemoccult smears. Subjects having at least one positive test underwent sigmoidoscopy and colonoscopy with or without barium enema and upper gastrointestinal tract assessment in selected cases.

The Sloan Kettering study involved approximately 22 000 subjects aged 40 years or more. Unlike the Minnesota study, this programme compared a test group which underwent sigmoidoscopy and occult blood screening with a control group having sigmoidoscopy alone. As in the Minnesota study, test-positive subjects underwent thorough colonic evaluation. Despite these differences the initial results from both studies tended to agree with each other. Thus compliance was approximately 75%. Using rehydration Haemoccult slides the overall positive rate was 3.5% (Minnesota) and 5.4% (Sloan Kettering). The predictive values of a positive test were 8% and 12% for a carcinoma and 29% and 36% for polyps respectively. In both studies the predictive value of a positive test increased with the patient's age. Most of the detected cancers had a favourable Dukes' stage.

The Minnesota Group were the first to publish mortality figures and found a one-third reduction in colorectal cancer mortality (from 0.9% to 0.6%) in patients randomized to annual screening (Table 30.15) (Mandel et al, 1993). However, the study was criticized because of the high false positive rate. The lack of specificity resulted in almost 40% of annually screened patients undergoing colonoscopy, and it seems reasonable to suggest that the reduction in cancer-related mortality resulted as much from the large number of colonoscopies performed as it did from the occult blood testing *per se* (Lang and Ransohoff, 1994).

The data from Nottingham are just as optimistic as the studies from the USA. This trial commenced in 1984 and finally reported in 1996 (Hardcastle et al, 1986, 1996), but differed from the Minnesota study in several ways. Subjects in the Nottingham study underwent biennial rather than annual occult blood testing. Slides were not rehydrated before testing, and some patients with weakly positive tests underwent immediate retesting to reduce the number of false positive results. Patients aged 45–74 years were identified from family practitioner age/sex registers and were randomly allocated into test and control groups. At completion of the trial, 150 251 individuals had been randomized and it was the largest study of its kind. The test group used the faecal occult blood test as the only screening investigation, and because of the modifications described above the test positivity rate was only 2.1% for initial screening and 1.2% for subsequent screening, while only 4% of subjects required colonoscopic or radiological investigation. Overall, there were 60 fewer deaths relating to colorectal cancer in the test group compared with controls, a 15% reduction in colorectal cancer-related mortality. Although not surprisingly there were a greater proportion of Dukes' A cancers in the screened group (29% versus 11%), the percentage of advanced metastatic Dukes' D cancers was almost identical in the two groups (22% test, 21% control). The reduction in mortality seemed to be due to a shift from regional (Dukes' C) to local (stage A) disease. A negative aspect of the study was the high rate of interval cancers (28%) compared with screen-detected cancers (26%) in the test group. This arose partly because of the relatively low sensitivity of occult blood tests for cancer, but also because the authors considered that only those cancers arising after a negative test were potentially 'missed' lesions even when they were diagnosed more than two years after a negative screening.

The results from Funen (Kronborg et al, 1996) were remarkably similar to those from Nottingham,

Table 30.15 Randomised controlled trials of faecal occult blood testing in populations at average risk.

Study	*Place of study*	*n*	*Positive slides (%)*	*Percentage of stage A cancers*		*Decrease in cancer-related mortality in screened group (%)*
				*Test**	*Control*	
Kewenter et al (1994)	Goteborg, Sweden	68 308	4.7†	26	9	NA
Kronborg et al (1996)	Funen, Denmark	61 933	1.0	22	11	18‡
Mandel et al (1993)	Minnesota, USA	46 551	9.8†	30§	22	33§
Hardcastle et al (1996)	Nottingham, UK	150 251	2.1¶	20	11	15‡

* Includes interval cancers and cancers in non-participants as well as screen-detected cancers. † Most slides rehydrated before testing. ‡ Biennial screening. § Annual screening. ¶ Percentage positive at initial screen (1.2% of subjects positive during later screening) rounds. NA, not available.
From Mulcahy et al (1997).

despite the smaller numbers. A total of 61 933 subjects were randomized; 22% of cancers were Dukes' A in the screened group compared with 11% in the control group, and the proportion of stage D lesions were similar in both groups. Mortality was reduced by 18% in the screened group, again because of a shift from locoregional to local disease (Table 30.15).

The results from Sweden (Kewenter et al, 1994) are similar with regard to detection of earlier tumours, although the mortality rates are not yet known. However, the interim results showed that 36% of screen-detected cancers were Dukes' A tumours compared with 9% of those in controls and 9% were incurable at diagnosis (25% in controls).

Compliance

No screening programme can be successful unless the target population is cooperative. The rate of compliance with faecal occult blood testing varies between 15% and 98% (see Table 30.14). High rates are uncommon and are usually obtained in small, particularly highly motivated groups. The more common situation within the general population is represented by the disappointing results in the large studies of Elwood et al (1978), Sontag et al (1983) and Winchester et al (1980) in which the overall compliance rates were 15%, 22% and 25% respectively. Compliance rates with flexible sigmoidoscopic screening programmes have occasionally been reported to be as high as 70% (Foley et al, 1987). However, in uncontrolled studies levels rarely rise above 30% (Bejes and Marvel, 1992).

The reasons for non-compliance are complex and involve demographic factors such as age, sex and social class as well as individual beliefs and motivations (Halper et al, 1980; Morrow et al, 1982; Dent et al, 1983; Farrands et al, 1984; Hart et al, 1995; Lieberman, 1995). A study of the subjects in the Sloan Kettering programme surprisingly revealed relatively few major differences between those who complied and those who did not (Halper et al, 1980). Farrands et al (1984) in a study in Nottingham made the following observations: those who accepted screening had a more positive attitude towards preventative health care, they were better informed about various illnesses, and were more optimistic and less frightened about cancer. The reasons most commonly volunteered for non-participation were indifference and procrastination. Only 15% of the non-participants said they did not carry out the test because of fear of cancer or worry about what the test might show. There was also a significant difference in compliance between social class I (professional) and social class III (skilled workers). Some individuals also feel that the process of testing faecal specimens is degrading and unacceptable (Hunter et al, 1991).

One of the major problems that many authors have found (Elwood et al, 1978; Farrands et al, 1981; Million et al, 1982; Morrow et al, 1982; Hardcastle et al, 1983; Hardcastle, 1990) is that the elderly are less compliant than middle-aged subjects. This is particularly unfortunate since the very individuals who are most likely to be helped by screening are paradoxically least likely to cooperate.

Another major problem encountered by several groups (Hastings, 1974; Goodman, 1979; Sterchi, 1979; Winchester et al, 1980) is the fact that a proportion of patients who have a positive test refuse to have further investigations. The reason is not always reluctance by the patient; in some cases there is an element of ignorance on the physician's part. Thus Macrae et al (1982) found that fewer than 60% of Australian physicians would advise subjects with a positive occult blood test to have sigmoidoscopy and only 33% would recommend any further investigation. Compliance can be improved considerably if medical consultation precedes the invitation to participate in screening. Thus Faivre (1990) in the Burgundy region of France found that when the doctor explained the importance of screening to individuals 83.1% participated, whereas only 35.5% responded to a postal invitation.

Cost-effectiveness

The issues involved in cost-effectiveness are extremely complex. On the face of it occult blood testing seems relatively cheap. Although the Haemoccult slides cost very little, the bulk of the expense lies in the investigation of false positive results and the massive organization required to run a programme.

It is estimated that faecal occult blood testing and subsequent colonic evaluation of those with positive results would cost the USA at least 1.2 billion dollars a year at 1991 costs (Ransohoff and Lang, 1991) rising to 2.5 billion dollars by the year 2000 (Brown, 1993). Regular sigmoidoscopy starting at 50 years of age is even more expensive than faecal occult blood testing and would increase America's screening costs by over 5 billion dollars a year (Eddy, 1990).

Apart from these obvious financial costs there are hidden costs (Simon, 1985) in terms of patient time and inconvenience, the physical hazard of unnecessary colonic investigations, emotional agony due to fear of malignancy and stress from undergoing complex tests. All of these costs must be weighed against the savings that would accrue from success of the screening programme. Earlier surgical intervention might decrease expenses from treating advanced malignancy, increase a productive life-span, and minimize grief and suffering. As mentioned previously, in the Nottingham study the high proportion of screen-detected Dukes' A lesions resulted in 24% of patients being treated endoscopically rather than by surgical resection. In terms of cost of therapy, treatment of early lesions is likely to be cheaper than treatment of advanced lesions, with fewer days of employment being lost by the patient.

Future developments and conclusions

The results of current trials, particularly those using faecal occult blood testing, are promising. There is little doubt that in a screened population tumours can be detected at an earlier stage and mortality from cancer can be reduced. However, it remains to be seen how cost-effective such screening programmes will be. The answer to this question will determine whether major population screening will be introduced into many countries. The cost-effectiveness of flexible sigmoidoscopic screening would increase if medically qualified endoscopists were replaced by nurse endoscopists. Several studies have shown that nurse practitioners can perform flexible sigmoidoscopy safely and accurately (Marks et al, 1979; Maule, 1994).

The cost-effectiveness of faecal occult blood testing needs to be improved. The sensitivity and specificity of current techniques are relatively low, so some tumours are overlooked and normal subjects are investigated needlessly. Compliance is relatively poor and the organization and cost of investigating false positive tests makes screening a more costly exercise than is generally realized. The introduction of new tests may improve matters. Haemoccult II Sensa (SmithKline Diagnostics) is a modification of the Haemoccult II test, while Haemselect (SmithKline Diagnostics) is an immunoassay for human haemoglobin. Both have been shown to have a higher sensitivity than the standard technique (Lance, 1993; St John et al, 1993; Robinson et al, 1995; Allison et al, 1996). Increased sensitivity without a corresponding loss of specificity might substantially improve the performance of faecal occult blood testing and enhance its cost-effectiveness.

Molecular biological techniques are increasingly being investigated as a means of screening. Sidransky et al (1992) and Smith Raven et al (1995) have isolated K-*ras* mutations in faeces and have suggested that such a technique could be used for screening. The advantage of screening for gene alterations rather than occult blood is that DNA is extremely stable, whereas blood – especially in the right colon – may be degraded by bacteria and result in a false negative result. However, although mutations are highly specific for neoplasia, the range that can be detected at present is too limited for routine use (Sidransky et al, 1992; Smith Raven et al, 1995; Eguchi et al, 1996). Nevertheless, with the rapid development of molecular biology, a non-invasive, sensitive and specific genetic screening test for colorectal cancer may become available in the near future.

REFERENCES

Abrams HL (1950) Skeletal metastases in carcinoma. *Radiology* **55**: 534.

Ackerman LV & Del Regato JA (1970) *Cancer: Diagnosis, Treatment and Prognosis*, 4th edn, p 484. St Louis: CV Mosby.

Adam IJ, Mohamdee MO, Martin IG et al (1994) Role of circumferential margin involvement in the local recurrence of rectal cancer. *Lancet* **344**: 707–711.

Adami H-O, Melrik O, Gustavsson S, Nyren O & Krusems U-B (1983) Colorectal cancer after cholecystectomy: absence of risk increase within 11–14 years. *Gastroenterology* **85**: 859–865.

Atkin WS, Morson BC & Cuzick J (1992) Long-term risk of colorectal cancer after excision of rectosigmoid adenomas. *N Engl J Med* **326**: 658–662.

Atkin WS, Cuzick J, Northover JMA & Whynes DK (1996) Pilot study for a multicentre randomized trial of 'once only' flexible sigmoidoscopy for prevention of bowel cancer. *Gut* **38**: A9.

Alberts DS, Einsphar J, Rees-McGee S et al (1990) Effects of dietary wheat bran fiber on rectal epithelial cell proliferation in patients with resection for colorectal cancers. *J Natl Cancer Inst* **82**: 1280–1285.

Alberts DS, Rees-McGee S, Einsphar J et al (1992) Double-blind placebo-controlled study of wheat bran fiber versus calcium carbonate in patients with resected adenomatous polyps. *Pro Am Assoc Cancer Res* **33**: 207.

Alexander RJT, Jaques BC & Mitchell KG (1993) Laparoscopically assisted colectomy and wound recurrence (letter). *Lancet* **341**: 249–250.

Ali MH, Satti MB & Al-Nafussi A (1984) Multiple benign colonic polypi at the site of ureterosigmoidostomy. *Cancer* **53**: 1006–1010.

Allende HD, Ona FV & Davis HT (1984) Gall bladder disease: risk factor for colorectal carcinoma. *J Clin Gastroenterol* **6**: 51–56.

Allison JE, Tekawa IS, Ransom LJ & Adrian AL (1996) A comparison of fecal occult blood tests for colorectal cancer screening. *N Engl J Med* **334**: 155–159.

Anderson DE & Romsdahl MM (1977) Family history a criterion for selective screening. In Mulvihill JJ, Miller RM & Praumeni JF Jr (eds) *Progress in Cancer Research and Therapy. Genetics of Human Cancer*, Vol. 3, p 235. New York: Raven Press.

Armitage NC & Hardcastle JD (1984) Flexible fibreoptic sigmoidoscopy in an outpatient setting. *Gut* **25**: 562.

Armitage NC, Robins RA, Evans DP et al (1985) The influence of tumour cell DNA abnormalities on survival in colorectal cancer. *Br J Surg* **72**: 828–830.

Armitage NC, Rooney PS, Gifford K-A et al (1995) The effect of calcium supplements on rectal mucosal proliferation. *Br J Cancer* **71**: 186–190.

Armstrong BK & Doll R (1975) Environmental factors and cancer incidence and mortality in different countries with special reference to dietary practices. *Int J Cancer* **15**: 167–172.

Astler VB & Coller FA (1954) The prognostic significance of direct extension of carcinoma of the colon and rectum. *Ann Surg* **139**: 846.

Auvinen A, Isola J, Visakorpi T et al (1994) Overexpression of p53 and long-term survival in colon carcinoma. *Br J Cancer* **70**: 293–296.

Axtell LM & Chiazzi L (1966) Changing relative frequency of cancer of the colon and rectum in the United States. *Cancer* **19**: 750–754.

Bacon HE & Jackson CC (1953) Visceral metastases from carcinoma of the distal colon and rectum. *Surgery (St Louis)* **33**: 495.

Bailar JC (1963) The incidence of independent tumours among uterine cancer patients. *Cancer* **16**: 842–853.

Baker JW, Margetts LH & Schutt RP (1955) The distal and proximal margin of resection in carcinoma of the pelvic colon and rectum. *Ann Surg* **141**: 693–706.

Baker S, Fearon E, Nigro J et al (1989) Chromosome 17 deletions and p53 gene mutations in colorectal carcinomas. *Science* **244**: 217–222.

Baretton GB, Vogt M, Muller C et al (1996) Prognostic significance of p53 expression, chromosome 17 copy number, and DNA-ploidy in non-metastasized colorectal carcinomas (stages IB and II). *Scand J Gastroenterol* **31**: 481–489.

Barillari P, Ramacciato G, De Angelis R et al (1990) Effect of preoperative colonoscopy on the incidence of synchronous and metachronous neoplasms. *Acta Chir Scand* **156**: 163–166.

Barker GM, Radley S, Bain I et al (1994). Biliary bile acid profiles in patients with familial adenomatous polyposis before and after colectomy. *Br J Surg* **81**(3): 441–444.

Barrows GH, Burton RM, Jarrett DD et al (1978) Immunochemical detection of human blood in faeces. *Am J Clin Pathol* **69**: 342–346.

Barsoum AL & Bhavanandan VP (1989) Detection of glycophorin A-like glycoproteins on the surface of cultured human cells. *Int J Biochem* **21**: 635–643.

Barsoum GH, Hendrickse C, Winslet MC et al (1992a) Reduction of mucosal crypt cell proliferation in patients with colorectal adenomatous polyps by dietary calcium supplementation. *Br J Surg* **79**: 481–583.

Barsoum GH, Thompson H, Neoptolemos JP & Keighley MRB (1992b) Dietary calcium does not reduce experimental colorectal carcinogenesis after small bowel resection, despite reducing cellular proliferation. *Gut* **33**: 1515–1520.

Bayerdorffer E, Mannes GA, Ochsenkuhn T, Dirschedl P & Paumgartner G (1994) Variation of serum bile acids in patients with colorectal adenomas during a one-year follow-up. *Digestion* **55**: 121–129.

Bayerdorffer E, Mannes GA, Ochsenkuhn T et al (1995) Unconjugated secondary bile acids in the serum of patients with colorectal adenomas. *Gut* **36**: 268–273.

Beal JM & Cornell GW (1956) A study of the problem of recurrence of carcinoma at the anastomotic site following resection of the colon for carcinoma. *Ann Surg* **143**: 1–7.

Beart RW Jr, Van Heerden JA & Beahrs OH (1978) Evolution in the pathologic staging of carcinoma of the colon. *Surg Gynecol Obstet* **146**: 257.

Bejes C & Marvel MK (1992) Attempting the improbable: offering colorectal cancer screening to all appropriate patients. *Fam Pract Res J* **12**: 83–90.

Beland FA & Kadlubar FF (1985) Formation and persistence of arylamine DNA adducts *in vivo*. *Environ Health Perspect* **62**: 19–30.

Bell SM, Kelly SA, Hoyle JA et al (1991) c-Ki-*ras* gene mutations in dysplasia and carcinomas complicating ulcerative colitis. *Br J Cancer* **64**: 174–178.

Berends FJ, Kazemier G, Bonjer HJ & Lange JF (1994) Subcutaneous metastases after laparoscopic colectomy (letter). *Lancet* **344**: 58.

Berman IR (1995) Laparoscopic colectomy for cancer: some cause for pause (editorial). *Ann Surg Oncol* **2**: 1–2.

Besbeas S & Stearns MW (1978) Osseous metastases from carcinomas of the colon and rectum. *Dis Colon Rectum* **21**: 266–268.

Bjelke E (1973) Epidemiologic studies of cancer of the stomach, colon and rectum with special emphasis on the role of diets. Vols I–IV. Thesis, University of Minnesota.

Black WA & Waugh JM (1948) The intramural extension of carcinoma of the descending colon, sigmoid and rectosigmoid: a pathologic study. *Surg Cynecol Obstet* **87**: 457–464.

Black WC & Ackerman LV (1965) Carcinoma of the large intestine as a late complication of pelvic radiotherapy. *Clin Radiol* **16**: 278–281.

Blanco D, Ross RK, Paganini-Hill A & Henerson BE (1984) Cholecystectomy and colonic cancer. *Dis Colon Rectum* **27**: 290–292.

Blot WJ, Fraumeni JF, Stone BJ & McKay FW (1976) Geographic patterns of large bowel cancer in the United States. *J Natl Cancer Inst* **57**: 1225.

Boley SJ, Schwartz S, Lash J & Sternhill V (1963) Reversible vascular occlusions of the colon. *Surg Gynecol Obstet* **116**: 53.

Booth SN, King JPG, Leonard JC & Dykes PW (1973) Serum carcinoembryonic antigen in clinical disorders. *Gut* **14**: 704–709.

Bordes M, Michiels R & Martin F (1973) Detection by immunofluorescence of carcinoembryonic antigen in colonic carcinoma, other malignant or benign tumours, and non-cancerous tissues. *Digestion* **9**: 106–115.

Boring CC, Squires TS & Tong T (1992) Cancer statistics. *CA Cancer J Clin* 42: 19–38.

Bostick RM, Potter JD, Fosdick L et al (1993) Calcium and colorectal epithelial cell proliferation: a preliminary randomized, double-blinded placebo-controlled clinical trial. *J Natl Cancer Inst* **85**: 132–141.

Botsford TW, Aliopoulios MA & Curtis LE (1965) Results of treatment of colorectal cancer at the Peter Brent Brigham Hospital. *Am J Surg* **109**: 566–567.

Boulez J & Herriot E (1994) Multicentric analysis of laparoscopic colorectal surgery in FDCL group: 274 cases. *Br J Surg* **81**: 527.

Boulos PB, Karamanolis DG, Salmon PR & Clarke CG (1984) Is colonoscopy necessary in diverticular disease? *Lancet* **i**: 95–96.

Bouvy ND, Marquet RL, Jeekel J et al (1996) Impact of gas (less) laparoscopy and laparotomy on peritoneal tumor growth and abdominal wall metastases. *Surg Endosc* **10**: 551.

Brady AP, Stevenson GW & Stevenson I (1994) Colorectal cancer overlooked at barium enema examination and colonoscopy: a continuing perceptual problem. *Radiology* **192**: 373–378.

Bralow SP & Kopel J (1979) Hemoccult screening for colorectal cancer: an impact study on Sarasola, Florida. *J Fla Med Assoc* **66**: 915–919.

Bramkamp RC (1939) Benzidine reaction: some observations relating to its clinical application. *J Lab Clin Med* **14**: 1987–1991.

Breslow NE & Enstrom JE (1974) Geographic correlations between cancer mortality rates and alcohol–tobacco consumption in the United States. *J Natl Cancer Inst* **53**: 631–639.

Broders AC (1925) The grading of carcinoma. *Minn Med* **8**: 726.

Brown ML (1993) Screening for colorectal cancer. *N Engl J Med* **329**: 1352–1353.

Buirge RE (1941) Carcinoma of the large intestine: review of 416 autopsy records. *Arch Surg* **42**: 801.

Bulow S (1980) Colorectal cancer in patients less than 40 years of age in Denmark 1943–1967. *Dis Colon Rectum* **23**: 327–336.

Bundred NJ, Whitfield BCS, Stanton E et al (1985) Gastric surgery and the risk of subsequent colorectal cancer. *Br J Surg* **72**: 618–619.

Burkitt DP (1971) Epidemiology of cancer of the colon and rectum. *Cancer* **28**: 3–13.

Burt RW, Bishop DT, Cannon-Albright L et al (1992) Hereditary aspects of colorectal cancer. *Cancer* **70**: 1296–1299.

Burton RM, Landreth KS, Barrows GH et al (1976) Appearance, properties and origin of altered human haemoglobin in faeces. *Lab Invest* **35**: 111–115.

Cady B, Pearson AV, Manson DO et al (1974) Changing patterns of colorectal carcinoma. *Cancer* **33**: 422.

Cameron AD (1960) Gastrointestinal blood loss measured by radioactive chromium. *Gut* **1**: 177–182.

Campo E, de la Calle-Martin O, Miquel R et al (1991) Loss of heterozygosity of p53 gene and p53 protein expression in human colorectal carcinomas. *Cancer Res* **51**: 4436–4442.

Carpenter S, Broughton M & Marks CG (1995) A screening clinic for relatives of patients with colorectal cancer in a district general hospital. *Gut* **36**: 90–92.

Castro CE (1987) Nutrient effects on DNA and chromatin structure. *Annual Rev Nutr* **7**: 407–421.

Castro EB, Rowen PP & Quan SAQ (1973) Carcinoma of large intestine in patients irradiated for carcinoma of cervix and uterus. *Surg Gynecol Obstet* **31**: 45–52.

Cats A, Kleibeuker JH, van der Meer R et al (1995) Randomized double-blinded placebo-controlled intervention study with supplemental calcium in families with hereditary nonpolyposis colorectal cancer. *J Natl Cancer Inst* **87**: 598–603.

Cawkwell L, Lewis FA & Quirke P (1994) Frequency of allele loss of DCC, p53, Rb1, WT1, NF1, NM23 and APC/MCC in colorectal cancer assayed by fluorescent multiplex polymerase chain reaction. *Br J Cancer* **70**: 813–818.

Caygill CPJ, Hill MJ, Hall CN, Kirkham JS & Northfield TC (1987) Increased risk of cancer at multiple sites after gastric surgery for peptic ulcer. *Gut* **28**: 924–928.

Caygill CPJ, Hill MJ, Kirkham JS & Northfield TC (1988) Mortality from colorectal and breast cancer in gastric surgery patients. *Int J Colorectal Dis* **74**: 1066.

Cedermark BJ, Shultz SS, Bakshi S et al (1977) The value of liver scan in the follow-up study of patients with adenocarcinoma of the colon and rectum. *Surg Gynecol Obstet* **144**: 745.

Chambers KJ & Morgan BP (1980) Colorectal cancer and Hemoccult. *Aust NZ J Surg* **50**: 464–467.

Chapman MA, Hardcastle JD & Armitage NC (1995) Five-year prospective study of DNA tumor ploidy and colorectal cancer survival. *Cancer* **76**: 383–387.

Chapuis PH, Newland RC, Jennifer C et al (1981) The distribution of colorectal carcinoma and the relationship of tumour site to the survival of patients following resection. *Aust NZ J Surg* **51**: 127.

Charneau J, D'Aubigny N, Burtin P et al (1990) Rectal micropolyps after total colectomy for familial polyposis: effectiveness of sulindac therapy. *Gastroenterol Clin Biol* **14**: 153–157.

Cheng MC, Chuang CY, Chan PY et al (1980) Evolution of colorectal cancer in schistosomiasis: transitional mucosal changes adjacent to larger intestinal carcinoma in colectomy specimens. *Cancer* **46**: 1661–1670.

Cheng MC, Chuang CY, Wung FP et al (1981) Colorectal cancer and schistosomiasis. *Lancet* **ii**: 971–973.

Chu KC, Tarone RE, Chow WH, Hankey BF & Ries LA (1994) Temporal patterns in colorectal cancer incidence, survival, and mortality from 1950 through 1990. *J Natl Cancer Inst* **86**: 997–1006.

Cipolla R & Garcia RI (1984) Colonic polyps and adenocarcinoma complicating ureterosigmoidostomy: report of a case. *Am J Gastroenterol* **79**: 453–457.

Cirocco WC, Schwartzman A & Golub RW (1994) Abdominal wall recurrence after laparoscopic colectomy for colon cancer. *Surgery* **116**: 842–846.

Cleave (1974) *The Saccharine Disease*, pp 28–43. Bristol: Wright.

Clemmesen J (1977) Statistical studies in the aetiology of malignant neoplasms. V: Trends and risks in Denmark 1942–72. *Acta Pathol Microbiol Immunol Scand Suppl:* 261.

Clogg HE (1908) Cancer of the colon: a study of 22 cases. *Lancet* **ii**: 1007.

Coffey RJ & Cardenas F (1964) Cancer of the bowel in the young adult. *Dis Colon Rectum* **7**: 491–492.

Cohen SM & Wexner SM (1994) Laparoscopic colorectal surgery: are we being honest with our patients? *Dis Colon Rectum* **37**: 858–861.

Cohn I Jr, Floyd E & Atik M (1963) Control of tumour implantation during operations on the colon. *Ann Surg* **157**: 825.

Cohn KH, Wang F, Desoto-Lapaix F et al (1991) Association of nm23-H1 allelic deletions with distant metastases in colorectal carcinoma. *Lancet* **338**: 722–724.

Colacchio TA & Memoli VA (1986) Chemoprevention of colorectal neoplasms: ascorbic acid and beta-carotene. *Arch Surg* **121**: 1421–1424.

Colacchio TA, Memoli VA & Hildebrandt L (1989) Antioxidants versus carotenoids: inhibitors or promoters of experimental colorectal cancers. *Arch Surg* **124**: 217–221.

Cole PP (1913) The intramural spread of rectal carcinoma. *BMJ* **1**: 431–433.

Cole WH, Packard D & Southwick HW (1954) Carcinoma of the colon with special reference to prevention of recurrence. *JAMA* **155**: 1549.

Coller FA, Kay EB & Maclntyre RS (1940) Regional lymphatic metastases of carcinoma of the rectum. *Surgery (St Louis)* **8**: 294.

Coller FA, Kay AB & Maclntyre RS (1941) Regional lymphatic metastases of carcinoma of the colon. *Ann Surg* **114**: 156.

Collins VP (1962) Time of occurrence of pulmonary metastases from carcinoma of colon and rectum. *Cancer* **15**: 387–395.

Connell JE Jr & Rottino A (1949) Retrograde spread of carcinoma of the rectum and rectosigmoid. *Arch Surg* **59**: 807–813.

Cook MG & McNamara P (1980) Effect of dietary vitamin E on dimethylhydrazine-induced colonic tumors in mice. *Cancer Res* **40**: 1329–1331.

Copeland EM, Millar LD & Jones RS (1968) Prognostic factors in carcinoma of the colon and rectum. *Am J Surg* **116**: 875–881.

Corman ML (1984) *Colon and Rectal Surgery*. London: Lippincott.

Costanza ME, Das S, Nathanson L, Rale A & Schwartz RS (1974) Carcinoembryonic antigen: report of a screening study. *Cancer* **33**: 583–590.

Court Brown WM & Doll R (1965) Mortality from cancer and other causes after radiotherapy for ankylosing spondylitis. *BMJ* **ii**: 1327–1332.

CRC (Cancer Research Campaign) (1993) *Facts on Cancer*. Fact Sheets 18.1–18.4.

Crowley MI, Freeman LD, Mottet MD et al (1983) Sensitivity of guaiac impregnated cards for the detection of colorectal neoplasia. *J Clin Gastroenterol* **5**: 127–130.

Crowther JS, Drasar BJ, Hill MJ et al (1976) Faecal steroids and bacteria and large bowel cancer in Hong Kong by socioeconomic groups. *Br J Cancer* **34**: 191–196.

Cruse JP, Lewin MR & Clark CC (1978) Failure of bran to protect against experimental colon cancer in rats. *Lancet* **ii**: 1278–1279.

Culp CE & Carlson HC (1984) Is there a safe interval between diagnostic invasive procedure and the barium enema study of the colorectum? *Gastrointest Radiol* **9**: 69–72.

Cummack DH (1969) *Gastrointestinal X-ray Diagnosis: A Descriptive Atlas*. Edinburgh: Livingstone.

Dales LG, Friedman GD, Ramcharan S et al (1973) Multiphase check-up evaluation study: outpatient clinic utilisation, hospitalisation and mortality experience after 7 years. *Prev Med* **2**: 211.

Dales LG, Friedman GD, Ury HK et al (1978) A case–control study of relationships of diet and other traits to colorectal cancer in American Blacks. *Am J Epidemiol* **109**: 132–144.

Davies RJ & Daly JM (1984) Potassium depletion and malignant transformation of villous adenomas of the colon and rectum. *Cancer* **53**: 1260–1264.

Davis NC & Newland RC (1982) The reporting of colorectal cancer: the Australian clinicopathological staging system. *Aust NZ J Surg* **52**: 395.

De Cosse JJ, Miller HH & Lesser ML (1989) Effect of wheat fiber and vitamins C and E on rectal polyps in patients with familial adenomatous polyposis. *J Natl Cancer Inst* **81**: 1290–1297.

de Mascarel A, Loindre JM, de Mascarel I et al (1981) The prognostic significance of specific histologic features of carcinoma of the colon and rectum. *Surg Gynecol Obstet* **153**: 511.

Debinski HS, Spigelman AD, Hatfield A, Williams CB & Phillips RKS (1995) Upper intestinal surveillance in familial adenomatous polyposis. *Eur J Cancer* **31A**: 1149–1153.

Deddish MR & Stearns MW (1961) Anterior resection for carcinoma of the rectum and rectosigmoid area. *Ann Surg* **154**: 961–966.

Dent OF, Bartrop R, Goulston KJ et al (1983) Participation in faecal occult blood screening for colorectal cancer. *Soc Sci Med* **17**: 17–23.

Deveroede G (1980) Risk of cancer in inflammatory bowel disease. In Winawer SJ, Sherlock P & Schottenfeld P (eds) *Colorectal Cancer: Prevention, Epidemiology and Screening*. New York: Raven Press.

Devitt SE, Roth Mayo LA & Brown FN (1969) The significance of multiple adenocarcinomas of the colon and rectum. *Ann Surg* **169**: 364–367.

Diamente M & Bacon HE (1966) Primary multiple malignancy of the colon and rectum: report of 230 cases. *Dis Colon Rectum* **9**: 441–446.

Dimmette RH, Elwi A & Sproat HF (1956) Relationship of schistosomiasis to polyposis and adenocarcinoma of the large intestine. *Am J Clin Path* **26**: 266.

Donald P, Fitzgerald Frazer JS & Wilkinson SP (1985) Sigmoidoscopy/proctoscopy clinic with open access to general practitioners. *BMJ* **290**: 759–761.

Doran J & Hardcastle JD (1982) Bleeding patterns in colorectal cancer: the effect of aspirin and the implications for faecal occult blood testing. *Br J Surg* **69**: 711–713.

Dorudi S, Kinrade E, Marshall NC et al (1998). Genetic defection of lymph node micrometastases in patients with colorectal cancer. *Br J Surg* **85**: 98–100.

dos Santos Silva I & Swerdlow AJ (1996) Sex differences in time trends of colorectal cancer in England and Wales: the possible effect of female hormonal factors. *Br J Cancer* **73**: 692–697.

Drasar BS & Irving D (1973) Environmental factors and cancer of the colon and breast. *Br J Cancer* **27**: 167–172.

Drasar BS & Jenkins DJA (1976) Bacteria, diet and large bowel cancer. *Am J Clin Nutr* **29**: 1410–1416.

Drasar BS, Goddard P, Heaton S et al (1976) Clostridia isolated from faeces. *J Med Microbiol* **9**: 63–72.

Dukes CE (1930) The spread of cancer of the rectum. *Br J Surg* **17**: 643–648.

Dukes CE (1940) Cancer of the rectum on analysis of 1000 cases. *J Path Bact* **50**: 527.

Dukes CE (1945) Discussion on the pathology and treatment of carcinoma of the colon. *Proc R Soc Med* **38**: 381.

Dukes CE (1951) The surgical pathology of tumours of the colon. *Med Press* 226: 512.

Dukes CE & Bussey HJR (1958) The spread of rectal cancer and its effect on prognosis. *Br J Cancer* **12**: 309.

Durdey P, Weston P & Williams NS (1987) Barium enema or colonoscopy as the initial investigation for colonic disease. *Lancet* **ii**: 549–551.

Durkin K & Haagensen CD (1980) An improved technique for the study of lymph nodes in surgical specimens. *Ann Surg* **191**: 419.

Eardley A & Wakefield J (1976) Long consultation by women with a lump in the breast. *Clin Oncol* **2**: 33–39.

Earnest DL, Hixson LJ, Fennerty MB et al (1991) Inhibition of prostaglandin synthesis: potential for chemoprevention of human colon cancer. *Cancer Bull* **43**: 561–568.

Eddy DM (1990) Screening for colorectal cancer. *Ann Intern Med* **113**: 373–384.

Eguchi S, Kohara N, Komuta K & Kanematsu T (1996) Mutations of the p53 gene in the stool of patients with resectable colorectal cancer. *Cancer* **77**: 1707–1710.

Ehrlich CP, Hall FM & Joffe N (1984) Post endoscopic perforation of normal colon in an area remote from instrumentation with secondary tension pneumoperitoneum. *Gastrointest Endosc* **30**: 190–191.

Eide TJ (1986) The age, sex and site specific occurrence of adenomas and carcinomas of the large intestine within a defined population. *Scand J Gastroenterol* **21**: 1083–1088.

Ekelund GR & Pihl B (1974) Multiple carcinomas of the colon and rectum. *Cancer* **35**: 1630–1634.

Elwood TW, Brickson A & Leiberman S (1978) Comparative educational approaches to screening for colorectal cancer. *Am J Publ Health* **68**: 135–138.

Enstrom JE (1975) Colorectal cancer and consumption of beef and fat. *Br J Cancer* **32**: 432–437.

Euchs CS, Giovannucci EL, Colditz GA et al (1994) A prospective study of family history and the risk of colorectal cancer. *N Engl J Med* **331**: 1669–1674.

Faivre J (1990) Preliminary results of a mass screening program for colorectal cancer in France. In Hardcastle JD (ed) *UKCCCR Screening for Colorectal Cancer*. Hamburg: Normed.

Faivre J, Doyon F & Boutron MC for the European Cancer Prevention Colon Group (1991) The ECP calcium fiber polyp prevention study. *Eur J Cancer Prev* **1** (Suppl 2): 83–89.

Faivre J, Boutron MC, Doyon F et al (1993) The ECP calcium fibre polyp prevention study preliminary report. *Eur J Cancer Prev* **2** (Suppl 2): 99–106.

Falterman KW, Hill CB, Markey JC et al (1974) Cancer of the colon, rectum and anus: a review of 2313 cases. *Cancer* **34**: 951–959.

Farrands PA & Britton DC (1985) Intervention in large bowel carcinogenesis: does screening improve prognosis? *Acta Chir Scand (Scand J Gastroenterol Suppl)* **101**: 151–159.

Farrands PA, Griffiths RL & Britton DC (1981) The Frome experiment: value of screening for colorectal cancer. *Lancet* **i**: 1231–1232.

Farrands PA, Vellacott JD, Amar SS, Balfour TW & Hardcastle JD (1983) Flexible fibreoptic sigmoidoscopy and double contrast barium enema examination in the identification of adenomas and carcinoma of the colon. *Dis Colon Rectum* **26**: 725–727.

Farrands PA, Hardcastle JD, Chamberlain J & Moss S (1984) Factors affecting compliance with screening for colorectal cancer. *Commum Med* **6**: 12–19.

Fearon E & Vogelstein B (1990) A genetic model for colorectal tumorigenesis. *Cell* **61**; 759–767.

Fearon E, Cho K, Nigro J et al (1990) Identification of a chromosome 18q gene that is altered in colorectal cancers. *Science* **247**: 49–56.

Feinberg A & Vogelstein B (1983) Hypomethylation of *ras* oncogenes in primary human cancers. *Biochem Biophys Res Commun* **111**: 47–54.

Fernandez-Banares F, Esteve M et al (1996) Changes of the mucosal n3 and n6 fatty acid status occur early in the colorectal adenoma–carcinoma sequence. *Gut* **38**: 254–259.

Fielding GA, Lumley J, Nathanson L, et al. (1997) Laparoscopic colectomy. *Surg Endosc.* **11**(7): 745–749.

Fingerhut A (1995) Laparoscopic colectomy: the French experience. In Jager R & Wexner SD (eds) *Laparoscopic Colorectal Surgery*. New York: Churchill Livingstone.

Finlay JG, Meek DR, Gray HW, Duncan JG & McArdle CS (1982) Incidence and detection of occult hepatic metastases in colorectal carcinoma. *BMJ* **284**: 803–805.

Floyd CE, Stirling CT & Cohn J Jr (1966) Cancer of the colon, rectum and anus: review of 1687 cases. *Ann Surg* **163**: 829–837.

Foggi E & Carbognani P (1993) The value of ploidy in the prognosis of the colorectal cancer. *Acta Biomed Ateneo Parmense* **64**: 185–194.

Foley DP, Dunne P, O'Brien M et al (1987) Left-sided colonoscopy as screening procedure for colorectal neoplasia in asymptomatic patients. *Gut* **28**: A1367.

Fraser J (1938) Malignant disease of the large intestine. *Br J Surg* **25**: 647.

Friend WG (1990) Sulindac suppression of colorectal polyps in Gardner's syndrome. *Am Fam Physician* **41**: 891–894.

Fruhmorgen P & Demling L (1978) Early detection of colorectal carcinoma with a modified quaiac test: a screening examination in 6000 humans. *Acta Gastroenterol Belg* **41**: 682–687.

Fusco MA & Paluzzi MW (1993) Abdominal wall recurrence after laparoscopic-assisted colectomy for adenocarcinoma of the colon: report of a case. *Dis Colon Rectum* **36**: 858–861.

Gabriel WB, Dukes C & Bussey HJR (1935) Lymphatic spread in cancer of the rectum. *Br J Surg* **23**: 395.

Ganauck R, Macrea FA & Fleisher M (1984) How to perform the faecal occult blood test. *CA* **34**: 134–147.

Garrick DP, Close JR & McMurray W (1977) Detection of occult blood in faeces (letter). *Lancet* **ii**: 820–821.

Gilbertsen VA (1974) Proctosigmoidoscopy and polypectomy in reducing the incidence of rectal cancer. *Cancer* **34**: 436–439.

Gilbertsen VA (1979) The earlier detection of colorectal cancers. In Brodie DR (ed) *Screening and Early Detection of Colorectal Cancer*, pp 211–215. NIH Publication 80–2075. Washington: US Dept of Health, Education and Welfare.

Gilbertsen VA & Nelms JM (1978) The prevention of invasive cancer of the rectum. *Cancer* **41**: 1137–1139.

Gilbertsen VA, Church TR & Grewe FJ (1980a) The design of a study to assess occult blood screening for colon cancer. *J Chron Dis* **33**: 107–114.

Gilbertsen VA, McHugh RB, Schuman LM et al (1980b) Colon cancer control study: an interim report. In Winawer SJ, Schottenfeld D & Sherlock P (eds) *Colorectal Cancer: Prevention, Epidemiology and Screening*, pp 261–266. New York: Raven Press.

Gilchrist RK & David VC (1947) A consideration of pathological factors influencing five year survival in radical resection of the large bowel and rectum for carcinoma. *Ann Surg* **126**: 421.

Giovannucci E, Colditz GA, Stampfer MJ et al (1994a) A prospective study of cigarette smoking and risk of colorectal adenoma and colorectal cancer in US women. *J Natl Cancer Inst* **86**: 192–199.

Giovannucci E, Rimm EB, Stampfer MJ et al (1994b) A prospective study of cigarette smoking and risk of colorectal adenoma and colorectal cancer in US men. *J Natl Cancer Inst* **86**: 183–191.

Giovannucci E, Rimm EB, Ascherio A et al (1995) Alcohol, low-methionine low-folate diets, and risk of colon cancer in men. *J Natl Cancer Inst* **87**: 265–273.

Glover RP & Waugh JM (1945) Retrograde lymphatic spread of carcinoma of the 'rectosigmoid' region: its influence on surgical procedures. *Surg Gynecol Obstet* **80**: 434.

Glynn SA, Albanes D, Pietinen P et al (1996) Alcohol consumption and risk of colorectal cancer in a cohort of Finnish men. *Cancer Causes Control* **7**: 214–223.

Gnauck R (1980) Occult blood tests (letter). *Lancet* **i**: 822.

Goligher JC (1941) The operability of carcinoma of the rectum. *BMJ* **2**: 393.

Goligher JC (1984) *Surgery of the Anus, Rectum and Colon*, p 468. London: Baillière Tindall.

Goligher JC & Smiddy FC (1957) The treatment of acute obstruction or perforation with carcinoma of the colon and rectum. *Br J Surg* **45**: 270.

Goligher JC, Dukes CB & Bussey NJR (1951) Local recurrences after sphincter saving excision for carcinoma of the rectum and rectosigmoid. *Br J Surg* **39**: 199.

Goodman MJ (1977) Mass screening for colorectal cancer. *Cancer* **40**: 945–949.

Goodman MJ (1979) Colorectal cancer screening (letter). *JAMA* **242**: 140.

Goulston K (1980) Role of diet in screening with faecal occult blood tests. In Winawer SJ, Schottenfeld D & Sherlock P (eds) *Colorectal Cancer: Prevention, Epidemiology and Screening*, pp 271–274. New York: Raven Press.

Graham DY, Sackman JW, Wallis CH & Melnich JL (1984) The Hemomatic analyser: a new occult blood testing device. *Am J Gastroenterol* **79**: 117–121.

Graham S, Dayal JI, Swanson M et al (1978) Diet in the epidemiology of cancer of the colon and rectum. *J Natl Cancer Inst* **61**: 709–714.

Greegor DH (1967) Diagnosis of large bowel cancer in the asymptomatic patient. *JAMA* **201**: 943.

Green SE, Chapman PD, Burn J, Bishop DT & Varma JS (1995) Clinical impact of colonoscopic screening in first-degree relatives of patients with hereditary non-polyposis colon cancer. *Br J Surg* **82**: 1338–1340.

Greenberg ER, Baron JA, Freeman DH Jr et al (1993) Reduced risk of large-bowel adenomas among aspirin users. *J Natl Cancer Res* **85**: 912–916.

Greenson JK, Isenhart CE, Rice R et al (1994) Identification of occult micrometastases in pericolic lymph nodes of Dukes' B colorectal cancer patients using monoclonal antibodies against cytokeratin and CC49: correlation with long-term survival. *Cancer* **73**: 563–569.

Greenwald P & Kelloff GJ (1993) The chemoprevention of cancer. In General Motors Research Foundation (eds) *Accomplishments in Cancer Research, 1992*, pp 242–265. Philadelphia: JB Lippincott.

Greenwald P, Kelloff GJ, Boone CW & McDonald SS (1995a) Genetic and cellular changes in colorectal cancer: proposed targets of chemopreventive agents (review). *Cancer Epidemiol Biomarkers Prev* **4**: 691–702.

Greenwald P, Kelloff GJ, Burch-Whitman C & Kramer BS (1995b) Chemoprevention. *CA Cancer J Clin* **45**: 31–49.

Gridley G, Mclaughlin JK, Ekbom A et al (1993) Incidence of cancer among patients with rheumatoid arthritis. *J Natl Cancer Inst* **85**: 307–311.

Griffith CDM, Turner DJ & Saunders JH (1981) False negative results of Hemoccult test in colorectal cancer. *BMJ* **283**: 4.

Grinnell RS (1939) The grading and prognosis of carcinoma of the colon and rectum. *Ann Surg* **109**: 500.

Grinnell RS (1954) Distal intramural spread of carcinoma of the rectum and rectosigmoid. *Surg Gynecol Obstet* **99**: 421–430.

Guillem JG & Weinstein IB (1990) The role of protein kinase C in colon neoplasia. In Herrera L (ed) *Familial Adenomatous Polyposis*, pp 325–332. New York: Alan R Liss.

Guillou PJ, Darzi A & Monson JRT (1993) Experience with laparoscopic colorectal surgery for malignant disease. *Surg Oncol* **2** (Suppl 1): 43–49.

Habba SJ & Doyle JS (1983) Colorectal cancer screening of asymptomatic patients in Ireland. *Ir J Med Sci* **152**: 121–124.

Haenszel W & Correa P (1971) Cancer of the colon and rectum and adenomatous polyps: a review of epidemiologic findings. *Cancer* **28**: 14–24.

Haenszel W, Berg JW, Segi M et al (1973) Large bowel cancer in Hawaiian Japanese. *J Natl Cancer Inst* **51**: 1765–1779.

Hague A, Manning AM, Hanlon KA et al (1993) Sodium butyrate induces apoptosis in human colonic tumour cell lines in a p53-independent pathway: implications for the possible role of dietary fibre in the prevention of large bowel cancer. *Int J Cancer* **55**: 498–505.

Hall C, Youngs D & Keighley MRB (1992) Crypt cell production rates at various sites around the colon in Wistar rats and humans. *Gut* **33**: 1528–1531.

Halper MS, Winawer SJ, Brody RS et al (1980) Issues of patient compliance. In Winawer SJ, Schottenfeld D & Sherlock P (eds) *Colorectal Cancer: Prevention, Epidemiology and Screening*, pp 299–310. New York: Raven Press.

Hamelin R, Laurent-Puig P, Olschwang S et al (1994) Association of p53 mutations with short survival in colorectal cancer. *Gastroenterology* **106**: 42–48.

Handley WS (1910) The surgery of the lymphatic system. *BMJ* **1**: 922–928.

Hansen HJ, Snyder JJ, Miller E et al (1974) Carcinoembryonic antigen (CEA) assay: a laboratory adjunct in the diagnosis and management of cancer. *Hum Pathol* **5**: 139–147.

Hardcastle JD (1987) Neoplasms: screening and diagnosis. *Curr Opin Gastroenterol* **3**: 16–20.

Hardcastle JD (1990) Population screening for colorectal cancer. In Hardcastle JD (ed) *UKCCR Screening for Colorectal Cancer*, pp 102–110. Hamburg: Normed.

Hardcastle JD, Farrands PA, Balfour TW et al (1983) Controlled trial of faecal occult blood testing in the detection of colorectal cancer. *Lancet* **ii**: 1–4.

Hardcastle JD, Armitage NC, Chamberlain J et al (1986) Faecal occult blood screening for colorectal cancer in the general population: results of a controlled trial. *Cancer* **58**: 397–403.

Hardcastle JD, Chamberlain JO, Robinson MHE et al (1996) Randomized controlled trial of faecal occult blood screening for colorectal cancer. *Lancet* **348**: 1472–1477.

Harford FJ, Fazio VW, Hpstein LM & Hewitt CB (1984) Rectosigmoid carcinoma occurring after ureterosigmoidostomy. *Dis Colon Rectum* **27**: 321–324.

Harned RK, Consigny PM, Cooper NB, Williams SM & Woltjen AJ (1982) Barium enema examination following biopsy of the rectum or colon. *Radiology* **145**: 11–16.

Hart AR, Wicks AC & Mayberry JF (1995) Colorectal cancer screening in asymptomatic populations. *Gut* **36**: 590–598.

Hastings JB (1974) Mass screening for colorectal cancer. *Am J Surg* **127**: 228–233.

Hauser A, Quigley ML, Driever CW et al (1981) More on false positive Hemoccult reaction with cimetidine (letter). *N Engl J Med* **304**: 847–848.

Havelaar IJ, Sugarbaker PH, Vermes M & Miller D (1984) Rate of growth of intra-abdominal metastases from colorectal cancer. *Cancer* **54**: 163–171.

Hayashi N, Ito I, Yanagisawa A et al (1995) Genetic diagnosis of lymph-node metastasis in colorectal cancer. *Lancet* **345**: 1257–1259.

Heald RJ & Bussey HJR (1975) Clinical experiences at St Mark's Hospital with multiple synchronous cancers of the colon and rectum. *Dis Colon Rectum* **18**: 6–10.

Heald RJ, Husband EM & Ryall RD (1982) The mesorectum in rectal cancer surgery: the clue to pelvic recurrence? *Br J Surg* **69**: 613–616

Heeb MA & Ahlvin RC (1978) Screening for colorectal carcinoma in a rural area. *Surgery* **83**: 540–541.

Heineman EF, Zahm SH, McLaughlin JK & Vaught JB (1995) Increased risk of colorectal cancer among smokers: results of a 26-year follow-up of US veterans and a review. *Int J Cancer* **59**: 728–738.

Heinrich HC & Icagic F (1980) Comparative studies on the *in vivo* sensitivity of four commercial pseudoperoxide-based faecal occult blood tests in relation to actual blood losses as calculated from measured whole body 59Fe-elimination rates. *Klin Wochenschr* **58**: 1283–1297.

Helfrich GB, Petrucel P & Webb H (1977) Mass screening for colorectal cancer. *JAMA* **238**: 1502–1503.

Henderson M & Kessel D (1977) Alterations in plasma sialyltransferase levels in patients with neoplastic disease. *Cancer* **39**: 1129–1134.

Hendrickse CW, Radley S, Davis A et al (1991) Fatty acids in the phospholipid and neutral lipid fractions in colorectal cancer. *Gut* **32**: A1241.

Hendrickse RG (1991) Clinical implications of food contaminated by aflatoxins. *Ann Acad Med (Sing)* **20**: 84–90.

Henson DE, Hutter RVP, Sobin LH et al (1994) Protocol for the examination of specimens removed from patients with colorectal carcinoma: a basis for check lists. *Arch Pathol Lab Med* **118**: 122–125

Hertz RE (1980) The management of adenomas of the large gut. In Stearns MW Jr (ed) *Neoplasms of the Colon, Rectum and Anus*, p 63. New York: Wiley.

Hertz RE, Deddish MR & Day E (1960) Value of periodic examinations in detecting cancer of the rectum and colon. *Postgrad Med* **27**: 290–292.

Herzog P & Holtermuller KH (1981) Oral cimetidine does not cause false positive test for blood in stools (letter). *N Engl J Med* **305**: 644–645.

Herzog P, Holtermuller KH, Preiss J et al (1982) Faecal blood loss in patients with colonic polyps: a comparison of measurements with ^{51}chromium-labelled erythrocytes and with Haemoccult test. *Gastroenterology* **83**: 957–962.

Hewett PJ, Thomas WN, King G et al (1996) Intraperitoneal cell movement during abdominal carbon dioxide insufflation and laparoscopy. *Dis Colon Rectum* **39**: 562–566.

Hill MJ (1975) The role of colon anacrobes in the metabolism of bile acids and steroids and its relation to colon cancer. *Cancer* **36**: 2387–2400.

Hill MJ (1983) Bile bacteria and bowel cancer. *Gut* **24**: 871–875.

Hill MJ, Drasar BS, Aries V et al (1971) Bacteria and the aetiology of cancer of the large bowel. *Lancet* **i**: 95–100.

Hill MJ, Drasar BS, Williams RR et al (1975) Faecal bile acids and clostridia in patients with cancer of the large bowel. *Lancet* **i**: 535–538.

Hoffman RM (1984) Altered methionine metabolism, DNA methylation and oncogene expression in carcinogenesis. *Biochem Biophys Acta* **738**: 49–87.

Hofstad B, Vatn M, Hoff G et al (1992) Growth of colorectal polyps: design of a prospective, randomized, placebo-controlled intervention study in patients with colorectal polyps. *Eur J Cancer Prev* **1**: 415–422.

Hojo K, Koyam Y & Moriya Y (1982) Lymphatic spread and its prognostic value in patients with rectal cancer. *Am J Surg* **144**: 350.

Holiday HW & Hardcastle JD (1979) Delay in diagnosis and treatment of symptomatic colorectal cancer. *Lancet* **i**: 309.

Houghton PW, Mortensen NJ & Williamson RC (1987) Effect of duodenogastric reflux on gastric mucosal proliferation after gastric surgery. *Br J Surg* **74**: 288–291.

Houlston RS, Murday V, Harocopos C, Williams CB & Slack J (1990) Screening and genetic counselling for relatives of patients with colorectal cancer in a family cancer clinic. *BMJ* **301**: 366–368.

Howe GR, Benito E, Castellato R et al (1992) Dietary intake of fiber and decreased risk of cancers of the colon and rectum: evidence from the combined analysis of 13 case–control studies. *J Natl Cancer Inst* **84**: 1887–1896.

Howell MA (1976) The association between colorectal cancer and breast cancer. *J Chron Dis* **29**: 243.

Hsu Y-H & Guzman LG (1982) Carcinoma of the colon, rectum and anal canal in young adults. *Am J Proctol Gastroenterol Colon Rect Surg* **33**(4): 7–12.

Huang TH-M, Quesenberry JT, Martin MB, Loy S & Diaz-Arias AA (1993) Loss of heterozygosity detected in formalin-fixed, paraffin-embedded tissue of colorectal carcinoma using a microsatellite located within the deleted-in-colorectal-carcinoma gene. *Diagn Mol Pathol* **2**: 90–93.

Hughes ES, McDermott FT, Poliglase AI & Johnson WR (1983) Tumor recurrence in the abdominal wall scar after large bowel cancer surgery. *Dis Colon Rectum* **26**: 571–572.

Humphreys F, Hewetson KA & Dellpiani AW (1984) Massive subcutaneous emphysema following colonoscopy. *Endoscopy* **16**: 160–161.

Hunter W, Farmer A, Mant D et al (1991) The effect of self-administered faecal occult blood tests on compliance with screening for colorectal cancer: results of a survey of those invited. *Fam Pract* **8**: 367–372.

Huntsman RG & Liddell J (1961) Paper tests for occult blood faeces and some observations on the fate of swallowed red cells. *J Clin Pathol* **14**: 436–438.

Iacopetta B, DiGrandi S, Dix B et al (1994) Loss of heterozygosity of tumour suppressor gene loci in human colorectal carcinoma. *Eur J Cancer* **30A**: 664–670.

Iliyasu Y, Ladipo JK, Akang EE et al (1996) A twenty-year review of malignant colorectal neoplasms at University College Hospital, Ibadan, Nigeria. *Dis Colon Rectum* **39**: 536–540.

Illingworth DG (1965) Influence of diet on occult blood tests. *Gut* **6**: 595–598.

Imray C, Sakaguchi M, Davis A et al (1990) Reduction of low density lipoprotein by N-3 fats is associated with impaired growth of human colonic cancer cell growth *in vivo*. *Gut* **31**: A1162.

Inokuchi K, Toludome S, Ipeka M et al (1984) Mortality from carcinoma after partial gastrectomy. *Jpn J Cancer Res (Gann)* **75**: 588–594.

Ionov Y, Peinado MA, Malkhosyan S, Shibata D & Perucho M (1993) Ubiquitous somatic mutations in simple repeated sequences reveal a new mechanism for colonic carcinogenesis. *Nature* **363**: 558–561.

Irons GV & Kirsner JB (1965) Routine chemical tests of the stool for occult blood: an evaluation. *Am J Med Sci* **249**: 247–260.

Jacobi C, Keller HW & Said S (1994) Implantation metastasis of unsuspected gallbladder carcinoma after laparoscopy. *Br J Surg* **81** (Suppl): 82 (abstract).

Jaffe RM, Kasten B, Young DS et al (1975) False negative stool circuit blood tests caused by ingestion of ascorbic acid (vitamin C). *Ann Intern Med* **83**: 824–826.

Jaquet P, Averbach AM & Jaquet N (1995) Abdominal wall metastasis and peritoneal carcinomatosis after laparoscopic-assisted colectomy for colon cancer (review). *Eur J Surg Oncol* **21**: 568–570.

Jarvinen H & Franssila KO (1984) Familial juvenile polyposis coli: increased risk of colo-rectal cancer. *Gut* **25**: 792–800.

Jarvinen HJ, Mecklin JP & Sistonen P (1995) Screening reduces colorectal cancer rate in families with hereditary non-polyposis colorectal cancer. *Gastroenterology* **108**: 1405–1411.

Jass JR & Sobin LH (eds) (1989) *International Histological Classification of Tumors*. Berlin: Springer Verlag.

Jass JR, Atkin WS, Cuzick J et al (1986) The grading of rectal cancer: historical perspectives and a multivariate analysis of 447 cases. *Histopathology* **10**: 437–459.

Jass JR, Love SB & Northover JMA (1987) A new classification of rectal cancer. *Lancet* **i**: 1303–1306.

Jeffers MD, O'Dowd GM, Mulcahy H et al (1994) The prognostic significance of immunohistochemically detected lymph-node micrometastases in colorectal carcinoma. *J Pathol* **172**: 183–187.

Jen J, Powell SM, Papadopoulos N et al (1994) Molecular determinants of dysplasia in colorectal lesions. *Cancer Res* **54**: 5523–5526.

Jensen OM & MacLennan R (1979) Dietary factors and colorectal cancer in Scandinavia. *Israel J Med Sci* **15**: 329–334.

Jinnai D (1982) quoted in Goligher JC (ed, 1984) *Surgery of the Anus, Rectum and Colon*, 4th edn, p 447. London: Baillière Tindall.

Johnson JW, Judd ES & Dahlin DC (1959) Malignant neoplasms of the colon and rectum in young patients. *Arch Surg (Chicago)* **79**: 365.

Jones DB, Guo LW, Reinhard MK et al (1995) Impact of pneumoperitoneum on trocar site implantation of colon cancer in hamster model. *Dis Colon Rectum* **38**: 1182–1188.

Judd ES (1924) A consideration of lesions of the colon treated surgically. *5th Med J (Nashville)* **17**: 75.

Kalra PA, Price WR, Jones BJM & Hamlyn AN (1988) Open access fibre sigmoidoscopy: a comparison audit of efficacy. *BMJ* **296**: 1095–1096.

Kelloff GJ, Boone CW, Steele VE et al (1994) Progress in cancer chemoprevention: perspectives on agent selection and short-term clinical intervention trials. *Cancer Res* **54**: S2015–2024.

Kelloff GJ, Johnson JR, Crowell JA et al (1995) Approaches to the development and marketing approval of drugs that prevent cancer. *Cancer Epidemiol Biomarkers Prev* **4**: 1–10.

Kewenter J, Brevinge H, Engaras B, Haglind E & Ahren C (1994) Results of screening, rescreening and follow-up in a prospective randomized study for detection of colorectal cancer by fecal occult blood testing: results for 63,308 subjects. *Scand J Gastroenterol* **29**: 468–473.

Khalili TM, Fleshner PR, Hiatt JR et al (1998) Colorectal cancer: comparison of laparoscopic with open approaches. *Dis Colon Rectum* **41**(7): 832–838.

Kikuchi-Yanoshita R, Konishi M, Ito S et al (1992) Genetic changes of both p53 alleles associated with the conversion from colorectal adenoma to early carcinoma in familial adenomatous polyposis and non-familial adenomatous polyposis patients. *Cancer Res* **52**; 3965–3971.

Kille JN & Glick S (1967) Neoplasia complicating uretero-sigmoidostomy. *BMJ* **3**: 783.

Killingback M, Wilson E & Hughes ESR (1965) Anal metastases from carcinoma of the rectum and colon. *Aust NZ J Surg* **34**: 178.

Kim HJ, Choi ES & Wade AE (1990) Effect of dietary fat on the induction of hepatic microsomal cytochrome P450 isozymes by phenobarbital. *Biochem Pharmacol* **39**: 1423–1430.

Kim HJ, Jen J, Vogelstein B et al (1994) Clinical and pathological characteristics of sporadic colorectal carcinoma with DNA replication errors in microsatellite sequences. *Am J Pathol* **145**: 148–156.

Kinzler K, Nilbert M, Vogelstein B et al (1991) Identification of a gene located at chromosome 5q21 that is mutated in colorectal cancers. *Science* **251**: 1366–1370.

Kirklin JW, Dockerty MB & Waugh JM (1949) The role of peritoneal reflection in the prognosis of carcinoma of the rectum and sigmoid colon. *Surg Gynecol Obstet* **88**: 326.

Kleibeuker JH, Nagengast FM & R van der Meer (1996) Carcinogenesis in the colon: In Young GP, Rozen P, Levin B (eds) *Prevention and Early Detection of Colorectal Cancer*, Ch 3, p. 57. London: WB Saunders.

Koha M, Wikstrom B & Brismar B (1992) Colorectal carcinoma: DNA ploidy pattern and prognosis with reference to tumor DNA heterogeneity. *Anal Quant Cytol Histol* **14**: 367–372.

Kokal W, Sheibain K, Terz J & Harrada JR (1986) Tumour DNA content in the prognosis of colorectal carcinoma. *JAMA* **255**: 3123–3127.

Kotanagi H, Fukuoka T, Shibata Y et al (1995) Blood vessel invasion in metastatic nodes for development of liver metastases in colorectal cancer. *Hepatogastroenterology* **42**: 771–774.

Kouri M, Nordling S, Kuusela P & Pyrhonen S (1993) Poor prognosis associated with elevated serum CA 19-9 level in advanced colorectal carcinoma, independent of DNA ploidy or SPF. *Eur J Cancer* **29A**: 1691–1696.

Kronborg O, Fenger C, Søndorgaard O, Pedensen KM & Olsen J (1987) Initial mass screening for colorectal cancer with faecal occult blood test: a prospective randomised study at Funen in Denmark. *Scand J Gastroenterol* **22**: 677–686.

Kronborg O, Fenger C, Olsen J, Bech K & Søndergaard O (1989) Repeated screening for colorectal cancer with faecal occult blood test. *Scand J Gastroenterol* **24**: 599–606.

Kronborg O, Fenger C, Olsen J, Jorgensen OD & Søndergaard (1996) Randomized study of screening for colorectal cancer with faecal occult blood test. *Lancet* **348**: 1467–1471.

Kune GA, Kune S, Watson LF & Brough HW (1988a) Peptic ulcer surgery and colorectal cancer risk. *Br J Surg* **75**: 187.

Kune GA, Kune S & Watson LF (1988b) Colorectal cancer risk, chronic illnesses, operations, and medications: case control from the Melbourne colorectal cancer study. *Cancer Res* **48**: 4399–4404.

Kurnick JB, Walley LB, Jacob HH et al (1980) Colorectal cancer detection in a community hospital screening program. *JAMA* **243**: 2056–2057.

Labayle D, Fischer D, Vielh P et al (1991) Sulindac causes regression of rectal polyps in familial adenomatous polyposis. *Gastroenterology* **101**: 635–639.

Lacy AM, Delgado S, Garcia-Valdecasas JC et al (1998) Port site metastases and recurrence after laparoscopic colectomy. A randomized trial. *Surg Endosc* **12**(8): 1039–1042.

Lance P (1993) Faecal occult blood tests: what's new? *Gastroenterology* **104**: 1852–1855.

Lang CA & Ransohoff DE (1994) Fecal occult blood screening for colorectal cancer: is mortality reduced by chance selection for screening colonoscopy? *JAMA* **271**: 1011–1013.

Langevin JM & Nivatvongs S (1984) The true incidence of synchronous cancer of the large bowel. *Am J Surg* **147**: 330–334.

Larkin KK (1980) Mass screening in colorectal cancer. *Aust NZ J Surg* **50**: 467–469.

Lasser A (1978) Synchronous primary adenocarcinomas of the colon and rectum. *Dis Colon Rectum* **21**: 20–22.

Lauer JD, Carlson HL & Wollaeger EE (1965) Accuracy of roentgenologic examination in detecting carcinoma of the colon. *Dis Colon Rectum* **8**: 190.

Laurent-Puig P, Olschwang S, Delattre O et al (1992) Survival and acquired genetic alterations in colorectal cancer. *Gastroenterology* **102**: 1136–1141

Lauroy J, Champault G, Risk N & Boutelier P (1994) Metastatic recurrence at the cannula site: should digestive carcinomas still be managed by laparoscopy? *Br J Surg* **81** (Suppl): 31 (abstract).

Levin B & Murphy GP (1992) Revision in American Cancer Society recommendations for the early detection of colorectal cancer. *CA Cancer J Clin* **42**: 296–299.

Lieberman DA (1995) Cost-effectiveness model for colorectal cancer screening. *Gastroenterology* **109**: 1781–1790.

Lifton LJ & Kreiser J (1982) False positive stool occult blood tests caused by iron preparations: a controlled study and review of literature. *Gastroenterology* **83**: 860–863.

Linos DA, Beard CM, O'Fallon WM et al (1981) Cholecystectomy and carcinoma of the colon. *Lancet* **ii**: 379–381.

Lipkin M & Newmark H (1995) Calcium and the prevention of colon cancer (review). *J Cell Biochem Suppl* **22**: 65–73.

Lipshutz GR, Katon RM, McCool MF et al (1979) Flexible sigmoidoscopy as a screening procedure for neoplasm of the colon. *Surg Gynecol Obstet* **148**: 19–22.

Loffeld R, Putten A & Balk A (1996) Changes in the localization of colorectal cancer: implications for clinical practice. *J Gastroenterol Hepatol* **11**: 47–50.

Lofgren EP, Waugh JM & Dockerty MB (1957) Local recurrence of carcinoma after anterior resection of the rectum and the sigmoid. *Arch Surg* **74**: 825–838.

Logan RFA, Little J, Hawtin PG & Hardcastle JD (1993) Effect of aspirin and non-steroidal anti-inflammatory drugs on colorectal adenomas: case–control study of subjects participating in the Nottingham faecal occult blood screening programme. *BMJ* **307**: 285–289.

Long L, Jonasson O, Robertson S et al (1960) Cancer cells in blood: results of a simplified isolation technique. *Arch Surg (Chicago)* **80**: 910.

Lothe RA, Fossli T, Danielsen HE et al (1992) Molecular genetic studies of tumor suppressor gene regions on chromosomes 13 and 17 in colorectal tumours. *J Natl Cancer Inst* **84**: 1100–1108.

Lovett E (1976) Family studies in cancers of the colon and rectum. *Br J Surg* **63**: 13–18.

Luchtefeld MA, Syverson D, Solfelt M et al (1991) Is colonoscopic screening appropriate in asymptomatic patients with a family history of colon cancer? *Dis Colon Rectum* **34**: 763–768.

Lundy S, Welch JP & Berman M (1983) Colorectal cancer in patients under 40 years of age. *J Surg Oncol* **24**: 11–14.

Lynch HT, Lynch J & Lynch P (1977) Management and control of familial cancer. In Mulvihill JJ, Miller RM & Fraumeni JF Jr (eds) *Progress in Cancer Research and Therapy. Genetics of Human Cancer*, Vol. 3, p 235. New York: Raven Press.

Lynch HT, Smyrk TC, Watson P et al (1993) Genetics, natural history, tumour spectrum and pathology of hereditary non-polyposis colorectal cancer: an updated review. *Gastroenterology* **104**: 1535–1549.

MacCarty RL (1992) Colorectal cancer: the case for barium enema (review). *Mayo Clin Proc* **67**: 253–257.

MacLennan R, Macrae F, Bain C et al (1995) Australian Polyp Prevention Project: Randomized trial of intake of fat, fiber, and beta-carotene to prevent colorectal adenomas. *J Natl Cancer Inst* **87**: 1760–1766.

Macrae FA & St John DJB (1982) Relationship between patterns of bleeding and Haemoccult sensitivity in patients with colorectal cancers or adenomas. *Gastroenterology* **82**: 891–898.

Macrae FA, Hill DJ, Dent O et al (1982) Colorectal cancer: knowledge and attitudes of doctors in Victoria. *Aust NZ J Med* **12**: 278–283.

Mandel JS, Bond JH, Church JR et al (1993) Reducing mortality from colorectal cancer by screening for faecal occult blood. *N Engl J Med* **328**: 1365–1371.

Mannes AG, Weinzierl M, Stellard F et al (1984) Adenomas of the large intestine after cholecystectomy. *Gut* **25**: 863–866.

Manson PN, Corman ML, Collar JA et al (1976) Anterior resection for adenocarcinoma: Lahey Clinic experience 1963–69. *Am J Surg* **131**: 434–443.

Marble K, Banerjee S & Greenwald L (1992) Colorectal carcinoma in young patients. *J Surg Oncol* **51**: 179–182.

Marks G, Boggs HW, Castro AF et al (1979) Sigmoidoscopic examinations with rigid and flexible fibreoptic sigmoidoscopies in the surgeon's office: a comparative study of effectiveness in 1,012 cases. *Dis Colon Rectum* **22**: 162–168.

Marnett LJ (1992) Aspirin and the potential role of prostaglandins in colon cancer. *Cancer Res* **52**: 5575–5589.

Marshall N, Kinrade E, Onwu D et al (1997) Haematogenous and lymphatic micrometastases in colorectal carcinoma. *Br J Surg* Suppl **84**: 39.

Mauie WF (1994) Screening for colorectal cancer by nurse endocopists. *N Engl J Med* **33**: 183–187.

Mayo CW & Pagtalunan RSG (1963) Malignancy of colon and rectum in patients under 30 years of age. *Surgery (St Louis)* **53**: 711.

McCallum RW, Meyer CT, Marignani P & Cane Contino C (1984) Flexible sigmoidoscopy diagnostic yield in 1015 patients. *Am J Gastroenterol* **79**: 433–437.

McCormack PM & Attiyeh FF (1979) Resected pulmonary metastases from colorectal cancer. *Dis Colon Rectum* **22**: 553–557.

McCoy GF & Parks TG (1984) Colorectal carcinoma in young patients. *J R Coll Surg Edinb* **29**: 130–133.

McDermott FT (1983) In Hughes ESR, Cuthbertson AM & Killingback MK (eds) *Colorectal Surgery*, p 336. Edinburgh: Churchill Livingstone.

McDermott FT, Hughes PSR, Pihl E, Milne BJ & Price AB (1981) Comparative results of surgical management of single carcinomas of the colon and rectum: a series of 1939 patients managed by one surgeon. *Br J Surg* **68**: 850–855.

McKeown-Eyssen GE, Bright-See E, Bruce WR & Jazmaji V (1994) Toronto Polyp Prevention Group: A randomized trial of a low-fat high-fibre diet in the recurrence of colorectal polyps. *J Clin Epidemiol* **47**: 525–536.

McKinley AJ, Wyllie AH & Dunlop MG (1997) Development of a genetic detection assay for colorectal cancer micrometastases. *Br J Surg* **84**: 715 (Abstract).

McMichael AJ & Bonnet T (1981) Cancer profiles of British and Southern European migrants: exploring South Australia's Cancer Registry data. *Med J Austr* **1**: 229–232.

Meigs J, Synder D, Heston J & Flannery J (1977) Changes in site distribution of colorectal carcinoma in Connecticut 1940–73. *Dig Dis Sci* **22**: 791–797.

Mercer PM, Reid FD, Harrison M & Bates T (1995) The relationship between cholecystectomy, unoperated gallstone disease, and colorectal cancer: a necropsy study. *Scand J Gastroenterol* **30**: 1017–1020.

Miles WE (1910) The radical abdomino-perineal operation for cancer of the rectum of the pelvic colon. *BMJ* **2**: 941.

Miles WE (1920) Discussion on the surgical treatment of cancer of the rectum. *BMJ* **2**: 730–742.

Miles WE (1926) *Cancer of the Rectum*. London: Harrison.

Miles WE (1931) The pathology of the spread of cancer of the rectum and its bearing upon the surgery of the cancerous rectum. *Surg Gynecol Obstet* **52**: 350–359.

Miller AB (1983) Trends in cancer mortality and epidemiology. *Cancer* **51**: 2413–2418.

Miller SF & Knight AR (1977) The early detection of colorectal cancer. *Cancer* **40**: 945–949.

Million R, Howarth J, Turnberg E et al (1982) Faecal occult blood testing for colorectal cancer in general practice. *Practitioner* **226**: 659–663.

Modan B (1979) Patterns of gastrointestinal neoplasms in Israel. *Israel J Med Sci* **15**: 301–304.

Modan B, Barell V, Lubin F et al (1975) Low fibre intake as an aetiological factor in cancer of the colon. *J Natl Cancer Inst* **55**: 15–18.

Moertel CG, Bargwen JA & Dockerty MB (1958) Multiple carcinoma of the large intestine: a review of the literature and a study of 261 cases. *Gastroenterology* **34**: 85–98.

Moertel CG, Hill JR & Dockerty MB (1966) The routine proctoscopic examination: a second look. *Mayo Clin Pro* **41**: 368–374.

Mogg RA (1977) Neoplasms at the site of ureterocolic anastomosis. *Br J Surg* **64**: 758.

Monroe CW (1949) Lymphatic spread of carcinoma of the breast. *Arch Surg (Chicago)* **57**: 479.

Moore GE & Sako K (1959) The spread of carcinoma of the colon and rectum: a study of invasion of blood vessels, lymph nodes and the peritoneum by tumour cells. *Dis Colon Rectum* **2**: 92.

Moore GE, Sandberg A & Schubarg JR (1957) Clinical and experimental observations on the occurrence and fate of tumour cells in the blood stream. *Ann Surg* **76**: 755.

Moore GE, Sako K, Kondo T et al (1961) Assessment of the exfoliation of tumour cells into the body cavities. *Surg Gynecol Obstet* **112**: 469.

Morgan JN (1950) Discussion on conservative resection in carcinoma of the rectum. *Proc R Soc Med* **43**: 701.

Morganstern L & Lee SE (1978) Spatial distribution of colonic carcinoma. *Arch Surg* **113**: 1141.

Mori M, Mimori K, Inoue H et al (1995) Detection of cancer micrometastases in lymph nodes by reverse transcriptase–polymerase chain reaction. *Cancer Res* **55**: 3417–3420.

Morotomi M, Guillem J, LoGerfo P & Weinstein IB (1990) Production of diacylglycerol, an activator of protein kinase C, by human intestinal microflora. *Cancer Res* **50**: 3595–3599.

Morris DW, Hansell JR, Ostron D et al (1976) Reliability of chemical tests for faecal occult blood in hospitalised patients. *Dig Dis Sci* **21**: 845–852.

Morrow GR, Way J, Hoagland AC et al (1982) Patient compliance with self-directed Hemoccult testing. *Prev Med* **11**: 512–520.

Morson BC & Dawson IMP (1990) *Gastrointestinal Pathology*, 3rd edn. Oxford: Blackwell Scientific.

Morson BC, Vaughan EG & Bussey HJR (1963) Pelvis recurrence after exclsion of rectum for carcinoma. *BMJ* **2**: 13.

Mulcahy HE, Farthing MJG & O'Donoghue DP (1997) Screening for asymptomatic colorectal cancer. *BMJ* **314**: 285–290

Mullan FJ, Wilson HK & Majury CW (1990) Bile acids and the increased risk of colorectal tumours after truncal vagotomy. *Br J Surg* **77**: 1085–1090.

Nagengast FM, Grubben MJ & van Munster IP (1995) Role of bile acids in colorectal carcinogenesis (review). *Eur J Cancer* **31A**: 1067–1070.

Nduka CC, Monson JRT, Menzies-Gow N & Darzi A (1994) Abdominal wall metastases following laparoscopy. *Br J Surg* **81**: 648–652.

Nelson RL (1984) Is the changing pattern of colorectal cancer caused by selenium deficiency? *Dis Colon Rectum* **27**: 459–461.

Newcomb PA, Norfleet RG, Storer BE, Surawicz TS & Marcus PM (1992) Screening sigmoidoscopy and colorectal cancer mortality. *J Natl Cancer Inst* **84**: 1572–1575.

Newmark HI, Wargovich MJ & Bruce WR (1984) Colon cancer and dietary fat, phosphate and calcium: a hypothesis. *J Natl Cancer Inst* **72**: 1323–1326.

Ng IOL, Luk ISC, Yuen ST et al (1993) Surgical lateral clearance in resected rectal carcinomas: a multivariate analysis of clinicopathological features. *Cancer* **71**: 1972–1976.

Nicholls RJ, Mason AY, Morson BC, Dixon AK & Kelsey Fry I (1982) The clinical staging of rectal cancer. *Br J Surg* **69**: 404–409.

Nicosia S & Patrono C (1989) Eicosanoid biosynthesis and action: novel opportunities for pharmacological intervention. *FASEB J* **3**: 1941–1948.

Nigro ND & Bull AW (1987) The impact of dietary fat and fiber on intestinal carcinogenesis. *Prev Med* **16**: 554–558.

Nishisho I, Nakamura Y, Miyoshi Y et al (1991) Mutations of chromosome 5g21 genes in FAP and colorectal cancer patients. *Science* **253**: 665–669.

Nivatvongs S, Gilbertsen VA, Goldberg SM et al (1982) Distribution of large bowel cancers detected by occult blood test in asymptomatic patients. *Dis Colon Rectum* **25**: 420–421.

Norfleet RG & Rhodes RA (1982) Cimetidine therapy does not affect faecal occult blood testing. *J Clin Gastroenterol* **4**: 419–420.

Norfleet RG, Rhodes RA & Savage K (1980) False positive 'Hemoccult' reaction with cimetidine (letter). *N Engl J Med* **302**: 467.

Nottle PD, Polgrase AL, Hughes ESN et al (1983) Synchronous carcinoma of the large intestine. *Aust NZ J Surg* **53**: 329–332.

Nugent KP, Farmer KCR, Spigelman AD et al (1993) Randomized controlled trial of the effect of sulindac on duodenal and rectal polyposis and cell proliferation in patients with familial adenomatous polyposis. *Br J Surg* **80**: 1618–1619.

O'Rourke N, Price PM, Kelly S & Sikora K (1993) Tumour inoculation during laparoscopy (letter). *Lancet* **342**: 368.

Obrecht WR Jr, Wu WC, Gelfand PW & Ott DJ (1984) The extent of successful colonoscopy: a second assessment using modern equipment. *Gastrointest Radiol* **9**: 161–162.

Okada Y, Kusano S & Endo T (1994) Double-contrast barium enema study with computed radiography: assessment in detection of colorectal polyps. *J Digit Imaging* **7**: 154–159.

Ookawa K, Sakamoto M, Hirohashi S et al (1993) Concordant p53 and DCC alterations and allelic losses on chromosomes 13q and 14q associated with liver metastases of colorectal carcinoma. *Int J Cancer* **53**: 382–387.

OPCS (Office of Population Censuses and Surveys) (1992) *Cancer Mortality Statistics: Review of the Registrar-General on Deaths in England and Wales, 1990* (DHI–24). London: HMSO.

Owen RW, Weisgerber UM, Spiegelhalder B & Bartsch H (1996) Faecal phytic acid and its relation to other putative markers of risk for colorectal cancer. *Gut* **38**: 591–597

Palmer JP & Spratt DW (1956) Pelvic carcinoma following irradiation of benign gynecologic diseases. *Am J Obstet Gynecol* **62**: 497–505.

Passman MA, Pommier RF & Vetto JT (1996) Synchronous colon primaries have the same prognosis as solitary colon cancers. *Dis Colon Rectum* **39**: 329–334.

Peleg I, Maibach HT & Wilcox CM (1993) Aspirin and non-steroidal anti-inflammatory drug use and the risk of subsequent colorectal polyps. *Gastroenterology* **104**: A440.

Peleg I, Maibach HT, Brown SH & Wilcox CM (1994) Aspirin and nonsteroidal anti-inflammatory drug use and the risk of subsequent colorectal cancer. *Arch Intern Med* **154**: 394–399.

Penfold JB (1974) A comparison of restorative resection of carcinoma of the middle third of the rectum with abdomino-perineal excision. *Aust NZ J Surg* **44**: 354–356.

Pickren JW (1956) Lymph node metastasis in carcinoma of the female mammary gland. *Bull Roswell Park Mem Inst* **1**: 79.

Pietra N, Sarli L, Sansebastiano G, Jotti GS & Peracchia A (1996) Prognostic value of ploidy, cell proliferation kinetics, and conventional clinicopathologic criteria in patients with colorectal carcinoma: a prospective study. *Dis Colon Rectum* **39**: 494–503.

Pitluk H & Poticha SM (1983) Carcinoma of the colon and rectum in patients less than 40 years of age. *Surg Gynecol Obstet* **157**: 335–337.

Podolsky DK, Weiser MW, Isselbacher KJ & Cohen AM (1978) A cancer associated galactosyltransferase isoenzyme. *N Engl J Med* **229**: 703–705.

Pollett WJ & Nicholls RJ (1981) Does the extent of distal clearance effect survival after radical anterior resection for carcinoma of the rectum? *Gut* **22**: 872.

Pomeranz AA & Garlock JH (1955) Postoperative recurrence of cancer of the colon due to desquamated malignant cells. *JAMA* **158**: 1434.

Potter JD (1996) Epidemiologic, environmental and lifestyle issues in colorectal cancer. In Young GP, Rozen P & Levin B (eds) *Prevention and Detection of Early Colorectal Cancer*, pp 23–43. London: WB Saunders.

Potter JD, Slattery ML, Bostick RM & Gapstur SM (1993) Colon cancer: a review of the epidemiology. *Epidemiol Rev* **15**: 499–545.

Powell SM, Zilz N, Beazer-Barclay Y et al (1992) APC mutations occur early during colorectal tumorigenesis. *Nature* **359**: 235–237.

Prasad A, Avery C & Foley RJE (1994) Abdominal wall metastases following laparoscopy (letter). *Br J Surg* **81**: 1697.

Quan SHQ (1959) Cul de sac smears for cancer cells. *Surgery (St Louis)* **45**: 258.

Quer RA, Dablin DC & Mayo CW (1953) Retrograde intramural spread of carcinoma of the rectum and rectosigmoid. *Surg Gynecol Obstet* **96**: 24–30.

Quirke P & Scott N (1992) The pathologist's role in the assessment of local recurrence in rectal carcinoma. *Surg Oncol Clin N Am* **1**: 1–17

Quirke P & Shepherd N (1997) Guidance notes on pathological

assessment and reporting. In *Handbook for the Clinico-Pathological Assessment and Staging of Colorectal Cancer*. London: UKCCCR.
Quirke P, Durdey P, Dixon MF & Williams NS (1986) Local recurrence of rectal adenocarcinoma due to inadequate surgical resection: a histopathological study of lateral tumour spread and surgical excision. *Lancet* **ii**: 993–996.
Rainey JB, Maeda M, Williams C & Williamson RCN (1984) The co-carcinogenic effect of intrarectal deoxycholate in rats is reduced by oral metronidazole. *Br J Cancer* **49**: 631–636.
Ramos JM, Gupta S, Anthone GJ et al (1994) Laparoscopy and colon cancer: is the port site at risk? A preliminary report. *Arch Surg* **129**: 897–899.
Rankin FW (1933) Curability of cancer of the colon, rectosigmoid and rectum. *JAMA* **101**: 491.
Ransohoff DF & Lang CA (1991) Screening for colorectal cancer. *N Engl J Med* **325**: 37–41.
Reddy BS & Wynder EL (1973) Large bowel carcinogenesis: faecal constituents of populations with diverse incidence rates of colon cancer. *J Natl Cancer Inst* **50**: 1437–1442.
Reddy BS & Wynder EL (1977) Metabolic epidemiology of colon cancer: faecal bile acids and neutral steroids in colon cancer patients and patients with adenomatous polyps. *Cancer* **39**: 2533–2539.
Reddy BS, Weisburger JH & Wynder EL (1974) Faecal bacterial B glucuronidase: control by diet. *Science* **183**: 416–417.
Reddy BS, Narisawa T & Weinberger JH (1976) Effect of diet with high levels of protein and fat on colon carcinogenesis in F344 rats treated with 112-dimethylhydrazine. *J Natl Cancer Inst* **57**: 567–569.
Reddy BS, Hirota N & Kayayama S (1982) Effect of dietary sodium ascorbate on 1,2-dimethylhydrazine- or methylnitrosourea-induced colon carcinogenesis in rats. *Carcinogenesis* **3**: 1097–1099.
Redston MS, Papadopoulos N, Caldas C et al (1995) Common occurrence of APC and K-*ras* gene mutations in the spectrum of colitis-associated neoplasias. *Gastroenterology* **108**: 383–392.
Reid FD, Mercer PM, Harrison M & Bates T (1996) Cholecystectomy as a risk factor for colorectal cancer: a meta-analysis. *Scand J Gastroenterol* **31**: 160–169.
Reilly JC, Rusin LC & Theuerkauf FJ Jr (1982) Colonoscopy: its role in cancer of the colon and rectum. *Dis Colon Rectum* **25**: 532–538.
ReillyWT, Nelson H, Schroeder G et al (1996) Wound recurrence following conventional treatment of colorectal cancer. A rare but perhaps underestimated problem. *Dis Colon Rectum* **39**: 200–207.
Rex DK, Lehman GA, Ulbright TM, Smith JJ & Hawes RH (1994) The yield of second-screening flexible sigmoidoscopy in average-risk persons after one negative examination. *Gastroenterolgy* **106**: 593–595.
Rhodes FB, Holmes FF & Clark GM (1977) Changing distribution of primary cancers in the large bowel. *JAMA* **238**: 1641–1643.
Ribet A, Frexinos J, Escourron J et al (1980) Occult blood tests and colorectal tumours. *Lancet* **i**: 417.
Riches M, Perez-Giminez ME, Layrisse M et al (1957) Study of urinary and faecal excretion of radioactive chromium Cr^{51} in man: its use in the measurement of intestinal blood loss associated with hookworm infection. *J Clin Invest* **36**: 1183–1193.
Robinson MHE, Kronoberg O, Williams CB et al (1995) Faecal occult blood testing and colonoscopy in the surveillance of subjects at high risk of colorectal neoplasia. *Br J Surg* **82**: 318–320.
Rosato FE & Marks G (1981) Changing site distribution patterns of colorectal cancer at Thomas Jefferson University Hospital. *Dis Colon Rectum* **24**: 93.
Rosato FE, Shelley WB, Fitts WT et al (1969) Non-metastatic cutaneous manifestations of cancer of the colon. *Am J Surg* **177**: 277–281.
Rosen L, Abel ME, Gordon PH et al (1992) Practice parameters for the detection of colorectal neoplasms: supporting documentation. *Dis Colon Rectum* **35**: 391–394
Rosenberg IL (1979) The aetiology of colonic suture line recurrence. *Ann R Coll Surg* **61**: 251–257.
Rosenberg L, Palmer JR, Zauber AG et al (1991) A hypothesis: nonsteroidal anti-inflammatory drugs reduce the incidence of large-bowel cancer. *J Natl Cancer Inst* **83**: 355–358.
Rosenfield RE, Kochwa S, Kaczera Z et al (1979) Non-uniform distribution of occult blood in faeces. *Am J Clin Pathol* **71**: 204–209.
Rosenthal MD (1987) Fatty acid metabolism of isolated mammalian cells. *Prog Lipid Res* **26**: 87–124.
Ross AHMCC, Smith MA, Anderson JR & Small WP (1982) Late mortality after surgery for peptic ulcer. *N Engl J Med* **307**: 519–522.
Rossouw JE, Finnegan LP, Harlan WR et al (1995) The evolution of the Women's Health Initiative: perspective for the NIH. *J Am Med Women's Assoc* **50**: 50–55.
Rowntree AC, Allardice JT, Woods WW et al (1993) Prospective clinical trial to determine the influence of sulindac on the formation of recurrent colonic adenomatous polyps. *Br J Surg* **80**: 1477 (Abstract).
Rozen P (1992) An evaluation of rectal epithelial proliferation measurement as biomarker of risk for colorectal neoplasia and response in intervention studies. *Eur J Cancer Prev* **1**: 215–224.
Rutten AAJJL & Flake HE (1987) Influence of high dietary levels of fat on rat hepatic phase I and II biotransformation enzyme activities. *Nutr Rep Int* **36**: 109.
Ryall C (1907) Cancer infection and cancer recurrence: a danger to avoid in cancer operations. *Lancet* **ii**: 1311.
Ryall C (1908) The technique of cancer operations with reference to the danger of cancer infection. *BMJ* **2**: 1005.
Sandler RS & Sandler DP (1983) Radiation induced cancers of the colon and rectum: assessing the risks. *Gastroenterology* **84**: 51–57.
Saner FD (1946) A case of carcinoma coli in a child. *Br J Surg* **33**: 398.
Sanguedolce R, Brumarescu I, Dardanoni G et al (1995) Thymidylate synthase level and DNA-ploidy pattern as possible prognostic factors in human colorectal cancer: a preliminary study. *Anticancer Res* **15**: 901–906.
Sauer L & Bacon HE (1952) A new approach for excision of carcinoma of the lower portion of the rectum and anal canal. *Surg Gynecol Obstet* **94**: 229.
Schatzkin A (1996) Dietary prevention of colorectal cancer. In Young GP, Rozen P & Levin B (eds) *Prevention and Early Detection of Colorectal Cancer*. London: WB Saunders.
Schatzkin A, Lanza E & Ballard-Barbash R (1990) The case for a dietary intervention study of large bowel polyps. *Cancer Prev* **1**: 84–90.
Schoenberg BS & Christine BW (1979) The association of neoplasms of the colon and rectum with primary malignancies of other sites. *Am J Proctol* **25**: 41–60.
Schoenberg BS, Greenberg RA & Eisenberg H (1969) Occurrence of certain multiple primary cancers in females. *J Natl Cancer Inst* **43**: 15–32.
Schottenfeld DM, Berg JW & Bilsky B (1969) Incidence of multiple primary cancers. II: Index cancers in the stomach and lower digestive system. *J Natl Cancer Inst* **43**: 77–86.
Schreinemachers DM & Everson RB (1994) Aspirin use and

lung, colon, and breast cancer incidence in a prospective study. *Epidemiology* **5**: 138–146.

Schulten MF, Heiskell CA & Shields TW (1976) The incidence of solitary pulmonary metastases from carcinoma of the large intestine. *Surg Gynecol Obstet* **143**: 727–729.

Schussheim A, Gold DM & Levine JJ (1993) Sulindac-induced regression of adenomatous colonic polyps in a child with a history of hepatoblastoma. *J Pediatr Gastroenterol Nutr* **17**: 445–448.

Schwartz FW, Holstein H & Brocht JG (1980) Preliminary report of faecal occult blood testing in Germany. In Winawer SJ, Schottenfeld D & Sherlock P (eds) *Colorectal Cancer: Prevention, Epidemiology and Screening*, pp 267–270. New York: Raven Press.

Scott N, Sagar P, Stewart J et al (1991) p53 in colorectal cancer: clinicopathological correlation and prognostic significance. *Br J Cancer* **63**: 317–319.

Scott N, Bell SM, Sagar P et al (1993) p53 expression and K-*ras* mutation in colorectal adenomas. *Gut* **34**: 621–624

Scott N, Jackson P, al-Jaberi T et al (1995) Total mesorectal excision and local recurrence: a study of tumour spread in the mesorectum distal to rectal cancer. *Br J Surg* **82**: 1031–1033

Selby JV, Friedman GD, Quesenbery CP & Weiss NS (1992) A case–control study of screening sigmoidoscopy and mortality from colorectal cancer. *N Engl J Med* **326**: 653–657.

Sellwood RA, Kaper SWA, Burn JI & Wallace EN (1965) Circulating cancer cells: the influence of surgical operation. *Br J Surg* **52**: 69 (abstract).

Shapiro S (1992) Case–control studies of colorectal cancer mortality: is the case made for screening sigmoidoscopy? *J Natl Cancer Inst* **84**: 1546–1547.

Shepherd NA, Baxter KJ & Love SB (1995) Influence of local peritoneal involvement on pelvic recurrence and prognosis in rectal cancer. *J Clin Pathol* **48**: 849–855.

Sherlock P & Winawer SJ (1977) The role of early diagnosis in controlling large bowel cancer. *Cancer* **40**: 2609–2615.

Shibata D, Peinado MA, Ionov Y, Malkhosyan S & Perucho M (1994) Genomic instability in repeated sequences is an early somatic event in colorectal tumorigenesis that persists after transformation. *Nature Genet* **6**: 273–281.

Siba S (1983) Experience with Haemoccult screening in Hungary: a multicentre trial. *Hepatogastroenterology* **30**: 27–29.

Sidransky D, Tokino T, Hamilton SR et al (1992) Identification of *ras* oncogene mutations in the stool of patients with curable colorectal tumours. *Science* **256**: 102–105.

Silverberg E (1981) *Cancer Statistics*. New York: American Cancer Society.

Silvestrini R, D'Agnano I, Faranda A et al (1993) Flow cytometric analysis of ploidy in colorectal cancer: a multicentric experience. *Br J Cancer* **67**: 1042–1046.

Simon JB (1985) Occult blood screening for colorectal carcinoma: a critical review. *Gastroenterology* **88**: 820–837.

Simpson WC & Mayo CW (1939) The mural penetration of the carcinoma cell in the colon: anatomical and clinical study. *Surg Gynecol Obstet* **68**: 872.

Slanetz CA, Herter FP & Grinnell RS (1972) Anterior resection versus abdomino-perineal resection for cancer of the rectum and rectosigmoid. *Am J Surg* **123**: 110–117.

Slater GI, Haber RH & Aufses AH (1984) Changing distribution of carcinomas of the colon and rectum. *Surg Gynecol Obstet* **158**: 216–218.

Smiddy FG & Goligher JC (1957) Results of surgery in treatment of cancer of the large intestine. *BMJ* **i**: 793.

Smith PG & Doll R (1976) Late effects of X-irradiation in patients treated for metropathic haemorrhagia. *Br J Radiol* **49**: 224–232.

Smith Raven J, England J, Talbot IC & Bodmer W (1995) Detection of c-Ki-*ras* mutations in faecal samples from sporadic colorectal cancer patients. *Gut* **36**: 81–86.

Songster CL, Barrows GH & Jarrett DD (1980) Immunochemical detection of faecal occult blood: the faecal smear punch-disc test – a new non-invasive screening test for colo-rectal cancer. *Cancer* **45**: 1099–1102.

Sontag SJ, Durczak C, Aranha GV et al (1983) Faecal occult blood screening for colorectal cancer in a Veterans Administration hospital. *Am J Surg* **145**: 89–93.

Spagnesi MT, Tonelli F, Dolara P et al (1994) Rectal proliferation and polyp occurrence in patients with familial adenomatous polyposis after sulindac treatment. *Gastroenterology* **106**: 362–366.

Spigelman AD, Williams CB, Talbot IC, Domizio P & Phillips RKS (1989) Upper gastrointestinal cancer in patients with familial adenomatous polyposis. *Lancet* **ii**: 783–785.

Spratt JJ & Spjut HJ (1976) Prevalence and prognosis of individual clinical and pathological variables associated with colorectal carcinoma. *Cancer* **20**: 1967.

St John JB, Young GP, Alexeyeff MA & Deacon MC (1993) Evaluation of new occult blood tests for detection of colorectal neoplasia. *Gastroenterology* **104**; 1661–1668.

Stander RW (1957) Irradiation castration: a follow-up study of results in benign pelvic disease. *Obstet Gynecol* **10**: 323–329.

Staszewski J, McCall MG & Stenhouse NS (1971) Cancer mortality in 1962–66 among Polish migrants to Australia. *Br J Cancer* **25**: 599.

Steeg PS, Bevilacqua G, Kopper L et al (1998) Evidence for a novel gene associated with low tumour metastatic potential. *J Natl Cancer Inst* **80**: 200–204.

Steiner J (1865) Areolan Krebs des pickolams beweinem neunjahrlgen Knaben. *Jahrb Kitdcrh* **7**: 61–64.

Steinmetz K & Potter J (1991) Vegetables, fruit, and cancer. II: Mechanisms. *Cancer Causes Control* **2**: 427–442.

Stemmerman GN (1979) Patterns of disease among Japanese living in Hawaii. *Arch Envir Health* **20**: 260.

Stemmerman GN, Nomura AMY, Mower H & Glober G (1981) Clues to the origin of colorectal cancer. In De Cosse JJ (ed) *Large Bowel Cancer*. Edinburgh: Churchill Livingstone.

Sterchi JM (1979) Screening for colorectal cancer. *South Med J* **72**: 1144–1146.

Stewart M, Macrae FA & Williams CB (1982) Neoplasia and ureterosigmoidostomy: a colonoscopy survey. *Br J Surg* **69**: 414–416.

Stewart MJ (1931) Precancerous lesions of the alimentary canal. *Lancet* **ii**: 669–674.

Stower MJ & Hardcastle JP (1985) The results of 1115 patients with colorectal cancer treated over an 8-year period in a single hospital. *Eur J Surg Oncol* **11**: 119–123.

Stroehlein JR, Fairbanks VF, McGill DB et al (1976) Haemoccult detection of faecal occult blood quantitated by radioassay. *Dig Dis Sci* **21**: 841–844.

Stuart M, Killingback MJ, Sakker S et al (1981) Hemoccult II test: routine screening procedure for colorectal neoplasm? *Med J Aust* **i**: 629–631.

Stubbs RS (1983) The aetiology of colorectal cancer. *Br J Surg* **70**: 313–316.

Suh O, Mettlin C & Petrelli NJ (1993) Aspirin use, cancer, and polyps of the large bowel. *Cancer* **72**: 1171–1177.

Summerton J, Flynn M, Cooke T & Taylor I (1983) Bile acid receptors in colorectal cancer. *Br J Surg* **70**: 549–551.

Sun X-F, Carstensen JM, Zhang H et al (1992) Prognostic significance of cytoplasmic p53 oncoprotein in colorectal adenocarcinoma. *Lancet* **340**: 1369–1373.

Swinton NW & Pashley PF (1962) Multiple cancers of the colon and rectum. *Dis Colon Rectum* **5**: 378–380.

Takahashi T & Kajitani T (1982) Some considerations on the lateral lymphatic metastases from rectal cancer. Quoted in Goligher JC (1984) *Surgery of the Anus, Rectum and Colon*. London: Baillière Tindall.

Talbot IC, Ritchje S, Leighton MH et al (1980) The clinical significance of invasion of veins by rectal cancer. *Br J Surg* **67**: 439.

Tang R, Ho YS, You YT et al (1995) Prognostic evaluation of DNA flow cytometric and histopathologic parameters of colorectal cancer. *Cancer* **76**: 1724–1730.

Taylor HW, Boyle M, Smith SC, Bustin S & Williams NS (1993) Expression of p53 in colorectal cancer and dysplasia complicating ulcerative colitis. *Br J Surg* **80**: 442–444.

Thibodeau SN, Bren G & Schaid D (1993) Microsatellite instability in cancer of the proximal colon. *Science* **260**: 816–819.

Thomas GPIJ, Dixon MF, Smeeton NC & Williams NS (1983) Observer variation in the histological grading of rectal carcinoma. *J Clin Pathol* **36**: 385–391.

Thompson PM, Hill JT & Packham DA (1979) Colonic carcinoma at the site of ureterosigmoidostomy: what is the risk? *Br J Surg* **66**: 65.

Thornton GHM & Illingworth DG (1955) An evaluation of the benzidine test for occult blood in the faeces. *Gastroenterology* **28**: 593–605.

Thun MJ, Namboodiri MM, Heath CW Jr (1991) Aspirin use and reduced risk of colon cancer. *N Engl J Med* **325**: 1593–1596.

Thun MJ, Calle EE, Namboodiri MM et al (1992) Risk factors for fatal colon cancer in a large prospective study. *J Natl Cancer Inst* **84**: 1491–1500.

Thun MJ, Namboodiri MM, Calle EE et al (1993) Aspirin use and risk of fatal cancer. *Cancer Res* **53**: 1322–1327.

Toft Gaard C (1987) Risk of colorectal cancer after surgery for benign peptic ulceration. *Br J Surg* **74**: 513–515.

Traviesco CR, Knoepp LF & Hanley PH (1972) Multiple adenocarcinomas of the colon and rectum. *Dis Colon Rectum* **15**: 1–6.

Tsuchiya A, Ando Y, Ishii Y, Yoshida T & Abe R (1992) Flow cytometric DNA analysis in Japanese colorectal cancer: a multivariate analysis. *Eur J Surg Oncol* **18**: 585–590.

Tsuchiya A, Ando Y, Kikuchi Y et al (1995) Venous invasion as a prognostic factor in colorectal cancer. *Surg Today* **25**: 950–953.

Turjman N, Guldry C, Jaegar B & Nair PP (1982) Faecal bile acids and neutral steroids in Seventh-Day Adventists and the general population of California. In Kaspar H & Goebell H (eds) *Colon and Nutrition*, pp 291–298. Lancaster: MTP Press.

Turnbull RB, Kyle K, Watson FB & Spratt J (1967) Cancer of the colon: the influence of the no-touch isolation technique of survival rates. *Ann Surg* **166**: 420.

Uff CR & Phillips RK (1993) Effect of suture material on tumor cell adherence at sites of colonic injury. *Br J Surg* **80**: 1354.

Umpleby HC, Femor B, Symes MO & Williamson RCN (1984) Viability of exfoliated colorectal carcinoma cells. *Br J Surg* **71**: 659–663.

Urdaneta LF, Duffell D, Creevy CD & Aust JB (1966) Late development of primary carcinoma following ureterosigmoidostomy: report of three cases and literature review. *Ann Surg* **164**: 503.

Utsunomiya J, Iwama T & Hirayama R (1981) Familial large bowel cancer. In De Cosse JJ (ed) *Large Bowel Cancer*, pp 16–33. Edinburgh: Churchill Livingstone.

Vahouny GV, Satchithandams S, Lightfoot F et al (1984) Morphological disruption of colonic mucosa by free or cholestyramine-bound bile acids. *Dig Dis Sci* **29**: 432–442.

Van den Berg FM, Tigges AJ, Schipper MEI et al (1989) Expression of the nuclear oncogene p53 in colon tumours. *J Pathol* **157**: 193–199.

Vasen HFA, Mecklin JP, Watson P et al (1993) Surveillance in hereditary non-polyposis colorectal cancer: an international cooperative study of 165 families. *Dis Colon Rectum* **36**: 1–4.

Vasen HFA, Nagengast FM & Meera Khan P (1995) Interval cancers in hereditary non-polyposis colorectal cancer (Lynch syndrome). *Lancet* **345**: 1183–1184.

Vellacott KD, Amar SS & Hardcastle JD (1982) Comparison of rigid and flexible sigmoidoscopy with double contrast barium enemas. *Br J Surg* **69**: 399–400.

Vellacott KD, Roe AM & Mortensen NJMcC (1987) An evaluation of a direct access flexible fibre optic sigmoidoscopy service. *Ann R Coll Surg Engl* **69**: 149–152.

Vernick LJ & Kuller LH (1981) Cholecystectomy and right-sided colon cancer: an epidemiologic study. *Lancet* **ii**: 381–383.

Vijayan V, Ho J & Goh HS (1995) Comparison study of DNA content of primary and metastatic lymph node lesions of colorectal cancer. *Ann Acad Med Singapore* **24**: 347–352.

Vink M (1954) Local recurrence of cancer in the large bowel: a role of implantation metastases and bowel disinfection. *Br J Surg* **41**: 431.

Vogelstein B, Fearon ER, Hamilton SR et al (1988) Genetic alterations during colorectal tumour development. *N Engl J Med* **319**: 525–532.

Vogelstein B, Fearon E, Kern S et al (1989) Allelotype of colorectal carcinomas. *Science* **244**: 207–212.

Waddell WR, Ganser GF, Cerise EJ & Loughry RW (1989) Sulindac for polyposis of the colon. *Am J Surg* **157**: 175–179.

Wade TP, Comitalo JB, Andrus CH, Goodwin MN & Kaminski DL (1994) Laparoscopic cancer surgery: lessons from gallbladder cancer. *Surg Endosc* **8**: 698–701.

Walsh DCA, Wattchow DA & Wilson TG (1993) Subcutanous metastases after laparoscopic resection of malignancy. *Aust NZ J Surg* **63**: 563–565.

Wang L, Patal U, Ghosh L, Chen H-C & Banerjee S (1993) Mutation in the mn23 gene is associated with metastasis in colorectal cancer. *Cancer Res* **53**: 717–720.

Wargovich MJ, Eng VWS, Newmark HI & Bruce WR (1983) Calcium ameliorates the toxic effect of deoxycholic acid on colonic epithelium. *Carcinogenesis* **4**: 1205–1207.

Warren S & Gates O (1932) Multiple primary malignant tumours: a survey of the literature and a statistical study. *Am J Cancer* **16**: 1358–1414.

Waterhouse JAH, Muir CS, Carrea P & Powell J (eds) (1976) *Cancer Incidence in Five Continents*, Vol. 3 (IARC Scientific Publications 15). Lyon: International Agency for Research in Cancer.

Watt PCH, Patterson CC & Kennedy TI (1984) Late mortality after vagotomy and drainage for duodenal ulcer. *BMJ* **228**: 1335–1338.

Wattenberg LW (1971) Studies of polycyclic hydrocarbon hydroxylases of the intestine possibly related to cancer. *Cancer* **28**: 99–102.

Wattenberg LW (1977) Inhibition of carcinogenic effects of polycyclic hydrocarbons by benzyl isothiocyanate and related compounds. *J Natl Cancer Inst* **58**: 395–398.

Wattenberg LW (1978) Inhibition of chemical carcinogenesis. *J Natl Cancer Inst* **60**: 11–18.

Weber J (1996) Cancer surveillance recommendations adopted for HNPCC. *Lancet* **348**: 465.

Weiss W, Hanak H & Hubar A (1977) Effizienz der rektal-digitaten Untersuchung zur Früherkennung des Dick-darmkarzinoms. *Wien Klin Wochenschr* **89**: 654–656.

Welch JP (1979) Trends in the anatomic distribution of colorectal cancer. *Conn Med* **43**: 457.

Welch JP (1981) Multiple colorectal tumours: an appraisal of natural history and therapeutic options. *Am J Surg* **142**: 274–280.

Welin S, Youker J & Spratt JS (1963) The rates and patterns of growth of 375 tumours of the large intestine and rectum observed serially by double contrast enema study (Malmo technique). *AJR* **90**: 673–687.

Westhues H (1930) Uber die Enlstehung and Vermeldung des localen Rektumkarzinom-Rezidius. *Arch Klin Chir* **161**: 582.

Westhues H (1934) *Die Pathologisch-anatomischen Grundlagen der Chirurgie des Rektumkarzinomas*. Leipzig: Thieme.

Wexner SD & Cohen SM (1995) Port site metastases after laparoscopic colorectal surgery for cure of malignancy. *Br J Surg* **82**: 295–298.

Whitaker RH, Puch RCB & Dow D (1971) Colonic tumours following ureterosigmoidostomy. *Br J Urol* **43**: 562.

Williams CB (1985) Colonoscopy. *Curr Opin Gastroenterol* **1**: 54–59.

Williams NS, Dixon MF & Johnston D (1983) Reappraisal of the 5 cm rule of distal excision for carcinoma of the rectum: a study of distal intramural spread and of patients' survival. *Br J Surg* **70**: 150–154.

Williams NS, Durdey P, Quirke P et al (1985) Preoperative staging of rectal neoplasm and its impact on clinical management. *Br J Surg* **72**: 868–874.

Williams NS, Jass J & Hardcastle SH (1988) Clinicopathological assessment and staging of colorectal cancer. *Br J Surg* **78**: 648–652.

Williams RD, Yurko AA, Kerr G et al (1966) Comparison of anterior and abdomino-perineal resections for low pelvic colon and rectal carcinoma. *Am J Surg* **11**: 114–119.

Wilpart M, Mainguet P, Maskens A & Roberfroid M (1983) Mutagenicity of 12 dimethylhydrazine towards *Salmonella typhimurium*: co-mutagenic effect of secondary bile acids. *Carcinogenesis* **4**: 45–48.

Wilson JP, Hoffman GC, Baker JW, Fichett CW & Vansant JH (1994) Laparoscopic-assisted colectomy: initial experience. *Ann Surg* **219**: 732–743.

Wilson SM & Beahrs OH (1976) The curative treatment of carcinoma of the sigmoid, rectosigmoid and rectum. *Ann Surg* **183**: 556–565.

Winawer SJ (1976) Faecal occult blood testing. *Am J Dig Dis* **21**: 885.

Winawer SJ (1979) Progress report of controlled trial of screening with faecal occult blood testing. In Brodie DR (ed) *Screening and Early Detection of Colorectal Cancer* (NIH Publication 80-2075), pp 193–210. Washington: US Dept of Health, Education and Welfare.

Winawer SJ (1980) Screening for colorectal cancer: an overview. *Cancer* **45**: 1093.

Winawer SJ (1981) Screening and diagnosis. In De Cosse JJ (ed) *Large Bowel Cancer*, p 46. Edinburgh: Churchill Livingstone.

Winawer SJ (1983) Detection and diagnosis of colorectal cancer. *Cancer* **51**: 2519–2524.

Winawer SJ, Sherlock P, Schottenfeld D & Miller DG (1976) Screening for colon cancer. *Gastroenterology* **70**: 783.

Winawer SJ, Miller DG, Schottenfeld D et al (1977) Feasibility of faecal occult blood testing for detection of colorectal neoplasia. *Cancer* **40**: 2616–2619.

Winawer SJ, Andrews M, Flehinger B et al (1980a) Progress report on controlled trial of faecal occult blood testing for detection of colorectal neoplasia. *Cancer* **45**: 2959–2964.

Winawer SJ, Andrews M & Miller C (1980b) Review of screening with faecal occult blood. In Winawer SJ, Sherlock P & Schottenfeld D (eds) *Colorectal Cancer: Prevention, Epidemiology and Screening*, pp 46–62. New York: Raven Press.

Winawer SJ, Fleisher M, Baldwin M & Sherlock P (1982) Current status of faecal occult blood testing in screening for colorectal cancer. *CA* **32**: 3–15.

Winawer SJ, Schottenfeld D & Flehinger BJ (1991) Colorectal cancer screening. *J Natl Acad Sci* **83**: 243–251.

Winchester DP, Shull JH, Scanion EH et al (1980) A mass screening program for colorectal cancer using chemical testing for occult blood in the stool. *Cancer* **45**: 2955–2958.

Winde G, Gumbinger HG, Osswald H et al (1993) The NŚAID sulindac reverses rectal adenomas in colectomized patients with familial adenomatous polyposis: clinical results of a dose-finding study on rectal sulindac administration. *Int J Colorect Dis* **8**: 13–17.

Wolley RC, Schreiber K, Koss LG, Karas M & Sherman A (1982) DNA distribution in human colon carcinomas and its relationship to clinical behaviour. *J Natl Cancer Inst* **69**: 15–22.

Wood DA, Robbins GF, Zippin C, Lum D & Stearns MW Jr (1979) Staging cancer of the colon and rectum. *Cancer* **43**: 961–968.

Wood WQ & Wilkie DPD (1933) Carcinoma of rectum on anatomic pathological study. *Edinb Med J* **40**: 321–343.

Wynder EL & Reddy ES (1974) Metabolic epidemiology of colorectal cancer. *Cancer* **34**: 801–806.

Yamaguchi A, Urano T, Fushida S et al (1993) Inverse association of nm23-H1 expression by colorectal cancer with liver metastasis. *Br J Cancer* **68**: 1020–1024.

Yamazoe Y, Maetani S, Nishikawa T et al (1994) The prognostic role of the DNA ploidy pattern in colorectal cancer analysis using paraffin-embedded tissue by an improved method. *Surg Today* **24**: 30–36.

Yudkin J (1972) *Pure White and Deadly*. London: Davis–Poynter.

Yunis JJ & Soreng AL (1984) Constitutive fragile sites and cancer. *Science* **226**: 1199–1204.

Zaky SA & Hashem M (1962) Distribution of bilharzial lesions and complications in various organs: a study of 1220 autopsies of bilharzial cases. *Gros Kasr-el-Ainy Fac Med* **30**: 15.

Zaras OI, Curti G, Cooke TG et al (1994) Prognostic value of ploidy of primary tumour and nodal secondaries in colorectal cancers. *Surg Oncol* **3**: 345–349.

31

SURGICAL MANAGEMENT OF CARCINOMA OF THE COLON AND RECTUM (WITH PARTICULAR REFERENCE TO COLON CANCER)

The treatment of colorectal carcinoma is in a state of flux at present. Although surgery remains the cornerstone of therapy, the realization that the prognosis has remained static over 50 years (Dukes, 1957; Eisenberg et al, 1967; Lockhart-Mummery et al, 1976) has encouraged surgeons and oncologists to investigate the use of adjuvant therapy. Numerous controlled trials have been performed or are in progress, the results of which are now affecting management of patients. One particular problem which has an important bearing on the results of these trials is that patients are inadequately staged before being admitted to them. Major efforts are now being made to provide more precise staging criteria for colorectal cancer. With advances in technology it is possible to define the degree of spread of these tumours more accurately. Such information should not only help rationalize adjuvant therapy but also allow the surgeon to tailor the surgery to the individual patient.

PREOPERATIVE ASSESSMENT

The patient should be assessed preoperatively with two aspects in mind: fitness for treatment, and the degree of spread of the tumour.

Fitness for treatment

Assessment of the patient's fitness for treatment is similar whether the patient has a colonic or a rectal carcinoma. It involves a thorough clinical examination, paying particular attention to the respiratory and cardiovascular systems and the general nutritional state of the patient. The surgeon needs to have details of previous illness or surgery. Common diseases such as diabetes and hypertension may need attention before operation, and it is always advisable to obtain the advice of the appropriate specialist. A previous deep venous thrombosis or pulmonary embolus may require special prophylactic measures. Anaemia should be corrected by blood transfusion if necessary. For patients with rectal and left-sided colonic lesions, a careful urological assessment is necessary. A patient with prostatic problems before operation is likely to have micturition difficulties after operation, particularly if there has been a pelvic dissection. An intravenous urogram may be useful in this regard. This investigation also has the advantage in determining if a rectal or left-sided lesion has invaded one or both ureters.

The nutritional status of the patient is also important and any deficit is perhaps best corrected before surgery. Assessment depends on a detailed history and physical examination supported by a few basic measurements. Weight loss is of major importance. Changes in weight over very short periods reflect alterations in fluid balance, but changes over weeks or months indicate loss of body tissue. Assessment of weight loss relies on an accurate recall of well weight but this may be difficult in the elderly patient with colorectal cancer. However, using recalled well weight is evidently more accurate than using standard tables of predicted weight for height (Morgan et al, 1980). Physical examination should aim to estimate the nutritional reserves of the patient; signs of hypermetabolism should be looked for, and the state of hydration needs assessment. Fat stores are estimated by gently pinching the skinfolds on the arms, back and abdomen to feel the amount of subcutaneous fat present. Muscle wasting is best observed in muscles around the scapula and in the temporal fossa, the interosseus muscles and the muscle bellies on the upper arm. Hydration needs to be assessed by examining for oedema in the lower legs and assessment of skin turgor. Nutritional assessment is incomplete without a few basic measurements. Plasma urea and electrolyte measurements are invaluable in assessing electrolyte and acid–base balance. Plasma albumin estimation may be useful in that a low concentration reflects protein losses, alterations in protein turnover and changes in intravascular distribution of albumin and water (Golden, 1982).

The above assessment should detect all patients with marked nutritional deficits. Lesser degrees of deficiency, however, will not be as evident, and this is relevant to patients with colorectal carcinoma who often do not lose weight. Much effort has been expended on assessing the values of nutritional markers so that subclinical malnutrition can be detected. The serum concentrations of pre-albumin and retinol-binding protein, immunological assessment, calorimetry and body composition analysis have all been investigated. Most of these measurements need complex and expensive equipment and there is considerable debate about their value. The busy surgeon will still have to rely on clinical acumen to decide which patients with colorectal carcinoma have nutritional deficits and which of them will require preoperative nutrition (see Chapter 4).

Assessment of spread

Assessment of the degree of spread of the tumour has previously relied on clinical examination together with simple radiographic evaluation. Recent advances in imaging, however, have allowed a more comprehensive preoperative assessment to be made.

Clinical examination

Clinical examination should include an attempt to determine if metastases have occurred. The presence of hepatomegaly (with or without jaundice) suggests liver involvement, particularly if the contour of the liver is irregular and hard. Ascites is strongly suggestive of peritoneal seedings. Multiple skin nodules particularly at the umbilicus (Sister Joseph's nodule) are diagnostic of dissemination. Enlarged lymph nodes in the axillae or supraclavicular fossa are occasionally present in a patient with widespread malignancy.

In the case of a colonic lesion it may be possible to

palpate the tumour per abdomen and useful information about its fixity to local structures may be obtained. Rectal examination may be of use in colonic tumours since sometimes a tumour in the sigmoid colon may be palpable through the rectal wall or – perhaps of greater importance – metastases in the pouch of Douglas may be detected.

Rectal examination is important in attempting to assess the degree of local spread of rectal carcinoma, although its accuracy in achieving this aim is debatable (Williams et al, 1985). Ideally this examination should be conducted under anaesthesia. Although it is usually possible to determine if a growth is fixed or mobile on digital examination, it is impossible in the case of a fixed tumour to be sure whether this is due to an inflammatory reaction or neoplastic infiltration.

Chest radiography

Chest radiography is mandatory to exclude secondary pulmonary lesions and rarely osseous metastases.

Intravenous urogram

The value of an intravenous urogram (IVU) is debatable. Some surgeons always require one in patients with lesions of the left colon and rectum (Cameron, 1977), while others believe that the information obtained is of such little value that a routine IVU is not justified (Phillips et al, 1983; Kettlewell, 1988). We take the view that an IVU can be useful and we recommend its use in cases where one or both ureters might be at risk. In practice, the number of tumours where there may be ureteric involvement is small, and these cases can usually be first identified using ultrasound. An IVU tells us whether there is encroachment of the tumour on to the ureter, and if so its degree of involvement can be assessed. Perhaps more importantly, it shows whether the contralateral kidney is functioning satisfactorily, information that is of crucial importance if a nephrectomy becomes necessary during the operation. Although similar information can be obtained by on-table techniques, these require prior organization and expenditure of time. We believe it is preferable for the surgeon to be forewarned so the scope of the operation can be planned well in advance.

Ultrasound examination

In patients with colorectal cancer it is now routine to assess the presence of liver metastases preoperatively by ultrasonography. Using the grey-scale machines, accuracy of detection is quoted to be approximately 85% (Lamb and Taylor, 1982). Our own experience has been somewhat less encouraging (Williams et al, 1985): false-positive rates were high, thus although specificity and accuracy were 86% and 80% respectively, sensitivity was only 57% (Table 31.1).

It is generally accepted that bowel gas will interfere with or completely prevent ultrasound scanning in approximately 10–15% of patients; the wider use and improved resolution of real-time scanners has greatly helped to reduce this problem (Figure 31.1).

All studies attempting to identify liver metastases are hampered by the fact that imaging is compared with laparotomy findings. The surgeon invariably underestimates the presence of overt liver metastases at operation. Thus Goligher (1941) found that of 31 patients who were judged to have a normal liver at laparotomy and subsequently came to postmortem examination within 1 month of operation, five (16%) had deep-seated hepatic metastases.

However, with careful bimanual palpation surgeons can improve their ability to detect overt hepatic metastases. Thus Gray (1980) had a false-positive rate of 8% and a false-negative rate of 6%, and Hogg and Pack (1955) had an overall accuracy of 95%. Both of these studies were of particular interest since they compared the findings at operation with those at post-mortem. Another important defect of studies designed to assess the accuracy of imaging is the fact that the liver undoubtedly contains metastases that are too small for the surgeon to detect no matter how thorough the examination (Finlay et al, 1982). Such 'occult' metastases are unlikely to be seen on ultrasound examination.

It is appropriate at this point to mention the use of intraoperative ultrasound examination of the liver. We used this technique in a consecutive series of 50 patients with a primary colorectal carcinoma (Johnston et al, 1989). Using a specially designed T-shaped 5 MHz probe we were able to detect 10 patients with hepatic metastases greater than 0.5 cm

Table 31.1 Detection of liver metastases by ultrasound and CT scan in 45 patients with rectal cancer.

	Sensitivity (%)	*Specificity (%)*	*Accuracy (%)*
Ultrasound	57	86	80
CT scan	100	90	97

$P < 0.05$.
From Williams et al (1985).

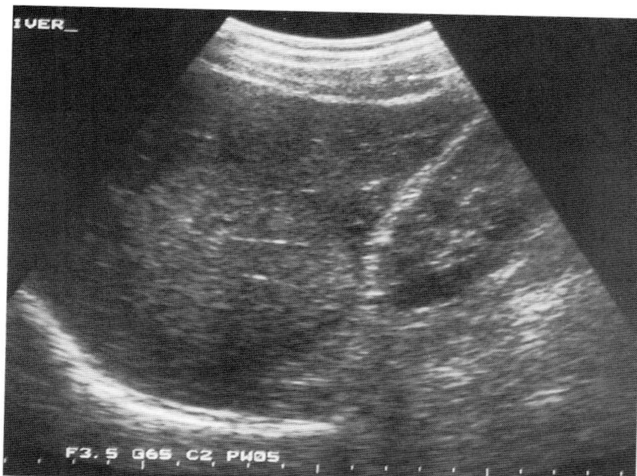

Figure 31.1 Ultrasound scan of liver showing large metastasis from a primary colonic tumour.

diameter (Figure 31.2). Preoperative ultrasound and computed tomographic scans confirmed the presence of metastases in only seven of these patients, thus indicating the greater accuracy of the intra-operative technique. Others have since confirmed the high sensitivity and specificity of intra-operative ultrasonography (Boldrini et al, 1987; Russo et al, 1989; Olsen, 1990; Machi et al, 1991; Charnley et al, 1991; Paul et al, 1994). Although it has been recommended for use routinely during all resections for colorectal tumours, its use is justified only if it changes treatment policy (Stone et al, 1994). It cannot detect metastases less than 5 mm diameter (Paul et al, 1996). It remains to be seen, therefore, how this technique will influence management of the disease in the future, but at present it is only an essential tool when liver resection is contemplated for metastases (Clarke et al, 1989; Parker et al, 1989; Rafaelsen et al, 1995).

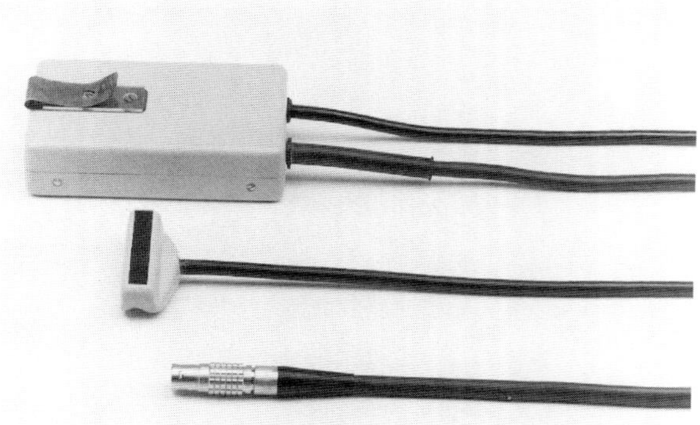

Figure 31.2 Ultrasound probe for intraoperative detection of liver metastases.

Ultrasound is now also being used to assess the degree of local spread of rectal carcinoma (Hildebrandt and Feifel, 1985; Romano et al, 1985; Benyon et al, 1986a,b; Anderson et al, 1994). Using an ultrasound probe designed originally for urological investigation, it is possible to determine the extent of spread through the rectal wall. The rectum exhibits a five-layer pattern which is composed of reflection at tissue interfaces as well as from tissue layers (Figure 31.3):

1. A bright reflection from the interface with the mucosa.
2. A hypoechoic layer from deep mucosa.
3. A hyperechoic layer from sub-mucosa. A bright interface from the muscularis mucosae may contribute to this layer, which also appears thicker sonographically than it is histologically. This is due to a prominent interface reflection from between the submucosa and the muscularis propria extending into the muscle layer (Kimmey et al, 1989). The thickness of the interface reflection relates to the axial resolution of the transducer.
4. A hypoechoic layer from the muscularis propria layer. With high-resolution transducers (10 MHz or above), the fascia between the inner circular and outer longitudinal layer may be visible, so that this layer appears split into two.
5. A bright reflection from the interface between the muscularis propria and adventitia (Bartram and Reznek, 1996).

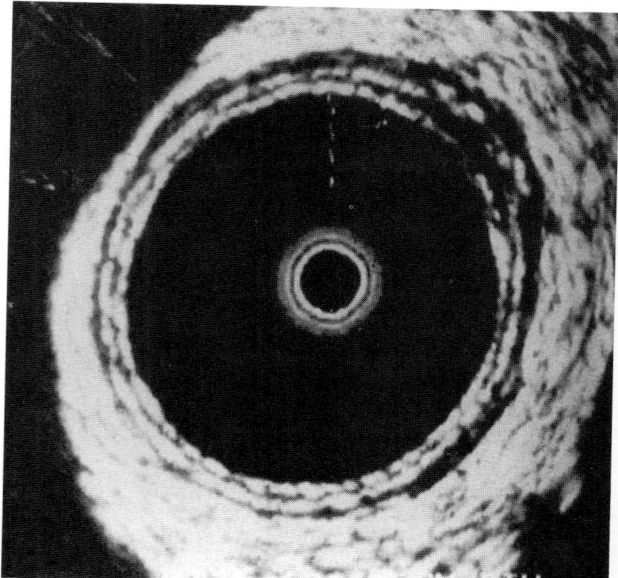

Figure 31.3 Endoluminal rectal ultrasound. Normal scan showing probe in centre of rectum and five layers of rectal wall.

Tumours can therefore be T-staged according to their depth of penetration through these layers. They are poorly reflective and seen as a hypoechoic mass (Figure 31.4). A T_2 lesion involves the fourth echopoor muscularis propria layer becoming a T_3 lesion when this layer is breached. In the early stages, this is seen as interruption of the fifth bright interface with small peg-like projections out into the perirectal fat.

Comparisons with histological staging suggest a 79–96% accuracy for endosonographic T-staging (Goldman et al, 1991; Thaler et al, 1994; Hildebrandt et al, 1994). Lesions low in the rectal ampulla may be incorrectly staged if not visualized at right-angles by the ultrasound beam. T_2 lesions may be overstaged owing to an inflammatory response around the tumour (Katsura et al, 1992) which cannot be distinguished sonographically from tumour invasion.

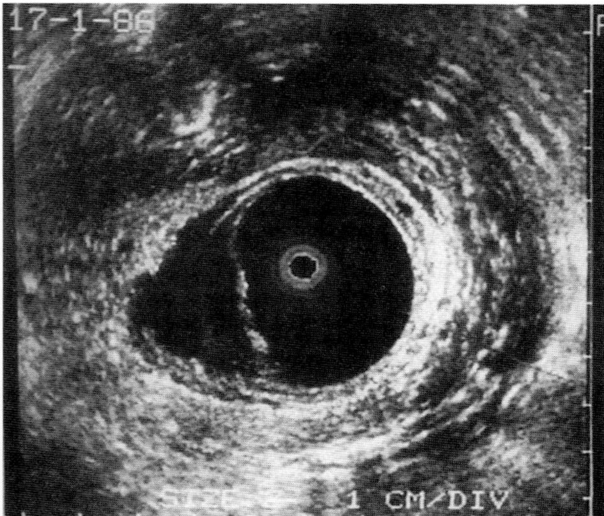

Figure 31.4 Endoluminal rectal ultrasound showing rectal cancer on right lateral wall invading through all layers of the rectal wall.

Bladder and prostatic involvement can be demonstrated, but lymph node involvement and spread within the pelvic cavity cannot yet be clearly identified. Although enlarged lymph nodes can be detected and hypoechogenicity is suggestive of metastatic invasion, the investigator cannot be sure that the image is not due to non-specific inflammation (Hildebrandt et al, 1990; Solomon et al, 1994; Detry et al, 1996). Similarly, microscopic invasion cannot be ruled out in nodes that appear normal on scanning.

Despite the drawbacks some authors have found the technique to be more accurate than computed tomography in the assessment of rectal wall penetration (Table 31.2). However, it should be noted that radiotherapy increases the reflectivity of the primary tumour and renders sonographic staging less accurate (Glaser et al, 1993). The technique of endoluminal ultrasound has been considerably refined and can be used during colonoscopy to assess the depth of invasion of colonic tumours (Aibe, 1984; Hildebrandt et al, 1990).

Computed tomography

Conventional computed tomography (CT) of the liver is very accurate in the detection of liver metastases greater than 1.5 cm diameter (Levitt et al,

Table 31.2 Accuracy of the assessment of rectal wall penetration by endorectal sonography and computed tomography.

Principal investigators	*n*	*Sensitivity (%)*	*Specificity (%)*	*PPV*	*NPV*
Endorectal sonography					
Romano et al (1985)	23	86.7	100	100	80
Benyon et al (1986b)	42	94	87	97	78
Rifkin and Wechsler (1986)	81	83	84	76	90
Hildebrandt et al (1990)		100	75	92.5	100
Goldman et al (1991)	32	90	67	82	81
Herzog et al (1993)	87	98.3	75	89.2	95.4
Computed tomography					
Romano et al (1985)	23	86.7	100	100	80
Benyon et al (1986b)	42	86	62	91	50
Rifkin and Wechsler (1986)	81	55	79	64	50
Hildebrandt et al (1990)		91.9	33.3	80.9	57.1
Goldman et al (1991)	32	67	27	60	33
Herzog et al (1993)	87	68.9	86.2	90.9	58.1

All data are percentages. PPV, positive predictive value; NPV, negative predictive value.

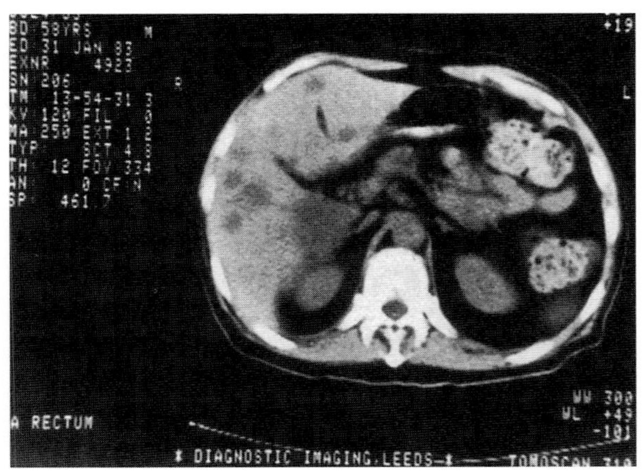

Figure 31.5 CT scan of liver showing multiple metastases from primary colonic cancer.

1977) (Figure 31.5). Overall accuracy in our own series of rectal carcinomas was 97% when the findings on the scan were compared with those at laparotomy (Williams et al, 1985). Similar results were obtained by others (Thoeni et al, 1981). The accuracy of the scan depends on the thickness of the slices taken (12 mm in our study) and whether it is enhanced or not. One advantage of CT scanning is that a biopsy or aspiration needle can be guided to the site of the suspected hepatic metastasis and a tissue diagnosis can be made.

The introduction of helical CT scanning has significantly improved visualization of liver metastases by making acquisition of the images more rapid during intravenous contrast injection. Ideally, the liver should be scanned before the equilibrium phase of contrast redistribution between the intravascular and extravascular compartments. The attenuation differences between normal parenchyma and metastases will then be maximal, whereas afterwards these differences may be minimal and metastatic disease may not be visualized. Using the helical CT technique, 100 mL of non-ionic contrast is injected intravenously with the first slice at 40 s after the start of injection. Scans are performed at 5–8 mm collimation at a pitch of 1 or 1.3 (Bartram and Reznek 1996).

It is possible using a technique known as planimetry to quantify from the CT images the percentage of the liver occupied by metastatic disease. Such a method was devised by our group and applied to patients with metastases from colorectal cancer (Purkiss and Williams, 1992). We obtained contiguous hepatic CT images at a slice thickness of 0.9–1.8 cm. Contrast enhancement was performed for all patients and a conventional CT machine was used (Phillips Tomoscan 350, Phillips Eindhoven, Holland). A digitizing tablet and mouse (TDS LC series II, Terminal Display Systems Ltd, Blackburn, UK) were used to plot a series of points on the perimeters of liver and metastases from the CT images (Figure 31.6a,b). A personal computer was used to calculate the cross-sectional areas of liver (L) and metastases (M) for each sequential slice of the scan. Percentage hepatic replacement (PHR) was calculated using the formula

$$PHR = (M/L) \times 100\%.$$

We demonstrated a linear correlation between the natural logarithm of PHR and survival in those

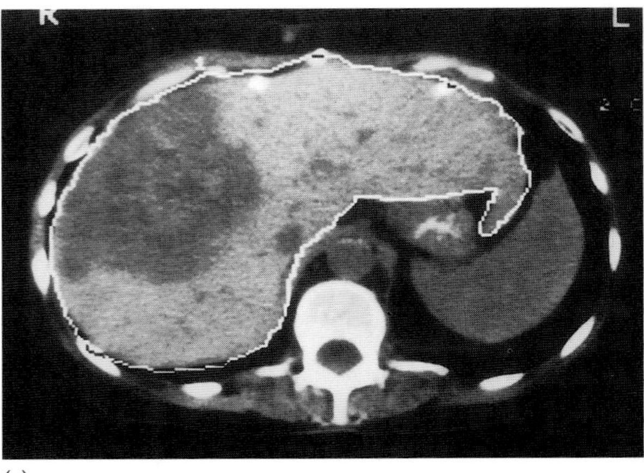

(a)

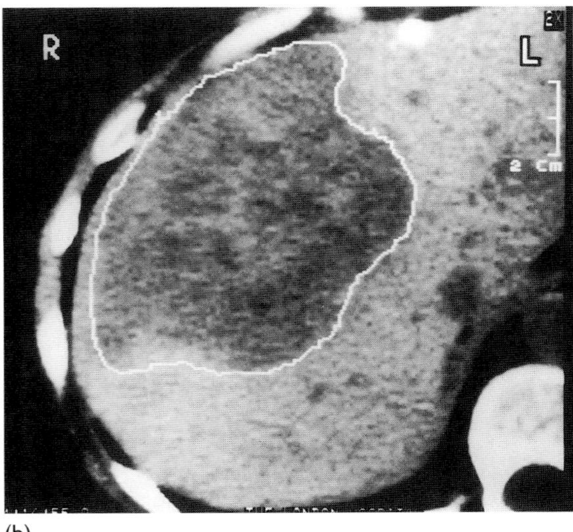

(b)

Figure 31.6a,b Technique of planimetry to measure percentage hepatic replacement (PHR). The perimeters of the liver (a) and the metastasis (b) are drawn around on each CT slice. The cross-sectional areas of liver and metastasis are calculated by the computer and the sums used to calculate PHR.

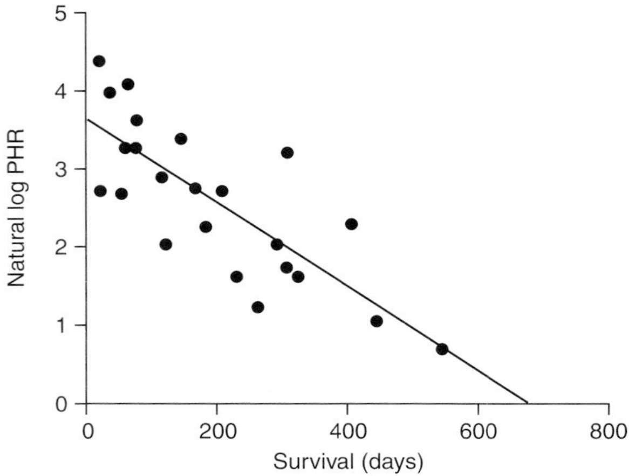

Figure 31.7 Plot of percentage hepatic replacement (PHR) as determined by planimetry and the survival of patients, from CT examination of the liver for patients without extrahepatic disease ($r = -0.76$; $P < 0.001$) (Purkiss and Williams, 1992).

patients without extrahepatic disease (Figure 31.7). This technique is thus useful in accurately determining the amount of liver occupied by metastases and may have a future particularly in studies assessing the effect of therapy on such disease.

Metastases smaller than 1.5 cm – so-called occult metastases – have been detected preoperatively using conventional CT, but their presence could only be confirmed by follow-up scans at regular intervals after operation (Finlay et al, 1982). The false-positive rate on the initial scans was 33% (IG Finlay, personal communication, 1985), and such inaccuracy makes conventional CT of little clinical value for the detection of occult metastases. Whether helical CT will improve the detection of these smaller metastases remains to be seen.

Despite this relative inability to detect very small liver metastases, CT seems to be superior to conventional ultrasound (Wernecke et al, 1991); ultrasound, however, is superior to radio-isotope scans (Bryan et al, 1977; Finlay et al, 1982; Williams et al, 1985). Both ultrasound and CT techniques are nevertheless complementary. Technetium-99m sulphur colloid scans are now no longer employed for routine detection of metastases. Pelvic CT has also been used for the detection of local spread of rectal cancer (Figure 31.8). However, individual bowel wall layers are not visible on CT, so that staging of T_2 and early T_3 tumours is less accurate than endosonography (Goldman et al, 1991). CT is most helpful in defining pelvic spread of rectal tumours. Its accuracy, as with most imaging techniques, depends on the available equipment and the skill and experience of the operator (Table 31.3).

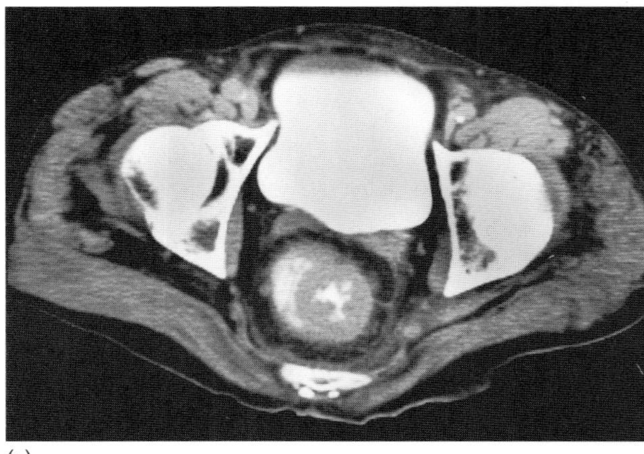

(a)

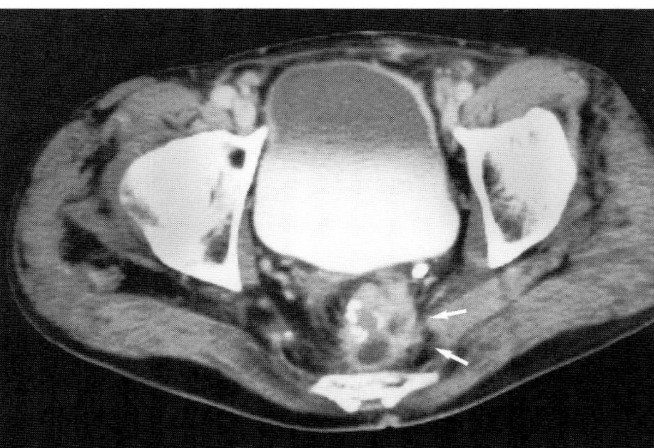

(b)

Figure 31.8a,b Pelvic CT scans of rectal carcinoma. (a) Nodularity in pelvic rectal fat indicative of extrarectal spread. (b) Rectal carcinoma has extended into the surrounding tissues and is invading the pelvic side wall.

Table 31.3 Assessment of tumour penetration depth by computed tomography.

Principal investigators	*n*	*Accuracy (%)*
Dixon et al (1981)	47	77
Thoeni et al (1981)	39	92
Zaubauer et al (1981)	11	100
van Waes et al (1983)	21	81
Grabbe et al (1985)	155	79
Thompson et al (1986)	25	79
Herzog et al (1993)	87	74.7

There is general agreement that CT can detect extensive spread more accurately than clinical examination. Nicholls et al (1982) showed that pathologically determined extensive spread was correctly demonstrated by CT in 89% of cases compared with 53% as assessed on clinical examination (mean of three examiners). Using more modern equipment we were able to detect minor spread with a fair degree of accuracy. Our overall accuracy rate for all depths of spread was 93% (Williams et al, 1985). Computed tomography also has the advantage (unlike digital palpation) of enabling all rectal cancers to be assessed irrespective of their position in the rectum. We have also used CT to determine whether fixation of a rectal tumour was caused by neoplastic infiltration or by inflammation.

When using pelvic CT to detect extrarectal spread, contrast medium is administered to demarcate the large bowel and intravenous contrast is used to differentiate vessels from lymph nodes. Bowel cleansing with gas insufflation of the colon has been recommended to define colonic tumours (Amin et al, 1996). Cancers appear as an irregular focal mass with some enhancement. CT allows accurate measurement of the tumour mass. The radial extent may be categorized as:

- confined to the lumen and bowel wall
- spread through the wall into the perirectal fat but not invading the perirectal fascia
- invading the perirectal fascia but not other pelvic structures
- involving either sacrum/coccyx, bladder, prostate, seminal vesicles, vagina, uterus, pelvic side wall, pelvic floor musculature or ureter.

Enlarged lymph nodes can also be visualized on CT but (as with ultrasound examination) it is not possible to determine if the enlargement is due to malignant infiltration (Table 31.4). Gross enlargement suggests malignant infiltration, but in the pelvis lymph node enlargement greater than 1.5 cm can be reactive. The maximum short-axis diameter of pelvic nodes is 10 mm (Vinnicombe et al, 1995). Nodes <10 mm are probably normal, those 10–15 mm are equivocal, and those >15 mm are abnormal. The size and number of nodes should be recorded:

- within the perirectal fascia
- outside the perirectal fascia
- along the internal iliac chain
- along the external iliac chain
- nodal groups around the aorta and IVC (Bartram and Reznek, 1996).

The overall accuracy of CT is in the range 65–75% for T-staging and 25–73% for N- (node) staging (Mehta et al, 1994). Endorectal ultrasound is more accurate for early T-staging and in defining mesorectal nodes, but is less accurate in advanced tumours as the side wall of the pelvis is not seen and a stenotic lesion may prevent a complete examination. Ultrasound will also miss those nodes around major vessels which are present in about 14% of tumours localized to the bowel wall.

Table 31.4 Assessment of lymph node metastases by computed tomography.

Principal investigators	*n*	*Sensitivity (%)*	*Specificity (%)*
Dixon et al (1981)	47	36	96
Zaubauer et al (1981)	11	100	100
Grabbe et al (1985)	154	34	92
Thompson et al (1986)	25	22	75

Magnetic resonance imaging

Nuclear magnetic resonance imaging (MRI) has recently been introduced to assess the pelvic spread of rectal cancer. A variety of scanning techniques can be used which map out the hydrogen nuclei density and molecular environment. Most studies have used body coil techniques for image acquisition, the results of which are summarized in Table 31.5. The reports with high accuracy rates tend to suffer from low patient numbers and a predominance of advanced tumours. Studies with over 30 patients show accuracy figures of 48–80%. In all studies two problems were identified: (1) bowel wall layers, and by extension breaches of the serosa, were not clearly seen; and (2) lymph nodes involved by tumour lacked any characteristic MRI features (Hadfield et al, 1997). It is hoped that the use of endorectal coils will improve the signal-to-noise ratio which is a feature of body coil techniques (Mehta et al, 1994). However, at present MRI cannot be recommended for use in the staging of rectal cancer.

Arteriography

Occasionally an arteriogram may be useful. Hepatic metastases derive their blood supply mainly from the hepatic artery. Hepatic arteriography, preferably using the digital vascular imaging technique, can demonstrate very small metastases. Its main indication, however, is to exclude portal vein involvement and the presence of anomalous vessels such as a right hepatic artery from the superior mesenteric artery, should hepatic resection, embolization or hepatic arterial infusions be considered (Bartram, 1985).

Dynamic hepatic scintigraphy

Dynamic hepatic scintigraphy has been described as a method of enhancing diagnostic specificity and

Table 31.5 Results of published series of magnetic resonance imaging staging using MRI body coil techniques.

		Accuracy (%)		*Detection of involved lymph nodes*		
Reference	*n*	*Overall*	*T-stage*	*Accuracy (%)*	*Sensitivity (%)*	*Specificity (%)*
Hodgman et al (1986)	27	59		39	13	88
Butch et al (1986)	16	94		94		
Guinet et al (1990)	19	79		84	40	100
Waizer et al (1991)	13	77				
Okizuka et al (1993)	33		88	88	57	95
Ou (1992)	35	74				
Golfieri et al (1993)	18	44		83	57	100
McNicholas et al (1994)	20	95		95		
Cova et al (1994)	22	67		90	89	92
Thaler et al (1994)	34	48	82	60	36	91
Kusunoki et al (1994)	33	88		58	40	

From Hadfield et al, 1997.

sensitivity of hepatic imaging (Sarper et al, 1981; Wraight et al, 1982). It is based on the premise that when tumours develop in the liver they are dependent for growth and viability on arterial blood. This produces an altered flow pattern associated with an increased proportion of arterial blood perfusing the liver (Breedis and Young, 1953). Using a scintigraphic method it is possible to assess the ratio of arterial flow to total hepatic blood flow and the hepatic perfusion index (HPI) can be calculated (Fleming et al, 1981; Sarper et al, 1981; Carter et al, 1996). Leveson et al (1985) used this technique for prospective assessment of the liver in 150 patients with gastrointestinal cancer, 112 of whom had a colorectal neoplasm. A group of 100 patients with no evidence of overt hepatic metastases at laparotomy were followed prospectively over a 12-month period. At one year the specificity and sensitivity of HPI in identifying patients who subsequently developed liver metastases were 72% and 96% respectively. The authors thus concluded that not only could the technique detect established metastases, but it could also identify patients who harbour occult metastases. Unfortunately, repeat studies from the same centre with longer follow-up periods cast doubt on the initial promise of HPI (Finan, 1990). Both Ballentyne et al (1990) and Carter et al (1996) also found that HPI was a sensitive technique in detecting established metastases, but long-term studies to assess its accuracy for micrometastases were not available. Thus the final verdict has not yet been passed on the use of HPI.

Monoclonal antibodies

Considerable research is being focused on the development of monoclonal antibodies specifically directed against the patient's tumour. Eventually it is hoped to combine these antibodies with chemotherapeutic agents and thus provide a form of targeted therapy; initial work, however, is directed to labelling the antibodies with radio-isotope so that the tumour and its metastases can be visualized by external photoscanning. Numerous groups are involved in this research and several have chosen colorectal cancer as their model (Mach et al, 1983; Zalcberg et al, 1983; Armitage et al, 1984; Rilinger et al, 1991; Yamaguchi et al, 1991; Yiu et al, 1991; Granowska et al, 1993; Behr et al, 1995). Although considerable progress has been made, the antibodies produced so far have not been sufficiently specific for routine clinical use.

Positron emission tomography (PET)

This is a relatively non-invasive scanning method that has recently been developed to study regional tissue function. Gamma-ray (positron-emitting) radio-isotopes are used to label biochemical or pharmaceutical compounds of interest, which are then introduced into the body and their spatial distribution is measured by external radiation detectors. The image thus obtained can be considered as *in vivo* autoradiography. Although PET can be used as a simple imaging device for detection, the aim is to measure biological differences between tumours and normal tissue. The technique has been used for the detection of hepatic metastases from colorectal cancer, as such tumours have been shown to have an increased uptake of 2-deoxyglucose (Strauss et al, 1989). ^{18}F-labelled 2-fluoro-2-deoxyglucose (FDG) has been the isotope most commonly used for colorectal tumour detection.

Early studies suggest that PET is a very accurate method of imaging metastases, and may have a role in the early detection of local recurrence in rectal cancer. However, it remains to be seen whether it will enter into routine clinical practice (Bohdiewicz et al, 1995).

Carcinoembryonic antigen and acute phase proteins

Preoperative serum concentrations of carcinoembryonic antigen (CEA) reflect the extent of tumour spread (Lewi et al, 1984; Logerfo and Herter, 1975; Herrera et al, 1976; Wanebo et al, 1978a). In a study by Lewi et al (1984) only 25% of patients who underwent curative surgery had elevated CEA values compared with 56% of those who received palliative treatment. Similarly 25% of patients with Dukes' B or C tumours had elevated preoperative CEA values compared with 70% of patients with Dukes' D lesions.

In our own study (Williams et al, 1985) a CEA level of over 45 ng/L was associated with extensive local spread or overt hepatic metastases, or both. Thus a serum CEA concentration of this value in the absence of CT or ultrasonographic evidence of local spread very strongly suggests that the patient has hepatic metastases.

Despite its ability to detect tumour burden there is some dispute as to whether preoperative serum CEA evaluation is a valuable guide to prognosis. In the study by Wanebo et al (1978a), 78% of patients with a CEA level of less than 5 μg/L were disease-free 30 months after curative resection of a Dukes' B tumour compared with 44% of patients with elevated levels. Similar findings were evident with Dukes' C lesions. Lewi et al (1984), on the other hand, were unable to relate preoperative levels with prognosis and explained their findings on the inability of serum CEA assessment to detect patients with occult metastases; as we have seen, these are patients who may have favourable lesions at operation and on conventional pathological examination but who die from hepatic metastases at an early stage after operation.

Certain acute phase proteins, in particular α_1-glycoprotein and C-reactive protein, have been shown to be useful in the detection of local spread (Durdey et al, 1984). They may also assist in discrimination between tumours that are fixed or partially fixed by an inflammatory reaction and those that are fixed by malignant infiltration. It would appear, however, that these serum markers have their greatest value in clarifying the findings obtained by imaging and can rarely be interpreted accurately in isolation.

Detection of synchronous neoplasms

Synchronous carcinomas occur in 3–9% of patients with a primary colorectal carcinoma whereas the incidence of synchronous adenoma may be as high as 30% (Travieso et al, 1972; Ekelund and Pihl, 1974; Lasser, 1978; Reilly et al, 1982; Cunliffe et al, 1984; Kaibara et al, 1984; Chu et al, 1986; Finan et al, 1987, Greig and Miller, 1989). Since these lesions (especially polyps) may be missed at operation, authors in the past have recommended preoperative barium enema supplemented by peroperative colonoscopy in all cases of colorectal cancer (Deddish and Hertz, 1955; Bacon and Peale, 1956).

In a previous era barium enema was performed by the single-contrast method and it is perhaps not surprising therefore that Deddish and Hertz (1955) found it was an unsatisfactory technique for the detection of polyps. This is the reason they supported the use of routine peroperative colonoscopy as advocated by Bacon and Peale (1956). The latter technique, however, was rather crude in that a rigid sterile sigmoidoscope was passed into the open end of bowel after resection of the carcinoma and before the anastomosis was completed. This was far from satisfactory; not only was a limited length of colon visualized, but there was inevitable spillage of faeces with a high risk of sepsis (Kleinfeld and Gump, 1960). Fortunately, with improvements in radiological techniques, in particular the advent of double-contrast barium enema and also the introduction of the colonoscope, it is rarely necessary to perform peroperative examination of the bowel.

The policy in many units is still that all patients have a double-contrast barium enema before operation (Figure 31.9). This applies particularly to patients with distal sigmoid lesions and rectal lesions, which are often diagnosed on sigmoidoscopy and these patients therefore may not routinely undergo a diagnostic radiological examination. If a carcinoma or a polyp is detected or the findings are equivocal the patient is submitted to colonoscopy.

It is our belief that a colonoscopy should be performed preoperatively in all cases, and only if a complete examination is unsuccessful should a barium enema be performed; however, it must be said that this view is not accepted by all (Durdey et al, 1987). The colon proximal to a tumour cannot always be visualized satisfactorily by either barium enema or colonoscopy, particularly if the bowel lumen is constricted by the tumour. Although failure to examine the proximal colon is stated to be a problem in 50% of cases (Finan et al, 1987; Tate et al, 1988), we have found the incidence to be nearer to 25%. In these cases a careful palpation of the bowel at operation is required, with all its accepted limitations; and if doubt exists, ideally a peroperative colonoscopic examination should be performed.

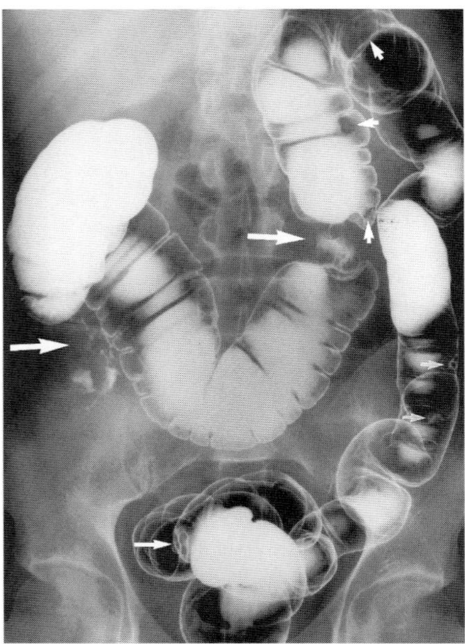

Figure 31.9 Double-contrast barium enema showing two large synchronous carcinomas (large arrows), a large polyp in the sigmoid (long arrow) and several smaller polyps (small arrows).

The latter is best achieved after peroperative colonic irrigation (Dudley et al, 1980). In patients in whom a synchronous tumour cannot be palpated or a peroperative colonoscopy has not been performed, it is essential to carry out a colonoscopy within 6 months of the operation.

Conclusions

Considerable progress has been made in the preoperative assessment of colorectal cancer. It is not yet clear, however, what impact such careful staging will have on clinical management. More research is required on larger numbers of patients, in particular concentrating on the new methods of imaging; only by so doing can we hope to see an improvement in survival. No matter how accurate investigations such as MRI and endoluminal ultrasound are, it is unlikely that all hospitals will have easy access to such facilities and associated expertise and some may argue that their provision is not cost-effective. It may be argued that availability of specialized investigative facilities is a reason for referral to centres of excellence, but because of the high incidence of the disease such an arrangement would be impractical and largely unsupported. It appears, therefore, that in many hospitals reliance will still have to be on clinical examination supported by routine radiology, ultrasound examination and perhaps computed tomography of the liver.

In response to a national cancer appraisal scheme, we in Birmingham have created a *multidisciplinary rapid-access facility* for the diagnoisis and management of colorectal cancer. The team consists of five surgeons, two support gastroenterologists, two oncologists (one with a special interest in radiotherapy), two dedicated radiologists, two histopathologists, two Macmillan nurses and stomacare nurses/counsellors. Patients with symptoms are seen within a week. Those with suspicious symptoms receive fast-track endoscopy or radiology within a week. All radiology and histopathology is reviewed on a weekly basis before the clinic so that the nursing staff are aware who will be attending and what form of counselling will be needed. Case conferences provide an excellent forum for undergraduate teaching and postgraduate training. At the end of the weekly clinic there is a journal club. All patient data is entered into an audit. There are protocols of management, patient information booklets and on-going research. There are parallel clinics for individuals found to have inflammatory bowel disease or family cancer syndromes, oncology clinics for treatment, and a functional bowel disease clinic. There are close links with palliative care.

In order to improve the assessment of patients with colorectal carcinoma, the United Kingdom Coordinating Committee for Cancer Research (UKCCCR) set up a working party in 1988 with the aim of standardizing the clinical and pathological parameters that need to be recorded. The aim was to produce practical recommendations which could be applied throughout the country, in most hospitals. The committee examined the clinical assessment of patients during the preoperative and operative periods together with pathological criteria. This was subsequently updated in 1996 and the conclusions concerning the preoperative assessment of patients with colorectal carcinoma are listed in Table 31.6. It should be emphasized that when staging a patient with this disease the preoperative assessment must not be taken in isolation but must be considered in conjunction with the operative and pathological findings.

Selection of patients for operation

The general philosophy in the treatment of colorectal cancer is that nearly all patients should be considered for operation. Even if the patient has metastases, removal of the primary tumour will usually alleviate some of the symptoms. If the primary tumour cannot be removed, operation may allow a short-circuiting manoeuvre to be performed

Table 31.6 Preoperative clinical assessment: recommendations of the UKCCCR Sub-Committee on Staging of Colorectal Cancer (1996).

1–5 are applicable to rectal cancer only

1. *Palpation* should be performed in the conscious state, and under anaesthetic only if it is deemed that an adequate examination is not possible with the patient awake.
2. *The distance of the lower margin of the tumour from the anal verge* should be determined using a rigid sigmoidoscope with the patient conscious and lying in the left lateral position.
3. *Circumferential involvement.* The number and position of quadrants of the bowel circumference which are involved should be indicated.
4. *Fixity.* Fixity on palpation should be classified as:
   (a) mobile (confined within the wall)
   (b) tethered (extending through the wall and partially fixed)
   (c) fixed (to adjacent structures and immobile).
   Examination under anaesthesia may be necessary here.
5. *Assessment of local spread by scanning techniques.*
   Whenever available, computerized tomography (CT), magnetic resonance imaging (MRI), rectal endosonography or endoluminal MRI should be used to assess the degree of local spread if the tumour feels fixed or is very large, with abdominal CT performed as part of the same examination.
   Rectal endosonography should be used if local excision is being considered.
6. *Histological grade of tumour.*
   (a) The biopsy should be stated as being adenocarcinoma or not.
   (b) The degree of differentiation should be classified as 'poor' or 'other'
7. *Assessment of lung fields.* A routine chest X-ray should be obtained and the presence of any pulmonary metastases noted. If there is indeterminate abnormality on chest X-ray, CT or MRI scanning should be considered.
8. *Detection of liver metastases.*
   (a) The liver should be scanned in all patients with colorectal cancer.
   (b) Scanning should preferably be by CT or MRI. Ultrasound should be used if CT or MRI are not feasible.
   (c) After scanning, the liver should be classified as one of the following:
      (i) definite hepatic metastases present
      (ii) equivocal
      (iii) hepatic metastases not present.
   (d) Serum carcinoembryonic antigen (CEA) concentration should be determined if facilities are available. A high level (>50 ng/mL) suggests metastatic disease even if liver imaging is negative.
9. *Assessment of established liver metastases.*
   (a) The number of liver metastases should be expressed as 'solitary' or 'multiple'. If solitary, it should be stated if the metastasis is in the right or in the left lobe. If multiple, it should be stated if they are uni- or bi-lobar.
   (b) The percentage of liver involved on scanning should be quantified by the radiologist as:
      0 0%
      1 <50%
      2 >50%
   If symptoms which are probably related to liver metastases are present, the symbol 'S' should be appended to each grade.
10. *Exclusion of synchronous lesions.* All patients with a colorectal carcinoma should have the remainder of the large bowel assessed, preferably by colonoscopy prior to surgery; but if colonoscopy is not available or is technically impossible (e.g. a stenotic lesion is present), a double-contrast barium enema should be performed.
    If preoperative assessment cannot rule out synchronous lesions, these should be sought by:
    (a) intraoperative palpation supplemented, if deemed appropriate, by on-table colonoscopy (however, either of these may be unreliable or unsatisfactory)
    (b) postoperative colonoscopy or barium enema within 6 months.
11. *Assessment of the urological tract.* A preoperative intravenous urogram is not routinely required, but may be indicated in exceptional circumstances.

or a defunctioning stoma to be created, which will prevent the development of intestinal obstruction.

There are, however, cases where the patient is so ill and the disease so advanced that any procedure no matter how simple is thought by the surgeon to be contraindicated. Each case has to be considered on its own merits and no hard and fast rules can be made.

The new imaging techniques, which seem to be relatively accurate in the detection of hepatic metastases, are gradually changing surgical philosophy; thus the demonstration of metastases by these techniques significantly affects our attitude to the extent of the procedure to be performed. In the case of a patient with a small, low rectal cancer who has multiple metastases in the liver on scanning, we would be tempted to perform some form of local manoeuvre which is associated with a much lower mortality and morbidity than rectal excision. Similarly, if in a patient with colonic carcinoma it is known that dissemination has occurred, a more limited resection is likely to be performed. The main use of the new imaging techniques, however, is likely to be in the selection of patients for adjuvant therapy rather than primary surgical treatment.

PREOPERATIVE PREPARATION

The patient should be in the best possible physical and mental state before operation. They should have been thoroughly counselled about their disease. Any underlying medical condition should be treated as energetically as possible. Specific aspects of preoperative preparation include bowel preparation, antibiotic prophylaxis, stoma advice and counselling.

Bowel preparation

Bowel preparation has been discussed at length in Chapter 3, but there are some points which are worth emphasizing in preparing the bowel in patients with carcinoma.

Most authors are agreed that whole-gut irrigation via a nasogastric tube produces a better bowel preparation than conventional methods (Crapp et al, 1975; Marti and Pouret, 1976; Chung et al, 1979; Gilmore et al, 1981; Raahave et al, 1981), but many patients find the procedure most disagreeable. Downing et al (1979) and Minervini et al (1980) found that 30% of their patients refused to submit themselves to the same procedure again, another 38% found it distinctly unpleasant and would agree to its administration a second time only if it were deemed to be absolutely necessary. Our own experience is similar: the main complaints of patients are the nausea, abdominal distension and pain frequently induced after several litres of fluid have been introduced down the nasogastric tube. Hence osmotic agents such as polyethylene glycol (PEG), electrolyte solutions (Golytely), sodium phosphate (Fleet Phospho-soda) and sodium picosulphate (Picolax) taken orally have become more popular (Davis et al, 1980; Thomson et al, 1996) particularly in elderly patients with carcinoma.

Another point to be stressed in relation to patients with carcinoma is the risk of inducing intestinal obstruction in those with constricting growths. Thus if the patient complains of symptoms of chronic obstruction, or if the barium enema or colonoscopy examination reveals a narrow lesion, vigorous bowel preparation and in particular whole-gut irrigation is contraindicated.

Despite the above disadvantages, whole-gut irrigation via a nasogastric tube has one important advantage, in that it can be carried out within a relatively short time. This is useful not only from an organizational point of view, but also because it probably reduces the risk of complications such as deep venous thrombosis and bronchopneumonia which are prevalent in elderly patients who are relatively sedentary while awaiting their operation. Up to recently, Golytely and other balanced electrolyte solutions taken orally (Adler et al, 1984) were generally the preferred options, but because of their taste they were unpopular with patients who also found that they could not drink the volume required to obtain an adequate catharsis. These preparations have therefore been superseded by oral sodium phosphate or sodium picosulphate, which have been shown in randomized controlled trials to be more tolerable for patients (Wolters et al, 1994; Afridi et al, 1995; Golub et al, 1995; Henderson et al, 1995; Thomson et al, 1996).

For the elderly patient with carcinoma in whom vigorous bowel preparation is contraindicated, a conventional 'old-fashioned' bowel preparation regimen may be used. There are numerous combinations of purgative drugs, enemas, washouts and suppositories. No data as far as we know suggest that one regimen is superior to the others. We occasionally use the following regimen. On day 1, magnesium sulphate 10 mL is given orally twice or three times a day. If the lesion is producing a marked narrowing on radiological examination, the magnesium sulphate is replaced by liquid paraffin which softens the faeces accumulated above the lesion and increases their chance of passing through it. This regimen continues up to the day of the operation. Forty-eight hours prior to surgery the patient is placed on a liquid diet and receives enemas consisting of 50 mg oxyphenisatin in 1 L of water morning and evening. The rectum is also washed out on the evening before the operation, or first thing in the morning if the operation is scheduled in the afternoon.

If at operation the bowel preparation is found to be inadequate, intraoperative irrigation using the method described by Dudley et al (1980) can be employed. Indeed this is now regarded by many as the optimum indication for on-table lavage. It is always a good idea to have this facility readily available when operating on patients with a colorectal carcinoma.

Antimicrobial prophylaxis

The role of intestinal antimicrobials, wound antiseptics and systemic antibiotics are discussed in Chapter 5. Patients operated on for carcinoma do not differ from other groups in their requirements for these prophylactic measures.

Prophylaxis against deep venous thrombosis and pulmonary embolus

Much has been written on this subject and it is beyond the scope of this book to present the arguments for and against the various regimens. It should be stressed that patients with colorectal cancer are at particular risk of developing venous thrombosis. They are usually elderly and often spend several days in hospital before their operation for investigation and sometimes protracted bowel preparation if they have subacute obstruction. The carcinoma itself also constitutes another important risk factor (Kakkar et al, 1970). Patients with carcinoma of the rectum or sigmoid colon are perhaps at even greater risk as they are often placed in positions on the operating table which may result in calf compression.

There are two approaches to the prophylaxis of deep venous thrombosis, one involving physical methods and the other the use of anticoagulants. Physical methods include activity by exercises, leg elevation, use of elastic stockings and early ambulation after surgery. During the operative procedure galvanic stimulation to produce contraction of calf muscles or motorized foot manoeuvres may be used, but we prefer intermittent external calf compression with a pneumatic sleeve. Anticoagulant prophylaxis takes various forms but can be divided into prothrombin depressants, platelet function suppressants and low-dose heparin. Prothrombin depressants are the vitamin K antagonists warfarin and phenindione derivatives. Platelet function suppressants include dextran, aspirin, sulphinpyrazone and hydroxychloroquine dipyridamole. Only two of these agents have been shown to be effective in the prevention of pulmonary embolism as distinct from deep venous thrombosis: they are low-dose unfractioned heparin and dextran 70 (Kline et al, 1975; Kakkar et al, 1977). Dextran is as effective as heparin against pulmonary embolus but not as useful in the prevention of deep venous thrombosis as detected by ^{125}I-labelled fibrinogen. For these reasons we use subcutaneous heparin for prophylaxis in colorectal cancer; however, since heparin carries an increased risk of wound haematoma (Gruber et al, 1980) when given as 5000 units three times a day, we prefer to give it twice a day. We also prefer to use low-molecular-weight heparin (LMWH) since a large randomized trial in patients undergoing abdominal surgery has shown that although LMWH is of similar efficacy to standard heparin, bleeding-related complications are less common (Kakker et al, 1993). As there are no data yet to support a better regimen, this is now our preferred method of prophylaxis (Ruckley, 1985).

Since these patients are at risk throughout their stay in hospital, it is probably best to start the regimen on admission and continue until they are fully mobilized after operation. If the patient is particularly at risk from bleeding and heparin is contraindicated, we require the patient to wear TED stockings (Kendall) throughout their hospital stay (Scurr et al, 1977; Bolton, 1978) and intermittent pneumatic calf compression is applied during the operation. All patients are encouraged to mobilize as quickly as possible after operation.

SURGICAL TREATMENT OF CARCINOMA OF THE COLON

Background

Reybard of Lyon in 1833 appears to be the first on record to have performed a successful resection and anastomosis for large bowel cancer, but he was severely criticized for this (Rankin, 1926). As a consequence a palliative defunctioning colostomy was, for some time, advocated as the only surgical procedure possible for the treatment of the disease. Later, resection and double-barrel colostomy were used and in some cases intestinal continuity was achieved by crushing the spur. However, as more surgeons obtained experience with intestinal suture an increasing number of colonic resections were performed. The mortality for intra-abdominal resection and anastomosis gradually decreased but it was still approximately 40% at the end of the nineteenth century (Morgan, 1952). The problems were intra-abdominal leakage and sepsis.

In 1894 in Copenhagen, Bloch in an attempt to prevent these intra-abdominal complications introduced the concept of extraperitoneal resection and anastomosis. He reported two cases in which the loop of colon containing the carcinoma had been mobilized and brought out through the abdominal wall. A tube was inserted into the proximal limb of the loop for drainage purposes. After several days when the colon was firmly adherent to the abdominal wall, the loop containing the cancer was excised. The resulting double-barrel colostomy was closed some time later by use of an enterotome. The same manoeuvre was also independently described by von Mikulicz of Breslau (von Mikulicz, 1903). Paul of Liverpool also described a very similar manoeuvre (Paul, 1895), but in his operation the protruding loop was excised at the time of exteriorization and special large, right-angled glass tubes were tied into the lumina of the distal and proximal ends of the colon. After some time the colostomy was closed using a crushing enterotome. This procedure became known as the Paul–Mikulicz procedure (although Bloch's name should have been added) and was popular throughout the world.

The mortality rate of colonic resection fell significantly as a result of this innovation. The main problem, however, was that because only a limited resection of the mesentery was feasible the lymphatic drainage of the cancer was not dealt with adequately. This often resulted in local recurrence within the wound (Rankin, 1926; Sistrunk, 1928) as involved nodes were cut across or cancer cells were implanted. For this reason some surgeons still persisted with intraperitoneal anastomosis and various modifications were introduced in an attempt to make the procedure safer. One such technique was to perform an aseptic manoeuvre in which neither lumen of the bowel was opened until union was virtually complete. The hope was that if crushing clamps occluded the bowel for as long as possible, minimal intraperitoneal contamination would occur. Another method of reducing intra-abdominal sepsis at the time of anastomosis was to perform a defunctioning stoma several weeks prior to the resection. Devine (1931, 1935) was the main proponent of this approach. His rationale was that diversion of faeces and irrigation of the distal colon would leave a 'defunctioned and debacterilized' bowel suitable for resection and anastomosis.

Although these techniques did achieve their aim of reducing intra-abdominal contamination at the time of anastomosis, they appear to have done little to reduce mortality rates. The breakthrough that gave surgeons the confidence to perform intra-abdominal colonic anastomosis was the introduction of sulphonamides and antibiotics, making it possible to sterilize the gut lumen prior to surgery and to treat septic complications more successfully. This advance coupled with improvements in anaesthesia, the introduction of blood transfusions and the greater understanding of fluid and electrolyte balance caused a revolution in the surgical treatment of colonic cancer. Surgeons abandoned the staged procedures described by Bloch, Mikulicz and Paul in favour of immediate resection and intra-abdominal anastomosis (Lloyd Davies et al, 1953).

Principles of modern surgery

Much of what follows also applies to the surgical treatment of rectal cancer but for the sake of clarity we have concentrated in this section on colon cancer.

The principles of surgery for carcinoma of the colon as carried out today are simple but depend to some extent on whether the operation is being performed in the belief that cure is possible (radical) or whether it is considered that cure cannot be obtained (palliative). A radical procedure requires that the tumour is removed with an adequate margin of normal colon together with the associated vascular pedicle and as many of the corresponding lymph-bearing structures as possible. A palliative procedure can be a limited excision of the tumour or a bypass or defunctioning procedure, each of which is designed to alleviate the patient's symptoms. These principles apply irrespective of whether the resection is performed as an open or as a laparoscopic procedure. Nevertheless, the potential for palliation without conventional laparotomy is a departure from current practice which is likely to be explored with great vigour over the next decades.

Following excision of the tumour-bearing colon, gastrointestinal continuity is restored by anastomosis between the proximal and distal bowel; the exact technique varies according to the individual surgeon's preference and according to which method appears to be most expedient or technically feasible at the time. No matter which procedure is performed it should, if possible, be carried out on a well-prepared bowel and with the minimum amount of spillage. Tissues should be handled with care, haemostasis must be absolute and apposition of tissue must be accurate. There is no room for complacency in this type of surgery since leakage from a colonic anastomosis is a potentially lethal complication.

Scope of radical resection

The exact extent of colonic resection is largely determined by the blood vessels that require division in order to remove the lymphatic drainage of the tumour-bearing part of the colon. The more radical the surgeon is in dealing with the lymphatic drainage, the greater the length of colon that will need to be resected. There are few reports of controlled studies to assist the surgeon in making these decisions, and inevitably there are differences of opinion as to how extensive the resection should be.

For tumours of the right colon (Figure 31.10) – that is, the caecum, ascending colon, hepatic flexure and proximal half of the transverse colon – the ileocolic artery, right colic artery and the right branch of the middle colic artery are usually divided, and resection of the distal 10 cm of ileum, the caecum, ascending colon and proximal one-third of the transverse colon is carried out. This is the standard right hemicolectomy. Some surgeons believe, however, that if a truly radical operation is required, the main branch of the middle colic artery must be divided as close to the superior mesenteric vessels as possible. The result of this manoeuvre (extended right hemicolectomy) is to increase the length of resection of the transverse colon leaving only its distal third available for anastomosis. This more radical manoeuvre ensures that the entire lymph drainage from the right colon is included but only circumstantial data suggest that this approach is more efficacious than the standard technique (Gall, 1991). Nevertheless, in an uncontrolled comparison from Erlangan the overall 5-year survival was improved by extended right hemicolectomy from 55% to 67%.

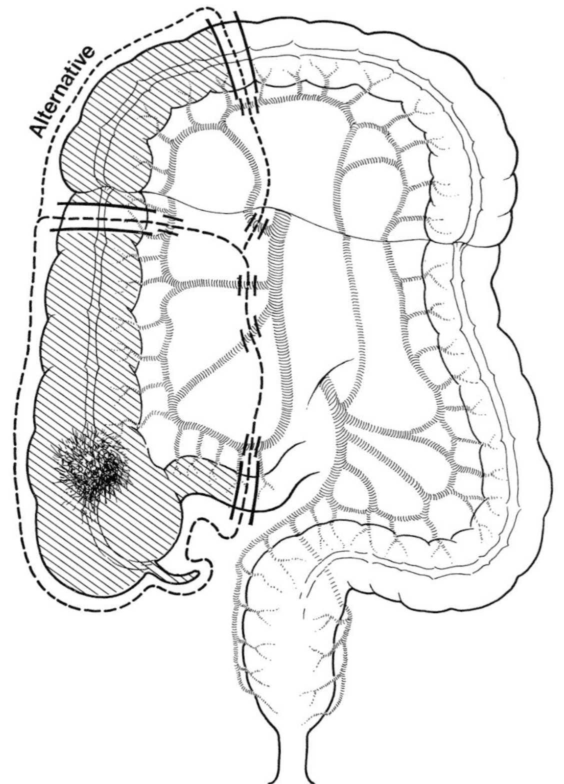

Figure 31.10 Extent of resection in standard right hemicolectomy and the alternative of extended right hemicolectomy.

Conversely, others believe that resection for carcinoma of the caecum should be even more conservative than the standard procedure (Lockhart-Mummery, 1983). These surgeons prefer to retain the hepatic flexure in patients with this tumour (Figure 31.10), although they do accept that the hepatic flexure should be sacrificed for growths of the ascending colon.

For growths of the caecum and ascending colon, the authors' practice is to divide the ileocolic, right colic and right branch of the middle colic arteries as close to their origin as possible. The length of colon that needs to be resected is then determined by the viability of the bowel that remains. The latter will vary from case to case; sometimes with a caecal lesion the hepatic flexure can be retained, and sometimes this is not possible. For tumours of the hepatic flexure the middle colic artery is divided together with the right colic artery, but the ileocolic artery is retained. Once again the length of resection depends on the viable bowel that remains.

For all tumours of the left colon, which include those of the distal half of the transverse colon, the splenic flexure and the descending and sigmoid colon, we prefer to divide the inferior mesenteric artery as close to the aorta as possible so that the proximal colon is anastomosed to the rectum; this relies on an intact marginal artery with perfusion of the left colon based on the middle colic artery (Figure 31.11). Others, however, are more selective. Thus for growths of the left half of the transverse colon, splenic flexure and proximal descending colon, the ascending left colic and descending left colic arteries are divided together with the left branch of the middle colic artery, and an anastomosis is constructed between the proximal transverse colon and proximal sigmoid colon. Those not practising high ligation similarly advise that for a tumour in the midpart of the descending colon the

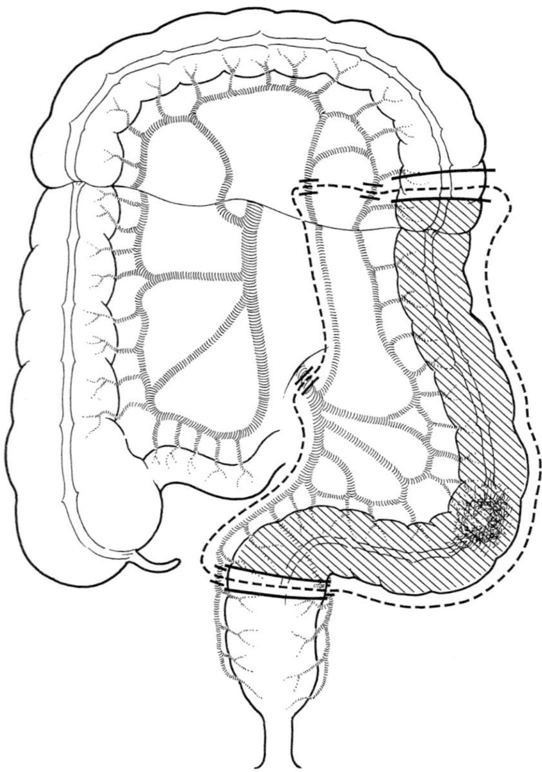

Figure 31.11 Extent of resection in a standard left hemicolectomy performed for a tumour in the sigmoid colon. The inferior mesenteric artery is divided as close to the aorta as possible. If the tumour was more proximal the hepatic flexure would also be resected.

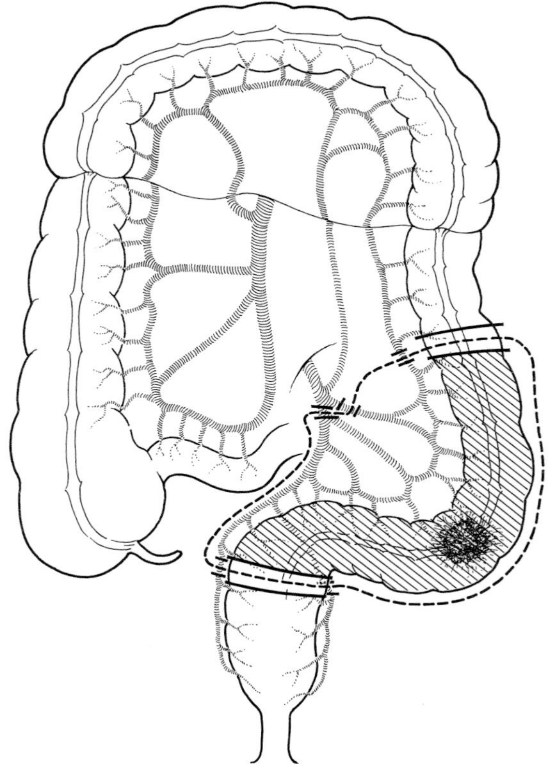

Figure 31.12 Extent of resection in limited resection for a tumour in the sigmoid colon. The sigmoid branches of the inferior mesenteric are divided distal to its main trunk.

same vessels are divided together with one or two sigmoid branches of the inferior mesenteric artery, but the left branch of the middle colic is left intact. The anastomosis is then constructed between the distal transverse colon and lower sigmoid colon. Those adopting the more selective approach for a tumour in the sigmoid colon merely divide the sigmoid branches of the inferior mesenteric artery so that the descending colon is anastomosed to the upper rectum (Figure 31.12).

The more radical procedure by which the inferior mesenteric artery is divided flush with the abdominal aorta under cover of the third part of the duodenum is preferred by many surgeons no matter where the tumour is sited in the left colon (Figure 31.11). Since the inferior mesenteric vessels supply the distal sigmoid colon and upper rectum through the superior rectal artery, the distal anastomosis is usually at the level of the upper rectum in the pelvis. The exact level depends on the adequacy of blood supply from the middle rectal vessels and marginal artery, which can be checked at operation using a tissue oximeter or by laser Doppler ultrasonography. Either way the dissection required is far greater than that needed for the more limited resection. Some surgeons (Goligher, 1984), including ourselves, therefore prefer the radical procedure whenever possible, but in older and more infirm patients tend to use the more limited resection.

It should be stressed at this point that no prospective data exist demonstrating that radical left hemicolectomy is superior in terms of survival and recurrence to the more limited resection. Indeed there are now data which suggest that the reverse might be the case. Busuttil and his colleagues treated 107 patients with carcinoma of the sigmoid colon or rectosigmoid junction between 1955 and 1970. Sixteen were treated by left hemicolectomy and 91 by segmental resection; the groups were similar with regard to age of the patients and the degree of spread of the tumour. Patients treated by limited resection had a shorter hospital stay, lower operative mortality rate and improved 5-year survival rate compared with those treated by the radical operation.

Table 31.7 Results of randomized trial between left hemicolectomy and left segmental resection for patients with left-sided colonic carcinoma.

	Left hemicolectomy (*n* = 131)	*Left segmental resection* (*n* = 129)
Postoperative mortality	8 (6%)	3 (2.3%)
Patients with one or more complications	27 (20.6%)	29 (22.5%)
Median duration of hospital stay (days)	14 (10.7%)	14 (10.9%)
10-year survival	47%	54%
Patients with two or more bowel actions daily at 12 months	7 (5.3%)	1 (0.8%)

From Rouffet et al (1994).

That group's retrospective data have now been supported by a prospective controlled multicentre trial conducted by the French Association for Surgical Research (Rouffet et al, 1994). Between 1980 and 1985, 270 consecutive patients with left colonic carcinoma were randomly allocated to undergo either left hemicolectomy or left segmental colectomy. After elimination of 10 patients for protocol violations, 131 patients with left hemicolectomy and 129 with left segmental resection were analysed. The only difference between the groups was the extra length of bowel removed in the left hemicolectomy patients. There was no significant difference in survival between the two groups. However, patients who underwent left hemicolectomy had a significant increase in bowel frequency (Table 31.7).

It is also interesting in this context to note that survival and recurrence after surgery for rectal cancer is not influenced by whether there has been a high or low ligation of the inferior mesenteric artery (Pezim and Nicholls, 1984). In addition, the no-touch isolation technique in which the vascular supply to a tumour is divided before the tumour is handled has been tested in a randomized controlled trial and shown to confer no statistically significant advantage (Wiggers et al, 1988).

Apart from the colon and its tumour it is often necessary to remove *en bloc* part or all of adjacent organs that appear to be invaded by tumour. Thus a tumour of the transverse colon may involve the greater curve of the stomach, or a tumour of the splenic flexure may invade the spleen, kidney, pancreas and diaphragm. Tumours of the right or left colon may involve the anterior or more commonly the posterior abdominal wall. Not infrequently a loop of small bowel becomes adherent to the colonic lesion. Further distally the bladder, the ureters, the uterus or ovaries may be involved. If at all possible attempts should be made to remove the adjacent organ in continuity with the colon and its tumour. The surgeon should be prepared to be as radical as possible, for it is a common finding that a tumour that appears to be invading another structure is bound to it by an inflammatory reaction only (Cooke, 1956; Jensen et al, 1970a; Ellis, 1971) and in the latter case the prognosis is so much better (Bonfanti et al, 1982; Durdey and Williams, 1984). Even if tumours invade local tissues by malignant infiltration, the lymph nodes are not necessarily involved and a radical local excision may be curative.

Radical or palliative resection?

As noted above, even in the presence of apparent invasion into local structures it is worth performing a radical resection provided there is no evidence of further spread. Where this philosophy was applied, 28.5% of patients who had tumours with malignant fixation lived for at least 5 years after operation (Durdey and Williams, 1984).

The presence of peritoneal seedings on the other hand is an indication for a palliative procedure, as is the presence of multiple liver metastases. In the case of peritoneal involvement it is always worth performing a frozen-section histological examination to confirm that the nodules are truly metastatic. This is particularly necessary when the patient is known to have undergone a previous laparotomy. It is possible to mistake starch granulomas from glove powder for carcinomatous deposits in the peritoneum.

The presence of multiple liver metastases is usually obvious; they appear on the surface of the liver as pearly grey lesions which are often umbilicated. Sometimes they are quite small and there is doubt in the mind of the surgeon as to their nature. Once more, frozen-section or fine-needle aspiration cytology will be useful and occasionally a negative result is a pleasant surprise, provided it is clear that there is no sampling error. Although the presence of multiple hepatic metastases is an absolute indication for a palliative procedure, the existence of a solitary deposit may sway the surgeon towards a more radical procedure (see later).

Direct involvement of the ovaries by spread from

a carcinoma in the upper rectum or sigmoid colon is also not necessarily a contraindication to radical resection. If, however, the ovaries are involved as a result of spread from a carcinoma in a part of the colon away from the pelvis (Krukenberg's tumour) palliation is usually all that can be hoped for. Approximately 2–6% of women with colorectal carcinoma will have macroscopic ovarian metastases at the time of laparotomy (Stearns and Deddish, 1959; Burt, 1960; MacKeigan and Ferguson, 1979; Blamey et al, 1981). In addition, approximately another 2% will have microscopic metastases.

These data were obtained from a few series in which the ovaries were removed routinely as part of the operation for colorectal cancer (Quan and Sehdev, 1974; MacKeigan and Ferguson, 1979). Prophylactic oophorectomy in all female patients with colorectal cancer is a contentious subject. As is so often the case in the surgical treatment of this condition, there are no prospective data to assist in making the decision. If such a policy was to be routinely adopted then perhaps one or two patients in every hundred might be cured. It is not known, however, if such benefit would be counterbalanced by a greater morbidity and mortality from prophylactic oophorectomy. We think this may be the case, and would caution against prophylactic oophorectomy until more reliable data become available.

The presence of multiple pulmonary metastases is another indication for a palliative procedure as opposed to a radical resection. Few data exist on the incidence of pulmonary metastases at the time of initial presentation of a colonic tumour. Although Bacon and Jackson (1953) found that 5% of their 600 cases of carcinoma of the distal colon and upper rectum had concomitant lung metastases, our experience suggests that the incidence is considerably lower. Although there are certain authors who advocate the removal of solitary lung metastases in patients with colorectal cancer (Schulten et al, 1976; Attiyeh, 1980; Muhe et al, 1981; Takita et al, 1981), virtually all the data were collected from patients who developed their lung manifestation several months or years after the initial resection. It is unknown, therefore, how patients with such a lesion at the time of initial presentation would fare, since it is generally agreed that the longer the time interval between resection and development of the pulmonary metastasis the better the prognosis. It would seem from the available literature that provided the lung secondary is small and truly solitary, concomitant resection may be worthwhile. We have no data to support this statement but have carried out this policy in the few patients that have presented in the way described.

Once a decision has been made to palliate, the manoeuvre designed to give the maximum relief should be carried out. If at all possible, the best policy is to remove the primary tumour, usually by a limited resection. However, it must be realized that there is no evidence that this approach improves survival (Baigrie and Berry, 1994). Occasionally the degree of dissemination is so great that it seems pointless to perform such a procedure when the patient is unlikely to survive long enough to experience relief and improved quality of life. If the patient is symptomatic and it is technically impossible to remove the tumour, a bypass or defunctioning procedure will be necessary. When a patient presents with metastases from a silent colonic tumour it is sometimes difficult to know whether palliative treatment of the primary lesion should be performed. Each case has to be considered on its own merits, but in general if the colonic tumour is asymptomatic we prefer to wait until symptoms develop and then perform the most appropriate manoeuvre.

Resection of synchronous hepatic metastases

If at operation the patient has a solitary hepatic metastasis or a closely clustered group of small metastases, which occur in 8–25% of patients (Babineau and Steele, 1996), consideration should be given to some form of hepatic resection combined with the colectomy. If the hepatic lesion is situated near the liver edge, a wedge resection can often be performed. Alternatively, local excision of each metastasis may be sufficient. Failing this a right or left hepatectomy may need to be carried out. Since these procedures – particularly right hepatectomy – carry a risk even in expert hands, it is necessary to examine if the risk is worth taking and if so whether the liver resection should be carried out at the same time as the colonic resection.

Several early reports described individual cases where right or left hepatectomy was performed successfully *pari passu* with the colonic resection (Lloyd Davies, 1947; Morgan, 1957). Peden and Blalock (1963) recorded one patient who survived for 5 years following right hepatectomy. The first substantial series of cases reported seems to be that from Brunschwig (1961) who performed seven left hepatectomies and seven right hepatectomies for associated liver metastases. There were three operative deaths and one patient managed to survive for 27 months. One of the most influential reports to date has been that from Wilson and Adson (1976). They reported on 60 patients at the Mayo Clinic who during 1949–72 inclusive underwent concomitant resection of liver metastases together with colonic resection. In 40 patients the metastases were solitary and in the remaining 20 they were multiple. In over 75% of patients the metastases were 5 cm or less in diameter. Wedge resection was performed in 39 patients, 10 patients required segmental resection and 11 patients underwent either right or left hepatectomy. Only one patient died, an operative mortality rate of 1.7%, and patients were followed up for a minimum of 2 years. None of the patients with multiple metastases survived longer than 5 years, whereas 15 of the 36 with alleged solitary metastases were alive 5 years after surgery and eight of these patients survived for 10 years or more. This report is important because the authors also attempted to compare this group of patients with a control group who did not undergo any form of hepatic resection for their metastases; although the latter group was composed of 'historical' control subjects, it was similar in composition to the group of patients who had undergone a liver resection. None of the control subjects survived for 5 years.

Similar encouraging results were reported by Wanebo et al (1978b) and Foster and Berman (1977). Many recent reports support these previous findings (Table 31.8) and in addition have helped to clarify the factors that seem to be significantly associated with a successful outcome from hepatic resection (August et al, 1985; Petrelli et al, 1985). Thus the prospect of cure does not seem to be influenced by the grade of malignancy or the Dukes' stage of the colonic tumour. Patients with two or three metastases (in the same lobe) have a similar prognosis to those with solitary deposits, but those with four or more metastases do badly. Patients treated by simple wedge excision have fared as well as those submitted to a formal partial hepatectomy. The absence of a disease-free margin in the specimen of excised liver is a bad prognostic finding (Bradpiece et al, 1987) (Figure 31.13). If the immediate mortality is going to be low, the liver resection must be performed by a surgeon with experience in this type of work.

Until recently the decision whether or not to deal with synchronous liver metastases by resection had to be made at the time of the original exploration. The standard teaching (Goligher, 1984) was that if a metastasis appeared to be solitary, or if only three or four were present and if they were in a close cluster, wedge resection should be performed at the time of the colonic resection if technically feasible. This policy was only advised if the metastasis was at or near the liver edge and the patient was fit enough to undergo the additional trauma. If these technical criteria were not met and the metastasis although solitary was sited deep within the liver structure, it

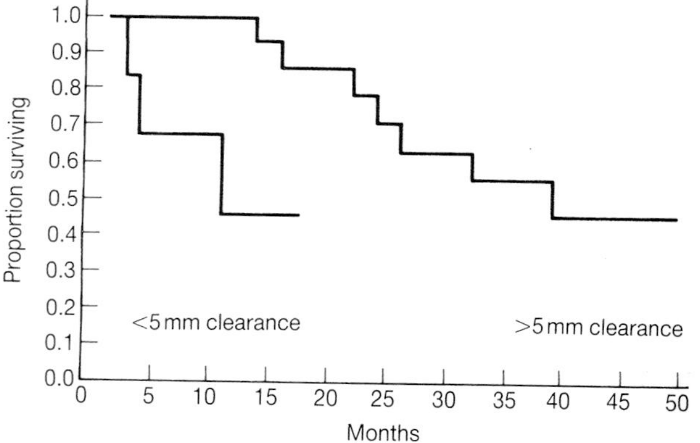

Figure 31.13 Actuarial survival curves for patients with and without complete metastatic clearance at the time of liver resection (Bradpiece et al, 1987).

Table 31.8 Results of liver resection for colorectal metastases.

Authors	*n*	*Operative mortality* (%)	*Survival* (%)	*Survival* (Years)
Bengmark and Hafstrom (1969)	39	5	23	3
Foster and Berman (1977)	88	—	18	5
Wanebo et al (1978b)	25	10	92	1
Fortner et al (1979)	65	7	57	3
Adson and van Heerden (1980)	34	59	82	1
Morrow et al (1980)	38	10	36	2
Steele et al (1984)	30	—	65	3
August et al (1985)	33	0	91	1
Doci et al (1995)	219	—	24	5
Jatzko et al (1995)	66*	4.5	29.6	5
Isenberg et al (1996)	17	—	47	5

*40 performed synchronously.

was advised not to proceed to liver resection but to perform a second laparotomy after appropriate scans had been performed and the definitive pathology of the colonic tumour had been ascertained.

At the present time most surgeons obtain at least an ultrasound or CT examination of the liver before exploration, so it is usually known preoperatively if a liver metastasis exists and whether or not it is present in isolation. If doubt exists a CT scan should help clarify the situation. Such information is of immense value to the surgeon, who can plan the resection well in advance and need not make uninformed judgements at the time of initial operation. In addition, this judgement can be further enhanced by the use of intra-operative ultrasound (Stewart et al, 1993; Stone et al, 1994). Furthermore, since the pathology of the colonic tumour does not influence the prognosis after liver resection (Adson, 1983), it is not necessary to await the definitive pathological report.

Since the results of liver resection for liver metastases in recent years have gradually improved, so we are changing our philosophy. Thus if the tumour is in direct continuity with the liver edge, a wedge resection is performed *en bloc* with the primary tumour. If three or four small metastases or a truly solitary metastasis are conveniently situated at the liver edge, again a wedge resection is performed provided preoperative scans show no evidence of other metastases. If a metastasis is truly solitary and is deep-seated, and is confirmed to be so on both ultrasound and CT scans, we will occasionally advise a lobectomy together with the colonic resection provided the patient is fit enough. We have been particularly impressed recently – as have others (Machi et al, 1987; Olsen, 1990; Stone et al, 1994) – with intraoperative ultrasonography and now regard this technique as essential when dealing with these patients. The intraoperative scan ensures we are dealing with a truly solitary hepatic metastasis and in addition helps in delineating the margins of excision. A preoperative arteriogram may also be of value in these cases. If there is any doubt about staging and exclusion of other disseminated disease, we do not advise synchronous excision of the liver metastases, preferring to refer the patient to a hepatic surgeon so that a second laparotomy can be performed at a later date when further information has been obtained. However, despite improvements in hepatic surgery, it should be remembered that only a small selected group of patients will be eligible for liver resection with the prospect of cure. The techniques and further results of hepatic resection for colorectal liver metastases are discussed in Chapter 33.

Scope of resection for synchronous carcinomas and polyps

If a synchronous neoplasm is detected either before or during operation, the operative strategy will depend on whether the second lesion is benign or malignant. If polyps are found, their number and site will dictate the type of resection required. A second or third synchronous carcinoma is usually to be found at a considerable distance from the primary carcinoma. For this reason, and also because colonic mucosa that has already produced more than one carcinoma is unstable and at greater risk of producing another, a total colectomy and ileorectal anastomosis is recommended provided the patient is fit enough to withstand this more extensive procedure. Very occasionally two carcinomas are present in one segment of colon: then the surgeon can conveniently remove both by a radical and possibly extended right hemicolectomy, transverse colectomy or left hemicolectomy, depending on their site. Whether such a manoeuvre is as curative as a total colectomy is difficult to say, as no data are available to answer the question. With the availability of colonoscopic surveillance this approach is probably justified in most patients. Perhaps the more radical approach of colectomy and ileorectal anastomosis should still be adopted for younger patients particularly if there are multiple polyps, since there is a long potential life-span and only the rectum has to be kept under endoscopic review.

The procedure to be adopted in patients with synchronous polyps is somewhat more controversial. The polyp population of the colon is not static, so that even if all the polyps at the time of operation were removed, others might develop later and be transformed into carcinoma. Thus Bussey et al (1967) found that 5% of those patients who had undergone resection for a carcinoma and who had polyps present at the time of operation developed a metachronous carcinoma when followed up for 20 years. For this reason various authors, including Lillehei and Wangensteen (1955), Teicher and Abrahams (1956) and Rosenthal and Baronofsky (1960), advocated total colectomy and ileorectal anastomosis when synchronous polyps were present. However, with the development of flexible endoscopy opinion has changed. In addition, although the risk of metachronous carcinoma in these patients is high after 20 years of follow-up, many patients are elderly when first diagnosed and may not be exposed to this degree of risk, and the morbidity of diarrhoea and potential incontinence is not justified. Bussey et al (1967) found that the incidence of carcinoma at 10 years was only 0.7%.

For these reasons it is our practice to remove synchronous polyps by colonoscopic snaring usually before operation if it is envisaged that the subsequent resection will not encompass them. We have adopted this policy when one to five polyps are present (singly) at intervals throughout the colon, provided they are less than 2 cm diameter. Occasionally a greater number are to be found, but too few (less than 100) for a diagnosis of familial adenomatous polyposis to be made; in these few cases it has been our policy to perform total colectomy and ileorectal anastomosis, particularly in younger patients.

Clearly patients with polyps and carcinoma treated by resection and colonoscopic polypectomy will need very careful colonoscopic surveillance. If the patient is likely to default from regular follow-up and the prognosis of the carcinoma is favourable, consideration must be given to a more radical operation. The same policy should also be adopted in the young patient (under 40 years old), particularly if there is a strong family history of large bowel malignancy.

Operative details

Incisions and position on the operating table

A urinary catheter is introduced before the start of the operation and left *in situ*, and an intravenous infusion is commenced in the upper limb. If there is coexisting severe cardiorespiratory or renal disease, a central venous pressure line is positioned together with an arterial line. A minimum of two units of cross-matched blood should be available in the theatre suite. Some patients now prefer autologous blood transfusion and in such patients who are not anaemic a unit of blood can be taken off two weeks before elective resection which may be transferred back during or soon after the operation if needed. In our view this policy seems unnecessary since most of these patients have low blood transfusion requirements and will be bled needlessly. It is a good idea, however, to have two units available from the blood bank as well, just in case a more radical resection with adjacent structures is needed.

For most procedures the patient is positioned supine on the operating table. It is an advantage when operating on the right or left colon to have the patient tilted 20–25 degrees to the opposite side. This tilt allows loops of small bowel to gravitate away from the uppermost half of the abdomen. The surgeon stands on the left side of the patient if the tumour is situated in the left colon and on the right side for tumours elsewhere. These guidelines are not rigid; for instance, it is not uncommon for the surgeon to change sides, from left to right, when mobilizing the splenic flexure.

For growths of the distal sigmoid colon or rectosigmoid region, it is preferable to place the patient in the Lloyd Davies position which allows ready access to the pelvis (Figure 31.14). Some would advocate the Lloyd Davies position for all tumours of the left colon if high ligation is practised, since the colorectal anastomosis may be constructed using the circular stapling device, for which access is required.

No matter where the carcinoma is sited within the colon, we employ a midline abdominal incision and

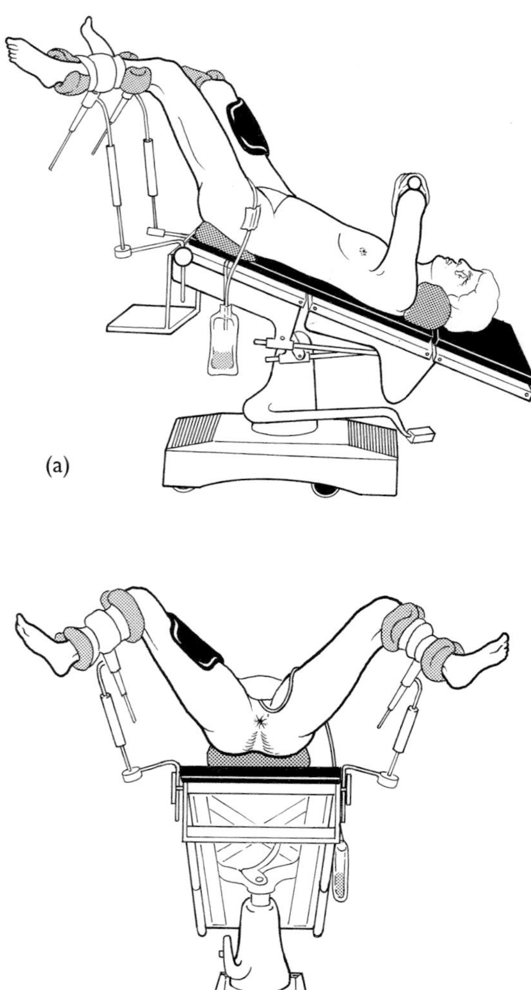

Figure 31.14a,b Lloyd Davies position to be used for patients with growths of the distal sigmoid colon or rectosigmoid regions.

adjust its length according to the site of the carcinoma and the build of the patient. The choice of abdominal incision is a very personal one. A midline incision has the advantages of simplicity and speed; in addition it allows a covering stoma to be sited on either side of the abdomen. The main fear has always been that the wound is less strong than its main alternative, the standard paramedian incision. This fear is based only on anecdotal evidence. In a controlled, prospective randomized trial, Ellis and colleagues from the Westminster Hospital were unable to show any significant difference in either dehiscence or incisional hernia rates between midline and paramedian incisions when both were closed using the same mass nylon closure technique (Ellis et al, 1984). On the other hand, Guillou et al (1980) showed that a very lateral paramedian incision (i.e. one placed at least 5 cm from the midline) had a significantly lower incidence of incisional hernia associated with it compared with a midline incision. The disadvantages of the lateral paramedian incision are that it is tedious to perform and it seems to be associated with a higher incidence of wound infection; for these reasons it is not an incision that has gained popularity for large bowel surgery.

While most surgeons prefer a vertical incision of some type, others have in the past favoured either a long oblique muscle-cutting incision (Lockhart-Mummery, 1934; Turner, 1955) or a transverse incision (Douglas, 1969; Goldberg et al, 1980). The former has lost some of its initial popularity, for although it gives excellent access to the splenic and hepatic flexures it gives a less satisfactory exposure of the main vessels. The transverse incision on the other hand still has its devotees, who consider that it produces a much stronger and more comfortable wound compared with either type of standard vertical incision. Again, the evidence from controlled trials does not support this contention. Thus both Greenall et al (1980a,b) and Ellis et al (1984) were unable to demonstrate any benefit from the transverse incision compared with a vertical incision (see Chapter 6).

Exploration of the abdomen and assessment of resectability

On first opening the abdominal cavity the surgeon should pass a hand over the surface of the liver and both its lobes should be carefully examined for the presence of metastases. Palpation should preferably be bimanual, for assiduous examination ensures that most large, overt metastases are detected (Cedermark et al, 1977; Williams et al, 1985). No matter how thoroughly hepatic assessment is conducted at operation, the surgeon may still miss small metastases and even larger ones situated deep within the liver substance. Reliance may have to be placed on the preoperative CT and ultrasound scans, but increasingly intraoperative ultrasound scans are being used at laparotomy to detect liver involvement. These imaging techniques are now being used to decide on the optimum surgical treatment.

After the liver has been examined all other organs should be carefully assessed. Particular attention should be paid to the presence of ascites, peritoneal seedings, omental deposits or secondary deposits on the surface of any other structure. The colon containing the neoplasm should be left to the last; adherence to such a plan ensures that distant spread is fully assessed. Finally the colon is carefully examined for the presence of synchronous tumours, and then the growth itself is assessed. Its position, size and mobility are noted. If it is adherent, the degree of fixity is assessed together with the structure or structures to which it is adherent. It is customary to see whether any lymph nodes in the vicinity of the tumour are enlarged. Caution must be exercised when interpreting the significance of enlarged nodes and it must not be assumed automatically that they are replaced by tumour. As with fixity, it is not unusual for an enlarged lymph node to be due to inflammation rather than malignant involvement.

A decision is next taken as to whether the tumour can be resected, and if so whether the procedure can be performed in a radical or palliative manner. It is rare indeed these days to deem a colonic tumour technically non-resectable. Other factors, however, such as age and general health of the patient come into consideration. Thus although a very large tumour of caecum or sigmoid colon which is invading both ureters might be resectable from a technical point of view with subsequent reimplantation of the ureters into the bladder, few surgeons are likely to submit an elderly patient with severe coexisting medical disease to such a formidable procedure. So saying, it is generally a good policy to resect the lesion if at all possible, even if there is evidence of distant spread. There is no doubt that resection is the best form of palliation and indeed wide resection of a locally invasive carcinoma may be curative. If for whatever reason the surgeon considers it is impossible or unwise to resect the tumour, consideration should be given to some form of bypass manoeuvre or defunctioning stoma. A stoma should be considered only if symptoms are severe and if it is envisaged that the patient's quality of life will be better with a stoma than without. This

Table 31.9 Intraoperative assessment: recommendations of the UKCCCR Sub-Committee on Staging of Colorectal Cancer (1996).

The surgeon should record the following details.

1a. *The indication* for performing the operation should be stated:
  (a) elective
  (b) emergency.
  If emergency, the reason should be stated (e.g. perforation, obstruction, haemorrhage, other).
1b. *ASA grade.*
2. *Tumour site.* If rectal, whether it is (a) above or (b) below the peritoneal reflection.
3. *Presence of synchronous carcinomas or polyps.*
4. *Fixity of tumour:*
  (a) mobile
  (b) tethered
  (c) fixed.
  If tethered or fixed the structure(s) to which the tumour is adherent should be specified. The surgeon must also specify if a biopsy has been taken from the area of invasion/adherence.
5. *Tumour associated with local abscess/operative perforation or ascites.*
6. *Peritoneal metastases.* If deemed to be present, a biopsy must be taken.
7. *Enlargement* of pre-aortic (mesenteric) lymph nodes and any other lymph nodes. Biopsy should be taken if the enlarged nodes are not to be included in the resection.
8. *Liver metastases.* Site and number should be specified and a *biopsy taken.*
9. *Other organs.* Description of other organs invaded, and whether removed in part or totally *en bloc.*
10. *Curative or palliative.* Statement as to whether the operative procedure is curative or palliative must be made based on the surgeon's impression as to whether all macroscopic tumour has been removed, or not. If there is any doubt, the uncertainty should be stated. If residual tumour is thought to remain, it must be biopsied.
11. *Blood.* Statement as to whether a blood transfusion was given, and if so what volume.

difficult decision can be made only after careful assessment of the patient's physical, emotional and social situation.

In order to standardize the operative findings, the UKCCCR subcommittee on the staging of colorectal cancer made certain recommendations in the hope of improving reporting standards (Williams et al, 1988). These recommendations have been updated (UKCCCR, 1996) and are listed in Table 31.9. Applying them together with the preoperative and pathological findings, an operation should then be deemed to be either curative, non-curative or indeterminate for cure.

Right hemicolectomy

Once it has been decided that a tumour of the right colon can be resected, mobilization of the caecum, ascending colon and hepatic flexure is commenced. The colon is retracted towards the midline and the peritoneal reflection along the right paracolic gutter is divided (Figure 31.15a). The peritoneum has small blood vessels in its interstices and it is our practice to electrocoagulate these before cutting them. In the more obese patient this may be impossible because the vessels cannot be visualized easily, in which case it may be best to divide the peritoneum between artery forceps. Peritoneal division commences at the caecal pole and continues around to the hepatic flexure (Figure 31.15a). Distal to the hepatic flexure the dissection is continued by entering the lesser sac.

The stomach is then grasped and put on traction by pulling the omentum down so that the greater omentum can be divided beyond the gastro-epiploic arcade to a point at which the bowel will be divided (Figure 31.15b). This part of the mobilization usually continues approximately to the junction between the proximal third and distal two-thirds of the transverse colon.

The right colon is then drawn towards the midline so that it is suspended by the medial leaf of peritoneum and colic vessels (Figure 31.15c). Mobilization is continued by gently pushing the adventitial tissue beneath the peritoneum away from the operator with a 'swab on a stick'. The spermatic (ovarian) vessels, the ureter and the second part of the duodenum are usually visualized during this procedure and care must be taken not to damage them (Figure 31.15c). Sometimes the tumour is adherent to one or more of these structures and it is not possible to separate the tumour from them. In this case an *en bloc* excision of the colon, together with part of the structure it is adherent to, may be required. The need for subsequent reconstitution of anatomy and the method by which this may be achieved depend on what remains after radical excision.

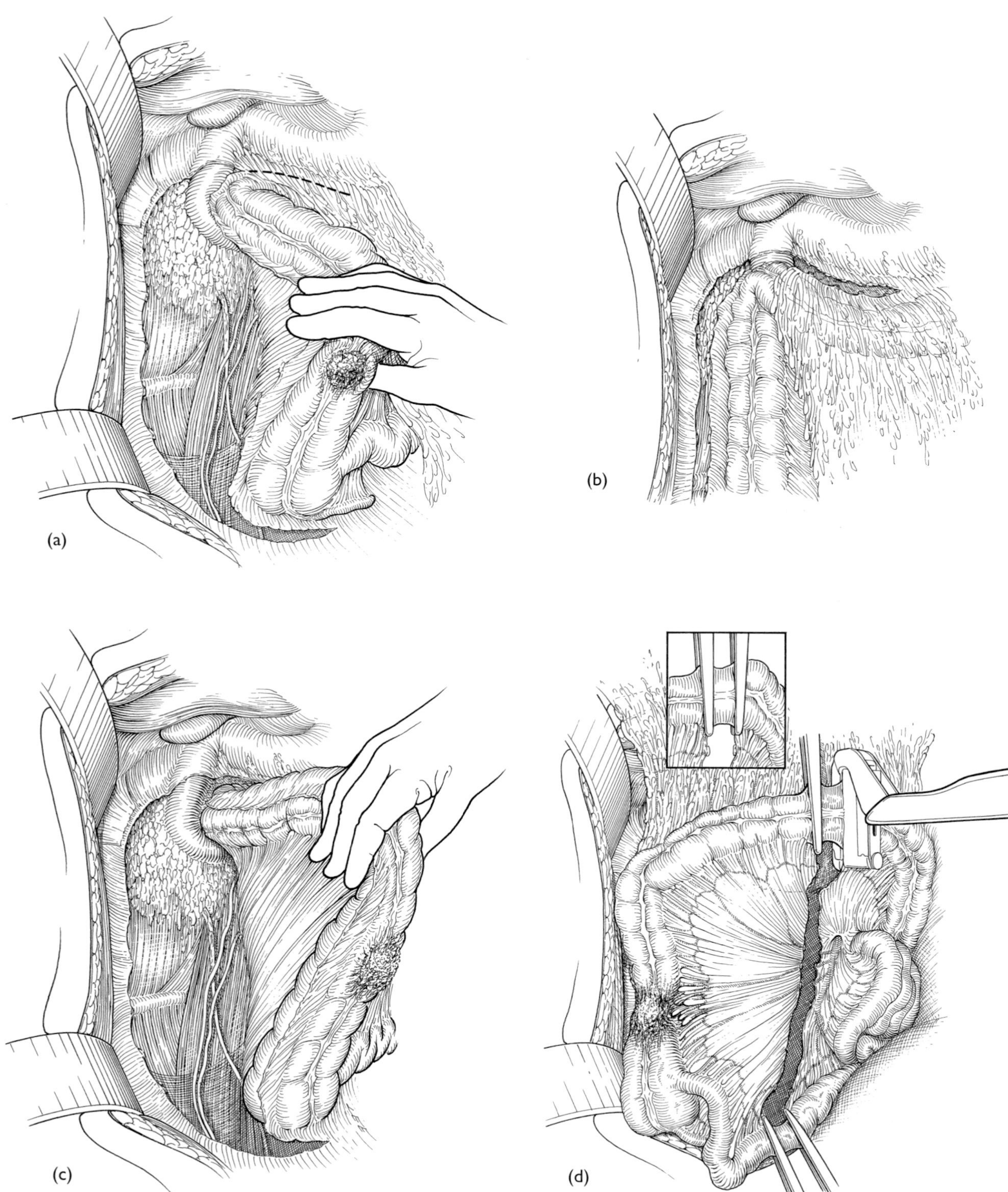

Figure 31.15a–d Right hemicolectomy. (a) The caecum and ascending colon are retracted to the patient's left side and the peritoneum divided from the pole of the caecum upwards and around the hepatic flexure. (b) The omentum distal to the hepatic flexure is divided and the lesser sac is entered. (c) The caecum, ascending colon and hepatic flexure have been fully mobilized revealing the duodenum, spermatic vessels and right ureter. (d) The mesentery together with the ileocolic, right colic and middle colic vessels is divided and ligated appropriately. The transverse colon is divided by transversely stapling its distal side or alternatively it is divided between crushing clamps (inset). Similarly the ileum is divided between crushing clamps.

Once the colon has been fully mobilized the mesentery and colic vessels are divided. This manoeuvre is helped considerably by transillumination of the mesentery so that the main vessels can be divided as near to their origin as possible. The ileocolic, the right colic and the middle colic arteries are divided between artery forceps and doubly ligated with non-absorbable material. The intervening mesentery is similarly dealt with but usually only single ligation is necessary, and sometimes in thin patients it can be divided with impunity. The mesenteric division is continued to the point on the ileum at which it is intended to be divided, usually 10–15 cm proximal to the ileocaecal valve. During the process it is necessary to divide the communicating arcade between the ileal branches of the superior mesenteric artery and the ileocolic artery (Figure 31.15d). Similarly, the mesentery is divided close to the transverse colon, during which procedure the marginal vessel between the two branches of the middle colic artery or that between the middle and ascending left colic arteries is divided and secured.

The ileum is next divided between crushing clamps (Figure 31.15d) or staples and if an end-to-end anastomosis is envisaged the clamps are applied obliquely to ensure as wide an anastomotic lumen as possible. Before transection of the transverse colon it may be necessary to complete the division of the greater omentum to the point of transection. The colon is then divided and the anastomotic technique will depend on which form of reconstruction is preferred.

Our preference at the Royal London Hospital has been to construct an end-to-side anastomosis (end of ileum to side of transverse colon). In this technique transection of the transverse colon takes place between a proximal crushing clamp and the TA 55 stapling instrument (Figure 31.15d). After the bowel has been divided the stapling instrument is released and the closed stapled end of transverse colon is oversewn with interrupted 2/0 polygalactin sutures so as to bury the staples. An anastomosis is then constructed approximately 2–3 cm distal to the closed end of colon. We use a two-layered technique (Figure 31.16). First, interrupted seromuscular polygalactin or monofilament polyglyconate sutures are inserted between the ileum and transverse colon and tied so as to approximate the two portions of bowel. A transverse incision is then made in the serosa of the transverse colon using cutting diathermy after first applying soft non-crushing clamps to the distal ileum and transverse colon. The length of the incision is matched exactly with the diameter of the ileum available for anastomosis. The mucosa of the colon is then incised and any colonic contents sucked out. The crushing clamp on the distal ileum is removed by incising the ileum immediately below the inferior border of the clamp. The contents of the open ileum are gently swabbed or sucked out and its lumen and that of the colon are irrigated with an antiseptic or antibiotic solution. A continuous 2/0 chromic catgut suture is then inserted through all layers of the posterior wall of the anastomosis which is continued on its anterior aspect as a Connell suture. The anastomosis is completed with interrupted seromuscular sutures of 2/0 polygalactin or monofilament polyglyconate on the anterior wall.

After the anastomosis is completed the mesenteric defect is closed in the customary way using interrupted chromic catgut sutures, taking care to avoid transfixion of blood vessels.

Recently, we have also used the functional end-to-end anastomosis using two enterotomies to construct a side-to-side stapled line. The tumour and the two enterotomies are then divided using a linear staple cutter (Figure 31.17).

Variations in ileotransverse anastomotic technique

The end-to-side anastomosis may be performed without the use of the stapling instrument, the end of the colon being closed with two layers of sutures.

An end-to-side anastomosis has a considerable advantage over the end-to-end variety in that technical problems related to disparity in size between the colon and ileum are overcome. Nevertheless, some surgeons prefer to use the end-to-end technique. Minor disparity can be dealt with by adjusting the gaps between the needle insertions. When there is gross disparity in size it is recommended by some (Lockhart-Mummery, 1983) that the antimesenteric half of the colon should be closed in two layers and an end-to-end anastomosis between the ileum and the remaining end of colon be carried out (Figure 31.18). Although we do not have experience in this technique we cannot recommend it, since it would seem to create unnecessary weakness at the junction of the superior part of the anastomosis and the transverse closure of the colon. This is comparable with the 'angle of sorrow' between a gastrojejunostomy and the lesser curve closure which is created during a partial gastrectomy. Our preferred alternative for constructing an end-to-end anastomosis is to increase the available diameter of the ileum by dividing it obliquely as demonstrated in Figure 31.19.

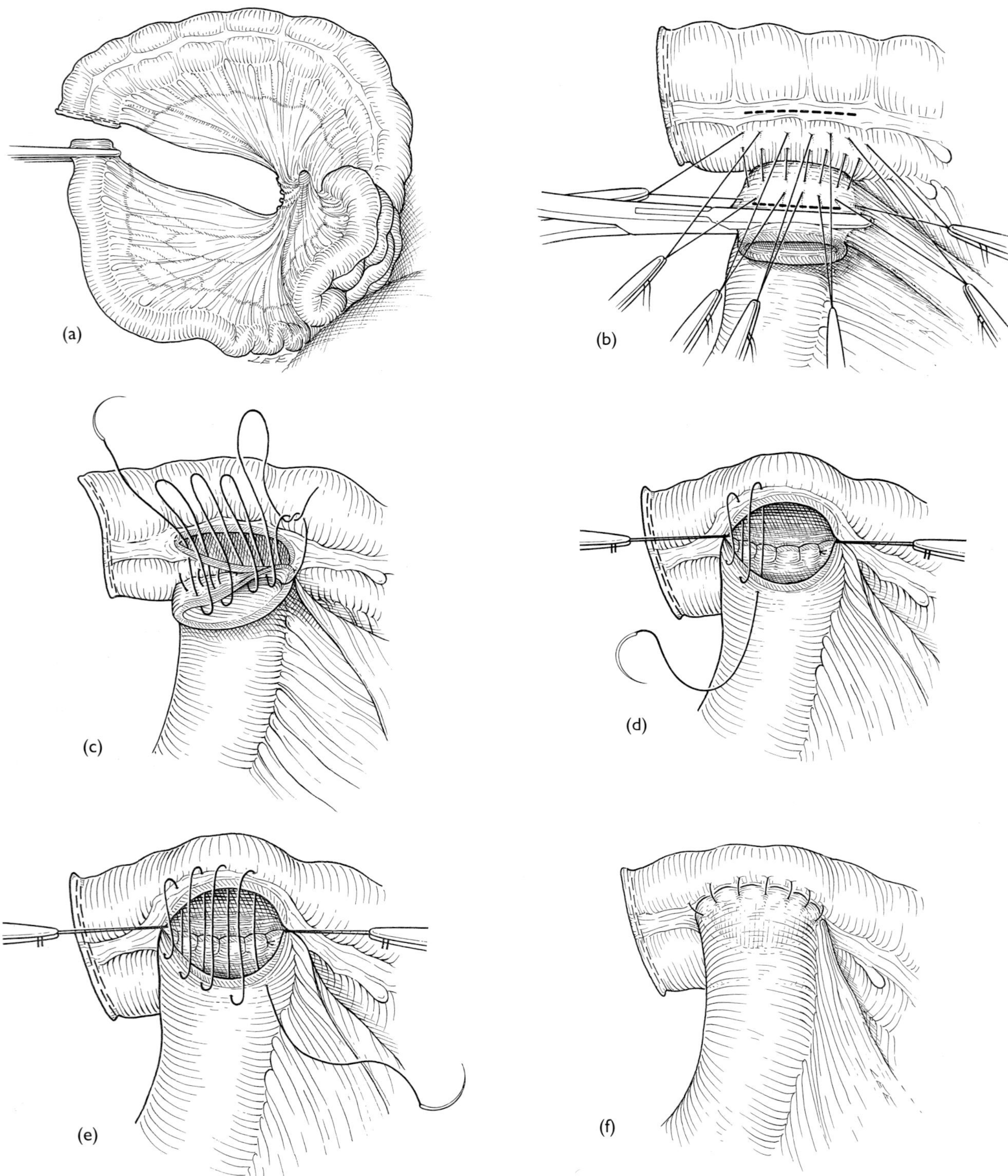

Figure 31.16a–f Right hemicolectomy with end-to-side anastomosis. (a) The caecum, ascending colon and hepatic flexure have been removed and the end of ileum is approximated to the side of the transverse colon. (b) Interrupted seromuscular sutures are placed between colon and ileum and are then tied. A transverse incision will be made in the colon (dotted line) and the crushing clamp will be cut off the ileum prior to insertion of the continuous inner layer of sutures. (c) A continuous 2/0 catgut suture is inserted through all layers of the posterior wall. (d) Insertion of continuous, all-layers anterior wall suture. This can be done using a continuous over-and-over inverting suture (as depicted) or a loop on mucosa Connell suture. (e) Insertion of interrupted seromuscular sutures on the anterior wall completes the anastomosis (f).

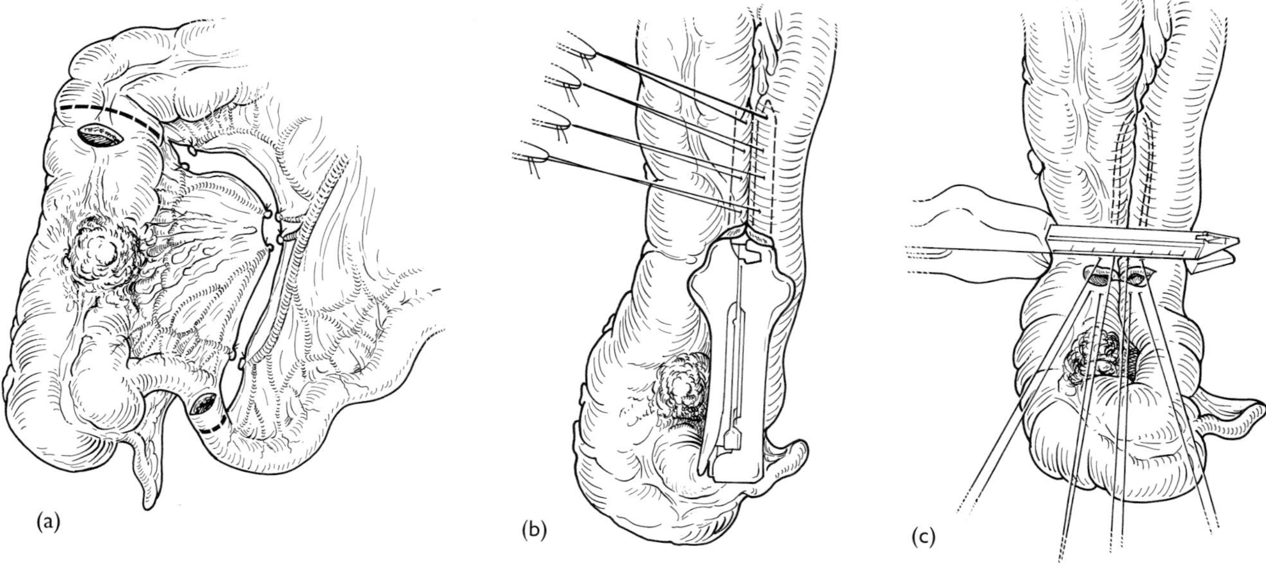

Figure 31.17a–c Right hemicolectomy using a linear staple cutter to form a functional end-to-end anastomosis.

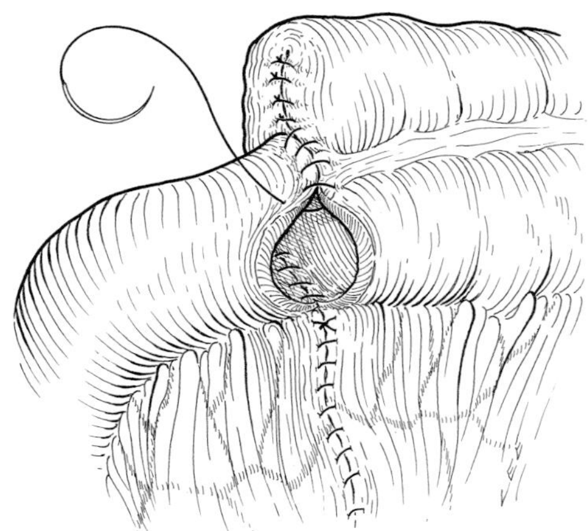

Figure 31.18 Right hemicolectomy: technique to overcome disparity between luminal sizes when performing an end-to-end ileocolic anastomosis. The antimesenteric half of the colon has been closed and the ileum is anastomosed to the remaining colonic lumen (Lockhart-Mummery, 1983).

In order to overcome gross disparity in size and to prevent the risk of intestinal obstruction when the distal ileum is of small calibre, some surgeons prefer to use a side-to-side anastomosis (Figure 31.20). In this technique both the distal end of the ileum and the proximal end of the transverse colon are closed either by staples or by hand. The anastomosis is then constructed manually in the usual way after making transverse incisions in both ileum and colon which are matched equally for length. All the anastomoses described above can be performed in one layer rather than two layers. Interrupted non-absorbable sutures are usually used. The arguments for or against these two types of anastomoses are set out in Chapter 6.

There has been a vogue of late to construct colonic anastomoses entirely by mechanical means. Thus each of the anastomoses discussed above – end-to-side, end-to-end or side-to-side – can be constructed using a variety of stapling instruments. Both the end-to-side and the end-to-end varieties require the use of the circular stapling gun. To insert the latter requires a separate enterotomy. For this reason we prefer a functional end-to-end anastomosis using the linear staple cutter to effect a side-to-side ileocolonic anastomosis while closing the two enterotomies with a second cartridge of the linear staple cutter or a transverse stapler. The technical details for these anastomoses are described in Chapter 6.

Transverse colectomy

Growths of the hepatic flexure are dealt with by radical right hemicolectomy and those of the splenic flexure by left hemicolectomy. Those in between require a transverse colectomy or an extended right or left hemicolectomy. The aims of transverse colectomy are the removal of the greater parts of the transverse colon, the attached greater omentum and

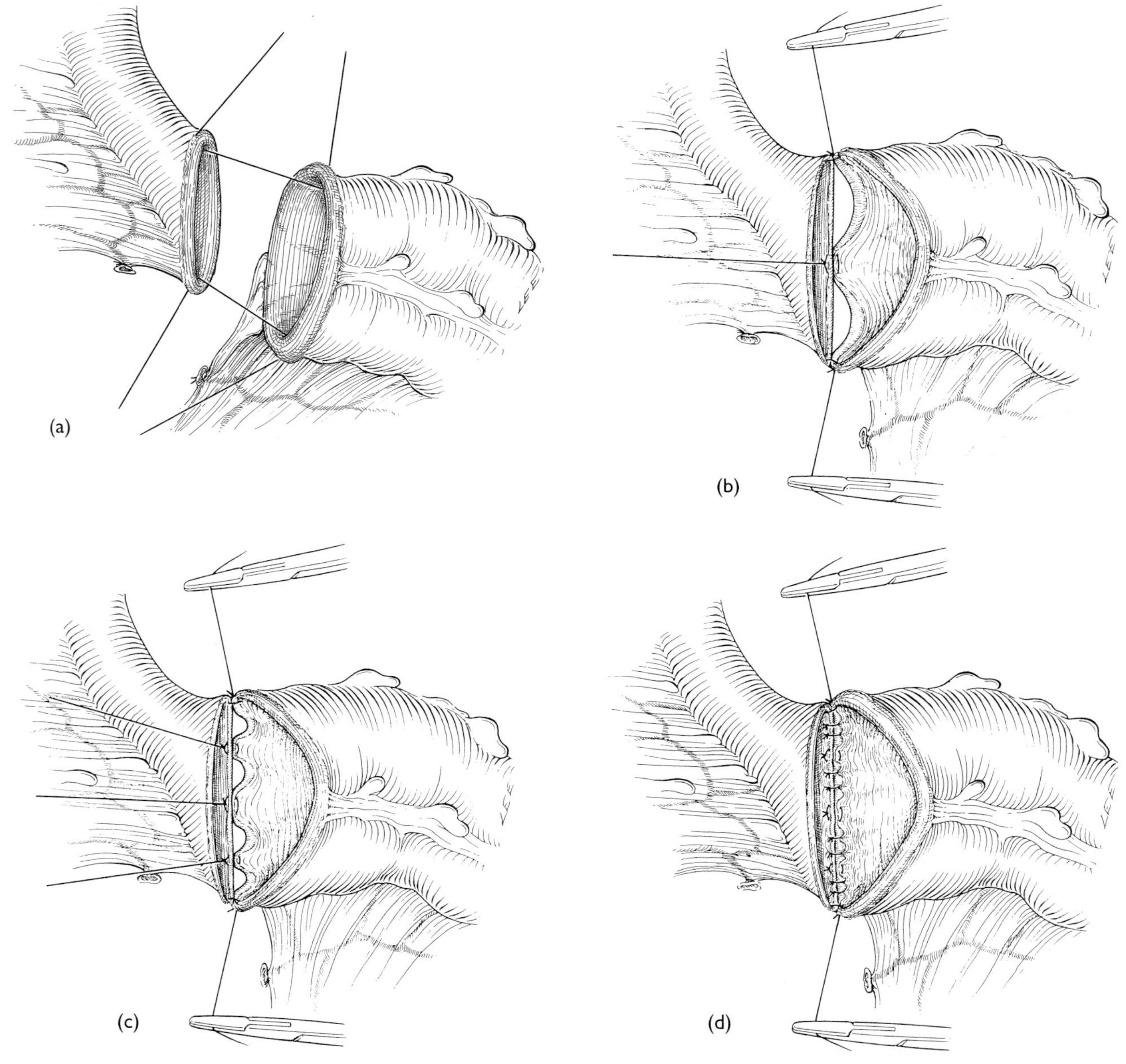

Figure 31.19a–d Right hemicolectomy with end-to-end ileocolic anastomosis. The ileum has been divided obliquely to overcome disparity between the size of the two lumina. The anastomosis can be constructed in one layer using interrupted non-absorbable sutures as depicted, or in two layers as for an end-to-side anastomosis.

the lymphatic field lying in the drainage of the middle colic artery.

The omentum is first detached from the greater curvature of the stomach, and the dissection continues around to both flexures of the colon (Figure 31.21a). The peritoneum forming the phrenicocolic ligaments is divided as each flexure is displaced downwards and medially. When dealing with the splenic flexure it is usually necessary to have the upper left lateral part of the wound powerfully retracted to obtain adequate access. Occasionally if there is a long, redundant transverse colon and a less than radical resection is to be performed, such mobilization is unnecessary. The middle colic artery is next divided close to its origin and the mesocolon is separated from its attachment to the posterior abdominal wall. The sites of transection are then selected carefully to ensure that both ends of the bowel have an adequate blood supply.

The mesocolon and marginal vessels are divided

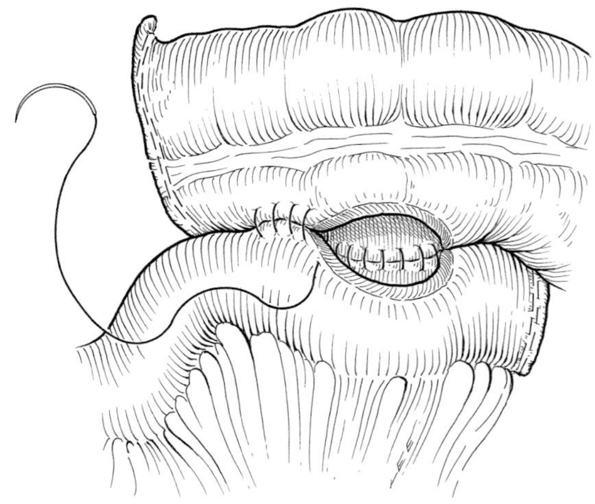

Figure 31.20 Right hemicolectomy with side-to-side ileocolic anastomosis.

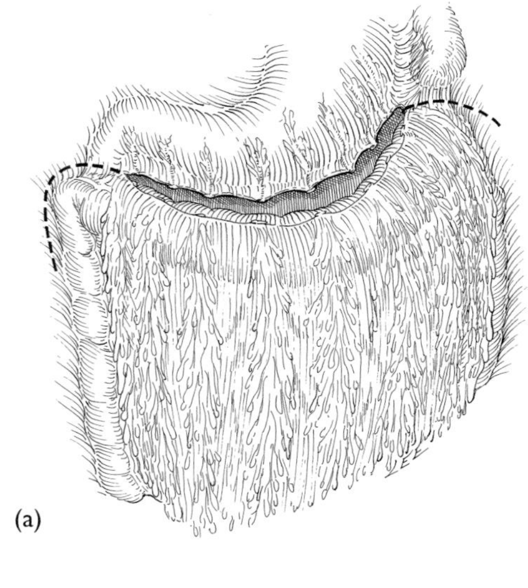

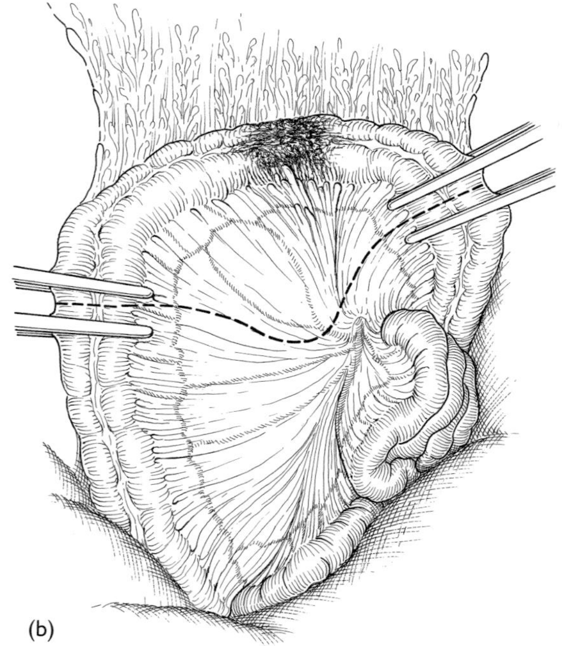

Figure 31.21a,b Transverse colectomy. (a) The omentum is detached from the greater curvature of the stomach and the dissection is continued around both flexures. (b) The mesocolon and marginal vessels are divided and the colon is transected between crushing clamps.

and ligated up to the colonic wall (Figure 31.21b), which is subsequently transected between crushing clamps. Since there is usually no disparity between the two ends of colon, except if some element of obstruction has occurred, an end-to-end anastomosis in two layers can usually be performed with ease. The defect in the mesocolon is then closed. If gross disparity does exist between the two ends, then one end of the transverse colon can be divided obliquely and an end-to-end anastomosis constructed; or failing this, an end-to-side or side-to-side anastomosis can be performed. Once again it is feasible (although expensive) to construct the anastomosis using stapling instruments.

Radical left hemicolectomy

Mobilization of the left colon normally commences at the level of the sigmoid colon. The peritoneal reflection on the lateral side of the colon is divided and the bowel is gradually mobilized medially (Figure 31.22a).

During the early part of mobilization the left ureter should be sought and swept laterally. If there is any doubt as to its subsequent course it is wise to place a sling of latex rubber around it and by so doing its course can be traced more easily. Mobilization of the descending colon and sigmoid colon reveals the perinephric fat, the ovarian or spermatic vessels, the lowest part of the aorta and the left common iliac artery in addition to the left ureter and left iliac vein (Figure 31.22b). The mesocolic vessels can now be seen usually running in the mesentery.

The next step involves freeing the entire splenic flexure. This is approached by first dividing the gastrocolic omentum beyond the gastro-epiploic arcade commencing opposite the junction of the middle and distal thirds of the transverse colon so that the omentum can be resected with the colon

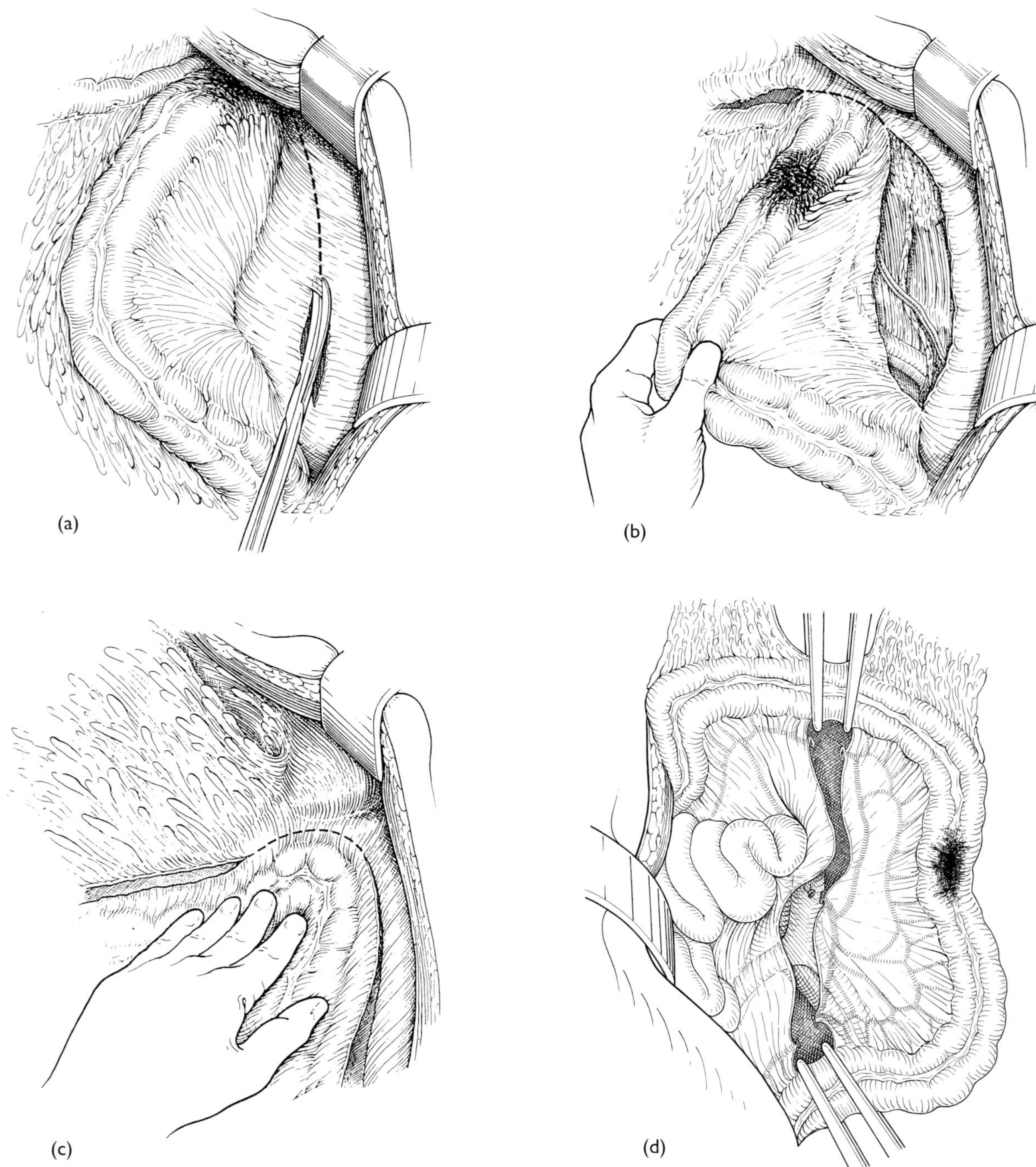

Figure 31.22a–d Left hemicolectomy. (a) The peritoneal reflection on the lateral side of the colon is divided. (b) Mobilization of the colon and splenic flexure continues by dividing the gastrocolic omentum and the peritoneal reflection to the lateral aspect of the splenic flexure (dotted line). The gonadal vessels, the left ureter, and the left common iliac artery and vein will be seen on the posterior abdominal wall. (c) Mobilization of the splenic flexure is highlighted illustrating the proximity of the spleen and the need for strong retraction of the left costal margin. (d) The posterior parietal peritoneum overlying the aorta is incised and the mesenteric artery and vein are divided at the level of the origin of the artery. The peritoneal incision is carried upwards exposing and dividing the left colic and marginal vessels on its way to reach the mid-transverse colon which is then clamped and divided. Similarly the distal sigmoid colon is clamped and divided.

(Figure 31.22b). This reflection of peritoneum is divided below the gastroepiploic vessels. The dissection is continued laterally towards the spleen. The splenic flexure must be taken down with great care as it is often very closely applied to the spleen. Rough handling can easily produce a tear in the splenic capsule which might result in severe haemorrhage and necessitate splenectomy. Rough handling of the splenic flexure may also damage the marginal artery upon which the proximal colon is dependent.

The left costal margin must be retracted with vigour and the light must be directed to the upper left quadrant (Figure 31.22c). Any vessels running between the spleen and the colon must be carefully electrocoagulated, or clamped and ligated. It is sometimes possible to create a pedicle of peritoneum and vessels by retracting the colon downwards and medially and creating a plane beneath the peritoneum which still remains intact between the colon and the spleen. This pedicle, which often contains the inferior mesenteric vein draining into the splenic vein, can gently be clamped between long artery forceps, divided and then ligated. The whole of the left colon is then freely mobile and remains attached to the posterior abdominal wall by the left end of the transverse mesocolon, the medial leaf of the peritoneum of the descending colon and the sigmoid mesocolon. The main vessels can now be seen running in this 'mesentery'.

The posterior parietal peritoneum over the aorta is next divided, commencing at the lower border of the third part of the duodenum taking down the duodenojejunal flexure and continuing downwards below the level of the aortic bifurcation. This division exposes the inferior mesenteric vessels (Figure 31.22d). The vessels are dealt with separately, the artery being divided flush with the aorta while the inferior mesenteric vein is ligated flush with the splenic vein if it has not already been ligated during mobilization of the splenic flexure. Both vessels are doubly ligated with a strong, non-absorbable ligature. After division of these vessels it is possible to displace them together with their associated lymph nodes forward off the aorta. Further dissection of the para-aortic lymph nodes may then take place if this is indicated.

The upper end of the peritoneal dissection is continued upwards around the lateral side of the duodenojejunal flexure to enter the transverse mesocolon. The peritoneal incision continues upwards parallel with the middle colic vessels and then the marginal artery is divided at the most appropriate level. The colon is next clamped and divided at this point (Figure 31.22d). The site of division of the marginal vessels and colon depends on the exact site of the growth. Thus if the lesion is at the splenic flexure, division is usually performed at the midpoint of the transverse colon. For tumours in the descending colon division of the transverse colon either at or just proximal to the splenic flexure is all that is required.

The peritoneal division is continued in a distal direction from the aortic bifurcation to the sacral promontory and then proceeds forwards in both leaves of the mesorectum to the level of the rectosigmoid junction. Division of the mesorectum is performed between clamps so that the superior rectal vessels may be divided. This part of the dissection may prove tedious in patients with a bulky, fat-laden mesorectum. Smaller vessels may be difficult to control if they retract into the mesorectum. To improve access during this part of the operation it may be necessary to position the patient in a 20-degree head-down tilt. This allows the rest of the bowel to be packed off with ease. The rectosigmoid junction is divided between crushing clamps or staples and the tumour-bearing colon is removed. An end-to-end anastomosis is constructed according to the preference of the surgeon; usually a single- or two-layer suture technique or a circular stapling instrument is employed, in a manner similar to that used for anterior resection, but being at an even higher level the anastomosis can easily be hand sutured. It is our practice to construct this in two layers as previously described for right hemicolectomy, but a one-layer anastomosis is quite acceptable.

Sigmoid colectomy

Most cases of carcinoma of the sigmoid colon can be removed by a less extensive procedure than radical left hemicolectomy (Figure 31.23). The technique is very similar, but only the superior rectal and sigmoid vessels are divided at their origin from the inferior mesenteric artery (i.e. just below the left colic artery). This ensures an excellent blood supply to most of the left colon which is then anastomosed to the upper rectum at the level of the sacral promontory in the manner previously described.

Additional manoeuvres

Peroperative irrigation of colon

During elective resections of the colon the lumen should be empty of faeces but there are times when bowel preparation is far from ideal. In these cases the best course of action is to perform on-table

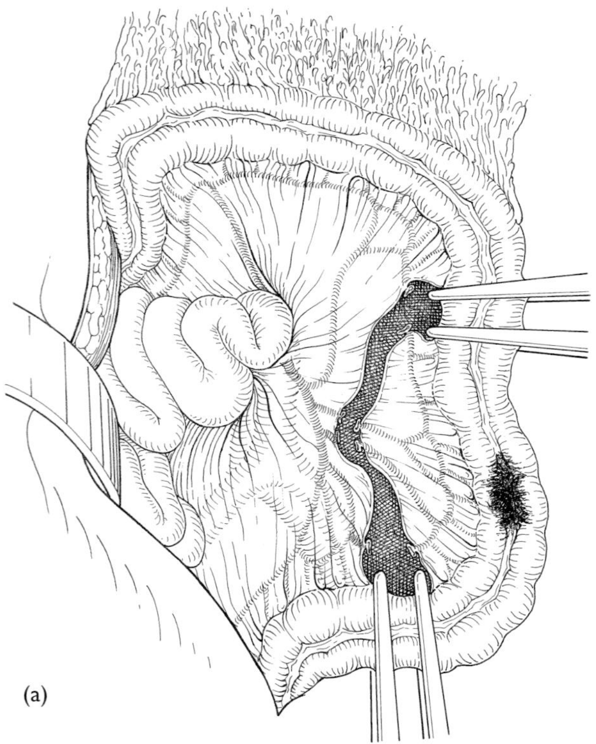

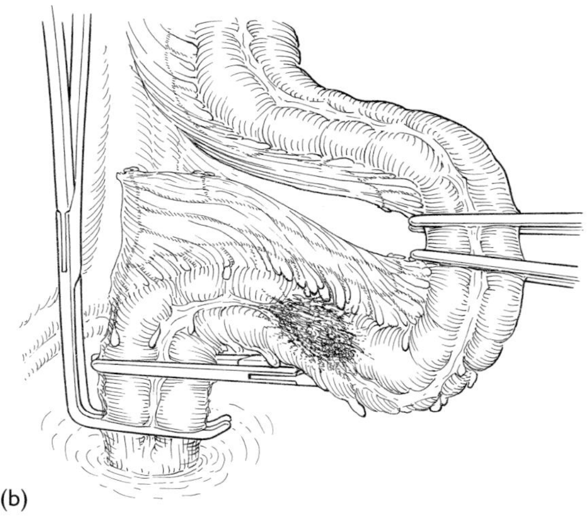

Figure 31.23a,b More restricted left hemicolectomy or sigmoid colectomy with preservation of the main inferior mesenteric artery and division of the left colic and first sigmoid arteries close to the main vessels.

irrigation of the colon. If the technique is performed accurately spillage of faeces should not occur (see Chapter 3).

After full mobilization of the colonic segment to be resected, a transverse incision is made between clamps in the colon just proximal to the proposed proximal division of the bowel (Figure 31.24a). Anaesthetic scavenger tubing is inserted through the colotomy. The tube is tied into place using tape; scavenger tubing is ideal since it contains grooves around its circumference which allow it to be tied securely into the bowel lumen. The distal end of the tube is placed by a non-sterile attendant into a container well away from the operating table, or a black plastic bag is tied to the tube. A purse-string suture is then placed in the ileum (or the appendix stump after appendicectomy). A large Foley catheter (about 24F) is passed through the purse-string into the caecum (Figure 31.24b). The balloon on the catheter is then inflated and the catheter is pulled back, and the purse-string suture is tied. The proximal end of the catheter is attached to an infusion set containing 1 L of Hartmann's solution. Approximately 3–4 L of fluid are run into the colon and by pressure and careful manipulation the colon is washed out. When clear fluid emanates from the distal end of the colon through the scavenger tubing, the irrigation is stopped and the colon is doubly clamped above the tubing and divided. The anastomosis then proceeds in the routine manner. At the end of the operation the Foley catheter is either removed or is brought out through the abdominal wall as a caecostomy.

Need for covering stoma

A covering stoma of any kind is rarely necessary after any type of colectomy for colon cancer when the procedure has been performed electively. Occasionally, however, even after peroperative irrigation of the colon, bowel preparation remains so poor that the surgeon feels it necessary to defunction the anastomosis. The usual practice is to perform a transverse loop colostomy for left-sided anastomoses or a loop ileostomy or caecostomy for right-sided ones. The pros and cons of these additional procedures are discussed elsewhere.

Other techniques for loaded colon

Other techniques for dealing with a loaded colon are rarely necessary during elective resection now that intraoperative irrigation can be performed so easily and efficiently. Certainly there is no justifica-

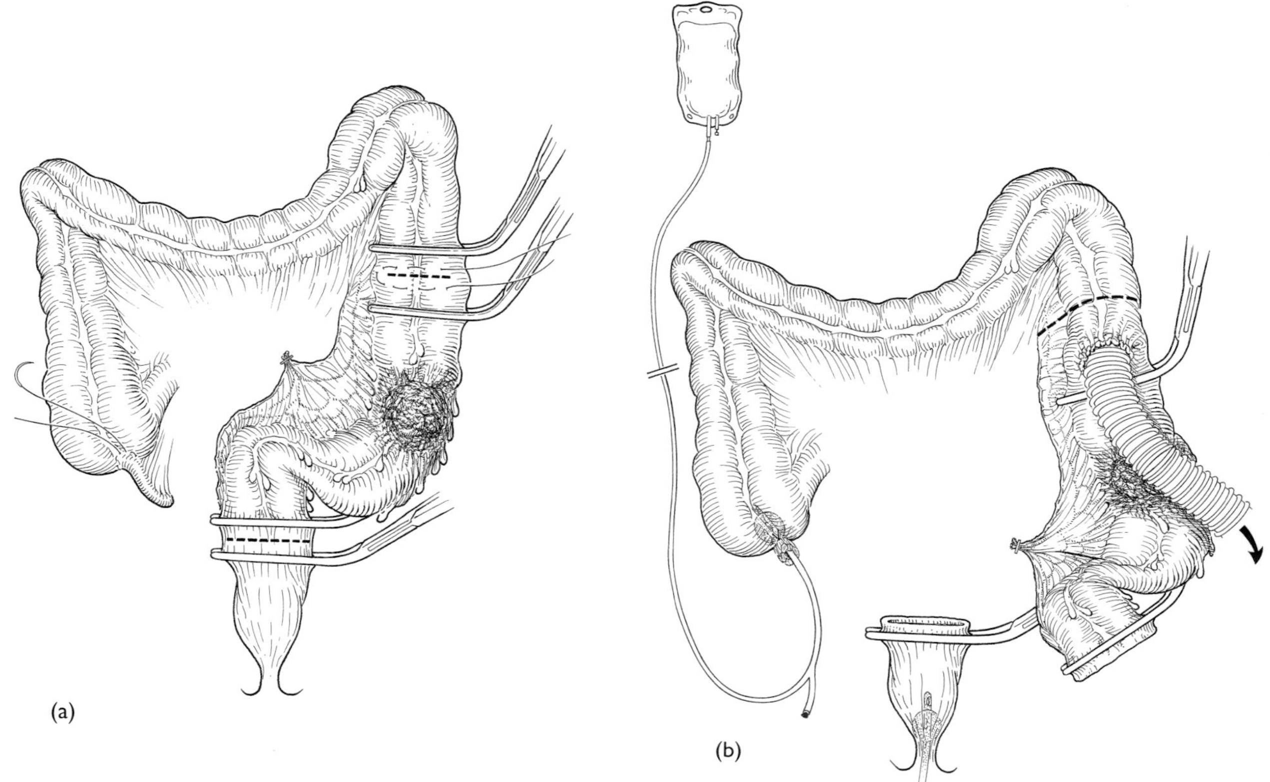

Figure 31.24a,b Peroperative, on-table colonic lavage. (a) After full mobilization of the colonic segment to be resected, a transverse incision is made between the proximal clamps after first inserting a purse-string suture. (b) Anaesthetic scavenger tubing is inserted through the colotomy and the purse-string suture is tied. The tubing is further secured using Nylon tape around the bowel. A large Foley catheter is inserted through the appendix stump into the caecum and secured by a purse-string suture. The catheter is attached to the infusion set and 3–4 L of fluid are then run into the colon.

tion these days for performing a subtotal colectomy or total colectomy with ileorectal or ileosigmoid anastomosis for this reason. Similarly, we cannot see the need for a preliminary transverse colostomy with resection of the tumour at a later stage. Occasionally a Hartmann's procedure may be needed for left-sided lesions, particularly if there has been contamination of the operative site by spillage of faeces or if sepsis is present.

Resection of other structures

Various structures may be invaded by the tumour or be adherent to it. In the case of tumours adherent to other structures, it is never wise to peel the lesion off the adjacent organ if a radical procedure is feasible. It is always advisable to assume that invasion of the structure has occurred so that an *en bloc* resection can be performed.

The most common structures invaded by tumours of the caecum and ascending colon are the right ureter, kidney, duodenum, liver, small intestine and the abdominal wall. Invasion of the right ureter may require a right nephrectomy. Occasionally after resection of the involved area the defect in the ureter can be repaired in some way and renal function on that side can be preserved. The actual type of repair will naturally depend on the surgeon's own experience and prejudices. It is our practice in these situations to discuss management with our urological colleagues. A ureterocystostomy (using either the 'psoas hitch' technique or the Boari flap) is invariably the first consideration. If this is not technically feasible, an end-to-end ureteric anastomosis, a transuretero-ureterostomy or a uretero-ileocystostomy will be considered. Sometimes none of these procedures is technically feasible, and provided renal function on the opposite side is adequate a nephrectomy is performed.

If the patient is in a poor condition an 'intubated ureterostomy' offers a safe, temporary way out of trouble. A suitable splinting catheter (e.g. a double J stent or Silastic tube) is tied in the proximal ureter. To ligate the ureter is to invite the risk of obstruction and infection in the first few postoperative days. The management of these urological complications is discussed in detail in Chapter 70.

En bloc resection of the small intestine usually presents no problems, but the same cannot be said for involvement of the duodenum. If duodenal invasion is extensive then radical resection is usually out of the question, although very occasionally a Whipple's procedure may be possible. With moderate invasion, it may be possible to perform a wedge resection of the duodenum together with the colectomy. Closure of the duodenal defect in these circumstances may, however, present a problem. End-to-end anastomosis may not be feasible owing to tension at the anastomotic line. Under these circumstances consideration should be given to suturing the duodenal defect to the side of a Roux loop of jejunum, or repairing it with a jejunal patch. Our preference is to use a Roux loop.

If there is direct invasion of the liver by a carcinoma of the hepatic flexure, transverse colon or splenic flexure, it may be possible to perform an *en bloc* resection taking a wedge out of the right or left lobes (see above). Invasion into the gallbladder alone can similarly be dealt with by concomitant cholecystectomy. However, involvement of the extrabiliary ducts or pancreatic head makes a radical procedure unlikely.

Tumours of the transverse colon not infrequently invade the stomach. In these circumstances the greater curve and/or antrum are usually implicated and often an *en bloc* resection with a distal two-thirds gastric resection is feasible. Gastrointestinal continuity is then best achieved as for a Polya gastrectomy. Invasion of the spleen, by a splenic flexure tumour, usually presents no problems since this organ can be removed concomitantly with the colonic segment. If the tail of the pancreas is also involved it can be dealt with in a similar manner, but the pancreatic duct will need to be ligated and the capsule of the pancreas closed with care.

Carcinomas of the descending colon and sigmoid colon are more likely to involve the ureter and kidney than tumours of the right colon. If retroperitoneal involvement does occur the tumours are dealt with by *en bloc* excision in the same manner. Not infrequently a bulky neoplasm may invade the psoas, quadratus lumborum, transversus abdominis or iliacus muscles. Involved muscle should be widely excised with the primary tumour. Sigmoid and rectosigmoid neoplasms may invade the bladder, and in the female the uterus or ovaries. Usually the dome of the bladder is involved and a wedge resection or partial cystectomy can be performed, the bladder being closed in two layers and a catheter then left *in situ* for at least seven days postoperatively.

Invasion of an ovary requires oophorectomy and salpingectomy, whereas if the uterus is involved concomitant hysterectomy is mandatory. Since invasion of pelvic organs is more likely in patients with carcinoma of the rectum, these additional manoeuvres are discussed at greater length in Chapter 32.

Preliminary ligation of colic vessels and isolation of tumour-bearing segment (no-touch technique of Turnbull)

Although customarily referred to as the Turnbull technique, the preliminary ligation of colic vessels and isolation of the tumour between tapes was first suggested by Cole et al (1954). The rationale propounded by Cole and by others (Miles, 1926; Fisher and Turnbull, 1955; Long et al, 1960) was that when a tumour is handled during mobilization, it releases into the circulation and bowel lumen large numbers of carcinoma cells which then have the propensity to spread throughout the body, seed and grow into metastases. Ligation of the vessels feeding and draining the tumour and placing tapes around the bowel above and below the tumour with injection of a cytocidal agent into the lumen as a first step should prevent this release. This is the theory, but by no means all coloproctologists are convinced of its veracity.

From the scientific point of view, the possibility of malignant cells being released into the circulation from a colorectal cancer does exist, but this phenomenon seems to occur throughout the life of the tumour and does not seem to be exaggerated by manipulation (Engell, 1955; Moore and Sako, 1959; Sellwood et al, 1965). If numerous cells are released into the circulation under normal conditions, the prevention during surgery of the release of a relatively small number of cancer cells seems unlikely to make much difference. Another point to consider is the viability of these cells; efforts to grow them in tissue culture have not always been successful (Moore, 1960).

The clinical evidence to support preliminary ligation of vessels also remains unconvincing. Most data have come from retrospective studies, of which that of Turnbull et al (1967) looks the most convincing. In this study the results of Turnbull's own cases treated by preliminary ligation were compared with those of his five colleagues at the same institution who did not practise this technique. The overall crude 5-year survival rate in the no-touch technique patients was 68.5% compared with 52.1% in patients treated in the more conventional manner. The difference for Dukes' C cases was even more striking: 57.8% for the no-touch technique versus 28.1% for the conventional method. However, such a comparison is not very informative: not only was the study not conducted in a prospective randomized manner, but the performance of five surgeons, each with their own individual technique, was compared with that of one surgeon. However, in a prospective randomized trial of 236 patients operated on for colon cancer, Wiggers et al (1988) demonstrated that in those patients who underwent preliminary ligation of vessels, liver metastases appeared later although no overall benefit in survival was demonstrated.

Omental wrap to reinforce anastomosis

Many surgeons believe that reinforcement of the anastomosis with a pedicled omental graft reduces the risk of leakage. Indeed, this procedure has been recommended for anastomoses constructed during oesophagectomy and various urological manoeuvres in addition to colorectal procedures (Turner-Warwick et al, 1967; Localio and Eng, 1975; Turner-Warwick, 1976; Goldsmith, 1977). Despite strong feelings expressed in favour of this manoeuvre, no objective data to support its use in humans are yet available. Experimental studies are similarly scanty and remain inconclusive. Thus Carter et al (1972) showed in rabbits that a free graft of omentum actually increased the chances of leakage, while a pedicled graft did not improve the survival rate of the animals. McLachlin and Denton (1973) confirmed in dogs the inadequacy of a free graft, but they did show in further experiments (McLachlin et al, 1976) that a pedicled graft when wrapped around a devascularized anastomosis of small bowel reduced the risk of leakage. Although it is to be hoped that all colonic anastomoses have an adequate blood supply, some may be marginally ischaemic. In these circumstances it could be argued that an omental wrap might be beneficial.

The technique of omental wrap should present little difficulty if the omentum is well developed and can reach the anastomosis without tension. For low anastomoses in the pelvis a pedicled graft has to be prepared, detaching the omentum from the transverse colon and greater curve of the stomach in such a way that it receives a blood supply from the right epiploic artery. It is usual to wrap the omental tail circumferentially around the anastomosis and secure its position by a few serosal sutures. In most patients having a colectomy, a segment of the omentum may have been resected with the tumour which could present difficulties if reinforcement is needed in the pelvis.

Drainage of the peritoneal cavity

While there have been several prospective controlled studies which demonstrate no benefit for draining the peritoneal cavity after cholecystectomy (Gordon et al, 1976; Stone et al, 1978; Johnson and Gilsdorf, 1981), scanty data are available for the benefit or otherwise of drainage after colonic resection (Lennox, 1984). Studies that have been performed have in the main used laboratory animals, and have demonstrated that open drainage instead of being a useful adjunct may be deleterious (Berliner et al, 1964; Manz et al, 1970). Certain materials such as latex rubber seem to be more of a problem than others (Smith et al, 1982). The few studies performed in humans show no appreciable difference in complications between patients in whom the abdomen is drained and those in whom it is not (Goligher, 1984).

It is clear from conversations with colleagues that despite the results of these studies opinion is firmly divided. Surgeons who routinely drain the abdomen after colonic resections believe that the drain serves several functions: it prevents the accumulation of possibly infected fluid, and if the anastomosis should break down it provides a route for egress of faecal material. Although drains may prevent the accumulation of fluid, the belief that drains minimize the consequences of anastomotic leak is only likely if the drain is left *in situ* for at least 5 or 6 days. Surgeons who advise against drainage suggest that the presence of an open drain may be deleterious as it can allow infection to gain entry to the peritoneal cavity, and by promoting an inflammatory reaction may encourage anastomotic dehiscence. Closed suction drains reduce the risk of accumulation of blood which if left *in situ* might cause an infected haematoma and an abscess.

It is our belief that closed drainage does have a useful role. The Vygon or Redivac suction drains seem to be the most efficient and least likely to produce reaction. Since a slight increase in the diameter of the tube will cause an enormous increase in flow rate (Evans, 1982), at the Royal London Hospital we use a no. 18 Portavac drain which is the largest available. In most cases the drain is left *in situ* no longer than 3 days and its principal role is to drain intraperitoneal fluid. In the few patients in whom there is concern about the future integrity of the anastomosis, the drain may be left in place for longer so that a track will form which will act as a conduit if faecal material escapes. Under these circumstances it is wise to leave the drain off suction and enclosed in a stoma bag to minimize exogenous bacterial contamination.

Injury to the spleen

Mobilization of the left colon and splenic flexure during colectomy may occasionally lead to splenic damage despite the most careful precautions. Injuries are most often caused by traction on the splenic peritoneal attachments, resulting in iatrogenic capsular avulsions. This is especially true in the area of insertion of the spleno-omental ligament which is often hidden under a fold of the gastrosplenic attachments (Kusminsky et al, 1984). The incidence of splenic damage during colonic operations seems to be approximately 2% (Devlin et al, 1969; Langevin et al, 1984).

Traditionally, surgeons have considered that any injury to the spleen – no matter how trivial – must be treated by splenectomy. Opinion in recent years has changed with the realization that the spleen has an important immunological role, and attempts are now made to preserve the spleen if at all possible. Tears of the splenic capsule can usually be easily dealt with by use of one of the several topical haemostatic agents now available, such as gelatine sponge or oxycellulose or by spray diathermy. Deep hilar injuries may be managed by first mobilizing the spleen. The injury can then be better assessed and the splenic artery temporarily occluded. Blood loss will be reduced and splenic blood pressure should fall sufficiently to allow haemostasis to be achieved by topical haemostatic agents or by splenorrhaphy (Langevin et al, 1984). It must be emphasized, however, that despite the feasibility of conserving the spleen after injury during colonic resection, if there is any doubt concerning the safety of such a manoeuvre, splenectomy should be performed forthwith. It is our practice to preserve the spleen only in cases with relatively minor tears of the capsule. If the spleen has to be removed the patient should receive pneumococcal vaccine for prophylaxis against pneumococcal septicaemia.

Faecal contamination of the peritoneal cavity

Faecal contamination may occur during the course of a colonic resection for carcinoma, particularly if the anastomosis is constructed using an open as opposed to a closed technique. In the main, however, spillage is minor. Occasionally more serious contamination results when the bowel is heavily loaded with faeces or is accidentally perforated. Such a complication greatly increases the risks of infection (Rosenberg et al, 1971) and every effort must be made to remove all faecal matter from the peritoneal cavity (Hau and Simmons, 1978; Hau et al, 1978). This aim may be achieved by irrigation of the peritoneal cavity with approximately 5–8 L of fluid.

Debate still thrives as to the optimum irrigating fluid. Three types of irrigant have been used: normal saline, antibiotic solutions and antiseptic solutions. The numerous antibiotic solutions which have been utilized include neomycin (0.5% or 1%) (Poth, 1953; Hoffman, 1959), tetracycline (Cohn, 1960; Poth, 1963; Stewart and Matheson, 1978; Stewart, 1980), cephalothin (Peloso et al, 1973), gentamicin and lincomycin (Stewart, 1980). Each has its supporters but trials are very difficult to assess, since patients almost always have received antibiotics systemically which usually achieve high concentrations in peritoneal fluid anyway. The two antiseptics most frequently used for peritoneal irrigation have been noxythiolin (Noxyflex) (Browne and Stoller, 1970) and povidone-iodine (Gilmore and Sanderson, 1975). Noxythiolin is claimed also to have the advantage of being cytotoxic to cancer cells (Jamieson, 1972) and to reduce the formation of adhesions (Rosin et al, 1978); the latter claim has not been substantiated (Rafferty, 1979). Although povidone-iodine may have an antibacterial effect, there is evidence that it may induce a metabolic acidosis (Lores et al, 1981). For this reason it is not to be recommended.

It is our belief that irrigation of the contaminated peritoneal cavity may be beneficial. Provided that the patient is on systemic antibiotics, irrigation with normal saline is all that is required. After instillation the fluid should be removed as completely as possible by suction. In addition the peritoneal cavity should be drained with closed suction drains. Although there may be a difference of opinion among surgeons concerning the necessity of draining the peritoneal cavity when there has been no faecal contamination, drainage is generally advised after major contamination. We use large suction drains; one is usually positioned in the pelvis and the other is sited near the anastomosis if appropriate. The drains are brought out through separate stab wounds as far from the main wound as possible.

Nowadays all patients undergoing colonic resection should have received prophylactic systemic antibiotics so that they will have high blood concentrations of the drug at the time of operation. If major faecal contamination occurs at the time of surgery, it is now generally accepted that the same antibiotic regimen should be continued for 2–3 days after the usual perioperative doses have been given.

Closure of the abdominal wound

Descriptions of abdominal wound closure are given in detail in Chapter 6. We prefer the technique of mass suture which involves the insertion of wide stitches (a minimum of 1 cm from the wound edge) through the entire musculoaponeurotic layers of the abdominal wall including the peritoneum but not the subcutaneous fat or skin. Either interrupted or continuous sutures may be used.

The type of suture material is also open to debate. Most surgeons use a non-absorbable material such as monofilament nylon or polypropylene. Such material, however, may result in persistent wound infection with resulting sinus formation, and in order to avoid this complication absorbable materials such as polyglycolic acid and polydioxan have more recently been utilized. These materials have the advantage that although absorbable they take a considerable period (2–3 months) to disappear and tend to maintain their strength during the interim. However, they are weaker than the non-absorbable materials and although dehiscence rates are similar incisional herniation may be more common. Our preference is to use a double loop of continuous 1/0 monofilament nylon.

Classification of operation

It is important after the operation to know whether the procedure has been curative or palliative. Until recently this distinction has been subjective, based primarily on the surgeon's view as to whether all the tumour had been removed. Sometimes this was supported by histological confirmation, but often it was not. In order to standardize the operative procedure, the UKCCCR subcommittee on colorectal cancer issued certain recommendations. Based on the standardized preoperative, operative and histological assessments an operation for colorectal cancer should be classified as curative, non-curative or indeterminate for cure (Williams et al, 1988; UKCCCR, 1996).

Non-curative operations

These are operations in which tumour has been left behind. The procedures should be categorized into two groups:

- *Non-curative owing to the presence of distant metastases*. Whenever possible this must be supported by histological confirmation. The latter proviso may be waived when metastases are convincingly demonstrated on imaging but biopsy is not feasible (e.g. lung metastases detected on chest radiography).
- *Non-curative owing to the presence of residual local disease*. This must be confirmed by histological examination. Included in this category are patients whose operative specimens on histological examination show tumour at any margin of excision.

Curative operations

Curative operations are defined as procedures in which metastases have been excluded by preoperative imaging and the surgeon has removed all tumour, as confirmed by postoperative histological examination of the specimen.

Indeterminate for cure

If there is any doubt the patient should be classified as having an operation which is indeterminate for cure. Procedures during which the specimen has been perforated either spontaneously or operatively should be classified as indeterminate for cure. The definition of 'curative' can be applied only to operations in which the tumour has been resected together with a segment of bowel and its associated area of lymphatic drainage. Procedures in which the tumour is removed by local excision can be classified only as either non-curative or indeterminate.

Postoperative care

Postoperative care following resection of the colon for malignant disease does not differ appreciably from any other major intra-abdominal procedure in which the gastrointestinal tract has been manipulated and entered. Analgesics (usually of the opiate variety) are administered systemically fairly regularly and we now prefer to give these via an infusion pump controlled by the patient (PCA). The patient is encouraged to mobilize as quickly as possible. These patients are often elderly and invariably require active physiotherapy for their chest and legs. The patient is examined daily for the presence of wound and chest sepsis, deep venous thrombosis and paralytic ileus. The urethral catheter should remain *in situ* for several days until the patient is fully mobilized. Intravenous fluids should be administered until the patient is able to drink *ad libitum*. A 0.18% solution of saline with 4% dextrose is used normally. The volume of intravenous fluid per 24 hours is reduced as the volume taken by mouth increases. Whereas in the past it was usual to keep a nasogastric tube *in situ* until flatus was passed per anum, the policy is now either to dispense with a tube altogether or to remove it within the first 24 hours after the operation. A nasogastric tube is uncomfortable for the patient and may impair respiratory function and mobilization. A randomized controlled trial (Olesen et al, 1984) compared the postoperative course of patients who had undergone colorectal procedures and who were treated with or without nasogastric decompression; 97 patients were included in the trial. Flatus was passed earlier in the patients without tubes. No significant differences were found between the two groups with respect to duration and severity of postoperative ileus as measured by occurrence and duration of nausea and vomiting, postoperative oral fluid intake and time until defecation. It has therefore been our policy to dispense with routine nasogastric decompression postoperatively in most patients.

Normally flatus is passed on the third or fourth postoperative day; sometimes it is necessary to encourage movement within the colon by use of one or two glycerine suppositories. Enemas are clearly contraindicated. If drainage tubes have been inserted they are left *in situ* for several days until drainage ceases. If all is well the subcuticular polypropylene skin suture is removed on or about the tenth day.

Postoperative complications

Resection of the colon for carcinoma may be followed by any of the local and general complications that can occur after major abdominal surgery. Since the patients are often elderly, the complication rate tends to be higher than after other procedures. Each of the various complications are discussed in detail elsewhere in this book. It is, however, pertinent to discuss anastomotic breakdown in relation to colonic anastomoses at this point.

Anastomotic breakdown

The causes for anastomotic breakdown after resection for malignancy are numerous and include both general and local factors. General factors which may be present include protein-energy deficiency, vitamin C deficiency, uraemia, steroid dependence and diabetes. Particular general factors that are more prevalent in this group of patients are age, anaemia and the malignant process itself. Local factors include the presence of infection in the operative field or the construction of an anastomosis under tension or in the presence of obstruction. An inadequate blood supply to the proximal or distal ends of the anastomosis is another important reason for dehiscence. Several studies have demonstrated that the blood supply under normal circumstances is considerably reduced at an anastomosis and if it is compromised in any other way by platelet aggregation, hypotension or hypovolaemia, dehiscence is almost inevitable.

Local trauma and infection depress the collagen content and tensile strength at the anastomotic site (Irvin and Hunt, 1974). Previous radiation therapy may also predispose to anastomotic disruption.

Clinical features

Anastomotic breakdown is more common than is clinically obvious. Thus Goligher et al (1970) using sigmoidoscopy, barium enema and digital examination detected a 40% leak rate in 47 patients who had undergone a high anterior resection and a leakage rate no less than 69% in 26 patients after low anterior resection. Although no comparable data are available for colonic resections alone, it is likely that there will be a higher rate of subclinical leaks compared with clinical leaks. Fielding et al (1980) in a large, multicentre study found that anastomotic leakage of clinical importance occurred in about 10% of all large-bowel anastomoses.

Anastomotic dehiscence may present in a variety of ways and may begin insidiously. Prodromal signs include abdominal pain, distension, and increasing pyrexia and pulse rate. Local peritonitis, diffuse peritonitis or a frank faecal fistula may supervene. The patient with local peritonitis often remains surprisingly well, but develops increasing pain and tenderness usually in the vicinity of the wound and the temperature remains elevated. Associated paralytic ileus is common. At this stage it is sometimes difficult to distinguish a localized leak from a simple wound infection. Often, there follows a discharge of pus and later faecal matter either through the wound, along the drain site or per rectum, and the patient's general condition may then improve.

The patient with generalized peritonitis may have all the signs and symptoms that are generally attributable to this condition: severe, generalized abdominal pain, diffuse tenderness, board-like rigidity and absent bowel sounds. Although there may be a gradual progression from non-specific clinical features to an obvious picture of dehiscence, this course of events is not always followed. Thus a patient may discharge faecal material through the abdominal wall with no evidence of a previous systemic illness or local signs. Similarly, the patient may suddenly collapse with shock and generalized peritonitis after appearing to have progressed well after the operation. Evidence of peritonitis may be lacking in patients who develop Gram-negative shock. Sometimes the patient never develops signs of an obvious dehiscence but continues to exhibit non-specific clinical features which cause a gradual deterioration in health. For these reasons it is essential to consider that dehiscence of the anastomosis may have occurred in any patient who does not progress satisfactorily after colonic resection. The onus on the surgeon, no matter how senior, is to prove that the patient has not suffered this complication. Only by accepting that dehiscence is always a possibility will the diagnosis be reached swiftly and prompt treatment instituted.

Investigations

The investigations that may help to achieve the diagnosis of dehiscence and their usefulness will depend to some extent on the clinical features. The white blood cell count will invariably be raised indicating the presence of intra-abdominal sepsis. Occasionally when the patient has collapsed from endotoxic shock the white cell count may be unusually low. A plain radiological examination of the abdomen in the erect and supine positions may be very helpful in resolving the dilemma. Distended large and small bowel with fluid levels will confirm the presence of a paralytic ileus. Gas under the diaphragm will almost certainly be present but its amount may be critical. After a laparotomy air within the peritoneal cavity is inevitable; however, it begins to be absorbed after several days and by the tenth day has usually disappeared entirely. Dehiscence usually takes place at a time when it is expected that little air will remain in the peritoneal cavity. The presence therefore of large quantities of air 7–10 days after colectomy in a patient with signs suggestive of leak is convincing evidence that dehiscence has occurred. However, anastomotic breakdown can occur without an increase in intraperitoneal gas.

It is sometimes difficult to distinguish clinically the patient who has a dehiscence from one with an intraperitoneal abscess alone, but abdominal ultrasonography can often determine which of the two entities is present.

If the diagnosis remains uncertain and provided the patient's general condition allows it, a Gastrografin or Urografin enema may be useful. This should be performed by an experienced radiologist with a member of the surgical team in attendance to ensure that excessive distension of the colon causing high intraluminal pressures is avoided. Many colonic anastomoses will show some radiological evidence of a leak, but this does not necessarily mean that it is the cause of the problem. However, in a patient with clinical signs of dehiscence who has a large amount of contrast medium escaping from the anastomotic area, it is highly likely that this is the cause of the problem. A normal Gastrografin enema is extremely helpful negative information. Nevertheless, we have seen clinically apparent anastomotic dehiscence develop after a normal contrast study, indicating that this examination may not demonstrate all leaks and may be responsible for anastomotic breakdown.

It should be stressed that if the clinical picture is clearly one of anastomotic dehiscence and the patient's general condition is poor, the surgeon must not waste time on investigations that will delay appropriate treatment. Often in these cases a swift repeat laparotomy can be life-saving.

Treatment of anastomotic breakdown

Treatment depends on the clinical manifestations of the dehiscence. Patients can broadly be divided into those with generalized peritonitis and those with localized peritonitis.

Generalized peritonitis

The patient with generalized peritonitis as a result of an anastomotic leak may be *in extremis* and the first priority will be resuscitation. A central venous pressure line should be established as quickly as possible. Infusion of plasma expanders will be necessary through a separate intravenous line. Effective systemic antibiotics must be given immediately: we usually give metronidazole and gentamicin. If the blood pressure still remains low, large doses of hydrocortisone may be required together with pressor agents such as dopamine. As soon as the patient is stable a laparotomy should be performed. The exact timing of the surgical intervention may be difficult. Prolonged attempts to resuscitate the patient may be time wasted, since the collapse is usually caused by faecal material in the peritoneal cavity. Until the contamination is resolved improvement in the patient's condition may not be possible. It is our policy in these circumstances to continue aggressive resuscitation for no more than an hour; the patient is then transferred to the operating theatre even if no improvement has occurred (see Chapter 66).

The abdomen is opened through the previous incision and the presence of peritonitis is confirmed. The small and large bowel tend to be matted together by fibrinous adhesions. These can easily be broken down and with care the site of the anastomosis can be visualized. The extent of the dehiscence can then be determined. Postoperative peritonitis may be due to various causes and if the anastomosis appears to be circumferentially intact another cause should be sought. In these circumstances particular attention should be paid to the detection of inadvertent damage to another part of the intestine, or to the presence of a perforated stress ulcer of the stomach or duodenum.

If an anastomotic dehiscence is detected, soft clamps should be placed across the bowel approximately 5 cm distal and proximal to the anastomosis to prevent further leakage. No matter how small the defect at the anastomosis, the surgeon must resist the temptation simply to suture it. Attempted closure of an anastomotic leak is doomed to failure. Some have recommended, in patients with a small leak who are considered to be in a good general condition and where minimal contamination has occurred, that the anastomosis can be resected and a reanastomosis performed (White and Harrison, 1975). We strongly advise against this course of action.

The safest treatment is to break down the anastomosis completely, resect both ends of bowel, and if there is sufficient length exteriorize them, the proximal end as a stoma (ileostomy or colostomy) and the distal end as a mucous fistula. If possible the two ends should be exteriorized as close together as possible on the abdominal wall since this will allow subsequent closure to be achieved more easily. Sometimes owing to tethering of the bowel and its mesentery it is not possible to exteriorize the distal end of colon; this is particularly true of left-sided colonic anastomoses. Under these circumstances it is acceptable to close the distal end of the colon and replace it within the peritoneal cavity.

After the anastomotic site has been dealt with, attention must be turned to dealing with the peritonitis. The peritoneal cavity should be irrigated with a fluid of the surgeon's choice. At the Royal London Hospital we prefer to use a solution of cefuroxime (750 mg dissolved in 1 L of normal saline). Some groups (Hudspeth, 1975; Hau and Simmons, 1978) also advocate the excision of all fibrinous deposits on the peritoneum on the grounds that they act as a nidus for continual bacterial growth. This we have always considered to be unnecessary, a view verified in a controlled clinical trial performed by Polk and Fry (1980).

Drainage is always used following laparotomy for dehiscence but the need for continuous postoperative peritoneal lavage is debatable. There has been some enthusiasm for this form of therapy in patients with faecal peritonitis (McKenna et al, 1970; Stephens and Loewenthal, 1979; O'Brien, 1981). Despite these reports, there are no controlled trials to support them and until such studies have shown the merits of this technique we remain sceptical.

Localized peritonitis

It may be best to treat patients who exhibit signs of localized peritonitis conservatively. Certainly, in patients with little systemic illness who are relatively comfortable, there may be considerable merit in pursuing a non-operative policy. This regimen is particularly attractive in the elderly patient. If this policy is adopted the patient must be carefully observed on a regular basis and if there is the slightest hint of deterioration without a collection of pus that may be drained percutaneously urgent laparotomy should be undertaken.

Part of the conservative management consists of establishing early parenteral nutritional support, which allows the patient to be maintained in a positive nitrogen balance. Progressive hypoalbuminaemia, however, suggests the presence of localized sepsis which should be drained. Parenteral nutrition is a relatively new addition to therapy which has allowed more patients with this complication to be treated without surgical intervention. Oral fluids are discontinued and a nasogastric tube is passed if there is an associated paralytic ileus. Systemic antibiotics are also commenced. Ultrasound and CT scans are very useful at this stage, and if they demonstrate a localized abscess, radiographically guided percutaneous drainage should be attempted. If pus is located the radiologist should leave an indwelling tube in the cavity (see Chapter 66).

Sometimes percutaneous drainage is not possible or is contraindicated, and after several days pus and faeces may drain from the wound or previous drain site resulting in a faecal fistula. Usually under these circumstances the patient's general condition improves and if so the therapeutic regimen should be continued. Provided there is no distal obstruction the fistula will usually close spontaneously.

Sometimes despite spontaneous drainage of

purulent material the patient's condition does not improve and the establishment of more efficient drainage becomes necessary. Similarly if the patient's condition deteriorates or if there is evidence that the abscess surrounding a dehiscence is no longer localized, urgent surgical intervention is necessary. Under these circumstances not only is drainage required but the anastomosis should be taken down in the manner previously described.

RESULTS OF ELECTIVE SURGICAL TREATMENT OF COLONIC CARCINOMA

Of the numerous publications on the results of surgical treatment for colorectal carcinoma, relatively few draw the distinction between carcinoma of the colon and carcinoma of the rectum. Since it appears that these tumours may behave differently, the results related to colonic cancer only are considered in this section. Hence the data presented here represent only a small proportion of that available for large bowel cancer.

Resectability and operative mortality

Improvements in anaesthesia, intensive therapy care and the introduction of modern antibiotic treatment have been responsible for the improved immediate results of surgery for colonic carcinoma. During the period 1910–60 the resectability rate steadily increased while the operative mortality rate decreased (Table 31.10). According to some authors (Grinnell, 1953) the resectability rate increased from approximately 50% to 90%, whereas the operative mortality was frequently reduced to about one-sixth of its former rate. Between 1950 and 1980 mortality rates appeared to reach a plateau (Table 31.11).

Pihl et al (1980), reporting on their series of 615 patients operated on between 1950 and 1977 at Monash University, Melbourne, had an operative mortality rate of 7.2%. Similarly Abrams (1980) recorded an overall mortality rate of 6.5% in 516 patients with colonic carcinoma operated on between 1971 and 1975 in Vermont. In this study the mortality rate for right colectomy (6.8%) did not differ significantly from that of left colectomy (6.1%). Of the 215 patients with colonic cancer treated by resection, Turunen and Peltokallio (1983) reported an operative mortality rate of 5%; again, there was no significant difference between right-sided and left-sided resections. Similar results were achieved by other authors (Miller and Allbritten, 1976; Corman et al, 1979). In a more recent study conducted in a region of Scotland, 490 paients had a colonic resection for a colon cancer over a 2-year period, and the operative mortality was 4.8% (Lothian and Borders, 1995). Sales and Parc (1994) in Paris found that their mortality in 1981 was 4.3%. Bokey et al (1995) in Australia found that between 1971 and 1991 their operative mortality was 3.6% in 971 patients who underwent elective resection for colon cancer, and there was no difference between patients who underwent right or left colonic resections.

Table 31.10 Resectability and operative mortality rates for colonic carcinoma between 1910 and 1960.

Authors	*Period*	*Resectability rate (%)*	*Mortality rate (%)*
Allen et al (1947)	1925–1942	51	17.5
	1943–1946	95	2
McKittrick (1948)	1932–1941		11
	1942–1949		5.4
Grinnell (1953)	1915–1920	50	31.3
	1945–1950	92	5.3
Morgan (1957)	1928–1942		14.9
	1943–1955		7.4
Smiddy and Goligher (1957)	1938–1943	41	21
	1947–1955	55	9.5

Only one left-sided colonic tumour included.

Table 31.11 Operative mortality for colonic cancer 1950–1980.

Authors	*n*	*Mortality* (%)
Pihl et al (1980)	615	7.2
Abrams (1980)	516	6.5
Turunen and Peltokallio (1983)	215	5.0

While it is not always possible to determine the resectability rate from all the recent studies, they average 90%. Although these rates have remained relatively static over the last 10–15 years, the age of the patients operated on for this condition has generally increased. Another difficulty is that some authors have not differentiated between palliative and radical excisions. While this distinction has been somewhat subjective on the part of the surgeon, the fact that it was made by some and not by others makes interpretation difficult. This criticism also applies to survival data.

When assessing these results it is important to take into consideration that they have usually been achieved in specialized centres where emergency cases have invariably been excluded. When the operative mortality and resectability rates are examined for regions in which every patient operated upon for carcinoma of colon is included in the statistics, the situation is somewhat different. Thus data from the Connecticut Tumour Registry, which had details of 12 727 patients operated on for carcinoma of colon since 1935, showed that the resectability rate although increasing over the years was only 77% in 1960–62 (Eisenberg et al, 1967). The data from the South Western Regional Cancer Bureau in the UK were even less encouraging, for between 1962 and 1964 only 59% of the 2023 patients who were registered to have carcinoma of the colon underwent a resection of their tumours. Similarly Slaney (1971) found that of the 6694 patients registered with colon cancer in the Birmingham Cancer Registry only 46.2% underwent radical surgery, and 23.3% had only a palliative procedure of some form. More recent data from Birmingham showed no improvement in operability between 1940 and 1985 (Slaney, 1971; West Midlands Cancer Registry, 1990; Allum et al, 1994). In the two largest audits of patients with colorectal cancer carried out recently in the UK, in the Trent/Wales and Wessex regions, the overall rates of curative resection were 60% and 53% respectively. It is also of interest that in these audits the rate of curative resection varied from 31% to 72% between districts (Royal College of Surgeons, 1996).

Thus in the UK it is apparent even today that, when all patients are considered, approximately half to one-third do not undergo a radical resection for their carcinoma. Presumably the main reason for this relates to the fact that patients present too late in the course of their illness for such treatment to be feasible. It would also appear that this happens more often outside specialized referral centres. With the emphasis on screening programmes and open-access endoscopy and fast track clinics, it is to be hoped that earlier diagnosis, increased resection rates and improved survival rates will be achieved in the future.

Morbidity

As might be expected with improvement in operative mortality, the postoperative morbidity rates following resection for colonic carcinoma have also decreased substantially.

Perhaps the most dramatic effect has been the reduction in wound sepsis. The ability to obtain a clean, empty bowel has certainly made some impact in this direction (Keighley, 1977), although there are data which dispute this assertion (Irving and Scrimgeour, 1987). Perhaps the major advance responsible for this improvement has been the introduction of systemic antibiotics administered in such a way that maximum serum concentrations are achieved at the time of operation and in the immediate postoperative period. In addition the introduction, from around 1975, of effective antianaerobic therapy has helped greatly to reduce sepsis rates (Goldring et al, 1975). If suitable antibiotics are given at the appropriate time, it appears that wound infection rates of between 2.5% and 10% can be obtained for patients undergoing elective operations for colorectal disease (Lewis et al, 1983; Aberg et al, 1984; Lindhagen et al, 1984; Peck et al, 1984; Matheson et al, 1985; Rowe-Jones et al, 1990; Page et al, 1993). This compares with the 40–70% rates frequently seen in bygone eras (Shorey, 1979). Similarly, the overall sepsis rates including intra-abdominal abscess formation are also reduced.

As with data concerning resection rates, it is unusual for authors to divide their results into colonic and rectal cases. However, it would be surprising if abdominal wound sepsis rates were not similar in the two subgroups of patients.

Similarly, it is difficult to determine the anastomotic dehiscence rates for resections performed for colonic cancer alone. Studies that have assessed this demonstrate a clinical dehiscence rate in elective cases of between 1% and 5% (Bokey et al, 1995;

Docherty et al, 1995; Flyger et al, 1995; Lothian and Borders, 1995). Where right and left colectomies have been compared, there do not appear to have been significant differences. Most studies have involved hand-sewn anastomoses, but where stapled colonic anastomoses have been compared postoperatively with hand-sewn anastomoses, there has also been no significant difference in clinical leak rates, although radiological leak rates have been significantly higher after the hand-sewn anastomoses (Docherty et al, 1995).

Survival

There are many problems in determining the accurate survival rates of patients operated on for colonic carcinoma. Studies abound which present their data as crude 5-year survival rates (Table 31.12). This method determines the percentage of patients from a given cohort who are alive at the end of a 5-year period. It includes patients who died from causes other than carcinoma and it makes no allowance for patients lost to follow-up.

In order to overcome the problem of deaths from other causes, 'corrected' 5-year survival rates have been reported. Using appropriate tables, the normal life-span for persons of the same age and sex as the patients can be determined and this allows a correction to be applied to the survival data. This method is, of course, a mathematical trick to derive the data. In order to achieve greater accuracy, other authors have used cancer-specific survival rates. This technique would seem to be the most accurate, but it can only be so if the cause of death is known with certainty for each patient. Clearly this is not always possible despite the most stringent follow-up. Postmortem examination will not have been performed on each patient and the information on death certificates cannot always be relied upon for its accuracy.

As can be seen, each of the methods used to calculate survival, whether crude, corrected or cancer-specific, has its inadequacies. No matter which technique is selected, correction for patients lost to follow-up seems desirable. To overcome this difficulty, survival curves derived by methods similar to those of Kaplan and Meier (1978) should be generated. It is also advisable when comparing survival between groups of patients to analyse the complete curves and not just the 5-year results. Statistical methods such as that described by Gehan (1965) are available to do this. Unfortunately it is only relatively recently that the need to assess survival by these sophisticated methods has been fully appreciated.

Another difficulty when results are compared between different centres relates to the inclusion or otherwise of patients who die in the immediate postoperative period. Whereas most authors exclude these deaths from their data, others – particularly those quoting data from cancer registries – do not. It is not surprising, therefore, that registry statistics present a more gloomy picture of prognosis following colectomy for colonic cancer. In addition some studies include patients in whom a palliative procedure was performed.

It can be seen that studies on survival following resection for colonic cancer express their data in a variety of ways, each of which has its imperfections. These factors must be considered when interpreting the results and drawing conclusions.

Crude 5-year survival rates in series that included only patients who survived the postoperative period and had potentially curative resections vary from 50% to 70%. These rates do not seem to have altered very much over the last few decades.

When corrected survival rates or cancer-specific survival rates are examined in similar groups of patients who have survived a radical operation, life expectancy appears more favourable. Pihl et al (1980) reported that the cancer-specific survival rates at 5, 10, 15 and 20 years for curative resections were 76%, 73%, 71% and 67% respectively in the 434 patients who survived operation. Similarly, the corrected 5-year survival rate in a report from Bristol was approximately 65% (Umpleby et al, 1984). On the other hand, when 5-year survival rates that include patients who died in the postoperative period are considered, a more depressing picture emerges, especially when palliative cases are also included. Thus Turunen and Peltokallio (1983)

Table 31.12 Crude 5-year survival rates following 'potentially curative' resections for colonic cancer.

Authors	*Five-year survival* (%)
Rankin and Olsen (1933)	51
Grinnell (1953)	<55.2
Gilbertsen (1959)	60
Hughes (1966)	62.2
Turnbull et al (1967)	68.8
Murray et al (1975)	64
Welch and Donaldson (1974a,b)	50
Miller and Allbritten (1976)	54
Wield et al (1985)	47
Allum et al (1994)	56.2
Hall et al (1996)	80
Diaz-Plasencia et al (1996)	53
Tominaga et al (1996)	76.3

reported a survival rate of 42% in their 305 patients undergoing both radical and palliative resections. On a much larger scale the data from the cancer registries is similar. Milnes Walker (1971), reporting the results of the South Western Regional Cancer Bureau, recorded a crude 5-year survival rate of 37% in 1194 patients undergoing palliative and radical resection. Similarly Slaney (1971) found that 42.3% of the 3094 patients undergoing radical resection and recorded in the Birmingham Cancer Registry survived for 5 years (corrected 5-year survival rate was 52.1%). More recent data from Birmingham collected between 1981 and 1985 showed a crude 5-year survival rate of 39% (West Midlands Cancer Registry, 1990; Slaney et al, 1991; Allum et al, 1994).

When the crude 5-year survival rates of *all* patients irrespective of whether they undergo surgery are examined, the situation is even more depressing. Grinnell (1953) found an overall or absolute 5-year survival rate of 30.8% between 1941 and 1945 at the Presbyterian Hospital, New York. This result was obtained despite a 92.1% resection rate in a specialized unit. When the results from regions, which include both specialized and non-specialized units, are examined the survival rates are even worse. Thus Milnes Walker (1971) reported an absolute survival rate of 22% for 2036 patients treated in south-western England, and Slaney's data from the Birmingham Cancer Register were remarkably similar, with a 20.5% crude 5-year survival between 1950 and 1961 from a total number of 6694 patients (corrected rate 27%) (Slaney, 1971).

The figures from the USA seem to be superior to those in the UK. The Connecticut Tumour Registry records that 1582 men and 1824 women were registered with colonic carcinoma between 1955 and 1959, with survival rates of 38.4% and 44.8% respectively. However, data from the USA are not strictly comparable with those from the UK since the rates are corrected and are not crude. Nevertheless, it does appear that in the 1950s and 1960s surgeons in the UK were failing to match the overall results achieved in the USA. One of the main problems seemed to be that UK patients were often referred late or had not consulted a surgeon. More recent data from the Cancer Research Campaign in the UK suggests an improvement with an overall 5-year survival for colorectal cancer of 38% (CRC, 1993). Nevertheless, these are still depressing data, and it is to be hoped that with the emphasis on screening and more awareness of the problem by both the public and the medical profession, overall survival will be improved.

Age

It is generally accepted that young patients with the disease have a poorer prognosis than their older counterparts. While this appears to be the case, it should be remembered that these data emanate from retrospective studies and little attempt has usually been made to compare patients who have similar personal and tumour characteristics. Another important criticism is that the number of young patients with the disease is small and this further complicates any comparative study.

Despite these criticisms there is little doubt that the prognosis for younger patients is appalling in some centres. Miller and Liechty (1967) found a crude 5-year survival rate of 18.2% in their 33 patients under the age of 30 years. Similarly Recalde et al (1974) reported a 5-year survival rate of 13% in 40 patients below the age of 35 years. These authors also found that there were no survivors in patients who had involved lymph nodes or in whom the tumour was 5 cm or more in diameter. Even more depressing is the 5-year survival rate of 7% recorded by Mills and Allen (1979) in patients below 30 years of age. Other authors, however, although accepting that these patients have a reduced survival rate compared with the average, report a more optimistic picture. Sanfelippo and Beahrs (1974) reported on 118 patients under the age of 40 years with an overall 5-year survival rate of 39%. Patients with Dukes' C lesions had a 5-year survival rate of 21%. Mayo and Pagtalunan (1963) found that 35% of their patients at the Mayo Clinic who were under the age of 30 years and underwent a radical excision survived 5 years or more.

A summary of the results in younger patients is given in Table 31.13. It should be remembered that these data relate to patients with rectal as well as colonic tumours.

Although the criticisms that apply to studies in younger patients are frequently applicable to those in the elderly (above 70 years of age), there is far less doubt that the elderly do have a very poor prognosis. This fact comes as no surprise since in the elderly there is a lower resectability rate and a higher operative mortality rate. A fair proportion of elderly patients never reach the surgeon, or present with an acute complication relating to their tumour; consequently mortality and morbidity rates are high. If the prognosis is considered in elderly patients with carcinoma of the colon who undergo elective surgery and survive the immediate post-operative period, the results are more comparable with those in younger age groups. Jensen et al (1970b) found crude and corrected 5-year survival

Table 31.13 Selected studies of colorectal carcinoma in younger patients.

Authors	*Maximum age of patients (years)*	*No. of patients*	*Five-year survival (%)*	*Five-year cure (%)*
Elzo et al (1958)	39	32	<22	
Mayo and Pagtalunan (1963)	29	126	54	
Coffey and Cardenas (1964)	40	86	<35	<16
Rosato et al (1969)	35	35	40	34
Miller and Liechty (1967)	29	33	18	
Sanfelippo and Beahrs (1974)	39	118	39	
Recalde et al (1974)	35	38	13	11
Howard et al (1975)	39	137	31	
Walton et al (1976)	39	70	41	
Walton et al (1976) review of world literature	39	717	28	
Scarpa and Hartmann (1976)	40	46	37	
Vezzoni et al (1977)	29	28	<28	
Simstein et al (1978)	39	41	24	
Mosley et al (1979)	30	14	34	
Mills and Allen (1979)	30	16	7	7
Bulow (1980)	40	951	32	
recent (1963–7) subgroup		181	39	
Fantelli and Sebek (1980)	39	78	43	42
Ahlberg et al (1980)	30	27	41	
Bedikian et al (1981)	39	183	31	
Martin et al (1981)	40	37	57	
Klempa et al (1981)	35	29	22	
Ohman (1982)	39	40	33	
Beckman et al (1984)	39	69	59	51

rates of 42.3% and 53.8% respectively in their patients over the age of 70 years, and these results were only slightly inferior to the rates in patients under this age. Similarly, Whittle et al (1992) found that the crude 2-year survival rate in patients over the age of 65 years who had undergone colonic resection for carcinoma was 63%. Thus it would appear that, provided elderly patients survive the operation, there is no reason to believe that their life expectancy from the cancer point of view will be much reduced compared with their younger counterparts, all other factors remaining equal.

The development of a carcinoma of colon in a child is a rarity, but in children the colon is the most likely structure of the gastrointestinal tract to develop a carcinoma. The prognosis when such a tumour does occur in a child is particularly poor, so much so that Pemberton (1970) could not find a single long-term survivor in the literature apart from the patient he reported.

Pathological characteristics of the carcinoma

Most of the work correlating stage and histological grade of tumour to the patient's ultimate survival has been performed on patients with carcinoma of rectum or of both colon and rectum. However, the data that are available on patients with colonic carcinoma alone tend to agree with these other studies. Although there are difficulties in accurately determining the pathological stage of a colorectal tumour and there are discrepancies in classification, if Dukes' original classification is used it is clear that patients with Dukes' A and B carcinoma survive significantly longer than patients with Dukes' C1 and C2 lesions. Thus Hawley (1972) found that the crude and corrected 5-year survival rates for patients with Dukes' A colonic tumours were respectively 82% and 99.3%, Dukes' B 69% and 84.4%, Dukes' C1 59.6% and 66.3%, and Dukes' C2 26.3% and 35.1%. These findings were similar to those reported by Shepherd and Jones (1971) and Murray et al (1975).

More recent papers using more sophisticated methods of analysis have also confirmed the findings of earlier studies. Pihl et al (1980), analysing Hughes' 1966 data using cancer-specific survival curves, admirably demonstrated the effect of pathological stage on survival (Figure 31.25). Similarly, the data from the Birmingham Cancer Registry between 1977 and 1981 showed that, after curative resection, 5-year age-adjusted survival rates for colon cancer were 85%, 67% and 37% for Dukes' A, B and C stages respectively (Slaney et al, 1991; Allum et al, 1994).

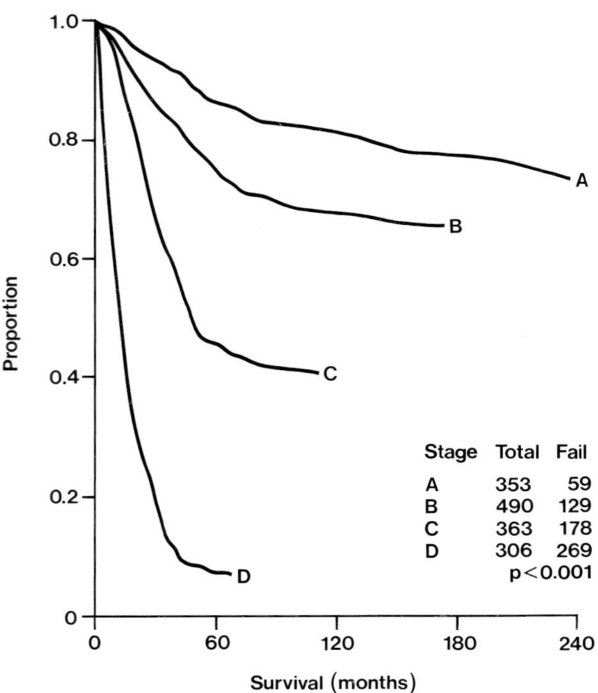

Figure 31.25 Cancer-specific survival rates for patients with colonic cancer according to Dukes' stage (Pihl et al, 1980).

The studies previously cited that have also examined the effect of histological grade of tumour on survival reach similar conclusions; that is, patients with poorly differentiated lesions fare significantly worse than patients with tumours of average or good differentiation. Histological grade, however, is a highly subjective parameter and, as noted previously, there is considerable interobserver variation which tends to make classification inaccurate and not uniform. For this reason various investigators have looked for alternative cellular factors which can be measured and which carry prognostic significance. One such factor is the cellular content of DNA. Flow cytometry can determine whether the cells of a particular tumour contain the normal content of DNA (diploid tumour) or an abnormal amount (non-diploid or aneuploid tumour). Several workers including ourselves (Quirke et al, 1987) demonstrated that patients with colorectal tumours of the diploid variety had a significantly better survival rate than those with aneuploid tumours (Wooley et al, 1982; Armitage et al, 1984; Nori et al, 1996).

Another pathological characteristic that appears to have a particularly detrimental effect on survival is venous invasion. Although various reports – notably that by Talbot et al (1980) – have emphasized this factor in colorectal tumours, few studies have examined colonic cancers alone. Those that have done so (e.g. Wield et al, 1985) report identical findings. It is also of interest that these investigators found that nerve invasion carried the same adverse prognosis. These two characteristics are perhaps the reason why colorectal carcinomas that are fixed by malignancy to local structures have a significantly worse prognosis than those that are not, irrespective of whether the lymph nodes are involved (Jensen et al, 1970a; Habib et al, 1983; Durdey and Williams, 1984).

The recent explosion in understanding of the genetic changes which occur in sporadic colorectal cancer development has led to numerous studies linking these changes with prognosis. Thus, p53 mutation and over-expression have been found to correlate with poor survival, although this does not appear to be an independent marker (Sun et al, 1992; Auvinen et al, 1994; Hamelin et al, 1994). Microsatellite instability also appears to confer a better prognosis (Lothe et al, 1992; Thibodeau et al, 1993). Other aberrant genes such as NM23, a putative metastasis suppresser gene (Steeg et al, 1988; Cohn et al, 1991) and the DCC gene (Fearon and Vogelstein, 1990) may well be important in prognosis, but further studies are awaited. This area is further reviewed extensively in Chapters 27 and 30.

Site of the tumour

There has always been controversy over whether the site of the tumour in the colon has an influence on survival. When survival data first became available there was a suggestion that right-sided lesions had a superior prognosis compared with left-sided growths (Rankin and Olsen, 1933; Gilbertsen, 1959). Later reports also tended to support this concept (Hughes, 1966; Irvin and Greaney, 1977). Throughout this period, however, contradictory data have been presented, most notably from Morgan (1957), Shepherd and Jones (1971), Slaney (1971) and Welch and Donaldson (1974b). Although some of these studies may be criticized on the grounds of inappropriate analysis, it is interesting to note that more recent data using life-table analysis also produced conflicting results. Thus Pihl et al (1980) were unable to show any significant difference in survival between left-sided and right-sided lesions when cancer-specific survival curves were analysed. On the other hand, Umpleby et al (1984) in their analysis of patients treated in Bristol demonstrated a significant benefit in the corrected survival rates of patients with tumours situated in the left colon as compared with those in the right side. There is also some evidence from the St Mary's Large Bowel Cancer project that tumours situated in the splenic flexure represent a group with an independent prognostic variable associated with a poor outcome (Fielding et al, 1986).

In view of these conflicting reports it would seem that if the anatomical site of the tumour does play a role in the survival of the patient it is not a major one.

Clinical features

Various authors have demonstrated that the longer the history the better the prognosis (Copeland et al, 1969; Slaney, 1971; Umpleby et al, 1984). On the other hand, asymptomatic patients seem to do significantly better than patients with symptoms (Mzabi et al, 1976). Also, patients who present with rectal bleeding seem to have a more favourable prognosis than those who do not (Mzabi et al, 1976; Umpleby et al, 1984).

The mode of presentation – elective or emergency – has tremendous prognostic significance. The operative mortality is significantly worse for patients who present with acute obstruction or perforation of their tumour. In addition, the long-term survival rate of patients after apparently curative resection for obstruction is lower than for patients undergoing an elective resection for cure (Welch and Donaldson, 1974b; Kronborg et al, 1975; Peloquin, 1975; Dutton et al, 1976; Irvin and Greaney, 1977; Turunen, 1983; Runkel et al, 1991) (Figure 31.26).

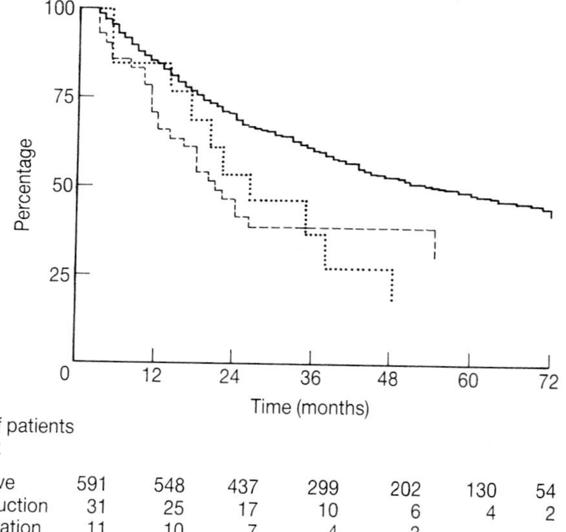

Figure 31.26 Overall survival curves (Kaplan–Meier estimates) for colorectal surgery following elective surgery (——) or emergency surgery for obstruction (– – –) or for perforation (. . . . .) (Runkel et al, 1991).

The difference in prognosis is maintained when patients with similar staged tumours are compared. Willet et al (1984) found that the 5-year survival rate of patients undergoing a curative resection for an obstructing lesion was only half that of patients undergoing an elective resection for apparent cure, owing to rapid intra-abdominal and systemic spread which suggested a peculiar biological behaviour of obstructing tumours. Similarly, the 5-year survival rate of patients who have undergone resection for perforated colorectal cancer is about 20% lower than that of patients undergoing elective surgery for apparent cure (Figure 31.26) (Donaldson, 1958; Miller et al, 1966; Glenn and McSherry, 1971; Raftery and Samson, 1980; Kelley et al, 1981; Ravo, 1988).

Extent of resection

Although many surgeons believe that removal of the lymphatic drainage of a tumour should be as wide as possible, there are no data available from prospective, controlled trials to validate this approach. The retrospective data available for colonic carcinoma suggest that a limited resection may be just as effective as a more radical resection.

Busuttil et al (1977) compared the results of left hemicolectomy with those following local segmental resection when used to treat tumours of the sigmoid colon and upper rectum. Although the groups were similar with regard to age and sex distribution, there was unfortunately a marked disparity in the number of patients in each group. Thus 16 patients had undergone a left hemicolectomy and 91 had undergone sigmoid colectomy. Such a difference makes analysis of results very difficult, but it is worth noting that the 5-year survival rate following left hemicolectomy was 56.3% and the rate following sigmoid colectomy was 70.3%. However, a prospective controlled multi-centre trial from the French Association of Surgical Research showed no significant difference in mortality or survival between left hemicolectomy compared with sigmoid resection (Rouffet et al, 1994).

More radical excision of lymphatic drainage may be more effective for carcinoma of the rectum. However, this has not been borne out as far as proximal lymphatic spread has been concerned if data from retrospective studies are to be believed. Thus, studies which have compared high tie of the inferior mesenteric artery with low tie in the resection of rectal cancer have demonstrated no survival advantage in either group (Surtees et al, 1990). Although Japanese studies have demonstrated improved survival for lateral pelvic lymphadenectomy, these have not been proven in controlled trials (see Chapter 32).

As previously emphasized, it is always worth excising *en bloc* structures into which the carcinoma has extended provided such a manoeuvre is technically feasible. In a percentage of such tumours – approximately 20% in our own series (Durdey and Williams, 1984) – infiltration is non-malignant, but even if it is malignant radical excision is the only hope of cure for the patient (Schiessel et al, 1986). Once more there are no controlled trials to prove the value of local radical excision, and it is doubtful on ethical grounds whether there ever will be. Although most of the available data suggest that tumours that are locally extensive have a very poor prognosis despite radical excision (Jensen et al, 1970a; Wood et al, 1981; Bonfanti et al, 1982), other reports are more optimistic. Pittam et al (1984) examined the results in 57 patients with tumours that were locally advanced and were invading neighbouring organs (including the abdominal wall) and who underwent extended *en bloc* resection. This study has the particular advantage that it compares the results after the extended resections with those of a similar group of patients with similar Dukes' stage tumours who did not require extended resection. The authors demonstrated that, although operative mortality was increased in the extended resection group, there was no significant difference in survival rates between the two groups as calculated by life-table methods.

Blood transfusion and survival

There are data to suggest that perioperative blood transfusion, possibly because of its immunosuppressive properties, may be associated with an increased risk of recurrence after surgery for colorectal cancer (Parrott et al, 1986; Voogt et al, 1987; Creasy, 1987; Benyon et al, 1989). Marsh et al (1990) suggested that this risk was associated with plasma proteins rather than the cellular components of whole blood. However, it must be emphasized that others have found no evidence for this increase in tumour recurrence following transfusion (Nathanson et al, 1985; Wieden et al, 1987; Jakobson et al, 1990).

REFERENCES

Aberg C, Olin B, Oresland J et al (1984) Comparison of metronidazole with doxycycline prophylaxis in elective colorectal surgery: a prospective randomized multicentre study. *Acta Chir Scand* **150**: 79–83.

Abrams JS (1980) Elective resection for colorectal cancer in Vermont 1971–75. *Am J Surg* **139**: 78–83.

Adler M, Quendeon M, Evenadin D et al (1984) Whole gut lavage for colonoscopy: a comparison between two solutions. *Gastrointest Endosc* **30**: 65–67.

Adson M (1983) Hepatic metastases in perspective. *Am J Roengen* **140**: 695–700.

Adson MA & Van Heerden JA (1980) Major hepatic resections for metastatic colorectal cancer. *Ann Surg* **191**: 576–583.

Afridi SA, Barthel JS, King PD, Pineda JJ & Marshall JB (1995) Prospective randomized trial comparing a new sodium phosphate–bisacodyl regimen with conventional PEG–ES lavage for outpatient colonoscopy preparation. *Gastrointest Endosc* **41**: 485–489.

Ahlberg J, Bergstrand O, Holmstrom B, Ullman J & Wallberg P (1980) Malignant tumours of the colon and rectum in patients aged 30 and younger. *Acta Chir Scand* **500** (Suppl): 29–31.

Aibe T (1984) A study on the structure of layers of the gastrointestinal wall visualised by means of ultrasonic endoscope. 2: The structure of layers of the oesophageal wall and colonic wall. *Gastrointest Endosc* **26**: 1447–1464.

Allen AW, Welch CE & Donaldson GA (1947) Carcinoma of the colon: effect of recent advances on the surgical management. *Ann Surg* **126**: 19.

Allum WH, Slaney G, McConkey CC & Powell J (1994) Cancer of the colon and rectum in the West MIdlands, 1957–81. *Br J Surg* **81**: 1060–1063

Amin Z, Boulos PB & Lees WR (1996) Technical report: spiral CT pneumocolon for suspected colonic neoplasms. *Clin Radiol* **51**: 56–61.

Anderson BO, Hann LE, Enker WE et al (1994) Transrectal ultrasonography and operative selection for early carcinoma of the rectum. *J Am Coll Surg* **179**: 513–517.

Armitage NC, Perkins MV, Pimm MV et al (1984) The localisation of an antitumour monoclonal antibody (791T/36) in gastrointestinal tumours. *Br J Surg* **71**: 407–412.

Attiyeh FF (1980) Surgery for metastasis from carcinoma of the rectum and colon. In Stearns M (ed) *Neoplasms of the Colon, Rectum and Anus*. New York: John Wiley.

August DA, Sugarbaker PH, Ottow RT, Gianola FJ & Schneier PD (1985) Hepatic resection of colorectal metastases: influence of clinical factors and adjuvant intraperitoneal 5-fluorouracil via Tenkoff catheter on survival. *Ann Surg* **201**: 210–217.

Auvinen A, Isola J, Visakorpi T et al (1994) Overexpression of p53 and long-term survival in colon carcinoma. *Br J Cancer* **70**; 293–296.

Babineau TJ & Steele Jr G (1996) Treatment of colorectal liver metastases. In Williams NS (ed) *Colorectal Cancer*. London: Churchill Livingstone.

Bacon HE & Jackson CC (1953) Visceral metastases from carcinoma of the distal colon and rectum. *Surgery (St Louis)* **33**: 495.

Bacon HE & Peale AR (1956) Appraisal of adenomatous polyps of the colon, their histopathology and surgical management. *Ann Surg* **144**: 9.

Baigrie RJ & Berry AR (1994) Management of advanced rectal cancer. *Br J Surg* **81**: 343–352.

Ballantyne KC, Charnley RM, Perkins AC et al (1990) Hepatic perfusion index in the diagnosis of overt metastatic colorectal cancer. *Nucl Med Commun* **11**: 23–28.

Bartram I (1985) Imaging. *Br J Surg* **72** (Suppl): 549–550.

Bartram I & Reznek RH (1996) Imaging techniques in preoperative assessment. In *Handbook for the Clinicopathological Assessment and Staging of Colorectal Cancer*. UKCCCR Sub-Committee for Colorectal Cancer.

Beckman EN, Gathright JB & Ray JE (1984) A potentially brighter prognosis for colon carcinoma in the third and fourth decades. *Cancer* **54**: 1478–1481.

Bedikian AY, Kantarijian H, Nelson RB, Stroehlein JR & Bodey GP (1981) Colorectal carcinoma in young adults. *South Med J* **74**: 920–923.

Behr T, Becker W, Hannappel E, Goldenberg DM & Wolf F (1995) Targeting of liver metastases of colorectal cancer with IgG, F(ab')2, and Fab' anti-carcinoembryonic antigen antibodies labeled with 99mTc: the role of metabolism and kinetics. *Cancer Res* **55** (Suppl 23): 5777–5785.

Bengmark S & Hafstrom L (1969) The natural history of primary and secondary malignant tumours of the liver. 1: The prognosis of patients with hepatic metastases from colonic and rectal carcinoma by laparotomy. *Cancer* **23**: 198–202.

Benyon J, Foy DMA, Roe AM et al (1986a) Endoluminal ultrasound in the assessment of local invasion of rectal cancer. *Br J Surg* **73**: 474–477.

Benyon J, McMortensen NJ, Foy DMA et al (1986b) Preoperative assessment of local invasion in rectal cancer: digital examination, endoluminal sonography or computed tomography? *Br J Surg* **73**: 1015–1017.

Benyon J, Davies PW, Billings PJ et al (1989) Perioperative blood transfusion increases the risk of recurrence in colorectal cancer. *Dis Colon Rectum* **29**: 975–979.

Berliner SD, Burson LC & Lear PE (1964) The use and abuse of intraperitoneal drains in colon surgery. *Arch Surg* **89**: 686–690.

Blamey S, McDermott F, Pihl E et al (1981) Ovarian involvement in adenocarcinoma of the colon and rectum. *Surg Gynecol Obstet* **153**: 42.

Bloch O (1894) Extra-abdominal resektion of hele colon descendens og et stykke of colon transversoum for cancer. *Hosp Tid Kjøbehn* **4**(ii): 1053.

Bohdiewicz PJ, Scott GC, Juni JE et al (1995) Indium-111 OncoScint CR/OV and F-18 FDG in colorectal and ovarian carcinoma recurrences: early observations. *Clin Nucl Med* **20**: 230–236.

Bokey EL, Chapuis PH, Fung C et al (1995) Postoperative morbidity following resection of the colon and rectum for cancer. *Dis Colon Rectum* **38**: 480–486; discussion 486–487.

Boldrini G, de Gaetano AM, Giovannini I et al (1987) The systematic use of operative ultrasound for detection of liver metastases during colorectal surgery. *World J Surg* **11**: 622–627.

Bolton J (1978) The prevention of postoperative deep venous thrombosis by graduated compression stockings. *Scot Med J* **23**: 333–337.

Bonfanti G, Rozetti F, Doci R et al (1982) Results of extended surgery for cancer of the rectum and sigmoid. *Br J Surg* **69**: 305–307.

Bradpiece HA, Benjamin IS, Halevy A & Blumgart LH (1987) Major hepatic resection for colorectal liver metastases. *Br J Surg* **74**: 324–326.

Breedis C & Young G (1953) The blood supply of neoplasms in the liver. *Am J Pathol* **30**: 227–232.

Browne MK & Stoller JL (1970) Intraperitoneal noxythiolin in faecal peritonitis. *Br J Surg* **57**: 37.

Brunschwig A (1961) Radical surgical management of cancer of the colon spread to tissues and organs beyond the colon. *Dis Colon Rectum* **4**: 83.

Bryan PJ, Dinn MW, Grossman ZP et al (1977) Correlation of computed tomography, gray scale ultrasonography and radionuclide imaging of the liver in detecting space occupying processes. *Radiology* **124**: 387–393.

Bulow S (1980) Colorectal cancer in patients less than 40 years of age in Denmark, 1943–67. *Dis Colon Rectum* **23**: 327–336.

Burt CAV (1960) Carcinoma of the ovaries secondary to cancer of the colon and rectum. *Dis Colon Rectum* **3**: 352.

Bussey HJR, Wallace MH & Morson BC (1967) Metachronous carcinoma of the large intestine and intestinal polyps. *Proc R Soc Med* **60**: 208.

Busuttil RW, Foglia RP & Longmire WP Jr (1977) Treatment of carcinoma of the sigmoid colon and upper rectum. *Arch Surg* **112**: 920.

Butch RJ, Stark DD, Wittenberg J et al (1986) Staging rectal cancer by MR and CT. *Am J Roentgenol* **146**: 1155–1160.

Cameron A (1977) Left colon resection. *Br J Hosp Med* **17**: 281–289.

Carter DC, Jenkins DHR & Whitfield HN (1972) Omental reinforcement of intestinal anastomoses. *Br J Surg* **39**: 10.

Carter R, Hemingway D, Cooke TG et al (1996) A prospective study of six methods for detection of hepatic colorectal metastases. *Ann R Coll Surg Engl* **78**: 27–30.

Cedermark BJ, Schultz SS, Bakshi S et al (1977) The value of liver scan in the follow-up study of patients with adenocarcinoma of the colon and rectum. *Surg Gynecol Obstet* **144**: 745–748.

Charnley RM, Morris DL, Dennison AR et al (1991) Detection of colorectal metastases using intraoperative ultrasonography. *Br J Surg* **78**: 45–48.

Chu DZJ, Giacco G, Martin RG & Guinee VF (1986) The significance of synchronous carcinoma and polyps in the colon and rectum. *Cancer* **71**: 941–943.

Chung RS, Gurll NJ & Berlund EM (1979) A controlled clinical trial of whole gut lavage as a method of bowel preparation for colonic operations. *Am J Surg* **137**: 75.

Clarke MP, Kane RA, Steele G Jr et al (1989) Prospective comparison of preoperative imaging and intraoperative ultrasonography in the detection of liver tumors. *Surgery* **106**: 849–855.

Coffey RJ & Cardenas F (1964) Cancer of the bowel in the young adult. *Dis Colon Rectum* **7**: 491–492.

Cohn I (1960) Dangers of intestinal antisepsis. *Dis Colon Rectum* **3**: 305.

Cohn KH, Wang F, Desoto-Lapaix F et al (1991) Association of nm23-H1 allelic deletions with distant metastases in colorectal carcinoma. *Lancet* **338**: 722–724.

Cole WH, Packard D & Southwick HW (1954) Carcinoma of the colon with special reference to the prevention of recurrence. *JAMA* **155**: 1549.

Cooke RV (1956) Advanced carcinoma of the colon with emphasis on the inflammatory factor. *Ann R Coll Surg Engl* **18**: 46.

Copeland EM, Miller LD & Jones RJ (1969) Prognostic factors in carcinoma of the colon and rectum. *Am J Surg* **116**: 875.

Corman ML, Veidenheimer MC & Coller JA (1979) Colorectal carcinoma: a decade of experience at the Lahey Clinic. *Dis Colon Rectum* **22**: 477–479.

Cova M, Frezza F, Pozzi-Mucelli RS et al (1994) Computed tomography and magnetic resonance in the preoperative staging of the spread of rectal cancer: a correlation with the anatomicopathological aspects. *Radiol Med (Torino)* **87**: 82–89.

Crapp AR, Tillotson P, Powis SJA, Cooke WI & Alexander-Williams J (1975) Preparation of the bowel by whole gut irrigation. *Lancet* **ii**: 1239–1240.

CRC (Cancer Research Campaign) (1993) *Facts on Cancer* factsheets 18.1–18.4

Creasy TS, Veitch PS & Bell PR (1987) A relationship between perioperative blood transfusion and recurrence of carcinoma of the sigmoid colon following potentially curative surgery. *Ann R Coll Surg Engl* **69**: 100–103.

Cunliffe WJ, Hasleton PS, Tweedle DEF & Schofield PF (1984) Incidence of synchronous and metachronous colorectal carcinoma. *Br J Surg* **71**: 941–943.

Davis GR, Santa Ana CA, Morawski SG & Fordtran JS (1980) Development of a lavage solution associated with minimal water and electrolyte absorption or secretion. *Gastroenterology* **78**: 991–995.

Deddish MR & Hertz RE (1955) Colostomy and colonoscopy in the management of mucosal polyps and cancer of the colon. *Am J Surg* **90**: 846.

Detry RJ, Kartheuser AH, Lagneaux G & Rahier J (1996) Preoperative lymph node staging in rectal cancer: a difficult challenge. *Int J Colorect Dis* **11**: 217–221

Devine HB (1931) Safer colon surgery. *Lancet* **i**: 627.

Devine HB (1935) Carcinoma of the colon. *BMJ* **2**: 1245.

Devlin HB, Evans DS & Birkhead JS (1969) The incidence and morbidity of accidental injury occurring during abdominal surgery. *Br J Surg* **56**: 446–448.

Diaz-Plasencia J, Tantalean E, Urtecho F, Guzman C & Angulo M (1996) Colorectal cancer: its clinical picture and survival (in Spanish). *Rev Gastroenterol (Peru)* **16**: 48–56.

Dixon AK, Fry IK, Morson BC, Nicholls RJ & Mason AY (1981) Preoperative computed tomography of carcinoma of the rectum. *Br J Radiol* **54**: 655–659.

Docherty JG, McGregor JR, Akyol AM, Murray GD & Galloway DJ (1995) West of Scotland and Highlands Anastomosis Study Group: comparison of manually constructed and stapled anastomoses in colorectal surgery. *Ann Surg* **221**: 176–184.

Doci R, Bignami P, Montalto F & Gennari L (1995) Prognostic factors for survival and disease-free survival in hepatic metastases from colorectal cancer treated by resection. *Tumori* **81** (Suppl 3): 143–146.

Donaldson CA (1958) The management of perforated carcinoma of the colon. *N Engl J Med* **258**: 201–207.

Douglas DM (1969) Right hemicolectomy with anastomosis. In Rob C & Smith R (eds) *Operative Surgery: Abdomen and Rectum and Anus*, Part II, pp 648–654. London: Butterworth.

Downing R, Dorricott NJ, Keighley MRB et al (1979) Whole gut irrigation: a survey of patient opinion. *Br J Surg* **66**: 201.

Dudley HAF, Radcliffe AG & McGeehan D (1980) Intraoperative irrigation of the colon to permit primary anastomosis. *Br J Surg* **67**: 80.

Dukes CE (1957) Discussion on major surgery in carcinoma of the rectum with or without colostomy excluding the anal canal and including the rectosigmoid. *Proc R Soc Med* **50**: 1031–1035.

Durdey P & Williams NS (1984) The effect of malignant and inflammatory fixation of rectal carcinoma on prognosis after rectal excision. *Br J Surg* **71**: 787–790.

Durdey P, Williams NS & Brown DA (1984) Serum carcinoembryonic antigen and acute phase reactant proteins in the preoperative detection of fixation of colorectal tumours. *Br J Surg* **71**: 881–884.

Durdey P, Weston PMT & Williams NS (1987) Colonoscopy or barium enema as initial investigation of colonic disease. *Lancet* **ii**: 549–551.

Dutton JW, Hreno A & Hampson LG (1976) Mortality and prognosis of obstructing carcinoma of the large bowel. *Am J Surg* **131**: 36–41.

Eisenberg H, Sullivan PD & Foote FM (1967) Trends of survival of digestive system cancer patients in Connecticut 1935–62. *Gastroenterology* **53**: 528–546.

Ekelund GR & Pihl B (1974) Multiple carcinomas of the colon and rectum. *Cancer* **33**: 1630–1634.

Ellis H (1971) Curative and palliative surgery in advanced carcinoma of the large bowel. *BMJ* **3**: 29.

Ellis H, Coleridge-Smith PD, Joyce AD et al (1984) Abdominal incisions: vertical or transverse? *Postgrad Med J* **60**: 407–410.

Elzo JA, Sullivan MD & Mack RE (1958) Carcinoma of the colon under the age of 40. *Ann Intern Med* **49**: 321–325.

Engell HC (1955) Cancer cells in the circulating blood: a clinical study on the occurrence of cancer cells in the peripheral blood and in venous blood draining the tumour area at operation. *Acta Chir Scand* **201** (Suppl).

Evans G (1982) Comment on drainage after cholecystectomy. *Ann R Coll Surg Engl* **64**: 428.

Fantelli FJ & Sebek BA (1980) Adenocarcinoma of the colon and rectum in the young adult. *Lab Invest* **42**: 19 (abstract).

Fearon ER & Vogelstein B (1990) A genetic model for colorectal tumorigenesis. *Cell* **61**; 759–767.

Fielding LP, Phillips RKS, Fry JS & Huttinger R (1986) Prediction of outcome after curative resection for large bowel cancer. *Lancet* **ii**: 904–907.

Fielding LP, Stewart-Brown S, Blesovsky L & Kearney G (1980) Anastomotic integrity after operations for large bowel cancer: a multicentre study. *BMJ* **281**: 411–414.

Finan PJ (1990) The hepatic perfusion index. In *Principles of Colon and Rectal Surgery*. University of Minnesota.

Finan PJ, Ritchie JK & Hawley PR (1987) Synchronous and early metachronous carcinomas of the colon and rectum. *Br J Surg* **74**: 945–947.

Finlay IG, Meek DR, Gray HW, Duncan JG & McArdle CS (1982) Incidence and detection of occult hepatic metastases in colorectal carcinoma. *BMJ* **284**: 803–805.

Fisher ER & Turnbull RB (1955) The cytologic demonstration and significance of tumour cells in the mesenteric venous blood in patients with colorectal carcinoma. *Surg Gynecol Obstet* **100**: 102.

Fleming J Sr, Humphries NLM, Farran SJ et al (1981) *In vivo* assessment of hepatic arterial and portal venous components of liver perfusion. *J Nucl Med* **22**: 18–21.

Flyger HL, Hakansson TU & Jensen LP (1995) Single-layer colonic anastomosis with a continuous absorbable monofilament polyglyconate suture. *Eur J Surg* **161**: 911–913.

Fortner JG, Kim DK, Barrett MK et al (1979) Eight years' experience with surgical management of 321 patients with liver tumours. In Fox BW (ed) *Advances in Medical Oncology Research and Education. Vol. 5: Basis for Cancer Therapy*, pp 257–261. Oxford: Pergamon.

Foster JH & Berman M (1977) Solid liver tumours. *Maj Probl Clin Surg* **22**: 1.

Gall FP (1991) Cancer of the rectum: local excision. *Int J Colorect Dis* **6**: 84–85.

Gehan EA (1965) Generalised Wilcoxon Test for comparing arbitrarily censored samples. *Biometrika* **52**: 203.

Gilbertsen VA (1959) Adenocarcinoma of the large bowel: 1340 cases with 100 per cent follow-up. *Surgery (St Louis)* **46**: 1027.

Gilmore IT, Ellis WR, Barrett GS et al (1981) A comparison of two methods of whole gut lavage for colonoscopy. *Br J Surg* **68**: 388.

Gilmore OJA & Sanderson PJ (1975) Prophylactic intraparietal povidone iodine in abdominal surgery. *Br J Surg* **62**: 792–799.

Glaser F, Kuntz C, Schlag P & Herfarth C (1993) Endorectal ultrasound for control of preoperative radiotherapy of rectal cancer. *Ann Surg* **217**: 64–71.

Glenn G & McSherry CK (1971) Obstruction and perforation in colorectal cancer. *Ann Surg* **173**: 983–992.

Goldberg SM, Gordon PH & Nivatvongs S (1980) *Essentials of Anorectal Surgery*. Philadelphia: Lippincott.

Golden MHN (1982) Transport proteins as indices of protein status. *Am J Clin Nutr* **35**: 1159–1165.

Goldman S, Arvidsson H, Norming U et al (1991) Transrectal ultrasound and computed tomography in preoperative staging of lower rectal adenocarcinoma. *Gastrointest Radiol* **16**: 259–263.

Goldring J, Scott A, McNaught W & Gillespie G (1975) Prophylactic oral antimicrobial agents in elective colonic surgery. *Lancet* **ii**: 997–999.

Goldsmith HS (1977) Protection of low rectal anastomosis with intact omentum. *Surg Gynecol Obstet* **144**: 584.

Golfieri R, Giampalma E, Leo P et al (1993) Comparison of magnetic resonance (0.5 T), computed tomography, and endorectal electrosonography in the preoperative staging of neoplasms of the rectum–sigma: correlation with surgical and anatomopathologic findings. *Radiol Med (Torino)* **85**: 773–783.

Goligher JC (1941) The operability of carcinoma of the rectum. *BMJ* **ii**: 393–397.

Goligher JC (1984) *Surgery of the Anus, Rectum and Colon*, 4th edn. London: Baillière Tindall.

Goligher JC, Graham NG, De Dombal FT et al (1970) Anastomotic dehiscence after anterior resection of rectum and colon. *Br J Surg* **57**: 109–118.

Golub RW, Kerner BA, Wise WE Jr et al (1995) Colonoscopic bowel preparations – which one? A blinded, prospective, randomized trial. *Dis Colon Rectum* **38**: 594–599.

Gordon AB, Bates T & Fiddian RV (1976) A controlled trial of drainage after cholecystectomy. *Br J Surg* **63**: 278–282.

Grabbe E, Bucheler E & Winkler R (1985) Stellenwert der Computertomographie in der Diagnostik und Verlaufskontrolle des Rektumkarzinoms. *Zentralbl Chir* **110**: 80–88 (Engl. abstract).

Granowska M, Britton KE, Mather SJ et al (1993) Radioimmunoscintigraphy with technetium-99m labelled monoclonal antibody, 1A3, in colorectal cancer. *Eur J Nucl Med* **20**: 690–698.

Gray B (1980) Surgeon accuracy in the diagnosis of liver metastases at laparotomy. *Aust NZ J Surg* **50**: 524–526.

Greenall MJ, Evans M & Pollock AV (1980a) Midline or transverse laparotomy? A random controlled clinical trial. 1: Influence on healing. *Br J Surg* **67**: 188.

Greenall MJ, Evans M & Pollock AV (1980b) Midline or transverse laparotomy? A random controlled clinical trial. 2: Influence on postoperative pulmonary complications. *Br J Surg* **67**: 191.

Greig JD & Miller DF (1989) Synchronous and early metachronous carcinomas of the colon and rectum. *Acta Chir Scand* **155**: 287–289.

Grinnell RS (1953) Results in treatment of carcinoma of the colon and rectum. *Surg Gynecol Obstet* **96**: 31.

Gruber UF, Saldeen T, Brokopt Eklof B et al (1980) Incidence of fatal postoperative pulmonary embolism with dextran 70 and low-dose heparin: an international multicentre study. *BMJ* **280**: 69–72.

Guillou PJ, Hall TJ, Donaldson D et al (1980) Vertical abdominal incisions: a choice. *Br J Surg* **67**: 395.

Guinet C, Buy JN, Ghossain M et al (1990) Comparison of magnetic resonance imaging and computed tomography in the preoperative staging of rectal cancer. *Arch Surg* **125**: 385–388.

Habib NA, Peck MA, Sawyer CN, Blaxland JW & Luck RJ (1983) Does fixity affect prognosis in colorectal tumours? *Br J Surg* **70**: 423–424.

Hadfield MB, Nicholson AA, MacDonald AW et al (1997) Preoperative staging of rectal carcinoma by magnetic resonance imaging with a pelvic phased-array coil. *Br J Surg* **84**: 529–531.

Hall NR, Tsang CS, Brown T, Al Jaberi T & Finan PJ (1996) Eight-year colorectal cancer audit: breaking the myth that rectal cancer carries a poorer prognosis than colon cancer. *Int J Colorectal Dis* **11**: 137 (abstract)

Hamelin R, Laurent-Puig P, Olschwang S et al (1994) Association of p53 mutations with short survival in colorectal cancer. *Gastroenterology* **106**: 42–48.

Hau T & Simmons RL (1978) Heparin in the treatment of experimental peritonitis. *Ann Surg* **187**: 294.

Hau T, Hoffmann R & Simmons RL (1978) Mechanisms of the adjuvant effect of haemoglobin in experimental peritonitis. *Surgery (St Louis)* **83**: 223.

Hawley PR (1972) Quoted in Goligher JC (1984) *Surgery of the Anus, Rectum and Colon*, 4th edn, p. 549. London: Baillière Tindall.

Henderson JM, Barnett JL, Turgeon DK et al (1995) Single-day, divided-dose oral sodium phosphate laxative versus intestinal lavage as preparation for colonoscopy: efficacy and patient tolerance. *Gastrointest Endosc* **42**: 238–243.

Herrera MA, Chu TM & Holyoke ED (1976) Carcinoembryonic antigen (CEA) as a prognostic and monitoring test in clinically complete resection of colorectal carcinoma. *Ann Surg* **183**: 5–9.

Herzog U, von Flue M, Tondelli P & Schuppisser JP (1993) How accurate is endorectal ultrasound in the preoperative staging of rectal cancer? *Dis Colon Rectum* **36**: 127–134.

Hildebrandt U & Feifel G (1985) Preoperative staging of rectal cancer by intrarectal ultrasound. *Dis Colon Rectum* **28**: 42–46.

Hildebrandt U, Benyon J, Feifel G & McMortensen NJ (1990) Endorectal sonography. In Feifel G, Hildebrandt U & McMortensen NJ (eds) *Endosonography in Gastroenterology, Gynecology and Urology*, pp 81–129. Berlin: Springer.

Hildebrandt U, Schuder G & Feifel G (1994) Preoperative staging of rectal and colonic cancer. *Endoscopy* **26**: 810–812.

Hodgman CG, MacCarty RJ, Wolff BG et al (1986) Preoperative staging of rectal carcinoma by computed tomography and 0.15 T magnetic resonance imaging. *Dis Colon Rectum* **29**: 446–450.

Hoffman E (1959) Intraperitoneal and extraperitoneal neomycin as a topical and irrigating agent. *Am J Surg* **25**: 170.

Hogg L & Pack GT (1955) Diagnostic accuracy of hepatic metastases at laparotomy. *Arch Surg* **72**: 251–252.

Howard EW, Cavallo C, Hovey LM & Nelson TG (1975) Colon and rectal carcinoma in the young adult. *Am Surg* **41**: 260–265.

Hudspeth AS (1975) Radical surgical debridement in the treatment of generalised bacterial peritonitis. *Arch Surg* **110**: 1233.

Hughes ESR (1966) Carcinoma of the right colon, upper left colon and sigmoid colon. *Aust NZ J Surg* **35**: 183.

Irvin TT & Greaney MG (1977) The treatment of colonic cancer presenting with intestinal obstruction. *Br J Surg* **64**: 741–744.

Irvin TT & Hunt TK (1974) The effect of trauma on colonic healing. *Br J Surg* **61**: 430.

Irving AD & Scrimgeour D (1987) Mechanical bowel preparation for colonic resection and anastomosis. *Br J Surg* **74**: 580–581.

Isenberg J, Fischbach R, Kruger I & Keller HW (1996) Treatment of liver metastases from colorectal cancer. *Anticancer Res* **16**(3A): 1291–1295.

Jakobsen EB, Eickhoff JH, Andersen J, Lundvall L & Stenderup JK (1990) Perioperative blood transfusion and recurrence and death after resection for cancer of the colon and rectum. *Scand J Gastroenterol* **25**: 435–442.

Jamieson CW (1972) Inhibition of the growth of tumour cells by noxythiolin. *Br J Surg* **59**: 108.

Jatzko GR, Lisborg PH, Stettner HM & Klimpfinger MH (1995) Hepatic resection for metastases from colorectal carcinoma: a survival analysis. *Eur J Cancer* **31A**: 41–46.

Jensen HE, Balslev I & Nielson J (1970a) Extensive surgery in the treatment of carcinoma of the colon. *Acta Chir Scand* **136**: 431–434.

Jensen HE, Nielsen J & Balslev I (1970b) Carcinoma of the colon in old age. *Ann Surg* **171**: 107.

Johnson G & Gilsdorf R (1981) Routine versus selective drainage of the gall bladder bed after cholecystectomy. *Am J Surg* **142**: 6.

Johnston D, Williams N, Durdey P & Blacklay P (1989) Assessment of intraoperative ultrasonography by a surgeon for detection of colorectal liver disease (abstract). Meeting of the Association of Surgeons, Edinburgh.

Kaibara N, Koga S & Jinnai D (1984) Synchronous and metachronous malignancies of the colon and rectum in Japan with special reference to a coexisting early cancer. *Cancer* **54**: 1870–1874.

Kakkar VV, Howe CT, Micolaides AN, Renney JTG & Clarke MB (1970) Deep vein thrombosis of the leg: is there a high-risk group? *Am J Surg* **120**: 527–530.

Kakkar VV, Corrigan TP, Fossard DP, Sutherland K & Thirwell J (1977) Prevention of fatal postoperative pulmonary embolism by low doses of heparin: reappraisal of results of international multicentre trial. *Lancet* **i**: 567–569.

Kakkar VV, Cohen AT, Edmonson RA et al (1993) Low-molecular-weight versus standard heparin for prevention of venous thromboembolism after major abdominal surgery. The Thromboprophylaxis Collaborative Group. *Lancet* **341**: 259–265

Kaplan EL & Meier P (1978) Non-parametric estimation from incomplete observations. *J Am Stat Assoc* **53**: 457.

Katsura Y, Yamada K, Ishizawa T, Yoshinaka H & Shimazu H (1992) Endorectal ultrasonography for the assessment of wall invasion and lymph node metastasis in rectal cancer. *Dis Colon Rectum* **35**: 362–368.

Keighley MRB (1977) Prevention of wound sepsis in gastrointestinal surgery. *Br J Surg* **64**: 315–321.

Kelley WE Jr, Brown PW, Laurence W Jr & Terz JJ (1981) Penetrating, obstructing and perforating carcinomas of the colon and rectum. *Arch Surg* **116**: 381–384.

Kettlewell MGW (1988) Neoplasm: present surgical treatment. Current opinion. *Gastroenterology* **4**: 19–27.

Kimmey MB, Martin RW, Haggit RC et al (1989) Histologic correlates of gastrointestinal ultrasound images. *Gastroenterology* **96**: 433–441.

Kleinfeld G & Gump FE (1960) Complications of colotomy and polypectomy. *Surg Gynecol Obstet* **111**: 726.

Klempa I, Menzel J & Rheinheimer R (1981) Das Kolorectalkarzinom des Jungen erwachsene unter 35 Jahre. *Zentralbl Chir* **106**: 1033–1041.

Kline A, Hughes LF, Campbell H et al (1975) Dextron 70 in prophylaxis thromboembolic disease after surgery: a clinically orientated randomised double blind trial. *BMJ* **ii**: 109–112.

Kronborg O, Backer O & Sprechler M (1975) Acute obstruction in cancer of colon and rectum. *Dis Colon Rectum* **18**: 22–27.

Kusminsky RE, Perry LG, Rushden RO, Medina S & Boland JP (1984) Colonic surgery: the splenic connection. *Dis Colon Rectum* **38**: 35–37.

Kusunoki M, Yanagi H, Kamikonya N et al (1994) Preoperative detection of local extension of carcinoma of the rectum using magnetic resonance imaging. *J Am Coll Surg* **179**: 653–656.

Lamb G & Taylor I (1982) An assessment of ultrasound scanning in the recognition of colorectal liver metastases. *Ann R Coll Surg Engl* **64**: 391–393.

Langevin JM, Rothenberger DA & Goldberg SM (1984) Accidental splenic injury during surgical treatment of the colon and rectum. *Surg Gynecol Obstet* **159**: 139–143.

Lasser A (1978) Synchronous primary adenocarcinomas of the colon and rectum. *Dis Colon Rectum* **21**: 20–22.

Lennox MS (1984) Prophylactic drainage of colonic anastomoses. *Br J Surg* **71**: 10–11.

Leveson SH, Wiggins PA, Giles GR, Parkin A & Robinson PJ (1985) Deranged liver blood flow patterns in the detection of liver metastases. *Br J Surg* **72**: 128–130.

Levitt RG, Dagel SS, Stanley RJ & Jost RG (1977) Accuracy of computed tomography of the liver and biliary tract. *Radiology* **124**: 123–128.

Lewi H, Blumgart LH, Carter DC et al (1984) Preoperative carcinoembryonic antigen and survival in patients with colorectal cancer. *Br J Surg* **71**: 206–208.

Lewis RT, Allan CM, Goodall RG et al (1983) Are first generation cephalosporins effective for antibiotic prophylaxis in elective surgery of the colon? *Can J Surg* **26**: 504–507.

Lillehei RC & Wangensteen OH (1955) Bowel function after colectomy for cancer, polyps and diverticulitis. *JAMA* **159**: 163.

Lindhagen J, Andaker L & Hojer H (1984) Comparison of systemic prophylaxis with metronidazole/placebo and metronidazole/fosfomycin in colorectal surgery: a clinical study demonstrating the need for additional anti-aerobic prophylactic cover. *Acta Chir Scand* **150**: 317–323.

Lloyd Davies OV (1947) Carcinoma of the rectum with a single secondary in the liver: synchronous combined excision and left hepatectomy. *Proc R Soc Med* **40**: 875.

Lloyd Davies OV, Morgan CN & Goligher JC (1953) The treatment of carcinoma of the colon. In Roch Carling E & Paterson Ross J (eds) *British Surgical Practice: Progress Volume*, p 71. London: Butterworth.

Localio SA & Eng K (1975) Malignant tumours of the rectum. *Curr Probl Surg* **12**: 1.

Lockhart-Mummery H (1983) Colectomy for malignant disease. In Todd IP & Fielding LP (eds) *Rob & Smith's Operative Surgery. Vol. 3: Colon, Rectum and Anus*, 4th edn, pp 283–292. London: Butterworth.

Lockhart-Mummery HE, Ritchie JK & Hawley PR (1976) The results of surgical treatment for carcinoma of the rectum at St Mark's Hospital 1948–72. *Br J Surg* **63**: 673–677.

Lockhart-Mummery JP (1934) *Disease of the Rectum and Colon*, 2nd edn. London: Baillière Tindall.

Logerfo P & Herter FP (1975) Carcinoembryonic antigen and prognosis in patients with colon cancer. *Ann Surg* **181**: 81–84.

Long L, Jonasson O, Roberts, S et al (1960) Cancer cells in blood: results of simplified polation technique. *Arch Surg* **80**: 910.

Lores ME, Ortiz JR & Rosello PJ (1981) Peritoneal lavage with povidone iodine solution in experimentally induced peritonitis. *Surg Gynecol Obstet* **153**: 33–35.

Lothe RA, Fossli T, Danielsen HE et al (1992) Molecular genetic studies of tumor suppressor gene regions on chromosomes 13 and 17 in colorectal tumours. *J Natl Cancer Inst* **84**: 1100–1108.

Lothian and Borders (consultant surgeons and pathologists of the Lothian and Borders health boards) (1995) Lothian and Borders large bowel cancer project: immediate outcome after surgery. *Br J Surg* **82**: 888–890.

Mach JP, Chatal JF, Lumbrusco JP et al (1983) Tumour

localisation in patients by radiolabelled monoclonal antibodies against colon carcinoma. *Cancer Res* **43**: 5593–5600.

Machi J, Isomoto H, Yamashita K et al (1987) Intraoperative ultrasonography in screening for liver metastases from colorectal cancer: comparative accuracy with traditional procedures. *Surgery* **101**: 678–684.

Machi J, Isomoto H, Kurohiji T et al (1991) Accuracy of intraoperative ultrasonography in diagnosing liver metastasis from colorectal cancer: evaluation with postoperative follow-up results. *World J Surg* **15**: 551–557.

MacKeigan JM & Ferguson IA (1979) Prophylactic oophorectomy and colorectal cancer in premenopausal patients. *Dis Colon Rectum* **222**: 401.

Manz CW, La Tendresse C & Sako Y (1970) The detrimental effects of drains on colonic anastomoses: an experimental study. *Dis Colon Rectum* **13**: 17.

Marsh J, Donnan PT & Hamer-Hodges DW (1990) Association between transfusions with plasma and the recurrence of colorectal carcinoma. *Br J Surg* **77**: 623–626.

Marti MC & Pouret JP (1976) La préparation colique rapide. *Chirurgie* **102**: 330.

Martin EW, Joyce S, Lucas J, Clauren K & Cooperman M (1981) Colorectal carcinoma in patients less than 40 years of age. *Dis Colon Rectum* **24**: 25–28.

Matheson NA, McIntosh CA & Krukowski ZH (1985) Continuing experience with single-layer appositional anastomosis in the large bowel. *Br J Surg* **72**: 104–106

Mayo CW & Pagtalunan RJG (1963) Malignancy of colon and rectum in patients under 30 years of age. *Surgery (St Louis)* **53**: 711.

McKenna JP, Currie DJ, Mahoney LJ et al (1970) The use of continuous postoperative peritoneal lavage in the management of diffuse peritonitis. *Surg Gynecol Obstet* **130**: 254.

McKittrick LS (1948) Principles old and new of resection of colon for carcinomas. *Surg Gynec Obst* **87**: 15–25.

McLachlin AD & Denton DW (1973) Omental protection of intestinal anastomoses. *Am J Surg* **125**: 134.

McLachlin AD, Olsson LS & Pitt DF (1976) Anterior anastomosis of the rectosigmoid colon: an experimental study. *Surgery (St Louis)* **80**: 306.

McNicholas MMJ, Joyce WP, Dolan J et al (1994) Magnetic resonance imaging of rectal carcinoma: a prospective study. *Br J Surg* **81**: 911–914.

Mehta S, Johnson RJ & Schofield PF (1994) Staging of colorectal cancer. *Clin Radiol* **49**: 515–523.

Miles WE (1926) *Cancer of the Rectum*. London: Harrison.

Miller DR & Allbritten FF (1976) Carcinoma of the colon and rectum. *Arch Surg* **111**: 692–696.

Miller FE & Liechty RD (1967) Adenocarcinomas of the colon and rectum in persons under thirty years of age. *Am J Surg* **113**: 507.

Miller LD, Borouchow IB & Fitts WT (1966) An analysis of 284 patients with perforated carcinoma of the colon. *Surg Gynecol Obstet* **123**: 1212–1218.

Mills SE & Allen MS Jr (1979) Colorectal carcinoma in the first three decades of life. *Am J Surg Pathol* **3**: 443–448.

Milnes Walker R (1971) *Annual Report of South Western Regional Cancer Bureau*. Bristol: South Western Regional Board.

Minervini S, Alexander-Williams J, Donovan IA et al (1980) Comparison of three methods of whole bowel irrigation. *Am J Surg* **140**: 400.

Moore GE & Sako K (1959) The spread of carcinoma of the colon and rectum: a study of invasion of blood vessels, lymph nodes and the peritoneum by tumour cells. *Dis Colon Rectum* **2**: 92.

Moore GE (1960) The circulating cancer cell. *Lancet* **ii**: 814.

Morgan CN (1952) The management of carcinoma of the colon. *Ann R Coll Surg Engl* **10**: 305–323.

Morgan CN (1957) In Jones A (ed) *Modern Trends in Gastroenterology*, 2nd edn, p 340. London: Butterworth.

Morgan DB, Hill GL & Burkinshaw L (1980) The assessment of weight loss from a single measurement of body weight: the problems and limitations. *Am J Clin Nutr* **33**: 2101–2105.

Morrow CE, Vassilopoulos PP & Grage TB (1980) Surgical resection for metastatic neoplasm of the lung. *Cancer* **45**: 2981–2985.

Mosley EL, Chung EB, Cornwell EE, Anderson J & Leffal LD (1979) Colorectal carcinoma in young persons: experience at Howard University Hospital 1955–77. *J Natl Med Assoc* **71**: 449–451.

Muhe E, Gall EP & Angermann B (1981) Surgical treatment of metastases to the lung and liver. *Surg Gynecol Obstet* **152**: 2111.

Muir EG (1968) Safety in colonic resection. *Proc R Soc Med* **61**: 401.

Murray D, Hreno A, Dutton J et al (1975) Prognosis in colon cancer: a pathologic reassessment. *Arch Surg* **110**: 908–913.

Mzabi R, Himal HS, Demers R et al (1976) A multiparameter computer analysis of carcinoma of the colon. *Surg Gynecol Obstet* **143**: 959–964.

Nathanson SD, Tilley BC, Schultz L & Smith RF (1985) Perioperative allogeneic blood transfusions: survival in patients with resected carcinomas of the colon and rectum. *Arch Surg* **120**: 734–738.

Nicholls RJ, Mason AY, Morson BC, Dixon AK & Kelsey FRY (1982) The clinical staging of rectal cancer. *Br J Surg* **69**: 404–409.

Nori D, Merimsky O, Saw D et al (1996) Tumor ploidy as a risk factor for disease recurrence and short survival in surgically treated Dukes' B2 colon cancer patients. *Tumor Biol* **17**: 75–80.

O'Brien PE (1981) Continuous lavage of the contaminated peritoneum. In Watts JM, McDonald PJ & O'Brien RE (eds) *Infection in Surgery*. Edinburgh: Churchill Livingstone.

Ohman U (1982) Colorectal carcinoma in patients less than 40 years of age. *Dis Colon Rectum* **25**: 209–214.

Okizuka H, Sugimura K & Ishida T (1993) Preoperative local staging of rectal carcinoma with MR imaging and a rectal balloon. *J Magn Reson Imaging* **3**: 329–335.

Olesen KL, Birth M, Bardram L & Burcharth F (1984) Value of nasogastric tube after colorectal surgery. *Acta Chir Scand* **150**: 251–253.

Olsen AK (1990) Intraoperative ultrasonography and the detection of liver metastases in patients with colorectal cancer. *Br J Surg* **77**: 998–1002.

Ou YH (1992) Value of MR imaging in the staging of rectal carcinoma. *Chung-Hua Chung Liu Tsa Chih* **13**: 442–445.

Page CP, Bohnen JMA, Fletcher JR et al (1993) Antimicrobial prophylaxis for surgical wounds: guidelines for critical care. *Arch Surg* **128**: 79–88

Parker GA, Lawrence W Jr, Horsley JS III et al (1989) Intraoperative ultrasound of the liver affects operative decision making. **209**: 569–577.

Parrott NR, Lennard TWJ, Taylor RMR et al (1986) Effect of perioperative blood transfusion on recurrence of colorectal cancer. *Br J Surg* **73**: 970–975.

Paul FT (1895) Colectomy. *BMJ* **i**: 1136.

Paul MA, Mulder LS, Cuesta MA et al (1994) Impact of intraoperative ultrasonography on treatment strategy for colorectal cancer. *Br J Surg* **81**: 1660–1663.

Paul MA, Blomjous JGA, Cuesta MA & Meijer S (1996) Prognostic value of negative intraoperative ultrasonography in primary colorectal cancer. *Br J Surg* **83**: 1741–1743

Peck IJ, Fuchs PC & Gustafson ME (1984) Anti-microbial prophylaxis in elective colon surgery: experience of 1035 operations in a community hospital. *Am J Surg* **147**: 633–637.

Peden OA & Blalock AL (1963) Right hepatic lobectomy for metastatic carcinoma of the large bowel: 5 year survival. *Cancer* **16**: 1133.

Peloquin AB (1975) Factors influencing survival with complete obstruction and free perforation of colorectal cancers. *Dis Colon Rectum* **18**: 11–21.

Peloso OA, Floyd VT & Wilkinson LH (1973) Treatment of peritonitis with continuous postoperative peritoneal lavage using cephalothin. *Am J Surg* **126**: 742.

Pemberton M (1970) Carcinoma of the large intestine with survival in a child of nine and his father: a study of carcinoma of the colon with particular reference to children. *Br J Surg* **57**: 841–846.

Petrelli NJ, Nambisan RN, Herrara L et al (1985) Hepatic resection for isolated metastases from colorectal carcinoma. *Am J Surg* **149**: 205–209.

Pezim ME & Nicholls RJ (1984) Survival after high or low ligation of the inferior mesenteric artery during curative surgery for rectal cancer. *Ann Surg* **200**: 729–733.

Phillips R, Hittinger R, Saunder V et al (1983) Preoperative urography in large bowel cancer: a useless investigation. *Br J Surg* **70**: 425–427.

Pihl E, Hughes ESR, McDermott FT et al (1980) Carcinoma of the colon: cancer-specific long-term survival in a series of 615 patients treated by one surgeon. *Ann Surg* **192**: 114–117.

Pittam MR, Thornton H & Ellis H (1984) Survival after extended resection for locally advanced carcinomas of the colon and rectum. *Ann R Coll Surg* **66**: 81–84.

Polk HC & Fry DE (1980) Radical peritoneal debridement for established peritonitis. *Ann Surg* **192**: 350.

Poth EJ (1953) Intestinal antiseptics in surgery. *JAMA* **153**: 1516.

Poth EJ (1963) Intestinal antisepsis: interim report. *Dis Colon Rectum* **6**: 45.

Purkiss SF & Williams NS (1992) Accurate method to measure the percentage hepatic replacement by tumour and its use in prognosis of patients with advanced colorectal cancer. *Br J Surg* **79**: 136–138.

Quan SH & Sehdev MK (1974) Pelvic surgery concomitant with bowel resection for carcinoma. *Surg Clin North Am* **54**: 881.

Quirke P, Dixon MF, Clayden AD et al (1987) Prognostic significance of DNA aneuploidy and cell proliferation in rectal adenocarcinomas. *J Pathol* **151**: 287–291.

Raahave D, Hansen OH, Cartensen HE & Frits Moller A (1981) Septic wound complications after whole bowel irrigation before colorectal operations. *Acta Chir Scand* **147**: 125.

Rafaelsen SR, Kronborg O, Larsen C & Fenger C (1995) Intraoperative ultrasonography in detection of hepatic metastases from colorectal cancer. *Clin Radiol* **49**: 515–523.

Rafferty AT (1979) Noxythiolin (Noxyflux), aprotinin (Trasylol) and peritoneal adhesion formation: an experimental study in the rat. *Br J Surg* **66**: 654.

Raftery TL & Samson N (1980) Carcinoma of the colon: a clinical correlation between presenting symptoms and survival. *Am Surg* **46**: 600–606.

Rankin FW (1926) *Surgery of the Colon*. New York: Appleton.

Rankin FW & Olsen PF (1933) The hopeful prognosis in cases of carcinoma of the colon. *Surg Gynecol Obstet* **56**: 366.

Ravo B (1988) Colorectal anastomotic healing and intracolonic bypass procedure. *Surg Clin North Am* **68**: 1264–1294.

Recalde M, Hoyyoke ED & Elias EG (1974) Carcinoma of the colon, rectum and anal canal in young patients. *Surg Gynecol Obstet* **139**: 909–913.

Reilly JC, Rusin LC & Theuerkauf FJ (1982) Colonoscopy: its role in cancer of the colon and rectum. *Dis Colon Rectum* **25**: 532–538.

Rifkin MD & Wechsler RJ (1986) A comparison of computed tomography and endorectal ultrasound in staging rectal cancer. *Int J Colorectal Dis* **1**: 219–223.

Rilinger N, Munz DL, Neimann H, Illiger HJ & Halbfass HJ (1991) Immunoscintigraphy using different methods of applying a 99mTc labeled monoclonal anti-CEA-antibody in the staging of patients with liver metastases before partial hepatectomy. *Int J Rad Appl Instrum B* **18**: 65–68.

Romano G, De Rosa P, Vallone G et al (1985) Intrarectal ultrasound and computed tomography in pre and postoperative assessment of patients with rectal cancer. *Br J Surg* (Suppl): S117–S119.

Rosato FE, Frazier TG, Copeland EM & Miller LP (1969) Carcinoma of the colon in young people. *Surg Gynecol Obstet* **129**: 29.

Rosenberg IL, Graham MG, De Dombal FT & Goligher JC (1971) Preparation of the intestine in patients undergoing major large bowel surgery mainly for neoplasms of the colon and rectum. *Br J Surg* **58**: 288.

Rosenthal I & Baronofsky IK (1960) Prognostic and therapeutic implications of polyps in metachronous colic carcinoma. *JAMA* **172**: 37.

Rosin RD, Exarchakos G, Gilmore OJA et al (1978) Topical noxythiolin in colonic healing. *Br J Surg* **65**: 603.

Rouffet F, Hay JM, Vacher B et al (1994) Curative resection for left colonic carcinoma: hemicolectomy versus segmental colectomy. A prospective, controlled, multicentre trial for the French Association for Surgical Research. *Dis Colon Rectum* **37**: 651–659.

Rowe-Jones DC, Peel ALG, Kingston RD et al (1990) Single-dose cefotaxime plus metronidazole versus three-dose cefuroxime plus metronidazole as prophylaxis against wound infection in colorectal surgery: multicentre prospective randomised study. *BMJ* **300**: 18–22.

Royal College of Surgeons (1996) *Guidelines for the Management of Colorectal Cancer*. London: RCS.

Ruckley CV (1985) Protection against thromboembolism. *Br J Surg* **72**: 421–422 (leading article).

Runkel NS, Schlag P, Schwarz V & Herfarth C (1991) Outcome after emergency surgery for cancer of the large intestine. *Br J Surg* **78**: 183–188.

Russo A, Sparacino G, Plaja S et al (1989) Role of intraoperative ultrasound in the screening of liver metastases from colorectal carcinoma: initial experiences. *J Surg Oncol* **42**: 249–255.

Sales JP & Parc R (1994) Did the stage of diagnosis and the surgical management of colonic cancers change over the last ten years: a look at 303 patients (in French). *Ann Chir* **48**: 591–595.

Sanfelippo PM & Beahrs OH (1974) Carcinoma of the colon in patients under forty years of age. *Surg Gynecol Obstet* **138**: 169–176.

Sarper R, Fajman WA, Tarcan YA & Nixon DW (1981) Enhanced detection of metastatic liver disease by computerised flow scintigrams. *J Nucl Med* **22**: 318–321.

Scarpa FJ & Hartmann WH (1976) Adenocarcinoma of the colon and rectum in young adults. *South Med J* **69**: 24–27.

Schiessel R, Wunderlich M & Herbst F (1986) Local recurrence of colorectal cancer: effect of early detection and aggressive surgery. *Br J Surg* **73**: 342–344

Schulten MF, Heiskell CA & Shields TW (1976) The incidence of solitary pulmonary metastases from carcinoma of the large intestine. *Surg Gynecol Obstet* **143**: 722.

Scurr JH, Ibrahim SZ, Faber RG & Le Quesne CP (1977) The efficacy of graduated compression stockings in the prevention of deep vein thrombosis. *Br J Surg* **64**: 371–373.

Sellwood RA, Kaper SWA, Burn JI & Wallace EN (1965) Circulating cancer cells: the influence of surgical operation. *Br J Surg* **52**: 69.

Shepherd JM & Jones JSP (1971) Adenocarcinoma of the large bowel. *Br J Cancer* **25**: 680.

Shorey BA (1979) Systemic antibiotic prophylaxis. In Strachan CJL & Wise R (eds) *Gastrointestinal Surgery in Surgical Sepsis*. New York: Grune & Stratton.

Simstein NL, Kovalcik PJ & Cross GH (1978) Colorectal carcinoma in patients less than 40 years old. *Dis Colon Rectum* **21**: 169–171.

Sistrunk WE (1928) Mikulicz operation for resection of the colon and rectum: its advantages and disadvantages. *Ann Surg* **88**: 563.

Slaney G (1971) Results of treatment of carcinoma of the colon and rectum. In Irvine WT (ed) *Modern Trends in Surgery*, 3rd edn. London: Butterworth.

Slaney G et al (eds) (1991) *Cancer of the Large Bowel*. Basingstoke: Macmillan.

Smiddy FG & Goligher JC (1957) Results of surgery in the treatment of cancer of the large intestine. *BMJ* **i**: 793.

Smith SRG, Connolly P, Crane PW et al (1982) The effect of surgical drainage materials on colonic healing. *Br J Surg* **60**: 153.

Solomon MJ, McLeod RS, Cohen EK, Simons ME & Wilson S (1994) Reliability and validity studies of endoluminal ultrasonography for anorectal disorders. *Dis Colon Rectum* **37**: 546–551.

Stearns MW Jr & Deddish MR (1959) Five year results of abdominopelvic lymph node dissection for carcinoma of the colon and rectum. *Dis Colon Rectum* **2**: 169.

Steeg PS, Bevilacqua G, Kopper L et al (1988) Evidence for a novel gene associated with low tumor metastatic potential. *J Natl Cancer Inst* **80**: 200–204.

Steele G Jr, Osteen RT, Wilson RE et al (1984) Patterns of failure after surgical cure of large liver tumours: a change in the proximate cause of death and a need for effective systemic adjuvant therapy. *Am J Surg* **147**: 554–560.

Stephens M & Loewenthal J (1979) Continuing peritoneal lavage in high risk peritonitis. *Surgery* **85**: 603.

Stewart DJ & Matheson NA (1978) Peritoneal lavage in faecal peritonitis in the rat. *Br J Surg* **65**: 57.

Stewart DJ (1980) Generalised peritonitis. *J R Coll Surg Edinb* **25**: 80.

Stewart PJ, Chu JM, Kos SC, Chapuis PH & Bokey EL (1993) Intraoperative ultrasound for the detection of hepatic metastases from colorectal cancer. *Aust NZ J Surg* **63**: 530–534.

Stone HH, Hooper CA & Millikan WJ (1978) Abdominal drainage following appendicectomy and cholecystectomy. *Am J Surg* **187**: 606–610.

Stone MD, Kane R, Bothe A Jr et al (1994) Intraoperative ultrasound imaging of the liver at the time of colorectal cancer resection. *Arch Surg* **129**: 431–436.

Strauss LG, Clorius JH, Schlag P et al (1989) Recurrence of colorectal tumours PET evaluation. *Radiology* **170**: 329–332

Sun X-F, Carstensen JM, Zhang H et al (1992) Prognostic significance of cytoplasmic p53 oncoprotein in colorectal adenocarcinoma. *Lancet* **340**: 1369–1373.

Surtees P, Ritchie JK & Phillips RKS (1990) High versus low ligation of the inferior mesenteric artery in rectal cancer. *Br J Surg* **77**: 618–621.

Takita H, Edgerton F, Karakouss C et al (1981) Surgical management of metastases to the lung. *Surg Gynecol Obstet* **152**: 191.

Talbot IC, Ritchie S, Leighton MH et al (1980) The clinical significance of invasion of veins by rectal cancer. *Br J Surg* **67**: 439.

Tate JJT, Rawlinson J, Royle GT, Brunton FJ & Taylor I (1988) Preoperative or postoperative colonic examination for synchronous lesions in colorectal cancer. *Br J Surg* **75**: 1016–1018.

Teicher I & Abrahams JI (1956) The treatment of selected cases of multiple polyps, familial polyposis and diverticular disease of the colon by subtotal colectomy and ileoproctostomy. *Surg Gynecol Obstet* **103**: 136.

Thaler W, Watzka S, Martin F et al (1994) Preoperative staging of rectal cancer by endoluminal ultrasound versus magnetic resonance imaging: preliminary results of a prospective, comparative study. *Dis Colon Rectum* **37**: 1189–1193.

Thibodeau SN, Bren G & Schaid D (1993) Microsatellite instability in cancer of the proximal colon. *Science* **260**: 816–819.

Thoeni RF, Moss AA, Schnyder P & Marguld AR (1981) Detection and staging of primary rectal and rectosigmoid cancer by computed tomography. *Radiology* **141**: 135–138.

Thompson WM, Halvorsen RA, Foster WL Jr, Roberts L & Gibbons R (1986) Preoperative and postoperative CT staging of rectosigmoid carcinoma. *Am J Roentgen* **146**: 703–710.

Thomson A, Naidoo P & Crotty B (1996) Bowel preparation for colonoscopy: a randomized prospective trial comparing sodium phosphate and polyethylene glycol in a predominantly elderly population. *J Gastroenterol Hepatol* **11**: 103–107.

Tominaga T, Sakabe T, Koyama Y et al (1996) Prognostic factors for patients with colon or rectal carcinoma treated with resection only: five-year follow-up report. *Cancer* **78**: 403–408.

Travieso CR, Knoepp LF & Hanley PH (1972) Multiple adenocarcinomas of the colon and rectum. *Dis Colon Rectum* **15**: 1–6.

Turnbull RB Jr, Kyle K & Watson FR (1967) Cancer of the colon: the influence of the no-touch isolation technic on survival rates. *Ann Surg* **166**: 420.

Turner GG (1955) Operations for intestinal obstruction. In *Modern Operative Surgery*, 4th edn, Vol 1, p 1017. London: Cassell.

Turner-Warwick RT (1976) The use of the omental pedicle graft in urinary tract reconstruction. *J Urol* **116**: 341.

Turner-Warwick RT, Wynne EJC & Handley Ashken M (1967) The use of the omental pedicle graft in the repair and reconstruction of the urinary tract. *Br J Surg* **54**: 55.

Turunen MJ & Peltokallio P (1983) Surgical results in 657 patients with colorectal cancer. *Dis Colon Rectum* **26**: 606–612.

Turunen MJ (1983) Colorectal cancer obstruction: a challenge to improve prognosis. *Ann Chir Gynaecol* **72**: 317–323.

UKCCCR Sub-Committee on Staging of Colorectal Cancer (1996) *Handbook for the Clinicopathological Assessment and Staging of Colorectal Cancer*, 2nd edn (available from PO Box 123, Lincoln's Inn Fields, London WC2A 3PX).

Umpleby HC, Bristol JB, Rainey JB & Williamson RCN (1984) Survival of 727 patients with single carcinomas of the large bowel. *Dis Colon Rectum* **27**: 803–809.

van Waes PF, Koehler PR & Feldberg MA (1983) Management of rectal carcinoma: impact of computed tomography. *Am J Roentgen* **140**: 1137–1142.

Vezzoni P, Clemente C & Gennari L (1977) Adenocarcinoma of the large intestine in young adults. *Tumori* **63**: 565–573.

Vinnicombe SJ, Norman AR, Nicolson V & Husband JE (1995) Normal pelvic lymph nodes: evaluation with CT after bipedal lymphangiography. *Radiology* **194**: 349–355.

von Mikulicz J (1903) Small contributions to the surgery of the intestinal tract. *Boston Med Surg J* **148**: 608.

Voogt PJ, van de Velde CJ, Brand A et al (1987) Perioperative blood transfusion and cancer prognosis: different aspects of blood transfusion on prognosis of colon and breast cancer patients. *Cancer* **59**: 836–834.

Waizer A, Powsner E, Russo I et al (1991) Prospective comparative study of magnetic resonance imaging versus transrectal ultrasound for preoperative staging and follow-up of rectal cancer: preliminary report. *Dis Colon Rectum* **34**: 1068–1072.

Walton WW, Hagihara PF & Griffin WO (1976) Colorectal adenocarcinoma in patients less than 40 years old. *Dis Colon Rectum* **19**: 529–534.

Wanebo HJ, Bhaskar R, Pinsey CM et al (1978a) Preoperative carcinoembryonic antigen level as a prognostic indicator in colorectal cancer. *N Engl J Med* **299**: 448–451.

Wanebo HJ, Semogou C, Attiyeh F & Stearns M (1978b) Surgical management of patients with primary operable colorectal cancer and synchronous liver metastases. *Am J Surg* **135**: 81.

Welch JP & Donaldson GA (1974a) Recent experience in the management of cancer of the colon and rectum. *Am J Surg* **127**: 258–265.

Welch JP & Donaldson GA (1974b) Management of severe obstruction of the large bowel due to malignant disease. *Am J Surg* **127**: 492–521.

Wernecke K, Rummeny E, Bongartz G et al (1991) Detection of hepatic masses in patients with carcinoma: comparative sensitivities of sonography, CT and MR imaging. *Am J Roentgenol* **157**: 731–739.

West Midlands Cancer Registry (1990) *Cancer in the West Midlands 1981–85*, pp 37–50.

White TT & Harrison RC (1975) *Reoperative Gastrointestinal Surgery*, 2nd edn, p 286. Boston: Little, Brown.

Whittle J, Steinberg EP, Anderson GF & Herbert R (1992) Results of colectomy in elderly patients with colon cancer, based on Medicare claims data. *Am J Surg* **163**: 572–576.

Wieden PL, Bean MA & Scultz P (1987) Perioperative blood transfusion does not increase the rate of colorectal cancer recurrence. *Cancer* **60**: 870–875.

Wield U, Nilsson T, Knudsen JB, Sprechler M & Johansen AA (1985) Postoperative survival of patients with potentially curable cancer of the colon. *Dis Colon Rectum* **28**: 332–335.

Wiggers T, Jeekel J, Arends JW et al (1988) No-touch isolation technique in colon cancer: a controlled prospective trial. *Br J Surg* **75**: 409–415

Willet CG, Tepper JE, Cohen AM, Orlow E & Welch CE (1984) Failure patterns following curative resection of colonic carcinoma. *Ann Surg* **200**: 685–690.

Williams NS, Durdey P & Quirk P (1985) Preoperative staging of rectal neoplasm and its impact on clinical management. *Br J Surg* **72**: 868–874.

Williams NS, Jass JR & Hardcastle DJD (1988) Clinicopathological assessment and staging of colorectal cancer. *Br J Surg* **75**: 649–652.

Wilson SM & Adson MA (1976) Surgical treatment of hepatic metastases from colorectal causes. *Arch Surg* **111**: 329.

Wolters U, Keller HW, Sorgatz S, Raab A & Pichlmaier H (1994) Prospective randomized study of properative bowel cleansing for patients undergoing colorectal surgery. *Br J Surg* **81**: 598–600.

Wood CB, Gillis CR, Hole D et al (1981) Local tumour invasion as a prognostic factor in colorectal cancer. *Br J Surg* **68**: 326–328.

Wooley RC, Schreiber K, Koss LG, Karas M & Sherman A (1982) DNA distribution in human colon carcinoma and its relation to clinical behaviour. *J Natl Cancer Inst* **69**: 15–22.

Wraight EP, Barber RW & Ritson A (1982) Relative hepatic arterial and portal flow in liver scintigraphy. *Nucl Med Commun* **3**: 273–279.

Yamaguchi A, Kurosaka Y, Ishida T et al (1991) Clinical significance of tumour markers NCC-JT 439 in large bowel cancers. *Dis Colon Rectum* **34**: 921–927.

Yiu CY, Baker LA & Boulos PB (1991) Antiepithelial monoclonal antibodies and radioimmunolocalisation of colorectal cancer. *Br J Surg* **35**: 3523–3525.

Zalcberg JR, Thompson CH, Lichenstein M, Andrews J & McKenzie IFC (1983) Localisation of human colorectal tumour xenografts in the nude mouse with the use of radiolabelled monoclonal antibody. *J Natl Cancer Inst* **71**: 801–808.

Zaubauer W, Haertel M & Fuchs WA (1981) Computed tomography in carcinoma of the rectum. *Gastrointest Radiol* **15**: 79–84.

32

SURGICAL TREATMENT OF RECTAL CANCER

DEVELOPMENT OF SURGICAL TECHNIQUES

Abdominoperineal excision of the rectum

The earliest surgical approaches to carcinoma of the rectum were via the perineum by Faget (1739), Lisfranc (1826) and Verneuil (1873). The technique used was entirely extraperitoneal, but despite this approach patients rarely survived the operation and perineal sepsis made life unbearable for those who did. Great strides were made by Allingham (Allingham, 1879; Allingham and Allingham, 1901) who used an inguinal colostomy to control sepsis, and also by Lockhart-Mummery (1926) who not only employed a colostomy but also applied aseptic principles to the operative procedure.

The operation as evolved at St Mark's Hospital was therefore performed in two parts. The initial establishment of a loop colostomy in the left iliac fossa allowed the peritoneal cavity to be explored for the presence of metastases and the operability of the rectal tumour to be assessed. The perineal resection was then performed 2–3 weeks later after the colon and rectum had been cleansed by repeated irrigation via the colostomy. The perineal procedure was performed with the patient in the left lateral position. The rectum was delivered after mobilization and the superior rectal vessels were ligated as high as possible. An attempt was made to resect as much of the rectum as possible from below (usually 20–25 cm). The cut distal end of the rectosigmoid was closed with an inverting stitch and the inguinal colostomy was left as a permanent feature.

There were two main disadvantages of this operation which were perceived at the time. First, it failed to deal adequately with tumours of the upper third of the rectum. Second, the closed-off distal end of the colon would frequently leak as faeces passed down into the blind end of the bowel. Despite these objections, perineal excision of the rectum became the standard operation for rectal carcinoma both in the UK and USA until the early 1930s. Its main advantage in the era before blood transfusions and antibiotics was its relative simplicity and safety. In 1932 Gabriel reported that this technique had an operability rate of 50%, a mortality rate of 11.6% and a crude 5-year survival rate of 40% (Gabriel, 1932).

The most important step in the evolution of the surgical treatment of carcinoma of the rectum was taken by Ernest Miles, a young surgeon and anatomist at St Mark's Hospital who was a contemporary of Allingham's. He was alarmed by the finding that 95% of his patients who underwent perineal resection developed recurrence; this stimulated him to investigate the precise pathological nature of spread of the tumour. In his now classical pathological studies which were based on specimens obtained in the operating theatre and post-mortem room, he found that lymphatic spread could occur in three directions – upwards, laterally and downwards (Miles, 1910, 1926). He concluded that to prevent recurrence it was necessary to remove the entire rectum, anal canal and sphincters, much of the levator ani muscles and the ischiorectal fat, most of the sigmoid colon and mesocolon including the glands lying in its base and the superior haemorrhoidal and inferior mesenteric vessels, and a portion of the pelvic peritoneum (Miles, 1908). To accomplish this it was necessary to remove the rectum by both an abdominal and a perineal approach. Thus was born the operation of abdominoperineal excision which was often referred to as the 'Miles operation'.

Although the principles seemed sound when Miles first described the procedure, it took some time before it became accepted as the operation of first choice for carcinoma of the rectum. This was no doubt due to the extent of surgical trauma inflicted on the patient in the course of the procedure; 22 of the first 61 patients (36.2%) treated by Miles died either on the operating table or shortly afterwards. Miles performed the abdominal part of the operation before the perineal part; it was for this reason that Gabriel (1934) developed the perineoabdominal excision. Perineoabdominal excision consisted of an extraperitoneal mobilization of the rectum via the perineum as in the perineal method previously described; the superior haemorrhoidal vessels, however, were not ligated during this stage but were dealt with via the abdominal approach which enabled the upward lymphatic spread to be dealt with adequately. This procedure was found to be very safe (Gabriel, 1957) because virtually all of the dissection and mobilization of the rectum was carried out from below outside the peritoneal cavity; intra-abdominal dissection was minimal.

Despite these apparent advantages, the operation never attained popularity, mainly because with the advances in anaesthesia and postoperative care a more extensive abdominal dissection became feasible. Since mobilization of the rectum was easier to perform via the abdominal route, the abdominoperineal resection as described by Miles slowly gained favour.

Abdominoperineal excision became even more refined by the subsequent development of the synchronous combined excision of the rectum, in which the abdominal and perineal phases were performed simultaneously by two separate surgeons. Kirschner (1934) was the first to demonstrate that a synchronous combined approach was feasible, but he subsequently abandoned it owing to the high mortality rate that occurred in the pretransfusion era. Although Devine (1937) reintroduced the technique to the UK and USA, Lloyd Davies (1939) was responsible for its subsequent popularity. Among many other technical modifications, he devised adjustable leg rests which enabled the patient to be supported in the lithotomy–Trendelenburg position necessary for a synchronous approach to abdomen and perineum. The combined technique considerably reduced the operating time and made removal of advanced tumours easier.

Those still opposed to the synchronous combined approach, however, claimed that the position of the patient on the operating table made the approach to the abdomen and perineum difficult. It was also considered by some that the combined approach was more 'shocking' for the patient compared with the two-stage procedure. As time progressed, however, these criticisms were dropped. Surgeons became used to the lithotomy–Trendelenburg position and did not find it an inconvenience; the introduction of safe blood transfusion and epidural anaesthesia made the procedure relatively safe. The operation thus became the procedure of first choice in the UK for the surgical treatment of all rectal carcinomas, irrespective of their height from the anal verge. In the USA the synchronous combined technique, known there as the 'two-team technique', never attained the same popularity as in the UK.

Surgeons in North America tended to adhere to the same technique originally described by Miles in which the abdominal procedure was performed in the first instance and was then followed by the perineal dissection.

Trans-sacral excision

In Europe events took a different course. Instead of approaching the rectum from the perineum, surgeons employed the sacral route. Originally described by Kocher in 1875, the technique was popularized by Kraske (1885). The patient was placed on the side and a vertical incision was made from behind the anus and over the sacrum, usually inclining to one or other side of the mid-line. The coccyx and one or two pieces of sacrum were removed and good access was obtained to the back of the rectum above the levator muscles. The peritoneum was then opened on one side of the bowel which was drawn downwards as far as possible and the superior rectal vessels were divided and ligated. Inferiorly the dissection was carried out as far as necessary. In the early days the rectum and the anal canal were excised *in toto* and the distal colon was brought out in the sacral region as a 'sacral anus'. Various modifications in the way the rectum was approached were introduced by a variety of surgeons including Bordenheuer, Rose, Hochenegg, Billroth, Rehn, Heineke and Rydygier (Rankin et al, 1932), and this operation rapidly became the procedure of first choice on the continent of Europe.

It was not long, however, before it was realized that with a tumour situated high in the rectum, the anal canal and sphincters could be technically retained and gastrointestinal continuity might be achieved. This realization led indirectly to the development of sphincter-saving resections.

Sphincter-saving resection

It was Kraske himself who was the first to attempt an anastomosis between colon and anorectal stump after the rectum had been removed via the sacral route. He initially attached the sigmoid colon to one-third of the circumference of the rectal stump; the resulting faecal fistula was closed several weeks later and thus continuity was restored. Although the same procedure was repeated by several other surgeons, it usually terminated in disaster because the anastomosis invariably broke down and the resulting faecal fistula was difficult to close.

In order to improve the chances of success, Hochenegg (1888, 1889) devised a procedure designed to obtain a safe union between colon and anorectal stump. The rectum with the cancer was excised in the usual way via the sacral route and the anorectal stump was everted through the anus. The proximal colon was then mobilized down through the everted anorectum and an anastomosis was fashioned between the colon and the anal canal outside the anus. Although this method was more successful than that of Kraske, the anastomosis still broke down with alarming regularity. This led Hochenegg to devise the *Durchzug* method (Hochenegg, 1900), in which the anorectum was once again everted through the anal canal but was stripped of its mucosa and returned to the pelvis. The colon was then delivered through the denuded anorectum and was sutured to the skin of the anal verge. It was hoped that the denuded anorectum would achieve a particularly firm union with the colonic serosa.

The relative success of this approach was documented by Mandl (1922, 1929) who found an overall mortality rate of 11.6% in 984 patients treated by sacral excision in Hochenegg's clinic; half of these patients had gastrointestinal continuity restored. Unfortunately the operation had a poor 5-year survival rate, which was 30% in Mandl's series, with a high local recurrence rate. The reason was the failure of the operation to deal adequately with the upward spread of the cancer, and as abdominoperineal excision became safer so the sacral operations were abandoned. The concept of sphincter preservation never died, but because of Miles' work on the spread of carcinoma it was considered unwise to leave any of the anorectum behind. An abdominal approach ensured that upward spread was dealt with adequately but it was considered that lateral and downward spread could be removed only if the anorectum was excised via the perineum.

The pathological observations of Miles on lymphatic spread of rectal carcinoma dominated treatment of rectal carcinoma for the next 30 years. They ensured that no matter where the carcinoma was situated in the rectum, the patient underwent an abdominoperineal excision of the rectum with the establishment of a permanent end colostomy. These views remained unchallenged until several authors demonstrated that Miles' original observations were not entirely correct (Dukes, 1930; Westhues, 1930, 1934; Wood and Wilkie, 1933; Gabriel et al, 1935; Gilchrist and David, 1938; Coller et al, 1940).

In meticulous studies carried out on rectal specimens removed at operation by the sacral, perineal or abdominoperineal routes, these investigators were seldom able to demonstrate the presence of lateral or downward spread. They agreed with Miles' finding that upward spread was common, but differed from Miles in that they found that upward spread progressed in an orderly manner from the pararectal glands on the posterior aspect of the rectum adjacent to the growth, to the glands along the main superior haemorrhoidal vessels and thence to the inferior mesenteric glands, eventually reaching the para-aortic glands. Spread was rarely discontinuous. In rare cases in which lateral and downward spread could be demonstrated, there was evidence that the growth was extremely advanced and that the lymphatics along the superior rectal vessels were choked with tumour, which presumably allowed retrograde flow of lymph to occur. The rarity of downward spread was later emphasized both by Glover and Waugh (1946) and by Goligher et al (1951). Goligher and others found that out of 1500 abdominoperineal excision specimens only 30 patients (2%) had evidence of distal lymphatic spread and most of these also had appreciable upward spread (Goligher et al, 1951).

As a result of these pathological studies it was soon appreciated that it was not always necessary to treat rectal carcinoma by excision of the anorectum with sacrifice of the anal sphincters. Thus in the early 1940s there was a proliferation of new techniques and a reappraisal of older methods which restored gastrointestinal continuity and preserved the anal sphincter. At this time, however, the philosophy of sphincter preservation was considered appropriate only for growths of the rectosigmoid region and upper third of the rectum. The reason for this was that at least 6–8 cm of residual anorectum was considered necessary for continence to be preserved. In addition, although distal lymphatic spread was considered a rarity, microscopic distal *intramural* spread was thought to be more frequent. In order to deal adequately with this potential problem, it was believed that a rectal carcinoma must be resected with a minimum distal clearance of 5 cm of macroscopically normal bowel if cure was to be achieved. These two objectives (i.e. a distal resection of at least 5 cm and the retention of 6–8 cm of anorectum, were incompatible for most tumours situated in the lower two-thirds of the rectum.

The techniques devised at this time to conserve gastrointestinal continuity and continence were certainly most ingenious and they laid the foundation for modern practice.

Since the earliest attempts at sphincter preservation had been made via the sacral approach it is not surprising that this route was once more employed. With the appreciation, however, that it was essential to deal adequately with the upward lymphatic spread an abdominal component was combined with the sacral approach and thus the *abdomino-sacral resection* was born. The technique was popularized by Finsterer (1941), Goetze (1944) and d'Allaines (1956) in Europe and by Pannett (1935) in the UK. The abdominal part was performed first in the same manner as for the Miles operation. The main vessels were ligated and divided and the rectum was mobilized, but the distal sigmoid colon was not divided. The colon was instead pushed down into the pelvis and the pelvic peritoneum was closed over it. The patient was then turned on the side and the rectum approached via the sacral route as previously described. The rectal excision was then performed and an end-to-end anastomosis constructed.

Despite the fact that this approach proved to be an adequate 'cancer operation' it did not gain universal popularity. There still remained the risk of faecal fistula through the sacral wound which itself caused considerable discomfort. The procedure was resurrected in the 1970s mainly by Localio of New York (Localio and Stahl, 1969; Localio and Baron, 1973; Localio and Eng, 1975; Localio et al, 1978). He modified the operation slightly so that it could be performed with the patient lying in the same position on their right side throughout the procedure. Despite Localio's excellent results the development of other techniques has tended to make this an obsolete operation, certainly in the UK.

The other main technique which was developed at about the same time as the abdominosacral operation was *anterior resection with sutured anastomosis*. Unsuccessful attempts had been made previously to re-establish intestinal continuity after rectal excision by the abdominal route. Rutherford Morrison (Turner, 1943), Balfour (1910) and Lockhart-Mummery (1934) had tried a 'telescopic' technique whereby a stout tube of metal or rubber had been tied into the proximal colon and this had been delivered down through the anorectal stump. While traction was exerted on this tube through the anus, sutures were placed between the serosa of the colon and the cut edge of the rectum. This technique proved disastrous and it was not until Dixon and his colleagues at the Mayo Clinic (Dixon, 1939, 1940) devised the modern technique of anterior resection that anastomosis via the abdominal approach was feasible. After rectal excision the proximal colon was sutured end-to-end with the rectal stump, usually in two layers. The operation, known for many years as the Mayo Clinic operation, gradually gained in popularity until it became the operation of choice for carcinomas of the rectosigmoid region and upper third of the rectum. Numerous studies have since shown that the procedure is as safe and curative as abdominoperineal excision for growths at this level (Morgan, 1955; Waugh et al, 1955; Mayo and Fly, 1956; Mayo et al, 1958; Lockhart-Mummery et al, 1976; Whittaker and Goligher, 1976; Wilson and Beahrs, 1976).

Once confidence had been gained in the use of anterior resection for growths of the upper third of the rectum, it was only natural that use of the technique should be extended to the treatment of suitable tumours situated at a lower level. This was facilitated by the realization that the anastomosis could also safely be performed using one layer of sutures (Everett, 1975).

Pari passu with the development of low anterior resection came the development of the *abdomino-anal pull-through techniques*. These procedures tended to be reserved for suitable patients in whom intestinal continuity could not be achieved by a standard Dixon anterior resection after rectal excision. The principle of the operation was to bring the colon into continuity with the anorectal stump by pulling it through the anus from below. Techniques differed in the exact way in which the colon was coapted to the anorectum. Thus in the procedure developed by Sebrechts (1935), Rayner (1935), Babcock (1939, 1947) and Bacon (1945), the lining of the anal canal was removed and the mobilized colon was brought down through the anal canal leaving about 50 cm projecting (Figure 32.1). The anal sphincters which had previously been divided were then sutured to the protruding colon. After approximately 10 days the excess colon was removed. In the modification described by Black (1952) the anal sphincter was not divided but was dilated manually (Figure 32.2).

In the Maunsell–Weir operation (Maunsell, 1892; Weir, 1901) the anorectal stump was everted through the anus and the colon was drawn down through it, so that the free edges of both stumps lay opposite each other and were then sutured together outside the anus (Figure 32.3). Yet another variation was the operation devised independently by Turnbull and Cuthbertson (1961) and by Cutait and Figlioni (1961) which was known as the Turnbull–Cutait operation. It was really the same technique as that described by Maunsell and Weir but was performed in two stages. In the first stage the colon was drawn through the everted anorectal stump and left for 10–14 days. At the second stage the redundant colon was resected and the cut edges of the colon and the anal canal were sutured; the anastomosis was then allowed to recede through the anus back into the pelvis.

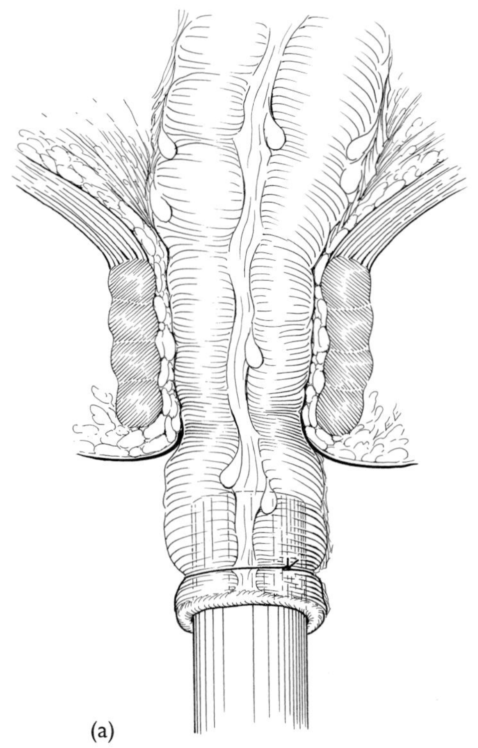

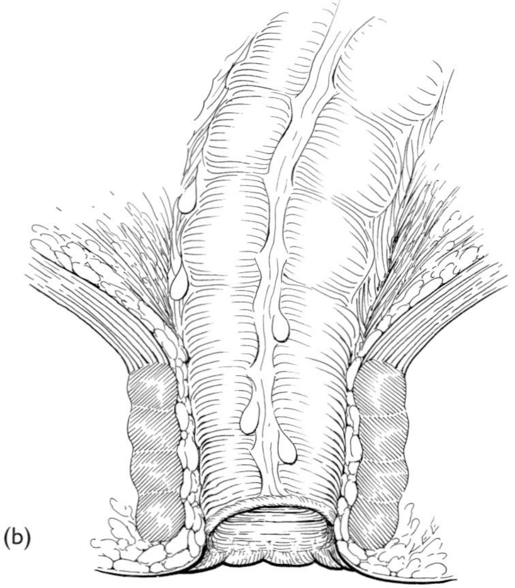

Figure 32.1a,b Abdominoanal pull-through resection described by Bacon. (a) After rectal excision the lining of the anal canal was removed and the mobilized colon was brought down through the anal canal leaving about 50 cm projecting. The anal sphincters which had previously been divided were sutured around the protruding colon. (b) After 2–3 weeks the protruding colon was excised, leaving the coloanal anastomosis.

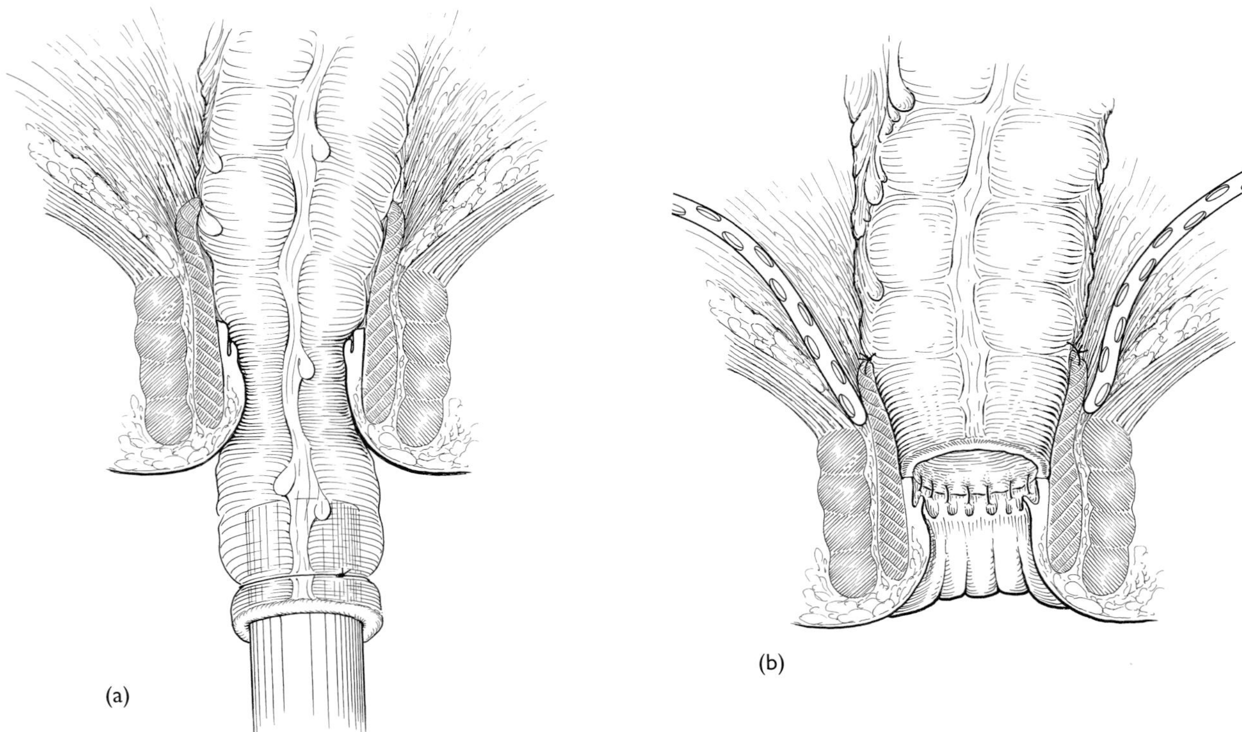

Figure 32.2a,b (a) Abdominoanal pull-through resection described by Black. Both the anal canal lining and sphincters were preserved although the canal was stretched to facilitate the pull-through manoeuvre. (b) The final situation after excision of the redundant colon.

Although the abdominoanal pull-through procedures described above could deal with tumours at a lower level in the pelvis than anterior resection, they never achieved universal acceptance. They were technically difficult to perform and the poor function achieved by many patients did not justify the risks and difficulties involved. In 1972 Mann demonstrated just how poor these results could be even in the hands of expert technicians (Mann, 1972). He studied a group of patients at St Mark's Hospital treated by the Maunsell–Weir and Babcock–Bacon operations between 1937 and 1970. The operative mortality was 13% and only 28% of patients convalesced without serious morbidity. The main complications encountered were pelvic abscess in 41% of patients, anastomotic breakdown in 31%, stricture formation in 26%, local recurrence of carcinoma in 24% and faecal incontinence in 10%. Other workers reported similar disappointing results with the Turnbull–Cutait operation (Cutait and Figlioni, 1961; Turnbull and Cuthbertson, 1961). It was for these reasons that most surgeons (apart from devotees) abandoned pull-through procedures, preferring to perform an abdominoperineal excision when an anterior resection was not technically feasible.

There was little change in technique during the late 1950s and 1960s. The policy in most units with a particular colorectal interest was relatively standard during this period. For tumours of the upper third of the rectum (above 12 cm from the anal verge) an anterior resection with a manual anastomosis was used whenever feasible, provided a distal margin of clearance of 5 cm could be obtained and a reasonable length of anorectal stump remained. The application of this policy, however, was very much dependent on the individual unit. At one extreme were surgeons who were prepared to push anterior resection to the limit and in some instances break the rules concerning distal margin of clearance in order to achieve a low anastomosis. Other surgeons considered that if an anterior resection could not be performed comfortably in two layers the patient must have an abdominoperineal excision. Most surgeons did, however, agree that for tumours of the lower third of the rectum an abdominoperineal excision was mandatory.

Between 1970 and 1980 technical innovations

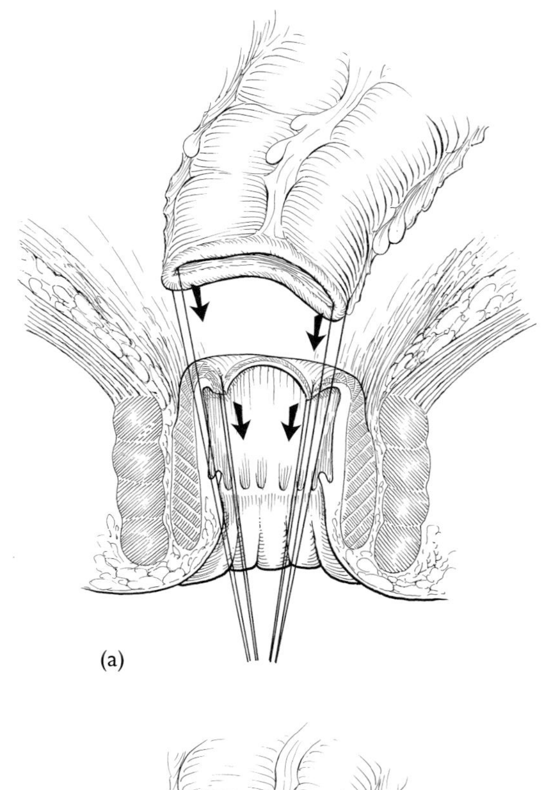

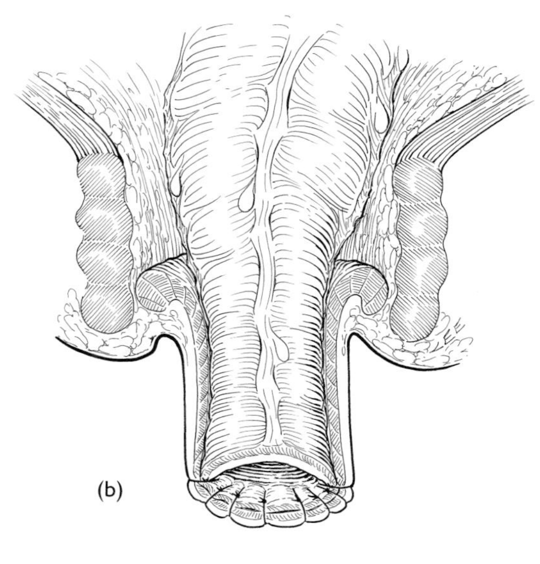

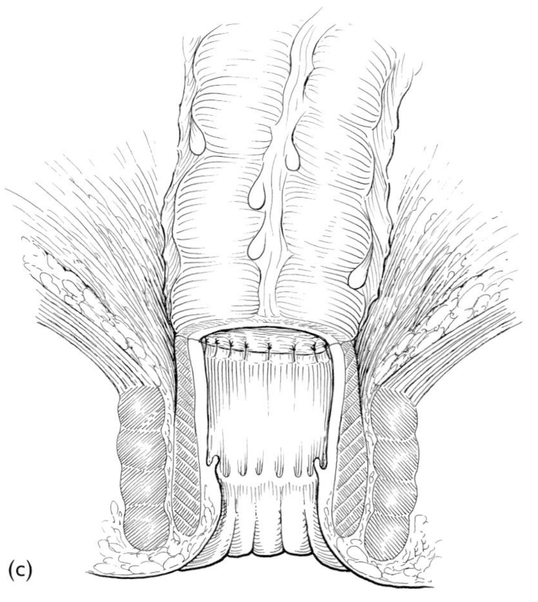

Figure 32.3a–c Abdominoanal pull-through resection of the Maunsell–Weir type. (a) The rectum with the cancer was excised and the anorectal stump was everted. The colon was pulled through the everted stump, and (b) the two were anastomosed externally. (c) The completed anastomosis and everted anorectal stump were returned to the pelvis.

began to change the aforementioned policy. In 1972 Parks described an important modification of the abdominoanal pull-through technique (Parks, 1972). In his *abdominotransanal technique* the anastomosis of the colon to the anorectum was performed through a dilated anal canal, thereby avoiding the potentially damaging eversion required in previous pull-through procedures (Figure 32.4). Not only was this a technical advance, but it also demonstrated that even if the whole of the rectum was removed and the colon was anastomosed directly to the anal canal continence could still be achieved (Lane and Parks, 1977). This finding was of immense importance since it demonstrated that retention of an anorectal stump of 6–8 cm in length was not always necessary for continence to be preserved. Further work demonstrated that the receptors for continence lay outside the rectum: not in the rectal wall but in the pelvic floor musculature (Lane and Parks, 1977; Williams et al, 1980b). If the pelvic floor muscles were not damaged in the course of the operation then continence could usually be attained.

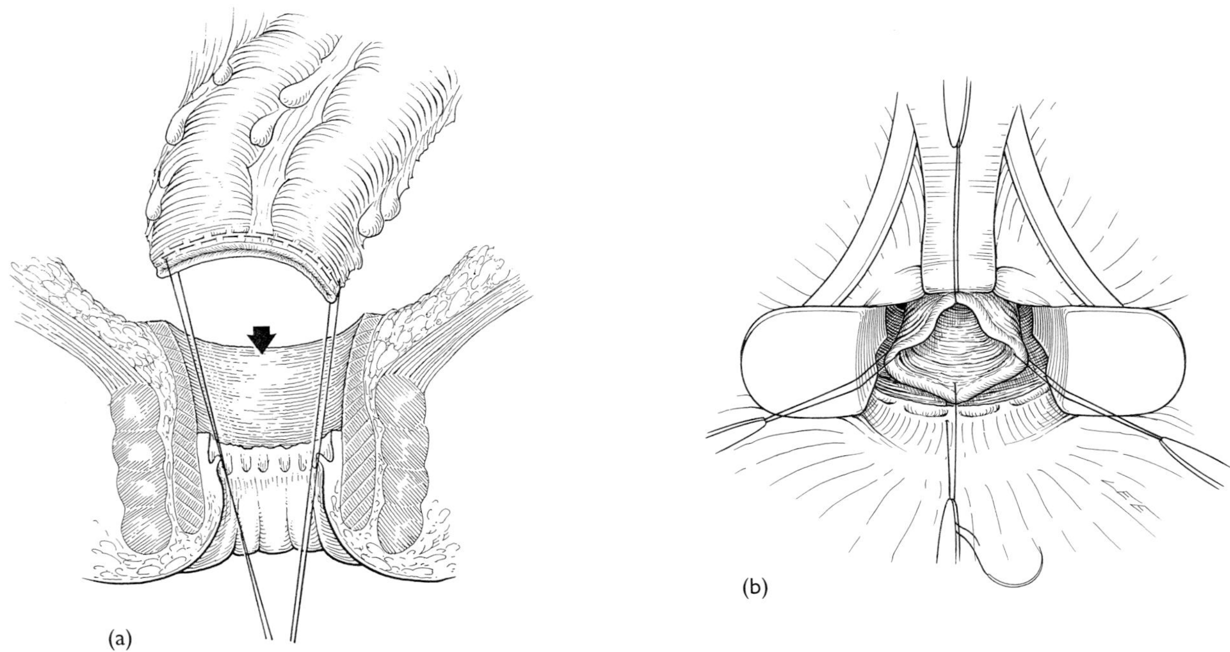

Figure 32.4a,b Principle of the Parks' abdominotransanal technique. (a) The rectum with the cancer has been excised down to the level of the levators. The upper part of the anal canal has been denuded of its mucosa by transanal stripping. The colon pulled through the denuded anal canal (b) is anastomosed at the dentate line by a transanal technique.

At the same time York Mason described a modification of the abdominosacral resection designed to produce a very low anastomosis (Mason, 1976). In this operation, termed *abdominotrans-sphincteric excision of the rectum*, the external anal sphincter and levator ani muscle were divided and the lower rectum exposed (Figure 32.5). The rectum, having been previously partially mobilized via the abdomen, was then freed from its attachments and resected down to the top of the intact internal anal sphincter. An anastomosis was constructed between the colon and anal canal. The levator ani and external anal sphincter were then carefully sutured in layers. Although Mason (1976, 1977) reported enthusiastically on its efficacy, the operation was never widely adopted.

Of much greater significance was the introduction of the automatic circular stapling instrument. Fain and his colleagues were the first to introduce this instrument to the English-speaking world in 1975 (Fain et al, 1975). They had used the Russian model 249 circular suturing device to construct a colorectal anastomosis in 169 patients with rectal carcinoma operated on between 1967 and 1972 in the Moscow Proctological Institute. Not all of the operations were low anastomoses but nevertheless a proportion

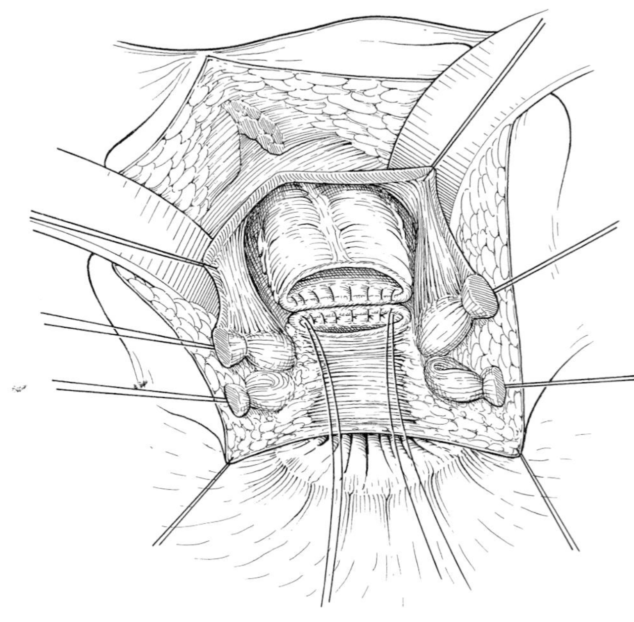

Figure 32.5 Principle of abdominotrans-sphincteric excision. The rectum has been excised and access posteriorly to the anal canal is achieved by division of the sphincters. The colon is then anastomosed to the anal canal and the transected sphincter mechanism is carefully repaired in layers.

were. They reported six cases of anastomotic dehiscence; two of these patients died but four recovered completely. Interestingly, there were no instances of anastomotic stenosis or late stricture formation.

In a similar number of patients, Goligher et al (1979) obtained comparable results using the same instrument. He emphasized that the instrument produced colorectal anastomoses that were as secure as those performed by hand. He was also able to show that these anastomoses could be performed at much lower levels in the pelvis than had previously been possible manually via the abdominal approach. Heald (1980) also demonstrated that these results could be reproduced outside a major centre when he reported on the successful use of the Russian SPTU gun in a group of patients treated in a district general hospital. These findings were extremely important since they showed that it was possible, using this new instrument, for most surgeons to construct a low sphincter-saving anastomosis. With the introduction of the American EEA gun, and since then various disposable instruments, the technique has become even more reliable. The availability of these instruments and the realization that such low anastomoses were compatible with continence and normal bowel function caused surgeons to re-evaluate their criteria for performing sphincter-saving resections, leading to a dramatic change in the treatment of carcinoma of the lower two-thirds of the rectum; we are now able to offer life without a colostomy to far more patients than was previously possible.

SURGICAL OPTIONS FOR THE RADICAL TREATMENT OF RECTAL CANCER

It is now accepted that the operation of choice for carcinoma of the upper third of the rectum (above 12 cm from the anal verge) is anterior resection. Most surgeons achieve the anastomosis by hand suture techniques in one or two layers, but some use the stapling instrument. Numerous studies have shown that anterior resection is as safe and curative as abdominoperineal excision of the rectum for growths at this level (Morgan, 1955; Waugh et al, 1955; Mayo and Fly, 1956; Mayo et al, 1958; Cullen and Mayo, 1963; Lockhart-Mummery et al, 1976; Whittaker and Goligher, 1976; Wilson and Beahrs, 1976). With tumours at this level it is invariably possible to resect the growth with a minimum distal clearance margin of 5 cm and a lateral clearance equivalent to that of an abdominoperineal excision.

Since approximately 1980, it has been the treatment of tumours of the middle third and upper part of the lower third of the rectum that has caused the most controversy. As discussed previously, it is technically possible to treat most of these tumours by a sphincter-saving resection of some type. In order to do this, however, it is sometimes necessary to reduce the margin of distal clearance to less than the customarily accepted 'safe' distance of 5 cm. This, combined with the belief that lateral clearance could not be as extensive as in an abdominoperineal excision, led to the fear that recurrence would be greater and survival reduced compared with the more conventional procedure. There was also concern that no matter how efficient the sphincter-saving technique or how proficient the surgeon, an anastomosis deep in the pelvis was likely to leak and hence morbidity and mortality rates would be high. In addition there was a widely held view that although an abdominoperineal excision resulted in a permanent colostomy the quality of life for the patient was not seriously affected. It was for these reasons that some surgeons performed sphincter-saving operations relatively sparingly for tumours at this level. The only way of being certain that the wider use of sphincter-saving resection was justified would have been to perform a prospective, controlled trial comparing it with abdominoperineal excision. Since such a trial was fraught with ethical constraints it was and will, now, never be performed. As a consequence the policy in many units has been governed by the data available from retrospective studies. When these data are critically examined as below, there is every reason to believe that a policy of sphincter preservation, wherever technically feasible, is justified.

Survival and recurrence: pathological considerations

Differences in survival and recurrence after sphincter-saving resection and abdominoperineal excision are thought to depend on how much tissue invaded by tumour is removed. Rectal carcinoma spreads in three directions: upwards, downwards and laterally (Miles, 1926). There is no disagreement that both abdominoperineal excision and sphincter-saving resection deal adequately with upward spread; it is the ability of sphincter-saving resection to deal with distal and lateral spread that is disputed.

Intramural distal spread

The recommendation that a distal margin of clearance of at least 5 cm should be achieved when resecting a rectal cancer was based on early pathological studies which demonstrated that in a few patients with rectal cancer distal microscopic spread occurred for a distance of 5 cm or more. Table 32.1 summarizes the main pathological studies that addressed this problem.

It appears that distal intramural spread is rare, but when it does occur it usually extends less than 1 cm from the macroscopic lower margin of the tumour. When spread occurs for a greater distance the tumours are very advanced lesions and carry a poor prognosis. In our own study in which we carried out a meticulous search for intramural spread in 50 specimens from abdominoperineal excision procedures (Williams et al, 1983), all of the five patients (10%) with spread greater than 1 cm were dead or dying of metastases a mean of 2 years postoperatively. Of even greater significance was the fact that each of these patients had undergone abdominoperineal excision with a distal margin of clearance of at least 5 cm. Similarly, Pollet and Nicholls (1983) could find no case in the literature even treated by total rectal excision where the patient survived for 5 years when distal spread was greater than 1.5 cm. These patients also died from distant metastases before they developed local recurrence.

Extramural distal (lymphatic) spread

Distal microscopic spread within the bowel wall is not the only theoretical reason for adherence to the '5 cm rule'. If distal extramural lymphatic spread is not dealt with, survival may also be compromised. Review of the literature reveals that the argument pertaining to distal intramural spread also holds for lymphatic spread. Thus Goligher et al (1951) carefully dissected 1500 operative specimens from abdominoperineal excision procedures. Metastatic involvement of glands below the level of the primary tumour was found in 98 (6.5%) of the cases. In 68 specimens the glands concerned lay within 6 mm of the lower margin of the growth and only 30 of the 98 (2% of the total) showed significant retrograde spread to 20 mm or more below the primary growth. Practically all these cases had very extensive lymphatic spread in an upward direction. Dukes (1943) recorded very similar results in the 1500 abdominoperineal excision specimens he studied. In 4.5% the involved nodes were located within 6 mm of the tumour and in only 2% of cases were metastases found 18 mm or more below it. These tumours were once again advanced lesions. Glover and Waugh (1946) recorded similar results even in patients with advanced growths. Thus in only three of their 100 cases (3%) was a distal lymph node involved with tumour. The results of our study (Williams et al, 1983), albeit in a smaller group of patients, agreed with these previous

Table 32.1 Microscopic distal intramural spread.

	No. of cases	*No. with spread*	*Distance of spread* (cm)
Clogg (1904)	25	0	–
Handley (1910)	10	2	NS
Cole (1913)	20	1	NS
Westhues (1934)	74	0	–
Block and Waugh (1948)	103	4	All < 1.2
Quer et al (1953)	91	5	2: 0–1.5 3: > 1.5
Grinnell (1954)	76	9	7: 0–1 2: 1–4
Williams et al (1983)	50	12	5: 0–1 3: 1–2 4: 2–5
Total	449	33 (7.4%)	> 2 in 11 cases* (2.5%)

*Includes three NS cases.
NS, not stated.

Table 32.2 Comparison of distal margin of clearance with local recurrence and 5-year survival rates.

Authors	Length of clearance			
	<4 cm	>4 cm	<5 cm	>5 cm
Recurrence				
Deddish and Stearns (1961)	4/62 (6.5%)	4/39 (10%)		
Manson et al (1976)			9/76 (11.8%)	3/30 (10%)
Wilson and Beahrs (1976)			56/400 (14%)	20/156 (13%)
Pollett and Nicholls (1983)			15/32 (6.5%)	8/102 (7.8%)
Williams et al (1983)			7/48 (15%)	3/31 (10%)
Crude 5-year survival rates				
Copeland et al (1968)			46/141 (32.6%)	86/206 (41.8%)
Pollett and Nicholls (1983)			159/232 (68.5%)	71/102 (69.6%)
Williams et al (1983)			33/48 (69%)	18/31 (58%)

meticulous studies. In only 3 of 50 cases (6%) was a distal lymph node involved and each of these patients had advanced tumours with the involved node being less than 2 cm from the distal margin of the tumour.

The pathological data thus suggested that transgression of the 5 cm rule in the course of sphincter-saving resections would not result in excessive recurrence rates. Clinical data supported this conclusion. Table 32.2 summarizes those studies of anterior resections that have compared the incidence of recurrence with the distal margin of clearance. No significant difference could be demonstrated between cases in which a distal clearance of more than 5 cm had been obtained and cases in which the margin was less than this. Thus it appeared that if in the course of a sphincter-saving resection a margin of clearance of 5 cm would make the re-establishment of gastrointestinal continuity impossible, the margin could safely be reduced to a minimum of 2 cm.

Lateral spread

Lateral spread, defined as the spread of a tumour to the lateral pelvic wall including the iliac lymph nodes, was considered by Miles (1926) to be of great importance. Sauer and Bacon (1952) confirmed this was the case for extraperitoneal tumours. They showed that the internal iliac lymph nodes were involved in 6 of 21 patients with tumours below the peritoneal reflection, whereas 11 patients with intraperitoneal lesions had no lateral spread. These findings contrasted with those of Westhues (1930), Gabriel et al (1935) and Wood and Wilkie (1933), who found in their exhaustive pathological studies of abdominoperineal excision specimens that very few lateral lymph nodes were involved by tumour. In specimens in which these nodes were involved the carcinomas were considerably advanced. In addition these lateral nodes were either at the same level as the carcinoma or above it. Thus, although lateral spread to lymph nodes undoubtedly occurs (Gilchrist and David, 1940, 1947; Sauer and Bacon, 1952) they are rarely removed in the course of a routine abdominoperineal excision of the rectum.

Lateral spread to lymph nodes, however, is not the only means of spread: direct invasion is important. In a study performed by our group (Quirke et al, 1986) we searched for lateral direct spread in 52 low rectal cancers by taking multiple serial lateral sections. This meticulous search was carried out in operative specimens removed by both abdominoperineal and sphincter-saving procedures. Direct lateral spread was found in 14 cases (27%), and was equally distributed between the two procedures. Thus lateral spread does occur by both the direct and lymphatic routes, but modern sphincter-saving techniques seem just as capable of removing this form of spread as is abdominoperineal excision, particularly if a total mesorectal excision (TME) is performed (Heald and Karanjia, 1992). It follows that recurrence resulting from failure to remove lateral extension of the disease is just as likely to occur after abdominoperineal excision of the rectum as after sphincter-saving resection. Some may argue (Sauer and Bacon, 1952) that lateral spread can only be adequately dealt with by extending the scope of the dissection to include the internal iliac lymph nodes. If this was shown to be beneficial, as suggested by some authors (Stearns, 1978; Enker et al, 1979), it would be possible to extend the pelvic dissection of a sphincter-saving resection to include these nodes. However, excision of internal iliac nodes is associated with a high incidence of complications such as impotence.

Survival and recurrence: clinical studies

There are many inherent difficulties associated with studies that attempt to compare the clinical outcomes of sphincter-saving resection and abdominoperineal excision of the rectum. As emphasized, reliance has to be made on retrospective data. It is impossible in studies of this nature to obtain groups with identical characteristics. Inevitably surgeons have been selective in the procedure they perform. The decision has usually involved various factors. The patient's build and sex and the surgeon's previous experience are clearly important. The extent of local spread and the histological differentiation of the tumour have also, in the past, been major factors in decision-making. A tumour that exhibits extensive local spread on clinical assessment is more likely to have been treated by abdominoperineal excision of the rectum. Similarly, since the risk of local recurrence is greater the lower the tumour is situated in the rectum (Stearns and Binkley, 1953; Gilbertsen, 1962), comparisons between operations that do not take into account the height of the tumour from the anal verge will be biased against abdominoperineal excision.

Clearly, then, not all the factors discussed above can be taken into account when comparing the results of the two types of operation. Nevertheless there are some studies available that contain the necessary data for reasonable comparison to be made.

Survival

Table 32.3 lists series in which the two operations have been compared for tumours of similar pathological characteristics below 15 cm from the anal verge. The sphincter-saving technique in the earlier studies was invariably anterior resection with a manual anastomosis constructed in either one or two layers. There was no significant difference in overall survival rates between the two operations. Each of these studies categorized the cases according to Dukes' stage, and when they were compared in this way, still no significant difference emerged. Two studies (Nicholls et al, 1979; Williams and Johnston, 1984) also looked at more than one pathological variable and still no significant difference was discernible.

Most of the series listed in Table 32.3 dealt primarily with tumours situated in the middle third of the rectum and were reported during the era when the more modern techniques of sphincter preservation were not yet available.

The limited amount of data now available on these more modern operations tend to confirm the previous findings. Thus the 3-year crude survival rate for 30 patients who had undergone abdominotransanal resection by Parks at St Mark's Hospital was 70% (Parks and Percy, 1982). A substantial proportion of these patients had tumours situated 4–8 cm from the anal verge. This survival rate compares very favourably with the 3-year survival of 67.9% achieved in 2083 patients who had undergone abdominoperineal excision for rectal cancer at the same institution (Lockhart-Mummery et al, 1976).

Localio (1978) reported on his 10 years' experience with abdominosacral resection and although this operation is practised infrequently elsewhere the principles with regard to cancer clearance are the same as in other techniques; his findings thus have important implications. He compared his

Table 32.3 Five-year survival rates for abdominoperineal excision of the rectum (APER) and sphincter-saving resection (SSR) when used to treat mid-rectal tumours.

Authors	*Distance of tumour from anal verge* (cm)	APER % (*n*)	SSR % (*n*)
Mayo et al (1958)	6–9	69 (108)	72 (46)
Deddish and Stearns (1961)	6–10	62 (106)	65 (33)
Williams et al (1966)	6–15	57	46
Slanetz et al (1972)	8–13	47 (106)	56 (61)
Patel et al (1977)	<10	56 (279)	64 (105)
Strauss et al (1978)	7–15	44 (34)	55 (49)
†Nicholls et al (1979)	8–12	57 (106)	73 (81)
Jones and Thomson (1982)	<15	52 (73)	67 (125)
†McDermott et al (1982)	6–11	71 (141)	68 (170)
†Williams and Johnston (1984)	7.5–12	62 (78)	74 (66)
Dixon et al (1991)	Low	52 (215)	64 (224)
Konn et al (1993)	Low	68 (100)	80 (203)
Alleman et al (1994)	5–10	54 (37)	53 (40)

**n*, number of patients who survived operation.
†Indicates cancer-specific survival rates; the remainder are crude 5-year survival rates.

results with those achieved after abdominoperineal excision and anterior resection. The comparative 5-year survival figures for curative resections were 67.3% after anterior resection, 58.3% after abdominosacral resection and 50% after abdominoperineal excision. These groups were not strictly comparable since patients who had undergone abdominoperineal excision had tumours that were situated at a significantly lower level in the rectum than those who had undergone abdominosacral resection. However, 30 cases had undergone resection for tumours 5–8.5 cm from the anal verge; 5-year survival rates were 61% for abdominosacral resection and 58.3% for abdominoperineal excision. When patients were compared with respect to whether the lymph nodes were involved or not, although the numbers were small, no significant difference between the two operations was demonstrated.

In a study by our group (Williams et al, 1985), we compared survival in our patients with tumours of the lower two-thirds of the rectum (3–12 cm from the anal verge) treated by modern sphincter-saving techniques during the period 1978–82 with a similar group of retrospective control patients treated by abdominoperineal excision prior to 1977. All patients had undergone a radical operation. During the more recent period our policy (like that of many other units) had changed in so far as most patients with tumours above the anal sphincter were considered for sphincter-saving resection provided a minimum distal clearance of 2 cm could be obtained. Selection was not made on the grounds of the degree of histological differentiation of the tumour, and although extensive local invasion was a relative contraindication it did not preclude a sphincter-saving resection. The build and sex of the patient occasionally influenced the decision but were not as important a consideration as previously. An attempt was made to match the abdominoperineal excision patients with the sphincter-saving group as accurately as possible with regard to age, sex, pathological characteristics of the tumour and degree of spread. In the sphincter-saving resection group, 66 patients had undergone an anterior resection, of whom 35 (47%) had a stapled anastomosis and 32 (43%) had a manual anastomosis. Transanal coloanal anastomosis had been performed in seven patients (9%) and an abdominotrans-sacral procedure conducted in one patient (1%). There were 74 subjects who had undergone a synchronous combined abdominoperineal excision of the rectum ('controls'). As can be seen from Figure 32.6 using corrected 5-year survival curves, there was no significant difference between the two groups. The overall 5-year survival rate was 68% after abdominoperineal excision and 74% after sphincter-saving resection.

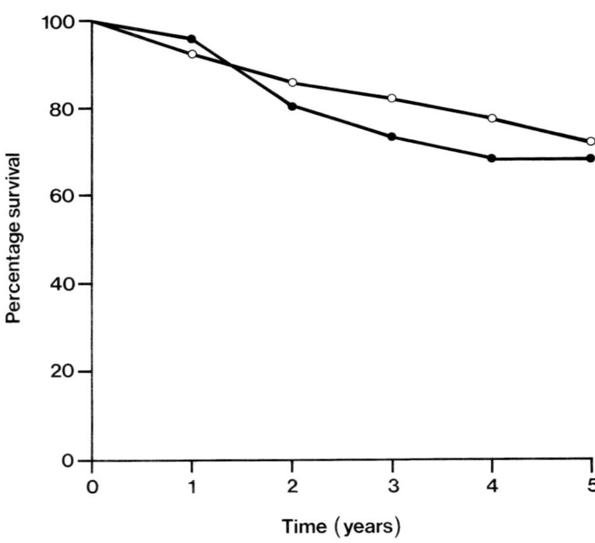

Figure 32.6 Comparison of cumulative 5-year survival rates between patients who had undergone sphincter saving resection and those who had undergone abdominoperineal excision (Williams et al, 1985). ○—○, SSR; ●—●, APER.

Similar conclusions have been reached by Wolmark and Fisher (1986), who analysed the results of the National Surgical Adjuvant Breast and Bowel Project prospective adjuvant therapy trial for rectal cancer. In this study 232 patients underwent abdominoperineal excision and 181 underwent sphincter-saving resection. The proportion of patients with low rectal cancers was not discussed but approximately 50% of the sphincter-saving resection group had a stapled anastomosis. There was no significant difference in survival rates between the two operative groups.

Recurrence

Studies that attempt to examine recurrence rates are fraught with difficulties. Patients may have silent metastases which cannot be detected by clinical or conventional radiological methods. Even after death it may not be possible to determine the extent and pattern of spread unless a meticulous post-mortem is carried out in each patient, and clearly this is impractical. Computed tomography (CT) enhances the detection of recurrence in both the liver and pelvis (Adalsteinsson et al, 1981; James et al, 1983) but it is unlikely that data from future studies will be more accurate even if serial scans are performed. At present such studies comparing the two procedures with sequential CT or MRI scanning have not been reported.

With these reservations in mind, examination of the available comparative data reveals in the main no significant difference in local recurrence rates between the two operations. Table 32.4 summarizes the results from authors who compared the results in patients with tumours of the middle third of the rectum (7.0–13 cm from the anal verge).

Nevertheless, there are two studies which demonstrate a higher rate of local recurrence after SSR than after APER. Thus, Phillips et al (1984a,b) found an 18% local recurrence rate after SSR compared with 12% after APER ($P < 0.05$). However, more alarming, Neville et al (1987) found a 32% incidence after SSR compared with a 13% rate after APER. These two studies bear closer inspection. Both reviewed the experience of a large number of surgeons in different types of hospitals. Many of these were general surgeons who did not specialize in colorectal surgery. It is also not clear whether irrigation of the rectal stump to prevent the implantation of free tumour cells was routinely employed. Nor is it clear whether there was any difference in the extent of local spread of tumours between the two groups. However, of particular concern is the high incidence of local recurrence in the SSR group, particularly in Neville et al's paper (32%). This rate is far higher than that recorded for SSRs in the other series in Table 32.4. Similarly, if one examines the recent data on recurrence rates after low SSR for tumours below 7.5 cm from the anal verge in non-comparative series (Table 32.5), Neville's data are at the upper end of the scale. Indeed, their nearest

Table 32.4 Incidence of local recurrence after abdominoperineal excision of the rectum (APER) and sphincter saving resection (SSR) for mid-rectal cancers.

	Patients (n)		*Local recurrence*	
Authors	*APER*	*SSR*	*APER*	*SSR*
Morson et al (1963)	1596	177	155 (9.7)	13 (7.3)
Slanetz et al (1972)				
Dukes' B	–	–	(25)	(23)
Dukes' C	–	–	(38)	(33)
Patel et al (1977)	326	142	52 (16.0)	23 (16.2)
Williams and Johnston (1984)	83	71	7 (8)	8 (11)
Phillips et al (1984a,b)	478	370	57 (12)	67 (18.1)
Neville et al (1987)			(13)	(32)
Fick et al (1990)	27	31	4 (15)	4 (13)
Amato et al (1991)	69	78	7 (10)	9 (12)
Dixon et al (1991)	61	150	3 (5)	6 (4.0)
Konn et al (1993)	100	203	(83.5)	(9)

Values in parentheses are percentages.

Table 32.5 Incidence of local recurrence after sphincter saving resection for carcinomas of the low rectum since 1980.

Author	*Operative method**	*Period of follow-up (yrs)*	*Number of cases treated*	*Number with recurrence*
Keighley and Matheson (1980)	Abd-transanal	1–3	7	3 (43)
Hurst et al (1982)	Ant resection with stapler	½–2	34	11 (32)
Parks and Percy (1982)	Abd-transanal	1–5	73	6 (8)
Andersberg et al (1983a,b)	Ant resection with stapler	?	39	9 (24)
Luke et al (1983)	Ant resection with stapler	2½–5	44	10 (22.7)
Goligher (1984)	Abd-transanal	2–5	18	2 (11)
Lasson et al (1984)	Ant resection with stapler	½–3	40	8 (20)
Reid et al (1984)	Ant resection with stapler	2–6	29	8 (28)
Oates (1985)	Ant resection with stapler	½–4	60	4 (7)
Heald and Ryall (1986)	Ant resection with stapler	½–6½	115	3 (2.6)
Braun et al (1992)	Most anterior resection with stapler	1–14	401	(11)
Liguori et al (1992)	Anterior resection with stapler	–	147	(16)†
Leo et al (1994)	Coloanal anastomosis with pouch	1–3	47	6 (15)
Paty et al (1994a,b)	Coloanal anastomosis with stapler	Median 4 years	144	13 (11)
Cavaliere et al (1995)	Coloanal anastomosis with stapler	4–14	117	8 (7)

Values in parentheses are percentages.
* Abd, abdomino; Ant, anterior. † Refers only to tumours 4–8 cm.

'rival' is the study from Hurst et al (1982), who recorded a local recurrence of 33% in a small number of patients operated on early in their experience with the stapling gun.

This wide discrepancy in recurrence rates in our view suggests that the differences are surgeon related and are not related to the type of procedure employed, and eloquently makes the point for specialization. Differences in case mix are unlikely to be the explanation. One aspect of technique which might account for the surgeon variability, and which has recently been highlighted, is the avoidance of 'coning' where the plane of dissection during SSR may be closer to the rectum than in APER (Andersberg et al, 1983b; Reid et al, 1984). Coning leaves behind elements of the mesorectum which may contain micrometastases which if left will lead to local recurrence. Such a risk can be considerably reduced if the dissection is carried out in the so-called 'holy plane' described by Heald (1988) which allows the whole of the mesorectum to be excised *en bloc* with the rectum.

Very few of the recent studies examining local recurrence after low SSR have compared their recurrence rates with a similar group of patients treated by abdominoperineal excision. Our previously mentioned study (Williams et al, 1985) attempted to do this as patients were operated on by similar techniques and were matched carefully. There was no significant difference demonstrated between the two operations as far as local recurrence was concerned. After 2 years, ten patients (14%) who had undergone low sphincter-saving resection developed a local recurrence compared with 14 patients (19%) who had undergone abdominoperineal excision. For tumours below 9 cm from the anal verge the numbers of patients with local recurrence were 4 of 36 (11%) after low sphincter-saving resection and 8 of 40 (20%) following abdominoperineal excision. Cumulative local recurrence rates for up to 5 years were similar in both groups (Figure 32.7). The incidence of proven distant recurrence 2 years postoperatively was also similar: 15% after sphincter-saving techniques compared with 20% after abdominoperineal excision. While it is appreciated that follow-up was still less than 5 years in some of the sphincter-saving resection patients (27%), we considered that these data were still valid for the following reasons. Firstly, 80–90% of recurrences after rectal excision occur in the first 24 months after operation (Goligher et al, 1951; Morson et al, 1963); and secondly, use of cumulative rates of recurrence helps to correct for those subjects not followed up for the full 5-year period.

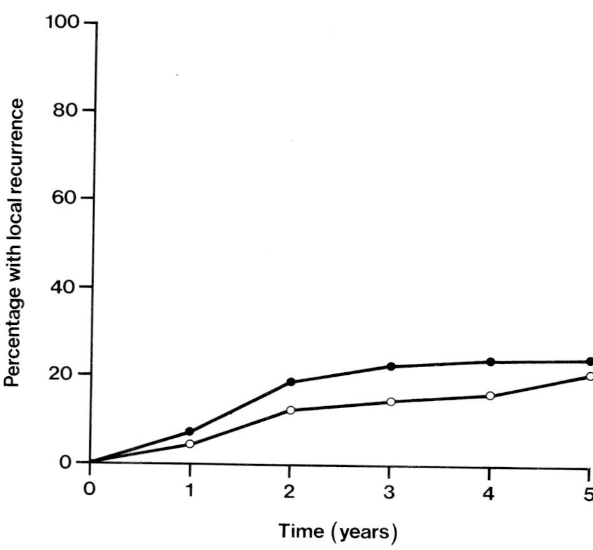

Figure 32.7 Comparison of cumulative local recurrence rates between patients who had undergone sphincter-saving resection and those who had undergone abdominoperineal excision (Williams et al, 1985). ○—○, SSR; ●—●, APER.

Mortality and morbidity

Numerous studies have analysed the operative mortality rates of either abdominoperineal excision or sphincter-saving resection with respect to low rectal cancers, but few have directly compared the two procedures. Thus, between 1947 and 1954 Deddish and Stearns (1961) performed an anterior resection with manual anastomosis on 65 patients with tumours 6–10 cm from the anal verge. The operative mortality was 9% (six patients). For tumours 11–13 cm from the anal verge the mortality rate was 4% (3 of 80). The comparable figures for abdominoperineal excision were not quoted, although their overall operative mortality rate for the latter procedure was less than 2%. Similarly, Goligher (1977) had a 7.3% mortality rate in a personal series of 535 cases treated by anterior resection. Although stating that slightly less than two-fifths of his patients underwent low resections he did not indicate the mortality rate in this group. The mortality rate in his 876 cases treated by abdominoperineal excision was 6.7% (Goligher, 1977). The results from St Mark's Hospital reported by Lockhart-Mummery et al (1976) also indicated that the two types of operation could be performed with a similar degree of safety: between 1958 and 1972, the operative mortality was 1.9% for abdominoperineal excision of the rectum and 2.9%

for sphincter-saving resection. In this study, however, comparisons were not made between patients with tumours at similar heights from the anal verge. More comparable data were recorded in the four papers discussed below.

Williams et al (1966) reviewed 182 patients with carcinomas between 6 cm and 15 cm from the anal verge. Between 1950 and 1961 a total of 89 patients underwent anterior resection with a hand-sewn anastomosis and 93 had an abdominoperineal excision. The median tumour size for each group was 5 cm and the Dukes' classifications were virtually identical. The operative mortality, although not statistically significant, was lower after anterior resection. In addition 53% of patients after abdominoperineal excision had one or more complications and 40% had problems after sphincter-saving resection. The higher incidence of complications after abdominoperineal excision was due to a greater frequency of urinary tract problems.

In a similar but much larger study, Slanetz et al (1972) analysed the results of 524 procedures: 277 consecutive abdominoperineal excisions and 247 anterior resections performed between 1944 and 1963. All tumours were situated between 8 cm and 18 cm from the anal verge. Both operations were found to have a mortality of 5.4% over the 24-year period. It was interesting to note that there had been a gradual increase in mortality from abdominoperineal excision of the rectum during this interval (3.5% from 1944 to 1950, and 6.8% from 1956 to 1963) while the mortality from anterior resection declined significantly during the same period (from 7.9% to 2.4%). With respect to morbidity only 32% of patients after abdominoperineal excision had no postoperative complications, compared with 44% following anterior resection.

Similar results were recorded by Jones and Thomson (1982), who reviewed the results of 271 patients who had undergone radical rectal excision for carcinoma below 15 cm from the anal verge. The overall mortality rate in the sphincter-saving resection group was 3 of 177 patients (1.7%) and in the abdominoperineal excision group was 4 of 92 (4.4%). There was no significant difference between the two groups with regard to Dukes' stage. Anterior resection with manual anastomosis had been the principal method of sphincter-saving resection, although ten patients had undergone coloanal anastomosis. One hundred patients had undergone sphincter-saving resection for carcinomas between 2 cm and 7 cm from the anal verge, but there were no separate details for this group.

Our results (Williams and Johnston, 1984) in a much smaller group of patients with tumours between 7.5 cm and 12 cm from the anal verge also showed no difference in mortality between the two operations.

Table 32.6 Mortality and anastomotic leak rate after stapled low colorectal anastomosis.

Authors	*Total no. of patients*	*Height of tumour or anastomosis from anal verge (cm)*	*Mortality*	*Leak*	
				Clinical	*Subclinical*
Fain et al (1975)	165	7–16	4 (2.4)	6 (3.6)	NS
Goligher et al (1979)	24	low	1 (4)	0	6 (25)
Ling et al (1979)	18	Below 5	0	3 (17)	6 (33)
Adolff et al (1980)	26	Mean 12	1 (3.8)	2 (7.7)	NS
Bolton and Britton (1980)	22	Mean 14	0	1 (4.5)	NS
Kirkegaard et al (1980)	30	7–12	1 (3.3)	2 (6.7)	3 (10)
Beart and Kelly (1981)	35*	Mean 13	1 (2.9)	1 (2.9)	NS
	10	Below 6	0	1 (10)	NS
Cade et al (1981)	32	Below 8	NS	3 (9.4)	NS
Heald and Leicester (1981)	73*	2.5–12	NS	13 (17.8)	4 (5.4)
Kirwan (1981)		Mean 8	1 (3.3)	NS	6 (20)
Shahinian et al (1981)	29*	Low	0	1 (3.4)	NS
Blamey and Lee (1982)		8–14	NS	3 (6)	5 (10)
Brennan et al (1982)	10	Low	0	1 (10)	4 (40)
Lazorthes and Chiotasso (1986)	57	Below 8	NS	3 (5.3)	3 (5.3)
Braun et al (1992)	389	Low	(4.6)	16 (4.3)	NS
Laxamana et al (1995)	189	Mid and low	3 (1.6)	14 (7.3)	NS

*Includes some patients with diverticular disease.
NS, not stated.
Figures in parentheses are percentages.

Table 32.7 Operative mortality after SSR and APER for low rectal cancer.

	Patients (n)		*Mortality*	
Author	*APER*	*SSR*	*APER*	*SSR*
Liguori et al (1992)	71	147	7 (9.9)	5 (3.4)
Konn et al (1993)	100	203	1 (1)	3 (1.5)

Figures in parentheses are percentages.

In the studies described above, the anastomoses had usually been constructed by hand. Although several authors have since reported mortality and morbidity rates after stapling, few have compared these rates with complication rates after abdominoperineal excision. Table 32.6 lists the mortality rates of recent series which utilized the stapling instrument for low sphincter-saving resections. The overall mortality was approximately 2.5%, which compares very favourably with that reported for abdominoperineal excision when used by other authors for tumours at similar sites in the rectum. Table 32.7 compares operative mortality between APER and low SSR in the few recent studies where these data are available. SSR seems be just as safe as APER in these studies.

The most serious complication that can befall a patient after a low sphincter-saving resection is breakdown of the anastomosis. The incidence of clinical leak after stapled anastomosis is between 3% and 18%, but clearly it has not dramatically increased the mortality rate (Table 32.6). Morbidity following this complication is difficult to quantify but is unlikely to differ significantly from the incidence of pelvic and perineal sepsis which occurs after abdominoperineal excision. Although stricture and late disruption of stapled anastomoses have also been recorded, the incidence is low in most series.

Quality of life

Many studies have documented the considerable psychological trauma and social problems experienced by patients after abdominoperineal excision (Bukh, 1954; Grier et al, 1964; Druss et al, 1969; Prudden, 1971; Pryse-Phillips, 1971; Balslev, 1973; Morrow, 1976; Williams and Johnston, 1983), many of which are caused by the presence of a colostomy. A low sphincter-saving resection eliminates the need for a permanent stoma, but such a procedure would be of little benefit to the patient if it caused incontinence; replacing an abdominal colostomy with an anal one would be of little use. In the past fear was expressed that if the anorectal stump was less then 6–8 cm in length incontinence was bound to occur. We now know that with modern techniques the whole rectum can be removed and the colon anastomosed to the anal canal with preservation of continence. Furthermore, anorectal function is usually acceptable. Table 32.8 lists several series which have documented detailed information about anorectal function after very low sphincter-saving resections.

Virtually all patients achieve continence for solid faeces although some have deficiencies in the control of flatus and liquid faeces. There is also a period of adaptation lasting 6–18 months during which normal function is regained. Many patients initially suffer from frequency of bowel action, but this usually improves with time (Williams et al, 1985). Nevertheless, there are patients who continue to suffer from urgency, frequency of bowel action and occasional incontinence, the so-called *anterior resection syndrome* (Paty et al, 1994a,b). This is more prevalent the closer the anastomosis is to the anal canal (McDonald and Heald, 1983; Carmona and Ortiz, 1991; Batignani et al, 1991). The incidence of this problem after 2 years of follow-up is difficult to determine, but in our experience it is small and most patients prefer gastrointestinal continuity, despite the symptoms, to a life with a permanent colostomy. In addition, the formation of a colonic pouch may ameliorate many of these symptoms (see later).

The difficulties that patients experience after abdominoperineal excision of the rectum were only fully appreciated following publication of a comprehensive study by Devlin et al (1971). In the 83 patients who had undergone abdominoperineal excision, these authors found that a very high proportion had significant problems with regard to employment, housing, diet, social isolation and psychosexual behaviour. The authors compared these patients with those who had had restorative operations and concluded that the latter had far fewer problems. Since this study was performed over 30 years ago it is likely that the anterior resections were performed for tumours situated at a higher level than those in the abdominoperineal excision patients. In an attempt to rectify this defect we conducted a study (Williams and Johnston, 1983) comparing a group of patients after abdominoperineal excision with a similar group after low sphincter-saving resection. Both groups had tumours at between 5 cm and 12 cm from the anal verge. The findings of Devlin et al (1971) were confirmed in every way (Table 32.9).

Table 32.8 Continence after low sphincter saving resection.

	Total no. of patients	Height of tumour or anastomosis from anal verge (cm)	Continence		
			Complete	Partial	Absent
Stapled anastomosis					
Cade et al (1981)	50	8–13* (32 below 8)	48 (96)	—	2
Heald (1980)	40	3–8*	39 (98)	1	—
Goligher et al (1979)	24	Below 7*	5	3	2
		7.7–10*	14 (79)	—	—
Kirkegaard et al (1981)	29	7–12*	29 (100)	0	0
Horgan et al (1989)	15	5–12*	12 (80)	2	1
Ekkehard et al (1995)	55	3–10*	12 (22)	23	20
Combination of stapled and hand-sewn anastomosis					
Williams and Johnston (1983)	40	5-12	30 (75)	10†	—
Enker et al (1985)	41	6.7 (mean)	18 (64)	?	?
Paty et al (1994a,b)	81	—	41 (51)	36‡	4
Transanal coloanal anastomosis					
Parks and Percy (1982)	70	Most below 12	69 (99)	—	1
Sweeney et al (1989)	60	Low	43	9	8
Keighley and Matheson (1980)	6	—	4 (66.7)	1	1
Castrini et al (1985)	17	—	17 (100)	0	0
Drake et al (1987)	25	—	21 (84)	4	0
Hautefeuille et al (1988)	31	—	30 (97)	—	—
Bernard et al (1989)	30	—	26 (87)	2	2
Abdominotrans-sacral anastomosis					
Localio et al (1978)	100	5.5–11	100 (100)	—	—

* Height of anastomosis. † Includes 4 incontinent for flatus alone.
Figures in parentheses are percentages.
‡ 17 incontinent for gas only.

Table 32.9 Quality of life of patients with low rectal cancer treated by abdominoperineal excision of the rectum (APER) or sphincter saving resection (SSR).

	APER (*n* = 38)		SSR (*n* = 40)	
	n	%	*n*	%
Bowel function				
>3 actions/24 hours	21	55	14	35
Excess flatus	19*	50	6	15
Odour	24*	63	8	20
Dietary restriction				
Items restricted:				
0–2	16*	42	30	75
3–5	16	42	6	15
>6	6	16	4	10
Psychological assessment				
Depression scores	4.6 ± 3.6*		2.8 ± 2.9	
Anxiety scores	4.0 ± 3.2		3.8 ± 3.9	
Change in body image	25* (66%)		2 (5%)	

* $P = 0.05$.
From Williams and Johnston (1983).

Conclusions

There are now various operative techniques available for the treatment of carcinoma of the middle third of the rectum and the upper half of the lower third of the rectum which allow gastrointestinal continuity to be restored and continence to be preserved. These operations can be performed relatively safely with mortality and morbidity rates comparable with those after abdominoperineal excision. The lifestyle of patients who have undergone these procedures seems far superior to that of patients after abdominoperineal excision. The most important and contentious issue that has not been entirely resolved is the relative recurrence and survival rates. However, all the comparative data that relate to middle-third carcinomas show no significant difference between sphincter-saving and abdominoperineal excision procedures. Furthermore, the rapidly expanding data available covering growths at a lower level point to similar conclusions.

While it is true that local recurrence rates after sphincter-saving resection for low rectal cancers vary enormously from series to series, it must be remembered that such studies have rarely compared the results of sphincter-saving resection with those obtained after abdominoperineal resection. Wide variation in results is not an unusual phenomenon when new techniques are introduced. Indeed, in the surgery of colorectal carcinoma such variation is commonplace even after well-established procedures (Phillips et al, 1984a,b; McArdle and Hole, 1991); the fault seems to lie with the surgeon rather than with the operation.

In our present state of knowledge it seems reasonable to pursue the following policy for carcinoma of the lower two-thirds of the rectum. All patients should be considered for a sphincter-saving resection of some form provided that the tumour does not involve the anal sphincter and provided that clinical examination or imaging does not indicate a fixed lesion. A trial dissection should be performed with complete mobilization of the rectum together with its tumour and the mesorectum, care if possible being taken to avoid damage to the autonomic nerves. The upward and lateral dissection should be as wide as possible. If after mobilization of the tumour, the rectum can be resected with a margin of distal clearance of 5 cm and restoration of continuity can be achieved, all well and good. If, however, such a procedure is not feasible the distal margin of transection of the rectal wall can be reduced to a minimum of 2 cm. In these circumstances, all the mesorectum distal to division of the 'gut tube' can still be removed, although this does increase the potential risk of ischaemia and a future anastomotic leak (see later). In such circumstances, therefore, a covering stoma is mandatory.

Continuity should then be achieved either by manual anastomosis from above or by a mechanical stapling instrument. The exact technique will depend on the height of the anastomosis and the preference of the surgeon. These days most surgeons favour the stapling instrument regardless of the height of the anastomosis to be constructed. Failing this, consideration should be given to one of the more specialized techniques: we favour abdominotransanal coloanastomosis. If the latter is not possible an abdominoperineal excision should be performed.

Occasionally it is obvious from the outset that a sphincter-saving resection is contraindicated. Few would argue that the patient with a bulky tumour which exhibits extensive local spread and which is situated deep in the pelvis should undergo abdominoperineal resection, preferably preceded by a course of radiotherapy. However, few patients have tumours in this category. We wish to emphasize that a patient should not be denied the chance of a sphincter-saving resection on clinical examination alone; only after laparotomy and full mobilization of the rectum can a decision be made. A tumour which at first appears to be too low in the pelvis may rise several centimetres after mobilization, making a sphincter-saving resection technically feasible. Another group of patients in whom a low sphincter-saving resection would be contraindicated are those with a weak anal sphincter. For this reason we usually perform anorectal manometry routinely on patients who are being considered for a sphincter-saving procedure. Some argue that since digital examination may be as sensitive as manometry (Hallan et al, 1989) in assessing external anal sphincter function, clinical examination may be sufficient for selection purposes. However, clinical examination is subjective, there is considerable observer variation, assessment of sphincter function requires years of experience, and correlation with manometry is not perfect.

Influence of extensive local or distant disease on sphincter preservation

The presence of a solitary hepatic metastasis is an indication to consider liver resection as part of a radical operation aimed at achieving cure. This subject is discussed at length in Chapter 31. However, most patients with hepatic involvement do not fall into this category. Cure cannot be contemplated in a patient with multiple metastases but palliation is a necessity and must be striven for.

The principle of excision of the tumour whenever possible (particularly if this does not involve a permanent stoma) is a good one and will ideally be achieved by anterior resection with colorectal anastomosis. The limit to which the surgeon goes to achieve gastrointestinal continuity in these patients will depend on many factors. The stimulus to avoid a colostomy is naturally very great in a patient whose prognosis is poor because of either disseminated disease or coexisting medical disease. There are two factors, however, that the surgeon needs to consider carefully when advising the restoration of intestinal continuity in a patient with a low rectal tumour which has metastasized.

- Firstly, an anterior resection with either a one-layer manual or stapled anastomosis or more frequently with an abdominotransanal procedure may require a covering stoma. The patient may never be fit enough to have the stoma closed and thus might have undergone the procedure unnecessarily.
- Secondly, no matter how carefully a low sphincter-saving resection is performed, bowel function is often impaired initially, with the patient having frequent loose bowel actions and occasional episodes of incontinence. Although function invariably improves with time it may take 6–18 months for it to do so. The patient with liver metastases may not survive long enough to enjoy the benefits of sphincter preservation or stoma closure, and therefore it is quite wrong to advise a two-stage operation or one where function is poor in the last remaining weeks of life.

The extent to which the surgeon should strive to achieve continuity must be an individual decision based on personal experience and patient preference. If the tumour could be removed and yet achieving gastrointestinal continuity is thought to be difficult and hazardous, the patient would be best served by a Hartmann's procedure. Although palliative abdominoperineal excision has been recommended (Goligher, 1984) we can see little use for it as a palliative procedure except where the tumour is so low and so extensive that adequate local control cannot be achieved by a Hartmann's procedure. Certainly it is most undesirable to leave behind tumour in the pelvis which can lead to distressing symptoms before the patient succumbs. In practice, however, there are few tumours in the rectum that cannot be removed adequately by a Hartmann's operation. An abdominoperineal excision leaves behind a perineal wound which can be very uncomfortable especially if wound breakdown takes place. It is the surgeon's duty to these patients to reduce their discomfort to a minimum and whenever possible to allow them to live the remainder of their lives with dignity.

DETAILS OF OPERATIVE TECHNIQUES

Sphincter-saving resections

Anterior resection

The patient is placed in the modified lithotomy–Trendelenburg position known as the Lloyd Davies position. A small sandbag should be placed under the sacrum to elevate it from the table. The end portion of the table should be removed and the patient's legs placed in stirrups, the latter being placed level with the end of the table. This allows the legs to be raised but the hip joint can then be abducted and flexed to a minimum degree. A large neurosurgical type of overtable is placed above the head of the operating area. Once this position has been achieved a urethral catheter is passed and the table is placed in a head-down tilt of at least 15 degrees. Shoulder restraints must be placed to prevent the patient from slipping off the table. An intravenous cannula for infusion of fluid is placed in one arm, but this is not outstretched on an arm board for fear of injury to the brachial plexus. Both arms are placed by the patient's sides and held in place by special arm rests. (The anaesthetist also usually places a central venous catheter *in situ*.) All pressure points are carefully padded. The catheter and the tube leading from it are taped to the patient in such a way as to remove it from the operative field. The genitalia are also taped in such a manner as to prevent them intruding into the perineal field. The urinary collecting bag must be sited so that the anaesthetist can see it throughout the operation and so measure urinary output with ease.

A urethral urinary catheter is used in most centres, but in order to reduce the risk of urinary tract infection some surgeons advocate the use of the subrapubic route for placement of the catheter (Rasmussen et al, 1977). The latter can be inserted using the 'Supracath' technique when the patient is anaesthetized but prior to the abdominal incision being made. Some surgeons, although recommending the suprapubic route for catheter insertion, favour the insertion of a larger catheter which can only be placed under direct vision after the abdomen has been opened (Christensen and Kronberg, 1981).

The abdomen and perineum are cleansed in the normal manner. Towelling is then commenced, and the legs are covered by special leggings. After the legs and the abdomen have been draped the perineum is covered to allow the assistant to assume a position between the legs of the patient and thus assist in retraction when dissection is taking place deep in the pelvis.

The lithotomy–Trendelenburg position is recommended for this operation since it has the advantage that if an anastomosis cannot be performed by the abdominal route, the surgeon has access to the anal region without having to reposition the patient. A transanal anastomosis or (if that is contraindicated) an abdominoperineal excision can thus be performed.

Incision

Either a long midline incision or a paramedian incision is employed. The incision should extend from the pubis to at least 5 cm above the umbilicus (Figure 32.8). We prefer a midline incision, but if a paramedian incision is to be used consideration should be given to whether this should be to the right or the left of the midline. When it is certain preoperatively that a restorative resection can be performed, a left paramedian incision is preferable. However, when there is uncertainty as to the possible need for an abdominoperineal excision a right paramedian incision is recommended. These approaches will assist the siting of the colostomy which is destined to be in the left iliac fossa. The further the main wound lies from the colostomy, the less is the risk of wound infection.

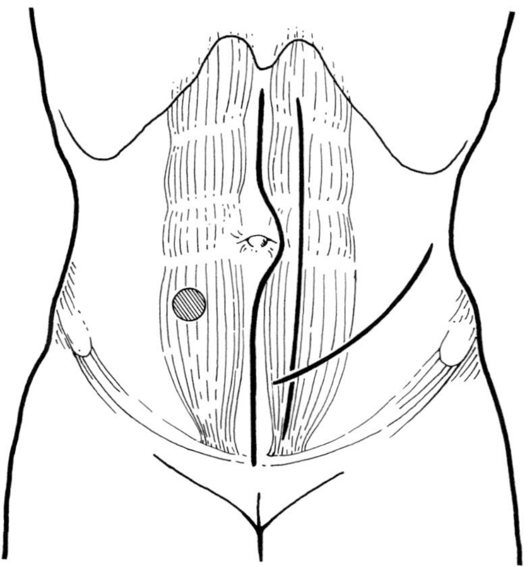

Figure 32.8 Midline and left paramedian incisions normally used for sphincter-saving resections. Occasionally a left oblique incision is used. The figure also shows the site for a defunctioning ileostomy.

An alternative is the oblique muscle-cutting incision sited in the left iliac fossa. Although popular with some surgeons in the past (Bacon, 1945; d'Allaines, 1956) it has never gained universal popularity. Access to the depths of the pelvis is compromised, a self-retaining retractor is difficult to use with it, and if an abdominoperineal excision is necessary the wound is very prone to colostomy herniation (Goligher, 1984).

A transverse incision has in the recent past been strongly recommended for these procedures (Goldberg, 1980). Although the transverse incision is cosmetically more acceptable and may produce a strong wound, postoperative discomfort is greater in our experience compared with a midline incision, access to the pelvis is restricted, and both potential stoma sites may be compromised.

Abdominal exploration and assessment of operability

As in operations for colonic carcinomas, the abdomen needs to be explored carefully to detect metastatic spread. In particular the liver requires careful bimanual palpation and on-table ultrasound examination if possible. Any suspicious areas should be biopsied and sent for histological examination. It is often useful to examine frozen sections from suspected liver metastases so that the surgeon knows at the time of the procedure whether it is to be radical or palliative. Similarly, the whole of the peritoneal cavity should be searched for the presence of metastases and a biopsy should be taken of any suspicious lesions. Enlarged lymph nodes should be sought in the mesentery and lateral pelvic side walls, although it must be realized that such enlargement does not necessarily mean that the node is involved with metastic tumour. If doubt exists, frozen-section or imprint cytology will resolve the dilemma.

Attention should next be turned to the rectal tumour itself. Its site within the rectum should be noted, in particular whether it is above or below the peritoneal reflection. If it is below the reflection it may not be possible to palpate the lesion via the abdominal approach until the rectum has been mobilized. The degree of mobility should be assessed, for if the lesion is fully mobile it will be possible to remove it and provided there are no distant metastases the excision should be radical. If, on the other hand, the tumour is fixed to other tissues radical excision is less likely. Nevertheless, it is always worth attempting to remove a lesion no matter how fixed it is to other structures. Fixation in approximately 25% of cases is due to inflammatory and not neoplastic infiltration (Durdey and Williams, 1984). An appraisal of the structures to which the tumour is adherent is essential in order to plan excision and reconstruction. On occasion the degree of local spread particularly in the depths of the pelvis seems so great that the removal of the tumour is thought to be impossible. In these cases a trial dissection should be commenced; but if this fails it is a good idea to eliminate the small bowel from the pelvis with omentum or a sheet of inert material so that a course of postoperative radiotherapy can be offered. It is unusual for a surgeon with experience in this type of surgery not to be able to remove most rectal cancers, no matter how fixed they first appear to be. The next problem is to decide whether a sphincter-saving procedure is feasible. Indeed, in patients with easily resected tumours this decision can often only be finally made after the tumour has been removed.

If it has been decided preoperatively that a sphincter-saving technique is a possibility, the surgeon should not be deflected from this course because on abdominal exploration the lesion is found to be very low within the pelvis. After full mobilization of the rectum many tumours become accessible so that some form of sphincter-saving technique is then feasible.

Mobilization of colon

After the abdominal exploration a self-retaining abdominal retractor should be positioned to provide maximum exposure. When the rectal tumour itself is examined the small bowel has to be removed from the pelvis: this can be done in one of two ways. Loops of bowel can be packed away in the upper abdomen and prevented from emerging into the operative field by insertion of the third blade of the self-retaining retractor. Alternatively the whole of the small bowel can be lifted out of the abdomen and placed under warm packs, or it can be inserted into a plastic Aldon bag.

The iliac portion of the colon is then mobilized by incising the congenital peritoneal folds attached to the lateral aspect of its mesentery (Figure 32.9). This is best achieved with the assistant grasping the sigmoid colon and drawing it to the right so as to put the tissues on the stretch. The peritoneal incision normally commences at the level of the proximal sigmoid colon and continues to the splenic flexure. After incision of the peritoneum the underlying left ureter can be seen, distinguishable from the more laterally lying spermatic or ovarian vessels by its characteristic vermicular movement – best displayed by 'pinching' the ureter lightly with non-toothed forceps. Once seen, the left ureter should be gently swept laterally away from the vascular pedicle. In some cases where it is difficult to determine the course of the ureter it is a good idea to place a latex sling around it. Traction on the sling allows the ureter to be traced more easily as it enters the pelvis.

In some cases with high rectal cancers the left ureter becomes displaced medially by retroperitoneal tumour infiltration or by adhesions. In these circumstances careful sharp dissection is required to release the ureter. On other occasions the growth directly invades the ureter and in such a case radical tumour ablation will involve excision of a segment of ureter as well. If mobilization of the whole of the left colon is necessary, a Kelly retractor is placed under the left costal margin and the assistant retracts upwards and outwards, revealing the splenic flexure. The colon is then displaced gently downwards and medially by the surgeon and the peritoneal incision is continued on the lateral side of the splenic flexure (Figure 32.10). Great care must be exercised to prevent injury to the spleen. This part of the mobilization may continue to the midpoint of the transverse colon by separating the greater omentum from the transverse mesocolon. It is our policy to mobilize the splenic flexure of the colon in all cases of radical sphincter-saving resection. It is only in this way that a wide anastomosis can be constructed between the descending colon and the rectum. Furthermore, if high ligation is practised, the supply to the sigmoid colon from the middle colic artery and the arcade is tenuous and the sigmoid must be resected.

After division of the lateral peritoneal reflection the sigmoid colon is retracted to the left by the surgeon and the peritoneum is incised to the right of the midline. This incision is extended upwards to the lower border of the third part of the duodenum (Figure 32.11). The incision is deepened and opened up to expose the front of the right common iliac artery and the aorta. The vascular supply of the rectum can now be approached from either side of the mesentery.

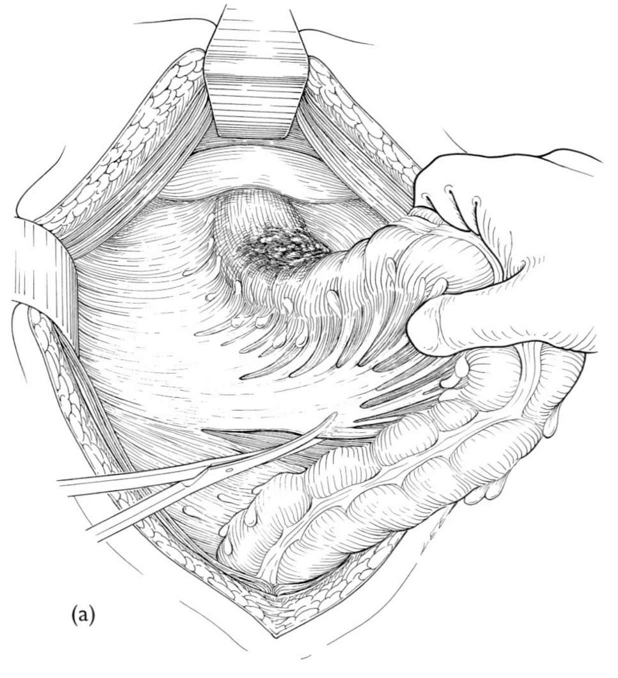

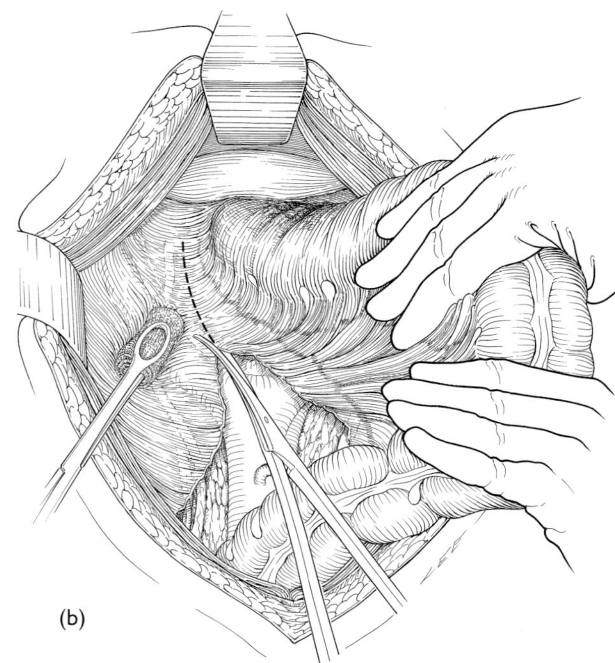

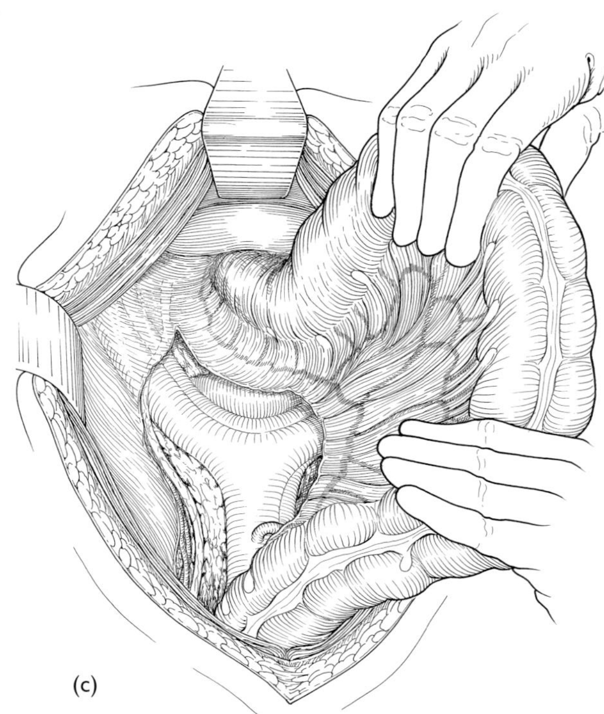

Figure 32.9a–c Mobilization of the left colon during sphincter-saving resection. (a) Division of developmental adhesions on the lateral side of the iliac colon and mesocolon. (b) The peritoneum on the left side of the base of the mesosigmoid is opened. As this incision is deepened (c) the ureter is visualized and can be pushed laterally or can be retracted by using a latex sling.

There are some surgeons (Goligher, 1984) who advocate that the proximal colon should be tied off with a stout Nylon tie prior to its mobilization; this is in the belief that tumour cells shed intraluminally may be viable, and may seed and thus cause anastomotic recurrence. Although such cells have been shown to be viable (Umpleby et al, 1984b), the inference that they cause recurrence is circumstantial. It is doubtful whether such a precaution is necessary and at present we do not use such a ligature. We do, however, accept that there is no contraindication for this manoeuvre and it may have benefits.

Ligation of vascular pedicle

The vascular pedicle can be tied either 'high' (i.e. flush with the aorta) or 'low'. It is our policy to try to employ a high tie if the aim is a radical operation. A low tie is reserved for obviously palliative procedures, when the patient is a poor risk and there is a need to be as swift as possible, and in patients with extensive arterial disease in whom the origin of the middle colic artery may be occluded. It should be stated, however, that the benefit of a high ligation to achieve cure is controversial, and there are those who argue that apical node involvement carries a poor prognosis anyway.

If a high tie is to be used, the surgeon's left index and middle fingers are passed to the patient's left between the inferior mesenteric vessels and the

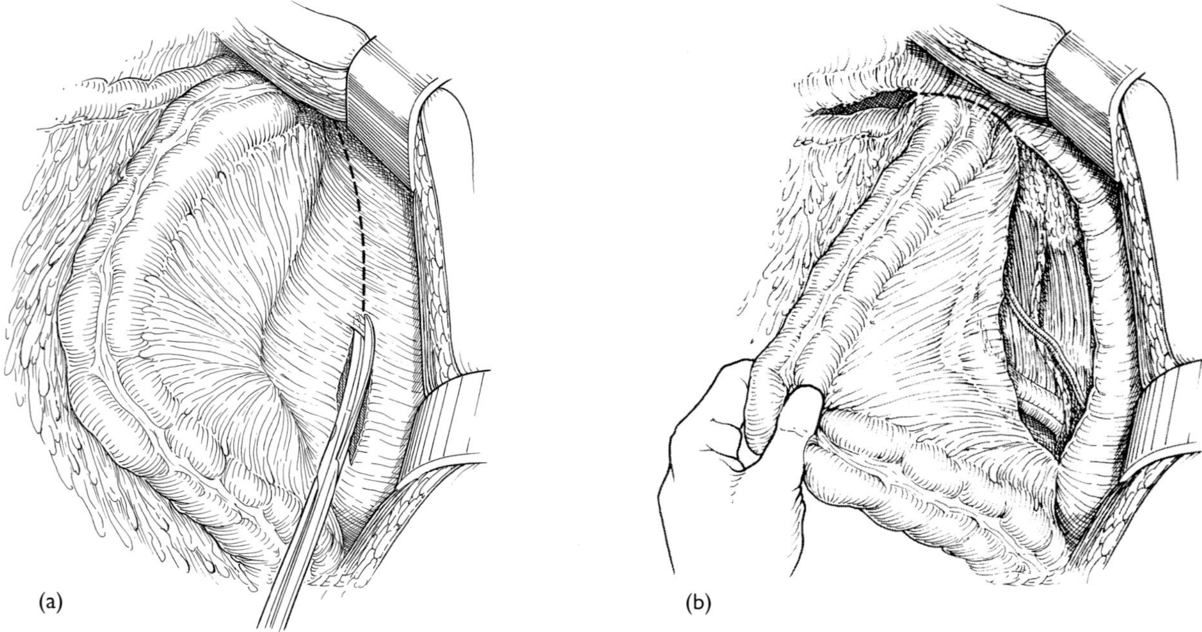

Figure 32.10 Mobilization of splenic flexure during sphincter-saving resection.

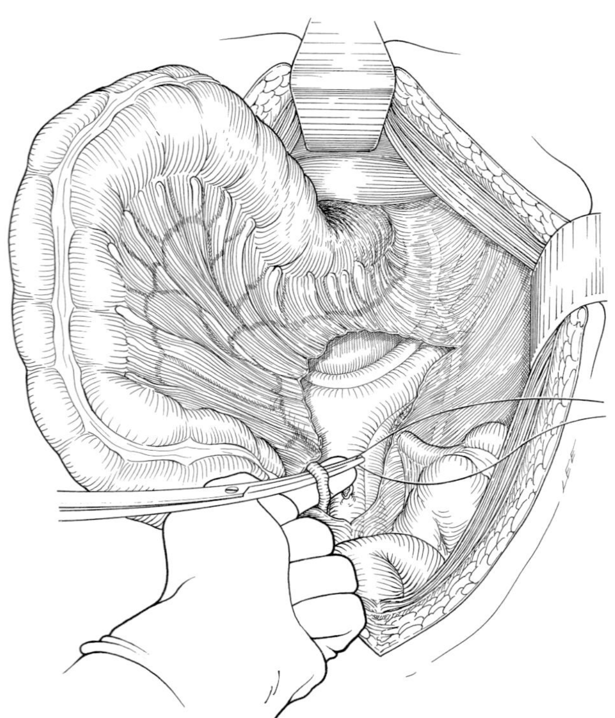

Figure 32.11 Exposure and division of inferior mesenteric vessels flush with aorta (high tie).

aorta (Figure 32.11). Initially the tips of the fingers are inserted through the gap which is then gradually enlarged to take the full breadth of the metacarpals. With the vessels gently clasped between the thumb anteriorly and the index and middle fingers posteriorly, a short transverse incision is made over the peritoneum at a point where it is thought that the inferior mesenteric artery emerges from the aorta. During this manoeuvre it is possible that the central root of the presacral nerve may be torn or stripped off with the vessels, but if care is exercised this nerve can be preserved. If, however, enlarged lymph nodes are obvious, it is unwise to jeopardize their removal by leaving the nerve intact, in which case it should be sacrificed.

Once the vessels have been identified they are doubly ligated with stout linen, silk or polygalactin ligatures flush with the aorta (Figure 32.11). Each vessel must be dealt with separately since the inferior mesenteric vein lies well to the left of the artery in its course towards the splenic vein. The vein is ligated under the pancreas after mobilization of the duodenojejunal flexure. This manoeuvre greatly facilitates mobilization of the splenic flexure. Division of the vessels should always leave approximately 0.5–1 cm of vessel distal to the tie to reduce the risk of the ligature slipping. Before clamping and division of the vascular pedicles it is always wise to check the position of the left ureter, and make sure it cannot be injured during this procedure.

In those patients in whom a low tie is deemed advisable (Figure 32.12), the ligature is usually applied to the inferior mesenteric vessels just below the origin of the left colic artery or first sigmoid branch. The index finger of the left hand is insinuated under the vascular pedicle and the peritoneum is incised over the vessels. A ligature is then placed around each vessel with the aid of an appropriate instrument, such as a Lahey dissector or cholecystectomy forceps. After doubly ligating each vessel and taking care to avoid damage to the left ureter, the vessels are divided.

Division of the colon

Division of the colon may take place at this point or may be accomplished after the pelvic dissection is complete. We prefer to divide at this stage.

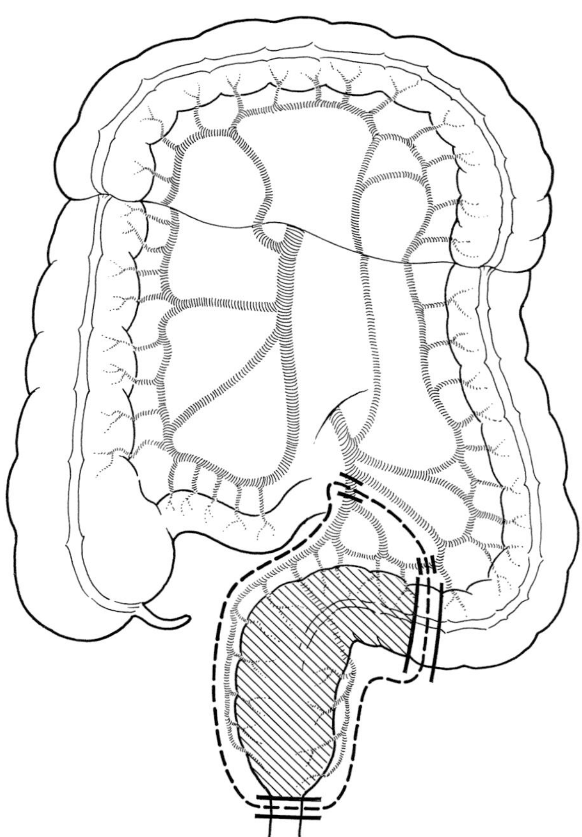

Figure 32.12 Site of division of inferior mesentery vessels for low tie. The shaded area represents the amount of tissue to be resected. The colon can be divided at the level of the distal sigmoid.

The sigmoid mesocolon is divided obliquely from the point of ligation of the inferior mesenteric vessels to the site of proposed transection of the left colon (Figure 32.13). During division of the mesocolon three vessels will need to be divided if a low tie is used. These are the ascending left colic artery running to the splenic flexure, the left colic artery, and the marginal artery between the left colic artery and the first sigmoid vessels. If a high ligation is used only the marginal artery will have to be divided.

Once these vessels have been divided and ligated the colon is transected between Parker–Kerr clamps or similar crushing clamps. Alternatively, a linear staple cutter may be used. Clamps should be applied from antimesenteric to mesenteric borders of the colon. It is then necessary to ensure firstly that the blood supply to the transected proximal end of the colon is adequate, and secondly that it will reach easily into the pelvis so that an anastomosis can be constructed without tension. Retention of the normal pink colour of the colon is usually sufficient evidence of an adequate blood supply. However, if there is doubt one of the small mural arteries of the colon at the point of intended anastomosis can be pricked with a hypodermic needle to observe if it gives rise to arterial bleeding. Some surgeons deliberately divide the marginal artery opposite the

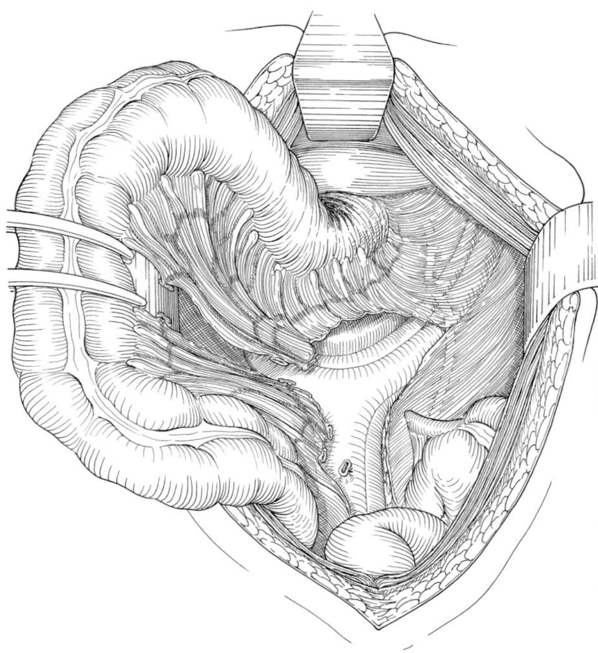

Figure 32.13 Division of the sigmoid mesocolon. Two crushing clamps have been placed at the site of division of the colon.

point of proposed colonic transection to ensure that it bleeds vigorously before ligation. If the blood supply is inadequate the proximal limit of excision will have to be taken to a higher level. A point is then selected in the descending colon where the blood supply is adequate and transection is performed.

If after division of the colon at the usual site (i.e. the distal descending colon) the proximal colon will not reach the pubis when gently stretched downwards, it is unlikely that a satisfactory anastomosis can be achieved. In this situation it is necessary to ensure that the left colon has been fully mobilized right around to the mid-transverse colon. If there is still inadequate length, the hepatic flexure must be completely mobilized so that the only fixed structure is the origin of the superior mesenteric vessels. In this way the left colon can be almost always brought down to the pelvis without tension.

The pelvic dissection

The extent of the pelvic dissection will depend on the height of the tumour from the anal verge. There follows a description of the technique used to mobilize the rectum when the tumour lies at a low level in the pelvis. However, it should be realized that this is not required in all cases; thus, the lateral ligaments do not always need to be divided for tumours in the upper third of the rectum.

At the commencement of the rectal dissection in the female it is useful to suture the uterus and fallopian tubes to the abdominal wall as depicted in Figure 32.14. This makes access to the rectum – particularly the anterolateral planes – much easier. The posterior rectal dissection is commenced by continuing the peritoneal incisions on each side of the rectum to the level of the seminal vesicles or the rectovaginal septum (Figure 32.15). The rectosigmoid region is then displaced anteriorly and gentle traction is exerted in this direction with the surgeon's left hand (Figure 32.16). The rectosigmoid mesentery containing the divided and ligated vascular pedicle is divided from the front of the lower aorta, the right common iliac vein and the fifth lumbar vertebra to the promontory of the sacrum. Great care should be exercised during this manoeuvre as the right common iliac vein can be damaged by overzealous dissection.

If the presacral nerve has been divided previously this nerve will be lifted forwards with the mesentery. If the nerve has not been sacrificed, there is a risk that it will be damaged during the next part of the procedure at the pelvic brim where the nerve divides into two branches; at this point the main trunk tends to adhere close to the rectum before the branches separate to run towards the sides of the pelvis. Both these branches should be identified and pushed gently off the posterior wall of the rectum.

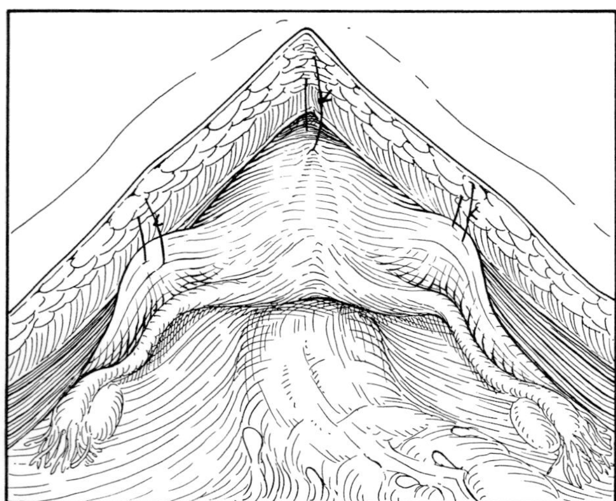

Figure 32.14 Access to the female rectum is improved by stitching the uterus and fallopian tubes to the lower part of the incision.

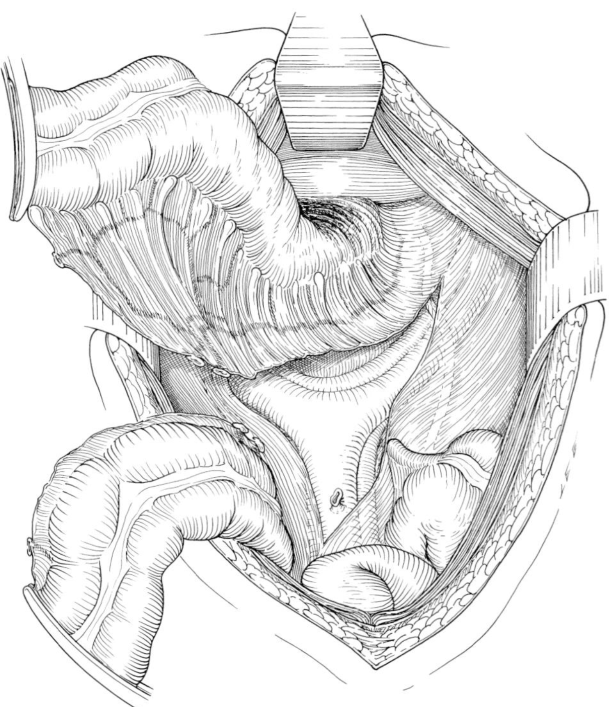

Figure 32.15 Sphincter-saving resection, pelvic dissection. The peritoneal incisions are continued down on each side of the rectum.

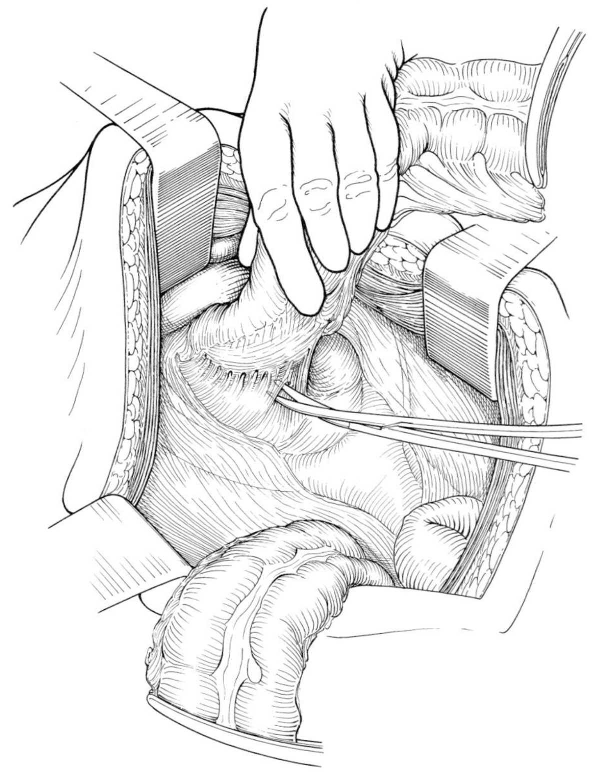

Figure 32.16 Freeing the ligated mesosigmoid pedicle and mesorectum from the aorta and sacrum.

Following this manoeuvre a pair of blunt-ended scissors should be inserted in the midline downwards and backwards immediately in front of the first piece of the sacrum and behind the mesorectum. This manoeuvre opens up the presacral space and allows the dissection of the rectum and mesorectum from the presacral fascia. This is best done using long, curved Nelson scissors. Any small veins that traverse the presacral space running between the posterior rectal wall and entering the middle sacral veins should be electrocoagulated before division.

The posterior dissection should continue downwards as far as the coccyx so that the entire mesorectum can be removed with the specimen. Sometimes it is not possible to complete the posterior rectal dissection under direct vision. In these circumstances the hand may have to be introduced into the presacral space (Figure 32.17) and the rectum gently pushed forward from the front of the presacral fascia and the sides of the pelvis as far down as the coccyx. Provided the plane of dissection remains anterior to the presacral fascia, the manoeuvre should be relatively bloodless.

Occasionally during the posterior dissection, particularly when the growth is situated posteriorly and is adherent to the sacrum, the middle sacral veins may themselves be damaged. Haemostasis in these circumstances may be more difficult and underrunning of the vessels may be required.

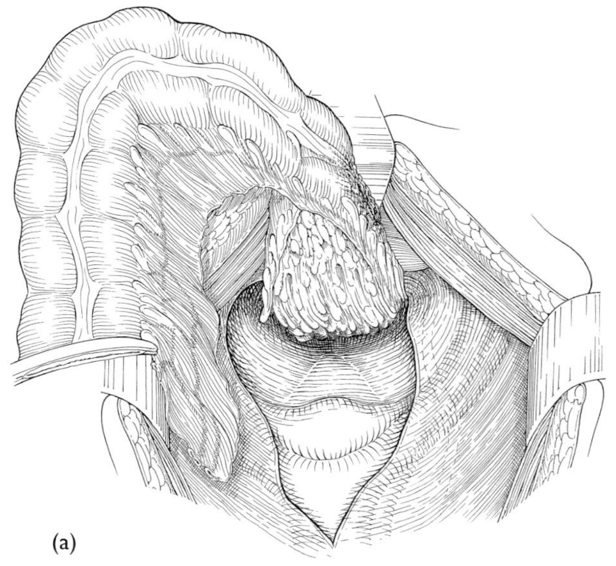

(a)

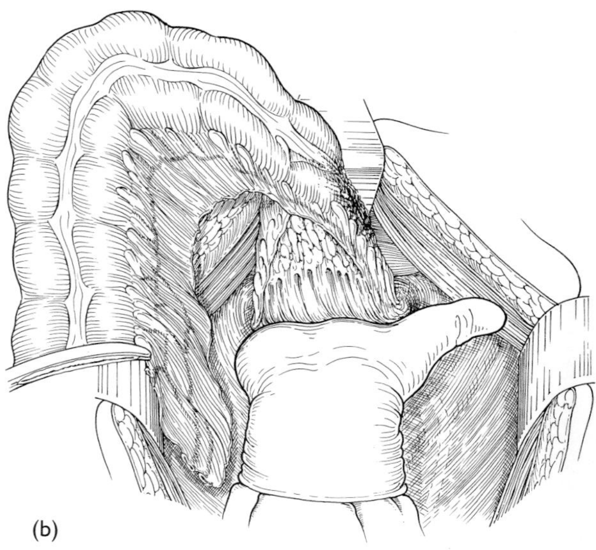

(b)

Figure 32.17a,b (a) The posterior rectal dissection down to the coccyx should be under direct vision. (b) However, in certain circumstances a hand may need to be inserted posterior to the rectum so as to displace it anteriorly.

Sometimes the vein retracts into a sacral foramen and bleeding can be controlled only by plugging the foramen with bone wax or a sterile drawing pin.

Once the posterior rectal dissection is complete, attention is turned towards the anterior dissection. The operating light is adjusted if a head lamp is not used, and the deep pelvic retractor is inserted between the anterior rectal wall and the posterior wall of the bladder. Deep dissection in the pelvis is unsatisfactory without the Lloyd Davies deep pelvic retractors. The bladder can then be lifted forwards by the second assistant who is positioned between the abducted legs of the patient. The peritoneal and subperitoneal tissues which have been incised on each side are now joined anteriorly by dividing the peritoneal reflection 1–2 cm in front of the lowest part of the peritoneal pouch (Figure 32.18).

The anterior plane of dissection between the posterior wall of the bladder and the anterior wall of the rectum is developed by scissor dissection (Figure 32.19a). It is useful at the start of dissection to pick up the edges of the cut pelvic peritoneum with two or three long artery forceps; traction upwards by the assistant can considerably improve exposure. The plane is gradually deepened until the base of the bladder and both seminal vesicles or the vaginal wall are reached. The long pelvic retractor with a lipped end is then reinserted into the plane, and by positioning it so that the assistant pulls it

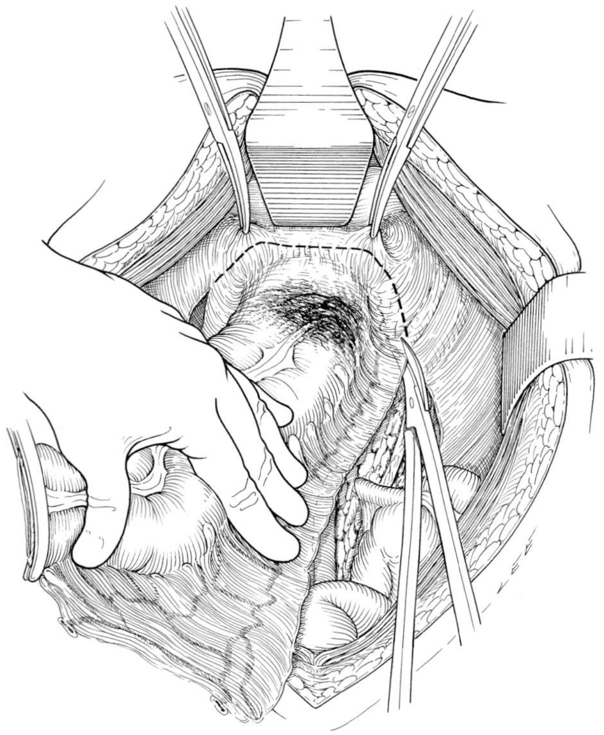

Figure 32.18 Commencing the anterior plane of dissection by joining the peritoneal incisions on both sides between the anterior rectal wall and the posterior wall of the bladder.

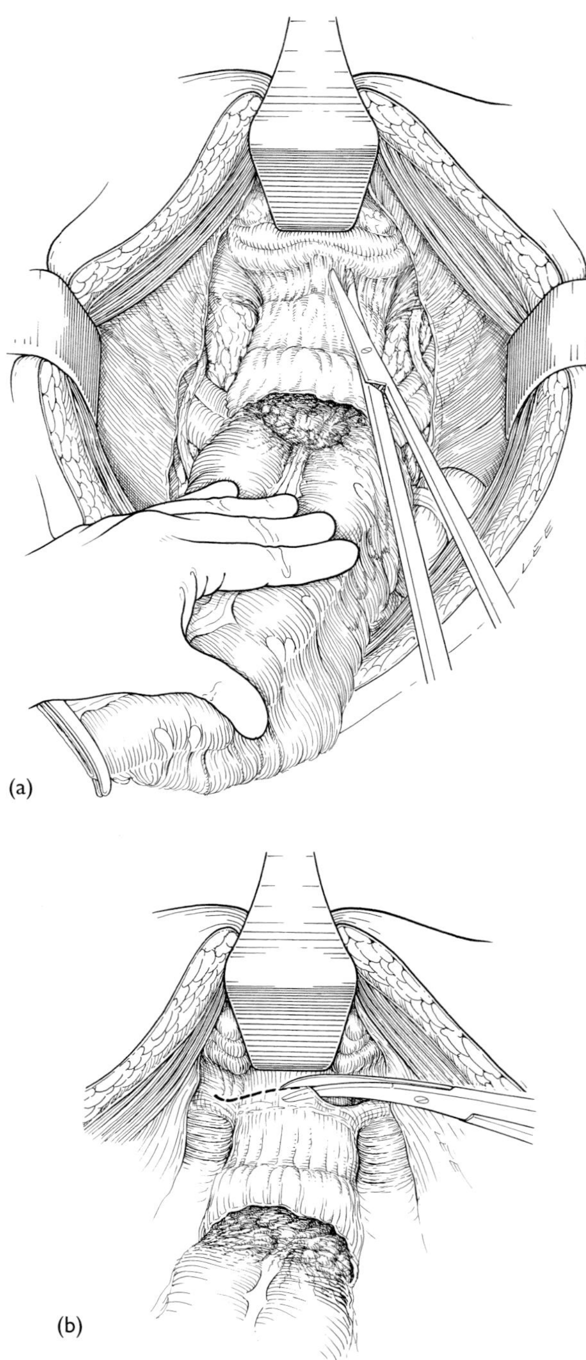

Figure 32.19a,b (a) The anterior plane of dissection between the rectum and bladder is developed. (b) Just below the level of the seminal vesicles the fascia of Denonvilliers is divided.

anteriorly and upwards, the fascia of Denonvilliers is exposed lying between the anterior rectal wall and the prostate. Denonvilliers' fascia is then incised transversely (Figure 32.19b), and the middle and index fingers or fine pledgets on Roberts forceps are used to find a line of cleavage extending as far as the apex of the prostate. Equally, this dissection may be accomplished entirely using the curved, blunt-edged Lloyd Davies scissors. While in this space the fingers or a pledget are swept laterally and the anterior border of the lateral ligament is defined. Dissection in this plane can cause troublesome haemorrhage, particularly from the back of the prostate, if the plane of dissection trespasses too far forwards. Careful diathermy may be required to control this bleeding and this may be difficult unless exposure and lighting are optimum.

Division of the lateral ligaments

Division of the lateral ligaments is often aided by the insertion of a second pelvic retractor which is positioned to allow access to the depths of the lateral side of the pelvis. The term 'lateral ligaments' relates to the areolar tissue which binds the rectum to the lateral pelvic side walls. 'Ligaments' is a misnomer for these structures, which, in addition to containing the middle rectal vessels, contain branches of the pelvic autonomic nerves. It appears that 'lateral ligaments' form part of the mesorectum. In older textbooks, the advice was to render the ligaments taut by drawing the rectum firmly upwards and towards the opposite side. After ensuring that the ureter was out of the field, the recommendation was to clamp the lateral ligaments, divide them and then ligate them. Nowadays, we prefer to divide this tissue piecemeal using a combination of scissor dissection and diathermy. It is first important to ensure that the ureters are not injured during this dissection. This is particularly important in the case of patients with bulky tumours situated in the mid-pelvis. In such cases both ureters should be exposed throughout their course to the bladder, to avoid injury. If there is any doubt as to the position of the ureters, it is a good policy for a cystoscopy to be performed so that both ureters can be catheterized and the catheters left *in situ* to aid identification during dissection.

The rectum is then drawn firmly upwards and towards the opposite side, a manoeuvre which puts the 'lateral ligaments' under stretch. A careful dissection of this tissue is carried out using long scissors (Figure 32.20) as close to the pelvic side wall as possible. All bleeding points are carefully diathermied and care is taken to avoid damage to any pelvic autonomic nerves that are visualized if this is feasible. The middle rectal artery may require separate division and ligation. The dissection proceeds from behind working forwards. Much of the tissue which in the past was labelled as lateral ligament is in fact the lateral component of the mesorectum. It is possible to fillet out the entire bilobed lipoma of the mesorectum in a completely bloodless plane leaving only the two middle rectal pedicles, which incidentally are anterolateral just peripheral to the anorectal junction. This manoeuvre has now been termed *total mesorectal excision* (TME).

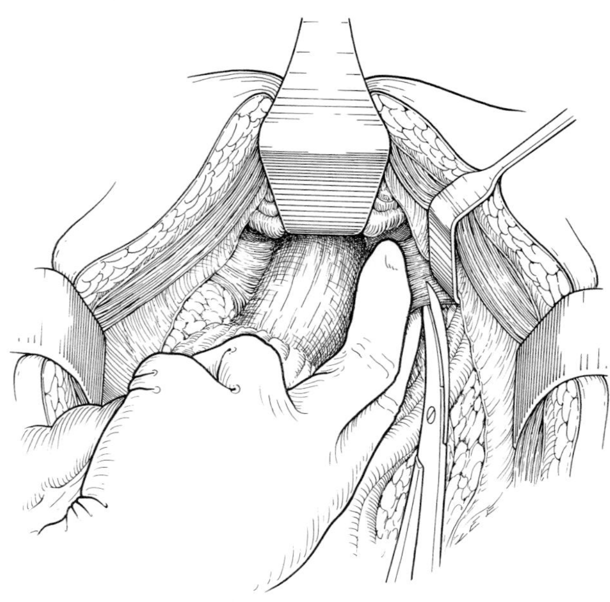

Figure 32.20 Division of the patient's right lateral ligament.

After division of the 'lateral ligaments' on both sides the rectum is fully mobilized, and attention can then be turned to completing the rectal excision.

'Extended' lateral pelvic dissection

The description above refers to the conventional technique of pelvic dissection and division of the lateral ligaments as practised in most units in western Europe and the USA. As discussed elsewhere, there are data to suggest that the lymph nodes lying on the iliac vessels may be involved with carcinoma. A few centres, therefore, advocate an extended lateral pelvic dissection in which the base of the lateral ligament is dissected off the structures of the pelvic side wall, removing the internal iliac and other lateral nodes in the process (Enker, 1978; Hojo and Koyama, 1982) (Figure 32.21). The technique is as follows.

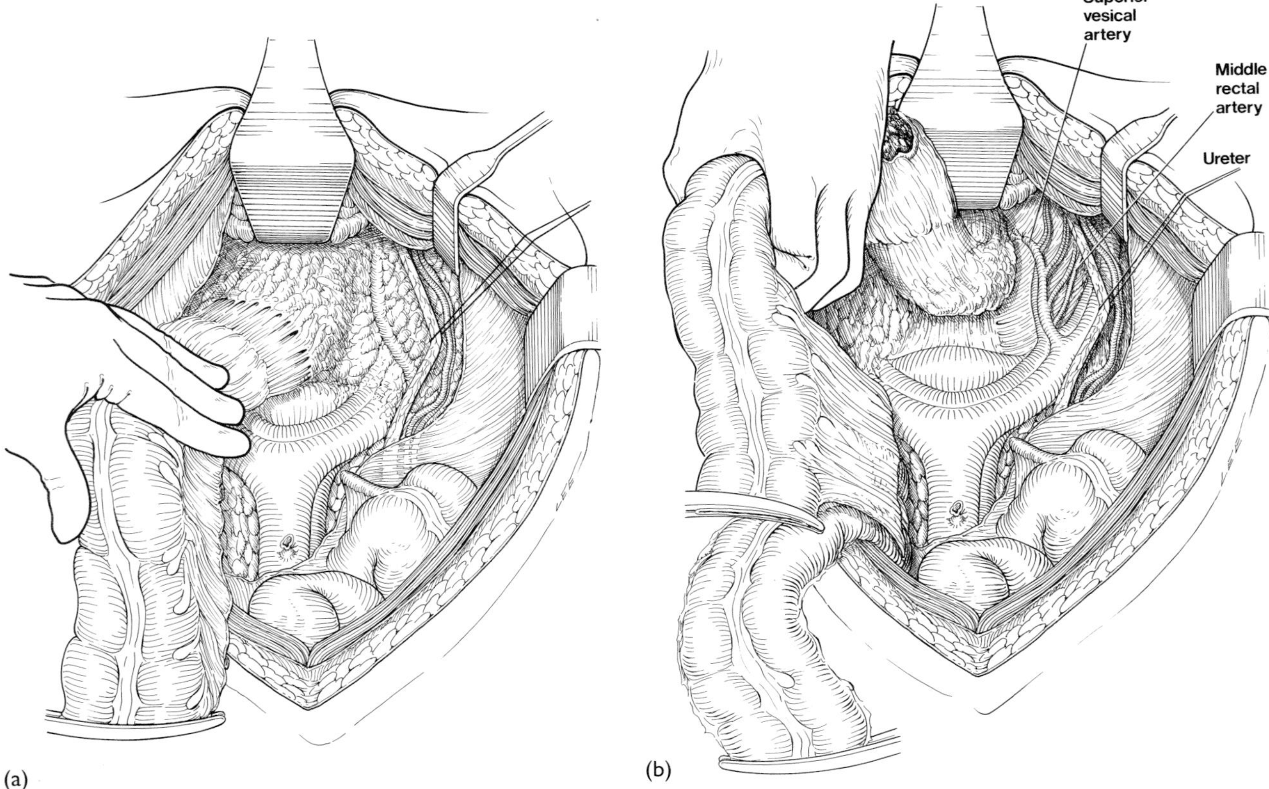

Figure 32.21a,b Extended lateral pelvic dissection. (a) The right lateral leaf of pelvic peritoneum is elevated and retracted outwards to expose the common iliac artery with the ureter crossing its bifurcation. Further downwards and backwards, fascial and fatty tissues cover the external and internal iliac vessels and will next be dissected off these structures and the pelvic side wall. (b) The process of separating the base of the lateral ligament from the pelvic side wall has been carried out down into the pelvis, exposing the external and internal iliac arteries, the middle rectal and superior vesical arteries, and the obturator nerve and obturator internus muscle.

The surgeon may start on either side; if on the right, the right lateral leaf of pelvic peritoneum is dissected upwards and retracted laterally to expose the ureter as it lies on the psoas muscle and runs down to cross the bifurcation of the common iliac artery. The ureter is mobilized and a sling of latex rubber is placed around it (Figure 32.21a). The ureter can then be retracted in such a way that the fibrofatty tissue overlying the common, external and internal iliac vessels and pelvic side wall can be dissected from them. The dissection proceeds downwards and backwards (Figure 32.21b). The middle rectal artery is first seen emerging from the internal iliac artery and is ligated and divided. The next vessel to be visualized is the superior vesical artery and this is carefully preserved. Gradually all the vessels are bared of tissue. As the pelvic side wall is cleared the obturator nerve is seen lying on the obturator internus muscle and is also preserved. The dissection continues until the upper surface of the levator muscles is seen. At this point the whole of the lateral ligament should be free and together with the rectum can be displaced to the other side. The pelvic side wall and vessels are then inspected to ensure that haemostasis is secure and that no tissue remains. The procedure is repeated on the left side.

Distal division of the rectum

With the rectum drawn upwards towards the operator and under minimal tension, the mesorectum below the growth is divided. For easily accessible tumours the mesorectum is divided at the same level as the proposed transection of the bowel wall. The latter is usually at least 5 cm distal to the lower border of the tumour. For less accessible tumours the margin of distal clearance of bowel wall can, in our view, be safely reduced to 2 cm, if by so doing a sphincter-saving resection can be performed. In the past we contented ourselves with dividing the mesorectum in these patients at the same level as the proposed site of the transection of the bowel wall. However, Heald et al (1982) and others (Scott et al, 1995) describe patients who have minute foci of adenocarcinoma in the mesorectum several centimetres distal to the lower edge of a rectal cancer; these observations have persuaded us to perform total mesorectal excision (TME) in all cases of low rectal cancer and even for mid-rectal cancers.

In this technique the distal mesorectum is dissected off the back of the muscular tube of the rectum with scissors while it is drawn upwards with a dry swab. The angle is thus emptied of the last remnants of fatty lymphovascular tissue (Figure 32.22). The rectal wall 2 cm below the tumour is then transected. This leaves behind a few centimetres of distal rectum denuded of its mesorectum to be used in the anastomosis. If this option is taken, a covering stoma is mandatory owing to the increased risk of anastomotic dehiscence.

If the mesorectum is to be transected rather than excised it may be quite bulky and is often best divided between artery forceps if feasible, otherwise diathermy will be necessary (Figure 32.23). Once the rectal wall has been bared of mesentery, a right-angled or curved aortic clamp is applied across it from right to left at the appropriate distance from the lower edge of the tumour (Figure 32.24). Some surgeons prefer to apply this clamp in the anteroposterior or sagittal plane; as a routine we do not believe this confers any particular advantage but it may be necessary in individual cases. Once the clamp is in place an assistant inserts a proctoscope into the anorectal stump for purposes of irrigation (Figure 32.25). A large-calibre catheter

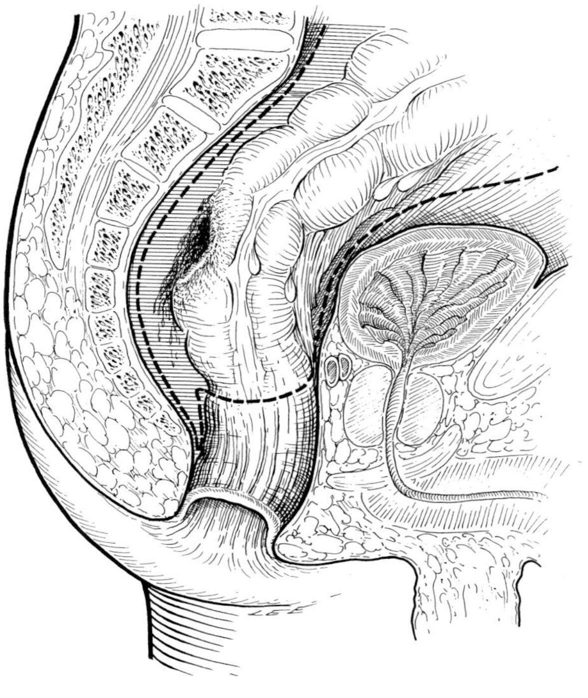

Figure 32.22 Plane of dissection for total mesorectal excision.

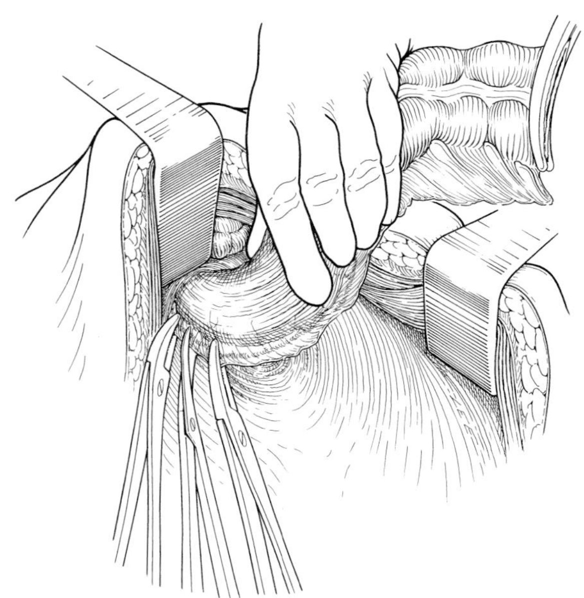

Figure 32.23 Transection of the mesorectum.

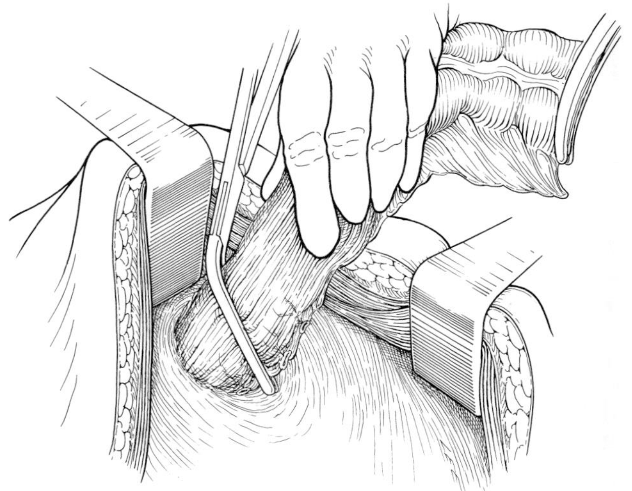

Figure 32.24 Cross-clamping the rectum below the tumour after the mesorectum has been transected, using a right-angled crushing clamp.

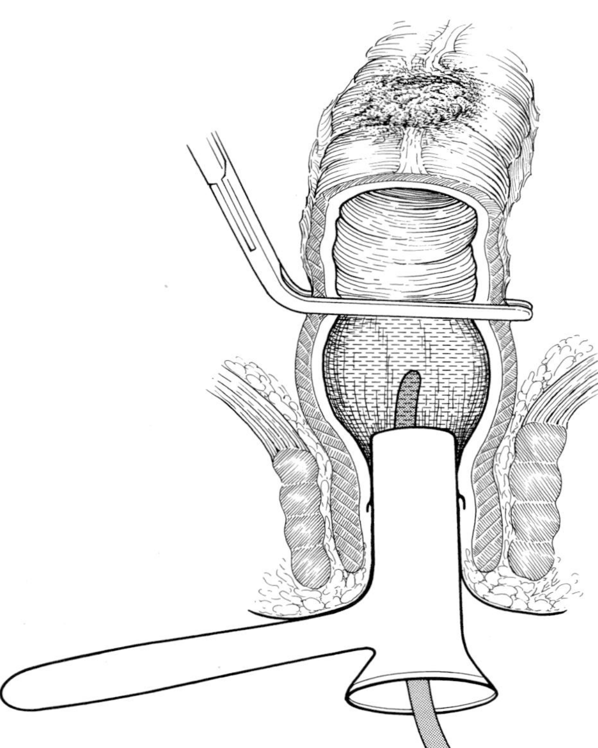

Figure 32.25 Irrigation of the rectal stump with a cancericidal solution.

attached to an irrigating set containing 1% cetrimide solution is inserted through the proctoscope into the rectum. The rectum is then irrigated with 1 L of this solution followed by 1 L of normal saline, and finally swabbed dry. This manoeuvre is designed to kill any viable cancer cells which may be present within the rectal lumen.

The anastomosis

There are three methods of achieving the anastomosis between the proximal colon and the anorectal stump via the abdominal route. These are:

- the two-layer manual suture technique
- the one-layer manual suture technique
- the technique with a circular stapling instrument.

The optimum method of anastomosis is open to debate but there are a few points worth making. Of the controlled trials that have been performed comparing one-layered and two-layered inverting sutured anastomoses, none has reported any statistical difference between the two (Everett, 1975; Goligher et al, 1977). Despite these findings, Goligher et al (1977) believed that a two-layered technique was safer. Several trials have compared manual anastomoses with those achieved by the stapler. The evidence to date suggests that a stapled anastomosis is as safe as a hand anastomosis for anastomoses low in the pelvis (McGinn et al, 1985; West of Scotland and Highland Anastomosis Study Group, 1991; Fingerhut et al, 1994). There is, however, a suggestion that stapled anastomoses at this level are less pliable and more likely to cause stenosis than those that are sutured. One of the chief advantages of the stapling technique is that an anastomosis can often be performed at a level in the pelvis at which it is impossible to perform a manual anastomosis of any kind.

It is for these reasons that we have evolved the following approach. Where the growth is high in the rectum and an anastomosis is considered straightforward, we perform a single- or two-layer inverting sutured anastomosis. For growths at a lower level we now use a triple stapling technique (Moran, 1996).

Two-layer sutured anastomosis

The proximal colon and rectum above the right-angled or aortic clamp are pulled upwards and out of the abdominal cavity. The clamp is steadied and everted so that the serosal surface of the anorectal stump faces the surgeon looking down from above into the pelvis. The Parker–Kerr or Schumacker clamp controlling the proximal colonic stump is rested on the left edge of the abdominal wound with its mesenteric border directed posteriorly and separated by a distance of 10–12 cm from the rectum. Prior to performing the anastomosis some surgeons like to inject the colonic stump with a cancericidal agent to ensure that any shed neoplastic cells are dealt with. They do this by clamping the colonic stump 10 cm from its end with a spring clamp. The cancericidal agent is then injected into this closed distal segment and is left in place as the anastomosis proceeds, eventually being evacuated by suction when the terminal crushing clamp is removed.

Until recently we considered that even if malignant cells were shed from a rectal cancer in the course of the operation they could not reach the proximal extent of resection; hence irrigation of the colonic stump was deemed to be unnecessary. Umpleby et al (1984b) contradicts this belief, however, and viable cells shed from a rectal neoplasm seem capable of travelling a considerable distance proximally. These findings have modified our practice, and although we do not routinely inject the distal colon, we ensure that the open end of the bowel is irrigated with 1% cetrimide solution during the construction of the anastomosis.

Once the ends of the bowel are aligned correctly the anastomosis proceeds. The posterior layer of mattress Lembert sutures is now inserted (Figure 32.26): 3/0 silk or linen sutures are traditionally used for this part of the procedure, but we now prefer to use 3/0 Vicryl or Maxon sutures since these materials have strength yet are still eventually absorbed. Each suture is waxed or lubricated prior to insertion to ensure it glides through the tissues. The sutures are placed without being tied, each being clamped with a mosquito artery forceps which is then threaded on to the shaft of a larger forceps (usually Roberts forceps). The reason for this manoeuvre is to ensure that the sutures do not become twisted on each other and are tied in order. Each serosal stitch is placed approximately 1 cm from the controlling clamps and at 0.5 cm intervals. When the posterior row of sutures has been inserted the proximal colon is slid down into the pelvis so that its posterior wall is apposed to that of the rectum. The Lembert sutures are then tied, the first and last sutures are left long and reclamped, and those in the middle are cut. The two long serosal sutures allow traction to be exerted on the anastomosis so that it can be visualized more easily.

The right-angled clamp is now pulled upwards and steadied, and is cut off from the distal anorectal stump with a long-handled scalpel, taking great care not to cut any of the serosal sutures which have just been placed (Figure 32.27). The same procedure is used to excise the straight clamp on the colon stump after a non-crushing clamp has been placed across the colon 10 cm proximally.

It is a good policy just before the clamps are removed to ensure that the anastomosis is surrounded by packs which are able to absorb any spillage of faeces should this occur. Furthermore, not only do we irrigate the bowel lumen with 1%

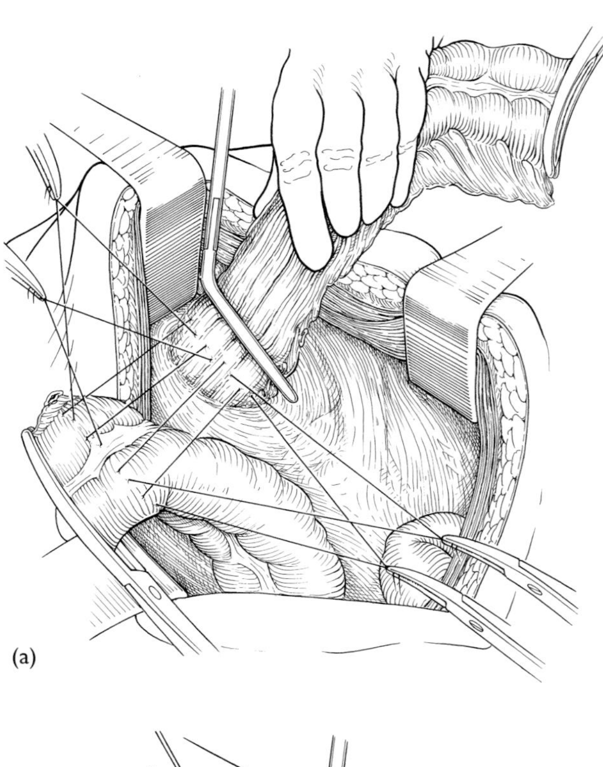

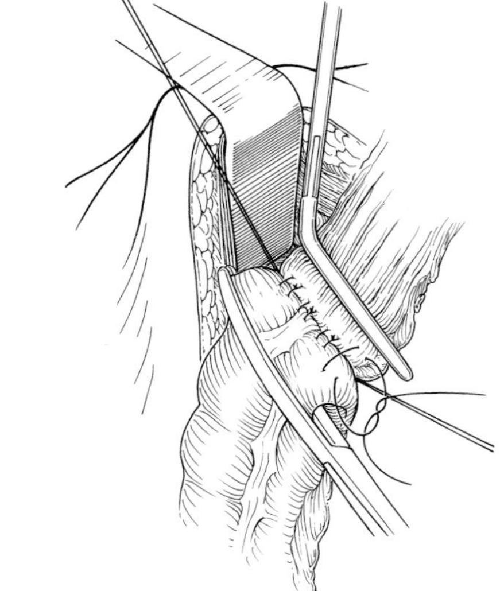

Figure 32.26a,b Anterior resection with two-layered sutured anastomosis. (a) Insertion of posterior seromuscular Lembert sutures. (b) The colon is approximated to the rectal stump and the posterior seromuscular sutures are tied and cut.

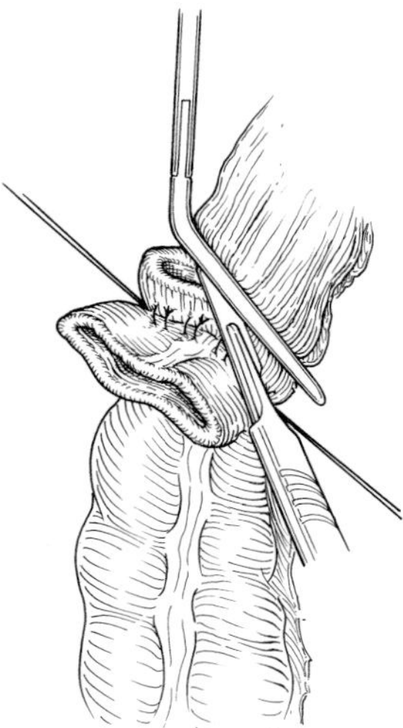

Figure 32.27 The clamps are cut from the colon and anorectal stump.

cetrimide as a cancericidal agent, but we follow this with an antibiotic solution (cefuroxime) in the hope that bacterial counts will be reduced.

Once the specimen has been removed it is opened by an associate and shown to the surgeon. This is done to ensure that there is at least a distal margin of clearance of 2 cm. If satisfied, the surgeon continues with the anastomosis.

The next layer to be inserted is the full-thickness, through-and-through layer (Figure 32.28). This can be achieved by either a continuous or an interrupted technique, using either absorbable or non-absorbable material. It is our preference to use a continuous layer of 2/0 or 3/0 chromic catgut on a fine, half-circle atraumatic needle.

This layer is commenced on the anterior or antimesenteric poles and the suture is inserted from the outer aspect of the rectum through the wall of the rectum and colon to the peritoneal aspect of the colon, thereby traversing the full thickness of the bowel walls. The knot is then tied on the outer surface of the bowel lumen. It is tied in such a way as to leave an end which is long enough (10–15 cm) for tying the knot when the layer is completed; this end is clipped with a small artery forceps. The needle is then introduced back into the bowel lumen and the posterior wall of the anastomosis is constructed uniting the posterior walls of the rectum and colon with a continuous over-and-over suture. Although it is not our preference to lock this suture, other surgeons do so. When the lateral apical suture on the mesenteric side is reached, the type of suture changes to a Connell or 'loop on mucosa' suture. This has the advantage of inverting the mucosa as it is continued on the anterior wall of the anastomosis until the lateral apical suture on the antimesenteric pole is reached. The suture is then tied to its proximal end which has been left long specifically for this purpose. The anastomosis is then completed by the insertion of a row of Lembert sutures on the anterior wall (Figure 32.29). These are placed as mattress sutures so as to secure a better grip on the rectal wall. The tails of each suture are left long and held by an assistant so as to assist in the insertion of the next suture.

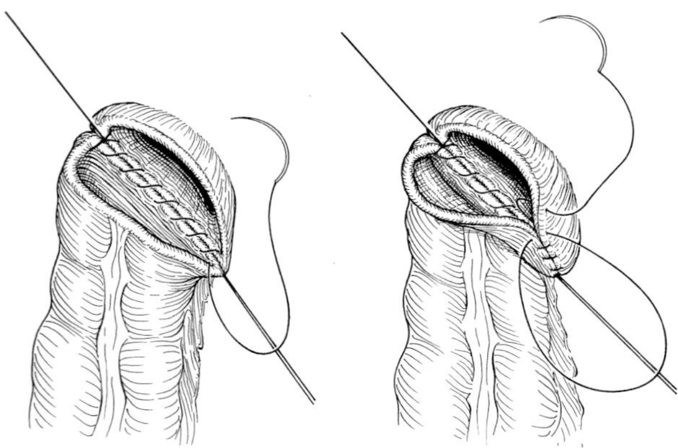

Figure 32.28a,b (a) Insertion of full-thickness, continuous through-and-through posterior layer. (b) The full-thickness, through-and-through suture continues on the anterior wall.

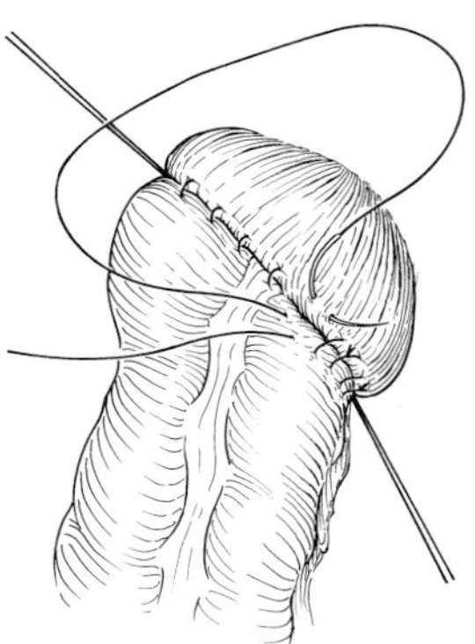

Figure 32.29 Insertion of anterior seromuscular sutures.

One-layer suture technique

Prior to the creation of a one-layer sutured anastomosis, two stay sutures are inserted in the lateral walls of the anorectal stump well below the right-angled clamp. This allows some traction to be exerted on the short stump once the clamp has been removed, and assists the placement of sutures. The right-angled clamp on the anorectal stump is then cut off, as is the Parker–Kerr clamp from the proximal colon. Some bleeding usually takes place from both ends of bowel and this is naturally a comforting sight for the surgeon. Nevertheless, it is important to control this haemorrhage with fine diathermy forceps. Both bowel lumina are irrigated with 1% cetrimide and cefuroxime solutions.

The sutures are then inserted individually between the two ends of bowel (Figure 32.30). The principle is to insert those sutures that will bring the posterior one-half to two-thirds of each lumen together while the ends of bowel are apart. The colonic stump can then be slid into the pelvis on these sutures and this makes completion of the anterior wall of the anastomosis relatively straightforward.

Most surgeons consider it essential to use non-absorbable material such as Ethiflex, Tevdek, silk, linen, etc. for this anastomosis. Despite an absence

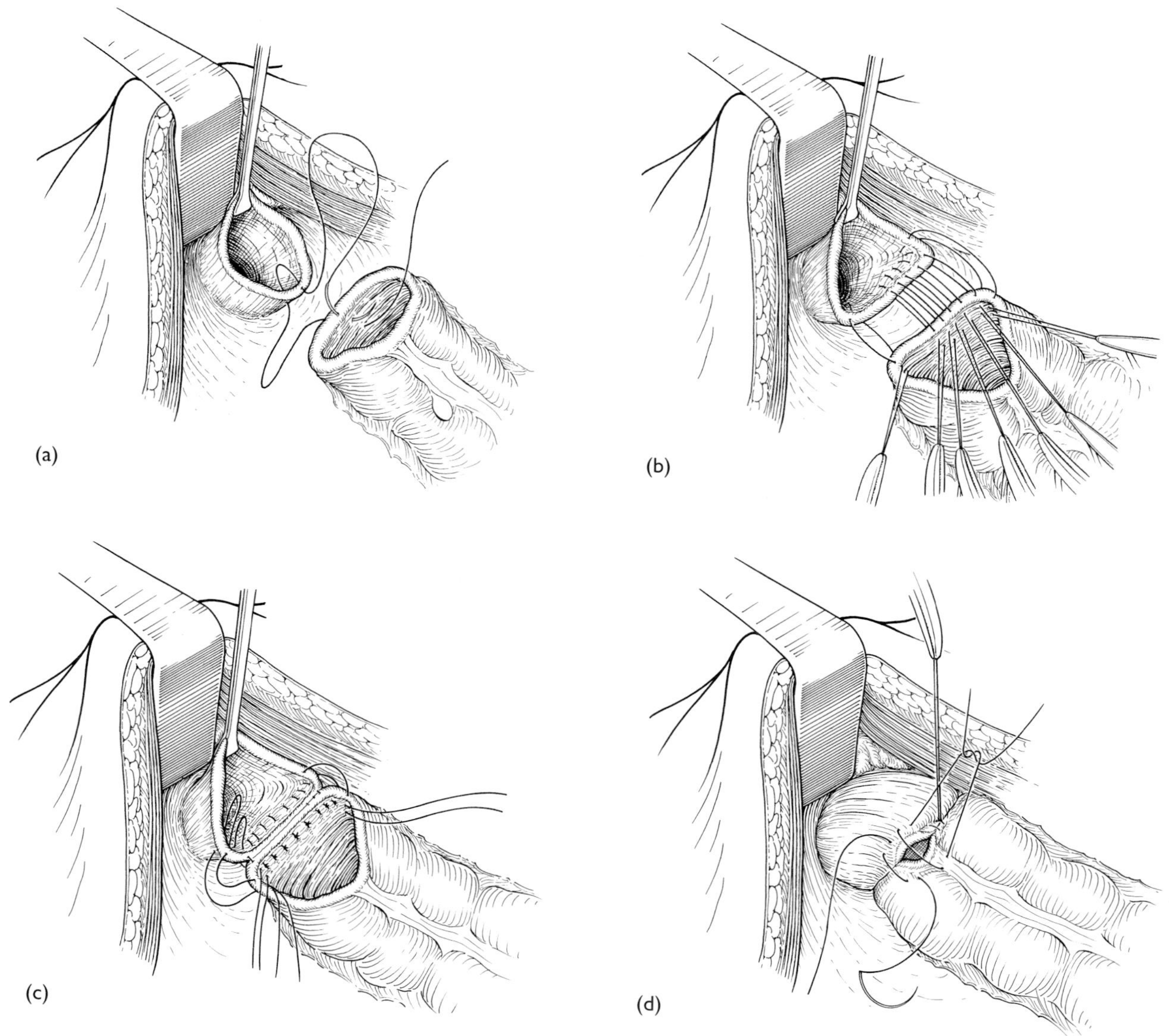

Figure 32.30a–d Anterior resection with one-layer sutured anastomosis. (a) Insertion of first all-coats interrupted mattress suture in the midline posteriorly. (b) Insertion of remaining sutures in the posterior two-thirds of the bowel circumference. (c) The colonic stump is slid down on to the rectal stump and the sutures are tied with the knots on the colonic mucosa. (d) Completion of the anterior layer.

of data, it has been suggested that chromic catgut is quite suitable. We compromise, using 2/0 or 3/0 Vicryl or Maxon which combine strength with eventual degradability. As in the two-layered technique, all sutures are waxed to allow them to glide through the tissues. The first stitch is placed in the midline posteriorly, corresponding to the mesenteric border of both the colonic and rectal stumps. The needle is inserted on the mucosal aspect of the colon 5 mm or so from the cut edge; it passes through the colonic wall and then through the rectal wall to emerge on the mucosal aspect of the rectum at a similar distance from the cut edge. It returns from rectum to colon by picking up the edges of first the colonic mucosa and then the rectal mucosa. The ends of the suture are then grasped in the tips of small artery forceps and the needle is cut off. Although this type of mattress suture is the most popular, some surgeons believe that it is preferable not to traverse the mucosa; they insert their sutures in a similar way through the muscle and seromuscular walls but not through the mucosa.

Once the midline suture has been inserted, two sutures are placed on either side of it approximately one-third of the way around the circumference. The gaps between these sutures are then filled in with exactly the same type of suture, each separated by a distance of 4–5 mm. When the sutures of the posterolateral two-thirds of the proposed anastomosis are in place they are held taut in the surgeon's left hand and the colonic stump is gently slid down into the pelvis where it is apposed to the rectal stump. The sutures are then tied, starting with the one in the midline. After all the sutures have been tied a defect remains in the anterior one-third of the circumference. This is then closed using interrupted sutures of the Gambee variety. Sometimes it is impossible to insert the latter sutures in the correct manner but Lembert sutures of horizontal mattress type will suffice.

After the anastomosis is thought to be complete it is rotated so that the posterior aspect can be inspected and any defect repaired. The stay sutures are then removed.

Technique with circular stapling device

Since Fain et al (1975) introduced to the Western surgical world the concept of using a stapling gun to effect a low colorectal anastomosis, it has gradually become the most popular method of anastomosis.

The original instrument used by Fain was the Russian SPTU gun. Its main disadvantage was that each staple had to be loaded into the instrument by hand, which was a tedious manoeuvre. Thus although cheap to use, the instrument was rapidly superseded by the American version, the EEA instrument marketed by United States Surgical Corporation (USSC). This proved to be a reliable instrument and because it had a disposable anvil and cartridge section eliminated the need for manual loading of the staples. Its other advantage over the Russian instrument was that it achieved an anastomosis with two layers of staples as opposed to one layer. It must be stated, however, that in the only controlled trial comparing the two types of instruments both were found to be equally reliable (Blamey and Lee, 1982). The main drawback of the American instrument has been its cost. The metal EEA gun with disposable anvil and cartridge section was then superseded by completely disposable instruments. The completely disposable EEA gun marketed by USSC came in two designs, one with a straight shaft and one with a curved shaft, the latter being designed to negotiate the sacral hollow. Ethicon also marketed a completely disposable instrument, the Proximate ILS. There were a variety of sizes of gun depending on the outside diameter of the shoulder piece: the ILS design had four sizes (21 mm, 25 mm, 29 mm and 33 mm), whereas the EEA design had only three sizes (26 mm, 28 mm and 31 mm). The equipment also came with 'sizers' which could be inserted into the bowel lumen prior to insertion of the gun and would indicate which size of anvil was required. With the disposable gun marketed by Ethicon the height of the staples could be varied.

In an attempt to improve this form of instrumentation further, USSC introduced another design, the Premium CEEA. This has a completely detachable anvil which is connected to its shaft or cartridge section as an integral unit. This allows the proximal bowel lumen to be more easily positioned over the anvil and allows the purse-string suture to be tied more securely (see below). The most recent modification of the Premium CEEA instrument is the Premium Plus CEEA which has a spring-loaded anvil that flips to the horizontal position when fired. Such a design aids removal after the instrument has been fired. A similar modification has been introduced by Ethicon with a steel central pin and a detachable anvil which clips over the central pin. These designs of gun have superseded all other designs and are illustrated in Figure 32.31.

All designs of stapling gun consist of an anvil and a shoulder piece with the cartridge section, both mounted on to the distal end of the instrument (Figure 32.31a). These are connected by the shaft of the instrument to the handle rotating wheel at its proximal end. The anvil can be unscrewed from the tip of the shaft. The shoulder piece contains a circular knife on its inner circumference and the staples on its outer circumference. The gap between the anvil and shoulder piece can be closed or opened depending on the direction in which the rotating wheel is moved. In the CEEA instrument there is an automatic check device which prevents the gap between anvil and shoulder piece being reduced to less than 2.0 mm and thus prevents damage by pressure to the walls of the colon and rectum. One refinement of the ILS instrument is that the gap between the anvil and shoulder piece can be varied according to the amount of tissue between them. The latter can be measured using a special device. There are no data as yet to show whether this refinement is an advantage.

The instrument is inserted closed through the anus and then by means of the rotating wheel is racked open so that the anvil and shoulder piece become separated. Both the proximal and distal bowel edges are tied circumferentially to the shaft of the instrument using purse-string sutures which have previously been inserted into the

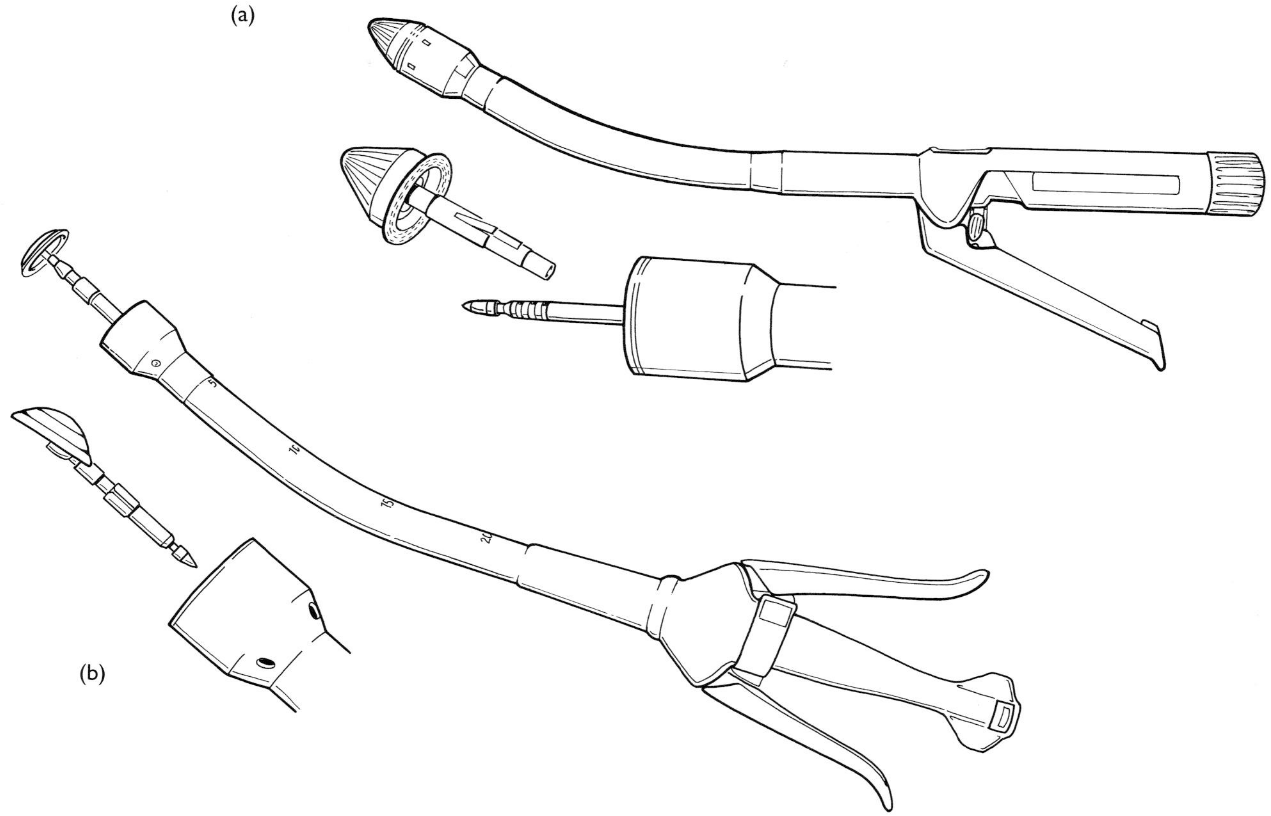

Figure 32.31a,b (a) Ethicon ILS circular stapling gun with detachable anvil. (b) Autosuture Premium Plus CEEA instrument with detachable 'tilt top' anvil.

circumference of the colon and rectum. The gap between the anvil and shoulder piece is then closed to the appropriate distance. The safety catch is released and the gun fired by compressing the handle. During firing the circular knife within the shoulder piece moves upwards and cuts off the bowel edge contained in the purse-string from both the rectal and colonic ends. It should do this in such a way that the cut edge of the bowel remains intact circumferentially and when removed from the instrument is doughnut shaped. Simultaneously with the movement of the knife, the staples emerge from their housing in the circumference of the shoulder piece. They are positioned in the shoulder piece opened with their prongs facing upwards towards the anvil. As they emerge from their housing they transfix both edges of the colon and rectum before becoming impaled in an individual small depression in the anvil. The force of collision with the anvil forces each staple prong to bend inwards and it then resembles a capital letter B lying on its side. In this way the circumferences of the colon and rectum are stapled together to form the anastomosis. The anvil and shoulder piece containing the retracted circular knife and 'doughnuts' of tissue are very slightly opened, the whole instrument is gently twisted until free within the lumen and it is then gently withdrawn.

With the Premium CEEA and Premium plus CEEA the anvil of the instrument and its attached shaft can be completely separated from the shoulder piece. The anvil can then be inserted into the proximal bowel lumen and the purse-string suture tied around it. The anvil and its shaft are inserted into the hollow shaft of the shoulder piece. The latter occupies the centre of the shoulder piece and can be advanced or retracted by turning the rotating wheel. Often the Premium instrument is used when the rectal stump has been transected using a transverse stapling instrument (i.e. the double stapling technique). In this situation the shoulder piece is inserted through the anal canal with its hollow shaft containing a trocar connection fully retracted. The trocar point is then advanced through the apex of the closed rectal stump by turning the rotating wheel in the appropriate direction. The trocar is removed and the anvil shaft pushed home into the hollow shaft of the shoulder piece. The two components of the gun are then racked together as with the earlier designed instrument. The gun is 'fired' in the usual way. Essentially the same process is used with the Ethicon detachable anvil, the only difference being that the trocar is not removed so that the anvil and shaft (which is hollow) engage over the trocar (Figure 32.31b). As in the ILS, the distance between the shoulder piece and anvil can be varied according to the thickness of bowel within it.

Operative details

Using the conventional technique, the rectum is divided above the clamp as described for the one-layer manual anastomosis. Haemostasis is obtained and a purse-string suture is inserted circumferentially into the cut edge of the rectal stump. A variety of materials may be used for this crucial suture: whichever is chosen should glide through the tissues with ease and be strong enough so that there is no risk of snapping at the critical time when the knot is tied. For these reasons we prefer to use a 1/0 polypropylene suture on an atraumatic small needle. Occasionally if the wall of the rectum is thin we use a 0/0 suture. We also lubricate this suture to be absolutely certain that it will 'run' when the purse-string is tied. If the rectal stump is very low and difficult to reach for the placement of the purse-string suture, its wall may have to be grasped with Babcock or Allis tissue forceps, but we try to avoid this if at all possible as there is a real risk that the rectal wall may be torn by overzealous traction.

The purse-string suture should be commenced in the midline anteriorly; this greatly facilitates subsequent tying of the purse-string. The needle is inserted from outside the lumen to inside 5 mm from the cut edge. The end of the suture is left long and clipped with artery forceps. The needle then is passed from inside the lumen to outside and then from outside to inside as a series of transverse mattress sutures approximately 4–5 mm apart (Figure 32.32a). This stitch continues around the whole circumference of the rectal wall until it reaches the point of commencement. The suture is then continued just past the starting point so that there is some overlap. The needle should then finish up on the outside of the bowel lumen. Gentle traction must be exerted on the two ends of the suture to ensure that it will run freely and to assess how easy it will be to tie the purse-string (Figure 32.32b). This is important, for once the gun lies within the lumen failure of the rectal stump purse-string suture to run and tighten may result in technical failure. If the purse-string is tested prior to gun insertion and seems unsatisfactory, it should be cut out and reinserted.

All layers of the bowel wall should be included in the purse-string suture, but deep bites should not be taken since too much tissue bulk within the lumen of the bowel may cause problems for the circular knife. Some surgeons prefer to place their suture as an over-and-over whip stitch rather than using the transverse mattress suture. Bokey and Pheils (1980) prefer to place the distal purse-string suture before they excise the growth. They leave a large open sigmoidoscope within the rectal lumen to assist them

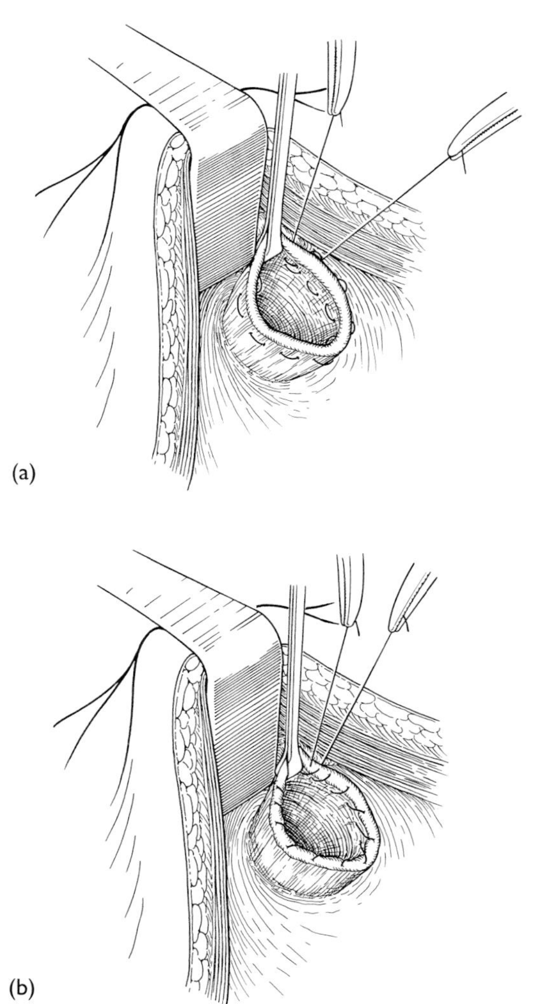

Figure 32.32a,b (a) Insertion of purse-string suture in the rectal stump. This should be continued past the starting point so there is some overlap. (b) The purse-string is pulled taut to demonstrate it glides easily through the tissues and will be capable of occluding the lumen round the shaft of the stapling instrument.

in the placement of the suture. The bowel wall is then cut off just above the stitch. The only disadvantage of such methods is that they fail to invert the mucosa and this may cause problems with the circular knife. One advantage, however, of Bokey and Pheils' technique is that the presence of the sigmoidoscope helps elevate a very low rectal stump and assists the placement of the purse-string.

Another method (which we prefer) for insertion of the suture into a low rectal stump is to insert each stitch into the bowel wall as the bowel below the right-angle clamp is gradually divided from the anorectal stump. This allows traction upwards to be exerted on the rectal stump thus elevating it from the pelvis. However, this manoeuvre may be difficult in the presence of a bulky tumour. Another trick for insertion of the difficult purse-string is to obtain the services of the most robust assistant. If he clenches his fist and inserts it with all his might into the perineum between the ischial tuberosities, the pelvic floor and rectal stump will be elevated 2–3 cm. With such a prolonged isometric contraction of the arm muscles, however, he must be allowed to rest from time to time!

In the very difficult case it is feasible to insert the rectal purse-string from below. This can be done either transanally with the use of a trivalve speculum or by eversion of the anorectal stump. Both these methods have their disadvantages since both cause disruption or considerable stretching of the anorectal ring. It must be said that the endoanal method can be technically extremely difficult. In addition, tying the purse-string in such cases tends to be a blind procedure. The main criticism of the eversion technique is the potential damage caused to the anal sphincter, for to evert the anal stump requires complete mobilization and downward traction. In our experience if the purse-string suture cannot be inserted via the abdominal route under direct vision, it is safer to consider performing a manual transanal coloanal anastomosis.

The stapling gun used to come with a double Furniss clamp, and if a straight needle and 2/0 polypropylene stitch are placed through the holes at each end of the clamp (Figure 32.33) a purse-string suture may be inserted into the rectal stump. Such a technique sounds simple and straightforward, but in practice it is virtually impossible to use deep in the pelvis. We never use this method for the rectal stump, even with the newer improved clamps, since where it is feasible to use it – that is to say within the abdominal cavity – we prefer to use a manual anastomosis and not a stapled one.

Once the rectal purse-string is in place the colonic purse-string is inserted. We prefer to use a transverse mattress stitch as for the rectal stump, but it is quite reasonable to use the Furniss clamp or its modern counterparts in this situation.

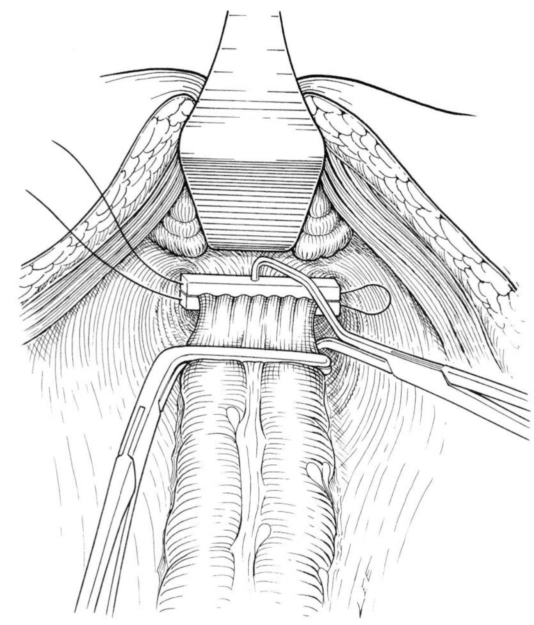

Figure 32.33 Insertion of the rectal purse-string suture using a Furniss clamp.

The size of anvil and cartridge section for the gun is next chosen. It is always desirable to use the largest size possible; i.e. 33 mm (ILS) or 31 mm (CEEA). In practice the size is limited by the diameter of the colonic lumen. This is one of the strongest arguments for mobilizing the splenic flexure and excising all the sigmoid and lower descending colon with the tumour so that as wide as possible a colonic lumen is used for the anastomosis. Although the latter is invariably smaller than the rectal lumen, the colon may go into spasm when transected especially if the blood supply is tenuous. If this occurs the diameter is much smaller than appreciated by the inexperienced operator. The more cavalier surgeon wishing to use the larger head may split the colonic wall. Conversely, the more timid may use too small a head with the greater risk of subsequent anastomotic stricture formation and staple failure, owing to there being insufficient bowel wall between the shaft and the circle of staples. In order to overcome these problems, at the Royal London Hospital we dilate the colonic stump using Hegar's dilators gradually to size 22 or 24F. This can usually be performed without damage. The largest Hegar's dilator is left *in situ* for a few minutes. The middle sizer is then inserted into the colonic lumen, followed by the largest if feasible, and this is left *in situ* until the head of the gun is ready for insertion. In Birmingham we always take down the splenic flexure so that the wider descending colon is used for anastomosis, and dilate the colonic purse-string site with a Foley catheter whose balloon is inflated to the same diameter as the anvil.

If the ILS gun is to be used, the manufacturers recommend that the thickness of the bowel walls should be measured prior to insertion of the instrument. This is achieved using their tissue measuring device which is closed across the anteroposterior aspect of the rectum so that the walls are apposed firmly. The measurement is then recorded as a double thickness of bowel wall. The colon is also measured and this value is added to that obtained for the rectum, and the sum divided by two. The width between the anvil and the shoulder piece of the gun should be adjusted to accommodate the width of bowel derived from this measurement. The manufacturers suggest that if this width is less than 1.0 mm or greater than 3.0 mm a stapled anastomosis should not be performed. It should be pointed out that the degree of error of the method has never been determined, but our observations suggest that it is relatively high, particularly since the measurement is made prior to tying the purse-string.

Preparations are complete for the insertion of the gun once the rectal stump has been washed out with 1% cetrimide. The introduction of the Premium CEEA and the Ethicon ILS circular stapling instruments with their detachable anvils have made the older designs virtually obsolete.

The head, shoulder piece and upper part of the shaft of the instrument are well lubricated with K-Y jelly and the instrument is closed. It is then inserted through the anus after the anal sphincter has been gently dilated. The assistant who inserts and fires the gun should be properly trained in the technique. The instrument is advanced upwards through the anorectal stump until its head just emerges from the top (Figure 32.34). It may be necessary for the abdominal operator to assist its passage around the sacral hollow by placing a hand behind the anorectum and moving both it and the instrument anteriorly. Once the top of the anvil of the instrument is glimpsed by the abdominal operator, the assistant is told to stop advancing the instrument and to open it as fully as possible by rotating the knob or wheel at the base of the shaft in an anticlockwise direction. This manoeuvre separates the anvil from the shoulder piece by 6–8 cm above the rectal stump and ensures that the upper margin of the shoulder piece and cartridge lies still within the stump.

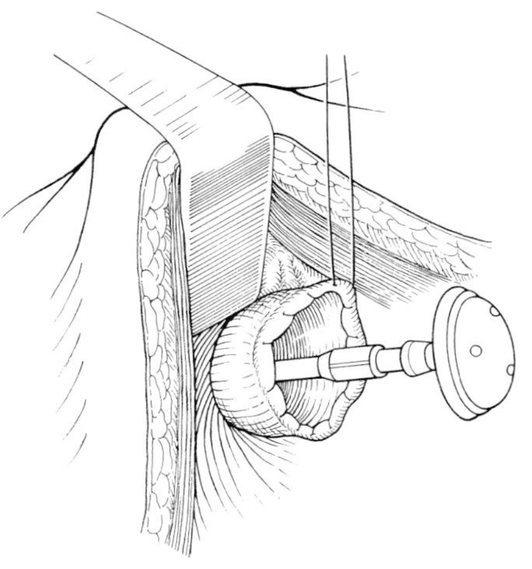

Figure 32.34 The stapling gun has been inserted through the anal canal to emerge through the open rectal stump. The instrument is opened so that the anvil advances into the pelvis.

Angulation of the whole instrument forwards by the assistant, depressing the shaft backwards, allows easy access to the anvil.

The anvil section is then detached from the shaft of the instrument and inserted into the lumen of the colon. This is done by first removing the sizer or Foley catheter and then applying three long-handled Babcock or Allis tissue forceps equidistantly on the cut edge of the bowel wall (Figure 32.35). One forceps is sited on the anterior antimesenteric border and the others on the two posterolateral walls. Traction of these forceps opens up the lumen sufficiently for the anvil to be gently inserted into the lumen. The purse-string is then tied on the shaft of the instrument. The rectal purse-string should then be tied on to the shaft. Great care is needed during this manoeuvre to close the purse-string completely and yet avoid snapping the suture or tying a poor knot which might slip.

The shaft, which is connected to the anvil as one unit, is then pushed into the hollow shaft of the shoulder piece, or over the trochar in the case of the Ethicon instrument (Figure 32.36). It is important to push this home firmly until it clicks into place. Care should also be taken during this manoeuvre not to press the button on the side of the anvil, since by so doing the anvil can become detached from its shaft.

When both purse-string sutures have been tied, the space between the anvil and shoulder piece is closed by turning the wheel or knob at the end of the shaft in a clockwise direction. It is essential

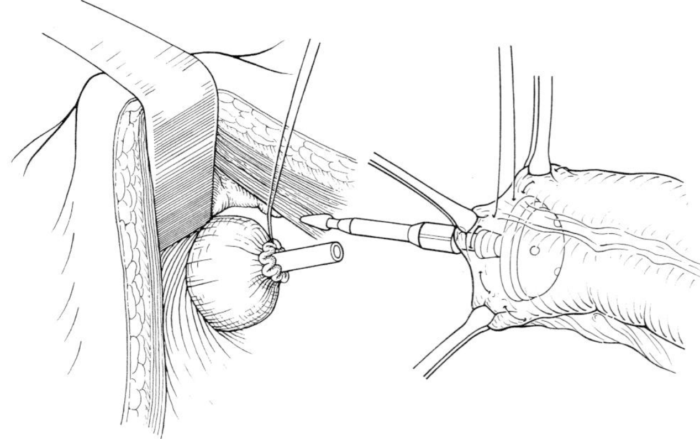

Figure 32.35 The anvil is separated from the shaft and is inserted into the open lumen of the proximal colon using three Allis or Babcock tissue forceps. Once in place the purse suture is tied securely round the shaft of the instrument, as is the rectal purse-string.

during this procedure to ensure that only the bowel wall is included in the gap, and in particular that the vagina does not become trapped within the gun. To this end the assistant gently pushes the whole instrument upwards so that the apex of the rectal stump is stretched outwards radially from the tied purse-string round the shaft. Similarly the surgeon exerts upwards traction on the colon and stretches the colonic apex over the shoulder piece (Figure 32.36). The instrument is closed by turning the wing nut of the CEEA instrument in a clockwise direction until the green dot located in the tissue approximation indicator is partially visible within the black markings. Similarly, the ILS instrument is closed by rotating the knob in a clockwise direction until the black line on the gap adjusting scale lies within the green markings.

The gun is now ready for firing. The safety catch is released, and while the shaft of the instrument is held firm with one hand, the handle is approximated to the shaft with the other hand in a steady, firm movement. There is a crunching sound which can also be felt as the staples cross the bowel wall and impinge on the anvil, and the circular knife cuts through the inverted bowel edges and the two purse-string polypropylene sutures. Once the operator is satisfied that firing has occurred, which is confirmed by both polypropylene sutures being cut, the gun is opened slightly and then rotated clockwise and anticlockwise until it feels free and can be withdrawn. However, occasionally the gun cannot be withdrawn easily and the anastomosis can be seen to intussuscept into the rectal stump as withdrawal takes place. In these circumstances the surgeon should not exert force. The instrument should be returned to its former position and rotated some more, and then the anastomosis should be grasped with a dry gauze swab around its whole circumference. The assistant should then attempt to withdraw while the surgeon exerts some upward traction. Sometimes it is advisable for the surgeon to take the shaft of the gun in the left hand and the anastomosis in the right hand so that both, under the control of one person, can be gently disengaged. These manoeuvres are usually sufficient to release most instruments.

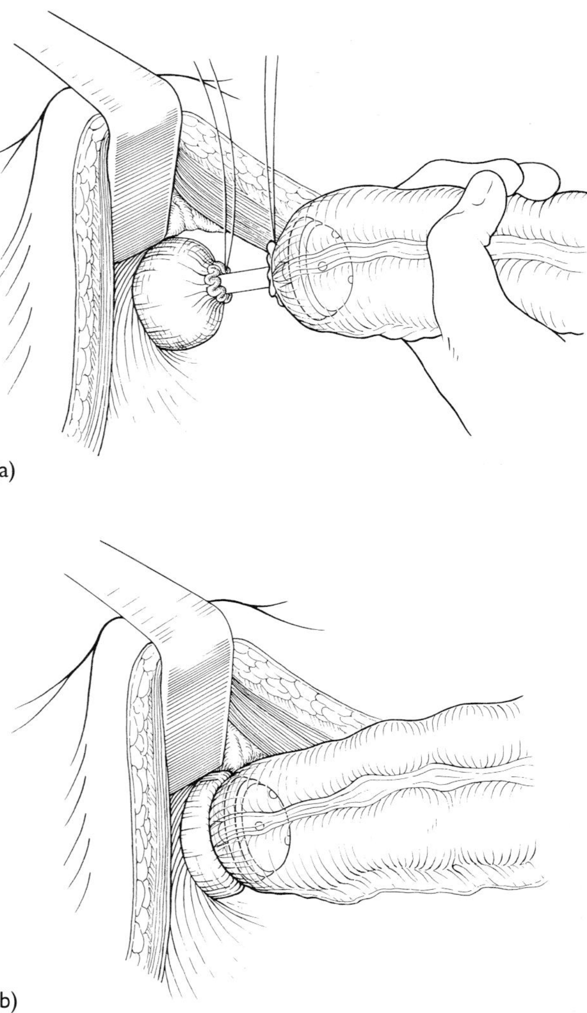

Figure 32.36a,b (a) The shaft of the anvil is inserted into the hollow shaft of the shoulder piece. (b) The instrument is then closed while gentle traction is exerted on the colon in an upwards direction and it is ensured that no extraneous tissue insinuates itself between the two ends. The instrument is completely closed, fired and then removed.

If the gun still cannot be withdrawn, a short colotomy may have to be made above the anastomosis so that the anvil of the instrument is accessible; it can then be unscrewed and the shaft can safely be removed. The colotomy can then be closed. We have fortunately never had to perform this manoeuvre but would imagine that by the time the colotomy is made, the anastomosis would be so unsatisfactory that it would either have to be repeated or abandoned. Although not experiencing this particular misfortune, we have in the past certainly had other difficulties; the most notable ones include failure of the gun to fire and missing staples. However, with the most recent designs, these problems seem to have disappeared.

After the withdrawal of the instrument it is essential to make sure that the anastomosis is complete and that there are no defects. Some suggestion of how satisfactory the anastomosis will be is obtained by examination of the 'doughnuts'. These can be retrieved by unscrewing the anvil and digging them out from the anvil and shoulder piece. They are laid out on a flat surface and the purse-string sutures are cut (Buchmann and Uhlschmid, 1980) (Figure 32.37). If both 'doughnuts' are intact the surgeon can be reasonably happy that the anastomosis is secure. If, however, one or both 'doughnuts' are not complete it is certain that there will be a defect in the anastomosis.

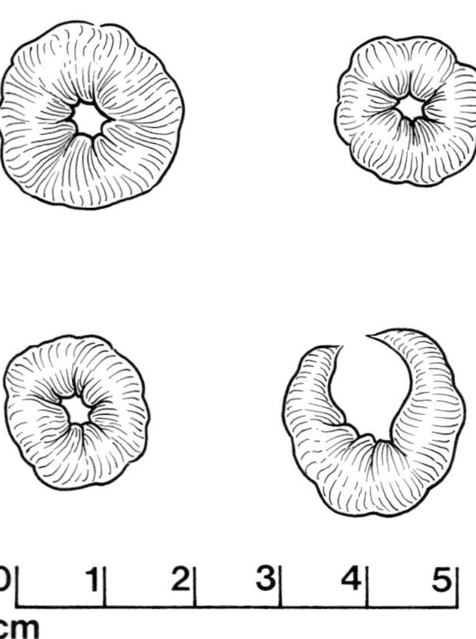

Figure 32.37 After firing and removal of the gun the 'doughnuts' should be retrieved. An incomplete 'doughnut' indicates a defect in the anastomosis.

The anastomosis should be inspected if possible for the site of a defect. Unfortunately, it is not usually possible in these low anastomoses to obtain a satisfactory view of the whole circumference. One method of testing the integrity of the anastomosis is to fill the pelvis with saline or sterile water. Air is then injected via a small catheter into the anorectal stump with a soft, non-crushing clamp above the anastomosis; if an anastomotic defect exists air bubbles will be seen to emerge from it. This we term a 'Jacuzzi' positive test. After the defect has been identified it should be reinforced by seromuscular sutures from above if possible. Occasionally this is impossible but it may be possible to insert through-and-through sutures transanally into the defect in these cases. After the anastomosis has been reinforced it should be tested again under water. If despite forceful distensions of the rectum with air no air leak is observed, it may not be absolutely necessary to raise a proximal stoma. However, as a general rule, any patient in whom there has been a technical problem and in whom the surgeon cannot be sure about the integrity of the anastomosis, should have a covering stoma performed (see later).

Cross stapling technique using the gun

An alternative technique to the one described above (Knight and Griffen, 1980; Yule and Fiddian, 1983) is to staple across the rectal stump with a TA55 (Autosuture) or TL60 or TL30 (Ethicon) stapling instrument or the Roticulator (Autosuture) or Articulating linear stapling (Ethicon) instrument. The TA30 or TL30 can sometimes be used, but only if the anus is transected. Some surgeons now routinely excise the entire mesorectum in middle and lower-third rectal cancer, and thus prefer to cross-staple the anus on the basis that there is less risk of anastomotic breakdown. If this is the case, the TL30 instrument is ideally suited, especially in a narrow male pelvis. The Roticulator or Articulating linear stapler is particularly useful since the transverse stapling component can be angulated on the shaft of the instrument making application much easier (Figure 32.38). However, these instruments are difficult to use low in the male pelvis.

Once the transverse stapler has been fired, a right-angled clamp is placed approximately 1 cm above it. Using a long-handled knife, the rectum is transected cutting directly on to the stapling instrument. After the specimen has been removed, the transverse stapling instrument is disengaged from the rectal stump leaving it stapled transversely. The Premium CEEA or the Ethicon equivalent can be used (Figure 32.39). These instruments were designed specifi-

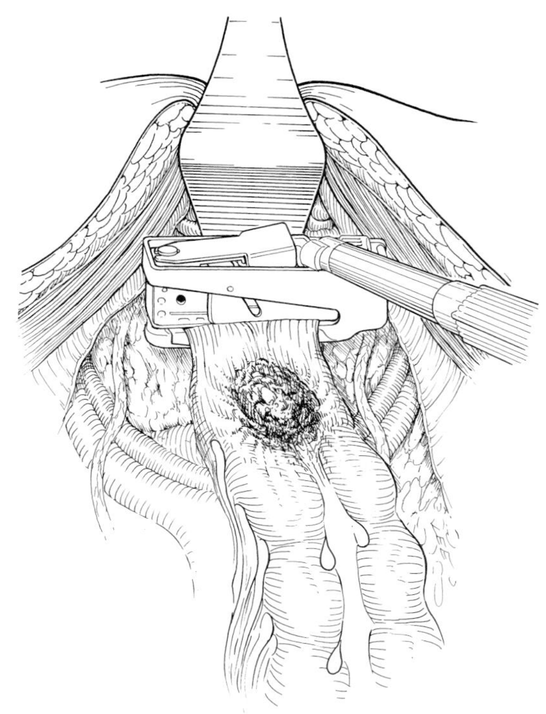

Figure 32.38 Cross-stapling of the rectum below the tumour using a Roticulator instrument prior to anastomosis using the Premium CEEA instrument.

cally for this procedure. The shoulder piece without the anvil is gently introduced into the anal canal and advanced up to the transverse stapled line. Great care must be exercised during this part of the procedure. If excessive force is applied to push the shoulder piece towards the pelvis, the staple line may split. The instrument is opened and the trocar of the shoulder piece is used to pierce the apex of the stapled rectal stump (Figure 32.39a). The trocar is then removed from its hollow shaft (in the case of the Premium CEEA) or left *in situ* (the Ethicon instrument). The anvil is inserted into the colonic lumen and the purse-string suture tied around its attached shaft. The anvil is then inserted into the hollow shaft of the shoulder piece, or slid over the trocar in the case of the Ethicon instrument, and pushed home (Figure 32.39b). The gun is then closed in the usual way and fired (Figure 32.39c).

Such a technique eliminates the need for the insertion of the distal rectal purse-string but has the disadvantage that two staple lines are juxtaposed and there is the theoretical risk of ischaemia developing between them. However, we now use this technique virtually exclusively and have not noticed an increase in our leak rate. There are now a number of reports attesting to the feasibility and safety of the technique (Feinberg et al, 1986; Nogueras et al, 1991; Griffen et al, 1992; Redmond et al, 1993; Moran et al, 1994). However, Moran (1996) in an excellent review of stapling techniques could only find one randomized trial in the literature. In this study 70 patients were randomized to single or double stapling. There was no significant difference in all parameters examined, but there was a trend towards a lower leak rate after double stapling (Moritz et al, 1991).

Another possible theoretical objection to this technique in malignant disease is that even when a cytocidal washout has been used before transecting the rectum, viable cells could be introduced into the crushed tissue, causing early pelvic recurrence. Ideally, the rectal stump should be irrigated below an occlusion clamp before stapling.

If a double-stapling technique is used, it is often difficult to apply the linear staple below the clamp, especially in a narrow pelvis. A new technique has been described (Moran et al, 1994). The linear stapler TA 30,55 (Autosuture) TL30,60 (Ethicon) is placed distal to the tumour after full mobilization of the rectum; it is then closed and fired. The stapler is unlocked and removed to leave an occlusive row of staples. The rectum is irrigated and may be inspected if desired. A further cartridge is loaded on the TA55 which is then reapplied across the cleaned rectum distal to the proximal occlusion staple line and fired (Figure 32.40). The rectum is sectioned above the TA55 stapler and standard double stapling is then performed. This technique has been termed 'triple stapling' (Moran, 1996) and is the one we usually recommend; but if the washout can be performed with a clamp across the bowel below the tumour, we often simply use the double-stapling method.

Additional manoeuvres after completion of anastomosis

Following completion of a low anastomosis, by whatever technique, the need for additional techniques requires consideration.

First is the question of closure of the pelvic peritoneum. For many years it was usual practice to ensure that the pelvic peritoneum was closed above the anastomosis. The logic behind this manoeuvre was that if a leak occurred from the anastomosis it would remain outside the peritoneal cavity and be less dangerous to the patient. However, most surgeons today leave the peritoneum open and as a consequence this allows small intestine and omentum to descend into the pelvis around the anastomosis. It is believed by some that the presence of these struc-

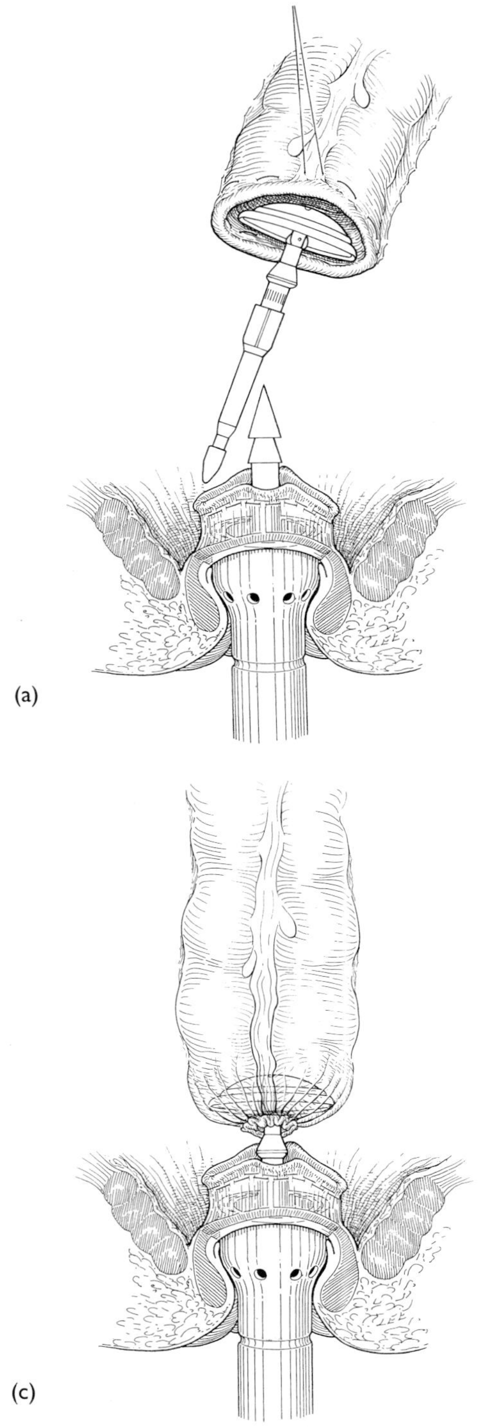

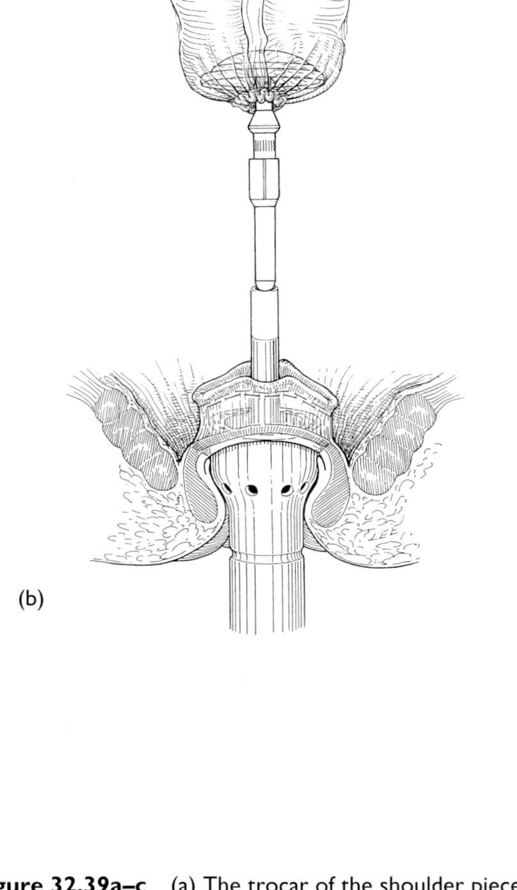

Figure 32.39a–c (a) The trocar of the shoulder piece of the Premium CEEA instrument is inserted through the apex of the stapled rectal stump. The detachable anvil is inserted into the colonic lumen and the purse-string suture is tied. (b) The trocar is removed from the shoulder piece and the stem of the anvil is inserted into the hollow shaft of the shoulder piece. (c) The gun is then closed so that the colonic stump is approximated to the rectal stump.

tures in close association with the anastomosis aids the healing process. It is impossible to support or refute either of these beliefs as no controlled trials have yet been performed. Although we keep an open mind on the subject we do not routinely close the pelvic peritoneum. This policy is adhered to not because of any firm beliefs, but because as a result of our lateral dissection during rectal excision precious little peritoneum remains that can be closed. Wrapping of omentum around the anastomosis is also believed by some to aid healing of the anastomosis and reduce leakage. As discussed elsewhere, there is insufficient information on this topic to recommend routine adoption of the technique.

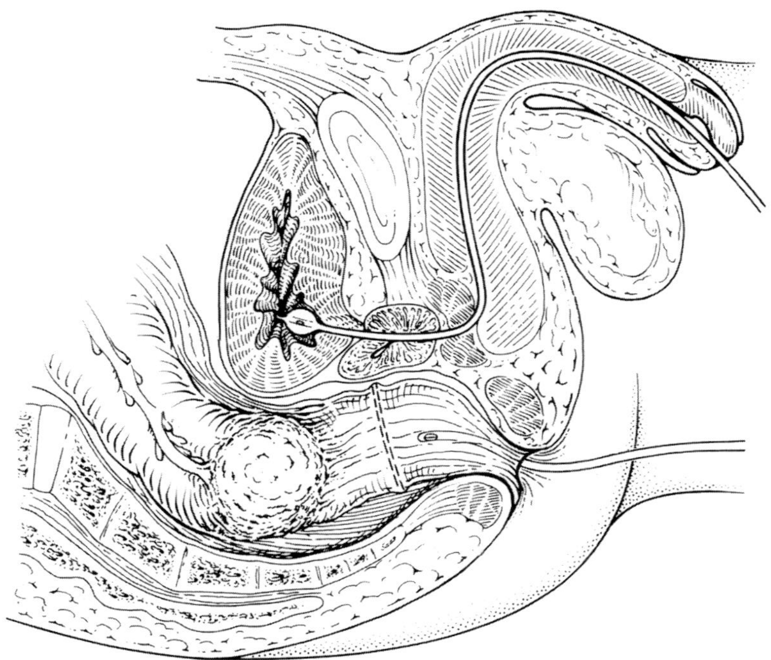

Figure 32.40 The triple-stapling technique. The rectum has been cross-stapled below the tumour and the rectal stump is irrigated peranally with a cytocidal solution. The cleansed rectal stump is then cross-stapled below the occlusion staple line and the rectum is divided proximal to the distal staple line, before standard double stapling.

It is agreed by most surgeons that it is preferable to drain the pelvis after low anterior resection. There is considerable debate, however, as to which is the best method of doing so. A variety of techniques are available, including the combination of irrigation and sump suction popular at the Cleveland Clinic (Fazio, 1978) and suprapubic drainage using sump drains. Our preference is to use a closed suction system of the Portavac variety.

Some surgeons in the past recommended anal dilatation at the completion of the operation (Mayo et al, 1958) in order to paralyse the anal sphincter and so prevent the build-up of flatus or faeces in the rectum which might disrupt the anastomosis. Such a manoeuvre in our view should be avoided, especially for low anastomoses. Damage to the anal sphincter, no matter how mild, may cause serious problems with continence in these patients. Although damage may only be temporary, in some cases it can be permanent and may be quite demoralizing for the patient.

The need for a covering stoma to protect the anastomosis after anterior resection is a contentious issue. There are some who believe that a covering stoma makes no difference to the incidence of leakage and is unnecessary (Bolton and Britton, 1980; Cady et al, 1980; Mittal and Cortez, 1980). Others, however, believe that for all anastomoses below the peritoneal reflection a covering stoma is mandatory (Kirwan, 1981; Goligher, 1984; MacFarlane et al, 1993). We prefer to take a middle line: if there is doubt as to the integrity of the anastomosis, we construct a covering proximal stoma; if the procedure has progressed smoothly, intraoperative testing shows no sign of a leak and (in the case of stapled anastomoses) both 'doughnuts' are intact, a stoma is not constructed. It would appear that this policy is widely adopted in other units (Beart and Kelly, 1981; Weakley, 1981; Blamey and Lee, 1982; Mealy et al, 1992; Grabham et al, 1995), particularly now that considerable experience has been gained with the stapling gun.

Once a covering stoma is decided upon, most surgeons in the past constructed a transverse loop colostomy. We, however, now prefer a loop ileostomy to defunction the anastomosis. We have found this to be aesthetically more pleasing for the patient, easier to manage and as safe as a transverse colostomy (Williams et al, 1986) (Table 32.10), as have other authors (Fasth and Hulten, 1984; HB Devlin, 1986, personal communication).

To avoid the need for a covering stoma, Ravo and his colleagues described the use of an intracolonic bypass (Ravo and Ger, 1985), which is known as the

Table 32.10 Complications related to stoma management: transverse loop colostomy compared with loop ileostomy.

	Colostomy (n = 20)	*Ileostomy* (n = 19)
Bleeding	6 (30%)	2 (11%)
Prolapse	2 (10%)	1 (5%)
Skin excoriation	10 (50%)	5 (26%)
Leakage	8 (40%)	7 (37%)
Odour	13 (65%)*	0
Frequency of appliance change: median (range)	2 days† (1–5)	3 days (1–4)

* $P < 0.01$.
† $P < 0.05$.
From Williams et al (1986).

Coloshield device (Derknatel Pfizer Hospital Products Co Inc). The procedure was designed to protect an anastomosis from the faecal stream without interrupting gastrointestinal continuity (Figure 32.41). A latex tube is sewn into the colonic lumen above the anastomosis and the tube is brought down past the anastomosis and out through the anal canal to the exterior. The end of the tube is inserted into an incontinence bag. The tube remains in place for 15–30 days and faecal contents are collected in the bag. In theory this allows time for the anastomosis to heal and the tube is either removed or becomes detached. The device can be used either with a manual anastomosis or with a stapled anastomosis. Ravo described its use in 29 patients: only three had a complicated postoperative course, and in only one patient was this ascribed to the device.

Keane et al (1988) also described its use in six patients with left-sided colonic obstruction treated by resection and primary anastomosis. The device was passed spontaneously a mean of 13 days postoperatively and there were no leaks or complications associated with the device. We have no experience with this technique. However, since the publication of the first edition of this textbook, we have read of no controlled trials using the device. Similarly, colleagues around the world seem not to employ the technique, and we suspect it has become obsolete.

Abdominotransanal coloanal anastomosis

The principles of this operation are to resect the rectal cancer in the usual way and to re-establish gastrointestinal continuity by bringing the proximal colon through the anorectal stump, the upper part of which is denuded of mucosa as a 'sleeve' anastomosis. The colon is anastomosed to the anal canal via the transanal route, without eversion of the

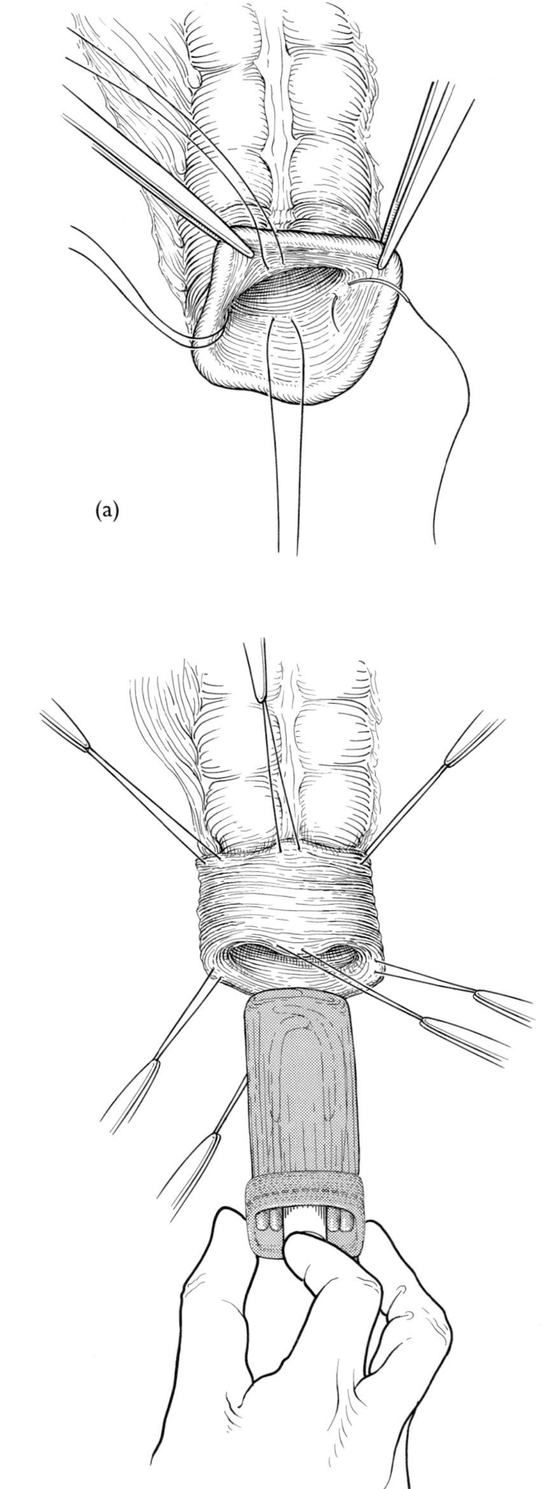

Figure 32.41a–f Coloshield intracolonic bypass procedure. (a) The lumen of the proximal colon is everted 7–10 cm using four stay sutures. (b) The intraluminal tube is lubricated and inserted into the colon. (*Continued*)

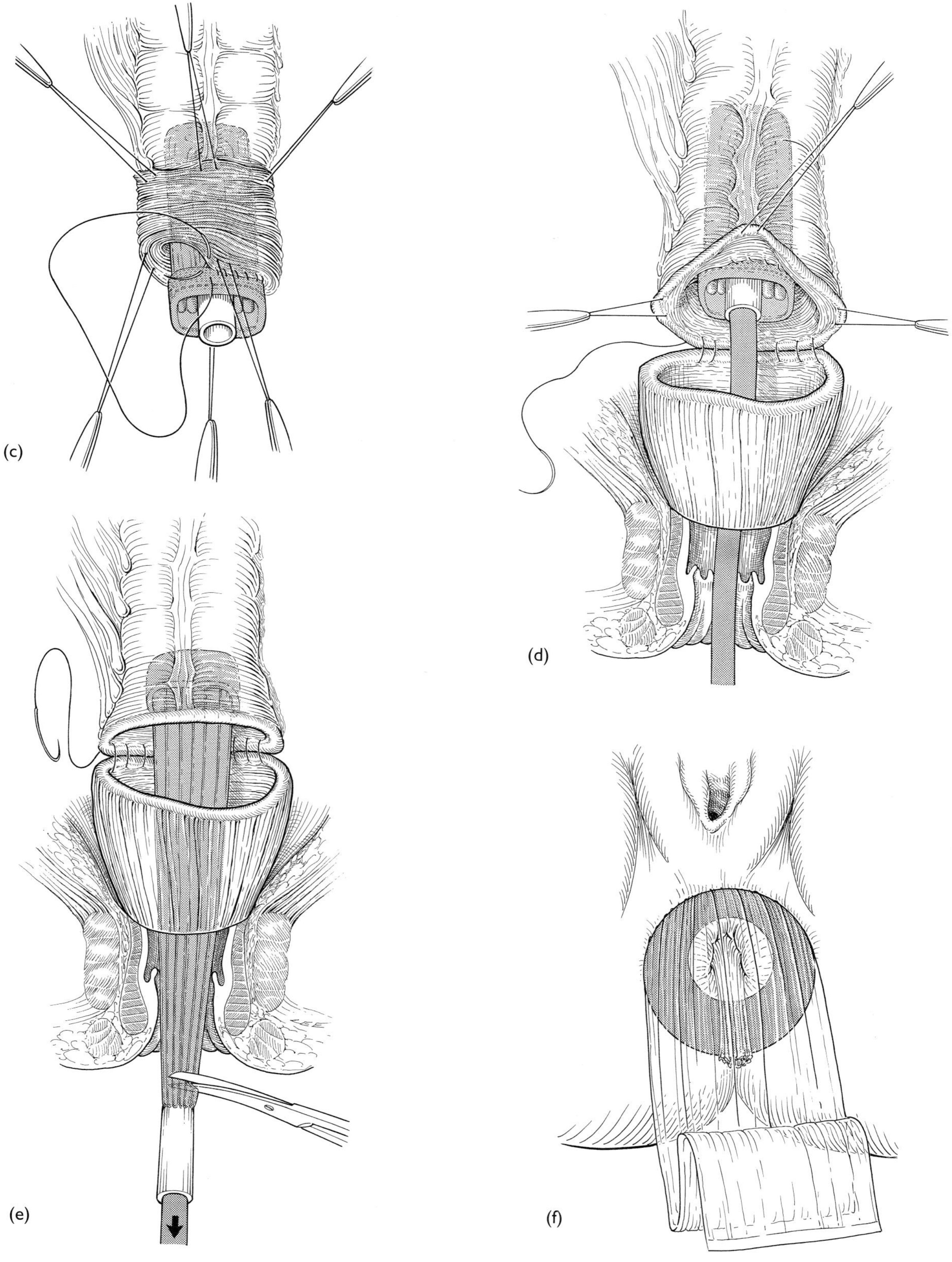

Figure 32.41a–f (*Continued*) (c) The Dacron cuff of the device is sutured to the colon with a running absorbable stitch. (d) The posterior layer of the manual anastomosis is completed and the rectal tube is passed into the Coloshield and the tube is pulled through the anastomosis, which is then completed. (e) The tube is brought out through the anus, its terminal connector is cut off and its end is inserted into the effluent collection bag (f) which is affixed to the perianal skin.

anorectum. Since this manoeuvre causes minimal damage to the sphincteric mechanism, and since receptors responsible for continence seem to lie outside the rectum, normal function can be achieved. Although the ideal is to have enough anorectal stump to produce a sleeve anastomosis, this is not essential and an anastomosis can be performed directly between the colon and the top of the anal canal. The preparation and position of the patient on the table are exactly the same as for a low anterior resection.

Abdominal phase

Adequate mobilization of the colon is essential for this operation. The descending colon should normally be used for the anastomosis and not the sigmoid colon. The latter has a tendency to undergo necrosis in the early postoperative period (particularly if 'high' pedicle ligation is performed) because it is more prone to ischaemia, especially when pulled down into the pelvis. In order therefore to obtain enough length to reach the anal canal, mobilization of the splenic flexure and distal transverse colon is essential and sometimes the hepatic flexure must be mobilized as well. As in anterior resection, the marginal artery should be carefully preserved.

It is important that the colon to be brought down into the pelvis contains no faecal material, for this will result in serious contamination during construction of the anastomosis. If preoperative bowel preparation has been inadequate the best course of action is to perform intraoperative irrigation (Dudley et al, 1980).

When the colon has been thoroughly mobilized, instead of applying a crushing clamp at the proposed transection point we prefer to staple the colon using the TA55 or TL60 stapling instrument. This allows the colon to be brought down to the pelvis while still sealed. If a crushing clamp is used this has to be removed prior to delivery of the colon down into the pelvis and any fluid left within its lumen will contaminate the pelvic tissue and thus increase the risk of sepsis.

The technique of mobilization and resection of the rectum is identical to that used for low anterior resection. Mobilization must extend down to the level of the levator ani muscle so that the upper anal canal is reached (Figure 32.42). In the female the dissection is easier since the rectovaginal plane can be readily opened down to the anal canal. It is important, however, to preserve the integrity of the vagina because a rectovaginal fistula may occur if the vaginal mucosa is exposed. The bowel is clamped and the anal canal is irrigated with a cancericidal agent. The anorectum is transected below the clamp at the level of the levator ani, which should be just below the anorectal junction.

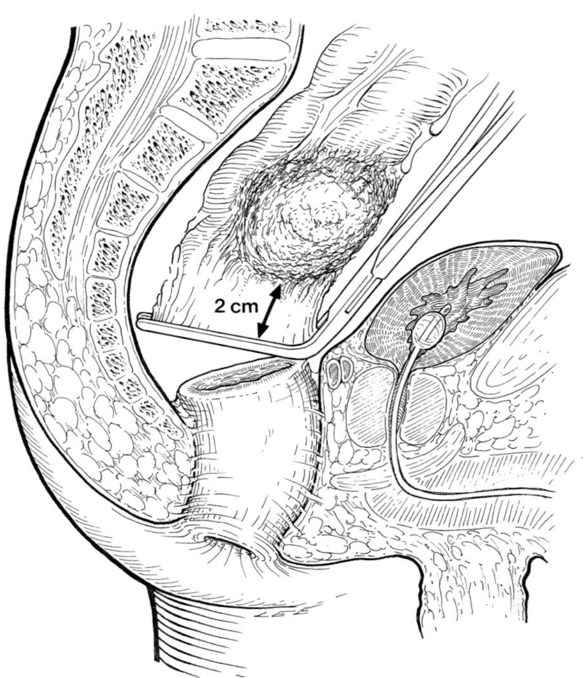

Figure 32.42 The abdominal phase of the abdomino-transanal procedure. The rectum is transected at the level of the pelvic floor a minimum of 2 cm below the carcinoma.

Two stay sutures are placed through the lateral corners of the stapled end of the colon which is to be brought down into the pelvis. These sutures should be of different colours for ease of identification, to prevent rotation of the colon when it is drawn down through the anorectal stump. The perineal operator then takes over and prepares the anal stump for the anastomosis; meanwhile the assistant may construct the defunctioning ileostomy, which is always required to protect this anastomosis.

Perineal phase

The surgeon moves to the perineum. A Parks' self-retaining transanal retractor is inserted into the canal to expose its wall together with any residual rectum (Figure 32.43a). If only the upper anal canal is left, it may be necessary to perform a 'butt-end' anastomosis. However, the ideal is an overlapping or 'sleeve' anastomosis. To this end it is necessary to denude the mucosa from the remnants of the anorectal stump. The submucosal plane just above

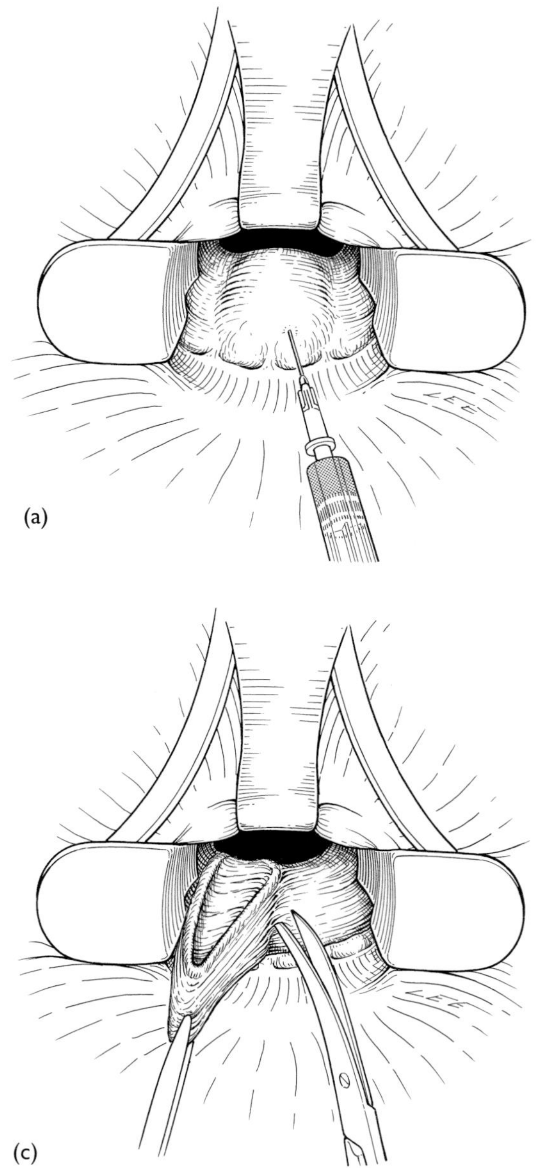

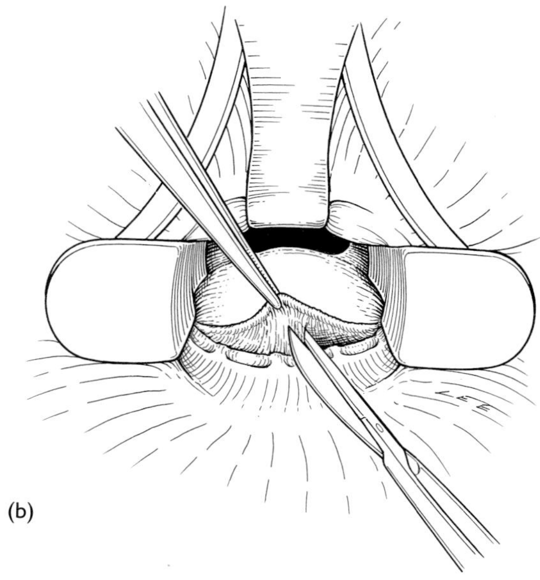

Figure 32.43a–c Perineal phase of the abdominotransanal technique. (a) A Parks self-retaining retractor is inserted into the anal canal and the submucosal plane is infiltrated with a 1 in 300 000 adrenaline saline solution. (b,c) The anorectal mucosa is stripped from the rectal muscle by dissecting in the submucosal plane. The dissection commences at the dentate line and the mucosa is removed as a complete cylinder.

the dentate line is infiltrated with saline and adrenaline solution (1 in 300 000) (Figure 32.43a). The mucosa is then excised with sharp pointed scissors. Parks did this in three or four strips but we prefer to remove the mucosa as a cylinder of tissue (Figure 32.43b,c). This technique ensures that all mucosa is removed. There is a theoretical risk that if nests of mucosal cells remain they will develop cysts between the rectal muscular cuff and the colonic wall which could have an adverse effect on subsequent anorectal function. Although the dissection should be performed as close to the mucosa as possible to avoid submucosal vessels, some bleeding is inevitable. Meticulous haemostasis is crucial to the success of the operation.

The colon is now brought into the pelvis and delivered through the denuded anorectal stump. In order to do this the stay sutures are passed down into the pelvis, grasped by the perineal operator using long artery forceps and gently pulled down through the stump in such a way that the colon is not rotated or twisted (Figure 32.44). The colon must reach the perineum without tension; this is rarely a problem if mobilization of the colon has included the splenic flexure and distal transverse colon. Prior to opening the colon we place four interrupted sutures between the serosa of the colon and the rectal muscle; these sutures are placed, one in each quadrant, by retracting the colon and anal sphincters in opposite directions using thin-bladed

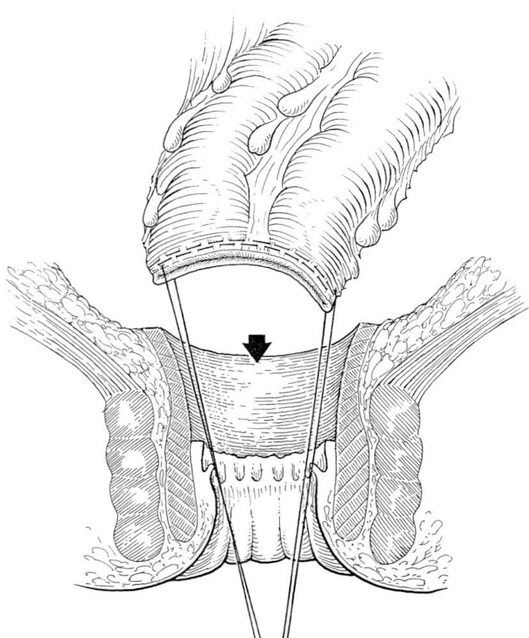

Figure 32.44 Abdominotransanal technique. The stapled end of the colon is brought down through the denuded anorectal cuff using the long stay sutures.

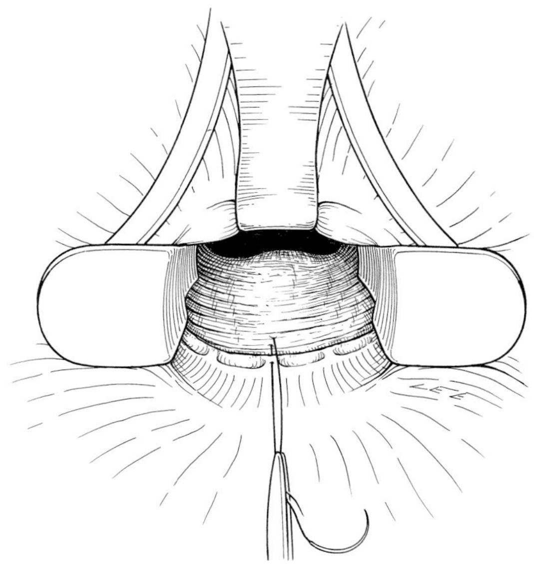

Figure 32.45 Placement of sutures in rectal muscle and cut anal mucosa prior to bringing the colon down. One suture is placed in each quadrant and the needle is left intact.

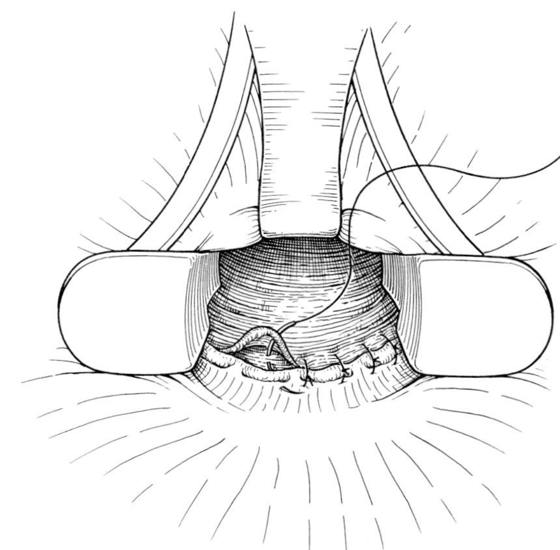

Figure 32.46 The coloanal anastomosis is performed via the transanal route. Note that each suture picks up the underlying rectal muscle.

Lane's or Langenbeck retractors. It is preferable if these sutures are placed in the rectal muscle prior to bringing the colon down (Figure 32.45). If they are left long with the needle attached, it is a relatively simple matter to complete the suture by passing the needle through the colonic serosa. These 'serosal' sutures anchor the colon in the muscular tube and make the mucosa-to-mucosa anastomosis easier. The stapled end of the colon is then excised and any remaining fluid within the lumen is sucked out.

The anastomosis is constructed by first placing four interrupted sutures at each quadrant, each suture traversing the full thickness of the cut edge of the colon and taking a deep bite of the rectal muscle and then traversing the cut edge of the anal canal mucosa (Figure 32.46). These sutures are left untied until they have all been placed. In order to facilitate the anastomosis it is useful to have a thin-bladed retractor within the colonic lumen. Parks used his self-retaining transanal retractor. At the Royal London Hospital we found this rather cumbersome and prefer to use a Sims gynaecological right-angled retractor which an assistant manipulates to retract the wall opposite to that being sutured. Once the four quadrant sutures are in place the anterior one is tied, the right (or left) lateral one is then retracted downwards and the gap between the two is filled in with four or five sutures. When these have all been placed they are tied, and the next quadrant is dealt with in the same manner until the whole circumference has been sutured. A variety of suture materials can be used for this anastomosis; our preference is 2/0 Vicryl on a 25 mm, strong half-circle needle.

In Birmingham we construct the sutured coloanal anastomosis using a slightly different technique. A Parks retractor is placed inside the anal canal with the blades at 3 and 9 o'clock. The open descending colon is delivered through the anal retractor and the anterior and posterior suture lines are completed, leaving the sutures untied until they have been correctly placed. The sutures, which pass through the entire wall of the colon and through the mucosa and internal sphincter of the anus, are then tied except for the four lateral sutures whose ends are left long. The Parks retractor is then withdrawn, closed and rotated through 90 degrees so that the blades are gently inserted into the colon over the completed anterior and posterior suture lines. The retractor is opened to display both lateral aspects of the colon. The anastomosis is then completed in a similar manner between the four corner sutures which have been left long.

Increasingly we both now simply use two Gelpi retractors set at right-angles to one another (Figure 32.47). This allows excellent visualization of the divided anal canal, and affords good exposure for a direct coloanal anastomosis, either as a sleeve anastomosis between the divided colon and the dentate line or a direct end-to-end anastomosis between the extramucosal colonic wall to the internal anal sphincter. Alternatively, the Lone Star retractor may be used for the same technique (Figure 32.48).

At the completion of the anastomosis the abdominal operator leaves the colon lying to the right of the small intestine, attaching its mesentery and mesocolon to the posterior abdominal wall peritoneum (Figure 32.49); this manoeuvre may reduce tension. Suction drainage of the pelvis is essential. In addition, a defunctioning stoma should be constructed in all cases. Our preference is a loop ileostomy. Parks originally used a caecostomy but we have found that no matter how carefully this is managed postoperatively, it invariably ceases to function within a few days. A transverse colostomy should never be used in this operation since its construction will often be difficult and the blood supply to the distal colon and anastomosis may be jeopardized owing to abdominal wall compression of the marginal artery upon which the viability of the colon depends.

The coloanal anastomosis may be constructed using the double-stapling technique by transecting the anus with a TA or TL30 and completing the coloanal anastomosis with the Premium CEEA or the Ethicon equivalent as described for anterior resection. Using this technique the entire rectum is removed with the tumour. If the colon is long enough, the option of a stapled colonic J pouch may provide better reservoir function.

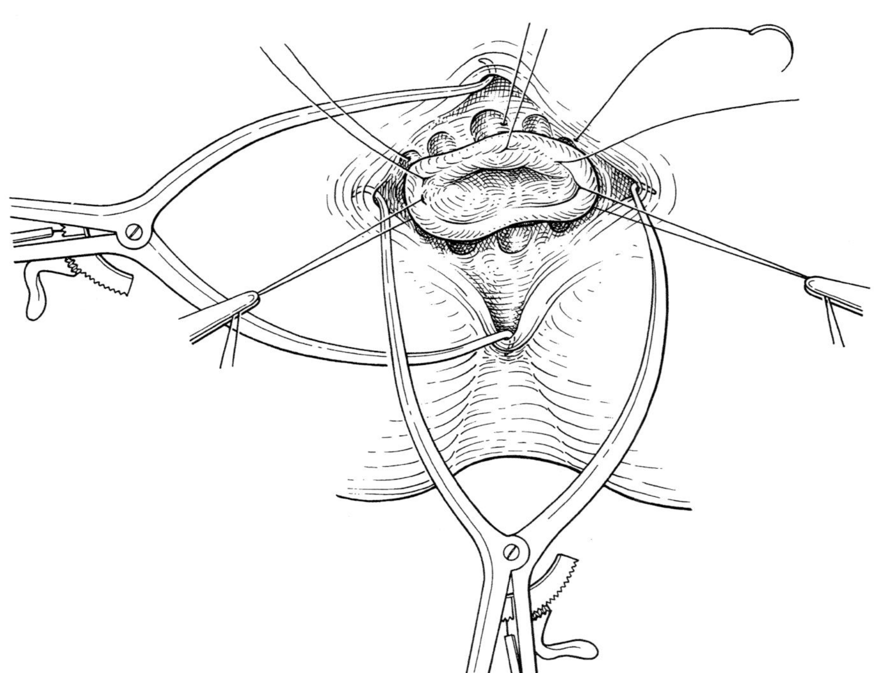

Figure 32.47 Transanal coloanal anastomosis using two Gelpi retractors at right-angles.

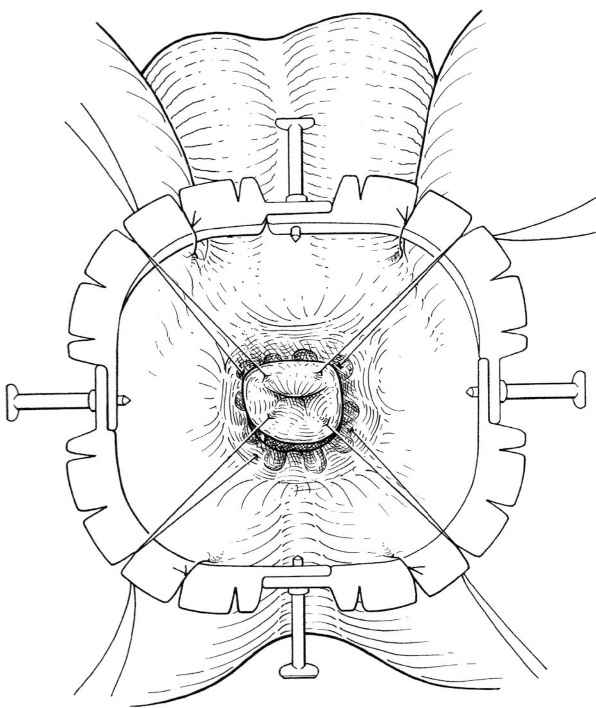

Figure 32.48 Transanal coloanal anastomosis using Lone Star retractor.

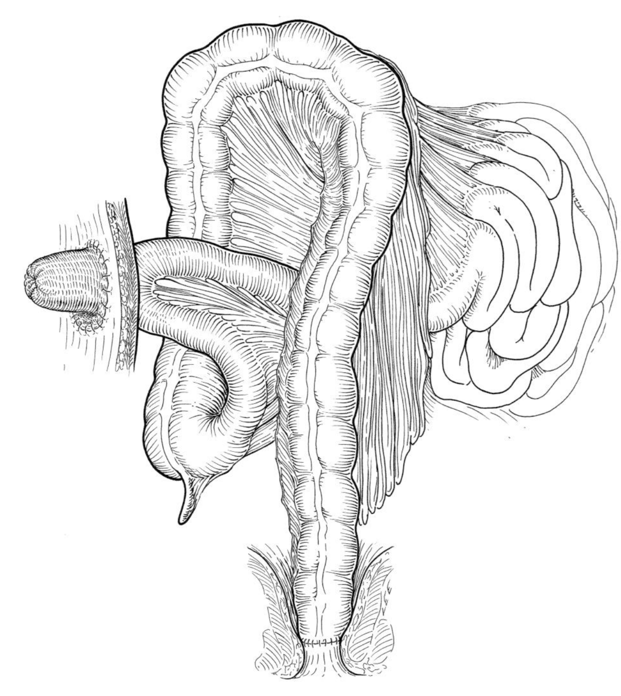

Figure 32.49 Completion of abdominotransanal operation. The colon is left to the right of the small intestine and a covering loop ileostomy is established.

Alternative sphincter-saving resection techniques

There are a variety of pull-through procedures described in the literature, each with its own minor technical differences. Pull-through procedures are now rarely performed and are really of historical interest. Although they were all technically feasible, function tended to be so unsatisfactory that surgeons who tried these techniques usually returned to abdominoperineal excision. These techniques invariably necessitated eversion of the anorectum with subsequent traction and damage to the sphincteric mechanisms; however, they paved the way for the abdominotransanal anastomosis which does result in satisfactory function because the anorectum is not everted. Technical details of these pull-through procedures are not described here; if interested, the reader is encouraged to refer to the excellent descriptions of these operations in their original form (Cutait and Figlioni, 1961; Turnbull and Cuthbertson, 1961).

Two other procedures are briefly described here: the abdominotrans-sacral and abdominotrans-sphincteric procedures. Both have their advocates, but neither is performed with any degree of regularity outside a few centres. We believe that they should be used only when it is impossible to use the stapling instrument, that is in situations that we normally reserve for an abdominotransanal procedure. Nevertheless, Localio and his colleagues from New York (Localio and Eng, 1985) considered that the abdominosacral resection was superior to anterior resection for low rectal growths and should be performed routinely. They maintained that greater distal and lateral clearance of the tumour is possible and that a more accurate anastomosis can be constructed via this approach than with an anterior resection. Despite these affirmations, this operation has never achieved universal popularity.

Abdominotrans-sacral resection

The patient is placed in the right lateral position with the back and buttocks at the edge of the table. An indwelling catheter is placed in the bladder, and the rectum is irrigated with normal saline. The incisions are marked, the skin prepared and the patient is draped to provide simultaneous access to the abdominal and posterior wounds.

Abdominal approach

The abdomen is opened through an oblique incision starting between the left costal margin and the iliac crest, running parallel to the inguinal ligament and curving across the rectus muscles above the pubis. The incision is carried through all layers of the abdominal wall. The abdominal phase of the operation is identical to that described for low anterior resection, but the surgeon has to reorientate from the vertical to the horizontal plane.

The oblique incision affords excellent exposure of the splenic flexure and the pelvic organs. After complete exploration of the abdomen the small bowel is delivered from the abdomen and mobilization of the left colon begins. This is performed from the splenic flexure downwards, by dividing first the phrenicocolic ligament and then the peritoneal reflection on the lateral side of the colon. The omentum is separated from the transverse mesocolon by sharp dissection which is carried far enough to the right to allow the transverse colon to rotate on the middle colic artery. Adhesions between the omentum and spleen can be divided at this time to allow the omentum to reach the pelvis if the surgeon wishes to use it to reinforce the anastomosis at a later stage. The left colon is then drawn downwards to the patient's right and its lateral peritoneal attachments are divided in the usual way. During this manoeuvre the left gonadal vessels and ureter are recognized and preserved.

The colon is then retracted upwards and to the patient's left side and the right leaf of the sigmoid mesentery is incised at its base. The right ureter is sought during this manoeuvre and is swept laterally. The sigmoid mesentery containing the superior haemorrhoidal vessels and lymphatics is now dissected free from the aorta and the inferior mesenteric artery is clamped, divided and ligated usually just below the origin of the left colic artery. After the left colon has been completely mobilized, the surgeon should ensure that the mobilization is sufficient to allow the descending colon to reach the pelvis without tension. If further mobilization is required the left colic artery can be divided at its origin; in this case, great care must be taken to preserve the marginal artery since the blood supply is now based on the middle colic artery.

The sigmoid mesocolon is now divided and ligated to the site selected for the proximal part of the anastomosis. The colon may be clamped at this point and divided. De Martel's or Potts' clamps should be used to allow the proximal colon to be delivered with ease through a relatively small sacral wound. Alternatively the TA stapler which ensures a hermetic seal to the colon may be used. The left border of the colon is marked with a stitch to prevent its rotation when it is delivered through the posterior wound. Some do not divide the proximal colon, preferring to do this later after the colon has been delivered through the posterior wound. The rectum is then mobilized in exactly the same way as for anterior resection. Since the patient is rotated with the right side dependent it is easier to divide the left lateral ligament before the right. The rectum is mobilized as thoroughly as possible via the abdominal route. The access is usually sufficient to allow the seminal vesicles or upper vagina to be visible. The tip of the coccyx and levator ani diaphragm and puborectalis muscle sling are usually palpable. Before proceeding to the posterior dissection, the pelvis is irrigated with saline and meticulous haemostasis is achieved.

Posterior approach

A transverse incision is made over the sacrococcygeal joint (Figure 32.50). The tip of the coccyx is depressed to define the cartilaginous junction. The sacrococcygeal joint is then disarticulated and the coccyx is grasped with strong forceps and retracted posteriorly. The posterior attachments of the levator muscles are separated from the coccyx with scissors and the presacral space is entered (Figure 32.50a). The coccyx is then excised. The opening into the presacral space is enlarged by blunt dissection, splitting the levator muscles in the direction of their fibres. If necessary the transverse incision can be lengthened and the gluteal muscles split for further exposure.

The lower rectum is now mobilized as much as possible. The lowest component of the lateral ligaments are divided from the side walls of the pelvis. The anterior rectal wall is freed from the prostate or lower vaginal wall and the posterior surface of the rectum is dissected off the puborectalis sling.

The rectum with the tumour is then retracted out of the wound and its wall cleared of fat down to the bare longitudinal muscle at a point where the proposed transection is to take place. The distal margin of clearance will vary depending on the surgeon's philosophy. As discussed elsewhere we believe that the distal margin of clearance should be as extensive as possible, but 2 cm should suffice if any longer would jeopardize the anastomosis and sphincter apparatus. A right-angled crushing clamp is applied at the point of distal transection (Figure 32.50b). The proximal colon is then delivered through the posterior wound and divided between crushing clamps if this has not been previously

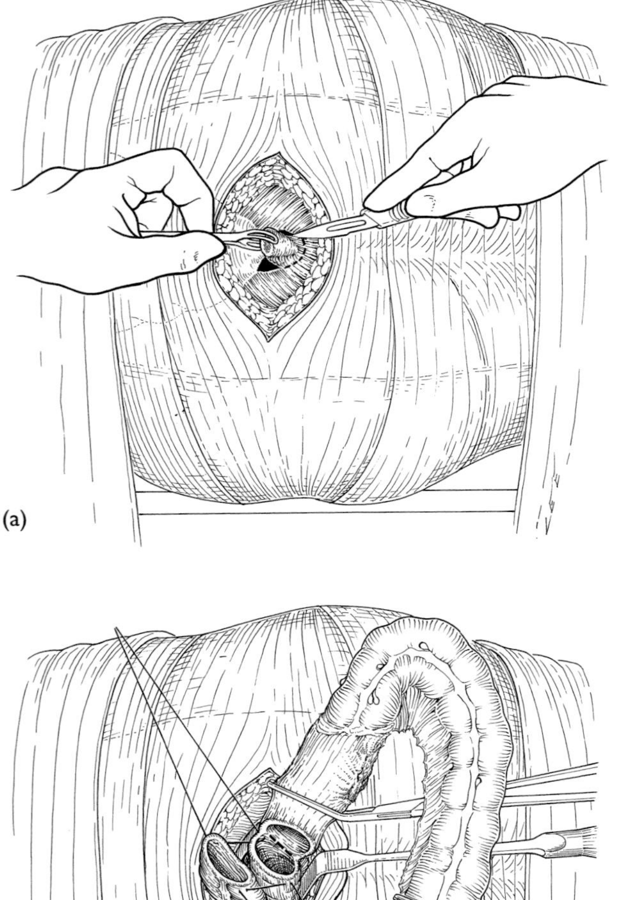

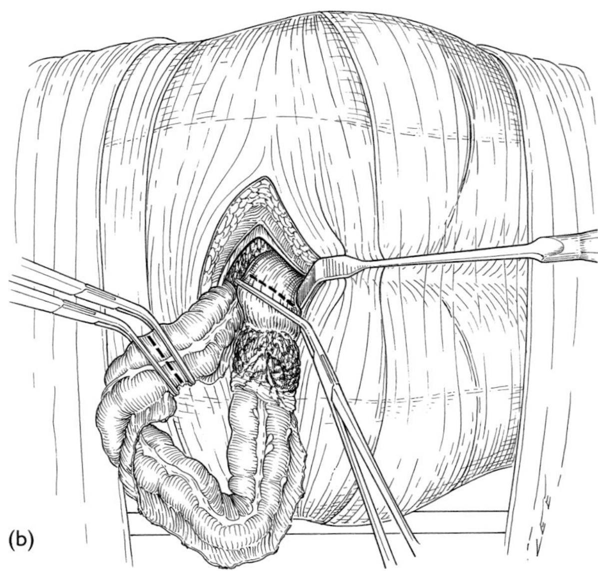

Figure 32.50a–c Abdominotrans-sacral technique. (a) A transverse incision is made over the sacrococcygeal joint. The attachments of the levator ani are separated from the coccyx which is then removed. Access is thus gained to the presacral space. (b) The mobilized colon and rectum are delivered through the posterior incision and the appropriate resection is performed. (c) The colorectal anastomosis is performed in one layer using interrupted sutures.

done via the abdominal route. If division of the proximal colon has been previously accomplished, the clamped or stapled proximal colonic stump is delivered through the wound taking care to avoid rotation of the bowel; the marking stitch is useful in preventing this. An extra 3–4 cm of proximal colon is pulled through the posterior wound to make suturing of the anastomosis easier.

The anastomosis can be constructed in a variety of ways; in the few operations of this type that we have performed we have used a standard two-layered anastomosis (Figure 32.50c).

The pelvic and sacral wounds are thoroughly irrigated with saline and haemostasis is secured. At this point the omentum can be delivered through the posterior wound and wrapped around the anastomosis if the surgeon so wishes, its position being maintained by several sutures to the levator ani.

The defect in the pelvic peritoneum is not closed but the pelvis is drained with a closed suction system. Before closing the abdomen consideration should be given to the addition of a covering stoma.

Abdominotrans-sphincteric resection

The abdominal phase of the operation proceeds in exactly the same way as that described for anterior resection up to the point of rectal excision. After excision of the diseased rectum a Foley catheter is inserted through the anal canal and rectal stump into the proximal colon. The end of the colon is closed around the shaft of the catheter with a purse-string suture. The balloon of the catheter is inflated and by traction downwards the colonic stump is brought into contact with the upper part of the anorectal stump. Attention must be paid to ensuring that the colon is correctly oriented and is free from tension. The abdomen is then closed with appropriate drainage to the pelvis. The patient is then repositioned prone on the operating table and the anorectal stump is displayed using the trans-sphincteric dissection as described for the management of villous adenoma in Chapter 28. After the sphincters have been divided and the rectum sectioned, two stay sutures are inserted into the sides of the proximal colon. The invaginated end of the colon is trimmed away to release the balloon catheter. An end-to-end anastomosis can then be constructed under direct vision, as either a single- or two-layer technique (Figure 32.51).

A modification of the technique is particularly useful for bulky growths which make mobilization and distal rectal transection via the abdominal approach particularly difficult. In such cases the mobilized colon and rectum are left in the peritoneal cavity with the chosen site for proximal transection marked with stay sutures to ensure correct orientation. The abdomen is then closed and the patient placed prone. The somatic and the visceral muscle tubes are opened. This manoeuvre enables the lower end of the carcinoma to be visualized so that the anorectal stump can be accurately transected below it. Further dissection of the lesion and the rectum can then be achieved from below upwards, which is particularly useful for very low anterior lesions. Once the rectum has been fully mobilized it is delivered into the wound until the marking sutures on the colon come into view. The rectum containing the tumour is excised and an anastomosis is then constructed in the usual manner.

The muscle layers of the external anal sphincter and puborectalis are then meticulously repaired, ensuring that accurate apposition is achieved.

We should emphasize that with the introduction of stapling instruments this technique is hardly ever performed for rectal carcinoma and we now consider it obsolete.

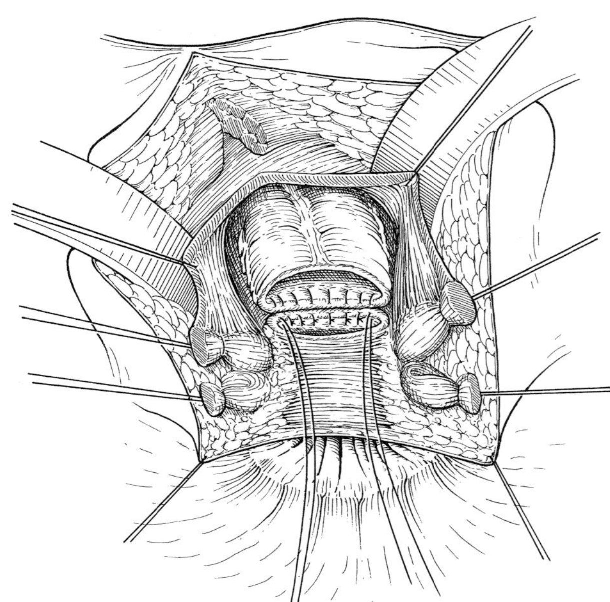

Figure 32.51 Abdominotrans-sphincteric technique. The sphincters have been dissected and the colon has been brought down to the anal canal; a coloanal anastomosis is constructed in one layer using interrupted sutures.

Abdominoperineal excision of the rectum

Despite the recent advances in technology which make sphincter-saving resection more feasible than hitherto, there is still a residuum of patients with lesions that require removal by abdominoperineal excision of the rectum. The percentage of patients with tumours of the lower two-thirds of the rectum who are submitted for this procedure will vary depending on the surgeon's beliefs. Our growing confidence in the new techniques of sphincter-saving resection has enabled us to reduce the rate of abdominoperineal excision by two-thirds (Williams et al, 1985). It appears that gradually colorectal surgeons have slowly accepted the rationale for sphincter-saving resections for low rectal cancer. Thus, in a recent report from the Birmingham Cancer Registry, the proportion of rectal tumours treated by abdominoperineal excision between 1957 and 1981 was 68% (Allum et al, 1994); whereas an audit in the Trent/Wales Region of the UK between 1992 and 1993 recorded an APER rate of 37% (RCS/AC, 1996).

The most popular variation of abdominoperineal excision is the synchronous combined technique, described below.

Position of patient

The patient is placed in the lithotomy–Trendelenburg position with Lloyd Davies leg supports and a pad is placed under the sacrum. An indwelling urinary catheter is inserted. The catheter and scrotum in the male are strapped to the right thigh to enable the perineal surgeon to have a clear field. The skin of the abdomen and perineum is prepared in the usual way, after which the drapes and leggings are applied.

Abdominal phase

A full laparotomy is performed through either a long paramedian or more commonly a midline incision (Figure 32.52) and the left colon and rectum are mobilized in exactly the same manner as described for low anterior resection, except that the splenic flexure need not be mobilized. The pelvic dissection continues down to the levator ani. The posterior dissection must be executed by the abdominal surgeon; once complete, it is usual for the abdominal and perineal dissections to meet behind the mesorectum, at the anorectal junction, the rectum having been completely freed posteriorly from above. The anterior dissection then continues in the plane between the anterior rectal wall and the base of the bladder (or uterus). This dissection continues down from above to the level of both seminal vesicles or the vaginal wall. A lipped St Mark's pelvic retractor is then inserted behind the vesicles which are displaced upwards exposing the fascia of Denonvilliers on the anterior rectal wall. This fascia is then incised transversely and the dissection continues down to the apex of the prostate, usually with the aid of the fingers or long, blunt-ended Lloyd Davies scissors. While in this plane the fingers or a pledget on a Roberts forceps are swept laterally to define the anterior border of the 'lateral ligaments'. The 'lateral ligaments' are then divided. Each ligament in turn is put on the stretch by displacing the rectum to the opposite side with the left hand, and 'the ligament' is divided as far laterally as possible on the side wall of the pelvis. Occasionally in the slim patient it is possible to encompass most of 'the ligament' in a clamp; division and ligation are then considerably simplified. Usually, however, each 'ligament' is divided with scissors and any bleeding vessel is picked up later and ligated; the middle rectal vessels are invariably dealt with in this way. Although most of 'the lateral ligaments' will be divided from above, a variable portion often needs division from below by the perineal operator.

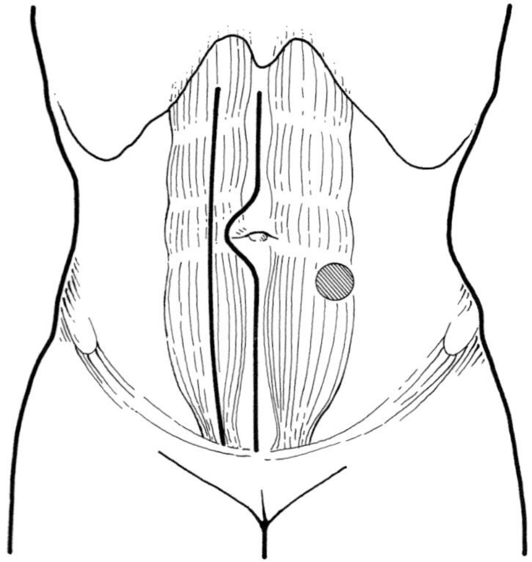

Figure 32.52 Abdominoperineal excision. The abdomen is normally opened using a long midline incision; however, when it is certain from the beginning that an abdominoperineal excision is to be performed, a right paramedian incision has the advantage that the colostomy site is well clear of the wound.

The colon is transected at approximately the midpoint of the sigmoid colon after division of the vascular arcade between the left colic artery and the first sigmoid artery. It is essential to ensure that there is sufficient viable colon to bring out through the abdominal wall as a colostomy. The bowel is best divided between small clamps such as those of Zachary Cope. These will enable the end of the colon destined for the colostomy to be brought out through the abdominal wall without the clamp having to be removed; such a manoeuvre reduces the risk of sepsis. Alternatively a transverse stapling device can be used and this is now our preference. Following division of the colon and after the perineal dissection is complete, the excised colon and the rectum are withdrawn through the perineal wound.

The trephine for the colostomy is next fashioned (Figure 32.53). This is best carried out at the site that has been preselected by the patient in consultation with the stoma care nurse. The site should have been marked on the skin prior to operation with an indelible marker (see Figure 32.52). If this has not been done the surgeon should choose a site approximately one-third of the way along a line from the anterior superior iliac spine to the umbilicus through the rectus muscle. In obese subjects it is best to site the colostomy 6–8 cm above this level so that it will be visible to the patient.

The skin is elevated with Littlewood or Allis tissue forceps and a disc of skin and subcutaneous

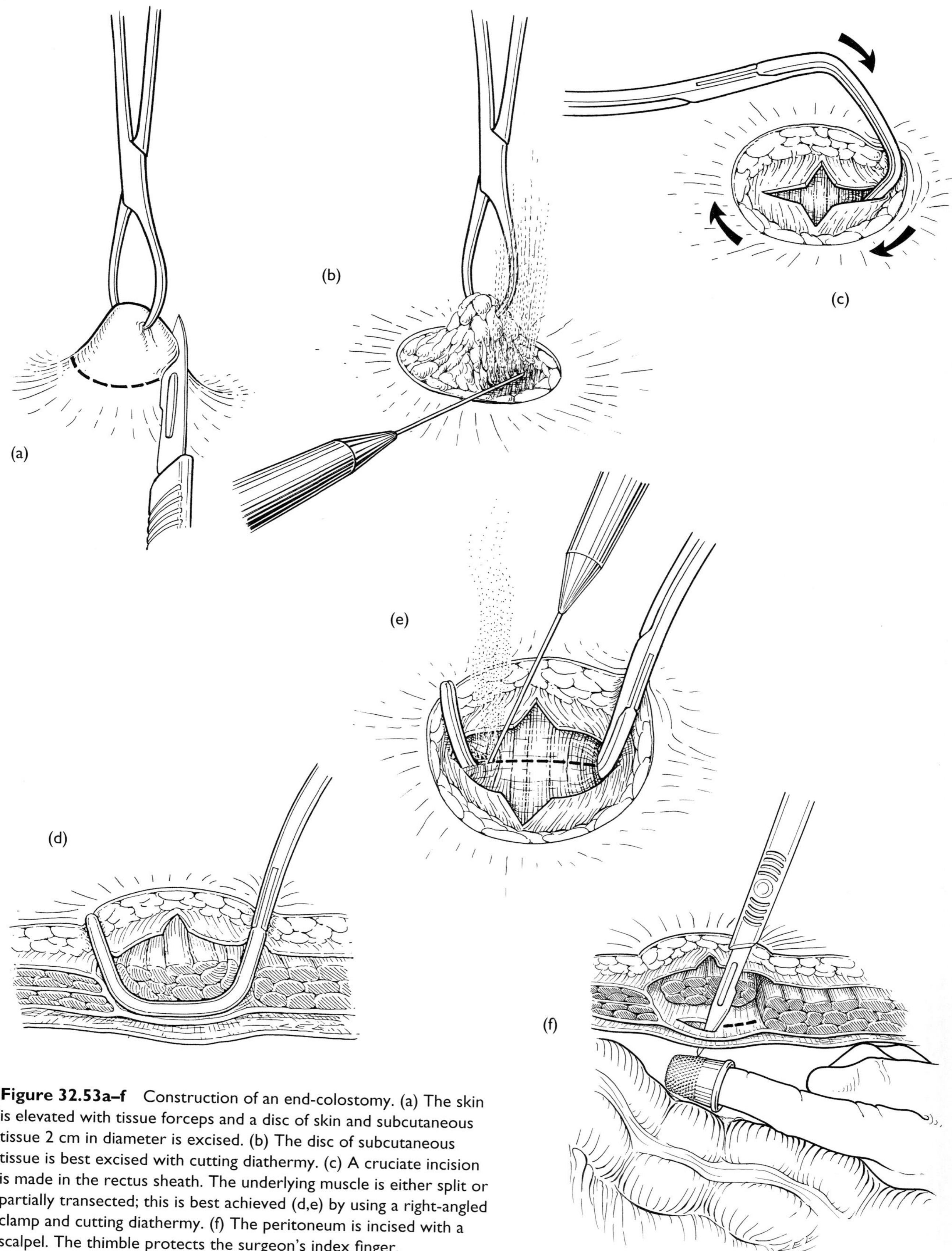

Figure 32.53a–f Construction of an end-colostomy. (a) The skin is elevated with tissue forceps and a disc of skin and subcutaneous tissue 2 cm in diameter is excised. (b) The disc of subcutaneous tissue is best excised with cutting diathermy. (c) A cruciate incision is made in the rectus sheath. The underlying muscle is either split or partially transected; this is best achieved (d,e) by using a right-angled clamp and cutting diathermy. (f) The peritoneum is incised with a scalpel. The thimble protects the surgeon's index finger.

tissue approximately 2 cm diameter is excised. The rectus sheath is opened using a cruciate incision, the rectus muscle is either split in the line of its fibres or partially transected, and the peritoneum is divided in a cruciate manner. It is useful during this manoeuvre to have the index finger of the non-cutting hand protected by a thimble, exerting pressure from within outwards. This helps to guide the incision through the abdominal wall as well as protecting the finger. When the defect has been created in the manner described it is usually necessary to stretch it so as to be sure it takes two fingers comfortably; this will in most cases prevent constriction of the colon.

Prior to exteriorization of the colon, most surgeons still close the lateral space (Figure 32.54). This is best done in the following manner. The left border of the laparotomy wound is elevated by passing a long forceps such as a Roberts or Moynihan forceps through the colostomy incision and out through the main abdominal wound. Strong elevation of the tip of this instrument with retraction medially of the sigmoid will display the left paracolic gutter adequately. A purse-string suture is then inserted into the parietal peritoneum from the inner edge of the colostomy wound to the lateral edge of the sigmoid stump just proximal to the clamp or staple line, the length depending on the depth of the abdominal wall. Care must be taken to insert the suture into the seromuscular layer of the colon and not into the lumen. Alternatively, interrupted sutures may be used. When these sutures are tied the lateral space is completely closed and this will prevent small bowel herniation. The clamp on the colostomy stump is then passed through the defect so that 3–4 cm of colon protrudes through the abdominal wall. Four seromuscular sutures are then placed between the colon and rectus sheath, to anchor the colostomy at this level.

The alternative method of exteriorization of the colostomy is the extraperitoneal technique (Figure 32.55). This has the advantage of eliminating the need for lateral space closure and also is said to prevent colostomy prolapse. In order to perform this technique the upper part of the left leaf of the peritoneum (which has already been divided during colonic mobilization) is grasped with long artery forceps. Using finger and scissor dissection an extraperitoneal space is created from the peritoneal cavity to the lateral border of the proposed colostomy incision (Figure 32.55a,b). The tunnel thus formed is stretched so that it can take the colon comfortably. The colostomy incision is performed in the manner described but with the index finger, guarded with a thimble, passed through the

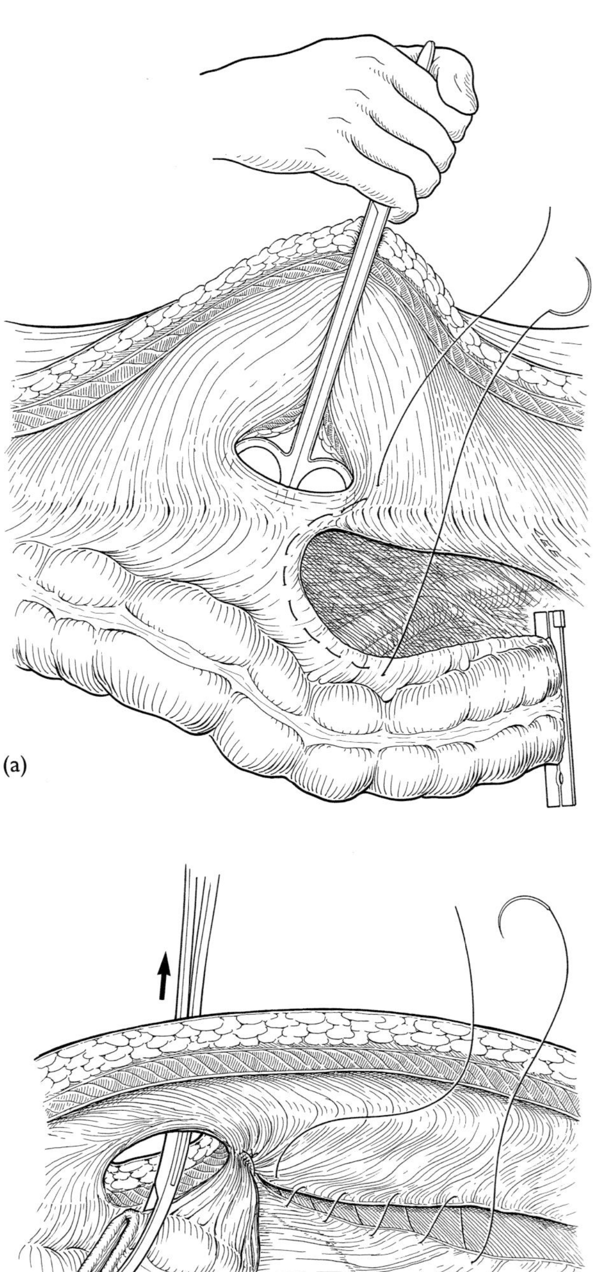

Figure 32.54a,b Closure of the lateral space by purse-string suture. (a) View of the inside of the left iliac region as seen from the right side. While the left edge of the main wound is elevated by scissors threaded through the colostomy trephine, a purse-string suture is placed around the lateral space. (b) The purse-string suture is tied and the remaining space between the mesocolon and cut edge of the peritoneum is closed. The colostomy is then exteriorized.

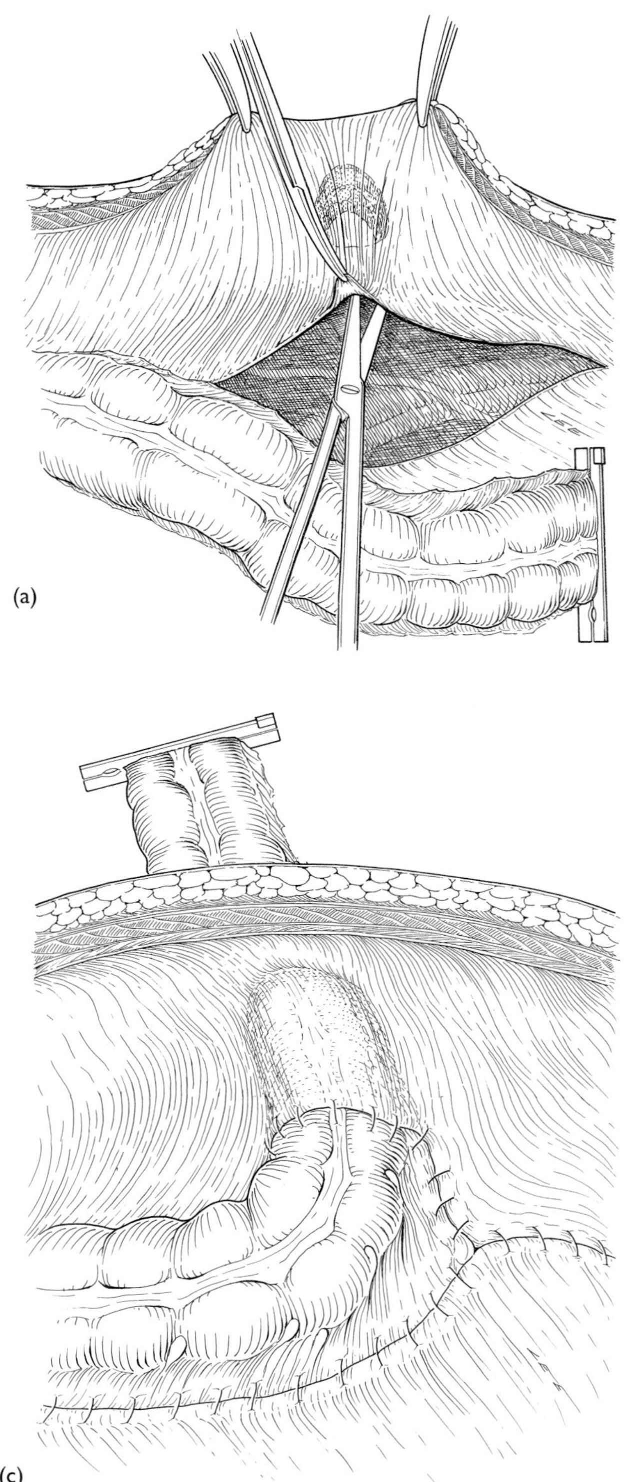

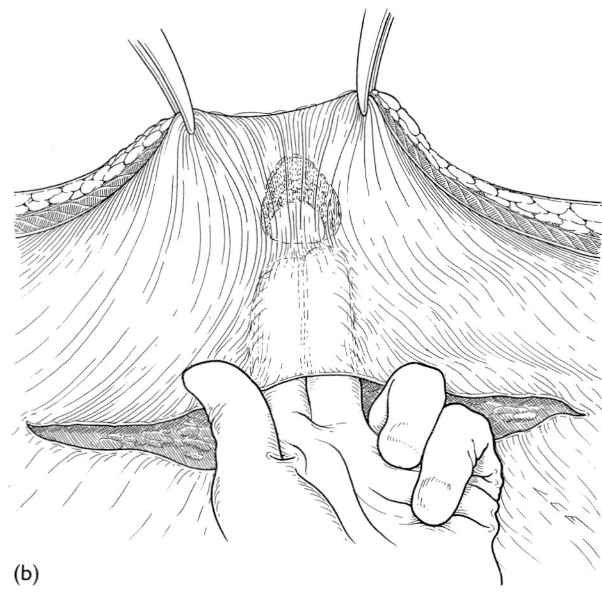

Figure 32.55a–c Exteriorization of colostomy using the extraperitoneal technique. View of the inside of the left iliac region as seen from the right side. (a,b) Making the extraperitoneal tunnel using scissors and finger dissection. (c) The colon is passed through the tunnel and exteriorized, and the peritoneal defect is repaired.

extraperitoneal space. The colostomy incision should then enter the extraperitoneal space instead of opening into the peritoneal cavity. The colon is passed through the retroperitoneal tunnel and through the defect in the abdominal wall (Figure 32.55c). A few tacking sutures are placed between the seromuscular layer of the colon and the rectus sheath as previously described. The defect in the peritoneum is closed using a continuous suture of chromic catgut.

We have used this technique on several occasions but find it tedious to perform, and although no data are available we do not have the impression that it is superior to the more conventional method.

Some surgeons make no attempt to close the lateral gutter, believing that if the defect is large small bowel is unlikely to become entrapped in the space. There are no data on the incidence of parastomal small bowel obstruction which would permit the three methods of colostomy construction to be compared.

Perineal phase

The perineal phase of the operation is commenced only when the abdominal surgeon has performed the laparotomy and is convinced that the tumour is operable. The moment when it is considered appropriate for the perineal dissection to commence will vary from surgeon to surgeon. Provided it is considered from the beginning that a sphincter-saving resection is impossible, it is the practice of many

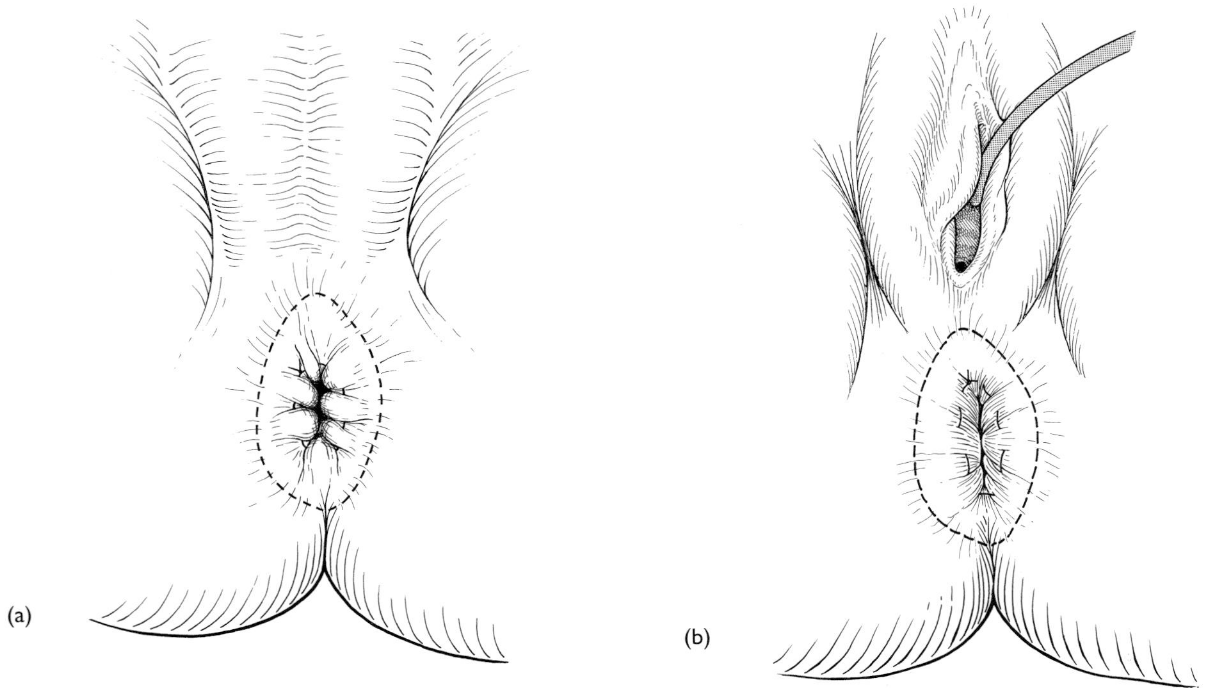

Figure 32.56a,b Incision for perineal dissection of synchronous combined excision of the rectum. Such an incision is suitable in the male (a) and in the female (b) provided the posterior vaginal wall does not need to be excised.

surgeons to commence when the abdominal surgeon is beginning the rectal mobilization. However, our policy has completely changed in the practice of abdominoperineal excision. We have abandoned the struggle between two groups of surgeons trying synchronously to remove the rectum. We now adopt a policy of performing as much as possible of the rectal dissection from above, leaving the assistant to construct the colostomy after dividing the bowel between clamps or staples. The abdominal surgeon then moves to the perineum to remove the tumour with a reasonable margin of surrounding tissue. Wide clearance is achieved using diathermy extensively and removing adjacent tissue and organs if necessary. Planes of dissection are confirmed with the abdominal surgeon at the level of the pelvic floor to achieve 'en bloc' excision. The dissection that is described does not differ from the surgical practice now adopted, only that the lead surgeon is the person who both performs the pelvic dissection and then continues the excision as the perineal operator, since he is then certain just what has been mobilized from above.

The anal orifice is first closed, using one or even two thick linen sutures on a hand needle. The purse-string suture is placed in the subcutaneous tissue and completely encircles the anal orifice. After the knot has been tied the ends of the suture are clipped and left long. Traction on this suture allows the loose perineal skin to be put on stretch; this makes the perineal incision easier and assists in the subsequent dissection. Alternatively the skin of the closed anal orifice may be grasped with two or three Littlewood forceps. An elliptical incision is made which encircles the anal verge; it commences midway between the anus and the posterior fourchette or bulb of the urethra anteriorly and extends posteriorly to the sacrococcygeal articulation (Figure 32.56). The incision is deepened to expose the lobulated fat in the ischiorectal fossae and the coccyx; the latter may then be disarticulated. If disarticulation is to be carried out the coccyx is more clearly defined by scalpel dissection and is then flexed strongly forwards by pressure on its tip with the thumb of the left hand (Figure 32.57). This manoeuvre exposes one of the intercoccygeal joints which is then completely divided with the scalpel. The terminal piece of coccyx is either displaced forwards or more usually excised completely from its muscular attachments. During disarticulation of the coccyx in this manner it is usual to encounter bleeding from the middle or lateral sacral vessels. This can be dealt with by diathermy or ligature.

Alternatively, the coccyx need not be disarticulated. It is our preference to incise the anococcygeal

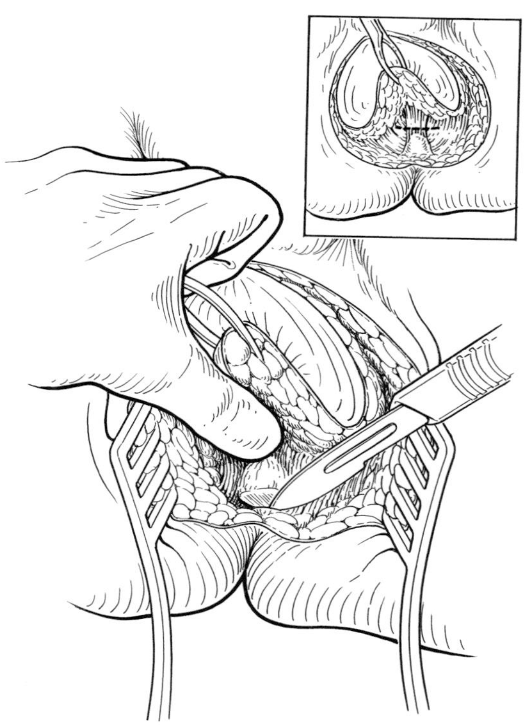

Figure 32.57 Dissection of the terminal part of the coccyx. The inset shows an alternative, now more common, method of cutting across the anococcygeal raphe.

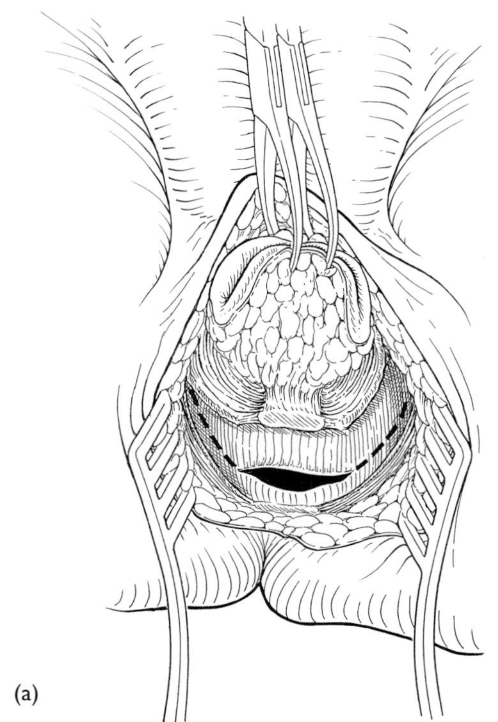

(a)

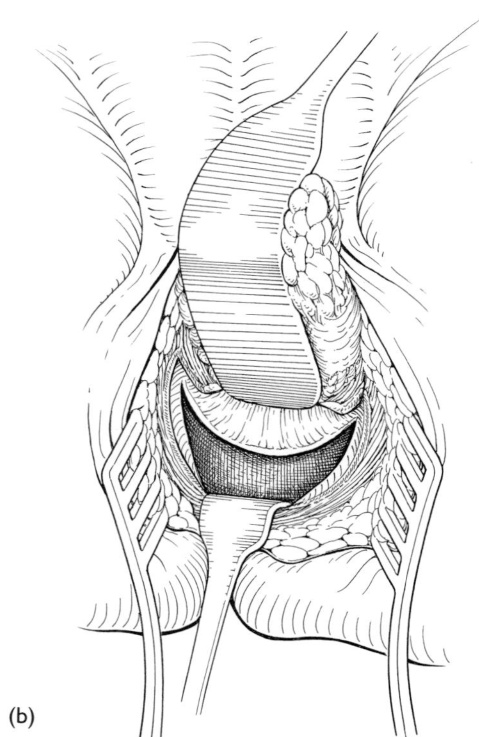

(b)

Figure 32.58 Division of the fascia of Waldeyer.

raphe in front of the bone to gain access to the pelvis (Figure 32.57 inset). Care must be taken to ensure that the rectum is not entered during this manoeuvre. It is our view that if the coccyx is retained the patient is more comfortable following the procedure. Excision of the bone is not necessary for eradication of the growth, it only makes subsequent access to the pelvis easier.

The closed anal orifice and surrounding skin are clipped with Littlewood tissue forceps and are retracted to the right of the patient. The left wound edge is picked up by similar tissue forceps and retracted to the left side of the patient. Small lateral incisions are made on each side of the coccyx through the fibrous attachment of the coccygeus muscle and a finger is inserted on each side in a forward and outward direction to separate the levator muscles from the underlying fascia of Waldeyer. The overlying fat in the ischiorectal fossa and the iliococcygeus muscle are divided well out to the lateral pelvic side wall. The inferior rectal vessels are secured during this manoeuvre.

After this has been performed on both sides, a St Mark's or laminectomy self-retaining retractor is inserted into the wound (Figure 32.58). The anal canal and rectum are then strongly retracted anteriorly displaying the fascia of Waldeyer behind the rectum. This fascia is incised transversely with scalpel or scissors just in front of the divided coccyx, extending the incision around each side of the rectum (Figure 32.58b). Failure to divide the fascia results in the presacral fascia being stripped from the sacrum, producing pelvic nerve damage and haemorrhage from the presacral venous plexus.

After complete incision of the fascia – which may be quite thick – the fingers of the right hand are inserted through it so that the rectum with the mesorectum is lifted forward off the front of the sacrum. It is usually at this stage that the abdominal and perineal operators meet. Often the operators are not working in exactly the same plane and some blunt dissection by each is necessary before they come into contact. To aid this dissection it is useful for the abdominal operator to thrust the index and second fingers as far down as possible in the posterior plane of dissection. The two fingers should be slightly separated and the perineal operator can thus cut carefully between them to establish continuum. The rectum is now completely free posteriorly.

Attention next turns to the anterior dissection. The anal canal is retracted posteriorly and the anterior part of the incision is deepened by scissor dissection to the central point of the perineum. Transverse incisions are then made on each side to expose the superficial and then the deep transverse perineal muscles (Figure 32.59). The plane of dissection must be behind these muscles to avoid injury to the urethra or the vagina, if this is being preserved. The transverse perineal muscles are separated from the front of the external anal sphincter. Afterwards the longitudinal fibres of the anterior rectal wall will be seen.

The next layer of muscles to be encountered run in an anteroposterior direction from the pubic ramus to the rectum, and around the urethra or vagina to the coccyx. They comprise the pubococcygeus and puborectalis part of the levator ani on either side, the rectourethralis muscle in the centre and undescribed muscle fibres from the pubis to the rectum. A finger is now inserted between the superior borders of the pubococcygeus and puborectalis muscles (Figure 32.60). Separation of these muscles from the underlying pelvic fascia facilitates their wide division from their origins on each side. The underlying fascia is then divided to expose the rectal wall. The prostate will be felt anteriorly and the plane between it and the rectum can be defined. Failure to cut the fascial layer as described will result in dissection occurring in the wrong plane, with resulting haemorrhage.

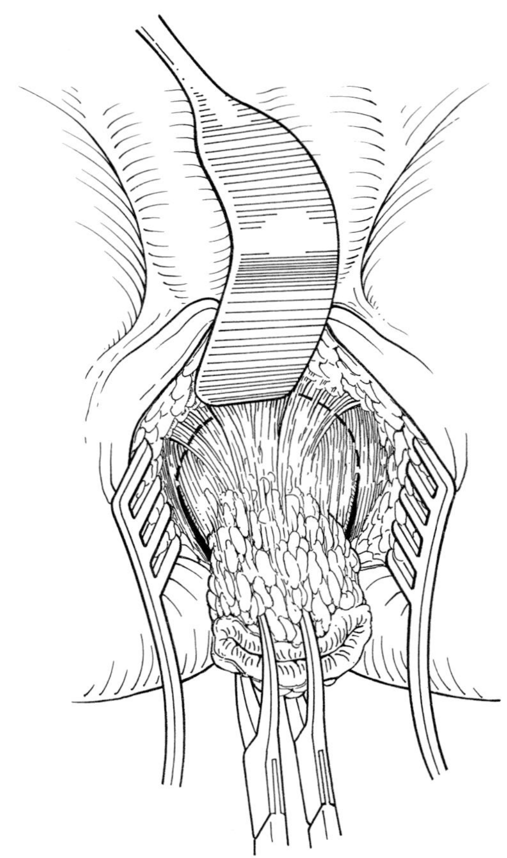

Figure 32.59 Anterior dissection during the perineal phase. The dotted line represents the transverse incisions which are made to expose the superficial and then the deep transverse perineal muscles.

The rectum is now left tethered anteriorly by a band of muscle which runs from the anterior rectal wall at the level of the anorectal angle to the apex of the prostate and membranous urethra and the pelvic side wall. This comprises the inferior borders of the inner fibres of the puborectalis muscles and the rectourethralis muscle. The next part of the dissection should be performed with caution as it is relatively easy to enter the rectum or damage the urethra. Failure to appreciate that the rectum is sharply angulated at this point can result in damage. In order to prevent this problem the anterior muscular barrier is separated into two bundles by blunt dissection with an artery forceps (Figure 32.61). The forceps are then directed towards the apex of the prostate which is located with the index finger of the left hand and must lie parallel with the posterior aspect of the gland to avoid injury to the urethra. The separated muscular bundles are divided in turn and the capsule of the prostate is

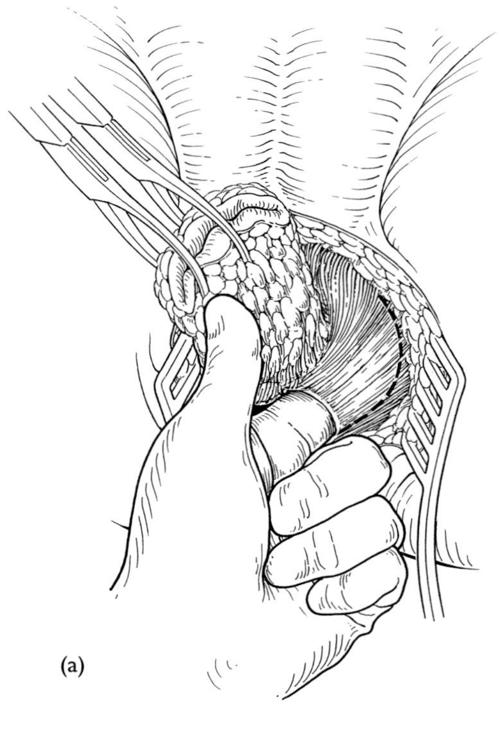

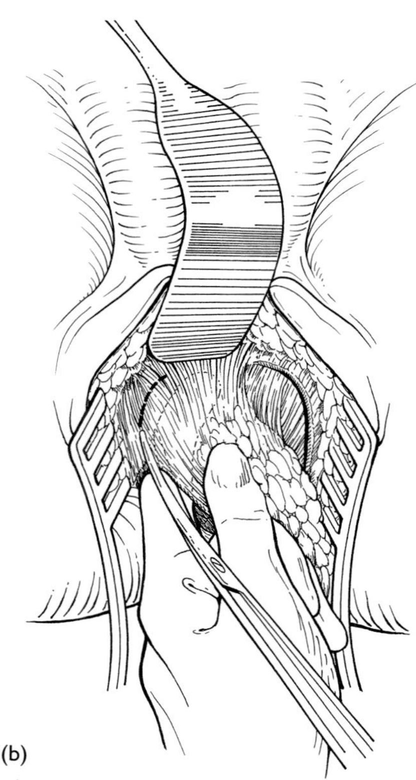

Figure 32.60 Separation and division of the pubococcygeus and puborectalis muscles.

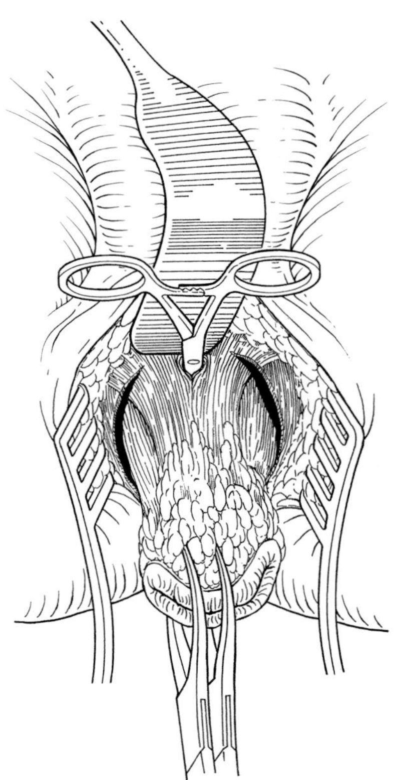

Figure 32.61 Separation and division of the anterior fibromuscular bundle.

exposed. Sometimes the prostatic capsule is still covered by longitudinal strands of muscle which obscure its view and these will need careful division if injury to the rectum is to be avoided.

The visceral pelvic fascia of Denonvilliers which is condensed anteriorly and passes forward to the lateral aspects of the prostate is divided. This allows an unhindered view of the posterior aspect of the prostate and seminal vesicles. It is at this point that the abdominal and perineal operators meet anteriorly (Figure 32.62). The majority of the retroprostatic dissection should be performed from below.

The rectum has now been freed anteriorly and posteriorly. In a thin patient with a broad pelvis the mesorectal tissue comprising the 'lateral ligaments' will usually have been divided completely from above and thus the rectum will be free at this stage. Usually, however, it is necessary for the perineal operator to complete the mobilization by dividing the remainder of the 'lateral ligaments' from below (Figure 32.63). The rectum is alternatively retracted to the opposite side and the stretched 'ligament' is divided close to the pelvic wall. Once free, the anorectum and sigmoid colon, if previously divided, are passed down through the perineal

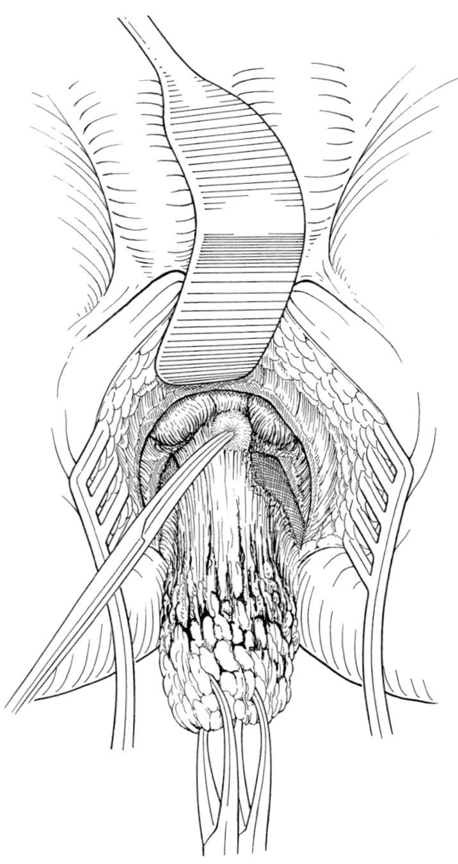

Figure 32.62 Division and separation of the fascia of Denonvilliers anteriorly brings the posterior aspect of the prostate and seminal vesicles into view. At this stage the abdominal and perineal operators meet.

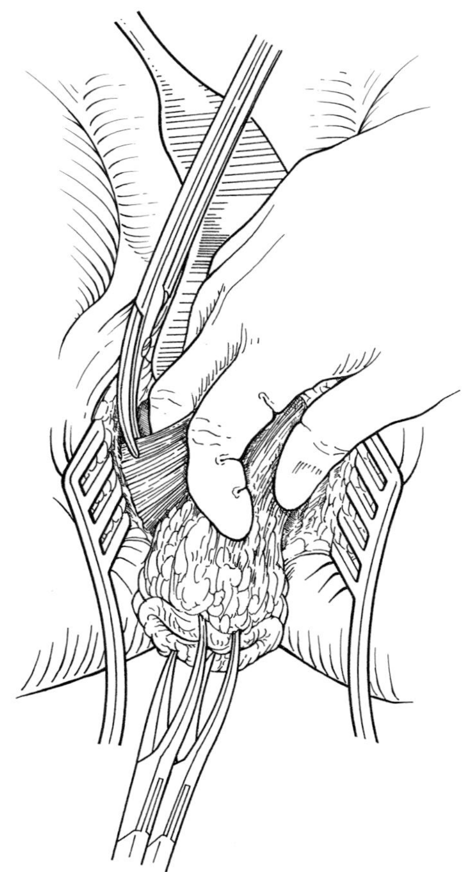

Figure 32.63 The rectum is freed by dividing what remains of the lateral ligaments.

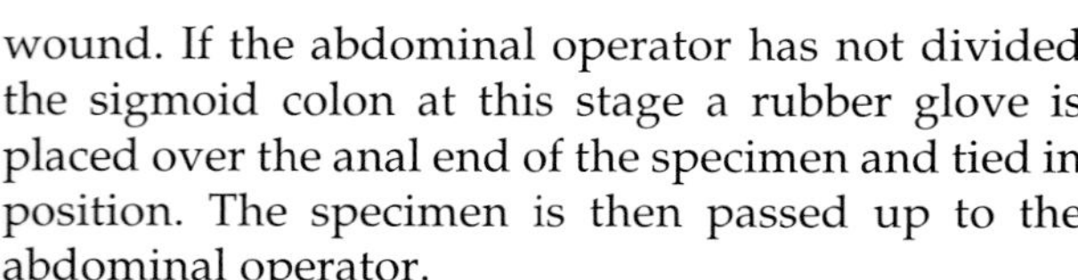

wound. If the abdominal operator has not divided the sigmoid colon at this stage a rubber glove is placed over the anal end of the specimen and tied in position. The specimen is then passed up to the abdominal operator.

Haemostasis in the pelvis and perineum is then secured from both above and below. It is quite usual to have some bleeding from the back of the prostate when a growth has been adherent to it. A careful search will usually display the bleeding points and after they are secured the perineal wound is closed.

Perineal dissection in the female

The perineal phase of the operation in the female differs from that described above only during the anterior dissection of the rectum from the posterior vaginal wall. These two structures are adherent and care is needed in separating them without buttonholing the vaginal wall. If the tumour is situated anteriorly or is in any way abutting on the vagina, the posterior vaginal wall should be excised in continuity with the anorectum to the level of the cervix. We do not subscribe, however, to the view that the posterior vaginal wall should be excised routinely in the course of an abdominoperineal excision (Goligher, 1984). If the posterior vaginal wall is to be excised, the perineal incision extends from the posterolateral aspects of the labia around the anus to the coccyx. Excision of the rectum continues as in the male until the anterior part of the dissection is reached. The anterior incisions are then carried upwards through the lateral aspects of the vagina as far as the posterior fornix (Figure 32.64). A transverse incision is then made through the posterior fornix to join the two lateral incisions. This incision is deepened to expose the rectal wall at which point the abdominal and perineal operator meet anteriorly. The 'lateral ligaments' are then divided and the specimen removed. Reconstruction of the

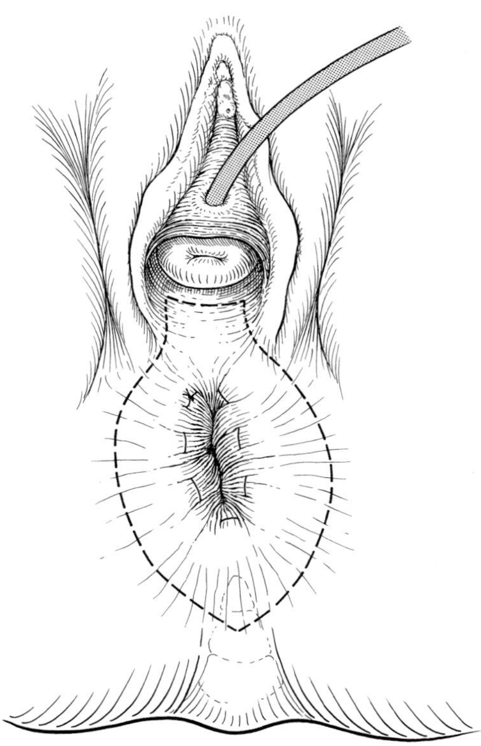

Figure 32.64 Perineal incision in the female when the posterior vaginal wall requires excision.

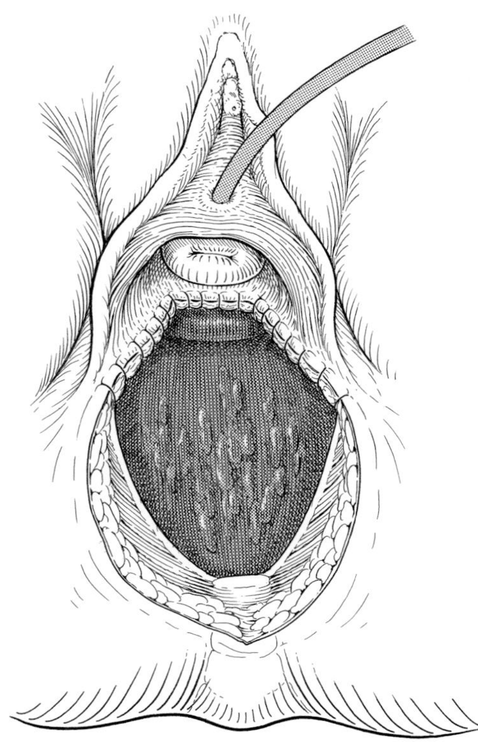

Figure 32.65 Oversewing of the cut vaginal wall to achieve haemostasis.

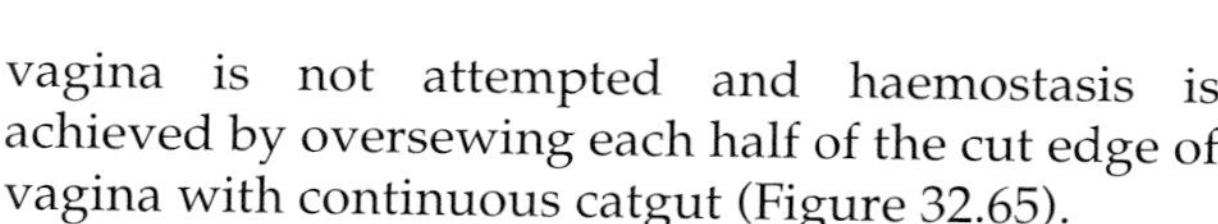

vagina is not attempted and haemostasis is achieved by oversewing each half of the cut edge of vagina with continuous catgut (Figure 32.65).

Closure of the perineal wound

In the past there has been considerable controversy concerning the best means of dealing with the perineal wound after abdominoperineal excision. The argument has revolved around whether the wound should be closed primarily with drainage, or should be partially or completely left open and either packed or drained. The majority view (which includes our own) is for primary closure of the wound whenever possible with suction drainage provided from above. This technique is more comfortable for the patient and shortens hospital stay. Provided that haemostasis is achieved, faecal contamination has not occurred and the patient is receiving systemic antibiotic prophylaxis, perineal wound breakdown is far less common than previously thought. Nevertheless, even recent antibiotic studies report over 40% breakdown rates in perineal wounds (see Chapter 5). If, however, haemostasis is inadequate and cannot be achieved completely or there has been faecal contamination, there should be no hesitation in leaving the wound open.

Primary closure is achieved usually with two layers of catgut or polygalactin sutures for the fat and one layer of polypropylene or nylon for the skin (Figure 32.66). It is impossible to close the pelvic floor muscles. At least two suction or sump drains are placed in the pelvic cavity and brought out either through the perineum itself or preferably through separate stab wounds in the suprapubic region. A refinement of this technique is that recommended by Kelly (1977) in which irrigation is combined with suction. Two large-bore tubes are inserted from the abdomen into the pelvic cavity and are exteriorized, one on each side of the perineal wound. Continuous irrigation with an antibiotic solution is carried out through one tube while continuous suction is applied to the other. The irrigation system involves open drains, hence we prefer to use closed suction drainage from above.

If it has been decided to leave the perineal wound open, the cavity may be packed with a wide gauze roll or it may be drained from below using a wide corrugated drain. It is usual in these circumstances to partially close the wound anteriorly and posteriorly.

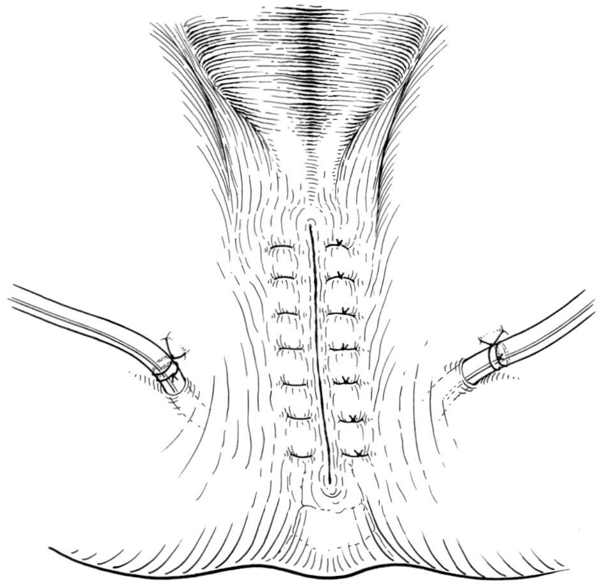

Figure 32.66 Primary closure of the perineal wound in the male. Note the suction drains.

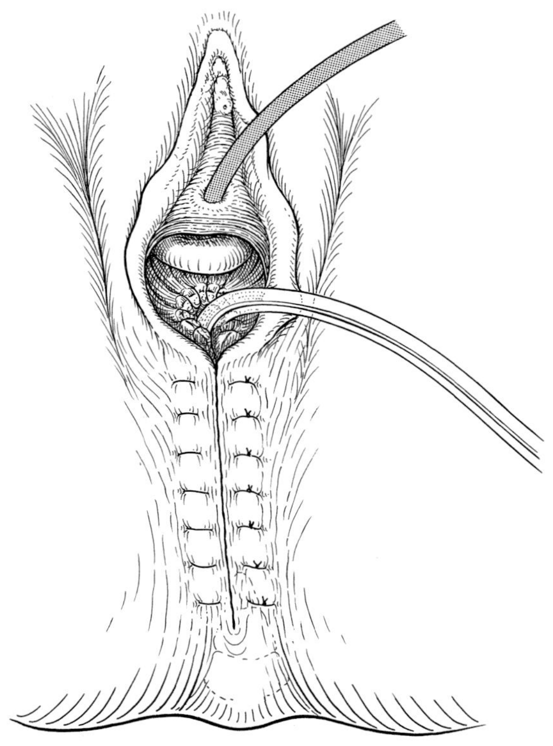

Figure 32.67 Primary closure of the perineal wound in the female when the posterior vaginal wall has been removed.

In the female when the posterior vaginal wall has been excised, primary closure is achieved by placing interrupted mattress sutures as far forward as the cut edges of the labia which are approximated (Figure 32.67). A corrugated drain may be used for drainage, placed into the pelvic cavity through the reformed vaginal orifice; but as previously stated we prefer closed suction drains from above.

Abdominal closure and completion of colostomy

It is common practice at the end of the abdominal and perineal phases of the operation to irrigate the pelvis with a cancericidal agent such as 1% cetrimide. If it is feasible the pelvic peritoneum is closed over the empty pelvis by an invaginating continuous suture of 2/0 chromic catgut (Figure 32.68). The main vascular pedicle is covered during this process and the suture is continued laterally between the free edge of the mesocolon and the peritoneum of the left iliac fossa to the point of exit of the colon.

The need to close the pelvic peritoneum, if primary perineal closure is performed, is debatable. Some surgeons prefer to leave it open in the hope that the small bowel and omentum will prolapse into the pelvis and fill the dead space, thus reducing the chance of haematoma formation. A modification of this technique (Ruckley et al, 1970) is to mobilize the omentum and stitch it in place within the pelvis. Our concern has always been the fear that small intestine may become obstructed if allowed to descend into the pelvis, and that is why we prefer to close the pelvic peritoneum whenever possible. However, it should be pointed out that often because of the wider lateral dissection now performed, there is little pelvic peritoneum left to close. In the only controlled trial on the subject, Irvin and Goligher (1975) found no significant difference with regard to any postoperative complications whether the peritoneum was closed or left open. If postoperative radiotherapy is contemplated, however, some method of excluding loops of small bowel from the pelvis may be desirable. Our preference is to use the omentum where possible to achieve this objective (see Figure 10.21).

The abdominal wound is closed in the normal way and is dressed to prevent contamination during the construction of the colostomy.

The clamp on the colon or the stapled transection line which has been brought out to form the colostomy is excised and the colon is trimmed to leave 1.5–2 cm projecting above the skin surface.

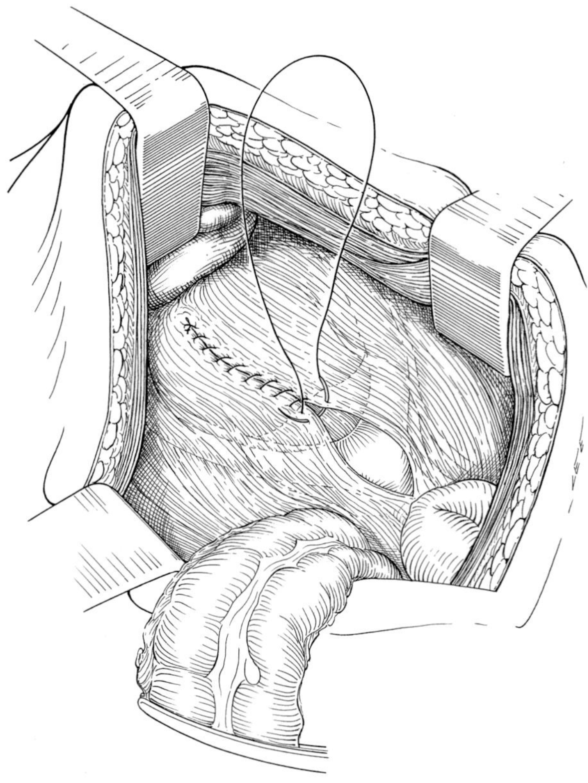

Figure 32.68 Closure of the pelvic peritoneum.

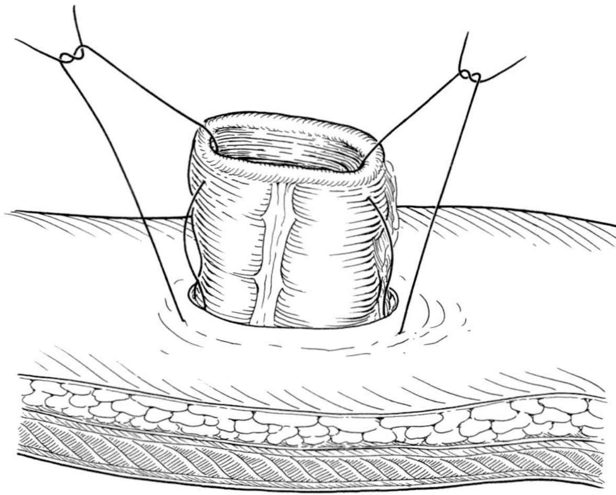

Figure 32.69 Completion of colostomy construction by mucocutaneous suture.

The edges of all coats of the colon are carefully sutured to the surrounding skin forming a mucocutaneous junction (Figure 32.69). Interrupted 2/0 chromic catgut or polygalactin sutures on a tapercut needle or 4/0 polypropylene sutures are commonly used for this manoeuvre. Four sutures are first placed, one in each quadrant, and are left untied. The spaces between them are gradually filled in until the whole circumference has been dealt with.

Hartmann's procedure

Occasionally in patients with a rectal carcinoma it is not feasible or desirable to perform either an abdominoperineal excision of the rectum or a sphincter-saving resection. For instance, it is unwise to construct an anastomosis following a high anterior resection for a carcinoma of the upper third of the rectum in the presence of pus. Similarly, it is probably unwise and unkind to perform either abdominoperineal excision of the rectum or a sphincter-saving resection in the presence of extensive local spread of a rectal cancer, when it is obvious that recurrence is inevitable and life expectancy is considerably reduced. Under these circumstances excision of the rectum with closure of the rectal stump and an end colostomy may be the operation of choice.

The technique for Hartmann's procedure is similar to that described above: the rectum is mobilized and removed in exactly the same manner as for an anterior resection, and the end colostomy is constructed in the same way as in an abdominoperineal excision of the rectum. The rectal stump is closed by one of several methods. A TA or RL stapling instrument can be used, or the closure can be sutured manually. Suturing is usually performed in two layers. One method is to insert a continuous suture of chromic catgut below the right-angled clamp as a mattress suture (Figure 32.70a). The clamp is then cut off and the suture line buried with interrupted non-absorbable sutures (Figure 32.70b). Alternatively, two layers of interrupted sutures can be inserted. Use of the TA or TL instrument or the Roticulator (Figure 32.71) allows the stump to be closed at a very low level in the pelvis if this is required. Very occasionally it is not possible to close the rectal stump and in these cases a tube drain should be inserted through the open stump and out through the anal canal.

Re-anastomosis following a Hartmann's procedure for carcinoma is not often performed, because the operation is usually considered to be the definitive procedure. Nevertheless, sometimes it is

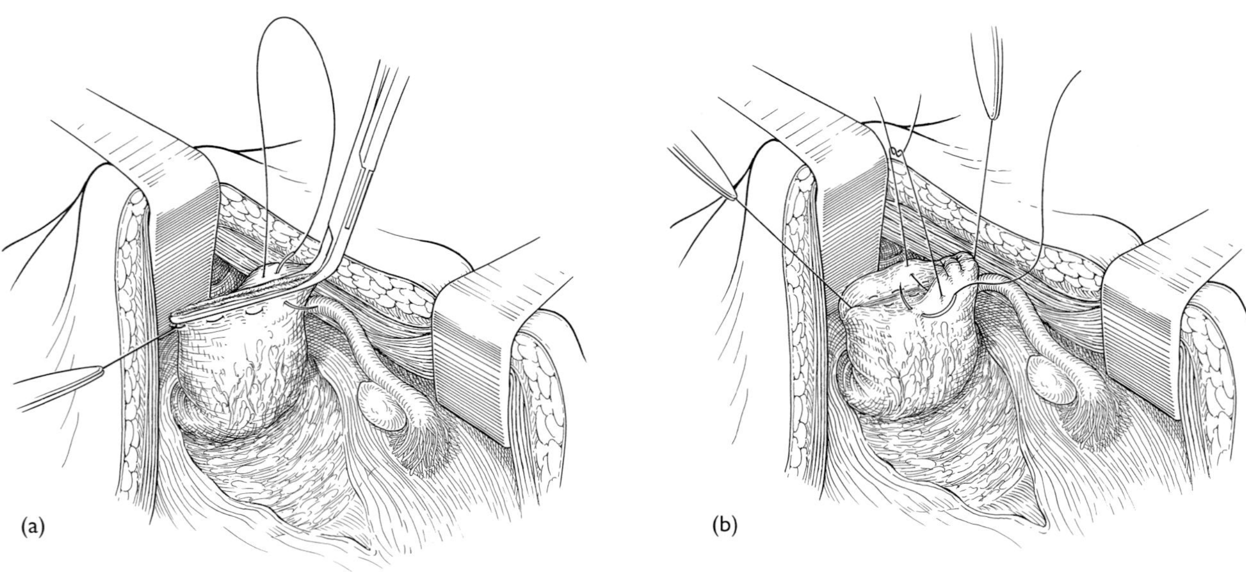

Figure 32.70 Closure of the rectal stump in Hartmann's procedure using the manual technique.

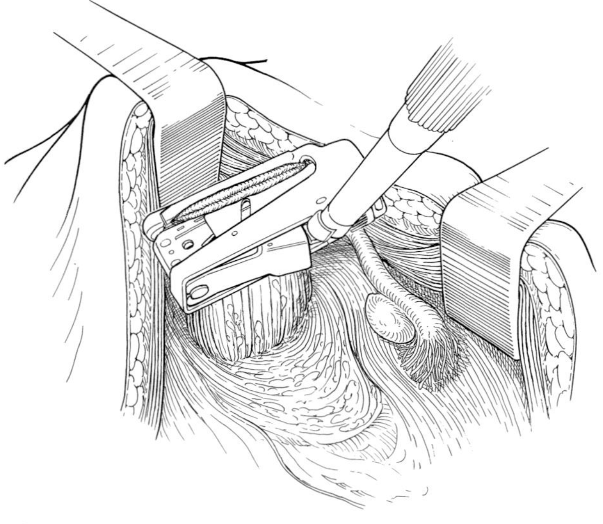

Figure 32.71 Closure of the rectal stump using the Roticulator.

possible to restore continuity and the techniques for doing so are the same as those considered in the section on diverticular disease (see Chapter 37).

New techniques of sphincter-saving resection

Colonic pouches

Function following low anterior resection – whether the anastomosis is constructed manually or stapled – is variable. With very low anastomoses, especially those performed by a transanal technique, patients do suffer from urgency and occasional incontinence. Our own investigations (Williams et al, 1980b) have shown that the main reasons for poor function are a neorectum of low capacity and a reduced resting anal pressure.

Several workers have attempted to increase the capacity of the neorectum by constructing a colonic pouch. Both Lazorthes et al (1986) and Parc et al (1986) in Toulouse and Paris respectively constructed a J colonic pouch with the GIA stapler and effected the anastomosis via a transanal approach. Originally they used 12 cm limbs of colon. They found that the technique reduced the frequency of diarrhoea and lessened the incidence of incontinence in the early postoperative months compared with the state after a straight coloanal anastomosis. However, of the 24 patients treated by Parc et al (1986), one quarter had difficulty in securing spontaneous defecation and had to resort to enemas and suppositories to empty their reservoirs. Parc then reduced the length of the colonic limbs to 6 cm and spontaneous evacuation was achieved more frequently (R Parc, 1989, personal communication).

We also performed J colonic pouches for very low rectal cancers. Our philosophy at the Royal London Hospital was somewhat different from that of Parc and Lazorthes. While the colonic pouch corrected the loss of reservoir capacity, the transanal coloanal anastomosis did nothing to prevent the damage to the internal anal sphincter. Sphincter damage was also aggravated by the stretching of the anal canal necessary to complete the anastomosis. To reduce this damage, we elected to preserve the anal canal and staple the pouch to the top of it. The technique we initially used avoided purse-string sutures completely (Williams, 1989) (Figure 32.72).

The rectum was dissected down to the pelvic floor as described for a low anterior resection. The anal canal was transected and stapled transversely using an appropriate instrument; the Roticulator stapling gun was ideal for this purpose if the low rectum was transected, but the TA or TL30 was preferred if the anus was transected. A J colonic pouch

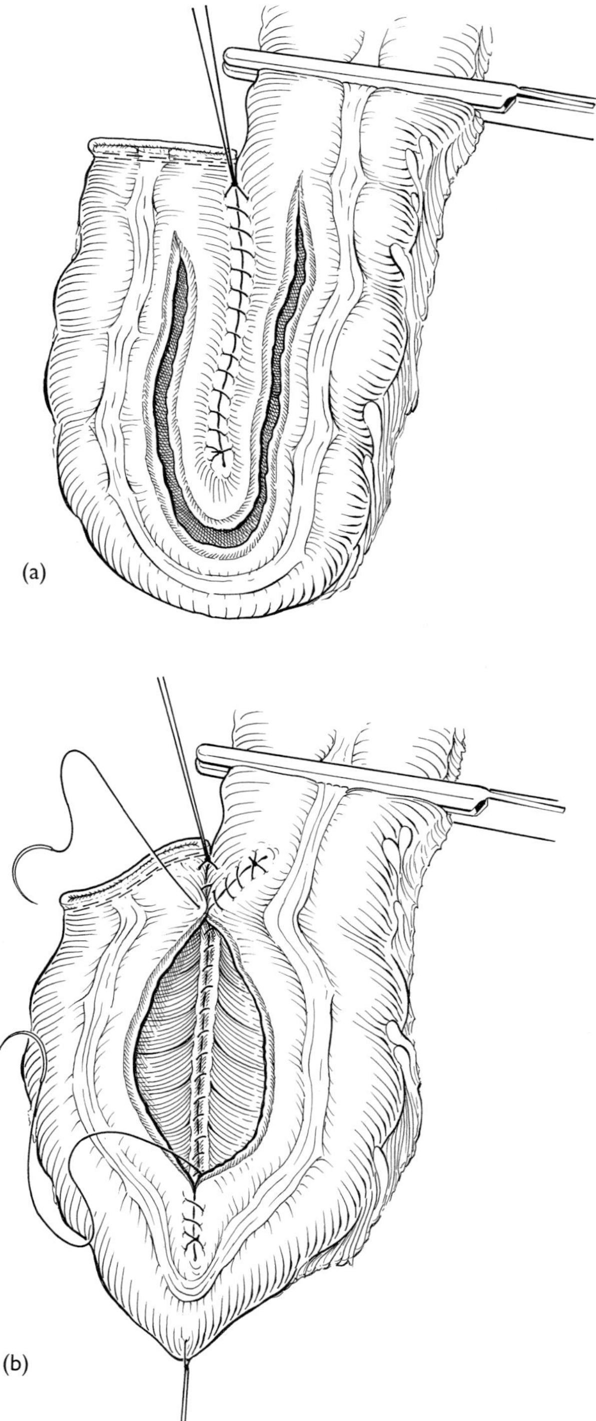

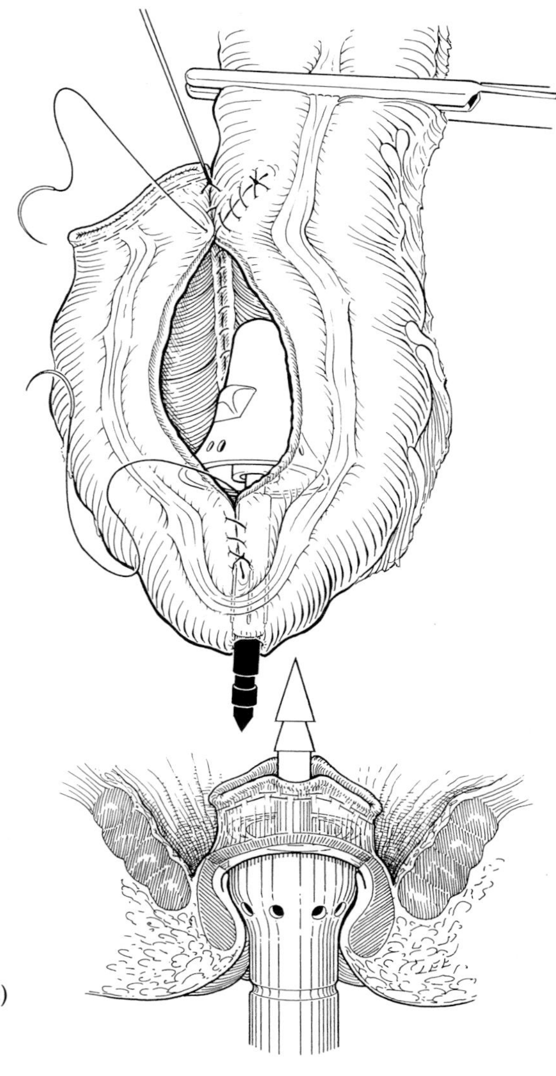

Figure 32.72a–f Construction of J colonic pouch and anal-pouch anastomosis without purse-string sutures. (a,b) A J colonic pouch is constructed manually but the anterior wall is left open. (c) The anvil of the Premium CEEA instrument is inserted into the pouch through the anterior wall defect. The anvil spike is thrust through the apex of the pouch away from the suture lines. (*Continued*)

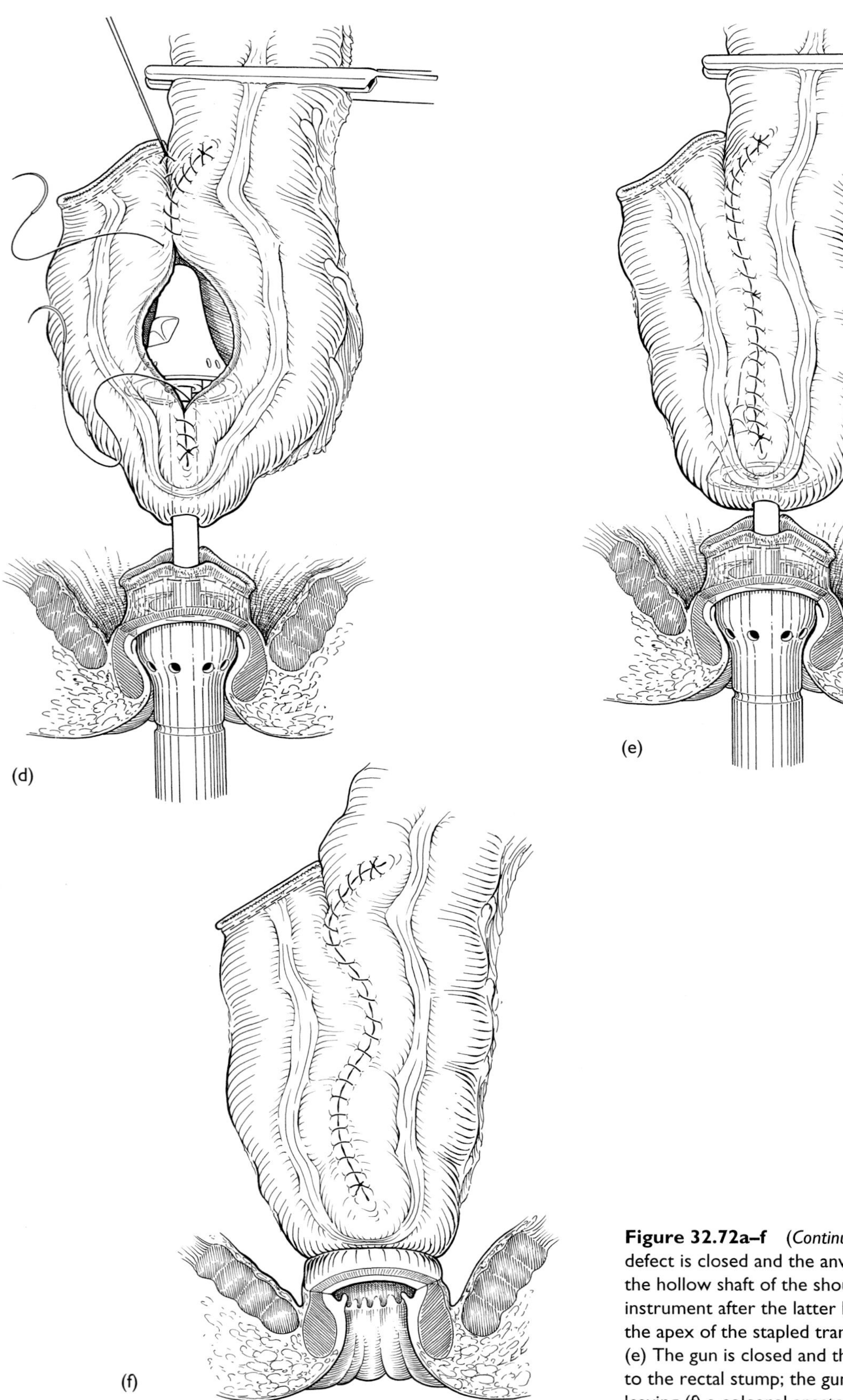

Figure 32.72a–f (*Continued*) (d) The anterior wall defect is closed and the anvil spike is inserted into the hollow shaft of the shoulder piece of the instrument after the latter has been thrust through the apex of the stapled transected rectal stump. (e) The gun is closed and the pouch is approximated to the rectal stump; the gun is fired and removed, leaving (f) a coloanal anastomosis.

was fashioned manually in two layers, but the anterior wall was not completed in its central part. The anvil and shaft of a Premium CEEA instrument was inserted into the interior of the pouch and the shaft was thrust through its apex, well away from the suture lines. An interrupted suture was placed on either side of the anvil and tied to prevent disruption of the suture lines. The defect in the anterior wall of the pouch was then closed. The cartridge section of the gun with its spike retracted was inserted into the anal canal. The trocar was advanced so that it pierced the anorectal stump. The trocar spike was removed and the shaft with the anvil of the instrument was inserted into the hollow shaft of the cartridge section. The gun was then closed, fired and removed in the usual way. The 'doughnuts' were checked and with the colon cross-clamped just above the pouch, the integrity of the anastomosis and suture lines of the pouch were tested by injection of air through the anal canal after filling the pelvis with saline. A loop ileostomy was then raised in the right iliac fossa to defunction the distal colon.

The technique we now use is the same as above, apart from the construction of the J pouch. We now construct the pouch using the GIA stapler, the apex of the pouch being anastomosed to the anorectal stump using the Premium CEEA instrument as described above (Figure 32.73).

At the Royal London Hospital we (like Parc) initially used two 10–12 cm limbs of colon. Three of the eight patients who underwent this procedure had great difficulty in evacuating their pouch. Dynamic proctography showed that these patients could not empty the pouch satisfactorily because its large volume caused the pouch to fall back in the pelvis and made the anal–pouch angle so acute that evacuation was impossible. As a result we reduced the length of the colonic limbs to 6 cm and ensured that the anastomosis was sited at the top of the anal canal.

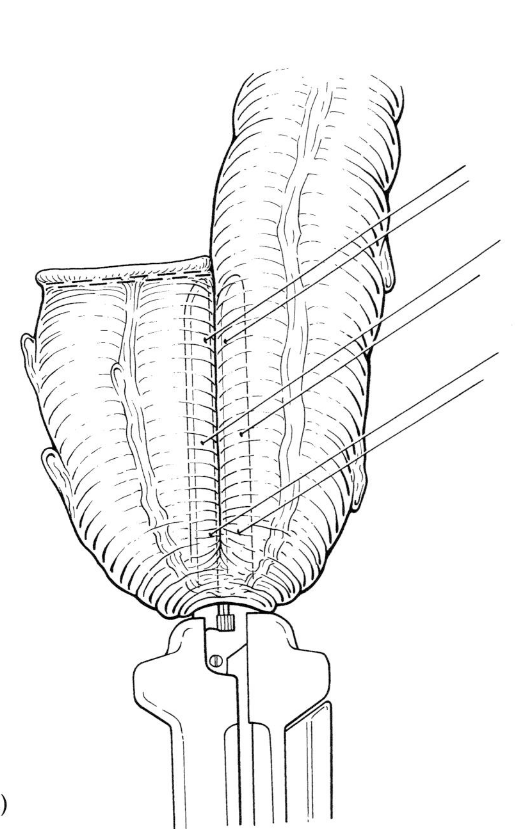

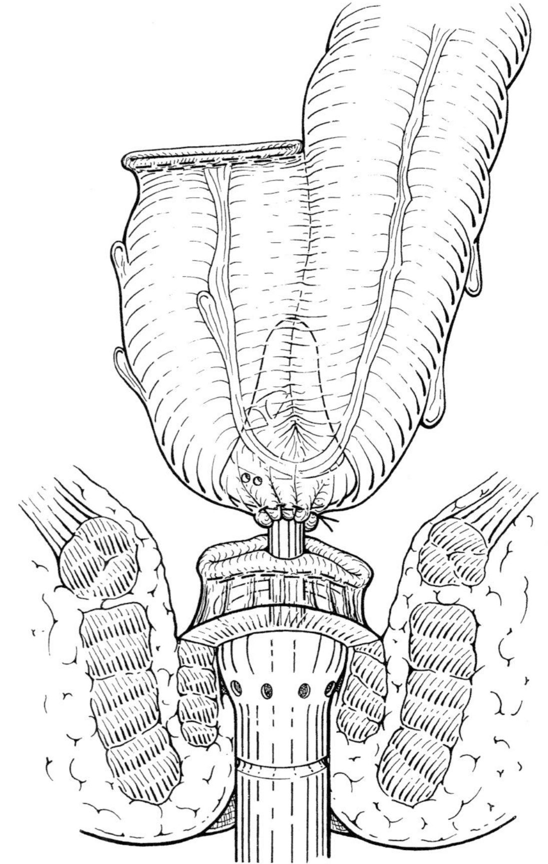

Figure 32.73 A side-to-side colocolic anastomosis is performed to achieve a J pouch. Two 6 cm lengths of colon are approximated by stay sutures. A small enterotomy is made in the apex of the J loop. A linear staple cutter is advanced between the two limbs of the bowel to achieve the side-to-side anastomosis.

This manoeuvre improved function, but evacuation has still remained a problem with a substantial proportion of patients requiring the regular use of enemas and suppositories. Several further studies have examined the use of a colonic pouch and coloanal anastomosis (Nicholls et al, 1988; Leo et al, 1993; Seow-Choen, 1993; Gross and Amir-Kabirian, 1994; von Flue et al, 1994; Mortensen et al, 1995). In most, the pouch and anastomosis have been constructed using the stapler.

Some have compared the results retrospectively with those after straight coloanal anastomosis (Table 32.11). As far as we are aware, there have been three randomized controlled trials (Hallbook et al, 1995; Seow-Choen, 1996; Ho et al, 1996; Lazorthes et al, 1997). The conclusions from these studies are that frequency of defecation, urgency and continence are improved with a pouch. However, it is acknowledged that some patients may develop evacuation difficulty, but this can be minimized by using no more than 12–16 cm of colon for the two-loop construction. Importantly, the morbidity and mortality rates do not seem to have increased.

Nevertheless, it is our view at the Royal London Hospital that before a colonic pouch is added as a routine to low anterior resection we need the results from larger randomized trials. At present, we reserve the pouch for selected patients who because of age and/or impaired anal sphincter function are likely to have significant frequency and urgency after a straight coloanal anastomosis. Our view in Birmingham is that pouch patients have a lower frequency of defecation and less soiling than patients having a straight coloanal anastomosis. Admittedly some studies report impaired evacuation, but we have not found this to be a problem when the pouch is no more than 7–8 cm long and constructed with a 7.5 cm linear staple cutter (Nicholls et al, 1988; Berger et al, 1992; Pélissier et al, 1992; Mortensen et al, 1995; Seow-Choen, 1996).

Total anorectal reconstruction using an electrically stimulated neoanal sphincter

Various workers have attempted to restore gastrointestinal continuity after abdominoperineal excision of the rectum for carcinoma. Simonsen et al (1976) and Wong and Wee (1984) described a procedure of coloperineal anastomosis and gracilis transposition in order to achieve this aim. Although they claimed some success, the procedure never gained universal acceptance. Cavina and his colleagues in Pisa tried a similar procedure, but modified it by applying electrical stimulation to the gracilis muscle via exteriorized electrodes for a short period after the operation. The stimulus was applied for approximately 10 minutes once or twice a day, the hope being to restore tone to the transposed muscle (Cavina et al, 1985).

It is unlikely that the transposed gracilis muscle alone will be able to function as a neoanal sphincter. This muscle is a fast twitch muscle which fatigues easily. An anal sphincter needs to be composed of slow twitch fibres so that it can contract continuously without fatigue, yet relax sufficiently to allow evacuation to proceed. Evidence is available, primarily from animal experiments, which shows that fast twitch fatiguable muscle fibres can be converted to slow twitch non-fatiguable muscle fibres by

Table 32.11 Functional outcome after colonic pouch and straight coloanal anastomosis (SCA).

Author	*Patients (n)*	*Continence*			*Mean bowel frequency per 24 h*
		Perfect	*Minor defects*	*Poor*	
Lazorthes et al (1986)					
SCA	15	12	3	0	3
Pouch	36	28	8	0	1.7
Nicholls et al (1988)					
SCA	15	9	6	1	2.3
Pouch	13	10	3	0	1.4
Gross and Amir-Kabirian (1994)					
SCA	11	2	7	2	6
Pouch	10	9	0	1	3
Hallbook et al (1995)*			*Median continence score†*		
SCA	51		5		3.6
Pouch	47		1		1.6

* Randomized prospective study; results at 1 year.
† Incontinence score 0–18; 0 = continence.

chronic low-frequency electrical stimulation. Much of this work in the past has concentrated on the development of a cardiac assist device capable of augmenting or replacing a failing heart. The latissimus dorsi muscle was used for this purpose. Chronic stimulation of the thoracodorsal nerve in the dog at a frequency of 2–10 Hz for a period of 6 weeks was capable of converting this predominantly fast twitch muscle to a slow twitch muscle with greater fatigue resistance (Mannion et al, 1986).

Most studies were performed in experimental animals, but some case reports in humans described the replacement of myocardial defects by electrically stimulated pedicles of latissimus dorsi (Carpentier and Chachques, 1985; Magovern et al, 1986). The success of this work encouraged us at the Royal London Hospital to apply chronic electrical stimulation to create a neoanal sphincter. In initial experiments in animals (Hallan et al, 1990) we showed that this approach was feasible and therefore proceeded to use it in patients who were incontinent despite conventional therapy. After achieving modest success in this group of patients (Williams et al, 1991) we applied the technique to patients who had undergone an abdominoperineal excision (Williams et al, 1990a,b).

Our initial technique was briefly as follows. A standard abdominoperineal excision of the rectum was performed; the distal end of the transected colon which had been transversely stapled was brought down to the perineum and a coloperineal anastomosis was constructed in the position previously occupied by the anal orifice (Figure 32.74a,b). The remainder of the perineal wound was sutured in the usual manner. A covering loop ileostomy was constructed in the right iliac fossa. After completion of the main part of the operation, the distal half of the gracilis muscle which was to be used for the neosphincter was mobilized by dividing the two or three vascular pedicles which supply it (Figure 32.74c). This procedure was carried out to enhance the blood supply to the distal part of the muscle when it was subsequently transposed. Our anatomical studies had shown that the blood supply to the gracilis was segmental (Patel et al, 1991), and division of the distal vessels at the same time as

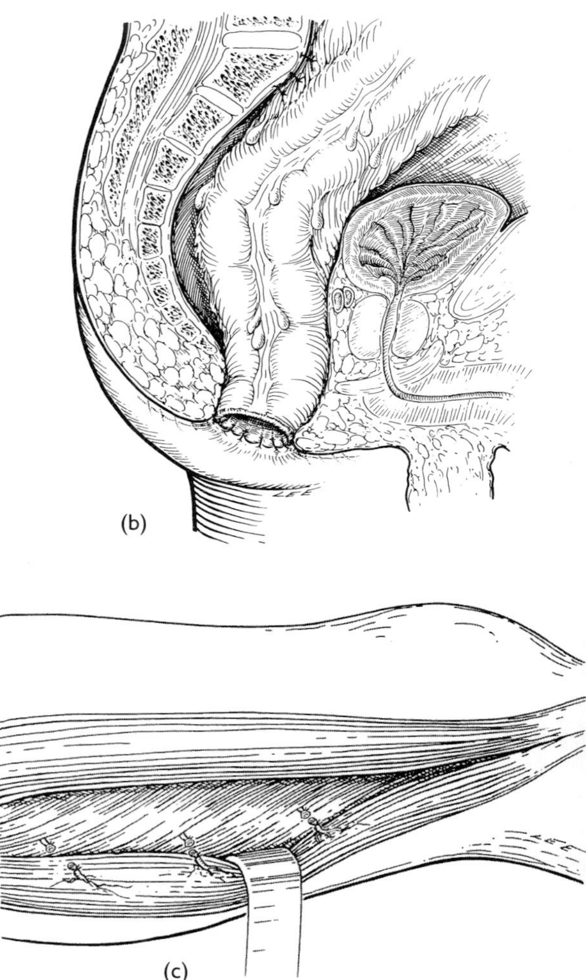

Figure 32.74a–c Total anorectal reconstruction (TAR) after abdominoperineal excision of the rectum by coloperineal anastomosis and an electrically stimulated gracilis neosphincter. (a,b) In the first stage the rectum is removed and the colon is brought down to the perineum and anastomosed. (c) In the second stage the distal two or three vascular pedicles to the gracilis are divided and the distal tendon is next transected close to its insertion.

transposition was thought to lead to ischaemia of the muscle. Our cadaver dissections also showed that there were tenuous arterioarterial connections between the segmental vessels. Division of the segmental vessels and delay in transposition allowed these arterioarterial anastomoses to open up, ensuring the viability of the muscle when it was subsequently transposed. The second stage was performed when the perineal wound and coloperineal anastomosis were healed. This usually took 4–6 weeks. However, other surgeons have since used gracilis transposition without a delay procedure and have not produced ischaemia in the distal part of the muscle. There are now numerous reports which seem to confirm that such a delay manoeuvre is not necessary. As a result, we have eliminated the initial division of the distal vessels, without ischaemic consequences.

At the second stage the gracilis muscle was mobilized from the thigh down to its insertion into the tibia and the tendon divided as low as possible. The proximal neurovascular bundle was carefully identified and preserved at the posterolateral border of the muscle at the junction of its proximal third and distal two-thirds. After the main nerve to the muscle had been identified using a nerve stimulator, the purpose-built electrode (initially NICE Inc, FL, USA; now Medtronic MN, USA) was positioned over the main trunk of the nerve (Figure 32.75a). The position of the electrode was adjusted until a point was identified where the voltage threshold for the contraction of the whole muscle was at its lowest (usually 2 V, 0.2 ms, 1–2 pulses per second). When this position was localized the electrode plate was sutured into position with interrupted fine silk sutures, taking care not to damage the nerve or blood supply of the muscle. A 3 cm vertical incision was made with its lower end overlying the left ischial tuberosity. The incision was deepened until the fascia between the thigh and perineum was reached. This fascia required division with scissors to create a large enough defect to allow the gracilis to be brought into the perineum without constriction. After infiltration with adrenaline and saline solution, a short circumanal incision was made approximately 3 cm from the left lateral margin of the anal canal. This incision was deepened through the subcutaneous fat into the ischiorectal fossa. A similar incision was made on the opposite side exactly adjacent to the previous incision. A circumferential track was then made around the neoanal canal by a mixture of blunt and sharp dissection. This track must be wide and deep enough to accommodate the transposed muscle without constriction.

A subcutaneous tunnel was also created between the thigh and the perineal wound and the mobilized gracilis muscle was brought into the perineum and passed round the neoanal canal in the manner depicted in Figure 32.75b. With the left leg adducted the tendon of gracilis was sutured to the periosteum overlying the right ischial tuberosity with two or three interrupted 0 Ethibond sutures. The wires from the electrode were then tunnelled subcutaneously to the site where the implanted stimulator was to be positioned – initially overlying the eighth and ninth ribs in the mid-clavicular line, but now in the upper outer quadrant of the abdomen. At this site a subcutaneous pocket was created by blunt dissection and the stimulator (initially Neuromed Inc, FL, USA; now Medtronic Inc, MN, USA) was connected to the electrode wires and inserted into the pocket (Figure 32.75c). Once the patient had recovered and the wounds were healed, the stimulator was programmed to deliver a pulse of 2 V, 0.2 ms pulse width at a frequency of 12 pulses per second. The patient was discharged from hospital and the chronic low-frequency stimulation was continued until evidence of conversion had been demonstrated. With a pressure microtransducer within the anal canal, the frequency of contraction of the neoanal sphincter could be determined. The stimulus frequency could be gradually increased until a fixed, tetanic contraction was produced (Figure 32.75d). The minimum frequency to produce this tetanic contraction is known as the fusion frequency. Before starting low-frequency stimulation, the fusion frequency is normally 25 pulses per second. After 6–8 weeks of low-frequency stimulation, the fusion frequency usually falls to approximately 15 pulses per second and the fatigue interval is significantly prolonged. Such findings indicate some degree of conversion to slow twitch muscle. When this had been achieved, the covering stoma was closed and the stimulator was reprogrammed to produce a subtetanic contraction of the neoanal sphincter which was sufficient to produce occlusion of the neoanal canal. When defecation was required the patient turned the stimulator off with the magnet, the neoanal sphincter relaxed, evacuation occurred and the stimulator was turned on once again with the magnet (see Chapter 20).

We initially performed this procedure in 12 patients (Mander et al, 1996) with rectal or anal canal neoplasms in whom a sphincter-saving operation was contraindicated. Eight patients had their defunctioning stomas closed. In seven of the eight patients complete physiological measurements were taken. Median basal and maximum neosphincter pressures were 30 and 122 cmH_2O at the start of stimulation and 22.5 and 76.2 cmH_2O

after one year. Median functioning neosphincter pressure was 36 cmH_2O at one year. All of the patients had some degree of incontinence to solid stool and wore pads. However, despite imperfect continence, no patient wished to go back to life with a stoma.

Throughout this period, modifications to the neosphincter technique were made. Initially, the peripheral nerves to the gracilis were stimulated. However, we now, as described above, stimulate the main nerve which has the considerable advantage of producing an *en masse* contraction of the neosphincter, ensuring that more type 2 fibres are converted to type 1 fibres, and thus increasing the neosphincter pressure. This modification alone should in future make the operation more successful. However, the technique suffers from other defects which mar the functional outcome. Thus,

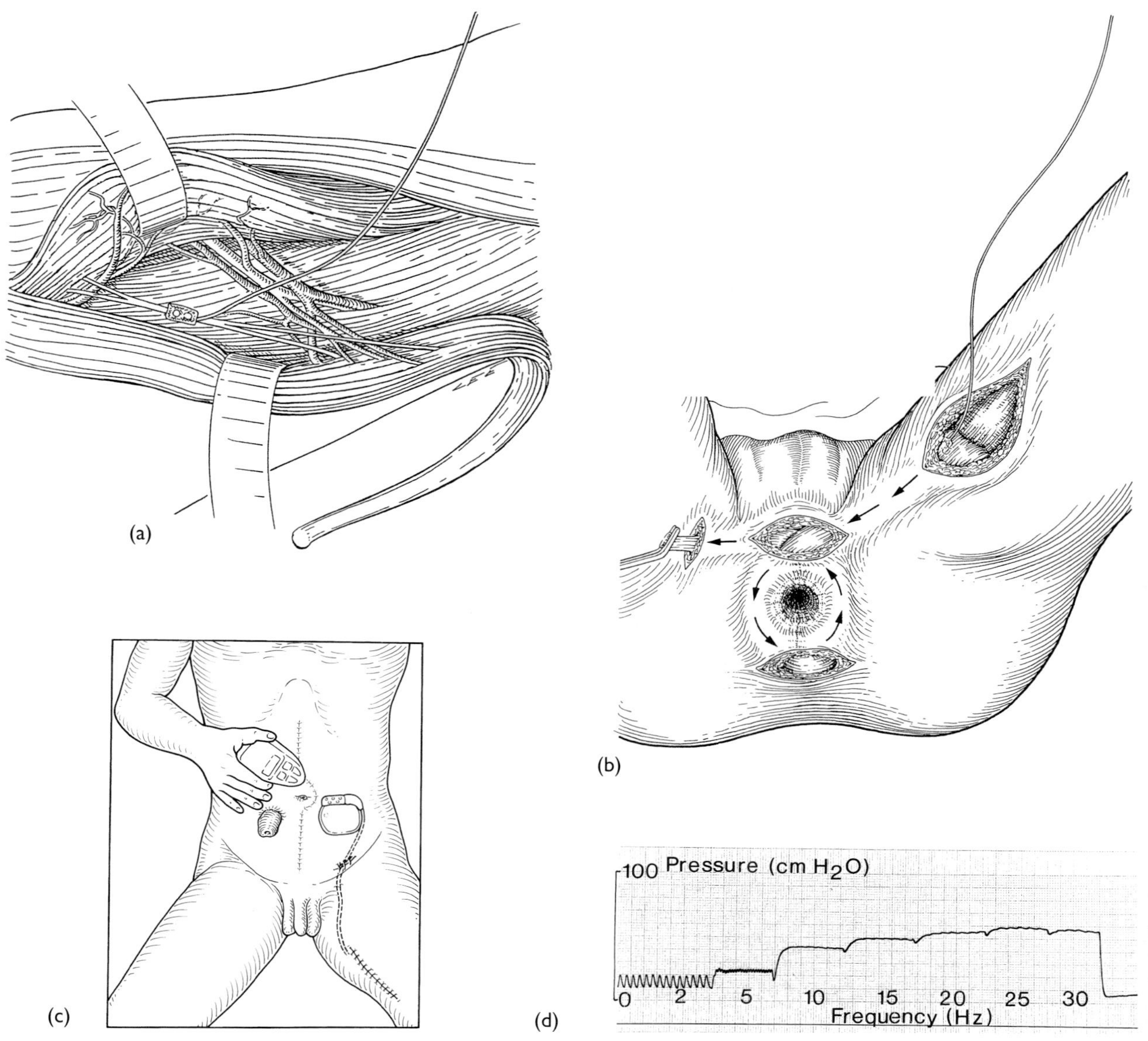

Figure 32.75a–d TAR. (a) The gracilis is mobilized, more proximally the main nerve is identified lying on the adductor brevis muscle, and the purpose-built electrode (Medtronic) is sutured over it. (b) The muscle is transposed around the neoanal canal in a 'gamma' configuration and sutured to the opposite inferior pubic ramus. (c) The electrode lead is connected to the stimulator which is implanted subcutaneously in the right iliac fossa. (d) With a microtransducer in the neoanal canal, the frequency of stimulation can be increased. The minimum frequency that can produce a fused, tetanic contraction is known as the 'tetanic fusion frequency', which in this patient was 25 Hz.

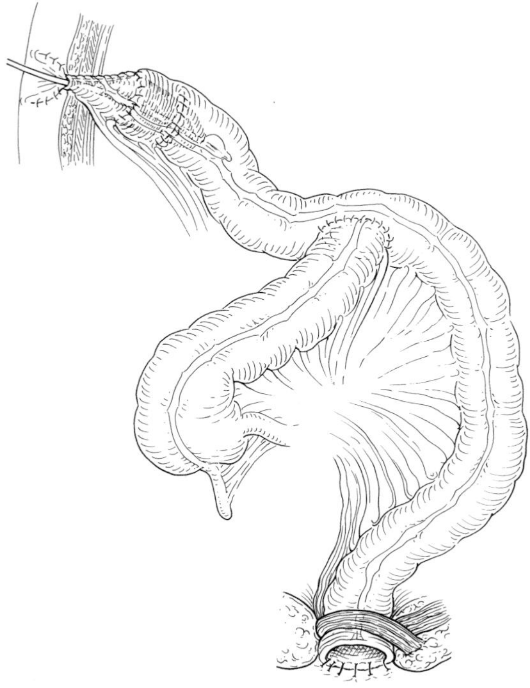

Figure 32.76 TAR, coloperineal anastomosis, electrically stimulated neosphincter and transverse colonic conduit. The neosphincter maintains continence while antegrade irrigation via the conduit achieves evacuation.

normal sensation is lost (Abercrombie et al, 1994) and patients cannot appreciate either the call to stool or when the neorectum is completely empty. All eight patients described previously reported difficulty in evacuation.

As a consequence, we have modified the operation of total anorectal reconstruction by the addition of a continent colonic conduit (see also Chapter 21). This conduit is intubated on a regular basis so that the neorectum can be evacuated by antegrade colonic lavage (Williams et al, 1994; Hughes and Williams, 1995). The conduit is constructed using the proximal transverse colon (Figure 32.76). Continence is provided by an intussuscepted valve which is akin to that used in the Kock pouch. It is stabilized by a mixture of staples and sutures (see Figure 21.26). The aperture on the abdominal wall is constructed using skin flaps to prevent stenosis (see Figure 21.31a–c).

The combination of the colonic conduit and the electrically stimulated neosphincter as part of total anorectal reconstruction has dramatically improved the results of this procedure. Provided patients are prepared to accept further surgery, there is now another option to life with a permanent colostomy. It remains to be seen how beneficial this new procedure will be compared with the more conventional approach. A prospective study has been set up to evaluate this further.

Postoperative care after excisional surgery

Postoperative care is similar to that given for any major abdominal operation. There are, however, some differences worth noting after sphincter-saving resection and abdominoperineal excision, particularly if a colostomy has been constructed.

Analgesia is given regularly and in adequate doses. The actual type will depend on the preferences of the surgeon and anaesthetist, but some form of morphine derivative delivered by a patient-controlled syringe driver is usually prescribed. A nasogastric tube is not normally retained in the postoperative period. The patient is not allowed food or fluids initially, and adequate hydration is maintained with an intravenous infusion of 4% dextrose and 0.18% saline with added potassium. Approximately 48–72 hours postoperatively oral fluids are gradually introduced. Usually the patient starts on 25–50 mL of clear fluid every hour which is built up gradually to free fluids provided nausea or vomiting does not occur. Usually by the time fluids are taken *ad libitum* flatus has been passed through the anus or colostomy. Food can then be introduced, starting usually with semisolids before going on to solids. If the patient required total parenteral nutrition before operation, the subclavian line is heparinized and occluded during the operation and in the first 48 hours afterwards. Once the risk of line sepsis from systemic bacteraemia is over, it is usual to recommence the feeding regimen in the postoperative period. Antibiotic policy will vary between individual surgeons but our normal practice is to give one or two further doses of antibiotic 6 hours or 12 hours after operation in addition to the one dose given with the premedication, depending on the severity of the operation and the pharmokinetics of the agents used. If there has been contamination of the operative site with faecal material, the course of antibiotics is continued for 3–5 days postoperatively.

Patients after anterior resection are best nursed in the low sitting position. After abdominoperineal excision it is preferable for the patient to be nursed on the side since this protects the perineal wound, and if the patient's position is changed at 4-hourly to 6-hourly intervals from one side to the other, pressure sores are unlikely to occur.

Urinary catheter drainage is maintained for several days after the operation and is not removed until the patient is relatively mobile. After removal spontaneous micturition usually proceeds normally, but if it does not recatheterization may be necessary, following a trial of autonomic stimulation using 0.25 mg carbachol (provided there has been no recent intestinal anastomosis when such measures may be contraindicated; see Chapter 70).

Closed suction drains will be removed as soon as they no longer drain blood. If return of peristalsis is delayed, parenteral fluid administration will have to continue and the provision of energy may be needed if the ileus continues. Although suppository administration may be tried, on no account must an enema or a stimulant suppository be given to these patients in an attempt to stimulate evacuation. If the patient with an end colostomy still fails to produce either flatus or faeces from the stoma, a finger should gently be inserted into the lumen to ensure there is no stenosis. Removal of the finger is often accompanied by a gush of fluid and flatus and this solves the problem.

It is current practice to place an *ileostomy* adherent drainage bag over the stoma at the completion of the operation. This is used because the effluent in the early postoperative period tends to be fluid rather than solid. As the days pass the effluent thickens, and the patient and stoma care nurse can then decide which is the optimum appliance. The patient should be encouraged at the earliest stage to take an interest in the stoma and under supervision be taught how to change the appliance.

Management of the perineal wound after abdominoperineal excision

Management depends on whether the perineal wound has been closed primarily or whether it has been left open and packed. If it has been closed, the suction drains are removed when drainage of blood ceases, usually after 2–3 days. The wound is observed daily to ensure that a haematoma or infection is not developing. In an uncomplicated convalescence the sutures are removed between the eighth and tenth days postoperatively. If a haematoma or sepsis develops it is necessary to take out one or two sutures prematurely in order to establish drainage. If adequate drainage is not established in this way the patient may have to be anaesthetized and returned to the theatre. After removal of all sutures the cavity can be cleared of haematoma and irrigated. The resulting wound is then packed and managed in the same way as if it were left open in the first place.

If a decision has been taken to leave the wound open, management involves packing with wide ribbon gauze soaked in an antiseptic which will not dry and stick to the wound edges; we prefer proflavine in liquid paraffin. The original packing is removed 48–72 hours after operation. This may be a painful manoeuvre and consequently should be done after giving the patient a hefty dose of strong analgesia. A mixture of nitrous oxide and air can also be inhaled during changing of the pack; but we prefer to bring the patient back to the theatre for the first change of dressing on the next available operating list. Once the pack has been removed the cavity is irrigated with a litre of dilute hydrogen peroxide solution followed by a litre of saline. The cavity is then lightly repacked and the manoeuvre is repeated daily in the ward. During this period the cavity contracts and granulates. There is a danger during this process that the central part of the cavity may constrict, closing off a space above it which may become infected. To prevent this happening it is essential for the surgeon to examine the cavity every 4–5 days and break down any adhesions within it with a finger. Regular baths are encouraged after removing the pack and before replacing it with a new one, as soon as the patient is mobile.

Once the patient is ambulant and the wound is shallower, the patient may be discharged for daily packing and irrigation as an outpatient or at home. An alternative, which we both advise routinely, is to use a foam elastomer stent (Wood et al, 1977; Macfie and McMahon, 1980). The liquid is inserted into the perineal cavity using a large bladder syringe, with the patient in the prone knee-elbow position, about 10–14 days postoperatively. The catalyst sets the polymer so that a sponge dressing is constructed which conforms to the size and shape of the cavity. The patient can be taught to remove the foam stent and to replace it after bathing. The foam is absorbent and since the patient can remove and replace it unaided there is no need for regular packing by the nursing staff.

In women in whom the posterior vaginal wall has been removed and the perineum has been closed primarily, the final result is most satisfactory provided the perineal wound heals by first intention. In these cases it is necessary to examine the cavity regularly through the vagina and break down any adhesions with the finger. The cavity usually fills up rapidly with granulation tissue and the posterior vaginal wall regenerates quickly. If the perineal wound breaks down the result is not as satisfactory. An anterior dehiscence results in a large introitus. If the wound breaks down in the middle or posteriorly a fistula results from the vagina to the perineum. It is then necessary to open the perineal wound back to the site of the fistula. The wound is then packed in the usual way and heals by secondary intention. If once healed the introitus remains large, some form of vaginoplasty may be required at a later date.

If the posterior vaginal wall is left intact a defect may develop between the vagina and the perineal wound during the postoperative period. The recto-vaginal septum is very thin at its midpoint and it is not unusual for necrosis to occur, presumably as a result of diathermy or operative trauma. A fistula between the perineum and vagina may never heal unless it is laid open by dividing the posterior vaginal wall and perineal tissue down to the exit of the fistula. In this way a cavity is formed by the lower part of the vagina and perineal wound which can be irrigated and packed as previously described.

Additional techniques

If the growth extends into local structures it may be possible to combine rectal excision with excision of the invaded organs. It is sometimes technically feasible to perform a sphincter-saving resection after such a manoeuvre, but in practice it is more likely that abdominoperineal excision will be performed or the surgeon will be content with a Hartmann's procedure, leaving a very short rectal stump.

Concomitant hysterectomy

Frequently, bulky anterior rectal tumours invade some part of the female genital tract, usually the uterus, broad ligaments or ovaries. An *en bloc* excision of rectum, uterus, ovaries, fallopian tubes and broad ligament should therefore be performed.

After mobilization of the left colon and identification of the left ureter, the left uterine appendages are grasped with long artery forceps at their junction with the body of the uterus and these structures are drawn upwards and to the right so as to render taut the round ligament and ovarian ligament (Figure 32.77). These structures are divided and ligatured and the pelvic peritoneum between them is incised.

The peritoneal incision is carried anteriorly to reach the midline between the bladder and anterior vaginal wall and posteriorly to the left side of the sigmoid mesocolon. The left ureter is identified and a sling is placed around its upper end so that it can be traced down into the pelvis. The ureter passes forwards under the uterine vessels which can be seen passing from the internal iliac pedicle to the

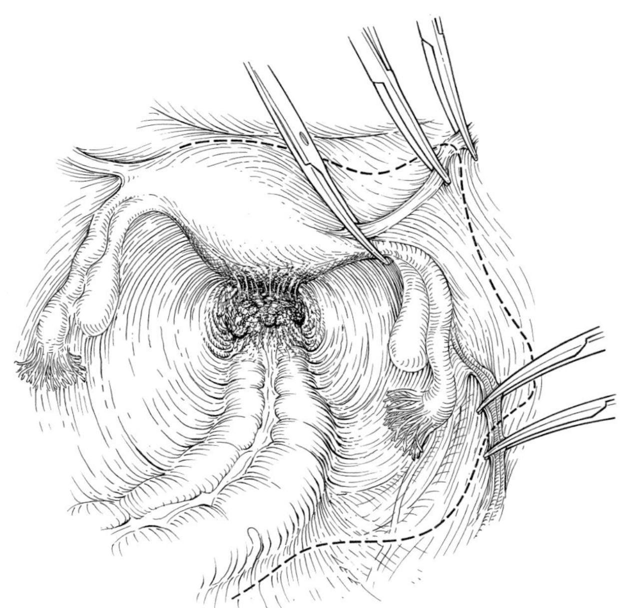

Figure 32.77 Combined total hysterectomy and rectal excision. The uterine appendages on one side have been grasped with artery forceps and drawn upwards and to the opposite side. The round ligament and ovarian ligament have been clipped and the line of peritoneal incision is indicated.

lateral wall of the uterus (Figure 32.78a). At this point the uterine vessels are clamped, divided and ligatured under direct vision (Figure 32.78b). The ureter can then be traced further forward to the point at which it enters the trigone of the bladder. Exactly the same manoeuvre is performed on the right side. The rest of the base of the broad ligament usually has to be divided by transfixion. The anterior plane is further developed down to the level of the vagina.

If an anterior resection or Hartmann's procedure is being performed it is usual to transect the vagina completely at this point below the cervix and the tumour. If, on the other hand, an abdominoperineal excision is in progress, the posterior vaginal wall will need to be excised. Under these circumstances a transverse incision is made in the anterior vaginal wall just below the cervix, taking care to avoid damage to the ureters (Figure 32.79a). From both ends of this incision longitudinal cuts are made in the lateral vaginal walls as far down as possible (Figure 32.79b). The perineal operator will then be able to complete excision of the posterior vaginal wall from below.

The rectum is now mobilized in the usual way and can be removed *en bloc* with the uterine structures.

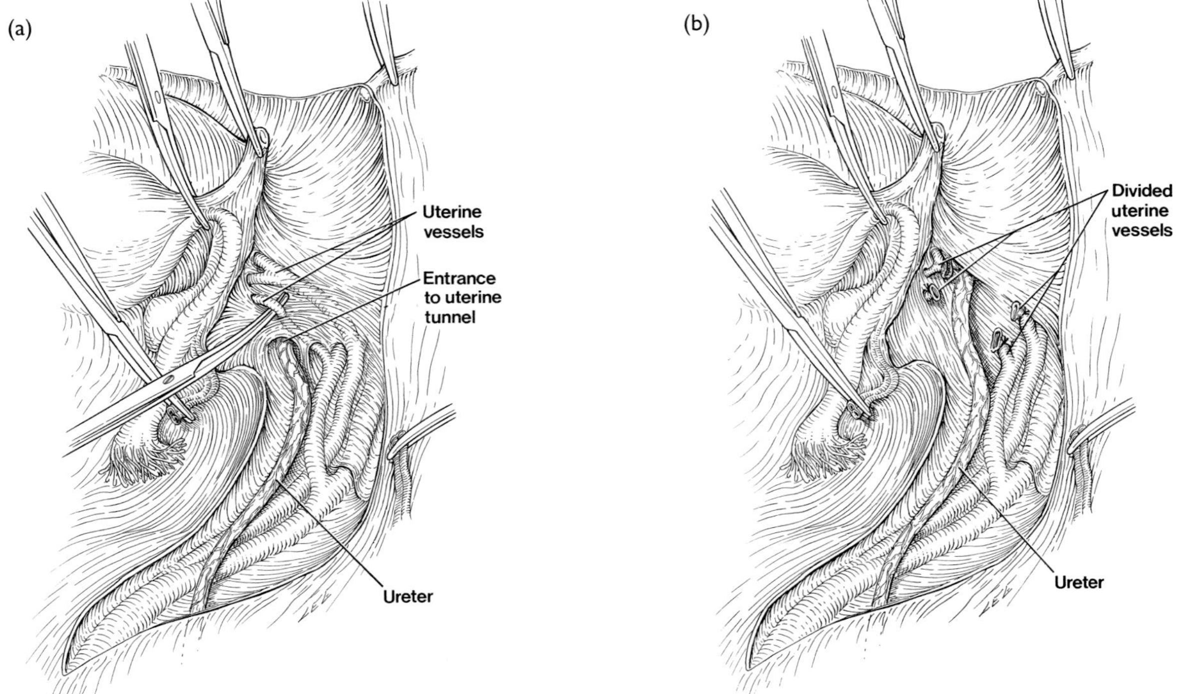

Figure 32.78a,b Combined total hysterectomy and rectal excision: exposing the ureter and uterine artery. (a) The round ligament and ovarian vessels are divided and the tissue spaces are opened up to display the ureter and uterine artery as it crosses in the uterine canal. (b) Complete exposure of the ureter down to the bladder after division of the uterine vessels.

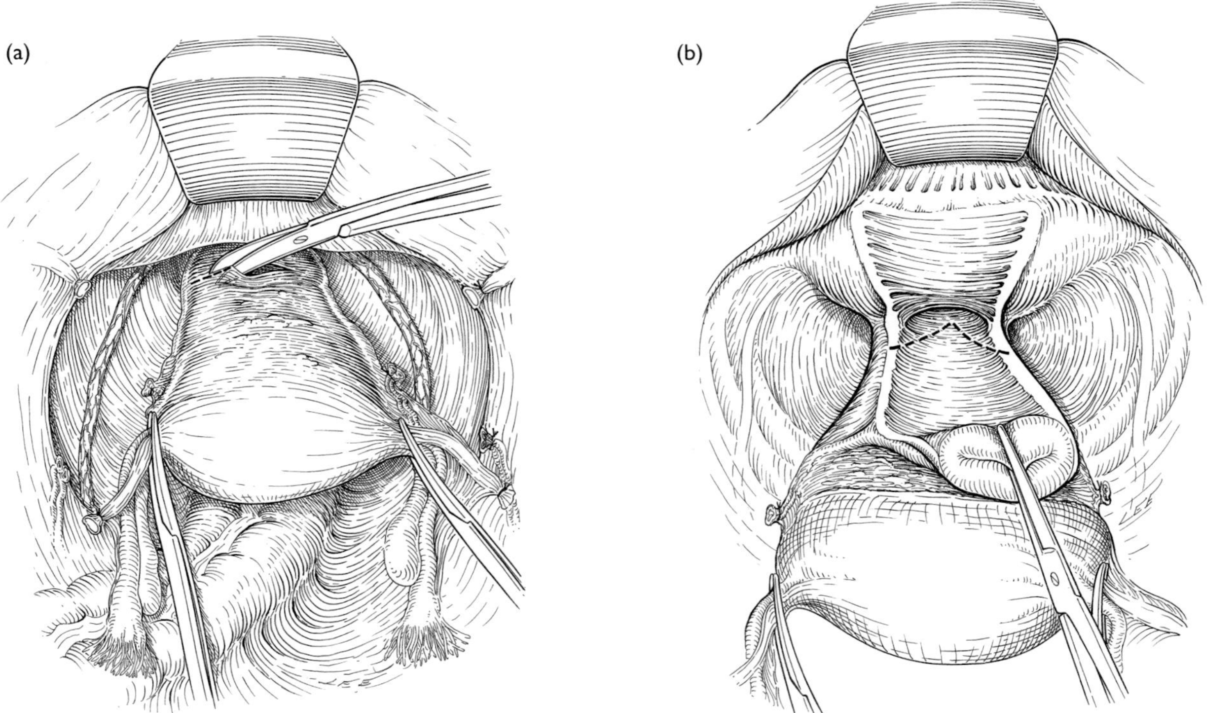

Figure 32.79a,b Combined total hysterectomy and rectal excision. (a) Opening the vagina from the front. (b) Extending the cut dividing the vagina into anterior and posterior halves.

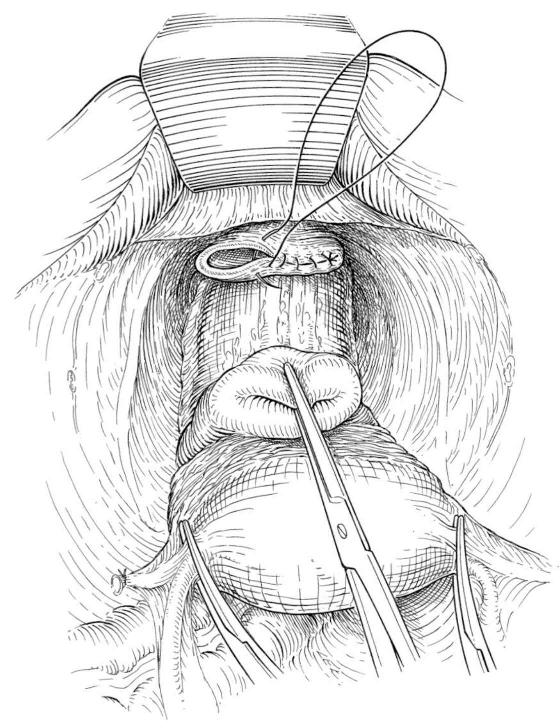

Figure 32.80 Combined total hysterectomy and anterior resection. The vaginal tube has been cut across and the fascia of Denonvilliers has been incised. The rectum has been mobilized and the vagina is being closed.

If the vagina has been transected completely the vault is closed with continuous or interrupted chromic catgut sutures on a 30 mm or 40 mm, strong, cutting half-circle needle, and buried beneath the pelvic peritoneum (Figure 32.80). If the posterior wall has been excised, the anterior wall is left open and its edges are oversewn to obtain haemostasis.

Extended lymph node dissection or radical lymphadenectomy

These terms refer to wide removal of the lateral and superior lymphatic system. This includes a high ligation of the inferior mesenteric artery flush with the aorta and an extended periaortic and pelvic lymph node dissection beginning at the duodenum and extending down to take in the periaortic and lateral iliac nodes (Orkin, 1992). The main proponents of this technique are the Japanese surgeons, whereas in the West it remains a highly controversial manoeuvre, principally because of the high morbidity rates, for what is perceived as a marginal gain. The technique requires that the iliac vessels and their branches be denuded or partially resected, which means the automatic sacrifice of several nerve branches responsible for bladder and sexual function (Hojo et al, 1989).

However, in recent years the National Cancer Center Hospital in Tokyo has presented some compelling supportive data forcing surgeons in the West to look again at the technique. The results of radical lymphadenectomy are critically discussed later in this chapter.

The procedure described below is that practised at the National Cancer Center Hospital in Tokyo and is used in patients in whom there are expected to be major lymph node metastases in the pelvis. If the suspicion of major locoregional metastatic spread is less, then the procedure will not be as radical as described, and attempts will be made to preserve the pelvic autonomic nerves. There follows a description of the technique which has been taken from the excellent thesis of Willem Hans Steup (1994).

The sigmoid colon is mobilized in the usual way and retracted to the right, thus exposing the left retroperitoneal space. The left renal vein serves as the upper border of the dissection. The inferior mesenteric vein is next identified and ligated at this level, and all fatty tissue is dissected and removed working in a caudal direction. In this way, the adventitial layers of the aorta and vena cava are exposed anteriorly and laterally and in between the vessels the pre-vertebral fascia is exposed, while the lumbar vessels are carefully preserved to prevent haemorrhage. As a consequence of this dissection, the sympathetic trunk is excised.

Working toward the right (or left) lateral side first, the ovarian or testicular vessels are identified to serve as the lateral border of the upward dissection. During this phase, the sigmoid colon should be retracted well to the right, in order to achieve exposure to the left retroperitoneum. On the right, the border for upward dissection is much more relative because of the different position of the ovarian or testicular vessels; resection beyond this point is not necessary. Before dissecting all the fatty tissue, it is advisable to identify the right ureter. Care must be taken not to strip the ureters and slings should be placed around them to help in their manipulation for better exposure of underlying structures. The vascular connections (usually four or five) between the ureteric vascular sheet and the gonadal vessels should be identified, dissected and ligated.

Working downward, the inferior mesenteric artery is identified and ligated flush to its origin with the aorta (Figure 32.81). At this point, it is wise to dissect the mesocolon after establishing the level

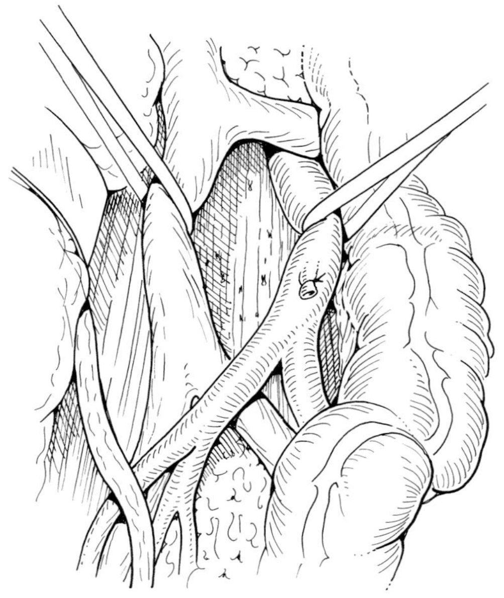

Figure 32.81 Radical lymphadenectomy: upward dissection and aortic caval stripping with ligation of the inferior mesenteric artery (IMA) at its origin.

of proximal transection, guaranteeing sufficient blood supply from the marginal artery by using transillumination of the mesocolon; to prevent the effects of traction on the anastomosis, the splenic flexure needs to be mobilized in the usual way. After sufficient length has been obtained, the sigmoid colon should be transected using a linear stapling device. It is recommended that the distal stump be sutured with a thick suture material, since the subsequent procedure includes frequent manipulation of the distal part of the bowel; therefore, this manoeuvre will decrease the risk of perforation and leakage of the distal stump. The connection between the right and left retroperitoneal dissection planes can now be completed.

After this, the surgeon works downwards, denuding the psoas muscles, vena cava and aorta, while preserving the genitofemoral nerve (overlying the psoas muscles and both ureters). The aortic bifurcation and insertion of the common iliac veins into the vena cava are freed from all surrounding tissues to the adventitial layer, and the sacral promontory is denuded to the level of the prevertebral fascia, and consequently the superior hypogastric nerve plexus is completely sacrificed.

The peritoneal vesicouterine fixation is divided close to the pelvic side walls on the left and right sides.

The retrorectal space is next opened under vision, applying traction to the distal rectal stump and using a rectangular-shaped retractor and blunt dissection. The median plane between the endopelvic fascia and the mesorectum is dissected down to the tip of the coccyx. The thin fascia of Waldeyer is incised, and using 'peanuts' the paravesical space is opened, first on the right and then on the left, exposing the deep levator ani muscle.

The right external iliac artery is exposed after placing slings around the ureter at this level and the internal iliac artery. All fatty tissue is removed from around these vessels. All the branches of the external iliac artery are ligated and divided. The superior vesical artery is preserved, but the internal iliac artery is ligated caudal to its origin.

Lateral to the internal iliac artery, the obturator fossa is opened and completely freed of all fatty tissue to the level of the obturator foramen, ligating the obturator artery and only preserving the obturator nerve (Figure 32.82).

The internal iliac veins on the right and left are ligated at their junction with the external iliac vein. Then the presacral fascia is opened, exposing the lumbosacral and sacral nerve roots. The gluteal vessels which penetrate these nerve plexuses are

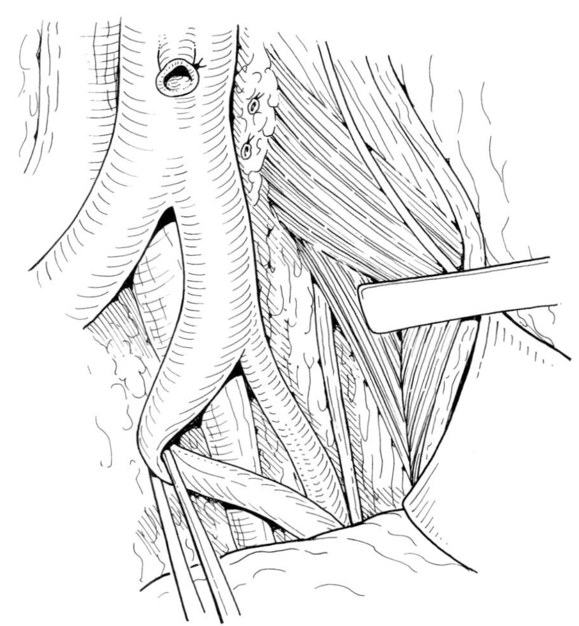

Figure 32.82 Radical lymphadenectomy: the result after complete dissection of the left obturator fossa clearly exposing the obturator nerve.

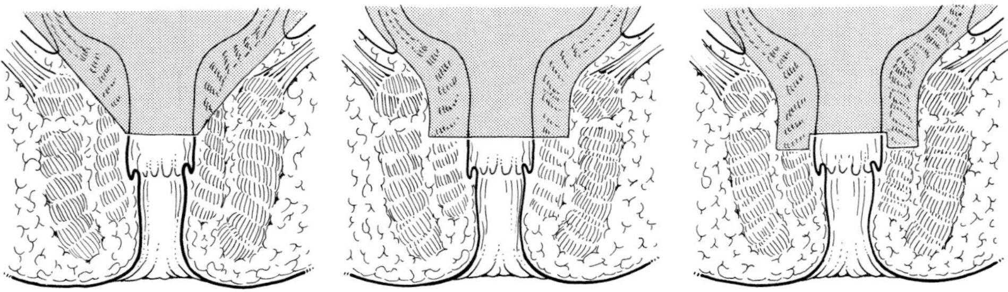

Figure 32.83 Radical lymphadenectomy: total mesorectal excision. A schematic view of possible extents of excision around the rectum within the pelvis in the saggital plane. The W-shaped method should be performed because the V and U dissections leave possible cancer deposits in the mesorectum (Konn et al, 1993).

ligated after identification under slight traction while carefully sparing the sacral nerve roots.

The rectum is then removed. When performing a sphincter-saving resection, the mesorectum is automatically excised totally provided the dissection is in the right plane and extends below the level of rectal transection to the level of the pelvic floor. The possible dissection methods of the mesorectum are illustrated in the sagittal view in Figure 32.83. The V-shaped and U-shaped types of dissection are not radical enough, and it is emphasized that the W-shaped dissection is the method to be employed so that a radical excision of all lymphovascular and fatty tissue is achieved. After transection of the rectal stump with a stapling device, a safe anastomosis can be performed.

In the case of abdominoperineal excision, the pudendal vessels – which represent the deepest point of dissection in the abdominal phase – are dissected. Using a wide perineal skin incision, the anus is excised. All ischiorectal fatty tissue is excised using diathermy and the inferior rectal vessels are identified and ligated on both sides as far lateral as possible. The fat to the level of the gluteal muscles is excised, including the fascia. The levator ani muscles are next transected to obtain communication with the pelvic cavity. The median fixation of the rectum to the sacrum is divided using diathermy close to the bone. The puborectalis is divided as close to the pelvic side wall as possible, and then the rectum is removed. Care has to be taken not to strip the distal part of the ureter of its vascularization and not to damage the prostate, posterior vaginal wall or urethra.

When there are lymph node metastases in the lateral compartment, the internal iliac artery can be excised and thus an extended lateral dissection can be performed (Figure 32.84). The psoas muscles, common and external iliac vessels, the right and left ureters and the lumbosacral and first and second sacral nerve roots (which unite to form the sciatic nerve) will be clearly exposed when an adequate extended radical dissection has been performed. This means total sacrifice of the superior hypogastric plexus, both the inferior hypogastric plexuses and the hypogastric nerves, resulting in 100% impotence in the male and severe loss of normal micturition in both male and female.

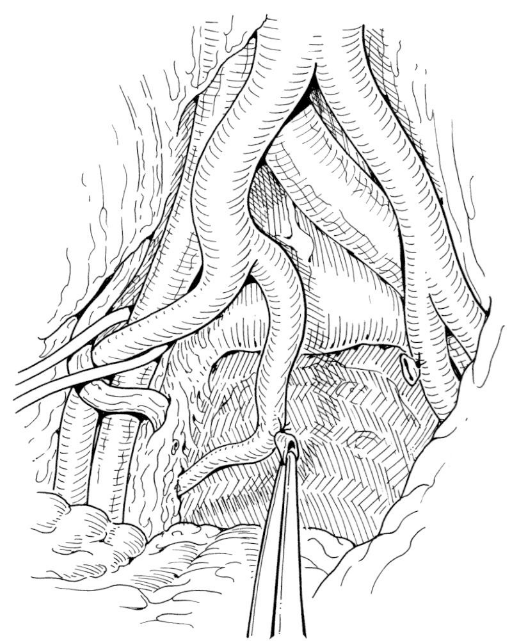

Figure 32.84 Radical lymphadenectomy: the result after complete extended right lateral pelvic dissection. A sling is placed around the external iliac artery. The forceps indicate the stump of the resected right internal iliac artery.

Concomitant excision of bladder and pelvic exenteration

Sometimes a tumour of the upper third of the rectum invades the upper part of the bladder. Under these circumstances it is a relatively simple manoeuvre to perform an *en bloc* excision of rectum and the affected part of the bladder. Gastrointestinal continuity can usually be achieved in these circumstances by an anterior resection performed either manually or by the stapling gun. The bladder is then closed in two layers and an indwelling catheter is left *in situ* for several days postoperatively.

If a tumour situated at a lower level invades the bladder it will usually involve the trigone and one or both ureters. *En bloc* resection will invariably require a total cystectomy and an abdominoperineal excision. The ureters are implanted into an isolated loop of ileum and one end of this ileal conduit is exteriorized as a urinary ileostomy.

The technique of total cystectomy has been well described by Pyrah and Raper (1955). The modifications which have been described over the last 40 years refer almost exclusively to techniques used to anastomose the ureter to the ileal loop (Nesbit, 1948; Cordonnier, 1950; Leadbetter, 1951; Goodwin et al, 1953). The basic principle of these variations in technique was to gain better apposition between ureteric and ileal mucosa than was the case with the original Coffey technique in which the ureters were merely pulled through the ileal wall (Coffey, 1931), leading invariably to stenosis. Using more modern methods of anastomosis and stents, ureteroileal stenosis is rare, although dilated upper tracts may still occur, perhaps due to stenosis at the site of exit of the ileal conduit through the abdominal wall (Neal et al, 1985).

Lesions that invade the sacrum may also be resectable when localized. Resection of the sacrum up to the S3 nerve roots is generally compatible with reasonable function. If one of these roots is left, acceptable urinary function may be retained; if both are sacrificed, function will be lost. If sacrectomy is combined with cystectomy, this concern is of course irrelevant. Further operative details on rectal excision combined with sacrectomy are described in relationship to local recurrence in Chapter 33.

These procedures are clearly formidable, and when combined with total cystectomy usually leave the patient with two stomas. There are no controlled data to demonstrate that they prolong life. However, although some would cast doubt on their widespread use, these procedures may be the only means of controlling local pelvic disease. In selected patients, particularly when the growth is shown only to be invading anteriorly with no evidence of distant metastases, the procedure may well be worth doing. Nevertheless, even in selected patients, there is likely to be considerable morbidity. Thus, Touran et al (1990) in a series of 20 patients, although having no operative deaths, found that 35% of their patients had urinary complications, 25% suffered wound disruption, and median blood loss was 1600 mL. Long-term survival was rare, but long-term control of local disease and palliation of symptoms was achieved in the majority of patients. Others have found a similarly high morbidity rate and poor survival (Eldar et al, 1985; Williams et al, 1988; Hafner et al, 1991; Yeung et al, 1993; Petros and Lopez, 1994). Liu et al (1994) were more optimistic provided the tumour was not invading the sacrum. Thus, 56% of 26 patients undergoing total pelvic exenteration of a primary tumour survived for 5 years.

In our opinion, anterior exenteration should be considered for relatively fit patients provided, of course, they are accepting of life with two stomas. However, considerable thought should be given to additional sacrectomy as the morbidity may outweigh the benefits. One way of reducing the psychological morbidity is to consider preserving the anal sphincter and performing a sphincter-saving resection with a colonic pouch (see later).

COMPLICATIONS OF MAJOR EXCISIONAL SURGERY

Any of the complications that may be associated with major abdominal surgery can occur after rectal excision. These include haemorrhage, respiratory infection, paralytic ileus, wound infection, wound dehiscence, urinary infection, deep venous thrombosis and pulmonary embolus. Only complications that are particularly common following rectal excision or are specific to it are considered here. Some of these problems are common to both abdominoperineal excision and sphincter-saving resection, whereas other problems are related to one or other of the procedures.

General complications

Intestinal obstruction

Intestinal obstruction may be due to paralytic ileus or mechanical causes. Ileus is invariable after these operations but rarely persists longer than 5–6 days. Treatment follows the usual conservative lines of nasogastric suction and intravenous infusion. Although stimulants such as parasympathomimetic drugs (Catchpole, 1969) have been suggested as a method of inducing normal peristalsis, experience suggests they are of little value. Prolonged ileus is usually due to some underlying cause such as a pelvic abscess or partial dehiscence of an anastomosis, ischaemia, metabolic disorders or coexisting medication. Provided these complications can be excluded the best policy is to continue conservative therapy for as long as it takes normal function to be re-established. This may necessitate the institution of total parenteral nutrition. Just occasionally oral intake reverses the process.

Mechanical obstruction occurs more commonly after rectal excision than after most abdominal operations. The reason probably relates to the fact that there are more areas in which the small bowel may become entrapped, particularly after abdominoperineal excision. Thus, bowel may pass between the side of the colostomy and the abdominal wall if the lateral space has not been closed adequately. Small intestine may become adherent to the pelvic peritoneal closure or a loop may escape through it into the pelvis. The terminal ileum may become twisted by the drag on an ileal band during suture of the pelvic peritoneal floor with resulting obstruction. After sphincter-saving resection a small dehiscence may occur at the anastomosis which becomes 'plugged' by a portion of small bowel. This prevents peritonitis but the small bowel may become obstructed in the process.

Diagnosis

In the early days following operation the distinction between paralytic ileus and mechanical obstruction is far from obvious. In both conditions the abdomen will become distended. Although classically mechanical obstruction is accompanied by abdominal pain and ileus is not, after operation this is rarely the case since other factors such as postoperative analgesia influence the symptoms. Mechanical obstruction should be strongly suspected if bowel function returns for a short period and then disappears. Straight abdominal radiography in both conditions will show distension of bowel with fluid levels. When air and fluid levels appear to be limited to the small bowel rather than involving the colon, mechanical obstruction should be suspected. In practice, however, it is often difficult to make this distinction.

Treatment

In most cases of obstruction, be it mechanical or paralytic, the treatment is conservative to start with provided strangulation of bowel is not suspected. Intravenous fluids restore water and electrolyte balance and nasogastric suction will usually reduce the abdominal distension. The patient must be examined at very frequent intervals until a decision has been reached as to whether the obstruction is mechanical or due to paralytic ileus. If it is mechanical and the patient is not responding to conservative measures, a laparotomy will be required. The type of procedure will depend on the findings at laparotomy. If obstruction has occurred through the lateral space (i.e. between the colostomy and the abdominal wall after abdominoperineal excision), it is usually an easy matter to reduce the bowel by pushing (not pulling) it back through the gap. If this is not possible due to distension of bowel, the obstructed loop can be deflated prior to its reduction. Other therapies which may be required include division of adhesions or resection of non-viable bowel.

Acute retention of urine

Acute retention of urine is a frequent problem following rectal excision. The usual scenario is that the urethral catheter is removed after 4–5 days when the patient is mobilizing, but the patient fails to pass urine despite all the usual simple remedies. The catheter is then replaced. Frequently after a further period of drainage normal micturition is established. In a proportion of cases, however, normal function is not regained. Often, even if the patients are able to pass urine per urethram after prolonged drainage they are troubled by severe urinary symptoms. The causes of this problem are varied and more than one factor is often contributory. The following should be considered.

Mechanical factors due to altered anatomy

A common explanation in the past for urinary dysfunction after abdominoperineal excision was that the bladder and prostatic urethra in the absence of the rectum fell backwards towards the sacrum and caused the urethra to be sharply angulated

(Konturri et al, 1974; Watson and Williams, 1952). Although this may be a factor in patients after abdominoperineal excision, it is clearly not the cause of the problem after sphincter-saving resection where the colon fills the space left by the rectum.

Prostatic enlargement

The patient who has prostatic symptoms prior to operation is very likely to become obstructed postoperatively. Frequently, however, patients with prostatic enlargement have had no symptoms attributable to it preoperatively, and were able to compensate quite well. After operation other factors combine to inhibit the normal compensatory mechanisms and the patient is unable to overcome the obstruction. Similarly, a moderately enlarged prostate may be present before operation but does not cause compression of the urethra. The pelvic dissection causes some oedema and fibrosis to occur both within the prostate and the membranous urethra and a complete obstruction to flow is produced. The incidence of prostatic obstruction is difficult to determine; few studies have investigated patients before and after operation. It is therefore difficult to determine which patients have true prostatic obstruction and which have a denervated bladder as a consequence of pelvic nerve damage.

Bladder denervation

Damage to the pelvic autonomic nerves in the course of rectal excision seems to be relatively common. The main problem results from parasympathetic injury rather than damage to sympathetic nerves. The parasympathetic nerve supply to the bladder and urethra is normally responsible for contraction of the detrusor muscle and relaxation of the bladder neck, as well as carrying the sensory fibres subserving bladder distension.

Injury is usually partial but the exact site is difficult to pinpoint. The parasympathetic nerve supply to the bladder originates from the nervi erigentes which arise from S2, S3 and S4. The nerves run laterally on each side and join the corresponding branch of the presacral nerve to form the pelvic plexus on the side wall of the pelvis. From this plexus mixed sympathetic and parasympathetic fibres pass medially to the various pelvic organs including the bladder, prostate and urethra. It is difficult to see how injury could occur to the nerves when they lie on the pelvic side wall unless the dissection was carried out far laterally and was accompanied by radical iliac lymph node excision. There is no evidence that patients with proven bladder denervation after rectal excision have had extensive lateral dissection. It is also unlikely that these nerves are damaged at the level of the nervi erigentes as these lie below the presacral fascia. It has been suggested that in some circumstances the perineal operator in the course of an abdominoperineal excision may enter the wrong plane from below. Instead of dividing the fascia of Waldeyer at the tip of the coccyx the operator may proceed upwards in the plane between the fascia and the sacrum and thus damage the nervi erigentes close to their origin from the sacral nerves. Although this may occur in a few instances it must be a rarity and does not explain why denervation occurs after sphincter-saving resection when the dissection is carried out completely from above. We would agree with Rankin, who considered that the most likely site of injury is where the nerves run forwards between the rectum and the posterior wall of the bladder and bladder neck (Rankin, 1969).

The degree of denervation will depend on the degree of neurogenic destruction, but complete denervation is rare. Initially the clinical picture is similar in most patients. After the catheter is withdrawn the patient is unable to pass urine and the bladder distends, usually without pain. If the patient is left untreated overflow incontinence results. As time progresses the patient may be able to initiate micturition by a combination of raised intra-abdominal pressure and residual detrusor muscular activity. The efficiency of voiding will depend on the degree of denervation, but the patient usually complains of difficulty in initiating micturition, poor stream and postmicturition dribbling. The patient will often be incontinent and a large residual volume leads to frequent urinary tract infections.

The incidence of both partial and complete bladder denervation following rectal excision is quoted as varying from 8% to 50% (Rankin, 1969; Eickenberg et al, 1976; Fowler et al, 1978; Gerstenberg et al, 1980). This wide variation is presumably accounted for by the retrospective nature of most of these studies and the different criteria used to define denervation. It is important to study each patient before and after surgery and demonstrate on both filling and voiding cystometrograms an absence of coordinated detrusor activity (Murnaghan et al, 1979). Applying these criteria we demonstrated that the incidence of bladder denervation after low sphincter-saving resection was 15% (Neal et al, 1981). Our previous data (Williams et al, 1980a) had suggested that patients undergoing this type of operation fared better than those undergoing abdominoperineal excision, but after further investigations it became clear that when the tumour was low in the pelvis the incidence of this problem increased and then was similar to that after abdominoperineal excision. Thus pelvic nerve damage seems to be related to the depth of pelvic dissection.

Management of retention of urine

Failure to pass urine following removal of the catheter is quite common after rectal excision even when the patient is mobilizing. Usually, however, after 12 hours normal micturition has been re-established. If this is not the case management should proceed along the conservative lines discussed in Chapter 70. If conservative therapy fails, a urological opinion should be sought and the patient investigated to determine the cause of the retention. The patient should ideally undergo cystoscopy with filling and voiding cystometrograms. An attempt should be made to establish whether the retention has a mechanical or a neurogenic cause. This is difficult and ideally requires that the key investigations be performed both before and after the operation, but this is rarely the case. Nevertheless, an experienced urologist with the aid of the postoperative investigations can usually determine which component is paramount.

Once the diagnosis has been established, management should continue along the lines discussed in Chapter 70.

Direct injuries to the urinary tract

Ureteric injuries

Perhaps the greatest fear for the surgeon performing rectal excision is that one or both ureters may be damaged in the course of the operation. Although such an injury is distressing, a normal functional result can be achieved provided the injury is recognized at the time and dealt with appropriately. Failure to detect the injury means that a delayed repair becomes necessary and the results from such treatment tend to be much worse than if the damage is corrected initially.

Injury to the ureters usually occurs at one of three places. One such is the point where the inferior mesenteric vascular pedicle is isolated, particularly if a mass pedicle ligature is used. The left ureter may be caught up with it and subsequently ligatured and divided. It is essential, therefore, to identify the left ureter at an early stage in the mobilization of the rectum and left colon and it should be swept laterally away from the vascular pedicle, which should involve separate isolated ligation and division of the inferior mesenteric vein and inferior mesenteric artery.

A second site where damage may occur to either ureter is deep in the pelvis when the 'lateral ligaments' are divided. The ureters are particularly at risk if a concomitant hysterectomy is performed. In this case, or if the pelvic dissection is particularly difficult (e.g. after previous surgery), it is a good policy to dissect the ureter out and follow its path down to its entry into the bladder. Occasionally in the really difficult case it may be necessary to catheterize the ureters with stents *in situ* prior to colonic mobilization.

Injury to the lower ureter is more likely to occur using the synchronous combined technique of abdominoperineal excision of the rectum than with the single-team approach or anterior resection (Graham and Goligher, 1954). If the lateral ligaments are divided from below or blind scissor dissection is employed the ureter can be injured without the surgeon realizing this has occurred.

The third site at which the ureters may be injured is the pelvic brim when the rectum is mobilized or alternatively when the pelvic peritoneum is closed at the end of the procedure. Both ureters may be divided as the peritoneum is elevated or they may be incorporated in a suture during the closure.

The incidence of ureteric injury is difficult to determine as surgeons are naturally reluctant to publish this type of data. Nevertheless the range seems to be between 0.7% and 6% (mean 3.7%) according to surgeons who have been bold enough to publish their results (Baumrucker and Shaw, 1953; Sankey and Heller, 1967; Thorsoe, 1971; Tank et al, 1972; Ward and Nay, 1972; Sakkas et al, 1974; Andersson and Bergdahl, 1976).

Of all ureteric injuries, 20–30% are recognized at the time of operation (Zinman et al, 1978). These recognized defects include ligature and complete or incomplete division.

Bladder injury

Injury to the bladder is uncommon in the course of rectal excision. The incidence is about 2% (Baumrucker and Shaw, 1953). It is most likely to occur when freeing an adherent growth from the posterior wall of the bladder in a male patient. Alternatively, the bladder is often damaged when excision or anastomosis of a very short rectal stump is attempted. Provided the surgeon is sure that there is no neoplastic infiltration into the bladder, the defect can be closed in two layers using 2/0 chromic or plain catgut. If there is neoplastic infiltration an *en bloc* excision will be required if feasible. When injury to the bladder neck or trigone has taken place, great care must be taken to avoid incorporating the distal ureters in the suture. Preliminary ureteric catheterization should prevent this complication. When the bladder has been closed primarily, it should be drained per urethram for 10–14 days. If there has been excessive haemorrhage or if the trigone has needed repair, a suprapubic cystostomy is required. In either case a drain should be left down to the suture line and brought out suprapubically.

Injury to the urethra

The membranous or prostatic urethra may be injured in a variety of ways during abdominoperineal excision. In an attempt to achieve haemostasis too vigorous electrocoagulation on the posterior aspect of the prostate may lead to subsequent urethral damage. Similarly, the urethra may be injured if the perineal surgeon inadvertently strikes the wrong plane during the anterior dissection, or if a tumour extends anteriorly and has to be shaved off the posterior aspect of the prostate. External trauma can lead to stricture. The latter may require dilatation, internal urethrotomy or urethroplasty depending on the severity and nature of the lesion (Zollinger and Sheppard, 1971). If part of the urethral wall is inadvertently opened or the urethra is completely transected and these injuries are noted at the time of operation, direct repair over an indwelling catheter is perhaps the best option. In other cases a urethroplasty may be required.

It is sometimes difficult to determine the incidence of urethral problems incurred as a result of operative damage during abdominoperineal excision of the rectum as it is not always clear how the injury occurred. Thus Ward and Nay (1972) described 3 of 150 (2%) patients who developed a urethral stricture following abdominoperineal excision. They could not totally exclude traumatic instrumentation either before or after the operation. Andersson and Bergdahl (1976) noted that 3 of 111 patients (2.7%) had the continuity of the urethra breached at the time of abdominoperineal excision. In both cases the injury was noted by the surgeon and treated primarily. One of these patients subsequently developed a stricture and the other a fistula which healed on conservative therapy. Overall the incidence of urethral injuries varies between 0.7% and 6.7% (Baumrucker and Shaw, 1953; Sankey and Heller, 1967; Thorsoe, 1971; Tank et al, 1972; Ward and Nay, 1972; Sakkas et al, 1974).

Urinary fistula

Failure to identify a direct injury to the ureter, bladder or urethra at the time of operation may lead to a collection of urine in the retroperitoneum or in the pelvis. Usually, however, urine will escape from one of the wounds or drain sites, resulting in a urinary fistula. In the early stages it is not always clear that the discharge is urine as it is often mixed with serosanguineous fluid. A persistent, high-volume discharge of fluid which gradually becomes clearer in colour should raise a suspicion of a urinary fistula. The diagnosis can usually be confirmed by measuring the urea and electrolyte concentrations in the discharge. Further management is discussed in Chapter 70.

Disorders of sexual function

The problems of sexual function that occur after abdominoperineal excision of the rectum are discussed at length in Chapter 11. Most complications are related to the colostomy and damage to the pelvic autonomic nerves. Damage to the nerves can occur whenever the rectum is mobilized extensively; hence sexual dysfunction may occur from nerve damage after sphincter-saving resection although the incidence seems to be lower than after abdominoperineal excision. Thus in one of our studies (Williams and Johnston, 1984) in which 70 patients with mid-rectal cancer who had undergone either abdominoperineal excision or sphincter-saving resection were carefully questioned about their sexual function, 67% who were sexually active preoperatively had problems after abdominoperineal excision compared with 30% after sphincter-saving resection ($P > 0.06$). Impotence occurred in 14% after sphincter-saving resection and 47% after abdominoperineal excision ($P < 0.05$). These results were similar to those from a study performed 10–12 years earlier by Devlin et al (1971). Both studies investigated patients in whom the tumours were situated in the upper two-thirds of the rectum. Currently more and more sphincter-saving resections are being performed for lesions in the upper half of the lower third of the rectum. With more extensive and deeper pelvic dissection we suspect that the incidence of sexual dysfunction caused by nerve damage will become more common after sphincter-saving resection.

Some centres have recognized these dangers and have modified their technique in an attempt to spare the autonomic nerve plexuses (Enker, 1992; Wang et al, 1992; Cosimelli et al, 1994). Thus, Enker (1992) performed autonomic nerve-preserving pelvic side wall dissections in 42 men undergoing sphincter-saving resections. Thirty-three (86.7%) of the 38 evaluable patients remained potent, and 29 (87.9%) of those had normal ejaculation. Deliberate sacrifice of the inferior hypogastric plexus caused only minor sexual dysfunction.

Complications specific to abdominoperineal excision

Perineal wound complications

Haemorrhage

Haemorrhage may be due to persistent bleeding at operation, or may be reactionary or secondary to infection.

Some minor bleeding from the perineum is common immediately after rectal excision, particularly if there is an open perineal wound. Provided vital signs are stable, the patient should be adequately sedated, extra blood should be cross-matched and the outer dressing should be changed as required. If the wound has been closed primarily, a careful watch on the amount of blood accumulating from the suction drains should be maintained and the perineum should be frequently observed to make sure it is not bulging owing to blood in the pelvis. If there is any change in the cardiovascular status of the patient or if the bleeding is considered to be excessive, the patient must be returned to the operating theatre forthwith, anaesthetized and placed in the lithotomy position. The perineal pack should be removed or the wound opened widely. The clot is evacuated from the cavity and irrigated with sterile saline. A careful search should be made for a bleeding vessel which if found is dealt with. Often, however, a gentle ooze is all that will be obvious. In these circumstances, evacuation of clot, irrigation and tight repacking with a naked gauze roll will, in our experience, invariably arrest the bleeding.

Secondary haemorrhage occurring 7–10 days after the operation is usually due to infection. In these circumstances it will be necessary to establish drainage of infected material, the cavity will need regular irrigation after arrest of the bleeding and a covering antibiotic is advisable.

Infection

Infection is probably the most frequent problem to affect the perineal wound. If the wound has been left open and packed, infection is the rule rather than the exception. It is usually managed quite satisfactorily by regular irrigation and repacking. The surgeon needs to keep a regular eye on progress. Removal of any accumulating slough is advisable as it inhibits healing. If the wound has been primarily sutured, mild infection will be indicated by redness around the sutures which may start to cut out. In these circumstances the sutures should be removed as soon as possible. More serious sepsis will be accompanied by swinging pyrexia and tenderness in the perineum. Some bulging of the perineal wound may occur with discharge of pus. Sometimes these signs are absent and the only indication of the complication is that the patient is not recovering as well as might be expected. Under these circumstances the perineal wound should be one of the first areas that the surgeon examines. Any tenderness or swelling should suggest the possibility of a perineal collection. Removal of a suture or two and the gentle insertion of sinus forceps will often confirm the diagnosis. When pus has been located in this manner it is wise to take the patient back to the operating theatre, open the wound widely, break down loculi, irrigate with hydrogen peroxide solution and pack the cavity. Occasionally severe synergistic gangrene may occur in the perineum, especially in diabetic patients. If this occurs, wide debridement is indicated urgently.

Pressure necrosis of the wound edges

Every attempt should be made to avoid pressure necrosis by frequent turning of the patient. No matter how meticulous the nursing staff, there are always some old, debilitated patients who develop this complication. Treatment is difficult and may require the excision of necrotic tissue.

Perineal sinus

It is quite common for the perineal wound not to heal completely, leaving a sinus. This track can be of variable diameter and length. Failure to heal is often idiopathic, but a sinus may be caused by the retention of a foreign body such as a swab, infection of the sacrum with sequestrum formation, or recurrence of the growth. Treatment consists of laying open the track, searching for any underlying cause and its removal. The wound is left open and packed in the usual manner. If the defect is very large a rectus flap might be indicated to fill the space and achieve primary healing (see Chapter 10).

Stenosis

The perineal wound may contract in its centre and cause an 'hourglass' deformity. This divides the wound into upper and lower cavities and may lead to pus accumulating in the upper recesses. It is for this reason the surgeon needs to assess the perineal wound regularly so as to prevent this complication. It is usually sufficient for the surgeon to insert an index finger into the wound to break down any adhesions that may form and to ensure that there is an adequate pathway for the egress of accumulated material.

Perineal hernia

Very occasionally a bulge appears in the perineal region after abdominoperineal excision which has a cough impulse and is due to herniation of bowel through a defect in the healed perineum. The patient may complain of a dragging feeling as well as the swelling. Sometimes symptoms and signs of subacute intestinal obstruction may be present. If possible the patient should be treated conservatively. Often the symptoms can be controlled by a firm pair of underpants or a T-bandage. Occasionally operative intervention may be justified.

A variety of repairs have been described, which have had variable success. The sac is either approached from the perineum (Gabriel, 1948; Ego-Aguirre et al, 1964), from the abdomen or via both routes. The sac is dissected and the gap in the perineum obliterated by a lattice of fascial strips, stainless steel wire or a mesh of polyglycolic acid or polypropylene. In women the defect may be obliterated by folding the uterus backwards and stitching the fundus to the sacrum and side walls of the pelvis (Bach-Nielson, 1967). Although the latter method seems ideal, in the few cases in which we have tried this technique the results have been disappointing.

'Phantom rectum'

'Phantom rectum' is a symptom analogous to the 'phantom limb' which follows amputation. The patient feels that the rectum is still present and often experiences discomfort which is similar to a desire to defecate as if the rectum was still intact. There is a spectrum of severity but it is not unusual for the patient to be considerably inconvenienced by the sensation. The incidence of this complication depends on how carefully the surgeon questions the patient, for it is not a symptom that is readily admitted to. The few in-depth studies of patients' quality of life after abdominoperineal excision have demonstrated an incidence of approximately 50% (Farley and Smith, 1968; Devlin et al, 1971; Williams and Johnston, 1984). The cause is unknown, and the only treatment is mild analgesia and reassurance.

Local recurrence

Local recurrence in the perineal wound and pelvis may be manifested by local pain or pain in the sacral or sciatic regions. Sometimes a swelling or some induration is present, or an abscess or discharging sinus develops. If the pelvis contains a large volume of tumour there may be bilateral leg oedema or urinary symptoms may develop as a result of infiltration into the bladder or prostate. The diagnosis should be strongly suspected if the patient develops any of these symptoms, in particular persistent perineal pain, although such pain can be due to causes other than recurrence. Proof of recurrence should always be sought by histological confirmation where possible. Thus any obvious lesion should be biopsied. Computed tomographic scanning (Figure 32.85) (Adalsteinsson et al, 1981; James et al, 1983) and magnetic resonance imaging have proved particularly useful in this area. Recurrence can often be seen as a soft-tissue mass; and by directing a needle into it under visual control, tissue can be obtained for histological purposes. Imaging has also demonstrated that local recurrence can be silent and hence its incidence is greater than generally realized. Routine imaging will, it is hoped, detect this form of recurrence at an early stage in the future and such an approach may improve the results of treatment for pelvic recurrence (see Chapter 33).

Colostomy complications

Colostomy complications are dealt with in Chapter 9.

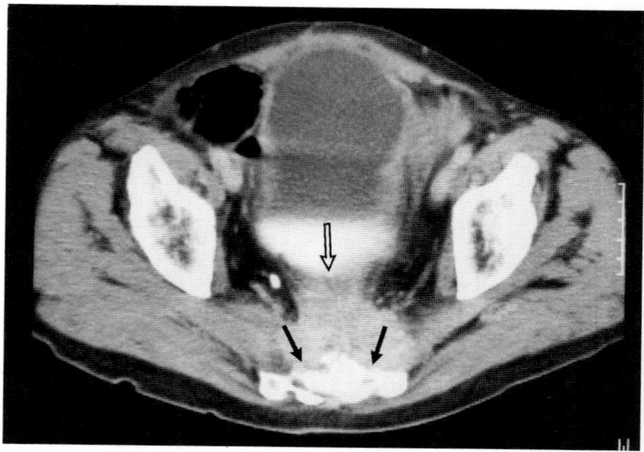

Figure 32.85 CT scan of the pelvis following previous abdominoperineal excision of the rectum. There is recurrent tumour (closed arrows) invading the sacrum and the bladder (open arrow).

Complications specific to sphincter-saving resection

Anterior resection (manual and stapled anastomosis)

Dehiscence of the anastomosis

Anastomotic leaks may present in a variety of ways. If there is a significant defect in the anastomosis it is likely that the peritoneal cavity will become contaminated by faecal material. The patient may therefore develop all the signs and symptoms of peritonitis. In the early postoperative period peritonitis may be manifested only by persistent paralytic ileus, other features being masked by postoperative analgesia. The leak may become walled off by adjacent small bowel, omentum and pelvic organs. In this case an abscess forms adjacent to the anastomosis. The patient will be toxic with persistent pelvic pain, although this is not always evident. Sometimes a pelvic abscess may perforate into the peritoneal cavity, resulting in peritonitis. On the other hand the pelvic abscess may drain spontaneously through the defect in the anastomosis and into the lumen of the rectum. This will result in an improvement in the toxic state of the patient and an offensive discharge per anum. If a gentle rectal examination is performed, the defect will be palpable in a low anastomosis and the finger can often be passed through this defect into the abscess cavity. The abscess may track to the skin and discharge either through the main wound or drain site. If this occurs the discharge of pus is sometimes followed by a discharge of faecal material and thus a fistula is established. Sometimes the abscess will point on the abdominal wall away from the main wound. Incision over it will allow pus and gas to escape but it soon becomes obvious that a fistula has formed.

If there is any doubt as to whether an anastomotic dehiscence has occurred and it is not in reach of the index finger, a Gastrografin or Urografin enema can be performed. It is not our practice in the early postoperative period to investigate the situation with either a rigid or a flexible endoscope; early instrumentation may make matters worse. There has been a vogue in recent years to make a routine check of the integrity of the anastomosis approximately 10 days after the operation with a Gastrografin enema; this policy detects an incidence of leakage four or five times greater than that detected clinically. Apart from the need for objectivity in controlled trials there must be some doubt about the rationale for routinely examining suture lines by radiography for anastomotic leak. Perhaps the only value afforded by such information is to assist the surgeon in deciding when to close a covering stoma if this has been constructed. Such information is probably best obtained 6–8 weeks after the operation, that is just before the stoma is due to be closed, rather than during the postoperative period. Apart from the cost of performing a routine Gastrografin enema in the immediate postoperative period, there is the risk of septicaemia. Despite taking every precaution, now and then a clinical anastomotic dehiscence results directly from a Gastrografin enema. In recent years we have seen two such cases.

Incidence

There are three ways in which the anastomosis can be constructed in the course of an anterior resection. A manual anastomosis can be performed in one or two layers, or alternatively a stapled anastomosis can be constructed. In the few controlled trials that have compared one-layer and two-layer manual anastomoses, differences have been recorded depending on whether the anastomosis was 'high' or 'low'; that is, above or below the peritoneal reflection. For high anastomosis there does not seen to be a significant difference between single- or two-layer anastomoses; on the other hand, anastomotic dehiscence occurred significantly more frequently with the two-layer technique when the anastomosis was low (Everett, 1975; Irvin and Goligher, 1975). This finding is not universal. Thus Goligher et al (1977) found a slight advantage for the two-layer technique for both high and low anastomoses. The suture material may also be important but few controlled trials have examined this point. Clark et al (1977) prospectively compared a two-layer anastomosis with catgut against a group in which Dexon was used. Dexon was associated with a significantly lower dehiscence rate compared with catgut.

Since the introduction of stapling instruments numerous uncontrolled series have been published suggesting that the clinical leak rate was approximately 8% and when routine radiological examination was used the rate doubled (Tables 32.12 and 32.13).

Retrospective studies using historical controls have compared manual with stapled anastomoses. A representative number are featured in Table 32.14.

From these data it seems that the stapler produces fewer leaks than do manual anastomoses. However, when the results of the more recent prospective controlled trials are examined, there does not seem to be any significant difference in leak rates. Thus Beart and Kelly (1981) used the EEA stapler and

Table 32.12 Incidence of leaks in stapled anastomoses.

Type of leak	*Stapler*	*Cases*	*Leaks*	*Percentage of cases*
Clinical only				
Fain et al (1975), Lepreau (1978), Bervar et al (1977), Beckers and Deldime (1978), Andalkar (1979), Polgalse et al (1979), Ravitch and Steichen (1979), Wheeless (1979), Adolff et al (1980), Bolton and Britton (1980), Cady et al (1980), Laitinen et al (1980), Mittall and Cortez (1980), Shahinian et al (1980), Beart and Kelly (1981), Cade et al (1981), Cutait et al (1985), Rothenberger and Finne (1990)	STPU EEA Total	235 465 700	21 30 51	9 7 7

Table 32.13 Incidence of leaks in stapled anastomoses – retrospective studies.

Type of leak	*Stapler*	*Cases*	*Leaks*	*Percentage of cases*
Combined radiological and clinical				
Goligher et al (1979)	SPTU	129	16	12
Ling et al (1979)				
Berthold et al (1980)	EEA	369	59	16
Buchmann and Uhlschmid (1980)				
Duch et al (1980)				
Kirkegaard et al (1980)				
Stoller et al (1980)				
Heald and Leicester (1981)				
Kirwan (1981)				
Blamey and Lee (1982)				
Killingback (1985)				
Tuson and Everett (1990)	Total	498	75	15

Table 32.14 Comparative leak rates, stapled versus sutured anastomoses – retrospective studies.

Author	*Sutured anastomosis*		*Stapled anastomosis*	
	No.	*Leaks*	*No.*	*Leaks*
Andalkar (1979)	6	1	10	—
Goligher et al (1979)	135	48	62	6
Adolff et al (1980)	25	4	20	1
Bolton and Britton (1980)	10	1	20	1
Buchmann and Uhlschmid (1980)	13	4	22	2
Cady et al (1980)	56	16	10	1
Killingback (1985)	87	16	57	5
All studies	332	90 (27%)	201	17 (8.5%)

compared this with a two-layer manual technique. The anastomoses were not assessed radiologically but there was no difference in clinical leak rates. More recent prospective controlled trials have also confirmed these findings (Brennan et al, 1982; Akyol et al, 1991; Sarker et al, 1994) (Table 32.15).

One such study performed by the West of Scotland and Highland Anastomosis Study Group (Akyol et al, 1991) randomized 224 patients undergoing a colorectal anastomosis; 113 patients had a manual sutured anastomosis and 111 patients had a stapled anastomosis. A clinical leak developed in five patients (4.4%) in the sutured group and nine (8.1%) in the stapled group, but this difference was not statistically significant. Only one study (McGinn et al, 1985) has demonstrated a significantly higher rate of leakage with stapled anastomoses compared with those performed by hand. One important point to emerge from all of these studies is that a stapled anastomosis can be achieved at a lower level in the pelvis than is possible by hand. In the prospective randomized trials, patients with low tumours were

Table 32.15 Randomized controlled trials of stapling versus suturing in low colorectal anastomosis.

	Staples			*Sutures*		
		No. of leaks			*No. of leaks*	
Authors	*Total*	*Clinical*	*Radiological*	*Total*	*Clinical*	*Radiological*
Beart and Kelly (1981)	35	1	–	35	1	–
Brennan et al (1982)	9	2	1	10	4	1
McGinn et al (1985)	58	7	14	60	2	4
Everett et al (1986)	44	0	7	50	2	6
West of Scotland and Highland Anastomosis Study Group (1991)	111	9	5	113	5	13
Fingerhut et al (1994)	54	2	4	59	5	6

excluded because a lower manual anastomosis was not deemed possible. It would thus seem, on balance, that a stapled anastomosis is at least as safe as a manual anastomosis where both are considered possible, but the stapler has the considerable advantage that an anastomosis can be constructed at a much lower level from above than is feasible by hand.

There has been recent concern that with the more widespread use of total mesorectal excision (TME) the incidence of anastomotic leakage from low stapled anastomosis will increase. Corder et al (1994) found that, in 219 patients undergoing TME, 24 patients (11.0%) developed major anastomotic leaks associated with peritonitis or a pelvic collection and 14 (6.4%) developed minor leaks that were asymptomatic and detected only by contrast enema. All major leaks occurred at an anastomotic height of less than 6 cm. The authors now recommend that all patients undergoing low colorectal anastomosis after TME should have a defunctioning stoma.

Management

Management of anastomotic dehiscence after anterior resection depends on the clinical picture. If the leak is demonstrated only on Gastrografin enema and the patient is entirely asymptomatic, no further action is required. If the patient has a defunctioning stoma it is wise to close it only after a repeat Gastrografin enema shows that the dehiscence has healed.

If there is discharge per anum but no other systemic symptoms, it may only be necessary to irrigate the cavity with an antiseptic solution via a catheter introduced through the anal canal at regular intervals. The cavity gradually shrinks down and the only evidence that leakage has occurred may be some puckering of the posterior aspect of the anastomosis. If healing does not occur it raises the possibility that the patient has an early recurrence. If a defunctioning stoma has not been constructed at the time of the initial operation it may be advisable to raise one at this stage. By preventing faeces flowing into the cavity through the anastomotic dehiscence healing will occur at a faster rate. Not all leaks of this nature, however, need to have a proximal diversion. Each case should be judged on its merits. If the patient develops pyrexia and the cavity is large and difficult to irrigate, a proximal stoma is clearly necessary. If, however, the patient is well and irrigation is achieving its objective, a stoma may be avoided. An intermediate measure is to place the patient on an elemental diet. This regimen acts as a medical colostomy and may considerably reduce the amount of residue in the colon.

In the past the development of a faecal fistula necessitated the immediate construction of a proximal colostomy if not already present. Many surgeons now merely stop oral intake and institute intravenous feeding. Using this regimen a large bowel fistula normally closes in 3–4 weeks, provided there is no distal obstruction. If the output from the fistula is not diminished during this period a proximal stoma should be constructed.

If an anastomosis leaks and forms a pelvic abscess this must be drained. In the case of a low colorectal anastomosis it is often possible to do this per anum. A finger is inserted through the gap in the anastomosis and loculi are broken down. The cavity is then irrigated regularly. With an anastomosis at a higher level this technique may not be possible. In the past a laparotomy might have been the only option both to drain the abscess and to provide a proximal diverting stoma. Today the alternative of using radiologically guided percutaneous drainage under either ultrasonographic or CT control has revolutionized abscess management (see Chapter 66). A catheter can be placed in the cavity for irrigation and a proximal stoma raised under local anaesthesia without laparotomy or laparoscopically if necessary. Nevertheless, even if pus is drained percutaneously, a laparotomy is still indicated if the patient remains ill.

Severe peritonitis complicating anastomotic dehiscence is a surgical emergency. The patient must be rapidly resuscitated, then an urgent operation is indicated (see Chapter 66). The peritoneal cavity will need to be washed out thoroughly, the anastomosis should be taken down, and the proximal colon should be brought out as an end colostomy leaving the anorectal stump open with a drain passing through it to the exterior via the anus. It is only in exceptional circumstances where the dehiscence is small and contamination is minor that it may be safe to oversew the leak or patch it with omentum and construct a defunctioning stoma. If there is any doubt, we would always recommend taking down the anastomosis.

Prevention and the need for a covering stoma

The principles related to the construction of any large intestinal anastomosis need to be adhered to when an anterior resection is performed. Bowel preparation should be satisfactory, the blood supply to both bowel ends must be adequate, and there should be no tension at the anastomosis.

The need for a covering colostomy is a debatable issue. Maingot (1969) believed that when the above principles could not be adhered to because of technical difficulties or when there was faecal contamination during construction of an anastomosis, a covering colostomy was mandatory. Although this advice seems sensible, Maingot produced no evidence to substantiate it. The feeling of many surgeons is not that a covering stoma prevents dehiscence, but that it facilitates management should dehiscence occur.

Surprisingly, only one controlled study has attempted to examine the benefit or harm that a temporary stoma may make in elective low colorectal anastomoses (Graffner et al, 1983). An end-to-end stapling device was used for all the anastomoses. The study showed that stomas provided no benefit when used to cover all anastomoses; furthermore they were found to be of questionable value even for the small number of patients in whom dehiscence was suspected. On the negative side, colostomy cover increased hospital stay and some patients developed complications after closure. In a retrospective study, Fielding et al (1984) also concluded that routine use of a covering stoma in low anastomoses was not necessary.

While we would agree that routine construction of a covering stoma is not required for all low colorectal anastomoses, we do believe that if there is doubt concerning the integrity of the anastomosis at the time of the operation or severe faecal contamination occurs, a stoma is required. With the availability of on-table irrigation, poor bowel preparation is no longer an indication for construction of a defunctioning stoma. Nevertheless, with the wider use of total mesorectal excision in which there appears to be a greater risk of anastomotic leak (Corder et al, 1994), there should be a lower threshold for the use of covering stomas.

Stricture of the anastomosis

Stenosis and stricture formation unrelated to local recurrence may occur after anterior resection. Often a colorectal anastomosis feels quite narrow at an early stage after operation, but with the passage of faeces through it the lumen gradually dilates. Sometimes the narrowing persists and certain patients develop a tight stenosis. This is particularly true in patients who have suffered an anastomotic breakdown with local sepsis, while in others it is due to ischaemia.

Few reports comment on stenosis after hand-sewn anterior resection. The use of the stapling instruments has resulted in a greater interest in this complication. There is a belief by some that staplers produce a higher incidence of stenosis. Analysis of the problem in the literature is difficult owing to a lack of definition of stenosis.

The overall stenosis rate after stapled colorectal anastomoses seems to be about 5–9% (Table 32.16). This compares with Goligher's report of 6 of 553 patients (0.6%) who required treatment for stenosis following a manual anastomosis (Goligher, 1984). From Table 32.16 it appears that the SPTU gun produced fewer problems than the EEA variety. This interpretation may be biased since the SPTU figures included data from Fain et al (1975) where there was some doubt as to whether follow-up was complete (Waxman, 1983). There is virtually no information collected in a carefully controlled, prospective manner as to whether stenosis is more common after stapled than manual anastomosis. The only study that has addressed this issue reported that stenosis rates did not differ (Akyol et al, 1991), but follow-up was short and the numbers were small.

The aetiology of anastomotic stenosis following circular stapling is unknown. Histological studies in experimental animals imply that it may be related to the healing by scar tissue of the exposed intraluminal seromuscular layer with poor epithelial bridging (Polglase et al, 1981), combined with the crushing of tissues and ischaemia. The suggestion that the incidence of stricture was lower with the

Table 32.16 Stenosis rate after stapled anterior resections.

Stapler	*Cases*	*Stenosis*	*Percentage of cases*
STPU	318	16	5
EEA	426	36	9
Total	744	52	7

Data from: Cutait and Figlioni (1961), Fain et al (1975), Beckers and Deldime (1978), Andalkar (1979), Goligher et al (1979), Ravitch and Steichen (1979), Adolff et al (1980), Bolton and Britton (1980), Duch et al (1980), Kirkegaard et al (1980), Shahinian et al (1980), Smith (1981), Cade et al (1981), Heald and Leicester (1981), Blamey and Lee (1982), Killingback (1985), Rothenberger and Finne (1990).

SPTU stapler may be related to the geometry of the cartridge, because the inversion annulus of tissue crushed was smaller than with the EEA and only a single layer of staples was inserted.

In a recent update, Waxman et al (1995) stated that the mean reported anastomotic stenosis rate was 8% in 33 studies of 2680 single-stapled circular anastomoses. They also noted that stenosis appeared more frequently following the use of a double row of staples compared with the single row of the old Russian guns. Waxman and colleagues hypothesized that the ideal circular stapler should apply one row of absorbable staples with a large luminal diameter. Even though luminal diameter does not appear to be a major factor in the incidence of stenosis following use of a circular stapler, we agree with Moran (1996) that it seems sensible to use the largest possible lumen size when constructing any anastomosis.

Treatment of anastomotic stricture is by dilatation, either blindly with Hegar's dilators or under visual control using a sigmoidoscope and gum elastic bougies (or a coaxial balloon). A surgical repair is rarely required.

Haemorrhage

Reactionary or secondary bleeding from a handsutured anastomosis is uncommon. The incidence is approximately 1% (Manson et al, 1976; Goligher, 1984). It may be due to inadequate haemostasis at the suture line itself or to a ruptured anastomosis. Inadequate haemostasis usually presents within the first 24 hours, whereas bleeding from anastomotic dehiscence usually does not become apparent for 10–14 days. Stapled anastomoses are thought to be more at risk from primary haemorrhage than handsewn anastomoses. Staples are designed not to be completely haemostatic but to allow blood to pass along the vessels in the tissues held by the staples. In fact bleeding has only been recorded in 0.5% of stapled colorectal anastomoses (Smith, 1981) so it would seem that in practice staples are just as haemostatic as sutures when used for colorectal anastomosis.

Treatment should be conservative in the first instance. If bleeding persists the patient should be returned to the operating theatre and anaesthetized. Using an anal retractor, clot should be removed and the anastomosis carefully inspected. The site of bleeding can often be seen and under-run with relative ease. If this is not possible the rectum should be packed tightly with gauze packs, or balloon tamponade is worth considering as a means of achieving local haemostasis.

Local recurrence

The causes of local recurrence after rectal excision are discussed in detail elsewhere (see Chapter 30). Suffice it to say that based on our histological study of lateral or circumferential spread (Quirke et al, 1986), we believe local recurrence is in the main due to microscopic disease left behind in the pelvis at the time of the original operation. Indeed, this belief has been further reinforced by a study which prospectively studied 190 patients with rectal cancer and confirmed the link between circumferential tumour involvement and local recurrence (Adam et al, 1994). In most patients with local recurrence after sphincter-saving resection the tumour has already penetrated the bowel wall. Only occasionally is a recurrent tumour seen solely at the anastomotic site in a tumour confined to the bowel wall. Anastomotic recurrence is almost always accompanied by extrarectal deposits.

The symptoms of local recurrence after sphincter-saving resection are similar to those occurring after abdominoperineal excision. The patient may complain of persistent pelvic pain which may radiate down the legs. If the bladder or urethra are involved urinary symptoms may be dominant. After sphincter-saving resection local recurrence may be heralded by a change in bowel habit or the passage of blood per rectum. Since the pelvis is more easily inspected after sphincter-saving resection than after abdominoperineal excision, it might be expected that local recurrence would be more common, since it will be diagnosed more easily. Despite this obvious advantage of sphincter-saving resection, the incidence of local recurrence does not differ significantly from the incidence after abdominoperineal excision.

Local recurrence rates are variable and seem to depend much on the surgeon's skill and the precautions taken (Phillips et al, 1984a,b; McArdle and Hole, 1991; Hermanek et al, 1995). With the introduction of the stapling instrument it was thought that local recurrence was bound to increase after low sphincter-saving resection, since less potentially involved tissue could be removed. The facts do not support this belief, as the recurrence rates even for low rectal tumours are similar to those achieved with abdominoperineal excision. The best way of avoiding local recurrence seems to be to ensure that the whole of the mesorectum is removed together with the tumour-bearing area of the rectum. The mesorectum may contain small satellite tumour deposits (Heald et al, 1982). Whether a wide pelvic excision with radical iliac lymphadenectomy as suggested by Enker et al (1979) would result in lower recurrence rates must remain debatable as no controlled data are available. Although there is no doubt that internal iliac nodes may be involved in some cases of middle and low rectal cancer (Hojo and Koyama, 1982), when this is the case the tumour is so advanced that, no matter how radical the surgery, cure cannot usually be achieved. There are more data, albeit retrospective, which support this view (Glass et al, 1986). The effect of total mesorectal excision (TME) and extended lymphadenectomy on survival and recurrence is discussed later in this chapter.

One means of preventing local recurrence may be irrigation of the anorectal stump with a cancericidal agent. Although it does appear that most local recurrence results from a failure to remove all the tumour, a small proportion of cases may be due to the implantation of viable neoplastic cells into and around the anastomosis. Although it had been accepted for some years that cells shed from the tumour were non-viable (Rosenberg et al, 1978), further evidence showed that this is not the case (Umpleby et al, 1984b). Such cells have the potential for seeding on to raw surfaces and growing. A variety of agents have been advocated for use as a cancericidal agent, including 1% cetrimide, 1–2% mustine hydrochloride and potassium perchloride. The most efficient and least toxic seems to be 1% cetrimide.

The other potential means of preventing local recurrence is to deal with microscopic distal intramural spread, and this topic is dealt with at length in Chapter 30.

In our view, patients should be followed up regularly, preferably with intraluminal ultrasonography, so that local recurrence can be detected at an early stage. The frequency of examination is debatable. We see our patients at 3-monthly intervals for the first 2 years and thereafter 6-monthly for 4–5 years. At each visit they have a sigmoidoscopic examination and any suspicious area is biopsied. The patient also undergoes colonoscopy once every 3 years to exclude metachronous lesions. If the history is suggestive, but no evidence of recurrence is detected on clinical examination including sigmoidoscopy, a pelvic CT or MRI scan (see Figure 32.85) or an endoluminal ultrasound scan is obtained. Although pelvic CT has been used most often, many centres have now found that endoluminal ultrasonography is easier and more reliable than CT for the detection of local recurrence after sphincter-saving resection (Benyon et al, 1986). A rise in serial serum concentrations of carcinoembryonic antigen (CEA) also suggests a recurrence, but we have found this a singularly unimpressive method of detecting local recurrence; by the time the CEA level rises the tumour burden is so great that there is no hope of cure – a view which is supported by the recent results from the CEA second-look trial (Northover, 1996, personal communication).

The treatment of local recurrence is discussed in detail in Chapter 33. Here it is worth noting that, although regular surveillance results in a greater yield of local recurrence, current available treatment is merely palliative and rarely results in cure. It could be argued at the moment that exhaustive follow-up is unlikely to have any impact on prognosis. However, it is to be hoped that with better CT and MRI resolution and more frequent use of CT, MRI and ultrasound scans, recurrence will be detected at an earlier stage and treatment will make some impact on survival.

Bowel frequency and incontinence

For a long time after the introduction of anterior resection it was accepted that incontinence was bound to occur unless the colon was anastomosed to at least 6–8 cm of anorectum. It was believed that the receptors necessary for continence were situated in the rectal wall and that without them control would be lost. Parks and his colleagues (Lane and Parks, 1977) showed, however, that it was possible to remove the whole of the rectum and join the colon to the anal canal and yet preserve continence. Physiological studies (Lane and Parks, 1977; Williams et al, 1980b) confirmed that the reflexes necessary for continence still remained, and it was demonstrated that the receptors which subserved this function were situated outside the rectum, presumably in the levator ani muscles.

It has now been demonstrated in thousands of patients that continence can be achieved when the anorectum is considerably less than 6–8 cm in length. Nevertheless, a proportion of patients after low anterior resection do experience episodes of incontinence.

In a detailed study which evaluated the quality of life in 40 of our patients with a colorectal anastomosis sited 10 cm or less from the anal verge, we found that six patients (15%) were incontinent of faeces occasionally and another four (10%) were incontinent of flatus (Williams and Johnston, 1983). All patients had increased frequency of bowel actions following the procedure, with a mean of three per 24 hours at a mean of 40 months postoperatively. However, these symptoms improved with time and patients were usually prepared to tolerate a situation which was not absolutely perfect so as to avoid a colostomy. Various authors have since confirmed these findings (Bernard et al, 1989; Vernava et al, 1989; Batignani et al, 1991; Carmona and Ortiz, 1991; Williamson et al, 1993, 1995; Ortiz and Armendariz, 1996). Indeed, the term *anterior resection syndrome* has been coined to describe the disturbed anorectal function which occurs postoperatively (Williamson et al, 1995; Ortiz and Armendariz, 1996).

Not surprisingly, frequency of bowel action is related to the level of the anastomosis from the anal verge (McDonald and Heald, 1983; Batignani et al, 1991; Carmona and Ortiz, 1991). Frequency is also related to impaired reservoir capacity of the neorectum and significantly reduced resting anal pressures. For these reasons, Parc and his colleagues in Paris and Lazorthes in Toulouse tried to increase reservoir capacity by constructing a colonic pouch anastomosed to the anal canal (Lazorthes et al, 1986; Parc et al, 1986). Their early results and those of others (Nicholls et al, 1988; Seow-Choen, 1993; Seow-Choen and Goh, 1995) suggest that this technique is superior from a functional point of view to the conventional technique, although evacuation may be a problem. However, the latter difficulty can be reduced if the pouch is no longer than 7–8 cm.

Complications of abdominotransanal anastomosis

Few reports have commented on the complications of abdominotransanal anastomosis. Parks and Percy (1982) found that only two of 76 patients (2.6%) developed a clinical leak after the operation, both of which were due to necrosis of the terminal colon. A further eight patients (11%) developed pelvic abscesses but it was unclear how many of these were due to anastomotic dehiscence. Six patients developed local recurrence but there were no data on the length of follow-up. Only one of the 70 patients whose bowel function was assessed was found to be incontinent (1.4%); 39 patients (56%) had entirely normal function, and 30 were continent but had irregular colonic activity with a frequency of defecation of three or four times per day. It was emphasized that many of these patients were assessed quite soon after operation, suggesting that over a period of time bowel function in some of them would improve. Indeed, in a follow-up report from the same institution, Sweeney et al (1989) reported that only 8% of their patients had a frequency of bowel action of more than three per day. However, in 28% of patients continence was disturbed. Long-term observations on the outcome of resection with straight or pouch coloanal reconstruction demonstrate that the advantages of the colonic pouch disappear after two years because of a gradual improvement in bowel function in the straight anastomosis group.

With the introduction of the stapling gun this operation is being used less often. Patients are thus carefully selected and only those with very low tumours are likely to be considered for the procedure. As a result function might be expected to be more impaired compared with other techniques. Nevertheless, provided a distal clearance of 2 cm can be obtained and the surgeon is sure that the patient has good anal sphincter function, the operation provides a realistic alternative to a permanent stoma. The introduction of a colonic reservoir may further increase the scope of the operation.

Complications of abdominotrans-sacral resection

The group with the most experience of abdominotrans-sacral resection is that led by Localio. They have reported their results over a 15-year period between 1966 and 1981 (Localio et al, 1983). The clinical anastomotic leak rate after 175 abdominosacral resections was 9.7% which compares with their leak rate of 1% in 320 anterior resections. These data are not comparable, however, because the abdominosacral resections were performed for lesions at a lower level in the rectum. The authors emphasized that the leak rate in their first 100 patients was 12% whereas in the last 74 patients it was only 6.7%. Most patients with anastomotic dehiscence developed a posterior fistula but four developed peritonitis and needed urgent laparotomy. Leaks were more common in men than in women. All patients were continent for faeces and flatus after operation but increased frequency of bowel action was common. Frequency largely disappeared within a 6–12 month period. The local recurrence rate was 14.6%, which compared with their rate of 13.2% in patients who underwent abdominoperineal excision of the rectum.

RESULTS OF MAJOR EXCISIONAL SURGERY

Operative mortality

Surgery for rectal cancer has gradually become safer during the last 70 years. The operative mortality (defined as death occurring within 30 days of the operation) and morbidity rates following the various types of operations have gradually decreased despite a simultaneous increase in the operability rates.

This is admirably demonstrated by the data emanating from St Mark's Hospital between the 1920s and 1970s (Lockhart-Mummery et al, 1976) (Table 32.17). Thus, in the 2948 patients with a primary adenocarcinoma of the rectum treated between 1948 and 1972, the operative mortality was 7.0% in the period 1948–52 and 2.1% in 1968–72, the operability rates being 92% and 95% respectively. These data include patients treated by both abdominoperineal excision and sphincter-saving resections. When the mortality rates were examined for each operation separately the same conclusions were reached. These data are indeed very creditable, but it must not be forgotten that they come from a specialized hospital which does not deal with emergency work. The mortality rates from hospitals with a more widespread workload tend to be higher. Whittaker and Goligher (1976) found that between 1955 and 1968, in one unit at the Leeds General Infirmary, 550 cases of carcinoma were treated with an overall mortality of 10.6%. For patients having an anterior resection the rate was 6.8%, and for those submitted for abdominoperineal excision of the rectum the rate was 12.5%. This difference between the two types of operation is difficult to interpret because each operation was performed for different indications.

Table 32.17 Operability rate and operative mortality of rectal cancer at St Mark's Hospital 1928–1972.

Period	*Percentage of patients accepted for excision (includes palliative excisions)*	*Operative mortality (%)*
1928–32	46.5	12.8
1933–37	57.6	11.0
1938–42	69.4	11.1
1943–47	79.0	7.9
1948–52	92.7	6.8
1953–57	93.2	4.0
1958–62		3.1
1963–67		2.3
1968–72		2.1

After Dukes (1957) and Lockhart-Mummery et al (1976).

The gradual improvement in mortality and morbidity rates over the years no doubt relates to the improvements in anaesthetic technique, the use of prophylactic antibiotics, prophylactic measures against deep venous thrombosis, the introduction of total parenteral nutrition, and improved diagnostic facilities for the early detection of complications. However, the older studies did not include patients with low rectal cancers treated by sphincter-saving resections. Despite these potentially higher risk cases, the mortality and morbidity rates have not been altered appreciably, presumably because of the introduction of modern stapling instruments.

Thus, when we looked at the results of patients treated by low sphincter-saving resection at Leeds General Infirmary 'post-Goligher' between 1978 and 1982, no significant difference in mortality rates was found between these patients and those operated on 'pre-Goligher' by abdominoperineal excision (Williams et al, 1985). Only those patients with tumours situated between 3 cm and 12 cm from the anal verge were included in the study. Of the 159 patients presenting, 153 underwent resection or excision, an operability rate of 96%. The overall mortality rate was 7%, and four patients died after sphincter-saving resections (5%). We compared our results for sphincter-saving resection with a carefully matched retrospective control group which had undergone abdominoperineal excision of the rectum prior to 1977, and there was no significant difference between them as far as mortality was concerned. The results of this study together with those extensively quoted elsewhere demonstrate that the swing towards sphincter preservation has not resulted in an increase in mortality.

Perhaps an even more accurate picture of the overall mortality for the treatment of rectal cancer is to be found in the St Mary's Large Bowel Cancer Project (Phillips et al, 1984a,b). This was a collaborative study set up to investigate prospectively the treatment and outcome of large bowel carcinoma in a variety of centres. Ninety-four surgeons in 23 hospitals in the UK included all their patients presenting with the disease. Between 1976 and 1980, a total of 4225 patients with an adenocarcinoma of the large bowel were included, of whom 1988 (47%) had a primary carcinoma in the rectum (1292 patients, 65%) or rectosigmoid region (696 patients, 35%). A resection of some kind was performed in 1700 patients; 778 (46%) had an abdominoperineal excision of the rectum and 598 (35%) had an anterior resection. The overall operative mortality for both procedures was 107 (6.3%); 63 patients (8%) died after abdominoperineal excision of the rectum and 44 (7%) died after sphincter-saving resection.

The causes of postoperative mortality are varied, with many of the older patients dying from cardiopulmonary problems. Thus in Whittaker and Goligher's study, 63% of their patients died from cardiopulmonary complications (Whittaker and Goligher, 1976). Major sepsis is the next most likely cause of death. It might be expected that this complication would be more common after sphincter-saving resection than after abdominoperineal excision of the rectum since there is a risk of anastomotic breakdown. However, this does not seem to be the case from the limited amount of data available; death due to sepsis occurred just as commonly after sphincter-saving resection as after abdominoperineal excision. Other factors, apart from operative technique, that are thought to be related to mortality are the age and sex of the patient and whether the operation is palliative or radical. Obviously, older patients are at greater risk of death than younger ones, but whether females are more at risk than males as suggested by Gabriel (1948) is doubtful.

Another variable which must influence mortality is the skill and experience of the individual surgeon. Although such data are difficult to accumulate, evidence is appearing which supports this view. The findings from the St Mary's Large Bowel Cancer project indicated that the experience of the surgeon was directly related to mortality, length of hospital stay, anastomosis leak rates, blood transfusion, local recurrence and survival (Fielding, personal communication). Similarly, in an audit from a Scottish region, 251 patients (96.5%) with rectal cancer underwent rectal resection, and intestinal continuity was restored in 179 (71.3%) (Lothian and Borders Large Bowel Cancer Project (1995)). Five of the 28 consultant surgeons involved in the study were responsible for half of these patients. Patients treated by these five consultants were no more likely to undergo an anastomosis, but when an anastomosis was performed it was far more unlikely to leak when compared with an anastomosis performed by one of the other 23 surgeons involved in the study.

The mortality figures in most studies include the results of both palliative and radical operations. This biases the data, since if the operation is purely palliative the patient has a higher risk of dying in the postoperative period than if the operation is performed for cure. Patients who undergo palliative manoeuvres are often in a poor physical state to start with. This is vividly demonstrated by Goligher's personal series of 896 abdominoperineal excisions of the rectum (Goligher, 1984). In 710 cases tumours were removed with a chance of cure and the operative mortality was 2.8%, while 186 were performed solely for palliation with a mortality of 21%.

Survival

Survival after operation for rectal carcinoma has been extensively reported. Unfortunately, much of the data are difficult to interpret. Until recently only crude 5-year survival rates were quoted. This is calculated by determining the number of patients still alive after 5 years and expressing it as a percentage of the number of patients treated initially. Crude survival rates therefore do not take into account death from other causes. Since many of the patients with rectal carcinoma are elderly and are likely to develop intercurrent disease, crude survival rates are particularly inaccurate. Corrected survival rates were introduced to overcome this problem. A mathematical correction is made from life table analyses which take into account the number of deaths from other illnesses in that group of individuals. Although this is a more accurate technique of analysis it is still an approximation and furthermore it does not take into account patients lost to follow-up.

The most accurate method of expressing and analysing survival is to plot the survival curves using corrected rates over at least a 5-year period. Most recent papers do this, so a more accurate picture of survival after surgery for rectal cancer is emerging. Another factor that needs to be assessed when examining the data is whether the radical procedures alone have been included or whether both radical and palliative procedures are included. Most studies analyse only the patients who undergo operation. Unfortunately we know from studies in Birmingham, Bristol and Connecticut that a substantial number of patients are never fit enough to undergo surgery. They are excluded from analysis and hence a biased picture emerges. In order to determine the true outcome of the disease all patients presenting for treatment should be included irrespective of whether they have undergone surgical treatment.

Despite these difficulties in the interpretation of survival data, comparative studies using the same methods may be useful provided the above pitfalls are recognized and allowed for.

Overall absolute survival rates

Grinnell (1953) seems to have been the first to document absolute survival rates of patients with rectal cancer. Between 1916 and 1945, a total of 1026 cases presented to the Presbyterian Hospital in New York. The resectability rate increased from 57.5% in the period 1916–20 to 68.3% in 1946–50, and the operative mortality declined from 40.9% to 6.7%. Absolute 5-year survival increased from 17.5% in 1916–20 to 28.6% in 1941–45.

A similar pattern emerged from examination of Cancer Registries. Data from the Connecticut Tumor Registry showed that the operability rates rose from approximately 35% in 1935–39 to approximately 72% in 1955–59 and the absolute corrected 5-year survival rate rose from 13% to 37% in the same periods (Eisenberg et al, 1967).

Similarly, the results from the Birmingham Regional Cancer Registry showed that 5800 cases of rectal cancer were entered between 1950 and 1961, and the crude and corrected 5-year survival rates for all these cases were 21.9% and 29.2% respectively (Slaney, 1971). The same story emerged from the South Western Regional Cancer Bureau; the crude 5-year survival rate for all 1346 patients entered was 23.5% (Milnes-Walker, 1971). More recent data from the West Midlands registry does not show any appreciable improvement in overall survival (West Midlands Cancer Registry, 1990; Slaney et al, 1991; Allum et al, 1994).

These data examine the outcome for all patients who present with rectal cancer irrespective of whether they have received an operation. Many of the patients are never in a fit enough state to undergo an operation. The picture is therefore excessively gloomy, especially when it is realized that the rates expressed do not even include patients who are unable to reach hospital.

Survival of patients undergoing surgery

When only the results of patients who undergo surgery are analysed a more optimistic picture emerges (Table 32.18).

Thus the data from Connecticut (Eisenberg et al, 1967) showed that the corrected 5-year survival rate of all patients submitted to operation rose from approximately 32% between 1935 and 1939 to 49% between 1955 and 1959 (cf absolute rates of 13% and 37% respectively). The Birmingham Cancer Registry showed that the crude and corrected 5-year survival rates for patients undergoing radical operation were 39.8% and 48.6% respectively (cf absolute rates of 21.9% and 29.2%) (Slaney, 1971). A further report from the Birmingham Cancer Registry between 1977 and 1981 indicated that after curative resection, corrected 5-year survival rates for rectal cancer were 80%, 55% and 32% for Dukes' A, B and C tumours (Slaney et al, 1991; Allum et al, 1994). The crude 5-year survival from the South Western Regional Cancer Bureau (Milnes-Walker, 1971) was 34.1% (cf absolute rate of 23.5%), but this includes patients who underwent a palliative procedure.

These registry figures illustrate the overall picture of survival after surgery for rectal cancer. They include data from specialized and non-specialized hospitals, from surgeons who perform the procedures on a regular basis and also from surgeons

Table 32.18 Overall survival of patients undergoing surgery for rectal cancer, including all patients submitted for radical and palliative surgery.

Authors	*Institution*	*Crude 5-year survival rate (%)*	*Corrected 5-year survival rate (%)*
Eisenberg et al (1967)	Specialized and non-specialized		49.0
Milnes-Walker (1971)	Specialized and non-specialized	34.1	
Slaney (1971)	Specialized and non-specialized	39.8	48.8
Lockhart-Mummery et al (1976)	Specialized	47.1	56.7
Whittaker and Goligher (1976)	Specialized	36.3	
McArdle et al (1990)	Non-specialized	36	

who perform them infrequently. Most of the reports also include patients who have undergone palliative and radical operations.

If the data from specialized centres are examined and the patients are divided into those that have had a radical resection and those that have had a palliative procedure the results are quite different from the registry data. In this respect the data reported by Lockhart-Mummery et al (1976) from St Mark's Hospital are most interesting. Between 1948 and 1967, a total of 2410 patients survived operation. The crude and corrected 5-year survival rates of the whole group were 47.1% and 56.7%. For the 1931 patients who survived a radical procedure, the corresponding rates were 56.6% and 68.4%. These figures include all patients undergoing surgery irrespective of the type. The data from Leeds General Infirmary between 1955 and 1968 demonstrated corresponding survival rates of approximately 10% less than St Mark's Hospital (Whittaker and Goligher, 1976). In 407 patients with rectal cancer who underwent a radical operation the crude and corrected 5-year survival rates were 48.8% and 56% respectively. The results from Hughes' unit in Melbourne were even more encouraging (McDermott et al, 1981); thus of the 867 patients presenting with rectal cancer, 67% underwent a radical procedure, the operative mortality was 5.2% and the corrected 5-year survival rate was 67% in men and 74% in women. In a smaller group of patients treated in Aberdeen, the results were even more creditable (Jones and Thomson, 1982): in 276 patients who underwent a radical excision the corrected 5-year survival rate was 84%.

The benefits of specialization are further highlighted by the study of McArdle and Hole (1991) who performed a prospective study of 645 patients with colorectal cancer treated from 1974 to 1979 by 13 surgeons. The proportion of patients undergoing apparently curative surgery varied among surgeons from 40% to 60%. Overall postoperative mortality was 8–30%, local recurrence was 0–21%, and 10-year corrected survival in patients who underwent curative resection was 20–63%. The authors concluded that some surgeons perform less than optimal surgery; some are less competent technically than their colleagues and some fail to supervise surgeons in training adequately. These factors may compromise survival and they strongly recommended specialization. Although this study included both colon and rectal cancer patients, there is agreement that greater skills are required for removing rectal tumours, and hence the argument for specialization is even greater.

The data from specialized units therefore indicate that prognosis should not be considered as hopeless as it appears from the registry figures. The registry data are likely to be improved by earlier diagnosis and earlier referral from family practitioner to consultant. To achieve this end both the public and general practitioners need to be more aware of the significance of symptoms such as rectal bleeding and change in bowel habit. The improvements in diagnostic services and their availability, particularly colonoscopy, should improve matters. Open access facilities for general practitioners might also assist; also, referral to consultants with a special interest in colorectal disease should result in a higher resection rate and a lower mortality nationwide.

Factors affecting survival

Type and extent of operation

The choice of operation is perhaps the most hotly debated issue, the crucial question being whether the recent vogue for sphincter-saving resection for carcinoma of the low rectum has jeopardized survival when compared with the results previously achieved by abdominoperineal excision of the rectum. This topic was discussed at length earlier in the chapter. There are some points, however, which bear emphasis.

First, there has as yet been no prospective study comparing the fate of patients with rectal cancer treated either by sphincter-saving resection or abdominoperineal excision of the rectum; only retrospective data are available. When the retrospective data are analysed carefully and patients with similar tumours situated at similar heights from the anal verge are compared, there is no significant difference between the two operations. Most of these studies, however, have not included tumours in the lower third of the rectum. In our own study we attempted to match patients with very low tumours treated by sphincter-saving resection between 1978 and 1982 with a similar group treated by abdominoperineal excision of the rectum before 1977 (Williams et al, 1985). On applying life table analysis to the two groups (see Figure 32.6), it was evident that there was no significant difference between them. Gradually, other studies have emerged in the literature which report the survival rates for sphincter-saving resection in low carcinomas. Thus Heald and Ryall (1986) from Basingstoke District Hospital performed a curative sphincter-saving resection in 115 patients, three of whom (2.6%) died postoperatively; 69 patients had an anastomosis less than 5 cm from the anal verge. The number undergoing sphincter-saving resection represented 86% of patients with rectal cancer who underwent operation. The corrected cumulative probability of survival at 5 years was 87% and patients with very low tumours did as well as those with high tumours when treated by sphincter-saving resection. Although these results were not compared with a control group of patients who had undergone abdominoperineal excision of the rectum, they are clearly exceptional and in fact better than any data in the literature reporting the results of abdominoperineal excision of the rectum for similar tumours. The authors stress the fact that the reason for their success is that the technique used necessitates the removal of the whole of the mesorectum since this may contain small microscopic deposits of carcinoma. This technique has been termed *total mesorectal excision* (TME) and has received considerable attention in recent years.

At first sight it appears impossible that anterior resection can lead to better results than abdominoperineal excision of the rectum. The authors explain this apparent paradox by the fact that parts of the mesorectum may still be left behind even with the apparently more radical procedure. Technical considerations such as manual extraction, lack of dissection under direct vision, lack of precise definable planes for the perineal operator, short operation times and a very large number of surgeons performing a relatively small number of operations are cited as the reasons for failure in other series. No matter what the explanation, it does appear from this work that survival after low sphincter-saving resection when performed radically and with care in a selected, well-motivated population is at least as good as that following abdominoperineal excision of the rectum. The results achieved by Heald and Ryall (1986) are those that we should all aspire to.

The impact that total mesorectal excision has had on the surgical treatment of rectal cancer and its effect on survival and recurrence bears further analysis and is discussed at the end of this section; suffice it to say at this point that TME does seem to have major advantages. Hence, it is not just the type of operation that might influence survival but also the extent of dissection. Another aspect which therefore has to be considered is whether the radical lateral lymph node dissection particularly recommended by the Japanese surgeons influences survival.

Most studies that have examined lateral lymph node clearance have done so when the dissection is combined with abdominoperineal excision. Enker and his colleagues (1979) and various surgeons in Japan have been the main proponents of extended lymph node dissection. Thus Takahashi and Kajitani (1982) found that 24% of the patients with metastases in the nodes on the pelvic side wall survived 5 or more years following radical excision. Similarly Koyama et al (1982) claimed a 20% increase in 5-year survival rate after 'extended' rectal excision for patients with Dukes' B and C lesions. Both studies used retrospective controls, so it is difficult to be certain about the comparability of the groups. Moriya et al (1989) in a more recent study of patients with rectal cancer who underwent radical pelvic lymphadenectomy in Japan reported a local recurrence rate of 5% and a disease-free survival rate of 69%. The latter was increased to 76% in patients undergoing bilateral 'extended' lymphadenectomy with localized pelvic disease. However, bilateral extended lymphadenectomy is performed in only 25% of patients with Dukes' B and C lesions (Scholefield and Northover, 1995) and the decision to perform it is subjective. Thus, patients are selected for the procedure, making comparison with the more conventional approach difficult.

The main disadvantage of extended lymphadenectomy, readily admitted by its proponents, is the increase in morbidity, particularly as a result of pelvic nerve destruction. Hojo's initial data in 1982 showed that 170 (39%) of 437 patients had long-term diffficulties in passing urine. Sexual dysfunction was more common: 76% of patients under the age of 60 years became impotent following surgery, and this rarely recovered (Hojo, 1989). The major site of injury leading to urinary difficulties is damage to the pelvic nerve plexus. However, if the anterior branch of S4 remains intact on one side, bladder sensation and hence voiding should not be significantly affected (Hojo et al, 1991). On the other hand, preservation of sexual function is much more difficult (Hojo et al, 1991). As a consequence of this disturbing morbidity, the Japanese have developed the 'nerve-sparing operation' which aims to preserve the hypogastric and pelvic plexuses without compromising tumour clearance. However, such a procedure has still resulted in 20% of patients requiring long-term use of a urinary catheter (Hojo, 1989; Hojo et al, 1989).

Colorectal surgeons in the West remain to be convinced that the increased morbidity related to extended lateral lymph node dissection justifies the results. In addition, there are similar retrospective studies which claim no benefit for the technique. Deddish and Stearns (1961) found no improvement in survival by lateral lymphadenectomy in their 442 patients who underwent anterior resection as well as abdominoperineal excision of the rectum. Glass et al (1985) from the Royal London Hospital failed to demonstrate any benefit in survival among 64 patients treated by lateral lymphadenectomy. Other authors describe similar results (Gall and Hermanek, 1988; Pol et al, 1989; Cavaliere et al, 1991). It is clear from the data so far collected on this subject that we do not know whether the increased morbidity associated with lateral node dissection is likely to result in an improvement in survival. Such a question can be answered only by a prospective controlled trial.

Another technical factor that may influence survival is the level at which the inferior mesenteric artery is ligated during the course of rectal excision. This subject has been discussed ever since Miles (1908) introduced the concept of the upward spread of carcinoma. Miles himself recommended division of the inferior mesenteric artery just distal to the left colic branch with subsequent *en bloc* excision of nodes and bowel below. Moynihan, however, argued that ligation and division of the inferior mesenteric artery should be flush with the aorta in order to remove even more proximal lymph nodes. When Dukes subsequently showed that upward lymphatic extension of cancer was confined with remarkable consistency to the glands intimately related to the inferior mesenteric artery right up to the aorta, Moynihan's 'high tie' became a logical extension of radical excision for rectal cancer (Dukes, 1930). Thus Moynihan's philosophy was supported by most colorectal surgeons up to the present time. Doubt was first cast on this approach by reports of poor survival after high ligation (Rosi et al, 1962; Grinnell, 1965). Those individuals with involved nodes above the left colic artery – precisely the ones for whom the high tie was supposed to have been most advantageous – did not appear to have any better prognosis than others treated more conservatively. More quantitative data supporting the same contention was provided by Pezim and Nicholls (1984). They reviewed 1370 patients treated by rectal excision; 784 patients had undergone low ligation of the inferior mesenteric artery and 586 patients had undergone high ligation. The two groups were similar with regard to histological grade of tumour and the degree of venous invasion. No difference in crude or corrected 5-year survival was found for patients with Dukes' A, B or C lesions. It would seem that once lymph nodes are involved up to the level of the aorta, wide dissemination of the tumour has occurred and the outcome will not be influenced by the level of inferior mesenteric artery ligation. Nevertheless, this must remain a tentative conclusion since no prospective study has yet been performed. Until a definitive answer is available we will continue to perform a high tie of the inferior mesenteric vessels, not only in the hope of improved survival but for more accurate staging and as an easier operative procedure.

Survival after the excision of involved contiguous structures also requires some comment. A tumour that has extended locally to involve other structures has a worse prognosis than a tumour that remains confined to the rectum. Nevertheless, some encouraging results have been reported from centres that have recorded the data of their extended procedures. Bonfanti et al (1982) claimed an 8.1% operative mortality in their 61 patients (abdominoperineal excision 41, sphincter-saving resection 18, Hartmann's procedure 2) who had *en bloc* resection of one or more organs in association with rectal excision. The actuarial 5-year survival was 32% in patients who had histological evidence of malignant invasion and 75% in those without. These figures underline the philosophy that an attempt should always be made to resect a tumour widely even if it appears to invade adjacent organs. In some tumours there will be no microscopic evidence of malignant invasion, while in others this is the only approach by which cure may be possible. Gilbertsen (1960), Cooke (1956), Van Prohaska et al (1953) and Pittam et al (1984) demonstrated similar results. Whether we should take this philosophy to its logical conclusion and perform complete pelvic clearance in extensive tumours is debatable. Brunschwig and Daniel (1960) showed that in their 21 cases of carcinoma treated by this operation the operative mortality was 5% and the 5-year survival rate was 31%. Similarly Ledesma et al (1981) from Roswell Park Hospital in Buffalo, New York, obtained equivalent results. Between 1955 and 1975 they performed a total pelvic exenteration in 30 patients with an overall postoperative mortality rate of 10% and a crude 5-year survival rate of 48%. Takagi et al (1985) using the same approach have treated 13 patients with advanced local spread. The operative mortality was 7.7% and the corrected 5-year survival rate was 38.5%. Shirouzu et al (1996) studied retrospectively 26 patients who underwent total pelvic exenteration for locally advanced rectal cancer. The operative mortality was 8% (two deaths). The 5-year survival rate in patients with locally advanced disease but no lymph node or other metastatic disease was 71%. Patients with metastatic disease not unexpectedly had a much reduced life-expectancy measured in months.

All these authors therefore conclude that total pelvic exenteration offers gains in quality of life by palliating symptoms and controlling disease and in selected patients cure can be achieved. It should be stressed that life with a double stoma may be irksome for some of these older patients. However, strides are now being taken in the treatment of younger patients to preserve sphincter function provided it does not compromise tumour ablation. It is also unknown whether less radical surgery combined with pelvic radiotherapy would achieve similar results. Perhaps the emphasis should remain on the careful selection of patients for such radical operations.

Age and sex of the patient

Several authors have demonstrated that women have a slightly superior prognosis than men. Early studies using crude 5-year survival data showed that the survival rate was approximately 5% better in women than in men for tumours in each of the various sites in the rectum and for each of the types of operation performed (Mayo and Fly, 1956; Dukes, 1957). These conclusions were supported by data from McDermott and his colleagues in Melbourne who found that the corresponding 5-year survival rates for women and men in their series were 57% and 51% respectively (McDermott et al, 1981). These data, however, included patients with carcinoma of colon in addition to those with rectal cancer. Fitzgibbons et al (1977) in their life table analysis of the results of abdominoperineal excision performed for rectal cancer also showed that females had a better prognosis than males. This difference could also not be explained by a higher incidence of more pathologically advanced tumours in the men compared with the women.

The influence of age on the prognosis of patients treated by rectal excision is perhaps a little more difficult to interpret. Since older patients die more frequently from intercurrent disease during follow-up than do younger patients, 5-year survival rates show that older patients have a worse prognosis. There are no data, however, to substantiate that older patients have tumours that are pathologically less favourable than those found in younger patients. At the other end of the spectrum, it is generally accepted that the tumours in the very young (i.e. below 30 years old) are particularly aggressive. Recent data, however, dispute this belief: Umpleby et al (1984a) could find no statistical difference in corrected 5-year survival rates in this group of patients compared with other age groups. Also, when McDermott et al (1981) looked at cancer-specific survival rates in their 1709 patients with rectal (and colonic) tumours, they found that patients under 40 years old had a significantly better prognosis than older patients.

Pathological characteristics of the tumour

Numerous studies have confirmed the original observations of Dukes that survival is directly correlated with the Dukes' stage of the tumour. In the 2256 patients collected by Dukes and treated by rectal excision, the corrected 5-year survival rates for Dukes' A, B and C lesions were approximately 97%, 79% and 32% respectively (Dukes, 1957).

As discussed in the pathology section of Chapter 30, many other factors also influence prognosis following surgery. Jass (1986) showed that prognosis was related to the number of involved lymph nodes and the presence of a lymphocytic infiltrate. The degree of histological differentiation, whether the tumour is diploid or aneuploid with respect to its cellular DNA content, the extent of local invasion, the degree of circumferential involvement and the presence of occult hepatic metastases are other important factors that have to be taken into consideration.

The site of the tumour in the rectum

Early studies which examined the impact of the site of primary tumours in relation to the prognosis found that patients with carcinomas of the extraperitoneal rectum fared better than those with tumours of the intraperitoneal rectum. The lower the tumour was sited in the rectum the worse the prognosis (Gilchrist and David, 1947; Waugh and Kirklin, 1949; Stearns and Binkley, 1953; Gilbertsen, 1960, 1962). Thus Stearns and Binkley (1953) from New York found that the 5-year survival rate for tumours 0–6 cm from the anal verge was 52.8%, at 6–11 cm it was 61.8% and above 11 cm it was 72.5%. Whittaker and Goligher (1976) confirmed that tumours in the lower third of the rectum had a worse prognosis than those sited in the upper two-thirds of the rectum (Table 32.19).

Studies by Quirke et al (1986) and Heald and Ryall (1986) may explain this difference. It appears that the incidence of microscopic spread of rectal cancer radially into the mesorectum is far more common than previously realized. Removal of this tissue when the tumour is in the upper third of the rectum is relatively simple and is usually performed. When the rectal carcinoma is deep in the pelvis the mesorectum is more difficult to remove. Furthermore, because the frequency of this mode of spread has not previously been realized, surgeons have perhaps not striven to remove all of it. With

Table 32.19 Crude 5-year survival rates after rectal excision related to height of tumour.

Height of growth	*Immediate survivors of operation*	*Patients alive at 5 years*	*Crude 5-year survival rate (%)*
Upper third (13–19 cm)	46	24	52.2
Middle third (7–12.5 cm)	200	111	55.5
Lower third (0–6.5 cm)	142	58	40.1

From Whittaker and Goligher (1976).

the introduction of total mesorectal excision, these differences in site-related survival may disappear.

Survival beyond 5 years

It is customary to express survival rates in terms of 5 years, the reason being that survival data over a longer period show that far fewer patients die from recurrent disease. Thus the overall corrected 5-year survival rate at St Mark's Hospital was 57.5%, at 10 years this fell to 51.4%, at 15 years it was 50.4%, and at 20 years it was 49.8%. So, fewer than 10% of patients died from their disease in the 15-year period following the initial 5 years (Bussey, 1963).

Recurrence

The incidence of recurrence after rectal excision for rectal carcinoma is difficult to determine. Ideally each case should have histological proof of recurrence, but in practice this is difficult to obtain. Often on clinical grounds there is a strong suspicion that recurrence is present but radiological investigation does not demonstrate the lesion and a biopsy is not practicable. This state of affairs is particularly common after abdominoperineal excision of the rectum where the pelvis is relatively inaccessible to examination. Recurrence may also be asymptomatic, detection being achieved only if a post-mortem is performed. With the more routine use of the modern imaging techniques such as CT scanning, endoluminal ultrasound examination and magnetic resonance imaging, it is hoped that detection of recurrence will be easier and also will be achieved at an earlier stage.

Even if a patient is found to have local recurrence it cannot always be determined if dissemination has occurred also. The only way of ensuring the exact incidence of recurrence is to perform a careful post-mortem examination on all patients who die, which is clearly impractical. The data available at the present time rely on a combination of clinical features, radiological appearances, sometimes biopsy data and post-mortem evidence. All studies no doubt underestimate the incidence of recurrence, and this point should always be borne in mind when reports on the subject are assessed.

Relative incidence of recurrence after different procedures

This subject has been dealt with earlier, but certain points bear repetition. The recurrence rates for similar tumours treated by sphincter-saving resection and abdominoperineal excision of the rectum are comparable, even for lesions in the lower part of the middle third and upper part of the lower third of the rectum (see Figure 32.7). The concept that low sphincter-saving resection is as effective as abdominoperineal excision of the rectum in the prevention of local recurrence is further underlined when it is realized that recurrence is harder to detect after abdominoperineal excision of the rectum. Such comparable recurrence rates are achieved only if the lateral margin of the excision is as wide as possible and there is at least a 2 cm margin of distal clearance. Tumours that are locally extensive are far more likely to recur than those that are mobile, no matter which type of procedure is performed.

The overall incidence of local recurrence attained throughout the UK was studied in the Large Bowel Cancer Project organized from St Mary's Hospital in London (Phillips et al, 1984a,b). This project included the results of operations carried out by a large number of surgeons in specialized hospitals, teaching hospitals and non-teaching district general hospitals. It was reported that 1376 patients underwent either an abdominoperineal excision of the rectum (788 patients) or a sphincter-saving resection (598 patients), and a 'curative' resection was performed in 897 patients (505 abdominoperineal excision of the rectum, 393 sphincter-saving resection). Local recurrence was detected in 124 patients (15%). Although a statistical difference existed in the rates of recurrence after abdominoperineal excision (12%) and sphincter-saving resection (18%), no data were given concerning the comparability of the patients for size, site and extent of the tumour, so the comparison is difficult to interpret. For instance, variations in local recurrence rates between individual surgeons were highlighted, but the relative rates with which these surgeons performed the two operations were not noted.

McCall et al (1995) reviewed the results of published surgical series of rectal cancer in which adjuvant therapy had not been used, between 1982 and 1992. Only those papers in which at least 50 patients had been treated were included. Specific information regarding the surgical procedure (sphincter-saving resection versus abdominoperineal excision) was available on 6188 patients. The pooled local recurrence rate for 3577 patients who underwent SSR was 16.2% (derived from 30 papers), and for 2601 patients who underwent abdominoperineal excision it was 19.3% (derived from 24 papers).

Other factors that influence recurrence

Although various hypotheses are suggested as the cause of local recurrence after rectal excision, by far the most important seems to be inadequate removal of the primary tumour. This is why tumours fixed by malignancy have a significantly greater incidence of recurrence than those that are mobile (Wood et al, 1981; Durdey and Williams, 1984). Although this mode of recurrence has been recognized for many years, recent evidence suggests that the problem is far more common than generally appreciated. The study by Quirke et al (1986) which looked at the extent of lateral spread around 52 rectal cancers has previously been alluded to. The extent that this mode of spread had been underestimated was largely due to imprecise histopathological examination of the resection specimen. In only 13 patients (21%) would lateral spread have been detected by taking one section through the macroscopically defined area of maximal tumour penetration. The practice of examining a single section through macroscopically involved lateral resection margins is routine practice for many pathologists when assessing lateral spread. The problem of recognizing lateral involvement cannot rest entirely with the pathologists, since 11 of the patients (52%) were classified at laparotomy by the surgeon as having undergone a curative excision. Our data also demonstrated that the extent of lateral spread was similar whether the patient had undergone an abdominoperineal excision of the rectum or a sphincter-saving resection. Another important point to emerge from the study was that there was no significant difference in the amount of tissue removed laterally during the course of an abdominoperineal excision of the rectum and a sphincter-saving resection. Both procedures were clearly as radical as each other with respect to the margin of lateral clearance.

All these findings have once more been confirmed in a larger prospective study performed by the Leeds group (Adam et al, 1994). Thus, in 190 patients with rectal cancer, the resected specimen was examined for circumferential spread. The technique used was simplified compared with the previous study. Tumour involvement of the circumferential margin was present in 35 of 141 (25%) of specimens for which the surgeon thought that the resection margin was potentially curative, and in 69 of 190 (36%) of all cases. After a median of 5 years' follow-up, the frequency of local recurrence after potentially curative resection was 25%. The frequency of local recurrence was significantly higher in patients who had circumferential involvement than in those without involvement (79% versus 10%). Circumferential margin involvement was an independent marker for local recurrence and survival after surgery for rectal cancer. Other authors, notably DeHass-Kock et al (1996), have confirmed these findings.

Most factors shown to influence survival also have a significant impact on recurrence rates. Thus Gilbertsen (1960, 1962) showed that the incidence of recurrence was related to Dukes' stage. The local and distant recurrence rates for Dukes' A cases were 9.1% and 13.6% respectively, for B cases they were 16.7% and 29%, and for C cases they were 40.8% and 28.5%. All patients had undergone abdominoperineal excision of the rectum, and the overall local and distant recurrence rates in Gilbertsen's series were 24% and 19.7% respectively. These findings were confirmed by Morson et al (1963) whose overall incidence of local recurrence was only 9.7%. Once again all patients had undergone abdominoperineal excision and the corresponding local recurrence rates for Dukes' A, B and C tumours were 0.8%, 5.2% and 16% respectively. McCall et al (1995), in a review of 51 papers, analysed the follow-up of 10 465 patients and found a median local recurrence rate of 18.5%; local recurrence rates were 8.5%, 16.3% and 28.6% in Dukes' A, B and C patients, respectively. Morson et al (1963) found that recurrence was influenced by the site of the lesion within the rectum, being 14.5% for tumours of the lower third, 8.3% for those in the middle third and 5.2% for those in the upper third. As might be expected, the incidence of recurrence was influenced by the extent of invasion beyond the rectum and was 0.9% in patients with no local extension, 5.9% in cases with slight spread and

16.8% in cases with extensive spread. In our own series (Durdey and Williams, 1984), the incidence of local recurrence after rectal excision (abdominoperineal excision and sphincter-saving resection) for patients with direct neoplastic spread was 41.3%, compared with 15% of patients with tumours which did not show extramural infiltration. This difference was statistically significant ($P < 0.01$).

The data from the St Mary's project also demonstrated the association between extent of local spread and recurrence. Other factors that served to influence recurrence and highlighted in the St Mary's project were tumour differentiation, obstruction and perforated carcinomas (Table 32.20). Differentiation, obstruction and perforation influenced recurrence irrespective of whether an abdominoperineal excision of the rectum or anterior resection had been performed. Another factor emphasized by this group, albeit not just for rectal cancers, was the effect of surgeon-related variables on the incidence of recurrence, which varied between 4% and 30%. In a similar study in Scotland, McArdle and Hole (1991) found that the local recurrence rates between 13 surgeons varied between nil and 21%; albeit these data were for colon and rectal carcinomas. Surgeon-related variables also had a significant effect on leak rates and wound sepsis. These figures argue strongly for the universal recognition of coloproctology as a speciality of its own where comprehensive and audited training is needed.

Length of follow-up also influences the incidence of recurrence. Nevertheless many studies indicate that 80–90% of local recurrences occur within the first 2 years after operation. Such a finding once again strongly supports the concept that most cases of local recurrence result from inadequate removal of the primary tumour. Despite this observation, local recurrence may occur initially at any time during the first 10 years of follow-up.

In the past the extent of distal clearance has been thought to influence local recurrence rates, particularly after sphincter-saving resection. There are abundant data, however, to show that provided the distal margin of clearance is at least 2 cm, local recurrence is not affected by the length of distal clearance (Pollett and Nicholls, 1981; Williams et al, 1983; Phillips et al, 1984a,b).

There has been a suggestion that stapled anastomoses are more likely to be associated with local recurrence than conventional manual anastomoses. Thus Rosen et al (1985), although finding no significant difference in recurrence between hand-sewn and stapled anastomoses for carcinomas of the upper and lower thirds of the rectum, did report that recurrence was more frequent when stapled rather than manual anastomoses were used for lesions of the middle third of the rectum.

Table 32.20 Factors influencing local recurrence in the St Mary's Large Bowel Cancer Project.

	APER		*AR*	
Variable	*No.*	*%*	*No.*	*%*
Dukes' stage:				
A	4	7.0	2	3.0
B	21	36.8	33	49.3
C	32	56.1	32	47.8
Tumour differentiation:				
Well	13	22.8	12	17.9
Moderate	33	57.9	45	67.2
Poor	11	19.3	10	14.9
Obstruction:				
Absent	57	100	63	94.0
Present	0	0	4	6.0
Perforation:				
Absent	54	94.7	65	97.0
Definite	1	1.8	0	0.0
Suspected	3	3.5	2	3.0
Tumour mobility:				
Mobile	30	52.6	50	74.6
Partially or completely fixed	27	47.4	17	25.4

APER, abdominoperineal excision of the rectum; AR, anterior resection.
From Phillips et al (1984b).

Nevertheless, Leff et al (1985), Bokey et al (1984), Williams et al (1985), Kennedy et al (1985) and Wolmark et al (1986) were unable to confirm these findings, although it has to be said that these comparisons were made on an uncontrolled basis. The fact that stapling instruments are used for low rectal cancers which previously could not have been treated by a manual sphincter-saving resection may explain why some authorities believe that local recurrence rates are higher with staples as opposed to hand suture. However, other mechanisms have been proposed, in particular the scraping of tumour cells by the intraluminal stapling gun and their deposition at the anastomosis (Rosen et al, 1985). In this context, it is of interest that one of the highest recorded recurrence rates of 32% (Hurst et al, 1982) occurred in a series in which the authors specified that they did not irrigate the rectal stump before introduction of the stapling instrument. Nevertheless, after appraising the literature in detail, we found that the use of stapling guns *per se* did not influence the local recurrence rate (Abulafi and Williams, 1994). However, it has to be said that the only way of ensuring that this statement is correct is to perform prospective controlled trials. The only prospective study which has examined this question was that conducted by surgeons in the West of Scotland (Akyol et al, 1991), and they included colon cancer patients. They found that the mean recurrence rates at 24 months follow-up were 29.4% after suturing and 19.1% after stapling ($P < 0.01$), thus indicating that stapling was less likely to result in recurrence! These data need to be confirmed or refuted by larger trials.

Total mesorectal excision (TME)

The introduction of total mesorectal excision for the surgery of rectal cancer is relatively new, and its impact deserves closer analysis. The technique and its rationale have been discussed earlier in this chapter.

Briefly, it consists of precise sharp dissection around the integral mesentery of the hindgut which envelopes the entire hindgut. By performing this manoeuvre, it is hoped that any micrometastases which might lie in the mesorectum will be removed *en bloc* with the rectum and its carcinoma (MacFarlane et al, 1993). With care, and provided the tumour is confined to the rectal wall, the operation can be performed with minimal injury to pelvic nerves (Havenga et al, 1996a).

The concept of TME was first introduced by Heald (Heald et al, 1982; Heald and Ryall, 1986) and from his point of view explains his extremely low recurrence rate. There has been some scepticism with regard to the technique as many colorectal surgeons believe they have for many years been carrying out the procedure in exactly the same way as Heald describes. While this may be true, there is no doubt that Heald and his disciples have concentrated the minds of all colorectal surgeons in ensuring a complete excision of the mesorectum under direct vision for most rectal cancers.

Independent analysis by MacFarlane et al (1993) of Heald's data over the 13-year period 1978–91 showed that the actuarial local recurrence rate after curative anterior resection at 5 years was 4% and the overall recurrence rate was 18%; 10-year figures were 4% and 19% (MacFarlane et al, 1993).

Data from Scandinavia highlight the impact that TME has made in that part of the world. Arbman et al (1996) from Norrkoping in Sweden compared their results for rectal cancer in the periods 1984–86 ('group 1') and 1990–92 ('group 2'), and during the second period they adopted the technique of TME. In group 1, there were 134 patients who had undergone anterior resection or abdominoperineal excision which was considered to be curative. In group 2, 128 curative rectal excisions had been performed. No differences were found between groups in stage distribution, rate of curative operations, postoperative mortality or complications. One year after the end of the study period, local recurrence had developed in 19 patients (14.3%) in group 1 and in 8 (6.3%) in group 2 ($P < 0.03$). Actuarial analysis showed a significant reduction in local recurrence rates ($P < 0.03$) and an increase in crude survival ($P < 0.03$) at 4 years in group 2 compared with group 1 (Figure 32.86).

Enker and colleagues from the Sloan Kettering Cancer Center found a local recurrence rate of 7.3% in a consecutive series of 246 patients with rectal cancer treated by TME. This recurrence rate included patients both with and without distant metastases and was considered to be significantly better than the rate achieved in their unit using a conventional surgical technique and combined modality adjuvant therapy (Enker et al, 1995).

In McCall et al's (1995) review of the literature, the median local recurrence rate was 18.5% after follow-up in 10 465 patients. Of these patients, 1033 had undergone TME (eight papers), and the local recurrence rate in this 'group' was 7.1%.

It does appear, therefore, that TME holds the promise of considerably reducing local recurrence, but attention to detail will be required to prevent complications. Provided the anatomy of the pelvic nerves are understood, bladder and sexual

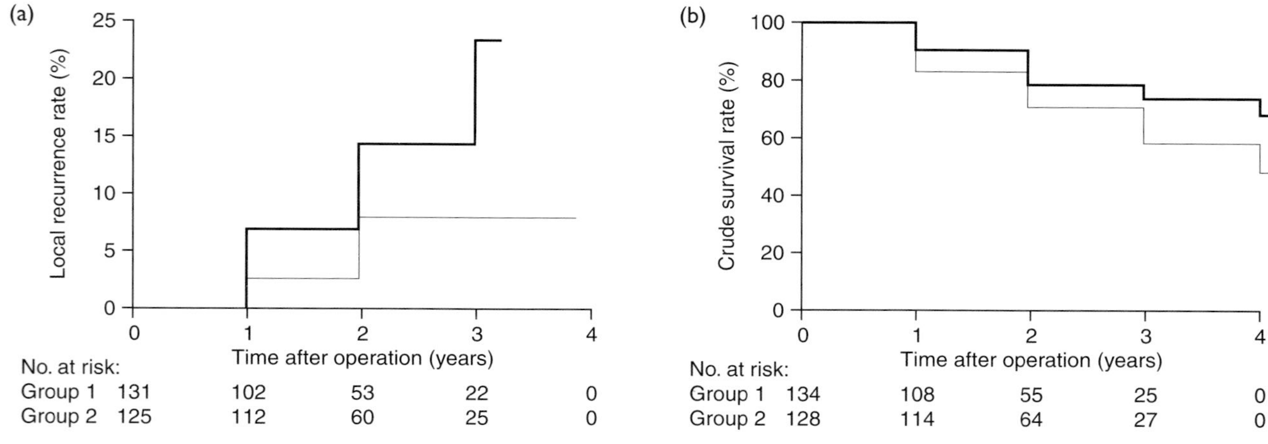

Figure 32.86a,b (a) Actuarial local recurrence rates before (——) and after (——) the introduction of TME. (b) Actuarial survival rates before (——) and after (——) the introduction of TME (Arbman et al, 1996).

dysfunction should be avoided. Readers are referred to an excellent review of this anatomy by Havenga et al (1996a). In a separate study, Havenga and colleagues showed that if these nerves are preserved 86% of men younger than 60 years of age will retain their potency (Havenga et al, 1996b).

One concern that has been raised is that TME may lead to a high incidence of anastomotic dehiscence. Thus, in Heald's series (Karanjia et al, 1994), there were 24 (11%) major anastomotic leaks in 219 patients undergoing low SSR with TME. In addition, a further 14 (6.4%) of asymptomatic leaks were found on contrast enemas. It may be that TME results in the devascularization of the anorectal stump. For this reason, a defunctioning stoma has been recommended as a routine addition when TME is used (Karanjia et al, 1991).

Opinion of the authors

We believe that TME should be performed for most tumours of the mid and lower rectum. This does *not* mean that the 'gut' tube requires to be divided at the same level in every case. Dissection of the distal mesorectum off the gut tube can be performed, so that the distal line of division of the bowel wall occurs at a minimum of 2 cm below the tumour if such a manoeuvre would ensure that the sphincters are preserved. However, such a manoeuvre is likely to increase the risk of anastomotic leakage because of the danger of rendering the anorectal stump ischaemic. Thus, a covering stoma should be employed routinely, but if the bowel is divided 2 cm from the dentate line, as in restorative proctocolectomy, the risk of leakage should be reduced and a covering stoma may not always be needed. In the upper third of the rectum and in some middle-third tumours, the mesorectum and gut tube can safely be divided 5 cm below the tumour without jeopardizing recurrence rates. By preserving as much anorectal remnant as possible in this way, postoperative function is likely to be enhanced without jeopardizing local recurrence rates.

LOCAL MANOEUVRES

Indications

Opinions differ as to the role of local procedures as an alternative to radical excision for the treatment of certain rectal cancers. The recent introduction of transanal endoscopic microsurgery (TEM) in particular has increased the debate. A small minority of early, small Dukes' A rectal cancers when first seen are suitable from the technical point of view for this form of therapy. Undoubtedly these patients would be cured by such a procedure. The problem in the minds of many surgeons is the accuracy of selection.

Clinical evaluation alone in these cases may be inaccurate and by embarking on local excision the patient may thus be denied a cure. Prior to the introduction of TEM those centres that particularly advocated local therapy stressed very strict selection criteria (Crile and Turnbull, 1972; Madden and

Kandalaft, 1971; Mason, 1976; Salvati and Rubin, 1976). Despite minor differences from centre to centre there was remarkable concordance for the criteria that were used to justify conventional local excision of rectal cancer. The tumour therefore had to be:

- small – less than 3 cm diameter
- located in an extraperitoneal region of the rectum
- mobile and limited to the bowel wall
- polypoid rather then ulcerated
- well or moderately differentiated (Weakley, 1983).

However, it was clear from our studies that assessment of mobility by clinical means and histological grade on preoperative biopsy were often inaccurate (Williams et al, 1985). Assessment of local spread can be improved by CT scanning (Nicholls et al, 1982; Williams et al, 1985), and endoluminal ultrasonography seems to be very effective in determining the depth of invasion of the cancer (Benyon et al, 1986). Similarly, preoperative histological grading can be improved by taking multiple biopsies, but interpretation is subjective and heterogeneity makes this parameter the least important for selection. Even if more sophisticated investigations were able to determine accurately the spread of the lesion through the rectal wall, the surgeon cannot be sure that lymph node invasion has not taken place. For these reasons the balance of opinion still favours local measures only for curative treatment in small, mobile T_1 lesions, or for patients with localized rectal cancer with or without metastases who are otherwise unfit for more radical surgery.

Our own view is that local excision, particularly using TEM, could be used more often as a curative operation but only in highly selected patients. This form of therapy is useful in the patient with a low, small, mobile lesion when the only other alternative is abdominoperineal excision and a permanent colostomy. Provided selection is made with the added benefit of pelvic CT or endoluminal ultrasonography and follow-up is meticulous, we have found conventional local excision to be an acceptable manoeuvre. Using TEM, the extent of local excision can be increased, although it is still confined to the extraperitoneal region of the rectum. This limits the maximal distance from the anal verge on the anterior wall to 12 cm, at the side walls to 15 cm, and on the posterior wall to 20 cm (Buess, 1996). The Boston group have explored the role of local excision with chemoradiotherapy for T_2 lesions. The 5-year results do support their view that this approach is an option in small tumours where patients are not eager to accept abdominoperineal excision (Bleday et al, 1997). Similar results have been achieved in Philadelphia (Fortunato et al, 1995).

There is less controversy over the use of local measures in the palliative treatment of rectal carcinoma. Local excision, fulguration, cryosurgery, laser therapy and TEM have all been used for palliation. With the more frequent use of liver ultrasound and CT scans more patients with disseminated disease are being detected. As a result a greater proportion of patients are eligible for this form of treatment.

Techniques

Conventional local excision

Local excision can be performed via the transanal or trans-sphincteric routes. The techniques are similar to those used for local excision of a villous adenoma (Chapter 28). However, the excisions performed for cancer involve full-thickness rather than submucosal excision.

Trans-sphincteric excision is now virtually an obsolete procedure. It was most suitable for a tumour situated on the anterior or anterolateral walls of the rectum 8–12 cm from the anal verge. It was performed with the patient in the prone jack-knife position. The posterior wall of the anorectum was opened longitudinally with stay sutures to mark the divided internal anal sphincter puborectalis and external sphincter. The tumour was resected with a 1–2 cm clearance taking the entire rectal wall. Once haemostasis was secured, the defect in the rectum was closed with interrupted Dexon or Vicryl sutures. The anorectum was then reconstituted in layers using interrupted Dexon or Vicryl sutures.

Conventional transanal excision is still used for small lesions within 8 cm of the anal verge, but higher lesions can be treated in this way provided they can be parachuted into the lower rectum. Posterior or posterolateral lesions are removed with the patient in the lithotomy position; when the lesion is situated anteriorly, the prone position is more suitable.

Technique of conventional transanal excision

The patient has a full bowel preparation, antibiotic cover and a stoma site is marked in case this is needed. Most operations are performed in the lithotomy position using general anaesthesia, but epidural or spinal anaesthesia has been used in our practice. If there is real doubt concerning the feasibility of local resection, the lithotomy–Trendelenburg position is used and both the abdomen and perineum are prepared.

The Parks' retractor is inserted so that eight stay sutures can be placed around the circumference of the lesion. Deep bites 1.5 cm from the edge of the growth are used as this minimizes damage to the lesion and ensures an adequate margin of clearance. The ends of the stay sutures are left long and twisted together to form a Chinese queue (Figure 32.87a). Traction on the eight stay sutures minimizes the risk of injury to the mucosa. The tumour in this manner

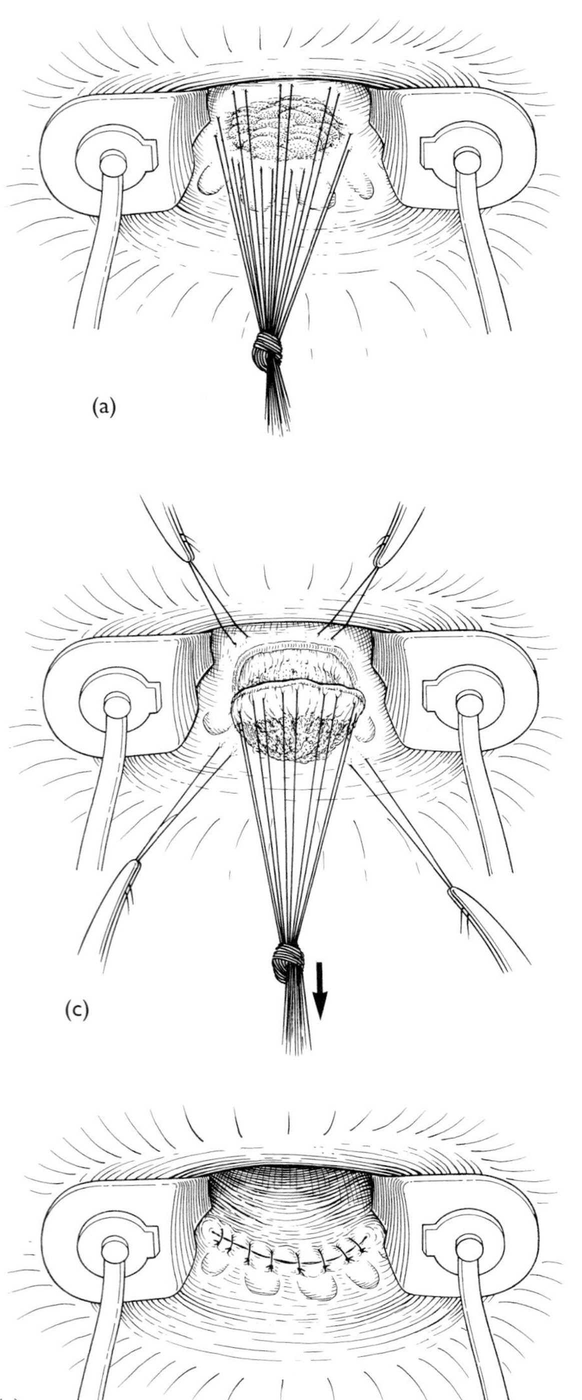

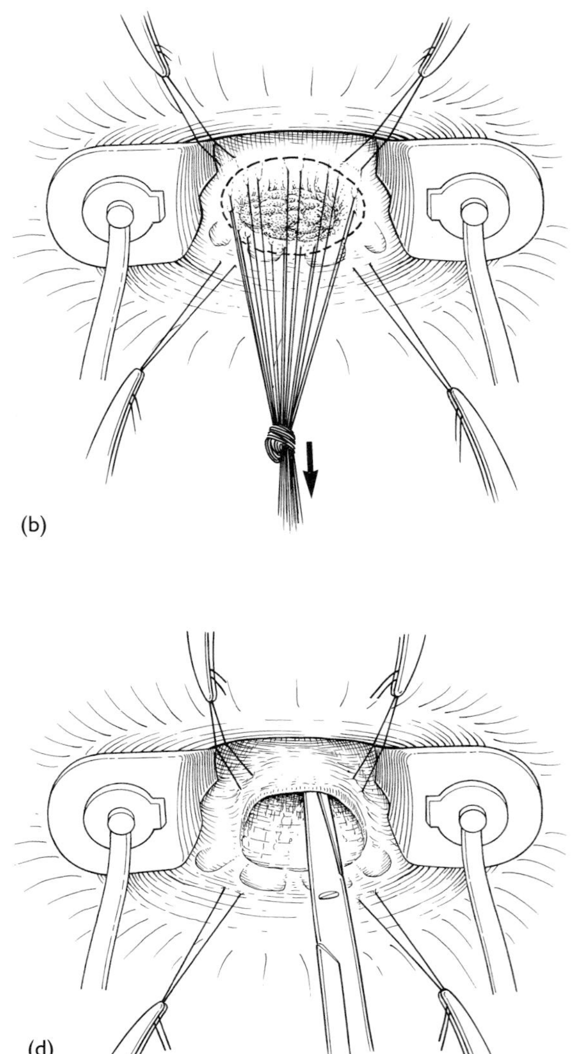

Figure 32.87 Transanal excision of rectal cancer (see text).

can be pulled down into the lower anal canal; if this is not possible it is likely that there is extensive extrarectal involvement and conventional local excision should be abandoned. Four stay sutures are placed 1–2 cm peripheral to the Chinese queue (Figure 32.87b) prior to division of the entire rectal wall out to extrarectal fat. We tend to divide the rectum with diathermy securing haemostasis during piecemeal division, since traction on the stays facilitates exposure (Figure 32.87c). Once the entire tumour has been excised there is a sizeable defect. The specimen should contain pararectal nodes and a segment of extrarectal fat.

Careful reconstruction of the rectum is crucial since closure can easily distort the rectal lumen, resulting in stenosis or contracture that causes disabling symptoms. The upper flap of the rectum should be mobilized so that the upper side of the defect can reach the distal margin of excision without tension (Figure 32.87d). The defect may be closed transversely in one or two layers. We prefer a continuous full-thickness closure, but interrupted sutures are sometimes preferred for large saucer-shaped defects (Figure 32.87e). Rectal washout with 1% cetrimide is advised prior to closing the defect. Once the suture line is completed the retractor is removed to permit digital examination and sigmoidoscopy, so that the surgeon can be sure that there is no rectal distortion.

A covering stoma is not normally necessary.

Transanal endoscopic microsurgery (TEM)

TEM was first introduced into clinical practice by Buess and his colleagues in Germany in 1983 (Buess et al, 1984). The reasons for the development of this technique were the invasiveness of the posterior approaches to the rectum and the limited view given by the conventional transanal approach.

The technique of TEM is complex and needs substantial training. The equipment which was developed by Buess is manufactured by Wolf (Knittlingen, Germany). It consists of an operating sigmoidoscope 12 or 20 cm in length and 4 cm in outer diameter which incorporates a high-quality binocular optical system providing up to 6× magnification. Rectal distension to a pressure of 10 mmHg with simultaneous continuous low-pressure suction is achieved by means of a combined endosurgical unit incorporating pressure-sensitive insufflation of carbon dioxide and a roller suction unit. Submucosal or full-thickness tumour excision is achieved by means of a diathermy knife and graspers introduced through gas-tight operating ports on the occlusive operating face-plate of the sigmoidoscope. The subsequent defect can then be closed with 3.0 polydioxanone using a purpose-designed needle holder and securing the suture by means of a silver clip.

Preoperative examination

Precise preoperative evaluation of the tumour is mandatory before using TEM. The location of the tumour, distance from the anal verge and the precise position on the circumference is essential in order to decide whether the tumour can be reached with the operating resectoscope and which positioning of the patient is necessary to perform the operation. The preoperative examination should include careful digital palpation if possible and inspection with a rigid sigmoidoscope. The upper tumour margin which can be reached is approximately 20 cm, but in case of angulation in a narrow sigmoid it might be difficult to reach this area. A basic rule is that a tumour which is easy to reach with a rigid sigmoidoscope can be operated on by TEM.

Positioning of the patient

The apparatus is supported by a multi-jointed Martin arm which allows repositioning of the sigmoidoscope during the procedure, but it is important to have the patient in the correct position from the outset. Depending on the location of the tumour, the patient is positioned so that the tumour lies at the bottom. This is because the instruments and the optics are designed to operate downwards. Thus, under general anaesthesia the patient with a tumour on the posterior wall is placed in the lithotomy or Lloyd Davis position, whereas for anterior lesions the patient is placed face down with the hips flexed and the legs apart. Occasionally, it is necessary to operate with the patient in the right or left lateral positions.

Operative details

The rectoscope is introduced into the rectum after first gently dilating the anal sphincter. The rectum is insufflated, the lesion identified and the instruments introduced (Figure 32.88). The margin of clearance is defined by marking dots using the high-frequency device. In the case of a proven or suspected cancer, a 10 mm margin is advised; for an adenoma a 5 mm margin is used.

The dissection is usually commenced at the lower edge of the lesion by circumcising the lower circumference. Coagulation of vessels is achieved by

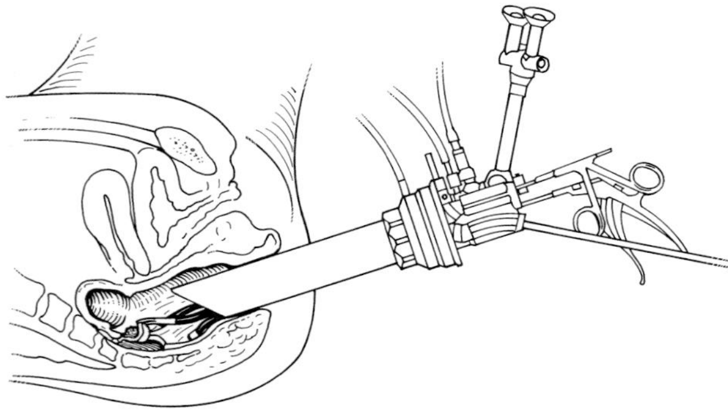

Figure 32.88 Transanal endoscopic microsurgery (TEM). The resectoscope is passed into the rectum, which is then insufflated, and the specially designed instruments are reintroduced.

diathermy as the dissection proceeds (Figure 32.89). The tumour is folded upwards so that the base is well exposed for dissection. Larger vessels in the perirectal fat can be dissected and coagulated before transection. Spurting vessels can be grasped with a forceps and their walls compressed before coagulation.

The plane of dissection in full-thickness excision is directly on the dorsal plane of the muscular layer. In the case of cancer on the posterior circumference, parts of the perirectal fat, including lymph nodes, can be resected with the specimen. Dissection of the superior margin of the tumour may be difficult owing to restricted vision. The marking dots help in defining the superior margin of resection, and if the incisions are made from marking dot to marking dot there is less risk of leaving tumour behind.

Once the tumour has been excised and removed, it is pinned out on a cork board to ensure that there is a healthy margin of macroscopic normal-looking mucosa. The rectal lumen is then irrigated with a cancercidal agent such as B-iodine to prevent implantation of cancer cells.

The defect is then closed with a transverse running suture. That used by Buess is a PDS suture in 5H needle size, and is shortened to a maximum length of 10 cm. As in conventional surgery, the suture is performed with a needle holder and forceps. Owing to restricted degrees of freedom of movement of the needle holder, some tricks are necessary to master the suturing technique. In some positions, for example, the needle holder is kept in position and the bowel tissue is pulled over the needle with the forceps. After a number of bites (5–8) of the suture needle, the suture material is put under tension and fixed using a silver clip which is pressed on it (Figure 32.90). The silver clip holds the suture safely, so that knotting, which is difficult, is not necessary. Semi-circumferential defects need about three continuous sutures, whereas complete segmental resections sometimes need up to eight.

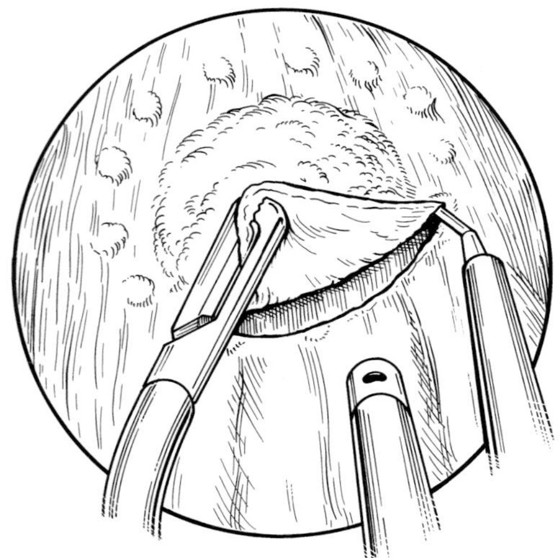

Figure 32.89 TEM. The margin of clearance is marked out using a series of dots created by the diathermy. The tumour is dissected by folding it upwards, and the vessels supplying it are divided using diathermy.

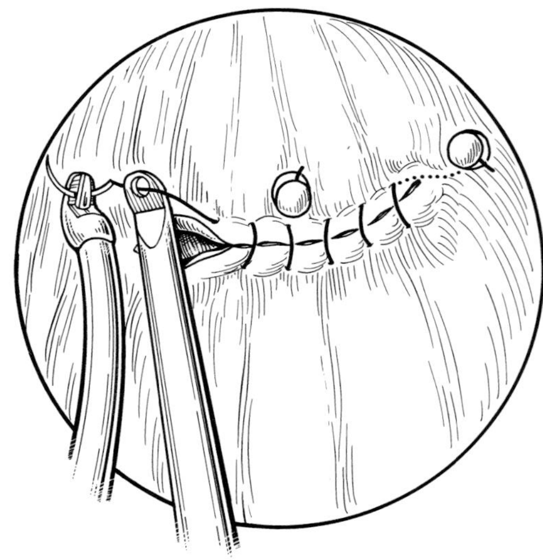

Figure 32.90 TEM. The defect can be closed using a continuous suture. Fixation of the suture is achieved using a silver clip as a substitute for a knot.

Postoperative course

Patients are mobilized as soon as anaesthesia allows. Postoperative pain occurs only when the excision is performed close to the dentate line. Higher localized excisions are usually completely pain-free, although sometimes a sense of pressure appears in the area of the sphincter because of the dilatation of the sphincter owing to the introduction of the 40 mm rectoscope. The same is, of course, true for the conventional transanal approach.

Complete oral nutrition is usually commenced on the fifth postoperative day if a full-thickness excision has been performed.

Studies on anorectal physiology suggest that the technique does not have any lasting adverse effect on continence (Jehle et al, 1992, 1995).

Electrocoagulation

Electrocoagulation may be an alternative to local excision but is usually reserved for larger tumours in patients who have either refused major abdominal surgery or are considered too unfit for it, or in whom palliative treatment only is being offered. The procedure can be performed under general, spinal or epidural anaesthesia.

Depending on the site of the tumour and the preference of the surgeon, the patient can be positioned in either the prone jack-knife or lithotomy position. Occasionally, it is necessary to have the patient in the left lateral position so as to expose the tumour with the operating sigmoidoscope. Usually, however, the procedure can be performed via a bivalve or trivalve anal retractor.

The diathermy blade is then applied to the surface of the tumour with the setting at medium power. Electrocoagulation of all of the superficial part of the tumour is performed by the surgeon, while the assistant uses the sucker to remove smoke and debris. The destroyed part of the tumour is then removed by curettage and the process is repeated. After each application the surgeon checks the progress with an index finger. Although the bulk of the lesion can be destroyed at one operation, it is usually necessary to bring the patient back 2–3 weeks later for a repeat treatment. On this occasion the area is examined digitally and suspicious areas are biopsied and sent for frozen-section histology; if positive, further coagulation is applied. This is the exception rather than the rule. It can be quite difficult to ensure that complete destruction has been achieved. Involved areas may still be present yet appear relatively normal on palpation.

Although some have used this technique as a curative manoeuvre, in our opinion it should be considered only as palliation (Madden and Kandalaft, 1967, 1971; Crile and Turnbull, 1972). The patient needs careful follow-up so that any recrudescence can be dealt with promptly.

Another method of applying electrocoagulation to the tumour has been described by Berry et al (1990). They modified a transurethral resectoscope which is inserted through the anal sphincter. The rectum is then distended with glycine solution, the obturator removed, and a diathermy loop inserted. Under direct vision the tumour is resected in a manner similar to transurethral resection of the prostate or bladder neck. We have used this technique in a few patients and find it a great improvement compared with conventional electrocoagulation.

Cryotherapy

Destruction of the growth by freezing is an alternative to electrocoagulation for palliative treatment. The patient is positioned as for a local excision, and the tip of a cryoprobe loaded with liquid nitrogen to approximately minus 20°C is applied to the centre of the tumour. The probe is left in contact with the tumour for approximately 60 seconds and is then applied to other parts of it.

Although some state that the procedure can be performed without general anaesthesia (Scholzell and Langer, 1981), we have found in the limited number of cases we have treated that some form of anaesthesia is essential. Although application of the probe to the tumour may not be too painful, the presence of the anal retractor is far too uncomfortable for the patient unless spinal or epidural anaesthesia is used.

After freezing, the tumour necroses over a period of weeks during which there is a copious discharge of mucus and debris per rectum. After approximately a month the lesion is reassessed and further treatment arranged if necessary.

We believe that this technique should be considered only as palliative. Despite its advocates, most specialists consider that even as a palliative technique it is inferior to the alternative methods available.

Laser and photodynamic treatment

Fleisher (1982) and Bown et al (1986) have described the use of a neodymium–yttrium aluminium garnet laser for the palliative treatment of symptomatic rectal cancer. The technique has been applied mainly to inoperable rectal carcinomas which are causing obstruction, discharge or incontinence owing to invasion of the sphincter. The laser beam has, generally, been used to increase the size of the lumen. Its ability to incise tissue while simultaneously providing haemostasis makes it an attractive alternative method for the excision of selected small primary tumours.

A similar technique which may be used for small rectal lesions is photodynamic therapy. In this form of treatment a photosensitizing drug, usually haematoporphyrin derivative (HpD), is administered intravenously 48 hours before therapy. This drug is preferentially taken up in neoplastic tissue. Red light generated from a tunable dye laser is then applied to the lesion which in turn releases singlet oxygen from the HpD which is cytotoxic. The advantage of this form of therapy is that the haematoporphyrin derivative is taken up selectively by the cancer cells and normal tissue is less likely to be damaged.

We have used this technique at the Royal London Hospital for palliative treatment of rectal cancer as an alternative to the Nd–YAG laser. Photodynamic therapy certainly improved symptoms in the few patients that we have treated, but since penetration of light is the limiting factor, we believe that the therapy is more suitable when the depth of the cancer is only a few millimetres. We have thus treated patients who after removal of a neoplastic polyp are known to have residual disease at the base yet are too unfit to undergo major surgery. Although these patients have suffered no untoward complications, it is too early to evaluate the success of the therapy. Further research is clearly indicated in this area.

Endocavitary radiation

This alternative method of local treatment is discussed in Chapter 33.

Complications

Complications of local procedures include both reactionary and secondary haemorrhage, perirectal infection with abscess formation, perforation of the rectum and rectal stricture. Local recurrence is almost inevitable when treatment is palliative. Sadly it is all too frequent when treatment is for cure, the complication being largely due to patient selection but may be caused by implantation of malignant cells. It is often impossible to determine whether this is true recurrence or recrudescence.

It is difficult to obtain the overall incidence of complications since series differ in their composition.

Crile and Turnbull (1972) using electrocoagulation claimed no morbidity and mortality in their 62 patients. Madden and Kandalaft (1971), on the other hand, had a 28.5% incidence of complications using the same technique. The most frequent problem was haemorrhage and a third of their patients needed re-operation to stop it. Perforation into the peritoneal cavity occurred in two patients (2.6%) and rectovaginal fistula developed in a further two patients. Similarly Hughes et al (1982) had five patients who needed transfusion as a result of haemorrhage; 8% of their patients also developed a rectal stricture. Cryosurgery is not without complications: Scholzell and Langer (1981) had 18 major complications in 184 patients (9.8%). Bleeding occurred in six (3%), perirectal abscess formation in two (1%) and perforation in three (1.5%) with subsequent rectal stricture in seven (3.8%).

As might be expected, the operative mortality rate for conventional transanal excision of rectal cancer approaches zero (Table 32.21). This also holds true for 'high-risk' operative patients who undergo local excision as a means of palliation. The morbidity rate for this procedure is not well described in the literature, but appears to be low. However, perforation and local sepsis are certainly possible, particularly with a tumour that is found to penetrate the rectal wall more deeply than was first thought.

The morbidity relating to transanal endoscopic microsurgery is also relatively low. Salm et al (1994) reported on the experiences of 44 clinics in Germany using TEM. In 1900 patients, 1411 adenomas and 433 carcinomas were resected. Of patients with cancer, 246 were resected with curative intent. Complications occurred in 6.3% of patients and 4% recovered with conservative treatment, surgical intervention being required in only 2.3%.

Within the first postoperative days, incontinence may occur following operations close to the

Table 32.21 Operative mortality for local transanal excision of rectal cancer.

	Operative mortality (%)
Morson et al (1977)	0
Cuthbertson and Kaye (1978)	0
Lock et al (1978)	0
Hager et al (1983)*	0
Grigg et al (1984)	0
Stearns et al (1984)*	6.1
Killingback (1985)	0
Whiteway et al (1985)*	0
Rothenberger and Finne (1990)	0

* Studies include high-risk patients treated palliatively.

sphincter region, and in elderly patients with preoperative existing continence problems. In a study by Steele et al (1996) of 100 patients treated with TEM in three centres, transient incontinence to liquid and gas occurred in only two patients (2%). The incontinence presumably relates to the lower resting anal pressure and loss of the rectoanal inhibitory reflex detected in these patients postoperatively (Banerjee et al, 1996). However, it should be noted that others have noticed no change in physiological measurements postoperatively (Jehle et al, 1992).

A rise in temperature up to 38°C is seen in most patients in the first 2–3 days after TEM. This could be due to bacterial contamination of the perirectal tissue during full-thickness excision. In most cases the pyrexia resolves after 2 days; if it does not, suture line dehiscence should be suspected. The latter can be confirmed by gentle sigmoidoscopy or a gastrografin enema. If this complication occurs, it is recommended that oral nutrition should cease, and intravenous infusion of fluids and antibiotics should commence. If such conservative measures fail, the establishment of a defunctioning stoma should be considered (Buess et al, 1996).

Minor postoperative bleeding is common, but in 1% this may be severe and require intervention. Such patients need to be returned to the operating theatre, the rectum needs to be irrigated and under direct vision the bleeder can be coagulated.

Late complications are rare as far as is known. Clearly, rectal stricture, particularly after excising a circumferential lesion, may be a potential problem. However, this complication seems to be uncommon in the literature so far. Steele et al (1996), for example, had only one case in their 100 patients, and this responded to dilatation.

Results

Conventional local excision

During the 1980s, owing largely to the powerful advocacy of Morson (1966) and Mason (1976), local excision either as a transanal procedure or via the posterior trans-sphincteric approach was proposed as primary treatment for certain small, sessile carcinomas of the lower rectum. These tumours were carefully selected on clinical and pathological grounds: they were small, were thought to be Dukes' A lesions, and on biopsy were determined as being well differentiated.

The results were variable. Hawley and Ritchie (1980) reported 42 cases with one operative death. Six patients had early re-operations for suspected incomplete removal. Of the remaining 36 cases, followed for 1–30 years, 20% recurred and 6% died from cancer.

Hermanek et al (1980) reported a local recurrence rate of 10% and a cancer-specific death rate of 2% in 48 patients. Stearns et al (1981) had disastrous results in 16 cases as 25% developed recurrence and the same percentage died from carcinoma.

Mason (1976) reported somewhat more gratifying results in that only 5 of 36 patients (14%) submitted to a potentially curative local resection had local recurrence, but three (8%) died from cancer. Killingback (1985) reported five local recurrences in 25 patients (18%) who had tumours confined to the rectal wall, while in 11 patients with tumours which had spread outside the rectal wall there were four recurrences (36%).

Nothiger (1985) followed up 62 patients who had had a local excision during a 10-year period. Twenty-four patients had tumours that extended into the muscle coat and 28 had tumours that were confined to the submucosa. Eight (13%) subsequently developed local recurrence, all of whom were patients who had ulcerating lesions invading the muscle coat.

Hermanek and Gall (1985) in a follow-up of 172 cases with purely submucosal carcinomas treated by local excision and followed for 2–8 years reported only nine patients with local recurrence (5.2%).

The variable results obtained by local excision were likely to be due to variation in selection. Furthermore, although a tumour may be entirely submucosal as far as direct spread is concerned, involved lymph nodes may still be present. Thus Cuthbertson et al (1984) have shown that 21% of those tumours which appear to be Dukes' A lesions and 13% of purely submucosal growths have associated involved nodes. Involvement of these nodes is virtually impossible to detect on clinical examination and is very difficult to find even with the more sophisticated endoluminal imaging techniques now available.

The results of the subsequent treatment of recurrence following local excision are extremely important, for if these local recurrences could always be effectively dealt with by a subsequent rectal excision, its development could be regarded as only a temporary inconvenience. However, the evidence on this point is somewhat conflicting and in the main disappointing. Of the nine cases reported by Killingback (1985) to have recurred after local excision, only five were deemed suitable for rectal excision and three of them recurred after this procedure. Four of eight patients with recurrence after local excision studied by Stearns et al (1984) came to rectal excision but only two survived any length of time. Seven out of Nothiger's eight recurrent cases were treated by abdominoperineal excision of the rectum but two developed further local recurrence (Nothiger, 1985).

The message therefore seems to be that conventional local excision should be performed for cure only in carefully selected patients. The tumours must be small, perhaps only 2–3 cm diameter; they should be exophytic and not ulcerated. They should be confined to the submucosa and be histologically well differentiated. Unfortunately the latter characteristics can be determined with certainty only after the excised specimen has been examined microscopically. Even if these guidelines are adhered to, up to 20% of these patients will have involved lymph nodes and will not therefore be cured. It is for this reason that most surgeons perform local excision only in highly selected favourable cases and when the patient is unfit for a more major procedure. However, with the advent of transanal endoscopic microsurgery (TEM) and improvements in imaging techniques which can improve the staging of the tumour, this policy may change.

Transanal endoscopic microsurgery (TEM)

Since this technique allows more accurate excision of the tumour, it is being used more frequently for larger and more advanced lesions than was the case with conventional local excision. Nevertheless, we agree with Steele et al (1996) that TEM with curative intent can be justified only for T_1 tumours at present. When used in this way, the results are reasonable, although follow-up is short.

Between 1989 and 1993, Buess operated on 34 patients with a T_1 lesion and detected local recurrence in only two patients (5.9%), although the mean length of follow-up was not stated (Mentges et al, 1994). In both of these patients, a subsequent radical resection with curative intent was performed. Similarly, in a much smaller group of seven patients with T_1 lesions, followed up for approximately 6 months, Steele et al (1996) found no recurrences. However, Stipa et al (1995) found a 9% local recurrence rate after treating 30 patients.

When the technique is used for more advanced lesions, the results are more worrying. Thus, Steele et al (1996) found that of the 14 patients with T_2 lesions, 13 had complete resections of their tumour, but within a mean of 6 months' follow-up two (15.4%) had recurred, the patient with the incomplete resection undergoing APER.

Whether the use of postoperative radiotherapy may improve the results in these more advanced lesions remains to be seen. However, we must emphasize that it is our strong belief, given the present state of knowledge, that even with this advanced technology only very carefully selected early cancers should be treated by TEM if the intention is cure, and preferably such patients should be treated within the confines of a clinical trial.

Electrocoagulation

Electrocoagulation has, in the main, been used as a palliative manoeuvre. It has also been used in certain patients who have been unfit for major surgery in the hope of securing a cure. Unfortunately, most reports do not separate the palliative from the curative cases and thus interpretation is difficult.

Wittoesch and Jackman (1958) were perhaps the first to describe the results of electrocoagulation in a large series of patients treated at the Mayo Clinic. During 1945–49 inclusive, of 2028 patients with rectal cancer who were treated, 128 underwent electrocoagulation. Fifty-four (42%) of this group of patients survived for more than 5 years. Similarly, Madden and Kandalaft (1971) described encouraging results in their 77 patients treated by the technique. Forty-two of their patients had been treated for 4–17 years, and of these, 20 (47%) were alive and well. Crile and Turnbull (1972) found that 42 (68%) of their 62 patients who were treated between 1952 and 1965 survived for at least 5 years. Eisenstat et al (1982) reported on the results of electrocoagulation in 48 patients treated with the hope of cure; 19 (39%) subsequently needed an abdominoperineal excision of the rectum for recurrence, of whom only five survived 5 years. Of the remaining 29 patients who were treated by electrocoagulation alone, 20 (68%) survived 5 years. The overall 5-year survival rate for the whole group was only 52%.

Hughes et al (1982) described the results of electrocoagulation in 39 patients treated by the technique for cure. In only 27 (69%) was there no evidence of recurrent disease at follow-up. They stressed that exophytic lesions did far better than ulcerated lesions. Thus of 24 patients with exophytic tumours, 22 (92%) were free from disease at follow-up compared with only five of 15 patients (33%) with ulcerated lesions.

The foregoing reported data do not indicate that electrocoagulation can be used as a curative form of therapy. As with local excision, however, patients need to be carefully selected. The general current view in both the UK and the USA is that electrocoagulation should be used only in patients with potentially curable lesions when they are unfit to undergo a more extensive procedure.

REFERENCES

Abercrombie JF, Rogers J & Williams NS (1994) Complete anorectal sensory loss following total anorectal reconstruction. *Br J Surg* **81**: 761.

Abulafi AM & Williams NS (1994). Local recurrence of colorectal cancer: the problem, mechanisms, management and adjuvant therapy. *Br J Surg* **81**: 7–19.

Adalsteinsson B, Glimelius B, Graffman S et al (1981) Computed tomography of recurrent rectal carcinoma. *Acta Radiol (Diagn) (Stockh)* **22**: 669–672.

Adam IJ, Mohamdee MO, Martin IG et al (1994) Role of circumferential margin involvement in the local recurrence of rectal cancer. *Lancet* **344**: 707–711.

Adolff M, Arnoud JP & Beehary S (1980) Stapled vs sutured colorectal anastomosis. *Arch Surg* **115**: 1436–1438.

Akyol AM, McGregor JR, Galloway OJ, Murray G & George WD (1991) Recurrence of colorectal cancer after sutured and stapled large bowel anastomosis. *Br J Surg* **78**: 1297–1300.

Alleman A, Barras JP & Wagner HE (1994) Low anterior resection versus rectum amputation for treatment of rectal cancer (in German). *Helv Chir Acta* **60**: 701–705.

Allingham W (1879) *Fistula, Haemorrhoids, Painful Ulcer Stricture, Prolapses and other Disease of the Rectum, their Diagnosis and Treatment*, 3rd edn. Philadelphia: Lindsay.

Allingham W & Allingham H (1901) *The Diagnosis and Treatment of Diseases of the Rectum*, 7th edn. London: Baillière.

Allum WH, Slaney G, McConkey CC & Powell J (1994) Cancer of the colon and rectum in the West Midlands. *Br J Surg* **81**: 1060–1063

Amato A, Pescatori M & Buti A (1991) Local recurrence following abdominoperineal excision and anterior resection for rectal carcinoma. *Dis Colon Rectum* **34**: 317–322.

Andalkar RR (1979) Comparative study of staple vs suture anastomosis in low anterior resection. *J Maine Med Assoc* **70**: 429–431.

Andersberg B, Enblad P, Sjodahl R & Wetterfors J (1983a) The EEA stapling device in anterior resection for carcinoma of the rectum. *Acta Chir Scand* **149**: 99–103.

Andersberg B, Enblad R & Sjodahl R (1983b) Recurrent rectal carcinoma after anterior resection and rectal stapling. *Br J Surg* **70**: 104.

Andersson A & Bergdahl L (1976) Urologic complications following abdominoperineal resection of the rectum. *Arch Surg* **111**: 969–971.

Arbman G, Nilsson E, Halbook O & Sjodahl R (1996) Local recurrence following total mesorectal excision for rectal cancer. *Br J Surg* **83**: 375–379.

Babcock WW (1939) Experiences with resection of the colon and the elimination of colostomy. *Am J Surg* **46**: 186–303.

Babcock WW (1947) Radical single-stage extirpation for cancer of the large bowel with retained functional anus. *Surg Gynecol Obstet* **85**: 1–7.

Bach-Nielson P (1967) New surgical method of repairing sacral hernia following abdominoperineal excision of the rectum. *Acta Chir Scand* **133**: 67.

Bacon HE (1945) Evolution of sphincter muscle preservation and re-establishment of continuity in the operative treatment of rectal and sigmoidal cancer. *Surg Gynecol Obstet* **81**: 113–127.

Balfour DC (1910) A method of anastomosis between sigmoid and rectum. *Am J Surg* **51**: 239.

Balslev IB (1973) Living with a colostomy. A long-term follow-up investigation of 110 patients submitted to operation for cancer of the rectum. *Ugeskr Laeger* **135**: 2799–2804.

Banerjee AK, Jehle EC, Kreis ME et al (1996). Prospective study of the proctographic and functional consequences of transanal endoscopic microsurgery. *Br J Surg* **83**: 211–213.

Batignani G, Monaci I, Ficari F & Tonelli F (1991) What affects continence after anterior resection of the rectum? *Dis Colon Rectum* **34**: 329–335.

Baumrucker GO & Shaw JW (1953) Urological complications following abdomino-perineal resection of the rectum. *Arch Surg* **67**: 502–513.

Beart RW & Kelly KA (1981) Randomised prospective evaluation of the EEA stapler for colorectal anastomoses. *Am J Surg* **141**: 143–147.

Beckers J & Deldime P (1978) A propos de 50 anastomoses colorectales basses par suture mécanique. *Acta Chir Belg* **77**: 327–333.

Benyon J, Foy DMA, Roe N, Temple LN & Mortensen NJM (1986) Endoluminal ultrasound in the assessment of local invasion in rectal cancer. *Br J Surg* **73**: 474–478.

Berger A, Tiret E, Parc R et al (1992) Excision of the rectum with colonic J pouch–anal anastomosis for adenocarcinoma of the low and mid rectum. *World J Surg* **16**: 470–477.

Bernard D, Morgan S, Tasse D & Wassef R (1989) Preliminary results of coloanal anastomosis. *Dis Colon Rectum* **32**: 580–584.

Berry AC, Souser RG, Cambell WB, Mortensen NJMcM & Kettlewell MGW (1990) Endoscopic transanal resection of rectal tumours: a preliminary report of its use. *Br J Surg* **77**: 134–137.

Berthold S, Alexander-Williams J, Hanni K & Eckmann L (1980) Erste Erfahrungen mit einem automatischen Klammernahtgerat fur enterale Anastomosen. *Chirurg* **51**: 671–674.

Bervar M, Petrovic M, Gugic B & Scekic M (1977) Nasa askustva sa primenom mechanickog samosivatelja kod niskih kolorektalnih anastomoza. *Vojnosanit Pregl* **34**: 266–268.

Black BM (1952) Combined abdomino–endorectal resection: technical aspects and indications. *Arch Surg (Chicago)* **65**: 406–416.

Blamey SL & Lee PWR (1982) A comparison of circular stapling devices in colorectal anastomoses. *Br J Surg* **69**: 19–22.

Bleday R, Breen E, Jessup M et al (1997) Prospective evaluation of local excision for small rectal cancers. *Dis Colon Rectum* **40**: 388–392.

Block WA & Waugh JM (1948) The intramural extension of carcinoma of the descending colon, sigmoid and rectosigmoid: a pathologic study. *Surg Gynecol Obstet* **87**: 457–464.

Bokey EL & Pheils MT (1980) An alternative technique of inserting the distal purse string for the EEA stapling device in a lower anterior resection. *Aust NZ J Surg* **50**: 311.

Bokey EL, Chapuis PH, Hughes WJ, Koorey SG & Dunn D (1984) Local recurrence following anterior resection for carcinoma of the rectum with a stapled anastomosis. *Acta Chir Scand* **150**: 683–686.

Bolton RA & Britton DC (1980) Restorative surgery of the rectum with circumferential stapler. *Lancet* **i**: 850–851.

Bonfanti G, Bozzetti F, Doci R et al (1982) Results of extended surgery for cancer of the rectum and sigmoid. *Br J Surg* **69**: 305.

Bown SG, Barr H, Matthewson K et al (1986) Endoscopic treatment of inoperable colorectal cancers with the Nd–YAG laser. *Br J Surg* **73**: 949–952.

Braun J, Pfingsten F, Schippers E & Schumpelick V (1992) Rectal cancer: results of continence-preserving resections (in German). *Leber Magen Darm* **22**(2): 59–66, 69–70.

Brennan SJ, Pickford IR, Evans M & Pollock AV (1982) Staples or sutures for colonic anastomoses: a controlled clinical trial. *Br J Surg* **69**: 722–724.

Brunschwig A & Daniel WD (1960) Pelvic exenteration operations with summary of sixty-six cases surviving more than five years. *Ann Surg* **151**: 571.

Buchmann P & Uhlschmid G (1980) When are EEA 'stapler doughnuts' really complete? *Lancet* **ii**: 94.

Buess GF (1996) Local procedures including endoscopic resection. In Williams NS (ed) *Colorectal Cancer*. Edinburgh: Churchill Livingstone.

Buess GF, Hutterer F, Theis J et al (1984) Das System fur die transanale endoskopische Rektumoperation. *Chirurg* **55**: 677–680.

Bukh H (1954) Clinical research on the permanent colostomy: its function and management. *Acta Chir Scand* **114** (Suppl): 190.

Bussey HJR (1963) The long term results of surgical treatment of cancer of the rectum. *Proc R Soc Med* **56**: 494.

Cade D, Gallagher P, Schofield PF & Turner L (1981) Complications of anterior resection of the rectum using the EEA stapling device. *Br J Surg* **68**: 339–340.

Cady J, Godfroy J, Sibaud O et al (1980) La désunion anastomotique en chirurgie colique et rectale: étude comparative des procédés de suture manuelle et mécanique à propos d'une serie de 149 resections. *Ann Chir* **34**: 350–356.

Carmona JA, Ortiz H & Perez-Cabanas I (1991) Alterations in anorectal function after anterior resection for cancer of the rectum. *Int J Colorect Dis* **6**: 108–110.

Carpentier A & Chachques JC (1985) Myocardial substitution with a stimulated skeletal muscle: first successful case. *Lancet* **i**: 1267.

Castrini G, Pappalardo G & Mobarhan S (1985). A new technique for ileoanal and coloanal anastomosis. *Surgery* **97**: 111–116.

Catchpole BW (1969) Ileus: use of sympathetic blocking agents in its treatment. *Surgery (St Louis)* **66**: 811.

Cavaliere F, Tedesco M, Giannarelli D et al (1991) Radical surgery in rectal cancer patients: what does it mean today? *J Surg Oncol* (Suppl 2): 24–31.

Cavaliere F, Pemberton JH, Cosimelli M, Fazio VW, Beart RW Jr (1995) Coloanal anastomosis for rectal cancer: long-term results at the Mayo and Cleveland Clinics. *Dis Colon Rectum* **38**: 807–812.

Cavina di E, Seccia M, Chiarugi M et al (1985) Contineza di colostomie perineale dopo operazione di Miles: neosfintere elettrosimolato. *Boll Soc It Chir* **6**: 3–4, 23–29.

Christensen PB & Kronberg O (1981) Suprapubic bladder drainage in colorectal surgery. *Br J Surg* **68**: 348.

Clark CG, Wyllie JH, Haggie SJ & Renton P (1977) Comparison of catgut and polyglycolic acid sutures in colonic anastomoses. *World J Surg* **1**: 501.

Clogg HS (1904) Some observations on carcinoma of the colon. *Practitioner* **72**: 525–544.

Coffey RC (1931) Transplantation of ureters into large intestine. *Br J Urol* **3**: 353.

Cole PP (1913) The intramural spread of rectal carcinoma. *BMJ* **i**: 431–433.

Coller FA, Kay EB & Macintyre RS (1940) Regional lymphatic metastases of carcinoma of the rectum. *Surgery* **8**: 294–311.

Cooke RV (1956) Advanced carcinoma of the colon with emphasis on the inflammatory factor. *Ann R Coll Surg Engl* **18**: 46.

Copeland EM, Miller LD & Jones RS (1968) Prognostic factors in carcinoma of the colon and rectum. *Am J Surg* **116**: 875–881.

Cordonnier JJ (1950) Ureterosigmoid anastomosis. *J Urol* **63**: 276.

Cosimelli M, Mannella E, Giannarelli D et al (1972) The role of electrocoagulation in the treatment of carcinoma of the rectum. *Surg Gynecol Obstet* **135**: 391.

Cosimelli M, Mannella E, Giannarelli D et al (1994) Nerve-sparing surgery in 302 resectable rectosigmoid cancer patients: genitourinary morbidity and 10-year survival. *Dis Colon Rectum* **37** (Suppl 2): S42–46.

Crile G Jr & Turnbull RB Jr (1972) The role of electrocoagulation in the treatment of carcinoma of the rectum. *Surg Gynaecol Obstet* **135**: 391–396.

Cullen PK Jr & Mayo CW (1963) A further evaluation of the one-stage low anterior resection. *Dis Colon Rectum* **6**: 415–421.

Cutait DE & Figlioni FJ (1961) A new method of colorectal anastomosis in abdominoperineal resection. *Dis Colon Rectum* **4**: 335–342.

Cutait DE, Cutait R, Ioshimoto et al (1985) Abdominoperineal endoanal pull through resection. *Dis Colon Rectum* **28**: 294.

Cuthbertson AM & Kaye AH (1978) Local excision of carcinomas of the rectum. *Aust NZ J Surg* **48**: 412–415.

Cuthbertson AM, Hughes ESR & Pihl E (1984) Metastatic 'early' colorectal cancer. *Aust NZ J Surg* **54**: 549–552.

d'Allaines F (1956) *Die Chirurgische Behandling des Rektumkarzinoms*. Leipzig: Borth.

Deddish MR & Stearns MW (1961) Anterior resection for carcinoma of the rectum and rectosigmoid area. *Ann Surg* **154**: 961–966.

DeHaas-Kock DFM, Baeten CGM, Jager JJ et al (1996) Prognostic significance of radial margins of clearance in rectal cancer. *Br J Surg* **83**: 781–785.

Devine H (1937) Excision of the rectum. *Br J Surg* **25**: 351.

Devlin HB, Plant JA & Griffen M (1971) Aftermath of surgery for anorectal cancer. *BMJ* **ii**: 413.

Dixon AR, Maxwell WA, Holmes JT & Thornton R (1991) Carcinoma of the rectum: a 10-year experience. *Br J Surg* **78**: 308–311.

Dixon CF (1939) Surgical removal of lesions occurring in sigmoid and rectosigmoid. *Am J Surg* **46**: 12–17.

Dixon CF (1940) Resection without permananent colostomy for carcinoma of the rectosigmoid and lower portion of the pelvic colon. In Pack GI & Livingstone EM (eds) *Treatment of Cancer and Allied Diseases*, Vol 2, p 1414. New York: PB Hoeber.

Drake DB, Pemberton JH, Beart RW Jr, Dozois RR & Wolff BG (1987) Coloanal anastomosis in the management of benign and malignant rectal disease. *Ann Surg* **206**: 600–605.

Druss RG, O'Connor JF & Stern LQ (1969) Psychological response to colectomy. II: Adjustment to a permanent colostomy. *Arch Gen Psychiat* **20**: 419–426.

Duch G, Axelsson CK & Ostergaard AH (1980) Kolorecktale anastomoser med autosuturapparat. *Ugeskr Laeger* **142**: 1914–1916.

Dudley HAF, Radcliffe AG & McGeechan D (1980) Intraoperative irrigation of the colon to permit primary anastomosis. *Br J Surg* **67**: 80–81.

Dukes CE (1930) The spread of cancer of the rectum (subsection in a paper by Gordon Watson C & Dukes CE). *Br J Surg* **17**: 643–648.

Dukes CE (1943) The surgical pathology of rectal cancer. *Proc R Soc Med* **37**: 131.

Dukes CE (1957) Discussion on major surgery in carcinoma of the rectum with or without colostomy, excluding the anal canal and including the rectosigmoid. *Proc R Soc Med* **50**: 1031.

Durdey P & Williams NS (1984) The effect of malignant and inflammatory fixation of rectal carcinoma on prognosis after rectal excision. *Br J Surg* **71**: 787–790.

Ego-Aguirre E, Spratt JS, Butcher HR & Bricker EM (1964) Repair of perineal hernias developing subsequent to pelvic exenteration. *Ann Surg* **159**: 66.

Eickenberg HU, Amin M, Klompus W & Lick R Jr (1976) Urologic complications following abdominoperineal excision of the rectum. *J Urol* **115**: 180–182.

Eisenberg H, Sullivan PD & Foote FM (1967) Trends in survival of digestive system cancer patients in Connecticut 1935–62. *Gastroenterology* **53**: 528.

Eisenstat TE, Deak ST, Rugin RJ et al (1982) Five year survival in patients with carcinoma of the rectum treated by electrocoagulation. *Am J Surg* **143**: 127.

Eldar S, Kemeny M & Terz JJ (1985) Extended resections for carcinoma of the colon and rectum. *Surg Gynecol Obstet* **161**: 319–322.

Enker WE (1978) Surgical treatment of large bowel cancer. In Enker WE (ed) *Carcinoma of the Colon and Rectum*, pp 73–106. Chicago: YearBook Medical.

Enker WE (1992) Potency, cure and local control in the operative treatment of rectal cancer (review). *Arch Surg* **127**: 1396–1401.

Enker WE, Laffer UT & Block GE (1979) Enhanced survival of patients with colon and rectal cancer is based upon wide anatomic resection. *Ann Surg* **190**: 350–358.

Enker WE, Stearns MW & Janov AJ (1985) Peranal coloanal anastomosis following low anterior resection for rectal carcinoma. *Dis Colon Rectum* **28**: 576–581.

Enker WE, Thaler HT, Cranor ML & Polyak T (1995). Total mesorectal excision in the operative treatment of carcinoma of the rectum. *J Am Coll Surg* **18**: 335–346

Everett WG (1975) A comparison of one layer and two layer techniques for colorectal anastomosis. *Br J Surg* **62**: 135–140.

Everett WG, Friend PJ & Forty J (1986) Comparison of stapling and hand-suture for left-sided large bowel anastomosis. *Br J Surg* **73**: 345–348.

Faget JL (1739) Quoted in Rankin FW, Barwen JA & Buie LA (1932) *The Colon, Rectum and Anus*, p 768. Philadelphia: WB Saunders.

Fain SN, Patin S & Morgenstern L (1975) Use of mechanical suturing apparatus in low colorectal anastomosis. *Arch Surg* **110**: 1079–1082.

Farley D & Smith I (1968) Phantom rectum after complete rectal excision. *Br J Surg* **55**: 40.

Fasth J & Hulten L (1984) Loop ileostomy: a superior diverting stoma in colorectal surgery. *World J Surg* **8**: 401–407.

Fazio VW (1978) Sump suction and irrigation of the presacral space. *Dis Colon Rectum* **21**: 401.

Feinberg SM, Parker F, Cohen Z et al (1986) The double stapling technique for low anterior resection of rectal carcinoma. *Dis Colon Rectum* **29**: 885–890.

Fick TE, Baeten CG, von Meyenfeldt MF & Obertop H (1990) Recurrence and survival after abdominoperineal and low anterior resection for rectal cancer without adjunctive therapy. *Eur J Surg Oncol* **16**: 105–108.

Fielding LP, Stewart Brown S, Hittinger R & Blesovsky L (1984) Covering stoma for elective anterior resection of the rectum: an outmoded operation. *Am J Surg* **147**: 524–530.

Fingerhut A, Elhadad A, Hay JM et al (1994) Infraperitoneal colorectal anastomosis: hand-sewn versus circular staples. A controlled clinical trial. *Surgery* **116**: 484–490

Finsterer H (1941) Zur chirgischen Behandlung des Rektumkarcinomas. *Arch Klin Chir* **202**: 15.

Fitzgibbons RJ, Harkrider WW & Cohn I (1977) Review of abdominoperineal resections for cancer. *Am J Surg* **134**: 624–629.

Fleisher DE (1982) The current status of gastrointestinal laser activity in the United States. *Gastointest Endosc* **281**: 157–161.

Fortunato L, Ahmad NR, Yeung RS et al (1995) Long-term follow-up of local incision and radiation therapy for invasive rectal cancer. *Dis Colon Rectum* **38**: 1193–1199.

Fowler JW, Bremner DN & Moffatt LEF (1978) The incidence and consequences of damage to the parasympathetic nerve supply to the bladder after abdominoperineal excision of the rectum for carcinoma. *Br J Urol* **50**: 95–98.

Gabriel WB (1932) The end results of perineal excision and of radium in the treatment of cancer of the rectum. *Br J Surg* **20**: 234–248.

Gabriel WB (1934) Perineo-abdominal excision of the rectum in one stage. *Lancet* **ii**: 69.

Gabriel WB (1948) *Principles and Practice of Rectal Surgery*, 4th edn. London: HK Lewis.

Gabriel WB (1957) Discussion on major surgery in carcinoma of the rectum with or without colostomy, excluding the anal canal and including the rectosigmoid. *Proc R Soc Med* **50**: 1041.

Gabriel WB, Dukes CE & Bussey HJR (1935) Lymphatic spread in cancer of the rectum. *Br J Surg* **23**: 395–413.

Gall FP & Hermanek P (1988) [Expanded lymph node dissection in stomach and colorectal cancer – uses and risks]. [in German]. *Chirurg* **59**: 202–210.

Gerstenberg TC, Nielson ML, Clausen S, Blaaber J & Lindberg J (1980) Bladder function after abdominoperineal excision of the rectum for anorectal carcinoma. *Ann Surg* **191**: 81–86.

Gilbertsen VA (1960) Adenocarcinoma of the rectum: a fifteen-year study with evaluation of the results of curative therapy. *Arch Surg (Chicago)* **80**: 135.

Gilbertsen VA (1962) The results of the surgical treatment of cancer of the rectum. *Surg Gynecol Obstet* **114**: 313–318.

Gilchrist RK & David VC (1938) Lymphatic spread or carcinoma of the rectum. *Ann Surg* **108**: 621–642.

Gilchrist RK & David VC (1940) Fundamental factors governing lateral spread of cancer of the rectum. *Ann Surg* **111**: 630.

Gilchrist RK & David VC (1947) A consideration of pathological factors influencing five-year survival in radical resection of the large bowel and rectum for carcinoma. *Ann Surg* **126**: 421.

Glass RE, Ritchie JL, Thompson HR & Mann CV (1985) The results of surgical treatment of cancer of the rectum by radical resection and extended abdomino-iliac lymphadenectomy. *Br J Surg* **72**: 599–601.

Glass RE, Fazio VW, Jagelman DG, Lavery IC, Weakley FL & Forsythe SR (1986) The results of surgical treatment of cancer of the colon at the Cleveland Clinic from 1965 to 1975: classification of the spread of colon cancer and long-term survival. *Int J Colorect Dis* **1**: 33–39.

Glover RP & Waugh JM (1946) Retrograde lymphatic spread of carcinoma of the 'rectosigmoid region': its influence on surgical procedures. *Surg Gynecol Obstet* **82**: 434–448.

Goetze O (1944) Die abdominosakrale Resektion des Mastdarms mit Wiederherstelling der naturlichen Kontinenz. *Arch Klin Chir* **206**: 293.

Goldberg SM (1980) Personal communication, cited in Goligher JC (1984) *Surgery of the Anus, Rectum and Colon*. London: Baillière Tindall.

Goligher JC (1977) Current trends in the medical management of carcinoma of the rectum. In Taylor S (ed) *Recent Advances in Surgery*, Vol 9, pp 1–32. Edinburgh: Churchill Livingstone.

Goligher JC (1984) *Surgery of the Anus, Rectum and Colon*. London: Baillière Tindall.

Goligher JC, Dukes CE & Bussey HJR (1951) Local recurrences after sphincter-saving excisions for carcinoma of the rectum and rectosigmoid. *Br J Surg* **39**: 199–211.

Goligher JC, Simpkins KC & Lintott DJ (1977) A controlled comparison of one and two layer technique of suture for high and low colorectal anastomoses. *Br J Surg* **64**: 609.

Goligher JC, Lee PWR, Macfie J & Lintott DJ (1979) Experience with the Russian model 249 suture gun for anastomosis of the rectum. *Surg Gynecol Obstet* **148**: 517–524.

Goodwin WE, Harris AP, Kaufman JJ & Beal JM (1953) Open transcolonic uretero-intestinal anastomosis. *Surg Gynecol Obstet* **97**: 295.

Gordon Watson C & Dukes C (1930) The treatment of carcinoma of the rectum with radium with an introduction on the spread of cancer of the rectum. *Br J Surg* **17**: 643–699.

Grabham JA, Moran BJ & Lane RHS (1995) Defunctioning colostomy for low anterior resection: a selective approach. *Br J Surg* **82**: 1331–1332.

Graffner H, Fredlund P, Olsen S et al (1983) Protective colostomy in low anterior resection of the rectum using the EEA stapling instrument: a randomized study. *Dis Colon Rectum* **26**: 87–90.

Graham JW & Goligher JC (1954) The management of accidental injuries and deliberate resections of the ureter during excision of the rectum. *Br J Surg* **42**: 151–160.

Grier W, Robson V, Postel AH et al (1964) An evaluation of colonic stoma management without irrigation. *Surg Gynecol Obstet* **118**: 1234–1242.

Griffen FD, Knight CD Sr & Knight CD Jr (1992) Results of the double stapling procedure in pelvic surgery. *World J Surg* **16**: 866–871.

Grigg ML, McDermott FT, Pihl EA et al (1984) Curative local excision in the treatment of carcinoma of the rectum. *Dis Colon Rectum* **27**: 81–83.

Grinnell RS (1953) Results in the treatment of carcinoma of the colon and rectum. *Surg Gynecol Obstet* **96**: 31.

Grinnell RS (1954) Distal intramural spread of carcinoma of the rectum and rectosigmoid. *Surg Gynecol Obstet* **99**: 421–429.

Grinnell RS (1965) Results of ligation of the inferior mesenteric artery at the aorta in resection of carcinoma of the descending and sigmoid colon and rectum. *Surg Gynecol Obstet* **120**: 1031.

Gross E & Amir-Kabirian H (1994) Coloanal pouch after total rectum resection (review in German). *Zentralbl Chir* **119**: 878–885.

Hafner GH, Herrrera L & Petrelli NJ (1991) Patterns of recurrence after pelvic exenteration for colorectal adenocarcinoma. *Arch Surg* **126**: 1510–1513.

Hager T, Gall FP & Hemanek P (1983) Local excision of cancer of the rectum. *Dis Colon Rectum* **26**: 149–151.

Hallan RI, Marzouk DE, Waldron DJ, Womack NR & Williams NS (1989) Comparison of digital and manometric assessment of anal sphincter function. *Br J Surg* **76**: 973–975.

Hallan RI, Williams NS & Hulten MRE (1990) Electrically stimulated sartorius neosphincter: canine model of activation and skeletal muscle transformation. *Br J Surg* **77**: 208–213.

Hallbook O, Pahlman L, Krog M et al (1996) Randomized comparison of straight and colonic J pouch anastomosis after low anterior resection. *Ann Surg* **224**: 58–65.

Handley WS (1910) The surgery of the lymphatic system. *BMJ* **i**: 922–928.

Hautefeuille P, Valleur P. Perniceni T et al (1988) Functional and oncological results after coloanal anastomosis for low rectal cancer. *Ann Surg* **207**: 61–64.

Havenga K, De-Ruiter MC, Enker WE & Welvaart K (1996a) Anatomical basis of autonomic nerve-preserving total mesorectal excision for rectal cancer. *Br J Surg* **83**: 384–388.

Havenga K, Enker WE, McDermott K, Cohen AM, Minsky BD, Guillem J (1996b) Male and female sexual and urinary function after total mesorectal excision with autonomic nerve preservation for carcinoma of the rectum. *J Am Coll Surg* **182**: 495–502.

Hawley PR & Ritchie JK (1980) Indications, technique and results of transanal tumour excision in cases of lower rectal carcinoma. In Reifferscheid H & Langer S (eds) *Der Mastdarmkrebs*. Stuttgart: Thieme.

Heald RJ (1980) Towards fewer colostomies: the impact of circular stapling devices on the surgery of rectal cancer in a district hospital. *Br J Surg* **60**: 198–200.

Heald RJ (1988) The 'holy plane' of rectal surgery. *J R Soc Med* **81**: 503–508.

Heald RJ & Karanjia ND (1992) Results of radical surgery for rectal cancer (review). *World J Surg* **16**: 848–857.

Heald RJ & Leicester RJ (1981) The low stapled anastomosis. *Br J Surg* **68**: 333–337.

Heald RJ & Ryall RDH (1986) Recurrence and survival after total mesorectal excision for rectal cancer. *Lancet* **i**: 1479–1482.

Heald RJ, Husband EM & Ryall RDH (1982) The mesorectum in rectal cancer surgery: the clue to pelvic recurrence. *Br J Surg* **69**: 613–616.

Hermanek P & Gall FP (1985) Early colorectal carcinoma. *Br J Surg* **72** (Suppl): S134.

Hermanek P, Altendorf A & Gunselman W (1980) Pathomorphologische Aspekte zu kontinen zerhaltenden Therapievarfahren bei Mastdarmkrebs. In Reifferscheid H & Langer S (eds) *Der Mastdarmkrebs*. Stuttgart: Thieme.

Hermanek P, Wiebelt H, Staimmer D et al (1995) Prognostic factors of rectal carcinoma: experience of the German multicentre study. *SGCRC Tumori* **81** (Suppl): 60–64

Ho Y-H, Tan M & Seow-Choen F (1996) Prospective randomized controlled study of clinical function and anorectal physiology after low anterior resection: comparison of straight and colonic J pouch anastomoses. *Br J Surg* **83**: 978–980.

Hochenegg J (1888) Die sakrale Method der Exstirpation van Mastdarmkrebsen bach Prof Kraske. *Wien Klin Wschr* **1**: 272–354.

Hochenegg J (1889) Beitrage zur Chirurgie des Rektums under der Beckenorgone. *Wien Klin Wschr* **2**: 578.

Hochenegg J (1900) Mein Operation ser folge bei rektum Karcinom. *Wien Klin Wschr* **13**: 399.

Hojo K (1989) Extended wide lymphadenectomy and preservatiuon of pelvic autonomic nerves in rectal cancer surgery. *G Chir* **10**: 149–153 (editorial).

Hojo K & Koyama Y (1982) The effectiveness of wide anatomical resection and radical lymphadenectomy for patients with rectal cancer. *Jap J Surg* **12**: 111.

Hojo K, Sawada T & Moriya Y (1989) An analysis of survival and voiding, sexual function after wide ileopelvic lymphadenectomy in patients with carcinoma of the rectum, compared with conventional lymphadenectomy. *Dis Colon Rectum* **32**: 128–133.

Hojo K, Vernava AM III, Sugihara K et al (1991) Preservation of urine voiding and sexual function after rectal cancer surgery. *Dis Colon Rectum* **34**: 532–539.

Horgan PG, O'Connell PR, Shinkwin CA & Kirwan WO (1989) Effect of anterior resection on anal sphincter function. *Br J Surg* **76**: 783–786.

Hughes SF & Williams NS (1995) Continent colonic conduit for the treatment of faecal incontinence associated with disordered evacuation. *Br J Surg* **82**: 1318–1320

Hughes EP, Veidenheimer MC, Corman ML & Coller JA (1982) Electrocoagulation of rectal cancer. *Dis Colon Rectum* **25**: 215–218.

Hurst PA, Prout WG, Kelly JM, Bannister JJ & Walker RT (1982) Local recurrence after low anterior resection using the staple gun. *Br J Surg* **69**: 275–276.

Irvin TT & Goligher JC (1975) A controlled trial of three methods of managing the perineal wound after abdominoperineal excision of the rectum. *Br J Surg* **62**: 287.

James RD, Johnson RJ, Eddlestone B, Zheng GL & Jones JM (1983) Prognostic factors in locally recurrent rectal carcinoma treated by radiotherapy. *Br J Surg* **70**: 469–472.

Jass JR (1986) Lymphocytic infiltration and survival in rectal cancer. *J Clin Pathol* **39**: 585–589.

Jehle EC, Starlinger MJ, Kreis ME et al (1992) Alterations of anal sphincter function following transanal endoscopic microsurgery (TEM) for rectal tumours. *Gastroenterology* **102**: 365–370.

Jehle EC, Haehnel T, Starlinger MJ & Becker HD (1995) Level of the anastomosis does not influence functional outcome after anterior rectal resection for rectal cancer. *Am J Surg* **169**: 147–152; discussion 152–153.

Jones PF & Thomson HJ (1982) Long term results of a consistent policy of sphincter preservation in the treatment of carcinoma of the rectum. *Br J Surg* **69**: 564–568.

Karanjia ND, Corder AP, Holdsworth PJ & Heald RJ (1991) Risk of peritonitis and fatal septicaemia and the need to defunction the low anastomosis. *Br J Surg* **78**: 196–198.

Karanjia ND, Corder AP, Bearn P & Heald RJ (1994) Leakage from stapled low anastomosis after total mesorectal excision for carcinoma of the rectum. *Br J Surg* **8**: 1224–1226.

Keane PF, Ohri SK, Wood CB & Sackier JM (1988) Management of the obstucted left colon by the one stage intracolonic bypass procedure. *Dis Colon Rectum* **31**: 948–951.

Keighley MRB & Matheson D (1980) Functional results of rectal excision and endoanal anastomoses. *Br J Surg* **67**: 757–761.

Keighley MRB & Williams NS (1993) *Surgery of the Anus, Rectum and Colon*. London: WB Saunders.

Kelly KA (1977) Personal communication, cited by Goligher JC (1984) *Surgery of the Anus, Rectum and Colon*. London: Baillière Tindall.

Kennedy HL, Langevin JM, Goldberg SM et al (1985) Recurrence following stapled coloproctostomy for carcinomas of the mid portion of the rectum. *Surg Gynecol Obstet* **160**: 513–516.

Killingback MJ (1985) Indications for local excision of rectal cancer. *Br J Surg* **72** (Suppl): S54–S56.

Kirkegaard P, Christiansen J & Hjartrup A (1980) Anterior resection for mid rectal cancer with the EEA stapling instrument. *Am J Surg* **140**: 312–314.

Kirkegaard P, Hjortrup A & Sanders S (1981) Bladder dysfunction after low anterior resection of mid rectal cancer. *Am J Surg* **141**: 266–268.

Kirschner M (1934) Das synchrone kombinierte Verfahren bei der Radikalbehandlung des Mastdarmkrebes. *Arch Klin Chir* **180**: 296.

Kirwan WD (1981) Integrity of low colorectal EEA-stapled anastomosis. *Br J Surg* **68**: 539–540.

Knight CD & Griffen FD (1980) An improved technique for low sphincter resection of the rectum using the EEA stapler. *Surgery* **88**: 710.

Kocher T (1875) Quoted in Rankin FW, Bergen JA & Buie LA (eds) *The Colon, Rectum and Anus*. Philadelphia: WB Saunders.

Konn M, Morita T, Hada R et al (1993) Survival and recurrence after low anterior resection and abdominoperineal resection for rectal cancer: the results of a long-term study with a review of the literature. *Surg Today* **23**(1): 21–30.

Konturri M, Larmi TKI & Tuononen S (1974) Bladder dysfunction and its manifestations following abdominoperineal extirpation of the rectum. *Ann Surg* **179**: 179.

Koyama Y, Moriya Y & Hojo K (1982) Problems in the surgical treatment of rectal cancer. *Jpn J Cancer Clin* **28**: 632.

Kraske P (1885) Zur Exstirpation hochsitzender Mastdarmkrebse. *Verhdt Chir* **14**: 464.

Laitinen S, Huttunen R, Stahlberg M et al (1980) Experience with the EEA stapling instrument for colorectal anastomoses. *Ann Chir Gynaecol* **69**: 102–105.

Lane RHS & Parks AG (1977) Function of the anal sphincters following coloanal anastomosis. *Br J Surg* **64**: 596–599.

Lasson ALL, Ekelund GR & Lindstrom CG (1984) Recurrence risks after stapled anastomosis for rectal carcinoma. *Acta Chir Scand* **150**: 85–89.

Laxamana A, Solomon MJ, Cohen Z et al (1995) Long-term results of anterior resection using the double-stapling technique. *Dis Colon Rectum* **38**: 1246–1250.

Lazorthes F & Chiotasso P (1986) Stapled colorectal anastomoses: peroperative integrity of the anastomosis and rate of post operative leakage. *Int J Colorect Dis* **1**: 96–98.

Lazorthes F, Fages P, Chiotasso P, Lemozy J & Bloom E (1986) Resection of the rectum with construction of a colonic reservoir and coloanal anastomosis for carcinoma of the rectum. *Br J Surg* **73**: 136–138.

Lazorthes F, Chiotasso P, Gamagami RA, Istvan G & Chevreau P (1997) Late clinical outcome in a randomized prospective comparison of colonic J pouch and straight colorectal anastomosis. *Br J Surg* **84**: 1449–1451.

Leadbetter WF (1951) Consideration of problems incident to performance of ureteroenterostomy: report of a technique. *J Urol* **65**: 818.

Ledesma EJ, Bruno S & Mittelman A (1981) Total pelvic exenteration in colorectal disease: a 20-year experience. *Ann Surg* **194**: 701–703.

Leff EI, Shaver JO, Hoexte R et al (1985) Anastomotic recurrences after low anterior resection: stapled or hand sewn. *Dis Colon Rectum* **28**: 164–167.

Leo E, Belli F, Baldini MT et al (1993) Total rectal resection, colo-endoanal anastomosis and colic reservoir for cancer of the lower third of the rectum. *Eur J Surg Oncol* **19**: 283–293.

Leo E, Belli F, Baldini MT et al (1994) Total rectal resection and coloanal anastomosis with colonic reservoir for low rectal cancer. *J Colorect Dis* **9**: 82–86.

Lepreau FJ (1978) Low anterior resection of the colon and anastomosis with staples. *Arch Surg* **113**: 1479.

Liguori G, Roseano M, Balani A & Turoldo A (1992) Low anterior resection in the curative surgical treatment of rectal cancer. *Ann Ital Chir* **63**: 271–277.

Ling L, Broom A & Ryden S (1979) Low anterior resection using stapling instrument. *Acta Chir Scand* **145**: 487–489.

Lisfranc J (1826) Observation sur une affection cancereuse du rectume guérie par l'excision. *Rev Med Franc Etrang* **2**: 380.

Liu SY, Wang YN, Zhu WQ, Gu WL & Fu H (1994) Total pelvic exenteration for locally advanced rectal carcinoma. *Dis Colon Rectum* **37**: 172–174.

Lloyd Davies OV (1939) Lithotomy–Trendelenberg position for resection of rectum and lower pelvic colon. *Lancet* **ii**: 74.

Localio SA & Baron B (1973) Abdominotrans-sacral resection and anastomosis for mid-rectal cancer. *Ann Surg* **178**: 540–546.

Localio SA & Eng K (1975) Malignant tumours of the rectum. *Curr Prob Surg* **12**: 1–48.

Localio SA & Eng K (1985) Abdominosacral resection. In Schwartz SI & Ellis H (eds) *Maingot's Abdominal Operations*, 8th edn, Vol 2. Norwalk, CN: Appleton–Century–Crofts.

Localio SA & Stahl WM (1969) Simultaneous abdominotrans-sacral resection and anastomosis for mid rectal cancer. *Am J Surg* **117**: 282.

Localio SA, Eng K, Gouge TH & Ransome JHC (1978) Abdominosacral resection for carcinoma of the mid-rectum: 10 years' experience. *Ann Surg* **188**: 745–780.

Localio SA, Eng K & Coppa GF (1983) Abdomino-sacral resection for mid rectal cancer. *Ann Surg* **198**: 320–324.

Lock MR, Cairns DW, Ritchie JK et al (1978) The treatment of early colorectal cancer by local excision. *Br J Surg* **65**: 346–349.

Lockhart-Mummery HE, Ritchie JK & Hawley PR (1976) The results of surgical treatment for carcinoma of the rectum at St Mark's Hospital from 1948 to 1972. *Br J Surg* **63**: 673–677.

Lockhart-Mummery JP (1926) Two hundred cases of cancer of the rectum treated by perineal excision. *Br J Surg* **14**: 110–124.

Lockhart-Mummery JP (1934) *Diseases of the Rectum and Colon*, 2nd edn. London: Baillière.

Lothian and Borders (consultant surgeons and pathologists of the Lothian and Borders health boards) (1995) Lothian and Borders large bowel cancer project: immediate outcome after surgery. *Br J Surg* **82**: 888–890.

Luke M, Kirkegaard P, Lendorf A & Christiansen J (1983) Pelvic recurrence rate after abdominoperineal resection and low anterior resection for rectal cancer before and after introduction of the stapling technique. *World J Surg* **7**: 616–619.

MacFarlane JK, Ryall RD & Heald RJ (1993) Mesorectal excision for rectal cancer. *Lancet* **341**: 457–460.

Macfie J & McMahon MJ (1980) The management of the open perineal wound using a foam elastomer dressing: a prospective clinical trial. *Br J Surg* **67**: 85.

Madden JL & Kandalaft S (1967) Electrocoagulation: a primary and preferred method of treatment for cancer of the rectum. *Ann Surg* **166**: 413.

Madden JL & Kandalaft S (1971) Clinical evaluation of electrocoagulation in the treatment of cancer of the rectum. *Am J Surg* **122**: 347.

Magovern CJ, Park SB, Magovern CJ et al (1986) Latissimus dorsi as a functioning synchronously paced muscle component in the region of a left ventricular aneurysm. *Ann Thorac Surg* **41**: 116.

Maingot R (1969) *Abdominal Operations*. Norwalk, CN: Appleton–Century–Crofts.

Mander BJ, Abercrombie JF, George BD & Williams NS (1996). The electrically stimulated gracilis neosphincter incorporated as part of total anorectal reconstruction following abdominoperineal excision of the rectum. *Ann Surg* **224**: 702–709

Mandl F (1922) Uber den Mastdarmkrebs. *Dtsch Z Chirurg* **168**: 145.

Mandl F (1929) Uber 1000 sakrale Mastdarmkrebsexstirpationen (aus dem Hocheneggschen Material). *Dtsch Z Chirurg* **219**: 3.

Mann CV (1972) Results of 'pull-through' operations for carcinoma of the rectum. *Proc R Soc Med* **65**: 976.

Mannion JD, Bitto T, Hammond RL, Rubinstein A & Stephenson LW (1986) Histochemical and fatigue characteristics of conditioned canine latissimus dorsi muscle. *Circulat Res* **58**: 298–304.

Manson PN, Carmen ML, Collar JA & Veidenheimer MC (1976) Anterior resection for adenocarcinoma: Lahey Clinic experience from 1963 through 1969. *Am J Surg* **131**: 434–441.

Mason AY (1976) Selective surgery for carcinoma of the rectum. *Aust NZ J Surg* **46**: 322.

Mason AY (1977) In Matt R & Robinson F (eds) *Surgical Techniques Illustrated*, Vol 2, p 71. Boston: Little, Brown.

Maunsell HW (1892) A new method of excising the two upper portions of the rectum and the lower segment of the sigmoid flexure of the colon. *Lancet* **ii**: 473–476.

Mayo CW & Fly OA (1956) Analysis of five year survival in carcinoma of the rectum and rectosigmoid. *Surg Gynecol Obstet* **103**: 94.

Mayo CW, Laberge MY & Hardy WM (1958) Five year survival after anterior resection for carcinoma of the rectum and rectosigmoid. *Surg Gynecol Obstet* **106**: 695–698.

McArdle CS & Hole D (1991) Impact of variability among surgeons on postoperative morbidity and mortality and ultimate survival. *BMJ* **302**: 1501–1505

McArdle CS, Hole D, Hansell D, Blumgarth LH & Wood CB (1990) Prospective study of colorectal cancer in the West of Scotland: 10-year follow-up. *Br J Surg* **77**: 280–282.

McCall JL, Cox MR & Wattchow DA (1995) Analysis of local recurrence rates after surgery for rectal cancer. *Int J Colorect Dis* **10**: 126–132.

McDermott FT, Hughes ESR, Pihl E, Milne BJ & Price A (1981) Comparative results of surgical management of single carcinomas of the colon and rectum: a series of 1939 patients managed by one surgeon. *Br J Surg* **68**: 850–855.

McDermott FT, Hughes ESR, Pihl E, Milne BJ & Price A (1982) Long term results of restorative resection and total excision for carcinoma of the middle third of the rectum. *Surg Gynecol Obstet* **154**: 833–837.

McDonald PJ & Heald RJ (1983) A survey of postoperative function after rectal anastomosis with circular stapling devices. *Br J Surg* **70**: 727–729.

McGinn FP, Gartell PC, Clifford PC & Brunton FJ (1985) Staples or sutures for low colorectal anastomoses: a prospective randomised trial. *Br J Surg* **72**: 603–605.

Mealy K, Burke P & Hyland J (1992) Anterior resection without a defunctioning colostomy: questions of safety. *Br J Surg* **79**: 305–307.

Mentges B, Buess G, Raestrup H, Manncke F & Becker HD (1994) TEM results of the Tubingen Group. *Endosc Surg Allied Technol* **2**: 247–250.

Miles WE (1908) A method of performing abdomino-perineal excision for carcinoma of the rectum and of the terminal portion of the pelvic colon. *Lancet* **ii**: 1812–1813.

Miles WE (1910) The radical abdomino-perineal operation for cancer of the rectum and of the pelvic colon. *BMJ* **ii**: 941–942.

Miles WE (1926) *Cancer of the Rectum*. London: Harrison.

Milnes-Walker R (1971) *Annual Report of South Western Regional Cancer Bureau*. Bristol: South Western Regional Board.

Mittal VK & Cortez JA (1980) New techniques of gastrointestinal anastomoses using the EEA stapler. *Surgery* **88**: 715–718.

Moran BJ (1996) Stapling instruments for intestinal anastomosis in colorectal surgery. *Br J Surg* **83**: 902–909

Moran BJ, Docherty A & Finnis D (1994) Novel stapling technique to facilitate low anterior resection for rectal cancer. *Br J Surg* **81**: 1230.

Morgan LN (1955) Trends in the treatment of tumours of the rectum, rectosigmoid and left colon. *J R Coll Surg Edinb* **1**: 112–125.

Moritz E, Achleitner D, Holbling N et al (1991) Single versus double stapling technique in colorectal surgery: a prospective randomized trial. *Dis Colon Rectum* **34**: 495–497.

Moriya Y, Hojo K, Sawada T & Koyama Y (1989) Significance of lateral lymph node dissection for advanced rectal carcinoma at or below the peritoneal reflection. *Dis Colon Rectum* **32**: 307–315.

Morrow L (1976) Psychological problems following ileostomy and colostomy. *Mt Sinai J Med* **43**: 368–370.

Morson BC (1966) Factors influencing the prognosis of early cancer of the rectum. *Proc R Soc Med* **59**: 607.

Morson BC, Vaughan EG & Bussey HJR (1963) Pelvic recurrence after excision of rectum for carcinoma. *BMJ* **ii**: 13.

Morson BC, Bussey HJR & Soomorian S (1977) Policy of local excision for early cancer of the colorectum. *Gut* **18**: 1045–1050.

Mortensen NJM, Ramirez JM, Takeuchi N & Humphreys MMS (1995) Colonic J pouch–anal anastomosis after rectal incision for carcinoma: functional outcome. *Br J Surg* **82**: 611–613.

Moynihan BGA (1908) The surgical treatment of cancer of the sigmoid flexure and rectum. *Surg Gynecol Obstet* **6**: 463.

Murnaghan GF, Gowland SP, Rose M, Millard RJ & Stening WA (1979) Experimental neurogenic disorders of the bladder after section of cauda equina. *Br J Urol* **67**: 411.

Neal DE, Hawkins, T, Gallaugher AS, Essenhigh DM & Hall RA (1985) The role of the ileal conduit in the development of upper tract dilatation. *Br J Urol* **57**: 520–524.

Neal DE, Williams NS & Johnston D (1981) A prospective study of bladder function before and after sphincter-saving resection for low carcinoma of the rectum. *Br J Urol* **53**: 558–564.

Nesbit RM (1948) Ureterosigmoid anastomosis by direct elliptical connection: preliminary report. *Univ Hosp Bull (Mich)* **14**: 45.

Neville R, Fielding LP & Amendola C (1987) Local tumour recurrence after curative resection of rectal cancer: a ten-hospital review. *Dis Colon Rectum* **30**: 12–17.

Nicholls RJ, Ritchie JK, Wadsworth J et al (1979) Total excision or restorative resection for carcinoma of the middle third of the rectum. *Br J Surg* **66**: 625–627.

Nicholls RJ, Mason AY & Morson BC (1982) Clinical staging of the extent of rectal carcinoma. *Br J Surg* **60**: 404.

Nicholls RJ, Lubowski DZ & Donaldson DR (1988) Comparison of colonic reservoir and straight coloanal reconstruction after rectal excision. *Br J Surg* **75**: 318–320.

Nogueras JJ, Whelan RL, Lowry AC et al (1991) The double staple technique for colorectal anastomosis. *Dis Colon Rectum* **34**: 18–22.

Nothiger F (1985) Technique and results of peranal excision of the rectal malignoma. *Helv Chir Acta* **52**: 325–327.

Oates GC (1985) Cited in Goligher JC (1985) Neoplasms: surgical treatment. *Curr Opin Gastroenterol* **1**: 43.

Orkin B (1992) Rectal carcinoma: treatment. In Wexner S (ed) *Fundamentals of Anorectal Surgery*. New York: McGraw-Hill.

Ortiz H & Armendariz P (1996) Anterior resection: do the patients perceive any clinical benefit. *Int J Colorect Dis* **11**: 191–195

Pannett CA (1935) Resection of the rectum with restoration of continuity. *Lancet* **ii**: 423.

Parc R, Tiret E, Frileux P, Moszkowski E & Loygue J (1986) Resection and coloanal anastomosis with colonic reservoir for rectal carcinoma. *Br J Surg* **73**: 139–141.

Parks AG (1972) Transanal technique in low rectal anastomoses. *Proc R Soc Med* **65**: 975–976.

Parks AG & Percy JP (1982) Resection and sutured coloanal anastomosis for rectal carcinoma. *Br J Surg* **69**: 301–304.

Patel SC, Tovee BE & Langer B (1977) Twenty-five years of experience with radical surgical treatment of carcinoma of the extraperitoneal rectum. *Surgery* **82**: 460–465.

Patel J, Shanahan D, Riches DJ et al (1991) The arterial anatomy and surgical relevance of the human gracilis muscle. *J Anat* **176**: 270–272.

Paty PB, Enker WE, Cohen AM & Lauwers GY (1994a) Treatment of rectal cancer by low anterior resection with coloanal anastomosis. *Ann Surg* **219**: 365–373.

Paty PB, Enker WE, Cohen AM, Minsky BD & Friedlander-Klar H (1994b) Long-term functional results of coloanal anastomosis for rectal cancer. *Am J Surg* **167**: 90–94; discussion 94–95.

Pélissier EP, Blum D, Bachour A & Bosset JF (1992) Functional results of coloanal anastomosis with reservoir. *Dis Colon Rectum* **35**: 843–846.

Petros JG & Lopez MJ (1994) Pelvic exenteration for carcinoma of the colon and rectum. *Surg Oncol Clin N Am* **3**: 257–266.

Pezim ME & Nicholls RJ (1984) Survival after high or low ligation of the inferior mesenteric artery during curative surgery for rectal cancer. *Ann Surg* **200**: 729–733.

Phillips RKS, Hittinger R, Blesovsky L, Fry JS & Fielding LP (1984a) Local recurrence following curative surgery for large bowel cancer. I: The overall picture. *Br J Surg* **71**: 12–16.

Phillips RKS, Hittinger R, Blesovsky L, Fry JS & Fielding LP (1984b) Local recurrence following curative surgery for large bowel cancer. II: The rectum and rectosigmoid. *Br J Surg* **71**: 17–20.

Pittam MR, Thornton H & Ellis H (1984) Survival after extended resection for locally advanced carcinomas of the colon and rectum. *Ann R Coll Surg* **66**: 81–84.

Pol B, Brandone JM, Le Treut YP et al (1989) [Excision of colorectal cancers: what can be expected of lymph node excision?] [in French]. *Ann Chir* **43**: 68–72.

Polglase AL, Hughes ESR, Masterton JP & Waxman BP (1979) The autosuture surgical stapling instruments: preliminary experience. *Aust NZ J Surg* **49**: 111–116.

Polglase AL, Hughes ESR, McDermott FT et al (1981) A comparison of end-to-end staple and suture colorectal anastomosis in the dog. *Surg Gynecol Obstet* **152**: 792.

Pollett WG & Nicholls RJ (1981) Does the extent of distal clearance affect survival after radical anterior resection for carcinoma of the rectum? *Gut* **2**: 872.

Pollett WG & Nicholls RJ (1983) The relationship between the extent of distal clearance and survival and local recurrence rates after curative anterior resection for carcinoma of rectum. *Ann Surg* **70**: 159–163.

Prudden JF (1971) Psychological problems following ileostomy and colostomy. *Cancer* **38**: 236–238.

Pryse-Phillips W (1971) Follow-up study of patients with colostomies. *Am J Surg* **122**: 27–32.

Pyrah LH & Raper FP (1955) Some uses of an isolated loop of ileum in genitourinary surgery. *Br J Surg* **42**: 337.

Quer EA, Dahlin DC & Mayo CW (1953) Retrograde intramural spread of carcinoma of the rectum and rectosigmoid: a microscopic study. *Surg Gynecol Obstet* **96**: 24–30.

Quirke P, Dixon MF, Durdey P & Williams NS (1986) Local recurrence of rectal adenocarcinoma due to inadequate surgical resection. *Lancet* **i**: 996–998.

Rankin FW, Barwen JA & Buie LA (1932) *The Colon, Rectum and Anus*. Philadelphia: WB Saunders.

Rankin JT (1969) Urological complications of rectal surgery. *Br J Urol* **41**: 655–659.

Rasmussen OV, Korner B, Moller-Sorenson P & Kronberg O (1977) Suprapubic versus urethral bladder drainage following surgery for rectal cancer. *Acta Chir Scand* **143**: 371–374.

Ravitch MM & Steichen FM (1979) A stapling instrument for end-to-end anastomoses in the gastrointestinal tract. *Ann Surg* **189**: 791–797.

Ravo B & Ger R (1985) Temporary colostomy: an outmoded procedure. *Dis Colon Rectum* **28**: 904–907.

Rayner HH (1935) Discussion on the conservative surgery of carcinoma of the rectum. *Proc R Soc Med* **28**: 1563–1565.

RCS/AC (Royal College of Surgeons of England, and Association of Coloproctology of Great Britain and Ireland) (1996) *Guidelines for the Management of Colorectal Cancer*, June.

Redmond HP, Austin OMB, Clery AP & Deasy JM (1993) Safety of double-stapled anastomosis in low anterior resection. *Br J Surg* **80**: 924–927.

Reid JD, Robins RE & Atkinson KG (1984) Pelvic recurrence after anterior resection and EEA stapling anastomosis for potentially curable carcinoma of the rectum. *Am J Surg* **147**: 629–632.

Rosen CB, Beart RW & Ilstrup DM (1985) Local recurrence of rectal carcinoma after hand sewn and stapled anastomoses. *Dis Colon Rectum* **28**: 305–309.

Rosenberg IL, Russell CW & Giles GR (1978) Cell viability studies on the exfoliated colonic cancer cell. *Br J Surg* **65**: 188.

Rosi PA, Cahill WJ & Carey J (1962) Ten-year study of hemicolectomy in the treatment of carcinoma of the left half of the colon. *Surg Gynecol Obstet* **114**: 15–20.

Rothenberger DA & Finne CO (1990) Radical surgery for early rectal cancer: the case against it. In Simmons R & Udekwu A (eds) *Debates in Clinical Surgery*. Chicago: YearBook Medical.

Ruckley CV, Smith AV & Balfour TW (1970) Perineal closure by omental graft. *Surg Gynecol Obstet* **131**: 300.

Sakkas JL, Mandrekas A, Androulakis J et al (1974) Urologic complications in malignant disease of the rectosigmoid colon. *South Med J*, 287–291.

Salm R, Lampe H, Bustos A & Matern U (1994) Experience with TEM in Germany. *Endosc Surg Allied Technol* **2**: 251–254.

Salvati EP & Rubin RJ (1976) Electrocoagulation as primary therapy for rectal carcinoma. *Am J Surg* **132**: 583.

Sankey NE & Heller E (1967) The urologic complications of abdomino-perineal resection. *J Urol* **97**: 367–370.

Sarker SK, Chaudry R & Sinha VK (1994) A comparison of stapled versus handsewn anastomosis in anterior resection for carcinoma of the rectum. *Indian J Cancer* **31**: 133–137.

Sauer I & Bacon HE (1952) A new approach for excision of carcinomas of the lower portion of the rectum and anal canal. *Surg Gynecol Obstet* **95**: 229.

Scholefield JH & Northover JM (1995) Surgical management of rectal cancer. *Br J Surg* **82**: 745–748.

Scholzell E & Langer S (1981) Die Kryotherapie das Mastolarmkrebses. *Helv Chir Acta* **48**: 867.

Scott N, Jackson P, al-Jaberi T et al (1995) Total mesorectal excision and local recurrence: a study of tumour spread in the mesorectum distal to rectal cancer. *Br J Surg* **82**: 1031–1033.

Sebrechts J (1935) quoted by Rayner HH (1935) Discussions on the conservative surgery of carcinoma of the rectum. *Proc R Soc Med* **28**: 1563–1565.

Seow-Choen F (1993) Colonic pouch after low anterior resection of the distal third of the rectum. *Ann Acad Med (Sing)* **22**: 229–232

Seow-Choen F (1996) Colonic pouches in the treatment of low rectal cancer (leading article). *Br J Surg* **83**: 881–882.

Seow-Choen F & Goh HS (1995) Prospective randomized trial comparing J colonic pouch–anal anastomosis and straight coloanal reconstruction. *Br J Surg* **82**: 608–610.

Shahinian TK, Bowen JR, Dorman BA et al (1980) Experience with the EEA stapling device. *Am J Surg* **139**: 549–553.

Shahinian TK, Bowen JR, Dorman BA et al (1981) Experience with the EEA stapler for colorectal anastomosis. *Am J Surg* **140**: 325.

Shirouzu K, Isomoto H & Kakegawa T (1996) Total pelvic exenteration for locally advanced colorectal carcinoma. *Br J Surg* **83**: 32–35.

Simonsen OS, Stolf NAG, Aun F, Raia A & Habr-Gama A (1976) Rectal sphincter reconstruction in perineal colostomies after abdominoperineal resection for cancer. *Br J Surg* **63**: 389–391.

Slanetz CA, Herter FP & Grinnell RS (1972) Anterior resection versus abdominoperineal resection for cancer of the rectum and rectosigmoid. *Am J Surg* **123**: 110–115.

Slaney G (1971) Results of treatment of carcinoma of the colon and rectum. In Irvine WT (ed) *Modern Trends in Surgery*, 3rd edn. London: Butterworth.

Slaney G et al (eds) (1991) *Cancer of the Large Bowel*. Basingstoke: Macmillan.

Smith LE (1981) Anastomosis with EEA stapler after anterior colonic resection. *Dis Colon Rectum* **29**: 236–242.

Stearns MW Jr (1978) Benign and malignant neoplasms of the colon and rectum: diagnosis and management. *Surg Clin N Am* **58**: 605–618.

Stearns MW & Binkley GE (1953) The influence of location on prognosis in operable rectal cancer. *Surg Gynecol Obstet* **96**: 368.

Stearns MW Jr, Sternberg SS & De Cosse JJ (1981) Local treatment of rectal cancer. In De Cosse JJ (ed) *Large Bowel Cancer*. Edinburgh: Churchill Livingstone.

Stearns MW, Sternberg SS & De Cosse JJ (1984) Treatment alternatives: localised rectal cancer. *Cancer* **54**: 2691–2694.

Steele RJ, Hershman MJ, Mortensen NJ, Armitage NC & Scholefield JH (1996). Transanal endoscopic microsurgery: initial experience from three centres in the United Kingdom. *Br J Surg* **83**: 207–210

Steup WH (1994) *Colorectal Cancer Surgery with Emphasis on Lymphadenectomy*. MD thesis, the Hague, Netherlands.

Stipa S, Lucandri G, Stipa F, Chiavellati L & Sapienza P (1995) Local excision of rectal tumours and transanal endoscopic microsurgery. *Tumori* **81** (3 suppl): 50–56.

Stoller JL, Dowell AJ & Atkinson KG (1980) Colorectal anastomosis by transanal end-to-end stapling. *Can J Surg* **23**: 461–464.

Strauss RJ, Friedman M, Platt M & Wise L (1978) Surgical treatment of rectal carcinoma: results of anterior resection versus abdominoperineal resection at a community hospital. *Dis Colon Rectum* **21**: 269–275.

Sweeney JL, Ritchie JK & Hawley PR (1989) Resection and sutured per anal anastomosis for carcinoma of the rectum. *Dis Colon Rectum* **32**: 103–106.

Takagi H, Morimoto T, Yasue M et al (1985) Total pelvic exenteration for advanced carcinoma of the lower colon. *J Surg Oncol* **28**: 59–62.

Takahashi T & Kajitani T (1982) Some considerations on the lateral lymphatic metastases from rectal cancer. Personal communication, quoted in Goligher JC (1984) *Surgery of the Anus, Rectum and Colon*, 4th edn. London: Baillière Tindall.

Tank ES, Ernst CB, Woolson ST et al (1972) Urinary tract complications of anorectal surgery. *Am J Surg* **123**: 118–122.

Thorsoe H (1971) Urologiske Komplikationer til abdomino-perineal rectumeksstirpation. *Ugeskr Laeger* **133**: 739–743.

Touran T, Frost DB & O'Connell TX (1990) Sacral resection: operative technique and outcome. *Arch Surg* **125**: 911–913

Turnbull RB Jr & Cuthbertson FM (1961) Abdomino rectal pull-through resection for cancer and for Hirschprung's disease. *Cleveland Clin Quart* **28**: 109–115.

Turner GG (1943) *Modern Operative Surgery*, 3rd edn, Vol 1, p 960. London: Cassell.

Tuson JRD & Everett WG (1990) A retrospective study of colostomies leaks and structures after colorectal anastomosis. *Int J Colorectal Dis* **5**: 44–48.

Umpleby HC, Bristol JB, Rainey JB & Williamson RCN (1984a) Survival of 727 patients with single carcinomas of the large bowel. *Dis Colon Rectum* **27**: 803–810.

Umpleby HC, Fermor B, Symes MO & Williamson RCN (1984b) Viability of exfoliated colorectal carcinoma cells. *Br J Surg* **71**: 659–663.

Van Prohaska F, Govostis MC & Wasick M (1953) Multiple organ resection for advanced carcinoma of the colon and rectum. *Surg Gynecol Obstet* **97**: 177.

Vernava AM, Robbins PL & Brabbee GW (1989) Coloanal anastomosis for benign and malignant disease. *Dis Colon Rectum* **32**: 690–693.

Verneuil AA (1873) Quoted by Tuttle JP (1905) *A Treatise on Diseases of the Anus, Rectum and Pelvic Colon*, 2nd edn, p 963. New York: Appleton.

von Flue M, Rothenbuhler JM, Helwig A, Beglinger C & Harder

F (1994) The colon–J pouch anal reconstruction following total rectum resection: functional aspects (in German). *Schweiz Med Wochenschr* **124**: 1056–1063.

Wang HM, Chen SS, Liou TY & Chang MC (1992) Autonomic nerve-preserving operation for rectal carcinoma: preliminary postoperative urinary function in 15 cases (in Chinese). *Chung Hua I Hsueh Tsa Chih (Taipei)* **49**: 259–263.

Ward JN & Nay HR (1972) Immediate and delayed urologic complications associated with abdomino-perineal resection. *Am J Surg* **123**: 642–646.

Watson BC & Williams DI (1952) The urological complications of excision of the rectum. *Br J Surg* **40**: 19.

Waugh JM & Kirklin JW (1949) The importance of the level of the lesion in the prognosis and treatment of carcinoma of the rectum and low sigmoid colon. *Ann Surg* **129**: 22.

Waugh JM, Block MA & Gage RP (1955) Three and five year survivals following combined abdomino-perineal resection, abdomino-resection with sphincter preservation and anterior resection for carcinoma of the rectum and lower part of the sigmoid colon. *Ann Surg* **142**: 752–757.

Waxman BP (1983) Large bowel anastomoses. II: The circular staplers. *Br J Surg* **70**: 64–67.

Waxman BP, Yii MK & Pahlman L (1995) Stapling in colorectal surgery. In Mazier WP (ed) *Surgery of the Colon, Rectum and Anus*. Philadelphia: WB Saunders.

Weakley FL (1981) Symposium: The use and misuse of staples in colonic surgery. *Dis Colon Rectum* **24**: 231–246.

Weakley FL (1983) Cancer of the rectum: a review of surgical options. *Surg Clin N Am* **63**: 129–135.

Weir RF (1901) An improved method of treating high-seated cancers of the rectum. *Am J Surg Gynecol (St Louis)* **15**: 134–135.

West Midlands Cancer Registry (1990) *Cancer in the West Midlands 1981–85*, pp 37–50.

West of Scotland and Highland Anastomosis Study Group (1991) Suturing or stapling in gastrointestinal surgery: a prospective randomised study. *Br J Surg* **78**: 337–341.

Westhues H (1930) Uber die Enstehung und Vermeidung des lokalen Rektumkarzinom: Rezidivs. *Arch Klin Chir* **161**: 582.

Westhues H (1934) *Die Pathologisch-anatomischen Grundlagen der Chirurgie des Rektum Karzinomas*, p 68. Leipzig: Thieme.

Wheeless CR Jr (1979) Avoidance of permanent colostomy in pelvic malignancy using the surgical stapler. *Obstet Gynecol* **54**: 501–505.

Whiteway J, Nicholls RJ & Morson BC (1985) The role of surgical local excision in the treatment of rectal cancer. *Br J Surg* **72**: 694–697.

Whittaker M & Goligher JC (1976) The prognosis after surgical treatment for carcinoma of the rectum. *Br J Surg* **63**: 384–388.

Williams LF, Huddleston CB, Sawyers JL et al (1988) Is total pelvic exenteration reasonable primary treatment for rectal carcinoma? *Ann Surg* **207**: 670–678.

Williams NS (1989) Stapling technique for pouch anal anastomosis without the need for purse string sutures. *Br J Surg* **76**: 348–349.

Williams NS & Johnston D (1983) The quality of life after rectal excision for low rectal cancer. *Br J Surg* **70**: 460–462.

Williams NS & Johnston D (1984) Survival and recurrence after sphincter-saving resection and abdominoperineal resection for carcinoma of the middle third of the rectum. *Br J Surg* **71**: 278–282.

Williams NS, Neal DE & Johnston D (1980a) Bladder function after excision of the rectum for low rectal carcinoma. *Gut* **21**: A453–A454.

Williams NS, Price R & Johnston D (1980b) The long term effect of sphincter preserving operations for rectal carcinoma on the function of the anal sphincters in man. *Br J Surg* **67**: 203–208.

Williams NS, Dixon MF & Johnston D (1983) Reappraisal of the 5 cm rule of distal excision for carcinoma of the rectum: a study of distal intramural spread and of patients' survival. *Br J Surg* **70**: 150–154.

Williams NS, Durdey P & Johnston D (1985) The outcome following sphincter-saving resection and abdominoperineal resection for low rectal cancer. *Br J Surg* **72**: 595–598.

Williams NS, Nasmyth DG, Jones D & Smith AH (1986) Defunctioning stomas: a prospective controlled trial comparing loop ileostomy with loop transverse colostomy. *Br J Surg* **73**: 566–570.

Williams NS, Hallan RI, Koeze TH & Watkins EJ (1990a) Restoration of gastrointestinal continuity and continence after abdominoperineal excision of the rectum using an electrically stimulated neoanal sphincter. *Dis Colon Rectum* **33**: 561–565.

Williams NS, Hallan RI, Koeze TH, Pilot MA & Watkins EJ (1990b) Construction of a neoanal sphincter by transposition of the gracilis and prolonged neuromuscular stimulation for the treatment of faecal incontinence. *Ann R Coll Surg Engl* **72**: 108–113.

Williams NS, Patel J, George BD, Hallan RI, Watkins ES (1991) Development of an electrically stimulated neo-anal sphincter. *Lancet* **338**: 1166–1169.

Williams NS, Hughes SF & Stuchfield B (1994) Continent colonic conduit for rectal evacuation in severe constipation. *Lancet* **343**: 1321–1324.

Williams RD, Yurko AA, Kerr G & Zollinger RM (1966) Comparison of anterior and abdominoperineal resection for low pelvic colon and rectal cancer. *Am J Surg* **111**: 114–119.

Williamson MER, Lewis WG, Holdsworth PJ et al (1993) Changes in anorectal function after low anterior resection of the rectum: a continuous ambulatory study. *Dis Colon Rectum* **36**: 19.

Williamson M, Lewis W, Finan P et al (1995) Recovery of physiological and clinical function after low anterior resection of the rectum for carcinoma: myth or reality? *Dis Colon Rectum* **38**: 411–418.

Wilson SM & Beahrs OH (1976) The curative treatment of carcinoma of the sigmoid, rectosigmoid and rectum. *Ann Surg* **183**: 556–565.

Wittoesch JH & Jackman RS (1958) Results of conservative management of cancer of the rectum in poor risk patients. *Surg Gynecol Obstet* **107**: 648.

Wolmark N & Fisher B (1986) An analysis of survival and treatment failure following abdominoperineal and sphincter-saving resection in Dukes' B and C rectal carcinoma. *Ann Surg* **204**: 480–487.

Wolmark N, Gordon PH, Fisher B et al (1986) A comparison of stapled and hand-sewn anastomosis in patients undergoing resection for Dukes' B and C colorectal cancer: an analysis of disease-free survival and survival from the NSA BP prospective clinical trials. *Dis Colon Rectum* **29**: 344–350.

Wong SKC & Wee JTK (1984) Reconstruction of an orthotopic functional anus after abdominoperineal resection. *Aust NZ J Surg* **54**: 575–578.

Wood CB, Gillis CR, Hole D et al (1981) Local tumour invasion as a prognosis factor in colorectal cancer. *Br J Surg* **68**: 326–328.

Wood RAB & Hughes LE (1975) Silicone foam sponge for pilonidal sinus: a new technique for dressing open granulating wounds. *BMJ* **3**: 131.

Wood RAB, Williams RHP & Hughes LE (1977) Foam elastomer dressings in the management of open granulating wounds: experience with 250 patients. *Br J Surg* **64**: 551.

Wood WQ & Wilkie DPD (1933) Carcinoma of the rectum: an anatomic pathological study. *Edinb Med J* **40**: 321–343.

Yeung RS, Moffat FL & Falk RE (1993) Pelvic excenteration for recurrent and extensive primary colorectal adenocarcinoma. *Cancer* **72**: 1853–1858.

Yule AG & Fiddian RV (1983) 'Two gun' surgery: low anterior resection of the rectum avoiding the anorectal purse-string suture. *Br J Surg* **70**: 100–115.

Zinman LM, Libertino JA & Roth RA (1978) Management of operative ureteral injury. *Urology* **12**: 290–303.

Zollinger RM & Sheppard MH (1971) Carcinoma of the rectum and sigmoid: a review of 279 cases. *Arch Surg* **102**: 335–338.

33

RADIOTHERAPY AND CHEMOTHERAPY FOR PRIMARY COLORECTAL CANCER, SURVEILLANCE AND RECURRENCE

RADIOTHERAPY FOR COLORECTAL CANCER

Rectal cancer is more amenable to treatment by radiation than colonic cancer. Radiotherapy may be used in one of three ways:

- as a primary treatment
- as adjuvant therapy
- as a palliative manoeuvre.

Another form of palliative therapy includes treatment of local recurrence from both colonic and rectal cancer.

Primary treatment of rectal cancer: endocavitary radiation

Although radiotherapy has been employed as a palliative treatment of incurable or recurrent rectal cancer for many years, it is only relatively recently that radiation has been used as primary therapy. The term 'endocavitary irradiation' is applied to irradiation given by means of an X-ray or gamma-ray emitter located in the lumen of the rectum. There are two modalities of endocavitary irradiation: contact X-ray therapy and interstitial therapy.

Contact irradiation

Contact irradiation has been used since 1932 for the treatment of carcinoma of the uterine cervix (Schaeffer and Witte, 1932), but its use in rectal cancer was not described until the early 1970s. The pioneer of this approach was Jean Papillon from Lyon, France (Papillon, 1973), and together with his colleagues he acquired considerable experience with the technique. The principles of contact X-ray therapy were laid down by Chaoul (1936). Two conditions are required: (a) a short focal distance, i.e. distance between the X-ray focus and the object, and (b) soft radiation quality. In order to achieve these conditions the Phillips contact X-ray machine is used. This has a low voltage (50 V), a short focal distance (4 cm) and a high output (20 Gy/min in the air). The rays are delivered via a narrow tube (3 cm diameter) which can be inserted via a special proctoscope (Figure 33.1). The applicator and proctoscope can be moved over the surface of the tumour and at each site an area measuring 3 cm in diameter is treated. The absorption of the X-rays is limited to a depth of 2 cm. Papillon recommended a dose of 3–4 Gy at each treatment administered within 3 minutes (Papillon, 1974). Treatments are repeated 1–3 weeks later giving a total dose of 80–150 Gy over a period of 4–10 weeks. Most patients can be treated on an outpatient basis and anaesthesia is not usually required.

The advantage of intracavitary contact irradiation over the conventional technique of external irradiation is that radiation is delivered mainly to tumour tissue in a high dose. When irradiation is given externally normal tissue is irradiated and thus the energy is dissipated. In order for the technique to be successful careful selection of patients is necessary. Those patients who fulfil the requirements for treatment tend to be the same patients who could be treated satisfactorily by local excision. Papillon has laid down the following criteria for tumours suitable for this form of therapy:

- The whole of the lesion must be accessible to the 29 mm applicator, particularly the lesion's upper edge.
- The tumour must not be too large as each field of irradiation is only 3 cm diameter; but it is possible to use two overlapping fields for cancers of 5 cm length and 3 cm width.
- The surrounding rectal wall, especially above the tumour, must be intact and there must be no palpable lymph nodes.
- Tumours projecting into the lumen of the bowel are more suitable for this treatment than are infiltrative lesions.
- The tumour should be well-differentiated.

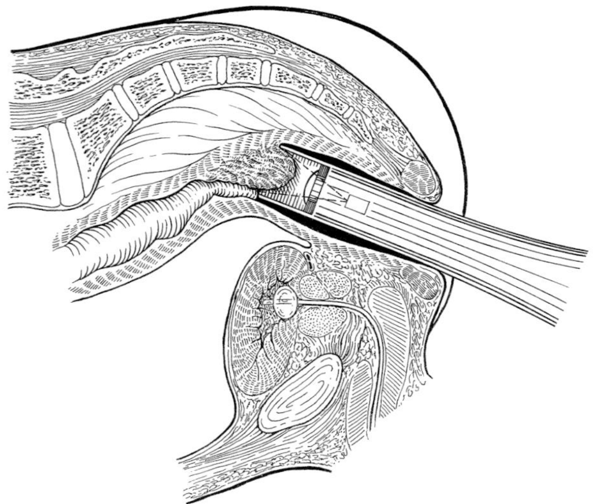

Figure 33.1 Papillon method of delivering endocavitary radiation to a rectal cancer.

Interstitial therapy

Insertion of radioactive needles into a tumour is termed 'interstitial therapy'. The first use of the technique in the treatment of rectal cancer was by Binkley (1938). He combined the technique with external irradiation for 3 weeks. After an interval of 2 weeks interstitial therapy was commenced using radium or radon needles. Binkley treated a variety of growths, many of them so advanced that they were beyond any form of therapy. His greatest success was achieved in 18 patients who had small tumours, but were considered to be high surgical risks; 15 of them were alive and well for periods varying from 15 months to 10 years. Ruff et al (1961) from the Mayo Clinic also reported the destruction of tumours by this technique in 10 of 96 patients treated. This method of therapy was largely abandoned because of the difficulty with dosimetry and safety experienced using radium and radon. With the introduction of new radioisotopes – particularly iridium-192 – these difficulties have been overcome. Papillon advocated the use of the technique when small remnants of tumour remain after contact irradiation (Papillon, 1982). It can also be used for the treatment of recurrence after local excision (Kozlova and Popova, 1977).

Papillon (1982) used the interstitial technique 6

weeks after the projecting part of the tumour had been destroyed. In this method the iridium needles are applied to the bed of the tumour which is still indurated. The needles consist of two wires of iridium-192 which are inserted down the prongs of a steel fork. The two prongs, 16 mm or 12 mm apart, are welded to a base plate (Figure 33.2). Each prong is preloaded with an iridium-192 wire 4 cm long. Through the special proctoscope the fork is implanted in the rectal wall at a distance of 1 cm below the site of the area to be treated. It is easily inserted upwards almost parallel with the axis of the rectal ampulla. The iridium fork is not sutured to the rectal wall but a rubber drain inserted through the anus is used to keep the fork in place. The rubber drain is sutured to the skin of the anal margin. The treatment time does not exceed 24 hours, after which the fork is removed.

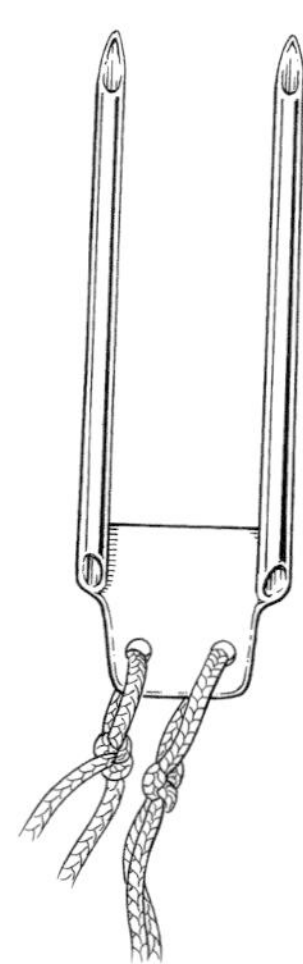

Figure 33.2 Interstitial technique of delivering radiation to a rectal cancer. The steel forks are inserted into the tumours. Each prong is preloaded with an iridium wire 4 cm long.

Results of endocavitary irradiation

In 1982 Papillon reported the results of 280 patients treated since 1951 by his team at the Centre Leon Berard (Papillon, 1982). He pointed out that during this time several changes had been instituted. In the first 10 years most tumours treated for cure were small polypoid lesions and the treatment consisted exclusively of contact X-ray therapy. Since 1960 more ulcerative lesions had been treated and interstitial therapy played a greater part as a supplement to contact therapy. After 1972, iridium-192 needles replaced radium needles for the interstitial approach.

Approximately 50% of the patients treated were poor surgical risks. The average age was 62 years (range 25–88). All tumours were true invasive carcinomas; *in situ* carcinomas, carcinomas in polyps and malignant villous adenomas were excluded. All tumours were well-differentiated or moderately well-differentiated on multiple biopsies. Colloid tumours were also excluded.

A total of 207 patients were followed for more than 5 years (Table 33.1). Of the lesions treated, 150 (72.5%) were 3 cm or less in diameter and were treated using only one field of contact X-ray therapy; 57 tumours (27.5%) exceeded 3 cm diameter and were treated by two overlapping fields of contact X-ray therapy during the first applications. Approximately 50% of patients in the last 20 years received combined treatment; i.e. contact and interstitial therapy. Of the 207 patients followed up for over 5 years, 153 were alive and well. This gives a crude 5-year survival rate of 73.9%. However, eight of these patients were not cured by irradiation and required surgery; the true crude 5-year survival rate must take these patients into consideration and this alters the rate slightly to 70%. Nevertheless the results were most impressive.

There was a relationship between the size of the tumour and the chance of cure. The 5-year survival rate for lesions 3 cm or less in diameter was 80%, whereas for lesions more than 3 cm diameter it was 61.5%.

All patients were followed up carefully; in addition to the usual clinical examination patients also had computed tomographic (CT) scans of the liver when considered necessary, and repeat cytology of the rectal mucosa was performed on a regular basis. Eleven patients (5.3%) were considered to be local failures in that they developed recurrent disease within the rectum. Most of these recurrences were detected within the first 2 years and were considered to be due to a failure of local control in the first instance. Of these 11 patients, three were considered to be unsuitable for further surgery but eight under-

Table 33.1 Intracavitary irradiation for cure of limited rectal cancers: results at 5 years from the Centre Léon Bérard.

	No. of cases	*Percentage*
Patients treated	207	100
Alive and well more than 5 years	153	73.9
Deaths	54	26.1
Death from cancer	22	10.6
Death from intercurrent disease	28	13.5
Postoperative death	4	2
Local failures	11	5.3
Nodal failures	12	5.8
Distant metastasis	6	2.9

From Papillon (1982).

went some form of 'salvage' rectal excision, of whom three patients survived for 5 years or more.

Another reason for unsuccessful treatment described by Papillon was nodal failure. He put great stress on the fact that involved nodes could be felt in the mesorectum on digital examination, and these nodes should be rechecked during follow-up. In 12 of the 207 cases (5.8%), indurated nodes were found either in the mesorectum (ten cases) or along the hypogastric chain against the pelvic wall (two cases). Ten of these 12 patients had no evidence of disease within the rectal wall. Six of these 12 patients were evidently inoperable and subsequently died, four subsequently underwent abdominoperineal excision of the rectum, and two had a procedure described as a perirectal lymphadenectomy.

Complications were said to be minimal. No death appeared to have been attributable to the irradiation itself. Narrowing or stricture formation of the rectal lumen was not described. After treatment rectal bleeding occurred from time to time from mucosal telangiectasia, but was rarely a problem.

Gérard et al (1994) recently updated Papillon's data. They described the results in 414 patients treated by endocavitary irradiation of small T1 and T2 adenocarcinomas of the rectum treated in Lyon between 1951 and 1993. Local control was achieved in 91%, and again complications were minimal. Very few groups have treated such a large number of patients with this form of therapy, so it is difficult to know whether Papillon's superb results are reproducible throughout the world.

Sischy and Remington (1975) reported on 25 patients treated by the technique. After approximately 2 years 23 patients had responded satisfactorily. Recurrence was found in only two patients (8%), both of whom were treated by abdominoperineal excision of the rectum. Fleshman et al (1985) had one failure in treating 8 patients (13%). However, perhaps the largest series treated by this technique outside of Lyon is that described by Hull et al (1994) from the Cleveland Clinic. Between 1973 and 1992 they treated 199 patients with endocavitary irradiation; 126 were treated with curative intent. Thirty-seven of the 126 patients treated curatively developed recurrence and the mean time to recurrence was 16.1 months (range 1–56); ten developed distant recurrence and 27 had local recurrence. The authors concluded that in selected patients endocavitary irradiation initially rendered 71% of patients free of disease. With additional treatment 11% were rendered free of disease. The 5-year recurrence rate was 32%, but after additional therapy this was reduced to 9%. Thus, although these results are not quite in the same league as those from the Lyon Group, they are relatively encouraging.

It seems, therefore, that with careful patient selection this method of therapy is practicable and good results can be achieved. Despite such encouraging results, however, the technique has never been popular in either the UK or the USA. This probably reflects differences in referral, in that patients with rectal bleeding are usually seen in clinics where primary treatment is usually operative. Tumours that are most suitable for endocavitary irradiation – that is to say less than 3 cm diameter – can also be excised locally without too much difficulty. Surgeons tend to prefer a form of therapy in which they feel that all the malignant tissue has been removed, and tend to be suspicious of techniques that do not achieve this aim.

Adjuvant radiotherapy for rectal cancer

The fact that 5-year survival rates have not improved over the last 40 years has stimulated many to explore forms of adjuvant therapy which might complement surgery. Radiotherapy has been used in this way, both before and after surgery (Fortier et al, 1986; Allen et al, 1987; Mendenhall, et al, 1987, 1988; Papillon, 1987; Taylor et al, 1987; Willett et al, 1987; Gérard et al, 1988; Reed et al, 1988; Kodner et al, 1989; Smith et al, 1989; Horn et al, 1990; Påhlman and Glimelius, 1990, 1992; Berard and Papillon, 1992; Klimberg et al, 1992).

Preoperative radiotherapy

Early work in this area was performed in animal models and one important observation was that the dose of radiation that could be used as adjuvant therapy with surgery was considerably less than the dose needed alone to treat animal tumours for cure. Powers and Tolmach (1964) demonstrated that a single dose of 5 Gy given immediately before excision of a transplanted murine lymphosarcoma improved the cure rate from 53% to 85%. This study was the main stimulus for the various clinical trials that have subsequently been performed, some of which are summarized below and in Tables 33.2 and 33.3.

Stearns et al (1974) reported on the results of a trial performed at the Memorial Hospital, New York. Patients were randomized to receive preoperative radiation therapy of 20 Gy in 2 weeks or surgical resection only. No improvement in overall 5-year survival or local recurrence was demonstrated.

The Veterans Administration Surgical Oncology

Table 33.2 Overall survival in patients undergoing preoperative radiation for adenocarcinoma of the rectum in non-randomized trials.

Study	Total dose (Gy)	No. of patients	Percentage 5-year survival	
			Radiation plus surgical resection	Surgical resection only
Memorial I	Variable	971	51	48
Cleveland	24	43	58	
Montpelier	40	116	59	44
Oregon	50–60	44	55	38

Table 33.3 Mortality in prospective randomized trials comparing adjuvant radiotherapy with no radiotherapy (including trial with identical chemotherapy for both treatment and control groups).

Trials	Dose (Gy)	Deaths/No. entered		Odds ratio* comparing treatment with control mortality rates
		Radiotherapy	Control	
Preoperative radiotherapy				
VASOG-20	20	225/347	251/353	
Yale	40	9/15	11/16	
Toronto	5	46/60	52/65	
MRC I	5/20	318/549	166/275	
EORTC-40761	34.5	55/201	61/209	
VASOG-28	31.5	121/180	114/181	
Stockholm	25	147/351	140/343	
Northwest	25	83/143	84/141	
MRC 2	40	60/129	73/132	
Total preoperative (observed–expected – 20.2, variance 206.9)		1064/1975	952/1715	Treatment better; 9%±7 Treatment worse
Postoperative radiotherapy				
Denmark	50	105/244	104/250	
GITSG-7175	40	49/101	63/110	
NSABP R-01	46.5	113/184	116/184	
MRC 3	40	23/180	39/189	
Total postoperative		290/709	322/733	Treatment better; 14%±11 Treatment worse
All radiotherapy trials (observed–expected – 31.8, variance 284.9)		1354/2684	1274/2448	Treatment better; 11%±6 Treatment worse
				Treatment effect 2P<0.06

*For each trial the observed odds reduction in the figures is represented by a black square, with its 99% confidence interval as a horizontal line. A diamond shape represents the odds reduction and 95% confidence interval for the overview of the individual trials.
From Gray et al (1991).

Group (VASOG) also carried out a randomized trial of preoperative radiation using 20 Gy over 2 weeks (Higgins et al, 1975). An additional 5 Gy over 2 weeks was given to any patient whose carcinoma was within 8 cm of the anal verge. Patients were included even if they had disseminated disease provided that resection of the primary tumour could be achieved. The most recent report on this study showed no significant improvement in 5-year survival between the irradiated group and the control group. However, three interesting findings did emerge. First, the patients who underwent abdominoperineal excision of the rectum and were irradiated had a significant 5-year survival advantage over those who were not irradiated: 41% compared with 28% ($P < 0.02$). There was, however, no significant survival difference in any other subgroup. The second point to emerge was that there was an apparent reduction in the number of lymph nodes involved by tumour after radiation, an apparent 'downgrading' of the tumour. Finally, there was a reduction in the incidence of pelvic recurrence after radiation in a subgroup who underwent postmortem examination.

The VASOG started a second trial limited to patients in whom abdominoperineal excision was planned (Higgins et al, 1981). The dose of radiation was 31.5 Gy over 3 weeks. However, 5-year survival rates did not differ significantly between the group receiving adjuvant radiotherapy compared with the group treated by surgery alone (50%) (Higgins et al, 1986).

In Toronto a trial was performed in which patients were randomized to receive either a single dose of 6 Gy or sham irradiation on the morning of operation (Rider et al, 1977). There was no difference in the overall 5-year survival rates (36% versus

38%) or local recurrence. However, in patients with tumour-involved lymph nodes, there was a significant 5-year survival benefit in the irradiated group (36% versus 18%, $P < 0.01$).

The Medical Research Council in Great Britain carried out a prospective trial in which patients were randomized to one of three groups. One group received a single dose of 5 Gy, the second group received a dose of 20 Gy over a 2-week period, and the third group acted as the control and did not receive adjuvant radiation (MRC Working Party, 1982, 1984). There was no significant difference in the 5-year survival rates or local recurrence rates between the three groups. However, in patients who received 20 Gy, there was a decrease in the number of involved nodes recovered from the resection specimen. In a second MRC trial, 279 patients were randomized to receive surgery alone ($n = 140$) or 40 Gy of preoperative radiotherapy ($n = 139$). At 5-year follow-up, 65 patients in the surgery-alone group had developed local recurrence compared with 50 patients in the radiotherapy group ($P < 0.04$) (Figure 33.3a); the corresponding numbers of patients with distant recurrence were 67 and 49 ($P < 0.02$) (Figure 33.3b). However, the survival results were equivocal (MRC Rectal Cancer Working Party, 1996a).

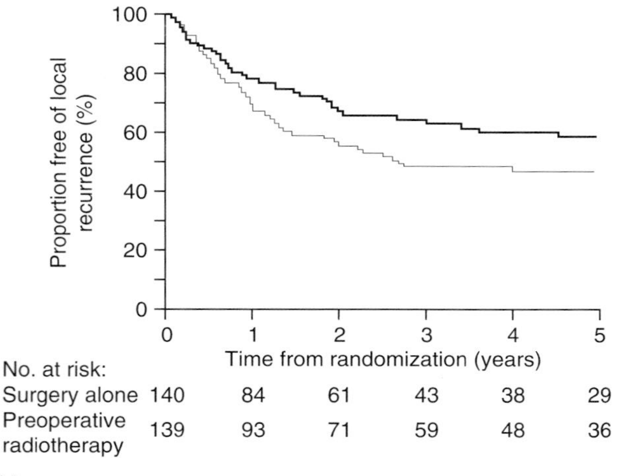

(a)

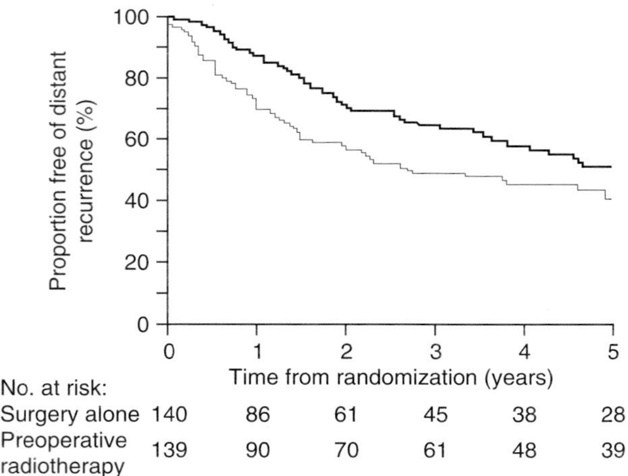

(b)

Figure 33.3a,b MRC study (1996) comparing preoperative radiotherapy (40 Gy) (bold lines) with surgery alone (fine lines) for fixed or tethered rectal cancer. (a) Local recurrence rates. (b) Distant recurrence rates.

The European Organization for Research on Treatment of Cancer (EORTC) used extended radiation fields to cover the pelvis and superior haemorrhoidal lymph nodes up to the level of the second lumbar vertebra (Gérard et al, 1985). The dose used was 34.50 Gy over a period of 3 weeks, surgery being preferred 2 weeks after completion of the radiotherapy. Although there was no significant difference in survival rates between the irradiated group and the control group, local recurrence at 5 years was significantly less in the irradiated group (65% versus 85%, $P < 0.001$).

A similar trial to the EORTC study above was performed by the Yale University group using an extended field of radiation and a dose of 46 Gy over a 4-week period (Kligerman et al, 1972); surgical resection was performed 4 weeks later. The 5-year survival rate was 41% in the irradiated group and 25% in the control group. This difference was not statistically significant, but since the number of patients in the trial ($n = 31$) was so small such statistical analysis is probably invalid.

The Stockholm Rectal Cancer Study Group randomized 694 patients with rectal cancer to receive either surgery alone or 25 Gy of preoperative radiotherapy over 5–7 days, and reported their findings in 1987. At a median follow-up period of 34 months the incidence of pelvic recurrence was significantly reduced but there was no significant difference in overall survival. This trial has since been updated (Stockholm Rectal Cancer Study Group, 1990). The significant reduction in local recurrence rates in the preoperative radiotherapy arm was confirmed (25% versus 11%), but there was still no benefit in 5-year survival rates (DXT 55%, controls 50%).

In a preoperative study conducted by the Imperial Cancer Research Fund (ICRF) in the UK, 468 patients were randomized to receive either a preoperative course of 25 Gy or surgery alone (Goldberg et al, 1994). There was a significant reduction in local recurrence in the irradiated group (17% versus 24%). Similarly, in a study in the North West of England 284 patients with locally advanced rectal cancer were randomized in a similar way to those in the ICRF trial (Marsh et al, 1994). There was again a significant reduction in local recurrence rates in the irradiated group (18% versus 41%).

The most recent and influential preoperative study to report is the Swedish Rectal Cancer Trial (1997). This randomized 1168 patients to receive either a short course of radiotherapy (25 Gy delivered in five fractions in one week), followed by surgery within one week, or to have surgery alone. After 5 years' follow-up, the rate of local recurrence was 11% (63 of 553 patients) in the group that received the preoperative radiotherapy and 27% (150 of 557) in the group treated by surgery alone ($P < 0.001$). This difference was found in all subgroups defined according to Dukes stage. The overall 5-year survival rate was 58% in the radiotherapy plus surgery group and 48% in the others ($P < 0.004$).

In addition to these prospective, controlled trials there have been several non-randomized studies. Stevens et al (1976) from Oregon, USA, used small radiation fields directed to the primary tumour only and delivered 50–60 Gy over 6–7 weeks followed by resection 4–7 weeks later. The 5-year survival rate was 55% compared with 38% in an historical control group. Several studies using short, intensive preoperative courses of radiation have been reported from the USA, Sweden and Russia (Rodriguez-Antunez et al, 1973; Simbirtseva et al, 1975; Dedkov and Zibina, 1976; Glimelius et al, 1982), all of which suggested that radiotherapy offers advantages in terms of survival and local control of disease compared with historical controls – a view supported by Duncan (1987) in a subsequent review of the subject.

Criticisms

Numerous criticisms can be levelled at the design of many of these trials. Several included insufficient numbers of patients to provide evidence of survival advantage because of a type II error. In some, large numbers of patients registered in the trial were excluded from analysis because of insufficient follow-up or protocol violations (Gérard et al, 1985). Stratification with regard to histological grade, distance from the anal verge and other well-known prognostic factors was not performed, although the MRC and EORTC trials did adjust statistical imbalances in prognostic factors between treatment groups (MRC Working Party, 1984; Gérard et al, 1985). Often there was no uniform definition of what length of bowel constituted the rectum, hence the criteria for inclusion varied greatly. The criteria by which a patient was assessed for possible surgery and included in the trial also varied. Thus, in some the tumour had to be clinically operable with no evidence of fixation (Rider et al, 1977), while in others both mobile and fixed lesions were eligible for entry (Duncan, 1981). Both the radiation dose given and the volume of tissue irradiated differed widely between studies. Operations were also not standardized, and although recent data suggest that survival after sphincter-saving resection and abdominoperineal excision is similar, the influence of surgical techniques and outcome has not been accounted for in the large, multicentre studies. The interval between cessation of radiotherapy and operation varied from study to study. Despite these obvious defects in design and the lack of uniformity in the various studies, certain conclusions can be drawn.

Conclusions

There is some evidence that in patients treated by preoperative radiation the size of the primary tumour and the number of involved lymph nodes are reduced. The extent to which this downgrading of the pathological stage of the tumour is achieved varies with the dose of radiation used. For instance, the *first* MRC trial (MRC Working Party, 1984) showed a statistically significant 30% decrease in the numbers of both involved and negative lymph nodes after a fractionated radiation dose of 20 Gy, whereas no difference was seen between the group that received a single dose of 5 Gy and the control group.

It might be expected that the improvement in pathological stage as a result of radiotherapy would improve survival and reduce local pelvic recurrence. Table 33.3 summarizes the survival results of most of the prospective randomized studies and Table 33.2 summarizes some of the larger, non-randomized comparisons. Overall there is little evidence from the randomized studies on any improvement in survival attributable to low-dose preoperative irradiation. However, the recent Swedish Rectal Cancer Trial (1997) is a notable exception with an increased overall survival rate of 58% compared with 48%. The higher-dose studies which use historical controls also suggest some improvement. When the patients are subdivided according to the histopathological characteristics of their tumour interesting trends emerge. Both the Toronto trial (Rider et al, 1977) and the VASOG study (Higgins et al, 1981) reported that survival in patients with involved lymph nodes was improved in those patients who had been irradiated. The first MRC trial, on the other hand, which used a similar radiation regimen, was unable to substantiate these findings. The MRC trial did suggest that the survival of patients with clinically fixed tumours who were irradiated was better than survival in patients with mobile lesions. On the strength of this finding the MRC commenced a trial of preoperative radiotherapy in patients with fixed tumours and increased the dose of radiation to 40 Gy but no improvement has been detected so far (MRC Working Party, 1996a).

The influence of preoperative radiotherapy on local pelvic recurrence is now more clear than previously. Many older studies failed to report sufficient information to enable detailed analysis of the sites or incidence of local relapse. However, in more recent studies this deficit has been corrected. Even so, the rates of pelvic and distant recurrence depend on the methods of detection and these vary considerably from study to study. Facilities such as computed tomography (CT) and endoluminal ultrasound may not generally be available and autopsy rates may differ. Despite these imperfections, most of the recent controlled studies show a reduction in local recurrence in the patients treated by preoperative, short-term, high-dose (25–40 Gy) irradiation (Table 33.4).

Another consistent finding is the ability of preoperative radiotherapy to reduce the size and extent of local spread of a locally advanced lesion sufficiently to make a surgical option feasible after radiotherapy. Hence an inoperable lesion can sometimes be rendered operable. Experience suggests that it is necessary to use 45–50 Gy over 14–16 fractions to treat T4 lesions, and in some patients chemotherapy may help. There is little doubt that a reduction in size of the tumour can be achieved in approximately one-third of patients and this allows surgery to proceed. However, the evidence from the previously cited MRC Trial (MRC Working Party, 1996) suggests that radiotherapy alone will not improve survival.

Concern is often expressed by surgeons as to the toxicity of radiotherapy. With a low-dose regimen increased postoperative morbidity has rarely been established. All studies using 30 Gy or more indicate that radiation-induced diarrhoea is common, but most patients responded well to symptomatic management. Deaths related to radiation alone are on the whole rare. Stevens described two patients (of 57 irradiated) who died from bowel perforation during or following radiation using 50 Gy or more (Stevens et al, 1976). In the most recent trials, mortality has not been increased in the irradiated arm despite the increased dose. However, in the Stockholm–Malmo trial (Stockholm Rectal Cancer Study Group, 1990) there was a significant increase in non-cancer deaths in patients over 75 years of age compared with controls. Most deaths were cardiovascular in nature and seemed to be due to an as yet unexplained effect of the combination of large radiation fractions with large field sizes. This toxic effect was abolished in subsequent trials by a reduction in field size (Swedish Rectal Cancer Trial, 1993).

Surprisingly, none of the studies so far has reported any increased technical difficulty of resection following irradiation to the pelvis. Similarly, healing of abdominal or perineal wounds has not been impaired to an unacceptable level. One group (Gary-Bobo et al, 1979) recommended that the perineum should not be closed primarily after irradiation and abdominoperineal excision when there was a short interval between the two. The EORTC group reported a mean delay of perineal wound healing of 60 days when abdominoperineal excision was performed within 14 days of patients receiving 34.5 Gy compared with 40 days in the control group (Gérard et al, 1985). Similarly, in the Swedish Rectal Cancer trial, there was a significant increase in perineal wound infections in the irradiated group (20% versus 10%, $P < 0.001$). Other groups (Kligerman et al, 1972; Stevens et al, 1976) using a 4-week or longer delay between irradiation and operation failed to observe any difficulty in perineal wound healing. Thus, provided sufficient time (a minimum of 4

Table 33.4 Local recurrence in patients having pre-operative radiotherapy for adenocarcinoma of the rectum.

**Trial*	*Dose (Gy)*	*No. of patients randomized*	*Local recurrence*		*P-value*
			**Radiotherapy*	*Surgery only*	
MRC1	5 or 20	824	235/549	112/275	NS
EORTC2	34.5	466	6/152	21/166	<0.01
			17/152	42/166	<0.01
VASOG2	31.5	361	37/180	40/181	NS
Stockholm	25	694	23/271	54/274	P<0.001
MRC2	40	261	41/129	50/132	NS
ICRF	25	468	31/185	51/210	P<0.05
North West	25	284	26/143	58/141	P<0.001
Swedish Rectal Cancer Trial	25	1168	63/553	150/557	P<0.001

* Data derived from Buvse et al (1988), except for MRC1 and 2 (MRC Working Party, 1984), Stockholm (Stockholm Rectal Cancer Study Group, 1990), North West (James et al, 1991) and Swedish Rectal Cancer Trial (1997). NS, not significant.

weeks) elapses between radiotherapy and operation, wound healing is not impaired.

Similar concern has been expressed about the healing of colorectal anastomoses after irradiation. Most of the older studies included patients who had mainly undergone abdominoperineal excision of the rectum so it was difficult to be totally reassured on this point. However, more recent studies have included more patients who have undergone sphincter-saving resections. Thus, in the first MRC trial (MRC Working Party, 1982), 21 of 70 control patients (30%) developed an anastomotic leak, compared with 4 of 53 (8%) in the group receiving 5 Gy and 8 of 52 (16%) in the group receiving 20 Gy. This apparent improvement in healing after irradiation is difficult to explain, but perhaps the surgeons took special care with the anastomosis when they knew the patients had received radiation. In the Swedish Rectal Cancer Trial (1993), 26 of 160 patients (11%) undergoing a sphincter-saving resection who received 25 Gy of preoperative radiotherapy developed an anastomotic dehiscence, compared with 17 of 165 patients (8%) in the surgery-alone arm.

In a non-randomized study with a dose of 45 Gy (25 fractions over 5 weeks) there were no anastomotic leaks in 24 patients who underwent a restorative anastomosis without a colostomy (Robertson et al, 1985). Stevens et al (1978), on the other hand, reported two leaks in nine patients who had a sphincter-saving resection without covering stoma after 50 Gy over 5 weeks. In their historical control group there was only one leak in 79 patients. They recommended, therefore, that all patients who were receiving a large dose of radiation and a sphincter-saving resection should have a temporary colostomy. There is insufficient information in most reports to know whether the anastomotic leaks were of clinical importance or whether they were found as a result of routine contrast enema examinations. The consensus is that patients who undergo sphincter-saving resection after receiving 45 Gy or more over a 4–5 week period should probably have a covering stoma.

Up to now, it appeared that preoperative radiation using doses of 25 Gy over 2 weeks were of no benefit with respect to survival. The results of the Swedish Rectal Cancer Trial (1997) have however, provided more optimism. There is also now good evidence from prospective controlled trials that using this and higher doses preoperatively reduces the incidence of local recurrence. With higher doses, complications of delayed wound healing and anastomotic dehiscence seem to be slightly increased. In SSR preoperative DXT is associated with higher bowel frequency, urgency and minor incontinence compared with controls. It remains to be seen whether the possible benefit achieved with local control will outweigh the toxicity of therapy. In the future it will be essential to stratify patients carefully according to their clinicopathological stage and to assess recurrence in a uniform manner using regular scanning techniques.

Postoperative adjuvant radiotherapy

It is perhaps more logical to give radiation after operation than before, since by then the disease will have been more accurately staged and treatment can be used selectively. In preoperative studies all patients were irradiated, some of whom had Dukes' A lesions while others had overt liver metastases. Radiation therapy in both these groups is unlikely to be justified. It would perhaps be better for the patients if only those who were thought to need radiation received it. This can probably be determined accurately only from operative and pathological findings; although with newer imaging techniques it is hoped that patients can be staged more accurately before operation than hitherto.

The results from controlled trials of postoperative adjuvant radiotherapy suggest only marginal improvement (Table 33.5). The Gastrointestinal Tumour Study Group conducted a trial in which postoperative radiation alone was included in one arm (GITSG, 1985). Patients with Duke's B and C lesions in whom the lower edge was within 12 cm of the anal verge were included in the trial. The control group received radical surgery alone; one group received radical surgery plus postoperative radiotherapy (44 or 48 Gy); one group received radical surgery and postoperative chemotherapy with fluorouracil and methyl-CCNU; while a fourth group received both radiation and chemotherapy in addition to surgery. A total of 227 patients were randomly assigned and data were available for 202 patients who had been followed for at least 5 years. The results of this trial are summarized in the section on adjuvant chemotherapy, but the results of the radiation-alone group are considered here. Of the 58 control subjects, 33 (55%) developed recurrence, of whom 20 (34%) developed distant recurrence and 12 (21%) developed local recurrence. In the group of 50 patients who received radiation only, 24 patients (48%) recurred – 15 distally (30%) and 9 locally (18%). Overall survival also did not differ significantly between the irradiated and non-irradiated groups.

Balslev et al (1986) from Denmark reported on their randomized postoperative radiotherapy trial: 494 patients with Dukes' B and C rectal cancer were randomized to receive either surgery alone or

Table 33.5 Mortality in prospective trials comparing postoperative adjuvant radiotherapy with no radiotherapy (including trial with identical chemotherapy for both treatment and control groups).

Trials	Dose (Gy)	Deaths/No. entered: Radiotherapy	Deaths/No. entered: Control	Odds ratio* comparing treatment with control mortality rates
Denmark	50	105/244	104/250	
GITSG-7175	40	49/101	63/110	
NSABP R-01	46	113/184	116/184	
MRC 3	40	23/180	39/189	
Total postoperative		290/709	322/733	14%±11
				Treatment better / Treatment better

* For each trial the observed odds reduction in the figures is represented by a black square, with its 99% confidence interval as a horizontal line. A diamond shape represents the odds reduction and 95% confidence interval for the overview of the individual trials.
(From Gray et al, 1991).

surgery plus 50 Gy of postoperative radiotherapy. Severe complications from the radiotherapy occurred in 10% of patients. Overall survival was not affected but patients with Dukes' C tumours had a reduced incidence of local recurrence. Fisher et al (1988) on behalf of the NSABP Group randomized 368 patients and detected no significant reduction in local recurrence or survival in those patients receiving 46.5 Gy postoperatively.

The most recent trial was that carried out in the United Kingdom by the MRC (MRC Working Party, 1996b). This was a relatively small trial in patients with mobile rectal cancers: 145 of 235 were allocated to surgery alone and 139 received postoperative radiotherapy. The dose of radiation was 40 Gy in 20 fractions of 2 Gy given over 4 weeks. At 5 years, 79 patients who received surgery alone and 49 who received radiotherapy developed local recurrence ($P < 0.001$). However, there was no difference in the development of distant metastases or survival.

Various non-randomized trials have been performed. Thus Mohiuddin et al (1981) reported on the results of 37 patients with Dukes' B and C lesions who were scheduled for postoperative therapy. Unfortunately only 21 of these patients received the prescribed radiation dose of 45 Gy, the remainder being withdrawn either by the surgeon or because the patient refused further therapy. In addition to postoperative treatment all patients received 5 Gy preoperatively. The results of this 'selective sandwich technique' are difficult to interpret as the numbers were so small and there was no adequate unselected control group (Marks et al, 1985, 1990; Mohiuddin et al, 1979, 1985). The authors chose to use the withdrawal group as a form of control. They reported that two of the 21 patients (9.5%) who received postoperative radiotherapy had recurrence but neither of these was a local pelvic recurrence. Of the 16 control patients, three (19%) developed pelvic recurrence and two (12.5%) developed distant metastases.

Other uncontrolled trials have reported similar encouraging results with regard to the incidence of pelvic recurrence. Thus, Hoskins et al (1985) reported from the Massachusetts General Hospital where 97 patients receiving a minimum of 50.4 Gy were compared with a group of 103 patients previously treated by surgery alone. The overall incidence of local failure was 39% in the surgery-alone group and 9% in the irradiated group. There was no difference in disease-free survival for node-negative patients. However, for node-positive patients there was a trend towards improved survival after 2 years. The complication rate also appeared to be comparable apart from diarrhoea and dysuria, which were more common following radiotherapy.

These uncontrolled studies thus suggest that pelvic recurrence can be reduced by postoperative radiotherapy, and this has been confirmed by at least one prospective study (MRC Working Party, 1996b). This difference may be even more evident if radiotherapy were confined to patients with proven residual microscopic disease and no distant metastasis. However, even if postoperative radiotherapy was found to be unequivocally as effective as preoperative, it is unlikely that it will prove to be popular. Patient compliance seems to be less when the radiotherapy is administered postoperatively, and earlier morbidity is greater. Thus, in the second MRC trial 90% of patients allocated preoperative radiotherapy received it in the scheduled period. The corresponding figure for the third MRC (postoperative) trial was 75% (MRC Working Party 1996b). In addition, twice as many patients experienced nausea, abdominal pain and urinary symptoms in this trial. There was an excess of diarrhoea (46% versus 33%) and of obstruction and colovesical fistula (James et al, 1996).

Adjuvant radiotherapy for colon cancer

The survival advantage reported by some authors using adjuvant radiotherapy for rectal cancer has led others to study adjuvant radiotherapy in colon cancer (Coltman, 1982; Moertel, 1982). Preliminary reports were encouraging (Balslev et al, 1986; Willett et al, 1987) but more data are needed. However, even if radiotherapy proved to be beneficial, morbidity from irradiation of the small intestine is likely to prove a problem which would restrict its use.

Adjuvant intraoperative radiotherapy

Intraoperative electron beam radiation therapy is being assessed in several centres in the USA, Japan and Europe in an attempt to achieve better local control of colorectal cancer, particularly in patients with extensive disease. Gunderson et al (1988) combined intraoperative radiotherapy (10–20 Gy) with external beam irradiation (45–55 Gy). They regarded local control to be acceptable; however, as might be expected, toxicity was high. Sischy and colleagues have also reported the use of intraoperative radiotherapy in a small number of patients (Sischy and Remington, 1975; Sischy, 1982, 1991; Sischy et al, 1985, 1988).

Kallinowski et al (1995) reported their experience in Heidelberg. They treated 40 primary and 20 recurrent adenocarcinomas of the rectum with intraoperative radiation. Treatment was combined with pre- and postoperative irradiation and 5FU and leucovorin therapy, and 42 tumours were completely excised. Residual disease was microscopically detectable in 10 patients. In eight patients, residual tumour was evident macroscopically. Postoperatively, wound infection occurred in six patients and anastomotic dehiscence in four. After follow-up at 26 months, 46 patients were free of disease. Local recurrence and distant metastases were detected in two patients each. Ten patients died of their disease.

Weinstein et al (1995) in Houston used an intraoperative dose of radiotherapy (10–20 Gy) in 11 patients with locally extensive rectal cancers. This again was combined with chemoirradiation. The authors claimed that this combination of therapy reduced local recurrence compared with historical controls, but the numbers treated were too small to draw any firm conclusions. As yet, no prospective controlled trials have been reported, so we do not know whether this form of treatment will be beneficial. However, we do know both from these early clinical studies and animal experiments (Seifert et al, 1995) that postoperative morbidity is increased.

Palliative radiotherapy for rectal cancer

Palliative radiotherapy may be used for rectal cancers that are considered at the outset to be inoperable, or for the treatment of local recurrence, particularly in the pelvis (Horiot, 1991; Gunderson et al, 1992; Papillon and Berard, 1992). In most centres it is rare for tumours to be considered inoperable, and hence radiotherapy is infrequently required outside clinical trials. Certain surgeons do use this modality in an attempt to convert an inoperable lesion to an operable one. There are also several reports of small series of patients with inoperable carcinoma who have been treated by radiotherapy alone. This has invariably been by external beam radiation as opposed to intracavitary therapy. Occasionally long-term survival is reported.

Wang and Schultz (1962) treated 16 patients by radiotherapy alone, two of whom survived 5 years. These authors noted that pain relief and arrest of bleeding could be achieved with 20–30 Gy, but a dose of 50 Gy was required to achieve regression of tumour masses. The duration of palliation was proportional to the dose administered. Stearns and Leaming (1975) suggested an alternative approach using lower doses of approximately 20 Gy, which could be repeated if necessary.

The largest series of patients with inoperable lesions treated by radiation alone was reported by Rider at the Princess Margaret Hospital in Toronto (Rider, 1975; Cummings et al, 1981): 123 patients were treated by radical external beam radiation therapy from 1970 to 1977. In the 67 patients who presented with tumour fixation, local control was achieved in only six cases (9%) and their 5-year survival rate was 8%. Of the 56 patients who presented with mobile cancers, but for reasons such as poor general health and the presence of metastases were considered to be inoperable, local control was achieved in 21 patients (38%) and the 5-year actuarial survival rate was 40%.

Bjerkeset and Dahl (1980) considered that 30 of their 130 consecutive patients (23%) had inoperable tumours, and treated them with external irradiation: 16 of the 30 (53%) after completion of the radiotherapy course were subsequently found to have operable tumours; 11 (37%) were considered permanently inoperable, but six of these patients had good palliation; but in two patients palliation of pain was only brief. Only one of these 11 patients was alive at the time the study was reported, the remainder dying an average of 12 months after irradiation.

In summary, palliative radiotherapy is perhaps best reserved for patients with locally advanced lesions with the aim of converting an inoperable lesion into an operable one. Rarely radiotherapy may be used when a patient is symptomatic and the tumour is too large for local excision, laser ablation or intracavitary radiotherapy, the patient is too sick to undergo any form of major surgery, or in individuals in whom metastases are present.

ADJUVANT CHEMOTHERAPY FOR COLORECTAL CANCER

In an attempt to improve the relatively static survival rates that have been achieved by surgery alone, various forms of adjuvant chemotherapy have been tried in colorectal carcinoma (Lawrence et al, 1978; Davis, 1982). Adjuvant chemotherapy has been tried for this condition since the 1950s. Much of the stimulus resulted from the work of Cole et al (1954). They confirmed previous observations that the peripheral blood of patients with carcinoma may carry cells closely resembling the neoplastic cells of the primary tumour and that during operative manipulation the number of tumour cells in the peripheral blood is greatly increased. A preponderance of these cells both singly and in clumps are in the venous blood draining the tumour area. Whether these cells are viable and whether they have the ability to seed and form metastases is debatable. Nevertheless the aim of adjuvant chemotherapy has been to kill these cells as they leave the tumour and pass round the circulation. In most studies adjuvant cytotoxic agents have been given at the end of the procedure and in the early postoperative period. Some studies, however, have attempted also to administer therapy during the operation (Taylor, 1978, 1981, 1982; Taylor et al, 1979a, 1985).

Studies using single agents

The first studies by Cole and his colleagues used mustine hydrochloride which was injected into a tributary of the portal vein and into a peripheral vein immediately after a curative procedure had been performed (Cruz et al, 1956; Mrazek et al, 1959). Controlled clinical trials, however, were first performed using thiotepa. Two large co-operative groups composed of Veterans Administration (VA) hospitals and university hospitals were involved using this agent (Holden et al, 1967; Dixon et al, 1971). The thiotepa was given intravenously and intraperitoneally at the conclusion of the operation and continued subsequently systemically during the postoperative period. Almost 1900 patients with colorectal cancer were entered into these two surgical trials, but no benefit was demonstrated from the adjuvant therapy.

After ending the entry of patients into these trials the VA surgical group next ran a study using 5-fluorodeoxyuridine. Three doses of 20 mg/kg were given intravenously daily on the first 3 days after operation, followed by a second course of five injections between the fourth and fifth weeks (Dwight et al, 1973). Once again, no significant survival benefit could be shown in this trial either overall or for the various subgroups.

After completing the accrual of patients to the previous trial the VA group began yet another using fluorouracil (Higgins et al, 1976). Fluorouracil (5FU) was given intravenously over 5 days beginning 1–2 weeks after operation with another 5-day course given 6 weeks later. Patients were divided into three separate groups on pathological criteria: these were curative resection, pathologically proven palliative resection, and clinically palliative resection. A total of 496 patients were thus randomized. In a further study the 'curative' patients were given 5-day courses of 5FU beginning as soon after operation as was possible and continued at 6-week intervals for 18 months; these patients were compared with controls. Patients with histological proof of residual disease also received the drug in the same dosage indefinitely and were compared with controls. A total of 685 patients were entered into this second study. Thus the 1181 patients entered into these two protocols actually participated in five separate trials and in every instance the survival rates of patients given chemotherapy were statistically superior to those treated by surgery alone (Table 33.6) (Higgins et al, 1978).

The Central Oncology Group also ran a randomized trial using 5FU in patients undergoing surgical resection (Grage et al, 1979). The drug was given in a dose of 12 mg/kg per day for 4 days, followed by 6 mg/kg per day on alternate days for a further 5 days; thereafter a weekly injection of 12 mg/kg was given for 1 year. For the 289 patients considered suitable for the final analysis, there was a small but consistent benefit to the patients receiving 5FU as regards their disease-free interval and survival rate. The benefit was pronounced in patients with positive lymph nodes and those with a primary lesion in the rectum.

Table 33.6 Survival data for 1159 patients with colorectal cancer treated by the VA Surgical Oncology Group within two trials of adjuvant chemotherapy using fluorouracil.

Patient group	n	Period of chemotherapy	Observed survival Treated (%)	Observed survival Control (%)
5FU trial				
'Curative' resection	308	5 years	58.2	48.0
Proven palliative	70	18 months	35.7	16.7
Clinically palliative	55	18 months	53.6	31.3
5FU PIT trial				
'Curative' resection	522	5 years	49.1	33.7
Proven palliative	163	18 months	37.7	26.8

Adapted from Higgins (1983).

Another study of adjuvant 5FU after curative resection was reported from the Nassau Hospital in Mineola, New York (Li and Ross, 1976). A substantial treatment benefit was demonstrated in patients receiving the drug, but these results must be treated with caution since historical controls from the same hospital were used.

Taylor and his colleagues from Southampton used adjuvant systemic 5FU treatment in a different way, infusing the drug directly into the portal vein and hence the liver during and after curative resection of colorectal cancer. Apart from killing cells released at the time of surgery into the circulation, it was hoped that this form of therapy would destroy any micrometastases that might have already established themselves within the liver. It is known that approximately 20% of patients who are thought by the surgeon to have undergone curative resection have micrometastases in the liver at the time of operation, from which they eventually die (Finlay and McArdle, 1982). These deposits have a high growth fraction and should thus be more sensitive to cytotoxic therapy than bulkier tumours. This trial was commenced in 1975 and a follow-up report appeared in 1985 (Taylor et al, 1979a, 1985; Taylor, 1981). At that stage 257 patients with a primary colorectal carcinoma but without obvious liver metastases had been randomized into the study. Before preoperative randomization all patients had either a technetium-99m sulphur colloid liver scan or ultrasound scan to exclude the presence of synchronous liver metastases. Following standard surgical resection of the primary tumour, patients were randomized to receive either surgery alone or surgery and adjuvant therapy using 1 g of 5FU with 5000 units of heparin in 5% dextrose perfused through the portal vein. Access to the portal vein was achieved by cannulation of the obliterated umbilical vein (Bayly and Garbalhaes, 1964). The infusion was commenced immediately and was continued for 24 hours each day for 7 days.

The patients were followed up at 3-monthly intervals for the first year and at 6-monthly intervals thereafter. Liver scans were obtained at each visit. After exclusions, 127 patients constituted the control group and 117 patients received adjuvant therapy. Overall survival and recurrence were significantly improved in the adjuvant chemotherapy group compared with the controls. When the groups were subdivided according to whether the cancer was rectal or colonic, there was no significant benefit for patients with rectal cancer. When the colonic cancers were subdivided according to Dukes' stage, although there appeared to be an advantage in the perfusion group this reached statistical significance only with the Dukes' B colon cancers (Figure 33.4).

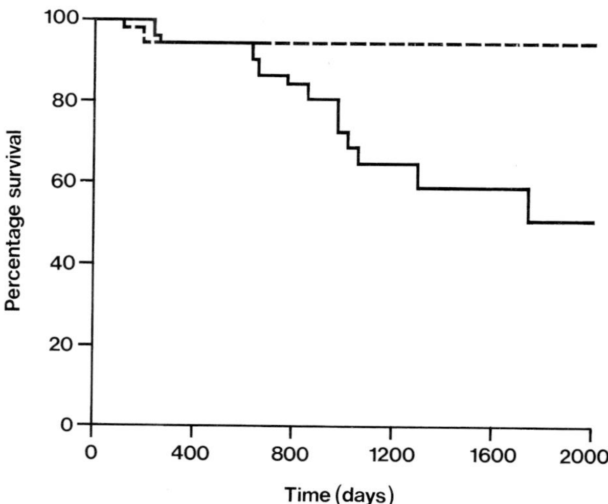

Figure 33.4 Survival analysis of patients with Dukes' B colon cancer in a study of portal perfusion of 5FU. ——, controls; - - -, perfusion; $P < 0.002$ (Taylor et al, 1985).

The technique of intraportal perfusion appeared to be relatively safe although there was one death in the perfusion group due to inadequate monitoring of the cytotoxic agent. Diarrhoea was common in the chemotherapy group but was invariably self-limiting. It did look as though this form of therapy might benefit some patients with colorectal cancer, particularly those with Dukes' B lesions. The authors, however, pointed out quite rightly that the numbers of patients were as yet quite small and before being certain of their findings they must be confirmed by larger, multicentre trials. As a consequence at least 10 subsequent studies were undertaken, some of which used additional agents apart from 5FU. A meta-analysis of some of these trials in 1991 (Gray et al, 1991; see Table 33.7) did show that, although the size of the mortality reduction originally reported by Taylor et al (1985) could not be confirmed, there appeared to be a survival benefit for portal vein infusion of 5FU. Subsequent reports have demonstrated this benefit, particularly for Dukes' C cases. Thus, the Swiss Group (SAKK, 1995) reported a 25% incidence of relapse confined to the liver in the control arm compared with 12% in the portal vein infusion group in node-positive patients. Overall, portal vein infusion reduced the risk of recurrence by 21% and the risk of death by 26%. The major risk reduction was in patients with Dukes' C disease, as indeed was the overall absolute survival improvement.

A meta-analysis of all 10 published trials of portal vein cytotoxic infusion, including a total of 3499 patients, has provided confirmatory evidence of benefit (Piedbois et al, 1995). Overall, portal vein infusion was associated with a mean 18% reduction in the annual risk of death from any cause with a 20% reduction in death from colorectal cancer (standard deviation 6% in each instance). The benefit was significantly greater for Dukes' C patients (54% versus 46.6%) than for Dukes' B patients (76.3% versus 71%).

The largest prospective trial (AXIS) mounted in the UK to test the benefit of portal vein infusion of 5FU has yet to report. So far 3500 patients have been randomized, the target being 4000. The results of this trial are eagerly awaited, as it should determine

Table 33.7 Mortality estimates in colorectal cancer trials comparing portal vein infusion of fluorouracil (sometimes in conjunction with mitomycin) with no adjuvant treatment.

	Deaths/No. entered		
Trials	*Radiotherapy*	*Control*	*Odds ratio* comparing treatment with control mortality rates*
First trial			
Liverpool/Southampton (Taylor et al, 1985)	26/117	54/127	60%±18
Subsequent trials			
Australia/NZ (Gray, 1990)	18/85	29/84	
SAKK† (Metzger et al, 1987)	66/236	88/233	
Rotterdam (Wereldsma et al, 1990)	28/99	35/102	
Virginia Mason†‡ (Ryan et al, 1988)	10/77	10/77	
NCCTG/Mayo (Beart, 1990)	37/110	32/109	
St Mary's‡ (Fielding et al, 1989)	22/145	26/130	
NSABP‡ (Wolmark et al, 1990)	65/438	85/461	
Subtotal of subsequent trials (observed–expected – 29.2, variance 102.7)	246/1190	305/1196	25%±9
All trials (observed–expected – 41.6, variance 116.6)	272/1307	359/1323	30%±8

Treatment better | Treatment worse

Treatment effect 2P<0.001
Test for heterogeneity: χ^2_7 = 9.8; NS

* For each trial the observed odds reduction in the figures is represented by a black square with its 99% confidence interval as a horizontal line. A diamond shape represents the odds reduction and 95% confidence interval for the overview of the individual trials.

† Fluorouracil plus mitomycin.

‡ Actual data not available: best estimate from available information.

From Gray et al (1991).

conclusively the benefits or otherwise of this form of therapy.

Intraluminal therapy

Rousselot et al (1972) studied an alternative method of delivering adjuvant therapy. They injected 5FU into the lumen of the segment of colon to be resected. The theory was that cells released into the lumen of the bowel might be destroyed, after which the drug would be absorbed through the veins draining the colonic segment into the portal system and there destroy cells that had been liberated from the tumour. In these workers' last report (Grossi et al, 1977) of 500 patients entered over 7 years, no significant difference was demonstrated in overall survival. However, patients with unfavourable prognostic signs, such as serosal penetration, Dukes' C stage or a combination of serosal involvement and positive lymph nodes, seemed to benefit from this form of adjuvant therapy. It is difficult to interpret this trial since comparisons were made with an historical control group.

Lawrence et al (1975) entered 203 patients in a similar trial to that of Rousselot and colleagues, but also gave the treatment group oral 5FU during the postoperative period. No significant difference in survival rates was observed between the groups. As far as we are aware, there have been no further reports on this form of therapy, and the reader should assume it is now obsolete.

Intraperitoneal chemotherapy

Sugarbaker and his group believed that intraperitoneal delivery of 5FU reduces the risk of recurrent peritoneal carcinomatosis and in this regard is more effective than intravenous adjuvant chemotherapy (Sugarbaker et al, 1985). It remains to be seen whether this route of administration will be more beneficial than any other route.

Studies using several agents

The VA Surgical Oncology Group performed a randomized trial using a combination of methyl-CCNU and fluorouracil as intermittent courses for 1 year (Higgins et al, 1984a,b). Patients were entered into the trial between 1973 and 1979; the study included patients in whom there was no microscopic evidence of residual disease but whose resected specimen showed evidence of disease spread (serosal penetration, invasion into perirectal fat, blood vessel invasion, lymphatic invasion, lymph node involvement and cancer in other organs included in the resection). These patients were randomized to receive either no adjuvant therapy or chemotherapy with 5FU and methyl-CCNU. Treated patients experienced a slightly more favourable survival rate than did controls. However, the difference appeared to be confined to patients with one to four positive lymph nodes in the resected specimen (treated group 5-year survival 51.3%; controls 31.0%).

The Gastrointestinal Tumour Study Group (GITSG, 1984) also reported an important study in which combination adjuvant chemotherapy (methyl-CCNU and 5FU) was compared with (a) surgical treatment alone, (b) immunotherapy in the form of methanol extraction residue of bacillus Calmette-Guerin (BCG), or (c) a combination of immunotherapy and chemotherapy. Only patients who had undergone 'curative' surgical resection were included. The patients were stratified according to anatomical localization of tumour and Dukes' stage, and they were followed up for a median period of 5 years. No significant difference in survival rates could be demonstrated between the groups. This finding was perhaps related to the fact that the 5-year survival rate was very high (68%) in the surgery-only group, which underlines the need in all trials of this kind to include a control group. One very important point to emerge from the study was that leukaemia developed in seven patients who had received chemotherapy alone. This worrying aspect of adjuvant combination chemotherapy was further highlighted by a study carried out by the VA Surgical Oncology Group (VASOG) (Boice et al, 1983). Among their 2067 patients who received methyl-CCNU as adjuvant therapy for gastrointestinal cancer, leukaemic disorders developed in 14 patients, whereas only one case of leukaemia occurred among 1566 patients given other therapies. It would seem, therefore, that the nitrosoureas are leukaemogenic in humans and that adjuvant chemotherapy with alkylating agents may increase the risk of leukaemia.

Both the GITSG and VASOG studies failed to demonstrate any overall worthwhile increase in survival for patients receiving combination adjuvant chemotherapy, although patients with one to four involved lymph nodes might have derived some benefit. When the results of most other studies are taken into consideration, it appears that the addition of methyl-CCNU to 5FU makes little difference to survival. Indeed, because of the potential risk of methyl-CCNU it was our view until recently that it should not be included in any adjuvant regimen. However, reports from the National Surgical Adjuvant Breast and Bowel Project Group (NSABP) in the USA (Wolmark et al, 1988) have caused us to rethink the situation.

In their first study, 1166 patients with Dukes' B and C colon cancers were randomized into one of three groups following curative surgery (Wolmark et al, 1983). One group had no further treatment; one received postoperative 5FU, methyl-CCNU and vincristine; and the remaining group received postoperative BCG. There was an overall significant improvement in both disease-free survival and recurrence in favour of the chemotherapy group. No improvement was evident in patients who received BCG. This was the first large, randomized study of its type to show an improvement in overall survival with systemic adjuvant chemotherapy. In the second study performed by the same group, 555 patients with Dukes' B and C rectal cancers were randomized to receive surgery alone, postoperative chemotherapy (the same regimen as for the colon study), or radiotherapy alone. There was a statistically significant benefit for adjuvant chemotherapy although this appeared to be restricted to males. Other studies still in progress also suggest a marginal benefit in survival for patients who receive prolonged systemic adjuvant therapy consisting of methyl-CCNU and 5FU, with or without vincristine (Table 33.8). These studies have therefore coloured our views concerning adjuvant combination chemotherapy; however, we still feel that the disadvantages of this form of therapy which utilizes methyl-CCNU outweigh the advantages and such treatment cannot be recommended.

The same may not be the case with combinations of 5FU and folinic acid. Folinic acid (FA) modulates the activity of 5FU by stabilizing the ternary complex of FdUMP with thymidylate synthetase, therefore increasing the degree of inhibition of the enzyme and enhancing the likelihood of cell death following thymidine depletion (Figure 33.5). Meta-analysis of the results in advanced disease has shown that the response rate for the 5FU/FA combination is 23% compared with 9% for single-agent FU, and there is a trend towards improved overall survival in the 5FU/FA groups (Advanced Colorectal Cancer Meta-analysis Project, 1992). Such data have led to the use of this combination in adjuvant therapy. More recent studies which recruited almost 3000 patients and compared a non-treatment control versus 6 months' treatment with the combination suggest a survival benefit. First, an overview of three randomized studies from Italy, France and Canada that had tested 6 months' of 5FU with high doses of FA (250 mg/m^2) reported a significant benefit of this combination in terms of recurrence-free survival, but not to date in survival (Zaniboni et al, 1993). Second, an American inter-group study of 5FU with much lower doses of FA (20 mg/m^2) has reported a significant reduction in recurrence-free survival, but not in survival (O'Connell et al, 1993). Finally, an NSABP study comparing 5FU and very-high-dose FA (500 mg/m^2) with combination methyl-CCNU + vincristine + 5FU (MOF) has

Table 33.8 Mortality in published trials comparing prolonged, adjuvant, systemic, multiple agent chemotherapy with no chemotherapy (including trials with identical radiotherapy for both treatment and control groups).

Trials	Treatment and duration	Deaths/No. entered: Chemotherapy	Deaths/No. entered: Control	O-E	Variance	Odds ratio* comparing treatment with control mortality rates
VASOG-27	5FU + MeCCNU 1 year	148/327	160/318	−8.1	40.3	
GITSG-6175	TFU + MeCCNU 16 months	70/156	71/159	0.2	19.5	
Vienna	5FU + MMC + AraC 3 months	25/59	21/62	2.6	7.2	
GITSG-7175	5FU + MeCCNU 18 months	30/58	37/62	−2.4	7.5	
SWOG-7510	5FU + MeCCNU 1 year	48/95	48/94	−0.3	11.9	
NSABP R-01	5FU + V + MeCCNU 18 months	78/187	95/184	−9.2	23.1	
NSABP C-01	5FU + V + MeCCNU 18 months	141/358	162/383	−5.4	44.8	
Subtotal: multiple agents		540/1240	594/1262	−22.5	154.3	14%±7 Treatment better / Treatment worse

AraC, arabinose; 5FU, fluorouracil; MeCCNU, methyl-CCNU; MMC, mitomycin; V, vincristine.

* For each trial the observed odds reduction in the figures is represented by a black square with its 95% confidence interval as a horizontal line. A diamond shape represents the odds reduction and 95% confidence interval for the overview of the individual trials.

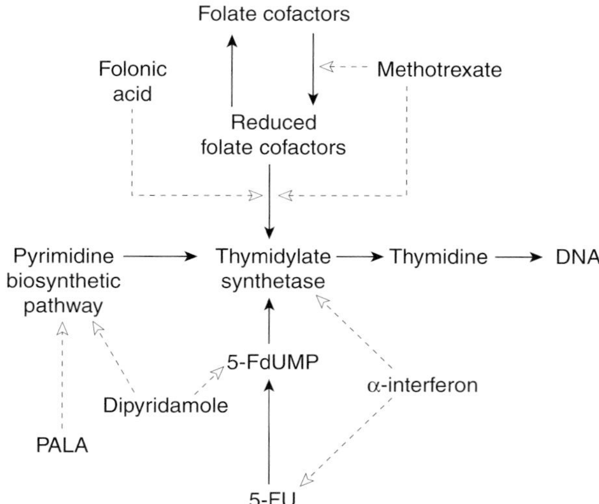

Figure 33.5 Biochemical modulation of 5-FU.

shown a significant improvement in recurrence-free survival and also a survival benefit for the 5FU/FA combination (Wolmark et al, 1993).

These early results are encouraging and suggest that the combination of 5FU and folinic acid is less toxic than combinations which include methyl-CCNU. However, it is not known whether low-dose FA is as effective as high-dose FA, or whether the addition of levamisole (see later) is of any benefit. In addition, there is still real doubt about the size of the survival benefit relative to toxicity, quality of life and health service resource usage (Kerr, 1995). A recent survey by the United Kingdom Co-ordinating Committee on Cancer Research (UKCCCR) suggested that less than 50% of clinicians polled in the UK offer adjuvant chemotherapy to colorectal cancer patients.

With these points in mind, the UKCCCR has instituted the QUASAR trial which attempts to answer some of these questions. Patients without metastases or apparent residual disease for whom there is substantial uncertainty over whether or not they should receive chemotherapy in addition to surgery are randomized equally between chemotherapy and control groups. Patients with a clear indication for chemotherapy, but for whom there is substantial uncertainty which regimen to use, are randomized between chemotherapy options. The chemotherapy tested is a practical outpatient regimen involving intravenous 5FU combined with either low-dose or high-dose L-folinic acid, and either levamisole or placebo. QUASAR aims to randomize 8000 patients with the aim of providing an opportunity for surgeons and oncologists to rationalize treatment options.

COMBINATION OF ADJUVANT RADIOTHERAPY AND CHEMOTHERAPY

Although the GITSG study showed that neither postoperative radiotherapy nor 5FU alone improved survival (GITSG, 1985), the combination of the two did appear to be beneficial in patients with rectal cancer (Figure 33.6). Both 5-year survival and disease-free interval were significantly better than in the control group and the other treatment groups. Nevertheless, the toxicity of the combined treatment was high (35%) and only 30 out of the 46 patients assigned to this therapy completed the regimen. Sparso et al (1984) experienced similar problems in their randomized trial using combined irradiation, 5FU and methotrexate. In fact these authors had to abandon the trial after the accrual of only 34 patients because of serious complications.

However, recent advances in the administration of adjuvant chemotherapy make the combination of radiotherapy and chemotherapy more feasible. In order for chemotherapy to improve the effectiveness of DXT, it must be present in the tumour at the time of DXT-inflicted DNA damage is being repaired. The biological half-life of 5FU is approxi-

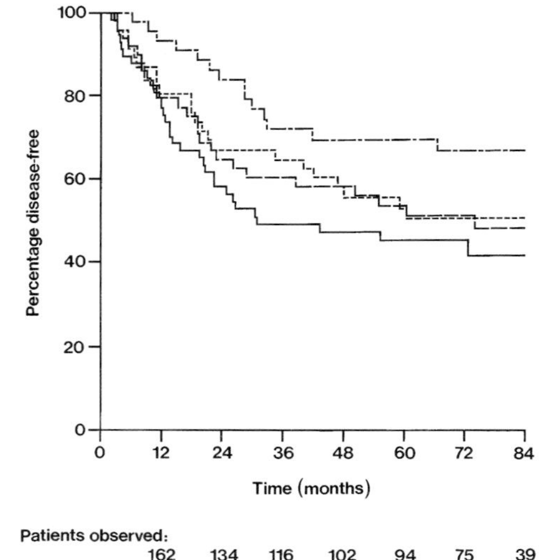

Figure 33.6 Gastrointestinal Tumour Study Group results showing significant improvement in survival of patients receiving a combination of adjuvant 5FU and methyl-CCNU chemotherapy and radiotherapy. ——, Controls; - - - , chemotherapy; – – –, radiotherapy; – - –, combined radiotherapy and chemotherapy.

mately 20 minutes, and thus the chemotherapy needs to be given while the patient is on the DXT machine. Such therapy is called *concomitant treatment*. Modern techniques of giving cytotoxics by continuous ambulatory infusion have made this more feasible. A North Central Cancer Treatment Group trial (NCCTG 86.47.51) is comparing the enhancement of postoperative DXT by concomitant 5FU delivered by bolus injection or continuous infusion. A planned interim analysis at 3 years (Gunderson, 1994) showed a significant advantage to infusion in terms of 3-year survival, local recurrence and distant metastases. If the chemotherapy is not intended as a specific radiosensitizer, it may be given at another time. Such sequential therapy is likely to be less toxic than concomitant therapy. Two further trials (G1 7175 and NCCTG 79-47-51) have shown a survival advantage in rectal cancer patients for postoperative DXT plus chemotherapy compared with postoperative DXT alone. Both trials used a combination of concomitant and sequential techniques (Krook et al, 1991, GITSG, 1992).

In contrast, an Eastern Co-operative Oncology Group trial (ECOG) showed no advantage for postoperative DXT plus chemotherapy when a sequential technique was used (Mansour et al, 1991). However, such a regime may downstage the tumour sufficiently to allow a less extensive operation to be performed.

ADJUVANT IMMUNOTHERAPY

Both the GITSG (1984) and the NSABP (Wolmark et al, 1988) studies included immunotherapy alone as one arm of the trial. This was in the form of methanol extraction residue (MER) of BCG. No benefit was derived from this form of therapy in either trial. Several other studies which have used similar immunotherapeutic agents as part of their adjuvant regimen for colorectal cancer have also reached similar conclusions. Thus patients with Dukes' C tumours treated at the Mayo Clinic or at the M. D. Anderson Hospital did not benefit from a combination of 5FU and immunotherapy (MER BCG or BCG) (Mavligit et al, 1976; Moertel, 1978).

Other immunotherapeutic agents than BCG are being used for adjuvant therapy. Thus *Corynebacterium parvum*, another non-specific immunostimulator, was investigated (Gill, 1980); however, preliminary results suggested that it was of little use. Animal experiments in a rat model of colorectal carcinoma suggested that levamisole might be a useful agent (House and Maley, 1983). Several clinical studies were therefore initiated using levamisole (Bancewicz et al, 1980; Laurie, 1982; Shiraki et al, 1982), and two (Windle et al, 1987; Moertel et al, 1990) demonstrated a significant survival advantage in patients treated with a combination of levamisole and 5FU.

The study by Moertel et al (1990) in the USA in particular excited both clinicians and the general public. In this study 1296 patients with colon cancer were randomized to levamisole and 5FU therapy, levamisole therapy alone, or a control group. The patients on levamisole alone continued their therapy for 1 year and those on the combination therapy continued for 2 years. The study showed that the combination of levamisole and 5FU significantly reduced the risk of recurrence by 41% (Figure 33.7); it also reduced the overall death rate by 33%, but only in patients with Dukes' C (stage III) carcinomas. In an updated analysis of this trial (median follow-up 5 years), the improvements in recurrence and survival have persisted at comparable levels of significance (Moertel, 1992, 1994). As a consequence the National Institutes of Health stated that adjuvant chemotherapy should be standard practice for patients with Dukes' C colonic carcinomas and that it was no longer justifiable to set up trials with the 'no treatment' control arm (NIH, 1990). This statement has resulted in most surgeons in the USA using 5FU and levamisole or folinic acid as adjuvant therapy for all patients with colonic cancer (Mayer, 1990; Vanchieri, 1990).

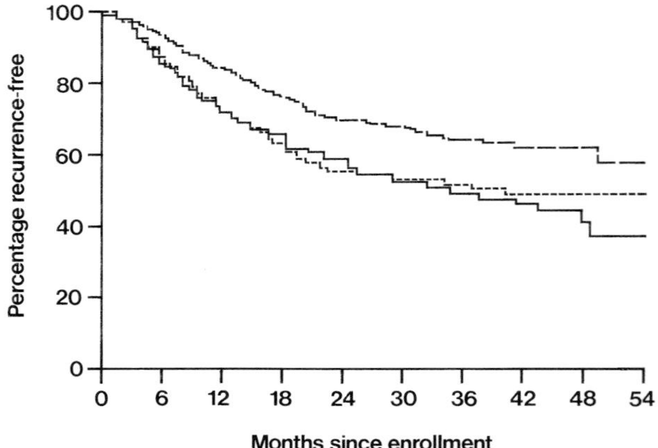

Figure 33.7 Study by Moertel and associates demonstrating significant improvement in recurrence-free interval of patients receiving adjuvant levamisole and 5FU. – – –, Levamisole + 5-FU; - - -, levamisole; ——, observation (Moertel et al, 1990).

The attitude in Europe is far more variable (Editorial, 1990; Wills and Wagener, 1990). Though most clinicians are now more optimistic in their attitude to adjuvant therapy for cancer of the colon, many believe that studies have not yet established that the reduction in mortality outweighs the toxicity and inconvenience of the treatment, and consider that trials should still include an untreated control arm (Slevin and Gray, 1991). The QUASAR study mentioned previously, which introduces the uncertainty principle into a clinical trial, caters for all views, and in our opinion solves the dilemma for clinicians.

A potentially exciting development in immunotherapy was the isolation and manufacture by recombinant technology of interleukin 2 (IL-2) and its subsequent use to generate lymphokine-activated killer cells (LAK) (Rosenberg et al, 1987). Although such adoptive immunotherapy seemed to be effective for melanoma and renal cell carcinoma, it was found to be not only ineffective but very toxic in patients with colorectal cancer.

Conclusions and future developments

Gradually optimism is being expressed concerning adjuvant chemotherapy and immunotherapy for colorectal cancer. Certainly it looks as if portal perfusion of 5FU and perhaps other agents delivered via this route during the perioperative period will have a role. Furthermore, the substantial benefit shown by Moertel's group with levamisole and 5FU seems promising, as do the studies with 5FU and folinic acid. Indeed, it now seems that the 5FU/FA combination is as effective as when 5FU is combined with levamisole (Haller et al, 1996). The combination of radiotherapy and portal infusion of 5FU for rectal cancer may also be beneficial and is the subject of the AXIS trial set up by the UK Co-ordinating Committee on Cancer Research. Until the results of this and other trials – particularly QUASAR – are known, we agree with the advice in the *Guidelines for the Management of Colorectal Cancer* published by the Royal College of Surgeons of England and the Association of Coloproctology of Great Britain and Ireland (RCS/ACGBI, 1996). Thus, it is recommended that patients with Dukes' C colorectal cancer who are medically and psychologically fit are either offered entry into a trial or are considered for 5-fluouracil containing adjuvant chemotherapy. To date, no trials have shown a convincing beneficial effect in stage B or A disease, and while entry of such patients into trials is ideal, no definite recommendations can be made. Despite these potential advances, further work needs to be carried out on other treatments and ways of targeting therapy more specifically.

In most studies there are certain groups of patients who respond to adjuvant therapy more positively than other groups (Gérard et al, 1986; Hafstrom et al, 1990); presumably if studies concentrated on these 'responders', overall results would be improved. This highlights the need to stage patients more accurately than hitherto.

Another method of selecting patients who might respond best to adjuvant therapy is to perform *in vitro* sensitivity tests in a similar manner to the way in which antibiotics are selected for treatment of bacterial infection. A variety of techniques have been evaluated. The most popular is the soft agar technique in which the patient's tumour is grown as a monolayer on agar which is impregnated with several antimitotic agents (Salmon et al, 1978). Nude mice tumour xenograft colonies may also be used (Carter, 1982), but both these techniques have limitations and are costly. A more practical *in vitro* system seems to be the use of tumour spheroids (Flowerdew et al, 1987; Britten et al, 1989). These are clumps of tumour cells which grow in culture and have the advantage that they simulate the parent tumour more closely than does the more artificial monolayer technique. Thus the spheroids have an anoxic centre with an outer layer of viable cells. We have demonstrated in rectal carcinomas that the flow cytometric characteristics (i.e. the DNA/RNA constitution) of spheroids are the same as in the parent tumour. Furthermore, when spheroids are injected into nude mice they are able to metastasize to the liver. The success rate of growing spheroids from colorectal cancers is approximately 70–75%, which is much higher than is usual for monolayer agar cultures. It remains to be seen how effective this technique will be in selecting patients for adjuvant therapy (Hunt et al, 1990).

Selection may be improved even more by the use of tumour-specific monoclonal antibodies either alone or conjugated with tumour-toxic agents, such as the vinca alkaloid indesine (Embleton et al, 1983; Ford et al, 1983), the plant toxin ricin, diphtheria toxin (Gilliland et al, 1980) and methotrexate and Adriamycin (Ghose et al, 1981). Each of these has been found to have limited tumour target specificity (Davies, 1981; Carter, 1982). Up to recently there was much scepticism as to the role of monoclonal antibodies in the treatment of colorectal cancer. There were and indeed remain some intellectual problems to be overcome, such as antihuman mouse antibody responses, poor tumour delivery and penetration of the therapeutic antibody, variation in antigen

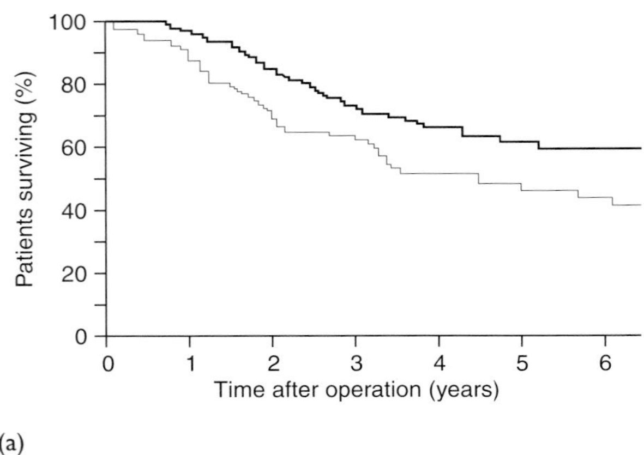

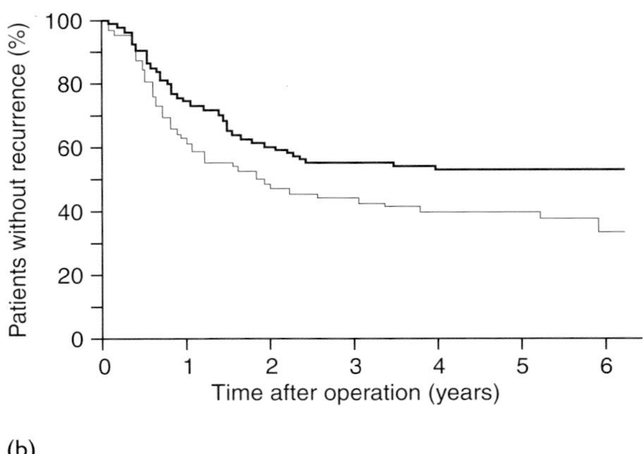

(a) (b)

Figure 33.8a,b (a) Survival curves in adjuvant immunotherapy trial using 17-1A monoclonal antibody. (b) Recurrence rates in adjuvant immunotherapy trial using 17-1A monoclonal antibody (Reithmuller et al, 1994). Bold lines, 17-1A monoclonal antibody; fine lines, surgery only.

expression and cross-reaction with normal tissues. However, a recent trial using the monoclonal antibody directed against 17-1A antigen has suggested there may be a role for this form of therapy. Thus, Reithmuller et al (1994) from Germany adopted a refreshingly different approach using this antibody. Previous studies with monoclonals had used patients with advanced disease. Reithmuller and colleagues argued first that such a large antigenic load and physiological barrier to delivery of antibodies limited their efficiency. Thus, micrometastases present at early stages of the cancer process would constitute more favourable targets. Second, and in particularly because these patients are clinically well, immunotoxins with potentially serious side-effects are not appropriate. Native antibodies, on the other hand, can lead to cellular destruction via complement-mediated lysis, antibody-dependent cellular cytotoxicity or opsonization of cells and subsequent phagocytosis, and in addition intravenous infusions of antibody are tolerated well. Third, a target antigen on normal epithelium may be partly shielded from antibody or accessory molecules and cells, whereas the same antigen may be readily accessible on a cancer cell within a micrometastasis in mesenchymal tissue (Nossal, 1994).

Accordingly, Riethmuller and associates randomized 189 patients with Dukes' C (UICC stage III) colorectal cancer who had undergone 'curative' surgery to receive either the murine $IgG_{2\alpha}$ monoclonal antibody 17-1A or surgery alone. Patients received 500 mg of antibody postoperatively and then 4-monthly infusions of 100 mg. After a median follow-up of 5 years, 51% of patients in the control group and 36% of patients in the treatment group had died, a statistically significant reduction. The treatment also reduced the 5-year recurrence rate from 66.5% to 48.7% (Figure 33.8). Toxic effects were minor, and easily controlled. The results of this study are thus very encouraging, and it has been speculated that if this monoclonal antibody was given in association with chemotherapy even greater benefit might accrue (Nossal, 1994).

Other innovative treatments are being developed for use as adjuvant therapy for colorectal cancer. Thus, there are several potent thymidylate synthetase inhibitors in phase II and III trials which might have a better therapeutic ratio than 5FU/FA. Novel molecular targets have been identified in the therapy of colorectal cancer: topoisomerase I, an enzyme involved in untwisting DNA during replication, isoforms of protein kinase C, and certain tyrosine kinases involved in growth factor–receptor–signal transduction pathways. It is hoped that small-molecular-weight inhibitors of these proteins can be developed (Kerr and Workman, 1994). Similarly, work is proceeding to develop gene therapy strategies against colorectal cancer (Huber et al, 1993).

SURVEILLANCE

There are few surgeons who do not recommend follow-up of all patients after operation for colorectal cancer. Nevertheless, there is no consensus as to the frequency of follow-up, the techniques that should be employed to detect recurrence, or even the benefits to be derived from earlier diagnosis of recurrent diseases. Indeed, there are some who seriously question the value of follow-up at all and maintain that most recurrences are identified between follow-up appointments. Even when recurrence is evident, early treatment has little impact on the natural history of disease. Various prospective studies are in progress which are designed to answer some of these questions.

The aims of follow-up after curative resections for colorectal cancer are the early diagnosis of synchronous neoplasms (if preoperative colonoscopy was not performed); early detection of metachronous disease; identification of local and disseminated recurrence of the original tumour; audit, which may or may not be part of therapeutic trials; and the general management and support of the patients and often their relatives (Killingback, 1986).

Follow-up regimens vary from clinical investigation alone at 3-monthly or 6-monthly intervals, to ultrasound and CT scans of liver and pelvis, serum carcinoembryonic antigen (CEA) measurements and full colonoscopic examination at regular intervals. The extent and aggressiveness of follow-up will vary depending on whether the surgeon believes that early detection and treatment of recurrence will alter prognosis, and whether the surgeon is involved in a clinical trial. Local availability particularly of scanning facilities will also alter the approach to follow-up. The Royal London Hospital has an aggressive follow-up policy; this is because the centre is involved in various trials rather than because of any firm conviction that earlier diagnosis of recurrence will inevitably lead to a better prognosis. The approach at Birmingham is quite different – we have set up an audit which involves our local primary care physicians, so that they have become extensively involved in management of colorectal cancer. We have open access so that these patients may be seen straight away if there are new symptoms. Apart from a postoperative check at 6 weeks, follow-up involves only a CT or liver ultrasound in Dukes' B and C lesions, at 12 months and at 2 years, provided the resection margins were clear.

Clinical evaluation during follow-up is undoubtedly inferior to the more specialized scanning investigations that are now available. Cochrane et al (1980) have illustrated the shortcomings of clinical follow-up: 180 patients were seen for outpatient follow-up over 15 years, involving 2319 visits. Only 42% of recurrences were detected during visits to the clinic, whereas 58% were diagnosed between visits by other clinicians as a result of new symptoms.

A strong argument for not following up any patients with colorectal cancer can be made by surgeons whose practice does not involve specific treatment (Steele, 1986). If a policy of no follow-up is adopted, the patient should be informed of the various symptoms that suggest recurrent or metachronous disease and may require investigation. If a patient develops what appears to be a symptomatic recurrence the appropriate investigations can be performed to delineate the nature of the recurrence so that palliative treatment can be instituted. Most surgeons, even if they do not believe in an aggressive follow-up regimen, are reluctant to discharge their patients immediately after operation. They prefer to see them regularly at least for the first 2–3 years for clinical examination, even though they accept that this is a poor method of detecting recurrence. The reasons for this policy are that it helps to support the patient psychologically, ensures that the surgeon and patient maintain contact, and that any stoma problems can be resolved. It also enables surgeons to maintain an accurate record of their results.

Prior to our involvement in the various clinical trials alluded to previously, we saw our patients every 3 months during the first year after resection, twice during the second year and thereafter annually. At each visit a full clinical examination was performed including rectal examination and rigid sigmoidoscopy, particularly after such operations as low anterior resection and local excision of rectal cancer. A barium enema or more recently a colonoscopy was performed once every 2 years to eliminate a metachronous carcinoma or polyp. Patients who complained of symptoms suggestive of recurrence were intensively investigated with chest radiography, CT scan of pelvis, and ultrasound and CT scans of liver.

Evaluation of intensive follow-up regimens

Tornquist et al (1982) compared two studies with follow-up performed by clinical examination, endoscopy, blood chemistry, chest radiography and barium enema. In the first study of 634 patients, which took 10 years to complete, patients were seen 3 months after operation and then at yearly intervals. These authors concluded that this form of follow-up was of little value in tracing curable recurrence. In a second study of 599 patients during a 5-year period, a more intensive follow-up programme was adopted using the same investigations. The patients were seen every 3 months for the first 2 years, every 6 months for the third and fourth years, and annually thereafter. It was found that the first, less intensive protocol was just as efficient as the second in that rates of potentially curative operations remained virtually the same (14% versus 13%). Thus if these modalities alone are to be used in follow-up, and detection of recurrence is the only aim, annual visits are probably all that is required.

Similar findings have resulted from several more recent studies which have employed more sophisticated imaging techniques – ultrasound, CT or MRI scan – to detect recurrence (Enker and Kramer, 1982; Schiessel et al, 1986; Böhm et al, 1993; Safi et al, 1993). Again, the results are disappointing. The number of patients available for a second operation for cure was very low (3–6%), and the survival after such a procedure was approximately 75% after 12 months, 50% after 24 months and under 25% after 5 years. The question therefore arises as to whether such patients could be cured if they were admitted some months later when they had developed symptoms (Påhlman, 1996).

Many studies in recent years have used repeated serum CEA measurements as a means of detecting recurrence at an early, potentially treatable stage. One of the earliest studies suggesting the benefits of this measurement was reported by Martin et al (1980) at the Ohio State University: 300 patients were followed from 1972 to 1975, of whom 22 (7.3%) had a further operation on the basis of a rise in CEA levels. These patients constituted a retrospective group, while a series of patients seen between 1976 and 1979 were classified as 'prospective'. In the initial group, CEA levels were measured every 3–6 months; in the prospective group, measurements were made at 4–6 weeks in the first year, 6–8 weeks in the second year and then at 3-monthly intervals until 5 years postoperatively. If the CEA value deviated from a normogram, patients underwent extensive non-operative staging and a very early 'second look' operation was then recommended. Of the 22 retrospective patients, 19 were found to have a recurrence but only six (30%) were resectable. In contrast, among the 38 prospective patients identified by a rise in CEA levels, 23 had resectable tumour, 14 had unresectable disease, and one patient had a negative laparotomy. While only two of the 22 retrospective patients were still alive at the time of the report, 22 of 38 patients remained alive in the prospective group. These authors concluded that the prospective use of serial CEA measurements to initiate 'second look' operations was worthwhile, but the long-term outcome in terms of survival advantages remained to be established (Martin et al, 1985).

At the Memorial Sloan Kettering Centre a similar favourable experience with the use of CEA assessment was encountered (Attiyeh and Stearns, 1981). Others have also demonstrated the benefit of such a regimen (Karesen et al, 1980; Pompecki and Winckler, 1980; Sakamoto et al, 1980; Stock et al, 1980). A less enthusiastic view has, however, been reported by others such as Junneman and Derra (1980), Orefice et al (1981) and Beart et al (1981) from the Mayo Clinic. The Mayo Clinic group reported that 34 of 149 patients (23%) who had undergone comprehensive prospective follow-up since 1976 developed recurrence of Dukes' B2 or C lesions within 1–3 years. Patients were seen at least every 15 weeks. Comprehensive physical, laboratory and invasive tests were carried out at regular intervals. Despite the frequency of visits and repeated CEA measurements, 29 of the 34 patients (85%) developed symptoms before or at the time the recurrence was detected by physical, biochemical or radiographic changes. In 25 of the 34 patients (74%) a rise in CEA levels greater than 5 ng/mL was noted at the time of recurrence. Twenty patients had both CEA elevation and symptoms, but nine patients had symptomatic recurrence without any elevation of CEA levels. In another study in which the CEA measurement was combined with comprehensive clinical follow-up, Wedell et al (1981) found that only 15 of 86 patients (17.4%) had raised CEA levels before clinical symptoms of recurrence. Of the 31 patients in whom a 'second look' operation was performed, only 15 had resectable disease. Furthermore, 12 of these 15 patients still had normal CEA values. The majority of patients (78%) had elevated CEA levels only at the time of symptomatic recurrence. Moreover, most resectable tumours were discovered by scanning when the patient's CEA value was still normal. In an attempt to make the CEA measurements more specific and assist in selection of patients for 'second look' procedures, several authors have concentrated on CEA slope analysis (Wood et al, 1980; Boey et al, 1984; Staab et al, 1985). These authors suggest that patients with a slow rise in CEA levels are more likely to have localized resectable disease.

Hence data on the value of CEA monitoring are contradictory and the case for regular CEA estimations remains to be proved. Although serum CEA measurement is not uniformly sensitive or specific it may be a reliable marker of recurrent disease (Northover, 1986). The problem that still remains to be elucidated is whether CEA estimation can detect recurrence at an early enough stage for treatment to be effective. Unfortunately none of the studies so far reported can convincingly answer this question, for none is a prospectively controlled study comparing a CEA-based policy with the usual conventional regimen (Meeker, 1978; Wood et al, 1980; Attiyeh and Stearns, 1981). Such a multicentre study was initiated in the UK under the auspices of the National Institutes of Health and the Cancer Research Campaign (Northover and Slack, 1984). The results have apparently shown that, although a rise in serum CEA concentration can detect recurrence reasonably accurately, early aggressive second-look laparotomy does not result in improved survival (J M Northover, personal communication, 1996). Other tumour markers, such as tissue polypeptide antigen (TPA) and monoclonal antibodies CA19 and CA50, have been shown to predict patients who might develop recurrence (Lindmark et al, 1994; Ståhle et al, 1988). However, no prospective randomized trial has evaluated the benefit of these markers.

Apart from the detection of early recurrence, one of the aims of intensive follow-up regimens is to detect metachronous lesions. Few studies are yet available that demonstrate the value of regular colonoscopic investigation. However, even in 1960 the beneficial value of regular barium enema examinations in detecting early metachronous carcinomas had been demonstrated (Hertz et al, 1960). In the current era of flexible endoscopy it should not only be possible to diagnose metachronous disease easily, but also if the adenoma–carcinoma sequence theory is accepted, the incidence of second primary colorectal cancers should be reduced markedly.

One trial in Funen, Denmark, was set up specifically to study the value of postoperative colonoscopy as well as follow-up in patients who had undergone surgery. Within 3 months postoperatively, all patients were subjected to a colonoscopy so that the remaining colon could be examined. After this 'clearing' procedure, patients were randomly allocated to have regular colonoscopies and follow-up (group 1) or no regular follow-up (group 2) (Kronborg et al, 1988; Kjeldsen et al, 1997). Metachronous cancer was detected in seven patients in group 1 and in two patients in group 2, but because of small numbers it was not possible to demonstrate a survival advantage.

The results of three randomized trials are now available which compare an intensive follow-up regimen with a more minimal routine follow-up regimen. These have all emanated from Scandinavia. Ohlsson et al (1995) randomized 107 patients to no follow-up or intensive follow-up consisting of clinical examination, liver function tests, CEA measurements, chest X-ray, rigid sigmoidoscopy and CT scan of the pelvis in patients undergoing abdominoperineal excision. Recurrence rates were similar in the two groups (33% versus 32%). Half the patients with recurrence in the intensive group were detected at an asymptomatic stage. However, there were no differences in curative resection or 5-year survival rates (67% versus 75%) between the two groups.

Makela et al (1995) randomized 106 patients to a conventional or intensive follow-up programme, which consisted of clinical examination, liver function tests, CEA measurements, faecal occult blood (FOB) chest X-ray, flexible sigmoidoscopy and colonoscopy. Ultrasound was performed every 6 months, and abdominal CT scan at yearly intervals. Recurrence was detected at an earlier stage (median 10 versus 15 months) in the intensive follow-up group; the proportion of asymptomatic and symptomatic recurrences were similar in the two groups. There was no difference in the number of curative re-operations between the two groups, and no significant difference in 5-year survival (54% versus 59%).

More recently, Kjeldsen et al (1997) reported on nearly 600 patients randomized to either 6-monthly follow-up or to follow-up visits at 5 and 10 years only. Investigations consisted of history and clinical examination, full blood count and liver enzymes, FOB chest X-ray and colonoscopy. Recurrence rates were similar in both groups (about 26%), but the tumour recurrences in the intensive group were detected on average 9 months earlier, often at an asymptomatic stage. Subsequently, more of these patients underwent re-operation with curative intent (22% versus 7%). However, there was no difference in overall survival between the two groups (68% versus 70% at 5 years). The authors concluded that such an intensive follow-up plan is not justified considering the small proportion of patients operated on for cure and the fact that no survival advantage was detected. However, as noted above, there might be an advantage for regular colonoscopies to detect metachronous tumours.

Conclusions and recommendations

No uniform opinion can yet be offered as to the frequency and intensity of follow-up after resection for colorectal cancer. Until the results of more prospective trials are available, surgeons must make up their own minds concerning a suitable follow-up regimen. We recommend that patients should be seen regularly for at least 5 years after operation, and that any symptom or sign of recurrent disease should be investigated thoroughly by the techniques available.

In the first 2–3 postoperative years, it is reasonable to offer liver imaging in favourable Dukes' B and C asymptomatic patients for the purpose of detecting liver metastases. Although there is no evidence that colonoscopic follow-up as yet improves survival, it has been shown to produce a reasonable yield of treatable tumours (Juhl et al, 1990; Kjeldsen et al, 1997). Thus we recommend that a clear colon should be examined by colonoscopy at least once every 3 years. These recommendations are broadly in agreement with the guidelines recently outlined by the Royal College of Surgeons and the Association of Coloproctology of Great Britain and Ireland.

RECURRENCE OF COLORECTAL CARCINOMA

Recurrence after surgery for colorectal cancer may be distant, local, or both. Local recurrence refers to a lesion which develops at or around the previous operation site; in the case of rectal carcinoma this term usually refers to disease that develops in the pelvis. Since pelvic recurrence tends to remain localized for some time, and since it has specific clinical features and treatment, it is dealt with as a separate topic in this section.

Diagnosis of recurrence is relatively straightforward when it is advanced, but at an early stage detection is difficult; hence the interest in CEA and other markers of early recurrence.

Distant recurrence

Clinical features

The development of metastases may be insidious, and the patient gradually deteriorates in energy and vigour. Such symptoms may be accompanied by dyspnoea or angina and other stigmata of anaemia. The patient may complain of pain in the upper quadrant on the right side of the abdomen as the liver enlarges and its capsule is stretched; alternatively the patient may notice liver enlargement and abdominal distension if ascites is present. If the metastases are widespread within the abdominal cavity they may lead to intestinal obstruction which usually affects the small intestine. Enlargement of lymph nodes round the porta hepatis may result in obstructive jaundice. Dissemination outside the abdominal cavity may produce a variety of symptoms and signs: thus pulmonary infiltration is likely to produce a cough, dyspnoea or haematemesis; skin involvement can present with nodules at any site. Occasionally a bony metastasis may cause a pathological fracture.

Diagnosis

When the patient presents with specific symptoms the diagnosis can usually be confirmed with relative ease. Thus if there is a complaint of pain in the right hypochondrium and the liver is enlarged and irregular, confirmation of the diagnosis is easily made by either an ultrasound scan or a CT scan of the liver. Similarly, if the patient's symptoms are suggestive of pulmonary metastases, the diagnosis usually can be made by a combination of chest radiography, bronchoscopy and sputum cytology. The diagnosis is a little more difficult when the patient has more nondescript symptoms with few or no clinical signs. Metastases in the liver less than 1 cm diameter are difficult to visualize even by modern imaging techniques. As previously discussed, a rise in serum CEA concentration may be helpful if this measurement is being performed regularly during the follow-up period.

Local pelvic recurrence

Clinical features

The clinical presentation of pelvic recurrence after operation for rectal carcinoma will depend to a certain extent on the type of procedure performed. The most common symptom independent of the type of operation is persistent perineal or sacral pain. If the sacral plexus is invaded the patient will often complain of sciatica which may be bilateral depending on the extent of infiltration. Involvement of the pelvic nerves may cause bladder dysfunction which can also result from direct bladder infiltration; rarely haematuria may be a presenting feature. Bilaterial leg oedema may occur as a result of lymphatic infiltration. After abdominoperineal excision of the rectum the patient may also develop induration, a mass or a persistent sinus in the perineum as a result of infiltration. Similar local signs may be present in the vagina.

After sphincter-saving resection, infiltration of the colorectal lumen by recurrent neoplasm is likely to cause a change in bowel habit and produce rectal bleeding, and in extreme cases intestinal obstruction may supervene. Since the pelvis is far more accessible to examination after sphincter-saving resection than after abdominoperineal excision of the rectum, detection of pelvic recurrence is easier. If there has been a true anastomotic recurrence or if recurrence within the pelvis has invaded the bowel lumen, it can usually be felt on rectal and vaginal examination and should be visualized and biopsied using the rigid or flexible sigmoidoscope. Barium enema is not a very useful investigation in this context, and several authors have pointed out the difficulties in interpreting the radiological appearances after a colorectal anastomosis (Cronquist, 1957; Agnew and Cooley, 1962). The clinical interpretation of abnormal tissue at the anastomosis on barium enema must be done with caution, as it is not unusual for a 'stitch granuloma' to develop at this site (Figure 33.9).

The result of the biopsy must be awaited before therapy is commenced and the patient and their relatives informed of the diagnosis. However, it may be difficult to confirm the diagnosis by biopsy since the recurrence tends to occur outside rather than in the lumen of the bowel; hence cross-sectional imaging is sometimes more helpful than biopsy (Figure 33.10). After local excision, fulguration or radiation, patients may develop local recurrence at the site of treatment. The symptoms will often be similar to those with which the patient first presented.

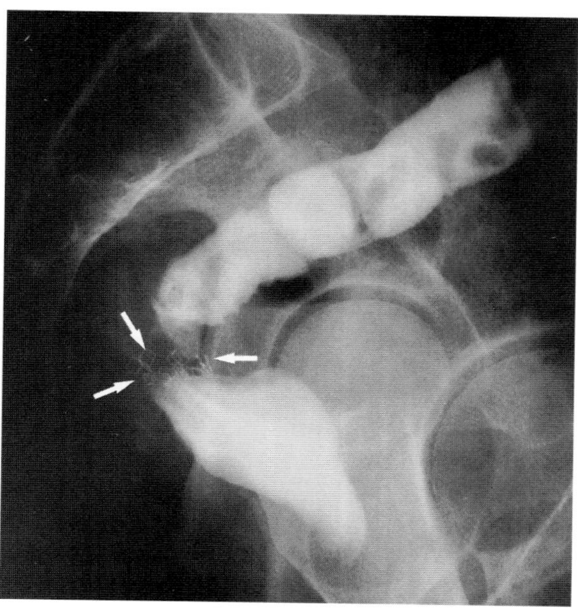

Figure 33.9 Barium enema in a patient following anterior resection. The stapled anastomosis (arrows) is disrupted and there appears to be recurrent tumour at the anastomotic site. Before proceeding with therapy it is important to perform a biopsy of the anastomotic area.

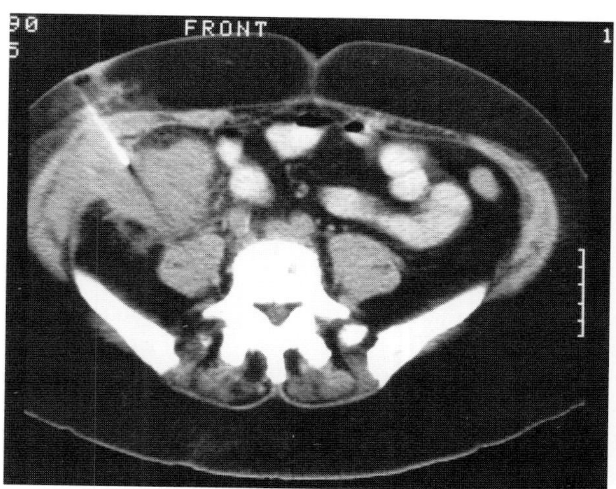

Figure 33.10 Computed tomographic scan of pelvis following anterior resection, showing recurrence, from which a biopsy is being taken by the percutaneous needle technique.

Diagnosis

Diagnosis of local recurrence can often be confirmed by biopsy via the bowel lumen as after sphincter-saving resection or a local manoeuvre. After abdominoperineal excision, histology may be obtained by biopsy of an infiltrated area or fistulous tract in the perineum or vagina. The difficulty arises when the patient complains of perineal pain, but no obvious external manifestation of recurrence is present. In these circumstances radiography of the pelvis and sacrum may be useful especially when the patient has sacral or sciatic pain, since destruction of the sacrum may be evident. Similarly a rise in serum CEA level may also be informative. Computed tomographic scans have proved to be a very useful method for the detection of metastatic disease in the pelvis (Figure 33.10). Not only can the recurrence be visualized, but also a biopsy needle can be guided into the area, so that histological confirmation can be obtained (Husband et al, 1980; Adalsteinsson et al, 1981; Lee et al, 1981; Moss et al, 1981; Zaunbauer et al, 1981).

Most studies evaluating CT scanning have investigated its use in patients who have developed symptoms suggestive of local recurrence. By the time symptoms have occurred, however, the tumour is often large and has invaded adjacent structures. Husband et al (1980) found that all pelvic recurrences demonstrated by CT were at least 5 cm in diameter, with invasion of adjacent muscle and other organs in 71% and 25% of patients respectively. Further studies, however, have emphasized the use of serial CT scans in the detection of asymptomatic pelvic recurrences (Kelvin et al, 1983; Reznek et al, 1983; Adalsteinsson et al, 1987). As normal postoperative changes within the pelvis can mimic recurrence it is essential that serial scans are performed. MRI is also now being used to detect pelvic recurrence, but it seems that this modality cannot easily distinguish between recurrence and fibrosis and inflammation (Ebner et al, 1988; Rafto et al, 1988). However, MRI can demonstrate the extent of a presacral mass well and guide percutaneous biopsy.

Whether the earlier detection of recurrence will influence the outcome remains to be determined. Such information is urgently required in order to ascertain if the expense associated with frequent CT scans is justified. A cheaper method which is applicable only for the detection of local recurrence after sphincter-saving resection is endoluminal ultrasonography (Benyon, 1988; Mascagni et al, 1989). In a series of 85 patients followed after surgical excision of rectal cancer, 22 developed local recurrence, all of whom were identified by endosonography (Beynon et al, 1989). Small extrarectal recurrences may be detected before there is evidence of luminal recurrence (Romano et al, 1985; Hildebrandt et al, 1986). An examination about 10–12 weeks after operation establishes a baseline, as organs such as the uterus and loops of bowel may fall to either side of the neorectum and may be mistakenly identified as recurrent tumours (Beynon et al, 1989). Detailed examination of the pelvis with endosonograpy yields additional information with which to plan further management, particularly if used with endosonographically directed transperineal biopsy. Its limitation, as for CT and MRI, is the persistent difficulty in differentiating between normal and abnormal lymph nodes (Rifkin and Wechsler, 1986).

Recently, positron emission tomography using 2-[F-18] fluoro-2-deoxy-D glucose (FDG) has been used to detect local recurrence and distant metastases, and has been compared with CT (Strauss et al, 1989; Beets et al, 1994; Scheipers et al, 1995; Ogunbiyi et al, 1997). In the study conducted by Ogunbiyi and associates, recurrent or advanced primary colorectal carcinoma were diagnosed in 40 and 11 patients respectively. The sensitivity and specificity of FDG–PET were 91% and 100% for detecting local recurrence and 95% and 100% for hepatic metastases. These results were significantly superior to CT, which had sensitivity and specificity of 52% and 82% for detecting pelvic recurrence, and 74% and 85% for hepatic metastases.

Immunoscintigraphy using a variety of monoclonal antibodies has been used to detect local recurrence both preoperatively and with a hand-held gamma counter probe at operation (Figure 33.11). The latter has been used as part of a second-look procedure. It may assist in the decision-making whereby unnecessary resections can be avoided and the extent of potentially curative resections may be expanded – so-called radio-immunoguided surgery (RIGS).

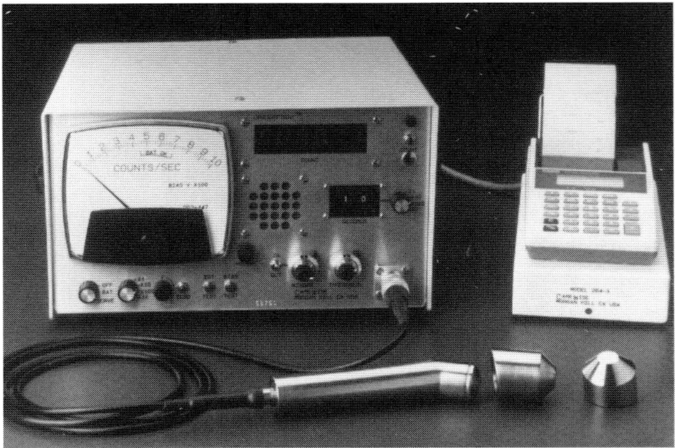

Figure 33.11 Carewise C TRAK probe used for intraoperative radioimmunodetection of colorectal cancer cells. Photograph courtesy Professor K Britton, St Bartholomew's Hospital and the Royal London School of Medicine and Dentistry.

A multicentre study using RIGS in 98 patients found that the tumour was localized in 63% of those with recurrent disease. However, one-third of patients with resectable disease were found to warrant more extensive resection than would have been carried out at traditional assessment (Cohen et al, 1991). The accuracy of this technique clearly depends on the specificity of the monoclonal antibody, and although this is improving it has not reached 100% accuracy. Nevertheless, there is optimism. Thus, indium III Cyt-103 immunoscintigraphy was used in a study of 19 patients suspected of having recurrent colorectal cancer (Doerr et al, 1993). Six patients had undergone curative excision of rectal cancer. Immunoscintigraphy revealed the site of recurrence in all six, three of whom were suitable for resection. Immunoscintigraphy has fared well in the detection of pelvic recurrence, achieving a rate of 74% compared with 57% for CT (Collier et al, 1992). As expected with a specific monoclonal antibody, immunoscintigraphy can detect normal-sized lymph nodes containing microscopic deposits (Neal and Abdel-Nabi, 1994).

Local recurrence after colonic resection

Local recurrence after colonic resection is much less common than after rectal excision. It appears that whereas pelvic recurrence can remain confined within the pelvis for a long time, recurrence within the abdominal cavity is often widespread by the time it is detected. Nevertheless, with more aggressive follow-up regimens and the wider use of CT and MRI scanning and colonoscopy, it is envisaged that true local recurrence confined to the previous operative site will be detected more often than hitherto. It should also be stressed that patients who present with new symptoms and signs following a resection for colorectal cancer must not automatically be assumed to have developed a recurrence. Thus Ellis (1978) demonstrated that approximately one-third of such patients have a benign cause for their symptoms or have developed another primary tumour.

Treatment of local recurrence

Palliative radiotherapy

Currently most patients with pelvic recurrence particularly after abdominoperineal excision are treated with radiotherapy, which is reasonably effective in controlling pain (Allum et al, 1987; Griffith et al, 1988). The dose used has varied from 20 Gy over a 2–3 week period to 60 Gy in 5–6 weeks. Goligher (1984) described 117 cases treated at Leeds General Infirmary, 75% of whom obtained good or fair relief of pain for the period prior to death. Villalon and Green (1981) had better results with a dose of 45 Gy. Boulware et al (1979) at the M D Anderson Hospital used single doses of 10 Gy separated by intervals of 4 weeks to a maximum of 30 Gy. Their patients were treated with opposed fields utilizing photon energies of 18–25 MV. An overall objective response rate of 40–50% was demonstrated and over half of these patients showed complete disappearance of local tumour. Pain and bleeding were successfully palliated in the majority of patients. Similar results were reported by Allum and his colleagues from Birmingham (Allum et al, 1987).

Surgical excision

The aim of an intense follow-up programme is to detect local disease at the earliest stage possible, preferably before symptoms develop. It remains to be seen whether detection of a rise in CEA levels will help to define patients with a small localized recurrence which would be amenable to further surgery, resulting in a survival advantage. However, preliminary results from a CEA 'second look' trial suggest that this will not be the case (J M Northover, 1998, personal communication). Much data has already been collected from centres which adopt a more aggressive approach to the treatment of patients with localized recurrence. Most patients included in these reports, however, complained of symptoms.

It is difficult to determine from these data if the results of surgery for recurrence after colonic resection differ from those after rectal excision, since most studies reported patients who suffered from both colonic and rectal cancer. Impressive results were claimed by Bacon and Berkeley (1959) who re-explored 93 patients who had local recurrence – 60 in the pelvis, 25 at an anastomotic resection site and eight in the abdominal wall. Further resection could be performed in 38 patients, and 15 of these (40%) survived 5 years or more.

Unfortunately, other authors have produced less impressive results. Berge et al (1973) found that 216 of their 638 patients developed recurrence, of whom 93 underwent a second laparotomy. Thirty of these 93 patients had a curative resection but only four (13%) were alive 4–5 years later. Ellis (1978) re-operated on 28 patients with recurrence but re-resection was deemed justified in only 17, of whom nine were alive 2 years later. Lewi et al (1981) found that 66 of 444 patients (14%) who had had an ostensibly curative resection for a colorectal cancer developed local recurrence which was amenable to further laparotomy. At operation nine of these 63 patients had benign disease, four had a new primary tumour and 50 had local recurrence. Of those with recurrent disease, 15 underwent re-resection with the hope of cure. There were two operative deaths, and three patients (20%) survived for 18 months.

These data together with those from the CEA studies show that some patients with local recurrence can benefit from laparotomy with a view to resection. Until the complete results of the CEA 'second look' trials are to hand, however, it is clear that only a few carefully selected patients should be submitted to re-operation. With the aid of sophisticated scanning the selection of patients who have localized disease should be improved.

Surgery of pelvic recurrence: principles

For many years a surgical approach to pelvic recurrence was considered not to be very profitable. However, there is now an appreciation that local recurrence, particularly after resection for rectal cancer, often remains localized without distant metastases in an otherwise fit patient. With improvements in surgical technique, intraoperative radiotherapy or brachytherapy and anaesthesia, so has come a more aggressive approach to local recurrence. Nevertheless, such surgery is not for the faint-hearted and patients need careful counselling concerning the likely pros and cons of often extensive surgery which may leave them with two stomas.

Different surgical strategies are required for different types of recurrence. The more extensive surgery will require a multidisciplinary team involving urologists, gynaecologists, plastic surgeons, neurosurgeons or even orthopaedic surgeons. Careful preoperative work-up is essential to rule out disseminated disease.

Local recurrence at or around the anastomosis

Occasionally it might be possible to resect the anastomosis and perform a second sphincter-saving procedure provided that there is no fixity of the recurrence to nearby structures. However, in our experience this is a very rare situation. Goligher (1984) considered that 14 of 28 patients with pelvic recurrence after sphincter-saving resection merited a laparotomy. In 12 it was possible to resect the recurrence, but only in two was it feasible to perform a sphincter-saving procedure. Guivarc'h et al (1993/94) also describe similar results. Thus most of these patients require conversion to an abdominoperineal excision. If the tumour is centrally situated and involving the bladder or prostate anteriorly, an *en bloc* resection will be required with construction of an ileal bladder. Improved margins may be obtained with entry into a fresh surgical plane by dissection in a plane lateral to the hypogastric vessels. Patients in whom the recurrence is isolated to one side after anterior resection may be suitable for *en bloc* resection of the rectum, a portion of the bladder and the dilated ureter. The transected ureter is then re-implanted into the reconstructed bladder. Recurrence that is fixed to the sacrum or pelvic side walls requires composite abdominosacral resection (Sagar and Pemberton, 1996).

Isolated perineal recurrence after abdominoperineal excision

Local excision of truly isolated perineal metastases has been performed by some authors and, although palliation has been achieved, cure is rare (Cohen and Minsky, 1990). Polk and Spratt (1971, 1979) recommended re-excision of the area with access being gained through a transverse incision at the sacrococcygeal junction. This approach resulted in a median survival of 12 months but no cure. We generally consider these approaches to be meddlesome. Perineal deposits are usually associated with tumour sited deeper in the pelvis and local excision will lead to wounds that are unlikely to heal, with other complications such as urinary or enterocutaneous fistulas.

Anterior pelvic recurrence

Anterior recurrences confined to the neorectum and anterior organs such as the bladder, prostate and vagina and uterus may be treated by a standard exenterative procedure with *en bloc* excision of the tumour and involved organs. Although such extensive surgery for primary rectal cancer has been a controversial subject for many years, for patients with recurrent tumour it provides another option (Brophy et al 1994; Sagar and Pemberton, 1996). Such an approach has been demonstrated to improve the quality of life in selected patients (Brophy et al, 1994). In addition, pelvic exenteration is associated with a median survival of 21–30% (Estes et al, 1993; Brophy et al, 1994) and 5-year survival rates of up to 50% (Eckhauser et al, 1979; Boey et al, 1982; Estes et al, 1993).

Pelvic exenteration for anterior pelvic recurrence must achieve clear margins of resection. This may be extremely difficult when the operation is performed for recurrence as opposed to when the procedure is carried out for an extensive, locally invasive, primary tumour. In recurrent disease, the planes of dissection are distorted, making the procedure technically very challenging. If pelvic exenteration cannot achieve clear margins, a sacrococcygectomy may also be required.

Technique of pelvic exenteration

The position of the patient on the table is a matter of preference. We prefer the modified Lloyd Davies position, but others prefer the traditional supine position for laparotomy, with transfer to an exaggerated lithotomy position when the necessity for a perineal phase becomes apparent.

After a careful laparotomy to ensure there are no widespread metastases, the dissection is begun by identifying both ureters, and incising the overlying peritoneum down into the pelvis and cephalad towards the duodenum. The underlying common iliac arteries are then exposed, and all of the tissues freed by pushing the finger cephalad on top of the artery first on one side, and then the other, until the aortic bifurcation is reached (Figure 33.12a).

The mesosigmoid containing the vascular bundle to the distal colon and rectum is elevated and skele-

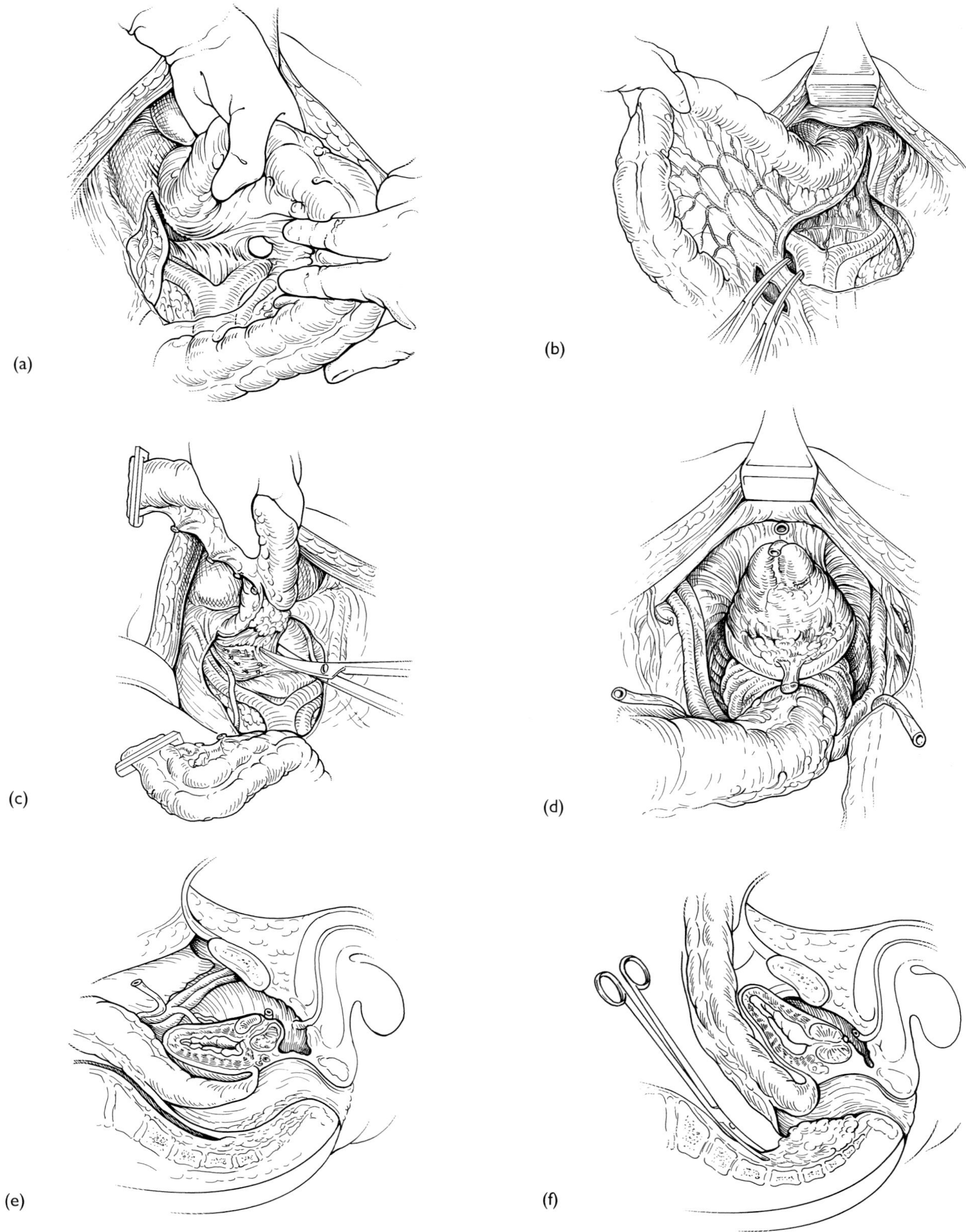

Figure 33.12a–f Pelvic exenteration (male) (see text).

tonized to either the origin of the inferior mesenteric or just below the left colic artery (Figure 33.12b). The mesosigmoid is divided to a point on the sigmoid selected for transection. Usually, the proximal end of the sigmoid will be used for an end-colostomy, but sometimes with a high lesion the proximal colon may be used for a colorectal anastomosis. Mobilization of the rectum continues by dissection of the tissues from the aortic bifurcation down to the presacral fascia and from the common iliac arteries and veins. Once the pre-sacral fascia is clearly identified, a combination of blunt and sharp dissection in an essentially bloodless field allows complete mobilization of the posterior and lateral attachments of the rectum, and mesorectum (Figure 33.12c). Sharp dissection should be used to free the medial aspect of the ureters and hypogastric vessels well down into the pelvis. Ligation of the hypogastric vessels at this point may lessen the bleeding associated with mobilization of the bladder.

Mobilization of the bladder at this point facilitates later posterior and lateral dissection. An incision is made in the anterior parietal peritoneum, and the urachus below the pubic ramus. The incision is connected with the peritoneal incisions over the ureters. The bladder and perivesical fat are mobilized from behind the pubis. The vas in males is identified and divided, as are the infundibulopelvic ligaments, ovarian vessels and round ligaments in women. The ureters are identified and transected with ligation of their distal stumps. The bladder is then mobilized down to the membranous urethra, which is readily identified by the previously placed catheter. The urethra may then be transected after withdrawal of the catheter (Figure 33.12d,e).

It is now usually advantageous to return to mobilization of the rectum by incising and dissecting Waldeyer's fascia, which is reflected from the back of the rectum on to the levator muscles (Figure 33.12f). The lateral attachments of the rectum, including the ureterosacral ligaments in women, are divided. Retraction of the specimen medially tents the ligaments between two fingers and helps to identify these structures, which are then divided close to the hypogastric vessels which represent the lateral extent of the dissection. The middle rectal artery can be clamped before division, but it will usually stop bleeding after complete division. Further mobilization from the lateral wall is continued until the specimen is fixed only by the vagina, rectum and urethra if the latter has not previously been divided. The membranous urethra is divided, as is the anterior vaginal wall in women. If the recurrent tumour is high in the rectum, the rectum can be transected 5 cm below the tumour, using a transverse stapling device and right-angled clamp. In women, the posterior vaginal wall should be divided and separated from the rectum before clamping.

However, more usually it is not possible to preserve the distal anorectum and sphincters. In this case, the specimen should be removed via the perineal approach after division of the urethra and anterior wall of the vagina. This part of the dissection is exactly the same as that described in Chapter 32 for abdominoperineal excision of the rectum.

Reconstruction involves restoration, if possible, of gastrointestinal continuity and formation of an ileal urinary conduit. The details of the latter are to be found in Chapter 70. However, we would stress that pelvic exenteration is a 'team procedure', and a urologist should be part of the team.

Composite abdominosacral resection for recurrent rectal cancer that involves the sacrum or pelvic side walls

Pelvic exenteration for recurrent rectal cancer has been shown to achieve disappointing results. The reason is thought to be due to involvement of the sacrum or pelvic side walls. The feasibility and safety of combining sacral resection with pelvic exenteration has, however, been demonstrated (Benotti et al, 1987; Temple and Ketcham, 1992; Wanebo et al, 1992). There are various approaches to this complex surgery.

The usual preoperative work-up to exclude disseminated disease is absolutely essential. Clinical examination should also include neuromuscular assessment of the lower limbs and careful pelvic, rectal and/or vaginal examinations. Plain films of the lumbosacral spine and a bone scan are useful to exclude upper sacral marrow involvement which would render the tumour inoperable (Turk and Wanebo, 1993). CT of the pelvis and abdomen with guided biopsy is essential, while MRI in the sagittal plane is useful to identify the level and depth of sacral involvement (Sagar and Pemberton, 1996).

Chemo-irradiation is also an important part of treatment. Thus, if the patient received no adjuvant radiotherapy after the first resection, then external beam radiotherapy is given before surgery. It is recommended that 50 Gy be given in 20–25 fractions combined with continuous infusion of sensitizing 5FU, 750 mg/m^2 per day (Wanebo et al, 1994). If the pelvis has been previously irradiated, 20 Gy is given in divided doses.

At laparotomy, provided extrapelvic disease is excluded, the presacral plane is entered and developed to a point below S2. If tumour is found to invade S2, on frozen section analysis, the patient is deemed to be inoperable (Temple and Ketcham, 1992). The sacrum is cleared 2 cm above the tumour to prepare it for later division, but no attempt is made to mobilize the tumour from the sacrum. If access is very difficult, then the central part of the pubis may be divided and the bony ring of the pelvis spread apart with a rib retractor (Patel et al, 1982). As the bladder is mobilized, the obturator nodes are swept medially with the specimen and both are resected *en bloc*. A urinary conduit and colostomy are constructed and an omental pedicle is mobilized for use in lining the raw pelvis.

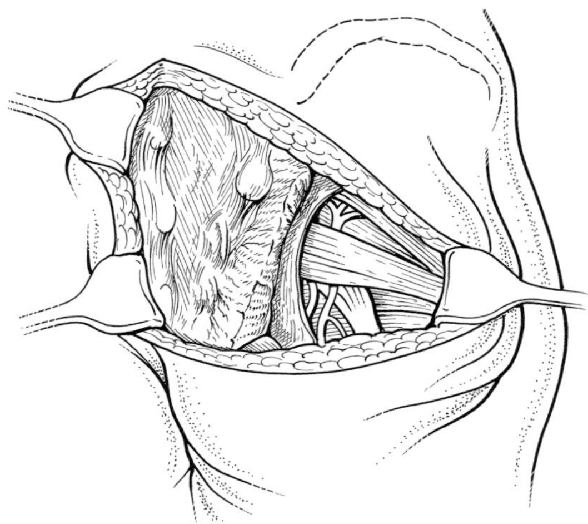

Figure 33.13 Composite abdominosacral resection for recurrent rectal cancer. The sacrum is exposed and the sciatic nerve and piriformis are identified.

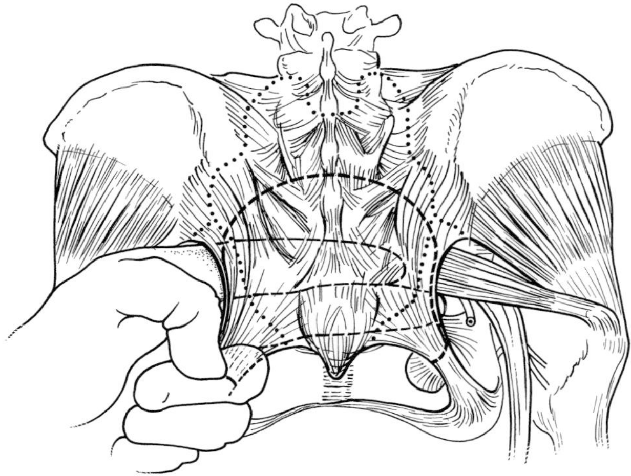

Figure 33.14 Composite abdominosacral resection for recurrent rectal cancer. The surgeon's fingers are inserted beneath piriformis and through the endopelvic fascia to reach the anterior surface of the sacrum. The level of transection of the sacrum, sacrospinous and sacrotuberous ligaments is indicated (– – – –).

Posterior procedures are performed with the patient in the prone jack-knife position. The sacrum is excised (Figures 33.13 and 33.14). The large perineal defect is closed with a rectus abdominus flap.

Radiotherapy may be given at operation, although as yet few centres have this capacity. Intraoperative radiotherapy (IORT) using an electron beam has the advantage of being localized to the tumour-bearing area. To reduce the expense of this approach, the isotope palladium-103 is currently under investigation for use as a permanent implant (Moigooni and Nath, 1989). Computerized remote afterloading brachytherapy techniques are also being used for pelvic irradiation boosting, which may be more practical than IORT (Kaufmann et al, 1989).

Results of surgery for pelvic recurrence

The results of several series of pelvic exenteration for recurrent rectal cancer are summarized in Table 33.9. As can be seen, in selected patients the procedures can be performed safely with long-term survival expected in approximately one-third of cases. Patients with preoperative CEA levels of less than 10 ng/mL have a survival rate of about 45%, while those with a CEA level greater than 10 ng/mL have a survival rate of about 15%. Bone marrow invasion, involvement of resection margins and metastatic deposits in pelvic nodes are all associated with a worse prognosis. Preoperative demonstration of bone marrow involvement or the intraoperative finding of lateral pelvic nodal involvement are therefore contraindications to resection (Wanebo et al, 1994).

It is difficult at this stage to know whether intraoperative radiotherapy (IORT) is beneficial. As expected, there are no controlled trials yet available. Suzuki et al (1995) from the Mayo Clinic have reported their experience in 106 patients with locally recurrent rectal cancer who underwent palliative surgical resections between 1981 and 1988. Forty-two patients received intraoperative electron beam irradiation. Gross residual disease remained after maximal surgical resection in 34 of these 42 patients, and in the remaining six patients who did not receive IORT. Most patients received a dose of 15–20 Gy. External beam irradiation was also administered to 41 of 42 patients. The 3-year cumulative probability of developing distant metastases was 60% in patients who received IORT and 54% in those who did not. However, the 3-year local relapse rate was 40% in the IORT group, compared with 93% of patients who did not receive IORT (Table 33.10). Despite these results, the authors con-

Table 33.9 Results of exenterative surgery for recurrent disease.

Authors	n	Curative/palliative	Operative mortality rate (%)	Operative morbidity rate (%)	Survival	Local recurrence (%)
Takagi et al (1986)	7	7/0	0	28	4 of 7 alive (3–36 months)	28
Benotti et al (1987)	29	15/14	3	25	80% at 1 year	54
Touran et al (1990)	12	12/0	0	35 (urine incontinence/retention) 25 (wound disruption)	63% at 1 year	41
Maetani et al (1992)	35	35/0	5.7	33 (wound infection)	23% at 5 years	69
Temple and Ketcham (1992)	9	9/0	9	NS	18% at 5 years	55
Wanebo et al (1992)	47	41/6	8.5	NS	24% at 5 years	
Estes et al (1993)	16	16/0	6.2	25 (wound infection)	49% at 5 years	NS
Hoffmann et al (1993)	19	19/0	0	NS	40% at 5 years	42
Pearlman (1993)	41	25/16	5	44	38% at 5 years	37
Tschmelitsch (1994)	20	9/11	0	10	Palliative 17 months* Curative 35.5 months*	55
Wanebo et al (1994)	53	47/6	8.5	38 (wound infection or separation)	33% at 4 years	18

* Median survival. NS Not stated.
From Sagar and Pemberton (1996).

Table 33.10 Results of surgery and intraoperative radiotherapy (IORT) in the treatment of local recurrence.

Regimen	Distant metastases at 3 years	Local recurrence at 3 years
IORT (*n* = 42)	60%	40%
No IORT (*n* = 64)	40%	93%

From Suzuki et al (1995).

cluded that further gains in treatment were necessary. Similar results have been achieved by Eble et al (1994) in Germany and Hoffman et al (1994) in Philadelphia.

Conclusions and author's view

It is essential to consider not only survival in patients with recurrent pelvic disease undergoing such extensive surgery, but also their quality of life. It is difficult to compare the quality of life of patients who develop such recurrence with those who undergo the surgery with its associated morbidity and risk of later recurrence. The surgery can take many hours and the transfusion requirements are usually high. The patient is often left with two stomas. Nevertheless, it has been shown that the quality of life in selected patients and life expectancy can be improved considerably by surgery (Temple and Ketcham, 1992). Such reports obviously emanate from centres which specialize in these approaches and one has to judge them in this light. However, there is little doubt that pelvic recurrence can be totally disabling and for a considerable length of time before dissemination of the tumour takes place. In addition, chemo-irradiation, although occasionally having a spectacular result, often does not work and will not produce cure. We think it is therefore appropriate to consider a surgical approach to locally recurrent disease provided the patient is otherwise fit and dissemination has been excluded. Clearly the patient must be motivated and have an understanding of what the surgery entails and the likely benefit. If agreeable, they should then be sent to a centre which specializes in this type of surgery and has the appropriate multidisciplinary team that is required. In addition, such centres should be encouraged to work together to carry out multicentre trials designed to determine if this aggressive approach is truly worthwhile.

Photodynamic therapy

Some groups are now treating extensive primary tumours by surgical excision followed by intraoperative radiotherapy. Such a technique can also be applied to recurrent tumours. Unfortunately the toxicity from this form of therapy is high.

An alternative method of destroying residual recurrent tumour after surgical excision is by the technique of intraoperative photodynamic therapy (PDT). This therapy involves a photosensitizing drug, initially haematoporphyrin derivative (HpD), which is given 48 hours before the operation. The patient then undergoes surgical resection where as much tumour as possible is removed. The photosensitizer should have selectively localized in tumour tissue and the area where residual tumour remains is irradiated with light at 635 nm generated from a dye laser. This has the effect of releasing singlet oxygen, which is cancericidal, from the photosensitizer. As a consequence of the selective uptake of the drug, only tumour is destroyed and normal tissue should be unaffected.

Since the operating theatre lights might activate HpD, and since some HpD does get taken up in normal tissue, there is a theoretical risk that normal tissue could be damaged. After extensive safety studies in mini-pigs using doses of HpD and light that would be therapeutically effective, we demonstrated that this mode of treatment was entirely safe provided certain precautions were adhered to (Allardice et al, 1992).

In a phase II study we have treated approximately ten patients with recurrent colorectal tumours with surgery and intraoperative PDT using HpD. In order to deliver light uniformly to the area of disease, special intraoperative light-delivery systems were devised (Allardice et al, 1992). The procedure appeared safe but the number of patients was too small to determine the effectiveness of the therapy (Ansell et al, 1996). Since this work commenced, a second-generation photosensitizer, meta-tetrahydroxyphenylchlorine (MTHPC) has been developed which appears to be more selective for cancer tissue than is HpD. In addition, it can be activated by a diode laser which can easily be transported (Abulafi et al, 1997). This contrasts with HpD, which requires a large immobile pumped dye laser for its activation. The combination of MTHPC and the practicality of treating more patients have encouraged us to continue to explore the value of intraoperative PDT for recurrent disease in a new trial.

Chemotherapy

Chemotherapy for local recurrence may be given systemically or via the intra-arterial route (Patt et al, 1985). Systemic chemotherapy is discussed later. The current revival of regional arterial therapy has led to its use in the management of some patients with recurrent rectal cancer. In patients with pelvic recurrence the usual approach is by simultaneous, bilateral, internal iliac artery infusion of 5FU or 5-fluorodeoxyuridine (5FUDR), or one of these drugs combined with mitomycin (Hickey et al, 1982).

The perfusion catheter is introduced either directly at laparotomy through the common iliac artery or, if an abdominal operation has not been performed, by a Seldinger technique through the femoral artery. Lawton (1965) using 5FU alone in combination with pelvic irradiation described 'excellent results' in several patients. A more objective report was provided by Hafström et al (1985) who used the retrograde route and infused 5FU; however, two of their 14 patients suffered from septicaemia through the infusion catheters. Three patients with partial ureteric obstruction to start with, progressed to complete obstruction during therapy. Nevertheless, 11 patients stated their pain was much improved and five had objective evidence of reduced tumour bulk. Hickey et al (1982) also suggested that the results of this form of treatment can be most impressive. These authors used a combination of 5FUDR and mitomycin. One important and evidently universal side-effect of this regimen, however, seemed to be a violaceous, confluent skin rash which developed in the perineal region shortly after commencement of the infusion. Although the rash could be controlled by concomitant administration of hydrocortisone, it produced severe infection and discomfort. Despite various optimistic reports one cannot help believe that a similar outcome could be achieved by simpler measures.

The management of pain

If the methods discussed above fail to relieve pain from local recurrence, further measures will be needed to control it. The multidisciplinary approach of a pain clinic is very helpful in evaluating these patients for treatment. The pain may be visceral due to tumour invading the intestines, bladder, uterus and prostate, and/or somatic with involvement of muscle, fascia, periosteum and nerves of the lumbar and sacral plexus. Generally, simpler methods of pain relief with little risk of side-effects are used first and for as long as possible, before proceeding to invasive and potentially destructive higher-risk procedures.

Drug therapy

Huber and Hill (1980) made the point that cancer pain of mild to moderate severity can usually be controlled by non-narcotic analgesics and non-steroidal anti-inflammatory drugs when these are administered in large doses and at short intervals. If the pain is not relieved (or is no longer controlled) by non-narcotic analgesics, then the narcotic analgesics that have morphine-like pharmacological action and bind to central nervous system receptors must be used. If these measures fail either because of tolerance or progression of the patient's disease, other forms of pain therapy must be considered.

Intrathecal injection of alcohol, phenol or morphine

Intrathecal injection is best performed by either a neurosurgeon or an anaesthetist skilled in spinal injections. The principle of using alcohol is that it is lighter than the cerebrospinal fluid, so that after the lumbar puncture needle has been inserted through the first lumbar intervertebral space, the patient is placed in a prone, head-down position so that the posterior sacral nerve roots are above the point of the needle and will be submerged in the alcohol. Phenol may be better than alcohol since it appears to have a selective affinity for sensory nerve fibres, so that the risk of motor nerve damage with resulting paralysis is reduced.

The identification of opiate receptor sites in the central nervous system in animals and humans, and successful analgesia in animals using morphine applied through chronic spinal catheters (Yaksh and Rudy, 1977), has led to the use of intraspinal or intraventricular opiates as a means of pain relief in pelvic cancer patients (Cousins et al, 1979; Samii et al, 1979; Wang et al, 1979; Tung et al, 1980). The technique seems to be very useful in selected patients but there is a risk of respiratory depression which fortunately is reversible by naloxone.

Neurosurgical techniques

Occasionally more intensive techniques are required for the control of chronic pelvic pain. These techniques have the disadvantage of being destructive and result in permanent changes in the nervous system, and should be used only when simpler methods of pain control have been exhausted.

- *Laminectomy and bilateral sacral root rhizotomy* can be effective for the relief of perineal and bilateral buttock and lower extremity pain due to carcinoma of the rectum. These patients may or may not have normal bladder function prior to rhizotomy. If bladder function is absent, sensory rhizotomy of S1 roots bilaterally and complete rhizotomy of S2–S5 are usually adequate in relieving pain and preserving function of the lower extremities until the disease progresses to involve the lumbar plexus. If the patient has normal bladder function and has intact S2 and S3 roots on one side prior to rhizotomy, these roots must be spared during bilateral rhizotomy to preserve bladder function.
- *Cordotomy* involves surgical interruption of the lateral spinothalamic tract of the spinal cord which carries pain and temperature sensory fibres. The tracts may be interrupted unilaterally or bilaterally depending on where the pain is sited. The operation may be performed as an open procedure or by a percutaneous radio-frequency stereotactic technique. In patients with pelvic pain only about 80% will be relieved with bilateral cordotomy because of anatomical variations and technical problems of localization (Schwartz, 1962). Cordotomy is suitable only for a few patients but it can be extremely successful. Hickey et al (1982) at the M D Anderson Hospital treated 18 patients with bilateral thoracic cordotomy. Not all patients had recurrent rectal cancers, but 11 of 18 patients experienced relief of pain lasting until death from disease; in three patients the pain recurred and four patients were lost to follow-up.
- *Commissural myelotomy* is another neurosurgical technique that may prove successful in a very small proportion of patients. Through a laminectomy the right and left pain fibres in the dorsal and ventral commissures of the spinal cord are sectioned. The procedure is lengthy and requires careful dissection with an operating microscope. Sourek (1969) and Lipert et al (1975) reported good results in some patients with rectal cancer, but not all authors are convinced of the benefit of this difficult technique (Cook and Kawakami, 1977).

Treatment of disseminated recurrent disease

Surgical resection for liver metastases

With the advance in hepatic surgery, resection of hepatic metastases from colorectal cancer is becoming more frequent. Nevertheless, it should be emphasized that careful selection of patients for surgical treatment is still essential if outcome is to be improved.

Progress in liver surgery has resulted from an understanding of the segmental anatomy of the liver, better perioperative care, improved anaesthesia and surgical techniques, including complete vascular isolation, improved blood salvage, modifications of the 'finger fracture' technique, and the use of the ultrasound aspirator and laser.

The presentation of liver metastases for primary cancer resection is variable, but usually takes one of three forms:

- discovered at initial laparotomy for the primary tumour – i.e. synchronous disease
- diagnosed later, either from regular scanning or as part of a work-up for an elevated serum CEA
- as a result of symptoms (Saenz et al, 1989).

Synchronous disease occurs in 8–25% of patients (Babineau and Steele, 1996) and its detailed surgical management is discussed in Chapter 31. If synchronous disease is suspected, it is usual nowadays to biopsy the lesion in the liver and then assess the extent of the disease more fully postoperatively, with a view to resecting the metastases if possible at a later date. An exception to this occurs in any patient found to have a single liver metastasis when the operation for the primary tumour has gone smoothly and when the hepatic resection represents a relatively minor additional procedure (i.e. 'wedge' resection). Even in this situation, however, it is wise to perform intraoperative ultrasonography before embarking on resection to eliminate any other suspected metastasis within the liver (Stone et al, 1994).

The number of patients who may be suitable for liver resection of their metastases is well illustrated by a recent review of the subject by Babineau and Steele (1996). In North America, only 9000 patients per year (less than 20% of patients who experience recurrence after resection of their primary tumour) will be diagnosed as having recurrence confined to the liver alone (GITSG, 1985; Steele, 1994a). Of these 9000, approximately 1000–1500 could be excluded from attempted surgical resection owing to comorbid disease. An additional 30–50% were found at laparotomy to be ineligible for resection owing to previous, unsuspected extrahepatic or profuse intrahepatic disease. Thus, 5000 patients may be suitable for hepatic resection in North America per year. However, assuming a 5% operative mortality and a 20–25% disease-free survival over 5–10 years, only 1000 patients might be expected to be cured. In addition, there is still some doubt that even these 1000 will be cured despite being rigorously selected. Recent updated follow-up of the only prospective multi-institutional liver resection trial has shown that there may be no plateau in the survival curve, even among the patients who have had curative resections (Steele, 1995). These data illustrate the clinical problem very clearly.

Despite the above points, it does appear that there are selected patients who can theoretically be cured of their liver metastases by surgical excision. However, this statement is not based on randomized controlled trials and the benefit of surgical excision cannot be unequivocally proven. The 'belief' is based on careful analysis of retrospective data comparing survival in patients who have undergone liver resection with those who have not (Foster and Berman, 1977; Hughes et al, 1986, 1988; Adson, 1987; Steele and Ravikumar, 1989).

Perhaps the best data come from the only prospective multicentre study organized by the Gastrointestinal Tumour Study Group (GITS 6584), which commenced in 1984. This group defined as their control group those patients who were found to have extrahepatic disease or unresectable disease within the liver at the time of laparotomy and did not undergo liver resection. The patients who did undergo resection were divided into two groups. Curative resections were defined as those in whom the margin of resection was confirmed by surgeon and pathologist to be free of disease. Non-curative resections were defined as those found by the pathologist to have tumour at or near to (<1 cm) the resection margin. Follow-up was for a minimum of 7 years. A total of 115 deaths were reported. Forty-four of the 69 patients (64%) who underwent curative resection died. Fourteen of the 18 patients (79%) who underwent non-curative resection died and 57 of the 63 (90%) non-resected group died. Median survival times for patients receiving curative and non-curative resections, and those receiving no resection at all, were estimated to be 35.7, 21.2 and 16.5 months respectively (Figure 33.15). There was no significant difference in the survival distribution between the patients in the non-curative versus the non-resected group. However, survival among the curatively resected patients was significantly superior ($P = 0.01$) to survival in the non-curatively resected and non-resected patients. Among the 25 surviving patients who underwent curative resection, 16 remained free of disease. Six patients were

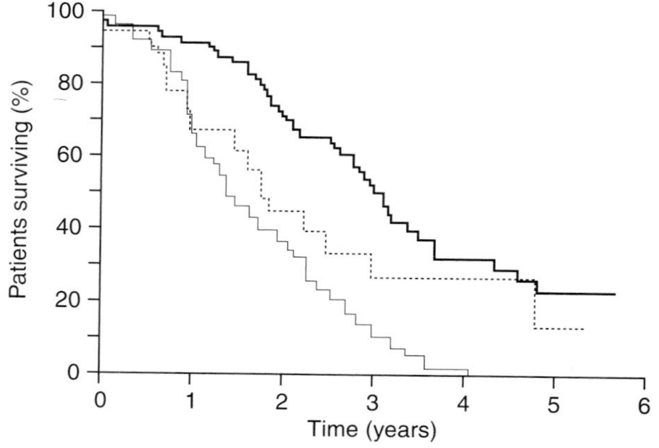

Figure 33.15 Survival following resection of liver metastases according to resection type (from GITSG study). Bold line, curative resection; dotted line, non-curative resection; fine line, no resection.

alive more than 5 years postoperatively and two of these six were disease-free. An estimate of the probable 5-year survival for patients undergoing curative resection is currently approximately 23%, although the slope of the survival curve continues on a downward trend. In this study, there were no preoperative factors which identified those patients in whom resection was possible.

Preoperative staging of liver metastases

It is essential to eliminate patients who will not obviously benefit by hepatic resection. A variety of modalities are now available for such assessment. Thus, if resection is clinically a possibility, the patient should undergo CT with vascular enhancement (Karl et al, 1993), in addition to an ultrasound scan. Approximately one-third to one-half of all patients suspected of having liver-only or liver-predominant colorectal cancer metastases staged by non-invasive diagnostic tests will be found at operation to have extrahepatic disease (Barbineau et al, 1994; Steele et al, 1991; Vaughn and Haller, 1993). In recent years, laparoscopy and intraoperative ultrasound, when used together, have proved useful in the selection process. Thus, this combination of investigations can detect satellite lesions smaller than 1–1.5 cm diameter, or lesions located deep within the liver parenchyma. Laparoscopy is also useful in demonstrating cirrhosis not suspected preoperatively, identifying satellite tumour deposits in the liver, and revealing previously unsuspected extrahepatic metastases (Babineau et al, 1994; Babineau and Steele, 1996).

Anatomical and technical considerations for hepatic resection

Hepatic resection should be performed only by surgeons who are regularly undertaking such procedures. In most colorectal units, this will mean referral to a surgeon who performs hepatic resections for indications other than colorectal metastases. Rapid strides in hepatic surgery have been made by the greater appreciation of liver anatomy and technical improvements. In 1957, Collinaud divided the liver into eight segments based primarily on the vascular supply as demonstrated by model casts produced by injections of the hepatic artery, portal vein and bile ducts. The right lobe contains segments 5–8, while the left lobe contains segments 1–4 (Figure 33.16). Although very elegant, these anatomical subdivisions are quite variable owing to extensive arborization of the intrahepatic vasculature. Hepatic resection primarily involves

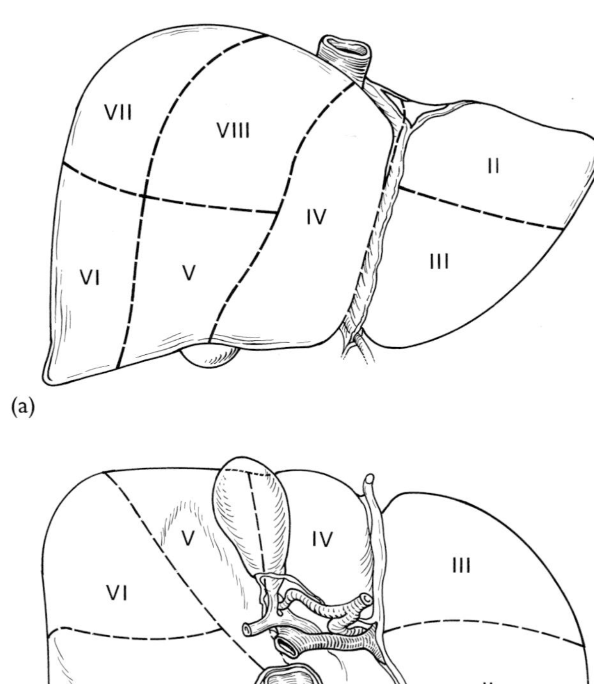

Figure 33.16a,b The liver divided into its segmental anatomy (Warren et al, 1991).

four distinct segments: the anatomic right lobe; the anatomic left lobe; the medial segment of the left lobe in conjunction with the right lobe (a right trisegmentectomy); and the lateral segment of the left lobe (Figure 33.17). Surgery that attempts to divide the liver along other planes increases the hazard and the blood loss.

The patient must be prepared meticulously before operation, particular care being paid to coagulation and nutritional defects. Age is not an absolute contraindication to hepatic surgery; often the 'physiological' age and performance of the patient are better measures of operability. Cirrhosis is a relative contraindication since the remaining liver after resection will have a decreased capacity to regenerate. Fortunately, however, colorectal cancer rarely metastasizes to a cirrhotic liver (Uetsuji et al, 1992).

Some liver surgeons recommend laparotomy in order to determine operability (Babineau and Steele, 1996). Thus, Babineau et al (1994) found that 48% of their patients about to undergo a planned laparotomy had unresectable liver disease.

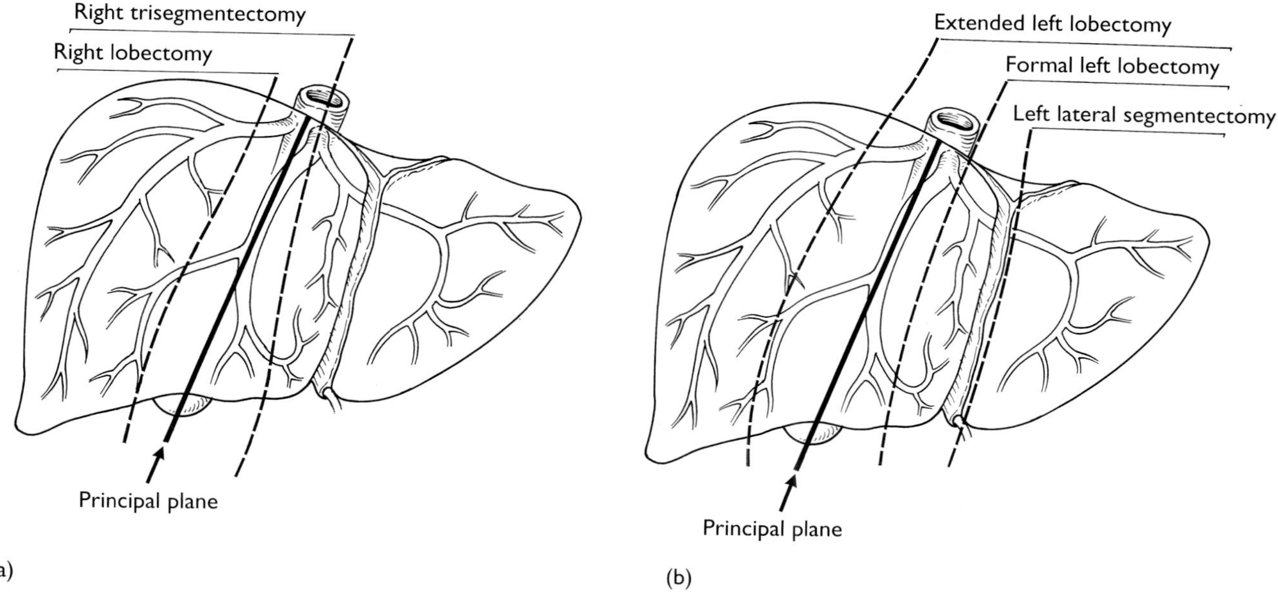

Figure 33.17a,b Hepatic venous anatomy and the options for (a) right lobectomy and (b) left lobectomy (Warren et al, 1991).

Technique of hepatic resection

The patient is usually placed supine with the right arm elevated and secured across the table. An exploratory right subcostal incision allows assessment of resectability by palpation of the liver and confirmation of the absence of peritoneal disease or fixed porta hepatic nodes. The incision is then extended from the midline to the tip of the twelfth rib and superiorly to the xiphisternum. An extension to the left of the midline is added in patients with a narrow costal margin. Occasionally with large tumours involving the right hepatic lobe, an extension of the incision into the right chest may be necessary to obtain control of the superior vena cava and hepatic veins. The liver is next mobilized by division of the falciform ligament to expose the superior vena cava, followed by division of the left and right triangular ligaments. Resectability is then confirmed by careful bimanual palpation and intraoperative ultrasound (Rees et al, 1996).

Large tumours adherent to the dome of the diaphragm are mobilized by *en bloc* resection of the involved diaphragm. Bleeding from the diaphragm is secured and the defect closed either by simple suturing or by polypropylene mesh.

The appropriate type of resection necessary to encompass the lesion(s) is next selected. The key technical factor is to obtain 1–2 cm of tumour-free margin, no matter what type of resection is required. The porta hepatis is dissected to isolate the hepatic artery, portal vein and bile duct (Figures 33.18–33.20). After the inflow to the liver is isolated, control of hepatic venous anatomy takes priority (Figure 33.21). Gaining access to the three hepatic veins constitutes the most technically demanding part of the operation and the various techniques for control are well described elsewhere (Warren et al, 1991).

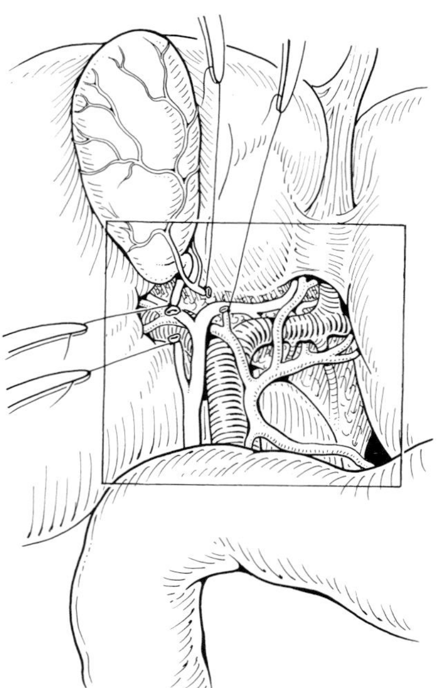

Figure 33.18 Liver resection. The porta hepatis is dissected to isolate the hepatic artery, portal vein and bile duct. The cystic duct and cystic artery are exposed, ligated and divided.

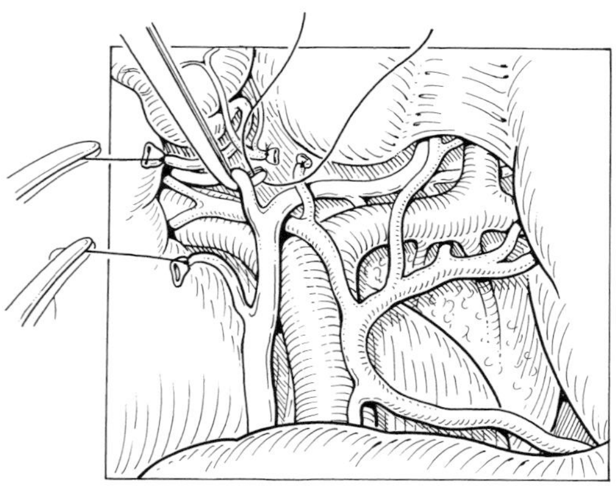

Figure 33.19 Liver resection, right lobectomy. The right hepatic duct is dissected, divided and ligated.

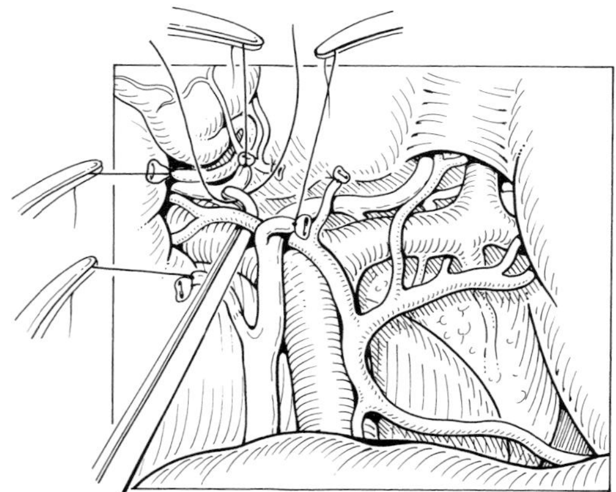

Figure 33.20 Liver resection, right lobectomy. The right hepatic artery is dissected, ligated and then divided.

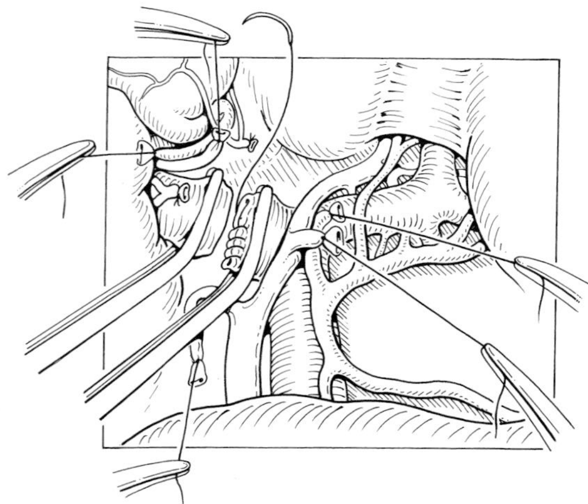

Figure 33.21 Liver resection, right lobectomy. The portal vein is exposed. The right branch of the portal vein is carefully dissected and divided between vascular clamps. The cut ends are oversewn.

Following the hepatic venous dissection, the actual transection of the liver may be performed in a number of ways. Some surgeons still prefer the 'finger fracture' technique, whereby the liver capsule is incised with diathermy and the parenchyma fractured away by the fingers, exposing the veins, ducts and arteries, which are subsequently ligated (Babineau and Steele, 1996) (Figures 33.22 and 33.23). Others prefer to use the ultrasonic aspirator (CUSA Valley Labs, London, or Selector, Surgical Technology Group, Andover, UK) (Hodgson et al, 1993), which removes the hepatic parenchyma while leaving the vascular structures and bile ducts intact so that they can be ligated and divided sepa-

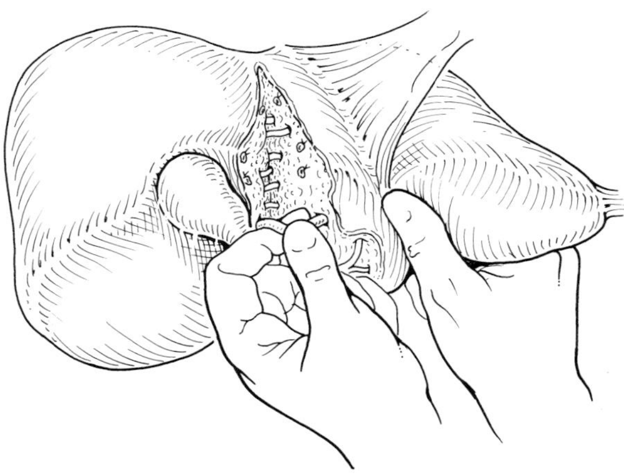

Figure 33.22 Liver resection, right lobectomy with the finger fracture technique. Once located, vessels and bile ducts are secured and ligated.

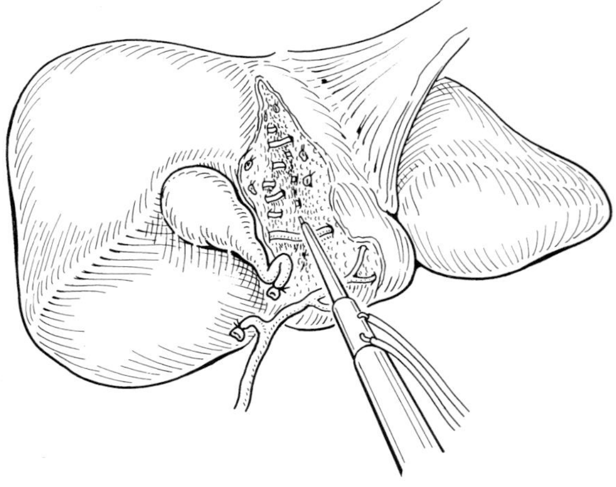

Figure 33.23 Liver resection – right lobectomy with diathermy along the lines of demarcation. The liver is then fractured between finger and thumb.

rately. The ultrasonic dissector can also be used in conjunction with the argon beam coagulator (Surgical Technology Group), which can coagulate small vascular branches.

If severe haemorrhage occurs intraoperatively, the liver can be completely isolated by applying a vascular clamp across the porta hepatis (Pringle's manoeuvre) and the vena cava can be compressed above and below the liver. Warm ischaemia will be tolerated by the liver for up to one hour. Using this time, the surgeon can sort out the technical problem. Ideally, if vascular isolation is required to perform a resection, it should be evident before the parenchymal dissection and planned for in an orderly fashion. Tumour in the caudate lobe or near the vena cava may best be resected in this way.

After removal of the specimen, the transected surface is observed carefully and small bleeding points are secured either by under-running or by argon beam coagulation if available. If there is still a problem with haemostasis, the surface can be covered with collagen sheets (Johnson & Johnson Medical, Ascot, UK) or the surface can be sprayed with coagulant glue (Tiseel Immuno, Sevenoaks, UK). Finally, the wound is closed, leaving multiple suction drains *in situ*, which are usually left for several days.

Clearly the above is not an exhaustive description of liver resection and the reader is urged to consult appropriate texts for more in-depth descriptions (Warren et al, 1991; Blumgart, 1994; Lygidakij et al, 1989).

Complications

Excessive bleeding is still the most common and lethal intraoperative complication and various measures have been devised to combat this problem. Intraoperative blood salvage techniques, such as the cell saver, are used and, along with preoperative autologous blood banking, the amount of bank blood used for transfusion can be reduced. Postoperatively, patients may need massive 'third space' requirements and, if they have required massive transfusion, metabolic alkalosis is invariable. The latter can be corrected with the central administration of 0.1N hydrochloric acid. Sepsis is the most common complication of liver resection; also, bleeding, bile leak and hepatic failure may occur. There is usually a transient rise in serum bilirubin and other liver function tests postoperatively, but these usually return to baseline within 10 days. A persistent elevation in liver enzymes suggests an infective complication or vascular injury, and a persistent elevation in serum bilirubin suggests a biliary obstruction with or without a leak.

Selection of procedure

The proper technique of resection is characterized by the single goal of removing all metastatic disease with a minimum of 1–1.5 cm margin of surrounding normal hepatic parenchyma. Anatomically defined lobectomy is not necessary if segmentectomy or wedge resection completely removes all metastatic deposits. Some authorities still claim that metastasectomy with an adequate surrounding shell of healthy liver is as effective as lobectomy or segmentectomy. Although the size of a solitary hepatic metastasis does not seem to be a prognostic indicator, the number of metastases seems to be important (Cady and McDermott, 1985; Hughes et al, 1988). Patients with more than three lesions have a shorter survival and some authors consider the presence of more than three lesions to be a contraindication to resection. It is possible to combine cryosurgical ablation with hepatic resection if more than one metastasis is present, particularly for bilobar lesions. However, the benefits of such a manoeuvre are not at all clear. Whether cryosurgery alone for solitary lesions can be as effective as hepatic resection remains to be seen, but there is no doubt that this technique is less traumatic and has a lower morbidity (see below).

Because of the relative success in treating a selected group of patients by liver resection, there has been a vogue in recent years to consider a second resection for recurrent metastases. This approach in very selected patients has been shown to be safe and can yield a few survivors at 5 years (Fowler et al, 1993; Que and Nagorney, 1994; Pinson et al, 1996).

Results (Table 33.11)

Nowadays liver resection for metastatic disease can be achieved with an operative mortality of below 5%. Indeed, there are surgeons with much lower rates (Rees et al, 1996). Nevertheless, the morbidity is still high. Approximately 25% of patients will have complications, and in one-third those complications will be major. If selection is careful, approximately 25% of patients undergoing resection can expect to survive for 5 years.

Cryosurgical ablation of liver metastases

Some lesions may be adequately treated with cryosurgical ablation, which is the destruction *in situ* of tumour using subzero temperatures. The technique involves ultrasonographic localization of the metastasis, placement of an encased liquid nitro-

Table 33.11 Hepatic resection for metastases from colorectal carcinomas: operative mortality and 5-year survival.

Author/year	*n*	*Operative mortality* (%)	*5-year survival* (%)
Wilson and Adson (1976)	60	2	28
Foster and Berman (1977)	126	–	22
Morrow et al (1982)	38	10	27
Adson et al (1984)	141	2	25*
August et al (1985)	33	0	35
Cady and McDermott (1985)	23	0	30
Butler et al (1986)†	62	10	34
Elkberg et al (1986)	72	–	16
Iwatsuki et al (1986)	60	0	45
Nordlinger et al (1987)	80	5	25
Attiyeh and Wichern (1988)	20	24	35
Fortner (1988)§	77	5	49
Hughes et al (1988)‡	859	–	33
Federov and Shelygin (1989)	71	5	26
Scheele et al (1990b)	183	5	31
Doci et al (1995)	219	–	24
Jatzko et al (1995)	66	4.5	29.6
Babineau and Steele (1996)	69¶	–	23**
Isenberg et al (1996)	17	–	47
Rees et al (1996)	150	0.7	–

* 46% patients without extrahepatic disease. † Recent operative mortality of 2%. ‡ Multi-institutional. § Highly selected. ¶ Curative resection only. ** Probability only.

gen probe within the lesion, and lowering of the tissue temperature to approximately –35°C for several minutes, followed by slow rewarming. This cycle is repeated two to three times.

The real-time monitoring of adequate freeze margins has resulted in several groups reporting low morbidity with effective ablation of liver tumour in large numbers of patients (Steele, 1994a,b; Fong et al, 1996; Morris and Ross, 1996; Adam et al, 1997; Korpan, 1997; Yeh et al, 1997). For patients with relatively small lesions in the depths of the right or left hepatic lobes, the avoidance of having to perform a major resection decreases the morbidity and mortality with no noticeable change in either pattern of recurrence or survival.

A contraindication to the technique is when the lesion to be treated is next to a major blood vessel. In these circumstances, a heat sink is created which may prevent cryosurgical destruction of all the tumour.

Provided the metastatic lesion can be treated with a 1–2 cm circumferential margin, cryodestruction of metastases is potentially a less invasive, and as effective, treatment as hepatic resection. However, time will tell whether it becomes the preferred option.

Laser destruction of liver metastases

Laser-induced thermotherapy can also be used as a local treatment for the destruction of liver metastases from colorectal cancer (Bown, 1983; Steger et al, 1992). The technique involves interstitial insertion of flexible bare wires into the metastases and inducing hyperthermia with a Nd-YAG laser. Using a bare fibre as the energy delivery system, well-defined spherically shaped areas of necrosis up to 16 mm diameter can be produced around the fibre tip (Matthewson et al, 1987). Several fibres can be placed either at laparotomy (Hashimoto et al, 1985) or percutaneously (Masters et al, 1992), and recently the laparoscopic approach has been explored (Germer et al, 1997). Photodynamic therapy can also be used in a similar way (Purkiss et al, 1993, 1994).

A problem with laser therapy is the limited dimensions of the inducible necrotic lesion that can be produced. At present, laser therapy can be used only for relatively small metastases and cryosurgery at present seems to be a better alternative.

Surgical resection of lung metastases

The lungs are the second most common site of metastatic disease from a colorectal primary tumour. Post-mortem studies reveal spread to the lungs in 30–50% of patients dying of colorectal cancer (Welch and Donaldson, 1979). Approximately 10% of patients will have their lung metastases detected during life and 10% of these metastases will be isolated. Therefore, about 1% of all patients with colorectal cancer may have resectable disease

(McCormack and Attiyeh, 1979; Welch and Donaldson, 1979; Hughes et al, 1982; Wilkins et al, 1985; Smith et al, 1992; Orkin, 1993; Gough et al, 1994). A solitary pulmonary nodule in a patient with a history of colorectal cancer will represent a metastasis in about one-half of cases and a primary neoplasm in the other half (Cahan et al, 1974).

CT scanning of the chest is the most accurate method of preoperative assessment. Exploration is indicated if the primary lesion has been controlled, if the pulmonary disease is isolated and if the patient is reasonably fit (Orkin, 1993).

The patient may be explored through a thoracotomy for single or monolateral lesions, although most thoracic surgeons favour a median sternotomy. This approach is said to be better tolerated than a thoracotomy and allows examination of both lungs (McCormack and Attiyeh, 1979). Bilateral examination is important because there is a high incidence of unsuspected bilateral lesions. However, if a unilateral approach is used, the other side can now be assessed by video thoracoscopy (Dowling et al, 1992; Landreneau et al, 1993).

Operative mortality seems to be low and 5-year survival in a highly selected group of patients averages 20–30% (Table 33.12). Long-term survival has been associated with a variety of prognostic factors but there seems to be no generalized agreement as to which factors are important.

Scheele et al (1990a,b) demonstrated a better long-term survival in patients with colon cancer as opposed to those with rectal cancer, but they stressed that this finding should not influence the decision-making process. Disease-free survival is often considered a major indicator of prognosis (Wilkins, 1978; Iwatsuki et al, 1983; Brister et al, 1988) but many authors have been unable to substantiate this finding (Wilkins et al, 1985; Greenway, 1988; Mori et al, 1991; McCormack et al, 1992; Yano et al, 1993). The number of resected metastases (single versus multiple) is usually considered the most important prognostic discriminant, but analysis of the largest series in the literature (McCormack et al, 1992) failed to confirm this finding. The size of the lesion does not necessarily indicate a better prognosis, although some would argue that the outcome following resection of lesions under 3 cm diameter is more favourable (Greenway, 1988; Shirouzu et al, 1995).

It is our experience that very few patients with pulmonary metastases are suitable for resection. Most have liver metastases and/or widespread bilateral disease. However, perhaps the colorectal surgeon should think about this possibility more than previously, particularly for a small solitary lesion in a patient free from disease elsewhere, who is otherwise fit.

Chemotherapy

Numerous treatment regimens have been tried in patients with disseminated colorectal cancer. Unfortunately none appears to be very effective. Without the confines of a clinical trial patients are best treated symptomatically. The various modalities which have been used are discussed below. In most reports no distinction has been made between disseminated rectal or colonic disease. It is also difficult to determine from these studies whether the metastases have developed synchronously or metachronously. In addition the efficacy of the treatment is impossible to determine as there are very few controlled trials.

Fluorouracil has become the standard chemotherapeutic agent for the treatment of advanced colorectal carcinoma, used either alone or in combination with other agents. Pitrelli and Mittelman (1984) reviewed the response rates in studies using 5FU alone in various dose schedules. They found that the response rate varied from 12% to 44%. One of the main problems in assessing the results of these studies is the lack of uniformity when defining response. Moertel (1978), in the light of his extensive experience in the field of gastrointestinal chemotherapy, listed the following criteria:

Table 33.12 Survival after resection of pulmonary metastases from colorectal carcinoma.

Author	*n*	*5-year survival (%)*
Cahan et al (1974)	31	30
Wilkins et al (1978)	34	27
McCormack & Attiyeh (1979)	35	22
Morrow et al (1981)	16	13
Mountain et al (1984)	28	28
Pihl et al (1987)	16	38
Brister et al (1988)	335	30
Goya et al (1989)	62	42
Scheele et al (1989)	45	44

- a reduction of the products of the longest perpendicular diameter of measurable known malignant disease by at least 50%
- no increase in size of other areas of malignant disease
- no new areas of malignant disease
- the results must be observed for at least 2 months after the onset of therapy.

Watkins et al (1970) listed two additional criteria which should be included in the assessment of hepatic disease:

- a significant decrease in the size of the liver accompanied by relief of symptoms and return of biochemical tests to normal or near-normal
- an improvement in functional capacity for normal activities prolonged for more than 3 months.

Many studies now also include performance indicators and an assessment of the quality of life for treatment of advanced disease.

Taylor (1982), reviewing the literature and applying the above criteria strictly, remained unconvinced that there was any evidence of benefit from a single chemotherapeutic agent in the management of disseminated metastases from colorectal cancer. Even if the criteria used are not as strict as those discussed above, it has to be admitted that response rates to 5FU alone in general are poor and a median survival for advanced disease remains at between 26 and 30 weeks.

The standard regimen for using 5FU was described by Rochlin et al (1965). They emphasized that it was essential to increase the dosage to the stage at which toxicity was produced. In addition they stressed the need to continue administration of the drug if a response had been achieved, either by using a maintenance dose or repeated courses of therapy to its toxic limits. The regimen was as follows:

- An initial loading dose consisted of a daily intravenous injection of 15 mg/kg bodyweight for 5 days.
- In the absence of toxic side-effects an additional intravenous injection of 7.5 mg/kg bodyweight was given every other day until toxicity developed.
- The end-point was determined when the white blood count fell below 4000/mm^3. Once this had occurred intravenous therapy was resumed at a level of 15 mg/kg bodyweight twice a week.

Since then 5FU has been administered by a variety of routes and in different dosages. The hope has been to reduce toxicity with an enhanced response rate. The conclusions that can be drawn from these various studies are as follows:

- Systemic therapy produces better response rates than oral administration (Hahn et al, 1975).
- Continuous intravenous administration is more effective than an intermittent regimen (Seifert et al, 1975), and with the use of ambulatory pumps, the patient no longer has to remain in hospital.
- Although weekly intravenous infusion is less effective than continuous infusion, it is less toxic (Ansfield et al, 1977).

This information, together with that about the enhancement of activity of 5FU by folinic acid has led, in certain quarters, to renewed optimism of the benefit of systemic chemotherapy for disseminated disease. Thus, in a small trial using 5FU, folinic acid and mitomycin, survival was shown to be improved compared with supportive care only (Scheithauer et al, 1993). A similar trial of 5FU and folinic acid in elderly patients reached the same conclusion (Beretta et al, 1994). In another study from the Nordic countries, patients with advanced but asymptomatic colorectal cancer were randomized for treatment with systemic methotrexate, leucovorin and 5FU either at the time of diagnosis or when symptoms developed. There was a significant improvement in survival and symptom-free period in the early-treatment group (Glimelius et al, 1991).

A new drug has recently emerged as an alternative to 5FU and folinic acid for the treatment of disseminated disease. Tomudex is a quinazoline antifolate. It is a direct and specific inhibitor of thymidylate synthase, and once it has entered the cell it is polyglutamated, leading to prolonged intracellular retention and increased enzyme inhibition. Tomudex has been compared with various combinations of 5FU folinic acid in three randomized trials in advanced colorectal cancer (Zeneca, personal communication 1997). Tomudex appears to produce the same slight survival benefit achieved by 5FU/FA, but with fewer side-effects.

It should be stressed, however, that all of these studies consisted of small numbers of patients and the results need to be confirmed in larger trials. Nevertheless, in selected patients, particularly in the younger group, it is wise for patients to discuss this option with a medical oncologist.

Infusion therapy with 5FU

Of particular interest is the intra-arterial delivery of 5FU (Johnson and Rivkin, 1985; Goldberg et al, 1990; Schlag et al, 1990). This type of therapy was first introduced for the treatment of advanced head and neck cancers. It was later adapted for use in patients with colorectal liver metastases (Watkins et al, 1970; Ansfield et al, 1977; Sundquist et al, 1978; Taylor, 1978; Grage et al, 1979; Presant et al, 1984; Oliver and Shorb, 1985; Cohen et al, 1986; Ramming and O'Toole, 1986). Fluorouracil or 5FUDR was perfused into the hepatic artery through catheters positioned either at laparotomy (via the gastroduodenal artery) or percutaneously (via the brachial or femoral artery). The majority of series have been confined to symptomatic metachronous tumours and no attempt was made to stage the extent of liver involvement. Ansfield et al (1977) had the largest experience (419 patients overall, 381 with colorectal primary tumours): 161 of the 419 patients were reported to have been improved symptomatically, but there was no objective assessment of reduced tumour burden. All reports suggested that the side-effects were severe and much worse than when the drug was administered intravenously.

Interest in the intra-arterial perfusion technique has recently been rekindled by the development of totally implantable pumps which can deliver the drug continuously and which do not require prolonged hospital admission (Hardy et al, 1984) (Figure 33.24).

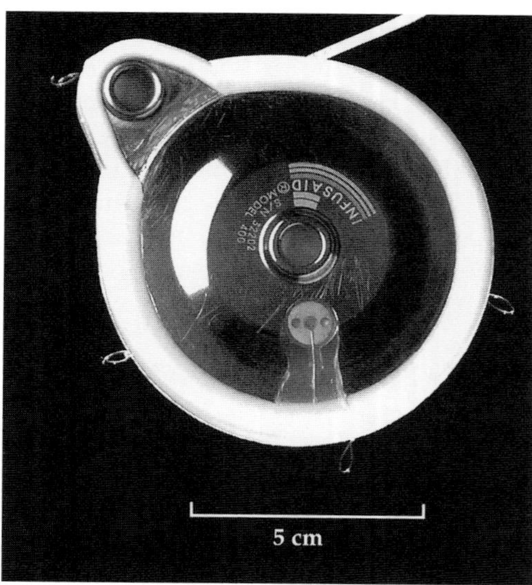

Figure 33.24 Infusaid model 400 infusion pump (Infusaid Norwood, MA, USA) for intrahepatic arterial chemotherapy. The pump is sited subcutaneously on the abdominal wall and the catheter (above) passes through the abdominal wall into the hepatic artery via the gastroduodenal artery. The pump is filled via the central septum, and the peripheral septum can be used for a flush injection through the catheter if required. Photograph courtesy Professor T G Allen-Mersh.

Neiderhuber et al (1984) described the results of hepatic arterial infusion of 5FUDR in 93 patients with liver metastases. The drug was delivered by the implantable Infusaid pump, and patients received cyclic therapy consisting of 5FUDR for 2 weeks alternating with 2 weeks' of saline infusion. This study was complicated in that patients who did not respond initially were given mitomycin in addition to the 5FUDR. Of the 50 patients with metastatic disease confined to the liver, 83% demonstrated a significant reduction in tumour size with a median duration of response of 13 months and a median survival of 25 months. Patients with extra-hepatic tumour recurrence did not experience a significant level of response. The results of this study and other, non-randomized studies, were equally encouraging (Cohen et al, 1983; Johnson et al, 1983; Weiss et al, 1983; Kemeny et al, 1984; Schwartz et al, 1985; Shepard et al, 1985; Balch and Urist, 1986; Curley et al, 1993; Kemeny et al, 1994a,b). This success in phase I trials resulted in the setting up of various randomized controlled trials; one of the first was that of Chang et al (1987), who compared continuous intra-arterial 5FUDR with intravenous 5FUDR in 62 patients with colorectal liver metastases. An improved response rate was noted in the intra-arterial group (63% versus 17%) but this was not mirrored by a significantly improved survival rate (2-year actuarial survival rate 22% versus 15%). However, patients without portal lymph node involvement did better with intra-arterial treatment than with intravenous treatment (2-year actuarial survival rate 47% versus 13%). Toxicity of intra-arterial 5FUDR was, however, considerable, including chemical hepatitis (79%), biliary sclerosis (21%) and peptic ulcer (17%). Since then at least six randomized studies have been performed using implantable pumps (Table 33.13). In these trials, hepatic arterial FUDR was delivered continuously for 2 weeks in 28-day cycles. These studies showed a greater response rate (more than two-fold higher), determined by imaging and/or serum markers to hepatic arterial chemotherapy. In all studies, although there appeared to be an improvement in median survival, this reached statistical significance in only two studies (Rougier et al, 1992; Allen-Mersh et al, 1994). The study by Allen-Mersh and associates was unique in that it demonstrated a significant improvement in quality of life in patients receiving pump chemotherapy compared with controls. Unfortunately, because of problems with

Table 33.13 Randomized studies of hepatic artery chemotherapy for irresectable hepatic colorectal metastases.

		Drug (mg per kg per day)		*Percentage response rate*			*Median survival in months*		
Authors	*n*	*Systemic*	*HAC*	*Systemic*	*HAC*	*P*	*Systemic*	*HAC*	*P*
Grage et al (1979)	61	5-FU (12)	5-FU (20)	23	34	NS	13	10	NS
Kemeny et al (1987)	162	FUDR (0.125)	FUDR (0.3)	20	50	0.001	12	17	NS
Chang et al (1987)	64	FUDR (0.125)	FUDR (0.3)	17	62	0.003	15	22	NS§
Hohn et al (1989)	143	FUDR (0.075)	FUDR (0.3)	10	42	0.0001	16	17	NS
Martin et al (1990)	69	5-FU (500)*	FUDR (0.3)	21	48	0.02	11	13	NS
Rougier et al (1992)	163	5-FU (500)*†	FUDR (0.3)	9	43	–	11	15	0.03
Allen-Mersh et al (1994)	100	‡	FUDR (0.2)	–	–	–	8	15	0.03

HAC, hepatic artery chemotherapy; 5-FU, 5-fluorouracil, FUDR, floxuridine. Dose mg/kg per day unless stated otherwise.
* mg/m². † Only half of patients received chemotherapy. ‡ Less than 25% of patients received systemic chemotherapy. NS, not significant.
§ $P < 0.03$ if patients with positive portal lymph nodes are excluded.
(From Vauthey et al, 1996).

study design, definitive conclusions cannot yet be made.

The portal vein has also been used for infusion of 5FU to treat colorectal hepatic metastases. Bevan (1973) used the obliterated umbilical vein for access in four patients with synchronous liver metastases and described a good response. Taylor (1978) described a technique of portal vein infusion with 5FU combined with hepatic artery ligation. These patients had an improved survival rate compared with a control group. Nevertheless, in a larger study (Taylor, 1981) employing stricter selection criteria, the difference was marginal and the author concluded that the slight improvement did not justify the routine use of the technique (Taylor, 1982).

Combination chemotherapy

In an attempt to improve response rates, 5FU has been combined with several other agents. The most popular regimen seems to have been 5FU, methyl-CCNU and vincristine, the so-called MOP regimen. This combination was greeted with particular enthusiasm when Moertel et al (1975) obtained a response rate of 43% using it. Unfortunately after more patients entered the trial no difference was demonstrated between MOP and 5FU alone (Moertel, 1978). Similar results were reported in Birmingham by Hine and Dykes (1984).

Engstrom et al (1984) reported an extensive study in which combination treatment regimens were compared with 5FU. The groups were (a) 5FU alone; (b) 5FU with hydroxyurea; (c) methyl-CCNU and docarbazine, (d) 5FU and hydroxyurea alternating with methyl-CCNU and docarbazine; (e) methyl-CCNU and razoxane; and (f) mitomycin and docarbazine. No clear survival advantage could be demonstrated for any one regimen over another, but the numbers of patients in the groups were small. As discussed previously, the combination of 5FU with its modulator folinic acid seems to be the most promising combination.

Leucovorin, dexamethasone, mitomycin and cisapride have also been studied in hepatic arterial chemotherapy. Although leucovorin has proved effective in combination with 5FU as systemic treatment, it must be used at a lower dosage when included in hepatic arterial chemotherapy to avoid excessive hepatobiliary toxicity (Kaplan et al, 1984; Kemeny et al, 1990; Patt et al, 1990; Kemeny and Sigurdson, 1994). The addition of dexamethasone to FUDR and leucovorin has resulted in fewer side-effects and a better response rate (Kemeny et al, 1994a). Mitomycin, cisplatin and bischoloethyl nitrosourea have been used variously in combination with FUDR in an effort to overcome resistance of tumour to FUDR alone (Niederhuber et al, 1984; Shepard et al, 1985; Patt et al, 1986), but without much success. Additional studies of FUDR in combination with interferon-γ (Jones et al, 1993), interleukin-2 (Mavligit et al, 1990a) and tumour necrosis factor (Mavligit et al, 1990b) have been reported. These regimens need further testing before phase 3 studies can be conducted.

Radiotherapy for advanced disease

There have been few studies using radiotherapy for metastatic colorectal carcinoma. However, the few that have been performed (Prasad et al, 1977; Sherman et al, 1978; Lightdale et al, 1979) claimed that patients developed significant relief of pain from hepatic metastases. Pain has also been alleviated when radiotherapy has been used to treat peritoneal metastases (Whiteley et al, 1970), as well as secondary deposits in lung, bones and brain (Stearns and Leaming, 1975). Another approach has been to introduce radioactive microspheres into the hepatic arterial tree of patients with liver metastases, and many authors claim good results (Ariel,

1965; Grady, 1979; Goldberg et al, 1988; Kerr et al, 1988). However, no study using radiotherapy has demonstrated any improvement in survival.

Combination of chemotherapy and radiotherapy

Moertel et al (1964) combined supervoltage radiotherapy with systemic 5FU therapy as treatment for advanced gastrointestinal carcinoma. Of the 44 patients treated in this manner, 37% obtained complete remission of their symptoms and a further 12% had some improvement. Byfield et al (1984) also reported a 4-year pilot study in 28 patients with colorectal cancer utilizing a combination of continuous intra-arterial chemotherapy with 5FUDR combined with whole-liver irradiation, the latter being started 3–7 days after the start of the chemotherapy. The authors concluded that treatment appeared to have improved the prognosis of these patients; however, no controlled trials have been performed using this form of therapy, so that it is difficult to draw firm conclusions.

Immunotherapy

Exciting developments in immunotherapy have occurred in recent years and various workers have used this therapy for the treatment of disseminated colorectal cancer. Perhaps the most promising area initially appeared to be the use of interleukin-2 and lymphokine activated killer (LAK) cells.

Interleukin-2 (IL-2) is a lymphokine which is now engineered by recombinant technology. When IL-2 is incubated with the patient's own lymphocytes, these are converted into killer cells which are capable of attacking the patient's tumour when reinfused. Rosenberg et al (1987), who pioneered the technique, treated 106 patients suffering from a variety of advanced cancers with LAK cells plus IL-2. Eight patients had a complete response and 15 had a partial response. Melanoma and renal cell tumours were the most responsive. Two patients with colorectal cancer had partial responses. One of the problems with systemic LAK therapy was the high incidence of toxicity. There were four treatment-related deaths and approximately one-third of patients needed intensive therapy care, particularly for ventilation purposes.

In the technique described by Rosenberg et al (1987) the lymphocytes were obtained by leucopheresis and the incubation with IL-2 occurs *in vitro*. Such a manoeuvre was time-consuming, expensive, and may have been the reason for some of the toxicity. We attempted to overcome these problems by using the peritoneal cavity as a LAK generating organ. A mixture of the patient's lymphocytes and IL-2 was infused through a Tenchoff catheter into the peritoneal cavity in 18 patients with advanced colorectal cancer (Johnson et al, 1989). Having confirmed that LAK cells could be generated within the peritoneal cavity, we subsequently inserted a peritoneovenous shunt ('Denver catheter') to transfer the LAK cells from the cavity to the systemic circulation. We were able to confirm that this technique was capable of transferring LAK activity satisfactorily into the systemic circulation without inducing the toxic effects seen in Rosenberg's cases. Of the 18 patients so treated, none required care in the intensive therapy unit. However, despite the reduction in toxicity, the response rate was not improved: only two of 18 patients had a partial response and only one patient was alive and asymptomatic 12 months after commencing therapy. We have now abandoned this form of therapy.

Another approach to immunotherapy is the use of monoclonal antibodies to which is attached a cancericidal agent – the 'magic bullet' approach. Hyams et al (1987) have used a CEA monoclonal antibody labelled with the potent beta-ray emitter yttrium-90 in diffuse intraperitoneal carcinomatoses in nude mice. Treated animals had a significant decrease in tumour load compared with untreated animals. As discussed previously in the adjuvant chemotherapy section, there remain several intellectual problems that need to be solved before this approach will be feasible in patients with disseminated disease. Nevertheless, progress continues particularly in the field of anti-idiotype antibodies (Goldenberg, 1993).

Other therapeutic manoeuvres for advanced disease

Hepatic arterial ligation

The growth of liver metastases depends primarily on an adequate blood supply. Breedis and Young (1954) originally demonstrated that the hepatic artery was the main blood supply to the established liver metastasis. This observation has since been confirmed *in vivo* both in experimental animals (Lien and Ackerman, 1970) and in humans (Gelin et al, 1968; Taylor et al, 1979b). It was hoped, therefore, that simple hepatic artery ligation might prolong survival. This hope has not been borne out in practice, for while the technique might palliate the pain that some patients experience (Larmi et al, 1974; Pitrelli et al, 1984), survival has not been influenced (Almersjo et al, 1972; Bengmark et al, 1974).

Hepatic dearterialization

Complete surgical division of the hepatic arterial supply has been used intermittently since 1972 in the management of liver tumours. Although some benefit has been recorded with primary liver neoplasms (Balasagaram, 1972), no great success has been reported for metastases. It is a technically difficult manoeuvre and the results in our opinion do not justify its use.

Hepatic arterial embolization

Hepatic arterial embolization is a relatively simple and potentially useful technique for the palliative treatment of liver metastases. Sterile absorbable gelatin sponge is injected either percutaneously at the time of angiography (Allison, 1978) or at laparotomy if synchronous liver metastases are being treated at the time of resection. Using embolization rather than simple ligation, the chance of forming collateral vessels is reduced, so theoretically the palliative effect might be more prolonged.

There are a few reports of the use of embolization for the treatment of metachronous liver metastases. Hunt et al (1990) evaluated hepatic artery embolization in a randomized study of 61 patients with hepatic metastases. Systemic treatment was compared with embolization with collagen and lyophilized dura, and chemoembolization with starch microspheres and 5FU repeated monthly via a subcutaneous chamber connected to the hepatic artery. The median survival times were no different between the groups (8, 7 and 11 months respectively). Apart from this study, there appear to be no others which have compared embolization with an appropriate control group; a more thorough evaluation is therefore needed before its place in therapy can be decided.

Conclusion

The treatment of advanced metastatic disease is difficult. Many claims have been made for various regimens but it has to be said that there is little evidence from controlled trials to establish the superiority of any one regimen. There is a real need for the discovery of a more effective chemotherapeutic agent than is available at present. If such a drug does become available it will be essential to perform carefully randomized, controlled clinical trials. If such trials had been carried out more often with currently available regimens a clearer picture of their efficacy might have emerged at an earlier date. Although the overall results of these methods of palliation are generally unrewarding, a few patients obtain spectacular results. It should always be remembered when deciding to treat these patients that the toxicity of the regimen may outstrip any potential benefit. The final decision in our opinion should only be taken after close consultation and counselling of each patient after fully informing them of the facts.

Other palliative manoeuvres

One of the most useful palliative surgical manoeuvres for patients with recurrent obstructing colorectal carcinoma is a bypass procedure or a defunctioning stoma. Whenever possible the aim should be to construct an enteroenteric anastomosis so that a stoma is avoided. However, sometimes a stoma is the only technique that can give relief, and if so it should be used in carefully selected patients who have been thoroughly counselled.

TREATMENT OF INOPERABLE RECTAL CANCER

A rectal carcinoma may be considered to be inoperable for several reasons. The patient may be too old, ill or frail to undergo a major procedure. The tumour may be so extensive locally that technically it cannot be removed. Lastly, dissemination may be so widespread that it is considered inappropriate to embark on major surgery as death is imminent. This situation is particularly pertinent if all that can be offered is an abdominoperineal excision of the rectum which would leave the patient with the added burden of a colostomy. Each case must be judged individually as there are several available options.

Thus if the patient has widespread metastases but the primary tumour is not causing serious problems the patient may be best managed with analgesia and good nursing care. If, on the other hand, the primary lesion is discharging blood and mucus and the patient complains of incapacitating diarrhoea or tenesmus, the best treatment may be a local manoeuvre such as electrocoagulation, cryotherapy, Nd-YAG laser treatment, external beam radiotherapy or/and a defunctioning stoma (Baigrie and Berry, 1994) (see also Chapter 32). If there is no evidence of dissemination but the surgeon considers that the lesion is so locally advanced that surgery cannot be performed, it may be preferable to treat the patient initially with a full course of radiotherapy in an attempt to shrink the lesion in the hope that it might become operable. If the tumour is causing pain which is uncontrolled by analgesia, intrathecal injection of alcohol or phenol or some type of neurosurgical procedure such as cordotomy may have to be considered in selected patients. If the lesion with widespread metastases is causing obstruction it is sometimes possible either by electrocoagulation or laser therapy to create a lumen through it and thus a colostomy and laparotomy can be avoided. In these circumstances stenting may prove useful for palliation.

We try to avoid a colostomy for inoperable rectal carcinoma if at all possible, as we do not think that this is generally good palliation when life expectancy is only a few months. Nevertheless, there are a few patients in whom a defunctioning procedure is justified. Thus if the tumour is invading the sphincters and causing serious incontinence, a colostomy will often be justified even though the prognosis is poor. Similarly, if a local manoeuvre fails to relieve intestinal obstruction or the patient presents with acute obstruction, a defunctioning stoma may be needed. Any stoma should be as close to the tumour as possible; most surgeons therefore recommend a left iliac fossa loop colostomy for a rectal cancer. An end-colostomy with closure of the distal rectum should be avoided, as the distal closure may leak in the presence of an obstructing tumour below it.

REFERENCES

Abulafi AM, de Jode ML, Allardice SJ, Ansell JK & Williams NS (1997) Adjuvant intraoperative photodynamic therapy in experimental cancer using a new photosensitizer. *Br J Surg* **84**: 368–371.

ACCMP (Advanced Colorectal Cancer Meta-analysis Project) (1992) Modulation of 5-FU by leucovorin in patients with advanced colorectal cancer: evidence in terms of response rates. *J Clin Oncol* **10**: 896–903.

Adalsteinsson B, Glimelius B, Graffman S et al (1981) Computed tomography of recurrent rectal cancer. *Acta Radiol (Diagn) (Stockh)* **22**: 669–672.

Adalsteinsson B, Påhlman A, Hemmingsson A, Glimelius B & Graffman S (1987) Computed tomography in early diagnosis of local recurrence of rectal carcinoma. *Acta Radiol* **28**: 41–46.

Adam R, Akpinar E, Johann M et al (1997) Place of cryosurgery in the treatment of malignant liver tumors. *Ann Surg* **225**: 39–48; discussion 48–50.

Adson MA (1987) Resection of liver metastases: when is it worthwhile? *World J Surg* **11**: 511–520.

Adson MA, Van Heerden JA, Adson MH, Wagner JS & Ilstrup DM (1984) Resection of hepatic metastases from colorectal cancer. *Arch Surg* **119**: 647–651.

Agnew CH & Cooley RN (1962) Barium enema study of postoperative recurrences of carcinoma of the colon. *JAMA* **179**: 331.

Allardice JT, Grahn MF, Rowland AC et al (1992) Safety studies for intraoperative photodynamic therapy. *Lasers Med Sci* **7**: 133–142.

Allen PIM, Fielding JWL, Middleton MD & Priestman TJ (1987) Rectal carcinoma: a new technique to allow safer postoperative irradiation of the pelvis. *Eur J Surg Oncol* **13**: 21–25.

Allen-Mersh TG, Earlam S, Fordy C et al (1994) Quality of life and survival with continuous hepatic-artery floxuridine infusion for colorectal liver metastases. *Lancet* **344**: 1255–1260.

Allison PJ (1978) Therapeutic embolisation. *Br J Hosp Med* **20**: 207–214.

Allum WH, Mack P, Priestman TJ & Fielding JWL (1987) Radiotherapy for pain relief in locally recurrent colorectal cancer. *Ann R Coll Surg Engl* **69**: 220–221.

Almersjo O, Bengmark S, Rudenstam CM et al (1972) Evaluation of hepatic de-arterialisation in primary and secondary cancer of the liver. *Am J Surg* **124**: 5–9.

Ansell J et al (1996) Abstract. *Br J Surg* **83**: 69.

Ansfield F, Klotz J, Nelaton T et al (1977) A phase III study comparing the clinical utility of four regimes of 5 fluorouracil. *Cancer* **39**: 34.

Ariel IM (1965) Treatment of inoperable primary pancreatic and liver cancer by intra-arterial administration of radioactive isotopes (Y-99 radiating microspheres). *Ann Surg* **162**: 267.

Attiyeh EF & Stearns MW (1981) Second-look laparotomy based on CEA elevations in colorectal cancer. *Cancer* **47**: 1229.

Attiyeh FF & Wichern WA Jr (1988) Hepatic resection for primary and metastatic tumors. *Am J Surg* **156**: 368–373.

August DA, Sugarbaker PH, Ottow RT, Gianola FJ & Schneider PD (1985) Hepatic resection of colorectal metastases: influence on survival of clinical factors and adjuvant intraperitoneal 5-FU via Tenckhoft catheter. *Ann Surg* **201**: 210–218.

Babineau TJ & Steele G, Jr (1996) Treatment of colorectal liver metastases. In: NS Williams (ed), *Colorectal Cancer*. Edinburgh: Churchill Livingstone.

Babineau TJ, Lewis WD, Jenkins RL et al (1994) Role of staging laparoscopy in the treatment of hepatic malignancy. *Am J Surg* **167**: 151–155.

Bacon HR & Berkeley JL (1959) The rationale of re-resection for recurrent cancer of the colon and rectum. *Dis Colon Rectum* **2**: 549.

Baigrie RJ & Berry AR (1994) Management of advanced rectal cancer. *Br J Surg* **81**: 343–352.

Balasagaram M (1972) Complete hepatic de-arterialisation for primary carcinomas of the liver: report of 24 patients. *Am J Surg* **124**: 340–345.

Balch CM & Urist MM (1986) Intraarterial chemotherapy for colorectal liver metastases and hepatomas using a totally implantable drug infusion pump. *Recent Results Cancer Res* **100**: 234–247.

Balch CM, Urist MM, Soong SJ & McGregor M (1983) A prospective phase II clinical trial of continuous FUDR regional chemotherapy for colorectal metastases to the liver using a totally implantable drug infusion pump. *Ann Surg* **198**: 567–573.

Balslev J, Pedersen M, Teglbjaerg PS et al (1986) Postoperative radiotherapy in Dukes B and C carcinoma of the rectum and rectosigmoid: a randomised multicentre study. *Cancer* **58**: 22–28.

Bancewicz J, Calman K, Macpherson SG, McArdle C, McVie JG & Soukop M (1980) Adjuvant chemotherapy and immunotherapy for colorectal cancer, preliminary communication. *J R Soc Med* **73**: 197–199.

Bayly JH & Garbalhaes OG (1964) The umbilical vein in the adult: diagnosis, treatment and research. *Am Surg* **30**: 56–60.

Beart RW (1990) Personal communication, cited by Gray R, James R & Mossman J (1991) Axis: a suitable case for treatment. AXIS: a suitable case for treatment. *Br J Cancer* **63**: 841–845.

Beart RW, Metzler PP, O'Connell MJ & Schutt AJ (1981) Postoperative screening of patients with carcinoma of the colon. *Dis Colon Rectum* **24**: 585.

Beets G, Penninckx F, Scheipers C et al (1994) Clinical value of whole-body positron emission tomography with FDG in recurrent colorectal cancer. *Br J Surg* **81**: 1666–1670.

Bengmark S, Fredlund P et al (1974) Present experiences with hepatic de-arterialisation in liver neoplasms. *Prog Surg* **13**: 141–166.

Benotti PN, Bothe A Jr, Eyre RC et al (1987) Management of recurrent pelvic tumors. *Arch Surg* **122**: 457–460.

Benyon J (1988) Endoluminal ultrasound in rectal cancer. MS Thesis, University of London.

Berard P & Papillon J (1992) Role of preoperative irradiation for anal preservation in cancer of the low rectum. *World J Surg* **16**: 502–509.

Beretta G, Bollina R, Martinnoni G et al (1994) Fluorouracil plus folates as standard treatment for advanced/metastatic gastrointestinal carcinomas. *Ann Oncol* **5** (Suppl 8): 48.

Berge T, Ekelund G, Meuner BP et al (1973) Carcinoma of the colon and rectum in a defined population: an epidemiological, clinical and post mortem investigation of colorectal carcinoma and coexisting benign polyps in Malmo. *Acta Chir Scand* **438** (Suppl): 1.

Bevan PG (1973) Cytotoxic perfusion of the liver via the umbilical vein for liver metastases in carcinoma of the colon. *Br J Surg* **60**: 369–375.

Beynon J, Mortensen NJM, Foy DMA et al (1989) The detection and evaluation of locally recurrent cancer with rectal endosonography. *Dis Colon Rectum* **32**: 509–517.

Binkley E (1938) Results of radiation therapy in primary operable rectal and anal cancer. *Radiology* **31**: 724–728.

Bjerkeset T & Dahl O (1980) Irradiation and surgery for primary inoperable rectal adenocarcinoma. *Dis Colon Rectum* **23**: 298–303.

Blumgart JH (1994) *Surgery of the Liver and Biliary Tract*, 2nd edn, pp 1557–1578. Edinburgh: Churchill Livingstone.

Blumgart JH, Drury JK & Wood CB (1979) Hepatic resection for trauma, tumour and biliary obstruction. *Br J Surg* **66**: 762–769.

Boey J, Wong J & Ong GB (1982) Pelvic exenteration for locally advanced colorectal carcinoma. *Ann Surg* **195**: 513–518.

Boey J, Cheung HC, Lai CK & Wong P (1984) A prospective evaluation of serum carcinoembryonic antigen (CRA) levels in the management of colorectal carcinoma. *World J Surg* **8**: 279–286.

Böhm B, Schwenk W, Hucke HP & Stock W (1993) Does methodic long-term follow-up affect survival after curative resection of colorectal cancer? *Dis Colon Rectum* **36**: 280–286.

Boice JD, Greene MH & Killen JY (1983) Leukaemia and pre leukaemia after adjuvant treatment of gastrointestinal cancer with Semustine (methyl CCNU). *N Engl J Med* **309**: 1074–1084.

Boulware RJ, Laderao JB, Pelcos L et al (1979) Whole pelvis megavoltage irradiation with single doses of 1000 rad to palliate advanced gynaecologic cancers. *Int J Radiat Oncol Biol Phys* **5**: 333–338.

Bown SG (1983) Phototherapy in tumors. *World J Surg* **7**: 700–709.

Breedis C & Young G (1954) The blood supply of neoplasms in the liver. *Am J Path* **30**: 969–977.

Brister SJ, deVarennes B, Gordon PH, Sheiner NM & Pym J (1988) Contemporary operative management of pulmonary metastases of colorectal origin. *Dis Colon Rectum* **31**: 786–792.

Britten AJ, Flowerdew DAS, Hunt TM, Taylor I, Ackery DM & Fleming JS (1989) A gamma camera method to monitor the use of degradable starch microspheres in hepatic arterial chemotherapy. *Eur J Nucl Med* **15**: 649–654.

Brophy PF, Hoffman JP & Eisenberg BL (1994) The role of palliative pelvic exenteration. *Am J Surg* **167**: 386–390.

Butler J, Attiyeh FF & Daly JM (1986) Hepatic resection for metastases of the colon and rectum. *Surg Gynecol Obstet* **162**: 109–113.

Buvse M, Zeleninch-Jacquottre A & Chalmers TC (1988) Adjuvant therapy of colorectal cancer: why we still don't know. *JAMA* **259**: 3571–3578.

Byfield JE, Barone RM, Frankel SS & Sharp TR (1984) Treatment with combined intra-arterial 5-FUDR infusion and whole liver radiation for colon carcinoma metastatic to the liver: preliminary results. *Am J Clin Oncol* **7**: 319–326.

Cady B & McDermott WV (1985) Major hepatic resection for metachronous metastases from colon cancer. *Ann Surg* **201**: 204–209.

Cahan WG, Castro El B & Hadju SI (1974) The significance of a solitary lung shadow in patients with colon carcinoma. *Cancer* **33**: 414–421.

Carter SK (1982) Future directions in the therapy for large bowel cancer. *Cancer* **50**: 2647–2656.

Chang AE, Schneider PD, Sugarbaker PH et al (1987) A prospective randomized trial of regional versus systemic continuous 5-fluorodeoxyuridine chemotherapy in the treatment of colorectal liver metastases. *Ann Surg* **206**: 685–693.

Chaoul H (1936) Die Behandlung operation freigelegter Rektumkarzinome mit der Rontgennahbestralung. *Med Wochenschr* **83**: 972.

Cochrane JPS, Williams JT, Faber RG & Slack WW (1980) Value of outpatient follow-up after curative surgery for carcinoma of the large bowel. *BMJ* **280**: 593–595.

Cohen AM & Minsky BD (1990) Aggressive surgical management of locally advanced primary and recurrent rectal cancer: current status and future directions. *Dis Colon Rectum* **33**: 432–438.

Cohen AM, Kaufman SD, Wood WC & Greenfield AJ (1983) Regional hepatic chemotherapy using an implantable drug infusion pump. *Am J Surg* **145**: 529–533.

Cohen AM, Schaeffer N & Higgins J (1986) Treatment of metastatic colorectal cancer with hepatic artery combination chemotherapy. *Cancer* **57**: 1115–1117.

Cohen AM, Martin EW Jr, Lavery I et al (1991) Radio-immunoguided surgery using iodine-125 B72.3 in patients with colorectal cancer. *Arch Surg* **126**: 349–352.

Cole WH, Packard D & Southwick HW (1954) Carcinoma of the colon with special reference to prevention of recurrence. *JAMA* **155**: 1549.

Collier BD, Abdel-Nabi H & Doerr RJ (1992) Immunoscintigraphy performed in In-111 labeled CYT-103 in the management of colorectal cancer: comparison with CT. *Radiology* **185**: 179–186.

Coltman CA (1982) *Compilation of Experimental Cancer Therapy Protocol Summaries*, edn 6PB, 82-158262, no 20121, p 120. Bethesda: National Institutes of Health.

Cook AW & Kawakami Y (1977) Commissural myeolotomy. *J Neurosurg* **47**: 1.

Cousins MJ, Mather LE, Glynn CJ, Wilson PR & Graham JR (1979) Selective spinal analgesia. *Lancet* **i**: 1141.

Cronquist S (1957) Changes in the colon following resection and end to end anastomosis. *Acta Radiol* **48**: 425.

Cruz EP, McDonald GO & Cole WH (1956) Prophylactic treatment of cancer: the use of chemotherapeutic agents to prevent tumour metastasis. *Surgery (St Louis)* **40**: 291.

Cummings BJ (1984) Adjuvant radiation therapy for rectal adenocarcinoma. *Dis Colon Rectum* **27**: 826–836.

Cummings BJ, Rider WD, Harwood AR, Keave TJ & Thomas GM (1981) Curative external radiation for adenocarcinoma of the rectum (ASTR Proceedings). *Int J Radiat Oncol Biol Phys* **1**: 1206.

Curley SA, Chase JL, Roh MS & Hohn DC (1993) Technical considerations and complications associated with the placement of 180 implantable hepatic arterial infusion devices. *Surgery* **114**: 928–935.

Davies J (1981) Magic bullets. *Nature* **289**: 12–13.

Davis HL (1982) Chemotherapy of large bowel cancer. *Cancer* **50**: 2638–2646.

Dedkov IP & Zibina MA (1976) Intensive preoperative gamma-therapy in combined treatment of cancer of the rectum. *Am J Proctol* **7**: 43–47.

Dixon WJ, Longmire WP Jr & Holden WD (1971) Use of thiotepa as an adjuvant to the surgical treatment of gastric and colorectal carcinoma: ten year follow-up. *Ann Surg* **173**: 26.

Doci R, Bignami P, Montalto F & Gennari L (1995) Prognostic factors for survival and disease-free survival in hepatic metastases from colorectal cancer treated by resection. *Tumori* **81** (Suppl): 143–146.

Doerr RJ, Herrera L & Abdel-Nabi H (1993) In-111 CYT-103 monoclonal antibody imaging in patients with suspected recurrent colorectal cancer. *Cancer* **71** (Suppl 12): 4241–4247.

Dowling RD, Keenan RJ, Ferson PF et al (1992) Video-assisted thoracoscopic resection of pulmonary metastases. *Ann Thorac Surg* **53**: 772–775.

Duncan WA (1981) A preliminary report on the MRC trial of preoperative radiotherapy in the management of rectal cancer. In Gerard A (ed) *Progress and Perspectives in the Treatment of Gastrointestinal Tumours*, pp 83–86. Oxford: Pergamon.

Duncan WA (1987) Preoperative radiotherapy in rectal cancer. *World J Surg* **11**: 439–445.

Dwight RW, Humphreys WE, Higgins GA et al (1973) FUDR as an adjuvant to surgery in cancer of the large bowel. *J Surg Oncol* **5**: 243.

Earhart RG, Moertel C, Hahn RG et al (1984) Phase II trial of PCNU in advanced colorectal carcinoma: an Eastern Cooperative Oncology Group pilot study. *Am J Oncol* **7**: 309–312.

Eble MJ, Kallinowski F, Wannenmacher MF & Herfarth C (1994) Intraoperative radiotherapy of locally advanced and recurrent rectal cancer (review, in German). *Chirurg* **65**: 585–592.

Ebner F, Kressel HY, Mintz MC et al (1988) Tumor recurrence versus fibrosis in the female pelvis: differentiation with MR imaging at 1.5 T. *Radiology* **166**: 333–340.

Eckhauser FE, Lindenauer SM & Morley GW (1979) Pelvic exenteration for advanced rectal carcinoma. *Am J Surg* **138**: 412–414.

Editorial (1990) Mixed European reactions to American colorectal data. *Ann Oncol* **1**: 239–240.

Editorial (1992) Advanced colorectal cancer meta-analysis project. Modulation of fluorouracil by leucovorin in patients with advanced colorectal cancer: evidence in terms of response rate. *J Clin Oncol* **10**: 896–903.

Elkberg H, Tranberg K-G, Andersson R et al (1986) Determinants of survival in liver resection for colorectal secondaries. *Br J Surg* **73**: 727–731.

Ellis H (1978) Advanced malignant disease. In Hadfield J & Hobsley M (eds) *Current Surgical Practice*, Vol 2. London: Edward Arnold.

Embleton MJ, Rowland GF, Simmonds RG et al (1983) Selective cytotoxicity against human tumour cells by a vindesine-monoclonal antibody conjugate. *Br J Cancer* **47**: 43–49.

Engstrom PF, MacIntyre JM, Mittelman A & Klassen DJ (1984) Chemotherapy of advanced colorectal carcinoma: fluorouracil alone vs two drug combinations using fluorouracil, hydroxyurea, semustine, dacarbazine, rozoxane and mitomycin. A phase III trial by the Eastern Cooperative Oncology Group. *Am J Clin Oncol* **7**: 313–318.

Enker WE & Kramer RG (1982) The follow-up of patients after definitive resection for large bowel cancer. *World J Surg* **6**: 578–584.

Estes NC, Thomas JH, Jewell WR, Beggs D & Hardin CA (1993) Pelvic exenteration: a treatment for failed rectal cancer surgery. *Am Surg* **59**: 420–422.

Federov V & Shelygin YA (1989) Treatment of patients with rectal cancer. *Dis Colon Rectum* **32**: 138–145.

Fielding LP, Hittinger R & Fry J (1989) Intraportal adjuvant chemotherapy for colorectal cancer. In Proceedings of Tripartite Meeting, Birmingham, 19–21 June (abstract).

Finlay IG & McArdle CS (1982) The identification of patients at high risk following curative resection for colorectal carcinoma. *Br J Surg* **69**: 583–584.

Fisher B, Wolmark N, Rockette H et al (1988) Postoperative adjuvant chemotherapy or radiation therapy for rectal cancer: results of NSABP Protocol R–01. *J Natl Cancer Inst* **80**: 21–29.

Fleshman JW, Kodner IJ, Fry RD et al (1985) Adenocarcinoma of the rectum: results of radiotherapy and resection, endocavitary irradiation, local excision and preoperative clinical staging. *Dis Colon Rectum* **28**: 810–815.

Flowerdew ADS, Richards HK & Taylor I (1987) Temporary blood flow stasis with degradable starch microspheres (DSM) for liver metastases in a rat model. *Gut* **28**: 1201–1207.

Fong Y, Kemeny N, Paty P, Blumgart LH & Cohen AM (1996) Treatment of colorectal cancer: hepatic metastases (review). *Semin Surg Oncol* **12**: 219–252.

Ford CHJ, Newman CE, Johnson JR et al (1983) Localization and toxicity study of a vindesine–anti-CEA conjugate in patients with advanced cancer. *Br J Cancer* **47**: 35–42.

Fortier GA, Constable WC, Meyers H & Wanebo HJ (1986) Preoperative radiation therapy for rectal cancer: an effective therapy in need of a clinical trial. *Arch Surg* **121**: 1380–1385.

Fortner JG (1988) Recurrence of colorectal cancer after hepatic resection. *Am J Surg* **155**: 378–382.

Foster JH & Berman MM (1977) Solid liver tumors. In *Major Problems in Clinical Surgery*, Vol 22, pp 1–342. Philadelphia: WB Saunders.

Fowler WC, Hoffman JP & Eisenberg BL (1993) Redo hepatic resection for metastatic colorectal carcinoma. *World J Surg* **17**: 658–662.

Gagache G, Dessant JP & Triboulet JP (1980) Indications for repeat operations for recurrence of colorectal cancer: contribution of serum carcino-embryonic antigen levels. *Chirurgie* **106**: 322.

Gary-Bobo J, Pyoc H, Solassol C, Broquerie JI & Nguyen M (1979) L'irradiation pré-operatoire du cancer rectal: résultats à 5 ans de 116 cas. *Bull Cancer* **66**: 491–496.

Gelin LE, Lewis DH & Nilsson L (1968) Liver blood flow in man during abdominal surgery. II: The effect of hepatic artery occlusion in the blood flow through metastatic tumour nodules. *Acta Hepatogastroenterol (Stuttgart)* **15**: 21–24.

Gérard A, Berrod J-L, Pene F et al (1985) Interim analysis of phase III study on preoperative radiation therapy in resectable rectal carcinoma. *Cancer* **55**: 2373–2379.

Gérard A, Berrod J-L & Loygue J (1986) EORTC trials in large bowel cancer. *Int J Colorectal Dis* **1**: 116–120.

Gérard A, Buyse M, Nordlinger B et al (1988) Preoperative radiotherapy as adjuvant treatment in rectal cancer: final results of a randomized study of the European Organization for Research and Treatment of Cancer (EORTC). *Ann Surg* **208**: 606–614.

Gérard JP, Coquard R, Fric D et al (1994) Curative endocavitary irradiation of small rectal cancers and preoperative radiotherapy in T2 T3 (T4) rectal cancer: a brief review of the Lyon experience. *Eur J Surg Oncol* **20**: 644–647.

Germer C-J, Albrecht D, Roggan A, Esbert C & Buhr HJ (1997) Experimental study of laparoscopy induced thermotherapy for liver tumours. *Br J Surg* **84**: 317–320.

Ghose T, Ramakrishnan S, Kulkarni P et al (1981) Use of antibodies against tumour associated antigens for cancer diagnosis and treatment. *Transplant Proc* **13**: 1970–1972.

Gill PG (1980) *Compilation of Cancer Therapy Protocol Summaries*, edn 4-PB, 80-151368, no 20124, p 125. Bethesda: National Institutes of Health.

Gilliland DG, Steplewski Z, Collier RJ et al (1980) Antibody-directed cytotoxic agents: use of monoclonal antibody to direct the action of toxin A chains to colorectal carcinoma cells. *Proc Natl Acad Sci* **77**: 4539–4543.

GITSG (Gastrointestinal Tumor Study Group) (1984) Adjuvant therapy of colon cancer: results of a prospectively randomized trial. *N Engl J Med* **310**: 737–743.

GITSG (Gastrointestinal Tumor Study Group) (1985) A controlled trial of adjuvant chemotherapy, radiation therapy or combined chemoradiation therapy following curative resection for rectal carcinoma. *N Engl J Med* **312**: 1465–1472.

GITSG (Gastrointestinal Tumor Study Group) (1992) Radiation and fluorouracil with or without semustine for the treatment of patients with surgical adjuvant adenocarcinoma of the rectum. *J Clin Onco* **10**: 549–557.

Glimelius B, Graffman S, Påhlman L, Rimsten A & Wilander E (1982) Preoperative irradiation with high-dose fractionation in adenocarcinoma of the rectum and rectosigmoid. *Acta Radiol Oncol* **21**: 373–379.

Glimelius B, for the Nordic Gastrointestinal Tumour Adjuvant Therapy Group (1991) Expectant or primary chemotherapy in patients with advanced asymptomatic colorectal cancer: a randomized trial. *Eur J Cancer* **27** (Suppl 2): S82.

Goldberg JA, Kerr DJ, Willmott N, McArdle CS, Murray T & Hilditch T (1988) Increased uptake of radio-labelled microspheres with angiotensin II in colorectal hepatic metastases. *Eur J Surg Oncol* **14**: 715.

Goldberg JA, Kerr DJ, Wilmott N, McKillop JH & McArdle CS (1990) Regional chemotherapy for colorectal liver metastases: a phase II evaluation of targeted hepatic arterial 5-fluorouracil for colorectal liver metastases. *Br J Surg* **77**: 1238–1240.

Goldberg JA, Nicholls RJ, Porter NH, Love S & Grimsey JE (1994) Long-term results of a randomized trial of short-course low-dose adjuvant preoperative radiotherapy for rectal cancer: reduction in local treatment failure. *Eur J Cancer* **30A**: 1602–1606.

Goldenberg D (1993) Monoclonal antibodies in cancer detection and therapy. *Am J Med* **94**: 297–312.

Goligher J (1984) *Surgery of the Anus, Rectum and Colon*. London: Baillière Tindall.

Gough DB, Donohue JH, Trastek VA & Nagorney DM (1994) Resection of hepatic and pulmonary metastases in patients with colorectal cancer. *Br J Surg* **81**: 94–96.

Goya T, Miyazawa N, Kondo H et al (1989) Surgical resection of pulmonary metastases from colorectal cancer: 10-year follow-up. *Cancer* **64**: 1418–1421.

Grady ED (1979) Internal radiation therapy of hepatic cancer. *Dis Colon Rectum* **22**: 371.

Grage TB, Vassilopoulos PP, Shingleton WW et al (1979) Results of a prospective randomized study of hepatic artery infusion with 5-fluorouracil versus intravenous 5-fluorouracil in patients with hepatic metastases from colorectal cancer: a Central Oncology Group study. *Surgery* **86**: 550–555.

Gray BN (1990) Personal communication, cited by Gray R, James R & Mossman J (1991) AXIS: a suitable case for treatment. *Br J Cancer* **63**: 841–845.

Gray R, James R, Mossman J & Stenning S (1991) AXIS: a suitable case for treatment. *Br J Cancer* **63**: 841–845.

Greenway B (1988) Hepatic metastases from colorectal cancer: resection or not? *Br J Surg* **75**: 513–519.

Griffith CDM, Ballantyne KC, Pollard S et al (1988) Radiotherapy for palliation of residual and recurrent rectal cancer. *J R Coll Surg Edinb* **33**: 25–27.

Grossi CE, Wolff WI, Nelson TF et al (1977) Intraluminal fluorouracil chemotherapy adjunct to surgical procedures for resectable carcinoma of the colon and rectum. *Surg Gynecol Obstet* **145**: 549–554.

Guivarc'h M, Sbai-Idrissi MS, Mosnier H & Roullet-Audy JC (1993/94) Re-operation for locoregional recurrence of cancer of the rectum (in French). *Chirurgie* **119**(1–2): 62–66.

Gunderson LL, Martin JK & Beart RW (1988) Intraoperative and external beam irradiation for locally advanced colorectal cancer. *Ann Surg* **207**: 52–60.

Gunderson LL, O'Connell MJ & Dozois RR (1992) The role of intra-operative irradiation in locally advanced primary and recurrent rectal adenocarcinoma. *World J Surg* **16**: 495–501.

Gunderson LL (1994) Adjuvant therapy for rectal cancer. In *ASCO Education Book*, American Society of Clinical Oncology, p 164.

Hafström L, Johnson RE, Landberg T et al (1979) Intra-arterial infusion chemotherapy (5-fluorouracil) in patients with inextirpable or locally recurrent rectal cancer. *Am J Surg* **137**: 757.

Hafström L, Rudenstam C-M, Domellöf L, for the Swedish Gastrointestinal Tumour Adjuvant Therapy Group (1985) A randomized trial of oral 5-fluorouracil versus placebo as adjuvant therapy in colorectal cancer Dukes' B and C: results after 5 years observation time. *Br J Surg* **72**: 138–141.

Hafström L, Domellöf L, Rudenstam C-M et al (1990) Adjuvant chemotherapy with 5-fluorouracil, vincristine and CCNU for patients with Dukes' C colorectal cancer. *Br J Surg* **77**: 1345–1348.

Hahn RG, Moertel CG, Schutt AJ et al (1975) A double-blind comparison of intensive course of 5-fluorouracil by oral vs intravenous route in the treatment of colorectal carcinoma. *Cancer* **35**: 1031.

Haller D et al (1996) Fluorouracil, leucovorin and levamisole adjuvant therapy in colon cancer. *Proc Am Soc Clin Oncol* **15**: x(A486).

Hardy TG, Aguilar PS, Plasencia G et al (1984) Adjuvant intrahepatic cytotoxic liver infusion for colon cancer: catheter placement technique. *Dis Colon Rectum* **27**: 495–497.

Hashimoto D, Takami M & Ideezuki Y (1985) In-depth radiation therapy by Nd–YAG laser for malignant tumours of the liver under ultrasound imaging. *Gastroenterology* **88**: 1663 (abstract).

Hertz RE, Deddish MR & Day E (1960) Value of periodic examination in detecting cancer of the rectum and colon. *Postgrad Med* **27**: 290.

Hickey RC, Romsdahl MM, Johnson DE et al (1982) Recurrent cancer and metastases. *World J Surg* **6**: 585–595.

Higgins GA (1983) Current status of adjuvant therapy in the treatment of large bowel cancer. Symposium on Colon and Rectal Surgery. *Surg Clin North Am* **63**: 137–151.

Higgins GA, Conn JH, Jordan PH Jr et al (1975) Preoperative radiotherapy for colorectal cancer. *Ann Surg* **181**: 624–631.

Higgins GA, Humphrey EW, Juler GL et al (1976) Adjuvant chemotherapy in the surgical treatment of large bowel cancer. *Cancer* **38**: 1461–1468.

Higgins GA, Lee LE, Dwight RW et al (1978) The case for adjuvant 5-fluorouracil in colorectal cancer. *Cancer Clin Trial* **1**: 35–41.

Higgins GA, Humphrey EW, Juler GL, Roswit B & Keehn RJ (1981) Adjuvant therapy for rectal cancer: update of Veterans Administration Surgical Oncology Group Trials. In Gerard A (ed) *Progress and Perspectives in the Treatment of Gastrointestinal Tumours*, pp 62–67. Oxford: Pergamon.

Higgins GA, Amadeo JH, McElhinney J et al (1984a) Efficacy of prolonged intermittent therapy with combined 5-fluorouracil and methyl CCNU following resection for carcinoma of the large bowel: a Veterans Administration Surgical Oncology Group report. *Cancer* **53**: 1–8.

Higgins GA, Donaldson RC, Rogers LS, Juler GL & Keehn RJ (1984b) Efficacy of MER immunotherapy when added to a regimen of 5-fluorouracil and methyl-CCNU following resection for carcinoma of the large bowel: a Veterans Administration Surgical Oncology Group report. *Cancer* **54**: 193–198.

Higgins GA, Humphrey EW, Dwight RW et al (1986) Preoperative radiation and surgery for cancer of the rectum: Veterans Administration Surgical Oncology Group Trial II. *Cancer* **58**: 352–359.

Hildebrandt U, Feifel G, Schwartz HP & Scherr O (1986) Endorectal ultrasound: instrumentation and clinical aspects. *Int J Colorect Dis* **1**: 203–207.

Hine KR & Dykes PW (1984) Prospective randomised trial of early cytotoxic therapy for recurrent colorectal carcinoma detected by serum CEA. *Gut* **25**: 682–688.

Hodgson WJ, Morgan J, Byrne D & Delguercio LR (1993) Hepatic resections for primary and metastatic tumours using the ultrasonic surgical dissector. *Am J Surg* **163**: 246–250.

Hoffman JP, Riley L, Carp NZ & Litwin S (1993) Isolated locally recurrent rectal cancer: a review of incidence, presentation and management. *Semin Oncol* **20**: 506–519.

Hohn DC, Stagg RJ, Friedman MA et al (1989) A randomized trial of continuous intravenous versus hepatic intraarterial floxuridine in patients with colorectal cancer metastatic to the liver: the Northern California Oncology Group trial. *J Clin Oncol* **7**: 1646–1654.

Holden WD, Dixon WJ & Kuzma JW (1967) The use of thiotepa as an adjuvant to the surgical treatment of colorectal carcinoma. *Ann Surg* **165**: 481.

Horiot J-C (1991) Local curative treatment of rectal cancer by radiotherapy alone. *Int J Colorectal Dis* **6**: 89–90.

Horn A, Halvorsen JF & Danl O (1990) Preoperative radiotherapy in operable rectal cancer. *Dis Colon Rectum* **33**: 823–828.

Hoskins RB, Gunderson LL, Posoretz DE et al (1985) Adjuvant postoperative radiotherapy in carcinoma of the rectum and rectosigmoid. *Cancer* **55**: 61–71.

House AK & Maley MAL (1983) Clinical and *in vivo* response following surgery or surgery plus adjuvant chemotherapy or immunotherapy for colorectal carcinoma in a rat model. *J R Soc Med* **76**: 833–840.

Huber BC, Austin EA, Good SS et al (1993) *In vivo* antitumour activity of 5-flucytosine on human colorectal cancer cells genetically modified to express cytosine deaminase. *Cancer Res* **53**: 4619–4626.

Huber SL & Hill CS (1980) Pharmacology management of cancer pain. *Cancer Bull* **32**: 183.

Hughes ES, McConchie IH, McDermott FT, Johnson WR & Price AB (1982) Resection of lung metastases in large bowel cancer. *Br J Surg* **69**: 410–412.

Hughes KS, Simon R, Songhorabodi S et al (1986) Resection of the liver for colorectal carcinoma metastases: a multi-institutional study of patterns of recurrence. *Surgery* **100**: 278–284.

Hughes KS, Simon R, Songhorabodi S et al (1988) Resection of the liver for colorectal carcinoma metastases: a multi-institutional study of long-term survivors. *Dis Colon Rectum* **31**: 1–4.

Hull TL, Lavery IC & Saxton JP (1994) Endocavity irradiation: an option in select patients with rectal cancer. *Dis Colon Rectum* **37**: 1266–1270.

Hunt TM, Flowerdew ADS, Birch SJ et al (1990) Prospective randomized controlled trial of hepatic arterial embolization or infusion chemotherapy with 5-fluorouracil and degradable starch microspheres for colorectal liver metastases. *Br J Surg* **77**: 779–782.

Husband JE, Hodson NJ & Parson CA (1980) The use of computed tomography in recurrent rectal tumours. *Radiology* **134**: 677–682.

Hyams DM, Esteban JM, Lollo CP, Beatty BG & Beatty JD (1987) Therapy of peritoneal carcinomatosis of colon cancer xenografts and yttrium-90 labelled anti carcinoembryonic antigen antibody ZCE025. *Arch Surg* **122**: 1333–1337.

Irvin TT, Vowles KDJ & Golby MG (1986) Fluorouracil in chemoprophylaxis of colorectal cancer: results of a controlled clinical trial. *Dis Colon Rectum* **29**: 704–706.

Isenberg J, Fishbach R, Kruger I & Keller HW (1996) Treatment of liver metastases from colorectal cancer. *Anticancer Res* **16**: 1291–1351.

Iwatsuki S, Esquivel CO, Gordon RD & Starzl TE (1986) Liver resection for metastatic colorectal cancer. *Surgery* **100**: 804–810.

Iwatsuki S, Shaw BW & Starzl T (1983) Experience with 150 liver resections. *Ann Surg* **197**: 247–253.

James RD (1996) Adjuvant radiotherapy. In Williams NS (ed) *Colorectal Cancer*. Edinburgh: Churchill Livingstone.

James RD, Haboubi N, Schofield PF et al (1991) Prognostic factors in colorectal carcinoma treated by preoperative radiotherapy and immediate surgery. *Dis Colon Rectum* **34**: 546–551.

Jatzko GR, Lisborg PH & Stettner HM (1995) Hepatic resection for metastases from colorectal carcinoma: a survival analysis. *Eur J Cancer* **31A**(1): 41–46.

Johnson DH, Williams NS, Newland AC et al (1989) Intraperitoneal production and systematic transfer of lymphokine activated killer (LAK) cells for treatment of disseminated gastrointestinal adenocarcinoma. *Br J Surg* **76**: 626.

Johnson LP & Rivkin SE (1985) The implanted pump in metastatic colorectal cancer of the liver: risk versus benefit. *Am J Surg* **149**: 595–598.

Johnson LP, Wasserman PB & Rivkin SE (1983) FUDR hepatic arterial infusions via an implantable pump for treatment of hepatic tumors. *Proc Am Soc Clin Oncol* **2**: 119.

Jones DV Jr, Patt YZ, Chase J et al (1993) A pilot study of 5-FU and recombinant human alpha interferon by hepatic arterial infusion for patients with colorectal cancer metastatic to the liver. *Proc Am Soc Clin Oncol* **12**: 216.

Juhl G, Larson GM, Mullins R, Bond S & Polk HC (1990) Six-year results of annual colonoscopy after resection of colorectal cancer. *World J Surg* **14**: 255–261.

Junneman A & Derra E (1980) Effectiveness of oncologic follow-up care of patients with colorectal carcinoma: report from Surgical Clinic, Dusseldorf University. *Therapie–Woche* **30**: 85–93.

Kallinowski F, Eble MJ, Buhr HJ, Wannenmacher M & Herfarth C (1995) Intraoperative radiotherapy for primary and recurrent rectal cancer. *Eur J Surg Oncol* **21**: 191–194.

Kaplan WD, Come SE, Takvorian RW et al (1984) Pulmonary uptake of technetium 99m macroaggregated albumin: a predictor of gastrointestinal toxicity during hepatic artery perfusion. *J Clin Oncol* **2**: 1266–1269.

Karesen R, Hertzberg J, Johannesen J, Thorlesen BO & Orjasaeter H (1980) Carcinoembryonic antigen in the diagnosis and follow up of colorectal carcinoma. *Am J Proctol Gastroenterol Colon Rectal Surg* **31**: 18–22.

Karl RC, Morse SS, Halper RD & Clark RA (1993) Preoperative evaluation of patients for liver resection: appropriate CT imaging. *Ann Surg* **217**: 226–232.

Kaufman N, Nori D, Shank B et al (1989) Remote afterloading intraluminal brachytherapy in the treatment of rectal, rectosigmoid and anal cancer: a feasibility study. *Int J Radiat Oncol Biol Phys* **17**: 663–668.

Kelvin FM, Kurobkin M, Heaston DK, Grant JP & Akwari O (1983) The pelvis after surgery for rectal carcinoma: serial CT observations with emphasis on non-neoplastic features. *AJR* **141**: 959–964.

Kemeny N & Sigurdson (1994) Intra-arterial chemotherapy for liver tumours. In Blumgart LH (ed) *Surgery of the Liver and Biliary Tract*, Vol 2, 2nd edn, pp 1473–1491. Edinburgh: Churchill Livingstone.

Kemeny N, Daly J, Oderman P et al (1984) Hepatic artery pump infusion: toxicity and results in patients with metastatic colorectal carcinoma. *J Clin Oncol* **2**: 595–600.

Kemeny N, Daly J, Reichman B et al (1987) Intrahepatic or systemic infusion of fluorodeoxyuridine in patients with liver metastases from colorectal carcinoma: a randomized trial. *Ann Intern Med* **107**: 459–465.

Kemeny N, Cohen A, Bertino JR et al (1990) Continuous intrahepatic infusion of floxuridine and leucovorin through an implantable pump for the treatment of hepatic metastases from colorectal carcinoma. *Cancer* **65**: 2446–2450.

Kemeny N, Conti JA, Cohen A et al (1994a) Phase II study of hepatic arterial floxuridine, leucovorin and dexamethasone for unresectable liver metastases from colorectal carcinoma. *J Clin Oncol* **12**: 2288–2295.

Kemeny N, Seiter K, Conti JA et al (1994b) Hepatic arterial floxuridine and leucovorin for unresectable liver metastases from colorectal carcinoma: new dose schedules and survival update. *Cancer* **73**: 1134–1142.

Kerr DJ (1995) Adjuvant chemotherapy and immunotherapy for colorectal cancer. In Williams NS (ed) *Colorectal Cancer*, pp 151–158. Edinburgh: Churchill Livingstone.

Kerr DJ & Workman P (1994) *New Molecular Targets for Cancer Chemotherapy*. Philadelphia: Cancer Reserach Campaign Press.

Kerr DJ, Willmott N, Lewi H & McArdle CS (1988) The pharmacokinetics and distribution of adriamycin-loaded albumin microspheres following intra-arterial administration. *Cancer* **62**: 878–882.

Killingback M (1986) Symposium: the management of recurrent colorectal cancer. *Int J Colorect Dis* **1**: 133–151.

Kjeldsen B, Kronberg O, Fenger C & Jorgensen (1997) A prospective randomized study of follow-up after radical surgery for colorectal cancer. *Br J Surg* **84**: 666–669.

Kligerman MM, Urdaneta N, Knowlton A et al (1972) Preoperative irradiation of rectosigmoid carcinoma including its regional lymph nodes. *AJR* **114**: 498–503.

Klimberg VS, Langston JD, Maners A et al (1992) Advantages of the Papillon protocol in the preoperative treatment of rectal carcinoma. *Am J Surg* **164**: 433–436.

Kodner IJ, Shemesh EI, Fry RD et al (1989) Preoperative irradiation for rectal cancer: improved local control and long-term survival. *Ann Surg* **209**: 194–199.

Korpan NN (1997) Hepatic cryosurgery for liver metastases: long-term follow-up. *Ann Surg* **225**: 193–201.

Kozlova AV & Popova TV (1977) Die Bedeutung der Strahlentherapie bein Rektumkarzinoma. *Radiobiol Radiother (Berlin)* **18**: 571–576.

Kronborg O, Fenger C, Deichgraeber E & Hansen L (1988) Follow-up after radical surgery for colorectal cancer: design of a randomized study. *Scand J Gastroenterol* **23**: 159–162.

Krook JE, Moertel CG, Gunderson LL et al (1991) Effective surgical adjuvant therapy for high-risk rectal carcinoma. *N Engl J Med* **324**: 709–715.

Landreneau RJ, Hazelrigg SR, Ferson PF et al (1993) Thorascopic resection of 85 pulmonary lesions. *Ann Thorac Surg* **54**: 415–419.

Larmi K, Karkola P, Klintrup HE et al (1974) Treatment of patients with hepatic tumours and jaundice by ligation of the hepatic artery. *Arch Surg* **108**: 178–183.

Laurie JA (1982) *Compilation of Experimental Cancer Therapy Protocol Summaries*, edn 6-PB, 82-158262, no 20101, p 112. Bethesda: National Institutes of Health.

Lawrence W, Terz JJ, Horsley S et al (1975) Chemotherapy as an adjuvant to surgery for colorectal cancer. *Ann Surg* **181**: 616–623.

Lawrence W, Terz JJ, Horsley JS, Brown PW & Romero C (1978) Chemotherapy as an adjuvant to surgery for colorectal cancer: a follow-up report. *Arch Surg* **113**: 164–168.

Lawton RL (1965) Cancer chemotherapy of the gastrointestinal tract with reference to intra-arterial infusion and irradiation. *Am J Surg* **109**: 47–53.

Lee JKT, Stanley RJ, Sagel SS, Levitt RG & McClennan BL (1981) CT appearances of the pelvis after abdominoperineal resection for rectal carcinoma. *Radiology* **141**: 737–741.

Lewi HJE, McArdle CS, Ratcliffe JG et al (1981) CEA and further laparotomy in symptomatic patients following treatment for colorectal cancer. *Br J Surg* **68**: 350.

Li MC & Ross ST (1976) Chemoprophylaxis for patients with colorectal cancer: postoperative study with five year follow up. *JAMA* **235**: 2825–2827.

Lien MW & Ackerman B (1970) The blood supply of experimental liver metastases. *Surgery* **68**: 334–340.

Lightdale CJ, Wasser J & Coleman M (1979) Anticoagulation and high dose liver radiation: a preliminary report. *Cancer* **43**: 174.

Lindmark G, Gerdin B, Påhlman L, Bergström R & Glimelius B (1994) Prognostic predictors in colorectal cancer. *Dis Colon Rectum* **37**: 1219–1227.

Lipert RG, Hosobuchi Y & Nielson SL (1975) Relief of pain by transcutaneous stimulation. *J Neurosurg* **42**: 308.

Little JM (1984) Hepatic secondaries: minimal tumour and resectable tumour. *World J Surg* **8**: 753–756.

Localio SA (1981) In discussion of Wanebo HH & Margrove RC (1981) Abdominal sacral resection of locally recurrent rectal cancer. *Ann Surg* **194**: 458.

Lygidakij NJ, Tytgut GNJ & Argner K (1989) *Hepatobiliary and Pancreatic Malignancies: Diagnosis, Medical and Surgical Management*. New York: Thieme Medical.

Maetani S, Nishikawa T, Iijima Y et al (1992) Extensive *en bloc* resection of regionally recurrent carcinoma of the rectum. *Cancer* **69**: 2876–2883.

Makela JT, Laitinen SO & Kairaluoma MI (1995) Five-year follow-up after radical surgery for colorectal cancer: results of a prospective randomized trial. *Arch Surg* **130**: 1062–1067.

Mansour EG, Letkopoulou M, Johnson R et al (1991) A comparison of postoperative adjuvant chemotherapy, radiotherapy or combination therapy in potentially curable resectable rectal carcinoma. *Proc Am Soc Clin Oncol* **10**: 154 (abstract).

Marks G, Mohiuddin M & Borenstein BD (1985) Preoperative radiation therapy and sphincter preservation by the combined abdomino-transsacral technique for selected rectal cancers. *Dis Colon Rectum* **28**: 565–571.

Marks G, Mohiuddin MM, Masoni L & Pecchioli L (1990) High-dose preoperative radiation and full-thickness local excision: a new option for patients with select cancers of the rectum. *Dis Colon Rectum* **33**: 735–739.

Marsh PJ, James RD & Schofield PF (1994) Adjuvant preoperative radiotherapy for locally advanced rectal carcinoma: results of a prospective randomized trial. *Dis Colon Rectum* **37**: 1205–1214.

Martin EW Jr, Cooperman M, Carey RC & Minton JD (1980) Sixty second look procedures indicated primarily by rise in serial carcinoembryonic antigen. *J Surg Res* **28**: 389.

Martin EW, Minton JP & Carey LC (1985) CEA directed second-look surgery in the asymptomatic patient after primary resection of colorectal carcinoma. *Ann Surg* **202**: 310–317.

Martin JK Jr, O'Connell MJ, Wieand HS et al (1990) Intra-arterial floxuridine versus systemic fluorouracil for hepatic metastases from colorectal cancer: a randomized trial. *Arch Surg* **125**: 1022–1027.

Mascagni D, Corellini L, Urciuolip DI & Matteo G (1989) Endoluminal ultrasound for early detection of local recurrence of rectal cancer. *Br J Surg* **76**: 1176–1180.

Masters A, Steger AC, Lees WR, Walmsley KM & Bown SG (1992) Interstitial laser hyperthermia: a new approach for treating liver metastases. *Br J Cancer* **66**: 518–522.

Matthewson K, Coleridge-Smith P, O'Sullivan JP, Northfield TC & Bown SG (1987) Biological effects of intrahepatic neodymium:yttrium aluminium garnet laser photocoagulation in rats. *Gastroenterology* **93**: 550–557.

Mavligit GM, Burgess MA, Seibert GB et al (1976) Prolongation of postoperative disease-free interval and survival in human colorectal cancer by BCG and BCG plus 5-fluorouracil. *Lancet* **i**: 871–885.

Mavligit GM, Zukiwski AA, Gutterman JU et al (1990a) Splenic versus hepatic artery infusion of interleukin-2 in patients with liver metastases. *J Clin Oncol* **8**: 319–324.

Mavligit GM, Zukiwski AA & Wallace (1990b) Tumor regression after hepatic arterial infusion of recombinant tumor necrosis factor in patients with colon carcinoma metastatic to the liver. *Proc Am Soc Clin Oncol* **9**: 118.

Mayer RJ (1990) Does adjuvant therapy work in colon cancer? *N Engl J Med* **322**: 399–401.

McCormack PM & Attiyeh FF (1979) Resected pulmonary metastases from colorectal cancer. *Dis Colon Rectum* **22**: 553–556.

McCormack PM, Burt ME, Bains MS et al (1992) Lung resection for colorectal metastases: 10-year results. *Arch Surg* **127**: 1403–1406.

Medical Research Council Rectal Cancer Working Party (1996a) Randomised trial of surgery alone versus surgery followed by radiotherapy for mobile cancer of the rectum. *Lancet* **348**: 1610–1614.

Medical Research Council Rectal Cancer Working Party (1996b) Randomised trial of surgery alone versus radiotherapy followed by surgery for potentially operable locally advanced rectal cancer. *Lancet* **348**: 1605–1610.

Meeker WR Jr (1978) The use and abuse of CRA test in clinical practice. *Cancer* **41**: 854–862.

Mendenhall WM, Bland KI, Pfaff WW, Million RR & Copeland EM (1987) Initially unresectable rectal adenocarcinoma treated with preoperative irradiation and surgery. *Ann Surg* **205**: 41–44.

Mendenhall WM, Bland KI, Rout WR et al (1988) Clinically resectable adenocarcinoma of the rectum treated with preoperative irradiation and surgery. *Dis Colon Rectum* **31**: 287–290.

Metzger U, Memillod B, Aeberhaard P et al (1987) Intraportal chemotherapy in colorectal carcinoma as an adjuvant modality. *World J Surg* **2**: 452–458.

Moertel CG (1978) Chemotherapy for colorectal cancer. In Grandmann E (ed) *Colon Cancer*, pp 207–216. New York: Fischer.

Moertel CG (1982) *Compilation of Experimental Cancer Therapy Protocol Summaries*, edn 6-PB, 82-158262, no 20081, p 104. Bethesda: National Institutes of Health.

Moertel CG (1994) Chemotherapy for colorectal cancer [Review]. *N Engl J Med* **330**: 1136–1142.

Moertel CG, Reitemeier RJ, Childs DS, Colby MY & Holbrook MA (1964) Combined 5-fluorouracil and supervoltage radiation therapy in the palliative management of advanced gastrointestinal cancer: a pilot study. *Mayo Clin Proc* **39**: 767.

Moertel CG, Schutt AJ, Hahn RG & Reitemeier RJ (1975) Therapy of advanced colorectal cancer with a combination of 5-fluorouracil, methyl-1,3-*cis*(2 chloroethyl)-1-nitrosurea and vincristine. *J Natl Cancer Inst* **54**: 69–71.

Moertel CG, Fleming TR & MacDonald JS (1990) Levamisole and fluorouracil for surgical adjuvant therapy of colon carcinoma. *N Engl J Med* **322**: 352–358.

Moertel C, Fleming T, MacDonald J, Haller D & Laurie JA (1992) The intergroup study of fluorouracil plus levamisole and levamisole alone as adjuvant therapy for stage C colon cancer: a final report. *Proc Am Soc Clin Oncol* **11**: 161 (abstract).

Mohiuddin M, Dobelbower RR, Turalba C, Kramer S & Marks G (1979) A selective sandwich technique of adjuvant radiotherapy in the treatment of rectal cancer: a preliminary experience. *Dis Colon Rectum* **22**: 3–4.

Mohiuddin M, Dobelbower RR, Kraker S & Marks G (1981) Adjuvant radiotherapy with selective sandwich technique in treatment of rectal cancer. *Dis Colon Rectum* **21**: 76–79.

Mohiuddin M, Derdel J, Marks G & Kramer S (1985) Results of adjuvant radiation therapy in cancer of the rectum: Thomas Jefferson University Hospital experience. *Cancer* **55**: 350–353.

Moigooni AS & Nath R (1989) Dosimetry of Pd-103 model 200 sources for intestinal brachytherapy. *Endocur Hypertherm Oncol* **5**: 64.

Mori M, Tomoda H, Ishida T et al (1991) Surgical resection of pulmonary metastases from colorectal adenocarcinoma: special reference to repeated pulmonary resections. *Arch Surg* **126**: 1297–1301.

Morris DL & Ross WB (1996) Australian experience of cryoablation of liver tumors: metastases (review). *Surg Oncol Clin N Am* **5**: 391–397.

Morrow CE, Vassilopoulos PP & Grage TB (1981) Surgical resection for metastatic neoplasms of the lung: experience at the University of Minnesota hospitals. *Cancer* **45**: 2981–2985.

Morrow CE, Grage CB, Sutherland DE & Najarian JS (1982) Hepatic resection for secondary neoplasms. *Surgery* **92**: 610–614.

Morton DL (1981) In discussion of paper by Wanebo and Margrove (1981) Abdominal sacral resection of locally recurrent rectal cancer. *Ann Surg* **194**: 458.

Moss AA, Thoeni RF, Schnyder P & Marguld AR (1981) Value of computed tomography in the detection and staging of recurrent rectal carcinomas. *J Comput Assist Tomogr* **5**: 870–874.

Mountain CF, McMurtrey MJ & Hermes KE (1984) Surgery for pulmonary metastases: a 20-year experience. *Ann Thorac Surg* **38**: 323–340.

Mrazek R, Economou S, McDonald GO, Slaughter DP & Cole WH (1959) Prophylactic and adjuvant use of nitrogen mustard in the surgical treatment of cancer. *Ann Surg* **150**: 745.

MRC Working Party (1982) A trial of preoperative radiotherapy in the management of operable rectal cancer. *Br J Surg* **69**: 513–519.

MRC Working Party Second Report (1984) The evaluation of low-dose preoperative x-ray therapy in the management of operable rectal cancer: results of a randomly controlled trial. *Br J Surg* **71**: 21–25.

Neal CE & Abdel-Nabi H (1994) Clinical immunoscintigraphy of recurrent colorectal carcinoma. *Appl Radiol* **23**: 32–39.

Neiderhuber JE, Ensminger W, Gyves J, Trall J, Walker S & Cozzi E (1984) Regional chemotherapy of colorectal cancer metastasis of the liver. *Cancer* **53**: 1336–1346.

Niederhuber JE, Ensminger W, Gyves J et al (1984) Regional chemotherapy of colorectal cancer metastatic to the liver. *Cancer* **53**: 1336–1343.

Niederle N, Kurschel B & Schmidt CG (1984) Biologic effect of recombinant leucocyte alpha2 interferon in metastatic colorectal carcinoma. *Dtsch Med Wochenschr* **109**: 779–782.

NIH (1990) NIH Consensus Conference. Adjuvant therapy for patients with colon and rectal cancer. *JAMA* **264**: 1444–1450.

Nordlinger B, Quilichini MA, Parc R et al (1987) Surgical resection of liver metastases from colorectal cancers. *Int Surg* **72**: 70–72.

Northover JMA & Slack WW (1984) A randomised controlled trial of CEA prompted second-look surgery in recurrent colorectal cancer: a preliminary report. *Dis Colon Rectum* **27**: 576.

Northover JMA (1986) Carcinoembryonic antigen and recurrent colorectal cancer. *Gut* **27**: 117–122.

Nossal GV (1994) Minimal residual disease as a target for immunotherapy of cancer. *Lancet* **343**: 1172–1174.

O'Connell M, Mailliard J, MacDonald J et al (1993) An intergroup trial of intensive course 5-FU and low-dose leucovorin as surgical adjuvant therapy for high-risk colon cancer. *Proc Am Soc Clin Oncol* **12**: 552 (abstract).

Ogunbiyi OA, Flanagan FL, Dehdashti F et al (1997) Detection of recurrent and metastatic colorectal cancer: comparison of positron emission tomography and computed tomography. *Ann Surg Oncol* **4**: 613–620.

Ohlsson B, Breland U, Ekberg H, Graffner H & Tranberg K (1995) Follow-up after curative surgery for colorectal carcinoma: randomized comparison with no follow-up. *Dis Colon Rectum* **38**: 619–626.

Oliver GC & Shorb PE (1985) The totally implantable infusion pump in treatment of metastatic colorectal cancer. *Dis Colon Rectum* **28**: 18–23.

Orefice S, Gennari L, Mor L & Costa D (1981) The value of the CEA test in the diagnosis of metastases of adenocarcinoma of the gastroenteric tract. *Tumori* **67**: 109.

Orkin BA (1993) Rectal carcinoma treatment. In Beck DE & Wexner SD (eds) *Fundamentals of Anorectal Surgery*, pp 260–369. New York: McGraw-Hill.

Påhlman L (1996) Surveillance and recurrence. In Williams NS (ed) *Colorectal Cancer*. Edinburgh: Churchill Livingstone.

Påhlman L & Glimelius B (1990) Pre- or postoperative radiotherapy in rectal and rectosigmoid carcinoma: report from a randomized multicenter trial. *Ann Surg* 211: 187–195.

Påhlman L & Glimelius B (1992) Preoperative and postoperative radiotherapy and rectal cancer. *World J Surg* 16: 858–865.

Papillon J (1973) Endocavitary irradiation of early rectal cancer for cure: a series of 123 cases. *Proc R Soc Med* **66**: 1179.

Papillon J (1974) Intracavitary irradiation in the curative treatment of early cancers. *Dis Colon Rectum* **17**: 172–180.

Papillon J (1982) *Rectal and Anal Cancers*. Berlin: Springer.

Papillon J (1987) The future of external beam irradiation as initial treatment of rectal cancer. *Br J Surg* **74**: 449–454.

Papillon J & Berard P (1992) Endocavitary irradiation in the conservative treatment of adenocarcinoma of the low rectum. *World J Surg* **16**: 451–457.

Patel UB, Ackerman NB & Waterhouse K (1982) The transpubic approach in the management of problems of the lower genitourinary and intestinal tracts. *Surg Gynecol Obstet* **155**: 97–101.

Patt YZ, Peters RE, Chuang VP et al (1985) Palliation of pelvic recurrence of colorectal cancer with intra-arterial 5-fluorouracil and mitomycin. *Cancer* **56**: 2175–2180.

Patt YZ, Boddie AW Jr, Charnsangavej C et al (1986) Hepatic arterial infusion with floxuridine and cisplatin: overriding importance of antitumor effect versus degree of tumor burden as determinants of survival among patients with colorectal cancer. *J Clin Oncol* **4**; 1356–1364.

Patt YZ, Roh M, Chase J et al (1990) A phase I trial of hepatic arterial infusion of floxuridine and folinic acid for colorectal cancer metastatic to the liver. *Proc Am Soc Clin Oncol* **9**: 118.

Pearlman NW (1993) Surgery for pelvic recurrences. In: Cohen AM, Winawer SJ, eds, *Cancer of the Colon, Rectum and Anus* pp 863–871. New Jersey: McGraw-Hill.

Piedbois P, Buyse M, Gray R et al (1995) Portal vein infusion as an effective adjuvant treatment for patients with colorectal cancer. *Proc Am Soc Clin Oncol* **14**: 192.

Pihl E, Hughes ES, McDermott FT, Johnson W & Katrivessis H (1987) Lung recurrence after curative surgery for colorectal cancer. *Dis Colon Rectum* **30**: 417–419.

Pilipshen SJ, Heilweil M, Quan SHQ, Sternberg SS & Enker WE (1984) Patterns of pelvic recurrence following definitive resections of rectal cancer. *Cancer* **53**: 1354–1362.

Pinson CW, Wright JK, Chapman WC et al (1996) Repeat hepatic surgery for colorectal cancer metastasis to the liver. *Ann Surg* **223**: 765–773; discussion 773–776.

Pitrelli NJ & Mittelman A (1984) An analysis of chemotherapy for colorectal carcinoma. *J Surg Oncol* **28**: 201–206.

Pitrelli NJ, Barcewicz PA, Evans JT et al (1984) Hepatic artery ligation for liver metastasis in colorectal carcinoma. *Cancer* **53**; 1347–1353.

Polk HC Jr & Spratt JS Jr (1971) Recurrent colorectal carcinoma: detection, treatment, and other considerations. *Surgery* **69**: 9–23.

Polk HC Jr & Spratt JS Jr (1979) The results of treatment of perineal recurrence of cancer of the rectum. *Cancer* **43**: 952–956.

Pompecki R & Winckler R (1980) Clinical significance of routine serum CEA determination in the postoperative control of rectal cancer. *Med Welt* **31**: 1780.

Powers WF & Tolmach LJ (1964) Preoperative radiation therapy: biological basis and experimental investigation. *Nature* **201**: 272–273.

Prasad B, Lee MS & Henrickson FR (1977) Irradiation of hepatic metastases. *Int J Radiat Oncol Biol Phys* **2**: 129.

Presant CA, Denes AF, Liu C & Bartolucci AA (1984) Prospective randomized reappraisal of 5-fluorouracil in metastatic colorectal carcinoma: a comparative trial with 6-thioguanine. *Cancer* **53**: 2610–2614.

Purkiss SF, Dean R, Allardice JT, Grahn M & Williams NS (1993) An interstitial light delivery system for photodynamic therapy within the liver. *Lasers Med Sci* **8**: 253–257.

Purkiss SF, Hutton M & Williams NS (1994) A comparison of photosensitizer administration routes for interstitial photodynamic therapy of the liver. *Lasers Med Sci* **9**: 291–296.

Que FG & Nagorney DM (1994) Resection of 'recurrent' colorectal metastases to the liver. *Br J Surg* **81**: 255–258.

Rafto SE, Amendola MA & Gefter WB (1988) MR imaging of recurrent colorectal carcinoma versus fibrosis. *J Comput Assist Tomogr* **12**: 521–523.

Ramming KP & O'Toole K (1986) The use of the implantable chemoinfusion pump in the treatment of hepatic metastases of colorectal cancer. *Arch Surg* **121**: 1440–1444.

RCS/ACGBI (Royal College of Surgeons & Association of Coloproctology of Great Britain and Ireland) (1996) *Guidelines for the Management of Colorectal Cancer*. RCS/ACGBI, June.

Reed WP, Garb JL, Park WC et al (1988) Long-term results and complication of preoperative radiation in the treatment of rectal cancer. *Surgery* **103**: 161–167.

Rees M, Plant G, Wells J & Bygrave S (1996) One hundred and fifty hepatic resections: evaluation of technique towards bloodless surgery. *Br J Surg* **83**: 1526–1529.

Reithmuller G, Schneider-Gadicke E, Schlimok G et al (1994) Randomized trial of monoclonal antibody for adjuvant therapy of resected Dukes' C colorectal carcinoma. *Lancet* **343**: 1117–1183.

Reznek RH, White FE, Young JWR et al (1983) The appearances on computed tomography after abdominoperineal resection for carcinoma of the rectum: a comparison between the normal appearances and those of recurrence. *Br J Radiol* **56**: 237–240.

Rider WD (1975) Is the Miles operation really necessary for the treatment of rectal cancer? *J Can Assoc Radiol* **36**: 167.

Rider WD, Palmer JA, Mahoney LJ & Robertson CT (1977) Preoperative irradiation in operable cancer of the rectum: report of the Toronto trial. *Can J Surg* **20**: 335–338.

Rifkin MD & Wechsler RJ (1986) A comparison of computed tomography and endorectal ultrasound in staging rectal cancer. *Int J Colorect Dis* **1**: 219–223.

Robertson SH, Heron HC, Kerman HE & Bloom TS (1985) Is anterior resection of the rectosigmoid safe after preoperative radiation? *Dis Colon Rectum* **28**: 254–259.

Rochlin DB, Smart CR & Silva A (1965) Chemotherapy of malignancies of the gastrointestinal tract. *Am J Surg* **109**: 43–46.

Rodriguez-Antunez A, Chernak FS, Jelden GL & Hunter TW (1973) Preoperative irradiation of carcinoma of the rectum. *Radiology* **108**: 689–690.

Romano G, deRosa P, Vallone G et al (1985) Intrarectal ultrasound and computed tomography in the pre- and post-operative assessment of patients with rectal cancer. *Br J Surg* **72** (Suppl): S117–119.

Rosenberg SA, Lotze MT, Muyl LM et al (1987) A progress report on the treatment of 157 patients with advanced cancer using lymphokine activated killer cells and interleukin 2 or high dose interleukin 2 alone. *N Engl J Med* **316**: 889–897.

Rougier P, Laplanche A, Huguier M et al (1992) Hepatic arterial infusion of floxuridine in patients with liver metastases from colorectal carcinoma: long-term results of a prospective randomized trial. *J Clin Oncol* **10**: 1112–1118.

Rousselot LM, Cole DR, Grossi CE et al (1972) Adjuvant chemotherapy with 5-fluorouracil in surgery for colorectal cancer: eight year progress report. *Dis Colon Rectum* **15**: 169.

Ruff C, Dockerty M, Fricke R & Waugh J (1961) Preoperative radiation therapy for adenocarcinoma of the rectum and rectosigmoid colon. *Radiology* **106**: 389–396.

Ryan J, Heiden P, Crowley J & Bloch K (1988) Adjuvant portal vein infusion for colorectal cancer: a 3-arm randomised trial (abstract 361). *Proc ASCO* **7**: 95.

Saenz NC, Cady B, McDermott WV & Steele GD Jr (1989) Experience with colorectal carcinoma metastatic to the liver. *Surg Clin N Am* **69**: 361–370.

Safi F, Link KH & Beger HG (1993) Is follow-up of colorectal cancer patients worthwhile? *Dis Colon Rectum* **36**: 636–644.

Sagar PM & Pemberton JH (1996) Surgical management of locally recurrent rectal cancer. *Br J Surg* **83**: 293–304.

Sakamoto M, Hirose T, Shita H et al (1980) Correlation between degree of advancement surgery and recurrence and carcinoembryonic antigen (CEA) values in cancer of the large intestine (follow up of 166 patients). *Nippan Shok Geka Gakk Z* **13**: 636.

SAKK (Swiss Group for Clinical Cancer Research) (1995) Long-term results of adjuvant intraportal chemotherapy for colorectal cancer. *Lancet* **345**: 349–353.

Salmon SE, Hamburger AW & Soehnlen B (1978) Quantitation of differential sensitivity of human-tumor stem cells to anticancer drugs. *N Engl J Med* **298**: 1321–1327.

Samii K, Feret J, Harari A & Viars P (1979) Selective spinal analgesia. *Lancet* **i**: 1142.

Schaeffer W & Witte E (1932) Uber eine neue Karperhohlenrantgenrohr zur Bestrahlung van Uterustumaren, *Strahlentherapie* **44**: 283.

Scheele J, Altendorf-Hofman A, Strangle R, Groite H & Gall FP (1989) Resection of lung metastases from colorectal cancer: indications and indication limits. *Zentralbl Chir* **114**: 639–654.

Scheele J, Altendorf-Hofman A, Stangl R & Gall FP (1990a) Pulmonary resection for metastic colon and upper rectum cancer. Is it useful? *Dis Colon Rectum* **33**: 745–752.

Scheele J, Stangl R & Altendorf-Hofman A (1990b) Hepatic metastases from colorectal carcinoma: impact of surgical resection on the natural history. *Br J Surg* **77**: 1241–1246.

Scheipers C, Penninckx F, De Valler N et al (1995) Contribution of PET in the diagnosis of recurrent colorectal cancer: comparison with conventional imaging. *Eur J Surg Oncol* **21**: 517–522.

Scheithauer W, Rosen H, Kornek GV, Sebesta C & Depisch D (1993) Randomized comparison of combination chemotherapy and supportive care alone in patients with metastatic colorectal cancer. *BMJ* **306**: 752–755.

Schiessel R, Wunderlich M & Herbst F (1986) Local recurrence of colorectal cancer: effect of early detection and aggressive surgery. *Br J Surg* **73**: 342–344.

Schlag P, Hohenberger P, Holting T et al (1990) Hepatic arterial infusion chemotherapy for liver metastases of colorectal cancer using 5-FU. *Eur J Surg Oncol* **16**: 99–104.

Schwartz AG (1962) High cervical cordotomy; techniques and results. *Clin Neurosurg* **8**: 282.

Schwartz SI, Jones LS, McCune CS (1985) Assessment of treatment of intrahepatic malignancies using chemotherapy via an implantable pump. *Ann Surg* **201**: 560–567.

Seifert TP, Baker HL, Reed ML et al (1975) Comparison of continuously infused 5-fluorouracil with bolus injection in treatment of patients with colorectal carcinoma. *Cancer* **36**: 123.

Seifert WF, Wobbes T, Hoogenhout J et al (1995) Intraoperative radiation delays anastomotic repair in rat colon. *Am J Surg* **170**: 256–261.

Shepard KV, Levin B, Karl RC et al (1985) Therapy for metastatic colorectal cancer with hepatic artery infusion chemotherapy using a subcutaneous implanted pump. *J Clin Oncol* **3**: 161–169.

Sherman DM, Weichselbaum R & Order SE (1978) Palliation of hepatic metastases. *Cancer* **41**: 2013.

Shiraki S, Mori H, Kadomoto N et al (1982) Adjuvant immunotherapy of carcinoma coli with levamisole: prevention of immune depression following surgical therapy and radiotherapy. *Int J Immunopharmacol* **4**: 73–80.

Shirouzu K, Isomoto H, Hayashi A et al (1995) Surgical treatment for patients with pulmonary metastases after resection of primary colorectal carcinoma. *Cancer* **76**: 393–398.

Simbirtseva LP, Sneshko LI & Smirov NM (1975) Results of intensive combined therapy for carcinoma of the rectum. *Vopr Onkol* **21**: 12–15.

Sischy B (1982) The place of radiotherapy in the management of rectal adenocarcinoma. *Cancer* **50**: 2631–2637.

Sischy B (1991) The role of endocavitary irradiation for limited lesions of the rectum. *Int J Colorectal Dis* **6**: 91–94.

Sischy B & Remington JH (1975) Treatment of carcinoma of the rectum by intracavitary irradiation. *Surg Gynecol Obstet* **141**: 562–564.

Sischy B, Graney MJ, Hinson EJ & Qazi R (1985) Preoperative radiation therapy with sensitizers in the management of carcinoma of the rectum. *Dis Colon Rectum* **28**: 56–57.

Sischy B, Hinson EJ & Wilkinson DR (1988) Definitive radiation therapy for selected cancers of the rectum. *Br J Surg* **75**: 901–903.

Slevin ML & Gray R (1991) Adjuvant therapy for cancer of the colon. *BMJ* **302**: 1100–1102.

Smith DE, Muff NS, Shetabi H, Stutz FH & Eiesland H (1989) Postoperative adjuvant chemotherapy and radiotherapy for cancer of the large bowel and rectum. *Am J Surg* **157**: 508–511.

Smith JW, Fortner JG & Burt M (1992) Resection of hepatic and pulmonary metastases from colorectal cancer. *Surg Oncol* **1**: 399–404.

Sourek K (1969) Commissural myelotomy. *J Neurosurg* **31**: 524.

Sparso BH, Van Der Maase H, Kristensen O et al (1984) Complications following postoperative combined radiation and chemotherapy in adenocarcinoma of the rectum and rectosigmoid: a randomized trial that failed. *Cancer* **54**: 2363–2366.

Spratt JS (1981) In discussion of paper by Wanebo HH & Margrove RC (1981) Abdominal sacral resection of locally recurrent rectal cancer. *Ann Surg* **194**: 458.

Staab HJ, Anderer FA, Strumpf F, Hornung A, Fischer R & Kieninger C (1985) Eighty-four potential second-look operations based on sequential carcinoembryonic antigen determinations and clinical investigations in patients with recurrent gastrointestinal cancer. *Am J Surg* **149**: 198–204.

Ståhle E, Glimelius B, Bergström R & Påhlman L (1988) Preoperative serum markers in carcinoma of the rectum and rectosigmoid. II: Prediction of prognosis. *Eur J Surg Oncol* **14**: 287–296.

Stearns MW Jr & Leaming RJ (1975) Irradiation in inoperable cancer. *JAMA* **231**: 1388.

Stearns MW, Leaming RH, Blanchard RT et al (1965) Treatment of patients with advanced cancer using Y-90 microspheres. *Cancer* **18**: 375.

Stearns MW Jr, Deddish MR, Quan SHQ & Leaming RH (1974) Preoperative roentgentherapy for cancer of the rectum and rectosigmoid. *Surg Gynecol Obstet* **138**: 584–586.

Steele GD Jr (1986) Symposium: The management of recurrent colorectal cancer. *Int J Colorect Dis* **1**: 133–157.

Steele GD Jr (1994a) Colorectal cancer. In McKenna RJ Sr & Murphy GP (eds) *Cancer Surgery*, pp 125–184. Philadelphia: JP Lippincott.

Steele GD Jr (1994b) Cryoablation in hepatic surgery. *Sem Liver Dis* **14**: 120–125.

Steele GD Jr (1995) The management of colorectal cancer metastatic to the liver. In Cameron JL (ed) *Current Surgical Therapy*, 5th edn. St Louis: Mosby Yearbook.

Steele GD Jr & Ravikumar TS (1989) Resection of hepatic metastases from colorectal cancer: biological perspectives. *Ann Surg* **210**: 127–138.

Steele GD Jr, Bleday R, Mayer RJ et al (1991) A prospective evaluation of hepatic resection for colorectal carcinoma metastases to the liver: Gastrointestinal Tumor Study Group protocol 6584. *J Clin Oncol* **9**: 1105–1112.

Steger AC, Lees WR, Shorvon P, Walmsley KM & Bown SG (1992) Multiple-fibre low-power interstitial laser hyperthermia: studies in the normal liver. *Br J Surg* **79**: 139–145.

Stevens KR Jr, Allen CV & Fletcher WS (1976) Preoperative radiotherapy for adenocarcinoma of the rectosigmoid. *Cancer* **37**: 2866–2874.

Stevens KR Jr, Fletcher WS & Allen CV (1978) Anterior resection and primary anastomosis following high dose preoperative irradiation for adenocarcinoma of the rectosigmoid. *Cancer* **41**: 2065–2071.

Stock W, Thielman-Jonen, Muller J & Wintzer G (1980) Follow-up of colorectal carcinoma. *Therapie Woche* **30**: 8595–8599.

Stockholm Rectal Cancer Study Group (1987) Short term preoperative radiotherapy for adenocarcinoma of the rectum: an interim analysis of a randomised multicentre trial. *Am J Clin Oncol* **10**: 369–375.

Stockholm Rectal Cancer Study Group (1990) Preoperative short-term radiation therapy in operable rectal carcinoma. *Cancer* **66**: 49–56.

Stone MD, Kane R, Bothe A Jr et al (1994) Intraoperative ultrasound imaging of the liver at the time of colorectal cancer resection. *Arch Surg* **129**: 431–435.

Strauss LG, Clorius JH, Schlag P et al (1989) Recurrence of colorectal tumours: FDG–PET evaluation. *Radiology* **170**: 329–332.

Sugarbaker PH, Gianola FJ, Speyer JC et al (1985) Prospective, randomized trial of intravenous versus intraperitoneal 5-fluorouracil in patients with advanced primary colon or rectal cancer. *Surgery* **98**: 414.

Sugarbaker PH, Gianola FJ, Barofsky I, Hancock SI & Wesley R (1986) 5-Fluorouracil chemotherapy and pelvic radiation in the treatment of large bowel cancer: decreased toxicity in combined treatment with 5-fluorouracil administration through the intraperitoneal route. *Cancer* **38**: 826–831.

Sundquist K, Häfstrom LO, Jonsson PE et al (1978) Treatment of liver carcinoma with regional intra-arterial 5FU infusions. *Am J Surg* **136**: 328–333.

Suzuki K, Gunderson LL, Devine RM et al (1995) Intraoperative radiation after palliative surgery for locally recurrent rectal cancer. *Cancer* **75**: 939–952.

Swedish Rectal Cancer Trial (1993) Initial report from a Swedish multicentre study examining the role of preoperative irradiation in the treatment of patients with resectable rectal carcinoma. *Br J Surg* **80**: 1333–1336.

Swedish Rectal Cancer Trial (1997) Improved survival with preoperative radiotherapy in resectable rectal cancer. *N Engl J Med* **336**: 980–987.

Takagi H, Morimoto T, Hara S, Suzuki R, Horio S (1986) Seven cases of pelvic exenteration combined with sacral resection for locally recurrent rectal cancer. *J Surg Oncol* **32**: 184–188.

Taylor I (1978) Cytotoxic perfusion for colorectal liver metastases. *Br J Surg* **65**: 109–114.

Taylor I (1981) Studies in the treatment and prevention of colorectal liver metastases. *Ann R Coll Surg Engl* **63**: 270–276.

Taylor I (1982) A critical review of the treatment of colorectal liver metastases. *Clin Oncol* **8**: 149–158.

Taylor I, Rowling J & West C (1979a) Adjuvant cytotoxic liver perfusion for colorectal cancer. *Br J Surg* **66**: 833–837.

Taylor I, Bennett R & Sherriff S (1979b) The blood supply of colorectal liver metastases. *Br J Cancer* **39**: 749–756.

Taylor I, Machin D, Mullee M, Trotter G, Cooke T & West C (1985) A randomized controlled trial of adjuvant portal vein cytotoxic perfusion in colorectal cancer. *Br J Surg* **72**: 359–364.

Taylor RE, Kerr GR & Arnott SJ (1987) External beam radiotherapy for rectal adenocarcinoma. *Br J Surg* **74**: 455–459.

Temple WJ & Ketcham AS (1992) Sacral resection for control of pelvic tumors. *Am J Surg* **163**: 370–374.

Tornquist A, Ekelund G & Leandder L (1982) The value of intensive follow-up after curative resection for colorectal carcinoma. *Br J Surg* **69**: 725–728.

Touran T, Frost DB & O'Connell TX (1990) Sacral resection: operative technique and outcome. *Arch Surg* **125**: 911–913.

Tschmelitsch J, Kronberger P, Glaser K, Klingler A & Bodner E (1994) Survival after surgical treatment of recurrent carcinoma of the rectum. *J Am Coll Surg* **179**: 54–58.

Tung A, Malianiak K, Tenkela R & Winter P (1980) Intrathecal morphine for intraoperative and postoperative analgesia. *JAMA* **244**: 2637.

Turk PS & Wanebo HJ (1993) Results of surgical treatment of nonhepatic recurrence of colorectal carcinoma. *Cancer* **71** (Suppl 12): 4267–4277.

Uetsuji S, Yamamura M, Yamamichi K et al (1992) Absence of colorectal cancer metastasis to the cirrhotic liver. *Am J Surg* **164**: 176–177.

Vanchieri C (1990) Colon cancer update triggers change in practice. *J Natl Cancer Inst* **82**: 898.

Vaughn DJ & Haller DG (1993) Nonsurgical management of recurrent colorectal cancer. *Cancer* **71** (Suppl 12): 4278–4292.

Vauthey J-N, Marsh de-W, Cendan JC, Chu N-M & Copeland EM (1996) Arterial therapy of hepatic colorectal metastases. *Br J Surg* **83**: 447–455.

Villalon AH & Green D (1981) The use of radiotherapy for pelvic recurrence following APER for carcinoma of the rectum: a 10 year experience. *Aust NZ J Surg* **55**: 149.

Wanebo HH & Margrove RC (1981) Abdominal sacral resection of locally recurrent rectal cancer. *Ann Surg* **194**: 458.

Wanebo HJ, Koness J, Turk PS & Cohen SI (1992) Composite resection of posterior pelvic malignancy. *Ann Surg* **215**: 685–695.

Wanebo HJ, Koness RJ, Vezeridis MP, Cohen SI & Wrobleski DE (1994) Pelvic resection of recurrent rectal cancer. *Ann Surg* **220**: 586–597.

Wang CC & Schultz MD (1962) The role of radiation therapy in the management of carcinoma of the sigmoid, rectosigmoid and rectum. *Radiology* **79**: 105.

Wang JK, Nauss LA & Thomas JE (1979) Pain relief by intrathecally applied morphine in man. *Anaesthesiology* **50**: 149.

Warren KW, Jenkins RL & Steele GD Jr (1991) *Atlas of Surgery of the Liver, Pancreas and Biliary Tract*, pp 236–290. Norwalk: Appleton & Lange.

Watkins E, Khazei AM & Wahra KS (1970) Surgical basis for arterial infusion chemotherapy of disseminated carcinoma of the liver. *Surg Gynecol Obstet* **130**: 581–605.

Wedell J, Meier zu Eissen P, Luu TH et al (1981) A retrospective study of serial CEA determinations in the early detection of recurrent colorectal cancer. *Dis Colon Rectum* **24**: 618–621.

Weinstein GD, Rich TA, Shumate CR et al (1995) Preoperative infusional chemoradiation and surgery with or without an electron beam intraoperative boost for advanced primary rectal cancer. *Int J Radiat Oncol Biol Phys* **32**: 197–204.

Weiss GR, Garnick MB, Osteen RT et al (1983) Long-term hepatic arterial infusion of 5-fluorodeoxyuridine for liver metastases using an implantable infusion pump. *J Clin Oncol* **1**: 337–344.

Welch JP & Donaldson GA (1979) The clinical correlation of an autopsy study of recurrent colorectal cancer. *Ann Surg* **189**: 496–502.

Wereldsma JCT, Bruggink EDM, Melser WJ et al (1990) Adjuvant portal liver infusion in colorectal cancer with 5-fluorouracil/heparin versus urokinase versus santrol. *Cancer* **65**: 425–432.

Whiteley HW, Stearns MW, Leaming RH et al (1970) Palliative radiation therapy in patients with cancer of the colon and rectum. *Cancer* **25**: 343.

Wilkins EJ Jr, Head JM & Burke JF (1978) Pulmonary resection for metastatic neoplasms in the lung: experience at the Massachusetts General Hospital. *Am J Surg* **135**: 480–483.

Wilkins EW Jr (1978) The status of pulmonary resection of metastases: experience at MGH. In Weiss L & Gilbert HA (eds) *Pulmonary Metastases*, pp 232–242. Boston: GK Hall.

Wilkins N, Petrelli NJ, Herrera L, Regal AM & Mittelman A (1985) Surgical resection of pulmonary metastases from colorectal adenocarcinoma. *Dis Colon Rectum* **28**: 562–564.

Willett CG, Tepper, JE, Skates SJ et al (1987) Adjuvant postoperative radiation therapy for colonic carcinoma. *Ann Surg* **206**: 694–698.

Wills J & Wagener DJTH (1990) Adjuvant treatment of colon cancer: where do we go from here? *Ann Oncol* **1**: 329–331.

Wilson SM & Adson MA (1976) Surgical treatment of hepatic metastases from colorectal cancers. *Arch Surg* **111**: 330–334.

Windle R, Bell PRF & Shaw D (1987) Five-year results of a randomized trial of adjuvant 5FU and levamisole in colorectal cancer. *Br J Surg* **74**: 569–572.

Wolmark N, Wieand HS, Rockette HE et al (1983) The prognostic significance of tumor location and bowel obstruction in Dukes' B and C colorectal cancer: fndings from the NSABP clinical trials. *Ann Surg* **198**: 743–752.

Wolmark N, Fisher B & Rockette H (1988) Postoperative adjuvant chemotherapy or BCL for colon cancer: results from NSABP protocol C-01. *J Natl Cancer Inst* **80**: 30–36.

Wolmark N, Rockette H, Wickerman DL et al (1990) Adjuvant therapy of Dukes' A, B and C adenocarcinoma of the colon with portal vein 5-FU hepatic infusion: preliminary results of NSABP protocol C-02. *J Clin Oncol* **8**: 1466–1475.

Wolmark N, Rockette H, Fisher B et al (1993) The benefit of leucovorin modulated fluorouracil as postoperative adjuvant therapy for primary colon cancer: results from the National Surgical Adjuvant Breast and Bowel Project protocol C-03. *J Clin Oncol* **1**: 1879–1887.

Wolmark N et al (1996) The relative efficiency of 5-FU and leucovorin, 5-FU + levamisole, and 5-FU + leucovorin + levamisole in patients with Dukes' B and C carcinoma of the colon: first report of NSABP C-04. *Proc Soc Clin Oncol* **15**: x(A460).

Wood CB, Radtcliffe JL, Burt RW, Malcolm AJH & Blumgart LH (1980) The clinical significance of the pattern of elevated serum carcinoembryonic antigen (CEA) levels in recurrent colorectal cancer. *Br J Surg* **67**: 46–48.

Yaksh IL & Rudy TA (1977) Studies on the direct spinal action of narcotics in the production of analgesia in the rat. *Pharmacol Exper Ther* **202**: 411.

Yano T, Hara N, Ichinose Y et al (1993) Result of pulmonary resection of metastatic colorectal cancer and its application. *J Thorac Cardiovasc Surg* **106**: 875–879.

Yeh KA, Fortunato L, Hoffman JP & Eisenberg BL (1997) Cryosurgical ablation of hepatic metastases from colorectal carcinomas. *Am Sur* **63**: 63–68.

Zalcberg J et al (1996) The role of 5-fluorouracil dose in the adjuvant therapy of colorectal cancer. *Ann Oncol* **7**: 41–46.

Zaniboni A, Ehrlichman C, Seitz JF et al (1993) FU/FA increased disease-free survival in resected B2C colon cancer: results of a prospective pooled analysis of three randomized trials. *Proc Am Soc Clin Oncol* **12**: 555 (abstract).

Zaunbauer W, Haertel M & Fuchs WA (1981) Computed tomography in carcinoma of the rectum. *Gastrointest Radiol* **6**: 79–84.

34

MALIGNANT TUMOURS OF THE ANAL CANAL AND ANUS

A variety of cancers may affect the anal canal and anus. They are rare, being 20–30 times less common than colorectal cancer. The most common primary tumour is epidermoid cancer; others include basal cell carcinoma and malignant melanoma. Secondary invasion from an adenocarcinoma of the rectum which descends into the anal canal may also occur.

EPIDERMOID CANCER OF THE ANUS

The pathological classification of epidermoid cancers has, in the past, been confusing, but World Health Organization recommendations have clarified matters. Thus, these tumours can be classified as squamous, basaloid or mucoepidermoid (Morson and Sobin, 1976).

Another area of confusion relates to the anatomical classification of these tumours. Anatomists consider the anal canal to be that part of the alimentary tract distal to the rectal ampulla (Williams and Warwick, 1980). Surgeons, on the other hand, have found that this definition does not correspond to the pathological features of tumours in that area (Greenall et al, 1985a). Both groups are agreed that the proximal end of the anal canal corresponds to the anorectal ring; there is, however, disagreement as to the distal limit of the anus. The dentate line was the limit chosen by Morson (1960), whereas Beahrs and Wilson (1976) referred to the anal verge. MacConnell (1970) used the terms 'upper' and 'lower anal canal', and others have used such ill-defined terms as 'mucocutaneous junction'

(Cortese, 1975) or have not even defined their terms at all (Welch and Malt, 1977; Frost et al, 1984).

Greenall et al (1985b), in an excellent review of the subject, advised against using terms such as 'mucocutaneous junction' and 'Hilton's line', since they have been used interchangeably and both have been ascribed to a variety of structures including the dentate line and anal verge (Ewing, 1954; Kuehn et al, 1968; Singh et al, 1981). Greenall et al (1985b) pointed out that the anatomical boundary used to distinguish the anal canal from its margin will determine the relative incidence of tumours at these two sites. Thus when the anal verge is used (Kuehn et al, 1968; Beahrs and Wilson, 1976; Papillon, 1982), less than 15% of cases are defined as being at the anal margin, whereas authors using the more proximal dentate line as their dividing line (Morson, 1960; Hardy et al, 1969; Al-Jurf et al, 1979; Greenall et al, 1985b) found that approximately 30% of cancers occur at this site. Ideally there should be agreement on the anatomical definition of the anal canal and anal margin. Until this is achieved it is important for authors to state clearly which definitions they use and for readers to be aware of the differences.

Pathology

Squamous cell carcinoma

Squamous cell carcinomas may be keratinizing or non-keratinizing. The well-differentiated type tends to arise from the skin of the anal margin, whereas the poorly differentiated tumours occur more frequently within the anal canal. According to Morson (1960), more than 80% of tumours of the margin produce keratin whereas only 50% of tumours in the anal canal do so. Gabriel (1941) in his series of 55 cases found that the tumours in males were more often of low-grade malignancy than the tumours in females.

Basaloid tumours

Basaloid tumours are derived from the cells of the anal transitional zone (Grodsky, 1969) and are also known as cloacogenic or transitional tumours (Grinvalsky and Helwig, 1956; Kheir et al, 1972). They account for 30–50% of all anal canal cancers (Singh et al, 1981; Boman et al, 1984; Greenall, 1988; Morson and Pang, 1968). These tumours may resemble carcinomas of anoepithelium or they may have patterns similar to those of basal cell carcinoma of the skin, hence the different names that have been applied to these tumours. The tumours that are termed 'basaloid' have cell nests with the cells at the periphery arranged in an orderly palisade fashion (Figure 34.1). Although they may resemble basal cell carcinoma of the skin they do not behave in the same way, since they frequently metastasize. The transitional cloacogenic tumours which appear more like anoepithelium are composed of islands or nests of cells that have indistinct borders and basal nuclei (Figure 34.2). Many of them show features of keratinization, but the tumour should be classified as squamous or basaloid according to the predominant cell type (Greenall et al, 1985b).

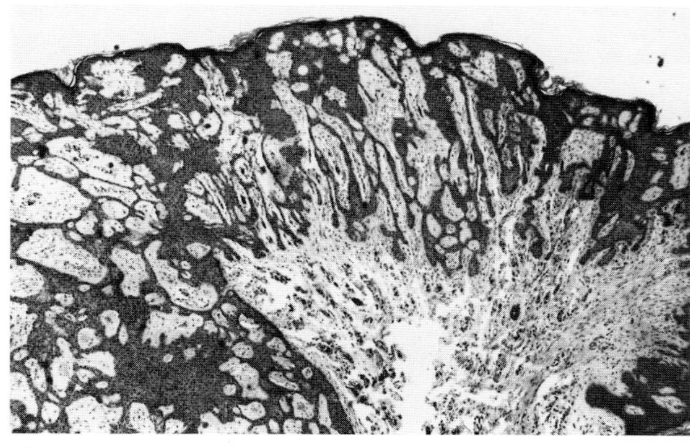
(a)

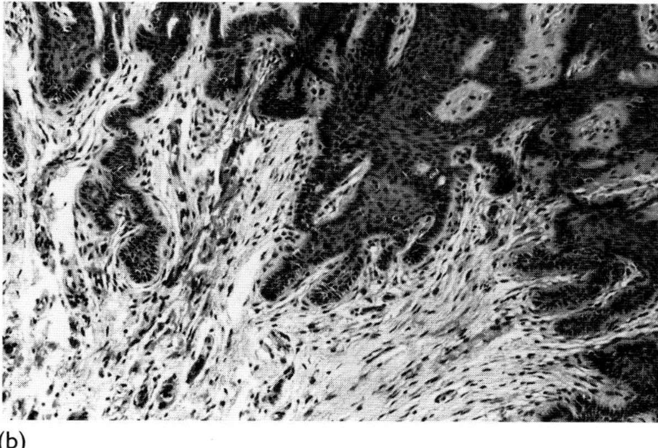
(b)

Figure 34.1 Basaloid carcinoma of the anus. (a) Trabeculae of dark-staining tumour cells extend beneath the epithelium (H&E, ×100) and (b) have a palisaded periphery (H&E, ×400).

Mucoepidermoid tumours

Mucoepidermoid tumours are rare. They occur in the anal canal and consist of squamous cells that produce both mucus and keratin (Morson, 1960;

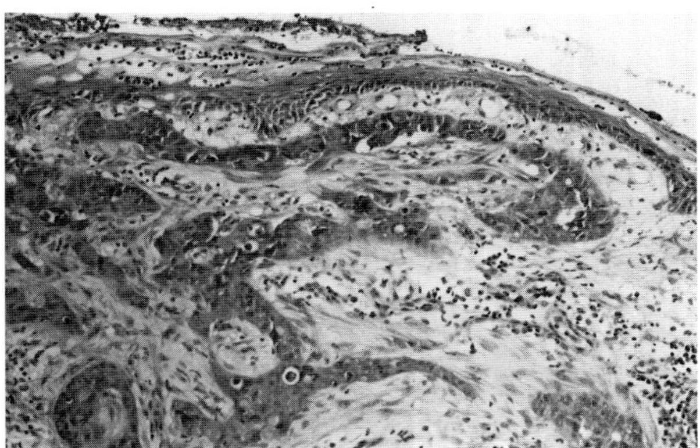

Figure 34.2 Transitional carcinoma of the anus. Strands of tumour are invading beneath the squamous epithelium and the tumour cells have a squamoid appearance (H&E, ×100).

Morson and Pang, 1968). A careful search using mucin stains may disclose a focus of mucin-producing cells in approximately 10–15% of patients with epidermoid cancers (Morson and Volkstadt, 1963b). These tumours behave in the same way as all other squamous cell carcinomas of the anus.

Spread

Direct spread of anal squamous cell carcinoma is preferentially in an upwards direction into the lower third of the rectum. The reason is said to be because the line of least resistance is upwards in the submucous layer (Morson and Dawson, 1990). Lymphatic spread commonly occurs to the inguinal nodes, but it is often not appreciated that spread to the superior haemorrhoidal lymph nodes and the nodes on the lateral wall of the pelvis is as common. Thus Morson (1960) found that in 43% of operative specimens the haemorrhoidal nodes were involved, and the inguinal nodes were involved in 36%. Indeed, there are studies that maintain that the inguinal nodes are involved at a later stage than the haemorrhoidal glands, the malignant cells possibly spreading backwards from within the pelvis (Gabriel, 1941; Morson, 1960; Hardcastle and Bussey, 1968; Morson and Pang, 1968). Such studies are flawed, however, by the fact that the data are derived from operative specimens supplemented by clinical observations. In these circumstances it is not possible to determine with accuracy the true incidence of lymph node involvement.

It has also been said that there is a relationship between the degree of histological differentiation and the incidence of lymph node metastases (Hardcastle and Bussey, 1968) since well-differentiated lesions rarely spread to the nodes. Although such a statement seems reasonable, in the absence of detailed microscopic examination of the inguinal nodes there are insufficient data to confirm this suggestion.

Squamous cell carcinoma of the anal margin spreads in a way similar to skin carcinoma, with direct spread deep to the dermis. Lymphatic spread to the inguinal nodes is said to occur in 40% of cases (Morson and Dawson, 1990).

Incidence

The reported incidence of epidermoid anal cancer in series of colorectal and anal carcinomas varies between 1% and 2.5% (Cattell and Williams, 1943; Grinnell, 1954; Sawyers et al, 1963; Beahrs and Wilson, 1976; Golden and Horsley, 1976).

Aetiology and clinical features

Epidermoid cancer can occur at almost any age but is most common in the sixth and seventh decades of life. Neither tumour site nor histology influences the age at presentation (Beahrs and Wilson, 1976). Anal canal tumours seem to be more common in women (Morson, 1960; Singh et al, 1981; Boman et al, 1984; Frost et al, 1984), whereas margin tumours, i.e. tumours extending up to the dentate line, occur more frequently in men (Morson, 1960; MacConnell, 1970; Goligher, 1984; Greenall, 1988). Tumour size is similar whether the lesion arose in the anal canal or from the anal margin. The mean diameter reported at presentation is approximately 3–4 cm (Cortese, 1975; Greenall et al, 1985b).

Symptoms include rectal bleeding, pruritus ani, mucous discharge, tenesmus, the sensation of a lump in the anus, incontinence and a change in bowel habit (Deans et al, 1994). Occasionally the patient may present with metastases in the inguinal lymph nodes before the primary tumour causes significant symptoms. The findings on examination of the anus are variable. The anal cancer may take the form of an ulcer, stricture or a proliferative lesion (Figure 34.3). There are often signs of other coexisting benign perianal conditions such as condylomata (Beahrs and Wilson, 1976; Welch and Malt, 1977; Sawyers, 1977), chronic fistula (Morson, 1960; Welch and Malt, 1977; Schraut et al, 1983), leucoplakia (Beahrs and Wilson, 1976) and the effects of previous irradiation (Sawyers, 1977; Singh et al, 1981; Goligher, 1984). The Sloan-Kettering group

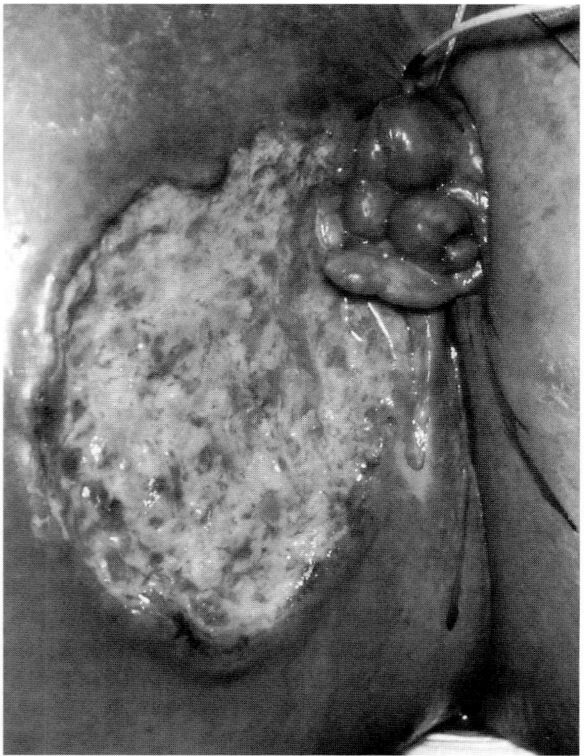

Figure 34.3 Large, ulcerated squamous cell carcinoma of the anal verge.

found that one or more of these features occurred in 60% of patients with margin cancer but in only 6% of those with canal tumours (Greenall et al, 1985b). Each of these associated conditions has been suggested as a possible cause of carcinoma of the margin, although conclusive proof is lacking.

Particular interest has recently focused on the association between condylomata acuminata and anal cancer (see Chapter 19). Since condylomata are caused by the human papillomavirus, it may be that this virus is involved in the pathogenesis of anal cancer and that the disease is sexually transmitted. Evidence is published to support the view that condylomata may become dysplastic and develop into frank carcinoma (Bogomoletz et al, 1985; Gillatt and Teasdale, 1985; Metcalfe and Dean, 1995). Furthermore, there is an association between anal squamous cell carcinoma, cervical cancer and other tumours of the genital tract which have been shown to contain DNA from human papillomavirus (HPV) types 16 and 18 in their genomes. Molecular biological techniques have also revealed that the majority of anal cancers harbour HPV DNA (Scholefield et al, 1990). These findings may explain the association between anal cancer and other sexually transmitted diseases, particularly human immunodeficiency virus (HIV) and syphilis (Judson et al, 1980; Daling et al, 1982; Schraut et al, 1983; Melbye et al, 1994; Harrison et al, 1995); hence a high incidence among the homosexual community (Cooper et al, 1979; Leach and Ellis, 1981; Lorenz et al, 1991; Metcalfe and Dean, 1995) (see Chapter 68). It is interesting that the incidence of anal cancer has increased *pari passu* with the AIDS epidemic and that HPV is found more frequently in individuals infected with HIV (Surawicz et al, 1993).

Much work has also centred on anal intraepithelial neoplasia (AIN) and the development of frank invasive carcinoma and the relationship between AIN, HPV and HIV infection. The term AIN has been coined to describe dysplastic changes which occur in the epithelium of the anal canal and in condylomata. There are three grades: AIN I, II and III, AIN I being low grade and AIN III being high grade. It is thought that AIN is probably induced by HPV infection (Surawicz et al, 1993, 1995) and will eventually progress through the grades to frank invasive carcinoma. AIN can be detected by cytology, anoscopy and biopsy, but it should be stressed that the natural history of AIN is not known, and further studies are being carried out to elucidate it (Scholefield et al, 1994). AIN is discussed in more detail later.

Several reports have suggested a significantly higher incidence of anal cancer in patients with Crohn's disease (Slater et al, 1984; Connell et al, 1994). Since anal lesions in such patients are often treated conservatively, it is good advice to periodically biopsy such lesions in Crohn's patients.

The patient may also present with synchronous inguinal lymph node involvement. The incidence of such spread was thought to be 25% (Klotz et al, 1967; Kuehn et al, 1968; Wolfe, 1968) but recent evidence suggests that this is an overestimate and that the true incidence is about 10% (Schraut et al, 1983; Greenall, 1988). Inguinal lymphatic involvement is probably much lower in patients with margin tumours (Schraut et al, 1983; Greenall et al, 1985b). Occasionally an anal cancer may be found incidentally during the histological examination of a specimen removed during a haemorrhoidectomy. This poses certain problems for the surgeon with regard to management (see below).

The differential diagnosis includes Bowen's disease, Paget's disease, condylomata acuminata, leucoplakia, melanoma, Crohn's disease, basal cell carcinoma and certain intrinsic skin disorders such as lichen sclerosis et atrophicus (Bender and Lechago, 1976; Lock et al, 1977a,b; Strauss and Fazio, 1979; Nielsen and Jensen, 1981; Sloan and Goepel, 1981; Quan, 1983). In fact, anal carcinoma has been described in association with all these diseases. It is thus important that any suspicious areas around the anus should be biopsied extensively and particular suspicion should be aroused if induration is present.

Staging

Staging of anal canal carcinoma has proved difficult. Dukes' stages cannot be applied as the tumour spreads to inguinal and iliac nodes which are not routinely removed at operation. The TNM system has been applied, but it can be criticized since it is difficult to distinguish tumours limited to the internal sphincter (T1) from those that involve the external sphincter (T2), and because extension into the rectum or perianal skin (T3) does not necessarily indicate a poor outcome (Papillon, 1982). Numerous modifications of the TNM system have been tried (Paradis et al, 1975; Singh et al, 1981; Papillon, 1982; Boman et al, 1984; Frost et al, 1984) but none has proved acceptable. There have been few attempts to stage margin tumours. One staging system recommended by the International Union Against Cancer (UICC) has been used occasionally (Papillon, 1982). In it T1 tumours are classified as less than 2 cm in diameter and are superficial or exophytic; T2 tumours are 2–5 cm in diameter with minimal infiltration; T3 tumours are 5 cm or greater in diameter; and T4 lesions infiltrate muscle or bone. The details of the UICC clinical staging systems for carcinoma of the anal canal and anal margin are illustrated in Figure 34.4.

Because of the relationship between stage and the results of therapy, attempts have been made to evaluate endoanal ultrasound in determining the depth of invasion. Early results suggest that this modality may have a place in the preoperative staging of anal carcinoma (Herzog et al, 1994; Roseau et al, 1994).

Treatment

Tumours of the anal canal

In the past, conventional treatment for anal carcinomas was abdominoperineal excision of the rectum, although local excision and radiotherapy were the preferred options for certain lesions. More recently the combination of chemotherapy and radiation has been used initially, with subsequent surgical excision being resorted to only if chemoirradiation fails. The introduction of chemoirradiation has made us critically appraise the overall treatment policy for this disease.

Abdominoperineal excision

Until recently, abdominoperineal excision was the standard initial procedure for the treatment of anal canal carcinoma. The technique was the same as that performed for a low rectal carcinoma except that a wide perineal phase was advised to prevent local recurrence (Klotz et al, 1967; Sawyers, 1977; Stearns et al, 1980; Goligher, 1984). Some advocated gluteal and perineal flaps to repair the perineal defect (Stearns et al, 1980). In women, excision of the posterior vaginal wall was often advised to obtain improved clearance (Klotz et al, 1967; Welch and Malt, 1977) but not all authors were convinced that this manoeuvre was necessary if the rectovaginal septum appeared free of disease (Stearns et al, 1980).

If the inguinal lymph nodes were involved with tumour, most authorities recommended that a block dissection of the groin was carried out 4–6 weeks after abdominoperineal excision of the rectum. Prophylactic inguinal lymphadenectomy was not to be recommended if the inguinal lymph nodes were not clinically affected, since the procedure had a high morbidity (Stearns and Quan, 1970; Beahrs and Wilson, 1976; Welch and Malt, 1977) and did not seem to improve survival. However, no controlled trial had been performed to assess the value of prophylactic block dissection of the groin.

Results

Five-year survival rates following abdominoperineal excision as a first option for anal canal carcinoma varied between 38% and 71% (Table 34.1). This variation was explained by differences in case selection and whether the data had been expressed as crude, corrected or actuarial survival rates (Greenall et al, 1985b). Survival seemed to be related to tumour size (Klotz et al, 1967; Boman et al, 1984; Greenall, 1988), histological grade (Klotz et al, 1967; Hardcastle and Bussey, 1968; Boman et al, 1984; Frost et al, 1984), depth of microscopic invasion (Frost et al, 1984; Greenall, 1988) and overall clinical staging (Klotz et al, 1967; Boman et al, 1984; Frost et al, 1984). The histological type of tumour, whether basaloid, mucoepidermoid or purely squamous, did not seem to influence survival (Welch and Malt, 1977; Schraut et al, 1983; Boman et al, 1984; Frost et al, 1984; Greenall, 1988).

Local recurrence, although difficult to detect after abdominoperineal excision, seemed to be the most

Figure 34.4 UICC clinical staging system for carcinoma of the anal canal and anal margin. The classification applies only to carcinoma. Histological verification of the diagnosis is necessary.

Definitions of anatomical regions and lymphatic spread

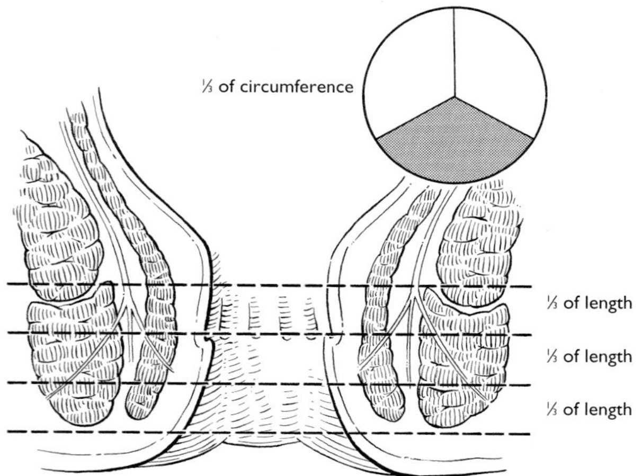

Anatomical regions. *Anal canal* with haemorrhoidal zone, crypts of Morgagni and Pecten and *anal orifice* (dermis).

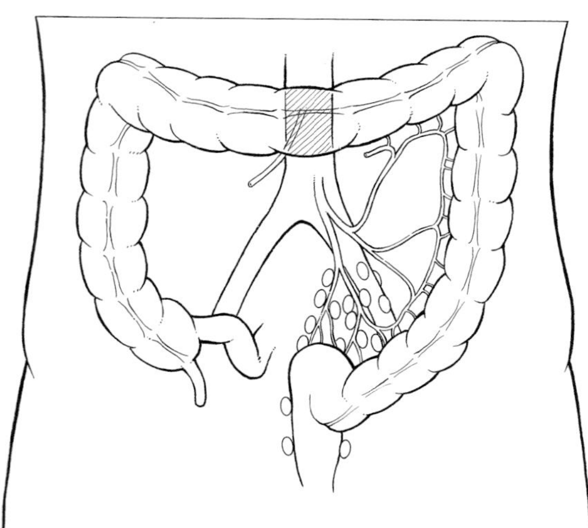

Regional lymph nodes. *Anal canal*: the regional lymph nodes are the perirectal nodes and the nodes distal to the origin of the inferior mesenteric artery.

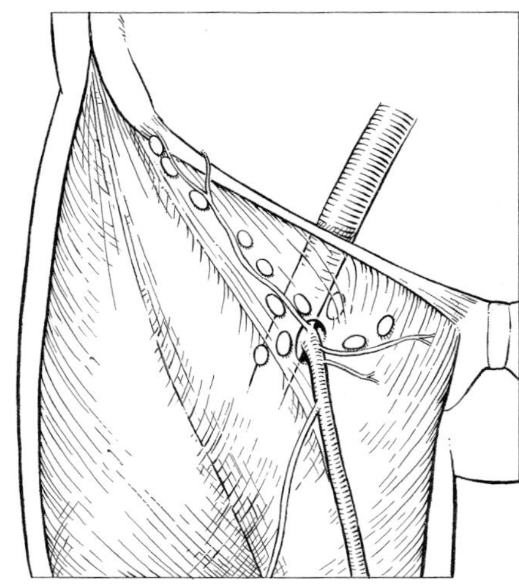

Regional lymph nodes. *Anal orifice*: the regional lymph nodes are the inguinal nodes.

Pretreatment clinical classification: TN

Anal canal

T = Primary tumour

- Tis Preinvasive carcinoma (carcinoma *in situ*).
- T0 No evidence of primary tumour.
- T1 Tumour occupying not more than one third of the circumference or length of the anal canal and not infiltrating the external sphincter muscle.
- T2 Tumour occupying more than one third of the circumference or length of the anal canal or tumour infiltrating the external sphincter muscle.
- T3 Tumour with extension to rectum or skin but not to other neighbouring structures.
- T4 Tumour with extension to other neighbouring structures.
- TX The minimum requirements to assess the primary tumour cannot be met.

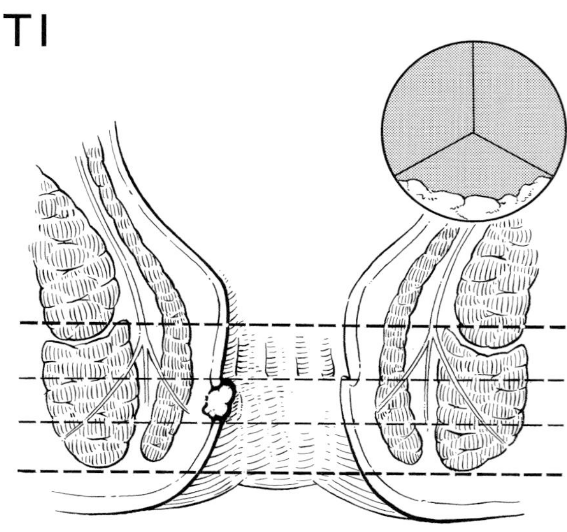

T2

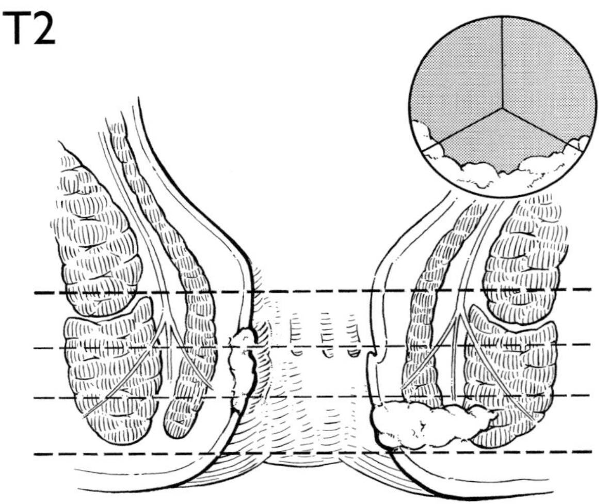

T4

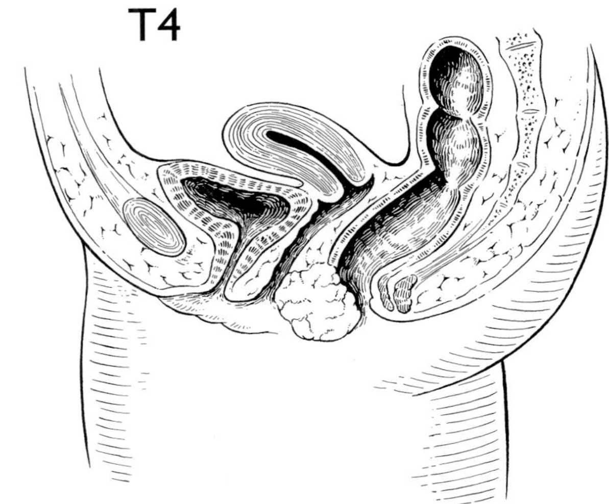

T3

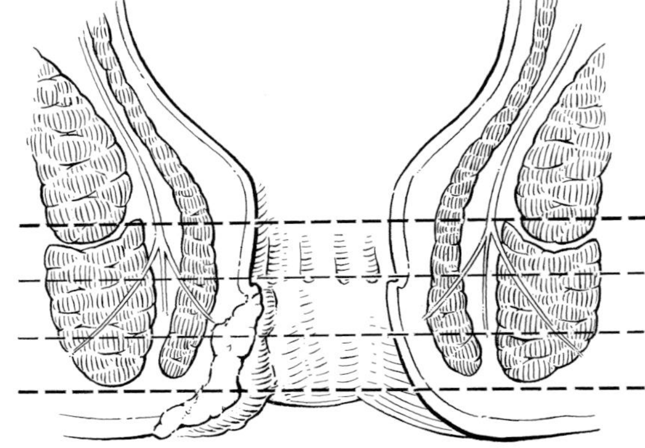

T3

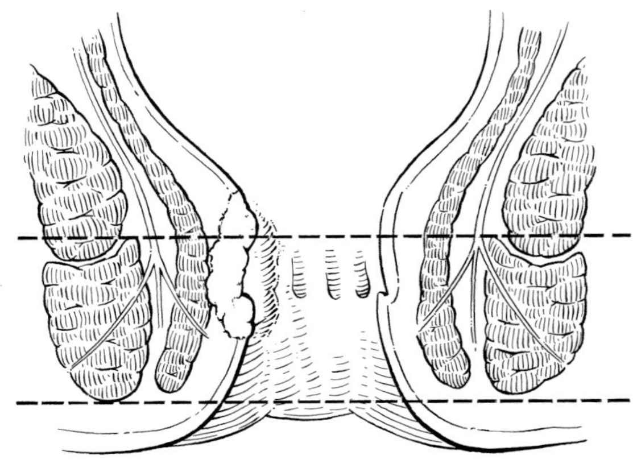

Anal canal

N = Regional lymph nodes

N0 No evidence of regional lymph node involvement.
N1 Evidence of involvement of regional lymph nodes.
NX The minimum requirements to assess the regional lymph nodes cannot be met.

N1

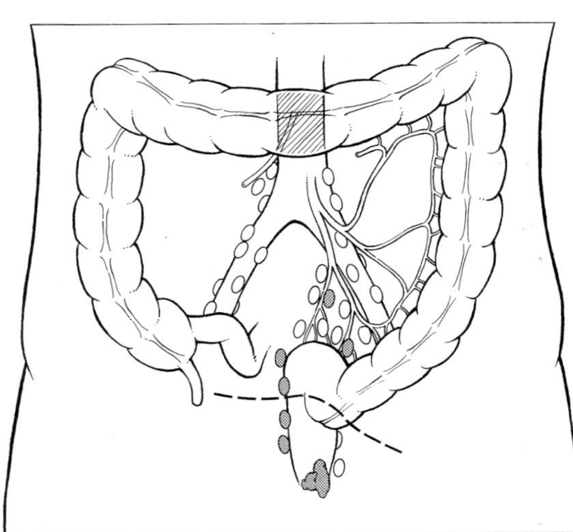

Pretreatment clinical classification: TN

Anal margin

T = Primary tumour

Tis	Preinvasive carcinoma (carcinoma *in situ*).
T0	No evidence of primary tumour.
T1	Tumour 2 cm or less in its greatest dimension strictly superficial or exophytic.
T2	Tumour more than 2 cm but not more than 5 cm in its greatest dimension or tumour with minimal infiltration of the dermis.
T3	Tumour more than 5 cm in its greatest dimension or tumour with deep infiltration of the dermis.
T4	Tumour with extensions to muscle and bone, etc.
TX	The minimum requirements to assess the primary tumour cannot be met.

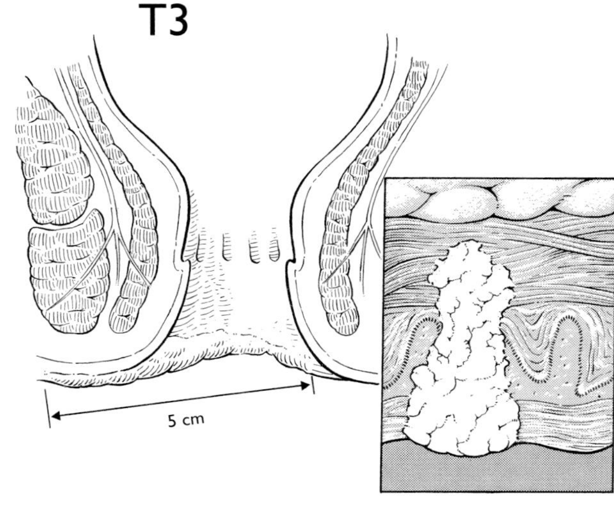

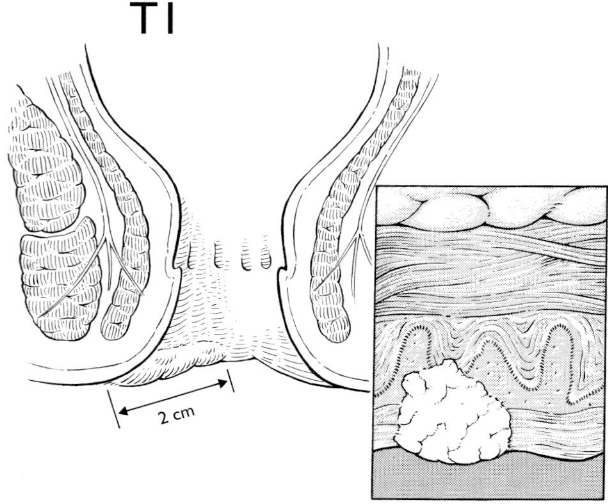

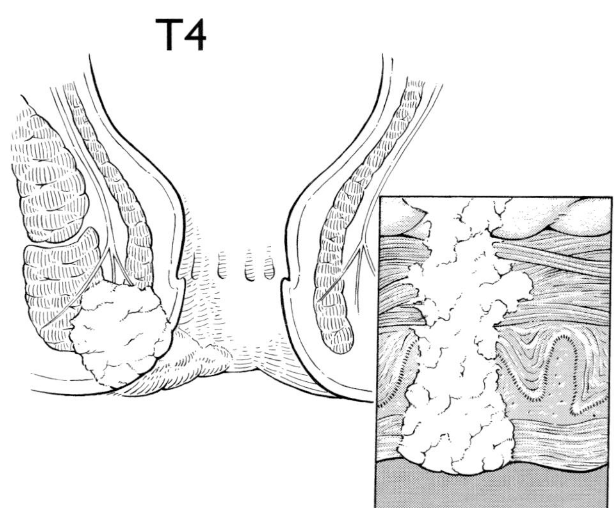

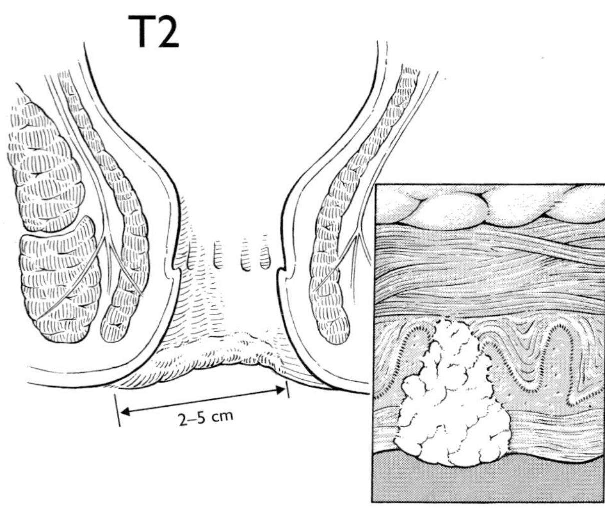

Anal margin

N = Regional lymph nodes

N0	No evidence of lymph node involvement.
N1	Evidence of involvement of movable unilateral regional lymph nodes.
N2	Evidence of involvement of movable regional lymph nodes.
N3	Evidence of involvement of fixed regional lymph nodes.
NX	The minimum requirements to assess the regional lymph nodes cannot be met.

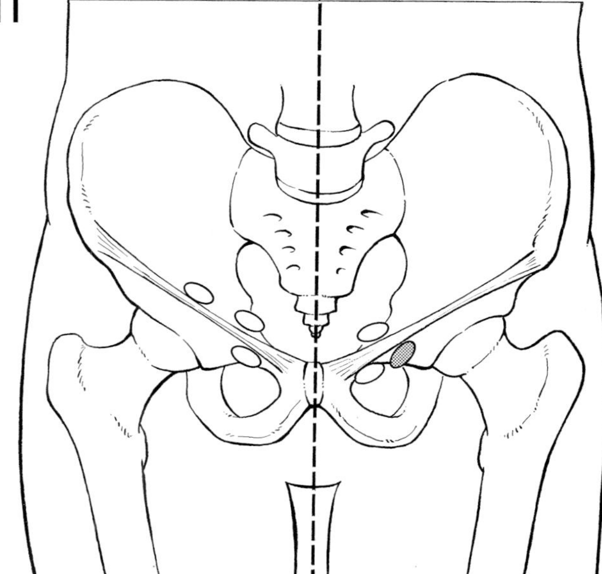

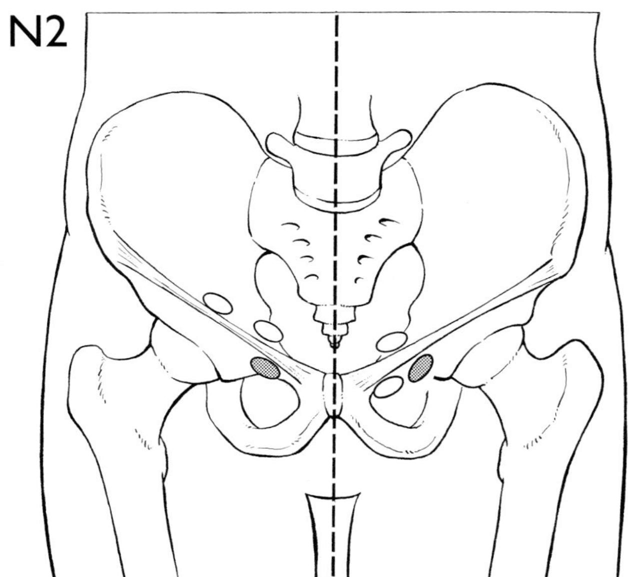

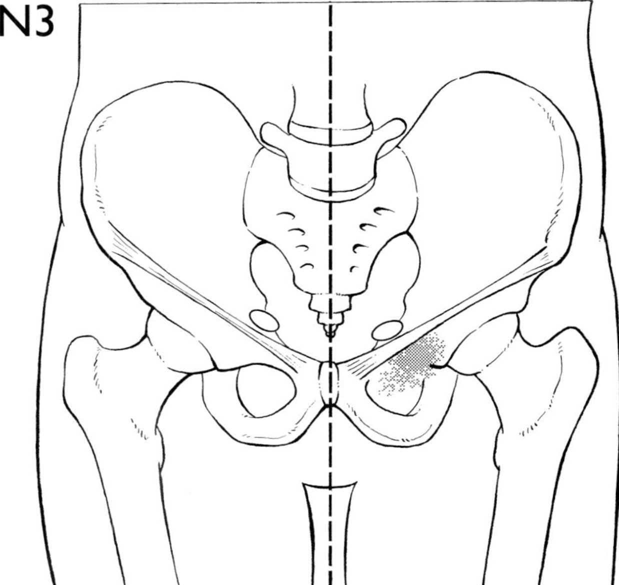

common reason for failure and only 10–20% of patients died from visceral metastases (Klotz et al, 1967; Boman et al, 1984; Frost et al, 1984; Greenall, 1988).

The time to recurrence was variable but the median seemed to be approximately 12 months (Boman et al, 1984; Frost et al, 1984; Greenall et al, 1986). Once recurrence had been detected in the pelvis or in the viscera, the prognosis was extremely poor. Greenall et al (1986) reported a median survival time of about 9 months for patients with pelvic or visceral recurrence. These forms of recurrence seemed to be resistant to treatment by surgery, radiotherapy or chemotherapy (Boman et al, 1984; Frost et al, 1984; Greenall, 1988), all of which had been tried.

Despite the gloomy outlook for patients with pelvic and visceral recurrence, the prognosis seemed to be better if the disease recurred in the inguinal lymph nodes. After radical block dissection of the groin 5-year survival rates between 40% and 70% were recorded (Kuehn et al, 1968; Wolfe, 1968;

Table 34.1 Abdominoperineal resection for epidermoid cancer in the anal canal.

Authors	*No. of patients treated*	*No. of 5-year survivors (%)*	*Distal limit of canal*
Klotz et al (1967)	194	97 (50)	Anal verge
Hardcastle and Bussey (1968)	83	40 (48)	Dentate line
O'Brien et al (1982)	21	8 (38)	Dentate line
Singh et al (1981)	47	25 (53)	Anal verge
Schraut et al (1983)	24	13 (54)	Anal verge
Boman et al (1984)	114	80 (71)	Anal verge
Greenall et al (1985b)	103	57 (55)	Dentate line
Total	586	320 (55)	

Sawyers, 1977; Frost et al, 1984; Greenall, 1988). This contrasted sharply with the poor survival rates when inguinal dissection was needed at the time of the original abdominoperineal excision (Grinnell, 1954; Judd and De Tar, 1955; Wolfe and Bussey, 1968; Stearns and Quan, 1970).

Local excision

Local excision has rarely been used as an initial procedure for anal canal carcinoma but analysis of the available data is confusing since the results are often combined with anal margin lesions. If local excision is to be used it is advisable to employ cutting diathermy with the aim of obtaining at least a 2.5-cm margin of clearance around all aspects of the growth. It will be appreciated that this aim cannot always be achieved for anal canal lesions as it is often not possible to reach the most proximal part of the lesion. With the introduction of chemoirradiation, it is our view that local excision should not now be used as an initial therapy for anal canal carcinoma.

Results

The results of local excision are difficult to interpret: in addition to problems of classification, authors often included patients who had received additional irradiation (Kuehn et al, 1968). As far as one can see from the available data, the 5-year survival was approximately 65% for carefully selected early lesions (Table 34.2).

However, despite these apparently good results, over 40% of patients developed local recurrence and eventually required an abdominoperineal excision. Even if the lesion was quite small, for instance less than 2 cm in diameter, and was limited to the submucosa, approximately 8% of patients had metastases within lymph nodes. Irrespective of size, approximately 30% of tumours confined to the submucosa will have nodal metastases and this figure is over 60% if the underlying muscle is involved. As it is usually necessary to resect part of the underlying external anal sphincter, anal function may be impaired.

The above data suggest that local excision for true anal canal carcinomas is not generally an effective method of treatment and cannot be recommended.

Radiotherapy

Radiotherapy has been employed for over 60 years as an alternative to surgery for this disease. A variety of techniques have been described which fall into three main types: interstitial radiation, external beam radiation and intracavitary radiation. The most common type of interstitial therapy up to the present time has been the implantation of radium

Table 34.2 Local excision (LE) for epidermoid cancer in the anal canal.

Authors	*Total no. treated*	*No. treated by LE*	*No. of 5-year survivors*	*No. with local recurrence*	*Distal limit of canal*
Klotz et al (1967)	373	33	20	11	Anal verge
Hardcastle and Bussey (1968)	127	8	6	2	Dentate line
Beahrs and Wilson (1976)	177	21	17	9	Anal verge
Singh et al (1981)	55	5	1	4	Anal verge
Schraut et al (1983)	31	7	5	2	Anal verge
Greenall et al (1985b)	126	11	5	7	Dentate line
Total	889	85 (10%)*	54 (64%)†	35 (41%)	

* Percentage of total number of cases treated for LE.
† Percentage of 5-year survivors after LE.

needles (Devois and Decker, 1960; Dalby and Pointon, 1961; Quan, 1983) but more recently iridium 192 has been used.

Interstitial therapy using radium has the theoretical advantage of providing high doses of radiation to the tumour and minimizing damage to normal tissue. However, it has the disadvantage of failing to deliver a homogeneous dose of radiation to the carcinoma, as well as failing to penetrate deep enough to treat malignant cells in pelvic lymphatics. In an attempt to improve results, fractionation techniques have been used: a high initial dose is followed by a lower dose several weeks later, the rationale being that the initial treatment shrinks the tumour sufficiently so that the second application has a greater chance of success (Papillon, 1982). Nowadays external beam radiation is delivered by megavoltage therapy or by electron and gamma irradiation from caesium 137 or cobalt 60. These forms of therapy have been used in a variety of dosages and over variable periods (Fenger, 1979; Cantril et al, 1983; Salmon et al, 1984).

Combinations of external beam, interstitial and intracavitary techniques have also been used. The first course is usually provided by external beam irradiation. This split course irradiation aims to prevent damage to normal tissue and allows more accurate dosage to be calculated on the basis of individual tumour radiosensitivity (Chrusčov et al, 1978; Papillon, 1982).

Results

The 5-year survival rates for all varieties of radiotherapy used in the treatment of anal canal carcinoma vary from 32% to 88% (Table 34.3). This variation is explained by the widely different definitions for patient inclusion. Thus some reports include patients with advanced disease, whereas others include small, superficial lesions. Furthermore they often do not state how many patients required subsequent surgery. Similar criticisms apply to the reporting of complications. No matter which type of radiotherapeutic technique is used, there is some degree of radionecrosis with the risk of anal stricture. However, such problems are not severe and only 5% of cases with strictures seem to require remedial surgery.

There is still controversy about radiotherapy if the patient presents with involved inguinal nodes. Papillon (1982) believed that complete cure of inguinal lymph node metastases could be obtained by irradiation with a dose of 45.0–45.4 Gy. This view is not universally held and many radiotherapists accept that a block dissection of involved nodes is more effective.

Combined radiotherapy and chemotherapy as initial treatment

Nigro et al (1974) were the first to introduce the concept and practice of radiotherapy combined with

Table 34.3 Radiation therapy for epidermoid cancer of the anal canal.

Authors	*n*	*Recurrence* (%)	*5-year survival* (%)	*Complication rate* (%)
Interstitial radiation				
Dalby and Pointon (1961)	28	23	32	23
Devois and Decker (1960)*	21	14	69	24
Papillon (1982)	88	14	69	5
Jones et al (1993)	20	40	40	40
Split course irradiation				
Chrusčov et al (1978)*	81	11	44	6
Papillon (1982)	97	8	67	6
External beam irradiation				
Seweg et al (1978)*	106	26	42	33
Cummings et al (1984)	51	20	59	31
Cantril et al (1983)*	33	12	79†	23
Salmon et al (1984)	183	34	59	15
Touboul et al (1995b)	147	29	58§	5
Jones et al 1993**	18	?	88	?

* May include margin cases.
† Actuarial survival.
§ 10-year survival.
** Also received interstitial treatment.

chemotherapy for this disease. They initially used combined therapy as preoperative adjuvant therapy before an abdominoperineal excision. Using this approach they soon discovered that they often could not find any evidence of residual carcinoma on pathological examination of the resection specimen. They postulated, therefore, that in many cases chemoirradiation might be all that was necessary to treat anal canal carcinoma. Their regimen involved fluorouracil and mitomycin since both drugs were not only cytotoxic to a variety of tumours but were also radiosensitizing agents (Nigro et al, 1974). Other workers used bleomycin, cisplatin and doxorubicin (Greenall et al, 1986).

Although the regimens have varied (Table 34.4), the basic plan in most of them has been to give mitomycin on day 1 as an intravenous bolus (10–15 mg/m^2) with fluorouracil as an intravenous infusion over 4–5 days, beginning on day 1 (750–1000 mg/m^2 each day). Radiotherapy is given over 3–7 weeks, beginning either on day 1 or immediately after the course of chemotherapy (day 6). The radiation dose varies from 30 Gy to 50 Gy. Most centres use parallel opposed pelvic fields, but others (Sischy et al, 1982) also administer a boost to the anus by a direct perineal port. The radiation field can be adjusted to include involved inguinal nodes if necessary.

The patients are then examined under anaesthesia 4–6 weeks after cessation of therapy. An abdominoperineal resection is only performed if there is obvious residual tumour. If there has been a good response to therapy, the scar tissue at the site of the original cancer is locally excised for histological scrutiny. If no microscopic carcinoma is present the patient is followed up carefully. If there is microscopic cancer in the excised specimen most authorities recommend radical excision (Nigro et al, 1983). Some centres, most notably Memorial Sloan-Kettering, suggest that patients with microscopic residual disease can be treated conservatively provided that they are followed up regularly (Greenall et al, 1986).

Such combined treatment cannot be considered lightly as it is associated with unpleasant side-effects. Leucopenia or thrombocytopenia occurs in 25% of patients 2–3 weeks after starting treatment, but is usually not severe and is reversible (Flam et al, 1983; Cummings et al, 1984). After radiotherapy, most patients experience proctitis and perianal dermatitis. Patients who receive fluorouracil should be warned about the development of alopecia; they often also develop stomatitis. Mitomycin can produce similar problems and can also cause the haemolytic uraemic syndrome (Gulati et al, 1980).

Results

Initial data using combined radiotherapy and chemotherapy appeared very promising. More than 90% of patients survived for more than 2 years (Table 34.5). At Sloan-Kettering there was a partial or complete response in 13 of 18 patients, all of whom had tumours proximal to the dentate line (Greenall, 1988). After examination under anaesthesia 11 were treated conservatively and seven required abdominoperineal excision of the rectum. The absolute 5-year survival rate was 78% and the corrected rate was 88%. These data were much better than the 58% corrected 5-year survival rate achieved by abdominoperineal excision of the rectum at the same institution. Preoperative chemoirradiation allowed preservation of the anal sphincter in about 50% of cases, whereas local excision without chemoirradiation was only applicable in 10% of cases and the 5-year survival rate for this group was only 45% (Greenall, 1988).

The results from Nigro et al (1983) were even better. They treated 28 patients: 24 patients had a complete response and four had a partial one. Of the 26 who had a pathological evaluation after therapy, 21

Table 34.4 Comparison of combined chemotherapy and radiotherapy regimens for anal canal carcinoma.

Treatment	*Nigro et al (1983)*	*Michaelson et al (1983)*	*Sischy et al (1982)*	*Cummings et al (1984)*
Mitomycin	15 mg/m^2 bolus (day 1)	15 mg/m^2 bolus (day 1)	10 mg/m^2 (day 1)	10 mg/m^2 (day 1)
Fluorouracil	1000 mg/m^2 cont. inf. (days 1–4)	750 mg/m^2 cont. inf. (days 1–5)	1000 mg/m^2 (days 1–4)	1000 mg/m^2 (days 1–4)
Radiotherapy	Day 1 (30 Gy in 3 weeks)	Begun day 6–8 (30 Gy in 3 weeks)	Day 1 (40–50 Gy in 5–6 weeks)	Day 1 (50 Gy in 4–8 weeks)
Surgery	After 4–6 weeks APR or LE	After 2–4 weeks APR or LE	None	None
Further chemotherapy	Fluorouracil only, 1 month later	In some patients with residual disease (mitomycin + fluorouracil)	1 month later	None

APR, abdominoperineal resection; cont. inf., continuous infusion; LE, local excision.

Table 34.5 Results of combined chemotherapy and irradiation for epidermoid cancer of the anal canal.

Authors	*n*	*CR*	*PR*	*Failure*	*LE*	*APR*	*Death from cancer*	*Follow-up (months)*
Sischy et al (1982)	19	18	—	1	14	5	1	?
Flam et al (1983)	12	12	—	0	12	0	0	4–24
Nigro et al (1983)	28	24	4	0	16	12	5	12–96
Cummings et al (1984)	30	28	—	2	1	4	1	8–50
Greenall et al (1985a)	18		13	5	11	7	2	60–120
Grabenbauer et al (1994)	139	96	–	43	–	45	21	60 minimum
Tanum (1993)	87	59	–	28	–	9	22	?
Zelnick et al (1992)	30	17	–	12	–	9	8	37
Johnson et al (1993)	24	18	–	6	–	–	–	41
Quan (1992)	42	9	20	4	23	23	8	7–156
Total	429	318		101	89	114	68	
Nigro et al (1974)*	104	97	7	0	62	31	13	24–132

APR, abdominoperineal resection; CR, complete response; LE, local excision or biopsy of remaining scar tissue; PR, partial response.
* Collected series.

had no evidence of microscopic disease; thus 22 of the 26 patients (85%) were considered eligible for sphincter-saving procedures. They reported that 22 of 28 patients were alive and free of disease 1–8 years after treatment. Failure of the regimen seemed to be related to the size of the tumour, those greater than 5 cm having a higher failure rate. It has been suggested that larger tumours should receive higher doses of radiation and chemotherapy, but no reliable data are available to show that such an approach is of benefit.

Several years ago it was not known whether chemoirradiation was superior to radiation alone for the treatment of anal canal carcinoma. Both the United Kingdom Co-ordinating Committee for Colorectal Cancer Research (UKCCCR) and the European Organization for Research in the Treatment of Cancer (EORTC) set up prospective randomized controlled trials to answer this question. The UKCCCR have now reported on their findings (UKCCCR Anal Cancer Trial Working Party, 1996). At the close of the trial in March 1994, 577 eligible paients had been randomized with a median follow-up of 42 months. Patient characteristics were similar in the two groups, although more patients in the combined modality arm (radiotherapy and fluorouracil and mitomycin C) were node palpable or stage T4 at the outset. The addition of chemotherapy did not impair the delivery of radiotherapy. The majority of assessable patients (92%) had a greater than 50% response to treatment at the 6-week assessment. In the long term there was a large and significant improvement in local control rates with the combined modality treatment compared to radiotherapy alone, and also a cancer-specific survival benefit (Figure 34.5). The reasons for the local treatment failure in the two groups are summarized in Table 34.6.

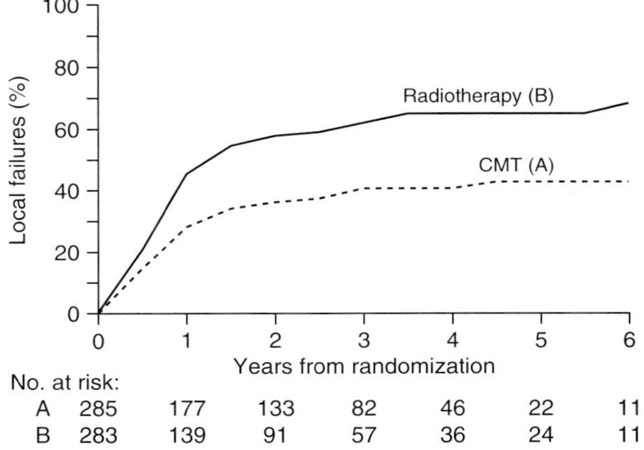

Figure 34.5 UKCCCR Anal Cancer Trial. Local treatment failure. CMT, combined modality treatment. Reproduced with permission from UKCCCR Anal Cancer Trial Working Party (1996).

Although no overall survival advantage was detected, a statistically significant reduction in the risk of dying of anal cancer was observed for patients receiving chemotherapy (Figures 34.6 and 34.7). The advantages of local control and cause-specific survival did not appear to be at the expense of undue morbidity, although there were several cases of treatment-related death. There were six deaths attributable to chemotherapy in the combined modality arm, and four deaths in the radiotherapy arm, two due to radiotherapy and two due to salvage surgery.

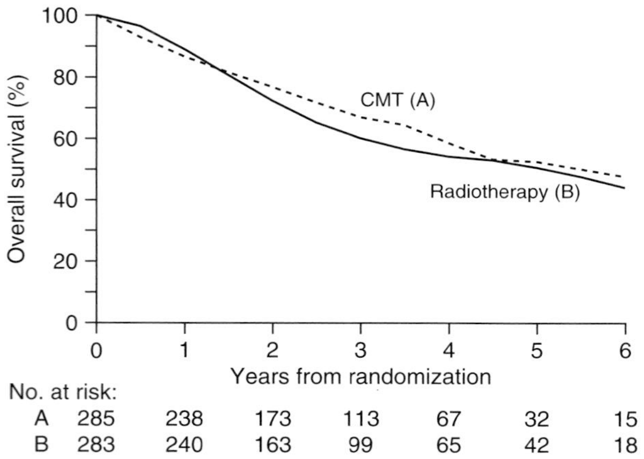

Figure 34.6 UKCCCR Anal Cancer Trial. Overall survival. CMT, combined modality treatment. Reproduced with permission from UKCCCR Anal Cancer Trial Working Party (1996).

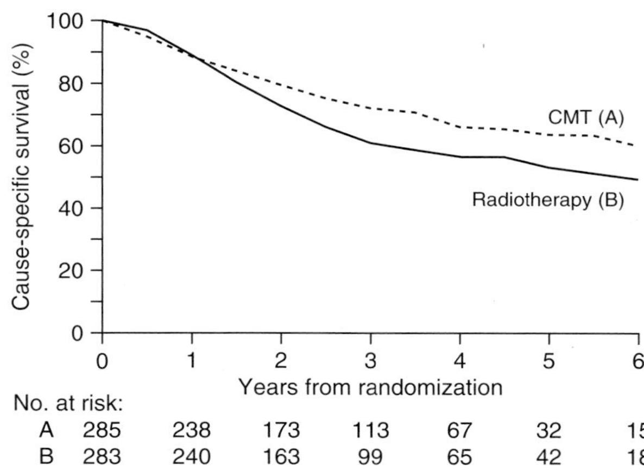

Figure 34.7 UKCCCR Anal Cancer Trial. Cancer-specific survival. CMT, combined modality treatment. Reproduced with permission from UKCCCR Anal Cancer Trial Working Party (1996).

Table 34.6 Reasons for local treatment failure in the UKCCCR Phase III Anal Cancer Trial (n = 577).

	Number of patients in whom treatment failed	
	Radiotherapy	*Combined modality*
Loco-regional disease		
Anorectal excision	90	43
Colostomy alone	7	6
No radical surgery	50	32
Surgery for morbidity		
Anorectal excision	6	2
Colostomy alone	4	8
Failure to close pretreatment colostomy	7	7
Anorectal excision tumour and radionecrosis-free	–	2
Reason not known – colostomy	–	1
Total	164	101

From UKCCCR Anal Cancer Trial Working Party (1996).

The EORTC study randomized 110 patients and used a virtually identical protocol to that of the UKCCCR study. It found a significant improvement in locoregional control and colostomy-free survival in the chemoirradiation arm (Bartelink et al, 1997). A similar trial by the RTOG ECOG Intergroup in the USA also obtained similar results, although toxicity was higher in patients receiving mitomycin (26% versus 7%, $P < 0.001$). There was also a greater difference in cause-specific survival compared with the UKCCCR study (John et al, 1995).

Since cisplatin may have a more specific effect on squamous cell carcinoma, consideration is being given to including this in the regime. Martenson et al (1996) recently reported on the treatment of 19 patients with radiotherapy (59.4 Gy) and concurrent fluorouracil (1000 mg/m^2) and cisplatin 75 mg/m^2. Of the 17 evaluable patients, 94% had a response, 12 had complete remission, 4 had a partial response and one had stable disease.

Salvage therapy after initial treatment failure

There is little information available concerning long-term follow-up of those patients who recur following multimodality therapy. Abdominoperineal excision is usually the preferred treatment provided the disease has remained relatively localized (Longo et al, 1995; Zelnick et al, 1992; UKCCCR Anal Cancer Trial Working Party, 1996). Thus, 265 of the 562 patients (47%) in the UKCCCR Anal Cancer Trial failed locally. Of the 265, 143 (54%) underwent abdominoperineal excision and 40 (15%) colostomy only, but no information is available on long-term follow-up (UKCCCR Anal Cancer Trial Working Party, 1996) (Table 34.7).

Longo et al (1995) found that 8 of 14 patients were alive a mean of 20 months after abdominoperineal excision for recurrence (Table 34.8). Others have demonstrated similar results (Zelnick et al, 1992). Other investigators have demonstrated that drugs known to be active in squamous cell carcinoma, such as cisplatin, bleomycin, vincristine and methotrexate, may be beneficial (Carey, 1984; Salem et al, 1985; Wilking et al, 1985; Hussain and Al-Sarraf, 1988; Ajani et al, 1989; Tanum, 1993) and of course such regimes can be combined wth radical surgery. Alternatively, consideration might be given to brachytherapy combined with further external radiation, provided the maximum allowable dose of radiation has not been previously administered (Martinez et al, 1985).

Table 34.7 Salvage surgery for locoregional recurrence in the UKCCCR Anal Cancer Trial Working Party (1996).

	Radiotherapy	*Combined modality*
Residual/recurrent locoregional disease	147	81
Abdominoperineal excision	90	43
Colostomy only	7	6
No colostomy-forming surgery	50	32

Table 34.8 Outcome of 14 patients with recurrence of anal canal cancer after multimodality therapy treated by salvage APER.

Initial TNM stage	*n*	*No. alive*	*Survival duration (months)*
I	4	2	16
II	10	6	20

From Longo et al (1995).

Conclusions

Unfortunately, there is still much confusion in the literature about the boundaries used for defining anal canal carcinomas. This needs to be clarified so that different studies can be compared. Similarly, we need a standardized staging system. As a result of the recent trials comparing chemoirradiation with radiation alone, there is little doubt that the former is superior. It remains to be seen whether the combination of mitomycin C and fluorouracil is the best. However, at present this must remain the standard initial treatment. Despite the outcome of recent trials, the other imponderable is whether chemoirradiation achieves a longer survival than initial radical excision. A controlled comparison between these two options is probably impossible to achieve in view of the impact of an inevitable stoma in one group. Even with the data so far available, such a controlled trial would be difficult to mount. At present therefore we recommend for all but the most extensive anal canal carcinomas that patients receive initial chemoirradiation. Radical excision should now only be regarded as a salvage manoeuvre in the treatment of residual or extensive disease.

TUMOURS OF THE ANAL MARGIN

Since the lymphatic drainage of the anal margin is exclusively to the inguinal glands, it has generally been accepted that epidermoid cancers of the anal margin may be treated by wide local excision. In fact few data are available for any other form of therapy.

The usual advice is to obtain a 2.5-cm margin around all aspects of the growth. Part of the external anal sphincter is usually excised but in most patients continence is not affected. However, if the lesion involves more than half the circumference of the anal verge the functional result is likely to be poor (Al-Jurf et al, 1979) and local excision alone is contraindicated. If a large skin defect does exist after excision and provided the sphincter has not been severely damaged, it can be covered by a split skin graft. It is safer to use skin grafts rather than to attempt primary wound closure under tension (Beahrs and Wilson, 1976; Al-Jurf et al, 1979; Schraut et al, 1983).

Local excision

From the few studies available on this subject, it appears that approximately 60% of margin tumours are suitable for local excision. The 5-year survival rate varies between 60% and 100% (Table 34.9). In some series the incidence of local recurrence is as high as 40% (Hardcastle and Bussey, 1968; Al-Jurf et al, 1979; Greenall et al, 1985b), but most of these patients can be salvaged by more radical local resection or by inguinal lymphadenectomy (Greenall et al, 1985a). Abdominoperineal excision may still be required but it is usually only recommended for extensive local recurrence (Greenall et al, 1985a). Some authors (Al-Jurf et al, 1979) recommend radical excision for patients who have presacral lymph node involvement as detected by rectal examination. Such nodes are, however, notoriously difficult to detect clinically, and until imaging techniques are sufficiently refined the operative decision cannot be based on clinical assessment of lymph node involvement. Indeed, it is disputed whether presacral node involvement occurs with anal margin lesions. Morson (1960) could find no case of anal margin carcinoma treated at St Mark's Hospital by abdominoperineal excision of the rectum where there was any involvement of the inferior mesen-

Table 34.9 Local excision for epidermoid cancer of the anal margin.

Authors	*No. treated*	*No. treated by local excision*	*No. of 5-year survivors*
Hardcastle and Bussey (1968)	53	30	18 (60)
MacConnell (1970)	42	21	17 (81)
Beahrs and Wilson (1976)	31	27	27 (100)
Schraut et al (1983)	16	11	9 (82)
Greenall et al (1985b)	48	31	21 (68)
Total	190	120 (63)	101 (78)

Values in parentheses are percentages.

teric lymph nodes, whereas Klotz et al (1967) found that there was nodal involvement in 15% of their cases with tumours below the dentate line.

Some authors would only recommend local excision for superficial growths of the anal margin (Schraut et al, 1983). Although prognosis is related to depth of invasion and some patients may have nodal invasion, there are no data to support the view that abdominoperineal excision of the rectum produces a longer survival than local excision. The 5-year survival of selected patients treated by abdominoperineal excision of the rectum varies between 20% and 80%. However, rational assessment is impossible because of patient selection and the small number of cases in each series (Hardy et al, 1969; Schraut et al, 1983).

Radiotherapy

Although irradiation has been used for some time as a primary treatment for anal margin cancers, accurate data on the results of radiotherapy are difficult to obtain. Since 1971 Papillon (1982) used a combination of cobalt 60 teletherapy with subsequent iridium 192 implantation, and a proportion of his patients also received fluorouracil and mitomycin. The overall 5-year survival rate was approximately 60%, and only one patient developed radionecrosis. This study was recently updated (Papillon and Chassard, 1992), and included a total of 54 patients. The crude and cancer-specific 5-year survival rates were 59.2% and 79.7% respectively. However, an acknowledgement was made that T4 lesions and mucoepidermoid tumours should also be treated by delayed surgery after the chemoirradiation.

Between 1973 and 1981, Touboul et al (1995a) used radiotherapy to treat 17 patients with anal margin carcinomas; nine of these patients had previously undergone incomplete surgery. Following treatment, 5- and 10-year cancer-specific survival rates were 86.2%, and 77.5% respectively. Severe complications occurred in two patients, resulting in loss of anorectal function.

Others have used radiotherapy as an adjunct to surgery (MacConnell, 1970; Beahrs and Wilson, 1976), but reliable information about its efficacy is scant.

Conclusion

Most anal margin tumours can be treated successfully by local excision provided a reasonable margin of clearance can be obtained. It is possible that the results from irradiation will be as good as local excision for many of these tumours, but until more data become available most surgeons, including ourselves, will continue to treat these lesions by surgery. Very few margin tumours require an abdominoperineal excision. If the tumour is so extensive that abdominoperineal excision of the rectum is considered necessary, a preoperative course of radiotherapy should be tried. Such treatment can reduce the size of the lesion and allow it to be treated by local excision instead of radical anorectal amputation. The routine use of preoperative chemoirradiation for most margin tumours seems excessive as the results of local excision are usually satisfactory.

ANAL INTRAEPITHELIAL NEOPLASIA (AIN)

AIN is defined as the presence of cellular and nuclear abnormalities in the perianal and anal epithelium without a breech of the epithelial basement membrane (Fenger and Nielson, 1981). It is a relatively recently described condition, and although, as discussed above, it seems to be a precursor to squamous cell carcinoma of the anus, its exact relationship and natural history remains to be determined (Ogunbiyi et al, 1994a).

Prevalence

The true prevalence of AIN is unknown; it was considered up to recently to be a rare condition. In some studies, the changes were reported to be detected during minor surgery to the anal margin in 0.2–4.4% of cases (Grodsky, 1968; Fenger and Nielsen, 1981; Nash et al, 1986). However, in at-risk groups, the rate is much higher. Thus, in immunosuppressed HIV-positive patients, the rate varies between 15% and 53% (Frazer et al, 1986; Palefsky et al, 1990; Caussy et al, 1990; Melbye et al, 1990; Kiviet et al, 1993; Williams et al, 1994). In women with high-grade genital intraepithelial or invasive neoplasia, the incidence varies between 19% and 47% (Scholefield et al, 1992; Ogunbiyi et al, 1994b). In patients with renal allografts, 24% seem to have AIN (Ogunbiyi et al, 1994c), and there appears to be a high incidence amongst patients of both sexes who have anogenital condylomata. The prevalence of AIN in control populations, on the other hand, is less than 1% (Ogunbiyi et al, 1995).

Pathological features

AIN is characterized by a loss of epithelial cellular maturation associated with nuclear hyperchromasia, pleomorphism, cellular crowding and abnormal mitoses within the anal epithelium. These features are identical to those of similar cervical and vulval lesions, and the classification is identical (Richart, 1973). Thus, in AIN I the cellular and nuclear abnormalities are restricted to the lower third of the epithelium. In AIN II and III, these changes affect the lower two-thirds and the full thickness of the epithelium respectively (Figure 34.8a,b).

Aetiology

AIN and squamous cell carcinoma of the anal region appear to share a common aetiology. Human papillomavirus (HPV) seems to be particularly involved. Thus, HPV 16 has been identified in 56–86% of patients with both squamous cell carcinoma and AIN (Zur Hausen et al, 1987; Scholefield et al, 1989; Caussy et al, 1990; Kiviat et al, 1993). AIN III lesions seem to contain HPV 16 more frequently than lower grades. However, it is unlikely that HPV alone is sufficient to produce and maintain the changes. It is probable that HPV acts synergistically with such viruses as HIV, herpes simplex virus 2 (HSV 2), Epstein–Barr virus (EBV) and cytomegalovirus (CMV) to produce AIN and anal carcinoma. Systemic immunosuppression also seems to play a role. Thus Ogunbiyi et al (1994c) demonstrated a prevalence rate of 24% (32/133) for

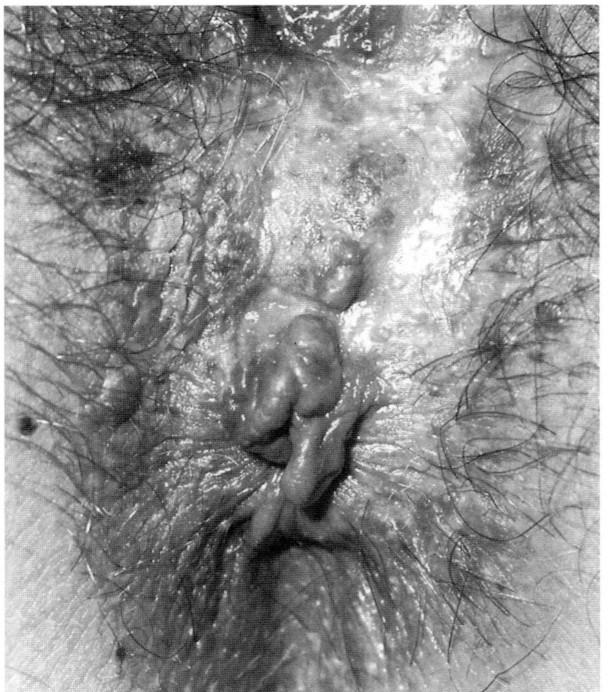

(a)

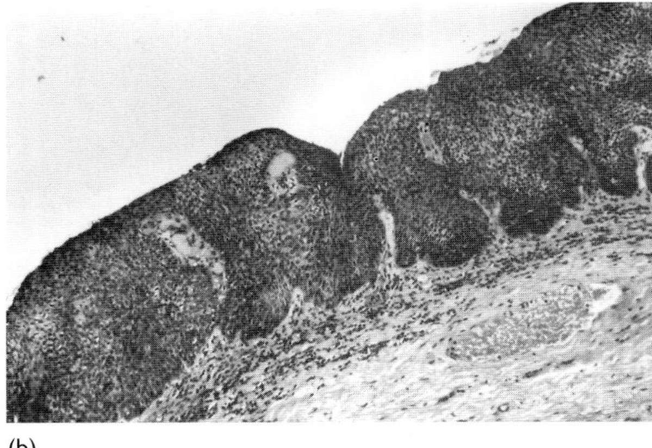

(b)

Figure 34.8 Anal intraepithelial neoplasia (AIN).
(a) Naked eye view of perianal high grade dysplasia with irregular anal pigmentation on skin tags and on the perianal skin. These areas are most marked at the one and two o'clock positions. These areas were confirmed to show high-grade AIN (AIN III) on biopsy. (b) Microscopic features of AIN III. There is no evidence of invasion in this lesion, but a marked mononuclear cell infiltrate is present in the connective tissue beneath the epithelium. (Illustrations provided by J H Scholefield, Nottingham.)

anal HPV infection and associated AIN in renal transplant patients. There are also several reports of the increased prevalence of AIN in immunosuppressed HIV-positive patients, and this is related to the degree of immunosuppression as determined by T helper/T suppressor cell ratios (Frazer et al, 1986; Palefsky et al, 1990; Caussy et al, 1990; Melbye et al, 1990; Beckmann et al, 1991; Williams et al, 1994).

Natural history and epidemiology

The natural history of AIN is unknown, but there is a certain degree of well-informed speculation based on the natural history of cervical dysplasia. Aetiological parallels with cervical intraepithelial neoplasia (CIN) and the histological appearances of AIN III suggest that AIN III may have malignant potential (Peters et al, 1984, Sherman et al, 1988, Melbye et al, 1991). Although Fenger and Nielson (1986) and others (Foust et al, 1991) showed that when AIN was found incidentally and patients were followed up for 6 years, anal cancer did not develop, they did demonstrate the presence of AIN III in a high proportion (about 80%) of cases of anal carcinoma. Scholefield and his colleagues in Sheffield found that of 32 patients with AIN III, 5 (15.5%) developed anal cancer within a median follow-up of 18 months (0.5–2 years) (Scholefield et al, 1992; Ogunbiyi et al, 1995). There is also evidence that AIN I and II may progress to AIN III. Thus Palefsky et al (1992) observed a significant progression (16%) of low-grade lesions to high-grade AIN lesions in 37 homosexual men with HIV followed up for 17 months.

Although the incidence of AIN and anal cancer is low, there is evidence that it is increasing. Thus Wexner et al (1987) demonstrated a 3-fold increase in the incidence of AIN and anal cancer between 1959 and 1986. Similar data from other centres in the USA and Scandinavia support this finding (Rabkin et al, 1992; Frisch et al, 1993; Melbye et al, 1994).

Clinical features

AIN and anal HPV infection are frequently asymptomatic (Scholefield et al, 1992; Surawicz et al, 1993). However, patients may present with perianal and anal canal condylomata, pruritus ani and bleeding. AIN is found not only in the perianal skin, but also, and evidently more commonly, in the anal transitional zone (Nash et al, 1986; Scholefield et al, 1989) and is invariably multifocal. Cytology and anoscopy can be used for detection. Anoscopy is the examination of the anal canal and perianal skin using a colposcope or operating microscope in conjunction with a proctoscope. Using criteria suggested for the colposcopic diagnosis of CIN by assessing the colour, vascular pattern and the appearance of the anal canal and perianal epithelium before and after application of 5% aqueous acetic acid, it is possible to make an assessment of the likelihood of HPV infection or AIN (Scholefield et al, 1989) (Figure 34.9). Since the extent of invasion cannot be demonstrated, suspicious areas detected by anoscopy must be biopsied.

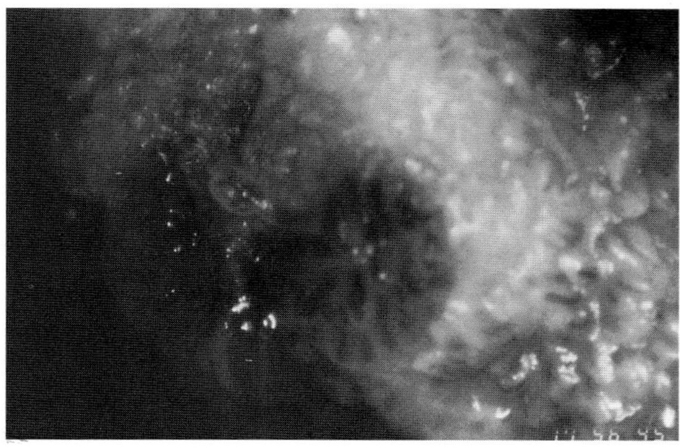

Figure 34.9 Photomicrograph obtained by anoscopy. An area of intense aceto-whitening in endoanal condylomatous tissue can be seen in response to the application of 5% aqueous acetic acid. The aceto-whitened area is less intense in the central area where the capillary loops are more pronounced. The central area was mildly dysplastic on biopsy and therefore shows the value of staining the tissue with 5% aqueous acetic acid. (Illustration provided by JH Scholefield, Nottingham.)

Management of AIN

Management is difficult because the natural history is unknown. Since AIN I and II seem unlikely to progress rapidly, a conservative approach of confirmatory biopsy and regular review seems appropriate. However, AIN III lesions pose a greater problem. On the one hand there is the risk of development of frank carcinoma, and on the other is the delay in healing and risk of infection in patients who are often immunocompromised.

If active treatment is deemed to be necessary, there are various options, including CO_2 laser vaporization, cryosurgery and surgical excision with grafting. While laser and cryosurgical techniques are less destructive, the experience of gynaecologists in treating vulval disease has shown that these modalities are often unsuccessful and rapid disease recurrence is not unusual (Centers for Disease Control, 1986; Ferenczy, 1987). Surgical excision may have to be relied upon, but should probably only be used in severe cases.

Surgical excision for AIN III will usually involve excision of all the anal canal mucosa. Resurfacing can then be accomplished by a double S-plasty technique (Oh and Albanese, 1992). In this technique an S-shaped incision is outlined as shown in Figure 12.48a. The length of each semicircular incision is about 12–13 cm. The base should be at least equal, but preferably longer than the length in the anterior/posterior axis. After the anal canal mucosa has been completely excised, a full-thickness incision is then made, and large skin flaps are constructed (Figure 12.48b). A layer of subcutaneous fat lobules is left on the entire undersurface of the skin in order to provide a good blood supply to the flap. The flap is then rotated into place, as shown in Figure 12.48c. The free skin edge is fixed to the mucosal edge by interrupted 2.0 chromic catgut sutures. In rotating the flaps to their new position, flap a to b covers one side and flap a^1 to b^1 covers the other side (Figure 12.48d). The remaining gap is approximated loosely without tension at the suture line with 3.0 Nylon sutures. Penrose drains are inserted under each flap and a pressure dressing is applied. It is wise then to construct a defunctioning stoma. An alternative to this is the double V-Y flap.

BASAL CELL CARCINOMA

Basal cell carcinoma (rodent ulcer) of the anal skin is rare. Even in major referral centres its incidence is only 0.1–0.4% of all anorectal malignancies (Buie and Brust, 1933; Armitage and Smith, 1954; Morson, 1960; Augey et al, 1994). The clinical presentation is usually identical to that of squamous cell carcinoma of the anal margin. However, since distant spread does not occur, the inguinal nodes are not involved. The inguinal nodes may be enlarged as a result of inflammation secondary to sepsis from the ulcerated lesion, but they do not feel hard on palpation. The lesion is usually ulcerated with an irregular outline and a hard or slightly raised edge, usually measuring no more than 2 cm in diameter. A lesion larger than 2 cm is unlikely to be a rodent ulcer.

Treatment

As with rodent ulcers elsewhere, there is little to choose between radiotherapy and local excision; since the cosmetic result is unimportant in this region, excision is preferred. Nielsen and Jensen (1981) reviewed the results of all patients with basal cell carcinoma treatment in Denmark between 1943 and 1974. There were 34 patients: initially 27 were treated by wide local excision, four by abdominoperineal excision and three by radiotherapy. Three patients developed local recurrence but no further recurrence occurred in them after additional treatment with local excision, abdominoperineal excision of the rectum or radiotherapy. The overall crude 5-year survival rate was 72.6%.

MALIGNANT MELANOMA

Malignant melanoma is a rare tumour, accounting for 3–15% of tumours arising in the anal canal. Only 1–1.5% of all malignant melanomas develop in the perianal region (Pyper and Parks, 1984; Lui et al, 1994) and up to 1982, 460 cases had been reported in the medical literature (Bolivar et al, 1982). Longo et al (1995) in a study of US Veterans found only eight patients (4%) with melanoma out of 204 patients (51%) who could be evaluated from a total of 405 patients with rare anal cancers. However, in certain countries, particularly Pakistan, the incidence seems to be higher. Thus Ahmad et al (1992) found that anorectal melanomas accounted for 14.2% of all primary malignant melanomas. The tumours are presumed to arise from melanocytes in the squamous mucosa of the lower anal canal. However, some authors are of the opinion that melanoma may arise primarily in the lower rectum as well as the anal canal (Alexander and Cone, 1977). The tumour seems to be more common in women and differs markedly in aetiology from cutaneous melanoma, indeed sun exposure may be protective (Weinstock, 1993).

Clinical features

The clinical features of pain, bleeding or an external mass are similar to those encountered in other anal neoplasms. A significant proportion of lesions are not pigmented (Morson and Volkstadt, 1963a; Sielezneff et al, 1993) (Figure 34.10). Antoniuk et al (1993) in a study of 15 patients at the Cleveland Clinic found that 25% were amelanotic. If the lesion is pigmented and polypoid it can resemble a thrombosed haemorrhoid and the clinician should be aware of this possibility (Rohr et al, 1992; Slingluff and Siegler, 1992). In advanced cases, a massive tumour may be present at the anus with enlarged, hard inguinal glands. Sometimes the primary tumour may remain small, with the patient presenting with evidence of widespread dissemination to lungs, liver, brain, skeleton, lymph glands and skin.

The diagnosis can only be confirmed on histological examination. Sometimes the true nature of the tumour is only revealed incidentally after histological examination of a presumed thrombosed pile removed as a minor procedure. It seems wise, therefore, to submit all tissue removed from the anus, including haemorrhoids, for histological examination.

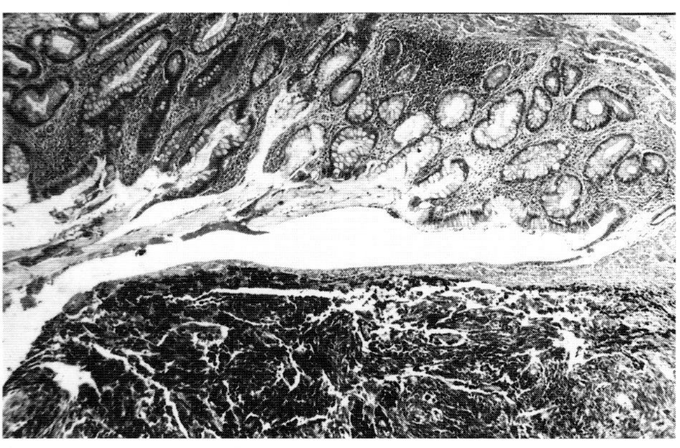

(a)

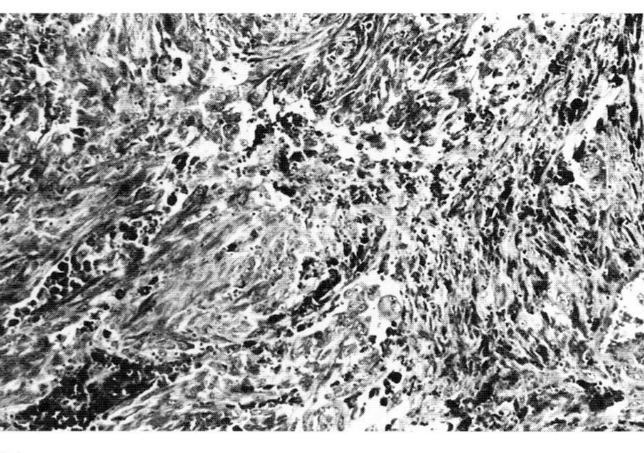

(b)

Figure 34.10 Malignant melanoma of anus. (a) An area of dark-staining cells has ulcerated close to the rectal mucosa (H&E, ×100). Higher magnification (b) shows a highly malignant tumour with much dark melanin pigment (H&E, ×400).

Treatment

It was customary to advise patients with malignant melanoma of the anal verge to undergo radical abdominoperineal excision with high ligation of the inferior mesenteric vessels. Some also advised block dissection of the inguinal nodes, but few patients survived. The other approach was to perform a local excision, the results of which were equally depressing. The poor outcome of treating the disease by either method was illustrated by Quan (1980). Of 49 cases treated at Memorial Sloan-Kettering Cancer Center between 1929 and 1975 only five (10%) were alive after 5 years. Brady et al (1995) updated these data and found that of 85 patients treated between 1929 and 1993 only 17% were alive at 5 years. Cooper et al (1982) also demonstrated in a review of a large number of cases that there was no difference in survival between those treated by abdominoperineal excision of the rectum and those treated by local excision. Similar results were found by Antonuik et al (1993) and Slingluff and Siegler (1992) in a smaller number of cases.

This being the case, there seems no point in subjecting all patients with anal melanoma to a radical operation which involves the construction of a permanent colostomy. It must be said, however, that the few long-term survivors in the literature had all been treated by abdominoperineal excision of the rectum. Wanebo et al (1981) reported that all three of their patients with tumours less than 2 mm in thickness had survived beyond 5 years and they had all undergone radical operations. Similar findings were observed in the study by Brady et al (1995). Whether these patients would have done as well with local excision is entirely speculative. Until more data are available it is probably wise to treat all suspicious malignant melanomas by wide local excision. If histology indicates that the tumour has penetrated less than 3 mm through the dermis we believe that the optimum surgical treatment is an abdominoperineal excision of the rectum, provided it can be demonstrated that widespread dissemination has not occurred.

PRIMARY (COLLOID) ADENOCARCINOMA OF THE ANAL REGION

Primary adenocarcinoma of the anal region is extremely rare (Dukes and Galvin, 1956; Zimberg and Kay, 1957; Wellman, 1962; Winkelman et al, 1964; Cabrera et al, 1966; Harrison et al, 1966; Hagihara et al, 1976; Sink et al, 1978) and its site of origin is still disputed. Many patients present initially with a chronic anal fistula. There is a suggestion that chronic sepsis leads to neoplastic change along a fistula track. This seems most unlikely and it is more likely that the tumour is responsible for the fistula and not vice versa. Another theory is that the adenocarcinoma arises from a congenital rectal reduplication. Dukes and Galvin (1956) found normal rectal epithelium in the fistula track adjacent to the colloid cancers in some of their patients, and in two cases the fistula track was surrounded by a smooth muscle coat. Another possible origin is the apocrine glands of the perianal skin (Grodsky, 1960; Nelson, 1960). Most current evidence favours the anal intermuscular glands as the principal origin of these tumours (Zimberg and Kay, 1957).

Clinical features and treatment

This tumour does not present as a lesion on the lining of the anal canal but grows extraluminally and tends to widely infiltrate the perianal tissues. Sometimes it penetrates the skin or presents occasionally as an area of eczema similar to Paget's disease of the nipple. Frequently the tumour presents as a chronic fistula-in-ano. The possibility of a colloid adenocarcinoma should be suspected if a fistula is associated with extensive granulation tissue at its external orifice or an indurated subcutaneous mass. The inguinal lymph nodes are often involved at the time of presentation. The fact that the carcinoma may mimic other primary dermatological problems highlights the need to take extensive biopsies from any suspicious lesion of the perianal region.

The only hope for cure seems to be abdominoperineal excision of the rectum with wide removal of the perianal tissues and block dissection of inguinal nodes if involved. The prognosis is generally poor and many patients present late with inoperable lesions. Extensive lesions may be best treated by irradiation.

ADENOCARCINOMA DESCENDING FROM THE RECTUM

Virtually all adenocarcinomas that present within the anal canal will have arisen from the rectum. Sigmoidoscopy will confirm that the tumour is at a higher level. Primary adenocarcinoma of the anal canal does not present within the bowel lumen.

VERRUCOUS SQUAMOUS CARCINOMA

Verrucous squamous carcinoma is a very rare variant of squamous cell carcinoma. It is also known as the tumour of Buschke and Loewenstein who originally described it in 1925. It may appear as a pale pink, cauliflower-like mass on the perianal skin or in the anal canal and can easily be confused with condylomata acuminata (Buschke and Loewenstein, 1925; Bertram et al, 1995) (see Chapter 18). Histological examination demonstrates a well-differentiated lesion, which may be considered initially to be a benign proliferative lesion of squamous epithelium until it is realized that there is invasion of underlying tissues. For this reason superficial biopsies cannot be relied upon for diagnosis and the base of the lesion should always be examined.

Treatment should be by wide local excision or abdominoperineal excision of the rectum if extensive invasion has occurred (Sturm et al, 1975; Lock et al, 1977b). Evidently irradiation therapy is of little value and may lead to a less differentiated and more aggressive cancer (Bertram et al, 1995).

BOWEN'S DISEASE OF THE ANAL REGION

Bowen (1912) was the first to describe a slowly growing intraepidermal squamous cell carcinoma which often mimics a chronic dermatosis. In 1979 only 112 cases had been described (Strauss and

Fazio, 1979). Bowen's disease can occur in the perianal skin and usually presents as pruritus ani. On examination it looks like psoriasis or senile keratosis, and should now be considered as a form of AIN III and treated as described previously (Scholefield and Amin, 1998).

PAGET'S DISEASE OF THE PERIANAL REGION

Cutaneous Paget's disease may occur in the perianal region. The lesions are similar to those that occur in the breast: they appear as red or whitish grey, elevated, crusty, scaly lesions. The appearances are similar to those of eczema but the histology is different (Figure 34.11a). Hyperkeratosis, parakeratosis and acanthosis are all present, together with the characteristic pale, vacuolated cells within the epidermis. If sections are stained with periodic acid-Schiff reagent (Figure 34.11b), sialomucin may be identified, which helps to distinguish the condition from Bowen's disease. Like Paget's disease of the breast, it is often associated with an underlying carcinoma. In Helwig and Graham's series of 40 patients with Paget's disease of the anogenital region, 13 had an underlying cutaneous carcinoma and another seven had a primary carcinoma elsewhere (Helwig and Graham, 1963). Of four cases described by Lock et al (1977a), three developed carcinoma. Other authors have also found a similar association with neoplastic disease (Arminski and Pollard, 1973; Jackson, 1975; Williams et al, 1976; Quan, 1978; Subbuswamy and Ribeiro, 1981; Goldman et al, 1992; Miller et al, 1992).

The treatment of Paget's disease depends on whether the underlying carcinoma is superficial or deep (Linder and Myers, 1970). If the tumour is non-infiltrative, wide local excision with or without grafting seems adequate. If, on the other hand, the tumour is more extensive, it is perhaps best to treat it in the same way as an anal canal carcinoma with initial chemoirradiation followed (if this approach fails) by abdominoperineal excision of the rectum.

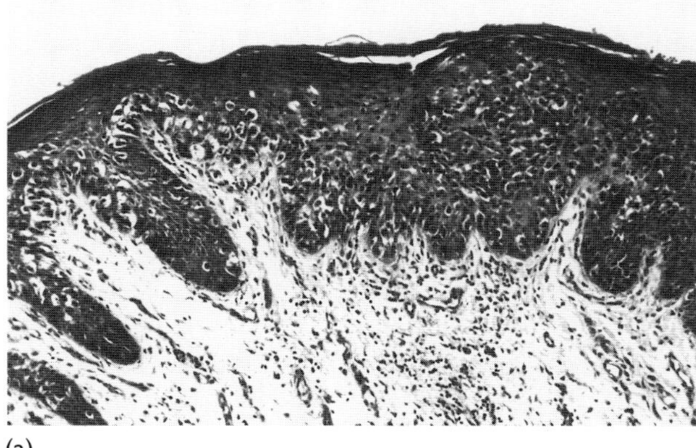

(a)

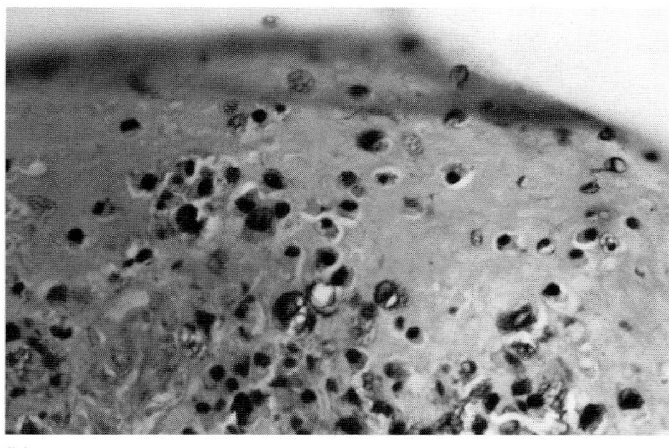

(b)

Figure 34.11 Paget's disease of perianal skin. (a) There are numerous large cells with clear cytoplasm throughout the full thickness of the epidermis (H&E, ×100). (b) Higher magnification shows mucin-containing large cells in the epidermis (PAS, ×400).

REFERENCES

Ahmad M, Mamoon N & Khan AH (1992) Anorectal melanoma in northern Pakistan. *JPMA J Pak Med Assoc* **42**: 155–157.

Ajani JA, Carrasco CH, Jackson DE & Wallace S (1989) Combination of cisplatin plus fluoropyrimidine chemotherapy effective against liver metastases from carcinoma of the anal canal. *Am J Med* **87**: 221–224.

Alexander RM & Cone LA (1977) Malignant melanoma of the rectal ampulla: report of a case and review of the literature. *Dis Colon Rectum* **20**: 53–55.

Al-Jurf AS, Turnbull RB & Fazio VW (1979) Local treatment of squamous cell carcinoma of the anus. *Surg Gynecol Obstet* **148**: 576–578.

Antoniuk PM. Tjandra JJ, Webb BW, Petras RE, Milsom JW & Fazio VW (1993) Anorectal malignant melanoma has a poor prognosis. *Int J Colorectal Dis* **8**: 81–86.

Arminski TC & Pollard RJ (1973) Paget's disease of the anus secondary to a malignant papillary adenoma of the rectum. *Dis Colon Rectum* **16**: 46–55.

Armitage G & Smith IB (1954) Rodent ulcer of the anus. *Br J Surg* **42**: 395.

Augey F, Cognat T, Balme B, Thomas L & Moulin G (1994) Perianal basal cell carcinoma. Apropos of 2 cases [in French]. *Ann Dermatol Venereol* **121**: 476–478.

Bartelink H, Roelofsen F, Eschwege F et al (1997) Concomitant radiotherapy and chemotherapy is superior to radiotherapy alone in the treatment of locally advanced anal cancer: results of a phase III randomized trial of the European Organization for Research and Treatment of Cancer Radiotherapy and Gastrointestinal Cooperative Groups. *J Clin Oncol* **15**: 2040–2049.

Beahrs OH & Wilson SM (1976) Carcinoma of the anus. *Ann Surg* **184**: 422–428.

Beckmann AM, Acker R, Christiansen AE & Sherman KJ (1991) Human papillomavirus infection in women with multicentric squamous cell neoplasia. *Am J Obstet Gynecol* **165**: 1431–1437.

Bender MD & Lechago J (1976) Leukoplakia of the anal canal. *Dig Dis Sci* **21**: 867–872.

Bertram P, Treutner KH, Rubben A, Hauptmann S & Schumpelick A (1995) Invasive squamous-cell carcinoma in giant anorectal condyloma (Buschke-Lowenstein tumor). *Langenbecks Arch Chir* **380**: 115–118.

Bogomoletz WV, Potet F & Molas G (1985) Condylomata acuminata, giant condyloma acuminatum (Buschke Loewenstein tumour) and verrucous squamous carcinoma of the perianal and ano rectal region: a continuous pre cancerous spectrum? *Histopathology* **9**: 1155–1170.

Bolivar JC, Harris JW, Branch W & Sherman RT (1982) Melanoma of the ano-rectal region. *Surg Gynecol Obstet* **154**: 337–341.

Boman BM, Moertel CG, O'Connell MJ et al (1984) Carcinoma of the anal canal. A clinical and pathologic study of 188 cases. *Cancer* **54**: 114–125.

Bowen JT (1912) Precancerous dermatoses; a study of two cases of atypical epithelial proliferation. *J Cutan Genito-urin Dis* **30**: 241.

Brady MS, Kavolius JP & Quan SH (1995) Anorectal melanoma. A 64-year experience at Memorial Sloan-Kettering Cancer Center. *Dis Colon Rectum* **38**: 146–151.

Buie LA & Brust JCM (1933) Malignant anal lesions of epithelial origin. *Lancet* **53**: 565.

Buschke A & Loewenstein L (1925) Condylomata acuminata simulating cancer on penis. *Klin Wochenschr* **4**: 1726–1728.

Cabrera A, Tsukada Y & Pickren JW (1966) Adenocarcinoma of the anal canal and perianal region. *Ann Surg* **164**: 152.

Cantril ST, Green JP, Schall GL & Schaupp WC (1983) Primary radiation therapy in the treatment of anal carcinoma. *Int J Radiat Oncol Biol Phys* **9**: 1271–1278.

Carey RW (1984) Regression of pulmonary metastases from cloacogenic carcinoma after cis-platinum/5 fluorouracil treatment. *J Clin Gastroenterol* **6**: 257–259.

Cattell RB & Williams AC (1943) Epidermoid carcinoma of the anus and rectum. *Arch Surg* **46**: 336–349.

Caussy D, Goedert JJ, Palefsky J et al (1990) Interaction of human immuodeficiency and papilloma viruses: Association with anal epithelial abnormality in homosexual men. *Int J Cancer* **46**: 214–219.

Centre for Disease Control (1986) Condylomata acuminatum, 1966–1983. *MMWR*, **33**: 81.

Chruščov MM, Semakina EP & Raifel BA (1978) Die Strahlentherapie des rektalen Epidermoidkarzinomas. *Radiobiol Radiother (Berlin)* **19**: 683–689.

Connell WR, Sheffield JP, Kamm MA. Ritchie JK, Hawley PR & Lennard-Jones JE (1994) Lower gastrointestinal malignancy in Crohn's disease. *Gut* **35**: 347–352.

Cooper HS, Patchefsky AS & Marks G (1979) Cloacogenic carcinoma of the anorectum in homosexual men: an observation of four cases. *Dis Colon Rectum* **22**: 557–558.

Cooper PH, Mills SE & Allen MS (1982) Malignant melanoma of the anus. Report of 12 patients and analysis of 255 additional cases. *Dis Colon Rectum* **25**: 692–703.

Cortese AF (1975) Surgical approach for treatment of epidermoid anal carcinoma. *Cancer* **36**: 1869–1875.

Cummings B, Keane, T, Thomas H, Harwood A & Rider W (1984) Results and toxicity of treatment of anal canal carcinoma by radiation therapy or radiation therapy and chemotherapy. *Cancer* **54**: 2062–2068.

Dalby JE & Pointon RS (1961) The treatment of anal carcinoma by interstitial irradiation. *AJR* **85**: 515–520.

Daling JR, Weiss NS, Klopfenstein LL, Cochran LE, Chow WH & Daifuku R (1982) Correlates of homosexual behaviour and the incidence of anal cancer. *JAMA* **247**: 1988–1990.

Deans GT, McAleer JJ & Spence RA (1994) Malignant anal tumours. *Br J Surg* **81**: 500–508.

Devois A & Decker R (1960) La Curiepuncture du cancer de l'anus. *Arch Fr Mal Appar Dig* **49**: 54–67.

Dukes GE & Galvin C (1956) Colloid carcinoma arising within fistulae in the anorectal region. *Ann R Coll Surg Engl* **18**: 246.

Ewing MR (1954) The white line of Hilton. *J R Soc Med* **47**: 525–530.

Fenger C (1979) The anal transitional zone. Location and extent. *Acta Pathol Microbiol Immunol Scand A* **87**: 379–386.

Fenger C & Nielson VT (1981) Dysplastic changes in the anal canal epithelium in minor surgical specimens. *Acta Pathol Microbiol Scand* **89**: 463–465.

Ferenczy A (1987) Laser treatment of patients with condylomata and squamous carcinoma precursors of the lower female genital tract. *CA-C Cancer J Clinic* **37**: 334–347.

Flam MS, John M, Lovalvo LJ et al (1983) Definitive nonsurgical therapy of epithelial malignancies of the anal canal. A report of 12 cases. *Cancer* **51**: 1378–1387.

Foust RL, Dean PJ, Stoler MH & Moinuddin SM (1991) Intraepithelian neoplasia of the anal canal in haemorrhoidal tissue: a study of 19 cases. *Hum Pathol* **22**: 529–534.

Frazer IH, Medley G, Crapper RM, Brown TC & Mackay IR (1986) Association between anorectal dysplasaia, human papillomavirus and human immunodeficiency virus infection in homosexual men. *Lancet* **ii**: 657–660.

Frisch M, Melbye M & Moiler H (1993) Trends in the incidence of anal cancer in Denmark. *Br Med J* **306**: 419–422.

Frost DB, Richards PC, Montague ED, Giacco GG & Martin RG (1984) Epidermoid cancer of the anorectum. *Cancer* **53**: 1285–1293.

Gabriel WB (1941) Squamous cell carcinoma of the anus and anal canal: an analysis of 55 cases. *Proc R Soc Med* **34**: 139.

Gillatt DA & Teasdale C (1985) Squamous cell carcinoma of the anus arising within condyloma acuminatum. *Eur J Surg Oncol* **11**: 369–371.

Golden PH & Horsley J (1976) Surgical management of epidermoid carcinoma of the anus. *Am J Surg* **141**: 280.

Goldman S, Ihre T, Lagerstedt U & Svensson C (1992) Perianal Paget's disease: report of five cases. *Int J Colorectal Dis* **7**: 167–169.

Goligher JC (1984) *Surgery of the Anus, Rectum and Colon.* Eastbourne: Baillière Tindall.

Grabenbauer GG, Panzer M, Hultenschmidt B et al (1994) The prognostic factors following the simultaneous radiochemotherapy of anal canal carcinoma in a multicenter series of 139 patients. *Strahlenther Onkol* **170**: 391–399.

Greenall MJ (1988) Epidermoid cancer of the anus. In Todd IP & DeCosse JJ (eds) *Ano Rectal Surgery*, Chapter 10, pp 157–170. Edinburgh: Churchill Livingstone.

Greenall MJ, Quan SHQ, Urmacher C & DeCosse JJ (1985a) Treatment of epidermoid cancer of the anal canal. *Surg Gynecol Obstet* **161**: 509–517.

Greenall MJ, Quan SHQ, Stearns MW, Urmacher C & DeCosse JJ (1985b) Epidermoid cancer of the anal margin: pathological features, treatment and clinical results. *Am J Surg* **149**: 95–101.

Greenall MJ, Magill E & DeCosse JJ (1986) Recurrent epidermoid cancer of the anus. *Cancer* **57**: 1437–1441.

Grinnell RS (1954) An analysis of 49 cases of squamous cell carcinoma of the anus. *Surg Gynecol Obstet* **98**: 29–39.

Grinvalsky HT & Helwig EB (1956) Carcinoma of the ano-rectal junction. *Cancer* **9**: 480.

Grodsky L (1960) Extramammary Paget's disease of the perianal region. *Dis Colon Rectum* **3**: 502.

Grodsky L (1968) Unsuspected anal cancer discovered after minor anorectal surgery. *Dis Colon Rectum* **10**: 471–479.

Grodsky L (1969) Current concepts on cloacogenic transitional cell ano-rectal cancers. *JAMA* **207**: 2057.

Gulati SC, Sordillo P, Kempin S et al (1980) Microangiopathic hemolytic anemia observed after treatment of epidermoid carcinoma with mitomycin C and 5-fluorouracil. *Cancer* **45**: 2252–2257.

Hagihara P, Vazquez MT, Parker JC & Griffen WO Jr (1976) Carcinoma of anal duct origin: report of a case. *Dis Colon Rectum* **19**: 694–701.

Hardcastle JD & Bussey HJR (1968) Results of surgical treatment of squamous cell carcinoma of the anal canal and anal margin seen at St Mark's Hospital 1928–66. *Proc R Soc Med* **61**: 27.

Hardy KJ, Hughes ESR & Cuthbertson AM (1969) Squamous cell carcinoma of the anal canal and anal margin. *Aust NZ J Surg* **38**: 301–305.

Harrison EG, Beahrs OH & Hill JR (1966) Anal and perianal malignant neoplasms: pathology and treatment. *Dis Colon Rectum* **9**: 255.

Harrison M, Tomlinson D & Stewart S (1995) Squamous cell carcinoma of the anus in patients with AIDS. *Clin Oncol* **7**: 50–51.

Helwig EB & Graham JH (1963) Anogenital (extramammary) Paget's disease. *Cancer* **16**: 387–403.

Herzog U, Boss M & Spichtin HP (1994) Endoanal ultrasonography in the follow-up of anal carcinoma. *Surg Endosc* **8**: 1186–1189.

Hussain M & Al-Sarraf M (1988) Anal carcinomas: new combined modality treatment approaches. *Oncology* **2**: 42–48.

Jackson BR (1975) Extramammary Paget's disease and anoplastic basaloid small cell carcinoma of the anus: report of a case. *Dis Colon Rectum* **18**: 339–345.

John MS et al (1995) Radiation and 5FU vs radiation, 5FU, mitomycin in the treatment of anal carcinoma: Results of a phase III randomised RTOG/ECOG Intergroup trial. American Society of Clinical Oncology, Abstract No. 443.

Johnson D, Lipsett J, Leong L, Wagman LD & Terz JJ (1993) Carcinoma of the anus treated with primary radiation therapy and chemotherapy. *Surg Gynecol Obstet* **177**: 329–334.

Jones RD, Symonds RP, Robertson AG & Thomas R (1993) Changes in the radiation treatment of cancer of the anus in Glasgow. *Br J Radiol* **66**: 797–800.

Judd ES Jr & De Tar BE Jr (1955) Squamous cell carcinoma of the anus: results of treatment. *Surgery (St Louis)* **37**: 282.

Judson FN, Penley KA, Robinson ME & Smith JK (1980) Comparative prevalence rates of sexually transmitted diseases in heterosexual and homosexual men. *Am J Epidemiol* **112**: 836–843.

Kheir S, Hickey RC, Martin RG, MacKay B & Gallagher HS (1972) Cloacogenic carcinoma of anal canal. *Arch Surg* **104**: 407.

Kiviat NB, Critchlow CW, Holmes KK et al (1993) Association of anal dysplasia and human papillomavirus with immunosuppression and HIV infection among homosexual men. *AIDS* **7**: 43–49.

Kiviat N, Rompalo A, Bowden R et al (1990) Anal human papillomavirus infection among human immunodeficiency virus seropositive and seronegative men. *J Infec Dis* **162**: 358–361.

Klotz RG, Pamukcoglu T & Souilliard DH (1967) Transitional cloacogenic carcinoma of the anal canal. *Cancer* **20**: 1727–1745.

Kuehn PG, Beckett R, Eisenberg H & Reed JF (1968) Epidermoid carcinoma of the perianal skin and anal canal. *Cancer* **22**: 932–938.

Leach RH & Ellis H (1981) Carcinoma of the rectum in male homosexuals. *J R Soc Med* **74**: 490–491.

Linder JH & Myers RT (1970) Perianal Paget's disease. *Am Surg* **36**: 342–345.

Liu YX, Hou M & Jiao SL (1994) Pathological and immunohistochemical study on anorectal melanoma. *Chung-hua Ping Li Hsueh Tsa Chih* **23**: 358–360.

Lock MR, Katz DR, Parks A & Thompson JPS (1977a) Perianal Paget's disease. *Postgrad Med J* **53**: 768–772.

Lock MR, Katz DR, Samooorian S et al (1977b) Giant condyloma of the rectum: report of a case. *Dis Colon Rectum* **20**: 154–157.

Longo WE, Vernava AM 3rd, Wade TP, Coplin MA, Virgo KS & Johnson FE (1995) Rare anal canal cancers in the US veteran: patterns of disease and results of treatment. *Am Surgeon* **61**: 495–500.

Lorenz HP, Wilson W, Leigh B et al (1991) Squamous cell carcinoma of the anus and HIV infection. *Dis Colon Rectum* **34**: 336–338.

MacConnell EM (1970) Squamous carcinoma of the anus – a review of 96 cases. *Br J Surg* **57**: 89–92.

Martenson JA, Lipsitz SR, Wagner H Jr, et al (1996) Initial results of a phase II trial of high dose radiation therapy, 5-fluorouracil, and cisplatin for patient with anal cancer (E4292): an Eastern Cooperative Oncology Group study. *Int J Radiat Oncol Biol Phys* **35**(4): 745–749.

Martinez A, Edmundson GK, Cox RJ et al (1985) Combination of external beam irridiation and multiple-site perineal applicator (MUPIT) for treatment of locally advanced or recurrent prostatic, anorectal and gynecologic malignancies. *Int J Radiat Oncol Biol Phys* **11**: 391–198.

Melbye M, Palefsky J, Gonzales J et al (1990) Immune status as a determinant of human papillomavirus detection and its association with anal epithelial abnormalities. *Int J Cancer* **46**: 203–206.

Melbye M & Sprogel P (1991) Aetiological parallel between anal cancer and cervical cancer. *Lancet* **338**: 657–659.

Melbye M, Cote TR, Kessler L, Gail M & Biggar RJ (1994) High incidence of anal cancer among AIDS patients. The AIDS/Cancer Working Group. *Lancet* **343**: 636–639.

Metcalfe AM & Dean T (1995) Risk of dysplasia in anal condyloma. *Surgery* **118**: 724–726.

Michaelson RA, Magill GB, Quan SH, Leaming RH, Nikrui M & Stearns MW (1983) Preoperative chemotherapy and radiation therapy in the management of anal epidermoid carcinoma. *Cancer* **51**: 390–395.

Miller LR, McCunniff AJ & Randall ME (1992) An immunohistochemical study of perianal Paget's disease. Possible origins and clinical implications. *Cancer* **69**: 2166–2171.

Morson BC (1960) The pathology and results of treatment of squamous cell carcinoma of the anal canal and anal margin. *Proc R Soc Med* **53**: 416–420.

Morson BC & Dawson IMP (1990) *Gastrointestinal Pathology*, 3rd edn. Oxford: Blackwell Scientific.

Morson BC & Pang LSC (1968) Pathology of anal cancer. *J Soc Med* **53**: 416–420.

Morson BC & Sobin LH (1976) *Histological Typing of Intestinal Tumours*, pp 62–65. Geneva: World Health Organization.

Morson BC & Volkstadt B (1963a) Malignant melanoma of the anal canal. *J Clin Pathol* **16**: 52–54.

Morson BC & Volkstadt H (1963b) Muco-epidermoid tumours of the anal canal. *J Clin Pathol* **16**: 200–205.

Nash G, Allen W & Nash S (1986) Atypical lesions of the anal mucosa in homosexual men. *JAMA* **256**: 873–876.

Nelson TF (1960) Perianal Paget's disease. *Dis Colon Rectum* **3**: 135.

Nielsen OV & Jensen SL (1981) Basal cell carcinoma of the anus – a clinical study of 34 cases. *Br J Surg* **68**: 856–857.

Nigro ND, Vaitkevicius VK & Considine BJ (1974) Combined therapy for cancer of the anal canal: a preliminary report. *Dis Colon Rectum* **17**: 354.

Nigro ND, Seydel HG, Considine B, Vaitkevicius VK, Leichman L & Kinzie JJ (1983) Combined preoperative radiation and chemotherapy for squamous cell carcinoma of the anal canal. *Cancer* **51**: 1826–1829.

O'Brien PH, Jenrette JM, Wallace KM & Metcalf JS (1982) Epidermoid carcinoma of the anus. *Surg Gynecol Obstet* **155**: 745–751.

Ogunbiyi OA, Scholefield JH, Robertson G et al (1994a) Anal human papillomavirus infection and squamous neoplasia in patients with invasive vulvar cancer. *Obstet Gynecol* **83**: 212–216.

Ogunbiyi OA, Scholefield JH, Raftery AT et al (1994b) Prevalence of anal human papillomavirus infection and intraepithelial neoplasia in renal allograft recipients. *Br J Surg* **81**: 365–367.

Ogunbiyi OA, Scholefield JH, Sharp F & Rogers K (1994c) Anal intra-epithelial neoplasia. Review. *Eur Cancer News* **7**: 7–12.

Oh C & Albanese C (1992) S-Plasty for various anal lesions. *Am J Surg* **163**: 606.

Palefsky JM, Gonzales J, Greenblatt RM, Ahn DK & Hollander H (1990) Anal intraepithelial neoplasia and anal papillomavirus infection among homosexual males with Group IV HIV disease. *JAMA* **263**: 2911–1916.

Palefsky JM, Holly EA, Gonzales J, Lamborn K & Hollander H (1992) Natural history of anal cytologic abnormalities and papillomavirus infection among homosexual men with Group IV HIV disease. *J Acquir Immune Defic Syndr* **5**: 1258–1265.

Papillon J (1982) *Rectal and Anal Cancers: Conservative Treatment by Irradiation – an Alternative to Radical Surgery*. Berlin: Springer.

Papillon J & Chassard JL (1992) Respective roles of radiotherapy and surgery in the management of epidermoid carcinoma of the anal margin. Series of 57 patients. *Dis Colon Rectum* **35**: 422–429.

Paradis P, Douglas HO Jr & Holyoke ED (1975) The clinical implications of a staging system for carcinoma of the anus. *Surg Gynecol Obstet* **141**: 411–416.

Peters RK, Mack TM & Bernstein L (1984) Parallels in the epidemiology of selected anogenital cancinomas. *J Natl Cancer Inst* **72**: 609–615.

Pyper PC & Parks TG (1984) Melanoma of the anal canal. *Br J Surg* **71**: 671–672.

Quan SHQ (1978) Anal and para anal tumours. *Surg Clin North Am* **58**: 591–603.

Quan SH (1980) Uncommon malignant anal and rectal tumours. In Stearns MW (ed.) *Neoplasms of the Colon, Rectum and Anus*. New York: Wiley.

Quan SHQ (1983) Carcinoma of the anus. *Int Adv Surg Oncol* **6**: 323–335.

Quan SHQ (1992) Anal cancers. Squamous and melanoma. *Cancer* **70**: 1384–1389.

Rabkin CS, Biggar RJ, Melbye M & Curtis RE (1992) Second primary cancers following anal and cervical carcinoma: evidence of shared aetiologic factors. *Am J Epidemiol* **136**: 54–58.

Richart RM (1973) Cervical intrapithelial neoplasia. In Sommers SC (ed.) *Pathology Annual*, pp 301–328. New York: Appleton-Century-Crofts.

Rohr S, Sadok H, Dai B & Meyer C (1992) Anorectal malignant melanomas. Apropos of 2 new cases [in French]. *J Chir (Paris)* **129**: 320–323.

Roseau G, Palazzo L, Colardelle P, Chaussade S, Couturier D & Paolaggi JA (1994) Endoscopic ultrasonography in the staging and follow-up of epidermoid carcinoma of the anal canal. *Gastrointest Endosc* **40**: 447–450.

Salem P, Habboubi N, Brihi ER et al (1985) Effectiveness of cisplatin in the treatment of anal squamous cell carcinoma. *Cancer Treat Rep* **69**: 891–893.

Salmon RJ, Fenton J, Asselain B et al (1984) Treatment of epidermoid anal canal cancer. *Am J Surg* **147**: 43–48.

Sawyers JL (1977) Current management of carcinoma of the anus and perianus. *Am Surg* **43**: 424–429.

Sawyers JL, Herrington JL & Main FB (1963) Surgical considerations in the treatment of epidermoid carcinoma of the anus. *Ann Surg* **157**: 817–824.

Scholefield JH & Amin S (1998) Anal intraepithelial neoplasia (AIN). *Colonews* **7**: 1–3.

Scholefield JH, Sonnex C, Talbot IC et al (1989) Anal and cervical intraepithelial neoplasia: possible parallel. *Lancet* **ii**: 765–768.

Scholefield JH, Palmer JG, Shepherd NA, Love S, Miller KJ & Northover JMA (1990) Clinical and pathological correlates of HPV Type 16 DNA in anal cancer. *Int J Colorectal Dis* **5**: 219–222.

Scholefield JH, Hickson WGE, Smith JHF, Rogers K & Sharp F (1992) Anal intraepitheial neoplasia: part of a multifocal disease process. *Lancet* **340**: 1271–1273.

Scholefield JH, Ogunbiyi OA, Smith JH, Rogers K & Sharp F (1994) Treatment of anal intraepithelial neoplasia. *Br J Surg* **81**: 1238–1240.

Schraut WH, Wang C, Dawson PJ & Block GE (1983) Depth of invasion, location and size of cancer of the anus dictate operative treatment. *Cancer* **51**: 1291–1296.

Sherman KJ, Daling JR, Chu J, McKnight B & Weiss NS (1988) Multiple primary tumours in women with vulvar neoplasms: A case control study. *Br J Cancer* **57**: 423–427.

Sielezneff I, Boutboul R, Thomas P, Henric A & Denis O (1993) Primary anorectal malignant melanomas: 2 cases [in French]. *Presse Medicale* **22**: 1999–2001.

Singh R, Nime F & Mittelman A (1981) Malignant epithelial tumors of the anal canal. *Cancer* **48**: 411–414.

Sink JD, Kramer SA, Copeland DD & Sieger HF (1978) Cloacogenic carcinoma. *Ann Surg* **188**: 53.

Sischy B, Remington JH, Hinson EJ, Sobel SH & Woll JE (1982) Definitive treatment of anal canal carcinoma by means of radiation therapy and chemotherapy. *Dis Colon Rectum* **25**: 685–688.

Slater G, Greenstein A & Aufses AH Jr (1984) Anal carcinoma in patients with Crohn's disease. *Ann Surg* **199**: 348–350.

Slingluff CL & Siegler HF (1992) Anorectal melanoma: clinical characteristics and the role of abdominoperineal resection. *Ann Plast Surg* **28**: 85–88.

Sloan PJM & Goepel J (1981) Lichen sclerosus et atrophicus and perianal carcinoma: a case report. *Clin Exp Dermatol* **6**: 399–402.

Stearns MW Jr & Quan SHQ (1970) Epidermoid carcinoma of the anorectum. *Surg Gynecol Obstet* **131**: 953.

Stearns MW, Urmacher C, Sternberg SS, Woodruff J & Attiyeh F (1980) Cancer of the anal canal. *Curr Probl Cancer* **4**: 1–44.

Strauss RJ & Fazio VW (1979) Bowen's disease of the anal and perianal area. A report and analysis of twelve cases. *Am J Surg* **137**: 231–234.

Sturm JT, Christenson CE, Uecker JH et al (1975) Squamous cell carcinoma of the anus arising in a giant condyloma acuminatum: report of a case. *Dis Colon Rectum* **18**: 147–151.

Subbuswamy SG & Ribeiro BF (1981) Perianal Paget's disease associated with cloacogenic carcinoma: report of a case. *Dis Colon Rectum* **24**: 535–538.

Surawicz CM, Kirby P, Critchlow C, Sayer J, Dunphy C & Kiviat N (1993) Anal dysplasia in homosexual men: role of anoscopy and biopsy. *Gastroenterology* **105**: 658–666.

Surawicz CM, Critchlow C, Sayer J, Hurt C et al (1995) High grade anal dysplasia in visually normal mucosa in homosexual men: seven cases. *Am J Gastroenterol* **90**: 1776–1778.

Tanum G (1993) Treatment of relapsing anal carcinoma. *Acta Oncol* **32**: 33–35.

Touboul E, Schlienger M, Buffat L et al (1995a) Epidermoid carcinoma of the anal margin: 17 cases treated with curative-intent radiation therapy. *Radiother Oncol* **34**: 195–202.

Touboul E, Schlienger M, Buffat L et al (1995b) Conservative versus nonconservative treatment of epidermoid carcinoma of the anal canal for tumors longer than or equal to 5 centimeters. A retrospective comparison. *Cancer* **75**: 786–793.

UKCCCR Anal Cancer Trial Working Party (1996) Epidermoid anal cancer: results from the UKCCCR randomized trial of radiotherapy alone versus radiotherapy, 5-fluorouracil and mitomycin C. *Lancet* **348**: 1049–1054.

Wanebo HJ, Woodruff JM, Farr GH & Quan SH (1981) Ano-rectal melanoma. *Cancer* **47**: 1891–1900.

Weinstock MA (1993) Epidemiology and prognosis of anorectal melanoma. *Gastroenterology* **104**: 174–178.

Welch JP & Malt RA (1977) Appraisal of the treatment of carcinoma of the anus and anal canal. *Surg Gynecol Obstet* **145**: 837–841.

Wellman KF (1962) Adenocarcinoma of anal duct origin. *Can J Surg* **5**: 311–318.

Wexner SD, Milsom JW & Dailey TH (1987) The demographics of anal cancers are changing: Identification of a high risk population. *Dis Colon Rectum* **30**: 942–946.

Wilking N, Petrelli N, Herrera L et al (1985) Phase II study of combination bleomycin, vincristine and high dose methotrexate (BOM) with leucovorin rescue in advanced squamous cell cancer of the anal canal. *Cancer Chemother Pharmacol* **15**: 300–302.

Williams AB, Darragh TM, Vranzian K et al (1994) Anal and cervical human papillomavirus infection and risk of anal and cervical epithelial abnormalities in human immunodeficiency virus-infected women. *Obstet Gynecol* **83**: 205–211.

Williams PL & Warwick R (1980) *Gray's Anatomy*, 36th edn, pp 1358–1361. Edinburgh: Churchill Livingstone.

Williams SL, Rogers LW & Quan SHQ (1976) Perianal Paget's disease: report of seven cases. *Dis Colon Rectum* **19**: 30–40.

Winkelman J, Grosfeld J & Bigelow B (1964) Colloid carcinoma of anal gland origin: report of a case and review of the literature. *Am J Clin Pathol* **42**: 395–401.

Wolfe HRI (1968) The management of metastatic inguinal adenitis in epidermoid cancer of the anus. *J R Soc Med* **61**: 626–628.

Wolfe HRI & Bussey HJR (1968) Squamous cell carcinoma of the anus. *Br J Surg* **55**: 295.

Zelnick RS, Haas PA, Ajlouni M, Szilagyi E & Fox TA (1992) Results of abdominoperineal resections for failures after combination chemotherapy and radiation therapy for anal canal cancers. *Dis Colon Rectum* **35**: 574–577.

Zimberg YH & Kay S (1957) Anorectal carcinomas of extramural origin. *Ann Surg* **145**: 344.

zur Hausen H & Schneider A (1987) The role of human papillomaviruses in human anogenital cancer. In Howley PM & Salzman NP (eds) *The Papillomaviruses*. New York: Plenum Publishing Corp., **2**: 245–263.

35 RARE TUMOURS OF THE COLON AND RECTUM

RARE BENIGN TUMOURS OF THE COLON AND RECTUM

Some benign tumours may form polypoid lesions and are therefore also considered in the section on polyps.

Benign lymphoma

Benign lymphoma is the most common non-epithelial benign tumour occurring in the large intestine, and is usually seen in the rectum as a single reddish-purple or grey, rounded polyp varying in diameter from a few millimetres to 3–4 cm. The appearances of this tumour on macroscopic and microscopic examination are similar to those of a malignant lymphoma. However, the benign tumour lacks the infiltrating and destructive characteristics of malignant lymphoma and does not metastasize. In benign lymphoma the cells form a follicular pattern and have a well-defined germinal centre, whereas in malignant lymphoma there is a haphazard pattern and no germinal centres are present (Price, 1978). The differentiation between benign and malignant lymphoma may be difficult. Thus approximately 50% of the 70 cases of benign lymphoma described by Helwig and Hansen (1951) were misdiagnosed originally.

If the pathologist is sure of the diagnosis it seems safe to treat these tumours by simple local excision. It is claimed that even if local excision is not complete there is no urgency to attempt further excision or more radical excision (Cornes et al, 1961).

Lipoma

A lipoma, although rare, appears to be the second most common non-epithelial benign tumour of the large bowel, with an incidence of 0.2–0.3% in autopsy studies (Weinberg and Feldman, 1955; Haller and Roberts, 1964). Most authors have found these tumours to be more common in the caecum and right colon (Pemberton and McCormack, 1937;

Castro and Stearns, 1972). The rectum is not a frequent site in either sex (Mayo et al, 1963). Lipomas arise from deposits of adipose tissue in the bowel wall. Most are situated in the submucosal layer but some lie subserosally. Patients are usually aged between 50 and 70 years and there does not seem to be any sex predilection. When, as is usual, the tumour grows submucosally, it is covered by mucosa and sometimes by the muscularis mucosae. A lipoma protrudes into the bowel lumen and may cause the mucosa overlying it to become stretched, atrophic and eventually necrotic and ulcerated (Figure 35.1).

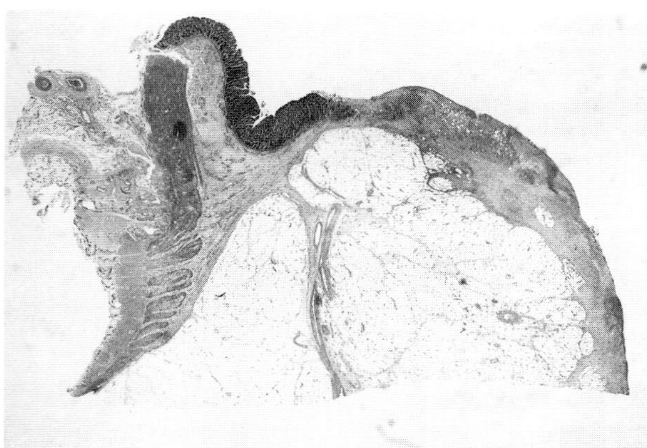

Figure 35.1 Lipoma of intestine showing superficial ulceration due to intussusception. This tumour was sited in the small intestine, but colonic lipomas have a similar appearance.

When the tumour begins in the subserosa it usually grows towards the peritoneal cavity. These lesions vary in size from a few millimetres to more than 6 cm. They are reputed never to turn malignant. Most often they occur singly but in some series up to 20% of patients had several lesions (Mayo et al, 1963).

The clinical picture varies. Most lipomas are asymptomatic, being discovered only on autopsy or at laparotomy for another condition. They may rarely cause intestinal obstruction owing to the lipoma forming the head of an intussusception (Marra, 1993; Siddiqui and Garnham, 1993; Wulff and Jesperson, 1995; Hackam et al, 1996). More commonly patients present with change in bowel habit, vague abdominal pain, bleeding per rectum or anaemia, symptoms that are indistinguishable from those associated with an adenocarcinoma.

Multiple lipomatosis needs to be differentiated from other polyposis syndromes. If this condition is suspected, radiological examination with a water-soluble enema may be useful. Using a low-kilovoltage technique which exploits the different absorption coefficients of fat and water, fat-containing lesions appear more radiolucent than other lesions. CT may also be useful (Rogy et al, 1991; Kakitsubata et al, 1993). The only sure way, however, of establishing the diagnosis is by colonoscopic biopsy.

If the lesion presents as a polypoid lesion on sigmoidoscopy or colonoscopy it can sometimes be removed by snare, although considerable care must be exercised to avoid perforation. If the histological examination confirms the diagnosis, no further action is required. Often the surgeon who finds an asymptomatic lipoma at laparotomy is unsure of the diagnosis. In these circumstances a partial colectomy will be needed to confirm the diagnosis and exclude a carcinoma. If the lipoma is causing symptoms, or after barium enema and colonoscopy there is doubt as to the diagnosis, partial resection is indicated.

Occasionally a lipoma develops in the rectum or in the perianal region and appears as a soft, smooth, lobulated yellow mass on rectal examination and proctoscopy. Symptoms will depend on its size, whether the internal anal sphincter is involved, and whether or not the overlying mucosa is ulcerated. If the lesion is pedunculated it can usually be excised by prolapsing it through the anus after transfixion of the base. Otherwise the rectal mucosa can be incised and the tumour enucleated via the transanal route.

Leiomyoma

Smooth muscle tumours of the large intestine are exceedingly rare. Stout (1955) found 30 leiomyomas in 200 benign tumours of the large intestine over a 50-year period, and Ferguson and Houston (1972) could only find two cases among 67 benign lesions. Kadakia et al (1992) found that only 3% of all gastrointestinal leiomyomas occurred in the colon. Leiomyomas are now classified as one category of stromal cell tumour. The latter include a wide range of non-epithelial neoplasms (Franquement, 1995). The largest category includes tumours showing differentiation to smooth muscle cells.

Leiomyomas arise in the muscle coat of the colon and may remain intramural or may grow into the lumen or into the peritoneal cavity. Sometimes they grow in both directions and form a dumb-bell type of tumour. They usually occur as single entities, and when small are rubbery, firm nodules; when large they form lobulated masses. On histological exami-

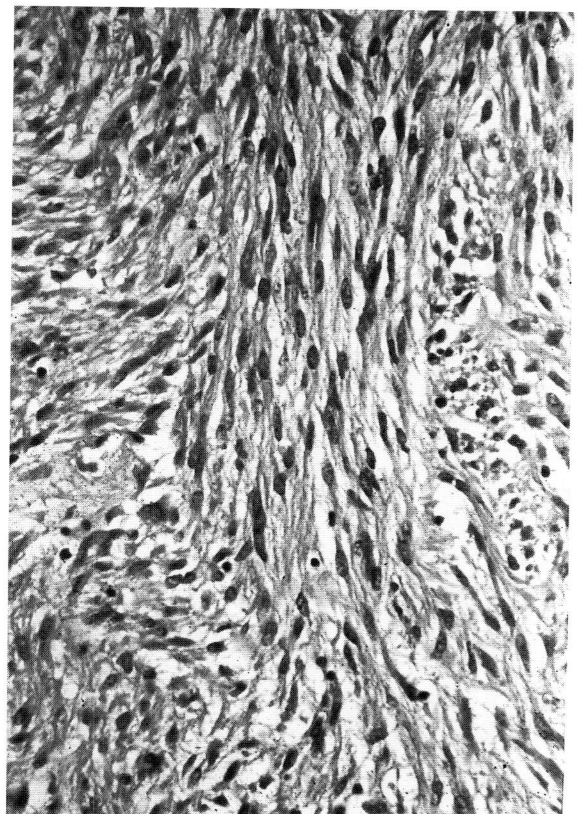

Figure 35.2 Leiomyoma of colon, consisting of spindle-shaped cells arranged in interlacing bundles with an admixture of fibrous tissue.

nation leiomyomas consist of spindle-shaped cells arranged in interlacing bundles with an admixture of fibrous tissue (Figure 35.2). Often (but not invariably) leiomyomas are encapsulated. Histologically the differentiation between benign and malignant smooth muscle tumours may be extremely difficult (Le Borgne et al, 1993–94). Most authorities regard size and a rapid mitotic rate as being the single most important criteria for the diagnosis of malignancy (Evans, 1919; Stout and Hill, 1958; Berg and McNeer, 1960; Botting et al, 1965). Other features indicating malignancy include variation in nuclear size and shape, hyperchromasia (Berg and McNeer, 1960), frequent bizarre cells and difficulty in identification of longitudinal myofibrils (Evans, 1919; Botting et al, 1965). Despite the presence or absence of these malignant characteristics, the final determinant of malignancy is based upon the ability of the tumour to metastasize.

According to Stout's data the colon seems to be affected more than the rectum (Stout, 1959), although the Mayo Clinic experience suggests the reverse (Anderson et al, 1950; Mackenzie et al, 1954). Within the colon, leiomyomas are most common in the sigmoid and transverse colon; the caecum is rarely involved (Lookanoff and Tsapralis, 1966).

The clinical features are similar to those of other benign tumours. The tumours may be entirely asymptomatic, being discovered only at autopsy or at operation. Colonic tumours may present with abdominal pain and bleeding, or the patient may notice an abdominal mass. Perforation and intussusception have both been reported but are rare (Murphy, 1973). Rectal leiomyomas may often present with symptoms identical to those of a rectal carcinoma.

Treatment is by surgical excision. Usually the preoperative diagnosis is uncertain, and because of the difficulty that the pathologist may have in interpreting the frozen sections it is advisable to perform a radical cancer operation. The only exception might be a small rectal leiomyoma which could be removed locally with ease under circumstances where otherwise a more radical operation would necessitate an abdominoperineal excision. However, a group of Russian surgeons appear to favour a more local approach. Vorobyov et al (1992) describe 36 patients with rectal leiomyomas operated on between 1972 and 1990. Electroexcision of tumours less than 1 cm in diameter was performed through the endoscope in 12 patients. Tumours with a diameter of 2.5–5.0 cm were removed transanally in 10 patients. Six patients underwent excision through the pararectal approach. Abdominoperineal excision and abdominoanal resection of the rectum was performed in seven patients for tumours measuring 8–20 cm. Recurrence occurred in nine of the patients who underwent local excision. In seven of them, malignant transformation occurred between 9 months and 9.5 years. If, after local excision, the lesion was considered to be benign, no further procedure would be adopted and the patient would merely be followed up carefully.

Fibroma

A fibroma consists of numerous spindle cells and may arise from any layer of the bowel wall (Aird, 1957). It may be mistaken for a leiomyoma, but differential tissue-staining techniques usually enable the two to be differentiated (Rose, 1972). There are few reports of colonic fibroma (Rose, 1972; Fayemi and Toker, 1974; Orda et al, 1976), but it would seem that resection is usually advisable (Vorobyov et al, 1995).

The so-called fibrous anal polyp is considered by

some (Corman, 1984) to be a type of fibroma. However, this lesion does not appear to be a neoplasm. The most likely explanation for its development is fibrous infiltration into a large, prolapsing haemorrhoid which has undergone several episodes of thrombosis without sloughing.

Other benign tumours

Haemangioma

Either capillary or cavernous haemangiomas may occur in either the colon or rectum. These tumours should be differentiated from angiodysplasia. Further details are to be found in the section on colonic haemorrhage (see Chapter 60).

Neurofibroma

Neurofibromas may occur within the large bowel either as part of neurofibromatosis (Von Recklinghausen's disease) or as a separate entity (Poate and Inglis, 1928; Levy and Khatib, 1960; Manley and Skyring, 1961). These tumours may arise in the submucosa or muscularis (Girdwood and Philip, 1971), eventually ulcerating through the overlying mucosa. Any patient with Von Recklinghausen's disease who bleeds per rectum or presents with an intussusception should be suspected of having a gastrointestinal neurofibroma. As malignant transformation may occur it is perhaps best that all neurofibromas should be treated by colorectal resection.

Other neurogenic tumours

Other neurogenic tumours include ganglioneuroma (Bibro et al, 1980) and granular cell tumour (Abrikossoff, 1926). Granular cell tumours are regarded by some as being derived from myoblasts (Klinge, 1928), while others suggest that they are regenerative in nature rather than neoplastic (Willis, 1960). As the constituent cells resemble Schwann cells, most believe that these tumours should be classified as neurogenic neoplasms. Granular cell tumours of the colon form yellowish-white, submucosal nodules often less than 2 cm in diameter, and are probably best treated by colonoscopic removal (Madiedo et al, 1980).

Another neurogenic tumour which has been found in the rectum is the gastrointestinal autonomic nerve tumour (GANT) which is a type of stromal tumour (Butler et al, 1997). Stromal cell tumours found in the gastrointestinal tract often differentiate to smooth muscle cells, i.e. to form a leiomyoma. However, such tumours can differentiate to neural elements and are then known as GANT tumours since their features have been likened to the neural cells in the autonomic myenteric plexus. Histologically, they appear to be low-grade neoplasms, and they have distinctive ultrastructural features on electron microscopy (King et al, 1996), and on immunohistochemical analysis they are commonly positive for neuron-specific enolase and/or S-100 protein (Hurlimann and Gardiol, 1991).

Lymphangioma

Lymphangioma is another rare benign tumour that has been described in the colon and rectum by Alvich and Lepow (1960), Arnett and Friedman (1956), Girdwood and Philip (1971), Greene et al (1962), Higgason (1958), Koenig et al (1955) and Ochsner et al (1959) (Figure 35.3).

Haemangiopericytoma

Haemangiopericytoma is a rare benign tumour arising from the pericytes of blood vessels (Ault et al, 1951; Genter et al, 1982).

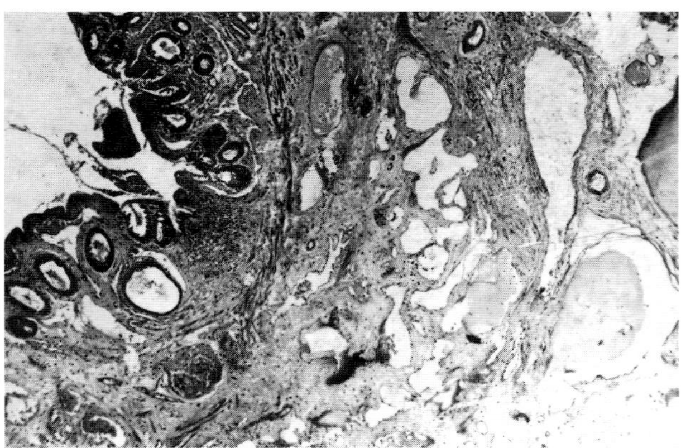

Figure 35.3 Lymphangioma (lymphangiectasia). Dilated lymphatic channels are present in the submucosa of the bowel (H&E, ×100).

RARE MALIGNANT TUMOURS OF THE COLON AND RECTUM

Leiomyosarcoma

Leiomyosarcoma is a rare smooth muscle tumour that may occur in either the colon or rectum. Approximately 215 cases had been described in the literature by 1994 with two-thirds occurring in the rectum (Anderson et al, 1950; Baker and Good, 1955; Swartzlander, 1955; Morson, 1960; Quan and Berg, 1962; Smith, 1963; Bacon, 1964; Bhargava et al, 1964; Asuncion, 1969; Roo and Vaas, 1969; Yoshikawa, 1969; Schumann, 1972; Calem and Keller, 1973; Astarjian et al, 1977; Eitan et al, 1978; Cho and Smith, 1980; Rao et al, 1980; Stavorovsky et al, 1980; Stair et al, 1983; Asbun et al, 1992; Lacava et al, 1992; Letessier et al, 1992; Tjandra et al, 1993; Wolf et al, 1994; Fallahzadeh, 1995; Witzigmann et al, 1995).

Rectal leiomyosarcoma

It is estimated that only 0.1–0.5% of all rectal tumours are leiomyosarcomas (Golden and Stout, 1941; Anderson et al, 1950; Nemer et al, 1977; Caffarena et al, 1993; Wolf et al, 1994). More than half of the smooth muscle tumours in the rectum are malignant, which is in contrast to the rest of the gastrointestinal tract where most smooth muscle tumours are benign. The tumour is invariably submucosal in location. Histologically it is composed of spindle-shaped cells in interlacing bundles and whorls (Figure 35.4). The nuclei may be vesicular with blunted edges and have enlarged, rounded nucleoli. Malignancy is best determined histologically by an increased mitotic index. Mucosal ulceration, submucosal spread and local infiltration are characteristic of the tumour. Distant metastases occur more often by haematogenous spread than by the lymphatic route. It is exceedingly difficult for histopathologists to determine whether a smooth muscle tumour of the large bowel is benign or malignant. The only sure way is to observe its behaviour. Consequently it is a wise policy for clinicians to treat such lesions from the beginning as though they were malignant.

Clinical features

The clinical manifestations of rectal leiomyosarcoma are often similar to those of adenocarcinoma of the rectum, usually rectal bleeding and change of bowel habit (Tjandra et al, 1993). At an early stage ulceration of the overlying mucosa may not have occurred, and thus any smooth, firm mass palpable per rectum with intact overlying mucosa should be suspected of being a leiomyosarcoma. More often, however, ulceration occurs, and the findings on rectal examination are indistinguishable from a rectal adenocarcinoma. Pain is said to be more common with malignant than benign lesions (Stair et al, 1983), but we regard this as an unreliable differentiating sign. The depth of invasion of the tumour through the rectal wall can be determined using endoluminal ultrasound (Wolf et al, 1994).

Treatment and results

Radical surgical excision seems to offer the only hope of cure. Local excision carries approximately an

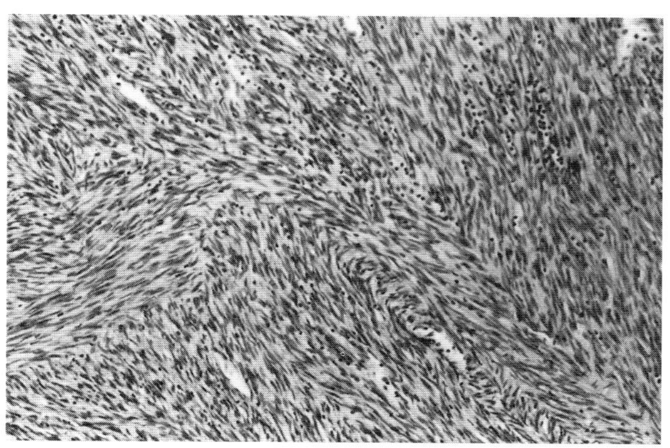

(a)

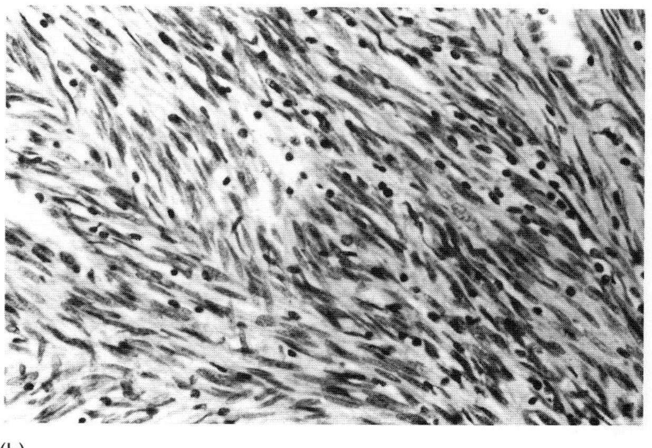

(b)

Figure 35.4 Leiomyosarcoma of rectum. (a) Spindle-shaped cells make up a herringbone pattern; a few lymphocytes reflect surface ulceration (H&E, ×100). (b) High-power view shows cellular tumour in which spindle cells with blunt-ended nuclei form a herringbone pattern; moderate pleomorphism and mitoses, not well seen here, were numerous (H&E, ×400).

80–85% chance of recurrence (Golden and Stout, 1941; Anderson et al, 1950; Nemer et al, 1977; Blatt et al, 1979). Since 80% of these tumours are low in the rectum, abdominoperineal excision has been the operation most frequently performed (Tjandra et al, 1993). However, with mid-rectal or upper rectal lesions restorative resection should achieve adequate local removal. The 5-year survival rate in most series seems to be 20–25% after radical surgery (Golden and Stout, 1941; Anderson et al, 1950; Diamente and Bacon, 1967; Nemer et al, 1977; Eitan et al, 1978; Blatt et al, 1979; Tjandra et al, 1993). With this poor prognosis there is little wonder that adjuvant therapy has been advised. The tumour is radioresistant and the results of radiation therapy are, not surprisingly, disappointing (Golden and Stout, 1941; Anderson et al, 1950; Sanger and Leckie, 1959; Sanders, 1961; Blatt et al, 1979) although local excision and brachytherapy with iridium 192 has recently been reported as an option (Minsky et al, 1991). Chemotherapy using combined drug therapy is advised but it is difficult to know from the literature the effectiveness of these regimens (Gottlieb et al, 1975; Wolfson and Oh, 1977). Some advocate CT surveillance in the belief (as yet unproven) that early recurrences can be resected with benefit.

Colonic leiomyosarcoma

Local infiltration tends to be less of a problem with colonic tumours than with rectal tumours (Rao et al, 1980), so complete excision is easier. Some authors have attempted to stage the disease to improve management (Astarjian et al, 1977). They describe three stages:

Stage I. Tumour confined to the intestinal wall with no invasion and no ulceration.
- (A) Submucosal tumours.
- (B) Subserosal tumours.

Stage II. Tumours extending beyond the wall of the colon.
- (A) Intraluminal ulceration.
- (B) Infiltration into adjacent extracolonic tissues.

Stage III. Tumours with distant metastases.

According to these authors, stage IA and B and stage IIA have an excellent prognosis; for stage IIB the prognosis is only fair, and patients in stage III have an exceedingly poor outlook. This seems an eminently sensible classification, but whether results of treatment will be improved as a result remains to be seen.

Carcinoid tumours

Carcinoid tumours arise from the Kulchitsky or basogranular enterochromaffin cells in the crypts of Lieberkühn (Masson, 1928), and are now classified as neuroendocrine tumours (Saclarides et al, 1994). The cells of origin are ectodermal and have an affinity for silver stains, hence the alternative term for these tumours is 'argentaffinoma' (Figure 35.5). There seems to be a variation in the histochemical, chemical and clinical properties of these tumours depending on their site of origin (Williams and Sandler, 1963; Black, 1968; Orloff, 1971). Carcinoids have been classified according to their anatomical site and their reactivity to silver incorporation by the cytoplasmic granules. The cells within the tumour may be either argyrophilic or argentaffin positive, or both. A positive argentaffin reaction means that the cytoplasmic granules are able to reduce ionic silver to metallic silver (Taxy et al, 1980). The granules within argyrophil cells tend to be small, whereas those present in argentaffin cells are large (Corman, 1984). Midgut carcinoids usually contain argyrophil and argentaffin-positive cells, they are multicentric in origin and are often associated with the carcinoid syndrome. Hindgut tumours seem to be different: they are far less com-

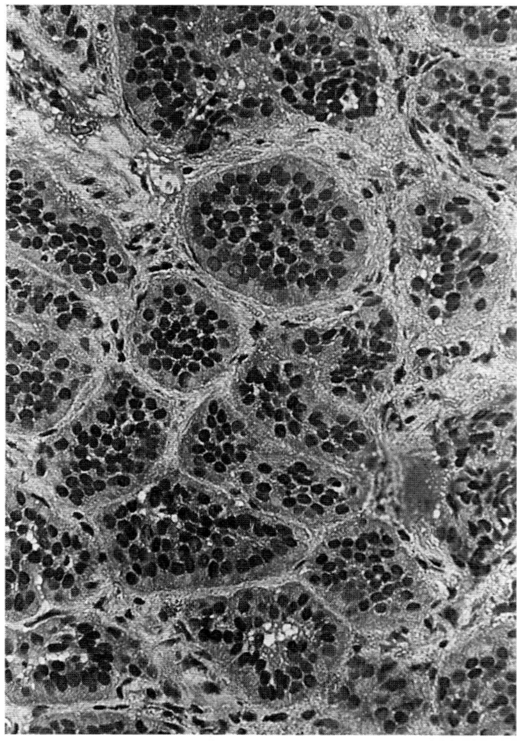

Figure 35.5 Carcinoid tumour or argentaffinoma. The cells contain large argentaffin-staining granules.

mon than those in the midgut and are unicentric in origin. Hindgut carcinoids are argyrophilic rather than argentaffin positive (Saegesser and Gross, 1969; Taxy et al, 1980); they rarely secrete 5-hydroxytryptamine (5HT), hence 5-hydroxyindoleacetic acid (5HIAA) is rarely identified in the urine (Black, 1968).

At present there is considerable confusion regarding the terminology of hormone-secreting intestinal epithelial tumours. The term carcinoid was originally meant to describe benign or very low-grade carcinoma-like tumours, yet it appears now to be given indiscriminately to a very diverse group of neoplasms. Included are cancers of all degrees of differentiation, endocrine and non-endocrine, functioning and non-functioning. Some authors believe the diagnosis of neuroendocrine tumour should be applied to any epithelial tumour capable of synthesizing, storing or secreting amines or neuropeptides, regardless of their degree of clinical activity (Saclarides et al, 1994). They believe that the term carcinoid should be limited to benign tumours or very low-grade, well-differentiated neuroendocrine tumours such as appendiceal tumours. Thus they consider the term neuroendocrine cancer should be used only for their high-grade, less well-differentiated counterparts. Such a classification seems eminently sensible, but has not yet been universally accepted, and we will therefore adhere to the more established meaning of the term carcinoid.

The large bowel is the third most common site for the development of carcinoid tumours after the appendix and small intestine. Up to 30% of all gastrointestinal carcinoids may occur in the colon and rectum (Cheek and Wilson, 1970; McDermott et al, 1994), the rectum or anus being the most frequent site (Jetmore et al, 1992) (Figure 35.6). In the large bowel the tumour usually occurs as a single growth, in contrast to the small intestine where multiple lesions are the rule. Initially the tumour forms a small, nodular thickening in the mucosa and submucosa. In its early stages a carcinoid tumour may appear similar to an adenomatous polyp, but it is usually paler in colour and sometimes has a yellowish tinge. As the carcinoid enlarges it produces a sessile lesion which, if allowed to progress, may become larger and ulcerate. For some time it tends to remain mobile on the deeper layers of the bowel wall. Occasionally it resembles a pedunculated polyp.

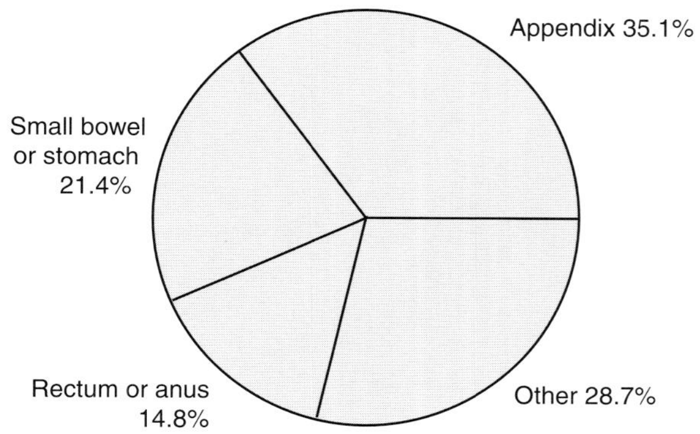

Figure 35.6 Site of primary gastrointestinal carcinoid tumour in 3763 patients in selected series. From McDermott et al (1994).

Clinical features and diagnosis

When carcinoid tumours arise in the colon they tend to remain asymptomatic for a considerable time (Spread et al, 1994). Even when they have grown to a large size they are less likely to cause intestinal obstruction or rectal bleeding than an adenocarcinoma. In a study reported by Orloff (1971), 53% of patients with colonic carcinoids were asymptomatic as far as the colonic carcinoid tumour was concerned. However, when symptoms do occur they do not differ from those produced by an adenocarcinoma.

In the rectum the tumour tends to be detected at an earlier stage, often on clinical examination for other complaints (Jetmore et al, 1992). In these circumstances it may be seen through a sigmoidoscope as a small, yellow submucosal nodule 1 cm or less in diameter.

A biopsy is needed to confirm the diagnosis of carcinoid, but it is very difficult to differentiate benign from malignant lesions. The usual criteria of malignancy such as mitotic activity or pyknotic nuclei are often missing (Corman, 1984). Hence the diagnosis of malignancy usually rests on the presence of local invasion or metastases. The incidence of malignancy using these criteria varies between 8% and 40% (Welch and Hedberg, 1975). Since carcinoids seem to be associated with a greater than normal incidence of gastrointestinal adenocarcinoma, the patient must have the rest of the gastrointestinal tract fully screened for malignancy (Bates, 1962; Caldarola et al, 1964; Quan et al, 1964; Gerstle et al, 1995).

Although midgut carcinoids secrete 5HT and foregut tumours secrete 5HT and histamine, hindgut carcinoids do not secrete 5HT and are not commonly associated with the carcinoid syndrome (cutaneous flushing, watery diarrhoea, bronchospasm and cardiopulmonary symptoms due to valvular heart lesions). For the syndrome to occur, sufficient bulk of disease needs to be present in the liver to overwhelm the normal detoxifying mechanisms of the various substances secreted, a rare phenomenon indeed for large bowel carcinoids.

Treatment

Carcinoid tumours are best treated by surgical resection. Preoperative assessment must attempt to identify metastatic disease, which is usually principally in the liver. Ultrasound and CT scanning are therefore essential. In the absence of dissemination a colonic carcinoid should be treated by the same radical resection used for an adenocarcinoma. If metastases are present a more limited resection may be undertaken, but as with adenocarcinoma the best palliation is resection. For rectal tumours without dissemination management is dictated by the size and the presence of local invasion. In 1959 Peskin and Orloff suggested that a rectal lesion less than 2 cm in diameter could be treated safely by local excision provided that on histological examination there was no local invasion into or beyond the muscle coat (Peskin and Orloff, 1959). All other lesions should be treated by radical excisional surgery, preferably retaining the anal sphincter if at all possible. Several authors have followed this advice and testify to its reliability (Morton and Johnstone, 1965; Morgan et al, 1973; Rothmund and Kisker, 1994).

Of the 23 patients with tumours smaller than 2 cm treated by Orloff (1971), all survived 5 years. Similarly, Jetmore et al (1992) treated 85 patients with rectal carcinoid tumours less than 2 cm in diameter by a variety of local measures, including transanal excision and fulguration. No local recurrence occurred during the 5-year follow-up. The same authors treated 10 patients with rectal tumours measuring 4 cm or more by radical surgery, but only one patient remained alive at 5 years. The average length of survival after resection of all colonic carcinoids seems to be about 2 years according to some authors (Berardi, 1972).

Spread et al (1994) resected 36 carcinoid tumours of the colon between 1964 and 1988. Two- and 5-year actuarial survival rates were 34% and 26%. The authors concluded that the outlook for colonic carcinoids was considerably worse than for carcinoids arising in the rectum and appendix. Indeed the prognosis of colonic carcinoids was inferior to adenocarcinoma of the colon. However, others (Welch and Donaldson, 1974; McDermott et al, 1994) reported that survival was comparable with that achieved after resection for colorectal adenocarcinoma. McDermott et al (1994), at the Memorial Sloan Kettering Cancer Center, found a 5-year survival rate of 44% in their cohort of patients with colorectal carcinoids. They found that women had a better prognosis than men, that survival was directly proportional to depth of invasion, tumour size, presence of involved lymph nodes or liver metastases, mode of discovery and operative intent. Caecal carcinoid seems to have a worse prognosis compared with carcinoids in the rest of the colon; this is associated with its greater metastasizing potential (Sanders and Axtell, 1964).

The treatment of hepatic metastases from a colorectal carcinoid may be difficult. Since metastatic disease from small bowel carcinoids can cause distressing symptoms due to the carcinoid syndrome, great efforts have been made to treat hepatic metastases with combinations of chemotherapy. Whether this approach is applicable to those colorectal carcinoids, whose metastases do not usually cause such symptoms, is arguable.

Chemotherapy

Various combinations of streptozotocin, fluorouracil, doxorubicin and cyclophosphamide have been tried. Usually the responses have been brief (Legha et al, 1977; Chernicoff et al, 1979; Moertel and Hanley, 1979). Moertel et al (1982), using a single agent, showed that partial response (defined as more than 50% regression) occurred in 26% of patients treated with fluorouracil, 21% with doxorubicin and 16% with streptozotocin. Combination therapy with fluorouracil and streptozotocin produced a 32% response rate (Moertel and Hanley, 1979), but the median duration of response was only 7 months and the median survival was only 21.7 months. Moertel et al (1982) confirmed this response rate and also pointed out that other drug combinations are equally ineffective.

Alternative therapies

Alternative therapies designed to reduce the blood supply to the metastatic deposits have been tried. They include local resection of metastases, operative ligation of the hepatic artery, and percutaneous embolization of the vessels supplying the metastases (Bengmark and Rosengren, 1970; Bengmark et al, 1982; Azizkhan et al, 1985; Kvols et al, 1986; Basson et al, 1993). Although these techniques have been shown to produce symptomatic relief in patients with the carcinoid syndrome, there is no evidence that they prolong survival, and morbidity is high. The mortality from operative hepatic artery ligation may be as high as 25% (Bengmark and Rosengren, 1970).

Since patients with metastases from large bowel carcinoid only rarely develop the carcinoid syndrome there seems little justification at present for prophylactic treatment. However, if patients do develop the carcinoid syndrome, treatment with the somatostatin analogue octreotide may be useful (McDermott et al, 1994).

Squamous cell carcinoma

Squamous cell carcinoma is an extremely rare tumour of the colon and rectum with approximately 72 cases described in the English medical literature up to 1992 (Schneider et al, 1992). A variety of theories have been suggested as to its aetiology. These include squamous metaplasia of existing adenomas or adenocarcinoma, embryonal rest cells, persistent damage to the mucosa by toxic chemical or radiation agents, basal cell anaplasia and metaplasia of glandular epithelium (Comer et al, 1971; Lyttle, 1983; Vezeridis et al, 1983). Long-standing ulcerative colitis, schistosomiasis and radiotherapy have all been implicated as predisposing factors (Comer et al, 1971; Vezeridis et al, 1983; Kulaylat et al, 1995).

The clinical features are exactly the same as those of adenocarcinoma. Furthermore, surgical treatment is the same as adenocarcinoma. However, if an abdominoperineal excision is contemplated for a squamous cell tumour of the rectum, it is worth considering a preoperative course of chemoirradiation as outlined for the treatment of anal canal carcinomas. Such a regimen may allow the tumour to regress sufficiently to permit a sphincter-saving resection. However, it does appear that the prognosis is worse than an adenocarcinoma (Vraux et al, 1994), although some patients have long-term survival after resection.

Malignant lymphoma

Although malignant lymphoma is the third most common malignant neoplasm of the large bowel after adenocarcinoma and carcinoid tumours, it is still unusual. Goligher saw only two in over 1500 cases of malignant tumours of the large bowel (Goligher, 1984). Other authorities have reported a slightly greater incidence of 0.5% of colonic neoplasms and 0.1% of rectal tumours (Sherlock et al, 1970). However, the tumour seems to occur more commonly in HIV, transplant patients and those receiving immunosuppression for inflammatory bowel disease (Cappell and Botros, 1994).

Site

The rectum and the caecum (Figure 35.7) seem to be the most common sites for malignant lymphoma (Stout, 1955; Montini et al, 1994), presumably because there is a greater accumulation of lymphoid tissue in these areas. The tumour may present at any age but patients are usually over 50 years old, and men seem to be more often afflicted than women (Wychulis et al, 1966; Moertel, 1973; Hwang et al, 1992; Habr-Gama et al, 1993).

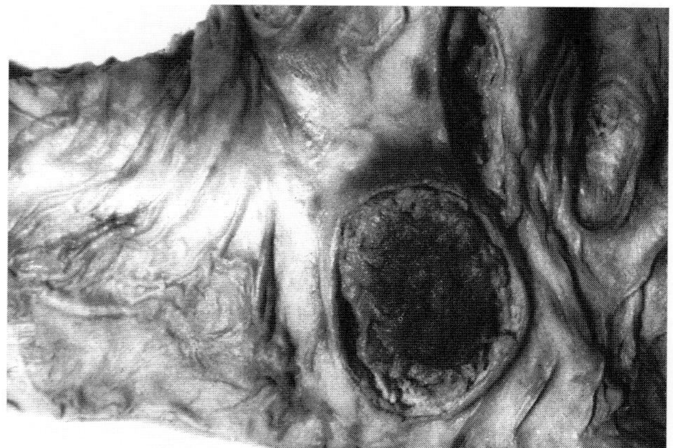

Figure 35.7 Ulcerated malignant lymphoma in caecum.

Pathology

The tumour may form a polypoid or ulcerated mass or may be more diffuse, extending over a large segment of the colon. In the colon the tumour may produce numerous polypoid excrescences, similar in appearance to multiple adenomatous polyposis

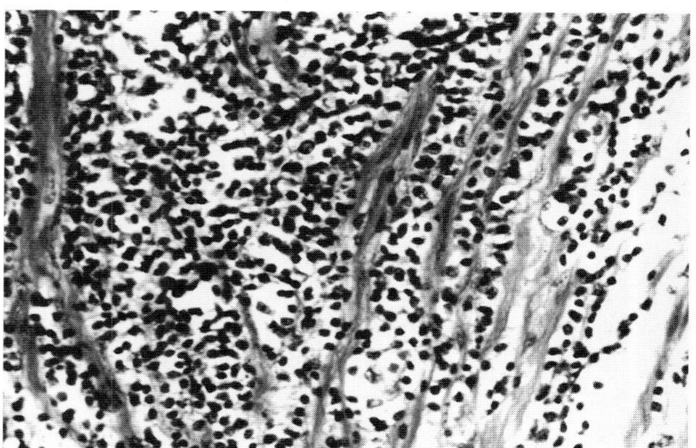

Figure 35.8 Malignant lymphoma of colon. Microscopic appearance shows a sparse infiltration of lymphocytic (B) cells in the bowel muscle (H&E, ×400).

(Cornes, 1961). The bowel wall is considerably thickened owing to the infiltration of closely packed tumour cells into the mucosa and submucosa. In contrast to lymphoma of the small bowel, superficial ulceration and necrosis of the colon may occur.

Like lymphomas elsewhere, colorectal lymphomas are classified according to their cellular morphology and immunological surface markers. Tumours may be of the typical Hodgkin's type; alternatively they may be T or B cell non-Hodgkin's lymphomas (Issacson and Wright, 1986) (Figure 35.8). Non-Hodgkin's lymphomas tend to be highly malignant and spread rapidly through the bowel wall in direct contiguity, and there is often extensive involvement of lymphatics. Approximately 50% of cases have lymph node involvement at operation. In addition to their histological and immunological classification, lymphomas may be classified according to their degree of spread.

Class I. Confined to bowel wall.
Class II. Regional lymph node involvement within the drainage area of the primary bowel disease.
Class III. Para-aortic node involvement and/or direct extension to adjacent viscera.

It seems that the prognosis of extranodal lymphoma in the colon and rectum is related to the stage of the disease rather than to its cell type (Wychulis et al, 1966; Saltzstein, 1969; Lewin et al, 1978).

Clinical features are in the main indistinguishable from those arising from an adenocarcinoma. A lymphoma of the rectum should be suspected when digital palpation reveals an intact mucosa overlying most of a tumour. Once ulceration has occurred, the tumour feels just like a rectal carcinoma. Although radiological appearances mimic those of an adenocarcinoma there are certain features suggestive of lymphoma (Halls, 1980). The diagnosis should be considered if there is a bulky extracolonic component, a concentric dilatation of the lumen or a polypoid filling defect of the terminal ileum and ileocaecal valve. The combination of barium enema and CT scan has been recommended as being particularly useful in the diagnosis of colorectal lymphomas (Wyatt et al, 1993). CT is also of use in staging the disease. With diffuse polypoid types of lymphoma, radiological appearances are similar to the other polyposis syndromes and must be differentiated from ulcerative colitis with pseudopolyps, Crohn's colitis, nodular lymphoid hyperplasia and schistosomiasis. Biopsy and histological examination should be diagnostic, but the differentiation between lymphoma and anaplastic carcinoma may be difficult using light microscopy alone. Appropriate staining for cell surface antigens is likely to clarify the diagnosis (Stansfield, 1985).

Malignant lymphoma may be associated with other diseases, particularly those with an altered immune status, or with the treatment of other diseases (Swanson and Schwartz, 1967; Doak et al, 1968; Fahey, 1971; Kim and Williams, 1972; Levy et al, 1976). There may be an overlap between colonic lymphoma and lymphocytic leukaemia (Waldenstrom, 1960). An association has also been observed between lymphoma, inflammatory bowel disease and coeliac disease (Lewin et al, 1978).

The treatment of gastrointestinal lymphoma is in a state of flux at present, but the general view is that the tumour should be removed surgically as for an adenocarcinoma of the colorectum if this is possible. If the lesion remains confined to the bowel wall, some would advocate adjuvant radiotherapy (Corman, 1984), whereas others would advise no further treatment. If lymph nodes are involved, the consensus is that one of the chemotherapeutic regimens used for the treatment of lymphoma should be given. Whether radiotherapy should also be administered is open to debate. There are as yet no controlled trials of therapy for large bowel lymphoma reported in the literature, which is not altogether surprising in view of the rarity of the disease. Survival data are therefore based on a variety of treatment regimens.

In a literature review, Moertel (1973) reported an overall 5-year survival rate of 55%. Contreary et al (1980) reported a 5-year survival rate of 50% for patients whose tumours were either confined to the bowel wall or in whom only local nodes were involved; however, if regional nodes were involved the survival rate was only 12%. The difference in survival rates between patients treated by surgery and adjuvant radiotherapy and those treated by surgery alone was 83% and 16% respectively. Hwang et al (1992) in Taiwan treated 14 patients with colorectal lymphomas by surgery followed by combination chemotherapy. Median follow-up was 38 months (range 2–82 months), 8 patients were alive with no evidence of metastases, whereas 6 patients died of their disease from 2 to 44 months after diagnosis. Further data are awaited on the use of adjuvant chemotherapy before firm recommendations can be made. We would generally recommend chemoradiotherapy in rectal lymphomas and chemotherapy alone in colonic tumours followed by early surgical resection unless there is a rapid and extensive initial response.

Fibrosarcoma

Fibrosarcoma seems to be the rarest of the sarcomas arising in the gastrointestinal tract. It arises most often within the rectum (Stoller and Weinstein, 1956). Approximately 30 cases are described in the literature, but only two of these tumours were found in the colon (Bassler and Peter, 1949; Hoehn et al, 1980) and one in the anal canal (Espinosa and Quan, 1975). The lesion should be treated in the same way as an adenocarcinoma. There is no information as to whether radiotherapy or chemotherapy is of any benefit.

Plasmacytoma

Plasmacytoma is a tumour composed of plasma cells that may occur as a primary tumour or as a secondary deposit in a patient with multiple myeloma (Hampton and Gandy, 1957; Goldstein and Poker, 1966; Sidani et al, 1983). Both types have been described in the large bowel but are exceedingly uncommon. In 1994 only eight cases had been published since 1972 (Wendum et al, 1994), and in that year a further two cases were described (Pais et al, 1994). In 1997, Holland et al claimed that 18 cases had been described in the English literature.

A patient with multiple myeloma requires general rather than local therapy. In such a patient a secondary deposit in the colon would only require resection if it were causing symptoms and were unresponsive to systemic therapy. A primary lesion should be excised in the usual way.

OTHER MALIGNANT TUMOURS

Other exceedingly rare tumours which may show malignant propensities are endothelioma (Morgan, 1932; Norbury, 1932), haemangiopericytoma (Ault et al, 1951; Genter et al, 1982), granular cell tumour (Abrikossoff, 1926) and rhabdomyosarcoma (Stout, 1959; Chetty and Bhathal, 1993; Marcus et al, 1996).

EXTRINSIC TUMOURS OF COLON AND RECTUM

Metastatic tumour

Metastatic tumour is the most frequent and important extrinsic neoplasm involving the colon. Spread from adjacent primary neoplasms is perhaps more common than blood-borne spread. Neoplastic disease of any intra-abdominal organ may be responsible. Blood-borne involvement occurs most frequently from primary carcinoma of the breast, lung or kidney and malignant melanoma. Symptoms may mimic a primary tumour of the colon and they may be the first sign of the underlying neoplasm. Often the clinical features are those of intestinal obstruction. A barium enema will usually reveal compression of the colonic lumen with no involvement of the mucosa. Sometimes the tumour invades the colonic mucosa and then it is impossible to differentiate a primary lesion from a secondary lesion.

The above comments apply equally to metastatic neoplasms that involve the rectum. When direct spread involves the rectum it invariably arises from a primary neoplasm of the uterus, ovaries, cervix, prostate or (very occasionally) the bladder. Sometimes a carcinoma in a mobile sigmoid colon can loop down into the pelvis and become adherent to the anterior wall of the rectum and form a fistula into it.

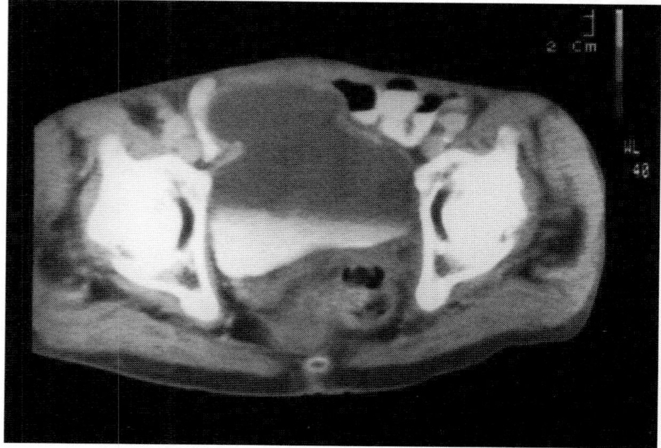

Figure 35.9 CT scan of pelvis showing large chordoma involving the lower sacrum and displacing the rectum to the left. The tumour extended to the bladder base and obstructed the right ureter.

Sacrococcygeal chordoma

Sacrococcygeal chordomas develop from the fetal notochord and lie posterior to the rectum in the sacral region (Figure 35.9). The sacrococcygeal variety represents 50% of all chordomas (Halls, 1980). They are extremely rare tumours and are slow growing. They may present at any age and in either sex, but seem most common in men aged above 50 years. The tumours invade by direct extension, and although they are considered to remain local it would appear that a proportion of tumours do metastasize. The exact proportion is difficult to determine, but the reported range is between 10% and 43% (Gentil and Coley, 1948; Higinbotham et al, 1967; Goligher, 1984; Jenkins and Colquhoun, 1995). Microscopically the tumour is composed of a syncytial mass of epithelial cells and swollen, bladder-like (physaliphoric) cells containing large vacuoles. Pain is the usual presenting symptom and tends to be chronic. Frequently the patient complains of backache, and as the sacral nerve roots become infiltrated sciatica may occur with appropriate localizing neurological signs. In addition bladder and anal sphincter dysfunction may develop. Constipation is also common. The tumour may become infected so the patient may complain of fever, chills, rigors and recurrent episodes of perianal suppuration. Large tumours may cause obstructed labour in females (Böhm et al, 1993).

On rectal examination the tumour is easily palpable as a rubbery, smooth, rounded, often lobulated swelling. Occasionally, there may be skin involvement. Thus Su et al (1993) found that of 207 cases of chordoma, 19 had skin involvement. The tumour is usually seen radiologically in the lateral plane of a straight pelvic radiograph; it appears as a soft tissue mass displacing the rectum anteriorly. Circular or oval areas of translucency in the sacrum corresponding to the lesion may be present, and trabeculation and calcification may be seen. Bony destruction may be evident and this is often more extensive than is apparent radiologically.

A useful method of diagnosis is by CT or MRI scanning; the chordoma is seen as a circumscribed mass which appears to arise from the sacrum and/or the coccyx (Figure 35.9) (Rosenthal et al, 1985; Suarez et al, 1990; Anson et al, 1994). Endominal ultrasound examination has also been shown to be a sensitive method of assessment in some centres (Böhm et al, 1993). Bone scintigraphy may also be useful, particularly using Tc99m HMDP and gallium. Thus a midline sacrococcygeal tumour showing reduced uptake or a cold lesion on bone scintigraphy and no increased accumulation on gallium scintigraphy could be a chordoma rather than another type of malignancy (Suga et al, 1992). Although needle aspiration cytology has been recommended for diagnosis (Hughes et al, 1992; Plate and Bittinger, 1992; Caballero and Fontaniere, 1993), most surgeons condemn this practice because of the risk of implantation of viable tumour cells along the needle track.

Treatment

Excision offers the best hope of cure, but there is some debate as to how radical this should be. Ideally the tumour should be removed en bloc with the sacrum; however, if the tumour is extensive a permanent neurological deficit will result. McCartey et al (1952) stated that the distal two (or even three) pieces of sacrum can be removed without serious neurological impairment, provided that the third sacral nerve on at least one side is preserved. Others, however, have removed all of the sacrum and coccyx apart from the first sacral segment without apparent neurological impairment (Localio et al, 1967, 1980). Removal of more than the lower three sacral segments may result in instability and collapse of the pelvis and descent of the lumbar spine (Beaugie et al, 1969; Pearlman and Friedman, 1970). The more extensive the resection, the greater the risk of permanent neurological handicap.

Localio et al (1980) reported good results after radical excision: 4 of 5 patients treated for cure using the abdominosacral approach were alive and well at a mean of 7.5 years after operation, the remaining patient having died from a coronary thrombosis 10 years after surgery. On the other hand, Adson (1980) reporting from the Mayo Clinic found that using a variety of approaches 60% of their 57 patients developed recurrence. Others have also found a high recurrence rate (Dahlin and McCartey, 1952; Higinbotham et al, 1967; Chambers and Schwinn, 1979; Böhm et al, 1993). One suspects that the incidence of local recurrence is related to the extent of resection. However, despite the view that the tumour is not radiosensitive, some claim that the combination of radical surgery and adjuvant radiotherapy can reduce recurrence. Thus, Samson et al (1993) operated on 21 patients using the posterior approach, 16 of whom received adjuvant radiotherapy. Four patients died, three of metastatic disease, but 15 (71.4%) were alive at an average of 4.5 years after surgery with no sign of recurrence.

Our own belief is that after careful assessment of the size and degree of tumour spread the situation must be fully discussed with the patient. The risks of impaired bladder, bowel and sexual function must be carefully explained. If the patient agrees, the aim should be a radical excision. We believe that the operation should be carried out with a neurosurgeon and if necessary an orthopaedic surgeon. The bladder should be catheterized and a pressure microtransducer should be inserted. This aids the identification of important sacral roots during the procedure, since stimulation of the roots supplying the bladder will cause an increase in intravesical pressure. The tumour should be approached initially via the trans-sacral route with the patient in the jack-knife position. If the chordoma is deemed operable the cauda equina should be opened and as many of the sacral roots should be dissected from the tumour as is possible with the aid of a nerve stimulator. The tumour, together with the lower two or three segments of the sacrum, are mobilized from the rectum anteriorly. The latter procedure can usually be carried out via the sacral approach as a plane invariably exists between the tumour and the posterior wall of the rectum. However, should this prove difficult the abdomen will need to be opened and the rectum will have to be mobilized. Once the tumour and the lower part of the sacrum have been fully mobilized they can be excised; this will usually require sacrifice of some sacral roots. We always aim to leave at least the third sacral root on one side, but invariably more can be retained.

Although some authors claim that these tumours are radiosensitive (Rosenquist and Saltzman, 1959; Windeyer, 1959), this is not our experience nor that of others (Goligher, 1984). Palliation for inoperable tumours or for recurrence after surgery is therefore a major problem, as severe pain is inevitable (Agular et al, 1994). Such patients may require cordotomy or similar manoeuvres to control their symptoms.

Sacrococcygeal teratoma

Sacrococcygeal teratoma has a solid or partly cystic consistency. It may be situated in front of or behind the sacrum, and the anteriorly placed tumours may encroach on the rectum. A sacrococcygeal teratoma usually remains well encapsulated and consists of tissue derived from all three embryonic layers. It is usually slow growing and may at times not grow at all. If left untreated, sarcomatous change may develop in approximately 12% (Killen and Jackson, 1963). Although sacrococcygeal teratomas occur most often in infants (Schropp et al, 1992) they have also been described in adults. A lateral pelvic radiograph may help in the diagnosis, especially if bone formation or teeth are evident. A pelvic CT or MRI scan (Bachmann et al, 1995) is also of value since it will show the tumour to be encapsulated, a feature that helps to differentiate a teratoma from a chordoma. The tumour may become infected and under these circumstances differentiation from a pelvic abscess may be difficult. There is also the risk that rupture of the tumour either into the rectum or into the peritoneal cavity may occur.

Clinical features are similar to those of chordoma, but since a teratoma tends to remain encapsulated, damage to the sacral nerves is less common, hence neurological symptoms are less frequent.

A teratoma should be excised, and it is usually possible to do this via a trans-sacral approach with the patient in the jack-knife position. If there is any doubt about the diagnosis, or in the case of large tumours, an abdominal approach should be used initially. A combined abdominosacral approach may subsequently be needed.

A sacrococcygeal teratoma should be differentiated from other pathological entities that might encroach on the posterior wall of the rectum, including chronic pelvic abscess, duplication (enterogenous) cysts, and soft tissue tumours which arise in the anorectal space such as lipoma, fibroma, neurofibroma and their malignant counterparts. A sacrococcygeal teratoma should also be differentiated from bony tumours of the sacrum and coccyx, and occasionally it may mimic a meningocele.

Ependymoma

These may arise in the region of the cauda equina, and are the most common tumours of glial origin in the region of the cauda equina. The tumour consists of a papillary neoplasm with cells containing relatively regular nuclei without significant mitotic activity. When Timmerman and Bubrick (1984) reviewed the literature in 1984, 17 cases were described in the postsacral space and 28 were presacral. A presacral ependymoma presents in a similar fashion to a chordoma. Wide local excision is recommended as recurrence is common. This may be done via a transverse posterior incision, which is the method recommended by Böhm et al (1993) (Figures 35.10 and 35.11).

Anterior sacral meningocele

This is a congenital cystic structure that may present as a presacral mass. Situated in the presacral space it

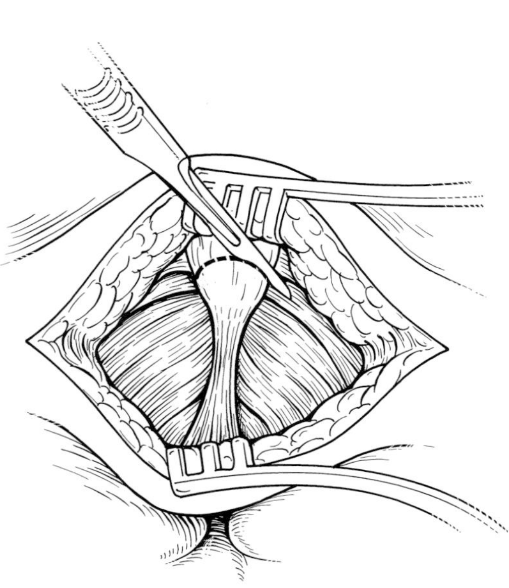

Figure 35.10 Excision of a small presacral developmental cyst via the posterior approach. The coccyx and anococcygeal ligament are exposed after a transverse incision has been made. The coccyx is excised. From Böhm et al (1993).

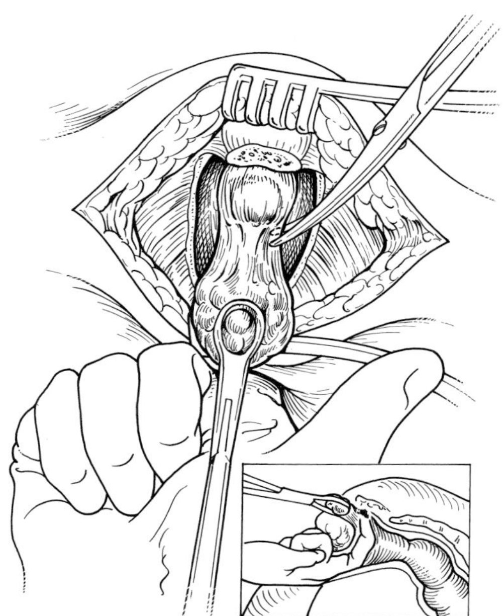

Figure 35.11 Excision of small presacral developmental cyst via posterior approach. The levator ani muscle is transected longitudinally to expose the tumour. To prevent injury of the rectal wall, the surgeon's finger is inserted transanally during mobilization of the tumour.

communicates with the dural sac through a narrow neck that passes through a much larger smooth defect (Kovalcik and Burke, 1988). Radiography of the pelvis may demonstrate the characteristic 'scimitar sign' (see Chapter 17, Figure 17.3b). Once again, treatment is by wide local excision, via a posterior sacral laminectomy.

PSEUDOTUMOURS OF THE COLORECTAL WALL

Pseudotumours are swellings that form in response to the retention of foreign material within the wall of the colon and rectum. The two substances that stimulate such a reaction most frequently are barium and oil. Colorectal duplication may cause similar swellings. Barium may gain access to the bowel wall through a break in the mucosa during radiological investigation. It produces a typical foreign body granulomatous reaction with giant cells. Barium granulomas most commonly occur in the lower rectum, presumably at the site where the enema catheter is introduced. Care in the introduction of the catheter should therefore avoid the problem. The granuloma appears as a submucosal white or yellow nodule or plaque, similar in appearance to a carcinoid tumour. It rarely produces symptoms but for diagnostic purposes it may have to be excised via the transanal route. A similar lesion may occur more proximally if a barium enema is performed soon after a sigmoidoscopic biopsy. For this reason many recommend a 2-week gap between biopsy and radiography (Margulis and Burhenne, 1967).

Mineral oil may enter the rectal wall either as a result of injection of haemorrhoids or when an oil enema is given to a constipated patient. Occasionally in these circumstances the oil initiates a marked foreign body reaction which is characterized by infiltration with mononuclear and epithelioid cells, eosinophils and giant cells surrounding large, clear spaces (Mazier et al, 1978). Under low-power microscopy the appearance resembles a Swiss cheese. An 'oleoma' is usually localized to the submucosa and produces a nodule with inflammation of the overlying mucosa. Excision may be required if the diagnosis is in doubt.

COLORECTAL DUPLICATION

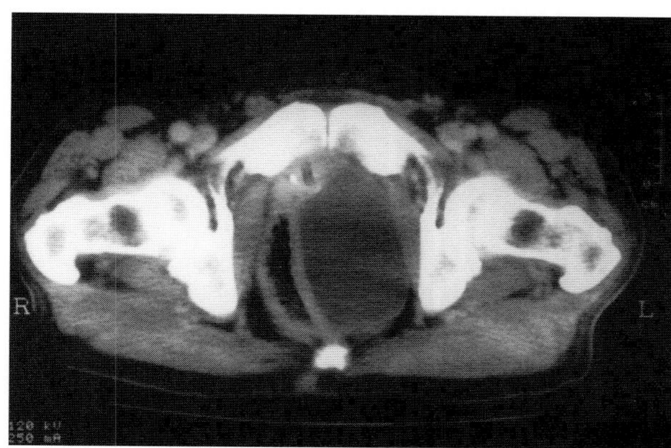

Figure 35.12 Enterogenous cyst. The CT shows a large cystic mass compressing the rectum. At operation, there was no direct communication with rectum, but the cyst was infected and excised locally.

Although not a tumour, a colonic duplication can be mistaken as such and is conveniently dealt with in this section. Colorectal duplications are uncommon congenital anomalies that usually present during infancy or early childhood. Their aetiology and clinical presentation during infancy are discussed in Chapters 71 and 72. Very occasionally they can present in adult life. Whereas obstruction and the presence of an abdominal mass are the clinical features usually apparent in infancy, progressive abdominal pain, bleeding and rarely perforation are characteristic of older children and adults.

True intestinal duplications should be differentiated from enterogenous cysts. The latter arise in the mesentery and retroperitoneal regions; their histology suggests an origin from the bowel, but this connection has generally been lost (Figure 35.12). True duplications are intimately attached to some part of the alimentary tract, and they have a smooth muscle coat and a mucosal lining similar to that of the stomach, small bowel or colon (Bass, 1980). Four subtypes have been described:

1. A tubular duplication branching into the mesenteric leaves.
2. A double-barrelled communicating structure.
3. A free-lying cystic dilatation connected to the gut by a thin mesenteric stalk.
4. A cystic duplication attached to the bowel by a common wall.

Stagnation in the blind pouch variety of duplication may lead to inflammation and stercoral ulceration which may cause pain, discharge if it bursts into the rectum or bleeding and anaemia. Distension of the pouch may cause reflex intestinal hurry and hence interfere with absorption. If the duplication is lined by gastric mucosa, peptic ulceration may occur causing pain and the complications of haemorrhage and perforation.

Plain abdominal radiography may demonstrate a soft tissue mass, evidence of small or large bowel obstruction and the presence of a gas-filled structure with an air fluid level on the erect film (Bass, 1980). Barium enema examination may demonstrate displacement of the bowel, compression by the mass or, in the case of a communicating pouch, an irregular double lumen. The condition is not uncommonly associated with other congenital anomalies such as malrotation, Meckel's diverticulum, lumbosacral anomalies and genitourinary problems. Treatment is governed by the fact that the blood supply to the two parts of the bowel is so intimately joined that separation at the common wall is impracticable. In adults an *en bloc* resection of the duplication and the normal colon is usually required. An alternative therapy for extensive lesions is to lay open the duplication, excise the lining mucosa, oversew the muscular wall and only resect the part of the bowel that bears the stoma leading into the duplication.

Duplication of the rectum is one case where laying open the common wall is perhaps the best option. By doing this a larger rectal structure is formed which functions well. The manoeuvre avoids a difficult pelvic dissection and avoids sacrifice of the rectum and sphincter mechanism in a situation in which the 'cyst' cannot be easily separated from the rectum.

REFERENCES

Abrikossoff AI (1926) Uber Myome, ausgehend von der quergestreften willkurlichen Muskalatur. *Virchows Arch (Path Anat)* **260**: 215–233.

Adson M (1980) In discussion of paper by Localio et al, 1980. *Ann Surg* **194**: 555.

Agular JL, Espachs P, Roca G, Samper D, Cubells C & Vidal F (1994) Difficult management of pain following sacrococcygeal chordoma: 13 months of subarachnoid infusion. *Pain* **59**: 317–320.

Aird I (1957) *A Companion in Surgical Studies*, 2nd edn, p 844. Edinburgh: E&S Livingstone.

Alvich JP & Lepow HI (1960) Cystic lymphangioma of hepatic flexure of colon: report of a case. *Ann Surg* **152**: 880–884.

Anderson PA, Dockerty MB & Buie LA (1950) Myomatous tumours of the rectum (leiomyomas and myosarcomas). *Surgery* **28**: 642–650.

Anson KM, Byrne PO, Robertson ID, Gullan RW & Montgomery ACV (1994) Radical excision of sacrococcygeal tumours. *Br J Surg* **81**: 460–461.

Arnett NL & Friedman PS (1956) Lymphangioma of the colon; roentgen aspects. A case report. *Radiology* **67**: 881–885.

Asbun J, Asbun HJ, Padilla A, Lang A & Bloch J (1992) Leiomyosarcoma of the rectum. *Am Surg* **58**: 311–314.

Astarjian NK, Tseng CH, Keating JA et al (1977) Leiomyosarcoma of the colon: report of a case. *Dis Colon Rectum* **20**: 139–143.

Asuncion CM (1969) Leiomyosarcoma of the rectum: report of two cases. *Dis Colon Rectum* **12**: 281–287.

Ault GW, Smith RS & Castro CF (1951) Hemangiopericytoma of the sigmoid colon: case report. *Surgery* **30**: 523–527.

Azizkhan RG, Tegtmeyer CJ & Wanebo HJ (1985) Malignant rectal carcinoid: a sequential multi-disciplinary approach for successful treatment of hepatic metastases. *Am J Surg* **149**: 210–214.

Bachmann G, Schuck R, Jovanovic V & Bauer T (1995) The MRI in pre- and postnatal diagnosis of congenital sacrococcygeal teratoma [in German]. *Radiologe* **35**: 504–507.

Bacon HE (1964) *Cancer of the Colon, Rectum and Anal Canal*, p 956. Philadelphia: Lippincott.

Baker HL Jr & Good CA (1955) Smooth-muscle tumours of the alimentary tract: their roentgen manifestations. *AJR* **74**: 246–255.

Bass EM (1980) Duplication of the colon. In Greenbourn EI (ed.) *Radiographic Atlas of Colon Disease*, pp 153–158. Chicago: Yearbook Medical.

Bassler A & Peter AG (1949) Fibrosarcoma, an unusual complication of ulcerative colitis, report of a case. *Arch Surg* **59**: 227–231.

Basson MD, Ahlman H, Wangberg B & Modlin IM (1993) Biology and management of the midgut carcinoid. *Am J Surg* **165**: 288–297.

Bates HR Jr (1962) Carcinoid tumours of the rectum. *Dis Colon Rectum* **5**: 270–280.

Beaugie JM, Mann CV & Butler EC (1969) Sacrococcygeal chordoma. *Br J Surg* **56**: 586–588.

Bengmark S & Rosengren K (1970) Angiographic study of the collateral circulation to the liver after ligation of the hepatic artery in man. *Am J Surg* **119**: 620–624.

Bengmark S, Ericsson M, Lunderguist A, Martensson H, Nobin A & Saho M (1982) Temporary liver de-arterialisation in patients with metastatic carcinoid disease. *World J Surg* **6**: 46–53.

Berardi RS (1972) Carcinoid tumours of the colon (exclusive of the rectum): review of the literature. *Dis Colon Rectum* **15**: 383–391.

Berg J & McNeer G (1960) Leiomyosarcoma of the stomach: a clinical and pathological study. *Cancer* **13**: 25–33.

Bhargava KS, Lahiri B, Gupta RC et al (1964) Leiomyosarcoma of the rectum. *J Indian Med Assoc* **42**: 228–230.

Bibro MC, Houlihan RK & Sheahan DG (1980) Colonic ganglioneuroma. *Arch Surg* **115**: 75–77.

Black WC III (1968) Enterochromaffin cell types and corresponding carcinoid tumours. *Lab Invest* **19**: 473–486.

Blatt JM, Kopolovic J, Gimmon Z & Rabinovici N (1979) Leiomyosarcoma of the rectum: diagnostic criteria and surgical approach. *Int Surg* **64**: 67–71.

Böhm B, Milsom JW, Fazio VW, Lavery IC, Church JM & Oakley JR (1993) Our approach to the management of congenital presacral tumors in adults. *Int J Colorectal Dis* **8**: 134–138.

Botting AJ, Soule EH & Brown AL Jr (1965) Smooth muscle tumours in children. *Cancer* **18**: 711–720.

Butler JD, Hershman MJ, Helliwell T, Garvey CJ & Myint S (1997) Stromal cell tumour of rectum treated by transanal endoscopic microsurgery. *J R Soc Med* **90**: 338–339.

Caballero C & Fontaniere B (1993) Sacrococcygeal chordoma: fine needle aspiration cytological findings and differential diagnosis. *Cytopathology* **4**: 311–313.

Caffarena PE, Martinelli M, Fratino G et al (1993) Leiomyosarcoma of the cecum in pediatric age: a case report and review of Italian reports. *Eur J Pediatr Surg* **3**: 306–308.

Caldarola VT, Jackman RJ, Moertel CG & Dockerty MB (1964) Carcinoid tumour of the rectum. *Am J Surg* **107**: 844–849.

Calem SH & Keller RJ (1973) Leiomyosarcoma of the sigmoid colon. *Mt Sinai J Med* **40**: 818–824.

Cappell MS & Botros N (1994) Predominantly gastrointestinal symptoms and signs in 11 consecutive AIDS patients with gastrointestinal lymphoma: a multicenter, multiyear study including 763 HIV-seropositive patients. *Am J Gastroenterol* **89**: 545–549.

Castro EB & Stearns MW (1972) Lipoma of the large intestine. A review of 45 cases. *Dis Colon Rectum* **15**: 441–444.

Chambers PW & Schwinn CP (1979) Chordoma: a clinicopathologic study of metastasis. *Am J Clin Pathol* **72**: 765–766.

Cheek RC & Wilson H (1970) Carcinoid tumours. *Curr Probl Surg* 4–31.

Chernicoff D, Bukowski RM, Groppel W & Hewlett JS (1979) Combination chemotherapy for islet cell carcinoma and metastatic carcinoid tumours with 5-fluorouracil and streptozotocin. *Cancer Treat Rep* **63**: 795–796.

Chetty R & Bhathal PS (1993) Caecal adenocarcinoma with rhabdoid phenotype: an immunohistochemical and ultrastructural analysis. *Virchows Arch A* **422**: 179–183.

Cho KC & Smith TR (1980) Multiple leiomyosarcoma of the transverse colon: report of a case and discussion. *Dis Colon Rectum* **23**: 118–121.

Comer TP, Beahrs OH & Dockerty MB (1971) Primary squamous cell carcinoma and adenoacanthoma of the colon. *Cancer* **28**: 1111–1117.

Contreary K, Nance FC & Becker WF (1980) Primary lymphoma of the gastrointestinal tract. *Ann Surg* **191**: 593–598.

Corman ML (1984) *Colon and Rectal Surgery*. Philadelphia: Lippincott.

Cornes JS (1961) Multiple lymphomatous polyposis of the gastrointestinal tract. *Cancer* **14**: 249.

Cornes JS, Wallace MH & Morson BC (1961) Benign lymphomas of the rectum and anal canal. A study of 100 cases. *J Pathol Bacteriol* **82**: 371–382.

Dahlin DC & McCartey CS (1952) Chordoma: a study of fifty-nine cases. *Cancer* **5**: 1170–1178.

Diamente M & Bacon HE (1967) Leiomyosarcoma of the rectum: report of a case. *Dis Colon Rectum* **10**: 347.

Doak PB, Montgomerie JZ, North JD et al (1968) Reticulum cell sarcoma after renal homotransplantation and azathioprine and prednisone therapy. *BMJ* **4**: 746–748.

Eitan N, Auslander L & Cohen Y (1978) Leiomyosarcoma of the rectum: report of three cases. *Dis Colon Rectum* **21**: 444–446.

Espinosa MH & Quan SHQ (1975) Anal fibrosarcoma: report of a case and review of literature. *Dis Colon Rectum* **18**: 522–527.

Evans N (1919) Malignant myomas and related tumours of the uterus (report of seventy-two cases occurring in a series of 4000 operations for uterine fibromyomas). *Coll Papers Mayo Clinic* **11**: 349–375.

Fahey JL (1971) Cancer in the immunosuppressed patient. *Ann Intern Med* **75**: 310–312.

Fallahzadeh H (1995) Leiomyosarcoma of colon: report of two cases. *Am Surg* **6**: 294–296.

Fayemi AO & Toker C (1974) Gastrointestinal fibroma. A clinicopathological study. *Am J Gastroenterol* **62**: 250–254.

Ferguson EF Jr & Houston CH (1972) Benign and malignant tumours of the colon and rectum. *South Med J* **65**: 1213–1220.

Franquement DW (1995) Differentiation and risk assessment of gastrointestinal stromal tumours. *Am J Clin Pathol* **103**: 41–47.

Genter B, Mir R, Strauss R et al (1982) Hemangiopericytoma of the colon. Report of a case and review of literature. *Dis Colon Rectum* **25**: 149–156.

Gentil F & Coley BL (1948) Sacrococcygeal chordoma. *Ann Surg* **127**: 432–455.

Gerstle JT, Kauffman GL Jr & Koltun WA (1995) The incidence, management, and outcome of patients with gastrointestinal carcinoids and second primary malignancies. *J Am Coll Surg* **180**: 427–432.

Girdwood TG & Philip LD (1971) Lymphatic cysts of the colon. *Gut* **12**: 933–935.

Golden T & Stout AP (1941) Smooth muscle tumours of the gastrointestinal tract and retroperitoneal tissues. *Surg Gynecol Obstet* **73**: 805–810.

Goldstein WB & Poker N (1966) Multiple myeloma involving the gastrointestinal tract. *Gastroenterology* **51**: 87–93.

Goligher J (1984) *Surgery of the Anus, Rectum and Colon*, 5th edn. London: Baillière Tindall.

Gottlieb JA, Baker LH & O'Bryan RM (1975) Adriamycin used alone and in combination for soft tissue and bony sarcomas. *Cancer Chemother Rep* **6**: 271.

Greene EI, Kirshen MM & Greene JM (1962) Lymphangioma of the transverse colon. *Am J Surg* **103**: 723–726.

Habr-Gama A, Campos FG, Ribeiro Junior U, Gansl R, da Silva JH & Pinotti HW (1993) Primary lymphomas of the large intestine [in Portuguese]. *Rev Hosp Clin Fac Med Sao Paulo* **48**: 272–277.

Hackam DJ, Saibil F, Wilson S & Litwin D (1996) Laparoscopic management of intussusception caused by colonic lipomata: a case report and review of the literature. *Surg Laparosc Endosc* **6**: 155–159.

Haller D & Roberts TW (1964) Lipomas of the colon. A clinicopathologic study of 20 cases. *Surgery* **55**: 773–781.

Halls JM (1980) Lymphomas of the large intestine. In Greenbaum EI (ed.) *Radiographic Atlas of Colon Disease*, pp 303–309. Chicago: Yearbook Medical.

Hampton JM & Gandy JR (1957) Plasmacytoma of the gastrointestinal tract. *Ann Surg* **145**: 415–422.

Helwig EB & Hansen MC (1951) Lymphoid polyps (benign lymphoma) and malignant lymphoma of the rectum and anus. *Surg Gynecol Obstet* **92**: 23.

Higgason JM (1958) Lymphatic cyst of the transverse colon. Report of a case. *AJR* **79**: 850–853.

Higinbotham NL, Phillips H, Farr W et al (1967) Chordoma: thirty-five year study at Memorial Hospital. *Cancer* **20**: 1841–1850.

Hoehn JL, Hamilton GH & Beltaos E (1980) Fibrosarcoma of the colon. *J Surg Oncol* **13**: 223–225.

Holland AJA, Kubacz GJ & Warren JR (1997) Plasmacytoma of the sigmoid colon associated with a diverticular stricture: case report and review of the literature. *J R Coll Surg Edinb* **42**: 47–49.

Hughes DE, Lamb J, Salter DM & al-Nafussi A (1992) Fine-needle aspiration cytology in a case of chordoma. *Cytopathology* **3**: 129–133.

Hurlimann J & Gardiol D (1991) Gastrointestinal stromal tumours. An immunohistochemical study of 165 cases. *Histopathology* **19**: 311–320.

Hwang WS, Yao JC, Cheng SS & Tseng HH (1992) Primary colorectal lymphoma in Taiwan. *Cancer* **70**: 575–580.

Issacson PG & Wright DH (1986) Immunocytochemistry of lymphoreticular tumours. In Poluk N & van Noorden S (eds) *Immunocytochemistry. Modern Methods and Applications*, 2nd edn. Bristol: Wright.

Jenkins CN & Colquhoun IR (1995) Case report: symptomatic metastasis from a sacrococcygeal chordoma. *Clin Radiol* **50**: 416–417.

Jetmore AB, Ray JE, Gathright JB Jr, McMullen KM, Hicks TC & Timmcke AE (1992) Rectal carcinoids: the most frequent carcinoid tumor. *Dis Colon Rectum* **35**: 717–725.

Kadakia SC, Kadakia AS & Seargent K (1992) Endoscopic removal of colonic leiomyoma. *J Clin Gastroenterol* **15**: 59–62.

Kakitsubata Y, Kakitsubata S, Nagatomo H, Mitsuo H, Yamada H & Watanabe K (1993) CT manifestations of lipomas of the small intestine and colon. *Clin Imaging* **17**: 179–182.

Killen DA & Jackson LM (1963) Sacrococcygeal teratoma in the adult. *Arch Surg (Chicago)* **88**: 425.

Kim HH & Williams NS (1972) Endometrioid carcinoma of the uterus and ovaries associated with immunosuppressive therapy and anticoagulation: report of a case. *Mayo Clin Proc* **47**: 39–41.

King R, Quinonez GE & Gough JC (1996) Fine needle aspiration biopsy diagnosis of a gastrointestinal stromal tumour utilizing transmission electron microscopy. *Acta Cytol* **40**: 581–584.

Klinge F (1928) Ueber die sogenannten ureifen, nicht guergestreften Myoblastenmyome. *Verh Dtsch Ges Pathol* **23**: 376–382.

Koenig RR, Claudon DB & Byrne RW (1955) Lymphatic cyst of the transverse colon. Report of a case radiographically simulating neoplastic polyp. *Arch Pathol* **60**: 431–434.

Kovalcik PJ & Burke JB (1988) Anterior sacral meningocoele and the Scimitar sign: Report of case. *Dis Colon Rectum* **31**: 806–807.

Kulaylat MN, Doerr R, Butler B, Stachidanand SK & Skingh A (1995) Squamous cell carcinoma complicating idiopathic inflammatory bowel disease. *J Surg Oncol* **59**: 48–55.

Kvols LK, Moertel CG, O'Connell MJ, Schutt AJ, Rubin J & Hahn RG (1986) Treatment of the malignant carcinoid syndrome. Evaluation of a long-acting somatostatin analogue. *N Engl J Med* **315**: 663–666.

Lacava N, Talarico F, Armaroli R et al (1992) Leiomyosarcoma of the rectum [in Italian]. *G Chir* **13**: 353–356.

Le Borgne J, Guiberteau-Canfrere V, Lehur PA et al (1993–94) Leiomyoma of the rectum [in French]. *Chirurgie* **119**: 212–215.

Legha SS, Valdiviescom M, Nelson RS, Benjamin RS & Bodey GP (1977) Chemotherapy for metastatic carcinoid tumours; experiences with 32 patients and a review of the literature. *Cancer Treat Rep* **61**: 703.

Letessier E, Hamy A, Bailly J, Paineau J & Visset J (1992) Leiomyosarcomas of the rectum. Amputation of the rectum or local resection? [in French]. *Ann Chir* **46**: 442–444.

Levy D & Khatib R (1960) Intestinal neurofibromatosis with malignant degeneration. Report of a case. *Dis Colon Rectum* **3**: 140–144.

Levy M, Stone AM & Platt N (1976) Reticulum cell sarcoma of the cecum and macroglobulinemia. A case report. *J Surg Oncol* **8**: 149–153.

Lewin KJ, Ranchod M & Dorfman RF (1978) Lymphomas of the gastrointestinal tract. A study of 117 cases presenting with gastrointestinal disease. *Cancer* **42**: 693–707.

Localio SA, Frances KC & Rossano PG (1967) Abdomino-sacral resection of sacrococcygeal chordoma. *Ann Surg* **166**: 394.

Localio SA, Eng K & Ransom JHC (1980) Abdomino-sacral approach for retrorectal tumours. *Ann Surg* **194**: 555.

Lookanoff VA & Tsapralis PC (1966) Smooth-muscle tumours of the colon. Report of a case involving the cecum and ascending colon. *JAMA* **198**: 206–207.

Lyttle JA (1983) Primary squamous carcinoma of the proximal large bowel. Report of a case and review of the literature. *Dis Colon Rectum* **26**: 279–282.

McCartey CS, Waugh JM, Mayo CW & Coventry MB (1952) Surgical treatment of presacral tumours: a combined problem. *Proc Staff Meet Mayo Clin* **27**: 23.

McDermott EWM, Guduric B & Brennan MF (1994) Prognostic variables in patients with gastrointestinal carcinoid tumours. *Br J Surg* **81**: 1007–1009.

Mackenzie D, McDonald JR & Waugh JM (1954) Leiomyoma and leiomyosarcoma of the colon. *Ann Surg* **139**: 67.

Madiedo G, Komorowski RA & Dhar GH (1980) Granular cell tumour (myoblastoma) of the large intestine removed by colonoscopy. *Gastrointest Endosc* **26**: 108–109.

Manley KA & Skyring AP (1961) Some heritable causes of gastrointestinal disease: special reference to hemorrhage. *Arch Intern Med* **107**: 182–203.

Marcus VA, Viloria J, Owen D & Tsao M-S (1996) Malignant rhabdoid tumor of the colon. Report of a case with molecular analysis. *Dis Colon Rectum* **39**: 1322–1326.

Margulis AR & Burhenne HJ (eds) (1967) *Alimentary Tract Roentgenology, Vol. 2*, p 730. St Louis: CV Mosby.

Marra B (1993) Intestinal occlusion due to a colonic lipoma. Apropos 2 cases [in Italian]. *Minerva Chir* **48**: 1035–1039.

Masson P (1928) Carcinoids and nerve hyperplasia of appendicular mucosa. *Am J Pathol* **4**: 131.

Mayo CW, Pagtalunan RJG & Brown DJ (1963) Lipoma of the alimentary tract. *Surgery (St Louis)* **53**: 598.

Mazier WP, Sun KM & Robertson WG (1978) Oil-induced granuloma (oleoma) of the rectum: report of four cases. *Dis Colon Rectum* **21**: 292–294.

Minsky BD, Cohen AM & Hajdu SI (1991) Conservative management of anal leiomyosarcoma. *Cancer* **68**: 1640–1643.

Moertel CG (1973) Large bowel. In Holland JF & Frei E III (eds) *Cancer Medicine*, pp 1597–1627. Philadelphia: Lea & Febiger.

Moertel CG & Hanley JA (1979) Combination chemotherapy trials in metastatic carcinoid tumour and the malignant carcinoid syndrome. *Cancer Clin Trials* **2**: 327–334.

Moertel CG, Martin J, O'Connell MJ et al (1982) Phase II trials in the treatment of malignant carcinoid and the carcinoid syndrome (abstr). *Proc Am Soc Clin Oncol* **23**: C547.

Montini F, Di Mascio DE, Fossaceca R, Frino F, Angelucci D & Errichi BM (1994) Primary non-Hodgkin's lymphomas of the colon: apropos of a case with double localization [in Italian]. *Chir Ital* **46**: 59–65.

Morgan CN (1932) Endothelioma of the rectum. *Proc R Soc Med* **25**: 1020.

Morgan JG, Marks C & Hearn D (1973) Carcinoid tumours of the gastrointestinal tract. *Ann Surg* **180**: 720.

Morson BC (1960) In Dukes DE (ed.) *Cancer of the Rectum, Vol. 3*, p 92. Edinburgh: E&S Livingstone.

Morton WA & Johnstone FRC (1965) Rectal carcinoids. *Br J Surg* **52**: 391.

Murphy B (1973) Leiomyoma of intestine. *J Ir Med Assoc* **66**: 153–154.

Nemer FD, Stoekinger JM & Evans OT (1977) Smooth-muscle rectal tumours: a therapeutic dilemma. *Dis Colon Rectum* **20**: 405–413.

Norbury LEC (1932) Specimen of endothelium of rectum. *Proc R Soc Med* **25**: 1021.

Ochsner SF, Ray JE & Clark WH Jr (1959) Lymphangioma of the colon: a case report. *Radiology* **72**: 423–425.

Orda R, Bawnik JB, Wiznitzer T et al (1976) Fibroma of the cecum: report of a case. *Dis Colon Rectum* **19**: 626–628.

Orloff MJ (1971) Carcinoid tumours of the rectum. *Cancer* **28**: 175–180.

Pais JR, Garcia-Segovia J, Rodriguez-Garcia JL, Alvarez-Baleriola I & Garcia-Gonzalez M (1994) Solitary plasmacytoma of the rectum: report of a case treated by endoscopic polypectomy and radiotherapy. *Eur J Surg Oncol* **20**: 592–594.

Pearlman AW & Friedman M (1970) Radial radiation therapy of chordoma. *AJR* **108**: 332–341.

Pemberton J & McCormack CJ (1937) Submucous lipomas of colon and rectum. *Am J Surg* **37**: 205–218.

Peskin GW & Orloff MJ (1959) A clinical study of 25 patients with carcinoid tumours of the rectum. *Surg Gynecol Obstet* **109**: 673.

Plate KH & Bittinger A (1992) Value of immunocytochemistry in aspiration cytology of sacrococcygeal chordoma. A report of two cases. *Acta Cytol* **36**: 87–90.

Poate H & Inglis K (1928) Ganglioneuromatosis of the alimentary tract. *Br J Surg* **16**: 221–225.

Price AB (1978) Benign lymphoid polyps and inflammatory polyps. In Morson BC (ed.) *The Pathogenesis of Colorectal Cancer*, pp 33–42. Philadelphia: WB Saunders.

Quan SH & Berg JW (1962) Leiomyoma and leiomyosarcoma of the rectum. *Dis Colon Rectum* **5**: 415–425.

Quan SH, Bader G & Berg JW (1964) Carcinoid tumours of the rectum. *Dis Colon Rectum* **7**: 197–206.

Rao BK, Kapur MM & Roy S (1980) Leiomyosarcoma of the colon. A case report and review of literature. *Dis Colon Rectum* **23**: 184–190.

Rogy MA, Miza D, Berlakovich G, Winkelbauer F & Rauhs R (1991) Submucous large-bowel lipomas – presentation and management. An 18-year study. *Eur J Surg* **157**: 51–55.

Roo T de & Vaas F (1969) Leiomyosarcoma of the transverse and descending colon. Two case reports and review. *Am J Gastroent* **52**: 150–156.

Rose TF (1972) True fibroma of the caecum. *Med J Austr* **1**: 532–533.

Rosenquist H & Saltzman GF (1959) Sacrococcygeal and vertebral chordomas and their treatment. *Acta Radiol* **52**: 177.

Rosenthal DI, Scott JA, Mankin HJ, Wismer GL & Brady TJ (1985) Sacrococcygeal chordoma: magnetic resonance imaging and computer tomography. *AJR Am J Roentgenol* **145**: 143–147.

Rothmund M & Kisker O (1994) Surgical treatment of carcinoid tumors of the small bowel, appendix, colon and rectum. *Digestion* **55** (Suppl 3): 86–91.

Saclarides TJ, Szeluga D & Staren ED (1994) Neuroendocrine cancers of the colon and rectum: results of a ten-year experience. *Dis Colon Rectum* **37**: 635–642.

Saegesser F & Gross M (1969) Carcinoid syndrome and carcinoid tumours of the rectum. *Am J Proctol* **20**: 27–32.

Saltzstein SL (1969) Extranodal malignant lymphomas and pseudolymphomas. *Pathol Ann* **4**: 159–184.

Samson IR, Springfield DS, Suit HD & Makin HJ (1993) Operative treatment of sacrococcygeal chordoma. A review of twenty-one cases. *J Bone Joint Surg Am* **75**: 1476–1484.

Sanders RJ (1961) Leiomyosarcoma of the rectum: report of six cases. *Ann Surg* **154** (Suppl): 150–154.

Sanders RJ & Axtell HK (1964) Carcinoids of the gastrointestinal tract. *Surg Gynecol Obstet* **119**: 369–380.

Sanger BJ & Leckie BD (1959) Plain muscle tumours of the rectum. *Br J Surg* **47**: 196–198.

Schneider TA, Birkett DH & Vernava AM (1992) Primary adenosquamous and squamous cell carcinoma of the colon and rectum. *Int J Colorectal Dis* **7**: 144–147.

Schropp KP, Lobe TE, Rao B et al (1992) Sacrococcygeal teratoma: the experience of four decades. *J Pediatr Surg* **27**: 1075–1078.

Schumann F (1972) Leiomyosarcoma of the colon: report of a case and review of treatment and prognosis. *Dis Colon Rectum* **15**: 211–216.

Sherlock P, Winawer SJ, Goldstein MJ et al (1970) Malignant lymphoma of the gastrointestinal tract. In Glass GB (ed.) *Progress in Gastroenterology, Vol. 2*, pp 367–391. New York: Grune & Stratton.

Sidani MS, Campos MM & Joseph JI (1983) Primary plasmacytomas of the colon. *Dis Colon Rectum* **26**: 182–187.

Siddiqui MN & Garnham JR (1993) Submucosal lipoma of the colon with intussusception. *Postgrad Med J* **69**: 497.

Smith G (1963) Leiomyosarcoma of the rectum. *Br J Surg* **50**: 633–635.

Spread C, Berkel H, Jewell L, Jenkins H & Yakimets W (1994) Colon carcinoid tumors: a population-based study. *Dis Colon Rectum* **37**: 482–491.

Stair MJ, Stevenson DR, Schaffer RF & Lang NP (1983) Leiomyosarcoma of the rectum: report of three cases. *J Surg Oncol* **24**: 180–183.

Stansfield AG (1985) *Lymph Node Biopsy Interpretation*. Edinburgh: Churchill Livingstone.

Stavorovsky M, Jaffa AJ, Papo J & Baratz M (1980) Leiomyosarcoma of the colon and rectum. *Dis Colon Rectum* **23**: 249–254.

Stoller R & Weinstein JJ (1956) Fibrosarcoma of the rectum. A review of the literature and the presentation of 2 additional cases. *Surgery* **39**: 565–573.

Stout AP (1955) Tumours of the colon and rectum (excluding carcinoma and adenoma). *Surg Clin North Am* **35**: 1283–1288.

Stout AP (1959) Tumours of the colon and rectum (excluding carcinoma and adenoma). In Turell R (ed.) *Diseases of the Colon and Ano-rectum*, p 295. Philadelphia: WB Saunders.

Stout AP & Hill WT (1958) Leiomyosarcoma of the superficial soft tissues. *Cancer* **11**: 844–854.

Su WP, Louback JB, Gagne EJ & Scheithauer BW (1993) Chordoma cutis: a report of nineteen patients with cutaneous involvement of chordoma. *J Am Acad Dermatol* **29**: 63–66.

Suarez R, Morrison D, Suarez V (1990) A pain in the rear. *Br J Radiol* **63**: 77–78.

Suga K, Tanaka N, Nakanishi T, Utsumi H & Yamada N (1992) Bone and gallium scintigraphy in sacral chordoma. Report of fours cases. *Clin Nucl Med* **17**: 206–212.

Swanson MA & Schwartz RS (1967) Immunosuppressive therapy. The relation between clinical response and immunologic competence. *N Engl J Med* **277**: 163–170.

Swartzlander FC (1955) *A Clinico-pathological Review of Submucosal Rectal Nodules*. Minnesota: University of Minnesota Press.

Taxy JB, Mendelsohn G & Gupta PK (1980) Carcinoid tumours of the rectum. Silver reactions, fluorescence and serotonin content of the cytoplasmic granules. *Am J Clin Pathol* **74**: 791–795.

Timmerman W & Bubrick MP (1984) Pre-sacral and post-sacral extraspinal ependymoma: a report of a case and review of the literature. *Dis Colon Rectum* **27**: 114–119

Tjandra JJ, Antoniuk PM, Webb B, Petras RE & Fazio VW (1993) Leiomyosarcoma of the rectum and anal canal. *Aust N Z J Surg* **63**: 703–709.

Vezeridis MP, Herrera LO, Lopez GE et al (1983) Squamous-cell carcinoma of the colon and rectum. *Dis Colon Rectum* **26**: 188–191.

Vorobyov GI, Odaryuk TS, Kapuller LL, Shelygin YA & Kornyak BS (1992) Surgical treatment of benign, myomatous rectal tumors. *Dis Colon Rectum* **35**: 328–331.

Vorobyov GI, Odariuk TS, Shelygin IuA et al (1995) Differential diagnosis of non-epithelial rectal neoplasms [in Russian]. *Khirugiia (Mosk)* **1**: 45–50.

Vraux H, Kartheuser A, Haot J et al (1994) Primary squamous-cell carcinoma of the colon: a case report. *Acta Chir Belg* **94**: 318–320.

Waldenstrom JG (1960) Studies on conditions associated with disturbed gamma globulin formation (gammopathies). *Harvey Lect 1960–1961* **56**: 211–231.

Weinberg T & Feldman M (1955) Lipomas of the gastrointestinal tract. *Am J Clin Pathol* **25**: 272–281.

Welch CE & Hedberg SE (1975) *Polypoid Lesions of the Gastrointestinal Tract*, 2nd edn, pp 121–143. Philadelphia: WB Saunders.

Welch JP & Donaldson GA (1974) Recent experience in the management of cancer of the colon and rectum. *Am J Surg* **127**: 258–266.

Wendum D, Vissuzaine C, Bellanger J, Le Goff JY, Behamou G & Potet F (1994) A case of polypoid solitary colonic plasmocytoma. [in French]. *Ann Pathol* **14**: 248–250.

Williams ED & Sandler M (1963) The classification of carcinoid tumours. *Lancet* **i**: 238–239.

Willis RA (1960) *The Borderland of Embryology and Pathology*, pp 348–350. London: Butterworth.

Windeyer BW (1959) Chordoma. *Proc R Soc Med* **52**: 1088.

Witzigmann H, Sagasser J, Leipprandt E & Witte J (1995) Leiomyosarcoma of the rectum [in German]. *Zentralbl Chir* **120**: 69–72.

Wolf O, Glaser F, Kuntz C & Lehnert T (1994) Endorectal ultrasound and leiomyosarcoma of the rectum. *Clin Invest* **72**: 381–384.

Wolfson P & Oh C (1977) Leiomyosarcoma of the anus: report of a case. *Dis Colon Rectum* **20**: 600–602.

Wulff C & Jespersen N (1995) Colo-colonic intussusception caused by lipoma. Case reports. *Acta Radiol* **36**: 478–480.

Wyatt SH, Fishman EK & Jones B (1993) Primary lymphoma of the colon and rectum: CT and barium enema correlation. *Abdom Imaging* **18**: 376–380.

Wychulis AR, Beahrs OH & Woolner LB (1966) Malignant lymphoma of the colon. A study of 69 cases. *Arch Surg* **93**: 215–225.

Yoshikawa O (1969) A case of leiomyosarcoma of the rectum. *Arch Jap Chir* **38**: 342–345.

36

LAPAROSCOPY FOR COLORECTAL CANCER

INTRODUCTION

Since the advent of laparoscopy, surgeons have been forced to re-evaluate almost every surgical procedure, from the most routine inguinal hernia to the most complicated cancer operations. Laparoscopy has become routinely employed for the treatment of both benign inflammatory and non-inflammatory conditions from cholecystectomy to appendicectomy and herniorrhaphy. Advantages of laparoscopy over laparotomy have been more clearly demonstrated for cholescystectomy than for appendicectomy or hernia repair (Spaw et al, 1991; Southern Surgeon's Club, 1991; Gees et al, 1992). Hopes of decreased pain, shorter hospitalization, earlier resumption of preoperative activity and improved cosmetic results have inspired enthusiastic acceptance of this technology both by physicians and by their patients. Many, if not all of these expectations, have been met by laparoscopic removal of the gallbladder and appendix and laparoscopic correction of hernia defects and gastro-oesophageal reflux (Cuschieri, 1992). It is therefore inevitable that laparoscopy should be attempted for colonic disease.

The teleological reasons for the initial use in colonic surgery were the avoidance of a long and often painful incision and more rapid postoperative recovery (Nogueras and Wexner, 1992). Aspiring to these goals, surgeons began performing laparoscopic colectomy for benign disease as early as 1990 (Schlinkert, 1991; Wexner et al, 1992). Almost immediately and prior to any evidence of the oncological merit of the procedure, surgeons reported the performance of laparoscopic colectomy for colorectal malignancy (Viamonte et al, 1994). The reasons for such an impulsive and potentially dangerous acceptance of the new technology were threefold. First, patients recognized the potential clinical benefit. Second, business managers in the healthcare system realized the potential financial savings and the advantages of earlier return of patients to the workforce. Finally, surgeons themselves recognized the need to maintain technological trends and patient and market demands in order to provide current and competitive care.

With respect to the application of this technology to malignancy, our enthusiasm must be tempered with scepticism. It is with such trepidation that in 1991, the Society of American Gastrointestinal

Endoscopic Surgeons (SAGES) recognized that the skills required for laparoscopic bowel surgery as compared to other laparoscopic procedures such as cholecystectomy or appendicectomy were unlike the skills required to perform these same procedures in the conventional fashion. Guidelines were offered for the granting of privileges for surgeons who wished to pursue these procedures (American Society of Colon and Rectal Surgeons, 1991). The potential for technology to supersede reason led the American Society of Colon and Rectal Surgeons (ASCRS) to recommend that laparoscopic surgery for colorectal malignancy should only be undertaken in the setting of a prospective data analysis in which the patient understood that this procedure for that indication remained investigational (Nogueras and Wexner, 1992; Beart et al, 1994).

The purpose of this chapter is not to discuss the feasibility of laparoscopic colectomy. The techniques and accomplishment of these procedures are considered elsewhere in this book (Chapters 6, 8 and 59) and in many articles (Jager and Wexner, 1996; Kok et al, 1996; Milsom and Bohm, 1996; Teoh and Wexner, 1996; Wu et al, 1997). Likewise, this chapter will not invoke laparoscopic colectomy as the new treatment of choice for cancer. Instead, it will critically evaluate the place of the laparoscopic approach in the treatment of colorectal cancer.

In a provocative editorial on laparoscopic surgery for colorectal cancer, Bergamaschi and Myrvold (1997) suggested that the best reason for a change of approach to radical surgery for colorectal cancer should be 'the proven superiority of the new approach to the treatment of benign diseases of the same viscera'. Sadly, this lofty but logical demand has not yet been fulfilled. Even the current prospective randomized National Institute of Health (NIH) trial does not seek to prove its technical superiority in either benign or malignant disease. It simply aims to prove equivalency to laparotomy. This chapter will analyse some of the data regarding laparoscopy for malignancy that may allow surgeons to compare these results to those reported for both conventional surgery for malignancy and laparoscopic colectomy for benign disease.

INDICATIONS AND CONTRAINDICATIONS

The general indications for laparoscopic surgery for colorectal malignancy do not differ from those of laparotomy for colorectal cancer. The most common indication for laparoscopic colectomy in most large series has been for colorectal tumours. The only caveat is that before attempting laparoscopic colectomy the tumour must be localized precisely. Methods for preoperative or intraoperative localization will be discussed in the next section.

Outside well-designed prospective trials, benign neoplasms and palliation for metastatic disease are the most widely accepted indications for laparoscopic bowel resection (Teoh and Wexner, 1996). Patients with multiple metastases have an extremely shortened survival and may benefit the most from the purported advantages of laparoscopic surgery. Removal of the segment of tumour-bearing colon without an extensive oncologic dissection will usually suffice from the palliative point of view. In addition, biopsies of the liver may be undertaken under direct vision with a Tru-cut needle percutaneously inserted with visual camera guidance. Milsom and Bohm (1996) have asserted that this method is the 'most feasible oncologic bowel resection' and that the laparoscopist should perform this type of evaluation prior to attempting curative resection. Bearing this in mind, the decision to operate on any patient with a malignancy should first be based on physician factors, primarily the surgeons' expertise in the performance of laparoscopic colectomy. As yet there are no data regarding the exact number of laparoscopic bowel resections that one must perform before a minimal level of competence is obtained. It is clear from urological data that complication rates are related to the experience of not only the surgeon performing the procedure, but also to the experience of the entire surgical team which assists with the procedure. See et al (1993) published a survey of 297 urological surgeons who had completed a standard laparoscopy-training course. Some of these surgeons sought additional training in advanced techniques. At 3 months, the surgeons who performed procedures without additional training were 3.39 times more likely to have had at least one complication when compared to their peers with the extra training ($P = 0.03$). A 12-month analysis of these surgeons revealed the importance of the 'laparoscopy team'; surgeons who had attended the training course alone, in solo practice, or who performed laparoscopic surgery with different assistants were 4.85, 7.74 and 4.80 times more likely, respectively, ($P = 0.004$, $P = 0.0008$, $P = 0.0015$) to have had a complication than were their counterparts who attended the course with a partner, were in a group practice, or operated with the same assistant (See et al, 1993). It is not unreasonable to extrapolate these data to the performance of laparoscopic colectomy; moreover, many authors have clearly demonstrated the decrease in morbidity with increasing experience.

Larach et al (1993a) reported their group's initial experience of performing a variety of laparoscopic-assisted colon resections on 18 of their patients in a 7-month period from October 1991 to April 1992. Eleven patients (62%) had undergone a previous abdominal procedure, usually an appendicectomy or cholecystectomy, and 13 of the 18 cases (72%) had cancer. The operative time was almost 50% longer than similar procedures carried out by laparotomy and the complication rate directly related to the laparoscopic procedure was 39% (7 of 18 patients). Included in the complication list were three episodes of bleeding, two bowel perforations (one related to the Babcock clamp), and resection of the wrong segment of bowel. Larach's critical analysis of their results led to some important conclusions. Mastery of the technique requires specialty training and should be performed by experienced surgeons who are well versed with the anatomy and the performance of these techniques via laparotomy. Second, the novice should begin by operating on a highly selected group of patients who are thin, have a 'virgin' abdomen and have minimal comorbid illness. With experience, both operating time and complication rates will fall. Hoffman et al (1994) performed 80 laparoscopic-assisted colectomies over a 14-month period and found that their conversion rate dropped from 30% in their first 40 cases to 15% in their last 40, giving them an overall conversion rate of 22.5%.

Hoffman's operative team included two board-certified general surgeons with advanced laparoscopic experience as well as a camera operator and a surgical nurse. The justification and logic of two trained surgeons is obvious: first, it broadens each individual's experience; second, it facilitates decision-making; finally, it allows improved exposure and reduces fatigue. For these reasons, these procedures should be attempted in centres with experienced surgeons and a dedicated support staff. This caveat is particularly true for malignancy where difficulties with intraoperative dissection can have devastating results; thus, operator inexperience should be an important contraindication.

Patient factors establish the principal indications and contraindications to laparoscopy. Not surprisingly, the pulmonary and haemodynamic sequelae of pneumoperitoneum have resulted in higher morbidity and mortality from laparoscopic surgery despite the potential benefits from reduced invasiveness and easier postoperative recovery. The physiological stresses associated with laparoscopic surgery may be more detrimental than those associated with laparotomy in this group of patients (Whitgen et al, 1993; Chiu et al, 1993; Safran and Orlando, 1994). Conversely, Safran et al (1993) showed with intensive monitoring that high-risk cardiac patients had no increase in postoperative cardiovascular complications following laparoscopic cholecystectomy. Laparoscopic colectomy differs, however, in the length of the procedure, the Lloyd Davies (lithotomy) position, prolonged periods of Trendelenburg and the extent of the dissection. Therefore, laparoscopic bowel surgery may impose a greater stress on the patient than does laparoscopic cholecystectomy and patients must be individualized and undergo extensive preoperative medical evaluation.

Other patient factors that generally serve as contraindications to laparoscopic surgery include access problems such as morbid obesity, intra-abdominal adhesions due to previous surgery, and intestinal obstruction with concomitant distension. These features may be viewed as relative contraindications and the experienced laparoscopist may begin to perform the procedure but should have a low threshold for conversion. Failure of the operation to progress within 2 hours or failure of any one portion to progress within 30 minutes are both indications to convert. Conversion should never be viewed as failure but rather as the exercise of common sense to ensure patient safety. Conversions generally occur in one of two scenarios: first, the surgeon recognizes a high likelihood of morbidity due to dense adhesions or unclear anatomy; secondly, an injury is sustained due to pursuit of the operation despite dense adhesions or unclear anatomy. Patients in the former group whose operations are converted to laparotomy can be expected to have outcomes approximating those of patients who undergo planned laparotomy. However, patients in the latter group can be expected to have a suboptimal outcome with significant increases in morbidity and length of hospitalization.

More absolute contraindications to laparoscopic colectomy may be concurrent pregnancy or portal hypertension with coagulopathy (Milsom and Bohm, 1996).

Certain features of the tumour may mitigate against laparoscopy for resection. Whether a tumour truly infiltrates or is merely attached to contiguous structures by an inflammatory response is an important consideration, since an en bloc resection must be undertaken in case tumour infiltration is ultimately proven. This type of operation offers the only potential for cure; laparotomy may be required for a multivisceral resection. Obstructing tumours that result in visceral distension should also preclude laparoscopic resection. Oedema of the bowel wall and its mesentery that result from the sequestration of fluid, combined with reduced visibility create a hazardous situation. Finally, large, bulky tumours can be extremely difficult to mobilize, which increases the risk of possible bowel injury and intraperitoneal spillage of tumour cells. These sizeable tumours require a large incision in order to extract the tumour from the abdominal cavity safely without damaging the bowel wall as can occur when removing a large specimen from a small wound. There is no exact size that absolutely contraindicates laparoscopic removal (Milsom and Bohm, 1996). The decision to resect these tumours laparoscopically should be based on the experience of the surgeon and a low threshold for conversion should be maintained. While we have considered any incision >5 cm indicative of a 'conversion', others have reported 'laparoscopic' resections through 25-cm incisions (Fleshman et al, 1996a).

TECHNIQUE

Preoperative evaluation and localization

As in any operation for cancer, adequate preoperative preparation and localization is essential. A thorough history and physical examination will suggest the need for a detailed medical examination or nutritional evaluation. The patient must be able to tolerate a somewhat lengthier procedure. Preoperative investigations should include a complete blood count, blood chemistry, carcinoembryonic antigen (CEA) level and coagulation profile, if indicated. While laparoscopic staging techniques are described and accurate for other pelvic and abdominal malignancies, the complete staging of colorectal cancer by laparoscopy is still evolving (Easter et al, 1992; Flowers et al, 1993). With the loss of tactile sensation, small liver lesions, particularly if they are within the liver substance, may not be recognized. Preoperative abdominal CT is still the best method of staging the liver prior to laparoscopic colectomy. Preoperative abdominal and pelvic CT scan is also useful for mid and low rectal cancer, although rectal ultrasound is even more important to stage lesions relative to depth of penetration and nodal involvement. Adjuvant therapy may be recommended contingent upon the results.

The most crucial factor in the preoperative evaluation is the exact localization of the tumour. In cases where localization has been inadequate, surgeons have reported high conversion rates or removal of the wrong colon segment (Monson et al, 1992; Corbitt, 1992; Larach et al, 1993a). Identification prior to resection may be accomplished in one of four ways: (1) preoperative contrast enema; (2) preoperative colonoscopy with dye injection; (3) intraoperative colonoscopy; or (4) direct visualization.

Large, infiltrative tumours are easily seen through the laparoscope and may not require further evaluation prior to removal, but not all large tumours will extend to the serosal surface. Furthermore, those same tumours may not be suitable for laparoscopic treatment due to increased rates of serosal tumour penetration and implantation. A water-soluble contrast enema is a simple, effective and inexpensive adjunct in such cases. As most colorectal surgeons are accomplished with the colonoscope and as cancer screening may help to identify smaller tumours, preoperative marking with india ink, indigo carmine, indocyanine green or methylene blue may allow visualization during laparoscopy. Finally, intraoperative colonoscopic identification of smaller tumours may help to avoid the removal of a normal colon segment (Monson et al, 1992; McDermott et al, 1994; Reissman et al, 1994; Vara-Thorbeck et al, 1994; Wexner et al, 1995). The colonoscope should be manipulated to the segment containing the tumour. In order to simplify this manoeuvre, a laparoscopic non-crushing bowel clamp is placed proximal to the lesion and colonoscopic progression visualized both through the colonoscope and the laparoscope. Once the lesion is confirmed, clips may be placed at the serosal surface to mark the site. The surgeon must be ready to use each tool in order to remove these tumours accurately and quickly. There have even been reports of laparoscopic bowel mobilization in order to facilitate colonoscopic polypectomy and avoid resection in benign but previously endoscopically inaccessible or unresectable polyps (Beck, 1996; Smedh et al, 1997; Beck and Beart, 1999).

Preoperative preparation

Like any other colon resection, adequate preoperative mechanical bowel preparation and antibiotic prophylaxis are essential (see Chapters 3 and 5). With regards to consent, the patient must be advised of the risks, benefits, potential complications and available alternatives. The patient should also be advised that the long-term benefits of this procedure for colorectal cancer remain as yet unproven. Currently, patients who do meet the inclusion criteria should be entered in prospective, randomized, controlled studies (Nelson et al, 1995).

Operative procedure

Patient positioning, port placement and the use of ureteric stents are discussed in Chapter 6. In addition, the generalities of laparoscopic-assisted colectomy (LAC) and the specifics of each type of resection have also been described in detail (Jager and Wexner, 1996; Milsom and Bohm, 1996; Wexner et al, 1997). The first step after placement of the ports is to perform a thorough search for metastatic deposits. The camera should make an extensive evaluation into the subdiaphragmatic recesses of the liver. One recent advance that may compensate for loss of tactile sensation, particularly in the area of the liver and porta hepatis, is the laparoscopic Doppler probe (Doppler System, Meadox Surgimed, Inc., Oakland, NJ, USA), This 20-MHz probe is 29 cm long and fits into a 5-mm port (Milsom and Bohm, 1996). During colectomy for carcinoma, intraoperative ultrasonography has proven highly specific and sensitive in detecting hepatic lesions (Charnley et al, 1990; Machi et al, 1991). Currently, the accuracy of laparoscopic ultrasonography in detecting liver metastases in patients with colorectal cancer is being compared to preoperative contrast-enhanced CT scan (Milsom and Bohm, 1996). Finally, the omentum is investigated and then the small bowel may be evaluated from the terminal ileum to the ligament of Treitz by a gentle two-handed technique.

In performing colorectal resections for cancer through the laparoscope, the surgeon must comply with all principles accumulated through experience with laparotomy. Complete mobilization of the colon from its attachments is done with as little manipulation of the tumour-bearing segment as possible (Figure 36.1). Turnbull et al (1967) proposed that forceful manipulation of the tumour during mobilization and resection would lead to increased shedding of viable cancer cells both locally and to distant sites; early isolation and exclusion of the lymphovascular pedicles prior to complete mobilization and removal prevents this. In a randomized, prospective trial from The Netherlands, the no-touch technique (NTT) was compared to conventional techniques by assessing the results of 236 resections for both local and distant recurrence (Wiggers et al, 1986). There was no difference in the local recurrence between the 117 patients who underwent NTT and the 119 patients who had conventional techniques. Distant metastases, however, did occur later and with less frequency in the NTT group, suggesting a benefit from this almost 30-year-old technique. As yet, there is no proof that laparoscopic bowel mobilization can absolutely adhere to the standards of NTT and prospective data are forthcoming. All of the technical descriptions of laparoscopic colectomy emphasize the importance of atraumatic manipulation of the tissue.

The next technical point is the proximal ligation of the lymphovascular pedicle. When done extracorporeally, the incision is made only after complete

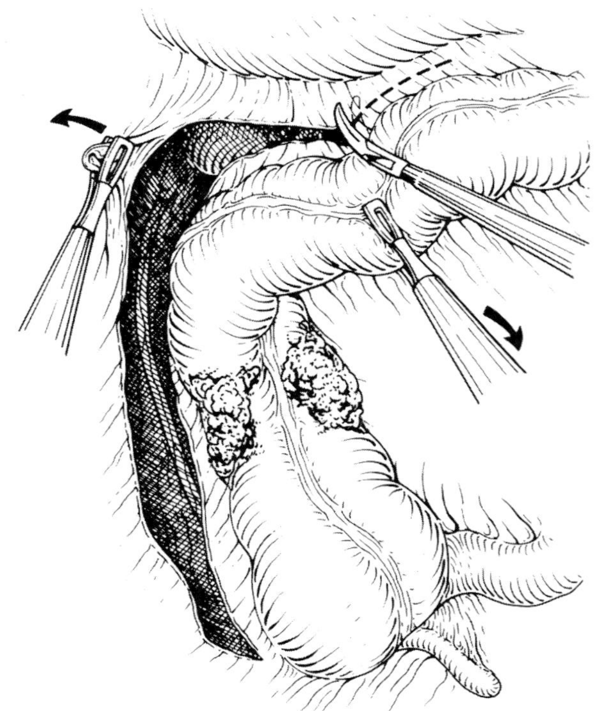

Figure 36.1 Laparoscopic right hemicolectomy. The ascending colon and transverse colon can be retracted in such a way (inferiorly and medially) that the omentum is separated from the colon relatively easily.

laparoscopic mobilization of the bowel (Figure 36.2a,b). This incision is much smaller than a laparotomy and the evisceration of the pathological segment can, at times, be challenging. The bowel should not be forced out of the abdomen as such uncontrolled force increases the likelihood of injury to the tumour, forcing malignant cells to local and distant sites. A simple 2-cm extension of the 1-cm umbilical port incision may be adequate to relieve the resistance and allow effortless removal of the segment. Once the bowel is exteriorized, the vessels are ligated as close to their origin as possible. A laparoscopic-assisted right colectomy is most efficiently accomplished in this fashion.

Left-sided lesions requiring left colectomy, sigmoidectomy, low anterior resection or abdominoperineal resections usually require the ligation of only two vessels, the inferior mesenteric artery (IMA) and veins; when applicable, the anastomosis is effected intracorporeally with a circular stapler (Figure 36.3a–d). For these reasons, the vessels for left-sided lesions are ligated using laparoscopic stapling devices. High ligation of the IMA for left colon, sigmoid and rectal tumours is controversial even in conventional surgery. Morgan and Griffiths (1959) advocated high ligation to include the left colic artery in 1959, over 50 years after WE Miles' (1908) original description. The Miles' operation included ligation of the IMA up to but not including its left colic branch. The controversy was revisited in the 1960s by Bacon and Khubchandani (1964), in the 1980s by Pezim and Nicholls (1984), and then by Surtees et al (1990). These data indicated that more proximal ligation of the IMA offered no survival advantage. However, such a level of ligation does facilitate the dissection including entry into the presacral space, and improves staging and sympathetic nerve identification. It also encourages a tension-free low anastomosis.

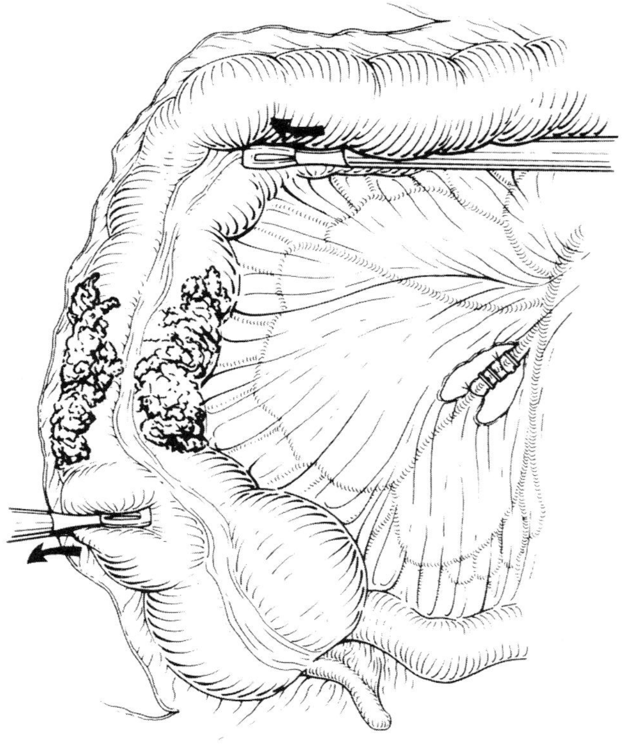

(a)

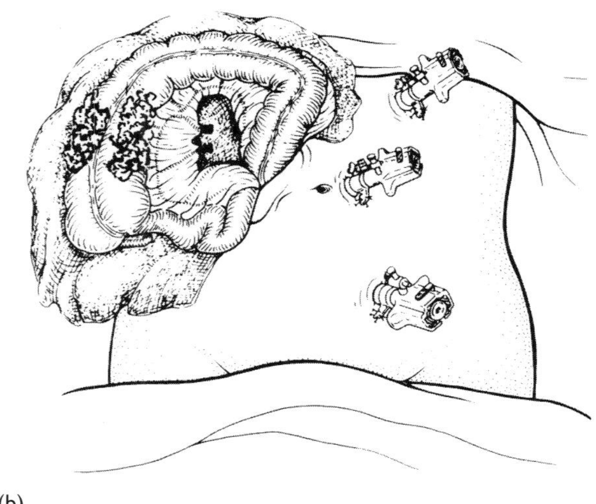

(b)

Figure 36.2 Laparoscopically assisted right hemicolectomy. (a) The mesentery is placed on tension, which facilitates identification of the superior mesenteric, ileocolic, right colic, and middle colic vessels. The primary vascular bundle that needs to be ligated laparoscopically is the ileocolic arcade. Vessels are double-clipped and endolooped. Once the ileocolic vascular pedicle is ligated, the bowel is fully mobile and is exteriorized easily. (b) Usually the mobile right colon reaches to the abdominal wall at the site of the right abdominal cannula; thus the 4- to 6-cm transverse incision should be made there. After bringing the bowel through the incision, the right branch of the middle colic artery may be easily ligated.

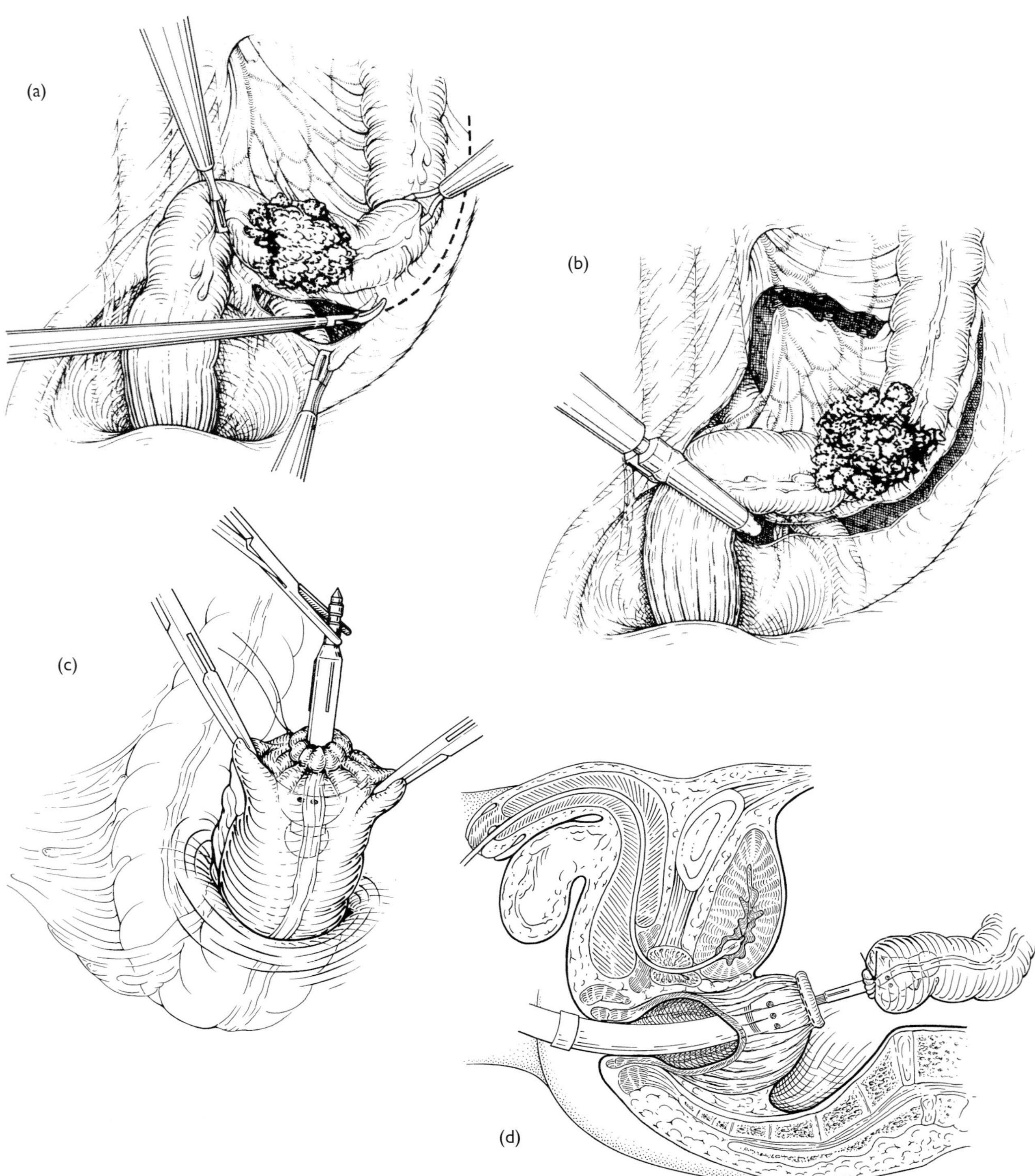

Figure 36.3 Laparoscopically assisted sigmoid resection. (a) The surgeon elevates the sigmoid colon in a cephalad direction and to the right using one hand, while the peritoneal attachments are divided with cautery using the other. The ureter is now identified. (b) Once the bowel is mobilized and the sigmoid/superior haemorrhoidal vascular pedicle ligated, the distal rectum is divided using one (or more) applications of the 60-mm linear stapler. A 20-mm cannula is required for this stapler and is placed through the right lower abdominal cannula site. The proximal bowel is then exteriorized, usually through a transverse incision no more than 6 cm long at the left mid-abdominal cannula site for placement of a purse string and resection. (c) After the bowel is resected, the anvil of a circular stapler is secured in the proximal bowel. The bowel and anvil are then returned to the abdominal cavity. (d) The circular stapler is then introduced per anus and a double-stapled anterior resection performed.

CLINICAL TRIALS OF LAPAROSCOPIC-ASSISTED COLECTOMY FOR MALIGNANCY

Retrospective data

The largest of the three retrospective analyses was performed by the Clinical Outcomes of Surgical Therapy (COST) Study Group. This included a review of 372 patients who had colorectal cancer laparoscopically resected by 32 surgeons chosen to participate in the national, prospective, randomized, controlled trial comparing laparoscopy and laparotomy for cure of colon carcinoma. This study hoped to gauge the adequacy and early success of this treatment by the potential trial participants during the beginning of the learning curve (Fleshman et al, 1996b). The data for each patient included follow-up information such as the presence of local, distant or trocar site recurrence and death attributable to the disease. Eighty-two per cent of the patients had curable lesions (TNM stage I, II or III) and over 80% of the cases were laparoscopically completed. The projected 3-year survivals in this study for stages I–IV were 93%, 72%, 53% and 10% respectively, comparing favourably to the results from conventional resection (Umpley et al, 1984). The operative mortality was only 2% and disease-related mortality in the patients treated for cure was only 3.6% (11 of 304 with one stage I, three stage II and eight stage III patients succumbing to their disease within 35 months). Finally, local recurrence was documented in 13 patients (3.5%) and trocar site and abdominal wall implants in four patients (1.3%) with curable lesions.

After laparotomy, the locoregional recurrence rates ranged from 5% to 19% for colon tumours and 7% to 45% for rectal lesions. These data therefore compare favourably with the results of the COST study and others (Turk and Wanebo, 1993). Similarly, abdominal wall recurrence has been reported after laparotomy for colorectal cancer with rates of 1% reported by Hughes et al (1983) and 1.5% noted by the North Central Cancer Treatment Group in 1996 (Reilly et al, 1996). However, excluding patients with carcinomatosis, the isolated wound implantation rates were less than 0.3%. These results indicated that laparoscopic-assisted colectomy could be safely completed with identical short-term survival. The study was able ethically to justify proceeding with the prospective randomized study on the basis of expected equivalence of the two procedures as highlighted by the low locoregional and trocar site metastases rates.

Three retrospective reviews assessed laparoscopic-assisted colectomies (LAC) for all indications, benign and malignant, and compared the results of the operation to either historical controls or to a control group comprised of the patients whose operations were converted to laparotomy. The first study, by Gellman et al (1996), was a single-institution survey of 104 attempted laparoscopic colectomies. Over half (58 of 104) of the cases were undertaken for cancer with very low morbidity and mortality, 4.8% and 1.0% respectively. Comparing their results to a group of historical controls from the same institution, the authors claimed that the lymph node retrieval (average of 9.5 in the laparotomy and 9.3 in the LAC groups) and early oncologic results were similar. They failed to identify any trocar site recurrences after resection of curable lesions and the only wound recurrence was noted 4 months after a sigmoid resection in an elderly man with carcinomatosis. This study did show a favourable decrease in length of stay in patients who underwent laparoscopic-assisted colectomy, an average of 5.7 days in the hospital, as compared to laparotomy, in which the average stay was about 11 days.

In another retrospective study, Senagore et al (1993), supported these findings when they compared 102 patients who had undergone laparotomy to 38 laparoscopic cases and found that bowel function returned sooner (3.0 days versus 4.9 days) and length of stay was significantly shorter (6.0 days versus 9.0 days) in the LAC group. The legitimacy of these results was flawed by the study design, and in fact the patients who underwent laparoscopic resection were probably treated more aggressively with regards to diet and activity than were patients after laparotomy; neither study directly addressed this issue.

A further retrospective study was a multicentre Italian study in which 146 of 200 patients had malignant lesions (Huscher et al, 1996). Almost 90% of the patients were operated upon laparoscopically; 37 patients (17.1%) had a complete laparoscopic procedure while 142 patients (71%) had a laparoscopic-assisted procedure. The 21 patients who had their procedure converted to laparotomy because of distorted anatomy (7 cases), adhesions (9 cases), obesity (3 cases), ureteral damage or instrument failure (1 case each) served as a 'control group' to assess return of intestinal function and length of hospitalization. The 'controls' were not used to scrutinize the oncologic integrity of the procedures. The majority of the lesions were Dukes' B or C tumours with a preponderance of left-sided neoplasms. The average proximal margin was 11.1 (range 3–35) cm and the average distal margin, 7.4 (range 1–32) cm; the average lymph node harvest varied from 9 nodes in rectal specimens to 12.6 nodes in right colon specimens. These figures were comparable to those published in the literature (Jass et al, 1986; Herrera-Ornelas et al, 1987; Scott and Grace, 1989; Cohen and Wexner, 1993) as was the local recurrence rate of 4% (6 of 142) and distant metastasis rate of 6% (9 of 142) with a maximum follow-up of almost 28 months. There were no reported cases of port site recurrence. Compared to the converted group, return of bowel function, as indicated by passage of flatus, occurred more than 24 hours earlier in the laparoscopic group (2.5 days versus 3.8 days). The first bowel movement, however, took place at approximately the same time period after operation (4.0 and 4.8 days in the laparoscopic and converted groups respectively). The average length of stay in the hospital was identical in the two groups even though the comparison group probably had lengthier operations. Thus, reports of earlier discharge were not substantiated by this study.

Prospective comparisons

The majority of the literature on laparoscopic surgery for colorectal malignancy has been in the form of prospective, non-randomized trials with or without historical controls. These studies can be subcategorized as those that discuss laparoscopic resection of malignancy incidentally within the framework of all laparoscopic colon resections; those that deal with all colorectal resections for cancer; and finally those that assess sigmoid and rectal resection, which undoubtedly comprise the majority of resections for cancer and may thus have the greatest impact.

Two studies, from Lumley et al (1996) and Fielding et al (1997) in Australia, are successive analyses of the results of laparoscopic colectomy for a variety of disorders. Malignancy constituted the primary indication in over 40% of the cases in both trials and the overall results were identical. Recurrence was reported in 5 of the first 103 resections and 10 of the total of 149 patients with two port site recurrences. One of the port site metastases occurred in a patient with a stage C lesion in the setting of concurrent para-aortic and liver disease and the second, in a patient with disseminated disease at the initial operation. The majority of resections were done for Dukes' B or C lesions with anterior resection as the most common operation performed. The authors remarked particularly upon the low incidence of leakage in the low circular stapled anastomosis in these studies, about 2.5%.

Phillips et al (1992) reported 51 laparoscopic colectomies for various indications including cancer. One concerning figure in their study was the 18% incidence of anastomosis dehiscence, being almost nine times greater than that seen during laparotomy (Lazorthes and Chiotassol, 1986). Although these authors were able to avert disaster by recognition of the problem, other less experienced surgeons may not have perceived the compromise in technique and thus may have endangered their patients. The Australian experience reassures us that, after appropriate experience has been obtained, results comparable to conventional resection can be expected.

The study from Phillips et al (1992) also revealed the existence of rather unorthodox laparoscopic practices. Sixteen per cent of their patients (8 out of 51) underwent laparoscopic colotomy and wedge resection of polyps. Likewise, Lauroy et al (1994) described a wound metastasis after laparoscopic colotomy for excision of a dysplastic villous tumour. This procedure is mentioned only to be condemned, as local recurrence rates have been shown to be unacceptably high after such operations, even when performed by open operation (Goligher, 1980; Wexner, 1991). This technique is an obvious departure from conventional surgical practice in order to facilitate an otherwise difficult technology. The incidence of malignant change in larger sessile polyps is high. As such, a standard cancer operation is mandatory and must be undertaken independent of the technical approach used or the preoperative awareness of the existence of malignancy within the lesion (Haggitt et al, 1985; Nivatvongs et al, 1991).

Another unorthodox feature of laparoscopic colectomy is the loss of tactile ability and this has forced some laparoscopic procedures to be aborted. Corbitt (1992) was only able to complete 15 of 18 laparoscopic-assisted colectomies due to an inability to laparoscopically identify the lesion. Others, such as Larach et al (1993b) and Monson et al (1992), have reported the laparoscopic removal of the wrong segment of bowel. Both Vara-Thorbeck et al (1994) and McDermott et al (1994) had to re-operate upon patients who obstructed from preoperatively unrecognized proximal synchronous malignancies. In fact, in a 1994 postal survey of the members of the American Society of Colon and Rectal Surgeons, 18 additional instances of incorrect segmental resection were recorded (Wexner et al, 1995). Over two-thirds of these respondents advocated routine use of either intraoperative colonoscopy or preoperative ink 'tattooing' of the lesion to avoid such problems.

Recently, there have been multiple prospective reports on the feasibility and obvious worldwide acceptance of this technology for a variety of indications that, at least initially, included a majority of benign colorectal conditions. Now, however, malignancy is by far the most common primary indication for laparoscopic colectomy in most series including those from The Netherlands (67 of 116 patients from three institutions with carcinoma), Spain (53 patients with cancer from a personal series of 64 operations) and Germany (235 of 504 patients from 17 different centres). Combined, these studies admit conversion rates of 7% to 17%, with operative mortality ranging from 0 to 1.7% and morbidity ranging from 8% to 14% (Jansen et al, 1994; Cruz-Vigo et al, 1996; Kockerling et al, 1997). There were no control groups and little follow-up so that no discussion about the oncologic outcome of their patients was included from any of these countries.

Quattlebaum et al (1993) reported on 40 laparoscopically assisted colon resections for indications including cancer, diverticular disease, and a variety of other benign conditions. They performed the gamut of colon resections with most of the procedures completed within 90 (range 30–90) minutes and denied any intraoperative mortality or morbidity. They did report on the postoperative care of the cancer patients who, like the patients with benign disease, had return of gastrointestinal function within 2.5 days and were discharged home in a comparable length of time (average of 4.2 days and 4.6 days for benign and malignant disease respectively). These results are analogous to those reported by Scoggin et al (1993), whose patients had return of bowel function (patient passing flatus) within 1.9 days and tolerance of oral feeding within 2.3 days. Jacobs et al (1991) also reported clear liquids were tolerated by 18 of their 20 patients on the first postoperative day and 14 of these patients were home by day four. Interestingly, Quattlebaum (1993) did detail one early local recurrence in a patient one year after laparoscopic resection of a Dukes' C splenic flexure carcinoma. This local recurrence of a colonic, as opposed to a rectal, neoplasm must be regarded as a failure of the technique and reminds the surgeon both of the importance of an honest and detailed informed consent and the investigational nature of the procedure.

Despite the prospective nature of the studies discussed above, they focus on the general plausibility and results of laparoscopic surgery and suffer from the lack of a control group. The next group of studies, while non-randomized, concentrate solely on laparoscopic surgery for large bowel cancer. Kwok et al (1996) from Hong Kong analysed their results of laparoscopic-assisted colon and rectal resections over a 30-month period with a median follow-up of only 15.2 (range 2.5–32.7) months. They divided their experience into two phases. Phase one included the first 30 patients comprised only of individuals older than 65 years of age and/or those who required palliative resection. The only other exclusion criterion was a distal rectal tumour within 5 cm of the dentate line that was potentially amenable to a restorative procedure. Distal rectal tumours 5 cm or less from the anal verge underwent laparoscopic abdominoperineal resections. The conversion rate in this initial group of patients was 33.3%, forcing the authors to reassess these indications.

Phase two of this study included the next 70 patients consisting of all age groups requiring both curative and palliative resections and excluded the distal rectal tumours within 5 cm of the dentate line, bulky tumours (6 cm or larger), locally advanced disease, patients with previous major abdominal surgery and patients who presented with obstruction or perforation. With these constraints, the authors were able to reduce the conversion rate to 8.9%. The mean number of lymph nodes removed was 12.8 and all distal and lateral margins were negative, again supporting adequate oncologic clearance with minimally invasive techniques. There was one port site recurrence in a patient with widespread carcinomatosis, but no isolated port site metastases. There was also one abdominal wound recurrence that occurred after a palliative right hemicolectomy at the specimen extraction site through an extended port site incision. This problem occurred early in the group's experience and they subsequently encouraged the routine use of a plastic wound protector to avoid this complication.

Similar to the above experience, Lord et al (1996) reported a 32% conversion rate during the first 6 months of application of the laparoscope for colon and rectal surgery. This rate dropped to only 8% during the next 6 months. Eight of the 19 complications (14.5%) were directly related to the laparoscopic technique, including four vessel injuries, two trocar site hernias, one ureteric injury and one enterotomy. During their 16.7 month follow-up, they reported no port site recurrence, two distant recurrences after resection of Dukes' C2 lesions and one local recurrence after resection of a Dukes' B2 rectal cancer. In comparison to a matched group of control patients who had right hemicolectomies or anterior resections by laparotomy during the same time period, the laparoscopic node harvest and resection margins were as good or slightly better. There was no significant difference in the length of stay for the right hemicolectomy group, but the patients who had laparoscopic anterior resections were discharged significantly sooner than were their 'conventional' counterparts (5.3 days versus 8.6 days).

Other non-randomized studies have had similar success with regard to completion of the laparoscopic procedure with low complication and recurrence rates. In fact, Viamonte et al (1994) found no port site recurrences in the 91 patients who they were able to laparoscopically resect and Vertruyen et al (1996) stated no isolated parietal recurrence at trocar sites. In the latter study, two patients did develop port site metastases in the setting of widely disseminated disease. Although Viamonte's group stated the average overall specimen lengths, neither study provided data on resection margins or tumour heights.

In an attempt to better define their results, Franklin et al (1995) prospectively reviewed 194 patients diagnosed with resectable colorectal cancer, 110 of whom underwent open colon resection (OCR) and 94 of whom had a laparoscopic procedure (LCR). The patients were well-matched for gender, age and tumour stage. One notable feature of this study was the distribution of the cancers. Low anterior resection and APR represented over 65% of the cases and left-sided lesions comprised 85% of the cancers. Oncologically, the resections were the same in the two groups with 'adequate' margins on all specimens and the lymph node retrieval was slightly better in the LCR group. In a postoperative follow-up period of 2–36 months, 22 patients (21%) in the OCR group were lost to follow-up. Sixty-three of the assessable patients in this group (57%) were alive without recurrence; 8 (7%) were alive with recurrence and 16 (15%) were deceased. Only 8% of the patients in the LCR were lost to follow-up during the same period; 60 patients (71%) were alive without evidence of disease while 7 patients (8%) were alive with disease and 11 patients (13%) had died. The three anastomotic recurrences occurred in the OCR group and none of the laparoscopically resected group had local tumour spread or port site metastases.

In addition to the extraordinary laudable oncologic results that these authors were able to obtain, the LCR group also benefited from a significantly shorter hospital stay (7.3 days compared to 12.2 days in the OCR group) and significantly lower wound complication rate (one in the LCR group versus 14 in the OCR group). The shorter hospital stay was attributed to the decrease in postoperative pain allowing earlier mobilization and improved pulmonary function in the LCR group. Recalling the improved postoperative results that Lord et al (1996) were able to attain in the laparoscopic anterior resection group, the large number of left-sided lesions in the study by Franklin et al (1995) may have contributed to the differences in the length of hospital stay between the groups. There is a suggestion that patients after laparoscopic left colon and rectal resections have a tendency towards earlier recovery when compared to patients after right or left colectomy by laparotomy or laparoscopic right hemicolectomy. Whether this feature may be a result of less excessive handling, palpating or packing away of the bowel is conjecture. Smaller incisions, routine closure of port sites, reduction in abdominal wall trauma and the use of plastic wound protectors may explain the lower incidence of incisional hernia and infection in the laparoscopic groups.

In the prospective studies of Franklin et al (1995) and Guillou et al (1993), the majority of laparoscopic resections for malignancy were for left-sided lesions. The value of the laparoscopic approach in the dissection of the rectum for the purpose of either anterior resection or abdominoperineal resection explains the disproportionate number of prospective randomized studies reviewing the results of only these two operations. Rhodes et al (1996) confirmed the feasibility of laparoscopic anterior resection in a study of 84 of these resections in over 200 colorectal procedures. There was an 11% conversion rate, most of which were for failure of the case to progress. Procedure-related morbidity was quite high, with a 20% minor complication rate and a 12% major complication rate within 30 days. There was another 12% rate of delayed complications. Some of these early and late problems included three anastomotic leaks, two anastomotic strictures treated by pneumatic dilatation, three small bowel obstructions requiring laparotomy, and one colocutaneous fistula.

The problem in drawing any conclusions from these results is the absence of a control group. In a study performed by Tate et al (1993), laparoscopic anterior resection was compared to conventional resection in a prospective non-randomized fashion. The patient groups were almost identical in age, sex and presentation. Despite the fact that the mean operating time was significantly longer in the laparoscopic group (205 min versus 123 min; P = 0.01), the time to reinstitution of a normal diet (2.5 days versus 3.6 days; P = 0.01) and postoperative analgesia requirements (2.6 versus 7.4 doses of narcotic; $P = 0.01$) were significantly lower. The average length of hospital stay, 12.3 days in the laparoscopic group versus 14.3 days in the open group, although shorter, did not achieve statistical significance ($P = 0.08$). This study reported no long-term oncologic follow-up but the immediate results, based on histological analysis of the specimen, showed no difference. The number of nodes resected (10 versus 13), the length of the resection (14 cm versus 15 cm), and the distal margin (2.0 cm versus 2.5 cm), were almost identical for the laparoscopic and open groups respectively. Importantly, the minimum length of the distal margin, although 2.0 cm in the laparotomy group, was only 0.5 cm in the laparoscopy group. Clearly such an unacceptably short margin highlights the technical difficulty of low rectal transection by laparoscopic techniques. Another inherent difficulty is the inability to assess the tumour-free distal margin which can, during laparotomy, result in restorative proctectomy rather than sphincter excision.

Goh et al (1997), from Singapore, reported a prospective, non-randomized, controlled comparison of laparoscopic anterior resection (LAR) and open anterior resection (OAR) for rectosigmoid cancer. Other than the actual procedure performed, the pre- and postoperative care of the patients was standardized in order to compare the operative results and postoperative recovery. The median operating time was 90 (range 55–185) minutes in the LAR group compared to 73 (range 40–140) minutes for the OAR patients with no intraoperative complications and no conversions: these results attest to the importance of both patient selection (maintaining strict operative criteria but also alluding to the relative absence of obesity in the Singapore population) and technical prowess. They carefully selected favourable cases for laparoscopy and less favourable cases for laparotomy; there were 20 patients in each group. Patients were excluded from laparoscopy if they had a palpable tumour, a previous laparotomy, a 'low' or 'ultra low' level of anastomosis or a low tumour height. Furthermore, the tumour heights were not stated. The method of selection for patients in the laparotomy group was also not stated but presumably included all of those patients excluded from the laparotomy arm. They also stated their definition of conversion as 'if the open method became necessary for the safe completion'.

The mean incision length in the 20 patients in the laparoscopic group was 5.5 (range 4–13) cm; the mean incision length of the 20 patients who underwent laparotomy was 18 (range 8–25) cm. Pathological scrutiny revealed an average of 4 cm to 4.5 cm margins on the specimen with negative lateral margins and a median of 20 (range 7–49) and 19 (range 7–97) harvested lymph nodes in the LAR and OAR groups respectively. Despite weighting the study in favour of laparoscopy, none of the benefits of laparoscopic anterior resection noted in the previous studies were reproduced. The authors suggested that routine use of a small left iliac fossa incision in the OAR group and the subspecialized care of a tertiary referral unit as possible explanations for these disappointing results. Ultimately, the authors concluded that 'we have not been able to demonstrate a significantly improved postoperative function'. This conclusion was despite their best attempt to do so in terms of patient selection and data analysis.

In colon cancer, the adequacy of resection is measured in proximal and distal margins and in the removal of the lymph-bearing tissue. Local recurrence is fairly uncommon if these factors are taken into consideration. Conversely, in rectal cancer surgery, complete radial clearance of the tumour supersedes all other variables in the avoidance of local recurrence. In 1992, Sackier (1992) and Coller (1992) both described the technique of laparoscopic abdominoperineal resection (LAPR). The reports that the laparoscope provided a remarkably clear view of the pelvis and a more precise dissection of blood vessels and nerves (Larach et al, 1993b; Darzi et al, 1995), inspired the growth of LAPR for both rectal (Chindasub et al, 1994) and anal cancer (Targarona et al, 1993).

Since Heald's original description of total mesorectal excision in 1982 (Heald et al, 1982), many colorectal surgeons have adopted this technique for the resection of mid and distal rectal tumours (MacFarlane et al, 1993; Enker et al, 1995; Aitken, 1996; Arbman et al, 1996; Leo et al, 1996). LAPR is indicated for low rectal tumours at a level that would not permit a sphincter-preserving operation. The difficulty in assessing the possibility of restoring continuity after mobilization with either a straight or a colonic pouch anastomosis, limits the utility of laparoscopy for distal rectal lesions. Whether it is done laparoscopically or by laparotomy, abdominoperineal resection is a technically demanding procedure that is already described elsewhere (Chapter 32). APR is a technically gratifying operation, particularly as only limited vascular control is needed (the inferior mesenteric artery and vein and the marginal arcade), there is excellent magnification in the pelvis and no need for any abdominal incision other than the stoma site. Because of these factors, surgeons may be more inclined to perform a rapid, technically easier abdominoperineal resection rather than to struggle with a technically demanding, lengthy restorative resection. Furthermore, it is very difficult, if not impossible, to reassess the distal margin after mobilization using the laparoscopic technique. Thus, patients may be placed at higher risk of sphincter sacrifice merely due to technical limitations and surgeon's preferences. These biases are highlighted in the series by Lumley et al (1996) in which one-third of patients with rectal carcinomas underwent abdominoperineal resection. Although adverse selection in their population could have accounted for this aberrant result, technical factors could also have been contributory.

Decanini et al (1994) performed LAPR in 'fresh' cadavers and determined the length of the specimen, the number of involved lymph nodes, and the overall extent of the mesenteric and pelvic resection. They determined that one could technically duplicate an oncologic resection comparable to laparotomy. From these early experiences, several prospective series arose.

Wu et al (1997) performed LAPR on 21 patients for a variety of indications of whom 14 had rectal cancer, four had squamous cell cancer of the anus and one had rectal melanoma. Patients with rectal or anal cancer were all treated preoperatively with pelvic radiation with or without chemotherapy. They were able to complete the laparoscopic surgery in 81% of the patients in just less than 4 hours. The reasons for conversion were adhesions from prior surgery (one), iliac vein injury (one), obesity obscuring view (one) and extensive disease with local invasion (one). Using the four converted patients as a 'control' group, the authors noted that operative time, blood loss, and time to ambulation, flatus and bowel movement were identical in both groups. The number of days to assume a regular diet and to be discharged were significantly lower in the laparoscopic group; however, the authors agreed that it was impossible to draw any definitive conclusions from these differences because the patients who underwent conversion did so due to a series of complications. The specimen length ranged from 33 cm to 70 cm with a distal margin of 6 cm and a mean lymph node harvest of 13 nodes. With a follow-up of 1–44 months, there was one (7%) local recurrence and 2 (14%) distant recurrences in the patients with rectal adenocarcinoma. The patients with squamous cell carcinoma of the anus did not fare as well and while there were no local recurrences, two (50%) patients developed distant disease and were dead at 20 months postoperation; there were no reported trocar site metastases.

The authors concluded that LAPR is not only feasible but that early results support the use of this procedure for low rectal cancer. Seow-Choen et al (1997) compared 16 patients who underwent LAPR to 11 who underwent the same procedure by laparotomy. The length of surgery was similar between the two groups (mean 110 min (65–210) versus mean 100 min (80–185) respectively). Patients in the laparoscopy group were able to walk unassisted on a mean of the fourth postoperative day (range day 2 to day 7). This was statistically significantly better than the 5-day mean (range 3–11) in the laparotomy group. Similarly, discharge from hospital was significantly expedited to a mean of 6.5 (range 3–10) days in the laparoscopy group as compared to a mean of 8 (5–22) days in the laparotomy group (P = 0.006). Lateral margins were uninvolved in both groups. The respective mean and range of lymph node harvests were 10 (6–16) versus 10 (6–32). There was no intraoperative morbidity in either group. Postoperative morbidity was seen in 3 of 16 patients in the laparoscopy group and in 6 of 16 in the laparotomy group. All of these data led the authors to conclude that the procedures were equivalent.

The results of these studies confirmed those of an earlier study performed by Darzi et al (1995) who compared 12 prospectively evaluated patients who underwent LAPR to a retrospectively reviewed group of 16 patients who underwent open abdominoperineal resection (OAPR). None of these 28 patients had adjuvant therapy; there was no mortality in either group and the complication rates were also similar. The oncologic results were somewhat difficult to interpret. While the lymph node harvest was approximately the same in the two groups (9.5 in the LAPR and 6.0 in the OAPR), the mean radial margins were almost twice as great in the laparotomy group (0.9 cm versus 0.5 cm). Despite this finding, 2 of the 16 patients in the open group had histologically positive margins. The authors attributed this potentially important finding to an improved assessment of excision margins by the laparoscope. This claim may be true but cannot be assumed from a non-randomized comparison to retrospective controls. Randomized, prospective studies need to be performed in order to confirm or disprove the results of the studies that have preceded them.

Randomized, prospective trials

Only recently have randomized, prospective trials been undertaken. The aim of these studies is to make direct comparisons between laparoscopic and laparotomy techniques concerning survival, safety and cost-effectiveness. Many parameters can be immediately assessed including patient-related advantages of reduced hospital stay and early return of bowel function as well as the cost effectiveness. With regard to oncological issues, the thoroughness of the resection can be immediately reviewed; however, the long-term benefits of this operation relative to recurrence and survival will take a minimum of 8 years of follow-up.

A phase III trial comparing laparoscopic-assisted colectomy to open colectomy for cancer was proposed in 1993 and began in 1995 (Nelson et al, 1995). This multi-institutional trial is attempting to collect 1200 patients with colon cancer in the right, left, or sigmoid colon; patients are stratified according to tumour site, primary surgeon and ASA classification. In order to assure standardization, the participating surgeons must provide videotapes of the procedures. Furthermore, surgeons must prequalify by having performed at least 20 'cancer-type' laparoscopic resections. Video documentation of certain key facets of the operation, such as level of ligation, ureteric identification and liver exploration are prerequisites to participation. The study will attempt to analyse all the relevant issues surrounding laparoscopy for malignancy; in addition, quality of life questionnaires will be answered by the patients to determine the patients' self-reported symptoms, functional status and utilities both preoperatively and postoperatively, at 2 months and again at 18 months. Unfortunately, despite the participation of more than 60 surgeons, 3 years into the study fewer than 500 patients have been enrolled so far. Nevertheless, preliminary results are forthcoming

Numerous other national and international laparoscopic colectomy for cancer trials are underway. Some of these trials include the German-speaking countries (Germany, Austria, Switzerland), the Scandinavian, Australia/New Zealand countries combined with Holland, and the United Kingdom (Sackier and Wexner, 1999). Short-term results are available from two other randomized prospective studies. Lacy et al (1995) noted 51 patients, 25 of whom underwent laparoscopic-assisted colectomy (LAC) while the other 26 had 'open' colectomy (OC). There was a 16% conversion rate (four cases) in each patient as a result of tumour invasion of the small bowel. While the mean operating time was significantly longer in the LAC group (mean = 148.8 minutes) than in the OC group (mean = 110.6 minutes), the LAC patients still had an expedited postoperative recovery. In fact, the LAC group had earlier passage of flatus (35.5 hours versus 71.1 hours; $P = 0.0001$), earlier resumption of diet (50.9 hours versus 98.6 hours; $P = 0.0001$) and a shorter hospital stay (5.2 days versus 8.1 days; $P = 0.0006$). The postoperative morbidity was also much lower in the LAC group (8% versus 30.8%) as a result of reduced wound complications. The authors failed to identify any port site metastases during their short follow-up period of a small number of patients.

A recently published Danish study supported some of these findings. Stage et al (1997) prospectively randomized 34 patients to undergo either laparoscopic colectomy or colectomy by laparotomy. Patients who required conversion of their operation were eliminated from the analysis. The patients were matched and the excisions were identical, with equal lymph node harvests and margin length. Shorter hospital stay (5 days versus 8 days), decreased pain over the first 24 hours, and earlier return to self-care were characteristic of the laparoscopic group. Postoperative pulmonary function and blood requirements were no different between the two groups. An interesting facet of this study was the collection of blood at 1, 3 and 10 days postoperatively for the analysis of C-reactive protein (CRP) and interleukin 6 (IL-6) as measures of immune function. While other studies have shown a beneficial effect of laparoscopy with regards to immune function, the significantly higher levels of both IL-6 and CRP indicate that the laparoscopic group suffered a fairly pronounced immunodepression lasting from 3 to 10 days after surgery.

The immune effects of laparoscopic surgery will be discussed further, however, aside from this last finding, the immediate results of laparoscopic surgery for colorectal cancer in these prospective randomized studies seems to favour this technique. However, more meaningful data regarding survival will not be available for some time. Meanwhile, one must be honest with the patients who desire laparoscopic colectomy for malignancy. The procedure should still be offered for attempted cure of cancer only within peer-reviewed, externally monitored, prospective randomized trials.

THE ONCOLOGY OF LAPAROSCOPIC COLECTOMY

Margins

The eventual success of laparoscopic surgery for colon and rectal cancer will depend on the integrity of the procedure relative to adherence to standard oncological principles and on the integrity of the surgeon. Proximal margins are typically not an issue and, in laparoscopy as in laparotomy, are defined by the blood supply and the attempt at creation of tension-free anastomoses. Despite the intuitive emotions, there have been some surprisingly narrow proximal margins reported. Van Ye et al (1994) recorded a minimal proximal margin as small as 1.5 cm, and the narrowest proximal margin of Monson et al (1992) was 3 cm; furthermore, their smallest distal margin was only 1.5 cm.

Distal margins are of concern, particularly with anterior resections performed for rectal cancers. The minimal acceptable margin does not change in laparoscopic colectomy and remains 2 cm (Orkin, 1992; Williams et al, 1983). In the laparoscopic literature, most distal margins are reported as an average value of all the margins from all of the specimens. The interpretation of data is critical. For example, in the study by Tate et al (1993) of 'anterior resection' for cancer, the authors reported an average distal resection margin of 2.0 cm with an average tumour height of 20 cm in the laparoscopic group. However, the closest margin was only 0.5 cm for these sigmoid and upper rectal lesions. Despite this unacceptably short margin, they concluded that laparoscopic resection is appropriate for rectal cancers. It seems that some serious concessions are being made for the sake of laparoscopic completion of these procedures. Although these same authors did not encounter a 5 mm margin during laparotomy (the smallest margin was 2.0 cm), it is still laudable that this compromise was reported. In a series by Lord et al (1996), the average distal resection margins for laparoscopic anterior resection were greater than those seen in laparotomy (4.9 cm versus 2.5 cm); however, neither tumour height nor anastomotic height were stated. This biased observation is likely to be the result of non-randomization. Presumably patients with a preponderance of lower rectal tumours underwent laparotomy with smaller distal margins while patients with higher tumours resected via the laparoscope had greater margins.

Obviously, from the above discussion, margins are not a problem for the majority of laparoscopic procedures attempted, particularly the standard right, left or sigmoid resection. Appropriate concern for the distal or lateral resection margins for rectal tumours have already been addressed by several studies which have shown equivalent results to those achieved by open resection (Decanini et al, 1994; Rhodes et al, 1996; Goh et al, 1997; Wu et al, 1997). Radial margins are at least equally and may even be more important in the prevention of pelvic recurrence in rectal cancer than distal margins (Quirke et al, 1986). Reports of radial margins after laparoscopic-assisted abdominoperineal resection have shown a reduction in the accepted margins. Darzi et al (1995) reported an average radial margin of only 0.5 cm (range 0.1–1.5 cm) in their laparoscopic group compared to 0.9 cm (0.1–3.6 cm). Despite the improved view that the laparoscope offers in pelvic dissection (Decanini et al, 1994; Darzi et al, 1995) this 'coning' effect may be detrimental in terms of radial tumour clearance. Barrat et al (1996) showed that specimen length and margins obtained during laparoscopically assisted colectomy (21.6 cm and 8.4 cm respectively) were almost identical to those found in their laparotomy group (24.3 cm and 6.6 cm respectively). Both results were significantly better than those findings in the group who had a laparoscopic resection (14.3 cm and 4.1 cm respectively). They concluded, as have so many authors, that laparoscopic resection for colorectal malignancy should be performed under the auspices of a prospective randomized trial.

With good judgement and adequate training, margins should not be a controversial issue in the discussion between laparotomy and laparoscopy. For this reason, the oncological merit of these operations should focus on three, more controversial points. The first is the results and implications of the lymph node harvest; the second deals with immune function; and the final controversy concerns the incidence, aetiology and ramifications of port site recurrence.

Lymph nodes

In the absence of long-term survival data, most authors have used quantitative criteria such as the number of lymph nodes retrieved from the resection specimen as a means of comparing open with laparoscopic colectomy (Jacobs et al, 1991; Larach et al, 1993a; Guillou et al, 1993; Chindasub et al, 1994; Lacy et al, 1995; Fielding et al, 1997; Stage et al, 1997). An important caveat is that there is a tremendous variability in the lymph node harvest even after open colectomy (Cawthorn et al, 1986; Jass et al, 1986; Scott and Grace, 1989; Haboubi et al, 1992; Cohen et al, 1994; Rodriguez-Bigas et al, 1996; Hida et al, 1997).

The difference in the number of reported nodes depends upon several factors. First, there is no absolute value of lymph nodes. Patient factors such as the thickness of the mesentery can effect the ease of lymph node clearance. Second, and hopefully a more consistent factor, is the technique displayed by the surgeon in removal of the specimen as well as his or her desire to achieve high ligation. Jacobs (1992) compared the number of lymph nodes harvested by laparoscopic right colectomy or rectosigmoid resections with that harvested by laparotomy. In the right colectomy specimens, the nodal count was greater in the laparoscopic group (17 versus 14; P = NS) while it was reversed for the rectosigmoid resections (16 versus 10; P = NS). The study by Goh et al (1997), however, confirmed that equal nodal harvests could be achieved with left-sided lesions.

The third and most subjective aspect of lymph node evaluation is the pathologist's perseverance in extracting nodes. There is considerable variability in the quantification of lymph nodes from institution to institution (Blenkinsopp et al, 1981). The number of lymph nodes resected has varied from 0 to 84 depending upon the type of resection performed (Table 36.1). Specimens containing 0 to 2 nodes are obviously inadequate to allow prognostication. Even when authors report 'adequate' or 'equivalent' resection, the actual number of nodes may reflect only the paracolic nodes and lack any sampling of the more significant apical nodes.

Toyota et al (1995) retrospectively analysed survival with regards to rate and degree of lymph node metastases after curative resection for right colon cancer. They noted a survival advantage in patients who had had a resection that involved removal of at least 10 cm of bowel both proximal and distal to the lesion with removal of all regional lymph-bearing tissue along the main trunk artery, including the apical nodes. The majority of positive nodes were within 10 cm of the lesion, regardless of whether the cancer was based in the caecum, ascending colon or transverse colon. Less than 1% of the nodes were further than 10 cm from the cancer. The incidence of metastases to the main (apical) nodes was as high as 6%. This may offer some guide as to the extent of laparoscopic mobilization and lymph node dissection that can be considered adequate.

Location rather than total number of lymph nodes may be a more important determinant of survival and at least one study has identified as high as a 32% incidence of skip metastases with involvement of distant nodes along major vessels without local nodal involvement (Shida et al, 1993).

Table 36.1 Comparison of lymph node harvest using open surgery or laparoscopy.

	Mean node harvest	
Authors	*Open*	*Laparoscopy*
Bleday et al (1993)	9.5 11.0	10.57 8.0
Darzi et al (1995)	6.0	9.5
Dodson et al (1993)	7.0	4.2
Fine et al (1995)	NS	9.1
Franklin et al (1995)	14.7	15.8
Hoffman et al (1994)	8.0	6.1
Larach et al (1993a)	–	9.8
Lord et al (1996)	8.9	7.8
Musser et al (1994)	7.9	10.6
Peters and Bartels (1993)	8.5	7.9
Tate et al (1993)	10	13
Tucker et al (1995)	6.4	8.7
Van Ye et al (1994)	7.6	10.5
Cohen et al (1994)	–	19
Jacobs et al (1991)	NA	Right: 25.5 Left: 8
Zucker et al (1994)	–	Right: 28.4 Left: 7.7
Stage et al (1997)	8.0	7.0
Kwok et al (1996)	NS	12.8
Phillips et al (1992)	NS	10.0
Monson et al (1992)	NS	10.0
Vara-Thorbeck et al (1994)	NS	8.5
Lacy et al (1995)	12.5	13.0
Chindasub et al (1994)	NS	10.0
Puente et al (1994)	NS	11.0
Guillou et al (1993)	NS	9.0
Goh et al (1997)	19.0	20.0
Wu et al (1997)	NS	13.0

NS, not stated.

No study has as yet identified a survival advantage to the removal of all involved lymph nodes; however, there are some retrospective data that suggest there may be a benefit in terms of recurrence (Bernstein and Wexner, 1995). The prognostic significance of the lymph nodes certainly extends beyond the mere involvement of the nodes, and the actual number plays an equal role. A number of studies have demonstrated a decrease in survival rates once five or more lymph nodes are involved with metastases (Hojo et al, 1982; Bernstein and Wexner, 1995).

To avoid missing involved nodes, some authors have proposed modifications to the traditional step-sectioning of resected specimens (Gilchrist and David, 1938; Blenkinsopp et al, 1981; Jass et al, 1986; Herrera-Ornelas, 1987; Hyder et al, 1990). One such technique involves fat clearance of the specimen with xylene and alcohol (Cohen et al, 1994;

Cawthorn et al, 1986). In fact, Cawthorn et al (1986) employed this technique in a multi-institutional trial looking at adjuvant preoperative radiotherapy for rectal cancer. Using the xylene/alcohol mixture, they were able to identify a significantly greater number of nodes per resection specimen (mean 23.1) than could pathologists at either St Marks Hospital or any of the other seven centres participating in the study (mean 10.6). More importantly, they found a greater number of lymph nodes with metastases in the cleared compared with non-cleared specimens (mean 3.7 versus 1.9 respectively).

Scott and Grace (1989) discovered a three times larger harvest of nodes with fat clearance compared to step-sectioning (18.9 versus 6.1 nodes). When subtotal and total colectomy specimens were evaluated using the standard sectioning technique, the mean number of lymph nodes harvested was 13.3 and 53 respectively. After xylene clearance, an additional 3.9 and 14.5 nodes could be added to the total number of nodes removed from the corresponding colectomy. This increased yield, however, only translated into two Dukes' stage changes and the authors concluded that the clearance of fat by xylene or any other chemical is only of value if the pathologist does not perform meticulous step-sectioning of the resection specimens. An overview of the results of nodal clearance are shown in Table 36.2.

Table 36.2 Lymph node harvest with and without fat clearance.

	Number of nodes harvested	
Authors	*With clearance*	*Without clearance*
Rodriguez-Bigas (1996)	40	NS
Cawthorn et al (1986)	18.9	6.1
Scott and Grace (1989)	23.1	10.5
Hida et al (1997)	76.4	18.1
Cohen et al (1994)	17	13
Haboubi et al (1992)	48	NS
Jass et al (1986)	16	19

NS, not stated.

Immune concepts

The immune system has been implicated in both the development and the treatment of malignant disease. It is natural to assume that the more one can do to enhance immune function, or rather, the less that one does to impair such function, would be of benefit in the care of patients with cancer. Even without scientific data, it seems reasonable to think of laparoscopic surgery as less stressful than laparotomy. Since the advent of the technique, animal and human studies have attempted to substantiate this assumption.

Cellular rather than humoral immunity has been implicated in limiting the establishment and spread of tumour cells. Cell-mediated immune functions such as lymphocyte and neutrophil chemotaxis, natural killer cell activity, and delayed-type hypersensitivity (DTH) responses have all been shown to be suppressed after major surgical procedures, the extent of impairment being proportional to the length and complexity of the operation (Lennard et al, 1985; Whelan et al, 1996a). Cancer patients with intact cell-mediated immunity as measured by normal DTH response were more often resectable (55% versus 20%) and had less recurrence or metastases on follow-up than non-responders (Eilber and Morton, 1970).

Bessler et al (1994) performed a series of animal studies to assess the effects of laparoscopic and open surgery on delayed-type hypersensitivity. Following 22 sigmoid resections (11 open and 11 laparoscopic) in pigs, DTH was tested by intradermal injection of a common antigenic preparation and measurement of the resultant wheals at 48 and 72 hours. The wheals in the laparoscopically treated animals were significantly larger at each time interval than those in the laparotomy group, suggesting that the laparoscopic technique may preserve cell-mediated immune functions (Figure 36.4).

Another approach to the analysis of immune function has been through the measurement of serum markers of physiological stress along with the assumption that the greater the concentrations of these markers, the more severe the stress. Cho et al (1994) reported the effect of laparoscopy on serum cytokine levels as a measure of surgical trauma. They measured interleukin 6 (IL-6) levels in three groups of patients who required operative intervention for biliary disease. The groups included patients undergoing laparoscopic cholecystectomy, open cholecystectomy, or laparoscopic cholecystectomy preceded by endoscopic retrograde cholangiopancreatography (ERCP). They found that IL-6 levels were 60% lower in the patients who had a laparoscopic cholecystectomy when compared to the open group. The addition of ERCP to the laparoscopic procedure increased the IL-6 levels from 3 to 6 times the values seen in either of the single procedures.

Collet et al (1995) analysed numerous other parameters of immune function such as serum tissue necrosis factor, bacterial clearance, phagocytosis and oxidative bursts of polymorphonuclear leuco-

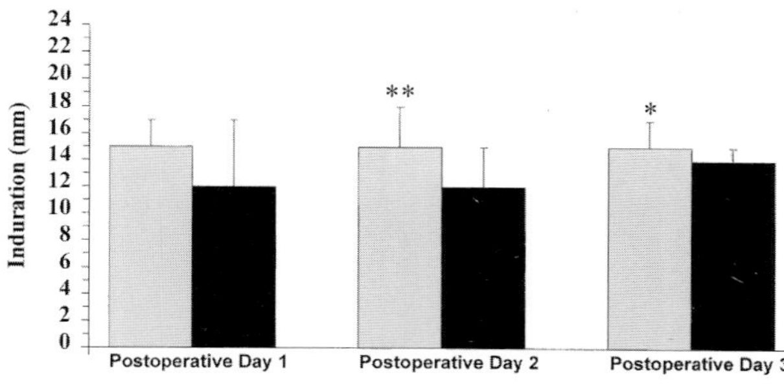

Figure 36.4 The wheals in the laparoscopically treated animals are significantly larger at each time interval than in laparotomy, suggesting that laparoscopy may preserve cell-mediated immune functions. Reproduced with permission from Bessler et al (1994).

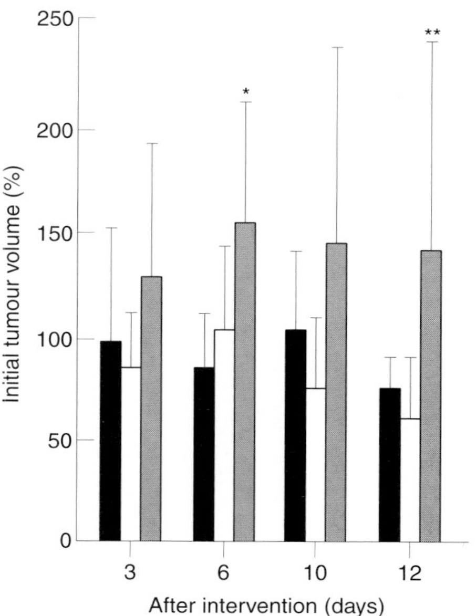

Figure 36.5 Tumour volumes assessed on postoperative days 3, 6, 10 and 12 showing a persistent increase in volume of tumour with laparotomy compared to a slow regression of tumour volume with the laparoscopic technique. Black bars, anaesthesia group; open bars, insufflation group; hatched bars, laparotomy group. * $P < 0.05$ versus insufflation and anaesthesia groups. ** $P < 0.05$ versus insufflation and anaesthesia groups. Reproduced with permission from Allendorf et al (1995).

cytes in pigs undergoing laparoscopic compared to open Nissen fundoplication. They also found less derangement of the immune system based on these parameters in the laparoscopic group.

Rather elegant tumour studies were also performed by Bessler et al (1994) as well as by another group from The Netherlands (Allendorf and Bessler, 1995; Bouvy et al, 1997). The first study looked simply at the growth and regression rates of established tumours (MC-2 mouse mammary carcinoma) in a control group of animals undergoing anaesthesia only, compared to two other groups of animals, the first having laparoscopy with insufflation and the second receiving a standard laparotomy. Tumour volumes assessed on postoperative days 3, 6, 10 and 12 revealed that while the control and insufflation groups showed a slow regression of tumour, the laparotomy group sustained a persistent increase in volume (Figure 36.5). Similarly, Bouvy et al (1997) implanted colon cancer cells in the intraperitoneal space and the renal subcapsular space of rats which underwent either laparoscopic or open small bowel resection or anaesthesia alone (controls). They found that there was less tumour growth in both the intraperitoneal and the subcapsular renal area in the laparoscopic group.

Dorrance et al (1996), looking for the effect of pneumoperitoneum on tumour growth, compared carbon dioxide and helium pneumoperitoneum to anaesthesia alone in a rat model. Tumours grew significantly larger in both omental and peritoneal surfaces in the laparoscopy groups and were independent of the type of gas used for insufflation. Southall et al (1997b) performed a similar experiment except that they analysed intradermal growth of tumour in animals with anaesthesia alone (controls), pneumoperitoneum alone, or laparotomy. The average tumour mass was similar between the laparoscopy and control groups but was significantly increased in only the laparotomy group. This finding suggests again that the trauma induced by the laparotomy promotes tumour growth. More importantly, the application of pneumoperitoneum by itself appears to be no more stressful than does a general anaesthetic.

These tumour growth studies confirm that operations, whether performed conventionally or by minimally invasive technique, represent a stress to the immune system. There is some suggestion that there may be less attenuation of immune defence mechanisms with minimally invasive techniques. The implication may become self-evident with a longer follow-up of the patients entered in the randomized prospective trials currently underway.

Port site recurrence

One of the most controversial and hotly debated issues is the link between laparoscopy and port site

Table 36.3 Port site recurrence.

Authors	Dukes' stage	Interval to recurrence (months)
Alexander et al (1993)	C	3
Walsh et al (1993)	C	6
Fusco and Paluzzi (1993)	C	10
Guillou et al (1993)	C	NS
O'Rourke et al (1993)	B	2.5
Cirocco et al (1994)	C	9
Nduka et al (1994)	C	3
Prasad et al (1994)	B	6
	A	26
Berends et al (1994)	B	NS
	C	NS
	D	NS
Lauroy et al (1994)	A	9
Boulez and Herriot (1994)	3 stages	NS
Ramos et al (1994)	C	NS
	C	NS
	C	NS
Kok et al (1996)	B	NS
Gionnone, 1994, pers commun	C	2
Gould, 1994, pers commun	NS	4
Newman et al, 1994, pers commun	C	6
Wexner and Cohen (1994)	B	3
	B	6
	C	6
	C	9
	C	12
Fingerhut (1995)	A	NS
	B	NS
	B	NS
Jacquet et al (1995)	C	1
	B	10
Drouard-Passone-Szerzyna, 1995, pers commun	A	9
	B	6
	B	6
	C	5
	C	1
	C	9
	D	2
Ugarte (1995)	C	10
Beck, 1995, pers commun	NS	NS
Lumley et al (1996)	D	NS
Molenaar et al (1998)	?	41
Kwok et al (1996)	D	NS
	C	NS
Vertruyen et al (1996)	D	6
	B	2

NS, not stated.

recurrence (PSR) (Table 36.3). Cirocco et al (1994) presented the fourth known case of abdominal wall recurrence, suggesting 'an alarming rate' of increase in the incidence of PSR that may 'carry ominous implications for the future of laparoscopic surgical procedures involving colorectal malignancy'. As far back as 1955, Ackerman and Wheat had noted several cases of tumour implantation following a variety of procedures involving many different neoplasms. A recent report of subcutaneous metastases after diagnostic laparoscopy for gastric adenocarcinoma with positive cytology also looked at several past case reports of neoplastic dissemination of tumour into tract sites. These authors tabulated subcutaneous metastases in everything from pleural biopsy for mesothelioma to percutaneous nephrostomy for retroperitoneal sarcoma to stereotaxic biopsy for cerebral lymphoma (Cava et al, 1990). Wound recurrence of colorectal cancer, first reported as early as 1928 by Sistrunk, occurred when colonic tumours were delivered through small incisions after either colotomy with polypectomy or limited resection.

The study by Hughes et al (1983) noted the occurrence of wound metastases in approximately 13 of 1600 laparotomies for colon cancer. Carcinomatosis coexisted in almost all cases of wound metastasis so that the actual incidence of isolated wound recurrence was only 0.2% of cases. Similarly, Reilly et al (1996) reported a 1.5% incidence of wound metastases in laparotomy for colon and rectal cancer (26 cases in 1711 patients with cancer). All of their patients had biopsy-proven recurrence and 18 of the 26 patients with recurrence underwent re-exploration. Nine of these patients had diffuse carcinomatosis and a total of 15 of the 18 patients had multiple sites of recurrence. In fact, only 3 of the 1711 patients (0.2%) had isolated abdominal wall recurrences. Thus there is no doubt, nor should it be any surprise that port site metastases occurs after laparoscopic colectomy (Table 36.3).

Aetiology of port site recurrence (PSR)

Although all unproven, speculations as to the origin of PSR are in abundance (Table 36.4). The most likely possibilities can be divided into technical factors, local factors and effect of pneumoperitoneum. Recurrence may occur early, as in the report by O'Rourke et al (1993) of two PSRs in one patient with a Dukes' B tumour 10 weeks after surgery. In tumours that recur early or early-stage tumours that recur, technical factors may be involved. Certainly, there is little question regarding the appearance of a subcutaneous nodule appearing at a cannula site 9 months after laparoscopic colotomy and polypectomy (Lauroy et al, 1994). This mishap represents a true breach of oncological principle and may reflect the experience, expertise and judgement of the surgeon. Alternatively, the finding of PSR in Dukes' A and B lesions after laparoscopic colectomy as in the report by O'Rourke et al (1993) suggests that factors inherent in the technical demands of the procedure

Table 36.4 Overview: aetiologic theories of port site recurrence.

Aetiologic theory	*Authors*
Pneumoperitoneum	Jones et al (1995); Knolmayer et al (1997); Wu et al (1997); Jacobi et al (1996); Tseng et al (1997); Bouvy et al (1997); Nduka and Darzi (1997)
Pneumoperitoneum increases portal tumour cells	Chen et al (1997)
Pneumoperitoneum has no effect	Whelan et al (1996a); Allardyce et al (1997); Hubens et al (1996)
Pneumoperitoneum has a protective effect	Southall et al (1997b)
Port or instrument contamination	Thomas et al (1996); Kockerling et al (1997); Allardyce et al (1997)
Ischaemia	Tseng et al (1997); Lee et al (1997); Bonjer et al (1997)
Exfoliated cells	Lumley et al (1996)
Gravity	Allardyce et al (1997)

may facilitate recurrence. Certainly, manipulation of colon cancer can cause exfoliation of viable tumour cells that may themselves have malignant potential (Weiss and Wexner, 1996). This feature is easy to explain with tumours that occur on the surface of the organ (e.g. ovarian cancer), but is harder to justify when tumours have an intraluminal location, unless the tumour has penetrated the serosal surface or where the lumen has somehow been violated.

Cook and Dehn (1996) assessed 46 patients, 6 of whom had colorectal carcinomas, 10 had gastric carcinomas and 30 had oesophageal carcinomas. The overall PSR rate was 11% (5 of 46 patients). They felt that the important mitigating factor was whether or not the serosa was invaded. Specifically, 5 of 20 patients in whom the tumours invaded through the serosa (25%) developed port site metastases, compared to none of the 26 patients in whom invasion was absent (0%). In laparoscopic colon surgery, retraction is difficult and careless handling may lead to microperforation and exposure of the peritoneum to malignant cells. These cells may then aerosolize within the established pneumoperitoneum and subsequently lodge into the subcutaneous tissue.

Jones et al (1995) confirmed the presence of such aerosolubilized droplets of tumour cells. In their hamster model of pneumoperitoneum, they were able to verify tumour deposits by histological identification of malignant cells within the caecal mesentery and at wound sites on the abdominal wall. While this study showed that implanted tumour cells within the peritoneal cavity could be spread by pneumoperitoneum, it does not prove that manipulation during laparoscopic colectomy leads to an increased inoculum of malignant cells into the peritoneal cavity. Although their initial study showed that pneumoperitoneum tripled the rate of tumour implantation, subsequent studies showed the phenomenon to be case-related.

Fritsch et al (1997) used a solitary caecal adenocarcinoma in a rat model using 12 mmHg pneumoperitoneum. They compared 24 rats who underwent laparotomy with 25 who underwent laparoscopy and 60 minutes of manipulation. The implant rate approximately doubled from 25% in the laparotomy group to 48% in the laparoscopy group at 14.5 ± 0.5 weeks. Unfortunately, due to their small sample size, this doubling was not stastistically significant.

A study by Kim et al (1997) hypothesized that, with laparoscopic techniques performed using accepted 'oncological principles', tumour cell spillage was comparable to that found in conventional surgery. Their preliminary results on the first 15 patients randomized to either laparoscopic or conventional colectomy included an equal number of right-sided and left-sided lesions as well as comparable T stages. During surgery, all fluids were collected before, during and after mobilization and resection of the tumour and then assessed for malignant cells. They were unable to detect tumour cells in either group in both the preresection and the postresection peritoneal fluids and thus concluded that laparoscopic surgery, in experienced hands, does not enhance malignant exfoliation of colon cancer.

Local factors may also play a role in the appearance of these PSRs. Surgical wounds offer a fertile environment for adhesion of tumour cells, particularly to damaged or ischaemic areas with impaired local defences. It is not surprising that tumours implant upon traumatized sites. Using a mouse model, Goldstein et al (1993) studied the effects of peritoneal injury at laparoscopy in relation to tumour cell implantation. They found that tumour inoculation and growth were increased at sites of peritoneal injury relative to uninjured areas, supporting the contention that if free tumour cells are present or shed during laparoscopy, then port sites serve as a convenient location for adherence. Wu et al (1998) found that the greater the inoculum of cells, the greater the chances of implantation. This certainly explains the greater than 50% incidence of PSRs that occur in diffuse carcinomatosis.

Other mechanisms must be sought to explain isolated wound metastases. One such explanation may be that the instruments themselves are responsible for the implantation of cancer cells. Using animal models, Hewett et al (1996) attempted to identify the culprit in the spread of malignant cells during laparoscopy. After injecting tumour cells into pigs and subjecting them to a laparoscopic procedure, they collected both filtered carbon dioxide gas and washings of the laparoscopic instruments for cellular analysis. The majority of cancer cells identified were either on the ports or laparoscopic instruments but not in the filtered gas. They found cells in one of 30 samples of carbon dioxide but in 20% of port washings and 40% of instrument washings. It may thus be concluded that the port site is contaminated by malignant cells due to the frequent passing of instruments in and out of the port during the procedure. They hypothesized that condensation of water vapour forms droplets that may harbour tumour cells. With port removal, these cells are then deposited within the wound, leading to implantation.

Similarly, Kockerling et al (1997) failed to isolate malignant cells within the carbon dioxide effluent of collected samples. They did, however, find that all instruments were contaminated using a monoclonal staining and polymerase chain reaction method of determination. Thomas et al (1996) supported the findings of Kockerling's group.

Allardyce et al (1996) used a chromium 51-labelled HeLa cell model of intraperitoneally injected cells in a swine model. Using gamma counting, cells were assessed for their presence on instruments, ports, security threads, in excised wounds, on margins and in filter pads which monitor leakage around otherwise sealed ports. They found that 64% of the operating surgeon's ports were contaminated with cells. They failed to find any tumour in the aerosol through the ports but there was indeed a chimney effect around the ports. Tumour cells were noted on threads and on instruments. The tumour cell accumulation at the rostral (surgeon's) port was 330% increased over other sites. Implantation of the ports was clearly adversely influenced by gravity and the Trendelenburg position and it was reduced but not eliminated by direct lavage.

In support of this conclusion Hubens (1998) used a CC531 colon cancer cell line in a rat model that was subjected to pneumoperitoneum. They found that pneumoperitoneum did not predispose to port site implantation when compared to controls.

One of the more attractive new theories is that ischaemia may play a role in the development of PSR. Using a rat model with power trocar leakage combined with crushing of the incisions on the one side to induce ischaemia, Tseng et al (1997) found an approximately 15-fold increase in the median tumour weight from 22 mg to 316 mg ($P = 0.007$). Leakage alone only increased the mean weight from 67 mg to 175 mg ($P = 0.005$). Thus, a combination of leakage and ischaemia at the port sites may well provide the nidus for tumour growth. Similarly, Lee et al (1997) crushed the peritoneum in an animal model. They found port site recurrence in 73% of animals in the control group, 71% in the pneumoperitoneum group, but in 95% in the ischaemic (crushed) plus pneumoperitoneum group. The percentage of port sites involved was 30%, 37% and 68% respectively. Jaap Bonjer et al (1997) also performed a study which lends credence to the local ischaemia theory. They found that the mean tumour weight in non-ischaemic sites was only 45 mg as compared to 320 mg in ischaemic port sites ($P = 0.003$).

Pneumoperitoneum is unique to laparoscopy and has been implicated in the promotion of tumour cell growth in several animal models. Using a murine hepatic metastases model, WS Chen et al (1997) injected colon cancer cells into the peritoneal cavity of mice: half of the animals then underwent helium insufflation to 15 cmH_2O and all the mice were then sacrificed except for five in each group that were observed for survival. They found that the pneumoperitoneum seemed to increase tumour cell spread from the portal system to the liver initially.

Knolmayer et al (1997) used a carbon dioxide dual collection system. They were unable to recover malignant cells from any of the patients in the control group. However, they were able to recover human caecal carcinoma cells in half of the laparoscopy group subjects. Despite this, there was no significant difference in long-term survival in the mice with or without gas insufflation.

Wu et al (1998) assessed the effect of pneumoperitoneum on trocar site implantation in hamsters that received decreasing inoculums of cancer cells. These animals were compared with a control group comprised of hamsters that had no gas insufflation. Pneumoperitoneum significantly increased the incidence and the size of the trocar site implants at higher concentrations of inoculum; this effect was not seen at the lower concentration. In a prior study, Wu et al (1997) found that pneumoperitoneum increased trocar site implantation from 50% to 71% ($P < 0.001$). It also increased positivity of four concomitant sites from 10% to 38% of the animals ($P < 0.02$). It increased probable tumours from 5% to 14% ($P < 0.01$) and increased the tumour mass from 0.2 g to 2.0 g ($P < 0.02$) as compared to no pneumoperitoneum.

Recent studies by Jacobi and colleagues from Germany have reaffirmed the findings of these previous studies. In their first study, Jacobi et al (1996) found a significant increase in the number of tumour cells after carbon dioxide pneumoperitoneum compared to a control group *in vitro* and in a rat model. In a follow-up study, these authors carefully measured both intraperitoneal and subcutaneous tumour growth of an adenocarcinoma cell line incubated in a rat model after laparotomy, laparoscopy with carbon dioxide or air and in a control group (Jacobi et al, 1997a). The intraperitoneal tumour weight increased significantly after both laparotomy (1203 ± 780 mg) and laparoscopy with CO_2 (718 ± 690 mg) or air (1085 ± 891 mg) relative to tumour growth in the control group (521 ± 221 mg). The interesting finding in this study was the relatively minor increase in tumour cell growth in the group of animals that had laparoscopy with CO_2 when compared to the groups that had either laparotomy or laparoscopy with air. This finding had not been noted *in vitro*, suggesting that host modification of tumour growth occurs *in vivo*. Subcutaneous tumour growth also increased after laparotomy (71 ± 35 mg) and laparoscopy with air (82 ± 45 mg) and CO_2 (99 ± 55 mg) compared to the control group (36 ± 33 mg).

Unlike the results with intraperitoneal tumours, CO_2 actually seems to promote tumour growth in the subcutaneous tissues. Jacobi et al (1997a) feel that this may be explained by the 'high solubility of carbon dioxide in subcutaneous tissue'. This feature is in accordance with the clinical findings that most PSRs do not occur in the abdominal wall but in the subcutaneous tissue underlying the trocar incisions (Cava et al, 1990; Walsh et al, 1993; Jacobi et al, 1995).

There is no overall agreement upon the adverse effect of pneumoperitoneum. Southall et al (1997a) utilized two separate tumour models, a C26 and a B26. In both groups, they found that the tumours actually were significantly smaller in the pneumoperitoneum than in the laparotomy group. They hypothesized that both the colon B26 adenocarcinoma and B16 melanoma tumours grew larger after laparotomy than after pneumoperitoneum and that the pneumoperitoneum therefore had a protective effect. It is difficult to assess how much of this effect is related to host response and alteration of immune function (Bessler et al, 1994).

Prevention of port site recurrence

Knowledge of port site metastases is the first step to prevention. The most effective method of prevention is simply to avoid any injury to the colon that may allow the escape of malignant cells. The importance of experience with the laparoscopic technique including atraumatic handling of the tissues and the use of good judgement have been stressed earlier in this chapter. The surgeon's ego should not prejudice the patient's cure and should PSR occur as a result of a transgression in technique, this constitutes a serious avoidable complication (Johnstone et al, 1996). Certainly, PSR rates after laparoscopic colectomy as high as 21% (Berends et al, 1994) are difficult to explain unless there has been some technical mishap. A more acceptable rate of PSR was reported by Ramos et al (1994) who evaluated the results of 208 laparoscopic colectomies in the ASCRS laparoscopic registry and found an overall PSR rate of 1.44% but only an 0.48% incidence in the absence of diffuse peritoneal carcinomatosis. A more recent update of this registry included 480 cases and a 1.1% overall incidence of wound recurrence at one year of follow-up (Vukasin et al, 1996).

In another review of PSR, Wexner and Cohen (1995) reported 33 incidences in six series of laparoscopic colectomy collected from many centres around the world. The incidence ranged from 1.5% to 21% (median: 3.5%; mean: 6.5%). The true rate may lie somewhere between the 1% and 6% range because 'the vast majority of surgeons do not routinely publish their results even when the results are exemplary' (Wexner et al, 1995). Thus, in assessing the true incidence, both the numerator and denominator are lacking.

Some authors have proposed that the pulling of large specimens through small wounds predisposes to subcutaneous metastases (Guillou et al, 1993; Jacquet et al, 1995). Thus others routinely use specimen bags or plastic wound protectors to prevent tumour inoculation (Goh et al, 1997; Murthy et al, 1989). However, Montorsi et al (1985) described a PSR in a patient with a Dukes' B lesion in whom the specimen was placed in a bag prior to removal and many authors have pointed out that these bags do not actually prevent wound metastases (Bouvy et al, 1996; Johnstone et al, 1996; Macias and Wexner, 1996).

In light of some of the evidence that pneumoperitoneum, specifically with carbon dioxide, may enhance the subcutaneous lodging and subsequent growth of tumour cells, some authors have suggested the use of gasless laparoscopy. In early experimental work, Bouvy et al (1996) found significantly less tumour growth at the port sites after gasless laparoscopic resection of colon cancer in the rat compared to the use of carbon dioxide pneumoperitoneum. In a direct comparison of the two techniques, Mathew et al (1997b) from Australia injected ^{51}Cr-labelled adenocarcinoma cells into a rat model and measured the radioactivity of the vented gas after both carbon dioxide insufflation and gasless laparoscopy. Significant transfer of tumour cells occurred only in the insufflation group, lending credence to the conclusion that gasless laparoscopy might prevent port site metastases. Data from Whelan et al (1996a) and others (Allendorf and Bessler, 1995; Allardyce et al, 1996) present contrary results and suggest that tumour adherence to the laparoscopic equipment is the cause of PSR so that gasless surgery may not prevent this occurrence. Comparison using animal models has its pitfalls, such as variability of host responses and peritoneal defences. A study of tumour implantation in a porcine model, for instance, cannot easily be compared to the same experiment in rodents.

Another potential problem is that of tumour inoculation: implantation patterns correspond to the number of viable cells introduced into the peritoneal cavity and studies differ with respect to concentration of tumour cell injected into the animal models (Mathew et al, 1997a). This dose–response curve will invariably interfere with the interpretation of the data.

Jacobi et al (1997b) measured tumour growth *in vitro* ($n = 60$), *ex vivo* ($n = 60$) and *in vivo* ($n = 60$), of colon adenocarcinoma DHD/K12/TRD in a rat model without insufflation (control) and after insufflation with both carbon dioxide and helium. They found that in all three settings, carbon dioxide promoted tumour growth compared to helium or controls. The difference was most pronounced in the *in vivo* group in whom the subcutaneous tumour growth after CO_2 insufflation (131 ± 55 mg) was about four times greater than after helium insufflation (35 ± 34 mg) or no insufflation at all (36 ± 33 mg).

Along the same lines, Dorrance et al (1997) tried utilizing helium instead of carbon dioxide for insufflation. Sixty animals were divided into a control group of 20, a carbon dioxide group of 20 and a helium group of 20. The mean and range tumour weight in grams for the three groups was 4.0 (range 3.2–5.9), 7.5 (5.8–8.8) and 6.1 (5.8–8.3). The absolute numbers of peritoneal nodules were 0 (0–10), 17 (10–20) and 19.5 (12.5–25.7) respectively.

There is little that one can do with extraluminal microscopic disease present at the time of resection as it is responsible for almost 50% of reported port site recurrences (Weiss and Wexner, 1996). In this group, PSR is a prognostic marker of advanced disease and decreased survival. The majority of these patients die from disseminated disease within one year of the recurrence (Cava et al, 1990; O'Rourke et al, 1993; Berends et al, 1994; Ramos et al, 1994; Cirocco et al, 1994; Johnstone et al, 1996). The situation, although desperate, is not hopeless and there have been reports of success with cytoreductive surgery combined with intraperitoneal chemotherapy as described by Jacquet et al (1995). The two patients in their case report were free of disease at 1.5 years after this therapy. The other 50% of patients with wound recurrence have it in isolation and they represent a small group that may benefit most from aggressive disease resection and intensive follow-up.

Hubens et al (1996) and more recently Wu et al (1999) suggested an obvious solution to the prevention of this problem, namely the excision of the trocar sites themselves. Their hypothesis is that pneumoperitoneum increases trocar site recurrence and they feel that excision of the port sites should prevent local recurrence. Wu et al (1999) used a WG39 human colon cancer cell line. Seventy-five hamsters underwent midline incision along with 10 minutes of pneumoperitoneum. A 4-mm radius was excised around each of the four ports and 7 weeks later, these sites were excised and examined. In the 35 animals who underwent excision, implants were noted in 89%, and palpable tumours in 44%. In the 35 animals in which the wounds had not been excised, the percentages were 78 and 61 respectively. Thus, excision reduced but did not eliminate implantation.

Another potential local means of eliminating port site recurrence was by irrigation (Jacobi et al, 1997b). Tumours were weighed in four groups of animals: a control group, a group which underwent heparin irrigation of the ports, a group which underwent taurolidine irrigation and a group in which both heparin and taurolidine were utilized. Tumour weights were 595 mg, 298 mg, 149 mg and 21.5 mg respectively. The differences were significant between heparin and the control ($P < 0.001$), taurolidine and control ($P < 0.05$) and both agents ($P < 0.001$). Thus, the combined irrigation reduced but did not eliminate port site recurrence. Similarly, Dorrance et al (1997) also tried wound irrigation to prevent port site implantation. Instead of heparin or taurolidine, they simply used normal saline and sterile water. They measured the median tumour nodules using interquartile ranges. Ten animals were in each of the four groups. Unfortunately, neither sterile water nor saline eliminated or even significantly reduced tumour cell implantation at the port sites. An overview of the results of studies looking at the prevention of PRS can be seen in Table 36.5.

Patients with isolated PSR represent approxi-

Table 36.5 Port site recurrence: methods of prevention.

Method of prevention	*Authors*	*Study specifics*	*Results*
Irrigation of port sites	Allardyce et al (1997)	NS	Reduction but not elimination
	Jacobi et al (1997a)	Heparin	Disappointing
	Jacobi et al (1997a)	Taurolaudine	Disappointing
	Jacobi et al (1997a)	Heparin and tauroladine	Reduction but not elimination
	Dorrance et al (1997)	Saline	No effect
	Dorrance et al (1997)	Water	No effect
Alternate method of abdominal insufflation	Mathew et al (1997b)	Gasless	Successful
	Jacobi et al (1996)	Helium	Reduction but not elimination
	Dorrance et al (1997)	Helium	Reduction but not elimination
Excision	Wu et al (1998)		Disappointing

mately 0.25–2% of the total number of laparoscopic colectomies performed for cure of colorectal cancer. As yet, the exact number has not been compiled. No one group of surgeons has a large enough experience with this phenomenon to have established a routine management plan for those patients. These individuals should be offered a wide local excision of the subcutaneous site after ruling out widely disseminated disease. Some of the questions that need to be answered include: (1) Is PSR a harbinger of later metastatic disease and if so, is early aggressive debulking and chemotherapy as proposed by Jacquet et al (1995) warranted? (2) Does PSR, in this second group of individuals, represent truly localized disease and, if so, can it be managed with local resection alone? (3) Finally, what is the natural history of patients with isolated wound metastases? It is likely that the cause of PSR is multifactorial and includes technique, insufflation, local factors present in the wound, the biology of the tumour and systemic factors that pertain to the immune system. The patients in whom PSR has the greatest impact are those with small, early-stage tumours that are resected for cure. The eventual acceptance of laparoscopic colectomy for colorectal cancer will depend upon the prevention of PSR in this group of patients. When PSR does occur, it should be reported so that a true estimation of incidence and standardization of treatment can be established.

LENGTH OF STAY AND COST ISSUES

Cost issues and the increased efficiency of health-care delivery have attained a prominent role in patient care even in the most industrialized and wealthy of countries of the world. Simple ways to save money are through the earlier discharge of patients from the hospital and containing equipment cost. In the case of cholecystectomy, the initial exorbitant cost of the laparoscopic equipment combined with the longer operating times for laparoscopists at the beginning of the learning curve was financially unattractive. Other financial factors such as an increased incidence of ductal injuries and delayed universal acceptance of the technique have taken time to change the market. However, laparoscopic cholecystectomy has now exceeded most expectations. When one considers the decreased hospital stay and earlier return to a preoperative functional level in what is usually a younger, working individual, the overall savings is generally worth the initial expense.

Laparoscopic colectomy has followed a similar, but much more arduous course. The initial novelty of this technique was followed by a wave of caution and criticism that arose as a reappraisal initiated by the complications and compromise following laparoscopic resections for cancer, particularly port site recurrence (Wexner and Cohen, 1994, 1995; Wexner and Reissman, 1994; Forde and Holten, 1996; Bergamaschi and Myrvold, 1997).

Ironically, cost analysis and comparison of length of stay in laparoscopy and conventional colectomy groups has forced a total reappraisal of the postoperative care of laparotomy patients (Tables 36.6 and 36.7).

Length of hospital stay in the postcolectomy patient is dependent on many factors, the most important being the resumption of a regular diet and the return of bowel function as indicated by a bowel movement. The teleological concept that laparoscopy was less of a traumatic insult to the patient led to early feeding of the laparoscopic

Table 36.6 Length of stay following laparotomy.

	Laparoscopy patients		*Open surgery patients*		
Authors	*n*	*Length of stay Mean (range) (days)*	*n*	*Length of stay (days)*	*Type of study*
Lointier et al (1993)	6	10 (7–16)	–	–	–
Zucker et al (1994)	65	4.4 (3–8)	–	–	–
Bauer et al (1994)	8	6.7 (5–10)	–	–	–
Phillips et al (1992)	51	4.6 (1–30)	–	–	–
Milsom et al (1993)	9	7 (5–12)	–	–	–
Monson et al (1992)	40	8 (NS)	–	–	–
Chindasub et al (1994)	10	8 (NS)	–	–	–
Puente et al (1994)	38	4.8 (3–14)	–	–	–
Van Ye et al (1994)	14	9.1 (4–9)	–	–	–
Senagore et al (1993)	38	7 (NS)	102	9.0	Retrospective
Corbitt (1992)	18	4 (3–6)	–	–	–
Etienne et al (1993)	35	9 (5–23)	–	–	–
Larach et al (1993a)	18	8.4 (NS)	–	–	–
Musser et al (1994)	24	8.5 (NS)	–	–	–
Vara-Thorbeck et al (1994)	18	7.6 (4–12)	–	–	–
Wexner et al (1993)	74	7.0 (2–40)	–	–	–
Sosa et al (1994)	14	6.3 (4–10)	–	–	–
Tucker et al (1995)	114	4.8 (NS)	–	–	–
Quattlebaum et al (1993)	20	4.4 (2–12)	–	–	–
Peters and Bartels (1993)	24	4.8 (NS)	33	8.2	Case
Scoggin et al (1993)	20	5.0 (2–31)	–	–	–
Darzi et al (1995)	12	4 (5–50)	16	17.5	Prospective, randomized
Wu et al (1997)	17	5 (NS)	4	10	Laparoscopic converted
Stage et al (1997)	15	5(3–12)	14	8.0	Prospective, randomized
Kwok et al (1996)	69	6 (2–33)	–	NS	–
Cruz-Vigo et al (1996)	52	6 (uncomplicated)	–	NS	–
	12	14 (complicated)	–	NS	–
Lacy et al (1995)	45	5.1	47	7.6	Prospective, randomized
Jansen et al (1994)	116	8.9 (NS)	–	NS	–
Lumley et al (1996)	248	7.0 (2–80)	–	NS	–
Rhodes et al (1996)	84	6.0 (2–33)	29	10	Historical
Tate et al (1993)	11	12.3 (NS)	14	14.3	Case (non-randomized)
Kockerling et al (1997)	504	15 (NS)	–	NS	–
Fielding et al (1997)	40	5.0 (3–33)	–	NS	–
Franklin et al (1995)	84	7.3 (NS)	110	12.2	Case (non-randomized)
Guillou et al (1993)	70	7.0 (3–31)	–	NS	–
Goh et al (1997)	20	5.0 (3–10)	20	5.5	Case (non-randomized)
Lord et al (1996)	33	5.8 (4–22)	14	8.2	Laparoscopic converted
Hoffman et al (1994)	62	5.2 (3–10)	18	6.5	Laparoscopic converted
			53	7.8	Open (non-randomized)
Molenaar et al (1998)	69	11	–	NS	–

NS, not stated.

patient, even before any evident return of bowel function. With this feature in mind, Binderow et al (1994) performed a prospective, randomized study on 64 consecutive patients undergoing laparotomy and resection after laparotomy. All nasogastric tubes were removed and the 32 patients (group I) were consigned to a traditional postoperative feeding regimen of solid food only after total resolution of the ileus as defined by bowel movements in the absence of nausea, vomiting or abdominal distension. The second group of 32 patients (group II) started a regular diet the first day after laparotomy. In both groups, relatively few patients required reinsertion of the nasogastric tube for symptoms (18.7% in group I and 12.5% in group II). In fact, the duration of the postoperative ileus was identical in the two groups (3.6 days and 3.4 days) and, of the 26 patients in group I that did not require a nasogastric tube, there was a trend towards a shorter hospital stay (6.7 days versus 8.0 days respectively).

Reissman et al (1995) prospectively evaluated the safety and tolerance of early oral feeding in 80 consecutive patients who underwent elective laparotomy and bowel resection. Early feeding was

Table 36.7 Cost studies (US$, unless stated otherwise).

Authors	*Laparoscopic*	*Open*	*Converted*
Falk et al (1993)*	12 000.00	12 500.00	15 000.00
Reiver et al (1994)	23 294.00	19 384.00	0
Senagore et al (1993)	12 131.00	14 496.00	17 583.00
Musser et al (1994)	9811.00	NS	11 207.00
Hoffman et al (1994)	12 464.00	10 213.00	13 956.00
Vayer et al (1993)	26 662.00	22 938.00	13 956.00
Pfeifer et al (1995)	29 636.00	26 903.00	19 702.00
Phillipson et al (1997) (Australian $)	9064.00	7881.00	NS

* Estimated costs for right hemicolectomy.
NS, not stated.

defined as the initiation of a clear liquid diet on the first postoperative day and advancement to a regular diet as tolerated. Eighty-one patients who were fed only after resolution of ileus served as a control group. None of these patients retained their nasogastric tubes immediately after operation and the tubes were reinserted only if the patient suffered two or more episodes of vomiting. In the absence of bowel function, there were no significant differences in the early and regular feeding groups with regard to rate of vomiting (21% versus 14% respectively), nasogastric tube reinsertion (11% versus 10% respectively), length of ileus (3.8 ± 0.1 days versus 4.1 ± 0.1 days respectively), length of hospitalization (6.2 ± 0.2 days versus 6.8 ± 0.2 days respectively), or overall complications (7.5% versus 6.1% respectively). Sixty-three patients (79%) in the early feeding group tolerated advancement to a regular diet within 24–48 hours after initiating liquids. These patients were taking a regular diet significantly earlier than the patients on a regular feeding schedule (2.6 ± 0.1 days versus 5 ± 0.1 days respectively; $P < 0.001$). Obviously, the method of feeding patients postoperatively must be taken into consideration when comparing the laparoscopic to the laparotomy patient.

Analysis of hospital care over the last decade has revealed a decline in the overall length of stay for colectomy patients. Rajagopal et al (1994) reviewed this trend and found that the average stay for colectomy patients in 1983 was 9.4 days and in 1993, the figure had come down to 6.3 days. At least part of this improvement was attributed to the rise of laparoscopic surgery and its influence on postoperative recovery. Crediting laparoscopy for this phenomenon may be a little presumptuous and the endeavour for earlier ambulation and feeding probably plays a larger role. In a study of 1300 patients who had undergone open segmental colectomy at the Cleveland Clinic in Florida between 1988 and 1996, Iroatulam et al (1997) found a significant decrease in the average postoperative hospital stay from 9.8 days at the beginning of this time period to 7.1 days towards the end. The simple comparison of the average length of stay over two time periods may or may not take into account other factors that impact hospital stay.

Schoetz et al (1997) retrospectively reviewed the records of 226 patients that had undergone an open colon resection between 1988 and 1995 in an attempt to identify some of these factors. As in the previous studies, there was a trend towards decreasing the average length of stay in recent years (11 days in 1988 versus 9 days in 1994). The authors indicated that age greater than 65 years, a stoma, the need for postoperative nasogastric decompression, and an emergency operation all significantly increased the average length of postoperative hospital stay. In these retrospective analyses, none of these variables were effectively controlled, which limits the accuracy of these time-period analyses.

HH Chen et al (1998) performed a case-control analysis of 71 patients who had laparoscopic colonic procedures for benign disorders including polyps, diverticular disease, Crohn's disease, and Hartman's reversal. The laparoscopic patients were well-matched with controls with regards to procedure, age and even perioperative complications. The authors found a significant ($P < 0.001$) reduction in disability in the laparoscopic group as determined by the study parameters, including length of hospitalization (6.3 days versus 9.0 days in the laparotomy group), return to partial activity (2.1 weeks versus 4.4 weeks), return to full activity (4.2 weeks versus 10.5 weeks) and time away from work (3.8 weeks versus 7.5 weeks). This same benefit may be more difficult to assess in patients undergoing laparoscopy for cancer. This patient group is generally older, retired and somewhat more sedentary than the individuals who require colectomy for benign indications. Return to a 'normal' activity status postoperatively may not be qualitatively different from that seen preoperatively and no cost benefit can be expected. However, decreasing hospital stay would definitely impact upon the immediate cost of the procedure.

Table 36.6 shows the lengths of stay from the various series of laparoscopic colectomy. Many of these series suffer from a lack of consistency regarding the analysis of hospital stay. Several studies compare length of stay for laparoscopic patients with either historical controls (Scoggin et al, 1993; Rhodes et al, 1996), case controls (Tate et al, 1993; Franklin et al, 1995; Goh et al, 1997), or even controls composed of laparoscopic patients who had their procedures converted to laparotomy for any number of reasons (Lord et al, 1996; Hoffman et al, 1994). Without stringent control of the postoperative variables that effect return of bowel function, comparison of the results of laparoscopy and laparotomy is inappropriate. Some of these variables have already been discussed and include early and consistent feeding regimens, early ambulation and the use of medications such as prokinetics, narcotics and anticholinergics that may alter bowel function.

Another variable that cannot be taken for granted is the current health-care climate throughout the world. In the United States, the impetus for reducing hospital stay has encouraged the development and use of short-term nursing facilities, skilled nursing centres, and home health-care nursing. Thus, early discharge from the hospital does not necessarily translate into a diminished need for care and it is likely that some of the patients in uncontrolled series have been discharged prior to the first bowel movement or while still on a liquid diet. Conversely, many of these options are not readily available in Europe and the length of stay is generally longer in studies from these countries (Tate et al, 1993; Darzi et al, 1995; Kockerling et al, 1997). Another factor that makes comparison between laparoscopy and laparotomy difficult is the inclusion of non-resectional laparoscopic procedures. The mean length of stay of 4.1 days (1–30 days) in the series by Phillips et al (1992) may be partially attributable to the addition of procedures such as colotomy and polypectomy.

In the ideal health-care system, cost issues would not dictate the medical care offered to an individual. Even in our non-ideal systems, cost does not preclude giving care that has truly been deemed superior no matter what the price. The superiority of laparoscopic colorectal surgery has yet to be realized, particularly for malignant indications. Most of the studies that have made cost comparisons between the laparoscopic and the open procedures have dealt with immediate costs. These charges are most easily quantifiable and include equipment cost, hospital stay, and operating room and anaesthesia time. The results of some of these studies are shown in Table 36.7. A recent retrospective cost comparison was performed by Phillipson et al (1997) who compared the cost of open right hemicolectomy (n = 33) to laparoscopic right hemicolectomy (n = 28). These authors were able to divide spending into direct costs (those specific to and incurred by the patient from the date of surgery to date of discharge) and indirect costs (administrative overhead). They further divided the direct costs into those related to the procedure (operating room and recovery room expenses) and those related to the postoperative care (ward expenses). The total cost (in Australian dollars) of laparoscopic right hemicolectomy was significantly greater than the open procedure ($9064 versus $7881 respectively; P < 0.001). The major expenses for the laparoscopic procedure were incurred during the operative phase as a result of the significantly longer operating room utilization time (261 min versus 203 min respectively; P < 0.001) and the greater cost of disposables ($854 versus $189 respectively; P < 0.001).

Pfeifer et al (1995) looked at cost in three groups of patients: (a) laparoscopic, (b) open, and (c) laparoscopic converted to open. The authors divided immediate costs into several components: surgery, anaesthesia, laboratory, radiology, respiratory, nursing and room to name a few. There were no significant differences in the overall costs in any of the three groups although the slightly increased expense of laparoscopy was ascribed to the increased operating room and anaesthetic costs.

In the series by Vayer et al (1993), the operating room time and equipment costs as well as the anaesthetic charges were significantly greater in the laparoscopic colectomy group ($4268, $5550 and $943 respectively) than in the open colectomy group ($3061, $2324 and $640 respectively). Most of the other studies concur regarding the slightly increased immediate cost of laparoscopic colectomy (Reiver et al, 1994; Hoffman et al, 1994). The delayed costs including work absence, productivity and port site recurrence are difficult to quantify but may be substantial. Certainly, if reduction of long-term disability was considerable and the incidence of port site recurrence remained negligible, then laparoscopy would appear to be cost effective. Should no difference in the cancer outcomes between the laparoscopic and open colectomy groups be noted in the current, prospective randomized trials, then cost analysis will be used to either justify or condemn the laparoscopic approach (Nelson et al, 1995).

CONCLUSION

There is very little that is actually conclusive about the results of laparoscopic colectomy for cancer, other than the improvements in cosmesis. Studies that have compared laparoscopic with open colectomy with regards to duration of ileus, length of hospital stay, metabolic response to stress and even postoperative analgesia are at best equivocal. Moreover, there is some real evidence for potential harm using laparoscopic resection as evidenced by the possible increase in wound metastases. In the United States, cancer continues to be the primary indication for laparoscopic colectomy in most of the prospective, non-randomized and randomized studies that are available for review. What may be even more disconcerting is the hypocrisy that underlies the apportioning of this new technology. In a survey of 600 surgeons who were asked about the impact of laparoscopy on their practice, 71% of the surgeons who replied attempted laparoscopic colectomy for patients with the diagnosis of carcinoma. Forty per cent of the same group of surgeons said that they themselves would undergo laparoscopic colectomy for a rectal villous tumour but only 6% would have an anterior resection for cancer performed laparoscopically (Wexner et al, 1995).

During mid-1997, questionnaires were sent to all American members of the American Society of Colon and Rectal Surgeons and the Society of American Gastrointestinal Endoscopic Surgeons (Mavrantonis et al, 1999). In over 3000 questionnaires, the results revealed that only 48% of surgeons performed laparoscopic colorectal surgery on 14% of their patients. Although 17% of surgeons performed more laparoscopic surgery than they did 3 years earlier, 27% of surgeons actually performed less. While 36% of surgeons had performed 1–10 curative cancer resections, only 8% had performed between 11 and 20 and only 14% more than 20 curative resections. When queried about specific pathology, 73% of surgeons used laparoscopic surgery for colonic polyps, 64% for villous adenomas, and only 37% for colonic cancer. Moreover, when asked specifically about cure of tumours of any stage, only 14% of surgeons utilized laparoscopy. The numbers decreased to 8.6% for upper rectal and 7.0% for lower rectal tumours. The future of laparoscopic colectomy for cancer appears dim if the surgeons who perform a particular procedure have such little faith in the safety or efficacy, such that they would not employ it on themselves. More importantly, if these surgeons offer laparoscopic colectomy to patients beyond the constraints of an externally monitored, peer-reviewed prospectively randomized trial, they are dealing in duplicity. Even if the future results of randomized, prospective studies do not support laparoscopy for colorectal cancer, the surgeons currently performing these operations should strive for a candid relationship with their patients and an honest reporting of their results.

Although we will have to await the results of large randomized trials before we can begin to understand the role of laparoscopic resection for colorectal cancer, there are certain points worth considering. At the moment, open surgery leaves much to be desired in terms of improving outcome, particularly with regard to rectal cancer. We must ensure that cancer is dealt with by colorectal specialists. Such individuals must be expert in techniques such as total mesorectal excision and reconstructive surgery, such as pouch formation. To become proficient, they must be fully trained to perform these operations in the open setting. Until we can improve the overall results of open surgery, laparoscopy seems to have little benefit, especially for rectal cancer, and there is considerable unease at present that it increases the risk of local recurrence and results in unnecessary sphincter ablation. Perhaps the rational way forward is to conduct prospective, randomized trials only in patients with tumours confined to the colon that do not involve other organs. When the results of such trials become available, and if indicated, we can then progress to trial the laparoscopic approach in rectal cancer, provided technical advances allow reconstructive procedures to be performed for low tumours.

REFERENCES

Ackerman LV & Wheat MW Jr (1955) Implantation of cancer: an avoidable surgical risk? *Surgery* **37**: 341–355.

Aitken RJ (1996) Mesorectal excision for rectal cancer. *Br J Surg* **83**: 214–216.

Alexander RJ, Jacques BC & Mitchell KG (1993) Laparoscopically assisted colectomy and wound recurrence (letter). *Lancet* **341**: 249–250.

Allardyce R, Morreau P & Bagshaw P (1996) Tumor cell distribution following laparoscopic colectomy in a porcine model. *Dis Colon Rectum* **39**: S47–S52.

Allardyce RA, Morreau P & Bagshaw PF (1997) Operative factors affecting tumor cell distribution following laparoscopic colectomy in a porcine model. *Dis Colon Rectum* **40**: 939–945.

Allendorf JDF & Bessler M (1995) Increased tumor establishment and growth after laparotomy versus laparoscopy. A murine model. *Arch Surg* **130**: 649–653.

Allendorf JD, Bessler M et al (1995) Increased tumor establishment and growth after laparotomy vs laparoscopy in a murine model [see comments]. *Arch Surg* **130**: 649–653.

American Society of Colon and Rectal Surgeons (1991) Position Statement in Laparoscopic Colectomy. Approved 15 May 1991.

Arbman G, Nilsson E, Hallbook O & Sjodahl R (1996) Local recurrence following total mesorectal excision for rectal cancer. *Br J Surg* **83**: 375–379.

Bacon HE & Khubchandani IT (1964) The rationale of aortoileopelvic lymphadenectomy and high ligation of the inferior mesenteric artery for carcinoma of the left colon and rectum. *Surg Gynecol Obstet* **919**: 503–508.

Barrat C, Turner R, Rizak N & Champault G (1996) Prospective comparison of laparoscopic and conventional colorectal surgery for cancer: lymph nodes and margins. *Br J Surg* **83** (Suppl): 23 (Abstract).

Bauer JJ, Harris MT, Gorfine SR, Gelert IM & Kreel I (1994) Laparoscopic assisted intestinal resection for Crohn's disease. *Surg Endosc* **119**: 503–508 (Abstract).

Beart RW, Ballantyne G, Fleshman JW et al (1994) Laparoscopic considerations in colon and rectal surgery. Expert exchange. *Perspect Colon Rectal Surg* **7**: 245–263.

Beck DE (1996) Laparoscopy and colonoscopy. In Jager R & Wexner SD (eds) *Laparoscopic Colorectal Surgery*, pp 143–148. New York: Churchill Livingstone.

Beck DE & Beart RW Jr (1999) Laparoscopic colectomy for polypoid disease. In Wexner SD & Sackier J (eds) *Protocols in General Surgery: Laparoscopic Colorectal Surgery*. New York: John Wiley (in press).

Berends FJ, Kazemier G, Bonjer HJ et al (1994) Subcutaneous metastases after laparoscopic colectomy. *Lancet* **344**: 58.

Bergamaschi R & Myrvold HE (1997) Laparoscopic surgery for cure of colorectal cancer. *Surg Endosc* **11**: 797–799.

Bernstein M & Wexner SD (1995) Laparoscopic resection for colorectal cancer: a USA perspective. *Semin Colon Rectal Surg* **2**: 216–223.

Bessler M, Whelan RL, Halverson A et al (1994) Is immune function better preserved after laparoscopic versus open colon resection? *Surg Endosc* **8**: 881–883.

Binderow SR, Cohen SM, Wexner SD et al (1994) Must early oral feeding be limited to laparoscopy? *Dis Colon Rectum* **37**: 584–589.

Bleday R, Babineau T & Forse RA (1993) Laparoscopic surgery for colon and rectal cancer. *Semin Surg Oncol* **9**: 59–64.

Blenkinsopp WK, Stewart-Brown S, Biesovsky L et al (1981) Histopathology reporting in large bowel cancer. *J Clin Pathol* **304**: 509–513.

Bonjer HJ, Lange JF, Jansen A et al (1997) Abdominal wall metastasis following removal of colorectal carcinomas. *Ned Tijdschr Geneesild* **141**: 1868–1870.

Boulez J & Herriot E (1994) Multicentric analysis of laparoscopic colorectal surgery in FDCL group: 274 cases. *Br J Surg* **81**: 527.

Bouvy ND, Marquet RL, Jeekel J et al (1996) Impact of gas (less) laparoscopy and laparotomy on peritoneal tumor growth and abdominal wall metastases. *Surg Endosc* **10**: 551.

Bouvy ND, Marquet RL, Jeekel J et al (1997) Laparoscopic surgery is associated with less tumor growth stimulation than conventional surgery: an experimental study. *Br J Surg* **84**: 358–361.

Cava A, Roman J, Gonzalez Quintela A et al (1990) Subcutaneous metastases following laparoscopy in gastric adenocarcinoma. *Eur J Surg Oncol* **16**: 63–67.

Cawthorn SJ, Gibbs NM, Marks CG (1986) Clearance technique for the detection of lymph nodes in colorectal cancer. *Br J Surg* 73: 58–60.

Charnley PM, Morris DL, Dennison AR et al (1990) Detection of colorectal liver metastases using intraoperative ultrasonography. *Br J Surg* 77: 998–999.

Chen WS, Lin WC, Kou YR et al (1997) Possible effect of pneumoperitoneum on the spreading of colon cancer tumor cells. *Dis Colon Rectum* **40**: 791–797.

Chen HH, Wexner SD, Weiss EG et al (1998) Laparoscopic colectomy for benign colorectal disease is associated with a significant reduction in disability compared with laparotomy. *Surg Endosc* **12**: 1397–1400.

Chindasub S, Charntaracharmnong C, Nimitvanit C, Akkaranurukul P & Santitarmmanon B (1994) Laparoscopic abdominoperineal resection. *J Laparoendosc Surg* **4**: 17–21.

Chiu PT, Gin T & Oh TE (1993) Anesthesia for laparoscopic general surgery. *Anesth Intensive Care* **21**: 163–167.

Cho JM, Laporta AJ, Clark JR et al (1994) Responses of serum cytokines in patients undergoing laparoscopic cholecystectomy. *Surg Endosc* **8**: 1380–1384.

Cirocco WC, Schwartzman A & Golub RW (1994) Abdominal wall recurrence after laparoscopic colectomy for colon cancer. *Surgery* **116**: 842–846.

Cohen SM & Wexner SD (1993) Laparoscopic colorectal resection for cancer: the Cleveland Clinic Florida experience. *Surg Oncol* **2**: 35–42.

Cohen SM, Wexner SD, Schmitt SL et al (1994) Does xylene mesenteric fat clearance improve lymph node harvest after colon resection? *Eur J Surg* **160**: 693–697.

Coller J (1992) Laparoscopic colectomy. *Laparosc Focus* **1**: 8.

Collet D, Vitale GC, Reynolds M et al (1995) Peritoneal host defenses are less impaired by laparoscopy than by open operation. *Surg Endosc* **9**: 1059–1064.

Cook TA, Dehn TCB (1996) Port site metastases in patients undergoing laparoscopy for gastrointestinal malignancy. *Br J Surg* **83**: 1419–1420.

Corbitt JD (1992) Preliminary experience with laparoscopic-guided colectomy. *Ann Surg* **216**: 703–707.

Cruz-Vigo JL, Pacho Valvuena S, Sanz Guadarrama O et al (1996) Colorectal laparoscopic surgery. *Surg Endosc* **10**: 557.

Cuschieri A (1992) The spectrum of laparoscopic surgery. *World J Surg* **16**: 1089–1097.

Darzi A, Lewis C, Menzies-Gow N, Guillou PJ & Monson JRT (1995) Laparoscopic abdominoperineal resection of the rectum. *Surg Endosc* **9**: 414–417.

Decanini C, Milsom JW, Bohm B & Fazio VW (1994) Laparoscopic oncologic abdominoperineal resection. *Dis Colon Rectum* **37**: 552–553.

Dodson RW, Cullado MJ, Tangen LE et al (1993) Laparoscopic assisted abdominoperineal resection. *Contemp Surg* **42**: 42–44.

Dorrance HR, Oein K & O'Dwyer PJ (1996) Laparoscopy promotes tumor growth in an animal model. *Surg Endosc* **5**: 559.

Dorrance HR, Oein K & O'Dwyer PJ (1997) Effect of laparoscopy, laparotomy and cytocidal agents on intraperitoneal tumor growth in an animal model. *Gastroenterology* **112**: A555 (Abstract).

Easter DN, Cuschieri A, Nathanson LK et al (1992) The utility of diagnostic laparoscopy for abdominal disorders. Audit of 120 patients. *Arch Surg* **127**: 379–383.

Eilber FR, Morton DL (1970) Impaired immunologic reactivity and recurrence following cancer surgery. *Cancer* **25**: 362–367.

Enker WE, Thaler HT, Cranor ML et al (1995) Total mesorectal excision in the operative treatment of carcinoma of the rectum. *J Am Coll Surg* **81**: 335–346.

Etienne J, Jehaes C, Karthauser A, de Neve S & Roden A (1993) Laparoscopic surgery for benign colorectal disease: a multicenter prospective study. *Br J Surg* **80**: S45 (Abstract).

Falk PM, Beart RW Jr, Wexner SD et al (1993) Laparoscopic colectomy: a critical appraisal. *Dis Colon Rectum* **36**: 28–33.

Fielding GA, Lumley J, Nathanson L et al (1997) Laparoscopic colectomy. *Surg Endosc* **11**: 745–749.

Fine AP, Lanasa S, Gannon MP, Cline CW & James R (1995) Laparoscopic colon surgery: report of a series. *Am Surg* **61**: 412–416.

Fingerhut A (1995) Laparoscopic colectomy. The French experience. In Jager R & Wexner SD (eds) *Laparoscopic Colorectal Surgery*, pp 253–257. New York: Churchill Livingstone.

Fleshman JW, Fry RD, Birnbaum EH & Kodner IJ (1996a) Laparoscopic assisted mini-laparotomy approaches to colorectal disease are similar in early outcome. *Dis Colon Rectum* **39**: 15–22.

Fleshman JW, Nelson H, Peters WR et al (1996b) Early results of laparoscopic surgery for colorectal cancer: retrospective analysis of 372 patients treated by clinical outcomes of surgical therapy (COST) study group. *Dis Colon Rectum* **39**: 553–558.

Flowers JL, Feldman J & Jacobs SC (1993) Laparoscopic pelvic lymphadenectomy. *Surg Laparosc Endosc* **3**: 184–190.

Forde KA & Holten L (1996) Laparoscopy in colorectal surgery. *Surg Endosc* **10**: 1039–1040.

Franklin ME, Rosenthal D & Norem RF (1995) Prospective evaluation of laparoscopic colon resection versus open colon resection for adenocarcinoma: a multicenter study. *Surg Endosc* **9**: 811–816.

Fritsch S, Gossot D, Lesourd A, Laborde F & Poupon MF (1997) Experimental abdominal wound metastases following laparoscopic versus open resection for colonic malignancy. *Surg Endosc* **11**: 552 (Abstract).

Fusco MA & Paluzzi MW (1993) Abdominal wall recurrence after laparoscopic assisted colectomy for adenocarcinoma of the colon. *Dis Colon Rectum* **36**: 858–861.

Gees WP, Miller CE, Kokoszka JS et al (1992) Laparoscopic appendectomy for acute appendicitis: rationale and technical aspects. *Contemp Surg* **40**: 13–19.

Gellman L, Salky B & Edye M (1996) Laparoscopic assisted colectomy. *Surg Endosc* **10**: 1041–1044.

Gilchrist RK & David VC (1938) Lymphatic spread of carcinoma of the rectum. *Ann Surg* **108**: 621–622.

Goh YC, Eu KW & Seow-Choen F (1997) Early postoperative results of a prospective series of laparoscopic versus open anterior resection for rectosigmoid cancer. *Dis Colon Rectum* **40**: 776–780.

Goldstein DS, Lu ML, Tomotaka H et al (1993) Inhibition of peritoneal tumor cell implantation: model for laparoscopic cancer surgery. *J Endocrinol* **7**: 237–241.

Goligher JC (1980) *Surgery of the Anus, Rectum and Colon*. Baillière-Tindall: London.

Guillou PJ, Darzi A & Monson JRT (1993) Experience with laparoscopic colorectal surgery for malignant disease. *Surg Oncol* **2**: 43–49.

Haboubi NY, Clark P, Kaftan SM & Schofield PF (1992) The importance of combining xylene clearance and immunohistochemistry in the accurate staging of colorectal carcinoma. *J R Soc Med* **85**: 386–388.

Haggitt RC, Glotzbach RE, Soffer EE et al (1985) Prognostic factors in colorectal carcinomas arising in adenomas: implications for lesions removed by endoscopic polypectomy. *Gastroenterology* **39**: 328–336.

Heald RJ, Husband EM & Ryall RDH (1982) The mesorectum in rectal cancer surgery: the clue to pelvic recurrence. *Br J Surg* **69**: 613–616.

Herrera-Ornelas L, Justiniano J, Castillo N et al (1987) Metastases in small lymph nodes from colon cancer. *Arch Surg* **122**: 1253–1256.

Hewett PJ, Thomas WM, King G et al (1996) Intraperitoneal cell movement during abdominal carbon dioxide insufflation and laparoscopy. *Dis Colon Rectum* **39**: 562–566.

Hida J, Yasutomi M, Maruyama T, Fujimoto K, Uchida T & Okuno K (1997) The extent of lymph node dissection for colon carcinoma: the potential impact on laparoscopic surgery. *Cancer* **80**: 188–192.

Hoffman GC, Baker JW, Fitchett CW et al (1994) Laparoscopic assisted colectomy: initial experience. *Ann Surg* **219**: 732–743.

Hojo K, Koyama Y & Moreya Y (1982) Lymphatic spread and its prognostic value in patients with rectal cancer. *Am J Surg* **144**: 350–354.

Hubens G (1998) Impact of CO_2 and gasless laparoscopy as well as laparotomy on peritoneal tumor growth and abdominal wall metastases (letter). *Ann Surg* **227**: 310–311.

Hubens G, Pauwels M, Hubens A, Vermeulen P, Van Marck E & Eyskens E (1996) The influence of pneumoperitoneum on the peritoneal implantation of free intraperitoneal colon cancer cells. *Surg Endosc* **10**: 809–812.

Hughes ES, McDermott FT, Poliglase AL et al (1983) Tumor recurrence in the abdominal wall scar tissue after large bowel cancer surgery. *Dis Colon Rectum* **26**: 571–572.

Huscher C, Silecchia G, Croce E et al (1996) Laparoscopic colorectal resection: a multicenter Italian study. *Surg Endosc* **10**: 875–879.

Hyder JW, Talbot TM & Maycroft TE (1990) A critical review of chemical lymph node clearance and staging of colon and rectal cancer at Ferguson Hospital, 1977 to 1982. *Dis Colon Rectum* **33**: 923–925.

Iroatulam AJN, Potenti FM, Chen HH et al (1997) A decrease in length of hospitalization after segmental non-laparoscopic colectomy over a nine year period. *Dis Colon Rectum* **40**: A43 (Abstract).

Jaap Bonjer H, Tseng L, Kazemier G & Marquet RL (1997) Port site metastasis: role of local ischemia. *Surg Endosc* **11**: 175 (Abstract).

Jacobi CA, Keller H, Monig S et al (1995) Implantation metastases of unsuspected gall bladder carcinoma after laparoscopy. *Surg Endosc* **9**: 351–352.

Jacobi CA, Ordemann J, Bohm B, Zieren HU, Volk HD & Muller JM (1996) Increased tumor growth after laparotomy and laparoscopy with air versus CO_2. *Surg Endosc* **10**: 551 (Abstract).

Jacobi CA, Ordemann J, Bohn B et al (1997a) The influence of laparotomy and laparoscopy on tumor growth in a rat model. *Surg Endosc* **11**: 618–621.

Jacobi CA, Sabat R, Zieren HU, Wenger F, Volk HD & Muller JM (1997b) Inhibition of tumor growth and trocar metastases in laparoscopic surgery in a rat model. *Surg Endosc* **11**: 552 (Abstract).

Jacobs M (1992) Laparoscopic colon resection: the Miami experience. In *Laparoscopic Colon and Rectal Seminar Syllabus*. Cincinnati, OH: Ethicon Endosurgery.

Jacobs S, Verdeja JC & Goldstein HC (1991) Minimally invasive colon resection (laparoscopic colectomy). *Surg Laparosc Endosc* **1**: 144–150.

Jacquet P, Averbach AM, Stephens AD et al (1995) Cancer recurrence following laparoscopic colectomy: report of two patients treated with heated intraperitoneal chemotherapy. *Dis Colon Rectum* **38**: 1110–1114.

Jager RM & Wexner SD (eds) (1996) *Laparoscopic Colorectal Surgery*. New York: Churchill Livingstone.

Jansen A, Cuesta MA, Go PNN, Bijnen AB & Lange JF (1994) Laparoscopic colon resection: the Dutch experience. *Surg Endosc* **8**: 251 (Abstract).

Jass JR, Miller K & Northover JM (1986) Fat clearance method versus manual dissection of lymph nodes in specimens of rectal cancer. *Int J Colorectal Dis* **1**: 155–156.

Johnstone PAS, Rohde DC, Swartz SE et al (1996) Port site recurrence after laparoscopic and thoracoscopic procedures in malignancy. *J Clin Oncol* **14**: 1950–1956.

Jones DB, Guo LW, Reinhold MD et al (1995) Impact of pneumoperitoneum on trocar site implantation of colon cancer in a hamster model. *Dis Colon Rectum* **38**: 1182–1188.

Kim S, Milsom J, Gramlich T et al (1997) Does laparoscopic versus conventional surgery increase exfoliated malignant cells in the peritoneal cavity during resection of colorectal cancer. *Dis Colon Rectum* **40**: A21 (Abstract).

Knolmayer TJ, Egan JC, Bowyer MW, Niemeyer DM & Asbun HJ (1997) Aerosolization of tumor cells during carbon dioxide insufflation. *Surg Endosc* **11**: 204 (Abstract).

Kockerling F, Schneider C, Reymond MA et al (1997) Multicenter study: laparoscopic colorectal surgery. Early results of 504 cases. *Surg Endosc* **11**: 181.

Kok KY, Ngoi SS, Kum CK, Tekant Y, Tasci I & Goh P (1996) Laparoscopic assisted large bowel resection. *Ann Acad Med Singapore* **25**: 650–652.

Kwok SP, Law WY, Carey PD et al (1996) Prospective evaluation of laparoscopically-assisted large bowel excision for cancer. *Ann Surg* **223**: 170–176.

Lacy AM, Garcia-Valdecasas JC, Pique JM et al (1995) Short term outcome analysis of a randomized study comparing laparoscopic versus open colectomy for colon cancer. *Surg Endosc* **9**: 1101–1105.

Larach SW, Vayer AG, Williamson PR & Goldstein E (1993a) Laparoscopic-assisted colectomy: experience during the learning curve. *Coloproctology* **15**: 38–41.

Larach SW, Salomon MC, Williamson PR & Goldstein E (1993b) Laparoscopic assisted abdominoperineal resection. *Surg Laparosc Endosc* **3**: 115–119.

Lauroy J, Champault G, Risk N et al (1994) Metastatic recurrence at the cannula site: should digestive carcinoma still be managed by laparoscopy? *Br J Surg* **81** (Suppl): 31.

Lazorthes F & Chiotassol P (1986) Stapled colorectal anastomosis: operative integrity of the anastomosis and risk of postoperative leakage. *Int J Colorectal Dis* **1**: 96–98.

Lee SW, Whelan R, Southall BA & Bessler M (1997) Pneumoperitoneum does not increase port site implantation rate of colon cancer in a murine model. *Surg Endosc* **11**: 174 (Abstract).

Lennard TWJ, Shenton BK, Borzotta A et al (1985) The influence of surgical operations in components of the human immune system. *Br J Surg* **72**: 771–776.

Leo E, Belli F, Andreola S et al (1996) Total mesorectal excision and coloendoanal anastomosis: a therapeutic option for the treatment of low rectal cancer. *Ann Surg Oncol* **3**: 336–343.

Lointier PH, Lautard M, Massoni C, Ferrier C & Dapoigny M (1993) Laparoscopic assisted subtotal colectomy. *J Laparoendosc Surg* **3**: 439–453.

Lord SA, Larach SW, Ferrara A et al (1996) Laparoscopic resection for colorectal carcinoma: a three year experience. *Dis Colon Rectum* **39**: 148–154.

Lumley JW, Fielding GA, Rhodes M et al (1996) Laparoscopic assisted colorectal surgery: lessons learned from 240 consecutive patients. *Dis Colon Rectum* **39**: 155–159.

McDermott J, Devereaux D & Caushaj P (1994) Pitfall of laparoscopic colectomy. An unrecognized synchronous carcinoma. *Dis Colon Rectum* **37**: 602–603.

MacFarlane JK, Ryall RDH & Heald RJ (1993) Mesorectal excision for rectal cancer. *Lancet* **2**: 1812–1813.

Machi J, Isomuto H, Kurohiji T et al (1991) Accuracy of intraoperative ultrasonography in diagnosing liver metastases from colorectal cancer: evaluation with postoperative follow up results. *World J Surg* **15**: 551–557.

Macias Rius J & Wexner SD (1996) Laparoscopic resection of rectal cancer: short and long term results. In Soreide O & Norstein J (eds) *Rectal Cancer Surgery*, pp 281–294. Berlin: Springer.

Mathew G, Watson DI, Ellis T et al (1997a) The effect of laparoscopy on the movement of tumor cells and metastases to surgical wounds. *Surg Endosc* **11**: 1163–1166.

Mathew G, Watson DJ, Rofe AM et al (1997b) Adverse impact of pneumoperitoneum on intraperitoneal implantation and growth of tumor cell suspension in an experimental model. *Aust N Z J Surg* **66**: 105–106.

Mavrantonis C, Potenti F & Wexner SD (1999) Laparoscopic colorectal surgery: have attitudes changed? *Dis Colon Rectum* (in press).

Miles WE (1908) A method of performing abdominoperineal excision for carcinoma of the rectum and of the terminal portion of the pelvic colon. *Lancet* **2**: 1812–1813.

Milsom JW & Bohm B (1996) *Laparoscopic Colorectal Surgery*. New York: Springer-Verlag.

Milsom JW, Lavery IC, Bohm B & Fazio VW (1993) Laparoscopic assisted ileocolectomy in Crohn's disease. *Surg Laparosc Endosc* **3**: 77–80.

Molenaar CBR, Bijnen AB & de Ruiter P (1998) Indication for laparoscopic colectomy: results from the medical center, Alkmaar, the Netherlands. *Surg Endosc* **12**: 42–45.

Monson JRT, Darzi A, Carey PD & Guillou PJ (1992) Prospective evaluation of laparoscopic assisted colectomy in an unselected group of patients. *Lancet* **340**: 831–833.

Montorsi M, Fumagaili U, Rosati R et al (1985) Early parietal recurrence of adenocarcinoma of the colon after laparoscopic colectomy. *Br J Surg* **82**: 1036–1037.

Morgan CN & Griffiths JD (1959) High ligation of the inferior mesenteric artery during operations for carcinoma of the distal colon and rectum. *Surg Gynecol Obstet* **108**: 641–650.

Murthy SM, Goldschmidt RA, Rao LN, Ammigati M, Buchmann T & Scanton EF (1989) The influence of surgical trauma on experimental metastases. *Cancer* **64**: 2035–2044.

Musser PJ, Boorse RC, Madera F & Reed FJ III (1994) Laparoscopic colectomy: at what cost? *Surg Laparosc Endosc* **4**: 1–5.

Nduka CC & Darzi A (1997) Port site metastases in patients undergoing laparoscopy for gastrointestinal malignancy (letter; comment). *Br J Surg* **84**: 583.

Nduka CC, Monson JRT, Menzies-Gow N & Darzi A (1994) Abdominal wall metastases following laparoscopy. *Br J Surg* **81**: 648–652.

Nelson H, Weeks JC & Wieand HS (1995) Proposed phase III trial comparing laparoscopic-assisted colectomy versus open colectomy for colon cancer. *J Natl Cancer Inst Monograph* **19**: 51–56.

Nivatvongs S, Rojanasakuz A, Reiman HM et al (1991) The risk of lymph node metastases in colorectal polyps with invasive adenocarcinoma. *Dis Colon Rectum* **34**: 323–328.

Nogueras JJ & Wexner SD (1992) Laparoscopic colon resection. *Perspect Colon Rectal Surg* **5**: 79–97.

O'Rourke N, Price PM, Kelly S et al (1993) Tumor innoculation during laparoscopy (letter). *Lancet* **342**: 368.

Orkin B (1992) Rectal carcinoma: treatment. In Beck DE & Wexner SD (eds) *Fundamentals of Anorectal Surgery*. New York: McGraw-Hill.

Peters WR & Bartels TL (1993) Minimally invasive colectomy: are the potential benefits realized? *Dis Colon Rectum* **36**: 751–756.

Pezim ME & Nicholls RJ (1984) Survival after high or low ligation of the inferior mesenteric artery during curative surgery for rectal cancer. *Ann Surg* **200**: 729–733.

Pfeifer J, Wexner SD, Reissman P et al (1995) Laparoscopic versus open colon surgery. Costs and outcome. *Surg Endosc* **9**: 1322–1326.

Phillips FH, Franklin M, Carroll BJ et al (1992) Laparoscopic colectomy. *Ann Surg* **216**: 703–707.

Phillipson BM, Bokey EL, Moore JWE, Chapuis PH & Bagge E (1997) Cost of open versus laparoscopically assisted right hemicolectomy for cancer. *World J Surg* **21**: 214–217.

Prasad A, Avery C & Foley RJE (1994) Abdominal wall metastases following laparoscopy (letter). *Br J Surg* **81**: 31.

Puente I, Sosa JL, Sleeman D, Desai U, Tranakas N & Hartmann R (1994) Laparoscopic assisted colorectal surgery. *J Laparoendosc Surg* **4**: 1–7.

Quattlebaum JK, Flanders HD & Usher CH (1993) Laparoscopically-assisted colectomy. *Surg Laparosc Endosc* **3**: 81–87.

Quirke P, Durdy P, Dixon MF et al (1986) Local recurrence of rectal adenocarcinoma due to inadequate surgical resection. *Lancet* **1**: 996–998.

Rajagopal AS, Thorson AG, Sentovich SM et al (1994) Decade trends in length of postoperative stay following abdominal colectomy. *Dis Colon Rectum* **37**: 26 (Abstract).

Ramos JM, Gupta S, Anthone GJ et al (1994) Laparoscopy and colon cancer. Is the port site at risk? A preliminary report. *Arch Surg* **129**: 897–899.

Reilly WT, Nelson H, Schroeder G et al (1996) Wound recurrence following conventional treatment of colorectal cancer. A rare but perhaps underestimated problem. *Dis Colon Rectum* **39**: 200–207.

Reissman P, Teoh T-A, Piccirillo M, Nogueras JJ & Wexner SD (1994) Colonoscopic assisted laparoscopic colectomy. *Surg Endosc* **8**: 1352–1353.

Reissman P, Teoh T-A, Weiss EG et al (1995) Is early oral feeding safe after elective colorectal surgery. *Ann Surg* **222**: 73–77.

Reiver D, Kmiot WA, Cohen SM, Weiss EG, Nogueras JJ & Wexner SD (1994) A prospective assessment of laparoscopic versus open procedures in colorectal surgery. *Dis Colon Rectum* **37**: A22 (Abstract).

Rhodes M, Rudd M, Nathanson L et al (1996) Laparoscopic anterior resection: a consecutive series of 84 patients. *Surg Laparosc Endosc* **6**: 213–217.

Rodriguez-Bigas MA, Maamoun S, Iber TK, Penetrante RB, Blumenson LE & Petrelli NJ (1996) Clinical significance of colorectal cancer metastases in lymph nodes. *Ann Surg Oncol* **3**: 124–130.

Sackier JM (1992) Laparoscopic abdominoperineal resection of the rectum. *Br J Surg* **79**: 1207–1208.

Sackier JM & Wexner SD (1999) *Protocols in General Surgery: Laparoscopic Colorectal Surgery*. New York: John Wiley (in press).

Safran DB & Orlando R III (1994) Physiologic effect of pneumoperitoneum. *Am J Surg* **167**: 231–239.

Safran DB, Sgambati S & Orlando R III (1993) Laparoscopy in high risk cardiac patients. *Gynecol Obstet* **176**: 548–554.

Schlinkert RT (1991) Laparoscopic-assisted hemicolectomy. *Dis Colon Rectum* **34**: 1030–1031.

Schoetz DJ, Bockler M, Rosenblatt MS et al (1997) 'Ideal' length of stay after colectomy. Whose ideal? *Dis Colon Rectum* **40**: 806–810.

Scoggin SD, Frazee RC, Snyder SK et al (1993) Laparoscopic assisted bowel surgery. *Dis Colon Rectum* **36**: 747–750.

Scott KWM & Grace RH (1989) Detection of lymph node metastases in colorectal carcinoma before and after fat clearance. *Br J Surg* **76**: 1165–1167.

See WA, Cooper CS & Fisher RJ (1993) Predictors of laparoscopic complications after formal training in laparoscopic surgery. *J Am Med Assoc* **73**: 2689–2692.

Senagore AL, Luchtefeld MA, MacKeigan JM et al (1993) Open colectomy versus laparoscopic colectomy: are there differences? *Am Surg* **59**: 549–554.

Seow-Choen F, Eu KW, Ho YH & Leong AF (1997) A preliminary comparison of a consecutive series of open versus laparoscopic abdominoperineal resection for rectal adenocarcinoma. *Int J Colorectal Dis* **12**: 88–90.

Shida J, Ban K, Mastumoto M et al (1993) Prognostic significance of location of lymph nodal metastases in colorectal cancer. *Dis Colon Rectum* **35**: 1046–1050.

Smedh K, Skullman S, Kald A et al (1997) Laparoscopic bowel mobilization combined with intraoperative colonoscopic polypectomy in patients with an inaccessible polyp of the colon. *Surg Endosc* **11**: 643–644.

Sosa JL, Sleeman D, Puente I, McKenney MG & Hartmann R (1994) Laparoscopic assisted colostomy closure after Hartmann's procedure. *Dis Colon Rectum* **37**: 149–152.

Southall J, Lee S, Allendorf J, Bessler M & Whelan R (1997a) Colon adenocarcinoma and B-16 melanoma grow larger after laparotomy versus laparoscopy in a murine model. *Dis Colon Rectum* **40**: A20 (Abstract)

Southall J, Lee S, Whelan R et al (1997b) The effect of peritoneal air exposure on postoperative tumor growth. *Surg Endosc* **11**: 176.

Southern Surgeon's Club (1991) A prospective analysis of 1518 laparoscopic cholecystectomies. *N Engl J Med* **324**: 1073–1078.

Spaw A, Reddick EJ & Olson DO (1991) Laparoscopic laser cholecystectomy: analysis of 500 procedures. *Surg Laparosc Endosc* **1**: 2–7.

Stage JG, Schulze S, Moller P et al (1997) Prospective randomized study of laparoscopic versus open colonic resection for adenocarcinoma. *Br J Surg* **84**: 391–396.

Surtees P, Ritchie JK & Phillips RKS (1990) High versus low ligation of the inferior mesenteric artery in rectal cancer. *Br J Surg* **77**: 618–621.

Targarona EM, Pons MJ, Anglada MT, Taura P & Trias M (1993) Laparoscopic abdominoperineal resection of the rectum. *Br J Surg* **80**: 535.

Tate JJT, Kwok S, Dawson JW et al (1993) Prospective comparison of laparoscopic and conventional anterior resection. *Br J Surg* **80**: 1396–1398.

Teoh T-A & Wexner SD (1996) Laparoscopic surgery. In Williams NS (ed.) *Colorectal Cancer*, pp 103–121. New York: Churchill Livingstone.

Thomas WM, Eaton MC & Hewett PJ (1996) A proposed model for the movement of cells within the abdominal cavity during CO_2 insufflation and laparoscopy. *Aust N Z J Surg* **66**: 105–106.

Toyota S, Ohta H & Anazawa S (1995) Rationale for extent of lymph node dissection for right colon cancer. *Dis Colon Rectum* **38**: 705–711.

Tseng LNL, Bouvy ND, Kazemier G, Marquet RL & Bonjer HJ (1997) 'Port site' metastasis: role of local ischemia and chimney effect. *Surg Endosc* **11**: 556 (Abstract).

Tucker JG, Ambrose WL, Orangio GR, Duncan TD, Mason EM & Lucas GW (1995) Laparoscopic assisted bowel surgery. *Surg Endosc* **2**: 297–300.

Turk PS & Wanebo HJ (1993) Results of surgical treatment of nonhepatic recurrence of colorectal carcinoma. *Cancer* **71**: 4267–4277.

Turnbull RB, Kyle K, Watson FR & Spratt J (1967) The influence of the no-touch isolation technique on survival. *Ann Surg* **166**: 420–425.

Ugarte F (1995) Laparoscopic cholecystectomy port seeding from a colon carcinoma. *Am Surg* **61**: 820–821.

Umpley HC, Brestol JB, Rainey JB et al (1984) Survival of 727 patients with single carcinoma of the large bowel. *Dis Colon Rectum* **27**: 803–810.

Van Ye TM, Carter RP & Henry LG (1994) Laparoscopically assisted colon resections compare favorably with open technique. *Surg Laparosc Endosc* **4**: 25–31.

Vara-Thorbeck C, Garcia-Caballero M, Salvi M et al (1994) Indications and advantages of laparoscopy-assisted colon resection for carcinoma in elderly patients. *Surg Laparosc Endosc* **4**: 110–118.

Vayer AJ, Larach SW, Williamson PR et al (1993) Cost effectiveness of laparoscopic colectomy. *Dis Colon Rectum* **36**: 34 (Abstract).

Vertruyen M, Cadiere GB, Himpens J, Bruyns J & Lemper JC (1996) Laparoscopic colectomy for cancer. *Br J Surg* **83**: 38 (Abstract).

Viamonte M, Plascencia G, Wiltz O & Jacobs M (1994) Laparoscopic colectomies in cancer. *Dis Colon Rectum* **37**: P5–P6 (Abstract).

Vukasin P, Ortega AE, Greene FL et al (1996) Wound recurrence following laparoscopic colon cancer resection. *Dis Colon Rectum* **39**: 520–523.

Walsh DCA, Wattchow DA & Wilson TG (1993) Subcutaneous metastases after laparoscopic resection for malignancy. *Aust N Z J Surg* **65**: 563–565.

Weiss EG & Wexner SD (1996) Laparoscopic port site recurrence in oncologic surgery – a review. *Ann Acad Med Singapore* **25**: 694–698.

Wexner SD (1991) Management of the malignant polyp. *Semin Colon Rectal Surg* **2**: 22–27.

Wexner SD & Cohen SM (1994) Laparoscopic colectomy for malignancy: advantages and limitations. *Surg Oncol Clin North Am* **3**: 634–643.

Wexner SD & Cohen SM (1995) Port site recurrence after laparoscopic surgery for cure of malignancy. *Br J Surg* **82**: 295–298.

Wexner SD & Reissman P (1994) Laparoscopic colorectal surgery: a provocative critique. *Int Surg* **79**: 235–239.

Wexner SD, Johansen OB, Nogueras JJ & Jagelman DG (1992) Laparoscopic total abdominal colectomy. A prospective trial. *Dis Colon Rectum* **35**: 641–645.

Wexner SD, Cohen SM, Johansen OB, Nogueras JJ & Jagelman DG (1993) Laparoscopic colorectal surgery: a prospective assessment and current perspective. *Br J Surg* **80**: 1602–1605.

Wexner SD, Cohen SM, Ulrich A & Reissman P (1995) Laparoscopic colorectal surgery: are we being honest with our patients? *Dis Colon Rectum* **38**: 723–727.

Wexner SD, Verzaro R & Agachan F (1997) Laparoscopic colorectal surgery. In Brune I (ed) *Laparoendoscopic Surgery*, pp 151–171. Oxford: Blackwell Scientific.

Whelan RL, Seller GJ, Allendorf JD et al (1996a) Trocar site recurrence is unlikely to result from aerosolization of tumor cells. *Dis Colon Rectum* **39**: S7–S13.

Whelan RL, Bessler M & Treat MR (1996b) Immune function after laparoscopy and laparotomy. In Jager RM & Wexner SD (eds) *Laparoscopic Colorectal Surgery*, pp 277–285. New York: Churchill Livingstone.

Whitgen CM, Andrus JP, Andrus CH et al (1993) Cholecystectomy. Which procedure is best for the high risk patient? *Surg Endosc* **7**: 395–397.

Wiggers T, Jeekal J, Arends J et al (1986) The no-touch isolation technique in colon cancer (a prospective controlled multicenter trial). *Surg Oncol Proc Assoc* **5**: 169–180.

Williams NS, Dixon MF & Johnson D (1983) Reappraisal of the 5 centimeter rule of distal excision for carcinoma of the rectum: a study of distal intramural spread and of patient's survival. *Br J Surg* **70**: 150–154.

Wu JS, Birnbaum EH & Fleshman JW (1997) Early experience with laparoscopic abdominoperineal resection. *Surg Endosc* **11**: 449–455.

Wu JS, Jones DB, Guo L-W et al (1998) Effects of pneumoperitoneum on tumor implantation with decreasing tumor inoculum. *Dis Colon Rectum* **41**: 141–146.

Wu JS, Guo L-W, Ruiz MB, Pfister SM, Connett JM & Fleshman JW (1999) Excision of trocar sites reduces tumor implantation in an animal model. *Dis Colon Rectum* (in press).

Zucker KA, Pitcher DE & Ford RS (1994) Laparoscopic assisted colon resection. *Surg Endosc* **8**: 12–18.

INDEX

Volume One pp. 1–1380; Volume Two pp. 1381–2702.

F

Q

R

T